2022

ICD-10-CM
FOR PHYSICIANS

Jackie L. Koesterman, CPC
Coding and Reimbursement Specialist
JDK Medical Coding EDU, LLC
Grand Forks, North Dakota

BUCK'S

INCLUDES
NETTER'S
ANATOMY
ART

ELSEVIER

Elsevier
3251 Riverport Lane
St. Louis, Missouri 63043

BUCK'S 2022 ICD-10-CM FOR PHYSICIANS   ISBN: 978-0-323-79035-2
Copyright © 2022 by Elsevier Inc. All rights reserved.

Previous editions copyrighted 2021, 2020, 2019, 2018, 2017, 2016, 2015, 2014, 2013, 2010.

International Standard Book Number 978-0-323-79035-2

Senior Content Strategist: Brandi Graham
Senior Content Development Manager: Luke E. Held
Senior Content Development Specialist: Joshua S. Rapplean
Publishing Services Manager: Shereen Jameel
Senior Project Manager: Kamatchi Madhavan
Senior Book Designer: Maggie Reid

Printed in India

Last digit is the print number: 9 8 7 6 5 4 3 2

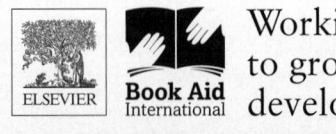

DEDICATION

To all the brave medical coders who transitioned the nation into a new coding system. Decades of waiting finally concluded with the implementation of I-10, and you have been the pioneers leading the way.

With greatest appreciations for your efforts!

Carol J. Buck, MS

CONTENTS

GUIDE TO USING THE 2022 ICD-10-CM FOR PHYSICIANS

Medical coding has long been a part of the health care profession. Through the years medical coding systems have become more complex and extensive. Today, medical coding is an intricate and immense process that is present in every health care setting. The increased use of electronic submissions for health care services only increases the need for coders who understand the coding process.

2022 ICD-10-CM for Physicians, Professional Edition was developed to help meet the needs of coding professionals at all levels by offering a comprehensive coding text at a reasonable price.

All material strictly adheres to the latest government versions available at the time of printing. Updates from the *Definitions of Medicare Code Edits* (MCE) will be posted to the companion website (www. codingupdates.com) when available.

Illustrations and Items

The ICD-10-CM Tabular List contains illustrations, pictures, and items to assist you in understanding difficult terminology, diseases/conditions, or coding in a specific category. Items are always printed in ▬▬▬▬ ink so that the added material is not mistaken for official notations or instructions. ▬▬▬▬ ink is used for other annotations in the text. Your ideas on what other descriptions or illustrations should be in future editions of this text are always appreciated.

Instructional Notations

Includes Notes

Includes
The word "Includes" appears immediately under certain categories to further define, or give examples of, the content of the category.

Excludes Notes

The ICD-10-CM has two types of excludes notes. Each note has a different definition for use, but they are both similar in that they indicate that codes excluded from each other are independent of each other.

Excludes1
A type 1 Excludes note is a pure excludes. It means "NOT CODED HERE!" An Excludes1 note indicates that the code excluded should never be used at the same time as the code above the Excludes1 note. An Excludes1 is for use when two conditions cannot occur together, such as a congenital form versus an acquired form of the same condition.

Excludes2
A type 2 Excludes note represents "NOT INCLUDED HERE." An Excludes2 note indicates that the condition excluded is not part of the condition it is excluded from, but a patient may have both conditions at the same time. When an Excludes2 note appears under a code, it is acceptable to use both the code and the excluded code together.

Code First/Use Additional Code notes (etiology/manifestation paired codes)

Certain conditions have both an underlying etiology and multiple body system manifestations due to the underlying etiology. For such conditions the ICD-10-CM has a coding convention that requires the underlying condition be sequenced first, followed by the manifestation. Wherever such a combination exists, there is a "use additional code" note at the etiology code, and a "code first" note at the manifestation code. These instructional notes indicate the proper sequencing order of the codes, etiology followed by manifestation.

In most cases the manifestation codes will have in the code title, "in diseases classified elsewhere." Codes with this title are a component of the etiology/manifestation convention. The code title indicates that it is a manifestation code. "In diseases classified elsewhere" codes are never permitted to be used as first-listed or principal diagnosis codes. They must be used in conjunction with an underlying condition code, and they must be listed following the underlying condition.

Use additional
The words indicate an instructional note that another code may be needed.

Code first
The words indicate an instructional note that directs the coder to sequence the underlying condition before the manifestation.

Code also
A "code also" note instructs that two codes may be required to fully describe a condition, but the sequencing of the two codes is discretionary, depending on the severity of the conditions and the reason for the encounter.

7th characters and placeholder X

For codes less than 6 characters that require a 7th character, a placeholder X should be assigned for all characters less than 6. The 7th character must always be the 7th character of a code.

Annotated

Throughout the manual, revisions, additions, and deleted codes or words are indicated by the following symbols:

⇒ **Revised:** Revisions within the line or code from the previous edition are indicated by the arrow.

▶ **New:** Additions to the previous edition are indicated by the triangle.

~~deleted~~ **Deleted:** Deletions from the previous edition are struck through.

ICD-10-CM Tabular List Symbols

● **Use Additional Character(s):** The red stop sign cautions that the code requires additional character(s) to ensure the greatest specificity.

X For codes less than 6 characters that require a 7th character, a placeholder X should be assigned for all characters less than 6. The 7th character must always be the 7th character of a code.

OGCR The *Official Guidelines for Coding and Reporting* symbol includes the placement of a portion of a guideline as that guideline pertains to the code by which it is located. The complete OGCR are located in Part I.

🏥 The **Hierarchical condition category (HCC)** was initiated in 2004 for the reimbursement for patients with Medicare Advantage plans (Medicare Part C). HCC is based on a list of chronic or severity of illness diagnosis codes that CMS uses to determine reimbursements to Medicare Advantage plans. The HCC risk adjustment factor data is calculated for an entire year for encounters of the patient's care.

◗ **Manifestation Code:** Describes the manifestation of an underlying disease, not the disease itself, and therefore should not be assigned as a principal diagnosis, according to the *Definitions of Medicare Code Edits* (MCE).

Age conflict: The *Definitions of Medicare Code Edits* (MCE) detects inconsistencies between a patient's age and diagnosis. For example, a 5-year-old patient with benign prostatic hypertrophy or a 78-year-old pregnant female.

The diagnosis is clinically and virtually impossible in a patient of the stated age. Therefore, either the diagnosis or the age is presumed to be incorrect. There are four age categories for diagnoses in the *Definitions of Medicare Code Edits* (MCE):

N • Newborn. Age of 0 years; a subset of diagnoses intended only for newborns and neonates (e.g., fetal distress, perinatal jaundice).

P • Pediatric. Age range is 0-17 years inclusive (e.g., Reye's syndrome, routine child health exam).

M • Maternity. Age range is 9-64 years inclusive (e.g., diabetes in pregnancy, antepartum pulmonary complication).

A • Adult. Age range is 15-124 years inclusive (e.g., senile delirium, mature cataract).

♀♂ **Sex conflict:** *Definitions of Medicare Code Edits* (MCE) detects inconsistencies between a patient's sex and any diagnosis or procedure on the patient's record. For example, a male patient with cervical cancer (diagnosis) or a female patient with a prostatectomy (procedure). In both instances, the indicated diagnosis or the procedure conflicts with the stated sex of the patient. Therefore, either the patient's diagnosis, procedure, or sex is presumed to be incorrect.

Key words
Highlight identifies key words within similar code descriptions in a particular category.

Coding Clinic Identifies the year, quarter, and page number that presents information about an ICD-10-CM code in the American Hospital Association's *Coding Clinic*® for ICD-10-CM.

Visit codingupdates.com for the full list of *2022* Present on Admission codes.

SYMBOLS AND CONVENTIONS

ICD-10-CM Tabular

Use Additional Character(s): The red stop sign cautions you that the code requires additional character(s) to ensure greatest specificity.

Volume 1, Tabular List

● **K22 Other diseases of esophagus**
    Excludes2   esophageal varices (I85.-)

X ● **V00.01 Pedestrian on foot injured in collision with roller-skater**

A02.20 Localized salmonella infection, unspecified

Placeholder X: The red X reminds you that for codes less than 6 characters that require a 7th character, a placeholder X should be assigned to all characters less than 6.

Unspecified: These codes are for use when the information in the medical record is insufficient to assign a more specific code. For those categories for which an unspecified code is not provided, the "other specified" code may represent both other and unspecified.

Use additional code: Located at the etiology code and directs you to assign a manifestation code.

A48.3 Toxic shock syndrome
    ▶ Use additional code to identify the organism (B95, B96)

Code first indicates the etiology code is to be first-listed before the manifestation code.

B39 Histoplasmosis
    ▶ *Code first associated AIDS (B20)*

Notes define terms or give coding instructions.

E34.0 Carcinoid syndrome
    ▶ **Note:** May be used as an additional code to identify functional activity associated with a carcinoid tumor.

Codes or index entries are for purposes of illustration only and may not be current.

OGCR Section I.C.6.B.5.

Neoplasm Related Pain Code G89.3 is assigned to pain documented as being related, associated or due to cancer, primary or secondary malignancy, or tumor. This code is assigned regardless of whether the pain is acute or chronic.

OGCR: The *Official Guidelines for Coding and Reporting* are placed near the codes to which they refer and are highlighted.

I70.2   **Atherosclerosis of native arteries of the extremities**
Mönckeberg's (medial) sclerosis
Use additional code, if applicable, to identify chronic total occlusion of artery of extremity (I70.92)

code, if applicable, directs the coder to other conditions that may be appropriate to report.

The word "and" should be interpreted to mean either "and" or "or" when it appears in a statement.

I74   **Arterial embolism and thrombosis**
Includes   embolic infarction
embolic occlusion
thrombotic infarction
thrombotic occlusion

Bold typeface is used on all codes and titles.

I83.001   **Varicose veins of unspecified lower extremity with ulcer of thigh**

"with" should be interpreted to mean "associated with" or "due to."

K73.2   **Chronic active hepatitis, not elsewhere classified**

"not elsewhere classified" or **NEC** identifies a code that is assigned only when the information at hand specifies a condition for which no more specific code is available.

"not otherwise specified" or **NOS** is equivalent to unspecified.

W13.9   **Fall from, out of or through building, not otherwise specified**

Codes or index entries are for purposes of illustration only and may not be current.

Excludes1 means "NOT CODED HERE!" An Excludes1 note indicates that the code excluded should never be assigned at the same time as the code above the Excludes1 note.

M19 Other and unspecified osteoarthritis
 Excludes1   polyarthritis (M15.-)
 Excludes2   arthrosis of spine (M47.-)
                 hallux rigidus (M20.2)
                 osteoarthritis of spine (M47.-)

Excludes2 represents "NOT INCLUDED HERE." An Excludes2 note indicates that the condition excluded is not part of the condition represented by the code, but a patient may have both conditions at the same time and it is acceptable to use both the code and the excluded code together, when appropriate.

Includes: This note appears immediately under a three-character code title to further define, or give examples of, the content.

A06 Amebiasis
 Includes   infection due to Entamoeba histolytica

E26.01 Conn's syndrome
    Code also adrenal adenoma (D35.0)

Code also instructs that two codes may be required to fully describe a condition, but this note does not provide sequencing direction.

Codes titled "other" or "other specified" are for use when the information in the medical record provides detail for which a specific code does not exist.

E25.8 Other adrenogenital disorders

O00.2 Ovarian pregnancy   M

Maternity DX (Diagnosis) for ages 9-64 according to the *Definitions of Medicare Code Edits* (MCE).

P02.20 Newborn (suspected to be) affected by unspecified morphological and functional abnormalities of placenta   N

Newborn, Age 0, according to the *Definitions of Medicare Code Edits* (MCE).

L21.0 Seborrhea capitis   P
         Cradle cap

Pediatric Age, 0-17, according to the *Definitions of Medicare Code Edits* (MCE).

G30.1 Alzheimer's disease with late onset   A

Adult Age, 15-124, according to the *Definitions of Medicare Code Edits* (MCE).

Females Only according to the *Definitions of Medicare Code Edits* (MCE).

B37.3 Candidiasis of vulva and vagina ♀

C60.1 Malignant neoplasm of glans penis ♂

Males Only according to the *Definitions of Medicare Code Edits* (MCE).

Codes or index entries are for purposes of illustration only and may not be current.

H22 *Disorders of iris and ciliary body in diseases classified elsewhere*

Code first underlying disease, such as:
gout (M1A-, M10.-)

Manifestation according to the *Definitions of Medicare Code Edits* (MCE).

F10.21 Alcohol dependence, in remission

Key Term Highlight identifies key words within similar code descriptions in a particular category.

Coding Clinic identifies the year, quarter, and page number that presents information about an ICD-10-PCS code in the American Hospital Association's *Coding Clinic®*.

B96.5 Pseudomonas (aeruginosa) (mallei) (pseudomallei) as the cause of diseases classified elsewhere
▶ Coding Clinic: 2015, Q1, P18

Codes or index entries are for purposes of illustration only and may not be current.

Alphabetic Index

Main terms are in **bold** typeface.

Aberrant (congenital) —*see also* Malposition, congenital
adrenal gland Q89.1

Etiology code first followed by the manifestation code in **brackets**. The code in brackets is always to be sequenced second.

Amyloid heart (disease) E85.4 *[I43]*

Amylophagia —*see* Pica

"see" indicates another term should be referenced.

Angiofibroma —*see also* Neoplasm, benign, by site

"see also" follows a main term and instructs that there is another main term that may also be referenced.

Appendicitis (pneumococcal) (retrocecal) K37
with
perforation NOS K35.32
peritoneal abscess K35.33

A default code is listed next to the main term and represents that condition most commonly associated with the main term. If a condition is documented in a medical record without any additional information, such as acute or chronic, the default code should be assigned.

Use Additional Character(s): The red stop sign cautions you that the code requires additional character(s) to ensure greatest specificity.

Abrasion T14.8
ankle S90.51-●

Codes or index entries are for purposes of illustration only and may not be current.

No Change **CHAPTER 1**

No Change **CERTAIN INFECTIOUS AND PARASITIC DISEASES (A00-B99)**

No Change **OTHER BACTERIAL DISEASES (A30-A49)**

No Change **A37** Whooping cough
No Change   **A37.0** Whooping cough due to Bordetella pertussis
No Change   **A37.00** **Whooping cough due to Bordetella pertussis without pneumonia**
Add   Paroxysmal cough due to Bordetella pertussis without pneumonia
No Change   **A37.01** **Whooping cough due to Bordetella pertussis with pneumonia**
Add   Paroxysmal cough due to Bordetella pertussis with pneumonia

No Change **RICKETTSIOSES (A75-A79)**

No Change **A77** Spotted fever [tick-borne rickettsioses]
No Change   **A77.4** Ehrlichiosis
No Change   **Excludes1**
Delete   Rickettsiosis due to Ehrlichia sennetsu (A79.81)
Add   anaplasmosis [A. phagocytophilum] (A79.82)
Add   rickettsiosis due to Ehrlichia sennetsu (A79.81)

No Change **A79** Other rickettsioses
No Change   **A79.8** Other specified rickettsioses
Add   **A79.82** **Anaplasmosis [A. phagocytophilum]**
Add   Transfusion transmitted A. phagocytophilum

No Change **VIRAL AND PRION INFECTIONS OF THE CENTRAL NERVOUS SYSTEM (A80-A89)**

No Change **A80** Acute poliomyelitis
Add   **Excludes1** acute flaccid myelitis (G04.82)

No Change **HELMINTHIASES (B65-B83)**

No Change **B74** Filariasis
No Change   **Excludes2**
Revise from   tropical (pulmonary) eosinophilia NOS (J82)
Revise to   tropical (pulmonary) eosinophilia NOS (J82.89)

No Change **SEQUELAE OF INFECTIOUS AND PARASITIC DISEASES (B90-B94)**

No Change **B94** Sequelae of other and unspecified infectious and parasitic diseases
No Change   **B94.9** Sequelae of unspecified infectious and parasitic disease
Add   **Excludes2** post COVID-19 condition (U09.9)

No Change **BACTERIAL AND VIRAL INFECTIOUS AGENTS (B95-B97)**

No Change **B97** Viral agents as the cause of diseases classified elsewhere
No Change   **B97.4** **Respiratory syncytial virus as the cause of diseases classified elsewhere**
Delete   **Excludes2** acute bronchiolitis due to respiratory syncytial virus (RSV) (J21.0)
Delete   acute bronchitis due to respiratory syncytial virus (RSV) (J20.5)
Delete   respiratory syncytial virus (RSV) pneumonia (J12.1)
Add   **Excludes1** acute bronchiolitis due to respiratory syncytial virus (RSV) (J21.0)
Add   acute bronchitis due to respiratory syncytial virus (RSV) (J20.5)
Add   respiratory syncytial virus (RSV) pneumonia (J12.1)

No Change **CHAPTER 2**

No Change **NEOPLASMS (C00-D49)**

No Change **MALIGNANT NEOPLASMS OF DIGESTIVE ORGANS (C15-C26)**

No Change **C25** Malignant neoplasm of pancreas
No Change   Code also
Revise from   exocrine pancreatic insufficiency (K86.81)
Revise to   if applicable exocrine pancreatic insufficiency (K86.81)

No Change **MALIGNANT NEOPLASMS OF RESPIRATORY AND INTRATHORACIC ORGANS (C30-C39)**

No Change **C30** Malignant neoplasm of nasal cavity and middle ear
No Change   **C30.0** Malignant neoplasm of nasal cavity
No Change   **Excludes1**
Revise from   other and unspecified malignant neoplasm of skin of nose C44.301, C44.311, C44.321, C44.391)
Revise to   other and unspecified malignant neoplasm of skin of nose (C44.301, C44.311, C44.321, C44.391)

No Change **MALIGNANT NEOPLASMS OF FEMALE GENITAL ORGANS (C51-C58)**

No Change **C56** Malignant neoplasm of ovary
Add   **C56.3** **Malignant neoplasm of bilateral ovaries**

No Change **MALIGNANT NEOPLASMS OF ILL-DEFINED, OTHER SECONDARY AND UNSPECIFIED SITES (C76-C80)**

No Change **C79** Secondary malignant neoplasm of other and unspecified sites
No Change   **C79.6** Secondary malignant neoplasm of ovary
Add   **C79.63** **Secondary malignant neoplasm of bilateral ovaries**

No Change			**MALIGNANT NEOPLASMS OF LYMPHOID, HEMATOPOIETIC AND RELATED TISSUE (C81-C96)**

No Change **C84** Mature T/NK-cell lymphomas
No Change   **C84.7** Anaplastic large cell lymphoma, ALK-negative
Add   **C84.7A** Anaplastic large cell lymphoma, ALK-negative, breast
Add   Breast implant associated anaplastic large cell lymphoma (BIA-ALCL)
Add   Use Additional code to identify:
Add   breast implant status (Z98.82)
Add   personal history of breast implant removal (Z98.86)

IN SITU NEOPLASMS (D00-D09)

No Change **D02** Carcinoma in situ of middle ear and respiratory system
No Change   **D02.3** Carcinoma in situ of other parts of respiratory system
No Change   **Excludes1**
Revise from   carcinoma in situ of nose NOS D09.8
Revise to   carcinoma in situ of nose NOS (D09.8)

NEOPLASMS OF UNCERTAIN BEHAVIOR, POLYCYTHEMIA VERA AND MYELODYSPLASTIC SYNDROMES (D37-D48)

No Change **D47** Other neoplasms of uncertain behavior of lymphoid, hematopoietic and related tissue
No Change   **D47.3** Essential (hemorrhagic) thrombocythemia
Add   Primary thrombocytosis
Add   **Excludes2** reactive thrombocytosis (D75.838)
Add   secondary thrombocytosis (D75.838)
Add   thrombocythemia NOS (D75.839)
Add   thrombocytosis NOS (D75.839)
No Change   **D47.Z** Other specified neoplasms of uncertain behavior of lymphoid, hematopoietic and related tissue
No Change   **D47.Z2** Castleman disease
No Change   Code also
Revise from   if applicable human herpesvirus 8 infection (B10.89)
Revise to   , if applicable, human herpesvirus 8 infection (B10.89)

No Change # CHAPTER 3

No Change # DISEASES OF THE BLOOD AND BLOOD-FORMING ORGANS AND CERTAIN DISORDERS INVOLVING THE IMMUNE MECHANISM (D50-D89)

HEMOLYTIC ANEMIAS (D55-D59)

No Change **D55** Anemia due to enzyme disorders
No Change   **D55.2** Anemia due to disorders of glycolytic enzymes
Delete   Hemolytic nonspherocytic (hereditary) anemia, type II
Delete   Hexokinase deficiency anemia
Delete   Pyruvate kinase [PK] deficiency anemia
Delete   Triose-phosphate isomerase deficiency anemia
Add   **D55.21** Anemia due to pyruvate kinase deficiency
Add   PK deficiency anemia
Add   Pyruvate kinase deficiency anemia
Add   **D55.29** Anemia due to other disorders of glycolytic enzymes
Add   Hexokinase deficiency anemia
Add   Triose-phosphate isomerase deficiency anemia

No Change **D57** Sickle-cell disorders
No Change   **D57.4** Sickle-cell thalassemia
No Change   **D57.41** Sickle-cell thalassemia, unspecified, with crisis
No Change   **D57.419** Sickle-cell thalassemia, unspecified, with crisis
Revise from   Sickle-cell thalassemia with vasoocclusive pain
Revise to   Sickle-cell thalassemia with vasoocclusive pain NOS
No Change   **D57.43** Sickle-cell thalassemia beta zero with crisis
No Change   **D57.439** Sickle-cell thalassemia beta zero with crisis, unspecified
Revise from   Sickle-cell thalassemia beta zero with vasoocclusive pain
Revise to   Sickle-cell thalassemia beta zero with vasoocclusive pain NOS
No Change   **D57.45** Sickle-cell thalassemia beta plus with crisis
No Change   **D57.459** Sickle-cell thalassemia beta plus with crisis, unspecified
Revise from   Sickle-cell thalassemia beta plus with vasoocclusive pain
Revise to   Sickle-cell thalassemia beta plus with vasoocclusive pain NOS

APLASTIC AND OTHER ANEMIAS AND OTHER BONE MARROW FAILURE SYNDROMES (D60-D64)

No Change **D64** Other anemias
No Change   **D64.8** Other specified anemias
No Change   **D64.81** Anemia due to antineoplastic chemotherapy
Delete   **Excludes1** aplastic anemia due to antineoplastic chemotherapy (D61.1)
Add   **Excludes2** aplastic anemia due to antineoplastic chemotherapy (D61.1)

COAGULATION DEFECTS, PURPURA AND OTHER HEMORRHAGIC CONDITIONS (D65-D69)

No Change **D68** Other coagulation defects
No Change   **D68.5** Primary thrombophilia
No Change   **Excludes1**
Revise from   thrombotic thrombocytopenic purpura (M31.1)
Revise to   thrombotic thrombocytopenic purpura (M31.19)

No Change **D69** Purpura and other hemorrhagic conditions
No Change   **Excludes1**
Revise from   thrombotic thrombocytopenic purpura (M31.1)
Revise to   thrombotic thrombocytopenic purpura (M31.19)

No Change **OTHER DISORDERS OF BLOOD AND BLOOD-FORMING ORGANS (D70-D77)**

No Change **D72** Other disorders of white blood cells
No Change   **D72.1** Eosinophilia
No Change   **Excludes2**
Revise from   Löffler's syndrome (J82)
Revise to   Löffler's syndrome (J82.89)
Revise from   pulmonary eosinophilia (J82)
Revise to   pulmonary eosinophilia (J82.-)

No Change **D75** Other and unspecified diseases of blood and blood-forming organs

No Change **D75.8** Other specified diseases of blood and blood-forming organs

Add **D75.83** Thrombocytosis

Add **Excludes2** essential thrombocythemia (D47.3)

Add **D75.838** Other thrombocytosis
Add Reactive thrombocytosis
Add Secondary thrombocytosis
Add Code also underlying condition, if known and applicable

Add **D75.839** Thrombocytosis, unspecified
Add Thrombocythemia NOS
Add Thrombocytosis NOS

No Change **CERTAIN DISORDERS INVOLVING THE IMMUNE MECHANISM (D8Ø-D89)**

No Change **D89** Other disorders involving the immune mechanism, not elsewhere classified

No Change **D89.4** Mast cell activation syndrome and related disorders

Add **D89.44** Hereditary alpha tryptasemia
Add Use additional code if applicable, for:
Add allergy status, other than to drugs and biological substances (Z91.Ø-)
Add personal history of anaphylaxis (Z87.892)

No Change **CHAPTER 4**

No Change **ENDOCRINE, NUTRITIONAL AND METABOLIC DISEASES (EØØ-E89)**

No Change **DISORDERS OF OTHER ENDOCRINE GLANDS (E2Ø-E35)**

No Change **E21** Hyperparathyroidism and other disorders of parathyroid gland

Delete **Excludes1** familial hypocalciuric hypercalcemia (E83.52)

Add **Excludes2** familial hypocalciuric hypercalcemia (E83.52)

No Change **OTHER NUTRITIONAL DEFICIENCIES (E5Ø-E64)**

No Change **E63** Other nutritional deficiencies
Delete **Excludes1** dehydration (E86.Ø)
Delete failure to thrive, adult (R62.7)
Delete failure to thrive, child (R62.51)
Delete feeding problems in newborn (P92.-)
Delete sequelae of malnutrition and other nutritional deficiencies (E64.-)

Add **Excludes2** dehydration (E86.Ø)
Add failure to thrive, adult (R62.7)
Add failure to thrive, child (R62.51)
Add feeding problems in newborn (P92.-)
Add sequelae of malnutrition and other nutritional deficiencies (E64.-)

No Change **METABOLIC DISORDERS (E7Ø-E88)**

Delete **Excludes1** Ehlers-Danlos syndromes (Q79.6-)

Add **Excludes2** Ehlers-Danlos syndromes (Q79.6-)

No Change **E75** Disorders of sphingolipid metabolism and other lipid storage disorders

No Change **E75.2** Other sphingolipidosis

No Change **E75.24** Niemann-Pick disease
Add Acid sphingomyelinase deficiency (ASMD)

No Change **E75.240** Niemann-Pick disease type A
Add Acid sphingomyelinase deficiency type A (ASMD type A)
Add Infantile neurovisceral acid sphingomyelinase deficiency

No Change **E75.241** Niemann-Pick disease type B
Add Acid sphingomyelinase deficiency type B (ASMD type B)
Add Chronic visceral acid sphingomyelinase deficiency

Add **E75.244** Niemann-Pick disease type A/B
Add Acid sphingomyelinase deficiency type A/B (ASMD type A/B)
Add Chronic neurovisceral acid sphingomyelinase deficiency

No Change **E75.249** Niemann-Pick disease, unspecified
Add Acid sphingomyelinase deficiency (ASMD) NOS

No Change **E87** Other disorders of fluid, electrolyte and acid-base balance

No Change **E87.2** Acidosis
No Change **Excludes1**
Revise from diabetic acidosis - see categories E08-E10, E13 with ketoacidosis
Revise to diabetic acidosis - see categories E08-E10, E11, E13 with ketoacidosis

No Change **CHAPTER 5**

No Change **MENTAL, BEHAVIORAL AND NEURODEVELOPMENTAL DISORDERS (FØ1-F99)**

No Change **MOOD [AFFECTIVE] DISORDERS (F3Ø-F39)**

Revise from **F32** Major depressive disorder, single episode
Revise to **F32** Depressive episode
No Change **F32.9** Major depressive disorder, single episode, unspecified
Delete Depression NOS
Delete Depressive disorder NOS

Add **F32.A** Depression, unspecified
Add Depression NOS
Add Depressive disorder NOS

No Change **BEHAVIORAL SYNDROMES ASSOCIATED WITH PHYSIOLOGICAL DISTURBANCES AND PHYSICAL FACTORS (F5Ø-F59)**

No Change **F5Ø** Eating disorders
Delete **Excludes1** feeding difficulties (R63.3)

Add **Excludes2** feeding difficulties (R63.3)

No Change **INTELLECTUAL DISABILITIES (F7Ø-F79)**

No Change **F78** Other intellectual disabilities
Add **F78.A** Other genetic related intellectual disabilities
Add **F78.A1** SYNGAP1-related intellectual disability
Add Code also, if applicable, any associated:
Add autism spectrum disorder (F84.Ø)
Add autistic disorder (F84.0)
Add encephalopathy (G93.4-)
Add epilepsy and recurrent seizures (G4Ø.-)
Add other pervasive developmental disorders (F84.8)
Add pervasive developmental disorder, NOS (F84.9)

Add	F78.A9	Other genetic related intellectual disability
Add		*Code also, if applicable, any associated disorders*

No Change **PERVASIVE AND SPECIFIC DEVELOPMENTAL DISORDERS (F80-F89)**

No Change F84	Pervasive developmental disorders	
Delete	Use Additional code to identify any associated medical condition and intellectual disabilities.	
Add	Code also any associated medical condition and intellectual disabilities	

No Change **BEHAVIORAL AND EMOTIONAL DISORDERS WITH ONSET USUALLY OCCURRING IN CHILDHOOD AND ADOLESCENCE (F90-F98)**

No Change F98	Other behavioral and emotional disorders with onset usually occurring in childhood and adolescence	
No Change	F98.2 Other feeding disorders of infancy and childhood	
Delete	**Excludes1** feeding difficulties (R63.3)	
Add	**Excludes2** feeding difficulties (R63.3)	

No Change **CHAPTER 6**

No Change **DISEASES OF THE NERVOUS SYSTEM (G00-G99)**

No Change **INFLAMMATORY DISEASES OF THE CENTRAL NERVOUS SYSTEM (G00-G09)**

No Change G02	Meningitis in other infectious and parasitic diseases classified elsewhere	
No Change	**Excludes1**	
Revise from		infectious mononucleosis complicated by meningitis (B27.- with fourth character 2)
Revise to		infectious mononucleosis complicated by meningitis (B27.- with fifth character 2)
No Change G04	Encephalitis, myelitis and encephalomyelitis	
No Change	**Excludes2**	
Revise from		toxic encephalitis (G92)
Revise to		toxic encephalitis (G92.8)
Revise from		toxic encephalopathy (G92)
Revise to		toxic encephalopathy (G92.8)
No Change	G04.8 Other encephalitis, myelitis and encephalomyelitis	
Add	G04.82 Acute flaccid myelitis	
Add	**Excludes1** transverse myelitis (G37.3)	
No Change G05	Encephalitis, myelitis and encephalomyelitis in diseases classified elsewhere	
Add	*Code first* congenital toxoplasmosis encephalitis, myelitis and encephalomyelitis (P37.1)	
Add	cytomegaloviral encephalitis, myelitis and encephalomyelitis (B25.8)	
Add	encephalitis, myelitis and encephalomyelitis (in) systemic lupus erythematosus (M32.19)	
Add	eosinophilic meningoencephalitis (B83.2)	
Delete	**Excludes1** congenital toxoplasmosis encephalitis, myelitis and encephalomyelitis (P37.1)	
Delete	cytomegaloviral encephalitis, myelitis and encephalomyelitis (B25.8)	
Delete	encephalitis, myelitis and encephalomyelitis (in) systemic lupus erythematosus (M32.19)	
Delete	eosinophilic meningoencephalitis (B83.2)	

No Change **DEMYELINATING DISEASES OF THE CENTRAL NERVOUS SYSTEM (G35-G37)**

No Change G37	Other demyelinating diseases of central nervous system	
No Change	G37.3 Acute transverse myelitis in demyelinating disease of central nervous system	
Add	**Excludes1** acute flaccid myelitis (G04.82)	

No Change **EPISODIC AND PAROXYSMAL DISORDERS (G40-G47)**

No Change G44	Other headache syndromes	
No Change	G44.8 Other specified headache syndromes	
Add	G44.86 Cervicogenic headache	
Add	Code also associated cervical spinal condition, if known	

No Change **NERVE, NERVE ROOT AND PLEXUS DISORDERS (G50-G59)**

No Change G55	Nerve root and plexus compressions in diseases classified elsewhere	
No Change	**Excludes1**	
Revise from		nerve root compression (due to) (in) spondylosis (M47.0-M47.2.-)
Revise to		nerve root compression (due to) (in) spondylosis (M47.0-, M47.2.-)

No Change **POLYNEUROPATHIES AND OTHER DISORDERS OF THE PERIPHERAL NERVOUS SYSTEM (G60-G65)**

No Change G63	Polyneuropathy in diseases classified elsewhere	
No Change	**Excludes1**	
Revise from		infectious mononucleosis (B27.0-B27.9 with 1)
Revise to		infectious mononucleosis complicated by polyneuropathy (B27.0-B27.9 with fifth character 1)

No Change **DISEASES OF MYONEURAL JUNCTION AND MUSCLE (G70-G73)**

No Change G71	Primary disorders of muscles	
No Change	G71.2 Congenital myopathies	
Revise from		G71.20 Congenital myopathy, unspecifed
Revise to		G71.20 Congenital myopathy, unspecified
No Change G73	Disorders of myoneural junction and muscle in diseases classified elsewhere	
No Change	G73.7 Myopathy in diseases classified elsewhere	
No Change	**Excludes1**	
Revise from		sicca syndrome [Sjögren] (M35.03)
Revise to		Sjögren syndrome (M35.03)

No Change **OTHER DISORDERS OF THE NERVOUS SYSTEM (G89-G99)**

No Change G89	Pain, not elsewhere classified	
No Change	**Excludes2**	
Revise from		lumbar region pain (M54.5)
Revise to		lumbar region pain (M54.5-)
No Change G92	Toxic encephalopathy	
Delete	Toxic encephalitis	
Delete	Toxic metabolic encephalopathy	
Delete	*Code first* , if applicable, drug induced (T36-T50) or use (T51-T65) to identify toxic agent	
Add	G92.0 Immune effector cell-associated neurotoxicity syndrome	
Add	*Code first* underlying cause such as:	
Add	complications of immune effector cellular therapy (T80.82)	
Add	Code also associated signs and symptoms, such as seizures and cerebral edema	
Add	Code also, if applicable:	
Add	cerebral edema (G93.6)	
Add	unspecified convulsions (R56.9)	

Add   G92.00 **Immune effector cell-associated neurotoxicity syndrome, grade unspecified**

Add   ICANS, grade unspecified

Add   G92.01 **Immune effector cell-associated neurotoxicity syndrome, grade 1**

Add   ICANS, grade 1

Add   G92.02 **Immune effector cell-associated neurotoxicity syndrome, grade 2**

Add   ICANS, grade 2

Add   G92.03 **Immune effector cell-associated neurotoxicity syndrome, grade 3**

Add   ICANS, grade 3

Add   G92.04 **Immune effector cell-associated neurotoxicity syndrome, grade 4**

Add   ICANS, grade 4

Add   G92.05 **Immune effector cell-associated neurotoxicity syndrome, grade 5**

Add   ICANS, grade 5

Add   G92.8 **Other toxic encephalopathy**

Add   Toxic encephalitis

Add   Toxic metabolic encephalopathy

Add   *Code first* poisoning due to drug or toxin, if applicable, (T36-T65 with fifth or sixth character 1-4 or 6)

Add   Use Additional code for adverse effect, if applicable, to identify drug (T36-T50 with fifth or sixth character 5)

Add   G92.9 **Unspecified toxic encephalopathy**

Add   *Code first* poisoning due to drug or toxin, if applicable, (T36-T65 with fifth or sixth character 1-4 or 6)

Add   Use Additional code for adverse effect, if applicable, to identify drug (T36-T50 with fifth or sixth character 5)

No Change **G93 Other disorders of brain**

No Change   G93.4 **Other and unspecified encephalopathy**

No Change   **Excludes2**

Revise from   toxic (metabolic) encephalopathy (G92)

Revise to   toxic (metabolic) encephalopathy (G92.8)

No Change   G93.5 **Compression of brain**

No Change   **Excludes1**

Delete   diffuse traumatic compression of brain (S06.2-)

Delete   focal traumatic compression of brain (S06.3-)

Add   traumatic compression of brain (S06.A-)

No Change **CHAPTER 7**

No Change **DISEASES OF THE EYE AND ADNEXA (H00-H59)**

No Change **DISORDERS OF CHOROID AND RETINA (H30-H36)**

No Change **H35 Other retinal disorders**

No Change   H35.0 **Background retinopathy and retinal vascular changes**

No Change   Code also

Revise from   any associated hypertension (I10.-)

Revise to   any associated hypertension (I10)

No Change **CHAPTER 9**

No Change **DISEASES OF THE CIRCULATORY SYSTEM (I00-I99)**

This chapter contains the following blocks:

Revise from	I30-I52	Other forms of heart disease
Revise to	I30-I5A	Other forms of heart disease

No Change **ISCHEMIC HEART DISEASES (I20-I25)**

Delete   Use Additional code to identify presence of hypertension (I10-I16)

Add   Code also the presence of hypertension (I10-I16)

No Change **I24 Other acute ischemic heart diseases**

Add   **Excludes2** non-ischemic myocardial injury (I5A)

No Change **I25 Chronic ischemic heart disease**

Add   **Excludes2** non-ischemic myocardial injury (I5A)

Delete **OTHER FORMS OF HEART DISEASE (I30-I52)**

Add **OTHER FORMS OF HEART DISEASE (I30-I5A)**

No Change **I50 Heart failure**

Delete   **Excludes1** neonatal cardiac failure (P29.0)

Add   **Excludes2** neonatal cardiac failure (P20.0)

Add   **I5A Non-ischemic myocardial injury (non-traumatic)**

Add   Acute (non-ischemic) myocardial injury

Add   Chronic (non-ischemic) myocardial injury

Add   Unspecified (non-ischemic) myocardial injury

Add   *Code first* the underlying cause, if known and applicable, such as:

Add   acute kidney failure (N17.-)

Add   acute myocarditis (I40.-)

Add   cardiomyopathy (I42.-)

Add   chronic kidney disease (CKD) (N18.-)

Add   heart failure (I50.-)

Add   hypertensive urgency (I16.0)

Add   nonrheumatic aortic valve disorders (I35.-)

Add   paroxysmal tachycardia (I47.-) pulmonary embolism (I26.-)

Add   pulmonary hypertension (I27.0, I27.2-)

Add   sepsis (A41.-)

Add   takotsubo syndrome (I51.81)

Add   **Excludes1** acute myocardial infarction (I21.-)

Add   injury of heart (S26.-)

Add   **Excludes2** other acute ischemic heart diseases (I24.-)

No Change **DISEASES OF VEINS, LYMPHATIC VESSELS AND LYMPH NODES, NOT ELSEWHERE CLASSIFIED (I80-I89)**

No Change **I83 Varicose veins of lower extremities**

Delete   **Excludes1** varicose veins complicating pregnancy (O22.0-)

Delete   varicose veins complicating the puerperium (O87.4)

Add   **Excludes2** varicose veins complicating pregnancy (O22.0-)

Add   varicose veins complicating the puerperium (O87.4)

No Change **CHAPTER 10**

No Change **DISEASES OF THE RESPIRATORY SYSTEM (J00-J99)**

No Change **ACUTE UPPER RESPIRATORY INFECTIONS (J00-J06)**

No Change **J05 Acute obstructive laryngitis [croup] and epiglottitis**

No Change   Code also

Revise from   , if present, such as:

Revise to   , influenza, if present, such as:

No Change	**CHRONIC LOWER RESPIRATORY DISEASES (J40-J47)**	

No Change J44   **Other chronic obstructive pulmonary disease**
No Change   **Includes:**
Revise from   chronic bronchitis with airways obstruction
Revise to   chronic bronchitis with airway obstruction

No Change J47   **Bronchiectasis**
No Change   J47.0   **Bronchiectasis with acute lower respiratory infection**
Delete   Use Additional code to identify the infection
Add   Code also to identify infection, if applicable

No Change	**OTHER DISEASES OF THE RESPIRATORY SYSTEM (J96-J99)**	

No Change J99   **Respiratory disorders in diseases classified elsewhere**
No Change   **Excludes1**
Revise from   sicca syndrome (M35.02)
Revise to   Sjögren syndrome (M35.02)

No Change **CHAPTER 11**

No Change **DISEASES OF THE DIGESTIVE SYSTEM (K00-K95)**

No Change	**DISEASES OF ORAL CAVITY AND SALIVARY GLANDS (K00-K14)**	

No Change K11   **Diseases of salivary glands**
No Change   K11.8   **Other diseases of salivary glands**
No Change   **Excludes1**
Revise from   sicca syndrome [Sjögren] (M35.0-)
Revise to   Sjögren syndrome (M35.0-)

No Change	**DISEASES OF ESOPHAGUS, STOMACH AND DUODENUM (K20-K31)**	

No Change K22   **Other diseases of esophagus**
No Change   K22.8   **Other specified diseases of esophagus**
Delete   Hemorrhage of esophagus NOS
Add   K22.81   **Esophageal polyp**
Add   **Excludes1** benign neoplasm of esophagus (D13.0)
Add   K22.82   **Esophagogastric junction polyp**
Add   **Excludes1** benign neoplasm of stomach (D13.1)
Add   K22.89   **Other specified disease of esophagus**
Add   Hemorrhage of esophagus NOS

No Change K31   **Other diseases of stomach and duodenum**
Add   K31.A   **Gastric intestinal metaplasia**
Add   K31.A0   **Gastric intestinal metaplasia, unspecified**
Add   Gastric intestinal metaplasia indefinite for dysplasia
Add   Gastric intestinal metaplasia NOS
Add   K31.A1   **Gastric intestinal metaplasia without dysplasia**
Add   K31.A11   **Gastric intestinal metaplasia without dysplasia, involving the antrum**
Add   K31.A12   **Gastric intestinal metaplasia without dysplasia, involving the body (corpus)**
Add   K31.A13   **Gastric intestinal metaplasia without dysplasia, involving the fundus**
Add   K31.A14   **Gastric intestinal metaplasia without dysplasia, involving the cardia**
Add   K31.A15   **Gastric intestinal metaplasia without dysplasia, involving multiple sites**
Add   K31.A19   **Gastric intestinal metaplasia without dysplasia, unspecified site**

Add   K31.A2   **Gastric intestinal metaplasia with dysplasia**
Add   K31.A21   **Gastric intestinal metaplasia with low grade dysplasia**
Add   K31.A22   **Gastric intestinal metaplasia with high grade dysplasia**
Add   K31.A29   **Gastric intestinal metaplasia with dysplasia, unspecified**

No Change	**DISEASES OF APPENDIX (K35-K38)**	

No Change K37   **Unspecified appendicitis**
No Change   **Excludes1**
Revise from   -unspecified appendicitis with peritonitis (K35.2-, K35.3-)
Revise to   unspecified appendicitis with peritonitis (K35.2-, K35.3-)

No Change	**NONINFECTIVE ENTERITIS AND COLITIS (K50-K52)**	

No Change K52   **Other and unspecified noninfective gastroenteritis and colitis**
No Change   K52.2   **Allergic and dietetic gastroenteritis and colitis**
Delete   **Excludes2** food protein-induced proctocolitis (K52.82)
No Change   K52.29   **Other allergic and dietetic gastroenteritis and colitis**
Add   Allergic proctocolitis
Add   Food-induced eosinophilic proctocolitis
Add   Food protein-induced proctocolitis
Add   Milk protein-induced proctocolitis
No Change   K52.8   **Other specified noninfective gastroenteritis and colitis**
No Change   K52.82   **Eosinophilic colitis**
Delete   Allergic proctocolitis
Delete   Food-induced eosinophilic proctocolitis
Delete   Food protein-induced proctocolitis
Delete   Milk protein-induced proctocolitis
Add   **Excludes2** allergic proctocolitis (K52.29)
Add   food-induced eosinophilic proctocolitis (K52.29)
Add   food protein-induced enterocolitis syndrome (FPIES) (K52.21)
Add   food protein-induced proctocolitis (K52.29)
Add   milk protein-induced proctocolitis (K52.29)

No Change	**OTHER DISEASES OF INTESTINES (K55-K64)**	

No Change K59   **Other functional intestinal disorders**
No Change   K59.0   **Constipation**
No Change   K59.03   **Drug induced constipation**
No Change   Use Additional
Revise from   code for adverse effect, if applicable, to identify drug (T36-T50 with fifth or sixth character 5
Revise to   code for adverse effect, if applicable, to identify drug (T36-T50 with fifth or sixth character 5)

No Change	**DISEASES OF LIVER (K70-K77)**	

No Change K72   **Hepatic failure, not elsewhere classified**
No Change   K72.1   **Chronic hepatic failure**
Add   End stage liver disease

No Change K77   **Liver disorders in diseases classified elsewhere**
Add   *Code first infectious mononucleosis with liver disease (B27.0-B27.9 with .9)*
Delete   **Excludes1** infectious mononucleosis with liver disease (B27.0-B27.9 with .9)

No Change **CHAPTER 12**

No Change
DISEASES OF THE SKIN AND SUBCUTANEOUS TISSUE (L00-L99)

No Change **DERMATITIS AND ECZEMA (L20-L30)**

No Change **L24** Irritant contact dermatitis

No Change **L24.A** Irritant contact dermatitis due to friction or contact with body fluids

Add **Excludes1** virritant contact dermatitis related to stoma or fistula (L24.B-)

Add **Excludes2** erythema intertrigo (L30.4)

Add **L24.A0** Irritant contact dermatitis due to friction or contact with body fluids, unspecified

Add **L24.A1** Irritant contact dermatitis due to saliva

Add **L24.A2** Irritant contact dermatitis due to fecal, urinary or dual incontinence

Add **Excludes1** diaper dermatitis (L22)

Add **L24.A9** Irritant contact dermatitis due friction or contact with other specified body fluids

Add Irritant contact dermatitis related to endotracheal tube

Add Wound fluids, exudate

Add **L24.B** Irritant contact dermatitis related to stoma or fistula

Add Use Additional code to identify any artificial opening status (Z93.-), if applicable, for contact dermatitis related to stoma secretions

Add **L24.B0** Irritant contact dermatitis related to unspecified stoma or fistula

Add Irritant contact dermatitis related to fistula NOS

Add Irritant contact dermatitis related to stoma NOS

Add **L24.B1** Irritant contact dermatitis related to digestive stoma or fistula

Add Irritant contact dermatitis related to gastrostomy

Add Irritant contact dermatitis related to jejunostomy

Add Irritant contact dermatitis related to saliva or spit fistula

Add **L24.B2** Irritant contact dermatitis related to respiratory stoma or fistula

Add Irritant contact dermatitis related to tracheostomy

Add **L24.B3** Irritant contact dermatitis related to fecal or urinary stoma or fistula

Add Irritant contact dermatitis related to colostomy

Add Irritant contact dermatitis related to enterocutaneous fistula

Add Irritant contact dermatitis related to ileostomy

No Change **OTHER DISORDERS OF THE SKIN AND SUBCUTANEOUS TISSUE (L80-L99)**

No Change **L89** Pressure ulcer

No Change **L89.0** Pressure ulcer of elbow

No Change **L89.01** Pressure ulcer of right elbow

No Change **L89.019** Pressure ulcer of right elbow, unspecified stage

Revise from Healing pressure right of elbow NOS

Revise to Healing pressure ulcer of right elbow NOS

Delete Healing pressure ulcer of right elbow, unspecified stage

No Change **L89.02** Pressure ulcer of left elbow

No Change **L89.029** Pressure ulcer of left elbow, unspecified stage

Revise from Healing pressure ulcer of left of elbow NOS

Revise to Healing pressure ulcer of left elbow NOS

Delete Healing pressure ulcer of left elbow, unspecified stage

No Change **L99** Other disorders of skin and subcutaneous tissue in diseases classified elsewhere

No Change **Excludes1**

Revise from skin disorders in diabetes (E08-E13 with .62)

Revise to skin disorders in diabetes (E08-E13 with .62-)

No Change **CHAPTER 13**

No Change
DISEASES OF THE MUSCULOSKELETAL SYSTEM AND CONNECTIVE TISSUE (M00-M99)

No Change **SYSTEMIC CONNECTIVE TISSUE DISORDERS (M30-M36)**

No Change **M31** Other necrotizing vasculopathies

No Change **M31.1** Thrombotic microangiopathy
Delete Thrombotic thrombocytopenic purpura

Add **M31.10** Thrombotic microangiopathy, unspecified

Add **M31.11** Hematopoietic stem cell transplantation-associated thrombotic microangiopathy [HSCT-TMA]

Add Transplant-associated thrombotic microangiopathy [TA-TMA]

Add *Code first* if applicable:

Add complications of bone marrow transplant (T86.0-)

Add complications of stem cell transplant (T86.5)

Add Use Additional code to identify specific organ dysfunction, such as:

Add acute kidney failure (N17.-)

Add acute respiratory distress syndrome (J80)

Add capillary leak syndrome (I78.8)

Add diffuse alveolar hemorrhage (R04.89)

Add encephalopathy (metabolic) (septic) (G93.41)

Add fluid overload, unspecified (E87.70)

Add graft versus host disease (D89.81-)

Add hemolytic uremic syndrome (D59.3)

Add hepatic failure (K72.-)

Add hepatic veno-occlusive disease (K76.5)

Add idiopathic interstitial pneumonia (J84.11-)

Add sinusoidal obstruction syndrome (K76.5)

Add **M31.19** Other thrombotic microangiopathy

Add Thrombotic thrombocytopenic purpura

No Change **M34** Systemic sclerosis [scleroderma]

No Change **M34.8** Other forms of systemic sclerosis

No Change **M34.81** Systemic sclerosis with lung involvement

Add Code also if applicable:

Add other interstitial pulmonary diseases (J84.89)

Add secondary pulmonary arterial hypertension (I27.21)

No Change	**M35**	**Other systemic involvement of connective tissue**
Revise from	**M35.0**	Sicca syndrome [Sjögren]
Revise to	**M35.0**	**Sjögren syndrome**
Add		Sicca syndrome
Add		Use Additional code to identify associated manifestations
Add		**Excludes1** dry mouth, unspecified (R68.2)
Revise from	**M35.00**	Sicca syndrome, unspecified
Revise to	**M35.00**	**Sjögren syndrome, unspecified**
Revise from	**M35.01**	Sicca syndrome with keratoconjunctivitis
Revise to	**M35.01**	**Sjögren syndrome with keratoconjunctivitis**
Revise from	**M35.02**	Sicca syndrome with lung involvement
Revise to	**M35.02**	**Sjögren syndrome with lung involvement**
Revise from	**M35.03**	Sicca syndrome with myopathy
Revise to	**M35.03**	**Sjögren syndrome with myopathy**
Revise from	**M35.04**	Sicca syndrome with tubulo-interstitial nephropathy
Revise to	**M35.04**	**Sjögren syndrome with tubulo-interstitial nephropathy**
Add	**M35.05**	**Sjögren syndrome with inflammatory arthritis**
Add	**M35.06**	**Sjögren syndrome with peripheral nervous system involvement**
Add	**M35.07**	**Sjögren syndrome with central nervous system involvement**
Add	**M35.08**	**Sjögren syndrome with gastrointestinal involvement**
Add	**M35.0A**	**Sjögren syndrome with glomerular disease**
Add	**M35.0B**	**Sjögren syndrome with vasculitis**
Add	**M35.0C**	**Sjögren syndrome with dental involvement**
Revise from	**M35.09**	Sicca syndrome with other organ involvement
Revise to	**M35.09**	**Sjögren syndrome with other organ involvement**
No Change	**M35.7**	**Hypermobility syndrome**
Delete		**Excludes1** Ehlers-Danlos syndromes (Q79.6-)
Add		**Excludes2** Ehlers-Danlos syndromes (Q79.6-)
No Change	**M35.8**	**Other specified systemic involvement of connective tissue**
No Change	**M35.81**	**Multisystem inflammatory syndrome**
No Change		Use Additional
Delete		sequelae of COVID-19 (B94.8)
Add		post COVID-19 condition (U09.9)

DEFORMING DORSOPATHIES (M40-M43)

No Change	**M40**	**Kyphosis and lordosis**
Add		*Code first* underlying disease
No Change	**M41**	**Scoliosis**
Delete		**Excludes1** postprocedural scoliosis (M96.-)
Add		**Excludes2** postprocedural scoliosis (M96.-)
No Change	**M41.5**	**Other secondary scoliosis**
Add		*Code first* underlying disease

SPONDYLOPATHIES (M45-M49)

No Change	**M45**	**Ankylosing spondylitis**
Add		**M45.A Non-radiographic axial spondyloarthritis**
Add		**M45.A0 Non-radiographic axial spondyloarthritis of unspecified sites in spine**
Add		**M45.A1 Non-radiographic axial spondyloarthritis of occipito-atlanto-axial region**
Add		**M45.A2 Non-radiographic axial spondyloarthritis of cervical region**

Add		**M45.A3 Non-radiographic axial spondyloarthritis of cervicothoracic region**
Add		**M45.A4 Non-radiographic axial spondyloarthritis of thoracic region**
Add		**M45.A5 Non-radiographic axial spondyloarthritis of thoracolumbar region**
Add		**M45.A6 Non-radiographic axial spondyloarthritis of lumbar region**
Add		**M45.A7 Non-radiographic axial spondyloarthritis of lumbosacral region**
Add		**M45.A8 Non-radiographic axial spondyloarthritis of sacral and sacrococcygeal region**
Add		**M45.AB Non-radiographic axial spondyloarthritis of multiple sites in spine**

No Change **OTHER DORSOPATHIES (M50-M54)**

No Change	**M54**	**Dorsalgia**
No Change	**M54.5**	**Low back pain**
Delete		Loin pain
Delete		Lumbago NOS
Add	**M54.50**	**Low back pain, unspecified**
Add		Loin pain
Add		Lumbago NOS
Add	**M54.51**	**Vertebrogenic low back pain**
Add		Low back vertebral endplate pain
Add	**M54.59**	**Other low back pain**
Add	**M54.8**	**Other dorsalgia**
No Change		**Excludes1**
Revise from		low back pain (M54.5)
Revise to		low back pain (M54.5-)

No Change # CHAPTER 14

No Change # DISEASES OF THE GENITOURINARY SYSTEM (N00-N99)

No Change **RENAL TUBULO-INTERSTITIAL DISEASES (N10-N16)**

No Change	**N16**	**Renal tubulo-interstitial disorders in diseases classified elsewhere**
No Change		**Excludes1**
Revise from		pyelonephritis and tubulo-interstitial nephritis in sicca syndrome [Sjogren's] (M35.04)
Revise to		pyelonephritis and tubulo-interstitial nephritis in Sjogren syndrome (M35.04)

No Change **OTHER DISEASES OF THE URINARY SYSTEM (N30-N39)**

Delete		**Excludes1** urinary infection (complicating):
Delete		abortion or ectopic or molar pregnancy (O00-O07, O08.8)
Delete		pregnancy, childbirth and the puerperium (O23.-, O75.3, O86.2-)
Add		**Excludes2** urinary infection (complicating):
Add		abortion or ectopic or molar pregnancy (O00-O07, O08.8)
Add		pregnancy, childbirth and the puerperium (O23.-, O75.3, O86.2-)
No Change	**N39**	**Other disorders of urinary system**
No Change	**N39.4**	**Other specified urinary incontinence**
No Change	**N39.44**	**Nocturnal enuresis**
Add		**Excludes2** nocturnal polyuria (R35.81)

No Change **NONINFLAMMATORY DISORDERS OF FEMALE GENITAL TRACT (N80-N98)**

No Change	**N97**	**Female infertility**
Delete		**Excludes1** female infertility associated with:
Delete		hypopituitarism (E23.0)
Delete		Stein-Leventhal syndrome (E28.2)
Add		**Excludes2** female infertility associated with:
Add		hypopituitarism (E23.0)
Add		Stein-Leventhal syndrome (E28.2)

No Change **CHAPTER 15**

No Change
PREGNANCY, CHILDBIRTH AND THE PUERPERIUM (O00-O9A)

No Change
OTHER MATERNAL DISORDERS PREDOMINANTLY RELATED TO PREGNANCY (O20-O29)

No Change **O22** Venous complications and hemorrhoids in pregnancy

No Change   **O22.3** Deep phlebothrombosis in pregnancy

No Change   Use Additional

Revise from   code to identify the deep vein thrombosis (I82.4-, I82.5-, I82.62-. I82.72-)

Revise to   code to identify the deep vein thrombosis (I82.4-, I82.5-, I82.62-, I82.72-)

No Change
COMPLICATIONS PREDOMINANTLY RELATED TO THE PUERPERIUM (O85-O92)

No Change **O87** Venous complications and hemorrhoids in the puerperium

No Change   **O87.1** Deep phlebothrombosis in the puerperium

No Change   Use Additional

Revise from   code to identify the deep vein thrombosis (I82.4-, I82.5-, I82.62-. I82.72-)

Revise to   code to identify the deep vein thrombosis (I82.4-, I82.5-, I82.62-, I82.72-)

No Change **CHAPTER 16**

No Change
CERTAIN CONDITIONS ORIGINATING IN THE PERINATAL PERIOD (P00-P96)

No Change
NEWBORN AFFECTED BY MATERNAL FACTORS AND BY COMPLICATIONS OF PREGNANCY, LABOR, AND DELIVERY (P00–P04)

No Change **P00** Newborn affected by maternal conditions that may be unrelated to present pregnancy

No Change   **P00.2** Newborn affected by maternal infectious and parasitic diseases

Add   **Excludes2** newborn affected by (positive) maternal group B streptococcus (GBS) colonization (P00.82)

No Change   **P00.8** Newborn affected by other maternal conditions

Add   **P00.82** Newborn affected by (positive) maternal group B streptococcus (GBS) colonization

Add   Contact with positive maternal group B streptococcus

No Change   **P00.89** Newborn affected by other maternal conditions

Add   **Excludes2** newborn affected by positive maternal group B streptococcus (GBS) colonization (P00.82)

No Change **P04** Newborn affected by noxious substances transmitted via placenta or breast milk

Add   *Code first any current condition in newborn, if applicable*

No Change
DISORDERS OF NEWBORN RELATED TO LENGTH OF GESTATION AND FETAL GROWTH (P05-P08)

No Change **P08** Disorders of newborn related to long gestation and high birth weight

No Change   **P08.1** Other heavy for gestational age newborn

No Change   **Excludes1**

Revise from   syndrome of infant of mother with gestational diabetes (P70.0).

Revise to   syndrome of infant of mother with gestational diabetes (P70.0)

No Change
ABNORMAL FINDINGS ON NEONATAL SCREENING (P09)

No Change **P09** Abnormal findings on neonatal screening

Delete   Use Additional code to identify signs, symptoms and conditions associated with the screening

Add   **Includes:** Abnormal findings on state mandated newborn screens

Add   Failed newborn screening

Add   **P09.1** Abnormal findings on neonatal screening for inborn errors of metabolism

Add   **P09.2** Abnormal findings on neonatal screening for congenital endocrine disease

Add   Abnormal findings on neonatal screening for congenital adrenal hyperplasia

Add   Abnormal findings on neonatal screening for hypothyroidism screen

Add   **P09.3** Abnormal findings on neonatal screening for congenital hematologic disorders

Add   Abnormal findings for hemoglobinothies screen

Add   Abnormal findings on red cell membrane defects screen

Add   Abnormal findings on sickle cell screen

Add   **P09.4** Abnormal findings on neonatal screening for cystic fibrosis

Add   **P09.5** Abnormal findings on neonatal screening for critical congenital heart disease

Add   Neonatal congenital heart disease screening failure

Add   **P09.6** Abnormal findings on neonatal screening for neonatal hearing loss

Add   **Excludes2** encounter for hearing examination following failed hearing screening (Z01.110)

Add   **P09.8** Other abnormal findings on neonatal screening

Add   **P09.9** Abnormal findings on neonatal screening, unspecified

No Change
RESPIRATORY AND CARDIOVASCULAR DISORDERS SPECIFIC TO THE PERINATAL PERIOD (P19-P29)

No Change **P29** Cardiovascular disorders originating in the perinatal period

Delete   **Excludes1** congenital malformations of the circulatory system (Q20-Q28)

Add   **Excludes2** congenital malformations of the circulatory system (Q20-Q28)

No Change
OTHER DISORDERS ORIGINATING IN THE PERINATAL PERIOD (P90-P96)

No Change **P92** Feeding problems of newborn

Delete   **Excludes1** feeding problems in child over 28 days old (R63.3)

Add   **Excludes2** feeding problems in child over 28 days old (R63.3)

No Change **CHAPTER 17**

No Change
CONGENITAL MALFORMATIONS, DEFORMATIONS AND CHROMOSOMAL ABNORMALITIES (Q00-Q99)

No Change
CONGENITAL MALFORMATIONS OF THE CIRCULATORY SYSTEM (Q20-Q28)

No Change   **Q21** Congenital malformations of cardiac septa

No Change   **Q21.8** Other congenital malformations of cardiac septa

No Change   Code also

Revise from   if applicable:

Revise to   , if applicable:

No Change	**CONGENITAL MALFORMATIONS OF THE URINARY SYSTEM (Q60-Q64)**	

No Change **Q61** Cystic kidney disease

No Change   **Q61.5** Medullary cystic kidney
Revise from   Nephronopthisis
Revise to   Nephronophthisis

No Change **CHAPTER 18**

No Change

SYMPTOMS, SIGNS AND ABNORMAL CLINICAL AND LABORATORY FINDINGS, NOT ELSEWHERE CLASSIFIED (R00-R99)

No Change **SYMPTOMS AND SIGNS INVOLVING THE CIRCULATORY AND RESPIRATORY SYSTEMS (R00-R09)**

No Change **R05** Cough
No Change   **Excludes1**
Delete   cough with hemorrhage (R04.2)
Add   paroxysmal cough due to Bordetella pertussis (A37.0-)
Add   **Excludes2** cough with hemorrhage (R04.2)
Add   **R05.1** Acute cough
Add   **R05.2** Subacute cough
Add   **R05.3** Chronic cough
Add   Persistent cough
Add   Refractory cough
Add   Unexplained cough
Add   **R05.4** Cough syncope
Add   *Code first* syncope and collapse (R55)
Add   **R05.8** Other specified cough
Add   **R05.9** Cough, unspecified

No Change **SYMPTOMS AND SIGNS INVOLVING THE GENITOURINARY SYSTEM (R30-R39)**

No Change **R35** Polyuria
No Change   **R35.8** Other polyuria
Delete   Polyuria NOS
Add   **R35.81** Nocturnal polyuria
Add   **Excludes2** nocturnal enuresis (N39.44)
Add   **R35.89** Other polyuria
Add   Polyuria NOS

No Change **SYMPTOMS AND SIGNS INVOLVING COGNITION, PERCEPTION, EMOTIONAL STATE AND BEHAVIOR (R40-R46)**

No Change **R45** Symptoms and signs involving emotional state
No Change   **R45.8** Other symptoms and signs involving emotional state
Add   **R45.88** Nonsuicidal self-harm
Add   Nonsuicidal self-injury
Add   Nonsuicidal self-mutilation
Add   Self-inflicted injury without suicidal intent
Add   Code also injury, if known

No Change **GENERAL SYMPTOMS AND SIGNS (R50-R69)**

No Change **R52** Pain, unspecified
No Change   **Excludes1**
Revise from   lumbar region pain (M54.5)
Revise to   lumbar region pain (M54.5-)

No Change **R57** Shock, not elsewhere classified
No Change   **Excludes1**
Delete   anesthetic shock (T88.3)
Add   shock due to anesthesia (T88.2)

No Change **R63** Symptoms and signs concerning food and fluid intake
No Change   **R63.3** Feeding difficulties
Delete   Feeding problem (elderly) (infant) NOS
Delete   Picky eater
Delete   **Excludes1** eating disorders (F50.-)
Delete   feeding problems of newborn (P92.-)
Delete   infant feeding disorder of nonorganic origin (F98.2-)
Add   **Excludes2** eating disorders (F50.-)
Add   feeding problems of newborn (P92.-)
Add   infant feeding disorder of nonorganic origin (F98.2-)
Add   **R63.30** Feeding difficulties, unspecified
Add   **R63.31** Pediatric feeding disorder, acute
Add   Pediatric feeding dysfunction, acute
Add   Code also, if applicable, associated conditions such as:
Add   aspiration pneumonia (J69.0)
Add   dysphagia (R13.1-)
Add   gastro-esophageal reflux disease (K21.-)
Add   malnutrition (E40-E46)
Add   **R63.32** Pediatric feeding disorder, chronic
Add   Pediatric feeding dysfunction, chronic
Add   Code also, if applicable, associated conditions such as:
Add   aspiration pneumonia (J69.0)
Add   dysphagia (R13.1-)
Add   gastro-esophageal reflux disease (K21.-)
Add   malnutrition (E40-E46)
Add   **R63.39** Other feeding difficulties
Add   Feeding problem (elderly) (infant) NOS
Add   Picky eater

No Change **R68** Other general symptoms and signs
No Change   **R68.2** Dry mouth, unspecified
No Change   **Excludes1**
Revise from   dry mouth due to sicca syndrome [Sjögren] (M35.0-)
Revise to   dry mouth due to Sjögren syndrome (M35.0-)

No Change **ABNORMAL FINDINGS ON EXAMINATION OF BLOOD, WITHOUT DIAGNOSIS (R70-R79)**

No Change **R79** Other abnormal findings of blood chemistry
No Change   **R79.8** Other specified abnormal findings of blood chemistry
Add   **R79.83** Abnormal findings of blood amino-acid level
Add   Homocysteinemia
Add   **Excludes1** disorders of amino-acid metabolism (E70-E72)

No Change **CHAPTER 19**

No Change

INJURY, POISONING AND CERTAIN OTHER CONSEQUENCES OF EXTERNAL CAUSES (S00-T88)

No Change **INJURIES TO THE HEAD (S00-S09)**

No Change **S00** Superficial injury of head
No Change   **S00.1** Contusion of eyelid and periocular area
No Change   **Excludes2**
Revise from   contusion of eyeball and orbital tissues (S05.1)
Revise to   contusion of eyeball and orbital tissues (S05.1-)

No Change	**S01**	**Open wound of head**
No Change	**S01.0**	**Open wound of scalp**
No Change		**Excludes1**
Revise from		avulsion of scalp (S08.0)
Revise to		avulsion of scalp (S08.0-)

No Change	**S06**	**Intracranial injury**
No Change	**S06.2**	**Diffuse traumatic brain injury**
Add		Use Additional code, if applicable, for traumatic brain compression or herniation (S06.A-)
No Change	**S06.3**	**Focal traumatic brain injury**
Add		Use Additional code, if applicable, for traumatic brain compression or herniation (S06.A-)
No Change	**S06.5**	**Traumatic subdural hemorrhage**
Add		Use Additional code, if applicable, for traumatic brain compression or herniation (S06.A-)
No Change	**S06.6**	**Traumatic subarachnoid hemorrhage**
Add		Use Additional code, if applicable, for traumatic brain compression or herniation (S06.A-)
Add	**S06.A**	**Traumatic brain compression and herniation**
Add		Traumatic cerebral compression
Add		*Code first the underlying traumatic brain injury, such as:*
Add		diffuse traumatic brain injury (S06.2-)
Add		focal traumatic brain injury (S06.3-)
Add		traumatic subdural hemorrhage (S06.5-)
Add		traumatic subarachnoid hemorrhage (S06.6-)
Add	**S06.A0**	**Traumatic brain compression without herniation**
Add		Traumatic brain compression NOS
Add		Traumatic cerebral compression NOS
Add	**S06.A1**	**Traumatic brain compression with herniation**
Add		Traumatic brain herniation
Add		Traumatic brainstem compression with herniation
Add		Traumatic cerebellar compression with herniation
Add		Traumatic cerebral compression with herniation

INJURIES TO THE THORAX (S20-S29)

No Change	**S23**	**Dislocation and sprain of joints and ligaments of thorax**
No Change	**S23.1**	**Subluxation and dislocation of thoracic vertebra**
No Change		Code also
Revise from		any associated
Revise to		any associated:

INJURIES TO THE KNEE AND LOWER LEG (S80-S89)

No Change	**S82**	**Fracture of lower leg, including ankle**
No Change		**Excludes2**
Revise from		periprosthetic fracture of prosthetic implant of knee (M97.0-)
Revise to		periprosthetic fracture around internal prosthetic implant of knee joint (M97.1-)

INJURIES TO THE ANKLE AND FOOT (S90-S99)

No Change	**S92**	**Fracture of foot and toe, except ankle**
Delete		**Excludes1** traumatic amputation of ankle and foot (S98.-)
Add		**Excludes2** traumatic amputation of ankle and foot (S98.-)

No Change			**POISONING BY, ADVERSE EFFECTS OF AND UNDERDOSING OF DRUGS, MEDICAMENTS AND BIOLOGICAL SUBSTANCES (T36-T50)**
No Change	**T40**		**Poisoning by, adverse effect of and underdosing of narcotics and psychodysleptics [hallucinogens]**
No Change		**T40.7**	**Poisoning by, adverse effect of and underdosing of cannabis (derivatives)**
Add		**T40.71**	**Poisoning by, adverse effect of and underdosing of cannabis (derivatives)**
Add			**T40.711 Poisoning by cannabis, accidental (unintentional)**
Add			**T40.712 Poisoning by cannabis, intentional self-harm**
Add			**T40.713 Poisoning by cannabis, assault**
Add			**T40.714 Poisoning by cannabis, undetermined**
Add			**T40.715 Adverse effect of cannabis**
Add			**T40.716 Underdosing of cannabis**
Add		**T40.72**	**Poisoning by, adverse effect of and underdosing of synthetic cannabinoids**
Add			**T40.721 Poisoning by synthetic cannabinoids, accidental (unintentional)**
Add			**T40.722 Poisoning by synthetic cannabinoids, intentional self-harm**
Add			**T40.723 Poisoning by synthetic cannabinoids, assault**
Add			**T40.724 Poisoning by synthetic cannabinoids, undetermined**
Add			**T40.725 Adverse effect of synthetic cannabinoids**
Add			**T40.726 Underdosing of synthetic cannabinoids**
Delete		**T40.7X**	**Poisoning by, adverse effect of and underdosing of cannabis (derivatives)**
Delete			**T40.7X1 Poisoning by cannabis (derivatives), accidental (unintentional)**
Delete			Poisoning by cannabis NOS
Delete			**T40.7X2 Poisoning by cannabis (derivatives), intentional self-harm**
Delete			**T40.7X3 Poisoning by cannabis (derivatives), assault**
Delete			**T40.7X4 Poisoning by cannabis (derivatives), undetermined**
Delete			**T40.7X5 Adverse effect of cannabis (derivatives)**
Delete			**T40.7X6 Underdosing of cannabis (derivatives)**
No Change	**T44**		**Poisoning by, adverse effect of and underdosing of drugs primarily affecting the autonomic nervous system**
No Change		**T44.8**	**Poisoning by, adverse effect of and underdosing of centrally-acting and adrenergic-neuron-blocking agents**
Delete			**Excludes1** poisoning by, adverse effect of and underdosing of clonidine (T46.5)
Delete			poisoning by, adverse effect of and underdosing of guanethidine (T46.5)
Add			**Excludes2** poisoning by, adverse effect of and underdosing of clonidine (T46.5)
Add			poisoning by, adverse effect of and underdosing of guanethidine (T46.5)

No Change		**TOXIC EFFECTS OF SUBSTANCES CHIEFLY NONMEDICINAL AS TO SOURCE (T51-T65)**				

No Change	T63	Toxic effect of contact with venomous animals and plants			
No Change		T63.6	Toxic effect of contact with other venomous marine animals		
Revise from			T63.61	Toxic effect of contact with Portugese Man-o-war	
Revise to			T63.61	Toxic effect of contact with Portuguese Man-o-war	
Revise from				T63.611	Toxic effect of contact with Portugese Man-o-war, accidental (unintentional)
Revise to				T63.611	Toxic effect of contact with Portuguese Man-o-war, accidental (unintentional)
Revise from				T63.612	Toxic effect of contact with Portugese Man-o-war, intentional self-harm
Revise to				T63.612	Toxic effect of contact with Portuguese Man-o-war, intentional self-harm
Revise from				T63.613	Toxic effect of contact with Portuguese Man-o-war, assault
Revise to				T63.613	Toxic effect of contact with Portuguese Man-o-war, assault
Revise from				T63.614	Toxic effect of contact with Portugese Man-o-war, undetermined
Revise to				T63.614	Toxic effect of contact with Portuguese Man-o-war, undetermined

No Change		**CERTAIN EARLY COMPLICATIONS OF TRAUMA (T79)**

No Change	T79	Certain early complications of trauma, not elsewhere classified	
No Change		T79.4 Traumatic shock	
No Change		Excludes1	
Delete			anesthetic shock (T88.2)
Add			shock due to anesthesia (T88.2)

No Change		**COMPLICATIONS OF SURGICAL AND MEDICAL CARE, NOT ELSEWHERE CLASSIFIED (T80-T88)**

No Change	T80	Complications following infusion, transfusion and therapeutic injection		
No Change		T80.8	Other complications following infusion, transfusion and therapeutic injection	
Add			T80.82	Complication of immune effector cellular therapy
Add				Complication of chimeric antigen receptor (CAR-T) cell therapy
Add				Complication of IEC therapy
Add				Excludes2 complication of bone marrow transplant (T86.0)
Add				complication of stem cell transplant (T86.5)
Add				Use Additional code to identify the
Add				specific complication, such as:
Add				cytokine release syndrome (D89.83-)
Add				immune effector cell-associated neurotoxicity syndrome (G92.0-)

No Change	T81	Complications of procedures, not elsewhere classified	
No Change		T81.1 Postprocedural shock	
No Change		Excludes1	
Delete			anesthetic shock (T88.2)
Add			shock due to anesthesia (T88.2)

No Change		T86 Complications of transplanted organs and tissue	
No Change		T86.2	Complications of heart transplant
No Change			Excludes1
Revise from			artificial heart device (T82.5)
Revise to			artificial heart device (T82.5-)
Revise from			heart-lung transplant (T86.3)
Revise to			heart-lung transplant (T86.3-)

No Change **CHAPTER 20**

No Change

EXTERNAL CAUSES OF MORBIDITY (V00-Y99)

No Change		**SLIPPING, TRIPPING, STUMBLING AND FALLS (W00-W19)**

No Change	W13	Fall from, out of or through building or structure	
No Change		W13.4 Fall from, out of or through window	
No Change		Excludes2	
Revise from			fall with subsequent striking against sharp glass (W01.110)
Revise to			fall with subsequent striking against sharp glass (W01.110-)

No Change		**EXPOSURE TO INANIMATE MECHANICAL FORCES (W20-W49)**

No Change	W25	Contact with sharp glass	
No Change		Excludes1	
Revise from			fall on same level due to slipping, tripping and stumbling with subsequent striking against sharp glass (W01.110)
Revise to			fall on same level due to slipping, tripping and stumbling with subsequent striking against sharp glass (W01.110-)
Revise from			striking against sharp glass with subsequent fall (W18.02)
Revise to			striking against sharp glass with subsequent fall (W18.02-)
No Change		Excludes2	
Revise from			glass embedded in skin (W45)
Revise to			glass embedded in skin (W45.-)

No Change	W26	Contact with other sharp objects	
No Change		Excludes2	
Revise from			sharp object(s) embedded in skin (W45)
Revise to			sharp object(s) embedded in skin (W45.-)

No Change		**LEGAL INTERVENTION, OPERATIONS OF WAR, MILITARY OPERATIONS, AND TERRORISM (Y35-Y38)**

No Change	Y35	Legal intervention		
No Change		Y35.8	Legal intervention involving other specified means	
No Change			Y35.89	Legal intervention involving other specified means
Add				Y35.899 Legal intervention involving other specified means, unspecified person injured

No Change **CHAPTER 21**

No Change

FACTORS INFLUENCING HEALTH STATUS AND CONTACT WITH HEALTH SERVICES (Z00-Z99)

No Change		**PERSONS ENCOUNTERING HEALTH SERVICES FOR EXAMINATIONS (Z00-Z13)**

No Change	Z01	Encounter for other special examination without complaint, suspected or reported diagnosis	
No Change		Z01.0	Encounter for examination of eyes and vision

No Change	Z01.02	Encounter for examination of eyes and vision following failed vision screening	
No Change		Excludes1	
Revise from		examination for examination of eyes and vision with abnormal findings (Z01.01)	
Revise to		encounter for examination of eyes and vision with abnormal findings (Z01.01)	
Revise from		examination for examination of eyes and vision without abnormal findings (Z01.00)	
Revise to		encounter for examination of eyes and vision without abnormal findings (Z01.00)	
No Change Z09		Encounter for follow-up examination after completed treatment for conditions other than malignant neoplasm	
No Change		Use Additional	
Revise from		code to identify any applicable history of disease code (Z86.-. Z87.-)	
Revise to		code to identify any applicable history of disease code (Z86.-, Z87.-)	
No Change Z13		Encounter for screening for other diseases and disorders	
No Change	Z13.2	Encounter for screening for nutritional, metabolic and other endocrine disorders	
No Change	Z13.29	Encounter for screening for other suspected endocrine disorder	
Delete		Excludes1 encounter for screening for diabetes mellitus (Z13.1)	
Add		Excludes2 encounter for screening for diabetes mellitus (Z13.1)	

PERSONS WITH POTENTIAL HEALTH HAZARDS RELATED TO COMMUNICABLE DISEASES (Z20-Z29)

No Change

No Change Z23	Encounter for immunization	
Add	Code also, if applicable, encounter for immunization safety counseling (Z71.85)	
No Change Z28	Immunization not carried out and underimmunization status	
Add	Code also, if applicable, encounter for immunization safety counseling (Z71.85)	

PERSONS ENCOUNTERING HEALTH SERVICES IN CIRCUMSTANCES RELATED TO REPRODUCTION (Z30-Z39)

No Change

No Change Z31	Encounter for procreative management	
Delete	Excludes1 complications associated with artificial fertilization (N98.-)	
Delete	female infertility (N97.-)	
Delete	male infertility (N46.-)	
Add	Excludes2 complications associated with artificial fertilization (N98.-)	
Add	female infertility (N97.-)	
Add	male infertility (N46.-)	
No Change Z3A	Weeks of gestation	
No Change	Code first	
Delete	complications of pregnancy, childbirth and the puerperium (O09-O9A)	
Add	obstetric condition or encounter for delivery (O09-O60, O80-O82)	

No Change	### ENCOUNTERS FOR OTHER SPECIFIC HEALTH CARE (Z40-Z53)		
No Change Z45	Encounter for adjustment and management of implanted device		
No Change	Z45.8	Encounter for adjustment and management of other implanted devices	
No Change		Z45.81	Encounter for adjustment or removal of breast implant
Revise from			Encounter removal of tissue expander with or without synchronous insertion of permanent implant
Revise to			Encounter for removal of tissue expander with or without synchronous insertion of permanent implant
No Change	### PERSONS WITH POTENTIAL HEALTH HAZARDS RELATED TO SOCIOECONOMIC AND PSYCHOSOCIAL CIRCUMSTANCES (Z55-Z65)		
No Change Z55	Problems related to education and literacy		
Add		Z55.5 Less than a high school diploma	
		No general equivalence degree (GED)	
Add	Z58	Problems related to physical environment	
Add		Excludes2 occupational exposure (Z57.-)	
Add		Z58.6 Inadequate drinking-water supply	
Add		Lack of safe drinking water	
Add		Excludes2 deprivation of water (T73.1)	
No Change Z59	Problems related to housing and economic circumstances		
No Change	Z59.0	Homelessness	
Add		Z59.00	Homelessness unspecified
Add		Z59.01	Sheltered homelessness
Add			Doubled up
Add			Living in a shelter such as: motel, scattered site housing, temporary or transitional living situation
Add		Z59.02	Unsheltered homelessness
Add			Residing in place not meant for human habitation such as: abandoned buildings, cars, parks, sidewalk
Add			Residing on the street
Revise from	Z59.4	Lack of adequate food and safe drinking water	
Revise to	Z59.4	Lack of adequate food	
Delete		Inadequate drinking water supply	
Delete		Excludes1 effects of hunger (T73.0)	
Delete		inappropriate diet or eating habits (Z72.4)	
Delete		malnutrition (E40-E46)	
Add		Excludes2 deprivation of food (T73.0)	
Add		effects of hunger (T73.0)	
Add		inappropriate diet or eating habits (Z72.4)	
Add		malnutrition (E40-E46)	
Add		Z59.41	Food insecurity
Add		Z59.48	Other specified lack of adequate food
Add			Inadequate food
Add			Lack of food
No Change	Z59.8	Other problems related to housing and economic circumstances	
Delete		Foreclosure on loan	
Delete		Isolated dwelling	
Delete		Problems with creditors	
Add		Z59.81	Housing instability, housed
Add			Foreclosure on home loan
Add			Past due on rent or mortgage
Add			Unwanted multiple moves in the last 12 months
Add			Z59.811 Housing instability, housed, with risk of homelessness
Add			Imminent risk of homelessness
Add			Z59.812 Housing instability, housed, homelessness in past 12 months
Add			Z59.819 Housing instability, housed unspecified

Add		Z59.89	**Other problems related to housing and economic circumstances**
Add			Foreclosure on loan
Add			Isolated dwelling
			Problems with creditors

No Change   **PERSONS ENCOUNTERING HEALTH SERVICES IN OTHER CIRCUMSTANCES (Z69-Z76)**

No Change	**Z71**	**Persons encountering health services for other counseling and medical advice, not elsewhere classified**	
No Change		Z71.8	**Other specified counseling**
Add			Z71.85 **Encounter for immunization safety counseling**
Add			Encounter for vaccine product safety counseling
Add			Code also, if applicable, encounter for immunization (Z23)
Add			Code also, if applicable, immunization not carried out (Z28.-)
Add			**Excludes1** encounter for health counseling related to travel (Z71.84)
No Change	**Z72**	**Problems related to lifestyle**	
No Change		Z72.4	**Inappropriate diet and eating habits**
No Change			**Excludes1**
Revise from			lack of adequate food (Z59.4)
Revise to			lack of adequate food (Z59.48)
No Change	**Z76**	**Persons encountering health services in other circumstances**	
No Change		Z76.4	**Other boarder to healthcare facility**
No Change			**Excludes1**
Revise from			homelessness (Z59.0)
Revise to			homelessness (Z59.0-)

No Change   **PERSONS WITH POTENTIAL HEALTH HAZARDS RELATED TO FAMILY AND PERSONAL HISTORY AND CERTAIN CONDITIONS INFLUENCING HEALTH STATUS (Z77-Z99)**

No Change	**Z79**	**Long term (current) drug therapy**	
No Change		Z79.4	**Long term (current) use of insulin**
Delete			**Excludes1** long term (current) use of oral antidiabetic drugs (Z79.84)
Delete			long term (current) use of oral hypoglycemic drugs (Z79.84)
Add			**Excludes2** long term (current) use of oral hypoglycemic drugs (Z79.84)
Add			long term (current) use of oral antidiabetic drugs (Z79.84)
No Change	**Z82**	**Family history of certain disabilities and chronic diseases (leading to disablement)**	
No Change		Z82.4	**Family history of ischemic heart disease and other diseases of the circulatory system**
Revise from			Conditions classifiable to I00-I52, I65-I99
Revise to			Conditions classifiable to I00-I5A, I65-I99
No Change	**Z86**	**Personal history of certain other diseases**	
No Change		Z86.1	**Personal history of infectious and parasitic diseases**
No Change			Z86.16 **Personal history of COVID-19**
Add			**Excludes1** post COVID-19 condition (U09.9)
No Change	**Z87**	**Personal history of other diseases and conditions**	
No Change		Z87.8	**Personal history of other specified conditions**
No Change			**Excludes2**
Revise from			personal history of self harm (Z91.5)
Revise to			personal history of self harm (Z91.5-)

No Change	**Z91**	**Personal risk factors, not elsewhere classified**	
No Change		Z91.0	**Allergy status, other than to drugs and biological substances**
No Change			Z91.01 **Food allergy status**
Add			Z91.014 **Allergy to mammalian meats**
Add			Allergy to beef
Add			Allergy to lamb
Add			Allergy to pork
Add			Allergy to red meats
No Change		Z91.5	**Personal history of self-harm**
Delete			Personal history of parasuicide
Delete			Personal history of self-poisoning
Delete			Personal history of suicide attempt
Add			Code also mental health disorder, if known
Add			Z91.51 **Personal history of suicidal behavior**
Add			Personal history of parasuicide
Add			Personal history of self-poisoning
Add			Personal history of suicide attempt
Add			Z91.52 **Personal history of nonsuicidal self-harm**
Add			Personal history of nonsuicidal self-injury
Add			Personal history of self-inflicted injury without suicidal intent
Add			Personal history of self-mutilation
No Change	**Z92**	**Personal history of medical treatment**	
No Change		Z92.2	**Personal history of drug therapy**
Revise from			Z92.25 **Personal history of immunosupression therapy**
Revise to			Z92.25 **Personal history of immunosuppression therapy**
No Change		Z92.8	**Personal history of other medical treatment**
Add			Z92.85 **Personal history of cellular therapy**
Add			Z92.850 **Personal history of Chimeric Antigen Receptor T-cell therapy**
Add			Personal history of CAR T-cell therapy
Add			Z92.858 **Personal history of other cellular therapy**
Add			Z92.859 **Personal history of cellular therapy, unspecified**
Add			Z92.86 **Personal history of gene therapy**
No Change	**Z99**	**Dependence on enabling machines and devices, not elsewhere classified**	
Delete			**Excludes1** cardiac pacemaker status (Z95.0)

No Change # CHAPTER 22

No Change # CODES FOR SPECIAL PURPOSES (U00-U85)

No Change   **PROVISIONAL ASSIGNMENT OF NEW DISEASES OF UNCERTAIN ETIOLOGY OR EMERGENCY USE (U00-U49)**

Add	**U09**	**Post COVID-19 condition**	
Add		U09.9	**Post COVID-19 condition, unspecified**
Add			**Note:** This code enables establishment of a link with COVID-19.
Add			This code is not to be used in cases that are still presenting with active COVID-19.
Add			However, an exception is made in cases of re-infection with COVID-19, occurring with a condition related to prior COVID-19.
Add			Post-acute sequela of COVID-19
Add			*Code first the specific condition related to COVID-19 if known, such as:*
Add			chronic respiratory failure (J96.1-)
Add			loss of smell (R43.8)
Add			loss of taste (R43.8)
Add			multisystem inflammatory syndrome (M35.81)
Add			pulmonary embolism (I26.-)
Add			pulmonary fibrosis (J84.10)

PART I

Introduction

ICD-10-CM Official Guidelines for Coding and Reporting FY2022
(October 1, 2021 - September 30, 2022)

Narrative changes appear in **bold** text
Items <u>underlined</u> have been moved within the guidelines since the 2021 version
Italics are used to indicate revisions to heading changes

The Centers for Medicare and Medicaid Services (CMS) and the National Center for Health Statistics (NCHS), two departments within the U.S. Federal Government's Department of Health and Human Services (DHHS), provide the following guidelines for coding and reporting using the International Classification of Diseases, 10th Revision, Clinical Modification (ICD-10-CM). These guidelines should be used as a companion document to the official version of the ICD-10-CM as published on the NCHS website. The ICD-10-CM is a morbidity classification published by the United States for classifying diagnoses and reason for visits in all health care settings. The ICD-10-CM is based on the ICD-10, the statistical classification of disease published by the World Health Organization (WHO).

These guidelines have been approved by the four organizations that make up the Cooperating Parties for the ICD-10-CM: the American Hospital Association (AHA), the American Health Information Management Association (AHIMA), CMS, and NCHS.

These guidelines are a set of rules that have been developed to accompany and complement the official conventions and instructions provided within the ICD-10-CM itself. The instructions and conventions of the classification take precedence over guidelines. These guidelines are based on the coding and sequencing instructions in the Tabular List and Alphabetic Index of ICD-10-CM, but provide additional instruction. Adherence to these guidelines when assigning ICD-10-CM diagnosis codes is required under the Health Insurance Portability and Accountability Act (HIPAA). The diagnosis codes (Tabular List and Alphabetic Index)

have been adopted under HIPAA for all health care settings. A joint effort between the health care provider and the coder is essential to achieve complete and accurate documentation, code assignment, and reporting of diagnoses and procedures. These guidelines have been developed to assist both the health care provider and the coder in identifying those diagnoses that are to be reported. The importance of consistent, complete documentation in the medical record cannot be overemphasized. Without such documentation accurate coding cannot be achieved. The entire record should be reviewed to determine the specific reason for the encounter and the conditions treated.

The term "encounter" is used for all settings, including hospital admissions. In the context of these guidelines, the term "provider" is used throughout the guidelines to mean physician or any qualified health care practitioner who is legally accountable for establishing the patient's diagnosis. Only this set of guidelines, approved by the Cooperating Parties, is official.

The guidelines are organized into sections. Section I includes the structure and conventions of the classification and general guidelines that apply to the entire classification, and chapter-specific guidelines that correspond to the chapters as they are arranged in the classification. Section II includes guidelines for selection of principal diagnosis for non-outpatient settings. Section III includes guidelines for reporting additional diagnoses in non-outpatient settings. Section IV is for outpatient coding and reporting. It is necessary to review all sections of the guidelines to fully understand all of the rules and instructions needed to code properly.

ICD-10-CM Official Guidelines for Coding and Reporting

Section I. Conventions, General Coding Guidelines and Chapter Specific Guidelines

A. Conventions for the ICD-10-CM
  1. The Alphabetic Index and Tabular List
  2. Format and Structure:
  3. Use of codes for reporting purposes
  4. Placeholder character
  5. 7th Characters
  6. Abbreviations
     a. Alphabetic Index abbreviations
     b. Tabular List abbreviations
  7. Punctuation
  8. Use of "and"
  9. Other and Unspecified codes
     a. "Other" codes
     b. "Unspecified" codes
  10. Includes Notes
  11. Inclusion terms
  12. Excludes Notes
     a. Excludes1
     b. Excludes2
  13. Etiology/manifestation convention ("code first", "use additional code" and "in diseases classified elsewhere" notes)
  14. "And"
  15. "With"
  16. "See" and "See Also"
  17. "Code also note"
  18. Default codes
  19. Code assignment and Clinical Criteria
B. General Coding Guidelines
  1. Locating a code in the ICD-10-CM
  2. Level of Detail in Coding
  3. Code or codes from A00.0 through T88.9, Z00-Z99.8, *U00-U85*
  4. Signs and symptoms
  5. Conditions that are an integral part of a disease process
  6. Conditions that are not an integral part of a disease process
  7. Multiple coding for a single condition
  8. Acute and Chronic Conditions
  9. Combination Code
  10. Sequela (Late Effects)
  11. Impending or Threatened Condition
  12. Reporting Same Diagnosis Code more than Once
  13. Laterality
  14. Documentation *by Clinicians Other than the Patient's Provider*
  15. Syndromes
  16. Documentation of Complications of Care
  17. Borderline Diagnosis
  18. Use of Sign/Symptom/Unspecified Codes
  19. Coding for Healthcare Encounters in Hurricane Aftermath
     a. Use of External Cause of Morbidity Codes
     b. Sequencing of External Causes of Morbidity Codes

c. Other External Causes of Morbidity Code Issues
  d. Use of Z codes
C. Chapter-Specific Coding Guidelines
  1. Chapter 1: Certain Infectious and Parasitic Diseases (A00-B99, U07.1, *U09.9*)
     a. Human Immunodeficiency Virus (HIV) Infections
     b. Infectious agents as the cause of diseases classified to other chapters
     c. Infections resistant to antibiotics
     d. Sepsis, Severe Sepsis, and Septic Shock *infection resistant to antibiotics*
     e. Methicillin Resistant *Staphylococcus aureus* (MRSA) Conditions
     f. Zika virus infection
     g. Coronavirus infections
  2. Chapter 2: Neoplasms (C00-D49)
     a. Treatment directed at the malignancy
     b. Treatment of secondary site
     c. Coding and sequencing of complications
     d. Primary malignancy previously excised
     e. Admissions/Encounters involving chemotherapy, immunotherapy and radiation therapy
     f. Admission/encounter to determine extent of malignancy
     g. Symptoms, signs, and abnormal findings listed in Chapter 18 associated with neoplasms
     h. Admission/encounter for pain control/ management
     i. Malignancy in two or more noncontiguous sites
     j. Disseminated malignant neoplasm, unspecified
     k. Malignant neoplasm without specification of site
     l. Sequencing of neoplasm codes
     m. Current malignancy versus personal history of malignancy
     n. Leukemia, Multiple Myeloma, and Malignant Plasma Cell Neoplasms in remission versus personal history
     o. Aftercare following surgery for neoplasm
     p. Follow-up care for completed treatment of a malignancy
     q. Prophylactic organ removal for prevention of malignancy
     r. Malignant neoplasm associated with transplanted organ
     s. Breast Implant Associated Anaplastic Large Cell Lymphoma
  3. Chapter 3: Disease of the Blood and Blood-Forming Organs and Certain Disorders Involving the Immune Mechanism (D50-D89)
  4. Chapter 4: Endocrine, Nutritional, and Metabolic Diseases (E00-E89)
     a. Diabetes mellitus
  5. Chapter 5: Mental, Behavioral, and Neurodevelopmental disorders (F01 – F99)
     a. Pain disorders related to psychological factors
     b. Mental and behavioral disorders due to psychoactive substance use
     c. Factitious Disorder
  6. Chapter 6: Diseases of the Nervous System (G00-G99)
     a. Dominant/nondominant side
     b. Pain - Category G89

Appendix I: Present on Admission Reporting Guidelines

Section I. Conventions, General Coding Guidelines, and Chapter Specific Guidelines

The conventions, general guidelines, and chapter-specific guidelines are applicable to all health care settings unless otherwise indicated. The conventions and instructions of the classification take precedence over guidelines.

A. **Conventions for the ICD-10-CM**
The conventions for the ICD-10-CM are the general rules for use of the classification independent of the guidelines. These conventions are incorporated within the Alphabetic Index and Tabular List of the ICD-10-CM as instructional notes.

1. **The Alphabetic Index and Tabular List**
The ICD-10-CM is divided into the Alphabetic Index, an alphabetical list of terms and their corresponding code, and the Tabular List, a structured list of codes divided into chapters based on body system or condition. The Alphabetic Index consists of the following parts: the Index of Diseases and Injury, the Index of External Causes of Injury, the Table of Neoplasms, and the Table of Drugs and Chemicals.
    See Section I.C2. General guidelines
    See Section I.C.19. Adverse effects, poisoning, underdosing and toxic effects

2. **Format and Structure:**
The ICD-10-CM Tabular List contains categories, subcategories and codes. Characters for categories, subcategories and codes may be either a letter or a number. All categories are 3 characters. A 3-character category that has no further subdivision is equivalent to a code. Subcategories are either 4 or 5 characters. Codes may be 3, 4, 5, 6 or 7 characters. That is, each level of subdivision after a category is a subcategory. The final level of subdivision is a code. Codes that have applicable 7th characters are still referred to as codes, not subcategories. A code that has an applicable 7th character is considered invalid without the 7th character.
    The ICD-10-CM uses an indented format for ease in reference

3. **Use of codes for reporting purposes**
For reporting purposes only codes are permissible, not categories or subcategories, and any applicable 7th character is required.

4. **Placeholder character**
The ICD-10-CM utilizes a placeholder character "X". The "X" is used as a placeholder at certain codes to allow for future expansion. An example of this is at the poisoning, adverse effect and underdosing codes, categories T36-T50. Where a placeholder exists, the X must be used in order for the code to be considered a valid code.

5. **7th Characters**
Certain ICD-10-CM categories have applicable 7th characters. The applicable 7th character is required for all codes within the category, or as the notes in the Tabular List instruct. The 7th character must always be the 7th character in the data field. If a

code that requires a 7th character is not 6 characters, a placeholder X must be used to fill in the empty characters.

6. **Abbreviations**

   a. **Alphabetic Index abbreviations**

   NEC "Not elsewhere classifiable"

   This abbreviation in the Alphabetic Index represents "other specified". When a specific code is not available for a condition the Alphabetic Index directs the coder to the "other specified" code in the Tabular List.

   NOS "Not otherwise specified"

   This abbreviation is the equivalent of unspecified.

   b. **Tabular List abbreviations**

   NEC "Not elsewhere classifiable"

   This abbreviation in the Tabular List represents "other specified". When a specific code is not available for a condition, the Tabular List includes an NEC entry under a code to identify the code as the "other specified" code.

   NOS "Not otherwise specified"

   This abbreviation is the equivalent of unspecified.

7. **Punctuation**

   [ ] Brackets are used in the Tabular List to enclose synonyms, alternative wording or explanatory phrases. Brackets are used in the Alphabetic Index to identify manifestation codes.

   ( ) Parentheses are used in both the Alphabetic Index and Tabular List to enclose supplementary words that may be present or absent in the statement of a disease or procedure without affecting the code number to which it is assigned. The terms within the parentheses are referred to as nonessential modifiers. The nonessential modifiers in the Alphabetic Index to Diseases apply to subterms following a main term except when a nonessential modifier and a subentry are mutually exclusive, the subentry takes precedence. For example, in the ICD-10-CM Alphabetic Index under the main term Enteritis, "acute" is a nonessential modifier and "chronic" is a subentry. In this case, the nonessential modifier "acute" does not apply to the subentry "chronic".

   : Colons are used in the Tabular List after an incomplete term which needs one or more of the modifiers following the colon to make it assignable to a given category.

8. **Use of "and".**

   See Section I.A.14. Use of the term "And"

9. **Other and Unspecified codes**

   a. **"Other" codes**

   Codes titled "other" or "other specified" are for use when the information in the medical record provides detail for which a specific code does not exist. Alphabetic Index entries with NEC in the line designate "other" codes in the Tabular List.

These Alphabetic Index entries represent specific disease entities for which no specific code exists so the term is included within an "other" code.

   b. **"Unspecified" codes**

   Codes titled "unspecified" are for use when the information in the medical record is insufficient to assign a more specific code. For those categories for which an unspecified code is not provided, the "other specified" code may represent both other and unspecified.

   See Section I.B.18 Use of signs/symptoms/unspecified codes

10. **Includes Notes**

    This note appears immediately under a 3-character code title to further define, or give examples of, the content of the category.

11. **Inclusion terms**

    List of terms is included under some codes. These terms are the conditions for which that code is to be used. The terms may be synonyms of the code title, or, in the case of "other specified" codes, the terms are a list of the various conditions assigned to that code. The inclusion terms are not necessarily exhaustive. Additional terms found only in the Alphabetic Index may also be assigned to a code.

12. **Excludes Notes**

    The ICD-10-CM has two types of excludes notes. Each type of note has a different definition for use, but they are all similar in that they indicate that codes excluded from each other are independent of each other.

    a. **Excludes1**

    A type 1 Excludes note is a pure excludes note. It means "NOT CODED HERE!" An Excludes1 note indicates that the code excluded should never be used at the same time as the code above the Excludes1 note. An Excludes1 is used when two conditions cannot occur together, such as a congenital form versus an acquired form of the same condition.

    An exception to the Excludes1 definition is the circumstance when the two conditions are unrelated to each other. If it is not clear whether the two conditions involving an Excludes1 note are related or not, query the provider. For example, code F45.8, Other somatoform disorders, has an Excludes1 note for "sleep related teeth grinding (G47.63)" because "teeth grinding" is an inclusion term under F45.8. Only one of these two codes should be assigned for teeth grinding. However, psychogenic dysmenorrhea is also an inclusion term under F45.8, and a patient could have both this condition and sleep-related teeth grinding. In this case, the two conditions are clearly unrelated to each other, and so it would be appropriate to report F45.8 and G47.63 together.

    b. **Excludes2**

    A Type 2 Excludes note represents "Not included here." An excludes2 note indicates that the condition excluded is not part of the condition represented by the code, but a patient may have both conditions at the same time. When an Excludes2 note appears under a code, it is acceptable to use both the code and the excluded code together, when appropriate.

13. **Etiology/manifestation convention ("code first", "use additional code" and "in diseases classified elsewhere" notes)**

Certain conditions have both an underlying etiology and multiple body system manifestations due to the underlying etiology. For such conditions, the ICD-10-CM has a coding convention that requires the underlying condition be sequenced first, if applicable, followed by the manifestation. Wherever such a combination exists, there is a "use additional code" note at the etiology code, and a "code first" note at the manifestation code. These instructional notes indicate the proper sequencing order of the codes, etiology followed by manifestation.

In most cases the manifestation codes will have in the code title, "in diseases classified elsewhere." Codes with this title are a component of the etiology/manifestation convention. The code title indicates that it is a manifestation code. "In diseases classified elsewhere" codes are never permitted to be used as first-listed or principal diagnosis codes. They must be used in conjunction with an underlying condition code and they must be listed following the underlying condition. See category F02, Dementia in other diseases classified elsewhere, for an example of this convention.

There are manifestation codes that do not have "in diseases classified elsewhere" in the title. For such codes, there is a "use additional code" note at the etiology code and a "code first" note at the manifestation code and the rules for sequencing apply.

In addition to the notes in the Tabular List, these conditions also have a specific Alphabetic Index entry structure. In the Alphabetic Index both conditions are listed together with the etiology code first followed by the manifestation codes in brackets. The code in brackets is always to be sequenced second.

An example of the etiology/manifestation convention is dementia in Parkinson's disease. In the Alphabetic Index, code G20 is listed first, followed by code F02.80 or F02.81 in brackets. Code G20 represents the underlying etiology, Parkinson's disease, and must be sequenced first, whereas code F02.80 and F02.81 represent the manifestation of dementia in diseases classified elsewhere, with or without behavioral disturbance.

"Code first" and "Use additional code" notes are also used as sequencing rules in the classification for certain codes that are not part of an etiology/manifestation combination.

See Section I.B.7. Multiple coding for a single condition.

14. **"And"**

The word "and" should be interpreted to mean either "and" or "or" when it appears in a title.

For example, cases of "tuberculosis of bones", "tuberculosis of joints" and "tuberculosis of bones

and joints" are classified to subcategory A18.0, Tuberculosis of bones and joints.

15. **"With"**

The word "with" or "in" should be interpreted to mean "associated with" or "due to" when it appears in a code title, the Alphabetic Index, (either under a main term or subterm) or an instructional note in the Tabular List. The classification presumes a causal relationship between the two conditions linked by these terms in the Alphabetic Index or Tabular List. These conditions should be coded as related even in the absence of provider documentation explicitly linking them, unless the documentation clearly states the conditions are unrelated or when another guideline exists that specifically requires a documented linkage between two conditions (e.g., sepsis guideline for "acute organ dysfunction that is not clearly associated with the sepsis").

For conditions not specifically linked by these relational terms in the classification or when a guideline requires that a linkage between two conditions be explicitly documented provider documentation must link the conditions in order to code them as related.

The word "with" in the Alphabetic Index is sequenced immediately following the main term or subterm, not in alphabetical order.

16. **"See" and "See Also"**

The "see" instruction following a main term in the Alphabetic Index indicates that another term should be referenced. It is necessary to go to the main term referenced with the "see" note to locate the correct code.

A "see also" instruction following a main term in the Alphabetic Index instructs that there is another main term that may also be referenced that may provide additional Alphabetic Index entries that may be useful. It is not necessary to follow the "see also" note when the original main term provides the necessary code.

17. **"Code also" note**

A "code also" note instructs that two codes may be required to fully describe a condition, but this note does not provide sequencing direction. The sequencing depends on the circumstances of the encounter.

18. **Default codes**

A code listed next to a main term in the ICD-10-CM Alphabetic Index is referred to as a default code. The default code represents that condition that is most commonly associated with the main term, or is the unspecified code for the condition. If a condition is documented in a medical record (for example, appendicitis) without any additional information, such as acute or chronic, the default code should be assigned.

19. **Code assignment and Clinical Criteria**

The assignment of a diagnosis code is based on the provider's diagnostic statement that the condition exists. The provider's statement that the patient has a particular condition is sufficient. Code assignment is not based on clinical criteria used by the provider to establish the diagnosis.

B. **General Coding Guidelines**

1. **Locating a code in the ICD-10-CM**

   To select a code in the classification that corresponds to a diagnosis or reason for visit documented in a medical record, first locate the term in the Alphabetic Index, and then verify the code in the Tabular List. Read and be guided by instructional notations that appear in both the Alphabetic Index and the Tabular List.

   It is essential to use both the Alphabetic Index and Tabular List when locating and assigning a code. The Alphabetic Index does not always provide the full code. Selection of the full code, including laterality and any applicable 7th character can only be done in the Tabular List. A dash (-) at the end of an Alphabetic Index entry indicates that additional characters are required. Even if a dash is not included at the Alphabetic Index entry, it is necessary to refer to the Tabular List to verify that no 7th character is required.

2. **Level of Detail in Coding**

   Diagnosis codes are to be used and reported at their highest number of characters available **and to the highest level of specificity documented in the medical record.**

   ICD-10-CM diagnosis codes are composed of codes with 3, 4, 5, 6, or 7 characters. Codes with three characters are included in ICD-10-CM as the heading of a category of codes that may be further subdivided by the use of 4th and/or 5th characters and/or 6th characters, which provide greater detail.

   A 3-character code is to be used only if it is not further subdivided. A code is invalid if it has not been coded to the full number of characters required for that code, including the 7th character, if applicable.

3. **Code or codes from A00.0 through T88.9, Z00-Z99.8, U00-U85**

   The appropriate code or codes from A00.0 through T88.9, Z00-Z99.8 and U00-U85 must be used to identify diagnoses, symptoms, conditions, problems, complaints or other reason(s) for the encounter/visit.

4. **Signs and symptoms**

   Codes that describe symptoms and signs, as opposed to diagnoses, are acceptable for reporting purposes when a related definitive diagnosis has not been established (confirmed) by the provider. Chapter 18 of ICD-10-CM, Symptoms, Signs, and Abnormal Clinical and Laboratory Findings, Not Elsewhere Classified (codes R00.0 - R99) contains many, but not all codes for symptoms.

   See Section I.B.18 Use of signs/symptoms/ unspecified codes

5. **Conditions that are an integral part of a disease process**

   Signs and symptoms that are associated routinely with a disease process should not be assigned as additional codes, unless otherwise instructed by the classification.

6. **Conditions that are not an integral part of a disease process**

   Additional signs and symptoms that may not be associated routinely with a disease process should be coded when present.

7. **Multiple coding for a single condition**

   In addition to the etiology/manifestation convention that requires two codes to fully describe a single condition that affects multiple body systems, there are other single conditions that also require more than one code. "Use additional code" notes are found in the Tabular List at codes that are not part of an etiology/manifestation pair where a secondary code is useful to fully describe a condition. The sequencing rule is the same as the etiology/manifestation pair, "use additional code" indicates that a secondary code should be added, if known.

   For example, for bacterial infections that are not included in Chapter 1, a secondary code from category B95, Streptococcus, Staphylococcus, and Enterococcus, as the cause of diseases classified elsewhere, or B96, Other bacterial agents as the cause of diseases classified elsewhere, may be required to identify the bacterial organism causing the infection. A "use additional code" note will normally be found at the infectious disease code, indicating a need for the organism code to be added as a secondary code.

   "Code first" notes are also under certain codes that are not specifically manifestation codes but may be due to an underlying cause. When there is a "code first" note and an underlying condition is present, the underlying condition should be sequenced first, if known.

   "Code, if applicable, any causal condition first," notes indicate that this code may be assigned as a principal diagnosis when the causal condition is unknown or not applicable. If a causal condition is known, then the code for that condition should be sequenced as the principal or first-listed diagnosis.

   Multiple codes may be needed for sequela, complication codes and obstetric codes to more fully describe a condition. See the specific guidelines for these conditions for further instruction.

8. **Acute and Chronic Conditions**

   If the same condition is described as both acute (subacute) and chronic, and separate subentries exist in the Alphabetic Index at the same indentation level, code both and sequence the acute (subacute) code first.

9. **Combination Code**

   A combination code is a single code used to classify:
   Two diagnoses, or
   A diagnosis with an associated secondary process (manifestation)
   A diagnosis with an associated complication
   Combination codes are identified by referring to subterm entries in the Alphabetic Index and by reading the inclusion and exclusion notes in the Tabular List.

Assign only the combination code when that code fully identifies the diagnostic conditions involved or when the Alphabetic Index so directs. Multiple coding should not be used when the classification provides a combination code that clearly identifies all of the elements documented in the diagnosis. When the combination code lacks necessary specificity in describing the manifestation or complication, an additional code should be used as a secondary code.

10. **Sequela (Late Effects)**
A sequela is the residual effect (condition produced) after the acute phase of an illness or injury has terminated. There is no time limit on when a sequela code can be used. The residual may be apparent early, such as in cerebral infarction, or it may occur months or years later, such as that due to a previous injury. Examples of sequela include: scar formation resulting from a burn, deviated septum due to a nasal fracture, and infertility due to tubal occlusion from old tuberculosis. Coding of sequela generally requires two codes sequenced in the following order: the condition or nature of the sequela is sequenced first. The sequela code is sequenced second.

An exception to the above guidelines are those instances where the code for the sequela is followed by a manifestation code identified in the Tabular List and title, or the sequela code has been expanded (at the 4th, 5th, or 6th character levels) to include the manifestation(s). The code for the acute phase of an illness or injury that led to the sequela is never used with a code for the late effect.

See Section I.C.9. Sequelae of cerebrovascular disease
See Section I.C.15. Sequelae of complication of pregnancy, childbirth and the puerperium
See Section I.C.19. Application of 7th characters for Chapter 19

11. **Impending or Threatened Condition**
Code any condition described at the time of discharge as "impending" or "threatened" as follows:
If it did occur, code as confirmed diagnosis.
If it did not occur, reference the Alphabetic Index to determine if the condition has a subentry term for "impending" or "threatened" and also reference main term entries for "Impending" and for "Threatened."
If the subterms are listed, assign the given code.
If the subterms are not listed, code the existing underlying condition(s) and not the condition described as impending or threatened.

12. **Reporting Same Diagnosis Code More Than Once**
Each unique ICD-10-CM diagnosis code may be reported only once for an encounter. This applies to bilateral conditions when there are no distinct codes identifying laterality or two different conditions classified to the same ICD-10-CM diagnosis code.

13. **Laterality**
Some ICD-10-CM codes indicate laterality, specifying whether the condition occurs on the left, right or is bilateral. If no bilateral code is provided and the condition is bilateral, assign separate codes for both the left and right side. If the side is not identified in the medical record, assign the code for the unspecified side.

When a patient has a bilateral condition and each side is treated during separate encounters, assign the "bilateral" code (as the condition still exists on both sides), including for the encounter to treat the first side. For the second encounter for treatment after one side has previously been treated and the condition no longer exists on that side, assign the appropriate unilateral code for the side where the condition still exists (e.g., cataract surgery performed on each eye in separate encounters). The bilateral code would not be assigned for the subsequent encounter, as the patient no longer has the condition in the previously-treated site. If the treatment on the first side did not completely resolve the condition, then the bilateral code would still be appropriate.

When laterality is not documented by the patient's provider, code assignment for the affected side may be based on medical record documentation from other clinicians. If there is conflicting medical record documentation regarding the affected side, the patient's attending provider should be queried for clarification. Codes for "unspecified" side should rarely be used, such as when the documentation in the record is insufficient to determine the affected side and it is not possible to obtain clarification.

14. **Documentation by Clinicians Other than the Patient's Provider**
Code assignment is based on the documentation by **the** patient's provider (i.e., physician or other qualified healthcare practitioner legally accountable for establishing the patient's diagnosis). There are a few exceptions **when** code assignment may be based on medical record documentation from clinicians who are not the patient's provider (i.e., physician or other qualified healthcare practitioner legally accountable for establishing the patient's diagnosis).

In this context, "clinicians" other than the patient's provider refer to healthcare professionals permitted, based on regulatory or accreditation requirements or internal hospital policies, to document in a patient's official medical record.

These exceptions include codes for:
- **Body Mass Index (BMI)**
- **Depth of non-pressure chronic ulcers**
- **Pressure ulcer stage**
- **Coma scale**
- **NIH stroke scale (NIHSS)**
- **Social determinants of health (SDOH)**
- **Laterality**
- **Blood alcohol level**

This information is typically, **or may be,** documented by other clinicians involved in the care of the patient (e.g., a dietitian often documents the BMI, a nurse often documents the pressure ulcer stages, and an emergency medical technician often documents the coma scale). However, the associated diagnosis (such as overweight, obesity, acute stroke, pressure ulcer, **or a condition classifiable to category F10, Alcohol related disorders**) must be documented by the patient's provider. If there is conflicting medical record documentation, either from the same clinician or different clinicians, the patient's attending provider should be queried for clarification.

The BMI, coma scale, and NIHSS **blood alcohol level** codes and **codes for social determinants of health** should only be reported as secondary diagnoses.

See Section I.C.21.c.17 for additional information regarding coding social determinants of health.

15. Syndromes

Follow the Alphabetic Index guidance when coding syndromes. In the absence of Alphabetic Index guidance, assign codes for the documented manifestations of the syndrome. Additional codes for manifestations that are not an integral part of the disease process may also be assigned when the condition does not have a unique code.

16. Documentation of Complications of Care

Code assignment is based on the provider's documentation of the relationship between the condition and the care or procedure, unless otherwise instructed by the classification. The guideline extends to any complications of care, regardless of the chapter the code is located in. It is important to note that not all conditions that occur during or following medical care or surgery are classified as complications. There must be a cause-and-effect relationship between the care provided and the condition, and an indication in the documentation that it is a complication. Query the provider for clarification, if the complication is not clearly documented.

17. Borderline Diagnosis

If the provider documents a "borderline" diagnosis at the time of discharge, the diagnosis is coded as confirmed, unless the classification provides a specific entry (e.g., borderline diabetes). If a borderline condition has a specific index entry in ICD-10-CM, it should be coded as such. Since borderline conditions are not uncertain diagnoses, no distinction is made between the care setting (inpatient versus outpatient). Whenever the documentation is unclear regarding a borderline condition, coders are encouraged to query for clarification.

18. Use of Sign/Symptom/Unspecified Codes

Sign/symptom and "unspecified" codes have acceptable, even necessary, uses. While specific diagnosis codes should be reported when they are supported by the available medical record documentation and clinical knowledge of the patient's health condition, there are instances when signs/symptoms or unspecified codes are the best

choices for accurately reflecting the healthcare encounter. Each healthcare encounter should be coded to the level of certainty known for that encounter.

As stated in the introductory section of these official coding guidelines, a joint effort between the healthcare provider and the coder is essential to achieve complete and accurate documentation, code assignment, and reporting of diagnoses and procedures. The importance of consistent, complete documentation in the medical record cannot be overemphasized. Without such documentation accurate coding cannot be achieved. The entire record should be reviewed to determine the specific reason for the encounter and the conditions treated.

If a definitive diagnosis has not been established by the end of the encounter, it is appropriate to report codes for sign(s) and/or symptom(s) in lieu of a definitive diagnosis. When sufficient clinical information isn't known or available about a particular health condition to assign a more specific code, it is acceptable to report the appropriate "unspecified" code (e.g., a diagnosis of pneumonia has been determined, but not the specific type). Unspecified codes should be reported when they are the codes that most accurately reflect what is known about the patient's condition at the time of that particular encounter. It would be inappropriate to select a specific code that is not supported by the medical record documentation or conduct medically unnecessary diagnostic testing in order to determine a more specific code.

19. Coding for Healthcare Encounters in Hurricane Aftermath

a. Use of External Cause of Morbidity Codes

An external cause of morbidity code should be assigned to identify the cause of the injury(ies) incurred as a result of the hurricane. The use of external cause of morbidity codes is supplemental to the application of ICD-10-CM codes. External cause of morbidity codes are never to be recorded as a principal diagnosis (first-listed in non-inpatient settings). The appropriate injury code should be sequenced before any external cause codes. The external cause of morbidity codes capture how the injury or health condition happened (cause), the intent (unintentional or accidental; or intentional, such as suicide or assault), the place where the event occurred, the activity of the patient at the time of the event, and the person's status (e.g., civilian, military). They should not be assigned for encounters to treat hurricane victims' medical conditions when no injury, adverse effect or poisoning is involved. External cause of morbidity codes should be assigned for each encounter for care and treatment of the injury. External cause of morbidity codes may be assigned in all health care settings. For the purpose of capturing complete and accurate ICD-10-CM data in the aftermath of the hurricane, a healthcare setting should be considered as any location where medical care is provided by licensed healthcare professionals.

b. Sequencing of External Causes of Morbidity Codes

Codes for cataclysmic events, such as a hurricane, take priority over all other external cause codes except child and adult abuse and terrorism and should be sequenced before other external cause of injury codes. Assign as many external cause of morbidity codes as necessary to fully explain each cause. For example, if an injury occurs as a result of a building collapse during the hurricane, external cause codes for both the hurricane and the building collapse should be assigned, with the external causes code for hurricane being sequenced as the first external cause code. For injuries incurred as a direct result of the hurricane, assign the appropriate code(s) for the injuries, followed by the code X37.0-, Hurricane (with the appropriate 7th character), and any other applicable external cause of injury codes. Code X37.0- also should be assigned when an injury is incurred as a result of flooding caused by a levee breaking related to the hurricane. Code X38.-, Flood (with the appropriate 7th character), should be assigned when an injury is from flooding resulting directly from the storm. Code X36.0.-, Collapse of dam or man-made structure, should not be assigned when the cause of the collapse is due to the hurricane. Use of code X36.0- is limited to collapses of man-made structures due to earth surface movements, not due to storm surges directly from a hurricane.

c. Other External Causes of Morbidity Code Issues

For injuries that are not a direct result of the hurricane, such as an evacuee that has incurred an injury as a result of a motor vehicle accident, assign the appropriate external cause of morbidity code(s) to describe the cause of the injury, but do not assign code X37.0-, Hurricane. If it is not clear whether the injury was a direct result of the hurricane, assume the injury is due to the hurricane and assign code X37.0-, Hurricane, as well as any other applicable external cause of morbidity codes. In addition to code X37.0-, Hurricane, other possible applicable external cause of morbidity codes include:

X30-	Exposure to excessive natural heat
X31-	Exposure to excessive natural cold
X38-	Flood

d. Use of Z codes

Z codes (other reasons for healthcare encounters) may be assigned as appropriate to further explain the reasons for presenting for healthcare services, including transfers between healthcare facilities **or provide additional information relevant to a patient encounter**. The ICD-10-CM Official Guidelines for Coding and Reporting identify which codes maybe assigned as principal or first-listed diagnosis only, secondary diagnosis only, or principal/first-listed or secondary (depending on the circumstances). Possible applicable Z codes include:

Z59.0-	Homelessness
Z59.1	Inadequate housing
Z59.5	Extreme poverty
Z75.1	Person awaiting admission to adequate facility elsewhere
Z75.3	Unavailability and inaccessibility of health-care facilities
Z75.4	Unavailability and inaccessibility of other helping agencies
Z76.2	Encounter for health supervision and care of other healthy infant and child
Z99.12	Encounter for respirator [ventilator] dependence during power failure

The external cause of morbidity codes and the Z codes listed above are not an all-inclusive list. Other codes may be applicable to the encounter based upon the documentation. Assign as many codes as necessary to fully explain each healthcare encounter. Since patient history information may be very limited, use any available documentation to assign the appropriate external cause of morbidity and Z codes.

C. Chapter-Specific Coding Guidelines

In addition to general coding guidelines, there are guidelines for specific diagnoses and/or conditions in the classification. Unless otherwise indicated, these guidelines apply to all health care settings. Please refer to Section II for guidelines on the selection of principal diagnosis.

1. Chapter 1: Certain Infectious and Parasitic Diseases (A00-B99, U07.1, *U09.9*)

a. Human Immunodeficiency Virus (HIV) Infections

1) Code only confirmed cases

Code only confirmed cases of HIV infection/illness. This is an exception to the hospital inpatient guideline Section II, H.

In this context, "confirmation" does not require documentation of positive serology or culture for HIV; the provider's diagnostic statement that the patient is HIV positive, or has an HIV-related illness is sufficient.

2) Selection and sequencing of HIV codes

(a) Patient admitted for HIV-related condition

If a patient is admitted for an HIV-related condition, the principal diagnosis should be B20, Human immunodeficiency virus [HIV] disease followed by additional diagnosis codes for all reported HIV-related conditions.

(b) Patient with HIV disease admitted for unrelated condition

If a patient with HIV disease is admitted for an unrelated condition (such as a traumatic injury), the code for the unrelated condition (e.g., the nature of injury code) should be the principal diagnosis. Other diagnoses would be B20 followed by additional diagnosis codes for all reported HIV-related conditions.

(c) Whether the patient is newly diagnosed

Whether the patient is newly diagnosed or has had previous admissions/encounters for HIV conditions is irrelevant to the sequencing decision.

(d) Asymptomatic human immunodeficiency virus

Z21, Asymptomatic human immunodeficiency virus [HIV] infection status, is to be applied when the patient without any documentation of symptoms is listed as being "HIV positive," "known HIV," "HIV test positive," or similar terminology. Do not use this code if the term "AIDS" **or "HIV disease"** is used or if the patient is treated for any HIV-related illness or is described as having any condition(s) resulting from his/her HIV positive status; use B20 in these cases.

(e) Patients with inconclusive HIV serology

Patients with inconclusive HIV serology, but no definitive diagnosis or manifestations of the illness, may be assigned code R75, Inconclusive laboratory evidence of human immunodeficiency virus [HIV].

(f) Previously diagnosed HIV-related illness

Patients with any known prior diagnosis of an HIV-related illness should be coded to B20. Once a patient has developed an HIV-related illness, the patient should always be assigned code B20 on every subsequent admission/encounter. Patients previously diagnosed with any HIV illness (B20) should never be assigned to R75 or Z21, Asymptomatic human immunodeficiency virus [HIV] infection status.

(g) HIV Infection in Pregnancy, Childbirth and the Puerperium

During pregnancy, childbirth or the puerperium, a patient admitted (or presenting for a health care encounter) because of an HIV-related illness should receive a principal diagnosis code of O98.7-, Human immunodeficiency [HIV] disease complicating pregnancy, childbirth and the puerperium, followed by B20 and the code(s) for the HIV-related illness(es). Codes from Chapter 15 always take sequencing priority.

Patients with asymptomatic HIV infection status admitted (or presenting for a health care encounter) during pregnancy, childbirth, or the puerperium should receive codes of O98.7- and Z21.

(h) Encounters for testing for HIV

If a patient is being seen to determine his/her HIV status, use code Z11.4, Encounter for screening for human immunodeficiency virus [HIV]. Use additional codes for any associated high-risk behavior, **if applicable.**

If a patient with signs or symptoms is being seen for HIV testing, code the signs and symptoms. An additional counseling code Z71.7, Human immunodeficiency virus [HIV] counseling, may be used if counseling is provided during the encounter for the test.

When a patient returns to be informed of his/her HIV test results and the test result is negative, use code Z71.7, Human immunodeficiency virus [HIV] counseling.

If the results are positive, see previous guidelines and assign codes as appropriate.

(i) History of HIV managed by medication

If a patient with documented history of HIV disease is currently managed on antiretroviral medications, assign code B20, Human immunodeficiency virus [HIV] disease. Code Z79.899, Other long term (current) drug therapy, may be assigned as an additional code to identify the long-term (current) use of antiretroviral medications.

b. Infectious agents as the cause of diseases classified to other chapters

Certain infections are classified in chapters other than Chapter 1 and no organism is identified as part of the infection code. In these instances, it is necessary to use an additional code from Chapter 1 to identify the organism. A code from category B95, Streptococcus, Staphylococcus, and Enterococcus as the cause of diseases classified to other chapters, B96, Other bacterial agents as the cause of diseases classified to other chapters, or B97, Viral agents as the cause of diseases classified to other chapters, is to be used as an additional code to identify the organism. An instructional note will be found at the infection code advising that an additional organism code is required.

c. Infections resistant to antibiotics

Many bacterial infections are resistant to current antibiotics. It is necessary to identify all infections documented as antibiotic resistant. Assign a code from category Z16, Resistance to antimicrobial drugs, following the infection code only if the infection code does not identify drug resistance.

d. Sepsis, Severe Sepsis, and Septic Shock

1) Coding of Sepsis and Severe Sepsis

(a) Sepsis

For a diagnosis of sepsis, assign the appropriate code for the underlying systemic infection. If the type of infection or causal organism is not further specified, assign code A41.9, Sepsis, unspecified organism.

A code from subcategory R65.2, Severe sepsis, should not be assigned unless severe sepsis or an associated acute organ dysfunction is documented.

(i) Negative or inconclusive blood cultures and sepsis
Negative or inconclusive blood cultures do not preclude a diagnosis of sepsis in patients with clinical evidence of the condition, however, the provider should be queried.

(ii) Urosepsis
The term urosepsis is a nonspecific term. It is not to be considered synonymous with sepsis. It has no default code in the Alphabetic Index. Should a provider use this

term, he/she must be queried for clarification.

   (iii) Sepsis with organ dysfunction
   If a patient has sepsis and associated acute organ dysfunction or multiple organ dysfunction (MOD), follow the instructions for coding severe sepsis.

   (iv) Acute organ dysfunction that is not clearly associated with the sepsis
   If a patient has sepsis and an acute organ dysfunction, but the medical record documentation indicates that the acute organ dysfunction is related to a medical condition other than the sepsis, do not assign a code from subcategory R65.2, Severe sepsis. An acute organ dysfunction must be associated with the sepsis in order to assign the severe sepsis code. If the documentation is not clear as to whether an acute organ dysfunction is related to the sepsis or another medical condition, query the provider.

(b) Severe sepsis

The coding of severe sepsis requires a minimum of 2 codes: first a code for the underlying systemic infection, followed by a code from subcategory R65.2, Severe sepsis. If the causal organism is not documented, assign code A41.9, Sepsis, unspecified organism, for the infection. Additional code(s) for the associated acute organ dysfunction are also required.

Due to the complex nature of severe sepsis, some cases may require querying the provider prior to assignment of the codes.

2) Septic shock

   (a) Septic shock generally refers to circulatory failure associated with severe sepsis, and therefore, it represents a type of acute organ dysfunction.

For all cases of septic shock, the code for the systemic infection should be sequenced first, followed by code R65.21, Severe sepsis with septic shock or code T81.12, Postprocedural septic shock. Any additional codes for the other acute organ dysfunctions should also be assigned. As noted in the sequencing instructions in the Tabular List, the code for septic shock cannot be assigned as a principal diagnosis.

3) Sequencing of severe sepsis

If severe sepsis is present on admission, and meets the definition of principal diagnosis, the underlying systemic infection should be assigned as principal diagnosis followed by the appropriate code from subcategory R65.2 as required by the sequencing rules in the Tabular List. A code from subcategory R65.2 can never be assigned as a principal diagnosis.

When severe sepsis develops during an encounter (it was not present on admission) the underlying systemic infection and the appropriate code from subcategory R65.2 should be assigned as secondary diagnoses.

Severe sepsis may be present on admission but the diagnosis may not be confirmed until sometime after admission. If the documentation is not clear whether severe sepsis was present on admission, the provider should be queried.

4) Sepsis or severe sepsis with a localized infection

If the reason for admission is sepsis or severe sepsis and a localized infection, such as pneumonia or cellulitis, a code(s) for the underlying systemic infection should be assigned first and the code for the localized infection should be assigned as a secondary diagnosis. If the patient has severe sepsis, a code from subcategory R65.2 should also be assigned as a secondary diagnosis. If the patient is admitted with a localized infection, such as pneumonia, and sepsis/severe sepsis doesn't develop until after admission, the localized infection should be assigned first, followed by the appropriate sepsis/severe sepsis codes.

5) Sepsis due to a postprocedural infection

   (a) Documentation of causal relationship
As with all postprocedural complications, code assignment is based on the provider's documentation of the relationship between the infection and the procedure.

   (b) Sepsis due to a postprocedural infection
For infections following a procedure, a code from T81.40, to T81.43. Infection following a procedure, or a code from O86.00 to O86.03, Infection of obstetric surgical wound, that identifies the site of the infection should be coded first, if known. Assign an additional code for sepsis following a procedure (T81.44) or sepsis following an obstetrical procedure (O86.04). Use an additional code to identify the infectious agent. If the patient has severe sepsis the appropriate code from subcategory R65.2 should also be assigned with the additional code(s) for any acute organ dysfunction.

For infections following infusion, transfusion, therapeutic injection, or immunization, a code from subcategory T80.2, Infections following infusion, transfusion, and therapeutic injection, or code T88.0-, Infection following immunization, should be coded first, followed by the code for the specific infection. If the patient has severe sepsis, the appropriate code from subcategory R65.2 should also be assigned, with the additional codes(s) for any acute organ dysfunction.

   (c) Postprocedural infection and postprocedural septic shock
If a postprocedural infection has resulted in postprocedural septic shock, assign the codes indicated above for sepsis due to a postprocedural infection, followed by code T81.12-, Postprocedural septic shock. Do not assign code R65.21, Severe sepsis with septic shock. Additional code(s) should

be assigned
for any acute organ dysfunction.

6) Sepsis and severe sepsis associated with a noninfectious process (condition)

In some cases a noninfectious process (condition), such as trauma, may lead to an infection which can result in sepsis or severe sepsis. If sepsis or severe sepsis is documented as associated with a noninfectious condition, such as a burn or serious injury, and this condition meets the definition for principal diagnosis, the code for the noninfectious condition should be sequenced first, followed by the code for the resulting infection. If severe sepsis is present, a code from subcategory R65.2 should also be assigned with any associated organ dysfunction(s) codes. It is not necessary to assign a code from subcategory R65.1, Systemic inflammatory response syndrome (SIRS) of non-infectious origin, for these cases.

If the infection meets the definition of principal diagnosis it should be sequenced before the non-infectious condition. When both the associated non-infectious condition and the infection meet the definition of principal diagnosis either may be assigned as principal diagnosis.

Only one code from category R65, Symptoms and signs specifically associated with systemic inflammation and infection, should be assigned. Therefore, when a non-infectious condition leads to an infection resulting in severe sepsis, assign the appropriate code from subcategory R65.2, Severe sepsis. Do not additionally assign a code from subcategory R65.1, Systemic inflammatory response syndrome (SIRS) of non-infectious origin.

See Section I.C.18. SIRS due to non-infectious process

7) Sepsis and septic shock complicating abortion, pregnancy, childbirth, and the puerperium

See Section I.C.15. Sepsis and septic shock complicating abortion, pregnancy, childbirth and the puerperium

8) Newborn sepsis

See Section I.C.16. f. Bacterial sepsis of Newborn

e. Methicillin Resistant Staphylococcus aureus (MRSA) Conditions

1) Selection and sequencing of MRSA codes

(a) Combination codes for MRSA infection

When a patient is diagnosed with an infection that is due to methicillin resistant *Staphylococcus aureus* (MRSA), and that infection has a combination code that includes the causal organism (e.g., sepsis, pneumonia) assign the appropriate combination code for the condition (e.g., code A41.02, Sepsis due to Methicillin resistant Staphylococcus aureus or code J15.212, Pneumonia due to Methicillin resistant Staphylococcus aureus). Do not assign code B95.62, Methicillin resistant Staphylococcus aureus infection as the cause of diseases classified elsewhere, as an additional code because the combination code includes the type of infection and the MRSA organism. Do not assign a code from

subcategory Z16.11, Resistance to penicillins, as an additional diagnosis.

See Section C.1. for instructions on coding and sequencing of sepsis and severe sepsis.

(b) Other codes for MRSA infection

When there is documentation of a current infection (e.g., wound infection, stitch abscess, urinary tract infection) due to MRSA, and that infection does not have a combination code that includes the causal organism, assign the appropriate code to identify the condition along with code B95.62, Methicillin resistant Staphylococcus aureus infection as the cause of diseases classified elsewhere for the MRSA infection. Do not assign a code from subcategory Z16.11, Resistance to penicillins.

(c) Methicillin susceptible Staphylococcus aureus (MSSA) and MRSA colonization

The condition or state of being colonized or carrying MSSA or MRSA is called colonization or carriage, while an individual person is described as being colonized or being a carrier. Colonization means that MSSA or MSRA is present on or in the body without necessarily causing illness. A positive MRSA colonization test might be documented by the provider as "MRSA screen positive" or "MRSA nasal swab positive".

Assign code Z22.322, Carrier or suspected carrier of Methicillin resistant Staphylococcus aureus, for patients documented as having MRSA colonization. Assign code Z22.321, Carrier or suspected carrier of Methicillin susceptible Staphylococcus aureus, for patients documented as having MSSA colonization. Colonization is not necessarily indicative of a disease process or as the cause of a specific condition the patient may have unless documented as such by the provider.

(d) MRSA colonization and infection

If a patient is documented as having both MRSA colonization and infection during a hospital admission, code Z22.322, Carrier or suspected carrier of Methicillin resistant Staphylococcus aureus, and a code for the MRSA infection may both be assigned.

f. Zika virus infections

1) Code only confirmed cases

Code only a confirmed diagnosis of Zika virus (A92.5, Zika virus disease) as documented by the provider. This is an exception to the hospital inpatient guideline Section II, H.

In this context, "confirmation" does not require documentation of the type of test performed; the provider's diagnostic statement that the condition is confirmed is sufficient. This code should be assigned regardless of the stated mode of transmission.

If the provider documents "suspected", "possible" or "probable" Zika, do not assign code A92.5. Assign a code(s) explaining the reason for encounter (such as fever, rash, or joint pain) or Z20.821, Contact with and (suspected) exposure to Zika virus.

g. Coronavirus infections

   1) COVID-19 infection (infection due to SARS-CoV-2)

     (a) Code only confirmed cases

Code only a confirmed diagnosis of the 2019 novel coronavirus disease (COVID-19) as documented by the provider, or documentation of a positive COVID-19 test result. For a confirmed diagnosis, assign code U07.1, COVID-19. This is an exception to the hospital inpatient guideline Section II, H. In this context, "confirmation" does not require documentation of a positive test result for COVID-19; the provider's documentation that the individual has COVID-19 is sufficient.

If the provider documents "suspected," "possible," "probable," or "inconclusive" COVID-19, do not assign code U07.1. Instead, code the signs and symptoms reported. See guideline I.C.1.g.1.g.

     (b) Sequencing of codes

When COVID-19 meets the definition of principal diagnosis, code U07.1, COVID-19, should be sequenced first, followed by the appropriate codes for associated manifestations, except when another guideline requires that certain codes be sequenced first, such as obstetrics, sepsis, or transplant complications.

For a COVID-19 infection that progresses to sepsis, see Section I.C.1.d. Sepsis, Severe Sepsis, and Septic Shock

See Section I.C.15.s. for COVID-19 infection in pregnancy, childbirth, and the puerperium

See Section I.C.16.h. for COVID-19 infection in newborn

For a COVID-19 infection in a lung transplant patient, see Section I.C.19.g.3.a. Transplant complications other than kidney.

     (c) Acute respiratory manifestations of COVID-19

When the reason for the encounter/admission is a respiratory manifestation of COVID-19, assign code U07.1, COVID-19, as the principal/first-listed diagnosis and assign code(s) for the respiratory manifestation(s) as additional diagnoses.

The following conditions are examples of common respiratory manifestations of COVID-19.

     (i) Pneumonia

For a patient with pneumonia confirmed as due to COVID-19, assign codes U07.1, COVID-19, and J12.89, Other viral pneumonia.

     (ii) Acute bronchitis

For a patient with acute bronchitis confirmed as due to COVID-19, assign codes U07.1, and J20.8, Acute bronchitis due to other specified organisms.

Bronchitis not otherwise specified (NOS) due to COVID-19 should be coded using code U07.1 and J40, Bronchitis, not specified as acute or chronic.

     (iii) Lower respiratory infection

If the COVID-19 is documented as being associated with a lower respiratory infection, not otherwise specified (NOS), or an acute respiratory infection, NOS, codes U07.1 and J22, Unspecified acute lower respiratory infection, should be assigned.

If the COVID-19 is documented as being associated with a respiratory infection, NOS, codes U07.1 and J98.8, Other specified respiratory disorders, should be assigned.

     (iv) Acute respiratory distress syndrome

For acute respiratory distress syndrome (ARDS) due to COVID-19, assign codes U07.1, and J80, Acute respiratory distress syndrome.

     (v) Acute respiratory failure

For acute respiratory failure due to COVID-19, assign code U07.1, and code J96.0-, Acute respiratory failure.

    (d) Non-respiratory manifestations of COVID-19

When the reason for the encounter/admission is a non-respiratory manifestation (e.g., viral enteritis) of COVID-19, assign code U07.1, COVID-19, as the principal/first-listed diagnosis and assign code(s) for the manifestation(s) as additional diagnoses.

    (e) Exposure to COVID-19

For asymptomatic individuals with actual or suspected exposure to COVID-19, assign code Z20.828, Contact with and (suspected) exposure to other viral communicable diseases.

For symptomatic individuals with actual or suspected exposure to COVID-19 and the infection has been ruled out, or test results are inconclusive or unknown, assign code Z20.828, Contact with and (suspected) exposure to other viral communicable diseases. See guideline I.C.21.c.1, Contact/Exposure, for additional guidance regarding the use of category Z20 codes.

If COVID-19 is confirmed, see guideline I.C.1.g.1.a.

    (f) Screening for COVID-19

During the COVID-19 pandemic, a screening code is generally not appropriate. For encounters for COVID-19 testing, including preoperative testing, code as exposure to COVID-19 (guideline I.C.1.g.1.e).

Coding guidance will be updated as new information concerning any changes in the pandemic status becomes available.

    (g) Signs and symptoms without definitive diagnosis of COVID-19

For patients presenting with any signs/symptoms associated with COVID-19 (such as fever, etc.) but a definitive diagnosis has not been established, assign the appropriate code(s) for each of the presenting signs and symptoms such as:
- R05.1, Acute cough, or R05.9, Cough, unspecified
- R06.02 Shortness of breath
- R50.9 Fever, unspecified

If a patient with signs/symptoms associated with COVID-19 also has an actual or suspected contact with or exposure to COVID-19, assign Z20.828, Contact with and (suspected) exposure to other viral communicable diseases, as an additional code.

(h) *Asymptomatic individuals who test positive for COVID-19*

For asymptomatic individuals who test positive for COVID-19, see guideline I.C.1.g.1.a. Although the individual is asymptomatic, the individual has tested positive and is considered to have the COVID-19 infection.

(i) *Personal history of COVID-19*

For patients with a history of COVID-19, assign code Z86.19, Personal history of other infectious and parasitic diseases.

(j) *Follow-up visits after COVID-19 infection has resolved*

For individuals who previously had COVID-19 without residual symptom(s) or condition(s), and are being seen for follow-up evaluation, and COVID-19 test results are negative, assign codes Z09, Encounter for follow-up examination after completed treatment for conditions other than malignant neoplasm, and Z86.19, Personal history of other infectious and parasitic diseases.

For follow-up visits for individuals with symptom(s) or condition(s) related to a previous COVID-19 infection, see guideline I.C.1.g.1.m.

See Section I.C.21.c.8, Factors influencing health states and contact with health services, Follow-up

(k) *Encounter for antibody testing*

For an encounter for antibody testing that is not being performed to confirm a current COVID-19 infection, nor is a follow-up test after resolution of COVID-19, assign Z01.84, Encounter for antibody response examination.

Follow the applicable guidelines above if the individual is being tested to confirm a current COVID-19 infection.

For follow-up testing after a COVID-19 infection, see guideline I.C.1.g.1.j.

(l) **Multisystem Inflammatory Syndrome**

For individuals with multisystem inflammatory syndrome (MIS) and COVID-19, assign code U07.1, COVID-19, as the principal/first-listed diagnosis and assign code M35.81, Multisystem inflammatory syndrome, as an additional diagnosis.

If an individual with a history of COVID-19 develops MIS, assign codes M35.81, Multisystem

inflammatory syndrome, and **U09.9, Post COVID-19 condition, unspecified.**

If an individual with a known or suspected exposure to COVID-19, and no current COVID-19 infection or history of COVID-19, develops MIS, assign codes M35.81, Multisystem inflammatory syndrome, and Z20.822, Contact with and (suspected) exposure to COVID-19.

Additional codes should be assigned for any associated complications of MIS.

(m) Post COVID-19 Condition

For sequela of COVID-19, or associated symptoms or conditions that develop following a previous COVID-19 infection, assign a code(s) for the specific symptom(s) or condition(s) related to the previous COVID-19 infection, if known, and code U09.9, Post COVID-19 condition, unspecified.

Code U09.9 should not be assigned for manifestations of an active (current) COVID-19 infection.

If a patient has a condition(s) associated with a previous COVID-19 infection and develops a new active (current) COVID-19 infection, code U09.9 may be assigned in conjunction with code U07.1, COVID-19, to identify that the patient also has a condition(s) associated with a previous COVID-19 infection. Code(s) for the specific condition(s) associated with the previous COVID-19 infection and code(s) for manifestation(s) of the new active (current) COVID-19 infection should also be assigned.

2. **Chapter 2: Neoplasms (C00-D49)**
General guidelines
Chapter 2 of the ICD-10-CM contains the codes for most benign and all malignant neoplasms. Certain benign neoplasms, such as prostatic adenomas, may be found in the specific body system chapters. To properly code a neoplasm it is necessary to determine from the record if the neoplasm is benign, in-situ, malignant, or of uncertain histologic behavior. If malignant, any secondary (metastatic) sites should also be determined.

Primary malignant neoplasms overlapping site boundaries

A primary malignant neoplasm that overlaps two or more contiguous (next to each other) sites should be classified to the subcategory/code .8 ("overlapping lesion"), unless the combination is specifically indexed elsewhere. For multiple neoplasms of the same site that are not contiguous such as tumors in different quadrants of the same breast, codes for each site should be assigned.

Malignant neoplasm of ectopic tissue
Malignant neoplasms of ectopic tissue are to be coded to the site of origin mentioned (e.g., ectopic pancreatic malignant neoplasms involving the stomach are coded to malignant neoplasm of pancreas, unspecified) (C25.9).

The neoplasm table in the Alphabetic Index should be referenced first. However, if the histological term is documented, that term should be referenced first, rather than going immediately to the Neoplasm Table, in order to determine which column in the Neoplasm Table is appropriate. For example, if the documentation indicates "adenoma," refer to the term in the Alphabetic Index to review the entries under this term and the instructional note to "see also neoplasm, by site, benign." The table provides the proper code based on the type of neoplasm and the site. It is important to select the proper column in the table that corresponds to the type of neoplasm. The Tabular List should then be referenced to verify that the correct code has been selected from the table and that a more specific site code does not exist.

See Section I.C.21. Factors influencing health status and contact with health services, Status, for information regarding Z15.0, codes for genetic susceptibility to cancer.

a. Treatment directed at the malignancy

If the treatment is directed at the malignancy, designate the malignancy as the principal diagnosis.

The only exception to this guideline is if a patient admission/encounter is solely for the administration of chemotherapy, immunotherapy or external beam radiation therapy, assign the appropriate Z51.— code as the first-listed or principal diagnosis, and the diagnosis or problem for which the service is being performed as a secondary diagnosis.

b. Treatment of secondary site

When a patient is admitted because of a primary neoplasm with metastasis and treatment is directed toward the secondary site only, the secondary neoplasm is designated as the principal diagnosis even though the primary malignancy is still present.

c. Coding and sequencing of complications

Coding and sequencing of complications associated with the malignancies or with the therapy thereof are subject to the following guidelines:

1) Anemia associated with malignancy

When admission/encounter is for management of an anemia associated with the malignancy, and the treatment is only for anemia, the appropriate code for the malignancy is sequenced as the principal or first-listed diagnosis followed by the appropriate code for the anemia (such as code D63.0, Anemia in neoplastic disease).

2) Anemia associated with chemotherapy, immunotherapy and radiation therapy

When the admission/encounter is for management of an anemia associated with an adverse effect of the administration of chemotherapy or immunotherapy and the only treatment is for the anemia, the anemia code is sequenced first followed by the appropriate codes for the neoplasm and the adverse effect (T45.1X5, Adverse effect of antineoplastic and immunosuppressive drugs).

When the admission/encounter is for management of an anemia associated with an adverse effect of radiotherapy, the anemia code should be sequenced first, followed by the appropriate neoplasm code and code Y84.2, Radiological procedure and radiotherapy as the cause of abnormal reaction of the patient, or of later complication, without mention of misadventure at the time of the procedure.

3) Management of dehydration due to the malignancy

When the admission/encounter is for management of dehydration due to the malignancy and only the dehydration is being treated (intravenous rehydration), the dehydration is sequenced first, followed by the code(s) for the malignancy.

4) Treatment of a complication resulting from a surgical procedure

When the admission/encounter is for treatment of a complication resulting from a surgical procedure, designate the complication as the principal or first-listed diagnosis if treatment is directed at resolving the complication.

d. Primary malignancy previously excised

When a primary malignancy has been previously excised or eradicated from its site and there is no further treatment directed to that site and there is no evidence of any existing primary malignancy, at that site a code from category Z85, Personal history of malignant neoplasm, should be used to indicate the former site of the malignancy. Any mention of extension, invasion, or metastasis to another site is coded as a secondary malignant neoplasm to that site. The secondary site may be the principal or first-listed diagnosis with the Z85 code used as a secondary code.

e. Admissions/Encounters involving chemotherapy, immunotherapy and radiation therapy

1) Episode of care involves surgical removal of neoplasm

When an episode of care involves the surgical removal of a neoplasm, primary or secondary site, followed by adjunct chemotherapy or radiation treatment during the same episode of care, the code for the neoplasm should be assigned as principal or first-listed diagnosis.

2) Patient admission/encounter solely for administration of chemotherapy, immunotherapy and radiation therapy

If a patient admission/encounter is solely for the administration of chemotherapy, immunotherapy or external beam radiation therapy assign code Z51.0, Encounter for antineoplastic radiation therapy, or Z51.11, Encounter for antineoplastic chemotherapy, or Z51.12, Encounter for antineoplastic immunotherapy as the first-listed or principal diagnosis. If a patient receives more than one of these therapies during the same admission more than one of these codes may be assigned, in any sequence.

The malignancy for which the therapy is being administered should be assigned as a secondary diagnosis.

If a patient admission/encounter is for the insertion or implantation of radioactive elements (e.g., brachytherapy) the appropriate code for the malignancy is sequenced as the principal or first-listed diagnosis. Code Z51.0 should not be assigned.

3) Patient admitted for radiation therapy, chemotherapy or immunotherapy and develops complications

When a patient is admitted for the purpose of external beam radiotherapy, immunotherapy or chemotherapy and develops complications such as uncontrolled nausea and vomiting or dehydration, the principal or first-listed diagnosis is Z51.0, Encounter for antineoplastic radiation therapy, or Z51.11, Encounter for antineoplastic chemotherapy, or Z51.12, Encounter for antineoplastic immunotherapy followed by any codes for the complications.

When a patient is admitted for the purpose of insertion or implantation of radioactive elements (e.g., brachytherapy) and develops complications such as uncontrolled nausea and vomiting or dehydration, the principal or first-listed diagnosis is the appropriate code for the malignancy followed by any codes for the complications.

f. Admission/encounter to determine extent of malignancy

When the reason for admission/encounter is to determine the extent of the malignancy, or for a procedure such as paracentesis or thoracentesis, the primary malignancy or appropriate metastatic site is designated as the principal or first-listed diagnosis, even though chemotherapy or radiotherapy is administered.

g. Symptoms, signs, and abnormal findings listed in Chapter 18 associated with neoplasms

Symptoms, signs, and ill-defined conditions listed in Chapter 18 characteristic of, or associated with, an existing primary or secondary site malignancy cannot be used to replace the malignancy as principal or first-listed diagnosis, regardless of the number of admissions or encounters for treatment and care of the neoplasm.

See Section I.C.21. Factors influencing health status and contact with health services, Encounter for prophylactic organ removal.

h. Admission/encounter for pain control/ management

See Section I.C.6. for information on coding admission/ encounter for pain control/management.

i. Malignancy in two or more noncontiguous sites

A patient may have more than one malignant tumor in the same organ. These tumors may represent different primaries or metastatic disease, depending on the site. Should the documentation be unclear,

the provider should be queried as to the status of each tumor so that the correct codes can be assigned.

j. Disseminated malignant neoplasm, unspecified

Code C80.0, Disseminated malignant neoplasm, unspecified, is for use only in those cases where the patient has advanced metastatic disease and no known primary or secondary sites are specified. It should not be used in place of assigning codes for the primary site and all known secondary sites.

k. Malignant neoplasm without specification of site

Code C80.1, Malignant (primary) neoplasm, unspecified, equates to Cancer, unspecified. This code should only be used when no determination can be made as to the primary site of a malignancy. This code should rarely be used in the inpatient setting.

l. Sequencing of neoplasm codes

1) Encounter for treatment of primary malignancy

If the reason for the encounter is for treatment of a primary malignancy, assign the malignancy as the principal/first-listed diagnosis. The primary site is to be sequenced first, followed by any metastatic sites.

2) Encounter for treatment of secondary malignancy

When an encounter is for a primary malignancy with metastasis and treatment is directed toward the metastatic (secondary) site(s) only, the metastatic site(s) is designated as the principal/ first-listed diagnosis. The primary malignancy is coded as an additional code.

3) Malignant neoplasm in a pregnant patient

When a pregnant **patient** has a malignant neoplasm, a code from subcategory O9A.1-, Malignant neoplasm complicating pregnancy, childbirth, and the puerperium, should be sequenced first, followed by the appropriate code from Chapter 2 to indicate the type of neoplasm.

4) Encounter for complication associated with a neoplasm

When an encounter is for management of a complication associated with a neoplasm, such as dehydration, and the treatment is only for the complication, the complication is coded first, followed by the appropriate code(s) for the neoplasm.

The exception to this guideline is anemia. When the admission/encounter is for management of an anemia associated with the malignancy, and the treatment is only for anemia, the appropriate code for the malignancy is sequenced as the principal or first-listed diagnosis followed by code D63.0, Anemia in neoplastic disease.

5) Complication from surgical procedure for treatment of a neoplasm

When an encounter is for treatment of a complication resulting from a surgical procedure performed for the treatment of the neoplasm, designate the complication as the principal/ first-listed diagnosis. See the guideline regarding the coding of a current malignancy versus personal history to determine if the code for the neoplasm should also be assigned.

6) Pathologic fracture due to a neoplasm

When an encounter is for a pathological fracture due to a neoplasm, and the focus of treatment is the fracture, a code from subcategory M84.5, Pathological fracture in neoplastic disease, should be sequenced first, followed by the code for the neoplasm.

If the focus of treatment is the neoplasm with an associated pathological fracture, the neoplasm code should be sequenced first, followed by a code from M84.5 for the pathological fracture.

m. Current malignancy versus personal history of malignancy

When a primary malignancy has been excised but further treatment, such as an additional surgery for the malignancy, radiation therapy or chemotherapy is directed to that site, the primary malignancy code should be used until treatment is completed.

When a primary malignancy has been previously excised or eradicated from its site, there is no further treatment (of the malignancy) directed to that site, and there is no evidence of any existing primary malignancy at that site, a code from category Z85, Personal history of malignant neoplasm, should be used to indicate the former site of the malignancy.

Codes from subcategories Z85.0 – Z85.85 should only be assigned for the former site of a primary malignancy, not the site of a secondary malignancy. Code Z85.89, may be assigned for the former site(s) of either a primary or secondary malignancy.

See Section I.C.21. Factors influencing health status and contact with health services, History (of)

n. Leukemia, Multiple Myeloma, and Malignant Plasma Cell Neoplasms in remission versus personal history

The categories for leukemia, and category C90, Multiple myeloma and malignant plasma cell neoplasms, have codes indicating whether or not the leukemia has achieved remission. There are also codes Z85.6, Personal history of leukemia, and Z85.79, Personal history of other malignant neoplasms of lymphoid, hematopoietic and related tissues. If the documentation is unclear, as to whether the leukemia has achieved remission, the provider should be queried.

See Section I.C.21. Factors influencing health status and contact with health services, History (of)

o. Aftercare following surgery for neoplasm

See Section I.C.21. Factors influencing health status and contact with health services, Aftercare

p. Follow-up care for completed treatment of a malignancy

See Section I.C.21. Factors influencing health status and contact with health services, Follow-up

q. Prophylactic organ removal for prevention of malignancy

See Section I.C. 21, Factors influencing health status and contact with health services, Prophylactic organ removal

r. Malignant neoplasm associated with transplanted organ

A malignant neoplasm of a transplanted organ should be coded as a transplant complication. Assign first the appropriate code from category T86.-, Complications of transplanted organs and tissue, followed by code C80.2, Malignant neoplasm associated with transplanted organ. Use an additional code for the specific malignancy.

s. Breast Implant Associated Anaplastic Large Cell Lymphoma

Breast implant associated anaplastic large cell lymphoma (BIA-ALCL) is a type of lymphoma that can develop around breast implants. Assign code C84.7A, Anaplastic large cell lymphoma, ALK-negative, breast, for BIA-ALCL. Do not assign a complication code from chapter 19.

3. **Chapter 3: Disease of the blood and blood-forming organs and certain disorders involving the immune mechanism (D50-D89)**

Reserved for future guideline expansion

4. **Chapter 4: Endocrine, Nutritional, and Metabolic Diseases (E00-E89)**

a. Diabetes mellitus

The diabetes mellitus codes are combination codes that include the type of diabetes mellitus, the body system affected, and the complications affecting that body system. As many codes within a particular category as are necessary to describe all of the complications of the disease may be used. They should be sequenced based on the reason for a particular encounter. Assign as many codes from categories E08 – E13 as needed to identify all of the associated conditions that the patient has.

1) Type of diabetes

The age of a patient is not the sole determining factor, though most type 1 diabetics develop the condition before reaching puberty. For this reason type 1 diabetes mellitus is also referred to as juvenile diabetes.

2) Type of diabetes mellitus not documented

If the type of diabetes mellitus is not documented in the medical record the default is E11.-, Type 2 diabetes mellitus.

3) Diabetes mellitus and the use of insulin, oral hypoglycemics, *and injectable non-insulin drugs*

If the documentation in a medical record does not indicate the type of diabetes but does indicate that the patient uses insulin, code E11, Type 2 diabetes mellitus, should be assigned. Additional code(s) should be assigned from category Z79 to identify the long-term (current) use of insulin or oral hypoglycemic drugs, **or injectable non-insulin antidiabetic, as follows:** If the patient is treated with both oral medications and insulin, **both code Z79.4, Long term (current) use of insulin, and code Z79.84, Long term (current) use of oral hypoglycemic drugs,** should be assigned. **If the patient is treated** with both insulin and an injectable non-insulin antidiabetic drug, assign codes Z79.4, Long-term (current) use of insulin, and Z79.899, Other long term (current) drug therapy. If the patient is treated with both oral hypoglycemic drugs and an injectable non-insulin antidiabetic drug, assign codes Z79.84, Long-term (current) use of oral hypoglycemic drugs, and Z79.899, Other long-term (current) drug therapy. Code Z79.4 should not be assigned if insulin is given temporarily to bring a type 2 patient's blood sugar under control during an encounter.

4) Diabetes mellitus in pregnancy and gestational diabetes

See Section I.C.15. Diabetes mellitus in pregnancy.
See Section I.C.15. Gestational (pregnancy induced) diabetes

5) Complications due to insulin pump malfunction

(a) Underdose of insulin due to insulin pump failure

An underdose of insulin due to an insulin pump failure should be assigned to a code from subcategory T85.6, Mechanical complication of other specified internal and external prosthetic devices, implants and grafts, that specifies the type of pump malfunction, as the principal or first-listed code, followed by code T38.3X6-, Underdosing of insulin and oral hypoglycemic [antidiabetic] drugs. Additional codes for the type of diabetes mellitus and any associated complications due to the underdosing should also be assigned.

(b) Overdose of insulin due to insulin pump failure

The principal or first-listed code for an encounter due to an insulin pump malfunction resulting in an overdose of insulin, should also be T85.6-, Mechanical complication of other specified internal and external prosthetic devices, implants and grafts, followed by code T38.3X1-, Poisoning by insulin and oral hypoglycemic [antidiabetic] drugs, accidental (unintentional).

6) Secondary diabetes mellitus

Codes under categories E08, Diabetes mellitus due to underlying condition, E09, Drug or chemical induced diabetes mellitus and E13, Other specified diabetes mellitus, identify complications/ manifestations associated with secondary diabetes mellitus. Secondary diabetes is always caused by another condition or event (e.g., cystic fibrosis, malignant neoplasm of pancreas, pancreatectomy, adverse effect of drug, or poisoning).

(a) Secondary diabetes mellitus and the use of insulin or hypoglycemic drugs

For patients with secondary diabetes mellitus who routinely use insulin or oral hypoglycemic drugs, **or injectable non-insulin drugs,** an additional code(s) from category Z79 should be assigned to identify the long-term (current) use of insulin or oral hypoglycemic drugs, **or non-injectable non-insulin drugs as follows:** If the patient is treated with both oral medications and insulin, **both code Z79.4, Long term (current) use of insulin, and code Z79.84, Long term (current) use of oral hypoglycemic drugs,** should be assigned. If the patient is treated with both insulin and an injectable non- insulin antidiabetic drug, assign codes Z79.4, Long- term (current) use of insulin, and Z79.899, Other long term (current) drug therapy. If the patient is treated with both oral hypoglycemic drugs and an injectable non-insulin antidiabetic drug, assign codes Z79.84, Long-term (current) use of oral hypoglycemic drugs, and Z79.899, Other long-term (current) drug therapy. Code Z79.4 should not be assigned if insulin is given temporarily to bring a type 2 patient's blood sugar under control during an encounter.

(b) Assigning and sequencing secondary diabetes codes and its causes

The sequencing of the secondary diabetes codes in relationship to codes for the cause of the diabetes is based on the Tabular List instructions for categories E08, E09 and E13.

(i) Secondary diabetes mellitus due to pancreatectomy
For postpancreatectomy diabetes mellitus (lack of insulin due to the surgical removal of all or part of the pancreas), assign code E89.1, Postprocedural hypoinsulinemia. Assign a code from category E13 and a code from subcategory Z90.41-, Acquired absence of pancreas, as additional codes.

(ii) Secondary diabetes due to drugs
Secondary diabetes may be caused by an adverse effect of correctly administered medications, poisoning or sequela of poisoning.

See Section I.C.19.e for coding of adverse effects and poisoning, and Section I.C.20 for external cause code reporting.

5. Chapter 5: Mental, Behavioral and Neurodevelopmental disorders (F01 – F99)

a. Pain disorders related to psychological factors

Assign code F45.41, for pain that is exclusively related to psychological disorders. As indicated by the Excludes1 note under category G89, a code from category G89 should not be assigned with code F45.41

Code F45.42, Pain disorders with related psychological factors, should be used with a code from category G89, Pain, not elsewhere classified, if there is documentation of a psychological component for a patient with acute or chronic pain.

See Section I.C.6. Pain

b. Mental and behavioral disorders due to psychoactive substance use

1) In Remission

Selection of codes for "in remission" for categories F10-F19, Mental and behavioral disorders due to psychoactive substance use (categories

F10-F19 with -11, -.21) requires the provider's clinical judgment. The appropriate codes for "in remission" are assigned only on the basis of provider documentation (as defined in the Official Guidelines for Coding and Reporting), unless otherwise instructed by the classification.

Mild substance use disorders in early or sustained remission are classified to the appropriate codes for substance abuse in remission, and moderate or severe substance use disorders in early or sustained remission are classified to the appropriate codes for substance dependence in remission.

2) Psychoactive Substance Use, Abuse and Dependence

When the provider documentation refers to use, abuse and dependence of the same substance (e.g., alcohol, opioid, cannabis, etc.), only one code should be assigned to identify the pattern of use based on the following hierarchy:

- If both use and abuse are documented, assign only the code for abuse
- If both abuse and dependence are documented, assign only the code for dependence
- If use, abuse and dependence are all documented, assign only the code for dependence
- If both use and dependence are documented, assign only the code for dependence.

3) Psychoactive Substance Use, Unspecified

As with all other unspecified diagnoses, the codes for unspecified psychoactive substance use disorders (F10.9-, F11.9-, F12.9-, F13.9-, F14.9-, F15.9-, F16.9-, F18.9-, F19.9-) should only be assigned based on provider documentation and when they meet the definition of a reportable diagnosis (see Section III, Reporting Additional Diagnoses). These codes are to be used only when the psychoactive substance use is associated 1with a **substance related disorder (chapter 5 such as sexual dysfunction and sleep disorder,** or a mental or behavioral disorder) **or medical condition**, and such a relationship is documented by the provider.

4) Medical Conditions Due to Psychoactive Substance Use, Abuse and Dependence

Medical conditions due to substance use, abuse, and dependence are not classified as substance-induced disorders. Assign the diagnosis code for the medical condition as directed by the Alphabetical Index along with the appropriate psychoactive substance use, abuse or dependence code. For example, for alcoholic pancreatitis due to alcohol dependence, assign the appropriate code from subcategory K85.2, Alcohol induced acute pancreatitis, and the appropriate code from subcategory F10.2, such as code F10.20, Alcohol dependence, uncomplicated. It would not be appropriate to assign code F10.288, Alcohol dependence with other alcohol-induced disorder.

5) Blood Alcohol Level

A code from category Y90, Evidence of alcohol involvement determined by blood alcohol level, may be assigned when this information is documented and the patient's provider has documented a condition classifiable to category F10, Alcohol related disorders. The blood alcohol level does not need to be documented by the patient's provider in order for it to be coded.

c. Factitious Disorder

Factitious disorder imposed on self or Munchausen's syndrome is a disorder in which a person falsely reports or causes his or her own physical or psychological signs or symptoms. For patients with documented factitious disorder on self or Munchausen's syndrome, assign the appropriate code from subcategory F68.1-, Factitious disorder imposed on self.

Munchausen's syndrome by proxy (MSBP) is a disorder in which a caregiver (perpetrator) falsely reports or causes an illness or injury in another person (victim) under his or her care, such as a child, an elderly adult, or a person who has a disability. The condition is also referred to as "factitious disorder imposed on another" or "factitious disorder by proxy." The perpetrator, not the victim, receives this diagnosis. Assign code F68.A, Factitious disorder imposed on another, to the perpetrator's record. For the victim of a patient suffering from MSBP, assign the appropriate code from categories T74, Adult and child abuse, neglect and other maltreatment, confirmed, or T76, Adult and child abuse, neglect and other maltreatment, suspected.

See Section I.C.19.f. Adult and child abuse, neglect and other maltreatment

6. Chapter 6: Diseases of the Nervous System (G00-G99)

a. Dominant/nondominant side

Codes from category G81, Hemiplegia and hemiparesis, and subcategories, G83.1, Monoplegia of lower limb, G83.2, Monoplegia of upper limb, and G83.3, Monoplegia, unspecified, identify whether the dominant or nondominant side is affected. Should the affected side be documented, but not specified as dominant or nondominant, and the classification system does not indicate a default, code selection is as follows:

- For ambidextrous patients, the default should be dominant.
- If the left side is affected, the default is non-dominant.
- If the right side is affected, the default is dominant.

b. Pain - Category G89

1) General coding information

Codes in category G89, Pain, not elsewhere classified, may be used in conjunction with codes from other categories and chapters to provide more detail about acute or chronic pain and neoplasm-related pain, unless otherwise indicated below.

If the pain is not specified as acute or chronic, post-thoracotomy, postprocedural, or neoplasm-related, do not assign codes from category G89.

A code from category G89 should not be assigned if the underlying (definitive) diagnosis is known, unless the reason for the encounter is pain control/management and not management of the underlying condition.

When an admission or encounter is for a procedure aimed at treating the underlying condition (e.g., spinal fusion, kyphoplasty), a code for the underlying condition (e.g., vertebral fracture, spinal stenosis) should be assigned as the principal diagnosis. No code from category G89 should be assigned.

(a) Category G89 Codes as Principal or First-Listed Diagnosis

Category G89 codes are acceptable as principal diagnosis or the first-listed code:

- When pain control or pain management is the reason for the admission/encounter (e.g., a patient with displaced intervertebral disc, nerve impingement and severe back pain presents for injection of steroid into the spinal canal). The underlying cause of the pain should be reported as an additional diagnosis, if known.
- When a patient is admitted for the insertion of a neurostimulator for pain control, assign the appropriate pain code as the principal or first-listed diagnosis. When an admission or encounter is for a procedure aimed at treating the underlying condition and a neurostimulator is inserted for pain control during the same admission/encounter, a code for the underlying condition should be assigned as the principal diagnosis and the appropriate pain code should be assigned as a secondary diagnosis.

(b) Use of Category G89 Codes in Conjunction with Site-Specific Pain Codes

(i) Assigning Category G89 and Site-Specific Pain Codes

Codes from category G89 may be used in conjunction with codes that identify the site of pain (including codes from Chapter 18) if the category G89 code provides additional information. For example, if the code describes the site of the pain, but does not fully describe whether the pain is acute or chronic, then both codes should be assigned.

(ii) Sequencing of Category G89 Codes with Site-Specific Pain Codes

The sequencing of category G89 codes with site-specific pain codes (including Chapter 18 codes), is dependent on the circumstances of the encounter/admission as follows:

- If the encounter is for pain control or pain management, assign the code from category G89 followed by the code identifying the specific site of pain (e.g., encounter for pain management for acute neck pain from trauma is assigned code G89.11, Acute pain due to trauma, followed by code M54.2, Cervicalgia, to identify the site of pain).
- If the encounter is for any other reason except pain control or pain management, and a related definitive diagnosis has not been established (confirmed) by the provider, assign the code for the specific site of pain first, followed by the appropriate code from category G89.

2) Pain due to devices, implants and grafts
See Section I.C.19. Pain due to medical devices

3) Postoperative Pain

The provider's documentation should be used to guide the coding of postoperative pain, as well as *Section III. Reporting Additional Diagnoses* and *Section IV. Diagnostic Coding and Reporting in the Outpatient Setting.*

The default for post-thoracotomy and other postoperative pain not specified as acute or chronic is the code for the acute form.

Routine or expected postoperative pain immediately after surgery should not be coded.

(a) Postoperative pain not associated with specific postoperative complication

Postoperative pain not associated with a specific postoperative complication is assigned to the appropriate postoperative pain code in category G89.

(b) Postoperative pain associated with specific postoperative complication

Postoperative pain associated with a specific postoperative complication (such as painful wire sutures) is assigned to the appropriate code(s) found in Chapter 19, Injury, poisoning, and certain other consequences of external causes. If appropriate, use additional code(s) from category G89 to identify acute or chronic pain (G89.18 or G89.28).

4) Chronic pain

Chronic pain is classified to subcategory G89.2. There is no time frame defining when pain becomes chronic pain. The provider's documentation should be used to guide use of these codes.

5) Neoplasm Related Pain

Code G89.3 is assigned to pain documented as being related, associated or due to cancer, primary or secondary malignancy, or tumor. This code is assigned regardless of whether the pain is acute or chronic.

This code may be assigned as the principal or first-listed code when the stated reason for the admission/encounter is documented as pain control/pain management. The underlying neoplasm should be reported as an additional diagnosis.

When the reason for the admission/encounter is management of the neoplasm and the pain associated with the neoplasm is also documented, code G89.3 may be assigned as an additional diagnosis. It is not necessary to assign an additional code for the site of the pain.

See Section I.C.2 for instructions on the sequencing of neoplasms for all other stated reasons for the admission/encounter (except for pain control/pain management).

6) Chronic pain syndrome

Central pain syndrome (G89.0) and chronic pain syndrome (G89.4) are different than the term "chronic pain," and therefore codes should only be used when the provider has specifically documented this condition.

See Section I.C.5. Pain disorders related to psychological factors

7. Chapter 7: Diseases of the Eye and Adnexa (H00-H59)

a. Glaucoma

1) Assigning Glaucoma Codes

Assign as many codes from category H40, Glaucoma, as needed to identify the type of glaucoma, the affected eye, and the glaucoma stage.

2) Bilateral glaucoma with same type and stage

When a patient has bilateral glaucoma and both eyes are documented as being the same type and stage, and there is a code for bilateral glaucoma, report only the code for the type of glaucoma, bilateral, with the seventh character for the stage.

When a patient has bilateral glaucoma and both eyes are documented as being the same type and stage, and the classification does not provide a code for bilateral glaucoma (i.e., subcategories H40.10, H40.11 and H40.20) report only one code for the type of glaucoma with the appropriate seventh character for the stage.

3) Bilateral glaucoma stage with different types or stages

When a patient has bilateral glaucoma and each eye is documented as having a different type or stage, and the classification distinguishes laterality, assign the appropriate code for each eye rather than the code for bilateral glaucoma.

When a patient has bilateral glaucoma and each eye is documented as having a different type, and the classification does not distinguish laterality (i.e., subcategories H40.10, H40.11 and H40.20), assign one code for each type of glaucoma with the appropriate 7th character for the stage.

When a patient has bilateral glaucoma and each eye is documented as having the same type, but different stage, and the classification does not distinguish laterality (i.e., subcategories H40.10, H40.11 and H40.20), assign a code for the type of glaucoma for each eye with the 7th character for the specific glaucoma stage documented for each eye.

4) Patient admitted with glaucoma and stage evolves during the admission

If a patient is admitted with glaucoma and the stage progresses during the admission, assign the code for highest stage documented.

5) Indeterminate stage glaucoma

Assignment of the 7th character "4" for "indeterminate stage" should be based on the clinical documentation. The 7th character "4" is used for glaucomas whose stage cannot be clinically determined. This 7th character should not be confused with the 7th character "0", unspecified, which should be assigned when there is no documentation regarding the stage of the glaucoma.

b. Blindness

If "blindness" or "low vision" of both eyes is documented but the visual impairment category is not documented, assign code H54.3, Unqualified visual loss, both eyes. If "blindness" or "low vision" in one eye is documented but the visual impairment category is not documented, assign a code from H54.6-, Unqualified visual loss, one eye. If "blindness" or "visual loss" is documented without any information about whether one or both eyes are affected, assign code H54.7, Unspecified visual loss.

8. Chapter 8: Diseases of the Ear and Mastoid Process (H60-H95)

Reserved for future guideline expansion

9. Chapter 9: Diseases of the Circulatory System (I00-I99)

a. Hypertension

The classification presumes a causal relationship between hypertension and heart involvement and between hypertension and kidney involvement, as the two conditions are linked by the term "with" in the Alphabetic Index. These conditions should be coded as related even in the absence of provider documentation explicitly linking them, unless the documentation clearly states the conditions are unrelated.

For hypertension and conditions not specifically linked by relational terms such as "with," "associated with" or "due to" in the classification, provider documentation must link the conditions in order to code them as related.

1) Hypertension with Heart Disease

Hypertension with heart conditions classified to I50.- or I51.4-I51.7, I51.89, I51.9, are assigned to, a code from category I11, Hypertensive heart disease. Use additional code(s) from category I50, Heart failure, to identify the type(s) of heart failure in those patients with heart failure.

The same heart conditions (I50.-, I51.4-I51.7, I51.89, I51.9) with hypertension are coded separately if the provider has documented they are unrelated to the hypertension. Sequence according to the circumstances of the admission/encounter.

2) Hypertensive Chronic Kidney Disease

Assign codes from category I12, Hypertensive chronic kidney disease, when both hypertension and a condition classifiable to category N18, Chronic kidney disease (CKD), are present. CKD should not be coded as hypertensive if the provider indicates the CKD is not related to the hypertension.

The appropriate code from category N18 should be used as a secondary code with a code from category I12 to identify the stage of chronic kidney disease.

See Section I.C.14. Chronic kidney disease.

If a patient has hypertensive chronic kidney disease and acute renal failure, the acute renal failure should also be coded. Sequence according to the circumstances of the admission/encounter.

3) Hypertensive Heart and Chronic Kidney Disease

Assign codes from combination category I13, Hypertensive heart and chronic kidney disease, when there is hypertension with both heart and kidney involvement. If heart failure is present, assign an additional code from category I50 to identify the type of heart failure.

The appropriate code from category N18, Chronic kidney disease, should be used as a secondary code with a code from category I13 to identify the stage of chronic kidney disease.

See Section I.C.14. Chronic kidney disease.

The codes in category I13, Hypertensive heart and chronic kidney disease, are combination codes that include hypertension, heart disease and chronic kidney disease. The Includes note at I13 specifies that the conditions included at I11 and I12 are included together in I13. If a patient has hypertension, heart disease and chronic kidney disease then a code from I13 should be used, not individual codes for hypertension, heart disease and chronic kidney disease, or codes from I11 or I12.

For patients with both acute renal failure and chronic kidney disease the acute renal failure should also be coded. Sequence according to the circumstances of the admission/encounter.

4) Hypertensive Cerebrovascular Disease

For hypertensive cerebrovascular disease, first assign the appropriate code from categories I60-I69, followed by the appropriate hypertension code.

5) Hypertensive Retinopathy

Subcategory H35.0, Background retinopathy and retinal vascular changes, should be used with a code from category I10 – I15, Hypertensive disease to include the systemic hypertension. The sequencing is based on the reason for the encounter.

6) Hypertension, Secondary

Secondary hypertension is due to an underlying condition. Two codes are required: one to identify the underlying etiology and one from category I15 to identify the hypertension. Sequencing of codes is determined by the reason for admission/encounter.

7) Hypertension, Transient

Assign code R03.0, Elevated blood pressure reading without diagnosis of hypertension, unless patient has an established diagnosis of hypertension. Assign code O13.-, Gestational [pregnancy-induced] hypertension without significant proteinuria, or O14.-, Pre-eclampsia, for transient hypertension of pregnancy.

8) Hypertension, Controlled

This diagnostic statement usually refers to an existing state of hypertension under control by therapy. Assign the appropriate code from categories I10-I15, Hypertensive diseases.

9) Hypertension, Uncontrolled

Uncontrolled hypertension may refer to untreated hypertension or hypertension not responding to current therapeutic regimen. In either case, assign the appropriate code from categories I10-I15, Hypertensive diseases.

10) Hypertensive Crisis

Assign a code from category I16, Hypertensive crisis, for documented hypertensive urgency, hypertensive emergency or unspecified hypertensive crisis. Code also any identified hypertensive disease (I10-I15). The sequencing is based on the reason for the encounter.

11) Pulmonary Hypertension

Pulmonary hypertension is classified to category I27, Other pulmonary heart diseases. For secondary pulmonary hypertension (I27.1, I27.2-), code also any associated conditions or adverse effects of drugs or toxins. The sequencing is based on the reason for the encounter, except for adverse effects of drugs.

See Section I.C.19.e

b. Atherosclerotic Coronary Artery Disease and Angina

ICD-10-CM has combination codes for atherosclerotic heart disease with angina pectoris. The subcategories for these codes are I25.11, Atherosclerotic heart disease of native coronary artery with angina pectoris and I25.7, Atherosclerosis of coronary artery bypass graft(s) and coronary artery of transplanted heart with angina pectoris.

When using one of these combination codes it is not necessary to use an additional code for angina pectoris. A causal relationship can be assumed in a patient with both atherosclerosis and angina pectoris, unless the documentation indicates the angina is due to something other than the atherosclerosis.

If a patient with coronary artery disease is admitted due to an acute myocardial infarction (AMI), the AMI should be sequenced before the coronary artery disease.

See Section I.C.9. Acute myocardial infarction (AMI)

c. Intraoperative and Postprocedural Cerebrovascular Accident

Medical record documentation should clearly specify the cause-and-effect relationship between the medical intervention and the cerebrovascular accident in order to assign a code for intraoperative or postprocedural cerebrovascular accident.

Proper code assignment depends on whether it was an infarction or hemorrhage and whether it occurred intraoperatively or postoperatively. If it was a cerebral hemorrhage, code assignment depends on the type of procedure performed.

d. Sequelae of Cerebrovascular Disease

GUIDELINES (ICD-10-CM)

1) Category I69, Sequelae of Cerebrovascular disease

Category I69 is used to indicate conditions classifiable to categories I60-I67 as the causes of sequela (neurologic deficits), themselves classified elsewhere. These "late effects" include neurologic deficits that persist after initial onset of conditions classifiable to categories I60-I67. The neurologic deficits caused by cerebrovascular disease may be present from the onset or may arise at any time after the onset of the condition classifiable to categories I60-I67.

Codes from category I69, Sequelae of cerebrovascular disease, that specify hemiplegia, hemiparesis and monoplegia identify whether the dominant or nondominant side is affected. Should the affected side be documented, but not specified as dominant or nondominant, and the classification system does not indicate a default, code selection is as follows:

- For ambidextrous patients, the default should be dominant.
- If the left side is affected, the default is non-dominant.
- If the right side is affected, the default is dominant.

2) Codes from category I69 with codes from I60-I67

Codes from category I69 may be assigned on a health care record with codes from I60-I67, if the patient has a current cerebrovascular disease and deficits from an old cerebrovascular disease.

3) Codes from category I69 and Personal history of transient ischemic attack (TIA) and cerebral infarction (Z86.73)

Codes from category I69 should not be assigned if the patient does not have neurologic deficits.

See Section I.C.21. 4. History (of) for use of personal history codes

e. Acute myocardial infarction (AMI)

1) Type 1 ST elevation myocardial infarction (STEMI) and non ST elevation myocardial infarction (NSTEMI)

The ICD-10-CM codes for type 1 acute myocardial infarction (AMI) identify the site, such as anterolateral wall or true posterior wall. Subcategories I21.0-I21.2 and code I21.3 are used for type 1 ST elevation myocardial infarction (STEMI). Code I21.4, Non-ST elevation (NSTEMI) myocardial infarction, is used for type 1 non ST elevation myocardial infarction (NSTEMI) and nontransmural MIs.

If a type 1 NSTEMI evolves to STEMI, assign the STEMI code. If a type 1 STEMI converts to NSTEMI due to thrombolytic therapy, it is still coded as STEMI.

For encounters occurring while the myocardial infarction is equal to, or less than, 4 weeks old, including transfers to another acute setting or a postacute setting, and the myocardial infarction meets the definition for "other diagnoses" (see Section III, Reporting Additional Diagnoses), codes from category I21 may continue to be reported. For encounters after the 4 week time frame and the patient is still receiving care related to the myocardial infarction, the appropriate aftercare code should be assigned, rather than a code from category I21. For old or healed myocardial infarctions not requiring further care, code I25.2, Old myocardial infarction, may be assigned.

2) Acute myocardial infarction, unspecified

Code I21.9, Acute myocardial infarction, unspecified, is the default for unspecified acute myocardial infarction or unspecified type. If only type 1 STEMI or transmural MI without the site is documented, assign code I21.3, ST elevation (STEMI) myocardial infarction of unspecified site.

3) AMI documented as nontransmural or subendocardial but site provided

If an AMI is documented as nontransmural or subendocardial, but the site is provided, it is still coded as a subendocardial AMI.

See Section I.C.21.3 for information on coding status post administration of tPA in a different facility within the last 24 hours.

4) Subsequent acute myocardial infarction

A code from category I22, Subsequent ST elevation (STEMI) and non ST elevation (NSTEMI) myocardial infarction, is to be used when a patient who has suffered a type 1 or unspecified AMI has a new AMI within the 4 week time frame of the initial AMI. A code from category I22 must be used in conjunction with a code from category I21. The sequencing of the I22 and I21 codes depends on the circumstances of the encounter.

Do not assign code I22 for subsequent myocardial infarctions other than type 1 or unspecified. For subsequent type 2 AMI assign only code I21.A1. For subsequent type 4 or type 5 AMI, assign only code I21.A9.

If a subsequent myocardial infarction of one type occurs within 4 weeks of a myocardial infarction of a different type, assign the appropriate codes from category I21 to identify each type. Do not assign a code from I22. Codes from category I22 should only be assigned if both the initial and subsequent myocardial infarctions are type 1 or unspecified.

5) Other Types of Myocardial Infarction

The ICD-10-CM provides codes for different types of myocardial infarction. Type 1 myocardial infarctions are assigned to codes I21.0-I21.4.

Type 2 myocardial infarction (myocardial infarction due to demand ischemia or secondary to ischemic imbalance) is assigned to code I21.A1, Myocardial infarction type 2 with the underlying cause coded first. Do not assign code I24.8, Other forms of acute ischemic heart disease, for the demand ischemia. If a type 2 AMI is described as NSTEMI or STEMI, only assign code I21.A1. Codes I21.01-I21.4 should only be assigned for type 1 AMIs.

Acute myocardial infarctions type 3, 4a, 4b, 4c, and 5 are assigned to code I21.A9, Other myocardial infarction type.

The "Code also" and "Code first" notes should be followed related to complications, and for coding of postprocedural myocardial infarctions during or following cardiac surgery.

10. **Chapter 10: Diseases of the Respiratory System (J00-J99,** *U07.1***)**

   a. **Chronic Obstructive Pulmonary Disease [COPD] and Asthma**

      1) **Acute exacerbation of chronic obstructive bronchitis and asthma**

The codes in categories J44 and J45 distinguish between uncomplicated cases and those in acute exacerbation. An acute exacerbation is a worsening or a decompensation of a chronic condition. An acute exacerbation is not equivalent to an infection superimposed on a chronic condition, though an exacerbation may be triggered by an infection.

   b. **Acute Respiratory Failure**

      1) **Acute respiratory failure as principal diagnosis**

A code from subcategory J96.0, Acute respiratory failure, or subcategory J96.2, Acute and chronic respiratory failure, may be assigned as a principal diagnosis when it is the condition established after study to be chiefly responsible for occasioning the admission to the hospital, and the selection is supported by the Alphabetic Index and Tabular List. However, chapter-specific coding guidelines (such as obstetrics, poisoning, HIV, newborn) that provide sequencing direction take precedence.

      2) **Acute respiratory failure as secondary diagnosis**

Respiratory failure may be listed as a secondary diagnosis if it occurs after admission, or if it is present on admission, but does not meet the definition of principal diagnosis.

      3) **Sequencing of acute respiratory failure and another acute condition**

When a patient is admitted with respiratory failure and another acute condition (e.g., myocardial infarction, cerebrovascular accident, aspiration pneumonia), the principal diagnosis will not be the same in every situation. This applies whether the other acute condition is a respiratory or nonrespiratory condition. Selection of the principal diagnosis will be dependent on the circumstances of admission. If both the respiratory failure and the other acute condition are equally responsible for occasioning the admission to the hospital, and there are no chapter-specific sequencing rules, the guideline regarding two or more diagnoses that equally meet the definition for principal diagnosis *(Section II, C.)* may be applied in these situations.

If the documentation is not clear as to whether acute respiratory failure and another condition are equally responsible for occasioning the admission, query the provider for clarification.

   c. **Influenza due to certain identified influenza viruses**

Code only confirmed cases of influenza due to certain identified influenza viruses (category J09), and due to other identified influenza virus (category J10). This is an exception to the hospital inpatient guideline Section II, H. (Uncertain Diagnosis).

In this context, "confirmation" does not require documentation of positive laboratory testing specific for avian or other novel influenza A or other identified influenza virus. However, coding should be based on the provider's diagnostic statement that the patient has avian influenza, or other novel influenza A, for category J09, or has another particular identified strain of influenza, such as H1N1 or H3N2, but not identified as novel or variant, for category J10.

If the provider records "suspected" or "possible" or "probable" avian influenza, or novel influenza, or other identified influenza, then the appropriate influenza code from category J11, Influenza due to unidentified influenza virus, should be assigned. A code from category J09, Influenza due to certain identified influenza viruses, should not be assigned nor should a code from category J10, Influenza due to other identified influenza virus.

   d. **Ventilator associated Pneumonia**

      1) **Documentation of Ventilator associated Pneumonia**

As with all procedural or postprocedural complications, code assignment is based on the provider's documentation of the relationship between the condition and the procedure.

Code J95.851, Ventilator associated pneumonia, should be assigned only when the provider has documented ventilator associated pneumonia (VAP). An additional code to identify the organism (e.g., Pseudomonas aeruginosa, code B96.5) should also be assigned. Do not assign an additional code from categories J12-J18 to identify the type of pneumonia.

Code J95.851 should not be assigned for cases where the patient has pneumonia and is on a mechanical ventilator and the provider has not specifically stated that the pneumonia is ventilator-associated pneumonia. If the documentation is unclear as to whether the patient has a pneumonia that is a complication attributable to the mechanical ventilator, query the provider.

      2) **Ventilator associated Pneumonia Develops after Admission**

A patient may be admitted with one type of pneumonia (e.g., code J13, Pneumonia due to Streptococcus pneumonia) and subsequently develop VAP. In this instance, the principal diagnosis would be the appropriate code from categories J12-J18 for the pneumonia diagnosed at the time of admission. Code J95.851, Ventilator associated pneumonia, would be assigned as an additional diagnosis when the provider has also documented the presence of ventilator associated pneumonia.

e. Vaping-related disorders

For patients presenting with condition(s) related to vaping, assign code U07.0, Vaping-related disorder, as the principal diagnosis. For lung injury due to vaping, assign only code U07.0. Assign additional codes for other manifestations, such as acute respiratory failure (subcategory J96.0-) or pneumonitis (code J68.0).

Associated respiratory signs and symptoms due to vaping, such as cough, shortness of breath, etc., are not coded separately, when a definitive diagnosis has been established. However, it would be appropriate to code separately any gastrointestinal symptoms, such as diarrhea and abdominal pain.

11. **Chapter 11: Diseases of the Digestive System (K00-K95)**
Reserved for future guideline expansion

12. **Chapter 12: Diseases of the Skin and Subcutaneous Tissue (L00-L99)**

a. **Pressure ulcer stage codes**

1) **Pressure ulcer stages**
Codes in category L89, Pressure ulcer, identify the site and stage of the pressure ulcer.

The ICD-10-CM classifies pressure ulcer stages based on severity, which is designated by stages 1-4, deep tissue pressure injury, unspecified stage, and unstageable.

Assign as many codes from category L89 as needed to identify all the pressure ulcers the patient has, if applicable.

See Section I.B.14 for pressure ulcer stage documentation by clinicians other than patient's provider

2) **Unstageable pressure ulcers**
Assignment of the code for unstageable pressure ulcer (L89.--0) should be based on the clinical documentation. These codes are used for pressure ulcers whose stage cannot be clinically determined (e.g., the ulcer is covered by eschar or has been treated with a skin or muscle graft). This code should not be confused with the codes for unspecified stage (L89.--9). When there is no documentation regarding the stage of the pressure ulcer, assign the appropriate code for unspecified stage (L89.9).

If during an encounter, the stage of an unstageable pressure ulcer is revealed after debridement, assign only the code for the stage revealed following debridement.

3) **Documented pressure ulcer stage**
Assignment of the pressure ulcer stage code should be guided by clinical documentation of the stage or documentation of the terms found in the Alphabetic Index. For clinical terms describing the stage that are not found in the Alphabetic Index, and there is no documentation of the stage, the provider should be queried.

4) **Patients admitted with pressure ulcers documented as healed**
No code is assigned if the documentation states that the pressure ulcer is completely healed at the time of admission.

5) **Pressure ulcers documented as healing**
Pressure ulcers described as healing should be assigned the appropriate pressure ulcer stage code based on the documentation in the medical record. If the documentation does not provide information about the stage of the healing pressure ulcer, assign the appropriate code for unspecified stage.

If the documentation is unclear as to whether the patient has a current (new) pressure ulcer or if the patient is being treated for a healing pressure ulcer, query the provider.

For ulcers that were present on admission but healed at the time of discharge, assign the code for the site and stage of the pressure ulcer at the time of admission.

6) **Patient admitted with pressure ulcer evolving into another stage during the admission**
If a patient is admitted to an inpatient hospital with a pressure ulcer at one stage and it progresses to a higher stage, two separate codes should be assigned: one code for the site and stage of the ulcer on admission and a second code for the same ulcer site and the highest stage reported during the stay.

7) **Pressure-induced deep tissue damage**
For pressure-induced deep tissue damage or deep tissue pressure injury, assign only the appropriate code for pressure-induced deep tissue damage (L89.--6).

b. **Non-Pressure Chronic Ulcers**

1) **Patients admitted with non-pressure ulcers documented as healed**
No code is assigned if the documentation states that the non-pressure ulcer is completely healed at the time of admission.

2) **Non-pressure ulcers documented as healing**
Non-pressure ulcers described as healing should be assigned the appropriate non-pressure ulcer code based on the documentation in the medical record. If the documentation does not provide information about the severity of the healing non-pressure ulcer, assign the appropriate code for unspecified severity.

If the documentation is unclear as to whether the patient has a current (new) non-pressure ulcer or if the patient is being treated for a healing non-pressure ulcer, query the provider.

For ulcers that were present on admission but healed at the time of discharge, assign the code for the site and severity of the non-pressure ulcer at the time of admission.

3) **Patient admitted with non-pressure ulcer that progresses to another severity level during the admission**

If a patient is admitted to an inpatient hospital with a non-pressure ulcer at one severity level and it progresses to a higher severity level, two separate codes should be assigned: one code for the site and severity level of the ulcer on admission and a second code for the same ulcer site and the highest severity level reported during the stay.

See Section I.B.14 for pressure ulcer stage documentation by clinicians other than patient's provider

13. **Chapter 13: Diseases of the Musculoskeletal System and Connective Tissue (M00-M99)**

    a. Site and laterality

    Most of the codes within Chapter 13 have site and laterality designations. The site represents the bone, joint or the muscle involved. For some conditions where more than one bone, joint or muscle is usually involved, such as osteoarthritis, there is a "multiple sites" code available. For categories where no multiple site code is provided and more than one bone, joint or muscle is involved, multiple codes should be used to indicate the different sites involved.

    1) Bone versus joint

    For certain conditions, the bone may be affected at the upper or lower end (e.g., avascular necrosis of bone, M87, Osteoporosis, M80, M81). Though the portion of the bone affected may be at the joint, the site designation will be the bone, not the joint.

    b. Acute traumatic versus chronic or recurrent musculoskeletal conditions

    Many musculoskeletal conditions are a result of previous injury or trauma to a site, or are recurrent conditions. Bone, joint or muscle conditions that are the result of a healed injury are usually found in Chapter 13. Recurrent bone, joint or muscle conditions are also usually found in Chapter 13. Any current, acute injury should be coded to the appropriate injury code from Chapter 19. Chronic or recurrent conditions should generally be coded with a code from Chapter 13. If it is difficult to determine from the documentation in the record which code is best to describe a condition, query the provider.

    c. Coding of Pathologic Fractures

    Seventh character A is for use as long as the patient is receiving active treatment for the fracture. While the patient may be seen by a new or different provider over the course of treatment for a pathological fracture, assignment of the 7th character is based on whether the patient is undergoing active treatment and not whether the provider is seeing the patient for the first time.

    Seventh character, D is to be used for encounters after the patient has completed active treatment for the fracture and is receiving routine care for the fracture during the healing or recovery phase. The other 7th characters, listed under each subcategory in the Tabular List, are to be used for subsequent encounters for treatment of problems associated with the healing, such as malunions, nonunions, and sequelae.

    Care for complications of surgical treatment for fracture repairs during the healing or recovery phase should be coded with the appropriate complication codes.

    See Section I.C.19. Coding of traumatic fractures

    d. Osteoporosis

    Osteoporosis is a systemic condition, meaning that all bones of the musculoskeletal system are affected. Therefore, site is not a component of the codes under category M81, Osteoporosis without current pathological fracture. The site codes under category M80, Osteoporosis with current pathological fracture, identify the site of the fracture, not the osteoporosis.

    1) Osteoporosis without pathological fracture

    Category M81, Osteoporosis without current pathological fracture, is for use for patients with osteoporosis who do not currently have a pathologic fracture due to the osteoporosis, even if they have had a fracture in the past. For patients with a history of osteoporosis fractures, status code Z87.310, Personal history of (healed) osteoporosis fracture, should follow the code from M81.

    2) Osteoporosis with current pathological fracture

    Category M80, Osteoporosis with current pathological fracture, is for patients who have a current pathologic fracture at the time of an encounter. The codes under M80 identify the site of the fracture. A code from category M80, not a traumatic fracture code, should be used for any patient with known osteoporosis who suffers a fracture, even if the patient had a minor fall or trauma, if that fall or trauma would not usually break a normal, healthy bone.

    e. Multisystem Inflammatory Syndrome

    See Section I.C.1.g.1.l for Multisystem Inflammatory Syndrome

14. **Chapter 14: Diseases of Genitourinary System (N00-N99)**

    a. Chronic kidney disease

    1) Stages of chronic kidney disease (CKD)

    The ICD-10-CM classifies CKD based on severity. The severity of CKD is designated by stages 1-5. Stage 2, code N18.2, equates to mild CKD; stage 3, codes N18.30-N18.32, equate to moderate CKD; and stage 4, code N18.4, equates to severe CKD. Code N18.6, End stage renal disease (ESRD), is assigned when the provider has documented end-stage-renal disease (ESRD).

    If both a stage of CKD and ESRD are documented, assign code N18.6 only.

    2) Chronic kidney disease and kidney transplant status

    Patients who have undergone kidney transplant may still have some form of chronic kidney disease (CKD) because the kidney transplant may not fully restore kidney function. Therefore, the presence of CKD alone does not constitute a transplant complication. Assign the appropriate N18 code for the patient's stage of CKD and code Z94.0, Kidney transplant status. If a transplant complication such as failure or rejection or other transplant complication is documented, see Section I.C.19.g for information on coding complications of a kidney transplant. If the documentation is unclear as to whether the patient has a complication of the transplant, query the provider.

3) Chronic kidney disease with other conditions

Patients with CKD may also suffer from other serious conditions, most commonly diabetes mellitus and hypertension. The sequencing of the CKD code in relationship to codes for other contributing conditions is based on the conventions in the Tabular List.

See I.C.9. Hypertensive chronic kidney disease.
See I.C.19. Chronic kidney disease and kidney transplant complications.

15. Chapter 15: Pregnancy, Childbirth, and the Puerperium (O00-O9A)

a. General Rules for Obstetric Cases

1) Codes from Chapter 15 and sequencing priority

Obstetric cases require codes from Chapter 15, codes in the range O00-O9A, Pregnancy, Childbirth, and the Puerperium. Chapter 15 codes have sequencing priority over codes from other chapters. Additional codes from other chapters may be used in conjunction with Chapter 15 codes to further specify conditions. Should the provider document that the pregnancy is incidental to the encounter, then code Z33.1, Pregnant state, incidental, should be used in place of any Chapter 15 codes. It is the provider's responsibility to state that the condition being treated is not affecting the pregnancy.

2) Chapter 15 codes used only on the maternal record

Chapter 15 codes are to be used only on the maternal record, never on the record of the newborn.

3) Final character for trimester

The majority of codes in Chapter 15 have a final character indicating the trimester of pregnancy. The time frames for the trimesters are indicated at the beginning of the chapter. If trimester is not a component of a code it is because the condition always occurs in a specific trimester, or the concept of trimester of pregnancy is not applicable. Certain codes have characters for only certain trimesters because the condition does not occur in all trimesters, but it may occur in more than just one.

Assignment of the final character for trimester should be based on the provider's documentation of the trimester (or number of weeks) for the current admission/encounter. This applies to the assignment of trimester for pre-existing conditions as well as those that develop during or are due to the pregnancy. The provider's documentation of the number of weeks may be used to assign the appropriate code identifying the trimester.

Whenever delivery occurs during the current admission, and there is an "in childbirth" option for the obstetric complication being coded, the "in childbirth" code should be assigned.

When the classification does not provide an obstetric code with an "in childbirth" option, it is appropriate to assign a code describing the current trimester.

4) Selection of trimester for inpatient admissions that encompass more than one trimester

In instances when a patient is admitted to a hospital for complications of pregnancy during one trimester and remains in the hospital into a subsequent trimester, the trimester character for the antepartum complication code should be assigned on the basis of the trimester when the complication developed, not the trimester of the discharge. If the condition developed prior to the current admission/encounter or represents a pre-existing condition, the trimester character for the trimester at the time of the admission/encounter should be assigned.

5) Unspecified trimester

Each category that includes codes for trimester has a code for "unspecified trimester." The "unspecified trimester" code should rarely be used, such as when the documentation in the record is insufficient to determine the trimester and it is not possible to obtain clarification.

6) 7th character for Fetus Identification

Where applicable, a 7th character is to be assigned for certain categories (O31, O32, O33.3 - O33.6, O35, O36, O40, O41, O60.1, O60.2, O64, and O69) to identify the fetus for which the complication code applies.

Assign 7th character "0":
- For single gestations
- When the documentation in the record is insufficient to determine the fetus affected and it is not possible to obtain clarification.
- When it is not possible to clinically determine which fetus is affected.

b. Selection of OB Principal or First-listed Diagnosis

1) Routine outpatient prenatal visits

For routine outpatient prenatal visits when no complications are present, a code from category Z34, Encounter for supervision of normal pregnancy, should be used as the first-listed diagnosis. These codes should not be used in conjunction with Chapter 15 codes.

2) Supervision of High-Risk Pregnancy

Codes from category O09, Supervision of high-risk pregnancy, are intended for use only during the prenatal period. For complications during the labor or delivery episode as a result of a high-risk pregnancy, assign the applicable complication codes from Chapter 15. If there are no complications during the labor or delivery episode, assign code O80, Encounter for full-term uncomplicated delivery.

For routine prenatal outpatient visits for patients with high-risk pregnancies, a code from category O09, Supervision of high-risk pregnancy, should be used as the first-listed diagnosis. Secondary Chapter 15 codes may be used in conjunction with these codes if appropriate.

3) Episodes when no delivery occurs
In episodes when no delivery occurs, the principal diagnosis should correspond to the principal complication of the pregnancy which necessitated the encounter. Should more than one complication exist, all of which are treated or monitored, any of the complication codes may be sequenced first.

4) When a delivery occurs
When an obstetric patient is admitted and delivers during that admission, the condition that prompted the admission should be sequenced as the principal diagnosis. If multiple conditions prompted the admission, sequence the one most related to the delivery as the principal diagnosis. A code for any complication of the delivery should be assigned as an additional diagnosis. In cases of cesarean delivery, if the patient was admitted with a condition that resulted in the performance of a cesarean procedure, that condition should be selected as the principal diagnosis. If the reason for the admission was unrelated to the condition resulting in the cesarean delivery, the condition related to the reason for the admission should be selected as the principal diagnosis.

5) Outcome of delivery
A code from category Z37, Outcome of delivery, should be included on every maternal record when a delivery has occurred. These codes are not to be used on subsequent records or on the newborn record.

c. Pre-existing conditions versus conditions due to the pregnancy
Certain categories in Chapter 15 distinguish between conditions of the mother that existed prior to pregnancy (pre-existing) and those that are a direct result of pregnancy. When assigning codes from Chapter 15, it is important to assess if a condition was pre-existing prior to pregnancy or developed during or due to the pregnancy in order to assign the correct code.

Categories that do not distinguish between pre-existing and pregnancy-related conditions may be used for either. It is acceptable to use codes specifically for the puerperium with codes complicating pregnancy and childbirth if a condition arises postpartum during the delivery encounter.

d. Pre-existing hypertension in pregnancy

Category O10, Pre-existing hypertension complicating pregnancy, childbirth and the puerperium, includes codes for hypertensive heart and hypertensive chronic kidney disease. When assigning one of the O10 codes that includes hypertensive heart disease or hypertensive chronic kidney disease, it is necessary to add a secondary code from the appropriate hypertension category to specify the type of heart failure or chronic kidney disease.

See Section I.C.9. Hypertension.

e. Fetal Conditions Affecting the Management of the Mother

1) Codes from categories O35 and O36
Codes from categories O35, Maternal care for known or suspected fetal abnormality and damage, and O36, Maternal care for other fetal problems, are assigned only when the fetal condition is actually responsible for modifying the management of the mother, i.e., by requiring diagnostic studies, additional observation, special care, or termination of pregnancy. The fact that the fetal condition exists does not justify assigning a code from this series to the mother's record.

2) In utero surgery
In cases when surgery is performed on the fetus, a diagnosis code from category O35, Maternal care for known or suspected fetal abnormality and damage, should be assigned identifying the fetal condition. Assign the appropriate procedure code for the procedure performed.

No code from Chapter 16, the perinatal codes, should be used on the mother's record to identify fetal conditions. Surgery performed in utero on a fetus is still to be coded as an obstetric encounter.

f. HIV Infection in Pregnancy, Childbirth and the Puerperium
During pregnancy, childbirth or the puerperium, a patient admitted because of an HIV-related illness should receive a principal diagnosis from subcategory O98.7-, Human immunodeficiency [HIV] disease complicating pregnancy, childbirth and the puerperium, followed by the code(s) for the HIV-related illness(es).

Patients with asymptomatic HIV infection status admitted during pregnancy, childbirth, or the puerperium should receive codes of O98.7- and Z21, Asymptomatic human immunodeficiency virus [HIV] infection status.

g. Diabetes mellitus in pregnancy
Diabetes mellitus is a significant complicating factor in pregnancy. Pregnant women who are diabetic should be assigned a code from category O24, Diabetes mellitus in pregnancy, childbirth, and the puerperium, first, followed by the appropriate diabetes code(s) (E08-E13) from Chapter 4.

h. Long-term use of insulin and oral hypoglycemics

See Section I.C.4.a.3 for information on the long term use of insulin and oral hypoglycemics.

i. Gestational (pregnancy induced) diabetes

Gestational (pregnancy induced) diabetes can occur during the second and third trimester of pregnancy in **patients** who were not diabetic prior to pregnancy. Gestational diabetes can cause complications in the pregnancy similar to those of pre-existing diabetes mellitus. It also puts the **patient** at greater risk of developing diabetes after the pregnancy. Codes for gestational diabetes are in subcategory O24.4, Gestational diabetes mellitus. No other code from category O24, Diabetes mellitus in pregnancy, childbirth, and the puerperium, should be used with a code from O24.4.

The codes under subcategory O24.4 include diet controlled, insulin controlled, and controlled by oral hypoglycemic drugs. If a patient with gestational diabetes is treated with both diet and insulin, only the code for insulin-controlled is required. If a patient with gestational diabetes is treated with both diet and oral hypoglycemic medications, only the code for "controlled by oral hypoglycemic drugs" is required. Code Z79.4, Long-term (current) use of insulin or code Z79.84, Long-term (current) use of oral hypoglycemic drugs, should not be assigned with codes from subcategory O24.4.

An abnormal glucose tolerance in pregnancy is assigned a code from subcategory O99.81, Abnormal glucose complicating pregnancy, childbirth, and the puerperium.

j. Sepsis and septic shock complicating abortion, pregnancy, childbirth and the puerperium

When assigning a Chapter 15 code for sepsis complicating abortion, pregnancy, childbirth, and the puerperium, a code for the specific type of infection should be assigned as an additional diagnosis. If severe sepsis is present, a code from subcategory R65.2, Severe sepsis, and code(s) for associated organ dysfunction(s) should also be assigned as additional diagnoses.

k. Puerperal sepsis

Code O85, Puerperal sepsis, should be assigned with a secondary code to identify the causal organism (e.g., for a bacterial infection, assign a code from category B95-B96, Bacterial infections in conditions classified elsewhere). A code from category A40, Streptococcal sepsis, or A41, Other sepsis, should not be used for puerperal sepsis. If applicable, use additional codes to identify severe sepsis (R65.2-) and any associated acute organ dysfunction.

Code O85 should not be assigned for sepsis following an obstetrical procedure (See Section I.C.1.d.5.b., Sepsis due to a postprocedural infection).

l. Alcohol, tobacco and drug use during pregnancy, childbirth and the puerperium

1) Alcohol use during pregnancy, childbirth and the puerperium

Codes under subcategory O99.31, Alcohol use complicating pregnancy, childbirth, and the puerperium, should be assigned for any pregnancy case when a mother uses alcohol during the pregnancy or postpartum. A secondary code from category F10, Alcohol related disorders, should also be assigned to identify manifestations of the alcohol use.

2) Tobacco use during pregnancy, childbirth and the puerperium

Codes under subcategory O99.33, Smoking (tobacco) complicating pregnancy, childbirth, and the puerperium, should be assigned for any pregnancy case when a mother uses any type of tobacco product during the pregnancy or postpartum. A secondary code from category F17, Nicotine dependence, should also be assigned to identify the type of nicotine dependence.

3) Drug use during pregnancy, childbirth and the puerperium

Codes under subcategory O99.32, Drug use complicating pregnancy, childbirth, and the puerperium, should be assigned for any pregnancy case when a mother uses drugs during the pregnancy or postpartum. This can involve illegal drugs, or inappropriate use or abuse of prescription drugs. Secondary code(s) from categories F11-F16 and F18-F19 should also be assigned to identify manifestations of the drug use.

m. Poisoning, toxic effects, adverse effects and underdosing in a pregnant patient

A code from subcategory O9A.2, Injury, poisoning and certain other consequences of external causes complicating pregnancy, childbirth, and the puerperium, should be sequenced first, followed by the appropriate injury, poisoning, toxic effect, adverse effect or underdosing code, and then the additional code(s) that specifies the condition caused by the poisoning, toxic effect, adverse effect or underdosing.

See Section I.C.19. Adverse effects, poisoning, underdosing and toxic effects.

n. Normal Delivery, Code O80

1) Encounter for full term uncomplicated delivery

Code O80 should be assigned when a woman is admitted for a full-term normal delivery and delivers a single, healthy infant without any complications antepartum, during the delivery, or postpartum during the delivery episode. Code O80 is always a principal diagnosis. It is not to be used if any other code from Chapter 15 is needed to describe a current complication of the antenatal, delivery, or postnatal period. Additional codes from other chapters may be used with code O80 if they are not related to or are in any way complicating the pregnancy.

2) Uncomplicated delivery with resolved antepartum complication

Code O80 may be used if the patient had a complication at some point during the pregnancy, but the complication is not present at the time of the admission for delivery.

3) Outcome of delivery for O80

Z37.0, Single live birth, is the only outcome of delivery code appropriate for use with O80.

o. The Peripartum and Postpartum Periods

1) Peripartum and Postpartum periods

The postpartum period begins immediately after delivery and continues for 6 weeks following delivery. The peripartum period is defined as the last month of pregnancy to 5 months postpartum.

2) Peripartum and postpartum complication

A postpartum complication is any complication occurring within the 6-week period.

3) Pregnancy-related complications after 6-week period

Chapter 15 codes may also be used to describe pregnancy-related complications after the peripartum or postpartum period if the provider documents that a condition is pregnancy related.

4) Admission for routine postpartum care following delivery outside hospital

When the mother delivers outside the hospital prior to admission and is admitted for routine postpartum care and no complications are noted, code Z39.0, Encounter for care and examination of mother immediately after delivery, should be assigned as the principal diagnosis.

5) Pregnancy associated cardiomyopathy

Pregnancy associated cardiomyopathy, code O90.3, is unique in that it may be diagnosed in the third trimester of pregnancy but may continue to progress months after delivery. For this reason, it is referred to as peripartum cardiomyopathy. Code O90.3 is only for use when the cardiomyopathy develops as a result of pregnancy in a woman who did not have pre-existing heart disease.

p. Code O94, Sequelae of complication of pregnancy, childbirth, and the puerperium

1) Code O94

Code O94, Sequelae of complication of pregnancy, childbirth, and the puerperium, is for use in those cases when an initial complication of a pregnancy develops a **sequela or** sequelae requiring care or treatment at a future date.

2) After the initial postpartum period

This code may be used at any time after the initial postpartum period.

3) Sequencing of Code O94

This code, like all sequela codes, is to be sequenced following the code describing the sequelae of the complication.

q. Termination of Pregnancy and Spontaneous abortions

1) Abortion with Liveborn Fetus

When an attempted termination of pregnancy results in a liveborn fetus assign code Z33.2, Encounter for elective termination of pregnancy and a code from category Z37, Outcome of Delivery.

2) Retained Products of Conception following an abortion

Subsequent encounters for retained products of conception following a spontaneous abortion or elective termination of pregnancy, without complications are assigned O03.4, Incomplete spontaneous, abortion without complication or codes O07.4, Failed attempted termination of pregnancy without complication. This advice is appropriate even when the patient was discharged previously with a discharge diagnosis of complete abortion. If the patient has a specific complication associated with the spontaneous abortion or elective termination of pregnancy in addition to retained products of conception, assign the appropriate complication code (e.g., O03.-, O04.-, O07.-) instead of code O03.4 or O07.4

3) Complications leading to abortion

Codes from Chapter 15 may be used as additional codes to identify any documented complications of the pregnancy in conjunction with codes in categories in O04, O07 and O08.

r. Abuse in a pregnant patient

For suspected or confirmed cases of abuse of a pregnant patient, a code(s) from subcategories O9A.3, Physical abuse complicating pregnancy, childbirth, and the puerperium, O9A.4, Sexual abuse complicating pregnancy, childbirth, and the puerperium, and O9A.5, Psychological abuse complicating pregnancy, childbirth, and the puerperium, should be sequenced first, followed by the appropriate codes (if applicable) to identify any associated current injury due to physical abuse, sexual abuse, and the perpetrator of abuse.

See Section I.C.19. Adult and child abuse, neglect and other maltreatment.

s. COVID-19 infection in pregnancy, childbirth, and the puerperium

During pregnancy, childbirth or the puerperium, when COVID-19 is the reason for admission/ encounter, code O98.5-, Other viral diseases complicating pregnancy, childbirth and the puerperium, should be sequenced as the principal/ first-listed diagnosis, and code U07.1, COVID-19, and the appropriate codes for associated manifestation(s) should be assigned as additional diagnoses. Codes from Chapter 15 always take sequencing priority.

If the reason for admission/encounter is unrelated to COVID-19 but the patient tests positive for COVID-19 during the admission/ encounter, the appropriate code for the reason for admission/encounter should be sequenced as the principal/first-listed diagnosis, and codes O98.5- and U07.1, as well as the appropriate codes for associated COVID-19 manifestations, should be assigned as additional diagnoses.

16. Chapter 16: Certain Conditions Originating in the Perinatal Period (P00-P96)

For coding and reporting purposes the perinatal period is defined as before birth through the 28th day following birth. The following guidelines are provided for reporting purposes

a. General Perinatal Rules

1) Use of Chapter 16 Codes

Codes in this chapter are never for use on the maternal record. Codes from Chapter 15, the obstetric chapter, are never permitted on the newborn record. Chapter 16 codes may be used throughout the life of the patient if the condition is still present.

2) Principal Diagnosis for Birth Record

When coding the birth episode in a newborn record, assign a code from category Z38, Liveborn infants according to place of birth and type of delivery, as the principal diagnosis. A code from category Z38 is assigned only once, to a newborn at the time of birth. If a newborn is transferred to another institution, a code from category Z38 should not be used at the receiving hospital.

A code from category Z38 is used only on the newborn record, not on the mother's record.

3) Use of Codes from other Chapters with Codes from Chapter 16

Codes from other chapters may be used with codes from Chapter 16 if the codes from the other chapters provide more specific detail. Codes for signs and symptoms may be assigned when a definitive diagnosis has not been established. If the reason for the encounter is a perinatal condition, the code from Chapter 16 should be sequenced first.

4) Use of Chapter 16 Codes after the Perinatal Period

Should a condition originate in the perinatal period, and continue throughout the life of the patient, the perinatal code should continue to be used regardless of the patient's age.

5) Birth process or community acquired conditions

If a newborn has a condition that may be either due to the birth process or community acquired and the documentation does not indicate which it is, the default is due to the birth process and the code from Chapter 16 should be used. If the condition is community-acquired, a code from Chapter 16 should not be assigned.

For COVID-19 infection in a newborn, see guideline I.C.16.h.

6) Code all clinically significant conditions

All clinically significant conditions noted on routine newborn examination should be coded. A condition is clinically significant if it requires:
- clinical evaluation; or
- therapeutic treatment; or
- diagnostic procedures; or
- extended length of hospital stay; or
- increased nursing care and/or monitoring; or
- has implications for future health care needs

Note: The perinatal guidelines listed above are the same as the general coding guidelines for "additional diagnoses", except for the final point regarding implications for future health care needs. Codes should be assigned for conditions that have been specified by the provider as having implications for future health care needs.

b. Observation and Evaluation of Newborns for Suspected Conditions not Found

1) Use of Z05 codes

Assign a code from category Z05, Observation and evaluation of newborns and infants for suspected conditions ruled out, to identify those instances when a healthy newborn is evaluated for a suspected condition that is determined after study not to be present. Do not use a code from category Z05 when the patient has identified signs or symptoms of a suspected problem; in such cases code the sign or symptom.

2) Z05 on other than the birth record

A code from category Z05 may also be assigned as a principal or first-listed code for readmissions or encounters when the code from category Z38 code no longer applies. Codes from category Z05 are for use only for healthy newborns and infants for which no condition after study is found to be present.

3) Z05 on a birth record

A code from category Z05 is to be used as a secondary code after the code from category Z38, Liveborn infants according to place of birth and type of delivery.

c. Coding Additional Perinatal Diagnoses

1) Assigning codes for conditions that require treatment

Assign codes for conditions that require treatment or further investigation, prolong the length of stay, or require resource utilization.

2) Codes for conditions specified as having implications for future health care needs

Assign codes for conditions that have been specified by the provider as having implications for future health care needs.

Note: This guideline should not be used for adult patients.

d. Prematurity and Fetal Growth Retardation

Providers utilize different criteria in determining prematurity. A code for prematurity should not be assigned unless it is documented. Assignment of codes in categories P05, Disorders of newborn related to slow fetal growth and fetal malnutrition, and P07, Disorders of newborn related to short gestation and low birth weight, not elsewhere classified, should be based on the recorded birth weight and estimated gestational age.

When both birth weight and gestational age are available, two codes from category P07 should be assigned, with the code for birth weight sequenced before the code for gestational age.

e. Low birth weight and immaturity status

Codes from category P07, Disorders of newborn related to short gestation and low birth weight, not elsewhere classified, are for use for a child or adult who was premature or had a low birth weight as a newborn and this is affecting the patient's current health status.

See Section I.C.21. Factors influencing health status and contact with health services, Status.

f. Bacterial Sepsis of Newborn
Category P36, Bacterial sepsis of newborn, includes congenital sepsis. If a perinate is documented as having sepsis without documentation of congenital or community acquired, the default is congenital and a code from category P36 should be assigned. If the P36 code includes the causal organism, an additional code from category B95, Streptococcus, Staphylococcus, and Enterococcus as the cause of diseases classified elsewhere, or B96, Other bacterial agents as the cause of diseases classified elsewhere, should not be assigned. If the P36 code does not include the causal organism, assign an additional code from category B96. If applicable, use additional codes to identify severe sepsis (R65.2-) and any associated acute organ dysfunction.

g. Stillbirth
Code P95, Stillbirth, is only for use in institutions that maintain separate records for stillbirths. No other code should be used with P95. Code P95 should not be used on the mother's record.

h. COVID-19 Infection in Newborn
For a newborn that tests positive for COVID-19, assign code U07.1, COVID-19, and the appropriate codes for associated manifestation(s) in neonates/newborns in the absence of documentation indicating a specific type of transmission. For a newborn that tests positive for COVID-19 and the provider documents the condition was contracted in utero or during the birth process, assign codes P35.8, Other congenital viral diseases, and U07.1, COVID-19. When coding the birth episode in a newborn record, the appropriate code from category Z38, Liveborn infants according to place of birth and type of delivery, should be assigned as the principal diagnosis.

17. **Chapter 17: Congenital Malformations, Deformations, and Chromosomal Abnormalities (Q00-Q99)**
Assign an appropriate code(s) from categories Q00-Q99, Congenital malformations, deformations, and chromosomal abnormalities when a malformation/deformation or chromosomal abnormality is documented. A malformation/deformation/or chromosomal abnormality may be the principal/first-listed diagnosis on a record or a secondary diagnosis.

When a malformation/deformation/or chromosomal abnormality does not have a unique code assignment, assign additional code(s) for any manifestations that may be present.

When the code assignment specifically identifies the malformation/deformation/or chromosomal abnormality, manifestations that are an inherent component of the anomaly should not be coded separately. Additional codes should be assigned for manifestations that are not an inherent component.

Codes from Chapter 17 may be used throughout the life of the patient. If a congenital malformation or deformity has been corrected, a personal history code should be used to identify the history of the malformation or deformity. Although present at birth, a malformation/deformation/or chromosomal abnormality may not be identified until later in life. Whenever the condition is diagnosed by the provider, it is appropriate to assign a code from codes Q00-Q99.

For the birth admission, the appropriate code from category Z38, Liveborn infants, according to place of birth and type of delivery, should be sequenced as the principal diagnosis, followed by any congenital anomaly codes, Q00-Q99.

18. **Chapter 18: Symptoms, Signs, and Abnormal Clinical and Laboratory Findings, Not Elsewhere Classified (R00-R99)**
Chapter 18 includes symptoms, signs, abnormal results of clinical or other investigative procedures, and ill-defined conditions regarding which no diagnosis classifiable elsewhere is recorded. Signs and symptoms that point to a specific diagnosis have been assigned to a category in other chapters of the classification.

a. Use of symptom codes
Codes that describe symptoms and signs are acceptable for reporting purposes when a related definitive diagnosis has not been established (confirmed) by the provider.

b. Use of a symptom code with a definitive diagnosis code
Codes for signs and symptoms may be reported in addition to a related definitive diagnosis when the sign or symptom is not routinely associated with that diagnosis, such as the various signs and symptoms associated with complex syndromes. The definitive diagnosis code should be sequenced before the symptom code.

Signs or symptoms that are associated routinely with a disease process should not be assigned as additional codes, unless otherwise instructed by the classification.

c. Combination codes that include symptoms
ICD-10-CM contains a number of combination codes that identify both the definitive diagnosis and common symptoms of that diagnosis. When using one of these combination codes, an additional code should not be assigned for the symptom.

d. Repeated falls
Code R29.6, Repeated falls, is for use for encounters when a patient has recently fallen and the reason for the fall is being investigated.

Code Z91.81, History of falling, is for use when a patient has fallen in the past and is at risk for future falls. When appropriate, both codes R29.6 and Z91.81 may be assigned together.

e. Coma

Code R40.20, Unspecified coma, may be assigned in conjunction with codes for any medical condition.

Do not report codes for **unspecified coma**, individual or total Glasgow coma scale scores for a patient with a medically induced coma or a sedated patient.

The coma scale codes (R40.21- to R40.24-) can be used in conjunction with traumatic brain injury codes. These codes are primarily for use by trauma registries, but they may be used in any setting where this information is collected. The coma scale codes should be sequenced after the diagnosis code(s).

These codes, one from each subcategory, are needed to complete the scale. The 7th character indicates when the scale was recorded. The 7th character should match for all three codes.

At a minimum, report the initial score documented on presentation at your facility. This may be a score from the emergency medicine technician (EMT) or in the emergency department. If desired, a facility may choose to capture multiple coma scale scores.

Assign code R40.24, Glasgow coma scale, total score, when only the total score is documented in the medical record and not the individual score(s).

If multiple coma scores are captured within the first 24 hours after hospital admission, assign only the code for the score at the time of admission. ICD-10-CM does not classify coma scores that are reported after admission but less than 24 hours later.

See Section I.B.14 for coma scale documentation by clinicians other than patient's provider

f. Functional quadriplegia
GUIDELINE HAS BEEN DELETED EFFECTIVE OCTOBER 1, 2017

g. SIRS due to Non-Infectious Process
The systemic inflammatory response syndrome (SIRS) can develop as a result of certain non-infectious disease processes, such as trauma, malignant neoplasm, or pancreatitis. When SIRS is documented with a noninfectious condition, and no subsequent infection is documented, the code for the underlying condition, such as an injury, should be assigned, followed by code R65.10, Systemic inflammatory response syndrome (SIRS) of non-infectious origin without acute organ dysfunction, or code R65.11, Systemic inflammatory response syndrome (SIRS) of non-infectious origin with acute organ dysfunction. If an associated acute organ dysfunction is documented, the appropriate code(s) for the specific type of organ dysfunction(s) should be assigned in addition to code R65.11. If acute organ dysfunction is documented, but it cannot be determined if the acute organ dysfunction is associated with SIRS or due to another condition (e.g., directly due to the trauma), the provider should be queried.

h. Death NOS

Code R99, Ill-defined and unknown cause of mortality, is only for use in the very limited circumstance when a patient who has already died is brought into an emergency department or other healthcare facility and is pronounced dead upon arrival. It does not represent the discharge disposition of death.

i. NIHSS Stroke Scale
The NIH stroke scale (NIHSS) codes (R29.7- -) can be used in conjunction with acute stroke codes (I63) to identify the patient's neurological status and the severity of the stroke. The stroke scale codes should be sequenced after the acute stroke diagnosis code(s).

At a minimum, report the initial score documented. If desired, a facility may choose to capture multiple stroke scale scores.

See Section I.B.14 for NIHSS stroke scale documentation by clinicians other than patient's provider

19. **Chapter 19: Injury, Poisoning, and Certain Other Consequences of External Causes (S00-T88)**

    a. Application of 7th Characters in Chapter 19
    Most categories in Chapter 19 have a 7th character requirement for each applicable code. Most categories in this chapter have three 7th character values (with the exception of fractures): A, initial encounter, D, subsequent encounter and S, sequela. Categories for traumatic fractures have additional 7th character values. While the patient may be seen by a new or different provider over the course of treatment for an injury, assignment of the 7th character is based on whether the patient is undergoing active treatment and not whether the provider is seeing the patient for the first time.

    For complication codes, active treatment refers to treatment for the condition described by the code, even though it may be related to an earlier precipitating problem. For example, code T84.50XA, Infection and inflammatory reaction due to unspecified internal joint prosthesis, initial encounter, is used when active treatment is provided for the infection, even though the condition relates to the prosthetic device, implant or graft that was placed at a previous encounter.

    7th character "A", initial encounter is used for each encounter where the patient is receiving active treatment for the condition.

    7th character "D" subsequent encounter is used for encounters after the patient has completed active treatment of the condition and is receiving routine care for the condition during the healing or recovery phase.

    The aftercare Z codes should not be used for aftercare for conditions such as injuries or poisonings, where 7th characters are provided to identify subsequent care. For example, for aftercare of an injury, assign the acute injury code with the 7th character "D" (subsequent encounter).

    7th character "S", sequela, is for use for complications or conditions that arise as a direct result of a condition, such as scar formation after a burn. The scars are sequelae of the burn. When using 7th character "S", it is necessary to use both the injury code that precipitated the sequela and the code for the sequela itself. The "S" is added only to the injury code, not the sequela code. The 7th character "S" identifies the injury responsible for the sequela. The specific type of sequela (e.g., scar) is sequenced first, followed by the injury code.

See Section I.B.10. Sequelae, (Late Effects)

b. Coding of Injuries

When coding injuries, assign separate codes for each injury unless a combination code is provided, in which case the combination code is assigned. Codes from category T07, Unspecified multiple injuries should not be assigned in the inpatient setting unless information for a more specific code is not available. Traumatic injury codes (S00-T14.9) are not to be used for normal, healing surgical wounds or to identify complications of surgical wounds.

The code for the most serious injury, as determined by the provider and the focus of treatment, is sequenced first.

1) Superficial injuries

Superficial injuries such as abrasions or contusions are not coded when associated with more severe injuries of the same site.

2) Primary injury with damage to nerves/ blood vessels

When a primary injury results in minor damage to peripheral nerves or blood vessels, the primary injury is sequenced first with additional code(s) for injuries to nerves and spinal cord (such as category S04), and/or injury to blood vessels (such as category S15). When the primary injury is to the blood vessels or nerves, that injury should be sequenced first.

3) Iatrogenic injuries

Injury codes from Chapter 19 should not be assigned for injuries that occur during, or as a result of, a medical intervention. Assign the appropriate complication code(s).

c. Coding of Traumatic Fractures

The principles of multiple coding of injuries should be followed in coding fractures. Fractures of specified sites are coded individually by site in accordance with both the provisions within categories S02, S12, S22, S32, S42, S49, S52, S59, S62, S72, S79, S82, S89, S92 and the level of detail furnished by medical record content.

A fracture not indicated as open or closed should be coded to closed. A fracture not indicated whether displaced or not displaced should be coded to displaced.

More specific guidelines are as follows:

1) Initial vs. subsequent encounter for fractures

Traumatic fractures are coded using the appropriate 7th character for initial encounter (A, B, C) for each encounter where the patient is receiving active treatment for the fracture. The appropriate 7th character for initial encounter should also be assigned for a patient who delayed seeking treatment for the fracture or nonunion.

Fractures are coded using the appropriate 7th character for subsequent care for encounters after

the patient has completed active treatment of the fracture and is receiving routine care for the fracture during the healing or recovery phase.

Care for complications of surgical treatment for fracture repairs during the healing or recovery phase should be coded with the appropriate complication codes.

Care of complications of fractures, such as malunion and nonunion, should be reported with the appropriate 7th character for subsequent care with nonunion (K, M, N,) or subsequent care with malunion (P, Q, R).

Malunion/nonunion: The appropriate 7th character for initial encounter should also be assigned for a patient who delayed seeking treatment for the fracture or nonunion.

The open fracture designations in the assignment of the 7th character for fractures of the forearm, femur and lower leg, including ankle are based on the Gustilo open fracture classification. When the Gustilo classification type is not specified for an open fracture, the 7th character for open fracture type I or II should be assigned (B, E, H, M, Q).

A code from category M80, not a traumatic fracture code, should be used for any patient with known osteoporosis who suffers a fracture, even if the patient had a minor fall or trauma, if that fall or trauma would not usually break a normal, healthy bone.

See Section I.C.13. Osteoporosis.

The aftercare Z codes should not be used for aftercare for traumatic fractures. For aftercare of a traumatic fracture, assign the acute fracture code with the appropriate 7th character.

2) Multiple fractures sequencing

Multiple fractures are sequenced in accordance with the severity of the fracture.

3) Physeal fractures

For physeal fractures, assign only the code identifying the type of physeal fracture. Do not assign a separate code to identify the specific bone that is fractured.

d. Coding of Burns and Corrosions

The ICD-10-CM makes a distinction between burns and corrosions. The burn codes are for thermal burns, except sunburns, that come from a heat source, such as a fire or hot appliance. The burn codes are also for burns resulting from electricity and radiation. Corrosions are burns due to chemicals. The guidelines are the same for burns and corrosions.

Current burns (T20-T25) are classified by depth, extent and by agent (X code). Burns are classified by depth as first degree (erythema), second degree (blistering), and third degree (full-thickness involvement). Burns of the eye and internal organs (T26-T28) are classified by site, but not by degree.

1) Sequencing of burn and related condition codes

Sequence first the code that reflects the highest degree of burn when more than one burn is present.

a. When the reason for the admission or encounter is for treatment of external multiple burns, sequence first the code that reflects the burn of the highest degree.

 b. When a patient has both internal and external burns, the circumstances of admission govern the selection of the principal diagnosis or first-listed diagnosis.

 c. When a patient is admitted for burn injuries and other related conditions such as smoke inhalation and/or respiratory failure, the circumstances of admission govern the selection of the principal or first-listed diagnosis.

2) Burns of the same anatomic site

Classify burns of the same anatomic site and on the same side but of different degrees to the subcategory identifying the highest degree recorded in the diagnosis (e.g., for second and third degree burns of right thigh, assign only code T24.311-).

3) Non-healing burns

Non-healing burns are coded as acute burns.

 Necrosis of burned skin should be coded as a non-healed burn.

4) Infected burn

For any documented infected burn site, use an additional code for the infection.

5) Assign separate codes for each burn site

When coding burns, assign separate codes for each burn site. Category T30, Burn and corrosion, body region unspecified is extremely vague and should rarely be used.

 Codes for burns of "multiple sites" should only be assigned when the medical record documentation does not specify the individual sites.

6) Burns and corrosions classified according to extent of body surface involved

Assign codes from category T31, Burns classified according to extent of body surface involved, or T32, Corrosions classified according to extent of body surface involved, **for acute burns or corrosions** when the site of the burn **or corrosion** is not specified or when there is a need for additional data. It is advisable to use category T31 as additional coding when needed to provide data for evaluating burn mortality, such as that needed by burn units. It is also advisable to use category T31 as an additional code for reporting purposes when there is mention of a third-degree burn involving 20 percent or more of the body surface. **Codes from categories T31 and T32 should not be used for sequelae of burns or corrosions.**

 Categories T31 and T32 are based on the classic "rule of nines" in estimating body surface involved: head and neck are assigned nine percent, each arm nine percent, each leg 18 percent, the anterior trunk 18 percent, posterior trunk 18 percent, and genitalia 1 percent. Providers may change these percentage assignments where necessary to accommodate infants and children who have proportionately larger heads than adults, and patients who have large buttocks, thighs, or abdomen that involve burns.

7) Encounters for treatment of sequela of burns

Encounters for the treatment of the late effects of burns or corrosions (i.e., scars or joint contractures) should be coded with a burn or corrosion code with the 7th character "S" for sequela.

8) Sequelae with a late effect code and current burn

When appropriate, both a code for a current burn or corrosion with 7th character "A" or "D" and a burn or corrosion code with 7th character "S" may be assigned on the same record (when both a current burn and sequelae of an old burn exist). Burns and corrosions do not heal at the same rate and a current healing wound may still exist with sequela of a healed burn or corrosion.

See Section I.B.10. Sequela, (Late Effects)

9) Use of an external cause code with burns and corrosions

An external cause code should be used with burns and corrosions to identify the source and intent of the burn, as well as the place where it occurred.

e. Adverse Effects, Poisoning, Underdosing and Toxic Effects

Codes in categories T36-T65 are combination codes that include the substance that was taken as well as the intent. No additional external cause code is required for poisonings, toxic effects, adverse effects and underdosing codes.

1) Do not code directly from the Table of Drugs

Do not code directly from the Table of Drugs and Chemicals. Always refer back to the Tabular List.

2) Use as many codes as necessary to describe

Use as many codes as necessary to describe completely all drugs, medicinal or biological substances.

3) If the same code would describe the causative agent

If the same code would describe the causative agent for more than one adverse reaction, poisoning, toxic effect or underdosing, assign the code only once.

4) If two or more drugs, medicinal or biological substances

If two or more drugs, medicinal or biological substances are taken, code each individually unless a combination code is listed in the Table of Drugs and Chemicals.

 If multiple unspecified drugs, medicinal or biological substances were taken, assign the appropriate code from subcategory T50.91, Poisoning by, adverse effect of and underdosing of multiple unspecified drugs, medicaments and biological substances.

5) The occurrence of drug toxicity is classified in ICD-10-CM as follows:

 (a) Adverse Effect

When coding an adverse effect of a drug that has been correctly prescribed and properly administered, assign the appropriate code for the nature of the adverse effect followed by the appropriate code for the adverse effect of the drug (T36-T50). The code for the drug should have a 5th or 6th character "5" (for example T36.0X5-) Examples of the nature of an adverse effect are tachycardia, delirium, gastrointestinal hemorrhaging, vomiting, hypokalemia, hepatitis, renal failure, or respiratory failure.

(b) Poisoning

When coding a poisoning or reaction to the improper use of a medication (e.g., overdose, wrong substance given or taken in error, wrong route of administration), first assign the appropriate code from categories T36-T50. The poisoning codes have an associated intent as their 5th or 6th character (accidental, intentional self-harm, assault and undetermined). If the intent of the poisoning is unknown or unspecified, code the intent as accidental intent. The undetermined intent is only for use if the documentation in the record specifies that the intent cannot be determined. Use additional code(s) for all manifestations of poisonings.

If there is also a diagnosis of abuse or dependence of the substance, the abuse or dependence is assigned as an additional code.

Examples of poisoning include:

(i) Error was made in drug prescription Errors made in drug prescription or in the administration of the drug by provider, nurse, patient, or other person.

(ii) Overdose of a drug intentionally taken If an overdose of a drug was intentionally taken or administered and resulted in drug toxicity, it would be coded as a poisoning.

(iii) Nonprescribed drug taken with correctly prescribed and properly administered drug.
If a nonprescribed drug or medicinal agent was taken in combination with a correctly prescribed and properly administered drug, any drug toxicity or other reaction resulting from the interaction of the two drugs would be classified as a poisoning.

(iv) Interaction of drug(s) and alcohol. When a reaction results from the interaction of a drug(s) and alcohol, this would be classified as poisoning.

See Section I.C.4. if poisoning is the result of insulin pump malfunctions.

(c) Underdosing

Underdosing refers to taking less of a medication than is prescribed by a provider or a manufacturer's instruction. Discontinuing the use of a prescribed medication on the patient's own initiative (not directed by the patient's provider) is also classified as an underdosing. For underdosing, assign the code from categories T36-T50 (5th or 6th character "6").

Codes for underdosing should never be assigned as principal or first-listed codes. If a patient has a relapse or exacerbation of the medical condition for which the drug is prescribed because of the reduction in dose, then the medical condition itself should be coded.

Noncompliance (Z91.12-, Z91.13- and Z91.14-) or complication of care (Y63.6-Y63.9) codes are to be used with an underdosing code to indicate intent, if known.

(d) Toxic Effects

When a harmful substance is ingested or comes in contact with a person, this is classified as a toxic effect. The toxic effect codes are in categories T51-T65.

Toxic effect codes have an associated intent: accidental, intentional self-harm, assault and undetermined.

f. Adult and child abuse, neglect and other maltreatment

Sequence first the appropriate code from categories T74 (Adult and child abuse, neglect and other maltreatment, confirmed) or T76 (Adult and child abuse, neglect and other maltreatment, suspected) for abuse, neglect and other maltreatment, followed by any accompanying mental health or injury code(s).

If the documentation in the medical record states abuse or neglect it is coded as confirmed (T74.-). It is coded as suspected if it is documented as suspected (T76.-).

For cases of confirmed abuse or neglect an external cause code from the assault section (X92-Y09) should be added to identify the cause of any physical injuries. A perpetrator code (Y07) should be added when the perpetrator of the abuse is known. For suspected cases of abuse or neglect, do not report external cause or perpetrator code.

If a suspected case of abuse, neglect or mistreatment is ruled out during an encounter code Z04.71, Encounter for examination and observation following alleged physical adult abuse, ruled out, or code Z04.72, Encounter for examination and observation following alleged child physical abuse, ruled out, should be used, not a code from T76.

If a suspected case of alleged rape or sexual abuse is ruled out during an encounter code Z04.41, Encounter for examination and observation following alleged adult rape or code Z04.42, Encounter for examination and observation following alleged child rape, should be used, not a code from T76.

If a suspected case of forced sexual exploitation or forced labor exploitation is ruled out during an encounter, code Z04.81, Encounter for examination and observation of victim following forced sexual exploitation, or code Z04.82, Encounter for examination and observation of victim following forced labor exploitation, should be used, not a code from T76.

See Section I.C.15. Abuse in a pregnant patient.

g. Complications of care

1) General guidelines for complications of care
(a) Documentation of complications of care
See Section I.B.16. for information on documentation of complications of care.

2) Pain due to medical devices
Pain associated with devices, implants or grafts left in a surgical site (for example painful hip prosthesis) is assigned to the appropriate code(s) found in Chapter 19, Injury, poisoning, and certain other consequences of external causes. Specific codes for pain due to medical devices are found in the T code section of the ICD-10-CM. Use additional code(s) from category G89 to identify acute or chronic pain due to presence of the device, implant or graft (G89.18 or G89.28).

3) Transplant complications
(a) Transplant complications other than kidney
Codes under category T86, Complications of transplanted organs and tissues, are for use for both complications and rejection of transplanted organs. A transplant complication code is only assigned if the complication affects the function of the transplanted organ. Two codes are required to fully describe a transplant complication: the appropriate code from category T86 and a secondary code that identifies the complication.

Pre-existing conditions or conditions that develop after the transplant are not coded as complications unless they affect the function of the transplanted organs.

See Section I.C.21. for transplant organ removal status
See Section I.C.2. for malignant neoplasm associated with transplanted organ.

(b) Kidney transplant complications
Patients who have undergone kidney transplant may still have some form of chronic kidney disease (CKD) because the kidney transplant may not fully restore kidney function. Code T86.1- should be assigned for documented complications of a kidney transplant, such as transplant failure or rejection or other transplant complication. Code T86.1- should not be assigned for post kidney transplant patients who have chronic kidney (CKD) unless a transplant complication such as transplant failure or rejection is documented. If the documentation is unclear as to whether the patient has a complication of the transplant, query the provider.

Conditions that affect the function of the transplanted kidney, other than CKD, should be assigned a code from subcategory T86.1, Complications of transplanted organ, Kidney, and a secondary code that identifies the complication.

For patients with CKD following a kidney transplant, but who do not have a complication such as failure or rejection, *see Section I.C.14. Chronic kidney disease and kidney transplant status.*

4) Complication codes that include the external cause
As with certain other T codes, some of the complications of care codes have the external cause included in the code. The code includes the nature of the complication as well as the type of procedure that caused the complication. No external cause code indicating the type of procedure is necessary for these codes.

5) Complications of care codes within the body system chapters
Intraoperative and postprocedural complication codes are found within the body system chapters with codes specific to the organs and structures of that body system. These codes should be sequenced first, followed by a code(s) for the specific complication, if applicable.

Complication codes from the body system chapters should be assigned for intraoperative and postprocedural complications (e.g., the appropriate complication code from Chapter 9 would be assigned for a vascular intraoperative or postprocedural complication) unless the complication is specifically indexed to a T code in Chapter 19.

20. Chapter 20: External Causes of Morbidity (V00-Y99)
The external causes of morbidity codes should never be sequenced as the first-listed or principal diagnosis.

External cause codes are intended to provide data for injury research and evaluation of injury prevention strategies. These codes capture how the injury or health condition happened (cause), the intent (unintentional or accidental; or intentional, such as suicide or assault), the place where the event occurred the activity of the patient at the time of the event, and the person's status (e.g., civilian, military).

There is no national requirement for mandatory ICD-10-CM external cause code reporting. Unless a provider is subject to a state-based external cause code reporting mandate or these codes are required by a particular payer, reporting of ICD-10-CM codes in Chapter 20, External Causes of Morbidity, is not required. In the absence of a mandatory reporting requirement, providers are encouraged to voluntarily report external cause codes, as they provide valuable data for injury research and evaluation of injury prevention strategies.

a. General External Cause Coding Guidelines
1) Used with any code in the range of A00.0-T88.9, Z00-Z99
An external cause code may be used with any code in the range of A00.0-T88.9, Z00-Z99, classification that represents a health condition due to an external cause. Though they are most applicable to injuries, they are also valid for use with such things as infections or diseases due to an external source, and other health conditions, such as a heart attack that occurs during strenuous physical activity.

2) External cause code used for length of treatment
Assign the external cause code, with the appropriate 7th character (initial encounter, subsequent

encounter or sequela) for each encounter for which the injury or condition is being treated.

Most categories in Chapter 20 have a 7th character requirement for each applicable code. Most categories in this chapter have three 7th character values: A, initial encounter, D, subsequent encounter and S, sequela. While the patient may be seen by a new or different provider over the course of treatment for an injury or condition, assignment of the 7th character for external cause should match the 7th character of the code assigned for the associated injury or condition for the encounter.

3) Use the full range of external cause codes
Use the full range of external cause codes to completely describe the cause, the intent, the place of occurrence and if applicable, the activity of the patient at the time of the event, and the patient's status, for all injuries, and other health conditions due to an external cause.

4) Assign as many external cause codes as necessary
Assign as many external cause codes as necessary to fully explain each cause. If only one external code can be recorded, assign the code most related to the principal diagnosis.

5) The selection of the appropriate external cause code
The selection of the appropriate external cause code is guided by the Alphabetic Index of External Causes and by Inclusion and Exclusion notes in the Tabular List.

6) External cause code can never be a principal diagnosis
An external cause code can never be a principal (first-listed) diagnosis.

7) Combination external cause codes
Certain of the external cause codes are combination codes that identify sequential events that result in an injury, such as a fall which results in striking against an object. The injury may be due to either event or both. The combination external cause code used should correspond to the sequence of events regardless of which caused the most serious injury.

8) No external cause code needed in certain circumstances
No external cause code from Chapter 20 is needed if the external cause and intent are included in a code from another chapter (e.g., T36.0X1- Poisoning by penicillins, accidental (unintentional)).

b. Place of Occurrence Guideline
Codes from category Y92, Place of occurrence of the external cause, are secondary codes for use after other external cause codes to identify the location of the patient at the time of injury or other condition.

Generally, a place of occurrence code is assigned only once, at the initial encounter for treatment. However, in the rare instance that a new injury occurs during hospitalization, an additional place of occurrence code may be assigned. No 7th characters are used for Y92. Only one code from Y92 should be recorded on a medical record.

Do not use place of occurrence code Y92.9 if the place is not stated or is not applicable.

c. Activity Code
Assign a code from category Y93, Activity code, to describe the activity of the patient at the time the injury or other health condition occurred.

An activity code is used only once, at the initial encounter for treatment. Only one code from Y93 should be recorded on a medical record.

The activity codes are not applicable to poisonings, adverse effects, misadventures or sequela.

Do not assign Y93.9, Unspecified activity, if the activity is not stated.

A code from category Y93 is appropriate for use with external cause and intent codes if identifying the activity provides additional information about the event.

d. Place of Occurrence, Activity, and Status Codes Used with other External Cause Code
When applicable, place of occurrence, activity, and external cause status codes are sequenced after the main external cause code(s). Regardless of the number of external cause codes assigned, there should be only one place of occurrence code, one activity code, and one external cause status code assigned to an encounter.

e. If the Reporting Format Limits the Number of External Cause Codes
If the reporting format limits the number of external cause codes that can be used in reporting clinical data, report the code for the cause/intent most related to the principal diagnosis. If the format permits capture of additional external cause codes, the cause/intent, including medical misadventures, of the additional events should be reported rather than the codes for place, activity, or external status.

f. Multiple External Cause Coding Guidelines
More than one external cause code is required to fully describe the external cause of an illness or injury. The assignment of external cause codes should be sequenced in the following priority:

If two or more events cause separate injuries, an external cause code should be assigned for each cause. The first-listed external cause code will be selected in the following order:

External codes for child and adult abuse take priority over all other external cause codes.
See Section I.C.19., Child and Adult abuse guidelines.
External codes for terrorism events take priority over all other external cause codes except child and adult abuse.

External cause codes for cataclysmic events take priority over all other external cause codes except child and adult abuse and terrorism.

External cause codes for transport accidents take priority over all other external cause codes except cataclysmic events, child and adult abuse and terrorism.

Activity and external cause status codes are assigned following all causal (intent) external cause codes.

The first-listed external cause code should correspond to the cause of the most serious diagnosis due to an assault, accident, or self-harm, following the order of hierarchy listed above.

g. Child and Adult Abuse Guideline

Adult and child abuse, neglect and maltreatment are classified as assault. Any of the assault codes may be used to indicate the external cause of any injury resulting from the confirmed abuse.

For confirmed cases of abuse, neglect and maltreatment, when the perpetrator is known, a code from Y07, Perpetrator of maltreatment and neglect, should accompany any other assault codes.

See Section I.C.19. Adult and child abuse, neglect and other maltreatment

h. Unknown or Undetermined Intent Guideline

If the intent (accident, self-harm, assault) of the cause of an injury or other condition is unknown or unspecified, code the intent as accidental intent. All transport accident categories assume accidental intent.

1) Use of undetermined intent

External cause codes for events of undetermined intent are only for use if the documentation in the record specifies that the intent cannot be determined.

i. Sequelae (Late Effects) of External Cause Guidelines

1) Sequelae external cause codes

Sequela are reported using the external cause code with the 7th character "S" for sequela. These codes should be used with any report of a late effect or sequela resulting from a previous injury.

See Section I.B.10. Sequela (Late Effects)

2) Sequela external cause code with a related current injury

A sequela external cause code should never be used with a related current nature of injury code.

3) Use of sequela external cause codes for subsequent visits

Use a late effect external cause code for subsequent visits when a late effect of the initial injury is being treated. Do not use a late effect external cause code for subsequent visits for follow-up care (e.g., to assess healing, to receive rehabilitative therapy) of the injury when no late effect of the injury has been documented.

j. Terrorism Guidelines

1) Cause of injury identified by the Federal Government (FBI) as terrorism

When the cause of an injury is identified by the Federal Government (FBI) as terrorism, the first-listed external cause code should be a code from category Y38, Terrorism. The definition of terrorism employed by the FBI is found at the inclusion note at the beginning of category Y38. Use additional code for place of occurrence (Y92.-). More than one Y38 code may be assigned if the injury is the result of more than one mechanism of terrorism.

2) Cause of an injury is suspected to be the result of terrorism

When the cause of an injury is suspected to be the result of terrorism a code from category Y38 should not be assigned. Suspected cases should be classified as assault.

3) Code Y38.9, Terrorism, secondary effects

Assign code Y38.9, Terrorism, secondary effects, for conditions occurring subsequent to the terrorist event. This code should not be assigned for conditions that are due to the initial terrorist act.

It is acceptable to assign code Y38.9 with another code from Y38 if there is an injury due to the initial terrorist event and an injury that is a subsequent result of the terrorist event.

k. External Cause Status

A code from category Y99, External cause status, should be assigned whenever any other external cause code is assigned for an encounter, including an Activity code, except for the events noted below. Assign a code from category Y99, External cause status, to indicate the work status of the person at the time the event occurred. The status code indicates whether the event occurred during military activity, whether a non-military person was at work, whether an individual including a student or volunteer was involved in a non-work activity at the time of the causal event.

A code from Y99, External cause status, should be assigned, when applicable, with other external cause codes, such as transport accidents and falls. The external cause status codes are not applicable to poisonings, adverse effects, misadventures or late effects.

Do not assign a code from category Y99 if no other external cause codes (cause, activity) are applicable for the encounter.

An external cause status code is used only once, at the initial encounter for treatment. Only one code from Y99 should be recorded on a medical record.

Do not assign code Y99.9, Unspecified external cause status, if the status is not stated.

21. Chapter 21: Factors Influencing Health Status and Contact with Health Services (Z00-Z99)

Note: The chapter-specific guidelines provide additional information about the use of Z codes for specified encounters.

a. Use of Z Codes in Any Healthcare Setting

Z codes are for use in any healthcare setting. Z codes may be used as either a first-listed (principal diagnosis code in the inpatient setting) or secondary code, depending on the circumstances of the encounter. Certain Z codes may only be used as first-listed or principal diagnosis.

b. Z Codes Indicate a Reason for an Encounter

Z codes are not procedure codes. A corresponding procedure code must accompany a Z code to describe any procedure performed.

c. Categories of Z Codes

1) Contact/Exposure

Category Z20 indicates contact with, and suspected exposure to, communicable diseases. These codes are for patients who are suspected to have been exposed to a disease by close personal contact with an infected individual or are in an area where a disease is epidemic.

Category Z77, Other contact with and (suspected) exposures hazardous to health, indicates contact with and suspected exposures hazardous to health.

Contact/exposure codes may be used as a first-listed code to explain an encounter for testing, or, more commonly, as a secondary code to identify a potential risk.

2) Inoculations and vaccinations

Code Z23 is for encounters for inoculations and vaccinations. It indicates that a patient is being seen to receive a prophylactic inoculation against a disease. Procedure codes are required to identify the actual administration of the injection and the type(s) of immunizations given. Code Z23 may be used as a secondary code if the inoculation is given as a routine part of preventive health care, such as a well-baby visit.

3) Status

Status codes indicate that a patient is either a carrier of a disease or has the sequelae or residual of a past disease or condition. This includes such things as the presence of prosthetic or mechanical devices resulting from past treatment. A status code is informative, because the status may affect the course of treatment and its outcome. A status code is distinct from a history code. The history code indicates that the patient no longer has the condition.

A status code should not be used with a diagnosis code from one of the body system chapters, if the diagnosis code includes the information provided by the status code. For example, code Z94.1, Heart transplant status, should not be used with a code from subcategory T86.2, Complications of heart transplant. The status code does not provide additional information. The complication code indicates that the patient is a heart transplant patient.

For encounters for weaning from a mechanical ventilator, assign a code from subcategory J96.1, Chronic respiratory failure, followed by code Z99.11, Dependence on respirator [ventilator] status.

The status Z codes/categories are:

Z14   Genetic carrier
       Genetic carrier status indicates that a person carries a gene, associated with a particular disease, which may be passed to offspring who may develop that disease. The person does not have the disease and is not at risk of developing the disease.

Z15   Genetic susceptibility to disease Genetic susceptibility indicates that a person has a gene that increases the risk of that person developing the disease.

Codes from category Z15 should not be used as principal or first-listed codes. If the patient has the condition to which he/she is susceptible, and that condition is the reason for the encounter, the code for the current condition should be sequenced first. If the patient is being seen for follow-up after completed treatment for this condition, and the condition no longer exists, a follow-up code should be sequenced first, followed by the appropriate personal history and genetic susceptibility codes. If the purpose of the encounter is genetic counseling associated with procreative management, code Z31.5, Encounter for genetic counseling, should be assigned as the first-listed code, followed by a code from category Z15. Additional codes should be assigned for any applicable family or personal history.

Z16   Resistance to antimicrobial drugs
       This code indicates that a patient has a condition that is resistant to antimicrobial drug treatment. Sequence the infection code first.

Z17   Estrogen receptor status

Z18   Retained foreign body fragments

Z19   Hormone sensitivity malignancy status

Z21   Asymptomatic HIV infection status This code indicates that a patient has tested positive for HIV but has manifested no signs or symptoms of the disease.

Z22   Carrier of infectious disease Carrier status indicates that a person harbors the specific organisms of a disease without manifest symptoms and is capable of transmitting the infection.

Z28.3   Underimmunization status

Z33.1   Pregnant state, incidental This code is a secondary code only for use when the pregnancy is in no way complicating the reason for visit. Otherwise, a code from the obstetric chapter is required.

Z66   Do not resuscitate
This code may be used when it is documented by the provider that a patient is on do not resuscitate status at any time during the stay.

Z67   Blood type

Z68   Body mass index (BMI)
       BMI codes should only be assigned when there is an associated reportable diagnosis (such as obesity). Do not assign BMI codes during pregnancy.

See Section I.B.14 for BMI documentation by clinicians other than the patient's provider.

Z74.01   Bed confinement status

Z76.82   Awaiting organ transplant status

Z78   Other specified health status
       Code Z78.1, Physical restraint status, may be used when it is documented by the provider that a patient has been put in restraints during the current encounter. Please note that this code should

not be reported when it is documented by the provider that a patient is temporarily restrained during a procedure.

Z79   Long-term (current) drug therapy

Codes from this category indicate a patient's continuous use of a prescribed drug (including such things as aspirin therapy) for the long-term treatment of a condition or for prophylactic use. It is not for use for patients who have addictions to drugs. This subcategory is not for use of medications for detoxification or maintenance programs to prevent withdrawal symptoms (e.g., methadone maintenance for opiate dependence). Assign the appropriate code for the drug use, abuse, or dependence instead.

Assign a code from Z79 if the patient is receiving a medication for an extended period as a prophylactic measure (such as for the prevention of deep vein thrombosis) or as treatment of a chronic condition (such as arthritis) or a disease requiring a lengthy course of treatment (such as cancer). Do not assign a code from category Z79 for medication being administered for a brief period of time to treat an acute illness or injury (such as a course of antibiotics to treat acute bronchitis).

Z88   Allergy status to drugs, medicaments and biological substances Except: Z88.9, Allergy status to unspecified drugs, medicaments and biological substances status

Z89   Acquired absence of limb

Z90   Acquired absence of organs, not elsewhere classified

Z91.0-   Allergy status, other than to drugs and biological substances

Z92.82   Status post administration of tPA (rtPA) in a different facility within the last 24 hours prior to admission to a current facility Assign code Z92.82, Status post administration of tPA (rtPA) in a different facility within the last 24 hours prior to admission to current facility, as a secondary diagnosis when a patient is received by transfer into a facility and documentation indicates they were administered tissue plasminogen activator (tPA) within the last 24 hours prior to admission to the current facility. This guideline applies even if the patient is still receiving the tPA at the time they are received into the current facility. The appropriate code for the condition for which the tPA was administered (such as cerebrovascular disease or myocardial infarction) should be assigned first. Code Z92.82 is only applicable to the receiving facility record and not to the transferring facility record.

Z93   Artificial opening status

Z94   Transplanted organ and tissue status

Z95   Presence of cardiac and vascular implants and grafts

Z96   Presence of other functional implants

Z97   Presence of other devices

Z98   Other postprocedural states

Assign code Z98.85, Transplanted organ removal status, to indicate that a transplanted organ has been previously removed. This code should not be assigned for the encounter in which the transplanted organ is removed. The complication necessitating removal of the transplant organ should be assigned for that encounter.

See Section I.C.19. for information on the coding of organ transplant complications.

Z99   Dependence on enabling machines and devices, not elsewhere classified

Note: Categories Z89-Z90 and Z93-Z99 are for use only if there are no complications or malfunctions of the organ or tissue replaced, the amputation site or the equipment on which the patient is dependent.

4) History (of)

There are two types of history Z codes, personal and family. Personal history codes explain a patient's past medical condition that no longer exists and is not receiving any treatment, but that has the potential for recurrence, and therefore may require continued monitoring.

Family history codes are for use when a patient has a family member(s) who has had a particular disease that causes the patient to be at higher risk of also contracting the disease.

Personal history codes may be used in conjunction with follow-up codes and family history codes may be used in conjunction with screening codes to explain the need for a test or procedure. History codes are also acceptable on any medical record regardless of the reason for visit. A history of an illness, even if no longer present, is important information that may alter the type of treatment ordered.

The reason for the encounter (for example, screening or counseling) should be sequenced first and the appropriate personal and/or family history code(s) should be assigned as additional diagnos(es).

The history Z code categories are:

Z80   Family history of primary malignant neoplasm

Z81   Family history of mental and behavioral disorders

Z82   Family history of certain disabilities and chronic diseases (leading to disablement)

Z83   Family history of other specific disorders

Z84   Family history of other conditions

Z85   Personal history of malignant neoplasm

Z86   Personal history of certain other diseases

Z87   Personal history of other diseases and conditions

Z91.4-   Personal history of psychological trauma, not elsewhere classified

Z91.5   Personal history of self-harm

Z91.81   History of falling

Z91.82   Personal history of military deployment

Z92   Personal history of medical treatment Except: Z92.0, Personal history of contraception Except: Z92.82, Status post administration of tPA (rtPA) in a different facility within the last 24 hours prior to admission to a current facility

5) Screening

Screening is the testing for disease or disease precursors in seemingly well individuals so that early detection and treatment can be provided for those who test positive for the disease (e.g., screening mammogram).

The testing of a person to rule out or confirm a suspected diagnosis because the patient has some sign or symptom is a diagnostic examination, not a screening. In these cases, the sign or symptom is used to explain the reason for the test.

A screening code may be a first-listed code if the reason for the visit is specifically the screening exam. It may also be used as an additional code if the screening is done during an office visit for other health problems. A screening code is not necessary if the screening is inherent to a routine examination, such as a pap smear done during a routine pelvic examination.

Should a condition be discovered during the screening then the code for the condition may be assigned as an additional diagnosis.

The Z code indicates that a screening exam is planned. A procedure code is required to confirm that the screening was performed.

The screening Z codes/categories:

Z11   Encounter for screening for infectious and parasitic diseases

Z12   Encounter for screening for malignant neoplasms

Z13   Encounter for screening for other diseases and disorders Except: Z13.9, Encounter for screening, unspecified

Z36   Encounter for antenatal screening for mother

6) Observation

There are three observation Z code categories. They are for use in very limited circumstances when a person is being observed for a suspected condition that is ruled out. The observation codes are not for use if an injury or illness or any signs or symptoms related to the suspected condition are present. In such cases the diagnosis/symptom code is used with the corresponding external cause code.

The observation codes are primarily to be used as a principal/first-listed diagnosis. An observation code may be assigned as a secondary diagnosis code when the patient is being observed for a condition that is ruled out and is unrelated to the principal/first-listed diagnosis (e.g., patient presents for treatment following injuries sustained in a motor vehicle accident and is also observed for suspected COVID-19 infection that is subsequently

ruled out). Also, when the principal diagnosis is required to be a code from category Z38, Liveborn infants according to place of birth and type of delivery, then a code from category Z05, Encounter for observation and evaluation of newborn for suspected diseases and conditions ruled out, is sequenced after the Z38 code. Additional codes may be used in addition to the observation code, but only if they are unrelated to the suspected condition being observed.

Codes from subcategory Z03.7 Encounter for suspected maternal and fetal conditions ruled out, may either be used as a first-listed or as an additional code assignment depending on the case. They are for use in very limited circumstances on a maternal record when an encounter is for a suspected maternal or fetal condition that is ruled out during that encounter (for example, a maternal or fetal condition may be suspected due to an abnormal test result). These codes should not be used when the condition is confirmed. In those cases, the confirmed condition should be coded. In addition, these codes are not for use if an illness or any signs or symptoms related to the suspected condition or problem are present. In such cases the diagnosis/symptom code is used.

Additional codes may be used in addition to the code from subcategory Z03.7, but only if they are unrelated to the suspected condition being evaluated.

Codes from subcategory Z03.7 may not be used for encounters for antenatal screening of mother. *See Section I.C.21. Screening.*

For encounters for suspected fetal condition that are inconclusive following testing and evaluation, assign the appropriate code from category O35, O36, O40 or O41.

The observation Z code categories:

Z03   Encounter for medical observation for suspected diseases and conditions ruled out

Z04   Encounter for examination and observation for other reasons Except: Z04.9, Encounter for examination and observation for unspecified reason

Z05   Encounter for observation and evaluation of newborn for suspected diseases and conditions ruled out

7) Aftercare

Aftercare visit codes cover situations when the initial treatment of a disease has been performed and the patient requires continued care during the healing or recovery phase, or for the long-term consequences of the disease. The aftercare Z code should not be used if treatment is directed at a current, acute disease. The diagnosis code is to be used in these cases.

Exceptions to this rule are codes Z51.0, Encounter for antineoplastic radiation therapy, and codes from subcategory Z51.1, Encounter for antineoplastic chemotherapy and immunotherapy. These codes are to be first-listed, followed by the diagnosis code when a patient's encounter is solely to receive radiation therapy, chemotherapy, or immunotherapy for the treatment of a neoplasm. If the reason for the encounter is more than one type of antineoplastic therapy, code Z51.0 and a code from subcategory Z51.1 may be assigned together, in which case one of these codes would be reported as a secondary diagnosis.

The aftercare Z codes should also not be used for aftercare for injuries. For aftercare of an injury, assign the acute injury code with the appropriate 7th character (for subsequent encounter).

The aftercare codes are generally first-listed to explain the specific reason for the encounter. An aftercare code may be used as an additional code when some type of aftercare is provided in addition to the reason for admission and no diagnosis code is applicable. An example of this would be the closure of a colostomy during an encounter for treatment of another condition.

Aftercare codes should be used in conjunction with other aftercare codes or diagnosis codes to provide better detail on the specifics of an aftercare encounter visit, unless otherwise directed by the classification. The sequencing of multiple aftercare codes depends on the circumstances of the encounter.

Certain aftercare Z code categories need a secondary diagnosis code to describe the resolving condition or sequelae. For others, the condition is included in the code title.

Additional Z code aftercare category terms include fitting and adjustment, and attention to artificial openings.

Status Z codes may be used with aftercare Z codes to indicate the nature of the aftercare. For example code Z95.1, Presence of aortocoronary bypass graft, may be used with code Z48.812, Encounter for surgical aftercare following surgery on the circulatory system, to indicate the surgery for which the aftercare is being performed. A status code should not be used when the aftercare code indicates the type of status, such as using Z43.0, Encounter for attention to tracheostomy, with Z93.0, Tracheostomy status.

The aftercare Z category/codes:

Z42 Encounter for plastic and reconstructive surgery following medical procedure or healed injury

Z43 Encounter for attention to artificial openings

Z44 Encounter for fitting and adjustment of external prosthetic device

Z45 Encounter for adjustment and management of implanted device

Z46 Encounter for fitting and adjustment of other devices

Z47 Orthopedic aftercare

Z48 Encounter for other postprocedural aftercare

Z49 Encounter for care involving renal dialysis

Z51 Encounter for other aftercare and medical care

8) Follow-up

The follow-up codes are used to explain continuing surveillance following completed treatment of a disease, condition, or injury. They imply that the condition has been fully treated and no longer exists. They should not be confused with aftercare codes, or injury codes with a 7th character for subsequent encounter, that explain ongoing care of a healing condition or its sequelae. Follow-up codes may be used in conjunction with history codes to provide the full picture of the healed condition and its treatment. The follow-up code is sequenced first, followed by the history code.

A follow-up code may be used to explain multiple visits. Should a condition be found to have recurred on the follow-up visit, then the diagnosis code for the condition should be assigned in place of the follow-up code.

The follow-up Z code categories:

Z08 Encounter for follow-up examination after completed treatment for malignant neoplasm

Z09 Encounter for follow-up examination after completed treatment for conditions other than malignant neoplasm

Z39 Encounter for maternal postpartum care and examination

9) Donor

Codes in category Z52, Donors of organs and tissues, are used for living individuals who are donating blood or other body tissue. These codes are only for individuals donating for others, **as well as** not for self-donations. They are not used to identify cadaveric donations.

10) Counseling

Counseling Z codes are used when a patient or family member receives assistance in the aftermath of an illness or injury, or when support is required in coping with family or social problems.

The counseling Z codes/categories:

Z30.0- Encounter for general counseling and advice on contraception

Z31.5 Encounter for procreative genetic counseling

Z31.6- Encounter for general counseling and advice on procreation

Z32.2 Encounter for childbirth instruction

Z32.3 Encounter for childcare instruction

Z69 Encounter for mental health services for victim and perpetrator of abuse

Z70 Counseling related to sexual attitude, behavior and orientation

Z71 Persons encountering health services for other counseling and medical advice, not elsewhere classified

Note: Code Z71.84, Encounter for health counseling related to travel, is to be used for health risk and safety counseling for future travel purposes.

Code Z71.85, Encounter for immunization safety counseling, is to be used for counseling of the patient or caregiver regarding the safety of a vaccine. This code should not be used for the provision of general information regarding risks and potential side effects during routine encounters for the administration of vaccines.

Z76.81 Expectant mother prebirth pediatrician visit

11) Encounters for Obstetrical and Reproductive Services
See Section I.C.15. Pregnancy, childbirth, and the puerperium, for further instruction on the use of these codes.

Z codes for pregnancy are for use in those circumstances when none of the problems or complications included in the codes from the Obstetrics chapter exist (a routine prenatal visit or postpartum care). Codes in category Z34, Encounter for supervision of normal pregnancy, are always first listed and are not to be used with any other code from the OB chapter.

Codes in category Z3A, Weeks of gestation, may be assigned to provide additional information about the pregnancy. Category Z3A codes should not be assigned for pregnancies with abortive outcomes (categories O00-O08), elective termination of pregnancy (code Z33.2), nor for postpartum conditions, as category Z3A is not applicable to these conditions. The date of the admission should be used to determine weeks of gestation for inpatient admissions that encompass more than one gestational week.

The outcome of delivery, category Z37, should be included on all maternal delivery records. It is always a secondary code. Codes in category Z37 should not be used on the newborn record.

Z codes for family planning (contraceptive) or procreative management and counseling should be included on an obstetric record either during the pregnancy or the postpartum stage, if applicable.

Z codes/categories for obstetrical and reproductive services:

Z30	Encounter for contraceptive management
Z31	Encounter for procreative management
Z32.2	Encounter for childbirth instruction
Z32.3	Encounter for childcare instruction
Z33	Pregnant state
Z34	Encounter for supervision of normal pregnancy
Z36	Encounter for antenatal screening of mother
Z3A	Weeks of gestation
Z37	Outcome of delivery
Z39	Encounter for maternal postpartum care and examination
Z76.81	Expectant mother prebirth pediatrician visit

12) Newborns and Infants

See Section I.C.16. Newborn (Perinatal) guidelines, for further instruction on the use of these codes.

Newborn Z codes/categories:

Z76.1	Encounter for health supervision and care of foundling
Z00.1-	Encounter for routine child health examination
Z38	Liveborn infants according to place of birth and type of delivery

13) Routine and Administrative Examinations
The Z codes allow for the description of encounters for routine examinations, such as, a general check-up, or, examinations for administrative purposes, such as, a pre-employment physical. The codes are not to be used if the examination is for diagnosis of a suspected condition or for treatment purposes. In such cases the diagnosis code is used. During a routine exam, should a diagnosis or condition be discovered, it should be coded as an additional code. Pre-existing and chronic conditions and history codes may also be included as additional codes as long as the examination is for administrative purposes and not focused on any particular condition.

Some of the codes for routine health examinations distinguish between "with" and "without" abnormal findings. Code assignment depends on the information that is known at the time the encounter is being coded. For example, if no abnormal findings were found during the examination, but the encounter is being coded before test results are back, it is acceptable to assign the code for "without abnormal findings." When assigning a code for "with abnormal findings," additional code(s) should be assigned to identify the specific abnormal finding(s).

Pre-operative examination and pre-procedural laboratory examination Z codes are for use only in those situations when a patient is being cleared for a procedure or surgery and no treatment is given.

The Z codes/categories for routine and administrative examinations:

Z00	Encounter for general examination without complaint, suspected or reported diagnosis
Z01	Encounter for other special examination without complaint, suspected or reported diagnosis
Z02	Encounter for administrative examination Except: Z02.9, Encounter for administrative examinations, unspecified
Z32.0-	Encounter for pregnancy test

14) Miscellaneous Z Codes
The miscellaneous Z codes capture a number of other health care encounters that do not fall into one of the other categories. Certain of these codes identify the reason for the encounter; others are for use as additional codes that provide useful information on circumstances that may affect a patient's care and treatment.

Prophylactic Organ Removal

For encounters specifically for prophylactic removal of an organ (such as prophylactic removal of breasts due to a genetic susceptibility to cancer or a family history of cancer), the principal or first-listed code should be a code from category Z40, Encounter for prophylactic surgery, followed by the appropriate codes to identify the associated risk factor (such as genetic susceptibility or family history).

If the patient has a malignancy of one site and is having prophylactic removal at another site to prevent either a new primary malignancy or metastatic disease, a code for the malignancy should also be assigned in addition to a code from subcategory Z40.0, Encounter for prophylactic surgery for risk factors related to malignant neoplasms. A Z40.0 code should not be assigned if the patient is having organ removal for treatment of a malignancy, such as the removal of the testes for the treatment of prostate cancer.

Miscellaneous Z codes/categories:

Z28	Immunization not carried out Except: Z28.3, Underimmunization status
Z29	Encounter for other prophylactic measures
Z40	Encounter for prophylactic surgery
Z41	Encounter for procedures for purposes other than remedying health state Except: Z41.9, Encounter for procedure for purposes other than remedying health state, unspecified
Z53	Persons encountering health services for specific procedures and treatment, not carried out
Z55	Problems related to education and literacy
Z56	Problems related to employment and unemployment
Z57	Occupational exposure to risk factors
Z58	Problems related to physical environment
Z59	Problems related to housing and economic circumstances
Z60	Problems related to social environment
Z62	Problems related to upbringing
Z63	Other problems related to primary support group, including family circumstances
Z64	Problems related to certain psychosocial circumstances
Z65	Problems related to other psychosocial circumstances
Z72	Problems related to lifestyle Note: These codes should be assigned only when the documentation specifies that the patient has an associated problem
Z73	Problems related to life management difficulty
Z74	Problems related to care provider dependency Except: Z74.01, Bed confinement status
Z75	Problems related to medical facilities and other health care

Z76.0	Encounter for issue of repeat prescription
Z76.3	Healthy person accompanying sick person
Z76.4	Other boarder to healthcare facility
Z76.5	Malingerer [conscious simulation]
Z91.1-	Patient's noncompliance with medical treatment and regimen
Z91.83	Wandering in diseases classified elsewhere
Z91.84-	Oral health risk factors
Z91.89	Other specified personal risk factors, not elsewhere classified

See Section I.B.14 for Z55-Z65 Persons with potential health hazards related to socioeconomic and psychosocial circumstances, documentation by clinicians other than the patient's provider

15) Nonspecific Z Codes

Certain Z codes are so non-specific, or potentially redundant with other codes in the classification, that there can be little justification for their use in the inpatient setting. Their use in the outpatient setting should be limited to those instances when there is no further documentation to permit more precise coding. Otherwise, any sign or symptom or any other reason for visit that is captured in another code should be used.

Nonspecific Z codes/categories:

Z02.9	Encounter for administrative examinations, unspecified
Z04.9	Encounter for examination and observation for unspecified reason
Z13.9	Encounter for screening, unspecified
Z41.9	Encounter for procedure for purposes other than remedying health state, unspecified
Z52.9	Donor of unspecified organ or tissue
Z86.59	Personal history of other mental and behavioral disorders
Z88.9	Allergy status to unspecified drugs, medicaments and biological substances status
Z92.0	Personal history of contraception

16) Z Codes That May Only be Principal/First-Listed Diagnosis

The following Z codes/categories may only be reported as the principal/first-listed diagnosis, except when there are multiple encounters on the same day and the medical records for the encounters are combined:

Z00	Encounter for general examination without complaint, suspected or reported diagnosis Except: Z00.6
Z01	Encounter for other special examination without complaint, suspected or reported diagnosis
Z02	Encounter for administrative examination
Z04	Encounter for examination and observation for other reasons
Z33.2	Encounter for elective termination of pregnancy

Z31.81   Encounter for male factor infertility in female patient

Z31.83   Encounter for assisted reproductive fertility procedure cycle

Z31.84   Encounter for fertility preservation procedure

Z34   Encounter for supervision of normal pregnancy

Z39   Encounter for maternal postpartum care and examination

Z38   Liveborn infants according to place of birth and type of delivery

Z40   Encounter for prophylactic surgery

Z42   Encounter for plastic and reconstructive surgery following medical procedure or healed injury

Z51.0   Encounter for antineoplastic radiation therapy

Z51.1-   Encounter for antineoplastic chemotherapy and immunotherapy

Z52   Donors of organs and tissues Except: Z52.9, Donor of unspecified organ or tissue

Z76.1   Encounter for health supervision and care of foundling

Z76.2   Encounter for health supervision and care of other healthy infant and child

Z99.12   Encounter for respirator [ventilator] dependence during power failure

17) Social Determinants of Health
Codes describing social determinants of health (SDOH) should be assigned when this information is documented.

For social determinants of health, such as information found in categories Z55-Z65, Persons with potential health hazards related to socioeconomic and psychosocial circumstances, code assignment may be based on medical record documentation from clinicians involved in the care of the patient who are not the patient's provider since this information represents social information, rather than medical diagnoses.

For example, coding professionals may utilize documentation of social information from social workers, community health workers, case managers, or nurses, if their documentation is included in the official medical record.

Patient self-reported documentation may be used to assign codes for social determinants of health, as long as the patient self-reported information is signed-off by and incorporated into the medical record by either a clinician or provider.

Social determinants of health codes are located primarily in these Z code categories:

Z55   Problems related to education and literacy

Z56   Problems related to employment and unemployment

Z57   Occupational exposure to risk factors

Z58   Problems related to physical environment

Z59   Problems related to housing and economic circumstances

Z60   Problems related to social environment

Z62   Problems related to upbringing

Z63   Other problems related to primary support group, including family circumstances

Z64   Problems related to certain psychosocial circumstances

Z65   Problems related to other psychosocial circumstances

See Section I.B.14. Documentation by Clinicians Other than the Patient's Provider.

22. Chapter 22: *Codes for Special Purposes (U00-U85)*

U07.0   Vaping-related disorder (see Section I.C.10.e., Vaping-related disorders)

U07.1   COVID-19 (see Section I.C.1.g.1., COVID-19 infection)

U09.9   Post COVID-19 condition, unspecified (see Section I.C.1.g.1.m)

Section II. Selection of Principal Diagnosis

The circumstances of inpatient admission always govern the selection of principal diagnosis. The principal diagnosis is defined in the Uniform Hospital Discharge Data Set (UHDDS) as "that condition established after study to be chiefly responsible for occasioning the admission of the patient to the hospital for care."

The UHDDS definitions are used by hospitals to report inpatient data elements in a standardized manner. These data elements and their definitions can be found in the July 31, 1985, Federal Register (Vol. 50, No, 147), pp. 31038-40.

Since that time, the application of the UHDDS definitions has been expanded to include all nonoutpatient settings (acute care, short term, long-term care and psychiatric hospitals; home health agencies; rehab facilities; nursing homes, etc. . .). The UHDDS definitions also apply to hospice services (all levels of care).

In determining principal diagnosis, coding conventions in the ICD-10-CM, the Tabular List and Alphabetic Index take precedence over these official coding guidelines.

(See Section I.A., Conventions for the ICD-10-CM)

The importance of consistent, complete documentation in the medical record cannot be overemphasized. Without such documentation the application of all coding guidelines is a difficult, if not impossible, task.

A. **Codes for symptoms, signs, and ill-defined conditions**

Codes for symptoms, signs, and ill-defined conditions from Chapter 18 are not to be used as principal diagnosis when a related definitive diagnosis has been established.

B. **Two or more interrelated conditions, each potentially meeting the definition for principal diagnosis.**

When there are two or more interrelated conditions (such as diseases in the same ICD-10-CM chapter or manifestations characteristically associated with a certain disease) potentially meeting the definition of principal diagnosis, either condition may be sequenced first, unless the circumstances of the admission, the therapy provided, the Tabular List, or the Alphabetic Index indicate otherwise.

C. Two or more diagnoses that equally meet the definition for principal diagnosis

In the unusual instance when two or more diagnoses equally meet the criteria for principal diagnosis as determined by the circumstances of admission, diagnostic workup and/or therapy provided, and the Alphabetic Index, Tabular List, or another coding guidelines does not provide sequencing direction, any one of the diagnoses may be sequenced first.

D. Two or more comparative or contrasting conditions.

In those rare instances when two or more contrasting or comparative diagnoses are documented as "either/or" (or similar terminology), they are coded as if the diagnoses were confirmed and the diagnoses are sequenced according to the circumstances of the admission. If no further determination can be made as to which diagnosis should be principal, either diagnosis may be sequenced first.

E. A symptom(s) followed by contrasting/ comparative diagnoses

GUIDELINE HAS BEEN DELETED EFFECTIVE OCTOBER 1, 2014

F. Original treatment plan not carried out

Sequence as the principal diagnosis the condition, which after study occasioned the admission to the hospital, even though treatment may not have been carried out due to unforeseen circumstances.

G. Complications of surgery and other medical care

When the admission is for treatment of a complication resulting from surgery or other medical care, the complication code is sequenced as the principal diagnosis. If the complication is classified to the T80-T88 series and the code lacks the necessary specificity in describing the complication, an additional code for the specific complication should be assigned.

H. Uncertain Diagnosis

If the diagnosis documented at the time of discharge is qualified as "probable," "suspected," "likely," "questionable," "possible," or "still to be ruled out," "compatible with," "consistent with," or other similar terms indicating uncertainty, code the condition as if it existed or was established. The bases for these guidelines are the diagnostic workup, arrangements for further workup or observation, and initial therapeutic approach that correspond most closely with the established diagnosis.

Note: This guideline is applicable only to inpatient admissions to short-term, acute, long-term care and psychiatric hospitals.

I. Admission from Observation Unit

1. Admission Following Medical Observation

When a patient is admitted to an observation unit for a medical condition, which either worsens or does not improve, and is subsequently admitted as an inpatient of the same hospital for this same medical condition, the principal diagnosis would be the medical condition which led to the hospital admission.

2. Admission Following Post-Operative Observation

When a patient is admitted to an observation unit to monitor a condition (or complication) that develops following outpatient surgery, and then is subsequently admitted as an inpatient of the same hospital, hospitals should apply the Uniform Hospital Discharge Data Set (UHDDS) definition of principal diagnosis as "that condition established after study to be chiefly responsible for occasioning the admission of the patient to the hospital for care."

J. Admission from Outpatient Surgery

When a patient receives surgery in the hospital's outpatient surgery department and is subsequently admitted for continuing inpatient care at the same hospital, the following guidelines should be followed in selecting the principal diagnosis for the inpatient admission:

- If the reason for the inpatient admission is a complication, assign the complication as the principal diagnosis.
- If no complication, or other condition, is documented as the reason for the inpatient admission, assign the reason for the outpatient surgery as the principal diagnosis.
- If the reason for the inpatient admission is another condition unrelated to the surgery, assign the unrelated condition as the principal diagnosis.

K. Admissions/Encounters for Rehabilitation

When the purpose for the admission/encounter is rehabilitation, sequence first the code for the condition for which the service is being performed. For example, for an admission/encounter for rehabilitation for right-sided dominant hemiplegia following a cerebrovascular infarction, report code I69.351, Hemiplegia and hemiparesis following cerebral infarction affecting right dominant side, as the first-listed or principal diagnosis.

If the condition for which the rehabilitation service is no longer present, report the appropriate aftercare code as the first-listed or principal diagnosis, unless the rehabilitation service is being provided following an injury. For rehabilitation services following active treatment of an injury, assign the injury code with the appropriate seventh character for subsequent encounter as the first-listed or principal diagnosis. For example, if a patient with severe degenerative osteoarthritis of the hip, underwent hip replacement and the current encounter/admission is for rehabilitation, report code Z47.1, Aftercare following joint replacement surgery, as the first-listed or principal diagnosis. If the patient requires rehabilitation post hip replacement for right intertrochanteric femur fracture, report code S72.141D, Displaced intertrochanteric fracture of right femur, subsequent encounter for closed fracture with routine healing, as the first-listed or principal diagnosis.

See Section I.C.21.c.7, Factors influencing health states and contact with health services, Aftercare.
See Section I.C.19.a, for additional information about the use of 7th characters for injury codes.

Section III. Reporting Additional Diagnoses

GENERAL RULES FOR OTHER (ADDITIONAL) DIAGNOSES

For reporting purposes the definition for "other diagnoses" is interpreted as additional conditions that affect patient care in terms of requiring:

    clinical evaluation; or
    therapeutic treatment; or
    diagnostic procedures; or
    extended length of hospital stay; or
    increased nursing care and/or monitoring.

The UHDDS item #11-b defines Other Diagnoses as "all conditions that coexist at the time of admission, that develop subsequently, or that affect the treatment received and/or the length of stay. Diagnoses that relate to an earlier episode which have no bearing on the current hospital stay are to be excluded." UHDDS definitions apply to inpatients in acute care, short-term, long term care and psychiatric hospital setting. The UHDDS definitions are used by acute care short-term hospitals to report inpatient data elements in a standardized manner. These data elements and their definitions can be found in the July 31, 1985, Federal Register (Vol. 50, No, 147), pp. 31038-40.

Since that time, the application of the UHDDS definitions has been expanded to include all nonoutpatient settings (acute care, short term, long term care and psychiatric hospitals; home health agencies; rehab facilities; nursing homes, etc. . .). The UHDDS definitions also apply to hospice services (all levels of care).

The following guidelines are to be applied in designating "other diagnoses" when neither the Alphabetic Index nor the Tabular List in ICD-10-CM provide direction. The listing of the diagnoses in the patient record is the responsibility of the attending provider.

A. Previous conditions

If the provider has included a diagnosis in the final diagnostic statement, such as the discharge summary or the face sheet, it should ordinarily be coded. Some providers include in the diagnostic statement resolved conditions or diagnoses and status-post procedures from previous admissions that have no bearing on the current stay. Such conditions are not to be reported and are coded only if required by hospital policy.

However, history codes (categories Z80-Z87) may be used as secondary codes if the historical condition or family history has an impact on current care or influences treatment.

B. Abnormal findings

Abnormal findings (laboratory, x-ray, pathologic, and other diagnostic results) are not coded and reported unless the provider indicates their clinical significance. If the findings are outside the normal range and the attending provider has ordered other tests to evaluate the condition or prescribed treatment, it is appropriate to ask the provider whether the abnormal finding should be added.

Please note: This differs from the coding practices in the outpatient setting for coding encounters for diagnostic tests that have been interpreted by a provider.

C. Uncertain Diagnosis

If the diagnosis documented at the time of discharge is qualified as "probable," "suspected," "likely," "questionable," "possible," or "still to be ruled out," "compatible with," "consistent with," or other similar terms indicating uncertainty, code the condition as if it existed or was established. The bases for these guidelines are the diagnostic workup, arrangements for further workup or observation, and initial therapeutic approach that correspond most closely with the established diagnosis.

Note: This guideline is applicable only to inpatient admissions to short-term, acute, long-term care and psychiatric hospitals.

Section IV. Diagnostic Coding and Reporting Guidelines for Outpatient Services

These coding guidelines for outpatient diagnoses have been approved for use by hospitals/ providers in coding and reporting hospital-based outpatient services and provider-based office visits. Guidelines in Section I, Conventions, general coding guidelines and chapter-specific guidelines, should also be applied for outpatient services and office visits.

Information about the use of certain abbreviations, punctuation, symbols, and other conventions used in the ICD-10-CM Tabular List (code numbers and titles), can be found in Section IA of these guidelines, under "Conventions Used in the Tabular List." Section I.B. contains general guidelines that apply to the entire classification. Section I.C. contains chapter-specific guidelines that correspond to the chapters as they are arranged in the classification. Information about the correct sequence to use in finding a code is also described in Section I.

The terms encounter and visit are often used interchangeably in describing outpatient service contacts and, therefore, appear together in these guidelines without distinguishing one from the other.

Though the conventions and general guidelines apply to all settings, coding guidelines for outpatient and provider reporting of diagnoses will vary in a number of instances from those for inpatient diagnoses, recognizing that:

The Uniform Hospital Discharge Data Set (UHDDS) definition of principal diagnosis does not apply to hospital-based outpatient services and provider-based office visits.

Coding guidelines for inconclusive diagnoses (probable, suspected, rule out, etc.) were developed for inpatient reporting and do not apply to outpatients.

A. Selection of first-listed condition

In the outpatient setting, the term first-listed diagnosis is used in lieu of principal diagnosis.

In determining the first-listed diagnosis the coding conventions of ICD-10-CM, as well as the general and disease specific guidelines take precedence over the outpatient guidelines.

Diagnoses often are not established at the time of the initial encounter/visit. It may take two or more visits before the diagnosis is confirmed.

The most critical rule involves beginning the search for the correct code assignment through the Alphabetic Index. Never begin searching initially in the Tabular List as this will lead to coding errors.

1. Outpatient Surgery

When a patient presents for outpatient surgery (same day surgery), code the reason for the surgery as the first-listed diagnosis (reason for the encounter), even if the surgery is not performed due to a contraindication.

2. Observation Stay

When a patient is admitted for observation for a medical condition, assign a code for the medical condition as the first-listed diagnosis.

When a patient presents for outpatient surgery and develops complications requiring admission to observation, code the reason for the surgery as the first reported diagnosis (reason for the encounter), followed by codes for the complications as secondary diagnoses.

B. Codes from A00.0 through T88.9, Z00-Z99, U00-U85

The appropriate code(s) from A00.0 through T88.9, Z00-Z99, **and U00-U85** must be used to identify diagnoses, symptoms, conditions, problems, complaints, or other reason(s) for the encounter/visit.

C. Accurate reporting of ICD-10-CM diagnosis codes

For accurate reporting of ICD-10-CM diagnosis codes, the documentation should describe the patient's condition, using terminology which includes specific diagnoses as well as symptoms, problems, or reasons for the encounter. There are ICD-10-CM codes to describe all of these.

D. Codes that describe symptoms and signs

Codes that describe symptoms and signs, as opposed to diagnoses, are acceptable for reporting purposes when a diagnosis has not been established (confirmed) by the provider. Chapter 18 of ICD-10-CM, Symptoms, Signs, and Abnormal Clinical and Laboratory Findings Not Elsewhere Classified (codes R00-R99) contains many, but not all codes for symptoms.

E. Encounters for circumstances other than a disease or injury

ICD-10-CM provides codes to deal with encounters for circumstances other than a disease or injury. The Factors Influencing Health Status and Contact with Health Services codes (Z00-Z99) are provided to deal with occasions when circumstances other than a disease or injury are recorded as diagnosis or problems.

See Section I.C.21., Factors influencing health status and contact with health services.

F. Level of Detail in Coding

1. ICD-10-CM codes with 3, 4, 5, 6 or 7 characters

ICD-10-CM is composed of codes with 3, 4, 5, 6 or 7 characters. Codes with three characters are included in ICD-10-CM as the heading of a category of codes that may be further subdivided by the use of 4th, 5th, 6th or 7th characters to provide greater specificity.

2. Use of full number of characters required for a code

A 3-character code is to be used only if it is not further subdivided. A code is invalid if it has not been coded to the full number of characters required for that code, including the 7th character, if applicable.

3. Highest level of specificity

Code to the highest level of specificity when supported by the medical record documentation.

G. ICD-10-CM code for the diagnosis, condition, problem, or other reason for encounter/visit

List first the ICD-10-CM code for the diagnosis, condition, problem, or other reason for encounter/visit shown in the medical record to be chiefly responsible for the services provided. List additional codes that describe any coexisting conditions. In some cases the first-listed diagnosis may be a symptom when a diagnosis has not been established (confirmed) by the provider.

H. Uncertain diagnosis

Do not code diagnoses documented as "probable," "suspected," "questionable," "ruled out," "compatible with," "consistent with," or "working diagnosis" or other similar terms indicating uncertainty. Rather, code the condition(s) to the highest degree of certainty for that encounter/visit, such as symptoms, signs, abnormal test results, or other reason for the visit.

Please note: This differs from the coding practices used by short-term, acute care, long-term care and psychiatric hospitals.

I. Chronic diseases

Chronic diseases treated on an ongoing basis may be coded and reported as many times as the patient receives treatment and care for the condition(s)

J. Code all documented conditions that coexist

Code all documented conditions that coexist at the time of the encounter/visit, and require or affect patient care treatment or management. Do not code conditions that were previously treated and no longer exist. However, history codes (categories Z80-Z87) may be used as secondary codes if the historical condition or family history has an impact on current care or influences treatment.

K. Patients receiving diagnostic services only

For patients receiving diagnostic services only during an encounter/visit, sequence first the diagnosis, condition, problem, or other reason for encounter/visit shown in the medical record to be chiefly responsible for the outpatient services provided during the encounter/visit. Codes for other diagnoses (e.g., chronic conditions) may be sequenced as additional diagnoses.

For encounters for routine laboratory/radiology testing in the absence of any signs, symptoms, or associated diagnosis, assign Z01.89, Encounter for other specified special examinations. If routine testing is performed during the same encounter as a test to evaluate a sign, symptom, or diagnosis, it is appropriate to assign both the Z code and the code describing the reason for the non-routine test.

For outpatient encounters for diagnostic tests that have been interpreted by a physician, and the final report is available at the time of coding, code any confirmed or definitive diagnosis(es) documented in the interpretation. Do not code related signs and symptoms as additional diagnoses.

Please note: This differs from the coding practice in the hospital inpatient setting regarding abnormal findings on test results.

L. **Patients receiving therapeutic services only**
For patients receiving therapeutic services only during an encounter/visit, sequence first the diagnosis, condition, problem, or other reason for encounter/visit shown in the medical record to be chiefly responsible for the outpatient services provided during the encounter/visit. Codes for other diagnoses (e.g., chronic conditions) may be sequenced as additional diagnoses.

The only exception to this rule is that when the primary reason for the admission/encounter is chemotherapy or radiation therapy, the appropriate Z code for the service is listed first, and the diagnosis or problem for which the service is being performed listed second.

M. **Patients receiving preoperative evaluations only**
For patients receiving preoperative evaluations only, sequence first a code from subcategory Z01.81, Encounter for pre-procedural examinations, to describe the pre-op consultations. Assign a code for the condition to describe the reason for the surgery as an additional diagnosis. Code also any findings related to the pre-op evaluation.

N. **Ambulatory surgery**
For ambulatory surgery, code the diagnosis for which the surgery was performed. If the postoperative diagnosis is known to be different from the preoperative diagnosis at the time the diagnosis is confirmed, select the postoperative diagnosis for coding, since it is the most definitive.

O. **Routine outpatient prenatal visits**
See Section I.C.15., Routine outpatient prenatal visits.

P. **Encounters for general medical examinations with abnormal findings**
The subcategories for encounters for general medical examinations, Z00.0- and encounter for routine child health examination, Z00.12-, provide codes for with and without abnormal findings. Should a general medical examination result in an abnormal finding, the code for general medical examination with abnormal finding should be assigned as the first-listed diagnosis. An examination with abnormal findings refers to a condition/diagnosis that is newly identified or a change in severity of a chronic condition (such as uncontrolled hypertension, or an acute exacerbation of chronic obstructive pulmonary disease) during a routine physical examination. A secondary code for the abnormal finding should also be coded.

Q. **Encounters for routine health screenings**
See Section I.C.21., Factors influencing health status and contact with health services, Screening

Appendix I
Present on Admission Reporting Guidelines

Introduction

These guidelines are to be used as a supplement to the *ICD-10-CM Official Guidelines for Coding and Reporting* to facilitate the assignment of the Present on Admission (POA) indicator for each diagnosis and external cause of injury code reported on claim forms (UB-04 and 837 Institutional).

These guidelines are not intended to replace any guidelines in the main body of the *ICD-10-CM Official Guidelines for Coding and Reporting*. The POA guidelines are not intended to provide guidance on when a condition should be coded, but rather, how to apply the POA indicator to the final set of diagnosis codes that have been assigned in accordance with Sections I, II, and III of the official coding guidelines. Subsequent to the assignment of the ICD-10-CM codes, the POA indicator should then be assigned to those conditions that have been coded.

As stated in the Introduction to the ICD-10-CM Official Guidelines for Coding and Reporting, a joint effort between the healthcare provider and the coder is essential to achieve complete and accurate documentation, code assignment, and reporting of diagnoses and procedures. The importance of consistent, complete documentation in the medical record cannot be overemphasized. Medical record documentation from any provider involved in the care and treatment of the patient may be used to support the determination of whether a condition was present on admission or not. In the context of the official coding guidelines, the term "provider" means a physician or any qualified healthcare practitioner who is legally accountable for establishing the patient's diagnosis.

These guidelines are not a substitute for the provider's clinical judgment as to the determination of whether a condition was/was not present on admission. The provider should be queried regarding issues related to the linking of signs/symptoms, timing of test results, and the timing of findings.

Please see the CDC website for the detailed list of ICD-10-CM codes that do not require the use of a POA indicator (https://www.cdc.gov/nchs/icd/icd10cm.htm) (https://www.cms.gov/Medicare/Coding/ICD10/2018-ICD-10-CM-and-GEMs.html). The codes and categories on this exempt list are for circumstances regarding the healthcare encounter or factors influencing health status that do not represent a current disease or injury or that describe conditions that are always present on admission.

General Reporting Requirements

All claims involving inpatient admissions to general acute care hospitals or other facilities that are subject to a law or regulation mandating collection of present on admission information.

Present on admission is defined as present at the time the order for inpatient admission occurs—conditions that develop during an outpatient encounter, including emergency department, observation, or outpatient surgery, are considered as present on admission.

POA indicator is assigned to principal and secondary diagnoses (as defined in Section II of the Official Guidelines for Coding and Reporting) and the external cause of injury codes.

Issues related to inconsistent, missing, conflicting or unclear documentation must still be resolved by the provider.

If a condition would not be coded and reported based on UHDDS definitions and current official coding guidelines, then the POA indicator would not be reported.

Reporting Options

Y - Yes

N - No

U - Unknown

W - Clinically undetermined

Unreported/Not used - (Exempt from POA reporting)

Reporting Definitions

Y = present at the time of inpatient admission

N = not present at the time of inpatient admission

U = documentation is insufficient to determine if condition is present on admission

W = provider is unable to clinically determine whether condition was present on admission or not

Timeframe for POA Identification and Documentation

There is no required timeframe as to when a provider (per the definition of "provider" used in these guidelines) must identify or document a condition to be present on admission. In some clinical situations, it may not be possible for a provider to make a definitive diagnosis (or a condition may not be recognized or reported by the patient) for a period of time after admission. In some cases it may be several days before the provider arrives at a definitive diagnosis. This does not mean that the condition was not present on admission. Determination of whether the condition was present on admission or not will be based on the applicable POA guideline as identified in this document, or on the provider's best clinical judgment.

If at the time of code assignment the documentation is unclear as to whether a condition was present on admission or not, it is appropriate to query the provider for clarification.

Assigning the POA Indicator

Condition is on the "Exempt from Reporting" list

Leave the "present on admission" field blank if the condition is on the list of ICD-10-CM codes for which this field is not applicable. This is the only circumstance in which the field may be left blank.

POA Explicitly Documented

Assign "Y" for any condition the provider explicitly documents as being present on admission.

Assign "N" for any condition the provider explicitly documents as not present at the time of admission.

Conditions diagnosed prior to inpatient admission

Assign "Y" for conditions that were diagnosed prior to admission (example: hypertension, diabetes mellitus, asthma)

Conditions diagnosed during the admission but clearly present before admission

Assign "Y" for conditions diagnosed during the admission that were clearly present but not diagnosed until after admission occurred.

Diagnoses subsequently confirmed after admission are considered present on admission if at the time of admission they are documented as suspected, possible, rule out, differential diagnosis, or constitute an underlying cause of a symptom that is present at the time of admission.

Condition develops during outpatient encounter prior to inpatient admission

Assign "Y" for any condition that develops during an outpatient encounter prior to a written order for inpatient admission.

Documentation does not indicate whether condition was present on admission

Assign "U" when the medical record documentation is unclear as to whether the condition was present on admission. "U" should not be routinely assigned and used only in very limited circumstances. Coders are encouraged to query the providers when the documentation is unclear.

Documentation states that it cannot be determined whether the condition was or was not present on admission

Assign "W" when the medical record documentation indicates that it cannot be clinically determined whether or not the condition was present on admission.

Chronic condition with acute exacerbation during the admission

If a single code identifies both the chronic condition and the acute exacerbation, see POA guidelines pertaining to codes that contain multiple clinical concepts.

If a single code only identifies the chronic condition and not the acute exacerbation (e.g., acute exacerbation of chronic leukemia), assign "Y."

Conditions documented as possible, probable, suspected, or rule out at the time of discharge

If the final diagnosis contains a possible, probable, suspected, or rule out diagnosis, and this diagnosis was based on signs, symptoms or clinical findings suspected at the time of inpatient admission, assign "Y."

If the final diagnosis contains a possible, probable, suspected, or rule out diagnosis, and this diagnosis was based on signs, symptoms or clinical findings that were not present on admission, assign "N".

Conditions documented as impending or threatened at the time of discharge

If the final diagnosis contains an impending or threatened diagnosis, and this diagnosis is based on symptoms or clinical findings that were present on admission, assign "Y".

If the final diagnosis contains an impending or threatened diagnosis, and this diagnosis is based on symptoms or clinical findings that were not present on admission, assign "N".

Acute and Chronic Conditions

Assign "Y" for acute conditions that are present at time of admission and "N" for acute conditions that are not present at time of admission.

Assign "Y" for chronic conditions, even though the condition may not be diagnosed until after admission.

If a single code identifies both an acute and chronic condition, see the POA guidelines for codes that contain multiple clinical concepts.

Codes That Contain Multiple Clinical Concepts

Assign "N" if at least one of the clinical concepts included in the code was not present on admission (e.g., COPD with acute exacerbation and the exacerbation was not present on admission; gastric ulcer that does not start bleeding until after admission; asthma patient develops status asthmaticus after admission).

Assign "Y" if all of the clinical concepts included in the code were present on admission (e.g., duodenal ulcer that perforates prior to admission).

For infection codes that include the causal organism, assign "Y" if the infection (or signs of the infection) were present on admission, even though the culture results may not be known until after admission (e.g., patient is admitted with pneumonia and the provider documents Pseudomonas as the causal organism a few days later).

Same Diagnosis Code for Two or More Conditions

When the same ICD-10-CM diagnosis code applies to two or more conditions during the same encounter (e.g., two separate conditions classified to the same ICD-10-CM diagnosis code):

Assign "Y" if all conditions represented by the single ICD-10-CM code were present on admission (e.g., bilateral unspecified age-related cataracts).

Assign "N" if any of the conditions represented by the single ICD-10-CM code was not present on admission (e.g., traumatic secondary and recurrent hemorrhage and seroma is assigned to a single code T79.2, but only one of the conditions was present on admission).

Obstetrical conditions

Whether or not the patient delivers during the current hospitalization does not affect assignment of the POA indicator. The determining factor for POA assignment is whether the pregnancy complication or obstetrical condition described by the code was present at the time of admission or not.

If the pregnancy complication or obstetrical condition was present on admission (e.g., patient admitted in preterm labor), assign "Y".

If the pregnancy complication or obstetrical condition was not present on admission (e.g., 2nd degree laceration during delivery, postpartum hemorrhage that occurred during current hospitalization, fetal distress develops after admission), assign "N".

If the obstetrical code includes more than one diagnosis and any of the diagnoses identified by the code were not present on admission assign "N".

GUIDELINES (ICD-10-CM)

(e.g., Category O11, Pre-existing hypertension with pre-eclampsia)

Perinatal conditions

Newborns are not considered to be admitted until after birth. Therefore, any condition present at birth or that developed in utero is considered present at admission and should be assigned "Y". This includes conditions that occur during delivery (e.g., injury during delivery, meconium aspiration, exposure to streptococcus B in the vaginal canal).

Congenital conditions and anomalies

Assign "Y" for congenital conditions and anomalies except for categories Q00-Q99, Congenital anomalies, which are on the exempt list. Congenital conditions are always considered present on admission.

External cause of injury codes

Assign "Y" for any external cause code representing an external cause of morbidity that occurred prior to inpatient admission (e.g., patient fell out of bed at home, patient fell out of bed in emergency room prior to admission).

Assign "N" for any external cause code representing an external cause of morbidity that occurred during inpatient hospitalization (e.g., patient fell out of hospital bed during hospital stay, patient experienced an adverse reaction to a medication administered after inpatient admission).

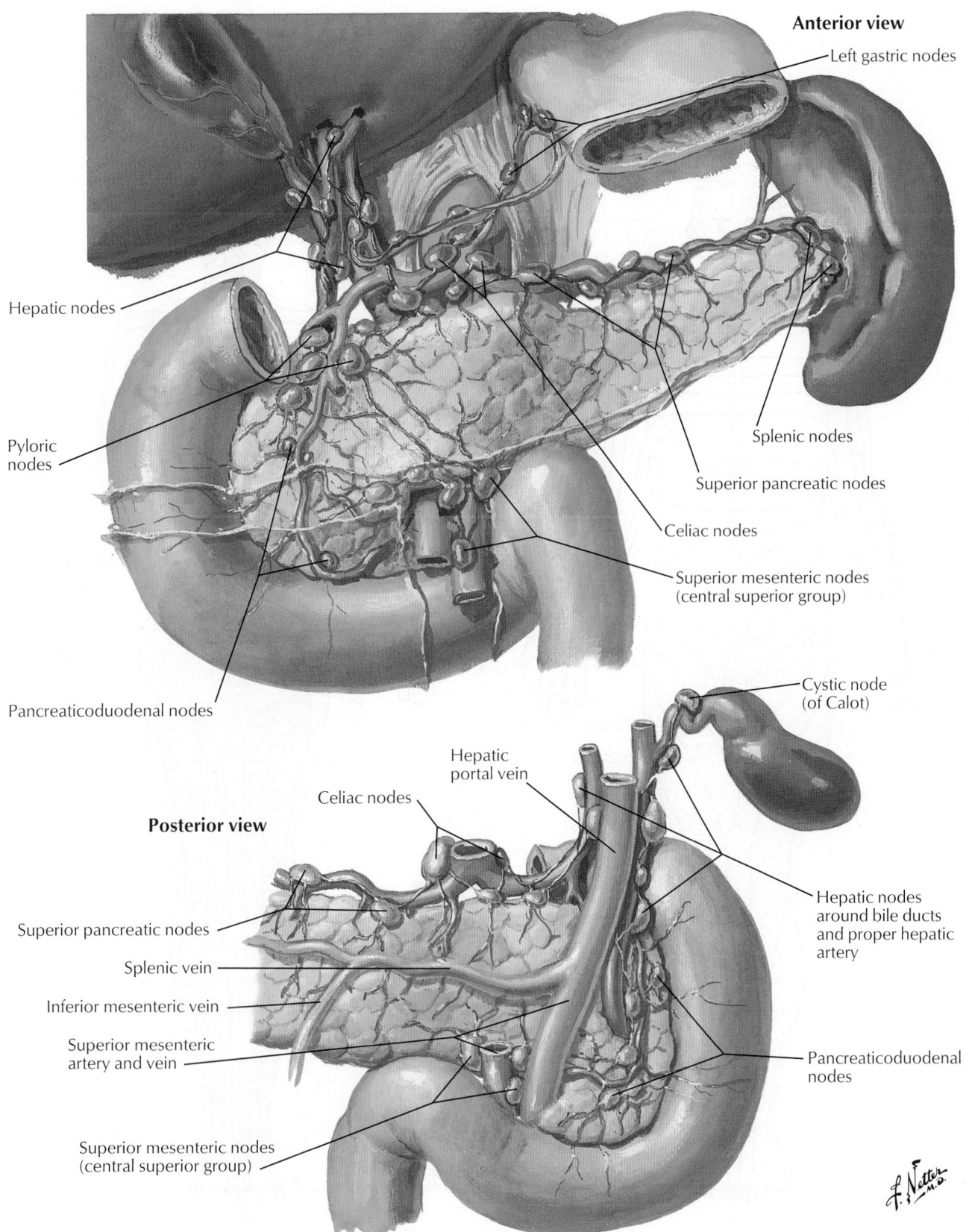

Anterior view

Left gastric nodes

Hepatic nodes

Pyloric nodes

Splenic nodes

Superior pancreatic nodes

Celiac nodes

Superior mesenteric nodes (central superior group)

Pancreaticoduodenal nodes

Cystic node (of Calot)

Hepatic portal vein

Celiac nodes

Posterior view

Hepatic nodes around bile ducts and proper hepatic artery

Superior pancreatic nodes

Splenic vein

Inferior mesenteric vein

Superior mesenteric artery and vein

Pancreaticoduodenal nodes

Superior mesenteric nodes (central superior group)

f. Netter M.D.

Plate 1 Lymph Vessels and Nodes of Pancreas. (Netter: Atlas of Human Anatomy, 4 ed, 2006, Saunders. Plate 315)

Levels of principal dermatomes

C5	Clavicles
C5, 6, 7	Lateral parts of upper limbs
C8, T1	Medial sides of upper limbs
C6	Thumb
C6, 7, 8	Hand
C8	Ring and little fingers
T4	Level of nipples
T10	Level of umbilicus
L1	Inguinal or groin regions
L1, 2, 3, 4	Anterior and inner surfaces of lower limbs
L4, 5, S1	Foot
L4	Medial side of great toe
S1, 2, L5	Posterior and other surfaces of lower limbs
S1	Lateral margin of foot and little toe
S2, 3, 4	Perineum

Plate 2 Schematic demarcation of Dermatomes. (Miller MD, Hart JA, MacKnight JM: Essential Orthopaedics, ed 2, Philadelphia, 2020, Elsevier.)

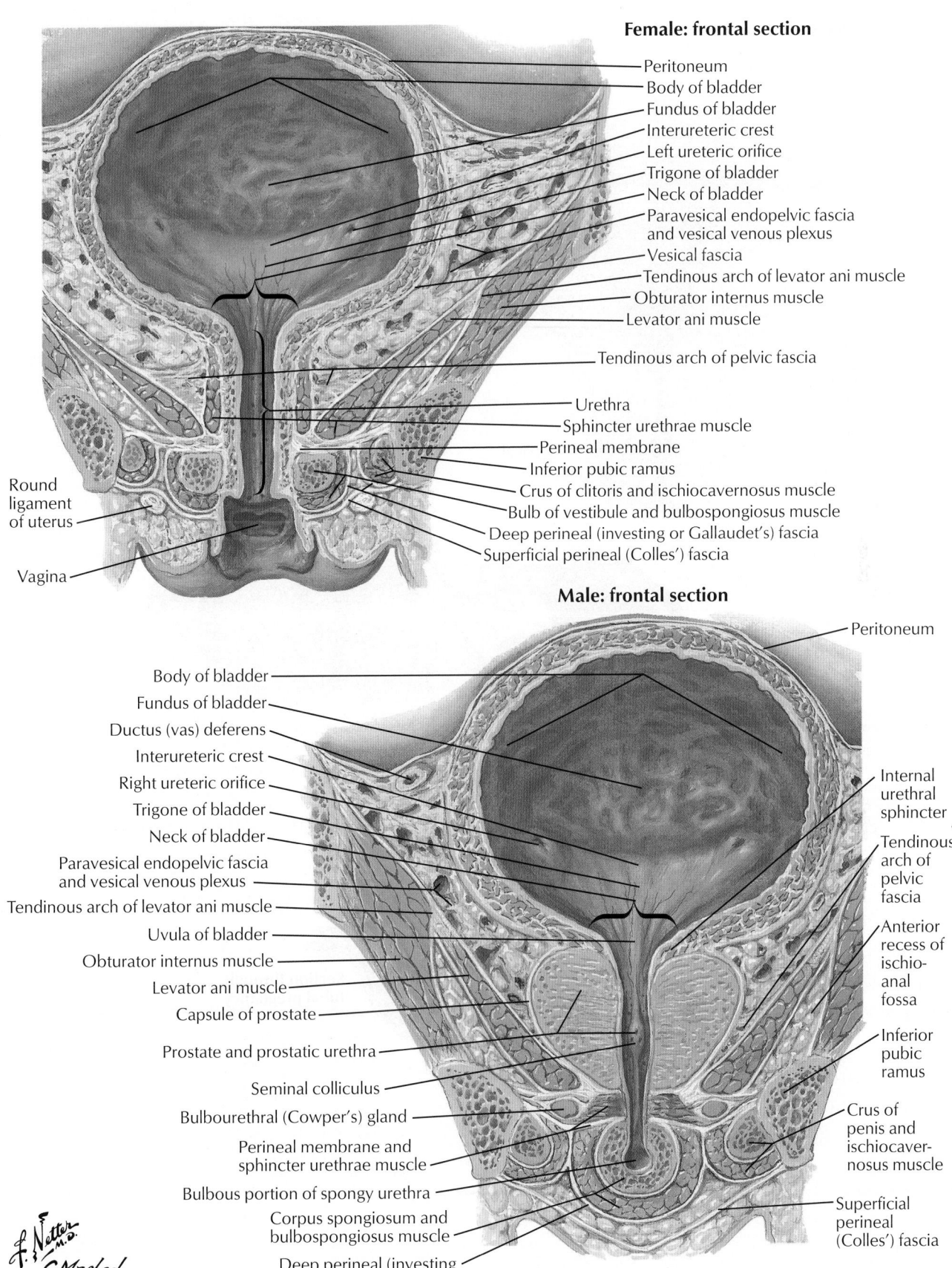

Female: frontal section

- Peritoneum
- Body of bladder
- Fundus of bladder
- Interureteric crest
- Left ureteric orifice
- Trigone of bladder
- Neck of bladder
- Paravesical endopelvic fascia and vesical venous plexus
- Vesical fascia
- Tendinous arch of levator ani muscle
- Obturator internus muscle
- Levator ani muscle
- Tendinous arch of pelvic fascia
- Urethra
- Sphincter urethrae muscle
- Perineal membrane
- Inferior pubic ramus
- Crus of clitoris and ischiocavernosus muscle
- Bulb of vestibule and bulbospongiosus muscle
- Deep perineal (investing or Gallaudet's) fascia
- Superficial perineal (Colles') fascia

Round ligament of uterus

Vagina

Male: frontal section

- Peritoneum
- Body of bladder
- Fundus of bladder
- Ductus (vas) deferens
- Interureteric crest
- Right ureteric orifice
- Trigone of bladder
- Neck of bladder
- Paravesical endopelvic fascia and vesical venous plexus
- Tendinous arch of levator ani muscle
- Uvula of bladder
- Obturator internus muscle
- Levator ani muscle
- Capsule of prostate
- Prostate and prostatic urethra
- Seminal colliculus
- Bulbourethral (Cowper's) gland
- Perineal membrane and sphincter urethrae muscle
- Bulbous portion of spongy urethra
- Corpus spongiosum and bulbospongiosus muscle
- Deep perineal (investing or Gallaudet's) fascia

- Internal urethral sphincter
- Tendinous arch of pelvic fascia
- Anterior recess of ischio-anal fossa
- Inferior pubic ramus
- Crus of penis and ischiocavernosus muscle
- Superficial perineal (Colles') fascia

ANATOMY ILLUSTRATIONS

Plate 3 Urinary Bladder: Female and Male. (Netter: Atlas of Human Anatomy, 4 ed, 2006, Saunders. Plate 366.)

Sites of ectopic implantation

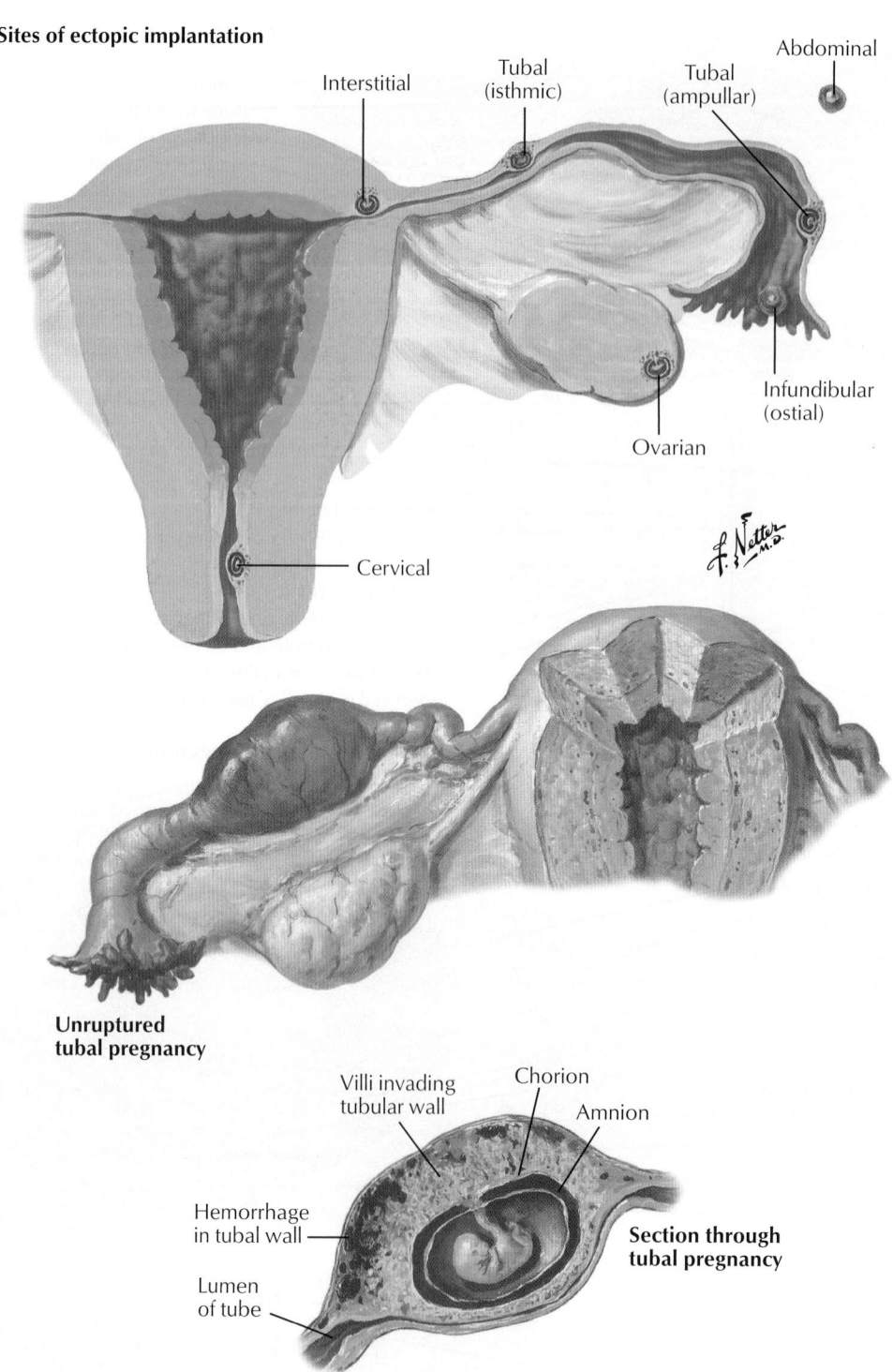

Interstitial

Tubal (isthmic)

Tubal (ampullar)

Abdominal

Infundibular (ostial)

Ovarian

Cervical

Unruptured tubal pregnancy

Villi invading tubular wall

Chorion

Amnion

Hemorrhage in tubal wall

Lumen of tube

Section through tubal pregnancy

Plate 4 Ectopic Pregnancy. (Netter: Atlas of Human Anatomy, 4 ed, 2006, Saunders. Plate 375)

Skin of penis

Superficial fascia of penis (Colles' fascia)

Deep (Buck's) fascia of penis

Testicular artery

Ductus deferens

Artery to ductus deferens

Genital branch of genitofemoral nerve

Pampiniform (venous) plexus

Epididymis

Appendix of epididymis

Appendix of testis

Testis (covered by visceral layer of tunica vaginalis)

Parietal layer of tunica vaginalis

Superficial inguinal ring

External spermatic fascia

Cremaster muscle and fascia

Septum of scrotum (formed by dartos fascia)

Superficial (dartos) fascia of scrotum

Skin of scrotum

Superficial (dartos) fascia of scrotum

External spermatic fascia

Cremaster muscle and fascia

Internal spermatic fascia

Parietal layer of tunica vaginalis

Epididymis

Testis (covered by visceral layer of tunica vaginalis)

Skin of scrotum

Plate 5   Scrotum and Contents. (Netter: Atlas of Human Anatomy, 4 ed, 2006, Saunders. Plate 387)

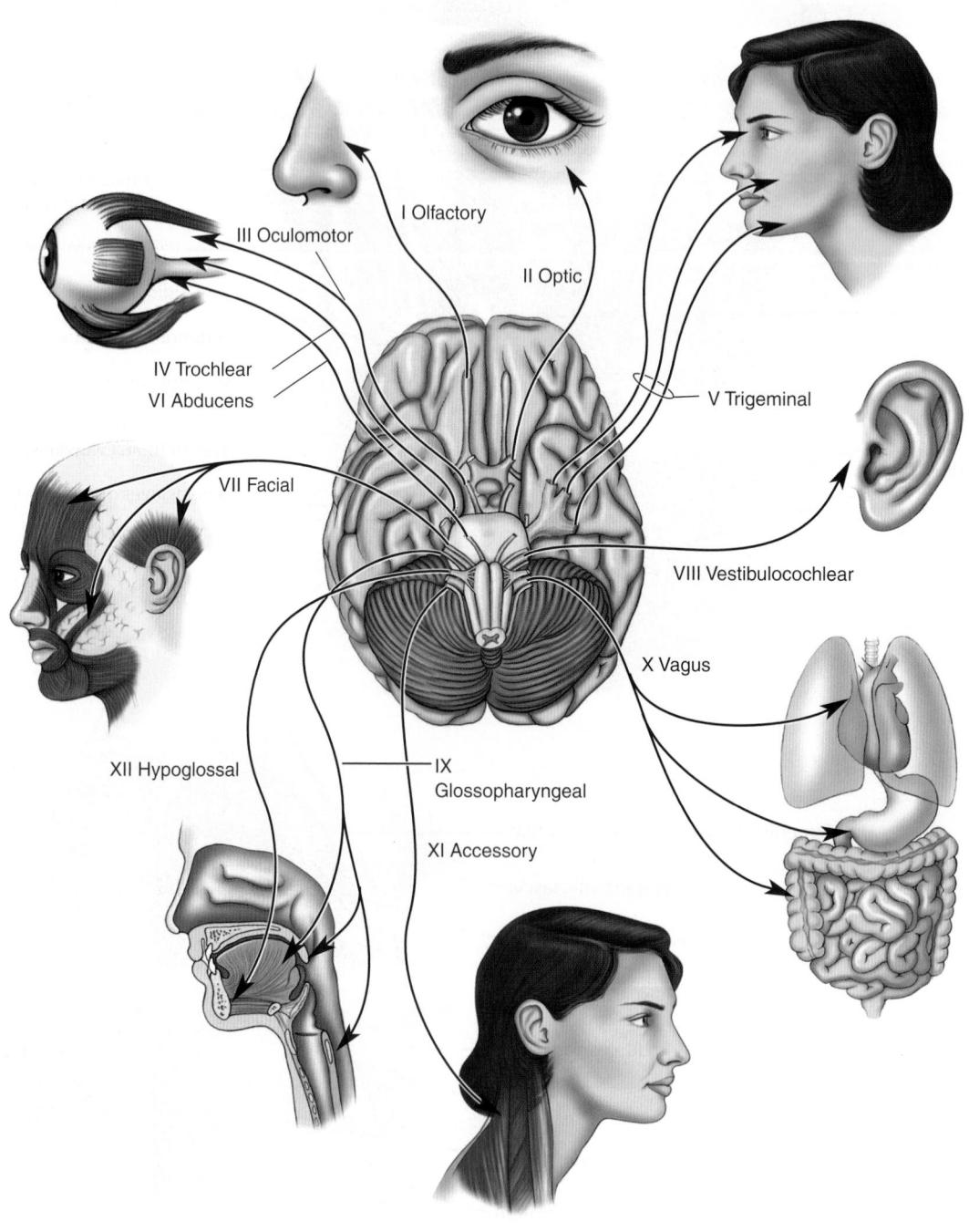

III Oculomotor

I Olfactory

II Optic

IV Trochlear
VI Abducens

V Trigeminal

VII Facial

VIII Vestibulocochlear

XII Hypoglossal

IX
Glossopharyngeal

XI Accessory

X Vagus

Plate 6 Cranial Nerves (12 pairs) are known by their numbers (Roman numerals) and names. (Herlihy BL: The Human Body in Health and Illness, ed 6, St. Louis, 2018, Elsevier.)

Superior view

Medial branch } Supraorbital nerve
Lateral branch

Supratrochlear nerve
Medial rectus muscle
Superior oblique muscle
Infratrochlear nerve
Nasociliary nerve
Trochlear nerve (IV)
Common tendinous ring
Ophthalmic nerve (V₁)
Optic nerve (II)
Internal carotid artery and nerve plexus
Oculomotor nerve (III)
Trochlear nerve (IV)
Abducent nerve (VI)
Tentorium cerebelli

Levator palpebrae superioris muscle
Superior rectus muscle
Lacrimal gland
Lacrimal nerve
Lateral rectus muscle
Frontal nerve
Maxillary nerve (V₂)
Meningeal branch of maxillary nerve
Mandibular nerve (V₃)
Lesser petrosal nerve
Meningeal branch of mandibular nerve
Greater petrosal nerve
Trigeminal (semilunar) ganglion
Tentorial (meningeal) branch of ophthalmic nerve

Superior view:
levator palpebrae superioris, superior rectus, and superior oblique muscles partially cut away

Supratrochlear nerve *(cut)*
Supraorbital nerve branches *(cut)*
Infratrochlear nerve
Anterior ethmoidal nerve
Optic nerve (II)
Posterior ethmoidal nerve
Superior branch of oculomotor nerve (III) *(cut)*
Nasociliary nerve
Internal carotid plexus
Trochlear nerve (IV) *(cut)*
Oculomotor nerve (III)
Abducent nerve (VI)

Long ciliary nerves
Short ciliary nerves
Lacrimal nerve
Ciliary ganglion
Parasympathetic root of ciliary ganglion (from inferior branch of oculomotor nerve)
Sympathetic root of ciliary ganglion (from internal carotid plexus)
Sensory root of ciliary ganglion (from nasociliary nerve)
Branches to inferior and medial rectus muscles
Abducent nerve (VI)
Inferior branch of oculomotor nerve (III)
Lacrimal nerve
Frontal nerve *(cut)*
Ophthalmic nerve (V₁)

Plate 7   Nerves of Orbit. (Netter: Atlas of Human Anatomy, 4 ed, 2006, Saunders. Plate 86)

Proper palmar digital nerves (median nerve)

Medial two lumbricals
innervated by ulnar nerve

Cutaneous innervation
of the median nerve in the hand

Cutaneous innervation
of the dorsal branch of
the ulnar nerve

Cutaneous innervation
of the palmar branch of
the median nerve

Palmar view

Dorsal view

Lateral two lumbricals
innervated by median nerve

Proper palmar
digital nerve
(ulnar nerve)

Intrinsic muscles
innervated by
ulnar nerve except
the thenar muscles
and the two lateral
lumbricals

Common palmar
digital nerve

Hypothenar
muscles
innervated by
ulnar nerve

Palmaris brevis

Deep branch of the
ulnar nerve

Superficial branch of the
ulnar nerve

Palmar branch of the
ulnar nerve

Ulnar nerve

Ulna

Common palmar digital nerves
(median nerve)

Cutaneous innervation
of the superficial branch of
the ulnar nerve in
the hand

Thenar muscles
innervated by median nerve

Recurrent branch of median nerve

Cutaneous innervation
of the palmar branch of
the ulnar nerve

Palmar view

Palmar branch of the
median nerve

Median nerve

Radius

Cutaneous innervation
of the median nerve in the hand

**Innervation of the hand, median and ulnar nerves
(palmar view)**

Dorsal view

Plate 8   Innervation of the Hand: Median and Ulnar Nerves (From Drake RL, Vogl AW, Mitchell AWM, Tibbitts RM, Richardson PE: Gray's Atlas of Anatomy, ed 2, Philadelphia, 2015, Churchill Livingstone.)

ANATOMY ILLUSTRATIONS

Biceps brachii

Posterior cutaneous nerve of forearm (cut) (from radial nerve)

Lateral cutaneous nerve of forearm (cut) (from musculocutaneous nerve)

Biceps brachii tendon

Radial artery

Brachioradialis

Radial artery

Palmaris longus tendon

Median nerve

Thenar muscles

Palmar branch of median nerve

Palmar aponeurosis

Ulnar nerve

Medial cutaneous nerve of forearm (from medial cord of brachial plexus)

Median nerve

Brachial artery

Medial epicondyle

Bicipital aponeurosis

Radial nerve

Brachial artery

Lateral epicondyle

Radial recurrent artery

Deep branch radial nerve

Radial artery

Supinator

Superficial branch radial nerve

Common interosseous artery

Posterior interosseous artery

Interosseous membrane

Pronator teres (cut)

Ulnar artery

Perforating branches of anterior interosseous artery

Brachioradialis tendon (cut)

Palmar branch of ulnar nerve

Hypothenar muscles

Median nerve

Flexor carpi radialis tendon (cut)

Flexor retinaculum

Superficial palmar branch of radial artery

Palmar branch of median nerve

Ulnar nerve

Median nerve

Recurrent interosseous artery

Ulnar nerve

Humeral head of pronator teres (cut)

Posterior interosseous artery

Anterior ulnar recurrent artery

Humeral head of flexor carpi ulnaris

Posterior ulnar recurrent artery

Ulnar head of pronator teres

Ulnar artery

Anterior interosseous nerve

Anterior interosseous artery

Radial artery

Interosseous membrane

Flexor digitorum superficialis (cut)

Flexor digitorum profundus

Superficial palmar branch of radial artery

Dorsal branch of ulnar nerve

Flexor carpi ulnaris tendon (cut)

Ulnar nerve

Palmar branch of ulnar nerve

Deep palmar branch of ulnar artery

Deep palmar arch

Superficial palmar arch

Superior ulnar collateral artery

Inferior ulnar collateral artery

Radial collateral artery

Brachial artery

Radial recurrent artery

Anterior ulnar recurrent artery

Posterior ulnar recurrent artery

Common interosseous artery

Anterior interosseous artery

Ulnar artery

Radius

Ulna

Superficial palmar branch of radial artery

Pisiform

Superficial palmar arch

Deep palmar arch

Arteries and nerves of forearm (anterior view)

ANATOMY ILLUSTRATIONS

Plate 9 Arteries and Nerves of the Forearm (Anterior View) (From Drake RL, Vogl AW, Mitchell AWM, Tibbitts RM, Richardson PE: Gray's Atlas of Anatomy, ed 2, Philadelphia, 2015, Churchill Livingstone.)

Lateral cutaneous branch of subcostal nerve

Inguinal ligament (Poupart's)

Superficial circumflex iliac vein

Femoral branches of genitofemoral nerve

Lateral femoral cutaneous nerve

Saphenous opening (fossa ovalis)

Fascia lata

Anterior cutaneous branches of femoral nerve

Patellar nerve plexus

Branches of lateral sural cutaneous nerve (from common fibular [peroneal] nerve)

Deep fascia of leg (crural fascia)

Superficial fibular (peroneal) nerve
Medial dorsal cutaneous branch

Intermediate dorsal cutaneous branch

Small saphenous vein and lateral dorsal cutaneous nerve (from sural nerve)

Lateral dorsal digital nerve and vein of 5th toe

Dorsal metatarsal veins

Dorsal digital nerves and veins

Superficial epigastric vein

Ilioinguinal nerve (scrotal branch) (usually passes through superficial inguinal ring)

Genital branch of genitofemoral nerve

Femoral vein

Superficial external pudendal vein

Accessory saphenous vein

Great saphenous vein

Cutaneous branches of obturator nerve

Infrapatellar branch of saphenous nerve

Saphenous nerve (terminal branch of femoral nerve)

Great saphenous vein

Dorsal digital nerves

Dorsal venous arch

Dorsal digital nerve and vein of medial side of great toe

Dorsal digital branch of deep fibular (peroneal) nerve

ANATOMY ILLUSTRATIONS

Plate 10 Superficial Nerves and Veins of Lower Limb: Anterior View. (Netter: Atlas of Human Anatomy, 4 ed, 2006, Saunders. Plate 544)

64

Lateral cutaneous branch of iliohypogastric nerve

Iliac crest

Medial cluneal nerves (from dorsal rami of S1, 2, 3)

Superior cluneal nerves (from dorsal rami of L1, 2, 3)

Inferior cluneal nerves (from posterior femoral cutaneous nerve)

Perforating cutaneous nerve (from dorsal rami of S1, 2, 3)

Branches of posterior femoral cutaneous nerve

Branches of lateral femoral cutaneous nerve

Accessory saphenous vein

Branch of femoral cutaneous nerve

Branch of cutaneous branch of femoral nerve

Terminal branches of posterior femoral cutaneous nerve

Great saphenous vein

Lateral sural cutaneous nerve (from common fibular [peroneal] nerve)

Small saphenous vein

Sural communicating nerve

Branches of saphenous nerve

Medial sural cutaneous nerve (from tibial nerve)

Sural nerve

Lateral calcaneal branches of sural nerve

Medial calcaneal branches of tibial nerve

Lateral dorsal cutaneous nerve (continuation of sural nerve)

Plantar cutaneous branches of medial plantar nerve

Plantar cutaneous branches of lateral plantar nerve

Plate 11 Superficial Nerves and Veins of Lower Limb: Posterior View. (Netter: Atlas of Human Anatomy, 4 ed, 2006, Saunders. Plate 545)

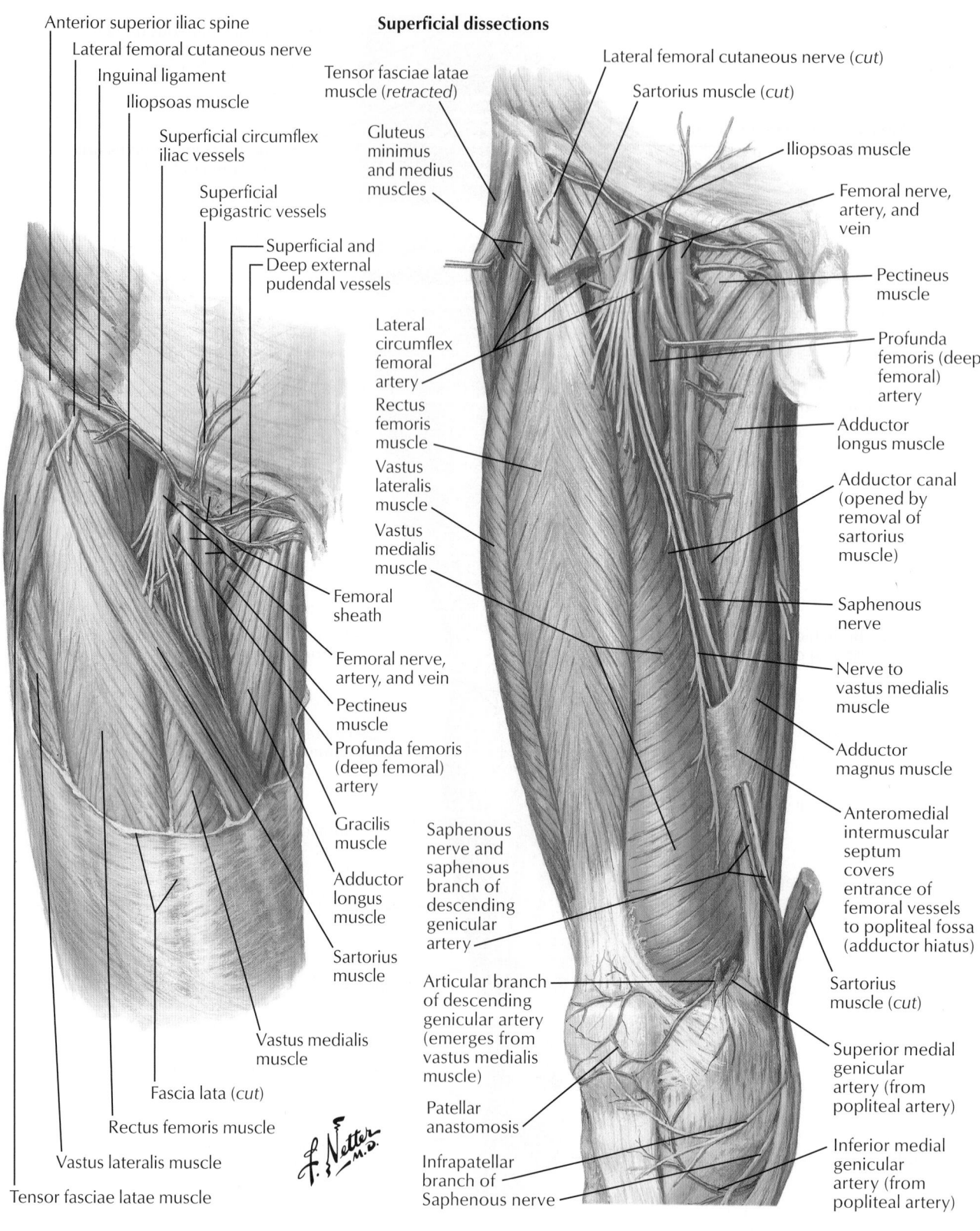

Superficial dissections

Anterior superior iliac spine

Lateral femoral cutaneous nerve

Inguinal ligament

Iliopsoas muscle

Superficial circumflex iliac vessels

Superficial epigastric vessels

Superficial and Deep external pudendal vessels

Tensor fasciae latae muscle (*retracted*)

Gluteus minimus and medius muscles

Lateral circumflex femoral artery

Rectus femoris muscle

Vastus lateralis muscle

Vastus medialis muscle

Femoral sheath

Femoral nerve, artery, and vein

Pectineus muscle

Profunda femoris (deep femoral) artery

Gracilis muscle

Adductor longus muscle

Sartorius muscle

Saphenous nerve and saphenous branch of descending genicular artery

Articular branch of descending genicular artery (emerges from vastus medialis muscle)

Patellar anastomosis

Infrapatellar branch of Saphenous nerve

Lateral femoral cutaneous nerve (*cut*)

Sartorius muscle (*cut*)

Iliopsoas muscle

Femoral nerve, artery, and vein

Pectineus muscle

Profunda femoris (deep femoral) artery

Adductor longus muscle

Adductor canal (opened by removal of sartorius muscle)

Saphenous nerve

Nerve to vastus medialis muscle

Adductor magnus muscle

Anteromedial intermuscular septum covers entrance of femoral vessels to popliteal fossa (adductor hiatus)

Sartorius muscle (*cut*)

Superior medial genicular artery (from popliteal artery)

Inferior medial genicular artery (from popliteal artery)

Vastus medialis muscle

Fascia lata (*cut*)

Rectus femoris muscle

Vastus lateralis muscle

Tensor fasciae latae muscle

Plate 12 Arteries and Nerves of Thigh: Anterior Views. (Netter: Atlas of Human Anatomy, 4 ed, 2006, Saunders. Plate 500)

Deep dissection

Deep circumflex iliac artery

Lateral femoral cutaneous nerve

Sartorius muscle (cut)

Iliopsoas muscle

Tensor fasciae latae muscle (retracted)

Gluteus medius and minimus muscles

Femoral nerve

Rectus femoris muscle (cut)

Ascending, transverse and descending branches of Lateral circumflex femoral artery

Medial circumflex femoral artery

Pectineus muscle (cut)

Profunda femoris (deep femoral) artery

Perforating branches

Adductor longus muscle (cut)

Vastus lateralis muscle

Vastus intermedius muscle

Rectus femoris muscle (cut)

Saphenous nerve

Anteromedial intermuscular septum (opened)

Vastus medialis muscle

Quadriceps femoris tendon

Patella and patellar anastomosis

Medial patellar retinaculum

Patellar ligament

External iliac artery and vein

Inguinal ligament (Poupart's)

Femoral artery and vein (cut)

Pectineus muscle (cut)

Obturator canal

Obturator externus muscle

Adductor longus muscle (cut)

Anterior branch and Posterior branch of obturator nerve

Quadratus femoris muscle

Adductor brevis muscle

Branches of posterior branch of obturator nerve

Adductor magnus muscle

Gracilis muscle

Cutaneous branch of obturator nerve

Femoral artery and vein (cut)

Descending genicular artery
Articular branch
Saphenous branch

Adductor hiatus

Sartorius muscle (cut)

Adductor magnus tendon

Adductor tubercle on medial epicondyle of femur

Superior medial genicular artery (from popliteal artery)

Infrapatellar branch of Saphenous nerve

Inferior medial genicular artery (from popliteal artery)

Plate 13 Arteries and Nerves of Thigh: Posterior View. (Netter: Atlas of Human Anatomy, 4 ed, 2006, Saunders. Plate 501)

Deep dissection

Superior cluneal nerves

Gluteus maximus muscle (*cut*)

Medial cluneal nerves

Inferior gluteal artery and nerve

Pudendal nerve

Nerve to obturator internus (and superior gemellus)

Posterior femoral cutaneous nerve

Sacrotuberous ligament

Ischial tuberosity

Inferior cluneal nerves (*cut*)

Adductor magnus muscle

Gracilis muscle

Sciatic nerve

Muscular branches of sciatic nerve

Semitendinosus muscle (*retracted*)

Semimembranosus muscle

Sciatic nerve

Articular branch

Adductor hiatus

Popliteal vein and artery

Superior medial genicular artery

Medial epicondyle of femur

Tibial nerve

Gastrocnemius muscle (medial head)

Medial sural cutaneous nerve

Small saphenous vein

Iliac crest

Gluteal aponeurosis and gluteus medius muscle (*cut*)

Superior gluteal artery and nerve

Gluteus minimus muscle

Tensor fasciae latae muscle

Piriformis muscle

Gluteus medius muscle (*cut*)

Superior gemellus muscle

Greater trochanter of femur

Obturator internus muscle

Inferior gemellus muscle

Gluteus maximus muscle (*cut*)

Quadratus femoris muscle

Medial circumflex femoral artery

Vastus lateralis muscle and iliotibial tract

Adductor minimus part of adductor magnus muscle

1st perforating artery (from profunda femoris artery)

Adductor magnus muscle

2nd and 3rd perforating arteries (from profunda femoris artery)

4th perforating artery (from profunda femoris artery)

Long head (*retracted*) ⎫
Short head   ⎬ Biceps femoris muscle
                    ⎭

Superior lateral genicular artery

Common fibular (peroneal) nerve

Plantaris muscle

Gastrocnemius muscle (lateral head)

Lateral sural cutaneous nerve

Plate 14   Arteries and Nerves of Thigh: Posterior View. (Netter: Atlas of Human Anatomy, 4 ed, 2006, Saunders. Plate 502)

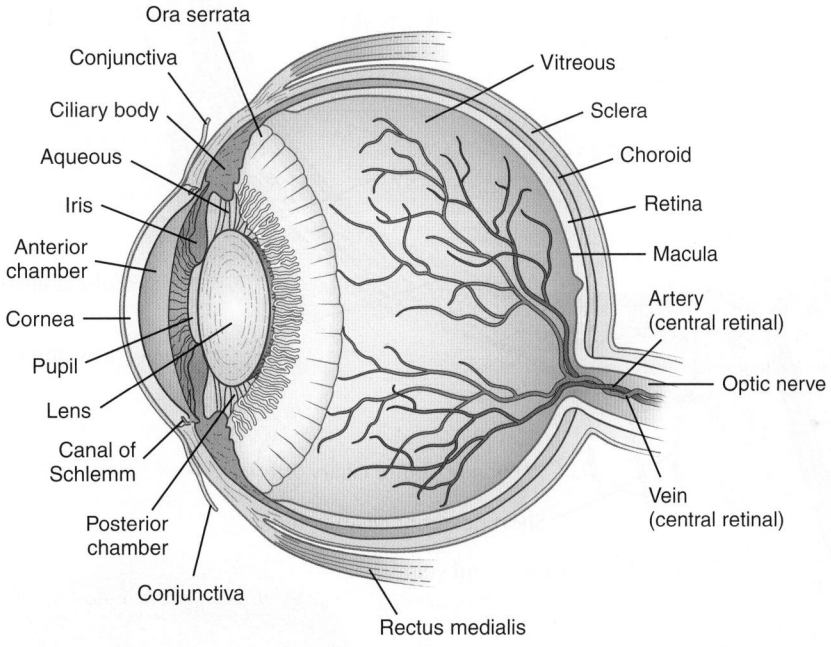

Ora serrata
Conjunctiva
Ciliary body
Aqueous
Iris
Anterior chamber
Cornea
Pupil
Lens
Canal of Schlemm
Posterior chamber
Conjunctiva
Rectus medialis

Vitreous
Sclera
Choroid
Retina
Macula
Artery (central retinal)
Optic nerve
Vein (central retinal)

Plate 15 Anatomy of the eye. (Dehn RW, Asprey DP: Essential Clinical Procedures, ed 3, Philadelphia, 2013, Saunders.)

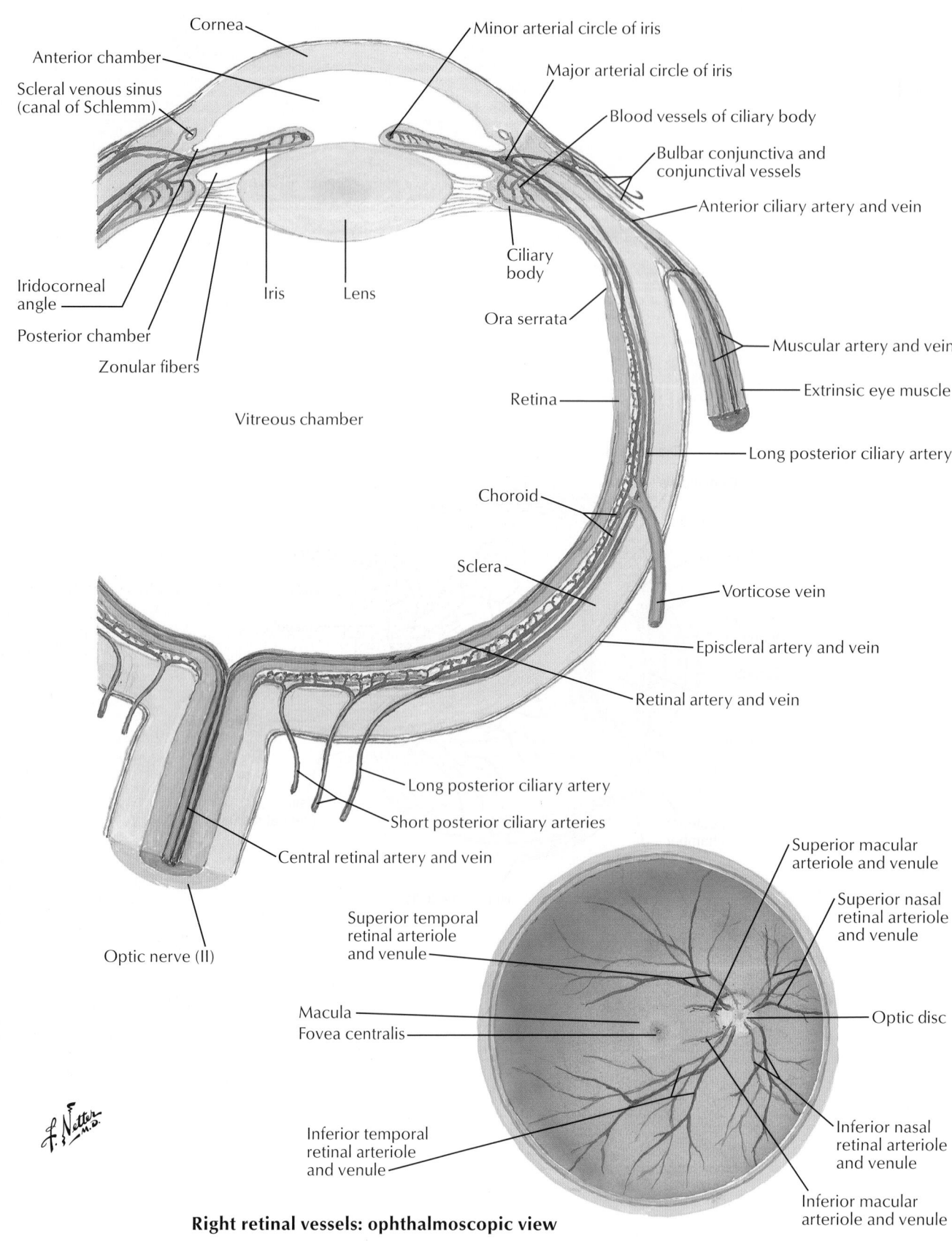

Cornea

Minor arterial circle of iris

Anterior chamber

Major arterial circle of iris

Scleral venous sinus (canal of Schlemm)

Blood vessels of ciliary body

Bulbar conjunctiva and conjunctival vessels

Anterior ciliary artery and vein

Iridocorneal angle

Iris

Lens

Ciliary body

Posterior chamber

Ora serrata

Zonular fibers

Muscular artery and vein

Extrinsic eye muscle

Vitreous chamber

Retina

Long posterior ciliary artery

Choroid

Sclera

Vorticose vein

Episcleral artery and vein

Retinal artery and vein

Long posterior ciliary artery

Short posterior ciliary arteries

Central retinal artery and vein

Optic nerve (II)

Superior macular arteriole and venule

Superior temporal retinal arteriole and venule

Superior nasal retinal arteriole and venule

Macula

Fovea centralis

Optic disc

Inferior nasal retinal arteriole and venule

Inferior temporal retinal arteriole and venule

Inferior macular arteriole and venule

Right retinal vessels: ophthalmoscopic view

Plate 16   Intrinsic Arteries and Veins of Eye. (Netter: Atlas of Human Anatomy, 4 ed, 2006, Saunders. Plate 90)

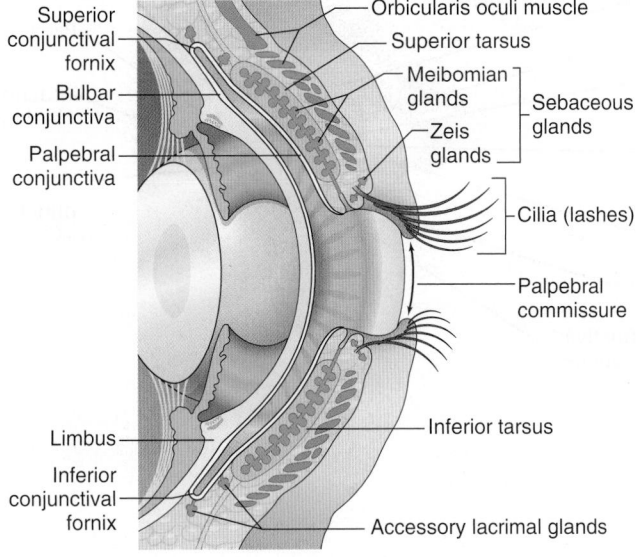

Plate 17 Anatomy of the conjunctiva and eyelids. (Kumar V, Abbas AK, Aster JC: Robbins and Cotran Pathologic Basis of Disease, ed 9, Philadelphia, 2015, Saunders.)

Superior palpebral conjunctiva: tarsal (meibomian) glands shining through

Seen through cornea { Pupil
Iris

Corneoscleral junction (corneal limbus)

Bulbar conjunctiva over sclera

Inferior conjunctival fornix

Inferior palpebral conjunctiva: tarsal glands shining through

Superior lacrimal papilla and punctum

Plica semilunaris

Lacrimal caruncle in lacrimal lake (lacus lacrimalis)

Inferior lacrimal papilla and punctum

Plate 18   Eyelid. (Netter: Atlas of Human Anatomy, 4 ed, 2006, Saunders. Plate 81, Upper)

Superior lacrimal papilla and punctum

Orbital part of lacrimal gland

Palpebral part of lacrimal gland

Excretory ducts of lacrimal gland

Plica semilunaris

Lacrimal caruncle

Inferior lacrimal papilla and punctum

Lacrimal canaliculi

Lacrimal sac

Nasolacrimal duct

Opening of nasolacrimal duct

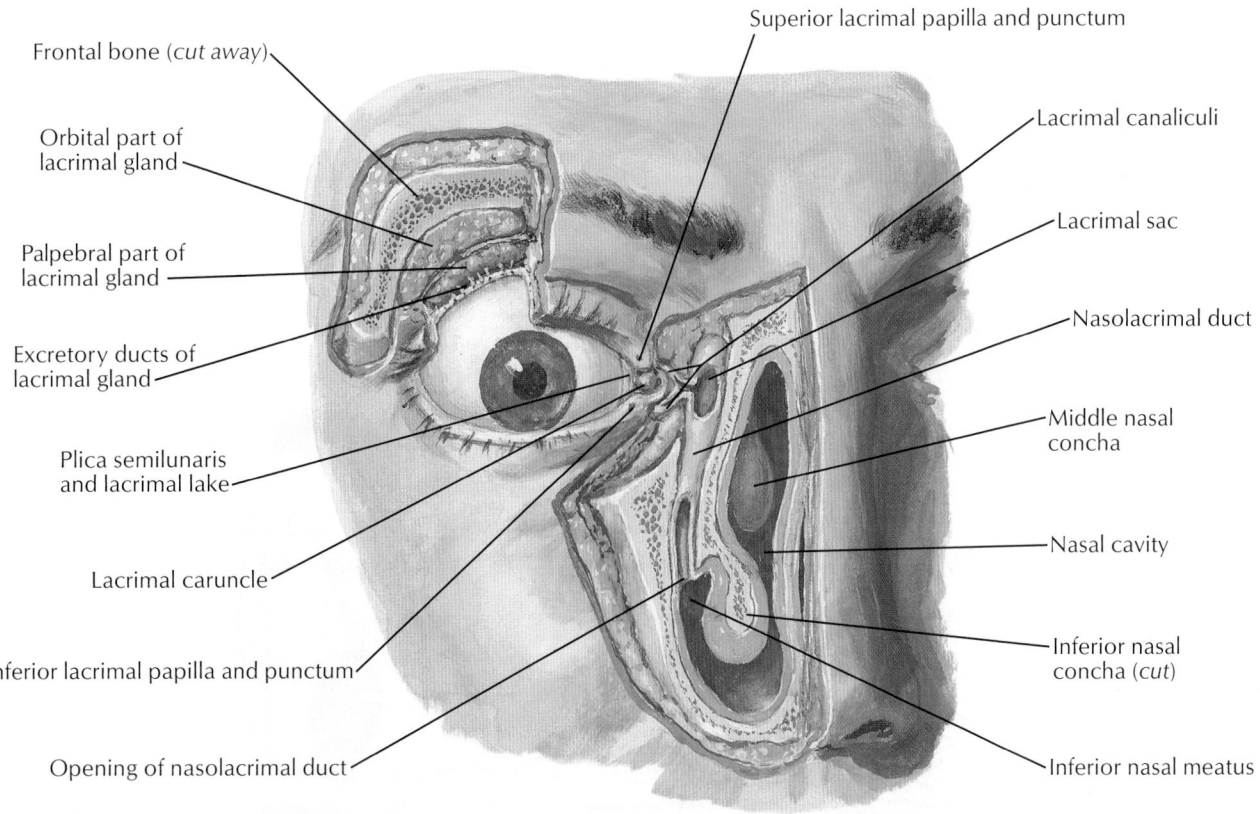

Frontal bone (cut away)

Orbital part of lacrimal gland

Palpebral part of lacrimal gland

Excretory ducts of lacrimal gland

Plica semilunaris and lacrimal lake

Lacrimal caruncle

Inferior lacrimal papilla and punctum

Opening of nasolacrimal duct

Superior lacrimal papilla and punctum

Lacrimal canaliculi

Lacrimal sac

Nasolacrimal duct

Middle nasal concha

Nasal cavity

Inferior nasal concha (cut)

Inferior nasal meatus

Plate 19 Lacrimal Apparatus. (Netter: Atlas of Human Anatomy, 4 ed, 2006, Saunders. Plate 82)

```
Pinna ──┐
  │      ├─ Outer ear
  ▼      │
External auditory canal ──┘

Tympanic membrane ──┐
  │                  │
  ▼                  │
Ossicles:            ├─ Middle ear
Malleus, incus, stapes │
  │                  │
  ▼                  │
Oval window ─────────┘

Cochlea ──┐
  │        ├─ Inner ear
  ▼        │
Auditory nerve ──┘

Cerebrum ── Brain
```

Plate 20   Pathway of Sound. (LaFleur Brooks D, LaFleur Brooks M: Basic Medical Language, ed 4, St. Louis, 2013, Mosby.)

Plate 21   Middle ear structures. (©Elsevier Collection.)

RIGHT TYMPANIC MEMBRANE

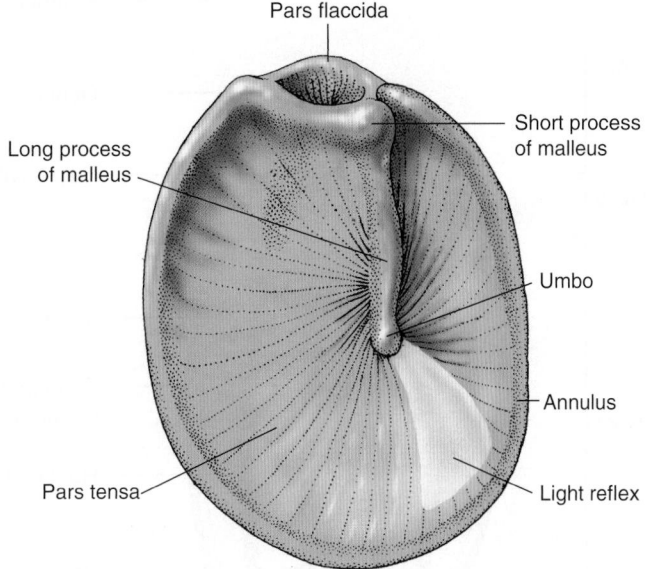

Pars flaccida

Short process
of malleus

Long process
of malleus

Umbo

Annulus

Pars tensa

Light reflex

Plate 22 Structural landmarks of tympanic membrane. (Ignatavicius DD, Workman ML: Medical-Surgical Nursing: Patient-Centered Collaborative Care, ed 7, St. Louis, 2013, Saunders.)

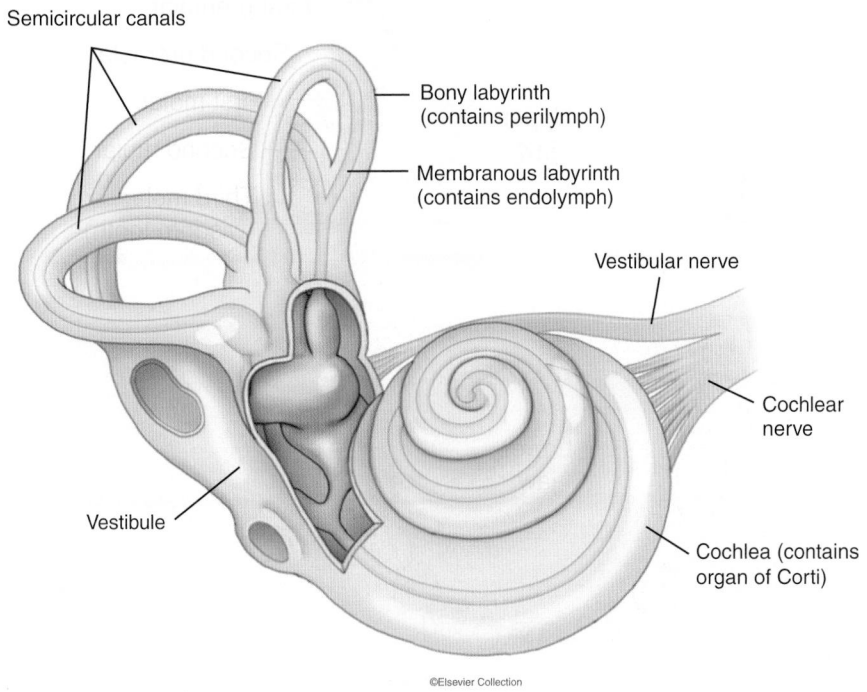

Semicircular canals

Bony labyrinth
(contains perilymph)

Membranous labyrinth
(contains endolymph)

Vestibular nerve

Cochlear
nerve

Vestibule

Cochlea (contains
organ of Corti)

©Elsevier Collection

Plate 23 Inner ear structures. (©Elsevier Collection.)

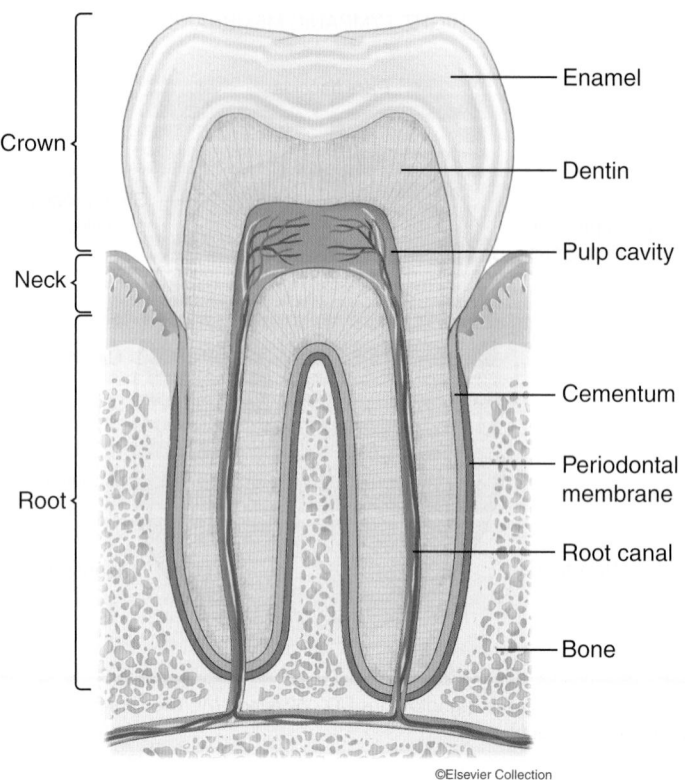

©Elsevier Collection

Plate 24 The Tooth. (©Elsevier Collection).

©Elsevier Collection

Plate 25 Adult Teeth. (©Elsevier Collection).

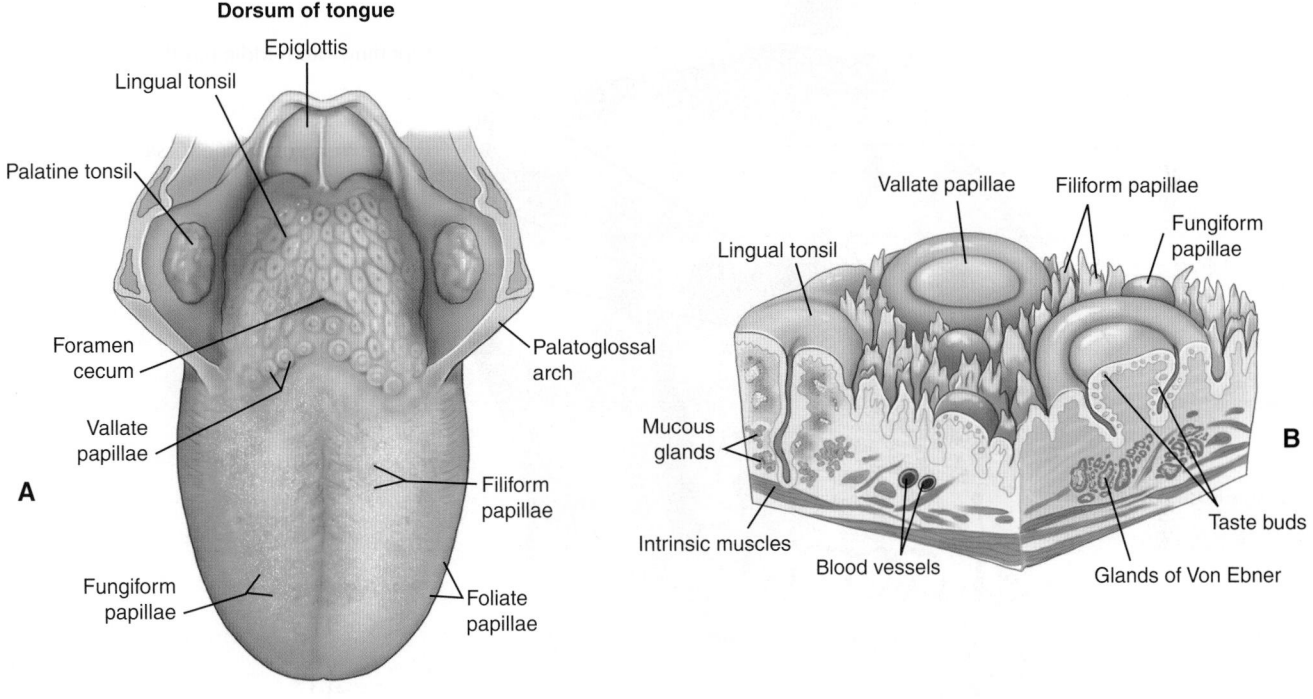

Dorsum of tongue

A

- Epiglottis
- Lingual tonsil
- Palatine tonsil
- Foramen cecum
- Vallate papillae
- Palatoglossal arch
- Filiform papillae
- Fungiform papillae
- Foliate papillae

B

- Vallate papillae
- Filiform papillae
- Fungiform papillae
- Lingual tonsil
- Mucous glands
- Intrinsic muscles
- Blood vessels
- Taste buds
- Glands of Von Ebner

© Elsevier Collection

Plate 26   A, Dorsal view of tongue showing the roughened large lingual tonsils on the posterior of the tongue and the foliate papillae on the side. B, Section of dorsal of the tongue showing a cutaway through lingual papillae and showing von Ebner's glands at the base of the vallate papilla. (Brand RW, Isselhard DE: Anatomy of Orofacial Structures: A Comprehensive Approach, ed 8, St. Louis, 2019, Elsevier.)

ANATOMY ILLUSTRATIONS

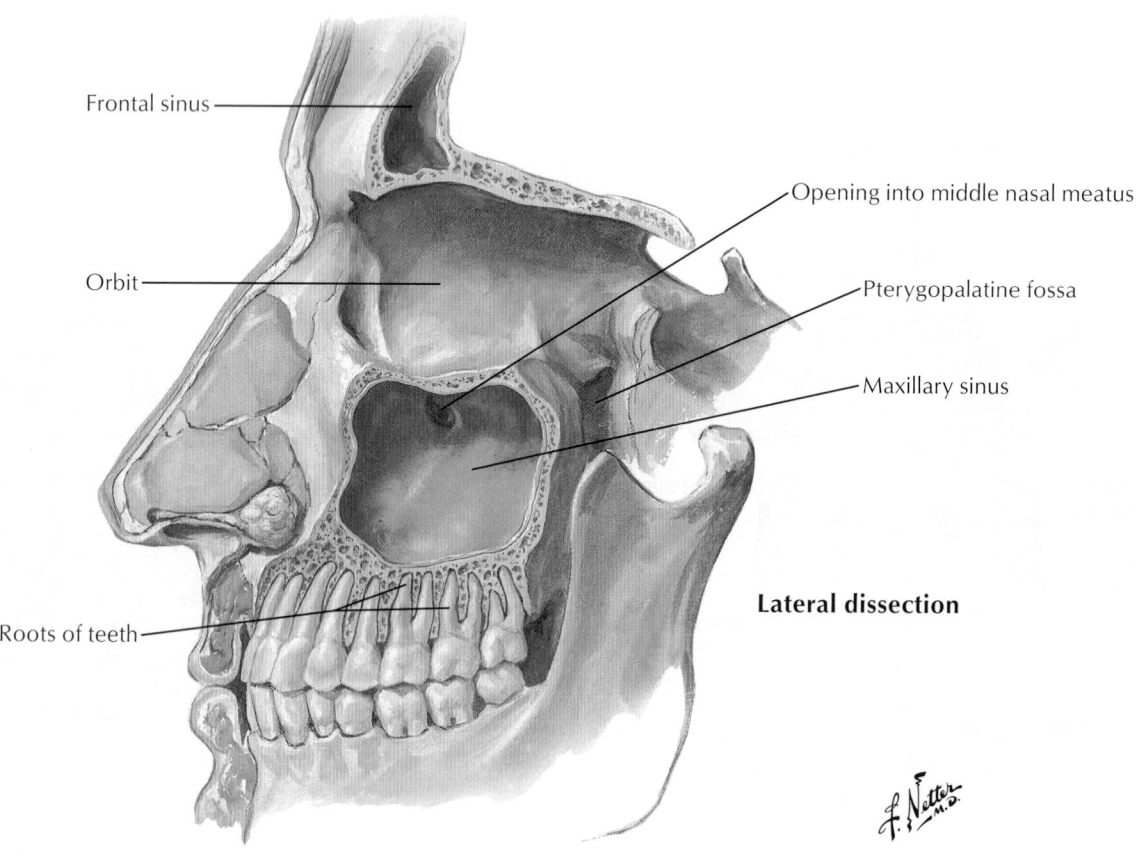

Frontal sinus

Orbit

Roots of teeth

Opening into middle nasal meatus

Pterygopalatine fossa

Maxillary sinus

Lateral dissection

Plate 27 Paranasal Sinuses. (Netter: Atlas of Human Anatomy, 4 ed, 2006, Saunders. Plate 49)

78

Superficial temporal artery and vein and auriculotemporal nerve

Branches of facial nerve

Transverse facial artery

Accessory parotid gland

Parotid duct

Buccinator muscle (*cut*)

Masseter muscle

Lingual nerve

Submandibular ganglion

Tongue

Frenulum of tongue

Sublingual fold with openings of sublingual ducts

Sublingual caruncle with opening of submandibular duct

Sublingual gland

Submandibular duct

Sublingual artery and vein

Mylohyoid muscle (*cut*)

Digastric muscle (anterior belly)

Submandibular gland

Facial artery and vein

Parotid gland

Retromandibular vein (anterior and posterior branches)

Digastric muscle (posterior belly)

Stylohyoid muscle

External jugular vein

Sternocleidomastoid muscle

Common trunk receiving facial, anterior branch of retromandibular, and lingual veins (common facial vein)

Internal jugular vein

External carotid artery

Hyoid bone

Parotid gland: totally serous

Submandibular gland: mostly serous, partially mucous

Sublingual gland: almost completely mucous

Plate 28   Salivary Glands. (Netter: Atlas of Human Anatomy, 4 ed, 2006, Saunders. Plate 61)

Coronary Arteries: Arteriographic Views

Right coronary artery: left anterior oblique view

Arteriogram

Sinuatrial (SA) nodal branch

Right coronary artery

Atrioventricular (AV) nodal branch

Branches to back of left ventricle

Right marginal branch

Posterior interventricular branch (posterior descending artery)

Right coronary artery: right anterior oblique view

Sinuatrial (SA) nodal branch

Conus (arteriosus) branch

Right coronary artery

Right marginal branch

Arteriogram

Atrioventricular (AV) nodal branch

Right posterolateral branches (to back of left ventricle)

Posterior interventricular branch (posterior descending artery)

Plate 29 Coronary Arteries: Arteriographic Views. (Netter: Atlas of Human Anatomy, 4 ed, 2006, Saunders. Plate 218)

Left coronary artery: left anterior oblique view

Left coronary artery

Circumflex branch

Arteriogram

Anterior interventricular branch (left anterior descending)

Diagonal branches of anterior interventricular branch

Atrioventricular branch of circumflex branch

Left (obtuse) marginal branch

Posterolateral branches

(Perforating) interventricular septal branches

Left coronary artery: right anterior oblique view

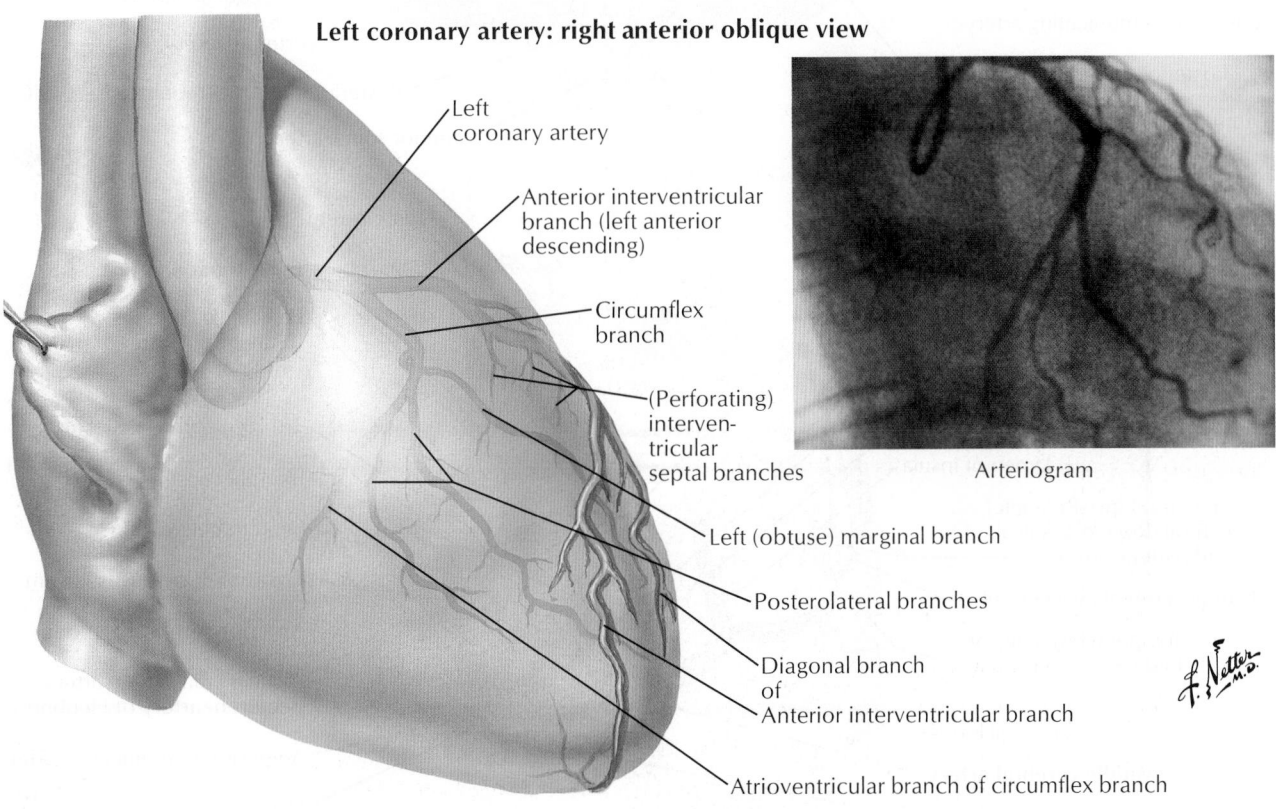

Left coronary artery

Anterior interventricular branch (left anterior descending)

Circumflex branch

(Perforating) interventricular septal branches

Arteriogram

Left (obtuse) marginal branch

Posterolateral branches

Diagonal branch of Anterior interventricular branch

Atrioventricular branch of circumflex branch

Plate 30 Coronary Arteries: Arteriographic Views. (Netter: Atlas of Human Anatomy, 4 ed, 2006, Saunders. Plate 219)

Corpus callosum

Anterolateral central
(lenticulostriate) arteries

Lateral frontobasal
(orbitofrontal) artery

Prefrontal artery

Precentral (pre-Rolandic)
and central (Rolandic)
sulcal arteries

Anterior parietal
(postcentral sulcal)
artery

Posterior parietal
artery

Branch to
angular gyrus

Temporal branches
(anterior, middle,
and posterior)

Middle cerebral artery
and branches
(deep in lateral cerebral
[Sylvian] sulcus)

Anterior communicating artery

Posterior communicating artery

Anterior inferior cerebellar artery (AICA)

Posterior spinal artery

Paracentral artery

Medial frontal branches

Pericallosal artery

Callosomarginal artery

Polar frontal artery

**Anterior cerebral
arteries**

Medial frontobasal
(orbitofrontal) artery

Distal medial striate
artery (recurrent
artery of Heubner)

Internal carotid
artery

Anterior choroidal
artery

**Posterior cerebral
artery**

Superior cerebellar artery

Basilar and pontine arteries

Labyrinthine (internal
acoustic) artery

Vertebral artery

Posterior inferior cerebellar artery (PICA)

Anterior spinal artery

Corpus striatum
(caudate and lentiform nuclei)

Anterolateral central
(lenticulostriate) arteries

Insula (island of Reil)

Limen of insula

Precentral (pre-Rolandic),
central (Rolandic) sulcal,
and parietal arteries

Lateral cerebral (Sylvian) sulcus

Temporal branches of
middle cerebral artery

Temporal lobe

Middle cerebral artery

Internal carotid artery

Falx cerebri

Callosomarginal arteries
and
Pericallosal arteries
(branches of anterior
cerebral arteries)

Trunk of corpus callosum

Internal capsule

Septum pellucidum

Rostrum of corpus callosum

Anterior cerebral arteries

Distal medial striate artery
(recurrent artery of Heubner)

Anterior communicating artery

Optic chiasm

Plate 31 Arteries of Brain: Frontal View and Section. (Netter: Atlas of Human Anatomy, 4 ed, 2006, Saunders. Plate 141)

82

ANATOMY ILLUSTRATIONS

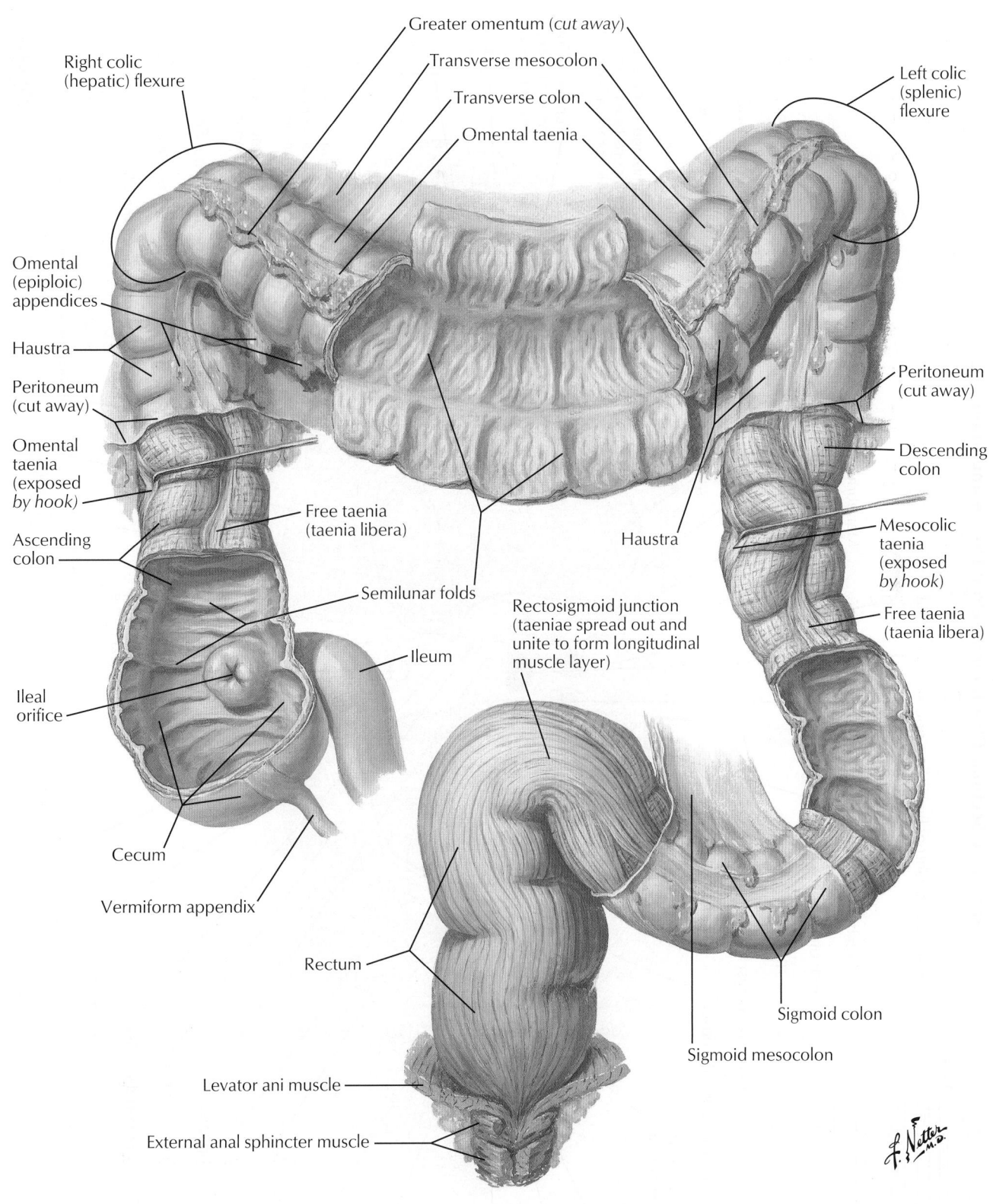

Greater omentum (*cut away*)

Transverse mesocolon

Transverse colon

Omental taenia

Right colic (hepatic) flexure

Left colic (splenic) flexure

Omental (epiploic) appendices

Haustra

Peritoneum (cut away)

Omental taenia (exposed *by hook*)

Ascending colon

Ileal orifice

Cecum

Vermiform appendix

Free taenia (taenia libera)

Semilunar folds

Ileum

Haustra

Peritoneum (cut away)

Descending colon

Mesocolic taenia (exposed *by hook*)

Free taenia (taenia libera)

Rectosigmoid junction (taeniae spread out and unite to form longitudinal muscle layer)

Rectum

Levator ani muscle

External anal sphincter muscle

Sigmoid colon

Sigmoid mesocolon

ANATOMY ILLUSTRATIONS

Plate 32 Mucosa and Musculature of Large Intestine. (Netter: Atlas of Human Anatomy, 4 ed, 2006, Saunders. Plate 284)

Transverse Section: T3–4 Intervertebral Disc, Manubrium

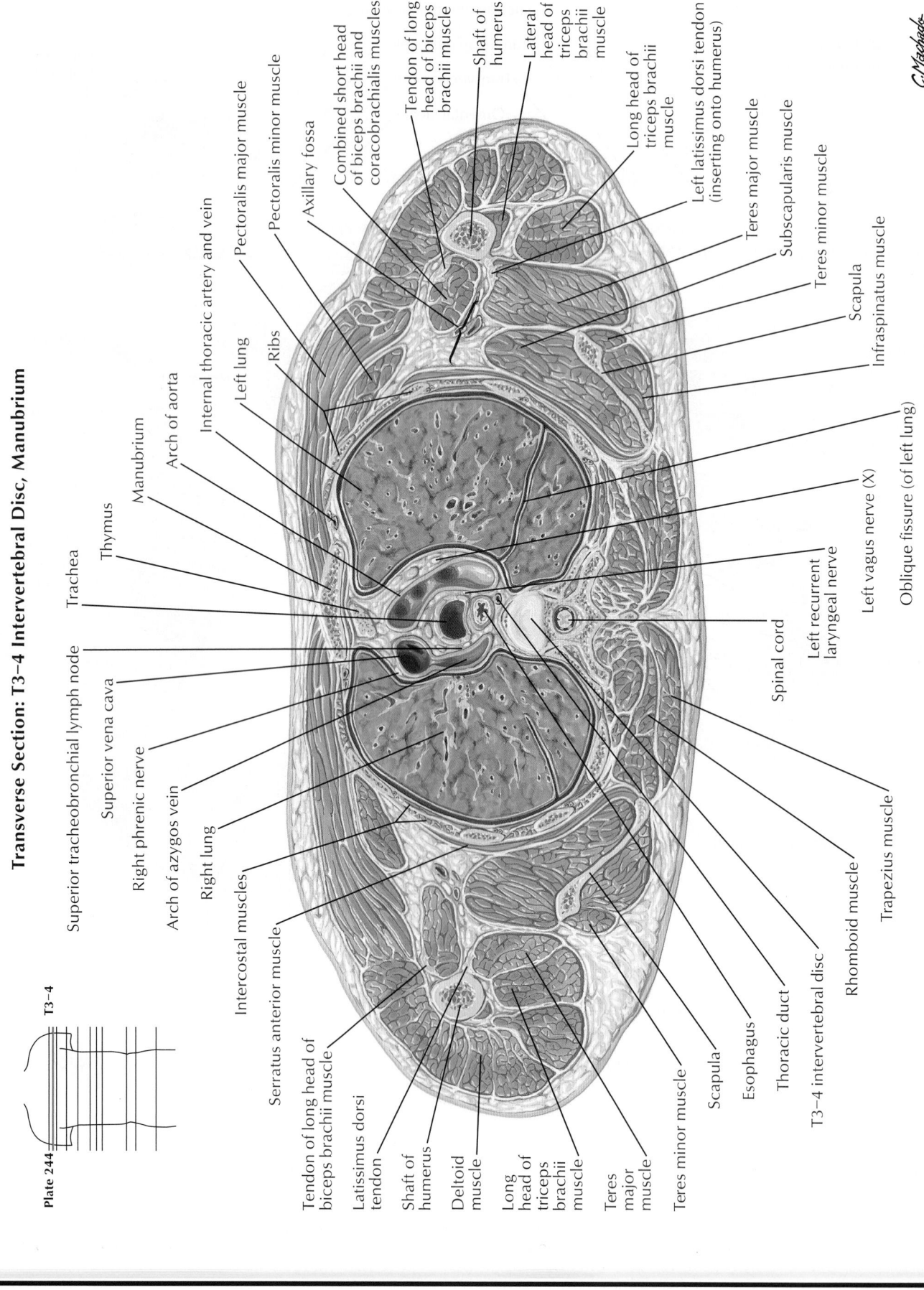

Plate 33 Cross Section of Thorax at T3-4 Disc Level. (Netter: Atlas of Human Anatomy, 4 ed, 2006, Saunders. Plate 244)

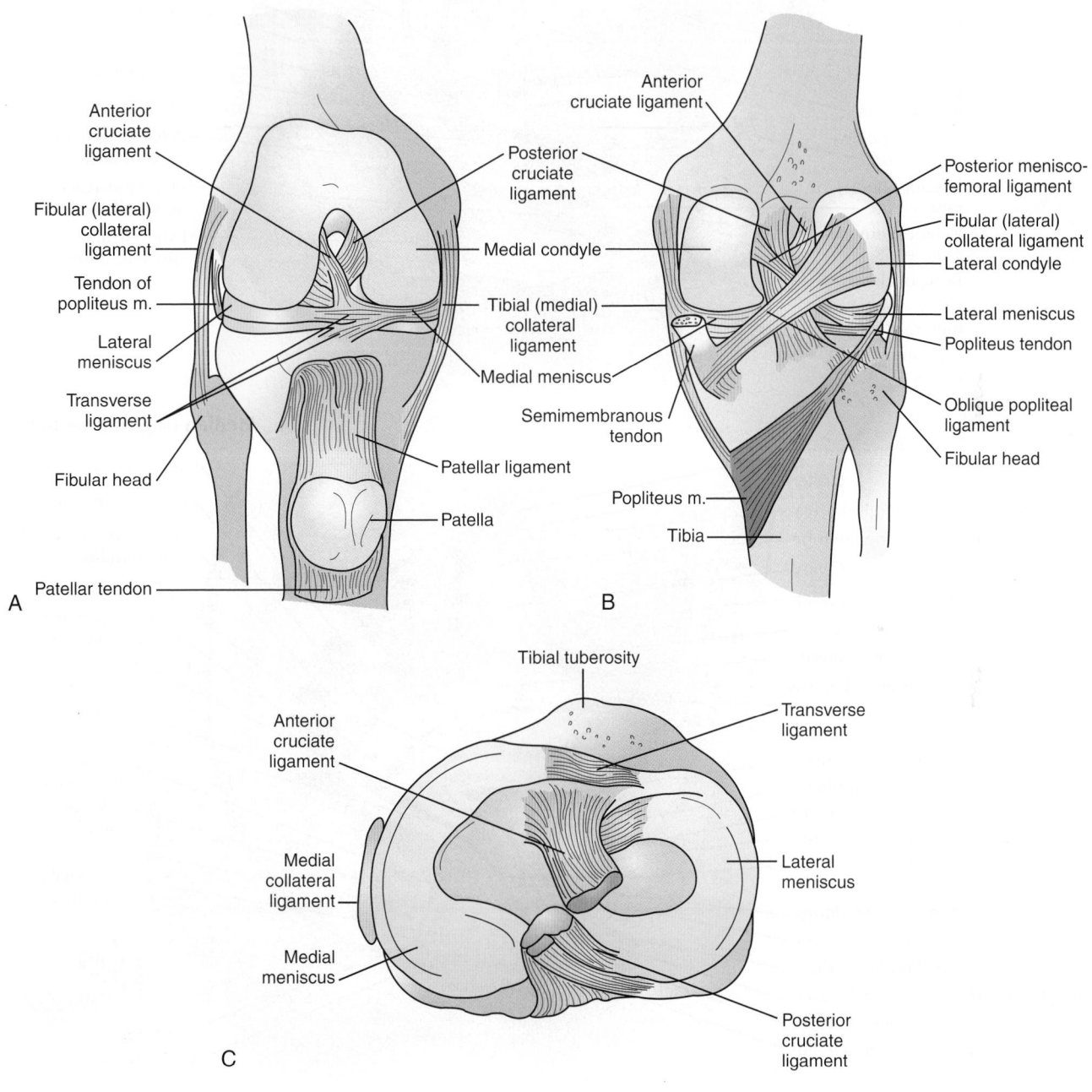

A — Anterior cruciate ligament

Fibular (lateral) collateral ligament

Tendon of popliteus m.

Lateral meniscus

Transverse ligament

Fibular head

Patellar tendon

Posterior cruciate ligament

Medial condyle

Tibial (medial) collateral ligament

Medial meniscus

Patellar ligament

Patella

B — Anterior cruciate ligament

Posterior menisco-femoral ligament

Fibular (lateral) collateral ligament

Lateral condyle

Lateral meniscus

Popliteus tendon

Oblique popliteal ligament

Fibular head

Semimembranous tendon

Popliteus m.

Tibia

C

Tibial tuberosity

Anterior cruciate ligament

Medial collateral ligament

Medial meniscus

Transverse ligament

Lateral meniscus

Posterior cruciate ligament

Plate 34 Knee joint opened; anterior, posterior, and proximal views. A, Anterior view of the knee joint, opened by folding the patella and patellar ligament inferiorly. On the lateral side is the fibular collateral ligament, separated by the popliteal tendon from the lateral meniscus. On the medial side, the tibial collateral ligament is attached to the medial meniscus. The anterior and posterior cruciate ligaments are seen between the femoral condyles. B, Posterior view of the opened knee joint with a more complete view of the posterior cruciate ligament. C, The femur is removed, showing the proximal (articular) end of the right tibia. On the medial side is the gently curved medial meniscus; on the lateral side is the more tightly curved lateral meniscus. The anterior end of the medial meniscus is anchored to the surface of the tibia by the transverse ligament. The cut ends of the anterior and posterior cruciate ligaments are shown, as well as the meniscofemoral ligament. (Fritz S: Mosby's Essential Sciences for Therapeutic Massage: Anatomy, Physiology, Biomechanics, and Pathology, ed 5, St. Louis, 2017, Elsevier.)

Paramedian (sagittal) dissection

Ureter

Uterine (fallopian) tube

Ovary

Ligament of ovary

Round ligament of uterus

Broad ligament (cut)

Superior pubic ramus (cut)

Inferior pubic ramus (cut)

Ischiocavernosus muscle

Body of clitoris

Labia minora

Labium majus

Rectouterine pouch (of Douglas)

Peritoneum (cut edge)

Vesicouterine pouch

Rectum

Ureter

Urinary bladder

Vagina

Pelvic diaphragm (levator ani muscle)

Deep transverse perineal muscle (cut)

External anal sphincter muscle

Median (sagittal) section

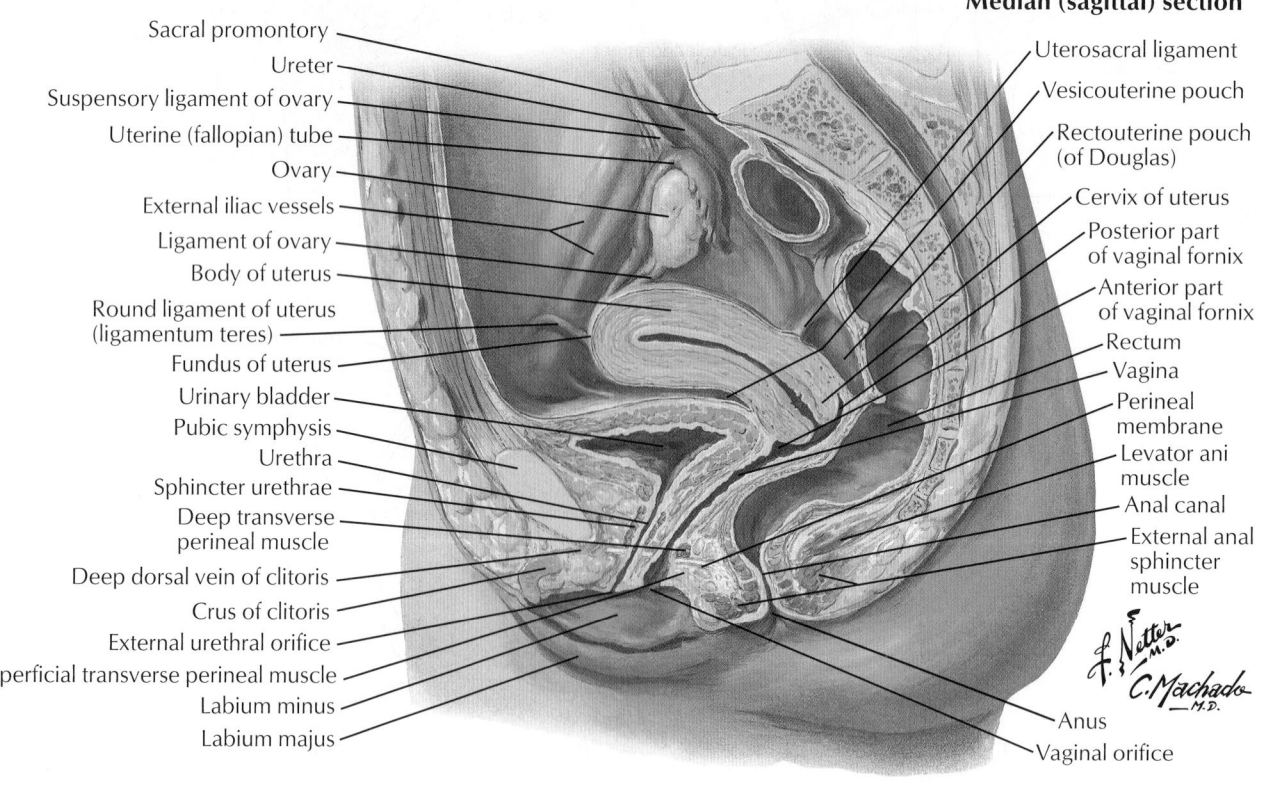

Sacral promontory

Ureter

Suspensory ligament of ovary

Uterine (fallopian) tube

Ovary

External iliac vessels

Ligament of ovary

Body of uterus

Round ligament of uterus (ligamentum teres)

Fundus of uterus

Urinary bladder

Pubic symphysis

Urethra

Sphincter urethrae

Deep transverse perineal muscle

Deep dorsal vein of clitoris

Crus of clitoris

External urethral orifice

Superficial transverse perineal muscle

Labium minus

Labium majus

Uterosacral ligament

Vesicouterine pouch

Rectouterine pouch (of Douglas)

Cervix of uterus

Posterior part of vaginal fornix

Anterior part of vaginal fornix

Rectum

Vagina

Perineal membrane

Levator ani muscle

Anal canal

External anal sphincter muscle

Anus

Vaginal orifice

Plate 35   Pelvic Viscera and Perineum: Female. (Netter: Atlas of Human Anatomy, 4 ed, 2006, Saunders. Plate 360)

PART II

Alphabetic Index

A

Aarskog's syndrome Q87.19
Abandonment —see Maltreatment
Abasia (-astasia) (hysterical) F44.4
Abderhalden-Kaufmann-Lignac syndrome
  (cystinosis) E72.04
Abdomen, abdominal —see also condition
  acute R10.0
  angina K55.1
  muscle deficiency syndrome Q79.4
Abdominalgia —see Pain, abdominal
Abduction contracture, hip or other joint —see
  Contraction, joint
Aberrant (congenital) —see also Malposition,
  congenital
  adrenal gland Q89.1
  artery (peripheral) Q27.8
    basilar NEC Q28.1
    cerebral Q28.3
    coronary Q24.5
    digestive system Q27.8
    eye Q15.8
    lower limb Q27.8
    precerebral Q28.1
    pulmonary Q25.79
    renal Q27.2
    retina Q14.1
    specified site NEC Q27.8
    subclavian Q27.8
    upper limb Q27.8
    vertebral Q28.1
  breast Q83.8
  endocrine gland NEC Q89.2
  hepatic duct Q44.5
  pancreas Q45.3
  parathyroid gland Q89.2
  pituitary gland Q89.2
  sebaceous glands, mucous membrane,
    mouth, congenital Q38.6
  spleen Q89.09
  subclavian artery Q27.8
  thymus (gland) Q89.2
  thyroid gland Q89.2
  vein (peripheral) NEC Q27.8
    cerebral Q28.3
    digestive system Q27.8
    lower limb Q27.8
    precerebral Q28.1
    specified site NEC Q27.8
    upper limb Q27.8
Aberration
  distantial —see Disturbance, visual
  mental F99
Abetalipoproteinemia E78.6
Abiotrophy R68.89
Ablatio, ablation
  retinae —see Detachment, retina
Ablepharia, ablepharon Q10.3
Abnormal, abnormality, abnormalities —see
  also Anomaly
  acid-base balance (mixed) E87.4
  albumin R77.0
  alphafetoprotein R77.2
  alveolar ridge K08.9
  anatomical relationship Q89.9
  apertures, congenital, diaphragm Q79.1
  auditory perception H93.29-●
    diplacusis —see Diplacusis
    hyperacusis —see Hyperacusis
    recruitment —see Recruitment, auditory
    threshold shift —see Shift, auditory
      threshold
  autosomes Q99.9
    fragile site Q95.5
  basal metabolic rate R94.8
  biosynthesis, testicular androgen
    E29.1
  bleeding time R79.1
▶blood amino-acid level R79.83

Abnormal, abnormality, abnormalities —
  (Continued)
  blood level (of)
    cobalt R79.0
    copper R79.0
    iron R79.0
    lithium R78.89
    magnesium R79.0
    mineral NEC R79.0
    zinc R79.0
  blood pressure
    elevated R03.0
    low reading (nonspecific) R03.1
  blood sugar R73.09
  blood-gas level R79.81
  bowel sounds R19.15
    absent R19.11
    hyperactive R19.12
  brain scan R94.02
  breathing R06.9
  caloric test R94.138
  cerebrospinal fluid R83.9
    cytology R83.6
    drug level R83.2
    enzyme level R83.0
    hormones R83.1
    immunology R83.4
    microbiology R83.5
    nonmedicinal level R83.3
    specified type NEC R83.8
  chemistry, blood R79.9
    C-reactive protein R79.82
    drugs —see Findings, abnormal, in blood
    gas level R79.81
    minerals R79.0
    pancytopenia D61.818
    PTT R79.1
    specified NEC R79.89
    toxins —see Findings, abnormal, in
      blood
  chest sounds (friction) (rales) R09.89
  chromosome, chromosomal Q99.9
    with more than three X chromosomes,
      female Q97.1
    analysis result R89.8
      bronchial washings R84.8
      cerebrospinal fluid R83.8
      cervix uteri NEC R87.89
      nasal secretions R84.8
      nipple discharge R89.8
      peritoneal fluid R85.89
      pleural fluid R84.8
      prostatic secretions R86.8
      saliva R85.89
      seminal fluid R86.8
      sputum R84.8
      synovial fluid R89.8
      throat scrapings R84.8
      vagina R87.89
      vulva R87.89
      wound secretions R89.8
    dicentric replacement Q93.2
    ring replacement Q93.2
    sex Q99.8
      female phenotype Q97.9
        specified NEC Q97.8
      male phenotype Q98.9
        specified NEC Q98.8
      structural male Q98.6
    specified NEC Q99.8
  clinical findings NEC R68.89
  coagulation D68.9
    newborn, transient P61.6
    profile R79.1
    time R79.1
  communication —see Fistula
  conjunctiva, vascular H11.41-●
  coronary artery Q24.5
  cortisol-binding globulin E27.8
  course, eustachian tube Q17.8

Abnormal, abnormality, abnormalities —
  (Continued)
  creatinine clearance R94.4
  cytology
    anus R85.619
      atypical squamous cells cannot
        exclude high grade squamous
        intraepithelial lesion (ASC-H)
        R85.611
      atypical squamous cells of undetermined
        significance (ASC-US) R85.610
      cytologic evidence of malignancy
        R85.614
      high grade squamous intraepithelial
        lesion (HGSIL) R85.613
      human papillomavirus (HPV) DNA test
        high risk positive R85.81
        low risk postive R85.82
      inadequate smear R85.615
      low grade squamous intraepithelial
        lesion (LGSIL) R85.612
      satisfactory anal smear but lacking
        transformation zone R85.616
      specified NEC R85.618
      unsatisfactory smear R85.615
    female genital organs —see Abnormal,
      Papanicolaou (smear)
  dark adaptation curve H53.61
  dentofacial NEC —see Anomaly, dentofacial
  development, developmental Q89.9
    central nervous system Q07.9
  diagnostic imaging
    abdomen, abdominal region NEC R93.5
    biliary tract R93.2
    bladder R93.41
    breast R92.8
    central nervous system NEC R90.89
    cerebrovascular NEC R90.89
    coronary circulation R93.1
    digestive tract NEC R93.3
    gastrointestinal (tract) R93.3
    genitourinary organs R93.89
    head R93.0
    heart R93.1
    intrathoracic organ NEC R93.89
    kidney R93.42-●
    limbs R93.6
    liver R93.2
    lung (field) R91.8
    musculoskeletal system NEC R93.7
    renal pelvis R93.41
    retroperitoneum R93.5
    site specified NEC R93.89
    skin and subcutaneous tissue R93.89
    skull R93.0
    testis R93.81-●
    urinary organs specified NEC R93.49
    ureter R93.41
  direction, teeth, fully erupted M26.30
  ear ossicles, acquired NEC H74.39-●
    ankylosis —see Ankylosis, ear ossicles
    discontinuity —see Discontinuity, ossicles,
      ear
    partial loss —see Loss, ossicles, ear (partial)
  Ebstein Q22.5
  echocardiogram R93.1
  echoencephalogram R90.81
  echogram —see Abnormal, diagnostic
    imaging
  electrocardiogram [ECG] [EKG] R94.31
  electroencephalogram [EEG] R94.01
  electrolyte —see Imbalance, electrolyte
  electromyogram [EMG] R94.131
  electro-oculogram [EOG] R94.110
  electrophysiological intracardiac studies
    R94.39
  electroretinogram [ERG] R94.111
  erythrocytes
    congenital, with perinatal jaundice D58.9
  feces (color) (contents) (mucus) R19.5

Abnormal, abnormality, abnormalities —
 (Continued)
 finding —see Findings, abnormal, without
  diagnosis
 fluid
  amniotic —see Abnormal, specimen,
   specified
  cerebrospinal —see Abnormal,
   cerebrospinal fluid
  peritoneal —see Abnormal, specimen,
   digestive organs
  pleural —see Abnormal, specimen,
   respiratory organs
  synovial —see Abnormal, specimen,
   specified
  thorax (bronchial washings) (pleural
   fluid) —see Abnormal, specimen,
   respiratory organs
  vaginal —see Abnormal, specimen, female
   genital organs
 form
  teeth K00.2
  uterus —see Anomaly, uterus
 function studies
  auditory R94.120
  bladder R94.8
  brain R94.09
  cardiovascular R94.30
  ear R94.128
  endocrine NEC R94.7
  eye NEC R94.118
  kidney R94.4
  liver R94.5
  nervous system
   central NEC R94.09
   peripheral NEC R94.138
  pancreas R94.8
  placenta R94.8
  pulmonary R94.2
  special senses NEC R94.128
  spleen R94.8
  thyroid R94.6
  vestibular R94.121
 gait —see Gait
  hysterical F44.4
 gastrin secretion E16.4
 globulin R77.1
  cortisol-binding E27.8
  thyroid-binding E07.89
 glomerular, minor —see also N00-N07 with
  fourth character .0 N05.0
 glucagon secretion E16.3
 glucose tolerance (test) (non-fasting)
  R73.09
 gravitational (G) forces or states (effect of)
  T75.81
 hair (color) (shaft) L67.9
  specified NEC L67.8
 hard tissue formation in pulp (dental)
  K04.3
 head movement R25.0
 heart
  rate R00.9
   specified NEC R00.8
  shadow R93.1
  sounds NEC R01.2
 hemoglobin (disease) —see also Disease,
  hemoglobin D58.2
  trait —see Trait, hemoglobin, abnormal
 histology NEC R89.7
 immunological findings R89.4
  in serum R76.9
   specified NEC R76.8
 increase in appetite R63.2
 involuntary movement —see Abnormal,
  movement, involuntary
 jaw closure M26.51
 karyotype R89.8
 kidney function test R94.4
 knee jerk R29.2
 leukocyte (cell) (differential) NEC D72.9

Abnormal, abnormality, abnormalities —
 (Continued)
⇒ liver function test (see also Elevated, liver
  function, test) R79.89
 loss of
  height R29.890
  weight R63.4
 mammogram NEC R92.8
  calcification (calculus) R92.1
  microcalcification R92.0
 Mantoux test R76.11
 movement (disorder) —see also Disorder,
  movement
  head R25.0
  involuntary R25.9
   fasciculation R25.3
   of head R25.0
   spasm R25.2
   specified type NEC R25.8
   tremor R25.1
 myoglobin (Aberdeen) (Annapolis) R89.7
⇒ neonatal screening P09.9
 ▶ for
  ▶congenital adrenal hyperplasia P09.2
  ▶congenital endocrine disease P09.2
  ▶congenital hematologic disorders P09.3
  ▶critical congenital heart disease P09.5
  ▶cystic fibrosis P09.4
  ▶hemoglobinothies P09.3
  ▶hypothyroidism P09.2
  ▶inborn errors of metabolism P09.1
  ▶neonatal hearing loss P09.6
  ▶red cell membrane defects P09.3
  ▶sickle cell P09.3
  ▶specified NEC P09.8
 oculomotor study R94.113
 palmar creases Q82.8
 Papanicolaou (smear)
  anus R85.619
   atypical squamous cells cannot
    exclude high grade squamous
    intraepithelial lesion (ASC-H)
    R85.611
   atypical squamous cells of undetermined
    significance (ASC-US) R85.610
   cytologic evidence of malignancy
    R85.614
   high grade squamous intraepithelial
    lesion (HGSIL) R85.613
   human papillomavirus (HPV) DNA test
    high risk positive R85.81
    low risk postive R85.82
   inadequate smear R85.615
   low grade squamous intraepithelial
    lesion (LGSIL) R85.612
   satisfactory anal smear but lacking
    transformation zone R85.616
   specified NEC R85.618
   unsatisfactory smear R85.615
  bronchial washings R84.6
  cerebrospinal fluid R83.6
  cervix R87.619
   atypical squamous cells cannot
    exclude high grade squamous
    intraepithelial lesion (ASC-H)
    R87.611
   atypical squamous cells of undetermined
    significance (ASC-US) R87.610
   cytologic evidence of malignancy
    R87.614
   high grade squamous intraepithelial
    lesion (HGSIL) R87.613
   inadequate smear R87.615
   low grade squamous intraepithelial
    lesion (LGSIL) R87.612
   non-atypical endometrial cells R87.618
   satisfactory cervical smear but lacking
    transformation zone R87.616
   specified NEC R87.618
   thin preparaton R87.619
   unsatisfactory smear R87.615

Abnormal, abnormality, abnormalities —
 (Continued)
 Papanicolaou (smear) (Continued)
  nasal secretions R84.6
  nipple discharge R89.6
  peritoneal fluid R85.69
  pleural fluid R84.6
  prostatic secretions R86.6
  saliva R85.69
  seminal fluid R86.6
  sites NEC R89.6
  sputum R84.6
  synovial fluid R89.6
  throat scrapings R84.6
  vagina R87.629
   atypical squamous cells cannot
    exclude high grade squamous
    intraepithelial lesion (ASC-H)
    R87.621
   atypical squamous cells of undetermined
    significance (ASC-US) R87.620
   cytologic evidence of malignancy
    R87.624
   high grade squamous intraepithelial
    lesion (HGSIL) R87.623
   inadequate smear R87.625
   low grade squamous intraepithelial
    lesion (LGSIL) R87.622
   specified NEC R87.628
   thin preparation R87.629
   unsatisfactory smear R87.625
  vulva R87.69
  wound secretions R89.6
 partial thromboplastin time (PTT) R79.1
 pelvis (bony) —see Deformity, pelvis
 percussion, chest (tympany) R09.89
 periods (grossly) —see Menstruation
 phonocardiogram R94.39
 plantar reflex R29.2
 plasma
  protein R77.9
   specified NEC R77.8
  viscosity R70.1
 pleural (folds) Q34.0
 posture R29.3
 product of conception O02.9
  specified type NEC O02.89
 prothrombin time (PT) R79.1
 pulmonary
  artery, congenital Q25.79
  function, newborn P28.89
  test results R94.2
 pulsations in neck R00.2
 pupillary H21.56-●
  function (reaction) (reflex) —see Anomaly,
   pupil, function
 radiological examination —see Abnormal,
  diagnostic imaging
 red blood cell(s) (morphology) (volume)
  R71.8
 reflex —see Reflex
 renal function test R94.4
 response to nerve stimulation R94.130
 retinal correspondence H53.31
 retinal function study R94.111
 rhythm, heart —see also Arrhythmia
 saliva —see Abnormal, specimen, digestive
  organs
 scan
  kidney R94.4
  liver R93.2
  thyroid R94.6
 secretion
  gastrin E16.4
  glucagon E16.3
 semen, seminal fluid —see Abnormal,
  specimen, male genital organs
 serum level (of)
  acid phosphatase R74.8
  alkaline phosphatase R74.8
  amylase R74.8

Abnormal, abnormality, abnormalities —
  (Continued)
  serum level (of) (Continued)
    enzymes R74.9
      specified NEC R74.8
    lipase R74.8
    triacylglycerol lipase R74.8
  shape
    gravid uterus —see Anomaly, uterus
  sinus venosus Q21.1
  size, tooth, teeth K00.2
  spacing, tooth, teeth, fully erupted M26.30
  specimen
    digestive organs (peritoneal fluid) (saliva)
      R85.9
      cytology R85.69
      drug level R85.2
      enzyme level R85.0
      histology R85.7
      hormones R85.1
      immunology R85.4
      microbiology R85.5
      nonmedicinal level R85.3
      specified type NEC R85.89
    female genital organs (secretions) (smears)
      R87.9
      cytology R87.69
        cervix R87.619
          human papillomavirus (HPV) DNA
            test
            high risk positive R87.810
            low risk positive R87.820
          inadequate (unsatisfactory) smear
            R87.615
          non-atypical endometrial cells
            R87.618
          specified NEC R87.618
        vagina R87.629
          human papillomavirus (HPV) DNA
            test
            high risk positive R87.811
            low risk positive R87.821
          inadequate (unsatisfactory) smear
            R87.625
        vulva R87.69
      drug level R87.2
      enzyme level R87.0
      histological R87.7
      hormones R87.1
      immunology R87.4
      microbiology R87.5
      nonmedicinal level R87.3
      specified type NEC R87.89
    male genital organs (prostatic secretions)
      (semen) R86.9
      cytology R86.6
      drug level R86.2
      enzyme level R86.0
      histological R86.7
      hormones R86.1
      immunology R86.4
      microbiology R86.5
      nonmedicinal level R86.3
      specified type NEC R86.8
    nipple discharge —see Abnormal,
      specimen, specified
    respiratory organs (bronchial washings)
      (nasal secretions) (pleural fluid)
      (sputum) R84.9
      cytology R84.6
      drug level R84.2
      enzyme level R84.0
      histology R84.7
      hormones R84.1
      immunology R84.4
      microbiology R84.5
      nonmedicinal level R84.3
      specified type NEC R84.8
    specified organ, system and tissue NOS
      R89.9
      cytology R89.6

Abnormal, abnormality, abnormalities —
  (Continued)
  specimen (Continued)
    specified organ, system and tissue NOS
      (Continued)
      drug level R89.2
      enzyme level R89.0
      histology R89.7
      hormones R89.1
      immunology R89.4
      microbiology R89.5
      nonmedicinal level R89.3
      specified type NEC R89.8
    synovial fluid —see Abnormal, specimen,
      specified
    thorax (bronchial washings) (pleural
      fluids) —see Abnormal, specimen,
      respiratory organs
    vagina (secretion) (smear) R87.629
    vulva (secretion) (smear) R87.69
    wound secretion —see Abnormal,
      specimen, specified
  spermatozoa —see Abnormal, specimen, male
    genital organs
  sputum (amount) (color) (odor) R09.3
  stool (color) (contents) (mucus) R19.5
    bloody K92.1
    guaiac positive R19.5
  synchondrosis Q78.8
  thermography —see also Abnormal,
    diagnostic imaging R93.89
  thyroid-binding globulin E07.89
  tooth, teeth (form) (size) K00.2
  toxicology (findings) R78.9
  transport protein E88.09
  tumor marker NEC R97.8
  ultrasound results —see Abnormal, diagnostic
    imaging
  umbilical cord complicating delivery O69.9
  urination NEC R39.198
  urine (constituents) R82.90
    bile R82.2
    cytological examination R82.89
    drugs R82.5
    fat R82.0
    glucose R81
    heavy metals R82.6
    hemoglobin R82.3
    histological examination R82.89
    ketones R82.4
    microbiological examination (culture) R82.79
    myoglobin R82.1
    positive culture R82.79
    protein —see Proteinuria
    specified substance NEC R82.998
      chromoabnormality NEC R82.91
    substances nonmedical R82.6
  uterine hemorrhage —see Hemorrhage, uterus
  vectorcardiogram R94.39
  visually evoked potential (VEP) R94.112
  white blood cells D72.9
    specified NEC D72.89
  X-ray examination —see Abnormal,
    diagnostic imaging
Abnormity (any organ or part) —see Anomaly
Abocclusion M26.29
  hemolytic disease (newborn) P55.1
  incompatibility reaction ABO —see
    Complication(s), transfusion,
    incompatibility reaction, ABO
Abolition, language R48.8
Aborter, habitual or recurrent —see Loss (of),
    pregnancy, recurrent
Abortion (complete) (spontaneous) O03.9
  with
    retained products of conception —see
      Abortion, incomplete
  attempted (elective) (failed) O07.4
    complicated by O07.30
      afibrinogenemia O07.1
      cardiac arrest O07.36

Abortion (Continued)
  attempted (Continued)
    complicated by (Continued)
      chemical damage of pelvic organ(s) O07.34
      circulatory collapse O07.31
      cystitis O07.38
      defibrination syndrome O07.1
      electrolyte imbalance O07.33
      embolism (air) (amniotic fluid) (blood
        clot) (fat) (pulmonary) (septic)
        (soap) O07.2
      endometritis O07.0
      genital tract and pelvic infection O07.0
      hemolysis O07.1
      hemorrhage (delayed) (excessive) O07.1
      infection
        genital tract or pelvic O07.0
        urinary tract tract O07.38
      intravascular coagulation O07.1
      laceration of pelvic organ(s) O07.34
      metabolic disorder O07.33
      oliguria O07.32
      oophoritis O07.0
      parametritis O07.0
      pelvic peritonitis O07.0
      perforation of pelvic organ(s) O07.34
      renal failure or shutdown O07.32
      salpingitis or salpingo-oophoritis O07.0
      sepsis O07.37
      shock O07.31
      specified condition NEC O07.39
      tubular necrosis (renal) O07.32
      uremia O07.32
      urinary tract infection O07.38
      venous complication NEC O07.35
        embolism (air) (amniotic fluid) (blood
          clot) (fat) (pulmonary) (septic)
          (soap) O07.2
  complicated (by) (following) O03.80
    afibrinogenemia O03.6
    cardiac arrest O03.86
    chemical damage of pelvic organ(s) O03.84
    circulatory collapse O03.81
    cystitis O03.88
    defibrination syndrome O03.6
    electrolyte imbalance O03.83
    embolism (air) (amniotic fluid) (blood clot)
      (fat) (pulmonary) (septic) (soap) O03.7
    endometritis O03.5
    genital tract and pelvic infection O03.5
    hemolysis O03.6
    hemorrhage (delayed) (excessive) O03.6
    infection
      genital tract or pelvic O03.5
      urinary tract O03.88
    intravascular coagulation O03.6
    laceration of pelvic organ(s) O03.84
    metabolic disorder O03.83
    oliguria O03.82
    oophoritis O03.5
    parametritis O03.5
    pelvic peritonitis O03.5
    perforation of pelvic organ(s) O03.84
    renal failure or shutdown O03.82
    salpingitis or salpingo-oophoritis O03.5
    sepsis O03.87
    shock O03.81
    specified condition NEC O03.89
    tubular necrosis (renal) O03.82
    uremia O03.82
    urinary tract infection O03.88
    venous complication NEC O03.85
      embolism (air) (amniotic fluid) (blood
        clot) (fat) (pulmonary) (septic)
        (soap) O03.7
  failed —see Abortion, attempted
  habitual or recurrent N96
    with current abortion —see categories
      O03-O04
    without current pregnancy N96
    care in current pregnancy O26.2-●

▶ New   ⇒ Revised   ~~deleted~~ Deleted   ● Use Additional Character(s)

Abortion (Continued)
incomplete (spontaneous) O03.4
complicated (by) (following) O03.30
afibrinogenemia O03.1
cardiac arrest O03.36
chemical damage of pelvic organ(s) O03.34
circulatory collapse O03.31
cystitis O03.38
defibrination syndrome O03.1
electrolyte imbalance O03.33
embolism (air) (amniotic fluid) (blood clot) (fat) (pulmonary) (septic) (soap) O03.2
endometritis O03.0
genital tract and pelvic infection O03.0
hemolysis O03.1
hemorrhage (delayed) (excessive) O03.1
infection
genital tract or pelvic O03.0
urinary tract O03.38
intravascular coagulation O03.1
laceration of pelvic organ(s) O03.34
metabolic disorder O03.33
oliguria O03.32
oophoritis O03.0
parametritis O03.0
pelvic peritonitis O03.0
perforation of pelvic organ(s) O03.34
renal failure or shutdown O03.32
salpingitis or salpingo-oophoritis O03.0
sepsis O03.37
shock O03.31
specified condition NEC O03.39
tubular necrosis (renal) O03.32
uremia O03.32
urinary infection O03.38
venous complication NEC O03.35
embolism (air) (amniotic fluid) (blood clot) (fat) (pulmonary) (septic) (soap) O03.2
induced (encounter for) Z33.2
complicated by O04.80
afibrinogenemia O04.6
cardiac arrest O04.86
chemical damage of pelvic organ(s) O04.84
circulatory collapse O04.81
cystitis O04.88
defibrination syndrome O04.6
electrolyte imbalance O04.83
embolism (air) (amniotic fluid) (blood clot) (fat) (pulmonary) (septic) (soap) O04.7
endometritis O04.5
genital tract and pelvic infection O04.5
hemolysis O04.6
hemorrhage (delayed) (excessive) O04.6
infection
genital tract or pelvic O04.5
urinary tract O04.88
intravascular coagulation O04.6
laceration of pelvic organ(s) O04.84
metabolic disorder O04.83
oliguria O04.82
oophoritis O04.5
parametritis O04.5
pelvic peritonitis O04.5
perforation of pelvic organ(s) O04.84
renal failure or shutdown O04.82
salpingitis or salpingo-oophoritis O04.5
sepsis O04.87
shock O04.81
specified condition NEC O04.89
tubular necrosis (renal) O04.82
uremia O04.82
urinary tract infection O04.88
venous complication NEC O04.85
embolism (air) (amniotic fluid) (blood clot) (fat) (pulmonary) (septic) (soap) O04.7
inevitable O03.4
missed O02.1

Abortion (Continued)
spontaneous —see Abortion (complete) (spontaneous)
threatened O20.0
threatened (spontaneous) O20.0
tubal O00.10-•
with intrauterine pregnancy O00.11-
Abortus fever A23.1
Aboulomania F60.7
Abrami's disease D59.8
Abramov-Fiedler myocarditis (acute isolated myocarditis) I40.1
Abrasion T14.8
abdomen, abdominal (wall) S30.811
alveolar process S00.512
ankle S90.51-•
antecubital space —see Abrasion, elbow
anus S30.817
arm (upper) S40.81-•
auditory canal —see Abrasion, ear
auricle —see Abrasion, ear
axilla —see Abrasion, arm
back, lower S30.810
breast S20.11-•
brow S00.81
buttock S30.810
calf —see Abrasion, leg
canthus —see Abrasion, eyelid
cheek S00.81
internal S00.512
chest wall —see Abrasion, thorax
chin S00.81
clitoris S30.814
cornea S05.0-•
costal region —see Abrasion, thorax
dental K03.1
digit(s)
foot —see Abrasion, toe
hand —see Abrasion, finger
ear S00.41-•
elbow S50.31-•
epididymis S30.813
epigastric region S30.811
epiglottis S10.11
esophagus (thoracic) S27.818
cervical S10.11
eyebrow —see Abrasion, eyelid
eyelid S00.21-•
face S00.81
finger(s) S60.41-•
index S60.41-•
little S60.41-•
middle S60.41-•
ring S60.41-•
flank S30.811
foot (except toe(s) alone) S90.81-•
toe —see Abrasion, toe
forearm S50.81-•
elbow only —see Abrasion, elbow
forehead S00.81
genital organs, external
female S30.816
male S30.815
groin S30.811
gum S00.512
hand S60.51-•
head S00.91
ear —see Abrasion, ear
eyelid —see Abrasion, eyelid
lip S00.511
nose S00.31
oral cavity S00.512
scalp S00.01
specified site NEC S00.81
heel —see Abrasion, foot
hip S70.21-•
inguinal region S30.811
interscapular region S20.419
jaw S00.81
knee S80.21-•
labium (majus) (minus) S30.814

Abrasion (Continued)
larynx S10.11
leg (lower) S80.81-•
knee —see Abrasion, knee
upper —see Abrasion, thigh
lip S00.511
lower back S30.810
lumbar region S30.810
malar region S00.81
mammary —see Abrasion, breast
mastoid region S00.81
mouth S00.512
nail
finger —see Abrasion, finger
toe —see Abrasion, toe
nape S10.81
nasal S00.31
neck S10.91
specified site NEC S10.81
throat S10.11
nose S00.31
occipital region S00.01
oral cavity S00.512
orbital region —see Abrasion, eyelid
palate S00.512
palm —see Abrasion, hand
parietal region S00.01
pelvis S30.810
penis S30.812
perineum
female S30.814
male S30.810
periocular area —see Abrasion, eyelid
phalanges
finger —see Abrasion, finger
toe —see Abrasion, toe
pharynx S10.11
pinna —see Abrasion, ear
popliteal space —see Abrasion, knee
prepuce S30.812
pubic region S30.810
pudendum
female S30.816
male S30.815
sacral region S30.810
scalp S00.01
scapular region —see Abrasion, shoulder
scrotum S30.813
shin —see Abrasion, leg
shoulder S40.21-•
skin NEC T14.8
sternal region S20.319
submaxillary region S00.81
submental region S00.81
subungual
finger(s) —see Abrasion, finger
toe(s) —see Abrasion, toe
supraclavicular fossa S10.81
supraorbital S00.81
temple S00.81
temporal region S00.81
testis S30.813
thigh S70.31-•
thorax, thoracic (wall) S20.91
back S20.41-•
front S20.31-•
throat S10.11
thumb S60.31-•
toe(s) (lesser) S90.416
great S90.41-•
tongue S00.512
tooth, teeth (dentifrice) (habitual) (hard tissues) (occupational) (ritual) (traditional) K03.1
trachea S10.11
tunica vaginalis S30.813
tympanum, tympanic membrane —see Abrasion, ear
uvula S00.512
vagina S30.814
vocal cords S10.11

Abrasion (Continued)
  vulva S30.814
  wrist S60.81- •
Abrism —see Poisoning, food, noxious, plant
Abruptio placentae O45.9- •
  with
    afibrinogenemia O45.01- •
    coagulation defect O45.00- •
      specified NEC O45.09- •
    disseminated intravascular coagulation
      O45.02- •
    hypofibrinogenemia O45.01- •
  specified NEC O45.8- •
Abruption, placenta —see Abruptio placentae
Abscess (connective tissue) (embolic) (fistulous)
    (infective) (metastatic) (multiple)
    (pernicious) (pyogenic) (septic) L02.91
  with
    diverticular disease (intestine) K57.80
      with bleeding K57.81
      large intestine K57.20
        with
          bleeding K57.21
          small intestine K57.40
            with bleeding K57.41
      small intestine K57.00
        with
          bleeding K57.01
          large intestine K57.40
            with bleeding K57.41
    lymphangitis - code by site under Abscess
  abdomen, abdominal
    cavity K65.1
    wall L02.211
  abdominopelvic K65.1
  accessory sinus —see Sinusitis
  adrenal (capsule) (gland) E27.8
  alveolar K04.7
    with sinus K04.6
  amebic A06.4
    brain (and liver or lung abscess) A06.6
    genitourinary tract A06.82
    liver (without mention of brain or lung
      abscess) A06.4
    lung (and liver) (without mention of brain
      abscess) A06.5
    specified site NEC A06.89
    spleen A06.89
  anerobic A48.0
  ankle —see Abscess, lower limb
  anorectal K61.2
  antecubital space —see Abscess, upper limb
  antrum (chronic) (Highmore) —see Sinusitis,
    maxillary
  anus K61.0
  apical (tooth) K04.7
    with sinus (alveolar) K04.6
  appendix K35.33
  areola (acute) (chronic) (nonpuerperal)
    N61.1
    puerperal, postpartum or gestational —see
      Infection, nipple
  arm (any part) —see Abscess, upper limb
  artery (wall) I77.89
  atheromatous I77.2
  auricle, ear —see Abscess, ear, external
  axilla (region) L02.41- •
    lymph gland or node L04.2
  back (any part, except buttock) L02.212
  Bartholin's gland N75.1
    with
      abortion —see Abortion, by type
        complicated by, sepsis
      ectopic or molar pregnancy O08.0
    following ectopic or molar pregnancy O08.0
  Bezold's —see Mastoiditis, acute
  bilharziasis B65.1
  bladder (wall) —see Cystitis, specified type
    NEC
  bone (subperiosteal) —see also Osteomyelitis,
    specified type NEC

Abscess (Continued)
  bone (Continued)
    accessory sinus (chronic) —see Sinusitis
    chronic or old —see Osteomyelitis, chronic
    jaw (lower) (upper) M27.2
    mastoid —see Mastoiditis, acute,
      subperiosteal
    petrous —see Petrositis
    spinal (tuberculous) A18.01
      nontuberculous —see Osteomyelitis,
        vertebra
  bowel K63.0
  brain (any part) (cystic) (otogenic) G06.0
    amebic (with abscess of any other site) A06.6
    gonococcal A54.82
    pheomycotic (chromomycotic) B43.1
    tuberculous A17.81
  breast (acute) (chronic) (nonpuerperal)
    N61.1
    newborn P39.0
    puerperal, postpartum, gestational —see
      Mastitis, obstetric, purulent
  broad ligament N73.2
    acute N73.0
    chronic N73.1
  Brodie's (localized) (chronic) M86.8X- •
  bronchi J98.09
  buccal cavity K12.2
  bulbourethral gland N34.0
  bursa M71.00
    ankle M71.07- •
    elbow M71.02- •
    foot M71.07- •
    hand M71.04- •
    hip M71.05- •
    knee M71.06- •
    multiple sites M71.09
    pharyngeal J39.1
    shoulder M71.01- •
    specified site NEC M71.08
    wrist M71.03- •
  buttock L02.31
  canthus —see Blepharoconjunctivitis
  cartilage —see Disorder, cartilage, specified
    type NEC
  cecum K35.33
  cerebellum, cerebellar G06.0
    sequelae G09
  cerebral (embolic) G06.0
    sequelae G09
  cervical (meaning neck) L02.11
    lymph gland or node L04.0
  cervix (stump) (uteri) —see Cervicitis
  cheek (external) L02.01
    inner K12.2
  chest J86.9
    with fistula J86.0
    wall L02.213
  chin L02.01
  choroid —see Inflammation, chorioretinal
  circumtonsillar J36
  cold (lung) (tuberculous) —see also
    Tuberculosis, abscess, lung
    articular —see Tuberculosis, joint
  colon (wall) K63.0
  colostomy K94.02
  conjunctiva —see Conjunctivitis, acute
  cornea H16.31- •
  corpus
    cavernosum N48.21
    luteum —see Oophoritis
  Cowper's gland N34.0
  cranium G06.0
  cul-de-sac (Douglas') (posterior) —see
    Peritonitis, pelvic, female
  cutaneous —see Abscess, by site
  dental K04.7
    with sinus (alveolar) K04.6
  dentoalveolar K04.7
    with sinus K04.6
  diaphragm, diaphragmatic K65.1

Abscess (Continued)
  Douglas' cul-de-sac or pouch —see
    Peritonitis, pelvic, female
  Dubois A50.59
  ear (middle) —see also Otitis, media,
    suppurative
    acute —see Otitis, media, suppurative,
      acute
    external H60.0- •
  entamebic —see Abscess, amebic
  enterostomy K94.12
  epididymis N45.4
  epidural G06.2
    brain G06.0
    spinal cord G06.1
  epiglottis J38.7
  epiploon, epiploic K65.1
  erysipelatous —see Erysipelas
  esophagus K20.80
  ethmoid (bone) (chronic) (sinus) J32.2
  external auditory canal —see Abscess, ear,
    external
  extradural G06.2
    brain G06.0
      sequelae G09
    spinal cord G06.1
  extraperitoneal K68.19
  eye —see Endophthalmitis, purulent
  eyelid H00.03- •
  face (any part, except ear, eye and nose) L02.01
  fallopian tube —see Salpingitis
  fascia M72.8
  fauces J39.1
  fecal K63.0
  femoral (region) —see Abscess, lower limb
  filaria, filarial —see Infestation, filarial
  finger (any) —see also Abscess, hand
    nail —see Cellulitis, finger
  foot L02.61- •
  forehead L02.01
  frontal sinus (chronic) J32.1
  gallbladder K81.0
  genital organ or tract
    female (external) N76.4
    male N49.9
      multiple sites N49.8
      specified NEC N49.8
  gestational mammary O91.11- •
  gestational subareolar O91.11- •
  gingival —see Periodontitis, localized
  gland, glandular (lymph) (acute) —see
    Lymphadenitis, acute
  gluteal (region) L02.31
  gonorrheal —see Gonococcus
  groin L02.214
  gum —see Periodontitis, localized
  hand L02.51- •
  head NEC L02.811
    face (any part, except ear, eye and nose)
      L02.01
  heart —see Carditis
  heel —see Abscess, foot
  helminthic —see Infestation, helminth
  hepatic (cholangitic) (hematogenic)
    (lymphogenic) (pylephlebitic) K75.0
    amebic A06.4
  hip (region) —see Abscess, lower limb
  horseshoe K61.31
  ileocecal K35.33
  ileostomy (bud) K94.12
  iliac (region) L02.214
    fossa K35.33
  infraclavicular (fossa) —see Abscess, upper
    limb
  inguinal (region) L02.214
    lymph gland or node L04.1
  intersphincteric K61.4
  intestine, intestinal NEC K63.0
    rectal K61.1
  intra-abdominal —see also Abscess,
    peritoneum K65.1

▶ New   ⇒ Revised   ~~deleted~~ Deleted   • Use Additional Character(s)

Abscess *(Continued)*
 intra-abdominal *(Continued)*
  following procedure T81.43
   obstetrical O86.03
  postprocedural T81.43
   retroperitoneal K68.11
 intracranial G06.0
 intramammary —*see* Abscess, breast
 intramuscular, following procedure
   T81.44
  obstetrical O86.02
 intraorbital —*see* Abscess, orbit
 intraperitoneal K65.1
 intrasphincteric (anus) K61.4
 intraspinal G06.1
 intratonsillar J36
 ischiorectal (fossa) (specified NEC) K61.39
 jaw (bone) (lower) (upper) M27.2
 joint —*see* Arthritis, pyogenic or pyemic
  spine (tuberculous) A18.01
   nontuberculous —*see* Spondylopathy,
     infective
 kidney N15.1
  with calculus N20.0
   with hydronephrosis N13.6
  puerperal (postpartum) O86.21
 knee —*see also* Abscess, lower limb
  joint M00.9
 labium (majus) (minus) N76.4
 lacrimal
  caruncle —*see* Inflammation, lacrimal,
    passages, acute
  gland —*see* Dacryoadenitis
  passages (duct) (sac) —*see* Inflammation,
    lacrimal, passages, acute
 lacunar N34.0
 larynx J38.7
 lateral (alveolar) K04.7
  with sinus K04.6
 leg (any part) —*see* Abscess, lower limb
 lens H27.8
 lingual K14.0
  tonsil J36
 lip K13.0
 Littre's gland N34.0
 liver (cholangitic) (hematogenic) (lymphogenic)
   (pylephlebitic) (pyogenic) K75.0
  amebic (due to Entamoeba histolytica)
    (dysenteric) (tropical) A06.4
   with
    brain abscess (and liver or lung
      abscess) A06.6
    lung abscess A06.5
 loin (region) L02.211
 lower limb L02.41-●
 lumbar (tuberculous) A18.01
  nontuberculous L02.212
 lung (miliary) (putrid) J85.2
  with pneumonia J85.1
   due to specified organism *(see*
     Pneumonia, in (due to))
  amebic (with liver abscess) A06.5
   with
    brain abscess A06.6
    pneumonia A06.5
 lymph, lymphatic, gland or node (acute) —*see
   also* Lymphadenitis, acute
  mesentery I88.0
 malar M27.2
 mammary gland —*see* Abscess, breast
 marginal, anus K61.0
 mastoid —*see* Mastoiditis, acute
 maxilla, maxillary M27.2
  molar (tooth) K04.7
   with sinus K04.6
  premolar K04.7
  sinus (chronic) J32.0
 mediastinum J85.3
 meibomian gland —*see* Hordeolum
 meninges G06.2
 mesentery, mesenteric K65.1
 mesosalpinx —*see* Salpingitis

Abscess *(Continued)*
 mons pubis L02.215
 mouth (floor) K12.2
 muscle —*see* Myositis, infective
 myocardium I40.0
 nabothian (follicle) —*see* Cervicitis
 nasal J32.9
 nasopharyngeal J39.1
 navel L02.216
  newborn P38.9
   with mild hemorrhage P38.1
   without hemorrhage P38.9
 neck (region) L02.11
  lymph gland or node L04.0
 nephritic —*see* Abscess, kidney
 nipple N61.1
  associated with
   lactation —*see* Pregnancy, complicated by
   pregnancy —*see* Pregnancy, complicated
     by
 nose (external) (fossa) (septum) J34.0
  sinus (chronic) —*see* Sinusitis
 omentum K65.1
 operative wound T81.49
 orbit, orbital —*see* Cellulitis, orbit
 otogenic G06.0
 ovary, ovarian (corpus luteum) —*see* Oophoritis
 oviduct —*see* Oophoritis
 palate (soft) K12.2
  hard M27.2
 palmar (space) —*see* Abscess, hand
 pancreas (duct) —*see* Pancreatitis, acute
 parafrenal N48.21
 parametric, parametrium N73.2
  acute N73.0
  chronic N73.1
 paranephric N15.1
 parapancreatic —*see* Pancreatitis, acute
 parapharyngeal J39.0
 pararectal K61.1
 parasinus —*see* Sinusitis
 parauterine *(see also* Disease, pelvis,
   inflammatory) N73.2
 paravaginal —*see* Vaginitis
 parietal region (scalp) L02.811
 parodontal —*see* Periodontitis, aggressive,
   localized
 parotid (duct) (gland) K11.3
  region K12.2
 pectoral (region) L02.213
 pelvis, pelvic
  female —*see* Disease, pelvis, inflammatory
  male, peritoneal K65.1
 penis N48.21
  gonococcal (accessory gland) (periurethral)
    A54.1
 perianal K61.0
 periapical K04.7
  with sinus (alveolar) K04.6
 periappendicular K35.33
 pericardial I30.1
 pericecal K35.33
 pericemental —*see* Periodontitis, aggressive,
   localized
 pericholecystic —*see* Cholecystitis, acute
 pericoronal —*see* Periodontitis, aggressive,
   localized
 peridental —*see* Periodontitis, aggressive,
   localized
 perimetric —*see also* Disease, pelvis,
   inflammatory N73.2
 perinephric, perinephritic —*see* Abscess,
   kidney
 perineum, perineal (superficial) L02.215
  urethra N34.0
 periodontal (parietal) —*see* Periodontitis,
   aggressive, localized
  apical K04.7
 periosteum, periosteal —*see also*
   Osteomyelitis, specified type NEC
  with osteomyelitis —*see also* Osteomyelitis,
    specified type NEC

Abscess *(Continued)*
 periosteum, periosteal *(Continued)*
  acute —*see* Osteomyelitis, acute
  chronic —*see* Osteomyelitis, chronic
 peripharyngeal J39.0
 peripleuritic J86.9
  with fistula J86.0
 periprostatic N41.2
 perirectal K61.1
 perirenal (tissue) —*see* Abscess, kidney
 perisinuous (nose) —*see* Sinusitis
 peritoneum, peritoneal (perforated)
   (ruptured) K65.1
  with appendicitis *(see also* Appendicitis)
    K35.33
  pelvic
   female —*see* Peritonitis, pelvic, female
   male K65.1
  postoperative T81.49
  puerperal, postpartum, childbirth O85
  tuberculous A18.31
 peritonsillar J36
 perityphlic K35.33
 periureteral N28.89
 periurethral N34.0
  gonococcal (accessory gland) (periurethral)
    A54.1
 periuterine —*see also* Disease, pelvis,
   inflammatory N73.2
 perivesical —*see* Cystitis, specified type NEC
 petrous bone —*see* Petrositis
 phagedenic NOS L02.91
  chancroid A57
 pharynx, pharyngeal (lateral) J39.1
 pilonidal L05.01
 pituitary (gland) E23.6
 pleura J86.9
  with fistula J86.0
 popliteal —*see* Abscess, lower limb
 postcecal K35.33
 postlaryngeal J38.7
 postnasal J34.0
 postoperative (any site) *(see also* Infection,
   postoperative wound) T81.49
  retroperitoneal K68.11
 postpharyngeal J39.0
 posttonsillar J36
 post-typhoid A01.09
 pouch of Douglas —*see* Peritonitis, pelvic,
   female
 premammary —*see* Abscess, breast
 prepatellar —*see* Abscess, lower limb
▶presacral K68.19
 prostate N41.2
  gonococcal (acute) (chronic) A54.22
 psoas muscle K68.12
 puerperal - code by site under Puerperal,
   abscess
 pulmonary —*see* Abscess, lung
 pulp, pulpal (dental) K04.01
  irreversible K04.02
  reversible K04.01
 rectovaginal septum K63.0
 rectovesical —*see* Cystitis, specified
   type NEC
 rectum K61.1
 renal —*see* Abscess, kidney
 retina —*see* Inflammation, chorioretinal
 retrobulbar —*see* Abscess, orbit
 retrocecal K65.1
 retrolaryngeal J38.7
 retromammary —*see* Abscess, breast
 retroperitoneal NEC K68.19
  postprocedural K68.11
 retropharyngeal J39.0
 retrouterine —*see* Peritonitis, pelvic, female
 retrovesical —*see* Cystitis, specified type NEC
 root, tooth K04.7
  with sinus (alveolar) K04.6
 round ligament —*see also* Disease, pelvis,
   inflammatory N73.2
 rupture (spontaneous) NOS L02.91

Abscess *(Continued)*
 sacrum (tuberculous)
  nontuberculous M46.28
 salivary (duct) (gland) K11.3
 scalp (any part) L02.811
 scapular —*see* Osteomyelitis, specified type
   NEC
 sclera —*see* Scleritis
 scrofulous (tuberculous) A18.2
 scrotum N49.2
 seminal vesicle N49.0
 septal, dental K04.7
  with sinus (alveolar) K04.6
 serous —*see* Periostitis
 shoulder (region) —*see* Abscess, upper limb
 sigmoid K63.0
 sinus (accessory) (chronic) (nasal) —*see also*
   Sinusitis
  intracranial venous (any) G06.0
 Skene's duct or gland N34.0
 skin —*see* Abscess, by site
 specified site NEC L02.818
 spermatic cord N49.1
 sphenoidal (sinus) (chronic) J32.3
 spinal cord (any part) (staphylococcal) G06.1
  tuberculous A17.81
 spine (column) (tuberculous) A18.01
  epidural G06.1
  nontuberculous —*see* Osteomyelitis, vertebra
 spleen D73.3
  amebic A06.89
 stitch T81.41
  following an obstetrical procedure O86.01
 subarachnoid G06.2
  brain G06.0
  spinal cord G06.1
 subareolar —*see* Abscess, breast
 subcecal K35.33
 subcutaneous —*see also* Abscess, by site
  following procedure T81.41
   obstetrical O86.01
  pheomycotic (chromomycotic) B43.2
 subdiaphragmatic K65.1
 subdural G06.2
  brain G06.0
   sequelae G09
  spinal cord G06.1
 sub-fascial, following an obstetrical
   procedure O86.02
 subgaleal L02.811
 subhepatic K65.1
 sublingual K12.2
  gland K11.3
 submammary —*see* Abscess, breast
 submandibular (region) (space) (triangle) K12.2
  gland K11.3
 submaxillary (region) L02.01
  gland K11.3
 submental L02.01
  gland K11.3
 subperiosteal —*see* Osteomyelitis, specified
   type NEC
 subphrenic K65.1
  following an obstetrical procedure O86.03
  postoperative T81.43
 suburethral N34.0
 sudoriparous L75.8
 supraclavicular (fossa) —*see* Abscess, upper
   limb
 supralevator K61.5
 suprapelvic, acute N73.0
 suprarenal (capsule) (gland) E27.8
 sweat gland L74.8
 tear duct —*see* Inflammation, lacrimal,
   passages, acute
 temple L02.01
 temporal region L02.01
 temporosphenoidal G06.0
 tendon (sheath) M65.00
  ankle M65.07-●
  foot M65.07-●
  forearm M65.03-●
  hand M65.04-●

Abscess *(Continued)*
 tendon (sheath) *(Continued)*
  lower leg M65.06-●
  pelvic region M65.05-●
  shoulder region M65.01-●
  specified site NEC M65.08
  thigh M65.05-●
  upper arm M65.02-●
 testis N45.4
 thigh —*see* Abscess, lower limb
 thorax J86.9
  with fistula J86.0
 throat J39.1
 thumb —*see also* Abscess, hand
  nail —*see* Cellulitis, finger
 thymus (gland) E32.1
 thyroid (gland) E06.0
 toe (any) —*see also* Abscess, foot
  nail —*see* Cellulitis, toe
 tongue (staphylococcal) K14.0
 tonsil(s) (lingual) J36
 tonsillopharyngeal J36
 tooth, teeth (root) K04.7
  with sinus (alveolar) K04.6
  supporting structures NEC —*see*
    Periodontitis, aggressive, localized
 trachea J39.8
 trunk L02.219
  abdominal wall L02.211
  back L02.212
  chest wall L02.213
  groin L02.214
  perineum L02.215
  umbilicus L02.216
 tubal —*see* Salpingitis
 tuberculous —*see* Tuberculosis, abscess
 tubo-ovarian —*see* Salpingo-oophoritis
 tunica vaginalis N49.1
 umbilicus L02.216
 upper
  limb L02.41-●
  respiratory J39.8
 urethral (gland) N34.0
 urinary N34.0
 uterus, uterine (wall) —*see also* Endometritis
  ligament —*see also* Disease, pelvis,
    inflammatory N73.2
  neck —*see* Cervicitis
 uvula K12.2
 vagina (wall) —*see* Vaginitis
 vaginorectal —*see* Vaginitis
 vas deferens N49.1
 vermiform appendix K35.33
 vertebra (column) (tuberculous) A18.01
  nontuberculous —*see* Osteomyelitis,
    vertebra
 vesical —*see* Cystitis, specified type NEC
 vesico-uterine pouch —*see* Peritonitis, pelvic,
   female
 vitreous (humor) —*see* Endophthalmitis,
   purulent
 vocal cord J38.3
 von Bezold's —*see* Mastoiditis, acute
 vulva N76.4
 vulvovaginal gland N75.1
 web space —*see* Abscess, hand
 wound T81.49
 wrist —*see* Abscess, upper limb
Absence (of) (organ or part) (complete or
   partial)
 adrenal (gland) (congenital) Q89.1
  acquired E89.6
 albumin in blood E88.09
 alimentary tract (congenital) Q45.8
  upper Q40.8
 alveolar process (acquired) —*see* Anomaly,
   alveolar
 ankle (acquired) Z89.44-●
 anus (congenital) Q42.3
  with fistula Q42.2
 aorta (congenital) Q25.41
 appendix, congenital Q42.8

Absence *(Continued)*
 arm (acquired) Z89.20-●
  above elbow Z89.22-●
   congenital (with hand present) —*see*
     Agenesis, arm, with hand present
     and hand —*see* Agenesis, forearm,
     and hand
  below elbow Z89.21-●
   congenital (with hand present) —*see*
     Agenesis, arm, with hand present
     and hand —*see* Agenesis, forearm,
     and hand
  congenital —*see* Defect, reduction, upper
    limb
  shoulder (following explantation of
    shoulder joint prosthesis) (joint) (with
    or without presence of antibiotic-
    impregnated cement spacer) Z89.23-●
   congenital (with hand present) —*see*
     Agenesis, arm, with hand present
 artery (congenital) (peripheral) Q27.8
  brain Q28.3
  coronary Q24.5
  pulmonary Q25.79
  specified NEC Q27.8
  umbilical Q27.0
 atrial septum (congenital) Q21.1
 auditory canal (congenital) (external) Q16.1
 auricle (ear), congenital Q16.0
 bile, biliary duct, congenital Q44.5
 bladder (acquired) Z90.6
  congenital Q64.5
 bowel sounds R19.11
 brain Q00.0
  part of Q04.3
 breast(s) (and nipple(s)) (acquired) Z90.1-●
  congenital Q83.8
 broad ligament Q50.6
 bronchus (congenital) Q32.4
 canaliculus lacrimalis, congenital Q10.4
 cerebellum (vermis) Q04.3
 cervix (acquired) (with uterus) Z90.710
  with remaining uterus Z90.712
  congenital Q51.5
 chin, congenital Q18.8
 cilia (congenital) Q10.3
  acquired —*see* Madarosis
 clitoris (congenital) Q52.6
 coccyx, congenital Q76.49
 cold sense R20.8
 congenital
  lumen —*see* Atresia
  organ or site NEC —*see* Agenesis
  septum —*see* Imperfect, closure
 corpus callosum Q04.0
 cricoid cartilage, congenital Q31.8
 diaphragm (with hernia), congenital Q79.1
 digestive organ(s) or tract, congenital Q45.8
  acquired NEC Z90.49
  upper Q40.8
 ductus arteriosus Q28.8
 duodenum (acquired) Z90.49
  congenital Q41.0
 ear, congenital Q16.9
  acquired H93.8-●
  auricle Q16.0
  external Q16.0
  inner Q16.5
  lobe, lobule Q17.8
  middle, except ossicles Q16.4
   ossicles Q16.3
  ossicles Q16.3
 ejaculatory duct (congenital) Q55.4
 endocrine gland (congenital) NEC Q89.2
  acquired E89.89
 epididymis (congenital) Q55.4
  acquired Z90.79
 epiglottis, congenital Q31.8
 esophagus (congenital) Q39.8
  acquired (partial) Z90.49
 eustachian tube (congenital) Q16.2
 extremity (acquired) Z89.9
  congenital Q73.0

▶ New   ⇒ Revised   ~~deleted~~ Deleted   ● Use Additional Character(s)

Absence *(Continued)*
  extremity (acquired) *(Continued)*
    knee (following explanation of knee joint
        prosthesis) (joint) (with or without
        presence of antibiotic-impregnated
        cement spacer) Z89.52-●
    lower (above knee) Z89.619
        below knee Z89.51-●
    upper —*see* Absence, arm
  eye (acquired) Z90.01
    congenital Q11.1
    muscle (congenital) Q10.3
  eyeball (acquired) Z90.01
  eyelid (fold) (congenital) Q10.3
    acquired Z90.01
  face, specified part NEC Q18.8
  fallopian tube(s) (acquired) Z90.79
    congenital Q50.6
  family member (causing problem in home)
      NEC —*see also* Disruption, family Z63.32
  femur, congenital —*see* Defect, reduction,
      lower limb, longitudinal, femur
  fibrinogen (congenital) D68.2
    acquired D65
  finger(s) (acquired) Z89.02-●
    congenital —*see* Agenesis, hand
  foot (acquired) Z89.43-●
    congenital —*see* Agenesis, foot
  forearm (acquired) —*see* Absence, arm, below
      elbow
  gallbladder (acquired) Z90.49
    congenital Q44.0
  gamma globulin in blood D80.1
    hereditary D80.0
  genital organs
    acquired (female) (male) Z90.79
    female, congenital Q52.8
        external Q52.71
        internal NEC Q52.8
    male, congenital Q55.8
  genitourinary organs, congenital NEC
    female Q52.8
    male Q55.8
  globe (acquired) Z90.01
    congenital Q11.1
  glottis, congenital Q31.8
  hand and wrist (acquired) Z89.11-●
    congenital —*see* Agenesis, hand
  head, part (acquired) NEC Z90.09
  heat sense R20.8
  hip (following explantation of hip joint
      prosthesis) (joint) (with or without
      presence of antibiotic-impregnated
      cement spacer) Z89.62-●
  hymen (congenital) Q52.4
  ileum (acquired) Z90.49
    congenital Q41.2
  immunoglobulin, isolated NEC D80.3
    IgA D80.2
    IgG D80.3
    IgM D80.4
  incus (acquired) —*see* Loss, ossicles, ear
    congenital Q16.3
  inner ear, congenital Q16.5
  intestine (acquired) (small) Z90.49
    congenital Q41.9
        specified NEC Q41.8
    large Z90.49
        congenital Q42.9
            specified NEC Q42.8
  iris, congenital Q13.1
  jejunum (acquired) Z90.49
    congenital Q41.1
  joint
    acquired
        hip (following explantation of hip joint
            prosthesis) (with or without
            presence of antibiotic-impregnated
            cement spacer) Z89.62-●
        knee (following explantation of knee
            joint prosthesis) (with or without
            presence of antibiotic-impregnated
            cement spacer) Z89.52-●

Absence *(Continued)*
  joint *(Continued)*
    acquired *(Continued)*
        shoulder (following explantation of
            shoulder joint prosthesis) (with or
            without presence of antibiotic-
            impregnated cement spacer) Z89.23-●
    congenital NEC Q74.8
  kidney(s) (acquired) Z90.5
    congenital Q60.2
        bilateral Q60.1
        unilateral Q60.0
  knee (following explantation of knee joint
      prosthesis) (joint) (with or without
      presence of antibiotic-impregnated
      cement spacer) Z89.52-●
  labyrinth, membranous Q16.5
  larynx (congenital) Q31.8
    acquired Z90.02
  leg (acquired) (above knee) Z89.61-●
    below knee (acquired) Z89.51-●
    congenital —*see* Defect, reduction, lower
        limb
  lens (acquired) —*see also* Aphakia
    congenital Q12.3
    post cataract extraction Z98.4-●
  limb (acquired) —*see* Absence, extremity
  lip Q38.6
  liver (congenital) Q44.7
  lung (fissure) (lobe) (bilateral) (unilateral)
      (congenital) Q33.3
    acquired (any part) Z90.2
  menstruation —*see* Amenorrhea
  muscle (congenital) (pectoral) Q79.8
    ocular Q10.3
  neck, part Q18.8
  neutrophil —*see* Agranulocytosis
  nipple(s) (with breast(s)) (acquired) Z90.1-●
    congenital Q83.2
  nose (congenital) Q30.1
    acquired Z90.09
  organ
    of Corti, congenital Q16.5
    or site, congenital NEC Q89.8
        acquired NEC Z90.89
  osseous meatus (ear) Q16.4
  ovary (acquired)
    bilateral Z90.722
    congenital
        bilateral Q50.02
        unilateral Q50.01
    unilateral Z90.721
  oviduct (acquired)
    bilateral Z90.722
    congenital Q50.6
    unilateral Z90.721
  pancreas (congenital) Q45.0
    acquired Z90.410
        complete Z90.410
        partial Z90.411
        total Z90.410
  parathyroid gland (acquired) E89.2
    congenital Q89.2
  patella, congenital Q74.1
  penis (congenital) Q55.5
    acquired Z90.79
  pericardium (congenital) Q24.8
  pituitary gland (congenital) Q89.2
    acquired E89.3
  prostate (acquired) Z90.79
    congenital Q55.4
  pulmonary valve Q22.0
  punctum lacrimale (congenital) Q10.4
  radius, congenital —*see* Defect, reduction,
      upper limb, longitudinal, radius
  rectum (congenital) Q42.1
    with fistula Q42.0
    acquired Z90.49
  respiratory organ NOS Q34.9
  rib (acquired) Z90.89
    congenital Q76.6
  sacrum, congenital Q76.49

Absence *(Continued)*
  salivary gland(s), congenital Q38.4
  scrotum, congenital Q55.29
  seminal vesicles (congenital) Q55.4
    acquired Z90.79
  septum
    atrial (congenital) Q21.1
    between aorta and pulmonary artery Q21.4
    ventricular (congenital) Q20.4
  sex chromosome
    female phenotype Q97.8
    male phenotype Q98.8
  skull bone (congenital) Q75.8
    with
        anencephaly Q00.0
        encephalocele —*see* Encephalocele
        hydrocephalus Q03.9
            with spina bifida —*see* Spina bifida, by
                site, with hydrocephalus
        microcephaly Q02
  spermatic cord, congenital Q55.4
  spine, congenital Q76.49
  spleen (congenital) Q89.01
    acquired Z90.81
  sternum, congenital Q76.7
  stomach (acquired) (partial) Z90.3
    congenital Q40.2
  superior vena cava, congenital Q26.8
  teeth, tooth (congenital) K00.0
    acquired (complete) K08.109
        class I K08.101
        class II K08.102
        class III K08.103
        class IV K08.104
        due to
            caries K08.139
                class I K08.131
                class II K08.132
                class III K08.133
                class IV K08.134
            periodontal disease K08.129
                class I K08.121
                class II K08.122
                class III K08.123
                class IV K08.124
            specified NEC K08.199
                class I K08.191
                class II K08.192
                class III K08.193
                class IV K08.194
            trauma K08.119
                class I K08.111
                class II K08.112
                class III K08.113
                class IV K08.114
    partial K08.409
        class I K08.401
        class II K08.402
        class III K08.403
        class IV K08.404
        due to
            caries K08.439
                class I K08.431
                class II K08.432
                class III K08.433
                class IV K08.434
            periodontal disease K08.429
                class I K08.421
                class II K08.422
                class III K08.423
                class IV K08.424
            specified NEC K08.499
                class I K08.491
                class II K08.492
                class III K08.493
                class IV K08.494
            trauma K08.419
                class I K08.411
                class II K08.412
                class III K08.413
                class IV K08.414
  tendon (congenital) Q79.8

Absence *(Continued)*
 testis (congenital) Q55.0
  acquired Z90.79
 thumb (acquired) Z89.01-•
  congenital —*see* Agenesis, hand
 thymus gland Q89.2
 thyroid (gland) (acquired) E89.0
  cartilage, congenital Q31.8
  congenital E03.1
 toe(s) (acquired) Z89.42-•
  with foot —*see* Absence, foot and ankle
  congenital —*see* Agenesis, foot
   great Z89.41-•
 tongue, congenital Q38.3
 trachea (cartilage), congenital Q32.1
 transverse aortic arch, congenital Q25.49
 tricuspid valve Q22.4
 umbilical artery, congenital Q27.0
 upper arm and forearm with hand present,
   congenital —*see* Agenesis, arm, with
   hand present
 ureter (congenital) Q62.4
  acquired Z90.6
 urethra, congenital Q64.5
 uterus (acquired) Z90.710
  with cervix Z90.710
  with remaining cervical stump Z90.711
  congenital Q51.0
 uvula, congenital Q38.5
 vagina, congenital Q52.0
 vas deferens (congenital) Q55.4
  acquired Z90.79
 vein (peripheral) congenital NEC Q27.8
  cerebral Q28.3
  digestive system Q27.8
  great Q26.8
  lower limb Q27.8
  portal Q26.5
  precerebral Q28.1
  specified site NEC Q27.8
  upper limb Q27.8
 vena cava (inferior) (superior), congenital
   Q26.8
 ventricular septum Q20.4
 vertebra, congenital Q76.49
 vulva, congenital Q52.71
 wrist (acquired) Z89.12-•
Absorbent system disease I87.8
Absorption
 carbohydrate, disturbance K90.49
 chemical —*see* Table of Drugs and Chemicals
  through placenta (newborn) P04.9
   environmental substance P04.6
   nutritional substance P04.5
   obstetric anesthetic or analgesic drug P04.0
 drug NEC —*see* Table of Drugs and Chemicals
  addictive
   through placenta (newborn) *(see also*
    Newborn, affected by, maternal,
    use of) P04.40
    cocaine P04.41
    hallucinogens P04.42
    specified drug NEC P04.49
  medicinal
   through placenta (newborn) P04.19
  through placenta (newborn) P04.19
   obstetric anesthetic or analgesic drug P04.0
 fat, disturbance K90.49
  pancreatic K90.3
 noxious substance —*see* Table of Drugs and
   Chemicals
 protein, disturbance K90.49
 starch, disturbance K90.49
 toxic substance —*see* Table of Drugs and
   Chemicals
 uremic —*see* Uremia
Abstinence symptoms, syndrome
 alcohol F10.239
  with delirium F10.231
 cocaine F14.23
 neonatal P96.1
 nicotine —*see* Dependence, drug, nicotine,
   with, withdrawal

Abstinence symptoms, syndrome *(Continued)*
 opioid F11.93
  with dependence F11.23
 psychoactive NEC F19.939
  with
   delirium F19.931
   dependence F19.239
    with
     delirium F19.231
     perceptual disturbance F19.232
    uncomplicated F19.230
   perceptual disturbance F19.932
  uncomplicated F19.930
 sedative F13.939
  with
   delirium F13.931
   dependence F13.239
    with
     delirium F13.231
     perceptual disturbance F13.232
    uncomplicated F13.230
   perceptual disturbance F13.932
  uncomplicated F13.930
 stimulant NEC F15.93
  with dependence F15.23
Abulia R68.89
Abulomania F60.7
Abuse
 adult —*see* Maltreatment, adult
  as reason for
   couple seeking advice (including
     offender) Z63.0
 alcohol (non-dependent) F10.10
  with
   anxiety disorder F10.180
   intoxication F10.129
    with delirium F10.121
    uncomplicated F10.120
   mood disorder F10.14
   other specified disorder F10.188
   psychosis F10.159
    delusions F10.150
    hallucinations F10.151
   sexual dysfunction F10.181
   sleep disorder F10.182
   unspecified disorder F10.19
   withdrawal F10.139
    with
     perceptual disturbance F10.132
    delirium F10.131
    uncomplicated F10.130
  counseling and surveillance Z71.41
  in remission (early) (sustained) F10.11
 amphetamine (or related substance) —*see also*
   Abuse, drug, stimulant NEC
  stimulant NEC F15.10
   with
    anxiety disorder F15.180
    intoxication F15.129
     with
      delirium F15.121
      perceptual disturbance F15.122
    withdrawal F15.13
 analgesics (non-prescribed) (over the counter)
   F55.8
 antacids F55.0
 antidepressants —*see* Abuse, drug,
   psychoactive NEC
 anxiolytic —*see* Abuse, drug, sedative
 barbiturates —*see* Abuse, drug, sedative
 caffeine —*see* Abuse, drug, stimulant NEC
 cannabis, cannabinoids —*see* Abuse, drug,
   cannabis
 child —*see* Maltreatment, child
 cocaine —*see* Abuse, drug, cocaine
 drug NEC (non-dependent) F19.10
  with sleep disorder F19.182
  amphetamine type —*see* Abuse, drug,
    stimulant NEC
  analgesics (non-prescribed) (over the
    counter) F55.8
  antacids F55.0
  antidepressants —*see* Abuse, drug,
    psychoactive NEC

Abuse *(Continued)*
 drug NEC *(Continued)*
  anxiolytics —*see* Abuse, drug, sedative
  barbiturates —*see* Abuse, drug, sedative
  caffeine —*see* Abuse, drug, stimulant NEC
  cannabis F12.10
   with
    anxiety disorder F12.180
    intoxication F12.129
     with
      delirium F12.121
      perceptual disturbance F12.122
     uncomplicated F12.120
    other specified disorder F12.188
    psychosis F12.159
     delusions F12.150
     hallucinations F12.151
    unspecified disorder F12.19
    withdrawal F12.13
   in remission (early) (sustained) F12.11
  cocaine F14.10
   with
    anxiety disorder F14.180
    intoxication F14.129
     with
      delirium F14.121
      perceptual disturbance F14.122
     uncomplicated F14.120
    mood disorder F14.14
    other specified disorder F14.188
    psychosis F14.159
     delusions F14.150
     hallucinations F14.151
    sexual dysfunction F14.181
    sleep disorder F14.182
    unspecified disorder F14.19
    withdrawal F14.13
   in remission (early) (sustained) F14.11
  counseling and surveillance Z71.51
  hallucinogen F16.10
   with
    anxiety disorder F16.180
    flashbacks F16.183
    intoxication F16.129
     with
      delirium F16.121
      perceptual disturbance F16.122
     uncomplicated F16.120
    mood disorder F16.14
    other specified disorder F16.188
    perception disorder, persisting F16.183
    psychosis F16.159
     delusions F16.150
     hallucinations F16.151
    unspecified disorder F16.19
   in remission (early) (sustained) F16.11
  hashish —*see* Abuse, drug, cannabis
  herbal or folk remedies F55.1
  hormones F55.3
  hypnotics —*see* Abuse, drug, sedative
  inhalant F18.10
   with
    anxiety disorder F18.180
    dementia, persisting F18.17
    intoxication F18.129
     with delirium F18.121
     uncomplicated F18.120
    mood disorder F18.14
    other specified disorder F18.188
    psychosis F18.159
     delusions F18.150
     hallucinations F18.151
    unspecified disorder F18.19
   in remission (early) (sustained) F18.11
  in remission (early) (sustained) F19.11
  laxatives F55.2
  LSD —*see* Abuse, drug, hallucinogen
  marihuana —*see* Abuse, drug, cannabis
  morphine type (opioids) —*see* Abuse, drug,
    opioid

► New   ⇒ Revised   ~~deleted~~ Deleted   • Use Additional Character(s)

Abuse *(Continued)*
  drug NEC *(Continued)*
    opioid F11.10
      with
        intoxication F11.129
          with
            delirium F11.121
            perceptual disturbance F11.122
          uncomplicated F11.120
        mood disorder F11.14
        other specified disorder F11.188
        psychosis F11.159
          delusions F11.150
          hallucinations F11.151
        sexual dysfunction F11.181
        sleep disorder F11.182
        unspecified disorder F11.19
        withdrawal F11.13
      in remission (early) (sustained) F11.11
    PCP (phencyclidine) (or related substance) —
      see Abuse, drug, hallucinogen
    psychoactive NEC F19.10
      with
        amnestic disorder F19.16
        anxiety disorder F19.180
        dementia F19.17
        intoxication F19.129
          with
            delirium F19.121
            perceptual disturbance F19.122
          uncomplicated F19.120
        mood disorder F19.14
        other specified disorder F19.188
        psychosis F19.159
          delusions F19.150
          hallucinations F19.151
        sexual dysfunction F19.181
        sleep disorder F19.182
        unspecified disorder F19.19
        withdrawal F19.139
          with
            perceptual disturbance F19.132
          delirium F19.131
          uncomplicated F19.130
    sedative, hypnotic or anxiolytic F13.10
      with
        anxiety disorder F13.180
        intoxication F13.129
          with delirium F13.121
          uncomplicated F13.120
        mood disorder F13.14
        other specified disorder F13.188
        psychosis F13.159
          delusions F13.150
          hallucinations F13.151
        sexual dysfunction F13.181
        sleep disorder F13.182
        unspecified disorder F13.19
        withdrawal F13.139
          with
            perceptual disturbance F13.132
          delirium F13.131
          uncomplicated F13.130
      in remission (early) (sustained) F13.11
    solvent —*see* Abuse, drug, inhalant
    steroids F55.3
    stimulant NEC F15.10
      with
        anxiety disorder F15.180
        intoxication F15.129
          with
            delirium F15.121
            perceptual disturbance F15.122
          uncomplicated F15.120
        mood disorder F15.14
        other specified disorder F15.188
        psychosis F15.159
          delusions F15.150
          hallucinations F15.151
        sexual dysfunction F15.181
        sleep disorder F15.182
        unspecified disorder F15.19
        withdrawal F15.13
      in remission (early) (sustained) F15.11

Abuse *(Continued)*
  drug NEC *(Continued)*
    tranquilizers —*see* Abuse, drug, sedative
    vitamins F55.4
  hallucinogens —*see* Abuse, drug, hallucinogen
  hashish —*see* Abuse, drug, cannabis
  herbal or folk remedies F55.1
  hormones F55.3
  hypnotic —*see* Abuse, drug, sedative
  inhalant —*see* Abuse, drug, inhalant
  laxatives F55.2
  LSD —*see* Abuse, drug, hallucinogen
  marihuana —*see* Abuse, drug, cannabis
  morphine type (opioids) —*see* Abuse, drug,
    opioid
  non-psychoactive substance NEC F55.8
    antacids F55.0
    folk remedies F55.1
    herbal remedies F55.1
    hormones F55.3
    laxatives F55.2
    steroids F55.3
    vitamins F55.4
  opioids —*see* Abuse, drug, opioid
  PCP (phencyclidine) (or related substance) —
    see Abuse, drug, hallucinogen
  physical (adult) (child) —*see* Maltreatment
  psychoactive substance —*see* Abuse, drug,
    psychoactive NEC
  psychological (adult) (child) —*see* Maltreatment
  sedative —*see* Abuse, drug, sedative
  sexual —*see* Maltreatment
  solvent —*see* Abuse, drug, inhalant
  steroids F55.3
  vitamins F55.4
Acalculia R48.8
  developmental F81.2
Acanthamebiasis (with) B60.10
  conjunctiva B60.12
  keratoconjunctivitis B60.13
  meningoencephalitis B60.11
  other specified B60.19
Acanthocephaliasis B83.8
Acanthocheilonemiasis B74.4
Acanthocytosis E78.6
Acantholysis L11.9
Acanthosis (acquired) (nigricans) L83
  benign Q82.8
  congenital Q82.8
  seborrheic L82.1
    inflamed L82.0
  tongue K14.3
Acapnia E87.3
Acarbia E87.2
Acardia, acardius Q89.8
Acardiacus amorphus Q89.8
Acardiotrophia I51.4
Acariasis B88.0
  scabies B86
Acarodermatitis (urticarioides) B88.0
Acarophobia F40.218
Acatalasemia, acatalasia E80.3
Acathisia (drug induced) G25.71
Accelerated atrioventricular conduction I45.6
Accentuation of personality traits (type A) Z73.1
Accessory (congenital)
  adrenal gland Q89.1
  anus Q43.4
  appendix Q43.4
  atrioventricular conduction I45.6
  auditory ossicles Q16.3
  auricle (ear) Q17.0
  biliary duct or passage Q44.5
  bladder Q64.79
  blood vessels NEC Q27.9
    coronary Q24.5
  bone NEC Q79.8
  breast tissue, axilla Q83.1
  carpal bones Q74.0
  cecum Q43.4
  chromosome(s) NEC (nonsex) Q92.9

Accessory *(Continued)*
  chromosome(s) NEC (nonsex) *(Continued)*
    with complex rearrangements NEC Q92.5
      seen only at prometaphase Q92.8
    13 —*see* Trisomy, 13
    18 —*see* Trisomy, 18
    21 —*see* Trisomy, 21
    partial Q92.9
    sex
      female phenotype Q97.8
  coronary artery Q24.5
  cusp(s), heart valve NEC Q24.8
    pulmonary Q22.3
  cystic duct Q44.5
  digit(s) Q69.9
  ear (auricle) (lobe) Q17.0
  endocrine gland NEC Q89.2
  eye muscle Q10.3
  eyelid Q10.3
  face bone(s) Q75.8
  fallopian tube (fimbria) (ostium) Q50.6
  finger(s) Q69.0
  foreskin N47.8
  frontonasal process Q75.8
  gallbladder Q44.1
  genital organ(s)
    female Q52.8
      external Q52.79
      internal NEC Q52.8
    male Q55.8
  genitourinary organs NEC Q89.8
    female Q52.8
    male Q55.8
  hallux Q69.2
  heart Q24.8
    valve NEC Q24.8
      pulmonary Q22.3
  hepatic ducts Q44.5
  hymen Q52.4
  intestine (large) (small) Q43.4
  kidney Q63.0
  lacrimal canal Q10.6
  leaflet, heart valve NEC Q24.8
  ligament, broad Q50.6
  liver Q44.7
    duct Q44.5
  lobule (ear) Q17.0
  lung (lobe) Q33.1
  muscle Q79.8
  navicular of carpus Q74.0
  nervous system, part NEC Q07.8
  nipple Q83.3
  nose Q30.8
  organ or site not listed —*see* Anomaly, by site
  ovary Q50.31
  oviduct Q50.6
  pancreas Q45.3
  parathyroid gland Q89.2
  parotid gland (and duct) Q38.4
  pituitary gland Q89.2
  preauricular appendage Q17.0
  prepuce N47.8
  renal arteries (multiple) Q27.2
  rib Q76.6
    cervical Q76.5
  roots (teeth) K00.2
  salivary gland Q38.4
  sesamoid bones Q74.8
    foot Q74.2
    hand Q74.0
  skin tags Q82.8
  spleen Q89.09
  sternum Q76.7
  submaxillary gland Q38.4
  tarsal bones Q74.2
  teeth, tooth K00.1
  tendon Q79.8
  thumb Q69.1
  thymus gland Q89.2
  thyroid gland Q89.2
  toes Q69.2

A

Accessory *(Continued)*
  tongue Q38.3
  tooth, teeth K00.1
  tragus Q17.0
  ureter Q62.5
  urethra Q64.79
  urinary organ or tract NEC Q64.8
  uterus Q51.28
  vagina Q52.10
  valve, heart NEC Q24.8
    pulmonary Q22.3
  vertebra Q76.49
  vocal cords Q31.8
  vulva Q52.79
Accident
  birth —*see* Birth, injury
  cardiac —*see* Infarct, myocardium
  cerebral I63.9
  cerebrovascular (embolic) (ischemic)
    (thrombotic) I63.9
    aborted I63.9
    hemorrhagic —*see* Hemorrhage,
      intracranial, intracerebral
    old (without sequelae) Z86.73
      with sequelae (of) —*see* Sequelae,
        infarction, cerebral
  coronary —*see* Infarct, myocardium
  craniovascular I63.9
  vascular, brain I63.9
Accidental —*see* condition
Accommodation (disorder) —*see also* condition
  hysterical paralysis of F44.89
  insufficiency of H52.4
  paresis —*see* Paresis, of accommodation
  spasm —*see* Spasm, of accommodation
Accouchement —*see* Delivery
Accreta placenta O43.21-●
Accretio cordis (nonrheumatic) I31.0
Accretions, tooth, teeth K03.6
Acculturation difficulty Z60.3
Accumulation secretion, prostate N42.89
Acephalia, acephalism, acephalus, acephaly
  Q00.0
Acephalobrachia monster Q89.8
Acephalochirus monster Q89.8
Acephalogaster Q89.8
Acephalostomus monster Q89.8
Acephalothorax Q89.8
Acerophobia F40.298
Acetonemia R79.89
  in Type 1 diabetes E10.10
    with coma E10.11
Acetonuria R82.4
Achalasia (cardia) (esophagus) K22.0
  congenital Q39.5
  pylorus Q40.0
  sphincteral NEC K59.89
Ache(s) —*see* Pain
Acheilia Q38.6
Achillobursitis —*see* Tendinitis, Achilles
Achillodynia —*see* Tendinitis, Achilles
Achlorhydria, achlorhydric (neurogenic) K31.83
  anemia D50.8
  diarrhea K31.83
  psychogenic F45.8
  secondary to vagotomy K91.1
Achluophobia F40.228
Acholia K82.8
Acholuric jaundice (familial)
  (splenomegalic) —*see also* Spherocytosis
  acquired D59.8
Achondrogenesis Q77.0
Achondroplasia (osteosclerosis congenita)
  Q77.4
Achroma, cutis L80
Achromat (ism), achromatopsia (acquired)
  (congenital) H53.51
Achromia, congenital —*see* Albinism
Achromia parasitica B36.0
Achylia gastrica K31.89
  psychogenic F45.8

Acid
  burn —*see* Corrosion
  deficiency
    amide nicotinic E52
    ascorbic E54
    folic E53.8
    nicotinic E52
    pantothenic E53.8
  intoxication E87.2
  peptic disease K30
  phosphatase deficiency E83.39
  stomach K30
    psychogenic F45.8
Acidemia E87.2
  argininosuccinic E72.22
  isovaleric E71.110
  metabolic (newborn) P19.9
    first noted before onset of labor P19.0
    first noted during labor P19.1
    noted at birth P19.2
  methylmalonic E71.120
  pipecolic E72.3
  propionic E71.121
Acidity, gastric (high) K30
  psychogenic F45.8
Acidocytopenia —*see* Agranulocytosis
Acidocytosis D72.10
Acidopenia —*see* Agranulocytosis
Acidosis (lactic) (respiratory) E87.2
  in Type 1 diabetes E10.10
    with coma E10.11
  kidney, tubular N25.89
  lactic E87.2
  metabolic NEC E87.2
    hyperchloremic, of newborn P74.421
    with respiratory acidosis E87.4
    late, of newborn P74.0
  mixed metabolic and respiratory, newborn P84
  newborn P84
  renal (hyperchloremic) (tubular) N25.89
  respiratory E87.2
    complicated by
      metabolic
        acidosis E87.4
        alkalosis E87.4
Aciduria
  4-hydroxybutyric E72.81
  argininosuccinic E72.22
  gamma-hydroxybutyric E72.81
  glutaric (type I) E72.3
    type II E71.313
    type III E71.5-●
  orotic (congenital) (hereditary) (pyrimidine
    deficiency) E79.8
    anemia D53.0
Acladiosis (skin) B36.0
Aclasis, diaphyseal Q78.6
Acleistocardia Q21.1
Aclusion —*see* Anomaly, dentofacial,
  malocclusion
Acne L70.9
  artificialis L70.8
  atrophica L70.2
  cachecticorum (Hebra) L70.8
  conglobata L70.1
  cystic L70.0
  decalvans L66.2
  excoriée (des jeunes filles) L70.5
  frontalis L70.2
  indurata L70.0
  infantile L70.4
  keloid L73.0
  lupoid L70.2
  necrotic, necrotica (miliaris) L70.2
  neonatal L70.4
  nodular L70.0
  occupational L70.8
  picker's L70.5
  pustular L70.0
  rodens L70.2
  rosacea L71.9

Acne *(Continued)*
  specified NEC L70.8
  tropica L70.3
  varioliformis L70.2
  vulgaris L70.0
Acnitis (primary) A18.4
Acosta's disease T70.29
Acoustic —*see* condition
Acousticophobia F40.298
ACPO (acute colonic pseudo-obstruction) K59.81
Acquired —*see also* condition
  immunodeficiency syndrome (AIDS) B20
Acrania Q00.0
Acroangiodermatitis I78.9
Acroasphyxia, chronic I73.89
Acrobystitis N47.7
Acrocephalopolysyndactyly Q87.0
Acrocephalosyndactyly Q87.0
Acrocephaly Q75.0
Acrochondrohyperplasia —*see* Syndrome,
  Marfan's
Acrocyanosis I73.89
  newborn P28.2
    meaning transient blue hands and feet -
      omit code
Acrodermatitis L30.8
  atrophicans (chronica) L90.4
  continua (Hallopeau) L40.2
  enteropathica (hereditary) E83.2
  Hallopeau's L40.2
  infantile papular L44.4
  perstans L40.2
  pustulosa continua L40.2
  recalcitrant pustular L40.2
Acrodynia —*see* Poisoning, mercury
Acromegaly, acromegalia E22.0
Acromelalgia I73.81
Acromicria, acromikria Q79.8
Acronyx L60.0
Acropachy, thyroid —*see* Thyrotoxicosis
Acroparesthesia (simple) (vasomotor) I73.89
Acropathy, thyroid —*see* Thyrotoxicosis
Acrophobia F40.241
Acroposthitis N47.7
Acroscleriasis, acroscleroderma,
  acrosclerosis —*see* Sclerosis, systemic
Acrosphacelus I96
Acrospiroma, eccrine —*see* Neoplasm, skin,
  benign
Acrostealgia —*see* Osteochondropathy
Acrotrophodynia —*see* Immersion
ACTH ectopic syndrome E24.3
Actinic —*see* condition
Actinobacillosis, actinobacillus A28.8
  mallei A24.0
  muris A25.1
Actinomyces israelii (infection) —*see*
  Actinomycosis
Actinomycetoma (foot) B47.1
Actinomycosis, actinomycotic A42.9
  with pneumonia A42.0
  abdominal A42.1
  cervicofacial A42.2
  cutaneous A42.89
  gastrointestinal A42.1
  pulmonary A42.0
  sepsis A42.7
  specified site NEC A42.89
Actinoneuritis G62.82
Action, heart
  disorder I49.9
  irregular I49.9
    psychogenic F45.8
Activated protein C resistance D68.51
Activation
  mast cell (disorder) (syndrome) D89.40
    idiopathic D89.42
    monoclonal D89.41
    secondary D89.43
    specified type NEC D89.49
Active —*see* condition

▶ New   ⇒ Revised   ~~deleted~~ Deleted   ● Use Additional Character(s)

Acute —*see also* condition
  abdomen R10.0
  gallbladder —*see* Cholecystitis, acute
Acyanotic heart disease (congenital) Q24.9
Acystia Q64.5
Adair-Dighton syndrome (brittle bones and
    blue sclera, deafness) Q78.0
Adamantinoblastoma —*see* Ameloblastoma
Adamantinoma —*see also* Cyst, calcifying
    odontogenic
  long bones C40.90
    lower limb C40.2-•
    upper limb C40.0-•
  malignant C41.1
    jaw (bone) (lower) C41.1
      upper C41.0
  tibial C40.2-•
Adamantoblastoma —*see* Ameloblastoma
Adams-Stokes (-Morgagni) disease or
    syndrome I45.9
Adaption reaction —*see* Disorder, adjustment
Addiction —*see also* Dependence F19.20
  alcohol, alcoholic (ethyl) (methyl) (wood)
      (without remission) F10.20
    with remission F10.21
  drug —*see* Dependence, drug
  ethyl alcohol (without remission) F10.20
    with remission F10.21
  heroin —*see* Dependence, drug, opioid
  methyl alcohol (without remission) F10.20
    with remission F10.21
  methylated spirit (without remission) F10.20
    with remission F10.21
  morphine(-like substances) —*see*
    Dependence, drug, opioid
  nicotine —*see* Dependence, drug, nicotine
  opium and opioids —*see* Dependence, drug,
    opioid
  tobacco —*see* Dependence, drug, nicotine
Addisonian crisis E27.2
Addison's
  anemia (pernicious) D51.0
  disease (bronze) or syndrome E27.1
    tuberculous A18.7
  keloid L94.0
Addison-Biermer anemia (pernicious) D51.0
Addison-Schilder complex E71.528
Additional —*see also* Accessory
  chromosome(s) Q99.8
    21 —*see* Trisomy, 21
    sex —*see* Abnormal, chromosome, sex
Adduction contracture, hip or other joint —*see*
    Contraction, joint
Adenitis —*see also* Lymphadenitis
  acute, unspecified site L04.9
  axillary I88.9
    acute L04.2
    chronic or subacute I88.1
  Bartholin's gland N75.8
  bulbourethral gland —*see* Urethritis
  cervical I88.9
    acute L04.0
    chronic or subacute I88.1
  chancroid (Hemophilus ducreyi) A57
  chronic, unspecified site I88.1
  Cowper's gland —*see* Urethritis
  due to Pasteurella multocida (P. septica) A28.0
  epidemic, acute B27.09
  gangrenous L04.9
  gonorrheal NEC A54.89
  groin I88.9
    acute L04.1
    chronic or subacute I88.1
  infectious (acute) (epidemic) B27.09
  inguinal I88.9
    acute L04.1
    chronic or subacute I88.1
  lymph gland or node, except mesenteric I88.9
    acute —*see* Lymphadenitis, acute
    chronic or subacute I88.1
  mesenteric (acute) (chronic) (nonspecific)
    (subacute) I88.0

Adenitis (Continued)
  parotid gland (suppurative) —*see*
    Sialoadenitis
  salivary gland (any) (suppurative) —*see*
    Sialoadenitis
  scrofulous (tuberculous) A18.2
  Skene's duct or gland —*see* Urethritis
  strumous, tuberculous A18.2
  subacute, unspecified site I88.1
  sublingual gland (suppurative) —*see*
    Sialoadenitis
  submandibular gland (suppurative) —*see*
    Sialoadenitis
  submaxillary gland (suppurative) —*see*
    Sialoadenitis
  tuberculous —*see* Tuberculosis, lymph gland
  urethral gland —*see* Urethritis
  Wharton's duct (suppurative) —*see*
    Sialoadenitis
Adenoacanthoma —*see* Neoplasm, malignant,
    by site
Adenoameloblastoma —*see* Cyst, calcifying
    odontogenic
Adenocarcinoid (tumor) —*see* Neoplasm,
    malignant, by site
Adenocarcinoma —*see also* Neoplasm,
    malignant, by site
  acidophil
    specified site —*see* Neoplasm, malignant,
      by site
    unspecified site C75.1
  adrenal cortical C74.0-•
  alveolar —*see* Neoplasm, lung, malignant
  apocrine
    breast —*see* Neoplasm, breast, malignant
    in situ
      breast D05.8-•
      specified site NEC —*see* Neoplasm, skin,
        in situ
      unspecified site D04.9
    specified site NEC —*see* Neoplasm, skin,
      malignant
    unspecified site C44.99
  basal cell
    specified site —*see* Neoplasm, skin,
      malignant
    unspecified site C08.9
  basophil
    specified site —*see* Neoplasm, malignant,
      by site
    unspecified site C75.1
  bile duct type C22.1
    liver C22.1
    specified site NEC —*see* Neoplasm,
      malignant, by site
    unspecified site C22.1
  bronchiolar —*see* Neoplasm, lung,
    malignant
  bronchioloalveolar —*see* Neoplasm, lung,
    malignant
  ceruminous C44.29-•
  cervix, in situ (*see also* Carcinoma, cervix
    uteri, in situ) D06.9
  chromophobe
    specified site —*see* Neoplasm, malignant,
      by site
    unspecified site C75.1
  diffuse type
    specified site —*see* Neoplasm, malignant,
      by site
    unspecified site C16.9
  duct
    infiltrating
      with Paget's disease —*see* Neoplasm,
        breast, malignant
      specified site —*see* Neoplasm,
        malignant, by site
      unspecified site (female) C50.91-•
        male C50.92-•
    specified site —*see* Neoplasm, malignant,
      by site

Adenocarcinoma (Continued)
  duct (Continued)
    unspecified site
      female C56.9
      male C61
  eosinophil
    specified site —*see* Neoplasm, malignant,
      by site
    unspecified site C75.1
  follicular
    with papillary C73
    moderately differentiated C73
    specified site —*see* Neoplasm, malignant,
      by site
    trabecular C73
    unspecified site C73
    well differentiated C73
  Hurthle cell C73
  in
    adenomatous
      polyposis coli C18.9
  infiltrating duct
    with Paget's disease —*see* Neoplasm,
      breast, malignant
    specified site —*see* Neoplasm,
      malignant, by site
    unspecified site (female)
      C50.91-•
      male C50.92-•
  inflammatory
    specified site —*see* Neoplasm,
      malignant, by site
    unspecified site (female)
      C50.91-•
      male C50.92-•
  intestinal type
    specified site —*see* Neoplasm,
      malignant, by site
    unspecified site C16.9
  intracystic papillary
  intraductal
    breast D05.1-•
    noninfiltrating
      breast D05.1-•
      papillary
        with invasion
          specified site —*see* Neoplasm,
            malignant, by site
          unspecified site (female)
            C50.91-•
            male C50.92-•
        breast D05.1-•
        specified site NEC —*see* Neoplasm, in
          situ, by site
        unspecified site D05.1-•
      specified site NEC —*see* Neoplasm, in
        situ, by site
      unspecified site D05.1-•
    papillary
      with invasion
        specified site —*see* Neoplasm,
          malignant, by site
        unspecified site (female)
          C50.91-•
          male C50.92-•
      breast D05.1-•
      specified site —*see* Neoplasm, in situ,
        by site
      unspecified site D05.1-•
    specified site NEC —*see* Neoplasm, in situ,
      by site
    unspecified site D05.1-•
  islet cell
    with exocrine, mixed
      specified site —*see* Neoplasm,
        malignant, by site
      unspecified site C25.9
    pancreas C25.4
    specified site NEC —*see* Neoplasm,
      malignant, by site
    unspecified site C25.4

Adenocarcinoma (Continued)
  lobular
    in situ
      breast D05.0-●
      specified site NEC —see Neoplasm, in
        situ, by site
      unspecified site D05.0-●
    specified site —see Neoplasm, malignant,
      by site
    unspecified site (female) C50.91-●
      male C50.92-●
  mucoid —see also Neoplasm, malignant,
    by site
    cell
      specified site —see Neoplasm,
        malignant, by site
      unspecified site C75.1
  nonencapsulated sclerosing C73
  papillary
    with follicular C73
    follicular variant C73
    intraductal (noninfiltrating)
      with invasion
        specified site —see Neoplasm,
          malignant, by site
        unspecified site (female) C50.91-●
          male C50.92-●
      breast D05.1-●
      specified site NEC —see Neoplasm, in
        situ, by site
      unspecified site D05.1-●
    serous
      specified site —see Neoplasm,
        malignant, by site
      unspecified site C56.9
  papillocystic
    specified site —see Neoplasm, malignant,
      by site
    unspecified site C56.9
  pseudomucinous
    specified site —see Neoplasm, malignant,
      by site
    unspecified site C56.9
  renal cell C64-●
  sebaceous —see Neoplasm, skin, malignant,
    by site
  serous —see also Neoplasm, malignant, by site
    papillary
      specified site —see Neoplasm,
        malignant, by site
      unspecified site C56.9
  sweat gland —see Neoplasm, skin, malignant
  water-clear cell C75.0
Adenocarcinoma-in-situ —see also Neoplasm,
  in situ, by site
  breast D05.9-●
Adenofibroma
  clear cell —see Neoplasm, benign, by site
  endometrioid D27.9
    borderline malignancy D39.10
    malignant C56-●
  mucinous
    specified site —see Neoplasm, benign, by
      site
    unspecified site D27.9
  papillary
    specified site —see Neoplasm, benign, by
      site
    unspecified site D27.9
  prostate —see Enlargement, enlarged,
    prostate
  serous
    specified site —see Neoplasm, benign, by
      site
    unspecified site D27.9
  specified site —see Neoplasm, benign,
    by site
  unspecified site D27.9
Adenofibrosis
  breast —see Fibroadenosis, breast
  endometrioid N80.0

Adenoiditis (chronic) J35.02
  with tonsillitis J35.03
  acute J03.90
    recurrent J03.91
    specified organism NEC J03.80
      recurrent J03.81
    staphylococcal J03.80
      recurrent J03.81
    streptococcal J03.00
      recurrent J03.01
Adenoids —see condition
Adenolipoma —see Neoplasm, benign,
  by site
Adenolipomatosis, Launois-Bensaude E88.89
Adenolymphoma
  specified site —see Neoplasm, benign, by site
  unspecified site D11.9
Adenoma —see also Neoplasm, benign, by site
  acidophil
    specified site —see Neoplasm, benign, by
      site
    unspecified site D35.2
  acidophil-basophil, mixed
    specified site —see Neoplasm, benign, by
      site
    unspecified site D35.2
  adrenal (cortical) D35.00
    clear cell D35.00
    compact cell D35.00
    glomerulosa cell D35.00
    heavily pigmented variant D35.00
    mixed cell D35.00
  alpha-cell
    pancreas D13.7
    specified site NEC —see Neoplasm, benign,
      by site
    unspecified site D13.7
  alveolar D14.30
  apocrine
    breast D24-●
    specified site NEC —see Neoplasm, skin,
      benign, by site
    unspecified site D23.9
  basal cell D11.9
  basophil
    specified site —see Neoplasm, benign,
      by site
    unspecified site D35.2
  basophil-acidophil, mixed
    specified site —see Neoplasm, benign, by
      site
    unspecified site D35.2
  beta-cell
    pancreas D13.7
    specified site NEC —see Neoplasm, benign,
      by site
    unspecified site D13.7
  bile duct D13.4
    common D13.5
    extrahepatic D13.5
    intrahepatic D13.4
    specified site NEC —see Neoplasm, benign,
      by site
    unspecified site D13.4
  black D35.00
  bronchial D38.1
    cylindroid type —see Neoplasm, lung,
      malignant
  ceruminous D23.2-●
  chief cell D35.1
  chromophobe
    specified site —see Neoplasm, benign, by
      site
    unspecified site D35.2
  colloid
    specified site —see Neoplasm, benign, by
      site
    unspecified site D34
  ~~duct~~
  eccrine, papillary —see Neoplasm, skin,
    benign

Adenoma (Continued)
  endocrine, multiple
    single specified site —see Neoplasm,
      uncertain behavior, by site
    two or more specified sites D44-●
    unspecified site D44.9
  endometrioid —see also Neoplasm, benign
    borderline malignancy —see Neoplasm,
      uncertain behavior, by site
  eosinophil
    specified site —see Neoplasm, malignant,
      by site
    unspecified site D35.2
  fetal
    specified site —see Neoplasm, benign, by
      site
    unspecified site D34
  follicular
    specified site —see Neoplasm, benign, by
      site
    unspecified site D34
  hepatocellular D13.4
  Hurthle cell D34
  islet cell
    pancreas D13.7
    specified site NEC —see Neoplasm, benign,
      by site
    unspecified site D13.7
  liver cell D13.4
  macrofollicular
    specified site —see Neoplasm, benign, by site
    unspecified site D34
  malignant, malignum —see Neoplasm,
    malignant, by site
  microcystic
    pancreas D13.6
    specified site NEC —see Neoplasm, benign,
      by site
    unspecified site D13.6
  microfollicular
    specified site —see Neoplasm, benign, by
      site
    unspecified site D34
  mucoid cell
    specified site —see Neoplasm, benign, by
      site
    unspecified site D35.2
  multiple endocrine
    single specified site —see Neoplasm,
      uncertain behavior, by site
    two or more specified sites D44-●
    unspecified site D44.9
  nipple D24-●
  papillary —see also Neoplasm, benign, by site
    eccrine —see Neoplasm, skin, benign, by
      site
  Pick's tubular
    specified site —see Neoplasm, benign, by
      site
    unspecified site
      female D27.9
      male D29.20
  pleomorphic
    carcinoma in —see Neoplasm, salivary
      gland, malignant
      specified site —see Neoplasm,
        malignant, by site
      unspecified site C08.9
  polypoid —see also Neoplasm, benign
    adenocarcinoma in —see Neoplasm,
      malignant, by site
    adenocarcinoma in situ —see Neoplasm, in
      situ, by site
  prostate —see Neoplasm, benign, prostate
  rete cell D29.20
  sebaceous —see Neoplasm, skin, benign
  Sertoli cell
    specified site —see Neoplasm, benign, by site
    unspecified site
      female D27.9
      male D29.20

  ▶ New   ⇒ Revised   ~~deleted~~ Deleted   ● Use Additional Character(s)

Adenoma *(Continued)*
skin appendage —*see* Neoplasm, skin, benign
sudoriferous gland —*see* Neoplasm, skin, benign
sweat gland —*see* Neoplasm, skin, benign
testicular
  specified site —*see* Neoplasm, benign, by site
  unspecified site
    female D27.9
    male D29.20
tubular —*see also* Neoplasm, benign, by site
  adenocarcinoma in —*see* Neoplasm, malignant, by site
  adenocarcinoma in situ —*see* Neoplasm, in situ, by site
  Pick's
    specified site —*see* Neoplasm, benign
    unspecified site
      female D27.9
      male D29.20
tubulovillous —*see also* Neoplasm, benign, by site
  adenocarcinoma in —*see* Neoplasm, malignant, by site
  adenocarcinoma in situ —*see* Neoplasm, in situ, by site
villous —*see* Neoplasm, uncertain behavior, by site
  adenocarcinoma in —*see* Neoplasm, malignant, by site
  adenocarcinoma in situ —*see* Neoplasm, in situ, by site
water-clear cell D35.1
Adenomatosis
endocrine (multiple) E31.20
  single specified site —*see* Neoplasm, uncertain behavior, by site
erosive of nipple D24-●
pluriendocrine —*see* Adenomatosis, endocrine
pulmonary D38.1
  malignant —*see* Neoplasm, lung, malignant
specified site —*see* Neoplasm, benign, by site
unspecified site D12.6
Adenomatous
goiter (nontoxic) E04.9
  with hyperthyroidism —*see* Hyperthyroidism, with, goiter, nodular
  toxic —*see* Hyperthyroidism, with, goiter, nodular
Adenomyoma —*see also* Neoplasm, benign, by site
prostate —*see* Enlarged, prostate
Adenomyometritis N80.0
Adenomyosis N80.0
Adenopathy (lymph gland) R59.9
generalized R59.1
inguinal R59.0
localized R59.0
mediastinal R59.0
mesentery R59.0
syphilitic (secondary) A51.49
tracheobronchial R59.0
  tuberculous A15.4
    primary (progressive) A15.7
tuberculous —*see also* Tuberculosis, lymph gland
  tracheobronchial A15.4
    primary (progressive) A15.7
Adenosalpingitis —*see* Salpingitis
Adenosarcoma —*see* Neoplasm, malignant, by site
Adenosclerosis I88.8
Adenosis (sclerosing) **breast** —*see* Fibroadenosis, breast
Adenovirus, as cause of disease classified elsewhere B97.0
Adentia (complete) (partial) —*see* Absence, teeth

Adherent —*see also* Adhesions
labia (minora) N90.89
pericardium (nonrheumatic) I31.0
  rheumatic I09.2
placenta (with hemorrhage) O72.0
  without hemorrhage O73.0
prepuce, newborn N47.0
scar (skin) L90.5
tendon in scar L90.5
Adhesions, adhesive (postinfective) K66.0
with intestinal obstruction K56.50
  complete K56.52
  incomplete K56.51
  partial K56.51
abdominal (wall) —*see* Adhesions, peritoneum
appendix K38.8
bile duct (common) (hepatic) K83.8
bladder (sphincter) N32.89
bowel —*see* Adhesions, peritoneum
cardiac I31.0
  rheumatic I09.2
cecum —*see* Adhesions, peritoneum
cervicovaginal N88.1
  congenital Q52.8
  postpartal O90.89
  old N88.1
cervix N88.1
ciliary body NEC —*see* Adhesions, iris
clitoris N90.89
colon —*see* Adhesions, peritoneum
common duct K83.8
congenital —*see also* Anomaly, by site
  fingers —*see* Syndactylism, complex, fingers
  omental, anomalous Q43.3
  peritoneal Q43.3
  tongue (to gum or roof of mouth) Q38.3
conjunctiva (acquired) H11.21-●
  congenital Q15.8
cystic duct K82.8
diaphragm —*see* Adhesions, peritoneum
due to foreign body —*see* Foreign body
duodenum —*see* Adhesions, peritoneum
ear
  middle H74.1-●
epididymis N50.89
epidural —*see* Adhesions, meninges
epiglottis J38.7
eyelid H02.59
female pelvis N73.6
gallbladder K82.8
globe H44.89
heart I31.0
  rheumatic I09.2
ileocecal (coil) —*see* Adhesions, peritoneum
ileum —*see* Adhesions, peritoneum
intestine —*see also* Adhesions, peritoneum
  with obstruction K56.50
    complete K56.52
    incomplete K56.51
    partial K56.51
intra-abdominal —*see* Adhesions, peritoneum
iris H21.50-●
  anterior H21.51-●
  goniosynechiae H21.52-●
  posterior H21.54-●
  to corneal graft T85.898
joint —*see* Ankylosis
  knee M23.8X
  temporomandibular M26.61-●
labium (majus) (minus), congenital Q52.5
liver —*see* Adhesions, peritoneum
lung J98.4
mediastinum J98.59
meninges (cerebral) (spinal) G96.12
  congenital Q07.8
  tuberculous (cerebral) (spinal) A17.0
mesenteric —*see* Adhesions, peritoneum
nasal (septum) (to turbinates) J34.89
ocular muscle —*see* Strabismus, mechanical
omentum —*see* Adhesions, peritoneum

Adhesions, adhesive *(Continued)*
ovary N73.6
  congenital (to cecum, kidney or omentum) Q50.39
paraovarian N73.6
pelvic (peritoneal)
  female N73.6
    postprocedural N99.4
  male —*see* Adhesions, peritoneum
  postpartal (old) N73.6
  tuberculous A18.17
penis to scrotum (congenital) Q55.8
periappendiceal —*see also* Adhesions, peritoneum
pericardium (nonrheumatic) I31.0
  focal I31.8
  rheumatic I09.2
  tuberculous A18.84
pericholecystic K82.8
perigastric —*see* Adhesions, peritoneum
periovarian N73.6
periprostatic N42.89
perirectal —*see* Adhesions, peritoneum
perirenal N28.89
peritoneum, peritoneal (postinfective) K66.0
  with obstruction (intestinal) K56.50
    complete K56.52
    incomplete K56.51
    partial K56.51
  congenital Q43.3
  pelvic, female N73.6
    postprocedural N99.4
  postpartal, pelvic N73.6
  postprocedural K66.0
  to uterus N73.6
peritubal N73.6
periureteral N28.89
periuterine N73.6
perivesical N32.89
perivesicular (seminal vesicle) N50.89
pleura, pleuritic J94.8
  tuberculous NEC A15.6
pleuropericardial J94.8
postoperative (gastrointestinal tract) K66.0
  with obstruction —*see also* Obstruction, intestine, postoperative K91.30
  due to foreign body accidentally left in wound —*see* Foreign body, accidentally left during a procedure
  pelvic peritoneal N99.4
  urethra —*see* Stricture, urethra, postprocedural
  vagina N99.2
postpartal, old (vulva or perineum) N90.89
preputial, prepuce N47.5
pulmonary J98.4
pylorus —*see* Adhesions, peritoneum
sciatic nerve —*see* Lesion, nerve, sciatic
seminal vesicle N50.89
shoulder (joint) —*see* Capsulitis, adhesive
sigmoid flexure —*see* Adhesions, peritoneum
spermatic cord (acquired) N50.89
  congenital Q55.4
spinal canal G96.12
stomach —*see* Adhesions, peritoneum
subscapular —*see* Capsulitis, adhesive
temporomandibular M26.61-●
tendinitis —*see also* Tenosynovitis, specified type NEC
  shoulder —*see* Capsulitis, adhesive
testis N44.8
tongue, congenital (to gum or roof of mouth) Q38.3
  acquired K14.8
trachea J39.8
tubo-ovarian N73.6
tunica vaginalis N44.8
uterus N73.6
  internal N85.6
  to abdominal wall N73.6

Adhesions, adhesive (Continued)
vagina (chronic) N89.5
postoperative N99.2
vitreomacular H43.82-●
vitreous H43.89
vulva N90.89
Adiaspiromycosis B48.8
Adie (-Holmes) pupil or syndrome —see
Anomaly, pupil, function, tonic pupil
Adiponecrosis neonatorum P83.88
Adiposis —see also Obesity
cerebralis E23.6
dolorosa E88.2
Adiposity —see also Obesity
heart —see Degeneration, myocardial
localized E65
Adiposogenital dystrophy E23.6
Adjustment
disorder —see Disorder, adjustment
implanted device —see Encounter (for),
adjustment (of)
prosthesis, external —see Fitting
reaction —see Disorder, adjustment
Administration of tPA (rtPA) in a different
facility within the last 24 hours prior to
admission to current facility Z92.82
Admission (for) —see also Encounter (for)
adjustment (of)
artificial
arm Z44.00-●
complete Z44.01-●
partial Z44.02-●
eye Z44.2
leg Z44.10-●
complete Z44.11-●
partial Z44.12-●
brain neuropacemaker Z46.2
implanted Z45.42
breast
implant Z45.81
prosthesis (external) Z44.3
colostomy belt Z46.89
contact lenses Z46.0
cystostomy device Z46.6
dental prosthesis Z46.3
device NEC
abdominal Z46.89
implanted Z45.89
cardiac Z45.09
defibrillator (with synchronous
cardiac pacemaker) Z45.02
pacemaker (cardiac
resynchronization therapy
(CRT-P)) Z45.018
pulse generator Z45.010
resynchronization therapy
defibrillator (CRT-D) Z45.02
hearing device Z45.328
bone conduction Z45.320
cochlear Z45.321
infusion pump Z45.1
nervous system Z45.49
CSF drainage Z45.41
hearing device —see Admission,
adjustment, device, implanted,
hearing device
neuropacemaker Z45.42
visual substitution Z45.31
specified NEC Z45.89
vascular access Z45.2
visual substitution Z45.31
nervous system Z46.2
implanted —see Admission,
adjustment, device, implanted,
nervous system
orthodontic Z46.4
prosthetic Z44.9
arm —see Admission, adjustment,
artificial, arm
breast Z44.3
dental Z46.3

Admission (Continued)
adjustment (Continued)
device NEC (Continued)
prosthetic (Continued)
eye Z44.2
leg —see Admission, adjustment,
artificial, leg
specified type NEC Z44.8
substitution
auditory Z46.2
implanted —see Admission,
adjustment, device, implanted,
hearing device
nervous system Z46.2
implanted —see Admission,
adjustment, device, implanted,
nervous system
visual Z46.2
implanted Z45.31
urinary Z46.6
hearing aid Z46.1
implanted —see Admission, adjustment,
device, implanted, hearing device
ileostomy device Z46.89
intestinal appliance or device NEC Z46.89
neuropacemaker (brain) (peripheral nerve)
(spinal cord) Z46.2
implanted Z45.42
orthodontic device Z46.4
orthopedic (brace) (cast) (device) (shoes)
Z46.89
pacemaker (cardiac resynchronization
therapy (CRT-P))
cardiac Z45.018
pulse generator Z45.010
nervous system Z46.2
implanted Z45.42
portacath (port-a-cath) Z45.2
prosthesis Z44.9
arm —see Admission, adjustment,
artificial, arm
breast Z44.3
dental Z46.3
eye Z44.2
leg —see Admission, adjustment,
artificial, leg
specified NEC Z44.8
spectacles Z46.0
aftercare (see also Aftercare) Z51.89
postpartum
immediately after delivery Z39.0
routine follow-up Z39.2
radiation therapy (antineoplastic) Z51.0
attention to artificial opening (of) Z43.9
artificial vagina Z43.7
colostomy Z43.3
cystostomy Z43.5
enterostomy Z43.4
gastrostomy Z43.1
ileostomy Z43.2
jejunostomy Z43.4
nephrostomy Z43.6
specified site NEC Z43.8
intestinal tract Z43.4
urinary tract Z43.6
tracheostomy Z43.0
ureterostomy Z43.6
urethrostomy Z43.6
breast augmentation or reduction Z41.1
breast reconstruction following mastectomy
Z42.1
change of
dressing (nonsurgical) Z48.00
neuropacemaker device (brain) (peripheral
nerve) (spinal cord) Z46.2
implanted Z45.42
surgical dressing Z48.01
circumcision, ritual or routine (in absence of
diagnosis) Z41.2
clinical research investigation (control)
(normal comparison) (participant) Z00.6

Admission (Continued)
contraceptive management Z30.9
cosmetic surgery NEC Z41.1
counseling (see also Counseling)
dietary Z71.3
gestational carrier Z31.7
HIV Z71.7
human immunodeficiency virus Z71.7
nonattending third party Z71.0
procreative management NEC Z31.69
delivery, full-term, uncomplicated O80
cesarean, without indication O82
desensitization to allergens Z51.6
dietary surveillance and counseling Z71.3
ear piercing Z41.3
examination at health care facility (adult) —
see also Examination Z00.00
with abnormal findings Z00.01
clinical research investigation (control)
(normal comparison) (participant)
Z00.6
dental Z01.20
with abnormal findings Z01.21
donor (potential) Z00.5
ear Z01.10
with abnormal findings NEC Z01.118
following failed vision screening
Z01.020
with abnormal findings Z01.021
eye Z01.00
with abnormal findings Z01.01
general, specified reason NEC Z00.8
hearing Z01.10
with abnormal findings NEC Z01.118
infant or child (over 28 days old) Z00.129
with abnormal findings Z00.121
postpartum checkup Z39.2
psychiatric (general) Z00.8
requested by authority Z04.6
vision Z01.00
with abnormal findings Z01.01
following failed vision screening
Z01.020
with abnormal findings Z01.021
infant or child (over 28 days old) Z00.129
with abnormal findings Z00.121
fitting (of)
artificial
arm —see Admission, adjustment,
artificial, arm
eye Z44.2
leg —see Admission, adjustment,
artificial, leg
brain neuropacemaker Z46.2
implanted Z45.42
breast prosthesis (external) Z44.3
colostomy belt Z46.89
contact lenses Z46.0
cystostomy device Z46.6
dental prosthesis Z46.3
dentures Z46.3
device NEC
abdominal Z46.89
nervous system Z46.2
implanted —see Admission,
adjustment, device, implanted,
nervous system
orthodontic Z46.4
prosthetic Z44.9
breast Z44.3
dental Z46.3
eye Z44.2
substitution
auditory Z46.2
implanted —see Admission,
adjustment, device, implanted,
hearing device
nervous system Z46.2
implanted —see Admission,
adjustment, device, implanted,
nervous system

▶ New   ⇒ Revised   ~~deleted~~ Deleted   ● Use Additional Character(s)

Admission *(Continued)*
  fitting (of) *(Continued)*
    device NEC *(Continued)*
      substitution *(Continued)*
        visual Z46.2
          implanted Z45.31
    hearing aid Z46.1
    ileostomy device Z46.89
    intestinal appliance or device NEC
      Z46.89
    neuropacemaker (brain) (peripheral nerve)
      (spinal cord) Z46.2
      implanted Z45.42
    orthodontic device Z46.4
    orthopedic device (brace) (cast) (shoes)
      Z46.89
    prosthesis Z44.9
      arm —*see* Admission, adjustment,
        artificial, arm
      breast Z44.3
      dental Z46.3
      eye Z44.2
      leg —*see* Admission, adjustment,
        artificial, leg
      specified type NEC Z44.8
    spectacles Z46.0
  follow-up examination Z09
  intrauterine device management Z30.431
    initial prescription Z30.014
  mental health evaluation Z00.8
    requested by authority Z04.6
  observation —*see* Observation
  Papanicolaou smear, cervix Z12.4
    for suspected malignant neoplasm
      Z12.4
  plastic and reconstructive surgery following
    medical procedure or healed injury NEC
    Z42.8
  plastic surgery, cosmetic NEC Z41.1
  postpartum observation
    immediately after delivery Z39.0
    routine follow-up Z39.2
  poststerilization (for restoration) Z31.0
    aftercare Z31.42
  procreative management Z31.9
  prophylactic (measure) —*see also* Encounter,
    prophylactic measures
    organ removal Z40.00
      breast Z40.01
      fallopian tube(s) Z40.03
        with ovary(s) Z40.02
      ovary(s) Z40.02
      specified organ NEC Z40.09
      testes Z40.09
    vaccination Z23
  psychiatric examination (general) Z00.8
    requested by authority Z04.6
  radiation therapy (antineoplastic) Z51.0
  reconstructive surgery following medical
    procedure or healed injury NEC Z42.8
  removal of
    cystostomy catheter Z43.5
    drains Z48.03
    dressing (nonsurgical) Z48.00
    implantable subdermal contraceptive Z30.46
    intrauterine contraceptive device Z30.432
    neuropacemaker (brain) (peripheral nerve)
      (spinal cord) Z46.2
      implanted Z45.42
    staples Z48.02
    surgical dressing Z48.01
    sutures Z48.02
    ureteral stent Z46.6
  respirator [ventilator] use during power
    failure Z99.12
  restoration of organ continuity
    (poststerilization) Z31.0
    aftercare Z31.42
  sensitivity test —*see also* Test, skin
    allergy NEC Z01.82
    Mantoux Z11.1

Admission *(Continued)*
  tuboplasty following previous sterilization
    Z31.0
    aftercare Z31.42
  vasoplasty following previous sterilization
    Z31.0
    aftercare Z31.42
  vision examination Z01.00
    with abnormal findings Z01.01
      following failed vision screening
        Z01.020
        with abnormal findings Z01.021
    infant or child (over 28 days old) Z00.129
      with abnormal findings Z00.121
  waiting period for admission to other facility
    Z75.1
Adnexitis (suppurative) —*see*
  Salpingo-oophoritis
Adolescent X-linked adrenoleukodystrophy
  E71.521
Adrenal (gland) —*see* condition
Adrenalism, tuberculous A18.7
Adrenalitis, adrenitis E27.8
  autoimmune E27.1
  meningococcal, hemorrhagic A39.1
Adrenarche, premature E27.0
Adrenocortical syndrome —*see* Cushing's,
  syndrome
Adrenogenital syndrome E25.9
  acquired E25.8
  congenital E25.0
  salt loss E25.0
Adrenogenitalism, congenital E25.0
Adrenoleukodystrophy E71.529
  neonatal E71.511
  X-linked E71.529
    Addison only phenotype E71.528
    Addison-Schilder E71.528
    adolescent E71.521
    adrenomyeloneuropathy E71.522
    childhood cerebral E71.520
    other specified E71.528
Adrenomyeloneuropathy E71.522
Adventitious bursa —*see* Bursopathy, specified
  type NEC
Adverse effect —*see* Table of Drugs and
  Chemicals, categories T36-T50, with 6th
  character 5
Advice —*see* Counseling
Adynamia (episodica) (hereditary) (periodic)
  G72.3
Aeration lung imperfect, newborn —*see*
  Atelectasis
Aerobullosis T70.3
Aerocele —*see* Embolism, air
Aerodermectasia
  subcutaneous (traumatic) T79.7
Aerodontalgia T70.29
Aeroembolism T70.3
Aerogenes capsulatus infection A48.0
Aero-otitis media T70.0
Aerophagy, aerophagia (psychogenic) F45.8
Aerophobia F40.228
Aerosinusitis T70.1
Aerotitis T70.0
Affection —*see* Disease
Afibrinogenemia —*see also* Defect, coagulation
  D68.8
  acquired D65
  congenital D68.2
  following ectopic or molar pregnancy
    O08.1
  in abortion —*see* Abortion, by type,
    complicated by, afibrinogenemia
  puerperal O72.3
African
  sleeping sickness B56.9
  tick fever A68.1
  trypanosomiasis B56.9
    gambian B56.0
    rhodesian B56.1

Aftercare —*see also* Care Z51.89
  following surgery (for) (on)
    amputation Z47.81
    attention to
      drains Z48.03
      dressings (nonsurgical) Z48.00
        surgical Z48.01
      sutures Z48.02
    circulatory system Z48.812
    delayed (planned) wound closure Z48.1
    digestive system Z48.815
    explantation of joint prosthesis (staged
      procedure)
      hip Z47.32
      knee Z47.33
      shoulder Z47.31
    genitourinary system Z48.816
    joint replacement Z47.1
    neoplasm Z48.3
    nervous system Z48.811
    oral cavity Z48.814
    organ transplant
      bone marrow Z48.290
      heart Z48.21
      heart-lung Z48.280
      kidney Z48.22
      liver Z48.23
      lung Z48.24
      multiple organs NEC Z48.288
      specified NEC Z48.298
    orthopedic NEC Z47.89
    planned wound closure Z48.1
    removal of internal fixation device Z47.2
    respiratory system Z48.813
    scoliosis Z47.82
    sense organs Z48.810
    skin and subcutaneous tissue Z48.817
    specified body system
      circulatory Z48.812
      digestive Z48.815
      genitourinary Z48.816
      nervous Z48.811
      oral cavity Z48.814
      respiratory Z48.813
      sense organs Z48.810
      skin and subcutaneous tissue Z48.817
      teeth Z48.814
    specified NEC Z48.89
    spinal Z47.89
    teeth Z48.814
  fracture — code to fracture with seventh
    character D
  involving
    removal of
      drains Z48.03
      dressings (nonsurgical) Z48.00
      staples Z48.02
      surgical dressings Z48.01
      sutures Z48.02
  neuropacemaker (brain) (peripheral nerve)
    (spinal cord) Z46.2
    implanted Z45.42
  orthopedic NEC Z47.89
  postprocedural —*see* Aftercare, following
    surgery
After-cataract —*see* Cataract, secondary
Agalactia (primary) O92.3
  elective, secondary or therapeutic O92.5
Agammaglobulinemia (acquired (secondary))
  (nonfamilial) D80.1
  with
    immunoglobulin-bearing B-lymphocytes
      D80.1
    lymphopenia D81.9
  autosomal recessive (Swiss type) D80.0
  Bruton's X-linked D80.0
  common variable (CVAgamma) D80.1
  congenital sex-linked D80.0
  hereditary D80.0
  lymphopenic D81.9
  Swiss type (autosomal recessive) D80.0

Agammaglobulinemia *(Continued)*
  X-linked (with growth hormone deficiency)
    (Bruton) D80.0
Aganglionosis (bowel) (colon) Q43.1
Age (old) —*see* Senility
Agenesis
  adrenal (gland) Q89.1
  alimentary tract (complete) (partial) NEC
      Q45.8
    upper Q40.8
  anus, anal (canal) Q42.3
    with fistula Q42.2
  aorta Q25.41
  appendix Q42.8
  arm (complete) Q71.0-•
    with hand present Q71.1-•
  artery (peripheral) Q27.9
    brain Q28.3
    coronary Q24.5
    pulmonary Q25.79
    specified NEC Q27.8
    umbilical Q27.0
  auditory (canal) (external) Q16.1
  auricle (ear) Q16.0
  bile duct or passage Q44.5
  bladder Q64.5
  bone Q79.9
  brain Q00.0
    part of Q04.3
  breast (with nipple present) Q83.8
    with absent nipple Q83.0
  bronchus Q32.4
  canaliculus lacrimalis Q10.4
  carpus —*see* Agenesis, hand
  cartilage Q79.9
  cecum Q42.8
  cerebellum Q04.3
  cervix Q51.5
  chin Q18.8
  cilia Q10.3
  circulatory system, part NOS Q28.9
  clavicle Q74.0
  clitoris Q52.6
  coccyx Q76.49
  colon Q42.9
    specified NEC Q42.8
  corpus callosum Q04.0
  cricoid cartilage Q31.8
  diaphragm (with hernia) Q79.1
  digestive organ(s) or tract (complete) (partial)
      NEC Q45.8
    upper Q40.8
  ductus arteriosus Q28.8
  duodenum Q41.0
  ear Q16.9
    auricle Q16.0
    lobe Q17.8
  ejaculatory duct Q55.4
  endocrine (gland) NEC Q89.2
  epiglottis Q31.8
  esophagus Q39.8
  eustachian tube Q16.2
  eye Q11.1
    adnexa Q15.8
  eyelid (fold) Q10.3
  face
    bones NEC Q75.8
    specified part NEC Q18.8
  fallopian tube Q50.6
  femur —*see* Defect, reduction, lower limb,
      longitudinal, femur
  fibula —*see* Defect, reduction, lower limb,
      longitudinal, fibula
  finger (complete) (partial) —*see* Agenesis,
      hand
  foot (and toes) (complete) (partial) Q72.3-•
  forearm (with hand present) —*see* Agenesis,
      arm, with hand present
    and hand Q71.2-•
  gallbladder Q44.0
  gastric Q40.2

Agenesis *(Continued)*
  genitalia, genital (organ(s))
    female Q52.8
      external Q52.71
      internal NEC Q52.8
    male Q55.8
  glottis Q31.8
  hair Q84.0
  hand (and fingers) (complete) (partial) Q71.3-•
  heart Q24.8
    valve NEC Q24.8
      pulmonary Q22.0
  hepatic Q44.7
  humerus —*see* Defect, reduction, upper limb
  hymen Q52.4
  ileum Q41.2
  incus Q16.3
  intestine (small) Q41.9
    large Q42.9
      specified NEC Q42.8
  iris (dilator fibers) Q13.1
  jaw M26.09
  jejunum Q41.1
  kidney(s) (partial) Q60.2
    bilateral Q60.1
    unilateral Q60.0
  labium (majus) (minus) Q52.71
  labyrinth, membranous Q16.5
  lacrimal apparatus Q10.4
  larynx Q31.8
  leg (complete) Q72.0-•
    with foot present Q72.1-•
    lower leg (with foot present) —*see*
        Agenesis, leg, with foot present
      and foot Q72.2-•
  lens Q12.3
  limb (complete) Q73.0
    lower —*see* Agenesis, leg
    upper —*see* Agenesis, arm
  lip Q38.0
  liver Q44.7
  lung (fissure) (lobe) (bilateral) (unilateral)
      Q33.3
  mandible, maxilla M26.09
  metacarpus —*see* Agenesis, hand
  metatarsus —*see* Agenesis, foot
  muscle Q79.8
    eyelid Q10.3
    ocular Q15.8
  musculoskeletal system NEC Q79.8
  nail(s) Q84.3
  neck, part Q18.8
  nerve Q07.8
  nervous system, part NEC Q07.8
  nipple Q83.2
  nose Q30.1
  nuclear Q07.8
  organ
    of Corti Q16.5
    or site not listed —*see* Anomaly, by site
  osseous meatus (ear) Q16.1
  ovary
    bilateral Q50.02
    unilateral Q50.01
  oviduct Q50.6
  pancreas Q45.0
  parathyroid (gland) Q89.2
  parotid gland(s) Q38.4
  patella Q74.1
  pelvic girdle (complete) (partial) Q74.2
  penis Q55.5
  pericardium Q24.8
  pituitary (gland) Q89.2
  prostate Q55.4
  punctum lacrimale Q10.4
  radioulnar —*see* Defect, reduction, upper
      limb
  radius —*see* Defect, reduction, upper limb,
      longitudinal, radius
  rectum Q42.1
    with fistula Q42.0

Agenesis *(Continued)*
  renal Q60.2
    bilateral Q60.1
    unilateral Q60.0
  respiratory organ NEC Q34.8
  rib Q76.6
  roof of orbit Q75.8
  round ligament Q52.8
  sacrum Q76.49
  salivary gland Q38.4
  scapula Q74.0
  scrotum Q55.29
  seminal vesicles Q55.4
  septum
    atrial Q21.1
    between aorta and pulmonary artery
        Q21.4
    ventricular Q20.4
  shoulder girdle (complete) (partial)
      Q74.0
  skull (bone) Q75.8
    with
      anencephaly Q00.0
      encephalocele —*see* Encephalocele
      hydrocephalus Q03.9
        with spina bifida —*see* Spina bifida, by
            site, with hydrocephalus
      microcephaly Q02
  spermatic cord Q55.4
  spinal cord Q06.0
  spine Q76.49
  spleen Q89.01
  sternum Q76.7
  stomach Q40.2
  submaxillary gland(s) (congenital) Q38.4
  tarsus —*see* Agenesis, foot
  tendon Q79.8
  testicle Q55.0
  thymus (gland) Q89.2
  thyroid (gland) E03.1
    cartilage Q31.8
  tibia —*see* Defect, reduction, lower limb,
      longitudinal, tibia
  tibiofibular —*see* Defect, reduction, lower
      limb, specified type NEC
  toe (and foot) (complete) (partial) —*see*
      Agenesis, foot
  tongue Q38.3
  trachea (cartilage) Q32.1
  ulna —*see* Defect, reduction, upper limb,
      longitudinal, ulna
  upper limb —*see* Agenesis, arm
  ureter Q62.4
  urethra Q64.5
  urinary tract NEC Q64.8
  uterus Q51.0
  uvula Q38.5
  vagina Q52.0
  vas deferens Q55.4
  vein(s) (peripheral) Q27.9
    brain Q28.3
    great NEC Q26.8
    portal Q26.5
  vena cava (inferior) (superior) Q26.8
  vermis of cerebellum Q04.3
  vertebra Q76.49
  vulva Q52.71
Ageusia R43.2
Agitated —*see* condition
Agitation R45.1
Aglossia (congenital) Q38.3
Aglossia-adactylia syndrome Q87.0
Aglycogenosis E74.00
Agnosia (body image) (other senses) (tactile)
    R48.1
  developmental F88
  verbal R48.1
    auditory R48.1
      developmental F80.2
    developmental F80.2
  visual (object) R48.3

▶ New   ⇒ Revised   ~~deleted~~ Deleted   • Use Additional Character(s)

Agoraphobia F40.00
  with panic disorder F40.01
  without panic disorder F40.02
Agrammatism R48.8
Agranulocytopenia —*see* Agranulocytosis
Agranulocytosis (chronic) (cyclical) (genetic)
    (infantile) (periodic) (pernicious) (*see also*
    Neutropenia) D70.9
  congenital D70.0
  cytoreductive cancer chemotherapy sequela
    D70.1
  drug-induced D70.2
    due to cytoreductive cancer chemotherapy
      D70.1
  due to infection D70.3
  secondary D70.4
    drug-induced D70.2
      due to cytoreductive cancer
        chemotherapy D70.1
Agraphia (absolute) R48.8
  with alexia R48.0
  developmental F81.81
Ague (dumb) —*see* Malaria
Agyria Q04.3
Ahumada-del Castillo syndrome E23.0
Aichomophobia F40.298
AIDS (related complex) B20
Ailment heart —*see* Disease, heart
Ailurophobia F40.218
Ainhum (disease) L94.6
AIN —*see* Neoplasia, intraepithelial, anal
AIPHI (acute idiopathic pulmonary hemorrhage
    in infants (over 28 days old)) R04.81
Air
  anterior mediastinum J98.2
  compressed, disease T70.3
  conditioner lung or pneumonitis J67.7
  embolism (artery) (cerebral) (any site)
      T79.0
    with ectopic or molar pregnancy O08.2
    due to implanted device NEC —*see*
      Complications, by site and type,
      specified NEC
    following
      abortion —*see* Abortion by type,
        complicated by, embolism
      ectopic or molar pregnancy O08.2
      infusion, therapeutic injection or
        transfusion T80.0
    in pregnancy, childbirth or puerperium —
      see Embolism, obstetric
    traumatic T79.0
  hunger, psychogenic F45.8
  rarefied, effects of —*see* Effect, adverse, high
    altitude
  sickness T75.3
Airplane sickness T75.3
Akathisia (drug-induced) (treatment- induced)
    G25.71
  neuroleptic induced (acute) G25.71
  tardive G25.71
Akinesia R29.898
Akinetic mutism R41.89
Akureyri's disease G93.3
Alactasia, congenital E73.0
Alagille's syndrome Q44.7
Alastrim B03
Albers-Schönberg syndrome Q78.2
Albert's syndrome —*see* Tendinitis,
    Achilles
Albinism, albino E70.30
  with hematologic abnormality E70.339
    Chédiak-Higashi syndrome E70.330
    Hermansky-Pudlak syndrome E70.331
    other specified E70.338
  I E70.320
  II E70.321
  ocular E70.319
    autosomal recessive E70.311
    other specified E70.318
    X-linked E70.310

Albinism, albino (*Continued*)
  oculocutaneous E70.329
    other specified E70.328
    tyrosinase (ty) negative E70.320
    tyrosinase (ty) positive E70.321
  other specified E70.39
Albinismus E70.30
Albright (-McCune)(-Sternberg) syndrome
    Q78.1
Albuminous —*see* condition
Albuminuria, albuminuric (acute) (chronic)
    (subacute) —*see also* Proteinuria R80.9
  complicating pregnancy —*see* Proteinuria,
      gestational
    with
      gestational hypertension —*see*
        Pre-eclampsia
      pre-existing hypertension —*see*
        Hypertension, complicating
        pregnancy, pre-existing, with,
        pre-eclampsia
  gestational —*see* Proteinuria, gestational
    with
      gestational hypertension —*see*
        Pre-eclampsia
      pre-existing hypertension —*see*
        Hypertension, complicating
        pregnancy, pre-existing, with,
        pre-eclampsia
  orthostatic R80.2
  postural R80.2
  pre-eclamptic —*see* Pre-eclampsia
  scarlatinal A38.8
Albuminurophobia F40.298
Alcaptonuria E70.29
Alcohol, alcoholic, alcohol-induced
  addiction (without remission) F10.20
    with remission F10.21
  amnestic disorder, persisting F10.96
    with dependence F10.26
  anxiety disorder F10.980
  bipolar and related disorder F10.94
  brain syndrome, chronic F10.97
    with dependence F10.27
  cardiopathy I42.6
  counseling and surveillance
      Z71.41
    family member Z71.42
  delirium (acute) (tremens) (withdrawal)
      F10.231
    with intoxication F10.921
    in
      abuse F10.121
      dependence F10.221
  dementia F10.97
    with dependence F10.27
  depressive disorder F10.94
  deterioration F10.97
    with dependence F10.27
  hallucinosis (acute) F10.951
    in
      abuse F10.151
      dependence F10.251
  insanity F10.959
  intoxication (acute) (without dependence)
      F10.129
    with
      delirium F10.121
      dependence F10.229
        with delirium F10.221
        uncomplicated F10.220
      uncomplicated F10.120
  jealousy F10.988
  Korsakoff's, Korsakov's, Korsakow's F10.26
  liver K70.9
    acute —*see* Disease, liver, alcoholic,
      hepatitis
  major neurocognitive disorder, amnestic-
    confabulatory type F10.96
  major neurocognitive disorder, nonamnestic-
    confabulatory type F10.97

Alcohol, alcoholic, alcohol-induced (*Continued*)
  mania (acute) (chronic) F10.959
  mild neurocognitive disorder F10.988
  paranoia, paranoid (type) psychosis F10.950
  pellagra E52
  poisoning, accidental (acute) NEC —*see*
      Table of Drugs and Chemicals, alcohol,
      poisoning
  psychosis —*see* Psychosis, alcoholic
  psychotic disorder F10.959
  sexual dysfunction F10.981
  sleep disorder F10.982
  withdrawal (without convulsions) F10.239
    with delirium F10.231
Alcoholism (chronic) (without remission) F10.20
  with
    psychosis —*see* Psychosis, alcoholic
    remission F10.21
  Korsakov's F10.96
    with dependence F10.26
Alder (-Reilly) anomaly or syndrome
    (leukocyte granulation) D72.0
Aldosteronism E26.9
  familial (type I) E26.02
  glucocorticoid-remediable E26.02
  primary (due to (bilateral) adrenal
    hyperplasia) E26.09
  primary NEC E26.09
  secondary E26.1
  specified NEC E26.89
Aldosteronoma D44.10
Aldrich(-Wiskott) syndrome (eczema-
    thrombocytopenia) D82.0
Alektorophobia F40.218
Aleppo boil B55.1
Aleukemic —*see* condition Aleukia
  congenital D70.0
  hemorrhagica D61.9
    congenital D61.09
  splenica D73.1
Alexia R48.0
  developmental F81.0
  secondary to organic lesion R48.0
Algoneurodystrophy M89.00
  ankle M89.07-●
  foot M89.07-●
  forearm M89.03-●
  hand M89.04-●
  lower leg M89.06-●
  multiple sites M89.0-●
  shoulder M89.01-●
  specified site NEC M89.08
  thigh M89.05-●
  upper arm M89.02-●
Algophobia F40.298
Alienation, mental —*see* Psychosis
Alkalemia E87.3
Alkalosis E87.3
  metabolic E87.3
    with respiratory acidosis E87.4
  of newborn P74.41
  respiratory E87.3
Alkaptonuria E70.29
Allen-Masters syndrome N83.8
Allergy, allergic (reaction) (to) T78.40
  air-borne substance NEC (rhinitis) J30.89
  alveolitis (extrinsic) J67.9
    due to
      Aspergillus clavatus J67.4
      Cryptostroma corticale J67.6
      organisms (fungal, thermophilic
        actinomycete) growing in
        ventilation (air conditioning)
        systems J67.7
    specified type NEC J67.8
  anaphylactic reaction or shock T78.2
  angioneurotic edema T78.3
  animal (dander) (epidermal) (hair) (rhinitis)
    J30.81
  bee sting (anaphylactic shock) —*see* Toxicity,
    venom, arthropod, bee

Allergy, allergic *(Continued)*
  biological —*see* Allergy, drug
  colitis —*see also* Colitis, allergic K52.29
  dander (animal) (rhinitis) J30.81
  dandruff (rhinitis) J30.81
  dental restorative material (existing) K08.55
  dermatitis —*see* Dermatitis, contact, allergic
  diathesis —*see* History, allergy
  drug, medicament & biological (any)
    (external) (internal) T78.40
    correct substance properly administered —
      see Table of Drugs and Chemicals, by
      drug, adverse effect
    wrong substance given or taken NEC (by
      accident) —*see* Table of Drugs and
      Chemicals, by drug, poisoning
    due to pollen J30.1
  dust (house) (stock) (rhinitis) J30.89
    with asthma —*see* Asthma, allergic extrinsic
  eczema —*see* Dermatitis, contact, allergic
  epidermal (animal) (rhinitis) J30.81
  feathers (rhinitis) J30.89
  food (any) (ingested) NEC T78.1
    anaphylactic shock —*see* Shock,
      anaphylactic, due to food
    dermatitis —*see* Dermatitis, due to, food
    dietary counseling and surveillance Z71.3
    in contact with skin L23.6
    rhinitis J30.5
    status (without reaction) Z91.018
      ▶beef Z91.014
      eggs Z91.012
      ▶lamb Z91.014
      ▶mammalian meats Z91.014
      milk products Z91.011
      peanuts Z91.010
      ▶pork Z91.014
      ▶red meats Z91.014
      seafood Z91.013
      specified NEC Z91.018
  gastrointestinal —*see also* specific type of
    allergic reaction
    meaning colitis —*see also* Colitis, allergic)
      K52.29
    meaning gastroenteritis —*see also*
      Gastroenteritis, allergic) K52.29
    meaning other adverse food reaction not
      elsewhere classified T78.1
  grain J30.1
  grass (hay fever) (pollen) J30.1
    asthma —*see* Asthma, allergic extrinsic
  hair (animal) (rhinitis) J30.81
  history (of) —*see* History, allergy
  horse serum —*see* Allergy, serum
  inhalant (rhinitis) J30.89
    pollen J30.1
  kapok (rhinitis) J30.89
  medicine —*see* Allergy, drug
  milk protein —*see also* Allergy, food Z91.011
    anaphylactic reaction T78.07
    dermatitis L27.2
    enterocolitis syndrome K52.21
    enteropathy K52.22
    gastroenteritis K52.29
    gastroesophageal reflux —*see also* Reaction,
      adverse, food) K21.9
      with esophagitis without bleeding K21.00
        with bleeding K21.01
    ➡proctocolitis K52.29
  nasal, seasonal due to pollen J30.1
  pneumonia J82.89
  pollen (any) (hay fever) J30.1
    asthma —*see* Asthma, allergic extrinsic
  primrose J30.1
  primula J30.1
  ➡proctocolitis K52.29
  purpura D69.0
  ragweed (hay fever) (pollen) J30.1
    asthma —*see* Asthma, allergic extrinsic
  rose (pollen) J30.1
  seasonal NEC J30.2

Allergy, allergic *(Continued)*
  Senecio jacobae (pollen) J30.1
  serum —*see also* Reaction, serum T80.69
    anaphylactic shock T80.59
  shock (anaphylactic) T78.2
    due to
      administration of blood and blood
        products T80.51
      adverse effect of correct medicinal
        substance properly administered
        T88.6
      immunization T80.52
      serum NEC T80.59
      vaccination T80.52
    specific NEC T78.49
  tree (any) (hay fever) (pollen) J30.1
    asthma —*see* Asthma, allergic extrinsic
  upper respiratory J30.9
  urticaria L50.0
  vaccine —*see* Allergy, serum
  wheat —*see* Allergy, food
Allescheriasis B48.2
Alligator skin disease Q80.9
Allocheiria, allochiria R20.8
Almeida's disease —*see*
  Paracoccidioidomycosis
Alopecia (hereditaria) (seborrheica) L65.9
  androgenic L64.9
    drug-induced L64.0
    specified NEC L64.8
  areata L63.9
    ophiasis L63.2
    specified NEC L63.8
    totalis L63.0
    universalis L63.1
  cicatricial L66.9
    specified NEC L66.8
  circumscripta L63.9
  congenital, congenitalis Q84.0
  due to cytotoxic drugs NEC L65.8
  mucinosa L65.2
  postinfective NEC L65.8
  postpartum L65.0
  premature L64.8
  specific (syphilitic) A51.32
  specified NEC L65.8
  syphilitic (secondary) A51.32
  totalis (capitis) L63.0
  universalis (entire body) L63.1
  X-ray L58.1
Alpers' disease G31.81
Alpine sickness T70.29
Alport syndrome Q87.81
ALTE (apparent life threatening event) in
  newborn and infant R68.13
Alteration (of), **Altered**
  awareness
    transient R40.4
    unintended under general anesthesia,
      during procedure T88.53
  mental status R41.82
  pattern of family relationships affecting child
    Z62.898
  sensation
    following
      cerebrovascular disease I69.998
        cerebral infarction I69.398
        intracerebral hemorrhage I69.198
        nontraumatic intracranial hemorrhage
          NEC I69.298
        specified disease NEC I69.898
        subarachnoid hemorrhage I69.098
Alternating —*see* condition
Altitude, high (effects) —*see* Effect, adverse,
  high altitude
Aluminosis (of lung) J63.0
Alveolitis
  allergic (extrinsic) —*see* Pneumonitis,
    hypersensitivity
  due to
    Aspergillus clavatus J67.4
    Cryptostroma corticale J67.6

Alveolitis *(Continued)*
  fibrosing (cryptogenic) (idiopathic) J84.112
  jaw M27.3
  sicca dolorosa M27.3
Alveolus, alveolar —*see* condition
Alymphocytosis D72.810
  thymic (with immunodeficiency) D82.1
Alymphoplasia, thymic D82.1
Alzheimer's disease or sclerosis —*see* Disease,
  Alzheimer's
Amastia (with nipple present) Q83.8
  with absent nipple Q83.0
Amathophobia F40.228
Amaurosis (acquired) (congenital) —*see also*
  Blindness
  fugax G45.3
  hysterical F44.6
  Leber's congenital H35.50
  uremic —*see* Uremia
Amaurotic idiocy (infantile) (juvenile) (late)
  E75.4
Amaxophobia F40.248
Ambiguous genitalia Q56.4
Amblyopia (congenital) (ex anopsia) (partial)
  (suppression) H53.00-●
  anisometropic —*see* Amblyopia, refractive
  deprivation H53.01-●
  hysterical F44.6
  nocturnal —*see also* Blindness, night
    vitamin A deficiency E50.5
  refractive H53.02-●
  strabismic H53.03-●
  suspect H53.04-●
  tobacco H53.8
  toxic NEC H53.8
  uremic —*see* Uremia
Ameba, amebic (histolytica) —*see also* Amebiasis
  abscess (liver) A06.4
Amebiasis A06.9
  with abscess —*see* Abscess, amebic
  acute A06.0
  chronic (intestine) A06.1
    with abscess —*see* Abscess, amebic
  cutaneous A06.7
  cutis A06.7
  cystitis A06.81
  genitourinary tract NEC A06.82
  hepatic —*see* Abscess, liver, amebic
  intestine A06.0
  nondysenteric colitis A06.2
  skin A06.7
  specified site NEC A06.89
Ameboma (of intestine) A06.3
Amelia Q73.0
  lower limb —*see* Agenesis, leg
  upper limb —*see* Agenesis, arm
Ameloblastoma —*see also* Cyst, calcifying
  odontogenic
  long bones C40.9-●
    lower limb C40.2-●
    upper limb C40.0-●
  malignant C41.1
    jaw (bone) (lower) C41.1
      upper C41.0
  tibial C40.2-●
Amelogenesis imperfecta K00.5
  nonhereditaria (segmentalis) K00.4
Amenorrhea N91.2
  hyperhormonal E28.8
  primary N91.0
  secondary N91.1
Amentia —*see* Disability, intellectual
  Meynert's (nonalcoholic) F04
American
  leishmaniasis B55.2
  mountain tick fever A93.2
Ametropia —*see* Disorder, refraction
AMH (asymptomatic microscopic hematuria)
  R31.21
Amianthosis J61
Amimia R48.8

Amino-acid disorder E72.9
  anemia D53.0
Aminoacidopathy E72.9
Aminoaciduria E72.9
Amnes (t)ic syndrome (post-traumatic) F04
  induced by
    alcohol F10.96
      with dependence F10.26
    psychoactive NEC F19.96
      with
        abuse F19.16
        dependence F19.26
    sedative F13.96
      with dependence F13.26
Amnesia R41.3
  anterograde R41.1
  auditory R48.8
  dissociative F44.0
    with dissociative fugue F44.1
  hysterical F44.0
  postictal in epilepsy —see Epilepsy
  psychogenic F44.0
  retrograde R41.2
  transient global G45.4
Amnion, amniotic —see condition
Amnionitis —see Pregnancy, complicated by
Amok F68.8
Amoral traits F60.89
Amphetamine (or other stimulant) —
    induced
  anxiety disorder F15.980
  bipolar and related disorder F15.94
  delirium F15.921
  depressive disorder F15.94
  obsessive-compulsive and related disorder
    F15.988
  psychotic disorder F15.959
  sexual dysfunction F15.981
  sleep disorder F15.982
  stimulant withdrawal F15.23
Ampulla
  ➠lower esophagus K22.89
  ➠phrenic K22.89
Amputation —see also Absence, by site,
    acquired
  neuroma (postoperative) (traumatic) —see
    Complications, amputation stump,
    neuroma
  stump (surgical)
    abnormal, painful, or with complication
      (late) —see Complications, amputation
      stump
    healed or old NOS Z89.9
  traumatic (complete) (partial)
    arm (upper) (complete) S48.91-●
      at
        elbow S58.01-●
          partial S58.02-●
        shoulder joint (complete) S48.01-●
          partial S48.02-●
      between
        elbow and wrist (complete) S58.11-●
          partial S58.12-●
        shoulder and elbow (complete)
          S48.11-●
          partial S48.12-●
      partial S48.92-●
    breast (complete) S28.21-●
      partial S28.22-●
    clitoris (complete) S38.211
      partial S38.212
    ear (complete) S08.11-●
      partial S08.12-●
    finger (complete) (metacarpophalangeal)
      S68.11-●
      index S68.11-●
      little S68.11-●
      middle S68.11-●
      partial S68.12-●
        index S68.12-●
        little S68.12-●

Amputation (Continued)
  traumatic (Continued)
    finger (Continued)
      partial (Continued)
        middle S68.12-●
        ring S68.12-●
      ring S68.11-●
      thumb —see Amputation, traumatic,
        thumb
      transphalangeal (complete) S68.61-●
        index S68.61-●
        little S68.61-●
        middle S68.61-●
        partial S68.62-●
          index S68.62-●
          little S68.62-●
          middle S68.62-●
          ring S68.62-●
        ring S68.61-●
    foot (complete) S98.91-●
      at ankle level S98.01-●
        partial S98.02-●
      midfoot S98.31-●
        partial S98.32-●
      partial S98.92-●
    forearm (complete) S58.91-●
      at elbow level (complete) S58.01-●
        partial S58.02-●
      between elbow and wrist (complete)
        S58.11-●
        partial S58.12-●
      partial S58.92-●
    genital organ(s) (external)
      female (complete) S38.211
        partial S38.212
      male
        penis (complete) S38.221
          partial S38.222
        scrotum (complete) S38.231
          partial S38.232
        testes (complete) S38.231
          partial S38.232
    hand (complete) (wrist level) S68.41-●
      finger(s) alone —see Amputation,
        traumatic, finger
      partial S68.42-●
      thumb alone —see Amputation,
        traumatic, thumb
      transmetacarpal (complete) S68.71-●
        partial S68.72-●
    head
      ear —see Amputation, traumatic, ear
      nose (partial) S08.812
        complete S08.811
      part S08.89
        scalp S08.0
    hip (and thigh) (complete) S78.91-●
      at hip joint (complete) S78.01-●
        partial S78.02-●
      between hip and knee (complete)
        S78.11-●
        partial S78.12-●
      partial S78.92-●
    labium (majus) (minus) (complete)
      S38.21-●
      partial S38.21-●
    leg (lower) S88.91-●
      at knee level S88.01-●
        partial S88.02-●
      between knee and ankle S88.11-●
        partial S88.12-●
      partial S88.92-●
    nose (partial) S08.812
      complete S08.811
    penis (complete) S38.221
      partial S38.222
    scrotum (complete) S38.231
      partial S38.232
    shoulder —see Amputation, traumatic, arm
      at shoulder joint —see Amputation,
        traumatic, arm, at shoulder joint

Amputation (Continued)
  traumatic (Continued)
    testes (complete) S38.231
      partial S38.232
    thigh —see Amputation, traumatic, hip
    thorax, part of S28.1
      breast —see Amputation, traumatic, breast
    thumb (complete) (metacarpophalangeal)
      S68.01-●
      partial S68.02-●
      transphalangeal (complete) S68.51-●
        partial S68.52-●
    toe (lesser) S98.13-●
      great S98.11-●
        partial S98.12-●
      more than one S98.21-●
        partial S98.22-●
      partial S98.14-●
    vulva (complete) S38.211
      partial S38.212
Amputee (bilateral) (old) Z89.9
Amsterdam dwarfism Q87.19
Amusia R48.8
  developmental F80.89
Amyelencephalus, amyelencephaly Q00.0
Amyelia Q06.0
Amygdalitis —see Tonsillitis
Amygdalolith J35.8
Amyloid heart (disease) E85.4 [I43]
Amyloidosis (generalized) (primary) E85.9
  with lung involvement E85.4 [J99]
  familial E85.2
  genetic E85.2
  heart E85.4 [I43]
  hemodialysis-associated E85.3
  light chain (AL) E85.81
  liver E85.4 [K77]
  localized E85.4
  neuropathic heredofamilial E85.1
  non-neuropathic heredofamilial E85.0
  organ limited E85.4
  Portuguese E85.1
  pulmonary E85.4 [J99]
  secondary systemic E85.3
  senile systemic (SSA) E85.82
  skin (lichen) (macular) E85.4 [L99]
  specified NEC E85.89
  subglottic E85.4 [J99]
  wild-type transthyretin-related (ATTR) E85.82
Amylopectinosis (brancher enzyme deficiency)
  E74.03
Amylophagia —see Pica
Amyoplasia congenita Q79.8
Amyotonia M62.89
  congenita G70.2
Amyotrophia, amyotrophy, amyotrophic G71.8
  congenita Q79.8
  diabetic —see Diabetes, amyotrophy
  lateral sclerosis G12.21
  neuralgic G54.5
  spinal progressive G12.25
Anacidity, gastric K31.83
  psychogenic F45.8
Anaerosis of newborn P28.89
Analbuminemia E88.09
Analgesia —see Anesthesia
Analphalipoproteinemia E78.6
Anaphylactic
  purpura D69.0
  shock or reaction —see Shock, anaphylactic
Anaphylactoid shock or reaction —see Shock,
  anaphylactic
Anaphylactoid syndrome of pregnancy
  O88.01-●
Anaphylaxis —see Shock, anaphylactic
Anaplasia cervix —see also Dysplasia, cervix
  N87.9
~~Anaplasmosis, human A77.49~~
▶Anaplasmosis [A. phagocytophilum]
  (transfusion transmitted) A79.82
▶human A77.49

Anarthria R47.1
Anasarca R60.1
  cardiac —*see* Failure, heart, congestive
  lung J18.2
  newborn P83.2
  nutritional E43
  pulmonary J18.2
  renal N04.9
Anastomosis
  aneurysmal —*see* Aneurysm
  arteriovenous ruptured brain I60.8
  intestinal K63.89
    complicated NEC K91.89
      involving urinary tract N99.89
  intracerebral I61.8
  intraparenchymal I61.8
  intraventricular I61.5
  retinal and choroidal vessels (congenital) Q14.8
  subarachnoid I60.8
Anatomical narrow angle H40.03- •
Ancylostoma, ancylostomiasis (braziliense)
  (caninum) (ceylanicum) (duodenale) B76.0
  Necator americanus B76.1
Andersen's disease (glycogen storage) E74.09
Anderson-Fabry disease E75.21
Andes disease T70.29
Andrews' disease (bacterid) L08.89
Androblastoma
  benign
    specified site —*see* Neoplasm, benign, by
      site
    unspecified site
      female D27.9
      male D29.20
  malignant
    specified site —*see* Neoplasm, malignant,
      by site
    unspecified site
      female C56.9
      male C62.90
  specified site —*see* Neoplasm, uncertain
    behavior, by site
  tubular
    with lipid storage
      specified site —*see* Neoplasm, benign,
        by site
      unspecified site
        female D27.9
        male D29.20
    specified site —*see* Neoplasm, benign, by site
    unspecified site
      female D27.9
      male D29.20
  unspecified site
    female D39.10
    male D40.10
Androgen insensitivity syndrome —*see also*
  Syndrome, androgen insensitivity E34.50
Androgen resistance syndrome —*see also*
  Syndrome, androgen insensitivity E34.50
Android pelvis Q74.2
  with disproportion (fetopelvic) O33.3
    causing obstructed labor O65.3
Androphobia F40.290
Anectasis, pulmonary (newborn) —*see* Atelectasis
Anemia (essential) (general) (hemoglobin
  deficiency) (infantile) (primary) (profound)
  D64.9
  with (due to) (in)
    disorder of
      ➡ anaerobic glycolysis D55.29
        pentose phosphate pathway D55.1
      koilonychia D50.9
  achlorhydric D50.8
  achrestic D53.1
  Addison (-Biermer) (pernicious) D51.0
  agranulocytic —*see* Agranulocytosis
  amino-acid-deficiency D53.0
  aplastic D61.9
    congenital D61.09
    drug-induced D61.1

Anemia *(Continued)*
  aplastic *(Continued)*
    due to
      drugs D61.1
      external agents NEC D61.2
      infection D61.2
      radiation D61.2
    idiopathic D61.3
    red cell (pure) D60.9
      chronic D60.0
      congenital D61.01
      specified type NEC D60.8
      transient D60.1
    specified type NEC D61.89
    toxic D61.2
  aregenerative
    congenital D61.09
  asiderotic D50.9
  atypical (primary) D64.9
  Baghdad spring D55.0
  Balantidium coli A07.0
  Biermer's (pernicious) D51.0
  blood loss (chronic) D50.0
    acute D62
  bothriocephalus B70.0 *[D63.8]*
  brickmaker's B76.9 *[D63.8]*
  cerebral I67.89
  childhood D58.9
  chlorotic D50.8
  chronic
    blood loss D50.0
    hemolytic D58.9
      idiopathic D59.9
    simple D53.9
  chronica congenita aregenerativa D61.09
  combined system disease NEC D51.0 *[G32.0]*
    due to dietary vitamin B12 deficiency
      D51.3 *[G32.0]*
  complicating pregnancy, childbirth
    or puerperium —*see* Pregnancy,
    complicated by (management affected
    by), anemia
  congenital P61.4
    aplastic D61.09
    due to isoimmunization NOS P55.9
    dyserythropoietic, dyshematopoietic D64.4
    following fetal blood loss P61.3
    Heinz body D58.2
    hereditary hemolytic NOS D58.9
    pernicious D51.0
    spherocytic D58.0
  Cooley's (erythroblastic) D56.1
  cytogenic D51.0
  deficiency D53.9
    ➡ 2, 3 diphosphoglycurate mutase D55.29
    ➡ 2, 3 PG D55.29
    6 phosphogluconate dehydrogenase D55.1
    6-PGD D55.1
    amino-acid D53.0
    combined B12 and folate D53.1
    enzyme D55.9
      drug-induced (hemolytic) D59.2
      glucose-6-phosphate dehydrogenase
        (G6PD) D55.0
    ➡ glycolytic D55.29
      nucleotide metabolism D55.3
      related to hexose monophosphate
        (HMP) shunt pathway NEC D55.1
      specified type NEC D55.8
    erythrocytic glutathione D55.1
    folate D52.9
      dietary D52.0
      drug-induced D52.1
    folic acid D52.9
      dietary D52.0
      drug-induced D52.1
    G SH D55.1
    G6PD D55.0
    GGS-R D55.1
    glucose-6-phosphate dehydrogenase D55.0
    glutathione reductase D55.1

Anemia *(Continued)*
  deficiency *(Continued)*
    ➡ glyceraldehyde phosphate dehydrogenase
      D55.29
    ➡ hexokinase D55.29
    iron D50.9
      secondary to blood loss (chronic) D50.0
    nutritional D53.9
      with
        poor iron absorption D50.8
        specified deficiency NEC D53.8
    ➡ phosphofructo-aldolase D55.29
    ➡ phosphoglycerate kinase D55.29
    ➡ PK D55.21
    protein D53.0
    ➡ pyruvate kinase D55.21
    transcobalamin II D55.22
    ➡ triose-phosphate isomerase D55.29
    vitamin B12 NOS D51.9
      dietary D51.3
      due to
        intrinsic factor deficiency D51.0
        selective vitamin B12 malabsorption
          with proteinuria D51.1
      pernicious D51.0
      specified type NEC D51.8
  Diamond-Blackfan (congenital hypoplastic)
    D61.01
  dibothriocephalus B70.0 *[D63.8]*
  dimorphic D53.1
  diphasic D53.1
  Diphyllobothrium (Dibothriocephalus) B70.0
    [D63.8]
  due to (in) (with)
    antineoplastic chemotherapy D64.81
    blood loss (chronic) D50.0
      acute D62
    chemotherapy, antineoplastic D64.81
    chronic disease classified elsewhere NEC
      D63.8
    chronic kidney disease D63.1
    deficiency
      amino-acid D53.0
      copper D53.8
      folate (folic acid) D52.9
        dietary D52.0
        drug-induced D52.1
      molybdenum D53.8
      protein D53.0
      zinc D53.8
    dietary vitamin B12 deficiency D51.3
    disorder of
      glutathione metabolism D55.1
      nucleotide metabolism D55.3
    drug —*see* Anemia, by type —*see also* Table
      of Drugs and Chemicals
    end stage renal disease D63.1
    enzyme disorder D55.9
    fetal blood loss P61.3
    fish tapeworm (D latum) infestation B70.0
      [D63.8]
    hemorrhage (chronic) D50.0
      acute D62
    impaired absorption D50.9
    loss of blood (chronic) D50.0
      acute D62
    myxedema E03.9 *[D63.8]*
    Necator americanus B76.1 *[D63.8]*
    prematurity P61.2
    selective vitamin B12 malabsorption with
      proteinuria D51.1
    transcobalamin II deficiency D51.2
  Dyke-Young type (secondary) (symptomatic)
    D59.19
  dyserythropoietic (congenital) D64.4
  dyshematopoietic (congenital) D64.4
  Egyptian B76.9 *[D63.8]*
  elliptocytosis —*see* Elliptocytosis
  enzyme-deficiency, drug-induced D59.2
  epidemic —*see also* Ancylostomiasis B76.9
    [D63.8]

    ▶ New   ➡ Revised   ~~deleted~~ Deleted   • Use Additional Character(s)

Anemia (Continued)
  erythroblastic
    familial D56.1
    newborn —see also Disease, hemolytic
        P55.9
    of childhood D56.1
  erythrocytic glutathione deficiency D55.1
  erythropoietin-resistant anemia (EPO
      resistant anemia) D63.1
  Faber's (achlorhydric anemia) D50.9
  factitious (self-induced blood letting) D50.0
  familial erythroblastic D56.1
  Fanconi's (congenital pancytopenia) D61.09
  favism D55.0
  fish tapeworm (D. latum) infestation B70.0
      [D63.8]
  folate (folic acid) deficiency D52.9
  glucose-6-phosphate dehydrogenase (G6PD)
      deficiency D55.0
  glutathione-reductase deficiency D55.1
  goat's milk D52.0
  granulocytic —see Agranulocytosis
  Heinz body, congenital D58.2
  hemolytic D58.9
    acquired D59.9
      with hemoglobinuria NEC D59.6
      autoimmune NEC D59.19
      infectious D59.4
      specified type NEC D59.8
      toxic D59.4
    acute D59.9
      due to enzyme deficiency specified type
          NEC D55.8
      Lederer's D59.19
    autoimmune D59.10
      cold D59.12
      drug-induced D59.0
      mixed D59.13
      warm D59.11
    chronic D58.9
      idiopathic D59.9
    cold type (secondary) (symptomatic)
        D59.12
    congenital (spherocytic) —see
        Spherocytosis
    due to
      cardiac conditions D59.4
      drugs (nonautoimmune) D59.2
        autoimmune D59.0
      enzyme disorder D55.9
        drug-induced D59.2
      presence of shunt or other internal
          prosthetic device D59.4
    familial D58.9
    hereditary D58.9
      due to enzyme disorder D55.9
        specified type NEC D55.8
      specified type NEC D58.8
    idiopathic (chronic) D59.9
    mechanical D59.4
    microangiopathic D59.4
    mixed type (primary) (secondary)
        (symptomatic) D59.13
    nonautoimmune D59.4
      drug-induced D59.2
    nonspherocytic
      congenital or hereditary NEC D55.8
        glucose-6-phosphate dehydrogenase
            deficiency D55.0
        ➠pyruvate kinase deficiency D55.21
        type
          I D55.1
          ➠II D55.29
      type
        I D55.1
        ➠II D55.29
    primary
      autoimmune
        cold type D59.12
        mixed type D59.13
        warm type D59.11

Anemia (Continued)
  hemolytic (Continued)
    secondary D59.4
      autoimmune
        cold type D59.12
        mixed type D59.13
        warm type D59.11
      specified (hereditary) type NEC D58.8
      Stransky-Regala type —see also
          Hemoglobinopathy D58.8
    symptomatic D59.4
      autoimmune
        cold type D59.12
        mixed type D59.13
        warm type D59.11
    toxic D59.4
    warm type (primary) (secondary)
        (symptomatic) D59.11
  hemorrhagic (chronic) D50.0
    acute D62
  Herrick's D57.1
  ➠hexokinase deficiency D55.29
  hookworm B76.9 [D63.8]
  hypochromic (idiopathic) (microcytic)
      (normoblastic) D50.9
    due to blood loss (chronic) D50.0
      acute D62
    familial sex-linked D64.0
    pyridoxine-responsive D64.3
    sideroblastic, sex-linked D64.0
  hypoplasia, red blood cells D61.9
    congenital or familial D61.01
  hypoplastic (idiopathic) D61.9
    congenital or familial (of childhood)
        D61.01
  hypoproliferative (refractive) D61.9
  idiopathic D64.9
    aplastic D61.3
    hemolytic, chronic D59.9
  in (due to) (with)
    chronic kidney disease D63.1
    end stage renal disease D63.1
    failure, kidney (renal) D63.1
    neoplastic disease —see also Neoplasm
        D63.0
  intertropical —see also Ancylostomiasis
      D63.8
  iron deficiency D50.9
    secondary to blood loss (chronic) D50.0
      acute D62
    specified type NEC D50.8
  Joseph-Diamond-Blackfan (congenital
      hypoplastic) D61.01
  Lederer's (hemolytic) D59.19
  leukoerythroblastic D61.82
  macrocytic D53.9
    nutritional D52.0
    tropical D52.8
  malarial (see also Malaria) B54 [D63.8]
  malignant (progressive) D51.0
  malnutrition D53.9
  marsh (see also Malaria) B54 [D63.8]
  Mediterranean (with other
      hemoglobinopathy) D56.9
  megaloblastic D53.1
    combined B12 and folate deficiency
        D53.1
    hereditary D51.1
    nutritional D52.0
    orotic aciduria D53.0
    refractory D53.1
    specified type NEC D53.1
  megalocytic D53.1
  microcytic (hypochromic) D50.9
    due to blood loss (chronic) D50.0
      acute D62
    familial D56.8
  microdrepanocytosis D57.40
  microelliptopoikilocytic (Rietti-Greppi-
      Micheli) D56.9
  miner's B76.9 [D63.8]

Anemia (Continued)
  myelodysplastic D46.9
  myelofibrosis D75.81
  myelogenous D64.89
  myelopathic D64.89
  myelophthisic D61.82
  myeloproliferative D47.Z9
  newborn P61.4
    due to
      ABO (antibodies, isoimmunization,
          maternal/fetal incompatibility)
          P55.1
      Rh (antibodies, isoimmunization,
          maternal/fetal incompatibility)
          P55.0
    following fetal blood loss P61.3
    posthemorrhagic (fetal) P61.3
  nonspherocytic hemolytic —see Anemia,
      hemolytic, nonspherocytic
  normocytic (infectional) D64.9
    due to blood loss (chronic) D50.0
      acute D62
    myelophthisic D61.82
  nutritional (deficiency) D53.9
    with
      poor iron absorption D50.8
      specified deficiency NEC D53.8
    megaloblastic D52.0
  of prematurity P61.2
  orotaciduric (congenital) (hereditary)
      D53.0
  osteosclerotic D64.89
  ovalocytosis (hereditary) —see Elliptocytosis
  paludal —see also Malaria B54 [D63.8]
  pernicious (congenital) (malignant)
      (progressive) D51.0
  pleochromic D64.89
    of sprue D52.8
  posthemorrhagic (chronic) D50.0
    acute D62
    newborn P61.3
  postoperative (postprocedural)
    due to (acute) blood loss D62
      chronic blood loss D50.0
  ➠specified NEC D64.89
  postpartum O90.81
  pressure D64.89
  progressive D64.9
    malignant D51.0
    pernicious D51.0
  protein-deficiency D53.0
  pseudoleukemica infantum D64.89
  pure red cell D60.9
    congenital D61.01
  pyridoxine-responsive D64.3
  ➠pyruvate kinase deficiency D55.21
  refractory D46.4
    with
      excess of blasts D46.20
        1 (RAEB 1) D46.21
        2 (RAEB 2) D46.22
        in transformation (RAEB T) —see
            Leukemia, acute myeloblastic
      hemochromatosis D46.1
      sideroblasts (ring) (RARS) D46.1
      without ring sideroblasts, so stated
          D46.0
    without sideroblasts without excess of
        blasts D46.0
    megaloblastic D53.1
    sideroblastic D46.1
    sideropenic D50.9
  Rietti-Greppi-Micheli D56.9
  scorbutic D53.2
  secondary to
    blood loss (chronic) D50.0
      acute D62
    hemorrhage (chronic) D50.0
      acute D62
  semiplastic D61.89
  sickle-cell —see Disease, sickle-cell

Anemia *(Continued)*
 sideroblastic D64.3
  hereditary D64.0
  hypochromic, sex-linked D64.0
  pyridoxine-responsive NEC D64.3
  refractory D46.1
  secondary (due to)
   disease D64.1
   drugs and toxins D64.2
   specified type NEC D64.3
 sideropenic (refractory) D50.9
  due to blood loss (chronic) D50.0
   acute D62
 simple chronic D53.9
 specified type NEC D64.89
 spherocytic (hereditary) —*see* Spherocytosis
 splenic D64.89
 splenomegalic D64.89
 stomatocytosis D58.8
 syphilitic (acquired) (late) A52.79 *[D63.8]*
 target cell D64.89
 thalassemia D56.9
 thrombocytopenic —*see* Thrombocytopenia
 toxic D61.2
 tropical B76.9 *[D63.8]*
  macrocytic D52.8
 tuberculous A18.89 *[D63.8]*
 vegan D51.3
 vitamin
  B6-responsive D64.3
  B12 deficiency (dietary) pernicious
   D51.0
 von Jaksch's D64.89
 Witts' (achlorhydric anemia) D50.8
Anemophobia F40.228
Anencephalus, anencephaly Q00.0
Anergasia —*see* Psychosis, organic
Anesthesia, anesthetic R20.0
 complication or reaction NEC —*see also*
  Complications, anesthesia T88.59
  due to
   correct substance properly
    administered —*see* Table of Drugs
    and Chemicals, by drug, adverse
    effect
   overdose or wrong substance given —*see*
    Table of Drugs and Chemicals, by
    drug, poisoning
   unintended awareness under general
    anesthesia during procedure
    T88.53
   personal history of Z92.84
 cornea H18.81-•
 dissociative F44.6
 functional (hysterical) F44.6
 hyperesthetic, thalamic G89.0
 hysterical F44.6
 local skin lesion R20.0
 sexual (psychogenic) F52.1
 shock (due to) T88.2
 skin R20.0
 testicular N50.9
Anetoderma (maculosum) (of) L90.8
 Jadassohn-Pellizzari L90.2
 Schweniger-Buzzi L90.1
Aneurin deficiency E51.9
Aneurysm (anastomotic) (artery) (cirsoid)
 (diffuse) (false) (fusiform) (multiple)
 (saccular) I72.9
 abdominal (aorta) I71.4
  ruptured I71.3
  syphilitic A52.01
 aorta, aortic (nonsyphilitic) I71.9
  abdominal I71.4
   ruptured I71.3
  arch I71.2
   ruptured I71.1
  arteriosclerotic I71.9
   ruptured I71.8
  ascending I71.2
   ruptured I71.1

Aneurysm *(Continued)*
 aorta, aortic (nonsyphilitic) *(Continued)*
  congenital Q25.43
  descending I71.9
   abdominal I71.4
    ruptured I71.3
   ruptured I71.8
   thoracic I71.2
    ruptured I71.1
  root Q25.43
  ruptured I71.8
  sinus, congenital Q25.43
  syphilitic A52.01
  thoracic I71.2
   ruptured I71.1
  thoracoabdominal I71.6
   ruptured I71.5
  thorax, thoracic (arch) I71.2
   ruptured I71.1
  transverse I71.2
   ruptured I71.1
  valve (heart) —*see also* Endocarditis, aortic
   I35.8
 arteriosclerotic I72.9
  cerebral I67.1
   ruptured —*see* Hemorrhage, intracranial,
    subarachnoid
 arteriovenous (congenital) —*see also*
  Malformation, arteriovenous
  acquired I77.0
   brain I67.1
    ruptured —*see* Aneurysm,
     arteriorvenous, brain, ruptured
   coronary I25.41
   pulmonary I28.0
  brain Q28.2
   ruptured I60.8
    intracerebral I61.8
    intraparenchymal I61.8
    intraventricular I61.5
    subarachnoid I60.8
  peripheral —*see* Malformation,
   arteriovenous, peripheral
  precerebral vessels Q28.0
  specified site NEC —*see also* Malformation,
   arteriovenous
   acquired I77.0
 basal —*see* Aneurysm, brain
 basilar (trunk) I72.5
 berry (congenital) (nonruptured) I67.1
  ruptured I60.7
 brain I67.1
  arteriosclerotic I67.1
   ruptured —*see* Hemorrhage, intracranial,
    subarachnoid
  arteriovenous (congenital) (nonruptured)
   Q28.2
   acquired I67.1
    ruptured —*see* Aneurysm,
     arteriorvenous, brain, ruptured
     I60.8-
   ruptured —*see* Aneurysm,
    arteriorvenous, brain, ruptured
    I60.8-
  berry (congenital) (nonruptured) I67.1
   ruptured —*see also* Hemorrhage,
    intracranial, subarachnoid I60.7
  congenital Q28.3
   aorta (root) (sinus) Q25.43
   ruptured I60.7
  meninges I67.1
   ruptured I60.8
  miliary (congenital) (nonruptured) I67.1
   ruptured —*see also* Hemorrhage,
    intracranial, subarachnoid I60.7
  mycotic I33.0
  ruptured —*see* Hemorrhage, intracranial,
   subarachnoid
  syphilitic (hemorrhage) A52.05
 cardiac (false) —*see also* Aneurysm, heart
  I25.3

Aneurysm *(Continued)*
 carotid artery (common) (external) I72.0
  internal (intracranial) I67.1
   extracranial portion I72.0
   ruptured into brain I60.0-•
  syphilitic A52.09
   intracranial A52.05
 cavernous sinus I67.1
  arteriovenous (congenital) (nonruptured)
   Q28.3
   ruptured I60.8
 celiac I72.8
 central nervous system, syphilitic A52.05
 cerebral —*see* Aneurysm, brain
 chest —*see* Aneurysm, thorax
 circle of Willis I67.1
  congenital Q28.3
   ruptured I60.6
  ruptured I60.6
 common iliac artery I72.3
 congenital (peripheral) Q27.8
  aorta (root) (sinus) Q25.43
  brain Q28.3
   ruptured I60.7
  coronary Q24.5
  digestive system Q27.8
  lower limb Q27.8
  pulmonary Q25.79
  retina Q14.1
  specified site NEC Q27.8
  upper limb Q27.8
 conjunctiva —*see* Abnormality, conjunctiva,
  vascular
 conus arteriosus —*see* Aneurysm, heart
 coronary (arteriosclerotic) (artery) I25.41
  arteriovenous, congenital Q24.5
  congenital Q24.5
  ruptured —*see* Infarct, myocardium
  syphilitic A52.06
  vein I25.89
 cylindroid (aorta) I71.9
  ruptured I71.8
  syphilitic A52.01
 ductus arteriosus Q25.0
 endocardial, infective (any valve) I33.0
 femoral (artery) (ruptured) I72.4
 gastroduodenal I72.8
 gastroepiploic I72.8
 heart (wall) (chronic or with a stated duration
  of over 4 weeks) I25.3
  valve —*see* Endocarditis
 hepatic I72.8
 iliac (common) (artery) (ruptured) I72.3
 infective I72.9
  endocardial (any valve) I33.0
 innominate (nonsyphilitic) I72.8
  syphilitic A52.09
 interauricular septum —*see* Aneurysm,
  heart
 interventricular septum —*see* Aneurysm,
  heart
 intrathoracic (nonsyphilitic) I71.2
  ruptured I71.1
  syphilitic A52.01
 lower limb I72.4
 lung (pulmonary artery) I28.1
 mediastinal (nonsyphilitic) I72.8
  syphilitic A52.09
 miliary (congenital) I67.1
  ruptured —*see* Hemorrhage, intracerebral,
   subarachnoid, intracranial
 mitral (heart) (valve) I34.8
 mural —*see* Aneurysm, heart
 mycotic I72.9
  endocardial (any valve) I33.0
  ruptured, brain —*see* Hemorrhage,
   intracerebral, subarachnoid
 myocardium —*see* Aneurysm, heart
 neck I72.0
 pancreaticoduodenal I72.8
 patent ductus arteriosus Q25.0

▶ New   ⇒ Revised   ~~deleted~~ Deleted   • Use Additional Character(s)

Aneurysm (Continued)
- peripheral NEC I72.8
  - congenital Q27.8
    - digestive system Q27.8
    - lower limb Q27.8
    - specified site NEC Q27.8
    - upper limb Q27.8
- popliteal (artery) (ruptured) I72.4
- precerebral
  - congenital (nonruptured) Q28.1
  - specified site, NEC I72.5
- pulmonary I28.1
  - arteriovenous Q25.72
    - acquired I28.0
  - syphilitic A52.09
  - valve (heart) —see Endocarditis, pulmonary
- racemose (peripheral) I72.9
  - congenital —see Aneurysm, congenital
- radial I72.1
- Rasmussen NEC A15.0
- renal (artery) I72.2
- retina —see also Disorder, retina,
      microaneurysms
  - congenital Q14.1
  - diabetic —see E08-E13 with .3-•
- sinus of Valsalva Q25.49
- specified NEC I72.8
- spinal (cord) I72.8
  - syphilitic (hemorrhage) A52.09
- splenic I72.8
- subclavian (artery) (ruptured) I72.8
  - syphilitic A52.09
- superior mesenteric I72.8
- syphilitic (aorta) A52.01
  - central nervous system A52.05
  - congenital (late) A50.54 [I79.0]
  - spine, spinal A52.09
- thoracoabdominal (aorta) I71.6
  - ruptured I71.5
  - syphilitic A52.01
- thorax, thoracic (aorta) (arch) (nonsyphilitic)
      I71.2
  - ruptured I71.1
  - syphilitic A52.01
- traumatic (complication) (early), specified
      site —see Injury, blood vessel
- tricuspid (heart) (valve) I07.8
- ulnar I72.1
- upper limb (ruptured) I72.1
- valve, valvular —see Endocarditis
- visceral NEC I72.8
- venous —see also Varix I86.8
  - congenital Q27.8
    - digestive system Q27.8
    - lower limb Q27.8
    - specified site NEC Q27.8
    - upper limb Q27.8
- ventricle —see Aneurysm, heart
- vertebral artery I72.6
- visceral NEC I72.8

Angelman syndrome Q93.51
Anger R45.4
Angiectasis, angiectopia I99.8
Angiitis I77.6
- allergic granulomatous M30.1
- hypersensitivity M31.0
- necrotizing M31.9
  - specified NEC M31.8
- nervous system, granulomatous I67.7
Angina (attack) (cardiac) (chest) (heart)
      (pectoris) (syndrome) (vasomotor) I20.9
- with
  - atherosclerotic heart disease —see
        Arteriosclerosis, coronary (artery)
  - documented spasm I20.1
- abdominal K55.1
- accelerated —see Angina, unstable
- agranulocytic —see Agranulocytosis
- angiospastic —see Angina, with documented
      spasm
- aphthous B08.5

Angina (Continued)
- crescendo —see Angina, unstable
- croupous J05.0
- cruris I73.9
- de novo effort —see Angina, unstable
- diphtheritic, membranous A36.0
- equivalent I20.8
- exudative, chronic J37.0
- following acute myocardial infarction I23.7
- gangrenous diphtheritic A36.0
- intestinal K55.1
- Ludovici K12.2
- Ludwig's K12.2
- malignant diphtheritic A36.0
- membranous J05.0
  - diphtheritic A36.0
  - Vincent's A69.1
- mesenteric K55.1
- monocytic —see Mononucleosis, infectious
- of effort —see Angina, specified NEC
- phlegmonous J36
  - diphtheritic A36.0
- post-infarctional I23.7
- pre-infarctional —see Angina, unstable
- Prinzmetal —see Angina, with documented
      spasm
- progressive —see Angina, unstable
- pseudomembranous A69.1
- pultaceous, diphtheritic A36.0
- spasm-induced —see Angina, with
      documented spasm
- specified NEC I20.8
- stable I20.8
- stenocardia —see Angina, specified NEC
- stridulous, diphtheritic A36.2
- tonsil J36
- trachealis J05.0
- unstable I20.0
- variant —see Angina, with documented spasm
- Vincent's A69.1
- worsening effort —see Angina, unstable
Angioblastoma —see Neoplasm, connective
      tissue, uncertain behavior
Angiocholecystitis —see Cholecystitis, acute
Angiocholitis —see also Cholecystitis, acute
      K83.09
Angiodysgenesis spinalis G95.19
Angiodysplasia (cecum) (colon) K55.20
- with bleeding K55.21
- duodenum (and stomach) K31.819
  - with bleeding K31.811
- stomach (and duodenum) K31.819
  - with bleeding K31.811
Angioedema (allergic) (any site) (with urticaria)
      T78.3
- episodic, with eosinophilia D72.118
- hereditary D84.1
Angioendothelioma —see Neoplasm, uncertain
      behavior, by site
- benign D18.00
  - intra-abdominal D18.03
  - intracranial D18.02
  - skin D18.01
  - specified site NEC D18.09
- bone —see Neoplasm, bone, malignant
- Ewing's —see Neoplasm, bone, malignant
Angioendotheliomatosis C85.8-•
Angiofibroma —see also Neoplasm, benign, by
      site
- juvenile
  - specified site —see Neoplasm, benign, by
        site
  - unspecified site D10.6
Angiohemophilia (A) (B) D68.0
Angioid streaks (choroid) (macula) (retina)
      H35.33
Angiokeratoma —see Neoplasm, skin, benign
- corporis diffusum E75.21
Angioleiomyoma —see Neoplasm, connective
      tissue, benign
Angiolipoma —see also Lipoma
- infiltrating —see Lipoma

Angioma —see also Hemangioma, by site
- capillary I78.1
- hemorrhagicum hereditaria I78.0
- intra-abdominal D18.03
- intracranial D18.02
- malignant —see Neoplasm, connective tissue,
      malignant
- plexiform D18.00
  - intra-abdominal D18.03
  - intracranial D18.02
  - skin D18.01
  - specified site NEC D18.09
- senile I78.1
- serpiginosum L81.7
- skin D18.01
- specified site NEC D18.09
- spider I78.1
- stellate I78.1
- venous Q28.3
Angiomatosis Q82.8
- bacillary A79.89
- encephalotrigeminal Q85.8
- hemorrhagic familial I78.0
- hereditary familial I78.0
- liver K76.4
Angiomyolipoma —see Lipoma
Angiomyoliposarcoma —see Neoplasm,
      connective tissue, malignant
Angiomyoma —see Neoplasm, connective
      tissue, benign
Angiomyosarcoma —see Neoplasm, connective
      tissue, malignant
Angiomyxoma —see Neoplasm, connective
      tissue, uncertain behavior
Angioneurosis F45.8
Angioneurotic edema (allergic) (any site) (with
      urticaria) T78.3
- hereditary D84.1
Angiopathia, angiopathy I99.9
- cerebral I67.9
  - amyloid E85.4 [I68.0]
- diabetic (peripheral) —see Diabetes,
      angiopathy
- peripheral I73.9
  - diabetic —see Diabetes, angiopathy
  - specified type NEC I73.89
- retinae syphilitica A52.05
- retinalis (juvenilis)
  - diabetic —see Diabetes, retinopathy
  - proliferative —see Retinopathy, proliferative
Angiosarcoma —see also Neoplasm, connective
      tissue, malignant
- liver C22.3
Angiosclerosis —see Arteriosclerosis
Angiospasm (peripheral) (traumatic) (vessel)
      I73.9
- brachial plexus G54.0
- cerebral G45.9
- cervical plexus G54.2
- nerve
  - arm —see Mononeuropathy, upper limb
    - axillary G54.0
    - median —see Lesion, nerve, median
    - ulnar —see Lesion, nerve, ulnar
  - axillary G54.0
  - leg —see Mononeuropathy, lower limb
  - median —see Lesion, nerve, median
  - plantar —see Lesion, nerve, plantar
  - ulnar —see Lesion, nerve, ulnar
Angiospastic disease or edema I73.9
Angiostrongyliasis
- due to
  - Parastrongylus
    - cantonensis B83.2
    - costaricensis B81.3
  - intestinal B81.3
Anguillulosis —see Strongyloidiasis
Angulation
- cecum —see Obstruction, intestine
- coccyx (acquired) —see also subcategory M43.8
  - congenital NEC Q76.49

Angulation (Continued)
   femur (acquired) —see also Deformity, limb,
      specified type NEC, thigh
      congenital Q74.2
   intestine (large) (small) —see Obstruction,
      intestine
   sacrum (acquired) —see also subcategory M43.8
      congenital NEC Q76.49
   sigmoid (flexure) —see Obstruction, intestine
   spine —see Dorsopathy, deforming,
      specified NEC
   tibia (acquired) —see also Deformity, limb,
      specified type NEC, lower leg
      congenital Q74.2
   ureter N13.5
      with infection N13.6
   wrist (acquired) —see also Deformity,
      limb, specified type NEC, forearm
      congenital Q74.0
Angulus infectiosus (lips) K13.0
Anhedonia R45.84
   sexual F52.0
Anhidrosis L74.4
Anhydration E86.0
Anhydremia E86.0
Anidrosis L74.4
Aniridia (congenital) Q13.1
Anisakiasis (infection) (infestation) B81.0
Anisakis larvae infestation B81.0
Aniseikonia H52.32
Anisocoria (pupil) H57.02
   congenital Q13.2
Anisocytosis R71.8
Anisometropia (congenital) H52.31
Ankle —see condition
Ankyloblepharon (eyelid) (acquired) —see also
   Blepharophimosis
   filiforme (adnatum) (congenital) Q10.3
   total Q10.3
Ankyloglossia Q38.1
Ankylosis (fibrous) (osseous) (joint) M24.60
   ankle M24.67-●
   arthrodesis status Z98.1
   cricoarytenoid (cartilage) (joint) (larynx) J38.7
   dental K03.5
   ear ossicles H74.31-●
   elbow M24.62-●
   foot M24.67-●
   hand M24.64-●
   hip M24.65-●
   incostapedial joint (infectional) —see
      Ankylosis, ear ossicles
   jaw (temporomandibular) M26.61-●
   knee M24.66-●
   lumbosacral (joint) M43.27
   postoperative (status) Z98.1
   produced by surgical fusion, status Z98.1
   sacro-iliac (joint) M43.28
   shoulder M24.61-●
   specified site NEC M24.69
   spine (joint) —see also Fusion, spine
      spondylitic —see Spondylitis, ankylosing
   surgical Z98.1
   temporomandibular M26.61-●
   tooth, teeth (hard tissues) K03.5
   wrist M24.63-●
Ankylostoma —see Ancylostoma
Ankylostomiasis —see Ancylostomiasis
Ankylurethria —see Stricture, urethra
Annular —see also condition
   detachment, cervix N88.8
   organ or site, congenital NEC —see Distortion
   pancreas (congenital) Q45.1
Anodontia (complete) (partial) (vera) K00.0
   acquired K08.10
Anomaly, anomalous (congenital) (unspecified
   type) Q89.9
   abdominal wall NEC Q79.59
   acoustic nerve Q07.8
   adrenal (gland) Q89.1
   Alder (-Reilly) (leukocyte granulation) D72.0

Anomaly, anomalous (Continued)
   alimentary tract Q45.9
      upper Q40.9
   alveolar M26.70
      hyperplasia M26.79
         mandibular M26.72
         maxillary M26.71
      hypoplasia M26.79
         mandibular M26.74
         maxillary M26.73
      ridge (process) M26.79
      specified NEC M26.79
   ankle (joint) Q74.2
   anus Q43.9
   aorta (arch) NEC Q25.40
      coarctation (preductal) (postductal) Q25.1
   aortic cusp or valve Q23.9
   appendix Q43.8
   apple peel syndrome Q41.1
   aqueduct of Sylvius Q03.0
      with spina bifida —see Spina bifida, with
         hydrocephalus
   arm Q74.0
   arteriovenous NEC
      coronary Q24.5
      gastrointestinal Q27.33
         acquired —see Angiodysplasia
   artery (peripheral) Q27.9
      basilar NEC Q28.1
      cerebral Q28.3
      coronary Q24.5
      digestive system Q27.8
      eye Q15.8
      great Q25.9
         specified NEC Q25.8
      lower limb Q27.8
      peripheral Q27.9
         specified NEC Q27.8
      pulmonary NEC Q25.79
      renal Q27.2
      retina Q14.1
      specified site NEC Q27.8
      subclavian Q27.8
        origin Q25.48
      umbilical Q27.0
      upper limb Q27.8
      vertebral NEC Q28.1
   aryteno-epiglottic folds Q31.8
   atrial
      bands or folds Q20.8
      septa Q21.1
   atrioventricular
      excitation I45.6
      septum Q21.0
   auditory canal Q17.8
   auricle
      ear Q17.8
         causing impairment of hearing Q16.9
      heart Q20.8
   Axenfeld's Q15.0
   back Q89.9
   band
      atrial Q20.8
      heart Q24.8
      ventricular Q24.8
   Bartholin's duct Q38.4
   biliary duct or passage Q44.5
   bladder Q64.70
      absence Q64.5
      diverticulum Q64.6
      exstrophy Q64.10
         cloacal Q64.12
         extroversion Q64.19
         specified type NEC Q64.19
         supravesical fissure Q64.11
      neck obstruction Q64.31
      specified type NEC Q64.79
   bone Q79.9
      arm Q74.0
      face Q75.9
      leg Q74.2

Anomaly, anomalous (Continued)
   bone (Continued)
      pelvic girdle Q74.2
      shoulder girdle Q74.0
      skull Q75.9
        with
           anencephaly Q00.0
           encephalocele —see Encephalocele
           hydrocephalus Q03.9
              with spina bifida —see Spina bifida,
                 by site, with hydrocephalus
           microcephaly Q02
   brain (multiple) Q04.9
      vessel Q28.3
   breast Q83.9
   broad ligament Q50.6
   bronchus Q32.4
   bulbus cordis Q21.9
   bursa Q79.9
   canal of Nuck Q52.4
   canthus Q10.3
   capillary Q27.9
   cardiac Q24.9
      chambers Q20.9
         specified NEC Q20.8
      septal closure Q21.9
         specified NEC Q21.8
      valve NEC Q24.8
         pulmonary Q22.3
   cardiovascular system Q28.8
   carpus Q74.0
   caruncle, lacrimal Q10.6
   cascade stomach Q40.2
   cauda equina Q06.3
   cecum Q43.9
   cerebral Q04.9
      vessels Q28.3
   cervix Q51.9
   Chédiak-Higashi(-Steinbrinck) (congenital
      gigantism of peroxidase granules)
      E70.330
   cheek Q18.9
   chest wall Q67.8
      bones Q76.9
   chin Q18.9
   chordae tendineae Q24.8
   choroid Q14.3
      plexus Q07.8
   chromosomes, chromosomal Q99.9
      D (1) —see condition, chromosome 13
      E (3) —see condition, chromosome 18
      G —see condition, chromosome 21
      sex
         female phenotype Q97.8
         gonadal dysgenesis (pure) Q99.1
         Klinefelter's Q98.4
         male phenotype Q98.9
         Turner's Q96.9
      specified NEC Q99.8
   cilia Q10.3
   circulatory system Q28.9
   clavicle Q74.0
   clitoris Q52.6
   coccyx Q76.49
   colon Q43.9
   common duct Q44.5
   communication
      coronary artery Q24.5
      left ventricle with right atrium Q21.0
   concha (ear) Q17.3
   connection
      portal vein Q26.5
      pulmonary venous Q26.4
         partial Q26.3
         total Q26.2
      renal artery with kidney Q27.2
   cornea (shape) Q13.4
   coronary artery or vein Q24.5
   cranium —see Anomaly, skull
   cricoid cartilage Q31.8
   cystic duct Q44.5

Anomaly, anomalous (Continued)
  dental
    alveolar —see Anomaly, alveolar
    arch relationship M26.20
      specified NEC M26.29
  dentofacial M26.9
    alveolar —see Anomaly, alveolar
    dental arch relationship M26.20
      specified NEC M26.29
    functional M26.50
      specified NEC M26.59
    jaw-cranial base relationship M26.10
      asymmetry M26.12
        maxillary M26.11
      specified type NEC M26.19
    jaw size M26.00
      macrogenia M26.05
      mandibular
        hyperplasia M26.03
        hypoplasia M26.04
      maxillary
        hyperplasia M26.01
        hypoplasia M26.02
      microgenia M26.06
      specified type NEC M26.09
    malocclusion M26.4
      dental arch relationship NEC M26.29
      jaw-cranial base relationship —see
        Anomaly, dentofacial, jaw-cranial
        base relationship
      jaw size —see Anomaly, dentofacial, jaw
        size
    specified type NEC M26.89
    temporomandibular joint M26.60-●
      adhesions M26.61-●
      ankylosis M26.61-●
      arthralgia M26.62-●
      articular disc M26.63-●
      specified type NEC M26.69
    tooth position, fully erupted M26.30
      specified NEC M26.39
  dermatoglyphic Q82.8
  diaphragm (apertures) NEC Q79.1
  digestive organ(s) or tract Q45.9
    lower Q43.9
    upper Q40.9
  distance, interarch (excessive) (inadequate)
    M26.25
  distribution, coronary artery Q24.5
  ductus
    arteriosus Q25.0
    botalli Q25.0
  duodenum Q43.9
  dura (brain) Q04.9
    spinal cord Q06.9
  ear (external) Q17.9
    causing impairment of hearing Q16.9
    inner Q16.5
    middle (causing impairment of hearing)
      Q16.4
    ossicles Q16.3
  Ebstein's (heart) (tricuspid valve) Q22.5
  ectodermal Q82.9
  Eisenmenger's (ventricular septal defect)
    Q21.8
  ejaculatory duct Q55.4
  elbow Q74.0
  endocrine gland NEC Q89.2
  epididymis Q55.4
  epiglottis Q31.8
  esophagus Q39.9
  eustachian tube Q17.8
  eye Q15.9
    anterior segment Q13.9
      specified NEC Q13.89
    posterior segment Q14.9
      specified NEC Q14.8
    ptosis (eyelid) Q10.0
    specified NEC Q15.8
  eyebrow Q18.8
  eyelid Q10.3
    ptosis Q10.0

Anomaly, anomalous (Continued)
  face Q18.9
    bone(s) Q75.9
  fallopian tube Q50.6
  fascia Q79.9
  femur NEC Q74.2
  fibula NEC Q74.2
  finger Q74.0
  fixation, intestine Q43.3
  flexion (joint) NOS Q74.9
    hip or thigh Q65.89
  foot NEC Q74.2
    varus (congenital) Q66.3-●
  foramen
    Botalli Q21.1
    ovale Q21.1
  forearm Q74.0
  forehead Q75.8
  form, teeth K00.2
  fovea centralis Q14.1
  frontal bone —see Anomaly, skull
  gallbladder (position) (shape) (size)
    Q44.1
  Gartner's duct Q52.4
  gastrointestinal tract Q45.9
  genitalia, genital organ(s) or system
    female Q52.9
      external Q52.70
      internal NOS Q52.9
    male Q55.9
      hydrocele P83.5
      specified NEC Q55.8
  genitourinary NEC
    female Q52.9
    male Q55.9
  Gerbode Q21.0
  glottis Q31.8
  granulation or granulocyte, genetic
    (constitutional) (leukocyte) D72.0
  gum Q38.6
  gyri Q07.9
  hair Q84.2
  hand Q74.0
  hard tissue formation in pulp K04.3
  head —see Anomaly, skull
  heart Q24.9
    auricle Q20.8
    bands or folds Q24.8
    fibroelastosis cordis I42.4
    obstructive NEC Q22.6
    patent ductus arteriosus (Botalli) Q25.0
    septum Q21.9
      auricular Q21.1
      interatrial Q21.1
      interventricular Q21.0
        with pulmonary stenosis or atresia,
          dextraposition of aorta and
          hypertrophy of right ventricle
          Q21.3
      specified NEC Q21.8
      ventricular Q21.0
        with pulmonary stenosis or atresia,
          dextraposition of aorta and
          hypertrophy of right ventricle
          Q21.3
    tetralogy of Fallot Q21.3
    valve NEC Q24.8
      aortic
        bicuspid valve Q23.1
        insufficiency Q23.1
        stenosis Q23.0
          subaortic Q24.4
      mitral
        insufficiency Q23.3
        stenosis Q23.2
      pulmonary Q22.3
        atresia Q22.0
        insufficiency Q22.2
        stenosis Q22.1
          infundibular Q24.3
          subvalvular Q24.3

Anomaly, anomalous (Continued)
  heart (Continued)
    valve NEC (Continued)
      tricuspid
        atresia Q22.4
        stenosis Q22.4
      ventricle Q20.8
  heel NEC Q74.2
  Hegglin's D72.0
  hemianencephaly Q00.0
  hemicephaly Q00.0
  hemicrania Q00.0
  hepatic duct Q44.5
  hip NEC Q74.2
  hourglass stomach Q40.2
  humerus Q74.0
  hydatid of Morgagni
    female Q50.5
    male (epididymal) Q55.4
      testicular Q55.29
  hymen Q52.4
  hypersegmentation of neutrophils, hereditary
    D72.0
  hypophyseal Q89.2
  ileocecal (coil) (valve) Q43.9
  ileum Q43.9
  ilium NEC Q74.2
  integument Q84.9
    specified NEC Q84.8
  interarch distance (excessive) (inadequate)
    M26.25
  intervertebral cartilage or disc Q76.49
  intestine (large) (small) Q43.9
    with anomalous adhesions, fixation or
      malrotation Q43.3
  iris Q13.2
  ischium NEC Q74.2
  jaw —see Anomaly, dentofacial
    alveolar —see Anomaly, alveolar
    jaw-cranial base relationship —see Anomaly,
      dentofacial, jaw-cranial base relationship
  jejunum Q43.8
  joint Q74.9
    specified NEC Q74.8
  Jordan's D72.0
  kidney(s) (calyx) (pelvis) Q63.9
    artery Q27.2
    specified NEC Q63.8
  Klippel-Feil (brevicollis) Q76.1
  knee Q74.1
  labium (majus) (minus) Q52.70
  labyrinth, membranous Q16.5
  lacrimal apparatus or duct Q10.6
  larynx, laryngeal (muscle) Q31.9
    web (bed) Q31.0
  lens Q12.9
  leukocytes, genetic D72.0
    granulation (constitutional) D72.0
  lid (fold) Q10.3
  ligament Q79.9
    broad Q50.6
    round Q52.8
  limb Q74.9
    lower NEC Q74.2
      reduction deformity —see Defect,
        reduction, lower limb
    upper Q74.0
  lip Q38.0
  liver Q44.7
    duct Q44.5
  lower limb NEC Q74.2
  lumbosacral (joint) (region) Q76.49
    kyphosis —see Kyphosis, congenital
    lordosis —see Lordosis, congenital
  lung (fissure) (lobe) Q33.9
  mandible —see Anomaly, dentofacial
  maxilla —see Anomaly, dentofacial
  May (-Hegglin) D72.0
  meatus urinarius NEC Q64.79
  meningeal bands or folds Q07.9
    constriction of Q07.8
    spinal Q06.9

Anomaly, anomalous (Continued)
  meninges Q07.9
    cerebral Q04.8
    spinal Q06.9
  meningocele Q05.9
  mesentery Q45.9
  metacarpus Q74.0
  metatarsus NEC Q74.2
  middle ear Q16.4
    ossicles Q16.3
  mitral (leaflets) (valve) Q23.9
    insufficiency Q23.3
    specified NEC Q23.8
    stenosis Q23.2
  mouth Q38.6
  Müllerian —see also Anomaly, by site
    uterus NEC Q51.818
  multiple NEC Q89.7
  muscle Q79.9
    eyelid Q10.3
  musculoskeletal system, except limbs Q79.9
  myocardium Q24.8
  nail Q84.6
  narrowness, eyelid Q10.3
  nasal sinus (wall) Q30.8
  neck (any part) Q18.9
  nerve Q07.9
    acoustic Q07.8
    optic Q07.8
  nervous system (central) Q07.9
  nipple Q83.9
  nose, nasal (bones) (cartilage) (septum)
    (sinus) Q30.9
    specified NEC Q30.8
  ocular muscle Q15.8
  omphalomesenteric duct Q43.0
  opening, pulmonary veins Q26.4
  optic
    disc Q14.2
    nerve Q07.8
  opticociliary vessels Q13.2
  orbit (eye) Q10.7
  organ Q89.9
    of Corti Q16.5
  origin
    artery
      innominate Q25.8
      pulmonary Q25.79
      renal Q27.2
      subclavian Q25.48
  osseous meatus (ear) Q16.1
  ovary Q50.39
  oviduct Q50.6
  palate (hard) (soft) NEC Q38.5
  pancreas or pancreatic duct Q45.3
  papillary muscles Q24.8
  parathyroid gland Q89.2
  paraurethral ducts Q64.79
  parotid (gland) Q38.4
  patella Q74.1
  Pelger-Huët (hereditary hyposegmentation)
    D72.0
  pelvic girdle NEC Q74.2
  pelvis (bony) NEC Q74.2
    rachitic E64.3
  penis (glans) Q55.69
  pericardium Q24.8
  peripheral vascular system Q27.9
  Peter's Q13.4
  pharynx Q38.8
  pigmentation L81.9
    congenital Q82.8
  pituitary (gland) Q89.2
  pleural (folds) Q34.0
  portal vein Q26.5
    connection Q26.5
  position, tooth, teeth, fully erupted M26.30
    specified NEC M26.39
  precerebral vessel Q28.1
  prepuce Q55.69
  prostate Q55.4

Anomaly, anomalous (Continued)
  pulmonary Q33.9
    artery NEC Q25.79
    valve Q22.3
      atresia Q22.0
      insufficiency Q22.2
      specified type NEC Q22.3
      stenosis Q22.1
        infundibular Q24.3
        subvalvular Q24.3
    venous connection Q26.4
      partial Q26.3
      total Q26.2
  pupil Q13.2
    function H57.00
      anisocoria H57.02
      Argyll Robertson pupil H57.01
      miosis H57.03
      mydriasis H57.04
      specified type NEC H57.09
      tonic pupil H57.05-●
  pylorus Q40.3
  radius Q74.0
  rectum Q43.9
  reduction (extremity) (limb)
    femur (longitudinal) —see Defect,
      reduction, lower limb, longitudinal,
      femur
    fibula (longitudinal) —see Defect,
      reduction, lower limb, longitudinal,
      fibula
    lower limb —see Defect, reduction, lower
      limb
    radius (longitudinal) —see Defect,
      reduction, upper limb, longitudinal,
      radius
    tibia (longitudinal) —see Defect, reduction,
      lower limb, longitudinal, tibia
    ulna (longitudinal) —see Defect, reduction,
      upper limb, longitudinal, ulna
    upper limb —see Defect, reduction, upper
      limb
  refraction —see Disorder, refraction
  renal Q63.9
    artery Q27.2
    pelvis Q63.9
      specified NEC Q63.8
  respiratory system Q34.9
    specified NEC Q34.8
  retina Q14.1
  rib Q76.6
    cervical Q76.5
  Rieger's Q13.81
  rotation —see Malrotation
    hip or thigh Q65.89
  round ligament Q52.8
  sacroiliac (joint) NEC Q74.2
  sacrum NEC Q76.49
    kyphosis —see Kyphosis, congenital
    lordosis —see Lordosis, congenital
  saddle nose, syphilitic A50.57
  salivary duct or gland Q38.4
  scapula Q74.0
  scrotum —see Malformation, testis and
    scrotum
  sebaceous gland Q82.9
  seminal vesicles Q55.4
  sense organs NEC Q07.8
  sex chromosomes NEC —see also Anomaly,
    chromosomes
    female phenotype Q97.8
    male phenotype Q98.9
  shoulder (girdle) (joint) Q74.0
  sigmoid (flexure) Q43.9
  simian crease Q82.8
  sinus of Valsalva Q25.49
  skeleton generalized Q78.9
  skin (appendage) Q82.9
  skull Q75.9
    with
      anencephaly Q00.0
      encephalocele —see Encephalocele

Anomaly, anomalous (Continued)
  skull (Continued)
    with (Continued)
      hydrocephalus Q03.9
        with spina bifida —see Spina bifida, by
          site, with hydrocephalus
      microcephaly Q02
    specified organ or site NEC Q89.8
  spermatic cord Q55.4
  spine, spinal NEC Q76.49
    column NEC Q76.49
      kyphosis —see Kyphosis, congenital
      lordosis —see Lordosis, congenital
    cord Q06.9
    nerve root Q07.8
  spleen Q89.09
    agenesis Q89.01
  stenonian duct Q38.4
  sternum NEC Q76.7
  stomach Q40.3
  submaxillary gland Q38.4
  tarsus NEC Q74.2
  tendon Q79.9
  testis —see Malformation, testis and scrotum
  thigh NEC Q74.2
  thorax (wall) Q67.8
    bony Q76.9
  throat Q38.8
  thumb Q74.0
  thymus gland Q89.2
  thyroid (gland) Q89.2
    cartilage Q31.8
  tibia NEC Q74.2
    saber A50.56
  toe Q74.2
  tongue Q38.3
  tooth, teeth K00.9
    eruption K00.6
    position, fully erupted M26.30
    spacing, fully erupted M26.30
  trachea (cartilage) Q32.1
  tragus Q17.9
  tricuspid (leaflet) (valve) Q22.9
    atresia or stenosis Q22.4
    Ebstein's Q22.5
  Uhl's (hypoplasia of myocardium, right
    ventricle) Q24.8
  ulna Q74.0
  umbilical artery Q27.0
  union
    cricoid cartilage and thyroid cartilage
      Q31.8
    thyroid cartilage and hyoid bone Q31.8
    trachea with larynx Q31.8
  upper limb Q74.0
  urachus Q64.4
  ureter Q62.8
    obstructive NEC Q62.39
      cecoureterocele Q62.32
      orthotopic ureterocele Q62.31
  urethra Q64.70
    absence Q64.5
    double Q64.74
    fistula to rectum Q64.73
    obstructive Q64.39
      stricture Q64.32
    prolapse Q64.71
    specified type NEC Q64.79
  urinary tract Q64.9
  uterus Q51.9
    with only one functioning horn Q51.4
  uvula Q38.5
  vagina Q52.4
  valleculae Q31.8
  valve (heart) NEC Q24.8
    coronary sinus Q24.5
    inferior vena cava Q24.8
    pulmonary Q22.3
    sinus coronario Q24.5
    venae cavae inferioris Q24.8
  vas deferens Q55.4

▶ New   ⇒ Revised   ~~deleted~~ Deleted   ● Use Additional Character(s)

Anomaly, anomalous *(Continued)*
  vascular Q27.9
    brain Q28.3
    ring Q25.45
  vein(s) (peripheral) Q27.9
    brain Q28.3
    cerebral Q28.3
    coronary Q24.5
    developmental Q28.3
    great Q26.9
      specified NEC Q26.8
  vena cava (inferior) (superior) Q26.9
  venous —*see* Anomaly, vein(s)
  venous return Q26.8
  ventricular
    bands or folds Q24.8
    septa Q21.0
  vertebra Q76.49
    kyphosis —*see* Kyphosis, congenital
    lordosis —*see* Lordosis, congenital
  vesicourethral orifice Q64.79
  vessel(s) Q27.9
    optic papilla Q14.2
    precerebral Q28.1
  vitelline duct Q43.0
  vitreous body or humor Q14.0
  vulva Q52.70
  wrist (joint) Q74.0
Anomia R48.8
Anonychia (congenital) Q84.3
  acquired L60.8
Anophthalmos, anophthalmus (congenital)
    (globe) Q11.1
  acquired Z90.01
Anopia, anopsia H53.46-●
  quadrant H53.46-●
Anorchia, anorchism, anorchidism Q55.0
Anorexia R63.0
  hysterical F44.89
  nervosa F50.00
    atypical F50.9
    binge-eating type F50.2
      with purging F50.02
    restricting type F50.01
Anorgasmy, psychogenic (female)
    F52.31
  male F52.32
Anosmia R43.0
  hysterical F44.6
  postinfectional J39.8
Anosognosia R41.89
Anosteoplasia Q78.9
Anovulatory cycle N97.0
Anoxemia R09.02
  newborn P84
Anoxia (pathological) R09.02
  altitude T70.29
  cerebral G93.1
    complicating
      anesthesia (general) (local) or other
        sedation T88.59
        in labor and delivery O74.3
        in pregnancy O29.21-●
        postpartum, puerperal O89.2
      delivery (cesarean) (instrumental)
        O75.4
    during a procedure G97.81
    newborn P84
    resulting from a procedure G97.82
  due to
    drowning T75.1
    high altitude T70.29
  heart —*see* Insufficiency, coronary
  intrauterine P84
  myocardial —*see* Insufficiency, coronary
  newborn P84
  spinal cord G95.11
  systemic (by suffocation) (low content in
    atmosphere) —*see* Asphyxia,
    traumatic
Anteflexion —*see* Anteversion

Antenatal
  care (normal pregnancy) Z34.90
  screening (encounter for) of mother —*see also*
    Encounter, antenatal screening Z36.9
Antepartum —*see* condition
Anterior —*see* condition
Antero-occlusion M26.220
Anteversion
  cervix —*see* Anteversion, uterus
  femur (neck), congenital Q65.89
  uterus, uterine (cervix) (postinfectional)
    (postpartal, old) N85.4
    congenital Q51.818
    in pregnancy or childbirth —*see* Pregnancy,
      complicated by
Anthophobia F40.228
Anthracosilicosis J60
Anthracosis (lung) (occupational) J60
  lingua K14.3
Anthrax A22.9
  with pneumonia A22.1
  cerebral A22.8
  colitis A22.2
  cutaneous A22.0
  gastrointestinal A22.2
  inhalation A22.1
  intestinal A22.2
  meningitis A22.8
  pulmonary A22.1
  respiratory A22.1
  sepsis A22.7
  specified manifestation NEC A22.8
Anthropoid pelvis Q74.2
  with disproportion (fetopelvic) O33.0
Anthropophobia F40.10
  generalized F40.11
Antibodies, maternal (blood group) —*see*
    Isoimmunization, affecting management of
    pregnancy
  anti-D —*see* Isoimmunization, affecting
    management of pregnancy, Rh
  newborn P55.0
Antibody
  anticardiolipin R76.0
    with
      hemorrhagic disorder D68.312
      hypercoagulable state D68.61
  antiphosphatidylglycerol R76.0
    with
      hemorrhagic disorder D68.312
      hypercoagulable state D68.61
  antiphosphatidylinositol R76.0
    with
      hemorrhagic disorder D68.312
      hypercoagulable state D68.61
  antiphosphatidylserine R76.0
    with
      hemorrhagic disorder D68.312
      hypercoagulable state D68.61
  antiphospholipid R76.0
    with
      hemorrhagic disorder D68.312
      hypercoagulable state D68.61
Anticardiolipin syndrome D68.61
Anticoagulant, circulating (intrinsic) —*see also* -
    Disorder, hemorrhagic D68.318
  drug-induced (extrinsic) —*see also* - Disorder,
    hemorrhagic D68.32
  iatrogenic D68.32
Antidiuretic hormone syndrome E22.2
Antimonial cholera —*see* Poisoning,
    antimony
Antiphospholipid
  antibody
    with hemorrhagic disorder D68.312
    syndrome D68.61
Antisocial personality F60.2
Antithrombinemia —*see* Circulating
    anticoagulants
Antithromboplastinemia D68.318
Antithromboplastinogenemia D68.318

Antitoxin complication or reaction —*see*
    Complications, vaccination
Antlophobia F40.228
Antritis J32.0
  maxilla J32.0
    acute J01.00
      recurrent J01.01
  stomach K29.60
    with bleeding K29.61
Antrum, antral —*see* condition
Anuria R34
  calculous (impacted) (recurrent) —*see also*
    Calculus, urinary N20.9
  following
    abortion —*see* Abortion by type
      complicated by, renal failure
    ectopic or molar pregnancy O08.4
  newborn P96.0
  postprocedural N99.0
  postrenal N13.8
  traumatic (following crushing) T79.5
Anus, anal —*see* condition
Anusitis K62.89
Anxiety F41.9
  depression F41.8
  episodic paroxysmal F41.0
  generalized F41.1
  hysteria F41.8
  neurosis F41.1
  panic type F41.0
  reaction F41.1
  separation, abnormal (of childhood) F93.0
  specified NEC F41.8
  state F41.1
Aorta, aortic —*see* condition
Aortectasia —*see* Ectasia, aorta
  with aneurysm —*see* Aneurysm, aorta
Aortitis (nonsyphilitic) (calcific) I77.6
  arteriosclerotic I70.0
  Doehle-Heller A52.02
  luetic A52.02
  rheumatic —*see* Endocarditis, acute,
    rheumatic
  specific (syphilitic) A52.02
  syphilitic A52.02
    congenital A50.54 *[I79.1]*
Apathetic thyroid storm —*see* Thyrotoxicosis
Apathy R45.3
Apeirophobia F40.228
Apepsia K30
  psychogenic F45.8
Aperistalsis, esophagus K22.0
Apertognathia M26.29
Apert's syndrome Q87.0
Aphagia R13.0
  psychogenic F50.9
Aphakia (acquired) (postoperative) H27.0-●
  congenital Q12.3
Aphasia (amnestic) (global) (nominal)
    (semantic) (syntactic) R47.01
  acquired, with epilepsy (Landau-Kleffner
    syndrome) —*see* Epilepsy, specified
    NEC
  auditory (developmental) F80.2
  developmental (receptive type) F80.2
    expressive type F80.1
    Wernicke's F80.2
  following
    cerebrovascular disease I69.920
      cerebral infarction I69.320
      intracerebral hemorrhage I69.120
      nontraumatic intracranial hemorrhage
        NEC I69.220
      specified disease NEC I69.820
      subarachnoid hemorrhage I69.020
  primary progressive G31.01 *[F02.80]*
    with behavioral disturbance G31.01
      [F02.81]
  progressive isolated G31.01 *[F02.80]*
    with behavioral disturbance G31.01
      [F02.81]

Aphasia *(Continued)*
  sensory F80.2
  syphilis, tertiary A52.19
  Wernicke's (developmental) F80.2
Aphonia (organic) R49.1
  hysterical F44.4
  psychogenic F44.4
Aphthae, aphthous —*see also* condition
  Bednar's K12.0
  cachectic K14.0
  epizootic B08.8
  fever B08.8
  oral (recurrent) K12.0
  stomatitis (major) (minor) K12.0
  thrush B37.0
  ulcer (oral) (recurrent) K12.0
    genital organ(s) NEC
      female N76.6
      male N50.89
    larynx J38.7
Apical —*see* condition
Apiphobia F40.218
Aplasia —*see also* Agenesis
  abdominal muscle syndrome Q79.4
  alveolar process (acquired) —*see* Anomaly,
    alveolar
    congenital Q38.6
  aorta (congenital) Q25.41
  axialis extracorticalis (congenita) E75.29
  bone marrow (myeloid) D61.9
    congenital D61.01
  brain Q00.0
    part of Q04.3
  bronchus Q32.4
  cementum K00.4
  cerebellum Q04.3
  cervix (congenital) Q51.5
  congenital pure red cell D61.01
  corpus callosum Q04.0
  cutis congenita Q84.8
  erythrocyte congenital D61.01
  extracortical axial E75.29
  eye Q11.1
  fovea centralis (congenital) Q14.1
  gallbladder, congenital Q44.0
  iris Q13.1
  labyrinth, membranous Q16.5
  limb (congenital) Q73.8
    lower —*see* Defect, reduction, lower limb
    upper —*see* Agenesis, arm
  lung, congenital (bilateral) (unilateral)
    Q33.3
  pancreas Q45.0
  parathyroid-thymic D82.1
  Pelizaeus-Merzbacher E75.29
  penis Q55.5
  prostate Q55.4
  red cell (with thymoma) D60.9
    acquired D60.9
      due to drugs D60.9
    adult D60.9
    chronic D60.0
    congenital D61.01
    constitutional D61.01
    due to drugs D60.9
    hereditary D61.01
    of infants D61.01
    primary D61.01
    pure D61.01
      due to drugs D60.9
    specified type NEC D60.8
    transient D60.1
  round ligament Q52.8
  skin Q84.8
  spermatic cord Q55.4
  spleen Q89.01
  testicle Q55.0
  thymic, with immunodeficiency D82.1
  thyroid (congenital) (with myxedema) E03.1
  uterus Q51.0
  ventral horn cell Q06.1

Apnea, apneic (of) (spells) R06.81
  newborn NEC P28.4
    obstructive P28.4
    sleep (central) (obstructive) (primary) P28.3
  prematurity P28.4
  sleep G47.30
    central (primary) G47.31
      idiopathic G47.31
      in conditions classified elsewhere G47.37
    obstructive (adult) (pediatric) G47.33
      hypopnea G47.33
    primary central G47.31
    specified NEC G47.39
Apneumatosis, newborn P28.0
Apocrine metaplasia (breast) —*see* Dysplasia,
  mammary, specified type NEC
Apophysitis (bone) —*see also*
  Osteochondropathy
  calcaneus M92.8
  juvenile M92.9
Apoplectiform convulsions (cerebral ischemia)
  I67.82
Apoplexia, apoplexy, apoplectic
  adrenal A39.1
  heart (auricle) (ventricle) —*see* Infarct,
    myocardium
  heat T67.01
  hemorrhagic (stroke) —*see* Hemorrhage,
    intracranial
  meninges, hemorrhagic —*see* Hemorrhage,
    intracranial, subarachnoid
  uremic N18.9 *[I68.8]*
Appearance
  bizarre R46.1
  specified NEC R46.89
  very low level of personal hygiene R46.0
Appendage
  epididymal (organ of Morgagni) Q55.4
  intestine (epiploic) Q43.8
  preauricular Q17.0
  testicular (organ of Morgagni) Q55.29
Appendicitis (pneumococcal) (retrocecal) K37
  with
    gangrene K35.891
    perforation NOS K35.32
    peritoneal abscess K35.33
    peritonitis NEC K35.33
      generalized (with perforation or
        rupture) K35.20
        with abscess K35.21
      localized K35.30
        with
          gangrene K35.32
          perforation K35.32
            and abscess K35.33
      ruptured NOS (with localized
        peritonitis) K35.32
  acute (catarrhal) (fulminating) (gangrenous)
    (obstructive) (retrocecal) (suppurative)
    K35.80
    with
      gangrene K35.891
      peritoneal abscess K35.33
      peritonitis NEC K35.33
        generalized (with perforation or
          rupture) K35.20
          with abscess K35.21
        localized K35.30
          with
            gangrene K35.32
            perforation K35.32
              and abscess K35.33
    specified NEC K35.890
      with gangrene K35.891
  amebic A06.89
  chronic (recurrent) K36
  exacerbation —*see* Appendicitis, acute
  gangrenous —*see* Appendicitis, acute
  healed (obliterative) K36
  interval K36
  neurogenic K36

Appendicitis *(Continued)*
  obstructive K36
  recurrent K36
  relapsing K36
    ruptured NOS (with localized peritonitis)
      K35.32
  subacute (adhesive) K36
  subsiding K36
  suppurative —*see* Appendicitis, acute
  tuberculous A18.32
Appendicopathia oxyurica B80
Appendix, appendicular —*see also* condition
  epididymis Q55.4
  Morgagni
    female Q50.5
    male (epididymal) Q55.4
      testicular Q55.29
  testis Q55.29
Appetite
  depraved —*see* Pica
  excessive R63.2
  lack or loss —*see also* Anorexia R63.0
    nonorganic origin F50.89
    psychogenic F50.89
  perverted (hysterical) —*see* Pica
Apple peel syndrome Q41.1
Apprehension state F41.1
Apprehensiveness, abnormal F41.9
Approximal wear K03.0
Apraxia (classic) (ideational) (ideokinetic)
  (ideomotor) (motor) (verbal) R48.2
  following
    cerebrovascular disease I69.990
      cerebral infarction I69.390
      intracerebral hemorrhage I69.190
      nontraumatic intracranial hemorrhage
        NEC I69.290
      specified disease NEC I69.890
      subarachnoid hemorrhage I69.090
  oculomotor, congenital H51.8
Aptyalism K11.7
Apudoma —*see* Neoplasm, uncertain behavior,
  by site
Aqueous misdirection H40.83-●
Arabicum elephantiasis —*see* Infestation, filarial
Arachnitis —*see* Meningitis
Arachnodactyly —*see* Syndrome, Marfan's
Arachnoiditis (acute) (adhesive) (basal) (brain)
  (cerebrospinal) —*see* Meningitis
Arachnophobia F40.210
Arboencephalitis, Australian A83.4
Arborization block (heart) I45.5
ARC (AIDS-related complex) B20
Arch
  aortic Q25.49
  bovine Q25.49
Arches —*see* condition
Arcuate uterus Q51.810
Arcuatus uterus Q51.810
Arcus (cornea) senilis —*see* Degeneration,
  cornea, senile
Arc-welder's lung J63.4
Areflexia R29.2
Areola —*see* condition
Argentaffinoma —*see also* Neoplasm, uncertain
  behavior, by site
  malignant —*see* Neoplasm, malignant, by site
  syndrome E34.0
Argininemia E72.21
Arginosuccinic aciduria E72.22
Argyll Robertson phenomenon, pupil or
  syndrome (syphilitic) A52.19
  atypical H57.09
  nonsyphilitic H57.09
Argyria, argyriasis
  conjunctival H11.13-●
  from drug or medicament —*see* Table of
    Drugs and Chemicals, by substance
Argyrosis, conjunctival H11.13-●
Arhinencephaly Q04.1
Ariboflavinosis E53.0

► New   ⇒ Revised   ~~deleted~~ Deleted   ● Use Additional Character(s)

Arm —*see* condition
Arnold-Chiari disease, obstruction or
    syndrome (type II) Q07.00
  with
    hydrocephalus Q07.02
      with spina bifida Q07.03
    spina bifida Q07.01
      with hydrocephalus Q07.03
  type III —*see* Encephalocele
  type IV Q04.8
Aromatic amino-acid metabolism disorder E70.9
  specified NEC E70.89
Arousals, confusional G47.51
Arrest, arrested
  cardiac I46.9
    complicating
      abortion —*see* Abortion, by type,
        complicated by, cardiac arrest
      anesthesia (general) (local) or other
        sedation —*see* Table of Drugs and
        Chemicals, by drug
      in labor and delivery O74.2
      in pregnancy O29.11-●
      postpartum, puerperal O89.1
      delivery (cesarean) (instrumental) O75.4
    due to
      cardiac condition I46.2
      specified condition NEC I46.8
    intraoperative I97.71-●
    newborn P29.81
    personal history, successfully resuscitated
      Z86.74
    postprocedural I97.12-●
      obstetric procedure O75.4
  cardiorespiratory —*see* Arrest, cardiac
  circulatory —*see* Arrest, cardiac
  deep transverse O64.0
  development or growth
    bone —*see* Disorder, bone, development or
      growth
    child R62.50
    tracheal rings Q32.1
  epiphyseal
    complete
      femur M89.15-●
      humerus M89.12-●
      tibia M89.16-●
      ulna M89.13-●
    forearm M89.13-●
      specified NEC M89.13-●
      ulna —*see* Arrest, epiphyseal, by type,
        ulna
    lower leg M89.16-●
      specified NEC M89.168
      tibia —*see* Arrest, epiphyseal, by type,
        tibia
    partial
      femur M89.15-●
      humerus M89.12-●
      tibia M89.16-●
      ulna M89.13-●
    specified NEC M89.18
  granulopoiesis —*see* Agranulocytosis
  growth plate —*see* Arrest, epiphyseal
  heart —*see* Arrest, cardiac
  legal, anxiety concerning Z65.3
  physeal —*see* Arrest, epiphyseal
  respiratory R09.2
    newborn P28.81
  sinus I45.5
  spermatogenesis (complete) —*see*
    Azoospermia
    incomplete —*see* Oligospermia
  transverse (deep) O64.0
Arrhenoblastoma
  benign
    specified site —*see* Neoplasm, benign, by
      site
    unspecified site
      female D27.9
      male D29.20

Arrhenoblastoma (*Continued*)
  malignant
    specified site —*see* Neoplasm, malignant,
      by site
    unspecified site
      female C56.9
      male C62.90
  specified site —*see* Neoplasm, uncertain
    behavior, by site
  unspecified site
    female D39.10
    male D40.10
Arrhythmia (auricle)(cardiac) (juvenile)(nodal)
  (reflex)(supraventricular)(transitory)
  (ventricle) I49.9
  block I45.9
  extrasystolic I49.49
  newborn
    bradycardia P29.12
    occurring before birth P03.819
      before onset of labor P03.810
      during labor P03.811
    tachycardia P29.11
  psychogenic F45.8
  sinus I49.8
  specified NEC I49.8
  vagal R55
  ventricular re-entry I47.0
Arrillaga-Ayerza syndrome (pulmonary
  sclerosis with pulmonary hypertension)
  I27.0
Arsenical pigmentation L81.8
  from drug or medicament —*see* Table of
    Drugs and Chemicals
Arsenism —*see* Poisoning, arsenic
Arterial —*see* condition
Arteriofibrosis —*see* Arteriosclerosis
Arteriolar sclerosis —*see* Arteriosclerosis
Arteriolith —*see* Arteriosclerosis
Arteriolitis I77.6
  necrotizing, kidney I77.5
  renal —*see* Hypertension, kidney
Arteriolosclerosis —*see* Arteriosclerosis
Arterionephrosclerosis —*see* Hypertension,
  kidney
Arteriopathy I77.9
  cerebral autosomal dominant,
    with subcortical infarcts and
    leukoencephalopathy
    (CADASIL) I67.850
Arteriosclerosis, arteriosclerotic (diffuse)
  (obliterans) (of) (senile) (with calcification)
  I70.90
  with
    chronic limb-threatening ischemia —*see*
      Arteriosclerosis, with critical limb
      ischemia
    critical limb ischemia
      bypass graft I70.329
        autologous vein graft I70.429
          leg I70.429
            with
              gangrene (and intermittent
                claudication, rest pain,
                and ulcer) I70.469
              rest pain (and intermittent
                claudication) I70.429
          bilateral I70.423
            with
              gangrene (and intermittent
                claudication, rest pain,
                and ulcer) I70.463
              rest pain (and intermittent
                claudication) I70.423
          left I70.422
            with
              gangrene (and intermittent
                claudication, rest pain,
                and ulcer) I70.462
              rest pain (and intermittent
                claudication) I70.422

Arteriosclerosis, arteriosclerotic (*Continued*)
  chronic limb-threatening ischemia
    (*Continued*)
    critical limb ischemia (*Continued*)
      bypass graft (*Continued*)
        autologous vein graft (*Continued*)
          leg (*Continued*)
            left (*Continued*)
              with (*Continued*)
                ulceration (and intermittent
                  claudication and rest
                  pain) I70.449
                ankle I70.443
                calf I70.442
                foot site NEC I70.445
                heel I70.444
                lower leg NEC I70.448
                mid foot I70.444
                thigh I70.441
            right I70.421
              with
                gangrene (and intermittent
                  claudication, rest pain,
                  and ulcer) I70.461
                rest pain (and intermittent
                  claudication) I70.421
                ulceration (and intermittent
                  claudication and rest
                  pain) I70.439
                ankle I70.433
                calf I70.432
                foot site NEC I70.435
                heel I70.434
                lower leg NEC I70.438
                midfoot I70.434
                thigh I70.431
          leg I70.329
            with
              gangrene (and intermittent
                claudication, rest pain, and
                ulcer) I70.369
              rest pain (and intermittent
                claudication) I70.329
          bilateral I70.323
            with
              gangrene (and intermittent
                claudication, rest pain,
                and ulcer) I70.363
             rest pain (and intermittent
                claudication) I70.323
          left I70.322
            with
              rest pain (and intermittent
                claudication) I70.322
              ulceration (and intermittent
                claudication and rest
                pain) I70.349
              ankle I70.343
              calf I70.342
              foot site NEC I70.345
              heel I70.344
              lower leg NEC I70.348
              midfoot I70.344
              thigh I70.341
          right I70.321
            with
              gangrene (and intermittent
                claudication, rest pain,
                and ulcer) I70.361
              rest pain (and intermittent
                claudication) I70.321
              ulceration (and intermittent
                claudication and rest
                pain) I70.339
              ankle I70.333
              calf I70.332
              foot site NEC I70.335
              heel I70.334
              lower leg NEC I70.338
              midfoot I70.334
              thigh I70.331

Arteriosclerosis, arteriosclerotic (Continued)
    chronic limb-threatening ischemia
        (Continued)
        critical limb ischemia (Continued)
            bypass graft (Continued)
                nonautologous biological graft I70.529
                    leg I70.529
                        with
                            gangrene (and intermittent
                                claudication, rest pain,
                                and ulcer) I70.569
                            rest pain (and intermittent
                                claudication) I70.529
                        bilateral I70.523
                            with
                                gangrene (and intermittent
                                    claudication, rest pain,
                                    and ulcer) I70.563
                                rest pain (and intermittent
                                    claudication) I70.523
                        left I70.522
                            with
                                gangrene (and intermittent
                                    claudication, rest pain,
                                    and ulcer) I70.562
                                rest pain (and intermittent
                                    claudication) I70.522
                                ulceration (and intermittent
                                    claudication and rest
                                    pain) I70.549
                                    ankle I70.543
                                    calf I70.542
                                    foot site NEC I70.545
                                    heel I70.544
                                    lower leg NEC I70.548
                                    midfoot I70.544
                                    thigh I70.541
                        right I70.521
                            with
                                gangrene (and intermittent
                                    claudication, rest pain,
                                    and ulcer) I70.561
                                rest pain (and intermittent
                                    claudication) I70.521
                                ulceration (and intermittent
                                    claudication and rest
                                    pain) I70.539
                                    ankle I70.533
                                    calf I70.532
                                    foot site NEC I70.535
                                    heel I70.534
                                    lower leg NEC I70.538
                                    midfoot I70.534
                                    thigh I70.531
                nonbiological graft I70.629
                    leg I70.629
                        with
                            gangrene (and intermittent
                                claudication, rest pain,
                                and ulcer) I70.669
                            rest pain (and intermittent
                                claudication) I70.629
                        bilateral I70.623
                            with
                                gangrene (and intermittent
                                    claudication, rest pain,
                                    and ulcer) I70.663
                                rest pain (and intermittent
                                    claudication) I70.623
                        left I70.622
                            with
                                gangrene (and intermittent
                                    claudication, rest pain,
                                    and ulcer) I70.662
                                rest pain (and intermittent
                                    claudication) I70.622
                                ulceration (and intermittent
                                    claudication and rest
                                    pain) I70.649
                                    ankle I70.643
                                    calf I70.642

Arteriosclerosis, arteriosclerotic (Continued)
    chronic limb-threatening ischemia
        (Continued)
        critical limb ischemia (Continued)
            bypass graft (Continued)
                nonbiological graft (Continued)
                    leg (Continued)
                        left (Continued)
                            with (Continued)
                                ulceration (Continued)
                                    foot site NEC I70.645
                                    heel I70.644
                                    lower leg NEC I70.648
                                    midfoot I70.644
                                    thigh I70.641
                        right I70.621
                            with
                                gangrene (and intermittent
                                    claudication, rest pain,
                                    and ulcer) I70.661
                                rest pain (and intermittent
                                    claudication) I70.621
                                ulceration (and intermittent
                                    claudication and rest
                                    pain) I70.639
                                    ankle I70.633
                                    calf I70.632
                                    foot site NEC I70.635
                                    heel I70.634
                                    lower leg NEC I70.638
                                    midfoot I70.634
                                    thigh I70.631
                specified graft NEC I70.729
                    leg I70.729
                        with
                            gangrene (and intermittent
                                claudication, rest pain,
                                and ulcer) I70.769
                            rest pain (and intermittent
                                claudication) I70.729
                        bilateral I70.723
                            with
                                gangrene (and intermittent
                                    claudication, rest pain,
                                    and ulcer) I70.763
                                rest pain (and intermittent
                                    claudication) I70.723
                        left I70.722
                            with
                                gangrene (and intermittent
                                    claudication, rest pain,
                                    and ulcer) I70.762
                                rest pain (and intermittent
                                    claudication) I70.722
                                ulceration (and intermittent
                                    claudication and rest
                                    pain) I70.749
                                    ankle I70.743
                                    calf I70.742
                                    foot site NEC I70.745
                                    heel I70.744
                                    lower leg NEC I70.748
                                    midfoot I70.744
                                    thigh I70.741
                        right I70.721
                            with
                                gangrene (and intermittent
                                    claudication, rest pain,
                                    and ulcer) I70.761
                                rest pain (and intermittent
                                    claudication) I70.721
                                ulceration (and intermittent
                                    claudication and rest
                                    pain) I70.739
                                    ankle I70.733
                                    calf I70.732
                                    foot site NEC I70.735
                                    heel I70.734
                                    lower leg NEC I70.738
                                    midfoot I70.734
                                    thigh I70.731

Arteriosclerosis, arteriosclerotic (Continued)
    chronic limb-threatening ischemia
        (Continued)
        critical limb ischemia (Continued)
            leg I70.229
                with
                    gangrene (and intermittent
                        claudication, rest pain, and
                        ulcer) I70.269
                    rest pain (and intermittent
                        claudication) I70.229
            bilateral I70.223
                with
                    gangrene (and intermittent
                        claudication, rest pain, and
                        ulcer) I70.263
                    rest pain (and intermittent
                        claudication) I70.223
            left I70.222
                with
                    gangrene (and intermittent
                        claudication, rest pain, and
                        ulcer) I70.262
                    rest pain (and intermittent
                        claudication) I70.222
                    ulceration (and intermittent
                        claudication and rest pain)
                        I70.249
                        ankle I70.243
                        calf I70.242
                        foot site NEC I70.245
                        heel I70.244
                        lower leg NEC I70.248
                        midfoot I70.244
                        thigh I70.241
            right I70.221
                with
                    gangrene (and intermittent
                        claudication, rest pain, and
                        ulcer) I70.261
                    rest pain (and intermittent
                        claudication) I70.221
                    ulceration (and intermittent
                        claudication and rest pain)
                        I70.239
                        ankle I70.233
                        calf I70.232
                        foot site NEC I70.235
                        heel I70.234
                        lower leg NEC I70.238
                        midfoot I70.234
                        thigh I70.231
    aorta I70.0
    arteries of extremities —see Arteriosclerosis,
        extremities
        with
            chronic limb-threatening ischemia —see
                Arteriosclerosis, with critical limb
                ischemia
            critical limb ischemia —see
                Arteriosclerosis, with critical limb
                ischemia
    brain I67.2
    bypass graft
        with
            chronic limb-threatening ischemia —see
                Arteriosclerosis, with critical limb
                ischemia
            critical limb ischemia —see
                Arteriosclerosis, with critical limb
                ischemia
        coronary —see Arteriosclerosis, coronary,
            bypass graft
        extremities —see Arteriosclerosis,
            extremities, bypass graft
    cardiac —see Disease, heart, ischemic,
        atherosclerotic
    cardiopathy —see Disease, heart, ischemic,
        atherosclerotic
    cardiorenal —see Hypertension,
        cardiorenal

▶ New   ⟿ Revised   ~~deleted~~ Deleted   • Use Additional Character(s)

Arteriosclerosis, arteriosclerotic *(Continued)*
  cardiovascular —*see* Disease, heart, ischemic,
    atherosclerotic
  carotid —*see also* Occlusion, artery, carotid
    I65.2-●
  central nervous system I67.2
  cerebral I67.2
  cerebrovascular I67.2
  coronary (artery) I25.10
    bypass graft I25.810
      with
        angina pectoris I25.709
          with documented spasm I25.701
          specified type NEC I25.708
          unstable I25.700
        ischemic chest pain I25.709
      autologous artery I25.810
        with
          angina pectoris I25.729
            with documented spasm
              I25.721
            specified type I25.728
            unstable I25.720
          ischemic chest pain I25.729
      autologous vein I25.810
        with
          angina pectoris I25.719
            with documented spasm
              I25.711
            specified type I25.718
            unstable I25.710
          ischemic chest pain I25.719
      nonautologous biological I25.810
        with
          angina pectoris I25.739
            with documented spasm
              I25.731
            specified type I25.738
            unstable I25.730
          ischemic chest pain I25.739
      specified type NEC I25.810
        with
          angina pectoris I25.799
            with documented spasm I25.791
            specified type I25.798
            unstable I25.790
          ischemic chest pain I25.799
    due to
      calcified coronary lesion (severely)
        I25.84
      lipid rich plaque I25.83
    native vessel
      with
        angina pectoris I25.119
          with documented spasm I25.111
          specified type NEC I25.118
          unstable I25.110
        ischemic chest pain I25.119
    transplanted heart I25.811
      bypass graft I25.812
        with
          angina pectoris I25.769
            with documented spasm I25.761
            specified type I25.768
            unstable I25.760
          ischemic chest pain I25.769
      native coronary artery I25.811
        with
          angina pectoris I25.759
            with documented spasm I25.751
            specified type I25.758
            unstable I25.750
          ischemic chest pain I25.759
  extremities (native arteries) I70.209
    with
      chronic limb-threatening ischemia —*see*
        Arteriosclerosis, with critical limb
        ischemia
      critical limb ischemia —*see*
        Arteriosclerosis, with critical limb
        ischemia

Arteriosclerosis, arteriosclerotic *(Continued)*
  extremities *(Continued)*
    bypass graft I70.309
      with
        chronic limb-threatening ischemia —
          see Arteriosclerosis, with critical
          limb ischemia
        critical limb ischemia —*see*
          Arteriosclerosis, with critical limb
          ischemia
    autologous vein graft I70.409
      leg I70.409
        with
          gangrene (and intermittent
            claudication, rest pain and
            ulcer) I70.469
          intermittent claudication I70.419
          rest pain (and intermittent
            claudication) I70.429
        bilateral I70.403
          with
            gangrene (and intermittent
              claudication, rest pain and
              ulcer) I70.463
            intermittent claudication
              I70.413
            rest pain (and intermittent
              claudication) I70.423
          specified type NEC I70.493
        left I70.402
          with
            gangrene (and intermittent
              claudication, rest pain and
              ulcer) I70.462
            intermittent claudication I70.412
            rest pain (and intermittent
              claudication) I70.422
            ulceration (and intermittent
              claudication and rest
              pain) I70.449
              ankle I70.443
              calf I70.442
              foot site NEC I70.445
              heel I70.444
              lower leg NEC I70.448
              midfoot I70.444
              thigh I70.441
          specified type NEC I70.492
        right I70.401
          with
            gangrene (and intermittent
              claudication, rest pain and
              ulcer) I70.461
            intermittent claudication
              I70.411
            rest pain (and intermittent
              claudication) I70.421
            ulceration (and intermittent
              claudication and rest
              pain) I70.439
              ankle I70.433
              calf I70.432
              foot site NEC I70.435
              heel I70.434
              lower leg NEC I70.438
              midfoot I70.434
              thigh I70.431
          specified type NEC I70.491
      specified type NEC I70.499
    specified NEC I70.408
      with
        gangrene (and intermittent
          claudication, rest pain and
          ulcer) I70.468
        intermittent claudication I70.418
        rest pain (and intermittent
          claudication) I70.428
        ulceration (and intermittent
          claudication and rest pain)
          I70.45
      specified type NEC I70.498

Arteriosclerosis, arteriosclerotic *(Continued)*
  extremities *(Continued)*
    bypass graft *(Continued)*
      leg I70.309
        with
          gangrene (and intermittent
            claudication, rest pain and
            ulcer) I70.369
          intermittent claudication I70.319
          rest pain (and intermittent
            claudication) I70.329
        bilateral I70.303
          with
            gangrene (and intermittent
              claudication, rest pain and
              ulcer) I70.363
            intermittent claudication I70.313
            rest pain (and intermittent
             claudication) I70.323
          specified type NEC I70.393
        left I70.302
          with
            gangrene (and intermittent
              claudication, rest pain and
              ulcer) I70.362
            intermittent claudication I70.312
            rest pain (and intermittent
             claudication) I70.322
            ulceration (and intermittent
              claudication and rest pain)
              I70.349
              ankle I70.343
              calf I70.342
              foot site NEC I70.345
              heel I70.344
              lower leg NEC I70.348
              midfoot I70.344
              thigh I70.341
          specified type NEC I70.392
        right I70.301
          with
            gangrene (and intermittent
              claudication, rest pain and
              ulcer) I70.361
            intermittent claudication
              I70.311
            rest pain (and intermittent
             claudication) I70.321
            ulceration (and intermittent
              claudication and rest pain)
              I70.339
              ankle I70.333
              calf I70.332
              foot site NEC I70.335
              heel I70.334
              lower leg NEC I70.338
              midfoot I70.334
              thigh I70.331
          specified type NEC I70.391
      specified type NEC I70.399
    nonautologous biological graft
      I70.509
      leg I70.509
        with
          gangrene (and intermittent
            claudication, rest pain and
            ulcer) I70.569
          intermittent claudication
            I70.519
          rest pain (and intermittent
            claudication) I70.529
        bilateral I70.503
          with
            gangrene (and intermittent
              claudication, rest pain and
              ulcer) I70.563
            intermittent claudication
              I70.513
            rest pain (and intermittent
             claudication) I70.523
          specified type NEC I70.593

Arteriosclerosis, arteriosclerotic *(Continued)*
  extremities *(Continued)*
    bypass graft *(Continued)*
      nonautologous biological graft
          (Continued)
        leg *(Continued)*
          left I70.502
            with
              gangrene (and intermittent
                  claudication, rest pain and
                  ulcer) I70.562
              intermittent claudication
                  I70.512
              rest pain (and intermittent
                  claudication) I70.522
              ulceration (and intermittent
                  claudication and rest
                  pain) I70.549
                ankle I70.543
                calf I70.542
                foot site NEC I70.545
                heel I70.544
                lower leg NEC I70.548
                midfoot I70.544
                thigh I70.541
              specified type NEC
                  I70.592
          right I70.501
            with
              gangrene (and intermittent
                  claudication, rest pain and
                  ulcer) I70.561
              intermittent claudication
                  I70.511
              rest pain (and intermittent
                  claudication) I70.521
              ulceration (and intermittent
                  claudication and rest
                  pain) I70.539
                ankle I70.533
                calf I70.532
                foot site NEC I70.535
                heel I70.534
                lower leg NEC I70.538
                midfoot I70.534
                thigh I70.531
              specified type NEC I70.591
          specified type NEC I70.599
        specified NEC I70.508
          with
            gangrene (and intermittent
                claudication, rest pain and
                ulcer) I70.568
            intermittent claudication
                I70.518
            rest pain (and intermittent
                claudication) I70.528
            ulceration (and intermittent
                claudication and rest pain)
                I70.55
            specified type NEC I70.598
      nonbiological graft I70.609
        leg I70.609
          with
            gangrene (and intermittent
                claudication, rest pain and
                ulcer) I70.669
            intermittent claudication
                I70.619
            rest pain (and intermittent
                claudication) I70.629
          bilateral I70.603
            with
              gangrene (and intermittent
                  claudication, rest pain and
                  ulcer) I70.663
              intermittent claudication
                  I70.613
              rest pain (and intermittent
                  claudication) I70.623
              specified type NEC I70.693

Arteriosclerosis, arteriosclerotic *(Continued)*
  extremities *(Continued)*
    bypass graft *(Continued)*
      nonbiological graft *(Continued)*
        leg *(Continued)*
          left I70.602
            with
              gangrene (and intermittent
                  claudication, rest pain and
                  ulcer) I70.662
              intermittent claudication
                  I70.612
              rest pain (and intermittent
                  claudication) I70.622
              ulceration (and intermittent
                  claudication and rest
                  pain) I70.649
                ankle I70.643
                calf I70.642
                foot site NEC I70.645
                heel I70.644
                lower leg NEC I70.648
                midfoot I70.644
                thigh I70.641
              specified type NEC I70.692
          right I70.601
            with
              gangrene (and intermittent
                  claudication, rest pain and
                  ulcer) I70.661
              intermittent claudication
                  I70.611
              rest pain (and intermittent
                  claudication) I70.621
              ulceration (and intermittent
                  claudication and rest
                  pain) I70.639
                ankle I70.633
                calf I70.632
                foot site NEC I70.635
                heel I70.634
                lower leg NEC I70.638
                midfoot I70.634
                thigh I70.631
              specified type NEC I70.691
          specified type NEC I70.699
        specified NEC I70.608
          with
            gangrene (and intermittent
                claudication, rest pain and
                ulcer) I70.668
            intermittent claudication I70.618
            rest pain (and intermittent
                claudication) I70.628
            ulceration (and intermittent
                claudication and rest pain)
                I70.65
            specified type NEC I70.698
      specified graft NEC I70.709
        leg I70.709
          with
            gangrene (and intermittent
                claudication, rest pain and
                ulcer) I70.769
            intermittent claudication I70.719
            rest pain (and intermittent
                claudication) I70.729
          bilateral I70.703
            with
              gangrene (and intermittent
                  claudication, rest pain and
                  ulcer) I70.763
              intermittent claudication I70.713
              rest pain (and intermittent
                  claudication) I70.723
              specified type NEC I70.793
          left I70.702
            with
              gangrene (and intermittent
                  claudication, rest pain and
                  ulcer) I70.762

Arteriosclerosis, arteriosclerotic *(Continued)*
  extremities *(Continued)*
    bypass graft *(Continued)*
      specified graft NEC *(Continued)*
        leg *(Continued)*
          left *(Continued)*
            with *(Continued)*
              intermittent claudication I70.712
              rest pain (and intermittent
                  claudication) I70.722
              ulceration (and intermittent
                  claudication and rest
                  pain) I70.749
                ankle I70.743
                calf I70.742
                foot site NEC I70.745
                heel I70.744
                lower leg NEC I70.748
                midfoot I70.744
                thigh I70.741
              specified type NEC I70.792
          right I70.701
            with
              gangrene (and intermittent
                  claudication, rest pain and
                  ulcer) I70.761
              intermittent claudication I70.711
              rest pain (and intermittent
                  claudication) I70.721
              ulceration (and intermittent
                  claudication and rest
                  pain) I70.739
                ankle I70.733
                calf I70.732
                foot site NEC I70.735
                heel I70.734
                lower leg NEC I70.738
                midfoot I70.734
                thigh I70.731
              specified type NEC I70.791
          specified type NEC I70.799
        specified NEC I70.708
          with
            gangrene (and intermittent
                claudication, rest pain and
                ulcer) I70.768
            intermittent claudication I70.718
            rest pain (and intermittent
                claudication) I70.728
            ulceration (and intermittent
                claudication and rest pain)
                I70.75
            specified type NEC I70.798
    specified NEC I70.308
      with
        gangrene (and intermittent
            claudication, rest pain and
            ulcer) I70.368
        intermittent claudication I70.318
        rest pain (and intermittent
            claudication) I70.328
        ulceration (and intermittent
            claudication and rest pain)
            I70.35
        specified type NEC I70.398
    leg I70.209
      with
        gangrene (and intermittent
            claudication, rest pain and ulcer)
            I70.269
        intermittent claudication I70.219
        rest pain (and intermittent
            claudication) I70.229
      bilateral I70.203
        with
          gangrene (and intermittent
              claudication, rest pain and
              ulcer) I70.263
          intermittent claudication I70.213
          rest pain (and intermittent
              claudication) I70.223
          specified type NEC I70.293

▶ New   ⇒ Revised   ~~deleted~~ Deleted   ● Use Additional Character(s)

Arteriosclerosis, arteriosclerotic *(Continued)*
  extremities *(Continued)*
    leg *(Continued)*
      left I70.202
        with
          gangrene (and intermittent
            claudication, rest pain and
            ulcer) I70.262
          intermittent claudication I70.212
          rest pain (and intermittent
            claudication) I70.222
          ulceration (and intermittent
            claudication and rest pain)
            I70.249
            ankle I70.243
            calf I70.242
            foot site NEC I70.245
            heel I70.244
            lower leg NEC I70.248
            midfoot I70.244
            thigh I70.241
        specified type NEC I70.292
      right I70.201
        with
          gangrene (and intermittent
            claudication, rest pain and
            ulcer) I70.261
          intermittent claudication I70.211
          rest pain (and intermittent
            claudication) I70.221
          ulceration (and intermittent
            claudication and rest pain)
            I70.239
            ankle I70.233
            calf I70.232
            foot site NEC I70.235
            heel I70.234
            lower leg NEC I70.238
            midfoot I70.234
            thigh I70.231
        specified type NEC I70.291
    specified type NEC I70.299
  specified site NEC I70.208
    with
      gangrene (and intermittent claudication,
        rest pain and ulcer) I70.268
      intermittent claudication I70.218
      rest pain (and intermittent
        claudication) I70.228
      ulceration (and intermittent
        claudication and rest pain) I70.25
    specified type NEC I70.298
  generalized I70.91
  heart (disease) —*see* Arteriosclerosis,
    coronary (artery)
  kidney —*see* Hypertension, kidney
  medial —*see* Arteriosclerosis, extremities
  mesenteric (artery) K55.1
  Mönckeberg's —*see* Arteriosclerosis,
    extremities
  myocarditis I51.4
  peripheral (of extremities) —*see*
    Arteriosclerosis, extremities
  pulmonary (idiopathic) I27.0
  renal (arterioles) —*see also* Hypertension,
    kidney
    artery I70.1
  retina (vascular) I70.8 [H35.0-●]
  specified artery NEC I70.8
  spinal (cord) G95.19
  vertebral (artery) I67.2
Arteriospasm I73.9
Arteriovenous —*see* condition
Arteritis I77.6
  allergic M31.0
  aorta (nonsyphilitic) I77.6
    syphilitic A52.02
  aortic arch M31.4
  brachiocephalic M31.4
  brain I67.7
    syphilitic A52.04

Arteritis *(Continued)*
  cerebral I67.7
    in
      diseases classified elsewhere I68.2
      systemic lupus erythematosus M32.19
    listerial A32.89
    syphilitic A52.04
    tuberculous A18.89
  coronary (artery) I25.89
    rheumatic I01.8
      chronic I09.89
    syphilitic A52.06
  cranial (left) (right), giant cell M31.6
  deformans —*see* Arteriosclerosis
  giant cell NEC M31.6
    with polymyalgia rheumatica M31.5
  necrosing or necrotizing M31.9
    specified NEC M31.8
  nodosa M30.0
  obliterans —*see* Arteriosclerosis
  pulmonary I28.8
  rheumatic —*see* Fever, rheumatic
  senile —*see* Arteriosclerosis
  suppurative I77.2
  syphilitic (general) A52.09
    brain A52.04
    coronary A52.06
    spinal A52.09
  temporal, giant cell M31.6
  young female aortic arch syndrome M31.4
Artery, arterial —*see also* condition
  abscess I77.89
  single umbilical Q27.0
Arthralgia (allergic) —*see also* Pain, joint
  in caisson disease T70.3
  temporomandibular M26.62
Arthritis, arthritic (acute) (chronic)
    (nonpyogenic) (subacute) M19.90
  allergic —*see* Arthritis, specified form NEC
  ankylosing (crippling) (spine) —*see also*
    Spondylitis, ankylosing
    sites other than spine —*see* Arthritis,
      specified form NEC
  atrophic —*see* Osteoarthritis
    spine —*see* Spondylitis, ankylosing
  back —*see* Spondylopathy, inflammatory
  blennorrhagic (gonococcal) A54.42
  Charcot's —*see* Arthropathy, neuropathic
    diabetic —*see* Diabetes, arthropathy,
      neuropathic
    syringomyelic G95.0
  chylous (filarial) —*see also* category M01 B74.9
  climacteric (any site) NEC —*see* Arthritis,
    specified form NEC
  crystal (-induced) —*see* Arthritis, in, crystals
  deformans —*see* Osteoarthritis
  degenerative —*see* Osteoarthritis
  due to or associated with
    acromegaly E22.0
    brucellosis —*see* Brucellosis
    caisson disease T70.3
    diabetes —*see* Diabetes, arthropathy
    dracontiasis —*see also* category M01 B72
    enteritis NEC
      regional —*see* Enteritis, regional
    erysipelas —*see also* category M01 A46
    erythema
      epidemic A25.1
      nodosum L52
    filariasis NOS B74.9
    glanders A24.0
    helminthiasis —*see also* category M01 B83.9
    hemophilia D66 [M36.2]
    Henoch-(Schönlein) purpura D69.0 [M36.4]
    human parvovirus —*see also* category M01
      B97.6
    infectious disease NEC —*see* category M01
    leprosy (*see also* category M01) —*see also*
      Leprosy A30.9
    Lyme disease A69.23
    mycobacteria —*see also* category M01 A31.8

Arthritis, arthritic *(Continued)*
  due to or associated with *(Continued)*
    parasitic disease NEC —*see also* category
      M01 B89
    paratyphoid fever (*see also* category M01)
      —*see also* Fever, paratyphoid A01.4
    rat bite fever —*see also* category M01 A25.1
    regional enteritis —*see* Enteritis, regional
    respiratory disorder NOS J98.9
    serum sickness —*see also* Reaction, serum
      T80.69
    syringomyelia G95.0
    typhoid fever A01.04
  epidemic erythema A25.1
▶ facet joint (*see also* Spondylosis) M47.819
  febrile —*see* Fever, rheumatic
  gonococcal A54.42
  gouty (acute) —*see* Gout
  in (due to)
    acromegaly —*see also* subcategory
      M14.8-● E22.0
    amyloidosis —*see also* subcategory
      M14.8-● E85.4
    bacterial disease —*see also* subcategory
      M01 A49.9
    Behçet's syndrome M35.2
    caisson disease —*see also* subcategory
      M14.8-● T70.3
    coliform bacilli (Escherichia coli) —*see*
      Arthritis, in, pyogenic organism NEC
    crystals M11.9
      dicalcium phosphate —*see* Arthritis, in,
        crystals, specified type NEC
      hydroxyapatite M11.0-●
      pyrophosphate —*see* Arthritis, in,
        crystals, specified type NEC
      specified type NEC M11.80
        ankle M11.87-●
        elbow M11.82-●
        foot joint M11.87-●
        hand joint M11.84-●
        hip M11.85-●
        knee M11.86-●
        multiple sites M11.8-●
        shoulder M11.81-●
        vertebrae M11.88
        wrist M11.83-●
    dermatoarthritis, lipoid E78.81
    dracontiasis (dracunculiasis) —*see also*
      category M01 B72
    endocrine disorder NEC —*see also*
      subcategory M14.8-● E34.9
    enteritis, infectious NEC —*see also* category
      M01 A09
      specified organism NEC —*see also*
        category M01 A08.8
    erythema
      multiforme —*see also* subcategory
        M14.8-● L51.9
      nodosum —*see also* subcategory M14.8-●
        L52
    gout —*see* Gout
    helminthiasis NEC —*see also* category M01
      B83.9
    hemochromatosis —*see also* subcategory
      M14.8-● E83.118
    hemoglobinopathy NEC D58.2 [M36.3]
    hemophilia NEC D66 [M36.2]
    Hemophilus influenzae M00.8-● [B96.3]
    Henoch(-Schönlein) purpura D69.0 [M36.4]
    hyperparathyroidism NEC —*see also*
      subcategory M14.8-● E21.3
    hypersensitivity reaction NEC T78.49
      [M36.4]
    hypogammaglobulinemia —*see also*
      subcategory M14.8-● D80.1
    hypothyroidism NEC —*see also*
      subcategory M14.8-● E03.9
    infection —*see* Arthritis, pyogenic or
      pyemic
      spine —*see* Spondylopathy, infective
    infectious disease NEC —*see* category M01

Arthritis, arthritic *(Continued)*
  in *(Continued)*
    leprosy —*see also* category M01 A30.9
    leukemia NEC C95.9-● *[M36.1]*
    lipoid dermatoarthritis E78.81
    Lyme disease A69.23
    Mediterranean fever, familial —*see also* subcategory M14.8-● M04.1
    Meningococcus A39.83
    metabolic disorder NEC —*see also* subcategory M14.8-● E88.9
    multiple myelomatosis C90.0-● *[M36.1]*
    mumps B26.85
    mycosis NEC —*see also* category M01 B49
    myelomatosis (multiple) C90.0-● *[M36.1]*
    neurological disorder NEC G98.0
    ochronosis —*see also* subcategory M14.8-● E70.29
    O'nyong-nyong —*see also* category M01 A92.1
    parasitic disease NEC —*see also* category M01 B89
    paratyphoid fever —*see also* category M01 A01.4
    Pseudomonas —*see* Arthritis, pyogenic, bacterial NEC
    psoriasis L40.50
    pyogenic organism NEC —*see* Arthritis, pyogenic, bacterial NEC
    Reiter's disease —*see* Reiter's disease
    respiratory disorder NEC —*see also* subcategory M14.8-● J98.9
    reticulosis, malignant —*see also* subcategory M14.8-● C86.0
    rubella B06.82
    Salmonella (arizonae) (cholerae-suis) (enteritidis) (typhimurium) A02.23
    sarcoidosis D86.86
    specified bacteria NEC —*see* Arthritis, pyogenic, bacterial NEC
    sporotrichosis B42.82
    syringomyelia G95.0
    thalassemia NEC D56.9 *[M36.3]*
    tuberculosis —*see* Tuberculosis, arthritis
    typhoid fever A01.04
    urethritis, Reiter's —*see* Reiter's disease
    viral disease NEC —*see also* category M01 B34.9
  infectious or infective —*see also* Arthritis, pyogenic or pyemic
    spine —*see* Spondylopathy, infective
  juvenile M08.90
    with systemic onset —*see* Still's disease
    ankle M08.97-●
    elbow M08.92-●
    foot joint M08.97-●
    hand joint M08.94-●
    hip M08.95-●
    knee M08.96-●
    multiple site M08.99
    pauciarticular M08.40
      ankle M08.47-●
      elbow M08.42-●
      foot joint M08.47-●
      hand joint M08.44-●
      hip M08.45-●
      knee M08.46-●
      shoulder M08.41-●
      specified site NEC M08.4A
      vertebrae M08.48
      wrist M08.43-●
    psoriatic L40.54
    rheumatoid —*see* Arthritis, rheumatoid, juvenile
    shoulder M08.91-●
    specified site NEC M08.9A
    specified type NEC M08.80
      ankle M08.87-●
      elbow M08.82-●
      foot joint M08.87-●

Arthritis, arthritic *(Continued)*
  juvenile *(Continued)*
    specified type NEC *(Continued)*
      hand joint M08.84-●
      hip M08.85-●
      knee M08.86-●
      multiple site M08.89
      shoulder M08.81-●
      specified joint NEC M08.88
      vertebrae M08.88
      wrist M08.83-●
    vertebra M08.98
    wrist M08.93-●
  meaning osteoarthritis —*see* Osteoarthritis
  meningococcal A39.83
  menopausal (any site) NEC —*see* Arthritis, specified form NEC
  mutilans (psoriatic) L40.52
  mycotic NEC —*see also* category M01 B49
  neuropathic (Charcot) —*see* Arthropathy, neuropathic
    diabetic —*see* Diabetes, arthropathy, neuropathic
    nonsyphilitic NEC G98.0
    syringomyelic G95.0
  ochronotic —*see also* subcategory M14.8-● E70.29
  palindromic (any site) —*see* Rheumatism, palindromic
  pneumococcal M00.10
    ankle M00.17-●
    elbow M00.12-●
    foot joint —*see* Arthritis, pneumococcal, ankle
    hand joint M00.14-●
    hip M00.15-●
    knee M00.16-●
    multiple site M00.19
    shoulder M00.11-●
    vertebra M00.18
    wrist M00.13-●
  postdysenteric —*see* Arthropathy, postdysenteric
  postmeningococcal A39.84
  postrheumatic, chronic —*see* Arthropathy, postrheumatic, chronic
  primary progressive —*see also* Arthritis, specified form NEC
    spine —*see* Spondylitis, ankylosing
  psoriatic L40.50
  purulent (any site except spine) —*see* Arthritis, pyogenic or pyemic
    spine —*see* Spondylopathy, infective
  pyogenic or pyemic (any site except spine) M00.9
    bacterial NEC M00.80
      ankle M00.87-●
      elbow M00.82-●
      foot joint —*see* Arthritis, pyogenic, bacterial NEC, ankle
      hand joint M00.84-●
      hip M00.85-●
      knee M00.86-●
      multiple site M00.89
      shoulder M00.81-●
      vertebra M00.88
      wrist M00.83-●
    pneumococcal —*see* Arthritis, pneumococcal
    spine —*see* Spondylopathy, infective
    staphylococcal —*see* Arthritis, staphylococcal
    streptococcal —*see* Arthritis, streptococcal NEC
      pneumococcal —*see* Arthritis, pneumococcal
  reactive —*see* Reiter's disease
  rheumatic —*see also* Arthritis, rheumatoid
    acute or subacute —*see* Fever, rheumatic

Arthritis, arthritic *(Continued)*
  rheumatoid M06.9
    with
      carditis —*see* Rheumatoid, carditis
      endocarditis —*see* Rheumatoid, carditis
      heart involvement NEC —*see* Rheumatoid, carditis
      lung involvement —*see* Rheumatoid, lung
      myocarditis —*see* Rheumatoid, carditis
      myopathy —*see* Rheumatoid, myopathy
      pericarditis —*see* Rheumatoid, carditis
      polyneuropathy —*see* Rheumatoid, polyneuropathy
      rheumatoid factor —*see* Arthritis, rheumatoid, seropositive
      splenoadenomegaly and leukopenia — *see* Felty's syndrome
      vasculitis —*see* Rheumatoid, vasculitis
      visceral involvement NEC —*see* Rheumatoid, arthritis, with involvement of organs NEC
    juvenile (with or without rheumatoid factor) M08.00
      with systemic onset —*see* Still's disease
      ankle M08.07-●
      elbow M08.02-●
      foot joint M08.07-●
      hand joint M08.04-●
      hip M08.05-●
      knee M08.06-●
      multiple site M08.09
      shoulder M08.01-●
      specified site NEC M08.0A
      vertebra M08.08
      wrist M08.03-●
    seronegative M06.00
      ankle M06.07-●
      elbow M06.02-●
      foot joint M06.07-●
      hand joint M06.04-●
      hip M06.05-●
      knee M06.06-●
      multiple sites M06.09
      shoulder M06.01-●
      specified site NEC M06.0A
      vertebra M06.08
      wrist M06.03-●
    seropositive M05.9
      without organ involvement M05.70
        ankle M05.77-●
        elbow M05.72-●
        foot joint M05.77-●
        hand joint M05.74-●
        hip M05.75-●
        knee M05.76-●
        multiple sites M05.79
        shoulder M05.71-●
        specified site NEC M05.7A
        vertebra —*see* Spondylitis, ankylosing
        wrist M05.73-●
    specified NEC M05.80
      ankle M05.87-●
      elbow M05.82-●
      foot joint M05.87-●
      hand joint M05.84-●
      hip M05.85-●
      knee M05.86-●
      multiple sites M05.89
      specified site NEC M05.8A
      shoulder M05.81-●
      vertebra —*see* Spondylitis, ankylosing
      wrist M05.83-●
    specified type NEC M06.80
      ankle M06.87-●
      elbow M06.82-●
      foot joint M06.87-●
      hand joint M06.84-●
      hip M06.85-●
      knee M06.86-●
      multiple site M06.89
      shoulder M06.81-●

▶ New   ⇒ Revised   ~~deleted~~ Deleted   ● Use Additional Character(s)

Arthritis, arthritic (Continued)
  rheumatoid (Continued)
    specified type NEC (Continued)
      specified site NEC M06.8A
      vertebra M06.88
      wrist M06.83-●
    spine —see Spondylitis, ankylosing
  rubella B06.82
  scorbutic —see also subcategory M14.8-● E54
  senile or senescent —see Osteoarthritis
  septic (any site except spine) —see Arthritis,
      pyogenic or pyemic
  spine —see Spondylopathy, infective
  serum (nontherapeutic) (therapeutic) —see
      Arthropathy, postimmunization
  specified form NEC M13.80
    ankle M13.87-●
    elbow M13.82-●
    foot joint M13.87-●
    hand joint M13.84-●
    hip M13.85-●
    knee M13.86-●
    multiple site M13.89
    shoulder M13.81-●
    specified joint NEC M13.88
    wrist M13.83-●
  spine —see also Spondylosis
    infectious or infective NEC —see
        Spondylopathy, infective
    Marie-Strümpell —see Spondylitis,
        ankylosing
    pyogenic —see Spondylopathy, infective
    rheumatoid —see Spondylitis, ankylosing
    traumatic (old) —see Spondylopathy,
        traumatic
    tuberculous A18.01
  staphylococcal M00.00
    ankle M00.07-●
    elbow M00.02-●
    foot joint —see Arthritis, staphylococcal,
        ankle
    hand joint M00.04-●
    hip M00.05-●
    knee M00.06-●
    multiple site M00.09
    shoulder M00.01-●
    vertebra M00.08
    wrist M00.03-●
  streptococcal NEC M00.20
    ankle M00.27-●
    elbow M00.22-●
    foot joint —see Arthritis, streptococcal, ankle
    hand joint M00.24-●
    hip M00.25-●
    knee M00.26-●
    multiple site M00.29
    shoulder M00.21 ●
    vertebra M00.28
    wrist M00.23-●
  suppurative —see Arthritis, pyogenic or
      pyemic
  syphilitic (late) A52.16
    congenital A50.55 [M12.80]
  syphilitica deformans (Charcot) A52.16
  temporomandibular joint M26.65-●
  toxic of menopause (any site) —see Arthritis,
      specified form NEC
  transient —see Arthropathy, specified form
      NEC
  traumatic (chronic) —see Arthropathy,
      traumatic
  tuberculous A18.02
    spine A18.01
  uratic —see Gout
  urethritica (Reiter's) —see Reiter's disease
  vertebral —see Spondylopathy, inflammatory
  villous (any site) —see Arthropathy, specified
      form NEC
Arthrocele —see Effusion, joint
Arthrodesis status Z98.1
Arthrodynia —see also Pain, joint

Arthrodysplasia Q74.9
Arthrofibrosis, joint —see Ankylosis
Arthrogryposis (congenital) Q68.8
  multiplex congenita Q74.3
Arthrokatadysis M24.7
Arthropathy (see also Arthritis) M12.9
  Charcot's —see Arthropathy, neuropathic
    diabetic —see Diabetes, arthropathy,
        neuropathic
    syringomyelic G95.0
  cricoarytenoid J38.7
  crystal(-induced) —see Arthritis, in, crystals
  diabetic NEC —see Diabetes, arthropathy
  distal interphalangeal, psoriatic L40.51
  enteropathic M07.60
    ankle M07.67-●
    elbow M07.62-●
    foot joint M07.67-●
    hand joint M07.64-●
    hip M07.65-●
    knee M07.66-●
    multiple site M07.69
    shoulder M07.61-●
    vertebra M07.68
    wrist M07.63-●
  ▶ facet joint (see also Spondylosis) M47.819
  following intestinal bypass M02.00
    ankle M02.07-●
    elbow M02.02-●
    foot joint M02.07-●
    hand joint M02.04-●
    hip M02.05-●
    knee M02.06-●
    multiple site M02.09
    shoulder M02.01-●
    vertebra M02.08
    wrist M02.03-●
  gouty —see also Gout
    in (due to)
      Lesch-Nyhan syndrome E79.1 [M14.8-●]
      sickle-cell disorders D57-● [M14.8-●]
  hemophilic NEC D66 [M36.2]
    in (due to)
      hyperparathyroidism NEC E21.3
          [M14.8-●]
      metabolic disease NOS E88.9 [M14.8-●]
  in (due to)
    acromegaly E22.0 [M14.8-●]
    amyloidosis E85.4 [M14.8-●]
    blood disorder NOS D75.9 [M36.3]
    diabetes —see Diabetes, arthropathy
    endocrine disease NOS E34.9 [M14.8-●]
    erythema
      multiforme L51.9 [M14.8-●]
      nodosum L52 [M14.8-●]
    hemochromatosis E83.118 [M14.8-●]
      hemoglobinopathy NEC D58.2 [M36.3]
      hemophilia NEC D66 [M36.2]
      Henoch-Schönlein purpura D69.0 [M36.4]
      hyperthyroidism E05.90 [M14.8-●]
      hypothyroidism E03.9 [M14.8-●]
      infective endocarditis I33.0 [M12.80]
      leukemia NEC C95.9-● [M36.1]
      malignant histiocytosis C96.A [M36.1]
      metabolic disease NOS E88.9 [M14.8-●]
      multiple myeloma C90.0-● [M36.1]
      neoplastic disease NOS (see also Neoplasm)
          D49.9 [M36.1]
      nutritional deficiency —see also
          subcategory M14.8-● E63.9
      psoriasis NOS L40.50
      sarcoidosis D86.86
      syphilis (late) A52.77
        congenital A50.55 [M12.80]
      thyrotoxicosis —see also subcategory
          M14.8-● E05.90
      ulcerative colitis K51.90 [M07.60]
      viral hepatitis (postinfectious) NEC B19.9
          [M12.80]
      Whipple's disease —see also subcategory
          M14.8-● K90.81

Arthropathy (Continued)
  Jaccoud —see Arthropathy, postrheumatic,
      chronic
  juvenile —see Arthritis, juvenile
    psoriatic L40.54
  mutilans (psoriatic) L40.52
  neuropathic (Charcot) M14.60
    ankle M14.67-●
    diabetic —see Diabetes, arthropathy,
        neuropathic
    elbow M14.62-●
    foot joint M14.67-●
    hand joint M14.64-●
    hip M14.65-●
    knee M14.66-●
    multiple site M14.69
    nonsyphilitic NEC G98.0
    shoulder M14.61-●
    syringomyelic G95.0
    vertebra M14.68
    wrist M14.63-●
  osteopulmonary —see Osteoarthropathy,
      hypertrophic, specified NEC
  postdysenteric M02.10
    ankle M02.17-●
    elbow M02.12-●
    foot joint M02.17-●
    hand joint M02.14-●
    hip M02.15-●
    knee M02.16-●
    multiple site M02.19
    shoulder M02.11-●
    vertebra M02.18
    wrist M02.13-●
  postimmunization M02.20
    ankle M02.27-●
    elbow M02.22-●
    foot joint M02.27-●
    hand joint M02.24-●
    hip M02.25-●
    knee M02.26-●
    multiple site M02.29
    shoulder M02.21-●
    vertebra M02.28
    wrist M02.23-●
  postinfectious NEC B99 [M12.80]
    in (due to)
      enteritis due to Yersinia enterocolitica
          A04.6 [M12.80]
      syphilis A52.77
      viral hepatitis NEC B19.9 [M12.80]
  postrheumatic, chronic (Jaccoud)
      M12.00
    ankle M12.07-●
    elbow M12.02-●
    foot joint M12.07-●
    hand joint M12.04-●
    hip M12.05-●
    knee M12.06-●
    multiple site M12.09
    shoulder M12.01-●
    specified joint NEC M12.08
    vertebrae M12.08
    wrist M12.03-●
  psoriatic NEC L40.59
    interphalangeal, distal L40.51
  reactive M02.9
    in (due to)
      infective endocarditis I33.0
          [M02.9]
    specified type NEC M02.80
      ankle M02.87-●
      elbow M02.82-●
      foot joint M02.87-●
      hand joint M02.84-●
      hip M02.85-●
      knee M02.86-●
      multiple site M02.89
      shoulder M02.81-●
      vertebra M02.88
      wrist M02.83-●

A

Arthropathy *(Continued)*
　specified form NEC M12.80
　　ankle M12.87-●
　　elbow M12.82-●
　　foot joint M12.87-●
　　hand joint M12.84-●
　　hip M12.85-●
　　knee M12.86-●
　　multiple site M12.89
　　shoulder M12.81-●
　　specified joint NEC M12.88
　　vertebrae M12.88
　　wrist M12.83-●
　syringomyelic G95.0
　tabes dorsalis A52.16
　tabetic A52.16
　temporomandibular joint M26.65-●
　transient —*see* Arthropathy, specified form
　　NEC
　traumatic M12.50
　　ankle M12.57-●
　　elbow M12.52-●
　　foot joint M12.57-●
　　hand joint M12.54-●
　　hip M12.55-●
　　knee M12.56-●
　　multiple site M12.59
　　shoulder M12.51-●
　　specified joint NEC M12.58
　　vertebrae M12.58
　　wrist M12.53-●
Arthropyosis —*see* Arthritis, pyogenic or
　pyemic
Arthrosis (deformans) (degenerative)
　(localized) —*see also* Osteoarthritis
　M19.90
　spine —*see* Spondylosis
Arthus' phenomenon or reaction T78.41
　due to
　　drug —*see* Table of Drugs and Chemicals,
　　　by drug
Articular —*see* condition
Articulation, reverse (teeth) M26.24
Artificial
　insemination complication —*see*
　　Complications, artificial, fertilization
　opening status (functioning) (without
　　complication) Z93.9
　　anus (colostomy) Z93.3
　　colostomy Z93.3
　　cystostomy Z93.50
　　　appendico-vesicostomy Z93.52
　　　cutaneous Z93.51
　　　specified NEC Z93.59
　　enterostomy Z93.4
　　gastrostomy Z93.1
　　ileostomy Z93.2
　　intestinal tract NEC Z93.4
　　jejunostomy Z93.4
　　nephrostomy Z93.6
　　specified site NEC Z93.8
　　tracheostomy Z93.0
　　ureterostomy Z93.6
　　urethrostomy Z93.6
　　urinary tract NEC Z93.6
　　vagina Z93.8
　vagina status Z93.8
Arytenoid —*see* condition
Asbestosis (occupational) J61
ASC-H (atypical squamous cells cannot exclude
　high grade squamous intraepithelial lesion
　on cytologic smear)
　anus R85.611
　cervix R87.611
　vagina R87.621
ASC-US (atypical squamous cells of
　undetermined significance on cytologic
　smear)
　anus R85.610
　cervix R87.610
　vagina R87.620

Ascariasis B77.9
　with
　　complications NEC B77.89
　　intestinal complications B77.0
　　pneumonia, pneumonitis B77.81
Ascaridosis, ascaridiasis —*see* Ascariasis
Ascaris (infection) (infestation)
　(lumbricoides) —*see* Ascariasis
Ascending —*see* condition
Aschoff's bodies —*see* Myocarditis, rheumatic
Ascites (abdominal) R18.8
　cardiac —*see also* Failure, heart, right I50.810
　chylous (nonfilarial) I89.8
　　filarial —*see* Infestation, filarial
　due to
　　cirrhosis, alcoholic K70.31
　　hepatitis
　　　alcoholic K70.11
　　　chronic active K71.51
　　S. japonicum B65.2
　heart —*see also* Failure, heart, right I50.810
　malignant R18.0
　pseudochylous R18.8
　syphilitic A52.74
　tuberculous A18.31
Aseptic —*see* condition
Asherman's syndrome N85.6
Asialia K11.7
Asiatic cholera —*see* Cholera
Asimultagnosia (simultanagnosia) R48.3
Askin's tumor —*see* Neoplasm, connective
　tissue, malignant
Asocial personality F60.2
Asomatognosia R41.4
Aspartylglucosaminuria E77.1
Asperger's disease or syndrome F84.5
Aspergilloma —*see* Aspergillosis
Aspergillosis (with pneumonia) B44.9
　bronchopulmonary, allergic B44.81
　disseminated B44.7
　generalized B44.7
　pulmonary NEC B44.1
　　allergic B44.81
　　invasive B44.0
　specified NEC B44.89
　tonsillar B44.2
Aspergillus (flavus) (fumigatus) (infection)
　(terreus) —*see* Aspergillosis
Aspermatogenesis —*see* Azoospermia
Aspermia (testis) —*see* Azoospermia
Asphyxia, asphyxiation (by) R09.01
　antenatal P84
　birth P84
　bunny bag —*see* Asphyxia, due to,
　　mechanical threat to breathing, trapped
　　in bed clothes
　crushing S28.0
　drowning T75.1
　gas, fumes, or vapor —*see* Table of Drugs and
　　Chemicals
　inhalation —*see* Inhalation
　intrauterine P84
　local I73.00
　　with gangrene I73.01
　mucus —*see also* Foreign body, respiratory
　　tract, causing asphyxia
　newborn P84
　pathological R09.01
　postnatal P84
　　mechanical —*see* Asphyxia, due to,
　　　mechanical threat to breathing
　prenatal P84
　reticularis R23.1
　strangulation —*see* Asphyxia, due to,
　　mechanical threat to breathing
　submersion T75.1
　traumatic T71.9
　　due to
　　　crushed chest S28.0
　　　foreign body (in) —*see* Foreign body,
　　　　respiratory tract, causing asphyxia

Asphyxia, asphyxiation *(Continued)*
　traumatic *(Continued)*
　　due to *(Continued)*
　　　low oxygen content of ambient air
　　　　T71.20
　　　　due to
　　　　　being trapped in
　　　　　　low oxygen environment
　　　　　　　T71.29
　　　　　　　in car trunk T71.221
　　　　　　　　circumstances undetermined
　　　　　　　　　T71.224
　　　　　　　　done with intent to harm by
　　　　　　　　　another person T71.223
　　　　　　　　　self T71.222
　　　　　　　in refrigerator T71.231
　　　　　　　　circumstances undetermined
　　　　　　　　　T71.234
　　　　　　　　done with intent to
　　　　　　　　　harm by
　　　　　　　　　another person T71.233
　　　　　　　　　self T71.232
　　　　cave-in T71.21
　　　mechanical threat to breathing
　　　　(accidental) T71.191
　　　　circumstances undetermined T71.194
　　　　done with intent to harm by
　　　　　another person T71.193
　　　　　self T71.192
　　　　hanging T71.161
　　　　　circumstances undetermined
　　　　　　T71.164
　　　　　done with intent to harm by
　　　　　　another person T71.163
　　　　　　self T71.162
　　　　plastic bag T71.121
　　　　　circumstances undetermined T71.124
　　　　　done with intent to harm by
　　　　　　another person T71.123
　　　　　　self T71.122
　　　　smothering
　　　　　in furniture T71.151
　　　　　　circumstances undetermined
　　　　　　　T71.154
　　　　　　done with intent to harm by
　　　　　　　another person T71.153
　　　　　　　self T71.152
　　　　　under
　　　　　　another person's body T71.141
　　　　　　　circumstances undetermined
　　　　　　　　T71.144
　　　　　　　done with intent to harm
　　　　　　　　T71.143
　　　　　pillow T71.111
　　　　　　circumstances undetermined
　　　　　　　T71.114
　　　　　　done with intent to harm by
　　　　　　　another person T71.113
　　　　　　　self T71.112
　　　　trapped in bed clothes T71.131
　　　　　circumstances undetermined
　　　　　　T71.134
　　　　　done with intent to harm by
　　　　　　another person T71.133
　　　　　　self T71.132
　vomiting, vomitus —*see* Foreign body,
　　respiratory tract, causing asphyxia
Aspiration
　amniotic (clear) fluid (newborn) P24.10
　　with
　　　pneumonia (pneumonitis) P24.11
　　　respiratory symptoms P24.11
　blood
　　newborn (without respiratory symptoms)
　　　P24.20
　　　with
　　　　pneumonia (pneumonitis) P24.21
　　　　respiratory symptoms P24.21
　　　specified age NEC —*see* Foreign body,
　　　　respiratory tract
　bronchitis J69.0

▶ New　⇒ Revised　~~deleted~~ Deleted　● Use Additional Character(s)

Aspiration (*Continued*)
➥food or foreign body —*see* Foreign body, by site
liquor (amnii) (newborn) P24.10
   with
      pneumonia (pneumonitis) P24.11
      respiratory symptoms P24.11
meconium (newborn) (without respiratory symptoms) P24.00
   with
      pneumonitis (pneumonitis) P24.01
      respiratory symptoms P24.01
milk (newborn) (without respiratory symptoms) P24.30
   with
      pneumonia (pneumonitis) P24.31
      respiratory symptoms P24.31
   specified age NEC —*see* Foreign body, respiratory tract
mucus —*see also* Foreign body, by site, causing asphyxia
   newborn P24.10
      with
         pneumonia (pneumonitis) P24.11
         respiratory symptoms P24.11
neonatal P24.9
   specific NEC (without respiratory symptoms) P24.80
      with
         pneumonia (pneumonitis) P24.81
         respiratory symptoms P24.81
newborn P24.9
   specific NEC (without respiratory symptoms) P24.80
      with
         pneumonia (pneumonitis) P24.81
         respiratory symptoms P24.81
pneumonia J69.0
pneumonitis J69.0
syndrome of newborn —*see* Aspiration, by substance, with pneumonia
vernix caseosa (newborn) P24.80
   with
      pneumonia (pneumonitis) P24.81
      respiratory symptoms P24.81
vomitus —*see also* Foreign body, respiratory tract
   newborn (without respiratory symptoms) P24.30
      with
         pneumonia (pneumonitis) P24.31
         respiratory symptoms P24.31
Asplenia (congenital) Q89.01
postsurgical Z90.81
Assam fever B55.0
Assault, sexual —*see* Maltreatment
Assmann's focus NEC A15.0
Astasia (-abasia) (hysterical) F44.4
Asteatosis cutis L85.3
Astereognosia, astereognosis R48.1
Asterixis R27.8
in liver disease K71.3
Asteroid hyalitis —*see* Deposit, crystalline
Asthenia, asthenic R53.1
cardiac —*see also* Failure, heart I50.9
   psychogenic F45.8
cardiovascular —*see also* Failure, heart I50.9
   psychogenic F45.8
heart —*see also* Failure, heart I50.9
   psychogenic F45.8
hysterical F44.4
myocardial —*see also* Failure, heart I50.9
   psychogenic F45.8
nervous F48.8
neurocirculatory F45.8
neurotic F48.8
psychogenic F48.8
psychoneurotic F48.8
psychophysiologic F48.8
reaction (psychophysiologic) F48.8
senile R54

Asthenopia —*see also* Discomfort, visual
hysterical F44.6
psychogenic F44.6
Asthenospermia —*see* Abnormal, specimen, male genital organs
Asthma, asthmatic (bronchial) (catarrh) (spasmodic) J45.909
with
   chronic obstructive bronchitis J44.9
      with
         acute lower respiratory infection J44.0
         exacerbation (acute) J44.1
   chronic obstructive pulmonary disease J44.9
      with
         acute lower respiratory infection J44.0
         exacerbation (acute) J44.1
   exacerbation (acute) J45.901
   hay fever —*see* Asthma, allergic extrinsic
   rhinitis, allergic —*see* Asthma, allergic extrinsic
   status asthmaticus J45.902
allergic extrinsic J45.909
   with
      exacerbation (acute) J45.901
      status asthmaticus J45.902
atopic —*see* Asthma, allergic extrinsic
cardiac —*see* Failure, ventricular, left
cardiobronchial I50.1
childhood J45.909
   with
      exacerbation (acute) J45.901
      status asthmaticus J45.902
chronic obstructive J44.9
   with
      acute lower respiratory infection J44.0
      exacerbation (acute) J44.1
collier's J60
cough variant J45.991
detergent J69.8
due to
   detergent J69.8
   inhalation of fumes J68.3
eosinophilic J82.83
extrinsic, allergic —*see* Asthma, allergic extrinsic
grinder's J62.8
hay —*see* Asthma, allergic extrinsic
heart I50.1
idiosyncratic —*see* Asthma, nonallergic
intermittent (mild) J45.20
   with
      exacerbation (acute) J45.21
      status asthmaticus J45.22
intrinsic, nonallergic —*see* Asthma, nonallergic
Kopp's E32.8
late-onset J45.909
   with
      exacerbation (acute) J45.901
      status asthmaticus J45.902
mild intermittent J45.20
   with
      exacerbation (acute) J45.21
      status asthmaticus J45.22
mild persistent J45.30
   with
      exacerbation (acute) J45.31
      status asthmaticus J45.32
Millar's (laryngismus stridulus) J38.5
miner's J60
mixed J45.909
   with
      exacerbation (acute) J45.901
      status asthmaticus J45.902
moderate persistent J45.40
   with
      exacerbation (acute) J45.41
      status asthmaticus J45.42

Asthma, asthmatic (*Continued*)
nervous —*see* Asthma, nonallergic
nonallergic (intrinsic) J45.909
   with
      exacerbation (acute) J45.901
      status asthmaticus J45.902
persistent
   mild J45.30
      with
         exacerbation (acute) J45.31
         status asthmaticus J45.32
   moderate J45.40
      with
         exacerbation (acute) J45.41
         status asthmaticus J45.42
   severe J45.50
      with
         exacerbation (acute) J45.51
         status asthmaticus J45.52
platinum J45.998
pneumoconiotic NEC J64
potter's J62.8
predominantly allergic J45.909
psychogenic F54
pulmonary eosinophilic J82.83
red cedar J67.8
Rostan's I50.1
sandblaster's J62.8
sequoiosis J67.8
severe persistent J45.50
   with
      exacerbation (acute) J45.51
      status asthmaticus J45.52
specified NEC J45.998
stonemason's J62.8
thymic E32.8
tuberculous —*see* Tuberculosis, pulmonary
Wichmann's (laryngismus stridulus) J38.5
wood J67.8
Astigmatism (compound) (congenital) H52.20-•
irregular H52.21-•
regular H52.22-•
Astraphobia F40.220
Astroblastoma
specified site —*see* Neoplasm, malignant, by site
unspecified site C71.9
Astrocytoma (cystic)
anaplastic
   specified site —*see* Neoplasm, malignant, by site
   unspecified site C71.9
fibrillary
   specified site —*see* Neoplasm, malignant, by site
   unspecified site C71.9
fibrous
   specified site —*see* Neoplasm, malignant, by site
   unspecified site C71.9
gemistocytic
   specified site —*see* Neoplasm, malignant, by site
   unspecified site C71.9
juvenile
   specified site —*see* Neoplasm, malignant, by site
   unspecified site C71.9
pilocytic
   specified site —*see* Neoplasm, malignant, by site
   unspecified site C71.9
piloid
   specified site —*see* Neoplasm, malignant, by site
   unspecified site C71.9
protoplasmic
   specified site —*see* Neoplasm, malignant, by site
   unspecified site C71.9

Astrocytoma (Continued)
  specified site NEC —see Neoplasm,
      malignant, by site
  subependymal D43.2
    giant cell
      specified site —see Neoplasm, uncertain
          behavior, by site
      unspecified site D43.2
    specified site —see Neoplasm, uncertain
        behavior, by site
    unspecified site D43.2
  unspecified site C71.9
Astroglioma
  specified site —see Neoplasm, malignant, by
      site
  unspecified site C71.9
Asymbolia R48.8
Asymmetry —see also Distortion
  between native and reconstructed breast N65.1
  face Q67.0
  jaw (lower) —see Anomaly, dentofacial, jaw-
      cranial base relationship, asymmetry
Asynergia, asynergy R27.8
  ventricular I51.89
Asystole (heart) —see Arrest, cardiac
At risk
  for
    dental caries Z91.849
      high Z91.843
      low Z91.841
      moderate Z91.842
    falling Z91.81
Ataxia, ataxy, ataxic R27.0
  acute R27.8
  autosomal recessive Friedreich G11.11
  brain (hereditary) G11.9
  cerebellar (hereditary) G11.9
    with defective DNA repair G11.3
    alcoholic G31.2
    early-onset G11.10
      with
        essential tremor G11.19
        myoclonus [Hunt's ataxia] G11.19
        retained tendon reflexes G11.19
      in
        alcoholism G31.2
        myxedema E03.9 [G13.2]
        neoplastic disease —see also Neoplasm
            D49.9 [G32.81]
        specified disease NEC G32.81
    late-onset (Marie's) G11.2
  cerebral (hereditary) G11.9
  congenital nonprogressive G11.0
  family, familial —see Ataxia, hereditary
  following
    cerebrovascular disease I69.993
      cerebral infarction I69.393
      intracerebral hemorrhage I69.193
      nontraumatic intracranial hemorrhage
          NEC I69.293
      specified disease NEC I69.893
      subarachnoid hemorrhage I69.093
  Friedreich's (heredofamilial) (cerebellar)
      (spinal) G11.11
  gait R26.0
    hysterical F44.4
  general R27.8
  gluten M35.9 [G32.81]
    with celiac disease K90.0 [G32.81]
  hereditary G11.9
    with neuropathy G60.2
    cerebellar —see Ataxia, cerebellar
    spastic G11.4
    specified NEC G11.8
    spinal (Friedreich's) G11.11
  heredofamilial —see Ataxia, hereditary
  Hunt's G11.19
  hysterical F44.4
  locomotor (progressive) (syphilitic) (partial)
      (spastic) A52.11
    diabetic —see Diabetes, ataxia

Ataxia, ataxy, ataxic (Continued)
  Marie's (cerebellar) (heredofamilial)
      (late- onset) G11.2
  nonorganic origin F44.4
  nonprogressive, congenital G11.0
  psychogenic F44.4
  Roussy-Lévy G60.0
  Sanger-Brown's (hereditary) G11.2
  spastic hereditary G11.4
  spinal
    hereditary (Friedreich's) G11.11
    progressive (syphilitic) A52.11
  spinocerebellar, X-linked recessive
      G11.19
  telangiectasia (Louis-Bar) G11.3
Ataxia-telangiectasia (Louis-Bar) G11.3
Atelectasis (massive) (partial) (pressure)
    (pulmonary) J98.11
  newborn P28.10
    due to resorption P28.11
    partial P28.19
    primary P28.0
    secondary P28.19
  primary (newborn) P28.0
  tuberculous —see Tuberculosis, pulmonary
Atelocardia Q24.9
Atelomyelia Q06.1
Atheroembolism
  of
    extremities
      lower I75.02-●
      upper I75.01-●
    kidney I75.81
    specified NEC I75.89
Atheroma, atheromatous —see also
    Arteriosclerosis I70.90
  aorta, aortic I70.0
    valve —see also Endocarditis,
        aortic I35.8
  aorto-iliac I70.0
  artery —see Arteriosclerosis
  basilar (artery) I67.2
  carotid (artery) (common) (internal)
      I67.2
  cerebral (arteries) I67.2
  coronary (artery) I25.10
    with angina pectoris —see Arteriosclerosis,
        coronary (artery)
  degeneration —see Arteriosclerosis
  heart, cardiac —see Disease, heart, ischemic,
      atherosclerotic
  mitral (valve) I34.8
  myocardium, myocardial —see Disease, heart,
      ischemic, atherosclerotic
  pulmonary valve (heart) —see also
      Endocarditis, pulmonary I37.8
  tricuspid (heart) (valve) I36.8
  valve, valvular —see Endocarditis
  vertebral (artery) I67.2
Atheromatosis —see Arteriosclerosis
Atherosclerosis —see also Arteriosclerosis
  coronary
    artery I25.10
      with angina pectoris —see
          Arteriosclerosis, coronary (artery),
      due to
        calcified coronary lesion (severely)
            I25.84
        lipid rich plaque I25.83
    transplanted heart I25.811
      bypass graft I25.812
        with angina pectoris —see
            Arteriosclerosis, coronary (artery)
      native coronary artery I25.811
        with angina pectoris —see
            Arteriosclerosis, coronary (artery)
Athetosis (acquired) R25.8
  bilateral (congenital) G80.3
  congenital (bilateral) (double) G80.3
  double (congenital) G80.3
  unilateral R25.8

Athlete's
  foot B35.3
  heart I51.7
Athrepsia E41
Athyrea (acquired) —see also Hypothyroidism
  congenital E03.1
Atonia, atony, atonic
  bladder (sphincter) (neurogenic) N31.2
  capillary I78.8
  cecum K59.89
    psychogenic F45.8
  colon —see Atony, intestine
  congenital P94.2
  ➡esophagus K22.89
  intestine K59.89
    psychogenic F45.8
  stomach K31.89
    neurotic or psychogenic F45.8
  uterus (during labor) O62.2
    with hemorrhage (postpartum) O72.1
    postpartum (with hemorrhage) O72.1
      without hemorrhage O75.89
Atopy —see History, allergy
Atransferrinemia, congenital E88.09
Atresia, atretic
  alimentary organ or tract NEC Q45.8
    upper Q40.8
  ani, anus, anal (canal) Q42.3
    with fistula Q42.2
  aorta (ring) Q25.29
  aortic (orifice) (valve) Q23.0
    arch Q25.21
    congenital with hypoplasia of ascending
        aorta and defective development of
        left ventricle (with mitral stenosis)
        Q23.4
    in hypoplastic left heart syndrome Q23.4
  aqueduct of Sylvius Q03.0
    with spina bifida —see Spina bifida, with
        hydrocephalus
  artery NEC Q27.8
    cerebral Q28.3
    coronary Q24.5
    digestive system Q27.8
    eye Q15.8
    lower limb Q27.8
    pulmonary Q25.5
    specified site NEC Q27.8
    umbilical Q27.0
    upper limb Q27.8
  auditory canal (external) Q16.1
  bile duct (common) (congenital) (hepatic)
      Q44.2
    acquired —see Obstruction, bile duct
  bladder (neck) Q64.39
    obstruction Q64.31
  bronchus Q32.4
  cecum Q42.8
  cervix (acquired) N88.2
    congenital Q51.828
    in pregnancy or childbirth —see Anomaly,
        cervix, in pregnancy or childbirth
      causing obstructed labor O65.5
  choana Q30.0
  colon Q42.9
    specified NEC Q42.8
  common duct Q44.2
  cricoid cartilage Q31.8
  cystic duct Q44.2
    acquired K82.8
      with obstruction K82.0
  digestive organs NEC Q45.8
  duodenum Q41.0
  ear canal Q16.1
  ejaculatory duct Q55.4
  epiglottis Q31.8
  esophagus Q39.0
    with tracheoesophageal fistula Q39.1
  eustachian tube Q17.8
  fallopian tube (congenital) Q50.6
    acquired N97.1

▶ New   ⇒ Revised   ~~deleted~~ Deleted   ● Use Additional Character(s)

Atresia, atretic (*Continued*)
  follicular cyst N83.0-●
  foramen of
    Luschka Q03.1
      with spina bifida —*see* Spina bifida, with
        hydrocephalus
    Magendie Q03.1
      with spina bifida —*see* Spina bifida, with
        hydrocephalus
  gallbladder Q44.1
  genital organ
    external
      female Q52.79
      male Q55.8
    internal
      female Q52.8
      male Q55.8
  glottis Q31.8
  gullet Q39.0
    with tracheoesophageal fistula Q39.1
  heart valve NEC Q24.8
    pulmonary Q22.0
    tricuspid Q22.4
  hymen Q52.3
    acquired (postinfective) N89.6
  ileum Q41.2
  intestine (small) Q41.9
    large Q42.9
      specified NEC Q42.8
  iris, filtration angle Q15.0
  jejunum Q41.1
  lacrimal apparatus Q10.4
  larynx Q31.8
  meatus urinarius Q64.33
  mitral valve Q23.2
    in hypoplastic left heart syndrome Q23.4
  nares (anterior) (posterior) Q30.0
  nasopharynx Q34.8
  nose, nostril Q30.0
    acquired J34.89
  organ or site NEC Q89.8
  osseous meatus (ear) Q16.1
  oviduct (congenital) Q50.6
    acquired N97.1
  parotid duct Q38.4
    acquired K11.8
  pulmonary (artery) Q25.5
    valve Q22.0
  pulmonic Q22.0
  pupil Q13.2
  rectum Q42.1
    with fistula Q42.0
  salivary duct Q38.4
    acquired K11.8
  sublingual duct Q38.4
    acquired K11.8
  submandibular duct Q38.4
    acquired K11.8
  submaxillary duct Q38.4
    acquired K11.8
  thyroid cartilage Q31.8
  trachea Q32.1
  tricuspid valve Q22.4
  ureter Q62.10
    pelvic junction Q62.11
    vesical orifice Q62.12
  ureteropelvic junction Q62.11
  ureterovesical orifice Q62.12
  urethra (valvular) Q64.39
    stricture Q64.32
  urinary tract NEC Q64.8
  uterus Q51.818
    acquired N85.8
  vagina (congenital) Q52.4
    acquired (postinfectional) (senile) N89.5
  vas deferens Q55.3
  vascular NEC Q27.8
    cerebral Q28.3
    digestive system Q27.8
    lower limb Q27.8
    specified site NEC Q27.8
    upper limb Q27.8

Atresia, atretic (*Continued*)
  vein NEC Q27.8
    digestive system Q27.8
    great Q26.8
    lower limb Q27.8
    portal Q26.5
    pulmonary Q26.4
      partial Q26.3
      total Q26.2
    specified site NEC Q27.8
    upper limb Q27.8
  vena cava (inferior) (superior) Q26.8
  vesicourethral orifice Q64.31
  vulva Q52.79
    acquired N90.5
Atrichia, atrichosis —*see* Alopecia
Atrophia —*see also* Atrophy
  cutis senilis L90.8
    due to radiation L57.8
  gyrata of choroid and retina H31.23
  senilis R54
    dermatological L90.8
      due to radiation (nonionizing) (solar)
        L57.8
  unguium L60.3
    congenita Q84.6
Atrophie blanche (en plaque) (de Milian) L95.0
Atrophoderma, atrophodermia (of) L90.9
  diffusum (idiopathic) L90.4
  maculatum L90.8
    et striatum L90.8
      due to syphilis A52.79
    syphilitic A51.39
  neuriticum L90.8
  Pasini and Pierini L90.3
  pigmentosum Q82.1
  reticulatum symmetricum faciei L66.4
  senile L90.8
    due to radiation (nonionizing) (solar) L57.8
  vermiculata (cheeks) L66.4
Atrophy, atrophic (of)
  adrenal (capsule) (gland) E27.49
    primary (autoimmune) E27.1
  alveolar process or ridge (edentulous) K08.20
  anal sphincter (disuse) N81.84
  appendix K38.8
  arteriosclerotic —*see* Arteriosclerosis
  bile duct (common) (hepatic) K83.8
  bladder N32.89
    neurogenic N31.8
  blanche (en plaque) (of Milian) L95.0
  bone (senile) NEC —*see also* Disorder, bone,
    specified type NEC
    due to
      tabes dorsalis (neurogenic) A52.11
  brain (cortex) (progressive) G31.9
    frontotemporal circumscribed G31.01
      [F02.80]
      with behavioral disturbance G31.01
        [F02.81]
    senile NEC G31.1
  breast N64.2
    obstetric —*see* Disorder, breast, specified
      type NEC
  buccal cavity K13.79
  cardiac —*see* Degeneration, myocardial
  cartilage (infectional) (joint) —*see* Disorder,
    cartilage, specified NEC
  cerebellar —*see* Atrophy, brain
  cerebral —*see* Atrophy, brain
  cervix (mucosa) (senile) (uteri) N88.8
    menopausal N95.8
  Charcot-Marie-Tooth G60.0
  choroid (central) (macular) (myopic) (retina)
    H31.10-●
    diffuse secondary H31.12-●
    gyrate H31.23
    senile H31.11-●
  ciliary body —*see* Atrophy, iris
  conjunctiva (senile) H11.89
  corpus cavernosum N48.89

Atrophy, atrophic (*Continued*)
  cortical —*see* Atrophy, brain
  cystic duct K82.8
  Déjérine-Thomas G23.8
  disuse NEC —*see* Atrophy, muscle
  Duchenne-Aran G12.21
  ear H93.8-●
  edentulous alveolar ridge K08.20
  endometrium (senile) N85.8
    cervix N88.8
  enteric K63.89
  epididymis N50.89
  eyeball —*see* Disorder, globe, degenerated
    condition, atrophy
  eyelid (senile) —*see* Disorder, eyelid,
    degenerative
  facial (skin) L90.9
  fallopian tube (senile) N83.32-●
    with ovary N83.33-●
  fascioscapulohumeral (Landouzy-Déjérine)
    G71.02
  fatty, thymus (gland) E32.8
  gallbladder K82.8
  gastric K29.40
    with bleeding K29.41
  gastrointestinal K63.89
  glandular I89.8
  globe H44.52-●
  gum —*see* Recession, gingival
  hair L67.8
  heart (brown) —*see* Degeneration, myocardial
  hemifacial Q67.4
    Romberg G51.8
  infantile E41
    paralysis, acute —*see* Poliomyelitis,
      paralytic
  intestine K63.89
  iris (essential) (progressive) H21.26-●
    specified NEC H21.29
  kidney (senile) (terminal) —*see also* Sclerosis,
    renal N26.1
    congenital or infantile Q60.5
      bilateral Q60.4
      unilateral Q60.3
    hydronephrotic —*see* Hydronephrosis
  lacrimal gland (primary) H04.14-●
    secondary H04.15-●
  Landouzy-Déjérine G71.02
  laryngitis, infective J37.0
  larynx J38.7
  Leber's optic (hereditary) H47.22
  lip K13.0
  liver (yellow) K72.90
    with coma K72.91
    acute, subacute K72.00
      with coma K72.01
    chronic K72.10
      with coma K72.11
  lung (senile) J98.4
  macular (dermatological) L90.8
    syphilitic, skin A51.39
      striated A52.79
  mandible (edentulous) K08.20
    minimal K08.21
    moderate K08.22
    severe K08.23
  maxilla K08.20
    minimal K08.24
    moderate K08.25
    severe K08.26
  muscle, muscular (diffuse) (general)
    (idiopathic) (primary) M62.50
    ankle M62.57-●
    Duchenne-Aran G12.21
    foot M62.57-●
    forearm M62.53-●
    hand M62.54-●
    infantile spinal G12.0
    lower leg M62.56-●
    multiple sites M62.59
    myelopathic —*see* Atrophy, muscle, spinal

Atrophy, atrophic *(Continued)*
  muscle, muscular *(Continued)*
    myotonic G71.11
    neuritic G58.9
    neuropathic (peroneal) (progressive) G60.0
    pelvic (disuse) N81.84
    peroneal G60.0
    progressive (bulbar) G12.21
      adult G12.1
      infantile (spinal) G12.0
      spinal G12.25
        adult G12.1
        infantile G12.0
    pseudohypertrophic G71.02
    shoulder region M62.51-●
    specified site NEC M62.58
    spinal G12.9
      adult form G12.1
      Aran-Duchenne G12.21
      childhood form, type II G12.1
      distal G12.1
      hereditary NEC G12.1
      infantile, type I (Werdnig-Hoffmann) G12.0
      juvenile form, type III (Kugelberg-Welander) G12.1
      progressive G12.25
      scapuloperoneal form G12.1
      specified NEC G12.8
    syphilitic A52.78
    thigh M62.55-●
    upper arm M62.52-●
  myocardium —*see* Degeneration, myocardial
  myometrium (senile) N85.8
    cervix N88.8
  myopathic NEC —*see* Atrophy, muscle
  myotonia G71.11
  nail L60.3
  nasopharynx J31.1
  nerve —*see also* Disorder, nerve
    abducens —*see* Strabismus, paralytic, sixth nerve
    accessory G52.8
    acoustic or auditory —*see* subcategory H93.3
    cranial G52.9
      eighth (auditory) —*see* subcategory H93.3
      eleventh (accessory) G52.8
      fifth (trigeminal) G50.8
      first (olfactory) G52.0
      fourth (trochlear) —*see* Strabismus, paralytic, fourth nerve
      second (optic) H47.20
      sixth (abducens) —*see* Strabismus, paralytic, sixth nerve
      tenth (pneumogastric) (vagus) G52.2
      third (oculomotor) —*see* Strabismus, paralytic, third nerve
      twelfth (hypoglossal) G52.3
    hypoglossal G52.3
    oculomotor —*see* Strabismus, paralytic, third nerve
    olfactory G52.0
    optic (papillomacular bundle)
      syphilitic (late) A52.15
        congenital A50.44
    pneumogastric G52.2
    trigeminal G50.8
    trochlear —*see* Strabismus, paralytic, fourth nerve
    vagus (pneumogastric) G52.2
  neurogenic, bone, tabetic A52.11
  nutritional E43
    with marasmus E41
  old age R54
  olivopontocerebellar G23.8
  optic (nerve) H47.20
    glaucomatous H47.23-●
    hereditary H47.22
    primary H47.21-●

Atrophy, atrophic *(Continued)*
  optic *(Continued)*
    specified type NEC H47.29-●
    syphilitic (late) A52.15
      congenital A50.44
  orbit H05.31-●
  ovary (senile) N83.31-●
    with fallopian tube N83.33-●
  oviduct (senile) —*see* Atrophy, fallopian tube
  palsy, diffuse (progressive) G12.22
  pancreas (duct) (senile) K86.89
  parotid gland K11.0
  pelvic muscle N81.84
  penis N48.89
  pharynx J39.2
  pluriglandular E31.8
    autoimmune E31.0
  polyarthritis M15.9
  prostate N42.89
  pseudohypertrophic (muscle) G71.02
  renal —*see also* Sclerosis, renal N26.1
  retina, retinal (postinfectional) H35.89
  rhinitis J31.0
  salivary gland K11.0
  scar L90.5
  sclerosis, lobar (of brain) G31.09 *[F02.80]*
    with behavioral disturbance G31.09 *[F02.81]*
  scrotum N50.89
  seminal vesicle N50.89
  senile R54
    due to radiation (nonionizing) (solar) L57.8
  skin (patches) (spots) L90.9
    degenerative (senile) L90.8
    due to radiation (nonionizing) (solar) L57.8
    senile L90.8
  spermatic cord N50.89
  spinal (acute) (cord) G95.89
    muscular —*see* Atrophy, muscle, spinal
    paralysis G12.20
      acute —*see* Poliomyelitis, paralytic
      meaning progressive muscular atrophy G12.25
  spine (column) —*see* Spondylopathy, specified NEC
  spleen (senile) D73.0
  stomach K29.40
    with bleeding K29.41
  striate (skin) L90.6
    syphilitic A52.79
  subcutaneous L90.9
  sublingual gland K11.0
  submandibular gland K11.0
  submaxillary gland K11.0
  Sudeck's —*see* Algoneurodystrophy
  suprarenal (capsule) (gland) E27.49
    primary E27.1
  systemic affecting central nervous system in
      myxedema E03.9 *[G13.2]*
      neoplastic disease —*see also* Neoplasm D49.9 *[G13.1]*
      specified disease NEC G13.8
  tarso-orbital fascia, congenital Q10.3
  testis N50.0
  thenar, partial —*see* Syndrome, carpal tunnel
  thymus (fatty) E32.8
  thyroid (gland) (acquired) E03.4
    with cretinism E03.1
    congenital (with myxedema) E03.1
  tongue (senile) K14.8
    papillae K14.4
  trachea J39.8
  tunica vaginalis N50.89
  turbinate J34.89
  tympanic membrane (nonflaccid) H73.82-●
    flaccid H73.81-●
  upper respiratory tract J39.8
  uterus, uterine (senile) N85.8
    cervix N88.8
    due to radiation (intended effect) N85.8
      adverse effect or misadventure N99.89

Atrophy, atrophic *(Continued)*
  vagina (senile) N95.2
  vas deferens N50.89
  vascular I99.8
  vertebra (senile) —*see* Spondylopathy, specified NEC
  vulva (senile) N90.5
  Werdnig-Hoffmann G12.0
  yellow —*see* Failure, hepatic
Attack, attacks
  with alteration of consciousness (with automatisms) —*see* Epilepsy, localization-related, symptomatic, with complex partial seizures
  without alteration of consciousness — *see* Epilepsy, localization-related, symptomatic, with simple partial seizures
  Adams-Stokes I45.9
  akinetic —*see* Epilepsy, generalized, specified NEC
  angina —*see* Angina
  atonic —*see* Epilepsy, generalized, specified NEC
  benign shuddering G25.83
  cataleptic —*see* Catalepsy
  coronary —*see* Infarct, myocardium
  cyanotic, newborn P28.2
  drop NEC R55
  epileptic —*see* Epilepsy
  heart —*see* infarct, myocardium
  hysterical F44.9
  jacksonian —*see* Epilepsy, localization-related, symptomatic, with simple partial seizures
  myocardium, myocardial —*see* Infarct, myocardium
  myoclonic —*see* Epilepsy, generalized, specified NEC
  panic F41.0
  psychomotor —*see* Epilepsy, localization-related, symptomatic, with complex partial seizures
  salaam —*see* Epilepsy, spasms
  schizophreniform, brief F23
  shuddering, benign G25.83
  Stokes-Adams I45.9
  syncope R55
  transient ischemic (TIA) G45.9
    specified NEC G45.8
  unconsciousness R55
    hysterical F44.89
  vasomotor R55
  vasovagal (paroxysmal) (idiopathic) R55
Attention (to)
  artificial
    opening (of) Z43.9
      digestive tract NEC Z43.4
        colon Z43.3
        ilium Z43.2
        stomach Z43.1
      specified NEC Z43.8
      trachea Z43.0
      urinary tract NEC Z43.6
        cystostomy Z43.5
        nephrostomy Z43.6
        ureterostomy Z43.6
        urethrostomy Z43.6
      vagina Z43.7
  colostomy Z43.3
  cystostomy Z43.5
  deficit disorder or syndrome F98.8
    with hyperactivity —*see* Disorder, attention-deficit hyperactivity
  gastrostomy Z43.1
  ileostomy Z43.2
  jejunostomy Z43.4
  nephrostomy Z43.6
  surgical dressings Z48.01
  sutures Z48.02
  tracheostomy Z43.0

▶ New   ⇒ Revised   ~~deleted~~ Deleted   ● Use Additional Character(s)

Attention (Continued)
  ureterostomy Z43.6
  urethrostomy Z43.6
Attrition
  gum —see Recession, gingival
  tooth, teeth (excessive) (hard tissues) K03.0
Atypical, atypism —see also condition
  cells (on cytolgocial smear) (endocervical)
    (endometrial) (glandular)
    cervix R87.619
    vagina R87.629
  cervical N87.9
  endometrium N85.9
    hyperplasia N85.00
  parenting situation Z62.9
Auditory —see condition
Aujeszky's disease B33.8
Aurantiasis, cutis E67.1
Auricle, auricular —see also condition
  cervical Q18.2
Auriculotemporal syndrome G50.8
Austin Flint murmur (aortic insufficiency)
  I35.1
Australian
  Q fever A78
  X disease A83.4
Autism, autistic (childhood) (infantile) F84.0
  atypical F84.9
  spectrum disorder F84.0
Autodigestion R68.89
Autoerythrocyte sensitization (syndrome)
  D69.2
Autographism L50.3
Autoimmune
  disease (systemic) M35.9
  inhibitors to clotting factors D68.311
  lymphoproliferative syndrome [ALPS]
    D89.82
  thyroiditis E06.3
Autointoxication R68.89
Automatism G93.89
  with temporal sclerosis G93.81
  epileptic —see Epilepsy, localization- related,
    symptomatic, with complex partial
    seizures
  paroxysmal, idiopathic —see Epilepsy,
    localization-related, symptomatic, with
    complex partial seizures

Autonomic, autonomous
  bladder (neurogenic) N31.2
  hysteria seizure F44.5
Autosensitivity, erythrocyte D69.2
Autosensitization, cutaneous L30.2
Autosome —see condition by chromosome
  involved
Autotopagnosia R48.1
Autotoxemia R68.89
Autumn —see condition
Avellis' syndrome G46.8
Aversion
⏵oral R63.39
    newborn P92.-•
    nonorganic origin F98.2
  sexual F52.1
Aviator's
  disease or sickness —see Effect, adverse, high
    altitude
  ear T70.0
Avitaminosis (multiple) —see also Deficiency,
  vitamin E56.9
  B E53.9
    with
      beriberi E51.11
      pellagra E52
  B2 E53.0
  B6 E53.1
  B12 E53.8
  D E55.9
    with rickets E55.0
  G E53.0
  K E56.1
  nicotinic acid E52
AVNRT (atrioventricular nodal re-entrant
  tachycardia) I47.1
AVRT (atrioventricular nodal re-entrant
  tachycardia) I47.1
Avulsion (traumatic)
  blood vessel —see Injury, blood vessel
  bone —see Fracture, by site
  cartilage —see also Dislocation, by site
    symphyseal (inner), complicating delivery
    O71.6
  external site other than limb —see Wound,
    open, by site
  eye S05.7-•

Avulsion (Continued)
  head (intracranial)
    external site NEC S08.89
    scalp S08.0
  internal organ or site —see Injury, by site
  joint —see also Dislocation, by site
    capsule —see Sprain, by site
  kidney S37.06-•
  ligament —see Sprain, by site
  limb —see also Amputation, traumatic,
    by site
    skin and subcutaneous tissue —see Wound,
      open, by site
  muscle —see Injury, muscle
  nerve (root) —see Injury, nerve
  scalp S08.0
  skin and subcutaneous tissue —see Wound,
    open, by site
  spleen S36.032
  symphyseal cartilage (inner), complicating
    delivery O71.6
  tendon —see Injury, muscle
  tooth S03.2
Awareness of heart beat R00.2
Axenfeld's
  anomaly or syndrome Q15.0
  degeneration (calcareous) Q13.4
Axilla, axillary —see also condition
  breast Q83.1
Axonotmesis —see Injury, nerve
Ayerza's disease or syndrome (pulmonary
  artery sclerosis with pulmonary
  hypertension) I27.0
Azoospermia (organic) N46.01
  due to
    drug therapy N46.021
    efferent duct obstruction N46.023
    infection N46.022
    radiation N46.024
    specified cause NEC N46.029
    systemic disease N46.025
Azotemia R79.89
  meaning uremia N19
Aztec ear Q17.3
Azygos
  continuation inferior vena cava Q26.8
  lobe (lung) Q33.1

A

B

Baastrup's disease —see Kissing spine
Babesiosis B60.00
  due to
    Babesia
      divergens B60.03
      duncani B60.02
      KO-1 B60.09
      microti B60.01
      MO-1 B60.03
      species
        unspecified B60.00
      venatorum B60.09
    specified NEC B60.09
Babington's disease (familial hemorrhagic
    telangiectasia) I78.0
Babinski's syndrome A52.79
Baby
  crying constantly R68.11
  floppy (syndrome) P94.2
Bacillary —see condition
Bacilluria R82.71
Bacillus —see also Infection, bacillus
  abortus infection A23.1
  anthracis infection A22.9
  coli infection —see also Escherichia coli B96.20
  Flexner's A03.1
  mallei infection A24.0
  Shiga's A03.0
  suipestifer infection —see Infection, salmonella
Back —see condition
Backache (postural) M54.9
  sacroiliac M53.3
  specified NEC M54.89
Backflow —see Reflux
Backward reading (dyslexia) F81.0
Bacteremia R78.81
  with sepsis —see Sepsis
Bactericholia —see Cholecystitis, acute
Bacterid, bacteride (pustular) L40.3
Bacterium, bacteria, bacterial
  agent NEC, as cause of disease classified
    elsewhere B96.89
  in blood —see Bacteremia
  in urine —see Bacteriuria
Bacteriuria, bacteruria R82.71
  asymptomatic R82.71
Bacteroides
  fragilis, as cause of disease classified
    elsewhere B96.6
Bad
  heart —see Disease, heart
  trip
    due to drug abuse —see Abuse, drug,
      hallucinogen
    due to drug dependence —see Dependence,
      drug, hallucinogen
Baelz's disease (cheilitis glandularis
    apostematosa) K13.0
Baerensprung's disease (eczema marginatum)
    B35.6
Bagasse disease or pneumonitis J67.1
Bagassosis J67.1
Baker's cyst —see Cyst, Baker's
Bakwin-Krida syndrome (metaphyseal
    dysplasia) Q78.5
Balancing side interference M26.56
Balanitis (circinata) (erosiva) (gangrenosa)
    (phagedenic) (vulgaris) N48.1
  amebic A06.82
  candidal B37.42
  due to Haemophilus ducreyi A57
  gonococcal (acute) (chronic) A54.23
  xerotica obliterans N48.0
Balanoposthitis N47.6
  gonococcal (acute) (chronic) A54.23
  ulcerative (specific) A63.8
Balanorrhagia —see Balanitis
Balantidiasis, balantidiosis A07.0
Bald tongue K14.4

Baldness —see also Alopecia
  male-pattern —see Alopecia, androgenic
Balkan grippe A78
Balloon disease —see Effect, adverse, high
    altitude
Balo's disease (concentric sclerosis) G37.5
Bamberger-Marie disease —see Osteoarthropathy,
    hypertrophic, specified type NEC
Bancroft's filariasis B74.0
Band(s)
  adhesive —see Adhesions, peritoneum
  anomalous or congenital —see also Anomaly,
    by site
    heart (atrial) (ventricular) Q24.8
    intestine Q43.3
    omentum Q43.3
  cervix N88.1
  constricting, congenital Q79.8
  gallbladder (congenital) Q44.1
  intestinal (adhesive) —see Adhesions,
    peritoneum
  obstructive
    intestine K56.50
      complete K56.52
      incomplete K56.51
      partial K56.51
     peritoneum K56.50
      complete K56.52
      incomplete K56.51
      partial K56.51
  periappendiceal, congenital Q43.3
  peritoneal (adhesive) —see Adhesions,
    peritoneum
  uterus N73.6
    internal N85.6
  vagina N89.5
Bandemia D72.825
Bandl's ring (contraction), complicating
    delivery O62.4
Bangkok hemorrhagic fever A91
Bang's disease (brucella abortus) A23.1
⇒Bankruptcy, anxiety concerning Z59.89
Bannister's disease T78.3
  hereditary D84.1
Banti's disease or syndrome (with cirrhosis)
    (with portal hypertension) K76.6
Bar, median, prostate —see Enlargement,
    enlarged, prostate
Barcoo disease or rot —see Ulcer, skin
Barlow's disease E54
Barodontalgia T70.29
Baron Münchausen syndrome —see Disorder,
    factitious
Barosinusitis T70.1
Barotitis T70.0
Barotrauma T70.29
  odontalgia T70.29
  otitic T70.0
  sinus T70.1
Barraquer (-Simons) disease or syndrome
    (progressive lipodystrophy) E88.1
Barré-Guillain disease or syndrome G61.0
Barré-Liéou syndrome (posterior cervical
    sympathetic) M53.0
Barrel chest M95.4
Barrett's
  disease —see Barrett's, esophagus
  esophagus K22.70
    with dysplasia K22.719
      high grade K22.711
      low grade K22.710
    without dysplasia K22.70
  syndrome —see Barrett's, esophagus
  ulcer K22.10
    with bleeding K22.11
    without bleeding K22.10
Barth syndrome E78.71
Bársony (-Polgár) (-Teschendorf) syndrome
    (corkscrew esophagus) K22.4
Bartholinitis (suppurating) N75.8
  gonococcal (acute) (chronic) (with abscess)
    A54.1

Bartonellosis A44.9
  cutaneous A44.1
  mucocutaneous A44.1
  specified NEC A44.8
  systemic A44.0
Barton's fracture S52.56-●
Bartter's syndrome E26.81
Basal —see condition
Basan's (hidrotic) ectodermal dysplasia Q82.4
Baseball finger —see Dislocation, finger
Basedow's disease (exophthalmic goiter) —see
    Hyperthyroidism, with, goiter
Basic —see condition
Basilar —see condition
Bason's (hidrotic) ectodermal dysplasia Q82.4
Basopenia —see Agranulocytosis
Basophilia D72.824
Basophilism (cortico-adrenal) (Cushing's)
    (pituitary) E24.0
Bassen-Kornzweig disease or syndrome E78.6
Bat ear Q17.5
Bateman's
  disease B08.1
  purpura (senile) D69.2
Bathing cramp T75.1
Bathophobia F40.248
Batten (-Mayou) disease E75.4
  retina E75.4 [H36]
Batten-Steinert syndrome G71.11
Battered —see Maltreatment
Battey Mycobacterium infection A31.0
Battle exhaustion F43.0
Battledore placenta O43.19-●
Baumgarten-Cruveilhier cirrhosis, disease or
    syndrome K74.69
Bauxite fibrosis (of lung) J63.1
Bayle's disease (general paresis) A52.17
Bazin's disease (primary) (tuberculous) A18.4
Beach ear —see Swimmer's, ear
Beaded hair (congenital) Q84.1
Béal conjunctivitis or syndrome B30.2
Beard's disease (neurasthenia) F48.8
Beat(s)
  atrial, premature I49.1
  ectopic I49.49
  elbow —see Bursitis, elbow
  escaped, heart I49.49
  hand —see Bursitis, hand
  knee —see Bursitis, knee
  premature I49.40
    atrial I49.1
    auricular I49.1
    supraventricular I49.1
Beau's
  disease or syndrome —see Degeneration,
    myocardial
  lines (transverse furrows on fingernails) L60.4
Bechterev's syndrome —see Spondylitis,
    ankylosing
Beck's syndrome (anterior spinal artery
    occlusion) I65.8
Becker's
  cardiomyopathy I42.8
  disease
    idiopathic mural endomyocardial disease
      I42.3
    myotonia congenita, recessive form G71.12
  dystrophy G71.01
  pigmented hairy nevus D22.5
Beckwith-Wiedemann syndrome Q87.3
Bed confinement status Z74.01
Bed sore —see Ulcer, pressure, by site
Bedbug bite(s) —see Bite(s), by site, superficial,
    insect
Bedclothes, asphyxiation or suffocation
    by —see Asphyxia, traumatic, due to,
    mechanical, trapped
Bednar's
  aphthae K12.0
  tumor —see Neoplasm, malignant, by site
Bedridden Z74.01

▶ New   ⇒ Revised   ~~deleted~~ Deleted   ● Use Additional Character(s)

Bedsore —see Ulcer, pressure, by site
Bedwetting —see Enuresis
Bee sting (with allergic or anaphylactic shock) —
    see Toxicity, venom, arthropod, bee
Beer drinker's heart (disease) I42.6
Begbie's disease (exophthalmic goiter) —see
    Hyperthyroidism, with, goiter
Behavior
    antisocial
        adult Z72.811
        child or adolescent Z72.810
    disorder, disturbance —see Disorder, conduct
    disruptive —see Disorder, conduct
    drug seeking Z76.5
    inexplicable R46.2
    marked evasiveness R46.5
    obsessive-compulsive R46.81
    overactivity R46.3
    poor responsiveness R46.4
    self-damaging (life-style) Z72.89
    sleep-incompatible Z72.821
    slowness R46.4
    specified NEC R46.89
    strange (and inexplicable) R46.2
    suspiciousness R46.5
    type A pattern Z73.1
    undue concern or preoccupation with
        stressful events R46.6
    verbosity and circumstantial detail obscuring
        reason for contact R46.7
Behcet's disease or syndrome M35.2
Behr's disease —see Degeneration, macula
Beigel's disease or morbus (white piedra)
    B36.2
Bejel A65
Bekhterev's syndrome —see Spondylitis,
    ankylosing
Belching —see Eructation
Bell's
    mania F30.8
    palsy, paralysis G51.0
        infant or newborn P11.3
    spasm G51.3-●
Bence Jones albuminuria or proteinuria NEC
    R80.3
Bends T70.3
Benedikt's paralysis or syndrome G46.3
Benign (see also condition)
    prostatic hyperplasia —see Hyperplasia,
        prostate
Bennett's fracture (displaced) S62.21-●
Benson's disease —see Deposit, crystalline
Bent
    back (hysterical) F44.4
    nose M95.0
        congenital Q67.4
Bereavement (uncomplicated) Z63.4
Bergeron's disease (hysterical chorea) F44.4
Berger's disease —see Nephropathy, IgA
Beriberi (dry) E51.11
    heart (disease) E51.12
    polyneuropathy E51.11
    wet E51.12
        involving circulatory system E51.11
Berlin's disease or edema (traumatic) S05.8X-●
Berlock (berloque) dermatitis L56.2
Bernard-Horner syndrome G90.2
Bernard-Soulier disease or thrombopathia D69.1
Bernhardt (-Roth) disease —see
    Mononeuropathy, lower limb, meralgia
    paresthetica
Bernheim's syndrome —see Failure, heart,
    right
Bertielliasis B71.8
Berylliosis (lung) J63.2
Besnier-Boeck (-Schaumann) disease —see
    Sarcoidosis
Besnier's
    lupus pernio D86.3
    prurigo L20.0
Bestiality F65.89
Best's disease H35.50

Beta-mercaptolactate-cysteine disulfiduria
    E72.09
Betalipoproteinemia, broad or floating E78.2
Betting and gambling Z72.6
    pathological (compulsive) F63.0
Bezoar T18.9
    intestine T18.3
    stomach T18.2
Bezold's abscess —see Mastoiditis, acute
Bianchi's syndrome R48.8
Bicornate or bicornis uterus Q51.3
    in pregnancy or childbirth O34.00
        causing obstructed labor O65.5
Bicuspid aortic valve Q23.1
Biedl-Bardet syndrome Q87.89
Bielschowsky (-Jansky) disease E75.4
Biermer's (pernicious) anemia or disease D51.0
Biett's disease L93.0
Bifid (congenital)
    apex, heart Q24.8
    clitoris Q52.6
    kidney Q63.8
    nose Q30.2
    patella Q74.1
    scrotum Q55.29
    toe NEC Q74.2
    tongue Q38.3
    ureter Q62.8
    uterus Q51.3
    uvula Q35.7
Biforis uterus (suprasimplex) Q51.3
Bifurcation (congenital)
    gallbladder Q44.1
    kidney pelvis Q63.8
    renal pelvis Q63.8
    rib Q76.6
    tongue, congenital Q38.3
    trachea Q32.1
    ureter Q62.8
    urethra Q64.74
    vertebra Q76.49
Big spleen syndrome D73.1
Bigeminal pulse R00.8
Bilateral —see condition
Bile
    duct —see condition
    pigments in urine R82.2
Bilharziasis —see also Schistosomiasis
    chyluria B65.0
    cutaneous B65.3
    galacturia B65.0
    hematochyluria B65.0
    intestinal B65.1
    lipemia B65.9
    lipuria B65.0
    oriental B65.2
    piarhemia B65.9
    pulmonary NOS B65.9 [J99]
        pneumonia B65.9 [J17]
    tropical hematuria B65.0
    vesical B65.0
Biliary —see condition
Bilirubin metabolism disorder E80.7
    specified NEC E80.6
Bilirubinemia, familial nonhemolytic E80.4
Bilirubinuria R82.2
Biliuria R82.2
Bilocular stomach K31.2
Binswanger's disease I67.3
Biparta, bipartite
    carpal scaphoid Q74.0
    patella Q74.1
    vagina Q52.10
Bird
    face Q75.8
    fancier's disease or lung J67.2
Birt-Hogg-Dube syndrome Q87.89
Birth
    complications in mother —see Delivery,
        complicated
    compression during NOS P15.9

Birth (Continued)
    defect —see Anomaly
    immature (less than 37 completed weeks) —
        see Preterm, newborn
        extremely (less than 28 completed
            weeks) —see Immaturity, extreme
    inattention, at or after —see Maltreatment,
        child, neglect
    injury NOS P15.9
        basal ganglia P11.1
        brachial plexus NEC P14.3
        brain (compression) (pressure) P11.2
        central nervous system NOS P11.9
        cerebellum P11.1
        cerebral hemorrhage P10.1
        external genitalia P15.5
        eye P15.3
        face P15.4
        fracture
            bone P13.9
                specified NEC P13.8
            clavicle P13.4
            femur P13.2
            humerus P13.3
            long bone, except femur P13.3
            radius and ulna P13.3
            skull P13.0
            spine P11.5
            tibia and fibula P13.3
        intracranial P11.2
            laceration or hemorrhage P10.9
                specified NEC P10.8
        intraventricular hemorrhage P10.2
        laceration
            brain P10.1
            by scalpel P15.8
            peripheral nerve P14.9
        liver P15.0
        meninges
            brain P11.1
            spinal cord P11.5
        nerve
            brachial plexus P14.3
            cranial NEC (except facial) P11.4
            facial P11.3
            peripheral P14.9
            phrenic (paralysis) P14.2
        paralysis
            facial nerve P11.3
            spinal P11.5
        penis P15.5
        rupture
            spinal cord P11.5
        scalp P12.9
        scalpel wound P15.8
        scrotum P15.5
        skull NEC P13.1
            fracture P13.0
        specified type NEC P15.8
        spinal cord P11.5
        spine P11.5
        spleen P15.1
        sternomastoid (hematoma) P15.2
        subarachnoid hemorrhage P10.3
        subcutaneous fat necrosis P15.6
        subdural hemorrhage P10.0
        tentorial tear P10.4
        testes P15.5
        vulva P15.5
    lack of care, at or after —see Maltreatment,
        child, neglect
    neglect, at or after —see Maltreatment, child,
        neglect
    palsy or paralysis, newborn, NOS (birth
        injury) P14.9
    premature (infant) —see Preterm, newborn
    shock, newborn P96.89
    trauma —see Birth, injury
    weight
        4000 grams to 4499 grams P08.1
        4500 grams or more P08.0

▶ New   ⇒ Revised   ~~deleted~~ Deleted   ● Use Additional Character(s)

Birth *(Continued)*
  weight *(Continued)*
    low (2499 grams or less) —*see* Low,
      birthweight
    extremely (999 grams or less) —*see* Low,
      birthweight, extreme
Birthmark Q82.5
Bisalbuminemia E88.09
Biskra's button B55.1
Bite(s) (animal) (human)
  abdomen, abdominal
    wall S31.159
      with penetration into peritoneal cavity
        S31.659
      epigastric region S31.152
        with penetration into peritoneal cavity
          S31.652
      left
        lower quadrant S31.154
          with penetration into peritoneal
            cavity S31.654
        upper quadrant S31.151
          with penetration into peritoneal
            cavity S31.651
      periumbilic region S31.155
        with penetration into peritoneal cavity
          S31.655
      right
        lower quadrant S31.153
          with penetration into peritoneal
            cavity S31.653
        upper quadrant S31.150
          with penetration into peritoneal
            cavity S31.650
      superficial NEC S30.871
        insect S30.861
  alveolar (process) —*see* Bite, oral cavity
  amphibian (venomous) —*see* Venom, bite,
    amphibian
  animal —*see also* Bite, by site
    venomous —*see* Venom
  ankle S91.05-●
    superficial NEC S90.57-●
      insect S90.56-●
  antecubital space —*see* Bite, elbow
  anus S31.835
    superficial NEC S30.877
      insect S30.867
  arm (upper) S41.15-●
    lower —*see* Bite, forearm
    superficial NEC S40.87-●
      insect S40.86-●
  arthropod NEC —*see* Venom, bite, arthropod
  auditory canal (external) (meatus) —
    see Bite, ear
  auricle, ear —*see* Bite, ear
  axilla —*see* Bite, arm
  back —*see also* Bite, thorax, back
    lower S31.050
      with penetration into retroperitoneal
        space S31.051
      superficial NEC S30.870
        insect S30.860
  bedbug —*see* Bite(s), by site, superficial,
    insect
  breast S21.05-●
    superficial NEC S20.17-●
      insect S20.16-●
  brow —*see* Bite, head, specified site NEC
  buttock S31.805
    left S31.825
    right S31.815
    superficial NEC S30.870
      insect S30.860
  calf —*see* Bite, leg
  canaliculus lacrimalis —*see* Bite, eyelid
  canthus, eye —*see* Bite, eyelid
  centipede —*see* Toxicity, venom, arthropod,
    centipede
  cheek (external) S01.45-●
    internal —*see* Bite, oral cavity
    superficial NEC S00.87
      insect S00.86

Bite *(Continued)*
  chest wall —*see* Bite, thorax
  chigger B88.0
  chin —*see* Bite, head, specified site NEC
  clitoris —*see* Bite, vulva
  costal region —*see* Bite, thorax
  digit(s)
    hand —*see* Bite, finger
    toe —*see* Bite, toe
  ear (canal) (external) S01.35-●
    superficial NEC S00.47-●
      insect S00.46-●
  elbow S51.05-●
    superficial NEC S50.37-●
      insect S50.36-●
  epididymis —*see* Bite, testis
  epigastric region —*see* Bite, abdomen
  epiglottis —*see* Bite, neck, specified site NEC
  esophagus, cervical S11.25
    superficial NEC S10.17
      insect S10.16
  eyebrow —*see* Bite, eyelid
  eyelid S01.15-●
    superficial NEC S00.27-●
      insect S00.26-●
  face NEC —*see* Bite, head, specified site NEC
  finger(s) S61.259
    with
      damage to nail S61.359
    index S61.258
      with
        damage to nail S61.358
      left S61.251
        with
          damage to nail S61.351
      right S61.250
        with
          damage to nail S61.350
      superficial NEC S60.478
        insect S60.46-●
    little S61.25-●
      with
        damage to nail S61.35-●
      superficial NEC S60.47-●
        insect S60.46-●
    middle S61.25-●
      with
        damage to nail S61.35-●
      superficial NEC S60.47-●
        insect S60.46-●
    ring S61.25-●
      with
        damage to nail S61.35-●
      superficial NEC S60.47-●
        insect S60.46-●
    superficial NEC S60.479
      insect S60.469
    thumb —*see* Bite, thumb
  flank —*see* Bite, abdomen, wall
  flea —*see* Bite, by site, superficial,
    insect
  foot (except toe(s) alone) S91.35-●
    superficial NEC S90.87-●
      insect S90.86-●
    toe —*see* Bite, toe
  forearm S51.85-●
    elbow only —*see* Bite, elbow
    superficial NEC S50.87-●
      insect S50.86-●
  forehead —*see* Bite, head, specified site
    NEC
  genital organs, external
    female S31.552
      superficial NEC S30.876
        insect S30.866
      vagina and vulva —*see* Bite, vulva
    male S31.551
      penis —*see* Bite, penis
      scrotum —*see* Bite, scrotum
      superficial NEC S30.875
        insect S30.865
      testes —*see* Bite, testis
  groin —*see* Bite, abdomen, wall

Bite *(Continued)*
  gum —*see* Bite, oral cavity
  hand S61.45-●
    finger —*see* Bite, finger
    superficial NEC S60.57-●
      insect S60.56-●
    thumb —*see* Bite, thumb
  head S01.95
    cheek —*see* Bite, cheek
    ear —*see* Bite, ear
    eyelid —*see* Bite, eyelid
    lip —*see* Bite, lip
    nose —*see* Bite, nose
    oral cavity —*see* Bite, oral cavity
    scalp —*see* Bite, scalp
    specified site NEC S01.85
      superficial NEC S00.87
        insect S00.86
    superficial NEC S00.97
      insect S00.96
    temporomandibular area —*see* Bite, cheek
  heel —*see* Bite, foot
  hip S71.05-●
    superficial NEC S70.27-●
      insect S70.26-●
  hymen S31.45
  hypochondrium —*see* Bite, abdomen, wall
  hypogastric region —*see* Bite, abdomen, wall
  inguinal region —*see* Bite, abdomen, wall
  insect —*see* Bite, by site, superficial, insect
  instep —*see* Bite, foot
  interscapular region —*see* Bite, thorax, back
  jaw —*see* Bite, head, specified site NEC
  knee S81.05-●
    superficial NEC S80.27-●
      insect S80.26-●
  labium (majus) (minus) —*see* Bite, vulva
  lacrimal duct —*see* Bite, eyelid
  larynx S11.015
    superficial NEC S10.17
      insect S10.16
  leg (lower) S81.85-●
    ankle —*see* Bite, ankle
    foot —*see* Bite, foot
    knee —*see* Bite, knee
    superficial NEC S80.87-●
      insect S80.86-●
    toe —*see* Bite, toe
    upper —*see* Bite, thigh
  lip S01.551
    superficial NEC S00.571
      insect S00.561
  lizard (venomous) —*see* Venom, bite, reptile
  loin —*see* Bite, abdomen, wall
  lower back —*see* Bite, back, lower
  lumbar region —*see* Bite, back, lower
  malar region —*see* Bite, head, specified site
    NEC
  mammary —*see* Bite, breast
  marine animals (venomous) —*see* Toxicity,
    venom, marine animal
  mastoid region —*see* Bite, head, specified site
    NEC
  mouth —*see* Bite, oral cavity
  nail
    finger —*see* Bite, finger
    toe —*see* Bite, toe
  nape —*see* Bite, neck, specified site NEC
  nasal (septum) (sinus) —*see* Bite, nose
  nasopharynx —*see* Bite, head, specified site
    NEC
  neck S11.95
    involving
      cervical esophagus —*see* Bite,
        esophagus, cervical
      larynx —*see* Bite, larynx
      pharynx —*see* Bite, pharynx
      thyroid gland S11.15
      trachea —*see* Bite, trachea
    specified site NEC S11.85
      superficial NEC S10.87
        insect S10.86

Bite *(Continued)*
  neck *(Continued)*
    superficial NEC S10.97
      insect S10.96
    throat S11.85
      superficial NEC S10.17
        insect S10.16
  nose (septum) (sinus) S01.25
    superficial NEC S00.37
      insect S00.36
  occipital region —*see* Bite, scalp
  oral cavity S01.552
    superficial NEC S00.572
      insect S00.562
  orbital region —*see* Bite, eyelid
  palate —*see* Bite, oral cavity
  palm —*see* Bite, hand
  parietal region —*see* Bite, scalp
  pelvis S31.050
    with penetration into retroperitoneal space S31.051
    superficial NEC S30.870
      insect S30.860
  penis S31.25
    superficial NEC S30.872
      insect S30.862
  perineum
    female —*see* Bite, vulva
    male —*see* Bite, pelvis
  periocular area (with or without lacrimal passages) —*see* Bite, eyelid
  phalanges
    finger —*see* Bite, finger
    toe —*see* Bite, toe
  pharynx S11.25
    superficial NEC S10.17
      insect S10.16
  pinna —*see* Bite, ear
  poisonous —*see* Venom
  popliteal space —*see* Bite, knee
  prepuce —*see* Bite, penis
  pubic region —*see* Bite, abdomen, wall
  rectovaginal septum —*see* Bite, vulva
  red bug B88.0
  reptile NEC —*see also* Venom, bite, reptile
    nonvenomous —*see* Bite, by site
    snake —*see* Venom, bite, snake
  sacral region —*see* Bite, back, lower
  sacroiliac region —*see* Bite, back, lower
  salivary gland —*see* Bite, oral cavity
  scalp S01.05
    superficial NEC S00.07
      insect S00.06
  scapular region —*see* Bite, shoulder
  scrotum S31.35
    superficial NEC S30.873
      insect S30.863
  sea-snake (venomous) —*see* Toxicity, venom, snake, sea snake
  shin —*see* Bite, leg
  shoulder S41.05-●
    superficial NEC S40.27-●
      insect S40.26-●
  snake —*see also* Venom, bite, snake
    nonvenomous —*see* Bite, by site
  spermatic cord —*see* Bite, testis
  spider (venomous) —*see* Toxicity, venom, spider
    nonvenomous —*see* Bite, by site, superficial, insect
  sternal region —*see* Bite, thorax, front
  submaxillary region —*see* Bite, head, specified site NEC
  submental region —*see* Bite, head, specified site NEC
  subungual
    finger(s) —*see* Bite, finger
    toe —*see* Bite, toe
  superficial —*see* Bite, by site, superficial
  supraclavicular fossa S11.85

Bite *(Continued)*
  supraorbital —*see* Bite, head, specified site NEC
  temple, temporal region —*see* Bite, head, specified site NEC
  temporomandibular area —*see* Bite, cheek
  testis S31.35
    superficial NEC S30.873
      insect S30.863
  thigh S71.15-●
    superficial NEC S70.37-●
      insect S70.36-●
  thorax, thoracic (wall) S21.95
    back S21.25-●
      with penetration into thoracic cavity S21.45-●
    breast —*see* Bite, breast
    front S21.15-●
      with penetration into thoracic cavity S21.35-●
    superficial NEC S20.97
      back S20.47-●
      front S20.37-●
      insect S20.96
        back S20.46-●
        front S20.36-●
  throat —*see* Bite, neck, throat
  thumb S61.05-●
    with
      damage to nail S61.15-●
    superficial NEC S60.37-●
      insect S60.36-●
  thyroid S11.15
    superficial NEC S10.87
      insect S10.86
  toe(s) S91.15-●
    with
      damage to nail S91.25-●
    great S91.15-●
      with
        damage to nail S91.25-●
    lesser S91.15-●
      with
        damage to nail S91.25-●
    superficial NEC S90.47-●
      great S90.47-●
      insect S90.46-●
        great S90.46-●
  tongue S01.552
  trachea S11.025
    superficial NEC S10.17
      insect S10.16
  tunica vaginalis —*see* Bite, testis
  tympanum, tympanic membrane —*see* Bite, ear
  umbilical region S31.155
  uvula —*see* Bite, oral cavity
  vagina —*see* Bite, vulva
  venomous —*see* Venom
  vocal cords S11.035
    superficial NEC S10.17
      insect S10.16
  vulva S31.45
    superficial NEC S30.874
      insect S30.864
  wrist S61.55-●
    superficial NEC S60.87-●
      insect S60.86-●
Biting, cheek or lip K13.1
Biventricular failure (heart) I50.82
Björck (-Thorson) syndrome (malignant carcinoid) E34.0
Black
  death A20.9
  eye S00.1-●
  hairy tongue K14.3
  heel (foot) S90.3-●
  lung (disease) J60
  palm (hand) S60.22-●
Blackfan-Diamond anemia or syndrome (congenital hypoplastic anemia) D61.01

Blackhead L70.0
Blackout R55
Bladder —*see* condition
Blast (air) (hydraulic) (immersion) (underwater)
  blindness S05.8X-●
  injury
    abdomen or thorax —*see* Injury, by site
    ear (acoustic nerve trauma) —*see* Injury, nerve, acoustic, specified type NEC
    syndrome NEC T70.8
Blastoma —*see* Neoplasm, malignant, by site
  pulmonary —*see* Neoplasm, lung, malignant
Blastomycosis, blastomycotic B40.9
  Brazilian —*see* Paracoccidioidomycosis
  cutaneous B40.3
  disseminated B40.7
  European —*see* Cryptococcosis
  generalized B40.7
  keloidal B48.0
  North American B40.9
  primary pulmonary B40.0
  pulmonary B40.2
    acute B40.0
    chronic B40.1
  skin B40.3
  South American —*see* Paracoccidioidomycosis
  specified NEC B40.89
Bleb(s) R23.8
  emphysematous (lung) (solitary) J43.9
  endophthalmitis H59.43
  filtering (vitreous), after glaucoma surgery Z98.83
  inflamed (infected), postprocedural H59.40
    stage 1 H59.41
    stage 2 H59.42
    stage 3 H59.43
  lung (ruptured) J43.9
    congenital —*see* Atelectasis
    newborn P25.8
  subpleural (emphysematous) J43.9
Blebitis, postprocedural H59.40
  stage 1 H59.41
  stage 2 H59.42
  stage 3 H59.43
Bleeder (familial) (hereditary) —*see* Hemophilia
Bleeding —*see also* Hemorrhage
  anal K62.5
  anovulatory N97.0
  atonic, following delivery O72.1
  capillary I78.8
    puerperal O72.2
  contact (postcoital) N93.0
  due to uterine subinvolution N85.3
  ear —*see* Otorrhagia
  excessive, associated with menopausal onset N92.4
  familial —*see* Defect, coagulation
  following intercourse N93.0
  gastrointestinal K92.2
  hemorrhoids —*see* Hemorrhoids
  intermenstrual (regular) N92.3
    irregular N92.1
  intraoperative —*see* Complication, intraoperative, hemorrhage
  irregular N92.6
  menopausal N92.4
  newborn, intraventricular —*see* Newborn, affected by, hemorrhage, intraventricular
  nipple N64.59
  nose R04.0
  ovulation N92.3
  perimenopausal N92.4
  postclimacteric N95.0
  postcoital N93.0
  postmenopausal N95.0
  postoperative —*see* Complication, postprocedural, hemorrhage
  preclimacteric N92.4
  pre-pubertal vaginal N93.1
  puberty (excessive, with onset of menstrual periods) N92.2

Bleeding (*Continued*)
rectum, rectal K62.5
newborn P54.2
tendencies —*see* Defect, coagulation
throat R04.1
tooth socket (post-extraction) K91.840
umbilical stump P51.9
uterus, uterine NEC N93.9
climacteric N92.4
dysfunctional or functional N93.8
menopausal N92.4
preclimacteric or premenopausal N92.4
unrelated to menstrual cycle N93.9
vagina, vaginal (abnormal) N93.9
dysfunctional or functional N93.8
newborn P54.6
pre-pubertal N93.1
vicarious N94.89
Blennorrhagia, blennorrhagic —*see* Gonorrhea
Blennorrhea (acute) (chronic) —*see also*
Gonorrhea
inclusion (neonatal) (newborn) P39.1
lower genitourinary tract (gonococcal) A54.00
neonatorum (gonococcal ophthalmia) A54.31
Blepharelosis —*see* Entropion
Blepharitis (angularis) (ciliaris) (eyelid)
(marginal) (nonulcerative) H01.009
herpes zoster B02.39
left H01.006
lower H01.005
upper H01.004
upper and lower H01.00B
right H01.003
lower H01.002
upper H01.001
upper and lower H01.00A
squamous H01.029
left H01.026
lower H01.025
upper H01.024
upper and lower H01.02B
right H01.023
lower H01.022
upper H01.021
upper and lower H01.02A
ulcerative H01.019
left H01.016
lower H01.015
upper H01.014
upper and lower H01.01B
right H01.013
lower H01.012
upper H01.011
upper and lower H01.01B
Blepharochalasis H02.30
congenital Q10.0
left H02.36
lower H02.35
upper H02.34
right H02.33
lower H02.32
upper H02.31
Blepharoclonus H02.59
Blepharoconjunctivitis H10.50-●
angular H10.52-●
contact H10.53-●
ligneous H10.51-●
Blepharophimosis (eyelid) H02.529
congenital Q10.3
left H02.526
lower H02.525
upper H02.524
right H02.523
lower H02.522
upper H02.521
Blepharoptosis H02.40-●
congenital Q10.0
mechanical H02.41-●
myogenic H02.42-●
neurogenic H02.43-●
paralytic H02.43-●
Blepharopyorrhea, gonococcal A54.39

Blepharospasm G24.5
drug induced G24.01
Blighted ovum O02.0
Blind —*see also* Blindness
bronchus (congenital) Q32.4
loop syndrome K90.2
congenital Q43.8
sac, fallopian tube (congenital) Q50.6
spot, enlarged —*see* Defect, visual field,
localized, scotoma, blind spot area
tract or tube, congenital NEC —*see* Atresia,
by site
Blindness (acquired) (congenital) (both eyes)
H54.0X-●
blast S05.8X-●
color —*see* Deficiency, color vision
concussion S05.8X-●
cortical H47.619
left brain H47.612
right brain H47.611
day H53.11
due to injury (current episode) S05.9-●
sequelae — code to injury with seventh
character S
eclipse (total) —*see* Retinopathy, solar
emotional (hysterical) F44.6
face H53.16
hysterical F44.6
legal (both eyes) (USA definition) H54.8
mind R48.8
night H53.60
abnormal dark adaptation curve H53.61
acquired H53.62
congenital H53.63
specified type NEC H53.69
vitamin A deficiency E50.5
one eye (other eye normal) H54.40
left (normal vision on right) H54.42-●
low vision on right H54.12-●
low vision, other eye H54.10
right (normal vision on left) H54.41-●
low vision on left H54.11-●
psychic R48.8
river B73.01
snow —*see* Photokeratitis
sun, solar —*see* Retinopathy, solar
transient —*see* Disturbance, vision, subjective,
loss, transient
traumatic (current episode) S05.9-●
word (developmental) F81.0
acquired R48.0
secondary to organic lesion R48.0
Blister (nonthermal)
abdominal wall S30.821
alveolar process S00.522
ankle S90.52-●
antecubital space —*see* Blister, elbow
anus S30.827
arm (upper) S40.82-●
auditory canal —*see* Blister, ear
auricle —*see* Blister, ear
axilla —*see* Blister, arm
back, lower S30.820
beetle dermatitis L24.89
breast S20.12-●
brow S00.82
calf —*see* Blister, leg
canthus —*see* Blister, eyelid
cheek S00.82
internal S00.522
chest wall —*see* Blister, thorax
chin S00.82
costal region —*see* Blister, thorax
digit(s)
foot —*see* Blister, toe
hand —*see* Blister, finger
due to burn —*see* Burn, by site, second degree
ear S00.42-●
elbow S50.32-●
epiglottis S10.12
esophagus, cervical S10.12
eyebrow —*see* Blister, eyelid

Blister (*Continued*)
eyelid S00.22-●
face S00.82
fever B00.1
finger(s) S60.429
index S60.42-●
little S60.42-●
middle S60.42-●
ring S60.42-●
foot (except toe(s) alone) S90.82-●
toe —*see* Blister, toe
forearm S50.82-●
elbow only —*see* Blister, elbow
forehead S00.82
fracture - omit code
genital organ
female S30.826
male S30.825
gum S00.522
hand S60.52-●
head S00.92
ear —*see* Blister, ear
eyelid —*see* Blister, eyelid
lip S00.521
nose S00.32
oral cavity S00.522
scalp S00.02
specified site NEC S00.82
heel —*see* Blister, foot
hip S70.22-●
interscapular region S20.429
jaw S00.82
knee S80.22-●
larynx S10.12
leg (lower) S80.82-●
knee —*see* Blister, knee
upper —*see* Blister, thigh
lip S00.521
malar region S00.82
mammary —*see* Blister, breast
mastoid region S00.82
mouth S00.522
multiple, skin, nontraumatic R23.8
nail
finger —*see* Blister, finger
toe —*see* Blister, toe
nasal S00.32
neck S10.92
specified site NEC S10.82
throat S10.12
nose S00.32
occipital region S00.02
oral cavity S00.522
orbital region —*see* Blister, eyelid
palate S00.522
palm —*see* Blister, hand
parietal region S00.02
pelvis S30.820
penis S30.822
periocular area —*see* Blister, eyelid
phalanges
finger —*see* Blister, finger
toe —*see* Blister, toe
pharynx S10.12
pinna —*see* Blister, ear
popliteal space —*see* Blister, knee
scalp S00.02
scapular region —*see* Blister, shoulder
scrotum S30.823
shin —*see* Blister, leg
shoulder S40.22-●
sternal region S20.329
submaxillary region S00.82
submental region S00.82
subungual
finger(s) —*see* Blister, finger
toe(s) —*see* Blister, toe
supraclavicular fossa S10.82
supraorbital S00.82
temple S00.82
temporal region S00.82
testis S30.823

▶ New ⇒ Revised ~~deleted~~ Deleted ● Use Additional Character(s)

Blister *(Continued)*
thermal —*see* Burn, second degree, by site
thigh S70.32-•
thorax, thoracic (wall) S20.92
  back S20.42-•
  front S20.32-•
throat S10.12
thumb S60.32-•
toe(s) S90.42-•
  great S90.42-•
tongue S00.522
trachea S10.12
tympanum, tympanic membrane —*see* Blister, ear
upper arm —*see* Blister, arm (upper)
uvula S00.522
vagina S30.824
vocal cords S10.12
vulva S30.824
wrist S60.82-•
Bloating R14.0
Bloch-Sulzberger disease or syndrome Q82.3
Block, blocked
alveolocapillary J84.10
arborization (heart) I45.5
arrhythmic I45.9
atrioventricular (incomplete) (partial) I44.30
  with atrioventricular dissociation I44.2
  complete I44.2
    congenital Q24.6
  congenital Q24.6
  first degree I44.0
  second degree (types I and II) I44.1
  specified NEC I44.39
  third degree I44.2
  types I and II I44.1
auriculoventricular —*see* Block, atrioventricular
bifascicular (cardiac) I45.2
bundle-branch (complete) (false) (incomplete) I45.4
  bilateral I45.2
  left I44.7
    with right bundle branch block I45.2
    hemiblock I44.60
      anterior I44.4
      posterior I44.5
    incomplete I44.7
      with right bundle branch block I45.2
  right I45.10
    with
      left bundle branch block I45.2
      left fascicular block I45.2
    specified NEC I45.19
  Wilson's type I45.19
cardiac I45.9
conduction I45.9
  complete I44.2
fascicular (left) I44.60
  anterior I44.4
  posterior I44.5
  right I45.0
  specified NEC I44.69
foramen Magendie (acquired) G91.1
  congenital Q03.1
    with spina bifida —*see* Spina bifida, by site, with hydrocephalus
heart I45.9
  bundle branch I45.4
    bilateral I45.2
  complete (atrioventricular) I44.2
  congenital Q24.6
  first degree (atrioventricular) I44.0
  second degree (atrioventricular) I44.1
  specified type NEC I45.5
  third degree (atrioventricular) I44.2
hepatic vein I82.0
intraventricular (nonspecific) I45.4
  bundle branch
    bilateral I45.2
kidney N28.9
  postcystoscopic or postprocedural N99.0

Block, blocked *(Continued)*
Mobitz (types I and II) I44.1
myocardial —*see* Block, heart
nodal I45.5
organ or site, congenital NEC —*see* Atresia, by site
portal (vein) I81
second degree (types I and II) I44.1
sinoatrial I45.5
sinoauricular I45.5
third degree I44.2
trifascicular I45.3
tubal N97.1
vein NOS I82.90
Wenckebach (types I and II) I44.1
Blockage —*see* Obstruction
Blocq's disease F44.4
Blood
constituents, abnormal R78.9
disease D75.9
donor —*see* Donor, blood
dyscrasia D75.9
  with
    abortion —*see* Abortion, by type, complicated by, hemorrhage
    ectopic pregnancy O08.1
    molar pregnancy O08.1
  following ectopic or molar pregnancy O08.1
  newborn P61.9
  puerperal, postpartum O72.3
flukes NEC —*see* Schistosomiasis
in
  feces K92.1
    occult R19.5
  urine —*see* Hematuria
mole O02.0
occult in feces R19.5
pressure
  decreased, due to shock following injury T79.4
  examination only Z01.30
  fluctuating I99.8
  high —*see* Hypertension
    borderline R03.0
    incidental reading, without diagnosis of hypertension R03.0
  low —*see also* Hypotension
    incidental reading, without diagnosis of hypotension R03.1
spitting —*see* Hemoptysis
staining cornea —*see* Pigmentation, cornea, stromal
transfusion
  reaction or complication —*see* Complications, transfusion
type
  A (Rh positive) Z67.10
    Rh negative Z67.11
  AB (Rh positive) Z67.30
    Rh negative Z67.31
  B (Rh positive) Z67.20
    Rh negative Z67.21
  O (Rh positive) Z67.40
    Rh negative Z67.41
  Rh (positive) Z67.90
    negative Z67.91
vessel rupture —*see* Hemorrhage
vomiting —*see* Hematemesis
Blood-forming organs, disease D75.9
Bloodgood's disease —*see* Mastopathy, cystic
Bloom (-Machacek)(-Torre) syndrome Q82.8
Blount disease or osteochondrosis M92.51-•
Blue
baby Q24.9
diaper syndrome E72.09
dome cyst (breast) —*see* Cyst, breast
dot cataract Q12.0
nevus D22.9

Blue *(Continued)*
sclera Q13.5
  with fragility of bone and deafness Q78.0
toe syndrome I75.02-•
Blueness —*see* Cyanosis
Blues, postpartal O90.6
baby O90.6
Blurring, visual H53.8
Blushing (abnormal) (excessive) R23.2
BMI —*see* Body, mass index
Boarder, hospital NEC Z76.4
accompanying sick person Z76.3
healthy infant or child Z76.2
  foundling Z76.1
Bockhart's impetigo L01.02
Bodechtel-Guttman disease (subacute sclerosing panencephalitis) A81.1
Boder-Sedgwick syndrome (ataxia-telangiectasia) G11.3
Body, bodies
Aschoff's —*see* Myocarditis, rheumatic
asteroid, vitreous —*see* Deposit, crystalline
cytoid (retina) —*see* Occlusion, artery, retina
drusen (degenerative) (macula) (retinal) —*see also* Degeneration, macula, drusen
optic disc —*see* Drusen, optic disc
foreign —*see* Foreign body
loose
  joint, except knee —*see* Loose, body, joint
    knee M23.4-•
  sheath, tendon —*see* Disorder, tendon, specified type NEC
mass index (BMI)
  adult
    19.9 or less Z68.1
    20.0-20.9 Z68.20
    21.0-21.9 Z68.21
    22.0-22.9 Z68.22
    23.0-23.9 Z68.23
    24.0-24.9 Z68.24
    25.0-25.9 Z68.25
    26.0-26.9 Z68.26
    27.0-27.9 Z68.27
    28.0-28.9 Z68.28
    29.0-29.9 Z68.29
    30.0-30.9 Z68.30
    31.0-31.9 Z68.31
    32.0-32.9 Z68.32
    33.0-33.9 Z68.33
    34.0-34.9 Z68.34
    35.0-35.9 Z68.35
    36.0-36.9 Z68.36
    37.0-37.9 Z68.37
    38.0-38.9 Z68.38
    39.0-39.9 Z68.39
    40.0-44.9 Z68.41
    45.0-49.9 Z68.42
    50.0-59.9 Z68.43
    60.0-69.9 Z68.44
    70 and over Z68.45
  pediatric
    5th percentile to less than 85th percentile for age Z68.52
    85th percentile to less than 95th percentile for age Z68.53
    greater than or equal to ninety-fifth percentile for age Z68.54
    less than fifth percentile for age Z68.51
Mooser's A75.2
rice —*see also* Loose, body, joint
  knee M23.4-•
rocking F98.4
Boeck's
disease or sarcoid —*see* Sarcoidosis
lupoid (miliary) D86.3
Boerhaave's syndrome (spontaneous esophageal rupture) K22.3
Boggy
cervix N88.8
uterus N85.8

Boil —*see also* Furuncle, by site
  Aleppo B55.1
  Baghdad B55.1
  Delhi B55.1
  lacrimal
    gland —*see* Dacryoadenitis
    passages (duct) (sac) —*see* Inflammation,
      lacrimal, passages, acute
  Natal B55.1
  orbit, orbital —*see* Abscess, orbit
  tropical B55.1
Bold hives —*see* Urticaria
Bombé, iris —*see* Membrane, pupillary
Bone —*see* condition
Bonnevie-Ullrich syndrome —*see also* Turner's
  syndrome Q87.19
Bonnier's syndrome —*see* subcategory H81.8
Bonvale dam fever T73.3
Bony block of joint —*see* Ankylosis
BOOP (bronchiolitis obliterans organized
  pneumonia) J84.89
Borderline
  diabetes mellitus R73.03
  hypertension R03.0
  osteopenia M85.8-●
  pelvis, with obstruction during labor O65.1
  personality F60.3
Borna disease A83.9
Bornholm disease B33.0
Boston exanthem A88.0
Botalli, ductus (patent) (persistent) Q25.0
Bothriocephalus latus infestation B70.0
Botulism (foodborne intoxication) A05.1
  infant A48.51
  non-foodborne A48.52
  wound A48.52
Bouba —*see* Yaws
Bouchard's nodes (with arthropathy) M15.2
Bouffée délirante F23
Bouillaud's disease or syndrome (rheumatic
  heart disease) I01.9
Bourneville's disease Q85.1
Boutonniere deformity (finger) —*see*
  Deformity, finger, boutonniere
Bouveret (-Hoffmann) syndrome (paroxysmal
  tachycardia) I47.9
Bovine heart —*see* Hypertrophy, cardiac
Bowel —*see* condition
Bowen's
  dermatosis (precancerous) —*see* Neoplasm,
    skin, in situ
  disease —*see* Neoplasm, skin, in situ
  epithelioma —*see* Neoplasm, skin, in situ
  type
    epidermoid carcinoma-in-situ —*see*
      Neoplasm, skin, in situ
    intraepidermal squamous cell carcinoma —
      see Neoplasm, skin, in situ
Bowing
  femur —*see also* Deformity, limb, specified
    type NEC, thigh
    congenital Q68.3
  fibula —*see also* Deformity, limb, specified
    type NEC, lower leg
    congenital Q68.4
  forearm —*see* Deformity, limb, specified type
    NEC, forearm
  leg(s), long bones, congenital Q68.5
  radius —*see* Deformity, limb, specified type
    NEC, forearm
  tibia —*see also* Deformity, limb, specified type
    NEC, lower leg
    congenital Q68.4
Bowleg(s) (acquired) M21.16-●
  congenital Q68.5
  rachitic E64.3
Boyd's dysentery A03.2
Brachial —*see* condition
Brachycardia R00.1
Brachycephaly Q75.0
Bradley's disease A08.19

Bradyarrhythmia, cardiac I49.8
Bradycardia (sinoatrial) (sinus) (vagal) R00.1
  neonatal P29.12
  reflex G90.09
  tachycardia syndrome I49.5
Bradykinesia R25.8
Bradypnea R06.89
Bradytachycardia I49.5
Brailsford's disease or osteochondrosis —*see*
  Osteochondrosis, juvenile, radius
Brain —*see also* condition
  death G93.82
  syndrome —*see* Syndrome, brain
Branched-chain amino-acid disorder E71.2
Branchial —*see* condition
  cartilage, congenital Q18.2
Branchiogenic remnant (in neck) Q18.0
Brandt's syndrome (acrodermatitis
  enteropathica) E83.2
Brash (water) R12
Bravais-Jacksonian epilepsy —*see* Epilepsy,
  localization-related, symptomatic, with
  simple partial seizures
Braxton Hicks contractions —*see* False, labor
Brazilian leishmaniasis B55.2
BRBPR K62.5
Break, retina (without detachment) H33.30-●
  with retinal detachment —*see* Detachment,
    retina
  horseshoe tear H33.31-●
  multiple H33.33-●
  round hole H33.32-●
Breakdown
  device, graft or implant —*see also*
    Complications, by site and type,
    mechanical T85.618
  arterial graft NEC —*see* Complication,
    cardiovascular device, mechanical,
    vascular
  breast (implant) T85.41
  catheter NEC T85.618
    cystostomy T83.010
    dialysis (renal) T82.41
      intraperitoneal T85.611
    Hopkins T83.018
    ileostomy T83.018
    infusion NEC T82.514
      cranial T85.610
      epidural T85.610
      intrathecal T85.610
      spinal T85.610
      subarachnoid T85.610
      subdural T85.610
    nephrostomy T83.012
    urethral indwelling T83.011
    urinary NEC T83.018
    urostomy T83.018
  electronic (electrode) (pulse generator)
    (stimulator)
    bone T84.310
    cardiac T82.119
      electrode T82.110
      pulse generator T82.111
      specified type NEC T82.118
    nervous system —*see* Complication,
      prosthetic device, mechanical,
      electronic nervous system stimulator
    urinary —*see* Complication,
      genitourinary, device, urinary,
      mechanical
  fixation, internal (orthopedic) NEC —
    see Complication, fixation device,
    mechanical
  gastrointestinal —*see* Complications,
    prosthetic device, mechanical,
    gastrointestinal device
  genital NEC T83.418
    intrauterine contraceptive device T83.31
    penile prosthesis (cylinder) (implanted)
      (pump) (resevoir) T83.410
    testicular prosthesis T83.411

Breakdown (*Continued*)
  device, graft or implant (*Continued*)
    heart NEC —*see* Complication,
      cardiovascular device, mechanical
    intrathecal infusion pump T85.615
    joint prosthesis —*see* Complications...,
      joint prosthesis, internal, mechanical, by site
    nervous system, specified device NEC
      T85.615
    ocular NEC —*see* Complications, prosthetic
      device, mechanical, ocular device
    orthopedic NEC —*see* Complication,
      orthopedic, device, mechanical
    specified NEC T85.618
    subcutaneous device pocket
      nervous system prosthetic device,
        implant, or graft T85.890
      other internal prosthetic device, implant,
        or graft T85.898
    sutures, permanent T85.612
      used in bone repair —*see* Complications,
        fixation device, internal
        (orthopedic), mechanical
    urinary NEC T83.118
      graft T83.21
      sphincter, implanted T83.111
      stent (ileal conduit) (nephroureteral)
        T83.113
      ureteral indwelling T83.112
    vascular NEC —*see* Complication,
      cardiovascular device, mechanical
    ventricular intracranial shunt T85.01
  nervous F48.8
  perineum O90.1
  respirator J95.850
    specified NEC J95.859
  ventilator J95.850
    specified NEC J95.859
Breast —*see also* condition
  buds E30.1
    in newborn P96.89
  dense R92.2
  nodule —*see also* Lump, breast N63.0
Breath
  foul R19.6
  holder, child R06.89
  holding spell R06.89
  shortness R06.02
Breathing
  labored —*see* Hyperventilation
  mouth R06.5
    causing malocclusion M26.5
  periodic R06.3
    high altitude G47.32
Breathlessness R06.81
Breda's disease —*see* Yaws
Breech presentation (mother) O32.1
  causing obstructed labor O64.1
  footling O32.8
    causing obstructed labor O64.8
  incomplete O32.8
    causing obstructed labor O64.8
Breisky's disease N90.4
Brennemann's syndrome I88.0
Brenner
  tumor (benign) D27.9
    borderline malignancy D39.1-●
    malignant C56
    proliferating D39.1
Bretonneau's disease or angina A36.0
Breus' mole O02.0
Brevicollis Q76.49
Brickmakers' anemia B76.9 [D63.8]
Bridge, myocardial Q24.5
Bright red blood per rectum (BRBPR)
  K62.5
Bright's disease —*see also* Nephritis
  arteriosclerotic —*see* Hypertension, kidney
Brill (-Zinsser) disease (recrudescent typhus)
  A75.1
Brill-Symmers' disease C82.90

▶ New ⇒ Revised ~~deleted~~ Deleted ● Use Additional Character(s)

Brion-Kayser disease —see Fever, parathyroid
Briquet's disorder or syndrome F45.0
Brissaud's
  infantilism or dwarfism E23.0
  motor-verbal tic F95.2
Brittle
  bones disease Q78.0
  nails L60.3
    congenital Q84.6
Broad —see also condition
  beta disease E78.2
  ligament laceration syndrome N83.8
Broad- or floating-betalipoproteinemia E78.2
Brock's syndrome (atelectasis due to enlarged
  lymph nodes) J98.19
Brocq-Duhring disease (dermatitis
  herpetiformis) L13.0
Brodie's abscess or disease M86.8X-●
Broken
  arches —see also Deformity, limb, flat foot
  arm (meaning upper limb) —see Fracture, arm
  back —see Fracture, vertebra
  bone —see Fracture
  implant or internal device —see
    Complications, by site and type,
    mechanical
  leg (meaning lower limb) —see Fracture, leg
  nose S02.2
  tooth, teeth —see Fracture, tooth
Bromhidrosis, bromidrosis L75.0
➡ Bromidism, bromism G92.8
  chronic (dependence) F13.20
  due to
    correct substance properly administered —
      see Table of Drugs and Chemicals, by
      drug, adverse effect
    overdose or wrong substance given
      or taken —see Table of Drugs and
      Chemicals, by drug, poisoning
Bromidrosiphobia F40.298
Bronchi, bronchial —see condition
Bronchiectasis (cylindrical) (diffuse) (fusiform)
  (localized) (saccular) J47.9
  with
    acute
      bronchitis J47.0
      lower respiratory infection J47.0
    exacerbation (acute) J47.1
  congenital Q33.4
  tuberculous NEC —see Tuberculosis,
    pulmonary
Bronchiolectasis —see Bronchiectasis
Bronchiolitis (acute) (infective) (subacute) J21.9
  with
    bronchospasm or obstruction J21.9
    influenza, flu or grippe —see Influenza,
      with, respiratory manifestations NEC
  chemical (chronic) J68.4
    acute J68.0
  chronic (fibrosing) (obliterative) J44.9
  due to
    external agent —see Bronchitis, acute,
      due to
    human metapneumovirus J21.1
    respiratory syncytial virus (RSV) J21.0
    specified organism NEC J21.8
  fibrosa obliterans J44.9
  influenzal —see Influenza, with, respiratory
    manifestations NEC
  obliterans J42
    with organizing pneumonia (BOOP) J84.89
  obliterative (chronic) (subacute) J44.9
    due to chemicals, gases, fumes or vapors
      (inhalation) J68.4
    due to fumes or vapors J68.4
  respiratory, interstitial lung disease J84.115
Bronchitis (diffuse) (fibrinous) (hypostatic)
  (infective) (membranous) J40
  with
    influenza, flu or grippe —see Influenza,
      with, respiratory manifestations NEC

Bronchitis (Continued)
  with (Continued)
    obstruction (airway) (lung) J44.9
    tracheitis (15 years of age and above) J40
      acute or subacute J20.9
      chronic J42
      under 15 years of age J20.9
  acute or subacute (with bronchospasm or
    obstruction) J20.9
    with
      bronchiectasis J47.0
      chronic obstructive pulmonary disease
        J44.0
    chemical (due to gases, fumes or vapors)
      J68.0
    due to
      fumes or vapors J68.0
      Haemophilus influenzae J20.1
      Mycoplasma pneumoniae J20.0
      radiation J70.0
      specified organism NEC J20.8
      Streptococcus J20.2
      virus
        coxsackie J20.3
        echovirus J20.7
        parainfluenzae J20.4
        respiratory syncytial (RSV) J20.5
        rhinovirus J20.6
    viral NEC J20.8
  allergic (acute) J45.909
    with
      exacerbation (acute) J45.901
      status asthmaticus J45.902
  arachidic T17.528
  aspiration (due to food and vomit) J69.0
  asthmatic J45.9
    chronic J44.9
      with
        acute lower respiratory infection J44.0
        exacerbation (acute) J44.1
  capillary —see Pneumonia, broncho
  caseous (tuberculous) A15.5
  Castellani's A69.8
  catarrhal (15 years of age and above) J40
    acute —see Bronchitis, acute
    chronic J41.0
    under 15 years of age J20.9
  chemical (acute) (subacute) J68.0
    chronic J68.4
    due to fumes or vapors J68.0
      chronic J68.4
  chronic J42
    with
      airways obstruction J44.9
      tracheitis (chronic) J42
    asthmatic (obstructive) J44.9
    catarrhal J41.0
    chemical (due to fumes or vapors) J68.4
    due to
      chemicals, gases, fumes or vapors
        (inhalation) J68.4
      radiation J70.0
      tobacco smoking J41.0
    emphysematous J44.9
    mucopurulent J41.1
    non-obstructive J41.0
    obliterans J44.9
    obstructive J44.9
    purulent J41.1
    simple J41.0
  croupous —see Bronchitis, acute
  due to gases, fumes or vapors (chemical)
    J68.0
  emphysematous (obstructive) J44.9
  exudative —see Bronchitis, acute
  fetid J41.1
  grippal —see Influenza, with, respiratory
    manifestations NEC
  in those under 15 years age —see Bronchitis,
    acute
    chronic —see Bronchitis, chronic

Bronchitis (Continued)
  influenzal —see Influenza, with, respiratory
    manifestations NEC
  mixed simple and mucopurulent J41.8
  moulder's J62.8
  mucopurulent (chronic) (recurrent) J41.1
    acute or subacute J20.9
    simple (mixed) J41.8
  obliterans (chronic) J44.9
  obstructive (chronic) (diffuse) J44.9
  pituitous J41.1
  pneumococcal, acute or subacute J20.2
  pseudomembranous, acute or subacute —see
    Bronchitis, acute
  purulent (chronic) (recurrent) J41.1
    acute or subacute —see Bronchitis, acute
  putrid J41.1
  senile (chronic) J42
  simple and mucopurulent (mixed) J41.8
  smokers' J41.0
  spirochetal NEC A69.8
  subacute —see Bronchitis, acute
  suppurative (chronic) J41.1
    acute or subacute —see Bronchitis, acute
  tuberculous A15.5
  under 15 years of age —see Bronchitis, acute
    chronic —see Bronchitis, chronic
  viral NEC, acute or subacute —see also
    Bronchitis, acute J20.8
Bronchoalveolitis J18.0
Bronchoaspergillosis B44.1
Bronchocele meaning goiter E04.0
Broncholithiasis J98.09
  tuberculous NEC A15.5
Bronchomalacia J98.09
  congenital Q32.2
Bronchomycosis NOS B49 [J99]
  candidal B37.1
Bronchopleuropneumonia —see Pneumonia,
  broncho
Bronchopneumonia —see Pneumonia, broncho
Bronchopneumonitis —see Pneumonia,
  broncho
Bronchopulmonary —see condition
Bronchopulmonitis —see Pneumonia, broncho
Bronchorrhagia (see Hemoptysis)
Bronchorrhea J98.09
  acute J20.9
  chronic (infective) (purulent) J42
Bronchospasm (acute) J98.01
  with
    bronchiolitis, acute J21.9
    bronchitis, acute (conditions in J20) —see
      Bronchitis, acute
  due to external agent —see condition,
    respiratory, acute, due to
  exercise induced J45.990
Bronchospirochetosis A69.8
  Castellani A69.8
Bronchostenosis J98.09
Bronchus —see condition
Brontophobia F40.220
Bronze baby syndrome P83.88
Brooke's tumor —see Neoplasm, skin, benign
Brown enamel of teeth (hereditary) K00.5
Brown's sheath syndrome H50.61-●
Brown-Séquard disease, paralysis or
  syndrome G83.81
Bruce sepsis A23.0
Brucellosis (infection) A23.9
  abortus A23.1
  canis A23.3
  dermatitis A23.9
  melitensis A23.0
  mixed A23.8
  sepsis A23.9
    melitensis A23.0
    specified NEC A23.8
  suis A23.2
Bruck-de Lange disease Q87.19
Bruck's disease —see Deformity, limb

BRUE (brief resolved unexplained event) R68.13
Brugsch's syndrome Q82.8
Bruise (skin surface intact) —see also Contusion
  with
    open wound —see Wound, open
    internal organ —see Injury, by site
  newborn P54.5
  scalp, due to birth injury, newborn P12.3
  umbilical cord O69.5
Bruit (arterial) R09.89
  cardiac R01.1
Brush burn —see Abrasion, by site
Bruton's X-linked agammaglobulinemia D80.0
Bruxism
  psychogenic F45.8
  sleep related G47.63
Bubbly lung syndrome P27.0
Bubo I88.8
  blennorrhagic (gonococcal) A54.89
  chancroidal A57
  climatic A55
  due to Haemophilus ducreyi A57
  gonococcal A54.89
  indolent (nonspecific) I88.8
  inguinal (nonspecific) I88.8
    chancroidal A57
    climatic A55
    due to H. ducreyi A57
    infective I88.8
  scrofulous (tuberculous) A18.2
  soft chancre A57
  suppurating —see Lymphadenitis, acute
  syphilitic (primary) A51.0
    congenital A50.07
  tropical A55
  virulent (chancroidal) A57
Bubonic plague A20.0
Bubonocele —see Hernia, inguinal
Buccal —see condition
Buchanan's disease or osteochondrosis M91.0
Buchem's syndrome (hyperostosis corticalis)
  M85.2
Bucket-handle fracture or tear (semilunar
  cartilage) —see Tear, meniscus
Budd-Chiari syndrome (hepatic vein
  thrombosis) I82.0
Budgerigar fancier's disease or lung
  J67.2
Buds
  breast E30.1
    in newborn P96.89
Buerger's disease (thromboangiitis obliterans)
  I73.1
Bulbar —see condition
Bulbus cordis (left ventricle) (persistent) Q21.8
Bulimia (nervosa) F50.2
  atypical F50.9
  normal weight F50.9
Bulky
  stools R19.5
  uterus N85.2
Bulla (e) R23.8
  lung (emphysematous) (solitary) J43.9
    newborn P25.8
Bullet wound —see also Wound, open
  fracture - code as Fracture, by site
  internal organ —see Injury, by site
Bundle
  branch block (complete) (false)
    (incomplete) —see Block, bundle-branch
  of His —see condition
Bunion M21.61-●
  tailor's M21.62-●
Bunionette M21.62-●
Buphthalmia, buphthalmos (congenital) Q15.0
Burdwan fever B55.0
Bürger-Grütz disease or syndrome E78.3
Buried
  penis (congenital) Q55.64
    acquired N48.83
  roots K08.3

Burke's syndrome K86.89
Burkitt
  cell leukemia C91.0-●
  lymphoma (malignant) C83.7-●
    small noncleaved, diffuse C83.7-●
    spleen C83.77
    undifferentiated C83.7-●
  tumor C83.7-●
  type
    acute lymphoblastic leukemia C91.0-●
    undifferentiated C83.7-●
Burn (electricity) (flame) (hot gas, liquid or hot
  object) (radiation) (steam) (thermal) T30.0
  abdomen, abdominal (muscle) (wall)
    T21.02
    first degree T21.12
    second degree T21.22
    third degree T21.32
  above elbow T22.039
    first degree T22.139
    left T22.032
      first degree T22.132
      second degree T22.232
      third degree T22.332
    right T22.031
      first degree T22.131
      second degree T22.231
      third degree T22.331
    second degree T22.239
    third degree T22.339
  acid (caustic) (external) (internal) —see
    Corrosion, by site
  alimentary tract NEC T28.2
    esophagus T28.1
    mouth T28.0
    pharynx T28.0
  alkaline (caustic) (external) (internal) —see
    Corrosion, by site
  ankle T25.019
    first degree T25.119
    left T25.012
      first degree T25.112
      second degree T25.212
      third degree T25.312
    multiple with foot —see Burn, lower, limb,
      multiple, ankle and foot
    right T25.011
      first degree T25.111
      second degree T25.211
      third degree T25.311
    second degree T25.219
    third degree T25.319
  anus —see Burn, buttock
  arm (lower) (upper) —see Burn, upper,
    limb
  axilla T22.049
    first degree T22.149
    left T22.042
      first degree T22.142
      second degree T22.242
      third degree T22.342
    right T22.041
      first degree T22.141
      second degree T22.241
      third degree T22.341
    second degree T22.249
    third degree T22.349
  back (lower) T21.04
    first degree T21.14
    second degree T21.24
    third degree T21.34
    upper T21.03
      first degree T21.13
      second degree T21.23
      third degree T21.33
  blisters - code as Burn, second degree, by site
  breast(s) —see Burn, chest wall
  buttock(s) T21.05
    first degree T21.15
    second degree T21.25
    third degree T21.35

Burn (Continued)
  calf T24.039
    first degree T24.139
    left T24.032
      first degree T24.132
      second degree T24.232
      third degree T24.332
    right T24.031
      first degree T24.131
      second degree T24.231
      third degree T24.331
    second degree T24.239
    third degree T24.339
  canthus (eye) —see Burn, eyelid
  caustic acid or alkaline —see Corrosion, by
    site
  cervix T28.3
  cheek T20.06
    first degree T20.16
    second degree T20.26
    third degree T20.36
  chemical (acids) (alkalines) (caustics) (external)
    (internal) —see Corrosion, by site
  chest wall T21.01
    first degree T21.11
    second degree T21.21
    third degree T21.31
  chin T20.03
    first degree T20.13
    second degree T20.23
    third degree T20.33
  colon T28.2
  conjunctiva (and cornea) —see Burn, cornea
  cornea (and conjunctiva) T26.1-●
    chemical —see Corrosion, cornea
  corrosion (external) (internal) —see
    Corrosion, by site
  deep necrosis of underlying tissue - code as
    Burn, third degree, by site
  dorsum of hand T23.069
    first degree T23.169
    left T23.062
      first degree T23.162
      second degree T23.262
      third degree T23.362
    right T23.061
      first degree T23.161
      second degree T23.261
      third degree T23.361
    second degree T23.269
    third degree T23.369
  due to ingested chemical agent —see
    Corrosion, by site
  ear (auricle) (external) (canal) T20.01
    first degree T20.11
    second degree T20.21
    third degree T20.31
  elbow T22.029
    first degree T22.129
    left T22.022
      first degree T22.122
      second degree T22.222
      third degree T22.322
    right T22.021
      first degree T22.121
      second degree T22.221
      third degree T22.321
    second degree T22.229
    third degree T22.329
  epidermal loss - code as Burn, second degree,
    by site
  erythema, erythematous - code as Burn, first
    degree, by site
  esophagus T28.1
  extent (percentage of body surface)
    less than 10 percent T31.0
    10-19 percent T31.10
      with 0-9 percent third degree burns
        T31.10
      with 10-19 percent third degree burns
        T31.11

▶ New   ⮕ Revised   ~~deleted~~ Deleted   ● Use Additional Character(s)

Burn *(Continued)*
  extent *(Continued)*
    20-29 percent T31.20
      with 0-9 percent third degree burns T31.20
      with 10-19 percent third degree burns T31.21
      with 20-29 percent third degree burns T31.22
    30-39 percent T31.30
      with 0-9 percent third degree burns T31.30
      with 10-19 percent third degree burns T31.31
      with 20-29 percent third degree burns T31.32
      with 30-39 percent third degree burns T31.33
    40-49 percent T31.40
      with 0-9 percent third degree burns T31.40
      with 10-19 percent third degree burns T31.41
      with 20-29 percent third degree burns T31.42
      with 30-39 percent third degree burns T31.43
      with 40-49 percent third degree burns T31.44
    50-59 percent T31.50
      with 0-9 percent third degree burns T31.50
      with 10-19 percent third degree burns T31.51
      with 20-29 percent third degree burns T31.52
      with 30-39 percent third degree burns T31.53
      with 40-49 percent third degree burns T31.54
      with 50-59 percent third degree burns T31.55
    60-69 percent T31.60
      with 0-9 percent third degree burns T31.60
      with 10-19 percent third degree burns T31.61
      with 20-29 percent third degree burns T31.62
      with 30-39 percent third degree burns T31.63
      with 40-49 percent third degree burns T31.64
      with 50-59 percent third degree burns T31.65
      with 60-69 percent third degree burns T31.66
    70-79 percent T31.70
      with 0-9 percent third degree burns T31.70
      with 10-19 percent third degree burns T31.71
      with 20-29 percent third degree burns T31.72
      with 30-39 percent third degree burns T31.73
      with 40-49 percent third degree burns T31.74
      with 50-59 percent third degree burns T31.75
      with 60-69 percent third degree burns T31.76
      with 70-79 percent third degree burns T31.77
    80-89 percent T31.80
      with 0-9 percent third degree burns T31.80
      with 10-19 percent third degree burns T31.81
      with 20-29 percent third degree burns T31.82
      with 30-39 percent third degree burns T31.83
      with 40-49 percent third degree burns T31.84

Burn *(Continued)*
  extent *(Continued)*
    80-89 percent T31.80 *(Continued)*
      with 50-59 percent third degree burns T31.85
      with 60-69 percent third degree burns T31.86
      with 70-79 percent third degree burns T31.87
      with 80-89 percent third degree burns T31.88
    90 percent or more T31.90
      with 0-9 percent third degree burns T31.90
      with 10-19 percent third degree burns T31.91
      with 20-29 percent third degree burns T31.92
      with 30-39 percent third degree burns T31.93
      with 40-49 percent third degree burns T31.94
      with 50-59 percent third degree burns T31.95
      with 60-69 percent third degree burns T31.96
      with 70-79 percent third degree burns T31.97
      with 80-89 percent third degree burns T31.98
      with 90 percent or more third degree burns T31.99
  extremity —*see* Burn, limb
  eye(s) and adnexa T26.4-●
    with resulting rupture and destruction of eyeball T26.2-●
    conjunctival sac —*see* Burn, cornea
    cornea —*see* Burn, cornea
    lid —*see* Burn, eyelid
    periocular area —*see* Burn, eyelid
    specified site NEC T26.3-●
  eyeball —*see* Burn, eye
  eyelid(s) T26.0-●
    chemical —*see* Corrosion, eyelid
  face —*see* Burn, head
  finger T23.029
    first degree T23.129
    left T23.022
      first degree T23.122
      second degree T23.222
      third degree T23.322
    multiple sites (without thumb) T23.039
      with thumb T23.049
        first degree T23.149
        left T23.042
          first degree T23.142
          second degree T23.242
          third degree T23.342
        right T23.041
          first degree T23.141
          second degree T23.241
          third degree T23.341
        second degree T23.249
        third degree T23.349
      first degree T23.139
      left T23.032
        first degree T23.132
        second degree T23.232
        third degree T23.332
      right T23.031
        first degree T23.131
        second degree T23.231
        third degree T23.331
      second degree T23.239
      third degree T23.339
    right T23.021
      first degree T23.121
      second degree T23.221
      third degree T23.321
    second degree T23.229
    third degree T23.329
  flank —*see* Burn, abdominal wall

Burn *(Continued)*
  foot T25.029
    first degree T25.129
    left T25.022
      first degree T25.122
      second degree T25.222
      third degree T25.322
    multiple with ankle —*see* Burn, lower, limb, multiple, ankle and foot
    right T25.021
      first degree T25.121
      second degree T25.221
      third degree T25.321
    second degree T25.229
    third degree T25.329
  forearm T22.019
    first degree T22.119
    left T22.012
      first degree T22.112
      second degree T22.212
      third degree T22.312
    right T22.011
      first degree T22.111
      second degree T22.211
      third degree T22.311
    second degree T22.219
    third degree T22.319
  forehead T20.06
    first degree T20.16
    second degree T20.26
    third degree T20.36
  fourth degree - code as Burn, third degree, by site
  friction —*see* Burn, by site
  from swallowing caustic or corrosive substance NEC —*see* Corrosion, by site
  full thickness skin loss - code as Burn, third degree, by site
  gastrointestinal tract NEC T28.2
    from swallowing caustic or corrosive substance T28.7
  genital organs
    external
      female T21.07
        first degree T21.17
        second degree T21.27
        third degree T21.37
      male T21.06
        first degree T21.16
        second degree T21.26
        third degree T21.36
    internal T28.3
      from caustic or corrosive substance T28.8
  groin —*see* Burn, abdominal wall
  hand(s) T23.009
    back —*see* Burn, dorsum of hand
    finger —*see* Burn, finger
    first degree T23.109
    left T23.002
      first degree T23.102
      second degree T23.202
      third degree T23.302
    multiple sites with wrist T23.099
      first degree T23.199
      left T23.092
        first degree T23.192
        second degree T23.292
        third degree T23.392
      right T23.091
        first degree T23.191
        second degree T23.291
        third degree T23.391
      second degree T23.299
      third degree T23.399
    palm —*see* Burn, palm
    right T23.001
      first degree T23.101
      second degree T23.201
      third degree T23.301

Burn (Continued)
  hand (Continued)
    second degree T23.209
    third degree T23.309
    thumb —see Burn, thumb
  head (and face) (and neck) T20.00
    cheek —see Burn, cheek
    chin —see Burn, chin
    ear —see Burn, ear
    eye(s) only —see Burn, eye
    first degree T20.10
    forehead —see Burn, forehead
    lip —see Burn, lip
    multiple sites T20.09
      first degree T20.19
      second degree T20.29
      third degree T20.39
    neck —see Burn, neck
    nose —see Burn, nose
    scalp —see Burn, scalp
    second degree T20.20
    third degree T20.30
  hip(s) —see Burn, thigh
  inhalation —see Burn, respiratory tract
    caustic or corrosive substance (fumes) —see
      Corrosion, respiratory tract
  internal organ(s) T28.40
    alimentary tract T28.2
      esophagus T28.1
    eardrum T28.41
    esophagus T28.1
    from caustic or corrosive substance
      (swallowing) NEC —see Corrosion,
      by site
    genitourinary T28.3
    mouth T28.0
    pharynx T28.0
    respiratory tract —see Burn, respiratory
      tract
    specified organ NEC T28.49
  interscapular region —see Burn, back,
    upper
  intestine (large) (small) T28.2
  knee T24.029
    first degree T24.129
    left T24.022
      first degree T24.122
      second degree T24.222
      third degree T24.322
    right T24.021
      first degree T24.121
      second degree T24.221
      third degree T24.321
    second degree T24.229
    third degree T24.329
  labium (majus) (minus) —see Burn, genital
    organs, external, female
  lacrimal apparatus, duct, gland or sac —see
    Burn, eye, specified site NEC
  larynx T27.0
    with lung T27.1
  leg(s) (lower) (upper) —see Burn, lower,
    limb
  lightning —see Burn, by site
  limb(s)
    lower (except ankle or foot alone) —see
      Burn, lower, limb
    upper —see Burn, upper limb
  lip(s) T20.02
    first degree T20.12
    second degree T20.22
    third degree T20.32
  lower
    back —see Burn, back
    limb T24.009
      ankle —see Burn, ankle
      calf —see Burn, calf
      first degree T24.109
      foot —see Burn, foot
      hip —see Burn, thigh
      knee —see Burn, knee

Burn (Continued)
  lower (Continued)
    limb (Continued)
      left T24.002
        first degree T24.102
        second degree T24.202
        third degree T24.302
      multiple sites, except ankle and foot
        T24.099
      ankle and foot T25.099
        first degree T25.199
        left T25.092
          first degree T25.192
          second degree T25.292
          third degree T25.392
        right T25.091
          first degree T25.191
          second degree T25.291
          third degree T25.391
        second degree T25.299
        third degree T25.399
      first degree T24.199
      left T24.092
        first degree T24.192
        second degree T24.292
        third degree T24.392
      right T24.091
        first degree T24.191
        second degree T24.291
        third degree T24.391
      second degree T24.299
      third degree T24.399
      right T24.001
        first degree T24.101
        second degree T24.201
        third degree T24.301
      second degree T24.209
      thigh —see Burn, thigh
      third degree T24.309
      toe —see Burn, toe
  lung (with larynx and trachea) T27.1
  mouth T28.0
  neck T20.07
    first degree T20.17
    second degree T20.27
    third degree T20.37
  nose (septum) T20.04
    first degree T20.14
    second degree T20.24
    third degree T20.34
  ocular adnexa —see Burn, eye
  orbit region —see Burn, eyelid
  palm T23.059
    first degree T23.159
    left T23.052
      first degree T23.152
      second degree T23.252
      third degree T23.352
    right T23.051
      first degree T23.151
      second degree T23.251
      third degree T23.351
    second degree T23.259
    third degree T23.359
  ~~partial thickness - code as Burn, degree, by site~~
  ▶ partial thickness - code as Burn, by site,
    second degree
  pelvis —see Burn, trunk
  penis —see Burn, genital organs, external,
    male
  perineum
    female —see Burn, genital organs, external,
      female
    male —see Burn, genital organs, external,
      male
  periocular area —see Burn, eyelid
  pharynx T28.0
  rectum T28.2
  respiratory tract T27.3
    larynx —see Burn, larynx
    specified part NEC T27.2
    trachea —see Burn, trachea

Burn (Continued)
  sac, lacrimal —see Burn, eye, specified site
    NEC
  scalp T20.05
    first degree T20.15
    second degree T20.25
    third degree T20.35
  scapular region T22.069
    first degree T22.169
    left T22.062
      first degree T22.162
      second degree T22.262
      third degree T22.362
    right T22.061
      first degree T22.161
      second degree T22.261
      third degree T22.361
    second degree T22.269
    third degree T22.369
  sclera —see Burn, eye, specified site NEC
  scrotum —see Burn, genital organs, external,
    male
  shoulder T22.059
    first degree T22.159
    left T22.052
      first degree T22.152
      second degree T22.252
      third degree T22.352
    right T22.051
      first degree T22.151
      second degree T22.251
      third degree T22.351
    second degree T22.259
    third degree T22.359
  stomach T28.2
  temple —see Burn, head
  testis —see Burn, genital organs, external, male
  thigh T24.019
    first degree T24.119
    left T24.012
      first degree T24.112
      second degree T24.212
      third degree T24.312
    right T24.011
      first degree T24.111
      second degree T24.211
      third degree T24.311
    second degree T24.219
    third degree T24.319
  thorax (external) —see Burn, trunk
  throat (meaning pharynx) T28.0
  thumb(s) T23.019
    first degree T23.119
    left T23.012
      first degree T23.112
      second degree T23.212
      third degree T23.312
    multiple sites with fingers T23.049
      first degree T23.149
      left T23.042
        first degree T23.142
        second degree T23.242
        third degree T23.342
      right T23.041
        first degree T23.141
        second degree T23.241
        third degree T23.341
      second degree T23.249
      third degree T23.349
    right T23.011
      first degree T23.111
      second degree T23.211
      third degree T23.311
    second degree T23.219
    third degree T23.319
  toe T25.039
    first degree T25.139
    left T25.032
      first degree T25.132
      second degree T25.232
      third degree T25.332

Burn *(Continued)*
  toe *(Continued)*
    right T25.031
      first degree T25.131
      second degree T25.231
      third degree T25.331
    second degree T25.239
    third degree T25.339
  tongue T28.0
  tonsil(s) T28.0
  trachea T27.0
    with lung T27.1
  trunk T21.00
    abdominal wall —*see* Burn, abdominal
      wall
    anus —*see* Burn, buttock
    axilla —*see* Burn, upper limb
    back —*see* Burn, back
    breast —*see* Burn, chest wall
    buttock —*see* Burn, buttock
    chest wall —*see* Burn, chest wall
    first degree T21.10
    flank —*see* Burn, abdominal wall
    genital
      female —*see* Burn, genital organs,
        external, female
      male —*see* Burn, genital organs, external,
        male
    groin —*see* Burn, abdominal wall
    interscapular region —*see* Burn, back,
      upper
    labia —*see* Burn, genital organs, external,
      female
    lower back —*see* Burn, back
    penis —*see* Burn, genital organs, external,
      male
    perineum
      female —*see* Burn, genital organs,
        external, female
      male —*see* Burn, genital organs, external,
        male
    scapula region —*see* Burn, scapular
      region
    scrotum —*see* Burn, genital organs,
      external, male
    second degree T21.20
    specified site NEC T21.09
      first degree T21.19
      second degree T21.29
      third degree T21.39
    testes —*see* Burn, genital organs, external,
      male
    third degree T21.30
    upper back —*see* Burn, back, upper
    vulva —*see* Burn, genital organs, external,
      female
  unspecified site with extent of body surface
    involved specified
    less than 10 percent T31.0
    10-19 percent (0-9 percent third degree)
      T31.10
      with 10-19 percent third degree
        T31.11
    20-29 percent (0-9 percent third degree)
      T31.20
      with
        10-19 percent third degree T31.21
        20-29 percent third degree T31.22
    30-39 percent (0-9 percent third degree)
      T31.30
      with
        10-19 percent third degree T31.31
        20-29 percent third degree T31.32
        30-39 percent third degree T31.33
    40-49 percent (0-9 percent third degree)
      T31.40
      with
        10-19 percent third degree T31.41
        20-29 percent third degree T31.42
        30-39 percent third degree T31.43
        40-49 percent third degree T31.44

Burn *(Continued)*
  unspecified site with extent of body surface
    involved specified *(Continued)*
    50-59 percent (0-9 percent third degree)
      T31.50
      with
        10-19 percent third degree T31.51
        20-29 percent third degree T31.52
        30-39 percent third degree T31.53
        40-49 percent third degree T31.54
        50-59 percent third degree T31.55
    60-69 percent (0-9 percent third degree)
      T31.60
      with
        10-19 percent third degree T31.61
        20-29 percent third degree T31.62
        30-39 percent third degree T31.63
        40-49 percent third degree T31.64
        50-59 percent third degree T31.65
        60-69 percent third degree T31.66
    70-79 percent (0-9 percent third degree)
      T31.70
      with
        10-19 percent third degree T31.71
        20-29 percent third degree T31.72
        30-39 percent third degree T31.73
        40-49 percent third degree T31.74
        50-59 percent third degree T31.75
        60-69 percent third degree T31.76
        70-79 percent third degree T31.77
    80-89 percent (0-9 percent third degree)
      T31.80
      with
        10-19 percent third degree T31.81
        20-29 percent third degree T31.82
        30-39 percent third degree T31.83
        40-49 percent third degree T31.84
        50-59 percent third degree T31.85
        60-69 percent third degree T31.86
        70-79 percent third degree T31.87
        80-89 percent third degree T31.88
    90 percent or more (0-9 percent third
      degree) T31.90
      with
        10-19 percent third degree T31.91
        20-29 percent third degree T31.92
        30-39 percent third degree T31.93
        40-49 percent third degree T31.94
        50-59 percent third degree T31.95
        60-69 percent third degree T31.96
        70-79 percent third degree T31.97
        80-89 percent third degree T31.98
        90-99 percent third degree T31.99
  upper limb T22.00
    above elbow —*see* Burn, above elbow
    axilla —*see* Burn, axilla
    elbow —*see* Burn, elbow
    first degree T22.10
    forearm —*see* Burn, forearm
    hand —*see* Burn, hand
    interscapular region —*see* Burn, back,
      upper
    multiple sites T22.099
      first degree T22.199
      left T22.092
        first degree T22.192
        second degree T22.292
        third degree T22.392
      right T22.091
        first degree T22.191
        second degree T22.291
        third degree T22.391
      second degree T22.299
      third degree T22.399
    scapular region —*see* Burn, scapular region
    second degree T22.20
    shoulder —*see* Burn, shoulder
    third degree T22.30
    wrist —*see* Burn, wrist
  uterus T28.3
  vagina T28.3

Burn *(Continued)*
  vulva —*see* Burn, genital organs, external,
    female
  wrist T23.079
    first degree T23.179
    left T23.072
      first degree T23.172
      second degree T23.272
      third degree T23.372
    multiple sites with hand T23.099
      first degree T23.199
      left T23.092
        first degree T23.192
        second degree T23.292
        third degree T23.392
      right T23.091
        first degree T23.191
        second degree T23.291
        third degree T23.391
      second degree T23.299
      third degree T23.399
    right T23.071
      first degree T23.171
      second degree T23.271
      third degree T23.371
    second degree T23.279
    third degree T23.379
Burnett's syndrome E83.52
Burning
  feet syndrome E53.9
  sensation R20.8
  tongue K14.6
Burn-out (state) Z73.0
Burns' disease or osteochondrosis —*see*
  Osteochondrosis, juvenile, ulna
Bursa —*see* condition
Bursitis M71.9
  Achilles —*see* Tendinitis, Achilles
  adhesive —*see* Bursitis, specified NEC
  ankle —*see* Enthesopathy, lower limb, ankle,
    specified type NEC
  calcaneal —*see* Enthesopathy, foot, specified
    type NEC
  collateral ligament, tibial —*see* Bursitis, tibial
    collateral
  due to use, overuse, pressure —*see also*
    Disorder, soft tissue, due to use,
    specified type NEC
    specified NEC —*see* Disorder, soft tissue,
      due to use, specified NEC
  Duplay's M75.0
  elbow NEC M70.3-●
    olecranon M70.2-●
  finger —*see* Disorder, soft tissue, due to use,
    specified type NEC, hand
  foot —*see* Enthesopathy, foot, specified type
    NEC
  gonococcal A54.49
  gouty —*see* Gout
  hand M70.1-●
  hip NEC M70.7-●
    trochanteric M70.6-●
  infective NEC M71.10
    abscess —*see* Abscess, bursa
    ankle M71.17-●
    elbow M71.12-●
    foot M71.17-●
    hand M71.14-●
    hip M71.15-●
    knee M71.16-●
    multiple sites M71.19
    shoulder M71.11-●
    specified site NEC M71.18
    wrist M71.13-●
  ischial —*see* Bursitis, hip
  knee NEC M70.5-●
    prepatellar M70.4-●
  occupational NEC —*see also* Disorder, soft
    tissue, due to, use
  olecranon —*see* Bursitis, elbow, olecranon
  pharyngeal J39.1

Bursitis *(Continued)*
  popliteal —*see* Bursitis, knee
  prepatellar M70.4-●
  radiohumeral M70.3-●
  rheumatoid M06.20
    ankle M06.27-●
    elbow M06.22-●
    foot joint M06.27-●
    hand joint M06.24-●
    hip M06.25-●
    knee M06.26-●
    multiple site M06.29
    shoulder M06.21-●
    vertebra M06.28
    wrist M06.23-●
  scapulohumeral —*see* Bursitis, shoulder
  semimembranous muscle (knee) —*see*
      Bursitis, knee
  shoulder M75.5-●
    adhesive —*see* Capsulitis, adhesive
  specified NEC M71.50
    ankle M71.57-●
    due to use, overuse or pressure —*see*
        Disorder, soft tissue, due to, use
    elbow M71.52-●
    foot M71.57-●
    hand M71.54-●

Bursitis *(Continued)*
  specified NEC *(Continued)*
    hip M71.55-●
    knee M71.56-●
    shoulder —*see* Bursitis, shoulder
    specified site NEC M71.58
    tibial collateral M76.4-●
    wrist M71.53-●
  subacromial —*see* Bursitis, shoulder
  subcoracoid —*see* Bursitis, shoulder
  subdeltoid —*see* Bursitis, shoulder
  syphilitic A52.78
  Thornwaldt, Tornwaldt J39.2
  tibial collateral M76.4-●
  toe —*see* Enthesopathy, foot, specified type
      NEC
  trochanteric (area) —*see* Bursitis, hip,
      trochanteric
  wrist —*see* Bursitis, hand
Bursopathy M71.9
  specified type NEC M71.80
    ankle M71.87-●
    elbow M71.82-●
    foot M71.87-●
    hand M71.84-●
    hip M71.85-●
    knee M71.86-●

Bursopathy *(Continued)*
  specified type NEC *(Continued)*
    multiple sites M71.89
    shoulder M71.81-●
    specified site NEC M71.88
    wrist M71.83-●
Burst stitches or sutures (complication of
    surgery) T81.31
  external operation wound T81.31
  internal operation wound T81.32
Buruli ulcer A31.1
Bury's disease L95.1
Buschke's
  disease —*see* Cryptococcosis by site
  scleredema —*see* Sclerosis, systemic
Busse-Buschke disease —*see* Cryptococcosis
    by site
Buttock —*see* condition
Button
  Biskra B55.1
  Delhi B55.1
  oriental B55.1
Buttonhole deformity (finger) —*see* Deformity,
    finger, boutonniere
Bwamba fever A92.8
Byssinosis J66.0
Bywaters' syndrome T79.5

C

Cachexia R64
  cancerous R64
  cardiac —see Disease, heart
  dehydration E86.0
  due to malnutrition R64
  exophthalmic —see Hyperthyroidism
  heart —see Disease, heart
  hypophyseal E23.0
  hypopituitary E23.0
  lead —see Poisoning, lead
  malignant R64
  marsh —see Malaria
  nervous F48.8
  old age R54
  paludal —see Malaria
  pituitary E23.0
▶ pulmonary R64
  renal N28.9
  saturnine —see Poisoning, lead
  senile R54
  Simmonds' E23.0
  splenica D73.0
  strumipriva E03.4
  tuberculous NEC —see Tuberculosis
CADASIL (cerebral autosomal dominant
    arteriopathy with subcortical infarcts
    and leukoencephalopathy) I67.850
Café au lait spots L81.3
Caffeine-induced
  anxiety disorder F15.980
  sleep disorder F15.982
Caffey's syndrome Q78.8
Caisson disease T70.3
Cake kidney Q63.1
Caked breast (puerperal, postpartum) O92.79
Calabar swelling B74.3
Calcaneal spur —see Spur, bone, calcaneal
Calcaneo-apophysitis M92.8
Calcareous —see condition
Calcicosis J62.8
Calciferol (vitamin D) deficiency E55.9
  with rickets E55.0
Calcification
  adrenal (capsule) (gland) E27.49
    tuberculous E35 [B90.8]
  aorta I70.0
  artery (annular) —see Arteriosclerosis
  auricle (ear) —see Disorder, pinna, specified
    type NEC
  basal ganglia G23.8
  bladder N32.89
    due to Schistosoma hematobium B65.0
  brain (cortex) —see Calcification, cerebral
  bronchus J98.09
  bursa M71.40
    ankle M71.47-●
    elbow M71.42-●
    foot M71.47-●
    hand M71.44-●
    hip M71.45-●
    knee M71.46-●
    multiple sites M71.49
    shoulder M75.3-●
    specified site NEC M71.48
    wrist M71.43-●
  cardiac —see Degeneration, myocardial
  cerebral (cortex) G93.89
    artery I67.2
  cervix (uteri) N88.8
  choroid plexus G93.89
  conjunctiva —see Concretion, conjunctiva
  corpora cavernosa (penis) N48.89
  cortex (brain) —see Calcification, cerebral
  dental pulp (nodular) K04.2
  dentinal papilla K00.4
  fallopian tube N83.8
  falx cerebri G96.198
  gallbladder K82.8
  general E83.59
  heart —see also Degeneration, myocardial
    valve —see Endocarditis

Calcification (Continued)
  idiopathic infantile arterial (IIAC) Q28.8
  intervertebral cartilage or disc
    (postinfective) —see Disorder, disc,
    specified NEC
  intracranial —see Calcification, cerebral
  joint —see Disorder, joint, specified type
    NEC
  kidney N28.89
    tuberculous N29 [B90.1]
  larynx (senile) J38.7
  lens —see Cataract, specified NEC
  lung (active) (postinfectional) J98.4
    tuberculous B90.9
  lymph gland or node (postinfectional) I89.8
    tuberculous —see also Tuberculosis, lymph
      gland B90.8
  mammographic R92.1
  massive (paraplegic) —see Myositis,
    ossificans, in, quadriplegia
  medial —see Arteriosclerosis, extremities
  meninges (cerebral) (spinal) G96.198
  metastatic E83.59
  Mönckeberg's —see Arteriosclerosis,
    extremities
  muscle M61.9
    due to burns —see Myositis, ossificans, in,
      burns
    paralytic —see Myositis, ossificans, in,
      quadriplegia
    specified type NEC M61.40
      ankle M61.47-●
      foot M61.47-●
      forearm M61.43-●
      hand M61.44-●
      lower leg M61.46-●
      multiple sites M61.49
      pelvic region M61.45-●
      shoulder region M61.41-●
      specified site NEC M61.48
      thigh M61.45-●
      upper arm M61.42-●
  myocardium, myocardial —see Degeneration,
    myocardial
  ovary N83.8
  pancreas K86.89
  penis N48.89
  periarticular —see Disorder, joint, specified
    type NEC
  pericardium —see also Pericarditis I31.1
  pineal gland E34.8
  pleura J94.8
    postinfectional J94.8
    tuberculous NEC B90.9
  pulpal (dental) (nodular) K04.2
  sclera H15.89
  spleen D73.89
  subcutaneous L94.2
  suprarenal (capsule) (gland) E27.49
  tendon (sheath) —see also Tenosynovitis,
    specified type NEC
    with bursitis, synovitis or tenosynovitis —
      see Tendinitis, calcific
  trachea J39.8
  ureter N28.89
  vitreous —see Deposit, crystalline
Calcified —see Calcification
Calcinosis (interstitial) (tumoral) (universalis)
    E83.59
  with Raynaud's phenomenon, esophageal
    dysfunction, sclerodactyly, telangiectasia
    (CREST syndrome) M34.1
  circumscripta (skin) L94.2
  cutis L94.2
Calciphylaxis —see also Calcification, by site
    E83.59
Calcium
  deposits —see Calcification, by site
  metabolism disorder E83.50
  salts or soaps in vitreous —see Deposit,
    crystalline

Calciuria R82.994
Calculi —see Calculus
Calculosis, intrahepatic —see Calculus, bile
    duct
Calculus, calculi, calculous
  ampulla of Vater —see Calculus, bile duct
  anuria (impacted) (recurrent) —see also
    Calculus, urinary N20.9
  appendix K38.1
  bile duct (common) (hepatic) K80.50
    with
      calculus of gallbladder —see Calculus,
        gallbladder and bile duct
      cholangitis K80.30
        with
          cholecystitis —see Calculus, bile
            duct, with cholecystitis
          obstruction K80.31
        acute K80.32
          with
            chronic cholangitis K80.36
              with obstruction K80.37
            obstruction K80.33
        chronic K80.34
          with
            acute cholangitis K80.36
              with obstruction K80.37
            obstruction K80.35
      cholecystitis (with cholangitis) K80.40
        with obstruction K80.41
        acute K80.42
          with
            chronic cholecystitis K80.46
              with obstruction K80.47
            obstruction K80.43
        chronic K80.44
          with
            acute cholecystitis K80.46
              with obstruction K80.47
            obstruction K80.45
      obstruction K80.51
    biliary —see also Calculus, gallbladder
      specified NEC K80.80
        with obstruction K80.81
    bilirubin, multiple —see Calculus,
      gallbladder
    bladder (encysted) (impacted) (urinary)
      (diverticulum) N21.0
    bronchus J98.09
    calyx (kidney) (renal) —see Calculus, kidney
    cholesterol (pure) (solitary) —see Calculus,
      gallbladder
    common duct (bile) —see Calculus, bile duct
    conjunctiva —see Concretion, conjunctiva
    cystic N21.0
      duct —see Calculus, gallbladder
    dental (subgingival) (supragingival)
      K03.6
    diverticulum
      bladder N21.0
      kidney N20.0
    epididymis N50.89
    gallbladder K80.20
      with
        bile duct calculus —see Calculus,
          gallbladder and bile duct
        cholecystitis K80.10
          with obstruction K80.11
          acute K80.00
            with
              chronic cholecystitis K80.12
                with obstruction K80.13
              obstruction K80.01
          chronic K80.10
            with
              acute cholecystitis K80.12
                with obstruction K80.13
              obstruction K80.11
        specified NEC K80.18
          with obstruction K80.19
        obstruction K80.21

Calculus, calculi, calculous *(Continued)*
    gallbladder and bile duct K80.70
        with
            cholecystitis K80.60
                with obstruction K80.61
                acute K80.62
                    with
                        chronic cholecystitis K80.66
                            with obstruction K80.67
                        obstruction K80.63
                    chronic K80.64
                        with
                            acute cholecystitis K80.66
                                with obstruction K80.67
                            obstruction K80.65
            obstruction K80.71
    hepatic (duct) —*see* Calculus, bile duct
    hepatobiliary K80.80
        with obstruction K80.81
    ileal conduit N21.8
    intestinal (impaction) (obstruction) K56.49
    kidney (impacted) (multiple) (pelvis)
            (recurrent) (staghorn) N20.0
        with calculus, ureter N20.2
        congenital Q63.8
    lacrimal passages —*see* Dacryolith
    liver (impacted) —*see* Calculus, bile duct
    lung J98.4
    mammographic R92.1
    nephritic (impacted) (recurrent) —*see*
            Calculus, kidney
    nose J34.89
    pancreas (duct) K86.89
    parotid duct or gland K11.5
    pelvis, encysted —*see* Calculus, kidney
    prostate N42.0
    pulmonary J98.4
    pyelitis (impacted) (recurrent) N20.0
        with hydronephrosis N13.6
    pyelonephritis (impacted) (recurrent) —*see*
            category N20
        with hydronephrosis N13.6
    renal (impacted) (recurrent) —*see* Calculus,
            kidney
    salivary (duct) (gland) K11.5
    seminal vesicle N50.89
    staghorn —*see* Calculus, kidney
    Stensen's duct K11.5
    stomach K31.89
    sublingual duct or gland K11.5
        congenital Q38.4
    submandibular duct, gland or region K11.5
    submaxillary duct, gland or region K11.5
    suburethral N21.8
    tonsil J35.8
    tooth, teeth (subgingival) (supragingival) K03.6
    tunica vaginalis N50.89
    ureter (impacted) (recurrent) N20.1
        with calculus, kidney N20.2
            with hydronephrosis N13.2
                with infection N13.6
    ureteropelvic junction N20.1
    urethra (impacted) N21.1
    urinary (duct) (impacted) (passage) (tract)
            N20.9
        with hydronephrosis N13.2
            with infection N13.6
        in (due to)
        lower N21.9
            specified NEC N21.8
    vagina N89.8
    vesical (impacted) N21.0
    Wharton's duct K11.5
    xanthine E79.8 [N22]
Calicectasis N28.89
Caliectasis N28.89
California
    disease B38.9
    encephalitis A83.5
Caligo cornea —*see* Opacity, cornea, central
Callositas, callosity (infected) L84

Callus (infected) L84
    bone —*see* Osteophyte
        excessive, following fracture - code as
            Sequelae of fracture
CALME (childhood asymmetric labium majus
        enlargement) N90.61
Calorie deficiency or malnutrition —*see also*
        Malnutrition E46
Calvé-Perthes disease —*see* Legg-Calve-Perthes
        disease
Calvé's disease —*see* Osteochondrosis, juvenile,
        spine
Calvities —*see* Alopecia, androgenic
Cameroon fever —*see* Malaria
Camptocormia (hysterical) F44.4
Camurati-Engelmann syndrome Q78.3
Canal —*see also* condition
    atrioventricular common Q21.2
Canaliculitis (lacrimal) (acute) (subacute)
        H04.33-●
    Actinomyces A42.89
    chronic H04.42-●
Canavan's disease E75.29
Canceled procedure (surgical) Z53.9
    because of
        contraindication Z53.09
            smoking Z53.01
        left against medical advice (AMA) Z53.29
        patient's decision Z53.20
            for reasons of belief or group pressure
                Z53.1
            specified reason NEC Z53.29
        specified reason NEC Z53.8
Cancer —*see also* Neoplasm, by site, malignant
    bile duct type, liver C22.1
    blood —*see* Leukemia
    breast —*see also* Neoplasm, breast, malignant
        C50.91-●
    hepatocellular C22.0
    lung —*see also* Neoplasm, lung, malignant
        C34.90-●
    ovarian —*see also* Neoplasm, ovary,
        malignant C56.9-●
    unspecified site (primary) C80.1
Cancer (o)phobia F45.29
Cancerous —*see* Neoplasm, malignant, by site
Cancrum oris A69.0
Candidiasis, candidal B37.9
    balanitis B37.42
    bronchitis B37.1
    cheilitis B37.83
    congenital P37.5
    cystitis B37.41
    disseminated B37.7
    endocarditis B37.6
    enteritis B37.82
    esophagitis B37.81
    intertrigo B37.2
    lung B37.1
    meningitis B37.5
    mouth B37.0
    nails B37.2
    neonatal P37.5
    onychia B37.2
    oral B37.0
    osteomyelitis B37.89
    otitis externa B37.84
    paronychia B37.2
    perionyxis B37.2
    pneumonia B37.1
    proctitis B37.82
    pulmonary B37.1
    pyelonephritis B37.49
    sepsis B37.7
    skin B37.2
    specified site NEC B37.89
    stomatitis B37.0
    systemic B37.7
    urethritis B37.41
    urogenital site NEC B37.49
    vagina B37.3
    vulva B37.3
    vulvovaginitis B37.3

Candidid L30.2
Candidosis —*see* Candidiasis
Candiru infection or infestation B88.8
Canities (premature) L67.1
    congenital Q84.2
Canker (mouth) (sore) K12.0
    rash A38.9
Cannabinosis J66.2
Cannabis induced
    anxiety disorder F12.980
    psychotic disorder F12.959
    sleep disorder F12.988
Canton fever A75.9
Cantrell's syndrome Q87.89
Capillariasis (intestinal) B81.1
    hepatic B83.8
Capillary —*see* condition
Caplan's syndrome —*see* Rheumatoid, lung
Capsule —*see* condition
Capsulitis (joint) —*see also* Enthesopathy
    adhesive (shoulder) M75.0-●
    hepatic K65.8
    labyrinthine —*see* Otosclerosis, specified NEC
    thyroid E06.9
Caput
    crepitus Q75.8
    medusae I86.8
    succedaneum P12.81
Car sickness T75.3
Carapata (disease) A68.0
Carate —*see* Pinta
Carbon lung J60
Carbuncle L02.93
    abdominal wall L02.231
    anus K61.0
    auditory canal, external —*see* Abscess, ear,
        external
    auricle ear —*see* Abscess, ear, external
    axilla L02.43-●
    back (any part) L02.232
    breast N61.1
    buttock L02.33
    cheek (external) L02.03
    chest wall L02.233
    chin L02.03
    corpus cavernosum N48.21
    ear (any part) (external) (middle) —*see*
        Abscess, ear, external
    external auditory canal —*see* Abscess, ear,
        external
    eyelid —*see* Abscess, eyelid
    face NEC L02.03
    femoral (region) —*see* Carbuncle, lower limb
    finger —*see* Carbuncle, hand
    flank L02.231
    foot L02.63-●
    forehead L02.03
    genital —*see* Abscess, genital
    gluteal (region) L02.33
    groin L02.234
    hand L02.53-●
    head NEC L02.831
    heel —*see* Carbuncle, foot
    hip —*see* Carbuncle, lower limb
    kidney —*see* Abscess, kidney
    knee —*see* Carbuncle, lower limb
    labium (majus) (minus) N76.4
    lacrimal
        gland —*see* Dacryoadenitis
        passages (duct) (sac) —*see* Inflammation,
            lacrimal, passages, acute
    leg —*see* Carbuncle, lower limb
    lower limb L02.43-●
    malignant A22.0
    navel L02.236
    neck L02.13
    nose (external) (septum) J34.0
    orbit, orbital —*see* Abscess, orbit
    palmar (space) —*see* Carbuncle, hand
    partes posteriores L02.33
    pectoral region L02.233
    penis N48.21

Carbuncle *(Continued)*
  perineum L02.235
  pinna —*see* Abscess, ear, external
  popliteal —*see* Carbuncle, lower limb
  scalp L02.831
  seminal vesicle N49.0
  shoulder —*see* Carbuncle, upper limb
  specified site NEC L02.838
  temple (region) L02.03
  thumb —*see* Carbuncle, hand
  toe —*see* Carbuncle, foot
  trunk L02.239
    abdominal wall L02.231
    back L02.232
    chest wall L02.233
    groin L02.234
    perineum L02.235
    umbilicus L02.236
  umbilicus L02.236
  upper limb L02.43-●
  urethra N34.0
  vulva N76.4
Carbunculus —*see* Carbuncle
Carcinoid (tumor) —*see* Tumor, carcinoid
Carcinoidosis E34.0
Carcinoma (malignant) —*see also* Neoplasm,
    by site, malignant
  acidophil
    specified site —*see* Neoplasm, malignant,
      by site
    unspecified site C75.1
  acidophil-basophil, mixed
    specified site —*see* Neoplasm, malignant,
      by site
    unspecified site C75.1
  adnexal (skin) —*see* Neoplasm, skin, malignant
  adrenal cortical C74.0-●
  alveolar —*see* Neoplasm, lung, malignant
    cell —*see* Neoplasm, lung, malignant
  ameloblastic C41.1
    upper jaw (bone) C41.0
  apocrine
    breast —*see* Neoplasm, breast, malignant
    specified site NEC —*see* Neoplasm, skin,
      malignant
    unspecified site C44.99
  basal cell (pigmented) *(see also* Neoplasm,
      skin, malignant) C44.91
    fibro-epithelial —*see* Neoplasm, skin,
      malignant
    morphea —*see* Neoplasm, skin, malignant
    multicentric —*see* Neoplasm, skin,
      malignant
  basaloid
  basal-squamous cell, mixed —*see* Neoplasm,
      skin, malignant
  basophil
    specified site —*see* Neoplasm, malignant,
      by site
    unspecified site C75.1
  basophil-acidophil, mixed
    specified site —*see* Neoplasm, malignant,
      by site
    unspecified site C75.1
  basosquamous —*see* Neoplasm, skin, malignant
  bile duct
    with hepatocellular, mixed C22.0
    liver C22.1
    specified site NEC —*see* Neoplasm,
      malignant, by site
    unspecified site C22.1
  branchial or branchiogenic C10.4
  bronchial or bronchogenic —*see* Neoplasm,
      lung, malignant
  bronchiolar —*see* Neoplasm, lung, malignant
  bronchioloalveolar —*see* Neoplasm, lung,
      malignant
  C cell
    specified site —*see* Neoplasm, malignant,
      by site
    unspecified site C73
  ceruminous C44.29-●

Carcinoma *(Continued)*
  cervix uteri
    in situ D06.9
      endocervix D06.0
      exocervix D06.1
      specified site NEC D06.7
  chorionic
    specified site —*see* Neoplasm, malignant,
      by site
    unspecified site
      female C58
      male C62.90
  chromophobe
    specified site —*see* Neoplasm, malignant,
      by site
    unspecified site C75.1
  cloacogenic
    specified site —*see* Neoplasm, malignant,
      by site
    unspecified site C21.2
  diffuse type
    specified site —*see* Neoplasm, malignant,
      by site
    unspecified site C16.9
  duct (cell)
    with Paget's disease —*see* Neoplasm,
      breast, malignant
    infiltrating
      with lobular carcinoma (in situ)
        specified site —*see* Neoplasm,
          malignant, by site
        unspecified site (female) C50.91-●
          male C50.92-●
      specified site —*see* Neoplasm,
        malignant, by site
      unspecified site (female) C50.91-●
        male C50.92-●
  ductal
    with lobular
      specified site —*see* Neoplasm,
        malignant, by site
      unspecified site (female) C50.91-●
        male C50.92-●
  ductular, infiltrating
    specified site —*see* Neoplasm, malignant,
      by site
    unspecified site (female) C50.91-●
      male C50.92-●
  embryonal
    liver C22.7
  endometrioid
    specified site —*see* Neoplasm, malignant,
      by site
    unspecified site
      female C56.9
      male C61
  eosinophil
    specified site —*see* Neoplasm, malignant,
      by site
    unspecified site C75.1
  epidermoid —*see also* Neoplasm, skin
      malignant
    in situ, Bowen's type —*see* Neoplasm, skin,
      in situ
  fibroepithelial, basal cell —*see* Neoplasm,
      skin, malignant
  follicular
    with papillary (mixed) C73
    moderately differentiated C73
    pure follicle C73
    specified site —*see* Neoplasm, malignant,
      by site
    trabecular C73
    unspecified site C73
    well differentiated C73
  generalized, with unspecified primary site
      C80.0
  glycogen-rich —*see* Neoplasm, breast,
      malignant
  granulosa cell C56-●
  hepatic cell C22.0

Carcinoma *(Continued)*
  hepatocellular C22.0
    with bile duct, mixed C22.0
    fibrolamellar C22.0
  hepatocholangiolitic C22.0
  Hurthle cell C73
  in
    adenomatous
      polyposis coli C18.9
    pleomorphic adenoma —*see* Neoplasm,
      salivary glands, malignant
    situ —*see* Carcinoma-in-situ
  infiltrating
    duct
      with lobular
        specified site —*see* Neoplasm,
          malignant, by site
        unspecified site (female) C50.91-●
          male C50.92-●
      with Paget's disease —*see* Neoplasm,
        breast, malignant
      specified site —*see* Neoplasm,
        malignant
      unspecified site (female) C50.91-●
        male C50.92-●
    ductular
      specified site —*see* Neoplasm,
        malignant
      unspecified site (female) C50.91-●
        male C50.92-●
    lobular
      specified site —*see* Neoplasm,
        malignant
      unspecified site (female) C50.91-●
        male C50.92-●
  inflammatory
    specified site —*see* Neoplasm, malignant
    unspecified site (female) C50.91-●
      male C50.92-●
  intestinal type
    specified site —*see* Neoplasm, malignant,
      by site
    unspecified site C16.9
  intracystic
    noninfiltrating —*see* Neoplasm, in situ,
      by site
  intraductal (noninfiltrating)
    with Paget's disease —*see* Neoplasm,
      breast, malignant
    breast D05.1-●
    papillary
      with invasion
        specified site —*see* Neoplasm,
          malignant, by site
        unspecified site (female) C50.91-●
          male C50.92-●
      breast D05.1-●
      specified site NEC —*see* Neoplasm,
        in situ, by site
      unspecified site (female) D05.1-●
    specified site NEC —*see* Neoplasm,
      in situ, by site
    unspecified site (female) D05.1-●
  intraepidermal —*see* Neoplasm, in situ
    squamous cell, Bowen's type —*see*
      Neoplasm, skin, in situ
  intraepithelial —*see* Neoplasm, in situ,
      by site
    squamous cell —*see* Neoplasm, in situ,
      by site
  intraosseous C41.1
    upper jaw (bone) C41.0
  islet cell
    with exocrine, mixed
      specified site —*see* Neoplasm,
        malignant, by site
      unspecified site C25.9
    pancreas C25.4
    specified site NEC —*see* Neoplasm,
      malignant, by site
    unspecified site C25.4

Carcinoma *(Continued)*
  juvenile, breast —*see* Neoplasm, breast,
    malignant
  large cell
    small cell
      specified site —*see* Neoplasm,
        malignant, by site
      unspecified site C34.90
  Leydig cell (testis)
    specified site —*see* Neoplasm, malignant,
      by site
    unspecified site
      female C56.9
      male C62.90
  lipid-rich (female) C50.91-●
    male C50.92-●
  liver cell C22.0
  liver NEC C22.7
  lobular (infiltrating)
    with intraductal
      specified site —*see* Neoplasm,
        malignant, by site
      unspecified site (female) C50.91-●
        male C50.92-●
    noninfiltrating
      breast D05.0-●
      specified site NEC —*see* Neoplasm, in
        situ, by site
      unspecified site D05.0-●
    specified site —*see* Neoplasm, malignant,
      by site
    unspecified site (female) C50.91-●
      male C50.92-●
  medullary
    with
      amyloid stroma
        specified site —*see* Neoplasm,
          malignant, by site
        unspecified site C73
      lymphoid stroma
        specified site —*see* Neoplasm,
          malignant, by site
        unspecified site (female) C50.91-●
          male C50.92-●
  Merkel cell C4A.9
    anal margin C4A.51
    anal skin C4A.51
    canthus C4A.1-●
    ear and external auricular canal C4A.2-●
    external auricular canal C4A.2-●
    eyelid, including canthus C4A.1-●
    face C4A.30
      specified NEC C4A.39
    hip C4A.7-●
    lip C4A.0
    lower limb, including hip C4A.7-●
    neck C4A.4
    nodal presentation C7B.1
    nose C4A.31
    overlapping sites C4A.8
    perianal skin C4A.51
    scalp C4A.4
    secondary C7B.1
    shoulder C4A.6-●
    skin of breast C4A.52
    trunk NEC C4A.59
    upper limb, including shoulder C4A.6-●
    visceral metastatic C7B.1
  metastatic —*see* Neoplasm, secondary
  metatypical —*see* Neoplasm, skin, malignant
  morphea, basal cell —*see* Neoplasm, skin,
    malignant
  mucoid
    cell
      specified site —*see* Neoplasm,
        malignant, by site
      unspecified site C75.1
  neuroendocrine —*see also* Tumor,
    neuroendocrine
    high grade, any site C7A.1
    poorly differentiated, any site C7A.1

Carcinoma *(Continued)*
  nonencapsulated sclerosing C73
  noninfiltrating
    intracystic —*see* Neoplasm, in situ, by site
    intraductal
      breast D05.1-●
      papillary
        breast D05.1-●
        specified site NEC —*see* Neoplasm, in
          situ, by site
        unspecified site D05.1-●
      specified site —*see* Neoplasm, in situ,
        by site
      unspecified site D05.1-●
    lobular
      breast D05.0-●
      specified site NEC —*see* Neoplasm, in
        situ, by site
      unspecified site (female) D05.0-●
  oat cell
    specified site —*see* Neoplasm, malignant,
      by site
    unspecified site C34.90
  odontogenic C41.1
    upper jaw (bone) C41.0
  papillary
    with follicular (mixed) C73
    follicular variant C73
    intraductal (noninfiltrating)
      with invasion
        specified site —*see* Neoplasm,
          malignant, by site
        unspecified site (female) C50.91-●
          male C50.92-●
      breast D05.1-●
      specified site NEC —*see* Neoplasm, in
        situ, by site
      unspecified site D05.1-●
    serous
      specified site —*see* Neoplasm,
        malignant, by site
      surface
        specified site —*see* Neoplasm,
          malignant, by site
        unspecified site C56.9
      unspecified site C56.9
  papillocystic
    specified site —*see* Neoplasm, malignant,
      by site
    unspecified site C56.9
  parafollicular cell
    specified site —*see* Neoplasm, malignant,
      by site
    unspecified site C73
  pilomatrix —*see* Neoplasm, skin, malignant
  pseudomucinous
    specified site —*see* Neoplasm, malignant,
      by site
    unspecified site C56.9
  renal cell C64-●
  Schmincke —*see* Neoplasm, nasopharynx,
    malignant
  Schneiderian
    specified site —*see* Neoplasm, malignant,
      by site
    unspecified site C30.0
  sebaceous —*see* Neoplasm, skin, malignant
  secondary —*see also* Neoplasm, secondary,
    by site
    Merkel cell C7B.1
  secretory, breast —*see* Neoplasm, breast,
    malignant
  serous
    papillary
      specified site —*see* Neoplasm,
        malignant, by site
      unspecified site C56.9
    surface, papillary
      specified site —*see* Neoplasm,
        malignant, by site
      unspecified site C56.9

Carcinoma *(Continued)*
  Sertoli cell
    specified site —*see* Neoplasm, malignant,
      by site
    unspecified site C62.90
      female C56.9
      male C62.90
  skin appendage —*see* Neoplasm, skin,
    malignant
  small cell
    fusiform cell
      specified site —*see* Neoplasm,
        malignant, by site
      unspecified site C34.90
    intermediate cell
      specified site —*see* Neoplasm,
        malignant, by site
      unspecified site C34.90
    large cell
      specified site —*see* Neoplasm,
        malignant, by site
      unspecified site C34.90
  solid
    with amyloid stroma
      specified site —*see* Neoplasm,
        malignant, by site
      unspecified site C73
    microinvasive
      specified site —*see* Neoplasm,
        malignant, by site
      unspecified site C53.9
  sweat gland —*see* Neoplasm, skin,
    malignant
  theca cell C56.-●
  thymic C37
  unspecified site (primary) C80.1
  water-clear cell C75.0
Carcinoma-in-situ —*see also* Neoplasm, in situ,
  by site
  breast NOS D05.9-●
    specified type NEC D05.8-●
  epidermoid —*see also* Neoplasm, in situ, by
    site
    with questionable stromal invasion
      cervix D06.9
      specified site NEC —*see* Neoplasm, in
        situ, by site
      unspecified site D06.9
    Bowen's type —*see* Neoplasm, skin,
      in situ
  intraductal
    breast D05.1-●
    specified site NEC —*see* Neoplasm, in situ,
      by site
    unspecified site D05.1-●
  lobular
    with
      infiltrating duct
        breast (female) C50.91-●
          male C50.92-●
        specified site NEC —*see* Neoplasm,
          malignant
        unspecified site (female) C50.91-●
          male C50.92-●
      intraductal
        breast D05.8-●
        specified site NEC —*see* Neoplasm, in
          situ, by site
        unspecified site (female) D05.8-●
    breast D05.0-●
    specified site NEC —*see* Neoplasm, in situ,
      by site
    unspecified site D05.0-●
  squamous cell —*see also* Neoplasm, in situ,
    by site
    with questionable stromal invasion
      cervix D06.9
      specified site NEC —*see* Neoplasm, in
        situ, by site
      unspecified site D06.9
Carcinomaphobia F45.29

▶ New   ⇒ Revised   ~~deleted~~ Deleted   ● Use Additional Character(s)

Carcinomatosis C80.0
  peritonei C78.6
  unspecified site (primary) (secondary) C80.0
Carcinosarcoma —*see* Neoplasm, malignant,
  by site
  embryonal —*see* Neoplasm, malignant, by site
Cardia, cardial —*see* condition
Cardiac —*see also* condition
  death, sudden —*see* Arrest, cardiac
  pacemaker
    in situ Z95.0
    management or adjustment Z45.018
  tamponade I31.4
Cardialgia —*see* Pain, precordial
Cardiectasis —*see* Hypertrophy, cardiac
Cardiochalasia K21.9
Cardiomalacia I51.5
Cardiomegalia glycogenica diffusa E74.02 *[143]*
Cardiomegaly —*see also* Hypertrophy, cardiac
  congenital Q24.8
  glycogen E74.02 *[143]*
  idiopathic I51.7
Cardiomyoliposis I51.5
Cardiomyopathy (familial) (idiopathic) I42.9
  alcoholic I42.6
  amyloid E85.4 *[143]*
    transthyretin-related (ATTR) familial E85.4
      [143]
  arteriosclerotic —*see* Disease, heart, ischemic,
    atherosclerotic
  beriberi E51.12
  cobalt-beer I42.6
  congenital I42.4
  congestive I42.0
  constrictive NOS I42.5
  dilated I42.0
  due to
    alcohol I42.6
    beriberi E51.12
    cardiac glycogenosis E74.02 *[143]*
    drugs I42.7
    external agents NEC I42.7
    Friedreich's ataxia G11.11
    myotonia atrophica G71.11 *[143]*
    progressive muscular dystrophy G71.09
      [143]
  glycogen storage E74.02 *[143]*
  hypertensive —*see* Hypertension, heart
  hypertrophic (nonobstructive) I42.2
    obstructive I42.1
      congenital Q24.8
  in
    Chagas' disease (chronic) B57.2
      acute B57.0
    sarcoidosis D86.85
  ischemic I25.5
  metabolic E88.9 *[143]*
    thyrotoxic E05.90 *[143]*
      with thyroid storm E05.91 *[143]*
  newborn I42.8
    congenital I42.4
  non-ischemic (*see also* by cause) I42.8
  nutritional E63.9 *[143]*
    beriberi E51.12
  obscure of Africa I42.8
  peripartum O90.3
  postpartum O90.3
  restrictive NEC I42.5
  rheumatic I09.0
  secondary I42.9
  specified NEC I42.8
  stress induced I51.81
  takotsubo I51.81
  thyrotoxic E05.90 *[143]*
    with thyroid storm E05.91 *[143]*
  toxic NEC I42.7
  transthyretin-related (ATTR) familial amyloid
    E85.4
  tuberculous A18.84
  viral B33.24
Cardionephritis —*see* Hypertension,
  cardiorenal

Cardionephropathy —*see* Hypertension,
  cardiorenal
Cardionephrosis —*see* Hypertension, cardiorenal
Cardiopathia nigra I27.0
Cardiopathy —*see also* Disease, heart I51.9
  idiopathic I42.9
  mucopolysaccharidosis E76.3 *[152]*
Cardiopericarditis —*see* Pericarditis
Cardiophobia F45.29
Cardiorenal —*see* condition
Cardiorrhexis —*see* Infarct, myocardium
Cardiosclerosis —*see* Disease, heart, ischemic,
  atherosclerotic
Cardiosis —*see* Disease, heart
Cardiospasm (esophagus) (reflex) (stomach)
  K22.0
  congenital Q39.5
    with megaesophagus Q39.5
Cardiostenosis —*see* Disease, heart
Cardiosymphysis I31.0
Cardiovascular —*see* condition
Carditis (acute) (bacterial) (chronic) (subacute)
  I51.89
  meningococcal A39.50
  rheumatic —*see* Disease, heart, rheumatic
  rheumatoid —*see* Rheumatoid, carditis
  viral B33.20
Care (of) (for) (following)
  child (routine) Z76.2
  family member (handicapped) (sick)
    creating problem for family Z63.6
    provided away from home for holiday
      relief Z75.5
    unavailable, due to
      absence (person rendering care)
        (sufferer) Z74.2
      inability (any reason) of person
        rendering care Z74.2
  foundling Z76.1
  holiday relief Z75.5
  improper —*see* Maltreatment
  lack of (at or after birth) (infant) —*see*
    Maltreatment, child, neglect
  lactating mother Z39.1
  palliative Z51.5
  postpartum
    immediately after delivery Z39.0
    routine follow-up Z39.2
  respite Z75.5
  unavailable, due to
    absence of person rendering care Z74.2
    inability (any reason) of person rendering
      care Z74.2
  well-baby Z76.2
Caries
  bone NEC A18.03
  dental (dentino enamel junction) (early
    childhood) (of dentine) (pre-eruptive)
    (recurrent) (to the pulp) K02.9
    arrested (coronal) (root) K02.3
    chewing surface
      limited to enamel K02.51
      penetrating into dentin K02.52
      penetrating into pulp K02.53
    coronal surface
      chewing surface
        limited to enamel K02.51
        penetrating into dentin K02.52
        penetrating into pulp K02.53
      pit and fissure surface
        limited to enamel K02.51
        penetrating into dentin K02.52
        penetrating into pulp K02.53
      smooth surface
        limited to enamel K02.61
        penetrating into dentin K02.62
        penetrating into pulp K02.63
    pit and fissure surface
      limited to enamel K02.51
      penetrating into dentin K02.52
      penetrating into pulp K02.53

Caries (*Continued*)
  dental (*Continued*)
    primary, cervical origin K02.52
    root K02.7
    smooth surface
      limited to enamel K02.61
      penetrating into dentin K02.62
      penetrating into pulp K02.63
  external meatus —*see* Disorder, ear, external,
    specified type NEC
  hip (tuberculous) A18.02
  initial (tooth)
    chewing surface K02.51
    pit and fissure surface K02.51
    smooth surface K02.61
  knee (tuberculous) A18.02
  labyrinth —*see* subcategory H83.8
  limb NEC (tuberculous) A18.03
  mastoid process (chronic) —*see* Mastoiditis,
    chronic
    tuberculous A18.03
  middle ear —*see* subcategory H74.8
  nose (tuberculous) A18.03
  orbit (tuberculous) A18.03
  ossicles, ear —*see* Abnormal, ear ossicles
  petrous bone —*see* Petrositis
  root (dental) (tooth) K02.7
  sacrum (tuberculous) A18.01
  spine, spinal (column) (tuberculous) A18.01
  syphilitic A52.77
    congenital (early) A50.02 *[M90.80]*
  tooth, teeth —*see* Caries, dental
  tuberculous A18.03
  vertebra (column) (tuberculous) A18.01
Carious teeth —*see* Caries, dental
Carneous mole O02.0
Carnitine insufficiency E71.40
Carotenemia (dietary) E67.1
Carotenosis (cutis) (skin) E67.1
Carotid body or sinus syndrome G90.01
Carotidynia G90.01
Carpal tunnel syndrome —*see* Syndrome,
  carpal tunnel
Carpenter's syndrome Q87.0
Carpopedal spasm —*see* Tetany
Carr-Barr-Plunkett syndrome Q97.1
Carrier (suspected) of
  amebiasis Z22.1
  bacterial disease NEC Z22.39
    diphtheria Z22.2
    intestinal infectious NEC Z22.1
      typhoid Z22.0
    meningococcal Z22.31
    sexually transmitted Z22.4
    specified NEC Z22.39
    staphylococcal (Methicillin susceptible)
      Z22.321
      Methicillin resistant Z22.322
    streptococcal Z22.338
      group B Z22.330
        complicating pregnancy or delivery
          O99.82-●
    typhoid Z22.0
  cholera Z22.1
  diphtheria Z22.2
  gastrointestinal pathogens NEC Z22.1
  genetic Z14.8
    cystic fibrosis Z14.1
    hemophilia A (asymptomatic) Z14.01
      symptomatic Z14.02
  gestational, pregnant Z33.1
  gonorrhea Z22.4
  HAA (hepatitis Australian-antigen) B18.8
  HB (c)(s)-AG B18.1
  hepatitis (viral) B18.9
    Australia-antigen (HAA) B18.8
    B surface antigen (HBsAg) B18.1
      with acute delta- (super)infection B17.0
    C B18.2
    specified NEC B18.8
  human T-cell lymphotropic virus type-1
    (HTLV-1) infection Z22.6

Carrier of *(Continued)*
  infectious organism Z22.9
    specified NEC Z22.8
  meningococci Z22.31
  Salmonella typhosa Z22.0
  serum hepatitis —*see* Carrier, hepatitis
  staphylococci (Methicillin susceptible) Z22.321
    Methicillin resistant Z22.322
  streptococci Z22.338
    group B Z22.330
      complicating pregnancy or delivery
        O99.82-●
  syphilis Z22.4
  typhoid Z22.0
  venereal disease NEC Z22.4
Carrion's disease A44.0
Carter's relapsing fever (Asiatic) A68.1
Cartilage —*see* condition
Caruncle (inflamed)
  conjunctiva (acute) —*see* Conjunctivitis, acute
  labium (majus) (minus) N90.89
  lacrimal —*see* Inflammation, lacrimal,
    passages
  myrtiform N89.8
  urethral (benign) N36.2
Cascade stomach K31.2
Caseation lymphatic gland (tuberculous) A18.2
Cassidy (-Scholte) **syndrome** (malignant
    carcinoid) E34.0
Castellani's disease A69.8
Castration, traumatic, male S38.231
Casts in urine R82.998
Cat
  cry syndrome Q93.4
  ear Q17.3
  eye syndrome Q92.8
Catabolism, senile R54
Catalepsy (hysterical) F44.2
  schizophrenic F20.2
Cataplexy (idiopathic) —*see* Narcolepsy
Cataract (cortical) (immature) (incipient) H26.9
  with
    neovascularization —*see* Cataract,
      complicated
  age-related —*see* Cataract, senile
  anterior
    and posterior axial embryonal Q12.0
    pyramidal Q12.0
  associated with
    galactosemia E74.21 *[H28]*
    myotonic disorders G71.19 *[H28]*
  blue Q12.0
  central Q12.0
  cerulean Q12.0
  complicated H26.20
    with
      neovascularization H26.21-●
      ocular disorder H26.22-●
      glaucomatous flecks H26.23-●
  congenital Q12.0
  coraliform Q12.0
  coronary Q12.0
  crystalline Q12.0
  diabetic —*see* Diabetes, cataract
  drug-induced H26.3-●
  due to
    ocular disorder —*see* Cataract, complicated
    radiation H26.8
  electric H26.8
  extraction status Z98.4-●
  glass-blower's H26.8
  heat ray H26.8
  heterochromic —*see* Cataract, complicated
  hypermature —*see* Cataract, senile,
    morgagnian type
  in (due to)
    chronic iridocyclitis —*see* Cataract,
      complicated
    diabetes —*see* Diabetes, cataract
    endocrine disease E34.9 *[H28]*
    eye disease —*see* Cataract, complicated

Cataract *(Continued)*
  in (due to) *(Continued)*
    hypoparathyroidism E20.9 *[H28]*
    malnutrition-dehydration E46 *[H28]*
    metabolic disease E88.9 *[H28]*
    myotonic disorders G71.19 *[H28]*
    nutritional disease E63.9 *[H28]*
  infantile —*see* Cataract, presenile
  irradiational —*see* Cataract, specified NEC
  juvenile —*see* Cataract, presenile
  malnutrition-dehydration E46 *[H28]*
  morgagnian —*see* Cataract, senile,
    morgagnian type
  myotonic G71.19 *[H28]*
  myxedema E03.9 *[H28]*
  nuclear
    embryonal Q12.0
    sclerosis —*see* Cataract, senile, nuclear
  presenile H26.00-●
    combined forms H26.06-●
    cortical H26.01-●
    lamellar —*see* Cataract, presenile, cortical
    nuclear H26.03-●
    specified NEC H26.09
    subcapsular polar (anterior) H26.04-●
      posterior H26.05-●
    zonular —*see* Cataract, presenile, cortical
  secondary H26.40
    Soemmering's ring H26.41-●
    specified NEC H26.49-●
    to eye disease —*see* Cataract, complicated
  senile H25.9
    brunescens —*see* Cataract, senile, nuclear
    combined forms H25.81-●
    coronary —*see* Cataract, senile, incipient
    cortical H25.01-●
    hypermature —*see* Cataract, senile,
      morgagnian type
    incipient (mature) (total) H25.09-●
      cortical —*see* Cataract, senile, cortical
      subcapsular —*see* Cataract, senile,
        subcapsular
    morgagnian type (hypermature) H25.2-●
    nuclear (sclerosis) H25.1-●
    polar subcapsular (anterior) (posterior) —
      see Cataract, senile, incipient
    punctate —*see* Cataract, senile, incipient
    specified NEC H25.89
    subcapsular polar (anterior) H25.03-●
      posterior H25.04-●
  snowflake —*see* Diabetes, cataract
  specified NEC H26.8
  toxic —*see* Cataract, drug-induced
  traumatic H26.10-●
    localized H26.11-●
    partially resolved H26.12-●
    total H26.13-●
  zonular (perinuclear) Q12.0
Cataracta —*see also* Cataract
  brunescens —*see* Cataract, senile, nuclear
  centralis pulverulenta Q12.0
  cerulea Q12.0
  complicata —*see* Cataract, complicated
  congenita Q12.0
  coralliformis Q12.0
  coronaria Q12.0
  diabetic —*see* Diabetes, cataract
  membranacea
    accreta —*see* Cataract, secondary
    congenita Q12.0
  nigra —*see* Cataract, senile, nuclear
  sunflower —*see* Cataract, complicated
Catarrh, catarrhal (acute) (febrile) (infectious)
    (inflammation) (—*see also* condition) J00
  bronchial —*see* Bronchitis
  chest —*see* Bronchitis
  chronic J31.0
  due to congenital syphilis A50.03
  enteric —*see* Enteritis
  eustachian H68.009
  fauces —*see* Pharyngitis

Catarrh, catarrhal *(Continued)*
  gastrointestinal —*see* Enteritis
  gingivitis K05.00
    nonplaque induced K05.01
    plaque induced K05.00
  hay —*see* Fever, hay
  intestinal —*see* Enteritis
  larynx, chronic J37.0
  liver B15.9
    with hepatic coma B15.0
  lung —*see* Bronchitis
  middle ear, chronic —*see* Otitis, media,
    nonsuppurative, chronic, serous
  mouth K12.1
  nasal (chronic) —*see* Rhinitis
  nasobronchial J31.1
  nasopharyngeal (chronic) J31.1
    acute J00
  pulmonary —*see* Bronchitis
  spring (eye) (vernal) —*see* Conjunctivitis,
    acute, atopic
  summer (hay) —*see* Fever, hay
  throat J31.2
  tubotympanal —*see also* Otitis, media,
    nonsuppurative
    chronic —*see* Otitis, media,
      nonsuppurative, chronic, serous
Catatonia (schizophrenic) F20.2
Catatonic
  disorder due to known physiologic condition
    F06.1
  schizophrenia F20.2
  stupor R40.1
Cat-scratch —*see also* Abrasion
  disease or fever A28.1
Cauda equina —*see* condition
Cauliflower ear M95.1-●
Causalgia (upper limb) G56.4-●
  lower limb G57.7-●
Cause
  external, general effects T75.89
Caustic burn —*see* Corrosion, by site
Cavare's disease (familial periodic paralysis)
    G72.3
Cave-in, injury
  crushing (severe) —*see* Crush
  suffocation —*see* Asphyxia, traumatic, due to
    low oxygen, due to cave-in
Cavernitis (penis) N48.29
Cavernositis N48.29
Cavernous —*see* condition
Cavitation of lung —*see also* Tuberculosis,
    pulmonary
  nontuberculous J98.4
Cavities, dental —*see* Caries, dental
Cavity
  lung —*see* Cavitation of lung
  optic papilla Q14.2
  pulmonary —*see* Cavitation of lung
Cavovarus foot, congenital Q66.1-●
Cavus foot (congenital) Q66.7-●
  acquired —*see* Deformity, limb, foot, specified
    NEC
Cazenave's disease L10.2
CDKL5 (Cyclin-Dependent Kinase-Like 5
    Deficiency Disorder) G40.42
Cecitis K52.9
  with perforation, peritonitis, or rupture K65.8
Cecoureterocele Q62.32
Cecum —*see* condition
Celiac
  artery compression syndrome I77.4
  disease (with steatorrhea) K90.0
  infantilism K90.0
Cell(s), cellular (—*see also* condition
  in urine R82.998
Cellulitis (diffuse) (phlegmonous) (septic)
    (suppurative) L03.90
  abdominal wall L03.311
  anaerobic A48.0
  ankle —*see* Cellulitis, lower limb
  anus K61.0

▶ New   ⟹ Revised   ~~deleted~~ Deleted   ● Use Additional Character(s)

Cellulitis *(Continued)*
arm —*see* Cellulitis, upper limb
auricle (ear) —*see* Cellulitis, ear
axilla L03.11-•
back (any part) L03.312
breast (acute) (nonpuerperal) (subacute)
   N61.0
  nipple N61.0
broad ligament
  acute N73.0
buttock L03.317
cervical (meaning neck) L03.221
cervix (uteri) —*see* Cervicitis
cheek (external) L03.211
  internal K12.2
chest wall L03.313
chronic L03.90
clostridial A48.0
corpus cavernosum N48.22
digit
  finger —*see* Cellulitis, finger
  toe —*see* Cellulitis, toe
Douglas' cul-de-sac or pouch
  acute N73.0
drainage site (following operation) T81.49
ear (external) H60.1-•
eosinophilic (granulomatous) L98.3
erysipelatous —*see* Erysipelas
external auditory canal —*see* Cellulitis, ear
eyelid —*see* Abscess, eyelid
face NEC L03.211
finger (intrathecal) (periosteal)
  (subcutaneous) (subcuticular) L03.01-•
foot —*see* Cellulitis, lower limb
gangrenous —*see* Gangrene
genital organ NEC
  female (external) N76.4
  male N49.9
    multiple sites N49.8
    specified NEC N49.8
gluteal (region) L03.317
gonococcal A54.89
groin L03.314
hand —*see* Cellulitis, upper limb
head NEC L03.811
  face (any part, except ear, eye and nose)
    L03.211
heel —*see* Cellulitis, lower limb
hip —*see* Cellulitis, lower limb
jaw (region) L03.211
knee —*see* Cellulitis, lower limb
labium (majus) (minus) —*see* Vulvitis
lacrimal passages —*see* Inflammation,
  lacrimal, passages
larynx J38.7
leg —*see* Cellulitis, lower limb
lip K13.0
lower limb L03.11-•
  toe —*see* Cellulitis, toe
mouth (floor) K12.2
multiple sites, so stated L03.90
nasopharynx J39.1
navel L03.316
  newborn P38.9
    with mild hemorrhage P38.1
    without hemorrhage P38.9
neck (region) L03.221
nipple (acute) (nonpuerperal) (subacute) N61.0
nose (septum) (external) J34.0
orbit, orbital H05.01-•
palate (soft) K12.2
pectoral (region) L03.313
pelvis, pelvic (chronic)
  female —*see also* Disease, pelvis,
    inflammatory N73.2
    acute N73.0
  following ectopic or molar pregnancy O08.0
  male K65.0
penis N48.22
perineal, perineum L03.315
periorbital L03.213

Cellulitis *(Continued)*
perirectal K61.1
peritonsillar J36
periurethral N34.0
periuterine —*see also* Disease, pelvis,
  inflammatory N73.2
  acute N73.0
pharynx J39.1
preseptal L03.213
rectum K61.1
retroperitoneal K68.9
round ligament
  acute N73.0
scalp (any part) L03.811
scrotum N49.2
seminal vesicle N49.0
shoulder —*see* Cellulitis, upper limb
specified site NEC L03.818
submandibular (region) (space) (triangle)
  K12.2
  gland K11.3
submaxillary (region) K12.2
  gland K11.3
thigh —*see* Cellulitis, lower limb
thumb (intrathecal) (periosteal)
  (subcutaneous) (subcuticular) —*see*
  Cellulitis, finger
toe (intrathecal) (periosteal) (subcutaneous)
  (subcuticular) L03.03-•
tonsil J36
trunk L03.319
  abdominal wall L03.311
  back (any part) L03.312
  buttock L03.317
  chest wall L03.313
  groin L03.314
  perineal, perineum L03.315
  umbilicus L03.316
tuberculous (primary) A18.4
umbilicus L03.316
upper limb L03.11-•
  axilla —*see* Cellulitis, axilla
  finger —*see* Cellulitis, finger
  thumb —*see* Cellulitis, finger
vaccinal T88.0
vocal cord J38.3
vulva —*see* Vulvitis
wrist —*see* Cellulitis, upper limb
Cementoblastoma, benign —*see* Cyst,
  calcifying odontogenic
Cementoma —*see* Cyst, calcifying odontogenic
Cementoperiostitis —*see* Periodontitis
Cementosis K03.4
Central auditory processing disorder H93.25
Central pain syndrome G89.0
Cephalematocele, cephal (o)hematocele
  newborn P52.8
    birth injury P10.8
  traumatic —*see* Hematoma, brain
Cephalematoma, cephalhematoma (calcified)
  newborn (birth injury) P12.0
  traumatic —*see* Hematoma, brain
Cephalgia, cephalalgia —*see also* Headache
  histamine G44.009
    intractable G44.001
    not intractable G44.009
  trigeminal autonomic (TAC) NEC G44.099
    intractable G44.091
    not intractable G44.099
Cephalic —*see* condition
Cephalitis —*see* Encephalitis
Cephalocele —*see* Encephalocele
Cephalomenia N94.89
Cephalopelvic —*see* condition
Cerclage (with cervical incompetence) in
  pregnancy —*see* Incompetence, cervix, in
  pregnancy
Cerebellitis —*see* Encephalitis
Cerebellum, cerebellar —*see* condition
Cerebral —*see* condition
Cerebritis —*see* Encephalitis

Cerebro-hepato-renal syndrome Q87.89
Cerebromalacia —*see* Softening, brain
  sequelae of cerebrovascular disease I69.398
Cerebroside lipidosis E75.22
Cerebrospasticity (congenital) G80.1
Cerebrospinal —*see* condition
Cerebrum —*see* condition
Ceroid-lipofuscinosis, neuronal E75.4
Cerumen (accumulation) (impacted) H61.2-•
Cervical —*see also* condition
  auricle Q18.2
  dysplasia in pregnancy —*see* Abnormal,
    cervix, in pregnancy or childbirth
  erosion in pregnancy —*see* Abnormal, cervix,
    in pregnancy or childbirth
  fibrosis in pregnancy —*see* Abnormal, cervix,
    in pregnancy or childbirth
  fusion syndrome Q76.1
  rib Q76.5
  shortening (complicating pregnancy) O26.87-•
Cervicalgia M54.2
Cervicitis (acute) (chronic) (nonvenereal)
  (senile (atrophic)) (subacute) (with
  ulceration) N72
  with
    abortion —*see* Abortion, by type complicated
      by genital tract and pelvic infection
    ectopic pregnancy O08.0
    molar pregnancy O08.0
  chlamydial A56.09
  gonococcal A54.03
  herpesviral A60.03
  puerperal (postpartum) O86.11
  syphilitic A52.76
  trichomonal A59.09
  tuberculous A18.16
Cervicocolpitis (emphysematosa) (*see also*
  Cervicitis) N72
Cervix —*see* condition
Cesarean delivery, previous, affecting
  management of pregnancy O34.219
  classical (vertical) scar O34.212
  isthmocele O34.22
  low transverse scar O34.211
  mid-transverse T incision O34.218
  scar
    defect (isthmocele) O34.22
    specified type NEC O34.218
Céstan (-Chenais) **paralysis or syndrome** G46.3
Céstan-Raymond syndrome I65.8
Cestode infestation B71.9
  specified type NEC B71.8
Cestodiasis B71.9
Chabert's disease A22.9
Chacaleh E53.8
Chafing L30.4
Chagas' (-Mazza) **disease** (chronic) B57.2
  with
    cardiovascular involvement NEC B57.2
    digestive system involvement B57.30
      megacolon B57.32
      megaesophagus B57.31
      other specified B57.39
    megacolon B57.32
    megaesophagus B57.31
    myocarditis B57.2
    nervous system involvement B57.40
      meningitis B57.41
      meningoencephalitis B57.42
      other specified B57.49
    specified organ involvement NEC B57.5
  acute (with) B57.1
    cardiovascular NEC B57.0
    myocarditis B57.0
Chagres fever B50.9
Chairridden Z74.09
Chalasia (cardiac sphincter) K21.9
Chalazion H00.19
  left H00.16
    lower H00.15
    upper H00.14

Chalazion *(Continued)*
  right H00.13
    lower H00.12
    upper H00.11
Chalcosis —*see also* Disorder, globe,
    degenerative, chalcosis
  cornea —*see* Deposit, cornea
  crystalline lens —*see* Cataract, complicated
  retina H35.89
Chalicosis (pulmonum) J62.8
Chancre (any genital site) (hard) (hunterian)
    (mixed) (primary) (seronegative)
    (seropositive) (syphilitic) A51.0
  congenital A50.07
  conjunctiva NEC A51.2
  Ducrey's A57
  extragenital A51.2
  eyelid A51.2
  lip A51.2
  nipple A51.2
  Nisbet's A57
  of
    carate A67.0
    pinta A67.0
    yaws A66.0
  palate, soft A51.2
  phagedenic A57
  simple A57
  soft A57
    bubo A57
    palate A51.2
  urethra A51.0
  yaws A66.0
Chancroid (anus) (genital) (penis) (perineum)
    (rectum) (urethra) (vulva) A57
Chandler's disease (osteochondritis dissecans,
    hip) —*see* Osteochondritis, dissecans, hip
Change(s) (in) (of) —*see also* Removal
  arteriosclerotic —*see* Arteriosclerosis
  bone —*see also* Disorder, bone
    diabetic —*see* Diabetes, bone change
  bowel habit R19.4
  cardiorenal (vascular) —*see* Hypertension,
    cardiorenal
  cardiovascular —*see* Disease, cardiovascular
  circulatory I99.9
  cognitive (mild) (organic) R41.89
  color, tooth, teeth
    during formation K00.8
    posteruptive K03.7
  contraceptive device Z30.433
  corneal membrane H18.30
    Bowman's membrane fold or rupture
      H18.31-●
    Descemet's membrane
      fold H18.32-●
      rupture H18.33-●
  coronary —*see* Disease, heart, ischemic
  degenerative, spine or vertebra —*see*
    Spondylosis
  dental pulp, regressive K04.2
  dressing (nonsurgical) Z48.00
    surgical Z48.01
  heart —*see* Disease, heart
  hip joint —*see* Derangement, joint, hip
  hyperplastic larynx J38.7
  hypertrophic
    nasal sinus J34.89
    turbinate, nasal J34.3
    upper respiratory tract J39.8
  indwelling catheter Z46.6
  inflammatory —*see also* Inflammation
    sacroiliac M46.1
  job, anxiety concerning Z56.1
  joint —*see* Derangement, joint
  life —*see* Menopause
  mental status R41.82
  minimal (glomerular) —*see also* N00-N07
    with fourth character .0 N05.0
  myocardium, myocardial —*see* Degeneration,
    myocardial - of life —*see* Menopause
  pacemaker Z45.018
    pulse generator Z45.010

Change *(Continued)*
  personality (enduring) F68.8
    due to (secondary to)
      general medical condition F07.0
    secondary (nonspecific) F60.89
  regressive, dental pulp K04.2
  renal —*see* Disease, renal
  retina H35.9
    myopic —*see also* Myopia, degenerative
      H44.2-●
  sacroiliac joint M53.3
  senile —*see also* condition R54
  sensory R20.8
  skin R23.9
    acute, due to ultraviolet radiation L56.9
      specified NEC L56.8
    chronic, due to nonionizing radiation L57.9
      specified NEC L57.8
    cyanosis R23.0
    flushing R23.2
    pallor R23.1
    petechiae R23.3
    specified change NEC R23.8
    swelling —*see* Mass, localized
    texture R23.4
  trophic
    arm —*see* Mononeuropathy, upper limb
    leg —*see* Mononeuropathy, lower limb
  vascular I99.9
  vasomotor I73.9
  voice R49.9
    psychogenic F44.4
    specified NEC R49.8
Changing sleep-work schedule, affecting sleep
  G47.26
Changuinola fever A93.1
Chapping skin T69.8
Charcot-Marie-Tooth disease, paralysis or
  syndrome G60.0
Charcot's
  arthropathy —*see* Arthropathy, neuropathic
  cirrhosis K74.3
  disease (tabetic arthropathy) A52.16
  joint (disease) (tabetic) A52.16
    diabetic —*see* Diabetes, with, arthropathy
    syringomyelic G95.0
  syndrome (intermittent claudication) I73.9
CHARGE association Q89.8
Charley-horse (quadriceps) M62.831
  traumatic (quadriceps) S76.11-●
Charlouis' disease —*see* Yaws
Cheadle's disease E54
Checking (of)
  cardiac pacemaker (battery) (electrode(s))
    Z45.018
    pulse generator Z45.010
  implantable subdermal contraceptive Z30.46
  intrauterine contraceptive device Z30.431
  wound Z48.0-●
    due to injury - code to Injury, by site, using
      appropriate seventh character for
      subsequent encounter
Check-up —*see* Examination
Chédiak-Higashi (-Steinbrinck) syndrome
  (congenital gigantism of peroxidase
  granules) E70.330
Cheek —*see* condition
Cheese itch B88.0
Cheese-washer's lung J67.8
Cheese-worker's lung J67.8
Cheilitis (acute) (angular) (catarrhal) (chronic)
  (exfoliative) (gangrenous) (glandular)
  (infectional) (suppurative) (ulcerative)
  (vesicular) K13.0
  actinic (due to sun) L56.8
    other than from sun L59.8
  candidal B37.83
Cheilodynia K13.0
Cheiloschisis —*see* Cleft, lip
Cheilosis (angular) K13.0
  with pellagra E52
  due to
    vitamin B2 (riboflavin) deficiency E53.0

Cheiromegaly M79.89
Cheiropompholyx L30.1
Cheloid —*see* Keloid
Chemical burn —*see* Corrosion, by site
Chemodectoma —*see* Paraganglioma,
  nonchromaffin
Chemosis, conjunctiva —*see* Edema,
  conjunctiva
Chemotherapy (session) (for)
  cancer Z51.11
  neoplasm Z51.11
Cherubism M27.8
Chest —*see* condition
Cheyne-Stokes breathing (respiration) R06.3
Chiari's
  disease or syndrome (hepatic vein
    thrombosis) I82.0
  malformation
    type I G93.5
    type II —*see* Spina bifida
    net Q24.8
Chicago disease B40.9
Chickenpox —*see* Varicella
Chiclero ulcer or sore B55.1
Chigger (infestation) B88.0
Chignon (disease) B36.8
  newborn (from vacuum extraction) (birth
    injury) P12.1
Chilaiditi's syndrome (subphrenic
  displacement, colon) Q43.3
Chilblain(s) (lupus) T69.1
Child
  custody dispute Z65.3
Childbirth —*see* Delivery
Childhood
  cerebral X-linked adrenoleukodystrophy
    E71.520
  period of rapid growth Z00.2
Chill(s) R68.83
  with fever R50.9
  without fever R68.83
  congestive in malarial regions B54
Chilomastigiasis A07.8
Chimera 46,XX/46,XY Q99.0
Chin —*see* condition
Chinese dysentery A03.9
Chionophobia F40.228
Chitral fever A93.1
Chlamydia, chlamydial A74.9
  cervicitis A56.09
  conjunctivitis A74.0
  cystitis A56.01
  endometritis A56.11
  epididymitis A56.19
  female
    pelvic inflammatory disease A56.11
    pelviperitonitis A56.11
  orchitis A56.19
  peritonitis A74.81
  pharyngitis A56.4
  proctitis A56.3
  psittaci (infection) A70
  salpingitis A56.11
  sexually-transmitted infection NEC A56.8
  specified NEC A74.89
  urethritis A56.01
  vulvovaginitis A56.02
Chlamydiosis —*see* Chlamydia
Chloasma (skin) (idiopathic) (symptomatic)
  L81.1
  eyelid H02.719
    hyperthyroid E05.90 *[H02.719]*
      with thyroid storm E05.91 *[H02.719]*
    left H02.716
      lower H02.715
      upper H02.714
    right H02.713
      lower H02.712
      upper H02.711
Chloroma C92.3-●
Chlorosis D50.9
  Egyptian B76.9 *[D63.8]*
  miner's B76.9 *[D63.8]*

Chlorotic anemia D50.8
Chocolate cyst (ovary) N80.1
Choked
    disc or disk —see Papilledema
    on food, phlegm, or vomitus NOS —see
        Foreign body, by site
    while vomiting NOS —see Foreign body, by
        site
Chokes (resulting from bends) T70.3
Choking sensation R09.89
Cholangiectasis K83.8
Cholangiocarcinoma
    with hepatocellular carcinoma, combined
        C22.0
    liver C22.1
    specified site NEC —see Neoplasm,
        malignant, by site
    unspecified site C22.1
Cholangiohepatitis K83.8
    due to fluke infestation B66.1
Cholangiohepatoma C22.0
Cholangiolitis (acute) (chronic) (extrahepatic)
        (gangrenous) (intrahepatic) K83.09
    paratyphoidal —see Fever, paratyphoid
    typhoidal A01.09
Cholangioma D13.4
    malignant —see Cholangiocarcinoma
Cholangitis (ascending) (primary) (recurrent)
        (sclerosing) (secondary) (stenosing)
        (suppurative) K83.09
    with calculus, bile duct —see Calculus, bile
        duct, with cholangitis
    chronic nonsuppurative destructive K74.3
    primary K83.09
        sclerosing K83.01
    sclerosing K83.09
Cholecystectasia K82.8
Cholecystitis K81.9
    with
        calculus, stones in
            bile duct (common) (hepatic) —
                see Calculus, bile duct, with
                cholecystitis
            cystic duct —see Calculus, gallbladder,
                with cholecystitis
            gallbladder —see Calculus, gallbladder,
                with cholecystitis
        choledocholithiasis —see Calculus, bile
            duct, with cholecystitis
        cholelithiasis —see Calculus, gallbladder,
            with cholecystitis
        gangrene of gallbladder K82.A1
        perforation of gallbladder K82.A2
    acute (emphysematous) (gangrenous)
        (suppurative) K81.0
        with
            calculus, stones in
                cystic duct —see Calculus, gallbladder,
                    with cholecystitis, acute
                gallbladder —see Calculus, gallbladder,
                    with cholecystitis, acute
            choledocholithiasis —see Calculus, bile
                duct, with cholecystitis, acute
            cholelithiasis —see Calculus, gallbladder,
                with cholecystitis, acute
        chronic cholecystitis K81.2
            with gallbladder calculus K80.12
                with obstruction K80.13
    chronic K81.1
        with acute cholecystitis K81.2
            with gallbladder calculus K80.12
                with obstruction K80.13
    emphysematous (acute) —see Cholecystitis,
        acute
    gangrenous —see Cholecystitis, acute
    paratyphoidal, current A01.4
    suppurative —see Cholecystitis, acute
    typhoidal A01.09
Cholecystolithiasis —see Calculus, gallbladder
Choledochitis (suppurative) K83.09
Choledocholith —see Calculus, bile duct

Choledocholithiasis (common duct) (hepatic
        duct) —see Calculus, bile duct
    cystic —see Calculus, gallbladder
    typhoidal A01.09
Cholelithiasis (cystic duct) (gallbladder)
        (impacted) (multiple) —see Calculus,
        gallbladder
    bile duct (common) (hepatic) —see Calculus,
        bile duct
    hepatic duct —see Calculus, bile duct
    specified NEC K80.80
        with obstruction K80.81
Cholemia —see also Jaundice
    familial (simple) (congenital) E80.4
    Gilbert's E80.4
Choleperitoneum, choleperitonitis K65.3
Cholera (Asiatic) (epidemic) (malignant) A00.9
    antimonial —see Poisoning, antimony
    classical A00.0
    due to Vibrio cholerae 01 A00.9
        biovar cholerae A00.0
        biovar eltor A00.1
        el tor A00.1
    el tor A00.1
Cholerine —see Cholera
Cholestasis NEC K83.1
    with hepatocyte injury K71.0
    due to total parenteral nutrition (TPN) K76.89
    pure K71.0
Cholesteatoma (ear) (middle) (with reaction)
        H71.9-●
    attic H71.0-●
    external ear (canal) H60.4-●
    mastoid H71.2-●
    postmastoidectomy cavity (recurrent) —see
        Complications, postmastoidectomy,
        recurrent cholesteatoma
    recurrent (postmastoidectomy) —see
        Complications, postmastoidectomy,
        recurrent cholesteatoma
    tympanum H71.1-●
Cholesteatosis, diffuse H71.3-●
Cholesteremia E78.00
Cholesterin in vitreous —see Deposit, crystalline
Cholesterol
    deposit
        retina H35.89
        vitreous —see Deposit, crystalline
    elevated (high) E78.00
        with elevated (high) triglycerides E78.2
        screening for Z13.220
    imbibition of gallbladder K82.4
Cholesterolemia (essential) (pure) E78.00
    familial E78.01
    hereditary E78.01
Cholesterolosis, cholesterosis (gallbladder)
        K82.4
    cerebrotendinous E75.5
Cholocolic fistula K82.3
Choluria R82.2
Chondritis M94.8X9
    aurical H61.03-●
    costal (Tietze's) M94.0
    external ear H61.03-●
    patella, posttraumatic —see Chondromalacia,
        patella
    pinna H61.03-●
    purulent M94.8X-●
    tuberculous NEC A18.02
        intervertebral A18.01
Chondroblastoma —see also Neoplasm, bone,
        benign
    malignant —see Neoplasm, bone, malignant
Chondrocalcinosis M11.20
    ankle M11.27-●
    elbow M11.22-●
    familial M11.10
        ankle M11.17-●
        elbow M11.12-●
        foot joint M11.17-●
        hand joint M11.14-●

Chondrocalcinosis (Continued)
    familial (Continued)
        hip M11.15-●
        knee M11.16-●
        multiple site M11.19
        shoulder M11.11-●
        vertebrae M11.18
        wrist M11.13-●
    foot joint M11.27-●
    hand joint M11.24-●
    hip M11.25-●
    knee M11.26-●
    multiple site M11.29
    shoulder M11.21-●
    specified type NEC M11.20
        ankle M11.27-●
        elbow M11.22-●
        foot joint M11.27-●
        hand joint M11.24-●
        hip M11.25-●
        knee M11.26-●
        multiple site M11.29
        shoulder M11.21-●
        vertebrae M11.28
        wrist M11.23-●
    vertebrae M11.28
    wrist M11.23-●
Chondrodermatitis nodularis helicis or
        anthelicis —see Perichondritis, ear
Chondrodysplasia Q78.9
    with hemangioma Q78.4
    calcificans congenita Q77.3
    fetalis Q77.4
    metaphyseal (Jansen's) (McKusick's)
        (Schmid's) Q78.8
    punctata Q77.3
Chondrodystrophy, chondrodystrophia
        (familial) (fetalis) (hypoplastic) Q78.9
    calcificans congenita Q77.3
    myotonic (congenital) G71.13
    punctata Q77.3
Chondroectodermal dysplasia Q77.6
Chondrogenesis imperfecta Q77.4
Chondrolysis M94.35-●
Chondroma —see also Neoplasm, cartilage,
        benign
    juxtacortical —see Neoplasm, bone, benign
    periosteal —see Neoplasm, bone, benign
Chondromalacia (systemic) M94.20
    acromioclavicular joint M94.21-●
    ankle M94.27-●
    elbow M94.22-●
    foot joint M94.27-●
    glenohumeral joint M94.21-●
    hand joint M94.24-●
    hip M94.25-●
    knee M94.26-●
        patella M22.4-●
    multiple sites M94.29
    patella M22.4-●
    rib M94.28
    sacroiliac joint M94.259
    shoulder M94.21-●
    sternoclavicular joint M94.21-●
    vertebral joint M94.28
    wrist M94.23-●
Chondromatosis —see also Neoplasm, cartilage,
        uncertain behavior
    internal Q78.4
Chondromyxosarcoma —see Neoplasm,
        cartilage, malignant
Chondro-osteodysplasia (Morquio-Brailsford
        type) E76.219
Chondro-osteodystrophy E76.29
Chondro-osteoma —see Neoplasm, bone, benign
Chondropathia tuberosa M94.0
Chondrosarcoma —see Neoplasm, cartilage,
        malignant
    juxtacortical —see Neoplasm, bone, malignant
    mesenchymal —see Neoplasm, connective
        tissue, malignant
    myxoid —see Neoplasm, cartilage, malignant

Chordee (nonvenereal) N48.89
  congenital Q54.4
  gonococcal A54.09
Chorditis (fibrinous) (nodosa) (tuberosa) J38.2
Chordoma —see Neoplasm, vertebral (column),
    malignant
Chorea (chronic) (gravis) (posthemiplegic)
    (senile) (spasmodic) G25.5
  with
    heart involvement I02.0
      active or acute (conditions in I01-•) I02.0
        rheumatic I02.9
          with valvular disorder I02.0
      rheumatic heart disease (chronic) (inactive)
        (quiescent) — code to rheumatic heart
        condition involved
  drug-induced G25.4
  habit F95.8
  hereditary G10
  Huntington's G10
  hysterical F44.4
  minor I02.9
    with heart involvement I02.0
  progressive G25.5
    hereditary G10
  rheumatic (chronic) I02.9
    with heart involvement I02.0
  Sydenham's I02.9
    with heart involvement —see Chorea, with
      rheumatic heart disease
    nonrheumatic G25.5
Choreoathetosis (paroxysmal) G25.5
Chorioadenoma (destruens) D39.2
Chorioamnionitis O41.12-•
Chorioangioma D26.7
Choriocarcinoma —see Neoplasm, malignant,
    by site
  combined with
    embryonal carcinoma —see Neoplasm,
      malignant, by site
    other germ cell elements —see Neoplasm,
      malignant, by site
    teratoma —see Neoplasm, malignant, by site
  specified site —see Neoplasm, malignant, by
    site
  unspecified site
    female C58
    male C62.90
Chorioencephalitis (acute) (lymphocytic)
    (serous) A87.2
Chorioepithelioma —see Choriocarcinoma
Choriomeningitis (acute) (lymphocytic)
    (serous) A87.2
Chorionepithelioma —see Choriocarcinoma
Chorioretinitis —see also Inflammation,
    chorioretinal
  disseminated —see also Inflammation,
    chorioretinal, disseminated
    in neurosyphilis A52.19
  Egyptian B76.9 [D63.8]
  focal —see also Inflammation, chorioretinal,
    focal
  histoplasmic B39.9 [H32]
  in (due to)
    histoplasmosis B39.9 [H32]
    syphilis (secondary) A51.43
      late A52.71
    toxoplasmosis (acquired) B58.01
      congenital (active) P37.1 [H32]
    tuberculosis A18.53
  juxtapapillary, juxtapapillaris —see
    Inflammation, chorioretinal, focal,
    juxtapapillary
  leprous A30.9 [H32]
  miner's B76.9 [D63.8]
  progressive myopia (degeneration) —see also
    Myopia, degenerative H44.2-•
  syphilitic (secondary) A51.43
    congenital (early) A50.01 [H32]
      late A50.32
    late A52.71
  tuberculous A18.53

Chorioretinopathy, central serous H35.71-•
Choroid —see condition
Choroideremia H31.21
Choroiditis —see Chorioretinitis
Choroidopathy —see Disorder, choroid
Choroidoretinitis —see Chorioretinitis
Choroidoretinopathy, central serous —see
    Chorioretinopathy, central serous
Christian-Weber disease M35.6
Christmas disease D67
Chromaffinoma —see also Neoplasm, benign,
    by site
  malignant —see Neoplasm, malignant, by site
Chromatopsia —see Deficiency, color vision
Chromhidrosis, chromidrosis L75.1
Chromoblastomycosis —see Chromomycosis
Chromoconversion R82.91
Chromomycosis B43.9
  brain abscess B43.1
  cerebral B43.1
  cutaneous B43.0
  skin B43.0
  specified NEC B43.8
  subcutaneous abscess or cyst B43.2
Chromophytosis B36.0
Chromosome —see condition by chromosome
    involved
  D (1) —see condition, chromosome 13
  E (3) —see condition, chromosome 18
  G —see condition, chromosome 21
Chromotrichomycosis B36.8
Chronic —see condition
  fracture —see Fracture, pathological
Churg-Strauss syndrome M30.1
Chyle cyst, mesentery I89.8
Chylocele (nonfilarial) I89.8
  filarial —see also Infestation, filarial B74.9
    [N51]
  tunica vaginalis N50.89
    filarial —see also Infestation, filarial B74.9
      [N51]
Chylomicronemia (fasting) (with
    hyperprebetalipoproteinemia) E78.3
Chylopericardium I31.3
  acute I30.9
⇒ Chylothorax (nonfilarial) J94.0
  filarial —see also Infestation, filarial B74.9 [J91.8]
Chylous —see condition
Chyluria (nonfilarial) R82.0
  due to
    bilharziasis B65.0
    Brugia (malayi) B74.1
      timori B74.2
    schistosomiasis (bilharziasis) B65.0
    Wuchereria (bancrofti) B74.0
  filarial —see Infestation, filarial
Cicatricial (deformity) —see Cicatrix
Cicatrix (adherent) (contracted) (painful)
    (vicious) —see also Scar L90.5
  adenoid (and tonsil) J35.8
  alveolar process M26.79
  anus K62.89
  auricle —see Disorder, pinna, specified type
    NEC
  bile duct (common) (hepatic) K83.8
  bladder N32.89
  bone —see Disorder, bone, specified type NEC
  brain G93.89
  cervix (postoperative) (postpartal) N88.1
  common duct K83.8
  cornea H17.9
    tuberculous A18.59
  duodenum (bulb), obstructive K31.5
  esophagus K22.2
  eyelid —see Disorder, eyelid function
  hypopharynx J39.2
  lacrimal passages —see Obstruction, lacrimal
  larynx J38.7
  lung J98.4
  middle ear —see subcategory H74.8
  mouth K13.79

Cicatrix (Continued)
  muscle M62.89
    with contracture —see Contraction, muscle
      NEC
  nasopharynx J39.2
  palate (soft) K13.79
  penis N48.89
  pharynx J39.2
  prostate N42.89
  rectum K62.89
  retina —see Scar, chorioretinal
  semilunar cartilage —see Derangement,
    meniscus
  seminal vesicle N50.89
  skin L90.5
    infected L08.89
    postinfective L90.5
    tuberculous B90.8
  specified site NEC L90.5
  throat J39.2
  tongue K14.8
  tonsil (and adenoid) J35.8
  trachea J39.8
  tuberculous NEC B90.9
  urethra N36.8
  uterus N85.8
  vagina N89.8
    postoperative N99.2
  vocal cord J38.3
  wrist, constricting (annular) L90.5
CIDP (chronic inflammatory demyelinating
    polyneuropathy) G61.81
CIN —see Neoplasia, intraepithelial, cervix
CINCA (chronic infantile neurological,
    cutaneous and articular syndrome)
    M04.2
Cinchonism —see Deafness, ototoxic
  correct substance properly administered —see
    Table of Drugs and Chemicals, by drug,
    adverse effect
  overdose or wrong substance given
    or taken —see Table of Drugs and
    Chemicals, by drug, poisoning
Circle of Willis —see condition
Circular —see condition
Circulating anticoagulants —see also - Disorder,
    hemorrhagic D68.318
  due to drugs —see also - Disorder,
    hemorrhagic D68.32
  following childbirth O72.3
Circulation
  collateral, any site I99.8
  defective (lower extremity) I99.9
    congenital Q28.9
  embryonic Q28.9
  failure (peripheral) R57.9
    newborn P29.89
  fetal, persistent P29.38
  heart, incomplete Q28.9
Circulatory system —see condition
Circulus senilis (cornea) —see Degeneration,
    cornea, senile
Circumcision (in absence of medical indication)
    (ritual) (routine) Z41.2
Circumscribed —see condition
Circumvallate placenta O43.11-•
Cirrhosis, cirrhotic (hepatic) (liver) K74.60
  alcoholic K70.30
    with ascites K70.31
  atrophic —see Cirrhosis, liver
  Baumgarten-Cruveilhier K74.69
  biliary (cholangiolitic) (cholangitic)
    (hypertrophic) (obstructive)
    (pericholangiolitic) K74.5
    due to
      Clonorchiasis B66.1
      flukes B66.3
    primary K74.3
    secondary K74.4
  cardiac (of liver) K76.1
  Charcot's K74.3

▶ New   ⇒ Revised   deleted Deleted   • Use Additional Character(s)

Cirrhosis, cirrhotic *(Continued)*
  cholangiolitic, cholangitic, cholestatic
      (primary) K74.3
  congestive K76.1
  Cruveilhier-Baumgarten K74.69
  cryptogenic (liver) K74.69
  due to
      hepatolenticular degeneration E83.01
      Wilson's disease E83.01
      xanthomatosis E78.2
  fatty K76.0
      alcoholic K70.0
  Hanot's (hypertrophic) K74.3
  hepatic —*see* Cirrhosis, liver
  hypertrophic K74.3
  Indian childhood K74.69
  kidney —*see* Sclerosis, renal
  Laennec's K70.30
      with ascites K70.31
      alcoholic K70.30
          with ascites K70.31
      nonalcoholic K74.69
  liver K74.60
      alcoholic K70.30
          with ascites K70.31
      fatty K70.0
      congenital P78.81
      syphilitic A52.74
  lung (chronic) J84.10
  macronodular K74.69
      alcoholic K70.30
          with ascites K70.31
  micronodular K74.69
      alcoholic K70.30
          with ascites K70.31
  mixed type K74.69
  monolobular K74.3
  nephritis —*see* Sclerosis, renal
  nutritional K74.69
      alcoholic K70.30
          with ascites K70.31
  obstructive —*see* Cirrhosis, biliary
  ovarian N83.8
  pancreas (duct) K86.89
  pigmentary E83.110
  portal K74.69
      alcoholic K70.30
          with ascites K70.31
  postnecrotic K74.69
      alcoholic K70.30
          with ascites K70.31
  pulmonary J84.10
  renal —*see* Sclerosis, renal
  spleen D73.2
  stasis K76.1
  Todd's K74.3
  unilobar K74.3
  xanthomatous (biliary) K74.5
      due to xanthomatosis (familial) (metabolic)
          (primary) E78.2
Cistern, subarachnoid R93.0
Citrullinemia E72.23
Citrullinuria E72.23
Civatte's disease or poikiloderma L57.3
Clam digger's itch B65.3
Clammy skin R23.1
Clap —*see* Gonorrhea
Clarke-Hadfield syndrome (pancreatic
      infantilism) K86.89
Clark's paralysis G80.9
Clastothrix L67.8
Claude Bernard-Horner syndrome G90.2
  traumatic —*see* Injury, nerve, cervical
      sympathetic
Claude's disease or syndrome G46.3
Claudicatio venosa intermittens I87.8
Claudication (intermittent) I73.9
  cerebral (artery) G45.9
  spinal cord (arteriosclerotic) G95.19
      syphilitic A52.09
  venous (axillary) I87.8

Claustrophobia F40.240
Clavus (infected) L84
Clawfoot (congenital) Q66.89
  acquired —*see* Deformity, limb, clawfoot
Clawhand (acquired) —*see also* Deformity, limb,
      clawhand
  congenital Q68.1
Clawtoe (congenital) Q66.89
  acquired —*see* Deformity, toe, specified NEC
Clay eating —*see* Pica
Cleansing of artificial opening —*see* Attention
      to, artificial, opening
Cleft (congenital) —*see also* Imperfect, closure
  alveolar process M26.79
  branchial (persistent) Q18.2
  cyst Q18.0
      fistula Q18.0
      sinus Q18.0
  cricoid cartilage, posterior Q31.8
  foot Q72.7
  hand Q71.6
  lip (unilateral) Q36.9
      with cleft palate Q37.9
          hard Q37.1
              with soft Q37.5
          soft Q37.3
              with hard Q37.5
      bilateral Q36.0
          with cleft palate Q37.8
              hard Q37.0
                  with soft Q37.4
              soft Q37.2
                  with hard Q37.4
      median Q36.1
  nose Q30.2
  palate Q35.9
      with cleft lip (unilateral) Q37.9
          bilateral Q37.8
      hard Q35.1
          with
              cleft lip (unilateral) Q37.1
                  bilateral Q37.0
              soft Q35.5
                  with cleft lip (unilateral) Q37.5
                      bilateral Q37.4
      medial Q35.5
      soft Q35.3
          with
              cleft lip (unilateral) Q37.3
                  bilateral Q37.2
              hard Q35.5
                  with cleft lip (unilateral) Q37.5
                      bilateral Q37.4
  penis Q55.69
  scrotum Q55.29
  thyroid cartilage Q31.8
  uvula Q35.7
Cleidocranial dysostosis Q74.0
Cleptomania F63.2
Clicking hip (newborn) R29.4
Climacteric (female) —*see also* Menopause
  arthritis (any site) NEC —*see* Arthritis,
      specified form NEC
  depression (single episode) F32.89
      recurrent episode F33.8
  male (symptoms) (syndrome) NEC N50.89
  melancholia (single episode) F32.89
      recurrent episode F33.8
  paranoid state F22
  polyarthritis NEC —*see* Arthritis, specified
      form NEC
  symptoms (female) N95.1
Clinical research investigation (clinical trial)
      (control subject) (normal comparison)
      (participant) Z00.6
Clitoris —*see* condition Cloaca (persistent)
      Q43.7
Clonorchiasis, clonorchis infection (liver)
      B66.1
Clonus R25.8
Closed bite M26.29

Clostridium (C.) perfringens, as cause of
      disease classified elsewhere B96.7
Closure
  congenital, nose Q30.0
  cranial sutures, premature Q75.0
  defective or imperfect NEC —*see* Imperfect,
      closure
  fistula, delayed —*see* Fistula
  foramen ovale, imperfect Q21.1
  hymen N89.6
  interauricular septum, defective Q21.1
  interventricular septum, defective Q21.0
  lacrimal duct —*see also* Stenosis, lacrimal,
      duct
      congenital Q10.5
  nose (congenital) Q30.0
      acquired M95.0
  of artificial opening —*see* Attention to,
      artificial, opening
  primary angle, without glaucoma damage
      H40.06-•
  vagina N89.5
  valve —*see* Endocarditis
  vulva N90.5
Clot (blood) —*see also* Embolism
  artery (obstruction) (occlusion) —*see*
      Embolism
  bladder N32.89
  brain (intradural or extradural) —*see*
      Occlusion, artery, cerebral
  circulation I74.9
  heart —*see also* Infarct, myocardium
      not resulting in infarction I51.3
  vein —*see* Thrombosis
Clouded state R40.1
  epileptic —*see* Epilepsy, specified NEC
  paroxysmal —*see* Epilepsy, specified NEC
Cloudy antrum, antra J32.0
Clouston's (hidrotic) ectodermal dysplasia
      Q82.4
Clubbed nail pachydermoperiostosis M89.40
      [L62]
Clubbing of finger(s) (nails) R68.3
Clubfinger R68.3
  congenital Q68.1
Clubfoot (congenital) Q66.89
  acquired —*see* Deformity, limb, clubfoot
  equinovarus Q66.0-•
  paralytic —*see* Deformity, limb, clubfoot
Clubhand (congenital) (radial) Q71.4-•
  acquired —*see* Deformity, limb, clubhand
Clubnail R68.3
  congenital Q84.6
Clump, kidney Q63.1
Clumsiness, clumsy child syndrome F82
Cluttering F98.81
Clutton's joints A50.51 [M12.80]
Coagulation, intravascular (diffuse)
      (disseminated) —*see also* Defibrination
      syndrome
  complicating abortion —*see* Abortion, by
      type, complicated by, intravascular
      coagulation
  following ectopic or molar pregnancy
      O08.1
Coagulopathy —*see also* Defect, coagulation
  consumption D65
  intravascular D65
  newborn P60
Coalition
  calcaneo-scaphoid Q66.89
  tarsal Q66.89
Coalminer's
  elbow —*see* Bursitis, elbow, olecranon
  lung or pneumoconiosis J60
Coalworker's lung or pneumoconiosis
      J60
Coarctation
  aorta (preductal) (postductal) Q25.1
  pulmonary artery Q25.71
Coated tongue K14.3

Coats' disease (exudative retinopathy) —see Retinopathy, exudative
Cocaine-induced
  anxiety disorder F14.980
  bipolar and related disorder F14.94
  depressive disorder F14.94
  obsessive-compulsive and related disorder F14.988
  psychotic disorder F14.959
  sleep disorder F14.982
  sexual dysfunction F14.981
Cocainism —see Disorder, cocaine use
Coccidioidomycosis B38.9
  cutaneous B38.3
  disseminated B38.7
  generalized B38.7
  meninges B38.4
  prostate B38.81
  pulmonary B38.2
    acute B38.0
    chronic B38.1
  skin B38.3
  specified NEC B38.89
Coccidioidosis —see Coccidioidomycosis
Coccidiosis (intestinal) A07.3
Coccydynia, coccygodynia M53.3
Coccyx —see condition
Cochin-China diarrhea K90.1
Cockayne's syndrome Q87.19
Cocked up toe —see Deformity, toe, specified NEC
Cock's peculiar tumor L72.3
Codman's tumor —see Neoplasm, bone, benign
Coenurosis B71.8
Coffee-worker's lung J67.8
Cogan's syndrome H16.32-●
  oculomotor apraxia H51.8
Coitus, painful (female) N94.10
  male N53.12
  psychogenic F52.6
Cold J00
  with influenza, flu, or grippe —see Influenza, with, respiratory manifestations NEC
  agglutinin disease or hemoglobinuria (chronic) D59.12
  bronchial —see Bronchitis
  chest —see Bronchitis
  common (head) J00
  effects of T69.9
    specified effect NEC T69.8
  excessive, effects of T69.9
    specified effect NEC T69.8
  exhaustion from T69.8
  exposure to T69.9
    specified effect NEC T69.8
  head J00
  injury syndrome (newborn) P80.0
  on lung —see Bronchitis
  rose J30.1
  sensitivity, auto-immune D59.12
  symptoms J00
  virus J00
Coldsore B00.1
Colibacillosis A49.8
  as the cause of other disease (see also Escherichia coli) B96.20
  generalized A41.50
Colic (bilious) (infantile) (intestinal) (recurrent) (spasmodic) R10.83
  abdomen R10.83
    psychogenic F45.8
  appendix, appendicular K38.8
  bile duct —see Calculus, bile duct
  biliary —see Calculus, bile duct
  common duct —see Calculus, bile duct
  cystic duct —see Calculus, gallbladder
  Devonshire NEC —see Poisoning, lead
  gallbladder —see Calculus, gallbladder
  gallstone —see Calculus, gallbladder
    gallbladder or cystic duct —see Calculus, gallbladder

Colic (Continued)
  hepatic (duct) —see Calculus, bile duct
  hysterical F45.8
  kidney N23
  lead NEC —see Poisoning, lead
  mucous K58.9
    with diarrhea K58.0
    psychogenic F54
  nephritic N23
  painter's NEC —see Poisoning, lead
  pancreas K86.89
  psychogenic F45.8
  renal N23
  saturnine NEC —see Poisoning, lead
  ureter N23
  urethral N36.8
    due to calculus N21.1
  uterus NEC N94.89
    menstrual —see Dysmenorrhea
  worm NOS B83.9
Colicystitis —see Cystitis
Colitis (acute) (catarrhal) (chronic) (noninfective) (hemorrhagic) (see also Enteritis) K52.9
  allergic K52.29
    with
      food protein-induced enterocolitis syndrome K52.21
      ⟣proctocolitis K52.29
  amebic (acute) —see also Amebiasis A06.0
    nondysenteric A06.2
  anthrax A22.2
  bacillary —see Infection, Shigella
  balantidial A07.0
  Clostridium difficile
    not specified as recurrent A04.72
    recurrent A04.71
  coccidial A07.3
  collagenous K52.831
  cystica superficialis K52.89
  dietary counseling and surveillance (for) Z71.3
  dietetic —see also Colitis, allergic K52.29
  drug-induced K52.1
  due to radiation K52.0
  eosinophilic K52.82
  food hypersensitivity —see also Colitis, allergic K52.29
  giardial A07.1
  granulomatous —see Enteritis, regional, large intestine
  infectious —see Enteritis, infectious
  indeterminate, so stated K52.3
  ischemic K55.9
    acute (subacute) —see also Ischemia, intestine, acute K55.039
    chronic K55.1
    due to mesenteric artery insufficiency K55.1
    fulminant (acute) —see also Ischemia, intestine, acute K55.039
  left sided K51.50
    with
      abscess K51.514
      complication K51.519
        specified NEC K51.518
      fistula K51.513
      obstruction K51.512
      rectal bleeding K51.511
  lymphocytic K52.832
  membranous
    psychogenic F54
  microscopic K52.839
    specified NEC K52.838
  mucous —see Syndrome, irritable, bowel
    psychogenic F54
  noninfective K52.9
    specified NEC K52.89
  polyposa —see Polyp, colon, inflammatory
  protozoal A07.9
  pseudomembranous
    not specified as recurrent A04.72
    recurrent A04.71

Colitis (Continued)
  pseudomucinous —see Syndrome, irritable, bowel
  regional —see Enteritis, regional, large intestine
    infectious A09
  segmental —see Enteritis, regional, large intestine
  septic —see Enteritis, infectious
  spastic K58.9
    with diarrhea K58.0
    psychogenic F54
  staphylococcal A04.8
    foodborne A05.0
  subacute ischemic —see also Ischemia, intestine, acute K55.039
  thromboulcerative —see also Ischemia, intestine, acute K55.039
  toxic NEC K52.1
    due to Clostridium difficile
      not specified as recurrent A04.72
      recurrent A04.71
  transmural —see Enteritis, regional, large intestine
  trichomonal A07.8
  tuberculous (ulcerative) A18.32
  ulcerative (chronic) K51.90
    with
      complication K51.919
        abscess K51.914
        fistula K51.913
        obstruction K51.912
        rectal bleeding K51.911
        specified complication NEC K51.918
    enterocolitis —see Enterocolitis, ulcerative
    ileocolitis —see Ileocolitis, ulcerative
    mucosal proctocolitis —see Proctocolitis, mucosal
    proctitis —see Proctitis, ulcerative
    pseudopolyposis —see Polyp, colon, inflammatory
    psychogenic F54
    rectosigmoiditis —see Rectosigmoiditis, ulcerative
    specified type NEC K51.80
      with
        complication K51.819
          abscess K51.814
          fistula K51.813
          obstruction K51.812
          rectal bleeding K51.811
          specified complication NEC K51.818
Collagenosis, collagen disease (nonvascular) (vascular) M35.9
  cardiovascular I42.8
  reactive perforating L87.1
  specified NEC M35.89
Collapse R55
  adrenal E27.2
  cardiorespiratory R57.0
  cardiovascular R57.0
    newborn P29.89
  circulatory (peripheral) R57.9
    during or after labor and delivery O75.1
    following ectopic or molar pregnancy O08.3
    newborn P29.89
  during or
    after labor and delivery O75.1
    resulting from a procedure, not elsewhere classified T81.10
  external ear canal —see Stenosis, external ear canal
  general R55
  heart —see Disease, heart
  heat T67.1
  hysterical F44.89
  labyrinth, membranous (congenital) Q16.5
  lung (massive) —see also Atelectasis J98.19
    pressure due to anesthesia (general) (local) or other sedation T88.2
    during labor and delivery O74.1
    in pregnancy O29.02-●
    postpartum, puerperal O89.09

Collapse (Continued)
  myocardial —see Disease, heart
  nervous F48.8
  neurocirculatory F45.8
  nose M95.0
  postoperative T81.10
  pulmonary —see also Atelectasis J98.19
    newborn —see Atelectasis
  trachea J39.8
  tracheobronchial J98.09
  valvular —see Endocarditis
  vascular (peripheral) R57.9
    during or after labor and delivery O75.1
    following ectopic or molar pregnancy O08.3
    newborn P29.89
  vertebra M48.50-●
    cervical region M48.52-●
    cervicothoracic region M48.53-●
    in (due to)
      metastasis —see Collapse, vertebra, in,
          specified disease NEC
      osteoporosis —see also Osteoporosis
          M80.88
        cervical region M80.88
        cervicothoracic region M80.88
        lumbar region M80.88
        lumbosacral region M80.88
        multiple sites M80.88
        occipito-atlanto-axial region M80.88
        sacrococcygeal region M80.88
        thoracic region M80.88
        thoracolumbar region M80.88
      specified disease NEC M48.50-●
        cervical region M48.52-●
        cervicothoracic region M48.53-●
        lumbar region M48.56-●
        lumbosacral region M48.57-●
        occipito-atlanto-axial region M48.51-●
        sacrococcygeal region M48.58-●
        thoracic region M48.54-●
        thoracolumbar region M48.55-●
    lumbar region M48.56-●
    lumbosacral region M48.57-●
    occipito-atlanto-axial region M48.51-●
    sacrococcygeal region M48.58-●
    thoracic region M48.54-●
    thoracolumbar region M48.55-●
Collateral —see also condition
  circulation (venous) I87.8
  dilation, veins I87.8
Colles' fracture S52.53-●
Collet (-Sicard) syndrome G52.7
Collier's asthma or lung J60
Collodion baby Q80.2
Colloid nodule (of thyroid) (cystic) E04.1
Coloboma (iris) Q13.0
  eyelid Q10.3
  fundus Q14.8
  lens Q12.2
  optic disc (congenital) Q14.2
    acquired H47.31-●
Coloenteritis —see Enteritis
Colon —see condition
Colonization
  MRSA (Methicillin resistant Staphylococcus
      aureus) Z22.322
  MSSA (Methicillin susceptible
      Staphylococcus aureus) Z22.321
  status —see Carrier (suspected) of
Coloptosis K63.4
Color blindness —see Deficiency, color vision
Colostomy
  attention to Z43.3
  fitting or adjustment Z46.89
  malfunctioning K94.03
  status Z93.3
Colpitis (acute) —see Vaginitis
Colpocele N81.5
Colpocystitis —see Vaginitis
Colpospasm N94.2
Column, spinal, vertebral —see condition

Coma R40.20
  with
    motor response (none) R40.231
      abnormal R40.233
      abnormal extensor posturing to pain or
          noxious stimuli (<2 years of age)
          R40.232
      abnormal flexure posturing to pain or
          noxious stimuli (0-5 years of age)
          R40.233
      extension R40.232
      extensor posturing to pain or noxious
          stimuli (2-5 years of age) R40.232
      flexion/decorticate posturing
          (<2 years of age) R40.233
      flexion withdrawal R40.234
      localizes pain (2-5 years of age) R40.235
      normal or spontaneous movement
          (<2 years of age) R40.236
      obeys commands (2-5 years of age)
          R40.236
      score of
        1 R40.231
        2 R40.232
        3 R40.233
        4 R40.234
        5 R40.235
        6 R40.236
      withdraws from pain or noxious stimuli
          (0-5 years of age) R40.234
      withdraws to touch (<2 years of age)
          R40.235
    opening of eyes (never) R40.211
      in response to
        pain R40.212
        sound R40.213
      score of
        1 R40.211
        2 R40.212
        3 R40.213
        4 R40.214
      spontaneous R40.214
    verbal response (none) R40.221
      confused conversation R40.224
      cooing or babbling or crying
          appropriately (<2 years of age)
          R40.225
      inappropriate crying or screaming
          (<2 years of age) R40.223
      inappropriate words R40.223
      inappropriate words (2-5 years of age)
          R40.224
      incomprehensible sounds (2-5 years of
          age) R40.222
      incomprehensible words R40.222
      irritable cries (<2 years of age) R40.224
      moans/grunts to pain; restless
          (<2 years old) R40.222
      oriented R40.225
      score of
        1 R40.221
        2 R40.222
        3 R40.223
        4 R40.224
        5 R40.225
      screaming (2-5 years of age) R40.223
      uses appropriate words (2-5 years of
          age) R40.225
  eclamptic —see Eclampsia
  epileptic —see Epilepsy
  Glasgow, scale score —see Glasgow coma
      scale
  hepatic —see Failure, hepatic, by type, with
      coma
  hyperglycemic (diabetic) —see Diabetes, by
      type, with hyperosmolarity, with coma
  hyperosmolar (diabetic) —see Diabetes, by
      type, with hyperosmolarity, with coma
  hypoglycemic (diabetic) —see Diabetes, by
      type, with hypoglycemia, with coma
      nondiabetic E15

Coma (Continued)
  in diabetes —see Diabetes, coma
  insulin-induced —see Coma, hypoglycemic
  ketoacidotic (diabetic) —see Diabetes, by
      type, with ketoacidosis, with coma
  myxedematous E03.5
  newborn P91.5
  persistent vegetative state R40.3
  specified NEC, without documented
      Glasgow coma scale score, or with
      partial Glasgow coma scale score
      reported R40.244
Comatose —see Coma
Combat fatigue F43.0
Combined —see condition
Comedo, comedones (giant) L70.0
Comedocarcinoma —see also Neoplasm, breast,
    malignant
  noninfiltrating
    breast D05.8-●
    specified site —see Neoplasm, in situ, by site
    unspecified site D05.8-●
Comedomastitis —see Ectasia, mammary duct
Comminuted fracture - code as Fracture, closed
Common
  arterial trunk Q20.0
  atrioventricular canal Q21.2
  atrium Q21.1
  cold (head) J00
  truncus (arteriosus) Q20.0 —see
  variable immunodeficiency —see
      Immunodeficiency, common variable
  ventricle Q20.4
Commotio, commotion (current)
  brain —see Injury, intracranial, concussion
  cerebri —see Injury, intracranial, concussion
  retinae S05.8X-●
  spinal cord —see Injury, spinal cord, by region
  spinalis —see Injury, spinal cord, by region
Communication
  between
    base of aorta and pulmonary artery Q21.4
    left ventricle and right atrium Q20.5
    pericardial sac and pleural sac Q34.8
    pulmonary artery and pulmonary vein,
        congenital Q25.72
  congenital between uterus and digestive or
      urinary tract Q51.7
Compartment syndrome (deep) (posterior)
    (traumatic) T79.A0
  abdomen T79.A3
  lower extremity (hip, buttock, thigh, leg, foot,
      toes) T79.A2
  nontraumatic
    abdomen M79.A3
    lower extremity (hip, buttock, thigh, leg,
        foot, toes) M79.A2-●
    specified site NEC M79.A9
    upper extremity (shoulder, arm, forearm,
        wrist, hand, fingers) M79.A1-●
  specified site NEC T79.A9
  upper extremity (shoulder, arm, forearm,
      wrist, hand, fingers) T79.A1
Compensation
  failure —see Disease, heart
  neurosis, psychoneurosis —see Disorder,
      factitious
Complaint —see also Disease
  bowel, functional K59.9
    psychogenic F45.8
  intestine, functional K59.9
    psychogenic F45.8
  kidney —see Disease, renal
  miners' J60
Complete —see condition
Complex
  Addison-Schilder E71.528
  cardiorenal —see Hypertension, cardiorenal
  Costen's M26.69
  disseminated mycobacterium avium-
      intracellulare (DMAC) A31.2

Complex (Continued)
Eisenmenger's (ventricular septal defect) I27.83
hypersexual F52.8
jumped process, spine —see Dislocation,
  vertebra
primary, tuberculous A15.7
Schilder-Addison E71.528
subluxation (vertebral) M99.19
  abdomen M99.19
  acromioclavicular M99.17
  cervical region M99.11
  cervicothoracic M99.11
  costochondral M99.18
  costovertebral M99.18
  head region M99.10
  hip M99.15
  lower extremity M99.16
  lumbar region M99.13
  lumbosacral M99.13
  occipitocervical M99.10
  pelvic region M99.15
  pubic M99.15
  rib cage M99.18
  sacral region M99.14
  sacrococcygeal M99.14
  sacroiliac M99.14
  specified NEC M99.19
  sternochondral M99.18
  sternoclavicular M99.17
  thoracic region M99.12
  thoracolumbar M99.12
  upper extremity M99.17
Taussig-Bing (transposition, aorta and
  overriding pulmonary artery) Q20.1
Complication(s) (from) (of)
accidental puncture or laceration during
  a procedure (of) —see Complications,
  intraoperative (intraprocedural),
  puncture or laceration
amputation stump (surgical) (late) NEC T87.9
  dehiscence T87.81
  infection or inflammation T87.40
    lower limb T87.4-●
    upper limb T87.4-●
  necrosis T87.50
    lower limb T87.5-●
    upper limb T87.5-●
  neuroma T87.30
    lower limb T87.3-●
    upper limb T87.3-●
  specified type NEC T87.89
anastomosis (and bypass) —see also
  Complications, prosthetic device or
  implant
  intestinal (internal) NEC K91.89
    involving urinary tract N99.89
  urinary tract (involving intestinal tract)
    N99.89
  vascular —see Complications,
    cardiovascular device or implant
anesthesia, anesthetic —see also Anesthesia,
  complication T88.59
  brain, postpartum, puerperal O89.2
  cardiac
    in
      labor and delivery O74.2
      pregnancy O29.19-●
    postpartum, puerperal O89.1
  central nervous system
    in
      labor and delivery O74.3
      pregnancy O29.29-●
    postpartum, puerperal O89.2
  difficult or failed intubation T88.4
    in pregnancy O29.6-●
  failed sedation (conscious) (moderate)
    during procedure T88.52
  general, unintended awareness during
    procedure T88.53
  hyperthermia, malignant T88.3
  hypothermia T88.51
  intubation failure T88.4

Complication (Continued)
anesthesia, anesthetic (Continued)
  malignant hyperthermia T88.3
  pulmonary
    in
      labor and delivery O74.1
      pregnancy NEC O29.09-●
    postpartum, puerperal O89.09
  shock T88.2
  spinal and epidural
    in
      labor and delivery NEC O74.6
        headache O74.5
      pregnancy NEC O29.5X-●
    postpartum, puerperal NEC O89.5
      headache O89.4
  unintended awareness under general
    anesthesia during procedure T88.53
anti-reflux device —see Complications,
  esophageal anti-reflux device
aortic (bifurcation) graft —see Complications,
  graft, vascular
aortocoronary (bypass) graft —see
  Complications, coronary artery
  (bypass) graft
aortofemoral (bypass) graft —see
  Complications, extremity artery
  (bypass) graft
arteriovenous
  fistula, surgically created T82.9
    embolism T82.818
    fibrosis T82.828
    hemorrhage T82.838
    infection or inflammation T82.7
    mechanical
      breakdown T82.510
      displacement T82.520
      leakage T82.530
      malposition T82.520
      obstruction T82.590
      perforation T82.590
      protrusion T82.590
    pain T82.848
    specified type NEC T82.898
    stenosis T82.858
    thrombosis T82.868
  shunt, surgically created T82.9
    embolism T82.818
    fibrosis T82.828
    hemorrhage T82.838
    infection or inflammation T82.7
    mechanical
      breakdown T82.511
      displacement T82.521
      leakage T82.531
      malposition T82.521
      obstruction T82.591
      perforation T82.591
      protrusion T82.591
    pain T82.848
    specified type NEC T82.898
    stenosis T82.858
    thrombosis T82.868
arthroplasty —see Complications, joint
  prosthesis
artificial
  fertilization or insemination N98.9
    attempted introduction (of)
      embryo in embryo transfer N98.3
      ovum following in vitro fertilization
        N98.2
    hyperstimulation of ovaries N98.1
    infection N98.0
    specified NEC N98.8
  heart T82.9
    embolism T82.817
    fibrosis T82.827
    hemorrhage T82.837
    infection or inflammation T82.7
    mechanical
      breakdown T82.512
      displacement T82.522
      leakage T82.532

Complication (Continued)
artificial (Continued)
  heart (Continued)
    mechanical (Continued)
      malposition T82.522
      obstruction T82.592
      perforation T82.592
      protrusion T82.592
    pain T82.847
    specified type NEC T82.897
    stenosis T82.857
    thrombosis T82.867
  opening
    cecostomy —see Complications, colostomy
    colostomy —see Complications, colostomy
    cystostomy —see Complications,
      cystostomy
    enterostomy —see Complications,
      enterostomy
    gastrostomy —see Complications,
      gastrostomy
    ileostomy —see Complications,
      enterostomy
    jejunostomy —see Complications,
      enterostomy
    nephrostomy —see Complications,
      stoma, urinary tract
    tracheostomy —see Complications,
      tracheostomy
    ureterostomy —see Complications,
      stoma, urinary tract
    urethrostomy —see Complications,
      stoma, urinary tract
balloon implant or device
  gastrointestinal T85.9
    embolism T85.818
    fibrosis T85.828
    hemorrhage T85.838
    infection and inflammation T85.79
    pain T85.848
    specified type NEC T85.898
    stenosis T85.858
    thrombosis T85.868
  vascular (counterpulsation) T82.9
    embolism T82.818
    fibrosis T82.828
    hemorrhage T82.838
    infection or inflammation T82.7
    mechanical
      breakdown T82.513
      displacement T82.523
      leakage T82.533
      malposition T82.523
      obstruction T82.593
      perforation T82.593
      protrusion T82.593
    pain T82.848
    specified type NEC T82.898
    stenosis T82.858
    thrombosis T82.868
bariatric procedure
  gastric band procedure K95.09
    infection K95.01
  specified procedure NEC K95.89
    infection K95.81
bile duct implant (prosthetic) T85.9
  embolism T85.818
  fibrosis T85.828
  hemorrhage T85.838
  infection and inflammation T85.79
  mechanical
    breakdown T85.510
    displacement T85.520
    malfunction T85.510
    malposition T85.520
    obstruction T85.590
    perforation T85.590
    protrusion T85.590
    specified NEC T85.590
  pain T85.848
  specified type NEC T85.898

Complication (*Continued*)
bile duct implant (*Continued*)
  stenosis T85.858
  thrombosis T85.868
bladder device (auxiliary) —*see*
  Complications, genitourinary, device or
  implant, urinary system
bleeding (postoperative) —*see* Complication,
  postoperative, hemorrhage
  intraoperative —*see* Complication,
    intraoperative, hemorrhage
blood vessel graft —*see* Complications, graft,
  vascular
bone
  device NEC T84.9
    embolism T84.81
    fibrosis T84.82
    hemorrhage T84.83
    infection or inflammation T84.7
    mechanical
      breakdown T84.318
      displacement T84.328
      malposition T84.328
      obstruction T84.398
      perforation T84.398
      protrusion T84.398
    pain T84.84
    specified type NEC T84.89
    stenosis T84.85
    thrombosis T84.86
  graft —*see* Complications, graft, bone
  growth stimulator (electrode) —*see*
    Complications, electronic stimulator
    device, bone
  marrow transplant —*see* Complications,
    transplant, bone, marrow
brain neurostimulator (electrode) —*see*
  Complications, electronic stimulator
  device, brain
breast implant (prosthetic) T85.9
  capsular contracture T85.44
  embolism T85.818
  fibrosis T85.828
  hemorrhage T85.838
  infection and inflammation T85.79
  mechanical
    breakdown T85.41
    displacement T85.42
    leakage T85.43
    malposition T85.42
    obstruction T85.49
    perforation T85.49
    protrusion T85.49
    specified NEC T85.49
  pain T85.848
  specified type NEC T85.898
  stenosis T85.858
  thrombosis T85.868
bypass —*see also* Complications, prosthetic
  device or implant
  aortocoronary —*see* Complications,
    coronary artery (bypass) graft
  arterial —*see also* Complications, graft,
    vascular
    extremity —*see* Complications, extremity
      artery (bypass) graft
cardiac —*see also* Disease, heart
  device, implant or graft T82.9
    embolism T82.817
    fibrosis T82.827
    hemorrhage T82.837
    infection or inflammation T82.7
      valve prosthesis T82.6
    mechanical
      breakdown T82.519
        specified device NEC T82.518
      displacement T82.529
        specified device NEC T82.528
      leakage T82.539
        specified device NEC T82.538
      malposition T82.529
        specified device NEC T82.528

Complication (*Continued*)
cardiac (*Continued*)
  device, implant or graft (*Continued*)
    mechanical (*Continued*)
      obstruction T82.599
        specified device NEC T82.598
      perforation T82.599
        specified device NEC T82.598
      protrusion T82.599
        specified device NEC T82.598
    pain T82.847
    specified type NEC T82.897
    stenosis T82.857
    thrombosis T82.867
cardiovascular device, graft or implant T82.9
  aortic graft —*see* Complications, graft,
    vascular
  arteriovenous
    fistula, artificial —*see* Complication,
      arteriovenous, fistula, surgically
      created
    shunt —*see* Complication, arteriovenous,
      shunt, surgically created
  artificial heart —*see* Complication,
    artificial, heart
  balloon (counterpulsation) device —*see*
    Complication, balloon implant,
    vascular
  carotid artery graft —*see* Complications,
    graft, vascular
  coronary bypass graft —*see* Complication,
    coronary artery (bypass) graft
  dialysis catheter (vascular) —*see*
    Complication, catheter, dialysis
  electronic T82.9
    electrode T82.9
      embolism T82.817
      fibrosis T82.827
      hemorrhage T82.837
      infection T82.7
      mechanical
        breakdown T82.110
        displacement T82.120
        leakage T82.190
        obstruction T82.190
        perforation T82.190
        protrusion T82.190
        specified type NEC T82.190
      pain T82.847
      specified NEC T82.897
      stenosis T82.857
      thrombosis T82.867
    embolism T82.817
    fibrosis T82.827
    hemorrhage T82.837
    infection T82.7
    mechanical
      breakdown T82.119
      displacement T82.129
      leakage T82.199
      obstruction T82.199
      perforation T82.199
      protrusion T82.199
      specified type NEC T82.199
    pain T82.847
    pulse generator T82.9
      embolism T82.817
      fibrosis T82.827
      hemorrhage T82.837
      infection T82.7
      mechanical
        breakdown T82.111
        displacement T82.121
        leakage T82.191
        obstruction T82.191
        perforation T82.191
        protrusion T82.191
        specified type NEC T82.191
      pain T82.847
      specified NEC T82.897
      stenosis T82.857
      thrombosis T82.867

Complication (*Continued*)
cardiovascular device, graft or implant
  (*Continued*)
  electronic (*Continued*)
    specified condition NEC T82.897
    specified device NEC T82.9
      embolism T82.817
      fibrosis T82.827
      hemorrhage T82.837
      infection T82.7
      mechanical
        breakdown T82.118
        displacement T82.128
        leakage T82.198
        obstruction T82.198
        perforation T82.198
        protrusion T82.198
        specified type NEC T82.198
      pain T82.847
      specified NEC T82.897
      stenosis T82.857
      thrombosis T82.867
    stenosis T82.857
    thrombosis T82.867
  extremity artery graft —*see* Complication,
    extremity artery (bypass) graft
  femoral artery graft —*see* Complication,
    extremity artery (bypass) graft
  heart
    transplant —*see* Complication,
      transplant, heart
    valve —*see* Complication, prosthetic
      device, heart valve
    graft —*see* Complication, heart, valve,
      graft
  heart-lung transplant —*see* Complication,
    transplant, heart, with lung
  infection or inflammation T82.7
  umbrella device —*see* Complication,
    umbrella device, vascular
  vascular graft (or anastomosis) —*see*
    Complication, graft, vascular
carotid artery (bypass) graft —*see*
  Complications, graft, vascular
catheter (device) NEC —*see also*
  Complications, prosthetic device or
  implant
  cranial infusion
    infection and inflammation T85.735
    mechanical
      breakdown T85.610
      displacement T85.620
      leakage T85.630
      malfunction T85.690
      malposition T85.620
      obstruction T85.690
      perforation T85.690
      protrusion T85.690
      specified NEC T85.690
  cystostomy T83.9
    embolism T83.81
    fibrosis T83.82
    hemorrhage T83.83
    infection and inflammation T83.510
    mechanical
      breakdown T83.010
      displacement T83.020
      leakage T83.030
      malposition T83.020
      obstruction T83.090
      perforation T83.090
      protrusion T83.090
      specified NEC T83.090
    pain T83.84
    specified type NEC T83.89
    stenosis T83.85
    thrombosis T83.86
  dialysis (vascular) T82.9
    embolism T82.818
    fibrosis T82.828
    hemorrhage T82.838

Complication (Continued)
  catheter NEC (Continued)
    dialysis (Continued)
      infection and inflammation T82.7
      intraperitoneal —see Complications,
        catheter, intraperitoneal
      mechanical
        breakdown T82.41
        displacement T82.42
        leakage T82.43
        malposition T82.42
        obstruction T82.49
        perforation T82.49
        protrusion T82.49
      pain T82.848
      specified type NEC T82.898
      stenosis T82.858
      thrombosis T82.868
    epidural infusion T85.9
      embolism T85.810
      fibrosis T85.820
      hemorrhage T85.830
      infection and inflammation T85.735
      mechanical
        breakdown T85.610
        displacement T85.620
        leakage T85.630
        malfunction T85.610
        malposition T85.620
        obstruction T85.690
        perforation T85.690
        protrusion T85.690
        specified NEC T85.690
      pain T85.840
      specified type NEC T85.890
      stenosis T85.850
      thrombosis T85.860
    intraperitoneal dialysis T85.9
      embolism T85.818
      fibrosis T85.828
      hemorrhage T85.838
      infection and inflammation T85.71
      mechanical
        breakdown T85.611
        displacement T85.621
        leakage T85.631
        malfunction T85.611
        malposition T85.621
        obstruction T85.691
        perforation T85.691
        protrusion T85.691
        specified NEC T85.691
      pain T85.848
      specified type NEC T85.898
      stenosis T85.858
      thrombosis T85.868
    intrathecal infusion
      infection and inflammation T85.735
      mechanical
        breakdown T85.610
        displacement T85.620
        leakage T85.630
        malfunction T85.690
        malposition T85.620
        obstruction T85.690
        perforation T85.690
        protrusion T85.690
        specified NEC T85.690
    intravenous infusion T82.9
      embolism T82.818
      fibrosis T82.828
      hemorrhage T82.838
      infection or inflammation T82.7
      mechanical
        breakdown T82.514
        displacement T82.524
        leakage T82.534
        malposition T82.524
        obstruction T82.594
        perforation T82.594
        protrusion T82.594
      pain T82.848

Complication (Continued)
  catheter NEC (Continued)
    intravenous infusion (Continued)
      specified type NEC T82.898
      stenosis T82.858
      thrombosis T82.868
    spinal infusion
      infection and inflammation T85.735
      mechanical
        breakdown T85.610
        displacement T85.620
        leakage T85.630
        malfunction T85.690
        malposition T85.620
        obstruction T85.690
        perforation T85.690
        protrusion T85.690
        specified NEC T85.690
    subarachnoid infusion
      infection and inflammation
        T85.735
      mechanical
        breakdown T85.610
        displacement T85.620
        leakage T85.630
        malfunction T85.690
        malposition T85.620
        obstruction T85.690
        perforation T85.690
        protrusion T85.690
        specified NEC T85.690
    subdural infusion T85.9
      embolism T85.810
      fibrosis T85.820
      hemorrhage T85.830
      infection and inflammation T85.735
      mechanical
        breakdown T85.610
        displacement T85.620
        leakage T85.630
        malfunction T85.610
        malposition T85.620
        obstruction T85.690
        perforation T85.690
        protrusion T85.690
        specified NEC T85.690
      pain T85.840
      specified type NEC T85.890
      stenosis T85.850
      thrombosis T85.860
    urethral T83.9
      displacement T83.028
      embolism T83.81
      fibrosis T83.82
      hemorrhage T83.83
      indwelling
        breakdown T83.011
        displacement T83.021
        infection and inflammation T83.511
        leakage T83.031
        specified complication NEC T83.091
      infection and inflammation T83.511
      leakage T83.038
      malposition T83.028
      mechanical
        breakdown T83.011
      obstruction (mechanical) T83.091
      pain T83.84
      perforation T83.091
      protrusion T83.091
      specified type NEC T83.091
      stenosis T83.85
      thrombosis T83.86
    urinary NEC
      breakdown T83.018
      displacement T83.028
      infection and inflammation T83.518
      leakage T83.038
      specified complication NEC T83.098
  cecostomy (stoma) —see Complications,
    colostomy

Complication (Continued)
  cesarean delivery wound NEC O90.89
    disruption O90.0
    hematoma O90.2
    infection (following delivery) O86.00
  chemotherapy (antineoplastic) NEC T88.7
 ►chimeric antigen receptor (CAR-T) cell
    therapy T80.82
  chin implant (prosthetic) —see Complication,
    prosthetic device or implant, specified
    NEC
  circulatory system I99.8
    intraoperative I97.88
    postprocedural I97.89
      following cardiac surgery —see also
        Infarct, myocardium, associated with
        revascularization procedure I97.19-●
      postcardiotomy syndrome I97.0
      hypertension I97.3
      lymphedema after mastectomy I97.2
      postcardiotomy syndrome I97.0
      specified NEC I97.89
  colostomy (stoma) K94.00
    hemorrhage K94.01
    infection K94.02
    malfunction K94.03
    mechanical K94.03
    specified complication NEC K94.09
  contraceptive device, intrauterine —
    see Complications, intrauterine,
    contraceptive device
  cord (umbilical) —see Complications,
    umbilical cord
  corneal graft —see Complications, graft, cornea
  coronary artery (bypass) graft T82.9
    atherosclerosis —see Arteriosclerosis,
      coronary (artery)
    embolism T82.818
    fibrosis T82.828
    hemorrhage T82.838
    infection and inflammation T82.7
    mechanical
      breakdown T82.211
      displacement T82.212
      leakage T82.213
      malposition T82.212
      obstruction T82.218
      perforation T82.218
      protrusion T82.218
      specified NEC T82.218
    pain T82.848
    specified type NEC T82.898
    stenosis T82.858
    thrombosis T82.868
  counterpulsation device (balloon), intra-
    aortic —see Complications, balloon
    implant, vascular
  cystostomy (stoma) N99.518
    catheter —see Complications, catheter,
      cystostomy
    hemorrhage N99.510
    infection N99.511
    malfunction N99.512
    specified type NEC N99.518
  delivery —see also Complications, obstetric
    O75.9
    procedure (instrumental) (manual)
      (surgical) O75.4
    specified NEC O75.89
  dialysis (peritoneal) (renal) —see also
    Complications, infusion
    catheter (vascular) —see Complication,
      catheter, dialysis
      peritoneal, intraperitoneal —see
        Complications, catheter,
        intraperitoneal
  dorsal column (spinal) neurostimulator —see
    Complications, electronic stimulator
    device, spinal cord
  drug NEC T88.7
  ear procedure —see also Disorder, ear
    intraoperative H95.88-●

▶ New   ⇥ Revised   ~~deleted~~ Deleted   ● Use Additional Character(s)

Complication *(Continued)*
  ear procedure *(Continued)*
    intraoperative *(Continued)*
      hematoma —*see* Complications,
        intraoperative, hematoma (of), ear
      hemorrhage —*see* Complications,
        intraoperative, hemorrhage (of), ear
      laceration —*see* Complications,
        intraoperative, puncture or
        laceration..., ear
      seroma —*see* Complications,
        postprocedural, seroma (of),
        mastoid process
      specified NEC H95.88-●
    postoperative H95.89-●
      external ear canal stenosis H95.81-●
      hematoma —*see* Complications,
        postprocedural, hemorrhage
        (hematoma) (of), ear
      hemorrhage —*see* Complications,
        postprocedural, hemorrhage
        (hematoma) (of), ear
      postmastoidectomy —*see* Complications,
        postmastoidectomy
      specified NEC H95.89-●
  ectopic pregnancy O08.9
    damage to pelvic organs O08.6
    embolism O08.2
    genital infection O08.0
    hemorrhage (delayed) (excessive) O08.1
    metabolic disorder O08.5
    renal failure O08.4
    shock O08.3
    specified type NEC O08.0
    venous complication NEC O08.7
  electronic stimulator device
    bladder (urinary) —*see* Complications,
      electronic stimulator device, urinary
    bone T84.9
      breakdown T84.310
      displacement T84.320
      embolism T84.81
      fibrosis T84.82
      hemorrhage T84.83
      infection or inflammation T84.7
      malfunction T84.310
      malposition T84.320
      mechanical NEC T84.390
      obstruction T84.390
      pain T84.84
      perforation T84.390
      protrusion T84.390
      specified type NEC T84.89
      stenosis T84.85
      thrombosis T84.86
    brain T85.9
      embolism T85.810
      fibrosis T85.820
      hemorrhage T85.830
      infection and inflammation T85.731
      mechanical
        breakdown T85.110
        displacement T85.120
        leakage T85.190
        malposition T85.120
        obstruction T85.190
        perforation T85.190
        protrusion T85.190
        specified NEC T85.190
      pain T85.840
      specified type NEC T85.890
      stenosis T85.850
      thrombosis T85.860
    cardiac (defibrillator) (pacemaker) —*see*
      Complications, cardiovascular device
      or implant, electronic
    generator (brain) (gastric) (peripheral)
      (sacral) (spinal)
      breakdown T85.113
      displacement T85.123
      leakage T85.193

Complication *(Continued)*
  electronic stimulator device *(Continued)*
    generator *(Continued)*
      malposition T85.123
      obstruction T85.193
      perforation T85.193
      protrusion T85.193
      specified type NEC T85.193
    muscle T84.9
      breakdown T84.418
      displacement T84.428
      embolism T84.81
      fibrosis T84.82
      hemorrhage T84.83
      infection or inflammation T84.7
      mechanical NEC T84.498
      pain T84.84
      specified type NEC T84.89
      stenosis T84.85
      thrombosis T84.86
    nervous system T85.9
      brain —*see* Complications, electronic
        stimulator device, brain
      cranial nerve —*see* Complications,
        electronic stimulator device,
        peripheral nerve
      embolism T85.810
      fibrosis T85.820
      gastric nerve —*see* Complications,
        electronic stimulator device,
        peripheral nerve
      hemorrhage T85.830
      infection and inflammation T85.738
      mechanical
        breakdown T85.118
        displacement T85.128
        leakage T85.199
        malposition T85.128
        obstruction T85.199
        perforation T85.199
        protrusion T85.199
        specified NEC T85.199
      pain T85.840
      peripheral nerve —*see* Complications,
        electronic stimulator device,
        peripheral nerve
      sacral nerve —*see* Complications, electronic
        stimulator device, peripheral nerve
      specified type NEC T85.890
      spinal cord —*see* Complications, electronic
        stimulator device, spinal cord
      stenosis T85.850
      thrombosis T85.860
      vagal nerve —*see* Complications, electronic
        stimulator device, peripheral nerve
    peripheral nerve T85.9
      embolism T85.810
      fibrosis T85.820
      hemorrhage T85.830
      infection and inflammation T85.732
      mechanical
        breakdown T85.111
        displacement T85.121
        leakage T85.191
        malposition T85.121
        obstruction T85.191
        perforation T85.191
        protrusion T85.191
        specified NEC T85.191
      pain T85.840
      specified type NEC T85.890
      stenosis T85.850
      thrombosis T85.860
    spinal cord T85.9
      embolism T85.810
      fibrosis T85.820
      hemorrhage T85.830
      infection and inflammation T85.733
      mechanical
        breakdown T85.112
        displacement T85.122

Complication *(Continued)*
  electronic stimulator device *(Continued)*
    spinal cord *(Continued)*
      mechanical *(Continued)*
        leakage T85.192
        malposition T85.122
        obstruction T85.192
        perforation T85.192
        protrusion T85.192
        specified NEC T85.192
      pain T85.840
      specified type NEC T85.890
      stenosis T85.850
      thrombosis T85.860
    urinary T83.9
      embolism T83.81
      fibrosis T83.82
      hemorrhage T83.83
      infection and inflammation T83.598
      mechanical
        breakdown T83.110
        displacement T83.120
        malposition T83.120
        perforation T83.190
        protrusion T83.190
        specified NEC T83.190
      pain T83.84
      specified type NEC T83.89
      stenosis T83.85
      thrombosis T83.86
  electroshock therapy T88.9
    specified NEC T88.8
  endocrine E34.9
    postprocedural
      adrenal hypofunction E89.6
      hypoinsulinemia E89.1
      hypoparathyroidism E89.2
      hypopituitarism E89.3
      hypothyroidism E89.0
      ovarian failure E89.40
        asymptomatic E89.40
        symptomatic E89.41
      specified NEC E89.89
      testicular hypofunction E89.5
  endodontic treatment NEC M27.59
  enterostomy (stoma) K94.10
    hemorrhage K94.11
    infection K94.12
    malfunction K94.13
    mechanical K94.13
    specified complication NEC K94.19
  episiotomy, disruption O90.1
  esophageal anti-reflux device T85.9
    embolism T85.818
    fibrosis T85.828
    hemorrhage T85.838
    infection and inflammation T85.79
    mechanical
      breakdown T85.511
      displacement T85.521
      malfunction T85.511
      malposition T85.521
      obstruction T85.591
      perforation T85.591
      protrusion T85.591
      specified NEC T85.591
    pain T85.848
    specified type NEC T85.898
    stenosis T85.858
    thrombosis T85.868
  esophagostomy K94.30
    hemorrhage K94.31
    infection K94.32
    malfunction K94.33
    mechanical K94.33
    specified complication NEC K94.39
  extracorporeal circulation T80.90
  extremity artery (bypass) graft T82.9
    arteriosclerosis —*see* Arteriosclerosis,
      extremities, bypass graft
    embolism T82.818
    fibrosis T82.828

Complication (Continued)
  extremity artery (bypass) graft (Continued)
    hemorrhage T82.838
    infection and inflammation T82.7
    mechanical
      breakdown T82.318
        femoral artery T82.312
      displacement T82.328
        femoral artery T82.322
      leakage T82.338
        femoral artery T82.332
      malposition T82.328
        femoral artery T82.322
      obstruction T82.398
        femoral artery T82.392
      perforation T82.398
        femoral artery T82.392
      protrusion T82.398
        femoral artery T82.392
    pain T82.848
    specified type NEC T82.898
    stenosis T82.858
    thrombosis T82.868
  eye H57.9
    corneal graft —see Complications, graft, cornea
    implant (prosthetic) T85.9
      embolism T85.818
      fibrosis T85.828
      hemorrhage T85.838
      infection and inflammation T85.79
      mechanical
        breakdown T85.318
        displacement T85.328
        leakage T85.398
        malposition T85.328
        obstruction T85.398
        perforation T85.398
        protrusion T85.398
        specified NEC T85.398
      pain T85.848
      specified type NEC T85.898
      stenosis T85.858
      thrombosis T85.868
    intraocular lens —see Complications, intraocular lens
    orbital prosthesis —see Complications, orbital prosthesis
  female genital N94.9
    device, implant or graft NEC —see Complications, genitourinary, device or implant, genital tract
  femoral artery (bypass) graft —see Complication, extremity artery (bypass) graft
  fixation device, internal (orthopedic) T84.9
    infection and inflammation T84.60
      arm T84.61-●
        humerus T84.61-●
        radius T84.61-●
        ulna T84.61-●
      leg T84.629
        femur T84.62-●
        fibula T84.62-●
        tibia T84.62-●
      specified site NEC T84.69
      spine T84.63
    mechanical
      breakdown
        limb T84.119
          carpal T84.210
          femur T84.11-●
          fibula T84.11-●
          humerus T84.11-●
          metacarpal T84.210
          metatarsal T84.213
          phalanx
            foot T84.213
            hand T84.210
          radius T84.11-●
          tarsal T84.213

Complication (Continued)
  fixation device, internal (Continued)
    mechanical (Continued)
      breakdown (Continued)
        limb (Continued)
          tibia T84.11-●
          ulna T84.11-●
        specified bone NEC T84.218
        spine T84.216
      displacement
        limb T84.129
          carpal T84.220
          femur T84.12-●
          fibula T84.12-●
          humerus T84.12-●
          metacarpal T84.220
          metatarsal T84.223
          phalanx
            foot T84.223
            hand T84.220
          radius T84.12-●
          tarsal T84.223
          tibia T84.12-●
          ulna T84.12-●
        specified bone NEC T84.228
        spine T84.226
      malposition —see Complications, fixation device, internal, mechanical, displacement
      obstruction —see Complications, fixation device, internal, mechanical, specified type NEC
      perforation —see Complications, fixation device, internal, mechanical, specified type NEC
      protrusion —see Complications, fixation device, internal, mechanical, specified type NEC
      specified type NEC
        limb T84.199
          carpal T84.290
          femur T84.19-●
          fibula T84.19-●
          humerus T84.19-●
          metacarpal T84.290
          metatarsal T84.293
          phalanx
            foot T84.293
            hand T84.290
          radius T84.19-●
          tarsal T84.293
          tibia T84.19-●
          ulna T84.19-●
        specified bone NEC T84.298
        vertebra T84.296
    specified type NEC T84.89
      embolism T84.81
      fibrosis T84.82
      hemorrhage T84.83
      pain T84.84
      specified complication NEC T84.89
      stenosis T84.85
      thrombosis T84.86
  following
    acute myocardial infarction NEC I23.8
      aneurysm (false) (of cardiac wall) (of heart wall) (ruptured) I23.3
      angina I23.7
      atrial
        septal defect I23.1
        thrombosis I23.6
      cardiac wall rupture I23.3
      chordae tendinae rupture I23.4
      defect
        septal
          atrial (heart) I23.1
          ventricular (heart) I23.2
      hemopericardium I23.0
      papillary muscle rupture I23.5
      rupture
        cardiac wall I23.3
          with hemopericardium I23.0

Complication (Continued)
  following (Continued)
    acute myocardial infarction NEC (Continued)
      rupture (Continued)
        chordae tendineae I23.4
        papillary muscle I23.5
      specified NEC I23.8
      thrombosis
        atrium I23.6
        auricular appendage I23.6
        ventricle (heart) I23.6
      ventricular
        septal defect I23.2
        thrombosis I23.6
    ectopic or molar pregnancy O08.9
      cardiac arrest O08.81
      sepsis O08.82
      specified type NEC O08.89
      urinary tract infection O08.83
    termination of pregnancy —see Abortion
  gastrointestinal K92.9
    bile duct prosthesis —see Complications, bile duct implant
    esophageal anti-reflux device —see Complications, esophageal anti-reflux device
    postoperative
      colostomy —see Complications, colostomy
      dumping syndrome K91.1
      enterostomy —see Complications, enterostomy
      gastrostomy —see Complications, gastrostomy
      malabsorption NEC K91.2
      obstruction —see also Obstruction, intestine, postoperative K91.30
      postcholecystectomy syndrome K91.5
      specified NEC K91.89
      vomiting after GI surgery K91.0
    prosthetic device or implant
      bile duct prosthesis —see Complications, bile duct implant
      esophageal anti-reflux device —see Complications, esophageal anti-reflux device
      specified type NEC
        embolism T85.818
        fibrosis T85.828
        hemorrhage T85.838
        mechanical
          breakdown T85.518
          displacement T85.528
          malfunction T85.518
          malposition T85.528
          obstruction T85.598
          perforation T85.598
          protrusion T85.598
          specified NEC T85.598
        pain T85.848
        specified complication NEC T85.898
        stenosis T85.858
        thrombosis T85.868
  gastrostomy (stoma) K94.20
    hemorrhage K94.21
    infection K94.22
    malfunction K94.23
    mechanical K94.23
    specified complication NEC K94.29
  genitourinary
    device or implant T83.9
      genital tract T83.9
        infection or inflammation T83.69
        intrauterine contraceptive device —see Complications, intrauterine, contraceptive device
        mechanical —see Complications, by device, mechanical
        mesh —see Complications, prosthetic device or implant, mesh
        penile prosthesis —see Complications, prosthetic device, penile

▶ New   ⮕ Revised   ~~deleted~~ Deleted   ● Use Additional Character(s)

Complication (Continued)
    genitourinary (Continued)
        device or implant (Continued)
            genital tract (Continued)
                specified type NEC T83.89
                    embolism T83.81
                    fibrosis T83.82
                    hemorrhage T83.83
                    pain T83.84
                    specified complication NEC T83.89
                    stenosis T83.85
                    thrombosis T83.86
                vaginal mesh —see Complications,
                    prosthetic device or implant, mesh
            urinary system T83.9
                cystostomy catheter —see
                    Complication, catheter,
                    cystostomy
                electronic stimulator —see
                    Complications, electronic
                    stimulator device, urinary
                indwelling urethral catheter —see
                    Complications, catheter, urethral,
                    indwelling
                infection or inflammation T83.598
                    indwelling urethral catheter T83.511
                kidney transplant —see Complication,
                    transplant, kidney
                organ graft —see Complication, graft,
                    urinary organ
                specified type NEC T83.89
                    embolism T83.81
                    fibrosis T83.82
                    hemorrhage T83.83
                    mechanical T83.198
                        breakdown T83.118
                        displacement T83.128
                        malfunction T83.118
                        malposition T83.128
                        obstruction T83.198
                        perforation T83.198
                        protrusion T83.198
                        specified NEC T83.198
                    sphincter, implanted T83.191
                    stent (ileal conduit) (nephroureteral)
                        T83.193
                        ureteral indwelling T83.192
                    pain T83.84
                    specified complication NEC T83.89
                    stenosis T83.85
                    thrombosis T83.86
                sphincter implant —see Complications,
                    implant, urinary sphincter
        postprocedural
            pelvic peritoneal adhesions N99.4
            renal failure N99.0
            specified NEC N99.89
            stoma —see Complications, stoma,
                urinary tract
            urethral stricture —see Stricture, urethra,
                postprocedural
            vaginal
                adhesions N99.2
                vault prolapse N99.3
    graft (bypass) (patch) —see also
        Complications, prosthetic device or
        implant
        aorta —see Complications, graft, vascular
        arterial —see Complication, graft, vascular
        bone T86.839
            failure T86.831
            infection T86.832
            mechanical T84.318
                breakdown T84.318
                displacement T84.328
                protrusion T84.398
                specified type NEC T84.398
            rejection T86.830
            specified type NEC T86.838
        carotid artery —see Complications, graft,
            vascular

Complication (Continued)
    graft (Continued)
        cornea T86.849-
            failure T86.841-
            infection T86.842-
            mechanical T85.398
                breakdown T85.318
                displacement T85.328
                protrusion T85.398
                specified type NEC T85.398
            rejection T86.840-
            retroprosthetic membrane T85.398
            specified type NEC T86.848-
        femoral artery (bypass) —see Complication,
            extremity artery (bypass) graft
        genital organ or tract —see Complications,
            genitourinary, device or implant,
            genital tract
        muscle T84.9
            breakdown T84.410
            displacement T84.420
            embolism T84.81
            fibrosis T84.82
            hemorrhage T84.83
            infection and inflammation T84.7
            mechanical NEC T84.490
            pain T84.84
            specified type NEC T84.89
            stenosis T84.85
            thrombosis T84.86
        nerve —see Complication, prosthetic device
            or implant, specified NEC
        skin —see Complications, prosthetic device
            or implant, skin graft
        tendon T84.9
            breakdown T84.410
            displacement T84.420
            embolism T84.81
            fibrosis T84.82
            hemorrhage T84.83
            infection and inflammation T84.7
            mechanical NEC T84.490
            pain T84.84
            specified type NEC T84.89
            stenosis T84.85
            thrombosis T84.86
        urinary organ T83.9
            embolism T83.81
            fibrosis T83.82
            hemorrhage T83.83
            infection and inflammation T83.598
                indwelling urethral catheter T83.511
            mechanical
                breakdown T83.21
                displacement T83.22
                erosion T83.24
                exposure T83.25
                leakage T83.23
                malposition T83.22
                obstruction T83.29
                perforation T83.29
                protrusion T83.29
                specified NEC T83.29
            pain T83.84
            specified type NEC T83.89
            stenosis T83.85
            thrombosis T83.86
        vascular T82.9
            embolism T82.818
            femoral artery —see Complication,
                extremity artery (bypass) graft
            fibrosis T82.828
            hemorrhage T82.838
            mechanical
                breakdown T82.319
                    aorta (bifurcation) T82.310
                    carotid artery T82.311
                    specified vessel NEC T82.318
                displacement T82.329
                    aorta (bifurcation) T82.320
                    carotid artery T82.321
                    specified vessel NEC T82.328

Complication (Continued)
    graft (Continued)
        vascular (Continued)
            mechanical (Continued)
                leakage T82.339
                    aorta (bifurcation) T82.330
                    carotid artery T82.331
                    specified vessel NEC T82.338
                malposition T82.329
                    aorta (bifurcation) T82.320
                    carotid artery T82.321
                    specified vessel NEC T82.328
                obstruction T82.399
                    aorta (bifurcation) T82.390
                    carotid artery T82.391
                    specified vessel NEC T82.398
                perforation T82.399
                    aorta (bifurcation) T82.390
                    carotid artery T82.391
                    specified vessel NEC T82.398
                protrusion T82.399
                    aorta (bifurcation) T82.390
                    carotid artery T82.391
                    specified vessel NEC T82.398
            pain T82.848
            specified complication NEC T82.898
            stenosis T82.858
            thrombosis T82.868
    heart I51.9
        assist device
            infection and inflammation T82.7
        following acute myocardial infarction —
            see Complications, following, acute
            myocardial infarction
        postoperative —see Complications,
            circulatory system
        transplant —see Complication, transplant,
            heart
            and lung(s) —see Complications,
                transplant, heart, with lung
        valve
            graft (biological) T82.9
                embolism T82.817
                fibrosis T82.827
                hemorrhage T82.837
                infection and inflammation T82.7
                mechanical T82.228
                    breakdown T82.221
                    displacement T82.222
                    leakage T82.223
                    malposition T82.222
                    obstruction T82.228
                    perforation T82.228
                    protrusion T82.228
                pain T82.847
                specified type NEC T82.897
                stenosis T82.857
                thrombosis T82.867
            prosthesis T82.9
                embolism T82.817
                fibrosis T82.827
                hemorrhage T82.837
                infection or inflammation T82.6
                mechanical T82.09
                    breakdown T82.01
                    displacement T82.02
                    leakage T82.03
                    malposition T82.02
                    obstruction T82.09
                    perforation T82.09
                    protrusion T82.09
                pain T82.847
                specified type NEC T82.897
                    mechanical T82.09
                stenosis T82.857
                thrombosis T82.867
        hematoma
            intraoperative —see Complication,
                intraoperative, hemorrhage
            postprocedural —see Complication,
                postprocedural, hematoma
        hemodialysis —see Complications, dialysis

Complication *(Continued)*
  hemorrhage
    intraoperative —*see* Complication,
      intraoperative, hemorrhage
    postprocedural —*see* Complication,
      postprocedural, hemorrhage
  ▶IEC (immune effector cellular) therapy T80.82
  ileostomy (stoma) —*see* Complications,
    enterostomy
  ▶immune effector cellular (IEC) therapy T80.82
  immunization (procedure) —*see*
    Complications, vaccination
  implant —*see also* Complications, by site and
    type
    urinary sphincter T83.9
      embolism T83.81
      fibrosis T83.82
      hemorrhage T83.83
      infection and inflammation T83.591
      mechanical
        breakdown T83.111
        displacement T83.121
        leakage T83.191
        malposition T83.121
        obstruction T83.191
        perforation T83.191
        protrusion T83.191
        specified NEC T83.191
      pain T83.84
      specified type NEC T83.89
      stenosis T83.85
      thrombosis T83.86
  infusion (procedure) T80.90
    air embolism T80.0
    blood —*see* Complications, transfusion
    catheter —*see* Complications, catheter
    infection T80.29
    pump —*see* Complications, cardiovascular,
      device or implant
    sepsis T80.29
    serum reaction —*see also* Reaction, serum
      T80.69
      anaphylactic shock —*see also* Shock,
        anaphylactic T80.59
    specified type NEC T80.89
  inhalation therapy NEC T81.81
  injection (procedure) T80.90
    drug reaction —*see* Reaction, drug
    infection T80.29
    sepsis T80.29
    serum (prophylactic) (therapeutic) —*see*
      Complications, vaccination
    specified type NEC T80.89
    vaccine (any) —*see* Complications,
      vaccination
  inoculation (any) —*see* Complications,
    vaccination
  insulin pump
    infection and inflammation T85.72
    mechanical
      breakdown T85.614
      displacement T85.624
      leakage T85.633
      malposition T85.624
      obstruction T85.694
      perforation T85.694
      protrusion T85.694
      specified NEC T85.694
  intestinal pouch NEC K91.858
  intraocular lens (prosthetic) T85.9
    embolism T85.818
    fibrosis T85.828
    hemorrhage T85.838
    infection and inflammation T85.79
    mechanical
      breakdown T85.21
      displacement T85.22
      malposition T85.22
      obstruction T85.29
      perforation T85.29
      protrusion T85.29
      specified NEC T85.29

Complication *(Continued)*
  intraocular lens *(Continued)*
    pain T85.848
    specified type NEC T85.898
    stenosis T85.858
    thrombosis T85.868
  intraoperative (intraprocedural)
    cardiac arrest —*see also* Infarct,
      myocardium, associated with
      revascularization procedure
      during cardiac surgery I97.710
      during other surgery I97.711
    cardiac functional disturbance NEC —*see*
      also Infarct, myocardium, associated
      with revascularization procedure
      during cardiac surgery I97.790
      during other surgery I97.791
    hemorrhage (hematoma) (of)
      circulatory system organ or structure
        during cardiac bypass I97.411
        during cardiac catheterization I97.410
        during other circulatory system
          procedure I97.418
        during other procedure I97.42
      digestive system organ
        during procedure on digestive system
          K91.61
        during procedure on other organ K91.62
      ear
        during procedure on ear and mastoid
          process H95.21
        during procedure on other organ
          H95.22
      endocrine system organ or structure
        during procedure on endocrine
          system organ or structure E36.01
        during procedure on other organ
          E36.02
      eye and adnexa
        during ophthalmic procedure H59.11-●
        during other procedure H59.12-●
      genitourinary organ or structure
        during procedure on genitourinary
          organ or structure N99.61
        during procedure on other organ
          N99.62
      mastoid process
        during procedure on ear and mastoid
          process H95.21
        during procedure on other organ
          H95.22
      musculoskeletal structure
        during musculoskeletal surgery
          M96.810
        during non-orthopedic surgery
          M96.811
        during orthopedic surgery M96.810
      nervous system
        during a nervous system procedure
          G97.31
        during other procedure G97.32
      respiratory system
        during other procedure J95.62
        during procedure on respiratory
          system organ or structure J95.61
      skin and subcutaneous tissue
        during a dermatologic procedure
          L76.01
        during a procedure on other organ
          L76.02
      spleen
        during a procedure on other organ
          D78.02
        during a procedure on the spleen
          D78.01
    puncture or laceration (accidental)
      (unintentional) (of)
      brain
        during a nervous system procedure
          G97.48
        during other procedure G97.49

Complication *(Continued)*
  intraoperative *(Continued)*
    puncture or laceration *(Continued)*
      circulatory system organ or structure
        during circulatory system procedure
          I97.51
        during other procedure I97.52
      digestive system
        during procedure on digestive system
          K91.71
        during procedure on other organ K91.72
      ear
        during procedure on ear and mastoid
          process H95.31
        during procedure on other organ
          H95.32
      endocrine system organ or structure
        during procedure on endocrine
          system organ or structure E36.11
        during procedure on other organ E36.12
      eye and adnexa
        during ophthalmic procedure H59.21-●
        during other procedure H59.22-●
      genitourinary organ or structure
        during procedure on genitourinary
          organ or structure N99.71
        during procedure on other organ
          N99.72
      mastoid process
        during procedure on ear and mastoid
          process H95.31
        during procedure on other organ
          H95.32
      musculoskeletal structure
        during musculoskeletal surgery
          M96.820
        during non-orthopedic surgery
          M96.821
        during orthopedic surgery M96.820
      nervous system
        during a nervous system procedure
          G97.48
        during other procedure G97.49
      respiratory system
        during other procedure J95.72
        during procedure on respiratory
          system organ or structure J95.71
      skin and subcutaneous tissue
        during a dermatologic procedure
          L76.11
        during a procedure on other organ
          L76.12
      spleen
        during a procedure on other organ
          D78.12
        during a procedure on the spleen
          D78.11
    specified NEC
      circulatory system I97.88
      digestive system K91.81
      ear H95.88
      endocrine system E36.8
      eye and adnexa H59.88
      genitourinary system N99.81
      mastoid process H95.88
      musculoskeletal structure M96.89
      nervous system G97.81
      respiratory system J95.88
      skin and subcutaneous tissue L76.81
      spleen D78.81
  intraperitoneal catheter (dialysis)
    ⇒(infusion) —*see* Complication(s),
    catheter, intraperitoneal dialysis
  intrathecal infusion pump
    infection and inflammation T85.738
    mechanical
      breakdown T85.615
      displacement T85.625
      leakage T85.635
      malfunction T85.695
      malposition T85.625
      obstruction T85.695

Complication (Continued)
  intrathecal infusion pump (Continued)
    mechanical (Continued)
      perforation T85.695
      protrusion T85.695
      specified NEC T85.695
  intrauterine
    contraceptive device
      embolism T83.81
      fibrosis T83.82
      hemorrhage T83.83
      infection and inflammation T83.69
      mechanical
        breakdown T83.31
        displacement T83.32
        malposition T83.32
        obstruction T83.39
        perforation T83.39
        protrusion T83.39
        specified NEC T83.39
      pain T83.84
      specified type NEC T83.89
      stenosis T83.85
      thrombosis T83.86
    procedure (fetal), to newborn P96.5
  jejunostomy (stoma) —see Complications,
      enterostomy
  joint prosthesis, internal T84.9
    breakage (fracture) T84.01-●
    dislocation T84.02-●
    fracture T84.01-●
    infection or inflammation T84.50
      hip T84.5-●
      knee T84.5-●
      specified joint NEC T84.59
    instability T84.02-●
    malposition —see Complications, joint
        prosthesis, mechanical, displacement
    mechanical
      breakage, broken T84.01-●
      dislocation T84.02-●
      fracture T84.01-●
      instability T84.02-●
      leakage —see Complications, joint
          prosthesis, mechanical, specified NEC
      loosening T84.039
        hip T84.03-●
        knee T84.03-●
        specified joint NEC T84.038
      obstruction —see Complications, joint
          prosthesis, mechanical, specified
          NEC
      perforation —see Complications, joint
          prosthesis, mechanical, specified
          NEC
      osteolysis T84.059
        hip T84.05-●
        knee T84.05-●
        other specified joint T84.058
      periprosthetic T84.059
    ▶ periprosthetic osteolysis T84.059
      protrusion —see Complications, joint
          prosthesis, mechanical, specified
          NEC
      specified complication NEC T84.099
        hip T84.09-●
        knee T84.09-●
        other specified joint T84.098
      subluxation T84.02-●
      wear of articular bearing surface T84.069
        hip T84.06-●
        knee T84.06-●
        other specified joint T84.068
    specified joint NEC T84.89
      embolism T84.81
      fibrosis T84.82
      hemorrhage T84.83
      pain T84.84
      specified complication NEC T84.89
      stenosis T84.85
      thrombosis T84.86
    subluxation T84.02-●

Complication (Continued)
  kidney transplant —see Complications,
      transplant, kidney
  labor O75.9
    specified NEC O75.89
  liver transplant (immune or nonimmune) —
      see Complications, transplant,
      liver
  lumbar puncture G97.1
    cerebrospinal fluid leak G97.0
    headache or reaction G97.1
  lung transplant —see Complications,
      transplant, lung
    and heart —see Complications, transplant,
        lung, with heart
  male genital N50.9
    device, implant or graft —see
        Complications, genitourinary,
        device or implant, genital tract
    postprocedural or postoperative —see
        Complications, genitourinary,
        postprocedural
    specified NEC N99.89
  mastoid (process) procedure
    intraoperative H95.88-●
      hematoma —see Complications,
          intraoperative, hemorrhage
          (hematoma) (of), mastoid process
      hemorrhage —see Complications,
          intraoperative, hemorrhage
          (hematoma) (of), mastoid process
      laceration —see Complications,
          intraoperative, puncture or
          laceration..., mastoid process
      specified NEC H95.88-●
    postmastoidectomy —see Complications,
        postmastoidectomy
    postoperative H95.89-●
      external ear canal stenosis H95.81-●
      hematoma —see Complications...,
          postprocedural, hematoma (of),
          mastoid process
      hemorrhage —see Complications...,
          postprocedural, hemorrhage (of),
          mastoid process
      postmastoidectomy —see Complications,
          postmastoidectomy
      seroma —see Complications,
          postprocedural, seroma (of),
          mastoid process
      specified NEC H95.89-●
  mastoidectomy cavity —see Complications,
      postmastoidectomy
  mechanical —see Complications, by site and
      type, mechanical
  medical procedures (see also Complication(s),
      intraoperative) T88.9
  metabolic E88.9
    postoperative E89.89
      specified NEC E89.89
  molar pregnancy NOS O08.9
    damage to pelvic organs O08.6
    embolism O08.2
    genital infection O08.0
    hemorrhage (delayed) (excessive) O08.1
    metabolic disorder O08.5
    renal failure O08.4
    shock O08.3
    specified type NEC O08.0
    venous complication NEC O08.7
  musculoskeletal system —see also
      Complication, intraoperative
      (intraprocedural), by site
    device, implant or graft NEC —see
        Complications, orthopedic, device or
        implant
    internal fixation (nail) (plate) (rod) —see
        Complications, fixation device,
        internal
    joint prosthesis —see Complications, joint
        prosthesis

Complication (Continued)
  musculoskeletal system (Continued)
    postoperative (postprocedural) M96.89
      with osteoporosis —see Osteoporosis
      fracture following insertion of device —
          see Fracture, following insertion of
          orthopedic implant, joint prosthesis
          or bone plate
      joint instability after prosthesis removal
          M96.89
      lordosis M96.4
      postlaminectomy syndrome NEC M96.1
        kyphosis M96.2
      pseudarthrosis M96.0
      specified complication NEC M96.89
    post radiation M96.89
      kyphosis M96.3
      scoliosis M96.5
      specified complication NEC M96.89
  nephrostomy (stoma) —see Complications,
      stoma, urinary tract, external NEC
  nervous system G98.8
    central G96.9
    device, implant or graft —see also
        Complication, prosthetic device or
        implant, specified NEC
      electronic stimulator (electrode(s)) —see
          Complications, electronic stimulator
          device
      specified NEC
        infection and inflammation T85.738
        mechanical T85.695
          breakdown T85.615
          displacement T85.625
          leakage T85.635
          malfunction T85.695
          malposition T85.625
          obstruction T85.695
          perforation T85.695
          protrusion T85.695
          specified NEC T85.695
      ventricular shunt —see Complications,
          ventricular shunt
    electronic stimulator (electrode(s)) —see
        Complications, electronic stimulator
        device
    postprocedural G97.82
      intracranial hypotension G97.2
      specified NEC G97.82
      spinal fluid leak G97.0
  newborn, due to intrauterine (fetal)
      procedure P96.5
  nonabsorbable (permanent) sutures —see
      Complication, sutures, permanent
  obstetric O75.9
    procedure (instrumental) (manual)
        (surgical) specified NEC O75.4
    specified NEC O75.89
    surgical wound NEC O90.89
      hematoma O90.2
      infection O86.00
  ocular lens implant —see Complications,
      intraocular lens
  ophthalmologic
    postprocedural bleb —see Blebitis
  orbital prosthesis T85.9
    embolism T85.818
    fibrosis T85.828
    hemorrhage T85.838
    infection and inflammation T85.79
    mechanical
      breakdown T85.31-●
      displacement T85.32-●
      malposition T85.32-●
      obstruction T85.39-●
      perforation T85.39-●
      protrusion T85.39-●
      specified NEC T85.39-●
    pain T85.848
    specified type NEC T85.898
    stenosis T85.858
    thrombosis T85.868

Complication *(Continued)*
  organ or tissue transplant (partial) (total) —
    see Complications, transplant
  orthopedic —*see also* Disorder, soft tissue
    device or implant T84.9
      bone
        device or implant —*see* Complication,
          bone, device NEC
        graft —*see* Complication, graft, bone
      breakdown T84.418
      displacement T84.428
      electronic bone stimulator —*see*
        Complications, electronic stimulator
        device, bone
      embolism T84.81
      fibrosis T84.82
      fixation device —*see* Complication,
        fixation device, internal
      hemorrhage T84.83
      infection or inflammation T84.7
      joint prosthesis —*see* Complication, joint
        prosthesis, internal
      malfunction T84.418
      malposition T84.428
      mechanical NEC T84.498
      muscle graft —*see* Complications, graft,
        muscle
      obstruction T84.498
      pain T84.84
      perforation T84.498
      protrusion T84.498
      specified complication NEC T84.89
      stenosis T84.85
      tendon graft —*see* Complications, graft,
        tendon
      thrombosis T84.86
    fracture (following insertion of device) —
      see Fracture, following insertion of
      orthopedic implant, joint prosthesis or
      bone plate
    postprocedural M96.89
      fracture —*see* Fracture, following
        insertion of orthopedic implant,
        joint prosthesis or bone plate
      postlaminectomy syndrome NEC M96.1
        kyphosis M96.3
        lordosis M96.4
      postradiation
        kyphosis M96.2
        scoliosis M96.5
      pseudarthrosis post-fusion M96.0
      specified type NEC M96.89
  pacemaker (cardiac) —*see* Complications,
    cardiovascular device or implant,
    electronic
  pancreas transplant —*see* Complications,
    transplant, pancreas
  penile prosthesis (implant) —*see*
    Complications, prosthetic device, penile
  perfusion NEC T80.90
  perineal repair (obstetrical) NEC O90.89
    disruption O90.1
    hematoma O90.2
    infection (following delivery) O86.09
  phototherapy T88.9
    specified NEC T88.8
  postmastoidectomy NEC H95.19-●
    cyst, mucosal H95.13-●
    granulation H95.12-●
    inflammation, chronic H95.11-●
    recurrent cholesteatoma H95.0-●
  postoperative —*see* Complications,
    postprocedural
    circulatory —*see* Complications, circulatory
      system
    ear —*see* Complications, ear
    endocrine —*see* Complications,
      endocrine
    eye —*see* Complications, eye
    lumbar puncture G97.1
      cerebrospinal fluid leak G97.0

Complication *(Continued)*
  postoperative *(Continued)*
    nervous system (central) (peripheral) —*see*
      Complications, nervous system
    respiratory system —*see* Complications,
      respiratory system
  postprocedural —*see also* Complications,
    surgical procedure
    cardiac arrest —*see also* Infarct,
      myocardium, associated with
      revascularization procedure
      following cardiac surgery I97.120
      following other surgery I97.121
    cardiac functional disturbance NEC —*see*
      also Infarct, myocardium, associated
      with revascularization procedure
      following cardiac surgery I97.190
      following other surgery I97.191
    cardiac insufficiency
      following cardiac surgery I97.110
      following other surgery I97.111
    chorioretinal scars following retinal
      surgery H59.81-●
    following cataract surgery
      cataract (lens) fragments H59.02-●
      cystoid macular edema H59.03-●
      specified NEC H59.09-●
      vitreous (touch) syndrome H59.01-●
    heart failure
      following cardiac surgery I97.130
      following other surgery I97.131
    hematoma (of)
      circulatory system organ or structure
        following cardiac bypass I97.631
        following cardiac catheterization
          I97.630
        following other circulatory system
          procedure I97.638
        following other procedure I97.621
      digestive system
        following procedure on digestive
          system K91.870
        following procedure on other organ
          K91.871
      ear
        following other procedure H95.52
        following procedure on ear and
          mastoid process H95.51
      endocrine system
        following endocrine system procedure
          E89.820
        following other procedure E89.821
      eye and adnexa
        following ophthalmic procedure
          H59.33-●
        following other procedure H59.34-●
      genitourinary organ or structure
        following procedure on genitourinary
          organ or structure N99.840
        following procedure on other organ
          N99.841
      mastoid process
        following other procedure H95.52
        following procedure on ear and
          mastoid process H95.51
      musculoskeletal structure
        following musculoskeletal surgery
          M96.840
        following non-orthopedic surgery
          M96.841
        following orthopedic surgery M96.840
      nervous system
        following nervous system procedure
          G97.61
        following other procedure G97.62
      respiratory system
        following other procedure J95.861
        following procedure on respiratory
          system organ or structure J95.860
      skin and subcutaneous tissue
        following dermatologic procedure
          L76.31

Complication *(Continued)*
  postprocedural *(Continued)*
    hematoma *(Continued)*
      skin and subcutaneous tissue *(Continued)*
        following procedure on other organ
          L76.32
      spleen
        following procedure on other organ
          D78.32
        following procedure on the spleen
          D78.31
    hemorrhage (of)
      circulatory system organ or structure
        following cardiac bypass I97.611
        following cardiac catheterization
          I97.610
        following other circulatory system
          procedure I97.618
        following other procedure I97.620
      digestive system
        following procedure on digestive
          system K91.840
        following procedure on other organ
          K91.841
      ear
        following other procedure H95.42
        following procedure on ear and
          mastoid process H95.41
      endocrine system
        following endocrine system procedure
          E89.810
        following other procedure E89.811
      eye and adnexa
        following ophthalmic procedure
          H59.31-●
        following other procedure H59.32-●
      genitourinary organ or structure
        following procedure on genitourinary
          organ or structure N99.820
        following procedure on other organ
          N99.821
      mastoid process
        following other procedure H95.42
        following procedure on ear and
          mastoid process H95.41
      musculoskeletal structure
        following musculoskeletal surgery
          M96.830
        following non-orthopedic surgery
          M96.831
        following orthopedic surgery M96.830
      nervous system
        following nervous system procedure
          G97.51
        following other procedure G97.52
      respiratory system
        following other procedure J95.831
        following procedure on respiratory
          system organ or structure J95.830
      skin and subcutaneous tissue
        following dermatologic procedure
          L76.21
        following a procedure on other organ
          L76.22
      spleen
        following procedure on other organ
          D78.22
        following procedure on the spleen
          D78.21
    seroma (of)
      circulatory system organ or structure
        following cardiac bypass I97.641
        following cardiac catheterization
          I97.640
        following other circulatory system
          procedure I97.648
        following other procedure I97.622
      digestive system
        following procedure on digestive
          system K91.872
        following procedure on other organ
          K91.873

▶ New   ⫸ Revised   ~~deleted~~ Deleted   ● Use Additional Character(s)

Complication *(Continued)*
  postprocedural *(Continued)*
    seroma *(Continued)*
      ear
        following other procedure H95.54
        following procedure on ear and
          mastoid process H95.53
      endocrine system
        following endocrine system procedure
          E89.822
        following other procedure E89.823
      eye and adnexa
        following ophthalmic procedure
          H59.35-●
        following other procedure H59.36-●
      genitourinary organ or structure
        following procedure on genitourinary
          organ or structure N99.842
        following procedure on other organ
          N99.843
      mastoid process
        following other procedure H95.54
        following procedure on ear and
          mastoid process H95.53
      musculoskeletal structure
        following musculoskeletal surgery
          M96.842
        following non-orthopedic surgery
          M96.843
        following orthopedic surgery M96.842
      nervous system
        following nervous system procedure
          G97.63
        following other procedure G97.64
      respiratory system
        following other procedure J95.863
        following procedure on respiratory
          system organ or structure J95.862
      skin and subcutaneous tissue
        following dermatologic procedure
          L76.33
        following procedure on other organ
          L76.34
      spleen
        following procedure on other organ
          D78.34
        following procedure on the spleen
          D78.33
    specified NEC
      circulatory system I97.89
      digestive K91.89
      ear H95.89
      endocrine E89.89
      eye and adnexa H59.89
      genitourinary N99.89
      mastoid process H95.89
      metabolic E89.89
      musculoskeletal structure M96.89
      nervous system G97.82
      respiratory system J95.89
      skin and subcutaneous tissue L76.82
      spleen D78.89
  pregnancy NEC —*see* Pregnancy,
    complicated by
  prosthetic device or implant T85.9
    bile duct —*see* Complications, bile duct
      implant
    breast —*see* Complications, breast
      implant
    bulking agent
      ureteral
        erosion T83.714
        exposure T83.724
      urethral
        erosion T83.713
        exposure T83.723
    cardiac and vascular NEC —*see*
      Complications, cardiovascular device
      or implant
    corneal transplant —*see* Complications,
      graft, cornea

Complication *(Continued)*
  prosthetic device or implant *(Continued)*
    electronic nervous system stimulator —*see*
      Complications, electronic stimulator
      device
    epidural infusion catheter —*see*
      Complications, catheter, epidural
    esophageal anti-reflux device —*see*
      Complications, esophageal anti-reflux
      device
    genital organ or tract —*see* Complications,
      genitourinary, device or implant,
      genital tract
      specified NEC T83.79
    heart valve —*see* Complications, heart,
      valve, prosthesis
    infection or inflammation T85.79
      intestine transplant T86.892
      liver transplant T86.43
      lung transplant T86.812
      pancreas transplant T86.892
      skin graft T86.822
    intraocular lens —*see* Complications,
      intraocular lens
  ➡ intraperitoneal (dialysis) catheter —*see*
      Complication(s), catheter,
      intraperitoneal dialysis
    joint —*see* Complications, joint prosthesis,
      internal
    mechanical NEC T85.698
      dialysis catheter (vascular) —*see also*
        Complication, catheter, dialysis,
        mechanical
      ➡ peritoneal —*see* Complication(s),
        catheter, intraperitoneal dialysis
      gastrointestinal device T85.598
      ocular device T85.398
      subdural (infusion) catheter T85.690
      suture, permanent T85.692
        that for bone repair —*see*
          Complications, fixation device,
          internal (orthopedic), mechanical
      ventricular shunt
        breakdown T85.01
        displacement T85.02
        leakage T85.03
        malposition T85.02
        obstruction T85.09
        perforation T85.09
        protrusion T85.09
        specified NEC T85.09
    mesh
      erosion (to surrounding organ or tissue)
        T83.718
        urethral (into pelvic floor muscles)
          T83.712
        vaginal (into pelvic floor muscles)
          T83.711
      exposure (into surrounding organ or
        tissue) T83.728
        urethral (through urethral wall)
          T83.722
        vaginal (into vagina) (through vaginal
          wall) T83.721
    orbital —*see* Complications, orbital
      prosthesis
    penile T83.9
      embolism T83.81
      fibrosis T83.82
      hemorrhage T83.83
      infection and inflammation T83.61
      mechanical
        breakdown T83.410
        displacement T83.420
        leakage T83.490
        malposition T83.420
        obstruction T83.490
        perforation T83.490
        protrusion T83.490
        specified NEC T83.490
      pain T83.84

Complication *(Continued)*
  prosthetic device or implant *(Continued)*
    penile *(Continued)*
      specified type NEC T83.89
      stenosis T83.85
      thrombosis T83.86
    prosthetic materials NEC
      erosion (to surrounding organ or tissue)
        T83.718
      exposure (into surrounding organ or
        tissue) T83.728
    skin graft T86.829
      artificial skin or decellularized
        allodermis
        embolism T85.818
        fibrosis T85.828
        hemorrhage T85.838
        infection and inflammation T85.79
        mechanical
          breakdown T85.613
          displacement T85.623
          malfunction T85.613
          malposition T85.623
          obstruction T85.693
          perforation T85.693
          protrusion T85.693
          specified NEC T85.693
        pain T85.848
        specified type NEC T85.898
        stenosis T85.858
        thrombosis T85.868
      failure T86.821
      infection T86.822
      rejection T86.820
      specified NEC T86.828
    sling
      urethral (female) (male)
        erosion T83.712
        exposure T83.722
    specified NEC T85.9
      embolism T85.818
      fibrosis T85.828
      hemorrhage T85.838
      infection and inflammation T85.79
      mechanical
        breakdown T85.618
        displacement T85.628
        leakage T85.638
        malfunction T85.618
        malposition T85.628
        obstruction T85.698
        perforation T85.698
        protrusion T85.698
        specified NEC T85.698
      pain T85.848
      specified type NEC T85.898
      stenosis T85.858
      thrombosis T85.868
    subdural infusion catheter —*see*
      Complications, catheter, subdural
    sutures —*see* Complications, sutures
    urinary organ or tract NEC —*see*
      Complications, genitourinary, device
      or implant, urinary system
    vascular —*see* Complications,
      cardiovascular device or implant
    ventricular shunt —*see* Complications,
      ventricular shunt (device)
  puerperium —*see* Puerperal
  puncture, spinal G97.1
    cerebrospinal fluid leak G97.0
    headache or reaction G97.1
  pyelogram N99.89
  radiation
    kyphosis M96.2
    scoliosis M96.5
  reattached
    extremity (infection) (rejection)
      lower T87.1X-●
      upper T87.0X-●
    specified body part NEC T87.2

Complication *(Continued)*
  reconstructed breast
    asymmetry between native and
      reconstructed breast N65.1
    deformity N65.0
    disproportion between native and
      reconstructed breast N65.1
    excess tissue N65.0
    misshappen N65.0
  reimplant NEC —*see also* Complications,
    prosthetic device or implant
    limb (infection) (rejection) —*see*
      Complications, reattached,
      extremity
    organ (partial) (total) —*see* Complications,
      transplant
    prosthetic device NEC —*see* Complications,
      prosthetic device
  renal N28.9
    allograft —*see* Complications, transplant,
      kidney
    dialysis —*see* Complications, dialysis
  respirator
    mechanical J95.850
      specified NEC J95.859
  respiratory system J98.9
    device, implant or graft —*see*
      Complication, prosthetic device or
      implant, specified NEC
    lung transplant —*see* Complications,
      prosthetic device or implant, lung
      transplant
    postoperative J95.89
      air leak J95.812
      Mendelson's syndrome (chemical
        pneumonitis) J95.4
      pneumothorax J95.811
      pulmonary insufficiency (acute) (after
        nonthoracic surgery) J95.2
        chronic J95.3
        following thoracic surgery J95.1
      respiratory failure (acute) J95.821
        acute and chronic J95.822
      specified NEC J95.89
      subglottic stenosis J95.5
      tracheostomy complication —*see*
        Complications, tracheostomy
    therapy T81.89
  sedation during labor and delivery O74.9
    cardiac O74.2
    central nervous system O74.3
    pulmonary NEC O74.1
  shunt —*see also* Complications, prosthetic
    device or implant
    arteriovenous —*see* Complications,
      arteriovenous, shunt
    ventricular (communicating) —*see*
      Complications, ventricular shunt
  skin
    graft T86.829
      failure T86.821
      infection T86.822
      rejection T86.820
      specified type NEC T86.828
  spinal
    anesthesia —*see* Complications, anesthesia,
      spinal
    catheter (epidural) (subdural) —*see*
      Complications, catheter
    puncture or tap G97.1
      cerebrospinal fluid leak G97.0
      headache or reaction G97.1
  stent
    bile duct —*see* Complications, bile duct
      prosthesis
    ureteral indwelling
      breakdown T83.112
      displacement T83.122
      leakage T83.192
      malposition T83.122

Complication *(Continued)*
  stent *(Continued)*
    ureteral indwelling *(Continued)*
      obstruction T83.192
      perforation T83.192
      protrusion T83.192
      specified NEC T83.192
    urinary (ileal conduit) (nephroureteral)
      T83.193
      embolism T83.81
      fibrosis T83.82
      hemorrhage T83.83
      infection and inflammation T83.593
      mechanical
        breakdown T83.113
        displacement T83.123
        leakage T83.193
        malposition T83.123
        obstruction T83.193
        perforation T83.193
        protrusion T83.193
        specified NEC T83.193
      pain T83.84
      specified type NEC T83.89
      stenosis T83.85
      thrombosis T83.86
    vascular
      end stent stenosis —*see* Restenosis,
        stent
      in stent stenosis —*see* Restenosis, stent
  stoma
    digestive tract
      colostomy —*see* Complications,
        colostomy
      enterostomy —*see* Complications,
        enterostomy
      esophagostomy —*see* Complications,
        esophagostomy
      gastrostomy —*see* Complications,
        gastrostomy
    urinary tract N99.528
      continent N99.538
        hemorrhage N99.530
        herniation N99.533
        infection N99.531
        malfunction N99.532
        specified type NEC N99.538
        stenosis N99.534
      cystostomy —*see* Complications,
        cystostomy
      external NOS N99.528
      hemorrhage N99.520
      herniation N99.523
      incontinent N99.528
        hemorrhage N99.520
        herniation N99.523
        infection N99.521
        malfunction N99.522
        specified type NEC N99.528
        stenosis N99.524
      infection N99.521
      malfunction N99.522
      specified type NEC N99.528
      stenosis N99.524
  stomach banding —*see* Complication(s),
    bariatric procedure
  stomach stapling —*see* Complication(s),
    bariatric procedure
  surgical material, nonabsorbable —*see*
    Complication, suture, permanent
  surgical procedure (on) T81.9
    amputation stump (late) —*see*
      Complications, amputation stump
    cardiac —*see* Complications, circulatory
      system
    cholesteatoma, recurrent —*see*
      Complications, postmastoidectomy,
      recurrent cholesteatoma
    circulatory (early) —*see* Complications,
      circulatory system

Complication *(Continued)*
  surgical procedure *(Continued)*
    digestive system —*see* Complications,
      gastrointestinal
    dumping syndrome (postgastrectomy)
      K91.1
    ear —*see* Complications, ear
    elephantiasis or lymphedema I97.89
      postmastectomy I97.2
    emphysema (surgical) T81.82
    endocrine —*see* Complications, endocrine
    eye —*see* Complications, eye
    fistula (persistent postoperative) T81.83
    foreign body inadvertently left in wound
      (sponge) (suture) (swab) —*see* Foreign
      body, accidentally left during a
      procedure
    gastrointestinal —*see* Complications,
      gastrointestinal
    genitourinary NEC N99.89
    hematoma
      intraoperative —*see* Complication,
        intraoperative, hemorrhage
      postprocedural —*see* Complication,
        postprocedural, hematoma
    hemorrhage
      intraoperative —*see* Complication,
        intraoperative, hemorrhage
      postprocedural —*see* Complication,
        postprocedural, hemorrhage
    hepatic failure K91.82
    hyperglycemia (postpancreatectomy) E89.1
    hypoinsulinemia (postpancreatectomy)
      E89.1
    hypoparathyroidism
      (postparathyroidectomy) E89.2
    hypopituitarism (posthypophysectomy)
      E89.3
    hypothyroidism (post-thyroidectomy)
      E89.0
    intestinal obstruction —*see also*
      Obstruction, intestine, postoperative
      K91.30
    intracranial hypotension following
      ventricular shunting
      (ventriculostomy) G97.2
    lymphedema I97.89
      postmastectomy I97.2
    malabsorption (postsurgical) NEC K91.2
      osteoporosis —*see* Osteoporosis,
        postsurgical malabsorption
    mastoidectomy cavity NEC —*see*
      Complications, postmastoidectomy
    metabolic E89.89
      specified NEC E89.89
    musculoskeletal —*see* Complications,
      musculoskeletal system
    nervous system (central) (peripheral) —*see*
      Complications, nervous system
    ovarian failure E89.40
      asymptomatic E89.40
      symptomatic E89.41
    peripheral vascular —*see* Complications,
      surgical procedure, vascular
    postcardiotomy syndrome I97.0
    postcholecystectomy syndrome K91.5
    postcommissurotomy syndrome I97.0
    postgastrectomy dumping syndrome K91.1
    postlaminectomy syndrome NEC M96.1
      kyphosis M96.3
    postmastectomy lymphedema syndrome
      I97.2
    postmastoidectomy cholesteatoma —*see*
      Complications, postmastoidectomy,
      recurrent cholesteatoma
    postvagotomy syndrome K91.1
    postvalvulotomy syndrome I97.0
    pulmonary insufficiency (acute) J95.2
      chronic J95.3
      following thoracic surgery J95.1

▶ New   ⇛ Revised   ~~deleted~~ Deleted   ● Use Additional Character(s)

Complication (Continued)
  vascular I99.9
    device or implant T82.9
      embolism T82.818
      fibrosis T82.828
      hemorrhage T82.838
      infection or inflammation T82.7
      mechanical
        breakdown T82.519
          specified device NEC T82.518
        displacement T82.529
          specified device NEC T82.528
        leakage T82.539
          specified device NEC T82.538
        malposition T82.529
          specified device NEC T82.528
        obstruction T82.599
          specified device NEC T82.598
        perforation T82.599
          specified device NEC T82.598
        protrusion T82.599
          specified device NEC T82.598
      pain T82.848
      specified type NEC T82.898
      stenosis T82.858
      thrombosis T82.868
    dialysis catheter —see Complication,
        catheter, dialysis
    following infusion, therapeutic injection or
        transfusion T80.1
    graft T82.9
      embolism T82.818
      fibrosis T82.828
      hemorrhage T82.838
      mechanical
        breakdown T82.319
          aorta (bifurcation) T82.310
          carotid artery T82.311
          specified vessel NEC T82.318
        displacement T82.329
          aorta (bifurcation) T82.320
          carotid artery T82.321
          specified vessel NEC T82.328
        leakage T82.339
          aorta (bifurcation) T82.330
          carotid artery T82.331
          specified vessel NEC T82.338
        malposition T82.329
          aorta (bifurcation) T82.320
          carotid artery T82.321
          specified vessel NEC T82.328
        obstruction T82.399
          aorta (bifurcation) T82.390
          carotid artery T82.391
          specified vessel NEC T82.398
        perforation T82.399
          aorta (bifurcation) T82.390
          carotid artery T82.391
          specified vessel NEC T82.398
        protrusion T82.399
          aorta (bifurcation) T82.390
          carotid artery T82.391
          specified vessel NEC T82.398
      pain T82.848
      specified complication NEC T82.898
      stenosis T82.858
      thrombosis T82.868
    postoperative —see Complications,
        postoperative, circulatory
    vena cava device (filter) (sieve) (umbrella) —
        see Complications, umbrella device,
        vascular
  ventilation therapy NEC T81.81
  ventilator
    mechanical J95.850
      specified NEC J95.859
  ventricular (communicating) shunt (device)
      T85.9
    embolism T85.810
    fibrosis T85.820
    hemorrhage T85.830
    infection and inflammation T85.730

Complication (Continued)
  ventricular shunt (Continued)
    mechanical
      breakdown T85.01
      displacement T85.02
      leakage T85.03
      malposition T85.02
      obstruction T85.09
      perforation T85.09
      protrusion T85.09
      specified NEC T85.09
    pain T85.840
    specified type NEC T85.890
    stenosis T85.850
    thrombosis T85.860
  wire suture, permanent (implanted) —see
      Complications, suture, permanent
Compressed air disease T70.3
Compression
  with injury - code by Nature of injury
  artery I77.1
    celiac, syndrome I77.4
  brachial plexus G54.0
  brain (stem) G93.5
    due to
      � (diffuse) (see also Injury,
          intracranial, diffuse) S06.A0
        ▶with herniation S06.A1
      ⤷focal (see also Injury, intracranial, focal)
          S06.A0
        ▶with herniation S06.A1
      ⤷injury NEC (see also Injury, intracranial,
          diffuse) S06.A0
    ▶nontraumatic G93.5
    ⤷traumatic (see also Injury, intracranial,
        diffuse) S06.A0
      ▶with herniation S06.A1
  bronchus J98.09
  cauda equina G83.4
  celiac (artery) (axis) I77.4
  cerebral —see Compression, brain
  cervical plexus G54.2
  cord
    spinal —see Compression, spinal
    umbilical —see Compression, umbilical cord
  cranial nerve G52.9
    eighth —see subcategory H93.3
    eleventh G52.8
    fifth G50.8
    first G52.0
    fourth —see Strabismus, paralytic, fourth
        nerve
    ninth G52.1
    second —see Disorder, nerve, optic
    seventh G51.8
    sixth —see Strabismus, paralytic, sixth nerve
    tenth G52.2
    third —see Strabismus, paralytic, third nerve
    twelfth G52.3
  diver's squeeze T70.3
  during birth (newborn) P15.9
  esophagus K22.2
  eustachian tube —see Obstruction, eustachian
      tube, cartilaginous
  facies Q67.1
  fracture
    nontraumatic NOS —see Collapse, vertebra
    pathological —see Fracture, pathological
    traumatic —see Fracture, traumatic
  heart —see Disease, heart
  intestine —see Obstruction, intestine
  laryngeal nerve, recurrent G52.2
    with paralysis of vocal cords and larynx
        J38.00
      bilateral J38.02
      unilateral J38.01
  lumbosacral plexus G54.1
  lung J98.4
  lymphatic vessel I89.0
  medulla —see Compression, brain
  nerve —see also Disorder, nerve G58.9
    arm NEC —see Mononeuropathy, upper limb

Compression (Continued)
  nerve (Continued)
    axillary G54.0
    cranial —see Compression, cranial nerve
    leg NEC —see Mononeuropathy, lower
        limb
    median (in carpal tunnel) —see Syndrome,
        carpal tunnel
    optic —see Disorder, nerve, optic
    plantar —see Lesion, nerve, plantar
    posterior tibial (in tarsal tunnel) —see
        Syndrome, tarsal tunnel
    root or plexus NOS (in) G54.9
      intervertebral disc disorder NEC —
          see Disorder, disc, with,
          radiculopathy
        with myelopathy —see Disorder, disc,
            with, myelopathy
      neoplastic disease —see also Neoplasm
          D49.9 [G55]
      spondylosis —see Spondylosis, with
          radiculopathy
    sciatic (acute) —see Lesion, nerve, sciatic
    sympathetic G90.8
    traumatic —see Injury, nerve
    ulnar —see Lesion, nerve, ulnar
    upper extremity NEC —see
        Mononeuropathy, upper limb
  spinal (cord) G95.20
    by displacement of intervertebral disc
        NEC —see also Disorder, disc, with,
        myelopathy
    nerve root NOS G54.9
      due to displacement of intervertebral
          disc NEC —see Disorder, disc, with,
          radiculopathy
        with myelopathy —see Disorder, disc,
            with, myelopathy
    specified NEC G95.29
    spondylogenic (cervical) (lumbar,
        lumbosacral) (thoracic) —see
        Spondylosis, with myelopathy NEC
    anterior —see Syndrome, anterior, spinal
        artery, compression
    traumatic —see Injury, spinal cord, by
        region
  subcostal nerve (syndrome) —see
      Mononeuropathy, upper limb, specified
      NEC
  sympathetic nerve NEC G90.8
  syndrome T79.5
  trachea J39.8
  ulnar nerve (by scar tissue) —see Lesion,
      nerve, ulnar
  umbilical cord
    complicating delivery O69.2
      cord around neck O69.1
      prolapse O69.0
      specified NEC O69.2
  ureter N13.5
  vein I87.1
  vena cava (inferior) (superior) I87.1
Compulsion, compulsive
  gambling F63.0
  neurosis F42.8
  personality F60.5
  states F42.8
  swearing F42.8
    in Gilles de la Tourette's syndrome F95.2
  tics and spasms F95.9
Concato's disease (pericardial polyserositis)
    A19.9
  nontubercular I31.1
  pleural —see Pleurisy, with effusion
Concavity chest wall M95.4
Concealed penis Q55.64
Concern (normal) about sick person in family
    Z63.6
Concrescence (teeth) K00.2
Concretio cordis I31.1
  rheumatic I09.2

▶ New   ⤷ Revised   ~~deleted~~ Deleted   • Use Additional Character(s)

INDEX TO DISEASES AND INJURIES / Consanguinity

Concretion —see also Calculus
  appendicular K38.1
  canaliculus —see Dacryolith
  clitoris N90.89
  conjunctiva H11.12-●
  eyelid —see Disorder, eyelid, specified type NEC
  lacrimal passages —see Dacryolith
  prepuce (male) N47.8
  salivary gland (any) K11.5
  seminal vesicle N50.89
  tonsil J35.8
Concussion (brain) (cerebral) (current)
    S06.0X9
  with
    loss of consciousness of 30 minutes or less
      S06.0X1
    loss of consciousness of unspecified
      duration S06.0X9
  blast (air) (hydraulic) (immersion)
      (underwater)
    abdomen or thorax —see Injury, blast, by
      site
    ear with acoustic nerve injury —see Injury,
      nerve, acoustic, specified type NEC
  cauda equina S34.3
  conus medullaris S34.02
  ocular S05.8X-●
  spinal (cord)
    cervical S14.0
    lumbar S34.01
    sacral S34.02
    thoracic S24.0
  syndrome F07.81
  without loss of consciousness S06.0X0
Condition —see also Disease
  post COVID-19 U09.9
Conditions arising in the perinatal period —
    see Newborn, affected by
Conduct disorder —see Disorder, conduct
Condyloma A63.0
  acuminatum A63.0
  gonorrheal A54.09
  latum A51.31
  syphilitic A51.31
    congenital A50.07
  venereal, syphilitic A51.31
Conflagration —see also Burn
  asphyxia (by inhalation of gases, fumes or
      vapors) —see also Table of Drugs and
      Chemicals T59.9-●
Conflict (with) —see also Discord
  family Z73.9
  marital Z63.0
    involving divorce or estrangement Z63.5
  parent-child Z62.820
    parent-adopted child Z62.821
    parent-biological child Z62.820
    parent-foster child Z62.822
  social role NEC Z73.5
Confluent —see condition
Confusion, confused R41.0
  epileptic F05
  mental state (psychogenic) F44.89
  psychogenic F44.89
  reactive (from emotional stress, psychological
      trauma) F44.89
Confusional arousals G47.51
Congelation T69.9
Congenital —see also condition
  aortic septum Q25.49
  intrinsic factor deficiency D51.0
  malformation —see Anomaly
Congestion, congestive
  bladder N32.89
  bowel K63.89
  brain G93.89
  breast N64.59
  bronchial J98.09
  catarrhal J31.0
  chest R09.89
  chill, malarial —see Malaria

Congestion, congestive (Continued)
  circulatory NEC I99.8
  duodenum K31.89
  eye —see Hyperemia, conjunctiva
  facial, due to birth injury P15.4
  general R68.89
  glottis J37.0
  heart —see Failure, heart, congestive
  hepatic K76.1
  hypostatic (lung) —see Edema, lung
  intestine K63.89
  kidney N28.89
  labyrinth —see subcategory H83.8
  larynx J37.0
  liver K76.1
  lung R09.89
    active or acute —see Pneumonia
  malaria, malarial —see Malaria
  nasal R09.81
  nose R09.81
  orbit, orbital —see also Exophthalmos
    inflammatory (chronic) —see Inflammation,
      orbit
  ovary N83.8
  pancreas K86.89
  pelvic, female N94.89
  pleural J94.8
  prostate (active) N42.1
  pulmonary —see Congestion, lung
  renal N28.89
  retina H35.81
  seminal vesicle N50.1
  spinal cord G95.19
  spleen (chronic) D73.2
  stomach K31.89
  trachea —see Tracheitis
  urethra N36.8
  uterus N85.8
    with subinvolution N85.3
  venous (passive) I87.8
  viscera R68.89
Congestive —see Congestion
Conical
  cervix (hypertrophic elongation) N88.4
  cornea —see Keratoconus
  teeth K00.2
Conjoined twins Q89.4
Conjugal maladjustment Z63.0
  involving divorce or estrangement Z63.5
Conjunctiva —see condition
Conjunctivitis (staphylococcal) (streptococcal)
    NOS H10.9
  Acanthamoeba B60.12
  acute H10.3-●
    atopic H10.1-●
    chemical —see also Corrosion, cornea
      H10.21-●
    mucopurulent H10.02-●
      follicular H10.01-●
    pseudomembranous H10.22-●
    serous except viral H10.23-●
      viral —see Conjunctivitis, viral
    toxic H10.21-●
  adenoviral (acute) (follicular) B30.1
  allergic (acute) —see Conjunctivitis, acute,
      atopic
    chronic H10.45
    vernal H10.44
  anaphylactic —see Conjunctivitis, acute,
      atopic
  Apollo B30.3
  atopic (acute) —see Conjunctivitis, acute,
      atopic
  Béal's B30.2
  blennorrhagic (gonococcal) (neonatorum)
      A54.31
  chemical (acute) —see also Corrosion, cornea
      H10.21-●
  chlamydial A74.0
    due to trachoma A71.1
    neonatal P39.1

Conjunctivitis (Continued)
  chronic (nodosa) (petrificans) (phlyctenular)
      H10.40-●
    allergic H10.45
      vernal H10.44
    follicular H10.43-●
      giant papillary H10.41-●
      simple H10.42-●
    vernal H10.44
  coxsackievirus 24 B30.3
  diphtheritic A36.86
  due to
    dust —see Conjunctivitis, acute, atopic
    filariasis B74.9
    mucocutaneous leishmaniasis B55.2
  enterovirus type 70 (hemorrhagic) B30.3
  epidemic (viral) B30.9
    hemorrhagic B30.3
  gonococcal (neonatorum) A54.31
  granular (trachomatous) A71.1
    sequelae (late effect) B94.0
  hemorrhagic (acute) (epidemic) B30.3
  herpes zoster B02.31
  in (due to)
    Acanthamoeba B60.12
    adenovirus (acute) (follicular) B30.1
    Chlamydia A74.0
    coxsackievirus 24 B30.3
    diphtheria A36.86
    enterovirus type 70 (hemorrhagic) B30.3
    filariasis B74.9
    gonococci A54.31
    herpes (simplex) virus B00.53
      zoster B02.31
    infectious disease NEC B99
    meningococci A39.89
    mucocutaneous leishmaniasis B55.2
    rosacea H10.82-●
    syphilis (late) A52.71
    zoster B02.31
  inclusion A74.0
  infantile P39.1
    gonococcal A54.31
  Koch-Weeks' —see Conjunctivitis, acute,
      mucopurulent
  light —see Conjunctivitis, acute, atopic
  ligneous —see Blepharoconjunctivitis,
      ligneous
  meningococcal A39.89
  mucopurulent —see Conjunctivitis, acute,
      mucopurulent
  neonatal P39.1
    gonococcal A54.31
  Newcastle B30.8
  of Béal B30.2
  parasitic
    filariasis B74.9
    mucocutaneous leishmaniasis B55.2
  Parinaud's H10.89
  petrificans H10.89
  rosacea H10.82-●
  specified NEC H10.89
  swimming-pool B30.1
  trachomatous A71.1
    acute A71.0
    sequelae (late effect) B94.0
  traumatic NEC H10.89
  tuberculous A18.59
  tularemic A21.1
  tularensis A21.1
  viral B30.9
    due to
      adenovirus B30.1
      enterovirus B30.3
    specified NEC B30.8
Conjunctivochalasis H11.82-●
Connective tissue —see condition
Conn's syndrome E26.01
Conradi (-Hunermann) disease Q77.3
Consanguinity Z84.3
  counseling Z71.89

▶ New   ⇒ Revised   deleted Deleted   ● Use Additional Character(s)   169

Conscious simulation (of illness) Z76.5
Consecutive —see condition
Consolidation lung (base) —see Pneumonia,
  lobar
Constipation (atonic) (neurogenic) (simple)
  (spastic) K59.00
  chronic K59.09
    idiopathic K59.04
  drug-induced K59.03
  functional K59.04
  outlet dysfunction K59.02
  psychogenic F45.8
  slow transit K59.01
  specified NEC K59.09
Constitutional —see also condition
  substandard F60.7
Constitutionally substandard F60.7
Constriction —see also Stricture
  auditory canal —see Stenosis, external ear
    canal
  bronchial J98.09
  duodenum K31.5
  esophagus K22.2
  external
    abdomen, abdominal (wall) S30.841
    alveolar process S00.542
    ankle S90.54-•
    antecubital space —see Constriction,
      external, forearm
    arm (upper) S40.84-•
    auricle —see Constriction, external, ear
    axilla —see Constriction, external, arm
    back, lower S30.840
    breast S20.14-•
    brow S00.84
    buttock S30.840
    calf —see Constriction, external, leg
    canthus —see Constriction, external, eyelid
    cheek S00.84
      internal S00.542
    chest wall —see Constriction, external,
      thorax
    chin S00.84
    clitoris S30.844
    costal region —see Constriction, external,
      thorax
    digit(s)
      foot —see Constriction, external, toe
      hand —see Constriction, external, finger
    ear S00.44-•
    elbow S50.34-•
    epididymis S30.843
    epigastric region S30.841
    esophagus, cervical S10.14
    eyebrow —see Constriction, external, eyelid
    eyelid S00.24-•
    face S00.84
    finger(s) S60.44-•
      index S60.44-•
      little S60.44-•
      middle S60.44-•
      ring S60.44-•
    flank S30.841
    foot (except toe(s) alone) S90.84-•
      toe —see Constriction, external, toe
    forearm S50.84-•
      elbow only —see Constriction, external,
        elbow
    forehead S00.84
    genital organs, external
      female S30.846
      male S30.845
    groin S30.841
    gum S00.542
    hand S60.54-•
    head S00.94
      ear —see Constriction, external, ear
      eyelid —see Constriction, external, eyelid
      lip S00.541
      nose S00.34
      oral cavity S00.542

Constriction (Continued)
  external (Continued)
    head (Continued)
      scalp S00.04
      specified site NEC S00.84
    heel —see Constriction, external, foot
    hip S70.24-•
    inguinal region S30.841
    interscapular region S20.449
    jaw S00.84
    knee S80.24-•
    labium (majus) (minus) S30.844
    larynx S10.14
    leg (lower) S80.84-•
      knee —see Constriction, external, knee
      upper —see Constriction, external, thigh
    lip S00.541
    lower back S30.840
    lumbar region S30.840
    malar region S00.84
    mammary —see Constriction, external, breast
    mastoid region S00.84
    mouth S00.542
    nail
      finger —see Constriction, external, finger
      toe —see Constriction, external, toe
    nasal S00.34
    neck S10.94
      specified site NEC S10.84
      throat S10.14
    nose S00.34
    occipital region S00.04
    oral cavity S00.542
    orbital region —see Constriction, external,
      eyelid
    palate S00.542
    palm —see Constriction, external, hand
    parietal region S00.04
    pelvis S30.840
    penis S30.842
    perineum
      female S30.844
      male S30.840
    periocular area —see Constriction, external,
      eyelid
    phalanges
      finger —see Constriction, external, finger
      toe —see Constriction, external, toe
    pharynx S10.14
    pinna —see Constriction, external, ear
    popliteal space —see Constriction, external,
      knee
    prepuce S30.842
    pubic region S30.840
    pudendum
      female S30.846
      male S30.845
    sacral region S30.840
    scalp S00.04
    scapular region —see Constriction,
      external, shoulder
    scrotum S30.843
    shin —see Constriction, external, leg
    shoulder S40.24-•
    sternal region S20.349
    submaxillary region S00.84
    submental region S00.84
    subungual
      finger(s) —see Constriction, external,
        finger
      toe(s) —see Constriction, external, toe
    supraclavicular fossa S10.84
    supraorbital S00.84
    temple S00.84
    temporal region S00.84
    testis S30.843
    thigh S70.34-•
    thorax, thoracic (wall) S20.94
      back S20.44-•
      front S20.34-•
    throat S10.14

Constriction (Continued)
  external (Continued)
    thumb S60.34-•
    toe(s) (lesser) S90.44-•
      great S90.44-•
    tongue S00.542
    trachea S10.14
    tunica vaginalis S30.843
    uvula S00.542
    vagina S30.844
    vulva S30.844
    wrist S60.84-•
  gallbladder —see Obstruction, gallbladder
  intestine —see Obstruction, intestine
  larynx J38.6
    congenital Q31.8
      specified NEC Q31.8
      subglottic Q31.1
  organ or site, congenital NEC —see Atresia,
    by site
  prepuce (acquired) (congenital) N47.1
  pylorus (adult hypertrophic) K31.1
    congenital or infantile Q40.0
    newborn Q40.0
  ring dystocia (uterus) O62.4
  spastic —see also Spasm
    ureter N13.5
  ureter N13.5
    with infection N13.6
  urethra —see Stricture, urethra
  visual field (peripheral) (functional) —see
    Defect, visual field
Constrictive —see condition
Consultation
  without complaint or sickness Z71.9
    feared complaint unfounded Z71.1
    specified reason NEC Z71.89
  medical —see Counseling, medical
  religious Z71.81
  specified reason NEC Z71.89
  spiritual Z71.81
Consumption —see Tuberculosis
Contact (with) —see also Exposure (to)
  acariasis Z20.7
  AIDS virus Z20.6
  air pollution Z77.110
  algae and algae toxins Z77.121
  algae bloom Z77.121
  anthrax Z20.810
  aromatic (hazardous) compounds NEC Z77.028
  aromatic amines Z77.020
  aromatic dyes NOS Z77.028
  arsenic Z77.010
  asbestos Z77.090
  bacterial disease NEC Z20.818
  benzene Z77.021
  blue-green algae bloom Z77.121
  body fluids (potentially hazardous) Z77.21
  brown tide Z77.121
  chemicals (chiefly nonmedicinal) (hazardous)
    NEC Z77.098
  cholera Z20.09
  chromium compounds Z77.018
  communicable disease Z20.9
    bacterial NEC Z20.818
    specified NEC Z20.89
    viral NEC Z20.828
    Zika virus Z20.821
  coronavirus (disease) (novel) 2019 Z20.822
  COVID-19 Z20.822
  cyanobacteria bloom Z77.121
  dyes Z77.098
  Escherichia coli (E. coli) Z20.01
  fiberglass —see Table of Drugs and
    Chemicals, fiberglass
  German measles Z20.4
  gonorrhea Z20.2
  hazardous metals NEC Z77.018
  hazardous substances NEC Z77.29
  hazards in the physical environment NEC
    Z77.128
  hazards to health NEC Z77.9

Contact (*Continued*)
  HIV Z20.6
  HTLV-III/LAV Z20.6
  human immunodeficiency virus (HIV) Z20.6
  infection Z20.9
    specified NEC Z20.89
  infestation (parasitic) NEC Z20.7
  intestinal infectious disease NEC Z20.09
    Escherichia coli (E. coli) Z20.01
  lead Z77.011
  meningococcus Z20.811
  mold (toxic) Z77.120
  nickel dust Z77.018
  noise Z77.122
  parasitic disease Z20.7
  pediculosis Z20.7
  pfiesteria piscicida Z77.121
  poliomyelitis Z20.89
  pollution
    air Z77.110
    environmental NEC Z77.118
    soil Z77.112
    water Z77.111
  polycyclic aromatic hydrocarbons Z77.028
▶ positive maternal group B streptococcus P00.82
  rabies Z20.3
  radiation, naturally occurring NEC Z77.123
  radon Z77.123
  red tide (Florida) Z77.121
  rubella Z20.4
  SARS-CoV-2 Z20.822
  sexually-transmitted disease Z20.2
  smallpox (laboratory) Z20.89
  syphilis Z20.2
  tuberculosis Z20.1
  uranium Z77.012
  varicella Z20.820
  venereal disease Z20.2
  viral disease NEC Z20.828
  viral hepatitis Z20.5
  water pollution Z77.111
  Zika virus Z20.821
Contamination, food —*see* Intoxication, foodborne
Contraception, contraceptive
  advice Z30.09
  counseling Z30.09
  device (intrauterine) (in situ) Z97.5
    causing menorrhagia T83.83
    checking Z30.431
    complications —*see* Complications,
      intrauterine, contraceptive device
    in place Z97.5
    initial prescription Z30.014
    reinsertion Z30.433
    removal Z30.432
    replacement Z30.433
  emergency (postcoital) Z30.012
  initial prescription Z30.019
    barrier Z30.018
    diaphragm Z30.018
    injectable Z30.013
    intrauterine device Z30.014
    pills Z30.011
    postcoital (emergency) Z30.012
    specified type NEC Z30.018
    subdermal implantable Z30.017
    transdermal patch hormonal Z30.016
    vaginal ring hormonal Z30.015
  maintenance Z30.40
    barrier Z30.49
    diaphragm Z30.49
    examination Z30.8
    injectable Z30.42
    intrauterine device Z30.431
    pills Z30.41
    specified type NEC Z30.49
    subdermal implantable Z30.46
    transdermal patch hormonal Z30.45
    vaginal ring hormonal Z30.44
  management Z30.9
    specified NEC Z30.8
  postcoital (emergency) Z30.012

Contraception, contraceptive (*Continued*)
  prescription Z30.019
    repeat Z30.40
  sterilization Z30.2
  surveillance (drug) —*see* Contraception,
    maintenance
Contraction(s), contracture, contracted
  Achilles tendon —*see also* Short, tendon,
    Achilles
    congenital Q66.89
  amputation stump (surgical) (flexion) (late)
    next proximal joint T87.89
  anus K59.89
  bile duct (common) (hepatic) K83.8
  bladder N32.89
    neck or sphincter N32.0
  bowel, cecum, colon or intestine, any part —
    see Obstruction, intestine
  Braxton Hicks —*see* False, labor
  breast implant, capsular T85.44
  bronchial J98.09
  burn (old) —*see* Cicatrix
  cervix —*see* Stricture, cervix
  cicatricial —*see* Cicatrix
  conjunctiva, trachomatous, active A71.1
    sequelae (late effect) B94.0
  Dupuytren's M72.0
  eyelid —*see* Disorder, eyelid function
  fascia (lata) (postural) M72.8
    Dupuytren's M72.0
    palmar M72.0
    plantar M72.2
  finger NEC —*see also* Deformity, finger
    congenital Q68.1
    joint —*see* Contraction, joint, hand
  flaccid —*see* Contraction, paralytic
  gallbladder K82.0
  heart valve —*see* Endocarditis
  hip —*see* Contraction, joint, hip
  hourglass
    bladder N32.89
      congenital Q64.79
    gallbladder K82.0
      congenital Q44.1
    stomach K31.89
      congenital Q40.2
      psychogenic F45.8
    uterus (complicating delivery) O62.4
  hysterical F44.4
  internal os —*see* Stricture, cervix
  joint (abduction) (acquired) (adduction)
    (flexion) (rotation) M24.50
    ankle M24.57-●
    congenital NEC Q68.8
      hip Q65.89
    elbow M24.52-●
    foot joint M24.57-●
    hand joint M24.54-●
    hip M24.55-●
      congenital Q65.89
    hysterical F44.4
    knee M24.56-●
    shoulder M24.51-●
    specified site NEC M24.59
    wrist M24.53-●
  kidney (granular) (secondary) N26.9
    congenital Q63.8
    hydronephritic —*see* Hydronephrosis
    Page N26.2
    pyelonephritic —*see* Pyelitis, chronic
    tuberculous A18.11
  ligament —*see also* Disorder, ligament
    congenital Q79.8
  muscle (postinfective) (postural) NEC M62.40
    with contracture of joint —*see* Contraction,
      joint
    ankle M62.47-●
    congenital Q79.8
      sternocleidomastoid Q68.0
    extraocular —*see* Strabismus
    eye (extrinsic) —*see* Strabismus
    foot M62.47-●

Contraction, contracture, contracted
  (*Continued*)
    muscle (*Continued*) forearm M62.43-●
      hand M62.44-●
      hysterical F44.4
      ischemic (Volkmann's) T79.6
      lower leg M62.46-●
      multiple sites M62.49
      pelvic region M62.45-●
      posttraumatic —*see* Strabismus, paralytic
      psychogenic F45.8
        conversion reaction F44.4
      shoulder region M62.41-●
      specified site NEC M62.48
      thigh M62.45-●
      upper arm M62.42-●
  neck —*see* Torticollis
  ocular muscle —*see* Strabismus
  organ or site, congenital NEC —*see* Atresia,
    by site
  outlet (pelvis) —*see* Contraction, pelvis
  palmar fascia M72.0
  paralytic
    joint —*see* Contraction, joint
    muscle —*see also* Contraction, muscle NEC
      ocular —*see* Strabismus, paralytic
  pelvis (acquired) (general) M95.5
    with disproportion (fetopelvic) O33.1
      causing obstructed labor O65.1
    inlet O33.2
    mid-cavity O33.3
    outlet O33.3
  plantar fascia M72.2
  premature
    atrium I49.1
    auriculoventricular I49.49
    heart I49.49
    junctional I49.2
    supraventricular I49.1
    ventricular I49.3
  prostate N42.89
  pylorus NEC —*see also* Pylorospasm
    psychogenic F45.8
  rectum, rectal (sphincter) K59.89
  ring (Bandl's) (complicating delivery) O62.4
  scar —*see* Cicatrix
  spine —*see* Dorsopathy, deforming
  sternocleidomastoid (muscle), congenital
    Q68.0
  stomach K31.89
    hourglass K31.89
      congenital Q40.2
      psychogenic F45.8
    psychogenic F45.8
  tendon (sheath) M62.40
    with contracture of joint —*see* Contraction,
      joint
    Achilles —*see* Short, tendon, Achilles
    ankle M62.47-●
      Achilles —*see* Short, tendon, Achilles
    foot M62.47-●
    forearm M62.43-●
    hand M62.44-●
    lower leg M62.46-●
    multiple sites M62.49
    neck M62.48
    pelvic region M62.45-●
    shoulder region M62.41-●
    specified site NEC M62.48
    thigh M62.45-●
    thorax M62.48
    trunk M62.48
    upper arm M62.42-●
  toe —*see* Deformity, toe, specified NEC
  ureterovesical orifice (postinfectional) N13.5
    with infection N13.6
  urethra —*see also* Stricture, urethra
    orifice N32.0
  uterus N85.8
    abnormal NEC O62.9
    clonic (complicating delivery) O62.4
    dyscoordinate (complicating delivery) O62.4

Contraction, contracture, contracted
  (Continued)
  uterus (Continued)
    hourglass (complicating delivery) O62.4
    hypertonic O62.4
    hypotonic NEC O62.2
    inadequate
      primary O62.0
      secondary O62.1
    incoordinate (complicating delivery) O62.4
    poor O62.2
    tetanic (complicating delivery) O62.4
  vagina (outlet) N89.5
  vesical N32.89
    neck or urethral orifice N32.0
  visual field —see Defect, visual field,
    generalized
  Volkmann's (ischemic) T79.6
Contusion (skin surface intact) T14.8
  abdomen, abdominal (muscle) (wall) S30.1
  adnexa, eye NEC S05.8X-●
  adrenal gland S37.812
  alveolar process S00.532
  ankle S90.0-●
  antecubital space —see Contusion, forearm
  anus S30.3
  arm (upper) S40.02-●
    lower (with elbow) —see Contusion,
      forearm
  auditory canal —see Contusion, ear
  auricle —see Contusion, ear
  axilla —see Contusion, arm, upper
  back —see also Contusion, thorax, back
    lower S30.0
  bile duct S36.13
  bladder S37.22
  bone NEC T14.8
  brain (diffuse) —see Injury, intracranial, diffuse
    focal —see Injury, intracranial, focal
  brainstem S06.38-●
  breast S20.0-●
  broad ligament S37.892
  brow S00.83
  buttock S30.0
  canthus, eye S00.1-●
  cauda equina S34.3
  cerebellar, traumatic S06.37-●
  cerebral S06.33-●
    left side S06.32-●
    right side S06.31-●
  cheek S00.83
    internal S00.532
  chest (wall) —see Contusion, thorax
  chin S00.83
  clitoris S30.23
  colon —see Injury, intestine, large, contusion
  common bile duct S36.13
  conjunctiva S05.1-●
    with foreign body (in conjunctival sac) —
      see Foreign body, conjunctival sac
  conus medullaris (spine) S34.139
  cornea —see Contusion, eyeball
    with foreign body —see Foreign body,
      cornea
  corpus cavernosum S30.21
  cortex (brain) (cerebral) —see Injury,
    intracranial, diffuse
    focal —see Injury, intracranial, focal
  costal region —see Contusion, thorax
  cystic duct S36.13
  diaphragm S27.802
  duodenum S36.420
  ear S00.43-●
  elbow S50.0-●
    with forearm —see Contusion, forearm
  epididymis S30.22
  epigastric region S30.1
  epiglottis S10.0
  esophagus (thoracic) S27.812
    cervical S10.0
  eyeball S05.1-●

Contusion (Continued)
  eyebrow S00.1-●
  eyelid (and periocular area) S00.1-●
  face NEC S00.83
  fallopian tube S37.529
    bilateral S37.522
    unilateral S37.521
  femoral triangle S30.1
  finger(s) S60.00
    with damage to nail (matrix) S60.10
    index S60.02-●
      with damage to nail S60.12-●
    little S60.05-●
      with damage to nail S60.15-●
    middle S60.03-●
      with damage to nail S60.13-●
    ring S60.04-●
      with damage to nail S60.14-●
    thumb —see Contusion, thumb
  flank S30.1
  foot (except toe(s) alone) S90.3-●
    toe —see Contusion, toe
  forearm S50.1-●
    elbow only —see Contusion, elbow
  forehead S00.83
  gallbladder S36.122
  genital organs, external
    female S30.202
    male S30.201
  globe (eye) —see Contusion, eyeball
  groin S30.1
  gum S00.532
  hand S60.22-●
    finger(s) —see Contusion, finger
    wrist —see Contusion, wrist
  head S00.93
    ear —see Contusion, ear
    eyelid —see Contusion, eyelid
    lip S00.531
    nose S00.33
    oral cavity S00.532
    scalp S00.03
    specified part NEC S00.83
  heart —see also Injury, heart S26.91
  heel —see Contusion, foot
  hepatic duct S36.13
  hip S70.0-●
  ileum S36.428
  iliac region S30.1
  inguinal region S30.1
  interscapular region S20.229
  intra-abdominal organ S36.92
    colon —see Injury, intestine, large, contusion
    liver S36.112
    pancreas —see Contusion, pancreas
    rectum S36.62
    small intestine —see Injury, intestine, small,
      contusion
    specified organ NEC S36.892
    spleen —see Contusion, spleen
    stomach S36.32
  iris (eye) —see Contusion, eyeball
  jaw S00.83
  jejunum S36.428
  kidney S37.01-●
    major (greater than 2 cm) S37.02-●
    minor (less than 2 cm) S37.01-●
  knee S80.0-●
  labium (majus) (minus) S30.23
  lacrimal apparatus, gland or sac S05.8X-●
  larynx S10.0
  leg (lower) S80.1-●
    knee —see Contusion, knee
  lens —see Contusion, eyeball
  lip S00.531
  liver S36.112
  lower back S30.0
  lumbar region S30.0
  lung S27.329
    bilateral S27.322
    unilateral S27.321

Contusion (Continued)
  malar region S00.83
  mastoid region S00.83
  membrane, brain —see Injury, intracranial,
    diffuse
    focal —see Injury, intracranial, focal
  mesentery S36.892
  mesosalpinx S37.892
  mouth S00.532
  muscle —see Contusion, by site
  nail
    finger —see Contusion, finger, with
      damage to nail
    toe —see Contusion, toe, with damage to
      nail
  nasal S00.33
  neck S10.93
    specified site NEC S10.83
    throat S10.0
  nerve —see Injury, nerve
  newborn P54.5
  nose S00.33
  occipital
    lobe (brain) —see Injury, intracranial,
      diffuse
      focal —see Injury, intracranial,
        focal
    region (scalp) S00.03
  orbit (region) (tissues) S05.1-●
  ovary S37.429
    bilateral S37.422
    unilateral S37.421
  palate S00.532
  pancreas S36.229
    body S36.221
    head S36.220
    tail S36.222
  parietal
    lobe (brain) —see Injury, intracranial,
      diffuse
      focal —see Injury, intracranial, focal
    region (scalp) S00.03
  pelvic organ S37.92
    adrenal gland S37.812
    bladder S37.22
    fallopian tube —see Contusion, fallopian
      tube
    kidney —see Contusion, kidney
    ovary —see Contusion, ovary
    prostate S37.822
    specified organ NEC S37.892
    ureter S37.12
    urethra S37.32
    uterus S37.62
  pelvis S30.0
  penis S30.21
  perineum
    female S30.23
    male S30.0
  periocular area S00.1-●
  peritoneum S36.81
  periurethral tissue —see Contusion,
    urethra
  pharynx S10.0
  pinna —see Contusion, ear
  popliteal space —see Contusion, knee
  prepuce S30.21
  prostate S37.822
  pubic region S30.1
  pudendum
    female S30.202
    male S30.201
  quadriceps femoris —see Contusion, thigh
  rectum S36.62
  retroperitoneum S36.892
  round ligament S37.892
  sacral region S30.0
  scalp S00.03
    due to birth injury P12.3
  scapular region —see Contusion, shoulder
  sclera —see Contusion, eyeball

▶ New   ⇒ Revised   ~~deleted~~ Deleted   ● Use Additional Character(s)

Contusion (Continued)
scrotum S30.22
seminal vesicle S37.892
shoulder S40.01-●
skin NEC T14.8
small intestine —see Injury, intestine, small,
    contusion
spermatic cord S30.22
spinal cord —see Injury, spinal cord,
    by region
  cauda equina S34.3
  conus medullaris S34.139
spleen S36.029
  major S36.021
  minor S36.020
sternal region S20.219
stomach S36.32
subconjunctival S05.1-●
subcutaneous NEC T14.8
submaxillary region S00.83
submental region S00.83
subperiosteal NEC T14.8
subungual
  finger —see Contusion, finger, with
      damage to nail
  toe —see Contusion, toe, with damage to
      nail
supraclavicular fossa S10.83
supraorbital S00.83
suprarenal gland S37.812
temple (region) S00.83
temporal
  lobe (brain) —see Injury, intracranial,
      diffuse
  focal —see Injury, intracranial, focal
  region S00.83
testis S30.22
thigh S70.1-●
thorax (wall) S20.20
  back S20.22-●
  front S20.21-●
throat S10.0
thumb S60.01-●
  with damage to nail S60.11-●
toe(s) (lesser) S90.12-●
  with damage to nail S90.22-●
  great S90.11-●
    with damage to nail S90.21-●
tongue S00.532
trachea (cervical) S10.0
  thoracic S27.52
tunica vaginalis S30.22
tympanum, tympanic membrane —see
    Contusion, ear
ureter S37.12
urethra S37.32
urinary organ NEC S37.892
uterus S37.62
uvula S00.532
vagina S30.23
vas deferens S37.892
vesical S37.22
vocal cord(s) S10.0
vulva S30.23
wrist S60.21-●
Conus (congenital) (any type) Q14.8
  cornea —see Keratoconus
  medullaris syndrome G95.81
Conversion hysteria, neurosis or reaction
    F44.9
Converter, tuberculosis (test reaction) R76.11
Conviction (legal), anxiety concerning
    Z65.0
  with imprisonment Z65.1
Convulsions (idiopathic) —see also Seizure(s)
    R56.9
  apoplectiform (cerebral ischemia) I67.82
  dissociative F44.5
  epileptic —see Epilepsy
  epileptiform, epileptoid —see Seizure,
      epileptiform

Convulsions (Continued)
ether (anesthetic) —see Table of Drugs and
    Chemicals, by drug
febrile R56.00
  with status epilepticus G40.901
  complex R56.01
    with status epilepticus G40.901
  simple R56.00
hysterical F44.5
infantile P90
  epilepsy —see Epilepsy
jacksonian —see Epilepsy, localization-
    related, symptomatic, with simple
    partial seizures
myoclonic G25.3
newborn P90
obstetrical (nephritic) (uremic) —see
    Eclampsia
paretic A52.17
post traumatic R56.1
psychomotor —see Epilepsy, localization-
    related, symptomatic, with complex
    partial seizures
recurrent R56.9
reflex R25.8
scarlatinal A38.8
tetanus, tetanic —see Tetanus
thymic E32.8
Convulsive —see also Convulsions
Cooley's anemia D56.1
Coolie itch B76.9
Cooper's
  disease —see Mastopathy, cystic
  hernia —see Hernia, abdomen, specified site
    NEC
Copra itch B88.0
Coprophagy F50.89
Coprophobia F40.298
Coproporphyria, hereditary E80.29
Cor
  biloculare Q20.8
  bovis, bovinum —see Hypertrophy, cardiac
  pulmonale (chronic) I27.81
    acute I26.09
  triatriatum, triatrium Q24.2
  triloculare Q20.8
    biatrium Q20.4
    biventriculare Q21.1
Corbus' disease (gangrenous balanitis) N48.1
Cord —see also condition
  around neck
    complicating delivery O69.81
    with compression O69.1
  bladder G95.89
    tabetic A52.19
Cordis ectopia Q24.8
Corditis (spermatic) N49.1
Corectopia Q13.2
Cori's disease (glycogen storage) E74.03
Corkhandler's disease or lung J67.3
Corkscrew esophagus K22.4
Corkworker's disease or lung J67.3
Corn (infected) L84
Cornea —see also condition
  donor Z52.5
  plana Q13.4
Cornelia de Lange syndrome Q87.19
Cornu cutaneum L85.8
Cornual gestation or pregnancy O00.80
  with intrauterine pregnancy O00.81
Coronary (artery) —see condition
Coronavirus (infection)
  as cause of disease classified elsewhere
    B97.29
  coronavirus-19 U07.1
  COVID-19 U07.1
  SARS-associated B97.21
Corpora —see also condition
  amylacea, prostate N42.89
  cavernosa —see condition
Corpulence —see Obesity

Corpus —see condition
Corrected transposition Q20.5
Corrosion (injury) (acid) (caustic) (chemical)
    (lime) (external) (internal) T30.4
  abdomen, abdominal (muscle) (wall)
    T21.42
    first degree T21.52
    second degree T21.62
    third degree T21.72
  above elbow T22.439
    first degree T22.539
    left T22.432
      first degree T22.532
      second degree T22.632
      third degree T22.732
    right T22.431
      first degree T22.531
      second degree T22.631
      third degree T22.731
    second degree T22.639
    third degree T22.739
  alimentary tract NEC T28.7
  ankle T25.419
    first degree T25.519
    left T25.412
      first degree T25.512
      second degree T25.612
      third degree T25.712
    multiple with foot —see Corrosion, lower,
        limb, multiple, ankle and foot
    right T25.411
      first degree T25.511
      second degree T25.611
      third degree T25.711
    second degree T25.619
    third degree T25.719
  anus —see Corrosion, buttock
  arm(s) (meaning upper limb(s)) —see
      Corrosion, upper limb
  axilla T22.449
    first degree T22.549
    left T22.442
      first degree T22.542
      second degree T22.642
      third degree T22.742
    right T22.441
      first degree T22.541
      second degree T22.641
      third degree T22.741
    second degree T22.649
    third degree T22.749
  back (lower) T21.44
    first degree T21.54
    second degree T21.64
    third degree T21.74
    upper T21.43
      first degree T21.53
      second degree T21.63
      third degree T21.73
  blisters - code as Corrosion, second degree,
      by site
  breast(s) —see Corrosion, chest wall
  buttock(s) T21.45
    first degree T21.55
    second degree T21.65
    third degree T21.75
  calf T24.439
    first degree T24.539
    left T24.432
      first degree T24.532
      second degree T24.632
      third degree T24.732
    right T24.431
      first degree T24.531
      second degree T24.631
      third degree T24.731
    second degree T24.639
    third degree T24.739
  canthus (eye) —see Corrosion, eyelid
  cervix T28.8

Corrosion *(Continued)*
  cheek T20.46
    first degree T20.56
    second degree T20.66
    third degree T20.76
  chest wall T21.41
    first degree T21.51
    second degree T21.61
    third degree T21.71
  chin T20.43
    first degree T20.53
    second degree T20.63
    third degree T20.73
  colon T28.7
  conjunctiva (and cornea) —*see* Corrosion,
      cornea
  cornea (and conjunctiva) T26.6-●
  deep necrosis of underlying tissue -
      code as Corrosion, third degree,
      by site
  dorsum of hand T23.469
    first degree T23.569
    left T23.462
      first degree T23.562
      second degree T23.662
      third degree T23.762
    right T23.461
      first degree T23.561
      second degree T23.661
      third degree T23.761
    second degree T23.669
    third degree T23.769
  ear (auricle) (external) (canal) T20.41
    drum T28.91
    first degree T20.51
    second degree T20.61
    third degree T20.71
  elbow T22.429
    first degree T22.529
    left T22.422
      first degree T22.522
      second degree T22.622
      third degree T22.722
    right T22.421
      first degree T22.521
      second degree T22.621
      third degree T22.721
    second degree T22.629
    third degree T22.729
  entire body —*see* Corrosion, multiple body
      regions
  epidermal loss - code as Corrosion, second
      degree, by site
  epiglottis T27.4
  erythema, erythematous - code as Corrosion,
      first degree, by site
  esophagus T28.6
  extent (percentage of body surface)
    less than 10 percent T32.0
    10-19 percent (0-9 percent third degree)
        T32.10
      with 10-19 percent third degree
          T32.11
    20-29 percent (0-9 percent third degree)
        T32.20
      with
        10-19 percent third degree T32.21
        20-29 percent third degree T32.22
    30-39 percent (0-9 percent third degree)
        T32.30
      with
        10-19 percent third degree T32.31
        20-29 percent third degree T32.32
        30-39 percent third degree T32.33
    40-49 percent (0-9 percent third degree)
        T32.40
      with
        10-19 percent third degree T32.41
        20-29 percent third degree T32.42
        30-39 percent third degree T32.43
        40-49 percent third degree T32.44

Corrosion *(Continued)*
  extent *(Continued)*
    50-59 percent (0-9 percent third degree)
        T32.50
      with
        10-19 percent third degree T32.51
        20-29 percent third degree T32.52
    50-59 percent *(Continued)*
      with *(Continued)*
        30-39 percent third degree T32.53
        40-49 percent third degree T32.54
        50-59 percent third degree T32.55
    60-69 percent (0-9 percent third degree)
        T32.60
      with
        10-19 percent third degree T32.61
        20-29 percent third degree T32.62
        30-39 percent third degree T32.63
        40-49 percent third degree T32.64
        50-59 percent third degree T32.65
        60-69 percent third degree T32.66
    70-79 percent (0-9 percent third degree)
        T32.70
      with
        10-19 percent third degree T32.71
        20-29 percent third degree T32.72
        30-39 percent third degree T32.73
        40-49 percent third degree T32.74
        50-59 percent third degree T32.75
        60-69 percent third degree T32.76
        70-79 percent third degree T32.77
    80-89 percent (0-9 percent third degree)
        T32.80
      with
        10-19 percent third degree T32.81
        20-29 percent third degree T32.82
        30-39 percent third degree T32.83
        40-49 percent third degree T32.84
        50-59 percent third degree T32.85
        60-69 percent third degree T32.86
        70-79 percent third degree T32.87
        80-89 percent third degree T32.88
    90 percent or more (0-9 percent third
        degree) T32.90
      with
        10-19 percent third degree T32.91
        20-29 percent third degree T32.92
        30-39 percent third degree T32.93
        40-49 percent third degree T32.94
        50-59 percent third degree T32.95
        60-69 percent third degree T32.96
        70-79 percent third degree T32.97
        80-89 percent third degree T32.98
        90-99 percent third degree T32.99
  extremity —*see* Corrosion, limb
  eye(s) and adnexa T26.9-●
    with resulting rupture and destruction of
        eyeball T26.7-●
    conjunctival sac —*see* Corrosion,
        cornea
    cornea —*see* Corrosion, cornea
    lid —*see* Corrosion, eyelid
    periocular area —*see* Corrosion eyelid
    specified site NEC T26.8-●
  eyeball —*see* Corrosion, eye
  eyelid(s) T26.5-●
  face —*see* Corrosion, head
  finger T23.429
    first degree T23.529
    left T23.422
      first degree T23.522
      second degree T23.622
      third degree T23.722
    multiple sites (without thumb)
        T23.439
      with thumb T23.449
        first degree T23.549
        left T23.442
          first degree T23.542
          second degree T23.642
          third degree T23.742

Corrosion *(Continued)*
  finger *(Continued)*
    multiple sites *(Continued)*
      with thumb *(Continued)*
        right T23.441
          first degree T23.541
          second degree T23.641
          third degree T23.741
        second degree T23.649
        third degree T23.749
      first degree T23.539
      left T23.432
        first degree T23.532
        second degree T23.632
        third degree T23.732
      right T23.431
        first degree T23.531
        second degree T23.631
        third degree T23.731
      second degree T23.639
      third degree T23.739
    right T23.421
      first degree T23.521
      second degree T23.621
      third degree T23.721
    second degree T23.629
    third degree T23.729
  flank —*see* Corrosion, abdomen
  foot T25.429
    first degree T25.529
    left T25.422
      first degree T25.522
      second degree T25.622
      third degree T25.722
    multiple with ankle —*see* Corrosion, lower,
        limb, multiple, ankle and foot
    right T25.421
      first degree T25.521
      second degree T25.621
      third degree T25.721
    second degree T25.629
    third degree T25.729
  forearm T22.419
    first degree T22.519
    left T22.412
      first degree T22.512
      second degree T22.612
      third degree T22.712
    right T22.411
      first degree T22.511
      second degree T22.611
      third degree T22.711
    second degree T22.619
    third degree T22.719
  forehead T20.46
    first degree T20.56
    second degree T20.66
    third degree T20.76
  fourth degree - code as Corrosion, third
      degree, by site
  full thickness skin loss - code as Corrosion,
      third degree, by site
  gastrointestinal tract NEC T28.7
  genital organs
    external
      female T21.47
        first degree T21.57
        second degree T21.67
        third degree T21.77
      male T21.46
        first degree T21.56
        second degree T21.66
        third degree T21.76
    internal T28.8
  groin —*see* Corrosion, abdominal wall
  hand(s) T23.409
    back —*see* Corrosion, dorsum of hand
    finger —*see* Corrosion, finger
    first degree T23.509
    left T23.402
      first degree T23.502
      second degree T23.602
      third degree T23.702

▶ New   ⇒ Revised   ~~deleted~~ Deleted   ● Use Additional Character(s)

Corrosion (Continued)
  toe T25.439
    first degree T25.539
    left T25.432
      first degree T25.532
      second degree T25.632
      third degree T25.732
    right T25.431
      first degree T25.531
      second degree T25.631
      third degree T25.731
    second degree T25.639
    third degree T25.739
  tongue T28.5
  tonsil(s) T28.5
  total body —see Corrosion, multiple body
      regions
  trachea T27.4
    with lung T27.5
  trunk T21.40
    abdominal wall —see Corrosion,
        abdominal wall
    anus —see Corrosion, buttock
    axilla —see Corrosion, upper limb
    back —see Corrosion, back
    breast —see Corrosion, chest wall
    buttock —see Corrosion, buttock
    chest wall —see Corrosion, chest wall
    first degree T21.50
    flank —see Corrosion, abdominal wall
    genital
      female —see Corrosion, genital organs,
          external, female
      male —see Corrosion, genital organs,
          external, male
    groin —see Corrosion, abdominal wall
    interscapular region —see Corrosion, back,
        upper
    labia —see Corrosion, genital organs,
        external, female
    lower back —see Corrosion, back
    penis —see Corrosion, genital organs,
        external, male
    perineum
      female —see Corrosion, genital organs,
          external, female
      male —see Corrosion, genital organs,
          external, male
    scapular region —see Corrosion, upper
        limb
    scrotum —see Corrosion, genital organs,
        external, male
    second degree T21.60
    shoulder —see Corrosion, upper limb
    specified site NEC T21.49
      first degree T21.59
      second degree T21.69
      third degree T21.79
    testes —see Corrosion, genital organs,
        external, male
    third degree T21.70
    upper back —see Corrosion, back, upper
    vagina T28.8
    vulva —see Corrosion, genital organs,
        external, female
  unspecified site with extent of body surface
      involved specified
    less than 10 percent T32.0
    10-19 percent (0-9 percent third degree)
        T32.10
      with 10-19 percent third degree T32.11
    20-29 percent (0-9 percent third degree)
        T32.20
      with
        10-19 percent third degree T32.21
        20-29 percent third degree T32.22
    30-39 percent (0-9 percent third degree)
        T32.30
      with
        10-19 percent third degree T32.31
        20-29 percent third degree T32.32
        30-39 percent third degree T32.33

Corrosion (Continued)
  unspecified site with extent of body surface
      involved specified (Continued)
    40-49 percent (0-9 percent third degree)
        T32.40
      with
        10-19 percent third degree T32.41
        20-29 percent third degree T32.42
        30-39 percent third degree T32.43
        40-49 percent third degree T32.44
    50-59 percent (0-9 percent third degree)
        T32.50
      with
        10-19 percent third degree T32.51
        20-29 percent third degree T32.52
        30-39 percent third degree T32.53
        40-49 percent third degree T32.54
        50-59 percent third degree T32.55
    60-69 percent (0-9 percent third degree)
        T32.60
      with
        10-19 percent third degree T32.61
        20-29 percent third degree T32.62
        30-39 percent third degree T32.63
        40-49 percent third degree T32.64
        50-59 percent third degree T32.65
        60-69 percent third degree T32.66
    70-79 percent (0-9 percent third degree)
        T32.70
      with
        10-19 percent third degree T32.71
        20-29 percent third degree T32.72
        30-39 percent third degree T32.73
        40-49 percent third degree T32.74
        50-59 percent third degree T32.75
        60-69 percent third degree T32.76
        70-79 percent third degree T32.77
    80-89 percent (0-9 percent third degree)
        T32.80
      with
        10-19 percent third degree T32.81
        20-29 percent third degree T32.82
        30-39 percent third degree T32.83
        40-49 percent third degree T32.84
        50-59 percent third degree T32.85
        60-69 percent third degree T32.86
        70-79 percent third degree T32.87
        80-89 percent third degree T32.88
    90 percent or more (0-9 percent third
        degree) T32.90
      with
        10-19 percent third degree T32.91
        20-29 percent third degree T32.92
        30-39 percent third degree T32.93
        40-49 percent third degree T32.94
        50-59 percent third degree T32.95
        60-69 percent third degree T32.96
        70-79 percent third degree T32.97
        80-89 percent third degree T32.98
        90-99 percent third degree T32.99
  upper limb (axilla) (scapular region) T22.40
    above elbow —see Corrosion, above elbow
    axilla —see Corrosion, axilla
    elbow —see Corrosion, elbow
    first degree T22.50
    forearm —see Corrosion, forearm
    hand —see Corrosion, hand
    interscapular region —see Corrosion, back,
        upper
    multiple sites T22.499
      first degree T22.599
      left T22.492
        first degree T22.592
        second degree T22.692
        third degree T22.792
      right T22.491
        first degree T22.591
        second degree T22.691
        third degree T22.791
      second degree T22.699
      third degree T22.799
    scapular region —see Corrosion, scapular
        region

Corrosion (Continued)
  upper limb (axilla) (scapular region) (Continued)
    second degree T22.60
    shoulder —see Corrosion, shoulder
    third degree T22.70
    wrist —see Corrosion, hand
  uterus T28.8
  vagina T28.8
  vulva —see Corrosion, genital organs,
      external, female
  wrist T23.479
    first degree T23.579
    left T23.472
      first degree T23.572
      second degree T23.672
      third degree T23.772
    multiple sites with hand T23.499
      first degree T23.599
      left T23.492
        first degree T23.592
        second degree T23.692
        third degree T23.792
      right T23.491
        first degree T23.591
        second degree T23.691
        third degree T23.791
      second degree T23.699
      third degree T23.799
    right T23.471
      first degree T23.571
      second degree T23.671
      third degree T23.771
    second degree T23.679
    third degree T23.779
Corrosive burn —see Corrosion
Corsican fever —see Malaria
Cortical —see condition
Cortico-adrenal —see condition
Coryza (acute) J00
  with grippe or influenza —see Influenza,
      with, respiratory manifestations NEC
  syphilitic
    congenital (chronic) A50.05
Costen's syndrome or complex M26.69
Costiveness —see Constipation
Costochondritis M94.0
Cot death R99
Cotard's syndrome F22
Cotia virus B08.8
Cotton wool spots (retinal) H35.81
Cotungo's disease —see Sciatica
Cough (affected) (epidemic) (nervous) R05.9
  with hemorrhage —see Hemoptysis
  acute R05.1
  bronchial R05.8
    with grippe or influenza —see Influenza,
        with, respiratory manifestations NEC
  chronic R05.3
  functional F45.8
  hysterical F45.8
  laryngeal, spasmodic R05.8
  paroxysmal, due to Bordetella pertussis
      (without pneumonia) A37.00
    with pneumonia A37.01
  persistent R05.3
  refractory R05.3
  psychogenic F45.8
  smokers' J41.0
  specified NEC R05.8
  subacute R05.2
  syncope R05.4
  tea taster's B49
  unexplained R05.3
Counseling (for) Z71.9
  abuse NEC
    perpetrator Z69.82
    victim Z69.81
  alcohol abuser Z71.41
    family Z71.42
  child abuse
    nonparental
      perpetrator Z69.021
      victim Z69.020

▶ New   ⇒ Revised   ~~deleted~~ Deleted   ● Use Additional Character(s)

Counseling (Continued)
  parental
    perpetrator Z69.011
    victim Z69.010
  consanguinity Z71.89
  contraceptive Z30.09
  dietary Z71.3
  drug abuser Z71.51
    family member Z71.52
  exercise Z71.82
  family Z71.89
  fertility preservation (prior to cancer therapy)
    (prior to removal of gonads) Z31.62
  for non-attending third party Z71.0
    related to sexual behavior or orientation Z70.2
  genetic
    nonprocreative Z71.83
    procreative NEC Z31.5
  gestational carrier Z31.7
  health (advice) (education) (instruction) —see
    Counseling, medical
    risk for travel (international) Z71.84
  human immunodeficiency virus (HIV) Z71.7
▶immunization safety Z71.85
  impotence Z70.1
  insulin pump use Z46.81
  medical (for) Z71.9
    boarding school resident Z59.3
    consanguinity Z71.89
    feared complaint and no disease found Z71.1
    human immunodeficiency virus (HIV) Z71.7
    institutional resident Z59.3
    on behalf of another Z71.0
      related to sexual behavior or orientation
        Z70.2
    person living alone Z60.2
    specified reason NEC Z71.89
  natural family planning
    procreative Z31.61
    to avoid pregnancy Z30.02
  perpetrator (of)
    abuse NEC Z69.82
    child abuse
      non-parental Z69.021
      parental Z69.011
    rape NEC Z69.82
    spousal abuse Z69.12
  procreative NEC Z31.69
    fertility preservation (prior to cancer therapy)
      (prior to removal of gonads) Z31.62
    using natural family planning Z31.61
  promiscuity Z70.1
  rape victim Z69.81
  religious Z71.81
  safety for travel (international) Z71.84
  sex, sexual (related to) Z70.9
    attitude(s) Z70.0
    behavior or orientation Z70.1
    combined concerns Z70.3
    non-responsiveness Z70.1
    on behalf of third party Z70.2
    specified reason NEC Z70.8
  specified reason NEC Z71.89
  spiritual Z71.81
  spousal abuse (perpetrator) Z69.12
    victim Z69.11
  substance abuse Z71.89
    alcohol Z71.41
    drug Z71.51
    tobacco Z71.6
  travel (international) Z71.84
  tobacco use Z71.6
  use (of)
    insulin pump Z46.81
▶vaccine product safety Z71.85
  victim (of)
    abuse Z69.81
    child abuse
      by parent Z69.010
      non-parental Z69.020
    rape NEC Z69.81
Coupled rhythm R00.8

Couvelaire syndrome or uterus (complicating
  delivery) O45.8X-●
COVID-19 U07.1
▶condition post U09.9
  contact (with) Z20.822
  exposure (to) Z20.822
  history of (personal) Z86.16
▶long (haul) U09.9
  pneumonia J12.82
  screening Z11.52
▶sequelae (post acute) U09.9
Cowperitis —see Urethritis
Cowper's gland —see condition
Cowpox B08.010
  due to vaccination T88.1
Coxa
  magna M91.4-●
  plana M91.2-●
  valga (acquired) —see also Deformity, limb,
    specified type NEC, thigh
    congenital Q65.81
    sequelae (late effect) of rickets E64.3
  vara (acquired) —see also Deformity, limb,
    specified type NEC, thigh
    congenital Q65.82
    sequelae (late effect) of rickets E64.3
Coxalgia, coxalgic (nontuberculous) —see also
  Pain, joint, hip
  tuberculous A18.02
Coxitis —see Monoarthritis, hip
Coxsackie (virus) (infection) B34.1
  as cause of disease classified elsewhere B97.11
  carditis B33.20
  central nervous system NEC A88.8
  endocarditis B33.21
  enteritis A08.39
  meningitis (aseptic) A87.0
  myocarditis B33.22
  pericarditis B33.23
  pharyngitis B08.5
  pleurodynia B33.0
  specific disease NEC B33.8
Crabs, meaning pubic lice B85.3
Crack baby P04.41
Cracked nipple N64.0
  associated with
    lactation O92.13
    pregnancy O92.11-●
    puerperium O92.12
Cracked tooth K03.81
Cradle cap L21.0
Craft neurosis F48.8
Cramp(s) R25.2
  abdominal —see Pain, abdominal
  bathing T75.1
  colic R10.83
    psychogenic F45.8
  due to immersion T75.1
  fireman T67.2
  heat T67.2
  immersion T75.1
  intestinal —see Pain, abdominal
    psychogenic F45.8
  leg, sleep related G47.62
  limb (lower) (upper) NEC R25.2
    sleep related G47.62
  linotypist's F48.8
    organic G25.89
  muscle (limb) (general) R25.2
    due to immersion T75.1
    psychogenic F45.8
  occupational (hand) F48.8
    organic G25.89
  salt-depletion E87.1
  sleep related, leg G47.62
  stoker's T67.2
  swimmer's T75.1
  telegrapher's F48.8
    organic G25.89
  typist's F48.8
    organic G25.89
  uterus N94.89
    menstrual —see Dysmenorrhea

Cramp(s) (Continued)
  writer's F48.8
    organic G25.89
Cranial —see condition
Craniocleidodysostosis Q74.0
Craniofenestria (skull) Q75.8
Craniolacunia (skull) Q75.8
Craniopagus Q89.4
Craniopathy, metabolic M85.2
Craniopharyngeal —see condition
Craniopharyngioma D44.4
Craniorachischisis (totalis) Q00.1
Cranioschisis Q75.8
Craniostenosis Q75.0
Craniosynostosis Q75.0
Craniotabes (cause unknown) M83.8
  neonatal P96.3
  rachitic E64.3
  syphilitic A50.56
Cranium —see condition
Craw-craw —see Onchocerciasis
Creaking joint —see Derangement, joint,
  specified type NEC
Creeping
  eruption B76.9
  palsy or paralysis G12.22
Crenated tongue K14.8
Creotoxism A05.9
Crepitus
  caput Q75.8
  joint —see Derangement, joint, specified type
    NEC
Crescent or conus choroid, congenital Q14.3
CREST syndrome M34.1
Cretin, cretinism (congenital) (endemic)
  (nongoitrous) (sporadic) E00.9
  pelvis
    with disproportion (fetopelvic) O33.0
      causing obstructed labor O65.0
  type
    hypothyroid E00.1
    mixed E00.2
    myxedematous E00.1
    neurological E00.0
Creutzfeldt-Jakob disease or syndrome (with
  dementia) A81.00
  familial A81.09
  iatrogenic A81.09
  specified NEC A81.09
  sporadic A81.09
  variant (vCJD) A81.01
Crib death R99
Cribriform hymen Q52.3
Cri-du-chat syndrome Q93.4
Crigler-Najjar disease or syndrome E80.5
Crime, victim of Z65.4
Crimean hemorrhagic fever A98.0
Criminalism F60.2
Crisis
  abdomen R10.0
  acute reaction F43.0
  addisonian E27.2
  adrenal (cortical) E27.2
  celiac K90.0
  Dietl's N13.8
  emotional —see also Disorder, adjustment
    acute reaction to stress F43.0
    specific to childhood and adolescence F93.8
  glaucomatocyclitic —see Glaucoma,
    secondary, inflammation
  heart —see Failure, heart
  nitritoid I95.2
    correct substance properly administered —
      see Table of Drugs and Chemicals, by
      drug, adverse effect
    overdose or wrong substance given
      or taken —see Table of Drugs and
      Chemicals, by drug, poisoning
  oculogyric H51.8
    psychogenic F45.8
  Pel's (tabetic) A52.11
  psychosexual identity F64.2
  renal N28.0

Crisis *(Continued)*
  sickle-cell D57.00
    with
      acute chest syndrome D57.01
      cerebral vascular involvement D57.03
      crisis (painful) D57.00
        with complication specified NEC D57.09
      splenic sequestration D57.02
      vasoocclusive pain D57.00
  state (acute reaction) F43.0
  tabetic A52.11
  thyroid —*see* Thyrotoxicosis with thyroid storm
  thyrotoxic —*see* Thyrotoxicosis with thyroid storm
Crocq's disease (acrocyanosis) I73.89
Crohn's disease —*see* Enteritis, regional
Crooked septum, nasal J34.2
Cross syndrome E70.328
Crossbite (anterior) (posterior) M26.24
Cross-eye —*see* Strabismus, convergent concomitant
Croup, croupous (catarrhal) (infectious) (inflammatory) (nondiphtheritic) J05.0
  bronchial J20.9
  diphtheritic A36.2
  false J38.5
  spasmodic J38.5
    diphtheritic A36.2
  stridulous J38.5
    diphtheritic A36.2
Crouzon's disease Q75.1
Crowding, tooth, teeth, fully erupted M26.31
CRST syndrome M34.1
Cruchet's disease A85.8
Cruelty in children —*see also* Disorder, conduct
Crural ulcer —*see* Ulcer, lower limb
Crush, crushed, crushing T14.8
  abdomen S38.1
  ankle S97.0-●
  arm (upper) (and shoulder) S47.-●
  axilla —*see* Crush, arm
  back, lower S38.1
  buttock S38.1
  cheek S07.0
  chest S28.0
  cranium S07.1
  ear S07.0
  elbow S57.0-●
  extremity
    lower
      ankle —*see* Crush, ankle
      below knee —*see* Crush, leg
      foot —*see* Crush, foot
      hip —*see* Crush, hip
      knee —*see* Crush, knee
      thigh —*see* Crush, thigh
      toe —*see* Crush, toe
    upper
      below elbow S67.9-●
      elbow —*see* Crush, elbow
      finger —*see* Crush, finger
      forearm —*see* Crush, forearm
      hand —*see* Crush, hand
      thumb —*see* Crush, thumb
      upper arm —*see* Crush, arm
      wrist —*see* Crush, wrist
  face S07.0
  finger(s) S67.1-●
    with hand (and wrist) —*see* Crush, hand, specified site NEC
    index S67.19-●
    little S67.19-●
    middle S67.19-●
    ring S67.19-●
    thumb —*see* Crush, thumb
  foot S97.8-●
    toe —*see* Crush, toe
  forearm S57.8-●
  genitalia, external
    female S38.002
      vagina S38.03
      vulva S38.03

Crush, crushed, crushing *(Continued)*
  genitalia, external *(Continued)*
    male S38.001
      penis S38.01
      scrotum S38.02
      testis S38.02
  hand (except fingers alone) S67.2-●
    with wrist S67.4-●
  head S07.9
    specified NEC S07.8
  heel —*see* Crush, foot
  hip S77.0-●
    with thigh S77.2-●
  internal organ (abdomen, chest, or pelvis) NEC T14.8
  knee S87.0-●
  labium (majus) (minus) S38.03
  larynx S17.0
  leg (lower) S87.8-●
    knee —*see* Crush, knee
  lip S07.0
  lower
    back S38.1
    leg —*see* Crush, leg
  neck S17.9
  nerve —*see* Injury, nerve
  nose S07.0
  pelvis S38.1
  penis S38.01
  scalp S07.8
  scapular region —*see* Crush, arm
  scrotum S38.02
  severe, unspecified site T14.8
  shoulder (and upper arm) —*see* Crush, arm
  skull S07.1
  syndrome (complication of trauma) T79.5
  testis S38.02
  thigh S77.1-●
    with hip S77.2-●
  throat S17.8
  thumb S67.0-●
    with hand (and wrist) —*see* Crush, hand, specified site NEC
  toe(s) S97.10-●
    great S97.11-●
    lesser S97.12-●
  trachea S17.0
  vagina S38.03
  vulva S38.03
  wrist S67.3-●
    with hand S67.4-●
Crusta lactea L21.0
Crusts R23.4
Crutch paralysis —*see* Injury, brachial plexus
Cruveilhier-Baumgarten cirrhosis, disease or syndrome K74.69
Cruveilhier's atrophy or disease G12.8
Crying (constant) (continuous) (excessive)
  child, adolescent, or adult R45.83
  infant (baby) (newborn) R68.11
Cryofibrinogenemia D89.2
Cryoglobulinemia (essential) (idiopathic) (mixed) (primary) (purpura) (secondary) (vasculitis) D89.1
  with lung involvement D89.1 *[J99]*
Cryptitis (anal) (rectal) K62.89
Cryptococcosis, cryptococcus (infection) (neoformans) B45.9
  bone B45.3
  cerebral B45.1
  cutaneous B45.2
  disseminated B45.7
  generalized B45.7
  meningitis B45.1
  meningocerebralis B45.1
  osseous B45.3
  pulmonary B45.0
  skin B45.2
  specified NEC B45.8
Cryptopapillitis (anus) K62.89
Cryptophthalmos Q11.2
  syndrome Q87.0

Cryptorchid, cryptorchism, cryptorchidism Q53.9
  bilateral Q53.20
    abdominal Q53.211
    perineal Q53.22
  unilateral Q53.10
    abdominal Q53.111
    perineal Q53.12
Cryptosporidiosis A07.2
  hepatobiliary B88.8
  respiratory B88.8
Cryptostromosis J67.6
Crystalluria R82.998
Cubitus
  congenital Q68.8
  valgus (acquired) M21.0-●
    congenital Q68.8
    sequelae (late effect) of rickets E64.3
  varus (acquired) M21.1-●
    congenital Q68.8
    sequelae (late effect) of rickets E64.3
Cultural deprivation or shock Z60.3
Curling esophagus K22.4
Curling's ulcer —*see* Ulcer, peptic, acute
Curschmann (-Batten) (-Steinert) disease or syndrome G71.11
Curse, Ondine's —*see* Apnea, sleep
Curvature
  organ or site, congenital NEC —*see* Distortion
  penis (lateral) Q55.61
  Pott's (spinal) A18.01
  radius, idiopathic, progressive (congenital) Q74.0
  spine (acquired) (angular) (idiopathic) (incorrect) (postural) —*see* Dorsopathy, deforming
    congenital Q67.5
    due to or associated with
      Charcot-Marie-Tooth disease —*see also* subcategory M49.8 G60.0
      osteitis
        deformans M88.88
        fibrosa cystica —*see also* subcategory M49.8 E21.0
      tuberculosis (Pott's curvature) A18.01
    sequelae (late effect) of rickets E64.3
    tuberculous A18.01
Cushingoid due to steroid therapy E24.2
  correct substance properly administered —*see* Table of Drugs and Chemicals, by drug, adverse effect
  overdose or wrong substance given or taken —*see* Table of Drugs and Chemicals, by drug, poisoning
Cushing's
  syndrome or disease E24.9
    drug-induced E24.2
    iatrogenic E24.2
    pituitary-dependent E24.0
    specified NEC E24.8
  ulcer —*see* Ulcer, peptic, acute
Cusp, Carabelli - omit code
Cut (external) —*see also* Laceration
  muscle —*see* Injury, muscle
Cutaneous —*see also* condition
  hemorrhage R23.3
  larva migrans B76.9
Cutis —*see also* condition
  hyperelastica Q82.8
    acquired L57.4
  laxa (hyperelastica) —*see* Dermatolysis
  marmorata R23.8
  osteosis L94.2
  pendula —*see* Dermatolysis
  rhomboidalis nuchae L57.2
  verticis gyrata Q82.8
    acquired L91.8
Cyanosis R23.0
  due to
    patent foramen botalli Q21.1
    persistent foramen ovale Q21.1
  enterogenous D74.8
  paroxysmal digital —*see* Raynaud's disease
    with gangrene I73.01
  retina, retinal H35.89

▶ New   ⇒ Revised   ~~deleted~~ Deleted   ● Use Additional Character(s)

Cyanotic heart disease I24.9
  congenital Q24.9
Cycle
  anovulatory N97.0
  menstrual, irregular N92.6
Cyclencephaly Q04.9
Cyclical vomiting, in migraine (see also
    Vomiting, cyclical) G43.A0
  psychogenic F50.89
Cyclitis —see also Iridocyclitis H20.9
  chronic —see Iridocyclitis, chronic
  Fuchs' heterochromic H20.81-●
  granulomatous —see Iridocyclitis, chronic
  lens-induced —see Iridocyclitis,
      lens-induced
  posterior H30.2-●
Cycloid personality F34.0
Cyclophoria H50.54
Cyclopia, cyclops Q87.0
Cyclopism Q87.0
Cyclosporiasis A07.4
Cyclothymia F34.0
Cyclothymic personality F34.0
Cyclotropia H50.41-●
Cylindroma —see also Neoplasm, malignant,
    by site
  eccrine dermal —see Neoplasm, skin, benign
  skin —see Neoplasm, skin, benign
Cylindruria R82.998
Cynanche
  diphtheritic A36.2
  tonsillaris J36
Cynophobia F40.218
Cynorexia R63.2
Cyphosis —see Kyphosis
Cyprus fever —see Brucellosis
Cyst (colloid) (mucous) (simple) (retention)
  adenoid (infected) J35.8
  adrenal gland E27.8
    congenital Q89.1
  air, lung J98.4
  allantoic Q64.4
  alveolar process (jaw bone) M27.40
  amnion, amniotic O41.8X-●
  aneurysmal M27.49
  anterior
    chamber (eye) —see Cyst, iris
    nasopalatine K09.1
  antrum J34.1
  anus K62.89
  apical (tooth) (periodontal) K04.8
  appendix K38.8
  arachnoid, brain (acquired) G93.0
    congenital Q04.6
  arytenoid J38.7
  Baker's M71.2-●
    ruptured M66.0
    tuberculous A18.02
  Bartholin's gland N75.0
  bile duct (common) (hepatic) K83.5
  bladder (multiple) (trigone) N32.89
  blue dome (breast) —see Cyst, breast
  bone (local) NEC M85.60
    aneurysmal M85.50
      ankle M85.57-●
      foot M85.57-●
      forearm M85.53-●
      hand M85.54-●
      jaw M27.49
      lower leg M85.56-●
      multiple site M85.59
      neck M85.58
      rib M85.58
      shoulder M85.51-●
      skull M85.58
      specified site NEC M85.58
      thigh M85.55-●
      toe M85.57-●
      upper arm M85.52-●
      vertebra M85.58
    solitary M85.40
      ankle M85.47-●
      fibula M85.46-●

Cyst (Continued)
  bone NEC (Continued)
    solitary (Continued)
      foot M85.47-●
      hand M85.44-●
      humerus M85.42-●
      jaw M27.49
      neck M85.48
      pelvis M85.45-●
      radius M85.43-●
      rib M85.48
      shoulder M85.41-●
      skull M85.48
      specified site NEC M85.48
      tibia M85.46-●
      toe M85.47-●
      ulna M85.43-●
      vertebra M85.48
    specified type NEC M85.60
      ankle M85.67-●
      foot M85.67-●
      forearm M85.63-●
      hand M85.64-●
      jaw M27.40
        developmental (nonodontogenic) K09.1
        odontogenic K09.0
        latent M27.0
      lower leg M85.66-●
      multiple site M85.69
      neck M85.68
      rib M85.68
      shoulder M85.61-●
      skull M85.68
      specified site NEC M85.68
      thigh M85.65-●
      toe M85.67-●
      upper arm M85.62-●
      vertebra M85.68
  brain (acquired) G93.0
    congenital Q04.6
    hydatid B67.99 [G94]
    third ventricle (colloid), congenital
        Q04.6
  branchial (cleft) Q18.0
  branchiogenic Q18.0
  breast (benign) (blue dome) (pedunculated)
      (solitary) N60.0-●
    involution —see Dysplasia, mammary,
        specified type NEC
    sebaceous —see Dysplasia, mammary,
        specified type NEC
  broad ligament (benign) N83.8
  bronchogenic (mediastinal) (sequestration)
      J98.4
    congenital Q33.0
  buccal K09.8
  bulbourethral gland N36.8
  bursa, bursal NEC M71.30
    with rupture —see Rupture, synovium
    ankle M71.37-●
    elbow M71.32-●
    foot M71.37-●
    hand M71.34-●
    hip M71.35-●
    multiple sites M71.39
    pharyngeal J39.2
    popliteal space —see Cyst, Baker's
    shoulder M71.31-●
    specified site NEC M71.38
    wrist M71.33-●
  calcifying odontogenic D16.5
    upper jaw (bone) (maxilla) D16.4
  canal of Nuck (female) N94.89
    congenital Q52.4
  canthus —see Cyst, conjunctiva
  carcinomatous —see Neoplasm, malignant,
      by site
  cauda equina G95.89
  cavum septi pellucidi —see Cyst, brain
  celomic (pericardium) Q24.8
  cerebellopontine (angle) —see Cyst, brain
  cerebellum —see Cyst, brain
  cerebral —see Cyst, brain

Cyst (Continued)
  cervical lateral Q18.0
  cervix NEC N88.8
    embryonic Q51.6
    nabothian N88.8
  chiasmal optic NEC —see Disorder, optic,
      chiasm
  chocolate (ovary) N80.1
  choledochus, congenital Q44.4
  chorion O41.8X-●
  choroid plexus G93.0
    congenital Q04.6
  ciliary body —see Cyst, iris
  clitoris N90.7
  colon K63.89
  common (bile) duct K83.5
  congenital NEC Q89.8
    adrenal gland Q89.1
    epiglottis Q31.8
    esophagus Q39.8
    fallopian tube Q50.4
    kidney Q61.00
      more than one (multiple) Q61.02
        specified as polycystic Q61.3
          adult type Q61.2
          infantile type NEC Q61.19
            collecting duct dilation Q61.11
      solitary Q61.01
    larynx Q31.8
    liver Q44.6
    lung Q33.0
    mediastinum Q34.1
    ovary Q50.1
    oviduct Q50.4
    periurethral (tissue) Q64.79
    prepuce Q55.69
    salivary gland (any) Q38.4
    sublingual Q38.6
    submaxillary gland Q38.6
    thymus (gland) Q89.2
    tongue Q38.3
    ureterovesical orifice Q62.8
    vulva Q52.79
  conjunctiva H11.44-●
  cornea H18.89-●
  corpora quadrigemina G93.0
  corpus
    albicans N83.29-●
    luteum (hemorrhagic) (ruptured) N83.1-●
  Cowper's gland (benign) (infected) N36.8
  cranial meninges G93.0
  craniobuccal pouch E23.6
  craniopharyngeal pouch E23.6
  cystic duct K82.8
  Cysticercus —see Cysticercosis
  Dandy-Walker Q03.1
    with spina bifida —see Spina bifida
  dental (root) K04.8
    developmental K09.0
    eruption K09.0
    primordial K09.0
  dentigerous (mandible) (maxilla) K09.0
  dermoid —see Neoplasm, benign, by site
    with malignant transformation C56.-●
    implantation
      external area or site (skin) NEC L72.0
      iris —see Cyst, iris, implantation
      vagina N89.8
      vulva N90.7
    mouth K09.8
    oral soft tissue K09.8
    sacrococcygeal —see Cyst, pilonidal
  developmental K09.1
    odontogenic K09.0
    oral region (nonodontogenic) K09.1
    ovary, ovarian Q50.1
  dura (cerebral) G93.0
    spinal G96.198
  ear (external) Q18.1
  echinococcal —see Echinococcus
  embryonic
    cervix uteri Q51.6
    fallopian tube Q50.4

Cyst (Continued)
  embryonic (Continued)
    vagina Q52.4
  endometrium, endometrial (uterus) N85.8
    ectopic —see Endometriosis
  enterogenous Q43.8
  epidermal, epidermoid (inclusion) (see also
      Cyst, skin) L72.0
    mouth K09.8
    oral soft tissue K09.8
  epididymis N50.3
  epiglottis J38.7
  epiphysis cerebri E34.8
  epithelial (inclusion) L72.0
  epoophoron Q50.5
  eruption K09.0
➡ esophagus K22.89
  ethmoid sinus J34.1
  external female genital organs NEC N90.7
  eye NEC H57.89
    congenital Q15.8
  eyelid (sebaceous) H02.829
    infected —see Hordeolum
    left H02.826
      lower H02.825
      upper H02.824
    right H02.823
      lower H02.822
      upper H02.821
  fallopian tube N83.8
    congenital Q50.4
  fimbrial (twisted) Q50.4
  fissural (oral region) K09.1
  follicle (graafian) (hemorrhagic) N83.0-●
    nabothian N88.8
  follicular (atretic) (hemorrhagic) (ovarian)
      N83.0-●
    dentigerous K09.0
    odontogenic K09.0
    skin L72.9
      specified NEC L72.8
  frontal sinus J34.1
  gallbladder K82.8
  ganglion —see Ganglion
  Gartner's duct Q52.4
  gingiva K09.0
  gland of Moll —see Cyst, eyelid
  globulomaxillary K09.1
  graafian follicle (hemorrhagic) N83.0-●
  granulosal lutein (hemorrhagic) N83.1-●
  hemangiomatous D18.00
    intra-abdominal D18.03
    intracranial D18.02
    skin D18.01
    specified site NEC D18.09
  hemorrhagic M27.49
  hydatid —see also Echinococcus B67.90
    brain B67.99 [G94]
    liver —see also Cyst, liver, hydatid B67.8
    lung NEC B67.99 [J99]
    Morgagni
      female Q50.5
      male (epididymal) Q55.4
        testicular Q55.29
    specified site NEC B67.99
  hymen N89.8
    embryonic Q52.4
  hypopharynx J39.2
  hypophysis, hypophyseal (duct) (recurrent)
      E23.6
    cerebri E23.6
  implantation (dermoid)
    external area or site (skin) NEC L72.0
    iris —see Cyst, iris, implantation
    vagina N89.8
    vulva N90.7
  incisive canal K09.1
  inclusion (epidermal) (epithelial)
      (epidermoid) (squamous) L72.0
    not of skin - code under Cyst, by site
  intestine (large) (small) K63.89
  intracranial —see Cyst, brain

Cyst (Continued)
  intraligamentous —see also Disorder, ligament
    knee —see Derangement, knee
  intrasellar E23.6
  iris H21.309
    exudative H21.31-●
    idiopathic H21.30-●
    implantation H21.32-●
    parasitic H21.33-●
    pars plana (primary) H21.34-●
      exudative H21.35-●
  jaw (bone) M27.40
    aneurysmal M27.49
    developmental (odontogenic) K09.0
    fissural K09.1
    hemorrhagic M27.49
    traumatic M27.49
  joint NEC —see Disorder, joint, specified type
      NEC
  kidney (acquired) N28.1
    calyceal —see Hydronephrosis
    congenital Q61.00
    more than one (multiple) Q61.02
      specified as polycystic Q61.3
        adult type (autosomal dominant)
            Q61.2
        infantile type (autosomal recessive)
            NEC Q61.19
          collecting duct dilation Q61.11
    pyelogenic —see Hydronephrosis
    simple N28.1
    solitary (single) Q61.01
      acquired N28.1
  labium (majus) (minus) N90.7
    sebaceous N90.7
  lacrimal —see also Disorder, lacrimal system,
      specified NEC
    gland H04.13-●
    passages or sac —see Disorder, lacrimal
        system, specified NEC
  larynx J38.7
  lateral periodontal K09.0
  lens H27.8
    congenital Q12.8
  lip (gland) K13.0
  liver (idiopathic) (simple) K76.89
    congenital Q44.6
    hydatid B67.8
      granulosus B67.0
      multilocularis B67.5
  lung J98.4
    congenital Q33.0
    giant bullous J43.9
  lutein N83.1-●
  lymphangiomatous D18.1
  lymphoepithelial, oral soft tissue K09.8
  macula —see Degeneration, macula, hole
  malignant —see Neoplasm, malignant, by site
  mammary gland —see Cyst, breast
  mandible M27.40
    dentigerous K09.0
    radicular K04.8
  maxilla M27.40
    dentigerous K09.0
    radicular K04.8
  medial, face and neck Q18.8
  median
    anterior maxillary K09.1
    palatal K09.1
  mediastinum, congenital Q34.1
  meibomian (gland) —see Chalazion
    infected —see Hordeolum
  membrane, brain G93.0
  meninges (cerebral) G93.0
    spinal G96.198
  meniscus, knee —see Derangement, knee,
      meniscus, cystic
  mesentery, mesenteric K66.8
    chyle I89.8
  mesonephric duct
    female Q50.5
    male Q55.4
  milk N64.89

Cyst (Continued)
  Morgagni (hydatid)
    female Q50.5
    male (epididymal) Q55.4
      testicular Q55.29
  mouth K09.8
  Müllerian duct Q50.4
    appendix testis Q55.29
    cervix Q51.6
    fallopian tube Q50.4
    female Q50.4
    male Q55.29
    prostatic utricle Q55.4
    vagina (embryonal) Q52.4
  multilocular (ovary) D39.10
    benign —see Neoplasm, benign, by site
  myometrium N85.8
  nabothian (follicle) (ruptured) N88.8
  nasoalveolar K09.1
  nasolabial K09.1
  nasopalatine (anterior) (duct) K09.1
  nasopharynx J39.2
  neoplastic —see Neoplasm, uncertain
      behavior, by site
    benign —see Neoplasm, benign, by site
  nerve root
    cervical G96.191
    lumbar G96.191
    sacral G96.191
    thoracic G96.191
  nervous system NEC G96.89
  neuroenteric (congenital) Q06.8
  nipple —see Cyst, breast
  nose (turbinates) J34.1
    sinus J34.1
  odontogenic, developmental K09.0
  omentum (lesser) K66.8
    congenital Q45.8
  ora serrata —see Cyst, retina, ora serrata
  oral
    region K09.9
      developmental (nonodontogenic) K09.1
      specified NEC K09.8
    soft tissue K09.9
      specified NEC K09.8
  orbit H05.81-●
  ovary, ovarian (twisted) N83.20-●
    adherent N83.20-●
    chocolate N80.1
    corpus
      albicans N83.29-●
      luteum (hemorrhagic) N83.1-●
    dermoid D27.9
    developmental Q50.1
    due to failure of involution NEC N83.20-●
    endometrial N80.1
    follicular (graafian) (hemorrhagic) N83.0-●
    hemorrhagic N83.20-●
    in pregnancy or childbirth O34.8-●
      with obstructed labor O65.5
    multilocular D39.10
    pseudomucinous D27.9
    retention N83.29-●
    serous N83.20-●
    specified NEC N83.29-●
    theca lutein (hemorrhagic) N83.1-●
    tuberculous A18.18
  oviduct N83.8
  palate (median) (fissural) K09.1
  palatine papilla (jaw) K09.1
  pancreas, pancreatic (hemorrhagic) (true) K86.2
    congenital Q45.2
    false K86.3
  paralabral
    hip M24.85-●
    shoulder S43.43-●
  paramesonephric duct Q50.4
    female Q50.4
    male Q55.29
  paranephric N28.1
  paraphysis, cerebri, congenital Q04.6
  parasitic B89
  parathyroid (gland) E21.4

▶ New   ➡ Revised   ~~deleted~~ Deleted   ● Use Additional Character(s)

Cyst *(Continued)*
 paratubal N83.8
 paraurethral duct N36.8
 paroophoron Q50.5
 parotid gland K11.6
 parovarian Q50.5
 pelvis, female N94.89
  in pregnancy or childbirth O34.8-●
   causing obstructed labor O65.5
 penis (sebaceous) N48.89
 periapical K04.8
 pericardial (congenital) Q24.8
  acquired (secondary) I31.8
 pericoronal K09.0
 perineural G96.191
 periodontal K04.8
  lateral K09.0
 peripelvic (lymphatic) N28.1
 peritoneum K66.8
  chylous I89.8
 periventricular, acquired, newborn P91.1
 pharynx (wall) J39.2
 pilar L72.11
 pilonidal (infected) (rectum) L05.91
  with abscess L05.01
  malignant C44.59-●
 pituitary (duct) (gland) E23.6
 placenta O43.19-●
 pleura J94.8
 popliteal —*see* Cyst, Baker's
 porencephalic Q04.6
  acquired G93.0
 postanal (infected) —*see* Cyst, pilonidal
 postmastoidectomy cavity (mucosal) —*see*
   Complications, postmastoidectomy, cyst
 preauricular Q18.1
 prepuce N47.4
  congenital Q55.69
 primordial (jaw) K09.0
 prostate N42.83
 pseudomucinous (ovary) D27.9
 pupillary, miotic H21.27-●
 radicular (residual) K04.8
 radiculodental K04.8
 ranular K11.8
 Rathke's pouch E23.6
 rectum (epithelium) (mucous) K62.89
 renal —*see* Cyst, kidney
 residual (radicular) K04.8
 retention (ovary) N83.29-●
  salivary gland K11.6
 retina H33.19-●
  ora serrata H33.11-●
  parasitic H33.12-●
 retroperitoneal K68.9
 sacrococcygeal (dermoid) —*see* Cyst,
   pilonidal
 salivary gland or duct (mucous extravasation
   or retention) K11.6
 Sampson's N80.1
 sclera H15.89
 scrotum L72.9
  sebaceous L72.3
 sebaceous (duct) (gland) L72.3
  breast —*see* Dysplasia, mammary, specified
    type NEC
  eyelid —*see* Cyst, eyelid
  genital organ NEC
   female N94.89
   male N50.89
  scrotum L72.3
 semilunar cartilage (knee) (multiple) —*see*
   Derangement, knee, meniscus, cystic
 seminal vesicle N50.89
 serous (ovary) N83.20-●
 sinus (accessory) (nasal) J34.1
 Skene's gland N36.8
 skin L72.9
  breast —*see* Dysplasia, mammary, specified
    type NEC
  epidermal, epidermoid L72.0
  epithelial L72.0
  eyelid —*see* Cyst, eyelid

Cyst *(Continued)*
 skin *(Continued)*
  genital organ NEC
   female N90.7
   male N50.89
  inclusion L72.0
  scrotum L72.9
  sebaceous L72.3
  sweat gland or duct L74.8
 solitary
  bone —*see* Cyst, bone, solitary
  jaw M27.40
  kidney N28.1
 spermatic cord N50.89
 sphenoid sinus J34.1
 spinal meninges G96.198
 spleen NEC D73.4
  congenital Q89.09
  hydatid —*see also* Echinococcus B67.99 [D77]
 Stafne's M27.0
 subarachnoid intrasellar R93.0
 subcutaneous, pheomycotic (chromomycotic)
   B43.2
 subdural (cerebral) G93.0
  spinal cord G96.198
 sublingual gland K11.6
 submandibular gland K11.6
 submaxillary gland K11.6
 suburethral N36.8
 suprarenal gland E27.8
 suprasellar —*see* Cyst, brain
 sweat gland or duct L74.8
 synovial —*see also* Cyst, bursa
  ruptured —*see* Rupture, synovium
 Tarlov G96.191
 tarsal —*see* Chalazion
 tendon (sheath) —*see* Disorder, tendon,
   specified type NEC
 testis N44.2
  tunica albuginea N44.1
 theca lutein (ovary) N83.1-●
 Thornwaldt's J39.2
 thymus (gland) E32.8
 thyroglossal duct (infected) (persistent) Q89.2
 thyroid (gland) E04.1
 thyrolingual duct (infected) (persistent) Q89.2
 tongue K14.8
 tonsil J35.8
 tooth —*see* Cyst, dental
 Tornwaldt's J39.2
 trichilemmal (proliferating) L72.12
 trichodermal L72.12
 tubal (fallopian) N83.8
  inflammatory —*see* Salpingitis, chronic
 tubo-ovarian N83.8
  inflammatory N70.13
 tunica
  albuginea testis N44.1
  vaginalis N50.89
 turbinate (nose) J34.1
 Tyson's gland N48.89
 urachus, congenital Q64.4
 ureter N28.89
 ureterovesical orifice N28.89
 urethra, urethral (gland) N36.8
 uterine ligament N83.8
 uterus (body) (corpus) (recurrent)
   N85.8
  embryonic Q51.818
   cervix Q51.6
 vagina, vaginal (implantation) (inclusion)
   (squamous cell) (wall) N89.8
  embryonic Q52.4
 vallecula, vallecular (epiglottis) J38.7
 vesical (orifice) N32.89
 vitreous body H43.89
 vulva (implantation) (inclusion) N90.7
  congenital Q52.79
  sebaceous gland N90.7
 vulvovaginal gland N90.7
 wolffian
  female Q50.5
  male Q55.4

Cystadenocarcinoma —*see* Neoplasm,
  malignant, by site
 bile duct C22.1
 endometrioid —*see* Neoplasm, malignant,
   by site
  specified site —*see* Neoplasm, malignant,
    by site
  unspecified site
   female C56.9
   male C61
 mucinous
  papillary
   specified site —*see* Neoplasm,
     malignant, by site
   unspecified site C56.9
  specified site —*see* Neoplasm, malignant,
    by site
  unspecified site C56.9
 papillary
  mucinous
   specified site —*see* Neoplasm,
     malignant, by site
   unspecified site C56.9
  pseudomucinous
   specified site —*see* Neoplasm,
     malignant, by site
   unspecified site C56.9
  serous
   specified site —*see* Neoplasm,
     malignant, by site
   unspecified site C56.9
  specified site —*see* Neoplasm, malignant,
    by site
  unspecified site C56.9
 pseudomucinous
  papillary
   specified site —*see* Neoplasm,
     malignant, by site
   unspecified site C56.9
  specified site —*see* Neoplasm, malignant,
    by site
  unspecified site C56.9
 serous
  papillary
   specified site —*see* Neoplasm,
     malignant, by site
   unspecified site C56.9
  specified site —*see* Neoplasm, malignant,
    by site
  unspecified site C56.9
Cystadenofibroma
 clear cell —*see* Neoplasm, benign, by site
 endometrioid D27.9
  borderline malignancy D39.1-●
  malignant C56.-●
 mucinous
  specified site —*see* Neoplasm, benign, by site
  unspecified site D27.9
 serous
  specified site —*see* Neoplasm, benign, by site
  unspecified site D27.9
 specified site —*see* Neoplasm, benign, by site
 unspecified site D27.9
Cystadenoma —*see also* Neoplasm, benign, by
  site
 bile duct D13.4
 endometrioid —*see* Neoplasm, benign, by site
  borderline malignancy —*see* Neoplasm,
    uncertain behavior, by site
 malignant —*see* Neoplasm, malignant, by site
 mucinous
  borderline malignancy
   ovary C56.-●
   specified site NEC —*see* Neoplasm,
     uncertain behavior, by site
   unspecified site C56.9
  papillary
   borderline malignancy
    ovary C56.-●
    specified site NEC —*see* Neoplasm,
      uncertain behavior, by site
    unspecified site C56.9

Cystadenoma *(Continued)*
  mucinous *(Continued)*
    papillary *(Continued)*
      specified site —*see* Neoplasm, benign,
        by site
      unspecified site D27.9
    specified site —*see* Neoplasm, benign, by site
    unspecified site D27.9
  papillary
    borderline malignancy
      ovary C56-•
      specified site NEC —*see* Neoplasm,
        uncertain behavior, by site
      unspecified site C56.9
    lymphomatosum
      specified site —*see* Neoplasm, benign,
        by site
      unspecified site D11.9
    mucinous
      borderline malignancy
        ovary C56.-•
        specified site NEC —*see* Neoplasm,
          uncertain behavior, by site
        unspecified site C56.9
      specified site —*see* Neoplasm, benign,
        by site
      unspecified site D27.9
    pseudomucinous
      borderline malignancy
        ovary C56.-•
        specified site NEC —*see* Neoplasm,
          uncertain behavior, by site
        unspecified site C56.9
      specified site —*see* Neoplasm, benign,
        by site
      unspecified site D27.9
    serous
      borderline malignancy
        ovary C56.-•
        specified site NEC —*see* Neoplasm,
          uncertain behavior, by site
        unspecified site C56.9
      specified site —*see* Neoplasm, benign,
        by site
      unspecified site D27.9
    specified site —*see* Neoplasm, benign, by site
    unspecified site D27.9
  pseudomucinous
    borderline malignancy
      ovary C56.-•
      specified site NEC —*see* Neoplasm,
        uncertain behavior, by site
      unspecified site C56.9
    papillary
      borderline malignancy
        ovary C56.-•
        specified site NEC —*see* Neoplasm,
          uncertain behavior, by site
        unspecified site C56.9
      specified site —*see* Neoplasm, benign,
        by site
      unspecified site D27.9
    specified site —*see* Neoplasm, benign, by site
    unspecified site D27.9
  serous
    borderline malignancy
      ovary C56.-•
      specified site NEC —*see* Neoplasm,
        uncertain behavior, by site
      unspecified site C56.9
    papillary
      borderline malignancy
        ovary C56.-•
        specified site NEC —*see* Neoplasm,
          uncertain behavior, by site
        unspecified site C56.9
      specified site —*see* Neoplasm, benign,
        by site
      unspecified site D27.9
    specified site —*see* Neoplasm, benign, by site
    unspecified site D27.9

Cystathionine synthase deficiency E72.11
Cystathioninemia E72.19
Cystathioninuria E72.19
Cystic —*see also* condition
  breast (chronic) —*see* Mastopathy, cystic
  corpora lutea (hemorrhagic) N83.1-•
  duct —*see* condition
  eyeball (congenital) Q11.0
  fibrosis —*see* Fibrosis, cystic
  kidney (congenital) Q61.9
    adult type Q61.2
    infantile type NEC Q61.19
      collecting duct dilatation Q61.11
    medullary Q61.5
  liver, congenital Q44.6
  lung disease J98.4
    congenital Q33.0
  mastitis, chronic —*see* Mastopathy, cystic
  medullary, kidney Q61.5
  meniscus —*see* Derangement, knee,
    meniscus, cystic
  ovary N83.20-•
Cysticercosis, cysticerciasis B69.9
  with
    epileptiform fits B69.0
    myositis B69.81
  brain B69.0
  central nervous system B69.0
  cerebral B69.0
  ocular B69.1
  specified NEC B69.89
Cysticercus cellulose infestation —*see*
  Cysticercosis
Cystinosis (malignant) E72.04
Cystinuria E72.01
Cystitis (exudative) (hemorrhagic) (septic)
  (suppurative) N30.90
  with
    fibrosis —*see* Cystitis, chronic, interstitial
    hematuria N30.91
    leukoplakia —*see* Cystitis, chronic,
      interstitial
    malakoplakia —*see* Cystitis, chronic,
      interstitial
    metaplasia —*see* Cystitis, chronic, interstitial
    prostatitis N41.3
  acute N30.00
    with hematuria N30.01
    of trigone N30.30
      with hematuria N30.31
  allergic —*see* Cystitis, specified type NEC
  amebic A06.81
  bilharzial B65.9 *[N33]*
  blennorrhagic (gonococcal) A54.01
  bullous —*see* Cystitis, specified type NEC
  calculous N21.0
  chlamydial A56.01
  chronic N30.20
    with hematuria N30.21
    interstitial N30.10
      with hematuria N30.11
    of trigone N30.30
      with hematuria N30.31
    specified NEC N30.20
      with hematuria N30.21
  cystic (a) —*see* Cystitis, specified type NEC
  diphtheritic A36.85
  echinococcal
    granulosus B67.39
    multilocularis B67.69
  emphysematous —*see* Cystitis, specified type
    NEC
  encysted —*see* Cystitis, specified type NEC
  eosinophilic —*see* Cystitis, specified type
    NEC
  follicular —*see* Cystitis, of trigone
  gangrenous —*see* Cystitis, specified type
    NEC
  glandularis —*see* Cystitis, specified type
    NEC

Cystitis *(Continued)*
  gonococcal A54.01
  incrusted —*see* Cystitis, specified type
    NEC
  interstitial (chronic) —*see* Cystitis, chronic,
    interstitial
  irradiation N30.40
    with hematuria N30.41
  irritation —*see* Cystitis, specified type
    NEC
  malignant —*see* Cystitis, specified type
    NEC
  of trigone N30.30
    with hematuria N30.31
  panmural —*see* Cystitis, chronic, interstitial
  polyposa —*see* Cystitis, specified type NEC
  prostatic N41.3
  puerperal (postpartum) O86.22
  radiation —*see* Cystitis, irradiation
  specified type NEC N30.80
    with hematuria N30.81
  subacute —*see* Cystitis, chronic
  submucous —*see* Cystitis, chronic, interstitial
  syphilitic (late) A52.76
  trichomonal A59.03
  tuberculous A18.12
  ulcerative —*see* Cystitis, chronic, interstitial
Cystocele (-urethrocele)
  female N81.10
    with prolapse of uterus —*see* Prolapse,
      uterus
    lateral N81.12
    midline N81.11
    paravaginal N81.12
  in pregnancy or childbirth O34.8-•
    causing obstructed labor O65.5
  male N32.89
Cystolithiasis N21.0
Cystoma —*see also* Neoplasm, benign, by site
  endometrial, ovary N80.1
  mucinous
    specified site —*see* Neoplasm, benign, by site
    unspecified site D27.9
  serous
    specified site —*see* Neoplasm, benign, by site
    unspecified site D27.9
  simple (ovary) N83.29-•
Cystoplegia N31.2
Cystoptosis N32.89
Cystopyelitis —*see* Pyelonephritis
Cystorrhagia N32.89
Cystosarcoma phyllodes D48.6-•
  benign D24-•
  malignant —*see* Neoplasm, breast, malignant
Cystostomy
  attention to Z43.5
  complication —*see* Complications, cystostomy
  status Z93.50
    appendico-vesicostomy Z93.52
    cutaneous Z93.51
    specified NEC Z93.59
Cystourethritis —*see* Urethritis
Cystourethrocele —*see also* Cystocele
  female N81.10
    with uterine prolapse —*see* Prolapse,
      uterus
    lateral N81.12
    midline N81.11
    paravaginal N81.12
  male N32.89
Cytomegalic inclusion disease
  congenital P35.1
Cytomegalovirus infection B25.9
Cytomycosis (reticuloendothelial) B39.4
Cytopenia D75.9
  refractory
    with multilineage dysplasia D46.A
      and ring sideroblasts (RCMD RS) D46.B
Czerny's disease (periodic hydrarthrosis of the
  knee) —*see* Effusion, joint, knee

▶ New   ⇒ Revised   ~~deleted~~ Deleted   • Use Additional Character(s)

D

Daae (-Finsen) disease (epidemic pleurodynia) B33.0
Dabney's grip B33.0
Da Costa's syndrome F45.8
Dacryoadenitis, dacryadenitis H04.00-●
  acute H04.01-●
  chronic H04.02-●
Dacryocystitis H04.30-●
  acute H04.32-●
  chronic H04.41-●
  neonatal P39.1
  phlegmonous H04.31-●
  syphilitic A52.71
    congenital (early) A50.01
  trachomatous, active A71.1
    sequelae (late effect) B94.0
Dacryocystoblenorrhea —see Inflammation, lacrimal, passages, chronic
Dacryocystocele —see Disorder, lacrimal system, changes
Dacryolith, dacryolithiasis H04.51-●
Dacryoma —see Disorder, lacrimal system, changes
Dacryopericystitis —see Dacryocystitis
Dacryops H04.11-●
Dacryostenosis —see also Stenosis, lacrimal
  congenital Q10.5
Dactylitis
  bone —see Osteomyelitis
  sickle-cell D57.00
    Hb C D57.219
    Hb SS D57.00
    specified NEC D57.819
  skin L08.9
  syphilitic A52.77
  tuberculous A18.03
Dactylolysis spontanea (ainhum) L94.6
Dactylosymphysis Q70.9
  fingers —see Syndactylism, complex, fingers
  toes —see Syndactylism, complex, toes
Damage
  arteriosclerotic —see Arteriosclerosis
  brain (nontraumatic) G93.9
    anoxic, hypoxic G93.1
      resulting from a procedure G97.82
    child NEC G80.9
    due to birth injury P11.2
  cardiorenal (vascular) —see Hypertension, cardiorenal
  cerebral NEC —see Damage, brain
  coccyx, complicating delivery O71.6
  coronary —see Disease, heart, ischemic
  deep tissue, pressure-induced —see also L89
    with final character .6
  eye, birth injury P15.3
  liver (nontraumatic) K76.9
    alcoholic K70.9
    due to drugs —see Disease, liver, toxic
    toxic —see Disease, liver, toxic
  lung
    dabbing (related) U07.0
    electronic cigarette (related) U07.0
    vaping (associated) (device) (product) (use) U07.0
  medication T88.7
  organ
    dabbing (related) U07.0
    electronic cigarette (related) U07.0
    vaping (associated) (device) (product) (use) U07.0
  pelvic
    joint or ligament, during delivery O71.6
    organ NEC
      during delivery O71.5
      following ectopic or molar pregnancy O08.6
  renal —see Disease, renal
  subendocardium, subendocardial —see Degeneration, myocardial
  vascular I99.9

Dana-Putnam syndrome (subacute combined sclerosis with pernicious anemia) —see Degeneration, combined
Danbolt (-Cross) syndrome (acrodermatitis enteropathica) E83.2
Dandruff L21.0
Dandy-Walker syndrome Q03.1
  with spina bifida —see Spina bifida
Danlos' syndrome (see also Syndrome, Ehler-Danlos) Q79.60
Darier (-White) disease (congenital) Q82.8
  meaning erythema annulare centrifugum L53.1
Darier-Roussy sarcoid D86.3
Darling's disease or histoplasmosis B39.4
Darwin's tubercle Q17.8
Dawson's (inclusion body) encephalitis A81.1
De Beurmann (-Gougerot) disease B42.1
De la Tourette's syndrome F95.2
De Lange's syndrome Q87.19
De Morgan's spots (senile angiomas) I78.1
De Quervain's
  disease (tendon sheath) M65.4
  syndrome E34.51
  thyroiditis (subacute granulomatous thyroiditis) E06.1
De Toni-Fanconi (-Debré) syndrome E72.09
  with cystinosis E72.04
Dead
  fetus, retained (mother) O36.4
    early pregnancy O02.1
  labyrinth —see subcategory H83.2
  ovum, retained O02.0
Deaf nonspeaking NEC H91.3
Deafmutism (acquired) (congenital) NEC H91.3
  hysterical F44.6
  syphilitic, congenital —see also subcategory H94.8 A50.09
Deafness (acquired) (complete) (hereditary) (partial) H91.9-●
  with blue sclera and fragility of bone Q78.0
  auditory fatigue —see Deafness, specified type NEC
  aviation T70.0
    nerve injury —see Injury, nerve, acoustic, specified type NEC
  boilermaker's —see subcategory H83.3
  central —see Deafness, sensorineural
  conductive H90.2
    and sensorineural
      mixed H90.8
        bilateral H90.6
    bilateral H90.0
    unilateral H90.1-●
      with restricted hearing on the contralateral side H90.A-●
  congenital H90.5
    with blue sclera and fragility of bone Q78.0
  due to toxic agents —see Deafness, ototoxic
  emotional (hysterical) F44.6
  functional (hysterical) F44.6
  high frequency H91.9-●
  hysterical F44.6
  low frequency H91.9-●
  mental R48.8
  mixed conductive and sensorineural H90.8
    bilateral H90.6
    unilateral H90.7-●
  nerve —see Deafness, sensorineural
  neural —see Deafness, sensorineural
  noise-induced —see also subcategory H83.3
    nerve injury —see Injury, nerve, acoustic, specified type NEC
  nonspeaking H91.3
  ototoxic —see subcategory H91.0
  perceptive —see Deafness, sensorineural
  psychogenic (hysterical) F44.6
  sensorineural H90.5
    and conductive
      mixed H90.8
        bilateral H90.6
    bilateral H90.3

Deafness (Continued)
  sensorineural (Continued)
    unilateral H90.4-●
      with restricted hearing on the contralateral side H90.A-●
  sensory —see Deafness, sensorineural
  specified type NEC —see subcategory H91.8
  sudden (idiopathic) H91.2-●
  syphilitic A52.15
  transient ischemic H93.01-●
  traumatic —see Injury, nerve, acoustic, specified type NEC
  word (developmental) H93.25
Death (cause unknown) (of) (unexplained) (unspecified cause) R99
  brain G93.82
  cardiac (sudden) (with successful resuscitation) — code to underlying disease
    family history of Z82.41
    personal history of Z86.74
  family member (assumed) Z63.4
Debility (chronic) (general) (nervous) R53.81
  congenital or neonatal NOS P96.9
  nervous R53.81
  old age R54
  senile R54
Débove's disease (splenomegaly) R16.1
Decalcification
  bone —see Osteoporosis
  teeth K03.89
Decapsulation, kidney N28.89
Decay
  dental —see Caries, dental
  senile R54
  tooth, teeth —see Caries, dental
Deciduitis (acute)
  following ectopic or molar pregnancy O08.0
Decline (general) —see Debility
  cognitive, age-associated R41.81
Decompensation
  cardiac (acute) (chronic) —see Disease, heart
  cardiovascular —see Disease, cardiovascular
  heart —see Disease, heart
  hepatic —see Failure, hepatic
  myocardial (acute) (chronic) —see Disease, heart
  respiratory J98.8
Decompression sickness T70.3
Decrease (d)
  absolute neutrophile count —see Neutropenia
  blood
    platelets —see Thrombocytopenia
    pressure R03.1
      due to shock following
        injury T79.4
        operation T81.19
  estrogen E28.39
    postablative E89.40
      asymptomatic E89.40
      symptomatic E89.41
  fragility of erythrocytes D58.8
  function
    lipase (pancreatic) K90.3
    ovary in hypopituitarism E23.0
    parenchyma of pancreas K86.89
    pituitary (gland) (anterior) (lobe) E23.0
      posterior (lobe) E23.0
  functional activity R68.89
  glucose R73.09
  hematocrit R71.0
  hemoglobin R71.0
  leukocytes D72.819
    specified NEC D72.818
  libido R68.82
  lymphocytes D72.810
  platelets D69.6
  respiration, due to shock following injury T79.4
  sexual desire R68.82
  tear secretion NEC —see Syndrome, dry eye

Decrease *(Continued)*
  tolerance
    fat K90.49
    glucose R73.09
    pancreatic K90.3
    salt and water E87.8
  vision NEC H54.7
  white blood cell count D72.819
    specified NEC D72.818
Decubitus (ulcer) —*see* Ulcer, pressure, by site
  cervix N86
Deepening acetabulum —*see* Derangement,
    joint, specified type NEC, hip
Defect, defective Q89.9
  3-beta-hydroxysteroid dehydrogenase E25.0
  11-hydroxylase E25.0
  21-hydroxylase E25.0
  abdominal wall, congenital Q79.59
  antibody immunodeficiency D80.9
  aorticopulmonary septum Q21.4
  atrial septal (ostium secundum type) Q21.1
    following acute myocardial infarction
        (current complication) I23.1
    ostium primum type Q21.2
  atrioventricular
    canal Q21.2
    septum Q21.2
  auricular septal Q21.1
  bilirubin excretion NEC E80.6
  biosynthesis, androgen (testicular) E29.1
  bulbar septum Q21.0
  catalase E80.3
  cell membrane receptor complex (CR3) D71
  circulation I99.9
    congenital Q28.9
    newborn Q28.9
  coagulation (factor) —*see also* Deficiency,
      factor D68.9
    with
      ectopic pregnancy O08.1
      molar pregnancy O08.1
    acquired D68.4
    antepartum with hemorrhage —*see*
        Hemorrhage, antepartum, with
        coagulation defect
    due to
      liver disease D68.4
      vitamin K deficiency D68.4
    hereditary NEC D68.2
    intrapartum O67.0
    newborn, transient P61.6
    postpartum O99.13
      with hemorrhage O72.3
    specified type NEC D68.8
  complement system D84.1
  conduction (heart) I45.9
    bone —*see* Deafness, conductive
  congenital, organ or site not listed —*see*
      Anomaly, by site
  coronary sinus Q21.1
  cushion, endocardial Q21.2
  degradation, glycoprotein E77.1
  dental bridge, crown, fillings —*see* Defect,
      dental restoration
  dental restoration K08.50
    specified NEC K08.59
  dentin (hereditary) K00.5
  Descemet's membrane, congenital Q13.89
  developmental —*see also* Anomaly
    cauda equina Q06.3
  diaphragm
    with elevation, eventration or hernia —*see*
        Hernia, diaphragm
    congenital Q79.1
      with hernia Q79.0
      gross (with hernia) Q79.0
  ectodermal, congenital Q82.9
  Eisenmenger's Q21.8
  enzyme
    catalase E80.3
    peroxidase E80.3

Defect, defective *(Continued)*
  esophagus, congenital Q39.9
  extensor retinaculum M62.89
  fibrin polymerization D68.2
  filling
    bladder R93.41
    kidney R93.42-●
    renal pelvis R93.41
    stomach R93.3
    ureter R93.41
    urinary organs, specified NEC R93.49
  GABA (gamma aminobutyric acid) metabolic
      E72.81
  Gerbode Q21.0
  glucose transport, blood-brain barrier E74.810
  glycoprotein degradation E77.1
  Hageman (factor) D68.2
  hearing —*see* Deafness
  high grade F70
  interatrial septal Q21.1
  interauricular septal Q21.1
  interventricular septal Q21.0
    with dextroposition of aorta, pulmonary
        stenosis and hypertrophy of right
        ventricle Q21.3
    in tetralogy of Fallot Q21.3
  learning (specific) —*see* Disorder, learning
  lymphocyte function antigen-1 (LFA-1) D84.0
  lysosomal enzyme, post-translational
      modification E77.0
  major osseous M89.70
    ankle M89.77-●
    carpus M89.74-●
    clavicle M89.71-●
    femur M89.75-●
    fibula M89.76-●
    fingers M89.74-●
    foot M89.77-●
    forearm M89.73-●
    hand M89.74-●
    humerus M89.72-●
    lower leg M89.76-●
    metacarpus M89.74-●
    metatarsus M89.77-●
    multiple sites M89.79
    pelvic region M89.75-●
    pelvis M89.75-●
    radius M89.73-●
    scapula M89.71-●
    shoulder region M89.71-●
    specified NEC M89.78
    tarsus M89.77-●
    thigh M89.75-●
    tibia M89.76-●
    toes M89.77-●
    ulna M89.73-●
  mental —*see* Disability, intellectual
  modification, lysosomal enzymes, post-
      translational E77.0
  obstructive, congenital
    renal pelvis Q62.39
    ureter Q62.39
      atresia —*see* Atresia, ureter
      cecoureterocele Q62.32
      megaureter Q62.2
      orthotopic ureterocele Q62.31
  osseous, major M89.70
    ankle M89.77-●
    carpus M89.74-●
    clavicle M89.71-●
    femur M89.75-●
    fibula M89.76-●
    fingers M89.74-●
    foot M89.77-●
    forearm M89.73-●
    hand M89.74-●
    humerus M89.72-●
    lower leg M89.76-●
    metacarpus M89.74-●
    metatarsus M89.77-●
    multiple sites M89.9

Defect, defective *(Continued)*
  osseous, major *(Continued)*
    pelvic region M89.75-●
    pelvis M89.75-●
    radius M89.73-●
    scapula M89.71-●
    shoulder region M89.71-●
    specified NEC M89.78
    tarsus M89.77-●
    thigh M89.75-●
    tibia M89.76-●
    toes M89.77-●
    ulna M89.73-●
  osteochondral NEC —*see also* Deformity
      M95.8-●
  ostium
    primum Q21.2
    secundum Q21.1
  peroxidase E80.3
  placental blood supply —*see* Insufficiency,
      placental
  platelets, qualitative D69.1
    constitutional D68.0
  postural NEC, spine —*see* Dorsopathy,
      deforming
  reduction
    limb Q73.8
      lower Q72.9-●
        absence —*see* Agenesis, leg
          foot —*see* Agenesis, foot
        longitudinal
          femur Q72.4-●
          fibula Q72.6-●
          tibia Q72.5-●
        specified type NEC Q72.89-●
        split foot Q72.7-●
      specified type NEC Q73.8
      upper Q71.9-●
        absence —*see* Agenesis, arm
          forearm —*see* Agenesis, forearm
          hand —*see* Agenesis, hand
        lobster-claw hand Q71.6-●
        longitudinal
          radius Q71.4-●
          ulna Q71.5-●
        specified type NEC Q71.89-●
  renal pelvis Q63.8
    obstructive Q62.39
  respiratory system, congenital Q34.9
  restoration, dental K08.50
    specified NEC K08.59
  retinal nerve bundle fibers H35.89
  septal (heart) NOS Q21.9
    acquired (atrial) (auricular) (ventricular)
        (old) I51.0
    atrial Q21.1
      concurrent with acute myocardial
          infarction —*see* Infarct,
          myocardium
      following acute myocardial infarction
          (current complication) I23.1
    ventricular —*see also* Defect, ventricular
        septal Q21.0
  sinus venosus Q21.1
  speech —*see* Disorder, speech
    developmental F80.9
    specified NEC R47.89
  Taussig-Bing (aortic transposition and
      overriding pulmonary artery)
      Q20.1
  teeth, wedge K03.1
  vascular (local) I99.9
    congenital Q27.9
  ventricular septal Q21.0
    concurrent with acute myocardial
        infarction —*see* Infarct,
        myocardium
    following acute myocardial infarction
        (current complication) I23.2
    in tetralogy of Fallot Q21.3
  vision NEC H54.7

▶ New   ⇒ Revised   ~~deleted~~ Deleted   ● Use Additional Character(s)

Defect, defective (Continued)
  visual field H53.40
    bilateral
      heteronymous H53.47
      homonymous H53.46-●
    generalized contraction H53.48-●
    localized
      arcuate H53.43-●
      scotoma (central area) H53.41-●
        blind spot area H53.42-●
      sector H53.43-●
      specified type NEC H53.45-●
  voice R49.9
    specified NEC R49.8
  wedge, tooth, teeth (abrasion) K03.1
Deferentitis N49.1
  gonorrheal (acute) (chronic) A54.23
Defibrination (syndrome) D65
  antepartum —see Hemorrhage, antepartum,
    with coagulation defect, disseminated
    intravascular coagulation
  following ectopic or molar pregnancy O08.1
  intrapartum O67.0
  newborn P60
  postpartum O72.3
Deficiency, deficient
  3-beta hydroxysteroid dehydrogenase E25.0
  11-hydroxylase E25.0
  21-hydroxylase E25.0
  5-alpha reductase (with male
    pseudohermaphroditism) E29.1
  AADC (aromatic L-amino acid
    decarboxylase) E70.81
  abdominal muscle syndrome Q79.4
  AC globulin (congenital) (hereditary) D68.2
    acquired D68.4
  accelerator globulin (Ac G) (blood) D68.2
  acid phosphatase E83.39
  ▶acid sphingomyelinase (ASMD) E75.249
    ▶type
      ▶A E75.240
      ▶A/B E75.244
      ▶B E75.241
  activating factor (blood) D68.2
  ADA2 (adenosine deaminase 2) D81.32
  adenosine deaminase (ADA) D81.30
    with severe combined immunodeficiency
      (SCID) D81.31
    partial (type 1) D81.39
    specified NEC D81.39
    type 1 (without SCID) (without severe
      combined immunodeficiency) D81.39
    type 2 D81.32
  aldolase (hereditary) E74.19
  alpha-1-antitrypsin E88.01
  amino-acids E72.9
  anemia —see Anemia
  aneurin E51.9
  antibody with
    hyperimmunoglobulinemia D80.6
    near-normal immunoglobins D80.6
  antidiuretic hormone E23.2
  anti-hemophilic
    factor (A) D66
      B D67
      C D68.1
    globulin (AHG) NEC D66
  antithrombin (antithrombin III) D68.59
  aromatic L-amino acid decarboxylase
    (AADC) E70.81
  ascorbic acid E54
  attention (disorder) (syndrome) F98.8
    with hyperactivity —see Disorder,
      attention-deficit hyperactivity
  autoprothrombin
    I D68.2
    II D67
    C D68.2
  beta-glucuronidase E76.29
  biotin E53.8
  biotin-dependent carboxylase D81.819
  biotinidase D81.810

Deficiency, deficient (Continued)
  brancher enzyme (amylopectinosis) E74.03
  C1 esterase inhibitor (C1-INH) D84.1
  calciferol E55.9
    with
      adult osteomalacia M83.8
      rickets —see Rickets
  calcium (dietary) E58
  calorie, severe E43
    with marasmus E41
      and kwashiorkor E42
  cardiac —see Insufficiency, myocardial
  carnitine E71.40
    due to
      hemodialysis E71.43
      inborn errors of metabolism E71.42
      Valproic acid therapy E71.43
    iatrogenic E71.43
    muscle palmityltransferase E71.314
    primary E71.41
    secondary E71.448
  carotene E50.9
  central nervous system G96.89
  ceruloplasmin (Wilson) E83.01
  choline E53.8
  Christmas factor D67
  chromium E61.4
  ▶chronic neurovisceral acid sphingomyelinase
    E75.244
  ▶chronic visceral acid sphingomyelinase
    E75.241
  clotting (blood) —see also Deficiency,
    coagulation factor D68.9
  clotting factor NEC (hereditary) —see also
    Deficiency, factor D68.2
  coagulation NOS D68.9
    with
      ectopic pregnancy O08.1
      molar pregnancy O08.1
    acquired (any) D68.4
    antepartum hemorrhage —see Hemorrhage,
      antepartum, with coagulation defect
    clotting factor NEC —see also Deficiency,
      factor D68.2
    due to
      hyperprothrombinemia D68.4
      liver disease D68.4
      vitamin K deficiency D68.4
    newborn, transient P61.6
    postpartum O72.3
    specified NEC D68.8
  cognitive F09
  color vision H53.50
    achromatopsia H53.51
    acquired H53.52
    deuteranomaly H53.53
    protanomaly H53.54
    specified type NEC H53.59
    tritanomaly H53.55
  combined glucocorticoid and
    mineralocorticoid E27.49
  contact factor D68.2
  copper (nutritional) E61.0
  corticoadrenal E27.40
    primary E27.1
  craniofacial axis Q75.0
  cyanocobalamin E53.8
  debrancher enzyme (limit dextrinosis) E74.03
  dehydrogenase
    long chain/very long chain acyl CoA
      E71.310
    medium chain acyl CoA E71.311
    short chain acyl CoA E71.312
  diet E63.9
  dihydropyrimidine dehydrogenase (DPD)
    E88.89
  disaccharidase E73.9
  edema —see Malnutrition, severe
  endocrine E34.9
  energy-supply —see Malnutrition
  enzymes, circulating NEC E88.09

Deficiency, deficient (Continued)
  ergosterol E55.9
    with
      adult osteomalacia M83.8
      rickets —see Rickets
  essential fatty acid (EFA) E63.0
  eye movements
    saccadic H55.81
    smooth pursuit H55.82
  factor —see also Deficiency, coagulation
    Hageman D68.2
    I (congenital) (hereditary) D68.2
    II (congenital) (hereditary) D68.2
    IX (congenital) (functional) (hereditary)
      (with functional defect) D67
    multiple (congenital) D68.8
      acquired D68.4
    V (congenital) (hereditary) D68.2
    VII (congenital) (hereditary) D68.2
    VIII (congenital) (functional) (hereditary)
      (with functional defect) D66
      with vascular defect D68.0
    X (congenital) (hereditary) D68.2
    XI (congenital) (hereditary) D68.1
    XII (congenital) (hereditary) D68.2
    XIII (congenital) (hereditary) D68.2
  femoral, proximal focal (congenital) —
    see Defect, reduction, lower limb,
    longitudinal, femur
  fibrin-stabilizing factor (congenital)
    (hereditary) D68.2
    acquired D68.4
  fibrinase D68.2
  fibrinogen (congenital) (hereditary) D68.2
    acquired D65
  folate E53.8
  folic acid E53.8
  foreskin N47.3
  fructokinase E74.11
  fructose 1,6-diphosphatase E74.19
  fructose-1-phosphate aldolase E74.19
  GABA (gamma aminobutyric acid)
    transaminase E72.81
  GABA-T (gamma aminobutyric acid
    transaminase) E72.81
  galactokinase E74.29
  galactose-1-phosphate uridyl transferase
    E74.29
  gammaglobulin in blood D80.1
    hereditary D80.0
  glass factor D68.2
  glucocorticoid E27.49
    mineralocorticoid E27.49
  glucose-6-phosphatase E74.01
  glucose-6-phosphate dehydrogenase anemia
    anemia D55.0
    without anemia D75.A
  glucose transporter protein type 1 E74.810
  glucuronyl transferase E80.5
  Glut1 E74.810
  glycogen synthetase E74.09
  gonadotropin (isolated) E23.0
  growth hormone (idiopathic) (isolated) E23.0
  Hageman factor D68.2
  hemoglobin D64.9
  hepatophosphorylase E74.09
  homogentisate 1,2-dioxygenase E70.29
  hormone
    anterior pituitary (partial) NEC E23.0
      growth E23.0
    growth (isolated) E23.0
    pituitary E23.0
    testicular E29.1
  hypoxanthine-(guanine)-
    phosphoribosyltransferase (HG-PRT)
    (total HG-PRT) E79.1
  immunity D84.9
    cell-mediated D84.89
      with thrombocytopenia and eczema
        D82.0
    combined D81.9

Deficiency, deficient *(Continued)*
  immunity *(Continued)*
    humoral D80.9
    IgA (secretory) D80.2
    IgG D80.3
    IgM D80.4
  immuno —*see* Immunodeficiency
  immunoglobulin, selective
    A (IgA) D80.2
    G (IgG) (subclasses) D80.3
    M (IgM) D80.4
  ▶infantile neurovisceral acid sphingomyelinase E75.240
  inositol (B complex) E53.8
  intrinsic
    factor (congenital) D51.0
    sphincter N36.42
      with urethral hypermobility N36.43
  iodine E61.8
    congenital syndrome —*see* Syndrome,
      iodine-deficiency, congenital
  iron E61.1
    anemia D50.9
  kalium E87.6
  kappa-light chain D80.8
  labile factor (congenital) (hereditary) D68.2
    acquired D68.4
  lacrimal fluid (acquired) —*see also* Syndrome,
    dry eye
    congenital Q10.6
  lactase
    congenital E73.0
    secondary E73.1
  Laki-Lorand factor D68.2
  lecithin cholesterol acyltransferase E78.6
  lipocaic K86.89
  lipoprotein (familial) (high density) E78.6
  liver phosphorylase E74.09
  lysosomal alpha-1, 4 glucosidase E74.02
  magnesium E61.2
  major histocompatibility complex
    class I D81.6
    class II D81.7
  manganese E61.3
  menadione (vitamin K) E56.1
    newborn P53
  mental (familial) (hereditary) —*see* Disability,
    intellectual
  methylenetetrahydrofolate reductase
    (MTHFR) E72.12
  mevalonate kinase M04.1
  mineral NEC E61.8
  mineralocorticoid E27.49
    with glucocorticoid E27.49
  molybdenum (nutritional) E61.5
  moral F60.2
  multiple nutrient elements E61.7
  multiple sulfatase (MSD) E75.26
  muscle
    carnitine (palmityltransferase) E71.314
    phosphofructokinase E74.09
  myoadenylate deaminase E79.2
  myocardial —*see* Insufficiency, myocardial
  myophosphorylase E74.04
  NADH diaphorase or reductase (congenital) D74.0
  NADH-methemoglobin reductase
    (congenital) D74.0
  natrium E87.1
  niacin (amide) (-tryptophan) E52
  nicotinamide E52
  nicotinic acid E52
  number of teeth —*see* Anodontia
  nutrient element E61.9
    multiple E61.7
    specified NEC E61.8
  nutrition, nutritional E63.9
    sequelae —*see* Sequelae, nutritional
      deficiency
    specified NEC E63.8
  of interleukin 1 receptor antagonist [DIRA] M04.8

Deficiency, deficient *(Continued)*
  ornithine transcarbamylase E72.4
  ovarian E28.39
  oxygen —*see* Anoxia
  pantothenic acid E53.8
  parathyroid (gland) E20.9
  perineum (female) N81.89
  phenylalanine hydroxylase E70.1
  phosphoenolpyruvate carboxykinase E74.4
  phosphofructokinase E74.19
  phosphomannomutuse E74.818
  phosphomannose isomerase E74.818
  phosphomannosyl mutase E74.818
  phosphorylase kinase, liver E74.09
  pituitary hormone (isolated) E23.0
  plasma thromboplastin
    antecedent (PTA) D68.1
    component (PTC) D67
  plasminogen (type 1) (type 2) E88.02
  platelet NEC D69.1
    constitutional D68.0
  polyglandular E31.8
    autoimmune E31.0
  potassium (K) E87.6
  prepuce N47.3
  proaccelerin (congenital) (hereditary) D68.2
    acquired D68.4
  proconvertin factor (congenital) (hereditary) D68.2
    acquired D68.4
  protein —*see also* Malnutrition E46
    anemia D53.0
    C D68.59
    S D68.59
  prothrombin (congenital) (heredItary) D68.2
    acquired D68.4
  Prower factor D68.2
  pseudocholinesterase E88.09
  PTA (plasma thromboplastin antecedent) D68.1
  PTC (plasma thromboplastin component) D67
  purine nucleoside phosphorylase (PNP) D81.5
  pyracin (alpha) (beta) E53.1
  pyridoxal E53.1
  pyridoxamine E53.1
  pyridoxine (derivatives) E53.1
  pyruvate
    carboxylase E74.4
    dehydrogenase E74.4
  riboflavin (vitamin B2) E53.0
  salt E87.1
  secretion
    ovary E28.39
    salivary gland (any) K11.7
    urine R34
  selenium (dietary) E59
  serum antitrypsin, familial E88.01
  short stature homeobox gene (SHOX)
    with
      dyschondrosteosis Q78.8
      short stature (idiopathic) E34.3
      Turner's syndrome Q96.9
  sodium (Na) E87.1
  SPCA (factor VII) D68.2
  sphincter, intrinsic N36.42
    with urethral hypermobility N36.43
  stable factor (congenital) (hereditary) D68.2
    acquired D68.4
  Stuart-Prower (factor X) D68.2
  succinic semialdehyde dehydrogenase E72.81
  sucrase E74.39
  sulfatase E75.26
  sulfite oxidase E72.19
  thiamin, thiaminic (chloride) E51.9
    beriberi (dry) E51.11
      wet E51.12
  thrombokinase D68.2
    newborn P53
  thyroid (gland) —*see* Hypothyroidism
  tocopherol E56.0
  tooth bud K00.0
  transcobalamine II (anemia) D51.2

Deficiency, deficient *(Continued)*
  vanadium E61.6
  vascular I99.9
  vasopressin E23.2
  vertical ridge K06.8
  viosterol —*see* Deficiency, calciferol
  vitamin (multiple) NOS E56.9
    A E50.9
      with
        Bitot's spot (corneal) E50.1
        follicular keratosis E50.8
        keratomalacia E50.4
        manifestations NEC E50.8
        night blindness E50.5
        scar of cornea, xerophthalmic E50.6
        xeroderma E50.8
        xerophthalmia E50.7
        xerosis
          conjunctival E50.0
            and Bitot's spot E50.1
          cornea E50.2
            and ulceration E50.3
      sequelae E64.1
    B (complex) NOS E53.9
      with
        beriberi (dry) E51.11
          wet E51.12
        pellagra E52
    B1 NOS E51.9
      beriberi (dry) E51.11
        with circulatory system
          manifestations E51.11
        wet E51.12
    B12 E53.8
    B2 (riboflavin) E53.0
    B6 E53.1
    C E54
      sequelae E64.2
    D E55.9
      with
        adult osteomalacia M83.8
        rickets —*see* Rickets
      25-hydroxylase E83.32
    E E56.0
    folic acid E53.8
    G E53.0
    group B E53.9
      specified NEC E53.8
    H (biotin) E53.8
    K E56.1
      of newborn P53
    nicotinic E52
    P E56.8
    PP (pellagra-preventing) E52
    specified NEC E56.8
    thiamin E51.9
      beriberi —*see* Beriberi
  zinc, dietary E60
Deficit —*see also* Deficiency
  attention and concentration R41.840
    following
      cerebral infarction I69.310
      cerebrovascular disease I69.910
        specified disease NEC I69.810
      nontraumatic
        intracerebral hemorrhage I69.110
        specified intracranial hemorrhage NEC I69.210
        subarachnoid hemorrhage I69.010
  disorder —*see* Attention, deficit
  cognitive
    communication R41.841
    emotional
      following
        cerebral infarction I69.315
        cerebrovascular disease I69.915
          specified disease NEC I69.815
        nontraumatic
          intracerebral hemorrhage I69.115
          specified intracranial hemorrhage NEC I69.215
          subarachnoid hemorrhage I69.015

Deficit *(Continued)*
  cognitive *(Continued)*
    following
      cerebral infarction I69.319
      cerebrovascular disease I69.919
        specified disease NEC I69.819
      nontraumatic
        intracerebral hemorrhage I69.119
        specified intracranial hemorrhage
          NEC I69.219
        subarachnoid hemorrhage I69.019
    social
      following
        cerebral infarction I69.315
        cerebrovascular disease I69.915
          specified disease NEC I69.815
        nontraumatic
          intracerebral hemorrhage I69.115
          specified intracranial hemorrhage
            NEC I69.215
          subarachnoid hemorrhage I69.015
  cognitive NEC R41.89
    following
      cerebral infarction I69.318
      cerebrovascular disease I69.918
        specified disease NEC I69.818
      nontraumatic
        intracerebral hemorrhage I69.118
        specified intracranial hemorrhage
          NEC I69.218
        subarachnoid hemorrhage I69.018
  concentration R41.840
  executive function R41.844
    following
      cerebral infarction I69.314
      cerebrovascular disease I69.914
        specified disease NEC I69.814
      nontraumatic
        intracerebral hemorrhage I69.114
        specified intracranial hemorrhage
          NEC I69.214
        subarachnoid hemorrhage I69.014
  frontal lobe R41.844
    following
      cerebral infarction I69.314
      cerebrovascular disease I69.914
        specified disease NEC I69.814
      nontraumatic
        intracerebral hemorrhage I69.114
        specified intracranial hemorrhage
          NEC I69.214
        subarachnoid hemorrhage I69.014
  memory
    following
      cerebral infarction I69.311
      cerebrovascular disease I69.911
        specified disease NEC I69.811
      nontraumatic
        intracerebral hemorrhage
          I69.111
        specified intracranial hemorrhage
          NEC I69.211
        subarachnoid hemorrhage I69.011
  neurologic NEC R29.818
    ischemic
      reversible (RIND) I63.9
        prolonged (PRIND) I63.9
  oxygen R09.02
  prolonged reversible ischemic neurologic
    (PRIND) I63.9
  psychomotor R41.843
    following
      cerebral infarction I69.313
      cerebrovascular disease I69.913
        specified disease NEC I69.813
      nontraumatic
        intracerebral hemorrhage I69.113
        specified intracranial hemorrhage
          NEC I69.213
        subarachnoid hemorrhage
          I69.013

Deficit *(Continued)*
  visuospatial R41.842
    following
      cerebral infarction I69.312
      cerebrovascular disease I69.912
        specified disease NEC I69.812
      nontraumatic
        intracerebral hemorrhage I69.112
        specified intracranial hemorrhage
          NEC I69.212
        subarachnoid hemorrhage
          I69.012
Deflection
  radius —*see* Deformity, limb, specified type
    NEC, forearm
  septum (acquired) (nasal) (nose) J34.2
  spine —*see* Curvature, spine
  turbinate (nose) J34.2
Defluvium
  capillorum —*see* Alopecia
  ciliorum —*see* Madarosis
  unguium L60.8
Deformity Q89.9
  abdomen, congenital Q89.9
  abdominal wall
    acquired M95.8
    congenital Q79.59
  acquired (unspecified site) M95.9
  adrenal gland Q89.1
  alimentary tract, congenital Q45.9
    upper Q40.9
  ankle (joint) (acquired) —*see also* Deformity,
    limb, lower leg
    abduction —*see* Contraction, joint, ankle
    congenital Q68.8
    contraction —*see* Contraction, joint, ankle
    specified type NEC —*see* Deformity, limb,
      foot, specified NEC
  anus (acquired) K62.89
    congenital Q43.9
  aorta (arch) (congenital) Q25.40
    acquired I77.89
  aortic
    arch, acquired I77.89
    cusp or valve (congenital) Q23.8
      acquired —*see also* Endocarditis, aortic
        I35.8
  arm (acquired) (upper) —*see also* Deformity,
    limb, upper arm
    congenital Q68.8
    forearm —*see* Deformity, limb, forearm
  artery (congenital) (peripheral) NOS Q27.9
    acquired I77.89
    coronary (acquired) I25.9
      congenital Q24.5
    umbilical Q27.0
  atrial septal Q21.1
  auditory canal (external) (congenital) —*see*
    also Malformation, ear, external
    acquired —*see* Disorder, ear, external,
      specified type NEC
  auricle
    ear (congenital) —*see also* Malformation,
      ear, external
      acquired —*see* Disorder, pinna,
        deformity
  back —*see* Dorsopathy, deforming
  bile duct (common) (congenital) (hepatic)
    Q44.5
    acquired K83.8
  biliary duct or passage (congenital) Q44.5
    acquired K83.8
  bladder (neck) (trigone) (sphincter)
    (acquired) N32.89
    congenital Q64.79
  bone (acquired) NOS M95.9
    congenital Q79.9
    turbinate M95.0
  brain (congenital) Q04.9
    acquired G93.89
    reduction Q04.3

Deformity *(Continued)*
  breast (acquired) N64.89
    congenital Q83.9
    reconstructed N65.0
  bronchus (congenital) Q32.4
    acquired NEC J98.09
  bursa, congenital Q79.9
  canaliculi (lacrimalis) (acquired) —*see also*
    Disorder, lacrimal system, changes
    congenital Q10.6
  canthus, acquired —*see* Disorder, eyelid,
    specified type NEC
  capillary (acquired) I78.8
  cardiovascular system, congenital Q28.9
  caruncle, lacrimal (acquired) —*see also*
    Disorder, lacrimal system, changes
    congenital Q10.6
  cascade, stomach K31.2
  cecum (congenital) Q43.9
    acquired K63.89
  cerebral, acquired G93.89
    congenital Q04.9
  cervix (uterus) (acquired) NEC N88.8
    congenital Q51.9
  cheek (acquired) M95.2
    congenital Q18.9
  chest (acquired) (wall) M95.4
    congenital Q67.8
    sequelae (late effect) of rickets E64.3
  chin (acquired) M95.2
    congenital Q18.9
  choroid (congenital) Q14.3
    acquired H31.8
    plexus Q07.8
      acquired G96.198
  cicatricial —*see* Cicatrix
  cilia, acquired —*see* Disorder, eyelid,
    specified type NEC
  clavicle (acquired) M95.8
    congenital Q68.8
  clitoris (congenital) Q52.6
    acquired N90.89
  clubfoot —*see* Clubfoot
  coccyx (acquired) —*see* subcategory
    M43.8
  colon (congenital) Q43.9
    acquired K63.89
  concha (ear), congenital —*see also*
    Malformation, ear, external
    acquired —*see* Disorder, pinna, deformity
  cornea (acquired) H18.70
    congenital Q13.4
    descemetocele —*see* Descemetocele
    ectasia —*see* Ectasia, cornea
    specified NEC H18.79-●
    staphyloma —*see* Staphyloma, cornea
  coronary artery (acquired) I25.9
    congenital Q24.5
  cranium (acquired) —*see* Deformity, skull
  cricoid cartilage (congenital) Q31.8
    acquired J38.7
  cystic duct (congenital) Q44.5
    acquired K82.8
  Dandy-Walker Q03.1
    with spina bifida —*see* Spina bifida
  diaphragm (congenital) Q79.1
    acquired J98.6
  digestive organ NOS Q45.9
  ductus arteriosus Q25.0
  duodenal bulb K31.89
  duodenum (congenital) Q43.9
    acquired K31.89
  dura —*see* Deformity, meninges
  ear (acquired) —*see also* Disorder, pinna,
    deformity
    congenital (external) Q17.9
      internal Q16.5
      middle Q16.4
        ossicles Q16.3
      ossicles Q16.3
  ectodermal (congenital) NEC Q84.9

Deformity *(Continued)*
ejaculatory duct (congenital) Q55.4
  acquired N50.89
elbow (joint) (acquired) —*see also* Deformity,
    limb, upper arm
  congenital Q68.8
  contraction —*see* Contraction, joint, elbow
endocrine gland NEC Q89.2
epididymis (congenital) Q55.4
  acquired N50.89
epiglottis (congenital) Q31.8
  acquired J38.7
esophagus (congenital) Q39.9
  ⇶acquired K22.89
eustachian tube (congenital) NEC Q17.8
eye, congenital Q15.9
eyebrow (congenital) Q18.8
eyelid (acquired) —*see also* Disorder, eyelid,
    specified type NEC
  congenital Q10.3
face (acquired) M95.2
  congenital Q18.9
fallopian tube, acquired N83.8
femur (acquired) —*see* Deformity, limb,
    specified type NEC, thigh
fetal
  with fetopelvic disproportion O33.7
    causing obstructed labor O66.3
finger (acquired) M20.00-●
  boutonniere M20.02-●
  congenital Q68.1
  flexion contracture —*see* Contraction, joint,
      hand
  mallet finger M20.01-●
  specified NEC M20.09-●
  swan-neck M20.03-●
flexion (joint) (acquired) —*see also* Deformity,
    limb, flexion M21.20
  congenital NOS Q74.9
    hip Q65.89
foot (acquired) —*see also* Deformity, limb,
    lower leg
  cavovarus (congenital) Q66.1-●
  congenital NOS Q66.9-●
    specified type NEC Q66.89
  specified type NEC —*see* Deformity, limb,
      foot, specified NEC
  valgus (congenital) Q66.6
    acquired —*see* Deformity, valgus, ankle
  varus (congenital) NEC Q66.3-●
    acquired —*see* Deformity, varus, ankle
forearm (acquired) —*see also* Deformity, limb,
    forearm
  congenital Q68.8
forehead (acquired) M95.2
  congenital Q75.8
frontal bone (acquired) M95.2
  congenital Q75.8
gallbladder (congenital) Q44.1
  acquired K82.8
gastrointestinal tract (congenital) NOS Q45.9
  acquired K63.89
genitalia, genital organ(s) or system NEC
  female (congenital) Q52.9
    acquired N94.89
    external Q52.70
  male (congenital) Q55.9
    acquired N50.89
globe (eye) (congenital) Q15.8
  acquired H44.89
gum, acquired NEC K06.8
hand (acquired) —*see* Deformity, limb, hand
  congenital Q68.1
head (acquired) M95.2
  congenital Q75.8
heart (congenital) Q24.9
  septum Q21.9
    auricular Q21.1
    ventricular Q21.0
  valve (congenital) NEC Q24.8
    acquired —*see* Endocarditis

Deformity *(Continued)*
heel (acquired) —*see* Deformity, foot
hepatic duct (congenital) Q44.5
  acquired K83.8
hip (joint) (acquired) —*see also* Deformity,
    limb, thigh
  congenital Q65.9
  due to (previous) juvenile
      osteochondrosis —*see* Coxa, plana
  flexion —*see* Contraction, joint, hip
hourglass —*see* Contraction, hourglass
humerus (acquired) M21.82-●
  congenital Q74.0
hypophyseal (congenital) Q89.2
ileocecal (coil) (valve) (acquired) K63.89
  congenital Q43.9
ileum (congenital) Q43.9
  acquired K63.89
ilium (acquired) M95.5
  congenital Q74.2
integument (congenital) Q84.9
intervertebral cartilage or disc (acquired) —
    see Disorder, disc, specified NEC
intestine (large) (small) (congenital) NOS
    Q43.9
  acquired K63.89
intrinsic minus or plus (hand) —*see*
    Deformity, limb, specified type NEC,
    forearm
iris (acquired) H21.89
  congenital Q13.2
ischium (acquired) M95.5
  congenital Q74.2
jaw (acquired) (congenital) M26.9
joint (acquired) NEC M21.90
  congenital Q68.8
  elbow M21.92-●
  hand M21.94-●
  hip M21.95-●
  knee M21.96-●
  shoulder M21.92-●
  wrist M21.93-●
kidney(s) (calyx) (pelvis) (congenital) Q63.9
  acquired N28.89
  artery (congenital) Q27.2
    acquired I77.89
Klippel-Feil (brevicollis) Q76.1
knee (acquired) NEC —*see also* Deformity,
    limb, lower leg
  congenital Q68.2
labium (majus) (minus) (congenital) Q52.79
  acquired N90.89
lacrimal passages or duct (congenital) NEC
    Q10.6
  acquired —*see* Disorder, lacrimal system,
      changes
larynx (muscle) (congenital) Q31.8
  acquired J38.7
  web (glottic) Q31.0
leg (upper) (acquired) NEC —*see also*
    Deformity, limb, thigh
  congenital Q68.8
  lower leg —*see* Deformity, limb, lower leg
lens (acquired) H27.8
  congenital Q12.9
lid (fold) (acquired) —*see also* Disorder,
    eyelid, specified type NEC
  congenital Q10.3
ligament (acquired) —*see* Disorder, ligament
  congenital Q79.9
limb (acquired) M21.90
  clawfoot M21.53-●
  clawhand M21.51-●
  clubfoot M21.54-●
  clubhand M21.52-●
  congenital, except reduction deformity
      Q74.9
  flat foot M21.4-●
  flexion M21.20
    ankle M21.27-●
    elbow M21.22-●

Deformity *(Continued)*
limb *(Continued)*
  flexion *(Continued)*
    finger M21.24-●
    hip M21.25-●
    knee M21.26-●
    shoulder M21.21-●
    toe M21.27-●
    wrist M21.23-●
  foot
    claw —*see* Deformity, limb, clawfoot
    club —*see* Deformity, limb, clubfoot
    drop M21.37-●
    flat —*see* Deformity, limb, flat foot
    specified NEC M21.6X-●
  forearm M21.93-●
  hand M21.94-●
  lower leg M21.96-●
  specified type NEC M21.80
    forearm M21.83-●
    lower leg M21.86-●
    thigh M21.85-●
    upper arm M21.82-●
  thigh M21.95-●
  unequal length M21.70
    short site is
      femur M21.75-●
      fibula M21.76-●
      humerus M21.72-●
      radius M21.73-●
      tibia M21.76-●
      ulna M21.73-●
    upper arm M21.92-●
  valgus —*see* Deformity, valgus
  varus —*see* Deformity, varus
  wrist drop M21.33-●
lip (acquired) NEC K13.0
  congenital Q38.0
liver (congenital) Q44.7
  acquired K76.89
lumbosacral (congenital) (joint) (region)
    Q76.49
  acquired —*see* subcategory M43.8
  kyphosis —*see* Kyphosis, congenital
  lordosis —*see* Lordosis, congenital
lung (congenital) Q33.9
  acquired J98.4
lymphatic system, congenital Q89.9
Madelung's (radius) Q74.0
mandible (acquired) (congenital) M26.9
maxilla (acquired) (congenital) M26.9
meninges or membrane (congenital) Q07.9
  cerebral Q04.8
    acquired G96.198
  ⇶spinal cord (congenital) Q06.-●
    acquired G96.198
metacarpus (acquired) —*see* Deformity, limb,
    forearm
  congenital Q74.0
metatarsus (acquired) —*see* Deformity, foot
  congenital Q66.9-●
middle ear (congenital) Q16.4
  ossicles Q16.3
mitral (leaflets) (valve) I05.8
  parachute Q23.2
  stenosis, congenital Q23.2
mouth (acquired) K13.79
  congenital Q38.6
multiple, congenital NEC Q89.7
muscle (acquired) M62.89
  congenital Q79.9
    sternocleidomastoid Q68.0
musculoskeletal system (acquired) M95.9
  congenital Q79.9
  specified NEC M95.8
nail (acquired) L60.8
  congenital Q84.6
nasal —*see* Deformity, nose
neck (acquired) M95.3
  congenital Q18.9
    sternocleidomastoid Q68.0

▶ New   ⇶ Revised   ~~deleted~~ Deleted   ● Use Additional Character(s)

Deformity (Continued)

nervous system (congenital) Q07.9
nipple (congenital) Q83.9
  acquired N64.89
nose (acquired) (cartilage) M95.0
  bone (turbinate) M95.0
  congenital Q30.9
    bent or squashed Q67.4
  saddle M95.0
    syphilitic A50.57
  septum (acquired) J34.2
    congenital Q30.8
  sinus (wall) (congenital) Q30.8
    acquired M95.0
  syphilitic (congenital) A50.57
    late A52.73
ocular muscle (congenital) Q10.3
  acquired —see Strabismus, mechanical
opticociliary vessels (congenital) Q13.2
orbit (eye) (acquired) H05.30
  atrophy —see Atrophy, orbit
  congenital Q10.7
  due to
    bone disease NEC H05.32-●
    trauma or surgery H05.33-●
  enlargement —see Enlargement, orbit
  exostosis —see Exostosis, orbit
organ of Corti (congenital) Q16.5
ovary (congenital) Q50.39
  acquired N83.8
oviduct, acquired N83.8
palate (congenital) Q38.5
  acquired M27.8
  cleft (congenital) —see Cleft, palate
pancreas (congenital) Q45.3
  acquired K86.89
parathyroid (gland) Q89.2
parotid (gland) (congenital) Q38.4
  acquired K11.8
patella (acquired) —see Disorder, patella,
    specified NEC
pelvis, pelvic (acquired) (bony) M95.5
  with disproportion (fetopelvic) O33.0
    causing obstructed labor O65.0
  congenital Q74.2
  rachitic sequelae (late effect) E64.3
penis (glans) (congenital) Q55.69
  acquired N48.89
pericardium (congenital) Q24.8
  acquired —see Pericarditis
pharynx (congenital) Q38.8
  acquired J39.2
pinna, acquired —see also Disorder, pinna,
    deformity
  congenital Q17.9
pituitary (congenital) Q89.2
posture —see Dorsopathy, deforming
prepuce (congenital) Q55.69
  acquired N47.8
prostate (congenital) Q55.4
  acquired N42.89
pupil (congenital) Q13.2
  acquired —see Abnormality, pupillary
pylorus (congenital) Q40.3
  acquired K31.89
rachitic (acquired), old or healed E64.3
radius (acquired) —see also Deformity, limb,
    forearm
  congenital Q68.8
rectum (congenital) Q43.9
  acquired K62.89
reduction (extremity) (limb), congenital (see
    also condition and site) Q73.8
  brain Q04.3
  lower —see Defect, reduction, lower limb
  upper —see Defect, reduction, upper limb
renal —see Deformity, kidney
respiratory system (congenital) Q34.9
rib (acquired) M95.4
  congenital Q76.6
    cervical Q76.5

Deformity (Continued)

rotation (joint) (acquired) —see Deformity,
    limb, specified site NEC
  congenital Q74.9
  hip —see Deformity, limb, specified type
      NEC, thigh
    congenital Q65.89
sacroiliac joint (congenital) Q74.2
  acquired —see subcategory M43.8
sacrum (acquired) —see subcategory M43.8
saddle
  back —see Lordosis
  nose M95.0
    syphilitic A50.57
salivary gland or duct (congenital) Q38.4
  acquired K11.8
scapula (acquired) M95.8
  congenital Q68.8
scrotum (congenital) —see also Malformation,
    testis and scrotum
  acquired N50.89
seminal vesicles (congenital) Q55.4
  acquired N50.89
septum, nasal (acquired) J34.2
shoulder (joint) (acquired) —see Deformity,
    limb, upper arm
  congenital Q74.0
  contraction —see Contraction, joint,
      shoulder
sigmoid (flexure) (congenital) Q43.9
  acquired K63.89
skin (congenital) Q82.9
skull (acquired) M95.2
  congenital Q75.8
    with
      anencephaly Q00.0
      encephalocele —see Encephalocele
      hydrocephalus Q03.9
        with spina bifida —see Spina bifida,
            by site, with hydrocephalus
      microcephaly Q02
soft parts, organs or tissues (of pelvis)
  in pregnancy or childbirth NEC O34.8-●
    causing obstructed labor O65.5
spermatic cord (congenital) Q55.4
  acquired N50.89
    torsion —see Torsion, spermatic cord
spinal —see Dorsopathy, deforming
  column (acquired) —see Dorsopathy,
      deforming
  congenital Q67.5
  cord (congenital) Q06.9
    acquired G95.89
  nerve root (congenital) Q07.9
spine (acquired) —see also Dorsopathy,
    deforming
  congenital Q67.5
  rachitic E64.3
  specified NEC —see Dorsopathy,
      deforming, specified NEC
spleen
  acquired D73.89
  congenital Q89.09
Sprengel's (congenital) Q74.0
sternocleidomastoid (muscle), congenital
    Q68.0
sternum (acquired) M95.4
  congenital NEC Q76.7
stomach (congenital) Q40.3
  acquired K31.89
submandibular gland (congenital) Q38.4
submaxillary gland (congenital) Q38.4
  acquired K11.8
talipes —see Talipes
testis (congenital) —see also Malformation,
    testis and scrotum
  acquired N44.8
    torsion —see Torsion, testis
thigh (acquired) —see also Deformity, limb,
    thigh
  congenital NEC Q68.8

Deformity (Continued)

thorax (acquired) (wall) M95.4
  congenital Q67.8
  sequelae of rickets E64.3
thumb (acquired) —see also Deformity, finger
  congenital NEC Q68.1
thymus (tissue) (congenital) Q89.2
thyroid (gland) (congenital) Q89.2
  cartilage Q31.8
    acquired J38.7
tibia (acquired) —see also Deformity, limb,
    specified type NEC, lower leg
  congenital NEC Q68.8
  saber (syphilitic) A50.56
toe (acquired) M20.6-●
  congenital Q66.9-●
  hallux rigidus M20.2-●
  hallux valgus M20.1-●
  hallux varus M20.3-●
  hammer toe M20.4-●
  specified NEC M20.5X-●
tongue (congenital) Q38.3
  acquired K14.8
tooth, teeth K00.2
trachea (rings) (congenital) Q32.1
  acquired J39.8
transverse aortic arch (congenital)
    Q25.49
tricuspid (leaflets) (valve) I07.8
  atresia or stenosis Q22.4
  Ebstein's Q22.5
trunk (acquired) M95.8
  congenital Q89.9
ulna (acquired) —see also Deformity, limb,
    forearm
  congenital NEC Q68.8
urachus, congenital Q64.4
ureter (opening) (congenital) Q62.8
  acquired N28.89
urethra (congenital) Q64.79
  acquired N36.8
urinary tract (congenital) Q64.9
  urachus Q64.4
uterus (congenital) Q51.9
  acquired N85.8
uvula (congenital) Q38.5
vagina (acquired) N89.8
  congenital Q52.4
valgus NEC M21.00
  ankle M21.07-●
  elbow M21.02-●
  hip M21.05-●
  knee M21.06-●
valve, valvular (congenital) (heart) Q24.8
  acquired —see Endocarditis
varus NEC M21.10
  ankle M21.17-●
  elbow M21.12-●
  hip M21.15
  knee M21.16-●
  tibia —see Osteochondrosis, juvenile, tibia
vas deferens (congenital) Q55.4
  acquired N50.89
vein (congenital) Q27.9
  great Q26.9
vertebra —see Dorsopathy, deforming
vertical talus (congenital) Q66.80
  left foot Q66.82
  right foot Q66.81
vesicourethral orifice (acquired) N32.89
  congenital NEC Q64.79
vessels of optic papilla (congenital) Q14.2
visual field (contraction) —see Defect, visual
    field
vitreous body, acquired H43.89
vulva (congenital) Q52.79
  acquired N90.89
wrist (joint) (acquired) —see also Deformity,
    limb, forearm
  congenital Q68.8
  contraction —see Contraction, joint, wrist

Degeneration, degenerative
adrenal (capsule) (fatty) (gland) (hyaline)
  (infectional) E27.8
amyloid —see also Amyloidosis E85.9
anterior cornua, spinal cord G12.29
anterior labral S43.49-●
aorta, aortic I70.0
  fatty I77.89
aortic valve (heart) —see Endocarditis,
  aortic
arteriovascular —see Arteriosclerosis
artery, arterial (atheromatous) (calcareous) —
  see also Arteriosclerosis
  cerebral, amyloid E85.4 [I68.0]
  medial —see Arteriosclerosis, extremities
articular cartilage NEC —see Derangement,
  joint, articular cartilage, by site
atheromatous —see Arteriosclerosis
basal nuclei or ganglia G23.9
  specified NEC G23.8
bone NEC —see Disorder, bone, specified
  type NEC
brachial plexus G54.0
brain (cortical) (progressive) G31.9
  alcoholic G31.2
  arteriosclerotic I67.2
  childhood G31.9
    specified NEC G31.89
  cystic G31.89
    congenital Q04.6
  in
    alcoholism G31.2
    beriberi E51.2
    cerebrovascular disease I67.9
    congenital hydrocephalus Q03.9
      with spina bifida —see also Spina
        bifida
    Fabry-Anderson disease E75.21
    Gaucher's disease E75.22
    Hunter's syndrome E76.1
    lipidosis
      cerebral E75.4
      generalized E75.6
    mucopolysaccharidosis —see
      Mucopolysaccharidosis
    myxedema E03.9 [G32.89]
    neoplastic disease —see also Neoplasm
      D49.6 [G32.89]
    Niemann-Pick disease E75.249 [G32.89]
    sphingolipidosis E75.3 [G32.89]
    vitamin B12 deficiency E53.8 [G32.89]
  senile NEC G31.1
breast N64.89
Bruch's membrane —see Degeneration,
  choroid
capillaries (fatty) I78.8
  amyloid E85.89 [I79.8]
cardiac —see also Degeneration, myocardial
  valve, valvular —see Endocarditis
cardiorenal —see Hypertension, cardiorenal
cardiovascular —see also Disease,
  cardiovascular
  renal —see Hypertension, cardiorenal
cerebellar NOS G31.9
  alcoholic G31.2
  primary (hereditary) (sporadic) G11.9
cerebral —see Degeneration, brain
cerebrovascular I67.9
  due to hypertension I67.4
cervical plexus G54.2
cervix N88.8
  due to radiation (intended effect) N88.8
    adverse effect or misadventure N99.89
chamber angle H21.21-●
changes, spine or vertebra —see Spondylosis
chorioretinal —see also Degeneration, choroid
  hereditary H31.20
choroid (colloid) (drusen) H31.10-●
  atrophy —see Atrophy, choroidal
  hereditary —see Dystrophy, choroidal,
    hereditary

Degeneration, degenerative *(Continued)*
ciliary body H21.22-●
cochlear —see subcategory H83.8
combined (spinal cord) (subacute) E53.8
  [G32.0]
  with anemia (pernicious) D51.0 [G32.0]
    due to dietary vitamin B12 deficiency
      D51.3 [G32.0]
  in (due to)
    vitamin B12 deficiency E53.8 [G32.0]
    anemia D51.9 [G32.0]
conjunctiva H11.10
  concretions —see Concretion, conjunctiva
  deposits —see Deposit, conjunctiva
  pigmentations —see Pigmentation,
    conjunctiva
  pinguecula —see Pinguecula
  xerosis —see Xerosis, conjunctiva
cornea H18.40
  calcerous H18.43
    band keratopathy H18.42-●
  familial, hereditary —see Dystrophy, cornea
  hyaline (of old scars) H18.49
  keratomalacia —see Keratomalacia
  nodular H18.45-●
  peripheral H18.46-●
  senile H18.41-●
  specified type NEC H18.49
cortical (cerebellar) (parenchymatous) G31.89
  alcoholic G31.2
  diffuse, due to arteriopathy I67.2
corticobasal G31.85
cutis L98.8
  amyloid E85.4 [L99]
dental pulp K04.2
disc disease —see Degeneration,
  intervertebral disc NEC
dorsolateral (spinal cord) —see Degeneration,
  combined
extrapyramidal G25.9
eye, macular —see also Degeneration, macula
  congenital or hereditary —see Dystrophy,
    retina
facet joints —see Spondylosis
fatty
  liver NEC K76.0
    alcoholic K70.0
grey matter (brain) (Alpers') G31.81
heart —see also Degeneration, myocardial
  amyloid E85.4 [I43]
  atheromatous —see Disease, heart,
    ischemic, atherosclerotic
  ischemic —see Disease, heart, ischemic
hepatolenticular (Wilson's) E83.01
hepatorenal K76.7
hyaline (diffuse) (generalized)
  localized —see Degeneration, by site
infrapatellar fat pad M79.4
intervertebral disc NOS
  with
    myelopathy —see Disorder, disc, with,
      myelopathy
    radiculitis or radiculopathy —see
      Disorder, disc, with, radiculopathy
  cervical, cervicothoracic —see Disorder,
    disc, cervical, degeneration
    with
      myelopathy —see Disorder, disc,
        cervical, with myelopathy
      neuritis, radiculitis or
        radiculopathy —see Disorder,
          disc, cervical, with neuritis
  lumbar region M51.36
    with
      myelopathy M51.06
      neuritis, radiculitis, radiculopathy or
        sciatica M51.16
  lumbosacral region M51.37
    with
      neuritis, radiculitis, radiculopathy or
        sciatica M51.17

Degeneration, degenerative *(Continued)*
intervertebral disc *(Continued)*
  sacrococcygeal region M53.3
  thoracic region M51.34
    with
      myelopathy M51.04
      neuritis, radiculitis, radiculopathy
        M51.14
  thoracolumbar region M51.35
    with
      myelopathy M51.05
      neuritis, radiculitis, radiculopathy
        M51.15
intestine, amyloid E85.4
iris (pigmentary) H21.23-●
ischemic —see Ischemia
joint disease —see Osteoarthritis
kidney N28.89
  amyloid E85.4 [N29]
  cystic, congenital Q61.9
  fatty N28.89
  polycystic Q61.3
    adult type (autosomal dominant)
      Q61.2
    infantile type (autosomal recessive) NEC
      Q61.19
      collecting duct dilatation Q61.11
Kuhnt-Junius —see also Degeneration, macula
  H35.32-●
lens —see Cataract
lenticular (familial) (progressive) (Wilson's)
  (with cirrhosis of liver) E83.01
liver (diffuse) NEC K76.89
  amyloid E85.4 [K77]
  cystic K76.89
    congenital Q44.6
  fatty NEC K76.0
    alcoholic K70.0
  hypertrophic K76.89
  parenchymatous, acute or subacute K72.00
    with coma K72.01
  pigmentary K76.89
  toxic (acute) K71.9
lung J98.4
lymph gland I89.8
  hyaline I89.8
macula, macular (acquired) (age-related)
  (senile) H35.30
  angioid streaks H35.33
  atrophic age-related H35.31-●
  congenital or hereditary —see Dystrophy,
    retina
  cystoid H35.35-●
  drusen H35.36-●
  dry age-related H35.31-●
  exudative H35.32-●
  hole H35.34-●
  nonexudative H35.31-●
  puckering H35.37-●
  toxic H35.38-●
  wet age-related H35.32-●
membranous labyrinth, congenital (causing
  impairment of hearing) Q16.5
meniscus —see Derangement, meniscus
mitral —see Insufficiency, mitral
Mönckeberg's —see Arteriosclerosis,
  extremities
motor centers, senile G31.1
multi-system G90.3
mural —see Degeneration, myocardial
muscle (fatty) (fibrous) (hyaline)
  (progressive) M62.89
  heart —see Degeneration, myocardial
myelin, central nervous system G37.9
myocardial, myocardium (fatty) (hyaline)
  (senile) I51.5
  with rheumatic fever (conditions in I00)
    I09.0
    active, acute or subacute I01.2
      with chorea I02.0
    inactive or quiescent (with chorea) I09.0

▶ New   ⟹ Revised   ~~deleted~~ Deleted   ● Use Additional Character(s)

Degeneration, degenerative *(Continued)*
 myocardial, myocardium *(Continued)*
  hypertensive —*see* Hypertension, heart
  rheumatic —*see* Degeneration, myocardial,
   with rheumatic fever
  syphilitic A52.06
 nasal sinus (mucosa) J32.9
  frontal J32.1
  maxillary J32.0
 nerve —*see* Disorder, nerve
 nervous system G31.9
  alcoholic G31.2
  amyloid E85.4 *[G99.8]*
  autonomic G90.9
  fatty G31.89
  specified NEC G31.89
 nipple N64.89
 olivopontocerebellar (hereditary) (familial)
   G23.8
 osseous labyrinth —*see* subcategory H83.8
 ovary N83.8
  cystic N83.20-●
  microcystic N83.20-●
 pallidal pigmentary (progressive) G23.0
 pancreas K86.89
  tuberculous A18.83
 penis N48.89
 pigmentary (diffuse) (general)
  localized —*see* Degeneration, by site
  pallidal (progressive) G23.0
 pineal gland E34.8
 pituitary (gland) E23.6
 popliteal fat pad M79.4
 posterolateral (spinal cord) —*see*
   Degeneration, combined
 pulmonary valve (heart) I37.8
 pulp (tooth) K04.2
 pupillary margin H21.24-●
 renal —*see* Degeneration, kidney
 retina H35.9
  hereditary (cerebroretinal) (congenital)
   (juvenile) (macula) (peripheral)
   (pigmentary) —*see* Dystrophy, retina
  Kuhnt-Junius —*see also* Degeneration,
   macula H35.32-●
  macula (cystic) (exudative) (hole)
   (nonexudative) (pseudohole) (senile)
   (toxic) —*see* Degeneration, macula
  peripheral H35.40
   lattice H35.41-●
   microcystoid H35.42-●
   paving stone H35.43-●
   secondary
    pigmentary H35.45-●
    vitreoretinal H35.46-●
   senile reticular H35.44-●
  pigmentary (primary) —*see also* Dystrophy,
   retina
  secondary —*see* Degeneration, retina,
   peripheral, secondary
  posterior pole —*see* Degeneration, macula
 saccule, congenital (causing impairment of
   hearing) Q16.5
 senile R54
  brain G31.1
  cardiac, heart or myocardium —*see*
   Degeneration, myocardial
  motor centers G31.1
  vascular —*see* Arteriosclerosis
  sinus (cystic) —*see also* Sinusitis
   polypoid J33.1
 skin L98.8
  amyloid E85.4 *[L99]*
  colloid L98.8
 spinal (cord) G31.89
  amyloid E85.4 *[G32.89]*
  combined (subacute) —*see* Degeneration,
   combined
  dorsolateral —*see* Degeneration, combined
  familial NEC G31.89
  fatty G31.89

Degeneration, degenerative *(Continued)*
 spinal *(Continued)*
  funicular —*see* Degeneration, combined
  posterolateral —*see* Degeneration,
   combined
  subacute combined —*see* Degeneration,
   combined
  tuberculous A17.81
 spleen D73.0
  amyloid E85.4 *[D77]*
 stomach K31.89
 striatonigral G23.2
 suprarenal (capsule) (gland) E27.8
 synovial membrane (pulpy) —*see* Disorder,
   synovium, specified type NEC
 tapetoretinal —*see* Dystrophy, retina
 thymus (gland) E32.8
  fatty E32.8
 thyroid (gland) E07.89
 tricuspid (heart) (valve) I07.9
 tuberculous NEC —*see* Tuberculosis
 turbinate J34.89
 uterus (cystic) N85.8
 vascular (senile) —*see* Arteriosclerosis
  hypertensive —*see* Hypertension
 vitreoretinal, secondary —*see* Degeneration,
   retina, peripheral, secondary, vitreoretinal
 vitreous (body) H43.81-●
 Wallerian —*see* Disorder, nerve
 Wilson's hepatolenticular E83.01
Deglutition
 paralysis R13.0
  hysterical F44.4
 pneumonia J69.0
Degos' disease I77.89
Dehiscence (of)
 amputation stump T87.81
 cesarean wound O90.0
 closure of
  cornea T81.31
  craniotomy T81.32
  fascia (muscular) (superficial) T81.32
  internal organ or tissue T81.32
  laceration (external) (internal) T81.33
  ligament T81.32
  mucosa T81.31
  muscle or muscle flap T81.32
  ribs or rib cage T81.32
  skin and subcutaneous tissue (full-
    thickness) (superficial) T81.31
  skull T81.32
  sternum (sternotomy) T81.32
  tendon T81.32
  traumatic laceration (external) (internal)
    T81.33
 episiotomy O90.1
 operation wound NEC T81.31
  external operation wound (superficial)
    T81.31
  internal operation wound (deep)
    T81.32
 perineal wound (postpartum) O90.1
 traumatic injury wound repair T81.33
 wound T81.30
  traumatic repair T81.33
Dehydration E86.0
 newborn P74.1
Déjérine-Roussy syndrome G93.89
Déjérine-Sottas disease or neuropathy
  (hypertrophic) G60.0
Déjérine-Thomas atrophy G23.8
Delay, delayed
 any plane in pelvis
  complicating delivery O66.9
 birth or delivery NOS O63.9
 closure, ductus arteriosus (Botalli) P29.38
 coagulation —*see* Defect, coagulation
 conduction (cardiac) (ventricular)
   I45.9
 delivery, second twin, triplet, etc
   O63.2

Delay, delayed *(Continued)*
 development R62.50
  global F88
  intellectual (specific) F81.9
  language F80.9
   due to hearing loss F80.4
  learning F81.9
  pervasive F84.9
  physiological R62.50
   specified stage NEC R62.0
  reading F81.0
  sexual E30.0
  speech F80.9
   due to hearing loss F80.4
  spelling F81.81
 ejaculation F52.32
 gastric emptying K30
 menarche E30.0
 menstruation (cause unknown) N91.0
 milestone R62.0
 passage of meconium (newborn)
   P76.0
 primary respiration P28.9
 puberty (constitutional) E30.0
 separation of umbilical cord P96.82
 sexual maturation, female E30.0
 sleep phase syndrome G47.21
 union, fracture —*see* Fracture, by site
 vaccination Z28.9
Deletion(s)
 autosome Q93.9
  identified by fluorescence in situ
    hybridization (FISH) Q93.89
  identified by in situ hybridization (ISH)
    Q93.89
 chromosome
  with complex rearrangements NEC
    Q93.7
  part of NEC Q93.59
  seen only at prometaphase Q93.89
  short arm
   4 Q93.3
   5p Q93.4
   22q11.2 Q93.81
  specified NEC Q93.89
 long arm chromosome 18 or 21 Q93.89
  with complex rearrangements NEC Q93.7
 microdeletions NEC Q93.88
Delhi boil or button B55.1
Delinquency (juvenile) (neurotic) F91.8
 group Z72.810
Delinquent immunization status Z28.3
Delirious (acute or subacute) (not alcohol or
   drug-induced) (with dementia) R41.0
 alcoholic (acute) (tremens) (withdrawal)
   F10.921
  with intoxication F10.921
   in
    abuse F10.121
    dependence F10.221
 due to (secondary to)
  alcohol
   intoxication F10.921
    in
     abuse F10.121
     dependence F10.221
   withdrawal F10.231
  amphetamine intoxication F15.921
   in
    abuse F15.121
    dependence F15.221
  anxiolytic
   intoxication F13.921
    in
     abuse F13.121
     dependence F13.221
   withdrawal F13.231
  cannabis intoxication (acute) F12.921
   in
    abuse F12.121
    dependence F12.221

Delirious (Continued)
  due to (Continued)
    cocaine intoxication (acute) F14.921
      in
        abuse F14.121
        dependence F14.221
    general medical condition F05
    hallucinogen intoxication F16.921
      in
        abuse F16.121
        dependence F16.221
    hypnotic
      intoxication F13.921
        in
          abuse F13.121
          dependence F13.221
      withdrawal F13.231
    inhalant intoxication (acute) F18.921
      in
        abuse F18.121
        dependence F18.221
    multiple etiologies F05
    opioid intoxication (acute) F11.921
      in
        abuse F11.121
        dependence F11.221
    other (or unknown) substance
        F19.921
    phencyclidine intoxication (acute)
        F16.921
      in
        abuse F16.121
        dependence F16.221
    psychoactive substance NEC intoxication
        (acute) F19.921
      in
        abuse F19.121
        dependence F19.221
    sedative
      intoxication F13.921
        in
          abuse F13.121
          dependence F13.221
      withdrawal F13.231
    unknown etiology R41.0
  exhaustion F43.0
  hysterical F44.89
  postprocedural (postoperative) F05
  puerperal F05
  thyroid —see Thyrotoxicosis with thyroid
      storm
  traumatic —see Injury, intracranial
  tremens (alcohol-induced) F10.231
    sedative-induced F13.231
Delivery (childbirth) (labor)
  arrested active phase O62.1
  cesarean (for)
    without indication O82
    abnormal
      pelvis (bony) (deformity) (major) NEC
          with disproportion (fetopelvic)
          O33.0
        with obstructed labor O65.0
      presentation or position O32.9
    abruptio placentae —see also Abruptio
        placentae Ø45.9-●
    acromion presentation O32.2
    atony, uterus O62.2
    breech presentation O32.1
      incomplete O32.8
    brow presentation O32.3
    cephalopelvic disproportion O33.9
    cerclage O34.3-●
    chin presentation O32.3
    cicatrix of cervix O34.4-●
    contracted pelvis (general)
      inlet O33.2
      outlet O33.3
    cord presentation or prolapse
        O69.0
    cystocele O34.8-●

Delivery (Continued)
  cesarean (Continued)
    deformity (acquired) (congenital)
      pelvic organs or tissues NEC O34.8-●
      pelvis (bony) NEC O33.0
    disproportion NOS O33.9
    eclampsia —see Eclampsia
    face presentation O32.3
    failed
      forceps O66.5
      induction of labor O61.9
        instrumental O61.1
        mechanical O61.1
        medical O61.0
        specified NEC O61.8
        surgical O61.1
      trial of labor NOS O66.40
        following previous cesarean delivery
            O66.41
      vacuum extraction O66.5
      ventouse O66.5
    fetal-maternal hemorrhage O43.01-●
    hemorrhage (intrapartum) O67.9
      with coagulation defect O67.0
      specified cause NEC O67.8
    high head at term O32.4
    hydrocephalic fetus O33.6
    incarceration of uterus O34.51-●
    incoordinate uterine action O62.4
    increased size, fetus O33.5
    inertia, uterus O62.2
      primary O62.0
      secondary O62.1
    isthmocele O34.22
    lateroversion, uterus O34.59-●
    mal lie O32.9
    malposition
      fetus O32.9
      pelvic organs or tissues NEC O34.8-●
      uterus NEC O34.59-●
    malpresentation NOS O32.9
    oblique presentation O32.2
    occurring after 37 completed weeks of
        gestation but before 39 completed
        weeks gestation due to (spontaneous)
        onset of labor O75.82
    oversize fetus O33.5
    pelvic tumor NEC O34.8-●
    placenta previa O44.0-●
      complete O44.0-●
        with hemorrhage O44.1-●
    placental insufficiency O36.51-●
    planned, occurring after 37 completed
        weeks of gestation but before 39
        completed weeks gestation due to
        (spontaneous) onset of labor O75.82
    polyp, cervix O34.4-●
      causing obstructed labor O65.5
    poor dilatation, cervix O62.0
    pre-eclampsia O14.94
      mild O14.04
      moderate O14.04
      severe O14.14
        with hemolysis, elevated liver
            enzymes and low platelet count
            (HELLP) O14.24
    previous
      cesarean delivery O34.219
        classical (vertical) scar O34.212
        isthmocele O34.22
        low transverse scar O34.211
        mid-transverse T incision O34.218
        scar
          defect (isthmocele) O34.22
          specified type NEC O34.218
      surgery (to)
        cervix O34.4-●
        gynecological NEC O34.8-●
        rectum O34.7-●
        uterus O34.29
        vagina O34.6-●

Delivery (Continued)
  cesarean (Continued)
    prolapse
      arm or hand O32.2
      uterus O34.52-●
    prolonged labor NOS O63.9
    rectocele O34.8-●
    retroversion
      uterus O34.53-●
    rigid
      cervix O34.4-●
      pelvic floor O34.8-●
      perineum O34.7-●
      vagina O34.6-●
      vulva O34.7-●
    sacculation, pregnant uterus O34.59-●
    scar(s)
      cervix O34.4-●
      cesarean delivery O34.219
        classical (vertical) O34.212
        isthmocele O34.22
        low transverse O34.211
        mid-transverse T incision O34.218
        scar
          defect (isthmocele) O34.22
          specified type NEC O34.218
      defect (isthmocele) O34.22
      transmural uterine O34.29
      uterus O34.29
    Shirodkar suture in situ O34.3-●
    shoulder presentation O32.2
    stenosis or stricture, cervix O34.4-●
    streptococcus group B (GBS) carrier state
        O99.824
    transmural uterine scar O34.29
    transverse presentation or lie O32.2
    tumor, pelvic organs or tissues NEC O34.8-●
      cervix O34.4-●
    umbilical cord presentation or prolapse
        O69.0
  completely normal case O80
  complicated O75.9
    by
      abnormal, abnormality (of)
        forces of labor O62.9
          specified type NEC O62.8
        glucose O99.814
        uterine contractions NOS O62.9
      abruptio placentae —see also Abruptio
          placentae O45.9-●
      abuse
        physical O9A.32
        psychological O9A.52
        sexual O9A.42
      adherent placenta O72.0
        without hemorrhage O73.0
      alcohol use O99.314
      anemia (pre-existing) O99.02
      anesthetic death O74.8
      annular detachment of cervix O71.3
      atony, uterus O62.2
      attempted vacuum extraction and
          forceps O66.5
      Bandl's ring O62.4
      bariatric surgery status O99.844
      biliary tract disorder O26.62
      bleeding —see Delivery, complicated by,
          hemorrhage
      blood disorder NEC O99.12
      cervical dystocia (hypotonic) O62.2
        primary O62.0
        secondary O62.1
      circulatory system disorder O99.42
      compression of cord (umbilical) NEC
          O69.2
      condition NEC O99.892
      contraction, contracted ring O62.4
      cord (umbilical)
        around neck
          with compression O69.1
          without compression O69.81

▶ New   ⇒ Revised   ~~deleted~~ Deleted   ● Use Additional Character(s)

Delivery (Continued)
  complicated (Continued)
    by (Continued)
      cord (Continued)
        bruising O69.5
        complication O69.9
          specified NEC O69.89
        compression NEC O69.2
        entanglement O69.2
          without compression O69.82
        hematoma O69.5
        presentation O69.0
        prolapse O69.0
        short O69.3
        thrombosis (vessels) O69.5
        vascular lesion O69.5
      Couvelaire uterus O45.8X-●
      damage to (injury to) NEC
        perineum O71.82
        periurethral tissue O71.82
        vulva O71.82
      delay following rupture of membranes
          (spontaneous) —see Pregnancy,
          complicated by, premature rupture
          of membranes
      depressed fetal heart tones O76
      diabetes O24.92
        gestational O24.429
          diet controlled O24.420
          insulin controlled O24.424
          oral drug controlled (antidiabetic)
              (hypoglycemic) O24.425
        pre-existing O24.32
          specified NEC O24.82
          type 1 O24.02
          type 2 O24.12
      diastasis recti (abdominis) O71.89
      dilatation
        bladder O66.8
        cervix incomplete, poor or slow O62.0
      disease NEC O99.892
      disruptio uteri —see Delivery,
          complicated by, rupture, uterus
      drug use O99.324
      dysfunction, uterus NOS O62.9
        hypertonic O62.4
        hypotonic O62.2
          primary O62.0
          secondary O62.1
        incoordinate O62.4
      eclampsia O15.1
      embolism (pulmonary) —see Embolism,
          obstetric
      endocrine, nutritional or metabolic
          disease NEC O99.284
      failed
        attempted vaginal birth after previous
            cesarean delivery O66.41
        induction of labor O61.9
          instrumental O61.1
          mechanical O61.1
          medical O61.0
          specified NEC O61.8
          surgical O61.1
        trial of labor O66.40
      female genital mutilation O65.5
      fetal
        abnormal acid-base balance O68
        acidemia O68
        acidosis O68
        alkalosis O68
        death, early O02.1
        deformity O66.3
        heart rate or rhythm (abnormal) (non-
            reassuring) O76
        hypoxia O77.8
        stress O77.9
          due to drug administration O77.1
          electrocardiographic evidence of
              O77.8
          specified NEC O77.8
          ultrasound evidence of O77.8

Delivery (Continued)
  complicated (Continued)
    by (Continued)
      fever during labor O75.2
      gastric banding status O99.844
      gastric bypass status O99.844
      gastrointestinal disease NEC O99.62
      gestational
        diabetes O24.429
          diet controlled O24.420
          insulin (and diet) controlled
              O24.424
          oral drug controlled (antidiabetic)
              (hypoglycemic) O24.425
        edema O12.04
          with proteinuria O12.24
        proteinuria O12.14
      gonorrhea O98.22
      hematoma O71.7
        ischial spine O71.7
        pelvic O71.7
        vagina O71.7
        vulva or perineum O71.7
      hemorrhage (uterine) O67.9
        associated with
          afibrinogenemia O67.0
          coagulation defect O67.0
          hyperfibrinolysis O67.0
          hypofibrinogenemia O67.0
        due to
          low implantation of placenta
              O44.5-●
          low-lying placenta O44.5-●
          placenta previa O44.1-●
            marginal O44.3-●
            partial O44.3-●
          premature separation of placenta
              (normally implanted) (see also
              Abruptio placentae) O45.9-●
          retained placenta O72.0
          uterine leiomyoma O67.8
        placenta NEC O67.8
        postpartum NEC (atonic) (immediate)
            O72.1
          with retained or trapped placenta
              O72.0
          delayed O72.2
          secondary O72.2
          third stage O72.0
      hourglass contraction, uterus O62.4
      hypertension, hypertensive (pre-
          existing) —see Hypertension,
          complicated by, childbirth (labor)
      hypotension O26.5-●
      incomplete dilatation (cervix)
          O62.0
      incoordinate uterus contractions
          O62.4
      inertia, uterus O62.2
        during latent phase of labor O62.0
        primary O62.0
        secondary O62.1
      infection (maternal) O98.92
        carrier state NEC O99.834
        gonorrhea O98.22
        human immunodeficiency virus (HIV)
            O98.72
        sexually transmitted NEC O98.32
        specified NEC O98.82
        syphilis O98.12
        tuberculosis O98.02
        viral hepatitis O98.42
        viral NEC O98.52
      injury (to mother) (see also Delivery,
          complicated, by, damage to)
          O71.9
        nonobstetric O9A.22
          caused by abuse —see Delivery,
              complicated by, abuse
      intrauterine fetal death, early O02.1
      inversion, uterus O71.2

Delivery (Continued)
  complicated (Continued)
    by (Continued)
      laceration (perineal) O70.9
        anus (sphincter) O70.4
          with third degree laceration —see
              also Delivery, complicated, by,
              laceration, perineum, third
              degree O70.20
            with mucosa O70.3
          without third degree laceration
              O70.4
        bladder (urinary) O71.5
        bowel O71.5
        cervix (uteri) O71.3
        fourchette O70.0
        hymen O70.0
        labia O70.0
        pelvic
          floor O70.1
          organ NEC O71.5
        perineum, perineal O70.9
          first degree O70.0
          fourth degree O70.3
          muscles O70.1
          second degree O70.1
          skin O70.0
          slight O70.0
          third degree O70.20
            with
              both external anal sphincter
                  (EAS) and internal anal
                  sphincter (IAS) torn (IIIc)
                  O70.23
              less than 50% of external anal
                  sphincter (EAS) thickness
                  torn (IIIa) O70.21
              more than 50% external anal
                  sphincter (EAS) thickness
                  torn (IIIb) O70.22
            IIIa O70.21
            IIIb O70.22
            IIIc O70.23
        peritoneum (pelvic) O71.5
        rectovaginal (septum) (without
            perineal laceration) O71.4
          with perineum —see also Delivery,
              complicated, by, laceration,
              perineum, third degree
              O70.20
            with anal or rectal mucosa
                O70.3
        specified NEC O71.89
        sphincter ani —see Delivery,
            complicated, by, laceration, anus
            (sphincter)
        urethra O71.5
        uterus O71.81
          before labor O71.81
        vagina, vaginal (deep) (high)
            (without perineal laceration)
            O71.4
          with perineum O70.0
            muscles, with perineum O70.1
        vulva O70.0
      liver disorder O26.62
      malignancy O9A.12
      malnutrition O25.2
      malposition, malpresentation
        without obstruction O32.9 —see
            also Delivery, complicated by,
            obstruction
        breech O32.1
        compound O32.6
        face (brow) (chin) O32.3
        footling O38.8
        high head O32.4
        oblique O32.2
        specified NEC O32.8
        transverse O32.2
        unstable lie O32.0

▶ New   ⇒ Revised   ~~deleted~~ Deleted   ● Use Additional Character(s)

Dementia *(Continued)*
  in *(Continued)*
    Alzheimer's disease —*see* Disease,
      Alzheimer's
    arteriosclerotic brain disease —*see*
      Dementia, vascular
    cerebral lipidoses E75.-● *[F02.80]*
      with behavioral disturbance
        E75.-● *[F02.81]*
    Creutzfeldt-Jakob disease —*see also*
      Creutzfeldt-Jakob disease or
      syndrome (with dementia) A81.00
    epilepsy G40.-● *[F02.80]*
      with behavioral disturbance
        G40.-● *[F02.81]*
    hepatolenticular degeneration E83.01
      [F02.80]
      with behavioral disturbance E83.01
        [F02.81]
    human immunodeficiency virus (HIV)
      disease B20 *[F02.80]*
      with behavioral disturbance B20 *[F02.81]*
    Huntington's disease or chorea G10 *[F02.80]*
      with behavioral disturbance G10 *[F02.81]*
    hypercalcemia E83.52 *[F02.80]*
      with behavioral disturbance E83.52
        [F02.81]
    hypothyroidism, acquired E03.9 *[F02.80]*
      with behavioral disturbance E03.9
        [F02.81]
      due to iodine deficiency E01.8 *[F02.80]*
        with behavioral disturbance E01.8
          [F02.81]
    inhalants F18.97
      with dependence F18.27
    multiple
      etiologies F03
      sclerosis G35 *[F02.80]*
        with behavioral disturbance G35
          [F02.81]
    neurosyphilis A52.17 *[F02.80]*
      with behavioral disturbance A52.17
        [F02.81]
      juvenile A50.49 *[F02.80]*
        with behavioral disturbance A50.49
          [F02.81]
    niacin deficiency E52 *[F02.80]*
      with behavioral disturbance E52 *[F02.81]*
    paralysis agitans G20 *[F02.80]*
      with behavioral disturbance G20 *[F02.81]*
    Parkinson's disease G20 *[F02.80]*
    pellagra E52 *[F02.80]*
      with behavioral disturbance E52 *[F02.81]*
    Pick's G31.01 *[F02.80]*
      with behavioral disturbance G31.01
        [F02.81]
    polyarteritis nodosa M30.0 *[F02.80]*
      with behavioral disturbance M30.0
        [F02.81]
    psychoactive drug F19.97
      with dependence F19.27
      inhalants F18.97
        with dependence F18.27
      sedatives, hypnotics or anxiolytics
        F13.97
        with dependence F13.27
    sedatives, hypnotics or anxiolytics
      F13.97
      with dependence F13.27
    systemic lupus erythematosus
      M32.-● *[F02.80]*
      with behavioral disturbance
        M32.-● *[F02.81]*
    trypanosomiasis
      African B56.9 *[F02.80]*
        with behavioral disturbance B56.9
          [F02.81]
    unknown etiology F03
    vitamin B12 deficiency E53.8 *[F02.80]*
      with behavioral disturbance E53.8
        [F02.81]

Dementia *(Continued)*
  vitamin B12 deficiency *(Continued)*
    volatile solvents F18.97
      with dependence F18.27
  infantile, infantilis F84.3
  Lewy body G31.83 *[F02.80]*
    with behavioral disturbance G31.83
      [F02.81]
  multi-infarct —*see* Dementia, vascular
  paralytica, paralytic (syphilitic) A52.17
    [F02.80]
    with behavioral disturbance A52.17
      [F02.81]
    juvenilis A50.45
  paretic A52.17
  praecox —*see* Schizophrenia
  presenile F03
    Alzheimer's type —*see* Disease,
      Alzheimer's, early onset
  primary degenerative F03
  progressive, syphilitic A52.17
  senile F03
    with acute confusional state F05
    Alzheimer's type —*see* Disease,
      Alzheimer's, late onset
    depressed or paranoid type F03
  vascular (acute onset) (mixed) (multi-infarct)
    (subcortical) F01.50
    with behavioral disturbance F01.51
Demineralization, bone —*see* Osteoporosis
Demodex folliculorum (infestation) B88.0
Demophobia F40.248
Demoralization R45.3
Demyelination, demyelinization
  central nervous system G37.9
    specified NEC G37.8
  corpus callosum (central) G37.1
  disseminated, acute G36.9
    specified NEC G36.8
  global G35
  in optic neuritis G36.0
Dengue (classical) (fever) A90
  hemorrhagic A91
  sandfly A93.1
Dennie-Marfan syphilitic syndrome
  A50.45
Dens evaginatus, in dente or invaginatus
  K00.2
Dense breasts R92.2
Density
  increased, bone (disseminated) (generalized)
    (spotted) —*see* Disorder, bone, density
    and structure, specified type NEC
  lung (nodular) J98.4
Dental —*see also* condition
  examination Z01.20
    with abnormal findings Z01.21
  restoration
    aesthetically inadequate or displeasing
      K08.56
    defective K08.50
      specified NEC K08.59
    failure of marginal integrity K08.51
    failure of periodontal anatomical integrity
      K08.54
Dentia praecox K00.6
Denticles (pulp) K04.2
Dentigerous cyst K09.0
Dentin
  irregular (in pulp) K04.3
  opalescent K00.5
  secondary (in pulp) K04.3
  sensitive K03.89
Dentinogenesis imperfecta K00.5
Dentinoma —*see* Cyst, calcifying odontogenic
Dentition (syndrome) K00.7
  delayed K00.6
  difficult K00.7
  precocious K00.6
  premature K00.6
  retarded K00.6

Dependence (on) (syndrome) F19.20
  with remission F19.21
  alcohol (ethyl) (methyl) (without remission)
    F10.20
    with
      amnestic disorder, persisting F10.26
      anxiety disorder F10.280
      dementia, persisting F10.27
      intoxication F10.229
        with delirium F10.221
        uncomplicated F10.220
      mood disorder F10.24
      psychotic disorder F10.259
        with
          delusions F10.250
          hallucinations F10.251
      remission F10.21
      sexual dysfunction F10.281
      sleep disorder F10.282
      specified disorder NEC F10.288
      withdrawal F10.239
        with
          delirium F10.231
          perceptual disturbance F10.232
        uncomplicated F10.230
    counseling and surveillance Z71.41
  ▶ in remission F10.21
  amobarbital —*see* Dependence, drug,
    sedative
  amphetamine(s) (type) —*see* Dependence,
    drug, stimulant NEC
  amytal (sodium) —*see* Dependence, drug,
    sedative
  analgesic NEC F55.8
  anesthetic (agent) (gas) (general) (local)
    NEC —*see* Dependence, drug,
    psychoactive NEC
  anxiolytic NEC —*see* Dependence, drug,
    sedative
  barbital(s) —*see* Dependence, drug, sedative
  barbiturate(s) (compounds) (drugs
    classifiable to T42) —*see* Dependence,
    drug, sedative
  benzedrine —*see* Dependence, drug,
    stimulant NEC
  bhang —*see* Dependence, drug, cannabis
  bromide(s) NEC —*see* Dependence, drug,
    sedative
  caffeine —*see* Dependence, drug, stimulant
    NEC
  cannabis (sativa) (indica) (resin) (derivatives)
    (type) —*see* Dependence, drug, cannabis
  chloral (betaine) (hydrate) —*see* Dependence,
    drug, sedative
  chlordiazepoxide —*see* Dependence, drug,
    sedative
  coca (leaf) (derivatives) —*see* Dependence,
    drug, cocaine
  cocaine —*see* Dependence, drug, cocaine
  codeine —*see* Dependence, drug, opioid
  combinations of drugs F19.20
  dagga —*see* Dependence, drug, cannabis
  demerol —*see* Dependence, drug, opioid
  dexamphetamine —*see* Dependence, drug,
    stimulant NEC
  dexedrine —*see* Dependence, drug, stimulant
    NEC
  dextromethorphan —*see* Dependence, drug,
    opioid
  dextromoramide —*see* Dependence, drug,
    opioid
  dextro-nor-pseudo-ephedrine —*see*
    Dependence, drug, stimulant NEC
  dextrorphan —*see* Dependence, drug,
    opioid
  diazepam —*see* Dependence, drug,
    sedative
  dilaudid —*see* Dependence, drug,
    opioid
  D-lysergic acid diethylamide —*see*
    Dependence, drug, hallucinogen

Dependence (Continued)
  drug NEC F19.20
    with sleep disorder F19.282
    cannabis F12.20
      with
        anxiety disorder F12.280
        intoxication F12.229
          with
            delirium F12.221
            perceptual disturbance F12.222
          uncomplicated F12.220
        other specified disorder F12.288
        psychosis F12.259
          delusions F12.250
          hallucinations F12.251
        unspecified disorder F12.29
        withdrawal F12.23
      in remission F12.21
    cocaine F14.20
      with
        anxiety disorder F14.280
        intoxication F14.229
          with
            delirium F14.221
            perceptual disturbance F14.222
          uncomplicated F14.220
        mood disorder F14.24
        other specified disorder F14.288
        psychosis F14.259
          delusions F14.250
          hallucinations F14.251
        sexual dysfunction F14.281
        sleep disorder F14.282
        unspecified disorder F14.29
        withdrawal F14.23
      in remission F14.21
      withdrawal symptoms in newborn P96.1
    counseling and surveillance Z71.51
    hallucinogen F16.20
      with
        anxiety disorder F16.280
        flashbacks F16.283
        intoxication F16.229
          with delirium F16.221
          uncomplicated F16.220
        mood disorder F16.24
        other specified disorder F16.288
        perception disorder, persisting F16.283
        psychosis F16.259
          delusions F16.250
          hallucinations F16.251
        unspecified disorder F16.29
      in remission F16.21
    in remission F19.21
    inhalant F18.20
      with
        anxiety disorder F18.280
        dementia, persisting F18.27
        intoxication F18.229
          with delirium F18.221
          uncomplicated F18.220
        mood disorder F18.24
        other specified disorder
          F18.288
        psychosis F18.259
          delusions F18.250
          hallucinations F18.251
        unspecified disorder F18.29
      in remission F18.21
    nicotine F17.200
      with disorder F17.209
        in remission F17.201
        specified disorder NEC
          F17.208
        withdrawal F17.203
      chewing tobacco F17.220
        with disorder F17.229
          in remission F17.221
          specified disorder NEC
            F17.228
          withdrawal F17.223

Dependence (Continued)
  drug NEC (Continued)
    nicotine (Continued)
      cigarettes F17.210
        with disorder F17.219
          in remission F17.211
          specified disorder NEC F17.218
          withdrawal F17.213
      specified product NEC F17.290
        with disorder F17.299
          remission F17.291
          specified disorder NEC F17.298
          withdrawal F17.293
    opioid F11.20
      with
        intoxication F11.229
          with
            delirium F11.221
            perceptual disturbance F11.222
          uncomplicated F11.220
        mood disorder F11.24
        other specified disorder F11.288
        psychosis F11.259
          delusions F11.250
          hallucinations F11.251
        sexual dysfunction F11.281
        sleep disorder F11.282
        unspecified disorder F11.29
        withdrawal F11.23
      in remission F11.21
    psychoactive NEC F19.20
      with
        amnestic disorder F19.26
        anxiety disorder F19.280
        dementia F19.27
        intoxication F19.229
          with
            delirium F19.221
            perceptual disturbance F19.222
          uncomplicated F19.220
        mood disorder F19.24
        other specified disorder F19.288
        psychosis F19.259
          delusions F19.250
          hallucinations F19.251
        sexual dysfunction F19.281
        sleep disorder F19.282
        unspecified disorder F19.29
        withdrawal F19.239
          with
            delirium F19.231
            perceptual disturbance F19.232
          uncomplicated F19.230
    sedative, hypnotic or anxiolytic F13.20
      with
        amnestic disorder F13.26
        anxiety disorder F13.280
        dementia, persisting F13.27
        intoxication F13.229
          with delirium F13.221
          uncomplicated F13.220
        mood disorder F13.24
        other specified disorder F13.288
        psychosis F13.259
          delusions F13.250
          hallucinations F13.251
        sexual dysfunction F13.281
        sleep disorder F13.282
        unspecified disorder F13.29
        withdrawal F13.239
          with
            delirium F13.231
            perceptual disturbance F13.232
          uncomplicated F13.230
      in remission F13.21
    stimulant NEC F15.20
      with
        anxiety disorder F15.280
        intoxication F15.229
          with
            delirium F15.221
            perceptual disturbance F15.222
          uncomplicated F15.220

Dependence (Continued)
  methyl (Continued)
    stimulant NEC (Continued)
      with (Continued)
        mood disorder F15.24
        other specified disorder F15.288
        psychosis F15.259
          delusions F15.250
          hallucinations F15.251
        sexual dysfunction F15.281
        sleep disorder F15.282
        unspecified disorder F15.29
        withdrawal F15.23
      in remission F15.21
  ethyl
    alcohol (without remission) F10.20
      with remission F10.21
    bromide —see Dependence, drug,
      sedative
    carbamate F19.20
    chloride F19.20
    morphine —see Dependence, drug, opioid
  ganja —see Dependence, drug, cannabis
  glue (airplane) (sniffing) —see Dependence,
    drug, inhalant
  glutethimide —see Dependence, drug,
    sedative
  hallucinogenics —see Dependence, drug,
    hallucinogen
  hashish —see Dependence, drug, cannabis
  hemp —see Dependence, drug, cannabis
  heroin (salt) (any) —see Dependence, drug,
    opioid
  hypnotic NEC —see Dependence, drug,
    sedative
  Indian hemp —see Dependence, drug,
    cannabis
  inhalants —see Dependence, drug, inhalant
  khat —see Dependence, drug, stimulant NEC
  laudanum —see Dependence, drug, opioid
  LSD (-25) (derivatives) —see Dependence,
    drug, hallucinogen
  luminal —see Dependence, drug, sedative
  lysergic acid —see Dependence, drug,
    hallucinogen
  maconha —see Dependence, drug, cannabis
  marihuana —see Dependence, drug, cannabis
  meprobamate —see Dependence, drug,
    sedative
  mescaline —see Dependence, drug,
    hallucinogen
  methadone —see Dependence, drug, opioid
  methamphetamine(s) —see Dependence,
    drug, stimulant NEC
  methaqualone —see Dependence, drug,
    sedative
  methyl
    alcohol (without remission) F10.20
      with remission F10.21
    bromide —see Dependence, drug, sedative
    morphine —see Dependence, drug, opioid
    phenidate —see Dependence, drug,
      stimulant NEC
    sulfonal —see Dependence, drug, sedative
  morphine (sulfate) (sulfite) (type) —see
    Dependence, drug, opioid
  narcotic (drug) NEC —see Dependence, drug,
    opioid
  nembutal —see Dependence, drug, sedative
  neraval —see Dependence, drug, sedative
  neravan —see Dependence, drug, sedative
  neurobarb —see Dependence, drug, sedative
  nicotine —see Dependence, drug, nicotine
  nitrous oxide F19.20
  nonbarbiturate sedatives and tranquilizers
    with similar effect —see Dependence,
    drug, sedative
  on
    artificial heart (fully implantable)
      (mechanical) Z95.812
    aspirator Z99.0

▶ New   ⇒ Revised   ~~deleted~~ Deleted   • Use Additional Character(s)

Dependence (Continued)
on (Continued)
  care provider (because of) Z74.9
    impaired mobility Z74.09
    need for
      assistance with personal care Z74.1
      continuous supervision Z74.3
    no other household member able to
      render care Z74.2
    specified reason NEC Z74.8
  machine Z99.89
    enabling NEC Z99.89
    specified type NEC Z99.89
  renal dialysis (hemodialysis) (peritoneal)
    Z99.2
  respirator Z99.11
  ventilator Z99.11
  wheelchair Z99.3
opiate —see Dependence, drug, opioid
opioids —see Dependence, drug, opioid
opium (alkaloids) (derivatives) (tincture) —
  see Dependence, drug, opioid
oxygen (long-term) (supplemental) Z99.81
paraldehyde —see Dependence, drug,
  sedative
paregoric —see Dependence, drug, opioid
PCP (phencyclidine) (or related substance) —
  see Dependence, drug, hallucinogen
pentobarbital —see Dependence, drug,
  sedative
pentobarbitone (sodium) —see Dependence,
  drug, sedative
pentothal —see Dependence, drug, sedative
peyote —see Dependence, drug, hallucinogen
phencyclidine (PCP) (or related substance) —
  see Dependence, drug, hallucinogen
phenmetrazine —see Dependence, drug,
  stimulant NEC
phenobarbital —see Dependence, drug,
  sedative
polysubstance F19.20
psilocibin, psilocin, psilocyn, psilocyline —see
  Dependence, drug, hallucinogen
psychostimulant NEC —see Dependence,
  drug, stimulant NEC
secobarbital —see Dependence, drug, sedative
seconal —see Dependence, drug, sedative
sedative NEC —see Dependence, drug,
  sedative
specified drug NEC —see Dependence, drug
stimulant NEC —see Dependence, drug,
  stimulant NEC
substance NEC —see Dependence, drug
supplemental oxygen Z99.81
tobacco —see Dependence, drug, nicotine
  counseling and surveillance Z71.6
tranquilizer NEC —see Dependence, drug,
  sedative
vitamin B6 E53.1
volatile solvents —see Dependence, drug,
  inhalant
Dependency
care-provider Z74.9
passive F60.7
reactions (persistent) F60.7
Depersonalization (in neurotic state) (neurotic)
  (syndrome) F48.1
Depletion
extracellular fluid E86.9
plasma E86.1
potassium E87.6
  nephropathy N25.89
salt or sodium E87.1
  causing heat exhaustion or prostration
    T67.4
  nephropathy N28.9
volume NOS E86.9
Deployment (current) (military) status Z56.82
in theater or in support of military war,
  peacekeeping and humanitarian
  operations Z56.82

Deployment (Continued)
personal history of Z91.82
  military war, peacekeeping and
    humanitarian deployment (current or
    past conflict) Z91.82
returned from Z91.82
Depolarization, premature I49.40
atrial I49.1
junctional I49.2
specified NEC I49.49
ventricular I49.3
Deposit
bone in Boeck's sarcoid D86.89
calcareous, calcium —see Calcification
cholesterol
  retina H35.89
  vitreous (body) (humor) —see Deposit,
    crystalline
conjunctiva H11.11-●
cornea H18.00-●
  argentous H18.02-●
  due to metabolic disorder H18.03-●
  Kayser-Fleischer ring H18.04-●
  pigmentation —see Pigmentation, cornea
crystalline, vitreous (body) (humor) H43.2-●
hemosiderin in old scars of cornea —see
  Pigmentation, cornea, stromal
metallic in lens —see Cataract, specified NEC
skin R23.8
tooth, teeth (betel) (black) (green) (materia
  alba) (orange) (tobacco) K03.6
urate, kidney —see Calculus, kidney
Depraved appetite —see Pica
Depressed
HDL cholesterol E78.6
⮑**Depression** (acute) (mental) F32.A
agitated (single episode) F32.2
anaclitic —see Disorder, adjustment
anxiety F41.8
  persistent F34.1
arches —see also Deformity, limb, flat foot
atypical (single episode) F32.89
  recurrent episode F33.8
basal metabolic rate R94.8
bone marrow D75.89
central nervous system R09.2
cerebral R29.818
  newborn P91.4
cerebrovascular I67.9
chest wall M95.4
climacteric (single episode) F32.89
  recurrent episode F33.8
endogenous (without psychotic symptoms)
  F33.2
  with psychotic symptoms F33.3
functional activity R68.89
hysterical F44.89
involutional (single episode) F32.89
  recurrent episode F33.8
major F32.9
  with psychotic symptoms F32.3
  recurrent —see Disorder, depressive,
    recurrent
manic-depressive —see Disorder, depressive,
  recurrent
masked (single episode) F32.89
medullary G93.89
menopausal (single episode) F32.89
  recurrent episode F33.8
metatarsus —see Depression, arches
monopolar F33.9
nervous F34.1
neurotic F34.1
nose M95.0
postnatal (NOS) F53.0
postpartum (NOS) F53.0
post-psychotic of schizophrenia F32.89
post-schizophrenic F32.89
psychogenic (reactive) (single episode)
  F32.9
psychoneurotic F34.1

Depression (Continued)
psychotic (single episode) F32.3
  recurrent F33.3
reactive (psychogenic) (single episode) F32.9
  psychotic (single episode) F32.3
recurrent —see Disorder, depressive, recurrent
respiratory center G93.89
seasonal —see Disorder, depressive, recurrent
senile F03
severe, single episode F32.2
situational F43.21
skull Q67.4
specified NEC (single episode) F32.89
sternum M95.4
visual field —see Defect, visual field
vital (recurrent) (without psychotic
  symptoms) F33.2
  with psychotic symptoms F33.3
  single episode F32.2
Deprivation
cultural Z60.3
effects NOS T73.9
  specified NEC T73.8
emotional NEC Z65.8
  affecting infant or child —see
    Maltreatment, child, psychological
food T73.0
protein —see Malnutrition
sleep Z72.820
social Z60.4
  affecting infant or child —see
    Maltreatment, child, psychological
specified NEC T73.8
vitamins —see Deficiency, vitamin
water T73.1
Derangement
ankle (internal) —see Derangement, joint,
  ankle
cartilage (articular) NEC —see Derangement,
  joint, articular cartilage, by site
  recurrent —see Dislocation, recurrent
cruciate ligament, anterior, current injury —
  see Sprain, knee, cruciate, anterior
elbow (internal) —see Derangement, joint,
  elbow
hip (joint) (internal) (old) —see Derangement,
  joint, hip
joint (internal) M24.9
  ankylosis —see Ankylosis
  articular cartilage M24.10
    ankle M24.17-●
    elbow M24.12-●
    foot M24.17-●
    hand M24.14-●
    hip M24.15-●
    knee NEC M23.9-●
    loose body —see Loose, body
    shoulder M24.11-●
    specified site NEC M24.19
    wrist M24.13-●
  contracture —see Contraction, joint
  current injury —see also Dislocation
    knee, meniscus or cartilage —see Tear,
      meniscus
  dislocation
    pathological —see Dislocation,
      pathological
    recurrent —see Dislocation, recurrent
  knee —see Derangement, knee
  ligament —see Disorder, ligament
  loose body —see Loose, body
  recurrent —see Dislocation, recurrent
  specified type NEC M24.80
    ankle M24.87-●
    elbow M24.82-●
    foot joint M24.87-●
    hand joint M24.84-●
    hip M24.85-●
    shoulder M24.81-●
    specified site NEC M24.89
    wrist M24.83-●
  temporomandibular M26.69

Derangement *(Continued)*
knee *(recurrent)* M23.9-●
    ligament disruption, spontaneous M23.60-●
        anterior cruciate M23.61-●
        capsular M23.67-●
        instability, chronic M23.5-●
        lateral collateral M23.64-●
        medial collateral M23.63-●
        posterior cruciate M23.62-●
    loose body M23.4-●
    meniscus M23.30-●
        cystic M23.00-●
            lateral M23.002
                anterior horn M23.04-●
                posterior horn M23.05-●
                specified NEC M23.06-●
            medial M23.005
                anterior horn M23.01-●
                posterior horn M23.02-●
                specified NEC M23.03-●
        degenerate —*see* Derangement, knee,
            meniscus, specified NEC
        detached —*see* Derangement, knee,
            meniscus, specified NEC
        due to old tear or injury M23.20-●
            lateral M23.20-●
                anterior horn M23.24-●
                posterior horn M23.25-●
                specified NEC M23.26-●
            medial M23.20-●
                anterior horn M23.21-●
                posterior horn M23.22-●
                specified NEC M23.23-●
        retained —*see* Derangement, knee,
            meniscus, specified NEC
        specified NEC M23.30-●
            lateral M23.30-●
                anterior horn M23.34-●
                posterior horn M23.35-●
                specified NEC M23.36-●
            medial M23.30-●
                anterior horn M23.31-●
                posterior horn M23.32-●
                specified NEC M23.33-●
    old M23.8X-●
    specified NEC —*see* subcategory M23.8
low back NEC —*see* Dorsopathy, specified NEC
meniscus —*see* Derangement, knee, meniscus
mental —*see* Psychosis
patella, specified NEC —*see* Disorder,
    patella, derangement NEC
semilunar cartilage (knee) —*see*
    Derangement, knee, meniscus,
    specified NEC
shoulder (internal) —*see* Derangement,
    joint, shoulder
Dercum's disease E88.2
Derealization (neurotic) F48.1
Dermal —*see* condition
Dermaphytid —*see* Dermatophytosis
Dermatitis (eczematous) L30.9
ab igne L59.0
acarine B88.0
actinic (due to sun) L57.8
    other than from sun L59.8
allergic —*see* Dermatitis, contact, allergic
ambustionis, due to burn or scald —*see* Burn
amebic A06.7
ammonia L22
arsenical (ingested) L27.8
artefacta L98.1
    psychogenic F54
atopic L20.9
    psychogenic F54
    specified NEC L20.89
autoimmune progesterone L30.8
berlock, berloque L56.2
blastomycotic B40.3
blister beetle L24.89
bullous, bullosa L13.9
    mucosynechial, atrophic L12.1
    seasonal L30.8
    specified NEC L13.8

Dermatitis *(Continued)*
calorica L59.0
    due to burn or scald —*see* Burn
caterpillar L24.89
cercarial B65.3
combustionis L59.0
    due to burn or scald —*see* Burn
congelationis T69.1
contact (occupational) L25.9
    allergic L23.9
        due to
            adhesives L23.1
            cement L23.5
            chemical products NEC L23.5
            chromium L23.0
            cosmetics L23.2
            dander (cat) (dog) L23.81
            drugs in contact with skin L23.3
            dyes L23.4
            food in contact with skin L23.6
            hair (cat) (dog) L23.81
            insecticide L23.5
            metals L23.0
            nickel L23.0
            plants, non-food L23.7
            plastic L23.5
            rubber L23.5
            specified agent NEC L23.89
        due to
            cement L25.3
            chemical products NEC L25.3
            cosmetics L25.0
            dander (cat) (dog) L23.81
            drugs in contact with skin L25.1
            dyes L25.2
            food in contact with skin L25.4
            hair (cat) (dog) L23.81
            plants, non-food L25.5
            specified agent NEC L25.8
    irritant L24.9
        due to
        ▶body fluids L24.A0
            ▶incontinence (dual) (fecal) (urinary)
                L24.A2
            ▶saliva L24.A1
            ▶specified NEC L24.A9
            cement L24.5
            chemical products NEC L24.5
            cosmetics L24.3
            detergents L24.0
            drugs in contact with skin L24.4
            food in contact with skin L24.6
            oils and greases L24.1
            plants, non-food L24.7
        ▶related to
            ▶colostomy L24.B3
            ▶endotracheal tube L24.A9
            ▶enterocutaneous
            ▶fistula L24.B3
            ▶gastrostomy L24.B1
            ▶ileostomy L24.B3
            ▶jejunostomy L24.B1
            ▶saliva or spit fistula L24.B1
            ▶stoma or fistula L24.B0
                ▶digestive L24.B1
                ▶fecal or urinary L24.B3
                ▶respiratory L24.B2
            ▶tracheostomy L24.B2
            solvents L24.2
            specified agent NEC L24.89
contusiformis L52
desquamative L30.8
diabetic —*see* E08-E13 with .620
diaper L22
diphtheritica A36.3
dry skin L85.3
due to
    acetone (contact) (irritant) L24.2
    acids (contact) (irritant) L24.5
    adhesive(s) (allergic) (contact) (plaster)
        L23.1
        irritant L24.5

Dermatitis *(Continued)*
due to *(Continued)*
    alcohol (irritant) (skin contact) (substances
        in category T51) L24.2
        taken internally L27.8
    alkalis (contact) (irritant) L24.5
    arsenic (ingested) L27.8
    carbon disulfide (contact) (irritant) L24.2
    caustics (contact) (irritant) L24.5
    cement (contact) L25.3
    cereal (ingested) L27.2
    chemical(s) NEC L25.3
        taken internally L27.8
    chlorocompounds L24.2
    chromium (contact) (irritant) L24.81
    coffee (ingested) L27.2
    cold weather L30.8
    cosmetics (contact) L25.0
        allergic L23.2
        irritant L24.3
    cyclohexanes L24.2
    dander (cat) (dog) L23.81
    Demodex species B88.0
    Dermanyssus gallinae B88.0
    detergents (contact) (irritant) L24.0
    dichromate L24.81
    drugs and medicaments (generalized)
        (internal use) L27.0
        external —*see* Dermatitis, due to, drugs,
            in contact with skin
        in contact with skin L25.1
            allergic L23.3
            irritant L24.4
        localized skin eruption L27.1
        specified substance —*see* Table of Drugs
            and Chemicals
    dyes (contact) L25.2
        allergic L23.4
        irritant L24.89
    epidermophytosis —*see* Dermatophytosis
    esters L24.2
    external irritant NEC L24.9
    fish (ingested) L27.2
    flour (ingested) L27.2
    food (ingested) L27.2
        in contact with skin L25.4
    fruit (ingested) L27.2
    furs (allergic) (contact) L23.81
    glues —*see* Dermatitis, due to, adhesives
    glycols L24.2
    greases NEC (contact) (irritant) L24.1
    hair (cat) (dog) L23.81
    hot
        objects and materials —*see* Burn
        weather or places L59.0
    hydrocarbons L24.2
    infrared rays L59.8
    ingestion, ingested substance L27.9
        chemical NEC L27.8
        drugs and medicaments —*see*
            Dermatitis, due to, drugs
        food L27.2
        specified NEC L27.8
    insecticide in contact with skin L24.5
    internal agent L27.9
        drugs and medicaments (generalized) —
            see Dermatitis, due to, drugs
        food L27.2
    irradiation —*see* Dermatitis, due to,
        radioactive substance
    ketones L24.2
    lacquer tree (allergic) (contact) L23.7
    light (sun) NEC L57.8
        acute L56.8
        other L59.8
    Liponyssoides sanguineus B88.0
    low temperature L30.8
    meat (ingested) L27.2
    metals, metal salts (contact) (irritant)
        L24.81
    milk (ingested) L27.2

▶ New   ⇛ Revised   ~~deleted~~ Deleted   ● Use Additional Character(s)

Dermatitis *(Continued)*
  due to *(Continued)*
    nickel (contact) (irritant) L24.81
    nylon (contact) (irritant) L24.5
    oils NEC (contact) (irritant) L24.1
    paint solvent (contact) (irritant) L24.2
    petroleum products (contact) (irritant)
      (substances in T52) L24.2
    plants NEC (contact) L25.5
      allergic L23.7
      irritant L24.7
    plasters (adhesive) (any) (allergic) (contact)
      L23.1
      irritant L24.5
    plastic (contact) L25.3
    preservatives (contact) —*see* Dermatitis,
      due to, chemical, in contact with skin
    primrose (allergic) (contact) L23.7
    primula (allergic) (contact) L23.7
    radiation L59.8
      nonionizing (chronic exposure) L57.8
      sun NEC L57.8
        acute L56.8
    radioactive substance L58.9
      acute L58.0
      chronic L58.1
    radium L58.9
      acute L58.0
      chronic L58.1
    ragweed (allergic) (contact) L23.7
    Rhus (allergic) (contact) (diversiloba)
      (radicans) (toxicodendron) (venenata)
      (verniciflua) L23.7
    rubber (contact) L24.5
    Senecio jacobaea (allergic) (contact) L23.7
    solvents (contact) (irritant) (substances in
      categories T52) L24.2
    specified agent NEC (contact) L25.8
      allergic L23.89
      irritant L24.89
    sunshine NEC L57.8
      acute L56.8
    tetrachlorethylene (contact) (irritant) L24.2
    toluene (contact) (irritant) L24.2
    turpentine (contact) L24.2
    ultraviolet rays (sun NEC) (chronic
      exposure) L57.8
      acute L56.8
    vaccine or vaccination L27.0
      specified substance —*see* Table of Drugs
        and Chemicals
    varicose veins —*see* Varix, leg, with,
      inflammation
    X-rays L58.9
      acute L58.0
      chronic L58.1
  dyshydrotic L30.1
  dysmenorrheica N94.6
  escharotica —*see* Burn
  exfoliative, exfoliativa (generalized) L26
    neonatorum L00
  eyelid —*(see also* Dermatosis, eyelid) H01.9
    allergic H01.119
      left H01.116
        lower H01.115
        upper H01.114
      right H01.113
        lower H01.112
        upper H01.111
    contact —*see* Dermatitis, eyelid, allergic
    due to
      Demodex species B88.0
      herpes (zoster) B02.39
        simplex B00.59
    eczematous H01.139
      left H01.136
        lower H01.135
        upper H01.134
      right H01.133
        lower H01.132
        upper H01.131
  specified NEC H01.8

Dermatitis *(Continued)*
  facta, factitia, factitial L98.1
    psychogenic F54
  flexural NEC L20.82
  friction L30.4
  fungus B36.9
    specified type NEC B36.8
  gangrenosa, gangrenous infantum L08.0
  harvest mite B88.0
  heat L59.0
  herpesviral, vesicular (ear) (lip) B00.1
  herpetiformis (bullous) (erythematous)
    (pustular) (vesicular) L13.0
    juvenile L12.2
    senile L12.0
  hiemalis L30.8
  hypostatic, hypostatica —*see* Varix, leg, with,
    inflammation
  infectious eczematoid L30.3
  infective L30.3
  irritant —*see* Dermatitis, contact, irritant
  Jacquet's (diaper dermatitis) L22
  Leptus B88.0
  lichenified NEC L28.0
  medicamentosa (generalized) (internal
    use) —*see* Dermatitis, due to drugs
  mite B88.0
  multiformis L13.0
    juvenile L12.2
  napkin L22
  neurotica L13.0
  nummular L30.0
  papillaris capillitii L73.0
  pellagrous E52
  perioral L71.0
  photocontact L56.2
  polymorpha dolorosa L13.0
  pruriginosa L13.0
  pruritic NEC L30.8
  psychogenic F54
  purulent L08.0
  pustular
    contagious B08.02
    subcorneal L13.1
  pyococcal L08.0
  pyogenica L08.0
  repens L40.2
  Ritter's (exfoliativa) L00
  Schamberg's L81.7
  schistosome B65.3
  seasonal bullous L30.8
  seborrheic L21.9
    infantile L21.1
    specified NEC L21.8
  sensitization NOS L23.9
  septic L08.0
  solare L57.8
  specified NEC L30.8
  stasis I87.2
    with
      varicose ulcer —*see* Varix, leg, with ulcer,
        with inflammation
      varicose veins —*see* Varix, leg, with,
        inflammation
    due to postthrombotic syndrome —*see*
      Syndrome, postthrombotic
  suppurative L08.0
  traumatic NEC L30.4
  trophoneurotica L13.0
  ultraviolet (sun) (chronic exposure) L57.8
    acute L56.8
  varicose —*see* Varix, leg, with, inflammation
  vegetans L10.1
  verrucosa B43.0
  vesicular, herpesviral B00.1
Dermatoarthritis, lipoid E78.81
Dermatochalasis, eyelid H02.839
  left H02.836
    lower H02.835
    upper H02.834
  right H02.833
    lower H02.832
    upper H02.831

Dermatofibroma (lenticulare) —*see* Neoplasm,
  skin, benign
  protuberans —*see* Neoplasm, skin, uncertain
    behavior
Dermatofibrosarcoma (pigmented)
  (protuberans) —*see* Neoplasm, skin,
  malignant
Dermatographia L50.3
Dermatolysis (exfoliativa) (congenital) Q82.8
  acquired L57.4
  eyelids —*see* Blepharochalasis
  palpebrarum —*see* Blepharochalasis
  senile L57.4
Dermatomegaly NEC Q82.8
Dermatomucosomyositis M33.10
  with
    myopathy M33.12
    respiratory involvement M33.11
    specified organ involvement NEC M33.19
Dermatomycosis B36.9
  furfuracea B36.0
  specified type NEC B36.8
Dermatomyositis (acute) (chronic) —*see also*
  Dermatopolymyositis
  adult —*see also* Dermatomyositis, specified
    NEC M33.10
  in (due to) neoplastic disease —*see also*
    Neoplasm D49.9 [M36.0]
  juvenile M33.00
    with
      myopathy M33.02
      respiratory involvement M33.01
      specified organ involvement NEC M33.09
    without myopathy M33.03
  specified NEC M33.10
    with
      myopathy M33.12
      respiratory involvement M33.11
      specified organ involvement NEC M33.19
    without myopathy M33.13
Dermatoneuritis of children —*see* Poisoning,
  mercury
Dermatophilosis A48.8
Dermatophytid L30.2
Dermatophytide —*see* Dermatophytosis
Dermatophytosis (epidermophyton) (infection)
  (Microsporum) (tinea) (Trichophyton) B35.9
  beard B35.0
  body B35.4
  capitis B35.0
  corporis B35.4
  deep-seated B35.8
  disseminated B35.8
  foot B35.3
  granulomatous B35.8
  groin B35.6
  hand B35.2
  nail B35.1
  perianal (area) B35.6
  scalp B35.0
  specified NEC B35.8
Dermatopolymyositis M33.90
  with
    myopathy M33.92
    respiratory involvement M33.91
    specified organ involvement NEC M33.99
  in neoplastic disease —*see also* Neoplasm
    D49.9 [M36.0]
  juvenile M33.00
    with
      myopathy M33.02
      respiratory involvement M33.01
      specified organ involvement NEC M33.09
  specified NEC M33.10
    myopathy M33.12
    respiratory involvement M33.11
    specified organ involvement NEC M33.19
  without myopathy M33.93
Dermatopolyneuritis —*see* Poisoning, mercury
Dermatorrhexis (*see also* Syndrome, Ehlers-
  Danlos) Q79.60
  acquired L57.4

Dermatosclerosis —see also Scleroderma
  localized L94.0
Dermatosis L98.9
  Andrews' L08.89
  Bowen's —see Neoplasm, skin, in situ
  bullous L13.9
    specified NEC L13.8
  exfoliativa L26
  eyelid (noninfectious) (see also Dermatitis,
    eyelid) H01.9
    dermatitis —see Dermatitis, eyelid
    discoid lupus erythematosus —see Lupus,
      erythematosus, eyelid
    xeroderma —see Xeroderma, acquired,
      eyelid
  factitial L98.1
  febrile neutrophilic L98.2
  gonococcal A54.89
  herpetiformis L13.0
    juvenile L12.2
  linear IgA L13.8
  menstrual NEC L98.8
  neutrophilic, febrile L98.2
  occupational —see Dermatitis, contact
  papulosa nigra L82.1
  pigmentary L81.9
    progressive L81.7
    Schamberg's L81.7
  psychogenic F54
  purpuric, pigmented L81.7
  pustular, subcorneal L13.1
  transient acantholytic L11.1
Dermographia, dermographism L50.3
Dermoid (cyst) —see also Neoplasm, benign,
  by site
  with malignant transformation C56-●
  due to radiation (nonionizing) L57.8
Dermopathy
  infiltrative with thyrotoxicosis —see
    Thyrotoxicosis
  nephrogenic fibrosing L90.8
Dermophytosis —see Dermatophytosis
Descemetocele H18.73-●
Descemet's membrane —see condition
Descending —see condition
Descensus uteri —see Prolapse, uterus
Desert
  rheumatism B38.0
  sore —see Ulcer, skin
Desertion (newborn) —see Maltreatment
Desmoid (extra-abdominal) (tumor) —see
  Neoplasm, connective tissue, uncertain
  behavior
  abdominal D48.1
Despondency F32.A
Desquamation, skin R23.4
Destruction, destructive —see also Damage
  articular facet —see also Derangement, joint,
    specified type NEC
    knee M23.8X-●
    vertebra —see Spondylosis
  bone —see also Disorder, bone, specified type
    NEC
    syphilitic A52.77
  joint —see also Derangement, joint, specified
    type NEC
    sacroiliac M53.3
  rectal sphincter K62.89
  septum (nasal) J34.89
  tuberculous NEC —see Tuberculosis
  tympanum, tympanic membrane
    (nontraumatic) —see Disorder, tympanic
    membrane, specified NEC
  vertebral disc —see Degeneration,
    intervertebral disc
Destructiveness —see also Disorder, conduct
  adjustment reaction —see Disorder, adjustment
Desultory labor O62.2
Detachment
  cartilage —see Sprain
  cervix, annular N88.8
    complicating delivery O71.3

Detachment (Continued)
  choroid (old) (postinfectional) (simple)
    (spontaneous) H31.40-●
    hemorrhagic H31.41-●
    serous H31.42-●
  ligament —see Sprain
  meniscus (knee) —see also Derangement,
    knee, meniscus, specified NEC
    current injury —see Tear, meniscus
    due to old tear or injury —see
      Derangement, knee, meniscus, due to
      old tear
  retina (without retinal break) (serous)
    H33.2-●
    with retinal:
      break H33.00-●
        giant H33.03-●
        multiple H33.02-●
        single H33.01-●
      dialysis H33.04-●
    pigment epithelium —see Degeneration,
      retina, separation of layers, pigment
      epithelium detachment
    rhegmatogenous —see Detachment, retina,
      with retinal, break
    specified NEC H33.8
    total H33.05-●
    traction H33.4-●
  vitreous (body) H43.81
Detergent asthma J69.8
Deterioration
  epileptic F06.8
  general physical R53.81
  heart, cardiac —see Degeneration,
    myocardial
  mental —see Psychosis
  myocardial, myocardium —see Degeneration,
    myocardial
  senile (simple) R54
Deuteranomaly (anomalous trichromat) H53.53
Deuteranopia (complete) (incomplete) H53.53
Development
  abnormal, bone Q79.9
  arrested R62.50
    bone —see Arrest, development or growth,
      bone
    child R62.50
    due to malnutrition E45
  defective, congenital —see also Anomaly, by
    site
    cauda equina Q06.3
    left ventricle Q24.8
      in hypoplastic left heart syndrome Q23.4
    valve Q24.8
      pulmonary Q22.3
  delayed (see also Delay, development) R62.50
    arithmetical skills F81.2
    language (skills) (expressive) F80.1
    learning skill F81.9
    mixed skills F88
    motor coordination F82
    reading F81.0
    specified learning skill NEC F81.89
    speech F80.9
    spelling F81.81
    written expression F81.81
  imperfect, congenital —see also Anomaly, by
    site
    heart Q24.9
    lungs Q33.6
  incomplete
    bronchial tree Q32.4
    organ or site not listed —see Hypoplasia,
      by site
    respiratory system Q34.9
  sexual, precocious NEC E30.1
  tardy, mental (see also Disability, intellectual)
    F79
Developmental —see condition
  testing, infant or child —see Examination,
    child

Devergie's disease (pityriasis rubra pilaris) L44.0
Deviation (in)
  conjugate palsy (eye) (spastic) H51.0
  esophagus (acquired) K22.89
  eye, skew H51.8
  midline (jaw) (teeth) (dental arch) M26.29
    specified site NEC —see Malposition
  nasal septum J34.2
    congenital Q67.4
  opening and closing of the mandible M26.53
  organ or site, congenital NEC —see
    Malposition, congenital
  septum (nasal) (acquired) J34.2
    congenital Q67.4
  sexual F65.9
    bestiality F65.89
    erotomania F52.8
    exhibitionism F65.2
    fetishism, fetishistic F65.0
      transvestism F65.1
    frotteurism F65.81
    masochism F65.51
    multiple F65.89
    necrophilia F65.89
    nymphomania F52.8
    pederosis F65.4
    pedophilia F65.4
    sadism, sadomasochism F65.52
    satyriasis F52.8
    specified type NEC F65.89
    transvestism F64.1
    voyeurism F65.3
  teeth, midline M26.29
  trachea J39.8
  ureter, congenital Q62.61
Device
  cerebral ventricle (communicating) in situ Z98.2
  contraceptive —see Contraceptive, device
  drainage, cerebrospinal fluid, in situ Z98.2
Devic's disease G36.0
Devil's
  grip B33.0
  pinches (purpura simplex) D69.2
Devitalized tooth K04.99
Devonshire colic —see Poisoning, lead
Dextraposition, aorta Q20.3
  in tetralogy of Fallot Q21.3
Dextrinosis, limit (debrancher enzyme
  deficiency) E74.03
Dextrocardia (true) Q24.0
  with
    complete transposition of viscera Q89.3
    situs inversus Q89.3
Dextrotransposition, aorta Q20.3
d-glycericacidemia E72.59
Dhat syndrome F48.8
Dhobi itch B35.6
Di George's syndrome D82.1
Di Guglielmo's disease C94.0-●
Diabetes, diabetic (mellitus) (sugar) E11.9
  with
    amyotrophy E11.44
    arthropathy NEC E11.618
    autonomic (poly)neuropathy E11.43
    cataract E11.36
    Charcot's joints E11.610
    chronic kidney disease E11.22
    circulatory complication NEC E11.59
    coma due to
      hyperosmolarity E11.01
      hypoglycemia E11.641
      ketoacidosis E11.11
    complication E11.8
      specified NEC E11.69
    dermatitis E11.620
    foot ulcer E11.621
    gangrene E11.52
    gastroparalysis E11.43
    gastroparesis E11.43
    glomerulonephrosis, intracapillary E11.21
    glomerulosclerosis, intercapillary E11.21
    hyperglycemia E11.65

Diabetes, diabetic *(Continued)*
　with *(Continued)*
　　hyperosmolarity E11.00
　　　with coma E11.01
　　hypoglycemia E11.649
　　　with coma E11.641
　　ketoacidosis E11.10
　　　with coma E11.11
　　kidney complications NEC E11.29
　　Kimmelsteil-Wilson disease E11.21
　　loss of protective sensation (LOPS) —*see*
　　　Diabetes, by type, with neuropathy
　　mononeuropathy E11.41
　　myasthenia E11.44
　　necrobiosis lipoidica E11.620
　　nephropathy E11.21
　　neuralgia E11.42
　　neurologic complication NEC E11.49
　　neuropathic arthropathy E11.610
　　neuropathy E11.40
　　ophthalmic complication NEC E11.39
　　oral complication NEC E11.638
　　osteomyelitis E11.69
　　periodontal disease E11.630
　　peripheral angiopathy E11.51
　　　with gangrene E11.52
　　polyneuropathy E11.42
　　renal complication NEC E11.29
　　renal tubular degeneration E11.29
　　retinopathy E11.319
　　　with macular edema E11.311
　　　　resolved following treatment
　　　　　E11.37
　　　nonproliferative E11.329
　　　　with macular edema E11.321
　　　　mild E11.329
　　　　　with macular edema E11.321
　　　　moderate E11.339
　　　　　with macular edema E11.331
　　　　severe E11.349
　　　　　with macular edema E11.341
　　　proliferative E11.359
　　　　with
　　　　　combined traction retinal
　　　　　　detachment and
　　　　　　rhegmatogenous retinal
　　　　　　detachment E11.354
　　　　　macular edema E11.351
　　　　　stable proliferative diabetic
　　　　　　retinopathy E11.355
　　　　　traction retinal detachment
　　　　　　involving the macula E11.352
　　　　　traction retinal detachment not
　　　　　　involving the macula E11.353
　　skin complication NEC E11.628
　　skin ulcer NEC E11.622
　brittle —*see* Diabetes, type 1
　bronzed E83.110
　complicating pregnancy —*see* Pregnancy,
　　complicated by, diabetes
　dietary counseling and surveillance Z71.3
　due to
　　autoimmune process —*see* Diabetes, type 1
　　immune mediated pancreatic islet
　　　beta-cell destruction —*see* Diabetes,
　　　type 1
　due to drug or chemical E09.9
　　with
　　　amyotrophy E09.44
　　　arthropathy NEC E09.618
　　　autonomic (poly)neuropathy E09.43
　　　cataract E09.36
　　　Charcot's joints E09.610
　　　chronic kidney disease E09.22
　　　circulatory complication NEC E09.59
　　　complication E09.8
　　　　specified NEC E09.69
　　　dermatitis E09.620
　　　foot ulcer E09.621
　　　gangrene E09.52
　　　gastroparalysis E09.43

Diabetes, diabetic *(Continued)*
　due to drug or chemical *(Continued)*
　　with *(Continued)*
　　　gastroparesis E09.43
　　　glomerulonephrosis, intracapillary
　　　　E09.21
　　　glomerulosclerosis, intercapillary E09.21
　　　hyperglycemia E09.65
　　　hyperosmolarity E09.00
　　　　with coma E09.01
　　　hypoglycemia E09.649
　　　　with coma E09.641
　　　ketoacidosis E09.10
　　　　with coma E09.11
　　　kidney complications NEC E09.29
　　　Kimmelsteil-Wilson disease E09.21
　　　mononeuropathy E09.41
　　　myasthenia E09.44
　　　necrobiosis lipoidica E09.620
　　　nephropathy E09.21
　　　neuralgia E09.42
　　　neurologic complication NEC E09.49
　　　neuropathic arthropathy E09.610
　　　neuropathy E09.40
　　　ophthalmic complication NEC E09.39
　　　oral complication NEC E09.638
　　　periodontal disease E09.630
　　　peripheral angiopathy E09.51
　　　　with gangrene E09.52
　　　polyneuropathy E09.42
　　　renal complication NEC E09.29
　　　renal tubular degeneration E09.29
　　　retinopathy E09.319
　　　　with macular edema E09.311
　　　　　resolved following treatment
　　　　　　E09.37
　　　　nonproliferative E09.329
　　　　　with macular edema E09.321
　　　　　mild E09.329
　　　　　　with macular edema E09.321
　　　　　moderate E09.339
　　　　　　with macular edema E09.331
　　　　　severe E09.349
　　　　　　with macular edema E09.341
　　　　proliferative E09.359
　　　　　with
　　　　　　combined traction retinal
　　　　　　　detachment and
　　　　　　　rhegmatogenous retinal
　　　　　　　detachment E09.354
　　　　　　macular edema E09.351
　　　　　　stable proliferative diabetic
　　　　　　　retinopathy E09.355
　　　　　　traction retinal detachment
　　　　　　　involving the macula
　　　　　　　E09.352
　　　　　　traction retinal detachment not
　　　　　　　involving the macula
　　　　　　　E09.353
　　　skin complication NEC E09.628
　　　skin ulcer NEC E09.622
　due to underlying condition E08.9
　　with
　　　amyotrophy E08.44
　　　arthropathy NEC E08.618
　　　autonomic (poly)neuropathy E08.43
　　　cataract E08.36
　　　Charcot's joints E08.610
　　　chronic kidney disease E08.22
　　　circulatory complication NEC E08.59
　　　complication E08.8
　　　　specified NEC E08.69
　　　dermatitis E08.620
　　　foot ulcer E08.621
　　　gangrene E08.52
　　　gastroparalysis E08.43
　　　gastroparesis E08.43
　　　glomerulonephrosis, intracapillary
　　　　E08.21
　　　glomerulosclerosis, intercapillary E08.21
　　　hyperglycemia E08.69

Diabetes, diabetic *(Continued)*
　due to underlying condition *(Continued)*
　　with *(Continued)*
　　　hyperosmolarity E08.00
　　　　with coma E08.01
　　　hypoglycemia E08.649
　　　　with coma E08.641
　　　ketoacidosis E08.10
　　　　with coma E08.11
　　　kidney complications NEC E08.29
　　　Kimmelsteil-WIlson disease E08.21
　　　mononeuropathy E08.41
　　　myasthenia E08.44
　　　necrobiosis lipoidica E08.620
　　　nephropathy E08.21
　　　neuralgia E08.42
　　　neurologic complication NEC E08.49
　　　neuropathic arthropathy E08.610
　　　neuropathy E08.40
　　　ophthalmic complication NEC
　　　　E08.39
　　　oral complication NEC E08.638
　　　periodontal disease E08.630
　　　peripheral angiopathy E08.51
　　　　with gangrene E08.52
　　　polyneuropathy E08.42
　　　renal complication NEC E08.29
　　　renal tubular degeneration E08.29
　　　retinopathy E08.319
　　　　with macular edema E08.311
　　　　　resolved following treatment
　　　　　　E08.37
　　　　nonproliferative E08.329
　　　　　with macular edema E08.321
　　　　　mild E08.329
　　　　　　with macular edema E08.321
　　　　　moderate E08.339
　　　　　　with macular edema E08.331
　　　　　severe E08.349
　　　　　　with macular edema E08.341
　　　　proliferative E08.359
　　　　　with
　　　　　　combined traction retinal
　　　　　　　detachment and
　　　　　　　rhegmatogenous retinal
　　　　　　　detachment E08.354
　　　　　　macular edema E08.351
　　　　　　stable proliferative diabetic
　　　　　　　retinopathy E08.355
　　　　　　traction retinal detachment
　　　　　　　involving the macula
　　　　　　　E08.352
　　　　　　traction retinal detachment not
　　　　　　　involving the macula
　　　　　　　E08.353
　　　skin complication NEC E08.628
　　　skin ulcer NEC E08.622
　gestational (in pregnancy) O24.419
　　affecting newborn P70.0
　　diet-controlled O24.410
　　in childbirth O24.429
　　　diet-controlled O24.420
　　　insulin (and diet) controlled O24.424
　　　oral drug controlled (antidiabetic)
　　　　(hypoglycemic) O24.425
　　insulin (and diet) controlled O24.414
　　oral drug controlled (antidiabetic)
　　　(hypoglycemic) O24.415
　　puerperal O24.439
　　　diet-controlled O24.430
　　　insulin (and diet) controlled O24.434
　　　oral drug controlled (antidiabetic)
　　　　(hypoglycemic) O24.435
　hepatogenous E13.9
　idiopathic —*see* Diabetes, type 1
　inadequately controlled — code to Diabetes,
　　by type, with hyperglycemia
　insipidus E23.2
　　nephrogenic N25.1
　　pituitary E23.2
　　vasopressin resistant N25.1

Diabetes, diabetic *(Continued)*
  insulin dependent — code to type of diabetes
  juvenile-onset —*see* Diabetes, type 1
  ketosis-prone —*see* Diabetes, type 1
  latent R73.03
  neonatal (transient) P70.2
  non-insulin dependent — code to type of
    diabetes
  out of control — code to Diabetes, by type,
    with hyperglycemia
  phosphate E83.39
  poorly controlled — code to Diabetes, by
    type, with hyperglycemia
  postpancreatectomy —*see* Diabetes, specified
    type NEC
  postprocedural —*see* Diabetes, specified type
    NEC
  secondary diabetes mellitus NEC —*see*
    Diabetes, specified type NEC
  specified type NEC E13.9
    with
      amyotrophy E13.44
      arthropathy NEC E13.618
      autonomic (poly)neuropathy E13.43
      cataract E13.36
      Charcot's joints E13.610
      chronic kidney disease E13.22
      circulatory complication NEC E13.59
      complication E13.8
        specified NEC E13.69
      dermatitis E13.620
      foot ulcer E13.621
      gangrene E13.52
      gastroparalysis E13.43
      gastroparesis E13.43
      glomerulonephrosis, intracapillary
        E13.21
      glomerulosclerosis, intercapillary E13.21
      hyperglycemia E13.65
      hyperosmolarity E13.00
        with coma E13.01
      hypoglycemia E13.649
        with coma E13.641
      ketoacidosis E13.10
        with coma E13.11
      kidney complications NEC E13.29
      Kimmelsteil-Wilson disease E13.21
      mononeuropathy E13.41
      myasthenia E13.44
      necrobiosis lipoidica E13.620
      nephropathy E13.21
      neuralgia E13.42
      neurologic complication NEC E13.49
      neuropathic arthropathy E13.610
      neuropathy E13.40
      ophthalmic complication NEC E13.39
      oral complication NEC E13.638
      periodontal disease E13.630
      peripheral angiopathy E13.51
        with gangrene E13.52
      polyneuropathy E13.42
      renal complication NEC E13.29
      renal tubular degeneration E13.29
      retinopathy E13.319
        with macular edema E13.311
          resolved following treatment
            E13.37
        nonproliferative E13.329
          with macular edema E13.321
          mild E13.329
            with macular edema E13.321
          moderate E13.339
            with macular edema E13.331
          severe E13.349
            with macular edema E13.341
        proliferative E13.359
          with
            combined traction retinal
              detachment and
              rhegmatogenous retinal
              detachment E13.354

Diabetes, diabetic *(Continued)*
  specified type NEC *(Continued)*
    with *(Continued)*
      retinopathy *(Continued)*
        proliferative *(Continued)*
          with *(Continued)*
            macular edema E13.351
            stable proliferative diabetic
              retinopathy E13.355
            traction retinal detachment
              involving the macula
              E13.352
            traction retinal detachment not
              involving the macula
              E13.353
      skin complication NEC E13.628
      skin ulcer E13.622
  steroid-induced —*see* Diabetes, due to, drug
    or chemical
  type 1 E10.9
    with
      amyotrophy E10.44
      arthropathy NEC E10.618
      autonomic (poly)neuropathy E10.43
      cataract E10.36
      Charcot's joints E10.610
      chronic kidney disease E10.22
      circulatory complication NEC E10.59
     ▶coma due to
      ▶hypoglycemia E11.641
      ▶ketoacidosis E11.11
      complication E10.8
        specified NEC E10.69
      dermatitis E10.620
      foot ulcer E10.621
      gangrene E10.52
      gastroparalysis E10.43
      gastroparesis E10.43
      glomerulonephrosis, intracapillary E10.21
      glomerulosclerosis, intercapillary E10.21
      hyperglycemia E10.65
      hypoglycemia E10.649
        with coma E10.641
      ketoacidosis E10.10
        with coma E10.11
      kidney complications NEC E10.29
      Kimmelsteil-Wilson disease E10.21
      mononeuropathy E10.41
      myasthenia E10.44
      necrobiosis lipoidica E10.620
      nephropathy E10.21
      neuralgia E10.42
      neurologic complication NEC E10.49
      neuropathic arthropathy E10.610
      neuropathy E10.40
      ophthalmic complication NEC E10.39
      oral complication NEC E10.638
      osteomyelitis E10.69
      periodontal disease E10.630
      peripheral angiopathy E10.51
        with gangrene E10.52
      polyneuropathy E10.42
      renal complication NEC E10.29
      renal tubular degeneration E10.29
      retinopathy E10.319
        with macular edema E10.311
          resolved following treatment E10.37
        nonproliferative E10.329
          with macular edema E10.321
          mild E10.329
            with macular edema E10.321
          moderate E10.339
            with macular edema E10.331
          severe E10.349
            with macular edema E10.341
        proliferative E10.359
          with
            combined traction retinal
              detachment and
              rhegmatogenous retinal
              detachment E13.354

Diabetes, diabetic *(Continued)*
  type 1 *(Continued)*
    with *(Continued)*
      retinopathy *(Continued)*
        proliferative *(Continued)*
          with *(Continued)*
            macular edema E13.351
            stable proliferative diabetic
              retinopathy E13.355
            traction retinal detachment
              involving the macula E13.352
            traction retinal detachment not
              involving the macula E13.353
      skin complication NEC E10.628
      skin ulcer NEC E10.622
  type 2 E11.9
    with
      amyotrophy E11.44
      arthropathy NEC E11.618
      autonomic (poly)neuropathy E11.43
      cataract E11.36
      Charcot's joints E11.610
      chronic kidney disease E11.22
      circulatory complication NEC E11.59
    ▶coma due to
      ▶hyperosmolarity E11.01
      ▶hypoglycemia E11.641
      ▶ketoacidosis E11.11
      complication E11.8
        specified NEC E11.69
      dermatitis E11.620
      foot ulcer E11.621
      gangrene E11.52
      gastroparalysis E11.43
      gastroparesis E11.43
      glomerulonephrosis, intracapillary E11.21
      glomerulosclerosis, intercapillary E11.21
      hyperglycemia E11.65
      hyperosmolarity E11.00
        with coma E11.01
      hypoglycemia E11.649
        with coma E11.641
      ketoacidosis E11.10
        with coma E11.11
      kidney complications NEC E11.29
      Kimmelsteil-Wilson disease E11.21
      mononeuropathy E11.41
      myasthenia E11.44
      necrobiosis lipoidica E11.620
      nephropathy E11.21
      neuralgia E11.42
      neurologic complication NEC E11.49
      neuropathic arthropathy E11.610
      neuropathy E11.40
      ophthalmic complication NEC E11.39
      oral complication NEC E11.638
      osteomyelitis E11.69
      periodontal disease E11.630
      peripheral angiopathy E11.51
        with gangrene E11.52
      polyneuropathy E11.42
      renal complication NEC E11.29
      renal tubular degeneration E11.29
      retinopathy E11.319
        with macular edema E11.311
          resolved following treatment E11.37
        nonproliferative E11.329
          with macular edema E11.321
          mild E11.329
            with macular edema E11.321
          moderate E11.339
            with macular edema E11.331
          severe E11.349
            with macular edema E11.341
        proliferative E11.359
          with
            combined traction retinal
              detachment and
              rhegmatogenous retinal
              detachment E11.354
            macular edema E11.351

▶ New   ⇒ Revised   ~~deleted~~ Deleted   ● Use Additional Character(s)

Diabetes, diabetic *(Continued)*
  type 2 *(Continued)*
    with *(Continued)*
      retinopathy *(Continued)*
        proliferative *(Continued)*
          with *(Continued)*
            stable proliferative diabetic
                retinopathy E11.355
            traction retinal detachment
                involving the macula E11.352
            traction retinal detachment not
                involving the macula E11.353
      skin complication NEC E11.628
      skin ulcer NEC E11.622
  uncontrolled
    meaning
      hyperglycemia —*see* Diabetes, by type,
          with, hyperglycemia
      hypoglycemia —*see* Diabetes, by type,
          with, hypoglycemia
Diacyclothrombopathia D69.1
Diagnosis deferred R69
Dialysis (intermittent) (treatment)
  noncompliance (with) Z91.15
  renal (hemodialysis) (peritoneal), status Z99.2
  retina, retinal —*see* Detachment, retina, with
      retinal, dialysis
Diamond-Blackfan anemia (congenital
    hypoplastic) D61.01
Diamond-Gardener syndrome
    (autoerythrocyte sensitization) D69.2
Diaper rash L22
Diaphoresis (excessive) R61
Diaphragm —*see* condition
Diaphragmalgia R07.1
Diaphragmatitis, diaphragmitis J98.6
Diaphysial aclasis Q78.6
Diaphysitis —*see* Osteomyelitis, specified type
    NEC
Diarrhea, diarrheal (disease) (infantile)
    (inflammatory) R19.7
  achlorhydric K31.83
  allergic K52.29
    due to
      colitis —*see* Colitis, allergic
      enteritis —*see* Enteritis, allergic
  amebic —*see also* Amebiasis A06.0
    with abscess —*see* Abscess, amebic
    acute A06.0
    chronic A06.1
    nondysenteric A06.2
  bacillary —*see* Dysentery, bacillary
  balantidial A07.0
  cachectic NEC K52.89
  Chilomastix A07.8
  choleriformis A00.1
  chronic (noninfectious) K52.9
  coccidial A07.3
  Cochin-China K90.1
    strongyloidiasis B78.0
  Dientamoeba A07.8
  dietetic —*see also* Diarrhea, allergic K52.29
  drug-induced K52.1
  due to
    bacteria A04.9
      specified NEC A04.8
    Campylobacter A04.5
    Capillaria philippinensis B81.1
    Clostridium difficile
      not specified as recurrent A04.72
      recurrent A04.71
    Clostridium perfringens (C) (F) A04.8
    Cryptosporidium A07.2
    drugs K52.1
    Escherichia coli A04.4
      enteroaggregative A04.4
      enterohemorrhagic A04.3
      enteroinvasive A04.2
      enteropathogenic A04.0
      enterotoxigenic A04.1
      specified NEC A04.4

Diarrhea, diarrheal *(Continued)*
  due to *(Continued)*
    food hypersensitivity —*see also* Diarrhea,
        allergic K52.29
    Necator americanus B76.1
    S. japonicum B65.2
    specified organism NEC A08.8
      bacterial A04.8
      viral A08.39
    Staphylococcus A04.8
    Trichuris trichiuria B79
    virus —*see* Enteritis, viral
    Yersinia enterocolitica A04.6
  dysenteric A09
  endemic A09
  epidemic A09
  flagellate A07.9
  Flexner's (ulcerative) A03.1
  functional K59.1
    following gastrointestinal surgery K91.89
    psychogenic F45.8
  Giardia lamblia A07.1
  giardial A07.1
  hill K90.1
  infectious A09
  malarial —*see* Malaria
  mite B88.0
  mycotic NEC B49
  neonatal (noninfectious) P78.3
  nervous F45.8
  neurogenic K59.1
  noninfectious K52.9
  postgastrectomy K91.1
  postvagotomy K91.1
  protozoal A07.9
    specified NEC A07.8
  psychogenic F45.8
  specified
    bacterium NEC A04.8
    virus NEC A08.39
  strongyloidiasis B78.0
  toxic K52.1
  trichomonal A07.8
  tropical K90.1
  tuberculous A18.32
  viral —*see* Enteritis, viral
Diastasis
  cranial bones M84.88
    congenital NEC Q75.8
  joint (traumatic) —*see* Dislocation
  muscle M62.00
    ankle M62.07-●
    congenital Q79.8
    foot M62.07-●
    forearm M62.03-●
    hand M62.04-●
    lower leg M62.06-●
    pelvic region M62.05-●
    shoulder region M62.01-●
    specified site NEC M62.08
    thigh M62.05-●
    upper arm M62.02-●
  recti (abdomen)
    complicating delivery O71.89
    congenital Q79.59
Diastema, tooth, teeth, fully erupted M26.32
Diastematomyelia Q06.2
Diataxia, cerebral G80.4
Diathesis
  allergic —*see* History, allergy
  bleeding (familial) D69.9
  cystine (familial) E72.00
  gouty —*see* Gout
  hemorrhagic (familial) D69.9
    newborn NEC P53
  spasmophilic R29.0
Diaz's disease or osteochondrosis (juvenile)
    (talus) —*see* Osteochondrosis, juvenile,
    tarsus
Dibothriocephalus, dibothriocephaliasis
    (latus) (infection) (infestation) B70.0
  larval B70.1

Dicephalus, dicephaly Q89.4
Dichotomy, teeth K00.2
Dichromat, dichromatopsia (congenital) —*see*
    Deficiency, color vision
Dichuchwa A65
Dicroceliasis B66.2
Didelphia, didelphys —*see* Double uterus
Didymytis N45.1
  with orchitis N45.3
Dietary
  inadequacy or deficiency E63.9
  surveillance and counseling Z71.3
Dietl's crisis N13.8
Dieulafoy lesion (hemorrhagic)
  duodenum K31.82
➠esophagus K22.89
  intestine (colon) K63.81
  stomach K31.82
Difficult, difficulty (in)
  acculturation Z60.3
➠feeding R63.30
    newborn P92.9
      breast P92.5
      specified NEC P92.8
    nonorganic (infant or child) F98.29
    ▶specified NEC R63.39
  intubation, in anesthesia T88.4
  mechanical, gastroduodenal stoma K91.89
    causing obstruction —*see also* Obstruction,
        intestine, postoperative K91.30
  micturition
    need to immediately re-void R39.191
    position dependent R39.192
    specified NEC R39.198
  reading (developmental) F81.0
    secondary to emotional disorders F93.9
  spelling (specific) F81.81
    with reading disorder F81.89
    due to inadequate teaching Z55.8
  swallowing —*see* Dysphagia
  walking R26.2
  work
    conditions NEC Z56.5
    schedule Z56.3
Diffuse —*see* condition
DiGeorge's syndrome (thymic hypoplasia) D82.1
Digestive —*see* condition
Dihydropyrimidine dehydrogenase disease
    (DPD) E88.89
Diktyoma —*see* Neoplasm, malignant, by site
Dilaceration, tooth K00.4
Dilatation
  anus K59.89
    venule —*see* Hemorrhoids
  aorta (focal) (general) —*see* Ectasia, aorta
    with aneurysm —*see* Aneurysm, aorta
    congenital Q25.44
  artery —*see* Aneurysm
  bladder (sphincter) N32.89
    congenital Q64.79
  blood vessel I99.8
  bronchial J47.9
    with
      exacerbation (acute) J47.1
      lower respiratory infection J47.0
➠calyx N28.89
    ▶due to obstruction —*see* Hydronephosis
  capillaries I78.8
  cardiac (acute) (chronic) —*see also*
      Hypertrophy, cardiac
    congenital Q24.8
      valve NEC Q24.8
        pulmonary Q22.3
    valve —*see* Endocarditis
  cavum septi pellucidi Q06.8
  cervix (uteri) —*see also* Incompetency, cervix
    incomplete, poor, slow complicating
        delivery O62.0
  colon K59.39
    congenital Q43.1
    psychogenic F45.8
    toxic K59.31

Dilatation *(Continued)*
  common duct (acquired) K83.8
    congenital Q44.5
  cystic duct (acquired) K82.8
    congenital Q44.5
  duct, mammary —*see* Ectasia, mammary duct
  duodenum K59.89
  esophagus K22.89
    congenital Q39.5
    due to achalasia K22.0
  eustachian tube, congenital Q17.8
  gallbladder K82.8
  gastric —*see* Dilatation, stomach
  heart (acute) (chronic) —*see also* Hypertrophy,
      cardiac
    congenital Q24.8
    valve —*see* Endocarditis
  ileum K59.89
    psychogenic F45.8
  jejunum K59.89
    psychogenic F45.8
  kidney (calyx) (collecting structures) (cystic)
      (parenchyma) (pelvis) (idiopathic) N28.89
    ▶due to obstruction —*see* Hydronephrosis
  lacrimal passages or duct —*see* Disorder,
      lacrimal system, changes
  lymphatic vessel I89.0
  mammary duct —*see* Ectasia, mammary duct
  Meckel's diverticulum (congenital) Q43.0
    malignant —*see* Table of Neoplasms, small
        intestine, malignant
  myocardium (acute) (chronic) —*see*
      Hypertrophy, cardiac organ or site,
      congenital NEC —*see* Distortion
  pancreatic duct K86.89
  pericardium —*see* Pericarditis
  pharynx J39.2
  prostate N42.89
  pulmonary
    artery (idiopathic) I28.8
    valve, congenital Q22.3
  pupil H57.04
  rectum K59.39
  saccule, congenital Q16.5
  salivary gland (duct) K11.8
  sphincter ani K62.89
  stomach K31.89
    acute K31.0
    psychogenic F45.8
  submaxillary duct K11.8
  trachea, congenital Q32.1
  ureter (idiopathic) N28.82
    congenital Q62.2
    due to obstruction N13.4
  urethra (acquired) N36.8
  vasomotor I73.9
  vein I86.8
  ventricular, ventricle (acute) (chronic) —*see
      also* Hypertrophy, cardiac
    cerebral, congenital Q04.8
  venule NEC I86.8
  vesical orifice N32.89
Dilated, dilation —*see* Dilatation
Diminished, diminution
  hearing (acuity) —*see* Deafness
  sense or sensation (cold) (heat) (tactile)
      (vibratory) R20.8
  vision NEC H54.7
  vital capacity R94.2
Diminuta taenia B71.0
Dimitri-Sturge-Weber disease Q85.8
Dimple
  congenital sacral Q82.6
  parasacral Q82.6
  pilonidal or postanal —*see* Cyst, pilonidal
Dioctophyme renalis (infection) (infestation)
    B83.8
Dipetalonemiasis B74.4
Diphallus Q55.69
Diphtheria, diphtheritic (gangrenous)
    (hemorrhagic) A36.9

Diphtheria, diphtheritic *(Continued)*
  carrier (suspected) Z22.2
  cutaneous A36.3
  faucial A36.0
  infection of wound A36.3
  laryngeal A36.2
  myocarditis A36.81
  nasal, anterior A36.89
  nasopharyngeal A36.1
  neurological complication A36.89
  pharyngeal A36.0
  specified site NEC A36.89
  tonsillar A36.0
Diphyllobothriasis (intestine) B70.0
  larval B70.1
Diplacusis H93.22-•
Diplegia (upper limbs) G83.0
  congenital (cerebral) G80.8
  facial G51.0
  lower limbs G82.20
  spastic G80.1
Diplococcus, diplococcal —*see* condition
Diplopia H53.2
Dipsomania F10.20
  with
    psychosis —*see* Psychosis, alcoholic
      remission F10.21
Dipylidiasis B71.1
DIRA (deficiency of interleukin 1 receptor
    antagonist) M04.8
Direction, teeth, abnormal, fully erupted M26.30
Dirofilariasis B74.8
Dirt-eating child F98.3
Disability, disabilities
  heart —*see* Disease, heart
  intellectual F79
    with
      autistic features F84.9
        ▶pathogenic CHAMP1 (genetic)
            (variant) F78.A9
        ▶pathogenic HNRNPH2 (genetic)
            (variant) F78.A9
        ▶pathogenic SATB2 (genetic) (variant)
            F78.A9
        ▶pathogenic SETBP1 (genetic) (variant)
            F78.A9
        ▶pathogenic STXBP1 (genetic) (variant)
            F78.A9
        ▶pathogenic SYNGAP1 (genetic)
            (variant) F78.A1
      ▶autosomal dominant F78.A9
      ▶autosomal recessive F78.A9
      ▶genetic related F78.A9
        ▶with
          ▶pathogenic CHAMP1 (variant) F78.
              A9
          ▶pathogenic HNRNPH2 (variant)
              F78.A9
          ▶pathogenic SATB2 (variant) F78.A9
            pathogenic SETBP1 (variant) F78.A9
          ▶pathogenic STXBP1 (variant) F78.A9
          ▶pathogenic SYNGAP1 (variant) F78.
              A1
          ▶specified NEC F78.A9
          ▶SYNGAP1-related F78.A1
      ▶in
        ▶autosomal dominant mental
            retardation F78.A9
        ▶autosomal recessive mental
            retardation F78.A9
        ▶SATB2-associated syndrome F78.A9
        ▶SETBP1 disorder F78.A9
        ▶STXBP1 encephalopathy with epilepsy
            (see also Encephalopathy; and
            see also Epilepsy) F78.A9
        ▶X-linked mental retardation
            (syndromic) (Bain type) F78.A9
    mild (I.Q. 50-69) F70
    moderate (I.Q. 35-49) F71
    profound (I.Q. under 20) F73
    severe (I.Q. 20-34) F72

Disability, disabilities *(Continued)*
  intellectual *(Continued)*
    ▶specified level NEC F78.A9
    ▶SYNGAP1-related F78.A1
    ▶X-linked (syndromic) (Bain type) F78.A9
    knowledge acquisition F81.9
    learning F81.9
    limiting activities Z73.6
    spelling, specific F81.81
Disappearance of family member Z63.4
Disarticulation —*see* Amputation
  meaning traumatic amputation —*see*
      Amputation, traumatic
Discharge (from)
  abnormal finding in —*see* Abnormal, specimen
  breast (female) (male) N64.52
  diencephalic autonomic idiopathic —*see*
      Epilepsy, specified NEC
  ear —*see also* Otorrhea
    blood —*see* Otorrhagia
  excessive urine R35.89
  nipple N64.52
  penile R36.9
  postnasal R09.82
  prison, anxiety concerning Z65.2
  urethral R36.9
    without blood R36.0
    hematospermia R36.1
  vaginal N89.8
Discitis, diskitis M46.40
  cervical region M46.42
  cervicothoracic region M46.43
  lumbar region M46.46
  lumbosacral region M46.47
  multiple sites M46.49
  occipito-atlanto-axial region M46.41
  pyogenic —*see* Infection, intervertebral
      disc, pyogenic
  sacrococcygeal region M46.48
  thoracic region M46.44
  thoracolumbar region M46.45
Discoid
  meniscus (congenital) Q68.6
  semilunar cartilage (congenital) —*see*
      Derangement, knee, meniscus,
      specified NEC
Discoloration
  nails L60.8
  teeth (posteruptive) K03.7
    during formation K00.8
Discomfort
  chest R07.89
  visual H53.14-•
Discontinuity, ossicles, ear H74.2-•
Discord (with)
  boss Z56.4
  classmates Z55.4
  counselor Z64.4
  employer Z56.4
  family Z63.8
  fellow employees Z56.4
  in-laws Z63.1
  landlord Z59.2
  lodgers Z59.2
  neighbors Z59.2
  probation officer Z64.4
  social worker Z64.4
  teachers Z55.4
  workmates Z56.4
Discordant connection
  atrioventricular (congenital) Q20.5
  ventriculoarterial Q20.3
Discrepancy
  centric occlusion maximum intercuspation
      M26.55
  leg length (acquired) —*see* Deformity, limb,
      unequal length
    congenital —*see* Defect, reduction, lower
        limb
  uterine size date O26.84-•
Discrimination
  ethnic Z60.5
  political Z60.5

▶ New   ▦ Revised   ~~deleted~~ Deleted   • Use Additional Character(s)

Discrimination (*Continued*)
racial Z60.5
religious Z60.5
sex Z60.5
Disease, diseased —*see also* Syndrome
absorbent system I87.8
acid-peptic K30
Acosta's T70.29
Adams-Stokes (-Morgagni) (syncope with heart block) I45.9
Addison's anemia (pernicious) D51.0
adenoids (and tonsils) J35.9
adrenal (capsule) (cortex) (gland) (medullary) E27.9
   hyperfunction E27.0
   specified NEC E27.8
ainhum L94.6
airway
   obstructive, chronic J44.9
      due to
         cotton dust J66.0
         specific organic dusts NEC J66.8
   reactive —*see* Asthma
akamushi (scrub typhus) A75.3
Albers-Schönberg (marble bones) Q78.2
Albert's —*see* Tendinitis, Achilles
alimentary canal K63.9
alligator-skin Q80.9
   acquired L85.0
alpha heavy chain C88.3
alpine T70.29
altitude T70.20
alveolar ridge
   edentulous K06.9
      specified NEC K06.8
alveoli, teeth K08.9
Alzheimer's G30.9 [F02.80]
   with behavioral disturbance G30.9 [F02.81]
   early onset G30.0 [F02.80]
      with behavioral disturbance G30.0 [F02.81]
   late onset G30.1 [F02.80]
      with behavioral disturbance G30.1 [F02.81]
   specified NEC G30.8 [F02.80]
      with behavioral disturbance G30.8 [F02.81]
amyloid —*see* Amyloidosis
Andersen's (glycogenosis IV) E74.09
Andes T70.29
Andrews' (bacterid) L08.89
angiospastic I73.9
   cerebral G45.9
   vein I87.8
anterior
   chamber H21.9
   horn cell G12.29
antiglomerular basement membrane (anti-GBM) antibody M31.0
   tubulo-interstitial nephritis N12
antral —*see* Sinusitis, maxillary
anus K62.9
   specified NEC K62.89
aorta (nonsyphilitic) I77.9
   syphilitic NEC A52.02
aortic (heart) (valve) I35.9
   rheumatic I06.9
Apollo B30.3
aponeuroses —*see* Enthesopathy
appendix K38.9
   specified NEC K38.8
aqueous (chamber) H21.9
Arnold-Chiari —*see* Arnold-Chiari disease
arterial I77.9
   occlusive —*see* Occlusion, by site
      due to stricture or stenosis I77.1
   peripheral I73.9
arteriocardiorenal —*see* Hypertension, cardiorenal
arteriolar (generalized) (obliterative) I77.9
arteriorenal —*see* Hypertension, kidney
arteriosclerotic —*see also* Arteriosclerosis
   cardiovascular —*see* Disease, heart, ischemic, atherosclerotic
   coronary (artery) —*see* Disease, heart, ischemic, atherosclerotic

Disease, diseased (*Continued*)
arteriosclerotic (*Continued*)
   heart —*see* Disease, heart, ischemic, atherosclerotic
artery I77.9
   cerebral I67.9
   coronary I25.10
      with angina pectoris —*see* Arteriosclerosis, coronary (artery)
   peripheral I73.9
arthropod-borne NOS (viral) A94
   specified type NEC A93.8
atticoantral, chronic H66.20
   left H66.22
      with right H66.23
   right H66.21
      with left H66.23
auditory canal —*see* Disorder, ear, external
auricle, ear NEC —*see* Disorder, pinna
Australian X A83.4
autoimmune (systemic) NOS M35.9
   hemolytic D59.10
      cold type (primary) (secondary) (symptomatic) D59.12
      drug-induced D59.0
      mixed type (primary) (secondary) (symptomatic) D59.13
      warm type (primary) (secondary) (symptomatic) D59.11
   thyroid E06.3
autoinflammatory M04.9
   NOD2-associated M04.8
   specified type NEC M04.8
aviator's —*see* Effect, adverse, high altitude
Ayerza's (pulmonary artery sclerosis with pulmonary hypertension) I27.0
Babington's (familial hemorrhagic telangiectasia) I78.0
bacterial A49.9
   specified NEC A48.8
   zoonotic A28.9
      specified type NEC A28.8
Baelz's (cheilitis glandularis apostematosa) K13.0
bagasse J67.1
balloon —*see* Effect, adverse, high altitude
Bang's (brucella abortus) A23.1
Bannister's T78.3
barometer makers' —*see* Poisoning, mercury
Barraquer (-Simons') (progressive lipodystrophy) E88.1
Barrett's —*see* Barrett's, esophagus
Bartholin's gland N75.9
basal ganglia G25.9
   degenerative G23.9
      specified NEC G23.8
   specified NEC G25.89
Basedow's (exophthalmic goiter) —*see* Hyperthyroidism, with, goiter (diffuse)
Bateman's B08.1
Batten-Steinert G71.11
Battey A31.0
Beard's (neurasthenia) F48.8
Becker
   idiopathic mural endomyocardial I42.3
   myotonia congenita G71.12
Begbie's (exophthalmic goiter) —*see* Hyperthyroidism, with, goiter (diffuse)
behavioral, organic F07.9
Beigel's (white piedra) B36.2
Benson's —*see* Deposit, crystalline
Bernard-Soulier (thrombopathy) D69.1
Bernhardt (-Roth) —*see* Mononeuropathy, lower limb, meralgia paresthetica
Biermer's (pernicious anemia) D51.0
bile duct (common) (hepatic) K83.9
   with calculus, stones —*see* Calculus, bile duct
   specified NEC K83.8
biliary (tract) K83.9
   specified NEC K83.8
Billroth's —*see* Spina bifida
bird fancier's J67.2
black lung J60

Disease, diseased (*Continued*)
bladder N32.9
   in (due to)
      schistosomiasis (bilharziasis) B65.0 [N33]
      specified NEC N32.89
bleeder's D66
blood D75.9
   forming organs D75.9
   vessel I99.9
Bloodgood's —*see* Mastopathy, cystic
Blount M92.51-●
Bodechtel-Guttmann (subacute sclerosing panencephalitis) A81.1
bone —*see also* Disorder, bone
   aluminum M83.4
   fibrocystic NEC
   jaw M27.49
bone-marrow D75.9
Borna A83.9
Bornholm (epidemic pleurodynia) B33.0
Bouchard's (myopathic dilatation of the stomach) K31.0
Bouillaud's (rheumatic heart disease) I01.9
Bourneville (-Brissaud) (tuberous sclerosis) Q85.1
Bouveret (-Hoffmann) (paroxysmal tachycardia) I47.9
bowel K63.9
   functional K59.9
      psychogenic F45.8
brain G93.9
   arterial, artery I67.9
   arteriosclerotic I67.2
   congenital Q04.9
   degenerative —*see* Degeneration, brain
   inflammatory —*see* Encephalitis
   organic G93.9
      arteriosclerotic I67.2
   parasitic NEC B71.9 [G94]
   senile NEC G31.1
   specified NEC G93.89
breast (*see also* Disorder, breast) N64.9
   cystic (chronic) —*see* Mastopathy, cystic
   fibrocystic —*see* Mastopathy, cystic
   Paget's
      female, unspecified side C50.91-●
      male, unspecified side C50.92-●
   specified NEC N64.89
Breda's —*see* Yaws
Bretonneau's (diphtheritic malignant angina) A36.0
Bright's —*see* Nephritis
   arteriosclerotic —*see* Hypertension, kidney
Brill's (recrudescent typhus) A75.1
Brill-Zinsser (recrudescent typhus) A75.1
Brion-Kayser —*see* Fever, paratyphoid
broad
   beta E78.2
   ligament (noninflammatory) N83.9
      inflammatory —*see* Disease, pelvis, inflammatory
      specified NEC N83.8
Brocq-Duhring (dermatitis herpetiformis) L13.0
Brocq's
   meaning
      dermatitis herpetiformis L13.0
      prurigo L28.2
bronchopulmonary J98.4
bronchus NEC J98.09
bronze Addison's E27.1
   tuberculous A18.7
budgerigar fancier's J67.2
Buerger's (thromboangiitis obliterans) I73.1
bullous L13.9
   chronic of childhood L12.2
   specified NEC L13.8
Bürger-Grütz (essential familial hyperlipemia) E78.3
bursa —*see* Bursopathy
caisson T70.3
California —*see* Coccidioidomycosis
capillaries I78.9
   specified NEC I78.8

Disease, diseased *(Continued)*
Carapata A68.0
cardiac —*see* Disease, heart
cardiopulmonary, chronic I27.9
cardiorenal (hepatic) (hypertensive) (vascular) —*see* Hypertension, cardiorenal
cardiovascular (atherosclerotic) I25.10
  with angina pectoris —*see* Arteriosclerosis, coronary (artery),
    congenital Q28.9
  hypertensive —*see* Hypertension, heart
  newborn P29.9
    specified NEC P29.89
  renal (hypertensive) —*see* Hypertension, cardiorenal
  syphilitic (asymptomatic) A52.00
cartilage —*see* Disorder, cartilage
Castellani's A69.8
Castleman (unicentric) (multicentric) D47.Z2
  HHV-8-associated —*see also* Herpesvirus, human, 8 D47.Z2
cat-scratch A28.1
Cavare's (familial periodic paralysis) G72.3
cecum K63.9
celiac (adult) (infantile) (with steatorrhea) K90.0
cellular tissue L98.9
central core G71.29
cerebellar, cerebellum —*see* Disease, brain
cerebral —*see also* Disease, brain
  degenerative —*see* Degeneration, brain
cerebrospinal G96.9
cerebrovascular I67.9
  acute I67.89
    embolic I63.4-●
    thrombotic I63.3-●
  arteriosclerotic I67.2
  hereditary NEC I67.858
  specified NEC I67.89
cervix (uteri) (noninflammatory) N88.9
  inflammatory —*see* Cervicitis
  specified NEC N88.8
Chabert's A22.9
Chandler's (osteochondritis dissecans, hip) — *see* Osteochondritis, dissecans, hip
Charlouis —*see* Yaws
Chédiak-Steinbrinck (-Higashi) (congenital gigantism of peroxidase granules) E70.330
chest J98.9
Chiari's (hepatic vein thrombosis) I82.0
Chicago B40.9
Chignon B36.8
chigo, chigoe B88.1
childhood granulomatous D71
Chinese liver fluke B66.1
chlamydial A74.9
  specified NEC A74.89
cholecystic K82.9
choroid H31.9
  specified NEC H31.8
Christmas D67
chronic bullous of childhood L12.2
chylomicron retention E78.3
ciliary body H21.9
  specified NEC H21.89
circulatory (system) NEC I99.8
  newborn P29.9
  syphilitic A52.00
    congenital A50.54
coagulation factor deficiency (congenital) — *see* Defect, coagulation
coccidioidal —*see* Coccidioidomycosis
cold
  agglutinin or hemoglobinuria D59.12
    paroxysmal D59.6
  hemagglutinin (chronic) D59.12
collagen NOS (nonvascular) (vascular) M35.9
  specified NEC M35.89
colon K63.9
  functional K59.9
    congenital Q43.2

Disease, diseased *(Continued)*
colon K63.9*(Continued)*
  ischemic —*see also* Ischemia, intestine, acute K55.039
colonic inflammatory bowel, unclassified (IBDU) K52.3
combined system —*see* Degeneration, combined
compressed air T70.3
Concato's (pericardial polyserositis) A19.9
  nontubercular I31.1
  pleural —*see* Pleurisy, with effusion
conjunctiva H11.9
  chlamydial A74.0
  specified NEC H11.89
  viral B30.9
    specified NEC B30.8
connective tissue, systemic (diffuse) M35.9
  in (due to)
    hypogammaglobulinemia D80.1 *[M36.8]*
    ochronosis E70.29 *[M36.8]*
  specified NEC M35.89
Conor and Bruch's (boutonneuse fever) A77.1
Cooper's —*see* Mastopathy, cystic
Cori's (glycogenosis III) E74.03
corkhandler's or corkworker's J67.3
cornea H18.9
  specified NEC H18.89-●
coronary (artery) —*see* Disease, heart, ischemic, atherosclerotic
  congenital Q24.5
  ostial, syphilitic (aortic) (mitral) (pulmonary) A52.03
corpus cavernosum N48.9
  specified NEC N48.89
Cotugno's —*see* Sciatica
COVID-19 U07.1
coxsackie (virus) NEC B34.1
cranial nerve NOS G52.9
Creutzfeldt-Jakob —*see* Creutzfeldt-Jakob disease or syndrome
Crocq's (acrocyanosis) I73.89
Crohn's —*see* Enteritis, regional
Curschmann G71.11
cystic
  breast (chronic) —*see* Mastopathy, cystic
  kidney, congenital Q61.9
  liver, congenital Q44.6
  lung J98.4
    congenital Q33.0
cytomegalic inclusion (generalized) B25.9
  with pneumonia B25.0
  congenital P35.1
cytomegaloviral B25.9
  specified NEC B25.8
Czerny's (periodic hydrarthrosis of the knee) —*see* Effusion, joint, knee
Daae (-Finsen) (epidemic pleurodynia) B33.0
Darling's —*see* Histoplasmosis capsulati
Débove's (splenomegaly) R16.1
deer fly —*see* Tularemia
Degos' I77.8
demyelinating, demyelinizating (nervous system) G37.9
  multiple sclerosis G35
  specified NEC G37.8
dense deposit —*see also* N00-N07 with fourth character .6 N05.6
deposition, hydroxyapatite —*see* Disease, hydroxyapatite deposition
de Quervain's (tendon sheath) M65.4
  thyroid (subacute granulomatous thyroiditis) E06.1
Devergie's (pityriasis rubra pilaris) L44.0
Devic's G36.0
diaphorase deficiency D74.0
diaphragm J98.6
diarrheal, infectious NEC A09
digestive system K92.9
  specified NEC K92.89
disc, degenerative —*see* Degeneration, intervertebral disc

Disease, diseased *(Continued)*
discogenic —*see also* Displacement, intervertebral disc NEC
  with myelopathy —*see* Disorder, disc, with, myelopathy
diverticular —*see* Diverticula
Dubois (thymus) A50.59 *[E35]*
Duchenne-Griesinger G71.01
Duchenne's
  muscular dystrophy G71.01
  pseudohypertrophy, muscles G71.01
ductless glands E34.9
Duhring's (dermatitis herpetiformis) L13.0
duodenum K31.9
  specified NEC K31.89
Dupré's (meningism) R29.1
Dupuytren's (muscle contracture) M72.0
Durand-Nicholas-Favre (climatic bubo) A55
Duroziez's (congenital mitral stenosis) Q23.2
ear —*see* Disorder, ear
Eberth's —*see* Fever, typhoid
Ebola (virus) A98.4
Ebstein's heart Q22.5
Echinococcus —*see* Echinococcus
echovirus NEC B34.1
Eddowes' (brittle bones and blue sclera) Q78.0
edentulous (alveolar) ridge K06.9
  specified NEC K06.8
Edsall's T67.2
Eichstedt's (pityriasis versicolor) B36.0
Eisenmenger's (irreversible) I27.83
Ellis-van Creveld (chondroectodermal dysplasia) Q77.6
end stage renal (ESRD) N18.6
  due to hypertension I12.0
endocrine glands or system NEC E34.9
endomyocardial (eosinophilic) I42.3
English (rickets) E55.0
enteroviral, enterovirus NEC B34.1
  central nervous system NEC A88.8
epidemic B99.9
  specified NEC B99.8
epididymis N50.9
Erb (-Landouzy) G71.02
Erdheim-Chester (ECD) E88.89
esophagus K22.9
  functional K22.4
  psychogenic F45.8
  specified NEC K22.89
Eulenburg's (congenital paramyotonia) G71.19
eustachian tube —*see* Disorder, eustachian tube
external
  auditory canal —*see* Disorder, ear, external
  ear —*see* Disorder, ear, external
extrapyramidal G25.9
  specified NEC G25.89
eye H57.9
  anterior chamber H21.9
  inflammatory NEC H57.89
  muscle (external) —*see* Strabismus
  specified NEC H57.89
  syphilitic —*see* Oculopathy, syphilitic
eyeball H44.9
  specified NEC H44.89
eyelid —*see* Disorder, eyelid
  specified NEC —*see* Disorder, eyelid, specified type NEC
eyeworm of Africa B74.3
facial nerve (seventh) G51.9
  newborn (birth injury) P11.3
Fahr (of brain) G23.8
Fahr Volhard (of kidney) I12.-●
fallopian tube (noninflammatory) N83.9
  inflammatory —*see* Salpingo-oophoritis
  specified NEC N83.8
familial periodic paralysis G72.3
Fanconi's (congenital pancytopenia) D61.09
fascia NEC —*see also* Disorder, muscle
  inflammatory —*see* Myositis
  specified NEC M62.89
Fauchard's (periodontitis) —*see* Periodontitis
Favre-Durand-Nicolas (climatic bubo) A55
Fede's K14.0

▶ New   ⇒ Revised   ~~deleted~~ Deleted   ● Use Additional Character(s)

Disease, diseased *(Continued)*
  Feer's —*see* Poisoning, mercury
  female pelvic inflammatory —*see also* Disease,
      pelvis, inflammatory N73.9
    syphilitic (secondary) A51.42
    tuberculous A18.17
  Fernels' (aortic aneurysm) I71.9
  fibrocaseous of lung —*see* Tuberculosis,
    pulmonary
  fibrocystic —*see* Fibrocystic disease
  Fiedler's (leptospiral jaundice) A27.0
  fifth B08.3
  file-cutter's —*see* Poisoning, lead
  fish-skin Q80.9
    acquired L85.0
  Flajani (-Basedow) (exophthalmic goiter) —
    see Hyperthyroidism, with, goiter (diffuse)
  flax-dresser's J66.1
  fluke —*see* Infestation, fluke
  foot and mouth B08.8
  foot process N04.9
  Forbes' (glycogenosis III) E74.03
  Fordyce-Fox (apocrine miliaria) L75.2
  Fordyce's (ectopic sebaceous glands) (mouth)
    Q38.6
  Forestier's (rhizomelic pseudopolyarthritis)
    M35.3
    meaning ankylosing hyperostosis —*see*
      Hyperostosis, ankylosing
  Fothergill's
    neuralgia —*see* Neuralgia, trigeminal
    scarlatina anginosa A38.9
  Fournier (gangrene) N49.3
    female N76.89
  fourth B08.8
  Fox (-Fordyce) (apocrine miliaria) L75.2
  Francis' —*see* Tularemia
  Franklin C88.2
  Frei's (climatic bubo) A55
  Friedreich's
    combined systemic or ataxia G11.11
    myoclonia G25.3
  frontal sinus —*see* Sinusitis, frontal
  fungus NEC B49
  Gaisböck's (polycythemia hypertonica) D75.1
  gallbladder K82.9
    calculus —*see* Calculus, gallbladder
    cholecystitis —*see* Cholecystitis
    cholesterolosis K82.4
    fistula —*see* Fistula, gallbladder
    hydrops K82.1
    obstruction —*see* Obstruction, gallbladder
    perforation K82.2
    specified NEC K82.8
  gamma heavy chain C88.2
  Gamna's (siderotic splenomegaly) D73.2
  Gamstorp's (adynamia episodica hereditaria)
    G72.3
  Gandy-Nanta (siderotic splenomegaly) D73.2
  ganister J62.8
  gastric —*see* Disease, stomach
  gastroesophageal reflux (GERD) K21.9
    with esophagitis (without bleeding) K21.00
      with bleeding K21.01
  gastrointestinal (tract) K92.9
    amyloid E85.4
    functional K59.9
      psychogenic F45.8
    specified NEC K92.89
  Gee (-Herter) (-Heubner) (-Thaysen)
    (nontropical sprue) K90.0
  genital organs
    female N94.9
    male N50.9
  Gerhardt's (erythromelalgia) I73.81
  Gibert's (pityriasis rosea) L42
  Gierke's (glycogenosis I) E74.01
  Gilles de la Tourette's (motor-verbal tic) F95.2
  gingiva K06.9
    plaque induced K05.00
    specified NEC K06.8
  gland (lymph) I89.9

Disease, diseased *(Continued)*
  Glanzmann's (hereditary hemorrhagic
    thrombasthenia) D69.1
  glass-blower's (cataract) —*see* Cataract,
    specified NEC
    salivary gland hypertrophy K11.1
  Glisson's —*see* Rickets
  globe H44.9
    specified NEC H44.89
  glomerular —*see also* Glomerulonephritis
    with edema —*see* Nephrosis
    acute —*see* Nephritis, acute
    chronic —*see* Nephritis, chronic
    minimal change N05.0
    rapidly progressive N01.9
  glycogen storage E74.00
    Andersen's E74.09
    Cori's E74.03
    Forbes' E74.03
    generalized E74.00
    glucose-6-phosphatase deficiency E74.01
    heart E74.02 *[I43]*
    hepatorenal E74.09
    Hers' E74.09
    liver and kidney E74.09
    McArdle's E74.04
    muscle phosphofructokinase E74.09
    myocardium E74.02 *[I43]*
    Pompe's E74.02
    Tauri's E74.09
    type 0 E74.09
    type I E74.01
    type II E74.02
    type III E74.03
    type IV E74.09
    type V E74.04
    type VI-XI E74.09
    Von Gierke's E74.01
  Goldstein's (familial hemorrhagic
    telangiectasia) I78.0
  gonococcal NOS A54.9
  graft-versus-host (GVH) D89.813
    acute D89.810
    acute on chronic D89.812
    chronic D89.811
  grainhandler's J67.8
  granulomatous (childhood) (chronic) D71
  Graves' (exophthalmic goiter) —*see*
    Hyperthyroidism, with, goiter (diffuse)
  Griesinger's —*see* Ancylostomiasis
  Grisel's M43.6
  Gruby's (tinea tonsurans) B35.0
  Guillain-Barré G61.0
  Guinon's (motor-verbal tic) F95.2
  gum K06.9
  gynecological N94.9
  H (Hartnup's) E72.02
  Haff —*see* Poisoning, mercury
  Hageman (congenital factor XII deficiency)
    D68.2
  hair (color) (shaft) L67.9
    follicles L73.9
      specified NEC L73.8
  Hamman's (spontaneous mediastinal
    emphysema) J98.2
  hand, foot and mouth B08.4
  Hansen's —*see* Leprosy
  Hantavirus, with pulmonary manifestations
    B33.4
    with renal manifestations A98.5
  Harada's H30.81-•
  Hartnup (pellagra-cerebellar ataxia-renal
    aminoaciduria) E72.02
  Hart's (pellagra-cerebellar ataxia-renal
    aminoaciduria) E72.02
  Hashimoto's (struma lymphomatosa) E06.3
  Hb —*see* Disease, hemoglobin
  heart (organic) I51.9
    with
      pulmonary edema (acute) —*see also*
        Failure, ventricular, left I50.1

Disease, diseased *(Continued)*
  heart *(Continued)*
    rheumatic fever (conditions in I00)
      active I01.9
        with chorea I02.0
        specified NEC I01.8
      inactive or quiescent (with chorea) I09.9
        specified NEC I09.89
    amyloid E85.4 *[I43]*
    aortic (valve) I35.9
    arteriosclerotic or sclerotic (senile) —*see*
      Disease, heart, ischemic, atherosclerotic
    artery, arterial —*see* Disease, heart,
      ischemic, atherosclerotic
    beer drinkers' I42.6
    beriberi (wet) E51.12
    black I27.0
    congenital Q24.9
      cyanotic Q24.9
      specified NEC Q24.8
    coronary —*see* Disease, heart, ischemic
    cryptogenic I51.9
    fibroid —*see* Myocarditis
    functional I51.89
      psychogenic F45.8
    glycogen storage E74.02 *[I43]*
    gonococcal A54.83
    hypertensive —*see* Hypertension, heart
    hyperthyroid —*see also* Hyperthyroidism
      E05.90 *[I43]*
      with thyroid storm E05.91 *[I43]*
    ischemic (chronic or with a stated duration
      of over 4 weeks) I25.9
      atherosclerotic (of) I25.10
        with angina pectoris —*see*
          Arteriosclerosis, coronary (artery)
        coronary artery bypass graft —*see*
          Arteriosclerosis, coronary (artery),
      cardiomyopathy I25.5
      diagnosed on ECG or other special
        investigation, but currently
        presenting no symptoms I25.6
      silent I25.6
      specified form NEC I25.89
    kyphoscoliotic I27.1
    meningococcal A39.50
      endocarditis A39.51
      myocarditis A39.52
      pericarditis A39.53
    mitral I05.9
      specified NEC I05.8
    muscular —*see* Degeneration, myocardial
    psychogenic (functional) F45.8
    pulmonary (chronic) I27.9
      in schistosomiasis B65.9 *[I52]*
      specified NEC I27.89
    rheumatic (chronic) (inactive) (old)
      (quiescent) (with chorea) I09.9
      active or acute I01.9
        with chorea (acute) (rheumatic)
          (Sydenham's) I02.0
      specified NEC I09.89
    senile —*see* Myocarditis
    syphilitic A52.06
      aortic A52.03
        aneurysm A52.01
      congenital A50.54 *[I52]*
    thyrotoxic —*see also* Thyrotoxicosis E05.90
      [I43]
      with thyroid storm E05.91 *[I43]*
    valve, valvular (obstructive)
      (regurgitant) —*see also* Endocarditis
      congenital NEC Q24.8
      pulmonary Q22.3
    vascular —*see* Disease, cardiovascular
  heavy chain NEC C88.2
    alpha C88.3
    gamma C88.2
    mu C88.2
  Hebra's
    pityriasis
      maculata et circinata L42
      rubra pilaris L44.0

Disease, diseased *(Continued)*
  Hebra's *(Continued)*
    prurigo L28.2
  hematopoietic organs D75.9
  hemoglobin or Hb
    abnormal (mixed) NEC D58.2
      with thalassemia D56.9
    AS genotype D57.3
    Bart's D56.0
    C (Hb-C) D58.2
      with other abnormal hemoglobin NEC
        D58.2
      elliptocytosis D58.1
      Hb-S D57.2-●
      sickle-cell D57.2-●
      thalassemia D56.8
    Constant Spring D58.2
    D (Hb-D) D58.2
    E (Hb-E) D58.2
    E-beta thalassemia D56.5
    elliptocytosis D58.1
    H (Hb-H) (thalassemia) D56.0
      with other abnormal hemoglobin NEC
        D56.9
      Constant Spring D56.0
    I thalassemia D56.9
    M D74.0
    S or SS D57.1
      with
        acute chest syndrome D57.01
        cerebral vascular involvement D57.03
        crisis (painful) D57.00
          with complication specified NEC
            D57.09
        splenic sequestration D57.02
        vasoocclusive pain D57.00
      beta plus D57.44
        with
          acute chest syndrome D57.451
          cerebral vascular involvement
            D57.453
          crisis D57.459
            with specified complication NEC
              D57.458
          splenic sequestration D57.452
          vasoocclusive pain D57.459
        without crisis D57.44
      beta zero D57.42
        with
          acute chest syndrome D57.431
          cerebral vascular involvement
            D57.433
          crisis D57.439
            with specified complication NEC
              D57.438
          splenic sequestration D57.432
          vasoocclusive pain D57.439
        without crisis D57.42
    SC D57.2-●
    SD D57.8-●
    SE D57.8-●
    spherocytosis D58.0
    unstable, hemolytic D58.2
  hemolytic (newborn) P55.9
    autoimmune D59.10
      cold type (primary) (secondary)
        (symptomatic) D59.12
      mixed type (primary) (secondary)
        (symptomatic) D59.13
      warm type (primary) (secondary)
        (symptomatic) D59.11
    drug-induced D59.0
    due to or with
      incompatibility
        ABO (blood group) P55.1
        blood (group) (Duffy) (K) (Kell)
          (Kidd) (Lewis) (M) (S) NEC P55.8
        Rh (blood group) (factor) P55.0
        Rh negative mother P55.0
      specified type NEC P55.8
    unstable hemoglobin D58.2
  hemorrhagic D69.9
    newborn P53

Disease, diseased *(Continued)*
  Henoch (-Schönlein) (purpura nervosa)
    D69.0
  hepatic —*see* Disease, liver
  hepatobiliary K83.9
    toxic K71.9
  hepatolenticular E83.01
  heredodegenerative NEC
    spinal cord G95.89
  herpesviral, disseminated B00.7
  Hers' (glycogenosis VI) E74.09
  Herter (-Gee) (-Heubner) (nontropical sprue)
    K90.0
  Heubner-Herter (nontropical sprue) K90.0
  high fetal gene or hemoglobin thalassemia
    D56.9
  Hildenbrand's —*see* Typhus
  hip (joint) M25.9
    congenital Q65.89
    suppurative M00.9
    tuberculous A18.02
  His (-Werner) (trench fever) A79.0
  Hodgson's I71.2
    ruptured I71.1
  Holla —*see* Spherocytosis
  hookworm B76.9
    specified NEC B76.8
  host-versus-graft D89.813
    acute D89.810
    acute on chronic D89.812
    chronic D89.811
  human immunodeficiency virus (HIV) B20
  Huntington's G10
    with dementia G10 *[F02.80]*
  Hutchinson's (cheiropompholyx) —*see*
    Hutchinson's disease
  hyaline (diffuse) (generalized)
    membrane (lung) (newborn) P22.0
      adult J80
  hydatid —*see* Echinococcus
  hydroxyapatite deposition M11.00
    ankle M11.07-●
    elbow M11.02-●
    foot joint M11.07-●
    hand joint M11.04-●
    hip M11.05-●
    knee M11.06-●
    multiple site M11.09
    shoulder M11.01-●
    vertebra M11.08
    wrist M11.03-●
  hyperkinetic —*see* Hyperkinesia
  hypertensive —*see* Hypertension
  hypophysis E23.7
  Iceland G93.3
  I-cell E77.0
  immune D89.9
  immunoproliferative (malignant) C88.9
    small intestinal C88.3
    specified NEC C88.8
  inclusion B25.9
    salivary gland B25.9
  infectious, infective B99.9
    congenital P37.9
      specified NEC P37.8
      viral P35.9
        specified type NEC P35.8
    specified NEC B99.8
  inflammatory
    penis N48.29
      abscess N48.21
      cellulitis N48.22
    prepuce N47.7
      balanoposthitis N47.6
    tubo-ovarian —*see* Salpingo-oophoritis
  intervertebral disc —*see also* Disorder, disc
    with myelopathy —*see* Disorder, disc, with,
      myelopathy
    cervical, cervicothoracic —*see* Disorder,
      disc, cervical
      with
        myelopathy —*see* Disorder, disc,
          cervical, with myelopathy

Disease, diseased *(Continued)*
  cervical, cervicothoracic *(Continued)*
    neuritis, radiculitis or
      radiculopathy —*see* Disorder,
        disc, cervical, with neuritis
    specified NEC —*see* Disorder, disc,
      cervical, specified type NEC
  lumbar (with)
    myelopathy M51.06
    neuritis, radiculitis, radiculopathy or
      sciatica M51.16
    specified NEC M51.86
  lumbosacral (with)
    neuritis, radiculitis, radiculopathy or
      sciatica M51.17
    specified NEC M51.87
  intervertebral disc *(Continued)*
    specified NEC —*see* Disorder, disc,
      specified NEC
    thoracic (with)
      myelopathy M51.04
      neuritis, radiculitis or radiculopathy
        M51.14
      specified NEC M51.84
    thoracolumbar (with)
      myelopathy M51.05
      neuritis, radiculitis or radiculopathy
        M51.15
      specified NEC M51.85
  intestine K63.9
    functional K59.9
      psychogenic F45.8
      specified NEC K59.89
    organic K63.9
    protozoal A07.9
    specified NEC K63.89
  iris H21.9
    specified NEC —*see* H21.89
  iron metabolism or storage E83.10
  island (scrub typhus) A75.3
  itai-itai —*see* Poisoning, cadmium
  Jakob-Creutzfeldt —*see* Creutzfeldt-Jakob
    disease or syndrome
  jaw M27.9
    fibrocystic M27.49
    specified NEC M27.8
  jigger B88.1
  joint —*see also* Disorder, joint
    Charcot's —*see* Arthropathy, neuropathic
      (Charcot)
    degenerative —*see* Osteoarthritis
      multiple M15.9
      spine —*see* Spondylosis
  ▶facet joint *(see also* Spondylosis) M47.819
    hypertrophic —*see* Osteoarthritis
    sacroiliac M53.3
    specified NEC —*see* Disorder, joint,
      specified type NEC
    spine NEC —*see* Dorsopathy
    suppurative —*see* Arthritis, pyogenic or
      pyemic
  Jourdain's (acute gingivitis) K05.00
    nonplaque induced K05.01
    plaque induced K05.00
  Kaschin-Beck (endemic polyarthritis) M12.10
    ankle M12.17-●
    elbow M12.12-●
    foot joint M12.17-●
    hand joint M12.14-●
    hip M12.15-●
    knee M12.16-●
    multiple site M12.19
    shoulder M12.11-●
    vertebra M12.18
    wrist M12.13-●
  Katayama B65.2
  Kedani (scrub typhus) A75.3
  Keshan E59
  kidney (functional) (pelvis) N28.9
    chronic N18.9
      hypertensive —*see* Hypertension, kidney
      stage 1 N18.1
      stage 2 (mild) N18.2

▶ New   ⇒ Revised   ~~deleted~~ Deleted   ● Use Additional Character(s)

Disease, diseased (Continued)
moldy hay J67.0
Monge's T70.29
Morgagni-Adams-Stokes (syncope with heart block) I45.9
Morgagni's (syndrome) (hyperostosis frontalis interna) M85.2
Morton's (with metatarsalgia) —see Lesion, nerve, plantar
Morvan's G60.8
motor neuron (bulbar) (mixed type) (spinal) G12.20
   amyotrophic lateral sclerosis G12.21
   familial G12.24
   progressive bulbar palsy G12.22
   specified NEC G12.29
moyamoya I67.5
mu heavy chain disease C88.2
multicore G71.29
multiminicore G71.29
muscle —see also Disorder, muscle
   inflammatory —see Myositis
   ocular (external) —see Strabismus
musculoskeletal system, soft tissue —see also Disorder, soft tissue
   specified NEC —see Disorder, soft tissue, specified type NEC
mushroom workers' J67.5
mycotic B49
myelodysplastic, not classified (see also Syndrome, myelodysplasia) C94.6
myeloproliferative, not classified C94.6
   chronic D47.1
myocardium, myocardial —see also Degeneration, myocardial I51.5
   primary (idiopathic) I42.9
myoneural G70.9
Naegeli's D69.1
nails L60.9
   specified NEC L60.8
Nairobi (sheep virus) A93.8
nasal J34.9
nemaline body G71.21
nerve —see Disorder, nerve
nervous system G98.8
   autonomic G90.9
   central G96.9
      specified NEC G96.89
   congenital Q07.9
   parasympathetic G90.9
   specified NEC G98.8
   sympathetic G90.9
   vegetative G90.9
neuromuscular system G70.9
Newcastle B30.8
Nicolas (-Durand)-Favre (climatic bubo) A55
nipple N64.9
   Paget's C50.01-•
      female C50.01-•
      male C50.02-•
Nishimoto (-Takeuchi) I67.5
nonarthropod-borne NOS (viral) B34.9
   enterovirus NEC B34.1
nonautoimmune hemolytic D59.4
   drug-induced D59.2
Nonne-Milroy-Meige (chronic hereditary edema) Q82.0
nose J34.9
nucleus pulposus —see Disorder, disc
nutritional E63.9
oast-house-urine E72.19
ocular
   herpesviral B00.50
   zoster B02.30
obliterative vascular I77.1
Ohara's —see Tularemia
Opitz's (congestive splenomegaly) D73.2
Oppenheim-Urbach (necrobiosis lipoidica diabeticorum) —see E08-E13 with .620
optic nerve NEC —see Disorder, nerve, optic
   orbit —see Disorder, orbit

Disease, diseased (Continued)
organ
   dabbing (related) U07.0
   electronic cigarette (related) U07.0
   vaping (associated) (device) (product) (use) U07.0
Oriental liver fluke B66.1
Oriental lung fluke B66.4
Ormond's N13.5
Oropouche virus A93.0
Osler-Rendu (familial hemorrhagic telangiectasia) I78.0
osteofibrocystic E21.0
Otto's M24.7
outer ear —see Disorder, ear, external
ovary (noninflammatory) N83.9
   cystic N83.20-•
   inflammatory —see Salpingo-oophoritis
   polycystic E28.2
   specified NEC N83.8
Owren's (congenital) —see Defect, coagulation
pancreas K86.9
   cystic K86.2
   fibrocystic E84.9
   specified NEC K86.89
panvalvular I08.9
   specified NEC I08.8
parametrium (noninflammatory) N83.9
parasitic B89
   cerebral NEC B71.9 [G94]
   intestinal NOS B82.9
   mouth B37.0
   skin NOS B88.9
   specified type —see Infestation
   tongue B37.0
parathyroid (gland) E21.5
   specified NEC E21.4
Parkinson's G20
parodontal K05.6
Parrot's (syphilitic osteochondritis) A50.02
Parry's (exophthalmic goiter) —see Hyperthyroidism, with, goiter (diffuse)
Parson's (exophthalmic goiter) —see Hyperthyroidism, with, goiter (diffuse)
Paxton's (white piedra) B36.2
pearl-worker's —see Osteomyelitis, specified type NEC
Pellegrini-Stieda (calcification, knee joint) —see Bursitis, tibial collateral
pelvis, pelvic
   female NOS N94.9
      specified NEC N94.89
   gonococcal (acute) (chronic) A54.24
   inflammatory (female) N73.9
      acute N73.0
      chlamydial A56.11
      chronic N73.1
      specified NEC N73.8
      syphilitic (secondary) A51.42
         late A52.76
      tuberculous A18.17
   organ, female N94.9
   peritoneum, female NEC N94.89
penis N48.9
   inflammatory N48.29
      abscess N48.21
      cellulitis N48.22
   specified NEC N48.89
periapical tissues NOS K04.90
periodontal K05.6
   specified NEC K05.5
periosteum —see Disorder, bone, specified type NEC
peripheral
   arterial I73.9
   autonomic nervous system G90.9
   nerves —see Polyneuropathy
   vascular NOS I73.9

Disease, diseased (Continued)
peritoneum K66.9
   pelvic, female NEC N94.89
   specified NEC K66.8
persistent mucosal (middle ear) H66.20
   left H66.22
      with right H66.23
   right H66.21
      with left H66.23
Petit's —see Hernia, abdomen, specified site NEC
pharynx J39.2
   specified NEC J39.2
Phocas' —see Mastopathy, cystic
photochromogenic (acid-fast bacilli) (pulmonary) A31.0
   nonpulmonary A31.9
Pick's G31.01 [F02.80]
   with behavioral disturbance G31.01 [F02.81]
   brain G31.01 [F02.80]
      with behavioral disturbance G31.01 [F02.81]
   of pericardium (pericardial pseudocirrhosis of liver) I31.1
pigeon fancier's J67.2
pineal gland E34.8
pink —see Poisoning, mercury
Pinkus' (lichen nitidus) L44.1
pinworm B80
Piry virus A93.8
pituitary (gland) E23.7
pituitary-snuff-taker's J67.8
pleura (cavity) J94.9
   specified NEC J94.8
pneumatic drill (hammer) T75.21
Pollitzer's (hidradenitis suppurativa) L73.2
polycystic
   kidney or renal Q61.3
      adult type Q61.2
      childhood type NEC Q61.19
         collecting duct dilatation Q61.11
   liver or hepatic Q44.6
   lung or pulmonary J98.4
      congenital Q33.0
   ovary, ovaries E28.2
   spleen Q89.09
polyethylene T84.05-•
Pompe's (glycogenosis II) E74.02
Posadas-Wernicke B38.9
Potain's (pulmonary edema) —see Edema, lung
prepuce N47.8
   inflammatory N47.7
      balanoposthitis N47.6
Pringle's (tuberous sclerosis) Q85.1
prion, central nervous system A81.9
   specified NEC A81.89
prostate N42.9
   specified NEC N42.89
protozoal B64
   acanthamebiasis —see Acanthamebiasis
   African trypanosomiasis —see African trypanosomiasis
   babesiosis —(see also Babesiosis) B60.00
   Chagas disease —see Chagas disease
   intestine, intestinal A07.9
   leishmaniasis —see Leishmaniasis
   malaria —see Malaria
   naegleriasis B60.2
   pneumocystosis B59
   specified organism NEC B60.8
   toxoplasmosis —see Toxoplasmosis
pseudo-Hurler's E77.0
psychiatric F99
psychotic —see Psychosis
Puente's (simple glandular cheilitis) K13.0
puerperal —see also Puerperal O90.89

▶ New   ⇒ Revised   ~~deleted~~ Deleted   • Use Additional Character(s)

Disease, diseased *(Continued)*
  pulmonary —*see also* Disease, lung
    artery I28.9
    chronic obstructive J44.9
      with
        acute bronchitis J44.0
        exacerbation (acute) J44.1
        lower respiratory infection (acute)
          J44.0
      decompensated J44.1
        with
          exacerbation (acute) J44.1
    heart I27.9
    specified NEC I27.89
    hypertensive (vascular) —*see also*
      Hypertension, pulmonary I27.20
    primary (idiopathic) I27.0
    valve I37.9
    rheumatic I09.89
  pulp (dental) NOS K04.90
  pulseless M31.4
  Putnam's (subacute combined sclerosis with
    pernicious anemia) D51.0
  Pyle (-Cohn) (metaphyseal dysplasia) Q78.5
  ragpicker's or ragsorter's A22.1
  Raynaud's —*see* Raynaud's disease
  reactive airway —*see* Asthma
  Reclus' (cystic) —*see* Mastopathy, cystic
  rectum K62.9
    specified NEC K62.89
  Refsum's (heredopathia atactica
    polyneuritiformis) G60.1
  renal (functional) (pelvis) —*see also* Disease,
    kidney N28.9
    with
      edema —*see* Nephrosis
      glomerular lesion —*see*
        Glomerulonephritis
        with edema —*see* Nephrosis
      interstitial nephritis N12
    acute N28.9
    chronic —*see also* Disease, kidney, chronic
      N18.9
    cystic, congenital Q61.9
    diabetic —*see* E08-E13 with .22
    end-stage (failure) N18.6
      due to hypertension I12.0
    fibrocystic (congenital) Q61.8
    hypertensive —*see* Hypertension, kidney
    lupus M32.14
    phosphate-losing (tubular) N25.0
    polycystic (congenital) Q61.3
      adult type Q61.2
      childhood type NEC Q61.19
        collecting duct dilatation Q61.11
    rapidly progressive N01.9
    subacute N01.9
  Rendu-Osler-Weber (familial hemorrhagic
    telangiectasia) I78.0
  renovascular (arteriosclerotic) —*see*
    Hypertension, kidney
  respiratory (tract) J98.9
    acute or subacute NOS J06.9
      due to
        chemicals, gases, fumes or vapors
          (inhalation) J68.3
        external agent J70.9
          specified NEC J70.8
        radiation J70.0
        smoke inhalation J70.5
      noninfectious J39.8
    chronic NOS J98.9
      due to
        chemicals, gases, fumes or vapors
          J68.4
        external agent J70.9
          specified NEC J70.8
        radiation J70.1
      newborn P27.9
        specified NEC P27.8

Disease, diseased *(Continued)*
  respiratory (tract) *(Continued)*
    due to
      chemicals, gases, fumes or vapors J68.9
        acute or subacute NEC J68.3
        chronic J68.4
      external agent J70.9
        specified NEC J70.8
    newborn P28.9
      specified type NEC P28.89
    upper J39.9
      acute or subacute J06.9
      noninfectious NEC J39.8
      specified NEC J39.8
      streptococcal J06.9
  retina, retinal H35.9
    Batten's or Batten-Mayou E75.4 *[H36]*
    specified NEC H35.89
  rheumatoid —*see* Arthritis, rheumatoid
  rickettsial NOS A79.9
    specified type NEC A79.89
  Riga (-Fede) (cachectic aphthae) K14.0
  Riggs' (compound periodontitis) —*see*
    Periodontitis
  Ritter's L00
  Rivalta's (cervicofacial actinomycosis) A42.2
  rod body G71.21
  Robles' (onchocerciasis) B73.01
  Roger's (congenital interventricular septal
    defect) Q21.0
  Rosenthal's (factor XI deficiency) D68.1
  Ross River B33.1
  Rossbach's (hyperchlorhydria) K31.89
    psychogenic F45.8
  Rotes Quérol —*see* Hyperostosis, ankylosing
  Roth (-Bernhardt) —*see* Mononeuropathy,
    lower limb, meralgia paresthetica
  Runeberg's (progressive pernicious anemia)
    D51.0
  sacroiliac NEC M53.3
  salivary gland or duct K11.9
    inclusion B25.9
    specified NEC K11.8
    virus B25.9
  sandworm B76.9
  Schimmelbusch's —*see* Mastopathy, cystic
  Schmorl's —*see* Schmorl's disease or nodes
  Schönlein (-Henoch) (purpura rheumatica)
    D69.0
  Schottmüller's —*see* Fever, paratyphoid
  Schultz's (agranulocytosis) —*see*
    Agranulocytosis
  Schwalbe-Ziehen-Oppenheim G24.1
  Schwartz-Jampel G71.13
  sclera H15.9
    specified NEC H15.89
  scrofulous (tuberculous) A18.2
  scrotum N50.9
  sebaceous glands L73.9
  semilunar cartilage, cystic —*see also*
    Derangement, knee, meniscus, cystic
  seminal vesicle N50.9
  serum NEC —*see also* Reaction, serum T80.69
  sexually transmitted A64
    anogenital
      herpesviral infection —*see* Herpes,
        anogenital
      warts A63.0
    chancroid A57
    chlamydial infection —*see* Chlamydia
    gonorrhea —*see* Gonorrhea
    granuloma inguinale A58
    specified organism NEC A63.8
    syphilis —*see* Syphilis
    trichomoniasis —*see* Trichomoniasis
  Sézary C84.1-●
  shimamushi (scrub typhus) A75.3
  shipyard B30.0
  sickle-cell D57.1
    with
      acute chest syndrome D57.01

Disease, diseased *(Continued)*
  sickle-cell *(Continued)*
    cerebral vascular involvement D57.03
    crisis (painful) D57.00
      with complication specified NEC
        D57.09
    splenic sequestration D57.02
    vasoocclusive pain D57.00
  elliptocytosis D57.8-●
  Hb-C D57.20
    with
      acute chest syndrome D57.211
      cerebral vascular involvement D57.213
      crisis (painful) D57.219
        with specified complication NEC
          D57.218
      splenic sequestration D57.212
      vasoocclusive pain D57.219
    without crisis D57.20
  Hb-SD D57.80
    with
      acute chest syndrome D57.811
      cerebral vascular involvement D57.813
      crisis (painful) D57.819
        with complication specified NEC
          D57.818
      splenic sequestration D57.812
      vasoocclusive pain D57.819
    without crisis D57.80
  Hb-SE D57.80
    with
      acute chest syndrome D57.811
      cerebral vascular involvement D57.813
      crisis (painful) D57.819
        with complication specified NEC
          D57.818
      splenic sequestration D57.812
      vasoocclusive pain D57.819
    without crisis D57.80
  specified NEC D57.80
    with
      acute chest syndrome D57.811
      cerebral vascular involvement
        D57.813
      crisis (painful) D57.819
        with complication specified NEC
          D57.818
      splenic sequestration D57.812
      vasoocclusive pain D57.819
    without crisis D57.80
  spherocytosis D57.80
    with
      acute chest syndrome D57.811
      cerebral vascular involvement D57.813
      crisis (painful) D57.819
        with complication specified NEC
          D57.818
      splenic sequestration D57.812
      vasoocclusive pain D57.819
    without crisis D57.80
  thalassemia D57.40
    with
      acute chest syndrome D57.411
      cerebral vascular involvement D57.413
      crisis (painful) D57.419
        with specified complication NEC
          D57.418
      splenic sequestration D57.412
      vasoocclusive pain D57.419
    beta plus D57.44
      with
        acute chest syndrome D57.451
        cerebral vascular involvement
          D57.453
        crisis D57.459
          with specified complication NEC
            D57.458
        splenic sequestration D57.452
        vasoocclusive pain D57.459
      without crisis D57.44

Disease, diseased *(Continued)*
  sickle-cell *(Continued)*
    thalassemia *(Continued)*
      beta zero D57.42
        with
          acute chest syndrome D57.431
          cerebral vascular involvement
            D57.433
          crisis D57.439
            with specified complication NEC
              D57.438
          splenic sequestration D57.432
          vasoocclusive pain D57.439
        without crisis D57.42
  silo-filler's J68.8
    bronchitis J68.0
    pneumonitis J68.0
    pulmonary edema J68.1
  simian B B00.4
  Simons' (progressive lipodystrophy) E88.1
  sin nombre virus B33.4
  sinus —see Sinusitis
  Sirkari's B55.0
  sixth B08.20
    due to human herpesvirus 6 B08.21
    due to human herpesvirus 7 B08.22
  skin L98.9
    due to metabolic disorder NEC
      E88.9 [L99]
    specified NEC L98.8
  slim (HIV) B20
  small vessel I73.9
  Sneddon-Wilkinson (subcorneal pustular
    dermatosis) L13.1
  South African creeping B88.0
  spinal (cord) G95.9
    congenital Q06.9
    specified NEC G95.89
  spine —see also Spondylopathy
    joint —see Dorsopathy
    tuberculous A18.01
  spinocerebellar (hereditary) G11.9
    specified NEC G11.8
  spleen D73.9
    amyloid E85.4 [D77]
    organic D73.9
    polycystic Q89.09
    postinfectional D73.89
  sponge-diver's —see Toxicity, venom, marine
    animal, sea anemone
  Startle Q89.8
  Steinert's G71.11
  Sticker's (erythema infectiosum) B08.3
  Stieda's (calcification, knee joint) —see
    Bursitis, tibial collateral
  Stokes' (exophthalmic goiter) —see
    Hyperthyroidism, with, goiter
    (diffuse)
  Stokes-Adams (syncope with heart block)
    I45.9
  stomach K31.9
    functional, psychogenic F45.8
    specified NEC K31.89
  stonemason's J62.8
  storage
    glycogen —see Disease, glycogen storage
    mucopolysaccharide —see
      Mucopolysaccharidosis
  striatopallidal system NEC G25.89
  Stuart-Prower (congenital factor X deficiency)
    D68.2
  Stuart's (congenital factor X deficiency)
    D68.2
  subcutaneous tissue —see Disease, skin
  supporting structures of teeth K08.9
    specified NEC K08.89
  suprarenal (capsule) (gland) E27.9
    hyperfunction E27.0
    specified NEC E27.8
  sweat glands L74.9
    specified NEC L74.8

Disease, diseased *(Continued)*
  Sweeley-Klionsky E75.21
  Swift (-Feer) —see Poisoning, mercury
  swimming-pool granuloma A31.1
  Sylvest's (epidemic pleurodynia) B33.0
  sympathetic nervous system G90.9
  synovium —see Disorder, synovium
  syphilitic —see Syphilis
  systemic tissue mast cell D47.02
  tanapox (virus) B08.71
  Tangier E78.6
  Tarral-Besnier (pityriasis rubra pilaris) L44.0
  Tauri's E74.09
  tear duct —see Disorder, lacrimal system
  tendon, tendinous —see also Disorder, tendon
    nodular —see Trigger finger
  terminal vessel I73.9
  testis N50.9
  thalassemia Hb-S —see Disease, sickle-cell,
    thalassemia
  Thaysen-Gee (nontropical sprue) K90.0
  Thomsen G71.12
  throat J39.2
    septic J02.0
  thromboembolic —see Embolism
  thymus (gland) E32.9
    specified NEC E32.8
  thyroid (gland) E07.9
    heart —see also Hyperthyroidism
      E05.90 [I43]
      with thyroid storm E05.91 [I43]
    specified NEC E07.8
  Tietze's M94.0
  tongue K14.9
    specified NEC K14.89
  tonsils, tonsillar (and adenoids) J35.9
  tooth, teeth K08.9
    hard tissues K03.9
      specified NEC K03.89
    pulp NEC K04.99
    specified NEC K08.89
  Tourette's F95.2
  trachea NEC J39.8
  tricuspid I07.9
    nonrheumatic I36.9
  triglyceride-storage E75.5
  trophoblastic —see Mole, hydatidiform
  tsutsugamushi A75.3
  tube (fallopian) (noninflammatory) N83.9
    inflammatory —see Salpingitis
    specified NEC N83.8
    tuberculous NEC —see Tuberculosis
  tubo-ovarian (noninflammatory) N83.9
    inflammatory —see Salpingo-oophoritis
    specified NEC N83.8
  tubotympanic, chronic —see Otitis, media,
    suppurative, chronic, tubotympanic
  tubulo-interstitial N15.9
    specified NEC N15.8
  tympanum —see Disorder, tympanic
    membrane
  Uhl's Q24.8
  Underwood's (sclerema neonatorum) P83.0
  Unverricht (-Lundborg) —see Epilepsy,
    generalized, idiopathic
  Urbach-Oppenheim (necrobiosis lipoidica
    diabeticorum) —see E08-E13 with .620
  ureter N28.9
    in (due to)
      schistosomiasis (bilharziasis)
        B65.0 [N29]
  urethra N36.9
    specified NEC N36.8
  urinary (tract) N39.9
    bladder N32.9
      specified NEC N32.89
    specified NEC N39.8
  uterus (noninflammatory) N85.9
    infective —see Endometritis
    inflammatory —see Endometritis
    specified NEC N85.8

Disease, diseased *(Continued)*
  uveal tract (anterior) H21.9
    posterior H31.9
  vagabond's B85.1
  vagina, vaginal (noninflammatory) N89.9
    inflammatory NEC N76.89
    specified NEC N89.8
  valve, valvular I38
    multiple I08.9
      specified NEC I08.8
  van Creveld-von Gierke (glycogenosis I)
    E74.01
  vas deferens N50.9
  vascular I99.9
    arteriosclerotic —see Arteriosclerosis
    ciliary body NEC —see Disorder, iris,
      vascular
    hypertensive —see Hypertension
    iris NEC —see Disorder, iris, vascular
    obliterative I77.1
    peripheral I73.9
    occlusive I99.8
    peripheral (occlusive) I73.9
      in diabetes mellitus —see E08-E13 with .51
  vasomotor I73.9
  vasospastic I73.9
  vein I87.9
  venereal —see also Disease, sexually
    transmitted A64
    chlamydial NEC A56.8
      anus A56.3
      genitourinary NOS A56.2
      pharynx A56.4
      rectum A56.3
    fifth A55
    sixth A55
    specified nature or type NEC A63.8
  vertebra, vertebral —see also Spondylopathy
    disc —see Disorder, disc
  vibration —see Vibration, adverse effects
  viral, virus —see also Disease, by type of virus
    B34.9
    arbovirus NOS A94
    arthropod-borne NOS A94
    congenital P35.9
      specified NEC P35.8
    Hanta (with renal manifestations)
      (Dobrava) (Puumala) (Seoul) A98.5
      with pulmonary manifestations (Andes)
        (Bayou) (Bermejo) (Black Creek
        Canal) (Choclo) (Juquitiba) (Laguna
        negra) (Lechiguanas) (New York)
        (Oran) (Sin nombre) B33.4
    Hantaan (Korean hemorrhagic fever) A98.5
    human immunodeficiency (HIV) B20
    Kunjin A83.4
    nonarthropod-borne NOS B34.9
    Powassan A84.81
    Rocio (encephalitis) A83.6
    Sin nombre (Hantavirus) (cardio)-
      pulmonary syndrome B33.4
    Tahyna B33.8
    vesicular stomatitis A93.8
  vitreous H43.9
    specified NEC H43.89
  vocal cord J38.3
  Volkmann's, acquired T79.6
  von Eulenburg's (congenital paramyotonia)
    G71.19
  von Gierke's (glycogenosis I) E74.01
  von Graefe's —see Strabismus, paralytic,
    ophthalmoplegia, progressive
  von Willebrand (-Jürgens) (angiohemophilia)
    D68.0
  Vrolik's (osteogenesis imperfecta) Q78.0
  vulva (noninflammatory) N90.9
    inflammatory NEC N76.89
    specified NEC N90.89
  Wallgren's (obstruction of splenic vein with
    collateral circulation) I87.8
  Wassilieff's (leptospiral jaundice) A27.0

▶ New   ⇒ Revised   ~~deleted~~ Deleted   ● Use Additional Character(s)

Disease, diseased (Continued)
wasting NEC R64
➡due to malnutrition E43
▶with marasmus E41
Waterhouse-Friderichsen A39.1
Wegner's (syphilitic osteochondritis) A50.02
Weil's (leptospiral jaundice of lung) A27.0
Weir Mitchell's (erythromelalgia) I73.81
Werdnig-Hoffmann G12.0
Wermer's E31.21
Werner-His (trench fever) A79.0
Werner-Schultz (neutropenic splenomegaly) D73.81
Wernicke-Posadas B38.9
whipworm B79
white blood cells D72.9
specified NEC D72.89
white matter R90.82
white-spot, meaning lichen sclerosus et atrophicus L90.0
penis N48.0
vulva N90.4
Wilkie's K55.1
Wilkinson-Sneddon (subcorneal pustular dermatosis) L13.1
Willis' —see Diabetes
Wilson's (hepatolenticular degeneration) E83.01
woolsorter's A22.1
yaba monkey tumor B08.72
yaba pox (virus) B08.72
Zika virus A92.5
zoonotic, bacterial A28.9
congenital P35.4
specified type NEC A28.8
Disfigurement (due to scar) L90.5
Disgerminoma —see Dysgerminoma
DISH (diffuse idiopathic skeletal hyperostosis) —see Hyperostosis, ankylosing
Disinsertion, retina —see Detachment, retina
Dislocatable hip, congenital Q65.6
Dislocation (articular)
with fracture —see Fracture
acromioclavicular (joint) S43.10-●
with displacement
100%-200% S43.12-●
more than 200% S43.13-●
inferior S43.14-●
posterior S43.15-●
ankle S93.0-●
astragalus —see Dislocation, ankle
atlantoaxial S13.121
atlantooccipital S13.111
atloidooccipital S13.111
breast bone S23.29
capsule, joint code by site under Dislocation
carpal (bone) —see Dislocation, wrist
carpometacarpal (joint) NEC S63.05-●
thumb S63.04-●
cartilage (joint) - code by site under Dislocation
cervical spine (vertebra) —see Dislocation, vertebra, cervical
chronic —see Dislocation, recurrent
clavicle —see Dislocation, acromioclavicular joint
coccyx S33.2
congenital NEC Q68.8
coracoid —see Dislocation, shoulder
costal cartilage S23.29
costochondral S23.29
cricoarytenoid articulation S13.29
cricothyroid articulation S13.29
dorsal vertebra —see Dislocation, vertebra, thoracic
ear ossicle —see Discontinuity, ossicles, ear
elbow S53.10-●
congenital Q68.8
pathological —see Dislocation, pathological NEC, elbow
radial head alone —see Dislocation, radial head

Dislocation (Continued)
elbow (Continued)
recurrent —see Dislocation, recurrent, elbow
traumatic S53.10-●
anterior S53.11-●
lateral S53.14-●
medial S53.13-●
posterior S53.12-●
specified type NEC S53.19-●
eye, nontraumatic —see Luxation, globe
eyeball, nontraumatic —see Luxation, globe
femur
distal end —see Dislocation, knee
proximal end —see Dislocation, hip
fibula
distal end —see Dislocation, ankle
proximal end —see Dislocation, knee
finger S63.25-●
index S63.25-●
interphalangeal S63.27-●
distal S63.29-●
index S63.29-●
little S63.29-●
middle S63.29-●
ring S63.29-●
index S63.27-●
little S63.27-●
middle S63.27-●
proximal S63.28-●
index S63.28-●
little S63.28-●
middle S63.28-●
ring S63.28-●
ring S63.27-●
little S63.25-●
metacarpophalangeal S63.26-●
index S63.26-●
little S63.26-●
middle S63.26-●
ring S63.26-●
middle S63.25-●
recurrent —see Dislocation, recurrent, finger
ring S63.25-●
thumb —see Dislocation, thumb
foot S93.30-●
recurrent —see Dislocation, recurrent, foot
specified site NEC S93.33-●
tarsal joint S93.31-●
tarsometatarsal joint S93.32-●
toe —see Dislocation, toe
fracture —see Fracture
glenohumeral (joint) —see Dislocation, shoulder
glenoid —see Dislocation, shoulder
habitual —see Dislocation, recurrent
hip S73.00-●
anterior S73.03-●
obturator S73.02-●
central S73.04-●
congenital (total) Q65.2
bilateral Q65.1
partial Q65.5
bilateral Q65.4
unilateral Q65.3-●
unilateral Q65.0-●
developmental M24.85-●
pathological —see Dislocation, pathological NEC, hip
posterior S73.01-●
recurrent —see Dislocation, recurrent, hip
humerus, proximal end —see Dislocation, shoulder
incomplete —see Subluxation, by site
incus —see Discontinuity, ossicles, ear
infracoracoid —see Dislocation, shoulder

Dislocation (Continued)
innominate (pubic junction) (sacral junction) S33.39
acetabulum —see Dislocation, hip
interphalangeal (joint(s))
finger S63.279
distal S63.29-●
index S63.29-●
little S63.29-●
middle S63.29-●
ring S63.29-●
index S63.27-●
little S63.27-●
middle S63.27-●
proximal S63.28-●
index S63.28-●
little S63.28-●
middle S63.28-●
ring S63.28-●
ring S63.27-●
foot or toe —see Dislocation, toe
thumb S63.12-●
jaw (cartilage) (meniscus) S03.0-●
joint prosthesis —see Complications, joint prosthesis, mechanical, displacement, by site
knee S83.106
cap —see Dislocation, patella
congenital Q68.2
old M23.8X-●
patella —see Dislocation, patella
pathological —see Dislocation, pathological NEC, knee
proximal tibia
anteriorly S83.11-●
laterally S83.14-●
medially S83.13-●
posteriorly S83.12-●
recurrent —see also Derangement, knee, specified NEC
specified type NEC S83.19-●
lacrimal gland H04.16-●
lens (complete) H27.10-●
anterior H27.12-●
congenital Q12.1
ocular implant —see Complications, intraocular lens
partial H27.11-●
posterior H27.13-●
traumatic S05.8X-●
ligament code by site under Dislocation
lumbar (vertebra) —see Dislocation, vertebra, lumbar
lumbosacral (vertebra) —see also Dislocation, vertebra, lumbar
congenital Q76.49
mandible S03.0-●
meniscus (knee) —see Tear, meniscus
other sites code by site under Dislocation
metacarpal (bone)
distal end —see Dislocation, finger
proximal end S63.06-●
metacarpophalangeal (joint)
finger S63.26-●
index S63.26-●
little S63.26-●
middle S63.26-●
ring S63.26-●
thumb S63.11-●
metatarsal (bone) —see Dislocation, foot
metatarsophalangeal (joint(s)) —see Dislocation, toe
midcarpal (joint) S63.03-●
midtarsal (joint) —see Dislocation, foot
neck S13.20
specified site NEC S13.29
vertebra —see Dislocation, vertebra, cervical
nose (septal cartilage) S03.1
occipitoatloid S13.111

Dislocation *(Continued)*
  old —*see* Derangement, joint, specified type
    NEC
  ossicles, ear —*see* Discontinuity, ossicles, ear
  partial —*see* Subluxation, by site
  patella S83.006
    congenital Q74.1
    lateral S83.01-●
    recurrent (nontraumatic) M22.0-●
      incomplete M22.1-●
    specified type NEC S83.09-●
  pathological NEC M24.30
    ankle M24.37-●
    elbow M24.32-●
    foot joint M24.37-●
    hand joint M24.34-●
    hip M24.35-●
    knee M24.36-●
    lumbosacral joint —*see* subcategory M53.2
    pelvic region —*see* Dislocation,
      pathological, hip
    sacroiliac —*see* subcategory M53.2
    shoulder M24.31-●
    specified site NEC M24.39
    wrist M24.33-●
  pelvis NEC S33.30
    specified NEC S33.39
  phalanx
    finger or hand —*see* Dislocation, finger
    foot or toe —*see* Dislocation, toe
  prosthesis, internal —*see* Complications,
    prosthetic device, by site, mechanical
  radial head S53.006
    anterior S53.01-●
    posterior S53.02-●
    specified type NEC S53.09-●
  radiocarpal (joint) S63.02-●
  radiohumeral (joint) —*see* Dislocation, radial
    head
  radioulnar (joint)
    distal S63.01-●
    proximal —*see* Dislocation, elbow
  radius
    distal end —*see* Dislocation, wrist
    proximal end —*see* Dislocation, radial head
  recurrent M24.40
    ankle M24.47-●
    elbow M24.42-●
    finger M24.44-●
    foot joint M24.47-●
    hand joint M24.44-●
    hip M24.45-●
    knee M24.46-●
      patella —*see* Dislocation, patella,
        recurrent
    patella —*see* Dislocation, patella,
      recurrent
    sacroiliac —*see* subcategory M53.2
    shoulder M24.41-●
    specified site NEC M24.49
    toe M24.47-●
    vertebra —*see also* subcategory M43.5
      atlantoaxial M43.4
        with myelopathy M43.3
    wrist M24.43-●
  rib (cartilage) S23.29
  sacrococcygeal S33.2
  sacroiliac (joint) (ligament) S33.2
    congenital Q74.2
    recurrent —*see* subcategory M53.2
  sacrum S33.2
  scaphoid (bone) (hand) (wrist) —*see*
    Dislocation, wrist
    foot —*see* Dislocation, foot
  scapula —*see* Dislocation, shoulder, girdle,
    scapula
  semilunar cartilage, knee —*see* Tear,
    meniscus
  septal cartilage (nose) S03.1
  septum (nasal) (old) J34.2
  sesamoid bone code by site under Dislocation

Dislocation *(Continued)*
  shoulder (blade) (ligament) (joint) (traumatic)
    S43.006
    acromioclavicular —*see* Dislocation,
      acromioclavicular
    chronic —*see* Dislocation, recurrent,
      shoulder
    congenital Q68.8
    girdle S43.30-●
      scapula S43.31-●
      specified site NEC S43.39-●
    humerus S43.00-●
      anterior S43.01-●
      inferior S43.03-●
      posterior S43.02-●
    pathological —*see* Dislocation, pathological
      NEC, shoulder
    recurrent —*see* Dislocation, recurrent,
      shoulder
    specified type NEC S43.08-●
  spine
    cervical —*see* Dislocation, vertebra, cervical
    congenital Q76.49
    due to birth trauma P11.5
    lumbar —*see* Dislocation, vertebra, lumbar
    thoracic —*see* Dislocation, vertebra,
      thoracic
  spontaneous —*see* Dislocation, pathological
  sternoclavicular (joint) S43.206
    anterior S43.21-●
    posterior S43.22-●
  sternum S23.29
  subglenoid —*see* Dislocation, shoulder
  symphysis pubis S33.4
  talus —*see* Dislocation, ankle
  tarsal (bone(s)) (joint(s)) —*see* Dislocation,
    foot
  tarsometatarsal (joint(s)) —*see* Dislocation,
    foot
  temporomandibular (joint) S03.0-●
  thigh, proximal end —*see* Dislocation, hip
  thorax S23.20
    specified site NEC S23.29
    vertebra —*see* Dislocation, vertebra
  thumb S63.10-●
    interphalangeal joint —*see* Dislocation,
      interphalangeal (joint), thumb
    metacarpophalangeal joint —*see*
      Dislocation, metacarpophalangeal
      (joint), thumb
  thyroid cartilage S13.29
  tibia
    distal end —*see* Dislocation, ankle
    proximal end —*see* Dislocation, knee
  tibiofibular (joint)
    distal —*see* Dislocation, ankle
    superior —*see* Dislocation, knee
  toe(s) S93.106
    great S93.10-●
      interphalangeal joint S93.11-●
      metatarsophalangeal joint S93.12-●
    interphalangeal joint S93.119
    lesser S93.106
      interphalangeal joint S93.11-●
      metatarsophalangeal joint S93.12-●
    metatarsophalangeal joint S93.12-●
  tooth S03.2
  trachea S23.29
  ulna
    distal end S63.07-●
    proximal end —*see* Dislocation, elbow
  ulnohumeral (joint) —*see* Dislocation, elbow
  vertebra (articular process) (body)
    (traumatic)
    cervical S13.101
      atlantoaxial joint S13.121
      atlantooccipital joint S13.111
      atloidooccipital joint S13.111
      joint between
        C0 and C1 S13.111
        C1 and C2 S13.121

Dislocation *(Continued)*
  vertebra *(Continued)*
    cervical *(Continued)*
      joint between *(Continued)*
        C2 and C3 S13.131
        C3 and C4 S13.141
        C4 and C5 S13.151
        C5 and C6 S13.161
        C6 and C7 S13.171
        C7 and T1 S13.181
      occipitoatloid joint S13.111
    congenital Q76.49
    lumbar S33.101
      joint between
        L1 and L2 S33.111
        L2 and L3 S33.121
        L3 and L4 S33.131
        L4 and L5 S33.141
    nontraumatic —*see* Displacement,
      intervertebral disc
    partial —*see* Subluxation, by site
    recurrent NEC —*see* subcategory
      M43.5
    thoracic S23.101
      joint between
        T1 and T2 S23.111
        T2 and T3 S23.121
        T3 and T4 S23.123
        T4 and T5 S23.131
        T5 and T6 S23.133
        T6 and T7 S23.141
        T7 and T8 S23.143
        T8 and T9 S23.151
        T9 and T10 S23.153
        T10 and T11 S23.161
        T11 and T12 S23.163
        T12 and L1 S23.171
  wrist (carpal bone) S63.006
    carpometacarpal joint —*see* Dislocation,
      carpometacarpal (joint)
    distal radioulnar joint —*see* Dislocation,
      radioulnar (joint), distal
    metacarpal bone, proximal —*see*
      Dislocation, metacarpal (bone),
      proximal end
    midcarpal —*see* Dislocation, midcarpal
      (joint)
    radiocarpal joint —*see* Dislocation,
      radiocarpal (joint)
    recurrent —*see* Dislocation, recurrent,
      wrist
    specified site NEC S63.09-●
    ulna —*see* Dislocation, ulna, distal end
  xiphoid cartilage S23.29
Disorder (of) —*see also* Disease
  acantholytic L11.9
    specified NEC L11.8
  acute
    psychotic —*see* Psychosis, acute
    stress F43.0
  adjustment (grief) F43.20
    with
      anxiety F43.22
        with depressed mood F43.23
      conduct disturbance F43.24
        with emotional disturbance
          F43.25
      depressed mood F43.21
        with anxiety F43.23
      other specified symptom F43.29
  adrenal (capsule) (gland) (medullary)
    E27.9
    specified NEC E27.8
  adrenogenital E25.9
    drug-induced E25.8
    iatrogenic E25.8
    idiopathic E25.8
  adult personality (and behavior) F69
    specified NEC F68.8
  affective (mood) —*see* Disorder, mood
  aggressive, unsocialized F91.1

▶ New   ⇒ Revised   ~~deleted~~ Deleted   ● Use Additional Character(s)

Disorder *(Continued)*
  alcohol-related F10.99
    with
      amnestic disorder, persisting
        F10.96
      anxiety disorder F10.980
      dementia, persisting F10.97
      intoxication F10.929
        with delirium F10.921
        uncomplicated F10.920
      mood disorder F10.94
      other specified F10.988
      psychotic disorder F10.959
        with
          delusions F10.950
          hallucinations F10.951
      sexual dysfunction F10.981
      sleep disorder F10.982
  alcohol use
    mild F10.10
      with
        alcohol-induced
          anxiety disorder F10.180
          bipolar and related disorder
            F10.14
          depressive disorder F10.14
          psychotic disorder F10.159
          sexual dysfunction F10.181
          sleep disorder F10.182
        alcohol intoxication F10.129
          delirium F10.121
      in remission (early) (sustained)
        F10.11
    moderate or severe F10.20
      with
        alcohol-induced
          anxiety disorder F10.280
          bipolar and related disorder
            F10.24
          depressive disorder F10.24
          major neurocognitive disorder,
            amnestic-confabulatory type
            F10.26
          major neurocognitive disorder,
            nonamnestic-confabulatory
            type F10.27
          mild neurocognitive disorder
            F10.288
          psychotic disorder F10.259
          sexual dysfunction F10.281
          sleep disorder F10.282
        alcohol intoxication F10.229
          delirium F10.221
      in remission (early) (sustained)
        F10.21
  allergic —*see* Allergy
  alveolar NEC J84.09
  amino-acid
    cystathioninuria E72.19
    cystinosis E72.04
    cystinuria E72.01
    glycinuria E72.09
    homocystinuria E72.11
    metabolism —*see* Disturbance,
      metabolism, amino-acid
      specified NEC E72.89
    neonatal, transitory P74.8
    renal transport NEC E72.09
    transport NEC E72.09
  amnesic, amnestic
    alcohol-induced F10.96
      with dependence F10.26
    due to (secondary to) general medical
      condition F04
    psychoactive NEC-induced F19.96
      with
        abuse F19.16
        dependence F19.26
    sedative, hypnotic or anxiolytic-●
      induced F13.96
      with dependence F13.26

Disorder *(Continued)*
  amphetamine-type substance use
    mild F15.10
      in remission (early) (sustained) F15.11
    moderate F15.20
      in remission (early) (sustained) F15.21
    severe F15.20
      in remission (early) (sustained) F15.21
  amphetamine (or other stimulant) use
    mild
      with
        amphetamine (or other stimulant)
          -induced
          anxiety disorder F15.180
          bipolar and related disorder F15.180
          depressive disorder F15.14
          obsessive-compulsive and related
            disorder F15.188
          psychotic disorder F15.159
          sexual dysfunction F15.181
        amphetamine, cocaine, or other
          stimulant intoxication
          with perceptual disturbances
            F15.122
          without perceptual disturbances
            F15.129
        intoxication delirium F15.121
    moderate or severe
      with
        amphetamine (or other stimulant)
          -induced
          anxiety disorder F15.280
          obsessive-compulsive and related
            disorder F15.288
          sexual dysfunction F15.281
          bipolar and related disorder F15.24
          depressive disorder F15.24
          psychotic disorder F15.259
        amphetamine, cocaine, or other
          stimulant intoxication
          with perceptual disturbances
            F15.222
          without perceptual disturbances
            F15.229
        intoxication delirium F15.221
▶ anaerobic glycolysis with anemia D55.29
  anxiety F41.9
    due to (secondary to)
      alcohol F10.980
        in
          abuse F10.180
          dependence F10.280
      amphetamine F15.980
        in
          abuse F15.180
          dependence F15.280
      anxiolytic F13.980
        in
          abuse F13.180
          dependence F13.280
      caffeine F15.980
        in
          abuse F15.180
          dependence F15.280
      cannabis F12.980
        in
          abuse F12.180
          dependence F12.280
      cocaine F14.980
        in
          abuse F14.180
          dependence F14.180
      general medical condition F06.4
      hallucinogen F16.980
        in
          abuse F16.180
          dependence F16.280
      hypnotic F13.980
        in
          abuse F13.180
          dependence F13.280

Disorder *(Continued)*
  anxiety *(Continued)*
    due to *(Continued)*
      inhalant F18.980
        in
          abuse F18.180
          dependence F18.280
      phencyclidine F16.980
        in
          abuse F16.180
          dependence F16.280
      psychoactive substance NEC
        F19.980
        in
          abuse F19.180
          dependence F19.280
      sedative F13.980
        in
          abuse F13.180
          dependence F13.280
      volatile solvents F18.980
        in
          abuse F18.180
          dependence F18.280
    generalized F41.1
    illness F45.21
    mixed
      with depression (mild) F41.8
      specified NEC F41.3
    organic F06.4
    phobic F40.9
      of childhood F40.8
    specified NEC F41.8
  aortic valve —*see* Endocarditis, aortic
  aromatic amino-acid metabolism E70.9
    specified NEC E70.89
  arteriole NEC I77.89
  artery NEC I77.89
  articulation —*see* Disorder, joint
  attachment (childhood)
    disinhibited F94.2
    reactive F94.1
  attention-deficit hyperactivity (adolescent)
    (adult) (child) F98.8
    combined
      presentation F90.2
      type F90.2
    hyperactive
      impulsive presentation F90.1
      type F90.1
    inattentive
      presentation F90.0
      type F90.0
    specified type NEC F90.8
  attention-deficit without hyperactivity
    (adolescent) (adult) (child) F90.0
  auditory processing (central) H93.25
  autism spectrum F84.0
  autistic F84.0
  autoimmune D89.89
  autonomic nervous system G90.9
    specified NEC G90.8
  avoidant
    child or adolescent F40.10
    restrictive food intake F50.82
  balance
    acid-base E87.8
      mixed E87.4
    electrolyte E87.8
    fluid NEC E87.8
  behavioral (disruptive) —*see* Disorder,
    conduct
  beta-amino-acid metabolism E72.89
  bile acid and cholesterol metabolism
    E78.70
    Barth syndrome E78.71
    other specified E78.79
    Smith-Lemli-Opitz syndrome
      E78.72
  bilirubin excretion E80.6
  binge eating F50.81

Disorder (Continued)
  binocular
    movement H51.9
      convergence
        excess H51.12
        insufficiency H51.11
      internuclear ophthalmoplegia —see
        Ophthalmoplegia, internuclear
      palsy of conjugate gaze H51.0
      specified type NEC H51.8
    vision NEC —see Disorder, vision, binocular
  bipolar (I) (type 1) F31.9
    and related due to a known physiological
      condition
      with
        manic features F06.33
        manic- or hypomanic-like episodes
          F06.33
        mixed features F06.34
    current (or most recent) episode
      depressed F31.9
        with psychotic features F31.5
        without psychotic features
          F31.30
          mild F31.31
          moderate F31.32
          severe (without psychotic features)
            F31.4
            with psychotic features
              F31.5
      hypomanic F31.0
      manic F31.9
        with psychotic features F31.2
        without psychotic features
          F31.10
          mild F31.11
          moderate F31.12
          severe (without psychotic features)
            F31.13
            with psychotic features
              F31.2
      mixed F31.60
        mild F31.61
        moderate F31.62
        severe (without psychotic features)
          F31.63
          with psychotic features F31.64
        severe depression (without psychotic
          features) F31.4
          with psychotic features F31.5
    II (type 2) F31.81
    in remission (currently) F31.70
      in full remission
        most recent episode
          depressed F31.76
          hypomanic F31.72
          manic F31.74
          mixed F31.78
      in partial remission
        most recent episode
          depressed F31.75
          hypomanic F31.71
          manic F31.73
          mixed F31.77
    organic F06.30
    single manic episode F30.9
      mild F30.11
      moderate F30.12
      hhsevere (without psychotic symptoms)
        F30.13
        with psychotic symptoms F30.2
    specified NEC F31.89
  bladder N32.9
    functional NEC N31.9
    in schistosomiasis B65.0 [N33]
    specified NEC N32.89
  bleeding D68.9
  blood D75.9
    in congenital early syphilis A50.09
      [D77]
  body dysmorphic F45.22

Disorder (Continued)
  bone M89.9
    continuity M84.9
      specified type NEC M84.80
        ankle M84.87-●
        fibula M84.86-●
        foot M84.87-●
        hand M84.84-●
        humerus M84.82-●
        neck M84.88
        pelvis M84.859
        radius M84.83-●
        rib M84.88
        shoulder M84.81-●
        skull M84.88
        thigh M84.85-●
        tibia M84.86-●
        ulna M84.83-●
        vertebra M84.88
    density and structure M85.9
      cyst —see also Cyst, bone, specified type
        NEC
        aneurysmal —see Cyst, bone,
          aneurysmal
        solitary —see Cyst, bone, solitary
      diffuse idiopathic skeletal
        hyperostosis —see Hyperostosis,
          ankylosing
      fibrous dysplasia (monostotic) —see
        Dysplasia, fibrous, bone
      fluorosis —see Fluorosis, skeletal
      hyperostosis of skull M85.2
      osteitis condensans —see Osteitis,
        condensans
      specified type NEC M85.8-●
        ankle M85.87-●
        foot M85.87-●
        forearm M85.83-●
        hand M85.84-●
        lower leg M85.86-●
        multiple sites M85.89
        neck M85.88
        rib M85.88
        shoulder M85.81-●
        skull M85.88
        thigh M85.85-●
        upper arm M85.82-●
        vertebra M85.88
    development and growth NEC M89.20
      carpus M89.24-●
      clavicle M89.21-●
      femur M89.25-●
      fibula M89.26-●
      finger M89.24-●
      humerus M89.22-●
      ilium M89.259
      ischium M89.259
      metacarpus M89.24-●
      metatarsus M89.27-●
      multiple sites M89.29
      neck M89.28
      radius M89.23-●
      rib M89.28
      scapula M89.21-●
      skull M89.28
      tarsus M89.27-●
      tibia M89.26-●
      toe M89.27-●
      ulna M89.23-●
      vertebra M89.28
    specified type NEC M89.8X-●
  brachial plexus G54.0
  branched-chain amino-acid metabolism E71.2
    specified NEC E71.19
  breast N64.9
    agalactia —see Agalactia
    associated with
      lactation O92.70
        specified NEC O92.79
      pregnancy O92.20
        specified NEC O92.29

Disorder (Continued)
  breast (Continued)
    associated with (Continued)
      puerperium O92.20
        specified NEC O92.29
    cracked nipple —see Cracked nipple
    galactorrhea —see Galactorrhea
    hypogalactia O92.4
    lactation disorder NEC O92.79
    mastitis —see Mastitis
    nipple infection —see Infection, nipple
    retracted nipple —see Retraction, nipple
    specified type NEC N64.89
  Briquet's F45.0
  bullous, in diseases classified elsewhere L14
  caffeine use
    mild
      with
        caffeine-induced
          anxiety disorder F15.180
          sleep disorder F15.182
    moderate or severe
      with
        caffeine-induced
          anxiety disorder F15.280
          sleep disorder F15.282
  cannabis use
    mild F12.10
      with
        cannabis-induced
          anxiety disorder F12.180
          psychotic disorder F12.159
          sleep disorder F12.188
        cannabis intoxication delirium
          F12.121
          with perceptual disturbances
            F12.122
          without perceptual disturbances
            F12.129
      in remission (early) (sustained) F12.11
    moderate or severe F12.20
      with
        cannabis-induced
          anxiety disorder F12.280
          psychotic disorder F12.259
          sleep disorder F12.288
        cannabis intoxication
          with perceptual disturbances
            F12.222
          without perceptual disturbances
            F12.229
          delirium F12.221
      in remission (early) (sustained) F12.21
  carbohydrate
    absorption, intestinal NEC E74.39
    metabolism (congenital) E74.9
      specified NEC E74.89
  cardiac, functional I51.89
  carnitine metabolism E71.40
  cartilage M94.9
    articular NEC —see Derangement, joint,
      articular cartilage
    chondrocalcinosis —see
      Chondrocalcinosis
    specified type NEC M94.8X-●
      articular —see Derangement, joint,
        articular cartilage
      multiple sites M94.8X0
  catatonia (due to known physiological
    condition) (with another mental
    disorder) F06.1
  catatonic
    due to (secondary to) known physiological
      condition F06.1
    organic F06.1
  central auditory processing H93.25
  cervical
    region NEC M53.82
    root (nerve) NEC G54.2
  character NOS F60.9
  childhood disintegrative NEC F84.3

▶ New   ⇒ Revised   ~~deleted~~ Deleted   ● Use Additional Character(s)

Disorder *(Continued)*
　cholesterol and bile acid metabolism E78.70
　　Barth syndrome E78.71
　　other specified E78.79
　　Smith-Lemli-Opitz syndrome E78.72
　choroid H31.9
　　atrophy —*see* Atrophy, choroid
　　degeneration —*see* Degeneration, choroid
　　detachment —*see* Detachment, choroid
　　dystrophy —*see* Dystrophy, choroid
　　hemorrhage —*see* Hemorrhage, choroid
　　rupture —*see* Rupture, choroid
　　scar —*see* Scar, chorioretinal
　　solar retinopathy —*see* Retinopathy, solar
　　specified type NEC H31.8
　ciliary body —*see* Disorder, iris
　　degeneration —*see* Degeneration, ciliary
　　　body
　coagulation (factor) (*see also* Defect,
　　coagulation) D68.9
　　newborn, transient P61.6
　cocaine use
　　mild F14.10
　　　with
　　　　amphetamine, cocaine, or other
　　　　　stimulant intoxication
　　　　　with perceptual disturbances
　　　　　　F14.122
　　　　　without perceptual disturbances
　　　　　　F14.129
　　　　cocaine-induced
　　　　　anxiety disorder F14.180
　　　　　bipolar and related disorder
　　　　　　F14.14
　　　　　depressive disorder F14.14
　　　　　obsessive-compulsive and related
　　　　　　disorder F14.188
　　　　　psychotic disorder F14.159
　　　　　sexual dysfunction F14.181
　　　　　sleep disorder F14.182
　　　　cocaine intoxication delirium F14.121
　　　in remission (early) (sustained) F14.11
　　moderate or severe F14.20
　　　with
　　　　amphetamine, cocaine, or other
　　　　　stimulant intoxication
　　　　　with perceptual disturbances
　　　　　　F14.222
　　　　　without perceptual disturbances
　　　　　　F14.229
　　　　cocaine-induced
　　　　　anxiety disorder F14.280
　　　　　bipolar and related disorder
　　　　　　F14.24
　　　　　depressive disorder F14.24
　　　　　obsessive-compulsive and related
　　　　　　disorder F14.288
　　　　　psychotic disorder F14.259
　　　　　sexual dysfunction F14.281
　　　　　sleep disorder F14.282
　　　　cocaine intoxication delirium F14.221
　　　in remission (early) (sustained) F14.21
　coccyx NEC M53.3
　cognitive F09
　　due to (secondary to) general medical
　　　condition F09
　　persisting R41.89
　　　due to
　　　　alcohol F10.97
　　　　　with dependence F10.27
　　　　anxiolytics F13.97
　　　　　with dependence F13.27
　　　　hypnotics F13.97
　　　　　with dependence F13.27
　　　　sedatives F13.97
　　　　　with dependence F13.27
　　　　specified substance NEC
　　　　　F19.97
　　　　　with
　　　　　　abuse F19.17
　　　　　　dependence F19.27

Disorder *(Continued)*
　communication F80.9
　　social pragmatic F80.82
　conduct (childhood) F91.9
　　adjustment reaction —*see* Disorder,
　　　adjustment
　　adolescent onset type F91.2
　　childhood onset type F91.1
　　compulsive F63.9
　　confined to family context F91.0
　　depressive F91.8
　　group type F91.2
　　hyperkinetic —*see* Disorder, attention-
　　　deficit hyperactivity
　　oppositional defiance F91.3
　　socialized F91.2
　　solitary aggressive type F91.1
　　specified NEC F91.8
　　unsocialized (aggressive) F91.1
　conduction, heart I45.9
　congenital glycosylation (CDG) E74.89
　conjunctiva H11.9
　　infection —*see* Conjunctivitis
　connective tissue, localized L94.9
　　specified NEC L94.8
　conversion (functional neurological symptom
　　disorder)
　　with
　　　abnormal movement F44.4
　　　anesthesia or sensory loss F44.6
　　　attacks or seizures F44.5
　　　mixed symptoms F44.7
　　　special sensory symptoms F44.6
　　　speech symptoms F44.4
　　　swallowing symptoms F44.4
　　　weakness or paralysis F44.4
　convulsive (secondary) —*see* Convulsions
　cornea H18.9
　　deformity —*see* Deformity, cornea
　　degeneration —*see* Degeneration, cornea
　　deposits —*see* Deposit, cornea
　　due to contact lens H18.82-●
　　　specified as edema —*see* Edema, cornea
　　edema —*see* Edema, cornea
　　keratitis —*see* Keratitis
　　keratoconjunctivitis —*see*
　　　Keratoconjunctivitis
　　membrane change —*see* Change, corneal
　　　membrane
　　neovascularization —*see*
　　　Neovascularization, cornea
　　scar —*see* Opacity, cornea
　　specified type NEC H18.89-●
　　ulcer —*see* Ulcer, cornea
　corpus cavernosum N48.9
　cranial nerve —*see* Disorder, nerve, cranial
　Cyclin-Dependent Kinase-Like 5 Deficiency
　　(CDKL5) G40.42
　cyclothymic F34.0
　defiant oppositional F91.3
　delusional (persistent) (systematized) F22
　　induced F24
　depersonalization F48.1
▶▶depressive F32.A
　　due to known physiological condition
　　　with
　　　　depressive features F06.31
　　　　major depressive-like episode F06.32
　　　　mixed features F06.34
　　major F32.9
　　　with psychotic symptoms F32.3
　　　in remission (full) F32.5
　　　　partial F32.4
　　　recurrent F33.9
　　　　with psychotic features F33.3
　　　single episode F32.9
　　　　mild F32.0
　　　　moderate F32.1
　　　　severe (without psychotic symptoms)
　　　　　F32.2
　　　　　with psychotic symptoms F32.3

Disorder *(Continued)*
　depressive *(Continued)*
　　organic F06.31
　　persistent F34.1
　　recurrent F33.9
　　　current episode
　　　　mild F33.0
　　　　moderate F33.1
　　　　severe (without psychotic symptoms)
　　　　　F33.2
　　　　　with psychotic symptoms F33.3
　　　in remission F33.40
　　　　full F33.42
　　　　partial F33.41
　　　specified NEC F33.8
　　single episode —*see* Episode, depressive
　　specified NEC F32.89
　developmental F89
　　arithmetical skills F81.2
　　coordination (motor) F82
　　expressive writing F81.81
　　language F80.9
　　　expressive F80.1
　　　mixed receptive and expressive
　　　　F80.2
　　　receptive type F80.2
　　　specified NEC F80.89
　　learning F81.9
　　　arithmetical F81.2
　　　reading F81.0
　　mixed F88
　　motor coordination or function F82
　　pervasive F84.9
　　　specified NEC F84.8
　　phonological F80.0
　　reading F81.0
　　scholastic skills —*see also* Disorder,
　　　learning
　　　mixed F81.89
　　specified NEC F88
　　speech F80.9
　　　articulation F80.0
　　　specified NEC F80.89
　　written expression F81.81
　diaphragm J98.6
　digestive (system) K92.9
　　newborn P78.9
　　　specified NEC P78.89
　　postprocedural —*see* Complication,
　　　gastrointestinal
　　psychogenic F45.8
　disc (intervertebral) M51.9
　　with
　　　myelopathy
　　　　cervical region M50.00
　　　　cervicothoracic region M50.03
　　　　high cervical region M50.01
　　　　lumbar region M51.06
　　　　mid-cervical region M50.020
　　　　sacrococcygeal region M53.3
　　　　thoracic region M51.04
　　　　thoracolumbar region M51.05
　　　radiculopathy
　　　　cervical region M50.10
　　　　cervicothoracic region M50.13
　　　　high cervical region M50.11
　　　　lumbar region M51.16
　　　　lumbosacral region M51.17
　　　　mid-cervical region M50.120
　　　　sacrococcygeal region M53.3
　　　　thoracic region M51.14
　　　　thoracolumbar region M51.15
　　cervical M50.90
　　　with
　　　　myelopathy M50.00
　　　　　C2-C3 M50.01
　　　　　C3-C4 M50.01
　　　　　C4-C5 M50.021
　　　　　C5-C6 M50.022
　　　　　C6-C7 M50.023
　　　　　C7-T1 M50.03

Disorder *(Continued)*
  disc *(Continued)*
    cervical *(Continued)*
      with *(Continued)*
        myelopathy *(Continued)*
          cervicothoracic region M50.03
          high cervical region M50.01
          mid-cervical region M50.020
        neuritis, radiculitis or radiculopathy
          M50.10
          C2-C3 M50.11
          C3-C4 M50.11
          C4-C5 M50.121
          C5-C6 M50.122
          C6-C7 M50.123
          C7-T1 M50.13
          cervicothoracic region M50.13
          high cervical region M50.11
          mid-cervical region M50.120
        C2-C3 M50.91
        C3-C4 M50.91
        C4-C5 M50.921
        C5-C6 M50.922
        C6-C7 M50.923
        C7-T1 M50.93
        cervicothoracic region M50.93
        degeneration M50.30
          C2-C3 M50.31
          C3-C4 M50.31
          C4-C5 M50.321
          C5-C6 M50.322
          C6-C7 M50.323
          C7-T1 M50.33
          cervicothoracic region M50.33
          high cervical region M50.31
          mid-cervical region M50.320
        displacement M50.20
          C2-C3 M50.21
          C3-C4 M50.21
          C4-C5 M50.221
          C5-C6 M50.222
          C6-C7 M50.223
          C7-T1 M50.23
          cervicothoracic region M50.23
          high cervical region M50.21
          mid-cervical region M50.220
        high cervical region M50.91
        mid-cervical region M50.920
        specified type NEC M50.80
          C2-C3 M50.81
          C3-C4 M50.81
          C4-C5 M50.821
          C5-C6 M50.822
          C6-C7 M50.823
          C7-T1 M50.83
          cervicothoracic region M50.83
          high cervical region M50.81
          mid-cervical region M50.820
    specified NEC
      lumbar region M51.86
      lumbosacral region M51.87
      sacrococcygeal region M53.3
      thoracic region M51.84
      thoracolumbar region M51.85
  disinhibited attachment (childhood) F94.2
  disintegrative, childhood NEC F84.3
  disruptive F91.9
    mood dysregulation F34.81
    specified NEC F91.8
  disruptive behavior —*see* Disorder, conduct
  dissocial personality F60.2
  dissociative F44.9
    affecting
      motor function F44.4
        and sensation F44.7
      sensation F44.6
        and motor function F44.7
    brief reactive F43.0
    due to (secondary to) general medical
      condition F06.8
    mixed F44.7

Disorder *(Continued)*
  dissociative *(Continued)*
    organic F06.8
    other specified NEC F44.89
  double heterozygous sickling —*see* Disease,
    sickle-cell
  dream anxiety F51.5
  drug induced hemorrhagic D68.32
  drug related F19.99
    abuse —*see* Abuse, drug
    dependence —*see* Dependence, drug
  dysmorphic body F45.22
  dysthymic F34.1
  ear H93.9-•
    bleeding —*see* Otorrhagia
    deafness —*see* Deafness
    degenerative H93.09-•
    discharge —*see* Otorrhea
    external H61.9-•
      auditory canal stenosis —*see* Stenosis,
        external ear canal
      exostosis —*see* Exostosis, external ear
        canal
      impacted cerumen —*see* Impaction,
        cerumen
      otitis —*see* Otitis, externa
      perichondritis —*see* Perichondritis, ear
      pinna —*see* Disorder, pinna
      specified type NEC H61.89-•
        in diseases classified elsewhere
          H62.8X-•
    inner H83.9-•
      vestibular dysfunction —*see* Disorder,
        vestibular function
    middle H74.9-•
      adhesive H74.1-•
      ossicle —*see* Abnormal, ear ossicles
      polyp —*see* Polyp, ear (middle)
      specified NEC, in diseases classified
        elsewhere H75.8-•
    postprocedural —*see* Complications, ear,
      procedure
    specified NEC, in diseases classified
      elsewhere H94.8-•
  eating (adult) (psychogenic) F50.9
    anorexia —*see* Anorexia
    binge F50.81
    bulimia F50.2
    child F98.29
      pica F98.3
      rumination disorder F98.21
    pica F50.89
      childhood F98.3
  electrolyte (balance) NEC E87.8
    with
      abortion —*see* Abortion by type
        complicated by specified condition
        NEC
      ectopic pregnancy O08.5
      molar pregnancy O08.5
    acidosis (metabolic) (respiratory) E87.2
    alkalosis (metabolic) (respiratory) E87.3
  elimination, transepidermal L87.9
    specified NEC L87.8
  emotional (persistent) F34.9
    of childhood F93.9
      specified NEC F93.8
  endocrine E34.9
    postprocedural E89.89
    specified NEC E89.89
  erectile (male) (organic) —*see also*
    Dysfunction, sexual, male, erectile N52.9
    nonorganic F52.21
  erythematous —*see* Erythema
  esophagus K22.9
    functional K22.4
    psychogenic F45.8
  eustachian tube H69.9-•
    infection —*see* Salpingitis, eustachian
    obstruction —*see* Obstruction, eustachian
      tube

Disorder *(Continued)*
  eustachian tube *(Continued)*
    patulous —*see* Patulous, eustachian tube
    specified NEC H69.8-•
  exhibitionistic F65.2
  extrapyramidal G25.9
    in diseases classified elsewhere —*see*
      category G26
    specified type NEC G25.89
  eye H57.9
    postprocedural —*see* Complication,
      postprocedural, eye
  eyelid H02.9
    cyst —*see* Cyst, eyelid
    degenerative H02.70
      chloasma —*see* Chloasma, eyelid
      madarosis —*see* Madarosis
      specified type NEC H02.79
      vitiligo —*see* Vitiligo, eyelid
      xanthelasma —*see* Xanthelasma
    dermatochalasis —*see* Dermato-chalasis
    edema —*see* Edema, eyelid
    elephantiasis —*see* Elephantiasis, eyelid
    foreign body, retained —*see* Foreign body,
      retained, eyelid
    function H02.59
      abnormal innervation syndrome —
        see Syndrome, abnormal
        innervation
      blepharochalasis —*see* Blepharochalasis
      blepharoclonus —*see* Blepharoclonus
      blepharophimosis —*see*
        Blepharophimosis
      blepharoptosis —*see* Blepharoptosis
      lagophthalmos —*see* Lagophthalmos
      lid retraction —*see* Retraction, lid
    hypertrichosis —*see* Hypertrichosis,
      eyelid
    specified type NEC H02.89
    vascular H02.879
      left H02.876
        lower H02.875
        upper H02.874
      right H02.873
        lower H02.872
        upper H02.871
  factitious
    by proxy F68.A
    imposed on another F68.A
    imposed on self F68.10
      with predominantly
        psychological symptoms F68.11
          with physical symptoms F68.13
        physical symptoms F68.12
          with psychological symptoms F68.13
  factor, coagulation —*see* Defect,
    coagulation
  fatty acid
    metabolism E71.30
      specified NEC E71.39
    oxidation
      LCAD E71.310
      MCAD E71.311
      SCAD E71.312
      specified deficiency NEC E71.318
  feeding (infant or child) —*see also* Disorder,
    ⯈eating R63.30
    or eating disorder F50.9
    ▶pediatric
      ▶acute R63.31
      ▶chronic R63.32
    specified NEC F50.9
  feigned (with obvious motivation)
    Z76.5
    without obvious motivation —
      see Disorder, factitious
  female
    hypoactive sexual desire F52.0
    orgasmic F52.31
    sexual interest/arousal F52.22
  fetishistic F65.0
  fibroblastic M72.9
    specified NEC M72.8

Disorder (Continued)
  fluency
    adult onset F98.5
    childhood onset F80.81
    following
      cerebral infarction I69.323
      cerebrovascular disease I69.923
        specified disease NEC I69.823
      intracerebral hemorrhage I69.123
      nontraumatic intracranial hemorrhage
          NEC I69.223
      subarachnoid hemorrhage I69.023
    in conditions classified elsewhere
        R47.82
  fluid balance E87.8
  follicular (skin) L73.9
    specified NEC L73.8
  frotteuristic F65.81
  fructose metabolism E74.10
    essential fructosuria E74.11
    fructokinase deficiency E74.11
    fructose-1, 6-diphosphatase deficiency
        E74.19
    hereditary fructose intolerance E74.12
    other specified E74.19
  functional polymorphonuclear neutrophils
      D71
  gallbladder, biliary tract and pancreas in
      diseases classified elsewhere K87
  gambling F63.0
  gamma aminobutyric acid (GABA)
      metabolism E72.81
  gamma-glutamyl cycle E72.89
  gastric (functional) K31.9
    motility K30
    psychogenic F45.8
    secretion K30
  gastrointestinal (functional) NOS K92.9
    newborn P78.9
    psychogenic F45.8
  gender-identity or -role F64.9
    childhood F64.2
    effect on relationship F66
    of adolescence or adulthood F64.0
      nontranssexual F64.8
    specified NEC F64.8
    uncertainty F66
  genito-pelvic pain penetration F52.6
  genitourinary system
    female N94.9
    male N50.9
    psychogenic F45.8
  globe H44.9
    degenerated condition H44.50
      absolute glaucoma H44.51-●
      atrophy H44.52-●
      leucocoria H44.53-●
    degenerative H44.30
      chalcosis H44.31-●
      myopia —see also Myopia, degenerative
          H44.2-●
      siderosis H44.32-●
      specified type NEC H44.39-●
    endophthalmitis —see Endophthalmitis
    foreign body, retained —see Foreign body,
        intraocular, old, retained
    hemophthalmos —see Hemophthalmos
    hypotony H44.40
      due to
        ocular fistula H44.42-●
        specified disorder NEC H44.43-●
      flat anterior chamber H44.41-●
      primary H44.44-●
    luxation —see Luxation, globe
    specified type NEC H44.89
  glomerular (in) N05.9
    amyloidosis E85.4 [N08]
    cryoglobulinemia D89.1 [N08]
    disseminated intravascular coagulation
        D65 [N08]
    Fabry's disease E75.21 [N08]

Disorder (Continued)
  glomerular (Continued)
    familial lecithin cholesterol acyltransferase
        deficiency E78.6 [N08]
    Goodpasture's syndrome M31.0
    hemolytic-uremic syndrome D59.3
    Henoch (-Schönlein) purpura D69.0
        [N08]
    malariae malaria B52.0
    microscopic polyangiitis M31.7 [N08]
    multiple myeloma C90.0-● [N08]
    mumps B26.83
    schistosomiasis B65.9 [N08]
    sepsis NEC A41.-● [N08]
      streptococcal A40.-● [N08]
    sickle-cell disorders D57.-● [N08]
    strongyloidiasis B78.9 [N08]
    subacute bacterial endocarditis I33.0
        [N08]
    syphilis A52.75
    systemic lupus erythematosus M32.14
➡ thrombotic thrombocytopenic purpura
        M31.19 [N08]
    Waldenström macroglobulinemia C88.0
        [N08]
    Wegener's granulomatosis M31.31
  gluconeogenesis E74.4
  glucosaminoglycan metabolism —
      see Disorder, metabolism,
      glucosaminoglycan
  glucose transport E74.819
    specified NEC E74.818
  glycine metabolism E72.50
    d-glycericacidemia E72.59
    hyperhydroxyprolinemia E72.59
    hyperoxaluria R82.992
      primary E72.53
    hyperprolinemia E72.59
    non-ketotic hyperglycinemia E72.51
    oxalosis E72.53
    oxaluria E72.53
    sarcosinemia E72.59
    trimethylaminuria E72.52
  glycoprotein metabolism E77.9
    specified NEC E77.8
  habit (and impulse) F63.9
    involving sexual behavior NEC F65.9
    specified NEC F63.89
  hallucinogen use
    mild F16.10
      with
        hallucinogen-induced
          anxiety disorder F16.180
          bipolar and related disorder
              F16.14
          depressive disorder F16.14
          psychotic disorder F16.159
        hallucinogen intoxication delirium
            F16.121
        other hallucinogen intoxication
            F16.129
      in remission (early) (sustained) F16.11
    moderate or severe F16.20
      with
        hallucinogen-induced
          anxiety disorder F16.280
          bipolar and related disorder
              F16.24
          depressive disorder F16.24
          psychotic disorder F16.259
        hallucinogen intoxication delirium
            F16.221
        other hallucinogen intoxication
            F16.229
      in remission (early) (sustained)
          F16.21
  heart action I49.9
  hematological D75.9
    newborn (transient) P61.9
      specified NEC P61.8
  hematopoietic organs D75.9

Disorder (Continued)
  hemorrhagic NEC D69.9
    drug-induced D68.32
    due to
      extrinsic circulating anticoagulants
          D68.32
      increase in
        anti-IIa D68.32
        anti-Xa D68.32
      intrinsic
        circulating anticoagulants D68.318
        increase in
          antithrombin D68.318
          anti-VIIIa D68.318
          anti-IXa D68.318
          anti-XIa D68.318
    following childbirth O72.3
  hemostasis —see Defect, coagulation
  histidine metabolism E70.40
    histidinemia E70.41
    other specified E70.49
  hoarding F42.3
  hyperkinetic —see Disorder, attention-deficit
      hyperactivity
  hyperleucine-isoleucinemia E71.19
  hypervalinemia E71.19
  hypoactive sexual desire F52.0
  hypochondriacal F45.20
    body dysmorphic F45.22
    neurosis F45.21
    other specified F45.29
  identity
    dissociative F44.81
    illness anxiety F45.21
    of childhood F93.8
  immune mechanism (immunity) D89.9
    specified type NEC D89.89
  impaired renal tubular function N25.9
    specified NEC N25.89
  impulse (control) F63.9
  inflammatory
    pelvic, in diseases classified elsewhere —
        see category N74
    penis N48.29
      abscess N48.21
      cellulitis N48.22
  inhalant use
    mild F18.10
      with
        inhalant-induced
          anxiety disorder F18.180
          depressive disorder F18.14
          major neurocognitive disorder
              F18.17
          mild neurocognitive disorder
              F18.188
          psychotic disorder F18.159
        inhalant intoxication F18.129
        inhalant intoxication delirium F18.121
      in remission (early) (sustained) F18.11
    moderate or severe F18.20
      with
        inhalant-induced
          anxiety disorder F18.280
          depressive disorder F18.24
          major neurocognitive disorder
              F18.27
          mild neurocognitive disorder
              F18.288
          psychotic disorder F18.259
        inhalant intoxication F18.229
        inhalant intoxication delirium F18.221
      in remission (early) (sustained) F18.21
  integument, newborn P83.9
    specified NEC P83.88
  intermittent explosive F63.81
  internal secretion pancreas —see Increased,
      secretion, pancreas, endocrine
  intestine, intestinal
    carbohydrate absorption NEC E74.39
      postoperative K91.2

Disorder *(Continued)*
  intestine, intestinal *(Continued)*
    functional NEC K59.9
      postoperative K91.89
    psychogenic F45.8
    vascular K55.9
      chronic K55.1
      specified NEC K55.8
  intraoperative (intraprocedural) *—see*
    Complications, intraoperative
  involuntary emotional expression (IEED) F48.2
  iris H21.9
    adhesions *—see* Adhesions, iris
    atrophy *—see* Atrophy, iris
    chamber angle recession *—see* Recession,
      chamber angle
    cyst *—see* Cyst, iris
    degeneration *—see* Degeneration, iris
    in diseases classified elsewhere H22
    iridodialysis *—see* Iridodialysis
    iridoschisis *—see* Iridoschisis
    miotic pupillary cyst *—see* Cyst, pupillary
    pupillary
      abnormality *—see* Abnormality, pupillary
      membrane *—see* Membrane, pupillary
    specified type NEC H21.89
    vascular NEC H21.1X-•
  iron metabolism E83.10
    specified NEC E83.19
  isovaleric acidemia E71.110
  jaw, developmental M27.0
    temporomandibular *—see also* Anomaly,
      dentofacial, temporomandibular joint
      M26.60-•
  joint M25.9
    derangement *—see* Derangement, joint
    effusion *—see* Effusion, joint
    fistula *—see* Fistula, joint
    hemarthrosis *—see* Hemarthrosis
    instability *—see* Instability, joint
    osteophyte *—see* Osteophyte
    pain *—see* Pain, joint
    psychogenic F45.8
    specified type NEC M25.80
      ankle M25.87-•
      elbow M25.82-•
      foot joint M25.87-•
      hand joint M25.84-•
      hip M25.85-•
      knee M25.86-•
      shoulder M25.81-•
      wrist M25.83-•
    stiffness *—see* Stiffness, joint
  ketone metabolism E71.32
  kidney N28.9
    functional (tubular) N25.9
    in
      schistosomiasis B65.9 *[N29]*
    tubular function N25.9
      specified NEC N25.89
  lacrimal system H04.9
    changes H04.69
    fistula *—see* Fistula, lacrimal
    gland H04.19
      atrophy *—see* Atrophy, lacrimal gland
      cyst *—see* Cyst, lacrimal, gland
      dacryops *—see* Dacryops
      dislocation *—see* Dislocation, lacrimal
        gland
      dry eye syndrome *—see* Syndrome, dry
        eye
      infection *—see* Dacryoadenitis
      granuloma *—see* Granuloma, lacrimal
      inflammation *—see* Inflammation, lacrimal
      obstruction *—see* Obstruction, lacrimal
      specified NEC H04.89
  lactation NEC O92.79
  language (developmental) F80.9
    expressive F80.1
    mixed receptive and expressive F80.2
    receptive F80.2

Disorder *(Continued)*
  late luteal phase dysphoric N94.89
  learning (specific) F81.9
    acalculia R48.8
    alexia R48.0
    mathematics F81.2
    reading F81.0
    specified
      with impairment in
        mathematics F81.2
        reading F81.0
        written expression F81.81
    specified NEC F81.89
    spelling F81.81
    written expression F81.81
  lens H27.9
    aphakia *—see* Aphakia
    cataract *—see* Cataract
    dislocation *—see* Dislocation, lens
    specified type NEC H27.8
  ligament M24.20
    ankle M24.27-•
    attachment, spine *—see* Enthesopathy,
      spinal
    elbow M24.22-•
    foot joint M24.27-•
    hand joint M24.24-•
    hip M24.25-•
    knee *—see* Derangement, knee, specified
      NEC
    shoulder M24.21-•
    specified site NEC M24.29
    vertebra M24.28
    wrist M24.23-•
  ligamentous attachments *—see also*
    Enthesopathy
    spine *—see* Enthesopathy, spinal
  lipid
    metabolism, congenital E78.9
    storage E75.6
      specified NEC E75.5
  lipoprotein
    deficiency (familial) E78.6
    metabolism E78.9
      specified NEC E78.89
  liver K76.9
    malarial B54 *[K77]*
  low back *—see also* Dorsopathy, specified NEC
  lumbosacral
    plexus G54.1
    root (nerve) NEC G54.4
  lung, interstitial, drug-induced J70.4
    acute J70.2
    chronic J70.3
    dabbing (related) U07.0
    e-cigarette (related) U07.0
    electronic cigarette (related) U07.0
    vaping (associated) (device) (product)
      (related) (use) U07.0
  lymphoproliferative, post-transplant (PTLD)
    D47.Z1
  lysine and hydroxylysine metabolism E72.3
  major neurocognitive *—see* Dementia, in
    (due to)
  male
    erectile (organic) *—see also* Dysfunction,
      sexual, male, erectile N52.9
      nonorganic F52.21
    hypoactive sexual desire F52.0
    orgasmic F52.32
  manic F30.9
    organic F06.33
  mast cell activation *—see* Activation, mast cell
  mastoid *—see also* Disorder, ear, middle
    postprocedural *—see* Complications, ear,
      procedure
  meninges, specified type NEC G96.198
  meniscus *—see* Derangement, knee,
    meniscus
  menopausal N95.9
    specified NEC N95.8

Disorder *(Continued)*
  menstrual N92.6
    psychogenic F45.8
    specified NEC N92.5
  mental (or behavioral) (nonpsychotic) F99
    due to (secondary to)
      amphetamine
        due to drug abuse *—see* Abuse, drug,
          stimulant
        due to drug dependence *—see*
          Dependence, drug, stimulant
      brain disease, damage and dysfunction
        F09
      caffeine use
        due to drug abuse *—see* Abuse, drug,
          stimulant
        due to drug dependence *—see*
          Dependence, drug, stimulant
      cannabis use
        due to drug abuse *—see* Abuse, drug,
          cannabis
        due to drug dependence *—see*
          Dependence, drug, cannabis
      general medical condition F09
      sedative or hypnotic use
        due to drug abuse *—see* Abuse, drug,
          sedative
        due to drug dependence *—see*
          Dependence, drug, sedative
      tobacco (nicotine) use *—see* Dependence,
        drug, nicotine
    following organic brain damage F07.9
      frontal lobe syndrome F07.0
      personality change F07.0
      postconcussional syndrome F07.81
      specified NEC F07.89
    infancy, childhood or adolescence F98.9
    neurotic *—see* Neurosis
    organic or symptomatic F09
    presenile, psychotic F03
    problem NEC
    psychoneurotic *—see* Neurosis
    psychotic *—see* Psychosis
    puerperal F53.0
    senile, psychotic NEC F03
  metabolic, amino acid, transitory, newborn
    P74.8
  metabolism NOS E88.9
    amino-acid E72.9
      aromatic E70.9
        albinism *—see* Albinism
        histidine E70.40
          histidinemia E70.41
          other specified E70.49
        hyperphenylalaninemia E70.1
          classical phenylketonuria E70.0
        other specified E70.89
        tryptophan E70.5
        tyrosine E70.20
          hypertyrosinemia E70.21
          other specified E70.29
      branched chain E71.2
        3-methylglutaconic aciduria E71.111
        hyperleucine-isoleucinemia E71.19
        hypervalinemia E71.19
        isovaleric acidemia E71.110
        maple syrup urine disease E71.0
        methylmalonic acidemia E71.120
        organic aciduria NEC E71.118
        other specified E71.19
        proprionate NEC E71.128
        proprionic acidemia E71.121
      glycine E72.50
        d-glycericacidemia E72.59
        hyperhydroxyprolinemia E72.59
        hyperoxaluria R82.992
          primary E72.53
        hyperprolinemia E72.59
        non-ketotic hyperglycinemia
          E72.51
        other specified E72.59

▶ New   ⇒ Revised   ~~deleted~~ Deleted   • Use Additional Character(s)

Disorder *(Continued)*
  metabolism *(Continued)*
    amino-acid *(Continued)*
      glycine *(Continued)*
        sarcosinemia E72.59
        trimethylaminuria E72.52
      hydroxylysine E72.3
      lysine E72.3
      ornithine E72.4
      other specified E72.89
        beta-amino acid E72.89
        gamma-glutamyl cycle E72.89
      straight-chain E72.89
      sulfur-bearing E72.10
        homocystinuria E72.11
        methylenetetrahydrofolate reductase
          deficiency E72.12
        other specified E72.19
    bile acid and cholesterol metabolism E78.70
    bilirubin E80.7
      specified NEC E80.6
    calcium E83.50
      hypercalcemia E83.52
      hypocalcemia E83.51
      other specified E83.59
    carbohydrate E74.9
      specified NEC E74.89
    cholesterol and bile acid metabolism
      E78.70
    congenital E88.9
    copper E83.00
      specified type NEC E83.09
      Wilson's disease E83.01
    cystinuria E72.01
    fructose E74.10
    galactose E74.20
    glucosaminoglycan E76.9
      mucopolysaccharidosis —*see*
        Mucopolysaccharidosis
      specified NEC E76.8
    glutamine E72.89
    glycine E72.50
    glycogen storage (hepatorenal) E74.09
    glycoprotein E77.9
      specified NEC E77.8
    glycosaminoglycan E76.9
      specified NEC E76.8
    in labor and delivery O75.89
    iron E83.10
    isoleucine E71.19
    leucine E71.19
    lipoid E78.9
    lipoprotein E78.9
      specified NEC E78.89
    magnesium E83.40
      hypermagnesemia E83.41
      hypomagnesemia E83.42
      other specified E83.49
    mineral E83.9
      specified NEC E83.89
    mitochondrial E88.40
      MELAS syndrome E88.41
      MERRF syndrome (myoclonic epilepsy
        associated with ragged-red fibers)
        E88.42
      other specified E88.49
    ornithine E72.4
    phosphatases E83.30
    phosphorus E83.30
      acid phosphatase deficiency E83.39
      hypophosphatasia E83.39
      hypophosphatemia E83.39
        familial E83.31
      other specified E83.39
      pseudovitamin D deficiency E83.32
    plasma protein NEC E88.09
    porphyrin —*see* Porphyria
    postprocedural E89.89
      specified NEC E89.89
    purine E79.9
      specified NEC E79.8

Disorder *(Continued)*
  metabolism *(Continued)*
    pyrimidine E79.9
      specified NEC E79.8
    pyruvate E74.4
    serine E72.89
    sodium E87.8
    specified NEC E88.89
    threonine E72.89
    valine E71.19
    zinc E83.2
  methylmalonic acidemia E71.120
  micturition NEC —*see also* Difficulty,
    micturition R39.198
    feeling of incomplete emptying R39.14
    hesitancy R39.11
    poor stream R39.12
    psychogenic F45.8
    split stream R39.13
    straining R39.16
    urgency R39.15
  mild neurocognitive G31.84
  mitochondrial metabolism E88.40
  mitral (valve) —*see* Endocarditis, mitral
  mixed
    anxiety and depressive F41.8
    of scholastic skills (developmental) F81.89
    receptive expressive language F80.2
  mood F39
    bipolar —*see* Disorder, bipolar
    depressive —*see* Disorder, depressive
    due to (secondary to)
      alcohol F10.94
      amphetamine F15.94
        in
          abuse F15.14
          dependence F15.24
      anxiolytic F13.94
        in
          abuse F13.14
          dependence F13.24
      cocaine F14.94
        in
          abuse F14.14
          dependence F14.24
      general medical condition F06.30
      hallucinogen F16.94
        in
          abuse F16.14
          dependence F16.24
      hypnotic F13.94
        in
          abuse F13.14
          dependence F13.24
      inhalant F18.94
        in
          abuse F18.14
          dependence F18.24
      opioid F11.94
        in
          abuse F11.14
          dependence F11.24
      phencyclidine (PCP) F16.94
        in
          abuse F16.14
          dependence F16.24
      physiological condition F06.30
        with
          depressive features F06.31
          major depressive-like episode
            F06.32
          manic features F06.33
          mixed features F06.34
      psychoactive substance NEC F19.94
        in
          abuse F19.14
          dependence F19.24
      sedative F13.94
        in
          abuse F13.14
          dependence F13.24

Disorder *(Continued)*
  mood *(Continued)*
    due to *(Continued)*
      volatile solvents F18.94
        in
          abuse F18.14
          dependence F18.24
    manic episode F30.9
      with psychotic symptoms F30.2
      without psychotic symptoms F30.10
        mild F30.11
        moderate F30.12
        severe F30.13
      in remission (full) F30.4
        partial F30.3
      specified type NEC F30.8
    organic F06.30
      right hemisphere F07.89
    persistent F34.9
      cyclothymia F34.0
      dysthymia F34.1
      specified type NEC F34.89
    recurrent F39
    right hemisphere organic F07.89
  movement G25.9
    drug-induced G25.70
      akathisia G25.71
      specified NEC G25.79
    hysterical F44.4
    in diseases classified elsewhere —*see*
      category G26
    periodic limb G47.61
      sleep related G47.61
    sleep related NEC G47.69
    specified NEC G25.89
    stereotyped F98.4
    treatment-induced G25.9
  multiple personality F44.81
  muscle M62.9
    attachment, spine —*see* Enthesopathy,
      spinal
    in trichinellosis —*see* Trichinellosis, with
      muscle disorder
    psychogenic F45.8
    specified type NEC M62.89
    tone, newborn P94.9
      specified NEC P94.8
  muscular
    attachments —*see also* Enthesopathy
      spine —*see* Enthesopathy, spinal
    urethra N36.44
  musculoskeletal system, soft tissue —*see*
    Disorder, soft tissue
    postprocedural M96.89
    psychogenic F45.8
  myoneural G70.9
    due to lead G70.1
    specified NEC G70.89
    toxic G70.1
  myotonic NEC G71.19
  nail, in diseases classified elsewhere L62
  neck region NEC —*see* Dorsopathy, specified
    NEC
  neonatal onset multisystemic inflammatory
    (NOMID) M04.2
  nerve G58.9
    abducent NEC —*see* Strabismus, paralytic,
      sixth nerve
    accessory G52.8
    acoustic —*see* subcategory H93.3
    auditory —*see* subcategory H93.3
    auriculotemporal G50.8
    axillary G54.0
    cerebral —*see* Disorder, nerve, cranial
    cranial G52.9
      eighth —*see* subcategory H93.3
      eleventh G52.8
      fifth G50.9
      first G52.0
      fourth NEC —*see* Strabismus, paralytic,
        fourth nerve

Disorder *(Continued)*
  nerve *(Continued)*
    cranial *(Continued)*
      multiple G52.7
      ninth G52.1
      second NEC —*see* Disorder, nerve, optic
      seventh NEC G51.8
      sixth NEC —*see* Strabismus, paralytic, sixth nerve
      specified NEC G52.8
      tenth G52.2
      third NEC —*see* Strabismus, paralytic, third nerve
      twelfth G52.3
    entrapment —*see* Neuropathy, entrapment
    facial G51.9
      specified NEC G51.8
    femoral —*see* Lesion, nerve, femoral
    glossopharyngeal NEC G52.1
    hypoglossal G52.3
    intercostal G58.0
    lateral
      cutaneous of thigh —*see* Mononeuropathy, lower limb, meralgia paresthetica
      popliteal —*see* Lesion, nerve, popliteal
    lower limb —*see* Mononeuropathy, lower limb
    medial popliteal —*see* Lesion, nerve, popliteal, medial
    median NEC —*see* Lesion, nerve, median
    multiple G58.7
    oculomotor NEC —*see* Strabismus, paralytic, third nerve
    olfactory G52.0
    optic NEC H47.09-●
      hemorrhage into sheath —*see* Hemorrhage, optic nerve
      ischemic H47.01-●
    peroneal —*see* Lesion, nerve, popliteal
    phrenic G58.8
    plantar —*see* Lesion, nerve, plantar
    pneumogastric G52.2
    posterior tibial —*see* Syndrome, tarsal tunnel
    radial —*see* Lesion, nerve, radial
    recurrent laryngeal G52.2
    root G54.9
      cervical G54.2
      lumbosacral G54.1
      specified NEC G54.8
      thoracic G54.3
    sciatic NEC —*see* Lesion, nerve, sciatic
    specified NEC G58.8
      lower limb —*see* Mononeuropathy, lower limb, specified NEC
      upper limb —*see* Mononeuropathy, upper limb, specified NEC
    sympathetic G90.9
    tibial —*see* Lesion, nerve, popliteal, medial
    trigeminal G50.9
      specified NEC G50.8
    trochlear NEC —*see* Strabismus, paralytic, fourth nerve
    ulnar —*see* Lesion, nerve, ulnar
    upper limb —*see* Mononeuropathy, upper limb
    vagus G52.2
  nervous system G98.8
    autonomic (peripheral) G90.9
      specified NEC G90.8
    central G96.9
      specified NEC G96.89
    parasympathetic G90.9
    specified NEC G98.8
    sympathetic G90.9
    vegetative G90.9

Disorder *(Continued)*
  neurocognitive R41.9
    major
      with
        aggressive behavior F01.51
        combative behavior F01.51
        violent behavior F01.51
      due to vascular disease, with behavioral disturbance F01.51
      in (due to) (other diseases classified elsewhere) —*see also* Dementia, in (due to) F02.80
        with
          aggressive behavior F02.81
          combative behavior F02.81
          violent behavior F02.81
        without behavioral disturbance F01.50
    mild G31.84
  neurodevelopmental F89
    specified NEC F88
  neurohypophysis NEC E23.3
  neurological NEC R29.818
  neuromuscular G70.9
    hereditary NEC G71.9
    specified NEC G70.89
    toxic G70.1
  neurotic F48.9
    specified NEC F48.8
  neutrophil, polymorphonuclear D71
  nightmare F51.5
  non-rapid eye movement sleep arousal
    sleep terror type F51.4
    sleepwalking type F51.3
  nose J34.9
    specified NEC J34.89
  obsessive-compulsive F42.9
    and related disorder due to a known physiological condition F06.8
  odontogenesis NOS K00.9
  opioid use
    with
      opioid-induced psychotic disorder F11.959
        with
          delusions F11.950
          hallucinations F11.951
    due to drug abuse —*see* Abuse, drug, opioid
    due to drug dependence —*see* Dependence, drug, opioid
    mild F11.10
      with
        opioid-induced
          anxiety disorder F11.188
          depressive disorder F11.14
          sexual dysfunction F11.181
        opioid intoxication
          with perceptual disturbances F11.122
          delirium F11.121
          without perceptual disturbances F11.129
      in remission (early) (sustained) F11.11
    moderate or severe F11.20
      with
        opioid-induced
          anxiety disorder F11.288
          anxiety disorder F11.988
          depressive disorder F11.24
          depressive disorder F11.94
          sexual dysfunction F11.281
          sexual dysfunction F11.981
        opioid intoxication
          with perceptual disturbances F11.222
          delirium F11.221
          without perceptual disturbances F11.229
      in remission (early) (sustained) F11.21
  oppositional defiant F91.3

Disorder *(Continued)*
  optic
    chiasm H47.49
      due to
        inflammatory disorder H47.41
        neoplasm H47.42
        vascular disorder H47.43
    disc H47.39-●
      coloboma —*see* Coloboma, optic disc
      drusen —*see* Drusen, optic disc
      pseudopapilledema —*see* Pseudopapilledema
    radiations —*see* Disorder, visual, pathway
    tracts —*see* Disorder, visual, pathway
  orbit H05.9
    cyst —*see* Cyst, orbit
    deformity —*see* Deformity, orbit
    edema —*see* Edema, orbit
    enophthalmos —*see* Enophthalmos
    exophthalmos —*see* Exophthalmos
    hemorrhage —*see* Hemorrhage, orbit
    inflammation —*see* Inflammation, orbit
    myopathy —*see* Myopathy, extraocular muscles
    retained foreign body —*see* Foreign body, orbit, old
    specified type NEC H05.89
  organic
    anxiety F06.4
    catatonic F06.1
    delusional F06.2
    dissociative F06.8
    emotionally labile (asthenic) F06.8
    mood (affective) F06.30
    schizophrenia-like F06.2
  orgasmic (female) F52.31
    male F52.32
  ornithine metabolism E72.4
  overanxious F41.1
    of childhood F93.8
  pain
    with related psychological factors F45.42
    exclusively related to psychological factors F45.41
    genito-pelvic penetration disorder F52.6
  pancreatic internal secretion E16.9
    specified NEC E16.8
  panic F41.0
    with agoraphobia F40.01
  papulosquamous L44.9
    in diseases classified elsewhere L45
    specified NEC L44.8
  paranoid F22
    induced F24
    shared F24
  paraphilic F65.9
    specified NEC F65.89
  parathyroid (gland) E21.5
    specified NEC E21.4
  parietoalveolar NEC J84.09
  paroxysmal, mixed R56.9
  patella M22.9-●
    chondromalacia —*see* Chondromalacia, patella
    derangement NEC M22.3X-●
    recurrent
      dislocation —*see* Dislocation, patella, recurrent
      subluxation —*see* Dislocation, patella, recurrent, incomplete
    specified NEC M22.8X-●
  patellofemoral M22.2X-●
  pedophilic F65.4
  pentose phosphate pathway with anemia D55.1
  perception, due to hallucinogens F16.983
    in
      abuse F16.183
      dependence F16.283
  peripheral nervous system NEC G64

▶ New   ⇒ Revised   ~~deleted~~ Deleted   ● Use Additional Character(s)

Disorder *(Continued)*
  peroxisomal E71.50
    biogenesis
      neonatal adrenoleukodystrophy E71.511
      specified disorder NEC E71.518
      Zellweger syndrome E71.510
    rhizomelic chondrodysplasia punctata E71.540
    specified form NEC E71.548
      group 1 E71.518
      group 2 E71.53
      group 3 E71.542
    X-linked adrenoleukodystrophy E71.529
      adolescent E71.521
      adrenomyeloneuropathy E71.522
      childhood E71.520
      specified form NEC E71.528
    Zellweger-like syndrome E71.541
  persistent
    (somatoform) pain F45.41
    affective (mood) F34.9
  personality —*see also* Personality F60.9
    affective F34.0
    aggressive F60.3
    amoral F60.2
    anankastic F60.5
    antisocial F60.2
    anxious F60.6
    asocial F60.2
    asthenic F60.7
    avoidant F60.6
    borderline F60.3
    change (secondary) due to general medical condition F07.0
    compulsive F60.5
    cyclothymic F34.0
    dependent (passive) F60.7
    depressive F34.1
    dissocial F60.2
    emotional instability F60.3
    expansive paranoid F60.0
    explosive F60.3
    following organic brain damage F07.9
    histrionic F60.4
    hyperthymic F34.0
    hypothymic F34.1
    hysterical F60.4
    immature F60.89
    inadequate F60.7
    labile F60.3
    mixed (nonspecific) F60.89
    moral deficiency F60.2
    narcissistic F60.81
    negativistic F60.89
    obsessional F60.5
    obsessive (-compulsive) F60.5
    organic F07.9
    overconscientious F60.5
    paranoid F60.0
    passive (-dependent) F60.7
    passive-aggressive F60.89
    pathological NEC F60.9
    pseudosocial F60.2
    psychopathic F60.2
    schizoid F60.1
    schizotypal F21
    self-defeating F60.7
    specified NEC F60.89
    type A F60.5
    unstable (emotional) F60.3
  pervasive, developmental F84.9
  phencyclidine use
    mild F16.10
      with
        phencyclidine-induced
          anxiety disorder F16.180
          bipolar and related disorder F16.14
          depressive disorder F16.14
          psychotic disorder F16.159

Disorder *(Continued)*
  phencyclidine use *(Continued)*
    mild *(Continued)*
      with *(Continued)*
        phencyclidine intoxication F16.129
        phencyclidine intoxication delirium F16.121
      in remission (early) (sustained) F16.11
    moderate or severe F16.20
      with
        phencyclidine-induced
          anxiety disorder F16.280
          bipolar and related disorder F16.24
          depressive disorder F16.24
          psychotic disorder F16.259
        phencyclidine intoxication F16.229
        phencyclidine intoxication delirium F16.221
      in remission (early) (sustained) F16.21
  phobic anxiety, childhood F40.8
  phosphate-losing tubular N25.0
  pigmentation L81.9
    choroid, congenital Q14.3
    diminished melanin formation L81.6
    iron L81.8
    specified NEC L81.8
  pinna (noninfective) H61.10-●
    deformity, acquired H61.11-●
    hematoma H61.12-●
    perichondritis —*see* Perichondritis, ear
    specified type NEC H61.19-●
  pituitary gland E23.7
    iatrogenic (postprocedural) E89.3
    specified NEC E23.6
  platelets D69.1
  plexus G54.9
    specified NEC G54.8
  polymorphonuclear neutrophils D71
  porphyrin metabolism —*see* Porphyria
  postconcussional F07.81
  posthallucinogen perception F16.983
    in
      abuse F16.183
      dependence F16.283
  postmenopausal N95.9
    specified NEC N95.8
  postprocedural (postoperative) —*see* Complications, postprocedural
  post-transplant lymphoproliferative D47.z1
  post-traumatic stress (PTSD) F43.10
    acute F43.11
    chronic F43.12
  premenstrual dysphoric (PMDD) F32.81
  prepuce N47.8
  propionic acidemia E71.121
  prostate N42.9
    specified NEC N42.89
  psychogenic NOS —*see also* condition F45.9
    anxiety F41.8
    appetite F50.9
    asthenic F48.8
    cardiovascular (system) F45.8
    compulsive F42.8
    cutaneous F54
    depressive F32.9
    digestive (system) F45.8
    dysmenorrheic F45.8
    dyspneic F45.8
    endocrine (system) F54
    eye NEC F45.8
    feeding —*see* Disorder, eating
    functional NEC F45.8
    gastric F45.8
    gastrointestinal (system) F45.8
    genitourinary (system) F45.8
    heart (function) (rhythm) F45.8
    hyperventilatory F45.8
    hypochondriacal —*see* Disorder, hypochondriacal
    intestinal F45.8
    joint F45.8

Disorder *(Continued)*
  psychogenic NOS *(Continued)*
    learning F81.9
    limb F45.8
    lymphatic (system) F45.8
    menstrual F45.8
    micturition F45.8
    monoplegic NEC F44.4
    motor F44.4
    muscle F45.8
    musculoskeletal F45.8
    neurocirculatory F45.8
    obsessive F42.8
    occupational F48.8
    organ or part of body NEC F45.8
    paralytic NEC F44.4
    phobic F40.9
    physical NEC F45.8
    rectal F45.8
    respiratory (system) F45.8
    rheumatic F45.8
    sexual (function) F52.9
    skin (allergic) (eczematous) F54
    sleep F51.9
    specified part of body NEC F45.8
    stomach F45.8
  psychological F99
    associated with
      disease classified elsewhere F54
      sexual
        development F66
        relationship F66
      uncertainty about gender identity F64.9
  psychomotor NEC F44.4
    hysterical F44.4
  psychoneurotic —*see also* Neurosis
    mixed NEC F48.8
  psychophysiologic —*see* Disorder, somatoform
  psychosexual F65.9
    development F66
    identity of childhood F64.2
  psychosomatic NOS —*see* Disorder, somatoform
    multiple F45.0
    undifferentiated F45.1
  psychotic —*see* Psychosis
    transient (acute) F23
  puberty E30.9
    specified NEC E30.8
  pulmonary (valve) —*see* Endocarditis, pulmonary
  purine metabolism E79.9
  pyrimidine metabolism E79.9
  pyruvate metabolism E74.4
  reactive attachment (childhood) F94.1
  reading R48.0
    developmental (specific) F81.0
  receptive language F80.2
  receptor, hormonal, peripheral —*see also* Syndrome, androgen insensitivity E34.50
  recurrent brief depressive F33.8
  reflex R29.2
  refraction H52.7
    aniseikonia H52.32
    anisometropia H52.31
    astigmatism —*see* Astigmatism
    hypermetropia —*see* Hypermetropia
    myopia —*see* Myopia
    presbyopia H52.4
    specified NEC H52.6
  relationship F68.8
    due to sexual orientation F66
  REM sleep behavior G47.52
  renal function, impaired (tubular) N25.9
  resonance R49.9
    specified NEC R49.8
  respiratory function, impaired —*see also* Failure, respiration
    postprocedural —*see* Complication, postoperative, respiratory system
    psychogenic F45.8

Disorder *(Continued)*
  retina H35.9
    angioid streaks H35.33
    changes in vascular appearance H35.01-●
    degeneration —*see* Degeneration, retina
    dystrophy (hereditary) —*see* Dystrophy,
        retina
    edema H35.81
    hemorrhage —*see* Hemorrhage, retina
    ischemia H35.82
    macular degeneration —*see* Degeneration,
        macula
    microaneurysms H35.04-●
    microvascular abnormality NEC H35.09
    neovascularization —*see*
        Neovascularization, retina
    retinopathy —*see* Retinopathy
    separation of layers H35.70
      central serous chorioretinopathy H35.71-●
      pigment epithelium detachment (serous)
          H35.72-●
        hemorrhagic H35.73-●
    specified type NEC H35.89
    telangiectasis —*see* Telangiectasis, retina
    vasculitis —*see* Vasculitis, retina
  retroperitoneal K68.9
  right hemisphere organic affective F07.89
  rumination (infant or child) F98.21
  sacrum, sacrococcygeal NEC M53.3
  schizoaffective F25.9
    bipolar type F25.0
    depressive type F25.1
    manic type F25.0
    mixed type F25.0
    specified NEC F25.8
  schizoid of childhood F84.5
  schizophrenia spectrum and other psychotic
      disorder F29
    specified NEC F28
  schizophreniform F20.81
    brief F23
  schizotypal (personality) F21
  secretion, thyrocalcitonin E07.0
  sedative, hypnotic, or anxiolytic use
    mild F13.10
      with
        sedative, hypnotic, or
            anxiolytic-induced
          anxiety disorder F13.180
          bipolar and related disorder F13.14
          depressive disorder F13.14
          psychotic disorder F13.159
          sexual dysfunction F13.181
          sedative, hypnotic, or anxiolytic
              intoxication F13.129
          sedative, hypnotic, or anxiolytic
              intoxication delirium F13.121
      in remission (early) (sustained) F13.11
    moderate or severe F13.20
      with
        sedative, hypnotic, or
            anxiolytic-induced
          anxiety disorder F13.280
          bipolar and related disorder F13.24
          depressive disorder F13.24
          major neurocognitive disorder
              F13.27
          mild neurocognitive disorder
              F13.288
          psychotic disorder F13.259
          sexual dysfunction F13.281
          sedative, hypnotic, or anxiolytic
              intoxication F13.229
          sedative, hypnotic, or anxiolytic
              intoxication delirium F13.221
      in remission (early) (sustained) F13.21
  seizure —*see also* Epilepsy G40.909
    intractable G40.919
      with status epilepticus G40.911
  semantic pragmatic F80.89
    with autism F84.0

Disorder *(Continued)*
  sense of smell R43.1
    psychogenic F45.8
  separation anxiety, of childhood F93.0
  sexual
    arousal, female F52.22
    aversion F52.1
    function, psychogenic F52.9
    interest/arousal, female F52.22
    masochism F65.51
    maturation F66
    nonorganic F52.9
    preference —*see also* Deviation, sexual
        F65.9
      fetishistic transvestism F65.1
    relationship F66
    sadism F65.52
  shyness, of childhood and adolescence F40.10
  sibling rivalry F93.8
  sickle-cell (sickling) (homozygous) —*see*
      Disease, sickle-cell
    heterozygous D57.3
    specified type NEC D57.8-●
    trait D57.3
  sinus (nasal) J34.9
    specified NEC J34.89
  skin L98.9
    atrophic L90.9
      specified NEC L90.8
    granulomatous L92.9
      specified NEC L92.8
    hypertrophic L91.9
      specified NEC L91.8
    infiltrative NEC L98.6
    newborn P83.9
      specified NEC P83.88
    picking F42.4
    psychogenic (allergic) (eczematous) F54
  sleep G47.9
    breathing-related —*see* Apnea, sleep
    circadian rhythm G47.20
      advance sleep phase type G47.22
      delayed sleep phase type G47.21
      due to
        alcohol
          abuse F10.182
          dependence F10.282
          use F10.982
        amphetamines
          abuse F15.182
          dependence F15.282
          use F15.982
        caffeine
          abuse F15.182
          dependence F15.282
          use F15.982
        cocaine
          abuse F14.182
          dependence F14.282
          use F14.982
        drug NEC
          abuse F19.182
          dependence F19.282
          use F19.982
        opioid
          abuse F11.182
          dependence F11.282
          use F11.982
        psychoactive substance NEC
          abuse F19.182
          dependence F19.282
          use F19.982
        sedative, hypnotic, or anxiolytic
          abuse F13.182
          dependence F13.282
          use F13.982
        stimulant NEC
          abuse F15.182
          dependence F15.282
          use F15.982
      free running type G47.24

Disorder *(Continued)*
  sleep *(Continued)*
    circadian rhythm *(Continued)*
      in conditions classified elsewhere
          G47.27
      irregular sleep wake type G47.23
      jet lag type G47.25
      non-24-hour sleep-wake type G47.24
      shift work type G47.26
      specified NEC G47.29
    due to
      alcohol
        abuse F10.182
        dependence F10.282
        use F10.982
      amphetamine
        abuse F15.182
        dependence F15.282
        use F15.982
      anxiolytic
        abuse F13.182
        dependence F13.282
        use F13.982
      caffeine
        abuse F15.182
        dependence F15.282
        use F15.982
      cocaine
        abuse F14.182
        dependence F14.282
        use F14.982
      drug NEC
        abuse F19.182
        dependence F19.282
        use F19.982
      hypnotic
        abuse F13.182
        dependence F13.282
        use F13.982
      opioid
        abuse F11.182
        dependence F11.282
        use F11.982
      psychoactive substance NEC
        abuse F19.182
        dependence F19.282
        use F19.982
      sedative
        abuse F13.182
        dependence F13.282
        use F13.982
      stimulant NEC
        abuse F15.182
        dependence F15.282
        use F15.982
    emotional F51.9
    excessive somnolence —*see* Hypersomnia
    hypersomnia type —*see* Hypersomnia
    initiating or maintaining —*see* Insomnia
    nightmares F51.5
    nonorganic F51.9
      specified NEC F51.8
    parasomnia type G47.50
    specified NEC G47.8
    terrors F51.4
    walking F51.3
  sleep-wake pattern or schedule —*see also*
      Disorder, sleep, circadian rhythm G47.9
    specified NEC G47.8
  social
    anxiety (of childhood) F40.10
      generalized F40.11
    functioning in childhood F94.9
      specified NEC F94.8
    pragmatic F80.82
  soft tissue M79.9
    ankle M79.9
    due to use, overuse and pressure M70.90
      ankle M70.97-●
      bursitis —*see* Bursitis
      foot M70.97-●

▶ New   ⇒ Revised   ~~deleted~~ Deleted   ● Use Additional Character(s)

Disorder *(Continued)*
  soft tissue *(Continued)*
    due to use, overuse and pressure
      (Continued)
      forearm M70.93-●
      hand M70.94-●
      lower leg M70.96-●
      multiple sites M70.99
      pelvic region M70.95-●
      shoulder region M70.91-●
      specified site NEC M70.98
      specified type NEC M70.80
        ankle M70.87-●
        foot M70.87-●
        forearm M70.83-●
        hand M70.84-●
        lower leg M70.86-●
        multiple sites M70.89
        pelvic region M70.85-●
        shoulder region M70.81-●
        specified site NEC M70.88
        thigh M70.85-●
        upper arm M70.82-●
      thigh M70.95-●
      upper arm M70.92-●
    foot M79.9
    forearm M79.9
    hand M79.9
    lower leg M79.9
    multiple sites M79.9
    occupational —*see* Disorder, soft tissue,
      due to use, overuse and pressure
    pelvic region M79.9
    shoulder region M79.9
    specified type NEC M79.89
    thigh M79.9
    upper arm M79.9
  somatic symptom F45.1
  somatization F45.0
  somatoform F45.9
    pain (persistent) F45.41
    somatization (multiple) (long-lasting)
      F45.0
    specified NEC F45.8
    undifferentiated F45.1
  somnolence, excessive —*see* Hypersomnia
  specific
    arithmetical F81.2
    developmental, of motor F82
    reading F81.0
    speech and language F80.9
    spelling F81.81
    written expression F81.81
  speech R47.9
    articulation (functional) (specific) F80.0
    developmental F80.9
    specified NEC R47.89
  speech-sound F80.0
  spelling (specific) F81.81
  spine —*see also* Dorsopathy
    ligamentous or muscular attachments,
      peripheral —*see* Enthesopathy, spinal
    specified NEC —*see* Dorsopathy, specified
      NEC
  stereotyped, habit or movement F98.4
  stimulant use (other) (unspecified)
    mild F15.10
      in remission (early) (sustained) F15.11
    moderate or severe F15.20
      in remission (early) (sustained) F15.21
  stomach (functional) —*see* Disorder, gastric
  stress F43.9
    acute F43.0
    post-traumatic F43.10
      acute F43.11
      chronic F43.12
  substance use (other) (unknown)
    mild F19.10
      with substance-induced
        anxiety disorder F19.180
        bipolar and related disorder F19.14

Disorder *(Continued)*
  substance use (other) (unknown) *(Continued)*
    mild *(Continued)*
      with substance-induced*(Continued)*
        depressive disorder F19.14
        major neurocognitive disorder F19.17
        mild neurocognitive disorder F19.188
        obsessive-compulsive and related
          disorder F19.188
        sexual dysfunction F19.181
      substance intoxication F19.129
      substance intoxication delirium F19.121
    moderate or severe F19.20
      with substance-induced
        anxiety disorder F19.280
        bipolar and related disorder F19.24
        depressive disorder F19.24
        major neurocognitive disorder F19.27
        mild neurocognitive disorder F19.288
        obsessive-compulsive and related
          disorder F19.288
        sexual dysfunction F19.281
      in remission (early) (sustained) F19.21
      substance intoxication F19.229
      substance intoxication delirium F19.221
  sulfur-bearing amino-acid metabolism
    E72.10
  sweat gland (eccrine) L74.9
    apocrine L75.9
      specified NEC L75.8
    specified NEC L74.8
  synovium M67.90
    acromioclavicular M67.91-●
    ankle M67.97-●
    elbow M67.92-●
    foot M67.97-●
    forearm M67.93-●
    hand M67.94-●
    hip M67.95-●
    knee M67.96-●
    multiple sites M67.99
    rupture —*see* Rupture, synovium
    shoulder M67.91-●
    specified type NEC M67.80
      acromioclavicular M67.81-●
      ankle M67.87-●
      elbow M67.82-●
      foot M67.87-●
      hand M67.84-●
      hip M67.85-●
      knee M67.86-●
      multiple sites M67.89
      wrist M67.83-●
    synovitis —*see* Synovitis
    upper arm M67.92-●
    wrist M67.93-●
  temperature regulation, newborn P81.9
    specified NEC P81.8
  temporomandibular joint M26.60-●
  tendon M67.90
    acromioclavicular M67.91-●
    ankle M67.97-●
    contracture —*see* Contracture, tendon
    elbow M67.92-●
    foot M67.97-●
    forearm M67.93-●
    hand M67.94-●
    hip M67.95-●
    knee M67.96-●
    multiple sites M67.99
    rupture —*see* Rupture, tendon
    shoulder M67.91-●
    specified type NEC M67.80
      acromioclavicular M67.81-●
      ankle M67.87-●
      elbow M67.82-●
      foot M67.87-●
      hand M67.84-●
      hip M67.85-●
      knee M67.86-●
      multiple sites M67.89

Disorder *(Continued)*
  tendon *(Continued)*
    specified type NEC *(Continued)*
      trunk M67.88
      wrist M67.83-●
    synovitis —*see* Synovitis
    tendinitis —*see* Tendinitis
    tenosynovitis —*see* Tenosynovitis
    trunk M67.98
    upper arm M67.92-●
    wrist M67.93-●
  thoracic root (nerve) NEC G54.3
  thyrocalcitonin hypersecretion E07.0
  thyroid (gland) E07.9
    function NEC, neonatal, transitory P72.2
    iodine-deficiency related E01.8
    specified NEC E07.89
  tic —*see* Tic
  tobacco use
    chewing tobacco (mild) (moderate) (severe)
      in remission (early) (sustained) F17.221
    cigarettes (mild) (moderate) (severe)
      in remission (early) (sustained) F17.211
    mild F17.200
      in remission (early) (sustained) F17.201
    moderate F17.200
      in remission (early) (sustained) F17.201
    severe F17.200
      in remission (early) (sustained) F17.201
    specified product NEC (mild) (moderate)
      (severe)
      in remission (early) (sustained) F17.291
  tooth K08.9
    development K00.9
      specified NEC K00.8
    eruption K00.6
  Tourette's F95.2
  trance and possession F44.89
  transvestic F65.1
  trauma and stressor-related F43.9
    other specified F43.8
  tricuspid (valve) —*see* Endocarditis, tricuspid
  tryptophan metabolism E70.5
  tubular, phosphate-losing N25.0
  tubulo-interstitial (in)
    brucellosis A23.9 *[N16]*
    cystinosis E72.04
    diphtheria A36.84
    glycogen storage disease E74.00 *[N16]*
    leukemia NEC C95.9-● *[N16]*
    lymphoma NEC C85.9-● *[N16]*
    mixed cryoglobulinemia D89.1 *[N16]*
    multiple myeloma C90.0-● *[N16]*
    Salmonella infection A02.25
    sarcoidosis D86.84
    sepsis A41.9 *[N16]*
      streptococcal A40.9 *[N16]*
    systemic lupus erythematosus M32.15
    toxoplasmosis B58.83
    transplant rejection T86.91 *[N16]*
    Wilson's disease E83.01 *[N16]*
  tubulo-renal function, impaired N25.9
    specified NEC N25.89
  tympanic membrane H73.9-●
    atrophy —*see* Atrophy, tympanic membrane
    infection —*see* Myringitis
    perforation —*see* Perforation, tympanum
    specified NEC H73.89-●
  unsocialized aggressive F91.1
  urea cycle metabolism E72.20
    argininemia E72.21
    arginosuccinic aciduria E72.22
    citrullinemia E72.23
    ornithine transcarbamylase deficiency
      E72.4
    other specified E72.29
  ureter (in) N28.9
    schistosomiasis B65.0 *[N29]*
    tuberculosis A18.11
  urethra N36.9
    specified NEC N36.8

Disorder (Continued)
 urinary system N39.9
  specified NEC N39.8
 valve, heart
  aortic —see Endocarditis, aortic
  mitral —see Endocarditis, mitral
  pulmonary —see Endocarditis, pulmonary
  rheumatic
   aortic —see Endocarditis, aortic,
    rheumatic
   mitral —see Endocarditis, mitral
   pulmonary —see Endocarditis,
    pulmonary, rheumatic
   tricuspid —see Endocarditis, tricuspid
  tricuspid —see Endocarditis, tricuspid
 vestibular function H81.9-●
  specified NEC —see subcategory H81.8
   in diseases classified elsewhere H82.-●
  vertigo —see Vertigo
 vision, binocular H53.30
  abnormal retinal correspondence H53.31
  diplopia H53.2
  fusion with defective stereopsis H53.32
  simultaneous perception H53.33
  suppression H53.34
 visual
  cortex
   blindness H47.619
    left brain H47.612
    right brain H47.611
   due to
    inflammatory disorder H47.629
     left brain H47.622
     right brain H47.621
    neoplasm H47.639
     left brain H47.632
     right brain H47.631
    vascular disorder H47.649
     left brain H47.642
     right brain H47.641
  pathway H47.9
   due to
    inflammatory disorder H47.51-●
    neoplasm H47.52-●
    vascular disorder H47.53-●
   optic chiasm —see Disorder, optic,
    chiasm
 vitreous body H43.9
  crystalline deposits —see Deposit,
   crystalline
  degeneration —see Degeneration, vitreous
  hemorrhage —see Hemorrhage, vitreous
  opacities —see Opacity, vitreous
  prolapse —see Prolapse, vitreous
  specified type NEC H43.89
 voice R49.9
  specified type NEC R49.8
 volatile solvent use
  due to drug abuse —see Abuse, drug,
   inhalant
  due to drug dependence —see Dependence,
   drug, inhalant
 voyeuristic F65.3
 white blood cells D72.9
  specified NEC D72.89
 withdrawing, child or adolescent
  F40.10
Disorientation R41.0
Displacement, displaced
 acquired traumatic of bone, cartilage, joint,
  tendon NEC —see Dislocation
 adrenal gland (congenital) Q89.1
 appendix, retrocecal (congenital) Q43.8
 auricle (congenital) Q17.4
 bladder (acquired) N32.89
  congenital Q64.19
 brachial plexus (congenital) Q07.8
 brain stem, caudal (congenital) Q04.8
 canaliculus (lacrimalis), congenital Q10.6
 cardia through esophageal hiatus (congenital)
  Q40.1

Displacement, displaced (Continued)
 cerebellum, caudal (congenital) Q04.8
 cervix —see Malposition, uterus
 colon (congenital) Q43.3
 device, implant or graft —see also
  Complications, by site and type,
  mechanical T85.628
  arterial graft NEC —see Complication,
   cardiovascular device, mechanical,
   vascular
  breast (implant) T85.42
  catheter NEC T85.628
   dialysis (renal) T82.42
    intraperitoneal T85.621
   infusion NEC T82.524
    spinal (epidural) (subdural) T85.620
   urinary
    cystostomy T83.020
    Hopkins T83.028
    ileostomy T83.028
    indwelling T83.021
    nephrostomy T83.022
    specified NEC T83.028
    urostomy T83.028
  electronic (electrode) (pulse generator)
   (stimulator) —see Complication,
   electronic stimulator
  fixation, internal (orthopedic) NEC —
   see Complication, fixation device,
   mechanical
  gastrointestinal —see Complications,
   prosthetic device, mechanical,
   gastrointestinal device
  genital NEC T83.428
   intrauterine contraceptive device (string)
    T83.32
   penile prosthesis (cylinder) (implanted)
    (pump) (resevoir) T83.420
   testicular prosthesis T83.421
  heart NEC —see Complication,
   cardiovascular device, mechanical
  joint prosthesis —see Complications, joint
   prosthesis, mechanical
  ocular —see Complications, prosthetic
   device, mechanical, ocular device
  orthopedic NEC —see Complication,
   orthopedic, device or graft,
   mechanical
  specified NEC T85.628
  urinary NEC T83.128
   graft T83.22
   sphincter, implanted T83.121
   stent (ileal conduit) (nephroureteral)
    T83.123
   ureteral indwelling T83.122
  vascular NEC —see Complication,
   cardiovascular device, mechanical
  ventricular intracranial shunt T85.02
 electronic stimulator
  bone T84.320
  cardiac —see Complications, cardiac
   device, electronic
  nervous system —see Complication,
   prosthetic device, mechanical,
   electronic nervous system
   stimulator
  urinary —see Complications, electronic
   stimulator, urinary
 esophageal mucosa into cardia of stomach,
  congenital Q39.8
 � esophagus (acquired) K22.89
  congenital Q39.8
 eyeball (acquired) (lateral) (old) —see
  Displacement, globe
  congenital Q15.8
  current —see Avulsion, eye
 fallopian tube (acquired) N83.4-●
  congenital Q50.6
  opening (congenital) Q50.6
 gallbladder (congenital) Q44.1
 gastric mucosa (congenital) Q40.2

Displacement, displaced (Continued)
 globe (acquired) (old) (lateral) H05.21-●
  current —see Avulsion, eye
 heart (congenital) Q24.8
  acquired I51.89
 hymen (upward) (congenital) Q52.4
 intervertebral disc NEC
  with myelopathy —see Disorder, disc, with,
   myelopathy
  cervical, cervicothoracic (with)
   M50.20
   myelopathy —see Disorder, disc,
    cervical, with myelopathy
   neuritis, radiculitis or radiculopathy —
    see Disorder, disc, cervical, with
    neuritis
  due to trauma —see Dislocation, vertebra
  lumbar region M51.26
   with
    neuritis, radiculitis, radiculopathy or
     sciatica M51.16
  lumbosacral region M51.27
   with
    myelopathy M51.07
    neuritis, radiculitis, radiculopathy or
     sciatica M51.17
  sacrococcygeal region M53.3
  thoracic region M51.24
   with
    myelopathy M51.04
    neuritis, radiculitis, radiculopathy
     M51.14
  thoracolumbar region M51.25
   with
    myelopathy M51.05
    neuritis, radiculitis, radiculopathy
     M51.15
 intrauterine device (string) T83.32
 kidney (acquired) N28.83
  congenital Q63.2
 lachrymal, lacrimal apparatus or duct
  (congenital) Q10.6
 lens, congenital Q12.1
 macula (congenital) Q14.1
 Meckel's diverticulum Q43.0
  malignant —see Table of Neoplasms, small
   intestine, malignant
 nail (congenital) Q84.6
  acquired L60.8
 opening of Wharton's duct in mouth Q38.4
 organ or site, congenital NEC —see
  Malposition, congenital
 ovary (acquired) N83.4-●
  congenital Q50.39
  free in peritoneal cavity (congenital)
   Q50.39
  into hernial sac N83.4-●
 oviduct (acquired) N83.4-●
  congenital Q50.6
 parathyroid (gland) E21.4
 parotid gland (congenital) Q38.4
 punctum lacrimale (congenital) Q10.6
 sacro-iliac (joint) (congenital) Q74.2
  current injury S33.2
  old —see subcategory M53.2
 salivary gland (any) (congenital) Q38.4
 spleen (congenital) Q89.09
 stomach, congenital Q40.2
 sublingual duct Q38.4
 tongue (downward) (congenital) Q38.3
 tooth, teeth, fully erupted M26.30
  horizontal M26.33
  vertical M26.34
 trachea (congenital) Q32.1
 ureter or ureteric opening or orifice
  (congenital) Q62.62
 uterine opening of oviducts or fallopian tubes
  Q50.6
 uterus, uterine —see Malposition, uterus
 ventricular septum Q21.0
  with rudimentary ventricle Q20.4

Disproportion
  between native and reconstructed breast
      N65.1
  fiber-type G71.20
      congenital G71.29
Disruptio uteri —*see* Rupture, uterus
Disruption (of)
  ciliary body NEC H21.89
  closure of
      cornea T81.31
      craniotomy T81.32
      fascia (muscular) (superficial) T81.32
      internal organ or tissue T81.32
      laceration (external) (internal) T81.33
      ligament T81.32
      mucosa T81.31
      muscle or muscle flap T81.32
      ribs or rib cage T81.32
      skin and subcutaneous tissue (full-
          thickness) (superficial) T81.31
      skull T81.32
      sternum (sternotomy) T81.32
      tendon T81.32
      traumatic laceration (external) (internal)
          T81.33
  family Z63.8
      due to
          absence of family member due to
              military deployment Z63.31
          absence of family member NEC
              Z63.32
          alcoholism and drug addiction in
              family Z63.72
          bereavement Z63.4
          death (assumed) or disappearance of
              family member Z63.4
          divorce or separation Z63.5
          drug addiction in family Z63.72
          return of family member from military
              deployment (current or past
              conflict) Z63.71
          stressful life events NEC Z63.79
  iris NEC H21.89
  ligament(s) —*see also* Sprain
      knee
          current injury —*see* Dislocation, knee
          old (chronic) —*see* Derangement, knee,
              ligament, instability, chronic
          spontaneous NEC —*see* Derangement,
              knee, disruption ligament
  ossicular chain —*see* Discontinuity, ossicles,
      ear
  pelvic ring (stable) S32.810
      unstable S32.811
  traumatic injury wound repair T81.33
  wound T81.30
      episiotomy O90.1
      operation T81.31
          cesarean O90.0
          external operation wound (superficial)
              T81.31
          internal operation wound (deep)
              T81.32
      perineal (obstetric) O90.1
  traumatic injury repair T81.33
Dissatisfaction with
  employment Z56.9
  school environment Z55.4
Dissecting —*see* condition
Dissection
  aorta I71.00
      abdominal I71.02
      thoracic I71.01
      thoracoabdominal I71.03
  artery I77.70
      basilar (trunk) I77.75
      carotid I77.71
      cerebral (nonruptured) I67.0
          ruptured —*see* Hemorrhage, intracranial,
              subarachnoid
      coronary I25.42

Dissection (Continued)
  artery (Continued)
      extremity
          lower I77.77
          upper I77.76
      iliac I77.72
      precerebral
          congenital (nonruptured) Q28.1
          specified site NEC I77.75
      renal I77.73
      specified NEC I77.79
      vertebral I77.74
  precerebral artery, congenital (nonruptured)
      Q28.1
      Heartland A93.8
  traumatic —*see* Wound, open, by site
  vascular I99.8
  wound —*see* Wound, open
Disseminated —*see* condition
Dissociation
  auriculoventricular or atrioventricular (AV)
      (any degree) (isorhythmic) I45.89
      with heart block I44.2
  interference I45.89
Dissociative reaction, state F44.9
Dissolution, vertebra —*see* Osteoporosis
Distension, distention
  abdomen R14.0
  bladder N32.89
  cecum K63.89
  colon K63.89
  gallbladder K82.8
  intestine K63.89
  kidney N28.89
  liver K76.89
  seminal vesicle N50.89
  stomach K31.89
      acute K31.0
      psychogenic F45.8
  ureter —*see* Dilatation, ureter
  uterus N85.8
Distoma hepaticum infestation B66.3
Distomiasis B66.9
  bile passages B66.3
  hemic B65.9
  hepatic B66.3
      due to Clonorchis sinensis B66.1
  intestinal B66.5
  liver B66.3
      due to Clonorchis sinensis B66.1
  lung B66.4
  pulmonary B66.4
Distomolar (fourth molar) K00.1
Disto-occlusion (Division I) (Division II)
      M26.212
Distortion(s) (congenital)
  adrenal (gland) Q89.1
  arm NEC Q68.8
  bile duct or passage Q44.5
  bladder Q64.79
  brain Q04.9
  cervix (uteri) Q51.9
  chest (wall) Q67.8
      bones Q76.8
  clavicle Q74.0
  clitoris Q52.6
  coccyx Q76.49
  common duct Q44.5
  coronary Q24.5
  cystic duct Q44.5
  ear (auricle) (external) Q17.3
      inner Q16.5
      middle Q16.4
          ossicles Q16.3
  endocrine NEC Q89.2
  eustachian tube Q17.8
  eye (adnexa) Q15.8
  face bone(s) NEC Q75.8
  fallopian tube Q50.6
  femur NEC Q68.8
  fibula NEC Q68.8

Distortion (Continued)
  finger(s) Q68.1
  foot Q66.9-•
  genitalia, genital organ(s)
      female Q52.8
          external Q52.79
          internal NEC Q52.8
  gyri Q04.8
  hand bone(s) Q68.1
  heart (auricle) (ventricle) Q24.8
      valve (cusp) Q24.8
  hepatic duct Q44.5
  humerus NEC Q68.8
  hymen Q52.4
  intrafamilial communications Z63.8
  jaw NEC M26.89
  labium (majus) (minus) Q52.79
  leg NEC Q68.8
  lens Q12.8
  liver Q44.7
  lumbar spine Q76.49
      with disproportion O33.8
          causing obstructed labor O65.0
  lumbosacral (joint) (region) Q76.49
      kyphosis —*see* Kyphosis, congenital
      lordosis —*see* Lordosis, congenital
  nerve Q07.8
  nose Q30.8
  organ
      of Corti Q16.5
      or site not listed —*see* Anomaly, by site
          ossicles, ear Q16.3
  oviduct Q50.6
  pancreas Q45.3
  parathyroid (gland) Q89.2
  pituitary (gland) Q89.2
  radius NEC Q68.8
  sacroiliac joint Q74.2
  sacrum Q76.49
  scapula Q74.0
  shoulder girdle Q74.0
  skull bone(s) NEC Q75.8
      with
          anencephalus Q00.0
          encephalocele —*see* Encephalocele
          hydrocephalus Q03.9
              with spina bifida —*see* Spina bifida,
                  with hydrocephalus
          microcephaly Q02
  spinal cord Q06.8
  spine Q76.49
      kyphosis —*see* Kyphosis, congenital
      lordosis —*see* Lordosis, congenital
  spleen Q89.09
  sternum NEC Q76.7
  thorax (wall) Q67.8
      bony Q76.8
  thymus (gland) Q89.2
  thyroid (gland) Q89.2
  tibia NEC Q68.8
  toe(s) Q66.9-•
  tongue Q38.3
  trachea (cartilage) Q32.1
  ulna NEC Q68.8
  ureter Q62.8
  urethra Q64.79
      causing obstruction Q64.39
  uterus Q51.9
  vagina Q52.4
  vertebra Q76.49
      kyphosis —*see* Kyphosis, congenital
      lordosis —*see* Lordosis, congenital
  visual —*see also* Disturbance, vision
      shape and size H53.15
  vulva Q52.79
  wrist (bones) (joint) Q68.8
Distress
  abdomen —*see* Pain, abdominal
  acute respiratory R06.03
      syndrome (adult) (child) J80
  epigastric R10.13

Distress *(Continued)*
  fetal P84
    complicating pregnancy —*see* Stress, fetal
  gastrointestinal (functional) K30
    psychogenic F45.8
  intestinal (functional) NOS K59.9
    psychogenic F45.8
  maternal, during labor and delivery O75.0
  relationship, with spouse or intimate partner
      Z63.0
  respiratory (adult) (child) R06.03
    newborn P22.9
      specified NEC P22.8
    orthopnea R06.01
    psychogenic F45.8
    shortness of breath R06.02
    specified type NEC R06.09
Distribution vessel, atypical Q27.9
  coronary artery Q24.5
  precerebral Q28.1
Districhiasis L68.8
Disturbance(s) —*see also* Disease
  absorption K90.9
    calcium E58
    carbohydrate K90.49
    fat K90.49
      pancreatic K90.3
    protein K90.49
    starch K90.49
    vitamin —*see* Deficiency, vitamin
  acid-base equilibrium E87.8
    mixed E87.4
  activity and attention (with hyperkinesis) —
      see Disorder, attention-deficit
      hyperactivity
  amino acid transport E72.00
  assimilation, food K90.9
  auditory nerve, except deafness —*see*
      subcategory H93.3
  behavior —*see* Disorder, conduct
  blood clotting (mechanism) —*see also* Defect,
      coagulation D68.9
  cerebral
    nerve —*see* Disorder, nerve, cranial
    status, newborn P91.9
      specified NEC P91.88
  circulatory I99.9
  conduct —*see also* Disorder, conduct F91.9
    adjustment reaction —*see* Disorder,
        adjustment
    compulsive F63.9
    disruptive F91.9
    hyperkinetic —*see* Disorder, attention-
        deficit hyperactivity
    socialized F91.2
    specified NEC F91.8
    unsocialized F91.1
  coordination R27.8
  cranial nerve —*see* Disorder, nerve, cranial
  deep sensibility —*see* Disturbance, sensation
  digestive K30
    psychogenic F45.8
  electrolyte —*see also* Imbalance, electrolyte
    newborn, transitory P74.49
      hyperammonemia P74.6
      hyperchloremia P74.421
      hyperchloremic metabolic acidosis
          P74.421
      hypochloremia P74.422
      potassium balance
        hyperkalemia P74.31
        hypokalemia P74.32
      sodium balance
        hypernatremia P74.21
        hyponatremia P74.22
      specified type NEC P74.49
  emotions specific to childhood and
      adolescence F93.9
    with
      anxiety and fearfulness NEC F93.8
      elective mutism F94.0

Disturbance *(Continued)*
  emotions specific to childhood and
      adolescence *(Continued)*
    with *(Continued)*
      oppositional disorder F91.3
      sensitivity (withdrawal) F40.10
      shyness F40.10
      social withdrawal F40.10
    involving relationship problems F93.8
    mixed F93.8
    specified NEC F93.8
  endocrine (gland) E34.9
    neonatal, transitory P72.9
      specified NEC P72.8
  equilibrium R42
  fructose metabolism E74.10
  gait —*see* Gait
    hysterical F44.4
    psychogenic F44.4
  gastrointestinal (functional) K30
    psychogenic F45.8
  habit, child F98.9
  hearing, except deafness and tinnitus —*see*
      Abnormal, auditory perception
  heart, functional (conditions in I44-I50)
    due to presence of (cardiac) prosthesis
        I97.19-●
    postoperative I97.89
      cardiac surgery —*see also* Infarct,
          myocardium, associated with
          revascularization procedure I97.19-●
  hormones E34.9
  innervation uterus (parasympathetic)
      (sympathetic) N85.8
  keratinization NEC
    gingiva K05.10
      nonplaque induced K05.11
      plaque induced K05.10
    lip K13.0
    oral (mucosa) (soft tissue) K13.29
    tongue K13.29
  learning (specific) —*see* Disorder, learning
  memory —*see* Amnesia
    mild, following organic brain damage F06.8
  mental F99
    associated with diseases classified
        elsewhere F54
  metabolism E88.9
    with
      abortion —*see* Abortion, by type with
          other specified complication
      ectopic pregnancy O08.5
      molar pregnancy O08.5
    amino-acid E72.9
      aromatic E70.9
      branched-chain E71.2
      straight-chain E72.89
      sulfur-bearing E72.10
    ammonia E72.20
    arginine E72.21
    arginosuccinic acid E72.22
    carbohydrate E74.9
    cholesterol E78.9
    citrulline E72.23
    cystathionine E72.19
    general E88.9
    glutamine E72.89
    histidine E70.40
    homocystine E72.19
    hydroxylysine E72.3
    in labor or delivery O75.89
    iron E83.10
    lipoid E78.9
    lysine E72.3
    methionine E72.19
    neonatal, transitory P74.9
      calcium and magnesium P71.9
        specified type NEC P71.8
      carbohydrate metabolism P70.9
        specified type NEC P70.8
      specified NEC P74.8

Disturbance *(Continued)*
  metabolism *(Continued)*
    ornithine E72.4
    phosphate E83.39
    sodium NEC E87.8
    threonine E72.89
    tryptophan E70.5
    tyrosine E70.20
    urea cycle E72.20
  motor R29.2
  nervous, functional R45.0
  neuromuscular mechanism (eye), due to
      syphilis A52.15
  nutritional E63.9
    nail L60.3
  ocular motion H51.9
    psychogenic F45.8
  oculogyric H51.8
    psychogenic F45.8
  oculomotor H51.9
    psychogenic F45.8
  olfactory nerve R43.1
  optic nerve NEC —*see* Disorder, nerve, optic
  oral epithelium, including tongue NEC
      K13.29
  perceptual due to
    alcohol withdrawal F10.232
    amphetamine intoxication F15.922
      in
        abuse F15.122
        dependence F15.222
    anxiolytic withdrawal F13.232
    cannabis intoxication (acute) F12.922
      in
        abuse F12.122
        dependence F12.222
    cocaine intoxication (acute) F14.922
      in
        abuse F14.122
        dependence F14.222
    hypnotic withdrawal F13.232
    opioid intoxication (acute) F11.922
      in
        abuse F11.122
        dependence F11.222
    phencyclidine intoxication (acute) F16.122
    sedative withdrawal F13.232
  personality (pattern) (trait) —*see also*
      Disorder, personality F60.9
    following organic brain damage F07.9
  polyglandular E31.9
    specified NEC E31.8
  potassium balance, newborn
    hyperkalemia P74.31
    hypokalemia P74.32
  psychogenic F45.9
  psychomotor F44.4
  psychophysical visual H53.16
  pupillary —*see* Anomaly, pupil, function
  reflex R29.2
  rhythm, heart I49.9
  salivary secretion K11.7
  sensation (cold) (heat) (localization) (tactile
      discrimination) (texture) (vibratory)
      NEC R20.9
    hysterical F44.6
    skin R20.9
      anesthesia R20.0
      hyperesthesia R20.3
      hypoesthesia R20.1
      paresthesia R20.2
      specified type NEC R20.8
    smell R43.9
      and taste (mixed) R43.8
      anosmia R43.0
      parosmia R43.1
      specified NEC R43.8
    taste R43.9
      and smell (mixed) R43.8
      parageusia R43.2
      specified NEC R43.8

▶ New   ⇒ Revised   ~~deleted~~ Deleted   ● Use Additional Character(s)

Disturbance *(Continued)*
  sensory —*see* Disturbance, sensation
  situational (transient) —*see also* Disorder,
      adjustment
    acute F43.0
  sleep G47.9
    nonorganic origin F51.9
  smell —*see* Disturbance, sensation, smell
  sociopathic F60.2
  sodium balance, newborn
    hypernatremia P74.21
    hyponatremia P74.22
  speech R47.9
    developmental F80.9
    specified NEC R47.89
  stomach (functional) K31.9
  sympathetic (nerve) G90.9
  taste —*see* Disturbance, sensation, taste
  temperature
    regulation, newborn P81.9
      specified NEC P81.8
    sense R20.8
      hysterical F44.6
  tooth
    eruption K00.6
    formation K00.4
    structure, hereditary NEC K00.5
  touch —*see* Disturbance, sensation
  vascular I99.9
    arteriosclerotic —*see* Arteriosclerosis
  vasomotor I73.9
  vasospastic I73.9
  vision, visual H53.9
    following
      cerebral infarction I69.398
      cerebrovascular disease I69.998
        specified NEC I69.898
      intracerebral hemorrhage I69.198
      nontraumatic intracranial hemorrhage
          NEC I69.298
      specified disease NEC I69.898
      subarachnoid hemorrhage I69.098
    psychophysical H53.16
    specified NEC H53.8
    subjective H53.10
      day blindness H53.11
      discomfort H53.14-●
      distortions of shape and size H53.15
      loss
        sudden H53.13-●
        transient H53.12-●
      specified type NEC H53.19
  voice R49.9
    psychogenic F44.4
    specified NEC R49.8
Diuresis R35.89
Diver's palsy, paralysis or squeeze T70.3
Diverticulitis (acute) K57.92
  bladder —*see* Cystitis
  ileum —*see* Diverticulitis, intestine, small
  intestine K57.92
    with
      abscess, perforation K57.80
        with bleeding K57.81
      bleeding K57.93
    congenital Q43.8
    large K57.32
      with
        abscess, perforation K57.20
          with bleeding K57.21
        bleeding K57.33
        small intestine K57.52
          with
            abscess, perforation K57.40
              with bleeding K57.41
            bleeding K57.53
    small K57.12
      with
        abscess, perforation K57.00
          with bleeding K57.01
        bleeding K57.13

Diverticulitis *(Continued)*
  intestine *(Continued)*
    small *(Continued)*
      with *(Continued)*
        large intestine K57.52
          with
            abscess, perforation K57.40
              with bleeding K57.41
            bleeding K57.53
Diverticulosis K57.90
  with bleeding K57.91
  large intestine K57.30
    with
      bleeding K57.31
      small intestine K57.50
        with bleeding K57.51
  small intestine K57.10
    with
      bleeding K57.11
      large intestine K57.50
        with bleeding K57.51
Diverticulum, diverticula (multiple) K57.90
  appendix (noninflammatory) K38.2
  bladder (sphincter) N32.3
    congenital Q64.6
  bronchus (congenital) Q32.4
    acquired J98.09
  calyx, calyceal (kidney) N28.89
  cardia (stomach) K31.4
  cecum —*see* Diverticulosis, intestine, large
    congenital Q43.8
  colon —*see* Diverticulosis, intestine, large
    congenital Q43.8
  duodenum —*see* Diverticulosis, intestine,
      small
    congenital Q43.8
  epiphrenic (esophagus) K22.5
  esophagus (congenital) Q39.6
    acquired (epiphrenic) (pulsion) (traction)
        K22.5
  eustachian tube —*see* Disorder, eustachian
      tube, specified NEC
  fallopian tube N83.8
  gastric K31.4
  heart (congenital) Q24.8
  ileum —*see* Diverticulosis, intestine, small
  jejunum —*see* Diverticulosis, intestine, small
  kidney (pelvis) (calyces) N28.89
    with calculus —*see* Calculus, kidney
  Meckel's (displaced) (hypertrophic) Q43.0
    malignant —*see* Table of Neoplasms, small
        intestine, malignant
  midthoracic K22.5
  organ or site, congenital NEC —*see* Distortion
  pericardium (congenital) (cyst) Q24.8
    acquired I31.8
  pharyngoesophageal (congenital) Q39.6
    acquired K22.5
  pharynx (congenital) Q38.7
  rectosigmoid —*see* Diverticulosis, intestine,
      large
    congenital Q43.8
  rectum —*see* Diverticulosis, intestine,
      large
    congenital Q43.8
  Rokitansky's K22.5
  seminal vesicle N50.89
  sigmoid —*see* Diverticulosis, intestine,
      large
    congenital Q43.8
  stomach (acquired) K31.4
    congenital Q40.2
  trachea (acquired) J39.8
  ureter (acquired) N28.89
    congenital Q62.8
  ureterovesical orifice N28.89
  urethra (acquired) N36.1
    congenital Q64.79
  ventricle, left (congenital) Q24.8
  vesical N32.3
    congenital Q64.6
  Zenker's (esophagus) K22.5

Division
  cervix uteri (acquired) N88.8
  glans penis Q55.69
  labia minora (congenital) Q52.79
  ligament (partial or complete) (current) —*see
      also* Sprain
    with open wound —*see* Wound, open
  muscle (partial or complete) (current) —*see
      also* Injury, muscle
    with open wound —*see* Wound, open
  nerve (traumatic) —*see* Injury, nerve
  spinal cord —*see* Injury, spinal cord,
      by region
  vein I87.8
Divorce, causing family disruption Z63.5
Dix-Hallpike neurolabyrinthitis —*see*
      Neuronitis, vestibular
Dizziness R42
  hysterical F44.89
  psychogenic F45.8
DMAC (disseminated mycobacterium avium-
      intracellulare complex) A31.2
DNR (do not resuscitate) Z66
Doan-Wiseman syndrome (primary splenic
      neutropenia) —*see* Agranulocytosis
Doehle-Heller aortitis A52.02
Dog bite —*see* Bite
Dohle body panmyelopathic syndrome D72.0
Dolichocephaly Q67.2
Dolichocolon Q43.8
Dolichostenomelia —*see* Syndrome, Marfan's
Donohue's syndrome E34.8
Donor (organ or tissue) Z52.9
  blood (whole) Z52.000
    autologous Z52.010
    specified component (lymphocytes)
        (platelets) NEC Z52.008
      autologous Z52.018
      specified donor NEC Z52.098
    specified donor NEC Z52.090
    stem cells Z52.001
      autologous Z52.011
      specified donor NEC Z52.091
  bone Z52.20
    autologous Z52.21
    marrow Z52.3
    specified type NEC Z52.29
  cornea Z52.5
  egg (Oocyte) Z52.819
    age 35 and over Z52.812
      anonymous recipient Z52.812
      designated recipient Z52.813
    under age 35 Z52.810
      anonymous recipient Z52.810
      designated recipient Z52.811
  kidney Z52.4
  liver Z52.6
  lung Z52.89
  lymphocyte —*see* Donor, blood, specified
      components NEC
  Oocyte —*see* Donor, egg
  platelets Z52.008
  potential, examination of Z00.5
  semen Z52.89
  skin Z52.10
    autologous Z52.11
    specified type NEC Z52.19
  specified organ or tissue NEC Z52.89
  sperm Z52.89
Donovanosis A58
Dorsalgia M54.9
  psychogenic F45.41
  specified NEC M54.89
Dorsopathy M53.9
  deforming M43.9
    specified NEC —*see* subcategory M43.8
  specified NEC M53.80
    cervical region M53.82
    cervicothoracic region M53.83
    lumbar region M53.86
    lumbosacral region M53.87

Dorsopathy *(Continued)*
  specified NEC *(Continued)*
    occipito-atlanto-axial region M53.81
    sacrococcygeal region M53.88
    thoracic region M53.84
    thoracolumbar region M53.85
Double
  albumin E88.09
  aortic arch Q25.45
  auditory canal Q17.8
  auricle (heart) Q20.8
  bladder Q64.79
  cervix Q51.820
    with doubling of uterus (and vagina)
        Q51.10
      with obstruction Q51.11
  inlet ventricle Q20.4
  kidney with double pelvis (renal) Q63.0
  meatus urinarius Q64.75
  monster Q89.4
  outlet
    left ventricle Q20.2
    right ventricle Q20.1
  pelvis (renal) with double ureter Q62.5
  tongue Q38.3
  ureter (one or both sides) Q62.5
    with double pelvis (renal) Q62.5
  urethra Q64.74
  urinary meatus Q64.75
  uterus Q51.28
    with
      doubling of cervix (and vagina) Q51.10
        with obstruction Q51.11
      complete Q51.21
    in pregnancy or childbirth O34.0-●
      causing obstructed labor O65.5
    partial Q51.22
    specified NEC Q51.28
  vagina Q52.10
    with doubling of uterus (and cervix)
        Q51.10
      with obstruction Q51.11
  vision H53.2
  vulva Q52.79
▶Doubled up Z59.01
Douglas' pouch, cul-de-sac —*see* condition
Down syndrome Q90.9
  meiotic nondisjunction Q90.0
  mitotic nondisjunction Q90.1
  mosaicism Q90.1
  translocation Q90.2
DPD (dihydropyrimidine dehydrogenase
    deficiency) E88.89
Dracontiasis B72
Dracunculiasis, dracunculosis B72
Dream state, hysterical F44.89
Drepanocytic anemia —*see* Disease,
    sickle-cell
Dresbach's syndrome (elliptocytosis)
    D58.1
Dreschlera (hawaiiensis) (infection)
    B43.8
Dressler's syndrome I24.1
Drift, ulnar —*see* Deformity, limb, specified
    type NEC, forearm
Drinking (alcohol)
  excessive, to excess NEC (without
      dependence) F10.10
    habitual (continual) (without remission)
        F10.20
      with remission F10.21
Drip, postnasal (chronic) R09.82
  due to
    allergic rhinitis —*see* Rhinitis, allergic
    common cold J00
    gastroesophageal reflux —*see* Reflux,
        gastroesophageal
    nasopharyngitis —*see* Nasopharyngitis
    other known condition — code to
        condition
    sinusitis —*see* Sinusitis

Droop
  facial R29.810
    cerebrovascular disease I69.992
      cerebral infarction I69.392
      intracerebral hemorrhage I69.192
      nontraumatic intracranial hemorrhage
          NEC I69.292
      specified disease NEC I69.892
      subarachnoid hemorrhage I69.092
Drop (in)
  attack NEC R55
  finger —*see* Deformity, finger
  foot —*see* Deformity, limb, foot, drop
  hematocrit (precipitous) R71.0
  hemoglobin R71.0
  toe —*see* Deformity, toe, specified NEC
  wrist —*see* Deformity, limb, wrist drop
Dropped heart beats I45.9
Dropsy, dropsical —*see also* Hydrops
  abdomen R18.8
  brain —*see* Hydrocephalus
  cardiac, heart —*see* Failure, heart, congestive
  gangrenous —*see* Gangrene
  heart —*see* Failure, heart, congestive
  kidney —*see* Nephrosis
  lung —*see* Edema, lung
  newborn due to isoimmunization P56.0
  pericardium —*see* Pericarditis
Drowned, drowning (near) T75.1
Drowsiness R40.0
Drug
  abuse counseling and surveillance Z71.51
  addiction —*see* Dependence
  dependence —*see* Dependence
  habit —*see* Dependence
  harmful use —*see* Abuse, drug
  induced fever R50.2
  overdose —*see* Table of Drugs and Chemicals,
      by drug, poisoning
  poisoning —*see* Table of Drugs and
      Chemicals, by drug, poisoning
  resistant organism infection —*see also*
      Resistant, organism, to, drug Z16.30
  therapy
    long term (current) (prophylactic) —*see*
        Therapy, drug long-term (current)
        (prophylactic)
    short term - omit code
  wrong substance given or taken in error —*see*
      Table of Drugs and Chemicals, by drug,
      poisoning
Drunkenness (without dependence) F10.129
  acute in alcoholism F10.229
  chronic (without remission) F10.20
    with remission F10.21
  pathological (without dependence) F10.129
    with dependence F10.229
  sleep F51.9
Drusen
  macula (degenerative) (retina) —*see*
      Degeneration, macula, drusen
  optic disc H47.32-●
Dry, dryness —*see also* condition
  larynx J38.7
  mouth R68.2
    due to dehydration E86.0
  nose J34.89
  socket (teeth) M27.3
  throat J39.2
DSAP L56.5
Duane's syndrome H50.81-●
Dubin-Johnson disease or syndrome E80.6
Dubois' disease (thymus gland) A50.59 *[E35]*
Dubowitz' syndrome Q87.19
Duchenne-Aran muscular atrophy G12.21
Duchenne-Griesinger disease G71.01
Duchenne's
  disease or syndrome
    motor neuron disease G12.22
    muscular dystrophy G71.01
  locomotor ataxia (syphilitic) A52.11

Duchenne's *(Continued)*
  paralysis
    birth injury P14.0
    due to or associated with
      motor neuron disease G12.22
      muscular dystrophy G71.01
Ducrey's chancre A57
Duct, ductus —*see* condition
Duhring's disease (dermatitis herpetiformis)
    L13.0
Dullness, cardiac (decreased) (increased) R01.2
Dumb ague —*see* Malaria
Dumbness —*see* Aphasia
Dumdum fever B55.0
Dumping syndrome (postgastrectomy) K91.1
Duodenitis (nonspecific) (peptic) K29.80
  with bleeding K29.81
Duodenocholangitis —*see* Cholangitis
Duodenum, duodenal —*see* condition
⇒Duplay's bursitis or periarthritis M75.0
Duplication, duplex —*see also* Accessory
  alimentary tract Q45.8
  anus Q43.4
  appendix (and cecum) Q43.4
  biliary duct (any) Q44.5
  bladder Q64.79
  cecum (and appendix) Q43.4
  cervix Q51.820
  chromosome NEC
    with complex rearrangements NEC Q92.5
    seen only at prometaphase Q92.8
  cystic duct Q44.5
  digestive organs Q45.8
  esophagus Q39.8
  frontonasal process Q75.8
  intestine (large) (small) Q43.4
  kidney Q63.0
  liver Q44.7
  pancreas Q45.3
  penis Q55.69
  respiratory organs NEC Q34.8
  salivary duct Q38.4
  spinal cord (incomplete) Q06.2
  stomach Q40.2
Dupré's disease (meningism) R29.1
Dupuytren's contraction or disease M72.0
Durand-Nicolas-Favre disease A55
Durotomy (inadvertent) (incidental) G97.41
Duroziez's disease (congenital mitral stenosis)
    Q23.2
Dutton's relapsing fever (West African)
    A68.1
Dwarfism E34.3
  achondroplastic Q77.4
  congenital E34.3
  constitutional E34.3
  hypochondroplastic Q77.4
  hypophyseal E23.0
  infantile E34.3
  Laron-type E34.3
  Lorain (-Levi) type E23.0
  metatropic Q77.8
  nephrotic-glycosuric (with
      hypophosphatemic rickets) E72.09
  nutritional E45
  pancreatic K86.89
  pituitary E23.0
  renal N25.0
  thanatophoric Q77.1
Dyke-Young anemia (secondary)
    (symptomatic) D59.19
Dysacusis —*see* Abnormal, auditory
    perception
Dysadrenocortism E27.9
  hyperfunction E27.0
Dysarthria R47.1
  following
    cerebral infarction I69.322
    cerebrovascular disease I69.922
      specified disease NEC I69.822
    intracerebral hemorrhage I69.122

Dysarthria *(Continued)*
  following *(Continued)*
    nontraumatic intracranial hemorrhage
      NEC I69.222
    subarachnoid hemorrhage I69.022
Dysautonomia (familial) G90.1
Dysbarism T70.3
Dysbasia R26.2
  angiosclerotica intermittens I73.9
  hysterical F44.4
  lordotica (progressiva) G24.1
  nonorganic origin F44.4
  psychogenic F44.4
Dysbetalipoproteinemia (familial) E78.2
Dyscalculia R48.8
  developmental F81.2
Dyschezia K59.00
Dyschondroplasia (with hemangiomata) Q78.4
Dyschromia (skin) L81.9
Dyscollagenosis M35.9
Dyscranio-pygo-phalangy Q87.0
Dyscrasia
  blood (with) D75.9
    antepartum hemorrhage —*see* Hemorrhage,
      antepartum, with coagulation defect
    intrapartum hemorrhage O67.0
    newborn P61.9
      specified type NEC P61.8
    puerperal, postpartum O72.3
  polyglandular, pluriglandular E31.9
Dysendocrinism E34.9
Dysentery, dysenteric (catarrhal) (diarrhea)
    (epidemic) (hemorrhagic) (infectious)
    (sporadic) (tropical) A09
  abscess, liver A06.4
  amebic —*see also* Amebiasis A06.0
    with abscess —*see* Abscess, amebic
    acute A06.0
    chronic A06.1
  arthritis —*see also* category M01 A09
    bacillary —*see also* category M01 A03.9
  bacillary A03.9
    arthritis —*see also* category M01 A03.9
    Boyd A03.2
    Flexner A03.1
    Schmitz (-Stutzer) A03.0
    Shiga (-Kruse) A03.0
    Shigella A03.9
      boydii A03.2
      dysenteriae A03.0
      flexneri A03.1
      group A A03.0
      group B A03.1
      group C A03.2
      group D A03.3
      sonnei A03.3
      specified type NEC A03.8
    Sonne A03.3
    specified type NEC A03.8
  balantidial A07.0
  Balantidium coli A07.0
  Boyd's A03.2
  candidal B37.82
  Chilomastix A07.8
  Chinese A03.9
  coccidial A07.3
  Dientamoeba (fragilis) A07.8
  Embadomonas A07.8
  Entamoeba, entamebic —*see* Dysentery,
    amebic
  Flexner-Boyd A03.2
  Flexner's A03.1
  Giardia lamblia A07.1
  Hiss-Russell A03.1
  Lamblia A07.1
  leishmanial B55.0
  malarial —*see* Malaria
  metazoal B82.0
  monilial B37.82
  protozoal A07.9
  Salmonella A02.0

Dysentery, dysenteric *(Continued)*
  schistosomal B65.1
  Schmitz (-Stutzer) A03.0
  Shiga (-Kruse) A03.0
  Shigella NOS —*see* Dysentery, bacillary
  Sonne A03.3
  strongyloidiasis B78.0
  trichomonal A07.8
  viral —*see also* Enteritis, viral A08.4
Dysequilibrium R42
Dysesthesia R20.8
  hysterical F44.6
Dysfibrinogenemia (congenital) D68.2
Dysfunction
  adrenal E27.9
    hyperfunction E27.0
  autonomic
    due to alcohol G31.2
    somatoform F45.8
  bladder N31.9
    neurogenic NOS —*see* Dysfunction,
      bladder, neuromuscular
    neuromuscular NOS N31.9
      atonic (motor) (sensory) N31.2
      autonomous N31.2
      flaccid N31.2
      nonreflex N31.2
      reflex N31.1
      specified NEC N31.8
      uninhibited N31.0
  bleeding, uterus N93.8
  cerebral G93.89
  colon K59.9
    psychogenic F45.8
  colostomy K94.03
  cystic duct K82.8
  cystostomy (stoma) —*see* Complications,
    cystostomy
  ejaculatory N53.19
    anejaculatory orgasm N53.13
    painful N53.12
    premature F52.4
    retarded N53.11
  endocrine NOS E34.9
  endometrium N85.8
  enterostomy K94.13
  erectile —*see* Dysfunction, sexual, male, erectile
▶ feeding, pediatric
▶   acute R63.31
▶   chronic R63.32
  gallbladder K82.8
  gastrostomy (stoma) K94.23
  gland, glandular NOS E34.9
    meibomian, of eyelid -see Dysfunction,
      meibomian gland
  heart I51.89
  hemoglobin D75.89
  hepatic K76.89
  hypophysis E23.7
  hypothalamic NEC E23.3
  ileostomy (stoma) K94.13
  jejunostomy (stoma) K94.13
  kidney —*see* Disease, renal
  labyrinthine —*see* subcategory H83.2
  left ventricular, following sudden emotional
    stress I51.81
  liver K76.89
  male —*see* Dysfunction, sexual, male
  meibomian gland, of eyelid H02.889
    left H02.886
      lower H02.885
      upper H02.884
      upper and lower eyelids H02.88B
    right H02.883
      lower H02.882
      upper H02.881
      upper and lower eyelids H02.88A
  orgasmic (female) F52.31
    male F52.32
  ovary E28.9
    specified NEC E28.8
  papillary muscle I51.89
  parathyroid E21.4

Dysfunction *(Continued)*
  physiological NEC R68.89
    psychogenic F59
  pineal gland E34.8
  pituitary (gland) E23.3
  platelets D69.1
  polyglandular E31.9
    specified NEC E31.8
  psychophysiologic F59
  psychosexual F52.9
    with
      dyspareunia F52.6
      premature ejaculation F52.4
      vaginismus F52.5
  pylorus K31.9
  rectum K59.9
    psychogenic F45.8
  reflex (sympathetic) —*see* Syndrome, pain,
    complex regional I
  segmental —*see* Dysfunction, somatic
  senile R54
  sexual (due to) R37
    alcohol F10.981
    amphetamine F15.981
      in
        abuse F15.181
        dependence F15.281
    anxiolytic F13.981
      in
        abuse F13.181
        dependence F13.281
    cocaine F14.981
      in
        abuse F14.181
        dependence F14.281
    excessive sexual drive F52.8
    failure of genital response (male) F52.21
      female F52.22
    female N94.9
      aversion F52.1
      dyspareunia N94.10
        psychogenic F52.6
      frigidity F52.22
      nymphomania F52.8
      orgasmic F52.31
      psychogenic F52.9
        aversion F52.1
        dyspareunia F52.6
        frigidity F52.22
        nymphomania F52.8
        orgasmic F52.31
        vaginismus F52.5
      vaginismus N94.2
        psychogenic F52.5
    hypnotic F13.981
      in
        abuse F13.181
        dependence F13.281
    inhibited orgasm (female) F52.31
      male F52.32
    lack
      of sexual enjoyment F52.1
      or loss of sexual desire F52.0
    male N53.9
      anejaculatory orgasm N53.13
      ejaculatory N53.19
        painful N53.12
        premature F52.4
        retarded N53.11
      erectile N52.9
        drug induced N52.2
        due to
          disease classified elsewhere N52.1
          drug N52.2
        postoperative (postprocedural) N52.39
          following
            cryotherapy N52.37
            interstitial seed therapy N52.36
            prostate ablative therapy N52.37
            prostatectomy N52.34
              radical N52.31

Dysfunction (Continued)
  sexual (Continued)
    male (Continued)
      erectile (Continued)
        postoperative (Continued)
          following (Continued)
            radiation therapy N52.35
            radical cystectomy N52.32
            ultrasound ablative therapy
              N52.37
            urethral surgery N52.33
        psychogenic F52.21
        specified cause NEC N52.8
        vasculogenic
          arterial insufficiency N52.01
            with corporo-venous occlusive
              N52.03
          corporo-venous occlusive N52.02
            with arterial insufficiency N52.03
      impotence —see Dysfunction, sexual,
        male, erectile
      psychogenic F52.9
        aversion F52.1
        erectile F52.21
        orgasmic F52.32
        premature ejaculation F52.4
        satyriasis F52.8
        specified type NEC F52.8
      specified type NEC N53.8
    nonorganic F52.9
      specified NEC F52.8
    opioid F11.981
      in
        abuse F11.181
        dependence F11.281
    orgasmic dysfunction (female) F52.31
      male F52.32
    premature ejaculation F52.4
    psychoactive substances NEC F19.981
      in
        abuse F19.181
        dependence F19.281
    psychogenic F52.9
    sedative F13.981
      in
        abuse F13.181
        dependence F13.281
    sexual aversion F52.1
    vaginismus (nonorganic) (psychogenic)
      F52.5
  sinoatrial node I49.5
  somatic M99.09
    abdomen M99.09
    acromioclavicular M99.07
    cervical region M99.01
    cervicothoracic M99.01
    costochondral M99.08
    costovertebral M99.08
    head region M99.00
    hip M99.05
    lower extremity M99.06
    lumbar region M99.03
    lumbosacral M99.03
    occipitocervical M99.00
    pelvic region M99.05
    pubic M99.05
    rib cage M99.08
    sacral region M99.04
    sacrococcygeal M99.04
    sacroiliac M99.04
    specified NEC M99.09
    sternochondral M99.08
    sternoclavicular M99.07
    thoracic region M99.02
    thoracolumbar M99.02
    upper extremity M99.07
  somatoform autonomic F45.8
  stomach K31.89
    psychogenic F45.8
  suprarenal E27.9
    hyperfunction E27.0

Dysfunction (Continued)
  symbolic R48.9
    specified type NEC R48.8
  temporomandibular (joint) M26.69
    joint-pain syndrome M26.62-●
  testicular (endocrine) E29.9
    specified NEC E29.8
  thymus E32.9
  thyroid E07.9
  ureterostomy (stoma) —see Complications,
    stoma, urinary tract
  urethrostomy (stoma) —see Complications,
    stoma, urinary tract
  uterus, complicating delivery O62.9
    hypertonic O62.4
    hypotonic O62.2
      primary O62.0
      secondary O62.1
  ventricular I51.9
    with congestive heart failure —see also
      Failure, heart I50.9
    left, reversible, following sudden
      emotional stress I51.81
Dysgenesis
  gonadal (due to chromosomal anomaly) Q96.9
    pure Q99.1
  renal Q60.5
    bilateral Q60.4
    unilateral Q60.3
  reticular D72.0
  tidal platelet D69.3
Dysgerminoma
  specified site —see Neoplasm, malignant,
    by site
  unspecified site
    female C56.9
    male C62.90
Dysgeusia R43.2
Dysgraphia R27.8
Dyshidrosis, dysidrosis L30.1
Dyskaryotic cervical smear R87.619
Dyskeratosis L85.8
  cervix —see Dysplasia, cervix
  congenital Q82.8
  uterus NEC N85.8
Dyskinesia G24.9
  biliary (cystic duct or gallbladder) K82.8
  drug induced
    orofacial G24.01
  esophagus K22.4
  hysterical F44.4
  intestinal K59.89
  nonorganic origin F44.4
  orofacial (idiopathic) G24.4
    drug induced G24.01
  psychogenic F44.4
  subacute, drug induced G24.01
  tardive G24.01
    neuroleptic induced G24.01
  trachea J39.8
  tracheobronchial J98.09
Dyslalia (developmental) F80.0
Dyslexia R48.0
  developmental F81.0
Dyslipidemia E78.5
  depressed HDL cholesterol E78.6
  elevated fasting triglycerides E78.1
Dysmaturity —see also Light for dates
  pulmonary (newborn) (Wilson-Mikity) P27.0
Dysmenorrhea (essential) (exfoliative) N94.6
  congestive (syndrome) N94.6
  primary N94.4
  psychogenic F45.8
  secondary N94.5
Dysmetabolic syndrome X E88.81
Dysmetria R27.8
Dysmorphism (due to)
  alcohol Q86.0
  exogenous cause NEC Q86.8
  hydantoin Q86.1
  warfarin Q86.2

Dysmorphophobia (nondelusional)
    F45.22
  delusional F22
Dysnomia R47.01
Dysorexia R63.0
  psychogenic F50.89
Dysostosis
  cleidocranial, cleidocranialis Q74.0
  craniofacial Q75.1
  Fairbank's (idiopathic familial generalized
    osteophytosis) Q78.9
  mandibulofacial (incomplete) Q75.4
  multiplex E76.01
  oculomandibular Q75.5
Dyspareunia (female) N94.10
  deep N94.12
  male N53.12
  nonorganic F52.6
  psychogenic F52.6
  secondary N94.19
  specified NEC N94.19
  superficial (introital) N94.11
Dyspepsia R10.13
  atonic K30
  functional (allergic) (congenital)
    (gastrointestinal) (occupational)
    (reflex) K30
  intestinal K59.89
  nervous F45.8
  neurotic F45.8
  psychogenic F45.8
Dysphagia R13.10
  cervical R13.19
  following
    cerebral infarction I69.391
    cerebrovascular disease I69.991
      specified NEC I69.891
    intracerebral hemorrhage I69.191
    nontraumatic intracranial hemorrhage
      NEC I69.291
    specified disease NEC I69.891
    subarachnoid hemorrhage I69.091
  functional (hysterical) F45.8
  hysterical F45.8
  nervous (hysterical) F45.8
  neurogenic R13.19
  oral phase R13.11
  oropharyngeal phase R13.12
  pharyngeal phase R13.13
  pharyngoesophageal phase R13.14
  psychogenic F45.8
  sideropenic D50.1
  spastica K22.4
  specified NEC R13.19
Dysphagocytosis, congenital D71
Dysphasia R47.02
  developmental
    expressive type F80.1
    receptive type F80.2
  following
    cerebrovascular disease I69.921
      cerebral infarction I69.321
      intracerebral hemorrhage I69.121
    nontraumatic intracranial hemorrhage NEC
      I69.221
      specified disease NEC I69.821
      subarachnoid hemorrhage I69.021
Dysphonia R49.0
  functional F44.4
  hysterical F44.4
  psychogenic F44.4
  spastica J38.3
Dysphoria
  gender F64.9
    in
      adolescence and adulthood
        F64.0
      children F64.2
    specified NEC F64.8
    postpartal O90.6
Dyspituitarism E23.3

▶ New   ⇒ Revised   ~~deleted~~ Deleted   ● Use Additional Character(s)

Dysplasia —see also Anomaly
　acetabular, congenital Q65.89
　alveolar capillary, with vein misalignment
　　　J84.843
　anus (histologically confirmed) (mild)
　　　(moderate) K62.82
　　severe D01.3
　arrhythmogenic right ventricular I42.8
　arterial, fibromuscular I77.3
　asphyxiating thoracic (congenital) Q77.2
　brain Q07.9
　bronchopulmonary, perinatal P27.1
　cervix (uteri) N87.9
　　mild N87.0
　　moderate N87.1
　　severe D06.9
　chondroectodermal Q77.6
　colon D12.6
　craniometaphyseal Q78.58
　dentinal K00.5
　diaphyseal, progressive Q78.3
　dystrophic Q77.5
　ectodermal (anhidrotic) (congenital)
　　　(hereditary) Q82.4
　　hydrotic Q82.8
　epithelial, uterine cervix —see Dysplasia,
　　　cervix
　eye (congenital) Q11.2
　fibrous
　　bone NEC (monostotic) M85.00
　　　ankle M85.07-●
　　　foot M85.07-●
　　　forearm M85.03-●
　　　hand M85.04-●
　　　lower leg M85.06-●
　　　multiple site M85.09
　　　neck M85.08
　　　rib M85.08
　　　shoulder M85.01-●
　　　skull M85.08
　　　specified site NEC M85.08
　　　thigh M85.05-●
　　　toe M85.07-●
　　　upper arm M85.02-●
　　　vertebra M85.08
　　diaphyseal, progressive Q78.3
　　jaw M27.8
　　polyostotic Q78.1
　florid osseous —see also Cyst, calcifying
　　　odontogenic
　high grade, focal D12.6
　hip, congenital Q65.89
　joint, congenital Q74.8
　kidney Q61.4
　　multicystic Q61.4
　leg Q74.2
　lung, congenital (not associated with short
　　　gestation) Q33.6
　mammary (gland) (benign) N60.9-●
　　cyst (solitary) —see Cyst, breast
　　cystic —see Mastopathy, cystic
　　duct ectasia —see Ectasia, mammary duct
　　fibroadenosis —see Fibroadenosis, breast
　　fibrosclerosis —see Fibrosclerosis, breast
　　specified type NEC N60.8-●
　metaphyseal Q78.5
　muscle Q79.8
　oculodentodigital Q87.0
　periapical (cemental) (cemento-osseous) —see
　　　Cyst, calcifying odontogenic
　periosteum —see Disorder, bone, specified
　　　type NEC
　polyostotic fibrous Q78.1
　prostate —see also Neoplasia, intraepithelial,
　　　prostate N42.30
　　severe D07.5
　　specified NEC N42.39
　renal Q61.4
　　multicystic Q61.4
　retinal, congenital Q14.1
　right ventricular, arrhythmogenic I42.8

Dysplasia (Continued)
　septo-optic Q04.4
　skin L98.8
　spinal cord Q06.1
　spondyloepiphyseal Q77.7
　thymic, with immunodeficiency D82.1
　vagina N89.3
　　mild N89.0
　　moderate N89.1
　　severe NEC D07.2
　vulva N90.3
　　mild N90.0
　　moderate N90.1
　　severe NEC D07.1
Dysplasminogenemia E88.02
Dyspnea (nocturnal) (paroxysmal) R06.00
　asthmatic (bronchial) J45.909
　　with
　　　bronchitis J45.909
　　　　with
　　　　　exacerbation (acute) J45.901
　　　　　status asthmaticus J45.902
　　　　chronic J44.9
　　　exacerbation (acute) J45.901
　　　status asthmaticus J45.902
　　cardiac —see Failure, ventricular, left
　cardiac —see Failure, ventricular, left
　functional F45.8
　hyperventilation R06.4
　hysterical F45.8
　newborn P28.89
　psychogenic F45.8
　shortness of breath R06.02
　specified type NEC R06.09
Dyspraxia R27.8
　developmental (syndrome) F82
Dysproteinemia E88.09
Dysreflexia, autonomic G90.4
Dysrhythmia
　cardiac I49.9
　　newborn
　　　bradycardia P29.12
　　　occurring before birth P03.819
　　　　before onset of labor P03.810
　　　　during labor P03.811
　　　tachycardia P29.11
　　postoperative I97.89
　cerebral or cortical —see Epilepsy
Dyssomnia —see Disorder, sleep
Dyssynergia
　biliary K83.8
　bladder sphincter N36.44
　cerebellaris myoclonica (Hunt's ataxia) G11.19
Dysthymia F34.1
Dysthyroidism E07.9
Dystocia O66.9
　affecting newborn P03.1
　cervical (hypotonic) O62.2
　　affecting newborn P03.6
　　primary O62.0
　　secondary O62.1
　contraction ring O62.4
　fetal O66.9
　　abnormality NEC O66.3
　　conjoined twins O66.3
　　oversize O66.2
　maternal O66.9
　positional O64.9
　shoulder (girdle) O66.0
　　causing obstructed labor O66.0
　uterine NEC O62.4
Dystonia G24.9
　cervical G24.3
　deformans progressiva G24.1
　drug induced NEC G24.09
　　acute G24.02
　　specified NEC G24.09
　familial G24.1
　idiopathic G24.1
　　familial G24.1
　　nonfamilial G24.2
　　orofacial G24.4

Dystonia (Continued)
　lenticularis G24.8
　musculorum deformans G24.1
　neuroleptic induced (acute) G24.02
　orofacial (idiopathic) G24.4
　oromandibular G24.4
　　due to drug G24.01
　specified NEC G24.8
　torsion (familial) (idiopathic) G24.1
　　acquired G24.8
　　genetic G24.1
　　symptomatic (nonfamilial) G24.2
Dystonic movements R25.8
Dystrophy, dystrophia
　adiposogenital E23.6
　autosomal recessive, childhood type,
　　　muscular dystrophy resembling
　　　Duchenne or Becker G71.01
　Becker's type G71.01
　cervical sympathetic G90.2
　choroid (hereditary) H31.20
　　central areolar H31.22
　　choroideremia H31.21
　　gyrate atrophy H31.23
　　specified type NEC H31.29
　cornea (hereditary) H18.50-●
　　endothelial H18.51-●
　　epithelial H18.52-●
　　granular H18.53-●
　　lattice H18.54-●
　　macular H18.55-●
　　specified type NEC H18.59-●
　Duchenne's type G71.01
　due to malnutrition E45
　Erb's G71.02
　Fuchs' H18.51-●
　Gower's muscular G71.01
　hair L67.8
　infantile neuraxonal G31.89
　Landouzy-Déjérine G71.02
　Leyden-Möbius G71.09
　muscular G71.00
　　autosomal recessive, childhood type,
　　　　muscular dystrophy resembling
　　　　Duchenne or Becker G71.01
　　benign (Becker type) G71.01
　　　scapuloperoneal with early contractures
　　　　[Emery-Dreifuss] G71.09
　　congenital (hereditary) (progressive) (with
　　　　specific morphological abnormalities
　　　　of the muscle fiber) G71.09
　　　myotonic G71.11
　　distal G71.09
　　Duchenne type G71.01
　　Emery-Dreifuss G71.09
　　Erb type G71.02
　　facioscapulohumeral G71.02
　　Gower's G71.01
　　hereditary (progressive) G71.09
　　Landouzy-Déjérine type G71.02
　　limb-girdle G71.09
　　myotonic G71.11
　　progressive (hereditary) G71.09
　　　Charcot-Marie (-Tooth) type G60.0
　　pseudohypertrophic (infantile) G71.01
　　scapulohumeral G71.02
　　scapuloperoneal G71.09
　　severe (Duchenne type) G71.01
　　specified type NEC G71.09
　myocardium, myocardial —see
　　　Degeneration, myocardial
　nail L60.3
　　congenital Q84.6
　nutritional E45
　ocular G71.09
　oculocerebrorenal E72.03
　oculopharyngeal G71.09
　ovarian N83.8
　polyglandular E31.8
　reflex (neuromuscular) (sympathetic) —
　　　see Syndrome, pain, complex regional I

Dystrophy, dystrophia *(Continued)*
   retinal (hereditary) H35.50
     in
       lipid storage disorders E75.6 *[H36]*
       systemic lipidoses E75.6 *[H36]*
     involving
       pigment epithelium H35.54
       sensory area H35.53
     pigmentary H35.52
     vitreoretinal H35.51

Dystrophy, dystrophia *(Continued)*
   Salzmann's nodular —*see* Degeneration,
     cornea, nodular
   scapuloperoneal G71.09
   skin NEC L98.8
   sympathetic (reflex) —*see* Syndrome, pain,
     complex regional I
     cervical G90.2
   tapetoretinal H35.54

Dystrophy, dystrophia *(Continued)*
   thoracic, asphyxiating Q77.2
   unguium L60.3
     congenital Q84.6
   vitreoretinal H35.51
   vulva N90.4
   yellow (liver) —*see* Failure, hepatic
Dysuria R30.0
   psychogenic F45.8

▶ New   ⇒ Revised   ~~deleted~~ Deleted   ● Use Additional Character(s)

E

Eales' disease H35.06-●
Ear —see also condition
  piercing Z41.3
  tropical NEC B36.9 [H62.40]
    in
      aspergillosis B44.89
      candidiasis B37.84
      moniliasis B37.84
  wax (impacted) H61.20
    left H61.22
      with right H61.23
    right H61.21
      with left H61.23
Earache —see subcategory H92.0
Early satiety R68.81
Eaton-Lambert syndrome—see Syndrome,
  Lambert-Eaton
Eberth's disease (typhoid fever) A01.00
Ebola virus disease A98.4
Ebstein's anomaly or syndrome (heart) Q22.5
Eccentro-osteochondrodysplasia E76.29
Ecchondroma —see Neoplasm, bone, benign
Ecchondrosis D48.0
Ecchymosis R58
  conjunctiva —see Hemorrhage, conjunctiva
  eye (traumatic) —see Contusion, eyeball
  eyelid (traumatic) —see Contusion, eyelid
  newborn P54.5
  spontaneous R23.3
  traumatic —see Contusion
Echinocicciasis —see Echinococcus
Echinococcosis —see Echinococcus
Echinococcus (infection) B67.90
  granulosus B67.4
    bone B67.2
    liver B67.0
    lung B67.1
    multiple sites B67.32
    specified site NEC B67.39
    thyroid B67.31
  liver NOS B67.8
    granulosus B67.0
    multilocularis B67.5
  lung NEC B67.99
    granulosus B67.1
    multilocularis B67.69
  multilocularis B67.7
    liver B67.5
    multiple sites B67.61
    specified site NEC B67.69
  specified site NEC B67.99
    granulosus B67.39
    multilocularis B67.69
  thyroid NEC B67.99
    granulosus B67.31
    multilocularis B67.69 [E35]
Echinorhynchiasis B83.8
Echinostomiasis B66.8
Echolalia R48.8
Echovirus, as cause of disease classified
  elsewhere B97.12
Eclampsia, eclamptic (coma) (convulsions)
  (delirium) (with hypertension) NEC O15.9
  complicating
    labor and delivery O15.1
    postpartum O15.2
    pregnancy O15.0-●
    puerperium O15.2
Economic circumstances affecting care Z59.9
Economo's disease A85.8
Ectasia, ectasis
  annuloaortic I35.8
  aorta I77.819
    with aneurysm —see Aneurysm, aorta
      abdominal I77.811
      thoracic I77.810
      thoracoabdominal I77.812
  breast —see Ectasia, mammary duct
  capillary I78.8
  cornea H18.71-●

Ectasia, ectasis (Continued)
  gastric antral vascular (GAVE) K31.819
    with hemorrhage K31.811
    without hemorrhage K31.819
  mammary duct N60.4-●
  salivary gland (duct) K11.8
  sclera —see Sclerectasia
Ecthyma L08.0
  contagiosum B08.02
  gangrenosum L08.0
  infectiosum B08.02
Ectocardia Q24.8
Ectodermal dysplasia (anhidrotic) Q82.4
Ectodermosis erosiva pluriorificialis
  L51.1
Ectopic, ectopia (congenital)
  abdominal viscera Q45.8
    due to defect in anterior abdominal wall
      Q79.59
  ACTH syndrome E24.3
  adrenal gland Q89.1
  anus Q43.5
  atrial beats I49.1
  beats I49.49
    atrial I49.1
    ventricular I49.3
  bladder Q64.10
  bone and cartilage in lung Q33.5
  brain Q04.8
  breast tissue Q83.8
  cardiac Q24.8
  cerebral Q04.8
  cordis Q24.8
  endometrium —see Endometriosis
  gastric mucosa Q40.2
  gestation —see Pregnancy, by site
  heart Q24.8
  hormone secretion NEC E34.2
  kidney (crossed) (pelvis) Q63.2
  lens, lentis Q12.1
  mole —see Pregnancy, by site
  organ or site NEC —see Malposition,
    congenital
  pancreas Q45.3
  pregnancy —see Pregnancy, ectopic
  pupil —see Abnormality, pupillary
  renal Q63.2
  sebaceous glands of mouth Q38.6
  spleen Q89.09
  testis Q53.00
    bilateral Q53.02
    unilateral Q53.01
  thyroid Q89.2
  tissue in lung Q33.5
  ureter Q62.63
  ventricular beats I49.3
  vesicae Q64.10
Ectromelia Q73.8
  lower limb —see Defect, reduction, limb,
    lower, specified type NEC
  upper limb —see Defect, reduction, limb,
    upper, specified type NEC
Ectropion H02.109
  cervix N86
    with cervicitis N72
  congenital Q10.1
  eyelid H02.109
    cicatricial H02.119
      left H02.116
        lower H02.115
        upper H02.114
      right H02.113
        lower H02.112
        upper H02.111
    congenital Q10.1
    left H02.106
      lower H02.105
      upper H02.104
    mechanical H02.129
      left H02.126
        lower H02.125
        upper H02.124

Ectropion (Continued)
  eyelid (Continued)
    mechanical (Continued)
      right H02.123
        lower H02.122
        upper H02.121
    paralytic H02.159
      left H02.156
        lower H02.155
        upper H02.154
      right H02.153
        lower H02.152
        upper H02.151
    right H02.103
      lower H02.102
      upper H02.101
    senile H02.139
      left H02.136
        lower H02.135
        upper H02.134
      right H02.133
        lower H02.132
        upper H02.131
    spastic H02.149
      left H02.146
        lower H02.145
        upper H02.144
      right H02.143
        lower H02.142
        upper H02.141
  iris H21.89
  lip (acquired) K13.0
    congenital Q38.0
  urethra N36.8
  uvea H21.89
Eczema (acute) (chronic) (erythematous)
    (fissum) (rubrum) (squamous) (see also
    Dermatitis) L30.9
  contact —see Dermatitis, contact
  dyshydrotic L30.1
  external ear —see Otitis, externa, acute,
    eczematoid
  flexural L20.82
  herpeticum B00.0
  hypertrophicum L28.0
  hypostatic —see Varix, leg, with,
    inflammation
  impetiginous L01.1
  infantile (due to any substance) L20.83
    intertriginous L21.1
    seborrheic L21.1
  intertriginous NEC L30.4
    infantile L21.1
  intrinsic (allergic) L20.84
  lichenified NEC L28.0
  marginatum (hebrae) B35.6
  pustular L30.3
  stasis I87.2
    with varicose veins —see Varix, leg, with,
      inflammation
  vaccination, vaccinatum T88.1
  varicose —see Varix, leg, with, inflammation
Eczematid L30.2
Eddowes (-Spurway) syndrome Q78.0
Edema, edematous (infectious) (pitting)
    (toxic) R60.9
  with nephritis —see Nephrosis
  allergic T78.3
  amputation stump (surgical) (sequelae
    (late effect)) T87.89
  angioneurotic (allergic) (any site) (with
    urticaria) T78.3
    hereditary D84.1
  angiospastic I73.9
  Berlin's (traumatic) S05.8X-●
  brain (cytotoxic) (vasogenic) G93.6
    due to birth injury P11.0
    newborn (anoxia or hypoxia) P52.4
      birth injury P11.0
    traumatic —see Injury, intracranial,
      cerebral edema
  cardiac —see Failure, heart, congestive

Edema, edematous (*Continued*)
cardiovascular —*see* Failure, heart, congestive
cerebral —*see* Edema, brain
cerebrospinal —*see* Edema, brain
cervix (uteri) (acute) N88.8
  puerperal, postpartum O90.89
chronic hereditary Q82.0
circumscribed, acute T78.3
  hereditary D84.1
conjunctiva H11.42-●
cornea H18.2-●
  idiopathic H18.22-●
  secondary H18.23-●
    due to contact lens H18.21-●
due to
  lymphatic obstruction I89.0
  salt retention E87.0
epiglottis —*see* Edema, glottis
essential, acute T78.3
  hereditary D84.1
extremities, lower —*see* Edema, legs
eyelid NEC H02.849
  left H02.846
    lower H02.845
    upper H02.844
  right H02.843
    lower H02.842
    upper H02.841
familial, hereditary Q82.0
famine —*see* Malnutrition, severe
generalized R60.1
glottis, glottic, glottidis (obstructive) (passive)
    J38.4
  allergic T78.3
    hereditary D84.1
heart —*see* Failure, heart, congestive
heat T67.7
hereditary Q82.0
inanition —*see* Malnutrition, severe
intracranial G93.6
iris H21.89
joint —*see* Effusion, joint
larynx —*see* Edema, glottis
legs R60.0
  due to venous obstruction I87.1
  hereditary Q82.0
localized R60.0
  due to venous obstruction I87.1
lower limbs —*see* Edema, legs
lung J81.1
  with heart condition or failure —*see*
      Failure, ventricular, left
  acute J81.0
    chemical (acute) J68.1
      chronic J68.1
    chronic J81.1
      due to
        chemicals, gases, fumes or vapors
            (inhalation) J68.1
        external agent J70.9
          specified NEC J70.8
        radiation J70.1
  due to
    chemicals, fumes or vapors (inhalation)
        J68.1
    external agent J70.9
      specified NEC J70.8
    high altitude T70.29
    near drowning T75.1
    radiation J70.0
  meaning failure, left ventricle I50.1
lymphatic I89.0
  due to mastectomy I97.2
macula H35.81
  cystoid, following cataract surgery —*see*
      Complications, postprocedural,
      following cataract surgery
  diabetic —*see* Diabetes, by type, with,
      retinopathy, with macular edema
malignant —*see* Gangrene, gas
Milroy's Q82.0

Edema, edematous (*Continued*)
nasopharynx J39.2
newborn P83.30
  hydrops fetalis —*see* Hydrops, fetalis
  specified NEC P83.39
nutritional —*see also* Malnutrition, severe
  with dyspigmentation, skin and hair E40
optic disc or nerve —*see* Papilledema
orbit H05.22-●
pancreas K86.89
papilla, optic —*see* Papilledema
penis N48.89
periodic T78.3
  hereditary D84.1
pharynx J39.2
pulmonary —*see* Edema, lung
Quincke's T78.3
  hereditary D84.1
renal —*see* Nephrosis
retina H35.81
  diabetic —*see* Diabetes, by type, with,
      retinopathy, with macular edema
salt E87.0
scrotum N50.89
seminal vesicle N50.89
spermatic cord N50.89
spinal (cord) (vascular) (nontraumatic) G95.19
starvation —*see* Malnutrition, severe
stasis —*see* Hypertension, venous, (chronic)
subglottic —*see* Edema, glottis
supraglottic —*see* Edema, glottis
testis N44.8
tunica vaginalis N50.89
vas deferens N50.89
vulva (acute) N90.89
Edentulism —*see* Absence, teeth, acquired
Edsall's disease T67.2
Educational handicap Z55.9
▶less than a high school diploma Z55.5
▶no general equivalence degree (GED) Z55.5
  specified NEC Z55.8
Edward's syndrome —*see* Trisomy, 18
Effect, adverse
  abnormal gravitational (G) forces or states
      T75.81
  abuse —*see* Maltreatment
  air pressure T70.9
    specified NEC T70.8
  altitude (high) —*see* Effect, adverse, high
      altitude
  anesthesia —*see also* Anesthesia T88.59
    in labor and delivery O74.9
    local, toxic
      in labor and delivery O74.4-●
      in pregnancy NEC O29.3-●
      postpartum, puerperal O89.3
    postpartum, puerperal O89.9
    specified NEC T88.59
      in labor and delivery O74.8
      postpartum, puerperal O89.8
    spinal and epidural T88.59
      headache T88.59
        in labor and delivery O74.5
        postpartum, puerperal O89.4
      specified NEC
        in labor and delivery O74.6
        postpartum, puerperal O89.5
  antitoxin —*see* Complications, vaccination
  atmospheric pressure T70.9
    due to explosion T70.8
    high T70.3
    low —*see* Effect, adverse, high altitude
    specified effect NEC T70.8
  biological, correct substance properly
      administered —*see* Effect, adverse, drug
  blood (derivatives) (serum) (transfusion) —
      see Complications, transfusion
  chemical substance —*see* Table of Drugs and
      Chemicals
  cold (temperature) (weather) T69.9
    chilblains T69.1
    frostbite —*see* Frostbite
    specified effect NEC T69.8

Effect, adverse (*Continued*)
drugs and medicaments T88.7
  specified drug —*see* Table of Drugs and
      Chemicals, by drug, adverse effect
  specified effect — code to condition
electric current, electricity (shock) T75.4
  burn —*see* Burn
exertion (excessive) T73.3
exposure —*see* Exposure
external cause NEC T75.89
foodstuffs T78.1
  allergic reaction —*see* Allergy, food
    causing anaphylaxis —*see* Shock,
        anaphylactic, due to food
  noxious —*see* Poisoning, food, noxious
gases, fumes, or vapors T59.9-●
  specified agent —*see* Table of Drugs and
      Chemicals
glue (airplane) sniffing
  due to drug abuse —*see* Abuse, drug,
      inhalant
  due to drug dependence —*see* Dependence,
      drug, inhalant
heat —*see* Heat
high altitude NEC T70.29
  anoxia T70.29
  on
    ears T70.0
    sinuses T70.1
  polycythemia D75.1
high pressure fluids T70.4
hot weather —*see* Heat
hunger T73.0
immersion, foot —*see* Immersion
immunization —*see* Complications,
    vaccination
immunological agents —*see* Complications,
    vaccination
infrared (radiation) (rays) NOS T66
  dermatitis or eczema L59.8
infusion —*see* Complications, infusion
lack of care of infants —*see* Maltreatment,
    child
lightning —*see* Lightning
medical care T88.9
  specified NEC T88.8
medicinal substance, correct, properly
    administered —*see* Effect, adverse, drug
motion T75.3
noise, on inner ear —*see* subcategory H83.3
overheated places —*see* Heat
psychosocial, of work environment Z56.5
radiation (diagnostic) (infrared) (natural
    source) (therapeutic) (ultraviolet) (X-ray)
    NOS T66
  dermatitis or eczema —*see* Dermatitis, due
      to, radiation
  fibrosis of lung J70.1
  pneumonitis J70.0
  pulmonary manifestations
    acute J70.0
    chronic J70.1
  skin L59.9
radioactive substance NOS
  dermatitis or eczema —*see* Radiodermatitis
reduced temperature T69.9
  immersion foot or hand —*see* Immersion
  specified effect NEC T69.8
serum NEC (*see also* Reaction, serum) T80.69
specified NEC T78.8
  external cause NEC T75.89
strangulation —*see* Asphyxia, traumatic
submersion T75.1
thirst T73.1
toxic —*see* Toxicity
transfusion —*see* Complications, transfusion
ultraviolet (radiation) (rays) NOS T66
  burn —*see* Burn
  dermatitis or eczema —*see* Dermatitis, due
      to, ultraviolet rays
    acute L56.8

▶ New   ⇨ Revised   ~~deleted~~ Deleted   ● Use Additional Character(s)

Effect, adverse (Continued)
vaccine (any) —see Complications, vaccination
vibration —see Vibration, adverse effects
water pressure NEC T70.9
specified NEC T70.8
weightlessness T75.82
whole blood —see Complications, transfusion
work environment Z56.5
Effect(s) (of) (from) —see Effect, adverse NEC
Effects, late —see Sequelae
Effluvium
anagen L65.1
telogen L65.0
Effort syndrome (psychogenic) F45.8
Effusion
⟹amniotic fluid —see Pregnancy, complicated by, premature rupture of membranes
brain (serous) G93.6
bronchial —see Bronchitis
cerebral G93.6
cerebrospinal —see also Meningitis
vessel G93.6
chest —see Effusion, pleura
chylous, chyliform (pleura) J94.0
intracranial G93.6
joint M25.40
ankle M25.47-•
elbow M25.42-•
foot joint M25.47-•
hand joint M25.44-•
hip M25.45-•
knee M25.46-•
shoulder M25.41-•
specified joint NEC M25.48
wrist M25.43-•
malignant pleural J91.0
meninges —see Meningitis
pericardium, pericardial (noninflammatory) I31.3
acute —see Pericarditis, acute
peritoneal (chronic) R18.8
pleura, pleurisy, pleuritic, pleuropericardial J90
chylous, chyliform J94.0
due to systemic lupus erythematosis M32.13
in conditions classified elsewhere J91.8
influenzal —see Influenza, with, respiratory manifestations NEC
malignant J91.0
newborn P28.89
tuberculous NEC A15.6
primary (progressive) A15.7
spinal —see Meningitis
thorax, thoracic —see Effusion, pleura
Egg shell nails L60.3
congenital Q84.6
EGPA (eosinophilic granulomatosis with polyangiitis) M30.1
Egyptian splenomegaly B65.1
Ehlers-Danlos syndrome (see also Syndrome, Ehlers-Danlos) Q79.60
Ehrlichiosis A77.40
due to
E. chafeensis A77.41
E. ewingii A77.49
E. muris euclairensis A77.49
E. sennetsu A79.81
specified organism NEC A77.49
Eichstedt's disease B36.0
Eisenmenger's
complex or syndrome I27.83
defect Q21.8
Ejaculation
delayed F52.32
painful N53.12
premature F52.4
retarded N53.11
retrograde N53.14
semen, painful N53.12
psychogenic F52.6

Ekbom's syndrome (restless legs) G25.81
Ekman's syndrome (brittle bones and blue sclera) Q78.0
Elastic skin Q82.8
acquired L57.4
Elastofibroma —see Neoplasm, connective tissue, benign
Elastoma (juvenile) Q82.8
Miescher's L87.2
Elastomyofibrosis I42.4
Elastosis
actinic, solar L57.8
atrophicans (senile) L57.4
perforans serpiginosa L87.2
senilis L57.4
Elbow —see condition
Electric current, electricity, effects (concussion) (fatal) (nonfatal) (shock) T75.4
burn —see Burn
Electric feet syndrome E53.8
Electrocution T75.4
from electroshock gun (taser) T75.4
Electrolyte imbalance E87.8
with
abortion —see Abortion by type, complicated by, electrolyte imbalance
ectopic pregnancy O08.5
molar pregnancy O08.5
Elephantiasis (nonfilarial) I89.0
arabicum —see Infestation, filarial
bancroftian B74.0
congenital (any site) (hereditary) Q82.0
due to
Brugia (malayi) B74.1
timori B74.2
mastectomy I97.2
Wuchereria (bancrofti) B74.0
eyelid H02.859
left H02.856
lower H02.855
upper H02.854
right H02.853
lower H02.852
upper H02.851
filarial, filariensis —see Infestation, filarial
glandular I89.0
graecorum A30.9
lymphangiectatic I89.0
lymphatic vessel I89.0
due to mastectomy I97.2
scrotum (nonfilarial) I89.0
streptococcal I89.0
surgical I97.89
postmastectomy I97.2
telangiectodes I89.0
vulva (nonfilarial) N90.89
Elevated, elevation
alanine transaminase (ALT) R74.01
ALT (alanine transaminase) R74.01
antibody titer R76.0
aspartate transaminase (AST) R74.01
AST (aspartate transaminase) R74.01
basal metabolic rate R94.8
blood pressure —see also Hypertension
reading (incidental) (isolated) (nonspecific), no diagnosis of hypertension R03.0
blood sugar R73.9
body temperature (of unknown origin) R50.9
C-reactive protein (CRP) R79.82
cancer antigen 125 [CA 125] R97.1
carcinoembryonic antigen [CEA] R97.0
cholesterol E78.00
with high triglycerides E78.2
conjugate, eye H51.0
diaphragm, congenital Q79.1
erythrocyte sedimentation rate R70.0
fasting glucose R73.01
fasting triglycerides E78.1
finding on laboratory examination —see Findings, abnormal, inconclusive, without diagnosis, by type of exam

Elevated, elevation (Continued)
GFR (glomerular filtration rate) —see Findings, abnormal, inconclusive, without diagnosis, by type of exam
glucose tolerance (oral) R73.02
immunoglobulin level R76.8
indoleacetic acid R82.5
lactic acid dehydrogenase (LDH) level R74.02
leukocytes D72.829
lipoprotein a (Lp(a)) level E78.41
liver function
study R94.5
test R79.89
alkaline phosphatase R74.8
aminotransferase R74.01
bilirubin R17
hepatic enzyme R74.8
lactate dehydrogenase R74.02
(Lp(a)) (lipoprotein(a)) E78.41
lymphocytes D72.820
prostate specific antigen [PSA] R97.20
Rh titer —see Complication(s), transfusion, incompatibility reaction, Rh (factor)
scapula, congenital Q74.0
sedimentation rate R70.0
SGOT R74.01
SGPT R74.01
transaminase level R74.01
triglycerides E78.1
with high cholesterol E78.2
troponin R77.8
tumor associated antigens [TAA] NEC R97.8
tumor specific antigens [TSA] NEC R97.8
urine level of
17-ketosteroids R82.5
catecholamine R82.5
indoleacetic acid R82.5
steroids R82.5
vanillylmandelic acid (VMA) R82.5
venous pressure I87.8
white blood cell count D72.829
specified NEC D72.828
Elliptocytosis (congenital) (hereditary) D58.1
Hb C (disease) D58.1
hemoglobin disease D58.1
sickle-cell (disease) D57.8-•
trait D57.3
Ellison-Zollinger syndrome E16.4
Ellis-van Creveld syndrome (chondroectodermal dysplasia) Q77.6
Elongated, elongation (congenital) —see also Distortion
bone Q79.9
cervix (uteri) Q51.828
acquired N88.4
hypertrophic N88.4
colon Q43.8
common bile duct Q44.5
cystic duct Q44.5
frenulum, penis Q55.69
labia minora (acquired) N90.69
ligamentum patellae Q74.1
petiolus (epiglottidis) Q31.8
tooth, teeth K00.2
uvula Q38.6
Eltor cholera A00.1
⟹**Emaciation** R64
▶due to manutrition E43
Embadomoniasis A07.8
Embedded tooth, teeth K01.0
root only K08.3
Embolic —see condition
Embolism (multiple) (paradoxical) I74.9
air (any site) (traumatic) T79.0
following
abortion —see Abortion by type, complicated by embolism
ectopic pregnancy O08.2
infusion, therapeutic injection or transfusion T80.0
molar pregnancy O08.2

Embolism *(Continued)*
  air *(Continued)*
    following *(Continued)*
      procedure NEC
        artery T81.719
          mesenteric T81.710
          renal T81.711
          specified NEC T81.718
        vein T81.72
    in pregnancy, childbirth or puerperium —
      see Embolism, obstetric
  amniotic fluid (pulmonary) —*see also*
    Embolism, obstetric
    following
      abortion —*see* Abortion by type
        complicated by embolism
      ectopic pregnancy O08.2
      molar pregnancy O08.2
  aorta, aortic I74.10
    abdominal I74.09
      saddle I74.01
    bifurcation I74.09
    saddle I74.01
    thoracic I74.11
  artery I74.9
    auditory, internal I65.8
    basilar —*see* Occlusion, artery, basilar
    carotid (common) (internal) —*see*
      Occlusion, artery, carotid
    cerebellar (anterior inferior) (posterior
      inferior) (superior) I66.3
    cerebral —*see* Occlusion, artery, cerebral
    choroidal (anterior) I65.8
    communicating posterior I65.8
    coronary —*see also* Infarct, myocardium
      not resulting in infarction I24.0
    extremity I74.4
      lower I74.3
      upper I74.2
    hypophyseal I65.8
    iliac I74.5
    limb I74.4
      lower I74.3
      upper I74.2
    mesenteric (with gangrene) —*see also*
      Ischemia, intestine, acute K55.09
    ophthalmic —*see* Occlusion, artery, retina
    peripheral I74.4
    pontine I65.8
    precerebral —*see* Occlusion, artery,
      precerebral
    pulmonary —*see* Embolism, pulmonary
    renal N28.0
    retinal —*see* Occlusion, artery, retina
    septic I76
    specified NEC I74.8
    vertebral —*see* Occlusion, artery, vertebral
  basilar (artery) I65.1
  blood clot
    following
      abortion —*see* Abortion by type
        complicated by embolism
      ectopic or molar pregnancy O08.2
    in pregnancy, childbirth or puerperium —
      see Embolism, obstetric
  brain —*see also* Occlusion, artery, cerebral
    following
      abortion —*see* Abortion by type
        complicated by embolism
      ectopic or molar pregnancy O08.2
    puerperal, postpartum, childbirth —*see*
      Embolism, obstetric
  capillary I78.8
  cardiac —*see also* Infarct, myocardium
    not resulting in infarction I51.3
  carotid (artery) (common) (internal) —*see*
    Occlusion, artery, carotid
  cavernous sinus (venous) —*see* Embolism,
    intracranial, venous sinus
  cerebral —*see* Occlusion, artery, cerebral
  cholesterol —*see* Atheroembolism

coronary (artery or vein) (systemic) —*see*
  Occlusion, coronary
due to device, implant or graft —*see also*
  Complications, by site and type,
  specified NEC
  arterial graft NEC T82.818
  breast (implant) T85.818
  catheter NEC T85.818
    dialysis (renal) T82.818
      intraperitoneal T85.818
    infusion NEC T82.818
      spinal (epidural) (subdural) T85.810
    urinary (indwelling) T83.81
  electronic (electrode) (pulse generator)
    (stimulator)
    bone T84.81
    cardiac T82.817
    nervous system (brain) (peripheral
      nerve) (spinal) T85.810
    urinary T83.81
  fixation, internal (orthopedic) NEC T84.81
  gastrointestinal (bile duct) (esophagus)
    T85.818
  genital NEC T83.81
  heart (graft) (valve) T82.817
  joint prosthesis T84.81
  ocular (corneal graft) (orbital implant)
    T85.818
  orthopedic (bone graft) NEC T86.838
  specified NEC T85.818
  urinary (graft) NEC T83.81
  vascular NEC T82.818
  ventricular intracranial shunt T85.810
extremities
  lower —*see* Embolism, vein, lower
    extremity
    arterial I74.3
  upper I74.2
eye H34.9
fat (cerebral) (pulmonary) (systemic) T79.1
  complicating delivery —*see* Embolism,
    obstetric
  following
    abortion —*see* Abortion by type
      complicated by embolism
    ectopic or molar pregnancy O08.2
following
  abortion —*see* Abortion by type
    complicated by embolism
  ectopic or molar pregnancy O08.2
  infusion, therapeutic injection or transfusion
    air T80.0
heart (fatty) —*see also* Infarct, myocardium
  not resulting in infarction I51.3
hepatic (vein) I82.0
in pregnancy, childbirth or puerperium —*see*
  Embolism, obstetric
intestine (artery) (vein) (with gangrene) —*see*
  also Ischemia, intestine, acute K55.039
intracranial —*see also* Occlusion, artery,
  cerebral
  venous sinus (any) G08
    nonpyogenic I67.6
intraspinal venous sinuses or veins G08
  nonpyogenic G95.19
kidney (artery) N28.0
lateral sinus (venous) —*see* Embolism,
  intracranial, venous sinus
leg —*see* Embolism, vein, lower extremity
  arterial I74.3
longitudinal sinus (venous) —*see* Embolism,
  intracranial, venous sinus
lung (massive) —*see* Embolism, pulmonary
meninges I66.8
mesenteric (artery) (vein) (with gangrene) —
  see also Ischemia, intestine, acute K55.059
obstetric (in) (pulmonary)
  childbirth O88.22
    air O88.02
    amniotic fluid O88.12

Embolism *(Continued)*
  obstetric *(Continued)*
    childbirth *(Continued)*
      blood clot O88.22
      fat O88.82
      pyemic O88.32
      septic O88.32
      specified type NEC O88.82
    pregnancy O88.21-●
      air O88.01-●
      amniotic fluid O88.11-●
      blood clot O88.21-●
      fat O88.81-●
      pyemic O88.31-●
      septic O88.31-●
      specified type NEC O88.81-●
    puerperal O88.23
      air O88.03
      amniotic fluid O88.13
      blood clot O88.23
      fat O88.83
      pyemic O88.33
      septic O88.33
      specified type NEC O88.83
  ophthalmic —*see* Occlusion, artery, retina
  penis N48.81
  peripheral artery NOS I74.4
  pituitary E23.6
  popliteal (artery) I74.3
  portal (vein) I81
  postoperative, postprocedural
    artery T81.719
      mesenteric T81.710
      renal T81.711
      specified NEC T81.718
    vein T81.72
  precerebral artery —*see* Occlusion, artery,
    precerebral
  puerperal —*see* Embolism, obstetric
  pulmonary (acute) (artery) (vein) I26.99
    with acute cor pulmonale I26.09
    chronic I27.82
    following
      abortion —*see* Abortion by type
        complicated by embolism
      ectopic or molar pregnancy O08.2
    healed or old Z86.711
    in pregnancy, childbirth or puerperium —
      see Embolism, obstetric
    multiple subsegmental without acute cor
      pulmonale I26.94
    personal history of Z86.711
    saddle I26.92
      with acute cor pulmonale I26.02
    septic I26.90
      with acute cor pulmonale I26.01
    single subsegmental without acute cor
      pulmonale I26.93
    subsegmental NOS I26.93
  pyemic (multiple) I76
    following
      abortion —*see* Abortion by type
        complicated by embolism
      ectopic or molar pregnancy O08.2
    Hemophilus influenzae A41.3
    pneumococcal A40.3
      with pneumonia J13
    puerperal, postpartum, childbirth
      (any organism) —*see* Embolism,
      obstetric
    specified organism NEC A41.89
    staphylococcal A41.2
    streptococcal A40.9
  renal (artery) N28.0
    vein I82.3
  retina, retinal —*see* Occlusion, artery,
    retina
  saddle
    abdominal aorta I74.01
    pulmonary artery I26.92
      with acute cor pulmonale I26.02

▶ New   ⇥ Revised   ~~deleted~~ Deleted   ● Use Additional Character(s)

Embolism (Continued)
  septic (arterial) I76
    complicating abortion —see Abortion, by
        type, complicated by, embolism
  sinus —see Embolism, intracranial, venous
      sinus
  soap complicating abortion —see Abortion,
      by type, complicated by, embolism
  spinal cord G95.19
    pyogenic origin G06.1
  spleen, splenic (artery) I74.8
  upper extremity I74.2
  vein (acute) I82.90
    antecubital I82.61-●
      chronic I82.71-●
    axillary I82.A1-●
      chronic I82.A2-●
    basilic I82.61-●
      chronic I82.71-●
    brachial I82.62-●
      chronic I82.72-●
    brachiocephalic (innominate) I82.290
      chronic I82.291
    cephalic I82.61-●
      chronic I82.71-●
    chronic I82.91
    deep (DVT) I82.40-●
      calf I82.4Z-●
        chronic I82.5Z-●
      lower leg I82.4Z-●
        chronic I82.5Z-●
      thigh I82.4Y-●
        chronic I82.5Y-●
      upper leg I82.4Y
        chronic I82.5y--●
    femoral I82.41-●
      chronic I82.51-●
    iliac (iliofemoral) I82.42-●
      chronic I82.52-●
    innominate I82.290
      chronic I82.291
    internal jugular I82.C1-●
      chronic I82.C2-●
    lower extremity
      deep I82.40-●
        chronic I82.50-●
        specified NEC I82.49-●
          chronic NEC I82.59-●
      distal
        deep I82.4Z-●
      proximal
        deep I82.4Y-●
          chronic I82.5Y-●
      superficial I82.81-●
    popliteal I82.43-●
      chronic I82.53-●
    radial I82.62-●
      chronic I82.72-●
    renal I82.3
    saphenous (greater) (lesser) I82.81-●
    specified NEC I82.890
      chronic NEC I82.891
    subclavian I82.B1-●
      chronic I82.B2-●
    thoracic NEC I82.290
      chronic I82.291
    tibial I82.44-●
      chronic I82.54-●
    ulnar I82.62-●
      chronic I82.72-●
    upper extremity I82.60-●
      chronic I82.70-●
      deep I82.62-●
        chronic I82.72-●
      superficial I82.61-●
        chronic I82.71-●
  vena cava
    inferior (acute) I82.220
      chronic I82.221
    superior (acute) I82.210
      chronic I82.211

Embolism (Continued)
  venous sinus G08
  vessels of brain —see Occlusion, artery,
      cerebral
Embolus —see Embolism
Embryoma —see also Neoplasm, uncertain
    behavior, by site
  benign —see Neoplasm, benign, by site
  kidney C64.-●
  liver C22.0
  malignant —see also Neoplasm, malignant,
      by site
    kidney C64.-●
    liver C22.0
    testis C62.9-●
      descended (scrotal) C62.1-●
      undescended C62.0-●
  testis C62.9-●
    descended (scrotal) C62.1-●
    undescended C62.0-●
Embryonic
  circulation Q28.9
  heart Q28.9
  vas deferens Q55.4
Embryopathia NOS Q89.9
Embryotoxon Q13.4
Emesis —see Vomiting
Emotional lability R45.86
Emotionality, pathological F60.3
Emotogenic disease —see Disorder,
    psychogenic
Emphysema (atrophic) (bullous) (chronic)
    (interlobular) (lung) (obstructive)
    (pulmonary) (senile) (vesicular) J43.9
  cellular tissue (traumatic) T79.7
    surgical T81.82
  centrilobular J43.2
  compensatory J98.3
  congenital (interstitial) P25.0
  conjunctiva H11.89
  connective tissue (traumatic) T79.7
    surgical T81.82
  due to chemicals, gases, fumes or vapors J68.4
  eyelid(s) —see Disorder, eyelid, specified type
      NEC
    surgical T81.82
    traumatic T79.7
  interstitial J98.2
    congenital P25.0
    perinatal period P25.0
  laminated tissue T79.7
    surgical T81.82
  mediastinal J98.2
    newborn P25.2
  orbit, orbital —see Disorder, orbit, specified
      type NEC
  panacinar J43.1
  panlobular J43.1
  specified NEC J43.8
  subcutaneous (traumatic) T79.7
    nontraumatic J98.2
    postprocedural T81.82
    surgical T81.82
  surgical T81.82
  thymus (gland) (congenital) E32.8
  traumatic (subcutaneous) T79.7
  unilateral J43.0
Empty nest syndrome Z60.0
Empyema (acute) (chest) (double) (pleura)
    (supradiaphragmatic) (thorax) J86.9
  with fistula J86.0
  accessory sinus (chronic) —see Sinusitis
  antrum (chronic) —see Sinusitis, maxillary
  brain (any part) —see Abscess, brain
  ethmoidal (chronic) (sinus) —see Sinusitis,
      ethmoidal
  extradural —see Abscess, extradural
  frontal (chronic) (sinus) —see Sinusitis, frontal
  gallbladder K81.0
  mastoid (process) (acute) —see Mastoiditis,
      acute
  maxilla, maxillary M27.2

Empyema (Continued)
  sinus (chronic) —see Sinusitis, maxillary
  nasal sinus (chronic) —see Sinusitis
  sinus (accessory) (chronic) (nasal) —see
      Sinusitis
  sphenoidal (sinus) (chronic) —see Sinusitis,
      sphenoidal
  subarachnoid —see Abscess, extradural
  subdural —see Abscess, subdural
  tuberculous A15.6
  ureter —see Ureteritis
  ventricular —see Abscess, brain
En coup de sabre lesion L94.1
Enamel pearls K00.2
Enameloma K00.2
Enanthema, viral B09
Encephalitis (chronic) (hemorrhagic)
    (idiopathic) (nonepidemic) (spurious)
    (subacute) G04.90
  acute —see also Encephalitis, viral A86
    disseminated G04.00
      infectious G04.01
      noninfectious G04.81
      postimmunization (postvaccination)
          G04.02
      postinfectious G04.01
    inclusion body A85.8
    necrotizing hemorrhagic G04.30
      postimmunization G04.32
      postinfectious G04.31
      specified NEC G04.39
  arboviral, arbovirus NEC A85.2
  arthropod-borne NEC (viral) A85.2
  Australian A83.4
  California (virus) A83.5
  Central European (tick-borne) A84.1
  Czechoslovakian A84.1
  Dawson's (inclusion body) A81.1
  diffuse sclerosing A81.1
  disseminated, acute G04.00
  due to
    cat scratch disease A28.1
    human immunodeficiency virus (HIV)
        disease B20 [G05.3]
    malaria —see Malaria
    rickettsiosis —see Rickettsiosis
    smallpox inoculation G04.02
    typhus —see Typhus
  Eastern equine A83.2
  endemic (viral) A86
  epidemic NEC (viral) A86
  equine (acute) (infectious) (viral) A83.9
    Eastern A83.2
    Venezuelan A92.2
    Western A83.1
  Far Eastern (tick-borne) A84.0
  following vaccination or other immunization
      procedure G04.02
  herpes zoster B02.0
  herpesviral B00.4
    due to herpesvirus 6 B10.01
    due to herpesvirus 7 B10.09
    specified NEC B10.09
  Ilheus (virus) A83.8
  in (due to)
    actinomycosis A42.82
    adenovirus A85.1
    African trypanosomiasis B56.9 [G05.3]
    Chagas' disease (chronic) B57.42
    cytomegalovirus B25.8
    enterovirus A85.0
    herpes (simplex) virus B00.4
      due to herpesvirus 6 B10.01
      due to herpesvirus 7 B10.09
      specified NEC B10.09
    infectious disease NEC B99 [G05.3]
    influenza —see Influenza, with,
        encephalopathy
    listeriosis A32.12
    measles B05.0
    mumps B26.2
    naegleriasis B60.2

Encephalitis *(Continued)*
 in *(Continued)*
  parasitic disease NEC B89 *[G05.3]*
  poliovirus A80.9 *[G05.3]*
  rubella B06.01
  syphilis
   congenital A50.42
   late A52.14
  systemic lupus erythematosus M32.19
  toxoplasmosis (acquired) B58.2
   congenital P37.1
  tuberculosis A17.82
  zoster B02.0
 inclusion body A81.1
 infectious (acute) (virus) NEC A86
 Japanese (B type) A83.0
 La Crosse A83.5
 lead —*see* Poisoning, lead
 lethargica (acute) (infectious) A85.8
 louping ill A84.89
 lupus erythematosus, systemic M32.19
 lymphatica A87.2
 Mengo A85.8
 meningococcal A39.81
 Murray Valley A83.4
 otitic NEC H66.40 *[G05.3]*
 parasitic NOS B71.9
 periaxial G37.0
 periaxialis (concentrica) (diffuse) G37.5
 postchickenpox B01.11
 postexanthematous NEC B09
 postimmunization G04.02
 postinfectious NEC G04.01
 postmeasles B05.0
 postvaccinal G04.02
 postvaricella B01.11
 postviral NEC A86
 Powassan A84.81
 Rasmussen G04.81
 Rio Bravo A85.8
 Russian
  autumnal A83.0
  spring-summer (taiga) A84.0
 saturnine —*see* Poisoning, lead
 specified NEC G04.81
 St. Louis A83.3
 subacute sclerosing A81.1
 summer A83.0
 suppurative G04.81
 tick-borne A84.9
 Torula, torular (cryptococcal) B45.1
⇒toxic NEC G92.8
 trichinosis B75 *[G05.3]*
 type
  B A83.0
  C A83.3
 van Bogaert's A81.1
 Venezuelan equine A92.2
 Vienna A85.8
 viral, virus A86
  arthropod-borne NEC A85.2
   mosquito-borne A83.9
    Australian X disease A83.4
    California virus A83.5
    Eastern equine A83.2
    Japanese (B type) A83.0
    Murray Valley A83.4
    specified NEC A83.8
    St. Louis A83.3
    type B A83.0
    type C A83.3
    Western equine A83.1
   tick-borne A84.9
    biundulant A84.1
    central European A84.1
    Czechoslovakian A84.1
    diphasic meningoencephalitis A84.1
    Far Eastern A84.0
    Russian spring-summer (taiga) A84.0
    specified NEC A84.89
   specified type NEC A85.8
   tick-borne, specified NEC A84.89
 Western equine A83.1

Encephalocele Q01.9
 frontal Q01.0
 nasofrontal Q01.1
 occipital Q01.2
 specified NEC Q01.8
Encephalocystocele —*see* Encephalocele
Encephaloduroarteriomyosynangiosis
 (EDAMS) I67.5
Encephalomalacia (brain) (cerebellar)
 (cerebral) —*see* Softening, brain
Encephalomeningitis —*see*
 Meningoencephalitis
Encephalomeningocele —*see* Encephalocele
Encephalomeningomyelitis —*see*
 Meningoencephalitis
Encephalomyelitis —*see also* Encephalitis G04.90
 acute disseminated G04.00
  infectious G04.01
  noninfectious G04.81
  postimmunization G04.02
  postinfectious G04.01
 acute necrotizing hemorrhagic G04.30
  postimmunization G04.32
  postinfectious G04.31
  specified NEC G04.39
 benign myalgic G93.3
 equine A83.9
  Eastern A83.2
  Venezuelan A92.2
  Western A83.1
 in diseases classified elsewhere G05.3
 myalgic, benign G93.3
 postchickenpox B01.11
 postinfectious NEC G04.01
 postmeasles B05.0
 postvaccinal G04.02
 postvaricella B01.11
 rubella B06.01
 specified NEC G04.81
 Venezuelan equine A92.2
Encephalomyelocele —*see* Encephalocele
Encephalomyelomeningitis —*see*
 Meningoencephalitis
Encephalomyelopathy G96.9
Encephalomyeloradiculitis (acute) G61.0
Encephalomyeloradiculoneuritis (acute)
 (Guillain-Barré) G61.0
Encephalomyeloradiculopathy G96.9
Encephalopathia hyperbilirubinemica,
 newborn P57.9
 due to isoimmunization (conditions in P55)
  P57.0
Encephalopathy (acute) G93.40
 acute necrotizing hemorrhagic G04.30
  postimmunization G04.32
  postinfectious G04.31
  specified NEC G04.39
 alcoholic G31.2
 anoxic —*see* Damage, brain, anoxic
 arteriosclerotic I67.2
 centrolobar progressive (Schilder) G37.0
 congenital Q07.9
 degenerative, in specified disease NEC G32.89
 due to
⇒ drugs (*see also* Table of Drugs and
   Chemicals) G92.8
 demyelinating callosal G37.1
 hepatic —*see* Failure, hepatic
 hyperbilirubinemic, newborn P57.9
  due to isoimmunization (conditions in P55)
   P57.0
 hypertensive I67.4
 hypoglycemic E16.2
 hypoxic —*see* Damage, brain, anoxic
 hypoxic ischemic P91.60
  mild P91.61
  moderate P91.62
  severe P91.63
 in (due to) (with)
  birth injury P11.1
  hyperinsulinism E16.1 *[G94]*

Encephalopathy *(Continued)*
 in *(Continued)*
  influenza —*see* Influenza, with,
   encephalopathy
  lack of vitamin (*see also* Deficiency, vitamin)
   E56.9 *[G32.89]*
  neoplastic disease (*see also* Neoplasm)
   D49.9 *[G13.1]*
  serum (*see also* Reaction, serum) T80.69
  syphilis A52.17
  trauma (postconcussional) F07.81
   current injury —*see* Injury, intracranial
  vaccination G04.02
 lead —*see* Poisoning, lead
 metabolic G93.41
⇒ drug induced G92.8
⇒ toxic G92.8
 myoclonic, early, symptomatic —*see* Epilepsy,
  generalized, specified NEC
 necrotizing, subacute (Leigh) G31.82
 neonatal P91.819
  in diseases classified elsewhere P91.811
 pellagrous E52 *[G32.89]*
 portosystemic —*see* Failure, hepatic
 postcontusional F07.81
  current injury —*see* Injury, intracranial,
   diffuse
 posthypoglycemic (coma) E16.1 *[G94]*
 postradiation G93.89
 saturnine —*see* Poisoning, lead
 septic G93.41
 specified NEC G93.49
 spongiform, subacute (viral) A81.09
⇒ toxic G92.8
⇒ metabolic G92.8
 traumatic (postconcussional) F07.81
  current injury —*see* Injury, intracranial
 vitamin B deficiency NEC E53.9 *[G32.89]*
  vitamin B1 E51.2
 Wernicke's E51.2
Encephalorrhagia —*see* Hemorrhage,
 intracranial, intracerebral
Encephalosis, posttraumatic F07.81
Enchondroma —*see also* Neoplasm, bone,
 benign
Enchondromatosis (cartilaginous) (multiple)
 Q78.4
Encopresis R15.9
 functional F98.1
 nonorganic origin F98.1
 psychogenic F98.1
Encounter (with health service) (for) Z76.89
 adjustment and management (of)
  breast implant Z45.81
  implanted device NEC Z45.89
  myringotomy device (stent) (tube)
   Z45.82
  neurostimulator (brain) (gastric)
   (peripheral nerve) (sacral nerve)
   (spinal cord) (vagus nerve) Z45.42
 administrative purpose only Z02.9
  examination for
   adoption Z02.82
   armed forces Z02.3
   disability determination Z02.71
   driving license Z02.4
   employment Z02.1
   insurance Z02.6
   medical certificate NEC Z02.79
   paternity testing Z02.81
   residential institution admission Z02.2
   school admission Z02.0
   sports Z02.5
  specified reason NEC Z02.89
 aftercare —*see* Aftercare
 antenatal screening Z36.9
  cervical length Z36.86
  chromosomal anomalies Z36.0
  congenital cardiac abnormalities Z36.83
  elevated maternal serum alphafetoprotein
   level Z36.1

▶ New   ⇒ Revised   ~~deleted~~ Deleted   ● Use Additional Character(s)

Encounter *(Continued)*
  antenatal screening *(Continued)*
    fetal growth retardation Z36.4
    fetal lung maturity Z36.84
    fetal macrosomia Z36.88
    hydrops fetalis Z36.81
    intrauterine growth restriction (IUGR)/
        small-for-dates Z36.4
    isoimmunization Z36.5
    large-for-dates Z36.88
    malformations Z36.3
    non-visualized anatomy on a previous scan
        Z36.2
    nuchal translucency Z36.82
    raised alphafetoprotein level Z36.1
    risk of pre-term labor Z36.86
    specified type NEC Z36.89
    specified follow-up NEC Z36.2
    specified genetic defects NEC Z36.8A
    Streptococcus B Z36.85
    suspected anomaly Z36.3
    uncertain dates Z36.87
  assisted reproductive fertility procedure cycle
      Z31.83
  blood typing Z01.83
    Rh typing Z01.83
  breast augmentation or reduction Z41.1
  breast implant exchange (different material)
      (different size) Z45.81
  breast reconstruction following mastectomy
      Z42.1
  check-up —*see* Examination
  chemotherapy for neoplasm Z51.11
  colonoscopy, screening Z12.11
  counseling —*see* Counseling
  delivery, full-term, uncomplicated O80
    cesarean, without indication O82
  desensitization to allergens Z51.6
  ear piercing Z41.3
  examination —*see* Examination
  expectant parent(s) (adoptive) pre-birth
      pediatrician visit Z76.81
  fertility preservation procedure (prior to
      cancer therapy) (prior to removal of
      gonads) Z31.84
  fitting (of) —*see* Fitting (and adjustment) (of)
  genetic
    counseling
      nonprocreative Z71.83
      procreative Z31.5
    testing —*see* Test, genetic
  hearing conservation and treatment Z01.12
  immunotherapy for neoplasm Z51.12
  in vitro fertilization cycle Z31.83
  instruction (in)
    child care (postpartal) (prenatal) Z32.3
    childbirth Z32.2
    natural family planning
      procreative Z31.61
      to avoid pregnancy Z30.02
  insulin pump titration Z46.81
  joint prosthesis insertion following prior
      explantation of joint prosthesis (staged
      procedure)
    hip Z47.32
    knee Z47.33
    shoulder Z47.31
  laboratory (as part of a general medical
      examination) Z00.00
    with abnormal findings Z00.01
  mental health services (for)
    abuse NEC
      perpetrator Z69.82
      victim Z69.81
    child abuse
      nonparental
        perpetrator Z69.021
        victim Z69.020
      parental
        perpetrator Z69.011
        victim Z69.010

Encounter *(Continued)*
  mental health services *(Continued)*
    child neglect
      nonparental
        perpetrator Z69.021
        victim Z69.020
      parental
        perpetrator Z69.011
        victim Z69.010
    child psychological abuse
      nonparental
        perpetrator Z69.021
        victim Z69.020
      parental
        perpetrator Z69.011
        victim Z69.010
    child sexual abuse
      nonparental
        perpetrator Z69.021
        victim Z69.020
      parental
        perpetrator Z69.011
        victim Z69.010
    non-spousal adult abuse
      perpetrator Z69.82
      victim Z69.81
    spousal or partner
      abuse
        perpetrator Z69.12
        victim Z69.11
      neglect
        perpetrator Z69.12
        victim Z69.11
      psychological abuse
        perpetrator Z69.12
        victim Z69.11
      violence
        perpetrator (physical) (sexual)
            Z69.12
        victim (physical) Z69.11
          sexual Z69.81
  observation (for) (ruled out)
    exposure to (suspected)
      anthrax Z03.810
      biological agent NEC Z03.818
  pediatrician visit, by expectant parent(s)
      (adoptive) Z76.81
  placental sample (taken vaginally) —*see also*
      Encounter, antenatal screening Z36.9
  plastic and reconstructive surgery following
      medical procedure or healed injury NEC
      Z42.8
  pregnancy
    supervision of —*see* Pregnancy,
        supervision of
    test Z32.00
      result negative Z32.02
      result positive Z32.01
  procreative management and counseling for
      gestational carrier Z31.7
  prophylactic measures Z29.9
    antivenin Z29.12
    fluoride administration Z29.3
    immunotherapy for respiratory syncytial
        virus (RSV) Z29.11
    rabies immune globin Z29.14
    Rho (D) immune globulin Z29.13
    specified NEC Z29.8
  radiation therapy (antineoplastic) Z51.0
  radiological (as part of a general medical
      examination) Z00.00
    with abnormal findings Z00.01
  reconstructive surgery following medical
      procedure or healed injury NEC
      Z42.8
  removal (of) —*see also* Removal
    artificial
      arm Z44.00-●
        complete Z44.01-●
        partial Z44.02-●
      eye Z44.2-●

Encounter *(Continued)*
  removal *(Continued)*
    artificial *(Continued)*
      leg Z44.10-●
        complete Z44.11-●
        partial Z44.12-●
    breast implant Z45.81
      tissue expander (with or without
          synchronous insertion of permanent
          implant) Z45.81
    device Z46.9
      specified NEC Z46.89
    external
      fixation device — code to fracture with
          seventh character D
      prosthesis, prosthetic device Z44.9
        breast Z44.3-●
        specified NEC Z44.8
    implanted device NEC Z45.89
    insulin pump Z46.81
    internal fixation device Z47.2
    myringotomy device (stent) (tube) Z45.82
    nervous system device NEC Z46.2
      brain neuropacemaker Z46.2
      visual substitution device Z46.2
        implanted Z45.31
    non-vascular catheter Z46.82
    orthodontic device Z46.4
    stent
      ureteral Z46.6
    urinary device Z46.6
  repeat cervical smear to confirm findings of
      recent normal smear following initial
      abnormal smear Z01.42
  respirator [ventilator] use during power
      failure (Z99.12)
  Rh typing Z01.83
  screening —*see* Screening
  specified NEC Z76.89
  sterilization Z30.2
  suspected condition, ruled out
    amniotic cavity and membrane Z03.71
    cervical shortening Z03.75
    fetal anomaly Z03.73
    fetal growth Z03.74
    maternal and fetal conditions NEC
        Z03.79
    oligohydramnios Z03.71
    placental problem Z03.72
    polyhydramnios Z03.71
  suspected exposure (to), ruled out
    anthrax Z03.810
    biological agents NEC Z03.818
  termination of pregnancy, elective Z33.2
  testing —*see* Test
  therapeutic drug level monitoring Z51.81
  titration, insulin pump Z46.81
  to determine fetal viability of pregnancy
      O36.80
  training
    insulin pump Z46.81
  X-ray of chest (as part of a general medical
      examination Z00.00)
    with abnormal findings Z00.01
Encystment —*see* Cyst
Endarteritis (bacterial, subacute) (infective)
    I77.6
  brain I67.7
  cerebral or cerebrospinal I67.7
  deformans —*see* Arteriosclerosis
  embolic —*see* Embolism
  obliterans —*see also* Arteriosclerosis
    pulmonary I28.8
  pulmonary I28.8
  retina —*see* Vasculitis, retina
  senile —*see* Arteriosclerosis
  syphilitic A52.09
    brain or cerebral A52.04
    congenital A50.54 *[I79.8]*
  tuberculous A18.89
Endemic —*see* condition

Endocarditis (chronic) (marantic) (nonbacterial) (thrombotic) (valvular) I38
  with rheumatic fever (conditions in I00)
    active —see Endocarditis, acute, rheumatic
    inactive or quiescent (with chorea) I09.1
  acute or subacute I33.9
    infective I33.0
    rheumatic (aortic) (mitral) (pulmonary) (tricuspid) I01.1
      with chorea (acute) (rheumatic) (Sydenham's) I02.0
  aortic (heart) (nonrheumatic) (valve) I35.8
    with
      mitral disease I08.0
        with tricuspid (valve) disease I08.3
        active or acute I01.1
          with chorea (acute) (rheumatic) (Sydenham's) I02.0
        rheumatic fever (conditions in I00)
          active —see Endocarditis, acute, rheumatic
          inactive or quiescent (with chorea) I06.9
      tricuspid (valve) disease I08.2
        with mitral (valve) disease I08.3
    acute or subacute I33.9
    arteriosclerotic I35.8
    rheumatic I06.9
      with mitral disease I08.0
        with tricuspid (valve) disease I08.3
        active or acute I01.1
          with chorea (acute) (rheumatic) (Sydenham's) I02.0
      active or acute I01.1
        with chorea (acute) (rheumatic) (Sydenham's) I02.0
      specified NEC I06.8
    specified cause NEC I35.8
    syphilitic A52.03
  arteriosclerotic I38
  atypical verrucous (Libman-Sacks) M32.11
  bacterial (acute) (any valve) (subacute) I33.0
  candidal B37.6
  congenital Q24.8
  constrictive I33.0
  Coxiella burnetii A78 [I39]
  Coxsackie B33.21
  due to
    prosthetic cardiac valve T82.6
    Q fever A78 [I39]
    Serratia marcescens I33.0
    typhoid (fever) A01.02
  gonococcal A54.83
  infectious or infective (acute) (any valve) (subacute) I33.0
  lenta (acute) (any valve) (subacute) I33.0
  Libman-Sacks M32.11
  listerial A32.82
  Löffler's I42.3
  malignant (acute) (any valve) (subacute) I33.0
  meningococcal A39.51
  mitral (chronic) (double) (fibroid) (heart) (inactive) (valve) (with chorea) I05.9
    with
      aortic (valve) disease I08.0
        with tricuspid (valve) disease I08.3
        active or acute I01.1
          with chorea (acute) (rheumatic) (Sydenham's) I02.0
      rheumatic fever (conditions in I00)
        active —see Endocarditis, acute, rheumatic
        inactive or quiescent (with chorea) I05.9
      tricuspid (valve) disease I08.1
        with aortic (valve) disease I08.3
    active or acute I01.1
      with chorea (acute) (rheumatic) (Sydenham's) I02.0
    bacterial I33.0

Endocarditis (Continued)
  mitral (Continued)
    arteriosclerotic I34.8
    nonrheumatic I34.8
      acute or subacute I33.9
    specified NEC I05.8
  monilial B37.6
  multiple valves I08.9
    specified disorders I08.8
  mycotic (acute) (any valve) (subacute) I33.0
  pneumococcal (acute) (any valve) (subacute) I33.0
  pulmonary (chronic) (heart) (valve) I37.8
    with rheumatic fever (conditions in I00)
      active —see Endocarditis, acute, rheumatic
      inactive or quiescent (with chorea) I09.89
        with aortic, mitral or tricuspid disease I08.8
    acute or subacute I33.9
      rheumatic I01.1
        with chorea (acute) (rheumatic) (Sydenham's) I02.0
    arteriosclerotic I37.8
    congenital Q22.2
    rheumatic (chronic) (inactive) (with chorea) I09.89
      active or acute I01.1
        with chorea (acute) (rheumatic) (Sydenham's) I02.0
    syphilitic A52.03
  purulent (acute) (any valve) (subacute) I33.0
  Q fever A78 [I39]
  rheumatic (chronic) (inactive) (with chorea) I09.1
    active or acute (aortic) (mitral) (pulmonary) (tricuspid) I01.1
      with chorea (acute) (rheumatic) (Sydenham's) I02.0
  rheumatoid —see Rheumatoid, carditis
  septic (acute) (any valve) (subacute) I33.0
  streptococcal (acute) (any valve) (subacute) I33.0
  subacute —see Endocarditis, acute
  suppurative (acute) (any valve) (subacute) I33.0
  syphilitic A52.03
  toxic I33.9
  tricuspid (chronic) (heart) (inactive) (rheumatic) (valve) (with chorea) I07.9
    with
      aortic (valve) disease I08.2
        mitral (valve) disease I08.3
      mitral (valve) disease I08.1
        aortic (valve) disease I08.3
      rheumatic fever (conditions in I00)
        active —see Endocarditis, acute, rheumatic
        inactive or quiescent (with chorea) I07.8
    active or acute I01.1
      with chorea (acute) (rheumatic) (Sydenham's) I02.0
    arteriosclerotic I36.8
    nonrheumatic I36.8
      acute or subacute I33.9
    specified cause, except rheumatic I36.8
  tuberculous —see Tuberculosis, endocarditis
  typhoid A01.02
  ulcerative (acute) (any valve) (subacute) I33.0
  vegetative (acute) (any valve) (subacute) I33.0
  verrucous (atypical) (nonbacterial) (nonrheumatic) M32.11
Endocardium, endocardial —see also condition
  cushion defect Q21.2
Endocervicitis —see also Cervicitis
  due to intrauterine (contraceptive) device T83.69
  hyperplastic N72
Endocrine —see condition
Endocrinopathy, pluriglandular E31.9

Endodontic
  overfill M27.52
  underfill M27.53
Endodontitis K04.01
  irreversible K04.02
  reversible K04.01
Endomastoiditis —see Mastoiditis
Endometrioma N80.9
Endometriosis N80.9
  appendix N80.5
  bladder N80.8
  bowel N80.5
  broad ligament N80.3
  cervix N80.0
  colon N80.5
  cul-de-sac (Douglas') N80.3
  exocervix N80.0
  fallopian tube N80.2
  female genital organ NEC N80.8
  gallbladder N80.8
  in scar of skin N80.6
  internal N80.0
  intestine N80.5
  lung N80.8
  myometrium N80.0
  ovary N80.1
  parametrium N80.3
  pelvic peritoneum N80.3
  peritoneal (pelvic) N80.3
  rectovaginal septum N80.4
  rectum N80.5
  round ligament N80.3
  skin (scar) N80.6
  specified site NEC N80.8
  stromal D39.0
  thorax N80.8
  umbilicus N80.8
  uterus (internal) N80.0
  vagina N80.4
  vulva N80.8
Endometritis (decidual) (nonspecific) (purulent) (senile) (atrophic) (suppurative) N71.9
  with ectopic pregnancy O08.0
  acute N71.0
  blenorrhagic (gonococcal) (acute) (chronic) A54.24
  cervix, cervical (with erosion or ectropion) — see also Cervicitis
    hyperplastic N72
  chlamydial A56.11
  chronic N71.1
  following
    abortion —see Abortion by type complicated by genital infection
    ectopic or molar pregnancy O08.0
  gonococcal, gonorrheal (acute) (chronic) A54.24
  hyperplastic —see also Hyperplasia, endometrial N85.00-•
    cervix N72
  puerperal, postpartum, childbirth O86.12
  subacute N71.0
  tuberculous A18.17
Endometrium —see condition
Endomyocardiopathy, South African I42.3
Endomyocarditis —see Endocarditis
Endomyofibrosis I42.3
Endomyometritis —see Endometritis
Endopericarditis —see Endocarditis
Endoperineuritis —see Disorder, nerve
Endophlebitis —see Phlebitis
Endophthalmia —see Endophthalmitis, purulent
Endophthalmitis (acute) (infective) (metastatic) (subacute) H44.009
  bleb associated H59.4 —see also Bleb, inflamed (infected), postprocedural
  gonorrheal A54.39
  in (due to)
    cysticercosis B69.1
    onchocerciasis B73.01
    toxocariasis B83.0

▶ New   ⇒ Revised   ~~deleted~~ Deleted   ● Use Additional Character(s)

Endophthalmitis *(Continued)*
  panuveitis —*see* Panuveitis
  parasitic H44.12-•
  purulent H44.00-•
    panophthalmitis —*see* Panophthalmitis
    vitreous abscess H44.02-•
  specified NEC H44.19
  sympathetic —*see* Uveitis, sympathetic
Endosalpingioma D28.2
Endosalpingiosis N94.89
Endosteitis —*see* Osteomyelitis
Endothelioma, bone —*see* Neoplasm, bone,
  malignant
Endotheliosis (hemorrhagic infectional)
  D69.8
Endotoxemia — code to condition
Endotrachelitis —*see* Cervicitis
Engelmann (-Camurati) syndrome Q78.3
English disease —*see* Rickets
Engman's disease L30.3
Engorgement
  breast N64.59
    newborn P83.4
    puerperal, postpartum O92.79
  lung (passive) —*see* Edema, lung
  pulmonary (passive) —*see* Edema, lung
  stomach K31.89
  venous, retina —*see* Occlusion, retina, vein,
    engorgement
Enlargement, enlarged —*see also* Hypertrophy
  adenoids J35.2
    with tonsils J35.3
  alveolar ridge K08.89
    congenital —*see* Anomaly, alveolar
  apertures of diaphragm (congenital)
    Q79.1
  gingival K06.1
  heart, cardiac —*see* Hypertrophy, cardiac
  labium majus, childhood asymmetric
    (CALME) N90.61
  lacrimal gland, chronic H04.03-•
  liver —*see* Hypertrophy, liver
  lymph gland or node R59.9
    generalized R59.1
    localized R59.0
  orbit H05.34-•
  organ or site, congenital NEC —*see* Anomaly,
    by site
  parathyroid (gland) E21.0
  pituitary fossa R93.0
  prostate N40.0
    with lower urinary tract symptoms (LUTS)
      N40.1
    without lower urinary tract symptoms
      (LUTS) N40.0
  sella turcica R93.0
  spleen —*see* Splenomegaly
  thymus (gland) (congenital) E32.0
  thyroid (gland) —*see* Goiter
  tongue K14.8
  tonsils J35.1
    with adenoids J35.3
  uterus N85.2
  vestibular aqueduct Q16.5
Enophthalmos H05.40-•
  due to
    orbital tissue atrophy H05.41-•
    trauma or surgery H05.42-•
Enostosis M27.8
Entamebic, entamebiasis —*see* Amebiasis
Entanglement
  umbilical cord(s) O69.82
    with compression O69.2
    around neck (with compression)
      O69.81
      with compression O69.1
      without compression O69.81
    of twins in monoamniotic sac O69.2
    without compression O69.82
Enteralgia —*see* Pain, abdominal
Enteric —*see* condition

Enteritis (acute) (diarrheal) (hemorrhagic)
  (noninfective) K52.9
  adenovirus A08.2
  aertrycke infection A02.0
  allergic K52.29
    with
      eosinophilic gastritis or gastroenteritis
        K52.81
      food protein-induced enterocolitis
        syndrome K52.21
      food protein-induced enteropathy K52.22
      FPIES K52.21
  amebic (acute) A06.0
    with abscess —*see* Abscess, amebic
    chronic A06.1
      with abscess —*see* Abscess, amebic
      nondysenteric A06.2
    nondysenteric A06.2
  astrovirus A08.32
  bacillary NOS A03.9
  bacterial A04.9
    specified NEC A04.8
  calicivirus A08.31
  candidal B37.82
  Chilomastix A07.8
  choleriformis A00.1
  chronic (noninfectious) K52.9
    ulcerative —*see* Colitis, ulcerative
  cicatrizing (chronic) —*see* Enteritis, regional,
    small intestine
  Clostridium
    botulinum (food poisoning) A05.1
    difficile
      not specified as recurrent A04.72
      recurrent A04.71
  coccidial A07.3
  coxsackie virus A08.39
  dietetic —*see also* Enteritis, allergic K52.29
  drug-induced K52.1
  due to
    astrovirus A08.32
    calicivirus A08.31
    coxsackie virus A08.39
    drugs K52.1
    echovirus A08.39
    enterovirus NEC A08.39
    food hypersensitivity —*see also* Enteritis,
      allergic K52.29
    infectious organism (bacterial) (viral) —*see*
      Enteritis, infectious
    torovirus A08.39
    Yersinia enterocolitica A04.6
  echovirus A08.39
  eltor A00.1
  enterovirus NEC A08.39
  eosinophilic K52.81
  epidemic (infectious) A09
  fulminant —*see also* Ischemia, intestine, acute
    K55.019
  gangrenous —*see* Enteritis, infectious
  giardial A07.1
  infectious NOS A09
    due to
      adenovirus A08.2
      Aerobacter aerogenes A04.8
      Arizona (bacillus) A02.0
      bacteria NOS A04.9
        specified NEC A04.8
      Campylobacter A04.5
      Clostridium difficile
        not specified as recurrent A04.72
        recurrent A04.71
      Clostridium perfringens A04.8
      Enterobacter aerogenes A04.8
      enterovirus A08.39
      Escherichia coli A04.4
        enteroaggregative A04.4
        enterohemorrhagic A04.3
        enteroinvasive A04.2
        enteropathogenic A04.0
        enterotoxigenic A04.1
        specified NEC A04.4

Enteritis *(Continued)*
  infectious NOS *(Continued)*
    due to *(Continued)*
      specified
        bacteria NEC A04.8
        virus NEC A08.39
      Staphylococcus A04.8
      virus NEC A08.4
        specified type NEC A08.39
      Yersinia enterocolitica A04.6
    specified organism NEC A08.8
  influenzal —*see* Influenza, with, digestive
    manifestations
  ischemic K55.9
    acute —*see also* Ischemia, intestine, acute
      K55.019
    chronic K55.1
  microsporidial A07.8
  mucomembranous, myxomembranous —*see*
    Syndrome, irritable bowel
  mucous —*see* Syndrome, irritable bowel
  necroticans A05.2
  necrotizing of newborn —*see* Enterocolitis,
    necrotizing, in newborn
  neurogenic —*see* Syndrome, irritable bowel
  newborn necrotizing —*see* Enterocolitis,
    necrotizing, in newborn
  noninfectious K52.9
  norovirus A08.11
  parasitic NEC B82.9
  paratyphoid (fever) —*see* Fever, paratyphoid
  protozoal A07.9
    specified NEC A07.8
  radiation K52.0
  regional (of) K50.90
    with
      complication K50.919
        abscess K50.914
        fistula K50.913
        intestinal obstruction K50.912
        rectal bleeding K50.911
        specified complication NEC K50.918
    colon —*see* Enteritis, regional, large
      intestine
    duodenum —*see* Enteritis, regional, small
      intestine
    ileum —*see* Enteritis, regional, small
      intestine
    jejunum —*see* Enteritis, regional, small
      intestine
    large bowel —*see* Enteritis, regional, large
      intestine
    large intestine (colon) (rectum) K50.10
      with
        complication K50.119
          abscess K50.114
          fistula K50.113
          intestinal obstruction K50.112
          rectal bleeding K50.111
          small intestine (duodenum) (ileum)
            (jejunum) involvement K50.80
            with
              complication K50.819
                abscess K50.814
                fistula K50.813
                intestinal obstruction
                  K50.812
                rectal bleeding K50.811
                specified complication NEC
                  K50.818
            specified complication NEC
              K50.118
    rectum —*see* Enteritis, regional, large
      intestine
    small intestine (duodenum) (ileum)
      (jejunum) K50.00
      with
        complication K50.019
          abscess K50.014
          fistula K50.013
          intestinal obstruction K50.012

Enteritis (Continued)
  regional (Continued)
    small intestine (Continued)
      with (Continued)
        complication (Continued)
          large intestine (colon) (rectum)
            involvement K50.80
            with
              complication K50.819
                abscess K50.814
                fistula K50.813
                intestinal obstruction
                  K50.812
                rectal bleeding K50.811
                specified complication NEC
                  K50.818
          rectal bleeding K50.011
          specified complication NEC
            K50.018
  rotaviral A08.0
  Salmonella, salmonellosis (arizonae)
    (cholerae-suis) (enteritidis)
    (typhimurium) A02.0
  segmental —see Enteritis, regional
  septic A09
  Shigella —see Infection, Shigella
  small round structured NEC A08.19
  spasmodic, spastic —see Syndrome, irritable
    bowel
  staphylococcal A04.8
    due to food A05.0
  torovirus A08.39
  toxic NEC K52.1
    due to Clostridium difficile
      not specified as recurrent A04.72
      recurrent A04.71
  trichomonal A07.8
  tuberculous A18.32
  typhosa A01.00
  ulcerative (chronic) —see Colitis, ulcerative
  viral A08.4
    adenovirus A08.2
    enterovirus A08.39
    Rotavirus A08.0
    small round structured NEC A08.19
    specified NEC A08.39
    virus specified NEC A08.39
Enterobiasis B80
Enterobius vermicularis (infection) (infestation)
  B80
Enterocele —see also Hernia, abdomen
  pelvic, pelvis (acquired) (congenital) N81.5
  vagina, vaginal (acquired) (congenital)
    NEC N81.5
Enterocolitis —see also Enteritis K52.9
  due to Clostridium difficile
    not specified as recurrent A04.72
    recurrent A04.71
  fulminant ischemic —see also Ischemia,
    intestine, acute K55.059
  granulomatous —see Enteritis, regional
  hemorrhagic (acute) —see also Ischemia,
    intestine, acute K55.059
    chronic K55.1
  infectious NEC A09
  ischemic K55.9
  necrotizing K55.30
    with
      perforation K55.33
      pneumatosis K55.32
      and perforation K55.33
    due to Clostridium difficile
      not specified as recurrent A04.72
      recurrent A04.71
    in non-newborn K55.30
      stage 1 (without pneumatosis, without
        perforation) K55.31
      stage 2 (with pneumatosis, without
        perforation) K55.32
      stage 3 (with pneumatosis, with
        perforation) K55.33

Enterocolitis (Continued)
  necrotizing (Continued)
    in newborn P77.9
      stage 1 (without pneumatosis, without
        perforation) P77.1
      stage 2 (with pneumatosis, without
        perforation) P77.2
      stage 3 (with pneumatosis, with
        perforation) P77.3
    without pneumatosis or perforation K55.31
  noninfectious K52.9
    newborn —see Enterocolitis, necrotizing, in
      newborn
  pseudomembranous (newborn)
    not specified as recurrent A04.72
    recurrent A04.71
  radiation K52.0
    newborn —see Enterocolitis, necrotizing, in
      newborn
  ulcerative (chronic) —see Pancolitis,
    ulcerative (chronic)
Enterogastritis —see Enteritis
Enteropathy K63.9
  celiac-gluten-sensitive K90.0
    non-celiac K90.41
  food protein-induced K52.22
  hemorrhagic, terminal —see also Ischemia,
    intestine, acute K55.059
  protein-losing K90.49
Enteroperitonitis —see Peritonitis
Enteroptosis K63.4
Enterorrhagia K92.2
Enterospasm —see also Syndrome, irritable,
  bowel
  psychogenic F45.8
Enterostenosis —see also Obstruction, intestine,
  specified NEC K56.699
Enterostomy
  complication —see Complication,
    enterostomy
  status Z93.4
Enterovirus, as cause of disease classified
  elsewhere B97.10
  coxsackievirus B97.11
  echovirus B97.12
  other specified B97.19
Enthesopathy (peripheral) M77.5-●
  Achilles tendinitis —see Tendinitis, Achilles
  ankle and tarsus M77.9
    specified type NEC —see Enthesopathy,
      foot, specified type NEC
  anterior tibial syndrome M76.81-●
  calcaneal spur —see Spur, bone, calcaneal
  elbow region M77.8
    lateral epicondylitis —see Epicondylitis,
      lateral
    medial epicondylitis —see Epicondylitis,
      medial
  foot NEC M77.8
    metatarsalgia —see Metatarsalgia
    specified type NEC M77.5-●
  forearm M77.8
  gluteal tendinitis —see Tendinitis, gluteal
  hand M77.8
  hip —see Enthesopathy, lower limb, specified
    type NEC
  iliac crest spur —see Spur, bone, iliac crest
  iliotibial band syndrome —see Syndrome,
    iliotibial band
  knee —see Enthesopathy, lower limb, lower
    leg, specified type NEC
  lateral epicondylitis —see Epicondylitis,
    lateral
  lower limb (excluding foot) M76.9
    Achilles tendinitis —see Tendinitis, Achilles
    ankle and tarsus M77.5-
      specified type NEC - see Enthesopathy,
        foot, specified type NEC
    anterior tibial syndrome M76.81-●
    gluteal tendinitis —see Tendinitis, gluteal
    iliac crest spur —see Spur, bone, iliac crest

Enthesopathy (Continued)
  lower limb (Continued)
    iliotibial band syndrome —see Syndrome,
      iliotibial band
    patellar tendinitis —see Tendinitis, patellar
    pelvic region —see Enthesopathy, lower
      limb, specified type NEC
    peroneal tendinitis —see Tendinitis,
      peroneal
    posterior tibial syndrome M76.82-●
    psoas tendinitis —see Tendinitis, psoas
    specified type NEC M76.89-●
    tibial collateral bursitis —see Bursitis, tibial
      collateral
  medial epicondylitis —see Epicondylitis,
    medial
  multiple sites M77.8
  patellar tendinitis —see Tendinitis, patellar
  pelvis M77.8
  periarthritis of wrist —see Periarthritis, wrist
  peroneal tendinitis —see Tendinitis, peroneal
  posterior tibial syndrome M76.82-●
  psoas tendinitis —see Tendinitis, psoas
  shoulder M77.8
  shoulder region —see Lesion, shoulder
  specified type NEC M77.8
  spinal M46.00
    cervical region M46.02
    cervicothoracic region M46.03
    lumbar region M46.06
    lumbosacral region M46.07
    multiple sites M46.09
    occipito-atlanto-axial region M46.01
    sacrococcygeal region M46.08
    thoracic region M46.04
    thoracolumbar region M46.05
  tibial collateral bursitis —see Bursitis, tibial
    collateral
  upper arm M77.8
  wrist and carpus NEC M77.8
    calcaneal spur —see Spur, bone, calcaneal
    periarthritis of wrist —see Periarthritis,
      wrist
Entomophobia F40.218
Entomophthoromycosis B46.8
Entrance, air into vein —see Embolism, air
Entrapment, nerve —see Neuropathy,
  entrapment
Entropion (eyelid) (paralytic) H02.009
  cicatricial H02.019
    left H02.016
      lower H02.015
      upper H02.014
    right H02.013
      lower H02.012
      upper H02.011
  congenital Q10.2
  left H02.006
    lower H02.005
    upper H02.004
  mechanical H02.029
    left H02.026
      lower H02.025
      upper H02.024
    right H02.023
      lower H02.022
      upper H02.021
  right H02.003
    lower H02.002
    upper H02.001
  senile H02.039
    left H02.036
      lower H02.035
      upper H02.034
    right H02.033
      lower H02.032
      upper H02.031
  spastic H02.049
    left H02.046
      lower H02.045
      upper H02.044

▶ New   ⇒ Revised   ~~deleted~~ Deleted   ● Use Additional Character(s)

Entropion (Continued)
  spastic (Continued)
    right H02.043
      lower H02.042
      upper H02.041
Enucleated eye (traumatic, current) S05.7-●
Enuresis R32
  functional F98.0
  habit disturbance F98.0
  nocturnal N39.44
    psychogenic F98.0
  nonorganic origin F98.0
  psychogenic F98.0
Eosinopenia —see Agranulocytosis
Eosinophilia (allergic) (idiopathic) (secondary)
    D72.10
  with
    angiolymphoid hyperplasia (ALHE)
      D18.01
  familial D72.19
  hereditary D72.19
  in disease classified elsewhere D72.18
  infiltrative —see Eosinophilia, pulmonary
  Löffler's J82.89
  peritoneal —see Peritonitis, eosinophilic
  pulmonary NEC J82.89
    acute J82.82
    asthmatic J82.83
    chronic J82.81
    specified NEC D72.19
  tropical (pulmonary) J82.89
Eosinophilia-myalgia syndrome M35.89
Ependymitis (acute) (cerebral) (chronic)
    (granular) —see Encephalomyelitis
Ependymoblastoma
  specified site —see Neoplasm, malignant, by
    site
  unspecified site C71.9
Ependymoma (epithelial) (malignant)
  anaplastic
    specified site —see Neoplasm, malignant,
      by site
    unspecified site C71.9
  benign
    specified site —see Neoplasm, benign, by
      site
    unspecified site D33.2
  myxopapillary D43.2
    specified site —see Neoplasm, uncertain
      behavior, by site
    unspecified site D43.2
  papillary D43.2
    specified site —see Neoplasm, uncertain
      behavior, by site
    unspecified site D43.2
  specified site —see Neoplasm, malignant, by
    site
  unspecified site C71.9
Ependymopathy G93.89
Ephelis, ephelides L81.2
Epiblepharon (congenital) Q10.3
Epicanthus, epicanthic fold (eyelid)
    (congenital) Q10.3
Epicondylitis (elbow)
  lateral M77.1-●
  medial M77.0-●
Epicystitis —see Cystitis
Epidemic —see condition
Epidermidalization, cervix —see Dysplasia,
    cervix
Epidermis, epidermal —see condition
Epidermodysplasia verruciformis B07.8
Epidermolysis
  bullosa (congenital) Q81.9
    acquired L12.30
      drug-induced L12.31
      specified cause NEC L12.35
    dystrophica Q81.2
    letalis Q81.1
    simplex Q81.0
    specified NEC Q81.8

Epidermolysis (Continued)
  necroticans combustiformis L51.2
    due to drug —see Table of Drugs and
      Chemicals, by drug
Epidermophytid —see Dermatophytosis
Epidermophytosis (infected) —see
    Dermatophytosis
Epididymis —see condition
Epididymitis (acute) (nonvenereal) (recurrent)
    (residual) N45.1
  with orchitis N45.3
  blennorrhagic (gonococcal) A54.23
  caseous (tuberculous) A18.15
  chlamydial A56.19
  filarial —see also Infestation, filarial B74.9
    [N51]
  gonococcal A54.23
  syphilitic A52.76
  tuberculous A18.15
Epididymo-orchitis —see also Epididymitis
    N45.3
Epidural —see condition
Epigastrium, epigastric —see condition
Epigastrocele —see Hernia, ventral
Epiglottis —see condition
Epiglottitis, epiglottiditis (acute) J05.10
  with obstruction J05.11
  chronic J37.0
Epignathus Q89.4
Epilepsia partialis continua —see also
    Kozhevnikof's epilepsy G40.1-●
Epilepsy, epileptic, epilepsia (attack) (cerebral)
    (convulsion) (fit) (seizure) G40.909

Note: the following terms are to be
considered equivalent to intractable:
pharmacoresistant (pharmacologically
resistant), treatment resistant, refractory
(medically) and poorly controlled

  with
    complex partial seizures —see Epilepsy,
      localization-related, symptomatic,
      with complex partial seizures
    grand mal seizures on awakening —
      see Epilepsy, generalized, specified
      NEC
    myoclonic absences —see Epilepsy,
      generalized, specified NEC
    myoclonic-astatic seizures —see Epilepsy,
      generalized, specified NEC
    simple partial seizures —see Epilepsy,
      localization-related, symptomatic,
      with simple partial seizures
  akinetic —see Epilepsy, generalized, specified
    NEC
  benign childhood with centrotemporal EEG
    spikes —see Epilepsy, localization-
    related, idiopathic
  benign myoclonic in infancy G40.80-●
  Bravais-jacksonian —see Epilepsy,
    localization-related, symptomatic,
    with simple partial seizures
  childhood
    with occipital EEG paroxysms —see
      Epilepsy, localization-related,
      idiopathic
    absence G40.A09
      intractable G40.A19
        with status epilepticus G40.A11
        without status epilepticus G40.A19
      not intractable G40.A09
        with status epilepticus G40.A01
        without status epilepticus G40.A09
  climacteric —see Epilepsy, specified NEC
  cysticercosis B69.0
  deterioration (mental) F06.8
  due to syphilis A52.19
  focal —see Epilepsy, localization-related,
    symptomatic, with simple partial
    seizures

Epilepsy, epileptic, epilepsia (Continued)
  generalized
    idiopathic G40.309
      intractable G40.319
        with status epilepticus G40.311
        without status epilepticus G40.319
      not intractable G40.309
        with status epilepticus G40.301
        without status epilepticus G40.309
    specified NEC G40.409
      intractable G40.419
        with status epilepticus G40.411
        without status epilepticus G40.419
      not intractable G40.409
        with status epilepticus G40.401
        without status epilepticus G40.409
  impulsive petit mal —see Epilepsy, juvenile
    myoclonic
  intractable G40.919
    with status epilepticus G40.911
    without status epilepticus G40.919
  juvenile absence G40.A09
    intractable G40.A19
      with status epilepticus G40.A11
      without status epilepticus G40.A19
    not intractable G40.A09
      with status epilepticus G40.A01
      without status epilepticus G40.A09
  juvenile myoclonic G40.B11
    intractable G40.B19
      with status epilepticus G40.B11
      without status epilepticus G40.B19
    not intractable G40.B09
      with status epilepticus G40.B01
      without status epilepticus G40.B09
  localization-related (focal) (partial)
    idiopathic G40.009
      with seizures of localized onset G40.009
        intractable G40.019
          with status epilepticus G40.011
          without status epilepticus G40.019
        not intractable G40.009
          with status epilepticus G40.001
          without status epilepticus G40.009
    symptomatic
      with complex partial seizures G40.209
        intractable G40.219
          with status epilepticus G40.211
          without status epilepticus G40.219
        not intractable G40.209
          with status epilepticus G40.201
          without status epilepticus
            G40.209
      with simple partial seizures G40.109
        intractable G40.119
          with status epilepticus G40.111
          without status epilepticus
            G40.119
        not intractable G40.109
          with status epilepticus G40.101
          without status epilepticus G40.109
  myoclonus, myoclonic —see also Epilepsy,
    generalized, specified NEC
  progressive —see Epilepsy, generalized,
    idiopathic
  severe, in infancy (SMEI) G40.83-●
  not intractable G40.909
    with status epilepticus G40.901
    without status epilepticus G40.909
  on awakening —see Epilepsy, generalized,
    specified NEC
  parasitic NOS B71.9 [G94]
  partialis continua —see also Kozhevnikof's
    epilepsy G40.1-●
  peripheral —see Epilepsy, specified NEC
  polymorphic, in infancy (PMEI) G40.83-●
  procursiva —see Epilepsy, localization-
    related, symptomatic, with simple
    partial seizures
  progressive (familial) myoclonic —see
    Epilepsy, generalized, idiopathic

Epilepsy, epileptic, epilepsia (Continued)
  reflex —see Epilepsy, specified NEC
  related to
    alcohol G40.509
      not intractable G40.509
        with status epilepticus G40.501
        without status epliepticus G40.509
    drugs G40.509
      not intractable G40.509
        with status epilepticus G40.501
        without status epliepticus G40.509
    external causes G40.509
      not intractable G40.509
        with status epilepticus G40.501
        without status epliepticus G40.509
    hormonal changes G40.509
      not intractable G40.509
        with status epilepticus G40.501
        without status epliepticus G40.509
    sleep deprivation G40.509
      not intractable G40.509
        with status epilepticus G40.501
        without status epliepticus G40.509
    stress G40.509
      not intractable G40.509
        with status epilepticus G40.501
        without status epliepticus G40.509
  somatomotor —see Epilepsy, localization-related, symptomatic, with simple partial seizures
  somatosensory —see Epilepsy, localization-related, symptomatic, with simple partial seizures
  spasms G40.822
    intractable G40.824
      with status epilepticus G40.823
      without status epilepticus G40.824
    not intractable G40.822
      with status epilepticus G40.821
      without status epilepticus G40.822
    specified NEC G40.802
      intractable G40.804
        with status epilepticus G40.803
        without status epilepticus G40.804
      not intractable G40.802
        with status epilepticus G40.801
        without status epilepticus G40.802
  syndromes
    generalized
      idiopathic G40.309
        intractable G40.319
          with status epilepticus G40.311
          without status epilepticus G40.319
        not intractable G40.309
          with status epilepticus G40.301
          without status epilepticus G40.309
      specified NEC G40.409
        intractable G40.419
          with status epilepticus G40.411
          without status epilepticus G40.419
        not intractable G40.409
          with status epilepticus G40.401
          without status epilepticus G40.409
    localization-related (focal) (partial)
      idiopathic G40.009
        with seizures of localized onset G40.009
        intractable G40.019
          with status epilepticus G40.011
          without status epilepticus G40.019
        not intractable G40.009
          with status epilepticus G40.001
          without status epilepticus G40.009
      symptomatic
        with complex partial seizures G40.209
        intractable G40.219
          with status epilepticus G40.211
          without status epilepticus G40.219

Epilepsy, epileptic, epilepsia (Continued)
  syndromes (Continued)
    localization-related (Continued)
      symptomatic (Continued)
        with complex partial seizures (Continued)
          not intractable G40.209
            with status epilepticus G40.201
            without status epilepticus G40.209
        with simple partial seizures G40.109
          intractable G40.119
            with status epilepticus G40.111
            without status epilepticus G40.119
          not intractable G40.109
            with status epilepticus G40.101
            without status epilepticus G40.109
      specified NEC G40.802
        intractable G40.804
          with status epilepticus G40.803
          without status epilepticus G40.804
        not intractable G40.802
          with status epilepticus G40.801
          without status epilepticus G40.802
    tonic (-clonic) —see Epilepsy, generalized, specified NEC
    twilight F05
    uncinate (gyrus) —see Epilepsy, localization-related, symptomatic, with complex partial seizures
    Unverricht (-Lundborg) (familial myoclonic) —see Epilepsy, generalized, idiopathic
    visceral —see Epilepsy, specified NEC
    visual —see Epilepsy, specified NEC
Epiloia Q85.1
Epimenorrhea N92.0
Epipharyngitis —see Nasopharyngitis
Epiphora H04.20-●
  due to
    excess lacrimation H04.21-●
    insufficient drainage H04.22-●
Epiphyseal arrest —see Arrest, epiphyseal
Epiphyseolysis, epiphysiolysis —see Osteochondropathy
Epiphysitis —see also Osteochondropathy
  juvenile M92.9
  syphilitic (congenital) A50.02
Epiplocele —see Hernia, abdomen
Epiploitis —see Peritonitis
Epiplosarcomphalocele —see Hernia, umbilicus
Episcleritis (suppurative) H15.10-●
  in (due to)
    syphilis A52.71
    tuberculosis A18.51
  nodular H15.12-●
  periodica fugax H15.11-●
    angioneurotic —see Edema, angioneurotic
  syphilitic (late) A52.71
  tuberculous A18.51
Episode
  affective, mixed F39
  depersonalization (in neurotic state) F48.1
  ➠depressive F32.A
    major F32.9
      mild F32.0
      moderate F32.1
      severe (without psychotic symptoms) F32.2
        with psychotic symptoms F32.3
      recurrent F33.9
      brief F33.8
      specified NEC F32.89
  hypomanic F30.8
  manic F30.9
    with
      psychotic symptoms F30.2
      remission (full) F30.4
      partial F30.3

Episode (Continued)
  manic (Continued)
    without psychotic symptoms F30.10
      mild F30.11
      moderate F30.12
      severe (without psychotic symptoms) F30.13
        with psychotic symptoms F30.2
    other specified F30.8
    recurrent F31.89
  psychotic F23
    organic F06.8
  schizophrenic (acute) NEC, brief F23
Epispadias (female) (male) Q64.0
Episplenitis D73.89
Epistaxis (multiple) R04.0
  hereditary I78.0
  vicarious menstruation N94.89
Epithelioma (malignant) —see also Neoplasm, malignant, by site
  adenoides cysticum —see Neoplasm, skin, benign
  basal cell —see Neoplasm, skin, malignant
  benign —see Neoplasm, benign, by site
  Bowen's —see Neoplasm, skin, in situ
  calcifying, of Malherbe —see Neoplasm, skin, benign
  external site —see Neoplasm, skin, malignant
  intraepidermal, Jadassohn —see Neoplasm, skin, benign
  squamous cell —see Neoplasm, malignant, by site
Epitheliomatosis pigmented Q82.1
Epitheliopathy, multifocal placoid pigment H30.14-●
Epithelium, epithelial —see condition
Epituberculosis (with atelectasis) (allergic) A15.7
Eponychia Q84.6
Epstein's
  nephrosis or syndrome —see Nephrosis
  pearl K09.8
Epulis (gingiva) (fibrous) (giant cell) K06.8
Equinia A24.0
Equinovarus (congenital) (talipes) Q66.0-●
  acquired —see Deformity, limb, clubfoot
Equivalent
  convulsive (abdominal) —see Epilepsy, specified NEC
  epileptic (psychic) —see Epilepsy, localization-related, symptomatic, with complex partial seizures
Erb (-Duchenne) paralysis (birth injury) (newborn) P14.0
Erb's
  disease G71.02
  palsy, paralysis (brachial) (birth) (newborn) P14.0
  spinal (spastic) syphilitic A52.17
  pseudohypertrophic muscular dystrophy G71.02
Erb-Goldflam disease or syndrome G70.00
  with exacerbation (acute) G70.01
  in crisis G70.01
Erdheim's syndrome (acromegalic macrospondylitis) E22.0
Erection, painful (persistent) —see Priapism
Ergosterol deficiency (vitamin D) E55.9
  with
    adult osteomalacia M83.8
    rickets —see Rickets
Ergotism —see also Poisoning, food, noxious, plant
  from ergot used as drug (migraine therapy) —see Table of Drugs and Chemicals
Erosio interdigitalis blastomycetica B37.2
Erosion
  artery I77.2
    without rupture I77.89
  bone —see Disorder, bone, density and structure, specified NEC

▶ New   ➠ Revised   ~~deleted~~ Deleted   ● Use Additional Character(s)

Erosion (Continued)
  bronchus J98.09
  cartilage (joint) —see Disorder, cartilage,
    specified type NEC
  cervix (uteri) (acquired) (chronic) (congenital)
    N86
    with cervicitis N72
  cornea (nontraumatic) —see Ulcer, cornea
    recurrent H18.83-●
    traumatic —see Abrasion, cornea
  dental (idiopathic) (occupational) (due to
    diet, drugs or vomiting) K03.2
  duodenum, postpyloric —see Ulcer,
    duodenum
  esophagus K22.10
    with bleeding K22.11
  gastric —see Ulcer, stomach
  gastrojejunal —see Ulcer, gastrojejunal
➩ implanted mesh —see Complications,
    prosthetic device or implant, mesh
  intestine K63.3
  lymphatic vessel I89.8
  pylorus, pyloric (ulcer) —see Ulcer, stomach
  spine, aneurysmal A52.09
  stomach —see Ulcer, stomach
  subcutaneous device pocket
    nervous system prosthetic device, implant,
      or graft T85.890
    other internal prosthetic device, implant, or
      graft T85.898
  teeth (idiopathic) (occupational) (due to diet,
    drugs or vomiting) K03.2
  urethra N36.8
  uterus N85.8
Erotomania F52.8
Error
  metabolism, inborn —see Disorder, metabolism
  refractive —see Disorder, refraction
Eructation R14.2
  nervous or psychogenic F45.8
Eruption
  creeping B76.9
  drug (generalized) (taken internally) L27.0
    fixed L27.1
    in contact with skin —see Dermatitis, due
      to drugs
    localized L27.1
  Hutchinson, summer L56.4
  Kaposi's varicelliform B00.0
  napkin L22
  polymorphous light (sun) L56.4
  recalcitrant pustular L13.8
  ringed R23.8
  skin (nonspecific) R21
    creeping (meaning hookworm) B76.9
    due to inoculation/vaccination
      (generalized) —see also Dermatitis,
        due to, vaccine L27.0
      localized L27.1
    erysipeloid A26.0
    feigned L98.1
    Kaposi's varicelliform B00.0
    lichenoid L28.0
    meaning dermatitis —see Dermatitis
    toxic NEC L53.0
  tooth, teeth, abnormal (incomplete) (late)
    (premature) (sequence) K00.6
  vesicular R23.8
Erysipelas (gangrenous) (infantile) (newborn)
    (phlegmonous) (suppurative) A46
  external ear A46 [H62.40]
  puerperal, postpartum O86.89
Erysipeloid A26.9
  cutaneous (Rosenbach's) A26.0
  disseminated A26.8
  sepsis A26.7
  specified NEC A26.8
Erythema, erythematous (infectional)
    (inflammation) L53.9
  ab igne L59.0

Erythema, erythematous (Continued)
  annulare (centrifugum) (rheumaticum) L53.1
  arthriticum epidemicum A25.1
  brucellum —see Brucellosis
  chronic figurate NEC L53.3
  chronicum migrans (Borrelia burgdorferi)
    A69.20
  diaper L22
  due to
    chemical NEC L53.0
      in contact with skin L24.5
    drug (internal use) —see Dermatitis, due
      to, drugs
  elevatum diutinum L95.1
  endemic E52
  epidemic, arthritic A25.1
  figuratum perstans L53.3
  gluteal L22
  heat - code by site under Burn, first degree
  ichthyosiforme congenitum bullosum
    Q80.3
  in diseases classified elsewhere L54
  induratum (nontuberculous) L52
    tuberculous A18.4
  infectiosum B08.3
  intertrigo L30.4
  iris L51.9
  marginatum L53.2
    in (due to) acute rheumatic fever I00
  medicamentosum —see Dermatitis, due to,
    drugs
  migrans A26.0
    chronicum A69.20
    tongue K14.1
  multiforme (major) (minor) L51.9
    bullous, bullosum L51.1
    conjunctiva L51.1
    nonbullous L51.0
    pemphigoides L12.0
    specified NEC L51.8
  napkin L22
  neonatorum P83.88
    toxic P83.1
  nodosum L52
    tuberculous A18.4
  palmar L53.8
  pernio T69.1
  rash, newborn P83.88
  scarlatiniform (recurrent) (exfoliative)
    L53.8
  solare L55.0
  specified NEC L53.8
  toxic, toxicum NEC L53.0
    newborn P83.1
  tuberculous (primary) A18.4
Erythematous, erythematosus —see condition
Erythermalgia (primary) I73.81
Erythralgia I73.81
Erythrasma L08.1
Erythredema (polyneuropathy) —see Poisoning,
    mercury
Erythremia (acute) C94.0-●
  chronic D45
  secondary D75.1
Erythroblastopenia —see also Aplasia, red cell
    D60.9
  congenital D61.01
Erythroblastophthisis D61.09
Erythroblastosis (fetalis) (newborn) P55.9
  due to
    ABO (antibodies) (incompatibility)
      (isoimmunization) P55.1
    Rh (antibodies) (incompatibility)
      (isoimmunization) P55.0
Erythrocyanosis (crurum) I73.89
Erythrocythemia —see Erythremia
Erythrocytosis (megalosplenic) (secondary)
    D75.1
  familial D75.0
  oval, hereditary —see Elliptocytosis

Erythrocytosis (Continued)
  secondary D75.1
  stress D75.1
Erythroderma (secondary) —see also Erythema
    L53.9
  bullous ichthyosiform, congenital Q80.3
  desquamativum L21.1
  ichthyosiform, congenital (bullous) Q80.3
  neonatorum P83.88
  psoriaticum L40.8
Erythrodysesthesia, palmar plantar (PPE)
    L27.1
Erythrogenesis imperfecta D61.09
Erythroleukemia C94.0-●
Erythromelalgia I73.81
Erythrophagocytosis D75.89
Erythrophobia F40.298
Erythroplakia, oral epithelium, and tongue
    K13.29
Erythroplasia (Queyrat) D07.4
  specified site —see Neoplasm, skin, in situ
  unspecified site D07.4
Escherichia coli (E. coli), as cause of disease
    classified elsewhere B96.20
  non-O157 Shiga toxin-producing (with
    known O group) B96.22
  non-Shiga toxin-producing B96.29
  O157 with confirmation of Shiga toxin when
    H antigen is unknown, or is not H7
    B96.21
  O157:H- (nonmotile) with confirmation of
    Shiga toxin B96.21
  Shiga toxin-producing (with unspecified O
    group) (STEC) B96.23
  O157 B96.21
  O157:H7 with or without confirmation of
    Shiga toxin-production B96.21
  specified NEC B96.29
Esophagismus K22.4
Esophagitis (acute) (alkaline) (chemical)
    (chronic) (infectional) (necrotic) (peptic)
    (postoperative) (without bleeding)
    K20.90
  with bleeding K20.91
  candidal B37.81
  due to gastrointestinal reflux disease (without
    bleeding) K21.00
    with bleeding K21.01
  eosinophilic K20.0
  reflux K21.00
  specified NEC (without bleeding) K20.80
    with bleeding K21.81
  tuberculous A18.83
  ulcerative K22.10
    with bleeding K22.11
Esophagocele K22.5
➩ **Esophagomalacia** K22.89
Esophagospasm K22.4
Esophagostenosis K22.2
Esophagostomiasis B81.8
Esophagotracheal —see condition
Esophagus —see condition
Esophoria H50.51
  convergence, excess H51.12
  divergence, insufficiency H51.8
Esotropia —see Strabismus, convergent
    concomitant
Espundia B55.2
Essential —see condition
Esthesioneuroblastoma C30.0
Esthesioneurocytoma C30.0
Esthesioneuroepithelioma C30.0
Esthiomene A55
Estivo-autumnal malaria (fever) B50.9
Estrangement (marital) Z63.5
  parent-child NEC Z62.890
Estriasis —see Myiasis
Ethanolism —see Alcoholism
Etherism —see Dependence, drug, inhalant
Ethmoid, ethmoidal —see condition

Ethmoiditis (chronic) (nonpurulent)
    (purulent) —see also Sinusitis, ethmoidal
  influenzal —see Influenza, with, respiratory
      manifestations NEC
  Woakes' J33.1
Ethylism —see Alcoholism
Eulenburg's disease (congenital paramyotonia)
    G71.19
Eumycetoma B47.0
Eunuchoidism E29.1
  hypogonadotropic E23.0
European blastomycosis —see Cryptococcosis
Eustachian —see condition
Evaluation (for) (of)
  development state
    adolescent Z00.3
    period of
      delayed growth in childhood Z00.70
        with abnormal findings Z00.71
      rapid growth in childhood Z00.2
    puberty Z00.3
  growth and developmental state (period of
      rapid growth) Z00.2
    delayed growth Z00.70
      with abnormal findings Z00.71
  mental health (status) Z00.8
    requested by authority Z04.6
  period of
    delayed growth in childhood Z00.70
      with abnormal findings Z00.71
    rapid growth in childhood Z00.2
  suspected condition —see Observation
Evans syndrome D69.41
Event
  apparent life threatening in newborn and
      infant (ALTE) R68.13
  brief resolved unexplained event (BRUE)
      R68.13
Eventration —see also Hernia, ventral
  colon into chest —see Hernia, diaphragm
  diaphragm (congenital) Q79.1
Eversion
  bladder N32.89
  cervix (uteri) N86
    with cervicitis N72
  foot NEC —see also Deformity, valgus, ankle
    congenital Q66.6
  punctum lacrimale (postinfectional) (senile)
      H04.52-●
  ureter (meatus) N28.89
  urethra (meatus) N36.8
  uterus N81.4
Evidence
  cytologic
    of malignancy on anal smear R85.614
    of malignancy on cervical smear R87.614
    of malignancy on vaginal smear R87.624
Evisceration
  birth injury P15.8
  traumatic NEC
    eye —see Enucleated eye
Evulsion —see Avulsion
Ewing's sarcoma or tumor —see Neoplasm,
    bone, malignant
Examination (for) (following) (general) (of)
    (routine) Z00.00
  with abnormal findings Z00.01
  abuse, physical (alleged), ruled out
    adult Z04.71
    child Z04.72
  adolescent (development state) Z00.3
  alleged rape or sexual assault (victim), ruled
      out
    adult Z04.41
    child Z04.42
  allergy Z01.82
  annual (adult) (periodic) (physical) Z00.00
    with abnormal findings Z00.01
    gynecological Z01.419
      with abnormal findings Z01.411
  antibody response Z01.84

Examination (Continued)
  blood —see Examination, laboratory
  blood pressure Z01.30
    with abnormal findings Z01.31
  cancer staging —see Neoplasm, malignant,
      by site
  cervical Papanicolaou smear Z12.4
    as part of routine gynecological
        examination Z01.419
      with abnormal findings Z01.411
  child (over 28 days old) Z00.129
    with abnormal findings Z00.121
    under 28 days old —see Newborn,
        examination
  clinical research control or normal
      comparison (control) (participant)
      Z00.6
  contraceptive (drug) maintenance (routine)
      Z30.8
    device (intrauterine) Z30.431
  dental Z01.20
    with abnormal findings Z01.21
  developmental —see Examination, child
  donor (potential) Z00.5
  ear Z01.10
    with abnormal findings NEC Z01.118
  eye Z01.00
    with abnormal findings Z01.01
    following failed vision screening Z01.020
      with abnormal findings Z01.021
  following
    accident NEC Z04.3
      transport Z04.1
      work Z04.2
    assault, alleged, ruled out
      adult Z04.71
      child Z04.72
    motor vehicle accident Z04.1
    treatment (for) Z09
      combined NEC Z09
        fracture Z09
        malignant neoplasm Z08
      malignant neoplasm Z08
      mental disorder Z09
      specified condition NEC Z09
  follow-up (routine) (following) Z09
    chemotherapy NEC Z09
      malignant neoplasm Z08
    fracture Z09
    malignant neoplasm Z08
    postpartum Z39.2
    psychotherapy Z09
    radiotherapy NEC Z09
      malignant neoplasm Z08
    surgery NEC Z09
      malignant neoplasm Z08
  forced sexual exploitation Z04.81
  forced labor exploitation Z04.82
  gynecological Z01.419
    with abnormal findings Z01.411
    for contraceptive maintenance Z30.8
  health —see Examination, medical
  hearing Z01.10
    with abnormal findings NEC Z01.118
    infant or child (over 28 days old) Z00.129
      with abnormal findings Z00.121
    following failed hearing screening
        Z01.110
  immunity status testing Z01.84
  laboratory (as part of a general medical
      examination) Z00.00
    with abnormal findings Z00.01
    preprocedural Z01.812
  lactating mother Z39.1
  medical (adult) (for) (of) Z00.00
    with abnormal findings Z00.01
    administrative purpose only Z02.9
      specified NEC Z02.89
    admission to
      armed forces Z02.3
      old age home Z02.2

Examination (Continued)
  medical (Continued)
    admission to (Continued)
      prison Z02.89
      residential institution Z02.2
      school Z02.0
        following illness or medical treatment
            Z02.0
      summer camp Z02.89
    adoption Z02.82
    blood alcohol or drug level Z02.83
    camp (summer) Z02.89
    clinical research, normal subject (control)
        (participant) Z00.6
    control subject in clinical research (normal
        comparison) (participant) Z00.6
    donor (potential) Z00.5
    driving license Z02.4
    general (adult) Z00.00
      with abnormal findings Z00.01
    immigration Z02.89
    insurance purposes Z02.6
    marriage Z02.89
    medicolegal reasons NEC Z04.89
    naturalization Z02.89
    participation in sport Z02.5
    paternity testing Z02.81
    population survey Z00.8
    pre-employment Z02.1
    pre-operative —see Examination,
        pre-procedural
    pre-procedural
      cardiovascular Z01.810
      respiratory Z01.811
      specified NEC Z01.818
    preschool children
      for admission to school Z02.0
    prisoners
      for entrance into prison Z02.89
    recruitment for armed forces Z02.3
    specified NEC Z00.8
    sport competition Z02.5
  medicolegal reason NEC Z04.89
    forced sexual exploitation Z04.81
    forced labor exploitation Z04.82
  newborn —see Newborn, examination
  pelvic (annual) (periodic) Z01.419
    with abnormal findings Z01.411
  period of rapid growth in childhood Z00.2
  periodic (adult) (annual) (routine) Z00.00
    with abnormal findings Z00.01
  physical (adult) —see also Examination,
      medical Z00.00
    sports Z02.5
  postpartum
    immediately after delivery Z39.0
    routine follow-up Z39.2
  pre-chemotherapy (antineoplastic) Z01.818
  prenatal (normal pregnancy) —see also
      Pregnancy, normal Z34.9-●
  pre-procedural (pre-operative)
    cardiovascular Z01.810
    laboratory Z01.812
    respiratory Z01.811
    specified NEC Z01.818
  prior to chemotherapy (antineoplastic) Z01.818
  psychiatric NEC Z00.8
    follow-up not needing further care Z09
    requested by authority Z04.6
  radiological (as part of a general medical
      examination) Z00.00
    with abnormal findings Z00.01
  repeat cervical smear to confirm findings of
      recent normal smear following initial
      abnormal smear Z01.42
  skin (hypersensitivity) Z01.82
  special —see also Examination, by type Z01.89
    specified type NEC Z01.89
  specified type or reason NEC Z04.89
  teeth Z01.20
    with abnormal findings Z01.21

Examination *(Continued)*
  urine —*see* Examination, laboratory
  vision Z01.00
    with abnormal findings Z01.01
    following failed vision screening Z01.020
      with abnormal findings Z01.021
    infant or child (over 28 days old) Z00.129
      with abnormal findings Z00.121
Exanthem, exanthema —*see also* Rash
  with enteroviral vesicular stomatitis B08.4
  Boston A88.0
  epidemic with meningitis A88.0 [G02]
  subitum B08.20
    due to human herpesvirus 6 B08.21
    due to human herpesvirus 7 B08.22
  viral, virus B09
    specified type NEC B08.8
Excess, excessive, excessively
  alcohol level in blood R78.0
  androgen (ovarian) E28.1
  attrition, tooth, teeth K03.0
  carotene, carotin (dietary) E67.1
  cold, effects of T69.9
    specified effect NEC T69.8
  convergence H51.12
  crying
    in child, adolescent, or adult R45.83
    in infant R68.11
  development, breast N62
  divergence H51.8
  drinking (alcohol) NEC (without
      dependence) F10.10
    habitual (continual) (without remission)
      F10.20
  eating R63.2
  estrogen E28.0
  fat —*see also* Obesity
    in heart —*see* Degeneration, myocardial
    localized E65
  foreskin N47.8
  gas R14.0
  glucagon E16.3
  heat —*see* Heat
  intermaxillary vertical dimension of fully
      erupted teeth M26.37
  interocclusal distance of fully erupted teeth
      M26.37
  kalium E87.5
  large
    colon K59.39
      congenital Q43.8
    infant P08.0
    organ or site, congenital NEC —*see*
      Anomaly, by site
  long
    organ or site, congenital NEC —*see*
      Anomaly, by site
  menstruation (with regular cycle) N92.0
    with irregular cycle N92.1
  napping Z72.821
  natrium E87.0
  number of teeth K00.1
  nutrient (dietary) NEC R63.2
  potassium (K) E87.5
  salivation K11.7
  secretion —*see also* Hypersecretion
    milk O92.6
    sputum R09.3
    sweat R61
  sexual drive F52.8
  short
    organ or site, congenital NEC —*see*
      Anomaly, by site
    umbilical cord in labor or delivery O69.3
  skin L98.7
    and subcutaneous tissue L98.7
    eyelid (acquired) —*see* Blepharochalasis
      congenital Q10.3
  sodium (Na) E87.0
  spacing of fully erupted teeth M26.32
  sputum R09.3

Excess, excessive, excessively *(Continued)*
  sweating R61
  thirst R63.1
    due to deprivation of water T73.1
  tuberosity of jaw M26.07
  vitamin
    A (dietary) E67.0
      administered as drug (prolonged
        intake) —*see* Table of Drugs and
        Chemicals, vitamins, adverse
        effect
      overdose or wrong substance given
        or taken —*see* Table of Drugs and
        Chemicals, vitamins, poisoning
    D (dietary) E67.3
      administered as drug (prolonged
        intake) —*see* Table of Drugs and
        Chemicals, vitamins, adverse
        effect
      overdose or wrong substance given
        or taken —*see* Table of Drugs and
        Chemicals, vitamins, poisoning
  weight
    gain R63.5
    loss R63.4
Excitability, abnormal, under minor stress
    (personality disorder) F60.3
Excitation
  anomalous atrioventricular I45.6
  psychogenic F30.8
  reactive (from emotional stress, psychological
    trauma) F30.8
Excitement
  hypomanic F30.8
  manic F30.9
  mental, reactive (from emotional stress,
    psychological trauma) F30.8
  state, reactive (from emotional stress,
    psychological trauma) F30.8
Excoriation (traumatic) —*see also* Abrasion
  neurotic L98.1
  skin picking disorder F42.4
Exfoliation
  due to erythematous conditions according to
      extent of body surface involved L49.0
    10-19 percent of body surface L49.1
    20-29 percent of body surface L49.2
    30-39 percent of body surface L49.3
    40-49 percent of body surface L49.4
    50-59 percent of body surface L49.5
    60-69 percent of body surface L49.6
    70-79 percent of body surface L49.7
    80-89 percent of body surface L49.8
    90-99 percent of body surface L49.9
    less than 10 percent of body surface L49.0
  teeth, due to systemic causes K08.0
Exfoliative —*see* condition
Exhaustion, exhaustive (physical NEC) R53.83
  battle F43.0
  cardiac —*see* Failure, heart
  delirium F43.0
  due to
    cold T69.8
    excessive exertion T73.3
    exposure T73.2
    neurasthenia F48.8
  heart —*see* Failure, heart
  heat —*see also* Heat, exhaustion T67.5
    due to
      salt depletion T67.4
      water depletion T67.3
  maternal, complicating delivery O75.81
  mental F48.8
  myocardium, myocardial —*see* Failure, heart
  nervous F48.8
  old age R54
  psychogenic F48.8
  psychosis F43.0
  senile R54
  vital NEC Z73.0
Exhibitionism F65.2

Exocervicitis —*see* Cervicitis
Exomphalos Q79.2
  meaning hernia —*see* Hernia, umbilicus
Exophoria H50.52
  convergence, insufficiency H51.11
  divergence, excess H51.8
Exophthalmos H05.2-•
  congenital Q15.8
  constant NEC H05.24-•
  displacement, globe —*see* Displacement,
    globe
  due to thyrotoxicosis (hyperthyroidism) —*see*
    Hyperthyroidism, with, goiter (diffuse)
  dysthyroid —*see* Hyperthyroidism, with,
    goiter (diffuse)
  goiter —*see* Hyperthyroidism, with, goiter
    (diffuse)
  intermittent NEC H05.25-•
  malignant —*see* Hyperthyroidism, with,
    goiter (diffuse)
  orbital
    edema —*see* Edema, orbit
    hemorrhage —*see* Hemorrhage, orbit
  pulsating NEC H05.26-•
  thyrotoxic, thyrotropic —*see*
    Hyperthyroidism, with, goiter (diffuse)
Exostosis —*see also* Disorder, bone
  cartilaginous —*see* Neoplasm, bone, benign
  congenital (multiple) Q78.6
  external ear canal H61.81-•
  gonococcal A54.49
  jaw (bone) M27.8
  multiple, congenital Q78.6
  orbit H05.35-•
  osteocartilaginous —*see* Neoplasm, bone,
    benign
  syphilitic A52.77
Exotropia —*see* Strabismus, divergent
  concomitant
Explanation of
  investigation finding Z71.2
  medication Z71.89
▶Exploitation
  ▶labor
    ▶confirmed
      ▶adult forced T74.61
      ▶child forced T74.62
    ▶suspected
      ▶adult forced T76.61
      ▶child forced T76.62
  ▶sexual
    ▶confirmed
      ▶adult forced T74.51
      ▶child T74.52
    ▶suspected
      ▶adult forced T76.51
      ▶child T76.52
Exposure (to) —*see also* Contact, with
    T75.89
  acariasis Z20.7
  AIDS virus Z20.6
  air pollution Z77.110
  algae and algae toxins Z77.121
  algae bloom Z77.121
  anthrax Z20.810
  aromatic amines Z77.020
  aromatic (hazardous) compounds NEC
    Z77.028
  aromatic dyes NOS Z77.028
  arsenic Z77.010
  asbestos Z77.090
  bacterial disease NEC Z20.818
  benzene Z77.021
  blue-green algae bloom Z77.121
  body fluids (potentially hazardous)
    Z77.21
  brown tide Z77.121
  chemicals (chiefly nonmedicinal) (hazardous)
    NEC Z77.098
  cholera Z20.09
  chromium compounds Z77.018

Exposure *(Continued)*
cold, effects of T69.9
  specified effect NEC T69.8
communicable disease Z20.9
  bacterial NEC Z20.818
  specified NEC Z20.89
  viral NEC Z20.828
  Zika virus Z20.821
▶coronavirus (disease) (novel) 2019 Z20.822
cyanobacteria bloom Z77.121
disaster Z65.5
discrimination Z60.5
dyes Z77.098
effects of T73.9
environmental tobacco smoke (acute)
    (chronic) Z77.22
Escherichia coli (E. coli) Z20.01
exhaustion due to T73.2
fiberglass —*see* Table of Drugs and
    Chemicals, fiberglass
German measles Z20.4
gonorrhea Z20.2
hazardous metals NEC Z77.018
hazardous substances NEC Z77.29
hazards in the physical environment NEC
    Z77.128
hazards to health NEC Z77.9
human immunodeficiency virus (HIV)
    Z20.6
human T-lymphotropic virus type-1 (HTLV-1)
    Z20.89
implanted
  mesh —*see* Complications, prosthetic
      device or implant, mesh
  prosthetic materials NEC —*see*
      Complications, prosthetic materials
      NEC
infestation (parasitic) NEC Z20.7
intestinal infectious disease NEC Z20.09
  Escherichia coli (E. coli) Z20.01
lead Z77.011
meningococcus Z20.811
mold (toxic) Z77.120
nickel dust Z77.018
noise Z77.122
occupational
  air contaminants NEC Z57.39
  dust Z57.2
  environmental tobacco smoke Z57.31
  extreme temperature Z57.6
  noise Z57.0

Exposure *(Continued)*
  radiation Z57.1
  risk factors Z57.9
    specified NEC Z57.8
  toxic agents (gases) (liquids) (solids)
      (vapors) in agriculture Z57.4
  toxic agents (gases) (liquids) (solids)
      (vapors) in industry NEC Z57.5
  vibration Z57.7
parasitic disease NEC Z20.7
pediculosis Z20.7
persecution Z60.5
pfiesteria piscicida Z77.121
poliomyelitis Z20.89
pollution
  air Z77.110
  environmental NEC Z77.118
  soil Z77.112
  water Z77.111
polycyclic aromatic hydrocarbons Z77.028
prenatal (drugs) (toxic chemicals) —*see*
    Newborn, affected by, noxious substances
    transmitted via placenta or breast milk
rabies Z20.3
radiation, naturally occurring NEC Z77.123
radon Z77.123
red tide (Florida) Z77.121
rubella Z20.4
second hand tobacco smoke (acute) (chronic)
    Z77.22
  in the perinatal period P96.81
sexually-transmitted disease Z20.2
smallpox (laboratory) Z20.89
syphilis Z20.2
terrorism Z65.4
torture Z65.4
tuberculosis Z20.1
uranium Z77.012
varicella Z20.820
venereal disease Z20.2
viral disease NEC Z20.828
war Z65.5
water pollution Z77.111
  Zika virus Z20.821
Exsanguination —*see* Hemorrhage
Exstrophy
  abdominal contents Q45.8
  bladder Q64.10
    cloacal Q64.12
    specified type NEC Q64.19
    supravesical fissure Q64.11

Extensive —*see* condition
Extra —*see also* Accessory
  marker chromosomes (normal individual)
    Q92.61
  in abnormal individual Q92.62
  rib Q76.6
    cervical Q76.5
Extrasystoles (supraventricular) I49.49
  atrial I49.1
  auricular I49.1
  junctional I49.2
  ventricular I49.3
Extrauterine gestation or pregnancy —*see*
    Pregnancy, by site
Extravasation
  blood R58
  chyle into mesentery I89.8
  pelvicalyceal N13.8
  pyelosinus N13.8
  urine (from ureter) R39.0
  vesicant agent
    antineoplastic chemotherapy T80.810
    other agent NEC T80.818
Extremity —*see* condition, limb
Extrophy —*see* Exstrophy
Extroversion
  bladder Q64.19
  uterus N81.4
    complicating delivery O71.2
    postpartal (old) N81.4
Extruded tooth (teeth) M26.34
Extrusion
  breast implant (prosthetic) T85.42
  eye implant (globe) (ball) T85.328
  intervertebral disc —*see* Displacement,
    intervertebral disc
  ocular lens implant (prosthetic) —*see*
    Complications, intraocular lens
  vitreous —*see* Prolapse, vitreous
Exudate
  pleural —*see* Effusion, pleura
  retina H35.89
▶wound fluids L24.A9
Exudative —*see* condition
Eye, eyeball, eyelid —*see* condition
Eyestrain —*see* Disturbance, vision, subjective
Eyeworm disease of Africa B74.3

▶ New   ⇒ Revised   ~~deleted~~ Deleted   ● Use Additional Character(s)

F

Faber's syndrome (achlorhydric anemia) D50.9
Fabry (-Anderson) disease E75.21
Facet syndrome M47.89-●
Faciocephalalgia, autonomic —see also
    Neuropathy, peripheral, autonomic G90.09
Factor(s)
  psychic, associated with diseases classified
    elsewhere F54
  psychological
    affecting physical conditions F54
    or behavioral
      affecting general medical condition F54
      associated with disorders or diseases
        classified elsewhere F54
Fahr disease (of brain) G23.8
Fahr Volhard disease (of kidney) I12.-●
Failure, failed
  abortion —see Abortion, attempted
  aortic (valve) I35.8
    rheumatic I06.8
  attempted abortion —see Abortion, attempted
  biventricular I50.82
    due to left heart failure I50.814
  bone marrow —see Anemia, aplastic
  cardiac —see Failure, heart
  cardiorenal (chronic) —see also Failure, renal,
    and Failure, heart I50.9
    hypertensive I13.2
  cardiorespiratory (see also Failure, heart) R09.2
  cardiovascular (chronic) —see Failure, heart
  cerebrovascular I67.9
  cervical dilatation in labor O62.0
  circulation, circulatory (peripheral) R57.9
    newborn P29.89
  compensation —see Disease, heart
  compliance with medical treatment or
    regimen —see Noncompliance
  congestive —see Failure, heart, congestive
  dental implant (endosseous) M27.69
    due to
      failure of dental prosthesis M27.63
      lack of attached gingiva M27.62
      occlusal trauma (poor prosthetic design)
        M27.62
      parafunctional habits M27.62
      periodontal infection (peri-implantitis)
        M27.62
      poor oral hygiene M27.62
    osseointegration M27.61
      due to
        complications of systemic disease
          M27.61
          poor bone quality M27.61
      iatrogenic M27.61
    post-osseointegration
      biological M27.62
      due to complications of systemic disease
        M27.62
      iatrogenic M27.62
      mechanical M27.63
    pre-integration M27.61
    pre-osseointegration M27.61
    specified NEC M27.69
  descent of head (at term) of pregnancy
    (mother) O32.4
  endosseous dental implant —see Failure,
    dental implant
  engagement of head (term of pregnancy)
    (mother) O32.4
  erection (penile) —see also Dysfunction,
    sexual, male, erectile N52.9
    nonorganic F52.21
  examination(s), anxiety concerning Z55.2
  expansion terminal respiratory units
    (newborn) (primary) P28.0
  forceps NOS (with subsequent cesarean
    delivery) O66.5
  gain weight (child over 28 days old) R62.51
    adult R62.7
    newborn P92.6

Failure, failed (Continued)
  genital response (male) F52.21
    female F52.22
  heart (acute) (senile) (sudden) I50.9
    with
      acute pulmonary edema —see Failure,
        ventricular, left
      decompensation I50.9
      ▶with
        ▶normal ejection fraction I50.33
        ▶preserved ejection fraction I50.33
        ▶reduced ejection fraction I50.23
          ▶with diastolic dysfunction I50.43
      ▶combined systolic and diastolic
        I50.43
      ▶diastolic I50.33
      ▶right I50.813
      ▶systolic I50.23
    dilatation —see Disease, heart
    hypertension —see Hypertension, heart
    normal ejection fraction —see Failure,
      heart, diastolic
    preserved ejection fraction —see Failure,
      heart, diastolic
    reduced ejection fraction —see Failure,
      heart, systolic
    arteriosclerotic I70.90
    biventricular I50.82
      due to left heart failure I50.814
    combined left-right sided I50.82
      due to left heart failure I50.814
    compensated —see also Failure, heart, by
      type as diastolic or systolic, chronic
      I50.9
    complicating
      anesthesia (general) (local) or other
        sedation
        in labor and delivery O74.2
        in pregnancy O29.12-●
        postpartum, puerperal O89.1
      delivery (cesarean) (instrumental) O75.4
    congestive I50.9
      with rheumatic fever (conditions in I00)
        active I01.8
        inactive or quiescent (with chorea)
          I09.81
      newborn P29.0
      rheumatic (chronic) (inactive) (with
        chorea) I09.81
        active or acute I01.8
          with chorea I02.0
    decompensated —see also Failure, heart, by
      type as diastolic or systolic, acute and
      chronic I50.9
    degenerative —see Degeneration, myocardial
    diastolic (congestive) (left ventricular) I50.30
      acute (congestive) I50.31
        and (on) chronic (congestive) I50.33
      chronic (congestive) I50.32
        and (on) acute (congestive) I50.33
      combined with systolic (congestive)
        I50.40
        acute (congestive) I50.41
          and (on) chronic (congestive) I50.43
        chronic (congestive) I50.42
          and (on) acute (congestive) I50.43
    due to presence of cardiac prosthesis I97.13-●
    end stage —see also Failure, heart, by type
      as diastolic or systolic, chronic I50.84
    following cardiac surgery I97.13-●
    high output NOS I50.83
    hypertensive —see Hypertension, heart
    left (ventricular) —see also Failure,
      ventricular, left
      combined diastolic and systolic —see
        Failure, heart, diastolic, combined
        with systolic
      diastolic —see Failure, heart, diastolic
      systolic —see Failure, heart, systolic
    low output (syndrome) NOS I50.9
    newborn P29.0
    organic —see Disease, heart
    peripartum O90.3

Failure, failed (Continued)
  heart (Continued)
    postprocedural I97.13-●
    rheumatic (chronic) (inactive) I09.9
    right (isolated) (ventricular) I50.810
      acute I50.811
        and (on) chronic I50.813
      chronic I50.812
        and acute I50.813
      secondary to left heart failure I50.814
    specified NEC I50.89

> Note: heart failure stages A, B, C, and
> D are based on the American College of
> Cardiology and American Heart Association
> stages of heart failure, which complement
> and should not be confused with the New
> York Heart Association Classification of
> Heart Failure, into Class I, Class II, Class III,
> and Class IV

    stage A Z91.89
    stage B (see also Failure, heart, by type as
      diastolic or systolic) I50.9
    stage C (see also Failure, heart, by type as
      diastolic or systolic) I50.9
    stage D (see also Failure, heart, by type
      as diastolic or systolic, chronic)
      I50.84
    systolic (congestive) (left ventricular)
      I50.20
      acute (congestive) I50.21
        and (on) chronic (congestive) I50.23
      chronic (congestive) I50.22
        and (on) acute (congestive) I50.23
      combined with diastolic (congestive)
        I50.40
        acute (congestive) I50.41
          and (on) chronic (congestive)
            I50.43
        chronic (congestive) I50.42
          and (on) acute (congestive) I50.43
    thyrotoxic (see also Thyrotoxicosis) E05.90
      [I43]
      with
        high output (see also Thyrotoxicosis)
          I50.83
        thyroid storm E05.91 [I43]
          high output (see also
            Thyrotoxicosis) I50.83
    valvular —see Endocarditis
  hepatic K72.90
    with coma K72.91
    acute or subacute K72.00
      with coma K72.01
      due to drugs K71.10
        with coma K71.11
    alcoholic (acute) (chronic) (subacute)
      K70.40
      with coma K70.41
    chronic K72.10
      with coma K72.11
      due to drugs (acute) (subacute) (chronic)
        K71.10
        with coma K71.11
    due to drugs (acute) (subacute) (chronic)
      K71.10
      with coma K71.11
    postprocedural K91.82
  hepatorenal K76.7
  induction (of labor) O61.9
    abortion —see Abortion, attempted
    by
      oxytocic drugs O61.0
      prostaglandins O61.0
    instrumental O61.1
    mechanical O61.1
    medical O61.0
    specified NEC O61.8
    surgical O61.1

Failure, failed (Continued)
  intubation during anesthesia T88.4
    in pregnancy O29.6-●
    labor and delivery O74.7
    postpartum, puerperal O89.6
  involution, thymus (gland) E32.0
  kidney —see also Disease, kidney, chronic N19
    acute —see also Failure, renal, acute N17.9-●
    diabetic —see E08-E13 with .22
  lactation (complete) O92.3
    partial O92.4
  Leydig's cell, adult E29.1
  liver —see Failure, hepatic
  menstruation at puberty N91.0
  mitral I05.8
  myocardial, myocardium —see also Failure,
      heart I50.9
    chronic —see also Failure, heart, congestive
        I50.9
    congestive —see also Failure, heart,
        congestive I50.9
▶newborn screening —see Abnormal, neonatal
      screening
▶neonatal congenital heart disease P09.5
  orgasm (female) (psychogenic) F52.31
    male F52.32
  ovarian (primary) E28.39
    iatrogenic E89.40
      asymptomatic E89.40
      symptomatic E89.41
    postprocedural (postablative)
        (postirradiation) (postsurgical) E89.40
      asymptomatic E89.40
      symptomatic E89.41
  ovulation causing infertility N97.0
  polyglandular, autoimmune E31.0
  prosthetic joint implant —see Complications,
      joint prosthesis, mechanical, breakdown,
      by site
  renal N19
    with
      tubular necrosis (acute) N17.0
    acute N17.9
      with
        cortical necrosis N17.1
        medullary necrosis N17.2
        tubular necrosis N17.0
      specified NEC N17.8
    chronic N18.9
      hypertensive —see Hypertension, kidney
    congenital P96.0
    end stage (chronic) N18.6
      due to hypertension I12.0
    following
      abortion —see Abortion by type
          complicated by specified
          condition NEC
      crushing T79.5
      ectopic or molar pregnancy O08.4
      labor and delivery (acute) O90.4
    hypertensive —see Hypertension, kidney
    postprocedural N99.0
  respiration, respiratory J96.90
    with
      hypercapnia J96.92
      hypercarbia J96.02
      hypoxia J96.91
    acute J96.00
      with
        hypercapnia J96.02
        hypercarbia J96.92
        hypoxia J96.01
    acute and (on) chronic J96.20
      with
        hypercapnia J96.22
        hypercarbia J96.22
        hypoxia J96.21
    center G93.89
    chronic J96.10
      with
        hypercapnia J96.12
        hypercarbia J96.12
        hypoxia J96.11

Failure, failed (Continued)
  respiration, respiratory (Continued)
    newborn P28.5
    postprocedural (acute) J95.821
      acute and chronic J95.822
  rotation
    cecum Q43.3
    colon Q43.3
    intestine Q43.3
    kidney Q63.2
  sedation (conscious) (moderate) during
      procedure T88.52
    history of Z92.83
  segmentation —see also Fusion
    fingers —see Syndactylism, complex,
        fingers
    vertebra Q76.49
      with scoliosis Q76.3
  seminiferous tubule, adult E29.1
  senile (general) R54
  sexual arousal (male) F52.21
    female F52.22
  testicular endocrine function E29.1
  to thrive (child over 28 days old) R62.51
    adult R62.7
    newborn P92.6
  transplant T86.92
    bone T86.831
      marrow T86.02
    cornea T86.841-●
    heart T86.22
      with lung(s) T86.32
    intestine T86.851
    kidney T86.12
    liver T86.42
    lung(s) T86.811
      with heart T86.32
    pancreas T86.891
    skin (allograft) (autograft) T86.821
    specified organ or tissue NEC T86.891
    stem cell (peripheral blood) (umbilical
        cord) T86.5
  trial of labor (with subsequent cesarean
      delivery) O66.40
    following previous cesarean delivery
        O66.41
  tubal ligation N99.89
  urinary —see Disease, kidney, chronic
  vacuum extraction NOS (with subsequent
      cesarean delivery) O66.5
  vasectomy N99.89
  ventouse NOS (with subsequent cesarean
      delivery) O66.5
  ventricular —see also Failure, heart I50.9
    left —see also Failure, heart, left I50.1
      with rheumatic fever (conditions
          in I00)
        active I01.8
          with chorea I02.0
        inactive or quiescent (with chorea)
            I09.81
      rheumatic (chronic) (inactive) (with
          chorea) I09.81
        active or acute I01.8
          with chorea I02.0
    right —see Failure, heart, right
  vital centers, newborn P91.88
Fainting (fit) R55
Fallen arches —see Deformity, limb, flat foot
Falling, falls (repeated) R29.6
  any organ or part —see Prolapse
Fallopian
  insufflation Z31.41
  tube —see condition
Fallot's
  pentalogy Q21.8
  tetrad or tetralogy Q21.3
  triad or trilogy Q22.3
False —see also condition
  croup J38.5
  joint —see Nonunion, fracture

False (Continued)
  labor (pains) O47.9
    at or after 37 completed weeks of gestation
        O47.1
    before 37 completed weeks of gestation
        O47.0-●
  passage, urethra (prostatic) N36.5
  pregnancy F45.8
Family, familial —see also condition
  disruption Z63.8
    involving divorce or separation
        Z63.5
  Li-Fraumeni (syndrome) Z15.01
  planning advice Z30.09
  problem Z63.9
    specified NEC Z63.8
  retinoblastoma C69.2-●
Famine (effects of) T73.0
  edema —see Malnutrition, severe
Fanconi (-de Toni)(-Debré) syndrome
    E72.09
  with cystinosis E72.04
Fanconi's anemia (congenital pancytopenia)
    D61.09
Farber's disease or syndrome E75.29
Farcy A24.0
Farmer's
  lung J67.0
  skin L57.8
Farsightedness —see Hypermetropia
Fascia —see condition
Fasciculation R25.3
Fasciitis M72.9
  diffuse (eosinophilic) M35.4
  infective M72.8
    necrotizing M72.6
  necrotizing M72.6
  nodular M72.4
  perirenal (with ureteral obstruction)
      N13.5
    with infection N13.6
  plantar M72.2
  specified NEC M72.8
  traumatic (old) M72.8
    current - code by site under Sprain
Fascioliasis B66.3
Fasciolopsis, fasciolopsiasis (intestinal)
    B66.5
Fascioscapulohumeral myopathy G71.02
Fast pulse R00.0
Fat
  embolism —see Embolism, fat
  excessive —see also Obesity
    in heart —see Degeneration, myocardial
  in stool R19.5
  localized (pad) E65
    heart —see Degeneration, myocardial
    knee M79.4
    retropatellar M79.4
  necrosis
    breast N64.1
    mesentery K65.4
    omentum K65.4
  pad E65
    knee M79.4
Fatigue R53.83
  auditory deafness —see Deafness
  chronic R53.82
  combat F43.0
  general R53.83
    psychogenic F48.8
  heat (transient) T67.6
  muscle M62.89
  myocardium —see Failure, heart
  neoplasm-related R53.0
  nervous, neurosis F48.8
  operational F48.8
  psychogenic (general) F48.8
  senile R54
  voice R49.8
Fatness —see Obesity

Fatty —*see also* condition
  apron E65
  degeneration —*see* Degeneration, fatty
  heart (enlarged) —*see* Degeneration,
    myocardial
  liver NEC K76.0
    alcoholic K70.0
    nonalcoholic K76.0
  necrosis —*see* Degeneration, fatty
Fauces —*see* condition
Fauchard's disease (periodontitis) —*see*
    Periodontitis
Faucitis J02.9
Favism (anemia) D55.0
Favus —*see* Dermatophytosis
Fazio-Londe disease or syndrome
    G12.1
Fear complex or reaction F40.9
Fear of —*see* Phobia
Feared complaint unfounded Z71.1
Febris, febrile —*see also* Fever
  flava —*see also* Fever, yellow A95.9
  melitensis A23.0
  pestis —*see* Plague
  recurrens —*see* Fever, relapsing
  rubra A38.9
Fecal
  incontinence R15.9
  smearing R15.1
  soiling R15.1
  urgency R15.2
Fecalith (impaction) K56.41
  appendix K38.1
  congenital P76.8
Fede's disease K14.0
Feeble rapid pulse due to shock following
    injury T79.4
Feeble-minded F70
Feeding
  difficulties R63.30
  problem (elderly) (infant) R63.39
    newborn P92.9
      specified NEC P92.8
    nonorganic (adult) —*see* Disorder,
      eating
Feeling (of)
  foreign body in throat R09.89
Feer's disease —*see* Poisoning, mercury
Feet —*see* condition
Feigned illness Z76.5
Feil-Klippel syndrome (brevicollis) Q76.1
Feinmesser's (hidrotic) ectodermal dysplasia
    Q82.4
Felinophobia F40.218
Felon —*see also* Cellulitis, digit
  with lymphangitis —*see* Lymphangitis,
    acute, digit
Felty's syndrome M05.00
  ankle M05.07-●
  elbow M05.02-●
  foot joint M05.07-●
  hand joint M05.04-●
  hip M05.05-●
  knee M05.06-●
  multiple site M05.09
  shoulder M05.01-●
  vertebra —*see* Spondylitis, ankylosing
  wrist M05.03-●
Female genital cutting status —*see* Female
    genital mutilation status (FGM)
Female genital mutilation status (FGM)
    N90.810
  specified NEC N90.818
  type I (clitorectomy status) N90.811
  type II (clitorectomy with excision
      of labia minora status)
      N90.812
  type III (infibulation status)
      N90.813
  type IV N90.818
Femur, femoral —*see* condition

Fenestration, fenestrated —*see also* Imperfect,
    closure
  aortico-pulmonary Q21.4
  cusps, heart valve NEC Q24.8
    pulmonary Q22.3
  pulmonic cusps Q22.3
Fernell's disease (aortic aneurysm) I71.9
Fertile eunuch syndrome E23.0
Fetid
  breath R19.6
  sweat L75.0
Fetishism F65.0
  transvestic F65.1
Fetus, fetal —*see also* condition
  alcohol syndrome (dysmorphic) Q86.0
  compressus O31.0-●
  hydantoin syndrome Q86.1
  lung tissue P28.0
  papyraceous O31.0-●
Fever (inanition) (of unknown origin)
    (persistent) (with chills) (with rigor) R50.9
  abortus A23.1
  Aden (dengue) A90
  African tick bite A77.8
  African tick-borne A68.1
  American
    mountain (tick) A93.2
    spotted A77.0
  aphthous B08.8
  arbovirus, arboviral A94
    hemorrhagic A94
    specified NEC A93.8
  Argentinian hemorrhagic A96.0
  Assam B55.0
  Australian Q A78
  Bangkok hemorrhagic A91
  Barmah forest A92.8
  Bartonella A44.0
  bilious, hemoglobinuric B50.8
  blackwater B50.8
  blister B00.1
  Bolivian hemorrhagic A96.1
  Bonvale dam T73.3
  boutonneuse A77.1
  brain —*see* Encephalitis
  Brazilian purpuric A48.4
  breakbone A90
  Bullis A77.0
  Bunyamwera A92.8
  Burdwan B55.0
  Bwamba A92.8
  Cameroon —*see* Malaria
  Canton A75.9
  catarrhal (acute) J00
    chronic J31.0
  cat-scratch A28.1
  Central Asian hemorrhagic A98.0
  cerebral —*see* Encephalitis
  cerebrospinal meningococcal A39.0
  Chagres B50.9
  Chandipura A92.8
  Changuinola A93.1
  Charcot's (biliary) (hepatic) (intermittent) —
    see Calculus, bile duct
  Chikungunya (viral) (hemorrhagic) A92.0
  Chitral A93.1
  Colombo —*see* Fever, paratyphoid
  Colorado tick (virus) A93.2
  congestive (remittent) —*see* Malaria
  Congo virus A98.0
  continued malarial B50.9
  Corsican —*see* Malaria
  Crimean-Congo hemorrhagic A98.0
  Cyprus —*see* Brucellosis
  dandy A90
  deer fly —*see* Tularemia
  dengue (virus) A90
    hemorrhagic A91
    sandfly A93.1
  desert B38.0
  drug induced R50.2

Fever (Continued)
  due to
    conditions classified elsewhere R50.81
    heat T67.01
  enteric A01.00
  enteroviral exanthematous (Boston
      exanthem) A88.0
  ephemeral (of unknown origin) R50.9
  epidemic hemorrhagic A98.5
  erysipelatous —*see* Erysipelas
  estivo-autumnal (malarial) B50.9
  famine A75.0
  five day A79.0
  following delivery O86.4
  Fort Bragg A27.89
  gastroenteric A01.00
  gastromalarial —*see* Malaria
  Gibraltar —*see* Brucellosis
  glandular —*see* Mononucleosis, infectious
  Guama (viral) A92.8
  Haverhill A25.1
  hay (allergic) J30.1
    with asthma (bronchial) J45.909
      with
        exacerbation (acute) J45.901
        status asthmaticus J45.902
    due to
      allergen other than pollen J30.89
      pollen, any plant or tree J30.1
  heat (effects) T67.01
  hematuric, bilious B50.8
  hemoglobinuric (malarial) (bilious) B50.8
  hemorrhagic (arthropod-borne) NOS A94
    with renal syndrome A98.5
    arenaviral A96.9
      specified NEC A96.8
    Argentinian A96.0
    Bangkok A91
    Bolivian A96.1
    Central Asian A98.0
    Chikungunya A92.0
    Crimean-Congo A98.0
    dengue (virus) A91
    epidemic A98.5
    Junin (virus) A96.0
    Korean A98.5
    Kyasanur forest A98.2
    Machupo (virus) A96.1
    mite-borne A93.8
    mosquito-borne A92.8
    Omsk A98.1
    Philippine A91
    Russian A98.5
    Singapore A91
    Southeast Asia A91
    Thailand A91
    tick-borne NEC A93.8
    viral A99
      specified NEC A98.8
  hepatic —*see* Cholecystitis
  herpetic —*see* Herpes
  icterohemorrhagic A27.0
  Indiana A93.8
  infective B99.9
    specified NEC B99.8
  intermittent (bilious) —*see also* Malaria
    of unknown origin R50.9
    pernicious B50.9
  iodide R50.2
  Japanese river A75.3
  jungle —*see also* Malaria
    yellow A95.0
  Junin (virus) hemorrhagic A96.0
  Katayama B65.2
  kedani A75.3
  Kenya (tick) A77.1
  Kew Garden A79.1
  Korean hemorrhagic A98.5
  Lassa A96.2
  Lone Star A77.0
  Machupo (virus) hemorrhagic A96.1

Fever *(Continued)*
  malaria, malarial —*see* Malaria
  Malta A23.9
  Marseilles A77.1
  marsh —*see* Malaria
  Mayaro (viral) A92.8
  Mediterranean —*see also* Brucellosis A23.9
    familial M04.1
    tick A77.1
  meningeal —*see* Meningitis
  Meuse A79.0
  Mexican A75.2
  mianeh A68.1
  miasmatic —*see* Malaria
  mosquito-borne (viral) A92.9
    hemorrhagic A92.8
  mountain —*see also* Brucellosis
    meaning Rocky Mountain spotted fever
      A77.0
    tick (American) (Colorado) (viral) A93.2
  Mucambo (viral) A92.8
  mud A27.9
  Neapolitan —*see* Brucellosis
  neutropenic D70.9
  newborn P81.9
    environmental P81.0
  Nine-Mile A78
  non-exanthematous tick A93.2
  North Asian tick-borne A77.2
  Omsk hemorrhagic A98.1
  O'nyong-nyong (viral) A92.1
  Oropouche (viral) A93.0
  Oroya A44.0
  pacific coast tick A77.8
  paludal —*see* Malaria
  Panama (malarial) B50.9
  Pappataci A93.1
  paratyphoid A01.4
    A A01.1
    B A01.2
    C A01.3
  parrot A70
  periodic (Mediterranean) M04.1
  persistent (of unknown origin) R50.9
  petechial A39.0
  pharyngoconjunctival B30.2
  Philippine hemorrhagic A91
  phlebotomus A93.1
  Piry (virus) A93.8
  Pixuna (viral) A92.8
  Plasmodium ovale B53.0
  polioviral (nonparalytic) A80.4
  Pontiac A48.2
  postimmunization R50.83
  postoperative R50.82
    due to infection T81.40
  posttransfusion R50.84
  postvaccination R50.83
  presenting with conditions classified
    elsewhere R50.81
  pretibial A27.89
  puerperal O86.4
  Q A78
  quadrilateral A78
  quartan (malaria) B52.9
  Queensland (coastal) (tick) A77.3
  quintan A79.0
  rabbit —*see* Tularemia
  rat-bite A25.9
    due to
      Spirillum A25.0
      Streptobacillus moniliformis A25.1
  recurrent —*see* Fever, relapsing
  relapsing (Borrelia) A68.9
    Carter's (Asiatic) A68.1
    Dutton's (West African) A68.1
    Koch's A68.9
    louse-borne A68.0
    Novy's
      louse-borne A68.0
      tick-borne A68.1

Fever *(Continued)*
  relapsing (Borrelia) *(Continued)*
    Obermeyer's (European) A68.0
    tick-borne A68.1
  remittent (bilious) (congestive) (gastric) —*see*
    Malaria
  rheumatic (active) (acute) (chronic) (subacute)
    I00
    with central nervous system involvement
      I02.9
    active with heart involvement —*see*
      category I01
    inactive or quiescent with
      cardiac hypertrophy I09.89
      carditis I09.9
      endocarditis I09.1
        aortic (valve) I06.9
          with mitral (valve) disease I08.0
        mitral (valve) I05.9
          with aortic (valve) disease I08.0
        pulmonary (valve) I09.89
        tricuspid (valve) I07.8
      heart disease NEC I09.89
      heart failure (congestive) (conditions in
        category I50.) I09.81
      left ventricular failure (conditions in
        I50.1-I50.4-) I09.81
      myocarditis, myocardial degeneration
        (conditions in I51.4) I09.0
      pancarditis I09.9
      pericarditis I09.2
  Rift Valley (viral) A92.4
  Rocky Mountain spotted A77.0
  rose J30.1
  Ross River B33.1
  Russian hemorrhagic A98.5
  San Joaquin (Valley) B38.0
  sandfly A93.1
  Sao Paulo A77.0
  scarlet A38.9
  seven day (leptospirosis) (autumnal)
    (Japanese) A27.89
  dengue A90
  shin-bone A79.0
  Singapore hemorrhagic A91
  solar A90
  Songo A98.5
  sore B00.1
  South African tick-bite A68.1
  Southeast Asia hemorrhagic A91
  spinal —*see* Meningitis
  spirillary A25.0
  splenic —*see* Anthrax
  spotted A77.9
    American A77.0
    Brazilian A77.0
    cerebrospinal meningitis A39.0
    Colombian A77.0
    due to Rickettsia
      africae (African tick bite fever) A77.8
      australis A77.3
      conorii A77.1
      parkeri A77.8
      rickettsii A77.0
      sibirica A77.2
      specified type NEC A77.8
    Ehrlichiosis A77.40
      due to
        E. chafeensis A77.41
        specified organism NEC A77.49
    Rocky Mountain A77.0
  steroid R50.2
  streptobacillary A25.1
  subtertian B50.9
  Sumatran mite A75.3
  sun A90
  swamp A27.9
  swine A02.8
  sylvatic, yellow A95.0
  Tahyna B33.8
  tertian —*see* Malaria, tertian

Fever *(Continued)*
  Thailand hemorrhagic A91
  thermic T67.01
  three-day A93.1
  tick
    American mountain A93.2
    Colorado A93.2
    Kemerovo A93.8
    Mediterranean A77.1
    mountain A93.2
    nonxanthematous A93.2
    Quaranfil A93.8
  tick-bite NEC A93.8
  tick-borne (hemorrhagic) NEC A93.8
  trench A79.0
  tsutsugamushi A75.3
  typhogastric A01.00
  typhoid (abortive) (hemorrhagic)
    (intermittent) (malignant) A01.00
    complicated by
      arthritis A01.04
      heart involvement A01.02
      meningitis A01.01
      osteomyelitis A01.05
      pneumonia A01.03
      specified NEC A01.09
  typhomalarial —*see* Malaria
  typhus —*see* Typhus (fever)
  undulant —*see* Brucellosis
  unknown origin R50.9
  uveoparotid D86.89
  valley B38.0
  Venezuelan equine A92.2
  vesicular stomatitis A93.8
  viral hemorrhagic —*see* Fever, hemorrhagic,
    by type of virus
  Volhynian A79.0
  Wesselsbron (viral) A92.8
  West
    African B50.8
    Nile (viral) A92.30
      with
        complications NEC A92.39
        cranial nerve disorders A92.32
        encephalitis A92.31
        encephalomyelitis A92.31
        neurologic manifestation NEC
          A92.32
        optic neuritis A92.32
        polyradiculitis A92.32
  Whitmore's —*see* Melioidosis
  Wolhynian A79.0
  worm B83.9
  yellow A95.9
    jungle A95.0
    sylvatic A95.0
    urban A95.1
  Zika virus A92.5
Fibrillation
  atrial or auricular (established) I48.91
    chronic I48.20
      persistent I48.19
    paroxysmal I48.0
    permanent I48.21
    persistent (chronic) (NOS) (other) I48.19
      longstanding I48.11
  cardiac I49.8
  heart I49.8
  muscular M62.89
  ventricular I49.01
Fibrin
  ball or bodies, pleural (sac) J94.1
  chamber, anterior (eye) (gelatinous
    exudate) —*see* Iridocyclitis, acute
Fibrinogenolysis —*see* Fibrinolysis
Fibrinogenopenia D68.8
  acquired D65
  congenital D68.2
Fibrinolysis (hemorrhagic) (acquired) D65
  antepartum hemorrhage —*see* Hemorrhage,
    antepartum, with coagulation defect

Fibrinolysis (Continued)
  following
    abortion —see Abortion by type
      complicated by hemorrhage
    ectopic or molar pregnancy O08.1
  intrapartum O67.0
  newborn, transient P60
  postpartum O72.3
Fibrinopenia (hereditary) D68.2
  acquired D68.4
Fibrinopurulent —see condition
Fibrinous —see condition
Fibroadenoma
  cellular intracanalicular D24-●
  giant D24-●
  intracanalicular
    cellular D24-●
    giant D24-●
    specified site —see Neoplasm, benign, by
      site
    unspecified site D24-●
  juvenile D24-●
  pericanalicular
    specified site —see Neoplasm, benign, by
      site
    unspecified site D24-●
  phyllodes D24-●
  prostate D29.1
  specified site NEC —see Neoplasm, benign,
    by site
  unspecified site D24-●
Fibroadenosis, breast (chronic) (cystic) (diffuse)
    (periodic) (segmental) N60.2-●
Fibroangioma —see also Neoplasm, benign, by
    site
  juvenile
    specified site —see Neoplasm, benign, by
      site
    unspecified site D10.6
Fibrochondrosarcoma —see Neoplasm,
    cartilage, malignant
Fibrocystic
  disease —see also Fibrosis, cystic
    breast —see Mastopathy, cystic
    jaw M27.49
    kidney (congenital) Q61.8
    liver Q44.6
    pancreas E84.9
  kidney (congenital) Q61.8
Fibrodysplasia ossificans progressiva —see
    Myositis, ossificans, progressiva
Fibroelastosis (cordis) (endocardial)
    (endomyocardial) I42.4
Fibroid (tumor) —see also Neoplasm, connective
    tissue, benign
  disease, lung (chronic) —see Fibrosis, lung
  heart (disease) —see Myocarditis
  in pregnancy or childbirth O34.1-●
    causing obstructed labor O65.5
  induration, lung (chronic) —see Fibrosis, lung
  lung —see Fibrosis, lung
  pneumonia (chronic) —see Fibrosis, lung
  uterus —see also Leiomyoma, uterus D25.9
Fibrolipoma —see Lipoma
Fibroliposarcoma —see Neoplasm, connective
    tissue, malignant
Fibroma —see also Neoplasm, connective tissue,
    benign
  ameloblastic —see Cyst, calcifying odontogenic
  bone (nonossifying) —see Disorder, bone,
    specified type NEC
    ossifying —see Neoplasm, bone, benign
  cementifying —see Neoplasm, bone, benign
  chondromyxoid —see Neoplasm, bone,
    benign
  desmoplastic —see Neoplasm, connective
    tissue, uncertain behavior
  durum —see Neoplasm, connective tissue,
    benign
  fascial —see Neoplasm, connective tissue,
    benign

Fibroma (Continued)
  invasive —see Neoplasm, connective tissue,
    uncertain behavior
  molle —see Lipoma
  myxoid —see Neoplasm, connective tissue,
    benign
  nasopharynx, nasopharyngeal (juvenile)
    D10.6
  nonosteogenic (nonossifying) —see Dysplasia,
    fibrous
  odontogenic (central) —see Cyst, calcifying
    odontogenic
  ossifying —see Neoplasm, bone, benign
  periosteal —see Neoplasm, bone, benign
  soft —see Lipoma
Fibromatosis M72.9
  abdominal —see Neoplasm, connective tissue,
    uncertain behavior
  aggressive —see Neoplasm, connective tissue,
    uncertain behavior
  congenital generalized —see Neoplasm,
    connective tissue, uncertain behavior
  Dupuytren's M72.0
  gingival K06.1
  palmar (fascial) M72.0
  plantar (fascial) M72.2
  pseudosarcomatous (proliferative)
    (subcutaneous) M72.4
  retroperitoneal D48.3
  specified NEC M72.8
Fibromyalgia M79.7
Fibromyoma —see also Neoplasm, connective
    tissue, benign
  uterus (corpus) —see also Leiomyoma, uterus
    in pregnancy or childbirth —see Fibroid, in
      pregnancy or childbirth
    causing obstructed labor O65.5
Fibromyositis M79.7
Fibromyxolipoma D17.9
Fibromyxoma —see Neoplasm, connective
    tissue, benign
Fibromyxosarcoma —see Neoplasm, connective
    tissue, malignant
Fibro-odontoma, ameloblastic —see Cyst,
    calcifying odontogenic
Fibro-osteoma —see Neoplasm, bone, benign
Fibroplasia, retrolental H35.17
Fibropurulent —see condition
Fibrosarcoma —see also Neoplasm, connective
    tissue, malignant
  ameloblastic C41.1
    upper jaw (bone) C41.0
  congenital —see Neoplasm, connective tissue,
    malignant
  fascial —see Neoplasm, connective tissue,
    malignant
  infantile —see Neoplasm, connective tissue,
    malignant
  odontogenic C41.1
    upper jaw (bone) C41.0
  periosteal —see Neoplasm, bone, malignant
Fibrosclerosis
  breast N60.3-●
  multifocal M35.5
  penis (corpora cavernosa) N48.6
Fibrosis, fibrotic
  adrenal (gland) E27.8
  amnion O41.8X-●
  anal papillae K62.89
  arteriocapillary —see Arteriosclerosis
  bladder N32.89
    interstitial —see Cystitis, chronic,
      interstitial
    localized submucosal —see Cystitis,
      chronic, interstitial
    panmural —see Cystitis, chronic, interstitial
  breast —see Fibrosclerosis, breast
  capillary —see also Arteriosclerosis I70.90
    lung (chronic) —see Fibrosis, lung
  cardiac —see Myocarditis
  cervix N88.8

Fibrosis, fibrotic (Continued)
  chorion O41.8X-●
  corpus cavernosum (sclerosing) N48.6
  cystic (of pancreas) E84.9
    with
      distal intestinal obstruction syndrome
        E84.19
      fecal impaction E84.19
      intestinal manifestations NEC E84.19
      pulmonary manifestations E84.0
      specified manifestations NEC E84.8
  due to device, implant or graft —see also
      Complications, by site and type,
      specified NEC T85.828
    arterial graft NEC T82.828
    breast (implant) T85.828
    catheter NEC T85.828
      dialysis (renal) T82.828
        intraperitoneal T85.828
      infusion NEC T82.828
        spinal (epidural) (subdural)
          T85.828
      urinary (indwelling) T83.82
    electronic (electrode) (pulse generator)
        (stimulator)
      bone T84.82
      cardiac T82.827
      nervous system (brain) (peripheral
        nerve) (spinal) T85.820
      urinary T83.82
    fixation, internal (orthopedic) NEC T84.82
    gastrointestinal (bile duct) (esophagus)
      T85.828
    genital NEC T83.82
    heart NEC T82.827
    joint prosthesis T84.82
    ocular (corneal graft) (orbital implant)
      NEC T85.828
    orthopedic NEC T84.82
    specified NEC T85.828
    urinary NEC T83.82
    vascular NEC T82.828
    ventricular intracranial shunt T85.820
  ejaculatory duct N50.89
  endocardium —see Endocarditis
  endomyocardial (tropical) I42.3
  epididymis N50.89
  eye muscle —see Strabismus, mechanical
  heart —see Myocarditis
  hepatic —see Fibrosis, liver
  hepatolienal (portal hypertension) K76.6
  hepatosplenic (portal hypertension) K76.6
  infrapatellar fat pad M79.4
  intrascrotal N50.89
  kidney N26.9
  liver K74.00
    with sclerosis K74.2
    advanced K74.02
    alcoholic K70.2
    early K74.01
    stage
      F1 or F2 K74.01
      F3 K74.02
  lung (atrophic) (chronic) (confluent)
      (massive) (perialveolar) (peribronchial)
      J84.10
    with
      anthracosilicosis J60
      anthracosis J60
      asbestosis J61
      bagassosis J67.1
      bauxite J63.1
      berylliosis J63.2
      byssinosis J66.0
      calcicosis J62.8
      chalicosis J62.8
      dust reticulation J64
      farmer's lung J67.0
      ganister disease J62.8
      graphite J63.3
      pneumoconiosis NOS J64

Fibrosis, fibrotic (Continued)
 lung (Continued)
  with (Continued)
   siderosis J63.4
   silicosis J62.8
  capillary J84.10
  congenital P27.8
  diffuse (idiopathic) J84.10
   chemicals, gases, fumes or vapors
    (inhalation) J68.4
   interstitial J84.10
    acute J84.114
   talc J62.0
  following radiation J70.1
  idiopathic J84.112
  postinflammatory J84.10
  silicotic J62.8
  tuberculous —see Tuberculosis, pulmonary
 lymphatic gland I89.8
 median bar —see Hyperplasia, prostate
 mediastinum (idiopathic) J98.59
 meninges G96.198
 myocardium, myocardial —see Myocarditis
 ovary N83.8
 oviduct N83.8
 pancreas K86.89
 penis NEC N48.6
 pericardium I31.0
 perineum, in pregnancy or childbirth O34.7-●
  causing obstructed labor O65.5
 pleura J94.1
 popliteal fat pad M79.4
 prostate (chronic) —see Hyperplasia, prostate
 pulmonary —see also Fibrosis, lung J84.10
  congenital P27.8
  idiopathic J84.112
 rectal sphincter K62.89
 retroperitoneal, idiopathic (with ureteral
   obstruction) N13.5
  with infection N13.6
 sclerosing mesenteric (idiopathic) K65.4
 scrotum N50.89
 seminal vesicle N50.89
 senile R54
 skin L90.5
 spermatic cord N50.89
 spleen D73.89
  in schistosomiasis (bilharziasis) B65.9 [D77]
 subepidermal nodular —see Neoplasm, skin,
   benign
 submucous (oral) (tongue) K13.5
 testis N44.8
  chronic, due to syphilis A52.76
 thymus (gland) E32.8
 tongue, submucous K13.5
 tunica vaginalis N50.89
 uterus (non-neoplastic) N85.8
 vagina N89.8
 valve, heart —see Endocarditis
 vas deferens N50.89
 vein I87.8
Fibrositis (periarticular) M79.7
 nodular, chronic (Jaccoud's) (rheumatoid) —
  see Arthropathy, postrheumatic, chronic
Fibrothorax J94.1
Fibrotic —see Fibrosis
Fibrous —see condition
Fibroxanthoma —see also Neoplasm, connective
  tissue, benign
 atypical —see Neoplasm, connective tissue,
   uncertain behavior
 malignant —see Neoplasm, connective tissue,
   malignant
Fibroxanthosarcoma —see Neoplasm,
  connective tissue, malignant
Fiedler's
 disease (icterohemorrhagic leptospirosis) A27.0
 myocarditis (acute) I40.1
Fifth disease B08.3
 venereal A55
Filaria, filarial, filariasis —see Infestation, filarial

Filatov's disease —see Mononucleosis, infectious
File-cutter's disease —see Poisoning, lead
Filling defect
 biliary tract R93.2
 bladder R93.41
 duodenum R93.3
 gallbladder R93.2
 gastrointestinal tract R93.3
 intestine R93.3
 kidney R93.42-●
 stomach R93.3
 ureter R93.41
 urinary organs, specified NEC R93.49
Fimbrial cyst Q50.4
Financial problem affecting care NOS Z59.9
⇒bankruptcy Z59.89
⇒foreclosure on loan Z59.89
▶home loan Z59.81-●
Findings, abnormal, inconclusive, without
  diagnosis —see also Abnormal
 17-ketosteroids, elevated R82.5
 acetonuria R82.4
 alcohol in blood R78.0
 anisocytosis R71.8
 antenatal screening of mother O28.9
  biochemical O28.1
  chromosomal O28.5
  cytological O28.2
  genetic O28.5
  hematological O28.0
  radiological O28.4
  specified NEC O28.8
  ultrasonic O28.3
 antibody titer, elevated R76.0
 anticardiolipin antibody R76.0
 antiphosphatidylglycerol antibody R76.0
 antiphosphatidylinositol antibody R76.0
 antiphosphatidylserine antibody R76.0
 antiphospholipid antibody R76.0
 bacteriuria R82.71
 bicarbonate E87.8
 bile in urine R82.2
 blood sugar R73.09
  high R73.9
  low (transient) E16.2
 body fluid or substance, specified NEC
   R88.8
 casts, urine R82.998
 catecholamines R82.5
 cells, urine R82.998
 chloride E87.8
 cholesterol E78.9
  high E78.00
   with high triglycerides E78.2
 chyluria R82.0
 cloudy
  dialysis effluent R88.0
  urine R82.90
 creatinine clearance R94.4
 crystals, urine R82.998
 culture
  blood R78.81
  positive —see Positive, culture
 echocardiogram R93.1
 electrolyte level, urinary R82.998
 function study NEC R94.8
  bladder R94.8
  endocrine NEC R94.7
   thyroid R94.6
  kidney R94.4
  liver R94.5
  pancreas R94.8
  placenta R94.8
  pulmonary R94.2
  spleen R94.8
 gallbladder, nonvisualization R93.2
 glucose (tolerance test) (non-fasting) R73.09
 glycosuria R81
 heart
  shadow R93.1
  sounds R01.2
 hematinuria R82.3

Findings, abnormal, inconclusive, without
  diagnosis (Continued)
 hematocrit drop (precipitous) R71.0
 hemoglobinuria R82.3
 human papillomavirus (HPV) DNA test
   positive
  cervix
   high risk R87.810
   low risk R87.820
  vagina
   high risk R87.811
   low risk R87.821
 in blood (of substance not normally found in
   blood) R78.9
  addictive drug NEC R78.4
  alcohol (excessive level) R78.0
  cocaine R78.2
  hallucinogen R78.3
  heavy metals (abnormal level) R78.79
  lead R78.71
  lithium (abnormal level) R78.89
  opiate drug R78.1
  psychotropic drug R78.5
  specified substance NEC R78.89
  steroid agent R78.6
 indoleacetic acid, elevated R82.5
 ketonuria R82.4
 lactic acid dehydrogenase (LDH) R74.02
⇒liver function test (see also Elevated, liver
   function, test) R79.89
 mammogram NEC R92.8
  calcification (calculus) R92.1
  inconclusive result (due to dense breasts)
    R92.2
  microcalcification R92.0
 mediastinal shift R93.89
 melanin, urine R82.998
 myoglobinuria R82.1
⇒neonatal screening —see Abnormal, neonatal
   screening
▶newborn screens, state mandated —see
   Abnormal, neonatal screening
 nonvisualization of gallbladder R93.2
 odor of urine NOS R82.90
 Papanicolaou cervix R87.619
  non-atypical endometrial cells R87.618
 pneumoencephalogram R93.0
 poikilocytosis R71.8
 potassium (deficiency) E87.6
  excess E87.5
 PPD R76.11
 radiologic (X-ray) R93.89
  abdomen R93.5
  biliary tract R93.2
  breast R92.8
  gastrointestinal tract R93.3
  genitourinary organs R93.89
  head R93.0
  inconclusive due to excess body fat of
    patient R93.9
  intrathoracic organs NEC R93.1
  musculoskeletal
   limbs R93.6
   other than limb R93.7
  placenta R93.89
  retroperitoneum R93.5
  skin R93.89
  skull R93.0
  subcutaneous tissue R93.89
  testis R93.81-●
 red blood cell (count) (morphology) (sickling)
   (volume) R71.8
 scan NEC R94.8
  bladder R94.8
  bone R94.8
  kidney R94.4
  liver R93.2
  lung R94.2
  pancreas R94.8
  placental R94.8
  spleen R94.8
  thyroid R94.6
 sedimentation rate, elevated R70.0

▶ New   ⇒ Revised   ~~deleted~~ Deleted   ● Use Additional Character(s)

Findings, abnormal, inconclusive, without diagnosis (Continued)
  SGOT R74.01
  SGPT R74.01
  sodium (deficiency) E87.1
    excess E87.0
  specified body fluid NEC R88.8
  stress test R94.39
  thyroid (function) (metabolic rate) (scan) (uptake) R94.6
  transaminase (level) R74.01
  triglycerides E78.9
    high E78.1
      with high cholesterol E78.2
  tuberculin skin test (without active tuberculosis) R76.11
  urine R82.90
    acetone R82.4
    bacteria R82.71
    bile R82.2
    casts or cells R82.998
    chyle R82.0
    culture positive R82.79
    glucose R81
    hemoglobin R82.3
    ketone R82.4
    sugar R81
  vanillylmandelic acid (VMA), elevated R82.5
  vectorcardiogram (VCG) R94.39
  ventriculogram R93.0
  white blood cell (count) (differential) (morphology) D72.9
  xerography R92.8
Finger —see condition
Fire, Saint Anthony's —see Erysipelas
Fire-setting
  pathological (compulsive) F63.1
Fish hook stomach K31.89
Fishmeal-worker's lung J67.8
Fissure, fissured
  anus, anal K60.2
    acute K60.0
    chronic K60.1
    congenital Q43.8
  ear, lobule, congenital Q17.8
  epiglottis (congenital) Q31.8
  larynx J38.7
    congenital Q31.8
  lip K13.0
    congenital —see Cleft, lip
  nipple N64.0
    associated with
      lactation O92.13
      pregnancy O92.11-●
      puerperium O92.12
  nose Q30.2
  palate (congenital) —see Cleft, palate
  skin R23.4
  spine (congenital) —see also Spina bifida
    with hydrocephalus —see Spina bifida, by site, with hydrocephalus
  tongue (acquired) K14.5
    congenital Q38.3
Fistula (cutaneous) L98.8
  abdomen (wall) K63.2
    bladder N32.2
    intestine NEC K63.2
    ureter N28.89
    uterus N82.5
  abdominorectal K63.2
  abdominosigmoidal K63.2
  abdominothoracic J86.0
  abdominouterine N82.5
    congenital Q51.7
  abdominovesical N32.2
  accessory sinuses —see Sinusitis
  actinomycotic —see Actinomycosis
  alveolar antrum —see Sinusitis, maxillary
  alveolar process K04.6
  anorectal K60.5
  antrobuccal —see Sinusitis, maxillary
  antrum —see Sinusitis, maxillary

Fistula (Continued)
  anus, anal (recurrent) (infectional) K60.3
    congenital Q43.6
      with absence, atresia and stenosis Q42.2
    tuberculous A18.32
  aorta-duodenal I77.2
  appendix, appendicular K38.3
  arteriovenous (acquired) (nonruptured) I77.0
    brain I67.1
      congenital Q28.2
        ruptured —see Fistula, arteriovenous, brain, ruptured
      ruptured I60.8
        intracerebral I61.8
        intraparenchymal I61.8
        intraventricular I61.5
        subarachnoid I60.8
    cerebral —see Fistula, arteriovenous, brain
    congenital (peripheral) —see also Malformation, arteriovenous
      brain Q28.2
        ruptured —see Fistula, arteriovenous, brain, ruptured
      coronary Q24.5
      pulmonary Q25.72
    coronary I25.41
      congenital Q24.5
    pulmonary I28.0
      congenital Q25.72
    surgically created (for dialysis) Z99.2
      complication —see Complication, arteriovenous, fistula, surgically created
    traumatic —see Injury, blood vessel
  artery I77.2
  aural (mastoid) —see Mastoiditis, chronic
  auricle —see also Disorder, pinna, specified type NEC
    congenital Q18.1
  Bartholin's gland N82.8
  bile duct (common) (hepatic) K83.3
    with calculus, stones —see also Calculus, bile duct K83.3
  biliary (tract) —see Fistula, bile duct
  bladder (sphincter) NEC —see also Fistula, vesico- N32.2
    into seminal vesicle N32.2
  bone —see also Disorder, bone, specified type NEC
    with osteomyelitis, chronic —see Osteomyelitis, chronic, with draining sinus
  brain G93.89
    arteriovenous (acquired) (see Fistula, arteriovenous, brain) I67.1
    congenital Q28.2
  branchial (cleft) Q18.0
  branchiogenous Q18.0
  breast N61.0
    puerperal, postpartum or gestational, due to mastitis (purulent) —see Mastitis, obstetric, purulent
  bronchial J86.0
  bronchocutaneous, bronchomediastinal, bronchopleural, bronchopleuromediastinal (infective) J86.0
    tuberculous NEC A15.5
  bronchoesophageal J86.0
    congenital Q39.2
      with atresia of esophagus Q39.1
  bronchovisceral J86.0
  buccal cavity (infective) K12.2
  cecosigmoidal K63.2
  cecum K63.2
  cerebrospinal (fluid) G96.08
  cervical, lateral Q18.1
  cervicoaural Q18.1
  cervicosigmoidal N82.4
  cervicovesical N82.1
  cervix N82.8
  chest (wall) J86.0

Fistula (Continued)
  cholecystenteric —see Fistula, gallbladder
  cholecystocolic —see Fistula, gallbladder
  cholecystocolonic —see Fistula, gallbladder
  cholecystoduodenal —see Fistula, gallbladder
  cholecystogastric —see Fistula, gallbladder
  cholecystointestinal —see Fistula, gallbladder
  choledochoduodenal —see Fistula, bile duct
  cholocolic K82.3
  coccyx —see Sinus, pilonidal
  colon K63.2
  colostomy K94.09
  colovesical N32.1
  common duct —see Fistula, bile duct
  congenital, site not listed —see Anomaly, by site
  coronary, arteriovenous I25.41
    congenital Q24.5
  costal region J86.0
  cul-de-sac, Douglas' N82.8
  cystic duct —see also Fistula, gallbladder
    congenital Q44.5
  dental K04.6
  diaphragm J86.0
  duodenum K31.6
  ear (external) (canal) —see Disorder, ear, external, specified type NEC
  enterocolic K63.2
  enterocutaneous K63.2
  enterouterine N82.4
    congenital Q51.7
  enterovaginal N82.4
    congenital Q52.2
    large intestine N82.3
    small intestine N82.2
  enterovesical N32.1
  epididymis N50.89
    tuberculous A18.15
  esophagobronchial J86.0
    congenital Q39.2
      with atresia of esophagus Q39.1
▶ esophagocutaneous K22.89
  esophagopleural-cutaneous J86.0
  esophagotracheal J86.0
    congenital Q39.2
      with atresia of esophagus Q39.1
▶ esophagus K22.89
    congenital Q39.2
      with atresia of esophagus Q39.1
  ethmoid —see Sinusitis, ethmoidal
  eyeball (cornea) (sclera) —see Disorder, globe, hypotony
  eyelid H01.8
  fallopian tube, external N82.5
  fecal K63.2
    congenital Q43.6
  from periapical abscess K04.6
  frontal sinus —see Sinusitis, frontal
  gallbladder K82.3
    with calculus, cholelithiasis, stones —see Calculus, gallbladder
  gastric K31.6
  gastrocolic K31.6
    congenital Q40.2
    tuberculous A18.32
  gastroenterocolic K31.6
  gastroesophageal K31.6
  gastrojejunal K31.6
  gastrojejunocolic K31.6
  genital tract (female) N82.9
    specified NEC N82.8
    to intestine NEC N82.4
    to skin N82.5
  hepatic artery-portal vein, congenital Q26.6
  hepatopleural J86.0
  hepatopulmonary J86.0
  ileorectal or ileosigmoidal K63.2
  ileovaginal N82.2
  ileovesical N32.1
  ileum K63.2
  in ano K60.3
    tuberculous A18.32

Fistula *(Continued)*
- inner ear (labyrinth) —*see* subcategory H83.1
- intestine NEC K63.2
- intestinocolonic (abdominal) K63.2
- intestinoureteral N28.89
- intestinouterine N82.4
- intestinovaginal N82.4
  - large intestine N82.3
  - small intestine N82.2
- intestinovesical N32.1
- ischiorectal (fossa) K61.39
- jejunum K63.2
- joint M25.10
  - ankle M25.17-•
  - elbow M25.12-•
  - foot joint M25.17-•
  - hand joint M25.14-•
  - hip M25.15-•
  - knee M25.16-•
  - shoulder M25.11-•
  - specified joint NEC M25.18
  - tuberculous —*see* Tuberculosis, joint
  - vertebrae M25.18
  - wrist M25.13-•
- kidney N28.89
- labium (majus) (minus) N82.8
- labyrinth —*see* subcategory H83.1
- lacrimal (gland) (sac) H04.61-•
- lacrimonasal duct —*see* Fistula, lacrimal
- laryngotracheal, congenital Q34.8
- larynx J38.7
- lip K13.0
  - congenital Q38.0
- lumbar, tuberculous A18.01
- lung J86.0
- lymphatic I89.8
- mammary (gland) N61.0
- mastoid (process) (region) —*see* Mastoiditis, chronic
- maxillary J32.0
- medial, face and neck Q18.8
- mediastinal J86.0
- mediastinobronchial J86.0
- mediastinocutaneous J86.0
- middle ear —*see* subcategory H74.8
- mouth K12.2
- nasal J34.89
  - sinus —*see* Sinusitis
- nasopharynx J39.2
- nipple N64.0
- nose J34.89
- oral (cutaneous) K12.2
  - maxillary J32.0
  - nasal (with cleft palate) —*see* Cleft, palate
- orbit, orbital —*see* Disorder, orbit, specified type NEC
- oroantral J32.0
- oviduct, external N82.5
- palate (hard) M27.8
- pancreatic K86.89
- pancreaticoduodenal K86.89
- parotid (gland) K11.4
  - region K12.2
- penis N48.89
- perianal K60.3
- pericardium (pleura) (sac) —*see* Pericarditis
- pericecal K63.2
- perineorectal K60.4 perineosigmoidal K63.2
- perineosigmoidal K63.2
- perineum, perineal (with urethral involvement) NEC N36.0
  - tuberculous A18.13
  - ureter N28.89
- perirectal K60.4
  - tuberculous A18.32
- peritoneum K65.9
- pharyngoesophageal J39.2
- pharynx J39.2
  - branchial cleft (congenital) Q18.0
- pilonidal (infected) (rectum) —*see* Sinus, pilonidal

Fistula *(Continued)*
- pleura, pleural, pleurocutaneous, pleuroperitoneal J86.0
  - tuberculous NEC A15.6
- pleuropericardial I31.8
- portal vein-hepatic artery, congenital Q26.6
- postauricular H70.81-•
- postoperative, persistent T81.83
  - specified site —*see* Fistula, by site
- preauricular (congenital) Q18.1
- prostate N42.89
- pulmonary J86.0
  - arteriovenous I28.0
    - congenital Q25.72
  - tuberculous —*see* Tuberculosis, pulmonary
- pulmonoperitoneal J86.0
- rectolabial N82.4
- rectosigmoid (intercommunicating) K63.2
- rectoureteral N28.89
- rectourethral N36.0
  - congenital Q64.73
- rectouterine N82.4
  - congenital Q51.7
- rectovaginal N82.3
  - congenital Q52.2
  - tuberculous A18.18
- rectovesical N32.1
  - congenital Q64.79
- rectovesicovaginal N82.3
- rectovulval N82.4
  - congenital Q52.79
- rectum (to skin) K60.4
  - congenital Q43.6
    - with absence, atresia and stenosis Q42.0
  - tuberculous A18.32
- renal N28.89
- retroauricular —*see* Fistula, postauricular
- salivary duct or gland (any) K11.4
  - congenital Q38.4
- scrotum (urinary) N50.89
  - tuberculous A18.15
- semicircular canals —*see* subcategory H83.1
- sigmoid K63.2
  - to bladder N32.1
- sinus —*see* Sinusitis
- skin L98.8
  - to genital tract (female) N82.5
- splenocolic D73.89
- stercoral K63.2
- stomach K31.6
- sublingual gland K11.4
- submandibular gland K11.4
- submaxillary (gland) K11.4
  - region K12.2
- thoracic J86.0
  - duct I89.8
- thoracoabdominal J86.0
- thoracogastric J86.0
- thoracointestinal J86.0
- thorax J86.0
- thyroglossal duct Q89.2
- thyroid E07.89
- trachea, congenital (external) (internal) Q32.1
- tracheoesophageal J86.0
  - congenital Q39.2
    - with atresia of esophagus Q39.1
  - following tracheostomy J95.04
- traumatic arteriovenous —*see* Injury, blood vessel, by site
- tuberculous - code by site under Tuberculosis
- typhoid A01.09
- umbilicourinary Q64.8
- urachus, congenital Q64.4
- ureter (persistent) N28.89
- ureteroabdominal N28.89
- ureterorectal N28.89
- ureterosigmoido-abdominal N28.89
- ureterovaginal N82.1
- ureterovesical N32.2
- urethra N36.0
  - congenital Q64.79
  - tuberculous A18.13

Fistula *(Continued)*
- urethroperineal N36.0
- urethroperineovesical N32.2
- urethrorectal N36.0
  - congenital Q64.73
- urethroscrotal N50.89
- urethrovaginal N82.1
- urethrovesical N32.2
- urinary (tract) (persistent) (recurrent) N36.0
- uteroabdominal N82.5
  - congenital Q51.7
- uteroenteric, uterointestinal N82.4
  - congenital Q51.7
- uterorectal N82.4
  - congenital Q51.7
- uteroureteric N82.1
- uterourethral Q51.7
- uterovaginal N82.8
- uterovesical N82.1
  - congenital Q51.7
- uterus N82.8
- vagina (postpartal) (wall) N82.8
- vaginocutaneous (postpartal) N82.5
- vaginointestinal NEC N82.4
  - large intestine N82.3
  - small intestine N82.2
- vaginoperineal N82.5
- vasocutaneous, congenital Q55.7
- vesical NEC N32.2
- vesicoabdominal N32.2
- vesicocervicovaginal N82.1
- vesicocolic N32.1
- vesicocutaneous N32.2
- vesicoenteric N32.1
- vesicointestinal N32.1
- vesicometrorectal N82.4
- vesicoperineal N32.2
- vesicorectal N32.1
  - congenital Q64.79
- vesicosigmoidal N32.1
- vesicosigmoidovaginal N82.3
- vesicoureteral N32.2
- vesicoureterovaginal N82.1
- vesicourethral N32.2
- vesicourethrorectal N32.1
- vesicouterine N82.1
  - congenital Q51.7
- vesicovaginal N82.0
- vulvorectal N82.4
  - congenital Q52.79

Fit R56.9
- epileptic —*see* Epilepsy
- fainting R55
- hysterical F44.5
- newborn P90

Fitting (and adjustment) (of)
- artificial
  - arm —*see* Admission, adjustment, artificial, arm
  - breast Z44.3
  - eye Z44.2
  - leg —*see* Admission, adjustment, artificial, leg
- automatic implantable cardiac defibrillator (with synchronous cardiac pacemaker) Z45.02
- brain neuropacemaker Z46.2
  - implanted Z45.42
- cardiac defibrillator —*see* Fitting (and adjustment) (of), automatic implantable cardiac defibrillator
- catheter, non-vascular Z46.82
- colostomy belt Z46.89
- contact lenses Z46.0
- CRT-D (resynchronization therapy defibrillator) Z45.02
- CRT-P (cardiac resynchronization therapy pacemaker) Z45.018
- pulse generator Z45.010
- cystostomy device Z46.6

▶ New   ⇒ Revised   ~~deleted~~ Deleted   • Use Additional Character(s)

Fitting (Continued)
  defibrillator, cardiac —*see* Fitting (and
      adjustment) (of), automatic implantable
      cardiac defibrillator
  dentures Z46.3
  device NOS Z46.9
    abdominal Z46.89
    gastrointestinal NEC Z46.59
    implanted NEC Z45.89
    nervous system Z46.2
      implanted —*see* Admission, adjustment,
          device, implanted, nervous system
    orthodontic Z46.4
    orthoptic Z46.0
    orthotic Z46.89
    prosthetic (external) Z44.9
      breast Z44.3
      dental Z46.3
      eye Z44.2
      specified NEC Z44.8
    specified NEC Z46.89
    substitution
      auditory Z46.2
        implanted —*see* Admission,
            adjustment, device, implanted,
            hearing device
      nervous system Z46.2
        implanted —*see* Admission,
            adjustment, device, implanted,
            nervous system
      visual Z46.2
        implanted Z45.31
    urinary Z46.6
  gastric lap band Z46.51
  gastrointestinal appliance NEC Z46.59
  glasses (reading) Z46.0
  hearing aid Z46.1
  ileostomy device Z46.89
  insulin pump Z46.81
  intestinal appliance NEC Z46.89
  myringotomy device (stent) (tube) Z45.82
  neuropacemaker Z46.2
    implanted Z45.42
  non-vascular catheter Z46.82
  orthodontic device Z46.4
  orthopedic device (brace) (cast) (corset)
      (shoes) Z46.89
  pacemaker (cardiac) (cardiac
      resynchronization therapy (CRT-P))
      Z45.018
    nervous system (brain) (peripheral nerve)
        (spinal cord) Z46.2
      implanted Z45.42
    pulse generator Z45.010
  portacath (port-a-cath) Z45.2
  prosthesis (external) Z44.9
    arm —*see* Admission, adjustment, artificial,
        arm
    breast Z44.3
    dental Z46.3
    eye Z44.2
    leg —*see* Admission, adjustment, artificial,
        leg
    specified NEC Z44.8
  spectacles Z46.0
  wheelchair Z46.89
Fitzhugh-Curtis syndrome
  due to
    Chlamydia trachomatis A74.81
    Neisseria gonorrhorea (gonococcal
        peritonitis) A54.85
Fitz's syndrome (acute hemorrhagic
    pancreatitis) —*see also* Pancreatitis,
    acute K85.80
Fixation
  joint —*see* Ankylosis
  larynx J38.7
  stapes —*see* Ankylosis, ear ossicles
    deafness —*see* Deafness, conductive
  uterus (acquired) —*see* Malposition, uterus
  vocal cord J38.3

Flabby ridge K06.8
Flaccid —*see also* condition
  palate, congenital Q38.5
Flail
  chest S22.5-●
    newborn (birth injury) P13.8
  joint (paralytic) M25.20
    ankle M25.27-●
    elbow M25.22-●
    foot joint M25.27-●
    hand joint M25.24-●
    hip M25.25-●
    knee M25.26-●
    shoulder M25.21-●
    specified joint NEC M25.28
    wrist M25.23-●
Flajani's disease —*see* Hyperthyroidism, with,
    goiter (diffuse)
Flap, liver K71.3
Flashbacks (residual to hallucinogen use)
    F16.283
Flat
  chamber (eye) —*see* Disorder, globe,
      hypotony, flat anterior chamber
  chest, congenital Q67.8
  foot (acquired) (fixed type) (painful)
      (postural) —*see also* Deformity, limb,
      flat foot
    congenital (rigid) (spastic (everted))
        Q66.5-●
    rachitic sequelae (late effect) E64.3
  organ or site, congenital NEC —*see* Anomaly,
      by site
  pelvis M95.5
    with disproportion (fetopelvic) O33.0
      causing obstructed labor O65.0
    congenital Q74.2
Flatau-Schilder disease G37.0
Flatback syndrome M40.30
  lumbar region M40.36
  lumbosacral region M40.37
  thoracolumbar region M40.35
Flattening
  head, femur M89.8X5
  hip —*see* Coxa, plana
  lip (congenital) Q18.8
  nose (congenital) Q67.4
    acquired M95.0
Flatulence R14.3
  psychogenic F45.8
Flatus R14.3
  vaginalis N89.8
Flax-dresser's disease J66.1
Flea bite —*see* Injury, bite, by site, superficial,
    insect
Flecks, glaucomatous (subcapsular) —*see*
    Cataract, complicated
Fleischer (-Kayser) ring (cornea) H18.04-●
Fleshy mole O02.0
Flexibilitas cerea —*see* Catalepsy
Flexion
  amputation stump (surgical) T87.89
  cervix —*see* Malposition, uterus
  contracture, joint —*see* Contraction, joint
  deformity, joint —*see also* Deformity, limb,
      flexion M21.20
    hip, congenital Q65.89
  uterus —*see also* Malposition, uterus
    lateral —*see* Lateroversion, uterus
Flexner-Boyd dysentery A03.2
Flexner's dysentery A03.1
Flexure —*see* Flexion
Flint murmur (aortic insufficiency) I35.1
Floater, vitreous —*see* Opacity, vitreous
Floating
  cartilage (joint) —*see also* Loose, body, joint
    knee —*see* Derangement, knee, loose body
  gallbladder, congenital Q44.1
  kidney N28.89
    congenital Q63.8
  spleen D73.89

Flooding N92.0
Floor —*see* condition
Floppy
  baby syndrome (nonspecific) P94.2
  iris syndrome (intraoperative) (IFIS) H21.81
  nonrheumatic mitral valve syndrome I34.1
Flu —*see also* Influenza
  avian —*see also* Influenza, due to, identified
      novel influenza A virus J09.X2
  bird —*see also* Influenza, due to, identified
      novel influenza A virus J09.X2
  intestinal NEC A08.4
  swine (viruses that normally cause infections
      in pigs) —*see also* Influenza, due to,
      identified novel influenza A virus J09.X2
Fluctuating blood pressure I99.8
Fluid
  abdomen R18.8
  chest J94.8
  heart —*see* Failure, heart, congestive
  joint —*see* Effusion, joint
  loss (acute) E86.9
  lung —*see* Edema, lung
  overload E87.70
    specified NEC E87.79
  peritoneal cavity R18.8
  pleural cavity J94.8
  retention R60.9
Flukes NEC —*see also* Infestation, fluke
  blood NEC —*see* Schistosomiasis
  liver B66.3
Fluor (vaginalis) N89.8
  trichomonal or due to Trichomonas
      (vaginalis) A59.00
Fluorosis
  dental K00.3
  skeletal M85.10
    ankle M85.17-●
    foot M85.17-●
    forearm M85.13-●
    hand M85.14-●
    lower leg M85.16-●
    multiple site M85.19
    neck M85.18
    rib M85.18
    shoulder M85.11-●
    skull M85.18
    specified site NEC M85.18
    thigh M85.15-●
    toe M85.17-●
    upper arm M85.12-●
    vertebra M85.18
Flush syndrome E34.0
Flushing R23.2
  menopausal N95.1
Flutter
  atrial or auricular I48.92
    atypical I48.4
    type I I48.3
    type II I48.4
    typical I48.3
  heart I49.8
    atrial or auricular I48.92
      atypical I48.4
      type I I48.3
      type II I48.4
      typical I48.3
    ventricular I49.02
  ventricular I49.02
FNHTR (febrile nonhemolytic transfusion
    reaction) R50.84
Fochier's abscess - code by site under Abscess
Focus, Assmann's —*see* Tuberculosis,
    pulmonary
Fogo selvagem L10.3
Foix-Alajouanine syndrome G95.19
Fold, folds (anomalous) —*see also* Anomaly,
    by site
  Descemet's membrane —*see* Change, corneal
      membrane, Descemet's, fold
  epicanthic Q10.3
  heart Q24.8

Folie à deux F24
Follicle
 cervix (nabothian) (ruptured) N88.8
 graafian, ruptured, with hemorrhage N83.0-●
 nabothian N88.8
Follicular —see condition
Folliculitis (superficial) L73.9
 abscedens et suffodiens L66.3
 cyst N83.0-●
 decalvans L66.2
 deep —see Furuncle, by site
 gonococcal (acute) (chronic) A54.01
 keloid, keloidalis L73.0
 pustular L01.02
 ulerythematosa reticulata L66.4
Folliculome lipidique
 specified site —see Neoplasm, benign, by site
 unspecified site
  female D27.9
  male D29.20
Følling's disease E70.0
Follow-up —see Examination, follow-up
Fong's syndrome (hereditary osteo-
  onychodysplasia) Q87.2
Food
 allergy L27.2
 asphyxia (from aspiration or inhalation) —see
  Foreign body, by site
 choked on —see Foreign body, by site
 deprivation T73.0
  specified kind of food NEC E63.8
▶insecurity Z59.41
 intoxication —see Poisoning, food
 lack of T73.0
 poisoning —see Poisoning, food
 rejection NEC —see Disorder, eating
 strangulation or suffocation —see Foreign
  body, by site
 toxemia —see Poisoning, food
Foot —see condition
Foramen ovale (nonclosure) (patent)
  (persistent) Q21.1
Forbes' glycogen storage disease E74.03
Fordyce-Fox disease L75.2
Fordyce's disease (mouth) Q38.6
Forearm —see condition
▶Foreclosure on loan Z59.89
Foreign body
 with
  laceration —see Laceration, by site, with
   foreign body
  puncture wound —see Puncture, by site,
   with foreign body
 accidentally left following a procedure
   T81.509
  aspiration T81.506
   resulting in
    adhesions T81.516
    obstruction T81.526
    perforation T81.536
    specified complication NEC
     T81.596
  cardiac catheterization T81.505
   resulting in
    acute reaction T81.60
     aseptic peritonitis T81.61
     specified NEC T81.69
    adhesions T81.515
    obstruction T81.525
    perforation T81.535
    specified complication NEC
     T81.595
  causing
   acute reaction T81.60
    aseptic peritonitis T81.61
    specified complication NEC T81.69
   adhesions T81.519
   aseptic peritonitis T81.61
   obstruction T81.529
   perforation T81.539
   specified complication NEC T81.599

Foreign body (Continued)
 accidentally left following a procedure
   (Continued)
  endoscopy T81.504
   resulting in
    adhesions T81.514
    obstruction T81.524
    perforation T81.534
    specified complication NEC T81.594
  immunization T81.503
   resulting in
    adhesions T81.513
    obstruction T81.523
    perforation T81.533
    specified complication NEC T81.593
  infusion T81.501
   resulting in
    adhesions T81.511
    obstruction T81.521
    perforation T81.531
    specified complication NEC T81.591
  injection T81.503
   resulting in
    adhesions T81.513
    obstruction T81.523
    perforation T81.533
    specified complication NEC T81.593
  kidney dialysis T81.502
   resulting in
    adhesions T81.512
    obstruction T81.522
    perforation T81.532
    specified complication NEC T81.592
  packing removal T81.507
   resulting in
    acute reaction T81.60
     aseptic peritonitis T81.61
     specified NEC T81.69
    adhesions T81.517
    obstruction T81.527
    perforation T81.537
    specified complication NEC T81.597
  puncture T81.506
   resulting in
    adhesions T81.516
    obstruction T81.526
    perforation T81.536
    specified complication NEC T81.596
  specified procedure NEC T81.508
   resulting in
    acute reaction T81.60
     aseptic peritonitis T81.61
     specified NEC T81.69
    adhesions T81.518
    obstruction T81.528
    perforation T81.538
    specified complication NEC T81.598
  surgical operation T81.500
   resulting in
    acute reaction T81.60
     aseptic peritonitis T81.61
     specified NEC T81.69
    adhesions T81.510
    obstruction T81.520
    perforation T81.530
    specified complication NEC T81.590
  transfusion T81.501
   resulting in
    adhesions T81.511
    obstruction T81.521
    perforation T81.531
    specified complication NEC T81.591
 alimentary tract T18.9
  anus T18.5
  colon T18.4
  esophagus —see Foreign body, esophagus
  mouth T18.0
  multiple sites T18.8
  rectosigmoid (junction) T18.5
  rectum T18.5
  small intestine T18.3

Foreign body (Continued)
 alimentary tract (Continued)
  specified site NEC T18.8
  stomach T18.2
 anterior chamber (eye) S05.5-●
 auditory canal —see Foreign body, entering
   through orifice, ear
 bronchus T17.508
  causing
   asphyxiation T17.500
    food (bone) (seed) T17.520
    gastric contents (vomitus) T17.510
    specified type NEC T17.590
   injury NEC T17.508
    food (bone) (seed) T17.528
    gastric contents (vomitus) T17.518
    specified type NEC T17.598
 canthus —see Foreign body, conjunctival sac
 ciliary body (eye) S05.5-●
 conjunctival sac T15.1-●
 cornea T15.0-●
 entering through orifice
  accessory sinus T17.0
  alimentary canal T18.9
   multiple parts T18.8
   specified part NEC T18.8
  alveolar process T18.0
  antrum (Highmore's) T17.0
  anus T18.5
  appendix T18.4
  auditory canal —see Foreign body, entering
    through orifice, ear
  auricle —see Foreign body, entering
    through orifice, ear
  bladder T19.1
  bronchioles —see Foreign body, respiratory
    tract, specified site NEC
  bronchus (main) —see Foreign body,
    bronchus
  buccal cavity T18.0
  canthus (inner) —see Foreign body,
    conjunctival sac
  cecum T18.4
  cervix (canal) (uteri) T19.3
  colon T18.4
  conjunctival sac —see Foreign body,
    conjunctival sac
  cornea —see Foreign body, cornea
  digestive organ or tract NOS T18.9
   multiple parts T18.8
   specified part NEC T18.8
  duodenum T18.3
  ear (external) T16.-●
  esophagus —see Foreign body, esophagus
  eye (external) NOS T15.9-●
   conjunctival sac —see Foreign body,
     conjunctival sac
   cornea —see Foreign body, cornea
   specified part NEC T15.8-●
  eyeball —see also Foreign body, entering
    through orifice, eye, specified part
    NEC
   with penetrating wound —see Puncture,
     eyeball
  eyelid —see also Foreign body, conjunctival
    sac
   with
    laceration —see Laceration, eyelid,
      with foreign body
    puncture —see Puncture, eyelid, with
      foreign body
    superficial injury —see Foreign body,
      superficial, eyelid
  gastrointestinal tract T18.9
   multiple parts T18.8
   specified part NEC T18.8
  genitourinary tract T19.9
   multiple parts T19.8
   specified part NEC T19.8
  globe —see Foreign body, entering through
    orifice, eyeball

▶ New   ⟹ Revised   ~~deleted~~ Deleted   ● Use Additional Character(s)

Foreign body *(Continued)*
  entering through orifice *(Continued)*
    gum T18.0
    Highmore's antrum T17.0
    hypopharynx —*see* Foreign body, pharynx
    ileum T18.3
    intestine (small) T18.3
      large T18.4
    lacrimal apparatus (punctum) —*see*
      Foreign body, entering through orifice,
      eye, specified part NEC
    large intestine T18.4
    larynx —*see* Foreign body, larynx
    lung —*see* Foreign body, respiratory tract,
      specified site NEC
    maxillary sinus T17.0
    mouth T18.0
    nasal sinus T17.0
    nasopharynx —*see* Foreign body, pharynx
    nose (passage) T17.1
    nostril T17.1
    oral cavity T18.0
    palate T18.0
    penis T19.4
    pharynx —*see* Foreign body, pharynx
    piriform sinus —*see* Foreign body, pharynx
    rectosigmoid (junction) T18.5
    rectum T18.5
    respiratory tract —*see* Foreign body,
      respiratory tract
    sinus (accessory) (frontal) (maxillary)
      (nasal) T17.0
      piriform —*see* Foreign body, pharynx
    small intestine T18.3
    stomach T18.2
    suffocation by —*see* Foreign body, by site
    tear ducts or glands —*see* Foreign body,
      entering through orifice, eye, specified
      part NEC
    throat —*see* Foreign body, pharynx
    tongue T18.0
    tonsil, tonsillar (fossa) —*see* Foreign body,
      pharynx
    trachea —*see* Foreign body, trachea
    ureter T19.8
    urethra T19.0
    uterus (any part) T19.3
    vagina T19.2
    vulva T19.2
  esophagus T18.108
    causing
      injury NEC T18.108
        food (bone) (seed) T18.128
        gastric contents (vomitus) T18.118
        specified type NEC T18.198
      tracheal compression T18.100
        food (bone) (seed) T18.120
        gastric contents (vomitus) T18.110
        specified type NEC T18.190
  feeling of, in throat R09.89
  fragment —*see* Retained, foreign body
    fragments (type of)
  genitourinary tract T19.9
    bladder T19.1
    multiple parts T19.8
    penis T19.4
    specified site NEC T19.8
    urethra T19.0
    uterus T19.3
      IUD Z97.5
    vagina T19.2
      contraceptive device Z97.5
    vulva T19.2
  granuloma (old) (soft tissue) —*see also*
    Granuloma, foreign body
    skin L92.3
  in
    laceration —*see* Laceration, by site, with
      foreign body
    puncture wound —*see* Puncture, by site,
      with foreign body
    soft tissue (residual) M79.5

Foreign body *(Continued)*
  inadvertently left in operation wound —*see*
    Foreign body, accidentally left during a
    procedure
  ingestion, ingested NOS T18.9
  inhalation or inspiration —*see* Foreign body,
    by site
  internal organ, not entering through a natural
    orifice - code as specific injury with
    foreign body
  intraocular S05.5-●
    old, retained (nonmagnetic) H44.70-●
      anterior chamber H44.71-●
      ciliary body H44.72-●
      iris H44.72-●
      lens H44.73-●
      magnetic H44.60-●
        anterior chamber H44.61-●
        ciliary body H44.62-●
        iris H44.62-●
        lens H44.63-●
        posterior wall H44.64-●
        specified site NEC H44.69-●
        vitreous body H44.65-●
      posterior wall H44.74-●
      specified site NEC H44.79-●
      vitreous body H44.75-●
  iris —*see* Foreign body, intraocular
  lacrimal punctum —*see* Foreign body,
    entering through orifice, eye, specified
    part NEC
  larynx T17.308
    causing
      asphyxiation T17.300
        food (bone) (seed) T17.320
        gastric contents (vomitus) T17.310
        specified type NEC T17.390
      injury NEC T17.308
        food (bone) (seed) T17.328
        gastric contents (vomitus) T17.318
        specified type NEC T17.398
  lens —*see* Foreign body, intraocular
  ocular muscle S05.4-●
    old, retained —*see* Foreign body, orbit, old
  old or residual
    soft tissue (residual) M79.5
  operation wound, left accidentally —*see*
    Foreign body, accidentally left during a
    procedure
  orbit S05.4-●
    old, retained H05.5-●
  pharynx T17.208
    causing
      asphyxiation T17.200
        food (bone) (seed) T17.220
        gastric contents (vomitus)
          T17.210
        specified type NEC T17.290
      injury NEC T17.208
        food (bone) (seed) T17.228
        gastric contents (vomitus)
          T17.218
        specified type NEC T17.298
  respiratory tract T17.908
    bronchioles —*see* Foreign body, respiratory
      tract, specified site NEC
    bronchus —*see* Foreign body, bronchus
    causing
      asphyxiation T17.900
        food (bone) (seed) T17.920
        gastric contents (vomitus) T17.910
        specified type NEC T17.990
      injury NEC T17.908
        food (bone) (seed) T17.928
        gastric contents (vomitus) T17.918
        specified type NEC T17.998
    larynx —*see* Foreign body, larynx
    lung —*see* Foreign body, respiratory tract,
      specified site NEC
    multiple parts —*see* Foreign body,
      respiratory tract, specified site NEC

Foreign body *(Continued)*
  respiratory tract *(Continued)*
    nasal sinus T17.0
    nasopharynx —*see* Foreign body,
      pharynx
    nose T17.1
    nostril T17.1
    pharynx —*see* Foreign body, pharynx
    specified site NEC T17.808
      causing
        asphyxiation T17.800
          food (bone) (seed) T17.820
          gastric contents (vomitus) T17.810
          specified type NEC T17.890
        injury NEC T17.808
          food (bone) (seed) T17.828
          gastric contents (vomitus) T17.818
          specified type NEC T17.898
    throat —*see* Foreign body, pharynx
    trachea —*see* Foreign body, trachea
  retained (old) (nonmagnetic) (in)
    anterior chamber (eye) —*see* Foreign body,
      intraocular, old, retained, anterior
      chamber
      magnetic —*see* Foreign body, intraocular,
        old, retained, magnetic, anterior
        chamber
    ciliary body —*see* Foreign body,
      intraocular, old, retained, ciliary body
      magnetic —*see* Foreign body, intraocular,
        old, retained, magnetic, ciliary body
    eyelid H02.819
      left H02.816
        lower H02.815
        upper H02.814
      right H02.813
        lower H02.812
        upper H02.811
    fragments —*see* Retained, foreign body
      fragments (type of)
    globe —*see* Foreign body, intraocular, old,
      retained
      magnetic —*see* Foreign body, intraocular,
        old, retained, magnetic
    intraocular —*see* Foreign body, intraocular,
      old, retained
      magnetic —*see* Foreign body, intraocular,
        old, retained, magnetic
    iris —*see* Foreign body, intraocular, old,
      retained, iris
      magnetic —*see* Foreign body, intraocular,
        old, retained, magnetic, iris
    lens —*see* Foreign body, intraocular, old,
      retained, lens
      magnetic —*see* Foreign body, intraocular,
        old, retained, magnetic, lens
    muscle —*see* Foreign body, retained, soft
      tissue
    orbit —*see* Foreign body, orbit, old
    posterior wall of globe —*see* Foreign body,
      intraocular, old, retained, posterior
      wall
      magnetic —*see* Foreign body, intraocular,
        old, retained, magnetic, posterior
        wall
    retrobulbar —*see* Foreign body, orbit, old,
      retrobulbar
    soft tissue M79.5
    vitreous —*see* Foreign body, intraocular,
      old, retained, vitreous body
      magnetic —*see* Foreign body, intraocular,
        old, retained, magnetic, vitreous
        body
  retina S05.5-●
  superficial, without open wound
    abdomen, abdominal (wall) S30.851
    alveolar process S00.552
    ankle S90.55-●
    antecubital space —*see* Foreign body,
      superficial, forearm
    anus S30.857

Foreign body *(Continued)*
  superficial, without open wound *(Continued)*
    arm (upper) S40.85-●
    auditory canal —*see* Foreign body,
      superficial, ear
    auricle —*see* Foreign body, superficial, ear
    axilla —*see* Foreign body, superficial, arm
    back, lower S30.850
    breast S20.15-●
    brow S00.85
    buttock S30.850
    calf —*see* Foreign body, superficial, leg
    canthus —*see* Foreign body, superficial,
      eyelid
    cheek S00.85
      internal S00.552
    chest wall —*see* Foreign body, superficial,
      thorax
    chin S00.85
    clitoris S30.854
    costal region —*see* Foreign body,
      superficial, thorax
    digit(s)
      foot —*see* Foreign body, superficial, toe
      hand —*see* Foreign body, superficial,
        finger
    ear S00.45-●
    elbow S50.35-●
    epididymis S30.853
    epigastric region S30.851
    epiglottis S10.15
    esophagus, cervical S10.15
    eyebrow —*see* Foreign body, superficial,
      eyelid
    eyelid S00.25-●
    face S00.85
    finger(s) S60.459
      index S60.45-●
      little S60.45-●
      middle S60.45-●
      ring S60.45-●
    flank S30.851
    foot (except toe(s) alone) S90.85-●
      toe —*see* Foreign body, superficial, toe
    forearm S50.85-●
      elbow only —*see* Foreign body,
        superficial, elbow
    forehead S00.85
    genital organs, external
      female S30.856
      male S30.855
    groin S30.851
    gum S00.552
    hand S60.55-●
    head S00.95
      ear —*see* Foreign body, superficial, ear
      eyelid —*see* Foreign body, superficial,
        eyelid
      lip S00.551
      nose S00.35
      oral cavity S00.552
      scalp S00.05
      specified site NEC S00.85
    heel —*see* Foreign body, superficial, foot
    hip S70.25-●
    inguinal region S30.851
    interscapular region S20.459
    jaw S00.85
    knee S80.25-●
    labium (majus) (minus) S30.854
    larynx S10.15
    leg (lower) S80.85-●
      knee —*see* Foreign body, superficial, knee
      upper —*see* Foreign body, superficial,
        thigh
    lip S00.551
    lower back S30.850
    lumbar region S30.850
    malar region S00.85
    mammary —*see* Foreign body, superficial,
      breast

Foreign body *(Continued)*
  superficial, without open wound *(Continued)*
    mastoid region S00.85
    mouth S00.552
    nail
      finger —*see* Foreign body, superficial,
        finger
      toe —*see* Foreign body, superficial, toe
    nape S10.85
    nasal S00.35
    neck S10.95
      specified site NEC S10.85
      throat S10.15
    nose S00.35
    occipital region S00.05
    oral cavity S00.552
    orbital region —*see* Foreign body,
      superficial, eyelid
    palate S00.552
    palm —*see* Foreign body, superficial,
      hand
    parietal region S00.05
    pelvis S30.850
    penis S30.852
    perineum
      female S30.854
      male S30.850
    periocular area —*see* Foreign body,
      superficial, eyelid
    phalanges
      finger —*see* Foreign body, superficial,
        finger
      toe —*see* Foreign body, superficial, toe
    pharynx S10.15
    pinna —*see* Foreign body, superficial, ear
    popliteal space —*see* Foreign body,
      superficial, knee
    prepuce S30.852
    pubic region S30.850
    pudendum
      female S30.856
      male S30.855
    sacral region S30.850
    scalp S00.05
    scapular region —*see* Foreign body,
      superficial, shoulder
    scrotum S30.853
    shin —*see* Foreign body, superficial, leg
    shoulder S40.25-●
    sternal region S20.359
    submaxillary region S00.85
    submental region S00.85
    subungual
      finger(s) —*see* Foreign body, superficial,
        finger
      toe(s) —*see* Foreign body, superficial,
        toe
    supraclavicular fossa S10.85
    supraorbital S00.85
    temple S00.85
    temporal region S00.85
    testis S30.853
    thigh S70.35-●
    thorax, thoracic (wall) S20.95
      back S20.45-●
      front S20.35-●
    throat S10.15
    thumb S60.35-●
    toe(s) (lesser) S90.456
      great S90.45-●
    tongue S00.552
    trachea S10.15
    tunica vaginalis S30.853
    tympanum, tympanic membrane —*see*
      Foreign body, superficial, ear
    uvula S00.552
    vagina S30.854
    vocal cords S10.15
    vulva S30.854
    wrist S60.85-●
  swallowed T18.9

Foreign body *(Continued)*
  trachea T17.408
    causing
      asphyxiation T17.400
        food (bone) (seed) T17.420
        gastric contents (vomitus) T17.410
        specified type NEC T17.490
      injury NEC T17.408
        food (bone) (seed) T17.428
        gastric contents (vomitus) T17.418
        specified type NEC T17.498
  type of fragment —*see* Retained, foreign body
    fragments (type of)
  vitreous (humor) S05.5-●
Forestier's disease (rhizomelic
  pseudopolyarthritis) M35.3-●
  meaning ankylosing hyperostosis —*see*
    Hyperostosis, ankylosing
Formation
  hyalin in cornea —*see* Degeneration, cornea
  sequestrum in bone (due to infection) —*see*
    Osteomyelitis, chronic
  valve
    colon, congenital Q43.8
    ureter (congenital) Q62.39
Formication R20.2
Fort Bragg fever A27.89
Fossa —*see also* condition
  pyriform —*see* condition
Foster-Kennedy syndrome H47.14-●
Fothergill's
  disease (trigeminal neuralgia) —*see also*
    Neuralgia, trigeminal
  scarlatina anginosa A38.9
Foul breath R19.6
Foundling Z76.1
Fournier disease or gangrene N49.3
  female N76.89
Fourth
  cranial nerve —*see* condition
  molar K00.1
Foville's (peduncular) disease or syndrome G46.3
Fox (-Fordyce) disease (apocrine miliaria) L75.2
FPIES (food protein-induced enterocolitis
  syndrome) K52.21
Fracture, burst —*see* Fracture, traumatic, by site
Fracture, chronic —*see* Fracture, pathological,
  by site
Fracture, insufficiency —*see* Fracture,
  pathological, by site
Fracture, nontraumatic, NEC
  atypical
    femur M84.750-●
      complete
        oblique M84.759
          left side M84.758
          right side M84.757
        transverse M84.756
          left side M84.755
          right side M84.754
      incomplete M84.753
        left side M84.752
        right side M84.751
Fracture, pathological (pathologic) —*see also*
  Fracture, traumatic M84.40
  ankle M84.47-●
  carpus M84.44-●
  clavicle M84.41-●
  compression (not due to trauma) —*see also*
    Collapse, vertebra M48.50-●
  dental implant M27.63
  dental restorative material K08.539
    with loss of material K08.531
    without loss of material K08.530
  due to
    neoplastic disease NEC —*see also*
      Neoplasm M84.50
      ankle M84.57-●
      carpus M84.54-●
      clavicle M84.51-●
      femur M84.55-●

▶ New   ⇒ Revised   ~~deleted~~ Deleted   ● Use Additional Character(s)

Fracture, pathological *(Continued)*
  due to *(Continued)*
    neoplastic disease NEC *(Continued)*
      fibula M84.56-●
      finger M84.54-●
      hip M84.559
      humerus M84.52-●
      ilium M84.550
      ischium M84.550
      metacarpus M84.54-●
      metatarsus M84.57-●
      neck M84.58
      pelvis M84.550
      radius M84.53-●
      rib M84.58
      scapula M84.51-●
      skull M84.58
      specified site NEC M84.58
      tarsus M84.57-●
      tibia M84.56-●
      toe M84.57-●
      ulna M84.53-●
      vertebra M84.58
    osteoporosis M80.00
      disuse —*see* Osteoporosis, specified type NEC, with pathological fracture
      drug-induced —*see* Osteoporosis, drug induced, with pathological fracture
      idiopathic —*see* Osteoporosis, specified type NEC, with pathological fracture
      postmenopausal —*see* Osteoporosis, postmenopausal, with pathological fracture
      postoophorectomy —*see* Osteoporosis, postoophorectomy, with pathological fracture
      postsurgical malabsorption —*see* Osteoporosis, specified type NEC, with pathological fracture
      specified cause NEC —*see* Osteoporosis, specified type NEC, with pathological fracture
    specified disease NEC M84.60
      ankle M84.67-●
      carpus M84.64-●
      clavicle M84.61-●
      femur M84.65-●
      fibula M84.66-●
      finger M84.64-●
      hip M84.65-●
      humerus M84.62-●
      ilium M84.650
      ischium M84.650
      metacarpus M84.64-●
      metatarsus M84.67-●
      neck M84.68
      radius M84.63-●
      rib M84.68
      scapula M84.61-●
      skull M84.68
      tarsus M84.67-●
      tibia M84.66-●
      toe M84.67-●
      ulna M84.63-●
      vertebra M84.68
  femur M84.45-●
  fibula M84.46-●
  finger M84.44-●
  hip M84.459
  humerus M84.42-●
  ilium M84.454
  ischium M84.454
  joint prosthesis —*see* Complications, joint prosthesis, mechanical, breakdown, by site
    periprosthetic —*see* Fracture, pathological, periprosthetic
  metacarpus M84.44-●
  metatarsus M84.47-●
  neck M84.48

Fracture, pathological *(Continued)*
  pelvis M84.454
  periprosthetic M97.9
    ankle M97.2-●
    elbow M97.4-●
    finger M97.8
    hip M97.0-●
    knee M97.1-●
    other specified joint M97.8
    shoulder M97.3-●
    spinal joint M97.8
    toe joint M97.8
    wrist joint M97.8
  radius M84.43-●
  restorative material (dental) K08.539
    with loss of material K08.531
    without loss of material K08.530
  rib M84.48
  scapula M84.41-●
  skull M84.48
  tarsus M84.47-●
  tibia M84.46-●
  toe M84.47-●
  ulna M84.43-●
  vertebra M84.48
Fracture, traumatic (abduction) (adduction) (separation) —*see also* Fracture, pathological T14.8
  acetabulum S32.40-●
    column
      anterior (displaced) (iliopubic) S32.43-●
        nondisplaced S32.436
      posterior (displaced) (ilioischial) S32.443
        nondisplaced S32.44-●
    dome (displaced) S32.48-●
      nondisplaced S32.48
    specified NEC S32.49-●
    transverse (displaced) S32.45-●
      with associated posterior wall fracture (displaced) S32.46-●
        nondisplaced S32.46-●
      nondisplaced S32.45-●
    wall
      anterior (displaced) S32.41-●
        nondisplaced S32.41-●
      medial (displaced) S32.47-●
        nondisplaced S32.47-●
      posterior (displaced) S32.42-●
      with associated transverse fracture (displaced) S32.46-●
        nondisplaced S32.46-●
      nondisplaced S32.42-●
  acromion —*see* Fracture, scapula, acromial process
  ankle S82.899
    bimalleolar (displaced) S82.84-●
      nondisplaced S82.84-●
    lateral malleolus only (displaced) S82.6-●
      nondisplaced S82.6-●
    medial malleolus (displaced) S82.5-●
      associated with Maisonneuve's fracture —*see* Fracture, Maisonneuve's
      nondisplaced S82.5-●
    talus —*see* Fracture, tarsal, talus
    trimalleolar (displaced) S82.85-●
      nondisplaced S82.85-●
  arm (upper) —*see also* Fracture, humerus, shaft
    humerus —*see* Fracture, humerus
    radius —*see* Fracture, radius
    ulna —*see* Fracture, ulna
  astragalus —*see* Fracture, tarsal, talus
  atlas —*see* Fracture, neck, cervical vertebra, first
  axis —*see* Fracture, neck, cervical vertebra, second
  back —*see* Fracture, vertebra
  Barton's —*see* Barton's fracture
  base of skull —*see* Fracture, skull, base

Fracture, traumatic *(Continued)*
  basicervical (basal) (femoral) S72.0
  Bennett's —*see* Bennett's fracture
  bimalleolar —*see* Fracture, ankle, bimalleolar
  blow-out S02.3-●
  bone NEC T14.8
    birth injury P13.9
    following insertion of orthopedic implant, joint prosthesis or bone plate —*see* Fracture, following insertion of orthopedic implant, joint prosthesis or bone plate
    in (due to) neoplastic disease NEC —*see* Fracture, pathological, due to, neoplastic disease
    pathological (cause unknown) —*see* Fracture, pathological
  breast bone —*see* Fracture, sternum
  buckle —*see* Fracture, by site, torus
  bucket handle (semilunar cartilage) —*see* Tear, meniscus
  burst —*see* Fracture, traumatic, by site
  calcaneus —*see* Fracture, tarsal, calcaneus
  carpal bone(s) S62.10-●
    capitate (displaced) S62.13-●
      nondisplaced S62.13-●
    cuneiform —*see* Fracture, carpal bone, triquetrum
    hamate (body) (displaced) S62.143
      hook process (displaced) S62.15-●
        nondisplaced S62.15-●
      nondisplaced S62.14-●
    larger multangular —*see* Fracture, carpal bones, trapezium
    lunate (displaced) S62.12-●
      nondisplaced S62.12-●
    navicular S62.00-●
      distal pole (displaced) S62.01-●
        nondisplaced S62.01-●
      middle third (displaced) S62.02-●
        nondisplaced S62.02-●
      proximal third (displaced) S62.03-●
        nondisplaced S62.03-●
      volar tuberosity —*see* Fracture, carpal bones, navicular, distal pole
    os magnum —*see* Fracture, carpal bones, capitate
    pisiform (displaced) S62.16-●
      nondisplaced S62.16-●
    semilunar —*see* Fracture, carpal bones, lunate
    smaller multangular —*see* Fracture, carpal bones, trapezoid
    trapezium (displaced) S62.17-●
      nondisplaced S62.17-●
    trapezoid (displaced) S62.18-●
      nondisplaced S62.18-●
    triquetrum (displaced) S62.11-●
      nondisplaced S62.11-●
    unciform —*see* Fracture, carpal bones, hamate
  cervical —*see* Fracture, vertebra, cervical
  clavicle S42.00-●
    acromial end (displaced) S42.03-●
      nondisplaced S42.03-●
    birth injury P13.4
    lateral end —*see* Fracture, clavicle, acromial end
    shaft (displaced) S42.02-●
      nondisplaced S42.02-●
    sternal end (anterior) (displaced) S42.01-●
      nondisplaced S42.01-●
      posterior S42.01-●
  coccyx S32.2
  collapsed —*see* Collapse, vertebra
  collar bone —*see* Fracture, clavicle
  Colles' —*see* Colles' fracture
  coronoid process —*see* Fracture, ulna, upper end, coronoid process
  corpus cavernosum penis S39.840

▶ New   ⇒ Revised   ~~deleted~~ Deleted   ● Use Additional Character(s)

Fracture, traumatic (Continued)
foot (Continued)
sesamoid S92.81-●
specified NEC S92.81-●
talus —see Fracture, tarsal, talus
tarsal —see Fracture, tarsal
toe —see Fracture, toe
forearm S52.9-●
radius —see Fracture, radius
ulna —see Fracture, ulna
fossa (anterior) (middle) (posterior) S02.19
fragility —see Fracture, pathological, due to
osteoporosis
frontal (bone) (skull) S02.0
sinus S02.19
glenoid (cavity) (scapula) —see Fracture,
scapula, glenoid cavity
greenstick —see Fracture, by site
hallux —see Fracture, toe, great
hand S62.9-●
carpal —see Fracture, carpal bone
finger (except thumb) —see Fracture,
finger
metacarpal —see Fracture, metacarpal
navicular (scaphoid) (hand) —see Fracture,
carpal bone, navicular
thumb —see Fracture, thumb
healed or old
with complications - code by Nature of the
complication
heel bone —see Fracture, tarsal, calcaneus
Hill-Sachs S42.29-●
hip —see Fracture, femur, neck
humerus S42.30-●
anatomical neck —see Fracture, humerus,
upper end
articular process —see Fracture, humerus,
lower end
capitellum —see Fracture, humerus, lower
end, condyle, lateral
distal end —see Fracture, humerus, lower
end
epiphysis
lower —see Fracture, humerus, lower
end, physeal
upper —see Fracture, humerus, upper
end, physeal
external condyle —see Fracture, humerus,
lower end, condyle, lateral
following insertion of implant, prosthesis
or plate M96.62-●
great tuberosity —see Fracture, humerus,
upper end, greater tuberosity
intercondylar —see Fracture, humerus,
lower end
internal epicondyle —see Fracture, humerus,
lower end, epicondyle, medial
lesser tuberosity —see Fracture, humerus,
upper end, lesser tuberosity
lower end S42.40-●
condyle
lateral (displaced) S42.45-●
nondisplaced S42.45-●
medial (displaced) S42.46-●
nondisplaced S42.46-●
epicondyle
lateral (displaced) S42.43-●
nondisplaced S42.43-●
medial (displaced) S42.44-●
incarcerated S42.44-●
nondisplaced S42.44-●
physeal S49.10-●
Salter-Harris
Type I S49.11-●
Type II S49.12-●
Type III S49.13-●
Type IV S49.14-●
specified NEC S49.19-●
specified NEC (displaced)
S42.49-●
nondisplaced S42.49-●

Fracture, traumatic (Continued)
humerus (Continued)
lower end (Continued)
supracondylar (simple) (displaced)
S42.41-●
with intercondylar fracture —see
Fracture, humerus, lower end
comminuted (displaced) S42.42-●
nondisplaced S42.42-●
nondisplaced S42.41-●
torus S42.48-●
transcondylar (displaced) S42.47-●
nondisplaced S42.47-●
proximal end —see Fracture, humerus,
upper end
shaft S42.30-●
comminuted (displaced) S42.35-●
nondisplaced S42.35-●
greenstick S42.31-●
oblique (displaced) S42.33-●
nondisplaced S42.33-●
segmental (displaced) S42.36-●
nondisplaced S42.36-●
specified NEC S42.39-●
spiral (displaced) S42.34-●
nondisplaced S42.34-●
transverse (displaced) S42.32-●
nondisplaced S42.32-●
supracondylar —see Fracture, humerus,
lower end
surgical neck —see Fracture, humerus,
upper end, surgical neck
trochlea —see Fracture, humerus, lower
end, condyle, medial
tuberosity —see Fracture, humerus, upper
end
upper end S42.20-●
anatomical neck —see Fracture,
humerus, upper end, specified NEC
articular head —see Fracture, humerus,
upper end, specified NEC
epiphysis —see Fracture, humerus,
upper end, physeal
greater tuberosity (displaced) S42.25-●
nondisplaced S42.25-●
lesser tuberosity (displaced) S42.26-●
nondisplaced S42.26-●
physeal S49.00-●
Salter-Harris
Type I S49.01-●
Type II S49.02-●
Type III S49.03-●
Type IV S49.04-●
specified NEC S49.09-●
specified NEC (displaced) S42.29-●
nondisplaced S42.29-●
surgical neck (displaced) S42.21-●
four-part S42.24-●
nondisplaced S42.21-●
three-part S42.23-●
two-part (displaced) S42.22-●
nondisplaced S42.22-●
torus S42.27-●
transepiphyseal —see Fracture, humerus,
upper end, physeal
hyoid bone S12.8
ilium S32.30-●
with disruption of pelvic ring —see
Disruption, pelvic ring
avulsion (displaced) S32.31-●
nondisplaced S32.31-●
specified NEC S32.39-●
impaction, impacted - code as Fracture, by
site
innominate bone —see Fracture, ilium
instep —see Fracture, foot
ischium S32.60-●
with disruption of pelvic ring —see
Disruption, pelvic ring
avulsion (displaced) S32.61-●
nondisplaced S32.61-●
specified NEC S32.69-●

Fracture, traumatic (Continued)
jaw (bone) (lower) —see Fracture, mandible
upper —see Fracture, maxilla
joint prosthesis —see Complications, joint
prosthesis, mechanical, breakdown,
by site
periprosthetic —see Fracture, traumatic,
periprosthetic
knee cap —see Fracture, patella
larynx S12.8
late effects —see Sequelae, fracture
leg (lower) S82.9-●
ankle —see Fracture, ankle
femur —see Fracture, femur
fibula —see Fracture, fibula
malleolus —see Fracture, ankle
patella —see Fracture, patella
specified site NEC S82.89-●
tibia —see Fracture, tibia
lumbar spine —see Fracture, vertebra, lumbar
lumbosacral spine S32.9
Maisonneuve's (displaced) S82.86-●
nondisplaced S82.86-●
malar bone —see also Fracture, maxilla
S02.400
left side S02.40B
right side S02.40A
malleolus —see Fracture, ankle
malunion —see Fracture, by site
mandible (lower jawbone) S02.609
alveolus S02.67-●
angle (of jaw) S02.65-●
body, unspecified S02.600-●
left side S02.602
right side S02.601
condylar process S02.61-●
coronoid process S02.63-●
ramus, unspecified S02.64-●
specified site NEC S02.69
subcondylar process S02.62-●
symphysis S02.66
manubrium (sterni) S22.21
dissociation from sternum S22.23
march —see Fracture, traumatic, stress, by site
maxilla, maxillary (bone) (sinus) (superior)
(upper jaw) S02.401
alveolus S02.42
inferior —see Fracture, mandible
LeFort I S02.411
LeFort II S02.412
LeFort III S02.413
left side S02.40D
right side S02.40C
metacarpal S62.309
base (displaced) S62.319
nondisplaced S62.349
fifth S62.30-●
base (displaced) S62.31-●
nondisplaced S62.34-●
neck (displaced) S62.33-●
nondisplaced S62.36-●
shaft (displaced) S62.32-●
nondisplaced S62.35-●
specified NEC S62.398
first S62.20-●
base NEC (displaced) S62.23-●
nondisplaced S62.23-●
Bennett's —see Bennett's fracture
neck (displaced) S62.25-●
nondisplaced S62.25-●
shaft (displaced) S62.24-●
nondisplaced S62.24-●
specified NEC S62.29-●
fourth S62.30-●
base (displaced) S62.31-●
nondisplaced S62.34-●
neck (displaced) S62.33-●
nondisplaced S62.36-●
shaft (displaced) S62.32-●
nondisplaced S62.35-●
specified NEC S62.39-●

Fracture, traumatic *(Continued)*
  metacarpal *(Continued)*
    neck (displaced) S62.33-●
    nondisplaced S62.36-●
    Rolando's —*see* Rolando's fracture
    second S62.30-●
      base (displaced) S62.31-●
        nondisplaced S62.34-●
      neck (displaced) S62.33-●
        nondisplaced S62.36-●
      shaft (displaced) S62.32-●
        nondisplaced S62.35-●
      specified NEC S62.39-●
    shaft (displaced) S62.32-●
      nondisplaced S62.35-●
    specified NEC S62.399
    third S62.30-●
      base (displaced) S62.31-●
        nondisplaced S62.34-●
      neck (displaced) S62.33-●
        nondisplaced S62.36-●
      shaft (displaced) S62.32-●
        nondisplaced S62.35-●
      specified NEC S62.39-●
  metaphyseal —*see* Fracture, traumatic, by
      site, shaft
  metastatic —*see* Fracture, pathological,
      due to, neoplastic disease —*see also*
      Neoplasm
  metatarsal bone S92.30-●
    fifth (displaced) S92.35-●
      nondisplaced S92.35-●
    first (displaced) S92.31-●
      nondisplaced S92.31-●
    fourth (displaced) S92.34-●
      nondisplaced S92.34-●
    physeal S99.10-●
      Salter-Harris
        Type I S99.11-●
        Type II S99.12-●
        Type III S99.13-●
        Type IV S99.14-●
      specified NEC S99.19-●
    second (displaced) S92.32-●
      nondisplaced S92.32-●
    third (displaced) S92.33-●
      nondisplaced S92.33-●
  Monteggia's —*see* Monteggia's fracture
  multiple
    hand (and wrist) NEC —*see* Fracture,
        by site
    ribs —*see* Fracture, rib, multiple
  nasal (bone(s)) S02.2
  navicular (scaphoid) (foot) —*see also* Fracture,
      tarsal, navicular
    hand —*see* Fracture, carpal, navicular
  neck S12.9
    cervical vertebra S12.9
      fifth (displaced) S12.400
        nondisplaced S12.401
        specified type NEC (displaced)
            S12.490
          nondisplaced S12.491
      first (displaced) S12.000
        burst (stable) S12.01
          unstable S12.02
        lateral mass (displaced)
            S12.040
          nondisplaced S12.041
        nondisplaced S12.001
        posterior arch (displaced)
            S12.030
          nondisplaced S12.031
        specified type NEC (displaced)
            S12.090
          nondisplaced S12.091
      fourth (displaced) S12.300
        nondisplaced S12.301
        specified type NEC (displaced)
            S12.390
          nondisplaced S12.391

Fracture, traumatic *(Continued)*
  neck *(Continued)*
    cervical vertebra *(Continued)*
      second (displaced) S12.100
        dens (anterior) (displaced) (type II)
            S12.110
          nondisplaced S12.112
          posterior S12.111
          specified type NEC (displaced)
              S12.120
            nondisplaced S12.121
        nondisplaced S12.101
        specified type NEC (displaced)
            S12.190
          nondisplaced S12.191
      seventh (displaced) S12.600
        nondisplaced S12.601
        specified type NEC (displaced)
            S12.690
          nondisplaced S12.691
      sixth (displaced) S12.500
        nondisplaced S12.501
        specified type NEC (displaced)
            S12.590
          nondisplaced S12.591
      third (displaced) S12.200
        nondisplaced S12.201
        specified type NEC (displaced)
            S12.290
          nondisplaced S12.291
    hyoid bone S12.8
    larynx S12.8
    specified site NEC S12.8
    thyroid cartilage S12.8
    trachea S12.8
  neoplastic NEC —*see* Fracture, pathological,
      due to, neoplastic disease
  neural arch —*see* Fracture, vertebra
  newborn —*see* Birth, injury, fracture
  nontraumatic —*see* Fracture, pathological
  nonunion —*see* Nonunion, fracture
  nose, nasal (bone) (septum) S02.2
  occiput —*see* Fracture, skull, base,
      occiput
  odontoid process —*see* Fracture, neck,
      cervical vertebra, second
  olecranon (process) (ulna) —*see* Fracture,
      ulna, upper end, olecranon process
  orbit, orbital (bone) (region) S02.85
    floor (blow-out) S02.3-●
    roof S02.12-●
    wall S02.85
      lateral S02.84-●
      medial S02.83-●
  os
    calcis —*see* Fracture, tarsal,
        calcaneus
    magnum —*see* Fracture, carpal,
        capitate
    pubis —*see* Fracture, pubis
  palate S02.8-●
  parietal bone (skull) S02.0
  patella S82.00-●
    comminuted (displaced) S82.04-●
      nondisplaced S82.04-●
    longitudinal (displaced) S82.02-●
      nondisplaced S82.02-●
    osteochondral (displaced) S82.01-●
      nondisplaced S82.01-●
    specified NEC S82.09-●
    transverse (displaced) S82.03-●
      nondisplaced S82.03-●
  pedicle (of vertebral arch) —*see* Fracture,
      vertebra
  pelvis, pelvic (bone) S32.9
    acetabulum —*see* Fracture, acetabulum
    circle —*see* Disruption, pelvic ring
    following insertion of implant, prosthesis
        or plate M96.65
    ilium —*see* Fracture, ilium
    ischium —*see* Fracture, ischium

Fracture, traumatic *(Continued)*
  pelvis, pelvic *(Continued)*
    multiple
      with disruption of pelvic ring (circle) —
          see Disruption, pelvic ring
      without disruption of pelvic ring (circle)
          S32.82
    pubis —*see* Fracture, pubis
    sacrum —*see* Fracture, sacrum
    specified site NEC S32.89
  periprosthetic, around internal prosthetic
      joint M97.9
    ankle M97.2-●
    elbow M97.4-●
    finger M97.8
    hip M97.0-●
    knee M97.1-●
    shoulder M97.3-●
    specified joint NEC M97.8
    spine M97.8
    toe M97.8
    wrist M97.8
  phalanx
    foot —*see* Fracture, toe
    hand —*see* Fracture, finger
  pisiform —*see* Fracture, carpal, pisiform
  pond —*see* Fracture, skull
  prosthetic device, internal —*see*
      Complications, prosthetic device, by site,
      mechanical
  pubis S32.50-●
    with disruption of pelvic ring —*see*
        Disruption, pelvic ring
    specified site NEC S32.59-●
    superior rim S32.59-●
  radius S52.9-●
    distal end —*see* Fracture, radius, lower end
    following insertion of implant, prosthesis
        or plate M96.63-●
    head —*see* Fracture, radius, upper end,
        head
    lower end S52.50-●
      Barton's —*see* Barton's fracture
      Colles' —*see* Colles' fracture
      extraarticular NEC S52.55-●
      intraarticular NEC S52.57-●
      physeal S59.20-●
        Salter-Harris
          Type I S59.21-●
          Type II S59.22-●
          Type III S59.23-●
          Type IV S59.24-●
        specified NEC S59.29-●
      Smith's —*see* Smith's fracture
      specified NEC S52.59-●
      styloid process (displaced) S52.51-●
        nondisplaced S52.51-●
      torus S52.52-●
    neck —*see* Fracture, radius, upper end
    proximal end —*see* Fracture, radius, upper
        end
    shaft S52.30-●
      bent bone S52.38-●
      comminuted (displaced) S52.35-●
        nondisplaced S52.35-●
      Galeazzi's —*see* Galeazzi's fracture
      greenstick S52.31-●
      oblique (displaced) S52.33-●
        nondisplaced S52.33-●
      segmental (displaced) S52.36-●
        nondisplaced S52.36-●
      specified NEC S52.39-●
      spiral (displaced) S52.34-●
        nondisplaced S52.34-●
      transverse (displaced) S52.32-●
        nondisplaced S52.32-●
    upper end S52.10-●
      head (displaced) S52.12-●
        nondisplaced S52.12-●
      neck (displaced) S52.13-●
        nondisplaced S52.13-●

▶ New   ⇒ Revised   ~~deleted~~ Deleted   ● Use Additional Character(s)

Fracture, traumatic *(Continued)*
   vertebra, vertebral *(Continued)*
     metastatic —*see* Collapse, vertebra, in,
       specified disease NEC —*see also*
       Neoplasm
     newborn (birth injury) P11.5
     sacrum S32.10
      specified NEC S32.19
      Type
       1 S32.14
       2 S32.15
       3 S32.16
       4 S32.17
      Zone
       I S32.119
        displaced (minimally) S32.111
         severely S32.112
        nondisplaced S32.110
       II S32.129
        displaced (minimally) S32.121
         severely S32.122
        nondisplaced S32.120
       III S32.139
        displaced (minimally) S32.131
         severely S32.132
        nondisplaced S32.130
     thoracic —*see* Fracture, thorax, vertebra
   vertex S02.0
   vomer (bone) S02.2
   wrist S62.10-●
     carpal —*see* Fracture, carpal bone
     navicular (scaphoid) (hand) —*see* Fracture,
       carpal, navicular
   xiphisternum, xiphoid (process) S22.24
   zygoma S02.442
     left side S02.40F
     right side S02.40E
Fragile, fragility
   autosomal site Q95.5
   bone, congenital (with blue sclera) Q78.0
   capillary (hereditary) D69.8
   hair L67.8
   nails L60.3
   non-sex chromosome site Q95.5
   X chromosome Q99.2
Fragilitas
   crinium L67.8
   ossium (with blue sclerae) (hereditary) Q78.0
   unguium L60.3
     congenital Q84.6
Fragments, cataract (lens), following cataract
     surgery H59.02-●
   retained foreign body —*see* Retained, foreign
     body fragments (type of)
Frailty (frail) R54
   mental R41.81
Frambesia, frambesial (tropica) —*see also* Yaws
   initial lesion or ulcer A66.0
   primary A66.0
Frambeside
   gummatous A66.4
   of early yaws A66.2
Frambesioma A66.1
Franceschetti-Klein (-Wildervanck) disease or
     syndrome Q75.4
Francis' disease —*see* Tularemia
Franklin disease C88.2
Frank's essential thrombocytopenia D69.3
Fraser's syndrome Q87.0
Freckle(s) L81.2
   malignant melanoma in —*see* Melanoma
   melanotic (Hutchinson's) —*see* Melanoma,
     in situ
   retinal D49.81
Frederickson's hyperlipoproteinemia, type
   I and V E78.3
   IIA E78.00
   IIB and III E78.2
   IV E78.1
Freeman Sheldon syndrome Q87.0
Freezing —*see also* Effect, adverse, cold T69.9

Freiberg's disease (infraction of metatarsal head
     or osteochondrosis) —*see* Osteochondrosis,
     juvenile, metatarsus
Frei's disease A55
Fremitus, friction, cardiac R01.2
Frenum, frenulum
   external os Q51.828
   tongue (shortening) (congenital) Q38.1
Frequency micturition (nocturnal) R35.0
   psychogenic F45.8
Frey's syndrome
   auriculotemporal G50.8
   hyperhidrosis L74.52
Friction
   burn —*see* Burn, by site
   fremitus, cardiac R01.2
   precordial R01.2
   sounds, chest R09.89
Friderichsen-Waterhouse syndrome or disease
     A39.1
Friedländer's B (bacillus) NEC —*see also*
     condition A49.8
Friedreich's
   ataxia G11.11
   combined systemic disease G11.11
   facial hemihypertrophy Q67.4
   sclerosis (cerebellum) (spinal cord)
     G11.11
Frigidity F52.22
Fröhlich's syndrome E23.6
Frontal —*see also* condition
   lobe syndrome F07.0
Frostbite (superficial) T33.90
   with
     partial thickness skin loss —*see* Frostbite
       (superficial), by site
     tissue necrosis T34.90
   abdominal wall T33.3
     with tissue necrosis T34.3
   ankle T33.81-●
     with tissue necrosis T34.81-●
   arm T33.4-●
     with tissue necrosis T34.4-●
     finger(s) —*see* Frostbite, finger
     hand —*see* Frostbite, hand
     wrist —*see* Frostbite, wrist
   ear T33.01-●
     with tissue necrosis T34.01-●
   face T33.09
     with tissue necrosis T34.09
   finger T33.53-●
     with tissue necrosis T34.53-●
   foot T33.82-●
     with tissue necrosis T34.82-●
   hand T33.52-●
     with tissue necrosis T34.52-●
   head T33.09
     with tissue necrosis T34.09
     ear —*see* Frostbite, ear
     nose —*see* Frostbite, nose
   hip (and thigh) T33.6-●
     with tissue necrosis T34.6-●
   knee T33.7-●
     with tissue necrosis T34.7-●
   leg T33.9-●
     with tissue necrosis T34.9-●
     ankle —*see* Frostbite, ankle
     foot —*see* Frostbite, foot
     knee —*see* Frostbite, knee
     lower T33.7-●
       with tissue necrosis T34.7-●
     thigh —*see* Frostbite, hip
     toe —*see* Frostbite, toe
   limb
     lower T33.99
       with tissue necrosis T34.99
     upper —*see* Frostbite, arm
   neck T33.1
     with tissue necrosis T34.1
   nose T33.02
     with tissue necrosis T34.02

Frostbite *(Continued)*
   pelvis T33.3
     with tissue necrosis T34.3
   specified site NEC T33.99
     with tissue necrosis T34.99
   thigh —*see* Frostbite, hip
   thorax T33.2
     with tissue necrosis T34.2
   toes T33.83-●
     with tissue necrosis T34.83-●
   trunk T33.99
     with tissue necrosis T34.99
   wrist T33.51-●
     with tissue necrosis T34.51-●
Frotteurism F65.81
Frozen —*see also* Effect, adverse, cold T69.9
   pelvis (female) N94.89
     male K66.8
   shoulder —*see* Capsulitis, adhesive
Fructokinase deficiency E74.11
Fructose 1,6 diphosphatase deficiency E74.19
Fructosemia (benign) (essential) E74.12
Fructosuria (benign) (essential) E74.11
Fuchs'
   black spot (myopic) —*see also* Myopia,
     degenerative H44.2-●
   dystrophy (corneal endothelium) H18.51-●
   heterochromic cyclitis —*see* Cyclitis, Fuchs'
     heterochromic
Fucosidosis E77.1
Fugue R68.89
   dissociative F44.1
   hysterical (dissociative) F44.1
   postictal in epilepsy —*see* Epilepsy
   reaction to exceptional stress (transient)
     F43.0
Fulminant, fulminating —*see* condition
Functional —*see also* condition
   bleeding (uterus) N93.8
Functioning, intellectual, borderline R41.83
Fundus —*see* condition
Fungemia NOS B49
Fungus, fungous
   cerebral G93.89
   disease NOS B49
   infection —*see* Infection, fungus
Funiculitis (acute) (chronic) (endemic)
     N49.1
   gonococcal (acute) (chronic) A54.23
   tuberculous A18.15
Funnel
   breast (acquired) M95.4
     congenital Q67.6
     sequelae (late effect) of rickets E64.3
   chest (acquired) M95.4
     congenital Q67.6
     sequelae (late effect) of rickets E64.3
   pelvis (acquired) M95.5
     with disproportion (fetopelvic) O33.3
       causing obstructed labor O65.3
     congenital Q74.2
FUO (fever of unknown origin) R50.9
Furfur L21.0
   microsporon B36.0
Furrier's lung J67.8
Furrowed K14.5
   nail(s) (transverse) L60.4
     congenital Q84.6
   tongue K14.5
     congenital Q38.3
Furuncle L02.92
   abdominal wall L02.221
   ankle —*see* Furuncle, lower limb
   antecubital space —*see* Furuncle, upper
     limb
   anus K61.0
   arm —*see* Furuncle, upper limb
   auditory canal, external —*see* Abscess, ear,
     external
   auricle (ear) —*see* Abscess, ear, external
   axilla (region) L02.42-●

Furuncle *(Continued)*
  back (any part) L02.222
  breast N61.1
  buttock L02.32
  cheek (external) L02.02
  chest wall L02.223
  chin L02.02
  corpus cavernosum N48.21
  ear, external —*see* Abscess, ear, external
  external auditory canal —*see* Abscess, ear,
      external
  eyelid —*see* Abscess, eyelid
  face L02.02
  femoral (region) —*see* Furuncle, lower
      limb
  finger —*see* Furuncle, hand
  flank L02.221
  foot L02.62-●
  forehead L02.02
  gluteal (region) L02.32
  groin L02.224
  hand L02.52-●
  head L02.821
      face L02.02
  hip —*see* Furuncle, lower limb
  kidney —*see* Abscess, kidney
  knee —*see* Furuncle, lower limb
  labium (majus) (minus) N76.4
  lacrimal
      gland —*see* Dacryoadenitis
      passages (duct) (sac) —*see* Inflammation,
          lacrimal, passages, acute
  leg (any part) —*see* Furuncle, lower limb
  lower limb L02.42-●
  malignant A22.0
  mouth K12.2
  navel L02.226
  neck L02.12
  nose J34.0
  orbit, orbital —*see* Abscess, orbit
  palmar (space) —*see* Furuncle, hand
  partes posteriores L02.32
  pectoral region L02.223
  penis N48.21
  perineum L02.225

Furuncle *(Continued)*
  pinna —*see* Abscess, ear, external
  popliteal —*see* Furuncle, lower limb
  prepatellar —*see* Furuncle, lower limb
  scalp L02.821
  seminal vesicle N49.0
  shoulder —*see* Furuncle, upper limb
  specified site NEC L02.828
  submandibular K12.2
  temple (region) L02.02
  thumb —*see* Furuncle, hand
  toe —*see* Furuncle, foot
  trunk L02.229
      abdominal wall L02.221
      back L02.222
      chest wall L02.223
      groin L02.224
      perineum L02.225
      umbilicus L02.226
  umbilicus L02.226
  upper limb L02.42-●
  vulva N76.4
Furunculosis —*see* Furuncle
Fused —*see* Fusion, fused
Fusion, fused *(congenital)*
  astragaloscaphoid Q74.2
  atria Q21.1
  auditory canal Q16.1
  auricles, heart Q21.1
  binocular with defective stereopsis H53.32
  bone Q79.8
  cervical spine M43.22
  choanal Q30.0
  commissure, mitral valve Q23.2
  cusps, heart valve NEC Q24.8
      mitral Q23.2
      pulmonary Q22.1
      tricuspid Q22.4
  ear ossicles Q16.3
  fingers Q70.0-●
  hymen Q52.3
  joint (acquired) —*see also* Ankylosis
      congenital Q74.8
  kidneys (incomplete) Q63.1
  labium (majus) (minus) Q52.5

Fusion, fused *(Continued)*
  larynx and trachea Q34.8
  limb, congenital Q74.8
      lower Q74.2
      upper Q74.0
  lobes, lung Q33.8
  lumbosacral (acquired) M43.27
      arthrodesis status Z98.1
      congenital Q76.49
      postprocedural status Z98.1
  nares, nose, nasal, nostril(s) Q30.0
  organ or site not listed —*see* Anomaly, by site
  ossicles Q79.9
      auditory Q16.3
  pulmonic cusps Q22.1
  ribs Q76.6
  sacroiliac (joint) (acquired) M43.28
      arthrodesis status Z98.1
      congenital Q74.2
      postprocedural status Z98.1
  spine (acquired) NEC M43.20
      arthrodesis status Z98.1
      cervical region M43.22
      cervicothoracic region M43.23
      congenital Q76.49
      lumbar M43.26
      lumbosacral region M43.27
      occipito-atlanto-axial region M43.21
      postoperative status Z98.1
      sacrococcygeal region M43.28
      thoracic region M43.24
      thoracolumbar region M43.25
  sublingual duct with submaxillary duct at
      opening in mouth Q38.4
  testes Q55.1
  toes Q70.2
  tooth, teeth K00.2
  trachea and esophagus Q39.8
  twins Q89.4
  vagina Q52.4
  ventricles, heart Q21.0
  vertebra (arch) —*see* Fusion, spine
  vulva Q52.5
Fusospirillosis (mouth) (tongue) (tonsil) A69.1
Fussy baby R68.12

▶ New   ⇒ Revised   ~~deleted~~ Deleted   ● Use Additional Character(s)

G

Gain in weight (abnormal) (excessive) —see also
 Weight, gain
Gaisböck's disease (polycythemia hypertonica)
 D75.1
Gait abnormality R26.9
 ataxic R26.0
 falling R29.6
 hysterical (ataxic) (staggering) F44.4
 paralytic R26.1
 spastic R26.1
 specified type NEC R26.89
 staggering R26.0
 unsteadiness R26.81
 walking difficulty NEC R26.2
Galactocele (breast) N64.89
 puerperal, postpartum O92.79
Galactokinase deficiency E74.29
Galactophoritis N61.0
 gestational, puerperal, postpartum O91.2-●
Galactorrhea O92.6
 not associated with childbirth N64.3
Galactosemia (classic) (congenital) E74.21
Galactosuria E74.29
Galacturia R82.0
 schistosomiasis (bilharziasis) B65.0
GALD (gestational alloimmune liver disease)
 P78.84
Galeazzi's fracture S52.37-●
Galen's vein —see condition
Galeophobia F40.218
Gall duct —see condition
Gallbladder —see also condition
 acute K81.0
Gallop rhythm R00.8
Gallstone (colic) (cystic duct) (gallbladder)
 (impacted) (multiple) —see also Calculus,
 gallbladder
 with
 cholecystitis —see Calculus, gallbladder,
 with cholecystitis
 bile duct (common) (hepatic) —see Calculus,
 bile duct
 causing intestinal obstruction K56.3
 specified NEC K80.80
 with obstruction K80.81
Gambling Z72.6
 pathological (compulsive) F63.0
Gammopathy (of undetermined significance
 [MGUS]) D47.2
 associated with lymphoplasmacytic dyscrasia
 D47.2
 monoclonal D47.2
 polyclonal D89.0
Gamna's disease (siderotic splenomegaly)
 D73.1
Gamophobia F40.298
Gampsodactylia (congenital) Q66.7-●
Gamstorp's disease (adynamia episodica
 hereditaria) G72.3
Gandy-Nanta disease (siderotic splenomegaly)
 D73.1
Gang
 membership offenses Z72.810
Gangliocytoma D36.10
Ganglioglioma —see Neoplasm, uncertain
 behavior, by site
Ganglion (compound) (diffuse) (joint) (tendon
 (sheath)) M67.40
 ankle M67.47-●
 foot M67.47-●
 forearm M67.43-●
 hand M67.44-●
 lower leg M67.46-●
 multiple sites M67.49
 of yaws (early) (late) A66.6
 pelvic region M67.45-●
 periosteal —see Periostitis
 shoulder region M67.41-●
 specified site NEC M67.48

Ganglion (Continued)
 thigh region M67.45-●
 tuberculous A18.09
 upper arm M67.42-●
 wrist M67.43-●
Ganglioneuroblastoma —see Neoplasm, nerve,
 malignant
Ganglioneuroma D36.10
 malignant —see Neoplasm, nerve, malignant
Ganglioneuromatosis D36.10
Ganglionitis
 fifth nerve —see Neuralgia, trigeminal
 gasserian (postherpetic) (postzoster)
 B02.21
 geniculate G51.1
 newborn (birth injury) P11.3
 postherpetic, postzoster B02.21
 herpes zoster B02.21
 postherpetic geniculate B02.21
Gangliosidosis E75.10
 GM1 E75.19
 GM2 E75.00
 other specified E75.09
 Sandhoff disease E75.01
 Tay-Sachs disease E75.02
 GM3 E75.19
 mucolipidosis IV E75.11
Gangosa A66.5
Gangrene, gangrenous (connective tissue)
 (dropsical) (dry) (moist) (skin) (ulcer) —see
 also Necrosis I96
➡ with diabetes (mellitus) —see Diabetes, with
 gangrene
 abdomen (wall) I96
 alveolar M27.3
 appendix K35.80
 with
 peritonitis, localized (see also
 Appendicitis) K35.31
 arteriosclerotic (general) (senile) —see
 Arteriosclerosis, extremities, with,
 gangrene
 auricle I96
 Bacillus welchii A48.0
 bladder (infectious) —see Cystitis, specified
 type NEC
 bowel, cecum, or colon —see Gangrene,
 intestine
 Clostridium perfringens or welchii A48.0
 cornea H18.89-●
 corpora cavernosa N48.29
 noninfective N48.89
 cutaneous, spreading I96
 decubital —see Ulcer, pressure, by site
➡ diabetic (any site) —see Diabetes, with gangrene
 emphysematous —see Gangrene, gas
 epidemic —see Poisoning, food, noxious,
 plant
 epididymis (infectional) N45.1
 erysipelas —see Erysipelas
 extremity (lower) (upper) I96
 Fournier N49.3
 female N76.89
 fusospirochetal A69.0
 gallbladder —see Cholecystitis, acute
 gas (bacillus) A48.0
 following
 abortion —see Abortion by type
 complicated by infection
 ectopic or molar pregnancy O08.0
 glossitis K14.0
 hernia —see Hernia, by site, with gangrene
 intestine, intestinal (hemorrhagic)
 (massive) —see also Infarct, intestine
 K55.069
 with
 mesenteric embolism —see also Infarct,
 intestine K55.069
 obstruction —see Obstruction, intestine
 laryngitis J04.0
 limb (lower) (upper) I96

Gangrene, gangrenous (Continued)
 lung J85.0
 spirochetal A69.8
 lymphangitis I89.1
 Meleney's (synergistic) —see Ulcer, skin
 mesentery —see also Infarct, intestine
 K55.069
 with
 embolism —see also Infarct, intestine
 K55.069
 intestinal obstruction —see Obstruction,
 intestine
 mouth A69.0
 ovary —see Oophoritis
 pancreas —see Pancreatitis, acute
 penis N48.29
 noninfective N48.89
 perineum I96
 pharynx —see also Pharyngitis
 Vincent's A69.1
 presenile I73.1
 progressive synergistic —see Ulcer, skin
 pulmonary J85.0
 pulpal (dental) K04.1
 quinsy J36
 Raynaud's (symmetric gangrene) I73.01
 retropharyngeal J39.2
 scrotum N49.3
 noninfective N50.89
 senile (atherosclerotic) —see Arteriosclerosis,
 extremities, with, gangrene
 spermatic cord N49.1
 noninfective N50.89
 spine I96
 spirochetal NEC A69.8
 spreading cutaneous I96
 stomatitis A69.0
 symmetrical I73.01
 testis (infectional) N45.2
 noninfective N44.8
 throat —see also Pharyngitis
 diphtheritic A36.0
 Vincent's A69.1
 thyroid (gland) E07.89
 tooth (pulp) K04.1
 tuberculous NEC —see Tuberculosis
 tunica vaginalis N49.1
 noninfective N50.89
 umbilicus I96
 uterus —see Endometritis
 uvulitis K12.2
 vas deferens N49.1
 noninfective N50.89
 vulva N76.89
Ganister disease J62.8
Ganser's syndrome (hysterical) F44.89
Gardner-Diamond syndrome (autoerythrocyte
 sensitization) D69.2
Gargoylism E76.01
Garré's disease, osteitis (sclerosing),
 osteomyelitis —see Osteomyelitis,
 specified type NEC
Garrod's pad, knuckle M72.1
Gartner's duct
 cyst Q52.4
 persistent Q50.6
Gas R14.3
 asphyxiation, inhalation, poisoning,
 suffocation NEC —see Table of Drugs
 and Chemicals
 excessive R14.0
 gangrene A48.0
 following
 abortion —see Abortion by type
 complicated by infection
 ectopic or molar pregnancy O08.0
 on stomach R14.0
 pains R14.1
Gastralgia —see also Pain, abdominal
Gastrectasis K31.0
 psychogenic F45.8

Gastric —see condition
Gastrinoma
  malignant
    pancreas C25.4
    specified site NEC —see Neoplasm,
      malignant, by site
    unspecified site C25.4
  specified site —see Neoplasm, uncertain
    behavior
  unspecified site D37.9
Gastritis (simple) K29.70
  with bleeding K29.71
  acute (erosive) K29.00
    with bleeding K29.01
  alcoholic K29.20
    with bleeding K29.21
  allergic K29.60
    with bleeding K29.61
  atrophic (chronic) K29.40
    with bleeding K29.41
  chronic (antral) (fundal) K29.50
    with bleeding K29.51
    atrophic K29.40
      with bleeding K29.41
    superficial K29.30
      with bleeding K29.31
  dietary counseling and surveillance Z71.3
  due to diet deficiency E63.9
  eosinophilic K52.81
  giant hypertrophic K29.60
    with bleeding K29.61
  granulomatous K29.60
    with bleeding K29.61
  hypertrophic (mucosa) K29.60
    with bleeding K29.61
  nervous F54
  spastic K29.60
    with bleeding K29.61
  specified NEC K29.60
    with bleeding K29.61
  superficial chronic K29.30
    with bleeding K29.31
  tuberculous A18.83
  viral NEC A08.4
Gastrocarcinoma —see Neoplasm, malignant,
  stomach
Gastrocolic —see condition
Gastrodisciasis, gastrodiscoidiasis B66.8
Gastroduodenitis K29.90
  with bleeding K29.91
  virus, viral A08.4
    specified type NEC A08.39
Gastrodynia —see Pain, abdominal
Gastroenteritis (acute) (chronic) (noninfectious)
  (see also Enteritis) K52.9
  allergic K52.29
  with
    eosinophilic gastritis or gastroenteritis
      K52.81
    food protein-induced enterocolitis
      syndrome K52.21
    food protein-induced enteropathy K52.22
  dietetic —see also Gastroenteritis, allergic
    K52.29
  drug-induced K52.1
  due to
    Cryptosporidium A07.2
    drugs K52.1
    food poisoning —see Intoxication,
      foodborne
    radiation K52.0
  eosinophilic K52.81
  epidemic (infectious) A09
  food hypersensitivity —see also
    Gastroenteritis, allergic K52.29
  infectious —see Enteritis, infectious
  influenzal —see Influenza, with
    gastroenteritis
  noninfectious K52.9
    specified NEC K52.89
  rotaviral A08.0

Gastroenteritis (Continued)
  Salmonella A02.0
  toxic K52.1
  viral NEC A08.4
    acute infectious A08.39
      type Norwalk A08.11
    infantile (acute) A08.39
    Norwalk agent A08.11
    rotaviral A08.0
    severe of infants A08.39
    specified type NEC A08.39
Gastroenteropathy —see also Gastroenteritis K52.9
  acute, due to Norovirus A08.11
  acute, due to Norwalk agent A08.11
  infectious A09
Gastroenteroptosis K63.4
Gastroesophageal laceration-hemorrhage
  syndrome K22.6
Gastrointestinal —see condition
Gastrojejunal —see condition
Gastrojejunitis —see also Enteritis K52.9
Gastrojejunocolic —see condition
Gastroliths K31.89
Gastromalacia K31.89
Gastroparalysis K31.84
  diabetic —see Diabetes, gastroparalysis
Gastroparesis K31.84
  diabetic —see Diabetes, by type, with
    gastroparesis
Gastropathy K31.9
  ➡congestive portal (see also, Hypertension,
    portal) K31.89
  erythematous K29.70
  exudative K90.89
  ➡portal hypertensive (see also, Hypertension,
    portal) K31.89
Gastroptosis K31.89
Gastrorrhagia K92.2
  psychogenic F45.8
Gastroschisis (congenital) Q79.3
Gastrospasm (neurogenic) (reflex) K31.89
  neurotic F45.8
  psychogenic F45.8
Gastrostaxis —see Gastritis, with bleeding
Gastrostenosis K31.89
Gastrostomy
  attention to Z43.1
  status Z93.1
Gastrosuccorrhea (continuous) (intermittent)
  K31.89
  neurotic F45.8
  psychogenic F45.8
Gatophobia F40.218
Gaucher's disease or splenomegaly (adult)
  (infantile) E75.22
Gee (-Herter)(-Thaysen) disease (nontropical
  sprue) K90.0
Gélineau's syndrome G47.419
  with cataplexy G47.411
Gemination, tooth, teeth K00.2
Gemistocytoma
  specified site —see Neoplasm, malignant, by
    site
  unspecified site C71.9
General, generalized —see condition
Genetic
  carrier (status)
    cystic fibrosis Z14.1
    hemophilia A (asymptomatic) Z14.01
      symptomatic Z14.02
    specified NEC Z14.8
  susceptibility to disease NEC Z15.89
    malignant neoplasm Z15.09
      breast Z15.01
      endometrium Z15.04
      ovary Z15.02
      prostate Z15.03
      specified NEC Z15.09
    multiple endocrine neoplasia Z15.81
Genital —see condition
Genito-anorectal syndrome A55

Genitourinary system —see condition
Genu
  congenital Q74.1
  extrorsum (acquired) —see also Deformity,
    varus, knee
    congenital Q74.1
    sequelae (late effect) of rickets E64.3
  introrsum (acquired) —see also Deformity,
    valgus, knee
    congenital Q74.1
    sequelae (late effect) of rickets E64.3
  rachitic (old) E64.3
  recurvatum (acquired) —see also Deformity,
    limb, specified type NEC, lower leg
    congenital Q68.2
    sequelae (late effect) of rickets E64.3
  valgum (acquired) (knock-knee) M21.06-●
    congenital Q74.1
    sequelae (late effect) of rickets E64.3
  varum (acquired) (bowleg) M21.16-●
    congenital Q74.1
    sequelae (late effect) of rickets E64.3
Geographic tongue K14.1
Geophagia —see Pica
Geotrichosis B48.3
  stomatitis B48.3
Gephyrophobia F40.242
Gerbode defect Q21.0
GERD (gastroesophageal reflux disease) K21.9
Gerhardt's
  disease (erythromelalgia) I73.81
  syndrome (vocal cord paralysis) J38.00
    bilateral J38.02
    unilateral J38.01
German measles —see also Rubella
  exposure to Z20.4
Germinoblastoma (diffuse) C85.9-●
  follicular C82.9-●
Germinoma —see Neoplasm, malignant, by site
Gerontoxon —see Degeneration, cornea, senile
Gerstmann-Sträussler-Scheinker syndrome
  (GSS) A81.82
Gerstmann's syndrome R48.8
  developmental F81.2
Gestation (period) —see also Pregnancy
  ectopic —see Pregnancy, by site
  multiple O30.9-●
    greater than quadruplets —see Pregnancy,
      multiple (gestation), specified NEC
    specified NEC —see Pregnancy, multiple
      (gestation), specified NEC
Gestational
  mammary abscess O91.11-●
  purulent mastitis O91.11-●
  subareolar abscess O91.11-●
Ghon tubercle, primary infection A15.7
Ghost
  teeth K00.4
  vessels (cornea) H16.41-●
Ghoul hand A66.3
Gianotti-Crosti disease L44.4
Giant
  cell
    epulis K06.8
    peripheral granuloma K06.8
  esophagus, congenital Q39.5
  kidney, congenital Q63.3
  urticaria T78.3
    hereditary D84.1
Giardiasis A07.1
Gibert's disease or pityriasis L42
Giddiness R42
  hysterical F44.89
  psychogenic F45.8
Gierke's disease (glycogenosis I) E74.01
Gigantism (cerebral) (hypophyseal) (pituitary)
  E22.0
  constitutional E34.4
Gilbert's disease or syndrome E80.4
Gilchrist's disease B40.9
Gilford-Hutchinson disease E34.8

▶ New   ➡ Revised   deleted Deleted   ● Use Additional Character(s)

Gilles de la Tourette's disease or syndrome
  (motor-verbal tic) F95.2
Gingivitis K05.10
  acute (catarrhal) K05.00
    necrotizing A69.1
    nonplaque induced K05.01
    plaque induced K05.00
  chronic (desquamative) (hyperplastic)
      (simple marginal) (pregnancy
      associated) (ulcerative) K05.10
    nonplaque induced K05.11
    plaque induced K05.10
  expulsiva —see Periodontitis
  necrotizing ulcerative (acute) A69.1
  pellagrous E52
    acute necrotizing A69.1
  Vincent's A69.1
Gingivoglossitis K14.0
Gingivopericementitis —see Periodontitis
Gingivosis —see Gingivitis, chronic
Gingivostomatitis K05.10
  herpesviral B00.2
  necrotizing ulcerative (acute) A69.1
Gland, glandular —see condition
Glanders A24.0
Glanzmann (-Naegeli) disease or
    thrombasthenia D69.1
Glasgow coma scale
  total score
    3-8 R40.243
    9-12 R40.242
    13-15 R40.241
Glass-blower's disease (cataract) —see
    Cataract, specified NEC
Glaucoma H40.9
  with
    increased episcleral venous pressure
        H40.81-●
    pseudoexfoliation of lens —see Glaucoma,
        open angle, primary, capsular
  absolute H44.51-●
  angle-closure (primary) H40.20-●
    acute (attack) (crisis) H40.21-●
    chronic H40.22-●
    intermittent H40.23-●
    residual stage H40.24-●
  borderline H40.00-●
  capsular (with pseudoexfoliation of lens) —
      see Glaucoma, open angle, primary,
      capsular
  childhood Q15.0
  closed angle —see Glaucoma, angle-closure
  congenital Q15.0
  corticosteroid-induced —see Glaucoma,
      secondary, drugs
  hypersecretion H40.82-●
  in (due to)
    amyloidosis E85.4 [H42]
    aniridia Q13.1 [H42]
    concussion of globe —see Glaucoma,
        secondary, trauma
    dislocation of lens —see Glaucoma,
        secondary
    disorder of lens NEC —see Glaucoma,
        secondary
    drugs —see Glaucoma, secondary, drugs
    endocrine disease NOS E34.9 [H42]
    eye
      inflammation —see Glaucoma,
          secondary, inflammation
      trauma —see Glaucoma, secondary,
          trauma
    hypermature cataract —see Glaucoma,
        secondary
    iridocyclitis —see Glaucoma, secondary,
        inflammation
    lens disorder —see Glaucoma, secondary,
        Lowe's syndrome E72.03 [H42]
    metabolic disease NOS E88.9 [H42]
    ocular disorders NEC —see Glaucoma,
        secondary

Glaucoma (Continued)
  in (due to) (Continued)
    onchocerciasis B73.02
    pupillary block —see Glaucoma, secondary
    retinal vein occlusion —see Glaucoma,
        secondary
    Rieger's anomaly Q13.81 [H42]
    rubeosis of iris —see Glaucoma, secondary
    tumor of globe —see Glaucoma, secondary
  infantile Q15.0
  low tension —see Glaucoma, open angle,
      primary, low-tension
  malignant H40.83-●
  narrow angle —see Glaucoma, angle-closure
  newborn Q15.0
  noncongestive (chronic) —see Glaucoma,
      open angle
  nonobstructive —see Glaucoma, open angle
  obstructive —see also Glaucoma,
      angle-closure
    due to lens changes —see Glaucoma,
        secondary
  open angle H40.10-●
    primary H40.11-●
      capsular (with pseudoexfoliation of lens)
          H40.14-●
      low-tension H40.12-●
      pigmentary H40.13-●
      residual stage H40.15-●
  phacolytic —see Glaucoma, secondary
  pigmentary —see Glaucoma, open angle,
      primary, pigmentary
  postinfectious —see Glaucoma, secondary,
      inflammation
  secondary (to) H40.5-●
    drugs H40.6-●
    inflammation H40.4-●
    trauma H40.3-●
  simple (chronic) H40.11-●
  simplex H40.11-●
  specified type NEC H40.89
  suspect H40.00-●
  syphilitic A52.71
  traumatic —see also Glaucoma, secondary,
      trauma
    newborn (birth injury) P15.3
  tuberculous A18.59
Glaucomatous flecks (subcapsular) —see
    Cataract, complicated
Glazed tongue K14.4
Gleet (gonococcal) A54.01
Glénard's disease K63.4
Glioblastoma (multiforme)
  with sarcomatous component
    specified site —see Neoplasm, malignant,
        by site
    unspecified site C71.9
  giant cell
    specified site —see Neoplasm, malignant,
        by site
    unspecified site C71.9
  specified site —see Neoplasm, malignant, by
      site
  unspecified site C71.9
Glioma (malignant)
  astrocytic
    specified site —see Neoplasm, malignant,
        by site
    unspecified site C71.9
  mixed
    specified site —see Neoplasm, malignant,
        by site
    unspecified site C71.9
  nose Q30.8
  specified site NEC —see Neoplasm,
      malignant, by site
  subependymal D43.2
    specified site —see Neoplasm, uncertain
        behavior, by site
    unspecified site D43.2
  unspecified site C71.9
Gliomatosis cerebri C71.0

Glioneuroma —see Neoplasm, uncertain
    behavior, by site
Gliosarcoma
  specified site —see Neoplasm, malignant, by
      site
  unspecified site C71.9
Gliosis (cerebral) G93.89
  spinal G95.89
Glisson's disease —see Rickets
Globinuria R82.3
Globus (hystericus) F45.8
Glomangioma D18.00
  intra-abdominal D18.03
  intracranial D18.02
  skin D18.01
  specified site NEC D18.09
Glomangiomyoma D18.00
  intra-abdominal D18.03
  intracranial D18.02
  skin D18.01
  specified site NEC D18.09
Glomangiosarcoma —see Neoplasm, connective
    tissue, malignant
Glomerular
  disease in syphilis A52.75
  nephritis —see Glomerulonephritis
Glomerulitis —see Glomerulonephritis
Glomerulonephritis —see also Nephritis N05.9
  with
    C3
      glomerulonephritis N05.A
      glomerulopathy N05.A
        with dense deposit disease N05.6
    edema —see Nephrosis
    minimal change N05.0
    minor glomerular abnormality N05.0
  acute N00.9
  chronic N03.9
  crescentic (diffuse) NEC —see also N00-N07
      with fourth character .7 N05.7
  dense deposit —see also N00-N07 with fourth
      character .6 N05.6
  diffuse
    crescentic —see also N00-N07 with fourth
        character .7 N05.7
    endocapillary proliferative —see also
        N00N07 with fourth character .4 N05.4
    membranous —see also N00-N07 with
        fourth character .2 N05.2
    mesangial proliferative —see also N00-N07
        with fourth character .3 N05.3
    mesangiocapillary —see also N00-N07 with
        fourth character .5 N05.5
    sclerosing N18.9
  endocapillary proliferative (diffuse) NEC —
      see also N00-N07 with fourth character
      .4 N05.4
  extracapillary NEC —see also N00-N07 with
      fourth character .7 N05.7
  focal (and segmental) —see also N00-N07 with
      fourth character .1 N05.1
  hypocomplementemic —
      see Glomerulonephritis,
      membranoproliferative
  IgA —see Nephropathy, IgA
  immune complex (circulating) NEC N05.8
  in (due to)
    amyloidosis E85.4 [N08]
    bilharziasis B65.9 [N08]
    cryoglobulinemia D89.1 [N08]
    defibrination syndrome D65 [N08]
    diabetes mellitus —see Diabetes,
        glomerulosclerosis
    disseminated intravascular coagulation
        D65 [N08]
    Fabry (-Anderson) disease E75.21 [N08]
    Goodpasture's syndrome M31.0
    hemolytic-uremic syndrome D59.3
    Henoch (-Schönlein) purpura D69.0 [N08]
    lecithin cholesterol acyltransferase
        deficiency E78.6 [N08]

Glomerulonephritis (Continued)
  in (Continued)
    microscopic polyangiitis M31.7 [N08]
    multiple myeloma C90.0- ● [N08]
    Plasmodium malariae B52.0
    schistosomiasis B65.9 [N08]
    sepsis A41.9- ● [N08]
      streptococcal A40- ● [N08]
    sickle-cell disorders D57.- ● [N08]
    strongyloidiasis B78.9 [N08]
    subacute bacterial endocarditis I33.0
      [N08]
    syphilis (late) congenital A50.59 [N08]
    systemic lupus erythematosus M32.14
➡️ thrombotic thrombocytopenic purpura
      M31.19 [N08]
    typhoid fever A01.09
    Waldenström macroglobulinemia C88.0
      [N08]
    Wegener's granulomatosis M31.31
  latent or quiescent N03.9
  lobular, lobulonodular —
      see Glomerulonephritis,
      membranoproliferative
  membranoproliferative (diffuse) (type 1
      or 3) —see also N00-N07 with fourth
      character .5 N05.5
    dense deposit (type 2) NEC —see also
      N00-N07 with fourth character .6
      N05.6
  membranous (diffuse) NEC —see also
      N00-N07 with fourth character .2 N05.2
  mesangial
    IgA/IgG —see Nephropathy, IgA
    proliferative (diffuse) NEC —see also
      N00-N07 with fourth character .3
      N05.3
  mesangiocapillary (diffuse) NEC —see also
      N00-N07 with fourth character .5 N05.5
  necrotic, necrotizing NEC —see also N00-N07
      with fourth character .8 N05.8
  nodular —see Glomerulonephritis,
      membranoproliferative
  poststreptococcal NEC N05.9
    acute N00.9
    chronic N03.9
    rapidly progressive N01.9
  proliferative NEC —see also N00-N07 with
      fourth character .8 N05.8
    diffuse (lupus) M32.14
  rapidly progressive N01.9
  sclerosing, diffuse N18.9
  specified pathology NEC —see also N00-N07
      with fourth character .8 N05.8
  subacute N01.9
Glomerulopathy —see Glomerulonephritis
Glomerulosclerosis —see also Sclerosis, renal
  intercapillary (nodular) (with diabetes) —see
      Diabetes, glomerulosclerosis
  intracapillary —see Diabetes, glomerulosclerosis
Glossagra K14.6
Glossalgia K14.6
Glossitis (chronic superficial) (gangrenous)
      (Moeller's) K14.0
  areata exfoliativa K14.1
  atrophic K14.4
  benign migratory K14.1
  cortical superficial, sclerotic K14.0
  Hunter's D51.0
  interstitial, sclerous K14.0
  median rhomboid K14.2
  pellagrous E52
  superficial, chronic K14.0
Glossocele K14.8
Glossodynia K14.6
  exfoliativa K14.4
Glossoncus K14.8
Glossopathy K14.9
Glossophytia K14.3
Glossoplegia K14.8
Glossoptosis K14.8

Glossopyrosis K14.6
Glossotrichia K14.3
Glossy skin L90.8
Glottis —see condition
Glottitis —see also Laryngitis J04.0
Glucagonoma
  pancreas
    benign D13.7
    malignant C25.4
    uncertain behavior D37.8
  specified site NEC
    benign —see Neoplasm, benign, by site
    malignant —see Neoplasm, malignant, by
      site
    uncertain behavior —see Neoplasm,
      uncertain behavior, by site
  unspecified site
    benign D13.7
    malignant C25.4
    uncertain behavior D37.8
Glucoglycinuria E72.51
Glucose-galactose malabsorption E74.39
Glue
  ear —see Otitis, media, nonsuppurative,
      chronic, mucoid
  sniffing (airplane) —see Abuse, drug, inhalant
    dependence —see Dependence, drug,
      inhalant
GLUT1 deficiency syndrome 1, infantile onset
      E74.810
GLUT1 deficiency syndrome 2, childhood
      onset E74.810
Glutaric aciduria E72.3
Glycinemia E72.51
Glycinuria (renal) (with ketosis) E72.09
Glycogen
  infiltration —see Disease, glycogen storage
  storage disease —see Disease, glycogen storage
Glycogenosis (diffuse) (generalized) —see also
      Disease, glycogen storage
  cardiac E74.02 [I43]
  diabetic, secondary —see Diabetes,
      glycogenosis, secondary
  pulmonary interstitial J84.842
Glycopenia E16.2
Glycosuria R81
  renal (familial) E74.818
Gnathostoma spinigerum (infection)
      (infestation), gnathostomiasis (wandering
      swelling) B83.1
Goiter (plunging) (substernal) E04.9
  with
    hyperthyroidism (recurrent) —see
      Hyperthyroidism, with, goiter
    thyrotoxicosis —see Hyperthyroidism,
      with, goiter
  adenomatous —see Goiter, nodular
  cancerous C73
  congenital (nontoxic) E03.0
    diffuse E03.0
    parenchymatous E03.0
    transitory, with normal functioning P72.0
  cystic E04.2
    due to iodine-deficiency E01.1
  due to
    enzyme defect in synthesis of thyroid
      hormone E07.1
    iodine-deficiency (endemic) E01.2
  dyshormonogenetic (familial) E07.1
  endemic (iodine-deficiency) E01.2
    diffuse E01.0
    multinodular E01.1
  exophthalmic —see Hyperthyroidism, with,
      goiter
  iodine-deficiency (endemic) E01.2
    diffuse E01.0
    multinodular E01.1
    nodular E01.1
  lingual Q89.2
  lymphadenoid E06.3
  malignant C73

Goiter (Continued)
  multinodular (cystic) (nontoxic) E04.2
    toxic or with hyperthyroidism E05.20
      with thyroid storm E05.21
  neonatal NEC P72.0
  nodular (nontoxic) (due to) E04.9
    with
      hyperthyroidism E05.20
        with thyroid storm E05.21
      thyrotoxicosis E05.20
        with thyroid storm E05.21
    endemic E01.1
    iodine-deficiency E01.1
    sporadic E04.9
    toxic E05.20
      with thyroid storm E05.21
  nontoxic E04.9
    diffuse (colloid) E04.0
    multinodular E04.2
    simple E04.0
    specified NEC E04.8
    uninodular E04.1
  simple E04.0
  toxic —see Hyperthyroidism, with, goiter
  uninodular (nontoxic) E04.1
    toxic or with hyperthyroidism E05.10
      with thyroid storm E05.11
Goiter-deafness syndrome E07.1
Goldberg syndrome Q89.8
Goldberg-Maxwell syndrome E34.51
Goldblatt's hypertension or kidney I70.1
Goldenhar (-Gorlin) syndrome Q87.0
Goldflam-Erb disease or syndrome G70.00
  with exacerbation (acute) G70.01
  in crisis G70.01
Goldscheider's disease Q81.8
Goldstein's disease (familial hemorrhagic
      telangiectasia) I78.0
Golfer's elbow —see Epicondylitis, medial
Gonadoblastoma
  specified site —see Neoplasm, uncertain
      behavior, by site
  unspecified site
    female D39.10
    male D40.10
Gonecystitis —see Vesiculitis
Gongylonemiasis B83.8
Goniosynechiae —see Adhesions, iris,
      goniosynechiae
Gonococcemia A54.86
Gonococcus, gonococcal (disease) (infection)
      —see also condition A54.9
  anus A54.6
  bursa, bursitis A54.49
  conjunctiva, conjunctivitis (neonatorum)
      A54.31
  endocardium A54.83
  eye A54.30
    conjunctivitis A54.31
    iridocyclitis A54.32
    keratitis A54.33
    newborn A54.31
    other specified A54.39
  fallopian tubes (acute) (chronic) A54.24
  genitourinary (organ) (system) (tract) (acute)
    lower A54.00
      with abscess (accessory gland)
        (periurethral) A54.1
    upper —see also condition A54.29
  heart A54.83
  iridocyclitis A54.32
  joint A54.42
  lymphatic (gland) (node) A54.89
  meninges, meningitis A54.81
  musculoskeletal A54.40
    arthritis A54.42
    osteomyelitis A54.43
    other specified A54.49
    spondylopathy A54.41
  pelviperitonitis A54.24
  pelvis (acute) (chronic) A54.24

▶ New   ➡️ Revised   ~~deleted~~ Deleted   ● Use Additional Character(s)

Gonococcus, gonococcal *(Continued)*
  pharynx A54.5
  proctitis A54.6
  pyosalpinx (acute) (chronic) A54.24
  rectum A54.6
  skin A54.89
  specified site NEC A54.89
  tendon sheath A54.49
  throat A54.5
  urethra (acute) (chronic) A54.01
    with abscess (accessory gland)
      (periurethral) A54.1
  vulva (acute) (chronic) A54.02
Gonocytoma
  specified site —*see* Neoplasm, uncertain
    behavior, by site
  unspecified site
    female D39.10
    male D40.10
Gonorrhea (acute) (chronic) A54.9
  Bartholin's gland (acute) (chronic) (purulent)
    A54.02
    with abscess (accessory gland)
      (periurethral) A54.1
  bladder A54.01
  cervix A54.03
  conjunctiva, conjunctivitis (neonatorum)
    A54.31
  contact Z20.2
  Cowper's gland (with abscess) A54.1
  exposure to Z20.2
  fallopian tube (acute) (chronic) A54.24
  kidney (acute) (chronic) A54.21
  lower genitourinary tract A54.00
    with abscess (accessory gland)
      (periurethral) A54.1
  ovary (acute) (chronic) A54.24
  pelvis (acute) (chronic) A54.24
    female pelvic inflammatory disease A54.24
  penis A54.09
  prostate (acute) (chronic) A54.22
  seminal vesicle (acute) (chronic) A54.23
  specified site not listed —*see also* Gonococcus
    A54.89
  spermatic cord (acute) (chronic) A54.23
  urethra A54.01
    with abscess (accessory gland)
      (periurethral) A54.1
  vagina A54.02
  vas deferens (acute) (chronic) A54.23
  vulva A54.02
Goodall's disease A08.19
Goodpasture's syndrome M31.0
Gopalan's syndrome (burning feet) E53.0
Gorlin-Chaudry-Moss syndrome Q87.0
Gottron's papules L94.4
Gougerot's syndrome (trisymptomatic) L81.7
Gougerot-Blum syndrome (pigmented
  purpuric lichenoid dermatitis) L81.7
Gougerot-Carteaud disease or syndrome
  (confluent reticulate papillomatosis) L83
Gouley's syndrome (constrictive pericarditis)
  I31.1
Goundou A66.6
Gout, chronic (*see also* Gout, gouty) M1A.9-•
  drug-induced M1A.20
    ankle M1A.27-•
    elbow M1A.22-•
    foot joint M1A.27-•
    hand joint M1A.24-•
    hip M1A.25-•
    knee M1A.26-•
    multiple site M1A.29-•
    shoulder M1A.21-•
    vertebrae M1A.28
    wrist M1A.23-•
  idiopathic M1A.00
    ankle M1A.07-•
    elbow M1A.02-•
    foot joint M1A.07-•
    hand joint M1A.04-•

Gout, chronic *(Continued)*
  idiopathic *(Continued)*
    hip M1A.05-•
    knee M1A.06-•
    multiple site M1A.09
    shoulder M1A.01-•
    vertebrae M1A.08
    wrist M1A.03-•
  in (due to) renal impairment M1A.30
    ankle M1A.37-•
    elbow M1A.32-•
    foot joint M1A.37-•
    hand joint M1A.34-•
    hip M1A.35-•
    knee M1A.36-•
    multiple site M1A.39
    shoulder M1A.31-•
    vertebrae M1A.38
    wrist M1A.33-•
  lead-induced M1A.10
    ankle M1A.17-•
    elbow M1A.12-•
    foot joint M1A.17-•
    hand joint M1A.14-•
    hip M1A.15-•
    knee M1A.16-•
    multiple site M1A.19
    shoulder M1A.11-•
    vertebrae M1A.18
    wrist M1A.13-•
  primary —*see* Gout, chronic, idiopathic
  saturnine —*see* Gout, chronic, lead-induced
  secondary NEC M1A.40
    ankle M1A.47-•
    elbow M1A.42-•
    foot joint M1A.47-•
    hand joint M1A.44-•
    hip M1A.45-•
    knee M1A.46-•
    multiple site M1A.49
    shoulder M1A.41-•
    vertebrae M1A.48
    wrist M1A.43-•
  syphilitic —*see also* subcategory M14.8-•
    A52.77
  tophi M1A.9
Gout, gouty (acute) (attack) (flare) —*see also*
  Gout, chronic M10.9-•
  drug-induced M10.20
    ankle M10.27-•
    elbow M10.22-•
    foot joint M10.27-•
    hand joint M10.24-•
    hip M10.25-•
    knee M10.26-•
    multiple site M10.29
    shoulder M10.21-•
    vertebrae M10.28
    wrist M10.23-•
  idiopathic M10.00
    ankle M10.07-•
    elbow M10.02-•
    foot joint M10.07-•
    hand joint M10.04-•
    hip M10.05-•
    knee M10.06-•
    multiple site M10.09
    shoulder M10.01-•
    vertebrae M10.08
    wrist M10.03-•
  in (due to) renal impairment M10.30
    ankle M10.37-•
    elbow M10.32-•
    foot joint M10.37-•
    hand joint M10.34-•
    hip M10.35-•
    knee M10.36-•
    multiple site M10.39
    shoulder M10.31-•
    vertebrae M10.38
    wrist M10.33-•

Gout, gouty *(Continued)*
  lead-induced M10.10
    ankle M10.17-•
    elbow M10.12-•
    foot joint M10.17-•
    hand joint M10.14-•
    hip M10.15-•
    knee M10.16-•
    multiple site M10.19
    shoulder M10.11-•
    vertebrae M10.18
    wrist M10.13-•
  primary —*see* Gout, idiopathic
  saturnine —*see* Gout, lead-induced
  secondary NEC M10.40
    ankle M10.47-•
    elbow M10.42-•
    foot joint M10.47-•
    hand joint M10.44-•
    hip M10.45-•
    knee M10.46-•
    multiple site M10.49
    shoulder M10.41-•
    vertebrae M10.48
    wrist M10.43-•
  syphilitic —*see also* subcategory M14.8-•
    A52.77
  tophi NEC —*see* Gout, chronic
Gower's
  muscular dystrophy G71.01
  syndrome (vasovagal attack) R55
Gradenigo's syndrome —*see* Otitis, media,
  suppurative, acute
Graefe's disease —*see* Strabismus, paralytic,
  ophthalmoplegia, progressive
Graft-versus-host disease D89.813
  acute D89.810
  acute on chronic D89.812
  chronic D89.811
Grain mite (itch) B88.0
Grainhandler's disease or lung J67.8
Grand mal —*see* Epilepsy, generalized,
  specified NEC
Grand multipara status only (not pregnant)
  Z64.1
  pregnant —*see* Pregnancy, complicated by,
    grand multiparity
Granite worker's lung J62.8
Granular —*see also* condition
  inflammation, pharynx J31.2
  kidney (contracting) —*see* Sclerosis, renal
  liver K74.69
Granulation tissue (abnormal) (excessive) L92.9
  postmastoidectomy cavity —*see*
    Complications, postmastoidectomy,
    granulation
Granulocytopenia (primary) (malignant) —*see*
  Agranulocytosis
Granuloma L92.9
  abdomen K66.8
    from residual foreign body L92.3
    pyogenicum L98.0
  actinic L57.5
  annulare (perforating) L92.0
  apical K04.5
  aural —*see* Otitis, externa, specified NEC
  beryllium (skin) L92.3
  bone
    eosinophilic C96.6
    from residual foreign body —*see*
      Osteomyelitis, specified type NEC
    lung C96.6
  brain (any site) G06.0
    schistosomiasis B65.9 *[G07]*
  canaliculus lacrimalis —*see* Granuloma,
    lacrimal
  candidal (cutaneous) B37.2
  cerebral (any site) G06.0
  coccidioidal (primary) (progressive) B38.7
    lung B38.1
    meninges B38.4

Granuloma (Continued)
colon K63.89
conjunctiva H11.22-●
dental K04.5
ear, middle —see Cholesteatoma
eosinophilic C96.6
  bone C96.6
  lung C96.6
  oral mucosa K13.4
  skin L92.2
eyelid H01.8
facial (e) L92.2
foreign body (in soft tissue) NEC M60.20
  ankle M60.27-●
  foot M60.27-●
  forearm M60.23-●
  hand M60.24-●
  in operation wound —see Foreign body,
    accidentally left during a procedure
  lower leg M60.26-●
  pelvic region M60.25-●
  shoulder region M60.21-●
  skin L92.3
  specified site NEC M60.28
  subcutaneous tissue L92.3
  thigh M60.25-●
  upper arm M60.22-●
gangraenescens M31.2
genito-inguinale A58
giant cell (central) (reparative) (jaw) M27.1
  gingiva (peripheral) K06.8
gland (lymph) I88.8
hepatic NEC K75.3
  in (due to)
    berylliosis J63.2 [K77]
    sarcoidosis D86.89
Hodgkin C81.9
ileum K63.89
infectious B99.9
  specified NEC B99.8
inguinale (Donovan) (venereal) A58
intestine NEC K63.89
intracranial (any site) G06.0
intraspinal (any part) G06.1
iridocyclitis —see Iridocyclitis, chronic
jaw (bone) (central) M27.1
  reparative giant cell M27.1
kidney —see also Infection, kidney N15.8
lacrimal H04.81-●
larynx J38.7
lethal midline (faciale) (e) M31.2
liver NEC —see Granuloma, hepatic
lung (infectious) —see also Fibrosis, lung
  coccidioidal B38.1
  eosinophilic C96.6
Majocchi's B35.8
malignant (facial (e)) M31.2
mandible (central) M27.1
midline (lethal) M31.2
monilial (cutaneous) B37.2
nasal sinus —see Sinusitis
operation wound T81.89
  foreign body —see Foreign body,
    accidentally left during a procedure
  stitch T81.89
  talc —see Foreign body, accidentally left
    during a procedure
oral mucosa K13.4
orbit, orbital H05.11-●
paracoccidioidal B41.8
penis, venereal A58
periapical K04.5
peritoneum K66.8
  due to ova of helminths NOS —see also
    Helminthiasis B83.9 [K67]
postmastoidectomy cavity —see
    Complications, postmastoidectomy,
    recurrent cholesteatoma
prostate N42.89
pudendi (ulcerating) A58
pulp, internal (tooth) K03.3

Granuloma (Continued)
pyogenic, pyogenicum (of) (skin) L98.0
  gingiva K06.8
  maxillary alveolar ridge K04.5
  oral mucosa K13.4
rectum K62.89
reticulohistiocytic D76.3
rubrum nasi L74.8
Schistosoma —see Schistosomiasis
septic (skin) L98.0
silica (skin) L92.3
sinus (accessory) (infective) (nasal) —see
    Sinusitis
skin L92.9
  from residual foreign body L92.3
  pyogenicum L98.0
spine
  syphilitic (epidural) A52.19
  tuberculous A18.01
stitch (postoperative) T81.89
suppurative (skin) L98.0
swimming pool A31.1
talc —see also Granuloma, foreign body
  in operation wound —see Foreign body,
    accidentally left during a procedure
telangiectaticum (skin) L98.0
tracheostomy J95.09
trichophyticum B35.8
tropicum A66.4
umbilical P83.81
umbilicus P83.81
urethra N36.8
uveitis —see Iridocyclitis, chronic
vagina A58
venereum A58
vocal cord J38.3
Granulomatosis L92.9
  with polyangiitis M31.3
  eosinophilic, with polyangiitis [EGPA] M30.1
  lymphoid C83.8-●
  miliary (listerial) A32.89
  necrotizing, respiratory M31.30
  progressive septic D71
  specified NEC L92.8
  Wegener's M31.30
    with renal involvement M31.31
Granulomatous tissue (abnormal) (excessive)
    L92.9
Granulosis rubra nasi L74.8
Graphite fibrosis (of lung) J63.3
Graphospasm F48.8
  organic G25.89
Grating scapula M89.8X1
Gravel (urinary) —see Calculus, urinary
Graves' disease —see Hyperthyroidism, with,
    goiter
Gravis —see condition
Grawitz tumor C64.-●
Gray syndrome (newborn) P93.0
Grayness, hair (premature) L67.1
  congenital Q84.2
Green sickness D50.8
Greenfield's disease
  meaning
    concentric sclerosis (encephalitis periaxialis
      concentrica) G37.5
    metachromatic leukodystrophy E75.25
Greenstick fracture - code as Fracture, by site
Grey syndrome (newborn) P93.0
Grief F43.21
  prolonged F43.29
  reaction —see also Disorder, adjustment F43.20
Griesinger's disease B76.0
Grinder's lung or pneumoconiosis J62.8
Grinding, teeth
  psychogenic F45.8
  sleep related G47.63
Grip
  Dabney's B33.0
  devil's B33.0
Grippe, grippal —see also Influenza
  Balkan A78
  summer, of Italy A93.1

Grisel's disease M43.6
Groin —see condition
Grooved tongue K14.5
Ground itch B76.9
Grover's disease or syndrome L11.1
Growing pains, children R29.898
Growth (fungoid) (neoplastic) (new) —see also
    Neoplasm
  adenoid (vegetative) J35.8
  benign —see Neoplasm, benign, by site
  malignant —see Neoplasm, malignant, by site
  rapid, childhood Z00.2
  secondary —see Neoplasm, secondary, by site
Gruby's disease B35.0
Gubler-Millard paralysis or syndrome G46.3
Guerin-Stern syndrome Q74.3
Guidance, insufficient anterior (occlusal) M26.54
Guillain-Barré disease or syndrome G61.0
  sequelae G65.0
Guinea worms (infection) (infestation) B72
Guinon's disease (motor-verbal tic) F95.2
Gull's disease E03.4
Gum —see condition
Gumboil K04.7
  with sinus K04.6
Gumma (syphilitic) A52.79
  artery A52.09
    cerebral A52.04
  bone A52.77
    of yaws (late) A66.6
  brain A52.19
  cauda equina A52.19
  central nervous system A52.3
  ciliary body A52.71
  congenital A50.59
  eyelid A52.71
  heart A52.06
  intracranial A52.19
  iris A52.71
  kidney A52.75
  larynx A52.73
  leptomeninges A52.19
  liver A52.74
  meninges A52.19
  myocardium A52.06
  nasopharynx A52.73
  neurosyphilitic A52.3
  nose A52.73
  orbit A52.71
  palate (soft) A52.79
  penis A52.76
  pericardium A52.06
  pharynx A52.73
  pituitary A52.79
  scrofulous (tuberculous) A18.4
  skin A52.79
  specified site NEC A52.79
  spinal cord A52.19
  tongue A52.79
  tonsil A52.73
  trachea A52.73
  tuberculous A18.4
  ulcerative due to yaws A66.4
  ureter A52.75
  yaws A66.4
    bone A66.6
Gunn's syndrome Q07.8
Gunshot wound —see also Puncture, open
  fracture - code as Fracture, by site
  internal organs —see Injury, by site
Gynandrism Q56.0
Gynandroblastoma
  specified site —see Neoplasm, uncertain
    behavior, by site
  unspecified site
    female D39.10
    male D40.10
Gynecological examination (periodic) (routine)
    Z01.419
  with abnormal findings Z01.411
Gynecomastia N62
Gynephobia F40.291
Gyrate scalp Q82.8

▶ New   ⇒ Revised   ~~deleted~~ Deleted   ● Use Additional Character(s)

H

H (Hartnup's) disease E72.02
Haas' disease or osteochondrosis (juvenile) (head of humerus) —see Osteochondrosis, juvenile, humerus
Habit, habituation
 bad sleep Z72.821
 chorea F95.8
 disturbance, child F98.9
 drug —see Dependence, drug
 irregular sleep Z72.821
 laxative F55.2
 spasm —see Tic
 tic —see Tic
Haemophilus (H.) influenzae, as cause of disease classified elsewhere B96.3
Haff disease —see Poisoning, mercury
Hageman's factor defect, deficiency or disease D68.2
Haglund's disease or osteochondrosis (juvenile) (os tibiale externum) —see Osteochondrosis, juvenile, tarsus
Hailey-Hailey disease Q82.8
Hair —see also condition
 plucking F63.3
  in stereotyped movement disorder F98.4
 tourniquet syndrome —see also Constriction, external, by site
  finger S60.44-●
  penis S30.842
  thumb S60.34-●
  toe S90.44-●
Hairball in stomach T18.2
Hair-pulling, pathological (compulsive) F63.3
Hairy black tongue K14.3
Half vertebra Q76.49
Halitosis R19.6
Hallerman-Streiff syndrome Q87.0
Hallervorden-Spatz disease G23.0
Hallopeau's acrodermatitis or disease L40.2
Hallucination R44.3
 auditory R44.0
 gustatory R44.2
 olfactory R44.2
 specified NEC R44.2
 tactile R44.2
 visual R44.1
Hallucinosis (chronic) F28
 alcoholic (acute) F10.951
  in
   abuse F10.151
   dependence F10.251
 drug-induced F19.951
  cannabis F12.951
  cocaine F14.951
  hallucinogen F16.151
  in
   abuse F19.151
    cannabis F12.151
    cocaine F14.151
    hallucinogen F16.151
    inhalant F18.151
    opioid F11.151
    sedative, anxiolytic or hypnotic F13.151
    stimulant NEC F15.151
   dependence F19.251
    cannabis F12.251
    cocaine F14.251
    hallucinogen F16.251
    inhalant F18.251
    opioid F11.251
    sedative, anxiolytic or hypnotic F13.251
    stimulant NEC F15.251
  inhalant F18.951
  opioid F11.951
  sedative, anxiolytic or hypnotic F13.951
  stimulant NEC F15.951
 organic F06.0

Hallux
 deformity (acquired) NEC M20.5X-●
 limitus M20.5X-●
 malleus (acquired) NEC M20.3-●
 rigidus (acquired) M20.2-●
  congenital Q74.2
  sequelae (late effect) of rickets E64.3
 valgus (acquired) M20.1-●
  congenital Q66.6
 varus (acquired) M20.3-●
  congenital Q66.3-●
Halo, visual H53.19
Hamartoma, hamartoblastoma Q85.9
 epithelial (gingival), odontogenic, central or peripheral —see Cyst, calcifying odontogenic
Hamartosis Q85.9
Hamman-Rich syndrome J84.114
Hammer toe (acquired) NEC —see also Deformity, toe, hammer toe
 congenital Q66.89
 sequelae (late effect) of rickets E64.3
Hand —see condition
Hand-foot syndrome L27.1
Handicap, handicapped
 educational Z55.9
  specified NEC Z55.8
Hand-Schüller-Christian disease or syndrome C96.5
Hanging (asphyxia) (strangulation) (suffocation) —see Asphyxia, traumatic, due to mechanical threat
Hangnail —see also Cellulitis, digit
 with lymphangitis —see Lymphangitis, acute, digit
Hangover (alcohol) F10.129
Hanhart's syndrome Q87.0
Hanot-Chauffard (-Troisier) syndrome E83.19
Hanot's cirrhosis or disease K74.3
Hansen's disease —see Leprosy
Hantaan virus disease (Korean hemorrhagic fever) A98.5
Hantavirus disease (with renal manifestations) (Dobrava) (Puumala) (Seoul) A98.5
 with pulmonary manifestations (Andes) (Bayou) (Bermejo) (Black Creek Canal) (Choclo) (Juquitiba) (Laguna negra) (Lechiguanas) (New York) (Oran) (Sin nombre) B33.4
Happy puppet syndrome Q93.59
Harada's disease or syndrome H30.81-●
Hardening
 artery —see Arteriosclerosis
 brain G93.89
Harelip (complete) (incomplete) —see Cleft, lip
Harlequin (newborn) Q80.4
Harley's disease D59.6
Harmful use (of)
 alcohol F10.10
 anxiolytics —see Abuse, drug, sedative
 cannabinoids —see Abuse, drug, cannabis
 cocaine —see Abuse, drug, cocaine
 drug —see Abuse, drug
 hallucinogens —see Abuse, drug, hallucinogen
 hypnotics —see Abuse, drug, sedative -
  opioids —see Abuse, drug, opioid
 PCP (phencyclidine) —see Abuse, drug, hallucinogen
 sedatives —see Abuse, drug, sedative
 stimulants NEC —see Abuse, drug, stimulant
Harris' lines —see Arrest, epiphyseal
Hartnup's disease E72.02
Harvester's lung J67.0
Harvesting ovum for in vitro fertilization Z31.83
Hashimoto's disease or thyroiditis E06.3
Hashitoxicosis (transient) E06.3
Hassal-Henle bodies or warts (cornea) H18.49
Haut mal —see Epilepsy, generalized, specified NEC
Haverhill fever A25.1

Hay fever —see also Fever, hay J30.1
Hayem-Widal syndrome D59.8
Haygarth's nodes M15.8
Haymaker's lung J67.0
Hb (abnormal)
 Bart's disease D56.0
 disease —see Disease, hemoglobin
 trait —see Trait
Head —see condition
Headache R51.9
 with
  orthostatic component NEC R51.0
  positional component NEC R51.0
 allergic NEC G44.89
 associated with sexual activity G44.82
▶cervicogenic G44.86
 chronic daily R51.9
 cluster G44.009
  chronic G44.029
   intractable G44.021
   not intractable G44.029
  episodic G44.019
   intractable G44.011
   not intractable G44.019
  intractable G44.001
  not intractable G44.009
 cough (primary) G44.83
 daily chronic R51.9
 drug-induced NEC G44.40
  intractable G44.41
  not intractable G44.40
 exertional (primary) G44.84
 histamine G44.009
  intractable G44.001
  not intractable G44.009
 hypnic G44.81
 lumbar puncture G97.1
 medication overuse G44.40
  intractable G44.41
  not intractable G44.40
 menstrual —see Migraine, menstrual
 migraine (type) —see also Migraine G43.909
 nasal septum R51.9
 neuralgiform, short lasting unilateral, with conjunctival injection and tearing (SUNCT) G44.059
  intractable G44.051
  not intractable G44.059
 new daily persistent (NDPH) G44.52
 orgasmic G44.82
 periodic syndromes in adults and children G43.C0
  with refractory migraine G43.C1
  intractable G43.C1
  not intractable G43.C0
  without refractory migraine G43.C0
 postspinal puncture G97.1
 post-traumatic G44.309
  acute G44.319
   intractable G44.311
   not intractable G44.319
  chronic G44.329
   intractable G44.321
   not intractable G44.329
  intractable G44.301
  not intractable G44.309
 pre-menstrual —see Migraine, menstrual
 preorgasmic G44.82
 primary
  cough G44.83
  exertional G44.84
  stabbing G44.85
  thunderclap G44.53
 rebound G44.40
  intractable G44.41
  not intractable G44.40
 short lasting unilateral neuralgiform, with conjunctival injection and tearing (SUNCT) G44.059
  intractable G44.051
  not intractable G44.059
 specified syndrome NEC G44.89

Headache *(Continued)*
  spinal and epidural anesthesia - induced T88.59
    in labor and delivery O74.5
    in pregnancy O29.4-●
    postpartum, puerperal O89.4
  spinal fluid loss (from puncture) G97.1
  stabbing (primary) G44.85
  tension (-type) G44.209
    chronic G44.229
      intractable G44.221
      not intractable G44.229
    episodic G44.219
      intractable G44.211
      not intractable G44.219
    intractable G44.201
    not intractable G44.209
  thunderclap (primary) G44.53
  vascular NEC G44.1
Healthy
  infant
    accompanying sick mother Z76.3
    receiving care Z76.2
  person accompanying sick person Z76.3
Hearing examination Z01.10
  with abnormal findings NEC Z01.118
  infant or child (over 28 days old) Z00.129
    with abnormal findings Z00.121
  following failed hearing screening Z01.110
  for hearing conservation and treatment Z01.12
Heart —*see* condition
Heart beat
  abnormality R00.9
    specified NEC R00.8
  awareness R00.2
  rapid R00.0
  slow R00.1
Heartburn R12
  psychogenic F45.8
Heartland virus disease A93.8
Heat (effects) T67.9
  apoplexy T67.01
  burn —*see also* Burn L55.9
  collapse T67.1
  cramps T67.2
  dermatitis or eczema L59.0
  edema T67.7
  erythema - code by site under Burn, first degree
  excessive T67.9
    specified effect NEC T67.8
  exhaustion T67.5
    anhydrotic T67.3
    due to
      salt (and water) depletion T67.4
      water depletion T67.3
        with salt depletion T67.4
  fatigue (transient) T67.6
  fever T67.01
  hyperpyrexia T67.01
  prickly L74.0
  prostration —*see* Heat, exhaustion
  pyrexia T67.01
  rash L74.0
  specified effect NEC T67.8
  stroke T67.01
    exertional T67.02
    specified NEC T67.09
  sunburn —*see* Sunburn
  syncope T67.1
Heavy-for-dates NEC (infant) (4000g to 4499g)
    P08.1
  exceptionally (4500g or more) P08.0
Hebephrenia, hebephrenic (schizophrenia) F20.1
Heberden's disease or nodes (with
    arthropathy) M15.1
Hebra's
  pityriasis L26
  prurigo L28.2
Heel —*see* condition
Heerfordt's disease D86.89
Hegglin's anomaly or syndrome D72.0
Heilmeyer-Schoner disease D45

Heine-Medin disease A80.9
Heinz body anemia, congenital D58.2
Heliophobia F40.228
Heller's disease or syndrome F84.3
HELLP syndrome (hemolysis, elevated liver
    enzymes and low platelet count) O14.2-●
  complicating
    childbirth O14.24
    puerperium O14.25
Helminthiasis —*see also* Infestation, helminth
  Ancylostoma B76.0
  intestinal B82.0
    mixed types (types classifiable to more
      than one of the titles B65.0-B81.3 and
      B81.8) B81.4
    specified type NEC B81.8
  mixed types (intestinal) (types classifiable to
    more than one of the titles B65.0-B81.3
    and B81.8) B81.4
  Necator (americanus) B76.1
  specified type NEC B83.8
Heloma L84
Hemangioblastoma —*see* Neoplasm,
    connective tissue, uncertain behavior
  malignant —*see* Neoplasm, connective tissue,
    malignant
Hemangioendothelioma —*see also* Neoplasm,
    uncertain behavior, by site
  benign D18.00
    intra-abdominal D18.03
    intracranial D18.02
    skin D18.01
    specified site NEC D18.09
  bone (diffuse) —*see* Neoplasm, bone,
    malignant
  epithelioid —*see also* Neoplasm, uncertain
    behavior, by site
    malignant —*see* Neoplasm, malignant, by
      site
  malignant —*see* Neoplasm, connective tissue,
    malignant
Hemangiofibroma —*see* Neoplasm, benign,
    by site
Hemangiolipoma —*see* Lipoma
Hemangioma D18.00
  arteriovenous D18.00
    intra-abdominal D18.03
    intracranial D18.02
    skin D18.01
    specified site NEC D18.09
  capillary I78.1
    intra-abdominal D18.03
    intracranial D18.02
    skin D18.01
    specified site NEC D18.09
  cavernous D18.00
    intra-abdominal D18.03
    intracranial D18.02
    skin D18.01
    specified site NEC D18.09
  epithelioid D18.00
    intra-abdominal D18.03
    intracranial D18.02
    skin D18.01
    specified site NEC D18.09
  histiocytoid D18.00
    intra-abdominal D18.03
    intracranial D18.02
    skin D18.01
    specified site NEC D18.09
  infantile D18.00
    intra-abdominal D18.03
    intracranial D18.02
    skin D18.01
    specified site NEC D18.09
  intra-abdominal D18.03
  intracranial D18.02
  intramuscular D18.00
    intra-abdominal D18.03
    intracranial D18.02
    skin D18.01
    specified site NEC D18.09

Hemangioma *(Continued)*
  intrathoracic structures D18.09
  juvenile D18.00
  malignant —*see* Neoplasm, connective tissue,
    malignant
  plexiform D18.00
    intra-abdominal D18.03
    intracranial D18.02
    skin D18.01
    specified site NEC D18.09
  racemose D18.00
    intra-abdominal D18.03
    intracranial D18.02
    skin D18.01
    specified site NEC D18.09
  sclerosing —*see* Neoplasm, skin, benign
  simplex D18.00
    intra-abdominal D18.03
    intracranial D18.02
    skin D18.01
    specified site NEC D18.09
  skin D18.01
  specified site NEC D18.09
  venous D18.00
    intra-abdominal D18.03
    intracranial D18.02
    skin D18.01
    specified site NEC D18.09
  verrucous keratotic D18.00
    intra-abdominal D18.03
    intracranial D18.02
    skin D18.01
    specified site NEC D18.09
Hemangiomatosis (systemic) I78.8
  involving single site —*see* Hemangioma
Hemangiopericytoma —*see also* Neoplasm,
    connective tissue, uncertain behavior
  benign —*see* Neoplasm, connective tissue,
    benign
  malignant —*see* Neoplasm, connective tissue,
    malignant
Hemangiosarcoma —*see* Neoplasm, connective
    tissue, malignant
Hemarthrosis (nontraumatic) M25.00
  ankle M25.07-●
  elbow M25.02-●
  foot joint M25.07-●
  hand joint M25.04-●
  hip M25.05-●
  in hemophilic arthropathy —*see* Arthropathy,
    hemophilic
  knee M25.06-●
  shoulder M25.01-●
  specified joint NEC M25.08
  traumatic —*see* Sprain, by site
  vertebrae M25.08
  wrist M25.03-●
Hematemesis K92.0
  with ulcer - code by site under Ulcer, with
    hemorrhage K27.4
  newborn, neonatal P54.0
    due to swallowed maternal blood
      P78.2
Hematidrosis L74.8
Hematinuria —*see also* Hemoglobinuria
  malarial B50.8
Hematobilia K83.8
Hematocele
  female NEC N94.89
    with ectopic pregnancy O00.90
      with intrauterine pregnancy O00.91
    ovary N83.8
  male N50.1
Hematochezia —*see also* Melena K92.1
Hematochyluria —*see also* Infestation, filarial
  schistosomiasis (bilharziasis) B65.0
Hematocolpos (with hematometra or
    hematosalpinx) N89.7
Hematocornea —*see* Pigmentation, cornea,
    stromal
Hematogenous —*see* condition

▶ New   ⇒ Revised   ~~deleted~~ Deleted   ● Use Additional Character(s)

Hematoma (traumatic) (skin surface intact) —
    see also Contusion
  with
    injury of internal organs —*see* Injury, by site
    open wound —*see* Wound, open
  amputation stump (surgical) (late) T87.89
  aorta, dissecting I71.00
    abdominal I71.02
    thoracic I71.01
    thoracoabdominal I71.03
  aortic intramural —*see* Dissection, aorta
  arterial (complicating trauma) —*see* Injury,
      blood vessel, by site
  auricle —*see* Contusion, ear
    nontraumatic —*see* Disorder, pinna,
      hematoma
  birth injury NEC P15.8
  brain (traumatic)
    with
      cerebral laceration or contusion
        (diffuse) —*see* Injury, intracranial,
        diffuse
      focal —*see* Injury, intracranial, focal
    cerebellar, traumatic S06.37-●
    intracerebral, traumatic —*see* Injury,
      intracranial, intracerebral hemorrhage
    newborn NEC P52.4
      birth injury P10.1
    nontraumatic —*see* Hemorrhage,
      intracranial
    subarachnoid, arachnoid, traumatic —*see*
      Injury, intracranial, subarachnoid
      hemorrhage
    subdural, traumatic —*see* Injury,
      intracranial, subdural hemorrhage
  breast (nontraumatic) N64.89
  broad ligament (nontraumatic) N83.7
    traumatic S37.892
  cerebellar, traumatic S06.37-●
  cerebral —*see* Hematoma, brain
  cerebrum S06.36-●
    left S06.35-●
    right S06.34-●
  cesarean delivery wound O90.2
  complicating delivery (perineal) (pelvic)
      (vagina) (vulva) O71.7
  corpus cavernosum (nontraumatic) N48.89
  epididymis (nontraumatic) N50.1
  epidural (traumatic) —*see* Injury, intracranial,
      epidural hemorrhage
    spinal —*see* Injury, spinal cord, by region
  episiotomy O90.2
  face, birth injury P15.4
  genital organ NEC (nontraumatic)
    female (nonobstetric) N94.89
      traumatic S30.202
    male N50.1
      traumatic S30.201
  internal organs —*see* Injury, by site
  intracerebral, traumatic —*see* Injury,
      intracranial, intracerebral hemorrhage
  intraoperative —*see* Complications,
      intraoperative, hemorrhage
  labia (nontraumatic) (nonobstetric) N90.8
  liver (subcapsular) (nontraumatic) K76.89
    birth injury P15.0
  mediastinum —*see* Injury, intrathoracic
  mesosalpinx (nontraumatic) N83.7
    traumatic S37.898
  muscle - code by site under Contusion
  nontraumatic
    muscle M79.81
    soft tissue M79.81
  obstetrical surgical wound O90.2
  orbit, orbital (nontraumatic) —*see also*
      Hemorrhage, orbit
    traumatic —*see* Contusion, orbit
  pelvis (female) (nontraumatic) (nonobstetric)
      N94.89
    obstetric O71.7
    traumatic —*see* Injury, by site

Hematoma *(Continued)*
  penis (nontraumatic) N48.89
    birth injury P15.5
  perianal (nontraumatic) K64.5
  perineal S30.23
    complicating delivery O71.7
  perirenal —*see* Injury, kidney
  pinna —*see* Contusion, ear
    nontraumatic —*see* Disorder, pinna,
      hematoma
  placenta O43.89-●
  postoperative (postprocedural) —*see*
      Complication, postprocedural,
      hematoma
  retroperitoneal (nontraumatic) K66.1
    traumatic S36.892
  scrotum, superficial S30.22
    birth injury P15.5
  seminal vesicle (nontraumatic) N50.1
    traumatic S37.892
  spermatic cord (traumatic) S37.892
    nontraumatic N50.1
  spinal (cord) (meninges) —*see also* Injury,
      spinal cord, by region
    newborn (birth injury) P11.5
  spleen D73.5
    intraoperative —*see* Complications,
      intraoperative, hemorrhage, spleen
    postprocedural (postoperative) —*see*
      Complications, postprocedural,
      hemorrhage, spleen
  sternocleidomastoid, birth injury P15.2
  sternomastoid, birth injury P15.2
  subarachnoid (traumatic) —*see* Injury,
      intracranial, subarachnoid hemorrhage
    newborn (nontraumatic) P52.5
      due to birth injury P10.3
    nontraumatic —*see* Hemorrhage,
      intracranial, subarachnoid
  subdural (traumatic) —*see* Injury, intracranial,
      subdural hemorrhage
    newborn (localized) P52.8
      birth injury P10.0
    nontraumatic —*see* Hemorrhage,
      intracranial, subdural
  superficial, newborn P54.5
  testis (nontraumatic) N50.1
    birth injury P15.5
  tunica vaginalis (nontraumatic) N50.1
  umbilical cord, complicating delivery O69.5
  uterine ligament (broad) (nontraumatic) N83.7
    traumatic S37.892
  vagina (ruptured) (nontraumatic) N89.8
    complicating delivery O71.7
  vas deferens (nontraumatic) N50.1
    traumatic S37.892
  vitreous —*see* Hemorrhage, vitreous
  vulva (nontraumatic) (nonobstetric) N90.89
    complicating delivery O71.7
    newborn (birth injury) P15.5
Hematometra N85.7
  with hematocolpos N89.7
Hematomyelia (central) G95.19
  newborn (birth injury) P11.5
  traumatic T14.8
Hematomyelitis G04.90
Hematoperitoneum —*see* Hemoperitoneum
Hematophobia F40.230
Hematopneumothorax (*see* Hemothorax)
Hematopoiesis, cyclic D70.4
Hematoporphyria —*see* Porphyria
Hematorachis, hematorrhachis G95.19
  newborn (birth injury) P11.5
Hematosalpinx N83.6
  with
    hematocolpos N89.7
    hematometra N85.7
      with hematocolpos N89.7
    infectional —*see* Salpingitis
Hematospermia R36.1
Hematothorax (*see* Hemothorax)

Hematuria R31.9
  benign (familial) (of childhood) —*see also*
      Hematuria, idiopathic
    essential microscopic R31.1
  due to sulphonamide, sulfonamide —*see* Table
      of Drugs and Chemicals, by drug
  endemic —*see also* Schistosomiasis B65.0
  gross R31.0
  idiopathic N02.9
    with glomerular lesion
      C3
        glomerulonephritis N02.A
        glomerulopathy N02.A
          with dense deposit disease N02.6
      crescentic (diffuse) glomerulonephritis
        N02.7
      dense deposit disease N02.6
      endocapillary proliferative
        glomerulonephritis N02.4
      focal and segmental hyalinosis or
        sclerosis N02.1
      membranoproliferative (diffuse) N02.5
      membranous (diffuse) N02.2
      mesangial proliferative (diffuse) N02.3
      mesangiocapillary (diffuse) N02.5
      minor abnormality N02.0
      proliferative NEC N02.8
      specified pathology NEC N02.8
  intermittent —*see* Hematuria, idiopathic
  malarial B50.8
  microscopic NEC (with symptoms) R31.29
    asymptomatic R31.21
    benign essential R31.1
  paroxysmal —*see also* Hematuria, idiopathic
    nocturnal D59.5
  persistent —*see* Hematuria, idiopathic
  recurrent —*see* Hematuria, idiopathic
  tropical —*see also* Schistosomiasis B65.0
  tuberculous A18.13
Hemeralopia (day blindness) H53.11
  vitamin A deficiency E50.5
Hemi-akinesia R41.4
Hemianalgesia R20.0
Hemianencephaly Q00.0
Hemianesthesia R20.0
Hemianopia, hemianopsia (heteronymous)
    H53.47
  homonymous H53.46-●
  syphilitic A52.71
Hemiathetosis R25.8
Hemiatrophy R68.89
  cerebellar G31.9
  face, facial, progressive (Romberg) G51.8
  tongue K14.8
Hemiballism (us) G25.5
Hemicardia Q24.8
Hemicephalus, hemicephaly Q00.0
Hemichorea G25.5
Hemicolitis, left —*see* Colitis, left sided
Hemicrania
  congenital malformation Q00.0
  continua G44.51
  meaning migraine —*see also* Migraine G43.909
  paroxysmal G44.039
    chronic G44.049
      intractable G44.041
      not intractable G44.049
    episodic G44.039
      intractable G44.031
      not intractable G44.039
    intractable G44.031
    not intractable G44.039
Hemidystrophy —*see* Hemiatrophy
Hemiectromelia Q73.8
Hemihypalgesia R20.8
Hemihypesthesia R20.1
Hemi-inattention R41.4
Hemimelia Q73.8
  lower limb —*see* Defect, reduction, lower
      limb, specified type NEC
  upper limb —*see* Defect, reduction, upper
      limb, specified type NEC

Hemiparalysis —see Hemiplegia
Hemiparesis —see Hemiplegia
Hemiparesthesia R20.2
Hemiparkinsonism G20
Hemiplegia G81.9-●
  alternans facialis G83.89
  ascending NEC G81.90
    spinal G95.89
  congenital (cerebral) G80.8
    spastic G80.2
  embolic (current episode) I63.4-●
  flaccid G81.0-●
  following
    cerebrovascular disease I69.959
      cerebral infarction I69.35-●
      intracerebral hemorrhage I69.15-●
      nontraumatic intracranial hemorrhage
        NEC I69.25-●
      specified disease NEC I69.85-●
      stroke NOS I69.35-●
      subarachnoid hemorrhage I69.05-●
  hysterical F44.4
  newborn NEC P91.88
    birth injury P11.9
  spastic G81.1-●
    congenital G80.2
  thrombotic (current episode) I63.3-●
Hemisection, spinal cord —see Injury, spinal
    cord, by region
Hemispasm (facial) R25.2
Hemisporosis B48.8
Hemitremor R25.1
Hemivertebra Q76.49
  failure of segmentation with scoliosis Q76.3
  fusion with scoliosis Q76.3
Hemochromatosis E83.119
  with refractory anemia D46.1
  due to repeated red blood cell transfusion
    E83.111
  hereditary (primary) E83.110
  neonatal P78.84
  primary E83.110
  specified NEC E83.118
Hemoglobin —see also condition
  abnormal (disease) —see Disease, hemoglobin
  AS genotype D57.3
  Constant Spring D58.2
  E-beta thalassemia D56.5
  fetal, hereditary persistence (HPFH) D56.4
  H Constant Spring D56.0
  low NOS D64.9
  S (Hb S), heterozygous D57.3
Hemoglobinemia D59.9
  due to blood transfusion T80.89
  paroxysmal D59.6
    nocturnal D59.5
Hemoglobinopathy (mixed) D58.2
  with thalassemia D56.8
  sickle-cell D57.1
    with thalassemia D57.40
      with
        acute chest syndrome D57.411
        cerebral vascular involvement
          D57.413
        crisis (painful) D57.419
          with specified complication NEC
            D57.418
        splenic sequestration D57.412
        vasoocclusive pain D57.419
      without crisis D57.40
Hemoglobinuria R82.3
  with anemia, hemolytic, acquired (chronic)
    NEC D59.6
  cold (paroxysmal) (with Raynaud's
    syndrome) D59.6
    agglutinin D59.12
  due to exertion or hemolysis NEC D59.6
  intermittent D59.6
  malarial B50.8
  march D59.6

Hemoglobinuria (Continued)
  nocturnal (paroxysmal) D59.5
  paroxysmal (cold) D59.6
    nocturnal D59.5
Hemolymphangioma D18.1
Hemolysis
  intravascular
    with
      abortion —see Abortion, by type,
        complicated by, hemorrhage
      ectopic or molar pregnancy O08.1
      hemorrhage
        antepartum —see Hemorrhage,
          antepartum, with coagulation
          defect
        intrapartum —see also Hemorrhage,
          complicating, delivery O67.0
      postpartum O72.3
  neonatal (excessive) P58.9
    specified NEC P58.8
Hemolytic —see condition
Hemopericardium I31.2
  following acute myocardial infarction
    (current complication) I23.0
  newborn P54.8
  traumatic —see Injury, heart, with
    hemopericardium
Hemoperitoneum K66.1
  infectional K65.9
  traumatic S36.899
    with open wound —see Wound, open,
      with penetration into peritoneal
      cavity
Hemophilia (classical) (familial) (hereditary)
    D66
  A D66
  B D67
  C D68.1
  acquired D68.311
  autoimmune D68.311
  calcipriva —see also Defect, coagulation
    D68.4
  nonfamilial —see also Defect, coagulation
    D68.4
  secondary D68.311
  vascular D68.0
Hemophthalmos H44.81-●
Hemopneumothorax —see also Hemothorax
  traumatic S27.2
Hemoptysis R04.2
  newborn P26.9
  tuberculous —see Tuberculosis, pulmonary
Hemorrhage, hemorrhagic (concealed) R58
  abdomen R58
  accidental antepartum —see Hemorrhage,
    antepartum
  acute idiopathic pulmonary, in infants
    R04.81
  adenoid J35.8
  adrenal (capsule) (gland) E27.49
    medulla E27.8
    newborn P54.4
  after delivery —see Hemorrhage,
    postpartum
  alveolar
    lung, newborn P26.8
    process K08.89
  alveolus K08.89
  amputation stump (surgical) T87.89
  anemia (chronic) D50.0
    acute D62
  antepartum (with) O46.90
    with coagulation defect O46.00-●
      afibrinogenemia O46.01-●
      disseminated intravascular coagulation
        O46.02-●
      hypofibrinogenemia O46.01-●
      specified defect NEC O46.09-●
    before 20 weeks gestation O20.9
      specified type NEC O20.8
      threatened abortion O20.0

Hemorrhage, hemorrhagic (Continued)
  antepartum (Continued)
    due to
      abruptio placenta —see also Abruptio
        placentae O45.9-●
      leiomyoma, uterus —see Hemorrhage,
        antepartum, specified cause NEC
      placenta previa O44.1-●
      specified cause NEC —see subcategory
        O46.8X-●
  anus (sphincter) K62.5
  apoplexy (stroke) —see Hemorrhage,
    intracranial, intracerebral
  arachnoid —see Hemorrhage, intracranial,
    subarachnoid
  artery R58
    brain —see Hemorrhage, intracranial,
      intracerebral
  basilar (ganglion) I61.0
  bladder N32.89
  bowel K92.2
    newborn P54.3
  brain (miliary) (nontraumatic) —see
      Hemorrhage, intracranial, intracerebral
    due to
      birth injury P10.1
      syphilis A52.05
    epidural or extradural (traumatic) —
      see Injury, intracranial, epidural
      hemorrhage
    newborn P52.4
      birth injury P10.1
    subarachnoid —see Hemorrhage,
      intracranial, subarachnoid
    subdural —see Hemorrhage, intracranial,
      subdural
  brainstem (nontraumatic) I61.3
    traumatic S06.38-●
  breast N64.59
  bronchial tube —see Hemorrhage, lung
  bronchopulmonary —see Hemorrhage, lung
  bronchus —see Hemorrhage, lung
  bulbar I61.5
  capillary I78.8
    primary D69.8
  cecum K92.2
  cerebellar, cerebellum (nontraumatic) I61.4
    newborn P52.6
    traumatic S06.37-●
  cerebral, cerebrum —see also Hemorrhage,
      intracranial, intracerebral
    lobe I61.1
    newborn (anoxic) P52.4
      birth injury P10.1
  cerebromeningeal I61.8
  cerebrospinal —see Hemorrhage, intracranial,
    intracerebral
  cervix (uteri) (stump) NEC N88.8
  chamber, anterior (eye) —see Hyphema
  childbirth —see Hemorrhage, complicating,
    delivery
  choroid H31.30-●
    expulsive H31.31-●
  ciliary body —see Hyphema
  cochlea —see subcategory H83.8
  colon K92.2
  complicating
    abortion —see Abortion, by type,
      complicated by, hemorrhage
    delivery O67.9
      associated with coagulation defect
        (afibrinogenemia) (DIC)
        (hyperfibrinolysis) O67.0
      specified cause NEC O67.8
    surgical procedure —see Hemorrhage,
      intraoperative
  conjunctiva H11.3-●
    newborn P54.8
  cord, newborn (stump) P51.9
  corpus luteum (ruptured) cyst N83.1-●
  cortical (brain) I61.1

▶ New   ⇒ Revised   ~~deleted~~ Deleted   ● Use Additional Character(s)

Hemorrhage, hemorrhagic *(Continued)*
  cranial —*see* Hemorrhage, intracranial
  cutaneous R23.3
    due to autosensitivity, erythrocyte D69.2
    newborn P54.5
  delayed
    following ectopic or molar pregnancy
      O08.1
    postpartum O72.2
  diathesis (familial) D69.9
  disease D69.9
    newborn P53
    specified type NEC D69.8
  due to or associated with
    afibrinogenemia or other coagulation defect
      (conditions in categories D65-D69)
      antepartum —*see* Hemorrhage,
        antepartum, with coagulation
        defect
      intrapartum O67.0
  dental implant M27.61
  device, implant or graft —*see also*
      Complications, by site and type,
      specified NEC T85.838
    arterial graft NEC T82.838
    breast T85.838
    catheter NEC T85.838
      dialysis (renal) T82.838
        intraperitoneal T85.838
      infusion NEC T82.838
        spinal (epidural) (subdural)
          T85.830
      urinary (indwelling) T83.83
    electronic (electrode) (pulse generator)
        (stimulator)
      bone T84.83
      cardiac T82.837
      nervous system (brain) (peripheral
        nerve) (spinal) T85.830
      urinary T83.83
    fixation, internal (orthopedic) NEC
        T84.83
    gastrointestinal (bile duct) (esophagus)
        T85.838
    genital NEC T83.83
    heart NEC T82.837
    joint prosthesis T84.83
    ocular (corneal graft) (orbital implant)
        NEC T85.838
    orthopedic NEC T84.83
      bone graft T86.838
    specified NEC T85.838
    urinary NEC T83.83
    vascular NEC T82.838
    ventricular intracranial shunt T85.838
  duodenum, duodenal K92.2
    ulcer —*see* Ulcer, duodenum, with
      hemorrhage
  dura mater —*see* Hemorrhage, intracranial,
    subdural
  endotracheal —*see* Hemorrhage, lung
  epicranial subaponeurotic (massive), birth
    injury P12.2
  epidural (traumatic) —*see also* Injury,
      intracranial, epidural hemorrhage
    nontraumatic I62.1
  esophagus K22.89
    varix I85.01
      secondary I85.11
  excessive, following ectopic gestation
    (subsequent episode) O08.1
  extradural (traumatic) —*see* Injury,
      intracranial, epidural hemorrhage
    birth injury P10.8
    newborn (anoxic) (nontraumatic) P52.8
    nontraumatic I62.1
  eye NEC H57.89
    fundus —*see* Hemorrhage, retina
    lid —*see* Disorder, eyelid, specified type
      NEC
  fallopian tube N83.6

Hemorrhage, hemorrhagic *(Continued)*
  fibrinogenolysis —*see* Fibrinolysis
  fibrinolytic (acquired) —*see* Fibrinolysis
  from
    ear (nontraumatic) —*see* Otorrhagia
    tracheostomy stoma J95.01
  fundus, eye —*see* Hemorrhage, retina
  funis —*see* Hemorrhage, umbilicus, cord
  gastric —*see* Hemorrhage, stomach
  gastroenteric K92.2
    newborn P54.3
  gastrointestinal (tract) K92.2
    newborn P54.3
  genital organ, male N50.1
  genitourinary (tract) NOS R31.9
  gingiva K06.8
  globe (eye) —*see* Hemophthalmos
  graafian follicle cyst (ruptured) N83.0-●
  gum K06.8
  heart I51.89
  hypopharyngeal (throat) R04.1
  intermenstrual (regular) N92.3
    irregular N92.1
  internal (organs) NEC R58
    capsule I61.0
    ear —*see* subcategory H83.8
    newborn P54.8
  intestine K92.2
    newborn P54.3
  intra-abdominal R58
  intra-alveolar (lung), newborn P26.8
  intracerebral (nontraumatic) —*see*
      Hemorrhage, intracranial,
      intracerebral
  intracranial (nontraumatic) I62.9
    birth injury P10.9
    epidural, nontraumatic I62.1
    extradural, nontraumatic I62.1
    intracerebral (nontraumatic) (in) I61.9
      brain stem I61.3
      cerebellum I61.4
      hemisphere I61.2
        cortical (superficial) I61.1
        subcortical (deep) I61.0
      intraoperative
        during a nervous system procedure
          G97.31
        during other procedure G97.32
      intraventricular I61.5
      multiple localized I61.6
      newborn P52.4
        birth injury P10.1
      postprocedural
        following a nervous system procedure
          G97.51
        following other procedure
          G97.52
      specified NEC I61.8
      superficial I61.1
      traumatic (diffuse) —*see* Injury,
        intracranial, diffuse
        focal —*see* Injury, intracranial, focal
    newborn P52.9
      specified NEC P52.8
    subarachnoid (nontraumatic) (from) I60.9
      intracranial (cerebral) artery I60.7
        anterior communicating I60.2
        basilar I60.4
        carotid siphon and bifurcation
          I60.0-●
        communicating I60.7
          anterior I60.2
          posterior I60.3-●
        middle cerebral I60.1-●
        posterior communicating I60.3-●
        specified artery NEC I60.6
        vertebral I60.5-●
      newborn P52.5
        birth injury P10.3
      specified NEC I60.8
      traumatic S06.6X-●

Hemorrhage, hemorrhagic *(Continued)*
  intracranial *(Continued)*
    subdural (nontraumatic) I62.00
      acute I62.01
      birth injury P10.0
      chronic I62.03
      newborn (anoxic) (hypoxic) P52.8
        birth injury P10.0
      spinal G95.19
      subacute I62.02
      traumatic —*see* Injury, intracranial,
        subdural hemorrhage
    traumatic —*see* Injury, intracranial, focal
      brain injury
  intramedullary NEC G95.19
  intraocular —*see* Hemophthalmos
  intraoperative, intraprocedural —*see*
      Complication, hemorrhage (hematoma),
      intraoperative (intraprocedural), by site
  intrapartum —*see* Hemorrhage, complicating,
    delivery
  intrapelvic
    female N94.89
    male K66.1
  intraperitoneal K66.1
  intrapontine I61.3
  intraprocedural —*see* Complication,
    hemorrhage (hematoma), intraoperative
    (intraprocedural), by site
  intrauterine N85.7
    complicating delivery —*see also* Hemorrhage,
      complicating, delivery O67.9
    postpartum —*see* Hemorrhage, postpartum
  intraventricular I61.5
    newborn (nontraumatic) —*see also* Newborn,
      affected by, hemorrhage P52.3
      due to birth injury P10.2
      grade
        1 P52.0
        2 P52.1
        3 P52.21
        4 P52.22
  intravesical N32.89
  iris (postinfectional) (postinflammatory)
    (toxic) —*see* Hyphema
  joint (nontraumatic) —*see* Hemarthrosis
  kidney N28.89
  knee (joint) (nontraumatic) —*see*
    Hemarthrosis, knee
  labyrinth —*see* subcategory H83.8
  lenticular striate artery I61.0
  ligature, vessel —*see* Hemorrhage,
    postoperative
  liver K76.89
  lung R04.89
    newborn P26.9
      massive P26.1
      specified NEC P26.8
    tuberculous —*see* Tuberculosis, pulmonary
  massive umbilical, newborn P51.0
  mediastinum —*see* Hemorrhage, lung
  medulla I61.3
  membrane (brain) I60.8
    spinal cord —*see* Hemorrhage, spinal cord
  meninges, meningeal (brain) (middle) I60.8
    spinal cord —*see* Hemorrhage, spinal cord
  mesentery K66.1
  metritis —*see* Endometritis
  mouth K13.79
  mucous membrane NEC R58
    newborn P54.8
  muscle M62.89
  nail (subungual) L60.8
  nasal turbinate R04.0
    newborn P54.8
  navel, newborn P51.9
  newborn P54.9
    specified NEC P54.8
  nipple N64.59
  nose R04.0
    newborn P54.8

Hemorrhage, hemorrhagic (Continued)
omentum K66.1
optic nerve (sheath) H47.02-•
orbit, orbital H05.23-•
ovary NEC N83.8
oviduct N83.6
pancreas K86.89
parathyroid (gland) (spontaneous) E21.4
parturition —see Hemorrhage, complicating, delivery
penis N48.89
pericardium, pericarditis I31.2
peritoneum, peritoneal K66.1
peritonsillar tissue J35.8
    due to infection J36
petechial R23.3
    due to autosensitivity, erythrocyte D69.2
pituitary (gland) E23.6
pleura —see Hemorrhage, lung
polioencephalitis, superior E51.2
polymyositis —see Polymyositis
pons, pontine I61.3
posterior fossa (nontraumatic) I61.8
    newborn P52.6
postmenopausal N95.0
postnasal R04.0
postoperative —see Complications, postprocedural, hemorrhage, by site
postpartum NEC (following delivery of placenta) O72.1
    delayed or secondary O72.2
    retained placenta O72.0
    third stage O72.0
pregnancy —see Hemorrhage, antepartum
preretinal —see Hemorrhage, retina
prostate N42.1
puerperal —see Hemorrhage, postpartum
    delayed or secondary O72.2
pulmonary R04.89
    newborn P26.9
        massive P26.1
        specified NEC P26.8
    tuberculous —see Tuberculosis, pulmonary
purpura (primary) D69.3
rectum (sphincter) K62.5
    newborn P54.2
recurring, following initial hemorrhage at time of injury T79.2
renal N28.89
respiratory passage or tract R04.9
    specified NEC R04.89
retina, retinal (vessels) H35.6-•
    diabetic —see Diabetes, retinal, hemorrhage
retroperitoneal R58
scalp R58
scrotum N50.1
secondary (nontraumatic) R58
    following initial hemorrhage at time of injury T79.2
seminal vesicle N50.1
skin R23.3
    newborn P54.5
slipped umbilical ligature P51.8
spermatic cord N50.1
spinal (cord) G95.19
    newborn (birth injury) P11.5
spleen D73.5
    intraoperative —see Complications, intraoperative, hemorrhage, spleen
    postprocedural —see Complications, postprocedural, hemorrhage, spleen
stomach K92.2
    newborn P54.3
    ulcer —see Ulcer, stomach, with hemorrhage
subarachnoid (nontraumatic) —see Hemorrhage, intracranial, subarachnoid
subconjunctival —see also Hemorrhage, conjunctiva
    birth injury P15.3
subcortical (brain) I61.0

Hemorrhage, hemorrhagic (Continued)
subcutaneous R23.3
subdiaphragmatic R58
subdural (acute) (nontraumatic) —see Hemorrhage, intracranial, subdural
subependymal
    newborn P52.0
        with intraventricular extension P52.1
            and intracerebral extension P52.22
subgaleal P12.2
subhyaloid —see Hemorrhage, retina
subperiosteal —see Disorder, bone, specified type NEC
subretinal —see Hemorrhage, retina
subtentorial —see Hemorrhage, intracranial, subdural
subungual L60.8
suprarenal (capsule) (gland) E27.49
    newborn P54.4
tentorium (traumatic) NEC —see Hemorrhage, brain
    newborn (birth injury) P10.4
testis N50.1
third stage (postpartum) O72.0
thorax —see Hemorrhage, lung
throat R04.1
thymus (gland) E32.8
thyroid (cyst) (gland) E07.89
tongue K14.8
tonsil J35.8
trachea —see Hemorrhage, lung
tracheobronchial R04.89
    newborn P26.0
traumatic — code to specific injury
    cerebellar —see Hemorrhage, brain
    intracranial —see Hemorrhage, brain
    recurring or secondary (following initial hemorrhage at time of injury) T79.2
tuberculous NEC —see also Tuberculosis, pulmonary A15.0
tunica vaginalis N50.1
ulcer - code by site under Ulcer, with hemorrhage K27.4
umbilicus, umbilical
    cord
        after birth, newborn P51.9
        complicating delivery O69.5
    newborn P51.9
        massive P51.0
        slipped ligature P51.8
    stump P51.9
urethra (idiopathic) N36.8
uterus, uterine (abnormal) N93.9
    climacteric N92.4
    complicating delivery —see Hemorrhage, complicating, delivery
    dysfunctional or functional N93.8
    intermenstrual (regular) N92.3
        irregular N92.1
    postmenopausal N95.0
    postpartum —see Hemorrhage, postpartum
    preclimacteric or premenopausal N92.4
    prepubertal N93.8
    pubertal N92.2
vagina (abnormal) N93.9
    newborn P54.6
vas deferens N50.1
vasa previa O69.4
ventricular I61.5
vesical N32.89
viscera NEC R58
    newborn P54.8
vitreous (humor) (intraocular) H43.1-•
vulva N90.89
Hemorrhoids (bleeding) (without mention of degree) K64.9
1st degree (grade/stage I) (without prolapse outside of anal canal) K64.0
2nd degree (grade/stage II) (that prolapse with straining but retract spontaneously) K64.1

Hemorrhoids (Continued)
3rd degree (grade/stage III) (that prolapse with straining and require manual replacement back inside anal canal) K64.2
4th degree (grade/stage IV) (with prolapsed tissue that cannot be manually replaced) K64.3
complicating
    pregnancy O22.4
    puerperium O87.2
external K64.4
    with
        thrombosis K64.5
internal (without mention of degree) K64.8
prolapsed K64.8
skin tags
    anus K64.4
    residual K64.4
specified NEC K64.8
strangulated —see also Hemorrhoids, by degree K64.8
thrombosed —see also Hemorrhoids, by degree K64.5
ulcerated —see also Hemorrhoids, by degree K64.8
Hemosalpinx N83.6
with
    hematocolpos N89.7
    hematometra N85.7
        with hematocolpos N89.7
Hemosiderosis (dietary) E83.19
pulmonary, idiopathic E83.1 [J84.03]
transfusion T80.89
Hemothorax (bacterial) (nontuberculous) J94.2
newborn P54.8
traumatic S27.1
    with pneumothorax S27.2
tuberculous NEC A15.6
Henoch (-Schönlein) **disease or syndrome** (purpura) D69.0
Henpue, henpuye A66.6
Hepar lobatum (syphilitic) A52.74
Hepatalgia K76.89
Hepatitis K75.9
acute B17.9
    with coma K72.01
    with hepatic failure —see Failure, hepatic
    alcoholic —see Hepatitis, alcoholic
    infectious B15.9
    non-viral K72.0
    viral B17.9
alcoholic (acute) (chronic) K70.10
    with ascites K70.11
amebic —see Abscess, liver, amebic
anicteric (viral) —see Hepatitis, viral
antigen-associated (HAA) —see Hepatitis, B
Australia-antigen (positive) —see Hepatitis, B
autoimmune K75.4
B B19.10
    with hepatic coma B19.11
    acute B16.9
        with
            delta-agent (coinfection) (without hepatic coma) B16.1
                with hepatic coma B16.0
            hepatic coma (without delta-agent coinfection) B16.2
    chronic B18.1
        with delta-agent B18.0
bacterial NEC K75.89
C (viral) B19.20
    with hepatic coma B19.21
    acute B17.10
        with hepatic coma B17.11
    chronic B18.2
catarrhal (acute) B15.9
    with hepatic coma B15.0
cholangiolitic K75.89
cholestatic K75.89

▶ New   ⇒ Revised   ~~deleted~~ Deleted   • Use Additional Character(s)

Hepatitis *(Continued)*
chronic K73.9
   active NEC K73.2
   lobular NEC K73.1
   persistent NEC K73.0
   specified NEC K73.8
cytomegaloviral B25.1
due to ethanol (acute) (chronic) —*see*
   Hepatitis, alcoholic
epidemic B15.9
   with hepatic coma B15.0
fulminant NEC (viral) —*see* Hepatitis, viral
granulomatous NEC K75.3
herpesviral B00.81
history of
   B Z86.19
   C Z86.19
homologous serum —*see* Hepatitis, viral,
   type B
in (due to)
   mumps B26.81
   toxoplasmosis (acquired) B58.1
      congenital (active) P37.1 *[K77]*
infectious, infective B15.9
   acute (subacute) B17.9
   chronic B18.9
inoculation —*see* Hepatitis, viral, type B
interstitial (chronic) K74.69
▶ischemia, ischemic K72.00
lupoid NEC K75.2
malignant NEC (with hepatic failure)
   K72.90
   with coma K72.91
neonatal giant cell P59.29
neonatal (idiopathic) (toxic) P59.29
newborn P59.29
postimmunization —*see* Hepatitis, viral,
   type B
post-transfusion —*see* Hepatitis, viral, type B
reactive, nonspecific K75.2
serum —*see* Hepatitis, viral, type B
▶shock K72.00
specified type NEC
   with hepatic failure —*see* Failure, hepatic
syphilitic (late) A52.74
   congenital (early) A50.08 *[K77]*
      late A50.59 *[K77]*
   secondary A51.45
toxic —*see also* Disease, liver, toxic K71.6
tuberculous A18.83
viral, virus B19.9
   with hepatic coma B19.0
   acute B17.9
   chronic B18.9
      specified NEC B18.8
      type
         B B18.1
            with delta-agent B18.0
         C B18.2
   congenital P35.3
   coxsackie B33.8 *[K77]*
   cytomegalic inclusion B25.1
   in remission, any type — code to Hepatitis,
      chronic, by type
   non-A, non-B B17.8
   specified type NEC (with or without coma)
      B17.8
   type
      A B15.9
         with hepatic coma B15.0
      B B19.10
         with hepatic coma B19.11
         acute B16.9
            with
               delta-agent (coinfection) (without
                  hepatic coma) B16.1
                  with hepatic coma B16.0
               hepatic coma (without delta-
                  agent coinfection) B16.2
         chronic B18.1
            with delta-agent B18.0

Hepatitis *(Continued)*
viral, virus *(Continued)*
   type *(Continued)*
      C B19.20
         with hepatic coma B19.21
         acute B17.10
            with hepatic coma B17.11
         chronic B18.2
      E B17.2
   non-A, non-B B17.8
Hepatization lung (acute) —*see* Pneumonia, lobar
Hepatoblastoma C22.2
Hepatocarcinoma C22.0
Hepatocholangiocarcinoma C22.0
Hepatocholangioma, benign D13.4
Hepatocholangitis K75.89
Hepatolenticular degeneration E83.01
Hepatoma (malignant) C22.0
   benign D13.4
   embryonal C22.0
Hepatomegaly —*see also* Hypertrophy, liver
   with splenomegaly R16.2
   congenital Q44.7
   in mononucleosis
      gammaherpesviral B27.09
      infectious specified NEC B27.89
Hepatoptosis K76.89
Hepatorenal syndrome following labor and
   delivery O90.4
Hepatosis K76.89
Hepatosplenomegaly R16.2
   hyperlipemic (Bürger-Grütz type) E78.3 *[K77]*
Hereditary —*see* condition
▶Hereditary alpha tryptasemia (syndrome) D89.44
Heredodegeneration, macular —*see* Dystrophy,
   retina
Heredopathia atactica polyneuritiformis G60.1
Heredosyphilis —*see* Syphilis, congenital
Herlitz' syndrome Q81.1
Hermansky-Pudlak syndrome E70.331
Hermaphrodite, hermaphroditism (true) Q56.0
   46,XX with streak gonads Q99.1
   46,XX/46,XY Q99.0
   46,XY with streak gonads Q99.1
   chimera 46,XX/46,XY Q99.0
Hernia, hernial (acquired) (recurrent) K46.9
   with
      gangrene —*see* Hernia, by site, with,
         gangrene
      incarceration —*see* Hernia, by site, with,
         obstruction
      irreducible —*see* Hernia, by site, with,
         obstruction
      obstruction —*see* Hernia, by site, with,
         obstruction
      strangulation —*see* Hernia, by site, with,
         obstruction
   abdomen, abdominal K46.9
      with
         gangrene (and obstruction) K46.1
         obstruction K46.0
      femoral —*see* Hernia, femoral
      incisional —*see* Hernia, incisional
      inguinal —*see* Hernia, inguinal
      specified site NEC K45.8
         with
            gangrene (and obstruction) K45.1
            obstruction K45.0
      umbilical —*see* Hernia, umbilical
      wall —*see* Hernia, ventral
   appendix —*see* Hernia, abdomen
   bladder (mucosa) (sphincter)
      congenital (female) (male) Q79.51
      female —*see* Cystocele
      male N32.89
   brain, congenital —*see* Encephalocele
   cartilage, vertebra —*see* Displacement,
      intervertebral disc
   cerebral, congenital —*see also* Encephalocele
      endaural Q01.8
   ciliary body (traumatic) S05.2-●

Hernia, hernial *(Continued)*
   colon —*see* Hernia, abdomen
   Cooper's —*see* Hernia, abdomen, specified
      site NEC
   crural —*see* Hernia, femoral
   diaphragm, diaphragmatic K44.9
      with
         gangrene (and obstruction) K44.1
         obstruction K44.0
      congenital Q79.0
   direct (inguinal) —*see* Hernia, inguinal
   diverticulum, intestine —*see* Hernia,
      abdomen
   double (inguinal) —*see* Hernia, inguinal,
      bilateral
   due to adhesions (with obstruction) K56.50
   epigastric —*see also* Hernia, ventral K43.9
   esophageal hiatus —*see* Hernia, hiatal
   external (inguinal) —*see* Hernia, inguinal
   fallopian tube N83.4-●
   fascia M62.89
   femoral K41.90
      with
         gangrene (and obstruction) K41.40
            not specified as recurrent K41.40
            recurrent K41.41
         obstruction K41.30
            not specified as recurrent K41.30
            recurrent K41.31
      bilateral K41.20
         with
            gangrene (and obstruction) K41.10
               not specified as recurrent K41.10
               recurrent K41.11
            obstruction K41.00
               not specified as recurrent K41.00
               recurrent K41.01
         not specified as recurrent K41.20
         recurrent K41.21
      not specified as recurrent K41.90
      recurrent K41.91
      unilateral K41.90
         with
            gangrene (and obstruction) K41.40
               not specified as recurrent K41.40
               recurrent K41.41
            obstruction K41.30
               not specified as recurrent K41.30
               recurrent K41.31
         not specified as recurrent K41.90
         recurrent K41.91
   foramen magnum G93.5
      congenital Q01.8
   funicular (umbilical) —*see also* Hernia,
      umbilicus
      spermatic (cord) —*see* Hernia, inguinal
   gastrointestinal tract —*see* Hernia, abdomen
   Hesselbach's —*see* Hernia, femoral, specified
      site NEC
   hiatal (esophageal) (sliding) K44.9
      with
         gangrene (and obstruction) K44.1
         obstruction K44.0
      congenital Q40.1
   hypogastric —*see* Hernia, ventral
   incarcerated —*see also* Hernia, by site, with
      obstruction
      with gangrene —*see* Hernia, by site, with
         gangrene
   incisional K43.2
      with
         gangrene (and obstruction) K43.1
         obstruction K43.0
   indirect (inguinal) —*see* Hernia, inguinal
   inguinal (direct) (external) (funicular)
      (indirect) (internal) (oblique) (scrotal)
      (sliding) K40.90
      with
         gangrene (and obstruction) K40.40
            not specified as recurrent K40.40
            recurrent K40.41

Hernia, hernial *(Continued)*
  inguinal *(Continued)*
    with *(Continued)*
      obstruction K40.30
        not specified as recurrent K40.30
        recurrent K40.31
      bilateral K40.20
        with
          gangrene (and obstruction) K40.10
            not specified as recurrent K40.10
            recurrent K40.11
          obstruction K40.00
            not specified as recurrent K40.00
            recurrent K40.01
        not specified as recurrent K40.20
        recurrent K40.21
      not specified as recurrent K40.90
      recurrent K40.91
      unilateral K40.90
        with
          gangrene (and obstruction) K40.40
            not specified as recurrent K40.40
            recurrent K40.41
          obstruction K40.30
            not specified as recurrent K40.30
            recurrent K40.31
        not specified as recurrent K40.90
        recurrent K40.91
  internal —*see also* Hernia, abdomen
    inguinal —*see* Hernia, inguinal
  interstitial —*see* Hernia, abdomen
  intervertebral cartilage or disc —*see* Displacement, intervertebral disc
  intestine, intestinal —*see* Hernia, by site
  intra-abdominal —*see* Hernia, abdomen
  iris (traumatic) S05.2-●
  irreducible —*see also* Hernia, by site, with obstruction
    with gangrene —*see* Hernia, by site, with gangrene
  ischiatic —*see* Hernia, abdomen, specified site NEC
  ischiorectal —*see* Hernia, abdomen, specified site NEC
  lens (traumatic) S05.2-●
  linea (alba) (semilunaris) —*see* Hernia, ventral
  Littre's —*see* Hernia, abdomen
  lumbar —*see* Hernia, abdomen, specified site NEC
  lung (subcutaneous) J98.4
  mediastinum J98.59
  mesenteric (internal) —*see* Hernia, abdomen
  midline —*see* Hernia, ventral
  muscle (sheath) M62.89
  nucleus pulposus —*see* Displacement, intervertebral disc
  oblique (inguinal) —*see* Hernia, inguinal
  obstructive —*see also* Hernia, by site, with obstruction
    with gangrene —*see* Hernia, by site, with gangrene
  obturator —*see* Hernia, abdomen, specified site NEC
  omental —*see* Hernia, abdomen
  ovary N83.4-●
  oviduct N83.4-●
  paraesophageal —*see also* Hernia, diaphragm
    congenital Q40.1
  parastomal K43.5
    with
      gangrene (and obstruction) K43.4
      obstruction K43.3
  paraumbilical —*see* Hernia, umbilicus
  perineal —*see* Hernia, abdomen, specified site NEC
  Petit's —*see* Hernia, abdomen, specified site NEC
  postoperative —*see* Hernia, incisional
  pregnant uterus —*see* Abnormal, uterus in pregnancy or childbirth
  prevesical N32.89

Hernia, hernial *(Continued)*
  properitoneal —*see* Hernia, abdomen, specified site NEC
  pudendal —*see* Hernia, abdomen, specified site NEC
  rectovaginal N81.6
  retroperitoneal —*see* Hernia, abdomen, specified site NEC
  Richter's —*see* Hernia, abdomen, with obstruction
  Rieux's, Riex's —*see* Hernia, abdomen, specified site NEC
  sac condition (adhesion) (dropsy) (inflammation) (laceration) (suppuration) - code by site under Hernia
  sciatic —*see* Hernia, abdomen, specified site NEC
  scrotum, scrotal —*see* Hernia, inguinal
  sliding (inguinal) —*see also* Hernia, inguinal
    hiatus —*see* Hernia, hiatal
  spigelian —*see* Hernia, ventral
  spinal —*see* Spina bifida
  strangulated —*see also* Hernia, by site, with obstruction
    with gangrene —*see* Hernia, by site, with gangrene
  subxiphoid —*see* Hernia, ventral
  supra-umbilicus —*see* Hernia, ventral
  tendon —*see* Disorder, tendon, specified type NEC
  Treitz's (fossa) —*see* Hernia, abdomen, specified site NEC
  tunica vaginalis Q55.29
  umbilicus, umbilical K42.9
    with
      gangrene (and obstruction) K42.1
      obstruction K42.0
  ureter N28.89
  urethra, congenital Q64.79
  urinary meatus, congenital Q64.79
  uterus N81.4
    pregnant —*see* Abnormal, uterus in pregnancy or childbirth
  vaginal (anterior) (wall) —*see* Cystocele
  Velpeau's —*see* Hernia, femoral
  ventral K43.9
    with
      gangrene (and obstruction) K43.7
      obstruction K43.6
    incisional K43.2
      with
        gangrene (and obstruction) K43.1
        obstruction K43.0
      recurrent —*see* Hernia, incisional
    specified NEC K43.9
      with
        gangrene (and obstruction) K43.7
        obstruction K43.6
  vesical
    congenital (female) (male) Q79.51
    female —*see* Cystocele
    male N32.89
  vitreous (into wound) S05.2-●
    into anterior chamber —*see* Prolapse, vitreous
Herniation —*see also* Hernia
  brain (stem) G93.5
  ▶nontraumatic G93.5
  ▶traumatic S06.A1
    ▶cerebellar S06.A1
    ▶subfalcine (cingulate) S06.A1
    ▶tonsillar S06.A1
    ▶transtentorial (central) (upward cerebellar) S06.A1
    ▶uncal S06.A1
  cerebral G93.5
  ▶nontraumatic G93.5
  ▶traumatic S06.A1
  mediastinum J98.59
  nucleus pulposus —*see* Displacement, intervertebral disc
Herpangina B08.5

Herpes, herpesvirus, herpetic B00.9
  anogenital A60.9
    perianal skin A60.1
    rectum A60.1
    urogenital tract A60.00
      cervix A60.03
      male genital organ NEC A60.02
      penis A60.01
      specified site NEC A60.09
      vagina A60.04
      vulva A60.04
  blepharitis (zoster) B02.39
    simplex B00.59
  circinatus B35.4
    bullosus L12.0
  conjunctivitis (simplex) B00.53
    zoster B02.31
  cornea B02.33
  encephalitis B00.4
    due to herpesvirus 6 B10.01
    due to herpesvirus 7 B10.09
    specified NEC B10.09
  eye (zoster) B02.30
    simplex B00.50
  eyelid (zoster) B02.39
    simplex B00.59
  facialis B00.1
  febrilis B00.1
  geniculate ganglionitis B02.21
  genital, genitalis A60.00
    female A60.09
    male A60.02
  gestational, gestationis O26.4-●
  gingivostomatitis B00.2
  human B00.9
    1 —*see* Herpes, simplex
    2 —*see* Herpes, simplex
    3 —*see* Varicella
    4 —*see* Mononucleosis, Epstein-Barr (virus)
    5 —*see* Disease, cytomegalic inclusion (generalized)
    6
      encephalitis B10.01
      specified NEC B10.81
    7
      encephalitis B10.09
      specified NEC B10.82
    8 B10.89
  infection NEC B10.89
    Kaposi's sarcoma associated B10.89
  iridocyclitis (simplex) B00.51
    zoster B02.32
  iris (vesicular erythema multiforme) L51.9
  iritis (simplex) B00.51
  Kaposi's sarcoma associated B10.89
  keratitis (simplex) (dendritic) (disciform) (interstitial) B00.52
    zoster (interstitial) B02.33
  keratoconjunctivitis (simplex) B00.52
    zoster B02.33
  labialis B00.1
  lip B00.1
  meningitis (simplex) B00.3
    zoster B02.1
  ophthalmicus (zoster) NEC B02.30
    simplex B00.50
  penis A60.01
  perianal skin A60.1
  pharyngitis, pharyngotonsillitis B00.2
  rectum A60.1
  scrotum A60.02
  sepsis B00.7
  simplex B00.9
    complicated NEC B00.89
    congenital P35.2
    conjunctivitis B00.53
    external ear B00.1
    eyelid B00.59
    hepatitis B00.81
    keratitis (interstitial) B00.52
    myleitis B00.82
    specified complication NEC B00.89
    visceral B00.89

▶ New   ⇒ Revised   ~~deleted~~ Deleted   ● Use Additional Character(s)

Herpes, herpesvirus, herpetic (*Continued*)
stomatitis B00.2
tonsurans B35.0
visceral B00.89
vulva A60.04
whitlow B00.89
zoster —*see also* condition B02.9
auricularis B02.21
complicated NEC B02.8
conjunctivitis B02.31
disseminated B02.7
encephalitis B02.0
eye(lid) B02.39
geniculate ganglionitis B02.21
keratitis (interstitial) B02.33
meningitis B02.1
myelitis B02.24
neuritis, neuralgia B02.29
ophthalmicus NEC B02.30
oticus B02.21
polyneuropathy B02.23
specified complication NEC B02.8
trigeminal neuralgia B02.22
Herpesvirus (human) —*see* Herpes
Herpetophobia F40.218
Herrick's anemia —*see* Disease, sickle-cell
Hers' disease E74.09
Herter-Gee syndrome K90.0
Herxheimer's reaction R68.89
Hesitancy
of micturition R39.11
urinary R39.11
Hesselbach's hernia —*see* Hernia, femoral, specified site NEC
Heterochromia (congenital) Q13.2
cataract —*see* Cataract, complicated
cyclitis (Fuchs) —*see* Cyclitis, Fuchs' heterochromic
hair L67.1
iritis —*see* Cyclitis, Fuchs' heterochromic
retained metallic foreign body
(nonmagnetic) —*see* Foreign body, intraocular, old, retained
magnetic —*see* Foreign body, intraocular, old, retained, magnetic
uveitis —*see* Cyclitis, Fuchs' heterochromic
Heterophoria —*see* Strabismus, heterophoria
Heterophyes, heterophyiasis (small intestine) B66.8
Heterotopia, heterotopic —*see also* Malposition, congenital
cerebralis Q04.8
Heterotropia —*see* Strabismus
Heubner-Herter disease K90.0
Hexadactylism Q69.9
HGSIL (cytology finding) (high grade squamous intraepithelial lesion on cytologic smear) (Pap smear finding)
anus R85.613
cervix R87.613
biopsy (histology) finding — *see* Neoplasia, intraepithelial, cervix, grade II or grade III
vagina R87.623
biopsy (histology) finding — *see* Neoplasia, intraepithelial, vagina, grade II or grade III
Hibernoma —*see* Lipoma
Hiccup, hiccough R06.6
epidemic B33.0
psychogenic F45.8
Hidden penis (congenital) Q55.64
acquired N48.83
Hidradenitis (axillaris) (suppurative) L73.2
Hidradenoma (nodular) —*see also* Neoplasm, skin, benign
clear cell —*see* Neoplasm, skin, benign
papillary —*see* Neoplasm, skin, benign
Hidrocystoma —*see* Neoplasm, skin, benign

High
altitude effects T70.20
anoxia T70.29
on
ears T70.0
sinuses T70.1
polycythemia D75.1
arch
foot Q66.7-●
palate, congenital Q38.5
arterial tension —*see* Hypertension
basal metabolic rate R94.8
blood pressure —*see also* Hypertension
borderline R03.0
reading (incidental) (isolated) (nonspecific), without diagnosis of hypertension R03.0
cholesterol E78.00
with high triglycerides E78.2
diaphragm (congenital) Q79.1
expressed emotional level within family Z63.8
head at term O32.4
palate, congenital Q38.5
risk
infant NEC Z76.2
sexual behavior (heterosexual) Z72.51
bisexual Z72.53
homosexual Z72.52
scrotal testis, testes
bilateral Q53.23
unilateral Q53.13
temperature (of unknown origin) R50.9
thoracic rib Q76.6
triglycerides E78.1
with high cholesterol E78.2
Hildenbrand's disease A75.0
Hilum —*see* condition
Hip —*see* condition
Hippel's disease Q85.8
Hippophobia F40.218
Hippus H57.09
Hirschsprung's disease or megacolon Q43.1
Hirsutism, hirsuties L68.0
Hirudiniasis
external B88.3
internal B83.4
Hiss-Russell dysentery A03.1
Histidinemia, histidinuria E70.41
Histiocytoma —*see also* Neoplasm, skin, benign
fibrous —*see also* Neoplasm, skin, benign
atypical —*see* Neoplasm, connective tissue, uncertain behavior
malignant —*see* Neoplasm, connective tissue, malignant
Histiocytosis D76.3
acute differentiated progressive C96.0
Langerhans' cell NEC C96.6
multifocal X
multisystemic (disseminated) C96.0
unisystemic C96.5
pulmonary, adult (adult PLCH) J84.82
unifocal (X) C96.6
lipid, lipoid D76.3
essential E75.29
malignant C96.A
mononuclear phagocytes NEC D76.1
Langerhans' cells C96.6
non-Langerhans cell D76.3
polyostotic sclerosing D76.3
sinus, with massive lymphadenopathy D76.3
syndrome NEC D76.3
X NEC C96.6
acute (progressive) C96.0
chronic C96.6
multifocal C96.5
multisystemic C96.0
unifocal C96.6
Histoplasmosis B39.9
with pneumonia NEC B39.2
African B39.5
American —*see* Histoplasmosis, capsulati

Histoplasmosis (*Continued*)
capsulati B39.4
disseminated B39.3
generalized B39.3
pulmonary B39.2
acute B39.0
chronic B39.1
Darling's B39.4
duboisii B39.5
lung NEC B39.2
History
family (of) —*see also* History, personal (of)
alcohol abuse Z81.1
allergy NEC Z84.89
anemia Z83.2
arthritis Z82.61
asthma Z82.5
blindness Z82.1
cardiac death (sudden) Z82.41
carrier of genetic disease Z84.81
chromosomal anomaly Z82.79
chronic
disabling disease NEC Z82.8
lower respiratory disease Z82.5
colonic polyps Z83.71
congenital malformations and deformations Z82.79
polycystic kidney Z82.71
consanguinity Z84.3
deafness Z82.2
diabetes mellitus Z83.3
disability NEC Z82.8
disease or disorder (of)
allergic NEC Z84.89
behavioral NEC Z81.8
blood and blood-forming organs Z83.2
cardiovascular NEC Z82.49
chronic disabling NEC Z82.8
digestive Z83.79
ear NEC Z83.52
elevated lipoprotein (a) (Lp(a)) Z83.430
endocrine NEC Z83.49
eye NEC Z83.518
glaucoma Z83.511
familial hypercholesterolemia Z83.42
genitourinary NEC Z84.2
glaucoma Z83.511
hematological Z83.2
immune mechanism Z83.2
infectious NEC Z83.1
ischemic heart Z82.49
kidney Z84.1
lipoprotein metabolism Z83.438
mental NEC Z81.8
metabolic Z83.49
musculoskeletal NEC Z82.69
neurological NEC Z82.0
nutritional Z83.49
parasitic NEC Z83.1
psychiatric NEC Z81.8
respiratory NEC Z83.6
skin and subcutaneous tissue NEC Z84.0
specified NEC Z84.89
drug abuse NEC Z81.3
elevated lipoprotein(a) (Lp (a)) Z83.430
epilepsy Z82.0
familial hypercholesterolemia Z83.42
genetic disease carrier Z84.81
glaucoma Z83.511
hearing loss Z82.2
human immunodeficiency virus (HIV) infection Z83.0
Huntington's chorea Z82.0
hyperlipidemia, familial combined Z83.438
intellectual disability Z81.0
leukemia Z80.6
lipidemia NEC Z83.438
malignant neoplasm (of) NOS Z80.9
bladder Z80.52
breast Z80.3
bronchus Z80.1

History *(Continued)*
  family *(Continued)*
    malignant neoplasm *(Continued)*
      digestive organ Z80.0
      gastrointestinal tract Z80.0
      genital organ Z80.49
        ovary Z80.41
        prostate Z80.42
        specified organ NEC Z80.49
        testis Z80.43
      hematopoietic NEC Z80.7
      intrathoracic organ NEC Z80.2
      kidney Z80.51
      lung Z80.1
      lymphatic NEC Z80.7
      ovary Z80.41
      prostate Z80.42
      respiratory organ NEC Z80.2
      specified site NEC Z80.8
      testis Z80.43
      trachea Z80.1
      urinary organ or tract Z80.59
        bladder Z80.52
        kidney Z80.51
    mental
      disorder NEC Z81.8
    multiple endocrine neoplasia (MEN)
      syndrome Z83.41
    osteoporosis Z82.62
    polycystic kidney Z82.71
    polyps (colon) Z83.71
    psychiatric disorder Z81.8
    psychoactive substance abuse NEC Z81.3
    respiratory condition NEC Z83.6
      asthma and other lower respiratory
        conditions Z82.5
    self-harmful behavior Z81.8
    SIDS (sudden infant death syndrome) Z84.82
    skin condition Z84.0
    specified condition NEC Z84.89
    stroke (cerebrovascular) Z82.3
    substance abuse NEC Z81.4
      alcohol Z81.1
      drug NEC Z81.3
      psychoactive NEC Z81.3
      tobacco Z81.2
    sudden
      cardiac death Z82.41
      infant death syndrome (SIDS) Z84.82
    tobacco abuse Z81.2
    violence, violent behavior Z81.8
    visual loss Z82.1
  personal (of) —*see also* History, family (of)
    abuse
      adult Z91.419
        forced labor or sexual exploitation
          Z91.42
        physical and sexual Z91.410
        psychological Z91.411
      childhood Z62.819
        forced labor or sexual exploitation in
          childhood Z62.813
        physical Z62.810
        psychological Z62.811
        sexual Z62.810
    alcohol dependence F10.21
    allergy (to) Z88.9
      analgesic agent NEC Z88.6
      anesthetic Z88.4
      antibiotic agent NEC Z88.1
      anti-infective agent NEC Z88.3
      contrast media Z91.041
      drugs, medicaments and biological
        substances Z88.9
        specified NEC Z88.8
      food Z91.018
        additives Z91.02
        ▶beef Z91.014
        eggs Z91.012
        ▶lamb Z91.014
        ▶mammalian meats Z91.014
        milk products Z91.011
        peanuts Z91.010

History *(Continued)*
  personal *(Continued)*
    allergy *(Continued)*
      food *(Continued)*
        ▶pork Z91.014
        ▶red meats Z91.014
        seafood Z91.013
        specified food NEC Z91.018
      insect Z91.038
        bee Z91.030
      latex Z91.040
      medicinal agents Z88.9
        specified NEC Z88.8
      narcotic agent NEC Z88.5
      nonmedicinal agents Z91.048
      penicillin Z88.0
      serum Z88.7
      specified NEC Z91.09
      sulfonamides Z88.2
      vaccine Z88.7
    anaphylactic shock Z87.892
    anaphylaxis Z87.892
    behavioral disorders Z86.59
    benign carcinoid tumor Z86.012
    benign neoplasm Z86.018
      brain Z86.011
      carcinoid Z86.012
      colonic polyps Z86.010
    brain injury (traumatic) Z87.820
    breast implant removal Z98.86
    calculi, renal Z87.442
    cancer —*see* History, personal (of),
      malignant neoplasm (of)
    cardiac arrest (death), successfully
      resuscitated Z86.74
    ▶CAR-T (Chimeric Antigen Receptor T-cell)
      therapy Z92.850
    ▶cellular therapy Z92.859
      ▶specified NEC Z92.858
    cerebral infarction without residual deficit
      Z86.73
    cervical dysplasia Z87.410
    chemotherapy for neoplastic condition
      Z92.21
    childhood abuse —*see* History, personal
      (of), abuse
    ▶Chimeric Antigen Receptor T-cell (CAR-T)
      therapy Z92.850
    cleft lip (corrected) Z87.730
    cleft palate (corrected) Z87.730
    collapsed vertebra (healed) Z87.311
      due to osteoporosis Z87.310
    combat and operational stress reaction
      Z86.51
    congenital malformation (corrected) Z87.798
      circulatory system (corrected) Z87.74
      digestive system (corrected) NEC
        Z87.738
      ear (corrected) Z87.721
      eye (corrected) Z87.720
      face and neck (corrected) Z87.790
      genitourinary system (corrected) NEC
        Z87.718
      heart (corrected) Z87.74
      integument (corrected) Z87.76
      limb(s) (corrected) Z87.76
      musculoskeletal system (corrected) Z87.76
      neck (corrected) Z87.790
      nervous system (corrected) NEC Z87.728
      respiratory system (corrected) Z87.75
      sense organs (corrected) NEC Z87.728
      specified NEC Z87.798
    contraception Z92.0
    coronavirus (disease) (novel) 2019 Z86.16
    COVID-19 Z86.16
    deployment (military) Z91.82
    diabetic foot ulcer Z86.31
    disease or disorder (of) Z87.898
      blood and blood-forming organs Z86.2
      circulatory system Z86.79
        specified condition NEC Z86.79
      connective tissue NEC Z87.39

History *(Continued)*
  personal *(Continued)*
    disease or disorder (of) *(Continued)*
      digestive system Z87.19
        colonic polyp Z86.010
        peptic ulcer disease Z87.11
        specified condition NEC Z87.19
      ear Z86.69
      endocrine Z86.39
        diabetic foot ulcer Z86.31
        gestational diabetes Z86.32
        specified type NEC Z86.39
      eye Z86.69
      genital (track) system NEC
        female Z87.42
        male Z87.438
      hematological Z86.2
      Hodgkin Z85.71
      immune mechanism Z86.2
      infectious Z86.19
        coronavirus (disease) (novel) 2019
          Z86.16
        COVID-19 Z86.16
        malaria Z86.13
        Methicillin resistant Staphylococcus
          aureus (MRSA) Z86.14
        poliomyelitis Z86.12
        SARS-CoV-2 Z86.16
        specified NEC Z86.19
        tuberculosis Z86.11
      mental NEC Z86.59
      metabolic Z86.39
        diabetic foot ulcer Z86.31
        gestational diabetes Z86.32
        specified type NEC Z86.39
      musculoskeletal NEC Z87.39
      nervous system Z86.69
      nutritional Z86.39
      parasitic Z86.19
      respiratory system NEC Z87.09
      sense organs Z86.69
      skin Z87.2
      specified site or type NEC Z87.898
      subcutaneous tissue Z87.2
      trophoblastic Z87.59
      urinary system NEC Z87.448
    drug dependence —*see* Dependence, drug,
      by type, in remission
    drug therapy
      antineoplastic chemotherapy Z92.21
      estrogen Z92.23
      ⇒immunosuppression Z92.25
      inhaled steroids Z92.240
      monoclonal drug Z92.22
      specified NEC Z92.29
      steroid Z92.241
      systemic steroids Z92.241
    dysplasia
      cervical (mild) (moderate) Z87.410
        severe (grade III) Z86.001
      prostatic Z87.430
      vaginal (mild) (moderate) Z87.411
        severe (grade III) Z86.002
      vulvar (mild) (moderate) Z87.412
        severe (grade III) Z86.002
    embolism (venous) Z86.718
      pulmonary Z86.711
    encephalitis Z86.61
    estrogen therapy Z92.23
    extracorporeal membrane oxygenation
      (ECMO) Z92.81
    failed conscious sedation Z92.83
    failed moderate sedation Z92.83
    fall, falling Z91.81
    forced labor or sexual exploitation Z91.42
      in childhood Z62.813
    fracture (healed)
      fatigue Z87.312
      fragility Z87.310
      osteoporosis Z87.310
      pathological NEC Z87.311
      stress Z87.312
      traumatic Z87.81

▶ New   ⇒ Revised   ~~deleted~~ Deleted   ● Use Additional Character(s)

History *(Continued)*
  personal *(Continued)*
    ▶gene therapy Z92.86
    gestational diabetes Z86.32
    hepatitis
      B Z86.19
      C Z86.19
    Hodgkin disease Z85.71
    hyperthermia, malignant Z88.4
    hypospadias (corrected) Z87.710
    hysterectomy Z90.710
    ➔immunosuppression therapy Z92.25
    in situ neoplasm
      breast Z86.000
      cervix uteri Z86.001
      digestive organs, specified NEC Z86.004
      esophagus Z86.003
      genital organs, specified NEC Z86.002
      melanoma Z86.006
      middle ear Z86.005
      oral cavity Z86.003
      respiratory system Z86.005
      skin Z86.007
      specified NEC Z86.008
      stomach Z86.003
    infection NEC Z86.19
      central nervous system Z86.61
      coronavirus (disease) (novel) 2019 Z86.16
      COVID-19 Z86.16
      latent tuberculosis Z86.15
      Methicillin resistant Staphylococcus
        aureus (MRSA) Z86.14
      SARS-CoV-2 Z86.16
      urinary (recurrent) (tract) Z87.41
    injury NEC Z87.828
    in utero procedure during pregnancy
      Z98.870
    in utero procedure while a fetus Z98.871
    irradiation Z92.3
    kidney stones Z87.442
    latent tuberculosis Z86.15
    leukemia Z85.6
    lymphoma (non-Hodgkin) Z85.72
    malignant melanoma (skin) Z85.820
    malignant neoplasm (of) Z85.9
      accessory sinuses Z85.22
      anus NEC Z85.048
        carcinoid Z85.040
      bladder Z85.51
      bone Z85.830
      brain Z85.841
      breast Z85.3
      bronchus NEC Z85.118
        carcinoid Z85.110
      carcinoid —*see* History, personal (of),
        malignant neoplasm, by site,
        carcinioid
      cervix Z85.41
      colon NEC Z85.038
        carcinoid Z85.030
      digestive organ Z85.00
        specified NEC Z85.09
      endocrine gland NEC Z85.858
      epididymis Z85.48
      esophagus Z85.01
      eye Z85.840
      gastrointestinal tract —*see* History,
        malignant neoplasm, digestive organ
      genital organ
        female Z85.40
          specified NEC Z85.44
        male Z85.45
          specified NEC Z85.49
      hematopoietic NEC Z85.79
      intrathoracic organ Z85.20-●
      kidney NEC Z85.528
        carcinoid Z85.520
      large intestine NEC Z85.038
        carcinoid Z85.030
      larynx Z85.21
      liver Z85.05
      lung NEC Z85.118
        carcinoid Z85.110

History *(Continued)*
  personal *(Continued)*
    malignant neoplasm (of) *(Continued)*
      mediastinum Z85.29
      Merkel cell Z85.821
      middle ear Z85.22
      nasal cavities Z85.22
      nervous system NEC Z85.848
        oral cavity Z85.819
        specified site NEC Z85.818
      ovary Z85.43
      pancreas Z85.07
      pelvis Z85.53
      pharynx Z85.819
        specified site NEC Z85.818
      pleura Z85.29
      prostate Z85.46
      rectosigmoid junction NEC Z85.048
        carcinoid Z85.040
      rectum NEC Z85.048
        carcinoid Z85.040
      respiratory organ Z85.20
      sinuses, accessory Z85.22
      skin NEC Z85.828
        melanoma Z85.820
        Merkel cell Z85.821
      small intestine NEC Z85.068
        carcinoid Z85.060
      soft tissue Z85.831
      specified site NEC Z85.89
      stomach NEC Z85.028
        carcinoid Z85.020
      testis Z85.47
      thymus NEC Z85.238
        carcinoid Z85.230
      thyroid Z85.850
      tongue Z85.810
      trachea Z85.12
      ureter Z85.54
      urinary organ or tract Z85.50
        specified NEC Z85.59
      uterus Z85.42
    maltreatment Z91.89
    medical treatment NEC Z92.89
    melanoma Z85.820
      in situ Z86.06
      malignant (skin) Z85.820
    meningitis Z86.61
    mental disorder Z86.59
    Merkel cell carcinoma (skin) Z85.821
    Methicillin resistant Staphylococcus aureus
      (MRSA) Z86.14
    military deployment Z91.82
    military war, peacekeeping and
      humanitarian deployment (current or
      past conflict) Z91.82
    myocardial infarction (old) I25.2
    neglect (in)
      adult Z91.412
      childhood Z62.812
    neoplasia
      anal intraepithelial, III [AIN III] Z86.004
      high-grade prostatic intraepithelial, III
        [HGPIN III] Z86.002
      vaginal intraepithelial, III [VAIN III]
        Z86.002
      vulvar intraepithelial, III [VIN III] Z86.002
    neoplasm
      benign Z86.018
        brain Z86.011
        colon polyp Z86.010
      in situ
        breast Z86.000
        cervix uteri Z86.001
        digestive organs, specified NEC Z86.004
        esophagus Z86.003
        genital organs, specified NEC Z86.002
        melanoma Z86.006
        middle ear Z86.005
        oral cavity Z86.003
        respiratory system Z86.005
        skin Z86.007
        specified NEC Z86.008

History *(Continued)*
  personal *(Continued)*
    neoplasm *(Continued)*
      in situ *(Continued)*
        stomach Z86.003
        malignant —*see* History of, malignant
          neoplasm
        uncertain behavior Z86.03
    nephrotic syndrome Z87.441
    nicotine dependence Z87.891
    noncompliance with medical treatment or
      regimen —*see* Noncompliance
    nutritional deficiency Z86.39
    obstetric complications Z87.59
      childbirth Z87.59
      pregnancy Z87.59
      pre-term labor Z87.51
      puerperium Z87.59
    osteoporosis fractures Z87.31
    ➔parasuicide (attempt) Z91.51
    physical trauma NEC Z87.828
      ➔self-harm or suicide attempt Z91.51
    pneumonia (recurrent) Z87.01
    poisoning NEC Z91.89
      ➔self-harm or suicide attempt Z91.51
    poor personal hygiene Z91.89
    preterm labor Z87.51
    procedure during pregnancy Z98.870
    procedure while a fetus Z98.871
    prolonged reversible ischemic neurologic
      deficit (PRINO) Z86.73
    prostatic dysplasia Z87.430
    psychiatric disorder NEC Z87.89
    psychological
      abuse
        adult Z91.411
        child Z62.811
      trauma, specified NEC Z91.49
    radiation therapy Z92.3
    removal
      implant
        breast Z98.86
    renal calculi Z87.442
    respiratory condition NEC Z87.09
    retained foreign body fully removed
      Z87.821
    risk factors NEC Z91.89
    SARS-CoV-2 infection Z86.16
    ➔self-harm
      ▶nonsuicidal Z91.52
      ▶suicidal Z91.51
    ▶self-inflicted injury without suicidal intent
      Z91.52
    ▶self-injury
      ▶nonsuicidal Z91.52
    ▶self-mutilation Z91.52
    ➔self-poisoning attempt Z91.51
      ▶suicidal behavior Z91.51
    sex reassignment Z87.890
    sleep-wake cycle problem Z72.821
    specified NEC Z87.898
    steroid therapy (systemic) Z92.241
      inhaled Z92.240
    stroke without residual deficits Z86.73
    substance abuse NEC F10-F19
    sudden cardiac arrest Z86.74
    sudden cardiac death successfully
      resuscitated Z86.74
    ➔suicide attempt Z91.51
    surgery NEC Z98.890
      with uterine scar Z98.891
      sex reassignment Z87.890
      transplant —*see* Transplant
    thrombophlebitis Z86.72
    thrombosis (venous) Z86.718
      pulmonary Z86.711
    tobacco dependence Z87.891
    transient ischemic attack (TIA) without
      residual deficits Z86.73
    trauma (physical) NEC Z87.828
      psychological NEC Z91.49
      ➔self-harm Z91.51
    traumatic brain injury Z87.820

History (Continued)
  personal (Continued)
    tuberculosis, latent infection Z86.15
    unhealthy sleep-wake cycle Z72.821
    unintended awareness under general
      anesthesia Z92.84
    urinary (recurrent) (tract) infection(s) Z87.440
    urinary calculi Z87.42
    uterine scar from previous surgery Z98.891
    vaginal dysplasia Z87.411
    venous thrombosis or embolism Z86.718
      pulmonary Z86.711
    vulvar dysplasia Z87.412
His-Werner disease A79.0
HIV —see also Human, immunodeficiency virus
  B20
  laboratory evidence (nonconclusive) R75
  nonconclusive test (in infants) R75
  positive, seropositive Z21
Hives (bold) —see Urticaria
Hoarseness R49.0
Hobo Z59.00
Hodgkin disease —see Lymphoma, Hodgkin
Hodgson's disease I71.2
  ruptured I71.1
Hoffa-Kastert disease E88.89
Hoffa's disease E88.89
Hoffmann-Bouveret syndrome I47.9
Hoffmann's syndrome E03.9 [G73.7]
Hole (round)
  macula H35.34-●
  retina (without detachment) —see Break,
    retina, round hole
    with detachment —see Detachment, retina,
      with retinal, break
Holiday relief care Z75.5
Hollenhorst's plaque —see Occlusion, artery,
  retina
Hollow foot (congenital) Q66.7-●
  acquired —see Deformity, limb, foot, specified
    NEC
Holoprosencephaly Q04.2
Holt-Oram syndrome Q87.2
Homelessness Z59.00
  sheltered Z59.01
  unsheltered Z59.02
Homesickness —see Disorder, adjustment
Homocysteinemia R79.83
Homocystinemia, homocystinuria E72.11
Homogentisate 1,2-dioxygenase deficiency
  E70.29
Homologous serum hepatitis (prophylactic)
  (therapeutic) —see Hepatitis, viral, type B
Honeycomb lung J98.4
  congenital Q33.0
Hooded
  clitoris Q52.6
  penis Q55.69
Hookworm (disease) (infection) (infestation) B76.9
  with anemia B76.9 [D63.8]
  specified NEC B76.8
Hordeolum (eyelid) (externum) (recurrent)
  H00.019
  internum H00.029
    left H00.026
      lower H00.025
      upper H00.024
    right H00.023
      lower H00.022
      upper H00.021
  left H00.016
    lower H00.015
    upper H00.014
  right H00.013
    lower H00.012
    upper H00.011
Horn
  cutaneous L85.8
  nail L60.2
    congenital Q84.6
Horner (-Claude Bernard) syndrome G90.2
  traumatic —see Injury, nerve, cervical
    sympathetic

Horseshoe kidney (congenital) Q63.1
Horton's headache or neuralgia G44.099
  intractable G44.091
  not intractable G44.099
Hospital hopper syndrome —see Disorder,
  factitious
Hospitalism in children —see Disorder,
  adjustment
Hostility R45.5
  towards child Z62.3
Hot flashes
  menopausal N95.1
Hourglass (contracture) —see also Contraction,
  hourglass
  stomach K31.89
    congenital Q40.2
    stricture K31.2
Household, housing circumstance affecting
  care Z59.9
  specified NEC Z59.89
Housemaid's knee —see Bursitis, prepatellar
HSCT-TMA (hematopoietic stem cell
  transplantation-associated thrombotic
  microangiopathy) M31.11
Hudson (-Ståhli) line (cornea) —see
  Pigmentation, cornea, anterior
Human
  bite (open wound) —see also Bite
    intact skin surface —see Bite, superficial
  herpesvirus —see Herpes
  immunodeficiency virus (HIV) disease
    (infection) B20
    asymptomatic status Z21
    contact Z20.6
    counseling Z71.7
    dementia B20 [F02.80]
      with behavioral disturbance B20 [F02.81]
    exposure to Z20.6
    laboratory evidence R75
    type-2 (HIV 2) as cause of disease classified
      elsewhere B97.35
  papillomavirus (HPV)
    DNA test positive
      high risk
        cervix R87.810
        vagina R87.811
      low risk
        cervix R87.820
        vagina R87.821
    screening for Z11.51
  T-cell lymphotropic virus
    type-1 (HTLV-I) infection B33.3
      as cause of disease classified elsewhere
        B97.33
      carrier Z22.6
    type-2 (HTLV-II) as cause of disease
      classified elsewhere B97.34
Humidifier lung or pneumonitis J67.7
Humiliation (experience) in childhood Z62.898
Humpback (acquired) —see Kyphosis
Hunchback (acquired) —see Kyphosis
Hunger T73.0
  air, psychogenic F45.8
Hungry bone syndrome E83.81
Hunner's ulcer —see Cystitis, chronic, interstitial
Hunter's
  glossitis D51.0
  syndrome E76.1
Huntington's disease or chorea G10
  with dementia G10 [F02.80]
    with behavioral disturbance G10 [F02.81]
Hunt's
  disease or syndrome (herpetic geniculate
    ganglionitis) B02.21
    dyssynergia cerebellaris myoclonica G11.19
  neuralgia B02.21
Hurler (-Scheie) disease or syndrome E76.02
Hurst's disease G36.1
Hurthle cell
  adenocarcinoma C73
  adenoma D34
  carcinoma C73
  tumor D34

Hutchinson-Boeck disease or syndrome —see
  Sarcoidosis
Hutchinson-Gilford disease or syndrome E34.8
Hutchinson's
  disease, meaning
    angioma serpiginosum L81.7
    pompholyx (cheiropompholyx) L30.1
    prurigo estivalis L56.4
    summer eruption or summer prurigo L56.4
  melanotic freckle —see Melanoma, in situ
    malignant melanoma in —see Melanoma
  teeth or incisors (congenital syphilis) A50.52
  triad (congenital syphilis) A50.53
Hyalin plaque, sclera, senile H15.89
Hyaline membrane (disease) (lung)
  (pulmonary) (newborn) P22.0
Hyalinosis
  cutis (et mucosae) E78.89
  focal and segmental (glomerular) —see also
    N00-N07 with fourth character .1 N05.1
Hyalitis, hyalosis, asteroid —see also Deposit,
  crystalline
  syphilitic (late) A52.71
Hydatid
  cyst or tumor —see Echinococcus
  mole —see Hydatidiform mole
  Morgagni
    female Q50.5
    male (epididymal) Q55.4
    testicular Q55.29
Hydatidiform mole (benign) (complicating
  pregnancy) (delivered) (undelivered) O01.9
  classical O01.0
  complete O01.0
  incomplete O01.1
  invasive D39.2
  malignant D39.2
  partial O01.1
Hydatidosis —see Echinococcus
Hydradenitis (axillaris) (suppurative) L73.2
Hydradenoma —see Hidradenoma
Hydramnios O40.-●
Hydrancephaly, hydranencephaly Q04.3
  with spina bifida —see Spina bifida, with
    hydrocephalus
Hydrargyrism NEC —see Poisoning, mercury
Hydrarthrosis —see also Effusion, joint
  gonococcal A54.42
  intermittent M12.40
    ankle M12.47-●
    elbow M12.42-●
    foot joint M12.47-●
    hand joint M12.44-●
    hip M12.45-●
    knee M12.46-●
    multiple site M12.49
    shoulder M12.41-●
    specified joint NEC M12.48
    wrist M12.43-●
  of yaws (early) (late) —see also subcategory
    M14.8-● A66.6
  syphilitic (late) A52.77
    congenital A50.55 [M12.80]
Hydremia D64.89
Hydrencephalocele (congenital) —see
  Encephalocele
Hydrencephalomeningocele (congenital) —see
  Encephalocele
Hydroa R23.8
  aestivale L56.4
  vacciniforme L56.4
Hydroadenitis (axillaris) (suppurative) L73.2
Hydrocalycosis —see Hydronephrosis
Hydrocele (spermatic cord) (testis) (tunica
  vaginalis) N43.3
  canal of Nuck N94.89
  communicating N43.2
    congenital P83.5
  congenital P83.5
  encysted N43.0
  female NEC N94.89
  infected N43.1
  newborn P83.5

Hydrocele *(Continued)*
  round ligament N94.89
  specified NEC N43.2
  spinalis —*see* Spina bifida
  vulva N90.89
Hydrocephalus (acquired) (external) (internal)
    (malignant) (recurrent) G91.9
  aqueduct Sylvius stricture Q03.0
  causing disproportion O33.6
    with obstructed labor O66.3
  communicating G91.0
  congenital (external) (internal) Q03.9
    with spina bifida Q05.4
      cervical Q05.0
      dorsal Q05.1
      lumbar Q05.2
      lumbosacral Q05.2
      sacral Q05.3
      thoracic Q05.1
      thoracolumbar Q05.1
    specified NEC Q03.8
  due to toxoplasmosis (congenital) P37.1
  foramen Magendie block (acquired) G91.1
    congenital —*see also* Hydrocephalus,
      congenital Q03.1
  in (due to)
    infectious disease NEC B89 *[G91.4]*
    neoplastic disease NEC (*see also* Neoplasm)
      G91.4
    parasitic disease B89 *[G91.4]*
  newborn Q03.9
    with spina bifida —*see* Spina bifida, with
      hydrocephalus
  noncommunicating G91.1
  normal pressure G91.2
    secondary G91.0
  obstructive G91.1
  otitic G93.2
  post-traumatic NEC G91.3
  secondary G91.4
    post-traumatic G91.3
  specified NEC G91.8
  syphilitic, congenital A50.49
Hydrocolpos (congenital) N89.8
Hydrocystoma —*see* Neoplasm, skin, benign
Hydroencephalocele (congenital) —*see*
    Encephalocele
Hydroencephalomeningocele (congenital) —
    see Encephalocele
Hydrohematopneumothorax —*see* Hemothorax
Hydromeningitis —*see* Meningitis
Hydromeningocele (spinal) —*see also* Spina bifida
  cranial —*see* Encephalocele
Hydrometra N85.8
Hydrometrocolpos N89.8
Hydromicrocephaly Q02
Hydromphalos (since birth) Q45.8
Hydromyelia Q06.4
Hydromyelocele —*see* Spina bifida
Hydronephrosis (atrophic) (early)
    (functionless) (intermittent) (primary)
    (secondary) NEC N13.30
  with
    infection N13.6
    obstruction (by) (of)
      renal calculus N13.2
        with infection N13.6
      ureteral NEC N13.1
        with infection N13.6
        calculus N13.2
          with infection N13.6
      ureteropelvic junction (congenital) Q62.11
        acquired N13.0
          with infection N13.6
      ureteral stricture NEC N13.1
        with infection N13.6
  congenital Q62.0
    due to acquired occlusion of ureteropelvic
      junction N13.0
  specified type NEC N13.39
  tuberculous A18.11
Hydropericarditis —*see* Pericarditis
Hydropericardium —*see* Pericarditis

Hydroperitoneum R18.8
Hydrophobia —*see* Rabies
Hydrophthalmos Q15.0
Hydropneumohemothorax —*see* Hemothorax
Hydropneumopericarditis —*see* Pericarditis
Hydropneumopericardium —*see* Pericarditis
Hydropneumothorax J94.8
  traumatic —*see* Injury, intrathoracic, lung
  tuberculous NEC A15.6
Hydrops R60.9
  abdominis R18.8
  articulorum intermittens —*see* Hydrarthrosis,
    intermittent
  cardiac —*see* Failure, heart, congestive
  causing obstructed labor (mother) O66.3
  endolymphatic H81.0-●
  fetal —*see* Pregnancy, complicated by,
    hydrops, fetalis
Hydrops *(Continued)*
  fetalis P83.2
    due to
      ABO isoimmunization P56.0
      alpha thalassemia D56.0
      hemolytic disease P56.90
        specified NEC P56.99
      isoimmunization (ABO) (Rh) P56.0
      other specified nonhemolytic disease
        NEC P83.2
      Rh incompatibility P56.0
    during pregnancy —*see* Pregnancy,
      complicated by, hydrops, fetalis
  gallbladder K82.1
  joint —*see* Effusion, joint
  labyrinth H81.0
  newborn (idiopathic) P83.2
    due to
      ABO isoimmunization P56.0
      alpha thalassemia D56.0
      hemolytic disease P56.90
        specified NEC P56.99
      isoimmunization (ABO) (Rh) P56.0
      Rh incompatibility P56.0
  nutritional —*see* Malnutrition, severe
  pericardium —*see* Pericarditis
  pleura —*see* Hydrothorax
  spermatic cord —*see* Hydrocele
Hydropyonephrosis N13.6
Hydrorachis Q06.4
Hydrorrhea (nasal) J34.89
  pregnancy —*see* Rupture, membranes,
    premature
Hydrosadenitis (axillaris) (suppurative) L73.2
Hydrosalpinx (fallopian tube) (follicularis) N70.11
Hydrothorax (double) (pleura) J94.8
  chylous (nonfilarial) I89.8
    filarial —*see also* Infestation, filarial B74.9
      [J91.8]
  traumatic —*see* Injury, intrathoracic
  tuberculous NEC (non primary) A15.6
Hydroureter —*see also* Hydronephrosis N13.4
  with infection N13.6
  congenital Q62.39
Hydroureteronephrosis —*see* Hydronephrosis
Hydrourethra N36.8
Hydroxykynureninuria E70.89
Hydroxylysinemia E72.3
Hydroxyprolinemia E72.59
Hygiene, sleep
  abuse Z72.821
  inadequate Z72.821
  poor Z72.821
Hygroma (congenital) (cystic) D18.1
  praepatellare, prepatellar —*see* Bursitis,
    prepatellar
Hymen —*see* condition
Hymenolepis, hymenolepiasis (diminuta)
    (infection) (infestation) (nana) B71.0
Hypalgesia R20.8
Hyperacidity (gastric) K31.89
  psychogenic F45.8
Hyperactive, hyperactivity F90.9
  basal cell, uterine cervix —*see* Dysplasia, cervix
  bowel sounds R19.12

Hyperactive, hyperactivity*(Continued)*
  cervix epithelial (basal) —*see* Dysplasia, cervix
  child F90.9
    attention deficit —*see* Disorder, attention-
      deficit hyperactivity
  detrusor muscle N32.81
  gastrointestinal K31.89
    psychogenic F45.8
  nasal mucous membrane J34.3
  stomach K31.89
  thyroid (gland) —*see* Hyperthyroidism
Hyperacusis H93.23-●
Hyperadrenalism E27.5
Hyperadrenocorticism E24.9
  congenital E25.0
  iatrogenic E24.2
    correct substance properly administered —
      see Table of Drugs and Chemicals, by
      drug, adverse effect
    overdose or wrong substance given
      or taken —*see* Table of Drugs and
      Chemicals, by drug, poisoning
  not associated with Cushing's syndrome E27.0
  pituitary-dependent E24.0
Hyperaldosteronism E26.9
  familial (type I) E26.02
  glucocorticoid-remediable E26.02
  primary (due to (bilateral) adrenal
    hyperplasia) E26.09
  primary NEC E26.09
  secondary E26.1
  specified NEC E26.89
Hyperalgesia R20.8
Hyperalimentation R63.2
  carotene, carotin E67.1
  specified NEC E67.8
  vitamin
    A E67.0
    D E67.3
Hyperaminoaciduria
  arginine E72.21
  cystine E72.01
  lysine E72.3
  ornithine E72.4
Hyperammonemia (congenital) E72.20
Hyperazotemia —*see* Uremia
Hyperbetalipoproteinemia (familial) E78.00
  with prebetalipoproteinemia E78.2
Hyperbilirubinemia
  constitutional E80.6
  familial conjugated E80.6
  neonatal (transient) —*see* Jaundice, newborn
Hypercalcemia, hypocalciuric, familial E83.52
Hypercalciuria, idiopathic R82.994
Hypercapnia R06.89
  newborn P84
Hypercarotenemia (dietary) E67.1
Hypercementosis K03.4
Hyperchloremia E87.8
Hyperchlorhydria K31.89
  neurotic F45.8
  psychogenic F45.8
Hypercholesterinemia —*see*
    Hypercholesterolemia
Hypercholesterolemia (essential) (primary)
    (pure) E78.00
  with hyperglyceridemia, endogenous E78.2
  dietary counseling and surveillance Z71.3
  familial E78.01
  hereditary E78.01
Hyperchylia gastrica, psychogenic F45.8
Hyperchylomicronemia (familial) (primary) E78.3
  with hyperbetalipoproteinemia E78.3
Hypercoagulable (state) D68.59
  activated protein C resistance D68.51
  antithrombin (III) deficiency D68.59
  factor V Leiden mutation D68.51
  primary NEC D68.59
  protein C deficiency D68.59
  protein S deficiency D68.59
  prothrombin gene mutation D68.52
  secondary D68.69
  specified NEC D68.69

Hypercoagulation (state) D68.59
Hypercorticalism, pituitary-dependent E24.0
Hypercorticosolism —*see* Cushing's, syndrome
Hypercorticosteronism E24.2
  correct substance properly administered —*see* Table of Drugs and Chemicals, by drug, adverse effect
  overdose or wrong substance given or taken —*see* Table of Drugs and Chemicals, by drug, poisoning
Hypercortisonism E24.2
  correct substance properly administered —*see* Table of Drugs and Chemicals, by drug, adverse effect
  overdose or wrong substance given or taken —*see* Table of Drugs and Chemicals, by drug, poisoning
Hyperekplexia Q89.8
Hyperelectrolytemia E87.8
Hyperemesis R11.10
  with nausea R11.2
  gravidarum (mild) O21.0
    with
      carbohydrate depletion O21.1
      dehydration O21.1
      electrolyte imbalance O21.1
      metabolic disturbance O21.1
    severe (with metabolic disturbance) O21.1
  projectile R11.12
  psychogenic F45.8
Hyperemia (acute) (passive) R68.89
  anal mucosa K62.89
  bladder N32.89
  cerebral I67.89
  conjunctiva H11.43-•
  ear internal, acute —*see* subcategory H83.0
  enteric K59.89
  eye —*see* Hyperemia, conjunctiva
  eyelid (active) (passive) —*see* Disorder, eyelid, specified type NEC
  intestine K59.89
  iris —*see* Disorder, iris, vascular
  kidney N28.89
  labyrinth —*see* subcategory H83.0
  liver (active) K76.89
  lung (passive) —*see* Edema, lung
  pulmonary (passive) —*see* Edema, lung
  renal N28.89
  retina H35.89
  stomach K31.89
Hyperesthesia (body surface) R20.3
  larynx (reflex) J38.7
    hysterical F44.89
  pharynx (reflex) J39.2
    hysterical F44.89
Hyperestrogenism (drug-induced) (iatrogenic) E28.0
Hyperexplexia Q89.8
Hyperfibrinolysis —*see* Fibrinolysis
Hyperfructosemia E74.19
Hyperfunction
  adrenal cortex, not associated with Cushing's syndrome E27.0
    medulla E27.5
      adrenomedullary E27.5
    virilism E25.9
      congenital E25.0
  ovarian E28.8
  pancreas K86.89
  parathyroid (gland) E21.3
  pituitary (gland) (anterior) E22.9
    specified NEC E22.8
  polyglandular E31.1
  testicular E29.0
Hypergammaglobulinemia D89.2
  polyclonal D89.0
  Waldenström D89.0
Hypergastrinemia E16.4
Hyperglobulinemia R77.1
Hyperglycemia, hyperglycemic (transient) R73.9
  coma —*see* Diabetes, by type, with coma
  postpancreatectomy E89.1

Hyperglyceridemia (endogenous) (essential) (familial) (hereditary) (pure) E78.1
  mixed E78.3
Hyperglycinemia (non-ketotic) E72.51
Hypergonadism
  ovarian E28.8
  testicular (primary) (infantile) E29.0
Hyperheparinemia D68.32
Hyperhidrosis, hyperidrosis R61
  focal
    primary L74.519
      axilla L74.510
      face L74.511
      palms L74.512
      soles L74.513
    secondary L74.52
  generalized R61
  localized
    primary L74.519
      axilla L74.510
      face L74.511
      palms L74.512
      soles L74.513
    secondary L74.52
  psychogenic F45.8
  secondary R61
    focal L74.52
Hyperhistidinemia E70.41
Hyperhomocysteinemia E72.11
Hyperhydroxyprolinemia E72.59
Hyperinsulinism (functional) E16.1
  with
    coma (hypoglycemic) E15
    encephalopathy E16.1 *[G94]*
  ectopic E16.1
  therapeutic misadventure (from administration of insulin) —*see* subcategory T38.3
Hyperkalemia E87.5
Hyperkeratosis —*see also* Keratosis L85.9
  cervix N88.0
  due to yaws (early) (late) (palmar or plantar) A66.3
  follicularis Q82.8
    penetrans (in cutem) L87.0
  palmoplantaris climacterica L85.1
  pinta A67.1
  senile (with pruritus) L57.0
  universalis congenita Q80.8
  vocal cord J38.3
  vulva N90.4
Hyperkinesia, hyperkinetic (disease) (reaction) (syndrome) (childhood) (adolescence) — *see also* Disorder, attention-deficit hyperactivity
  heart I51.89
Hyperleucine-isoleucinemia E71.19
Hyperlipemia, hyperlipidemia E78.5
  combined E78.2
    familial E78.49
  group
    A E78.00
    B E78.1
    C E78.2
    D E78.3
  mixed E78.2
  specified NEC E78.49
Hyperlipidosis E75.6
  hereditary NEC E75.5
Hyperlipoproteinemia E78.5
  Fredrickson's type
    I E78.3
    IIa E78.00
    IIb E78.2
    III E78.2
    IV E78.1
    V E78.3
  low-density-lipoprotein-type (LDL) E78.00
  very-low-density-lipoprotein-type (VLDL) E78.1
Hyperlucent lung, unilateral J43.0
Hyperlysinemia E72.3
Hypermagnesemia E83.41
  neonatal P71.8

Hypermenorrhea N92.0
Hypermethioninemia E72.19
Hypermetropia (congenital) H52.0-•
Hypermobility, hypermotility
  cecum —*see* Syndrome, irritable bowel
  coccyx —*see* subcategory M53.2
  colon —*see* Syndrome, irritable bowel
    psychogenic F45.8
  ileum K58.9
  intestine —*see also* Syndrome, irritable bowel K58.9
    psychogenic F45.8
  meniscus (knee) —*see* Derangement, knee, meniscus
  scapula —*see* Instability, joint, shoulder
  stomach K31.89
    psychogenic F45.8
  syndrome M35.7
  urethra N36.41
    with intrinsic sphincter deficiency N36.43
Hypernasality R49.21
Hypernatremia E87.0
Hypernephroma C64.-•
Hyperopia —*see* Hypermetropia
Hyperorexia nervosa F50.2
Hyperornithinemia E72.4
Hyperosmia R43.1
Hyperosmolality E87.0
Hyperostosis (monomelic) —*see also* Disorder, bone, density and structure, specified NEC
  ankylosing (spine) M48.10
    cervical region M48.12
    cervicothoracic region M48.13
    lumbar region M48.16
    lumbosacral region M48.17
    multiple sites M48.19
    occipito-atlanto-axial region M48.11
    sacrococcygeal region M48.18
    thoracic region M48.14
    thoracolumbar region M48.15
  cortical (skull) M85.2
    infantile M89.8X-•
  frontal, internal of skull M85.2
  interna frontalis M85.2
  skeletal, diffuse idiopathic —*see* Hyperostosis, ankylosing
  skull M85.2
    congenital Q75.8
  vertebral, ankylosing —*see* Hyperostosis, ankylosing
Hyperovarism E28.8
Hyperoxaluria (primary) R82.992
Hyperparathyroidism E21.3
  primary E21.0
  secondary (renal) N25.81
    non-renal E21.1
  specified NEC E21.2
  tertiary E21.2
Hyperpathia R20.8
Hyperperistalsis R19.2
  psychogenic F45.8
Hyperpermeability, capillary I78.8
Hyperphagia R63.2
Hyperphenylalaninemia NEC E70.1
Hyperphoria (alternating) H50.53
Hyperphosphatemia E83.39
Hyperpiesis, hyperpiesia —*see* Hypertension
Hyperpigmentation —*see also* Pigmentation
  melanin NEC L81.4
  postinflammatory L81.0
Hyperpinealism E34.8
Hyperpituitarism E22.9
Hyperplasia, hyperplastic
  adenoids J35.2
  adrenal (capsule) (cortex) (gland) E27.8
    with
      sexual precocity (male) E25.9
        congenital E25.0
      virilism, adrenal E25.9
        congenital E25.0
      virilization (female) E25.9
        congenital E25.0

▶ New   ⇒ Revised   ~~deleted~~ Deleted   • Use Additional Character(s)

Hyperplasia, hyperplastic (Continued)
  adrenal(Continued)
    congenital E25.0
      salt-losing E25.0
  adrenomedullary E27.5
  angiolymphoid, eosinophilia (ALHE) D18.01
  appendix (lymphoid) K38.0
  artery, fibromuscular I77.3
  bone —see also Hypertrophy, bone
    marrow D75.89
  breast —see also Hypertrophy, breast
    atypical, atypia N60.9-●
      ductal N60.9-●
      lobular N60.9-●
  C-cell, thyroid E07.0
  cementation (tooth) (teeth) K03.4
  cervical gland R59.0
  cervix (uteri) (basal cell) (endometrium)
    (polypoid) —see also Dysplasia, cervix
    congenital Q51.828
  clitoris, congenital Q52.6
  denture K06.2
  endocervicitis N72
  endometrium, endometrial (adenomatous)
    (cystic) (glandular) (glandular-cystic)
    (polypoid) N85.00
    with atypia N85.02
    benign N85.01
    cervix —see Dysplasia, cervix
    complex (without atypia) N85.01
    simple (without atypia) N85.01
  epithelial L85.9
    focal, oral, including tongue K13.29
    nipple N62
    skin L85.9
    tongue K13.29
    vaginal wall N89.3
  erythroid D75.89
  fibromuscular of artery (carotid) (renal) I77.3
  genital
    female NEC N94.89
    male N50.89
  gingiva K06.1
  glandularis cystica uteri (interstitialis) —see
    also Hyperplasia, endometrial N85.00-●
  gum K06.1
  hymen, congenital Q52.4
  irritative, edentulous (alveolar) K06.2
  jaw M26.09
    alveolar M26.79
    lower M26.03
      alveolar M26.72
    upper M26.01
      alveolar M26.71
  kidney (congenital) Q63.3
  labia N90.69
    epithelial N90.3
  liver (congenital) Q44.7
    nodular, focal K76.89
  lymph gland or node R59.9
  mandible, mandibular M26.03
    alveolar M26.72
    unilateral condylar M27.8
  maxilla, maxillary M26.01
    alveolar M26.71
  myometrium, myometrial N85.2
  neuroendocrine cell, of infancy J84.841
  nose
    lymphoid J34.89
    polypoid J33.9
  oral mucosa (irritative) K13.6
  organ or site, congenital NEC —see Anomaly,
    by site
  ovary N83.8
  palate, papillary (irritative) K13.6
  pancreatic islet cells E16.9
    alpha E16.8
      with excess
        gastrin E16.4
        glucagon E16.3
    beta E16.1
  parathyroid (gland) E21.0

Hyperplasia, hyperplastic (Continued)
  pharynx (lymphoid) J39.2
  prostate (adenofibromatous) (nodular)
    N40.0
    with lower urinary tract symptoms (LUTS)
      N40.1
    without lower urinary tract symptoms
      (LUTS) N40.0
  renal artery I77.89
  reticulo-endothelial (cell) D75.89
  salivary gland (any) K11.1
  Schimmelbusch's —see Mastopathy, cystic
  suprarenal capsule (gland) E27.8
  thymus (gland) (persistent) E32.0
  thyroid (gland) —see Goiter
  tonsils (faucial) (infective) (lingual)
    (lymphoid) J35.1
    with adenoids J35.3
  unilateral condylar M27.8
  uterus, uterine N85.2
    endometrium (glandular) —see also
      Hyperplasia, endometrial
      N85.00-●
  vulva N90.69
    epithelial N90.3
Hyperpnea —see Hyperventilation
Hyperpotassemia E87.5
Hyperprebetalipoproteinemia (familial)
  E78.1
Hyperprolactinemia E22.1
Hyperprolinemia (type I) (type II) E72.59
Hyperproteinemia E88.09
Hyperprothrombinemia, causing coagulation
  factor deficiency D68.4
Hyperpyrexia R50.9
  heat (effects) T67.01
  malignant, due to anesthetic T88.3
  rheumatic —see Fever, rheumatic
  unknown origin R50.9
Hyper-reflexia R29.2
Hypersalivation K11.7
Hypersecretion
  ACTH (not associated with Cushing's
    syndrome) E27.0
    pituitary E24.0
  adrenaline E27.5
  adrenomedullary E27.5
  androgen (testicular) E29.0
    ovarian (drug-induced) (iatrogenic) E28.1
  calcitonin E07.0
  catecholamine E27.5
  corticoadrenal E24.9
  cortisol E24.9
  epinephrine E27.5
  estrogen E28.0
  gastric K31.89
    psychogenic F45.8
  gastrin E16.4
  glucagon E16.3
  hormone(s)
    ACTH (not associated with Cushing's
      syndrome) E27.0
      pituitary E24.0
    antidiuretic E22.2
    growth E22.0
    intestinal NEC E34.1
    ovarian androgen E28.1
    pituitary E22.9
    testicular E29.0
    thyroid stimulating E05.80
      with thyroid storm E05.81
  insulin —see Hyperinsulinism
  lacrimal glands —see Epiphora
  medulloadrenal E27.5
  milk O92.6
  ovarian androgens E28.1
  salivary gland (any) K11.7
  thyrocalcitonin E07.0
  upper respiratory J39.8
Hypersegmentation, leukocytic, hereditary
  D72.0

Hypersensitive, hypersensitiveness,
  hypersensitivity —see also Allergy
  carotid sinus G90.01
  colon —see Irritable, colon
  drug T88.7
  gastrointestinal K52.29
    immediate K52.29
    psychogenic F45.8
  labyrinth —see subcategory H83.2
  pain R20.8
  pneumonitis —see Pneumonitis, allergic
  reaction T78.40
    upper respiratory tract NEC J39.3
Hypersomnia (organic) G47.10
  due to
    alcohol
      abuse F10.182
      dependence F10.282
      use F10.982
    amphetamines
      abuse F15.182
      dependence F15.282
      use F15.982
    caffeine
      abuse F15.182
      dependence F15.282
      use F15.982
    cocaine
      abuse F14.182
      dependence F14.282
      use F14.982
    drug NEC
      abuse F19.182
      dependence F19.282
      use F19.982
    medical condition G47.14
    mental disorder F51.13
    opioid
      abuse F11.182
      dependence F11.282
      use F11.982
    psychoactive substance NEC
      abuse F19.182
      dependence F19.282
      use F19.982
    sedative, hypnotic, or anxiolytic
      abuse F13.182
      dependence F13.282
      use F13.982
    stimulant NEC
      abuse F15.182
      dependence F15.282
      use F15.982
  idiopathic G47.11
    with long sleep time G47.11
    without long sleep time G47.12
  menstrual related G47.13
  nonorganic origin F51.11
    specified NEC F51.19
  not due to a substance or known
    physiological condition F51.11
    specified NEC F51.19
  primary F51.11
  recurrent G47.13
  specified NEC G47.19
Hypersplenia, hypersplenism D73.1
Hyperstimulation, ovaries (associated with
  induced ovulation) N98.1
Hypersusceptibility —see Allergy
Hypertelorism (ocular) (orbital) Q75.2
Hypertension, hypertensive (accelerated)
  (benign) (essential) (idiopathic)
  (malignant) (systemic) I10
  with
    heart failure (congestive) I11.0
    heart involvement (conditions in I50.-
      or I51.4-I51.7, I51.89, I51.9, due to
      hypertension) —see Hypertension,
      heart
    kidney involvement —see Hypertension,
      kidney

Hypertension, hypertensive (Continued)
  benign, intracranial G93.2
  borderline R03.0
  cardiorenal (disease) I13.10
    with heart failure I13.0
      with stage 1 through stage 4 chronic
        kidney disease I13.0
      with stage 5 or end stage renal disease
        I13.2
    without heart failure I13.10
      with stage 1 through stage 4 chronic
        kidney disease I13.10
      with stage 5 or end stage renal disease
        I13.11
  cardiovascular
    disease (arteriosclerotic) (sclerotic) —see
      Hypertension, heart
    renal (disease) —see Hypertension,
      cardiorenal
  chronic venous —see Hypertension, venous
    (chronic)
  complicating
    childbirth (labor) O16.4
      pre-existing O10.92
        with
          heart disease O10.12
            with renal disease O10.32
          pre-eclampsia O11.4
          renal disease O10.22
            with heart disease O10.32
          essential O10.02
          secondary O10.42
    pregnancy O16.-•
      with edema —see also Pre-eclampsia
        O14.9-•
      gestational (pregnancy induced)
        (without proteinuria) O13.-•
        with proteinuria O14.9-•
          mild pre-eclampsia O14.0-•
          moderate pre-eclampsia O14.0-•
          severe pre-eclampsia O14.1-•
            with hemolysis, elevated liver
              enzymes and low platelet
              count (HELLP) O14.2-•
      pre-existing O10.91-•
        with
          heart disease O10.11-•
            with renal disease O10.31-•
          pre-eclampsia —see category O11
          renal disease O10.21-•
            with heart disease O10.31-•
          essential O10.01-•
          secondary O10.41-•
        transient O13.-•
    puerperium pre-existing O16.5
      pre-existing
        with
          heart disease O10.13
            with renal disease O10.33
          pre-eclampsia O11.5
          renal disease O10.23
            with heart disease O10.33
          essential O10.03
      pregnancy-induced O13.9
      secondary O10.43
  crisis I16.9
  due to
    endocrine disorders I15.2
    pheochromocytoma I15.2
    renal disorders NEC I15.1
      arterial I15.0
    renovascular disorders I15.0
    specified disease NEC I15.8
  emergency I16.1
  encephalopathy I67.4
  gestational (without significant proteinuria)
      (pregnancy-induced) (transient) O13.-•
    with significant proteinuria —see
      Pre-eclampsia
    complicating
      delivery O13.4
      puerperium O13.5

Hypertension, hypertensive (Continued)
  Goldblatt's I70.1
  heart (disease) (conditions in I51.4-I51.9 due
      to hypertension) I11.9
    with
      heart failure (congestive) I11.0
      kidney disease (chronic) —see
        Hypertension, cardiorenal
  intracranial, benign G93.2
  kidney I12.9
    with
      heart disease —see Hypertension,
        cardiorenal
      stage 1 through stage 4 chronic kidney
        disease I12.9
      stage 5 chronic kidney disease (CKD) or
        end stage renal disease (ESRD) I12.0
  lesser circulation I27.0
  maternal O16.-•
  newborn P29.2
    pulmonary (persistent) P29.30
  ocular H40.05-•
  pancreatic duct — code to underlying
      condition
    with chronic pancreatitis K86.1
  portal (due to chronic liver disease)
      (idiopathic) K76.6
    gastropathy K31.89
    in (due to) schistosomiasis (bilharziasis)
      B65.9 [K77]
  postoperative I97.3
  psychogenic F45.8
  pulmonary NEC I27.20
    with
      cor pulmonale (chronic) I27.29
        acute I26.09
      right heart ventricular strain/failure
        I27.29
        acute I26.09
      right to left shunt related to congenital
        heart disease I27.83
      unclear multifactorial mechanisms
        I27.29
    arterial (associated) (drug-induced) (toxin-
      induced) I27.21
    chronic thromboembolic I27.24
    due to
      hematologic disorders I27.29
      ▶kyphoscoliotic heart disease I27.1
      left heart disease I27.22
      lung diseases and hypoxia I27.23
      metabolic disorders I27.29
      specified systemic disorders NEC I27.29
    group 1 (associated) (drug-induced) (toxin-
      induced) I27.21
    group 2 I27.22
    group 3 I27.23
    group 4 I27.24
    group 5 I27.29
    of newborn (persistent) P29.30
    secondary
      arterial I27.21
      specified NEC I27.29
    primary (idiopathic) I27.0
  renal —see Hypertension, kidney
  renovascular I15.0
  secondary NEC I15.9
    due to
      endocrine disorders I15.2
      pheochromocytoma I15.2
      renal disorders NEC I15.1
        arterial I15.0
      renovascular disorders I15.0
    specified NEC I15.8
  transient R03.0
    of pregnancy O13.•
  urgency I16.0
  venous (chronic)
    due to
      deep vein thrombosis —see Syndrome,
        postthrombotic

Hypertension, hypertensive (Continued)
  venous (Continued)
    idiopathic I87.309
      with
        inflammation I87.32-•
          with ulcer I87.33-•
        specified complication NEC I87.39-•
        ulcer I87.31-•
          with inflammation I87.33-•
      asymptomatic I87.30-•
Hypertensive urgency —see Hypertension
Hyperthecosis ovary E28.8
Hyperthermia (of unknown origin) —see also
      Hyperpyrexia
  malignant, due to anesthesia T88.3
  newborn P81.9
    environmental P81.0
Hyperthyroid (recurrent) —see Hyperthyroidism
Hyperthyroidism (latent) (pre-adult) (recurrent)
      E05.90
  with
    goiter (diffuse) E05.00
      with thyroid storm E05.01
      nodular (multinodular) E05.20
        with thyroid storm E05.21
        uninodular E05.10
          with thyroid storm E05.11
    storm E05.91
  due to ectopic thyroid tissue E05.30
    with thyroid storm E05.31
  neonatal, transitory P72.1
  specified NEC E05.80
    with thyroid storm E05.81
Hypertony, hypertonia, hypertonicity
  bladder N31.8
  congenital P94.1
  stomach K31.89
    psychogenic F45.8
  uterus, uterine (contractions) (complicating
      delivery) O62.4
Hypertrichosis L68.9
  congenital Q84.2
  eyelid H02.869
    left H02.866
      lower H02.865
      upper H02.864
    right H02.863
      lower H02.862
      upper H02.861
  lanuginosa Q84.2
    acquired L68.1
  localized L68.2
  specified NEC L68.8
Hypertriglyceridemia, essential E78.1
Hypertrophy, hypertrophic
  adenofibromatous, prostate —see
      Enlargement, enlarged, prostate
  adenoids (infective) J35.2
    with tonsils J35.3
  adrenal cortex E27.8
  alveolar process or ridge —see Anomaly,
      alveolar
  anal papillae K62.89
  artery I77.89
    congenital NEC Q27.8
      digestive system Q27.8
      lower limb Q27.8
      specified site NEC Q27.8
      upper limb Q27.8
  auricular —see Hypertrophy, cardiac
  Bartholin's gland N75.8
  bile duct (common) (hepatic) K83.8
  bladder (sphincter) (trigone) N32.89
  bone M89.30
    carpus M89.34-•
    clavicle M89.31-•
    femur M89.35-•
    fibula M89.36-•
    finger M89.34-•
    humerus M89.32-•
    ilium M89.359

Hypertrophy, hypertrophic (Continued)
 bone (Continued)
  ischium M89.359
  metacarpus M89.34-•
  metatarsus M89.37-•
  multiple sites M89.39
  neck M89.38
  radius M89.33-•
  rib M89.38
  scapula M89.31-•
  skull M89.38
  tarsus M89.37-•
  tibia M89.36-•
  toe M89.37-•
  ulna M89.33-•
  vertebra M89.38
 brain G93.89
 breast N62
  cystic —see Mastopathy, cystic
  newborn P83.4
  pubertal, massive N62
  puerperal, postpartum —see Disorder,
    breast, specified type NEC
  senile (parenchymatous) N62
 cardiac (chronic) (idiopathic) I51.7
  with rheumatic fever (conditions in I00)
   active I01.8
   inactive or quiescent (with chorea) I09.89
  congenital NEC Q24.8
  fatty —see Degeneration, myocardial
  hypertensive —see Hypertension, heart
  rheumatic (with chorea) I09.89
   active or acute I01.8
    with chorea I02.0
  valve —see Endocarditis
 cartilage —see Disorder, cartilage, specified
    type NEC
 cecum —see Megacolon
 cervix (uteri) N88.8
  congenital Q51.828
  elongation N88.4
 clitoris (cirrhotic) N90.89
  congenital Q52.6
 colon —see also Megacolon
  congenital Q43.2
 conjunctiva, lymphoid H11.89
 corpora cavernosa N48.89
 cystic duct K82.8
 duodenum K31.89
 endometrium (glandular) —see also
    Hyperplasia, endometrial N85.00-•
  cervix N88.8
 epididymis N50.89
 esophageal hiatus (congenital) Q79.1
  with hernia —see Hernia, hiatal
 eyelid —see Disorder, eyelid, specified type
    NEC
▶facet joint (see also Spondylosis) M47.819
 fat pad E65
  knee (infrapatellar) (popliteal) (prepatellar)
    (retropatellar) M79.4
 foot (congenital) Q74.2
 frenulum, frenum (tongue) K14.8
  lip K13.0
 gallbladder K82.8
 gastric mucosa K29.60
  with bleeding K29.61
 gland, glandular R59.9
  generalized R59.1
  localized R59.0
 gum (mucous membrane) K06.1
 heart (idiopathic) —see also Hypertrophy,
    cardiac
  valve —see also Endocarditis I38
 hemifacial Q67.4
 hepatic —see Hypertrophy, liver
 hiatus (esophageal) Q79.1
 hilus gland R59.0
 hymen, congenital Q52.4
 ileum K63.89
 intestine NEC K63.89
 jejunum K63.89

Hypertrophy, hypertrophic (Continued)
 kidney (compensatory) N28.81
  congenital Q63.3
 labium (majus) (minus) N90.60
 ligament —see Disorder, ligament
 lingual tonsil (infective) J35.1
  with adenoids J35.3
 lip K13.0
  congenital Q18.6
 liver R16.0
  acute K76.89
  cirrhotic —see Cirrhosis, liver
  congenital Q44.7
  fatty —see Fatty, liver
 lymph, lymphatic gland R59.9
  generalized R59.1
  localized R59.0
  tuberculous —see Tuberculosis, lymph
    gland
 mammary gland —see Hypertrophy, breast
 Meckel's diverticulum (congenital) Q43.0
  malignant —see Table of Neoplasms, small
    intestine, malignant
 median bar —see Hyperplasia, prostate
 meibomian gland —see Chalazion
 meniscus, knee, congenital Q74.1
 metatarsal head —see Hypertrophy, bone,
    metatarsus
 metatarsus —see Hypertrophy, bone,
    metatarsus
 mucous membrane
  alveolar ridge K06.2
  gum K06.1
  nose (turbinate) J34.3
 muscle M62.89
 muscular coat, artery I77.89
 myocardium —see also Hypertrophy, cardiac
  idiopathic I42.2
 myometrium N85.2
 nail L60.2
  congenital Q84.5
 nasal J34.89
  alae J34.89
  bone J34.89
  cartilage J34.89
  mucous membrane (septum) J34.3
  sinus J34.89
  turbinate J34.3
 nasopharynx, lymphoid (infectional) (tissue)
    (wall) J35.2
 nipple N62
 organ or site, congenital NEC —see Anomaly,
    by site - ovary N83.8
 palate (hard) M27.8
  soft K13.79
 pancreas, congenital Q45.3
 parathyroid (gland) E21.0
 parotid gland K11.1
 penis N48.89
 pharyngeal tonsil J35.2
 pharynx J39.2
  lymphoid (infectional) (tissue) (wall)
    J35.2
 pituitary (anterior) (fossa) (gland) E23.6
 prepuce (congenital) N47.8
  female N90.89
 prostate —see Enlargement, enlarged,
    prostate
  congenital Q55.4
 pseudomuscular G71.09
 pylorus (adult) (muscle) (sphincter) K31.1
  congenital or infantile Q40.0
 rectal, rectum (sphincter) K62.89
 rhinitis (turbinate) J31.0
 salivary gland (any) K11.1
  congenital Q38.4
 scaphoid (tarsal) —see Hypertrophy, bone,
    tarsus
 scar L91.0
 scrotum N50.89
 seminal vesicle N50.89

Hypertrophy, hypertrophic (Continued)
 sigmoid —see Megacolon
 skin L91.9
  specified NEC L91.8
 spermatic cord N50.89
 spleen —see Splenomegaly
 spondylitis —see Spondylosis
 stomach K31.89
 sublingual gland K11.1
 submandibular gland K11.1
 suprarenal cortex (gland) E27.8
 synovial NEC M67.20
  acromioclavicular M67.21-•
  ankle M67.27-•
  elbow M67.22-•
  foot M67.27-•
  hand M67.24-•
  hip M67.25-•
  knee M67.26-•
  multiple sites M67.29
  specified site NEC M67.28
  wrist M67.23-•
 tendon —see Disorder, tendon, specified type
    NEC
 testis N44.8
  congenital Q55.29
 thymic, thymus (gland) (congenital)
    E32.0
 thyroid (gland) —see Goiter
 toe (congenital) Q74.2
  acquired —see also Deformity, toe, specified
    NEC
 tongue K14.8
  congenital Q38.2
  papillae (foliate) K14.3
 tonsils (faucial) (infective) (lingual)
    (lymphoid) J35.1
  with adenoids J35.3
 tunica vaginalis N50.89
 ureter N28.89
 urethra N36.8
 uterus N85.2
  neck (with elongation) N88.4
  puerperal O90.89
 uvula K13.79
 vagina N89.8
 vas deferens N50.89
 vein I87.8
 ventricle, ventricular (heart) —see also
    Hypertrophy, cardiac
  congenital Q24.8
  in tetralogy of Fallot Q21.3
 verumontanum N36.8
 vocal cord J38.3
 vulva N90.60
  stasis (nonfilarial) N90.69
Hypertropia H50.2-•
Hypertyrosinemia E70.21
Hyperuricemia (asymptomatic) E79.0
Hyperuricosuria R82.993
Hypervalinemia E71.19
Hyperventilation (tetany) R06.4
 hysterical F45.8
 psychogenic F45.8
 syndrome F45.8
Hypervitaminosis (dietary) NEC E67.8
 A E67.0
  administered as drug (prolonged intake) —
    see Table of Drugs and Chemicals,
    vitamins, adverse effect
  overdose or wrong substance given
    or taken —see Table of Drugs and
    Chemicals, vitamins, poisoning
 B6 E67.2
 D E67.3
  administered as drug (prolonged intake) —
    see Table of Drugs and Chemicals,
    vitamins, adverse effect
  overdose or wrong substance given
    or taken —see Table of Drugs and
    Chemicals, vitamins, poisoning

Hypervitaminosis NEC (Continued)
K E67.8
administered as drug (prolonged intake) —
see Table of Drugs and Chemicals,
vitamins, adverse effect
overdose or wrong substance given
or taken —see Table of Drugs and
Chemicals, vitamins, poisoning
Hypervolemia E87.70
specified NEC E87.79
Hypesthesia R20.1
cornea —see Anesthesia, cornea
Hyphema H21.0-•
traumatic S05.1-•
Hypoacidity, gastric K31.89
psychogenic F45.8
Hypoadrenalism, hypoadrenia E27.40
primary E27.1
tuberculous A18.7
Hypoadrenocorticism E27.40
pituitary E23.0
primary E27.1
Hypoalbuminemia E88.09
Hypoaldosteronism E27.40
Hypoalphalipoproteinemia E78.6
Hypobarism T70.29
Hypobaropathy T70.29
Hypobetalipoproteinemia (familial) E78.6
Hypocalcemia E83.51
dietary E58
neonatal P71.1
due to cow's milk P71.0
phosphate-loading (newborn) P71.1
Hypochloremia E87.8
Hypochlorhydria K31.89
neurotic F45.8
psychogenic F45.8
Hypochondria, hypochondriac,
hypochondriasis (reaction) F45.21
sleep F51.03
Hypochondrogenesis Q77.0
Hypochondroplasia Q77.4
Hypochromasia, blood cells D50.8
Hypodontia —see Anodontia
Hypocitraturia R82.991
Hypoeosinophilia D72.89
Hypoesthesia R20.1
Hypofibrinogenemia D68.8
acquired D65
congenital (hereditary) D68.2
Hypofunction
adrenocortical E27.40
drug-induced E27.3
postprocedural E89.6
primary E27.1
adrenomedullary, postprocedural E89.6
cerebral R29.818
corticoadrenal NEC E27.40
intestinal K59.89
labyrinth —see subcategory H83.2
ovary E28.39
pituitary (gland) (anterior) E23.0
testicular E29.1
postprocedural (postsurgical)
(postirradiation) (iatrogenic) E89.5
Hypogalactia O92.4
Hypogammaglobulinemia —see also
Agammaglobulinemia D80.1
hereditary D80.0
nonfamilial D80.1
transient, of infancy D80.7
Hypogenitalism (congenital) —see
Hypogonadism
Hypoglossia Q38.3
Hypoglycemia (spontaneous) E16.2
coma E15
diabetic —see Diabetes, by type, with
hypoglycemia, with coma
diabetic —see Diabetes, hypoglycemia
dietary counseling and surveillance
Z71.3

Hypoglycemia (Continued)
drug-induced E16.0
with coma (nondiabetic) E15
due to insulin E16.0
with coma (nondiabetic) E15
therapeutic misadventure —see
subcategory T38.3
functional, nonhyperinsulinemic E16.1
iatrogenic E16.0
with coma (nondiabetic) E15
in infant of diabetic mother P70.1
gestational diabetes P70.0
infantile E16.1
leucine-induced E71.19
neonatal (transitory) P70.4
iatrogenic P70.3
reactive (not drug-induced) E16.1
transitory neonatal P70.4
Hypogonadism
female E28.39
hypogonadotropic E23.0
male E29.1
ovarian (primary) E28.39
pituitary E23.0
testicular (primary) E29.1
Hypohidrosis, hypoidrosis L74.4
Hypoinsulinemia, postprocedural E89.1
Hypokalemia E87.6
Hypoleukocytosis —see Agranulocytosis
Hypolipoproteinemia (alpha) (beta) E78.6
Hypomagnesemia E83.42
neonatal P71.2
Hypomania, hypomanic reaction F30.8
Hypomenorrhea —see Oligomenorrhea
Hypometabolism R63.8
Hypomotility
gastrointestinal (tract) K31.89
psychogenic F45.8
intestine K59.89
psychogenic F45.8
stomach K31.89
psychogenic F45.8
Hyponasality R49.22
Hyponatremia E87.1
Hypo-osmolality E87.1
Hypo-ovarianism, hypo-ovarism
E28.39
Hypoparathyroidism E20.9
familial E20.8
idiopathic E20.0
neonatal, transitory P71.4
postprocedural E89.2
specified NEC E20.8
Hypoperfusion (in)
newborn P96.89
Hypopharyngitis —see Laryngopharyngitis
Hypophoria H50.53
Hypophosphatemia, hypophosphatasia
(acquired) (congenital) (renal) E83.39
familial E83.31
Hypophyseal, hypophysis —see also
condition
dwarfism E23.0
gigantism E22.0
Hypopiesis —see Hypotension
Hypopinealism E34.8
Hypopituitarism (juvenile) E23.0
drug-induced E23.1
due to
hypophysectomy E89.3
radiotherapy E89.3
iatrogenic NEC E23.1
postirradiation E89.3
postpartum O99.285
postprocedural E89.3
Hypoplasia, hypoplastic
adrenal (gland), congenital Q89.1
alimentary tract, congenital Q45.8
upper Q40.8
anus, anal (canal) Q42.3
with fistula Q42.2

Hypoplasia, hypoplastic (Continued)
aorta, aortic Q25.42
ascending, in hypoplastic left heart
syndrome Q23.4
valve Q23.1
in hypoplastic left heart syndrome
Q23.4
areola, congenital Q83.8
arm (congenital) —see Defect, reduction,
upper limb
artery (peripheral) Q27.8
brain (congenital) Q28.3
coronary Q24.5
digestive system Q27.8
lower limb Q27.8
pulmonary Q25.79
functional, unilateral J43.0
retinal (congenital) Q14.1
specified site NEC Q27.8
umbilical Q27.0
upper limb Q27.8
auditory canal Q17.8
causing impairment of hearing Q16.9
biliary duct or passage Q44.5
bone NOS Q79.9
face Q75.8
marrow D61.9
megakaryocytic D69.49
skull —see Hypoplasia, skull
brain Q02
gyri Q04.3
part of Q04.3
breast (areola) N64.82
bronchus Q32.4
cardiac Q24.8
carpus —see Defect, reduction, upper limb,
specified type NEC
cartilage hair Q78.8
cecum Q42.8
cementum K00.4
cephalic Q02
cerebellum Q04.3
cervix (uteri), congenital Q51.821
clavicle (congenital) Q74.0
coccyx Q76.49
colon Q42.9
specified NEC Q42.8
corpus callosum Q04.0
cricoid cartilage Q31.2
digestive organ(s) or tract NEC Q45.8
upper (congenital) Q40.8
ear (auricle) (lobe) Q17.2
middle Q16.4
enamel of teeth (neonatal) (postnatal)
(prenatal) K00.4
endocrine (gland) NEC Q89.2
endometrium N85.8
epididymis (congenital) Q55.4
epiglottis Q31.2
erythroid, congenital D61.01
esophagus (congenital) Q39.8
eustachian tube Q17.8
eye Q11.2
eyelid (congenital) Q10.3
face Q18.8
bone(s) Q75.8
femur (congenital) —see Defect, reduction,
lower limb, specified type NEC
fibula (congenital) —see Defect, reduction,
lower limb, specified type NEC
finger (congenital) —see Defect, reduction,
upper limb, specified type NEC
focal dermal Q82.8
foot —see Defect, reduction, lower limb,
specified type NEC
gallbladder Q44.0
genitalia, genital organ(s)
female, congenital Q52.8
external Q52.79
internal NEC Q52.8
in adiposogenital dystrophy E23.6

▶ New   ⇒ Revised   ~~deleted~~ Deleted   • Use Additional Character(s)

Hypoplasia, hypoplastic (*Continued*)
glottis Q31.2
hair Q84.2
hand (congenital) —*see* Defect, reduction, upper limb, specified type NEC
heart Q24.8
humerus (congenital) —*see* Defect, reduction, upper limb, specified type NEC
intestine (small) Q41.9
  large Q42.9
    specified NEC Q42.8
jaw M26.09
  alveolar M26.79
  lower M26.04
    alveolar M26.74
  upper M26.02
    alveolar M26.73
kidney(s) Q60.5
  bilateral Q60.4
  unilateral Q60.3
labium (majus) (minus), congenital Q52.79
larynx Q31.2
left heart syndrome Q23.4
leg (congenital) —*see* Defect, reduction, lower limb
limb Q73.8
  lower (congenital) —*see* Defect, reduction, lower limb
  upper (congenital) —*see* Defect, reduction, upper limb
liver Q44.7
lung (lobe) (not associated with short gestation) Q33.6
  associated with immaturity, low birth weight, prematurity, or short gestation P28.0
mammary (areola), congenital Q83.8
mandible, mandibular M26.04
  alveolar M26.74
  unilateral condylar M27.8
maxillary M26.02
  alveolar M26.73
medullary D61.9
megakaryocytic D69.49
metacarpus —*see* Defect, reduction, upper limb, specified type NEC
metatarsus —*see* Defect, reduction, lower limb, specified type NEC
muscle Q79.8
nail(s) Q84.6
nose, nasal Q30.1
optic nerve H47.03-●
osseous meatus (ear) Q17.8
ovary, congenital Q50.39
pancreas Q45.0
parathyroid (gland) Q89.2
parotid gland Q38.4
patella Q74.1
pelvis, pelvic girdle Q74.2
penis (congenital) Q55.62
peripheral vascular system Q27.8
  digestive system Q27.8
  lower limb Q27.8
  specified site NEC Q27.8
  upper limb Q27.8
pituitary (gland) (congenital) Q89.2
pulmonary (not associated with short gestation) Q33.6
  artery, functional J43.0
  associated with short gestation P28.0
radioulnar —*see* Defect, reduction, upper limb, specified type NEC
radius —*see* Defect, reduction, upper limb
rectum Q42.1
  with fistula Q42.0
respiratory system NEC Q34.8
rib Q76.6
right heart syndrome Q22.6
sacrum Q76.49
scapula Q74.0
scrotum Q55.1

Hypoplasia, hypoplastic (*Continued*)
shoulder girdle Q74.0
skin Q82.8
skull (bone) Q75.8
  with
    anencephaly Q00.0
    encephalocele —*see* Encephalocele
    hydrocephalus Q03.9
      with spina bifida —*see* Spina bifida, by site, with hydrocephalus
    microcephaly Q02
spinal (cord) (ventral horn cell) Q06.1
spine Q76.49
sternum Q76.7
tarsus —*see* Defect, reduction, lower limb, specified type NEC
testis Q55.1
thymic, with immunodeficiency D82.1
thymus (gland) Q89.2
  with immunodeficiency D82.1
thyroid (gland) E03.1
  cartilage Q31.2
tibiofibular (congenital) —*see* Defect, reduction, lower limb, specified type NEC
toe —*see* Defect, reduction, lower limb, specified type NEC
tongue Q38.3
Turner's K00.4
ulna (congenital) —*see* Defect, reduction, upper limb
umbilical artery Q27.0
unilateral condylar M27.8
ureter Q62.8
uterus, congenital Q51.811
vagina Q52.4
vascular NEC peripheral Q27.8
  brain Q28.3
  digestive system Q27.8
  lower limb Q27.8
  specified site NEC Q27.8
  upper limb Q27.8
vein(s) (peripheral) Q27.8
  brain Q28.3
  digestive system Q27.8
  great Q26.8
  lower limb Q27.8
  specified site NEC Q27.8
  upper limb Q27.8
vena cava (inferior) (superior) Q26.8
vertebra Q76.49
vulva, congenital Q52.79
zonule (ciliary) Q12.8
Hypoplasminogenemia E88.02
Hypopnea, obstructive sleep apnea G47.33
Hypopotassemia E87.6
Hypoproconvertinemia, congenital (hereditary) D68.2
Hypoproteinemia E77.8
Hypoprothrombinemia (congenital) (hereditary) (idiopathic) D68.2
  acquired D68.4
  newborn, transient P61.6
Hypoptyalism K11.7
Hypopyon (eye) (anterior chamber) —*see* Iridocyclitis, acute, hypopyon
Hypopyrexia R68.0
Hyporeflexia R29.2
Hyposecretion
  ACTH E23.0
  antidiuretic hormone E23.2
  ovary E28.39
  salivary gland (any) K11.7
  vasopressin E23.2
Hyposegmentation, leukocytic, hereditary D72.0
Hyposideremia D50.9
Hypospadias Q54.9
  balanic Q54.0
  coronal Q54.0

Hypospadias (*Continued*)
glandular Q54.0
penile Q54.1
penoscrotal Q54.2
perineal Q54.3
specified NEC Q54.8
Hypospermatogenesis —*see* Oligospermia
Hyposplenism D73.0
Hypostasis pulmonary, passive —*see* Edema, lung
Hypostatic —*see* condition
Hyposthenuria N28.89
Hypotension (arterial) (constitutional) I95.9
chronic I95.89
drug-induced I95.2
due to (of) hemodialysis I95.3
iatrogenic I95.89
idiopathic (permanent) I95.0
intracranial G96.810
  following
    lumbar cerebrospinal fluid shunting G97.83
    specified procedure NEC G97.84
    ventricular shunting (ventriculostomy) G97.2
  specified NEC G96.819
  spontaneous G96.811
intra-dialytic I95.3
maternal, syndrome (following labor and delivery) O26.5-●
neurogenic, orthostatic G90.3
orthostatic (chronic) I95.1
  due to drugs I95.2
  neurogenic G90.3
postoperative I95.81
postural I95.1
specified NEC I95.89
Hypothermia (accidental) T68
due to anesthesia, anesthetic T88.51
low environmental temperature T68
neonatal P80.9
  environmental (mild) NEC P80.8
  mild P80.8
  severe (chronic) (cold injury syndrome) P80.0
  specified NEC P80.8
not associated with low environmental temperature R68.0
Hypothyroidism (acquired) E03.9
autoimmune —*see* Thyroiditis, autoimmune
congenital (without goiter) E03.1
  with goiter (diffuse) E03.0
due to
  exogenous substance NEC E03.2
  iodine-deficiency, acquired E01.8
    subclinical E02
  irradiation therapy E89.0
  medicament NEC E03.2
  P-aminosalicylic acid (PAS) E03.2
  phenylbutazone E03.2
  resorcinol E03.2
  sulfonamide E03.2
  surgery E89.0
  thiourea group drugs E03.2
iatrogenic NEC E03.2
iodine-deficiency (acquired) E01.8
  congenital —*see* Syndrome, iodine-deficiency, congenital
  subclinical E02
neonatal, transitory P72.2
postinfectious E03.3
postirradiation E89.0
postprocedural E89.0
postsurgical E89.0
specified NEC E03.8
subclinical, iodine-deficiency related E02
Hypotonia, hypotonicity, hypotony
bladder N31.2
congenital (benign) P94.2
eye —*see* Disorder, globe, hypotony
Hypotrichosis —*see* Alopecia

Hypotropia H50.2-●
Hypoventilation R06.89
  congenital central alveolar G47.35
  sleep related
    idiopathic nonobstructive alveolar
      G47.34
    in conditions classified elsewhere G47.36
Hypovitaminosis —*see* Deficiency, vitamin
Hypovolemia E86.1
  surgical shock T81.19
  traumatic (shock) T79.4

Hypoxemia R09.02
  newborn P84
  sleep related, in conditions classified
    elsewhere G47.36
Hypoxia —*see also* Anoxia R09.02
  cerebral, during a procedure NEC G97.81
    postprocedural NEC G97.82
  intrauterine P84
  myocardial —*see* Insufficiency, coronary
  newborn P84
  sleep-related G47.34

Hypsarhythmia —*see* Epilepsy, generalized,
  specified NEC
Hysteralgia, pregnant uterus O26.89-●
Hysteria, hysterical (conversion) (dissociative
  state) F44.9
  anxiety F41.8
  convulsions F44.5
  psychosis, acute F44.9
Hysteroepilepsy F44.5

▶ New   ⮕ Revised   ~~deleted~~ Deleted   ● Use Additional Character(s)

I

IBDU (colonic inflammatory bowel dissease unclassified) K52.3
▶ICANS (immune effector cell-associated neurotoxicity syndrome) —see Syndrome, immune effector cell-associated neurotoxicity
Ichthyoparasitism due to Vandellia cirrhosa B88.8
Ichthyosis (congenital) Q80.9
  acquired L85.0
  fetalis Q80.4
  hystrix Q80.8
  lamellar Q80.2
  lingual K13.29
  palmaris and plantaris Q82.8
  simplex Q80.0
  vera Q80.8
  vulgaris Q80.0
  X-linked Q80.1
Ichthyotoxism —see Poisoning, fish
  bacterial —see Intoxication, foodborne
Icteroanemia, hemolytic (acquired) D59.9
  congenital —see Spherocytosis
Icterus —see also Jaundice
  conjunctiva R17
  gravis, newborn P55.0
  hematogenous (acquired) D59.9
  hemolytic (acquired) D59.9
    congenital —see Spherocytosis
  hemorrhagic (acute) (leptospiral) (spirochetal) A27.0
    newborn P53
  infectious B15.9
    with hepatic coma B15.0
    leptospiral A27.0
    spirochetal A27.0
  neonatorum —see Jaundice, newborn
  newborn P59.9
  spirochetal A27.0
Ictus solaris, solis T67.01
Ideation
  homicidal R45.850
  suicidal R45.851
Identity disorder (child) F64.9
  gender role F64.2
  psychosexual F64.2
Idioglossia F80.0
Idiopathic —see condition
Idiot, idiocy (congenital) F73
  amaurotic (Bielschowsky(-Jansky)) (family) (infantile (late)) (juvenile (late)) (Vogt-Spielmeyer) E75.4
  microcephalic Q02
Id reaction (due to bacteria) L30.2
IgE asthma J45.909
IIAC (idiopathic infantile arterial calcification) Q28.8
Ileitis (chronic) (noninfectious) —see also Enteritis K52.9
  backwash —see Pancolitis, ulcerative (chronic)
  infectious A09
  regional (ulcerative) —see Enteritis, regional, small intestine
  segmental —see Enteritis, regional
  terminal (ulcerative) —see Enteritis, regional, small intestine
Ileocolitis —see also Enteritis K52.9
  infectious A09
  regional —see Enteritis, regional
  ulcerative K51.0-●
Ileostomy
  attention to Z43.2
  malfunctioning K94.13
  status Z93.2
    with complication —see Complications, enterostomy
Ileotyphus —see Typhoid
Ileum —see condition
Ileus (bowel) (colon) (inhibitory) (intestine) K56.7
  adynamic K56.0

Ileus (Continued)
  due to gallstone (in intestine) K56.3
  duodenal (chronic) K31.5
  gallstone K56.3
  mechanical NEC —see also Obstruction, intestine, specified K56.699
  meconium P76.0
    in cystic fibrosis E84.11
    meaning meconium plug (without cystic fibrosis) P76.0
  myxedema K59.89
  neurogenic K56.0
    Hirschsprung's disease or megacolon Q43.1
  newborn
    due to meconium P76.0
      in cystic fibrosis E84.11
      meaning meconium plug (without cystic fibrosis) P76.0
    transitory P76.1
  obstructive —see also Obstruction, intestine, specified K56.699
  paralytic K56.0
  postoperative K91.89
Iliac —see condition
Iliotibial band syndrome M76.3-●
Illiteracy Z55.0
Illness —see also Disease R69
  manic-depressive —see Disorder, bipolar
Imbalance R26.89
  autonomic G90.8
  constituents of food intake E63.1
  electrolyte E87.8
    with
      abortion —see Abortion by type, complicated by, electrolyte imbalance
      molar pregnancy O08.5
    due to hyperemesis gravidarum O21.1
    following ectopic or molar pregnancy O08.5
    neonatal, transitory NEC P74.49
      potassium
        hyperkalemia P74.31
        hypokalemia P74.32
      sodium
        hypernatremia P74.21
        hyponatremia P74.22
  endocrine E34.9
  eye muscle NOS H50.9
  hormone E34.9
  hysterical F44.4
  labyrinth —see subcategory H83.2
  posture R29.3
  protein-energy —see Malnutrition
  sympathetic G90.8
Imbecile, imbecility (I.Q. 35-49) F71
Imbedding, intrauterine device T83.39
Imbibition, cholesterol (gallbladder) K82.4
Imbrication, teeth, fully erupted M26.30
Imerslund (-Gräsbeck) syndrome D51.1
Immature —see also Immaturity
  birth (less than 37 completed weeks) —see Preterm, newborn
  extremely (less than 28 completed weeks) —see Immaturity, extreme
  personality F60.89
Immaturity (less than 37 completed weeks) —see also Preterm, newborn
  extreme of newborn (less than 28 completed weeks of gestation) (less than 196 completed days of gestation) (unspecified weeks of gestation) P07.20
    gestational age
      23 completed weeks (23 weeks, 0 days through 23 weeks, 6 days) P07.22
      24 completed weeks (24 weeks, 0 days through 24 weeks, 6 days) P07.23
      25 completed weeks (25 weeks, 0 days through 25 weeks, 6 days) P07.24
      26 completed weeks (26 weeks, 0 days through 26 weeks, 6 days) P07.25
      27 completed weeks (27 weeks, 0 days through 27 weeks, 6 days) P07.26
    less than 23 completed weeks P07.21

Immaturity (Continued)
  fetus or infant light-for-dates —see Light-for-dates
  lung, newborn P28.0
  organ or site NEC —see Hypoplasia
  pulmonary, newborn P28.0
  reaction F60.89
  sexual (female) (male), after puberty E30.0
Immersion T75.1
  foot T69.02-●
  hand T69.01-●
Immobile, immobility
  complete, due to severe physical disability or frailty R53.2
  intestine K59.89
  syndrome (paraplegic) M62.3
Immune reconstitution (inflammatory) syndrome [IRIS] D89.3
Immunization —see also Vaccination
  ABO —see Incompatibility, ABO
    in newborn P55.1
  appropriate for age
    child (over 28 days old) Z00.129
      with abnormal findings Z00.121
  complication —see Complications, vaccination
  encounter for Z23
  not done (not carried out) Z28.9
    because (of)
      acute illness of patient Z28.01
      allergy to vaccine (or component) Z28.04
      caregiver refusal Z28.82
      chronic illness of patient Z28.02
      contraindication NEC Z28.09
      delay in delivery of vaccine Z28.83
      group pressure Z28.1
      guardian refusal Z28.82
      immune compromised state of patient Z28.03
      lack of availability of vaccine Z28.83
      manufacturer delay of vaccine Z28.83
      parent refusal Z28.82
      patient's belief Z28.1
      patient had disease being vaccinated against Z28.81
      patient refusal Z28.21
      religious beliefs of patient Z28.1
      specified reason NEC Z28.89
        of patient Z28.29
      unavailability of vaccine Z28.83
      unspecified patient reason Z28.20
  Rh factor
    affecting management of pregnancy NEC O36.09-●
    anti-D antibody O36.01-●
    from transfusion —see Complication(s), transfusion, incompatibility reaction, Rh (factor)
Immunocompromised NOS D84.9
Immunocytoma C83.0-●
Immunodeficiency D84.9
  with
    adenosine-deaminase deficiency (see also Deficiency, adenosine deaminase) D81.30
    antibody defects D80.9
      specified type NEC D80.8
    hyperimmunoglobulinemia D80.6
    increased immunoglobulin M (IgM) D80.5
    major defect D82.9
      specified type NEC D82.8
    partial albinism D82.8
    short-limbed stature D82.2
    thrombocytopenia and eczema D82.0
  antibody with
    hyperimmunoglobulinemia D80.6
    near-normal immunoglobulins D80.6
  autosomal recessive, Swiss type D80.0

Immunodeficiency (Continued)
  combined D81.9
    biotin-dependent carboxylase D81.819
      biotinidase D81.810
      holocarboxylase synthetase D81.818
      specified type NEC D81.818
    severe (SCID) D81.9
      with
        low or normal B-cell numbers D81.2
        low T- and B-cell numbers D81.1
        reticular dysgenesis D81.0
    specified type NEC D81.89
  common variable D83.9
    with
      abnormalities of B-cell numbers and
        function D83.0
      autoantibodies to B- or T-cells D83.2
      immunoregulatory T-cell disorders
        D83.1
    specified type NEC D83.8
  due to
    conditions classified elsewhere D84.81
    drugs D84.821
    external causes D84.822
    medication (current or past) D84.821
  following hereditary defective response to
    Epstein-Barr virus (EBV) D82.3
  selective, immunoglobulin
    A (IgA) D80.2
    G (IgG) (subclasses) D80.3
    M (IgM) D80.4
  severe combined (SCID) D81.9
    due to adenosine deaminase deficiency
      D81.31
  specified type NEC D84.89
  X-linked, with increased IgM D80.5
Immunodeficient NOS D84.9
Immunosuppressed NOS D84.9
Immunotherapy (encounter for)
  antineoplastic Z51.12
Impaction, impacted
  bowel, colon, rectum —see also Impaction,
    fecal K56.49
    by gallstone K56.3
  calculus —see Calculus
  cerumen (ear) (external) H61.2-●
  cuspid —see Impaction, tooth
  dental (same or adjacent tooth) K01.1
  fecal, feces K56.41
  fracture —see Fracture, by site
  gallbladder —see Calculus, gallbladder
  gallstone(s) —see Calculus, gallbladder
    bile duct (common) (hepatic) —see
      Calculus, bile duct
    cystic duct —see Calculus, gallbladder
    in intestine, with obstruction (any part)
      K56.3
  intestine (calculous) NEC —see also
    Impaction, fecal K56.49
    gallstone, with ileus K56.3
  intrauterine device (IUD) T83.39
  molar —see Impaction, tooth
  shoulder, causing obstructed labor O66.0
  tooth, teeth K01.1
  turbinate J34.89
Impaired, impairment (function)
  auditory discrimination —see Abnormal,
    auditory perception
  cognitive, mild, so stated G31.84
  dual sensory Z73.82
  fasting glucose R73.01
  glucose tolerance (oral) R73.02
  hearing —see Deafness
  heart —see Disease, heart
  kidney N28.9
    disorder resulting from N25.9
      specified NEC N25.89
  liver K72.90
    with coma K72.91
  mastication K08.89
  mild cognitive, so stated G31.84

Impaired, impairment (Continued)
  mobility
    ear ossicles —see Ankylosis, ear ossicles
    requiring care provider Z74.09
  myocardium, myocardial —see Insufficiency,
    myocardial
  rectal sphincter R19.8
  renal (acute) (chronic) N28.9
    disorder resulting from N25.9
      specified NEC N25.89
  vision NEC H54.7
    both eyes H54.3
Impediment, speech (see also Disorder, speech)
    R47.9
  psychogenic (childhood) F98.8
  slurring R47.81
  specified NEC R47.89
Impending
  coronary syndrome I20.0
  delirium tremens F10.239
  myocardial infarction I20.0
Imperception auditory (acquired) —see also
    Deafness
  congenital H93.25
Imperfect
  aeration, lung (newborn) NEC —see
    Atelectasis
  closure (congenital)
    alimentary tract NEC Q45.8
      lower Q43.8
      upper Q40.8
    atrioventricular ostium Q21.2
    atrium (secundum) Q21.1
    branchial cleft NOS Q18.2
      cyst Q18.0
      fistula Q18.0
      sinus Q18.0
    choroid Q14.3
    cricoid cartilage Q31.8
    cusps, heart valve NEC Q24.8
      pulmonary Q22.3
    ductus
      arteriosus Q25.0
      Botalli Q25.0
    ear drum (causing impairment of hearing)
      Q16.4
    esophagus with communication to
      bronchus or trachea Q39.1
    eyelid Q10.3
    foramen
      botalli Q21.1
      ovale Q21.1
    genitalia, genital organ(s) or system
      female Q52.8
        external Q52.79
        internal NEC Q52.8
      male Q55.8
    glottis Q31.8
    interatrial ostium or septum Q21.1
    interauricular ostium or septum Q21.1
    interventricular ostium or septum Q21.0
    larynx Q31.8
    lip —see Cleft, lip
    nasal septum Q30.3
    nose Q30.2
    omphalomesenteric duct Q43.0
    optic nerve entry Q14.2
    organ or site not listed —see Anomaly,
      by site
    ostium
      interatrial Q21.1
      interauricular Q21.1
      interventricular Q21.0
    palate —see Cleft, palate
    preauricular sinus Q18.1
    retina Q14.1
    roof of orbit Q75.8
    sclera Q13.5
    septum
      aorticopulmonary Q21.4
      atrial (secundum) Q21.1

Imperfect (Continued)
  closure (Continued)
    septum (Continued)
      between aorta and pulmonary artery
        Q21.4
      heart Q21.9
      interatrial (secundum) Q21.1
      interauricular (secundum) Q21.1
      interventricular Q21.0
        in tetralogy of Fallot Q21.3
      nasal Q30.3
      ventricular Q21.0
        with pulmonary stenosis or atresia,
          dextraposition of aorta, and
          hypertrophy of right ventricle
          Q21.3
        in tetralogy of Fallot Q21.3
    skull Q75.0
      with
        anencephaly Q00.0
        encephalocele —see Encephalocele
        hydrocephalus Q03.9
          with spina bifida —see Spina bifida,
            by site, with hydrocephalus
        microcephaly Q02
    spine (with meningocele) —see Spina
      bifida
    trachea Q32.1
    tympanic membrane (causing impairment
      of hearing) Q16.4
    uterus Q51.818
    vitelline duct Q43.0
  erection —see Dysfunction, sexual, male,
    erectile
  fusion —see Imperfect, closure
  inflation, lung (newborn) —see Atelectasis
  posture R29.3
  rotation, intestine Q43.3
  septum, ventricular Q21.0
Imperfectly descended testis —see
    Cryptorchid
Imperforate (congenital) —see also Atresia
  anus Q42.3
    with fistula Q42.2
  cervix (uteri) Q51.828
  esophagus Q39.0
    with tracheoesophageal fistula Q39.1
  hymen Q52.3
  jejunum Q41.1
  pharynx Q38.8
  rectum Q42.1
    with fistula Q42.0
  urethra Q64.39
  vagina Q52.4
Impervious (congenital) —see also Atresia
  anus Q42.3
    with fistula Q42.2
  bile duct Q44.2
  esophagus Q39.0
    with tracheoesophageal fistula Q39.1
  intestine (small) Q41.9
    large Q42.9
      specified NEC Q42.8
  rectum Q42.1
    with fistula Q42.0
  ureter —see Atresia, ureter
  urethra Q64.39
Impetiginization of dermatoses L01.1
Impetigo (any organism) (any site) (circinate)
    (contagiosa) (simplex) (vulgaris) L01.00
  Bockhart's L01.02
  bullous, bullosa L01.03
  external ear L01.00 [H62.40]
  follicularis L01.02
  furfuracea L30.5
  herpetiformis L40.1
    nonobstetrical L40.1
  neonatorum L01.03
  nonbullous L01.01
  specified type NEC L01.09
  ulcerative L01.09

Impingement (on teeth)
  joint —*see* Disorder, joint, specified type NEC
  soft tissue
    anterior M26.81
    posterior M26.82
Implant, endometrial N80.9
Implantation
  anomalous —*see* Anomaly, by site
    ureter Q62.63
  cyst
    external area or site (skin) NEC L72.0
    iris —*see* Cyst, iris, implantation
    vagina N89.8
    vulva N90.7
  dermoid (cyst) —*see* Implantation, cyst
Impotence (sexual) N52.9
  counseling Z70.1
  organic origin —*see also* Dysfunction, sexual,
    male, erectile N52.9
  psychogenic F52.21
Impression, basilar Q75.8
Imprisonment, anxiety concerning Z65.1
Improper care (child) (newborn) —*see*
    Maltreatment
Improperly tied umbilical cord (causing
    hemorrhage) P51.8
Impulsiveness (impulsive) R45.87
Inability to swallow —*see* Aphagia
Inaccessible, inaccessibility
  health care NEC Z75.3
    due to
      waiting period Z75.2
        for admission to facility elsewhere Z75.1
    other helping agencies Z75.4
Inactive —*see* condition
Inadequate, inadequacy
  aesthetics of dental restoration K08.56
  biologic, constitutional, functional, or social
    F60.7
  development
    child R62.50
    genitalia
      after puberty NEC E30.0
      congenital
        female Q52.8
          external Q52.79
          internal Q52.8
        male Q55.8
    lungs Q33.6
      associated with short gestation P28.0
    organ or site not listed —*see* Anomaly, by
      site
  diet (causing nutritional deficiency)
    E63.9
▶drinking-water supply Z58.6
  eating habits Z72.4
  environment, household Z59.1
  family support Z63.8
⇒food (supply) NEC Z59.48
    hunger effects T73.0
  functional F60.7
  household care, due to
    family member
      handicapped or ill Z74.2
      on vacation Z75.5
      temporarily away from home Z74.2
    technical defects in home Z59.1
    temporary absence from home of person
      rendering care Z74.2
  housing (heating) (space) Z59.1
  income (financial) Z59.6
  intrafamilial communication Z63.8
  material resources Z59.9
  mental —*see* Disability, intellectual
  parental supervision or control of child
    Z62.0
  personality F60.7
  pulmonary
    function R06.89
      newborn P28.5
    ventilation, newborn P28.5

Inadequate, inadequacy (*Continued*)
  sample of cytologic smear
    anus R85.615
    cervix R87.615
    vagina R87.625
  social F60.7
    insurance Z59.7
    skills NEC Z73.4
  supervision of child by parent Z62.0
  teaching affecting education Z55.8
  welfare support Z59.7
Inanition R64
  with edema —*see* Malnutrition, severe
  due to
    deprivation of food T73.0
    malnutrition —*see* Malnutrition
  fever R50.9
Inappropriate
  change in quantitative human chorionic
    gonadotropin (hCG) in early pregnancy
    O02.81
  diet or eating habits Z72.4
  level of quantitative human chorionic
    gonadotropin (hCG) for gestational age
    in early pregnancy O02.81
  secretion
    antidiuretic hormone (ADH) (excessive)
      E22.2
      deficiency E23.2
    pituitary (posterior) E22.2
Inattention at or after birth —*see* Neglect
Incarceration, incarcerated
  enterocele K46.0
    gangrenous K46.1
  epiplocele K46.0
    gangrenous K46.1
  exomphalos K42.0
    gangrenous K42.1
  hernia —*see also* Hernia, by site, with
    obstruction
    with gangrene —*see* Hernia, by site, with
      gangrene
  iris, in wound —*see* Injury, eye, laceration,
    with prolapse
  lens, in wound —*see* Injury, eye, laceration,
    with prolapse
  omphalocele K42.0
  prison, anxiety concerning Z65.1
  rupture —*see* Hernia, by site
  sarcoepiplocele K46.0
    gangrenous K46.1
  sarcoepiplomphalocele K42.0
    with gangrene K42.1
  uterus N85.8
    gravid O34.51-●
      causing obstructed labor O65.5
Incised wound
  external —*see* Laceration
  internal organs —*see* Injury, by site
Incision, incisional
  hernia K43.2
    with
      gangrene (and obstruction) K43.1
      obstruction K43.0
    surgical, complication —*see* Complications,
      surgical procedure
    traumatic
      external —*see* Laceration
      internal organs —*see* Injury, by site
Inclusion
  azurophilic leukocytic D72.0
  blennorrhea (neonatal) (newborn)
    P39.1
  gallbladder in liver (congenital) Q44.1
Incompatibility
  ABO
    affecting management of pregnancy
      O36.11-●
      anti-A sensitization O36.11-●
      anti-B sensitization O36.19-●
      specified NEC O36.19-●

Incompatibility (*Continued*)
  ABO (*Continued*)
    infusion or transfusion reaction —*see*
      Complication(s), transfusion,
      incompatibility reaction, ABO
    newborn P55.1
  blood (group) (Duffy) (K) (Kell) (Kidd)
    (Lewis) (M) (S) NEC
    affecting management of pregnancy
      O36.11-●
      anti-A sensitization O36.11-●
      anti-B sensitization O36.19-●
    infusion or transfusion reaction
      T80.89
    newborn P55.8
  divorce or estrangement Z63.5
  Rh (blood group) (factor) Z31.82
    affecting management of pregnancy NEC
      O36.09-●
      anti-D antibody O36.01-●
    infusion or transfusion reaction —*see*
      Complication(s), transfusion,
      incompatibility reaction, Rh (factor)
    newborn P55.0
  rhesus —*see* Incompatibility, Rh
Incompetency, incompetent, incompetence
  annular
    aortic (valve) —*see* Insufficiency, aortic
    mitral (valve) I34.0
    pulmonary valve (heart) I37.1
  aortic (valve) —*see* Insufficiency, aortic
  cardiac valve —*see* Endocarditis
  cervix, cervical (os) N88.3
    in pregnancy O34.3-●
  chronotropic I45.89
    with
      autonomic dysfunction G90.8
      ischemic heart disease I25.89
      left ventricular dysfunction I51.89
      sinus node dysfunction I49.8
  esophagogastric (junction) (sphincter) K22.0
  mitral (valve) —*see* Insufficiency, mitral
  pelvic fundus N81.89
  pubocervical tissue N81.82
  pulmonary valve (heart) I37.1
    congenital Q22.3
  rectovaginal tissue N81.83
  tricuspid (annular) (valve) —*see* Insufficiency,
    tricuspid
  valvular —*see* Endocarditis
    congenital Q24.8
  vein, venous (saphenous) (varicose) —*see*
    Varix, leg
Incomplete —*see also* condition
  bladder, emptying R33.9
  defecation R15.0
  expansion lungs (newborn) NEC —*see*
    Atelectasis
  rotation, intestine Q43.3
Inconclusive
  diagnostic imaging due to excess body fat of
    patient R93.9
  findings on diagnostic imaging of breast NEC
    R92.8
  mammogram (due to dense breasts) R92.2
Incontinence R32
  anal sphincter R15.9
  coital N39.491
  feces R15.9
    nonorganic origin F98.1
  insensible (urinary) N39.42
  overflow N39.490
  postural (urinary) N39.492
  psychogenic F45.8
  rectal R15.9
  reflex N39.498
  stress (female) (male) N39.3
    and urge N39.46
  urethral sphincter R32
  urge N39.41
    and stress (female) (male) N39.46

Incontinence *(Continued)*
  urine (urinary) R32
    continuous N39.45
      due to cognitive impairment, or severe
        physical disability or immobility
        R39.81
    functional R39.81
    insensible N39.42
    mixed (stress and urge) N39.46
    nocturnal N39.44
    nonorganic origin F98.0
    overflow N39.490
    post dribbling N39.43
    postural N39.492
    reflex N39.498
    specified NEC N39.498
    stress (female) (male) N39.3
      and urge N39.46
    total N39.498
    unaware N39.42
    urge N39.41
      and stress (female) (male) N39.46
Incontinentia pigmenti Q82.3
Incoordinate, incoordination
  esophageal-pharyngeal (newborn) —*see*
    Dysphagia
  muscular R27.8
  uterus (action) (contractions) (complicating
    delivery) O62.4
Increase, increased
  abnormal, in development R63.8
  androgens (ovarian) E28.1
  anticoagulants (antithrombin) (anti-VIIIa)
    (anti-IXa) (anti-Xa) (anti-XIa) —*see*
    Circulating anticoagulants
  cold sense R20.8
  estrogen E28.0
  function
    adrenal
      cortex —*see* Cushing's, syndrome
      medulla E27.5
    pituitary (gland) (anterior) (lobe) E22.9
      posterior E22.2
  heat sense R20.8
  intracranial pressure (benign) G93.2
  permeability, capillaries I78.8
  pressure, intracranial G93.2
  secretion
    gastrin E16.4
    glucagon E16.3
    pancreas, endocrine E16.9
      growth hormone-releasing hormone
        E16.8
      pancreatic polypeptide E16.8
      somatostatin E16.8
      vasoactive-intestinal polypeptide
        E16.8
  sphericity, lens Q12.4
  splenic activity D73.1
  venous pressure I87.8
    portal K76.6
Increta placenta O43.22-●
Incrustation, cornea, foreign body (lead)
  (zinc) —*see* Foreign body, cornea
Incyclophoria H50.54
Incyclotropia —*see* Cyclotropia
Indeterminate sex Q56.4
India rubber skin Q82.8
Indigestion (acid) (bilious) (functional)
  K30
  catarrhal K31.89
  due to decomposed food NOS A05.9
  nervous F45.8
  psychogenic F45.8
Indirect —*see* condition
Induratio penis plastica N48.6
Induration, indurated
  brain G93.89
  breast (fibrous) N64.51
    puerperal, postpartum O92.29
  broad ligament N83.8

Induration, indurated *(Continued)*
  chancre
    anus A51.1
      congenital A50.07
    extragenital NEC A51.2
  corpora cavernosa (penis) (plastic) N48.6
  liver (chronic) K76.89
  lung (black) (chronic) (fibroid) —*see also*
    Fibrosis, lung J84.10
      essential brown J84.03
  penile (plastic) N48.6
  phlebitic —*see* Phlebitis
  skin R23.4
Inebriety (without dependence) —*see* Alcohol,
  intoxication
Inefficiency, kidney N28.9
Inelasticity, skin R23.4
Inequality, leg (length) (acquired) —*see also*
  Deformity, limb, unequal length
  congenital —*see* Defect, reduction, lower limb
  lower leg —*see* Deformity, limb, unequal
    length
Inertia
  bladder (neurogenic) N31.2
  stomach K31.89
    psychogenic F45.8
  uterus, uterine during labor O62.2
    during latent phase of labor O62.0
    primary O62.0
    secondary O62.1
  vesical (neurogenic) N31.2
Infancy, infantile, infantilism —*see also*
  condition
  celiac K90.0
  genitalia, genitals (after puberty) E30.0
  Herter's (nontropical sprue) K90.0
  intestinal K90.0
  Lorain E23.0
  pancreatic K86.89
  pelvis M95.5
    with disproportion (fetopelvic) O33.1
      causing obstructed labor O65.1
  pituitary E23.0
  renal N25.0
  uterus —*see* Infantile, genitalia
Infant(s) —*see also* Infancy
  excessive crying R68.11
  irritable child R68.12
  lack of care —*see* Neglect
  liveborn (singleton) Z38.2
    born in hospital Z38.00
      by cesarean Z38.01
    born outside hospital Z38.1
    multiple NEC Z38.8
      born in hospital Z38.68
        by cesarean Z38.69
      born outside hospital Z38.7
    quadruplet Z38.8
      born in hospital Z38.63
        by cesarean Z38.64
      born outside hospital Z38.7
    quintuplet Z38.8
      born in hospital Z38.65
        by cesarean Z38.66
      born outside hospital Z38.7
    triplet Z38.8
      born in hospital Z38.61
        by cesarean Z38.62
      born outside hospital Z38.7
    twin Z38.5
      born in hospital Z38.30
        by cesarean Z38.31
      born outside hospital Z38.4
  of diabetic mother (syndrome of) P70.1
    gestational diabetes P70.0
Infantile —*see also* condition
  genitalia, genitals E30.0
  os, uterine E30.0
  penis E30.0
  testis E29.1
  uterus E30.0

Infantilism —*see* Infancy
Infarct, infarction
  adrenal (capsule) (gland) E27.49
  appendices epiploicae —*see also* Infarct,
    intestine K55.069
  bowel —*see also* Infarct, intestine K55.069
  brain (stem) —*see* Infarct, cerebral
  breast N64.89
  brewer's (kidney) N28.0
  cardiac —*see* Infarct, myocardium
  cerebellar —*see* Infarct, cerebral
  cerebral (acute) (chronic) (*see also* Occlusion,
    artery cerebral or precerebral, with
    infarction) I63.9-●
    aborted I63.9
    cortical I63.9
    due to
      cerebral venous thrombosis,
        nonpyogenic I63.6
      embolism
        cerebral arteries I63.4-●
        precerebral arteries I63.1-●
      occlusion NEC
        cerebral arteries I63.5-●
        precerebral arteries I63.2-●
        small artery I63.81
      stenosis NEC
        cerebral arteries I63.5-●
        precerebral arteries I63.2-●
        small artery I63.81
      thrombosis
        cerebral artery I63.3-●
        precerebral artery I63.0-●
    intraoperative
      during cardiac surgery I97.810
      during other surgery I97.811
    neonatal P91.82-●
    perinatal (arterial ischemic) P91.82-●
    postprocedural
      following cardiac surgery I97.820
      following other surgery I97.821
    specified NEC I63.89
  colon (acute) (agnogenic) (embolic)
    (hemorrhagic) (nonocclusive)
    (nonthrombotic) (occlusive) (segmental)
    (thrombotic) (with gangrene) —*see also*
    Infarct, intestine K55.049
  coronary artery —*see* Infarct, myocardium
  embolic —*see* Embolism
  fallopian tube N83.8
  gallbladder K82.8
  heart —*see* Infarct, myocardium
  hepatic K76.3
  hypophysis (anterior lobe) E23.6
  impending (myocardium) I20.0
  intestine (acute) (agnogenic) (embolic)
    (hemorrhagic) (nonocclusive)
    (nonthrombotic) (occlusive) (thrombotic)
    (with gangrene) K55.069
    diffuse K55.062
    focal K55.061
    large K55.049
      diffuse K55.042
      focal K55.041
    small K55.029
      diffuse K55.022
      focal K55.021
  kidney N28.0
  lacunar I63.81
  liver K76.3
  lung (embolic) (thrombotic) —*see* Embolism,
    pulmonary
  lymph node I89.8
  mesentery, mesenteric (embolic) (thrombotic)
    (with gangrene) —*see also* Infarct,
    intestine K55.069
  muscle (ischemic) M62.20
    ankle M62.27-●
    foot M62.27-●
    forearm M62.23-●
    hand M62.24-●

▶ New ⇒ Revised ~~deleted~~ Deleted ● Use Additional Character(s)

Infarct, infarction (Continued)
  muscle (Continued)
    lower leg M62.26-●
    pelvic region M62.25-●
    shoulder region M62.21-●
    specified site NEC M62.28
    thigh M62.25-●
    upper arm M62.22-●
  myocardium, myocardial (acute) (with stated
      duration of 4 weeks or less) I21.9
    associated with revascularization
        procedure I21.A9
    diagnosed on ECG, but presenting no
        symptoms I25.2
    due to
      demand ischemia I21.A1
      ischemic imbalance I21.A1
    healed or old I25.2
    intraoperative —see also Infarct,
        myocardium, associated with
        revascularization procedure
      during cardiac surgery I97.790
      during other surgery I97.791
    non-Q wave I21.4
    non-ST elevation (NSTEMI) I21.4
      subsequent I22.2
    nontransmural I21.4
    past (diagnosed on ECG or other
        investigation, but currently presenting
        no symptoms) I25.2
    postprocedural —see also Infarct,
        myocardium, associated with
        revascularization procedure
      following cardiac surgery —see also Infarct,
          myocardium, type 4 or type 5 I97.190
      following other surgery I97.191
    Q wave —see also Infarct, myocardium, by
        site I21.3
    secondary to
      demand ischemia I21.A1
      ischemic imbalance I21.A1
    ST elevation (STEMI) I21.3
      anterior (anteroapical) (anterolateral)
          (anteroseptal) (Q wave) (wall) I21.09
        subsequent I22.0
      inferior (diaphragmatic) (inferolateral)
          (inferoposterior) (wall) NEC I21.19
        subsequent I22.1
      inferoposterior transmural (Q wave) I21.11
      involving
        coronary artery of anterior wall NEC
            I21.09
        coronary artery of inferior wall NEC
            I21.19
        diagonal coronary artery I21.02
        left anterior descending coronary
            artery I21.02
        left circumflex coronary artery I21.21
        left main coronary artery I21.01
        oblique marginal coronary artery I21.21
        right coronary artery I21.11
      lateral (apical-lateral) (basal-lateral)
          (high) I21.29
        subsequent I22.8
      posterior (posterobasal) (posterolateral)
          (posteroseptal) (true) I21.29
        subsequent I22.8
      septal I21.29
        subsequent I22.8
      specified NEC I21.29
        subsequent I22.8
    subsequent I22.9
      anterior (anteroapical) (anterolateral)
          (anteroseptal) (wall) I22.0
      diaphragmatic (wall) I22.1
      inferior (diaphragmatic) (inferolateral)
          (inferoposterior) (wall) I22.1
      lateral (apical-lateral) (basal-lateral)
          (high) I22.8
      non-ST elevation (NSTEMI) I22.2

Infarct, infarction (Continued)
  myocardium, myocardial (Continued)
    subsequent (Continued)
      posterior (posterobasal) (posterolateral)
          (posteroseptal) (true) I22.8
      septal I22.8
      specified NEC I22.8
      ST elevation I22.9
        anterior (anteroapical) (anterolateral)
            (anteroseptal) (wall) I22.0
        inferior (diaphragmatic) (inferolateral)
            (inferoposterior) (wall) I22.1
        specified NEC I22.8
      subendocardial I22.2
      transmural I21.3
        anterior (anteroapical) (anterolateral)
            (anteroseptal) (wall) I22.0
        diaphragmatic (wall) I22.1
        inferior (diaphragmatic) (inferolateral)
            (inferoposterior) (wall) I22.1
        lateral (apical-lateral) (basal-lateral)
            (high) I22.8
        posterior (posterobasal) (posterolateral)
            (posteroseptal) (true) I22.8
        specified NEC I22.8
      type 1 —see also Infarction, myocardial,
          subsequent, by site, or by ST
          elevation or non-ST elevation I22.9
      type 2 I21.A1
      type 3 I21.A9
      type 4 I21.A9
      type 5 I21.A9
    syphilitic A52.06
    transmural I21.9
      anterior (anteroapical) (anterolateral)
          (anteroseptal) (Q wave) (wall) NEC
          I21.09
      inferior (diaphragmatic) (inferolateral)
          (inferoposterior) (Q wave) (wall)
          NEC I21.19
      inferoposterior (Q wave) I21.11
      lateral (apical-lateral) (basal-lateral)
          (high) NEC I21.29
      posterior (posterobasal) (posterolateral)
          (posteroseptal) (true) NEC I21.29
      septal NEC I21.29
      specified NEC I21.29
      type 1 —see also Infarction, myocardial,
          by site, or by ST elevation or non-ST
          elevation I21.9
      type 2 I21.A1
      type 3 I21.A9
      type 4 (a) (b) (c) I21.A9
      type 5 I21.A9
    nontransmural I21.4
  omentum —see also Infarct, intestine
      K55.069
  ovary N83.8
  pancreas K86.89
  papillary muscle —see Infarct, myocardium
  parathyroid gland E21.4
  pituitary (gland) E23.6
  placenta O43.81-●
  prostate N42.89
  pulmonary (artery) (vein) (hemorrhagic) —
      see Embolism, pulmonary
  renal (embolic) (thrombotic) N28.0
  retina, retinal (artery) —see Occlusion, artery,
      retina
  spinal (cord) (acute) (embolic) (nonembolic)
      G95.11
  spleen D73.5
    embolic or thrombotic I74.8
  subendocardial (acute) (nontransmural) I21.4
  suprarenal (capsule) (gland) E27.49
  testis N50.1
  thrombotic —see also Thrombosis
    artery, arterial —see Embolism
  thyroid (gland) E07.89
  ventricle (heart) —see Infarct, myocardium
Infecting —see condition

Infection, infected, infective (opportunistic)
    B99.9
  with
    drug resistant organism —see Resistance
        (to), drug —see also specific organism
    lymphangitis —see Lymphangitis
    organ dysfunction (acute) R65.20
      with septic shock R65.21
  abscess (skin) - code by site under Abscess
  Absidia —see Mucormycosis
  Acanthamoeba —see Acanthamebiasis
  Acanthocheilonema (perstans) (streptocerca)
      B74.4
  accessory sinus (chronic) —see Sinusitis
  achorion —see Dermatophytosis
  Acremonium falciforme B47.0
  acromioclavicular M00.9
  Actinobacillus (actinomycetem-comitans)
      A28.8
    mallei A24.0
    muris A25.1
  Actinomadura B47.1
  Actinomyces (israelii) —see also
      Actinomycosis A42.9
  Actinomycetales —see Actinomycosis
  actinomycotic NOS —see Actinomycosis
  adenoid (and tonsil) J03.90
    chronic J35.02
  adenovirus NEC
    as cause of disease classified elsewhere
        B97.0
    unspecified nature or site B34.0
  aerogenes capsulatus A48.0
  aertrycke —see Infection, salmonella
  alimentary canal NOS —see Enteritis,
      infectious
  Allescheria boydii B48.2
  Alternaria B48.8
  alveolus, alveolar (process) K04.7
  Ameba, amebic (histolytica) —see Amebiasis
  amniotic fluid, sac or cavity O41.10-●
    chorioamnionitis O41.12-●
    placentitis O41.14-●
  amputation stump (surgical) —see
      Complication, amputation stump,
      infection
  Ancylostoma (duodenalis) B76.0
  Anisakiasis, Anisakis larvae B81.0
  anthrax —see Anthrax
  antrum (chronic) —see Sinusitis, maxillary
  anus, anal (papillae) (sphincter) K62.89
  arbovirus (arbor virus) A94
    specified type NEC A93.8
  artificial insemination N98.0
  Ascaris lumbricoides —see Ascariasis
  Ascomycetes B47.0
  Aspergillus (flavus) (fumigatus) (terreus) —
      see Aspergillosis
  atypical
    acid-fast (bacilli) —see Mycobacterium,
        atypical
    mycobacteria —see Mycobacterium, atypical
    virus A81.9
      specified type NEC A81.89
  auditory meatus (external) —see Otitis,
      externa, infective
  auricle (ear) —see Otitis, externa, infective
  axillary gland (lymph) L04.2
  Bacillus A49.9
    abortus A23.1
    anthracis —see Anthrax
    Ducrey's (any location) A57
    Flexner's A03.1
    Friedländer's NEC A49.8
    gas (gangrene) A48.0
    mallei A24.0
    melitensis A23.0
    paratyphoid, paratyphosus A01.4
      A A01.1
      B A01.2
      C A01.3

Infection, infected, infective (Continued)
 Bacillus (Continued)
  Shiga (-Kruse) A03.0
  suipestifer —see Infection, salmonella
  swimming pool A31.1
  typhosa A01.00
  welchii —see Gangrene, gas
 bacterial NOS A49.9
  as cause of disease classified elsewhere
    B96.89
   Bacteroides fragilis [B. fragilis] B96.6
   Clostridium perfringens [C. perfringens]
    B96.7
   Enterobacter sakazakii B96.89
   Enterococcus B95.2
   Escherichia coli [E. coli] (see also
    Escherichia coli) B96.20
   Helicobacter pylori [H.pylori] B96.81
   Hemophilus influenzae [H. influenzae]
    B96.3
   Klebsiella pneumoniae [K. pneumoniae]
    B96.1
   Mycoplasma pneumoniae [M.
    pneumoniae] B96.0
   Proteus (mirabilis) (morganii) B96.4
   Pseudomonas (aeruginosa) (mallei)
    (pseudomallei) B96.5
   Staphylococcus B95.8
    aureus (methicillin susceptible)
     (MSSA) B95.61
     methicillin resistant (MRSA) B95.62
    specified NEC B95.7
   Streptococcus B95.5
    group A B95.0
    group B B95.1
    pneumoniae B95.3
    specified NEC B95.4
   Vibrio vulnificus B96.82
  specified NEC A48.8
 Bacterium
  paratyphosum A01.4
   A A01.1
   B A01.2
   C A01.3
  typhosum A01.00
 Bacteroides NEC A49.8
  fragilis, as cause of disease classified
   elsewhere B96.6
 Balantidium coli A07.0
 Bartholin's gland N75.8
 Basidiobolus B46.8
 bile duct (common) (hepatic) —see
   Cholangitis
 bladder —see Cystitis
 Blastomyces, blastomycotic —see also
   Blastomycosis
  brasiliensis —see Paracoccidioidomycosis
  dermatitidis —see Blastomycosis
  European —see Cryptococcosis
  Loboi B48.0
  North American B40.9
  South American —see
    Paracoccidioidomycosis
 bleb, postprocedure —see Blebitis
 bone —see Osteomyelitis
 Bordetella —see Whooping cough
 Borrelia bergdorfi A69.20
 brain —see also Encephalitis G04.90
  membranes —see Meningitis
  septic G06.0
   meninges —see Meningitis, bacterial
 branchial cyst Q18.0
 breast —see Mastitis
 bronchus —see Bronchitis
 Brucella A23.9
  abortus A23.1
  canis A23.3
  melitensis A23.0
  mixed A23.8
  specified NEC A23.8
  suis A23.2

Infection, infected, infective (Continued)
 Brugia (malayi) B74.1
  timori B74.2
 bursa —see Bursitis, infective
 buttocks (skin) L08.9
 Campylobacter, intestinal A04.5
  as cause of disease classified elsewhere
    B96.81
 Candida (albicans) (tropicalis) —see
    Candidiasis
 candiru B88.8
 Capillaria (intestinal) B81.1
  hepatica B83.8
  philippinensis B81.1
 cartilage —see Disorder, cartilage, specified
    type NEC
 catheter-related bloodstream (CRBSI)
    T80.211
 cat liver fluke B66.0
 cellulitis - code by site under Cellulitis
 central line-associated T80.219
  bloodstream (CLABSI) T80.211
  specified NEC T80.218
 Cephalosporium falciforme B47.0
 cerebrospinal —see Meningitis
 cervical gland (lymph) L04.0
 cervix —see Cervicitis
 cesarean delivery wound (puerperal)
    O86.00
 cestodes —see Infestation, cestodes
 chest J22
 Chilomastix (intestinal) A07.8
 Chlamydia, chlamydial A74.9
  anus A56.3
  genitourinary tract A56.2
   lower A56.00
    specified NEC A56.19
  lymphogranuloma A55
  pharynx A56.4
  psittaci A70
  rectum A56.3
  sexually transmitted NEC A56.8
 cholera —see Cholera
 Cladosporium
  bantianum (brain abscess) B43.1
  carrionii B43.0
  castellanii B36.1
  trichoides (brain abscess) B43.1
  werneckii B36.1
 Clonorchis (sinensis) (liver) B66.1
 Clostridium NEC
  bifermentans A48.0
  botulinum (food poisoning) A05.1
   infant A48.51
   wound A48.52
  difficile
   as cause of disease classified elsewhere
     B96.89
   foodborne (disease)
    not specified as recurrent A04.72
    recurrent A04.71
   gas gangrene A48.0
   necrotizing enterocolitis
    not specified as recurrent A04.72
    recurrent A04.71
   sepsis A41.4
  gas-forming NEC A48.0
  histolyticum A48.0
  novyi, causing gas gangrene A48.0
  oedematiens A48.0
  perfringens
   as cause of disease classified elsewhere
     B96.7
   due to food A05.2
   foodborne (disease) A05.2
   gas gangrene A48.0
   sepsis A41.4
  septicum, causing gas gangrene
     A48.0
  sordellii, causing gas gangrene
     A48.0

Infection, infected, infective (Continued)
 Clostridium NEC (Continued)
  welchii
   as cause of disease classified elsewhere
     B96.7
   foodborne (disease) A05.2
   gas gangrene A48.0
   necrotizing enteritis A05.2
   sepsis A41.4
 Coccidioides (immitis) —see
    Coccidioidomycosis
 colon —see Enteritis, infectious
 colostomy K94.02
 common duct —see Cholangitis
 congenital P39.9
  Candida (albicans) P37.5
  cytomegalovirus P35.1
  hepatitis, viral P35.3
  herpes simplex P35.2
  infectious or parasitic disease P37.9
   specified NEC P37.8
  listeriosis (disseminated) P37.2
  malaria NEC P37.4
   falciparum P37.3
  Plasmodium falciparum P37.3
  poliomyelitis P35.8
  rubella P35.0
  skin P39.4
  toxoplasmosis (acute) (subacute) (chronic)
     P37.1
  tuberculosis P37.0
  urinary (tract) P39.3
  vaccinia P35.8
  virus P35.9
   specified type NEC P35.8
 Conidiobolus B46.8
 coronavirus-2019 U07.1
 coronavirus NEC B34.2
  as cause of disease classified elsewhere
     B97.29
  severe acute respiratory syndrome (SARS
    associated) B97.21
 corpus luteum —see Salpingo-oophoritis
 Corynebacterium diphtheriae —see
    Diphtheria
 cotia virus B08.8
 COVID-19 U07.1
 Coxiella burnetii A78
 coxsackie —see Coxsackie
 Cryptococcus neoformans —see
    Cryptococcosis
 Cryptosporidium A07.2
 Cunninghamella —see Mucormycosis
 cyst —see Cyst
 cystic duct —see also Cholecystitis K81.9
 Cysticercus cellulosae —see Cysticercosis
 cytomegalovirus, cytomegaloviral B25.9
  congenital P35.1
  maternal, maternal care for (suspected)
    damage to fetus O35.3
  mononucleosis B27.10
   with
    complication NEC B27.19
    meningitis B27.12
    polyneuropathy B27.11
 delta-agent (acute), in hepatitis B carrier
    B17.0
 dental (pulpal origin) K04.7
 Deuteromycetes B47.0
 Dicrocoelium dendriticum B66.2
 Dipetalonema (perstans) (streptocerca) B74.4
 diphtherial —see Diphtheria
 Diphyllobothrium (adult) (latum) (pacificum)
    B70.0
  larval B70.1
 Diplogonoporus (grandis) B71.8
 Dipylidium caninum B67.4
 Dirofilaria B74.8
 Dracunculus medinensis B72
 Drechslera (hawaiiensis) B43.8
 Ducrey Haemophilus (any location) A57

▶ New   ⇒ Revised   ~~deleted~~ Deleted   ● Use Additional Character(s)

Infection, infected, infective (Continued)
  due to or resulting from
    artificial insemination N98.0
    Babesia
      divergens (-like) strain B60.03
      duncani (-type) species B60.02
      microti B60.01
      species
        specified NEC B60.09
    central venous catheter T80.219
      bloodstream T80.211
      exit or insertion site T80.212
      localized T80.212
      port or reservoir T80.212
      specified NEC T80.218
      tunnel T80.212
    device, implant or graft —see also
      Complications, by site and type,
      infection or inflammation T85.79
      arterial graft NEC T82.7
      breast (implant) T85.79
      catheter NEC T85.79
        dialysis (renal) T82.7
          central line T80.211
          intraperitoneal T85.71
        infusion NEC T82.7
          cranial T85.735
          intrathecal T85.735
          spinal (epidural) (subdural) T85.735
          subarachnoid T85.735
        urinary T83.518
          cystostomy T83.510
          Hopkins T83.518
          ileostomy T83.518
          nephrostomy T83.512
          specified NEC T83.518
          urethral indwelling T83.511
          urostomy T83.518
      electronic (electrode) (pulse generator)
        (stimulator)
        bone T84.7
        cardiac T82.7
        nervous system T85.738
          brain T85.731
          cranial nerve T85.732
          gastric nerve T85.732
          generator pocket T85.734
          neurostimulator generator
            T85.734
          peripheral nerve T85.732
          sacral nerve T85.732
          spinal cord T85.733
          vagal nerve T85.732
        urinary T83.590
      fixation, internal (orthopedic) NEC —
        see Complication, fixation device,
        infection
      gastrointestinal (bile duct) (esophagus)
        T85.79
        neurostimulator electrode (lead)
          T85.732
      genital NEC T83.69
      heart NEC T82.7
        valve (prosthesis) T82.6
        graft T82.7
      joint prosthesis —see Complication, joint
        prosthesis, infection
      ocular (corneal graft) (orbital implant)
        NEC T85.79
      orthopedic NEC T84.7
      penile (cylinder) (pump) (resevoir)
        T83.61
      specified NEC T85.79
      testicular T83.62
      urinary NEC T83.598
        ileal conduit stent T83.593
        implanted neurostimulation T83.590
        implanted sphincter T83.591
        indwelling ureteral stent T83.592
        nephroureteral stent T83.593
        specified stent NEC T83.593

Infection, infected, infective (Continued)
  due to or resulting from (Continued)
    device, implant or graft (Continued)
      vascular NEC T82.7
      ventricular intracranial (communicating)
        shunt T85.730
    Hickman catheter T80.219
      bloodstream T80.211
      localized T80.212
      specified NEC T80.218
    immunization or vaccination
      T88.0
    infusion, injection or transfusion
      NEC T80.29
      acute T80.22
    injury NEC - code by site under Wound,
      open
    peripherally inserted central catheter
      (PICC) T80.219
      bloodstream T80.211
      localized T80.212
      specified NEC T80.218
    portacath (port-a-cath) T80.219
      bloodstream T80.211
      localized T80.212
      specified NEC T80.218
    protozoa of the order Piroplasmida NEC
      B60.09
    pulmonary artery catheter —see Infection,
      due to or resulting from, central
      venous catheter
    surgery T81.40
    Swan Ganz catheter —see Infection, due
      to or resulting from, central venous
      catheter
    triple lumen catheter T80.219
      bloodstream T80.211
      localized T80.212
      specified NEC T80.218
    umbilical venous catheter T80.219
      bloodstream T80.211
      localized T80.212
      specified NEC T80.218
  during labor NEC O75.3
  ear (middle) —see also Otitis media
    external —see Otitis, externa, infective
    inner —see subcategory H83.0
  Eberthella typhosa A01.00
  Echinococcus —see Echinococcus
  echovirus
    as cause of disease classified elsewhere
      B97.12
    unspecified nature or site B34.1
  endocardium I33.0
  endocervix —see Cervicitis
  Entamoeba —see Amebiasis
  enteric —see Enteritis, infectious
  Enterobacter sakazakii B96.89
  Enterobius vermicularis B80
  enterostomy K94.12
  enterovirus B34.1
    as cause of disease classified elsewhere
      B97.10
      coxsackievirus B97.11
      echovirus B97.12
      specified NEC B97.19
  Entomophthora B46.8
  Epidermophyton —see Dermatophytosis
  epididymis —see Epididymitis
  episiotomy (puerperal) O86.09
  Erysipelothrix (insidiosa) (rhusiopathiae) —
    see Erysipeloid
  erythema infectiosum B08.3
  Escherichia (E.) coli NEC A49.8
    as cause of disease classified elsewhere —
      see also Escherichia coli B96.20
    congenital P39.8
      sepsis P36.4
    generalized A41.51
    intestinal —see Enteritis, infectious, due to,
      Escherichia coli

Infection, infected, infective (Continued)
  ethmoidal (chronic) (sinus) —see Sinusitis,
    ethmoidal
  eustachian tube (ear) —see Salpingitis,
    eustachian
  external auditory canal (meatus) NEC —see
    Otitis, externa, infective
  eye (purulent) —see Endophthalmitis, purulent
  eyelid —see Inflammation, eyelid
  fallopian tube —see Salpingo-oophoritis
  Fasciola (gigantica) (hepatica) (indica) B66.3
  Fasciolopsis (buski) B66.5
  filarial —see Infestation, filarial
  finger (skin) L08.9
    nail L03.01-●
      fungus B35.1
  fish tapeworm B70.0
    larval B70.1
  flagellate, intestinal A07.9
  fluke —see Infestation, fluke
  focal
    teeth (pulpal origin) K04.7
    tonsils J35.01
  Fonsecaea (compactum) (pedrosoi) B43.0
  food —see Intoxication, foodborne
  foot (skin) L08.9
    dermatophytic fungus B35.3
  Francisella tularensis —see Tularemia
  frontal (sinus) (chronic) —see Sinusitis, frontal
  fungus NOS B49
    beard B35.0
    dermatophytic —see Dermatophytosis
    foot B35.3
    groin B35.6
    hand B35.2
    nail B35.1
    pathogenic to compromised host only B48.8
    perianal (area) B35.6
    scalp B35.0
    skin B36.9
      foot B35.3
      hand B35.2
      toenails B35.1
  Fusarium B48.8
  gallbladder —see Cholecystitis
  gas bacillus —see Gangrene, gas
  gastrointestinal —see Enteritis, infectious
  generalized NEC —see Sepsis
  generator pocket, implanted electronic
    neurostimulator T85.734
  genital organ or tract
    female —see Disease, pelvis, inflammatory
    male N49.9
      multiple sites N49.8
      specified NEC N49.8
  Ghon tubercle, primary A15.7
  Giardia lamblia A07.1
  gingiva (chronic) K05.10
    acute K05.00
      nonplaque induced K05.01
      plaque induced K05.00
    nonplaque induced K05.11
    plaque induced K05.10
  glanders A24.0
  glenosporopsis B48.0
  Gnathostoma (spinigerum) B83.1
  Gongylonema B83.8
  gonococcal —see Gonococcus
  gram-negative bacilli NOS A49.9
  guinea worm B72
  gum (chronic) K05.10
    acute K05.00
      nonplaque induced K05.01
      plaque induced K05.00
    nonplaque induced K05.11
    plaque induced K05.10
  Haemophilus —see Infection, Hemophilus
  heart —see Carditis
  Helicobacter pylori A04.8
    as cause of disease classified elsewhere
      B96.81

Infection, infected, infective (Continued)
helminths B83.9
    intestinal B82.0
        mixed (types classifiable to more than
            one of the titles B65.0-B81.3 and
            B81.8) B81.4
        specified type NEC B81.8
    specified type NEC B83.8
Hemophilus
    aegyptius, systemic A48.4
    ducrey (any location) A57
    generalized A41.3
    influenzae NEC A49.2
        as cause of disease classified elsewhere
            B96.3
herpes (simplex) —see also Herpes
    congenital P35.2
    disseminated B00.7
    zoster B02.9
herpesvirus, herpesviral —see Herpes
Heterophyes (heterophyes) B66.8
hip (joint) NEC M00.9
    due to internal joint prosthesis
        left T84.52
        right T84.51
    skin NEC L08.9
Histoplasma —see Histoplasmosis
    American B39.4
    capsulatum B39.4
hookworm B76.9
human
    papilloma virus A63.0
    T-cell lymphotropic virus type-1 (HTLV-1)
        B33.3
hydrocele N43.0
Hymenolepis B71.0
hypopharynx —see Pharyngitis
inguinal (lymph) glands L04.1
    due to soft chancre A57
intervertebral disc, pyogenic M46.30
    cervical region M46.32
    cervicothoracic region M46.33
    lumbar region M46.36
    lumbosacral region M46.37
    multiple sites M46.39
    occipito-atlanto-axial region M46.31
    sacrococcygeal region M46.38
    thoracic region M46.34
    thoracolumbar region M46.35
intestine, intestinal —see Enteritis, infectious
    specified NEC A08.8
intra-amniotic affecting newborn NEC P39.2
intrauterine inflammation O41.12-●
Isospora belli or hominis A07.3
Japanese B encephalitis A83.0
jaw (bone) (lower) (upper) M27.2
joint NEC M00.9
    due to internal joint prosthesis T84.50
kidney (cortex) (hematogenous) N15.9
    with calculus N20.0
        with hydronephrosis N13.6
    following ectopic gestation O08.83
    pelvis and ureter (cystic) N28.85
    puerperal (postpartum) O86.21
    specified NEC N15.8
Klebsiella (K.) pneumoniae NEC A49.8
    as cause of disease classified elsewhere
        B96.1
knee (joint) NEC M00.9
    due to internal joint prosthesis
        left T84.54
        right T84.53
    joint M00.9
    skin L08.9
Koch's —see Tuberculosis
labia (majora) (minora) (acute) —see Vulvitis
lacrimal
    gland —see Dacryoadenitis
    passages (duct) (sac) —see Inflammation,
        lacrimal, passages
lancet fluke B66.2

Infection, infected, infective (Continued)
larynx NEC J38.7
leg (skin) NOS L08.9
Legionella pneumophila A48.1
    nonpneumonic A48.2
Leishmania —see also Leishmaniasis
    aethiopica B55.1
    braziliensis B55.2
    chagasi B55.0
    donovani B55.0
    infantum B55.0
    major B55.1
    mexicana B55.1
    tropica B55.1
lentivirus, as cause of disease classified
    elsewhere B97.31
Leptosphaeria senegalensis B47.0
Leptospira interrogans A27.9
    autumnalis A27.89
    canicola A27.89
    hebdomadis A27.89
    icterohaemorrhagiae A27.0
    pomona A27.89
    specified type NEC A27.89
leptospirochetal NEC —see Leptospirosis
Listeria monocytogenes —see also Listeriosis
    congenital P37.2
Loa loa B74.3
    with conjunctival infestation B74.3
    eyelid B74.3
Loboa loboi B48.0
local, skin (staphylococcal) (streptococcal)
    L08.9
    abscess - code by site under Abscess
    cellulitis - code by site under Cellulitis
    specified NEC L08.89
    ulcer —see Ulcer, skin
Loefflerella mallei A24.0
lung —see also Pneumonia J18.9
    atypical Mycobacterium A31.0
    spirochetal A69.8
    tuberculous —see Tuberculosis, pulmonary
    virus —see Pneumonia, viral
lymph gland —see also Lymphadenitis, acute
    mesenteric I88.0
lymphoid tissue, base of tongue or posterior
    pharynx, NEC (chronic) J35.03
Madurella (grisea) (mycetomii) B47.0
major
    following ectopic or molar pregnancy
        O08.0
    puerperal, postpartum, childbirth O85
Malassezia furfur B36.0
Malleomyces
    mallei A24.0
    pseudomallei (whitmori) —see Melioidosis
mammary gland N61.0
Mansonella (ozzardi) (perstans) (streptocerca)
    B74.4
mastoid —see Mastoiditis
maxilla, maxillary M27.2
    sinus (chronic) —see Sinusitis, maxillary
mediastinum J98.51
Medina (worm) B72
meibomian cyst or gland —see Hordeolum
meninges —see Meningitis, bacterial
meningococcal —see also condition A39.9
    adrenals A39.1
    brain A39.81
    cerebrospinal A39.0
    conjunctiva A39.89
    endocardium A39.51
    heart A39.50
        endocardium A39.51
        myocardium A39.52
        pericardium A39.53
    joint A39.83
    meninges A39.0
    meningococcemia A39.4
        acute A39.2
        chronic A39.3

Infection, infected, infective (Continued)
meningococcal (Continued)
    myocardium A39.52
    pericardium A39.53
    retrobulbar neuritis A39.82
    specified site NEC A39.89
mesenteric lymph nodes or glands NEC
    I88.0
Metagonimus B66.8
metatarsophalangeal M00.9
methicillin
    resistant Staphylococcus aureus (MRSA)
        A49.02
    susceptible Staphylococcus aureus (MSSA)
        A49.01
Microsporum, microsporic —see
    Dermatophytosis
mixed flora (bacterial) NEC A49.8
Monilia —see Candidiasis
Monosporium apiospermum B48.2
mouth, parasitic B37.0
Mucor —see Mucormycosis
muscle NEC —see Myositis, infective
mycelium NOS B49
mycetoma B47.9
    actinomycotic NEC B47.1
    mycotic NEC B47.0
Mycobacterium, mycobacterial —see
    Mycobacterium
Mycoplasma NEC A49.3
    pneumoniae, as cause of disease classified
        elsewhere B96.0
mycotic NOS B49
    pathogenic to compromised host only
        B48.8
    skin NOS B36.9
myocardium NEC I40.0
nail (chronic)
    with lymphangitis —see Lymphangitis,
        acute, digit
    finger L03.01-●
        fungus B35.1
    ingrowing L60.0
    toe L03.03-●
        fungus B35.1
nasal sinus (chronic) —see Sinusitis
nasopharynx —see Nasopharyngitis
navel L08.82
Necator americanus B76.1
Neisseria —see Gonococcus
Neotestudina rosatii B47.0
newborn P39.9
    intra-amniotic NEC P39.2
    skin P39.4
    specified type NEC P39.8
nipple N61.0
    associated with
        lactation O91.03
        pregnancy O91.01-●
        puerperium O91.02
Nocardia —see Nocardiosis
obstetrical surgical wound (puerperal)
    O86.00
    incisional site
        deep O86.02
        superficial O86.01
    organ and space site O86.03
    surgical site specified NEC O86.09
Oesophagostomum (apiostomum)
    B81.8
Oestrus ovis —see Myiasis
Oidium albicans B37.9
Onchocerca (volvulus) —see Onchocerciasis -
    oncovirus, as cause of disease classified
        elsewhere B97.32
operation wound T81.49
Opisthorchis (felineus) (viverrini) B66.0
orbit, orbital —see Inflammation, orbit
orthopoxvirus NEC B08.09
ovary —see Salpingo-oophoritis
Oxyuris vermicularis B80

Infection, infected, infective *(Continued)*

pancreas (acute) —*see* Pancreatitis, acute
    abscess —*see* Pancreatitis, acute
    specified NEC —*see also* Pancreatitis, acute
       K85.80
papillomavirus, as cause of disease classified
    elsewhere B97.7
papovavirus NEC B34.4
Paracoccidioides brasiliensis —*see*
    Paracoccidioidomycosis
Paragonimus (westermani) B66.4
parainfluenza virus B34.8
parameningococcus NOS A39.9
parapoxvirus B08.60
    specified NEC B08.69
parasitic B89
Parastrongylus
    cantonensis B83.2
    costaricensis B81.3
    paratyphoid A01.4
       Type A A01.1
       Type B A01.2
       Type C A01.3
paraurethral ducts N34.2
parotid gland —*see* Sialoadenitis
parvovirus NEC B34.3
    as cause of disease classified elsewhere
       B97.6
Pasteurella NEC A28.0
    multocida A28.0
    pestis —*see* Plague
    pseudotuberculosis A28.0
    septica (cat bite) (dog bite) A28.0
    tularensis —*see* Tularemia
pelvic, female —*see* Disease, pelvis,
    inflammatory
Penicillium (marneffei) B48.4
penis (glans) (retention) NEC N48.29
periapical K04.5
peridental, periodontal K05.20
    generalized —*see* Periodontitis, aggressive,
       generalized
    localized —*see* Periodontitis, aggressive,
       localized
perinatal period P39.9
    specified type NEC P39.8
perineal repair (puerperal) O86.09
periorbital —*see* Inflammation, orbit
perirectal K62.89
perirenal —*see* Infection, kidney
peritoneal —*see* Peritonitis
periureteral N28.89
Petriellidium boydii B48.2
pharynx —*see also* Pharyngitis
    coxsackievirus B08.5
    posterior, lymphoid (chronic) J35.03
Phialophora
    gougerotii (subcutaneous abscess or cyst)
       B43.2
    jeanselmei (subcutaneous abscess or cyst)
       B43.2
    verrucosa (skin) B43.0
Piedraia hortae B36.3
pinta A67.9
    intermediate A67.1
    late A67.2
    mixed A67.3
    primary A67.0
pinworm B80
pityrosporum furfur B36.0
pleuro-pneumonia-like organism (PPLO)
    NEC A49.3
    as cause of disease classified elsewhere
       B96.0
pneumococcus, pneumococcal NEC A49.1
    as cause of disease classified elsewhere
       B95.3
    generalized (purulent) A40.3
       with pneumonia J13
Pneumocystis carinii (pneumonia) B59
Pneumocystis jiroveci (pneumonia) B59

Infection, infected, infective *(Continued)*

port or reservoir T80.212
postoperative T81.40
postoperative wound T81.49
postprocedural T81.40
    surgical site
       deep incisional T81.42
       organ and space T81.43
       specified NEC T81.49
       superficial incisional T81.41
postvaccinal T88.0
prepuce NEC N47.7
    with penile inflammation N47.6
prion —*see* Disease, prion, central nervous
    system
prostate (capsule) —*see* Prostatitis
Proteus (mirabilis) (morganii) (vulgaris) NEC
    A49.8
    as cause of disease classified elsewhere
       B96.4
protozoal NEC B64
    intestinal A07.9
       specified NEC A07.8
    specified NEC B60.8
Pseudoallescheria boydii B48.2
Pseudomonas NEC A49.8
    as cause of disease classified elsewhere
       B96.5
    mallei A24.0
    pneumonia J15.1
    pseudomallei —*see* Melioidosis
puerperal O86.4
    genitourinary tract NEC O86.89
    major or generalized O85
    minor O86.4
    specified NEC O86.89
pulmonary —*see* Infection, lung
purulent —*see* Abscess
Pyrenochaeta romeroi B47.0
Q fever A78
rectum (sphincter) K62.89
renal —*see also* Infection, kidney
    pelvis and ureter (cystic) N28.85
reovirus, as cause of disease classified
    elsewhere B97.5
respiratory (tract) NEC J98.8
    acute J22
    chronic J98.8
    influenzal (upper) (acute) —*see* Influenza,
       with, respiratory manifestations
       NEC
    lower (acute) J22
       chronic —*see* Bronchitis, chronic
    rhinovirus J00
    syncytial virus (RSV) —*see* Infection, virus,
       respiratory syncytial (RSV)
    upper (acute) NOS J06.9
       chronic J39.8
       streptococcal J06.9
       viral NOS J06.9
          due to respiratory syncytial virus
             (RSV) J06.9 *[B97.1]*
resulting from
    presence of internal prosthesis, implant,
       graft —*see* Complications, by site and
       type, infection
retortamoniasis A07.8
retroperitoneal NEC K68.9
retrovirus B33.3
    as cause of disease classified elsewhere
       B97.30
    human
       immunodeficiency, type 2 (HIV 2)
          B97.35
       T-cell lymphotropic
          type I (HTLV-I) B97.33
          type II (HTLV-II) B97.34
    lentivirus B97.31
    oncovirus B97.32
    specified NEC B97.39
Rhinosporidium (seeberi) B48.1

Infection, infected, infective *(Continued)*

rhinovirus
    as cause of disease classified elsewhere
       B97.89
    unspecified nature or site B34.8
Rhizopus —*see* Mucormycosis
rickettsial NOS A79.9
roundworm (large) NEC B82.0
    Ascariasis —*see also* Ascariasis B77.9
rubella —*see* Rubella
Saccharomyces —*see* Candidiasis
salivary duct or gland (any) —*see*
    Sialoadenitis
Salmonella (aertrycke) (arizonae)
    (callinarum) (cholerae-suis) (enteritidis)
    (suipestifer) (typhimurium) A02.9
    with
       (gastro) enteritis A02.0
       sepsis A02.1
       specified manifestation NEC
          A02.8
    due to food (poisoning) A02.9
    hirschfeldii A01.3
    localized A02.20
       arthritis A02.23
       meningitis A02.21
       osteomyelitis A02.24
       pneumonia A02.22
       pyelonephritis A02.25
       specified NEC A02.29
    paratyphi A01.4
       A A01.1
       B A01.2
       C A01.3
    schottmuelleri A01.2
    typhi, typhosa —*see* Typhoid
Sarcocystis A07.8
scabies B86
Schistosoma —*see* Infestation, Schistosoma
scrotum (acute) NEC N49.2
seminal vesicle —*see* Vesiculitis
septic
    localized, skin —*see* Abscess
sheep liver fluke B66.3
Shigella A03.9
    boydii A03.2
    dysenteriae A03.0
    flexneri A03.1
    group
       A A03.0
       B A03.1
       C A03.2
       D A03.3
    Schmitz (-Stutzer) A03.0
    schmitzii A03.0
    shigae A03.0
    sonnei A03.3
    specified NEC A03.8
shoulder (joint) NEC M00.9
    due to internal joint prosthesis
       T84.59
    skin NEC L08.9
sinus (accessory) (chronic) (nasal) —*see also*
    Sinusitis
    pilonidal —*see* Sinus, pilonidal
    skin NEC L08.89
Skene's duct or gland —*see* Urethritis
skin (local) (staphylococcal) (streptococcal)
    L08.9
    abscess - code by site under Abscess
    cellulitis - code by site under Cellulitis
    due to fungus B36.9
       specified type NEC B36.8
    mycotic B36.9
       specified type NEC B36.8
    newborn P39.4
    ulcer —*see* Ulcer, skin
slow virus A81.9
    specified NEC A81.89
Sparganum (mansoni) (proliferum) (baxteri)
    B70.1

Infection, infected, infective (Continued)
  specific —see also Syphilis
    to perinatal period —see Infection,
      congenital
  specified NEC B99.8
  spermatic cord NEC N49.1
  sphenoidal (sinus) —see Sinusitis,
    sphenoidal
  spinal cord NOS —see also Myelitis G04.91
    abscess G06.1
    meninges —see Meningitis
    streptococcal G04.89
  Spirillum A25.0
  spirochetal NOS A69.9
    lung A69.8
    specified NEC A69.8
  Spirometra larvae B70.1
  spleen D73.89
  Sporotrichum, Sporothrix (schenckii) —see
    Sporotrichosis
  staphylococcal, unspecified site
    aureus (methicillin susceptible) (MSSA)
      A49.01
      methicillin resistant (MRSA) A49.02
    as cause of disease classified elsewhere
      B95.8
      aureus (methicillin susceptible) (MSSA)
        B95.61
        methicillin resistant (MRSA)
          B95.62
      specified NEC B95.7
    food poisoning A05.0
    generalized (purulent) A41.2
    pneumonia —see Pneumonia,
      staphylococcal
  Stellantchasmus falcatus B66.8
  streptobacillus moniliformis A25.1
  streptococcal NEC A49.1
    as cause of disease classified elsewhere
      B95.5
    B genitourinary complicating
      childbirth O98.82
      pregnancy O98.81-●
      puerperium O98.83
    congenital
      sepsis P36.10
        group B P36.0
        specified NEC P36.19
    generalized (purulent) A40.9
  Streptomyces B47.1
  Strongyloides (stercoralis) —see
    Strongyloidiasis
  stump (amputation) (surgical) —see
    Complication, amputation stump,
    infection
  subcutaneous tissue, local L08.9
  suipestifer —see Infection, salmonella
  swimming pool bacillus A31.1
  Taenia —see Infestation, Taenia
  Taeniarhynchus saginatus B68.1
  tapeworm —see Infestation,
    tapeworm
  tendon (sheath) —see Tenosynovitis, infective
    NEC
  Ternidens diminutus B81.8
  testis —see Orchitis
  threadworm B80
  throat —see Pharyngitis
  thyroglossal duct K14.8
  toe (skin) L08.9
    cellulitis L03.03-●
      fungus B35.1
    nail L03.03-●
      fungus B35.1
  tongue NEC K14.0
    parasitic B37.0
  tonsil (and adenoid) (faucial) (lingual)
    (pharyngeal) —see Tonsillitis
  tooth, teeth K04.7
    irreversible K04.02
    periapical K04.7

Infection, infected, infective (Continued)
  tooth, teeth (Continued)
    peridental, periodontal K05.20
      generalized —see Periodontitis,
        aggressive, generalized
      localized —see Periodontitis, aggressive,
        localized
    pulp K04.01
      irreversible K04.02
      reversible K04.01
    TORCH —see Infection, congenital
      without active infection P00.2
    Torula histolytica —see Cryptococcosis
    Toxocara (canis) (cati) (felis) B83.0
    Toxoplasma gondii —see Toxoplasma
    trachea, chronic J42
    trematode NEC —see Infestation, fluke
    trench fever A79.0
    Treponema pallidum —see Syphilis
    Trichinella (spiralis) B75
    Trichomonas A59.9
      cervix A59.09
      intestine A07.8
      prostate A59.02
      specified site NEC A59.8
      urethra A59.03
      urogenitalis A59.00
      vagina A59.01
      vulva A59.01
    Trichophyton, trichophytic —see
      Dermatophytosis
    Trichosporon (beigelii) cutaneum B36.2
    Trichostrongylus B81.2
    Trichuris (trichiura) B79
    Trombicula (irritans) B88.0
    Trypanosoma
      brucei
        gambiense B56.0
        rhodesiense B56.1
      cruzi —see Chagas' disease
    tubal —see Salpingo-oophoritis
    tuberculous
      latent (LTBI) Z22.7
      NEC —see Tuberculosis
    tubo-ovarian —see Salpingo-oophoritis
    tunica vaginalis N49.1
    tunnel T80.212
    tympanic membrane NEC —see Myringitis
    typhoid (abortive) (ambulant) (bacillus) —see
      Typhoid
    typhus A75.9
      flea-borne A75.2
      mite-borne A75.3
      recrudescent A75.1
      tick-borne A77.9
        African A77.1
        North Asian A77.2
    umbilicus L08.82
    ureter —see Ureteritis
    urethra —see Urethritis
    urinary (tract) N39.0
      bladder —see Cystitis
      complicating
        pregnancy O23.4-●
          specified type NEC O23.3-●
      kidney —see Infection, kidney
      newborn P39.3
      puerperal (postpartum) O86.20
      tuberculous A18.13
      urethra —see Urethritis
    uterus, uterine —see Endometritis
    vaccination T88.0
    vaccinia not from vaccination B08.011
    vagina (acute) —see Vaginitis
    varicella B01.9
    varicose veins —see Varix
    vas deferens NEC N49.1
    vesical —see Cystitis
    Vibrio
      cholerae A00.0
        El Tor A00.1

Infection, infected, infective (Continued)
  Vibrio (Continued)
    parahaemolyticus (food poisoning)
      A05.3
    vulnificus
      as cause of disease classified elsewhere
        B96.82
      foodborne intoxication A05.5
  Vincent's (gum) (mouth) (tonsil) A69.1
  virus, viral NOS B34.9
    adenovirus
      as cause of disease classified elsewhere
        B97.0
      unspecified nature or site B34.0
    arborvirus, arbovirus arthropod-borne
      A94
    as cause of disease classified elsewhere
      B97.89
      adenovirus B97.0
      coronavirus B97.29
        SARS-associated B97.21
      coxsackievirus B97.11
      echovirus B97.12
      enterovirus B97.10
        coxsackievirus B97.11
        echovirus B97.12
        specified NEC B97.19
      human
        immunodeficiency, type 2 (HIV 2)
          B97.35
        metapneumovirus B97.81
        T-cell lymphotropic,
          type I (HTLV-I) B97.33
          type II (HTLV-II) B97.34
      papillomavirus B97.7
      parvovirus B97.6
      reovirus B97.5
      respiratory syncytial (RSV) —see
        Infection virus, respiratory
        syncytial (RSV)
      retrovirus B97.30
        human
          immunodeficiency, type 2 (HIV 2)
            B97.35
          T-cell lymphotropic,
            type I (HTLV-I) B97.33
            type II (HTLV-II) B97.34
        lentivirus B97.31
        oncovirus B97.32
        specified NEC B97.39
      specified NEC B97.89
    central nervous system A89
      atypical A81.9
        specified NEC A81.89
      enterovirus NEC A88.8
        meningitis A87.0
      slow virus A81.9
        specified NEC A81.89
      specified NEC A88.8
    chest J98.8
    cotia B08.8
    COVID-19 U07.1
    coxsackie —see also Infection, coxsackie
      B34.1
      as cause of disease classified elsewhere
        B97.11
    ECHO
      as cause of disease classified elsewhere
        B97.12
      unspecified nature or site B34.1
    encephalitis, tick-borne A84.9
    enterovirus, as cause of disease classified
      elsewhere B97.10
      coxsackievirus B97.11
      echovirus B97.12
      specified NEC B97.19
    exanthem NOS B09
    human metapneumovirus as cause of
      disease classified elsewhere B97.81
    human papilloma as cause of disease
      classified elsewhere B97.7

Infection, infected, infective (Continued)
  virus, viral NOS (Continued)
    intestine —see Enteritis, viral
    respiratory syncytial (RSV) —see Infection
        virus, respiratory syncytial (RSV)
      bronchiolitis J21.0
      bronchitis J20.5
      bronchopneumonia J12.1
      otitis media H65.- ● [B97.4]
      pneumonia J12.1
      upper respiratory infection J06.9
          [B97.4]
    rhinovirus
      as cause of disease classified elsewhere
          B97.89
      unspecified nature or site B34.8
    slow A81.9
      specified NEC A81.89
    specified type NEC B33.8
      as cause of disease classified elsewhere
          B97.89
      unspecified nature or site B34.8
    unspecified nature or site B34.9
    West Nile —see Virus, West Nile
  vulva (acute) —see Vulvitis
  West Nile —see Virus, West Nile
  whipworm B79
  worms B83.9
    specified type NEC B83.8
  Wuchereria (bancrofti) B74.0
    malayi B74.1
    yatapoxvirus B08.70
      specified NEC B08.79
  yeast (see also Candidiasis) B37.9
  yellow fever —see Fever, yellow
  Yersinia
    enterocolitica (intestinal) A04.6
    pestis —see Plague
    pseudotuberculosis A28.2
  Zeis' gland —see Hordeolum
  Zika virus A92.5
    congenital P35.4
  zoonotic bacterial NOS A28.9
  Zopfia senegalensis B47.0
Infective, infectious —see condition
Infertility
  female N97.9
    age-related N97.8
    associated with
      anovulation N97.0
      cervical (mucus) disease or anomaly
          N88.3
      congenital anomaly
        cervix N88.3
        fallopian tube N97.1
        uterus N97.2
        vagina N97.8
      dysmucorrhea N88.3
      fallopian tube disease or anomaly
          N97.1
      pituitary-hypothalamic origin
          E23.0
      specified origin NEC N97.8
      Stein-Leventhal syndrome E28.2
      uterine disease or anomaly N97.2
      vaginal disease or anomaly N97.8
    due to
      cervical anomaly N88.3
      fallopian tube anomaly N97.1
      ovarian failure E28.39
      Stein-Leventhal syndrome
          E28.2
      uterine anomaly N97.2
      vaginal anomaly N97.8
    nonimplantation N97.2
    origin
      cervical N88.3
      tubal (block) (occlusion) (stenosis)
          N97.1
      uterine N97.2
      vaginal N97.8

Infertility (Continued)
  male N46.9
    azoospermia N46.01
      extratesticular cause N46.029
        drug therapy N46.021
        efferent duct obstruction N46.023
        infection N46.022
        radiation N46.024
        specified cause NEC N46.029
        systemic disease N46.025
    oligospermia N46.11
      extratesticular cause N46.129
        drug therapy N46.121
        efferent duct obstruction N46.123
        infection N46.122
        radiation N46.124
        specified cause NEC N46.129
        systemic disease N46.125
    specified type NEC N46.8
Infestation B88.9
  Acanthocheilonema (perstans) (streptocerca)
      B74.4
  Acariasis B88.0
    demodex folliculorum B88.0
    sarcoptes scabiei B86
    trombiculae B88.0
  Agamofilaria streptocerca B74.4
  Ancylostoma, ankylostoma (braziliense)
      (caninum) (ceylanicum) (duodenale)
      B76.0
    americanum B76.1
    new world B76.1
  Anisakis larvae, anisakiasis B81.0
  arthropod NEC B88.2
  Ascaris lumbricoides —see Ascariasis
  Balantidium coli A07.0
  beef tapeworm B68.1
  Bothriocephalus (latus) B70.0
    larval B70.1
  broad tapeworm B70.0
    larval B70.1
  Brugia (malayi) B74.1
    timori B74.2
  candiru B88.8
  Capillaria
    hepatica B83.8
    philippinensis B81.1
  cat liver fluke B66.0
  cestodes B71.9
    diphyllobothrium —see Infestation,
        diphyllobothrium
    dipylidiasis B71.1
    hymenolepiasis B71.0
    specified type NEC B71.8
  chigger B88.0
  chigo, chigoe B88.1
  Clonorchis (sinensis) (liver) B66.1
  coccidial A07.3
  crab-lice B85.3
  Cysticercus cellulosae —see Cysticercosis
  Demodex (folliculorum) B88.0
  Dermanyssus gallinae B88.0
  Dermatobia (hominis) —see Myiasis
  Dibothriocephalus (latus) B70.0
    larval B70.1
  Dicrocoelium dendriticum B66.2
  Diphyllobothrium (adult) (latum) (intestinal)
      (pacificum) B70.0
    larval B70.1
  Diplogonoporus (grandis) B71.8
  Dipylidium caninum B67.4
  Distoma hepaticum B66.3
  dog tapeworm B67.4
  Dracunculus medinensis B72
  dragon worm B72
  dwarf tapeworm B71.0
  Echinococcus —see Echinococcus
  Echinostomum ilocanum B66.8
  Entamoeba (histolytica) —see Infection,
      Ameba
  Enterobius vermicularis B80

Infestation (Continued)
  eyelid
    in (due to)
      leishmaniasis B55.1
      loiasis B74.3
      onchocerciasis B73.09
      phthiriasis B85.3
    parasitic NOS B89
  eyeworm B74.3
  Fasciola (gigantica) (hepatica) (indica) B66.3
  Fasciolopsis (buski) (intestine) B66.5
  filarial B74.9
    bancroftian B74.0
    conjunctiva B74.9
    due to
      Acanthocheilonema (perstans)
          (streptocerca) B74.4
      Brugia (malayi) B74.1
        timori B74.2
      Dracunculus medinensis B72
      guinea worm B72
      loa loa B74.3
      Mansonella (ozzardi) (perstans)
          (streptocerca) B74.4
      Onchocerca volvulus B73.00
        eye B73.00
        eyelid B73.09
      Wuchereria (bancrofti) B74.0
    Malayan B74.1
    ozzardi B74.4
    specified type NEC B74.8
  fish tapeworm B70.0
    larval B70.1
  fluke B66.9
    blood NOS —see Schistosomiasis
    cat liver B66.0
    intestinal B66.5
    lancet B66.2
    liver (sheep) B66.3
      cat B66.0
      Chinese B66.1
      due to clonorchiasis B66.1
      oriental B66.1
    lung (oriental) B66.4
    sheep liver B66.3
    specified type NEC B66.8
  fly larvae —see Myiasis
  Gasterophilus (intestinalis) —see Myiasis
  Gastrodiscoides hominis B66.8
  Giardia lamblia A07.1
  Gnathostoma (spinigerum) B83.1
  Gongylonema B83.8
  guinea worm B72
  helminth B83.9
    angiostrongyliasis B83.2
      intestinal B81.3
    gnathostomiasis B83.1
    hirudiniasis, internal B83.4
    intestinal B82.0
      angiostrongyliasis B81.3
      anisakiasis B81.0
      ascariasis —see Ascariasis
      capillariasis B81.1
      cysticercosis —see Cysticercosis
      diphyllobothriasis —see Infestation,
          diphyllobothriasis
      dracunculiasis B72
      echinococcus —see Echinococcosis
      enterobiasis B80
      filariasis —see Infestation, filarial
      fluke —see Infestation, fluke
      hookworm —see Infestation, hookworm
      mixed (types classifiable to more than
          one of the titles B65.0-B81.3 and
          B81.8) B81.4
      onchocerciasis —see Onchocerciasis
      schistosomiasis —see Infestation,
          schistosoma
      specified
        cestode NEC —see Infestation, cestode
            type NEC B81.8

Infestation (Continued)
- helminth (Continued)
  - intestinal (Continued)
    - strongyloidiasis —see Strongyloidiasis
    - taenia —see Infestation, taenia
    - trichinellosis B75
    - trichostrongyliasis B81.2
    - trichuriasis B79
  - specified type NEC B83.8
  - syngamiasis B83.3
  - visceral larva migrans B83.0
- Heterophyes (heterophyes) B66.8
- hookworm B76.9
  - ancylostomiasis B76.0
  - necatoriasis B76.1
  - specified type NEC B76.8
- Hymenolepis (diminuta) (nana) B71.0
- intestinal NEC B82.9
- leeches (aquatic) (land) —see Hirudiniasis
- Leishmania —see Leishmaniasis
- lice, louse —see Infestation, Pediculus
- Linguatula B88.8
- Liponyssoides sanguineus B88.0
- Loa loa B74.3
  - conjunctival B74.3
  - eyelid B74.3
- louse —see Infestation, Pediculus
- maggots —see Myiasis
- Mansonella (ozzardi) (perstans) (streptocerca) B74.4
- Medina (worm) B72
- Metagonimus (yokogawai) B66.8
- microfilaria streptocerca —see Onchocerciasis
  - eye B73.00
  - eyelid B73.09
- mites B88.9
  - scabic B86
- Monilia (albicans) —see Candidiasis
- mouth B37.0
- Necator americanus B76.1
- nematode NEC (intestinal) B82.0
  - Ancylostoma B76.0
  - conjunctiva NEC B83.9
  - Enterobius vermicularis B80
  - Gnathostoma spinigerum B83.1
  - physaloptera B80
  - specified NEC B81.8
  - trichostrongylus B81.2
  - trichuris (trichuria) B79
- Oesophagostomum (apiostomum) B81.8
- Oestrus ovis —see also Myiasis B87.9
- Onchocerca (volvulus) —see Onchocerciasis
- Opisthorchis (felineus) (viverrini) B66.0
- orbit, parasitic NOS B89
- Oxyuris vermicularis B80
- Paragonimus (westermani) B66.4
- parasite, parasitic B89
  - eyelid B89
  - intestinal NOS B82.9
  - mouth B37.0
  - skin B88.9
  - tongue B37.0
- Parastrongylus
  - cantonensis B83.2
  - costaricensis B81.3
- Pediculus B85.2
  - body B85.1
  - capitis (humanus) (any site) B85.0
  - corporis (humanus) (any site) B85.1
  - head B85.0
  - mixed (classifiable to more than one of the titles B85.0-B85.3) B85.4
  - pubis (any site) B85.3
- Pentastoma B88.8
- Phthirus (pubis) (any site) B85.3
  - with any infestation classifiable to B85.0-B85.2 B85.4
- pinworm B80
- pork tapeworm (adult) B68.0

Infestation (Continued)
- protozoal NEC B64
  - intestinal A07.9
    - specified NEC A07.8
  - specified NEC B60.8
- pubic, louse B85.3
- rat tapeworm B71.0
- red bug B88.0
- roundworm (large) NEC B82.0
  - Ascariasis —see also Ascariasis B77.9
- sandflea B88.1
- Sarcoptes scabiei B86
- scabies B86
- Schistosoma B65.9
  - bovis B65.8
  - cercariae B65.3
  - haematobium B65.0
  - intercalatum B65.8
  - japonicum B65.2
  - mansoni B65.1
  - mattheei B65.8
  - mekongi B65.8
  - specified type NEC B65.8
  - spindale B65.8
- screw worms —see Myiasis
- skin NOS B88.9
- Sparganum (mansoni) (proliferum) (baxteri) B70.1
  - larval B70.1
- specified type NEC B88.8
- Spirometra larvae B70.1
- Stellantchasmus falcatus B66.8
- Strongyloides stercoralis —see Strongyloidiasis
- Taenia B68.9
  - diminuta B71.0
  - echinococcus —see Echinococcus
  - mediocanellata B68.1
  - nana B71.0
  - saginata B68.1
  - solium (intestinal form) B68.0
    - larval form —see Cysticercosis
- Taeniarhynchus saginatus B68.1
- tapeworm B71.9
  - beef B68.1
  - broad B70.0
    - larval B70.1
  - dog B67.4
  - dwarf B71.0
  - fish B70.0
    - larval B70.1
  - pork B68.0
  - rat B71.0
- Ternidens diminutus B81.8
- Tetranychus molestissimus B88.0
- threadworm B80
- tongue B37.0
- Toxocara (canis) (cati) (felis) B83.0
- trematode(s) NEC —see Infestation, fluke
- Trichinella (spiralis) B75
- Trichocephalus B79
- Trichomonas —see Trichomoniasis
- Trichostrongylus B81.2
- Trichuris (trichiura) B79
- Trombicula (irritans) B88.0
- Tunga penetrans B88.1
- Uncinaria americana B76.1
- Vandellia cirrhosa B88.8
- whipworm B79
- worms B83.9
  - intestinal B82.0
- Wuchereria (bancrofti) B74.0

Infiltrate, infiltration
- amyloid (generalized) (localized) —see Amyloidosis
- calcareous NEC R89.7
  - localized —see Degeneration, by site
- calcium salt R89.7
- cardiac
  - fatty —see Degeneration, myocardial
  - glycogenic E74.02 [I43]

Infiltrate, infiltration (Continued)
- corneal —see Edema, cornea
- eyelid —see Inflammation, eyelid
- glycogen, glycogenic —see Disease, glycogen storage
- heart, cardiac
  - fatty —see Degeneration, myocardial
  - glycogenic E74.02 [I43]
- inflammatory in vitreous H43.89
- kidney N28.89
- leukemic —see Leukemia
- liver K76.89
  - fatty —see Fatty, liver NEC
  - glycogen —see also Disease, glycogen storage E74.03 [K77]
- lung R91.8
  - eosinophilic —see Eosinophilia, pulmonary
- lymphatic —see also Leukemia, lymphatic C91.9-●
  - gland I88.9
- muscle, fatty M62.89
- myocardium, myocardial
  - fatty —see Degeneration, myocardial
  - glycogenic E74.02 [I43]
- on chest x-ray R91.8
- pulmonary R91.8
  - with eosinophilia —see Eosinophilia, pulmonary
- skin (lymphocytic) L98.6
- thymus (gland) (fatty) E32.8
- urine R39.0
- vesicant agent
  - antineoplastic chemotherapy T80.810
  - other agent NEC T80.818
- vitreous body H43.89
Infirmity R68.89
- senile R54
Inflammation, inflamed, inflammatory (with exudation)
- abducent (nerve) —see Strabismus, paralytic, sixth nerve
- accessory sinus (chronic) —see Sinusitis
- adrenal (gland) E27.8
- alveoli, teeth M27.3
  - scorbutic E54
- anal canal, anus K62.89
- antrum (chronic) —see Sinusitis, maxillary
- appendix —see Appendicitis
- arachnoid —see Meningitis
- areola N61.0
  - puerperal, postpartum or gestational —see Infection, nipple
- areolar tissue NOS L08.9
- artery —see Arteritis
- auditory meatus (external) —see Otitis, externa
- Bartholin's gland N75.8
- bile duct (common) (hepatic) or passage —see Cholangitis
- bladder —see Cystitis
- bone —see Osteomyelitis
- brain —see also Encephalitis
  - membrane —see Meningitis
- breast N61.0
  - puerperal, postpartum, gestational —see Mastitis, obstetric
- broad ligament —see Disease, pelvis, inflammatory
- bronchi —see Bronchitis
- catarrhal J00
- cecum —see Appendicitis
- cerebral —see also Encephalitis
  - membrane —see Meningitis
- cerebrospinal
  - meningococcal A39.0
- cervix (uteri) —see Cervicitis
- chest J98.8
- chorioretinal H30.9-●
  - cyclitis —see Cyclitis
  - disseminated H30.10-●
    - generalized H30.13-●
    - peripheral H30.12-●
    - posterior pole H30.11-●

▶ New   ⇒ Revised   ~~deleted~~ Deleted   ● Use Additional Character(s)

Inflammation, inflamed, inflammatory
(Continued)
  chorioretinal (Continued)
    epitheliopathy —see Epitheliopathy
    focal H30.00-●
      juxtapapillary H30.01-●
      macular H30.04-●
      paramacular —see Inflammation,
        chorioretinal, focal, macular
      peripheral H30.03-●
      posterior pole H30.02-●
      specified type NEC H30.89-●
    choroid —see Inflammation, chorioretinal
  chronic, postmastoidectomy cavity —see
    Complications, postmastoidectomy,
    inflammation
  colon —see Enteritis
  connective tissue (diffuse) NEC —see
    Disorder, soft tissue, specified type NEC
  cornea —see Keratitis
  corpora cavernosa N48.29
  cranial nerve —see Disorder, nerve, cranial
  Douglas' cul-de-sac or pouch (chronic) N73.0
  due to device, implant or graft —see also
    Complications, by site and type,
    infection or inflammation
    arterial graft T82.7
    breast (implant) T85.79
    catheter T85.79
      dialysis (renal) T82.7
        intraperitoneal T85.71
      infusion T82.7
        cranial T85.735
        intrathecal T85.735
        spinal (epidural) (subdural) T85.735
        subarachnoid T85.735
      urinary T83.518
        cystostomy T83.510
        Hopkins T83.518
        ileostomy T83.518
        nephrostomy T83.512
        specified NEC T83.518
        urethral indwelling T83.511
        urostomy T83.518
    electronic (electrode) (pulse generator)
      (stimulator)
      bone T84.7
      cardiac T82.7
      nervous system T85.738
        brain T85.731
        cranial nerve T85.732
        gastric nerve T85.732
        neurostimulator generator T85.734
        peripheral nerve T85.732
        sacral nerve T85.732
        spinal cord T85.733
        vagal nerve T85.732
      urinary T83.590
    fixation, internal (orthopedic) NEC —
      see Complication, fixation device,
      infection
    gastrointestinal (bile duct) (esophagus)
      T85.79
    neurostimulator electrode (lead) T85.732
    genital NEC T83.69
    heart NEC T82.7
      valve (prosthesis) T82.6
        graft T82.7
    joint prosthesis —see Complication, joint
      prosthesis, infection
    ocular (corneal graft) (orbital implant)
      NEC T85.79
    orthopedic NEC T84.7
    penile (cylinder) (pump) (resevoir) T83.61
    specified NEC T85.79
    testicular T83.62
    urinary NEC T83.598
      ileal conduit stent T83.593
      implanted neurostimulation T83.590
      implanted sphincter T83.591
      indwelling ureteral stent T83.592

Inflammation, inflamed, inflammatory
(Continued)
  due to device, implant or graft (Continued)
  (Continued)
    urinary NEC (Continued)
      nephroureteral stent T83.593
      specified stent NEC T83.593
    vascular NEC T82.7
    ventricular intracranial (communicating)
      shunt T85.730
  duodenum K29.80
    with bleeding K29.81
  dura mater —see Meningitis
  ear (middle) —see also Otitis, media
    external —see Otitis, externa
    inner —see subcategory H83.0
  epididymis —see Epididymitis
  esophagus —see Esophagitis
  ethmoidal (sinus) (chronic) —see Sinusitis,
    ethmoidal
  eustachian tube (catarrhal) —see Salpingitis,
    eustachian
  eyelid H01.9
    abscess —see Abscess, eyelid
    blepharitis —see Blepharitis
    chalazion —see Chalazion
    dermatosis (noninfectious) —see
      Dermatosis, eyelid
    hordeolum —see Hordeolum
    specified NEC H01.8
  fallopian tube —see Salpingo-oophoritis
  fascia —see Myositis
  follicular, pharynx J31.2
  frontal (sinus) (chronic) —see Sinusitis, frontal
  gallbladder —see Cholecystitis
  gastric —see Gastritis
  gastrointestinal —see Enteritis
  genital organ (internal) (diffuse)
    female —see Disease, pelvis, inflammatory
    male N49.9
      multiple sites N49.8
      specified NEC N49.8
  gland (lymph) —see Lymphadenitis
  glottis —see Laryngitis
  granular, pharynx J31.2
  gum K05.10
    nonplaque induced K05.11
    plaque induced K05.10
  heart —see Carditis
  hepatic duct —see Cholangitis
  ileoanal (internal) pouch K91.850
  ileum —see also Enteritis
    regional or terminal —see Enteritis, regional
  intestinal pouch K91.850
  intestine (any part) —see Enteritis
  jaw (acute) (bone) (chronic) (lower)
    (suppurative) (upper) M27.2
  joint NEC —see Arthritis
    sacroiliac M46.1
  kidney —see Nephritis
  knee (joint) M13.169
    tuberculous A18.02
  labium (majus) (minus) —see Vulvitis
  lacrimal
    gland —see Dacryoadenitis
    passages (duct) (sac) —see also Dacryocystitis
      canaliculitis —see Canaliculitis, lacrimal
  larynx —see Laryngitis
  leg NOS L08.9
  lip K13.0
  liver (capsule) —see also Hepatitis
    chronic K73.9
    suppurative K75.0
  lung (acute) —see also Pneumonia
    chronic J98.4
  lymphatic vessel —see Lymphangitis
  lymph gland or node —see Lymphadenitis
  maxilla, maxillary M27.2
    sinus (chronic) —see Sinusitis, maxillary
  membranes of brain or spinal cord —see
    Meningitis

Inflammation, inflamed, inflammatory
(Continued)
  meninges —see Meningitis
  mouth K12.1
  muscle —see Myositis
  myocardium —see Myocarditis
  nasal sinus (chronic) —see Sinusitis
  nasopharynx —see Nasopharyngitis
  navel L08.82
  ▷nerve NEC —see Neuritis
  nipple N61.0
    puerperal, postpartum or gestational —see
      Infection, nipple
  nose —see Rhinitis
  oculomotor (nerve) —see Strabismus,
    paralytic, third nerve
  optic nerve —see Neuritis, optic
  orbit (chronic) H05.10
    acute H05.00
      abscess —see Abscess, orbit
      cellulitis —see Cellulitis, orbit
      osteomyelitis —see Osteomyelitis, orbit
      periostitis —see Periostitis, orbital
      tenonitis —see Tenonitis, eye
    granuloma —see Granuloma, orbit
    myositis —see Myositis, orbital
  ovary —see Salpingo-oophoritis
  oviduct —see Salpingo-oophoritis
  pancreas (acute) —see Pancreatitis
  parametrium N73.0
  parotid region L08.9
  pelvis, female —see Disease, pelvis,
    inflammatory
  penis (corpora cavernosa) N48.29
  perianal K62.89
  pericardium —see Pericarditis
  perineum (female) (male) L08.9
  perirectal K62.89
  peritoneum —see Peritonitis
  periuterine —see Disease, pelvis, inflammatory
  perivesical —see Cystitis
  petrous bone (acute) (chronic) —see Petrositis
  pharynx (acute) —see Pharyngitis
  pia mater —see Meningitis
  pleura —see Pleurisy
  polyp, colon —see also Polyp, colon,
    inflammatory K51.40
  prostate —see also Prostatitis
    specified type NEC N41.8
  rectosigmoid —see Rectosigmoiditis
  rectum —see also Proctitis K62.89
  respiratory, upper —see also Infection,
    respiratory, upper J06.9
    acute, due to radiation J70.0
    chronic, due to external agent —see
      condition, respiratory, chronic, due to
    due to
      chemicals, gases, fumes or vapors
        (inhalation) J68.2
      radiation J70.1
  retina —see Chorioretinitis
  retrocecal —see Appendicitis
  retroperitoneal —see Peritonitis
  salivary duct or gland (any) (suppurative) —
    see Sialoadenitis
  scorbutic, alveoli, teeth E54
  scrotum N49.2
  seminal vesicle —see Vesiculitis
  sigmoid —see Enteritis
  sinus —see Sinusitis
  Skene's duct or gland —see Urethritis
  skin L08.9
  spermatic cord N49.1
  sphenoidal (sinus) —see Sinusitis, sphenoidal
  spinal
    cord —see Encephalitis
    membrane —see Meningitis
    nerve —see Disorder, nerve
  spine —see Spondylopathy, inflammatory
  spleen (capsule) D73.89
  stomach —see Gastritis

Injury *(Continued)*
  arm *(Continued)*
    nerve —*see* Injury, nerve, arm
    open —*see* Wound, open, arm
    specified type NEC S49.8-●
    superficial —*see* Injury, superficial, arm
  artery (complicating trauma) —*see also* Injury,
        blood vessel, by site
    cerebral or meningeal —*see* Injury,
        intracranial
  auditory canal (external) (meatus) S09.91
  auricle, auris, ear S09.91
  axilla —*see* Injury, shoulder
  back —*see* Injury, back, lower
  bile duct S36.13
  birth —*see also* Birth, injury P15.9
  bladder (sphincter) S37.20
    at delivery O71.5
    contusion S37.22
    laceration S37.23
    obstetrical trauma O71.5
    specified type NEC S37.29
  blast (air) (hydraulic) (immersion)
        (underwater) NEC T14.8
    acoustic nerve trauma —*see* Injury, nerve,
        acoustic
    bladder —*see* Injury, bladder
    brain —*see* Concussion
    colon —*see* Injury, intestine, large, blast
        injury
    ear (primary) S09.31-●
      secondary S09.39-●
    generalized T70.8
    lung —*see* Injury, intrathoracic, lung, blast
        injury
    multiple body organs T70.8
    peritoneum S36.81
    rectum S36.61
    retroperitoneum S36.898
    small intestine S36.419
      duodenum S36.410
      specified site NEC S36.418
    specified
      intra-abdominal organ NEC S36.898
      pelvic organ NEC S37.899
  blood vessel NEC T14.8
    abdomen S35.9-●
      aorta —*see* Injury, aorta, abdominal
      celiac artery —*see* Injury, blood vessel,
          celiac artery
      iliac vessel —*see* Injury, blood vessel, iliac
      laceration S35.91
      mesenteric vessel —*see* Injury, mesenteric
      portal vein —*see* Injury, blood vessel,
          portal vein
      renal vessel —*see* Injury, blood vessel,
          renal
      specified vessel NEC S35.8X-●
      splenic vessel —*see* Injury, blood vessel,
          splenic
      vena cava —*see* Injury, vena cava,
          inferior
    ankle —*see* Injury, blood vessel, foot
    aorta (abdominal) (thoracic) —*see* Injury,
        aorta
    arm (upper) NEC S45.90-●
      forearm —*see* Injury, blood vessel,
          forearm
      laceration S45.91-●
      specified
        site NEC S45.80-●
          laceration S45.81-●
          specified type NEC S45.89-●
        type NEC S45.99-●
      superficial vein S45.30-●
        laceration S45.31-●
        specified type NEC S45.39-●
    axillary
      artery S45.00-●
        laceration S45.01-●
        specified type NEC S45.09-●

Injury *(Continued)*
  blood vessel NEC *(Continued)*
    axillary *(Continued)*
      vein S45.20-●
        laceration S45.21-●
        specified type NEC S45.29-●
    azygos vein —*see* Injury, blood vessel,
        thoracic, specified site NEC
    brachial
      artery S45.10-●
        laceration S45.11-●
        specified type NEC S45.19-●
      vein S45.20-●
        laceration S45.219
        specified type NEC S45.29-●
    carotid artery (common) (external)
        (internal, extracranial) S15.00-●
      internal, intracranial S06.8-●
      laceration (minor) (superficial) S15.01-●
        major S15.02-●
      specified type NEC S15.09-●
    celiac artery S35.219
      branch S35.299
        laceration (minor) (superficial) S35.291
          major S35.292
        specified NEC S35.298
      laceration (minor) (superficial) S35.211
        major S35.212
      specified type NEC S35.218
    cerebral —*see* Injury, intracranial
    deep plantar —*see* Injury, blood vessel,
        plantar artery
    digital (hand) —*see* Injury, blood vessel,
        finger
    dorsal
      artery (foot) S95.00-●
        laceration S95.01-●
        specified type NEC S95.09-●
      vein (foot) S95.20-●
        laceration S95.21-●
        specified type NEC S95.29-●
    due to accidental laceration during
        procedure —*see* Laceration, accidental
        complicating surgery
    extremity —*see* Injury, blood vessel, limb
    femoral
      artery (common) (superficial) S75.00-●
        laceration (minor) (superficial) S75.01-●
          major S75.02-●
        specified type NEC S75.09-●
      vein (hip level) (thigh level) S75.10-●
        laceration (minor) (superficial) S75.11-●
          major S75.12-●
        specified type NEC S75.19-●
    finger S65.50-●
      index S65.50-●
        laceration S65.51-●
        specified type NEC S65.59-●
      laceration S65.51-●
      little S65.50-●
        laceration S65.51-●
        specified type NEC S65.59-●
      middle S65.50-●
        laceration S65.51-●
        specified type NEC S65.59-●
      specified type NEC S65.59-●
      thumb —*see* Injury, blood vessel, thumb
    foot S95.90-●
      dorsal
        artery —*see* Injury, blood vessel,
            dorsal, artery
        vein —*see* Injury, blood vessel, dorsal,
            vein
      laceration S95.91-●
      plantar artery —*see* Injury, blood vessel,
          plantar artery
      specified
        site NEC S95.80-●
          laceration S95.81-●
          specified type NEC S95.89-●
        specified type NEC S95.99-●

Injury *(Continued)*
  blood vessel NEC *(Continued)*
    forearm S55.90-●
      laceration S55.91-●
      radial artery —*see* Injury, blood vessel,
          radial artery
      specified
        site NEC S55.80-●
          laceration S55.81-●
          specified type NEC S55.89-●
        type NEC S55.99-●
      ulnar artery —*see* Injury, blood vessel,
          ulnar artery
      vein S55.20-●
        laceration S55.21-●
        specified type NEC S55.29-●
    gastric
      artery —*see* Injury, mesenteric, artery,
          branch
      vein —*see* Injury, blood vessel, abdomen
    gastroduodenal artery —*see* Injury,
        mesenteric, artery, branch
    greater saphenous vein (lower leg level)
        S85.30-●
      hip (and thigh) level S75.20-●
        laceration (minor) (superficial) S75.21-●
          major S75.22-●
        specified type NEC S75.29-●
      laceration S85.31-●
      specified type NEC S85.39-●
    hand (level) S65.90-●
      finger —*see* Injury, blood vessel, finger
      laceration S65.91-●
      palmar arch —*see* Injury, blood vessel,
          palmar arch
      radial artery —*see* Injury, blood vessel,
          radial artery, hand
      specified
        site NEC S65.80-●
          laceration S65.81-●
          specified type NEC S65.89-●
        type NEC S65.99-●
      thumb —*see* Injury, blood vessel, thumb
      ulnar artery —*see* Injury, blood vessel,
          ulnar artery, hand
    head S09.0
      intracranial —*see* Injury, intracranial
      multiple S09.0
    hepatic
      artery —*see* Injury, mesenteric, artery
      vein —*see* Injury, vena cava, inferior
    hip S75.90-●
      femoral artery —*see* Injury, blood vessel,
          femoral, artery
      femoral vein —*see* Injury, blood vessel,
          femoral, vein
      greater saphenous vein —*see* Injury, blood
          vessel, greater saphenous, hip level
      laceration S75.91-●
      specified
        site NEC S75.80-●
          laceration S75.81-●
          specified type NEC S75.89-●
        type NEC S75.99-●
    hypogastric (artery) (vein) —*see* Injury,
        blood vessel, iliac
    iliac S35.5-●
      artery S35.51-●
      specified vessel NEC S35.5-●
      uterine vessel —*see* Injury, blood vessel,
          uterine
      vein S35.51-●
    innominate —*see* Injury, blood vessel,
        thoracic, innominate
    intercostal (artery) (vein) —*see* Injury,
        blood vessel, thoracic, intercostal
    jugular vein (external) S15.20-●
      internal S15.30-●
        laceration (minor) (superficial) S15.31-●
          major S15.32-●
        specified type NEC S15.39-●

Injury *(Continued)*
  blood vessel NEC *(Continued)*
    jugular vein *(Continued)*
      laceration (minor) (superficial) S15.21-●
        major S15.22-●
      specified type NEC S15.29-●
    leg (level) (lower) S85.90-●
      greater saphenous —*see* Injury, blood vessel, greater saphenous
      laceration S85.91-●
      lesser saphenous —*see* Injury, blood vessel, lesser saphenous
      peroneal artery —*see* Injury, blood vessel, peroneal artery
      popliteal
        artery —*see* Injury, blood vessel, popliteal, artery
        vein —*see* Injury, blood vessel, popliteal, vein
      specified
        site NEC S85.80-●
          laceration S85.81-●
          specified type NEC S85.89-●
        type NEC S85.99-●
      thigh —*see* Injury, blood vessel, hip
      tibial artery —*see* Injury, blood vessel, tibial artery
    lesser saphenous vein (lower leg level) S85.40-●
      laceration S85.41-●
      specified type NEC S85.49-●
    limb
      lower —*see* Injury, blood vessel, leg
      upper —*see* Injury, blood vessel, arm
    lower back —*see* Injury, blood vessel, abdomen
      specified NEC —*see* Injury, blood vessel, abdomen, specified, site NEC
    mammary (artery) (vein) —*see* Injury, blood vessel, thoracic, specified site NEC
    mesenteric (inferior) (superior)
      artery —*see* Injury, mesenteric, artery
      vein —*see* Injury, mesenteric, vein
    neck S15.9
      specified site NEC S15.8
    ovarian (artery) (vein) —*see* subcategory S35.8
    palmar arch (superficial) S65.20-●
      deep S65.30-●
        laceration S65.31-●
        specified type NEC S65.39-●
      laceration S65.21-●
      specified type NEC S65.29-●
    pelvis —*see* Injury, blood vessel, abdomen
      specified NEC —*see* Injury, blood vessel, abdomen, specified, site NEC
    peroneal artery S85.20-●
      laceration S85.21-●
      specified type NEC S85.29-●
    plantar artery (deep) (foot) S95.10-●
      laceration S95.11-●
      specified type NEC S95.19-●
    popliteal
      artery S85.00-●
        laceration S85.01-●
        specified type NEC S85.09-●
      vein S85.50-●
        laceration S85.51-●
        specified type NEC S85.59-●
    portal vein S35.319
      laceration S35.311
      specified type NEC S35.318
    precerebral —*see* Injury, blood vessel, neck
    pulmonary (artery) (vein) —*see* Injury, blood vessel, thoracic, pulmonary
    radial artery (forearm level) S55.10-●
      hand and wrist (level) S65.10-●
        laceration S65.11-●
        specified type NEC S65.19-●
      laceration S55.11-●
      specified type NEC S55.19-●

Injury *(Continued)*
  blood vessel NEC *(Continued)*
    renal
      artery S35.40-●
        laceration S35.41-●
        specified NEC S35.49-●
      vein S35.40-●
        laceration S35.41-●
        specified NEC S35.49-●
    saphenous vein (greater) (lower leg level) —*see* Injury, blood vessel, greater saphenous
      hip and thigh level —*see* Injury, blood vessel, greater saphenous, hip level
      lesser —*see* Injury, blood vessel, lesser saphenous
    shoulder
      specified NEC —*see* Injury, blood vessel, arm, specified site NEC
      superficial vein —*see* Injury, blood vessel, arm, superficial vein
    specified NEC T14.8
    splenic
      artery —*see* Injury, blood vessel, celiac artery, branch
      vein S35.329
        laceration S35.321
        specified NEC S35.328
    subclavian —*see* Injury, blood vessel, thoracic, innominate
    thigh —*see* Injury, blood vessel, hip
    thoracic S25.90
      aorta S25.00
        laceration (minor) (superficial) S25.01
          major S25.02
        specified type NEC S25.09
      azygos vein —*see* Injury, blood vessel, thoracic, specified, site NEC
      innominate
        artery S25.10-●
          laceration (minor) (superficial) S25.11-●
            major S25.12-●
          specified type NEC S25.19-●
        vein S25.30-●
          laceration (minor) (superficial) S25.31-●
            major S25.32-●
          specified type NEC S25.39-●
      intercostal S25.50-●
        laceration S25.51-●
        specified type NEC S25.59-●
      laceration S25.91
      mammary vessel —*see* Injury, blood vessel, thoracic, specified, site NEC
      pulmonary S25.40-●
        laceration (minor) (superficial) S25.41-●
          major S25.42-●
        specified type NEC S25.49-●
      specified
        site NEC S25.80-●
          laceration S25.81-●
          specified type NEC S25.89-●
        type NEC S25.99
      subclavian —*see* Injury, blood vessel, thoracic, innominate
      vena cava (superior) S25.20
        laceration (minor) (superficial) S25.21
          major S25.22
        specified type NEC S25.29
    thumb S65.40-●
      laceration S65.41-●
      specified type NEC S65.49-●
    tibial artery S85.10-●
      anterior S85.13-●
        laceration S85.14-●
        specified injury NEC S85.15-●
      laceration S85.11-●

Injury *(Continued)*
  blood vessel NEC *(Continued)*
    tibial artery *(Continued)*
      posterior S85.16-●
        laceration S85.17-●
        specified injury NEC S85.18-●
      specified injury NEC S85.12-●
    ulnar artery (forearm level) S55.00-●
      hand and wrist (level) S65.00-●
        laceration S65.01-●
        specified type NEC S65.09-●
      laceration S55.01-●
      specified type NEC S55.09-●
    upper arm (level) —*see* Injury, blood vessel, arm
    superficial vein —*see* Injury, blood vessel, arm, superficial vein
    uterine S35.5-●
      artery S35.53-●
      vein S35.53-●
    vena cava —*see* Injury, vena cava
    vertebral artery S15.10-●
      laceration (minor) (superficial) S15.11-●
        major S15.12-●
      specified type NEC S15.19-●
    wrist (level) —*see* Injury, blood vessel, hand
  brachial plexus S14.3
    newborn P14.3
  brain (traumatic) S06.9-●
    diffuse (axonal) S06.2X-●
    focal S06.30-●
  brainstem S06.38-●
  breast NOS S29.9
  broad ligament —*see* Injury, pelvic organ, specified site NEC
  bronchus, bronchi —*see* Injury, intrathoracic, bronchus
  brow S09.90
  buttock S39.92
  canthus, eye S05.90
  cardiac plexus —*see* Injury, nerve, thorax, sympathetic
  cauda equina S34.3
  cavernous sinus —*see* Injury, intracranial
  cecum —*see* Injury, colon
  celiac ganglion or plexus —*see* Injury, nerve, lumbosacral, sympathetic
  cerebellum —*see* Injury, intracranial
  cerebral —*see* Injury, intracranial
  cervix (uteri) —*see* Injury, uterus
  cheek (wall) S09.93
  chest —*see* Injury, thorax
  childbirth (newborn) —*see also* Birth, injury
    maternal NEC O71.9
  chin S09.93
  choroid (eye) —*see* Injury, eye, specified site NEC
  clitoris S39.94
  coccyx —*see also* Injury, back, lower
    complicating delivery O71.6
  colon —*see* Injury, intestine, large
  common bile duct —*see* Injury, liver
  conjunctiva (superficial) —*see* Injury, eye, conjunctiva
  conus medullaris —*see* Injury, spinal, sacral cord
    spermatic (pelvic region) S37.898
      scrotal region S39.848
    spinal —*see* Injury, spinal cord, by region
  cornea —*see* Injury, eye, specified site NEC
    abrasion —*see* Injury, eye, cornea, abrasion
  cortex (cerebral) —*see also* Injury, intracranial
    visual —*see* Injury, nerve, optic
  costal region NEC S29.9
  costochondral NEC S29.9
  cranial
    cavity —*see* Injury, intracranial
    nerve —*see* Injury, nerve, cranial

▶ New   ⇒ Revised   ~~deleted~~ Deleted   ● Use Additional Character(s)

Injury *(Continued)*
  crushing —*see* Crush
  cutaneous sensory nerve
  cystic duct —*see* Injury, liver
  deep tissue —*see* Contusion, by site
    meaning pressure ulcer —*see* Ulcer,
      pressure L89 with final character .6
  delivery (newborn) P15.9
    maternal NEC O71.9
  Descemet's membrane —*see* Injury, eyeball,
    penetrating
  diaphragm —*see* Injury, intrathoracic,
    diaphragm
  duodenum —*see* Injury, intestine, small,
    duodenum
  ear (auricle) (external) (canal) S09.91
    abrasion —*see* Abrasion, ear
    bite —*see* Bite, ear
    blister —*see* Blister, ear
    bruise —*see* Contusion, ear
    contusion —*see* Contusion, ear
    external constriction —*see* Constriction,
      external, ear
    hematoma —*see* Hematoma, ear
    inner —*see* Injury, ear, middle
    laceration —*see* Laceration, ear
    middle S09.30-•
      blast —*see* Injury, blast, ear
      specified NEC S09.39-•
    puncture —*see* Puncture, ear
    superficial —*see* Injury, superficial, ear
  eighth cranial nerve (acoustic or auditory) —
    see Injury, nerve, acoustic
  elbow S59.90-•
    contusion —*see* Contusion, elbow
    dislocation —*see* Dislocation, elbow
    fracture —*see* Fracture, ulna, upper
      end
    open —*see* Wound, open, elbow
    specified NEC S59.80-•
    sprain —*see* Sprain, elbow
    superficial —*see* Injury, superficial,
      elbow
  eleventh cranial nerve (accessory) —*see*
    Injury, nerve, accessory
  epididymis S39.94
  epigastric region S39.91
  epiglottis NEC S19.89
  esophageal plexus —*see* Injury, nerve, thorax,
    sympathetic
  esophagus (thoracic part) —*see also* Injury,
    intrathoracic, esophagus
    cervical NEC S19.85
  eustachian tube S09.30-•
  eye S05.9-•
    avulsion S05.7-•
    ball —*see* Injury, eyeball
    conjunctiva S05.0-•
    cornea
      abrasion S05.0-•
    laceration S05.3-•
      with prolapse S05.2-•
    lacrimal apparatus S05.8X-•
    orbit penetration S05.4-•
    specified site NEC S05.8X-•
  eyeball S05.8X-•
    contusion S05.1-•
    penetrating S05.6-•
      with
        foreign body S05.5-•
        prolapse or loss of intraocular tissue
          S05.2-•
      without prolapse or loss of intraocular
        tissue S05.3-•
    specified type NEC S05.8-•
  eyebrow S09.93
  eyelid S09.93
    abrasion —*see* Abrasion, eyelid
    contusion —*see* Contusion, eyelid
    open —*see* Wound, open, eyelid
  face S09.93

Injury *(Continued)*
  fallopian tube S37.509
    bilateral S37.502
      blast injury S37.512
      contusion S37.522
      laceration S37.532
      specified type NEC S37.592
    blast injury (primary) S37.519
      bilateral S37.512
      secondary —*see* Injury, fallopian tube,
        specified type NEC
      unilateral S37.511
    contusion S37.529
      bilateral S37.522
      unilateral S37.521
    laceration S37.539
      bilateral S37.532
      unilateral S37.531
    specified type NEC S37.599
      bilateral S37.592
      unilateral S37.591
    unilateral S37.501
      blast injury S37.511
      contusion S37.521
      laceration S37.531
      specified type NEC S37.591
  fascia —*see* Injury, muscle
  fifth cranial nerve (trigeminal) —*see* Injury,
    nerve, trigeminal
  finger (nail) S69.9-•
    blood vessel —*see* Injury, blood vessel,
      finger
    contusion —*see* Contusion, finger
    dislocation —*see* Dislocation, finger
    fracture —*see* Fracture, finger
    muscle —*see* Injury, muscle, finger
    nerve —*see* Injury, nerve, digital, finger
    open —*see* Wound, open, finger
    specified NEC S69.8-•
    sprain —*see* Sprain, finger
    superficial —*see* Injury, superficial, finger
  first cranial nerve (olfactory) —*see* Injury,
    nerve, olfactory
  flank —*see* Injury, abdomen
  foot S99.92-•
    blood vessel —*see* Injury, blood vessel,
      foot
    contusion —*see* Contusion, foot
    dislocation —*see* Dislocation, foot
    fracture —*see* Fracture, foot
    muscle —*see* Injury, muscle, foot
    open —*see* Wound, open, foot
    specified type NEC S99.82-•
    sprain —*see* Sprain, foot
    superficial —*see* Injury, superficial, foot
  forceps NOS P15.9
  forearm S59.91-•
    blood vessel —*see* Injury, blood vessel,
      forearm
    contusion —*see* Contusion, forearm
    fracture —*see* Fracture, forearm
    muscle —*see* Injury, muscle, forearm
    nerve —*see* Injury, nerve, forearm
    open —*see* Wound, open, forearm
    specified NEC S59.81-•
    superficial —*see* Injury, superficial, forearm
  forehead S09.90
  fourth cranial nerve (trochlear) —*see* Injury,
    nerve, trochlear
  gallbladder S36.129
    contusion S36.122
    laceration S36.123
    specified NEC S36.128
  ganglion
    celiac, coeliac —*see* Injury, nerve,
      lumbosacral, sympathetic
    gasserian —*see* Injury, nerve, trigeminal
    stellate —*see* Injury, nerve, thorax,
      sympathetic
    thoracic sympathetic —*see* Injury, nerve,
      thorax, sympathetic

Injury *(Continued)*
  gasserian ganglion —*see* Injury, nerve,
    trigeminal
  gastric artery —*see* Injury, blood vessel, celiac
    artery, branch
  gastroduodenal artery —*see* Injury, blood
    vessel, celiac artery, branch
  gastrointestinal tract —*see* Injury,
    intra-abdominal
    with open wound into abdominal cavity —
      see Wound, open, with penetration
      into peritoneal cavity
    colon —*see* Injury, intestine, large
    rectum —*see* Injury, intestine, large, rectum
      with open wound into abdominal cavity
        S36.61
    small intestine —*see* Injury, intestine, small
    specified site NEC —*see* Injury, intra-
      abdominal, specified, site NEC
    stomach —*see* Injury, stomach
  genital organ(s)
    external S39.94
      specified NEC S39.848
    internal S37.90
      fallopian tube —*see* Injury, fallopian tube
      ovary —*see* Injury, ovary
      prostate —*see* Injury, prostate
      seminal vesicle —*see* Injury, pelvis,
        organ, specified site NEC
      uterus —*see* Injury, uterus
      vas deferens —*see* Injury, pelvis, organ,
        specified site NEC
    obstetrical trauma O71.9
  gland
    lacrimal laceration —*see* Injury, eye,
      specified site NEC
    salivary S09.93
    thyroid NEC S19.84
  globe (eye) S05.90
    specified NEC S05.8X-•
  groin —*see* Injury, abdomen
  gum S09.90
  hand S69.9-•
    blood vessel —*see* Injury, blood vessel,
      hand
    contusion —*see* Contusion, hand
    fracture —*see* Fracture, hand
    muscle —*see* Injury, muscle, hand
    nerve —*see* Injury, nerve, hand
    open —*see* Wound, open, hand
    specified NEC S69.8-•
    sprain —*see* Sprain, hand
    superficial —*see* Injury, superficial, hand
  head S09.90
    with loss of consciousness S06.9-•
    specified NEC S09.8-•
  ➨heart (traumatic) S26.90
    with hemopericardium S26.00
      contusion S26.01
      laceration (mild) S26.020
        major S26.022
        moderate S26.021
      specified type NEC S26.09
    without hemopericardium S26.10
      contusion S26.11
      laceration S26.12
      specified type NEC S26.19
    contusion S26.91
    laceration S26.92
    ▶non-traumatic (acute) (chronic) (non-
      ischemic) I5A
    specified type NEC S26.99
  heel —*see* Injury, foot
  hepatic
    artery —*see* Injury, blood vessel, celiac
      artery, branch
    duct —*see* Injury, liver
    vein —*see* Injury, vena cava, inferior
  hip S79.91-•
    blood vessel —*see* Injury, blood vessel, hip
    contusion —*see* Contusion, hip
    dislocation —*see* Dislocation, hip

Injury *(Continued)*
  hip *(Continued)*
    fracture —*see* Fracture, femur, neck
    muscle —*see* Injury, muscle, hip
    nerve —*see* Injury, nerve, hip
    open —*see* Wound, open, hip
    specified NEC S79.81-●
    sprain —*see* Sprain, hip
    superficial —*see* Injury, superficial, hip
  hymen S39.94
  hypogastric
    blood vessel —*see* Injury, blood vessel, iliac
    plexus —*see* Injury, nerve, lumbosacral,
      sympathetic
  ileum —*see* Injury, intestine, small
  iliac region S39.91
  instrumental (during surgery) —*see*
    Laceration, accidental complicating
    surgery
    birth injury —*see* Birth, injury
    nonsurgical —*see* Injury, by site
  obstetrical O71.9
    bladder O71.5
    cervix O71.3
    high vaginal O71.4
    perineal NOS O70.9
    urethra O71.5
    uterus O71.5
      with rupture or perforation O71.1
  internal T14.8
    aorta —*see* Injury, aorta
    bladder (sphincter) —*see* Injury, bladder
      with
        ectopic or molar pregnancy O08.6
        following ectopic or molar pregnancy
          O08.6
        obstetrical trauma O71.5
    bronchus, bronchi —*see* Injury,
      intrathoracic, bronchus
    cecum —*see* Injury, intestine, large
    cervix (uteri) —*see also* Injury, uterus
      with ectopic or molar pregnancy O08.6
      following ectopic or molar pregnancy
        O08.6
      obstetrical trauma O71.3
    chest —*see* Injury, intrathoracic
    gastrointestinal tract —*see* Injury,
      intra-abdominal
    heart —*see* Injury, heart
    intestine NEC —*see* Injury, intestine
    intrauterine —*see* Injury, uterus
    mesentery —*see* Injury, intra-abdominal,
      specified, site NEC
    pelvis, pelvic (organ) S37.90
      following ectopic or molar pregnancy
        (subsequent episode) O08.6
      obstetrical trauma NEC O71.5
        rupture or perforation O71.1
      specified NEC S39.83
    rectum —*see* Injury, intestine, large, rectum
    stomach —*see* Injury, stomach
    ureter —*see* Injury, ureter
    urethra (sphincter) following ectopic or
      molar pregnancy O08.6
    uterus —*see* Injury, uterus
  interscapular area —*see* Injury, thorax
  intestine
    large S36.509
      ascending (right) S36.500
        blast injury (primary) S36.510
          secondary S36.590
        contusion S36.520
        laceration S36.530
        specified type NEC S36.590
      blast injury (primary) S36.519
        ascending (right) S36.510
        descending (left) S36.512
        rectum S36.61
        sigmoid S36.513
        specified site NEC S36.518
        transverse S36.511

Injury *(Continued)*
  intestine *(Continued)*
    large *(Continued)*
      contusion S36.529
        ascending (right) S36.520
        descending (left) S36.522
        rectum S36.62
        sigmoid S36.523
        specified site NEC S36.528
        transverse S36.521
      descending (left) S36.502
        blast injury (primary) S36.512
          secondary S36.592
        contusion S36.522
        laceration S36.532
        specified type NEC S36.592
      laceration S36.539
        ascending (right) S36.530
        descending (left) S36.532
        rectum S36.63
        sigmoid S36.533
        specified site NEC S36.538
        transverse S36.531
      rectum S36.60
        blast injury (primary) S36.61
          secondary S36.69
        contusion S36.62
        laceration S36.63
        specified type NEC S36.69
      sigmoid S36.503
        blast injury (primary) S36.513
          secondary S36.593
        contusion S36.523
        laceration S36.533
        specified type NEC S36.593
      specified
        site NEC S36.508
          blast injury (primary)
            S36.518
            secondary S36.598
          contusion S36.528
          laceration S36.538
          specified type NEC S36.598
        type NEC S36.599
          ascending (right) S36.590
          descending (left) S36.592
          rectum S36.69
          sigmoid S36.593
          specified site NEC S36.598
          transverse S36.591
      transverse S36.501
        blast injury (primary) S36.511
          secondary S36.591
        contusion S36.521
        laceration S36.531
        specified type NEC S36.591
    small S36.409
      blast injury (primary) S36.419
        duodenum S36.410
        secondary S36.499
          duodenum S36.490
          specified site NEC S36.498
        specified site NEC S36.418
      contusion S36.429
        duodenum S36.420
        specified site NEC S36.428
      duodenum S36.400
        blast injury (primary) S36.410
          secondary S36.490
        contusion S36.420
        laceration S36.430
        specified NEC S36.490
      laceration S36.439
        duodenum S36.430
        specified site NEC S36.438
      specified
        site NEC S36.408
        type NEC S36.499
          duodenum S36.490
          specified site NEC
            S36.498

Injury *(Continued)*
  intra-abdominal S36.90
    adrenal gland —*see* Injury, adrenal gland
    bladder —*see* Injury, bladder
    colon —*see* Injury, intestine, large
    contusion S36.92
    fallopian tube —*see* Injury, fallopian tube
    gallbladder —*see* Injury, gallbladder
    intestine —*see* Injury, intestine
    kidney —*see* Injury, kidney
    laceration S36.93
    liver —*see* Injury, liver
    ovary —*see* Injury, ovary
    pancreas —*see* Injury, pancreas
    pelvic NOS S37.90
    peritoneum —*see* Injury, intra-abdominal,
      specified, site NEC
    prostate —*see* Injury, prostate
    rectum —*see* Injury, intestine, large, rectum
    retroperitoneum —*see* Injury, intra-
      abdominal, specified, site NEC
    seminal vesicle —*see* Injury, pelvis, organ,
      specified site NEC
    small intestine —*see* Injury, intestine, small
    specified
      pelvic S37.90
        specified
          site NEC S37.899
            specified type NEC S37.898
          type NEC S37.99
      site NEC S36.899
        contusion S36.892
        laceration S36.893
        specified type NEC S36.898
      type NEC S36.99
    spleen —*see* Injury, spleen
    stomach —*see* Injury, stomach
    ureter —*see* Injury, ureter
    urethra —*see* Injury, urethra
    uterus —*see* Injury, uterus
    vas deferens —*see* Injury, pelvis, organ,
      specified site NEC
  ➧intracranial (traumatic) (*see also*, if applicable,
    Compression, brain, traumatic) S06.9-●
    cerebellar hemorrhage, traumatic —*see*
      Injury, intracranial, focal
    cerebral edema, traumatic S06.1X-●
      diffuse S06.1X-●
      focal S06.1X-●
    diffuse (axonal) S06.2X-●
    epidural hemorrhage (traumatic) S06.4X-●
    focal brain injury S06.30-●
      contusion —*see* Contusion, cerebral
      laceration —*see* Laceration, cerebral
    intracerebral hemorrhage, traumatic
      S06.36-●
      left side S06.35-●
      right side S06.34-●
    subarachnoid hemorrhage, traumatic
      S06.6X-●
    subdural hemorrhage, traumatic
      S06.5X-●
  intraocular —*see* Injury, eyeball, penetrating
  intrathoracic S27.9
    bronchus S27.409
      bilateral S27.402
      blast injury (primary) S27.419
        bilateral S27.412
        secondary —*see* Injury, intrathoracic,
          bronchus, specified type NEC
        unilateral S27.411
      contusion S27.429
        bilateral S27.422
        unilateral S27.421
      laceration S27.439
        bilateral S27.432
        unilateral S27.431
      specified type NEC S27.499
        bilateral S27.492
        unilateral S27.491
      unilateral S27.401

▶ New   ➠ Revised   ~~deleted~~ Deleted   ● Use Additional Character(s)

Injury *(Continued)*
  intrathoracic *(Continued)*
    diaphragm S27.809
      contusion S27.802
      laceration S27.803
      specified type NEC S27.808
    esophagus (thoracic) S27.819
      contusion S27.812
      laceration S27.813
      specified type NEC S27.818
    heart —*see* Injury, heart
    hemopneumothorax S27.2
    hemothorax S27.1
    lung S27.309
      aspiration J69.0
      bilateral S27.302
      blast injury (primary) S27.319
        bilateral S27.312
        secondary —*see* Injury, intrathoracic,
          lung, specified type NEC
        unilateral S27.311
      contusion S27.329
        bilateral S27.322
        unilateral S27.321
      laceration S27.339
        bilateral S27.332
        unilateral S27.331
      specified type NEC S27.399
        bilateral S27.392
        unilateral S27.391
      unilateral S27.301
    pleura S27.60
      laceration S27.63
      specified type NEC S27.69
    pneumothorax S27.0
    specified organ NEC S27.899
      contusion S27.892
      laceration S27.893
      specified type NEC S27.898
    thoracic duct —*see* Injury, intrathoracic,
      specified organ NEC
    thymus gland —*see* Injury, intrathoracic,
      specified organ NEC
    trachea, thoracic S27.50
      blast (primary) S27.51
      contusion S27.52
      laceration S27.53
      specified type NEC S27.59
  iris —*see* Injury, eye, specified site NEC
    penetrating —*see* Injury, eyeball,
      penetrating
  jaw S09.93
  jejunum —*see* Injury, intestine, small
  joint NOS T14.8
    old or residual —*see* Disorder, joint,
      specified type NEC
  kidney S37.00-●
    acute (nontraumatic) N17.9
    contusion —*see* Contusion, kidney
    laceration —*see* Laceration, kidney
    specified NEC S37.09-●
  knee S89.9-●
    contusion —*see* Contusion, knee
    dislocation —*see* Dislocation, knee
    meniscus (lateral) (medial) —*see* Sprain,
      knee, specified site NEC
      old injury or tear —*see* Derangement,
        knee, meniscus, due to old injury
    open —*see* Wound, open, knee
    specified NEC S89.8-●
    sprain —*see* Sprain, knee
    superficial —*see* Injury, superficial, knee
  labium (majus) (minus) S39.94
  labyrinth, ear S09.30-●
  lacrimal apparatus, duct, gland, or sac —*see*
    Injury, eye, specified site NEC
  larynx NEC S19.81
  leg (lower) S89.9-●
    blood vessel —*see* Injury, blood vessel, leg
    contusion —*see* Contusion, leg
    fracture —*see* Fracture, leg

Injury *(Continued)*
  leg *(Continued)*
    muscle —*see* Injury, muscle, leg
    nerve —*see* Injury, nerve, leg
    open —*see* Wound, open, leg
    specified NEC S89.8-●
    superficial —*see* Injury, superficial, leg
  lens, eye —*see* Injury, eye, specified site
    NEC
    penetrating —*see* Injury, eyeball,
      penetrating
  limb NEC T14.8
  lip S09.93
  liver S36.119
    contusion S36.112
    laceration S36.113
      major (stellate) S36.116
      minor S36.114
      moderate S36.115
    specified NEC S36.118
  lower back S39.92
    specified NEC S39.82
  lumbar, lumbosacral (region) S39.92
    plexus —*see* Injury, lumbosacral plexus
  lumbosacral plexus S34.4
  lung —*see also* Injury, intrathoracic, lung
    aspiration J69.0
    dabbing (related) U07.0
    electronic cigarette (related) U07.0
    EVALI - [e-cigarette, or vaping, product
      use associated] U07.0
    transfusion-related (TRALI) J95.84
    vaping (associated) (device) (product) (use)
      U07.0
  lymphatic thoracic duct —*see* Injury,
    intrathoracic, specified organ NEC
  malar region S09.93
  mastoid region S09.90
  maxilla S09.93
  mediastinum —*see* Injury, intrathoracic,
    specified organ NEC
  membrane, brain —*see* Injury, intracranial
  meningeal artery —*see* Injury, intracranial,
    subdural hemorrhage
  meninges (cerebral) —*see* Injury, intracranial
  mesenteric
    artery
      branch S35.299
        laceration (minor) (superficial) S35.291
          major S35.292
        specified NEC S35.298
      inferior S35.239
        laceration (minor) (superficial) S35.231
          major S35.232
        specified NEC S35.238
      superior S35.229
        laceration (minor) (superficial) S35.221
          major S35.222
        specified NEC S35.228
    plexus (inferior) (superior) —*see* Injury,
      nerve, lumbosacral, sympathetic
    vein
      inferior S35.349
        laceration S35.341
        specified NEC S35.348
      superior S35.339
        laceration S35.331
        specified NEC S35.338
  mesentery —*see* Injury, intra-abdominal,
    specified site NEC
  mesosalpinx —*see* Injury, pelvic organ,
    specified site NEC
  middle ear S09.30-●
  midthoracic region NOS S29.9
  mouth S09.93
  multiple NOS T07
  muscle (and fascia) (and tendon)
    abdomen S39.001
      laceration S39.021
      specified type NEC S39.091
      strain S39.011

Injury *(Continued)*
  muscle *(Continued)*
    abductor
      thumb, forearm level —*see* Injury,
        muscle, thumb, abductor
    adductor
      thigh S76.20-●
        laceration S76.22-●
        specified type NEC S76.29-●
        strain S76.21-●
    ankle —*see* Injury, muscle, foot
    anterior muscle group, at leg level (lower)
      S86.20-●
      laceration S86.22-●
      specified type NEC S86.29-●
      strain S86.21-●
    arm (upper) —*see* Injury, muscle,
      shoulder
    biceps (parts NEC) S46.20-●
      laceration S46.22-●
      long head S46.10-●
        laceration S46.12-●
        specified type NEC S46.19-●
        strain S46.11-●
      specified type NEC S46.29-●
      strain S46.21-●
    extensor
      finger(s) (other than thumb) —*see* Injury,
        muscle, finger by site, extensor
      forearm level, specified NEC —*see*
        Injury, muscle, forearm, extensor
      thumb —*see* Injury, muscle, thumb,
        extensor
      toe (large) (ankle level) (foot level) —*see*
        Injury, muscle, toe, extensor
    finger
      extensor (forearm level) S56.40-●
        hand level S66.309
          laceration S66.329
          specified type NEC S66.399
          strain S66.319
        laceration S56.429
        specified type NEC S56.499
        strain S56.419
      flexor (forearm level) S56.10-●
        hand level S66.109
          laceration S66.129
          specified type NEC S66.199
          strain S66.119
        laceration S56.129
        specified type NEC S56.199
        strain S56.119
      index
        extensor (forearm level)
          hand level S66.308
            laceration S66.32-●
            specified type NEC S66.39-●
            strain S66.31-●
          specified type NEC S56.492-●
        flexor (forearm level)
          hand level S66.108
            laceration S66.12-●
            specified type NEC
              S66.19-●
            strain S66.11-●
          specified type NEC S56.19-●
          strain S56.11-●
        intrinsic S66.50-●
          laceration S66.52-●
          specified type NEC S66.59-●
          strain S66.51-●
      intrinsic S66.509
        laceration S66.529
        specified type NEC S66.599
        strain S66.519
      little
        extensor (forearm level)
          hand level S66.30-●
            laceration S66.32-●
            specified type NEC S66.39-●
            strain S66.31-●

Injury (Continued)
  muscle (Continued)
    finger (Continued)
      little (Continued)
        extensor (Continued)
          laceration S56.42-●
          specified type NEC S56.49-●
          strain S56.41-●
        flexor (forearm level)
          hand level S66.10-●
            laceration S66.12-●
            specified type NEC S66.19-●
            strain S66.11-●
          laceration S56.12-●
          specified type NEC S56.19-●
          strain S56.11-●
        intrinsic S66.50-●
          laceration S66.52-●
          specified type NEC S66.59-●
          strain S66.51-●
      middle
        extensor (forearm level)
          hand level S66.30-●
            laceration S66.32-●
            specified type NEC
              S66.39-●
            strain S66.31-●
          laceration S56.42-●
          specified type NEC
            S56.49-●
          strain S56.41-●
        flexor (forearm level)
          hand level S66.10-●
            laceration S66.12-●
            specified type NEC
              S66.19-●
            strain S66.11-●
          laceration S56.12-●
          specified type NEC S56.19-●
          strain S56.11-●
        intrinsic S66.50-●
          laceration S66.52-●
          specified type NEC S66.59-●
          strain S66.51-●
      ring
        extensor (forearm level)
          hand level S66.30-●
            laceration S66.32-●
            specified type NEC S66.39-●
            strain S66.31-●
          laceration S56.42-●
          specified type NEC S56.49-●
          strain S56.41-●
        flexor (forearm level)
          hand level S66.10-●
            laceration S66.12-●
            specified type NEC S66.19-●
            strain S66.11-●
          laceration S56.12-●
          specified type NEC S56.19-●
          strain S56.11-●
        intrinsic S66.50-●
          laceration S66.52-●
          specified type NEC S66.59-●
          strain S66.51-●
    flexor
      finger(s) (other than thumb) — see Injury,
        muscle, finger
      forearm level, specified NEC —
        see Injury, muscle, forearm,
        flexor
      thumb —see Injury, muscle, thumb,
        flexor
      toe (long) (ankle level) (foot level) —see
        Injury, muscle, toe, flexor
    foot S96.90-●
      intrinsic S96.20-●
        laceration S96.22-●
        specified type NEC S96.29-●
        strain S96.21-●
      laceration S96.92-●

Injury (Continued)
  muscle (Continued)
    foot (Continued)
      long extensor, toe —see Injury, muscle,
        toe, extensor
      long flexor, toe —see Injury, muscle, toe,
        flexor
      specified
        site NEC S96.80-●
          laceration S96.82-●
          specified type NEC S96.89-●
          strain S96.81-●
        type NEC S96.99-●
      strain S96.91-●
    forearm (level) S56.90-●
      extensor S56.50-●
        laceration S56.52-●
        specified type NEC S56.59-●
        strain S56.51-●
      flexor S56.20-●
        laceration S56.22-●
        specified type NEC S56.29-●
        strain S56.21-●
      laceration S56.92-●
      specified S56.99-●
        site NEC S56.80-●
          laceration S56.82-●
          strain S56.81-●
        type NEC S56.89-●
      strain S56.91-●
    hand (level) S66.90-●
      laceration S66.92-●
      specified
        site NEC S66.80-●
          laceration S66.82-●
          specified type NEC S66.89-●
          strain S66.81-●
        type NEC S66.99-●
      strain S66.91-●
    head S09.10
      laceration S09.12
      specified type NEC S09.19
      strain S09.11
    hip NEC S76.00-●
      laceration S76.02-●
      specified type NEC S76.09-●
      strain S76.01-●
    intrinsic
      ankle and foot level —see Injury, muscle,
        foot, intrinsic
      finger (other than thumb) —see Injury,
        muscle, finger by site, intrinsic
      foot (level) —see Injury, muscle, foot,
        intrinsic
      thumb —see Injury, muscle, thumb,
        intrinsic
    leg (level) (lower) S86.90-●
      Achilles tendon —see Injury, Achilles
        tendon
      anterior muscle group —see Injury,
        muscle, anterior muscle group
      laceration S86.92-●
      peroneal muscle group —see Injury,
        muscle, peroneal muscle group
      posterior muscle group —see Injury,
        muscle, posterior muscle group,
        leg level
      specified
        site NEC S86.80-●
          laceration S86.82-●
          specified type NEC S86.89-●
          strain S86.81-●
        type NEC S86.99-●
      strain S86.91-●
    long
      extensor toe, at ankle and foot level —see
        Injury, muscle, toe, extensor
      flexor, toe, at ankle and foot level —see
        Injury, muscle, toe, flexor
      head, biceps —see Injury, muscle, biceps,
        long head

Injury (Continued)
  muscle (Continued)
    lower back S39.002
      laceration S39.022
      specified type NEC S39.092
      strain S39.012
    neck (level) S16.9
      laceration S16.2
      specified type NEC S16.8
      strain S16.1
    pelvis S39.003
      laceration S39.023
      specified type NEC S39.093
      strain S39.013
    peroneal muscle group, at leg level (lower)
      S86.30-●
      laceration S86.32-●
      specified type NEC S86.39-●
      strain S86.31-●
    posterior muscle (group)
      leg level (lower) S86.10-●
        laceration S86.12-●
        specified type NEC S86.19-●
        strain S86.11-●
      thigh level S76.30-●
        laceration S76.32-●
        specified type NEC S76.39-●
        strain S76.31-●
    quadriceps (thigh) S76.10-●
      laceration S76.12-●
      specified type NEC S76.19-●
      strain S76.11-●
    shoulder S46.90-●
      laceration S46.92-●
      rotator cuff —see Injury, rotator cuff
      specified site NEC S46.80-●
        laceration S46.82-●
        specified type NEC S46.89-●
        strain S46.81-●
      specified type NEC S46.99-●
      strain S46.91-●
    thigh NEC (level) S76.90-●
      adductor —see Injury, muscle, adductor,
        thigh
      laceration S76.92-●
      posterior muscle (group) —see Injury,
        muscle, posterior muscle, thigh level
      quadriceps —see Injury, muscle,
        quadriceps
      specified
        site NEC S76.80-●
          laceration S76.82-●
          specified type NEC S76.89-●
          strain S76.81-●
        type NEC S76.99-●
      strain S76.91-●
    thorax (level) S29.009
      back wall S29.002
      front wall S29.001
      laceration S29.029
        back wall S29.022
        front wall S29.021
      specified type NEC S29.099
        back wall S29.092
        front wall S29.091
      strain S29.019
        back wall S29.012
        front wall S29.011
    thumb
      abductor (forearm level) S56.30-●
        laceration S56.32-●
        specified type NEC S56.39-●
        strain S56.31-●
      extensor (forearm level) S56.30-●
        hand level S66.20-●
          laceration S66.22-●
          specified type NEC S66.29-●
          strain S66.21-●
        laceration S56.32-●
        specified type NEC S56.39-●
        strain S56.31-●

  ▶ New   ⇒ Revised   deleted Deleted   ● Use Additional Character(s)

Injury *(Continued)*
  muscle *(Continued)*
    thumb *(Continued)*
      flexor (forearm level) S56.00-•
        hand level S66.00-•
          laceration S66.02-•
          specified type NEC S66.09-•
          strain S66.01-•
        laceration S56.02-•
        specified type NEC S56.09-•
        strain S56.01-•
        wrist level —*see* Injury, muscle, thumb, flexor, hand level
      intrinsic S66.40-•
        laceration S66.42-•
        specified type NEC S66.49-•
        strain S66.41-•
    toe —*see also* Injury, muscle, foot
      extensor, long S96.10-•
        laceration S96.12-•
        specified type NEC S96.19-•
        strain S96.11-•
      flexor, long S96.00-•
        laceration S96.02-•
        specified type NEC S96.09-•
        strain S96.01-•
    triceps S46.30-•
      laceration S46.32-•
      specified type NEC S46.39-•
      strain S46.31-•
    wrist (and hand) level —*see* Injury, muscle, hand
  musculocutaneous nerve —*see* Injury, nerve, musculocutaneous
  ►myocardial (acute) (chronic) (non-ischemic) (non-traumatic) I5A
    ►traumatic —*see* Injury, heart
  ⇒myocardium —*see also* Injury, heart
    ►non-traumatic —*see* Injury, myocardial
  nape —*see* Injury, neck
  nasal (septum) (sinus) S09.92
  nasopharynx S09.92
  neck S19.9
    specified NEC S19.80
      specified site NEC S19.89
  nerve NEC T14.8
    abdomen S34.9
      peripheral S34.6
      specified site NEC S34.8
    abducens S04.4-•
      contusion S04.4-•
      laceration S04.4-•
      specified type NEC S04.4-•
    abducent —*see* Injury, nerve, abducens
    accessory S04.7-•
      contusion S04.7-•
      laceration S04.7-•
      specified type NEC S04.7-•
    acoustic S04.6-•
      contusion S04.6-•
      laceration S04.6-•
      specified type NEC S04.6-•
    ankle S94.9-•
      cutaneous sensory S94.3-•
      specified site NEC —*see* subcategory S94.8
    anterior crural, femoral —*see* Injury, nerve, femoral
    arm (upper) S44.9-•
      axillary —*see* Injury, nerve, axillary
      cutaneous —*see* Injury, nerve, cutaneous, arm
      median —*see* Injury, nerve, median, upper arm
      musculocutaneous —*see* Injury, nerve, musculocutaneous
      radial —*see* Injury, nerve, radial, upper arm
      specified site NEC —*see* subcategory S44.8
      ulnar —*see* Injury, nerve, ulnar, arm
    auditory —*see* Injury, nerve, acoustic

Injury *(Continued)*
  nerve NEC *(Continued)*
    axillary S44.3-•
    brachial plexus —*see* Injury, brachial plexus
    cervical sympathetic S14.5
    cranial S04.9
      contusion S04.9
      eighth (acoustic or auditory) —*see* Injury, nerve, acoustic
      eleventh (accessory) —*see* Injury, nerve, accessory
      fifth (trigeminal) —*see* Injury, nerve, trigeminal
      first (olfactory) —*see* Injury, nerve, olfactory
      fourth (trochlear) —*see* Injury, nerve, trochlear
      laceration S04.9
      ninth (glossopharyngeal) —*see* Injury, nerve, glossopharyngeal
      second (optic) —*see* Injury, nerve, optic
      seventh (facial) —*see* Injury, nerve, facial
      sixth (abducent) —*see* Injury, nerve, abducens
      specified
        nerve NEC S04.89-•
          contusion S04.89-•
          laceration S04.89-•
          specified type NEC S04.89-•
        type NEC S04.9
      tenth (pneumogastric or vagus) —*see* Injury, nerve, vagus
      third (oculomotor) —*see* Injury, nerve, oculomotor
      twelfth (hypoglossal) —*see* Injury, nerve, hypoglossal
    cutaneous sensory
      ankle (level) S94.3-•
      arm (upper) (level) S44.5-•
      foot (level) —*see* Injury, nerve, cutaneous sensory, ankle
      forearm (level) S54.3-•
      hip (level) S74.2-•
      leg (lower level) S84.2-•
      shoulder (level) —*see* Injury, nerve, cutaneous sensory, arm
      thigh (level) —*see* Injury, nerve, cutaneous sensory, hip
    deep peroneal —*see* Injury, nerve, peroneal, foot
    digital
      finger S64.4-•
        index S64.49-•
        little S64.49-•
        middle S64.49-•
        ring S64.49-•
        thumb S64.3-•
      toe —*see* Injury, nerve, ankle, specified site NEC
    eighth cranial (acoustic or auditory) —*see* Injury, nerve, acoustic
    eleventh cranial (accessory) —*see* Injury, nerve, accessory
    facial S04.5-•
      contusion S04.5-•
      laceration S04.5-•
      newborn P11.3
      specified type NEC S04.5-•
    femoral (hip level) (thigh level) S74.1-•
    fifth cranial (trigeminal) —*see* Injury, nerve, trigeminal
    finger (digital) —*see* Injury, nerve, digital, finger
    first cranial (olfactory) —*see* Injury, nerve, olfactory
    foot S94.9-•
      cutaneous sensory S94.3-•
      deep peroneal S94.2-•
      lateral plantar S94.0-•

Injury *(Continued)*
  nerve NEC *(Continued)*
    foot *(Continued)*
      medial plantar S94.1-•
      specified site NEC —*see* subcategory S94.8
    forearm (level) S54.9-•
      cutaneous sensory —*see* Injury, nerve, cutaneous sensory, forearm
      median —*see* Injury, nerve, median
      radial —*see* Injury, nerve, radial
      specified site NEC —*see* subcategory S54.8
      ulnar —*see* Injury, nerve, ulnar
    fourth cranial (trochlear) —*see* Injury, nerve, trochlear
    glossopharyngeal S04.89-•
      specified type NEC S04.89-•
    hand S64.9-•
      median —*see* Injury, nerve, median, hand
      radial —*see* Injury, nerve, radial, hand
      specified NEC —*see* subcategory S64.8
      ulnar —*see* Injury, nerve, ulnar, hand
    hip (level) S74.9-•
      cutaneous sensory —*see* Injury, nerve, cutaneous sensory, hip
      femoral —*see* Injury, nerve, femoral
      sciatic —*see* Injury, nerve, sciatic
      specified site NEC —*see* subcategory S74.8
    hypoglossal S04.89-•
      specified type NEC S04.89-•
    lateral plantar S94.0-•
    leg (lower) S84.9-•
      cutaneous sensory —*see* Injury, nerve, cutaneous sensory, leg
      peroneal —*see* Injury, nerve, peroneal
      specified site NEC —*see* subcategory S84.8
      tibial —*see* Injury, nerve, tibial
      upper —*see* Injury, nerve, thigh
    lower
      back —*see* Injury, nerve, abdomen, specified site NEC
        peripheral —*see* Injury, nerve, abdomen, peripheral
      limb —*see* Injury, nerve, leg
    lumbar plexus —*see* Injury, nerve, lumbosacral, sympathetic
    ⇒lumbar spinal
    ►peripheral S34.6
      ►root S34.21
      ►sympathetic S34.5
    lumbosacral
      plexus —*see* Injury, nerve, lumbosacral, sympathetic
      sympathetic S34.5
    medial plantar S94.1-•
    median (forearm level) S54.1-•
      hand (level) S64.1-•
      upper arm (level) S44.1-•
      wrist (level) —*see* Injury, nerve, median, hand
    musculocutaneous S44.4-•
    musculospiral (upper arm level) —*see* Injury, nerve, radial, upper arm
    neck S14.9
      peripheral S14.4
      specified site NEC S14.8
      sympathetic S14.5
    ninth cranial (glossopharyngeal) —*see* Injury, nerve, glossopharyngeal
    oculomotor S04.1-•
      contusion S04.1-•
      laceration S04.1-•
      specified type NEC S04.1-•
    olfactory S04.81-•
      specified type NEC S04.81-•
    optic S04.01-•
      contusion S04.01-•
      laceration S04.01-•
      specified type NEC S04.01-•

Injury *(Continued)*
  nerve NEC *(Continued)*
    pelvic girdle —*see* Injury, nerve, hip
    pelvis —*see* Injury, nerve, abdomen, specified site NEC
    peripheral —*see* Injury, nerve, abdomen, peripheral
    peripheral NEC T14.8
      abdomen —*see* Injury, nerve, abdomen, peripheral
      lower back —*see* Injury, nerve, abdomen, peripheral
      neck —*see* Injury, nerve, neck, peripheral
      pelvis —*see* Injury, nerve, abdomen, peripheral
      specified NEC T14.8
    peroneal (lower leg level) S84.1-●
      foot S94.2-●
    plexus
      brachial —*see* Injury, brachial plexus
      celiac, coeliac —*see* Injury, nerve, lumbosacral, sympathetic
      mesenteric, inferior —*see* Injury, nerve, lumbosacral, sympathetic
      sacral —*see* Injury, lumbosacral plexus
      spinal
        brachial —*see* Injury, brachial plexus
        lumbosacral —*see* Injury, lumbosacral plexus
    pneumogastric —*see* Injury, nerve, vagus
    radial (forearm level) S54.2-●
      hand (level) S64.2-●
      upper arm (level) S44.2-●
      wrist (level) —*see* Injury, nerve, radial, hand
    root —*see* Injury, nerve, spinal, root
    sacral plexus —*see* Injury, lumbosacral plexus
    sacral spinal
      peripheral S34.6
      root S34.22
      sympathetic S34.5
    sciatic (hip level) (thigh level) S74.0-●
    second cranial (optic) —*see* Injury, nerve, optic
    self-inflicted, without suicidal intent R45.88
    seventh cranial (facial) —*see* Injury, nerve, facial
    shoulder —*see* Injury, nerve, arm
    sixth cranial (abducent) —*see* Injury, nerve, abducens
    spinal
      plexus —*see* Injury, nerve, plexus, spinal
      root
        cervical S14.2
        dorsal S24.2
        lumbar S34.21
        sacral S34.22
        thoracic —*see* Injury, nerve, spinal, root, dorsal
    splanchnic —*see* Injury, nerve, lumbosacral, sympathetic
    sympathetic NEC —*see* Injury, nerve, lumbosacral, sympathetic
      cervical —*see* Injury, nerve, cervical sympathetic
    tenth cranial (pneumogastric or vagus) —*see* Injury, nerve, vagus
    thigh (level) —*see* Injury, nerve, hip
      cutaneous sensory —*see* Injury, nerve, cutaneous sensory, hip
      femoral —*see* Injury, nerve, femoral
      sciatic —*see* Injury, nerve, sciatic
      specified NEC —*see* Injury, nerve, hip
    third cranial (oculomotor) —*see* Injury, nerve, oculomotor
    thorax S24.9
      peripheral S24.3
      specified site NEC S24.8
      sympathetic S24.4

Injury *(Continued)*
  nerve NEC *(Continued)*
    thumb, digital —*see* Injury, nerve, digital, thumb
    tibial (lower leg level) (posterior) S84.0-●
    toe —*see* Injury, nerve, ankle
    trigeminal S04.3-●
      contusion S04.3-●
      laceration S04.3-●
      specified type NEC S04.3-●
    trochlear S04.2-●
      contusion S04.2-●
      laceration S04.2-●
      specified type NEC S04.2-●
    twelfth cranial (hypoglossal) —*see* Injury, nerve, hypoglossal
    ulnar (forearm level) S54.0-●
      arm (upper) (level) S44.0-●
      hand (level) S64.0-●
      wrist (level) —*see* Injury, nerve, ulnar, hand
    vagus S04.89-●
      specified type NEC S04.89-●
    wrist (level) —*see* Injury, nerve, hand
  ninth cranial nerve (glossopharyngeal) —*see* Injury, nerve, glossopharyngeal
  nose (septum) S09.92
  obstetrical O71.9
    specified NEC O71.89
  occipital (region) (scalp) S09.90
    lobe —*see* Injury, intracranial
  optic chiasm S04.02
  optic radiation S04.03-●
  optic tract and pathways S04.03-●
  orbit, orbital (region) —*see* Injury, eye
    penetrating (with foreign body) —*see* Injury, eye, orbit, penetrating
    specified NEC —*see* Injury, eye, specified site NEC
  ovary, ovarian S37.409
    bilateral S37.402
      contusion S37.422
      laceration S37.432
      specified type NEC S37.492
    blood vessel —*see* Injury, blood vessel, ovarian
    contusion S37.429
      bilateral S37.422
      unilateral S37.421
    laceration S37.439
      bilateral S37.432
      unilateral S37.431
    specified type NEC S37.499
      bilateral S37.492
      unilateral S37.491
    unilateral S37.401
      contusion S37.421
      laceration S37.431
      specified type NEC S37.491
  palate (hard) (soft) S09.93
  pancreas S36.209
    body S36.201
      contusion S36.221
      laceration S36.231
        major S36.261
        minor S36.241
        moderate S36.251
      specified type NEC S36.291
    contusion S36.229
    head S36.200
      contusion S36.220
      laceration S36.230
        major S36.260
        minor S36.240
        moderate S36.250
      specified type NEC S36.290
    laceration S36.239
      major S36.269
      minor S36.249
      moderate S36.259
    specified type NEC S36.299
    tail S36.202
      contusion S36.222

Injury *(Continued)*
  pancreas *(Continued)*
    tail *(Continued)*
      laceration S36.232
        major S36.262
        minor S36.242
        moderate S36.252
      specified type NEC S36.292
  parietal (region) (scalp) S09.90
    lobe —*see* Injury, intracranial
  patellar ligament (tendon) S76.10-●
    laceration S76.12-●
    specified NEC S76.19-●
    strain S76.11-●
  pelvis, pelvic (floor) S39.93
    complicating delivery O70.1
    joint or ligament, complicating delivery O71.6
    organ S37.90
      with ectopic or molar pregnancy O08.6
      complication of abortion —*see* Abortion
      contusion S37.92
      following ectopic or molar pregnancy O08.6
      laceration S37.93
      obstetrical trauma NEC O71.5
      specified
        site NEC S37.899
          contusion S37.892
          laceration S37.893
          specified type NEC S37.898
        type NEC S37.99
    specified NEC S39.83
  penis S39.94
  perineum S39.94
  peritoneum S36.81
    laceration S36.893
  periurethral tissue —*see* Injury, urethra
    complicating delivery O71.82
  phalanges
    foot —*see* Injury, foot
    hand —*see* Injury, hand
  pharynx NEC S19.85
  pleura —*see* Injury, intrathoracic, pleura
  plexus
    brachial —*see* Injury, brachial plexus
    cardiac —*see* Injury, nerve, thorax, sympathetic
    celiac, coeliac —*see* Injury, nerve, lumbosacral, sympathetic
    esophageal —*see* Injury, nerve, thorax, sympathetic
    hypogastric —*see* Injury, nerve, lumbosacral, sympathetic
    lumbar, lumbosacral —*see* Injury, lumbosacral plexus
    mesenteric —*see* Injury, nerve, lumbosacral, sympathetic
    pulmonary —*see* Injury, nerve, thorax, sympathetic
  postcardiac surgery (syndrome) I97.0
  prepuce S39.94
  pressure
    injury —*see* Ulcer, pressure, by site
  prostate S37.829
    contusion S37.822
    laceration S37.823
    specified type NEC S37.828
  pubic region S39.94
  pudendum S39.94
  pulmonary plexus —*see* Injury, nerve, thorax, sympathetic
  rectovaginal septum NEC S39.83
  rectum —*see* Injury, intestine, large, rectum
  retina —*see* Injury, eye, specified site NEC
    penetrating —*see* Injury, eyeball, penetrating
  retroperitoneal —*see* Injury, intra-abdominal, specified site NEC

Injury *(Continued)*
rotator cuff (muscle(s)) (tendon(s)) S46.00-●
    laceration S46.02-●
    specified type NEC S46.09-●
    strain S46.01-●
round ligament —*see* Injury, pelvic organ,
    specified site NEC
sacral plexus —*see* Injury, lumbosacral
    plexus
salivary duct or gland S09.93
scalp S09.90
    newborn (birth injury) P12.9
        due to monitoring (electrode) (sampling
            incision) P12.4
        specified NEC P12.89
            caput succedaneum P12.81
scapular region —*see* Injury, shoulder
sclera —*see* Injury, eye, specified site NEC
    penetrating —*see* Injury, eyeball,
        penetrating
scrotum S39.94
second cranial nerve (optic) —*see* Injury,
    nerve, optic
seminal vesicle —*see* Injury, pelvic organ,
    specified site NEC
seventh cranial nerve (facial) —*see* Injury,
    nerve, facial
shoulder S49.9-●
    blood vessel —*see* Injury, blood vessel,
        arm
    contusion —*see* Contusion, shoulder
    dislocation —*see* Dislocation, shoulder
    fracture —*see* Fracture, shoulder
    muscle —*see* Injury, muscle, shoulder
    nerve —*see* Injury, nerve, shoulder
    open —*see* Wound, open, shoulder
    specified type NEC S49.8-●
    sprain —*see* Sprain, shoulder girdle
    superficial —*see* Injury, superficial,
        shoulder
sinus
    cavernous —*see* Injury, intracranial
    nasal S09.92
sixth cranial nerve (abducent) —*see* Injury,
    nerve, abducens
skeleton, birth injury P13.9
    specified part NEC P13.8
skin NEC T14.8
    surface intact —*see* Injury, superficial
skull NEC S09.90
specified NEC T14.8
spermatic cord (pelvic region) S37.898
    scrotal region S39.848
spinal (cord)
    cervical (neck) S14.109
        anterior cord syndrome S14.139
            C1 level S14.131
            C2 level S14.132
            C3 level S14.133
            C4 level S14.134
            C5 level S14.135
            C6 level S14.136
            C7 level S14.137
            C8 level S14.138
        Brown-Séquard syndrome S14.149
            C1 level S14.141
            C2 level S14.142
            C3 level S14.143
            C4 level S14.144
            C5 level S14.145
            C6 level S14.146
            C7 level S14.147
            C8 level S14.148
        C1 level S14.101
        C2 level S14.102
        C3 level S14.103
        C4 level S14.104
        C5 level S14.105
        C6 level S14.106
        C7 level S14.107
        C8 level S14.108

Injury *(Continued)*
    spinal *(Continued)*
        cervical *(Continued)*
            central cord syndrome
                S14.129
                C1 level S14.121
                C2 level S14.122
                C3 level S14.123
                C4 level S14.124
                C5 level S14.125
                C6 level S14.126
                C7 level S14.127
                C8 level S14.128
            complete lesion S14.119
                C1 level S14.111
                C2 level S14.112
                C3 level S14.113
                C4 level S14.114
                C5 level S14.115
                C6 level S14.116
                C7 level S14.117
                C8 level S14.118
            concussion S14.0
            edema S14.0
            incomplete lesion specified NEC
                S14.159
                C1 level S14.151
                C2 level S14.152
                C3 level S14.153
                C4 level S14.154
                C5 level S14.155
                C6 level S14.156
                C7 level S14.157
                C8 level S14.158
            posterior cord syndrome S14.159
                C1 level S14.151
                C2 level S14.152
                C3 level S14.153
                C4 level S14.154
                C5 level S14.155
                C6 level S14.156
                C7 level S14.157
                C8 level S14.158
        dorsal —*see* Injury, spinal, thoracic
        lumbar S34.109
            complete lesion S34.119
                L1 level S34.111
                L2 level S34.112
                L3 level S34.113
                L4 level S34.114
                L5 level S34.115
            concussion S34.01
            edema S34.01
            incomplete lesion S34.129
                L1 level S34.121
                L2 level S34.122
                L3 level S34.123
                L4 level S34.124
                L5 level S34.125
            L1 level S34.101
            L2 level S34.102
            L3 level S34.103
            L4 level S34.104
            L5 level S34.105
        nerve root NEC
            cervical —*see* Injury, nerve, spinal, root,
                cervical
            dorsal —*see* Injury, nerve, spinal, root,
                dorsal
            lumbar S34.21
            sacral S34.22
            thoracic —*see* Injury, nerve, spinal, root,
                dorsal
        plexus
            brachial —*see* Injury, brachial
                plexus
            lumbosacral —*see* Injury, lumbosacral
                plexus
        sacral S34.139
            complete lesion S34.131
            incomplete lesion S34.132

Injury *(Continued)*
    spinal *(Continued)*
        thoracic S24.109
            anterior cord syndrome S24.139
                T1 level S24.131
                T2-T6 level S24.132
                T7-T10 level S24.133
                T11-T12 level S24.134
            Brown-Séquard syndrome
                S24.149
                T1 level S24.141
                T2-T6 level S24.142
                T7-T10 level S24.143
                T11-T12 level S24.144
            complete lesion S24.119
                T1 level S24.111
                T2-T6 level S24.112
                T7-T10 level S24.113
                T11-T12 level S24.114
            concussion S24.0
            edema S24.0
            incomplete lesion specified NEC
                S24.159
                T1 level S24.151
                T2-T6 level S24.152
                T7-T10 level S24.153
                T11-T12 level S24.154
            posterior cord syndrome S24.159
                T1 level S24.151
                T2-T6 level S24.152
                T7-T10 level S24.153
                T11-T12 level S24.154
            T1 level S24.101
            T2-T6 level S24.102
            T7-T10 level S24.103
            T11-T12 level S24.104
    splanchnic nerve —*see* Injury, nerve,
        lumbosacral, sympathetic
    spleen S36.00
        contusion S36.029
            major S36.021
            minor S36.020
        laceration S36.039
            major (massive) (stellate) S36.032
            moderate S36.031
            superficial (capsular) (minor) S36.030
        specified type NEC S36.09
    splenic artery —*see* Injury, blood vessel, celiac
        artery, branch
    stellate ganglion —*see* Injury, nerve, thorax,
        sympathetic
    sternal region S29.9
    stomach S36.30
        contusion S36.32
        laceration S36.33
        specified type NEC S36.39
    subconjunctival —*see* Injury, eye, conjunctiva
    subcutaneous NEC T14.8
    submaxillary region S09.93
    submental region S09.93
    subungual
        fingers —*see* Injury, hand
        toes —*see* Injury, foot
    superficial NEC T14.8
        abdomen, abdominal (wall) S30.92
            abrasion S30.811
            bite S30.871
                insect S30.861
            contusion S30.1
            external constriction S30.841
            foreign body S30.851
        abrasion —*see* Abrasion, by site
        adnexa, eye NEC —*see* Injury, eye,
            specified site NEC
        alveolar process —*see* Injury, superficial,
            oral cavity
        ankle S90.91-●
            abrasion —*see* Abrasion, ankle
            bite —*see* Bite, ankle
            blister —*see* Blister, ankle
            contusion —*see* Contusion, ankle

Injury *(Continued)*
  superficial NEC *(Continued)*
    ankle *(Continued)*
      external constriction —*see* Constriction, external, ankle
      foreign body —*see* Foreign body, superficial, ankle
    anus S30.98
    arm (upper) S40.92-•
      abrasion —*see* Abrasion, arm
      bite —*see* Bite, superficial, arm
      blister —*see* Blister, arm (upper)
      contusion —*see* Contusion, arm
      external constriction —*see* Constriction, external, arm
      foreign body —*see* Foreign body, superficial, arm
    auditory canal (external) (meatus) —*see* Injury, superficial, ear
    auricle —*see* Injury, superficial, ear
    axilla —*see* Injury, superficial, arm
    back —*see also* Injury, superficial, thorax, back
      lower S30.91
        abrasion S30.810
        contusion S30.0
        external constriction S30.840
        superficial
          bite NEC S30.870
            insect S30.860
          foreign body S30.850
    bite NEC —*see* Bite, superficial NEC, by site
    blister —*see* Blister, by site
    breast S20.10-•
      abrasion —*see* Abrasion, breast
      bite —*see* Bite, superficial, breast
      contusion —*see* Contusion, breast
      external constriction —*see* Constriction, external, breast
      foreign body —*see* Foreign body, superficial, breast
    brow —*see* Injury, superficial, head, specified NEC
    buttock S30.91
    calf —*see* Injury, superficial, leg
    canthus, eye —*see* Injury, superficial, periocular area
    cheek (external) —*see* Injury, superficial, head, specified NEC
      internal —*see* Injury, superficial, oral cavity
    chest wall —*see* Injury, superficial, thorax
    chin —*see* Injury, superficial, head NEC
    clitoris S30.95
    conjunctiva —*see* Injury, eye, conjunctiva
      with foreign body (in conjunctival sac) —*see* Foreign body, conjunctival sac
    contusion —*see* Contusion, by site
    costal region —*see* Injury, superficial, thorax
    digit(s)
      hand —*see* Injury, superficial, finger
    ear (auricle) (canal) (external) S00.40-•
      abrasion —*see* Abrasion, ear
      bite —*see* Bite, superficial, ear
      contusion —*see* Contusion, ear
      external constriction —*see* Constriction, external, ear
      foreign body —*see* Foreign body, superficial, ear
    elbow S50.90-•
      abrasion —*see* Abrasion, elbow
      bite —*see* Bite, superficial, elbow
      blister —*see* Blister, elbow
      contusion —*see* Contusion, elbow
      external constriction —*see* Constriction, external, elbow
      foreign body —*see* Foreign body, superficial, elbow

Injury *(Continued)*
  superficial NEC *(Continued)*
    epididymis S30.94
    epigastric region S30.92
    epiglottis —*see* Injury, superficial, throat
    esophagus
      cervical —*see* Injury, superficial, throat
    external constriction —*see* Constriction, external, by site
    extremity NEC T14.8
    eyeball NEC —*see* Injury, eye, specified site NEC
    eyebrow —*see* Injury, superficial, periocular area
    eyelid S00.20-•
      abrasion —*see* Abrasion, eyelid
      bite —*see* Bite, superficial, eyelid
      contusion —*see* Contusion, eyelid
      external constriction —*see* Constriction, external, eyelid
      foreign body —*see* Foreign body, superficial, eyelid
    face NEC —*see* Injury, superficial, head, specified NEC
    finger(s) S60.949
      abrasion —*see* Abrasion, finger
      bite —*see* Bite, superficial, finger
      blister —*see* Blister, finger
      contusion —*see* Contusion, finger
      external constriction —*see* Constriction, external, finger
      foreign body —*see* Foreign body, superficial, finger
      index S60.94-•
      insect bite —*see* Bite, by site, superficial, insect
      little S60.94-•
      middle S60.94-•
      ring S60.94-•
    flank S30.92
    foot S90.92-•
      abrasion —*see* Abrasion, foot
      bite —*see* Bite, foot
      blister —*see* Blister, foot
      contusion —*see* Contusion, foot
      external constriction —*see* Constriction, external, foot
      foreign body —*see* Foreign body, superficial, foot
    forearm S50.91-•
      abrasion —*see* Abrasion, forearm
      bite —*see* Bite, forearm, superficial
      blister —*see* Blister, forearm
      contusion —*see* Contusion, forearm
      elbow only —*see* Injury, superficial, elbow
      external constriction —*see* Constriction, external, forearm
      foreign body —*see* Foreign body, superficial, forearm
    forehead —*see* Injury, superficial, head NEC
    foreign body —*see* Foreign body, superficial
    genital organs, external
      female S30.97
      male S30.96
    globe (eye) —*see* Injury, eye, specified site NEC
    groin S30.92
    gum —*see* Injury, superficial, oral cavity
    hand S60.92-•
      abrasion —*see* Abrasion, hand
      bite —*see* Bite, superficial, hand
      contusion —*see* Contusion, hand
      external constriction —*see* Constriction, external, hand
      foreign body —*see* Foreign body, superficial, hand

Injury *(Continued)*
  superficial NEC *(Continued)*
    head S00.90
      ear —*see* Injury, superficial, ear
      eyelid —*see* Injury, superficial, eyelid
      nose S00.30
      oral cavity S00.502
      scalp S00.00
      specified site NEC S00.80
    heel —*see* Injury, superficial, foot
    hip S70.91-•
      abrasion —*see* Abrasion, hip
      bite —*see* Bite, superficial, hip
      blister —*see* Blister, hip
      contusion —*see* Contusion, hip
      external constriction —*see* Constriction, external, hip
      foreign body —*see* Foreign body, superficial, hip
    iliac region —*see* Injury, superficial, abdomen
    inguinal region —*see* Injury, superficial, abdomen
    insect bite —*see* Bite, by site, superficial, insect
    interscapular region —*see* Injury, superficial, thorax, back
    jaw —*see* Injury, superficial, head, specified NEC
    knee S80.91-•
      abrasion —*see* Abrasion, knee
      bite —*see* Bite, superficial, knee
      blister —*see* Blister, knee
      contusion —*see* Contusion, knee
      external constriction —*see* Constriction, external, knee
      foreign body —*see* Foreign body, superficial, knee
    labium (majus) (minus) S30.95
    lacrimal (apparatus) (gland) (sac) —*see* Injury, eye, specified site NEC
    larynx —*see* Injury, superficial, throat
    leg (lower) S80.92-•
      abrasion —*see* Abrasion, leg
      bite —*see* Bite, superficial, leg
      contusion —*see* Contusion, leg
      external constriction —*see* Constriction, external, leg
      foreign body —*see* Foreign body, superficial, leg
      knee —*see* Injury, superficial, knee
    limb NEC T14.8
    lip S00.501
    lower back S30.91
    lumbar region S30.91
    malar region —*see* Injury, superficial, head, specified NEC
    mammary —*see* Injury, superficial, breast
    mastoid region —*see* Injury, superficial, head, specified NEC
    mouth —*see* Injury, superficial, oral cavity
    muscle NEC T14.8
    nail NEC T14.8
      finger —*see* Injury, superficial, finger
      toe —*see* Injury, superficial, toe
    nasal (septum) —*see* Injury, superficial, nose
    neck S10.90
      specified site NEC S10.80
    nose (septum) S00.30
    occipital region —*see* Injury, superficial, scalp
    oral cavity S00.502
    orbital region —*see* Injury, superficial, periocular area
    palate —*see* Injury, superficial, oral cavity
    palm —*see* Injury, superficial, hand
    parietal region —*see* Injury, superficial, scalp
    pelvis S30.91
      girdle —*see* Injury, superficial, hip

▶ New ⇒ Revised ~~deleted~~ Deleted • Use Additional Character(s)

Injury (Continued)
  superficial NEC (Continued)
    penis S30.93
    perineum
      female S30.95
      male S30.91
    periocular area S00.20-●
      abrasion —see Abrasion, eyelid
      bite —see Bite, superficial, eyelid
      contusion —see Contusion, eyelid
      external constriction —see Constriction,
        external, eyelid
      foreign body —see Foreign body,
        superficial, eyelid
    phalanges
      finger —see Injury, superficial, finger
      toe —see Injury, superficial, toe
    pharynx —see Injury, superficial, throat
    pinna —see Injury, superficial, ear
    popliteal space —see Injury, superficial,
      knee
    prepuce S30.93
    pubic region S30.91
    pudendum
      female S30.97
      male S30.96
    sacral region S30.91
    scalp S00.00
    scapular region —see Injury, superficial,
      shoulder
    sclera —see Injury, eye, specified site NEC
    scrotum S30.94
    shin —see Injury, superficial, leg
    shoulder S40.91-●
      abrasion —see Abrasion, shoulder
      bite —see Bite, superficial, shoulder
      blister —see Blister, shoulder
      contusion —see Contusion, shoulder
      external constriction —see Constriction,
        external, shoulder
      foreign body —see Foreign body,
        superficial, shoulder
    skin NEC T14.8
    sternal region —see Injury, superficial,
      thorax, front
    subconjunctival —see Injury, eye, specified
      site NEC
    subcutaneous NEC T14.8
    submaxillary region —see Injury,
      superficial, head, specified NEC
    submental region —see Injury, superficial,
      head, specified NEC
    subungual
      finger(s) —see Injury, superficial, finger
      toe(s) —see Injury, superficial, toe
    supraclavicular fossa —see Injury,
      superficial, neck
    supraorbital —see Injury, superficial, head,
      specified NEC
    temple —see Injury, superficial, head,
      specified NEC
    temporal region —see Injury, superficial,
      head, specified NEC
    testis S30.94
    thigh S70.92-●
      abrasion —see Abrasion, thigh
      bite —see Bite, superficial, thigh
      blister —see Blister, thigh
      contusion —see Contusion, thigh
      external constriction —see Constriction,
        external, thigh
      foreign body —see Foreign body,
        superficial, thigh
    thorax, thoracic (wall) S20.90
      abrasion —see Abrasion, thorax
      back S20.40-●
      bite —see Bite, thorax, superficial
      blister —see Blister, thorax
      contusion —see Contusion, thorax
      external constriction —see Constriction,
        external, thorax

Injury (Continued)
  superficial NEC (Continued)
    thorax, thoracic (Continued)
      foreign body —see Foreign body,
        superficial, thorax
      front S20.30-●
    throat S10.10
      abrasion S10.11
      bite S10.17
        insect S10.16
      blister S10.12
      contusion S10.0
      external constriction S10.14
      foreign body S10.15
    thumb S60.93-●
      abrasion —see Abrasion, thumb
      bite —see Bite, superficial, thumb
      blister —see Blister, thumb
      contusion —see Contusion, thumb
      external constriction —see Constriction,
        external, thumb
      foreign body —see Foreign body,
        superficial, thumb
      insect bite —see Bite, by site, superficial,
        insect
      specified type NEC S60.39-●
    toe(s) S90.93-●
      abrasion —see Abrasion, toe
      bite —see Bite, toe
      blister —see Blister, toe
      contusion —see Contusion, toe
      external constriction —see Constriction,
        external, toe
      foreign body —see Foreign body,
        superficial, toe
      great S90.93-●
    tongue —see Injury, superficial, oral cavity
    tooth, teeth —see Injury, superficial, oral
      cavity
    trachea S10.10
    tunica vaginalis S30.94
    tympanum, tympanic membrane —see
      Injury, superficial, ear
    uvula —see Injury, superficial, oral cavity
    vagina S30.95
    vocal cords —see Injury, superficial, throat
    vulva S30.95
    wrist S60.91-●
  supraclavicular region —see Injury, neck
  supraorbital S09.93
  suprarenal gland (multiple) —see Injury,
    adrenal
  surgical complication (external or internal
    site) —see Laceration, accidental
    complicating surgery
  temple S09.90
  temporal region S09.90
  tendon —see also Injury, muscle, by site
    abdomen —see Injury, muscle, abdomen
    Achilles —see Injury, Achilles tendon
    lower back —see Injury, muscle, lower
      back
    pelvic organs —see Injury, muscle, pelvis
  tenth cranial nerve (pneumogastric or
    vagus) —see Injury, nerve, vagus
  testis S39.94
  thigh S79.92-●
    blood vessel —see Injury, blood vessel, hip
    contusion —see Contusion, thigh
    fracture —see Fracture, femur
    muscle —see Injury, muscle, thigh
    nerve —see Injury, nerve, thigh
    open —see Wound, open, thigh
    specified NEC S79.82-●
    superficial —see Injury, superficial, thigh
  third cranial nerve (oculomotor) —see Injury,
    nerve, oculomotor
  thorax, thoracic S29.9
    blood vessel —see Injury, blood vessel,
      thorax
    cavity —see Injury, intrathoracic

Injury (Continued)
  thorax, thoracic (Continued)
    dislocation —see Dislocation, thorax
    external (wall) S29.9
      contusion —see Contusion, thorax
      nerve —see Injury, nerve, thorax
      open —see Wound, open, thorax
      specified NEC S29.8
      sprain —see Sprain, thorax
      superficial —see Injury, superficial,
        thorax
    fracture —see Fracture, thorax
    internal —see Injury, intrathoracic
    intrathoracic organ —see Injury,
      intrathoracic
    sympathetic ganglion —see Injury, nerve,
      thorax, sympathetic
  throat —see also Injury, neck S19.9
  thumb S69.9-●
    blood vessel —see Injury, blood vessel,
      thumb
    contusion —see Contusion, thumb
    dislocation —see Dislocation, thumb
    fracture —see Fracture, thumb
    muscle —see Injury, muscle, thumb
    nerve —see Injury, nerve, digital, thumb
    open —see Wound, open, thumb
    specified NEC S69.8-●
    sprain —see Sprain, thumb
    superficial —see Injury, superficial, thumb
  thymus (gland) —see Injury, intrathoracic,
    specified organ NEC
  thyroid (gland) NEC S19.84
  toe S99.92-●
    contusion —see Contusion, toe
    dislocation —see Dislocation, toe
    fracture —see Fracture, toe
    muscle —see Injury, muscle, toe
    open —see Wound, open, toe
    specified type NEC S99.82-●
    sprain —see Sprain, toe
    superficial —see Injury, superficial, toe
  tongue S09.93
  tonsil S09.93
  tooth S09.93
  trachea (cervical) NEC S19.82
    thoracic —see Injury, intrathoracic, trachea,
      thoracic
  transfusion-related acute lung (TRALI)
    J95.84
  tunica vaginalis S39.94
  twelfth cranial nerve (hypoglossal) —see
    Injury, nerve, hypoglossal
  ureter S37.10
    contusion S37.12
    laceration S37.13
    specified type NEC S37.19
  urethra (sphincter) S37.30
    at delivery O71.5
    contusion S37.32
    laceration S37.33
    specified type NEC S37.38
  urinary organ S37.899
    contusion S37.92
    laceration S37.93
    specified
      site NEC S37.899
        contusion S37.892
        laceration S37.893
        specified type NEC S37.898
      type NEC S37.99
  uterus, uterine S37.60
    with ectopic or molar pregnancy O08.6
    blood vessel —see Injury, blood vessel, iliac
    contusion S37.62
    laceration S37.63
      cervix at delivery O71.3
    rupture associated with obstetrics —see
      Rupture, uterus
    specified type NEC S37.69
  uvula S09.93

Injury *(Continued)*
- vagina S39.93
  - abrasion S30.814
  - bite S31.45
    - insect S30.864
    - superficial NEC S30.874
  - contusion S30.23
  - crush S38.03
  - during delivery —*see* Laceration, vagina, during delivery
  - external constriction S30.844
  - insect bite S30.864
  - laceration S31.41
    - with foreign body S31.42
  - open wound S31.40
  - puncture S31.43
    - with foreign body S31.44
  - superficial S30.95
    - foreign body S30.854
- vas deferens —*see* Injury, pelvic organ, specified site NEC
- vascular NEC T14.8
- vein —*see* Injury, blood vessel
- vena cava (superior) S25.20
  - inferior S35.10
    - laceration (minor) (superficial) S35.11
      - major S35.12
      - specified type NEC S35.19
  - laceration (minor) (superficial) S25.21
    - major S25.22
  - specified type NEC S25.29
- vesical (sphincter) —*see* Injury, bladder
- visual cortex S04.04-●
- vitreous (humor) S05.90
  - specified NEC S05.8X-●
- vocal cord NEC S19.83
- vulva S39.94
  - abrasion S30.814
  - bite S31.45
    - insect S30.864
    - superficial NEC S30.874
  - contusion S30.23
  - crush S38.03
  - during delivery —*see* Laceration, perineum, female, during delivery
  - external constriction S30.844
  - insect bite S30.864
  - laceration S31.41
    - with foreign body S31.42
  - open wound S31.40
  - puncture S31.43
    - with foreign body S31.44
  - superficial S30.95
    - foreign body S30.854
- whiplash (cervical spine) S13.4
- wrist S69.9-●
  - blood vessel —*see* Injury, blood vessel, hand
  - contusion —*see* Contusion, wrist
  - dislocation —*see* Dislocation, wrist
  - fracture —*see* Fracture, wrist
  - muscle —*see* Injury, muscle, hand
  - nerve —*see* Injury, nerve, hand
  - open —*see* Wound, open, wrist
  - specified NEC S69.8-●
  - sprain —*see* Sprain, wrist
  - superficial —*see* Injury, superficial, wrist
Inoculation —*see also* Vaccination
- complication or reaction —*see* Complications, vaccination
Insanity, insane —*see also* Psychosis
- adolescent —*see* Schizophrenia
- confusional F28
  - acute or subacute F05
- delusional F22
- senile F03
Insect
- bite —*see* Bite, by site, superficial, insect
- venomous, poisoning NEC (by) —*see* Venom, arthropod
▶**Insecurity, food** Z59.41

Insensitivity
- adrenocorticotropin hormone (ACTH) E27.49
- androgen E34.50
  - complete E34.51
  - partial E34.52
Insertion
- cord (umbilical) lateral or velamentous O43.12-●
- intrauterine contraceptive device (encounter for) —*see* Intrauterine contraceptive device
Insolation (sunstroke) T67.01
Insomnia (organic) G47.00
- without objective findings F51.02
- adjustment F51.02
- adjustment disorder F51.02
- behavioral, of childhood Z73.819
  - combined type Z73.812
  - limit setting type Z73.811
  - sleep-onset association type Z73.810
- childhood Z73.819
- chronic F51.04
  - somatized tension F51.04
- conditioned F51.04
- due to
  - alcohol
    - abuse F10.182
    - dependence F10.282
    - use F10.982
  - amphetamines
    - abuse F15.182
    - dependence F15.282
    - use F15.982
  - anxiety disorder F51.05
  - caffeine
    - abuse F15.182
    - dependence F15.282
    - use F15.982
  - cocaine
    - abuse F14.182
    - dependence F14.282
    - use F14.982
  - depression F51.05
  - drug NEC
    - abuse F19.182
    - dependence F19.282
    - use F19.982
  - medical condition G47.01
  - mental disorder NEC F51.05
  - opioid
    - abuse F11.182
    - dependence F11.282
    - use F11.982
  - psychoactive substance NEC
    - abuse F19.182
    - dependence F19.282
    - use F19.982
  - sedative, hypnotic, or anxiolytic
    - abuse F13.182
    - dependence F13.282
    - use F13.982
  - stimulant NEC
    - abuse F15.182
    - dependence F15.282
    - use F15.982
- fatal familial (FFI) A81.83
- idiopathic F51.01
- learned F51.3
- nonorganic origin F51.01
- not due to a substance or known physiological condition F51.01
  - specified NEC F51.09
- paradoxical F51.03
- primary F51.01
- psychiatric F51.05
- psychophysiologic F51.04
- related to psychopathology F51.05
- short-term F51.02
- specified NEC G47.09
- stress-related F51.02
- transient F51.02

Inspiration
- food or foreign body —*see* Foreign body, by site
- mucus —*see* Asphyxia, mucus
Inspissated bile syndrome (newborn) P59.1
Instability
- emotional (excessive) F60.3
▶housing
  - ▶housed Z59.819
    - ▶with risk of homelessness Z59.811
    - ▶homelessness in past 12 months Z59.812
- joint (post-traumatic) M25.30
  - ankle M25.37-●
  - due to old ligament injury —*see* Disorder, ligament
  - elbow M25.32-●
  - flail —*see* Flail, joint
  - foot M25.37-●
  - hand M25.34-●
  - hip M25.35-●
  - knee M25.36-●
  - lumbosacral —*see* subcategory M53.2
  - prosthesis —*see* Complications, joint prosthesis, mechanical, displacement, by site
  - sacroiliac —*see* subcategory M53.2
  - secondary to
    - old ligament injury —*see* Disorder, ligament
    - removal of joint prosthesis M96.89
  - shoulder (region) M25.31-●
  - specified site NEC M25.39
  - spine —*see* subcategory M53.2
  - wrist M25.33-●
- knee (chronic) M23.5-●
- lumbosacral —*see* subcategory M53.2
- nervous F48.8
- personality (emotional) F60.3
- spine —*see* Instability, joint, spine
- vasomotor R55
Institutional syndrome (childhood) F94.2
Institutionalization, affecting child Z62.22
- disinhibited attachment F94.2
Insufficiency, insufficient
- accommodation, old age H52.4
- adrenal (gland) E27.40
  - primary E27.1
- adrenocortical E27.40
  - drug-induced E27.3
  - iatrogenic E27.3
  - primary E27.1
- anatomic crown height K08.89
- anterior (occlusal) guidance M26.54
- anus K62.89
- aortic (valve) I35.1
  - with
    - mitral (valve) disease I08.0
      - with tricuspid (valve) disease I08.3
    - stenosis I35.2
    - tricuspid (valve) disease I08.2
      - with mitral (valve) disease I08.3
  - congenital Q23.1
  - rheumatic I06.1
    - with
      - mitral (valve) disease I08.0
        - with tricuspid (valve) disease I08.3
      - stenosis I06.2
        - with mitral (valve) disease I08.0
          - with tricuspid (valve) disease I08.3
      - tricuspid (valve) disease I08.2
        - with mitral (valve) disease I08.3
  - specified cause NEC I35.1
  - syphilitic A52.03
- arterial I77.1
  - basilar G45.0
  - carotid (hemispheric) G45.1
  - cerebral I67.81
  - coronary (acute or subacute) I24.8
  - mesenteric K55.1
  - peripheral I73.9
  - precerebral (multiple) (bilateral) G45.2
  - vertebral G45.0

▶ New   ⇒ Revised   ~~deleted~~ Deleted   ● Use Additional Character(s)

Insufficiency, insufficient *(Continued)*
- arteriovenous I99.8
- biliary K83.8
- cardiac —*see also* Insufficiency, myocardial
  - due to presence of (cardiac) prosthesis I97.11-●
    - postprocedural I97.11-●
- cardiorenal, hypertensive I13.2
- cardiovascular —*see* Disease, cardiovascular
- cerebrovascular (acute) I67.81
  - with transient focal neurological signs and symptoms G45.8
- circulatory NEC I99.8
  - newborn P29.89
- clinical crown length K08.89
- convergence H51.11
- coronary (acute or subacute) I24.8
  - chronic or with a stated duration of over 4 weeks I25.89
- corticoadrenal E27.40
  - primary E27.1
- dietary E63.9
- divergence H51.8
- food T73.0
- gastroesophageal K22.89
- gonadal
  - ovary E28.39
  - testis E29.1
- heart —*see also* Insufficiency, myocardial
  - newborn P29.0
  - valve —*see* Endocarditis
- hepatic —*see* Failure, hepatic
- idiopathic autonomic G90.09
- interocclusal distance of fully erupted teeth (ridge) M26.36
- kidney N28.9
  - acute N28.9
  - chronic N18.9
- lacrimal (secretion) H04.12-●
  - passages —*see* Stenosis, lacrimal
- liver —*see* Failure, hepatic
- lung —*see* Insufficiency, pulmonary
- mental (congenital) —*see* Disability, intellectual
- mesenteric K55.1
- mitral (valve) I34.0
  - with
    - aortic valve disease I08.0
      - with tricuspid (valve) disease I08.3
    - obstruction or stenosis I05.2
      - with aortic valve disease I08.0
    - tricuspid (valve) disease I08.1
      - with aortic (valve) disease I08.3
  - congenital Q23.3
  - rheumatic I05.1
    - with
      - aortic valve disease I08.0
        - with tricuspid (valve) disease I08.3
      - obstruction or stenosis I05.2
        - with aortic valve disease I08.0
          - with tricuspid (valve) disease I08.3
      - tricuspid (valve) disease I08.1
        - with aortic (valve) disease I08.3
    - active or acute I01.1
      - with chorea, rheumatic (Sydenham's) I02.0
  - specified cause, except rheumatic I34.0
- muscle —*see also* Disease, muscle
  - heart —*see* Insufficiency, myocardial
  - ocular NEC H50.9
- myocardial, myocardium (with arteriosclerosis) —*see also* Failure, heart I50.9
  - with
    - rheumatic fever (conditions in I00) I09.0
      - active, acute or subacute I01.2
        - with chorea I02.0
      - inactive or quiescent (with chorea) I09.0
  - congenital Q24.8

Insufficiency, insufficient *(Continued)*
- myocardial, myocardium *(Continued)*
  - hypertensive —*see* Hypertension, heart
  - newborn P29.0
  - rheumatic I09.0
    - active, acute, or subacute I01.2
  - syphilitic A52.06
- nourishment T73.0
- pancreatic K86.89
  - exocrine K86.81
- parathyroid (gland) E20.9
- peripheral vascular (arterial) I73.9
- pituitary E23.0
- placental (mother) O36.51-●
- platelets D69.6
- prenatal care affecting management of pregnancy O09.3-●
- progressive pluriglandular E31.0
- pulmonary J98.4
  - acute, following surgery (nonthoracic) J95.2
    - thoracic J95.1
  - chronic, following surgery J95.3
  - following
    - shock J98.4
    - trauma J98.4
  - newborn P28.89
  - valve I37.1
    - with stenosis I37.2
    - congenital Q22.2
    - rheumatic I09.89
      - with aortic, mitral or tricuspid (valve) disease I08.8
- pyloric K31.89
- renal (acute) N28.9
  - chronic N18.9
- respiratory R06.89
  - newborn P28.5
- rotation —*see* Malrotation
- sleep syndrome F51.12
- social insurance Z59.7
- suprarenal E27.40
  - primary E27.1
- tarso-orbital fascia, congenital Q10.3
- testis E29.1
- thyroid (gland) (acquired) E03.9
  - congenital E03.1
- tricuspid (valve) (rheumatic) I07.1
  - with
    - aortic (valve) disease I08.2
      - with mitral (valve) disease I08.3
    - mitral (valve) disease I08.1
      - with aortic (valve) disease I08.3
    - obstruction or stenosis I07.2
      - with aortic (valve) disease I08.2
        - with mitral (valve) disease I08.3
  - congenital Q22.8
  - nonrheumatic I36.1
    - with stenosis I36.2
- urethral sphincter R32
- valve, valvular (heart) I38
  - aortic —*see* Insufficiency, aortic (valve)
  - mitral —*see* Insufficiency, mitral (valve)
  - pulmonary —*see* Insufficiency, pulmonary, valve
  - tricuspid —*see* Insufficiency, tricuspid (valve)
  - congenital Q24.8
- vascular I99.8
  - intestine K55.9
    - acute —*see also* Ischemia, intestine, acute K55.059
  - mesenteric K55.1
  - peripheral I73.9
  - renal —*see* Hypertension, kidney
- velopharyngeal
  - acquired K13.79
  - congenital Q38.8
- venous (chronic) (peripheral) I87.2
- ventricular —*see* Insufficiency, myocardial
- welfare support Z59.7

Insufflation, fallopian Z31.41
Insular —*see* condition
Insulinoma
- pancreas
  - benign D13.7
  - malignant C25.4
  - uncertain behavior D37.8
- specified site
  - benign —*see* Neoplasm, by site, benign
  - malignant —*see* Neoplasm, by site, malignant
  - uncertain behavior —*see* Neoplasm, by site, uncertain behavior
- unspecified site
  - benign D13.7
  - malignant C25.4
  - uncertain behavior D37.8
Insuloma —*see* Insulinoma
Interference
- balancing side M26.56
- non-working side M26.56
Intermenstrual —*see* condition
Intermittent —*see* condition
Internal —*see* condition
Interrogation
- cardiac defibrillator (automatic) (implantable) Z45.02
- cardiac pacemaker Z45.018
- cardiac (event) (loop) recorder Z45.09
- infusion pump (implanted) (intrathecal) Z45.1
- neurostimulator Z46.2
Interruption
- aortic arch Q25.21
- phase-shift, sleep cycle —*see* Disorder, sleep, circadian rhythm
- sleep phase-shift, or 24 hour sleep-wake cycle —*see* Disorder, sleep, circadian rhythm
Interstitial —*see* condition
Intertrigo L30.4
- labialis K13.0
Intervertebral disc —*see* condition
Intestine, intestinal —*see* condition
Intolerance
- carbohydrate K90.49
- disaccharide, hereditary E73.0
- fat NEC K90.49
  - pancreatic K90.3
- food K90.49
  - dietary counseling and surveillance Z71.3
- fructose E74.10
  - hereditary E74.12
- glucose(-galactose) E74.39
- gluten K90.01
- lactose E73.9
  - specified NEC E73.8
- lysine E72.3
- milk NEC K90.49
  - lactose E73.9
- protein K90.49
- starch NEC K90.49
- sucrose (-isomaltose) E74.31
Intoxicated NEC (without dependence) —*see* Alcohol, intoxication
Intoxication
- acid E87.2
- alcoholic (acute) (without dependence) —*see* Alcohol, intoxication
- alimentary canal K52.1
- amphetamine (without dependence) —*see also* Abuse, drug, stimulant, with intoxication
  - stimulant NEC F15.10
    - with
      - anxiety disorder F15.180
      - intoxication F15.129
        - with
          - delirium F15.121
          - perceptual disturbance F15.122
      - with dependence —*see* Dependence, drug, stimulant, with intoxication

Intoxication *(Continued)*
  anxiolytic (acute) (without dependence) —*see*
    Abuse, drug, sedative, with intoxication
    with dependence —*see* Dependence, drug,
      sedative, with intoxication
  caffeine F15.929
    with dependence —*see* Dependence, drug,
      stimulant, with intoxication
  cannabinoids (acute) (without
      dependence) —*see* Use, cannabis, with
      intoxication
    with
      abuse —*see* Abuse, drug, cannabis, with
        intoxication
      dependence —*see* Dependence, drug,
        cannabis, with intoxication
  chemical —*see* Table of Drugs and
    Chemicals
    via placenta or breast milk —*see*
      Absorption, chemical, through
      placenta
  cocaine (acute) (without dependence) —*see*
    Abuse, drug, cocaine, with intoxication
    with dependence —*see* Dependence, drug,
      cocaine, with intoxication
  drug
    acute (without dependence) —*see* Abuse,
      drug, by type with intoxication
      with dependence —*see* Dependence,
        drug, by type with intoxication
    addictive
      via placenta or breast milk —*see*
        Absorption, drug, addictive,
        through placenta
    newborn P93.8
      gray baby syndrome P93.0
    overdose or wrong substance given
      or taken —*see* Table of Drugs and
      Chemicals, by drug, poisoning
  enteric K52.1
  foodborne A05.9
    bacterial A05.9
    classical (Clostridium botulinum)
      A05.1
    due to
      Bacillus cereus A05.4
      bacterium A05.9
        specified NEC A05.8
      Clostridium
        botulinum A05.1
        perfringens A05.2
        welchii A05.2
      Salmonella A02.9
        with
          (gastro) enteritis A02.0
          localized infection(s) A02.20
            arthritis A02.23
            meningitis A02.21
            osteomyelitis A02.24
            pneumonia A02.22
            pyelonephritis A02.25
            specified NEC A02.29
          sepsis A02.1
          specified manifestation NEC
            A02.8
      Staphylococcus A05.0
      Vibrio
        parahaemolyticus A05.3
        vulnificus A05.5
    enterotoxin, staphylococcal A05.0
    noxious —*see* Poisoning, food, noxious
  gastrointestinal K52.1
  hallucinogenic (without dependence) —
    see Abuse, drug, hallucinogen, with
    intoxication
    with dependence —*see* Dependence, drug,
      hallucinogen, with intoxication
  hypnotic (acute) (without dependence) —*see*
    Abuse, drug, sedative, with intoxication
    with dependence —*see* Dependence, drug,
      sedative, with intoxication

Intoxication *(Continued)*
  inhalant (acute) (without dependence) —*see*
    Abuse, drug, inhalant, with intoxication
    with dependence —*see* Dependence, drug,
      inhalant, with intoxication
  meaning
    inebriation —*see* category F10
    poisoning —*see* Table of Drugs and
      Chemicals
  methyl alcohol (acute) (without
      dependence) —*see* Alcohol, intoxication
  opioid (acute) (without dependence) —*see*
    Abuse, drug, opioid, with intoxication
    with dependence —*see* Dependence, drug,
      opioid, with intoxication
  pathologic NEC (without dependence) —*see*
    Alcohol, intoxication
  phencyclidine (without dependence) —*see*
    Abuse, drug, hallucinogen, with
    intoxication
    with dependence —*see* Dependence, drug,
      hallucinogen, with intoxication
  potassium (K) E87.5
  psychoactive substance NEC (without
      dependence) —*see* Abuse, drug,
      psychoactive NEC, with intoxication
    with dependence —*see* Dependence, drug,
      psychoactive NEC, with intoxication
  sedative (acute) (without dependence) —*see*
    Abuse, drug, sedative, with intoxication
    with dependence —*see* Dependence, drug,
      sedative, with intoxication
  serum —*see also* Reaction, serum T80.69
  uremic —*see* Uremia
  volatile solvents (acute) (without
      dependence) —*see* Abuse, drug,
      inhalant, with intoxication
    with dependence —*see* Dependence, drug,
      inhalant, with intoxication
  water E87.79
Intraabdominal testis, testes
  bilateral Q53.211
  unilateral Q53.111
Intracranial —*see* condition
Intrahepatic gallbladder Q44.1
Intraligamentous —*see* condition
Intrathoracic —*see also* condition
  kidney Q63.2
Intrauterine contraceptive device
  checking Z30.431
  in situ Z97.5
  insertion Z30.430
    immediately following removal
      Z30.433
  management Z30.431
  reinsertion Z30.433
  removal Z30.432
  replacement Z30.433
  retention in pregnancy O26.3-●
Intraventricular —*see* condition
Intrinsic deformity —*see* Deformity
Intubation, difficult or failed T88.4
Intumescence, lens (eye) (cataract) —*see*
  Cataract
Intussusception (bowel) (colon) (enteric)
    (ileocecal) (ileocolic) (intestine) (rectum)
    K56.1
  appendix K38.8
  congenital Q43.8
  ureter (with obstruction) N13.5
Invagination (bowel, colon, intestine or rectum)
  K56.1
Inversion
  albumin-globulin (A-G) ratio E88.09
  bladder N32.89
  cecum —*see* Intussusception
  cervix N88.8
  chromosome in normal individual
    Q95.1
  circadian rhythm —*see* Disorder, sleep,
    circadian rhythm

Inversion *(Continued)*
  nipple N64.59
    congenital Q83.8
    gestational —*see* Retraction, nipple
    puerperal, postpartum —*see* Retraction,
      nipple
  nyctohemeral rhythm —*see* Disorder, sleep,
    circadian rhythm
  optic papilla Q14.2
  organ or site, congenital NEC —*see* Anomaly,
    by site
  sleep rhythm —*see* Disorder, sleep, circadian
    rhythm
  testis (congenital) Q55.29
  uterus (chronic) (postinfectional) (postpartal,
    old) N85.5
    postpartum O71.2
  vagina (posthysterectomy) N99.3
  ventricular Q20.5
Investigation —*see also* Examination Z04.9
  clinical research subject (control) (normal
    comparison) (participant) Z00.6
Involuntary movement, abnormal R25.9
Involution, involutional —*see also* condition
  breast, cystic —*see* Dysplasia, mammary,
    specified type NEC
  depression (single episode) F32.89
    recurrent episode F33.9
  melancholia (single episode) F32.89
    recurrent episode F33.8
  ovary, senile —*see* Atrophy, ovary
  thymus failure E32.8
I.Q.
  under 20 F73
  20-34 F72
  35-49 F71
  50-69 F70
IRDS (type I) P22.0
  type II P22.1
Irideremia Q13.1
Iridis rubeosis —*see* Disorder, iris, vascular
Iridochoroiditis (panuveitis) —*see* Panuveitis
Iridocyclitis H20.9-●
  acute H20.0-●
    hypopyon H20.05-●
    primary H20.01-●
    recurrent H20.02-●
    secondary (noninfectious) H20.04-●
      infectious H20.03-●
  chronic H20.1-●
  due to allergy —*see* Iridocyclitis, acute,
    secondary
  endogenous —*see* Iridocyclitis, acute,
    primary
  Fuchs' —*see* Cyclitis, Fuchs' heterochromic
  gonococcal A54.32
  granulomatous —*see* Iridocyclitis, chronic
  herpes, herpetic (simplex) B00.51
    zoster B02.32
  hypopyon —*see* Iridocyclitis, acute,
    hypopyon
  in (due to)
    ankylosing spondylitis M45.9
    gonococcal infection A54.32
    herpes (simplex) virus B00.51
      zoster B02.32
    infectious disease NOS B99
    parasitic disease NOS B89 [H22]
    sarcoidosis D86.83
    syphilis A51.43
    tuberculosis A18.54
    zoster B02.32
  lens-induced H20.2-●
  nongranulomatous —*see* Iridocyclitis, acute
  recurrent —*see* Iridocyclitis, acute, recurrent
  rheumatic —*see* Iridocyclitis, chronic
  subacute —*see* Iridocyclitis, acute
  sympathetic —*see* Uveitis, sympathetic
  syphilitic (secondary) A51.43
  tuberculous (chronic) A18.54
  Vogt-Koyanagi H20.82-●

▶ New   ⇒ Revised   ~~deleted~~ Deleted   ● Use Additional Character(s)

Iridocyclochoroiditis (panuveitis) —*see*
    Panuveitis
Iridodialysis H21.53-●
Iridodonesis H21.89
Iridoplegia (complete) (partial) (reflex) H57.09
Iridoschisis H21.25-●
Iris —*see also* condition
    bombé —*see* Membrane, pupillary
Iritis —*see also* Iridocyclitis
    chronic —*see* Iridocyclitis, chronic
    diabetic —*see* E08-E13 with .39
    due to
        herpes simplex B00.51
        leprosy A30.9 [H22]
    gonococcal A54.32
    gouty —*see also* Gout, by type M10.9 [H22]
    granulomatous —*see* Iridocyclitis, chronic
    lens induced —*see* Iridocyclitis, lens-induced
    papulosa (syphilitic) A52.71
    rheumatic —*see* Iridocyclitis, chronic
    syphilitic (secondary) A51.43
        congenital (early) A50.01
        late A52.71
    tuberculous A18.54
Iron —*see* condition
Iron-miner's lung J63.4
Irradiated enamel (tooth, teeth) K03.89
Irradiation effects, adverse T66
Irreducible, irreducibility —*see* condition
Irregular, irregularity
    action, heart I49.9
    alveolar process K08.89
    bleeding N92.6
    breathing R06.89
    contour of cornea (acquired) —*see* Deformity,
        cornea
        congenital Q13.4
    contour, reconstructed breast N65.0
    dentin (in pulp) K04.3
    eye movements H55.89
        deficient
            saccadic H55.81
            smooth H55.82
        nystagmus —*see* Nystagmus
    labor O62.2
    menstruation (cause unknown) N92.6
    periods N92.6
    prostate N42.9
    pupil —*see* Abnormality, pupillary
    reconstructed breast N65.0
    respiratory R06.89
    septum (nasal) J34.2
    shape, organ or site, congenital NEC —*see*
        Distortion
    sleep-wake pattern (rhythm) G47.23
Irritable, irritability R45.4
    bladder N32.89
    bowel (syndrome) K58.9
        with
            constipation K58.1
            diarrhea K58.0
        mixed K58.2
        psychogenic F45.8
        specified NEC K58.8
    bronchial —*see* Bronchitis
    cerebral, in newborn P91.3
    colon —*see also* Irritable, bowel K58.9
        with diarrhea K58.0
        psychogenic F45.8
    duodenum K59.89
    heart (psychogenic) F45.8
    hip —*see* Derangement, joint, specified type
        NEC, hip
    ileum K59.89
    infant R68.12
    jejunum K59.89
    rectum K59.89
    stomach K31.89
        psychogenic F45.8
    sympathetic G90.8
    urethra N36.8

Irritation
    anus K62.89
    axillary nerve G54.0
    bladder N32.89
    brachial plexus G54.0
    bronchial —*see* Bronchitis
    cervical plexus G54.2
    cervix —*see* Cervicitis
    choroid, sympathetic —*see* Endophthalmitis
    cranial nerve —*see* Disorder, nerve, cranial
    gastric K31.89
        psychogenic F45.8
    globe, sympathetic —*see* Uveitis, sympathetic
    labyrinth —*see* subcategory H83.2
    lumbosacral plexus G54.1
    meninges (traumatic) —*see* Injury, intracranial
        nontraumatic —*see* Meningismus
    nerve —*see* Disorder, nerve
    nervous R45.0
    penis N48.89
    perineum NEC L29.3
    peripheral autonomic nervous system G90.8
    peritoneum —*see* Peritonitis
    pharynx J39.2
    plantar nerve —*see* Lesion, nerve, plantar
    spinal (cord) (traumatic) —*see also* Injury,
        spinal cord, by region
        nerve G58.9
            root NEC —*see* Radiculopathy
            nontraumatic —*see* Myelopathy
    stomach K31.89
        psychogenic F45.8
    sympathetic nerve NEC G90.8
    ulnar nerve —*see* Lesion, nerve, ulnar
    vagina N89.8
Ischemia, ischemic I99.8
    bowel (transient)
        acute —*see also* Ischemia, intestine, acute
            K55.059
        chronic K55.1
        due to mesenteric artery insufficiency
            K55.1
    brain —*see* Ischemia, cerebral
    cardiac (*see* Disease, heart, ischemic)
    cardiomyopathy I25.5
    cerebral (chronic) (generalized) I67.82
        arteriosclerotic I67.2
        intermittent G45.9
        newborn P91.0
        recurrent focal G45.8
        transient G45.9
    colon chronic (due to mesenteric artery
        insufficiency) K55.1
    coronary —*see* Disease, heart, ischemic
    demand (coronary) —*see also* Angina
        I24.8
        with myocardial infarction I21.A1
        resulting in myocardial infarction
            I21.A1
    heart (chronic or with a stated duration of
        over 4 weeks) I25.9
        acute or with a stated duration of 4 weeks
            or less I24.9
        subacute I24.9
    infarction, muscle —*see* Infarct, muscle
    intestine (large) (small) (transient) K55.9
        acute K55.059
            diffuse K55.052
            focal K55.051
            large K55.039
                diffuse K55.032
                focal K55.031
            small K55.019
                diffuse K55.012
                focal K55.011
        chronic K55.1
        due to mesenteric artery insufficiency
            K55.1
    kidney N28.0
    limb, critical —*see* Arteriosclerosis, with
        critical limb ischemia

Ischemia, ischemic *(Continued)*
    limb-threatening, chronic —*see*
        Arteriosclerosis, with critical limb
        ischemia
    mesenteric, acute —*see also* Ischemia,
        intestine, acute K55.059
    muscle, traumatic T79.6
    myocardium, myocardial (chronic or with
        a stated duration of over 4 weeks)
        I25.9
        acute, without myocardial infarction
            I51.3
        silent (asymptomatic) I25.6
        transient of newborn P29.4
    renal N28.0
    retina, retinal —*see* Occlusion, artery, retina
    small bowel
        acute K55.019
            diffuse K55.012
            focal K55.011
        chronic K55.1
        due to mesenteric artery insufficiency
            K55.1
    spinal cord G95.11
    subendocardial —*see* Insufficiency,
        coronary
    supply (coronary) —*see also* Angina
        I25.9
        due to vasospasm I20.1
Ischial spine —*see* condition
Ischialgia —*see* Sciatica
Ischiopagus Q89.4
Ischium, ischial —*see* condition
Ischuria R34
Iselin's disease or osteochondrosis —*see*
    Osteochondrosis, juvenile, metatarsus
Islands of
    parotid tissue in
        lymph nodes Q38.6
        neck structures Q38.6
    submaxillary glands in
        fascia Q38.6
        lymph nodes Q38.6
        neck muscles Q38.6
Islet cell tumor, pancreas D13.7
Isoimmunization NEC —*see also*
    Incompatibility
    affecting management of pregnancy (ABO)
        (with hydrops fetalis) O36.11-●
        anti-A sensitization O36.11-●
        anti-B sensitization O36.19-●
        anti-c sensitization O36.09-●
        anti-C sensitization O36.09-●
        anti-e sensitization O36.09-●
        anti-E sensitization O36.09-●
        Rh NEC O36.09-●
            anti-D antibody O36.01-●
        specified NEC O36.19-●
    newborn P55.9
        with
            hydrops fetalis P56.0
            kernicterus P57.0
        ABO (blood groups) P55.1
        Rhesus (Rh) factor P55.0
        specified type NEC P55.8
Isolation, isolated
▶dwelling Z59.89
    family Z63.79
    social Z60.4
Isoleucinosis E71.19
Isomerism atrial appendages (with asplenia or
    polysplenia) Q20.6
Isosporiasis, isosporosis A07.3
Isovaleric acidemia E71.110
Issue of
    medical certificate Z02.79
        for disability determination Z02.71
    repeat prescription (appliance) (glasses)
        (medicinal substance, medicament,
        medicine) Z76.0
        contraception —*see* Contraception

Itch, itching —*see also* Pruritus
  baker's L23.6
  barber's B35.0
  bricklayer's L24.5
  cheese B88.0
  clam digger's B65.3
  coolie B76.9
  copra B88.0
  dew B76.9
  dhobi B35.6
  filarial —*see* Infestation, filarial
  grain B88.0
  grocer's B88.0

Itch, itching (Continued)
  ground B76.9
  harvest B88.0
  jock B35.6
  Malabar B35.5
    beard B35.0
    foot B35.3
    scalp B35.0
  meaning scabies B86
  Norwegian B86
  perianal L29.0
  poultrymen's B88.0

Itch, itching (Continued)
  sarcoptic B86
  scabies B86
  scrub B88.0
  straw B88.0
  swimmer's B65.3
  water B76.9
  winter L29.8
Ivemark's syndrome (asplenia with congenital
    heart disease) Q89.01
Ivory bones Q78.2
Ixodiasis NEC B88.8

▶ New   ⇛ Revised   ~~deleted~~ Deleted   ● Use Additional Character(s)

J

Jaccoud's syndrome —*see* Arthropathy, postrheumatic, chronic
Jackson's
  membrane Q43.3
  paralysis or syndrome G83.89
  veil Q43.3
Jacquet's dermatitis (diaper dermatitis) L22
Jadassohn-Pellizari's disease or anetoderma L90.2
Jadassohn's
  blue nevus —*see* Nevus
  intraepidermal epithelioma —*see* Neoplasm, skin, benign
Jaffe-Lichtenstein (-Uehlinger) syndrome —*see* Dysplasia, fibrous, bone NEC
Jakob-Creutzfeldt disease or syndrome —*see* Creutzfeldt-Jakob disease or syndrome
Jaksch-Luzet disease D64.89
Jamaican
⇒ neuropathy G92.8
⇒ paraplegic tropical ataxic-spastic syndrome G92.8
Janet's disease F48.8
Janiceps Q89.4
Jansky-Bielschowsky amaurotic idiocy E75.4
Japanese
  B-type encephalitis A83.0
  river fever A75.3
Jaundice (yellow) R17
  acholuric (familial) (splenomegalic) —*see also* Spherocytosis
    acquired D59.8
  breast-milk (inhibitor) P59.3
  catarrhal (acute) B15.9
    with hepatic coma B15.0
  cholestatic (benign) R17
  due to or associated with
    delayed conjugation P59.8
      associated with (due to) preterm delivery P59.0
    preterm delivery P59.0
  epidemic (catarrhal) B15.9
    with hepatic coma B15.0
    leptospiral A27.0
    spirochetal A27.0
  familial nonhemolytic (congenital) (Gilbert) E80.4
    Crigler-Najjar E80.5
  febrile (acute) B15.9
    with hepatic coma B15.0
    leptospiral A27.0
    spirochetal A27.0
  hematogenous D59.9
  hemolytic (acquired) D59.9
    congenital —*see* Spherocytosis

Jaundice (Continued)
  hemorrhagic (acute) (leptospiral) (spirochetal) A27.0
  infectious (acute) (subacute) B15.9
    with hepatic coma B15.0
    leptospiral A27.0
    spirochetal A27.0
  leptospiral (hemorrhagic) A27.0
  malignant (without coma) K72.90
    with coma K72.91
  neonatal —*see* Jaundice, newborn
  newborn P59.9
    due to or associated with
      ABO
        antibodies P55.1
        incompatibility, maternal/fetal P55.1
        isoimmunization P55.1
      absence or deficiency of enzyme system for bilirubin conjugation (congenital) P59.8
      bleeding P58.1
      breast milk inhibitors to conjugation P59.3
        associated with preterm delivery P59.0
      bruising P58.0
      Crigler-Najjar syndrome E80.5
      delayed conjugation P59.8
        associated with preterm delivery P59.0
      drugs or toxins
        given to newborn P58.42
        transmitted from mother P58.41
      excessive hemolysis P58.9
        due to
          bleeding P58.1
          bruising P58.0
          drugs or toxins
            given to newborn P58.42
            transmitted from mother P58.41
          infection P58.2
          polycythemia P58.3
          swallowed maternal blood P58.5
        specified type NEC P58.8
      galactosemia E74.21
      Gilbert syndrome E80.4
      hemolytic disease P55.9
        ABO isoimmunization P55.1
        Rh isoimmunization P55.0
        specified NEC P55.8
      hepatocellular damage P59.20
        specified NEC P59.29
      hereditary hemolytic anemia P58.8
      hypothyroidism, congenital E03.1
      incompatibility, maternal/fetal NOS P55.9
      infection P58.2

Jaundice (Continued)
  newborn (Continued)
    due to or associated with (Continued)
      inspissated bile syndrome P59.1
      isoimmunization NOS P55.9
      mucoviscidosis E84.9
      polycythemia P58.3
      preterm delivery P59.0
      Rh
        antibodies P55.0
        incompatibility, maternal/fetal P55.0
        isoimmunization P55.0
      specified cause NEC P59.8
      swallowed maternal blood P58.5
    spherocytosis (congenital) D58.0
    nonhemolytic congenital familial (Gilbert) E80.4
    nuclear, newborn —*see also* Kernicterus of newborn P57.9
    obstructive —*see also* Obstruction, bile duct K83.1
    post-immunization —*see* Hepatitis, viral, type, B
    post-transfusion —*see* Hepatitis, viral, type, B
    regurgitation —*see also* Obstruction, bile duct K83.1
    serum (homologous) (prophylactic) (therapeutic) —*see* Hepatitis, viral, type, B
    spirochetal (hemorrhagic) A27.0
    symptomatic R17
      newborn P59.9
Jaw —*see* condition
Jaw-winking phenomenon or syndrome Q07.8
Jealousy
  alcoholic F10.988
  childhood F93.8
  sibling F93.8
Jejunitis —*see* Enteritis
Jejunostomy status Z93.4
Jejunum, jejunal —*see* condition
Jensen's disease —*see* Inflammation, chorioretinal, focal, juxtapapillary
Jerks, myoclonic G25.3
Jervell-Lange-Nielsen syndrome I45.81
Jeune's disease Q77.2
Jigger disease B88.1
Job's syndrome (chronic granulomatous disease) D71
Joint —*see also* condition
  mice —*see* Loose, body, joint
    knee M23.4-●
Jordan's anomaly or syndrome D72.0
Joseph-Diamond-Blackfan anemia (congenital hypoplastic) D61.01
Jungle yellow fever A95.0
Jüngling's disease —*see* Sarcoidosis
Juvenile —*see* condition

K

Kahler's disease C90.0-•
Kakke E51.11
Kala-azar B55.0
Kallmann's syndrome E23.0
Kanner's syndrome (autism) —*see* Psychosis, childhood
Kaposi's
  dermatosis (xeroderma pigmentosum) Q82.1
  lichen ruber L44.0
    acuminatus L44.0
  sarcoma
    colon C46.4
    connective tissue C46.1
    gastrointestinal organ C46.4
    lung C46.5-•
    lymph node (multiple) C46.3
    palate (hard) (soft) C46.2
    rectum C46.4
    skin (multiple sites) C46.0
    specified site NEC C46.7
    stomach C46.4
    unspecified site C46.9
  varicelliform eruption B00.0
    vaccinia T88.1
Kartagener's syndrome or triad (sinusitis, bronchiectasis, situs inversus) Q89.3
Karyotype
  with abnormality except iso (Xq) Q96.2
  45,X Q96.0
  46,X
    iso (Xq) Q96.1
  46,XX Q98.3
    with streak gonads Q50.32
    hermaphrodite (true) Q99.1
    male Q98.3
  46,XY
    with streak gonads Q56.1
    female Q97.3
    hermaphrodite (true) Q99.1
  47,XXX Q97.0
  47,XXY Q98.0
  47,XYY Q98.5
Kaschin-Beck disease —*see* Disease, Kaschin-Beck
Katayama's disease or fever B65.2
Kawasaki's syndrome M30.3
Kayser-Fleischer ring (cornea) (pseudosclerosis) H18.04-•
Kaznelson's syndrome (congenital hypoplastic anemia) D61.01
Kearns-Sayre syndrome H49.81-•
Kedani fever A75.3
Kelis L91.0
Kelly (-Patterson) syndrome (sideropenic dysphagia) D50.1
Keloid, cheloid L91.0
  acne L73.0
  Addison's L94.0
  cornea —*see* Opacity, cornea
  Hawkin's L91.0
  scar L91.0
Keloma L91.0
Kenya fever A77.1
Keratectasia —*see also* Ectasia, cornea
  congenital Q13.4
Keratinization of alveolar ridge mucosa
  excessive K13.23
  minimal K13.22
Keratinized residual ridge mucosa
  excessive K13.23
  minimal K13.22
Keratitis (nodular) (nonulcerative) (simple) (zonular) H16.9
  with ulceration (central) (marginal) (perforated) (ring) —*see* Ulcer, cornea
  actinic —*see* Photokeratitis
  arborescens (herpes simplex) B00.52
  areolar H16.11-•
  bullosa H16.8

Keratitis (Continued)
  deep H16.309
    specified type NEC H16.399
  dendritic (a) (herpes simplex) B00.52
  disciform (is) (herpes simplex) B00.52
    varicella B01.81
  filamentary H16.12-•
  gonococcal (congenital or prenatal) A54.33
  herpes, herpetic (simplex) B00.52
    zoster B02.33
  in (due to)
    acanthamebiasis B60.13
    adenovirus B30.0
    exanthema —*see also* Exanthem B09
    herpes (simplex) virus B00.52
    measles B05.81
    syphilis A50.31
    tuberculosis A18.52
    zoster B02.33
  interstitial (nonsyphilitic) H16.30-•
    diffuse H16.32-•
    herpes, herpetic (simplex) B00.52
      zoster B02.33
    sclerosing H16.33-•
    specified type NEC H16.39-•
    syphilitic (congenital) (late) A50.31
    tuberculous A18.52
  macular H16.11-•
  nummular H16.11-•
  oyster shuckers' H16.8
  parenchymatous —*see* Keratitis, interstitial
  petrificans H16.8
  postmeasles B05.81
  punctata
    leprosa A30.9 [H16.14-•]
    syphilitic (profunda) A50.31
  punctate H16.14-•
  purulent H16.8
  rosacea L71.8
  sclerosing H16.33-•
  specified type NEC H16.8
  stellate H16.11-•
  striate H16.11-•
  superficial H16.10-•
    with conjunctivitis —*see* Keratoconjunctivitis
    due to light —*see* Photokeratitis
  suppurative H16.8
  syphilitic (congenital) (prenatal) A50.31
  trachomatous A71.1
    sequelae B94.0
  tuberculous A18.52
  vesicular H16.8
  xerotic —*see also* Keratomalacia H16.8
    vitamin A deficiency E50.4
Keratoacanthoma L85.8
Keratocele —*see* Descemetocele
Keratoconjunctivitis H16.20-•
  Acanthamoeba B60.13
  adenoviral B30.0
  epidemic B30.0
  exanthema H16.21-•
  herpes, herpetic (simplex) B00.52
    zoster B02.33
  in exanthema —*see also* Exanthem B09
  infectious B30.0
  lagophthalmic —*see* Keratoconjunctivitis, specified type NEC
  neurotrophic H16.23-•
  phlyctenular H16.25-•
  postmeasles B05.81
  shipyard B30.0
  sicca (Sjogren's) M35.0-•
    not Sjogren's H16.22-•
  specified type NEC H16.29-•
  tuberculous (phlyctenular) A18.52
  vernal H16.26-•
Keratoconus H18.60-•
  congenital Q13.4
  stable H18.61-•
  unstable H18.62-•

Keratocyst (dental) (odontogenic) —*see* Cyst, calcifying odontogenic
Keratoderma, keratodermia (congenital) (palmaris et plantaris) (symmetrical) Q82.8
  acquired L85.1
    in diseases classified elsewhere L86
  climactericum L85.1
  gonococcal A54.89
  gonorrheal A54.89
  punctata L85.2
  Reiter's —*see* Reiter's disease
Keratodermatocele —*see* Descemetocele
Keratoglobus H18.79
  congenital Q15.8
    with glaucoma Q15.0
Keratohemia —*see* Pigmentation, cornea, stromal
Keratoiritis —*see also* Iridocyclitis
  syphilitic A50.39
  tuberculous A18.54
Keratoma L57.0
  palmaris and plantaris hereditarium Q82.8
  senile L57.0
Keratomalacia H18.44-•
  vitamin A deficiency E50.4
Keratomegaly Q13.4
Keratomycosis B49
  nigrans, nigricans (palmaris) B36.1
Keratopathy H18.9
  band H18.42-•
  bullous H18.1-•
  bullous (aphakic), following cataract surgery H59.01-•
Keratoscleritis, tuberculous A18.52
Keratosis L57.0
  actinic L57.0
  arsenical L85.8
  congenital, specified NEC Q80.8
  female genital NEC N94.89
  follicularis Q82.8
    acquired L11.0
    congenita Q82.8
    et parafollicularis in cutem penetrans L87.0
    spinulosa (decalvans) Q82.8
    vitamin A deficiency E50.8
  gonococcal A54.89
  male genital (external) N50.89
  nigricans L83
  obturans, external ear (canal) —*see* Cholesteatoma, external ear
  palmaris et plantaris (inherited) (symmetrical) Q82.8
    acquired L85.1
  penile N48.89
  pharynx J39.2
  pilaris, acquired L85.8
  punctata (palmaris et plantaris) L85.2
  scrotal N50.89
  seborrheic L82.1
    inflamed L82.0
  senile L57.0
  solar L57.0
  tonsillaris J35.8
  vagina N89.4
  vegetans Q82.8
  vitamin A deficiency E50.8
  vocal cord J38.3
Kerato-uveitis —*see* Iridocyclitis
Kerion (celsi) B35.0
Kernicterus of newborn (not due to isoimmunization) P57.9
  due to isoimmunization (conditions in P55.0-P55.9) P57.0
  specified type NEC P57.8
Kerunoparalysis T75.09
Keshan disease E59
Ketoacidosis E87.2
  diabetic —*see* Diabetes, by type, with ketoacidosis
Ketonuria R82.4

▶ New ⇒ Revised ~~deleted~~ Deleted • Use Additional Character(s)

Ketosis NEC E88.89
  diabetic —*see* Diabetes, by type, with
    ketoacidosis
Kew Garden fever A79.1
Kidney —*see* condition
Kienböck's disease —*see also* Osteochondrosis,
    juvenile, hand, carpal lunate
  adult M93.1
Kimmelstiel (-Wilson) disease —*see* Diabetes,
    Kimmelstiel (-Wilson) disease
Kimura disease D21.9
  specified site (*see* Neoplasm, connective
    tissue benign)
Kink, kinking
  artery I77.1
  hair (acquired) L67.8
  ileum or intestine —*see* Obstruction,
    intestine
  Lane's —*see* Obstruction, intestine
  organ or site, congenital NEC —*see* Anomaly,
    by site
  ureter (pelvic junction) N13.5
    with
      hydronephrosis N13.1
        with infection N13.6
      pyelonephritis (chronic) N11.1
    congenital Q62.39
  vein(s) I87.8
    caval I87.1
    peripheral I87.1
Kinnier Wilson's disease (hepatolenticular
    degeneration) E83.01
Kissing spine M48.20
  cervical region M48.22
  cervicothoracic region M48.23
  lumbar region M48.26
  lumbosacral region M48.27
  occipito-atlanto-axial region M48.21
  thoracic region M48.24
  thoracolumbar region M48.25
Klatskin's tumor C24.0
Klauder's disease A26.8
Klebs' disease —*see also* Glomerulonephritis
    N05.-●
Klebsiella (K.) pneumoniae, as cause of
    disease classified elsewhere B96.1
Klein (e)-Levin syndrome G47.13
Kleptomania F63.2
Klinefelter's syndrome Q98.4
  karyotype 47,XXY Q98.0
  male with more than two X chromosomes
    Q98.1
Klippel-Feil deficiency, disease, or syndrome
    (brevicollis) Q76.1
Klippel's disease I67.2
Klippel-Trenaunay (-Weber) syndrome
    Q87.2
Klumpke (-Déjerine) palsy, paralysis (birth)
    (newborn) P14.1
Knee —*see* condition
Knock knee (acquired) M21.06-●
  congenital Q74.1

Knot(s)
  intestinal, syndrome (volvulus) K56.2
    surfer S89.8-●
  umbilical cord (true) O69.2
Knotting (of)
  hair L67.8
  intestine K56.2
Knuckle pad (Garrod's) M72.1
Koch's
  infection —*see* Tuberculosis
  relapsing fever A68.9
Koch-Weeks' conjunctivitis —*see*
    Conjunctivitis, acute, mucopurulent
Köebner's syndrome Q81.8
Köenig's disease (osteochondritis dissecans) —
    see Osteochondritis, dissecans
Köhler-Pellegrini-Steida disease or syndrome
    (calcification, knee joint) —*see* Bursitis,
    tibial collateral
Köhler's disease
  patellar —*see* Osteochondrosis, juvenile,
    patella
  tarsal navicular —*see* Osteochondrosis,
    juvenile, tarsus
Koilonychia L60.3
  congenital Q84.6
Kojevnikov's, epilepsy —*see* Kozhevnikof's
    epilepsy
Koplik's spots B05.9
Kopp's asthma E32.8
Korsakoff's (Wernicke) disease, psychosis or
    syndrome (alcoholic) F10.96
  with dependence F10.26
  drug-induced
    due to drug abuse —*see* Abuse, drug, by
      type, with amnestic disorder
    due to drug dependence —*see* Dependence,
      drug, by type, with amnestic disorder
  nonalcoholic F04
Korsakov's disease, psychosis or syndrome —
    see Korsakoff's disease
Korsakow's disease, psychosis or syndrome —
    see Korsakoff's disease
Kostmann's disease or syndrome (infantile
    genetic agranulocytosis) —*see*
    Agranulocytosis
Kozhevnikof's epilepsy G40.109
  intractable G40.119
    with status epilepticus G40.111
    without status epilepticus G40.119
  not intractable G40.109
    with status epilepticus G40.101
    without status epilepticus G40.109
Krabbe's
  disease E75.23
  syndrome, congenital muscle hypoplasia
    Q79.8
Kraepelin-Morel disease —*see* Schizophrenia
Kraft-Weber-Dimitri disease Q85.8
Kraurosis
  ani K62.89
  penis N48.0

Kraurosis (*Continued*)
  vagina N89.8
  vulva N90.4
Kreotoxism A05.9
Krukenberg's
  spindle —*see* Pigmentation, cornea, posterior
  tumor C79.6-●
Kufs' disease E75.4
Kugelberg-Welander disease G12.1
Kuhnt-Junius degeneration —*see also*
    Degeneration, macula H35.32-●
Kümmell's disease or spondylitis —*see*
    Spondylopathy, traumatic
Kupffer cell sarcoma C22.3
Kuru A81.81
Kussmaul's
  disease M30.0
  respiration E87.2
    in diabetic acidosis —*see* Diabetes, by type,
      with ketoacidosis
Kwashiorkor E40
  marasmic, marasmus type E42
Kyasanur Forest disease A98.2
Kyphoscoliosis, kyphoscoliotic (acquired) —
    see also Scoliosis M41.9
  congenital Q67.5
  heart (disease) I27.1
  sequelae of rickets E64.3
  tuberculous A18.01
Kyphosis, kyphotic (acquired) M40.209
  cervical region M40.202
  cervicothoracic region M40.203
  congenital Q76.419
    cervical region Q76.412
    cervicothoracic region Q76.413
    occipito-atlanto-axial region Q76.411
    thoracic region Q76.414
    thoracolumbar region Q76.415
  Morquio-Brailsford type (spinal) —*see also*
    subcategory M49.8 E76.219
  postlaminectomy M96.3
  postradiation therapy M96.2
  postural (adolescent) M40.00
    cervicothoracic region M40.03
    thoracic region M40.04
    thoracolumbar region M40.05
  secondary NEC M40.10
    cervical region M40.12
    cervicothoracic region M40.13
    thoracic region M40.14
    thoracolumbar region M40.15
  sequelae of rickets E64.3
  specified type NEC M40.299
    cervical region M40.292
    cervicothoracic region M40.293
    thoracic region M40.294
    thoracolumbar region M40.295
  syphilitic, congenital A50.56
  thoracic region M40.204
  thoracolumbar region M40.205
  tuberculous A18.01
Kyrle disease L87.0

K

L

Labia, labium —*see* condition
Labile
 blood pressure R09.89
 vasomotor system I73.9
Labioglossal paralysis G12.29
Labium leporinum —*see* Cleft, lip
Labor —*see* Delivery
Labored breathing —*see* Hyperventilation
Labyrinthitis (circumscribed) (destructive)
 (diffuse) (inner ear) (latent) (purulent)
 (suppurative) (*see also* subcategory)
 H83.0
 syphilitic A52.79
Laceration
 with abortion —*see* Abortion, by type,
  complicated by laceration of pelvic
  organs
 abdomen, abdominal
  wall S31.119
   with
    foreign body S31.129
    penetration into peritoneal cavity
     S31.619
     with foreign body S31.629
   epigastric region S31.112
    with
     foreign body S31.122
     penetration into peritoneal cavity
      S31.612
      with foreign body S31.622
   left
    lower quadrant S31.114
     with
      foreign body S31.124
      penetration into peritoneal cavity
       S31.614
       with foreign body S31.624
    upper quadrant S31.111
     with
      foreign body S31.121
      penetration into peritoneal cavity
       S31.611
       with foreign body S31.621
   periumbilic region S31.115
    with
     foreign body S31.125
     penetration into peritoneal cavity
      S31.615
      with foreign body S31.625
   right
    lower quadrant S31.113
     with
      foreign body S31.123
      penetration into peritoneal cavity
       S31.613
       with foreign body S31.623
    upper quadrant S31.110
     with
      foreign body S31.120
      penetration into peritoneal cavity
       S31.610
       with foreign body S31.620
 accidental, complicating surgery —*see*
  Complications, surgical, accidental
  puncture or laceration
 Achilles tendon S86.02-•
 adrenal gland S37.813
 alveolar (process) —*see* Laceration, oral cavity
 ankle S91.01-•
  with
   foreign body S91.02-•
 antecubital space —*see* Laceration, elbow
 anus (sphincter) S31.831
  with
   ectopic or molar pregnancy O08.6
   foreign body S31.832
  complicating delivery —*see* Delivery,
   complicated, by, laceration, anus
   (sphincter)

Laceration *(Continued)*
 anus *(Continued)*
  following ectopic or molar pregnancy
   O08.6
  nontraumatic, nonpuerperal —*see* Fissure,
   anus
 arm (upper) S41.11-•
  with foreign body S41.12-•
  lower —*see* Laceration, forearm
 auditory canal (external) (meatus) —*see*
  Laceration, ear
 auricle, ear —*see* Laceration, ear
 axilla —*see* Laceration, arm
 back —*see also* Laceration, thorax, back
  lower S31.010
   with
    foreign body S31.020
     with penetration into
      retroperitoneal space S31.021
     penetration into retroperitoneal space
      S31.011
 bile duct S36.13
 bladder S37.23
  with ectopic or molar pregnancy O08.6
  following ectopic or molar pregnancy
   O08.6
  obstetrical trauma O71.5
 blood vessel —*see* Injury, blood vessel
 bowel —*see also* Laceration, intestine
  with ectopic or molar pregnancy O08.6
  complicating abortion —*see* Abortion,
   by type, complicated by, specified
   condition NEC
  following ectopic or molar pregnancy
   O08.6
  obstetrical trauma O71.5
 brain (any part) (cortex) (diffuse)
  (membrane) —*see also* Injury,
  intracranial, diffuse
  during birth P10.8
   with hemorrhage P10.1
  focal —*see* Injury, intracranial, focal brain
   injury
 brainstem S06.38-•
 breast S21.01-•
  with foreign body S21.02-•
 broad ligament S37.893
  with ectopic or molar pregnancy O08.6
  following ectopic or molar pregnancy
   O08.6
  laceration syndrome N83.8
  obstetrical trauma O71.6
  syndrome (laceration) N83.8
 buttock S31.801
  with foreign body S31.802
  left S31.821
   with foreign body S31.822
  right S31.811
   with foreign body S31.812
 calf —*see* Laceration, leg
 canaliculus lacrimalis —*see* Laceration,
  eyelid
 canthus, eye —*see* Laceration, eyelid
 capsule, joint —*see* Sprain
 causing eversion of cervix uteri (old) N86
 central (perineal), complicating delivery
  O70.9
 cerebellum, traumatic S06.37-•
 cerebral S06.33-•
  during birth P10.8
   with hemorrhage P10.1
  left side S06.32-•
  right side S06.31-•
 cervix (uteri)
  with ectopic or molar pregnancy O08.6
  following ectopic or molar pregnancy
   O08.6
  nonpuerperal, nontraumatic N88.1
  obstetrical trauma (current) O71.3
  old (postpartal) N88.1
  traumatic S37.63

Laceration *(Continued)*
 cheek (external) S01.41-•
  with foreign body S01.42-•
  internal —*see* Laceration, oral cavity
 chest wall —*see* Laceration, thorax
 chin —*see* Laceration, head, specified site
  NEC
 chordae tendinae NEC I51.1
  concurrent with acute myocardial
   infarction —*see* Infarct, myocardium
  following acute myocardial infarction
   (current complication) I23.4
 clitoris —*see* Laceration, vulva
 colon —*see* Laceration, intestine, large,
  colon
 common bile duct S36.13
 cortex (cerebral) —*see* Injury, intracranial,
  diffuse
 costal region —*see* Laceration, thorax
 cystic duct S36.13
 diaphragm S27.803
 digit(s)
  foot —*see* Laceration, toe
  hand —*see* Laceration, finger
 duodenum S36.430
 ear (canal) (external) S01.31-•
  with foreign body S01.32-•
  drum S09.2-•
 elbow S51.01-•
  with
   foreign body S51.02-•
 epididymis —*see* Laceration, testis
 epigastric region —*see* Laceration, abdomen,
  wall, epigastric region
➥esophagus K22.89
  traumatic
   cervical S11.21
    with foreign body S11.22
   thoracic S27.813
 eye (ball) S05.3-•
  with prolapse or loss of intraocular tissue
   S05.2-•
  penetrating S05.6-•
 eyebrow —*see* Laceration, eyelid
 eyelid S01.11-•
  with foreign body S01.12-•
 face NEC —*see* Laceration, head, specified
  site NEC
 fallopian tube S37.539
  bilateral S37.532
  unilateral S37.531
 finger(s) S61.219
  with
   damage to nail S61.319
    with
     foreign body S61.329
   foreign body S61.229
  index S61.218
   with
    damage to nail S61.318
     with
      foreign body S61.328
    foreign body S61.228
   left S61.211
    with
     damage to nail S61.311
      with
       foreign body S61.321
     foreign body S61.221
   right S61.210
    with
     damage to nail S61.310
      with
       foreign body S61.320
     foreign body S61.220
  little S61.218
   with
    damage to nail S61.318
     with
      foreign body S61.328
    foreign body S61.228

▶ New ⇒ Revised ~~deleted~~ Deleted • Use Additional Character(s)

Laceration *(Continued)*
finger *(Continued)*
little *(Continued)*
left S61.217
with
damage to nail S61.317
with
foreign body S61.327
foreign body S61.227
right S61.216
with
damage to nail S61.316
with
foreign body S61.326
foreign body S61.226
middle S61.218
with
damage to nail S61.318
with
foreign body S61.328
foreign body S61.228
left S61.213
with
damage to nail S61.313
with
foreign body S61.323
foreign body S61.223
right S61.212
with
damage to nail S61.312
with
foreign body S61.322
foreign body S61.222
ring S61.218
with
damage to nail S61.318
with
foreign body S61.328
foreign body S61.228
left S61.215
with
damage to nail S61.315
with
foreign body S61.325
foreign body S61.225
right S61.214
with
damage to nail S61.314
with
foreign body S61.324
foreign body S61.224
flank S31.119
with foreign body S31.129
foot (except toe(s) alone) S91.319
with foreign body S91.329
left S91.312
with foreign body S91.322
right S91.311
with foreign body S91.321
toe —*see* Laceration, toe
forearm S51.819
with
foreign body S51.829
elbow only —*see* Laceration, elbow
left S51.812
with
foreign body S51.822
right S51.811
with
foreign body S51.821
forehead S01.81
with foreign body S01.82
fourchette O70.0
with ectopic or molar pregnancy O08.6
complicating delivery O70.0
following ectopic or molar pregnancy O08.6
gallbladder S36.123

genital organs, external
female S31.512
with foreign body S31.522
vagina —*see* Laceration, vagina
vulva —*see* Laceration, vulva
male S31.511
with foreign body S31.521
penis —*see* Laceration, penis
scrotum —*see* Laceration, scrotum
testis —*see* Laceration, testis
groin —*see* Laceration, abdomen, wall
gum —*see* Laceration, oral cavity
hand S61.419
with
foreign body S61.429
finger —*see* Laceration, finger
left S61.412
with
foreign body S61.422
right S61.411
with
foreign body S61.421
thumb —*see* Laceration, thumb
head S01.91
with foreign body S01.92
cheek —*see* Laceration, cheek
ear —*see* Laceration, ear
eyelid —*see* Laceration, eyelid
lip —*see* Laceration, lip
nose —*see* Laceration, nose
oral cavity —*see* Laceration, oral cavity
scalp S01.01
with foreign body S01.02
specified site NEC S01.81
with foreign body S01.82
temporomandibular area —*see* Laceration, cheek
heart —*see* Injury, heart, laceration
heel —*see* Laceration, foot
hepatic duct S36.13
hip S71.019
with foreign body S71.029
left S71.012
with foreign body S71.022
right S71.011
with foreign body S71.021
hymen —*see* Laceration, vagina
hypochondrium —*see* Laceration, abdomen, wall
hypogastric region —*see* Laceration, abdomen, wall
ileum S36.438
inguinal region —*see* Laceration, abdomen, wall
instep —*see* Laceration, foot
internal organ —*see* Injury, by site
interscapular region —*see* Laceration, thorax, back
intestine
large
colon S36.539
ascending S36.530
descending S36.532
sigmoid S36.533
specified site NEC S36.538
rectum S36.63
transverse S36.531
small S36.439
duodenum S36.430
specified site NEC S36.438
intra-abdominal organ S36.93
intestine —*see* Laceration, intestine
liver —*see* Laceration, liver
pancreas —*see* Laceration, pancreas
peritoneum S36.81
specified site NEC S36.893
spleen —*see* Laceration, spleen
stomach —*see* Laceration, stomach

intracranial NEC —*see also* Injury, intracranial, diffuse
birth injury P10.9
jaw —*see* Laceration, head, specified site NEC
jejunum S36.438
joint capsule —*see* Sprain, by site
kidney S37.03-●
major (greater than 3 cm) (massive) (stellate) S37.06-●
minor (less than 1 cm) S37.04-●
moderate (1 to 3 cm) S37.05-●
multiple S37.06-●
knee S81.01-●
with foreign body S81.02-●
labium (majus) (minus) —*see* Laceration, vulva
lacrimal duct —*see* Laceration, eyelid
large intestine —*see* Laceration, intestine, large
larynx S11.011
with foreign body S11.012
leg (lower) S81.819
with foreign body S81.829
foot —*see* Laceration, foot
knee —*see* Laceration, knee
left S81.812
with foreign body S81.822
right S81.811
with foreign body S81.821
upper —*see* Laceration, thigh
ligament —*see* Sprain
lip S01.511
with foreign body S01.521
liver S36.113
major (stellate) S36.116
minor S36.114
moderate S36.115
loin —*see* Laceration, abdomen, wall
lower back —*see* Laceration, back, lower
lumbar region —*see* Laceration, back, lower
lung S27.339
bilateral S27.332
unilateral S27.331
malar region —*see* Laceration, head, specified site NEC
mammary —*see* Laceration, breast
mastoid region —*see* Laceration, head, specified site NEC
meninges —*see* Injury, intracranial, diffuse
meniscus —*see* Tear, meniscus
mesentery S36.893
mesosalpinx S37.893
mouth —*see* Laceration, oral cavity
muscle —*see* Injury, muscle, by site, laceration
nail
finger —*see* Laceration, finger, with damage to nail
toe —*see* Laceration, toe, with damage to nail
nasal (septum) (sinus) —*see* Laceration, nose
nasopharynx —*see* Laceration, head, specified site NEC
neck S11.91
with foreign body S11.92
involving
cervical esophagus S11.21
with foreign body S11.22
larynx —*see* Laceration, larynx
pharynx —*see* Laceration, pharynx
thyroid gland —*see* Laceration, thyroid gland
trachea —*see* Laceration, trachea
specified site NEC S11.81
with foreign body S11.82
nerve —*see* Injury, nerve
nose (septum) (sinus) S01.21
with foreign body S01.22
ocular NOS S05.3-●
adnexa NOS S01.11-●

Laceration (Continued)
oral cavity S01.512
   with foreign body S01.522
orbit (eye) —see Wound, open, ocular, orbit
ovary S37.439
   bilateral S37.432
   unilateral S37.431
palate —see Laceration, oral cavity
palm —see Laceration, hand
pancreas S36.239
   body S36.231
      major S36.261
      minor S36.241
      moderate S36.251
   head S36.230
      major S36.260
      minor S36.240
      moderate S36.250
   major S36.269
   minor S36.249
   moderate S36.259
   tail S36.232
      major S36.262
      minor S36.242
      moderate S36.252
pelvic S31.010
   with
      foreign body S31.020
         penetration into retroperitoneal cavity S31.021
      penetration into retroperitoneal cavity S31.011
   floor —see also Laceration, back, lower
      with ectopic or molar pregnancy O08.6
      complicating delivery O70.1
      following ectopic or molar pregnancy O08.6
      old (postpartal) N81.89
   organ S37.93
      with ectopic or molar pregnancy O08.6
      adrenal gland S37.813
      bladder S37.23
      fallopian tube —see Laceration, fallopian tube
      following ectopic or molar pregnancy O08.6
      kidney —see Laceration, kidney
      obstetrical trauma O71.5
      ovary —see Laceration, ovary
      prostate S37.823
      specified site NEC S37.893
      ureter S37.13
      urethra S37.33
      uterus S37.63
penis S31.21
   with foreign body S31.22
perineum
   female S31.41
      with
         ectopic or molar pregnancy O08.6
         foreign body S31.42
      during delivery O70.9
         first degree O70.0
         fourth degree O70.3
         second degree O70.1
         third degree —see also Delivery, complicated, by, laceration, perineum, third degree O70.20
      old (postpartal) N81.89
      postpartal N81.89
      secondary (postpartal) O90.1
   male S31.119
      with foreign body S31.129
periocular area (with or without lacrimal passages) —see Laceration, eyelid
peritoneum S36.893
periumbilic region —see Laceration, abdomen, wall, periumbilic

Laceration (Continued)
periurethral tissue —see Laceration, urethra
phalanges
   finger —see Laceration, finger
   toe —see Laceration, toe
pharynx S11.21
   with foreign body S11.22
pinna —see Laceration, ear
popliteal space —see Laceration, knee
prepuce —see Laceration, penis
prostate S37.823
pubic region S31.119
   with foreign body S31.129
pudendum —see Laceration, genital organs, external
rectovaginal septum —see Laceration, vagina
rectum S36.63
retroperitoneum S36.893
round ligament S37.893
sacral region —see Laceration, back, lower
sacroiliac region —see Laceration, back, lower
salivary gland —see Laceration, oral cavity
scalp S01.01
   with foreign body S01.02
scapular region —see Laceration, shoulder
scrotum S31.31
   with foreign body S31.32
seminal vesicle S37.893
shin —see Laceration, leg
shoulder S41.019
   with foreign body S41.029
   left S41.012
      with foreign body S41.022
   right S41.011
      with foreign body S41.021
small intestine —see Laceration, intestine, small
spermatic cord —see Laceration, testis
spinal cord (meninges) —see also Injury, spinal cord, by region
   due to injury at birth P11.5
   newborn (birth injury) P11.5
spleen S36.039
   major (massive) (stellate) S36.032
   moderate S36.031
   superficial (minor) S36.030
sternal region —see Laceration, thorax, front
stomach S36.33
submaxillary region —see Laceration, head, specified site NEC
submental region —see Laceration, head, specified site NEC
subungual
   finger(s) —see Laceration, finger, with damage to nail
   toe(s) —see Laceration, toe, with damage to nail
suprarenal gland —see Laceration, adrenal gland
temple, temporal region —see Laceration, head, specified site NEC
temporomandibular area —see Laceration, cheek
tendon —see Injury, muscle, by site, laceration
   Achilles S86.02-●
tentorium cerebelli —see Injury, intracranial, diffuse
testis S31.31
   with foreign body S31.32
thigh S71.11-●
   with foreign body S71.12-●
thorax, thoracic (wall) S21.91
   with foreign body S21.92
      back S21.22-●
         with penetration into thoracic cavity S21.42-●
      front S21.12-●
         with penetration into thoracic cavity S21.32-●

Laceration (Continued)
thorax, thoracic (Continued)
   back S21.21-●
      with
         foreign body S21.22-●
            with penetration into thoracic cavity S21.42-●
         penetration into thoracic cavity S21.41-●
   breast —see Laceration, breast
   front S21.11-●
      with
         foreign body S21.12-●
            with penetration into thoracic cavity S21.32-●
         penetration into thoracic cavity S21.31-●
thumb S61.019
   with
      damage to nail S61.119
         with
            foreign body S61.129
      foreign body S61.029
   left S61.012
      with
         damage to nail S61.112
            with
               foreign body S61.122
         foreign body S61.022
   right S61.011
      with
         damage to nail S61.111
            with
               foreign body S61.121
         foreign body S61.021
thyroid gland S11.11
   with foreign body S11.12
toe(s) S91.119
   with
      damage to nail S91.219
         with
            foreign body S91.229
      foreign body S91.129
   great S91.113
      with
         damage to nail S91.213
            with
               foreign body S91.223
         foreign body S91.123
      left S91.112
         with
            damage to nail S91.212
               with
                  foreign body S91.222
            foreign body S91.122
      right S91.111
         with
            damage to nail S91.211
               with
                  foreign body S91.221
            foreign body S91.121
   lesser S91.116
      with
         damage to nail S91.216
            with
               foreign body S91.226
         foreign body S91.126
      left S91.115
         with
            damage to nail S91.215
               with
                  foreign body S91.225
            foreign body S91.125
      right S91.114
         with
            damage to nail S91.214
               with
                  foreign body S91.224
            foreign body S91.124
tongue —see Laceration, oral cavity

▶ New   ➠ Revised   ~~deleted~~ Deleted   ● Use Additional Character(s)

Laceration *(Continued)*
trachea S11.021
　with foreign body S11.022
tunica vaginalis —*see* Laceration, testis
tympanum, tympanic membrane —*see*
　　Laceration, ear, drum
umbilical region S31.115
　with foreign body S31.125
ureter S37.13
urethra S37.33
　with or following ectopic or molar
　　pregnancy O08.6
　obstetrical trauma O71.5
urinary organ NEC S37.893
uterus S37.63
　with ectopic or molar pregnancy O08.6
　following ectopic or molar pregnancy O08.6
　nonpuerperal, nontraumatic N85.8
　obstetrical trauma NEC O71.81
　old (postpartal) N85.8
uvula —*see* Laceration, oral cavity
vagina S31.41
　with
　　ectopic or molar pregnancy O08.6
　　foreign body S31.42
　during delivery O71.4
　　with perineal laceration —*see* Laceration,
　　　perineum, female, during delivery
　following ectopic or molar pregnancy
　　O08.6
　nonpuerperal, nontraumatic N89.8
　old (postpartal) N89.8
vas deferens S37.893
vesical —*see* Laceration, bladder
vocal cords S11.031
　with foreign body S11.032
vulva S31.41
　with
　　ectopic or molar pregnancy O08.6
　　foreign body S31.42
　complicating delivery O70.0
　following ectopic or molar pregnancy
　　O08.6
　nonpuerperal, nontraumatic N90.89
　old (postpartal) N90.89
wrist S61.519
　with
　　foreign body S61.529
　left S61.512
　　with
　　　foreign body S61.522
　right S61.511
　　with
　　　foreign body S61.521
Lack of
achievement in school Z55.3
adequate
➠food Z59.48
　intermaxillary vertical dimension of fully
　　erupted teeth M26.36
　sleep Z72.820
appetite (*see* Anorexia) R63.0
awareness R41.9
care
　in home Z74.2
　of infant (at or after birth) T76.02
　　confirmed T74.02
cognitive functions R41.9
coordination R27.9
　ataxia R27.0
　specified type NEC R27.8
development (physiological) R62.50
　failure to thrive (child over 28 days old)
　　R62.51
　　adult R62.7
　　newborn P92.6
　short stature R62.52
　specified type NEC R62.59
energy R53.83
financial resources Z59.6

Lack of *(Continued)*
➠food Z59.48
growth R62.52
heating Z59.1
➠housing (permanent) (temporary) Z59.00
　adequate Z59.1
learning experiences in childhood Z62.898
leisure time (affecting life-style) Z73.2
material resources Z59.9
memory —*see also* Amnesia
　mild, following organic brain damage
　　F06.8
ovulation N97.0
parental supervision or control of child Z62.0
person able to render necessary care Z74.2
physical exercise Z72.3
play experience in childhood Z62.898
posterior occlusal support M26.57
relaxation (affecting life-style) Z73.2
▶safe drinking water Z58.6
sexual
　desire F52.0
　enjoyment F52.1
➠shelter Z59.02
sleep (adequate) Z72.820
supervision of child by parent Z62.0
support, posterior occlusal M26.57
water T73.1
▶safe drinking Z58.6
Lacrimal —*see* condition
Lacrimation, abnormal —*see* Epiphora
Lacrimonasal duct —*see* condition
Lactation, lactating (breast) (puerperal,
　postpartum)
associated
　cracked nipple O92.13
　retracted nipple O92.03
defective O92.4
disorder NEC O92.79
excessive O92.6
failed (complete) O92.3
　partial O92.4
mastitis NEC —*see* Mastitis, obstetric
mother (care and/or examination) Z39.1
nonpuerperal N64.3
Lacticemia, excessive E87.2
Lacunar skull Q75.8
Laennec's cirrhosis K70.30
　with ascites K70.31
　nonalcoholic K74.69
Lafora's disease —*see* Epilepsy, generalized,
　idiopathic
Lag, lid (nervous) —*see* Retraction, lid
Lagophthalmos (eyelid) (nervous) H02.209
bilateral, upper and lower eyelids H02.20C
cicatricial H02.219
　bilateral, upper and lower eyelids H02.21C
　left H02.216
　　lower H02.215
　　upper H02.214
　　upper and lower eyelids H02.21B
　right H02.213
　　lower H02.212
　　upper H02.211
　　upper and lower eyelids H02.21A
keratoconjunctivitis —*see* Keratoconjunctivitis
left H02.206
　lower H02.205
　upper H02.204
　upper and lower eyelids H02.20B
mechanical H02.229
　bilateral, upper and lower eyelids H02.22C
　left H02.226
　　lower H02.225
　　upper H02.224
　　upper and lower eyelids H02.22B
　right H02.223
　　lower H02.222
　　upper H02.221
　　upper and lower eyelids H02.22A

Lagophthalmos *(Continued)*
paralytic H02.239
　bilateral, upper and lower eyelids H02.23C
　left H02.236
　　lower H02.235
　　upper H02.234
　　upper and lower eyelids H02.23B
　right H02.233
　　lower H02.232
　　upper H02.231
　　upper and lower eyelids H02.23A
right H02.203
　lower H02.202
　upper H02.201
　upper and lower eyelids H02.20A
Laki-Lorand factor deficiency —*see* Defect,
　coagulation, specified type NEC
Lalling F80.0
Lambert-Eaton syndrome —*see* Syndrome,
　Lambert-Eaton
Lambliasis, lambliosis A07.1
Landau-Kleffner syndrome —*see* Epilepsy,
　specified NEC
Landouzy-Déjérine dystrophy or
　facioscapulohumeral atrophy G71.02
Landouzy's disease (icterohemorrhagic
　leptospirosis) A27.0
Landry-Guillain-Barré, syndrome or paralysis
　G61.0
Landry's disease or paralysis G61.0
Lane's
band Q43.3
kink —*see* Obstruction, intestine
syndrome K90.2
Langdon Down's syndrome —*see* Trisomy, 21
Lapsed immunization schedule status Z28.3
Large
baby (regardless of gestational age) (4000g to
　4499g) P08.1
ear, congenital Q17.1
physiological cup Q14.2
stature R68.89
Large-for-dates NEC (infant) (4000g to 4499g)
　P08.1
affecting management of pregnancy O36.6-●
exceptionally (4500g or more) P08.0
Larsen-Johansson disease
orosteochondrosis —*see* Osteochondrosis,
　juvenile, patella
Larsen's syndrome (flattened facies and
　multiple congenital dislocations) Q74.8
Larva migrans
cutaneous B76.9
　Ancylostoma B76.0
visceral B83.0
Laryngeal —*see* condition
Laryngismus (stridulus) J38.5
congenital P28.89
diphtheritic A36.2
Laryngitis (acute) (edematous) (fibrinous)
　(infective) (infiltrative) (malignant)
　(membranous) (phlegmonous)
　(pneumococcal) (pseudomembranous)
　(septic) (subglottic) (suppurative)
　(ulcerative) J04.0
with
　influenza, flu, or grippe —*see* Influenza,
　　with, laryngitis
　tracheitis (acute) —*see* Laryngotracheitis
atrophic J37.0
catarrhal J37.0
chronic J37.0
　with tracheitis (chronic) J37.1
diphtheritic A36.2
due to external agent —*see* Inflammation,
　respiratory, upper, due to
Hemophilus influenzae J04.0
H. influenzae J04.0
hypertrophic J37.0
influenzal —*see* Influenza, with, respiratory
　manifestations NEC

Laryngitis *(Continued)*
  obstructive J05.0
  sicca J37.0
  spasmodic J05.0
    acute J04.0
  streptococcal J04.0
  stridulous J05.0
  syphilitic (late) A52.73
    congenital A50.59 *[J99]*
      early A50.03 *[J99]*
  tuberculous A15.5
  Vincent's A69.1
Laryngocele (congenital) (ventricular) Q31.3
Laryngofissure J38.7
  congenital Q31.8
Laryngomalacia (congenital) Q31.5
Laryngopharyngitis (acute) J06.0
  chronic J37.0
  due to external agent —*see* Inflammation,
    respiratory, upper, due to
Laryngoplegia J38.00
  bilateral J38.02
  unilateral J38.01
Laryngoptosis J38.7
Laryngospasm J38.5
Laryngostenosis J38.6
Laryngotracheitis (acute) (Infectional)
    (infective) (viral) J04.2
  atrophic J37.1
  catarrhal J37.1
  chronic J37.1
  diphtheritic A36.2
  due to external agent —*see* Inflammation,
    respiratory, upper, due to
  Hemophilus influenzae J04.2
  hypertrophic J37.1
  influenzal —*see* Influenza, with, respiratory
    manifestations NEC
  pachydermic J38.7
  sicca J37.1
  spasmodic J38.5
    acute J05.0
  streptococcal J04.2
  stridulous J38.5
  syphilitic (late) A52.73
    congenital A50.59 *[J99]*
      early A50.03 *[J99]*
  tuberculous A15.5
  Vincent's A69.1
Laryngotracheobronchitis —*see* Bronchitis
Larynx, laryngeal —*see* condition
Lassa fever A96.2
Lassitude —*see* Weakness
Late
  talker R62.0
  walker R62.0
Late effect(s) —*see* Sequelae
Latent —*see* condition
Laterocession —*see* Lateroversion
Lateroflexion —*see* Lateroversion
Lateroversion
  cervix —*see* Lateroversion, uterus
  uterus, uterine (cervix) (postinfectional)
    (postpartal, old) N85.4
    congenital Q51.818
    in pregnancy or childbirth O34.59-●
Lathyrism —*see* Poisoning, food, noxious,
  plant
Launois' syndrome (pituitary gigantism) E22.0
Launois-Bensaude adenolipomatosis E88.89
Laurence-Moon (-Bardet)-Biedl syndrome
  Q87.89
Lax, laxity —*see also* Relaxation
  ligament (ous) —*see also* Disorder, ligament
    familial M35.7
    knee —*see* Derangement, knee
  skin (acquired) L57.4
    congenital Q82.8
Laxative habit F55.2
Lazy leukocyte syndrome D70.8
Lead miner's lung J63.6

Leak, leakage
  air NEC J93.82
    postprocedural J95.812
  amniotic fluid —*see* Rupture, membranes,
    premature
  blood (microscopic), fetal, into maternal
    circulation affecting management
    of pregnancy —*see* Pregnancy,
    complicated by
  cerebrospinal fluid G96.00
    cranial
      postoperative G96.08
      specified NEC G96.08
      spontaneous G96.01
      traumatic G96.08
    from spinal (lumbar) puncture G97.0
    spinal
      postoperative G96.09
      post-traumatic G96.09
      specified NEC G96.09
      spontaneous G96.02
    spontaneous
      from
        skull base G96.01
      spine G96.02
  CSF —*see* Leak, cerebrospinal fluid
  device, implant or graft —*see also*
    Complications, by site and type,
    mechanical
    arterial graft NEC —*see* Complication,
      cardiovascular device, mechanical,
      vascular
    breast (implant) T85.43
    catheter NEC T85.638
      dialysis (renal) T82.43
        intraperitoneal T85.631
      infusion NEC T82.534
        spinal (epidural) (subdural)
          T85.630
      urinary T83.038
        cystostomy T83.030
        Hopkins T83.038
        ileostomy T83.038
        indwelling T83.031
        nephrostomy T83.032
        specified NEC T83.038
        urostomy T83.038
    gastrointestinal —*see* Complications,
      prosthetic device, mechanical,
      gastrointestinal device
    genital NEC T83.498
      penile prosthesis (cylinder) (implanted)
        (pump) (resevoir) T83.490
      testicular prosthesis T83.491
    heart NEC —*see* Complication,
      cardiovascular device, mechanical
    joint prosthesis —*see* Complications, joint
      prosthesis, mechanical, specified NEC,
      by site
    ocular NEC —*see* Complications, prosthetic
      device, mechanical, ocular device
    orthopedic NEC —*see* Complication,
      orthopedic, device, mechanical
    persistent air J93.82
    specified NEC T85.638
    urinary NEC —*see also* Complication,
      genitourinary, device, urinary,
      mechanical
      graft T83.23
    vascular NEC —*see* Complication,
      cardiovascular device, mechanical
    ventricular intracranial shunt T85.03
  urine —*see* Incontinence
Leaky heart —*see* Endocarditis
Learning defect (specific) F81.9
Leather bottle stomach C16.9
Leber's
  congenital amaurosis H35.50
  optic atrophy (hereditary) H47.22
Lederer's anemia D59.19
Leeches (external) —*see* Hirudiniasis

Leg —*see* condition
Legg (-Calvé)-Perthes disease, syndrome or
  osteochondrosis M91.1-●
Legionellosis A48.1
  nonpneumonic A48.2
Legionnaires'
  disease A48.1
    nonpneumonic A48.2
    pneumonia A48.1
Leigh's disease G31.82
Leiner's disease L21.1
Leiofibromyoma —*see* Leiomyoma
Leiomyoblastoma —*see* Neoplasm, connective
  tissue, benign
Leiomyofibroma —*see also* Neoplasm,
  connective tissue, benign
  uterus (cervix) (corpus) D25.9
Leiomyoma —*see also* Neoplasm, connective
  tissue, benign
  bizarre —*see* Neoplasm, connective tissue,
    benign
  cellular —*see* Neoplasm, connective tissue,
    benign
  epithelioid —*see* Neoplasm, connective
    tissue, benign
  uterus (cervix) (corpus) D25.9
    intramural D25.1
    submucous D25.0
    subserosal D25.2
  vascular —*see* Neoplasm, connective tissue,
    benign
Leiomyoma, leiomyomatosis (intravascular) —
  see Neoplasm, connective tissue, uncertain
  behavior
Leiomyosarcoma —*see also* Neoplasm,
  connective tissue, malignant
  epithelioid —*see* Neoplasm, connective
    tissue, malignant
  myxoid —*see* Neoplasm, connective tissue,
    malignant
Leishmaniasis B55.9
  American (mucocutaneous) B55.2
    cutaneous B55.1
  Asian Desert B55.1
  Brazilian B55.2
  cutaneous (any type) B55.1
  dermal —*see also* Leishmaniasis, cutaneous
    post-kala-azar B55.0
  eyelid B55.1
  infantile B55.0
  Mediterranean B55.0
  mucocutaneous (American) (New World)
    B55.2
  naso-oral B55.2
  nasopharyngeal B55.2
  old world B55.1
  tegumentaria diffusa B55.1
  visceral B55.0
Leishmanoid, dermal —*see also* Leishmaniasis,
  cutaneous
  post-kala-azar B55.0
Lenegre's disease I44.2
Lengthening, leg —*see* Deformity, limb,
  unequal length
Lennert's lymphoma —*see* Lymphoma,
  Lennert's
Lennox-Gastaut syndrome G40.812
  intractable G40.814
    with status epilepticus G40.813
    without status epilepticus G40.814
  not intractable G40.812
    with status epilepticus G40.811
    without status epilepticus G40.812
Lens —*see* condition
Lenticonus (anterior) (posterior) (congenital)
  Q12.8
Lenticular degeneration, progressive E83.01
Lentiglobus (posterior) (congenital) Q12.8
Lentigo (congenital) L81.4
  maligna —*see also* Melanoma, in situ
    melanoma —*see* Melanoma

  ▶ New   ⟹ Revised   ~~deleted~~ Deleted   ● Use Additional Character(s)

Lentivirus, as cause of disease classified
    elsewhere B97.31
Leontiasis
  ossium M85.2
  syphilitic (late) A52.78
    congenital A50.59
Lepothrix A48.8
Lepra —see Leprosy
Leprechaunism E34.8
Leprosy A30.-•
  with muscle disorder A30.9 [M63.80]
    ankle A30.9 [M63.87-•]
    foot A30.9 [M63.87-•]
    forearm A30.9 [M63.83-•]
    hand A30.9 [M63.84-•]
    lower leg A30.9 [M63.86-•]
    multiple sites A30.9 [M63.89]
    pelvic region A30.9 [M63.85-•]
    shoulder region A30.9 [M63.81-•]
    specified site NEC A30.9 [M63.88]
    thigh A30.9 [M63.85-•]
    upper arm A30.9 [M63.82-•]
  anesthetic A30.9
  BB A30.3
  BL A30.4
  borderline (infiltrated) (neuritic) A30.3
    lepromatous A30.4
    tuberculoid A30.2
  BT A30.2
  dimorphous (infiltrated) (neuritic) A30.3
  I A30.0
  indeterminate (macular) (neuritic) A30.0
  lepromatous (diffuse) (infiltrated) (macular)
    (neuritic) (nodular) A30.5
  LL A30.5
  macular (early) (neuritic) (simple) A30.9
  maculoanesthetic A30.9
  mixed A30.3
  neural A30.9
  nodular A30.5
  primary neuritic A30.3
  specified type NEC A30.8
  TT A30.1
  tuberculoid (major) (minor) A30.1
Leptocytosis, hereditary D56.9
Leptomeningitis (chronic) (circumscribed)
  (hemorrhagic) (nonsuppurative) —see
  Meningitis
Leptomeningopathy G96.198
Leptospiral —see condition
Leptospirochetal —see condition
Leptospirosis A27.9
  canicola A27.89
  due to Leptospira interrogans serovar
    icterohaemorrhagiae A27.0
  icterohemorrhagica A27.0
  pomona A27.89
  Weil's disease A27.0
Leptus dermatitis B88.0
Leriche's syndrome (aortic bifurcation
  occlusion) I74.09
Leri's pleonosteosis Q78.8
Leri-Weill syndrome Q77.8
Lermoyez' syndrome —see Vertigo, peripheral
  NEC
Lesch-Nyhan syndrome E79.1
Leser-Trélat disease L82.1
  inflamed L82.0
Lesion(s) (nontraumatic)
  abducens nerve —see Strabismus, paralytic,
    sixth nerve
  alveolar process K08.9
  angiocentric immunoproliferative
    D47.Z9
  anorectal K62.9
  aortic (valve) I35.9
  auditory nerve —see subcategory
    H93.3
  basal ganglion G25.9
  bile duct —see Disease, bile duct
  biomechanical M99.9

Lesion (Continued)
  biomechanical (Continued)
    specified type NEC M99.89
      abdomen M99.89
      acromioclavicular M99.87
      cervical region M99.81
      cervicothoracic M99.81
      costochondral M99.88
      costovertebral M99.88
      head region M99.80
      hip M99.85
      lower extremity M99.86
      lumbar region M99.83
      lumbosacral M99.83
      occipitocervical M99.80
      pelvic region M99.85
      pubic M99.85
      rib cage M99.88
      sacral region M99.84
      sacrococcygeal M99.84
      sacroiliac M99.84
      specified NEC M99.89
      sternochondral M99.88
      sternoclavicular M99.87
      thoracic region M99.82
      thoracolumbar M99.82
      upper extremity M99.87
  bladder N32.9
  bone —see Disorder, bone
  brachial plexus G54.0
  brain G93.9
    congenital Q04.9
    vascular I67.9
      degenerative I67.9
      hypertensive I67.4
  buccal cavity K13.79
  calcified —see Calcification
  canthus —see Disorder, eyelid
  carate —see Pinta, lesions
  cardia K31.9
  cardiac —see also Disease, heart I51.9
    congenital Q24.9
    valvular —see Endocarditis
  cauda equina G83.4
  cecum K63.9
  cerebral —see Lesion, brain
  cerebrovascular I67.9
    degenerative I67.9
    hypertensive I67.4
  cervical (nerve) root NEC G54.2
  chiasmal —see Disorder, optic, chiasm
  chorda tympani G51.8
  coin, lung R91.1
  colon K63.9
  combined periodontic - endodontic K05.5
  congenital —see Anomaly, by site
  conjunctiva H11.9
  conus medullaris —see Injury, conus
    medullaris
  coronary artery —see Ischemia, heart
  cranial nerve G52.9
    eighth —see Disorder, ear
    eleventh G52.9
    fifth G50.9
    first G52.0
    fourth —see Strabismus, paralytic, fourth
      nerve
    seventh G51.9
    sixth —see Strabismus, paralytic, sixth nerve
    tenth G52.2
    twelfth G52.3
  cystic —see Cyst
  degenerative —see Degeneration
  duodenum K31.9
  edentulous (alveolar) ridge, associated with
    trauma, due to traumatic occlusion K06.2
  en coup de sabre L94.1
  eyelid —see Disorder, eyelid
  gasserian ganglion G50.8
  gastric K31.9
  gastroduodenal K31.9

Lesion (Continued)
  gastrointestinal K63.9
  gingiva, associated with trauma K06.2
  glomerular
    focal and segmental —see also N00-N07
      with fourth character .1 N05.1
    minimal change —see also N00-N07 with
      fourth character .0 N05.0
  heart (organic) —see Disease, heart
  hyperchromic, due to pinta (carate) A67.1
  hyperkeratotic —see Hyperkeratosis
  hypothalamic E23.7
  ileocecal K63.9
  ileum K63.9
  iliohypogastric nerve G57.8-•
  inflammatory —see Inflammation
  intestine K63.9
  intracerebral —see Lesion, brain
  intrachiasmal (optic) —see Disorder, optic,
    chiasm
  intracranial, space-occupying R90.0
  joint —see Disorder, joint
    sacroiliac (old) M53.3
  keratotic —see Keratosis
  kidney —see Disease, renal
  laryngeal nerve (recurrent) G52.2
  lip K13.0
  liver K76.9
  lumbosacral
    plexus G54.1
    root (nerve) NEC G54.4
  lung (coin) R91.1
  maxillary sinus J32.0
  mitral I05.9
  Morel-Lavallée —see Hematoma,
    by site
  motor cortex NEC G93.89
  mouth K13.79
  nerve G58.9
    femoral G57.2-•
    median G56.1-•
      carpal tunnel syndrome —see Syndrome,
        carpal tunnel
    plantar G57.6-•
    popliteal (lateral) G57.3-•
      medial G57.4-•
    radial G56.3-•
    sciatic G57.0-•
    spinal —see Injury, nerve, spinal
    ulnar G56.2-•
  nervous system, congenital Q07.9
  nonallopathic —see Lesion, biomechanical
  nose (internal) J34.89
  obstructive —see Obstruction
  obturator nerve G57.8-•
  oral mucosa K13.70
  organ or site NEC —see Disease, by site
  osteolytic —see Osteolysis
  peptic K27.9
  periodontal, due to traumatic occlusion K05.5
  pharynx J39.2
  pigment, pigmented (skin) L81.9
  pinta —see Pinta, lesions
  polypoid —see Polyp
  prechiasmal (optic) —see Disorder, optic,
    chiasm
  primary —see also Syphilis, primary A51.0
    carate A67.0
    pinta A67.0
    yaws A66.0
  pulmonary J98.4
    valve I37.9
  pylorus K31.9
  rectosigmoid K63.9
  retina, retinal H35.9
  sacroiliac (joint) (old) M53.3
  salivary gland K11.9
    benign lymphoepithelial K11.8
  saphenous nerve G57.8-•
  sciatic nerve G57.0-•
  secondary —see Syphilis, secondary

Lesion *(Continued)*
  shoulder (region) M75.9-●
    specified NEC M75.8-●
  sigmoid K63.9
  sinus (accessory) (nasal) J34.89
  skin L98.9
    suppurative L08.0
  SLAP S43.43-●
  spinal cord G95.9
    congenital Q06.9
  spleen D73.89
  stomach K31.9
  superior glenoid labrum S43.43-●
  syphilitic —*see* Syphilis
  tertiary —*see* Syphilis, tertiary
  thoracic root (nerve) NEC G54.3
  tonsillar fossa J35.9
  tooth, teeth K08.9
    white spot
      chewing surface K02.51
      pit and fissure surface K02.51
      smooth surface K02.61
  traumatic —*see* specific type of injury by site
  tricuspid (valve) I07.9
    nonrheumatic I36.9
  trigeminal nerve G50.9
  ulcerated or ulcerative —*see* Ulcer, skin
  uterus N85.9
  vagina N89.8
  vulva N90.89
  vagus nerve G52.2
  valvular —*see* Endocarditis
  vascular I99.9
    affecting central nervous system I67.9
    following trauma NEC T14.8
    umbilical cord, complicating delivery O69.5
  warty —*see* Verruca
  white spot (tooth)
    chewing surface K02.51
    pit and fissure surface K02.51
    smooth surface K02.61
▶Less than a high school diploma Z55.5
Lethargic —*see* condition
Lethargy R53.83
Letterer-Siwe's disease C96.0
Leukemia, leukemic C95.9-●
  acute basophilic C94.8-●
  acute bilineal C95.0-●
  acute erythroid C94.0-●
  acute lymphoblastic C91.0-●
  acute megakaryoblastic C94.2-●
  acute megakaryocytic C94.2-●
  acute mixed lineage C95.0-●
  acute monoblastic (monoblastic/monocytic)
    C93.0-●
  acute monocytic (monoblastic/monocytic)
    C93.0-●
  acute myeloblastic (minimal differentiation)
    (with maturation) C92.0-●
  acute myeloid, NOS C92.0-●
    with
      11q23-abnormality C92.6-●
      dysplasia of remaining hematopoesis
        and/or myelodysplastic disease in
        its history C92.A-●
      multilineage dysplasia C92.A-●
      variation of MLL-gene C92.6-●
    M6 (a)(b) C94.0-●
    M7 C94.2-●
  acute myelomonocytic C92.5-●
  acute promyelocytic C92.4-●
  adult T-cell (HTLV-1-associated) (acute
    variant) (chronic variant)
    (lymphomatoid variant) (smouldering
    variant) C91.5-●
  aggressive NK-cell C94.8-●
  AML (1/ETO) (M0) (M1) (M2) (without a
    FAB classification) C92.0-●
  AML M3 C92.4-●
  AML M4 (Eo with inv(16) or t(16;16)) C92.5-●
  AML M5 C93.0-●

Leukemia, leukemic *(Continued)*
  AML M5a C93.0-●
  AML M5b C93.0-●
  AML Me with t (15;17) and variants C92.4-●
  atypical chronic myeloid, BCR/ABL-negative
    C92.2-●
  biphenotypic acute C95.0-●
  blast cell C95.0-●
  Burkitt-type, mature B-cell C91.A-●
  chronic eosinophilic (*see also* Syndrome,
    hypereosinophilic, myeloid) C94.8-●
  chronic lymphocytic, of B-cell type C91.1-●
  chronic monocytic C93.1-●
  chronic myelogenous (Philadelphia
    chromosome (Ph1) positive) (t(9;22))
    (q34;q11) (with crisis of blast cells)
    C92.1-●
  chronic myeloid, BCR/ABL-positive C92.1-●
    atypical, BCR/ABL-negative C92.2-●
  chronic myelomonocytic C93.1-●
  chronic neutrophilic D47.1
  CMML (-1) (-2) (with eosinophilia) C93.1-●
  granulocytic —*see also* Category C92 C92.9-●
  hairy-cell C91.4-●
  juvenile myelomonocytic C93.3-●
  lymphoid C91.9-●
    specified NEC C91.Z-●
  mast cell C94.3-●
  mature B-cell, Burkitt-type C91.A-●
  monocytic (subacute) C93.9-●
    specified NEC C93.Z-●
  myelogenous —*see also* Category
    C92 C92.9-●
  myeloid C92.9-●
    specified NEC C92.Z-●
  plasma cell C90.1-●
  plasmacytic C90.1-●
  prolymphocytic
    of B-cell type C91.3-●
    of T-cell type C91.6-●
  specified NEC C94.8-●
  stem cell, of unclear lineage C95.0-●
  subacute lymphocytic C91.9-●
  T-cell large granular lymphocytic C91.Z-●
  unspecified cell type C95.9-●
    acute C95.0-●
    chronic C95.1-●
Leukemoid reaction —*see also* Reaction,
  leukemoid D72.823-●
Leukoaraiosis (hypertensive) I67.81
Leukoariosis —*see* Leukoaraiosis
Leukocoria —*see* Disorder, globe, degenerated
  condition, leucocoria
Leukocytopenia D72.819
Leukocytosis D72.829
  eosinophilic D72.19
Leukoderma, leukodermia NEC L81.5
  syphilitic A51.39
    late A52.79
Leukodystrophy E75.29
Leukoedema, oral epithelium K13.29
Leukoencephalitis G04.81
  acute (subacute) hemorrhagic G36.1
    postimmunization or postvaccinal
      G04.02
  postinfectious G04.01
  subacute sclerosing A81.1
  van Bogaert's (sclerosing) A81.1
Leukoencephalopathy —*see also*
  Encephalopathy G93.49
  Binswanger's I67.3
▶heroin vapor G92.8
  metachromatic E75.25
  multifocal (progressive) A81.2
  postimmunization and postvaccinal
    G04.02
  progressive multifocal A81.2
  reversible, posterior G93.6
  van Bogaert's (sclerosing) A81.1
  vascular, progressive I67.3
Leukoerythroblastosis D75.9

Leukokeratosis —*see also* Leukoplakia
  mouth K13.21
  nicotina palati K13.24
  oral mucosa K13.21
  tongue K13.21
  vocal cord J38.3
Leukokraurosis vulva (e) N90.4
Leukoma (cornea) —*see also* Opacity, cornea
  adherent H17.0-●
  interfering with central vision —*see* Opacity,
    cornea, central
Leukomalacia, cerebral, newborn P91.2
  periventricular P91.2
Leukomelanopathy, hereditary D72.0
Leukonychia (punctata) (striata) L60.8
  congenital Q84.4
Leukopathia unguium L60.8
  congenital Q84.4
Leukopenia D72.819
  basophilic D72.818
  chemotherapy (cancer) induced D70.1
  congenital D70.0
  cyclic D70.0
  drug induced NEC D70.2
    due to cytoreductive cancer chemotherapy
      D70.1
  eosinophilic D72.818
  familial D70.0
  infantile genetic D70.0
  malignant D70.9
  periodic D70.0
  transitory neonatal P61.5
Leukopenic —*see* condition
Leukoplakia
  anus K62.89
  bladder (postinfectional) N32.89
  buccal K13.21
  cervix (uteri) N88.0
▶esophagus K22.89
  gingiva K13.21
  hairy (oral mucosa) (tongue) K13.3
  kidney (pelvis) N28.89
  larynx J38.7
  lip K13.21
  mouth K13.21
  oral epithelium, including tongue (mucosa)
    K13.21
  palate K13.21
  pelvis (kidney) N28.89
  penis (infectional) N48.0
  rectum K62.89
  syphilitic (late) A52.79
  tongue K13.21
  ureter (postinfectional) N28.89
  urethra (postinfectional) N36.8
  uterus N85.8
  vagina N89.4
  vocal cord J38.3
  vulva N90.4
Leukorrhea N89.8
  due to Trichomonas (vaginalis)
    A59.00
  trichomonal A59.00
Leukosarcoma C85.9
Levocardia (isolated) Q24.1
  with situs inversus Q89.3
Levotransposition Q20.5
Lev's disease or syndrome (acquired complete
  heart block) I44.2
Levulosuria —*see* Fructosuria
Levurid L30.2
Lewy body (ies) (dementia) (disease)
  G31.83
Leyden-Moebius dystrophy G71.09
Leydig cell
  carcinoma
    specified site —*see* Neoplasm, malignant,
      by site
    unspecified site
      female C56.9-●
      male C62.9-●

    ▶ New   ⇒ Revised   ~~deleted~~ Deleted   ● Use Additional Character(s)

Leydig cell (Continued)
  tumor
    benign
      specified site —see Neoplasm, benign,
        by site
      unspecified site
        female D27.-●
        male D29.2-●
    malignant
      specified site —see Neoplasm,
        malignant, by site
      unspecified site
        female C56.-●
        male C62.9-●
    specified site —see Neoplasm, uncertain
      behavior, by site
    unspecified site
      female D39.1-●
      male D40.1-●
Leydig-Sertoli cell tumor
  specified site —see Neoplasm, benign,
    by site
  unspecified site
    female D27.-●
    male D29.2-●
LGSIL (Low grade squamous intraepithelial
  lesion on cytologic smear of)
  anus R85.612
  cervix R87.612
  vagina R87.622
Liar, pathologic F60.2
Libido
  decreased R68.82
Libman-Sacks disease M32.11
Lice (infestation) B85.2
  body (Pediculus corporis) B85.1
  crab B85.3
  head (Pediculus capitis) B85.0
  mixed (classifiable to more than one of the
    titles B85.0-B85.3) B85.4
  pubic (Phthirus pubis) B85.3
Lichen L28.0
  albus L90.0
    penis N48.0
    vulva N90.4
  amyloidosis E85.4 [L99]
  atrophicus L90.0
    penis N48.0
    vulva N90.4
  congenital Q82.8
  myxedematosus L98.5
  nitidus L44.1
  pilaris Q82.8
    acquired L85.8
  planopilaris L66.1
  planus (chronicus) L43.9
    annularis L43.8
    bullous L43.1
    follicular L66.1
    hypertrophic L43.0
    moniliformis L44.3
    of Wilson L43.9
    specified NEC L43.8
    subacute (active) L43.3
    tropicus L43.3
  ruber
    acuminatus L44.0
    moniliformis L44.3
    planus L43.9
  sclerosus (et atrophicus) L90.0
    penis N48.0
    vulva N90.4
  scrofulosus (primary) (tuberculous) A18.4
  simplex (chronicus) (circumscriptus)
    L28.0
  striatus L44.2
  urticatus L28.2
Lichenification L28.0
Lichenoides tuberculosis (primary) A18.4
Lichtheim's disease or syndrome D51.0
Lien migrans D73.89

Ligament —see condition
Light
  for gestational age —see Light for dates
  headedness R42
Light-for-dates (infant) P05.00
  with weight of
    499 grams or less P05.01
    500-749 grams P05.02
    750-999 grams P05.03
    1000-1249 grams P05.04
    1250-1499 grams P05.05
    1500-1749 grams P05.06
    1750-1999 grams P05.07
    2000-2499 grams P05.08
    2500 grams and over P05.09
  affecting management of pregnancy O36.59-●
  and small-for-dates —see Small for dates
  specified NEC P05.09
Lightning (effects) (stroke) (struck by) T75.00
  burn —see Burn
  foot E53.8
  shock T75.01
  specified effect NEC T75.09
Lightwood-Albright syndrome N25.89
Lightwood's disease or syndrome (renal
  tubular acidosis) N25.89
Lignac (-de Toni) (-Fanconi) (-Debré) disease or
  syndrome E72.09
  with cystinosis E72.04
Ligneous thyroiditis E06.5
Likoff's syndrome I20.8
Limb —see condition
Limbic epilepsy personality syndrome F07.0
Limitation, limited
  activities due to disability Z73.6
  cardiac reserve —see Disease, heart
  eye muscle duction, traumatic —see
    Strabismus, mechanical
  mandibular range of motion M26.52
Lindau (-von Hippel) disease Q85.8
Line(s)
  Beau's L60.4
  Harris' —see Arrest, epiphyseal
  Hudson's (cornea) —see Pigmentation,
    cornea, anterior
  Stähli's (cornea) —see Pigmentation, cornea,
    anterior
Linea corneae senilis —see Change, cornea,
  senile
Lingua
  geographica K14.1
  nigra (villosa) K14.3
  plicata K14.5
  tylosis K13.29
Lingual —see condition
Linguatulosis B88.8
Linitis (gastric) plastica C16.9
Lip —see condition
Lipedema —see Edema
Lipemia —see also Hyperlipidemia
  retina, retinalis E78.3
Lipidosis E75.6
  cerebral (infantile) (juvenile) (late) E75.4
  cerebroretinal E75.4
  cerebroside E75.22
  cholesterol (cerebral) E75.5
  glycolipid E75.21
  hepatosplenomegalic E78.3
  sphingomyelin —see Niemann-Pick disease
    or syndrome
  sulfatide E75.29
Lipoadenoma —see Neoplasm, benign, by site
Lipoblastoma —see Lipoma
Lipoblastomatosis —see Lipoma
Lipochondrodystrophy E76.01
Lipochrome histiocytosis (familial) D71
Lipodermatosclerosis —see Varix, leg, with,
  inflammation
  ulcerated —see Varix, leg, with, ulcer, with
    inflammation by site
Lipodystrophia progressiva E88.1

Lipodystrophy (progressive) E88.1
  insulin E88.1
  intestinal K90.81
  mesenteric K65.4
Lipofibroma —see Lipoma
Lipofuscinosis, neuronal (with ceroidosis)
  E75.4
Lipogranuloma, sclerosing L92.8
Lipogranulomatosis E78.89
Lipoid —see also condition
  histiocytosis D76.3
    essential E75.29
  nephrosis N04.9
  proteinosis of Urbach E78.89
Lipoidemia —see Hyperlipidemia
Lipoidosis —see Lipidosis
Lipoma D17.9
  fetal D17.9
    fat cell D17.9
  infiltrating D17.9
  intramuscular D17.9
  pleomorphic D17.9
  site classification
    arms (skin) (subcutaneous) D17.2-●
    connective tissue D17.30
      intra-abdominal D17.5
      intrathoracic D17.4
      peritoneum D17.79
      retroperitoneum D17.79
      specified site NEC D17.39
      spermatic cord D17.6
    face (skin) (subcutaneous) D17.0
    genitourinary organ NEC D17.72
    head (skin) (subcutaneous) D17.0
    intra-abdominal D17.5
    intrathoracic D17.4
    kidney D17.71
    legs (skin) (subcutaneous) D17.2-●
    neck (skin) (subcutaneous) D17.0
    peritoneum D17.79
    retroperitoneum D17.79
    skin D17.30
      specified site NEC D17.39
    specified site NEC D17.79
    spermatic cord D17.6
    subcutaneous D17.30
      specified site NEC D17.39
    trunk (skin) (subcutaneous) D17.1
    unspecified D17.9
  spindle cell D17.9
Lipomatosis E88.2
  dolorosa (Dercum) E88.2
  fetal —see Lipoma
  Launois-Bensaude E88.89
Lipomyoma —see Lipoma
Lipomyxoma —see Lipoma
Lipomyxosarcoma —see Neoplasm, connective
  tissue, malignant
Lipoprotein metabolism disorder E78.9
Lipoproteinemia E78.5
  broad-beta E78.2
  floating-beta E78.2
  hyper-pre-beta E78.1
Liposarcoma —see also Neoplasm, connective
  tissue, malignant
  dedifferentiated —see Neoplasm, connective
    tissue, malignant
  differentiated type —see Neoplasm,
    connective tissue, malignant
  embryonal —see Neoplasm, connective tissue,
    malignant
  mixed type —see Neoplasm, connective
    tissue, malignant
  myxoid —see Neoplasm, connective tissue,
    malignant
  pleomorphic —see Neoplasm, connective
    tissue, malignant
  round cell —see Neoplasm, connective tissue,
    malignant
  well differentiated type —see Neoplasm,
    connective tissue, malignant

Liposynovitis prepatellaris E88.89
Lipping, cervix N86
Lipschütz disease or ulcer N76.6
Lipuria R82.0
　schistosomiasis (bilharziasis) B65.0
Lisping F80.0
Lissauer's paralysis A52.17
Lissencephalia, lissencephaly Q04.3
Listeriosis, listerellosis A32.9
　congenital (disseminated) P37.2
　cutaneous A32.0
　neonatal, newborn (disseminated) P37.2
　oculoglandular A32.81
　specified NEC A32.89
Lithemia E79.0
Lithiasis —see Calculus
Lithosis J62.8
Lithuria R82.998
Litigation, anxiety concerning Z65.3
Little leaguer's elbow —see Epicondylitis, medial
Little's disease G80.9
Littre's
　gland —see condition
　hernia —see Hernia, abdomen
Littritis —see Urethritis
Livedo (annularis) (racemosa) (reticularis) R23.1
Liver —see condition
Living alone (problems with) Z60.2
　with handicapped person Z74.2
▶Living in a shelter (motel) (scattered site
　　housing) (temporary or transitional living
　　situation) Z59.01
Lloyd's syndrome —see Adenomatosis, endocrine
Loa loa, loaiasis, loasis B74.3
Lobar —see condition
Lobomycosis B48.0
Lobo's disease B48.0
Lobotomy syndrome F07.0
Lobstein (-Ekman) disease or syndrome Q78.0
Lobster-claw hand Q71.6-●
Lobulation (congenital) —see also Anomaly,
　　by site
　kidney, Q63.1
　liver, abnormal Q44.7
　spleen Q89.09
Lobule, lobular —see condition
Local, localized —see condition
Locked twins causing obstructed labor O66.1
Locked-in state G83.5
Locking
　joint —see Derangement, joint, specified type
　　NEC
　knee —see Derangement, knee
Lockjaw —see Tetanus
Löffler's
　endocarditis I42.3
　eosinophilia J82.89
　pneumonia J82.89
　syndrome (eosinophilic pneumonitis) J82.89
Loiasis (with conjunctival infestation) (eyelid)
　　B74.3
Lone Star fever A77.0
Long
　▶COVID (-19) (see also COVID-19) U09.9
　labor O63.9
　　first stage O63.0
　　second stage O63.1
　QT syndrome I45.81
Long-term (current) (prophylactic) drug
　　therapy (use of)
　agents affecting estrogen receptors and
　　estrogen levels NEC Z79.818
　anastrozole (Arimidex) Z79.811
　antibiotics Z79.2
　　short-term use - omit code
　anticoagulants Z79.01
　anti-inflammatory, non-steroidal (NSAID)
　　Z79.1
　antiplatelet Z79.02
　antithrombotics Z79.02
　aromatase inhibitors Z79.811
　aspirin Z79.82
　birth control pill or patch Z79.3

Long-term (Continued)
　bisphosphonates Z79.83
　contraceptive, oral Z79.3
　drug, specified NEC Z79.899
　estrogen receptor downregulators Z79.818
　Evista Z79.810
　exemestane (Aromasin) Z79.811
　Fareston Z79.810
　fulvestrant (Faslodex) Z79.818
　gonadotropin-releasing hormone (GnRH)
　　agonist Z79.818
　goserelin acetate (Zoladex) Z79.818
　hormone replacement Z79.890
　insulin Z79.4
　letrozole (Femara) Z79.811
　leuprolide acetate (leuprorelin) (Lupron)
　　Z79.818
　megestrol acetate (Megace) Z79.818
　methadone for pain management Z79.891
　Nolvadex Z79.810
▶non-insulin antidiabetic drug, injectable
　　Z79.899
　non-steroidal anti-inflammatories (NSAID)
　　Z79.1
　opiate analgesic Z79.891
　oral
　　antidiabetic Z79.84
　　contraceptive Z79.3
　　hypoglycemic Z79.84
　raloxifene (Evista) Z79.810
　selective estrogen receptor modulators
　　(SERMs) Z79.810
　steroids
　　inhaled Z79.51
　　systemic Z79.52
　tamoxifen (Nolvadex) Z79.810
　toremifene (Fareston) Z79.810
Longitudinal stripes or grooves, nails L60.8
　congenital Q84.6
Loop
　intestine —see Volvulus
　vascular on papilla (optic) Q14.2
Loose —see also condition
　body
　　joint M24.00
　　　ankle M24.07-●
　　　elbow M24.02-●
　　　hand M24.04-●
　　　hip M24.05-●
　　　knee M23.4-●
　　　shoulder (region) M24.01-●
　　　specified site NEC M24.08
　　　toe M24.07-●
　　　vertebra M24.08
　　　wrist M24.03-●
　　knee M23.4-●
　　sheath, tendon —see Disorder, tendon,
　　　specified type NEC
　cartilage —see Loose, body, joint
　skin and subcutaneous tissue (following
　　bariatric surgery weight loss) (following
　　dietary weight loss) L98.7
　tooth, teeth K08.89
Loosening
　aseptic
　　joint prosthesis —see Complications, joint
　　　prosthesis, mechanical, loosening,
　　　by site
　　epiphysis —see Osteochondropathy
　mechanical
　　joint prosthesis —see Complications, joint
　　　prosthesis, mechanical, loosening,
　　　by site
Looser-Milkman (-Debray) syndrome M83.8
Lop ear (deformity) Q17.3
Lorain (-Levi) short stature syndrome E23.0
Lordosis M40.50
　acquired —see Lordosis, specified type NEC
　congenital Q76.429
　　lumbar region Q76.426
　　lumbosacral region Q76.427
　　sacral region Q76.428
　　sacrococcygeal region Q76.428

Lordosis (Continued)
　congenital(Continued)
　　thoracolumbar region Q76.425
　lumbar region M40.56
　lumbosacral region M40.57
　postsurgical M96.4
　postural —see Lordosis, specified type NEC
　rachitic (late effect) (sequelae) E64.3
　sequelae of rickets E64.3
　specified type NEC M40.40
　　lumbar region M40.46
　　lumbosacral region M40.47
　　thoracolumbar region M40.45
　thoracolumbar region M40.55
　tuberculous A18.01
Loss (of)
　appetite (see Anorexia) R63.0
　　hysterical F50.89
　　nonorganic origin F50.89
　　psychogenic F50.89
　blood —see Hemorrhage
　bone —see Loss, substance of, bone
　consciousness, transient R55
　　traumatic —see Injury, intracranial
　control, sphincter, rectum R15.9
　　nonorganic origin F98.1
　elasticity, skin R23.4
　family (member) in childhood Z62.898
　fluid (acute) E86.9
　function of labyrinth —see subcategory H83.2
　hair, nonscarring —see Alopecia
　hearing —see also Deafness
　　central NOS H90.5
　　conductive H90.2
　　　bilateral H90.0
　　　unilateral
　　　　with
　　　　　restricted hearing on the
　　　　　　contralateral side H90.A1-●
　　　　　unrestricted hearing on the
　　　　　　contralateral side H90.1-●
　　mixed conductive and sensorineural
　　　hearing loss H90.8
　　　bilateral H90.6
　　　unilateral
　　　　with
　　　　　restricted hearing on the
　　　　　　contralateral side H90.A3-●
　　　　　unrestricted hearing on the
　　　　　　contralateral side H90.7-●
　　neural NOS H90.5
　　perceptive NOS H90.5
　　sensorineural NOS H90.5
　　　bilateral H90.3
　　　unilateral
　　　　with
　　　　　restricted hearing on the
　　　　　　contralateral side H90.A2-●
　　　　　unrestricted hearing on the
　　　　　　contralateral side H90.4-●
　　sensory NOS H90.5
　height R29.890
　limb or member, traumatic, current —see
　　Amputation, traumatic
　love relationship in childhood Z62.898
　memory —see also Amnesia
　　mild, following organic brain damage F06.8
　mind —see Psychosis
　occlusal vertical dimension of fully erupted
　　teeth M26.37
　organ or part —see Absence, by site, acquired
　ossicles, ear (partial) H74.32-●
　parent in childhood Z63.4
　pregnancy, recurrent N96
　　without current pregnancy N96
　　care in current pregnancy O26.2-●
　recurrent pregnancy —see Loss, pregnancy,
　　recurrent
　self-esteem, in childhood Z62.898
　sense of
　　smell —see Disturbance, sensation, smell
　　taste —see Disturbance, sensation, taste
　　touch R20.8

▶ New　⇒ Revised　~~deleted~~ Deleted　● Use Additional Character(s)

Loss *(Continued)*
 sensory R44.9
  dissociative F44.6
 sexual desire F52.0
 sight (acquired) (complete) (congenital) —*see*
  Blindness
 substance of
  bone —*see* Disorder, bone, density and
   structure, specified NEC
   horizontal alveolar K06.3
  cartilage —*see* Disorder, cartilage, specified
   type NEC
   auricle (ear) —*see* Disorder, pinna,
    specified type NEC
  vitreous (humor) H15.89
 tooth, teeth —*see* Absence, teeth, acquired
 vision, visual H54.7
  both eyes H54.3
  one eye H54.60
   left (normal vision on right) H54.62
   right (normal vision on left) H54.61
  specified as blindness —*see* Blindness
  subjective
   sudden H53.13-●
   transient H53.12-●
 vitreous —*see* Prolapse, vitreous
 voice —*see* Aphonia
 weight (abnormal) (cause unknown) R63.4
Louis-Bar syndrome (ataxia-telangiectasia)
 G11.3
Louping ill (encephalitis) A84.89
Louse, lousiness —*see* Lice
Low
 achiever, school Z55.3
▸back syndrome M54.50
 basal metabolic rate R94.8
 birthweight (2499 grams or less) P07.10
  with weight of
   1000-1249 grams P07.14
   1250-1499 grams P07.15
   1500-1749 grams P07.16
   1750-1999 grams P07.17
   2000-2499 grams P07.18
  extreme (999 grams or less) P07.00
   with weight of
    499 grams or less P07.01
    500-749 grams P07.02
    750-999 grams P07.03
  for gestational age —*see* Light for dates
 blood pressure —*see also* Hypotension
  reading (incidental) (isolated) (nonspecific)
   R03.1
 cardiac reserve —*see* Disease, heart
 function —*see also* Hypofunction
  kidney N28.9
 hematocrit D64.9
 hemoglobin D64.9
 income Z59.6
 level of literacy Z55.0
 lying
  kidney N28.89
  organ or site, congenital —*see* Malposition,
   congenital
 output syndrome (cardiac) —*see* Failure,
  heart
 platelets (blood) —*see* Thrombocytopenia
 reserve, kidney N28.89
 salt syndrome E87.1
 self esteem R45.81
 set ears Q17.4
 vision H54.2X-
  one eye (other eye normal) H54.50
   left (normal vision on right)
    H54.52A-
   other eye blind —*see* Blindness
   right (normal vision on left)
    H54.511-
Low-density-lipoprotein-type (LDL)
 hyperlipoproteinemia E78.00
Lowe's syndrome E72.03
Lown-Ganong-Levine syndrome I45.6

LSD reaction (acute) (without dependence)
 F16.90
 with dependence F16.20
L-shaped kidney Q63.8
LTBI (lantent tuberculosis infection) Z22.7
Ludwig's angina or disease K12.2
Lues (venerea), luetic —*see* Syphilis
Luetscher's syndrome (dehydration) E86.0
▸Lumbago, lumbalgia M54.50
 with sciatica M54.4-●
 due to intervertebral disc disorder
  M51.17
 due to displacement, intervertebral disc
  M51.27
  with sciatica M51.17
Lumbar —*see* condition
Lumbarization, vertebra, congenital Q76.49
Lumbermen's itch B88.0
Lump —*see also* Mass
 breast N63.0
  axillary tail
   left N63.32
   right N63.31
  left
   lower inner quadrant N63.24
   lower outer quadrant N63.23
   overlapping quadrants N63.25
   unspecified quadrant N63.20
   upper inner quadrant N63.22
   upper outer quadrant N63.21
  right
   lower inner quadrant N63.14
   lower outer quadrant N63.13
   overlapping quadrants N63.15
   unspecified quadrant N63.10
   upper inner quadrant N63.12
   upper outer quadrant N63.11
  subareolar
   left N63.42
   right N63.41
Lunacy —*see* Psychosis
Lung —*see* condition
Lupoid (miliary) of Boeck D86.3
Lupus
 anticoagulant D68.62
  with
   hemorrhagic disorder D68.312
   hypercoagulable state D68.62
  finding without diagnosis R76.0
 discoid (local) L93.0
 erythematosus (discoid) (local) L93.0
  disseminated —*see* Lupus, erythematosus,
   systemic
  eyelid H01.129
   left H01.126
    lower H01.125
    upper H01.124
   right H01.123
    lower H01.122
    upper H01.121
  profundus L93.2
  specified NEC L93.2
  subacute cutaneous L93.1
  systemic M32.9
   with organ or system involvement
    M32.10
    endocarditis M32.11
    lung M32.13
    pericarditis M32.12
    renal (glomerular) M32.14
     tubulo-interstitial M32.15
    specified organ or system NEC
     M32.19
   drug-induced M32.0
   inhibitor (presence of) D68.62
    with
     hemorrhagic disorder D68.312
     hypercoagulable state D68.62
    finding without diagnosis R76.0
   specified NEC M32.8
 exedens A18.4

Lupus *(Continued)*
 hydralazine M32.0
  correct substance properly administered —
   see Table of Drugs and Chemicals, by
   drug, adverse effect
  overdose or wrong substance given
   or taken —*see* Table of Drugs and
   Chemicals, by drug, poisoning
 nephritis (chronic) M32.14
 nontuberculous, not disseminated L93.0
 panniculitis L93.2
 pernio (Besnier) D86.3
 systemic —*see* Lupus, erythematosus,
  systemic
 tuberculous A18.4
  eyelid A18.4
 vulgaris A18.4
  eyelid A18.4
Luteinoma D27.-●
Lutembacher's disease or syndrome (atrial
 septal defect with mitral stenosis) Q21.1
Luteoma D27.-●
Lutz (-Splendore-de Almeida) disease —*see*
 Paracoccidioidomycosis
Luxation —*see also* Dislocation
 eyeball (nontraumatic) —*see* Luxation, globe
  birth injury P15.3
 globe, nontraumatic H44.82-●
 lacrimal gland —*see* Dislocation, lacrimal
  gland
 lens (old) (partial) (spontaneous)
  congenital Q12.1
  syphilitic A50.39
Lycanthropy F22
Lyell's syndrome L51.2
 due to drug L51.2
  correct substance properly administered —
   see Table of Drugs and Chemicals, by
   drug, adverse effect
  overdose or wrong substance given
   or taken —*see* Table of Drugs and
   Chemicals, by drug, poisoning
Lyme disease A69.20
Lymph
 gland or node —*see* condition
 scrotum —*see* Infestation, filarial
Lymphadenitis I88.9
 with ectopic or molar pregnancy O08.0
 acute L04.9
  axilla L04.2
  face L04.0
  head L04.0
  hip L04.3
  limb
   lower L04.3
   upper L04.2
  neck L04.0
  shoulder L04.2
  specified site NEC L04.8
  trunk L04.1
 anthracosis (occupational) J60
 any site, except mesenteric I88.9
  chronic I88.1
  subacute I88.1
 breast
  gestational —*see* Mastitis, obstetric
  puerperal, postpartum (nonpurulent)
   O91.22
 chancroidal (congenital) A57
 chronic I88.1
  mesenteric I88.0
 due to
  Brugia (malayi) B74.1
   timori B74.2
  chlamydial lymphogranuloma A55
  diphtheria (toxin) A36.89
  lymphogranuloma venereum A55
  Wuchereria bancrofti B74.0
 following ectopic or molar pregnancy O08.0
 gonorrheal A54.89
 infective —*see* Lymphadenitis, acute

Lymphadenitis *(Continued)*
  mesenteric (acute) (chronic) (nonspecific)
    (subacute) I88.0
    due to Salmonella typhi A01.09
    tuberculous A18.39
  mycobacterial A31.8
  purulent —*see* Lymphadenitis, acute
  pyogenic —*see* Lymphadenitis, acute
  regional, nonbacterial I88.8
  septic —*see* Lymphadenitis, acute
  subacute, unspecified site I88.1
  suppurative —*see* Lymphadenitis, acute
  syphilitic (early) (secondary) A51.49
    late A52.79
  tuberculous —*see* Tuberculosis, lymph gland
  venereal (chlamydial) A55
Lymphadenoid goiter E06.3
Lymphadenopathy (generalized) R59.1
  angioimmunoblastic, with dysproteinemia
    (AILD) C86.5
  due to toxoplasmosis (acquired) B58.89
    congenital (acute) (subacute) (chronic) P37.1
  localized R59.0
  syphilitic (early) (secondary) A51.49
Lymphadenosis R59.1
Lymphangiectasis I89.0
  conjunctiva H11.89
  postinfectional I89.0
  scrotum I89.0
Lymphangiectatic elephantiasis, nonfilarial
  I89.0
Lymphangioendothelioma D18.1
  malignant —*see* Neoplasm, connective tissue,
    malignant
Lymphangioleiomyomatosis J84.81
Lymphangioma D18.1
  capillary D18.1
  cavernous D18.1
  cystic D18.1
  malignant —*see* Neoplasm, connective tissue,
    malignant
Lymphangiomyoma D18.1
Lymphangiomyomatosis J84.81
Lymphangiosarcoma —*see* Neoplasm,
  connective tissue, malignant
Lymphangitis I89.1
  with
    abscess - code by site under Abscess
    cellulitis - code by site under Cellulitis
    ectopic or molar pregnancy O08.0
  acute L03.91
    abdominal wall L03.321
    ankle —*see* Lymphangitis, acute, lower
      limb
    arm —*see* Lymphangitis, acute, upper limb
    auricle (ear) —*see* Lymphangitis, acute, ear
    axilla L03.12-●
    back (any part) L03.322
    buttock L03.327
    cervical (meaning neck) L03.222
    cheek (external) L03.212
    chest wall L03.323
    digit
      finger —*see* Lymphangitis, acute, finger
      toe —*see* Lymphangitis, acute, toe
    ear (external) H60.1-●
    external auditory canal —*see*
      Lymphangitis, acute, ear
    eyelid —*see* Abscess, eyelid
    face NEC L03.212
    finger (intrathecal) (periosteal)
      (subcutaneous) (subcuticular)
      L03.02-●
    foot —*see* Lymphangitis, acute, lower limb
    gluteal (region) L03.327
    groin L03.324
    hand —*see* Lymphangitis, acute, upper
      limb
    head NEC L03.891
      face (any part, except ear, eye and nose)
        L03.212

Lymphangitis *(Continued)*
  acute *(Continued)*
    heel —*see* Lymphangitis, acute, lower limb
    hip —*see* Lymphangitis, acute, lower limb
    jaw (region) L03.212
    knee —*see* Lymphangitis, acute, lower limb
    leg —*see* Lymphangitis, acute, lower limb
    lower limb L03.12-●
      toe —*see* Lymphangitis, acute, toe
    navel L03.326
    neck (region) L03.222
    orbit, orbital —*see* Cellulitis, orbit
    pectoral (region) L03.323
    perineal, perineum L03.325
    scalp (any part) L03.891
    shoulder —*see* Lymphangitis, acute, upper
      limb
    specified site NEC L03.898
    thigh —*see* Lymphangitis, acute, lower
      limb
    thumb (intrathecal) (periosteal)
      (subcutaneous) (subcuticular) —*see*
      Lymphangitis, acute, finger
    toe (intrathecal) (periosteal) (subcutaneous)
      (subcuticular) L03.04-●
    trunk L03.329
      abdominal wall L03.321
      back (any part) L03.322
      buttock L03.327
      chest wall L03.323
      groin L03.324
      perineal, perineum L03.325
      umbilicus L03.326
    umbilicus L03.326
    upper limb L03.12-●
      axilla —*see* Lymphangitis, acute, axilla
      finger —*see* Lymphangitis, acute, finger
      thumb —*see* Lymphangitis, acute, finger
      wrist —*see* Lymphangitis, acute, upper
        limb
  breast
    gestational —*see* Mastitis, obstetric
  chancroidal A57
  chronic (any site) I89.1
  due to
    Brugia (malayi) B74.1
      timori B74.2
    Wuchereria bancrofti B74.0
  following ectopic or molar pregnancy
    O08.89
  penis
    acute N48.29
    gonococcal (acute) (chronic) A54.09
  puerperal, postpartum, childbirth O86.89
  strumous, tuberculous A18.2
  subacute (any site) I89.1
  tuberculous —*see* Tuberculosis, lymph gland
Lymphatic (vessel) —*see* condition
Lymphatism E32.8
Lymphectasia I89.0
Lymphedema (acquired) —*see also* Elephantiasis
  congenital Q82.0
  hereditary (chronic) (idiopathic) Q82.0
  postmastectomy I97.2
  praecox I89.0
  secondary I89.0
  surgical NEC I97.89
    postmastectomy (syndrome) I97.2
Lymphoblastic —*see* condition
Lymphoblastoma (diffuse) —*see* Lymphoma,
  lymphoblastic (diffuse)
  giant follicular —*see* Lymphoma,
    lymphoblastic (diffuse)
  macrofollicular —*see* Lymphoma,
    lymphoblastic (diffuse)
Lymphocele I89.8
Lymphocytic
  chorioencephalitis (acute) (serous) A87.2
  choriomeningitis (acute) (serous) A87.2
  meningoencephalitis A87.2
Lymphocytoma, benign cutis L98.8

Lymphocytopenia D72.810
Lymphocytosis (symptomatic) D72.820
  infectious (acute) B33.8
Lymphoepithelioma —*see* Neoplasm,
  malignant, by site
Lymphogranuloma (malignant) —*see also*
  Lymphoma, Hodgkin
  chlamydial A55
  inguinale A55
  venereum (any site) (chlamydial) (with
    stricture of rectum) A55
Lymphogranulomatosis (malignant) —*see also*
  Lymphoma, Hodgkin
  benign (Boeck's sarcoid) (Schaumann's)
    D86.1
Lymphohistiocytosis, hemophagocytic
  (familial) D76.1
Lymphoid —*see* condition
Lymphoma (of) (malignant) C85.90
  adult T-cell (HTLV-1-associated) (acute
    variant) (chronic variant)
    (lymphomatoid variant) (smouldering
    variant) C91.5-●
  anaplastic large cell
    ALK-negative C84.7-●
    ALK-positive C84.6-●
  ▶breast implant associated (BIA-ALCL)
    C84.7A
    CD30-positive C84.6-●
    primary cutaneous C86.6
  angioimmunoblastic T-cell C86.5
  BALT C88.4
  B-cell C85.1-●
  B-precursor C83.5-●
  blastic NK-cell C86.4
  blastic plasmacytoid dendritic cell neoplasm
    (BPDCN) C86.4
  bronchial-associated lymphoid tissue
    [BALT-lymphoma] C88.4
  Burkitt (atypical) C83.7-●
  Burkitt-like C83.7-●
  centrocytic C83.1-●
  cutaneous follicle center C82.6-●
  cutaneous T-cell C84.A-●
  diffuse follicle center C82.5-●
  diffuse large cell C83.3-●
    anaplastic C83.3-●
    B-cell C83.3-●
    CD30-positive C83.3-●
    centroblastic C83.3-●
    immunoblastic C83.3-●
    plasmablastic C83.3-●
    subtype not specified C83.3-●
    T-cell rich C83.3-●
  enteropathy-type (associated) (intestinal)
    T-cell C86.2
  extranodal marginal zone B-cell lymphoma
    of mucosa-associated lymphoid tissue
    [MALT-lymphoma] C88.4
  extranodal NK/T-cell, nasal type C86.0
  follicular C82.9-●
    grade
      I C82.0-●
      II C82.1-●
      III C82.2-●
      IIIa C82.3-●
      IIIb C82.4-●
    specified NEC C82.8-●
  hepatosplenic T-cell (alpha-beta) (gamma-
    delta) C86.1
  histiocytic C85.9-●
    true C96.A
  Hodgkin C81.9
    lymphocyte-rich (classical) C81.4-●
    lymphocyte depleted (classical) C81.3-●
    mixed cellularity (classical) C81.2-●
    nodular sclerosis (classical) C81.1-●
    specified NEC (classical) C81.7-●
    lymphocyte-rich classical C81.4-●
    lymphocyte depleted classical C81.3-●
    mixed cellularity classical C81.2-●

▶ New   ⇒ Revised   ~~deleted~~ Deleted   ● Use Additional Character(s)

Lymphoma *(Continued)*
  Hodgkin *(Continued)*
    nodular
      lymphocyte predominant C81.0-•
        sclerosis (classical) C81.1-•
  intravascular large B-cell C83.8-•
  Lennert's C84.4-•
  lymphoblastic (diffuse) C83.5-•
  lymphoblastic B-cell C83.5-•
  lymphoblastic T-cell C83.5-•
  lymphoepithelioid C84.4-•
  lymphoplasmacytic C83.0-•
    with IgM-production C88.0
  MALT C88.4
  mantle cell C83.1-•
  mature T-cell NEC C84.4-•
  mature T/NK-cell C84.9-•
    specified NEC C84.Z-•
  mediastinal (thymic) large B-cell
    C85.2-•
  Mediterranean C88.3

Lymphoma *(Continued)*
  mucosa-associated lymphoid tissue
    [MALT-lymphoma] C88.4
  NK/T cell C84.9-•
  nodal marginal zone C83.0-•
  non-follicular (diffuse) C83.9-•
    specified NEC C83.8-•
  non-Hodgkin —*see also* Lymphoma, by type
    C85.9-•
    specified NEC C85.8-•
  non-leukemic variant of B-CLL C83.0-•
  peripheral T-cell, not classified C84.4-•
  primary cutaneous
    anaplastic large cell C86.6
    CD30-positive large T-cell C86.6
  primary effusion B-cell C83.8-•
  SALT C88.4
  skin-associated lymphoid tissue
    [SALT-lymphoma] C88.4
  small cell B-cell C83.0-•
  splenic marginal zone C83.0-•

Lymphoma *(Continued)*
  subcutaneous panniculitis-like T-cell
    C86.3
  T-precursor C83.5-•
  true histiocytic C96.A
Lymphomatosis —*see* Lymphoma
Lymphopathia venereum, veneris A55
Lymphopenia D72.810
Lymphoplasmacytic leukemia —*see* Leukemia,
  chronic lymphocytic, B-cell type
Lymphoproliferation, X-linked disease D82.3
Lymphoreticulosis, benign (of inoculation)
  A28.1
Lymphorrhea I89.8
Lymphosarcoma (diffuse) —*see also* Lymphoma
  C85.9-•
Lymphostasis I89.8
Lypemania —*see* Melancholia
Lysine and hydroxylysine metabolism
  disorder E72.3
Lyssa —*see* Rabies

M

Macacus ear Q17.3
Maceration, wet feet, tropical (syndrome)
     T69.02-•
MacLeod's syndrome J43.0
Macrocephalia, macrocephaly Q75.3
Macrocheilia, macrochilia (congenital)Q18.6
Macrocolon —see also Megacolon Q43.1
Macrocornea Q15.8
   with glaucoma Q15.0
Macrocytic —see condition
Macrocytosis D75.89
Macrodactylia, macrodactylism (fingers)
     (thumbs) Q74.0
   toes Q74.2
Macrodontia K00.2
Macrogenia M26.05
Macrogenitosomia (adrenal) (male) (praecox)
     E25.9
   congenital E25.0
Macroglobulinemia (idiopathic) (primary)
     C88.0
   monoclonal (essential) D47.2
   Waldenström C88.0
Macroglossia (congenital) Q38.2
   acquired K14.8
Macrognathia, macrognathism (congenital)
     (mandibular) (maxillary) M26.09
Macrogyria (congenital) Q04.8
Macrohydrocephalus —see Hydrocephalus
Macromastia —see Hypertrophy, breast
Macrophthalmos Q11.3
   in congenital glaucoma Q15.0
Macropsia H53.15
Macrosigmoid K59.39
   congenital Q43.2
Macrospondylitis, acromegalic E22.0
Macrostomia (congenital) Q18.4
Macrotia (external ear) (congenital) Q17.1
Macula
   cornea, corneal —see Opacity, cornea
   degeneration (atrophic) (exudative)
        (senile) —see also Degeneration, macula
      hereditary —see Dystrophy, retina
Maculae ceruleae — B85.1
Maculopathy, toxic —see Degeneration, macula,
     toxic
Madarosis (eyelid) H02.729
   left H02.726
      lower H02.725
      upper H02.724
   right H02.723
      lower H02.722
      upper H02.721
Madelung's
   deformity (radius) Q74.0
   disease
      radial deformity Q74.0
      symmetrical lipomas, neck E88.89
Madness —see Psychosis
Madura
   foot B47.9
      actinomycotic B47.1
      mycotic B47.0
Maduromycosis B47.0
Maffucci's syndrome Q78.4
Magnesium metabolism disorder —see
     Disorder, metabolism, magnesium
Main en griffe (acquired) —see also Deformity,
     limb, clawhand
   congenital Q74.0
Maintenance (encounter for)
   antineoplastic chemotherapy Z51.11
   antineoplastic radiation therapy Z51.0
   methadone F11.20
Majocchi's
   disease L81.7
   granuloma B35.8
Major —see condition
Malabar itch (any site) B35.5

Malabsorption K90.9
   calcium K90.89
   carbohydrate K90.49
   disaccharide E73.9
   fat K90.49
   galactose E74.20
   glucose(-galactose) E74.39
   intestinal K90.9
      specified NEC K90.89
   isomaltose E74.31
   lactose E73.9
   methionine E72.19
   monosaccharide E74.39
   postgastrectomy K91.2
   postsurgical K91.2
   protein K90.49
   starch K90.49
   sucrose E74.39
   syndrome K90.9
      postsurgical K91.2
Malacia, bone (adult) M83.9
   juvenile —see Rickets
Malacoplakia
   bladder N32.89
   pelvis (kidney) N28.89
   ureter N28.89
   urethra N36.8
Malacosteon, juvenile —see Rickets
Maladaptation —see Maladjustment
Maladie de Roger Q21.0
Maladjustment
   conjugal Z63.0
      involving divorce or estrangement Z63.5
   educational Z55.4
   family Z63.9
   marital Z63.0
      involving divorce or estrangement Z63.5
   occupational NEC Z56.89
   simple, adult —see Disorder, adjustment
   situational —see Disorder, adjustment
   social Z60.9
      due to
         acculturation difficulty Z60.3
         discrimination and persecution
              (perceived) Z60.5
         exclusion and isolation Z60.4
         life-cycle (phase of life) transition Z60.0
         rejection Z60.4
         specified reason NEC Z60.8
Malaise R53.81
Malakoplakia —see Malacoplakia
Malaria, malarial (fever) B54
   with
      blackwater fever B50.8
         hemoglobinuric (bilious) B50.8
      hemoglobinuria B50.8
   accidentally induced (therapeutically) - code
        by type under Malaria
   algid B50.9
   cerebral B50.0 [G94]
   clinically diagnosed (without parasitological
        confirmation) B54
   congenital NEC P37.4
      falciparum P37.3
   congestion, congestive B54
   continued (fever) B50.9
   estivo-autumnal B50.9
   falciparum B50.9
      with complications NEC B50.8
         cerebral B50.0 [G94]
      severe B50.8
   hemorrhagic B54
   malariae B52.9
      with
         complications NEC B52.8
         glomerular disorder B52.0
   malignant (tertian) —see Malaria, falciparum
   mixed infections — code to first listed type
        in B50-B53
   ovale B53.0
   parasitologically confirmed NEC B53.8

Malaria, malarial (Continued)
   pernicious, acute —see Malaria, falciparum
   Plasmodium (P.)
      falciparum NEC —see Malaria, falciparum
      malariae NEC B52.9
         with Plasmodium
            falciparum (and or vivax) —see
                 Malaria, falciparum
            vivax —see also Malaria, vivax
                 and falciparum —see Malaria,
                      falciparum
      ovale B53.0
         with Plasmodium malariae —see also
              Malaria, malariae
            and vivax —see also Malaria, vivax
                 and falciparum —see Malaria,
                      falciparum
      simian B53.1
         with Plasmodium malariae —see also
              Malaria, malariae
            and vivax —see also Malaria, vivax
                 and falciparum —see Malaria,
                      falciparum
      vivax NEC B51.9
         with Plasmodium falciparum —see
              Malaria, falciparum
   quartan —see Malaria, malariae
   quotidian —see Malaria, falciparum
   recurrent B54
   remittent B54
   specified type NEC (parasitologically
        confirmed) B53.8
   spleen B54
   subtertian (fever) —see Malaria, falciparum
   tertian (benign) —see also Malaria, vivax
      malignant B50.9
   tropical B50.9
   typhoid B54
   vivax B51.9
      with
         complications NEC B51.8
         ruptured spleen B51.0
Malassez's disease (cystic) N50.89
Malassimilation K90.9
Mal de los pintos —see Pinta
Mal de mer T75.3
Maldescent, testis Q53.9
   bilateral Q53.20
      abdominal Q53.211
      perineal Q53.22
   unilateral Q53.10
      abdominal Q53.111
      perineal Q53.12
Maldevelopment —see also Anomaly
   brain Q07.9
   colon Q43.9
   hip Q74.2
      congenital dislocation Q65.2
         bilateral Q65.1
         unilateral Q65.0-•
   mastoid process Q75.8
   middle ear Q16.4
      except ossicles Q16.4
      ossicles Q16.3
   ossicles Q16.3
   spine Q76.49
   toe Q74.2
Male type pelvis Q74.2
   with disproportion (fetopelvic) O33.3
      causing obstructed labor O65.3
Malformation (congenital) —see also Anomaly
   adrenal gland Q89.1
   affecting multiple systems with skeletal
        changes NEC Q87.5
   alimentary tract Q45.9
      specified type NEC Q45.8
      upper Q40.9
         specified type NEC Q40.8
   aorta Q25.40
      absence Q25.41
      aneurysm, congenital Q25.43

▶ New   ⇒ Revised   ~~deleted~~ Deleted   • Use Additional Character(s)

Malformation (Continued)
  aorta (Continued)
    aplasia Q25.41
    atresia Q25.29
      aortic arch Q25.21
    coarctation (preductal) (postductal) Q25.1
    dilatation, congenital Q25.44
    hypoplasia Q25.42
    patent ductus arteriosus Q25.0
    specified type NEC Q25.49
    stenosis Q25.1
      supravalvular Q25.3
  aortic valve Q23.9
    specified NEC Q23.8
  arteriovenous, aneurysmatic (congenital)
      Q27.30
    brain Q28.2
      ruptured I60.8
        intracerebral I61.8
        intraparenchymal I61.8
        intraventricular I61.5
        subarachnoid I60.8
    cerebral (see Malformation, arteriovenous,
      brain) Q28.2
    peripheral Q27.30
      congenital Q27.33
      digestive system —see Angiodysplasia
      lower limb Q27.32
      other specified site Q27.39
      renal vessel Q27.34
      upper limb Q27.31
    precerebral vessels (nonruptured) Q28.0
  auricle
    ear (congenital) Q17.3
      acquired H61.119
        left H61.112
          with right H61.113
        right H61.111
          with left H61.113
  bile duct Q44.5
  bladder Q64.79
    aplasia Q64.5
    diverticulum Q64.6
    exstrophy —see Exstrophy, bladder
    neck obstruction Q64.31
  bone Q79.9
    face Q75.9
      specified type NEC Q75.8
    skull Q75.9
      specified type NEC Q75.8
  brain (multiple) Q04.9
    arteriovenous Q28.2
    specified type NEC Q04.8
  branchial cleft Q18.2
  breast Q83.9
    specified type NEC Q83.8
  broad ligament Q50.6
  bronchus Q32.4
  bursa Q79.9
  cardiac
    chambers Q20.9
      specified type NEC Q20.8
    septum Q21.9
      specified type NEC Q21.8
  cerebral Q04.9
    vessels Q28.3
  cervix uteri Q51.9
    specified type NEC Q51.828
  Chiari
    Type I G93.5
    Type II Q07.01
  choroid (congenital) Q14.3
    plexus Q07.8
  circulatory system Q28.9
  cochlea Q16.5
  cornea Q13.4
  coronary vessels Q24.5
  corpus callosum (congenital) Q04.0
  diaphragm Q79.1
  digestive system NEC, specified type NEC
    Q45.8

Malformation (Continued)
  dura Q07.9
    brain Q04.9
    spinal Q06.9
  ear Q17.9
    causing impairment of hearing Q16.9
    external Q17.9
      accessory auricle Q17.0
      causing impairment of hearing Q16.9
        absence of
          auditory canal Q16.1
          auricle Q16.0
      macrotia Q17.1
      microtia Q17.2
      misplacement Q17.4
      misshapen NEC Q17.3
      prominence Q17.5
      specified type NEC Q17.8
    inner Q16.5
    middle Q16.4
      absence of eustachian tube Q16.2
      ossicles (fusion) Q16.3
    ossicles Q16.3
    specified type NEC Q17.8
  epididymis Q55.4
  esophagus Q39.9
    specified type NEC Q39.8
  eye Q15.9
    lid Q10.3
    specified NEC Q15.8
  fallopian tube Q50.6
  genital organ —see Anomaly, genitalia
  great
    artery Q25.9
      aorta —see Malformation, aorta
      pulmonary artery —see Malformation,
        pulmonary, artery
      specified type NEC Q25.8
    vein Q26.9
      anomalous
        portal venous connection Q26.5
        pulmonary venous connection Q26.4
          partial Q26.3
          total Q26.2
      persistent left superior vena cava Q26.1
      portal vein-hepatic artery fistula Q26.6
      specified type NEC Q26.8
      vena cava stenosis, congenital Q26.0
  gum Q38.6
  hair Q84.2
  heart Q24.9
    specified type NEC Q24.8
  integument Q84.9
    specified type NEC Q84.8
  internal ear Q16.5
  intestine Q43.9
    specified type NEC Q43.8
  iris Q13.2
  joint Q74.9
    ankle Q74.2
    lumbosacral Q76.49
    sacroiliac Q74.2
    specified type NEC Q74.8
  kidney Q63.9
    accessory Q63.0
    giant Q63.3
    horseshoe Q63.1
    hydronephrosis Q62.0
    malposition Q63.2
    specified type NEC Q63.8
  lacrimal apparatus Q10.6
  lingual Q38.3
  lip Q38.0
  liver Q44.7
  lung Q33.9
  meninges or membrane (congenital) Q07.9
    cerebral Q04.8
    spinal (cord) Q06.9
  middle ear Q16.4
    ossicles Q16.3
  mitral valve Q23.9
    specified NEC Q23.8

Malformation (Continued)
  Mondini's (congenital) (malformation,
    cochlea) Q16.5
  mouth (congenital) Q38.6
  multiple types NEC Q89.7
  musculoskeletal system Q79.9
  myocardium Q24.8
  nail Q84.6
  nervous system (central) Q07.9
  nose Q30.9
    specified type NEC Q30.8
  optic disc Q14.2
  orbit Q10.7
  ovary Q50.39
  palate Q38.5
  parathyroid gland Q89.2
  pelvic organs or tissues NEC
    in pregnancy or childbirth O34.8-•
      causing obstructed labor O65.5
  penis Q55.69
    aplasia Q55.5
    curvature (lateral) Q55.61
    hypoplasia Q55.62
  pericardium Q24.8
  peripheral vascular system Q27.9
    specified type NEC Q27.8
  pharynx Q38.8
  precerebral vessels Q28.1
  prostate Q55.4
  pulmonary
    arteriovenous Q25.72
    artery Q25.9
      atresia Q25.5
      specified type NEC Q25.79
      stenosis Q25.6
    valve Q22.3
  renal artery Q27.2
  respiratory system Q34.9
  retina Q14.1
  scrotum —see Malformation, testis and scrotum
  seminal vesicles Q55.4
  sense organs NEC Q07.9
  skin Q82.9
  specified NEC Q89.8
  spinal
    cord Q06.9
    nerve root Q07.8
  spine Q76.49
    kyphosis —see Kyphosis, congenital
    lordosis —see Lordosis, congenital
  spleen Q89.09
  stomach Q40.3
    specified type NEC Q40.2
  teeth, tooth K00.9
  tendon Q79.9
  testis and scrotum Q55.20
    aplasia Q55.0
    hypoplasia Q55.1
    polyorchism Q55.21
    retractile testis Q55.22
    scrotal transposition Q55.23
    specified NEC Q55.29
  thorax, bony Q76.9
  throat Q38.8
  thyroid gland Q89.2
  tongue (congenital) Q38.3
    hypertrophy Q38.2
    tie Q38.1
  trachea Q32.1
  tricuspid valve Q22.9
    specified type NEC Q22.8
  umbilical cord NEC (complicating delivery)
    O69.89
  umbilicus Q89.9
  ureter Q62.8
    agenesis Q62.4
    duplication Q62.5
    malposition —see Malposition, congenital,
      ureter
    obstructive defect —see Defect, obstructive,
      ureter
    vesico-uretero-renal reflux Q62.7

Malformation (Continued)
 urethra Q64.79
  aplasia Q64.5
  duplication Q64.74
  posterior valves Q64.2
  prolapse Q64.71
  stricture Q64.32
 urinary system Q64.9
 uterus Q51.9
  specified type NEC Q51.818
 vagina Q52.4
 vascular system, peripheral Q27.9
 vas deferens Q55.4
  atresia Q55.3
 venous —see Anomaly, vein(s)
 vulva Q52.70
Malfunction —see also Dysfunction
 cardiac electronic device T82.119
  electrode T82.110
  pulse generator T82.111
  specified type NEC T82.118
 catheter device NEC T85.618
  cystostomy T83.010
  dialysis (renal) (vascular) T82.41
   intraperitoneal T85.611
  infusion NEC T82.514
   cranial T85.610
   epidural T85.610
   intrathecal T85.610
   spinal T85.610
   subarachnoid T85.610
   subdural T85.610
  urinary —see also Breakdown, device,
    catheter T83.018
 colostomy K94.03
  valve K94.03
 cystostomy (stoma) N99.512
  catheter T83.010
 enteric stoma K94.13
 enterostomy K94.13
 esophagostomy K94.33
 gastroenteric K31.89
 gastrostomy K94.23
 ileostomy K94.13
  valve K94.13
 intrathecal infusion pump T85.615
 jejunostomy K94.13
 nervous system device, implant or graft,
    specified NEC T85.615
 pacemaker —see Malfunction, cardiac
    electronic device
 prosthetic device, internal —see
    Complications, prosthetic device, by site,
    mechanical
 tracheostomy J95.03
 urinary device NEC —see Complication,
    genitourinary, device, urinary,
    mechanical
 valve
  colostomy K94.03
  heart T82.09
  ileostomy K94.13
 vascular graft or shunt NEC —see
    Complication, cardiovascular device,
    mechanical, vascular
 ventricular (communicating shunt) T85.01
Malherbe's tumor —see Neoplasm, skin,
  benign
Malibu disease L98.8-●
Malignancy —see also Neoplasm, malignant,
  by site
 unspecified site (primary) C80.1
Malignant —see condition
Malingerer, malingering Z76.5
Mallet finger (acquired) —see Deformity, finger,
  mallet finger
 congenital Q74.0
 sequelae of rickets E64.3
Malleus A24.0
Mallory's bodies R89.7
Mallory-Weiss syndrome K22.6

Malnutrition E46
 degree
  first E44.1
   mild (protein) E44.1
   moderate (protein) E44.0
  second E44.0
  severe (protein-energy) E43
   intermediate form E42
    with
     kwashiorkor (and marasmus) E42
     marasmus E41
  third E43
 following gastrointestinal surgery K91.2
 intrauterine
  light-for-dates —see Light for dates
  small-for-dates —see Small for dates
 lack of care, or neglect (child) (infant) T76.02
  confirmed T74.02
 malignant E40
 protein E46
  calorie E46
   mild E44.1
   moderate E44.0
   severe E43
    intermediate form E42
     with
      kwashiorkor (and marasmus)
       E42
      marasmus E41
  energy E46
   mild E44.1
   moderate E44.0
   severe E43
    intermediate form E42
     with
      kwashiorkor (and marasmus)
       E42
      marasmus E41
  severe (protein-energy) E43
   with
    kwashiorkor (and marasmus) E42
    marasmus E41
Malocclusion (teeth) M26.4
 Angle's M26.219
  class I M26.211
  class II M26.212
  class III M26.213
 due to
  abnormal swallowing M26.59
  mouth breathing M26.59
  tongue, lip or finger habits M26.59
 temporomandibular (joint) M26.69
Malposition
 cervix —see Malposition, uterus
 congenital
  adrenal (gland) Q89.1
  alimentary tract Q45.8
   lower Q43.8
   upper Q40.8
  aorta Q25.49
  appendix Q43.8
  arterial trunk Q20.0
  artery (peripheral) Q27.8
   coronary Q24.5
   digestive system Q27.8
   lower limb Q27.8
   pulmonary Q25.79
   specified site NEC Q27.8
   upper limb Q27.8
  auditory canal Q17.8
   causing impairment of hearing Q16.9
  auricle (ear) Q17.4
   causing impairment of hearing Q16.9
  cervical Q18.2
  biliary duct or passage Q44.5
  bladder (mucosa) —see Exstrophy,
    bladder
  brachial plexus Q07.8
  brain tissue Q04.8
  breast Q83.8
  bronchus Q32.4

Malposition (Continued)
 congenital (Continued)
  cecum Q43.8
  clavicle Q74.0
  colon Q43.8
  digestive organ or tract NEC Q45.8
   lower Q43.8
   upper Q40.8
  ear (auricle) (external) Q17.4
   ossicles Q16.3
  endocrine (gland) NEC Q89.2
  epiglottis Q31.8
  eustachian tube Q17.8
  eye Q15.8
  facial features Q18.8
  fallopian tube Q50.6
  finger(s) Q68.1
   supernumerary Q69.0
  foot Q66.9-●
  gallbladder Q44.1
  gastrointestinal tract Q45.8
  genitalia, genital organ(s) or tract
   female Q52.8
    external Q52.79
    internal NEC Q52.8
   male Q55.8
  glottis Q31.8
  hand Q68.1
  heart Q24.8
   dextrocardia Q24.0
    with complete transposition of viscera
     Q89.3
  hepatic duct Q44.5
  hip (joint) Q65.89
  intestine (large) (small) Q43.8
   with anomalous adhesions, fixation or
     malrotation Q43.3
  joint NEC Q68.8
  kidney Q63.2
  larynx Q31.8
  limb Q68.8
   lower Q68.8
   upper Q68.8
  liver Q44.7
  lung (lobe) Q33.8
  nail(s) Q84.6
  nerve Q07.8
  nervous system NEC Q07.8
  nose, nasal (septum) Q30.8
  organ or site not listed —see Anomaly,
    by site
  ovary Q50.39
  pancreas Q45.3
  parathyroid (gland) Q89.2
  patella Q74.1
  peripheral vascular system Q27.8
  pituitary (gland) Q89.2
  respiratory organ or system NEC
    Q34.8
  rib (cage) Q76.6
   supernumerary in cervical region
     Q76.5
  scapula Q74.0
  shoulder Q74.0
  spinal cord Q06.8
  spleen Q89.09
  sternum NEC Q76.7
  stomach Q40.2
  symphysis pubis Q74.2
  thymus (gland) Q89.2
  thyroid (gland) (tissue) Q89.2
   cartilage Q31.8
  toe(s) Q66.9-●
   supernumerary Q69.2
  tongue Q38.3
  trachea Q32.1
  ureter Q62.60
   deviation Q62.61
   displacement Q62.62
   ectopia Q62.63
   specified type NEC Q62.69

▶ New   ➡ Revised   ~~deleted~~ Deleted   ● Use Additional Character(s)

Malposition (Continued)
  congenital (Continued)
    uterus Q51.818
    vein(s) (peripheral) Q27.8
      great Q26.8
    vena cava (inferior) (superior) Q26.8
  device, implant or graft —see also
        Complications, by site and type,
        mechanical T85.628
    arterial graft NEC —see Complication,
        cardiovascular device, mechanical,
        vascular
    breast (implant) T85.42
    catheter NEC T85.628
      cystostomy T83.020
      dialysis (renal) T82.42
        intraperitoneal T85.621
      infusion NEC T82.524
        spinal (epidural) (subdural) T85.620
      urinary —see also Displacement, device,
          catheter, urinary T83.028
    electronic (electrode) (pulse generator)
        (stimulator)
      bone T84.320
      cardiac T82.129
        electrode T82.120
        pulse generator T82.121
        specified type NEC T82.128
      nervous system —see Complication,
          prosthetic device, mechanical,
          electronic nervous system
          stimulator
      urinary —see Complication,
          genitourinary, device, urinary,
          mechanical
    fixation, internal (orthopedic) NEC —
        see Complication, fixation device,
        mechanical
    gastrointestinal —see Complications,
        prosthetic device, mechanical,
        gastrointestinal device
    genital NEC T83.428
      intrauterine contraceptive device (string)
          T83.32
      penile prosthesis (cylinder) (implanted)
          (pump) (resevoir) T83.420
      testicular prosthesis T83.421
    heart NEC —see Complication,
        cardiovascular device, mechanical
    joint prosthesis —see Complication, joint
        prosthesis, mechanical
    ocular NEC —see Complications,
        prosthetic device, mechanical,
        ocular device
    orthopedic NEC —see Complication,
        orthopedic, device, mechanical
    specified NEC T85.628
    urinary NEC —see also Complication,
        genitourinary, device, urinary,
        mechanical
      graft T83.22
    vascular NEC —see Complication,
        cardiovascular device, mechanical
    ventricular intracranial shunt T85.02
  fetus —see Pregnancy, complicated by
      (management affected by), presentation,
      fetal
  gallbladder K82.8
  gastrointestinal tract, congenital Q45.8
  heart, congenital NEC Q24.8
  joint prosthesis —see Complications, joint
      prosthesis, mechanical, displacement,
      by site
  stomach K31.89
    congenital Q40.2
  tooth, teeth, fully erupted M26.30
  uterus (acute) (acquired) (adherent)
      (asymptomatic) (postinfectional)
      (postpartal, old) N85.4
    anteflexion or anteversion N85.4
      congenital Q51.818

Malposition (Continued)
  uterus (Continued)
    flexion N85.4
      lateral —see Lateroversion, uterus
    inversion N85.5
    lateral (flexion) (version) —see
        Lateroversion, uterus
      in pregnancy or childbirth —see
          subcategory O34.5
    retroflexion or retroversion —see
        Retroversion, uterus
Malposture R29.3
Malrotation
  cecum Q43.3
  colon Q43.3
  intestine Q43.3
  kidney Q63.2
Malta fever —see Brucellosis
Maltreatment
  adult
    abandonment
      confirmed T74.01
      suspected T76.01
    bullying
      confirmed T74.31
      suspected T76.31
    confirmed T74.91
    history of Z91.419
    intimidation (through social media)
      confirmed T74.31
      suspected T76.31
    neglect
      confirmed T74.01
      suspected T76.01
    physical abuse
      confirmed T74.11
      suspected T76.11
    psychological abuse
      confirmed T74.31
      history of Z91.411
      suspected T76.31
    sexual abuse
      confirmed T74.21
      suspected T76.21
    suspected T76.91
  child
    abandonment
      confirmed T74.02
      suspected T76.02
    bullying
      confirmed T74.32
      suspected T76.32
    confirmed T74.92
    history of —see History, personal (of),
        abuse
    intimidation (through social media)
      confirmed T74.32
      suspected T76.32
    neglect
      confirmed T74.02
      history of —see History, personal (of),
          abuse
      suspected T76.02
    physical abuse
      confirmed T74.12
      history of —see History, personal (of),
          abuse
      suspected T76.12
    psychological abuse
      confirmed T74.32
      history of —see History, personal (of),
          abuse
      suspected T76.32
    sexual abuse
      confirmed T74.22
      history of —see History, personal (of),
          abuse
      suspected T76.22
    suspected T76.92
  personal history of Z91.89
Maltworker's lung J67.4

Malunion, fracture —see Fracture, by site
Mammillitis N61.0
  puerperal, postpartum O91.02
Mammitis —see Mastitis
Mammogram (examination) Z12.39
  routine Z12.31
Mammoplasia N62
Management (of)
  bone conduction hearing device (implanted)
      Z45.320
  cardiac pacemaker NEC Z45.018
  cerebrospinal fluid drainage device Z45.41
  cochlear device (implanted) Z45.321
  contraceptive Z30.9
    specified NEC Z30.8
  implanted device Z45.9
    specified NEC Z45.89
  infusion pump Z45.1
  procreative Z31.9
    male factor infertility in female Z31.81
    specified NEC Z31.89
  prosthesis (external) —see also Fitting
      Z44.9
    implanted Z45.9
      specified NEC Z45.89
  renal dialysis catheter Z49.01
  vascular access device Z45.2
Mangled —see specified injury by site
Mania (monopolar) —see also Disorder, mood,
      manic episode
  with psychotic symptoms F30.2
  without psychotic symptoms F30.10
    mild F30.11
    moderate F30.12
    severe F30.13
  Bell's F30.8
  chronic (recurrent) F31.89
  hysterical F44.89
  puerperal F30.8
  recurrent F31.89
Manic depression F31.9
Manic-depressive insanity, psychosis, or
      syndrome —see Disorder, bipolar
Mannosidosis E77.1
Mansonelliasis, mansonellosis B74.4
Manson's
  disease B65.1
  schistosomiasis B65.1
Manual —see condition
Maple-bark-stripper's lung (disease) J67.6
Maple-syrup-urine disease E71.0
Marable's syndrome (celiac artery
      compression) I77.4
Marasmus E41
  due to malnutrition E41
  intestinal E41
  nutritional E41
  senile R54
  tuberculous NEC —see Tuberculosis
Marble
  bones Q78.2
  skin R23.8
Marburg virus disease A98.3
March
  fracture —see Fracture, traumatic, stress, by
      site
  hemoglobinuria D59.6
Marchesani (-Weill) syndrome Q87.0
Marchiafava (-Bignami) syndrome or disease
      G37.1
Marchiafava-Micheli syndrome D59.5
Marcus Gunn's syndrome Q07.8
Marfan's syndrome —see Syndrome, Marfan's
Marie-Bamberger disease —see
      Osteoarthropathy, hypertrophic, specified
      NEC
Marie-Charcot-Tooth neuropathic muscular
      atrophy G60.0
Marie's
  cerebellar ataxia (late-onset) G11.2
  disease or syndrome (acromegaly) E22.0

Marie-Strümpell arthritis, disease or
   spondylitis —see Spondylitis, ankylosing
Marion's disease (bladder neck obstruction)
   N32.0
Marital conflict Z63.0
Mark
   port wine Q82.5
   raspberry Q82.5
   strawberry Q82.5
   stretch L90.6
   tattoo L81.8
Marker heterochromatin —see Extra, marker
   chromosomes
Maroteaux-Lamy syndrome (mild) (severe)
   E76.29
Marrow (bone)
   arrest D61.9
   poor function D75.89
Marseilles fever A77.1
Marsh fever —see Malaria
Marshall's (hidrotic) ectodermal dysplasia
   Q82.4
Marsh's disease (exophthalmic goiter)
   E05.00
   with storm E05.01
Masculinization (female) with adrenal
   hyperplasia E25.9
   congenital E25.0
Masculinovoblastoma D27.-●
Masochism (sexual) F65.51
Mason's lung J62.8
Mass
   abdominal R19.00
      epigastric R19.06
      generalized R19.07
      left lower quadrant R19.04
      left upper quadrant R19.02
      periumbilic R19.05
      right lower quadrant R19.03
      right upper quadrant R19.01
      specified site NEC R19.09
   breast —see also Lump, breast N63.0
   chest R22.2
   cystic —see Cyst
   ear H93.8-●
   head R22.0
   intra-abdominal (diffuse) (generalized) —see
      Mass, abdominal
   kidney N28.89
   liver R16.0
   localized (skin) R22.9
      chest R22.2
      head R22.0
      limb
         lower R22.4-●
         upper R22.3-●
      neck R22.1
      trunk R22.2
   lung R91.8
   malignant —see Neoplasm, malignant,
      by site
   neck R22.1
   pelvic (diffuse) (generalized) —see Mass,
      abdominal
   specified organ NEC —see Disease, by site
   splenic R16.1
   substernal thyroid —see Goiter
   superficial (localized) R22.9
   umbilical (diffuse) (generalized) R19.09
Massive —see condition
Mast cell
   disease, systemic tissue D47.02
   leukemia C94.3-●
   neoplasm
      malignant C96.20
         specified type NEC C96.29
      of uncertain behavior NEC D47.09
   sarcoma C96.22
   tumor D47.09
Mastalgia N64.4
Masters-Allen syndrome N83.8

Mastitis (acute) (diffuse) (nonpuerperal)
   (subacute) N61.0
   with abscess N61.1
   chronic (cystic) —see Mastopathy, cystic
   cystic (Schimmelbusch's type) —see
      Mastopathy, cystic
   fibrocystic —see Mastopathy, cystic
   granulomatous N61.2-●
   infective N61.0
      newborn P39.0
   interstitial, gestational or puerperal —see
      Mastitis, obstetric
   neonatal (noninfective) P83.4
      infective P39.0
   obstetric (interstitial) (nonpurulent)
      associated with
         lactation O91.23
         pregnancy O91.21-●
         puerperium O91.22
      purulent
         associated with
            lactation O91.13
            pregnancy O91.11-●
            puerperium O91.12
   periductal —see Ectasia, mammary duct
   phlegmonous —see Mastopathy, cystic
   plasma cell —see Ectasia, mammary duct
   without abscess N61.0
Mastocytoma (extracutaneous) D47.09
   malignant C96.29
   solitary D47.01
Mastocytosis D47.09
   aggressive systemic C96.21
   cutaneous (diffuse) (maculopapular) D47.01
      congenital Q82.2
      of neonatal onset Q82.2
      of newborn onset Q82.2
   indolent systemic D47.02
   isolated bone marrow D47.02
   malignant C96.29
   systemic (indolent) (smoldering)
      with an associated hematological
         non-mast cell lineage disease (SM-
         AHNMD) D47.02
Mastodynia N64.4
Mastoid —see condition
Mastoidalgia —see subcategory H92.0
Mastoiditis (coalescent) (hemorrhagic)
   (suppurative) H70.9-●
   acute, subacute H70.00-●
      complicated NEC H70.09-●
      subperiosteal H70.01-●
   chronic (necrotic) (recurrent) H70.1-●
   in (due to)
      infectious disease NEC B99 [H75.0-●]
      parasitic disease NEC B89 [H75.0-●]
      tuberculosis A18.03
   petrositis —see Petrositis
   postauricular fistula —see Fistula,
      postauricular
   specified NEC H70.89-●
   tuberculous A18.03
Mastopathy, mastopathia N64.9
   chronica cystica —see Mastopathy, cystic
   cystic (chronic) (diffuse) N60.1
      with epithelial proliferation N60.3-●
   diffuse cystic —see Mastopathy, cystic
   estrogenic, oestrogenica N64.89
   ovarian origin N64.89
Mastoplasia, mastoplastia N62
Masturbation (excessive) F98.8
Maternal care (for) —see Pregnancy
   (complicated by) (management affected by)
Matheiu's disease (leptospiral jaundice) A27.0
Mauclaire's disease or osteochondrosis —see
   Osteochondrosis, juvenile, hand, metacarpal
Maxcy's disease A75.2
Maxilla, maxillary —see condition
May (-Hegglin) anomaly or syndrome D72.0
McArdle (-Schmid)-(-Pearson) disease
   (glycogen storage) E74.04

McCune-Albright syndrome Q78.1
McQuarrie's syndrome (idiopathic familial
   hypoglycemia) E16.2
Meadow's syndrome Q86.1
Measles (black) (hemorrhagic) (suppressed)
   B05.9
   with
      complications NEC B05.89
      encephalitis B05.0
      intestinal complications B05.4
      keratitis (keratoconjunctivitis) B05.81
      meningitis B05.1
      otitis media B05.3
      pneumonia B05.2
   French —see Rubella
   German —see Rubella
   Liberty —see Rubella
Meatitis, urethral —see Urethritis
Meatus, meatal —see condition
Meat-wrappers' asthma J68.9
Meckel-Gruber syndrome Q61.9
Meckel's diverticulitis, diverticulum
   (displaced) (hypertrophic) Q43.0
Meconium
   ileus, newborn P76.0
      in cystic fibrosis E84.11
      meaning meconium plug (without cystic
         fibrosis) P76.0
   obstruction, newborn P76.0
      due to fecaliths P76.0
      in mucoviscidosis E84.11
   peritonitis P78.0
   plug syndrome (newborn) NEC P76.0
Median —see also condition
   arcuate ligament syndrome I77.4
   bar (prostate) (vesical orifice) —see
      Hyperplasia, prostate
   rhomboid glossitis K14.2
Mediastinal shift R93.89
Mediastinitis (acute) (chronic) J98.51
   syphilitic A52.73
   tuberculous A15.8
Mediastinopericarditis —see also Pericarditis
   acute I30.9
   adhesive I31.0
   chronic I31.8
      rheumatic I09.2
Mediastinum, mediastinal —see condition
Medicine poisoning —see Table of Drugs and
   Chemicals, by drug, poisoning
Mediterranean
   fever —see Brucellosis
      familial M04.1
      tick A77.1
   kala-azar B55.0
   leishmaniasis B55.0
   tick fever A77.1
Medulla —see condition
Medullary cystic kidney Q61.5
Medullated fibers
   optic (nerve) Q14.8
   retina Q14.1
Medulloblastoma
   desmoplastic C71.6
   specified site —see Neoplasm, malignant, by
      site
   unspecified site C71.6
Medulloepithelioma —see also Neoplasm,
   malignant, by site
   teratoid —see Neoplasm, malignant, by site
Medullomyoblastoma
   specified site —see Neoplasm, malignant, by
      site
   unspecified site C71.6
Meekeren-Ehlers-Danlos syndrome —see also
   Syndrome, Ehlers-Danlos Q79.6
Megacolon (acquired) (functional) (not
   Hirschsprung's disease) (in) K59.39
   Chagas' disease B57.32
   congenital, congenitum (aganglionic) Q43.1
   Hirschsprung's (disease) Q43.1

▶ New   ⇒ Revised   ~~deleted~~ Deleted   ● Use Additional Character(s)

Megacolon *(Continued)*
 toxic NEC K59.31
  due to Clostridium difficile
   not specified as recurrent A04.72
   recurrent A04.71
Megaesophagus (functional) K22.0
 congenital Q39.5
 in (due to) Chagas' disease B57.31
Megalencephaly Q04.5
Megalerythema (epidemic) B08.3
Megaloappendix Q43.8
Megalocephalus, megalocephaly NEC Q75.3
Megalocornea Q15.8
 with glaucoma Q15.0
Megalocytic anemia D53.1
Megalodactylia (fingers) (thumbs) (congenital)
  Q74.0
 toes Q74.2
Megaloduodenum Q43.8
Megaloesophagus (functional) K22.0
 congenital Q39.5
Megalogastria (acquired) K31.89
 congenital Q40.2
Megalophthalmos Q11.3
Megalopsia H53.15
Megalosplenia —*see* Splenomegaly
Megaloureter N28.82
 congenital Q62.2
Megarectum K62.89
Megasigmoid K59.39
 congenital Q43.2
Megaureter N28.82
 congenital Q62.2
Megavitamin-B6 syndrome E67.2
Megrim —*see* Migraine
Meibomian
 cyst, infected —*see* Hordeolum
 gland —*see* condition
 sty, stye —*see* Hordeolum
Meibomitis —*see* Hordeolum
Meige-Milroy disease (chronic hereditary
  edema) Q82.0
Meige's syndrome Q82.0
Melalgia, nutritional E53.8
▶ Melancholia F32.A
 climacteric (single episode) F32.89
  recurrent episode F33.8
 hypochondriac F45.29
 intermittent (single episode) F32.89
  recurrent episode F33.8
 involutional (single episode) F32.89
  recurrent episode F33.8
 menopausal (single episode) F32.89
  recurrent episode F33.8
 puerperal F32.89
 reactive (emotional stress or trauma) F32.3
 recurrent F33.9
 senile F03
 stuporous (single episode) F32.89
  recurrent episode F33.8
Melanemia R79.89
Melanoameloblastoma —*see* Neoplasm, bone,
  benign
Melanoblastoma —*see* Melanoma
Melanocarcinoma —*see* Melanoma
Melanocytoma, eyeball D31.9-●
Melanocytosis, neurocutaneous Q82.8
Melanoderma, melanodermia L81.4
Melanodontia, infantile K03.89
Melanodontoclasia K03.89
Melanoepithelioma —*see* Melanoma
Melanoma (malignant) C43.9
 acral lentiginous, malignant —*see* Melanoma,
  skin, by site
 amelanotic —*see* Melanoma, skin, by site
 balloon cell —*see* Melanoma, skin, by site
 benign —*see* Nevus
 desmoplastic, malignant —*see* Melanoma,
  skin, by site
 epithelioid cell —*see* Melanoma, skin, by site
  with spindle cell, mixed —*see* Melanoma,
   skin, by site

Melanoma *(Continued)*
 in
  giant pigmented nevus —*see* Melanoma,
   skin, by site
  Hutchinson's melanotic freckle —*see*
   Melanoma, skin, by site
  junctional nevus —*see* Melanoma, skin,
   by site
  precancerous melanosis —*see* Melanoma,
   skin, by site
 in situ D03.9
  abdominal wall D03.59
  ala nasi D03.39
  ankle D03.7-●
  anus, anal (margin) (skin) D03.51
  arm D03.6-●
  auditory canal D03.2-●
  auricle (ear) D03.2-●
  auricular canal (external) D03.2-●
  axilla, axillary fold D03.59
  back D03.59
  breast D03.52
  brow D03.39
  buttock D03.59
  canthus (eye) D03.1-●
  cheek (external) D03.39
  chest wall D03.59
  chin D03.39
  choroid D03.8
  conjunctiva D03.8
  ear (external) D03.2-●
  external meatus (ear) D03.2-●
  eye D03.8
  eyebrow D03.39
  eyelid (lower) (upper) D03.1-●
  face D03.30
   specified NEC D03.39
  female genital organ (external) NEC D03.8
  finger D03.6-●
  flank D03.59
  foot D03.7-●
  forearm D03.6-●
  forehead D03.39
  foreskin D03.8
  gluteal region D03.59
  groin D03.59
  hand D03.6-●
  heel D03.7-●
  helix D03.2-●
  hip D03.7-●
  interscapular region D03.59
  iris D03.8
  jaw D03.39
  knee D03.7-●
  labium (majus) (minus) D03.8
  lacrimal gland D03.8
  leg D03.7-●
  lip (lower) (upper) D03.0
  lower limb NEC D03.7-●
  male genital organ (external) NEC D03.8
  nail D03.9
   finger D03.6-●
   toe D03.7-●
  neck D03.4
  nose (external) D03.39
  orbit D03.8
  penis D03.8
  perianal skin D03.51
  perineum D03.51
  pinna D03.2-●
  popliteal fossa or space D03.7-●
  prepuce D03.8
  pudendum D03.8
  retina D03.8
  retrobulbar D03.8
  scalp D03.4
  scrotum D03.8
  shoulder D03.6-●
  specified site NEC D03.8
  submammary fold D03.52
  temple D03.39

Melanoma *(Continued)*
 in situ *(Continued)*
  thigh D03.7-●
  toe D03.7-●
  trunk NEC D03.59
  umbilicus D03.59
  upper limb NEC D03.6-●
  vulva D03.8
 juvenile —*see* Nevus
 malignant, of soft parts except skin —*see*
   Neoplasm, connective tissue, malignant
 metastatic
  breast C79.81
  genital organ C79.82
  specified site NEC C79.89
 neurotropic, malignant —*see* Melanoma, skin,
   by site
 nodular —*see* Melanoma, skin, by site
 regressing, malignant —*see* Melanoma, skin,
   by site
 skin C43.9
  abdominal wall C43.59
  ala nasi C43.31
  ankle C43.7-●
  anus, anal (skin) C43.51
  arm C43.6-●
  auditory canal (external) C43.2-●
  auricle (ear) C43.2-●
  auricular canal (external) C43.2-●
  axilla, axillary fold C43.59
  back C43.59
  breast (female) (male) C43.52
  brow C43.39
  buttock C43.59
  canthus (eye) C43.1-●
  cheek (external) C43.39
  chest wall C43.59
  chin C43.39
  ear (external) C43.2-●
  elbow C43.6-●
  external meatus (ear) C43.2-●
  eyebrow C43.39
  eyelid (lower) (upper) C43.1-●
  face C43.30
   specified NEC C43.39
  female genital organ (external) NEC C51.9
  finger C43.6-●
  flank C43.59
  foot C43.7-●
  forearm C43.6-●
  forehead C43.39
  foreskin C60.0
  glabella C43.39
  gluteal region C43.59
  groin C43.59
  hand C43.6-●
  heel C43.7-●
  helix C43.2-●
  hip C43.7-●
  interscapular region C43.59
  jaw (external) C43.39
  knee C43.7-●
  labium C51.9
   majus C51.0
   minus C51.1
  leg C43.7-●
  lip (lower) (upper) C43.0
  lower limb NEC C43.7-●
  male genital organ (external) NEC C63.9
  nail
   finger C43.6-●
   toe C43.7-●
  nasolabial groove C43.39
  nates C43.59
  neck C43.4
  nose (external) C43.31
  overlapping site C43.8
  palpebra C43.1-●
  penis C60.9
  perianal skin C43.51
  perineum C43.51

M

Melanoma *(Continued)*
  skin *(Continued)*
    pinna C43.2-●
    popliteal fossa or space C43.7-●
    prepuce C60.0
    pudendum C51.9
    scalp C43.4
    scrotum C63.2
    shoulder C43.6-●
    skin NEC C43.9
    submammary fold C43.52
    temple C43.39
    thigh C43.7-●
    toe C43.7-●
    trunk NEC C43.59
    umbilicus C43.59
    upper limb NEC C43.6-●
    vulva C51.9
      overlapping sites C51.8
  spindle cell
    with epithelioid, mixed —*see* Melanoma,
      skin, by site
    type A C69.4-●
    type B C69.4-●
  superficial spreading —*see* Melanoma, skin,
    by site
Melanosarcoma —*see also* Melanoma
  epithelioid cell —*see* Melanoma
Melanosis L81.4
  addisonian E27.1
    tuberculous A18.7
  adrenal E27.1
  colon K63.89
  conjunctiva —*see* Pigmentation, conjunctiva
    congenital Q13.89
  cornea (presenile) (senile) —*see also*
    Pigmentation, cornea
    congenital Q13.4
  eye NEC H57.89
    congenital Q15.8
  lenticularis progressiva Q82.1
  liver K76.89
  precancerous —*see also* Melanoma, in situ
    malignant melanoma in —*see* Melanoma
  Riehl's L81.4
  sclera H15.89
    congenital Q13.89
  suprarenal E27.1
  tar L81.4
  toxic L81.4
Melanuria R82.998
MELAS syndrome E88.41
Melasma L81.1
  adrenal (gland) E27.1
  suprarenal (gland) E27.1
Melena K92.1
  with ulcer - code by site under Ulcer, with
    hemorrhage K27.4
  due to swallowed maternal blood P78.2
  newborn, neonatal P54.1
    due to swallowed maternal blood P78.2
Meleney's
  gangrene (cutaneous) —*see* Ulcer, skin
  ulcer (chronic undermining) —*see* Ulcer, skin
Melioidosis A24.9
  acute A24.1
  chronic A24.2
  fulminating A24.1
  pneumonia A24.1
  pulmonary (chronic) A24.2
    acute A24.1
    subacute A24.2
  sepsis A24.1
  specified NEC A24.3
  subacute A24.2
Melitensis, febris A23.0
Melkersson (-Rosenthal) syndrome G51.2
Mellitus, diabetes —*see* Diabetes
Melorheostosis (bone) —*see* Disorder, bone,
  density and structure, specified NEC
Meloschisis Q18.4

Melotia Q17.4
Membrana
  capsularis lentis posterior Q13.89
  epipapillaris Q14.2
Membranacea placenta O43.19-●
Membranaceous uterus N85.8
Membrane(s), membranous —*see also* condition
  cyclitic —*see* Membrane, pupillary
  folds, congenital —*see* Web
  Jackson's Q43.3
  over face of newborn P28.9
  premature rupture —*see* Rupture,
    membranes, premature
  pupillary H21.4-●
    persistent Q13.89
  retained (with hemorrhage) (complicating
    delivery) O72.2
    without hemorrhage O73.1
  secondary cataract —*see* Cataract, secondary
  unruptured (causing asphyxia) —*see*
    Asphyxia, newborn
  vitreous —*see* Opacity, vitreous, membranes
    and strands
Membranitis —*see* Chorioamnionitis
Memory disturbance, lack or loss —*see also*
  Amnesia
  mild, following organic brain damage F06.8
Menadione deficiency E56.1
Menarche
  delayed E30.0
  precocious E30.1
Mendacity, pathologic F60.2
Mendelson's syndrome (due to anesthesia) J95.4
  in labor and delivery O74.0
  in pregnancy O29.01-●
  obstetric O74.0
  postpartum, puerperal O89.01
Ménétrier's disease or syndrome K29.60
  with bleeding K29.61
Ménière's disease, syndrome or vertigo H81.0-●
Meninges, meningeal —*see* condition
Meningioma —*see also* Neoplasm, meninges,
  benign
  angioblastic —*see* Neoplasm, meninges,
    benign
  angiomatous —*see* Neoplasm, meninges,
    benign
  atypical —*see* Neoplasm, meninges, uncertain
    behavior
  endotheliomatous —*see* Neoplasm, meninges,
    benign
  fibroblastic —*see* Neoplasm, meninges,
    benign
  fibrous —*see* Neoplasm, meninges, benign
  hemangioblastic —*see* Neoplasm, meninges,
    benign
  hemangiopericytic —*see* Neoplasm,
    meninges, benign
  malignant —*see* Neoplasm, meninges,
    malignant
  meningiothelial —*see* Neoplasm, meninges,
    benign
  meningotheliomatous —*see* Neoplasm,
    meninges, benign
  mixed —*see* Neoplasm, meninges, benign
  multiple —*see* Neoplasm, meninges,
    uncertain behavior
  papillary —*see* Neoplasm, meninges,
    uncertain behavior
  psammomatous —*see* Neoplasm, meninges,
    benign
  syncytial —*see* Neoplasm, meninges, benign
  transitional —*see* Neoplasm, meninges,
    benign
Meningiomatosis (diffuse) —*see* Neoplasm,
  meninges, uncertain behavior
Meningism —*see* Meningismus
Meningismus (infectional) (pneumococcal) R29.1
  due to serum or vaccine R29.1
  influenzal —*see* Influenza, with,
    manifestations NEC

Meningitis (basal) (basic) (brain) (cerebral)
  (cervical) (congestive) (diffuse)
  (hemorrhagic) infantile) (membranous)
  (metastatic) (nonspecific) (pontine)
  (progressive) (simple) (spinal) (subacute)
  (sympathetic) (toxic) G03.9
  abacterial G03.0
  actinomycotic A42.81
  adenoviral A87.1
  arbovirus A87.8
  aseptic (acute) G03.0
  bacterial G00.9
    Escherichia coli (E. coli) G00.8
    Friedländer (bacillus) G00.8
    gram-negative G00.9
    H. influenzae G00.0
    Klebsiella G00.8
    pneumococcal G00.1
    specified organism NEC G00.8
    staphylococcal G00.3
    streptococcal (acute) G00.2
  benign recurrent (Mollaret) G03.2
  candidal B37.5
  caseous (tuberculous) A17.0
  cerebrospinal A39.0
  chronic NEC G03.1
  clear cerebrospinal fluid NEC G03.0
  coxsackievirus A87.0
  cryptococcal B45.1
  diplococcal (gram positive) A39.0
  echovirus A87.0
  enteroviral A87.0
  eosinophilic B83.2
  epidemic NEC A39.0
  Escherichia coli (E. coli) G00.8
  fibrinopurulent G00.9
    specified organism NEC G00.8
  Friedländer (bacillus) G00.8
  gonococcal A54.81
  gram-negative cocci G00.9
  gram-positive cocci G00.9
  Haemophilus (influenzae) G00.0
  H. influenzae G00.0
  in (due to)
    adenovirus A87.1
    African trypanosomiasis B56.9 *[G02]*
    anthrax A22.8
    bacterial disease NEC A48.8 *[G01]*
    Chagas' disease (chronic) B57.41
    chickenpox B01.0
    coccidioidomycosis B38.4
    Diplococcus pneumoniae G00.1
    enterovirus A87.0
    herpes (simplex) virus B00.3
      zoster B02.1
    infectious mononucleosis B27.92
    leptospirosis A27.81
    Listeria monocytogenes A32.11
    Lyme disease A69.21
    measles B05.1
    mumps (virus) B26.1
    neurosyphilis (late) A52.13
    parasitic disease NEC B89 *[G02]*
    poliovirus A80.9 *[G02]*
    preventive immunization, inoculation or
      vaccination G03.8
    rubella B06.02
    Salmonella infection A02.21
    specified cause NEC G03.8
    Streptococcal pneumoniae G00.1
    typhoid fever A01.01
    varicella B01.0
    viral disease NEC A87.8
    whooping cough A37.90
    zoster B02.1
  infectious G00.9
  influenzal (H. influenzae) G00.0
  Klebsiella G00.8
  leptospiral (aseptic) A27.81
  lymphocytic (acute) (benign) (serous) A87.2
  meningococcal A39.0

► New   ⇒ Revised   ~~deleted~~ Deleted   ● Use Additional Character(s)

Meningitis *(Continued)*
  Mima polymorpha G00.8
  Mollaret (benign recurrent) G03.2
  monilial B37.5
  mycotic NEC B49 *[G02]*
  Neisseria A39.0
  nonbacterial G03.0
  nonpyogenic NEC G03.0
  ossificans G96.198
  pneumococcal streptococcus pneumoniae
      G00.1
  poliovirus A80.9 *[G02]*
  postmeasles B05.1
  purulent G00.9
    specified organism NEC G00.8
  pyogenic G00.9
    specified organism NEC G00.8
  Salmonella (arizonae) (Cholerae-Suis)
      (enteritidis) (typhimurium) A02.21
  septic G00.9
    specified organism NEC G00.8
  serosa circumscripta NEC G03.0
  serous NEC G93.2
  specified organism NEC G00.8
  sporotrichosis B42.81
  staphylococcal G00.3
  sterile G03.0
  Streptococcal (acute) G00.2
    pneumoniae G00.1
  suppurative G00.9
    specified organism NEC G00.8
  syphilitic (late) (tertiary) A52.13
    acute A51.41
    congenital A50.41
    secondary A51.41
  Torula histolytica (cryptococcal) B45.1
  traumatic (complication of injury) T79.8
  tuberculous A17.0
  typhoid A01.01
  viral NEC A87.9
  Yersinia pestis A20.3
Meningocele (spinal) —*see also* Spina bifida
  with hydrocephalus —*see* Spina bifida, by
      site, with hydrocephalus
  acquired (traumatic) G96.198
  cerebral —*see* Encephalocele
Meningocerebritis —*see* Meningoencephalitis
Meningococcemia A39.4
  acute A39.2
  chronic A39.3
Meningococcus, meningococcal —*see also*
      condition A39.9
  adrenalitis, hemorrhagic A39.1
  carrier (suspected) of Z22.31
  meningitis (cerebrospinal) A39.0
Meningoencephalitis —*see also* Encephalitis
      G04.90
  acute NEC —*see also* Encephalitis, viral A86
  bacterial NEC G04.2
  California A83.5
  diphasic A84.1
  eosinophilic B83.2
  epidemic A39.81
  herpesviral, herpetic B00.4
    due to herpesvirus 6 B10.01
    due to herpesvirus 7 B10.09
    specified NEC B10.09
  in (due to)
    blastomycosis NEC B40.81
    diseases classified elsewhere G05.3
    free-living amebae B60.2
    Hemophilus influenzae (H. influenzae)
        G00.0
    herpes B00.4
      due to herpesvirus 6 B10.01
      due to herpesvirus 7 B10.09
      specified NEC B10.09
    H. influenzae G00.0
    Lyme disease A69.22
    mercury —*see* subcategory T56.1
    mumps B26.2

Meningoencephalitis *(Continued)*
  in (due to) *(Continued)*
    Naegleria (amebae) (organisms) (fowleri)
        B60.2
    Parastrongylus cantonensis B83.2
    toxoplasmosis (acquired) B58.2
      congenital P37.1
  infectious (acute) (viral) A86
  influenzal (H. influenzae) G00.0
  Listeria monocytogenes A32.12
  lymphocytic (serous) A87.2
  mumps B26.2
  parasitic NEC B89 *[G05.3]*
  pneumococcal G04.2
  primary amebic B60.2
  specific (syphilitic) A52.14
  specified organism NEC G04.81
  staphylococcal G04.2
  streptococcal G04.2
  syphilitic A52.14
➡ toxic NEC G92.8
    due to mercury —*see* subcategory T56.1
  tuberculous A17.82
  virus NEC A86
Meningoencephalocele —*see also*
      Encephalocele
  syphilitic A52.19
    congenital A50.49
Meningoencephalomyelitis —*see also*
      Meningoencephalitis
  acute NEC (viral) A86
    disseminated G04.00
      postimmunization or postvaccination
          G04.02
      postinfectious G04.01
  due to
    actinomycosis A42.82
    Torula B45.1
    Toxoplasma or toxoplasmosis (acquired)
        B58.2
      congenital P37.1
  postimmunization or postvaccination
      G04.02
Meningoencephalomyelopathy G96.9
Meningoencephalopathy G96.9
Meningomyelitis —*see also*
      Meningoencephalitis
  bacterial NEC G04.2
  blastomycotic NEC B40.81
  cryptococcal B45.1
  in diseases classified elsewhere G05.4
  meningococcal A39.81
  syphilitic A52.14
  tuberculous A17.82
Meningomyelocele —*see also* Spina bifida
  syphilitic A52.19
Meningomyeloneuritis —*see*
      Meningoencephalitis
Meningoradiculitis —*see* Meningitis
Meningovascular —*see* condition
Menkes' disease or syndrome E83.09
  meaning maple-syrup-urine disease E71.0
Menometrorrhagia N92.1
Menopause, menopausal (asymptomatic)
      (state) Z78.0
  arthritis (any site) NEC —*see* Arthritis,
      specified form NEC
  bleeding N92.4
  depression (single episode) F32.89
    agitated (single episode) F32.2
      recurrent episode F33.9
    psychotic (single episode) F32.89
      zrecurrent episode F33.8
    recurrent episode F33.9
    melancholia (single episode) F32.89
      recurrent episode F33.8
  paranoid state F22
  premature E28.319
    asymptomatic E28.319
      postirradiation E89.40
      postsurgical E89.40

Menopause, menopausal *(Continued)*
  premature *(Continued)*
    symptomatic E28.310
      postirradiation E89.41
      postsurgical E89.41
  psychosis NEC F28
  symptomatic N95.1
  toxic polyarthritis NEC —*see* Arthritis,
      specified form NEC
Menorrhagia (primary) N92.0
  climacteric N92.4
    menopausal N92.4
  menopausal N92.4
  perimenopausal N92.4
  postclimacteric N95.0
  postmenopausal N95.0
  preclimacteric or premenopausal N92.4
  pubertal (menses retained) N92.2
Menostaxis N92.0
Menses, retention N94.89
Menstrual —*see* Menstruation
Menstruation
  absent —*see* Amenorrhea
  anovulatory N97.0
  cycle, irregular N92.6
  delayed N91.0
  disorder N93.9
    psychogenic F45.8
  during pregnancy O20.8
  excessive (with regular cycle) N92.0
    with irregular cycle N92.1
    at puberty N92.2
  frequent N92.0
  infrequent —*see* Oligomenorrhea
  irregular N92.6
    specified NEC N92.5
  latent N92.5
  membranous N92.5
  painful —*see also* Dysmenorrhea N94.6
    primary N94.4
    psychogenic F45.8
    secondary N94.5
  passage of clots N92.0
  precocious E30.1
  protracted N92.5
  rare —*see* Oligomenorrhea
  retained N94.89
  retrograde N92.5
  scanty —*see* Oligomenorrhea
  suppression N94.89
  vicarious (nasal) N94.89
Mental —*see also* condition
  deficiency —*see* Disability, intellectual
  deterioration —*see* Psychosis
  disorder —*see* Disorder, mental
  exhaustion F48.8
  insufficiency (congenital) —*see* Disability,
      intellectual
  observation without need for further medical
      care Z03.89
  retardation —*see* Disability, intellectual
  subnormality —*see* Disability, intellectual
  upset —*see* Disorder, mental
Meralgia paresthetica G57.1-●
Mercurial —*see* condition
Mercurialism —*see* subcategory T56.1
MERRF syndrome (myoclonic epilepsy
      associated with ragged-red fiber) E88.42
Merkel cell tumor —*see* Carcinoma, Merkel cell
Merocele —*see* Hernia, femoral
Meromelia
  lower limb —*see* Defect, reduction, lower
      limb
    intercalary
      femur —*see* Defect, reduction, lower
          limb, specified type NEC
        tibiofibular (complete) (incomplete) —
            see Defect, reduction, lower limb
  upper limb —*see* Defect, reduction, upper
      limb
    intercalary, humeral, radioulnar —*see*
        Agenesis, arm, with hand present

Merzbacher-Pelizaeus disease E75.29
Mesaortitis —see Aortitis
Mesarteritis —see Arteritis
Mesencephalitis —see Encephalitis
Mesenchymoma —see also Neoplasm,
   connective tissue, uncertain behavior
  benign —see Neoplasm, connective tissue,
    benign
  malignant —see Neoplasm, connective tissue,
    malignant
Mesenteritis
  retractile K65.4
  sclerosing K65.4
Mesentery, mesenteric —see condition
Mesiodens, mesiodentes K00.1
Mesio-occlusion M26.213
Mesocolon —see condition
Mesonephroma (malignant) —see Neoplasm,
   malignant, by site
  benign —see Neoplasm, benign, by site
Mesophlebitis —see Phlebitis
Mesostromal dysgenesia Q13.89
Mesothelioma (malignant) C45.9
  benign
    mesentery D19.1
    mesocolon D19.1
    omentum D19.1
    peritoneum D19.1
    pleura D19.0
    specified site NEC D19.7
    unspecified site D19.9
  biphasic C45.9
    benign
      mesentery D19.1
      mesocolon D19.1
      omentum D19.1
      peritoneum D19.1
      pleura D19.0
      specified site NEC D19.7
      unspecified site D19.9
  cystic D48.4
  epithelioid C45.9
    benign
      mesentery D19.1
      mesocolon D19.1
      omentum D19.1
      peritoneum D19.1
      pleura D19.0
      specified site NEC D19.7
      unspecified site D19.9
  fibrous C45.9
    benign
      mesentery D19.1
      mesocolon D19.1
      omentum D19.1
      peritoneum D19.1
      pleura D19.0
      specified site NEC D19.7
      unspecified site D19.9
  site classification
    liver C45.7
    lung C45.7
    mediastinum C45.7
    mesentery C45.1
    mesocolon C45.1
    omentum C45.1
    pericardium C45.2
    peritoneum C45.1
    pleura C45.0
      parietal C45.0
    retroperitoneum C45.7
    specified site NEC C45.7
    unspecified C45.9
Metabolic syndrome E88.81
Metagonimiasis B66.8
Metagonimus infestation (intestine)
   B66.8
Metal
  pigmentation L81.8
  polisher's disease J62.8
Metamorphopsia H53.15

Metaplasia
  apocrine (breast) —see Dysplasia, mammary,
    specified type NEC
  cervix (squamous) —see Dysplasia, cervix
  endometrium (squamous) (uterus) N85.8
  esophagus K22.7-
▶gastric intestinal K31.A0
  ▶with dysplasia K31.A29
    ▶high grade K31.A22
    ▶low grade K31.A21
  ▶indefinite for dysplasia K31.A0
  ▶without dysplasia K31.A19
    ▶involving
      ▶antrum K31.A11
      ▶body (corpus) K31.A12
      ▶cardia K31.A14
      ▶fundus K31.A13
      ▶multiple sites K31.A15
  kidney (pelvis) (squamous) N28.89
  myelogenous D73.1
  myeloid (agnogenic) (megakaryocytic) D73.1
  spleen D73.1
  squamous cell, bladder N32.89
Metastasis, metastatic
  abscess —see Abscess
  calcification E83.59
  cancer
    from specified site —see Neoplasm,
      malignant, by site
    to specified site —see Neoplasm, secondary,
      by site
  deposits (in) —see Neoplasm, secondary, by site
  disease (see also Neoplasm, secondary, by site)
    C79.9
  spread (to) —see Neoplasm, secondary, by site
Metastrongyliasis B83.8
Metatarsalgia M77.4-●
  anterior G57.6-●
  Morton's G57.6-●
Metatarsus, metatarsal —see also condition
  adductus, congenital Q66.22-●
  valgus (abductus), congenital Q66.6
  varus (congenital) Q66.22-●
  primus Q66.21-●
Methadone use —see Use, opioid
Methemoglobinemia D74.9
  acquired (with sulfhemoglobinemia) D74.8
  congenital D74.0
  enzymatic (congenital) D74.0
  Hb M disease D74.0
  hereditary D74.0
  toxic D74.8
Methemoglobinuria —see Hemoglobinuria
Methioninemia E72.19
Methylmalonic acidemia E71.120
Metritis (catarrhal) (hemorrhagic) (septic)
    (suppurative) —see also Endometritis
  cervical —see Cervicitis
Metropathia hemorrhagica N93.8
Metroperitonitis —see Peritonitis, pelvic, female
Metrorrhagia N92.1
  climacteric N92.4
  menopausal N92.4
  perimenopausal N92.4
  postpartum NEC (atonic) (following delivery
    of placenta) O72.1
    delayed or secondary O72.2
  preclimacteric or premenopausal N92.4
  psychogenic F45.8
Metrorrhexis —see Rupture, uterus
Metrosalpingitis N70.91
Metrostaxis N93.8
Metrovaginitis —see Endometritis
Meyer-Schwickerath and Weyers syndrome
   Q87.0
Meynert's amentia (nonalcoholic) F04
  alcoholic F10.96
    with dependence F10.26
Mibelli's disease (porokeratosis) Q82.8
Mice, joint —see Loose, body, joint
  knee M23.4
Micrencephalon, micrencephaly Q02

Microalbuminuria R80.9
Microaneurysm, retinal —see also Disorder,
   retina, microaneurysms
  diabetic —see E08-E13 with .31
Microangiopathy (peripheral) I73.9
▶thrombotic M31.10
    ▶hematopoietic stem cell transplantation-
      associated [HSCT-TMA] M31.10
Microcalcifications, breast R92.0
Microcephalus, microcephalic, microcephaly
   Q02
  due to toxoplasmosis (congenital) P37.1
Microcheilia Q18.7
Microcolon (congenital) Q43.8
Microcornea (congenital) Q13.4
Microcytic —see condition D57.40
Microdeletions NEC Q93.88
Microdontia K00.2
Microdrepanocytosis D57.40
  with
    acute chest syndrome D57.411
    cerebral vascular involvement D57.413
    crisis (painful) D57.419
      with specified complication NEC D57.418
    splenic sequestration D57.412
    vasoocclusive pain D57.419
Microembolism
  atherothrombotic —see Atheroembolism
  retinal —see Occlusion, artery, retina
Microencephalon Q02
Microfilaria streptocerca infestation —see
   Onchocerciasis
Microgastria (congenital) Q40.2
Microgenia M26.06
Microgenitalia, congenital
  female Q52.8
  male Q55.8
Microglioma —see Lymphoma, non-Hodgkin,
   specified NEC
Microglossia (congenital) Q38.3
Micrognathia, micrognathism (congenital)
   (mandibular) (maxillary) M26.09
Microgyria (congenital) Q04.3
Microinfarct of heart —see Insufficiency, coronary
Microlentia (congenital) Q12.8
Microlithiasis, alveolar, pulmonary J84.02
Micromastia N64.82
Micromyelia (congenital) Q06.8
Micropenis Q55.62
Microphakia (congenital) Q12.8
Microphthalmos, microphthalmia (congenital)
   Q11.2
  due to toxoplasmosis P37.1
Micropsia H53.15
Microscopic polyangiitis (polyarteritis) M31.7
Microsporidiosis B60.8
  intestinal A07.8
Microsporon furfur infestation B36.0
Microsporosis —see also Dermatophytosis
  nigra B36.1
Microstomia (congenital) Q18.5
Microtia (congenital) (external ear) Q17.2
Microtropia H50.40
Microvillus inclusion disease (MVD) (MVID)
   Q43.8
Micturition
  disorder NEC —see also Difficulty, micturition
    R39.198
    psychogenic F45.8
  frequency R35.0
    psychogenic F45.8
  hesitancy R39.11
  incomplete emptying R39.14
  nocturnal R35.1
  painful R30.9
    dysuria R30.0
    psychogenic F45.8
    tenesmus R30.1
  poor stream R39.12
  position dependent R39.192
  split stream R39.13
  straining R39.16
  urgency R39.15

Mid plane —*see* condition
Middle
  ear —*see* condition
  lobe (right) syndrome J98.19
Miescher's elastoma L87.2
Mietens' syndrome Q87.2
Migraine (idiopathic) G43.909
  with refractory migraine G43.919
    with status migrainosus G43.911
    without status migrainosus G43.919
  with aura (acute-onset) (prolonged) (typical)
    (without headache) G43.109
    with refractory migraine G43.119
      with status migrainosus G43.111
      without status migrainosus G43.119
    intractable G43.119
      with status migrainosus G43.111
      without status migrainosus G43.119
    not intractable G43.109
      with status migrainosus G43.101
      without status migrainosus G43.109
    persistent G43.509
      with cerebral infarction G43.609
        with refractory migraine G43.619
          with status migrainosus G43.611
          without status migrainosus G43.619
        intractable G43.619
          with status migrainosus G43.611
          without status migrainosus G43.619
        not intractable G43.609
          with status migrainosus G43.601
          without status migrainosus G43.609
        without refractory migraine G43.609
          with status migrainosus G43.601
          without status migrainosus G43.609
      without cerebral infarction G43.509
        with refractory migraine G43.519
          with status migrainosus G43.511
          without status migrainosus G43.519
        intractable G43.519
          with status migrainosus G43.511
          without status migrainosus G43.519
        not intractable G43.509
          with status migrainosus G43.501
          without status migrainosus G43.509
        without refractory migraine G43.509
          with status migrainosus G43.501
          without status migrainosus G43.509
    without mention of refractory migraine
      G43.109
      with status migrainosus G43.101
      without status migrainosus G43.109
  abdominal G43.D0
    with refractory migraine G43.D1
    intractable G43.D1
    not intractable G43.D0
    without refractory migraine G43.D0
  basilar —*see* Migraine, with aura
  classical —*see* Migraine, with aura
  common —*see* Migraine, without aura
  complicated G43.109
  equivalents —*see* Migraine, with aura
  familiar —*see* Migraine, hemiplegic
  hemiplegic G43.409
    with refractory migraine G43.419
      with status migrainosus G43.411
      without status migrainosus G43.419
    intractable G43.419
      with status migrainosus G43.411
      without status migrainosus G43.419
    not intractable G43.409
      with status migrainosus G43.401
      without status migrainosus G43.409
    without refractory migraine G43.409
      with status migrainosus G43.401
      without status migrainosus G43.409
  intractable G43.919
    with status migrainosus G43.911
    without status migrainosus G43.919
  menstrual G43.829
    with refractory migraine G43.839
      with status migrainosus G43.831
      without status migrainosus G43.839

Migraine *(Continued)*
  menstrual *(Continued)*
    intractable G43.839
      with status migrainosus G43.831
      without status migrainosus G43.839
    not intractable G43.829
      with status migrainosus G43.821
      without status migrainosus G43.829
    without refractory migraine G43.829
      with status migrainosus G43.821
      without status migrainosus G43.829
  menstrually related —*see* Migraine, menstrual
  not intractable G43.909
    with status migrainosus G43.901
    without status migrainosus G43.919
  ophthalmoplegic G43.B0
    with refractory migraine G43.B1
    intractable G43.B1
    not intractable G43.B0
    without refractory migraine G43.B0
  persistent aura (with, without) cerebral
    infarction —*see* Migraine, with aura,
    persistent
  preceded or accompanied by transient focal
    neurological phenomena —*see* Migraine,
    with aura
  pre-menstrual —*see* Migraine, menstrual
  pure menstrual —*see* Migraine, menstrual
  retinal —*see* Migraine, with aura
  specified NEC G43.809
    intractable G43.819
      with status migrainosus G43.811
      without status migrainosus G43.819
    not intractable G43.809
      with status migrainosus G43.801
      without status migrainosus G43.809
  sporadic —*see* Migraine, hemiplegic
  transformed —*see* Migraine, without aura,
    chronic
  triggered seizures —*see* Migraine, with aura
  without aura G43.009
    with refractory migraine G43.019
      with status migrainosus G43.011
      without status migrainosus G43.019
    chronic G43.709
      with refractory migraine G43.719
        with status migrainosus G43.711
        without status migrainosus G43.719
      intractable
        with status migrainosus G43.711
        without status migrainosus G43.719
      not intractable
        with status migrainosus G43.701
        without status migrainosus G43.709
      without refractory migraine G43.709
        with status migrainosus G43.701
        without status migrainosus G43.709
    intractable
      with status migrainosus G43.011
      without status migrainosus G43.019
    not intractable
      with status migrainosus G43.001
      without status migrainosus G43.009
    without mention of refractory migraine
      G43.009
      with status migrainosus G43.001
      without status migrainosus G43.009
    without refractory migraine G43.909
      with status migrainosus G43.901
      without status migrainosus G43.919
➡ Migrant, social Z59.00
Migration, anxiety concerning Z60.3
Migratory, migrating —*see also* condition
➡ person Z59.00
  testis Q55.29
Mikity-Wilson disease or syndrome P27.0
Mikulicz' disease or syndrome K11.8
Miliaria L74.3
  alba L74.1
  apocrine L75.2
  crystallina L74.1
  profunda L74.2
  rubra L74.0

Miliaria *(Continued)*
  tropicalis L74.2
Miliary —*see* condition
Milium L72.0
  colloid L57.8
Milk
  crust L21.0
  excessive secretion O92.6
  poisoning —*see* Poisoning, food, noxious
  retention O92.79
  sickness —*see* Poisoning, food, noxious
  spots I31.0
Milk-alkali disease or syndrome E83.52
Milk-leg (deep vessels) (nonpuerperal) —*see*
  Embolism, vein, lower extremity
  complicating pregnancy O22.3-●
  puerperal, postpartum, childbirth O87.1
Milkman's disease or syndrome M83.8
Milky urine —*see* Chyluria
Millard-Gubler (-Foville) paralysis or
  syndrome G46.3
Millar's asthma J38.5
Miller-Fisher syndrome G61.0
Mills' disease —*see* Hemiplegia
Millstone maker's pneumoconiosis J62.8
Milroy's disease (chronic hereditary edema)
  Q82.0
Minamata disease T56.1-●
Miners' asthma or lung J60
Minkowski-Chauffard syndrome —*see*
  Spherocytosis
Minor —*see* condition
Minor's disease (hematomyelia) G95.19
Minot's disease (hemorrhagic disease),
  newborn P53
Minot-von Willebrand-Jurgens disease or
  syndrome (angiohemophilia) D68.0
Minus (and plus) hand (intrinsic) —*see* Deformity,
  limb, specified type NEC, forearm
Miosis (pupil) H57.03
Mirizzi's syndrome (hepatic duct stenosis)
  K83.1
Mirror writing F81.0
MIS-A M35.81
MIS-C M35.81
Misadventure (of) (prophylactic) (therapeutic) —
  see also Complications T88.9
  administration of insulin (by accident) —*see*
    subcategory T38.3
  infusion —*see* Complications, infusion
  local applications (of fomentations, plasters,
    etc.) T88.9
    burn or scald —*see* Burn
    specified NEC T88.8
  medical care (early) (late) T88.9
    adverse effect of drugs or chemicals —*see*
      Table of Drugs and Chemicals
    medical care (early) (late)
      burn or scald —*see* Burn
      specified NEC T88.8
    specified NEC T88.8
  surgical procedure (early) (late) —*see*
    Complications, surgical procedure
  transfusion —*see* Complications, transfusion
  vaccination or other immunological
    procedure —*see* Complications,
    vaccination
Miscarriage O03.9
Misdirection, aqueous H40.83-●
Misperception, sleep state F51.02
Misplaced, misplacement
  ear Q17.4
  kidney (acquired) N28.89
    congenital Q63.2
  organ or site, congenital NEC —*see*
    Malposition, congenital
Missed
  abortion O02.1
  delivery O36.4
Missing —*see also* Absence
  string of intrauterine contraceptive device
    T83.32

Misuse of drugs F19.99
Mitchell's disease (erythromelalgia) I73.81
Mite(s) (infestation) B88.9
  diarrhea B88.0
  grain (itch) B88.0
  hair follicle (itch) B88.0
  in sputum B88.0
Mitral —see condition
Mittelschmerz N94.0
Mixed —see condition
MMN (multifocal motor neuropathy) G61.82
MNGIE (Mitochondrial Neurogastrointestinal
    Encephalopathy) syndrome E88.49
Mobile, mobility
  cecum Q43.3
  excessive —see Hypermobility
  gallbladder, congenital Q44.1
  kidney N28.89
  organ or site, congenital NEC —see
      Malposition, congenital
Mobitz heart block (atrioventricular) I44.1
Moebius, Möbius
  disease (ophthalmoplegic migraine) —see
      Migraine, ophthalmoplegic
  syndrome Q87.0
    congenital oculofacial paralysis (with other
        anomalies) Q87.0
    ophthalmoplegic migraine —see Migraine,
        ophthalmoplegic
Moeller's glossitis K14.0
Mohr's syndrome (Types I and II) Q87.0
Mola destruens D39.2
Molar pregnancy O02.0
Molarization of premolars K00.2
Molding, head (during birth) - omit code
Mole (pigmented) —see also Nevus
  blood O02.0
  Breus' O02.0
  cancerous —see Melanoma
  carneous O02.0
  destructive D39.2
  fleshy O02.0
  hydatid, hydatidiform (benign) (complicating
      pregnancy) (delivered) (undelivered)
      O01.9
    classical O01.0
    complete O01.0
    incomplete O01.1
    invasive D39.2
    malignant D39.2
    partial O01.1
  intrauterine O02.0
  invasive (hydatidiform) D39.2
  malignant
    meaning
      malignant hydatidiform mole D39.2
      melanoma —see Melanoma
  nonhydatidiform O02.0
  nonpigmented —see Nevus
  pregnancy NEC O02.0
  skin —see Nevus
  tubal O00.10-
    with intrauterine pregnancy O00.11-
  vesicular —see Mole, hydatidiform
Molimen, molimina (menstrual) N94.3
Molluscum contagiosum (epitheliale) B08.1
Mönckeberg's arteriosclerosis, disease, or
    sclerosis —see Arteriosclerosis, extremities
Mondini's malformation (cochlea) Q16.5
Mondor's disease I80.8
Monge's disease T70.29
Monilethrix (congenital) Q84.1
Moniliasis —see also Candidiasis B37.9
  neonatal P37.5
Monitoring (encounter for)
  therapeutic drug level Z51.81
Monkey malaria B53.1
Monkeypox B04
Monoarthritis M13.10
  ankle M13.17-●
  elbow M13.12-●

Monoarthritis (Continued)
  foot joint M13.17-●
  hand joint M13.14-●
  hip M13.15-●
  knee M13.16-●
  shoulder M13.11-●
  wrist M13.13-●
Monoblastic —see condition
Monochromat (ism), monochromatopsia
    (acquired) (congenital) H53.51
Monocytic —see condition
Monocytopenia D72.818
Monocytosis (symptomatic) D72.821
Monomania —see Psychosis
Mononeuritis G58.9
  cranial nerve —see Disorder, nerve,
      cranial
  femoral nerve G57.2-●
  lateral
    cutaneous nerve of thigh G57.1-●
    popliteal nerve G57.3-●
  lower limb G57.9-●
    specified nerve NEC G57.8-●
  medial popliteal nerve G57.4-●
  median nerve G56.1-●
  multiplex G58.7
  plantar nerve G57.6-●
  posterior tibial nerve G57.5-●
  radial nerve G56.3-●
  sciatic nerve G57.0-●
  specified NEC G58.8
  tibial nerve G57.4-●
  ulnar nerve G56.2-●
  upper limb G56.9-●
    specified nerve NEC G56.8-●
  vestibular —see subcategory H93.3
Mononeuropathy G58.9
  carpal tunnel syndrome —see Syndrome,
      carpal tunnel
  diabetic NEC —see E08-E13 with .41
  femoral nerve —see Lesion, nerve, femoral
  ilioinguinal nerve G57.8-●
  in diseases classified elsewhere —see category
      G59
  intercostal G58.0
  lower limb G57.9-●
    causalgia —see Causalgia, lower limb
    femoral nerve —see Lesion, nerve,
        femoral
    meralgia paresthetica G57.1-●
    plantar nerve —see Lesion, nerve, plantar
    popliteal nerve —see Lesion, nerve,
        popliteal
    sciatic nerve —see Lesion, nerve, sciatic
    specified NEC G57.8-●
    tarsal tunnel syndrome —see Syndrome,
        tarsal tunnel
  median nerve —see Lesion, nerve, median
  multiplex G58.7
  obturator nerve G57.8-●
  popliteal nerve —see Lesion, nerve, popliteal
  radial nerve —see Lesion, nerve, radial
  saphenous nerve G57.8-●
  specified NEC G58.8
  tarsal tunnel syndrome —see Syndrome,
      tarsal tunnel
  tuberculous A17.83
  ulnar nerve —see Lesion, nerve, ulnar
  upper limb G56.9-●
    carpal tunnel syndrome —see Syndrome,
        carpal tunnel
    causalgia —see Causalgia
    median nerve —see Lesion, nerve, median
    radial nerve —see Lesion, nerve, radial
    specified site NEC G56.8-●
    ulnar nerve —see Lesion, nerve, ulnar
Mononucleosis, infectious B27.90
  with
    complication NEC B27.99
    meningitis B27.92
    polyneuropathy B27.91

Mononucleosis, infectious (Continued)
  cytomegaloviral B27.10
    with
      complication NEC B27.19
      meningitis B27.12
      polyneuropathy B27.11
  Epstein-Barr (virus) B27.00
    with
      complication NEC B27.09
      meningitis B27.02
      polyneuropathy B27.01
  gammaherpesviral B27.00
    with
      complication NEC B27.09
      meningitis B27.02
      polyneuropathy B27.01
  specified NEC B27.80
    with
      complication NEC B27.89
      meningitis B27.82
      polyneuropathy B27.81
Monoplegia G83.3-●
  congenital (cerebral) G80.8
    spastic G80.1
  embolic (current episode) I63.4-●
  following
    cerebrovascular disease
      cerebral infarction
        lower limb I69.34-●
        upper limb I69.33-●
      intracerebral hemorrhage
        lower limb I69.14-●
        upper limb I69.13-●
      lower limb I69.94-●
      nontraumatic intracranial hemorrhage
          NEC
        lower limb I69.24-●
        upper limb I69.23-●
      specified disease NEC
        lower limb I69.84-●
        upper limb I69.83-●
      stroke NOS
        lower limb I69.34-●
        upper limb I69.33-●
      subarachnoid hemorrhage
        lower limb I69.04-●
        upper limb I69.03-●
      upper limb I69.93-●
  hysterical (transient) F44.4
  lower limb G83.1-●
  psychogenic (conversion reaction) F44.4
  thrombotic (current episode) I63.3-●
  transient R29.818
  upper limb G83.2-●
Monorchism, monorchidism Q55.0
Monosomy —see also Deletion, chromosome
    Q93.9
  specified NEC Q93.89
  whole chromosome
    meiotic nondisjunction Q93.0
    mitotic nondisjunction Q93.1
    mosaicism Q93.1
  X Q96.9
Monster, monstrosity (single) Q89.7
  acephalic Q00.0
  twin Q89.4
Monteggia's fracture (-dislocation) S52.27-●
Mooren's ulcer (cornea) —see Ulcer, cornea,
    Mooren's
Moore's syndrome —see Epilepsy, specified
    NEC
Mooser-Neill reaction A75.2
Mooser's bodies A75.2
Morbidity not stated or unknown R69
Morbilli —see Measles
Morbus —see also Disease
  angelicus, anglorum E55.0
  Beigel B36.2
  caducus —see Epilepsy
  celiacus K90.0
  comitialis —see Epilepsy

► New   ⇒ Revised   ~~deleted~~ Deleted   ● Use Additional Character(s)

Morbus *(Continued)*
  cordis —*see also* Disease, heart I51.9
    valvulorum —*see* Endocarditis
  coxae senilis M16.9
    tuberculous A18.02
  hemorrhagicus neonatorum P53
  maculosus neonatorum P54.5
Morel (-Stewart)(-Morgagni) syndrome M85.2
Morel-Kraepelin disease —*see* Schizophrenia
Morel-Moore syndrome M85.2
Morgagni's
  cyst, organ, hydatid, or appendage
    female Q50.5
    male (epididymal) Q55.4
      testicular Q55.29
  syndrome M85.2
Morgagni-Stewart-Morel syndrome M85.2
Morgagni-Stokes-Adams syndrome I45.9
Morgagni-Turner (-Albright) syndrome Q96.9
Moria F07.0
Moron (I.Q. 50-69) F70
Morphea L94.0
Morphinism (without remission) F11.20
  with remission F11.21
Morphinomania (without remission) F11.20
  with remission F11.21
Morquio (-Ullrich)(-Brailsford) disease or syndrome —*see* Mucopolysaccharidosis
Mortification (dry) (moist) —*see* Gangrene
Morton's metatarsalgia (neuralgia)(neuroma) (syndrome) G57.6
Morvan's disease or syndrome G60.8
Mosaicism, mosaic (autosomal) (chromosomal)
  45,X/46,XX Q96.3
  45,X/other cell lines NEC with abnormal sex chromosome Q96.4
  sex chromosome
    female Q97.8
    lines with various numbers of X chromosomes Q97.2
    male Q98.7
  XY Q96.3
Moschowitz' disease M31.19
Mother yaw A66.0
Motion sickness (from travel, any vehicle) (from roundabouts or swings) T75.3
Mottled, mottling, teeth (enamel) (endemic) (nonendemic) K00.3
Mounier-Kuhn syndrome Q32.4
  with bronchiectasis J47.9
    exacerbation (acute) J47.1
    lower respiratory infection J47.0
  acquired J98.09
    with bronchiectasis J47.9
      with
        exacerbation (acute) J47.1
        lower respiratory infection J47.0
Mountain
  sickness T70.29
    with polycythemia , acquired (acute) D75.1
  tick fever A93.2
Mouse, joint —*see* Loose, body, joint
  knee M23.4-•
Mouth —*see* condition
Movable
  coccyx —*see* subcategory M53.2
  kidney N28.89
    congenital Q63.8
  spleen D73.89
Movements, dystonic R25.8
Moyamoya disease I67.5
MRSA (Methicillin resistant Staphylococcus aureus)
  infection A49.02
    as the cause of diseases classified elsewhere B95.62
  sepsis A41.02
MSD (multiple sulfatase deficiency) E75.26

MSSA (Methicillin susceptible Staphylococcus aureus)
  infection A49.01
    as the cause of diseases classified elsewhere B95.61
  sepsis A41.01
Mucha-Habermann disease L41.0
Mucinosis (cutaneous) (focal) (papular) (reticular erythematous) (skin) L98.5
  oral K13.79
Mucocele
  appendix K38.8
  buccal cavity K13.79
  gallbladder K82.1
  lacrimal sac, chronic H04.43-•
  nasal sinus J34.1
  nose J34.1
  salivary gland (any) K11.6
  sinus (accessory) (nasal) J34.1
  turbinate (bone) (middle) (nasal) J34.1
  uterus N85.8
Mucolipidosis
  I E77.1
  II, III E77.0
  IV E75.11
Mucopolysaccharidosis E76.3
  beta-gluduronidase deficiency E76.29
  cardiopathy E76.3 [I52]
  Hunter's syndrome E76.1
  Hurler's syndrome E76.01
  Hurler-Scheie syndrome E76.02
  Maroteaux-Lamy syndrome E76.29
  Morquio syndrome E76.219
    A E76.210
    B E76.211
    classic E76.210
  Sanfilippo syndrome E76.22
  Scheie's syndrome E76.03
  specified NEC E76.29
  type
    I
      Hurler's syndrome E76.01
      Hurler-Scheie syndrome E76.02
      Scheie's syndrome E76.03
    II E76.1
    III E76.22
    IV E76.219
    IVA E76.210
    IVB E76.211
    VI E76.29
    VII E76.29
Mucormycosis B46.5
  cutaneous B46.3
  disseminated B46.4
  gastrointestinal B46.2
  generalized B46.4
  pulmonary B46.0
  rhinocerebral B46.1
  skin B46.3
  subcutaneous B46.3
Mucositis (ulcerative) K12.30
  due to drugs NEC K12.32
  gastrointestinal K92.81
  mouth (oral) (oropharyngeal) K12.30
    due to antineoplastic therapy K12.31
    due to drugs NEC K12.32
    due to radiation K12.33
    specified NEC K12.39
    viral K12.39
  nasal J34.81
  oral cavity —*see* Mucositis, mouth
  oral soft tissues —*see* Mucositis, mouth
  vagina and vulva N76.81
Mucositis necroticans agranulocytica —*see* Agranulocytosis
Mucous —*see also* condition
  patches (syphilitic) A51.39
    congenital A50.07
Mucoviscidosis E84.9
  with meconium obstruction E84.11

Mucus
  asphyxia or suffocation —*see* Asphyxia, mucus
  in stool R19.5
  plug —*see* Asphyxia, mucus
Muguet B37.0
Mulberry molars (congenital syphilis) A50.52
Müllerian mixed tumor
  specified site —*see* Neoplasm, malignant, by site
  unspecified site C54.9
Multicystic kidney (development) Q61.4
Multiparity (grand) Z64.1
  affecting management of pregnancy, labor and delivery (supervision only) O09.4-•
  requiring contraceptive management —*see* Contraception
Multipartita placenta O43.19-•
Multiple, multiplex —*see also* condition
  digits (congenital) Q69.9
  endocrine neoplasia —*see* Neoplasia, endocrine, multiple [MEN]
  personality F44.81
Multisystem inflammatory syndrome (in adults) (in children) M35.81
Mumps B26.9
  arthritis B26.85
  complication NEC B26.89
  encephalitis B26.2
  hepatitis B26.81
  meningitis (aseptic) B26.1
  meningoencephalitis B26.2
  myocarditis B26.82
  oophoritis B26.89
  orchitis B26.0
  pancreatitis B26.3
  polyneuropathy B26.84
Mumu —*see also* Infestation, filarial B74.9 [N51]
Münchhausen's syndrome —*see* Disorder, factitious
Münchmeyer's syndrome —*see* Myositis, ossificans, progressiva
Mural —*see* condition
Murmur (cardiac) (heart) (organic) R01.1
  abdominal R19.15
  aortic (valve) —*see* Endocarditis, aortic
  benign R01.0
  diastolic —*see* Endocarditis
  Flint I35.1
  functional R01.0
  Graham Steell I37.1
  innocent R01.0
  mitral (valve) —*see* Insufficiency, mitral
  nonorganic R01.0
  presystolic, mitral —*see* Insufficiency, mitral
  pulmonic (valve) I37.8
  systolic R01.1
  tricuspid (valve) I07.9
  valvular —*see* Endocarditis
Murri's disease (intermittent hemoglobinuria) D59.6
Muscle, muscular —*see also* condition
  carnitine (palmityltransferase) deficiency E71.314
Musculoneuralgia —*see* Neuralgia
Mushroom-workers' (pickers') disease or lung J67.5
Mushrooming hip —*see* Derangement, joint, specified NEC, hip
Mutation(s)
  factor V Leiden D68.51
  surfactant, of lung J84.83
  prothrombin gene D68.52
Mutism —*see also* Aphasia
  deaf (acquired) (congenital) NEC H91.3
  elective (adjustment reaction) (childhood) F94.0
  hysterical F44.4
  selective (childhood) F94.0
MVD (microvillus inclusion disease) Q43.8
MVID (microvillus inclusion disease) Q43.8

Myalgia M79.10
  auxiliary muscles, head and neck M79.12
  epidemic (cervical) B33.0
  mastication muscle M79.11
  site specified NEC M79.18
  traumatic NEC T14.8
Myasthenia G70.9
  congenital G70.2
  cordis —see Failure, heart
  developmental G70.2
  gravis G70.00
    with exacerbation (acute) G70.01
    in crisis G70.01
    neonatal, transient P94.0
    pseudoparalytica G70.00
      with exacerbation (acute) G70.01
      in crisis G70.01
  stomach, psychogenic F45.8
  syndrome
    in
      diabetes mellitus —see E08-E13 with .44
      neoplastic disease —see also Neoplasm
        D49.9 [G73.3]
      pernicious anemia D51.0 [G73.3]
      thyrotoxicosis E05.90 [G73.3]
        with thyroid storm E05.91 [G73.3]
Myasthenic M62.81
Mycelium infection B49
Mycetismus —see Poisoning, food, noxious,
  mushroom
Mycetoma B47.9
  actinomycotic B47.1
  bone (mycotic) B47.9 [M90.80]
  eumycotic B47.0
  foot B47.9
    actinomycotic B47.1
    mycotic B47.0
  madurae NEC B47.9
    mycotic B47.0
  maduromycotic B47.0
  mycotic B47.0
  nocardial B47.1
Mycobacteriosis —see Mycobacterium
Mycobacterium, mycobacterial (infection)
    A31.9
  anonymous A31.9
  atypical A31.9
    cutaneous A31.1
    pulmonary A31.0
      tuberculous —see Tuberculosis,
        pulmonary
    specified site NEC A31.8
  avium (intracellulare complex) A31.0
  balnei A31.1
  Battey A31.0
  chelonei A31.8
  cutaneous A31.1
  extrapulmonary systemic A31.8
  fortuitum A31.8
  intracellulare (Battey bacillus) A31.0
  kakaferifu A31.8
  kansasii (yellow bacillus) A31.0
  kasongo A31.8
  leprae —see also Leprosy A30.9
  luciflavum A31.1
  marinum (M. balnei) A31.1
  nonspecific —see Mycobacterium, atypical
  pulmonary (atypical) A31.0
    tuberculous —see Tuberculosis, pulmonary
  scrofulaceum A31.8
  simiae A31.8
  systemic, extrapulmonary A31.8
  szulgai A31.8
  terrae A31.8
  triviale A31.8
  tuberculosis (human, bovine) —see
    Tuberculosis
  ulcerans A31.1
  xenopi A31.8
Mycoplasma (M.) pneumoniae, as cause of
  disease classified elsewhere B96.0

Mycosis, mycotic B49
  cutaneous NEC B36.9
  ear B36.9
    in
      aspergillosis B44.89
      candidiasis B37.84
      moniliasis B37.84
  fungoides (extranodal) (solid organ) C84.0-●
  mouth B37.0
  nails B35.1
  opportunistic B48.8
  skin NEC B36.9
  specified NEC B48.8
  stomatitis B37.0
  vagina, vaginitis (candidal) B37.3
Mydriasis (pupil) H57.04
Myelatelia Q06.1
Myelinolysis, pontine, central G37.2
Myelitis (acute) (ascending) (childhood)
    (chronic) (descending) (diffuse)
    (disseminated) (idiopathic) (pressure)
    (progressive) (spinal cord) (subacute) —see
    also Encephalitis G04.91
➡ flaccid G04.82
  herpes simplex B00.82
  herpes zoster B02.24
  in diseases classified elsewhere G05.4
  necrotizing, subacute G37.4
  optic neuritis in G36.0
  postchickenpox B01.12
  postherpetic B02.24
  postimmunization G04.02
  postinfectious NEC G04.89
  postvaccinal G04.02
  specified NEC G04.89
  syphilitic (transverse) A52.14
➡ toxic G92.9
  transverse (in demyelinating diseases of
    central nervous system) G37.3
  tuberculous A17.82
  varicella B01.12
Myeloblastic —see condition
Myeloblastoma
  granular cell —see also Neoplasm, connective
    tissue
    malignant —see Neoplasm, connective
      tissue, malignant
    tongue D10.1
Myelocele —see Spina bifida
Myelocystocele —see Spina bifida
Myelocytic —see condition
Myelodysplasia M46.9
  specified NEC D46.Z
  spinal cord (congenital) Q06.1
Myelodysplastic syndrome (see also Syndrome,
  myelodysplastic) D46.9
  with
    5q deletion D46.C
    isolated del (5q) chromosomal abnormality
      C46.C
  specified NEC D46.Z
Myeloencephalitis —see Encephalitis
Myelofibrosis D75.81
  with myeloid metaplasia D47.4
  acute C94.4-●
  idiopathic (chronic) D47.4
  primary D47.1
  secondary D75.81
    in myeloproliferative disease
      D47.4
Myelogenous —see condition
Myeloid —see condition
Myelokathexis D70.9
Myeloleukodystrophy E75.29
Myelolipoma —see Lipoma
Myeloma (multiple) C90.0-●
  monostotic C90.3
    plasma cell C90.0-●
  plasma cell C90.0-●
  solitary —see also Plasmacytoma, solitary
    C90.3-●

Myelomalacia G95.89
Myelomatosis C90.0-●
Myelomeningitis —see Meningoencephalitis
Myelomeningocele (spinal cord) —see Spina
  bifida
Myelo-osteo-musculodysplasia hereditaria
    Q79.8
Myelopathic
  anemia D64.89
  muscle atrophy —see Atrophy, muscle,
    spinal
  pain syndrome G89.0
Myelopathy (spinal cord) G95.9
  drug-induced G95.89
  in (due to)
    degeneration or displacement,
      intervertebral disc NEC —see
      Disorder, disc, with, myelopathy
    infection —see Encephalitis
    intervertebral disc disorder —see also
      Disorder, disc, with, myelopathy
    mercury —see subcategory T56.1
    neoplastic disease —see also Neoplasm
      D49.9 [G99.2]
    pernicious anemia D51.0 [G99.2]
    spondylosis —see Spondylosis, with
      myelopathy NEC
  necrotic (subacute) (vascular) G95.19
  radiation-induced G95.89
  spondylogenic NEC —see Spondylosis, with
    myelopathy NEC
  toxic G95.89
  transverse, acute G37.3
  vascular G95.19
  vitamin B12 E53.8 [G32.0]
Myelophthisis D61.82
Myeloradiculitis G04.91
Myeloradiculodysplasia (spinal)
    Q06.1
Myelosarcoma C92.3-●
Myelosclerosis D75.89
  with myeloid metaplasia D47.4
  disseminated, of nervous system
    G35
  megakaryocytic D47.4
    with myeloid metaplasia
      D47.4
Myelosis
  acute C92.0-●
  aleukemic C92.9-●
  chronic D47.1
  erythremic (acute) C94.0-●
  megakaryocytic C94.2-●
  nonleukemic D72.828
  subacute C92.9-●
Myiasis (cavernous) B87.9
  aural B87.4
  creeping B87.0
  cutaneous B87.0
  dermal B87.0
  ear (external) (middle) B87.4
  eye B87.2
  genitourinary B87.81
  intestinal B87.82
  laryngeal B87.3
  nasopharyngeal B87.3
  ocular B87.2
  orbit B87.2
  skin B87.0
  specified site NEC B87.89
  traumatic B87.1
  wound B87.1
Myoadenoma, prostate —see Hyperplasia,
  prostate
Myoblastoma
  granular cell —see also Neoplasm, connective
    tissue, benign
    malignant —see Neoplasm, connective
      tissue, malignant
  tongue D10.1
Myocardial —see condition

▶ New   ➡ Revised   ~~deleted~~ Deleted   ● Use Additional Character(s)

Myocardiopathy (congestive) (constrictive)
    (familial) (hypertrophic nonobstructive)
    (idiopathic) (infiltrative) (obstructive)
    (primary) (restrictive) (sporadic) —see also
    Cardiomyopathy I42.9
  alcoholic I42.6
  cobalt-beer I42.6
  glycogen storage E74.02 [I43]
  hypertrophic obstructive I42.1
  in (due to)
    beriberi E51.12
    cardiac glycogenosis E74.02 [I43]
    Friedreich's ataxia G11.11 [I43]
    myotonia atrophica G71.11 [I43]
    progressive muscular dystrophy G71.03
      [I43]
  obscure (African) I42.8
  secondary I42.9
  thyrotoxic E05.90 [I43]
    with storm E05.91 [I43]
  toxic NEC I42.7
Myocarditis (with arteriosclerosis) (chronic)
    (fibroid) (interstitial) (old) (progressive)
    (senile) I51.4
  with
    rheumatic fever (conditions in I00) I09.0
      active —see Myocarditis, acute,
        rheumatic
      inactive or quiescent (with chorea) I09.0
  active I40.9
    rheumatic I01.2
      with chorea (acute) (rheumatic)
        (Sydenham's) I02.0
  acute or subacute (interstitial) I40.9
    due to
      streptococcus (beta-hemolytic) I01.2
    idiopathic I40.1
    rheumatic I01.2
      with chorea (acute) (rheumatic)
        (Sydenham's) I02.0
    specified NEC I40.8
  aseptic of newborn B33.22
  bacterial (acute) I40.0
  Coxsackie (virus) B33.22
  diphtheritic A36.81
  eosinophilic I40.1
  epidemic of newborn (Coxsackie) B33.22
  Fiedler's (acute) (isolated) I40.1
  giant cell (acute) (subacute) I40.1
  gonococcal A54.83
  granulomatous (idiopathic) (isolated)
    (nonspecific) I40.1
  hypertensive —see Hypertension, heart
  idiopathic (granulomatous) I40.1
  in (due to)
    diphtheria A36.81
    epidemic louse-borne typhus A75.0 [I41]
    Lyme disease A69.29
    sarcoidosis D86.85
    scarlet fever A38.1
    toxoplasmosis (acquired) B58.81
    typhoid A01.02
    typhus NEC A75.9 [I41]
  infective I40.0
  influenzal —see Influenza, with, myocarditis
  isolated (acute) I40.1
  meningococcal A39.52
  mumps B26.82
  nonrheumatic, active I40.9
  parenchymatous I40.9
  pneumococcal I40.0
  rheumatic (chronic) (inactive) (with chorea)
    I09.0
    active or acute I01.2
      with chorea (acute) (rheumatic)
        (Sydenham's) I02.0
  rheumatoid —see Rheumatoid, carditis
  septic I40.0
  staphylococcal I40.0
  suppurative I40.0
  syphilitic (chronic) A52.06

Myocarditis (Continued)
  toxic I40.8
    rheumatic —see Myocarditis, acute,
      rheumatic
  tuberculous A18.84
  typhoid A01.02
  valvular —see Endocarditis
  virus, viral I40.0
    of newborn (Coxsackie) B33.22
Myocardium, myocardial —see condition
Myocardosis —see Cardiomyopathy
Myoclonus, myoclonic, myoclonia (familial)
    (essential) (multifocal) (simplex) G25.3
  drug-induced G25.3
  epilepsy —see also Epilepsy, generalized,
    specified NEC G40.4-●
    familial (progressive) G25.3
  epileptica G40.409
    with status epilepticus G40.401
  facial G51.3-●
  familial progressive G25.3
  Friedreich's G25.3
  jerks G25.3
  massive G25.3
  palatal G25.3
  pharyngeal G25.3
Myocytolysis I51.5
Myodiastasis —see Diastasis, muscle
Myoendocarditis —see Endocarditis
Myoepithelioma —see Neoplasm, benign, by
    site
Myofasciitis (acute) —see Myositis
Myofibroma —see also Neoplasm, connective
    tissue, benign
  uterus (cervix) (corpus) —see Leiomyoma
Myofibromatosis D48.1
  infantile Q89.8
Myofibrosis M62.89
  heart —see Myocarditis
  scapulohumeral —see Lesion, shoulder,
    specified NEC
Myofibrositis M79.7
  scapulohumeral —see Lesion, shoulder,
    specified NEC
Myoglobulinuria, myoglobinuria (primary)
    R82.1
Myokymia, facial G51.4
Myolipoma —see Lipoma
Myoma —see also Neoplasm, connective tissue,
    benign
  malignant —see Neoplasm, connective tissue,
    malignant
  prostate D29.1
  uterus (cervix) (corpus) —see Leiomyoma
Myomalacia M62.89
Myometritis —see Endometritis
Myometrium —see condition
Myonecrosis, clostridial A48.0
Myopathy G72.9
  acute
    necrotizing G72.81
    quadriplegic G72.81
  alcoholic G72.1
  benign congenital G71.20
  central core G71.29
  centronuclear G71.228
    autosomal (dominant) (recessive)
      G71.228
    other specified NEC G71.228
  congenital (benign) G71.20
  critical illness G72.81
  distal G71.09
  drug-induced G72.0
  endocrine NEC E34.9 [G73.7]
  extraocular muscles H05.82-●
  facioscapulohumeral G71.02
  hereditary G71.9
    specified NEC G71.8
  hyaline body G71.29
  myosin storage G71.29
  immune NEC G72.49

Myopathy (Continued)
  in (due to)
    Addison's disease E27.1 [G73.7]
    alcohol G72.1
    amyloidosis E85.0 [G73.7]
    cretinism E00.9 [G73.7]
    Cushing's syndrome E24.9 [G73.7]
    drugs G72.0
    endocrine disease NEC E34.9 [G73.7]
    giant cell arteritis M31.6 [G73.7]
    glycogen storage disease E74.00 [G73.7]
    hyperadrenocorticism E24.9 [G73.7]
    hyperparathyroidism NEC E21.3 [G73.7]
    hypoparathyroidism E20.9 [G73.7]
    hypopituitarism E23.0 [G73.7]
    hypothyroidism E03.9 [G73.7]
    infectious disease NEC B99 [G73.7]
    lipid storage disease E75.6 [G73.7]
    metabolic disease NEC E88.9 [G73.7]
    myxedema E03.9 [G73.7]
    parasitic disease NEC B89 [G73.7]
    polyarteritis nodosa M30.0 [G73.7]
    rheumatoid arthritis —see Rheumatoid,
      myopathy
    sarcoidosis D86.87
    scleroderma M34.82
    sicca syndrome M35.03
    Sjögren's syndrome M35.03
    systemic lupus erythematosus M32.19
    thyrotoxicosis (hyperthyroidism) E05.90
      [G73.7]
      with thyroid storm E05.91 [G73.7]
    toxic agent NEC G72.2
  inflammatory NEC G72.49
  intensive care (ICU) G72.81
  limb-girdle G71.09
  mitochondrial NEC G71.3
  myosin storage G71.29
  mytonic, proximal (PROMM) G71.11
  myotubular (centronuclear) G71.220
    X-linked G71.220
  nemaline G71.21
  ocular G71.09
  oculopharyngeal G71.09
  of critical illness G72.81
  primary G71.9
    specified NEC G71.8
  progressive NEC G72.89
  proximal myotonic (PROMM) G71.11
  rod (body) G71.21
  scapulohumeral G71.02
  specified NEC G72.89
  toxic G72.2
Myopericarditis —see also Pericarditis
  chronic rheumatic I09.2
Myopia (axial) (congenital) H52.1-●
  degenerative (malignant) H44.20
    with
      choroidal neovascularization H44.2A-●
      foveoschisis H44.2D-●
      macular hole H44.2B-●
      retinal detachment H44.2C-●
      specified maculopathy NEC H44.2E-●
    bilateral H44.23
    left eye H44.22
    right eye H44.21
  malignant —see also Myopia, degenerative
    H44.2-●
  pernicious —see also Myopia, degenerative
    H44.2-●
  progressive high (degenerative) —see also
    Myopia, degenerative H44.2-●
Myosarcoma —see Neoplasm, connective tissue,
    malignant
Myosis (pupil) H57.03
  stromal (endolymphatic) D39.0
Myositis M60.9
  clostridial A48.0
  due to posture —see Myositis, specified type
    NEC

Myositis *(Continued)*
  epidemic B33.0
  fibrosa or fibrous (chronic), Volkmann's T79.6
  foreign body granuloma —*see* Granuloma,
      foreign body
  in (due to)
    bilharziasis B65.9 *[M63.8-●]*
    cysticercosis B69.81
    leprosy A30.9 *[M63.8-●]*
    mycosis B49 *[M63.8-●]*
    sarcoidosis D86.87
    schistosomiasis B65.9 *[M63.8-●]*
    syphilis
      late A52.78
      secondary A51.49
    toxoplasmosis (acquired) B58.82
    trichinellosis B75 *[M63.8-●]*
    tuberculosis A18.09
  inclusion body [IBM] G72.41
  infective M60.009
    arm M60.002
      left M60.001
      right M60.000
    leg M60.005
      left M60.004
      right M60.003
    lower limb M60.005
      ankle M60.07-●
      foot M60.07-●
      lower leg M60.06-●
      thigh M60.05-●
      toe M60.07-●
    multiple sites M60.09
    specified site NEC M60.08
    upper limb M60.002
      finger M60.04-●
      forearm M60.03-●
      hand M60.04-●
      shoulder region M60.01-●
      upper arm M60.02-●
  interstitial M60.10
    ankle M60.17-●
    foot M60.17-●
    forearm M60.13-●
    hand M60.14-●
    lower leg M60.16-●
    multiple sites M60.19
    shoulder region M60.11-●
    specified site NEC M60.18
    thigh M60.15-●
    upper arm M60.12-●
  mycotic B49 *[M63.8-●]*
  ossificans or ossifying (circumscripta) —*see
      also* Ossification, muscle, specified NEC
    in (due to)
      burns M61.30
        ankle M61.37-●
        foot M61.37-●
        forearm M61.33-●
        hand M61.34-●
        lower leg M61.36-●

Myositis *(Continued)*
  ossificans or ossifying *(Continued)*
    in (due to) *(Continued)*
      burns *(Continued)*
        multiple sites M61.39
        pelvic region M61.35-●
        shoulder region M61.31-●
        specified site NEC M61.38
        thigh M61.35-●
        upper arm M61.32-●
      quadriplegia or paraplegia M61.20
        ankle M61.27-●
        foot M61.27-●
        forearm M61.23-●
        hand M61.24-●
        lower leg M61.26-●
        multiple sites M61.29
        pelvic region M61.25-●
        shoulder region M61.21-●
        specified site NEC M61.28
        thigh M61.25-●
        upper arm M61.22-●
    progressiva M61.10
      ankle M61.17-●
      finger M61.14-●
      foot M61.17-●
      forearm M61.13-●
      hand M61.14-●
      lower leg M61.16-●
      multiple sites M61.19
      pelvic region M61.15-●
      shoulder region M61.11-●
      specified site NEC M61.18
      thigh M61.15-●
      toe M61.17-●
      upper arm M61.12-●
    traumatica M61.00
      ankle M61.07-●
      foot M61.07-●
      forearm M61.03-●
      hand M61.04-●
      lower leg M61.06-●
      multiple sites M61.09
      pelvic region M61.05-●
      shoulder region M61.01-●
      specified site NEC M61.08
      thigh M61.05-●
      upper arm M61.02-●
  purulent —*see* Myositis, infective
  specified type NEC M60.80
    ankle M60.87-●
    foot M60.87-●
    forearm M60.83-●
    hand M60.84-●
    lower leg M60.86-●
    multiple sites M60.89
    pelvic region M60.85-●
    shoulder region M60.81-●
    specified site NEC M60.88
    thigh M60.85-●
    upper arm M60.82-●

Myositis *(Continued)*
  suppurative —*see* Myositis, infective
  traumatic (old) —*see* Myositis, specified type
      NEC
Myospasia impulsiva F95.2
Myotonia (acquisita) (intermittens) M62.89
  atrophica G71.11
  chondrodystrophic G71.13
  congenita (acetazolamide responsive)
      (dominant) (recessive) G71.12
  drug-induced G71.14
  dystrophica G71.11
  fluctuans G71.19
  levior G71.12
  permanens G71.19
  symptomatic G71.19
Myotonic pupil —*see* Anomaly, pupil, function,
    tonic pupil
Myriapodiasis B88.2
Myringitis H73.2-●
  with otitis media —*see* Otitis, media
  acute H73.00-●
    bullous H73.01-●
    specified NEC H73.09-●
  bullous —*see* Myringitis, acute, bullous
  chronic H73.1-●
Mysophobia F40.228
Mytilotoxism —*see* Poisoning, fish
Myxadenitis labialis K13.0
Myxedema (adult) (idiocy) (infantile)
      (juvenile) —*see also* Hypothyroidism
      E03.9
  circumscribed E05.90
    with storm E05.91
  coma E03.5
  congenital E00.1
  cutis L98.5
  localized (pretibial) E05.90
    with storm E05.91
  papular L98.5
Myxochondrosarcoma —*see* Neoplasm,
    cartilage, malignant
Myxofibroma —*see* Neoplasm, connective
    tissue, benign
  odontogenic —*see* Cyst, calcifying
    odontogenic
Myxofibrosarcoma —*see* Neoplasm, connective
    tissue, malignant
Myxolipoma D17.9
Myxoliposarcoma —*see* Neoplasm, connective
    tissue, malignant
Myxoma —*see also* Neoplasm, connective tissue,
    benign
  nerve sheath —*see* Neoplasm, nerve,
    benign
  odontogenic —*see* Cyst, calcifying
    odontogenic
Myxosarcoma —*see* Neoplasm, connective
    tissue, malignant

▶ New   ⇒ Revised   ~~deleted~~ Deleted   ● Use Additional Character(s)

N

Naegeli's
  disease Q82.8
  leukemia, monocytic C93.1-●
Naegleriasis (with meningoencephalitis)
    B60.2
Naffziger's syndrome G54.0
Naga sore —see Ulcer, skin
Nägele's pelvis M95.5
  with disproportion (fetopelvic) O33.0
    causing obstructed labor O65.0
Nail —see also condition
  biting F98.8
  patella syndrome Q87.2
Nanism, nanosomia —see Dwarfism
Nanophyetiasis B66.8
Nanukayami A27.89
Napkin rash L22
Narcolepsy G47.419
  with cataplexy G47.411
  in conditions classified elsewhere G47.429
    with cataplexy G47.421
Narcosis R06.89
Narcotism —see Dependence
NARP (Neuropathy, Ataxia and Retinitis
    pigmentosa) syndrome E88.49
Narrow
  anterior chamber angle H40.03-●
  gingival width (of periodontal soft tissue)
      K05.5
  pelvis —see Contraction, pelvis
Narrowing —see also Stenosis
  artery I77.1
    auditory, internal I65.8
    basilar —see Occlusion, artery, basilar
    carotid —see Occlusion, artery, carotid
    cerebellar —see Occlusion, artery, cerebellar
    cerebral —see Occlusion artery, cerebral
    choroidal —see Occlusion, artery,
        precerebral, specified NEC
    communicating posterior —see
        Occlusion, artery, precerebral,
        specified NEC
    coronary —see also Disease, heart, ischemic,
        atherosclerotic
      congenital Q24.5
        syphilitic A50.54 [I52]
      due to syphilis NEC A52.06
    hypophyseal —see Occlusion, artery,
        precerebral, specified NEC
    pontine —see Occlusion, artery, precerebral,
        specified NEC
    precerebral —see Occlusion, artery,
        precerebral
    vertebral —see Occlusion, artery, vertebral
  auditory canal (external) —see Stenosis,
      external ear canal
  eustachian tube —see Obstruction, eustachian
      tube
  eyelid —see Disorder, eyelid function
  larynx J38.6
  mesenteric artery —see also Ischemia,
      intestine, acute K55.059
  palate M26.89
  palpebral fissure —see Disorder, eyelid
      function
  ureter N13.5
    with infection N13.6
  urethra —see Stricture, urethra
Narrowness, abnormal, eyelid Q10.3
Nasal —see condition
Nasolachrymal, nasolacrimal —see condition
Nasopharyngeal —see also condition
  pituitary gland Q89.2
  torticollis M43.6
Nasopharyngitis (acute) (infective)
      (streptococcal) (subacute) J00
  chronic (suppurative) (ulcerative) J31.1
Nasopharynx, nasopharyngeal —see condition
Natal tooth, teeth K00.6

Nausea (without vomiting) R11.0
  with vomiting R11.2
  gravidarum —see Hyperemesis, gravidarum
  marina T75.3
  navalis T75.3
Navel —see condition
Neapolitan fever —see Brucellosis
Near drowning T75.1
Nearsightedness —see Myopia
Near-syncope R55
Nebula, cornea —see Opacity, cornea
Necator americanus infestation B76.1
Necatoriasis B76.1
Neck —see condition
Necrobiosis R68.89
  lipoidica NEC L92.1
    with diabetes —see E08-E13 with .620
Necrolysis, toxic epidermal L51.2
  due to drug
    correct substance properly administered —
        see Table of Drugs and Chemicals, by
        drug, adverse effect
    overdose or wrong substance given
        or taken —see Table of Drugs and
        Chemicals, by drug, poisoning
Necrophilia F65.89
Necrosis, necrotic (ischemic) —see also
      Gangrene
  adrenal (capsule) (gland) E27.49
  amputation stump (surgical) (late) T87.50
    arm T87.5-●
    leg T87.5-●
  antrum J32.0
  aorta (hyaline) —see also Aneurysm, aorta
    cystic medial —see Dissection, aorta
  artery I77.5
  bladder (aseptic) (sphincter) N32.89
  bone —see also Osteonecrosis M87.9
    aseptic or avascular —see Osteonecrosis
        idiopathic M87.00
    ethmoid J32.2
    jaw M27.2
    tuberculous —see Tuberculosis, bone
  brain I67.89
  breast (aseptic) (fat) (segmental) N64.1
  bronchus J98.09
  central nervous system NEC I67.89
  cerebellar I67.89
  cerebral I67.89
  colon —see also Infarct, intestine K55.049
  cornea H18.89-●
  cortical (acute) (renal) N17.1
  cystic medial (aorta) —see Dissection, aorta
  dental pulp K04.1
  esophagus K22.89
  ethmoid (bone) J32.2
  eyelid —see Disorder, eyelid, degenerative
  fat, fatty (generalized) —see also Disorder, soft
      tissue, specified type NEC
    abdominal wall K65.4
    breast (aseptic) (segmental) N64.1
    localized —see Degeneration, by site, fatty
    mesentery K65.4
    omentum K65.4
    pancreas K86.89
    peritoneum K65.4
    skin (subcutaneous), newborn P83.0
    subcutaneous, due to birth injury P15.6
  gallbladder —see Cholecystitis, acute
  heart —see Infarct, myocardium
  hip, aseptic or avascular —see Osteonecrosis,
      by type, femur
  intestine (acute) (hemorrhagic) (massive) —
      see also Infarct, intestine K55.069
  jaw M27.2
  kidney (bilateral) N28.0
    acute N17.9
    cortical (acute) (bilateral) N17.1
      with ectopic or molar pregnancy O08.4
    medullary (bilateral) (in acute renal failure)
        (papillary) N17.2

Necrosis, necrotic (Continued)
  kidney (Continued)
    papillary (bilateral) (in acute renal
        failure) N17.2
    tubular N17.0
      with ectopic or molar pregnancy
          O08.4
      complicating
        abortion —see Abortion, by type,
            complicated by, tubular necrosis
        ectopic or molar pregnancy O08.4
        pregnancy —see Pregnancy,
            complicated by, diseases of,
            specified type or system NEC
      following ectopic or molar pregnancy
          O08.4
    traumatic T79.5
  larynx J38.7
  liver (with hepatic failure) (cell) —see Failure,
      hepatic
    hemorrhagic, central K76.2
  lung J85.0
  lymphatic gland —see Lymphadenitis, acute
  mammary gland (fat) (segmental) N64.1
  mastoid (chronic) —see Mastoiditis, chronic
  medullary (acute) (renal) N17.2
  mesentery —see also Infarct, intestine
      K55.069
    fat K65.4
  mitral valve —see Insufficiency, mitral
  myocardium, myocardial —see Infarct,
      myocardium
  nose J34.0
  omentum (with mesenteric infarction) —see
      also Infarct, intestine K55.069
    fat K65.4
  orbit, orbital —see Osteomyelitis, orbit
  ossicles, ear —see Abnormal, ear ossicles
  ovary N70.92
  pancreas (aseptic) (duct) (fat) K86.89
    acute (infective) —see Pancreatitis, acute
    infective —see Pancreatitis, acute
  papillary (acute) (renal) N17.2
  perineum N90.89
  peritoneum (with mesenteric infarction) —see
      also Infarct, intestine K55.069
    fat K65.4
  pharynx J02.9
    in granulocytopenia —see Neutropenia
      Vincent's A69.1
  phosphorus —see subcategory T54.2
  pituitary (gland) E23.0
    postpartum O99.285
    Sheehan O99.285
  pressure —see Ulcer, pressure, by site
  pulmonary J85.0
  pulp (dental) K04.1
  radiation —see Necrosis, by site
  radium —see Necrosis, by site
  renal —see Necrosis, kidney
  sclera H15.89
  scrotum N50.89
  skin or subcutaneous tissue NEC I96
  spine, spinal (column) —see also
      Osteonecrosis, by type, vertebra
    cord G95.19
  spleen D73.5
  stomach K31.89
  stomatitis (ulcerative) A69.0
  subcutaneous fat, newborn P83.88
  subendocardial (acute) I21.4
    chronic I25.89
  suprarenal (capsule) (gland) E27.49
  testis N50.89
  thymus (gland) E32.8
  tonsil J35.8
  trachea J39.8
  tuberculous NEC —see Tuberculosis
  tubular (acute) (anoxic) (renal) (toxic)
      N17.0
    postprocedural N99.0

Necrosis, necrotic (Continued)
  vagina N89.8
  vertebra —see also Osteonecrosis, by type,
      vertebra
    tuberculous A18.01
  vulva N90.89
  X-ray —see Necrosis, by site
Necrospermia —see Infertility, male
Need (for)
  care provider because (of)
    assistance with personal care Z74.1
    continuous supervision required Z74.3
    impaired mobility Z74.09
    no other household member able to render
        care Z74.2
    specified reason NEC Z74.8
  immunization —see Vaccination
  vaccination —see Vaccination
Neglect
  adult
    confirmed T74.01
    history of Z91.412
    suspected T76.01
  child (childhood)
    confirmed T74.02
    history of Z62.812
    suspected T76.02
  emotional, in childhood Z62.898
  hemispatial R41.4
  left-sided R41.4
  sensory R41.4
  visuospatial R41.4
Neisserian infection NEC —see Gonococcus
Nelaton's syndrome G60.8
Nelson's syndrome E24.1
Nematodiasis (intestinal) B82.0
  Ancylostoma B76.0
Neonatal —see also Newborn
  acne L70.4
  bradycardia P29.12
  ▸screening, abnormal findings on —see
      Abnormal, neonatal screening P09
  tachycardia P29.11
  tooth, teeth K00.6
Neonatorum —see condition
Neoplasia
  endocrine, multiple (MEN) E31.20
    type I E31.21
    type IIA E31.22
    type IIB E31.23
  intraepithelial (histologically confirmed)
    anal (AIN) (histologically confirmed)
        K62.82
      grade I K62.82
      grade II K62.82
      severe D01.3
    cervical glandular (histologically
        confirmed) D06.9
    cervix (uteri) (CIN) (histologically
        confirmed) N87.9
      glandular D06.9
      grade I N87.0
      grade II N87.1
      grade III (severe dysplasia) —see also
          Carcinoma, cervix uteri, in situ
          D06.9
    prostate (histologically confirmed) (PIN)
        N42.31
      grade I N42.31
      grade II N42.31
      grade III (severe dysplasia) D07.5
    vagina (histologically confirmed) (VAIN)
        N89.3
      grade I N89.0
      grade II N89.1
      grade III (severe dysplasia) D07.2
    vulva (histologically confirmed) (VIN)
        N90.3
      grade I N90.0
      grade II N90.1
      grade III (severe dysplasia) D07.1

Neoplasm, neoplastic —see also Table of
    Neoplasms
  lipomatous, benign —see Lipoma
  malignant mast cell C96.20
    specified type NEC C96.29
  mast cell, of uncertain behavior NEC D47.09
Neovascularization
  ciliary body —see Disorder, iris, vascular
  cornea H16.40-●
    deep H16.44-●
    ghost vessels —see Ghost, vessels
    localized H16.43-●
    pannus —see Pannus
  iris —see Disorder, iris, vascular
  retina H35.05-●
Nephralgia N23
Nephritis, nephritic (albuminuric) (azotemic)
    (congenital) (disseminated) (epithelial)
    (familial) (focal) (granulomatous)
    (hemorrhagic) (infantile) (nonsuppurative,
    excretory) (uremic) N05.9
  with
    C3
      glomerulonephritis N05.A
      glomerulopathy N05.A
        with dense deposit disease N05.6
      dense deposit disease N05.6
      diffuse
        crescentic glomerulonephritis N05.7
        endocapillary proliferative
            glomerulonephritis N05.4
        membranous glomerulonephritis N05.2
        mesangial proliferative
            glomerulonephritis N05.3
        mesangiocapillary glomerulonephritis
            N05.5
    edema —see Nephrosis
    focal and segmental glomerular lesions
        N05.1
    foot process disease N04.9
    glomerular lesion
      diffuse sclerosing N05.8
      hypocomplementemic —see Nephritis,
          membranoproliferative
      IgA —see Nephropathy, IgA
      lobular, lobulonodular —see Nephritis,
          membranoproliferative
      nodular —see Nephritis,
          membranoproliferative
    lesion of
      glomerulonephritis, proliferative N05.8
      renal necrosis N05.9
    minor glomerular abnormality N05.0
    specified morphological changes NEC
        N05.8
  acute N00.9
    with
      C3
        glomerulonephritis N00.A
        glomerulopathy N00.A
          with dense deposit disease N00.6
        dense deposit disease N00.6
        diffuse
          crescentic glomerulonephritis N00.7
          endocapillary proliferative
              glomerulonephritis N00.4
          membranous glomerulonephritis
              N00.2
          mesangial proliferative
              glomerulonephritis N00.3
          mesangiocapillary glomerulonephritis
              N00.5
      focal and segmental glomerular lesions
          N00.1
      minor glomerular abnormality N00.0
      specified morphological changes NEC
          N00.8
  amyloid E85.4 [N08]
  antiglomerular basement membrane (anti-
      GBM) antibody NEC
    in Goodpasture's syndrome M31.0

Nephritis, nephritic (Continued)
  antitubular basement membrane (tubulo-
      interstitial) NEC N12
    toxic —see Nephropathy, toxic
  arteriolar —see Hypertension, kidney
  arteriosclerotic —see Hypertension, kidney
  ascending —see Nephritis, tubulo-interstitial
  atrophic N03.9
  Balkan (endemic) N15.0
  calculous, calculus —see Calculus,
      kidney
  cardiac —see Hypertension, kidney
  cardiovascular —see Hypertension,
      kidney
  chronic N03.9
    with
      C3
        glomerulonephritis N03.A
        glomerulopathy N03.A
          with dense deposit disease N03.6
        dense deposit disease N03.6
        diffuse
          crescentic glomerulonephritis
              N03.7
          endocapillary proliferative
              glomerulonephritis N03.4
          membranous glomerulonephritis
              N03.2
          mesangial proliferative
              glomerulonephritis N03.3
          mesangiocapillary glomerulonephritis
              N03.5
      focal and segmental glomerular lesions
          N03.1
      minor glomerular abnormality
          N03.0
      specified morphological changes
          NEC N03.8
    arteriosclerotic —see Hypertension,
        kidney
  cirrhotic N26.9
  complicating pregnancy O26.83-●
  croupous N00.9
  degenerative —see Nephrosis
  diffuse sclerosing N05.8
  due to
    diabetes mellitus —see E08-E13 with .21
    subacute bacterial endocarditis I33.0
    systemic lupus erythematosus (chronic)
        M32.14
    typhoid fever A01.09
  gonococcal (acute) (chronic) A54.21
  hypocomplementemic —see Nephritis,
      membranoproliferative
  IgA —see Nephropathy, IgA
  immune complex (circulating) NEC N05.8
  infective —see Nephritis, tubulo-interstitial
  interstitial —see Nephritis, tubulo-interstitial
  lead N14.3
  membranoproliferative (diffuse) (type 1
      or 3) —see also N00-N07 with fourth
      character .5 N05.5
    type 2 —see also N00-N07 with fourth
        character .6 N05.6
  minimal change N05.0
  necrotic, necrotizing NEC —see also N00-N07
      with fourth character .8 N05.8
  nephrotic —see Nephrosis
  nodular —see Nephritis,
      membranoproliferative
  polycystic Q61.3
    adult type Q61.2
    autosomal
      dominant Q61.2
      recessive NEC Q61.19
    childhood type NEC Q61.19
    infantile type NEC Q61.19
  poststreptococcal N05.9
    acute N00.9
    chronic N03.9
    rapidly progressive N01.9

▶ New   ⇒ Revised   ~~deleted~~ Deleted   ● Use Additional Character(s)

Nephritis, nephritic *(Continued)*
proliferative NEC —*see also* N00-N07 with
    fourth character .8 N05.8
purulent —*see* Nephritis, tubulo-interstitial
rapidly progressive N01.9
  with
    C3
      glomerulonephritis N01.A
      glomerulopathy N01.A
        with dense deposit disease N01.6
    dense deposit disease N01.6
    diffuse
      crescentic glomerulonephritis N01.7
      endocapillary proliferative
        glomerulonephritis N01.4
      membranous glomerulonephritis
        N01.2
      mesangial proliferative
        glomerulonephritis N01.3
      mesangiocapillary glomerulonephritis
        N01.5
    focal and segmental glomerular lesions
      N01.1
    minor glomerular abnormality N01.0
    specified morphological changes NEC
      N01.8
salt losing or wasting NEC N28.89
saturnine N14.3
sclerosing, diffuse N05.8
septic —*see* Nephritis, tubulo-interstitial
specified pathology NEC —*see also* N00-N07
  with fourth character .8 N05.8
subacute N01.9
suppurative —*see* Nephritis,
  tubulo-interstitial
syphilitic (late) A52.75
  congenital A50.59 *[N08]*
  early (secondary) A51.44
toxic —*see* Nephropathy, toxic
tubal, tubular —*see* Nephritis,
  tubulo-interstitial
tuberculous A18.11
tubulo-interstitial (in) N12
  acute (infectious) N10
  chronic (infectious) N11.9
    nonobstructive N11.8
      reflux-associated N11.0
    obstructive N11.1
    specified NEC N11.8
  due to
    brucellosis A23.9 *[N16]*
    cryoglobulinemia D89.1 *[N16]*
    glycogen storage disease E74.00 *[N16]*
  Sjögren's syndrome M35.04
vascular —*see* Hypertension, kidney
war N00.9
Nephroblastoma (epithelial) (mesenchymal)
  C64-●
Nephrocalcinosis E83.59 *[N29]*
Nephrocystitis, pustular —*see* Nephritis,
  tubulo-interstitial
Nephrolithiasis (congenital) (pelvis)
  (recurrent) —*see also* Calculus, kidney
Nephroma C64-●
  mesoblastic D41.0-●
Nephronephritis —*see* Nephrosis
Nephronophthisis Q61.5
Nephropathia epidemica A98.5
Nephropathy —*see also* Nephritis N28.9
  with
    edema —*see* Nephrosis
    glomerular lesion —*see*
      Glomerulonephritis
  amyloid, hereditary E85.0
  analgesic N14.0
    with medullary necrosis, acute N17.2
  Balkan (endemic) N15.0
  chemical —*see* Nephropathy, toxic
  diabetic —*see* E08-E13 with .21
  drug-induced N14.2
    specified NEC N14.1

Nephropathy *(Continued)*
focal and segmental hyalinosis or sclerosis
  N02.1
heavy metal-induced N14.3
hereditary NEC N07.9
  with
    C3
      glomerulonephritis N07.A
      glomerulopathy N07.A
        with dense deposit disease N07.6
    dense deposit disease N07.6
    diffuse
      crescentic glomerulonephritis N07.7
      endocapillary proliferative
        glomerulonephritis N07.4
      membranous glomerulonephritis
        N07.2
      mesangial proliferative
        glomerulonephritis N07.3
      mesangiocapillary glomerulonephritis
        N07.5
    focal and segmental glomerular lesions
      N07.1
    minor glomerular abnormality N07.0
    specified morphological changes NEC
      N07.8
hypercalcemic N25.89
hypertensive —*see* Hypertension, kidney
hypokalemic (vacuolar) N25.89
IgA N02.8
  with glomerular lesion N02.9
    focal and segmental hyalinosis or
      sclerosis N02.1
    membranoproliferative (diffuse) N02.5
    membranous (diffuse) N02.2
    mesangial proliferative (diffuse) N02.3
    mesangiocapillary (diffuse) N02.5
    proliferative NEC N02.8
    specified pathology NEC N02.8
lead N14.3
membranoproliferative (diffuse) N02.5
membranous (diffuse) N02.2
mesangial (IgA/IgG) —*see* Nephropathy, IgA
  proliferative (diffuse) N02.3
mesangiocapillary (diffuse) N02.5
obstructive N13.8
phenacetin N17.2
phosphate-losing N25.0
potassium depletion N25.89
pregnancy-related O26.83-●
proliferative NEC (*see also* N00-N07 with
  fourth character .8) N05.8
protein-losing N25.89
saturnine N14.3
sickle-cell D57.-● *[N08]*
toxic NEC N14.4
  due to
    drugs N14.2
      analgesic N14.0
      specified NEC N14.1
    heavy metals N14.3
vasomotor N17.0
water-losing N25.89
Nephroptosis N28.83
Nephropyosis —*see* Abscess, kidney
Nephrorrhagia N28.89
Nephrosclerosis (arteriolar) (arteriosclerotic)
  (chronic) (hyaline) —*see also* Hypertension,
  kidney
hyperplastic —*see* Hypertension, kidney
senile N26.9
Nephrosis, nephrotic (Epstein's) (syndrome)
  (congenital) N04.9
  with
    foot process disease N04.9
    glomerular lesion N04.1
    hypocomplementemic N04.5
  acute N04.9
  anoxic —*see* Nephrosis, tubular
  chemical —*see* Nephrosis, tubular
  cholemic K76.7

Nephrosis, nephrotic *(Continued)*
diabetic —*see* E08-E13 with .21
Finnish type (congenital) Q89.8
hemoglobin N10
hemoglobinuric —*see* Nephrosis, tubular
in
  amyloidosis E85.4 *[N08]*
  diabetes mellitus —*see* E08-E13 with .21
  epidemic hemorrhagic fever A98.5
  malaria (malariae) B52.0
ischemic —*see* Nephrosis, tubular
lipoid N04.9
lower nephron —*see* Nephrosis, tubular
malarial (malariae) B52.0
minimal change N04.0
myoglobin N10
necrotizing —*see* Nephrosis, tubular
osmotic (sucrose) N25.89
radiation N04.9
syphilitic (late) A52.75
toxic —*see* Nephrosis, tubular
tubular (acute) N17.0
  postprocedural N99.0
  radiation N04.9
Nephrosonephritis, hemorrhagic (endemic)
  A98.5
Nephrostomy
attention to Z43.6
status Z93.6
Nerve —*see also* condition
injury —*see* Injury, nerve, by body site
Nerves R45.0
Nervous —*see also* condition R45.0
heart F45.8
stomach F45.8
tension R45.0
Nervousness R45.0
Nesidioblastoma
pancreas D13.7
specified site NEC —*see* Neoplasm, benign,
  by site
unspecified site D13.7
Nettleship's syndrome —*see* Urticaria
  pigmentosa
Neumann's disease or syndrome L10.1
Neuralgia, neuralgic (acute) M79.2
accessory (nerve) G52.8
acoustic (nerve) —*see* subcategory H93.3
auditory (nerve) —*see* subcategory H93.3
ciliary G44.009
  intractable G44.001
  not intractable G44.009
cranial
  nerve —*see also* Disorder, nerve, cranial
    fifth or trigeminal —*see* Neuralgia,
      trigeminal
  postherpetic, postzoster B02.29
ear —*see* subcategory H92.0
facialis vera G51.1
Fothergill's —*see* Neuralgia, trigeminal
glossopharyngeal (nerve) G52.1
Horton's G44.099
  intractable G44.091
  not intractable G44.099
Hunt's B02.21
hypoglossal (nerve) G52.3
infraorbital —*see* Neuralgia, trigeminal
malarial —*see* Malaria
migrainous G44.009
  intractable G44.001
  not intractable G44.009
Morton's G57.6-●
nerve, cranial —*see* Disorder, nerve, cranial
nose G52.0
occipital M54.81
olfactory G52.0
penis N48.9
perineum R10.2
postherpetic NEC B02.29
  trigeminal B02.22
pubic region R10.2

Neuralgia, neuralgic (Continued)
scrotum R10.2
Sluder's G44.89
specified nerve NEC G58.8
spermatic cord R10.2
sphenopalatine (ganglion) G90.09
trifacial —see Neuralgia, trigeminal
trigeminal G50.0
posttherpetic, postzoster B02.22
vagus (nerve) G52.2
writer's F48.8
organic G25.89
Neurapraxia —see Injury, nerve
Neurasthenia F48.8
cardiac F45.8
gastric F45.8
heart F45.8
Neurilemmoma —see also Neoplasm, nerve,
benign
acoustic (nerve) D33.3
malignant —see also Neoplasm, nerve,
malignant
acoustic (nerve) C72.4
Neurilemmosarcoma —see Neoplasm, nerve,
malignant
Neurinoma —see Neoplasm, nerve, benign
Neurinomatosis —see Neoplasm, nerve,
uncertain behavior
Neuritis (rheumatoid) M79.2
abducens (nerve) —see Strabismus, paralytic,
sixth nerve
accessory (nerve) G52.8
acoustic (nerve) —see also subcategory H93.3
in (due to)
infectious disease NEC B99 [H94.0-●]
parasitic disease NEC B89 [H94.0-●]
syphilitic A52.15
alcoholic G62.1
with psychosis —see Psychosis, alcoholic
amyloid, any site E85.4 [G63]
auditory (nerve) —see subcategory H93.3
brachial —see Radiculopathy
due to displacement, intervertebral disc —
see Disorder, disc, cervical, with neuritis
cranial nerve
due to Lyme disease A69.22
eighth or acoustic or auditory —see
subcategory H93.3
eleventh or accessory G52.8
fifth or trigeminal G51.0
first or olfactory G52.0
fourth or trochlear —see Strabismus,
paralytic, fourth nerve
second or optic —see Neuritis, optic
seventh or facial G51.8
newborn (birth injury) P11.3
sixth or abducent —see Strabismus,
paralytic, sixth nerve
tenth or vagus G52.2
third or oculomotor —see Strabismus,
paralytic, third nerve
twelfth or hypoglossal G52.3
Déjérine-Sottas G60.0
diabetic (mononeuropathy) —see E08-E13
with .41
polyneuropathy —see E08-E13 with .42
due to
beriberi E51.11
displacement, prolapse or rupture,
intervertebral disc —see Disorder, disc,
with, radiculopathy
herniation, nucleus pulposus M51.9 [G55]
endemic E51.11
facial G51.8
newborn (birth injury) P11.3
general —see Polyneuropathy
geniculate ganglion G51.1
due to herpes (zoster) B02.21
gouty —see also Gout, by type M10.9 [G63]
hypoglossal (nerve) G52.3
ilioinguinal (nerve) G57.9-●
infectious (multiple) NEC G61.0

Neuritis (Continued)
interstitial hypertrophic progressive G60.0
lumbar M54.16
lumbosacral M54.17
multiple —see also Polyneuropathy
endemic E51.11
infective, acute G61.0
multiplex endemica E51.11
nerve root —see Radiculopathy
oculomotor (nerve) —see Strabismus,
paralytic, third nerve
olfactory nerve G52.0
optic (nerve) (hereditary) (sympathetic) H46.9
with demyelination G36.0
in myelitis G36.0
nutritional H46.2
papillitis —see Papillitis, optic
retrobulbar H46.1-●
specified type NEC H46.8
toxic H46.3
peripheral (nerve) G62.9
multiple —see Polyneuropathy
single —see Mononeuritis
pneumogastric (nerve) G52.2
posttherpetic, postzoster B02.29
progressive hypertrophic interstitial G60.0
retrobulbar —see also Neuritis, optic,
retrobulbar
in (due to)
late syphilis A52.15
meningococcal infection A39.82
meningococcal A39.82
syphilitic A52.15
sciatic (nerve) —see also Sciatica
due to displacement of intervertebral
disc —see Disorder, disc, with,
radiculopathy
serum —see also Reaction, serum T80.69
shoulder-girdle G54.5
specified nerve NEC G58.8
spinal (nerve) root —see Radiculopathy
syphilitic A52.15
thenar (median) G56.1-●
thoracic M54.14
toxic NEC G62.2
trochlear (nerve) —see Strabismus, paralytic,
fourth nerve
vagus (nerve) G52.2
Neuroastrocytoma —see Neoplasm, uncertain
behavior, by site
Neuroavitaminosis E56.9 [G99.8]
Neuroblastoma
olfactory C30.0
specified site —see Neoplasm, malignant, by
site
unspecified site C74.90
Neurochorioretinitis —see Chorioretinitis
Neurocirculatory asthenia F45.8
Neurocysticercosis B69.0
Neurocytoma —see Neoplasm, benign, by site
Neurodermatitis (circumscribed)
(circumscripta) (local) L28.0
atopic L20.81
diffuse (Brocq) L20.81
disseminated L20.81
Neuroencephalomyelopathy, optic G36.0
Neuroepithelioma —see also Neoplasm,
malignant, by site
olfactory C30.0
Neurofibroma —see also Neoplasm, nerve,
benign
melanotic —see Neoplasm, nerve, benign
multiple —see Neurofibromatosis
plexiform —see Neoplasm, nerve, benign
Neurofibromatosis (multiple) (nonmalignant)
Q85.00
acoustic Q85.02
malignant —see Neoplasm, nerve, malignant
specified NEC Q85.09
type 1 (von Recklinghausen) Q85.01
type 2 Q85.02

Neurofibrosarcoma —see Neoplasm, nerve,
malignant
Neurogenic —see also condition
bladder —see also Dysfunction, bladder,
neuromuscular N31.9
cauda equina syndrome G83.4
bowel NEC K59.2
heart F45.8
Neuroglioma —see Neoplasm, uncertain
behavior, by site
Neurolabyrinthitis (of Dix and Hallpike) —see
Neuronitis, vestibular
Neurolathyrism —see Poisoning, food, noxious,
plant
Neuroleprosy A30.9
Neuroma —see also Neoplasm, nerve, benign
acoustic (nerve) D33.3
amputation (stump) (traumatic) (surgical
complication) (late) T87.3-●
arm T87.3-●
leg T87.3-●
digital (toe) G57.6-●
interdigital G58.8
lower limb toe G57.8-●
upper limb G56.8-●
intermetatarsal G57.8-●
Morton's G57.6-●
nonneoplastic
arm G56.9-●
leg G57.9-●
lower extremity G57.9-●
upper extremity G56.9-●
optic (nerve) D33.3
plantar G57.6-●
plexiform —see Neoplasm, nerve,
benign
surgical (nonneoplastic)
arm G56.9-●
leg G57.9-●
lower extremity G57.9-●
upper extremity G56.9-●
Neuromyalgia —see Neuralgia
Neuromyasthenia (epidemic) (postinfectious)
G93.3
Neuromyelitis G36.9
ascending G61.0
optica G36.0
Neuromyopathy G70.9
paraneoplastic D49.9 [G13.0]
Neuromyotonia (Isaacs) G71.19
Neuronevus —see Nevus
Neuronitis G58.9
ascending (acute) G57.2-●
vestibular H81.2-●
Neuroparalytic —see condition
Neuropathy, neuropathic G62.9
acute motor G62.81
alcoholic G62.1
with psychosis —see Psychosis,
alcoholic
arm G56.9-●
autonomic, peripheral —see Neuropathy,
peripheral, autonomic
axillary G56.9-●
bladder N31.9
atonic (motor) (sensory) N31.2
autonomous N31.2
flaccid N31.2
nonreflex N31.2
reflex N31.1
uninhibited N31.0
brachial plexus G54.0
cervical plexus G54.2
chronic
progressive segmentally demyelinating
G62.89
relapsing demyelinating G62.89
Déjérine-Sottas G60.0
diabetic —see E08-E13 with .40
mononeuropathy —see E08-E13 with .41
polyneuropathy —see E08-E13 with .42

▶ New   ⇒ Revised   ~~deleted~~ Deleted   ● Use Additional Character(s)

Nevus *(Continued)*
  dysplastic —*see* Neoplasm, skin, benign
  eye D31.9-●
  flammeus Q82.5
  hemangiomatous D18.00
    intra-abdominal D18.03
    intracranial D18.02
    skin D18.01
    specified site NEC D18.09
  iris D31.4-●
  lacrimal gland D31.5-●
  lymphatic D18.1
  magnocellular
    specified site —*see* Neoplasm, benign, by
        site
    unspecified site D31.40
  malignant —*see* Melanoma
  meaning hemangioma D18.00
    intra-abdominal D18.03
    intracranial D18.02
    skin D18.01
    specified site NEC D18.09
  mouth (mucosa) D10.30
    specified site NEC D10.39
    white sponge Q38.6
  multiplex Q85.1
  non-neoplastic I78.1
  oral mucosa D10.30
    specified site NEC D10.39
    white sponge Q38.6
  orbit D31.6-●
  pigmented
    giant —*see also* Neoplasm, skin, uncertain
        behavior D48.5
      malignant melanoma in —*see* Melanoma
  portwine Q82.5
  retina D31.2-●
  retrobulbar D31.6-●
  sanguineous Q82.5
  senile I78.1
  skin D22.9
    abdominal wall D22.5
    ala nasi D22.39
    ankle D22.7-●
    anus, anal D22.5
    arm D22.6-●
    auditory canal (external) D22.2-●
    auricle (ear) D22.2-●
    auricular canal (external) D22.2-●
    axilla, axillary fold D22.5
    back D22.5
    breast D22.5
    brow D22.39
    buttock D22.5
    canthus (eye) D22.1-●
    cheek (external) D22.39
    chest wall D22.5
    chin D22.39
    ear (external) D22.2-●
    external meatus (ear) D22.2-●
    eyebrow D22.39
    eyelid (lower) (upper) D22.1-●
    face D22.30
      specified NEC D22.39
    female genital organ (external) NEC D28.0
    finger D22.6-●
    flank D22.5
    foot D22.7-●
    forearm D22.6-●
    forehead D22.39
    foreskin D29.0
    genital organ (external) NEC
      female D28.0
      male D29.9
    gluteal region D22.5
    groin D22.5
    hand D22.6-●
    heel D22.7-●
    helix D22.2-●
    hip D22.7-●
    interscapular region D22.5

Nevus *(Continued)*
  skin *(Continued)*
    jaw D22.39
    knee D22.7-●
    labium (majus) (minus) D28.0
    leg D22.7-●
    lip (lower) (upper) D22.0
    lower limb D22.7-●
    male genital organ (external) D29.9
    nail D22.9
      finger D22.6-●
      toe D22.7-●
    nasolabial groove D22.39
    nates D22.5
    neck D22.4
    nose (external) D22.39
    palpebra D22.1-●
    penis D29.0
    perianal skin D22.5
    perineum D22.5
    pinna D22.2-●
    popliteal fossa or space D22.7-●
    prepuce D29.0
    pudendum D28.0
    scalp D22.4
    scrotum D29.4
    shoulder D22.6-●
    submammary fold D22.5
    temple D22.39
    thigh D22.7-●
    toe D22.7-●
    trunk NEC D22.5
    umbilicus D22.5
    upper limb D22.6-●
    vulva D28.0
    specified site NEC —*see* Neoplasm, benign,
        by site
  spider I78.1
  stellar I78.1
  strawberry Q82.5
  Sutton's benign D22.9
  unius lateris Q82.5
  Unna's Q82.5
  vascular Q82.5
  verrucous Q82.5
Newborn (infant) (liveborn) (singleton)
      Z38.2
  abstinence syndrome P96.1
  acne L70.4
  affected by
    abnormalities of membranes P02.9
      specified NEC P02.8
    abruptio placenta P02.1
    amino-acid metabolic disorder, transitory
        P74.8
    amniocentesis (while in utero) P00.6
    amnionitis P02.78
    apparent life threatening event (ALTE)
        R68.13
    bleeding (into)
      cerebral cortex P52.22
      germinal matrix P52.0
      ventricles P52.1
    breech delivery P03.0
    cardiac arrest P29.81
    cardiomyopathy I42.8
      congenital I42.4
    cerebral ischemia P91.0
    Cesarean delivery P03.4
    chemotherapy agents P04.11
    chorioamnionitis P02.78
    cocaine (crack) P04.41
    complications of labor and delivery P03.9
      specified NEC P03.89
    compression of umbilical cord NEC P02.5
    contracted pelvis P03.1
    cyanosis P28.2
    delivery P03.9
      Cesarean P03.4
      forceps P03.2
      vacuum extractor P03.3

Newborn *(Continued)*
  affected by *(Continued)*
    drugs of addiction P04.40
      cocaine P04.41
      hallucinogens P04.42
      specified drug NEC P04.49
    entanglement (knot) in umbilical cord P02.5
    environmental chemicals P04.6
    fetal (intrauterine)
      growth retardation P05.9
      inflammatory response syndrome (FIRS)
          P02.70
      malnutrition not light or small for
          gestational age P05.2
    FIRS (fetal inflammatory response
        syndrome) P02.70
    forceps delivery P03.2
    heart rate abnormalities
      bradycardia P29.12
      intrauterine P03.819
        before onset of labor P03.810
        during labor P03.811
      tachycardia P29.11
    hemorrhage (antepartum) P02.1
      cerebellar (nontraumatic) P52.6
      intracerebral (nontraumatic) P52.4
      intracranial (nontraumatic) P52.9
        specified NEC P52.8
      intraventricular (nontraumatic) P52.3
        grade 1 P52.0
        grade 2 P52.1
        grade 3 P52.21
        grade 4 P52.22
      posterior fossa (nontraumatic) P52.6
      subarachnoid (nontraumatic) P52.5
      subependymal P52.0
        with intracerebral extension P52.22
        with intraventricular extension P52.1
          with enlargment of ventricles P52.21
        without intraventricular extension
            P52.0
    hypoxic ischemic encephalopathy [HIE]
        P91.60
      mild P91.61
      moderate P91.62
      severe P91.63
    induction of labor P03.89
    intestinal perforation P78.0
    intrauterine (fetal) blood loss P50.9
      due to (from)
        cut end of co-twin cord P50.5
        hemorrhage into
          co-twin P50.3
          maternal circulation P50.4
        placenta P50.2
        ruptured cord blood P50.1
        vasa previa P50.0
      specified NEC P50.8
    intrauterine (fetal) hemorrhage P50.9
    intrauterine (in utero) procedure P96.5
    malpresentation (malposition) NEC P03.1
    maternal (complication of) (use of)
      alcohol P04.3
      amphetamines P04.16
      analgesia (maternal) P04.0
      anesthesia (maternal) P04.0
      anticonvulsants P04.13
      antidepressants P04.15
      antineoplastic chemotherapy P04.11
      anxiolytics P04.1A
      blood loss P02.1
      cannabis P04.81
      circulatory disease P00.3
      condition P00.9
        specified NEC P00.89
      cytotoxic drugs P04.12
      delivery P03.9
        Cesarean P03.4
        forceps P03.2
        vacuum extractor P03.3
      diabetes mellitus (pre-existing) P70.1

▶ New   ⇒ Revised   ~~deleted~~ Deleted   ● Use Additional Character(s)

Newborn *(Continued)*
- affected by *(Continued)*
  - maternal *(Continued)*
    - disorder P00.9
      - specified NEC P00.89
    - drugs (addictive) (illegal) NEC P04.49
    - ectopic pregnancy P01.4
    - gestational diabetes P70.0
    - ▶ group B streptococcus (GBS)
      - colonization (positive) P00.82
    - hemorrhage P02.1
    - hypertensive disorder P00.0
    - incompetent cervix P01.0
    - infectious disease P00.2
    - injury P00.5
    - labor and delivery P03.9
    - malpresentation before labor P01.7
    - maternal death P01.6
    - medical procedure P00.7
    - medication P04.19
      - specified type NEC P04.18
    - multiple pregnancy P01.5
    - nutritional disorder P00.4
    - oligohydramnios P01.2
    - opiates P04.14
      - administered for procedures during pregnancy or labor and delivery P04.0
    - parasitic disease P00.2
    - periodontal disease P00.81
    - placenta previa P02.0
    - polyhydramnios P01.3
    - precipitate delivery P03.5
    - pregnancy P01.9
      - specified P01.8
    - premature rupture of membranes P01.1
    - renal disease P00.1
    - respiratory disease P00.3
    - sedative-hypnotics P04.17
    - surgical procedure P00.6
    - tranquilizers administered for procedures during pregnancy or labor and delivery P04.0
    - urinary tract disease P00.1
    - uterine contraction (abnormal) P03.6
  - meconium peritonitis P78.0
  - medication (legal) (maternal use) (prescribed) P04.19
  - membrane abnormalities P02.9
    - specified NEC P02.8
  - membranitis P02.78
  - methamphetamine(s) P04.49
  - mixed metabolic and respiratory acidosis P84
  - neonatal abstinence syndrome P96.1
  - noxious substances transmitted via placenta or breast milk P04.9
    - cannabis P04.81
    - specified NEC P04.89
  - nutritional supplements P04.5
  - placenta previa P02.0
  - placental
    - abnormality (functional) (morphological) P02.20
      - specified NEC P02.29
    - dysfunction P02.29
    - infarction P02.29
    - insufficiency P02.29
    - separation NEC P02.1
    - transfusion syndromes P02.3
  - placentitis P02.78
  - precipitate delivery P03.5
  - prolapsed cord P02.4
  - respiratory arrest P28.81
  - slow intrauterine growth P05.9
  - tobacco P04.2
  - twin to twin transplacental transfusion P02.3
  - umbilical cord (tightly) around neck P02.5
  - umbilical cord condition P02.60
    - short cord P02.69
    - specified NEC P02.69
  - uterine contractions (abnormal) P03.6
  - vasa previa P02.69
    - from intrauterine blood loss P50.0

Newborn *(Continued)*
- apnea P28.4
  - obstructive P28.4
  - primary P28.3
  - sleep (central) (obstructive) (primary) P28.3
- born in hospital Z38.00
  - by cesarean Z38.01
- born outside hospital Z38.1
- breast buds P96.89
- breast engorgement P83.4
- check-up —*see* Newborn, examination
- convulsion P90
- dehydration P74.1
- examination
  - 8 to 28 days old Z00.111
  - under 8 days old Z00.110
- fever P81.9
  - environmentally-induced P81.0
- hyperbilirubinemia P59.9
  - of prematurity P59.0
- hypernatremia P74.21
- hyponatremia P74.22
- infection P39.9
  - candidal P37.5
  - specified NEC P39.8
  - urinary tract P39.3
- jaundice P59.9
  - due to
    - breast milk inhibitor P59.3
    - hepatocellular damage P59.20
      - specified NEC P59.29
    - preterm delivery P59.0
  - of prematurity P59.0
  - specified NEC P59.8
- late metabolic acidosis P74.0
- mastitis P39.0
  - infective P39.0
  - noninfective P83.4
- multiple born NEC Z38.8
  - born in hospital Z38.68
    - by cesarean Z38.69
  - born outside hospital Z38.7
- omphalitis P38.9
  - with mild hemorrhage P38.1
  - without hemorrhage P38.9
- post-term P08.21
- prolonged gestation (over 42 completed weeks) P08.22
- quadruplet Z38.8
  - born in hospital Z38.63
    - by cesarean Z38.64
  - born outside hospital Z38.7
- quintuplet Z38.8
  - born in hospital Z38.65
    - by cesarean Z38.66
  - born outside hospital Z38.7
- seizure P90
- sepsis (congenital) P36.9
  - due to
    - anaerobes NEC P36.5
    - Escherichia coli P36.4
    - Staphylococcus P36.30
      - aureus P36.2
      - specified NEC P36.39
    - Streptococcus P36.10
      - group B P36.0
      - specified NEC P36.19
  - specified NEC P36.8
- triplet Z38.8
  - born in hospital Z38.61
    - by cesarean Z38.62
  - born outside hospital Z38.7
- twin Z38.5
  - born in hospital Z38.30
    - by cesarean Z38.31
  - born outside hospital Z38.4
- vomiting P92.09
  - bilious P92.01
- weight check Z00.111

Newcastle conjunctivitis or disease B30.8
Nezelof's syndrome (pure alymphocytosis) D81.4

Niacin (amide) deficiency E52
Nicolas (-Durand)-Favre disease A55
Nicotine —*see* Tobacco
Nicotinic acid deficiency E52
Niemann-Pick disease or syndrome E75.249
- specified NEC E75.248
- type
  - A E75.240
  - ▶ A/B E75.244
  - B E75.241
  - C E75.242
  - D E75.243

Night
- blindness —*see* Blindness, night
- sweats R61
- terrors (child) F51.4
Nightmares (REM sleep type) F51.5
NIHSS (National Institutes of Health Stroke Scale) score R29.7-●
Nipple —*see* condition
Nisbet's chancre A57
Nishimoto (-Takeuchi) disease I67.5
Nitritoid crisis or reaction —*see* Crisis, nitritoid
Nitrosohemoglobinemia D74.8
Njovera A65
▶ No general equivalence degree (GED) Z55.5
Nocardiosis, nocardiasis A43.9
- cutaneous A43.1
- lung A43.0
- pneumonia A43.0
- pulmonary A43.0
- specified site NEC A43.8
Nocturia R35.1
- psychogenic F45.8
Nocturnal —*see* condition
Nodal rhythm I49.8
Node(s) —*see also* Nodule
- Bouchard's (with arthropathy) M15.2
- Haygarth's M15.8
- Heberden's (with arthropathy) M15.1
- larynx J38.7
- lymph —*see* condition
- milker's B08.03
- Osler's I33.0
- Schmorl's —*see* Schmorl's disease
- singer's J38.2
- teacher's J38.2
- tuberculous —*see* Tuberculosis, lymph gland
- vocal cord J38.2
Nodule(s), nodular
- actinomycotic —*see* Actinomycosis
- breast NEC —*see also* Lump, breast N63.0
- colloid (cystic), thyroid E04.1
- cutaneous —*see* Swelling, localized
- endometrial (stromal) D26.1
- Haygarth's M15.8
- inflammatory —*see* Inflammation
- juxta-articular
  - syphilitic A52.77
  - yaws A66.7
- larynx J38.7
- lung, solitary (subsegmental branch of the bronchial tree) R91.1
  - multiple R91.8
- milker's B08.03
- prostate N40.2
  - with lower urinary tract symptoms (LUTS) N40.3
  - without lower urinary tract symptoms (LUTS) N40.2
- pulmonary, solitary (subsegmental branch of the bronchial tree) R91.1
- retrocardiac R09.89
- rheumatoid M06.30
  - ankle M06.37-●
  - elbow M06.32-●
  - foot joint M06.37-●
  - hand joint M06.34-●

Nodule(s), nodular *(Continued)*
  rheumatoid *(Continued)*
    hip M06.35-●
    knee M06.36-●
    multiple site M06.39
    shoulder M06.31-●
    vertebra M06.38
    wrist M06.33-●
  scrotum (inflammatory) N49.2
  singer's J38.2
  solitary, lung (subsegmental branch of the
    bronchial tree) R91.1
    multiple R91.8
  subcutaneous —*see* Swelling, localized
  teacher's J38.2
  thyroid (cold) (gland) (nontoxic) E04.1
    with thyrotoxicosis E05.20
      with thyroid storm E05.21
    toxic or with hyperthyroidism E05.20
      with thyroid storm E05.21
  vocal cord J38.2
Noma (gangrenous) (hospital) (infective)
  A69.0
  auricle I96
  mouth A69.0
  pudendi N76.89
  vulvae N76.89
Nomad, nomadism Z59.00
NOMID (neonatal onset multisystemic
  inflammatory disorder) M04.2
Nonadherence to medical treatment Z91.19
Nonautoimmune hemolytic anemia D59.4
  drug-induced D59.2
Nonclosure —*see also* Imperfect, closure
  ductus arteriosus (Botallo's) Q25.0
  foramen
    botalli Q21.1
    ovale Q21.1
Noncompliance Z91.19
  with
    dialysis Z91.15
    dietary regimen Z91.11
    medical treatment Z91.19
    medication regimen NEC Z91.14
      underdosing —*see also* Table of Drugs
        and Chemicals, categories T36-T50,
        with final character 6 Z91.14
        intentional NEC Z91.128
          due to financial hardship of patient
            Z91.120
        unintentional NEC Z91.138
          due to patient's age related debility
            Z91.130
    renal dialysis Z91.15
Nondescent (congenital) —*see also* Malposition,
  congenital
  cecum Q43.3
  colon Q43.3

Nondescent *(Continued)*
  testicle Q53.9
    bilateral Q53.20
      abdominal Q53.211
      perineal Q53.22
    unilateral Q53.10
      abdominal Q53.111
      perineal Q53.12
Nondevelopment
  brain Q02
    part of Q04.3
  heart Q24.8
  organ or site, congenital NEC —*see*
    Hypoplasia
Nonengagement
  head NEC O32.4
    in labor, causing obstructed labor
      O64.8
Nonexanthematous tick fever A93.2
Nonexpansion, lung (newborn) P28.0
Nonfunctioning
  cystic duct —*see also* Disease, gallbladder
    K82.8
  gallbladder —*see also* Disease, gallbladder
    K82.8
  kidney N28.9
  labyrinth —*see* subcategory H83.2
Non-Hodgkin lymphoma NEC —*see*
  Lymphoma, non-Hodgkin
Nonimplantation, ovum N97.2
Noninsufflation, fallopian tube N97.1
Non-ketotic hyperglycinemia E72.51
Nonne-Milroy syndrome Q82.0
Nonovulation N97.0
Non-palpable testicle(s)
  bilateral R39.84
  unilateral R39.83
Nonpatent fallopian tube N97.1
Nonpneumatization, lung NEC P28.0
Nonrotation —*see* Malrotation
Nonsecretion, urine —*see* Anuria
Nonunion
  fracture —*see* Fracture, by site
  joint, following fusion or arthrodesis
    M96.0
  organ or site, congenital NEC —*see*
    Imperfect, closure
  symphysis pubis, congenital Q74.2
Nonvisualization, gallbladder R93.2
Nonvital, nonvitalized tooth K04.99
Non-working side interference
  M26.56
Noonan's syndrome Q87.19
Normocytic anemia (infectional) due to
  blood loss (chronic) D50.0
  acute D62
Norrie's disease (congenital) Q15.8
North American blastomycosis B40.9

Norwegian itch B86
Nose, nasal —*see* condition
Nosebleed R04.0
Nose-picking F98.8
Nosomania F45.21
Nosophobia F45.22
Nostalgia F43.20
Notch of iris Q13.2
Notching nose, congenital (tip)
  Q30.2
Nothnagel's
  syndrome —*see* Strabismus, paralytic, third
    nerve
  vasomotor acroparesthesia I73.89
Novy's relapsing fever A68.9
  louse-borne A68.0
  tick-borne A68.1
Noxious
  foodstuffs, poisoning by —*see* Poisoning,
    food, noxious, plant
  substances transmitted through placenta or
    breast milk P04.9
Nucleus pulposus —*see* condition
Numbness R20.0
Nuns' knee —*see* Bursitis, prepatellar
Nursemaid's elbow S53.03-●
Nutcracker esophagus K22.4
Nutmeg liver K76.1
Nutrient element deficiency E61.9
  specified NEC E61.8
Nutrition deficient or insufficient —*see also*
  Malnutrition E46
  due to
    insufficient food T73.0
    lack of
      care (child) T76.02
        adult T76.01
      food T73.0
Nutritional stunting E45
Nyctalopia (night blindness) —*see* Blindness,
  night
Nycturia R35.1
  psychogenic F45.8
Nymphomania F52.8
Nystagmus H55.00
  benign paroxysmal —*see* Vertigo, benign
    paroxysmal
  central positional H81.4
  congenital H55.01
  dissociated H55.04
  latent H55.02
  miners' H55.09
  positional
    benign paroxysmal H81.4
    central H81.4
  specified form NEC H55.09
  visual deprivation H55.03

O

Obermeyer's relapsing fever (European) A68.0
Obesity E66.9
  with alveolar hypoventilation E66.2
  adrenal E27.8
  complicating
    childbirth O99.214
    pregnancy O99.21-•
    puerperium O99.215
  constitutional E66.8
  dietary counseling and surveillance Z71.3
  drug-induced E66.1
  due to
    drug E66.1
    excess calories E66.09
      morbid E66.01
      severe E66.01
  endocrine E66.8
  endogenous E66.8
  exogenous E66.09
  familial E66.8
  glandular E66.8
  hypothyroid —see Hypothyroidism
  hypoventilation syndrome (OHS) E66.2
  morbid E66.01
    with
      alveolar hypoventilation E66.2
      obesity hypoventilation syndrome (OHS) E66.2
    due to excess calories E66.01
  nutritional E66.09
  pituitary E23.6
  severe E66.01
  specified type NEC E66.8
Oblique —see condition
Obliteration
  appendix (lumen) K38.8
  artery I77.1
  bile duct (noncalculous) K83.1
  common duct (noncalculous) K83.1
  cystic duct —see Obstruction, gallbladder
  disease, arteriolar I77.1
  endometrium N85.8
  eye, anterior chamber —see Disorder, globe, hypotony
  fallopian tube N97.1
  lymphatic vessel I89.0
    due to mastectomy I97.2
  organ or site, congenital NEC —see Atresia, by site
  ureter N13.5
    with infection N13.6
  urethra —see Stricture, urethra
  vein I87.8
  vestibule (oral) K08.89
Observation (following) (for) (without need for further medical care) Z04.9
  accident NEC Z04.3
    at work Z04.2
    transport Z04.1
  adverse effect of drug Z03.6
  alleged rape or sexual assault (victim), ruled out
    adult Z04.41
    child Z04.42
  criminal assault Z04.89
  development state
    adolescent Z00.3
    period of rapid growth in childhood Z00.2
    puberty Z00.3
  disease, specified NEC Z03.89
  following work accident Z04.2
  forced sexual exploitation Z04.81
  forced labor exploitation Z04.82
  growth and development state —see Observation, development state
  injuries (accidental) NEC —see also Observation, accident

Observation (Continued)
  newborn (for)
    suspected condition, related to exposure from the mother or birth process —see Newborn, affected by, maternal
    ruled out Z05.9
      cardiac Z05.0
      connective tissue Z05.73
      gastrointestinal Z05.5
      genetic Z05.41
      genitourinary Z05.6
      immunologic Z05.43
      infectious Z05.1
      metabolic Z05.42
      musculoskeletal Z05.72
      neurological Z05.2
      respiratory Z05.3
      skin and subcutaneous tissue Z05.71
      specified condition NEC Z05.8
  postpartum
    immediately after delivery Z39.0
    routine follow-up Z39.2
  pregnancy (normal) (without complication) Z34.9-•
    high risk O09.9-•
  suicide attempt, alleged NEC Z03.89
    self-poisoning Z03.6
  suspected, ruled out —see also Suspected condition, ruled out
    abuse, physical
      adult Z04.71
      child Z04.72
    accident at work Z04.2
    adult battering victim Z04.71
    child battering victim Z04.72
    condition NEC Z03.89
      newborn —see also Observation, newborn (for), suspected condition, ruled out Z05.9
    drug poisoning or adverse effect Z03.6
    exposure (to)
      anthrax Z03.810
      biological agent NEC Z03.818
      foreign body
        aspirated (inhaled) Z03.822
        ingested Z03.821
        inserted (injected), in (eye) (orifice) (skin) Z03.823
      inflicted injury NEC Z04.89
      suicide attempt, alleged Z03.89
        self-poisoning Z03.6
      toxic effects from ingested substance (drug) (poison) Z03.6
    toxic effects from ingested substance (drug) (poison) Z03.6
Obsession, obsessional state F42.8
  mixed thoughts and acts F42.2
Obsessive-compulsive neurosis or reaction F42.8
Obstetric embolism, septic —see Embolism, obstetric, septic
Obstetric trauma (complicating delivery) O71.9
  with or following ectopic or molar pregnancy O08.6
  specified type NEC O71.89
Obstipation —see Constipation
Obstruction, obstructed, obstructive
  airway J98.8
    with
      allergic alveolitis J67.9
      asthma J45.909
        with
          exacerbation (acute) J45.901
          status asthmaticus J45.902
      bronchiectasis J47.9
        with
          exacerbation (acute) J47.1
          lower respiratory infection J47.0
      bronchitis (chronic) J44.9
      emphysema J43.9

Obstruction, obstructed, obstructive (Continued)
  airway (Continued)
    chronic J44.9
      with
        allergic alveolitis —see Pneumonitis, hypersensitivity
        bronchiectasis J47.9
          with
            exacerbation (acute) J47.1
            lower respiratory infection J47.0
      due to
        foreign body —see Foreign body, by site, causing asphyxia
        inhalation of fumes or vapors J68.9
        laryngospasm J38.5
  ampulla of Vater K83.1
  aortic (heart) (valve) —see Stenosis, aortic
  aortoiliac I74.09
  aqueduct of Sylvius G91.1
    congenital Q03.0
      with spina bifida —see Spina bifida, by site, with hydrocephalus
  Arnold-Chiari —see Arnold-Chiari disease
  artery (see also Atherosclerosis, artery) I70.9
    basilar (complete) (partial) —see Occlusion, artery, basilar
    carotid (complete) (partial) —see Occlusion, artery, carotid
    cerebellar —see Occlusion, artery, cerebellar
    cerebral (anterior) (middle) (posterior) —see Occlusion, artery, cerebral
    precerebral —see Occlusion, artery, precerebral
    renal N28.0
    retinal NEC —see Occlusion, artery, retina
    stent —see Restenosis, stent
    vertebral (complete) (partial) —see Occlusion, artery, vertebral
  band (intestinal) —see also Obstruction, intestine, specified NEC K56.699
  bile duct or passage (common) (hepatic) (noncalculous) K83.1
    with calculus K80.51
    congenital (causing jaundice) Q44.3
  biliary (duct) (tract) K83.1
    gallbladder K82.0
  bladder-neck (acquired) N32.0
    congenital Q64.31
    due to hyperplasia (hypertrophy) of prostate —see Hyperplasia, prostate
  bowel —see Obstruction, intestine
  bronchus J98.09
  canal, ear —see Stenosis, external ear canal
  cardia K22.2
  caval veins (inferior) (superior) I87.1
  cecum —see Obstruction, intestine
  circulatory I99.8
  colon —see Obstruction, intestine
  common duct (noncalculous) K83.1
  coronary (artery) —see Occlusion, coronary
  cystic duct —see also Obstruction, gallbladder
    with calculus K80.21
  device, implant or graft —see also Complications, by site and type, mechanical T85.698
    arterial graft NEC —see Complication, cardiovascular device, mechanical, vascular
    catheter NEC T85.628
      cystostomy T83.090
      dialysis (renal) T82.49
        intraperitoneal T85.691
      Hopkins T83.098
      ileostomy T83.098
      infusion NEC T82.594
        spinal (epidural) (subdural) T85.690
      nephrostomy T83.092
      urethral indwelling T83.091
      urinary T83.098
      urostomy T83.098

Obstruction, obstructed, obstructive
(Continued)
  device, implant or graft (Continued)
    due to infection T85.79
    gastrointestinal —see Complications,
      prosthetic device, mechanical,
      gastrointestinal device
    genital NEC T83.498
      intrauterine contraceptive device T83.39
      penile prosthesis (cylinder) (implanted)
        (pump) (resevoir) T83.490
      testicular prosthesis T83.491
    heart NEC —see Complication,
      cardiovascular device, mechanical
    joint prosthesis —see Complications, joint
      prosthesis, mechanical, specified NEC,
      by site
    orthopedic NEC —see Complication,
      orthopedic, device, mechanical
    specified NEC T85.628
    urinary NEC —see also Complication,
      genitourinary, device, urinary,
      mechanical
      graft T83.29
    vascular NEC —see Complication,
      cardiovascular device, mechanical
    ventricular intracranial shunt T85.09
  due to foreign body accidentally left in
    operative wound T81.529
  duodenum K31.5
  ejaculatory duct N50.89
  esophagus K22.2
  eustachian tube (complete) (partial) H68.10-●
    cartilagenous (extrinsic) H68.13-●
      intrinsic H68.12-●
      osseous H68.11-●
  fallopian tube (bilateral) N97.1
  fecal K56.41
    with hernia —see Hernia, by site, with
      obstruction
  foramen of Monro (congenital) Q03.8
    with spina bifida —see Spina bifida,
      by site, with hydrocephalus
  foreign body —see Foreign body
  gallbladder K82.0
    with calculus, stones K80.21
    congenital Q44.1
  gastric outlet K31.1
  gastrointestinal —see Obstruction, intestine
  hepatic K76.89
    duct (noncalculous) K83.1
  hepatobiliary K83.1
  ileum —see Obstruction, intestine
  iliofemoral (artery) I74.5
  intestine K56.609
    complete K56.601
    incomplete K56.600
    partial K56.600
    with
      adhesions (intestinal) (peritoneal) K56.50
        complete K56.52
        incomplete K56.51
        partial K56.51
    adynamic K56.0
    by gallstone K56.3
    congenital (small) Q41.9
      large Q42.9
        specified part NEC Q42.8
    neurogenic K56.0
      Hirschsprung's disease or megacolon
        Q43.1
    newborn P76.9
      due to
        fecaliths P76.8
        inspissated milk P76.2
        meconium (plug) P76.0
          in mucoviscidosis E84.11
      specified NEC P76.8
    postoperative K91.30
      complete K91.32
      incomplete K91.31
      partial K91.31

Obstruction, obstructed, obstructive
(Continued)
  intestine (Continued)
    reflex K56.0
    specified NEC K56.699
      complete K56.691
      incomplete K56.690
      partial K56.690
    volvulus K56.2
  intracardiac ball valve prosthesis T82.09
  jejunum —see Obstruction, intestine
  joint prosthesis —see Complications, joint
    prosthesis, mechanical, specified NEC,
    by site
⇒ kidney (calices) (see also Hydronephrosis)
    N28.89
  labor —see Delivery
  lacrimal (passages) (duct)
    by
      dacryolith —see Dacryolith
      stenosis —see Stenosis, lacrimal
    congenital Q10.5
    neonatal H04.53-●
  lacrimonasal duct —see Obstruction, lacrimal
  lacteal, with steatorrhea K90.2
  laryngitis —see Laryngitis
  larynx NEC J38.6
    congenital Q31.8
  lung J98.4
    disease, chronic J44.9
  lymphatic I89.0
  meconium (plug)
    newborn P76.0
      due to fecaliths P76.0
      in mucoviscidosis E84.11
  mitral —see Stenosis, mitral
  nasal J34.89
  nasolacrimal duct —see also Obstruction,
    lacrimal
    congenital Q10.5
  nasopharynx J39.2
  nose J34.89
  organ or site, congenital NEC —see Atresia,
    by site
  pancreatic duct K86.89
  parotid duct or gland K11.8
  pelviureteral junction N13.5
    with hydronephrosis N13.0
    congenital Q62.39
  pharynx J39.2
  portal (circulation) (vein) I81
  prostate —see also Hyperplasia, prostate
    valve (urinary) N32.0
  pulmonary valve (heart) I37.0
  pyelonephritis (chronic) N11.1
  pylorus
    adult K31.1
    congenital or infantile Q40.0
  rectosigmoid —see Obstruction, intestine
  rectum K62.4
⇒ renal (see also Hydronephrosis) N28.89
    outflow N13.8
    pelvis, congenital Q62.39
  respiratory J98.8
    chronic J44.9
  retinal (vessels) H34.9
  salivary duct (any) K11.8
    with calculus K11.5
  sigmoid —see Obstruction, intestine
  sinus (accessory) (nasal) J34.89
  Stensen's duct K11.8
  stomach NEC K31.89
    acute K31.0
    congenital Q40.2
    due to pylorospasm K31.3
  submandibular duct K11.8
  submaxillary gland K11.8
    with calculus K11.5
  thoracic duct I89.0
  thrombotic —see Thrombosis
  trachea J39.8

Obstruction, obstructed, obstructive
(Continued)
  tracheostomy airway J95.03
  tricuspid (valve) —see Stenosis, tricuspid
  upper respiratory, congenital Q34.8
  ureter (functional) (pelvic junction) NEC N13.5
    with
      hydronephrosis N13.1
        with infection N13.6
      ▶ congenital Q62.39
      pyelonephritis (chronic) N11.1
    congenital Q62.39
    due to calculus —see Calculus, ureter
  urethra NEC N36.8
    congenital Q64.39
  urinary (moderate) N13.9
    due to hyperplasia (hypertrophy) of
      prostate —see Hyperplasia, prostate
    organ or tract (lower) N13.9
    prostatic valve N32.0
    specified NEC N13.8
  uropathy N13.9
  uterus N85.8
  vagina N89.5
  valvular —see Endocarditis
  vein, venous I87.1
    caval (inferior) (superior) I87.1
    thrombotic —see Thrombosis
  vena cava (inferior) (superior) I87.1
  vesical NEC N32.0
  vesicourethral orifice N32.0
    congenital Q64.31
  vessel NEC I99.8
    stent —see Restenosis, stent
Obturator —see condition
Occlusal wear, teeth K03.0
Occlusio pupillae —see Membrane, pupillary
Occlusion, occluded
  anus K62.4
    congenital Q42.3
      with fistula Q42.2
  aortoiliac (chronic) I74.09
  aqueduct of Sylvius G91.1
    congenital Q03.0
      with spina bifida —see Spina bifida, by
        site, with hydrocephalus
  artery —see also Atherosclerosis, artery I70.9
    auditory, internal I65.8
    basilar I65.1
      with
        infarction I63.22
          due to
            embolism I63.12
            thrombosis I63.02
    brain or cerebral I66.9
      with infarction (due to) I63.5-●
        embolism I63.4-●
        thrombosis I63.3-●
    carotid I65.2-●
      with
        infarction I63.23-●
          due to
            embolism I63.13-●
            thrombosis I63.03-●
    cerebellar (anterior inferior) (posterior
      inferior) (superior) I66.3
      with infarction I63.54-●
        due to
          embolism I63.44-●
          thrombosis I63.34-●
    cerebral I66.9
      with infarction I63.50
        due to
          embolism I63.40
            specified NEC I63.49
          thrombosis I63.30
            specified NEC I63.39
      anterior I66.1-●
        with infarction I63.52-●
          due to
            embolism I63.42-●
            thrombosis I63.32-●

Occlusion, occluded *(Continued)*
  artery *(Continued)*
    cerebral *(Continued)*
      middle I66.0-•
        with infarction I63.51-•
          due to
            embolism I63.41-•
            thrombosis I63.31-•
      posterior I66.2-•
        with infarction I63.53-•
          due to
            embolism I63.43-•
            thrombosis I63.33-•
      specified NEC I66.8
        with infarction I63.59
          due to
            embolism I63.4-•
            thrombosis I63.3-•
    choroidal (anterior) —*see* Occlusion,
      artery, cerebral, specified NEC
    communicating posterior —*see* Occlusion,
      artery, precerebral, specified NEC
    complete
      coronary I25.82
      extremities I70.92
    coronary (acute) (thrombotic) (without
      myocardial infarction) I24.0
      with myocardial infarction —*see*
        Infarction, myocardium
      chronic total I25.82
      complete I25.82
      healed or old I25.2
      total (chronic) I25.82
    hypophyseal —*see* Occlusion, artery,
      precerebral, specified NEC
    iliac I74.5
    lower extremities due to stenosis or
      stricture I77.1
    mesenteric (embolic) (thrombotic) —*see also*
      Infarct, intestine K55.069
    perforating —*see* Occlusion, artery,
      cerebral, specified NEC
    peripheral I77.9
      thrombotic or embolic I74.4
    pontine —*see* Occlusion, artery, precerebral,
      specified NEC
    precerebral I65.9
      with infarction I63.20
        due to
          embolism I63.10
            specified NEC I63.19
          thrombosis I63.00
            specified NEC I63.09
        specified NEC I63.29
      basilar —*see* Occlusion, artery, basilar
      carotid —*see* Occlusion, artery, carotid
      puerperal O88.23
      specified NEC I65.8
        with infarction I63.29
          due to
            embolism I63.19
            thrombosis I63.09
      vertebral —*see* Occlusion, artery,
        vertebral
    renal N28.0
    retinal
      branch H34.23-•
      central H34.1-•
      partial H34.21-•
      transient H34.0-•
    spinal —*see* Occlusion, artery, precerebral,
      vertebral
    total (chronic)
      coronary I25.82
      extremities I70.92
    vertebral I65.0-•
      with
        infarction I63.21-•
          due to
            embolism I63.11-•
            thrombosis I63.01-•

Occlusion, occluded *(Continued)*
  basilar artery —*see* Occlusion, artery, basilar
  bile duct (common) (hepatic) (noncalculous)
    K83.1
  bowel —*see* Obstruction, intestine
  carotid (artery) (common) (internal) —*see*
    Occlusion, artery, carotid
  centric (of teeth) M26.59
    maximum intercuspation discrepancy
      M26.55
  cerebellar (artery) —*see* Occlusion, artery,
    cerebellar
  cerebral (artery) —*see* Occlusion, artery,
    cerebral
  cerebrovascular —*see also* Occlusion, artery,
    cerebral
    with infarction I63.5-•
  cervical canal —*see* Stricture, cervix
  cervix (uteri) —*see* Stricture, cervix
  choanal Q30.0
  choroidal (artery) —*see* Occlusion, artery,
    precerebral, specified NEC
  colon —*see* Obstruction, intestine
  communicating posterior artery —*see*
    Occlusion, artery, precerebral, specified
    NEC
  coronary (artery) (vein) (thrombotic) —*see*
    also Infarct, myocardium
    chronic total I25.82
    healed or old I25.2
    not resulting in infarction I24.0
    total (chronic) I25.82
  cystic duct —*see* Obstruction, gallbladder
  embolic —*see* Embolism
  fallopian tube N97.1
    congenital Q50.6
  gallbladder —*see also* Obstruction,
    gallbladder
    congenital (causing jaundice) Q44.1
  gingiva, traumatic K06.2
  hymen N89.6
    congenital Q52.3
  hypophyseal (artery) —*see* Occlusion, artery,
    precerebral, specified NEC
  iliac artery I74.5
  intestine —*see* Obstruction, intestine
  lacrimal passages —*see* Obstruction, lacrimal
  lung J98.4
  lymph or lymphatic channel I89.0
  mammary duct N64.89
  mesenteric artery (embolic) (thrombotic) —
    see also Infarct, intestine K55.069
  nose J34.89
    congenital Q30.0
  organ or site, congenital NEC —*see* Atresia,
    by site
  oviduct N97.1
    congenital Q50.6
  peripheral arteries
    due to stricture or stenosis I77.1
    upper extremity I74.2
  pontine (artery) —*see* Occlusion, artery,
    precerebral, specified NEC
  posterior lingual, of mandibular teeth M26.29
  precerebral artery —*see* Occlusion, artery,
    precerebral
  punctum lacrimale —*see* Obstruction,
    lacrimal
  pupil —*see* Membrane, pupillary
  pylorus, adult —*see also* Stricture, pylorus
    K31.1
  renal artery N28.0
  retina, retinal
    artery —*see* Occlusion, artery, retinal
    vein (central) H34.81-•
      engorgement H34.82-•
      tributary H34.83-•
      vessels H34.9
  spinal artery —*see* Occlusion, artery,
    precerebral, vertebral
  teeth (mandibular) (posterior lingual) M26.29

Occlusion, occluded *(Continued)*
  thoracic duct I89.0
  thrombotic —*see* Thrombosis, artery
  traumatic
    edentulous (alveolar) ridge K06.2
    gingiva K06.2
    periodontal K05.5
  tubal N97.1
  ureter (complete) (partial) N13.5
    congenital Q62.10
  ureteropelvic junction N13.5
    congenital Q62.11
  ureterovesical orifice N13.5
    congenital Q62.12
  urethra —*see* Stricture, urethra
  uterus N85.8
  vagina N89.5
  vascular NEC I99.8
  vein —*see* Thrombosis
    retinal —*see* Occlusion, retinal, vein
  vena cava (inferior) (superior) —*see*
    Embolism, vena cava
  ventricle (brain) NEC G91.1
  vertebral (artery) —*see* Occlusion, artery,
    vertebral
  vessel (blood) I99.8
  vulva N90.5
Occult
  blood in feces (stools) R19.5
Occupational
  problems NEC Z56.89
Ochlophobia —*see* Agoraphobia
Ochronosis (endogenous) E70.29
Ocular muscle —*see* condition
Oculogyric crisis or disturbance H51.8
  psychogenic F45.8
Oculomotor syndrome H51.9
Oculopathy
  syphilitic NEC A52.71
    congenital
      early A50.01
      late A50.30
    early (secondary) A51.43
    late A52.71
Oddi's sphincter spasm K83.4
Odontalgia K08.89
Odontoameloblastoma —*see* Cyst, calcifying
  odontogenic
Odontoclasia K03.89
Odontodysplasia, regional K00.4
Odontogenesis imperfecta K00.5
Odontoma (ameloblastic) (complex)
  (compound) (fibroameloblastic) —*see* Cyst,
  calcifying odontogenic
Odontomyelitis (closed) (open) K04.01
  irreversible K04.02
  reversible K04.01
Odontorrhagia K08.89
Odontosarcoma, ameloblastic C41.1
  upper jaw (bone) C41.0
Oestriasis —*see* Myiasis
Oguchi's disease H53.63
Ohara's disease —*see* Tularemia
OHS (obesity hypoventilation syndrome) E66.2

Oidiomycosis —*see* Candidiasis
Oidium albicans infection —*see* Candidiasis
Old (previous) **myocardial infarction**
  I25.2
Old age (without mention of debility) R54-•
  dementia F03
Olfactory —*see* condition
Oligemia —*see* Anemia
Oligoastrocytoma
  specified site —*see* Neoplasm, malignant,
    by site
  unspecified site C71.9
Oligocythemia D64.9
Oligodendroblastoma
  specified site —*see* Neoplasm, malignant
  unspecified site C71.9

Oligodendroglioma
  anaplastic type
    specified site —see Neoplasm, malignant,
      by site
    unspecified site C71.9
  specified site —see Neoplasm, malignant,
    by site
  unspecified site C71.9
Oligodontia —see Anodontia
Oligoencephalon Q02
Oligohidrosis L74.4
Oligohydramnios O41.0-•
Oligohydrosis L74.4
Oligomenorrhea N91.5
  primary N91.3
  secondary N91.4
Oligophrenia —see also Disability, intellectual
  phenylpyruvic E70.0
Oligospermia N46.11
  due to
    drug therapy N46.121
    efferent duct obstruction N46.123
    infection N46.122
    radiation N46.124
    specified cause NEC N46.129
    systemic disease N46.125
Oligotrichia —see Alopecia
Oliguria R34
  with, complicating or following ectopic or
    molar pregnancy O08.4
  postprocedural N99.0
Ollier's disease Q78.4
Omenotocele —see Hernia, abdomen, specified
  site NEC
Omentitis —see Peritonitis
Omentum, omental —see condition
Omphalitis (congenital) (newborn) P38.9
  with mild hemorrhage P38.1
  without hemorrhage P38.9
  not of newborn L08.82
  tetanus A33
Omphalocele Q79.2
Omphalomesenteric duct, persistent Q43.0
Omphalorrhagia, newborn P51.9
Omsk hemorrhagic fever A98.1
Onanism (excessive) F98.8
Onchocerciasis, onchocercosis B73.1
  with
    eye disease B73.00
      endophthalmitis B73.01
      eyelid B73.09
      glaucoma B73.02
      specified NEC B73.09
  eye NEC B73.00
  eyelid B73.09
Oncocytoma —see Neoplasm, benign, by site
Oncovirus, as cause of disease classified
  elsewhere B97.32
Ondine's curse —see Apnea, sleep
Oneirophrenia F23
Onychauxis L60.2
  congenital Q84.5
Onychia —see also Cellulitis, digit
  with lymphangitis —see Lymphangitis, acute,
    digit
  candidal B37.2
  dermatophytic B35.1
Onychitis —see also Cellulitis, digit
  with lymphangitis —see Lymphangitis, acute,
    digit
Onychocryptosis L60.0
Onychodystrophy L60.3
  congenital Q84.6
Onychogryphosis, onychogryposis L60.2
Onycholysis L60.1
Onychomadesis L60.8
Onychomalacia L60.3
Onychomycosis (finger) (toe) B35.1
Onycho-osteodysplasia Q87.2
Onychophagia F98.8
Onychophosis L60.8

Onychoptosis L60.8
Onychorrhexis L60.3
  congenital Q84.6
Onychoschizia L60.3
Onyxis (finger) (toe) L60.0
Onyxitis —see also Cellulitis, digit
  with lymphangitis —see Lymphangitis, acute,
    digit
Oophoritis (cystic) (infectional) (interstitial)
  N70.92
  with salpingitis N70.93
  acute N70.02
    with salpingitis N70.03
  chronic N70.12
    with salpingitis N70.13
  complicating abortion —see Abortion, by
    type, complicated by, oophoritis
Oophorocele N83.4-•
Opacity, opacities
  cornea H17.-•
    central H17.1-•
    congenital Q13.3
    degenerative —see Degeneration, cornea
    hereditary —see Dystrophy, cornea
    inflammatory —see Keratitis
    minor H17.81-•
    peripheral H17.82-•
    sequelae of trachoma (healed) B94.0
    specified NEC H17.89
  enamel (teeth) (fluoride) (nonfluoride) K00.3
  lens —see Cataract
  snowball —see Deposit, crystalline
  vitreous (humor) NEC H43.39-•
    congenital Q14.0
    membranes and strands H43.31-•
Opalescent dentin (hereditary) K00.5
Open, opening
  abnormal, organ or site, congenital —see
    Imperfect, closure
  angle with
    borderline
      findings
        high risk H40.02-•
        low risk H40.01-•
      intraocular pressure H40.00-•
    cupping of discs H40.01-•
    glaucoma (primary) —see Glaucoma, open
      angle
  bite
    anterior M26.220
    posterior M26.221
  false —see Imperfect, closure
  margin on tooth restoration K08.51
  restoration margins of tooth K08.51
  wound —see Wound, open
Operational fatigue F48.8
Operative —see condition
Operculitis —see Periodontitis
Operculum —see Break, retina
Ophiasis L63.2
Ophthalmia —see also Conjunctivitis H10.9
  actinic rays —see Photokeratitis
  allergic (acute) —see Conjunctivitis, acute,
    atopic
  blennorrhagic (gonococcal) (neonatorum)
    A54.31
  diphtheritic A36.86
  Egyptian A71.1
  electrica —see Photokeratitis
  gonococcal (neonatorum) A54.31
  metastatic —see Endophthalmitis, purulent
  migraine —see Migraine, ophthalmoplegic
  neonatorum, newborn P39.1
    gonococcal A54.31
  nodosa H16.24-•
  purulent —see Conjunctivitis, acute,
    mucopurulent
  spring —see Conjunctivitis, acute, atopic
  sympathetic —see Uveitis, sympathetic
Ophthalmitis —see Ophthalmia
Ophthalmocele (congenital) Q15.8

Ophthalmoneuromyelitis G36.0
Ophthalmoplegia —see also Strabismus, paralytic
  anterior internuclear —see Ophthalmoplegia,
    internuclear
  ataxia-areflexia G61.0
  diabetic —see E08-E13 with .39
  exophthalmic E05.00
    with thyroid storm E05.01
  external H49.88-•
    progressive H49.4-•
      with pigmentary retinopathy —see
        Kearns-Sayre syndrome
    total H49.3-•
  internal (complete) (total) H52.51-•
  internuclear H51.2-•
  migraine —see Migraine, ophthalmoplegic
  Parinaud's H49.88-•
  progressive external —see Ophthalmoplegia,
    external, progressive
  supranuclear, progressive G23.1
  total (external) —see Ophthalmoplegia,
    external, total
Opioid(s)
  abuse —see Abuse, drug, opioids
  dependence —see Dependence, drug, opioids
  induced, without use disorder
    anxiety disorder F11.988
    delirium F11.921
    depressive disorder F11.94
    sexual dysfunction F11.981
    sleep disorder F11.982
Opisthognathism M26.09
Opisthorchiasis (felineus) (viverrini) B66.0
Opitz' disease D73.2
Opiumism —see Dependence, drug, opioid
Oppenheim's disease G70.2
Oppenheim-Urbach disease (necrobiosis
  lipoidica diabeticorum) —see E08-E13 with
  .620
Optic nerve —see condition
Orbit —see condition
Orchioblastoma C62.9-•
Orchitis (gangrenous) (nonspecific) (septic)
  (suppurative) N45.2
  blennorrhagic (gonococcal) (acute) (chronic)
    A54.23
  chlamydial A56.19
  filarial —see also Infestation, filarial B74.9
    [N51]
  gonococcal (acute) (chronic) A54.23
  mumps B26.0
  syphilitic A52.76
  tuberculous A18.15
Orf (virus disease) B08.02
Organic —see also condition
  brain syndrome F09
  heart —see Disease, heart
  mental disorder F09
  psychosis F09
Orgasm
  anejaculatory N53.13
Oriental
  bilharziasis B65.2
  schistosomiasis B65.2
Orifice —see condition
Origin of both great vessels from right
  ventricle Q20.1
Ormond's disease (with ureteral obstruction)
  N13.5
  with infection N13.6
Ornithine metabolism disorder E72.4
Ornithinemia (Type I) (Type II) E72.4
Ornithosis A70
Orotaciduria, oroticaciduria (congenital)
  (hereditary) (pyrimidine deficiency) E79.8
  anemia D53.0
Orthodontics
  adjustment Z46.4
  fitting Z46.4
Orthopnea R06.01
Orthopoxvirus B08.09

Os, uterus —see condition
Osgood-Schlatter disease or osteochondrosis
   M92.52-•
Osler (-Weber)-Rendu disease I78.0
Osler's nodes I33.0
Osmidrosis L75.0
Osseous —see condition
Ossification
  artery —see Arteriosclerosis
  auricle (ear) —see Disorder, pinna, specified
    type NEC
  bronchial J98.09
  cardiac —see Degeneration, myocardial
  cartilage (senile) —see Disorder, cartilage,
    specified type NEC
  coronary (artery) —see Disease, heart,
    ischemic, atherosclerotic
  diaphragm J98.6
  ear, middle —see Otosclerosis
  falx cerebri G96.198
  fontanel, premature Q75.0
  heart —see also Degeneration, myocardial
    valve —see Endocarditis
  larynx J38.7
  ligament —see Disorder, tendon, specified
    type NEC
    posterior longitudinal —see
      Spondylopathy, specified NEC
  meninges (cerebral) (spinal) G96.198
  multiple, eccentric centers —see Disorder,
    bone, development or growth
  muscle —see also Calcification, muscle
    due to burns —see Myositis, ossificans, in,
      burns
    paralytic —see Myositis, ossificans, in,
      quadriplegia
    progressive —see Myositis, ossificans,
      progressiva
    specified NEC M61.50
      ankle M61.57-•
      foot M61.57-•
      forearm M61.53-•
      hand M61.54-•
      lower leg M61.56-•
      multiple sites M61.59
      pelvic region M61.55-•
      shoulder region M61.51-•
      specified site NEC M61.58
      thigh M61.55-•
      upper arm M61.52-•
    traumatic —see Myositis, ossificans,
      traumatica
  myocardium, myocardial —see Degeneration,
    myocardial
  penis N48.89
  periarticular —see Disorder, joint, specified
    type NEC
  pinna —see Disorder, pinna, specified type
    NEC
  rider's bone —see Ossification, muscle,
    specified NEC
  sclera H15.89
  subperiosteal, post-traumatic M89.8X-•
  tendon —see Disorder, tendon, specified
    type NEC
  trachea J39.8
  tympanic membrane —see Disorder, tympanic
    membrane, specified NEC
  vitreous (humor) —see Deposit, crystalline
Osteitis —see also Osteomyelitis
  alveolar M27.3
  condensans M85.30
    ankle M85.37-•
    foot M85.37-•
    forearm M85.33-•
    hand M85.34-•
    lower leg M85.36-•
    multiple site M85.39
    neck M85.38
    rib M85.38
    shoulder M85.31-•

Osteitis (Continued)
  condensans (Continued)
    skull M85.38
    specified site NEC M85.38
    thigh M85.35-•
    toe M85.37-•
    upper arm M85.32-•
    vertebra M85.38
  deformans M88.9
    in (due to)
      malignant neoplasm of bone
        C41.9 [M90.60]
      neoplastic disease —see also Neoplasm
        D49.9 [M90.60]
        carpus D49.9 [M90.64-•]
        clavicle D49.9 [M90.61-•]
        femur D49.9 [M90.65-•]
        fibula D49.9 [M90.66-•]
        finger D49.9 [M90.64-•]
        humerus D49.9 [M90.62-•]
        ilium D49.9 [M90.65-•]
        ischium D49.9 [M90.65-•]
        metacarpus D49.9 [M90.64-•]
        metatarsus D49.9 [M90.67-•]
        multiple sites D49.9 [M90.69]
        neck D49.9 [M90.68]
        radius D49.9 [M90.63-•]
        rib D49.9 [M90.68]
        scapula D49.9 [M90.61-•]
        skull D49.9 [M90.68]
        tarsus D49.9 [M90.67-•]
        tibia D49.9 [M90.66-•]
        toe D49.9 [M90.67-•]
        ulna D49.9 [M90.63-•]
        vertebra D49.9 [M90.68]
    skull M88.0
    specified NEC —see Paget's disease, bone,
      by site
    vertebra M88.1
  due to yaws A66.6
  fibrosa NEC —see Cyst, bone, by site
    circumscripta —see Dysplasia, fibrous,
      bone NEC
    cystica (generalisata) E21.0
    disseminata Q78.1
    osteoplastica E21.0
  fragilitans Q78.0
  Garr's (sclerosing) —see Osteomyelitis,
    specified type NEC
  jaw (acute) (chronic) (lower) (suppurative)
    (upper) M27.2
  parathyroid E21.0
  petrous bone (acute) (chronic) —see Petrositis
  sclerotic, nonsuppurative —see Osteomyelitis,
    specified type NEC
  tuberculosa A18.09
    cystica D86.89
    multiplex cystoides D86.89
Osteoarthritis M19.90
  ankle M19.07-•
  elbow M19.02-•
  foot joint M19.07-•
➠generalized (multiple joints) M15.9
    erosive M15.4
    primary M15.0
    specified NEC M15.8
  hand joint M19.04-•
    first carpometacarpal joint M18.9-•
  hip M16.1-•
    bilateral M16.0
    due to hip dysplasia (unilateral) M16.3-•
      bilateral M16.2
  interphalangeal
    distal (Heberden) M15.1
    proximal (Bouchard) M15.2
  knee M17.1-•
    bilateral M17.0
  post-traumatic NEC M19.92
    ankle M19.17-•
    elbow M19.12-•
    foot joint M19.17-•

Osteoarthritis (Continued)
  post-traumatic NEC (Continued)
    hand joint M19.14-•
      first carpometacarpal joint M18.3-•
        bilateral M18.2
    hip M16.5-•
      bilateral M16.4
    knee M17.3-•
      bilateral M17.2
    shoulder M19.11-•
    specified site NEC M19.19
    wrist M19.13-•
  primary M19.91
    ankle M19.07-•
    elbow M19.02-•
    foot joint M19.07-•
    hand joint M19.04-•
      first carpometacarpal joint M18.1-•
        bilateral M18.0
    hip M16.1-•
      bilateral M16.0
    knee M17.1-•
      bilateral M17.0
➠ multiple sites M15.9
    shoulder M19.01-•
    spine —see Spondylosis
    wrist M19.03-•
  secondary M19.93
    ankle M19.27-•
    elbow M19.22-•
    foot joint M19.27-•
    hand joint M19.24-•
      first carpometacarpal joint M18.5-•
        bilateral M18.4
    hip M16.7
      bilateral M16.6
    knee M17.5
      bilateral M17.4
    multiple M15.3
    shoulder M19.21-•
    specified site NEC M19.29
    spine —see Spondylosis
    wrist M19.23-•
  shoulder M19.01-•
  specified site NEC M19.09
  spine —see Spondylosis
  wrist M19.03-•
Osteoarthropathy (hypertrophic) M19.90
  ankle —see Osteoarthritis, primary, ankle
  elbow —see Osteoarthritis, primary, elbow
  foot joint —see Osteoarthritis, primary, foot
  hand joint —see Osteoarthritis, primary, hand
    joint
  knee joint —see Osteoarthritis, primary, knee
  multiple site —see Osteoarthritis, primary,
    multiple joint
  pulmonary —see also Osteoarthropathy,
    specified type NEC
    hypertrophic —see Osteoarthropathy,
      hypertrophic, specified type NEC
  secondary —see Osteoarthropathy, specified
    type NEC
  secondary hypertrophic —see
    Osteoarthropathy, specified type NEC
  shoulder —see Osteoarthritis, primary, shoulder
  specified joint NEC —see Osteoarthritis,
    primary, specified joint NEC
  specified type NEC M89.40
    carpus M89.44-•
    clavicle M89.41-•
    femur M89.45-•
    fibula M89.46-•
    finger M89.44-•
    humerus M89.42-•
    ilium M89.459
    ischium M89.459
    metacarpus M89.44-•
    metatarsus M89.47-•
    multiple sites M89.49
    neck M89.48
    radius M89.43-•

Osteoarthropathy (Continued)
  specified type NEC (Continued)
    rib M89.48
    scapula M89.41-●
    skull M89.48
    tarsus M89.47-●
    tibia M89.46-●
    toe M89.47-●
    ulna M89.43-●
    vertebra M89.48
  spine —see Spondylosis
  wrist —see Osteoarthritis, primary, wrist
Osteoarthrosis (degenerative) (hypertrophic)
    (joint) —see also Osteoarthritis
  deformans alkaptonurica E70.29 [M36.8]
  erosive M15.4
  generalized M15.9
    primary M15.0
  polyarticular M15.9
  spine —see Spondylosis
Osteoblastoma —see Neoplasm, bone, benign
  aggressive —see Neoplasm, bone, uncertain
    behavior
Osteochondroarthrosis deformans
    endemica —see Disease, Kaschin-Beck
Osteochondritis —see also Osteochondropathy,
    by site
  Brailsford's —see Osteochondrosis, juvenile,
    radius
  dissecans M93.20
    ankle M93.27-●
    elbow M93.22-●
    foot M93.27-●
    hand M93.24-●
    hip M93.25-●
    knee M93.26-●
    multiple sites M93.29
    shoulder joint M93.21-●
    specified site NEC M93.28
    wrist M93.23-●
  juvenile M92.9
    patellar —see Osteochondrosis, juvenile,
      patella
  syphilitic (congenital) (early) A50.02
      [M90.80]
    ankle A50.02 [M90.87-●]
    elbow A50.02 [M90.82-●]
    foot A50.02 [M90.87-●]
    forearm A50.02 [M90.83-●]
    hand A50.02 [M90.84-●]
    hip A50.02 [M90.85-●]
    knee A50.02 [M90.86-●]
    multiple sites A50.02 [M90.89]
    shoulder joint A50.02 [M90.81-●]
    specified site NEC A50.02 [M90.88]
Osteochondrodysplasia Q78.9
  with defects of growth of tubular bones and
    spine Q77.9
    specified NEC Q77.8
  specified NEC Q78.8
Osteochondrodystrophy E78.9
Osteochondrolysis —see Osteochondritis,
    dissecans
Osteochondroma —see Neoplasm, bone, benign
Osteochondromatosis D48.0
  syndrome Q78.4
Osteochondromyxosarcoma —see Neoplasm,
    bone, malignant
Osteochondropathy M93.90
  ankle M93.97-●
  elbow M93.92-●
  foot M93.97-●
  hand M93.94-●
  hip M93.95-●
  Kienböck's disease of adults M93.1
  knee M93.96-●
  multiple joints M93.99
  osteochondritis dissecans —see
    Osteochondritis, dissecans
  osteochondrosis —see Osteochondrosis
  shoulder region M93.91-●

Osteochondropathy (Continued)
  slipped upper femoral epiphysis —see
    Slipped, epiphysis, upper femoral
  specified joint NEC M93.98
  specified type NEC M93.80
    ankle M93.87-●
    elbow M93.82-●
    foot M93.87-●
    hand M93.84-●
    hip M93.85-●
    knee M93.86-●
    multiple joints M93.89
    shoulder region M93.81-●
    specified joint NEC M93.88
    wrist M93.83-●
  syphilitic, congenital
    early A50.02 [M90.80]
    late A50.56 [M90.80]
  wrist M93.93-●
Osteochondrosarcoma —see Neoplasm, bone,
    malignant
Osteochondrosis —see also Osteochondropathy,
    by site
  acetabulum (juvenile) M91.0
  adult —see Osteochondropathy, specified
    type NEC, by site
  astragalus (juvenile) —see Osteochondrosis,
    juvenile, tarsus
  Blount's —see Osteochondrosis, juvenile, tibia
  Blount M92.51-●
  Buchanan's M91.0
  Burns' —see Osteochondrosis, juvenile, ulna
  calcaneus (juvenile) —see Osteochondrosis,
    juvenile, tarsus
  capitular epiphysis (femur) (juvenile) —see
    Legg-Calvé-Perthes disease
  carpal (juvenile) (lunate) (scaphoid) —see
    Osteochondrosis, juvenile, hand, carpal
    lunate
    adult M93.1
  coxae juvenilis —see Legg-Calvé-Perthes
    disease
  deformans juvenilis, coxae —see Legg-Calvé-
    Perthes disease
  Diaz's —see Osteochondrosis, juvenile, tarsus
  dissecans (knee) (shoulder) —see
    Osteochondrosis, dissecans
  femoral capital epiphysis (juvenile) —see
    Legg-Calvé-Perthes disease
  femur (head), juvenile —see Legg-Calvé-
    Perthes disease
  fibula (juvenile) —see Osteochondrosis,
    juvenile, fibula
  foot NEC (juvenile) M92.8
  Freiberg's —see Osteochondrosis, juvenile,
    metatarsus
  Haas' (juvenile) —see Osteochondrosis,
    juvenile, humerus
  Haglund's —see Osteochondrosis, juvenile,
    tarsus
  hip (juvenile) —see Legg-Calvé-Perthes disease
  humerus (capitulum) (head) (juvenile) —see
    Osteochondrosis, juvenile, humerus
  ilium, iliac crest (juvenile) M91.0
  ischiopubic synchondrosis M91.0
  Iselin's —see Osteochondrosis, juvenile,
    metatarsus
  juvenile, juvenilis M92.9
    after congenital dislocation of hip
      reduction —see Osteochondrosis,
      juvenile, hip, specified NEC
    arm —see Osteochondrosis, juvenile, upper
      limb NEC
    capitular epiphysis (femur) —see Legg-
      Calvé-Perthes disease
    clavicle, sternal epiphysis —see
      Osteochondrosis, juvenile, upper limb
      NEC
    coxae —see Legg-Calvé-Perthes disease
    deformans M92.9
    fibula M92.50-●

Osteochondrosis (Continued)
  juvenile, juvenilis (Continued)
    foot NEC M92.8
    hand M92.20-●
      carpal lunate M92.21-●
      metacarpal head M92.22-●
      specified site NEC M92.29-●
    head of femur —see Legg-Calvé-Perthes
      disease
    hip and pelvis M91.9-●
      coxa plana —see Coxa, plana
      femoral head —see Legg-Calvé-Perthes
        disease
      pelvis M91.0
      pseudocoxalgia —see Pseudocoxalgia
      specified NEC M91.8-●
    humerus M92.0-●
    limb
      lower NEC M92.8
      upper NEC —see Osteochondrosis,
        juvenile, upper limb NEC
    medial cuneiform bone —see
      Osteochondrosis, juvenile, tarsus
    metatarsus M92.7-●
    patella M92.4-●
    radius M92.1-●
    specified
      site NEC M92.8
      type NEC M92.8
      tibia and fibula M92.59-●
    specified site NEC M92.8
    spine M42.00
      cervical region M42.02
      cervicothoracic region M42.03
      lumbar region M42.06
      lumbosacral region M42.07
      multiple sites M42.09
      occipito-atlanto-axial region
        M42.01
      sacrococcygeal region M42.08
      thoracic region M42.04
      thoracolumbar region M42.05
    tarsus M92.6-●
    tibia M92.50-●
      proximal M92.51-●
      tubercle M92.52-●
    ulna M92.1-●
    upper limb NEC M92.3-●
    vertebra (body) (epiphyseal plates)
      (Calvé's) (Scheuermann's) —see
      Osteochondrosis, juvenile, spine
  Kienböck's —see Osteochondrosis, juvenile,
    hand, carpal lunate
    adult M93.1
  Köhler's
    patellar —see Osteochondrosis, juvenile,
      patella
    tarsal navicular —see Osteochondrosis,
      juvenile, tarsus
  Legg-Perthes (-Calvé's) (-Waldenström) —see
    Legg-Calvé-Perthes disease
  limb
    lower NEC (juvenile) M92.8
      tibia and fibula M92.59-●
    upper NEC (juvenile) —see
      Osteochondrosis, juvenile, upper limb
      NEC
  lunate bone (carpal) (juvenile) —see also
    Osteochondrosis, juvenile, hand, carpal
    lunate
    adult M93.1
  Mauclaire's —see Osteochondrosis, juvenile,
    hand, metacarpal
  metacarpal (head) (juvenile) —see
    Osteochondrosis, juvenile, hand,
    metacarpal
  metatarsus (fifth) (head) (juvenile)
    (second) —see Osteochondrosis, juvenile,
    metatarsus
  navicular (juvenile) —see Osteochondrosis,
    juvenile, tarsus

▶ New ⇒ Revised ~~deleted~~ Deleted ● Use Additional Character(s)

Osteochondrosis (Continued)

os

calcis (juvenile) —see Osteochondrosis,
juvenile, tarsus

tibiale externum (juvenile) —see
Osteochondrosis, juvenile, tarsus

Osgood-Schlatter M92.52-●

Panner's —see Osteochondrosis, juvenile,
humerus

patellar center (juvenile) (primary)
(secondary) —see Osteochondrosis,
juvenile, patella

pelvis (juvenile) M91.0

Pierson's M91.0

radius (head) (juvenile) —see
Osteochondrosis, juvenile, radius

Scheuermann's —see Osteochondrosis,
juvenile, spine

Sever's —see Osteochondrosis, juvenile, tarsus

Sinding-Larsen —see Osteochondrosis,
juvenile, patella

spine M42.9

adult M42.10

cervical region M42.12

cervicothoracic region M42.13

lumbar region M42.16

lumbosacral region M42.17

multiple sites M42.19

occipito-atlanto-axial region M42.11

sacrococcygeal region M42.18

thoracic region M42.14

thoracolumbar region M42.15

juvenile —see Osteochondrosis, juvenile,
spine

symphysis pubis (juvenile) M91.0

syphilitic (congenital) A50.02

talus (juvenile) —see Osteochondrosis,
juvenile, tarsus

tarsus (navicular) (juvenile) —see
Osteochondrosis, juvenile, tarsus

tibia (proximal) (tubercle) (juvenile) —see
Osteochondrosis, juvenile, tibia

tuberculous —see Tuberculosis, bone

ulna (lower) (juvenile) —see Osteochondrosis,
juvenile, ulna

van Neck's M91.0

vertebral —see Osteochondrosis, spine

Osteoclastoma D48.0

malignant —see Neoplasm, bone, malignant

Osteodynia —see Disorder, bone, specified type
NEC

Osteodystrophy Q78.9

azotemic N25.0

congenital Q78.9

parathyroid, secondary E21.1

renal N25.0

Osteofibroma —see Neoplasm, bone, benign

Osteofibrosarcoma —see Neoplasm, bone,
malignant

Osteogenesis imperfecta Q78.0

Osteogenic —see condition

Osteolysis M89.50

carpus M89.54-●

clavicle M89.51-●

femur M89.55-●

fibula M89.56-●

finger M89.54-●

humerus M89.52-●

ilium M89.559

ischium M89.559

joint prosthesis (periprosthetic) —see
Complications, joint prosthesis,
mechanical, periprosthetic, osteolysis,
by site

metacarpus M89.54-●

metatarsus M89.57-●

multiple sites M89.59

neck M89.58

periprosthetic —see Complications, joint
prosthesis, mechanical, periprosthetic,
osteolysis, by site

Osteolysis (Continued)

radius M89.53-●

rib M89.58

scapula M89.51-●

skull M89.58

tarsus M89.57-●

tibia M89.56-●

toe M89.57-●

ulna M89.53-●

vertebra M89.58

Osteoma —see also Neoplasm, bone, benign

osteoid —see also Neoplasm, bone, benign

giant —see Neoplasm, bone, benign

Osteomalacia M83.9

adult M83.9

drug-induced NEC M83.5

due to

malabsorption (postsurgical) M83.2

malnutrition M83.3

specified NEC M83.8

aluminium-induced M83.4

infantile —see Rickets

juvenile —see Rickets

oncogenic E83.89

pelvis M83.8

puerperal M83.0

senile M83.1

vitamin-D-resistant in adults E83.31 [M90.8-●]

carpus E83.31 [M90.84-●]

clavicle E83.31 [M90.81-●]

femur E83.31 [M90.85-●]

fibula E83.31 [M90.86-●]

finger E83.31 [M90.84-●]

humerus E83.31 [M90.82-●]

ilium E83.31 [M90.859]

ischium E83.31 [M90.859]

metacarpus E83.31 [M90.84-●]

metatarsus E83.31 [M90.87-●]

multiple sites E83.31 [M90.89]

neck E83.31 [M90.88]

radius E83.31 [M90.83-●]

rib E83.31 [M90.88]

scapula E83.31 [M90.819]

skull E83.31 [M90.88]

tarsus E83.31 [M90.879]

tibia E83.31 [M90.869]

toe E83.31 [M90.879]

ulna E83.31 [M90.839]

vertebra E83.31 [M90.88]

Osteomyelitis (general) (infective)
(localized) (neonatal) (purulent)
(septic) (staphylococcal) (streptococcal)
(suppurative) (with periostitis) M86.9

acute M86.10

carpus M86.14-●

clavicle M86.11-●

femur M86.15-●

fibula M86.16-●

finger M86.14-●

hematogenous M86.00

carpus M86.04-●

clavicle M86.01-●

femur M86.05-●

fibula M86.06-●

finger M86.04-●

humerus M86.02-●

➠ ilium M86.08

➠ ischium M86.08

mandible M27.2

metacarpus M86.04-●

metatarsus M86.07-●

multiple sites M86.09

neck M86.08

orbit H05.02-●

petrous bone —see Petrositis

radius M86.03-●

rib M86.08

scapula M86.01-●

skull M86.08

tarsus M86.07-●

tibia M86.06-●

Osteomyelitis (Continued)

acute (Continued)

hematogenous (Continued)

toe M86.07-●

ulna M86.03-●

vertebra —see Osteomyelitis, vertebra

humerus M86.12-●

ilium M86.18

ischium M86.18

mandible M27.2

metacarpus M86.14-●

metatarsus M86.17-●

multiple sites M86.19

neck M86.18

orbit H05.02-●

petrous bone —see Petrositis

radius M86.13-●

rib M86.18

scapula M86.11-●

skull M86.18

tarsus M86.17-●

tibia M86.16-●

toe M86.17-●

ulna M86.13-●

vertebra —see Osteomyelitis, vertebra

chronic (or old) M86.60

with draining sinus M86.40

carpus M86.44-●

clavicle M86.41-●

femur M86.45-●

fibula M86.46-●

finger M86.44-●

humerus M86.42-●

ilium M86.459

ischium M86.459

mandible M27.2

metacarpus M86.44-●

metatarsus M86.47-●

multiple sites M86.49

neck M86.48

orbit H05.02-●

petrous bone —see Petrositis

radius M86.43-●

rib M86.48

scapula M86.41-●

skull M86.48

tarsus M86.47-●

tibia M86.46-●

toe M86.47-●

ulna M86.43-●

vertebra —see Osteomyelitis, vertebra

carpus M86.64-●

clavicle M86.61-●

femur M86.65-●

fibula M86.66-●

finger M86.64-●

hematogenous NEC M86.50

carpus M86.54-●

clavicle M86.51-●

femur M86.55-●

fibula M86.56-●

finger M86.54-●

humerus M86.52-●

ilium M86.559

ischium M86.559

mandible M27.2

metacarpus M86.54-●

metatarsus M86.57-●

multifocal M86.30

carpus M86.34-●

clavicle M86.31-●

femur M86.35-●

fibula M86.36-●

finger M86.34-●

humerus M86.32-●

ilium M86.359

ischium M86.359

metacarpus M86.34-●

metatarsus M86.37-●

multiple sites M86.39

neck M86.38

Osteomyelitis (Continued)
  chronic (Continued)
    hematogenous NEC (Continued)
      multifocal (Continued)
        radius M86.33-●
        rib M86.38
        scapula M86.31-●
        skull M86.38
        tarsus M86.37-●
        tibia M86.36-●
        toe M86.37-●
        ulna M86.33-●
        vertebra —see Osteomyelitis, vertebra
      multiple sites M86.59
      neck M86.58
      orbit H05.02-●
      petrous bone —see Petrositis
      radius M86.53-●
      rib M86.58
      scapula M86.51-●
      skull M86.58
      tarsus M86.57-●
      tibia M86.56-●
      toe M86.57-●
      ulna M86.53-●
      vertebra —see Osteomyelitis, vertebra
    humerus M86.62-●
    ilium M86.659
    ischium M86.659
    mandible M27.2
    metacarpus M86.64-●
    metatarsus M86.67-●
    multifocal —see Osteomyelitis, chronic,
      hematogenous, multifocal
    multiple sites M86.69
    neck M86.68
    orbit H05.02-●
    petrous bone —see Petrositis
    radius M86.63-●
    rib M86.68
    scapula M86.61-●
    skull M86.68
    tarsus M86.67-●
    tibia M86.66-●
    toe M86.67-●
    ulna M86.63-●
    vertebra —see Osteomyelitis, vertebra
  echinococcal B67.2
  Garré's —see Osteomyelitis, specified type NEC
  in diabetes mellitus —see E08-E13 with .69
  jaw (acute) (chronic) (lower) (neonatal)
    (suppurative) (upper) M27.2
  nonsuppurating —see Osteomyelitis,
    specified type NEC
  orbit H05.02-●
  petrous bone —see Petrositis
  Salmonella (arizonae) (cholerae-suis)
    (enteritidis) (typhimurium) A02.24
  sclerosing, nonsuppurative —see
    Osteomyelitis, specified type NEC
  specified type NEC —see also subcategory
    M86.8X-●
    mandible M27.2
    orbit H05.02-●
    petrous bone —see Petrositis
    vertebra —see Osteomyelitis, vertebra
  subacute M86.20
    carpus M86.24-●
    clavicle M86.21-●
    femur M86.25-●
    fibula M86.26-●
    finger M86.24-●
    humerus M86.22-●
    mandible M27.2
    metacarpus M86.24-●
    metatarsus M86.27-●
    multiple sites M86.29
    neck M86.28
    orbit H05.02-●
    petrous bone —see Petrositis
    radius M86.23-●

Osteomyelitis (Continued)
  subacute (Continued)
    rib M86.28
    scapula M86.21-●
    skull M86.28
    tarsus M86.27-●
    tibia M86.26-●
    toe M86.27-●
    ulna M86.23-●
    vertebra —see Osteomyelitis, vertebra
  syphilitic A52.77
    congenital (early) A50.02 [M90.80]
  tuberculous —see Tuberculosis, bone
  typhoid A01.05
  vertebra M46.20
    cervical region M46.22
    cervicothoracic region M46.23
    lumbar region M46.26
    lumbosacral region M46.27
    occipito-atlanto-axial region M46.21
    sacrococcygeal region M46.28
    thoracic region M46.24
    thoracolumbar region M46.25
Osteomyelofibrosis D47.4
Osteomyelosclerosis D75.89
Osteonecrosis M87.9
  due to
    drugs —see Osteonecrosis, secondary, due
      to, drugs
    trauma —see Osteonecrosis, secondary, due
      to, trauma
  idiopathic aseptic M87.00
    ankle M87.07-●
    carpus M87.03-●
    clavicle M87.01-●
    femur M87.05-●
    fibula M87.06-●
    finger M87.04-●
    humerus M87.02-●
    ilium M87.050
    ischium M87.050
    metacarpus M87.04-●
    metatarsus M87.07-●
    multiple sites M87.09
    neck M87.08
    pelvis M87.050
    radius M87.03-●
    rib M87.08
    scapula M87.01-●
    skull M87.08
    tarsus M87.07-●
    tibia M87.06-●
    toe M87.07-●
    ulna M87.03-●
    vertebra M87.08
  secondary NEC M87.30
    carpus M87.33-●
    clavicle M87.31-●
    due to
      drugs M87.10
        carpus M87.13-●
        clavicle M87.11-●
        femur M87.15-●
        fibula M87.16-●
        finger M87.14-●
        humerus M87.12-●
        ilium M87.159
        ischium M87.159
        jaw M87.180
        metacarpus M87.14-●
        metatarsus M87.17-●
        multiple sites M87.19
        neck M87.18
        radius M87.13-●
        rib M87.18
        scapula M87.11-●
        skull M87.18
        tarsus M87.17-●
        tibia M87.16-●
        toe M87.17-●
        ulna M87.13-●
        vertebra M87.18

Osteonecrosis (Continued)
  secondary NEC (Continued)
    due to (Continued)
      hemoglobinopathy NEC D58.2
        [M90.50]
        carpus D58.2 [M90.54-●]
        clavicle D58.2 [M90.51-●]
        femur D58.2 [M90.55-●]
        fibula D58.2 [M90.56-●]
        finger D58.2 [M90.54-●]
        humerus D58.2 [M90.52-●]
        ilium D58.2 [M90.55-●]
        ischium D58.2 [M90.55-●]
        metacarpus D58.2 [M90.54-●]
        metatarsus D58.2 [M90.57-●]
        multiple sites D58.2 [M90.58]
        neck D58.2 [M90.58]
        radius D58.2 [M90.53-●]
        rib D58.2 [M90.58]
        scapula D58.2 [M90.51-●]
        skull D58.2 [M90.58]
        tarsus D58.2 [M90.57-●]
        tibia D58.2 [M90.56-●]
        toe D58.2 [M90.57-●]
        ulna D58.2 [M90.53-●]
        vertebra D58.2 [M90.58]
      trauma (previous) M87.20
        carpus M87.23-●
        clavicle M87.21-●
        femur M87.25-●
        fibula M87.26-●
        finger M87.24-●
        humerus M87.22-●
        ilium M87.25-●
        ischium M87.25-●
        metacarpus M87.24-●
        metatarsus M87.27-●
        multiple sites M87.29
        neck M87.28
        radius M87.23-●
        rib M87.28
        scapula M87.21-●
        skull M87.28
        tarsus M87.27-●
        tibia M87.26-●
        toe M87.27-●
        ulna M87.23-●
        vertebra M87.28
  femur M87.35-●
  fibula M87.36-●
  finger M87.34-●
  humerus M87.32
  ilium M87.350
  in
    caisson disease T70.3 [M90.50]
      carpus T70.3 [M90.54-●]
      clavicle T70.3 [M90.51-●]
      femur T70.3 [M90.55-●]
      fibula T70.3 [M90.56-●]
      finger T70.3 [M90.54-●]
      humerus T70.3 [M90.52-●]
      ilium T70.3 [M90.55-●]
      ischium T70.3 [M90.55-●]
      metacarpus T70.3 [M90.54-●]
      metatarsus T70.3 [M90.57-●]
      multiple sites T70.3 [M90.59]
      neck T70.3 [M90.58]
      radius T70.3 [M90.53-●]
      rib T70.3 [M90.58]
      scapula T70.3 [M90.51-●]
      skull T70.3 [M90.58]
      tarsus T70.3 [M90.57-●]
      tibia T70.3 [M90.56-●]
      toe T70.3 [M90.57-●]
      ulna T70.3 [M90.53-●]
      vertebra T70.3 [M90.58]
  ischium M87.350
  metacarpus M87.34-●
  metatarsus M87.37-●
  multiple site M87.39
  neck M87.38

▶ New   ⟹ Revised   ~~deleted~~ Deleted   ● Use Additional Character(s)

Osteonecrosis *(Continued)*
  secondary NEC *(Continued)*
    radius M87.33-●
    rib M87.38
    scapula M87.319
    skull M87.38
    tarsus M87.379
    tibia M87.366
    toe M87.379
    ulna M87.33-●
    vertebra M87.38
  specified type NEC M87.80
    carpus M87.83-●
    clavicle M87.81-●
    femur M87.85-●
    fibula M87.86-●
    finger M87.84-●
    humerus M87.82-●
    ilium M87.85-●
    ischium M87.85-●
    metacarpus M87.84-●
    metatarsus M87.87-●
    multiple sites M87.89
    neck M87.88
    radius M87.83-●
    rib M87.88-●
    scapula M87.81-●
    skull M87.88
    tarsus M87.87-●
    tibia M87.86-●
    toe M87.87-●
    ulna M87.83-●
    vertebra M87.88
Osteo-onycho-arthro-dysplasia Q87.2
Osteo-onychodysplasia, hereditary Q87.2
Osteopathia condensans disseminata Q78.8
Osteopathy —*see also* Osteomyelitis,
  Osteonecrosis, Osteoporosis
  after poliomyelitis M89.60
    carpus M89.64-●
    clavicle M89.61-●
    femur M89.65-●
    fibula M89.66-●
    finger M89.64-●
    humerus M89.62-●
    ilium M89.659
    ischium M89.659
    metacarpus M89.64-●
    metatarsus M89.67-●
    multiple sites M89.69
    neck M89.68
    radius M89.63-●
    rib M89.68
    scapula M89.61-●
    skull M89.68
    tarsus M89.67-●
    tibia M89.66-●
    toe M89.67-●
    ulna M89.63-●
    vertebra M89.68
  in (due to)
    renal osteodystrophy N25.0
    specified diseases classified elsewhere —
      see subcategory M90.8
Osteopenia M85.8-●
  borderline M85.8-●
Osteoperiostitis —*see* Osteomyelitis, specified
  type NEC
Osteopetrosis (familial) Q78.2
Osteophyte M25.70
  ankle M25.77-●
  elbow M25.72-●
  foot joint M25.77-●
  hand joint M25.74-●
  hip M25.75-●
  knee M25.76-●
  shoulder M25.71-●
  spine M25.78
  vertebrae M25.78
  wrist M25.73-●
Osteopoikilosis Q78.8

Osteoporosis (female) (male) M81.0
  with current pathological fracture M80.00
  age-related M81.0
    with current pathologic fracture M80.00
      carpus M80.04-●
      clavicle M80.01-●
      fibula M80.06-●
      finger M80.04-●
      humerus M80.02-●
      ilium M80.05-●
      ischium M80.05-●
      metacarpus M80.04-●
      metatarsus M80.07-●
      pelvis M80.05-●
      radius M80.03-●
      scapula M80.01-●
      site specified NEC M80.0A
      tarsus M80.07-●
      tibia M80.06-●
      toe M80.07-●
      ulna M80.03-●
      vertebra M80.08
  disuse M81.8
    with current pathological fracture M80.80
      carpus M80.84-●
      clavicle M80.81-●
      fibula M80.86-●
      finger M80.84-●
      humerus M80.82-●
      ilium M80.85-●
      ischium M80.85-●
      metacarpus M80.84-●
      metatarsus M80.87-●
      pelvis M80.85-●
      radius M80.83-●
      scapula M80.81-●
      site specified NEC M80.8A
      tarsus M80.87-●
      tibia M80.86-●
      toe M80.87-●
      ulna M80.83-●
      vertebra M80.88
  drug-induced —*see* Osteoporosis, specified
    type NEC
  idiopathic —*see* Osteoporosis, specified type
    NEC
  involutional —*see* Osteoporosis, age-related
  Lequesne M81.6
  localized M81.6
  postmenopausal M81.0
    with pathological fracture M80.00
      carpus M80.04-●
      clavicle M80.01-●
      fibula M80.06-●
      finger M80.04-●
      humerus M80.02-●
      ilium M80.05-●
      ischium M80.05-●
      metacarpus M80.04-●
      metatarsus M80.07-●
      pelvis M80.05-●
      radius M80.03-●
      scapula M80.01-●
      site specified NEC M80.0A
      tarsus M80.07-●
      tibia M80.06-●
      toe M80.07-●
      ulna M80.03-●
      vertebra M80.08
  postoophorectomy —*see* Osteoporosis,
    specified type NEC
  postsurgical malabsorption —*see*
    Osteoporosis, specified type NEC
  post-traumatic —*see* Osteoporosis, specified
    type NEC
  senile —*see* Osteoporosis, age-related
  specified type NEC M81.8
    with pathological fracture M80.80
      carpus M80.84-●
      clavicle M80.81-●
      fibula M80.86-●

Osteoporosis *(Continued)*
  specified type NEC *(Continued)*
    with pathological fracture *(Continued)*
      finger M80.84-●
      humerus M80.82-●
      ilium M80.85-●
      ischium M80.85-●
      metacarpus M80.84-●
      metatarsus M80.87-●
      pelvis M80.85-●
      radius M80.83-●
      scapula M80.81-●
      site specified NEC M80.8A
      tarsus M80.87-●
      tibia M80.86-●
      toe M80.87-●
      ulna M80.83-●
      vertebra M80.88
Osteopsathyrosis (idiopathica) Q78.0
Osteoradionecrosis, jaw (acute) (chronic)
  (lower) (suppurative) (upper) M27.2
Osteosarcoma (any form) —*see* Neoplasm,
  bone, malignant
Osteosclerosis Q78.2
  acquired M85.8-●
  congenita Q77.4
  fragilitas (generalisata) Q78.2
  myelofibrosis D75.81
Osteosclerotic anemia D64.89
Osteosis
  cutis L94.2
  renal fibrocystic N25.0
Österreicher-Turner syndrome Q87.2
Ostium
  atrioventriculare commune Q21.2
  primum (arteriosum) (defect) (persistent) Q21.2
  secundum (arteriosum) (defect) (patent)
    (persistent) Q21.1
Ostrum-Furst syndrome Q75.8
Otalgia —*see* subcategory H92.0
Otitis (acute) H66.90
  with effusion —*see also* Otitis, media,
    nonsuppurative
    purulent —*see* Otitis, media, suppurative
  adhesive —*see* subcategory H74.1
  chronic —*see also* Otitis, media, chronic
    with effusion —*see also* Otitis, media,
      nonsuppurative, chronic
  externa H60.9-●
    abscess —*see* Abscess, ear, external
    acute (noninfective) H60.50-●
      actinic H60.51-●
      chemical H60.52-●
      contact H60.53-●
      eczematoid H60.54-●
      infective —*see* Otitis, externa, infective
      reactive H60.55-●
      specified NEC H60.59-●
    cellulitis —*see* Cellulitis, ear
    chronic H60.6-●
    diffuse —*see* Otitis, externa, infective, diffuse
    hemorrhagic —*see* Otitis, externa, infective,
      hemorrhagic
    in (due to)
      aspergillosis B44.89
      candidiasis B37.84
      erysipelas A46 [H62.40]
      herpes (simplex) virus infection B00.1
        zoster B02.8
      impetigo L01.00 [H62.40]
      infectious disease NEC B99 [H62.4-●]
      mycosis NEC B36.9 [H62.40]
      parasitic disease NEC B89 [H62.40]
      viral disease NEC B34.9 [H62.40]
      zoster B02.8
    infective NEC H60.39-●
      abscess —*see* Abscess, ear, external
      cellulitis —*see* Cellulitis, ear
      diffuse H60.31-●
      hemorrhagic H60.32-●
      swimmer's ear —*see* Swimmer's, ear

Otitis (Continued)
  externa (Continued)
    malignant H60.2-●
    mycotic NEC B36.9 [H62.40]
      in
        aspergillosis B44.89
        candidiasis B37.84
        moniliasis B37.84
    necrotizing —see Otitis, externa,
      malignant
    Pseudomonas aeruginosa —see Otitis,
      externa, malignant
    reactive —see Otitis, externa, acute,
      reactive
    specified NEC —see subcategory
      H60.8
    tropical NEC B36.9 [H62.40]
      in
        aspergillosis B44.89
        candidiasis B37.84
        moniliasis B37.84
  insidiosa —see Otosclerosis
  interna —see subcategory H83.0
  media (hemorrhagic) (staphylococcal)
    (streptococcal) H66.9-●
    with effusion (nonpurulent) —see Otitis,
      media, nonsuppurative
    acute, subacute H66.90
      allergic —see Otitis, media,
        nonsuppurative, acute, allergic
      exudative —see Otitis, media,
        suppurative, acute
      mucoid —see Otitis, media,
        nonsuppurative, acute
      necrotizing —see also Otitis, media,
        suppurative, acute
        in
          measles B05.3
          scarlet fever A38.0
      nonsuppurative NEC —see Otitis, media,
        nonsuppurative, acute
      purulent —see Otitis, media,
        suppurative, acute
      sanguinous —see Otitis, media,
        nonsuppurative, acute
      secretory —see Otitis, media,
        nonsuppurative, acute, serous
      seromucinous —see Otitis, media,
        nonsuppurative, acute
      serous —see Otitis, media,
        nonsuppurative, acute, serous
      suppurative —see Otitis, media,
        suppurative, acute
    allergic —see Otitis, media, nonsuppurative
    catarrhal —see Otitis, media,
      nonsuppurative
    chronic H66.90
      with effusion (nonpurulent) —see Otitis,
        media, nonsuppurative, chronic
      allergic —see Otitis, media,
        nonsuppurative, chronic, allergic
      benign suppurative —see Otitis, media,
        suppurative, chronic, tubotympanic
      catarrhal —see Otitis, media,
        nonsuppurative, chronic, serous
      exudative —see Otitis, media,
        suppurative, chronic
      mucinous —see Otitis, media,
        nonsuppurative, chronic, mucoid
      mucoid —see Otitis, media,
        nonsuppurative, chronic, mucoid
      nonsuppurative NEC —see Otitis, media,
        nonsuppurative, chronic
      purulent —see Otitis, media,
        suppurative, chronic
      secretory —see Otitis, media,
        nonsuppurative, chronic, mucoid
      seromucinous —see Otitis, media,
        nonsuppurative, chronic
      serous —see Otitis, media,
        nonsuppurative, chronic, serous

Otitis (Continued)
  media (Continued)
    chronic (Continued)
      suppurative —see Otitis, media,
        suppurative, chronic
      transudative —see Otitis, media,
        nonsuppurative, chronic, mucoid
    exudative —see Otitis, media,
      nonsuppurative
    in (due to) (with)
      influenza —see Influenza, with, otitis
        media
      measles B05.3
      scarlet fever A38.0
      tuberculosis A18.6
      viral disease NEC B34.-● [H67.-●]
    mucoid —see Otitis, media,
      nonsuppurative
    nonsuppurative H65.9-●
      acute or subacute NEC H65.19-●
        allergic H65.11-●
          recurrent H65.11-●
        recurrent H65.19-●
        secretory —see Otitis, media,
          nonsuppurative, serous
        serous H65.0-●
          recurrent H65.0-●
      chronic H65.49-●
        allergic H65.41-●
        mucoid H65.3-●
        serous H65.2-●
    postmeasles B05.3
    purulent —see Otitis, media, suppurative
    secretory —see Otitis, media,
      nonsuppurative
    seromucinous —see Otitis, media,
      nonsuppurative
    serous —see Otitis, media, nonsuppurative
    suppurative H66.4-●
      acute H66.00-●
        with rupture of ear drum H66.01-●
        recurrent H66.00-●
          with rupture of ear drum H66.01-●
      chronic —see also subcategory H66.3
        atticoantral H66.2-●
        benign —see Otitis, media,
          suppurative, chronic,
          tubotympanic
        tubotympanic H66.1-●
    transudative —see Otitis, media,
      nonsuppurative
    tuberculous A18.6
Otocephaly Q18.2
Otolith syndrome —see subcategory H81.8
Otomycosis (diffuse) NEC B36.9 [H62.40]
  in
    aspergillosis B44.89
    candidiasis B37.84
    moniliasis B37.84
Otoporosis —see Otosclerosis
Otorrhagia (nontraumatic) H92.2-●
  traumatic - code by Type of injury
Otorrhea H92.1-●
  cerebrospinal (fluid) G96.01
    postoperative G96.08
    specified NEC G96.08
    spontaneous G96.01
    traumatic G96.08
Otosclerosis (general) H80.9-●
  cochlear (endosteal) H80.2-●
  involving
    otic capsule —see Otosclerosis, cochlear
    oval window
      nonobliterative H80.0-●
      obliterative H80.1-●
    round window —see Otosclerosis, cochlear
  nonobliterative —see Otosclerosis, involving,
    oval window, nonobliterative
  obliterative —see Otosclerosis, involving, oval
    window, obliterative
  specified NEC H80.8-●

Otospongiosis —see Otosclerosis
Otto's disease or pelvis M24.7
Outcome of delivery Z37.9
  multiple births Z37.9
    all liveborn Z37.50
      quadruplets Z37.52
      quintuplets Z37.53
      sextuplets Z37.54
      specified number NEC Z37.59
      triplets Z37.51
    all stillborn Z37.7
    some liveborn Z37.60
      quadruplets Z37.62
      quintuplets Z37.63
      sextuplets Z37.64
      specified number NEC Z37.69
      triplets Z37.61
  single NEC Z37.9
    liveborn Z37.0
    stillborn Z37.1
  twins NEC Z37.9
    both liveborn Z37.2
    both stillborn Z37.4
    one liveborn, one stillborn Z37.3
Outlet —see condition
Ovalocytosis (congenital) (hereditary) —see
  Elliptocytosis
Ovarian —see Condition
Ovariocele N83.4-●
Ovaritis (cystic) —see Oophoritis
Ovary, ovarian —see also condition
  resistant syndrome E28.39
  vein syndrome N13.8
Overactive —see also Hyperfunction
  adrenal cortex NEC E27.0
  bladder N32.81
  hypothalamus E23.3
  thyroid —see Hyperthyroidism
Overactivity R46.3
  child —see Disorder, attention-deficit
    hyperactivity
Overbite (deep) (excessive) (horizontal)
  (vertical) M26.29
Overbreathing —see Hyperventilation
Overconscientious personality F60.5
Overdevelopment —see Hypertrophy
Overdistension —see Distension
Overdose, overdosage (drug) —see Table of
  Drugs and Chemicals, by drug, poisoning
Overeating R63.2
  nonorganic origin F50.89
  psychogenic F50.89
Overexertion (effects) (exhaustion) T73.3
Overexposure (effects) T73.9
  exhaustion T73.2
Overfeeding —see Overeating
  newborn P92.4
Overfill, endodontic M27.52
Overgrowth, bone —see Hypertrophy, bone
Overhanging of dental restorative material
  (unrepairable) K08.52
Overheated (places) (effects) —see Heat
Overjet (excessive horizontal) M26.23
Overlaid, overlying (suffocation) —see Asphyxia,
  traumatic, due to mechanical threat
Overlap, excessive horizontal (teeth) M26.23
Overl apping toe (acquired) —see also
  Deformity, toe, specified NEC
  congenital (fifth toe) Q66.89
Overload
  circulatory, due to transfusion (blood) (blood
    components) (TACO) E87.71
  fluid E87.70
    due to transfusion (blood) (blood
      components) E87.71
    specified NEC E87.79
  iron, due to repeated red blood cell
    transfusions E83.111
  potassium (K) E87.5
  sodium (Na) E87.0
Overnutrition —see Hyperalimentation

Overproduction —*see also* Hypersecretion
  ACTH E27.0
  catecholamine E27.5
  growth hormone E22.0
Overprotection, child by parent Z62.1
Overriding
  aorta Q25.49
  finger (acquired) —*see* Deformity, finger
    congenital Q68.1
  toe (acquired) —*see also* Deformity, toe,
      specified NEC
    congenital Q66.89

Overstrained R53.83
  heart —*see* Hypertrophy, cardiac
Overuse, muscle NEC
  M70.8-●
Overweight E66.3
Overworked R53.83
Oviduct —*see* condition
Ovotestis Q56.0
Ovulation (cycle)
  failure or lack of N97.0
  pain N94.0

Ovum —*see* condition
Owren's disease or syndrome (parahemophilia)
    D68.2
Ox heart —*see* Hypertrophy, cardiac
Oxalosis E72.53
Oxaluria E72.53
Oxycephaly, oxycephalic Q75.0
  syphilitic, congenital A50.02
Oxyuriasis B80
Oxyuris vermicularis (infestation) B80
Ozena J31.0

P

Pachyderma, pachydermia L85.9
  larynx (verrucosa) J38.7
Pachydermatocele (congenital) Q82.8
Pachydermoperiostosis —*see also*
    Osteoarthropathy, hypertrophic, specified
    type NEC
  clubbed nail M89.4Ø *[L62]*
Pachygyria Q04.3
Pachymeningitis (adhesive) (basal) (brain)
    (cervical) (chronic) (circumscribed)
    (external) (fibrous) (hemorrhagic)
    (hypertrophic) (internal) (purulent) (spinal)
    (suppurative) —*see* Meningitis
Pachyonychia (congenital) Q84.5
Pacinian tumor —*see* Neoplasm, skin, benign
Pad, knuckle or Garrod's M72.1
Paget-Schroetter syndrome I82.89Ø
Paget's disease
  with infiltrating duct carcinoma —*see*
    Neoplasm, breast, malignant
  bone M88.9
    carpus M88.84-●
    clavicle M88.81-●
    femur M88.85-●
    fibula M88.86-●
    finger M88.84-●
    humerus M88.82-●
    ilium M88.85-●
    in neoplastic disease —*see* Osteitis,
      deformans, in neoplastic disease
    ischium M88.85-●
    metacarpus M88.84-●
    metatarsus M88.87-●
    multiple sites M88.89
    neck M88.88
    radius M88.83-●
    rib M88.88
    scapula M88.81-●
    skull M88.Ø
    specified NEC M88.88
    tarsus M88.87-●
    tibia M88.86-●
    toe M88.87-●
    ulna M88.83-●
    vertebra M88.1
  breast (female) C5Ø.Ø1-●
    male C5Ø.Ø2-●
  extramammary —*see also* Neoplasm, skin,
    malignant
    anus C21.Ø
      margin C44.59Ø
      skin C44.59Ø
  intraductal carcinoma —*see* Neoplasm,
    breast, malignant
  malignant —*see* Neoplasm, skin, malignant
    breast (female) C5Ø.Ø1-●
      male C5Ø.Ø2-●
    unspecified site (female) C5Ø.Ø1-●
      male C5Ø.Ø2-●
  mammary —*see* Paget's disease, breast
  nipple —*see* Paget's disease, breast
  osteitis deformans —*see* Paget's disease, bone
Pain(s) —*see also* Painful R52
  abdominal R10.9
    colic R10.83
    generalized R10.84
      with acute abdomen R10.0
    lower R10.30
      left quadrant R10.32
      pelvic or perineal R10.2
      periumbilical R10.33
      right quadrant R10.31
    rebound —*see* Tenderness, abdominal,
      rebound
    severe with abdominal rigidity R10.0
    tenderness —*see* Tenderness, abdominal
    upper R10.10
      epigastric R10.13
      left quadrant R10.12
      right quadrant R10.11

Pain *(Continued)*
  acute R52
    due to trauma G89.11
    neoplasm related G89.3
    postprocedural NEC G89.18
    post-thoracotomy G89.12
    specified by site — code to Pain, by site
  adnexa (uteri) R10.2
  anginoid —*see* Pain, precordial
  anus K62.89
  arm —*see* Pain, limb, upper
  axillary (axilla) M79.62-●
  back (postural) M54.9
  bladder R39.89
    associated with micturition —*see*
      Micturition, painful
    chronic R39.82
  bone —*see* Disorder, bone, specified type NEC
  breast N64.4
  broad ligament R10.2
  cancer associated (acute) (chronic) G89.3
  cecum —*see* Pain, abdominal
  cervicobrachial M53.1
  chest (central) R07.9
    anterior wall R07.89
    atypical R07.89
    ischemic I20.9
    musculoskeletal R07.89
    non-cardiac R07.89
    on breathing R07.1
    pleurodynia R07.81
    precordial R07.2
    wall (anterior) R07.89
  chronic G89.29
    associated with significant psychosocial
      dysfunction G89.4
    due to trauma G89.21
    neoplasm related G89.3
    postoperative NEC G89.28
    postprocedural NEC G89.28
    post-thoracotomy G89.22
    specified NEC G89.29
  coccyx M53.3
  colon —*see* Pain, abdominal
  coronary —*see* Angina
  costochondral R07.1
  diaphragm R07.1
  due to cancer G89.3
  due to device, implant or graft —*see also*
    Complications, by site and type,
      specified NEC T85.848
    arterial graft NEC T82.848
    breast (implant) T85.848
    catheter NEC T85.848
      dialysis (renal) T82.848
        intraperitoneal T85.848
      infusion NEC T82.848
        spinal (epidural) (subdural) T85.840
      urinary (indwelling) T83.84
    electronic (electrode) (pulse generator)
      (stimulator)
      bone T84.84
      cardiac T82.847
      nervous system (brain) (peripheral
        nerve) (spinal) T85.840
      urinary T83.84
    fixation, internal (orthopedic) NEC T84.84
    gastrointestinal (bile duct) (esophagus)
      T85.848
    genital NEC T83.84
    heart NEC T82.847
    infusion NEC T85.848
    joint prosthesis T84.84
    ocular (corneal graft) (orbital implant)
      NEC T85.848
    orthopedic NEC T84.84
    specified NEC T85.848
    urinary NEC T83.84
    vascular NEC T82.848
    ventricular intracranial shunt T85.840
  due to malignancy (primary) (secondary) G89.3
  ear —*see* subcategory H92.0
  epigastric, epigastrium R10.13

Pain *(Continued)*
  eye —*see* Pain, ocular
  face, facial R51.9
    atypical G50.1
  female genital organs NEC N94.89
  finger —*see* Pain, limb, upper
  flank —*see* Pain, abdominal
  foot —*see* Pain, limb, lower
  gallbladder K82.9
  gas (intestinal) R14.1
  gastric —*see* Pain, abdominal
  generalized NOS R52
  genital organ
    female N94.89
    male N50.89
  groin —*see* Pain, abdominal, lower
  hand —*see* Pain, limb, upper
  head —*see* Headache
  heart —*see* Pain, precordial
  infra-orbital —*see* Neuralgia, trigeminal
  intercostal R07.82
  intermenstrual N94.0
  jaw R68.84
  joint M25.50
    ankle M25.57-●
    elbow M25.52-●
    finger M25.54-●
    foot M25.57-●
    hand M25.54-●
    hip M25.55-●
    knee M25.56-●
    shoulder M25.51-●
    specified site NEC M25.59
    toe M25.57-●
    wrist M25.53-●
  kidney N23
  laryngeal R07.0
  leg —*see* Pain, limb, lower
  limb M79.609
    lower M79.60-●
      foot M79.67-●
      lower leg M79.66-●
      thigh M79.65-●
      toe M79.67-●
    upper M79.60-●
      axilla M79.62-●
      finger M79.64-●
      forearm M79.63-●
      hand M79.64-●
      upper arm M79.62-●
  ➠loin M54.50
  ➠low back M54.50
    ▶specified NEC M54.59
    ▶vertebral end plate M54.51
    ▶vertebrogenic M54.51
  ➠lumbar region M54.50
    ▶vertebral end plate M54.51
    ▶vertebrogenic M54.51
  mandibular R68.84
  mastoid —*see* subcategory H92.0
  maxilla R68.84
  menstrual —*see also* Dysmenorrhea N94.6
  metacarpophalangeal (joint) —*see* Pain, joint,
    hand
  metatarsophalangeal (joint) —*see* Pain, joint,
    foot
  mouth K13.79
  muscle —*see* Myalgia
  musculoskeletal —*see also* Pain, by site M79.18
  myofascial M79.18
  nasal J34.89
  nasopharynx J39.2
  neck NEC M54.2
  nerve NEC —*see* Neuralgia
  neuromuscular —*see* Neuralgia
  nose J34.89
  ocular H57.1-●
  ophthalmic —*see* Pain, ocular
  orbital region —*see* Pain, ocular
  ovary N94.89
  over heart —*see* Pain, precordial
  ovulation N94.0

  ▶ New   ➠ Revised   ~~deleted~~ Deleted   ● Use Additional Character(s)

Pain *(Continued)*
  pelvic (female) R10.2
  penis N48.89
  pericardial —*see* Pain, precordial
  perineal, perineum R10.2
  pharynx J39.2
  pleura, pleural, pleuritic R07.81
  postoperative NOS G89.18
  postprocedural NOS G89.18
  post-thoracotomy G89.12
  precordial (region) R07.2
  premenstrual N94.3
  psychogenic (persistent) (any site) F45.41
  radicular (spinal) —*see* Radiculopathy
  rectum K62.89
  respiration R07.1
  retrosternal R07.2
  rheumatoid, muscular —*see* Myalgia
  rib R07.81
  root (spinal) —*see* Radiculopathy
  round ligament (stretch) R10.2
  sacroiliac M53.3
  sciatic —*see* Sciatica
  scrotum N50.82
  seminal vesicle N50.89
  shoulder M25.51-●
  spermatic cord N50.89
  spinal root —*see* Radiculopathy
  spine M54.9
    cervical M54.2
  ⮕low back M54.50
      with sciatica M54.4-●
      ▶vertebral end plate —*see* Pain,
        vertebrogenic
    thoracic M54.6
  stomach —*see* Pain, abdominal
  substernal R07.2
  temporomandibular (joint) M26.62-●
  testis N50.81-●
  thoracic spine M54.6
    with radicular and visceral pain M54.14
  throat R07.0
  tibia —*see* Pain, limb, lower
  toe —*see* Pain, limb, lower
  tongue K14.6
  tooth K08.89
  trigeminal —*see* Neuralgia, trigeminal
  tumor associated G89.3
  ureter N23
  urinary (organ) (system) N23
  uterus NEC N94.89
  vagina R10.2
  ⮕vertebrogenic M54.89
    ▶low back M54.51
    ▶lumbar M54.51
    ▶syndrome M54.89
  vesical R39.89
    associated with micturition —*see*
      Micturition, painful
  vulva R10.2
Painful —*see also* Pain
  coitus
    female N94.10
    male N53.12
      psychogenic F52.6
  ejaculation (semen) N53.12
    psychogenic F52.6
  erection —*see* Priapism
  feet syndrome E53.8
  joint replacement (hip) (knee) T84.84
  menstruation —*see* Dysmenorrhea
    psychogenic F45.8
  micturition —*see* Micturition, painful
  respiration R07.1
  scar NEC L90.5
  wire sutures T81.89
Painter's colic —*see* subcategory T56.0
Palate —*see* condition
Palatoplegia K13.79
Palatoschisis —*see* Cleft, palate
Palilalia R48.8
Palliative care Z51.5

Pallor R23.1
  optic disc, temporal —*see* Atrophy, optic
Palmar —*see also* condition
  fascia —*see* condition
Palpable
  cecum K63.89
  kidney N28.89
  ovary N83.8
  prostate N42.9
  spleen —*see* Splenomegaly
Palpitations (heart) R00.2
  psychogenic F45.8
Palsy —*see also* Paralysis G83.9
  atrophic diffuse (progressive) G12.22
  Bell's —*see also* Palsy, facial
    newborn P11.3
  brachial plexus NEC G54.0
    newborn (birth injury) P14.3
  brain —*see* Palsy, cerebral
  bulbar (progressive) (chronic) G12.22
    of childhood (Fazio-Londe) G12.1
    pseudo NEC G12.29
    supranuclear (progressive) G23.1
  cerebral (congenital) G80.9
    ataxic G80.4
    athetoid G80.3
    choreathetoid G80.3
    diplegic G80.8
      spastic G80.1
    dyskinetic G80.3
      athetoid G80.3
      choreathetoid G80.3
      distonic G80.3
    dystonic G80.3
    hemiplegic G80.8
      spastic G80.2
    mixed G80.8
    monoplegic G80.8
      spastic G80.1
    paraplegic G80.8
      spastic G80.1
    quadriplegic G80.8
      spastic G80.0
    spastic G80.1
      diplegic G80.1
      hemiplegic G80.2
      monoplegic G80.1
      quadriplegic G80.0
      specified NEC G80.1
      tetrapelgic G80.0
    specified NEC G80.8
    syphilitic A52.12
      congenital A50.49
    tetraplegic G80.8
      spastic G80.0
  cranial nerve —*see also* Disorder, nerve,
    cranial
    multiple G52.7
      in
        infectious disease B99 *[G53]*
        neoplastic disease —*see also* Neoplasm
          D49.9 *[G53]*
        parasitic disease B89 *[G53]*
        sarcoidosis D86.82
  creeping G12.22
  diver's T70.3
  Erb's P14.0
  facial G51.0
    newborn (birth injury) P11.3
  glossopharyngeal G52.1
  Klumpke (-Déjérine) P14.1
  lead —*see* subcategory T56.0
  median nerve (tardy) G56.1-●
  nerve G58.9
    specified NEC G58.8
  peroneal nerve (acute) (tardy) G57.3-●
  progressive supranuclear G23.1
  pseudobulbar NEC G12.29
  radial nerve (acute) G56.3-●
  seventh nerve —*see also* Palsy, facial
    newborn P11.3
  shaking —*see* Parkinsonism
  spastic (cerebral) (spinal) G80.1

Palsy*(Continued)*
  ulnar nerve (tardy) G56.2-●
  wasting G12.29
Paludism —*see* Malaria
Panangiitis M30.0
Panaris, panaritium —*see also* Cellulitis, digit
  with lymphangitis —*see* Lymphangitis, acute,
    digit
Panarteritis nodosa M30.0
  brain or cerebral I67.7
Pancake heart R93.1
  with cor pulmonale (chronic) I27.81
Pancarditis (acute) (chronic) I51.89
  rheumatic I09.89
    active or acute I01.8
Pancoast's syndrome or tumor C34.1-●
Pancolitis, ulcerative (chronic) K51.00
  with
    abscess K51.014
    complication K51.019
    fistula K51.013
    obstruction K51.012
    rectal bleeding K51.011
    specified complication NEC K51.018
Pancreas, pancreatic —*see* condition
Pancreatitis (annular) (apoplectic) (calcareous)
    (edematous) (hemorrhagic) (malignant)
    (subacute) (suppurative) K85.90
  with necrosis (uninfected) K85.91
    infected K85.92
  acute (without necrosis or infection)
      K85.90
    with necrosis (uninfected) K85.91
      infected K85.92
    alcohol induced (without necrosis or
        infection) K85.20
      with necrosis (uninfected) K85.21
        infected K85.22
    biliary (without necrosis or infection)
        K85.10
      with necrosis (uninfected) K85.11
        infected K85.12
    drug induced (without necrosis or
        infection) K85.30
      with necrosis (uninfected) K85.31
        infected K85.32
    gallstone (without necrosis or infection)
        K85.10
      with necrosis (uninfected) K85.11
        infected K85.12
    idiopathic (without necrosis or infection)
        K85.00
      with necrosis (uninfected) K85.01
        infected K85.02
    specified NEC (without necrosis or
        infection) K85.80
      with necrosis (uninfected) K85.81
        infected K85.82
  chronic (infectious) K86.1
    alcohol-induced K86.0
    recurrent K86.1
    relapsing K86.1
  cystic (chronic) K86.1
  cytomegaloviral B25.2
  fibrous (chronic) K86.1
  gallstone (without necrosis or infection)
      K85.10
    with necrosis (uninfected) K85.11
      infected K85.12
  gangrenous —*see* Pancreatitis, acute
  interstitial (chronic) K86.1
    acute —*see also* Pancreatitis, acute K85.80
  mumps B26.3
  recurrent
  ⮕acute —*see* Pancreatitis, acute by type
    chronic
    relapsing, chronic K86.1
  syphilitic A52.74
Pancreatoblastoma —*see* Neoplasm, pancreas,
    malignant
Pancreolithiasis K86.89
Pancytolysis D75.89

Pancytopenia (acquired) D61.818
  with
    malformations D61.09
    myelodysplastic syndrome —see
      Syndrome, myelodysplastic
    antineoplastic chemotherapy induced
      D61.810
  congenital D61.09
  drug-induced NEC D61.811
PANDAS (pediatric autoimmune
    neuropsychiatric disorders associated with
    streptococcal infections syndrome) D89.89
Panencephalitis, subacute, sclerosing
    A81.1
Panhematopenia D61.9
  congenital D61.09
  constitutional D61.09
  splenic, primary D73.1
Panhemocytopenia D61.9
  congenital D61.09
  constitutional D61.09
Panhypogonadism E29.1
Panhypopituitarism E23.0
  prepubertal E23.0
Panic (attack) (state) F41.0
  reaction to exceptional stress (transient) F43.0
Panmyelopathy, familial, constitutional D61.09
Panmyelophthisis D61.82
  congenital D61.09
Panmyelosis (acute) (with myelofibrosis)
    C94.4-●
Panner's disease —see Osteochondrosis,
    juvenile, humerus
Panneuritis endemica E51.11
Panniculitis (nodular) (nonsuppurative) M79.3
  back M54.00
    cervical region M54.02
    cervicothoracic region M54.03
    lumbar region M54.06
    lumbosacral region M54.07
    multiple sites M54.09
    occipito-atlanto-axial region M54.01
    sacrococcygeal region M54.08
    thoracic region M54.04
    thoracolumbar region M54.05
  lupus L93.2
  mesenteric K65.4
  neck M54.02
    cervicothoracic region M54.03
    occipito-atlanto-axial region M54.01
  relapsing M35.6
Panniculus adiposus (abdominal) E65
Pannus (allergic) (cornea) (degenerativus)
    (keratic) H16.42-●
  abdominal (symptomatic) E65
  trachomatosus, trachomatous (active) A71.1
Panophthalmitis H44.01-●
Pansinusitis (chronic) (hyperplastic)
    (nonpurulent) (purulent) J32.4
  acute J01.40
    recurrent J01.41
  tuberculous A15.8
Panuveitis (sympathetic) H44.11-●
Panvalvular disease I08.9
  specified NEC I08.8
PAPA (pyogenic arthritis, pyoderma
    gangrenosum, and acne syndrome) M04.8
Papanicolaou smear, cervix Z12.4
  as part of routine gynecological examination
      Z01.419
    with abnormal findings Z01.411
  for suspected neoplasm Z12.4
  nonspecific abnormal finding R87.619
  routine Z01.419
    with abnormal findings Z01.411
Papilledema (choked disc) H47.10
  associated with
    decreased ocular pressure H47.12
    increased intracranial pressure H47.11
    retinal disorder H47.13
  Foster-Kennedy syndrome H47.14-●

Papillitis H46.00
  anus K62.89
  chronic lingual K14.4
  necrotizing, kidney N17.2
  optic H46.0-●
  rectum K62.89
  renal, necrotizing N17.2
  tongue K14.0
Papilloma —see also Neoplasm, benign,
    by site
  acuminatum (female) (male) (anogenital)
      A63.0
  basal cell L82.1
    inflamed L82.0
  benign pinta (primary) A67.0
  bladder (urinary) (transitional cell) D41.4
  choroid plexus (lateral ventricle) (third
      ventricle) D33.0
    anaplastic C71.5
    fourth ventricle D33.1
    malignant C71.5
  renal pelvis (transitional cell) D41.1-●
    benign D30.1-●
  Schneiderian
    specified site —see Neoplasm, benign, by
        site
    unspecified site D14.0
  serous surface
    borderline malignancy
      specified site —see Neoplasm, uncertain
          behavior, by site
      unspecified site D39.10
    specified site —see Neoplasm, benign, by
        site
    unspecified site D27.9
  transitional (cell)
    bladder (urinary) D41.4
    inverted type —see Neoplasm, uncertain
        behavior, by site
    renal pelvis D41.1-●
    ureter D41.2-●
  ureter (transitional cell) D41.2-●
    benign D30.2-●
  urothelial —see Neoplasm, uncertain
      behavior, by site
  villous —see Neoplasm, uncertain behavior,
      by site
    adenocarcinoma in —see Neoplasm,
        malignant, by site
    in situ —see Neoplasm, in situ
  yaws, plantar or palmar A66.1
Papillomata, multiple, of yaws A66.1
Papillomatosis —see also Neoplasm, benign,
    by site
  confluent and reticulated L83
  cystic, breast —see Mastopathy, cystic
  ductal, breast —see Mastopathy, cystic
  intraductal (diffuse) —see Neoplasm, benign,
      by site
  subareolar duct D24-●
Papillomavirus, as cause of disease classified
    elsewhere B97.7
Papillon-Léage and Psaume syndrome
    Q87.0
Papule(s) R23.8
  carate (primary) A67.0
  fibrous, of nose D22.39
  Gottron's L94.4
  pinta (primary) A67.0
Papulosis
  lymphomatoid C86.6
  malignant I77.89
Papyraceous fetus O31.0-●
Para-albuminemia E88.09
Paracephalus Q89.7
Parachute mitral valve Q23.2
Paracoccidioidomycosis B41.9
  disseminated B41.7
  generalized B41.7
  mucocutaneous-lymphangitic B41.8
  pulmonary B41.0

Paracoccidioidomycosis (Continued)
  specified NEC B41.8
  visceral B41.8
Paradentosis K05.4
Paraffinoma T88.8
Paraganglioma D44.7
  adrenal D35.0-●
    malignant C74.1-●
  aortic body D44.7
    malignant C75.5
  carotid body D44.6
    malignant C75.4
  chromaffin —see also Neoplasm, benign, by
      site
    malignant —see Neoplasm, malignant, by
        site
  extra-adrenal D44.7
    malignant C75.5
      specified site —see Neoplasm,
          malignant, by site
      unspecified site C75.5
    specified site —see Neoplasm, uncertain
        behavior, by site
    unspecified site D44.7
  gangliocytic D13.2
    specified site —see Neoplasm, benign, by
        site
    unspecified site D13.2
  glomus jugulare D44.7
    malignant C75.5
  jugular D44.7
  malignant C75.5
    specified site —see Neoplasm, malignant,
        by site
    unspecified site C75.5
  nonchromaffin D44.7
    malignant C75.5
      specified site —see Neoplasm,
          malignant, by site
      unspecified site C75.5
    specified site —see Neoplasm, uncertain
        behavior, by site
    unspecified site D44.7
  parasympathetic D44.7
    specified site —see Neoplasm, uncertain
        behavior, by site
    unspecified site D44.7
  specified site —see Neoplasm, uncertain
      behavior, by site
  sympathetic D44.7
    specified site —see Neoplasm, uncertain
        behavior, by site
    unspecified site D44.7
  unspecified site D44.7
Parageusia R43.2
  psychogenic F45.8
Paragonimiasis B66.4
Paragranuloma, Hodgkin —see Lymphoma,
    Hodgkin, specified NEC
Parahemophilia —see also Defect, coagulation
    D68.2
Parakeratosis R23.4
  variegata L41.0
Paralysis, paralytic (complete) (incomplete)
    G83.9
  with
    syphilis A52.17
  abducens, abducent (nerve) —see Strabismus,
      paralytic, sixth nerve
  abductor, lower extremity G57.9-●
  accessory nerve G52.8
  accommodation —see also Paresis, of
      accommodation
    hysterical F44.89
  acoustic nerve (except Deafness) —see
      subcategory H93.3
  agitans —see also Parkinsonism G20
    arteriosclerotic G21.4
  alternating (oculomotor) G83.89
  amyotrophic G12.21

▶ New   ⇒ Revised   ~~deleted~~ Deleted   ● Use Additional Character(s)

Paralysis, paralytic *(Continued)*
ankle G57.9-•
anus (sphincter) K62.89
arm —*see* Monoplegia, upper limb
ascending (spinal), acute G61.0
association G12.29
asthenic bulbar G70.00
  with exacerbation (acute) G70.01
  in crisis G70.01
ataxic (hereditary) G11.9
  general (syphilitic) A52.17
atrophic G58.9
  infantile, acute —*see* Poliomyelitis, paralytic
  progressive G12.22
  spinal (acute) —*see* Poliomyelitis, paralytic
axillary G54.0
Babinski-Nageotte's G83.89
Bell's G51.0
  newborn P11.3
Benedikt's G46.3
birth injury P14.9
  spinal cord P11.5
bladder (neurogenic) (sphincter)
    N31.2
bowel, colon or intestine K56.0
brachial plexus G54.0
  birth injury P14.3
  newborn (birth injury) P14.3
brain G83.9
  diplegia G83.0
  triplegia G83.89
bronchial J98.09
Brown-Séquard G83.81
bulbar (chronic) (progressive) G12.22
  infantile —*see* Poliomyelitis, paralytic
  poliomyelitic —*see* Poliomyelitis, paralytic
  pseudo G12.29
bulbospinal G70.00
  with exacerbation (acute) G70.01
  in crisis G70.01
cardiac —*see also* Failure, heart I50.9
cerebrocerebellar, diplegic G80.1
cervical
  plexus G54.2
  sympathetic G90.09
Céstan-Chenais G46.3
Charcot-Marie-Tooth type G60.0
Clark's G80.9
colon K56.0
compressed air T70.3
compression
  arm G56.9-•
  leg G57.9-•
  lower extremity G57.9-•
  upper extremity G56.9-•
congenital (cerebral) —*see* Palsy, cerebral
conjugate movement (gaze) (of eye) H51.0
  cortical (nuclear) (supranuclear) H51.0
cordis —*see* Failure, heart
cranial or cerebral nerve G52.9
creeping G12.22
crossed leg G83.89
crutch —*see* Injury, brachial plexus
deglutition R13.0
  hysterical F44.4
dementia A52.17
descending (spinal) NEC G12.29
diaphragm (flaccid) J98.6
  due to accidental dissection of phrenic
    nerve during procedure —*see*
    Puncture, accidental complicating
    surgery
digestive organs NEC K59.89
diplegic —*see* Diplegia
divergence (nuclear) H51.8
diver's T70.3
Duchenne's
  birth injury P14.0
  due to or associated with
    motor neuron disease G12.22
    muscular dystrophy G71.01

Paralysis, paralytic *(Continued)*
due to intracranial or spinal birth injury —*see*
    Palsy, cerebral
embolic (current episode) I63.4-•
Erb (-Duchenne) (birth) (newborn) P14.0
Erb's syphilitic spastic spinal A52.17
esophagus K22.89
eye muscle (extrinsic) H49.9
  intrinsic —*see also* Paresis, of
    accommodation
facial (nerve) G51.0
  birth injury P11.3
  congenital P11.3
  following operation NEC —*see* Puncture,
    accidental complicating surgery
  newborn (birth injury) P11.3
familial (recurrent) (periodic) G72.3
  spastic G11.4
fauces J39.2
finger G56.9-•
gait R26.1
gastric nerve (nondiabetic) G52.2
gaze, conjugate H51.0
general (progressive) (syphilitic) A52.17
  juvenile A50.45
glottis J38.00
  bilateral J38.02
  unilateral J38.01
gluteal G54.1
Gubler (-Millard) G46.3
hand —*see* Monoplegia, upper limb
heart —*see* Arrest, cardiac
hemiplegic —*see* Hemiplegia
hyperkalemic periodic (familial) G72.3
hypoglossal (nerve) G52.3
hypokalemic periodic G72.3
hysterical F44.4
ileus K56.0
infantile —*see also* Poliomyelitis, paralytic
  A80.30
  bulbar —*see* Poliomyelitis, paralytic
  cerebral —*see* Palsy, cerebral
  spastic —*see* Palsy, cerebral, spastic
infective —*see* Poliomyelitis, paralytic
inferior nuclear G83.9
internuclear —*see* Ophthalmoplegia,
    internuclear
intestine K56.0
iris H57.09
  due to diphtheria (toxin) A36.89
ischemic, Volkmann's (complicating trauma)
    T79.6
Jackson's G83.89
jake —*see* Poisoning, food, noxious, plant
Jamaica ginger (jake) G62.2
juvenile general A50.45
Klumpke (-Déjérine) (birth) (newborn) P14.1
labioglossal (laryngeal) (pharyngeal) G12.29
Landry's G61.0
laryngeal nerve (recurrent) (superior)
    (unilateral) J38.00
  bilateral J38.02
  unilateral J38.01
larynx J38.00
  bilateral J38.02
  due to diphtheria (toxin) A36.2
  unilateral J38.01
lateral G12.23
lead —*see* subcategory T56.0
left side —*see* Hemiplegia
leg G83.1-•
  both —*see* Paraplegia
  crossed G83.89
  hysterical F44.4
  psychogenic F44.4
  transient or transitory R29.818
    traumatic NEC —*see* Injury, nerve, leg
levator palpebrae superioris —*see*
    Blepharoptosis, paralytic
limb —*see* Monoplegia
lip K13.0

Paralysis, paralytic *(Continued)*
Lissauer's A52.17
lower limb —*see* Monoplegia, lower limb
  both —*see* Paraplegia
lung J98.4
median nerve G56.1-•
medullary (tegmental) G83.89
mesencephalic NEC G83.89
  tegmental G83.89
middle alternating G83.89
Millard-Gubler-Foville G46.3
monoplegic —*see* Monoplegia
motor G83.9
muscle, muscular NEC G72.89
  due to nerve lesion G58.9
  eye (extrinsic) H49.9
    intrinsic —*see* Paresis, of accommodation
    oblique —*see* Strabismus, paralytic,
      fourth nerve
  iris sphincter H21.9
  ischemic (Volkmann's) (complicating
    trauma) T79.6
  progressive G12.21
  progressive, spinal G12.25
  pseudohypertrophic G71.02
  spinal progressive G12.25
musculocutaneous nerve G56.9-•
musculospiral G56.9-•
nerve —*see also* Disorder, nerve
  abducent —*see* Strabismus, paralytic, sixth
    nerve
  accessory G52.8
  auditory (except Deafness) —*see*
    subcategory H93.3
  birth injury P14.9
  cranial or cerebral G52.9
  facial G51.0
    birth injury P11.3
    congenital P11.3
    newborn (birth injury) P11.3
  fourth or trochlear —*see* Strabismus,
    paralytic, fourth nerve
  newborn (birth injury) P14.9
  oculomotor —*see* Strabismus, paralytic,
    third nerve
  phrenic (birth injury) P14.2
  radial G56.3-•
  seventh or facial G51.0
    newborn (birth injury) P11.3
  sixth or abducent —*see* Strabismus,
    paralytic, sixth nerve
  syphilitic A52.15
  third or oculomotor —*see* Strabismus,
    paralytic, third nerve
  trigeminal G50.9
  trochlear —*see* Strabismus, paralytic,
    fourth nerve
  ulnar G56.2-•
normokalemic periodic G72.3
ocular H49.9
  alternating G83.89
oculofacial, congenital (Moebius) Q87.0
oculomotor (external bilateral) (nerve) —*see*
    Strabismus, paralytic, third nerve
palate (soft) K13.79
paratrigeminal G50.9
periodic (familial) (hyperkalemic)
    (hypokalemic) (myotonic)
    (normokalemic) (potassium sensitive)
    (secondary) G72.3
peripheral autonomic nervous system —*see*
    Neuropathy, peripheral, autonomic
peroneal (nerve) G57.3-•
pharynx J39.2
phrenic nerve G56.8-•
plantar nerve(s) G57.6-•
pneumogastric nerve G52.2
poliomyelitis (current) —*see* Poliomyelitis,
    paralytic
popliteal nerve G57.3-•
postepileptic transitory G83.84

Paralysis, paralytic *(Continued)*
  progressive (atrophic) (bulbar) (spinal)
    G12.22
    general A52.17
    infantile acute —*see* Poliomyelitis, paralytic
    supranuclear G23.1
  pseudobulbar G12.29
  pseudohypertrophic (muscle) G71.09
  psychogenic F44.4
  quadriceps G57.9-●
  quadriplegic —*see* Tetraplegia
  radial nerve G56.3-●
  rectus muscle (eye) H49.9
  recurrent isolated sleep G47.53
  respiratory (muscle) (system) (tract) R06.81
    center NEC G93.89
    congenital P28.89
    newborn P28.89
  right side —*see* Hemiplegia
  saturnine —*see* subcategory T56.0
  sciatic nerve G57.0-●
  senile G83.9
  shaking —*see* Parkinsonism
  shoulder G56.9-●
  sleep, recurrent isolated G47.53
  spastic G83.9
    cerebral —*see* Palsy, cerebral, spastic
    congenital (cerebral) —*see* Palsy, cerebral,
      spastic
    familial G11.4
    hereditary G11.4
    quadriplegic G80.0
    syphilitic (spinal) A52.17
  sphincter, bladder —*see* Paralysis, bladder
  spinal (cord) G83.9
    accessory nerve G52.8
    acute —*see* Poliomyelitis, paralytic
    ascending acute G61.0
    atrophic (acute) —*see also* Poliomyelitis,
      paralytic
      spastic, syphilitic A52.17
    congenital NEC —*see* Palsy, cerebral
    hereditary G95.89
    infantile —*see* Poliomyelitis, paralytic
    progressive G12.21
    muscle G12.25
    sequelae NEC G83.89
  sternomastoid G52.8
  stomach K31.84
    diabetic —*see* Diabetes, by type, with
      gastroparesis
    nerve G52.2
      diabetic —*see* Diabetes, by type, with
        gastroparesis
  stroke —*see* Infarct, brain
  subcapsularis G56.8-●
  supranuclear (progressive) G23.1
  sympathetic G90.8
    cervical G90.09
    nervous system —*see* Neuropathy,
      peripheral, autonomic
  syndrome G83.9
    specified NEC G83.89
  syphilitic spastic spinal (Erb's) A52.17
  thigh G57.9-●
  throat J39.2
    diphtheritic A36.0
    muscle J39.2
  thrombotic (current episode) I63.3-●
  thumb G56.9-●
  tick —*see* Toxicity, venom, arthropod,
    specified NEC
  Todd's (postepileptic transitory paralysis)
    G83.84
  toe G57.6-●
  tongue K14.8
  transient R29.5
    arm or leg NEC R29.818
    traumatic NEC —*see* Injury, nerve
  trapezius G52.8
  traumatic, transient NEC —*see* Injury, nerve

Paralysis, paralytic *(Continued)*
  trembling —*see* Parkinsonism
  triceps brachii G56.9-●
  trigeminal nerve G50.9
  trochlear (nerve) —*see* Strabismus, paralytic,
    fourth nerve
  ulnar nerve G56.2-●
  upper limb —*see* Monoplegia, upper limb
  uremic N18.9 [G99.8]
  uveoparotitic D86.89
  uvula K13.79
    postdiphtheritic A36.0
  vagus nerve G52.2
  vasomotor NEC G90.8
  velum palati K13.79
  vesical —*see* Paralysis, bladder
  vestibular nerve (except Vertigo) —*see*
    subcategory H93.3
  vocal cords J38.00
    bilateral J38.02
    unilateral J38.01
  Volkmann's (complicating trauma)
    T79.6
  wasting G12.29
  Weber's G46.3
  wrist G56.9-●
Paramedial urethrovesical orifice
  Q64.79
Paramenia N92.6
Parametritis —*see also* Disease, pelvis,
  inflammatory N73.2
  acute N73.0
  complicating abortion —*see* Abortion, by
    type, complicated by, parametritis
Parametrium, parametric —*see* condition
Paramnesia —*see* Amnesia
Paramolar K00.1
Paramyloidosis E85.89
Paramyoclonus multiplex G25.3
Paramyotonia (congenita) G71.19
Parangi —*see* Yaws
Paranoia (querulans) F22
  senile F03
Paranoid
  dementia (senile) F03
    praecox —*see* Schizophrenia
  personality F60.0
  psychosis (climacteric) (involutional)
    (menopausal) F22
    psychogenic (acute) F23
    senile F03
  reaction (acute) F23
    chronic F22
  schizophrenia F20.0
  state (climacteric) (involutional)
    (menopausal) (simple) F22
    senile F03
  tendencies F60.0
  traits F60.0
  trends F60.0
  type, psychopathic personality F60.0
Paraparesis —*see* Paraplegia
Paraphasia R47.02
Paraphilia F65.9
Paraphimosis (congenital) N47.2
  chancroidal A57
Paraphrenia, paraphrenic (late) F22
  schizophrenia F20.0
Paraplegia (lower) G82.20
  ataxic —*see* Degeneration, combined, spinal
    cord
  complete G82.21
  congenital (cerebral) G80.8
    spastic G80.1
  familial spastic G11.4
  functional (hysterical) F44.4
  hereditary, spastic G11.4
  hysterical F44.4
  incomplete G82.22
  Pott's A18.01
  psychogenic F44.4

Paraplegia *(Continued)*
  spastic
    Erb's spinal, syphilitic A52.17
    hereditary G11.4
    tropical G04.1
  syphilitic (spastic) A52.17
  traumatic
    current injury - code to injury with seventh
      character A
    sequela of previous injury - code to
      injury with seventh character S
  tropical spastic G04.1
Parapoxvirus B08.60
  specified NEC B08.69
Paraproteinemia D89.2
  benign (familial) D89.2
  monoclonal D47.2
  secondary to malignant disease D47.2
Parapsoriasis L41.9
  en plaques L41.4
  guttata L41.1
  large plaque L41.4
  retiform, retiformis L41.5
  small plaque L41.3
  specified NEC L41.8
  varioliformis (acuta) L41.0
Parasitic —*see also* condition
  disease NEC B89
  stomatitis B37.0
  sycosis (beard) (scalp) B35.0
  twin Q89.4
Parasitism B89
  intestinal B82.9
  skin B88.9
  specified —*see* Infestation
Parasitophobia F40.218
Parasomnia G47.50
  due to
    alcohol
      abuse F10.182
      dependence F10.282
      use F10.982
    amphetamines
      abuse F15.182
      dependence F15.282
      use F15.982
    caffeine
      abuse F15.182
      dependence F15.282
      use F15.982
    cocaine
      abuse F14.182
      dependence F14.282
      use F14.982
    drug NEC
      abuse F19.182
      dependence F19.282
      use F19.982
    opioid
      abuse F11.182
      dependence F11.282
      use F11.982
    psychoactive substance NEC
      abuse F19.182
      dependence F19.282
      use F19.982
    sedative, hypnotic, or anxiolytic
      abuse F13.182
      dependence F13.282
      use F13.982
    stimulant NEC
      abuse F15.182
      dependence F15.282
      use F15.982
  in conditions classified elsewhere
    G47.54
  nonorganic origin F51.8
  organic G47.50
  specified NEC G47.59
Paraspadias Q54.9
Paraspasmus facialis G51.8

▶ New   ⇒ Revised   ~~deleted~~ Deleted   ● Use Additional Character(s)

Parasuicide (attempt)
➡ history of (personal) Z91.51
 in family Z81.8
Parathyroid gland —see condition
Parathyroid tetany E20.9
Paratrachoma A74.0
Paratyphilitis —see Appendicitis
Paratyphoid (fever) —see Fever, paratyphoid
Paratyphus —see Fever, paratyphoid
Paraurethral duct Q64.79
Paraurethritis —see also Urethritis
 gonococcal (acute) (chronic) (with abscess)
  A54.1
Paravaccinia NEC B08.04
Paravaginitis —see Vaginitis
Parencephalitis —see also Encephalitis
 sequelae G09
Parent-child conflict —see Conflict, parent-child
 estrangement NEC Z62.890
Paresis —see also Paralysis
 accommodation —see Paresis, of
  accommodation
 Bernhardt's G57.1-●
 bladder (sphincter) —see also Paralysis, bladder
  tabetic A52.17
 bowel, colon or intestine K56.0
 extrinsic muscle, eye H49.9
 general (progressive) (syphilitic) A52.17
  juvenile A50.45
 heart —see Failure, heart
 insane (syphilitic) A52.17
 juvenile (general) A50.45
 of accommodation H52.52-●
 peripheral progressive (idiopathic) G60.3
 pseudohypertrophic G71.09
 senile G83.9
 syphilitic (general) A52.17
  congenital A50.45
 vesical NEC N31.2
Paresthesia —see also Disturbance, sensation,
 skin R20.2
 Bernhardt G57.1-●
Paretic —see condition
Parinaud's
 conjunctivitis H10.89
 oculoglandular syndrome H10.89
 ophthalmoplegia H49.88
Parkinsonism (idiopathic) (primary) G20
 with neurogenic orthostatic hypotension
  (symptomatic) G90.3
 arteriosclerotic G21.4
 dementia G31.83 [F02.80]
  with behavioral disturbance G31.83 [F02.81]
 due to
  drugs NEC G21.19
   neuroleptic G21.11
  medication-induced NEC G21.19
 neuroleptic induced G21.11
 postencephalitic G21.3
 secondary G21.9
  due to
   arteriosclerosis G21.4
   drugs NEC G21.19
    neuroleptic G21.11
   encephalitis G21.3
   external agents NEC G21.2
   syphilis A52.19
  specified NEC G21.8
 syphilitic A52.19
 treatment-induced NEC G21.19
 vascular G21.4
Parkinson's disease, syndrome or tremor —see
 Parkinsonism
Parodontitis —see Periodontitis
Parodontosis K05.4
Paronychia —see also Cellulitis, digit
 with lymphangitis —see Lymphangitis, acute,
  digit
 candidal (chronic) B37.2
 tuberculous (primary) A18.4
Parorexia (psychogenic) F50.89

Parosmia R43.1
 psychogenic F45.8
Parotid gland —see condition
Parotitis, parotiditis (allergic) (nonspecific
 toxic) (purulent) (septic) (suppurative) —
 see also Sialoadenitis
 epidemic —see Mumps
 infectious —see Mumps
 postoperative K91.89
 surgical K91.89
Parrot fever A70
Parrot's disease (early congenital syphilitic
 pseudoparalysis) A50.02
Parry-Romberg syndrome G51.8
Parry's disease or syndrome E05.00
 with thyroid storm E05.01
Pars planitis —see Cyclitis
Parsonage (-Aldren)-Turner syndrome G54.5
Parson's disease (exophthalmic goiter) E05.00
 with thyroid storm E05.01
Particolored infant Q82.8
Parturition —see Delivery
Parulis K04.7
 with sinus K04.6
Parvovirus, as cause of disease classified
 elsewhere B97.6
Pasini and Pierini's atrophoderma L90.3
Passage
 false, urethra N36.5
 meconium (newborn) during delivery P03.82
 of sounds or bougies —see Attention to,
  artificial, opening
Passive —see condition
 smoking Z77.22
▶ Past due on rent or mortgage Z59.81- ●
Pasteurella septica A28.0
Pasteurellosis —see Infection, Pasteurella
PAT (paroxysmal atrial tachycardia) I47.1
Patau's syndrome —see Trisomy, 13
Patches
 mucous (syphilitic) A51.39
  congenital A50.07
 smokers' (mouth) K13.24
Patellar —see condition
Patent —see also Imperfect, closure
 canal of Nuck Q52.4
 cervix N88.3
 ductus arteriosus or Botallo's Q25.0
 foramen
  botalli Q21.1
  ovale Q21.1
 interauricular septum Q21.1
 interventricular septum Q21.0
 omphalomesenteric duct Q43.0
 os (uteri) —see Patent, cervix
 ostium secundum Q21.1
 urachus Q64.4
 vitelline duct Q43.0
Paterson (-Brown)(-Kelly) syndrome or web
 D50.1
Pathologic, pathological —see also condition
 asphyxia R09.01
 fire-setting F63.1
 gambling F63.0
 ovum O02.0
 resorption, tooth K03.3
 stealing F63.2
Pathology (of) —see Disease
 periradicular, associated with previous
  endodontic treatment NEC M27.59
Pattern, sleep-wake, irregular G47.23
Patulous —see also Imperfect, closure
 (congenital)
 alimentary tract Q45.8
  lower Q43.8
  upper Q40.8
 eustachian tube H69.0-●
Pause, sinoatrial I49.5
Paxton's disease B36.2
Pearl(s)
 enamel K00.2
 Epstein's K09.8

Pearl-worker's disease —see Osteomyelitis,
 specified type NEC
Pectenosis K62.4
Pectoral —see condition
Pectus
 carinatum (congenital) Q67.7
  acquired M95.4
  rachitic sequelae (late effect) E64.3
 excavatum (congenital) Q67.6
  acquired M95.4
  rachitic sequelae (late effect) E64.3
 recurvatum (congenital) Q67.6
Pedatrophia E41
Pederosis F65.4
Pediatric inflammatory multisystem syndrome
 M35.81
Pediculosis (infestation) B85.2
 capitis (head-louse) (any site) B85.0
 corporis (body-louse) (any site) B85.1
 eyelid B85.0
 mixed (classifiable to more than one of the
  titles B85.0-B85.3) B85.4
 pubis (pubic louse) (any site) B85.3
 vestimenti B85.1
 vulvae B85.3
Pediculus (infestation) —see Pediculosis
Pedophilia F65.4
Peg-shaped teeth K00.2
Pelade —see Alopecia, areata
Pelger-Huët anomaly or syndrome D72.0
Peliosis (rheumatica) D69.0
 hepatis K76.4
  with toxic liver disease K71.8
Pelizaeus-Merzbacher disease E75.29
Pellagra (alcoholic) (with polyneuropathy)
 E52
Pellagra-cerebellar-ataxia-renal aminoaciduria
 syndrome E72.02
Pellegrini (-Stieda) disease or syndrome —see
 Bursitis, tibial collateral
Pellizzi's syndrome E34.8
Pel's crisis A52.11
Pelvic —see also condition
 examination (periodic) (routine) Z01.419
  with abnormal findings Z01.411
 kidney, congenital Q63.2
Pelviolithiasis —see Calculus, kidney
Pelviperitonitis —see also Peritonitis, pelvic
 gonococcal A54.24
 puerperal O85
Pelvis —see condition or type
Pemphigoid L12.9
 benign, mucous membrane L12.1
 bullous L12.0
 cicatricial L12.1
 juvenile L12.2
 ocular L12.1
 specified NEC L12.8
Pemphigus L10.9
 benign familial (chronic) Q82.8
 Brazilian L10.3
 circinatus L13.0
 conjunctiva L12.1
 drug-induced L10.5
 erythematosus L10.4
 foliaceous L10.2
 gangrenous —see Gangrene
 neonatorum L01.03
 ocular L12.1
 paraneoplastic L10.81
 specified NEC L10.89
 syphilitic (congenital) A50.06
 vegetans L10.1
 vulgaris L10.0
 wildfire L10.3
Pendred's syndrome E07.1
Pendulous
 abdomen, in pregnancy —see Pregnancy,
  complicated by, abnormal, pelvic organs
  or tissues NEC
 breast N64.89

Penetrating wound —*see also* Puncture
　with internal injury —*see* Injury, by site
　eyeball —*see* Puncture, eyeball
　orbit (with or without foreign body) —*see*
　　　Puncture, orbit
　uterus by instrument with or following
　　　ectopic or molar pregnancy O08.6
Penicillosis B48.4
Penis —*see* condition
Penitis N48.29
Pentalogy of Fallot Q21.8
Pentasomy X syndrome Q97.1
Pentosuria (essential) E74.89
Percreta placenta O43.23-●
Peregrinating patient —*see* Disorder, factitious
Perforation, perforated (nontraumatic) (of)
　accidental during procedure (blood vessel)
　　　(nerve) (organ) —*see* Complication,
　　　accidental puncture or laceration
　antrum —*see* Sinusitis, maxillary
　appendix K35.22
　　with localized peritonitis K35.32
　atrial septum, multiple Q21.1
　attic, ear —*see* Perforation, tympanum, attic
　bile duct (common) (hepatic) K83.2
　　cystic K82.2
　bladder (urinary)
　　with or following ectopic or molar
　　　pregnancy O08.6
　　obstetrical trauma O71.5
　　traumatic S37.29
　　　at delivery O71.5
　bowel K63.1
　　with or following ectopic or molar
　　　pregnancy O08.6
　　newborn P78.0
　　obstetrical trauma O71.5
　　traumatic —*see* Laceration, intestine
　broad ligament N83.8
　　with or following ectopic or molar
　　　pregnancy O08.6
　　obstetrical trauma O71.6
　by
　　device, implant or graft —*see also*
　　　Complications, by site and type,
　　　mechanical T85.628
　　　arterial graft NEC —*see* Complication,
　　　　cardiovascular device, mechanical,
　　　　vascular
　　　breast (implant) T85.49
　　　catheter NEC T85.698
　　　　cystostomy T83.090
　　　　dialysis (renal) T82.49
　　　　　intraperitoneal T85.691
　　　　infusion NEC T82.594
　　　　　spinal (epidural) (subdural) T85.690
　　　　urinary —*see also* Complications,
　　　　　catheter, urinary T83.098
　　　electronic (electrode) (pulse generator)
　　　　(stimulator)
　　　　bone T84.390
　　　　cardiac T82.199
　　　　　electrode T82.190
　　　　　pulse generator T82.191
　　　　　specified type NEC T82.198
　　　　nervous system —*see* Complication,
　　　　　prosthetic device, mechanical,
　　　　　electronic nervous system
　　　　　stimulator
　　　　urinary —*see* Complication,
　　　　　genitourinary, device, urinary,
　　　　　mechanical
　　　fixation, internal (orthopedic) NEC —
　　　　see Complication, fixation device,
　　　　mechanical
　　　gastrointestinal —*see* Complications,
　　　　prosthetic device, mechanical,
　　　　gastrointestinal device
　　　genital NEC T83.498
　　　　intrauterine contraceptive device
　　　　　T83.39
　　　　penile prosthesis T83.490

Perforation, perforated *(Continued)*
　by *(Continued)*
　　device, implant or graft *(Continued)*
　　　heart NEC —*see* Complication,
　　　　cardiovascular device, mechanical
　　　joint prosthesis —*see* Complications,
　　　　joint prosthesis, mechanical,
　　　　specified NEC, by site
　　　ocular NEC —*see* Complications,
　　　　prosthetic device, mechanical,
　　　　ocular device
　　　orthopedic NEC —*see* Complication,
　　　　orthopedic, device, mechanical
　　　specified NEC T85.628
　　　urinary NEC —*see also* Complication,
　　　　genitourinary, device, urinary,
　　　　mechanical
　　　　graft T83.29
　　　vascular NEC —*see* Complication,
　　　　cardiovascular device, mechanical
　　　ventricular intracranial shunt T85.09
　　foreign body left accidentally in
　　　operative wound T81.539
　　instrument (any) during a procedure,
　　　accidental —*see* Puncture, accidental
　　　complicating surgery
　cecum K35.22
　　with localized peritonitis K35.32
　cervix (uteri) N88.8
　　with or following ectopic or molar
　　　pregnancy O08.6
　　obstetrical trauma O71.3
　colon K63.1
　　newborn P78.0
　　obstetrical trauma O71.5
　　traumatic —*see* Laceration, intestine, large
　common duct (bile) K83.2
　cornea (due to ulceration) —*see* Ulcer,
　　cornea, perforated
　cystic duct K82.2
　diverticulum (intestine) K57.80
　　with bleeding K57.81
　　large intestine K57.20
　　　with
　　　　bleeding K57.21
　　　　small intestine K57.40
　　　　　with bleeding K57.41
　　small intestine K57.00
　　　with
　　　　bleeding K57.01
　　　　large intestine K57.40
　　　　　with bleeding K57.41
　ear drum —*see* Perforation, tympanum
　esophagus K22.3
　ethmoidal sinus —*see* Sinusitis, ethmoidal
　frontal sinus —*see* Sinusitis, frontal
　gallbladder K82.2
　heart valve —*see* Endocarditis
　ileum K63.1
　　newborn P78.0
　　obstetrical trauma O71.5
　　traumatic —*see* Laceration, intestine, small
　instrumental, surgical (accidental) (blood
　　vessel) (nerve) (organ) —*see* Puncture,
　　accidental complicating surgery
　intestine NEC K63.1
　　with ectopic or molar pregnancy O08.6
　　newborn P78.0
　　obstetrical trauma O71.5
　　traumatic —*see* Laceration, intestine
　　ulcerative NEC K63.1
　　　newborn P78.0
　jejunum, jejunal K63.1
　　obstetrical trauma O71.5
　　traumatic —*see* Laceration, intestine, small
　　ulcer —*see* Ulcer, gastrojejunal, with
　　　perforation
　joint prosthesis —*see* Complications, joint
　　prosthesis, mechanical, specified NEC,
　　by site
　mastoid (antrum) (cell) —*see* Disorder,
　　mastoid, specified NEC

Perforation, perforated *(Continued)*
　maxillary sinus —*see* Sinusitis, maxillary
　membrana tympani —*see* Perforation,
　　tympanum
　nasal
　　septum J34.89
　　　congenital Q30.3
　　　syphilitic A52.73
　　sinus J34.89
　　　congenital Q30.8
　　　due to sinusitis —*see* Sinusitis
　palate —*see also* Cleft, palate Q35.9
　　syphilitic A52.79
　palatine vault —*see also* Cleft, palate, hard Q35.1
　　syphilitic A52.79
　　congenital A50.59
　pars flaccida (ear drum) —*see* Perforation,
　　tympanum, attic
　pelvic
　　floor S31.030
　　　with
　　　　ectopic or molar pregnancy O08.6
　　　　penetration into retroperitoneal space
　　　　　S31.031
　　　　retained foreign body S31.040
　　　　　with penetration into
　　　　　　retroperitoneal space S31.041
　　　following ectopic or molar pregnancy
　　　　O08.6
　　　obstetrical trauma O70.1
　　organ S37.99
　　　adrenal gland S37.818
　　　bladder —*see* Perforation, bladder
　　　fallopian tube S37.599
　　　　bilateral S37.592
　　　　unilateral S37.591
　　　kidney S37.09-●
　　　obstetrical trauma O71.5
　　　ovary S37.499
　　　　bilateral S37.492
　　　　unilateral S37.491
　　　prostate S37.828
　　　specified organ NEC S37.898
　　　ureter —*see* Perforation, ureter
　　　urethra —*see* Perforation, urethra
　　　uterus —*see* Perforation, uterus
　perineum —*see* Laceration, perineum
　pharynx J39.2
　rectum K63.1
　　newborn P78.0
　　obstetrical trauma O71.5
　　traumatic S36.63
　root canal space due to endodontic treatment
　　M27.51
　sigmoid K63.1
　　newborn P78.0
　　obstetrical trauma O71.5
　　traumatic S36.533
　sinus (accessory) (chronic) (nasal) J34.89
　sphenoidal sinus —*see* Sinusitis, sphenoidal
　surgical (accidental) (by instrument) (blood
　　vessel) (nerve) (organ) —*see* Puncture,
　　accidental complicating surgery
　traumatic
　　external —*see* Puncture
　　eye —*see* Puncture, eyeball
　　internal organ —*see* Injury, by site
　tympanum, tympanic (membrane) (persistent
　　post-traumatic) (postinflammatory)
　　H72.9-●
　　attic H72.1-●
　　　multiple —*see* Perforation, tympanum,
　　　　multiple
　　　total —*see* Perforation, tympanum, total
　　central H72.0-●
　　　multiple —*see* Perforation, tympanum,
　　　　multiple
　　　total —*see* Perforation, tympanum, total
　　marginal NEC —*see* subcategory H72.2
　　multiple H72.81-●
　　pars flaccida —*see* Perforation, tympanum,
　　　attic

▶ New　⇒ Revised　~~deleted~~ Deleted　● Use Additional Character(s)

Perforation, perforated *(Continued)*
  tympanum, tympanic *(Continued)*
    total H72.82-●
    traumatic, current episode S09.2-●
  typhoid, gastrointestinal —*see* Typhoid
  ulcer —*see* Ulcer, by site, with perforation
  ureter N28.89
    traumatic S37.19
  urethra N36.8
    with ectopic or molar pregnancy O08.6
    following ectopic or molar pregnancy O08.6
    obstetrical trauma O71.5
    traumatic S37.39
      at delivery O71.5
  uterus
    with ectopic or molar pregnancy O08.6
    by intrauterine contraceptive device T83.39
    following ectopic or molar pregnancy
        O08.6
    obstetrical trauma O71.1
    traumatic S37.69
      obstetric O71.1
  uvula K13.79
    syphilitic A52.79
  vagina
    obstetrical trauma O71.4
    other trauma - *see* Puncture, vagina
Periadenitis mucosa necrotica recurrens K12.0
Periappendicitis (acute) —*see* Appendicitis
Periarteritis nodosa (disseminated) (infectious)
    (necrotizing) M30.0
Periarthritis (joint) —*see also* Enthesopathy
  Duplay's M75.0-●
  gonococcal A54.42
  humeroscapularis —*see* Capsulitis, adhesive
  scapulohumeral —*see* Capsulitis, adhesive
  shoulder —*see* Capsulitis, adhesive
  wrist M77.2-●
Periarthrosis (angioneural) —*see* Enthesopathy
Pericapsulitis, adhesive (shoulder) —*see*
    Capsulitis, adhesive
Pericarditis (with decompensation) (with
    effusion) I31.9
  with rheumatic fever (conditions in I00)
    active —*see* Pericarditis, rheumatic
    inactive or quiescent I09.2
  acute (hemorrhagic) (nonrheumatic) (Sicca)
      I30.9
    with chorea (acute) (rheumatic)
        (Sydenham's) I02.0
    benign I30.8
    nonspecific I30.0
    rheumatic I01.0
      with chorea (acute) (Sydenham's) I02.0
  adhesive or adherent (chronic) (external)
      (internal) I31.0
    acute —*see* Pericarditis, acute
    rheumatic I09.2
  bacterial (acute) (subacute) (with serous or
      seropurulent effusion) I30.1
  calcareous I31.1
  cholesterol (chronic) I31.8
    acute I30.9
  chronic (nonrheumatic) I31.9
    rheumatic I09.2
  constrictive (chronic) I31.1
  coxsackie B33.23
  fibrinocaseous (tuberculous) A18.84
  fibrinopurulent I30.1
  fibrinous I30.8
  fibrous I31.0
  gonococcal A54.83
  idiopathic I30.0
  in systemic lupus erythematosus M32.12
  infective I30.1
  meningococcal A39.53
  neoplastic (chronic) I31.8
    acute I30.9
  obliterans, obliterating I31.0
  plastic I31.0
  pneumococcal I30.1

Pericarditis *(Continued)*
  postinfarction I24.1
  purulent I30.1
  rheumatic (active) (acute) (with effusion)
      (with pneumonia) I01.0
    with chorea (acute) (rheumatic)
        (Sydenham's) I02.0
    chronic or inactive (with chorea) I09.2
  rheumatoid —*see* Rheumatoid, carditis
  septic I30.1
  serofibrinous I30.8
  staphylococcal I30.1
  streptococcal I30.1
  suppurative I30.1
  syphilitic A52.06
  tuberculous A18.84
  uremic N18.9 *[I32]*
  viral I30.1
Pericardium, pericardial —*see* condition
Pericellulitis —*see* Cellulitis
Pericementitis (chronic) (suppurative) —*see also*
    Periodontitis
  acute K05.20
    generalized —*see* Periodontitis, aggressive,
        generalized
    localized —*see* Periodontitis, aggressive,
        localized
Perichondritis
  auricle —*see* Perichondritis, ear
  bronchus J98.09
  ear (external) H61.00-●
    acute H61.01-●
    chronic H61.02-●
  external auditory canal —*see* Perichondritis,
      ear
  larynx J38.7
    syphilitic A52.73
    typhoid A01.09
  nose J34.89
  pinna —*see* Perichondritis, ear
  trachea J39.8
Periclasia K05.4
Pericoronitis —*see* Periodontitis
Pericystitis N30.90
  with hematuria N30.91
Peridiverticulitis (intestine) K57.92
  cecum —*see* Diverticulitis, intestine, large
  colon —*see* Diverticulitis, intestine, large
  duodenum —*see* Diverticulitis, intestine,
      small
  intestine —*see* Diverticulitis, intestine
  jejunum —*see* Diverticulitis, intestine, small
  rectosigmoid —*see* Diverticulitis, intestine,
      large
  rectum —*see* Diverticulitis, intestine, large
  sigmoid —*see* Diverticulitis, intestine, large
Periendocarditis —*see* Endocarditis
Periepididymitis N45.1
Perifolliculitis L01.02
  abscedens, caput, scalp L66.3
  capitis, abscedens (et suffodiens) L66.3
  superficial pustular L01.02
Perihepatitis K65.8
Perilabyrinthitis (acute) —*see* subcategory H83.0
Perimeningitis —*see* Meningitis
Perimetritis —*see* Endometritis
Perimetrosalpingitis —*see* Salpingo-oophoritis
Perineocele N81.81
Perinephric, perinephritic —*see* condition
Perinephritis —*see also* Infection, kidney
  purulent —*see* Abscess, kidney
Perineum, perineal —*see* condition
Perineuritis NEC —*see* Neuralgia
Periodic —*see* condition
Periodontitis (chronic) (complex) (compound)
    (local) (simplex) K05.30
  acute K05.20
    generalized K05.229
      moderate K05.222
      severe K05.223
      slight K05.221

Periodontitis *(Continued)*
  acute *(Continued)*
    localized K05.219
      moderate K05.212
      severe K05.213
      slight K05.211
  apical K04.5
    acute (pulpal origin) K04.4
  generalized K05.329
    moderate K05.322
    severe K05.323
    slight K05.321
  localized K05.319
    moderate K05.312
    severe K05.313
    slight K05.311
Periodontoclasia K05.4
Periodontosis (juvenile) K05.4
Periods —*see also* Menstruation
  heavy N92.0
  irregular N92.6
  shortened intervals (irregular) N92.1
Perionychia —*see also* Cellulitis, digit
  with lymphangitis —*see* Lymphangitis, acute,
      digit
Perioophoritis —*see* Salpingo-oophoritis
Periorchitis N45.2
Periosteum, periosteal —*see* condition
Periostitis (albuminosa) (circumscribed)
    (diffuse) (infective) (monomelic) —*see also*
    Osteomyelitis
  alveolar M27.3
  alveolodental M27.3
  dental M27.3
  gonorrheal A54.43
  jaw (lower) (upper) M27.2
  orbit H05.03-●
  syphilitic A52.77
    congenital (early) A50.02 *[M90.80]*
    secondary A51.46
  tuberculous —*see* Tuberculosis, bone
  yaws (hypertrophic) (early) (late) A66.6
      [M90.80]
Periostosis (hyperplastic) —*see also* Disorder,
    bone, specified type NEC
  with osteomyelitis —*see* Osteomyelitis,
      specified type NEC
Peripartum
  cardiomyopathy O90.3
Periphlebitis —*see* Phlebitis
Periproctitis K62.89
Periprostatitis —*see* Prostatitis
Perirectal —*see* condition
Perirenal —*see* condition
Perisalpingitis —*see* Salpingo-oophoritis
Perisplenitis (infectional) D73.89
Peristalsis, visible or reversed R19.2
Peritendinitis —*see* Enthesopathy
Peritoneum, peritoneal —*see* condition
Peritonitis (adhesive) (bacterial) (fibrinous)
    (hemorrhagic) (idiopathic) (localized)
    (perforative) (primary) (with adhesions)
    (with effusion) K65.9
  with or following
    abscess K65.1
    appendicitis
      with perforation or rupture K35.32
      generalized *(see also* Appendicitis) K35.20
      localized *(see also* Appendicitis) K35.30
    diverticular disease (intestine) K57.80
      with bleeding K57.81
    ectopic or molar pregnancy O08.0
    large intestine K57.20
      with
        bleeding K57.21
        small intestine K57.40
          with bleeding K57.41
    small intestine K57.00
      with
        bleeding K57.01
        large intestine K57.40
          with bleeding K57.41

Peritonitis (Continued)
  acute (generalized) K65.0
  aseptic T81.61
  bile, biliary K65.3
  chemical T81.61
  chlamydial A74.81
  chronic proliferative K65.8
  complicating abortion —see Abortion, by
      type, complicated by, pelvic peritonitis
  congenital P78.1
  diaphragmatic K65.0
  diffuse K65.0
  diphtheritic A36.89
  disseminated K65.0
  due to
    bile K65.3
    foreign
      body or object accidentally left during
          a procedure (instrument) (sponge)
          (swab) T81.599
      substance accidentally left during a
          procedure (chemical) (powder)
          (talc) T81.61
    talc T81.61
    urine K65.8
  eosinophilic K65.8
    acute K65.0
  fibrocaseous (tuberculous) A18.31
  fibropurulent K65.0
  following ectopic or molar pregnancy
      O08.0
  general (ized) K65.0
  gonococcal A54.85
  meconium (newborn) P78.0
  neonatal P78.1
    meconium P78.0
  pancreatic K65.0
  paroxysmal, familial E85.0
    benign E85.0
  pelvic
    female N73.5
      acute N73.3
      chronic N73.4
        with adhesions N73.6
    male K65.0
  periodic, familial E85.0
  proliferative, chronic K65.8
  puerperal, postpartum, childbirth O85
  purulent K65.0
  septic K65.0
  specified NEC K65.8
  spontaneous bacterial K65.2
  subdiaphragmatic K65.0
  subphrenic K65.0
  suppurative K65.0
  syphilitic A52.74
    congenital (early) A50.08 [K67]
  talc T81.61
  tuberculous A18.31
  urine K65.8
Peritonsillar —see condition
Peritonsillitis J36
Perityphlitis K37
Periureteritis N28.89
Periurethral —see condition
Periurethritis (gangrenous) —see Urethritis
Periuterine —see condition
Perivaginitis —see Vaginitis
Perivasculitis, retinal H35.06-●
Perivasitis (chronic) N49.1
Perivesiculitis (seminal) —see Vesiculitis
Perlèche NEC K13.0
  due to
    candidiasis B37.83
    moniliasis B37.83
    riboflavin deficiency E53.0
    vitamin B2 (riboflavin) deficiency E53.0
Pernicious —see condition
Pernio, perniosis T69.1
Perpetrator (of abuse) —see Index to External
    Causes of Injury, Perpetrator

Persecution
  delusion F22
  social Z60.5
Perseveration (tonic) R48.8
Persistence, persistent (congenital)
  anal membrane Q42.3
    with fistula Q42.2
  arteria stapedia Q16.3
  atrioventricular canal Q21.2
  branchial cleft NOS Q18.2
    cyst Q18.0
    fistula Q18.0
    sinus Q18.0
  bulbus cordis in left ventricle Q21.8
  canal of Cloquet Q14.0
  capsule (opaque) Q12.8
  cilioretinal artery or vein Q14.8
  cloaca Q43.7
  communication —see Fistula, congenital
  convolutions
    aortic arch Q25.46
    fallopian tube Q50.6
    oviduct Q50.6
    uterine tube Q50.6
  double aortic arch Q25.45
  ductus arteriosus (Botalli) Q25.0
  fetal
    circulation P29.38
    form of cervix (uteri) Q51.828
    hemoglobin, hereditary (HPFH) D56.4
  foramen
    Botalli Q21.1
    ovale Q21.1
  Gartner's duct Q52.4
  hemoglobin, fetal (hereditary) (HPFH)
      D56.4
  hyaloid
    artery (generally incomplete) Q14.0
    system Q14.8
  hymen, in pregnancy or childbirth —see
      Pregnancy, complicated by, abnormal,
      vulva
  lanugo Q84.2
  left
    posterior cardinal vein Q26.8
    root with right arch of aorta Q25.49
    superior vena cava Q26.1
  Meckel's diverticulum Q43.0
    malignant —see Table of Neoplasms, small
        intestine, malignant
  mucosal disease (middle ear) —see
      Otitis, media, suppurative, chronic,
      tubotympanic
  nail(s), anomalous Q84.6
  omphalomesenteric duct Q43.0
  organ or site not listed —see Anomaly, by site
  ostium
    atrioventriculare commune Q21.2
    primum Q21.2
    secundum Q21.1
  ovarian rests in fallopian tube Q50.6
  pancreatic tissue in intestinal tract Q43.8
  primary (deciduous)
    teeth K00.6
    vitreous hyperplasia Q14.0
  pupillary membrane Q13.89
  rhesus (Rh)titer —see Complication(s),
      transfusion, incompatibility reaction, Rh
      (factor)
  right aortic arch Q25.47
  sinus
    urogenitalis
      female Q52.8
      male Q55.8
    venosus with imperfect incorporation in
        right auricle Q26.8
  thymus (gland) (hyperplasia) E32.0
  thyroglossal duct Q89.2
  thyrolingual duct Q89.2
  truncus arteriosus or communis Q20.0
  tunica vasculosa lentis Q12.2

Persistence, persistent (Continued)
  umbilical sinus Q64.4
  urachus Q64.4
  vitelline duct Q43.0
Person (with)
  admitted for clinical research, as a
      control subject (normal comparison)
      (participant) Z00.6
  awaiting admission to adequate facility
      elsewhere Z75.1
  concern (normal) about sick person in family
      Z63.6
  consulting on behalf of another Z71.0
  feigning illness Z76.5
  living (in)
    without
      adequate housing (heating) (space) Z59.1
    ➠housing (permanent) (temporary) Z59.00
      person able to render necessary care
          Z74.2
    ➠shelter Z59.02
    alone Z60.2
    boarding school Z59.3
    residential institution Z59.3
  on waiting list Z75.1
  sick or handicapped in family Z63.6
Personality (disorder) F60.9
  accentuation of traits (type A pattern) Z73.1
  affective F34.0
  aggressive F60.3
  amoral F60.2
  anacastic, anankastic F60.5
  antisocial F60.2
  anxious F60.6
  asocial F60.2
  asthenic F60.7
  avoidant F60.6
  borderline F60.3
  change due to organic condition (enduring)
      F07.0
  compulsive F60.5
  cycloid F34.0
  cyclothymic F34.0
  dependent F60.7
  depressive F34.1
  dissocial F60.2
  dual F44.81
  eccentric F60.89
  emotionally unstable F60.3
  expansive paranoid F60.0
  explosive F60.3
  fanatic F60.0
  haltlose type F60.89
  histrionic F60.4
  hyperthymic F34.0
  hypothymic F34.1
  hysterical F60.4
  immature F60.89
  inadequate F60.7
  labile (emotional) F60.3
  mixed (nonspecific) F60.89
  morally defective F60.2
  multiple F44.81
  narcissistic F60.81
  obsessional F60.5
  obsessive (-compulsive) F60.5
  organic F07.0
  overconscientious F60.5
  paranoid F60.0
  passive (-dependent) F60.7
  passive-aggressive F60.89
  pathologic F60.9
  pattern defect or disturbance F60.9
  pseudopsychopathic (organic) F07.0
  pseudoretarded (organic) F07.0
  psychoinfantile F60.4
  psychoneurotic NEC F60.89
  psychopathic F60.2
  querulant F60.0
  sadistic F60.89
  schizoid F60.1

Personality (Continued)
  self-defeating F60.89
  sensitive paranoid F60.0
  sociopathic (amoral) (antisocial) (asocial)
      (dissocial) F60.2
  specified NEC F60.89
  type A Z73.1
  unstable (emotional) F60.3
Perthes' disease —see Legg-Calvé-Perthes
    disease
Pertussis (see also Whooping cough) A37.90
Perversion, perverted
  appetite F50.89
    psychogenic F50.89
  function
    pituitary gland E23.2
      posterior lobe E22.2
  sense of smell and taste R43.8
    psychogenic F45.8
  sexual —see Deviation, sexual
Pervious, congenital —see also Imperfect, closure
    ductus arteriosus Q25.0
Pes (congenital) —see also Talipes
  acquired —see also Deformity, limb, foot,
      specified NEC
  planus —see Deformity, limb, flat foot
  adductus Q66.89
  cavus Q66.7-●
  deformity NEC, acquired —see Deformity,
      limb, foot, specified NEC
  planus (acquired) (any degree) —see also
      Deformity, limb, flat foot
    rachitic sequelae (late effect) E64.3
  valgus Q66.6
Pest, pestis —see Plague
Petechia, petechiae R23.3
  newborn P54.5
Petechial typhus A75.9
Peter's anomaly Q13.4
Petit mal seizure —see Epilepsy, childhood,
    absence
Petit's hernia —see Hernia, abdomen, specified
    site NEC
Petrellidosis B48.2
Petrositis H70.20-●
  acute H70.21-●
  chronic H70.22-●
Peutz-Jeghers disease or syndrome Q85.8
Peyronie's disease N48.6
PFAPA (periodic fever, aphthous stomatitis,
    pharyngitis, and adenopathy syndrome)
    M04.8
Pfeiffer's disease —see Mononucleosis,
    infectious
Phagedena (dry) (moist) (sloughing) —see also
    Gangrene
  geometric L88
  penis N48.29
  tropical —see Ulcer, skin
  vulva N76.6
Phagedenic —see condition
Phakoma H35.89
Phakomatosis —see also specific eponymous
    syndromes Q85.9
  Bourneville's Q85.1
  specified NEC Q85.8
Phantom limb syndrome (without pain) G54.7
  with pain G54.6
Pharyngeal pouch syndrome D82.1
Pharyngitis (acute) (catarrhal) (gangrenous)
      (infective) (malignant) (membranous)
      (phlegmonous) (pseudomembranous)
      (simple) (subacute) (suppurative)
      (ulcerative) (viral) J02.9
  with influenza, flu, or grippe —see Influenza,
      with, pharyngitis
  aphthous B08.5
  atrophic J31.2
  chlamydial A56.4
  chronic (atrophic) (granular) (hypertrophic)
      J31.2

Pharyngitis (Continued)
  coxsackievirus B08.5
  diphtheritic A36.0
  enteroviral vesicular B08.5
  follicular (chronic) J31.2
  fusospirochetal A69.1
  gonococcal A54.5
  granular (chronic) J31.2
  herpesviral B00.2
  hypertrophic J31.2
  infectional, chronic J31.2
  influenzal —see Influenza, with, respiratory
      manifestations NEC
  lymphonodular, acute (enteroviral) B08.8
  pneumococcal J02.8
  purulent J02.9
  putrid J02.9
  septic J02.0
  sicca J31.2
  specified organism NEC J02.8
  staphylococcal J02.8
  streptococcal J02.0
  syphilitic, congenital (early) A50.03
  tuberculous A15.8
  vesicular, enteroviral B08.5
  viral NEC J02.8
Pharyngoconjunctivitis, viral B30.2
Pharyngolaryngitis (acute) J06.0
  chronic J37.0
Pharyngoplegia J39.2
Pharyngotonsillitis, herpesviral B00.2
Pharyngotracheitis, chronic J42
Pharynx, pharyngeal —see condition
Phencyclidine-induced
  anxiety disorder F16.980
  bipolar and related disorder F16.94
  depressive disorder F16.94
  psychotic disorder F16.959
Phenomenon
  Arthus' —see Arthus' phenomenon
  jaw-winking Q07.8
  lupus erythematosus (LE) cell M32.9
  Raynaud's (secondary) I73.00
    with gangrene I73.01
  vasomotor R55
  vasospastic I73.9
  vasovagal R55
  Wenckebach's I44.1
Phenylketonuria E70.1
  classical E70.0
  maternal E70.1
Pheochromoblastoma
  specified site —see Neoplasm, malignant, by
      site
  unspecified site C74.10
Pheochromocytoma
  malignant
    specified site —see Neoplasm, malignant,
        by site
    unspecified site C74.10
  specified site —see Neoplasm, benign, by site
  unspecified site D35.00
Pheohyphomycosis —see Chromomycosis
Pheomycosis —see Chromomycosis
Phimosis (congenital) (due to infection) N47.1
  chancroidal A57
Phlebectasia —see also Varix
  congenital Q27.4
Phlebitis (infective) (pyemic) (septic)
      (suppurative) I80.9
  antepartum —see Thrombophlebitis,
      antepartum
  blue —see Phlebitis, leg, deep
  breast, superficial I80.8
  calf muscular vein (NOS) I80.25-●
  cavernous (venous) sinus —see Phlebitis,
      intracranial (venous) sinus
  cerebral (venous) sinus —see Phlebitis,
      intracranial (venous) sinus
  chest wall, superficial I80.8
  cranial (venous) sinus —see Phlebitis,
      intracranial (venous) sinus

Phlebitis (Continued)
  deep (vessels) —see Phlebitis, leg, deep
  due to implanted device —see Complications,
      by site and type, specified NEC
  during or resulting from a procedure T81.72
  femoral vein (superficial) I80.1-●
  femoropopliteal vein I80.0-●
  gastrocnemial vein I80.25-●
  gestational —see Phlebopathy, gestational
  hepatic veins I80.8
  iliac vein (common) (external) (internal)
      I80.21-●
  iliofemoral —see Phlebitis, femoral vein
  intracranial (venous) sinus (any) G08
    nonpyogenic I67.6
  intraspinal venous sinuses and veins G08
    nonpyogenic G95.19
  lateral (venous) sinus —see Phlebitis,
      intracranial (venous) sinus
  leg I80.3
    antepartum —see Thrombophlebitis,
        antepartum
    deep (vessels) NEC I80.20-●
      iliac I80.21-●
      popliteal vein I80.22-●
      specified vessel NEC I80.29-●
      tibial vein (anterior) (posterior) I80.23-●
    femoral vein (superficial) I80.1-●
    superficial (vessels) I80.0-●
  longitudinal sinus —see Phlebitis, intracranial
      (venous) sinus
  lower limb —see Phlebitis, leg
  migrans, migrating (superficial) I82.1
  pelvic
    with ectopic or molar pregnancy O08.0
    following ectopic or molar pregnancy O08.0
    puerperal, postpartum O87.1
  peroneal vein I80.24-●
  popliteal vein —see Phlebitis, leg, deep,
      popliteal
  portal (vein) K75.1
  postoperative T81.72
  pregnancy —see Thrombophlebitis,
      antepartum
  puerperal, postpartum, childbirth O87.0
    deep O87.1
    pelvic O87.1
    superficial O87.0
  retina —see Vasculitis, retina
  saphenous (accessory) (great) (long)
      (small) —see Phlebitis, leg, superficial
  sinus (meninges) —see Phlebitis, intracranial
      (venous) sinus
  soleal vein I80.25-●
  specified site NEC I80.8
  syphilitic A52.09
  tibial vein —see Phlebitis, leg, deep, tibial
  ulcerative I80.9
    leg —see Phlebitis, leg
  umbilicus I80.8
  uterus (septic) —see Endometritis
  varicose (leg) (lower limb) —see Varix, leg,
      with, inflammation
Phlebofibrosis I87.8
Phleboliths I87.8
Phlebopathy
  gestational O22.9-●
  puerperal O87.9
Phlebosclerosis I87.8
Phlebothrombosis —see also Thrombosis
  antepartum —see Thrombophlebitis,
      antepartum
  pregnancy —see Thrombophlebitis,
      antepartum
  puerperal —see Thrombophlebitis, puerperal
Phlebotomus fever A93.1
Phlegmasia
  alba dolens O87.1
    nonpuerperal —see Phlebitis, femoral vein
  cerulea dolens —see Phlebitis, leg, deep
Phlegmon —see Abscess
Phlegmonous —see condition

Phlyctenulosis (allergic) (keratoconjunctivitis) (nontuberculous) —see also Keratoconjunctivitis
  cornea —see Keratoconjunctivitis
  tuberculous A18.52
Phobia, phobic F40.9
  animal F40.218
    spiders F40.210
  examination F40.298
  reaction F40.9
  simple F40.298
  social F40.10
    generalized F40.11
  specific (isolated) F40.298
    animal F40.218
      spiders F40.210
    blood F40.230
    injection F40.231
    injury F40.233
    men F40.290
    natural environment F40.228
      thunderstorms F40.220
    situational F40.248
      bridges F40.242
      closed in spaces F40.240
      flying F40.243
      heights F40.241
    specified focus NEC F40.298
    transfusion F40.231
    women F40.291
  specified NEC F40.8
    medical care NEC F40.232
  state F40.9
Phocas' disease —see Mastopathy, cystic
Phocomelia Q73.1
  lower limb —see Agenesis, leg, with foot present
  upper limb —see Agenesis, arm, with hand present
Phoria H50.50
Phosphate-losing tubular disorder N25.0
Phosphatemia E83.39
Phosphaturia E83.39
Photodermatitis (sun) L56.8
  chronic L57.8
  due to drug L56.8
  light other than sun L59.8
Photokeratitis H16.13-●
Photophobia H53.14-●
Photophthalmia —see Photokeratitis
Photopsia H53.19
Photoretinitis —see Retinopathy, solar
Photosensitivity, photosensitization (sun) skin L56.8
  light other than sun L59.8
Phrenitis —see Encephalitis
Phrynoderma (vitamin A deficiency) E50.8
Phthiriasis (pubis) B85.3
  with any infestation classifiable to B85.0-B85.2 B85.4
Phthirus infestation —see Phthiriasis
Phthisis —see also Tuberculosis
  bulbi (infectional) —see Disorder, globe, degenerated condition, atrophy
  eyeball (due to infection) —see Disorder, globe, degenerated condition, atrophy
Phycomycosis —see Zygomycosis
Physalopteriasis B81.8
Physical restraint status Z78.1
Phytobezoar T18.9
  intestine T18.3
  stomach T18.2
Pian —see Yaws
Pianoma A66.1
Pica F50.89
  in adults F50.89
  infant or child F98.3
Picking, nose F98.8
Pick-Niemann disease —see Niemann-Pick disease or syndrome

Pick's
  cerebral atrophy G31.01 [F02.80]
    with behavioral disturbance G31.01 [F02.81]
  disease or syndrome (brain) G31.01 [F02.80]
    with behavioral disturbance G31.01 [F02.81]
    brain G31.01 [F02.80]
      with behavioral disturbance G31.01 [F02.81]
    pericardium (pericardial pseudocirrhosis of liver) I31.1
  syndrome
    brain G31.01 [F02.80]
      with behavioral disturbance G31.01 [F02.81]
    of heart (pericardial pseudocirrhosis of liver) I31.1
Pickwickian syndrome E66.2
Piebaldism E70.39
Piedra (beard) (scalp) B36.8
  black B36.3
  white B36.2
Pierre Robin deformity or syndrome Q87.0
Pierson's disease or osteochondrosis M91.0
Pig-bel A05.2
Pigeon
  breast or chest (acquired) M95.4
    congenital Q67.7
    rachitic sequelae (late effect) E64.3
  breeder's disease or lung J67.2
  fancier's disease or lung J67.2
  toe —see Deformity, toe, specified NEC
Pigmentation (abnormal) (anomaly) L81.9
  conjunctiva H11.13-●
  cornea (anterior) H18.01-●
    posterior H18.05-●
    stromal H18.06-●
  diminished melanin formation NEC L81.6
  iron L81.8
  lids, congenital Q82.8
  limbus corneae —see Pigmentation, cornea
  metals L81.8
  optic papilla, congenital Q14.2
  retina, congenital (grouped) (nevoid) Q14.1
  scrotum, congenital Q82.8
  tattoo L81.8
Piles —see also Hemorrhoids K64.9
Pili
  annulati or torti (congenital) Q84.1
  incarnati L73.1
Pill roller hand (intrinsic) —see Parkinsonism
Pilomatrixoma —see Neoplasm, skin, benign
  malignant —see Neoplasm, skin, malignant
Pilonidal —see condition
Pimple R23.8
PIMS M35.81
PIN —see Neoplasia, intraepithelial, prostate
Pinched nerve —see Neuropathy, entrapment
Pindborg tumor —see Cyst, calcifying odontogenic
Pineal body or gland —see condition
Pinealoblastoma C75.3
Pinealoma D44.5
  malignant C75.3
Pineoblastoma C75.3
Pineocytoma D44.5
Pinguecula H11.15-●
Pingueculitis H10.81-●
Pinhole meatus —see also Stricture, urethra N35.919
Pink
  disease —see subcategory T56.1
  eye —see Conjunctivitis, acute, mucopurulent
Pinkus' disease (lichen nitidus) L44.1
Pinpoint
  meatus —see Stricture, urethra
  os (uteri) —see Stricture, cervix
Pins and needles R20.2
Pinta A67.9
  cardiovascular lesions A67.2
  chancre (primary) A67.0

Pinta (Continued)
  erythematous plaques A67.1
  hyperchromic lesions A67.1
  hyperkeratosis A67.1
  lesions A67.9
    cardiovascular A67.2
    hyperchromic A67.1
    intermediate A67.1
    late A67.2
    mixed A67.3
    primary A67.0
    skin (achromic) (cicatricial) (dyschromic) A67.2
      hyperchromic A67.1
      mixed (achromic and hyperchromic) A67.3
  papule (primary) A67.0
  skin lesions (achromic) (cicatricial) (dyschromic) A67.2
    hyperchromic A67.1
    mixed (achromic and hyperchromic) A67.3
  vitiligo A67.2
Pintids A67.1
Pinworm (disease) (infection) (infestation) B80
Piroplasmosis (see also Babesiosis) B60.00
  specified NEC B60.09
Pistol wound —see Gunshot wound
Pitchers' elbow —see Derangement, joint, specified type NEC, elbow
Pithecoid pelvis Q74.2
  with disproportion (fetopelvic) O33.0
    causing obstructed labor O65.0
Pithiatism F48.8
Pitted —see Pitting
Pitting —see also Edema R60.9
  lip R60.0
  nail L60.8
  teeth K00.4
Pituitary gland —see condition
Pituitary-snuff-taker's disease J67.8
Pityriasis (capitis) L21.0
  alba L30.5
  circinata (et maculata) L42
  furfuracea L21.0
  Hebra's L26
  lichenoides L41.0
    chronica L41.1
    et varioliformis (acuta) L41.0
  maculata (et circinata) L30.5
  nigra B36.1
  pilaris, Hebra's L44.0
  rosea L42
  rotunda L44.8
  rubra (Hebra) pilaris L44.0
  simplex L30.5
  specified type NEC L30.5
  streptogenes L30.5
  versicolor (scrotal) B36.0
Placenta, placental —see Pregnancy, complicated by (care of) (management affected by), specified condition
Placentitis O41.14-●
Plagiocephaly Q67.3
Plague A20.9
  abortive A20.8
  ambulatory A20.8
  asymptomatic A20.8
  bubonic A20.0
  cellulocutaneous A20.1
  cutaneobubonic A20.1
  lymphatic gland A20.0
  meningitis A20.3
  pharyngeal A20.8
  pneumonic (primary) (secondary) A20.2
  pulmonary, pulmonic A20.2
  septicemic A20.7
  tonsillar A20.8
    septicemic A20.7
Planning, family
  contraception Z30.9
  procreation Z31.69

▶ New   ⇛ Revised   ~~deleted~~ Deleted   ● Use Additional Character(s)

Plaque(s)
  artery, arterial —see Arteriosclerosis
  calcareous —see Calcification
  coronary, lipid rich I25.83
  epicardial I31.8
  erythematous, of pinta A67.1
  Hollenhorst's —see Occlusion, artery, retina
  lipid rich, coronary I25.83
  pleural (without asbestos) J92.9
    with asbestos J92.0
  tongue K13.29
Plasmacytoma C90.3-●
  extramedullary C90.2-●
  medullary C90.0-●
  solitary C90.3-●
Plasmacytopenia D72.818
Plasmacytosis D72.822
Plaster ulcer —see Ulcer, pressure, by site
Plateau iris syndrome (post-iridectomy)
    (postprocedural) (without glaucoma)
    H21.82
  with glaucoma H40.22-●
Platybasia Q75.8
Platyonychia (congenital) Q84.6
  acquired L60.8
Platypelloid pelvis M95.5
  with disproportion (fetopelvic) O33.0
    causing obstructed labor O65.0
  congenital Q74.2
Platyspondylisis Q76.49
Plaut (-Vincent) disease —see also Vincent's
    A69.1
Plethora R23.2
  newborn P61.1
Pleura, pleural —see condition
Pleuralgia R07.81
Pleurisy (acute) (adhesive) (chronic) (costal)
    (diaphragmatic) (double) (dry) (fibrinous)
    (fibrous) (interlobar) (latent) (plastic)
    (primary) (residual) (sicca) (sterile)
    (subacute) (unresolved) R09.1
  with
    adherent pleura J86.0
    effusion J90
      chylous, chyliform J94.0
      tuberculous (non primary) A15.6
        primary (progressive) A15.7
      tuberculosis —see Pleurisy, tuberculous
        (non primary)
  encysted —see Pleurisy, with effusion
  exudative —see Pleurisy, with effusion
  fibrinopurulent, fibropurulent —see
    Pyothorax
  hemorrhagic —see Hemothorax
  pneumococcal J90
  purulent —see Pyothorax
  septic —see Pyothorax
  serofibrinous —see Pleurisy, with effusion
  seropurulent —see Pyothorax
  serous —see Pleurisy, with effusion
  staphylococcal J86.9
  streptococcal J90
  suppurative —see Pyothorax
  traumatic (post) (current) —see Injury,
    intrathoracic, pleura
  tuberculous (with effusion) (non primary)
    A15.6
    primary (progressive) A15.7
Pleuritis sicca —see Pleurisy
Pleurobronchopneumonia —see Pneumonia,
    broncho
Pleurodynia R07.81
  epidemic B33.0
  viral B33.0
Pleuropericarditis —see also Pericarditis
  acute I30.9
Pleuropneumonia (acute) (bilateral) (double)
    (septic) —see also Pneumonia J18.8
  chronic —see Fibrosis, lung
Pleuro-pneumonia-like-organism (PPLO), as
    cause of disease classified elsewhere B96.0

Pleurorrhea —see Pleurisy, with effusion
Plexitis, brachial G54.0
Plica
  polonica B85.0
  syndrome, knee M67.5
  tonsil J35.8
Plicated tongue K14.5
Plug
  bronchus NEC J98.09
  meconium (newborn) NEC syndrome
    P76.0
  mucus —see Asphyxia, mucus
Plumbism —see subcategory T56.0
Plummer's disease E05.20
  with thyroid storm E05.21
Plummer-Vinson syndrome D50.1
Pluricarential syndrome of infancy E40
Plus (and minus) hand (intrinsic) —see
    Deformity, limb, specified type NEC,
    forearm
PMEI (polymorphic epilepsy in infancy)
    G40.83-●
Pneumathemia —see Air, embolism
Pneumatic hammer (drill) syndrome T75.21
Pneumatocele (lung) J98.4
  intracranial G93.89
  tension J44.9
Pneumatosis
  cystoides intestinalis K63.89
  intestinalis K63.89
  peritonei K66.8
Pneumaturia R39.89
Pneumoblastoma —see Neoplasm, lung,
    malignant
Pneumocephalus G93.89
Pneumococcemia A40.3
Pneumococcus, pneumococcal —see condition
Pneumoconiosis (due to) (inhalation of) J64
  with tuberculosis (any type in A15) J65
  aluminum J63.0
  asbestos J61
  bagasse, bagassosis J67.1
  bauxite J63.1
  beryllium J63.2
  coal miners' (simple) J60
  coalworkers' (simple) J60
  collier's J60
  cotton dust J66.0
  diatomite (diatomaceous earth) J62.8
  dust
    inorganic NEC J63.6
    lime J62.8
    marble J62.8
    organic NEC J66.8
  fumes or vapors (from silo) J68.9
  graphite J63.3
  grinder's J62.8
  kaolin J62.8
  mica J62.8
  millstone maker's J62.8
  mineral fibers NEC J61
  miner's J60
  moldy hay J67.0
  potter's J62.8
  rheumatoid —see Rheumatoid, lung
  sandblaster's J62.8
  silica, silicate NEC J62.8
    with carbon J60
  stonemason's J62.8
  talc (dust) J62.0
Pneumocystis carinii pneumonia B59
Pneumocystis jiroveci (pneumonia) B59
Pneumocystosis (with pneumonia) B59
Pneumohemopericardium I31.2
Pneumohemothorax J94.2
  traumatic S27.2
Pneumohydropericardium —see Pericarditis
Pneumohydrothorax —see Hydrothorax
Pneumomediastinum J98.2
  congenital or perinatal P25.2
Pneumomycosis B49 [J99]

Pneumonia (acute) (double) (migratory)
    (purulent) (septic) (unresolved) J18.9
  with
    influenza —see Influenza, with, pneumonia
    lung abscess J85.1
      due to specified organism —see
        Pneumonia, in (due to)
  2019 (novel) coronavirus J12.82
  adenoviral J12.0
  adynamic J18.2
  alba A50.04
  allergic (see also Pneumonitis,
      hypersensitivity) J82.89
  alveolar —see Pneumonia, lobar
  anaerobes J15.8
  anthrax A22.1
  apex, apical —see Pneumonia, lobar
  Ascaris B77.81
  aspiration J69.0
    due to
      aspiration of microorganisms
        bacterial J15.9
        viral J12.9
      food (regurgitated) J69.0
      gastric secretions J69.0
      milk (regurgitated) J69.0
      oils, essences J69.1
      solids, liquids NEC J69.8
      vomitus J69.0
    newborn P24.81
      amniotic fluid (clear) P24.11
      blood P24.21
      food (regurgitated) P24.31
      liquor (amnii) P24.11
      meconium P24.01
      milk P24.31
      mucus P24.11
      specified NEC P24.81
      stomach contents P24.31
    postprocedural J95.4
  atypical NEC J18.9
  bacillus J15.9
    specified NEC J15.8
  bacterial J15.9
    specified NEC J15.8
  Bacteroides (fragilis) (oralis)
      (melaninogenicus) J15.8
  basal, basic, basilar —see Pneumonia, by type
  bronchiolitis obliterans organized (BOOP)
      J84.89
  broncho-, bronchial (confluent) (croupous)
      (diffuse) (disseminated) (hemorrhagic)
      (involving lobes) (lobar) (terminal) J18.0
    allergic (see also Pneumonitis,
        hypersensitivity) J82.89
    aspiration —see Pneumonia, aspiration
    bacterial J15.9
      specified NEC J15.8
    chronic —see Fibrosis, lung
    diplococcal J13
    Eaton's agent J15.7
    Escherichia coli (E. coli) J15.5
    Friedländer's bacillus J15.0
    Hemophilus influenzae J14
    hypostatic J18.2
    inhalation —see also Pneumonia, aspiration
      due to fumes or vapors (chemical) J68.0
      of oils or essences J69.1
    Klebsiella (pneumoniae) J15.0
    lipid, lipoid J69.1
      endogenous J84.89
    Mycoplasma (pneumoniae) J15.7
    pleuro-pneumonia-like-organisms (PPLO)
        J15.7
    pneumococcal J13
    Proteus J15.6
    Pseudomonas J15.1
    Serratia marcescens J15.6
    specified organism NEC J16.8
    staphylococcal —see Pneumonia,
        staphylococcal

Pneumonia (Continued)
  broncho-, bronchial (Continued)
    streptococcal NEC J15.4
      group B J15.3
      pneumoniae J13
    viral, virus —see Pneumonia, viral
  Butyrivibrio (fibriosolvens) J15.8
  Candida B37.1
  caseous —see Tuberculosis, pulmonary
  catarrhal —see Pneumonia, broncho
  chlamydial J16.0
    congenital P23.1
  cholesterol J84.89
  cirrhotic (chronic) —see Fibrosis, lung
  Clostridium (haemolyticum) (novyi) J15.8
  confluent —see Pneumonia, broncho
  congenital (infective) P23.9
    due to
      bacterium NEC P23.6
      Chlamydia P23.1
      Escherichia coli P23.4
      Haemophilus influenzae P23.6
      infective organism NEC P23.8
      Klebsiella pneumoniae P23.6
      Mycoplasma P23.6
      Pseudomonas P23.5
      Staphylococcus P23.2
      Streptococcus (except group B) P23.6
        group B P23.3
      viral agent P23.0
    specified NEC P23.8
  coronavirus (novel) (disease) 2019 J12.82
  COVID-19 J12.82
  croupous —see Pneumonia, lobar
  cryptogenic organizing J84.116
  cytomegalic inclusion B25.0
  cytomegaloviral B25.0
  deglutition —see Pneumonia, aspiration
  desquamative interstitial J84.117
  diffuse —see Pneumonia, broncho
  diplococcal, diplococcus (broncho-) (lobar) J13
  disseminated (focal) —see Pneumonia, broncho
  Eaton's agent J15.7
  embolic, embolism —see Embolism,
      pulmonary
  Enterobacter J15.6
  eosinophilic J82.81
    acute J82.82
    chronic J82.81
  Escherichia coli (E. coli) J15.5
  Eubacterium J15.8
  fibrinous —see Pneumonia, lobar
  fibroid, fibrous (chronic) —see Fibrosis, lung
  Friedländer's bacillus J15.0
  Fusobacterium (nucleatum) J15.8
  gangrenous J85.0
  giant cell (measles) B05.2
  gonococcal A54.84
  gram-negative bacteria NEC J15.6
    anaerobic J15.8
  Hemophilus influenzae (broncho) (lobar) J14
  human metapneumovirus J12.3
  hypostatic (broncho) (lobar) J18.2
  in (due to)
    actinomycosis A42.0
    adenovirus J12.0
    anthrax A22.1
    ascariasis B77.81
    aspergillosis B44.9
    Bacillus anthracis A22.1
    Bacterium anitratum J15.6
    candidiasis B37.1
    chickenpox B01.2
    Chlamydia J16.0
      neonatal P23.1
    coccidioidomycosis B38.2
      acute B38.0
      chronic B38.1
    cytomegalovirus disease B25.0
    Diplococcus (pneumoniae) J13
    Eaton's agent J15.7

Pneumonia (Continued)
  in (Continued)
    Enterobacter J15.6
    Escherichia coli (E. coli) J15.5
    Friedländer's bacillus J15.0
    fumes and vapors (chemical) (inhalation)
        J68.0
    gonorrhea A54.84
    Hemophilus influenzae (H. influenzae) J14
    Herellea J15.6
    histoplasmosis B39.2
      acute B39.0
      chronic B39.1
    human metapneumovirus J12.3
    Klebsiella (pneumoniae) J15.0
    measles B05.2
    Mycoplasma (pneumoniae) J15.7
    nocardiosis, nocardiasis A43.0
    ornithosis A70
    parainfluenza virus J12.2
    pleuro-pneumonia-like-organism (PPLO)
        J15.7
    pneumococcus J13
    pneumocystosis (Pneumocystis carinii)
        (Pneumocystis jiroveci) B59
    Proteus J15.6
    Pseudomonas NEC J15.1
      pseudomallei A24.1
    psittacosis A70
    Q fever A78
    respiratory syncytial virus (RSV) J12.1
    rheumatic fever I00 [J17]
    rubella B06.81
    Salmonella (infection) A02.22
      typhi A01.03
    schistosomiasis B65.9 [J17]
    Serratia marcescens J15.6
    specified
      bacterium NEC J15.8
      organism NEC J16.8
    spirochetal NEC A69.8
    Staphylococcus J15.20
      aureus (methicillin susceptible) (MSSA)
          J15.211
        methicillin resistant (MRSA) J15.212
      specified NEC J15.29
    Streptococcus J15.4
      group B J15.3
      pneumoniae J13
      specified NEC J15.4
    toxoplasmosis B58.3
    tularemia A21.2
    typhoid (fever) A01.03
    varicella B01.2
    virus —see Pneumonia, viral
    whooping cough A37.91
      due to
        Bordetella parapertussis A37.11
        Bordetella pertussis A37.01
        specified NEC A37.81
    Yersinia pestis A20.2
  inhalation of food or vomit —see Pneumonia,
      aspiration
  interstitial J84.9
    chronic J84.111
    desquamative J84.117
    due to
      collagen vascular disease J84.178
      known underlying cause J84.178
    idiopathic NOS J84.111
    in disease classified elsewhere J84.178
    lymphocytic (due to collagen vascular
        disease) (in diseases classified
        elsewhere) J84.178
    lymphoid J84.2
    non-specific J84.89
      due to
        collagen vascular disease J84.178
        known underlying cause J84.178
      idiopathic J84.113
      in diseases classified elsewhere J84.178

Pneumonia (Continued)
  interstitial (Continued)
    plasma cell B59
    pseudomonas J15.1
    usual J84.112
      due to collagen vascular disease J84.178
      idiopathic J84.112
      in diseases classified elsewhere J84.178
  Klebsiella (pneumoniae) J15.0
  lipid, lipoid (exogenous) J69.1
    endogenous J84.89
  lobar (disseminated) (double) (interstitial)
      J18.1
    bacterial J15.9
      specified NEC J15.8
    chronic —see Fibrosis, lung
    Escherichia coli (E. coli) J15.5
    Friedländer's bacillus J15.0
    Hemophilus influenzae J14
    hypostatic J18.2
    Klebsiella (pneumoniae) J15.0
    pneumococcal J13
    Proteus J15.6
    Pseudomonas J15.1
    specified organism NEC J16.8
    staphylococcal —see Pneumonia,
        staphylococcal
    streptococcal NEC J15.4
    Streptococcus pneumoniae J13
    viral, virus —see Pneumonia, viral
  lobular —see Pneumonia, broncho
  Löffler's J82.89
  lymphoid interstitial J84.2
  massive —see Pneumonia, lobar
  meconium P24.01
  MRSA (Methicillin resistant Staphylococcus
      aureus) J15.212
  MSSA (methicillin susceptible Staphylococcus
      aureus) J15.211
  multilobar —see Pneumonia, by type
  Mycoplasma (pneumoniae) J15.7
  necrotic J85.0
  neonatal P23.9
    aspiration —see Aspiration, by substance,
        with pneumonia
  nitrogen dioxide J68.0
  organizing J84.89
    due to
      collagen vascular disease J84.178
      known underlying cause J84.178
    in diseases classified elsewhere J84.178
  orthostatic J18.2
  parainfluenza virus J12.2
  parenchymatous —see Fibrosis, lung
  passive J18.2
  patchy —see Pneumonia, broncho
  Peptococcus J15.8
  Peptostreptococcus J15.8
  plasma cell (of infants) B59
  pleurolobar —see Pneumonia, lobar
  pleuro-pneumonia-like organism (PPLO) J15.7
  pneumococcal (broncho) (lobar) J13
  Pneumocystis (carinii) (jiroveci) B59
  postinfectional NEC B99 [J17]
  postmeasles B05.2
  Proteus J15.6
  Pseudomonas J15.1
  psittacosis A70
  radiation J70.0
    respiratory syncytial virus (RSV) J12.1
  resulting from a procedure J95.89
  rheumatic I00 [J17]
  Salmonella (arizonae) (cholerae-suis)
      (enteritidis) (typhimurium) A02.22
    typhi A01.03
    typhoid fever A01.03
  SARS-associated coronavirus J12.81
  SARS-CoV-2 J12.82
  segmented, segmental —see Pneumonia,
      broncho-•
  Serratia marcescens J15.6

Pneumonia *(Continued)*
  specified NEC J18.8
    bacterium NEC J15.8
    organism NEC J16.8
    virus NEC J12.89
  spirochetal NEC A69.8
  staphylococcal (broncho) (lobar) J15.20
    aureus (methicillin susceptible) (MSSA)
      J15.211
      methicillin resistant (MRSA) J15.212
    specified NEC J15.29
  static, stasis J18.2
  streptococcal NEC (broncho) (lobar) J15.4
    group
      A J15.4
      B J15.3
      specified NEC J15.4
  Streptococcus pneumoniae J13
  syphilitic, congenital (early) A50.04
  traumatic (complication) (early) (secondary)
    T79.8
  tuberculous (any) —*see* Tuberculosis,
    pulmonary
  tularemic A21.2
  varicella B01.2
  Veillonella J15.8
  ventilator associated J95.851
  viral, virus (broncho) (interstitial) (lobar) J12.9
    adenoviral J12.0
    congenital P23.0
    human metapneumovirus J12.3
    parainfluenza J12.2
    respiratory syncytial (RSV) J12.1
    SARS-associated coronavirus J12.81
    specified NEC J12.89
  white (congenital) A50.04
Pneumonic —*see* condition
Pneumonitis (acute) (primary) —*see also*
    Pneumonia
  air-conditioner J67.7
  allergic (due to) J67.9
    organic dust NEC J67.8
    red cedar dust J67.8
    sequoiosis J67.8
    wood dust J67.8
  aspiration J69.0
    due to
      anesthesia J95.4
        during
          labor and delivery O74.0
          pregnancy O29.01-●
          puerperium O89.01
      fumes or gases J68.0
      obstetric O74.0
  chemical (due to gases, fumes or vapors)
    (inhalation) J68.0
    due to anesthesia J95.4
  cholesterol J84.89
  chronic —*see* Fibrosis, lung
  congenital rubella P35.0
  crack (cocaine) J68.0
  due to
    beryllium J68.0
    cadmium J68.0
    crack (cocaine) J68.0
    detergent J69.8
    fluorocarbon-polymer J68.0
    food, vomit (aspiration) J69.0
    fumes or vapors J68.0
    gases, fumes or vapors (inhalation) J68.0
    inhalation
      blood J69.8
      essences J69.1
      food (regurgitated), milk, vomit J69.0
      oils, essences J69.1
      saliva J69.0
      solids, liquids NEC J69.8
    manganese J68.0
    nitrogen dioxide J68.0
    oils, essences J69.1
    solids, liquids NEC J69.8

Pneumonitis *(Continued)*
  due to *(Continued)*
    toxoplasmosis (acquired) B58.3
      congenital P37.1
    vanadium J68.0
    ventilator J95.851
  eosinophilic J82.81
    acute J82.82
    chronic J82.81
  hypersensitivity J67.9
    air conditioner lung J67.7
    bagassosis J67.1
    bird fancier's lung J67.2
    farmer's lung J67.0
    maltworker's lung J67.4
    maple bark-stripper's lung J67.6
    mushroom worker's lung J67.5
    specified organic dust NEC J67.8
    suberosis J67.3
  interstitial (chronic) J84.89
    acute J84.114
    lymphoid J84.2
    non-specific J84.89
      idiopathic J84.113
  lymphoid, interstitial J84.2
  meconium P24.01
  postanesthetic J95.4
    correct substance properly administered —
      see Table of Drugs and Chemcials, by
      drug, adverse effect
    in labor and delivery O74.0
    in pregnancy O29.01-●
    obstetric O74.0
    overdose or wrong substance given or taken
      (by accident) —*see* Table of Drugs and
      Chemicals, by drug, poisoning
    postpartum, puerperal O89.01
  postoperative J95.4
    obstetric O74.0
  radiation J70.0
  rubella, congenital P35.0
  ventilation (air-conditioning) J67.7
  ventilator associated J95.851
  wood-dust J67.8
Pneumonoconiosis —*see* Pneumoconiosis
Pneumoparotid K11.8
Pneumopathy NEC J98.4
  alveolar J84.09
  due to organic dust NEC J66.8
  parietoalveolar J84.09
Pneumopericarditis —*see also* Pericarditis
  acute I30.9
Pneumopericardium —*see also* Pericarditis
  congenital P25.3
  newborn P25.3
  traumatic (post) —*see* Injury, heart
Pneumophagia (psychogenic) F45.8
Pneumopleurisy, pneumopleuritis —*see also*
    Pneumonia J18.8
Pneumopyopericardium I30.1
Pneumopyothorax —*see* Pyopneumothorax
  with fistula J86.0
Pneumorrhagia —*see also* Hemorrhage, lung
  tuberculous —*see* Tuberculosis, pulmonary
Pneumothorax NOS J93.9
  acute J93.83
  chronic J93.81
  congenital P25.1
  perinatal period P25.1
  postprocedural J95.811
  specified NEC J93.83
  spontaneous NOS J93.83
    newborn P25.1
    primary J93.11
    secondary J93.12
    tension J93.0
  tense valvular, infectional J93.0
  tension (spontaneous) J93.0
  traumatic S27.0
    with hemothorax S27.2
  tuberculous —*see* Tuberculosis, pulmonary

Podagra —*see also* Gout M10.9
Podencephalus Q01.9
Poikilocytosis R71.8
Poikiloderma L81.6
  Civatte's L57.3
  congenital Q82.8
  vasculare atrophicans L94.5
Poikilodermatomyositis M33.10
  with
    myopathy M33.12
    respiratory involvement M33.11
    specified organ involvement NEC M33.19
Pointed ear (congenital) Q17.3
Poison ivy, oak, sumac or other plant
    dermatitis (allergic) (contact) L23.7
Poisoning (acute) —*see also* Table of Drugs and
    Chemicals
  algae and toxins T65.82-●
  Bacillus B (aertrycke) (cholerae (suis))
    (paratyphosus) (suipestifer) A02.9
    botulinus A05.1
  bacterial toxins A05.9
  berries, noxious —*see* Poisoning, food,
    noxious, berries
  botulism A05.1
  ciguatera fish T61.0-●
  Clostridium botulinum A05.1
  death-cap (Amanita phalloides) (Amanita
    verna) —*see* Poisoning, food, noxious,
    mushrooms
  drug —*see* Table of Drugs and Chemicals, by
    drug, poisoning
  epidemic, fish (noxious) —*see* Poisoning,
    seafood
    bacterial A05.9
  fava bean D55.0
  fish (noxious) T61.9-●
    bacterial —*see* Intoxication, foodborne, by
      agent
    ciguatera fish —*see* Poisoning, ciguatera
      fish
    scombroid fish —*see* Poisoning, scombroid
      fish
    specified type NEC T61.77-●
  food NEC A05.9
    bacterial —*see* Intoxication, foodborne, by
      agent
    due to
      Bacillus (aertrycke) (choleraesuis)
        (paratyphosus) (suipestifer) A02.9
        botulinus A05.1
      Clostridium (perfringens) (Welchii)
        A05.2
      salmonella (aertrycke) (callinarum)
        (choleraesuis) (enteritidis)
        (paratyphi) (suipestifer) A02.9
        with
          gastroenteritis A02.0
          sepsis A02.1
      staphylococcus A05.0
      Vibrio
        parahaemolyticus A05.3
        vulnificus A05.5
    noxious or naturally toxic T62.9-●
      berries —*see* subcategory T62.1-●
      fish —*see* Poisoning, seafood
      mushrooms —*see* subcategory T62.0X-●
      plants NEC —*see* subcategory T62.2X-●
      seafood —*see* Poisoning, seafood
      specified NEC —*see* subcategory
        T62.8X-●
  ichthyotoxism —*see* Poisoning, seafood
  kreotoxism, food A05.9
  latex T65.81-●
  lead T56.0-●
  mushroom —*see* Poisoning, food, noxious,
    mushroom
  mussels —*see also* Poisoning, shellfish
    bacterial —*see* Intoxication, foodborne, by
      agent
  nicotine (tobacco) T65.2-●

Poisoning (Continued)
  noxious foodstuffs —see Poisoning, food,
    noxious
  plants, noxious —see Poisoning, food,
    noxious, plants NEC
  ptomaine —see Poisoning, food
  radiation J70.0
  Salmonella (arizonae) (cholerae-suis)
    (enteritidis) (typhimurium) A02.9
  scombroid fish T61.1-•
  seafood (noxious) T61.9-•
    bacterial —see Intoxication, foodborne, by
      agent
    fish —see Poisoning, fish
    shellfish —see Poisoning, shellfish
    specified NEC —see subcategory T61.8X-•
  shellfish (amnesic) (azaspiracid) (diarrheic)
    (neurotoxic) (noxious) (paralytic)
    T61.78-•
    bacterial —see Intoxication, foodborne, by
      agent
    ciguatera mollusk —see Poisoning,
      ciguatera fish
  specified substance NEC T65.891
  Staphylococcus, food A05.0
  tobacco (nicotine) T65.2-•
  water E87.79
Poker spine —see Spondylitis, ankylosing
Poland syndrome Q79.8
Polioencephalitis (acute) (bulbar) A80.9
  inferior G12.22
  influenzal —see Influenza, with,
    encephalopathy
  superior hemorrhagic (acute) (Wernicke's)
    E51.2
  Wernicke's E51.2
Polioencephalomyelitis (acute) (anterior) A80.9
  with beriberi E51.2
Polioencephalopathy, superior hemorrhagic
  E51.2
  with
    beriberi E51.11
    pellagra E52
Poliomeningoencephalitis —see
  Meningoencephalitis
Poliomyelitis (acute) (anterior) (epidemic) A80.9
  with paralysis (bulbar) —see Poliomyelitis,
    paralytic
  abortive A80.4
  ascending (progressive) —see Poliomyelitis,
    paralytic
  bulbar (paralytic) —see Poliomyelitis,
    paralytic
  congenital P35.8
  nonepidemic A80.9
  nonparalytic A80.4
  paralytic A80.30
    specified NEC A80.39
    vaccine-associated A80.0
    wild virus
      imported A80.1
      indigenous A80.2
  spinal, acute A80.9
Poliosis (eyebrow) (eyelashes) L67.1
  circumscripta, acquired L67.1
Pollakiuria R35.0
  psychogenic F45.8
Pollinosis J30.1
Pollitzer's disease L73.2
Polyadenitis —see also Lymphadenitis
  malignant A20.0
Polyalgia M79.89
Polyangiitis M30.0
  microscopic M31.7
  overlap syndrome M30.8
Polyarteritis
  microscopic M31.7
  nodosa M30.0
    with lung involvement M30.1
    juvenile M30.2
    related condition NEC M30.8

Polyarthralgia —see Pain, joint
Polyarthritis, polyarthropathy —see also
  Arthritis M13.0
  due to or associated with other specified
    conditions —see Arthritis
  epidemic (Australian) (with exanthema) B33.1
  infective —see Arthritis, pyogenic or pyemic
  inflammatory M06.4
  juvenile (chronic) (seronegative) M08.3
  migratory M13.8-•
  rheumatic, acute —see Fever, rheumatic
Polyarthrosis M15.9
  post-traumatic M15.3
  primary M15.0
  specified NEC M15.8
Polycarential syndrome of infancy E40
Polychondritis (atrophic) (chronic) —see also
  Disorder, cartilage, specified type NEC
  relapsing M94.1
Polycoria Q13.2
Polycystic (disease)
  degeneration, kidney Q61.3
    autosomal dominant (adult type) Q61.2
    autosomal recessive (infantile type) NEC
      Q61.19
  kidney Q61.3
    autosomal
      dominant Q61.2
      recessive NEC Q61.19
    autosomal dominant (adult type) Q61.2
    autosomal recessive (childhood type) NEC
      Q61.19
    infantile type NEC Q61.19
  liver Q44.6
  lung J98.4
    congenital Q33.0
  ovary, ovaries E28.2
  spleen Q89.09
Polycythemia (secondary) D75.1
  acquired D75.1
  benign (familial) D75.0
  due to
    donor twin P61.1
    erythropoietin D75.1
    fall in plasma volume D75.1
    high altitude D75.1
    maternal-fetal transfusion P61.1
    stress D75.1
  emotional D75.1
  erythropoietin D75.1
  familial (benign) D75.0
  Gaisböck's (hypertonica) D75.1
  high altitude D75.1
  hypertonica D75.1
  hypoxemic D75.1
  neonatorum P61.1
  nephrogenous D75.1
  relative D75.1
  secondary D75.1
  spurious D75.1
  stress D75.1
  vera D45
Polycytosis cryptogenica D75.1
Polydactylism, polydactyly Q69.9
  toes Q69.2
Polydipsia R63.1
Polydystrophy, pseudo-Hurler E77.0
Polyembryoma —see Neoplasm, malignant,
  by site
Polyglandular
  deficiency E31.0
  dyscrasia E31.9
  dysfunction E31.9
  syndrome E31.8
Polyhydramnios O40.-•
Polymastia Q83.1
Polymenorrhea N92.0
Polymyalgia M35.3
  arteritica, giant cell M31.5
  rheumatica M35.3
    with giant cell arteritis M31.5

Polymyositis (acute) (chronic) (hemorrhagic)
  M33.20
  with
    myopathy M33.22
    respiratory involvement M33.21
    skin involvement —see
      Dermatopolymyositis
    specified organ involvement NEC M33.29
  ossificans (generalisata) (progressiva) —see
    Myositis, ossificans, progressiva
Polyneuritis, polyneuritic —see also
  Polyneuropathy
  acute (post-)infective G61.0
  alcoholic G62.1
  cranialis G52.7
  demyelinating, chronic inflammatory (CIDP)
    G61.81
  diabetic —see Diabetes, polyneuropathy
  diphtheritic A36.83
  due to lack of vitamin NEC E56.9 [G63]
  endemic E51.11
  erythredema —see subcategory T56.1
  febrile, acute G61.0
  hereditary ataxic G60.1
  idiopathic, acute G61.0
  infective (acute) G61.0
  inflammatory, chronic demyelinating (CIDP)
    G61.81
  nutritional E63.9 [G63]
  postinfective (acute) G61.0
  specified NEC G62.89
Polyneuropathy (peripheral) G62.9
  alcoholic G62.1
  amyloid (Portuguese) E85.1 [G63]
    transthyretin-related (ATTR) familial E85.1
  arsenical E85.1 [G63]
  critical illness G62.81
  demyelinating, chronic inflammatory (CIDP)
    G61.81
  diabetic —see Diabetes, polyneuropathy
  drug-induced G62.0
  hereditary G60.9
    specified NEC G60.8
  idiopathic G60.9
    progressive G60.3
  in (due to)
    alcohol G62.1
      sequelae G65.2
    amyloidosis, familial (Portuguese) E85.1
      [G63]
    antitetanus serum G61.1
    arsenic G62.2
      sequelae G65.2
    avitaminosis NEC E56.9 [G63]
    beriberi E51.11
    collagen vascular disease NEC M35.9 [G63]
    deficiency (of)
      B (-complex) vitamins E53.9 [G63]
      vitamin B6 E53.1 [G63]
    diabetes —see Diabetes, polyneuropathy
    diphtheria A36.83
    drug or medicament G62.0
      correct substance properly
        administered —see Table of Drugs
        and Chemicals, by drug, adverse
        effect
      overdose or wrong substance given
        or taken —see Table of Drugs and
        Chemicals, by drug, poisoning
    endocrine disease NEC E34.9 [G63]
    herpes zoster B02.23
    hypoglycemia E16.2 [G63]
    infectious
      disease NEC B99 [G63]
      mononucleosis B27.91
    lack of vitamin NEC E56.9 [G63]
    lead G62.2
      sequelae G65.2
    leprosy A30.9 [G63]
    Lyme disease A69.22
    metabolic disease NEC E88.9 [G63]

▶ New   ⇒ Revised   ~~deleted~~ Deleted   • Use Additional Character(s)

Polyneuropathy (Continued)
in (Continued)
microscopic polyangiitis M31.7 [G63]
mumps B26.84
neoplastic disease —see also Neoplasm
D49.9 [G63]
nutritional deficiency NEC E63.9 [G63]
organophosphate compounds G62.2
sequelae G65.2
parasitic disease NEC B89 [G63]
pellagra E52 [G63]
polyarteritis nodosa M30.0
porphyria E80.20 [G63]
radiation G62.82
rheumatoid arthritis —see Rheumatoid,
polyneuropathy
sarcoidosis D86.89
serum G61.1
syphilis (late) A52.15
congenital A50.43
systemic
connective tissue disorder M35.9 [G63]
lupus erythematosus M32.19
toxic agent NEC G62.2
sequelae G65.2
transthyretin-related (ATTR) familial
amyloid E85.1
triorthocresyl phosphate G62.2
sequelae G65.2
tuberculosis A17.89
uremia N18.9 [G63]
vitamin B12 deficiency E53.8 [G63]
with anemia (pernicious) D51.0 [G63]
due to dietary deficiency D51.3 [G63]
zoster B02.23
inflammatory G61.9
chronic demyelinating (CIDP) G61.81
sequelae G65.1
specified NEC G61.89
lead G62.2
sequelae G65.2
nutritional NEC E63.9 [G63]
postherpetic (zoster) B02.23
progressive G60.3
radiation-induced G62.82
sensory (hereditary) (idiopathic) G60.8
specified NEC G62.89
syphilitic (late) A52.15
congenital A50.43
Polyopia H53.8
Polyorchism, polyorchidism Q55.21
Polyosteoarthritis —see also Osteoarthritis,
generalized M15.9-•
post-traumatic M15.3
specified NEC M15.8
Polyostotic fibrous dysplasia Q78.1
Polyotia Q17.0
Polyp, polypus
accessory sinus J33.8
adenocarcinoma in —see Neoplasm,
malignant, by site
adenocarcinoma in situ in —see Neoplasm, in
situ, by site
adenoid tissue J33.0
adenomatous —see also Neoplasm, benign,
by site
adenocarcinoma in —see Neoplasm,
malignant, by site
adenocarcinoma in situ in —see Neoplasm,
in situ, by site
carcinoma in —see Neoplasm, malignant,
by site
carcinoma in situ in —see Neoplasm, in
situ, by site
multiple —see Neoplasm, benign
adenocarcinoma in —see Neoplasm,
malignant, by site
adenocarcinoma in situ in —see
Neoplasm, in situ, by site
antrum J33.8
anus, anal (canal) K62.0
Bartholin's gland N84.3
bladder D41.4

Polyp, polypus (Continued)
carcinoma in —see Neoplasm, malignant, by
site
carcinoma in situ in —see Neoplasm, in situ,
by site
cecum D12.0
cervix (uteri) N84.1
in pregnancy or childbirth —see Pregnancy,
complicated by, abnormal, cervix
mucous N84.1
nonneoplastic N84.1
choanal J33.0
cholesterol K82.4
clitoris N84.3
colon K63.5
adenomatous D12.6
ascending D12.6
cecum D12.0
descending D12.4
▶ascending K63.5
▶sigmoid D12.5
▶transverse D12.3
▶cecum K63.5
▶descending K63.5
inflammatory K51.40
with
abscess K51.414
complication K51.419
specified NEC K51.418
fistula K51.413
intestinal obstruction K51.412
rectal bleeding K51.411
sigmoid D12.5
transverse D12.3
corpus uteri N84.0
dental K04.01
irreversible K04.02
reversible K04.01
duodenum K31.7
ear (middle) H74.4-•
endometrium N84.0
▶esophageal K22.81
▶esophagogastric junction K22.82
ethmoidal (sinus) J33.8
fallopian tube N84.8
female genital tract N84.9
specified NEC N84.8
frontal (sinus) J33.8
gallbladder K82.4
gingiva, gum K06.8
hyperplastic, (any site) K63.5
labia, labium (majus) (minus) N84.3
larynx (mucous) J38.1
adenomatous D14.1
malignant —see Neoplasm, malignant, by site
maxillary (sinus) J33.8
middle ear —see Polyp, ear (middle)
myometrium N84.0
nares
anterior J33.9
posterior J33.0
nasal (mucous) J33.9
cavity J33.0
septum J33.0
nasopharyngeal J33.0
nose (mucous) J33.9
oviduct N84.8
pharynx J39.2
placenta O90.89
prostate —see Enlargement, enlarged,
prostate
pudenda, pudendum N84.3
pulpal (dental) K04.01
irreversible K04.02
reversible K04.01
rectum (nonadenomatous) K62.1
adenomatous —see Polyp, adenomatous
septum (nasal) J33.0
sinus (accessory) (ethmoidal) (frontal)
(maxillary) (sphenoidal) J33.8
sphenoidal (sinus) J33.8
stomach K31.7
adenomatous D13.1

Polyp, polypus (Continued)
tube, fallopian N84.8
turbinate, mucous membrane J33.8
umbilical, newborn P83.6
ureter N28.89
urethra N36.2
uterus (body) (corpus) (mucous) N84.0
cervix N84.1
in pregnancy or childbirth —see Pregnancy,
complicated by, tumor, uterus
vagina N84.2
vocal cord (mucous) J38.1
vulva N84.3
Polyphagia R63.2
Polyploidy Q92.7
Polypoid —see condition
Polyposis —see also Polyp
coli (adenomatous) D12.6
adenocarcinoma in C18.9
adenocarcinoma in situ in —see Neoplasm,
in situ, by site
carcinoma in C18.9
colon (adenomatous) D12.6
familial D12.6
adenocarcinoma in situ in —see Neoplasm,
in situ, by site
intestinal (adenomatous) D12.6
malignant lymphomatous C83.1
multiple, adenomatous —see also Neoplasm,
benign D36.9
Polyradiculitis —see Polyneuropathy
Polyradiculoneuropathy (acute) (postinfective)
(segmentally demyelinating) G61.0
Polyserositis
due to pericarditis I31.1
pericardial I31.1
periodic, familial E85.0
tuberculous A19.9
acute A19.1
chronic A19.8
Polysplenia syndrome Q89.09
Polysyndactyly —see also Syndactylism,
syndactyly Q70.4
Polytrichia L68.3
Polyunguia Q84.6
➡Polyuria R35.89
➡nocturnal R35.81
psychogenic F45.8
▶specified NEC R35.89
Pompe's disease (glycogen storage) E74.02
Pompholyx L30.1
Poncet's disease (tuberculous rheumatism)
A18.09
Pond fracture —see Fracture, skull
Ponos B55.0
Pons, pontine —see condition
Poor
aesthetic of existing restoration of tooth
K08.56
contractions, labor O62.2
gingival margin to tooth restoration K08.51
personal hygiene R46.0
prenatal care, affecting management of
pregnancy —see Pregnancy, complicated
by, insufficient, prenatal care
sucking reflex (newborn) R29.2
urinary stream R39.12
vision NEC H54.7
Poradenitis, nostras inguinalis or venerea
A55
Porencephaly (congenital) (developmental)
(true) Q04.6
acquired G93.0
nondevelopmental G93.0
traumatic (post) F07.89
Porocephaliasis B88.8
Porokeratosis Q82.8
Poroma, eccrine —see Neoplasm, skin, benign
Porphyria (South African) E80.20
acquired E80.20
acute intermittent (hepatic) (Swedish)
E80.21

Porphyria (Continued)
  cutanea tarda (hereditary) (symptomatic) E80.1
  due to drugs E80.20
    correct substance properly administered —
      see Table of Drugs and Chemicals, by
      drug, adverse effect
    overdose or wrong substance given
      or taken —see Table of Drugs and
      Chemicals, by drug, poisoning
  erythropoietic (congenital) (hereditary) E80.0
  hepatocutaneous type E80.1
  secondary E80.20
  toxic NEC E80.20
  variegata E80.20
Porphyrinuria —see Porphyria
Porphyruria —see Porphyria
Portal —see condition
Port wine nevus, mark, or stain Q82.5
Posadas-Wernicke disease B38.9
Positive
  culture (nonspecific)
    blood R78.81
    bronchial washings R84.5
    cerebrospinal fluid R83.5
    cervix uteri R87.5
    nasal secretions R84.5
    nipple discharge R89.5
    nose R84.5
      staphylococcus (Methicillin susceptible)
        Z22.321
        Methicillin resistant Z22.322
    peritoneal fluid R85.5
    pleural fluid R84.5
    prostatic secretions R86.5
    saliva R85.5
    seminal fluid R86.5
    sputum R84.5
    synovial fluid R89.5
    throat scrapings R84.5
    urine R82.79
    vagina R87.5
    vulva R87.5
    wound secretions R89.5
  PPD (skin test) R76.11
  serology for syphilis A53.0
    with signs or symptoms - code as Syphilis,
      by site and stage
    false R76.8
  skin test, tuberculin (without active
    tuberculosis) R76.11
  test, human immunodeficiency virus (HIV)
    R75
  VDRL A53.0
    with signs or symptoms - code by site and
      stage under Syphilis A53.9
  Wassermann reaction A53.0
▶ **Post COVID-19 condition, unspecified** U09.9
Postcardiotomy syndrome I97.0
Postcaval ureter Q62.62
Postcholecystectomy syndrome K91.5
Postclimacteric bleeding N95.0
Postcommissurotomy syndrome I97.0
Postconcussional syndrome F07.81
Postcontusional syndrome F07.81
Postcricoid region —see condition
Post-dates (40-42 weeks) (pregnancy) (mother)
  O48.0
  more than 42 weeks gestation O48.1
Postencephalitic syndrome F07.89
Posterior —see condition
Posterolateral sclerosis (spinal cord) —see
  Degeneration, combined
Postexanthematous —see condition
Postfebrile —see condition
Postgastrectomy dumping syndrome K91.1
Posthemiplegic chorea —see Monoplegia
Posthemorrhagic anemia (chronic) D50.0
  acute D62
  newborn P61.3
Postherpetic neuralgia (zoster) B02.29
  trigeminal B02.22

Posthitis N47.7
Postimmunization complication or reaction —
  see Complications, vaccination
Postinfectious —see condition
Postlaminectomy syndrome NEC M96.1
Postleukotomy syndrome F07.0
Postmastectomy lymphedema (syndrome) I97.2
Postmaturity, postmature (over 42 weeks)
  maternal (over 42 weeks gestation) O48.1
  newborn P08.22
Postmeasles complication NEC —see also
  condition B05.89
Postmenopausal
  endometrium (atrophic) N95.8
    suppurative —see also Endometritis N71.9
  osteoporosis —see Osteoporosis,
    postmenopausal
Postnasal drip R09.82
  due to
    allergic rhinitis —see Rhinitis, allergic
    common cold J00
    gastroesophageal reflux —see Reflux,
      gastroesophageal
    nasopharyngitis —see Nasopharyngitis
    other know condition — code to condition
    sinusitis —see Sinusitis
Postnatal —see condition
Postoperative (postprocedural) —see
  Complication, postoperative
  pneumothorax, therapeutic Z98.3
  state NEC Z98.890
Postpancreatectomy hyperglycemia E89.1
Postpartum —see Puerperal
Postphlebitic syndrome —see Syndrome,
  postthrombotic
Postpolio (myelitic) **syndrome** G14
Postpoliomyelitic —see also condition
  osteopathy —see Osteopathy, after
    poliomyelitis
Postprocedural —see also Postoperative
  hypoinsulinemia E89.1
Postschizophrenic depression F32.89
Postsurgery status —see also Status (post)
  pneumothorax, therapeutic Z98.3
Post-term (40-42 weeks) (pregnancy) (mother)
  O48.0
  infant P08.21
  more than 42 weeks gestation (mother) O48.1
Post-traumatic brain syndrome, nonpsychotic
  F07.81
Post-typhoid abscess A01.09
Postures, hysterical F44.2
Postvaccinal reaction or complication —see
  Complications, vaccination
Postvalvulotomy syndrome I97.0
Potain's
  disease (pulmonary edema) —see Edema, lung
  syndrome (gastrectasis with dyspepsia) K31.0
Potter's
  asthma J62.8
  facies Q60.6
  lung J62.8
  syndrome (with renal agenesis) Q60.6
Pott's
  curvature (spinal) A18.01
  disease or paraplegia A18.01
  spinal curvature A18.01
  tumor, puffy —see Osteomyelitis, specified
    type NEC
Pouch
  bronchus Q32.4
  Douglas' —see condition
  esophagus, esophageal, congenital Q39.6
    acquired K22.5
  gastric K31.4
  Hartmann's K82.8
  pharynx, pharyngeal (congenital) Q38.7
Pouchitis K91.850
Poultrymen's itch B88.0
Poverty NEC Z59.6
  extreme Z59.5

Poxvirus NEC B08.8
Prader-Willi syndrome Q87.11
Prader-Willi-like syndrome Q87.11
Preauricular appendage or tag Q17.0
Prebetalipoproteinemia (acquired) (essential)
  (familial) (hereditary) (primary)
  (secondary) E78.1
  with chylomicronemia E78.3
Precipitate labor or delivery O62.3
Preclimacteric bleeding (menorrhagia) N92.4
Precocious
  adrenarche E30.1
  menarche E30.1
  menstruation E30.1
  pubarche E30.1
  puberty E30.1
    central E22.8
  sexual development NEC E30.1
  thelarche E30.8
Precocity, sexual (constitutional) (cryptogenic)
  (female) (idiopathic) (male) E30.1
  with adrenal hyperplasia E25.9
    congenital E25.0
Precordial pain R07.2
Predeciduous teeth K00.2
Prediabetes, prediabetic R73.03
  complicating
    pregnancy —see Pregnancy, complicated
      by, diseases of, specified type or
      system NEC
    puerperium O99.893
Predislocation status of hip at birth Q65.6
Pre-eclampsia O14.9-●
  with pre-existing hypertension —see
    Hypertension, complicating pregnancy,
    pre-existing, with, pre-eclampsia
  complicating
    childbirth O14.94
    puerperium O14.95
  mild O14.0-●
    complicating
      childbirth O14.04
      puerperium O14.05
  moderate O14.0-●
    complicating
      childbirth O14.04
      puerperium O14.05
  severe O14.1-●
    with hemolysis, elevated liver enzymes
      and low platelet count (HELLP)
      O14.2-●
      complicating
        childbirth O14.24
        puerperium O14.25
    complicating
      childbirth O14.14
      puerperium O14.15
Pre-eruptive color change, teeth, tooth K00.8
Pre-excitation atrioventricular conduction I45.6
Preglaucoma H40.00-●
Pregnancy (single) (uterine) —see also Delivery
  and Puerperal Z33.1

Note: The Tabular must be reviewed for
assignment of the appropriate character
indicating the trimester of the pregnancy

Note: The Tabular must be reviewed for
assignment of appropriate seventh character
for multiple gestation codes in Chapter 15

---

  abdominal (ectopic) O00.00
    with intrauterine pregnancy O00.01
      with viable fetus O36.7-●
  ampullar O00.10-●
    with intrauterine pregnancy O00.11-●
  biochemical O02.81
  broad ligament O00.80
    with intrauterine pregnancy O00.81
  cervical O00.80
    with intrauterine pregnancy O00.81

Pregnancy *(Continued)*
 chemical O02.81
 complicated NOS O26.9-●
 complicated by (care of) (management
    affected by)
  abnormal, abnormality
   cervix O34.4-●
    causing obstructed labor O65.5
   cord (umbilical) O69.9
   fetal heart rate or rhythm O36.83-●
   findings on antenatal screening of
       mother O28.9
    biochemical O28.1
    chromosomal O28.5
    cytological O28.2
    genetic O28.5
    hematological O28.0
    radiological O28.4
    specified NEC O28.8
    ultrasonic O28.3
   glucose (tolerance) NEC O99.810
   pelvic organs O34.9-●
    specified NEC O34.8-●
     causing obstructed labor O65.5
   pelvis (bony) (major) NEC O33.0
   perineum O34.7-●
   position
    placenta O44.0-●
     with hemorrhage O44.1-●
    uterus O34.59-●
   uterus O34.59-●
    causing obstructed labor O65.5
    congenital O34.0-●
   vagina O34.6-●
    causing obstructed labor O65.5
   vulva O34.7-●
    causing obstructed labor O65.5
  abruptio placentae —*see* Abruptio
      placentae
  abscess or cellulitis
   bladder O23.1-●
   breast O91.11-●
   genital organ or tract O23.9-●
  abuse
   physical O9A.31-●
   psychological O9A.51-●
   sexual O9A.41-●
  adverse effect anesthesia O29.9-●
   aspiration pneumonitis O29.01-●
   cardiac arrest O29.11-●
   cardiac complication NEC O29.19-●
   cardiac failure O29.12-●
   central nervous system complication
       NEC O29.29-●
   cerebral anoxia O29.21-●
   failed or difficult intubation O29.6-●
   inhalation of stomach contents or
       secretions NOS O29.01-●
   local, toxic reaction O29.3X
   Mendelson's syndrome O29.01-●
   pressure collapse of lung O29.02-●
   pulmonary complications NEC O29.09-●
   specified NEC O29.8X
   spinal and epidural type NEC O29.5X
    induced headache O29.4-●
  albuminuria —*see also* Proteinuria,
      gestational O12.1-●
  alcohol use O99.31-●
  amnionitis O41.12-●
  anaphylactoid syndrome of pregnancy
      O88.01-●
  anemia (conditions in D50-D64) (pre-
      existing) O99.01-●
   complicating the puerperium O99.03
  antepartum hemorrhage O46.9-●
   with coagulation defect —*see*
       Hemorrhage, antepartum, with
       coagulation defect
   specified NEC O46.8X-●
  appendicitis O99.61-●
  atrophy (yellow) (acute) liver (subacute)
      O26.61-●

Pregnancy *(Continued)*
 complicated by *(Continued)*
  bariatric surgery status O99.84-●
  bicornis or bicornuate uterus O34.0-●
  biliary tract problems O26.61-●
  breech presentation O32.1
  cardiovascular diseases (conditions in
      I00-I09, I20-I52, I70-I99) O99.41-●
  cerebrovascular disorders (conditions in
      I60-I69) O99.41-●
  cervical shortening O26.87-●
  cervicitis O23.51-●
  cesarean scar defect (isthmocele) O34.22
  chloasma (gravidarum) O26.89-●
  cholecystitis O99.61-●
  cholestasis (intrahepatic) O26.61-●
  chorioamnionitis O41.12-●
  circulatory system disorder (conditions in
      I00-I09, I20-I99, O99.41-●)
  compound presentation O32.6
  conjoined twins O30.02-●
  connective system disorders (conditions in
      M00-M99) O99.891
  contracted pelvis (general) O33.1
   inlet O33.2
   outlet O33.3
  convulsions (eclamptic) (uremic) —*see also*
      Eclampsia O15.9-●
  cracked nipple O92.11-●
  cystitis O23.1-●
  cystocele O34.8-●
  death of fetus (near term) O36.4
   early pregnancy O02.1
   of one fetus or more in multiple
       gestation O31.2-●
  deciduitis O41.14-●
  decreased fetal movement O36.81-●
  dental problems O99.61-●
  diabetes (mellitus) O24.91-●
   gestational (pregnancy induced) —*see*
       Diabetes, gestational
   pre-existing O24.31-●
    specified NEC O24.81-●
    type 1 O24.01-●
    type 2 O24.11-●
  digestive system disorders (conditions in
      K00-K93) O99.61-●
  diseases of —*see* Pregnancy, complicated
      by, specified body system disease
   biliary tract O26.61-●
   blood NEC (conditions in D65-D77)
       O99.11-●
   liver O26.61-●
   specified NEC O99.891
  disorders of —*see* Pregnancy, complicated
      by, specified body system disorder
   amniotic fluid and membranes
       O41.9-●
    specified NEC O41.8X-●
   biliary tract O26.61-●
   ear and mastoid process (conditions in
       H60-H95) O99.891
   eye and adnexa (conditions in H00-H59)
       O99.891
   liver O26.61-●
   skin (conditions in L00-L99) O99.71-●
   specified NEC O99.891
  displacement, uterus NEC O34.59-●
   causing obstructed labor O65.5
  disproportion (due to) O33.9
   fetal (ascites) (hydrops)
       (meningomyelocele) (sacral
       teratoma) (tumor) deformities NEC
       O33.7
   generally contracted pelvis O33.1
   hydrocephalic fetus O33.6
   inlet contraction of pelvis O33.2
   mixed maternal and fetal origin O33.4
   specified NEC O33.8
  double uterus O34.0-●
   causing obstructed labor O65.5
  drug use (conditions in F11-F19) O99.32-●

Pregnancy *(Continued)*
 complicated by *(Continued)*
  eclampsia, eclamptic (coma) (convulsions)
      (delirium) (nephritis) (uremia) (*see also*
      Eclampsia) O15-●
  ectopic pregnancy —*see* Pregnancy, ectopic
  edema O12.0-●
   with
    gestational hypertension, mild —*see
        also* Pre-eclampsia O14.0-●
    proteinuria O12.2-●
  effusion, amniotic fluid —*see* Pregnancy,
      complicated by, premature rupture of
      membranes
  elderly
   multigravida O09.52-●
   primigravida O09.51-●
  embolism —*see also* Embolism, obstetric,
      pregnancy O88.-●
  endocrine diseases NEC O99.28-●
  endometritis O86.12
  excessive weight gain O26.0-●
  exhaustion O26.81-●
   during labor and delivery O75.81
  face presentation O32.3
  failed induction of labor O61.9
  failed or difficult intubation for anesthesia
      O29.6-●
   instrumental O61.1
   mechanical O61.1
   medical O61.0
   specified NEC O61.8
   surgical O61.1
  false labor (pains) O47.9
   at or after 37 completed weeks of
       pregnancy O47.1
   before 37 completed weeks of pregnancy
       O47.0-●
  fatigue O26.81-●
   during labor and delivery O75.81
  fatty metamorphosis of liver O26.61-●
  female genital mutilation O34.8-● [N90.81-●]
  fetal (maternal care for)
   abnormality or damage O35.9
    acid-base balance O68
    specified type NEC O35.8
   acidemia O68
   acidosis O68
   alkalosis O68
   anemia and thrombocytopenia O36.82-●
   anencephaly O35.0
   bradycardia O36.83-●
   chromosomal abnormality (conditions in
       Q90-Q99) O35.1
   conjoined twins O30.02-●
   damage from
    amniocentesis O35.7
    biopsy procedures O35.7
    drug addiction O35.5
    hematological investigation O35.7
    intrauterine contraceptive device O35.7
    maternal
     alcohol addiction O35.4
     cytomegalovirus infection O35.3
     disease NEC O35.8
     drug addiction O35.5
     listeriosis O35.8
     rubella O35.3
     toxoplasmosis O35.8
     viral infection O35.3
    medical procedure NEC O35.7
    radiation O35.6
   death (near term) O36.4
    early pregnancy O02.1
   decreased movement O36.81-●
   depressed heart rate tones O36.83-●
   disproportion due to deformity (fetal)
       O33.7
   excessive growth (large for dates) O36.6-●
   growth retardation O36.59-●
    light for dates O36.59-●
    small for dates O36.59-●

Pregnancy *(Continued)*
  complicated by *(Continued)*
    fetal *(Continued)*
      heart rate irregularity (abnormal
          variability) (bradycardia)
          (decelerations) (tachycardia)
          O36.83-●
      hereditary disease O35.2
      hydrocephalus O35.Ø
      intrauterine death O36.4
      non-reassuring heart rate or rhythm
          O36.83-●
      poor growth O36.59-●
        light for dates O36.59-●
        small for dates O36.59-●
      problem O36.9-●
        specified NEC O36.89-●
      reduction (elective) O31.3-●
      selective termination O31.3-●
      spina bifida O35.Ø
      thrombocytopenia O36.82-●
    fibroid (tumor) (uterus) O34.1-●
    fissure of nipple O92.11-●
    gallstones O99.61-●
    gastric banding status O99.84-●
    gastric bypass status O99.84-●
    genital herpes (asymptomatic) (history of)
        (inactive) O98.3-●
    genital tract infection O23.9-●
    glomerular diseases (conditions in
        NØØ-NØ7) O26.83-●
      with hypertension, pre-existing —*see*
          Hypertension, complicating,
          pregnancy, pre-existing, with, renal
          disease
    gonorrhea O98.21-●
    grand multiparity OØ9.4
    habitual aborter —*see* Pregnancy,
        complicated by, recurrent pregnancy
        loss
    HELLP syndrome (hemolysis, elevated
        liver enzymes and low platelet count)
        O14.2-●
    hemorrhage
      antepartum —*see* Hemorrhage,
          antepartum
      before 2Ø completed weeks gestation
          O2Ø.9
        specified NEC O2Ø.8
      due to premature separation, placenta —
          see also Abruptio placentae O45.9-●
      early O2Ø.9
        specified NEC O2Ø.8
      threatened abortion O2Ø.Ø
    hemorrhoids O22.4-●
    hepatitis (viral) O98.41-●
    herniation of uterus O34.59-●
    high
      head at term O32.4
      risk —*see* Supervision (of) (for),
          high-risk
    history of in utero procedure during
        previous pregnancy OØ9.82-●
    HIV O98.71-●
    human immunodeficiency virus (HIV)
        disease O98.71-●
    hydatidiform mole —*see also* Mole,
        hydatidiform OØ1.9-●
    hydramnios O4Ø.-●
    hydrocephalic fetus (disproportion) O33.6
    hydrops
      amnii O4Ø.-●
      fetalis O36.2-●
        associated with isoimmunization —*see
            also* Pregnancy, complicated by,
            isoimmunization O36.11-●
    hydrorrhea O42.9Ø
    hyperemesis (gravidarum) (mild) —*see also*
        Hyperemesis, gravidarum O21.Ø-●
    hypertension —*see* Hypertension,
        complicating pregnancy

Pregnancy *(Continued)*
  complicated by *(Continued)*
    hypertensive
      heart and renal disease, pre-existing —
          see Hypertension, complicating,
          pregnancy, pre-existing, with, heart
          disease, with renal disease
      heart disease, pre-existing —*see*
          Hypertension, complicating,
          pregnancy, pre-existing, with, heart
          disease
      renal disease, pre-existing —*see*
          Hypertension, complicating,
          pregnancy, pre-existing, with, renal
          disease
    hypotension O26.5-●
    immune disorders NEC (conditions in
        D8Ø-D89) O99.11-●
    incarceration, uterus O34.51-●
    incompetent cervix O34.3-●
    inconclusive fetal viability O36.8Ø
    infection(s) O98.91-●
      amniotic fluid or sac O41.1Ø-●
      bladder O23.1-●
      carrier state NEC O99.83Ø
        streptococcus B O99.82Ø
      genital organ or tract O23.9-●
        specified NEC O23.59-●
      genitourinary tract O23.9-●
      gonorrhea O98.21-●
      hepatitis (viral) O98.41-●
      HIV O98.71-●
      human immunodeficiency virus (HIV)
          O98.71-●
      ▶intrauterine O41.12
      kidney O23.Ø-●
      nipple O91.Ø1-●
      parasitic disease O98.91-●
        specified NEC O98.81-●
      protozoal disease O98.61-●
      sexually transmitted NEC O98.31-●
      specified type NEC O98.81-●
      syphilis O98.11-●
      tuberculosis O98.Ø1-●
      urethra O23.2-●
      urinary (tract) O23.4-●
        specified NEC O23.3-●
      viral disease O98.51-●
    ▶inflammation
      ▶intrauterine O41.12
    injury or poisoning (conditions in SØØ-T88)
        O9A.21-●
      due to abuse
        physical O9A.31-●
        psychological O9A.51-●
        sexual O9A.41-●
    insufficient
      prenatal care OØ9.3-●
      weight gain O26.1-●
    insulin resistance O26.89
    intrauterine fetal death (near term) O36.4
      early pregnancy OØ2.1
      multiple gestation (one fetus or more)
          O31.2-●
    isoimmunization O36.11-●
      anti-A sensitization O36.11-●
      anti-B sensitization O36.19-●
      Rh O36.Ø9-●
        anti-D antibody O36.Ø1-●
      specified NEC O36.19-●
    laceration of uterus NEC O71.81
    malformation
      placenta, placental (vessel) O43.1Ø-●
        specified NEC O43.19-●
      uterus (congenital) O34.Ø-●
    malnutrition (conditions in E4Ø-E46) O25.1-●
    maternal hypotension syndrome O26.5-●
    mental disorders (conditions in FØ1-FØ9,
        F2Ø-F52 and F54-F99) O99.34-●
      alcohol use O99.31-●
      drug use O99.32-●
      smoking O99.33-●
    mentum presentation O32.3

Pregnancy *(Continued)*
  complicated by *(Continued)*
    metabolic disorders O99.28-●
    missed
      abortion OØ2.1
      delivery O36.4
    multiple gestations O3Ø.9-●
      conjoined twins O3Ø.Ø2-●
      quadruplet —*see* Pregnancy, quadruplet
      specified complication NEC O31.8X-●
      specified number of multiples NEC —*see*
          Pregnancy, multiple (gestation),
          specified NEC
      triplet —*see* Pregnancy, triplet
      twin —*see* Pregnancy, twin
    musculoskeletal condition (conditions is
        MØØ-M99) O99.891
    necrosis, liver (conditions in K72) O26.61-●
    neoplasm
      benign
        cervix O34.4-●
        corpus uteri O34.1-●
        uterus O34.1-●
      malignant O9A.11-●
    nephropathy NEC O26.83-●
    nervous system condition (conditions in
        GØØ-G99) O99.35-●
    nutritional diseases NEC O99.28-●
    obesity (pre-existing) O99.21-●
    obesity surgery status O99.84-●
    oblique lie or presentation O32.2
    older mother —*see* Pregnancy, complicated
        by, elderly
    oligohydramnios O41.Ø-●
      with premature rupture of
          membranes —*see also* Pregnancy,
          complicated by, premature rupture
          of membranes O42-●
    onset (spontaneous) of labor after 37
        completed weeks of gestation but
        before 39 completed weeks gestation,
        with delivery by (planned) cesarean
        section O75.82
    oophoritis O23.52-●
    overdose, drug —*see also* Table of Drugs
        and Chemicals, by drug, poisoning
        O9A.21-●
    oversize fetus O33.5
    papyraceous fetus O31.Ø-●
    pelvic inflammatory disease O99.891
    periodontal disease O99.61-●
    peripheral neuritis O26.82-●
    peritoneal (pelvic) adhesions O99.891
    phlebitis O22.9-●
    phlebopathy O22.9-●
    phlebothrombosis (superficial) O22.2-●
      deep O22.3-●
    placenta accreta O43.21-●
    placenta increta O43.22-●
    placenta percreta O43.23-●
    placenta previa O44.Ø-●
      complete O44.Ø-●
        with hemorrhage O44.1-●
      marginal O44.2-●
        with hemorrhage O44.3-●
      partial O44.2-●
        with hemorrhage O44.3-●
    placental disorder O43.9-●
      specified NEC O43.89-●
    placental dysfunction O43.89-●
    placental infarction O43.81-●
    placental insufficiency O36.51-●
    placental transfusion syndromes
      fetomaternal O43.Ø1-●
      fetus to fetus O43.Ø2-●
      maternofetal O43.Ø1-●
    placentitis O41.14-●
    pneumonia O99.51-●
    poisoning —*see also* Table of Drugs and
        Chemicals O9A.21-●
    polyhydramnios O4Ø-●

▶ New   ⇒ Revised   ~~deleted~~ Deleted   ● Use Additional Character(s)

Pregnancy *(Continued)*
  complicated by *(Continued)*
    polymorphic eruption of pregnancy O26.86
    poor obstetric history NEC O09.29-•
    postmaturity (post-term) (40 to 42 weeks)
        O48.0
      more than 42 completed weeks gestation
          (prolonged) O48.1
    pre-eclampsia O14.9-•
      mild O14.0-•
      moderate O14.0-•
      severe O14.1-•
        with hemolysis, elevated liver
            enzymes and low platelet count
            (HELLP) O14.2-•
    premature labor —*see* Pregnancy,
        complicated by, preterm labor
    premature rupture of membranes O42.90
      full-term, unspecified as to length of
          time between rupture and onset of
          labor O42.92
      with onset of labor
        within 24 hours O42.00
          at or after 37 weeks gestation, onset
              of labor within 24 hours of
              rupture O42.02
          pre-term (before 37 completed
              weeks of gestation)
              O42.01-•
        after 24 hours O42.10
          at or after 37 weeks gestation,
              onset of labor more than
              24 hours following rupture
              O42.12
          pre-term (before 37 completed
              weeks of gestation) O42.11-•
      at or after 37 weeks gestation,
          unspecified as to length of time
          between rupture and onset of labor
          O42.92
      pre-term (before 37 completed weeks of
          gestation) O42.91-•
    premature separation of placenta —*see also*
        Abruptio placentae O45.9-•
    presentation, fetal —*see* Delivery,
        complicated by, malposition
    preterm delivery O60.10
    preterm labor
      with delivery O60.10
        preterm O60.10
        term O60.20
      second trimester
        with preterm delivery
          second trimester O60.12
          third trimester O60.13
        with term delivery O60.22
        without delivery O60.02
      third trimester
        with term delivery O60.23
        with third trimester preterm delivery
            O60.14
        without delivery O60.03
      without delivery O60.00
        second trimester O60.02
        third trimester O60.03
    previous history of —*see* Pregnancy,
        supervision of, high-risk
    prolapse, uterus O34.52-•
    proteinuria (gestational) —*see also*
        Proteinuria, gestational O12.1-•
      with edema O12.2-•
    pruritic urticarial papules and plaques of
        pregnancy (PUPPP) O26.86
    pruritus (neurogenic) O26.89-•
    psychosis or psychoneurosis (puerperal)
        F53.1
    ptyalism O26.89-•
    PUPPP (pruritic urticarial papules and
        plaques of pregnancy) O26.86
    pyelitis O23.0-•
    recurrent pregnancy loss O26.2-•

Pregnancy *(Continued)*
  complicated by *(Continued)*
    renal disease or failure NEC O26.83-•
      with secondary hypertension, pre-
          existing —*see* Hypertension,
          complicating, pregnancy, pre-
          existing, secondary
      hypertensive, pre-existing —*see*
          Hypertension, complicating,
          pregnancy, pre-existing, with, renal
          disease
    respiratory condition (conditions in
        J00-J99) O99.51-•
    retained, retention
      dead ovum O02.0
      intrauterine contraceptive device
          O26.3-•
    retroversion, uterus O34.53-•
    Rh immunization, incompatibility or
        sensitization NEC O36.09-•
      anti-D antibody O36.01-•
    rupture
      amnion (premature) —*see also*
          Pregnancy, complicated by,
          premature rupture of membranes
          O42-•
      membranes (premature) —*see also*
          Pregnancy, complicated by,
          premature rupture of membranes
          O42-•
      uterus (during labor) O71.1
        before onset of labor O71.0-•
    salivation (excessive) O26.89-•
    salpingitis O23.52-•
    salpingo-oophoritis O23.52-•
    sepsis (conditions in A40, A41) O98.81-•
    size date discrepancy (uterine) O26.84-•
    skin condition (conditions in L00-L99)
        O99.71-•
    smoking (tobacco) O99.33-•
    social problem O09.7-•
    specified condition NEC O26.89-•
    spotting O26.85-•
    streptococcus group B (GBS) carrier state
        O99.820
    subluxation of symphysis (pubis) O26.71-•
    syphilis (conditions in A50-A53) O98.11-•
    threatened
      abortion O20.0
      labor O47.9
        at or after 37 completed weeks of
            gestation O47.1
        before 37 completed weeks of
            gestation O47.0-•
    thrombophlebitis (superficial) O22.2-•
    thrombosis O22.9-•
      cerebral venous O22.5-•
      cerebrovenous sinus O22.5-•
      deep O22.3-•
    tobacco use disorder (smoking) O99.33-•
    torsion of uterus O34.59-•
    toxemia O14.9-•
    transverse lie or presentation O32.2
    tuberculosis (conditions in A15-A19)
        O98.01-•
    tumor (benign)
      cervix O34.4-•
      malignant O9A.11-•
      uterus O34.1-•
    unstable lie O32.0
    upper respiratory infection O99.51-•
    urethritis O23.2-•
    uterine size date discrepancy O26.84-•
    vaginitis or vulvitis O23.59-•
    varicose veins (lower extremities) O22.0-•
      genitals O22.1-•
      legs O22.0-•
      perineal O22.1-•
      vaginal or vulval O22.1-•
    venereal disease NEC (conditions in A63.8)
        O98.31-•

Pregnancy *(Continued)*
  complicated by *(Continued)*
    venous disorders O22.9-•
      specified NEC O22.8X-•
    very young mother —*see* Pregnancy,
        complicated by, young mother
    viral diseases (conditions in A80-B09,
        B25-B34) O98.51-•
    vomiting O21.9
      due to diseases classified elsewhere O21.8
      hyperemesis gravidarum (mild) —*see
          also* Hyperemesis, gravidarum
          O21.0-•
      late (occurring after 20 weeks of
          gestation) O21.2
    young mother
      multigravida O09.62-•
      primigravida O09.61-•
  concealed O09.3-•
  continuing following
    elective fetal reduction of one or more fetus
        O31.3-•
    intrauterine death of one or more fetus
        O31.2-•
    spontaneous abortion of one or more fetus
        O31.1-•
  cornual O00.80
    with intrauterine pregnancy O00.81
  ectopic (ruptured) O00.90
    with intrauterine pregnancy O00.91
    abdominal O00.00
      with
        intrauterine pregnancy O00.01
        viable fetus O36.7-•
    cervical O00.80
      with intrauterine pregnancy O00.81
    complicated (by) O08.9
      afibrinogenemia O08.1
      cardiac arrest O08.81
      chemical damage of pelvic organ(s)
          O08.6
      circulatory collapse O08.3
      defibrination syndrome O08.1
      electrolyte imbalance O08.5
      embolism (amniotic fluid) (blood clot)
          (pulmonary) (septic) O08.2
      endometritis O08.0
      genital tract and pelvic infection O08.0
      hemorrhage (delayed) (excessive) O08.1
      infection
        genital tract or pelvic O08.0
        kidney 008.83
        urinary tract O08.83
      intravascular coagulation O08.1
      laceration of pelvic organ(s)
          O08.6
      metabolic disorder O08.5
      oliguria O08.4
      oophoritis O08.0
      parametritis O08.0
      pelvic peritonitis O08.0
      perforation of pelvic organ(s)
          O08.6
      renal failure or shutdown O08.4
      salpingitis or salpingo-oophoritis
          O08.0
      sepsis O08.82
      shock O08.83
        septic O08.82
      specified condition NEC O08.89
      tubular necrosis (renal) O08.4
      uremia O08.4
      urinary infection O08.83
      venous complication NEC O08.7
        embolism O08.2
    cornual O00.80
      with intrauterine pregnancy
          O00.81
    intraligamentous O00.80
      with intrauterine pregnancy
          O00.81

Pregnancy *(Continued)*
  ectopic *(Continued)*
    mural O00.80
      with intrauterine pregnancy O00.81
    ovarian O00.20-•
      with intrauterine pregnancy O00.21-•
    specified site NEC O00.80
      with intrauterine pregnancy O00.81
    tubal (ruptured) O00.10-•
      with intrauterine pregnancy O00.11-•
  examination (normal) Z34.9-•
    first Z34.0-•
    high-risk —*see* Pregnancy, supervision of,
      high-risk
    specified Z34.8-•
  extrauterine —*see* Pregnancy, ectopic
  fallopian O00.10-•
    with intrauterine pregnancy O00.11-•
  false F45.8
  gestational carrier Z33.3
  heptachorionic, hepta-amniotic (septuplets)
    O30.83-•
  hexachorionic, hexa-amniotic (sextuplets)
    O30.83-•
  hidden O09.3-•
  high-risk —*see* Pregnancy, supervision of,
    high-risk
  incidental finding Z33.1
  interstitial O00.80
    with intrauterine pregnancy O00.81
  intraligamentous O00.80
    with intrauterine pregnancy O00.81
  intramural O00.80
    with intrauterine pregnancy O00.81
  intraperitoneal O00.00
    with intrauterine pregnancy O00.01
  isthmian O00.10-•
    with intrauterine pregnancy O00.11-•
  mesometric (mural) O00.80
    with intrauterine pregnancy O00.81
  molar NEC O02.0
    complicated (by) O08.9
      afibrinogenemia O08.1
      cardiac arrest O08.81
      chemical damage of pelvic organ(s) O08.6
      circulatory collapse O08.3
      defibrination syndrome O08.1
      electrolyte imbalance O08.5
      embolism (amniotic fluid) (blood clot)
        (pulmonary) (septic) O08.2
      endometritis O08.0
      genital tract and pelvic infection O08.0
      hemorrhage (delayed) (excessive) O08.1
      infection
        genital tract or pelvic O08.0
        kidney O08.83
        urinary tract O08.83
      intravascular coagulation O08.1
      laceration of pelvic organ(s) O08.6
      metabolic disorder O08.5
      oliguria O08.4
      oophoritis O08.0
      parametritis O08.0
      pelvic peritonitis O08.0
      perforation of pelvic organ(s) O08.6
      renal failure or shutdown O08.4
      salpingitis or salpingo-oophoritis O08.0
      sepsis O08.82
      shock O08.3
        septic O08.82
      specified condition NEC O08.89
      tubular necrosis (renal) O08.4
      uremia O08.4
      urinary infection O08.83
      venous complication NEC O08.7
        embolism O08.2
    hydatidiform —*see also* Mole, hydatidiform
      O01.9-•
  multiple (gestation) O30.9-•
    greater than quadruplets —*see* Pregnancy,
      multiple (gestation), specified NEC

Pregnancy *(Continued)*
  multiple (gestation) *(Continued)*
    specified NEC O30.80-•
      with
        two or more monoamniotic fetuses
          O30.82-•
        two or more monochorionic fetuses
          O30.81-•
      number of chorions and amnions are
        both equal to the number of fetuses
        O30.83-•
      two or more monoamniotic fetuses
        O30.82-•
      two or more monochorionic fetuses
        O30.81-•
      unable to determine number of placenta
        and number of amniotic sacs
        O30.89-•
      unspecified number of placenta and
        unspecified number of amniotic
        sacs O30.80-•
  mural O00.80
    with intrauterine pregnancy O00.81
  normal (supervision of) Z34.9-•
    first Z34.0-•
    high-risk —*see* Pregnancy, supervision of,
      high-risk
    specified Z34.8-•
  ovarian O00.20-•
    with intrauterine pregnancy O00.21-•
  pentachorionic, penta-amniotic (quintuplets)
    O30.83-•
  postmature (40 to 42 weeks) O48.0
    more than 42 weeks gestation O48.1
  post-term (40 to 42 weeks) O48.0
  prenatal care only Z34.9-•
    first Z34.0-•
    high-risk —*see* Pregnancy, supervision of,
      high-risk
    specified Z34.8-•
  prolonged (more than 42 weeks gestation)
    O48.1
  quadruplet O30.20-•
    with
      two or more monoamniotic fetuses
        O30.22-•
      two or more monochorionic fetuses
        O30.21-•
    quadrachorionic/quadra-amniotic O30.23-•
    two or more monoamniotic fetuses O30.22-•
    two or more monochorionic fetuses
      O30.21-•
    unable to determine number of placenta
      and number of amniotic sacs O30.29-•
    unspecified number of placenta and
      unspecified number of amniotic sacs
      O30.20-•
  quintuplet —*see* Pregnancy, multiple
    (gestation), specified NEC
  sextuplet —*see* Pregnancy, multiple
    (gestation), specified NEC
  supervision of
    concealed pregnancy O09.3-•
    elderly mother
      multigravida O09.52-•
      primigravida O09.51-•
    hidden pregnancy O09.3-•
    high-risk O09.9-•
      due to (history of)
        ectopic pregnancy O09.1-•
        elderly —*see* Pregnancy, supervision,
          elderly mother
        grand multiparity O09.4
        infertility O09.0-•
        insufficient prenatal care O09.3-•
        in utero procedure during previous
          pregnancy O09.82-•
        in vitro fertilization O09.81-•
        molar pregnancy O09.A-•
        multiple previous pregnancies O09.4-•
        older mother —*see* Pregnancy,
          supervision of, elderly mother

Pregnancy *(Continued)*
  supervision of *(Continued)*
    high-risk *(Continued)*
      due to *(Continued)*
        poor reproductive or obstetric history
          NEC O09.29-•
        pre-term labor O09.21-•
        previous
          neonatal death O09.29-•
        social problems O09.7-•
        specified NEC O09.89-•
        very young mother —*see* Pregnancy,
          supervision, young mother
      resulting from in vitro fertilization
        O09.81-•
    normal Z34.9-•
      first Z34.0-•
      specified NEC Z34.8-•
    young mother
      multigravida O09.62-•
      primigravida O09.61-•
  triplet O30.10-•
    with
      two or more monoamniotic fetuses
        O30.12-•
      two or more monochorionic fetuses
        O30.11-•
    trichorionic/triamniotic O30.13-•
    two or more monoamniotic fetuses O30.12-•
    two or more monochorionic fetuses O30.11-•
    unable to determine number of placenta
      and number of amniotic sacs O30.19-•
    unspecified number of placenta and
      unspecified number of amniotic sacs
      O30.10-•
  tubal (with abortion) (with rupture) O00.10-•
    with intrauterine pregnancy O00.11-•
  twin O30.00-•
    conjoined O30.02-•
    dichorionic/diamniotic (two placenta, two
      amniotic sacs) O30.04-•
    monochorionic/diamniotic (one placenta,
      two amniotic sacs) O30.03-•
    monochorionic/monoamniotic (one
      placenta, one amniotic sac) O30.01-•
    unable to determine number of placenta
      and number of amniotic sacs O30.09-•
    unspecified number of placenta and
      unspecified number of amniotic sacs
      O30.00-•
  unwanted Z64.0
  weeks of gestation
    8 weeks Z3A.08
    9 weeks Z3A.09
    10 weeks Z3A.10
    11 weeks Z3A.11
    12 weeks Z3A.12
    13 weeks Z3A.13
    14 weeks Z3A.14
    15 weeks Z3A.15
    16 weeks Z3A.16
    17 weeks Z3A.17
    18 weeks Z3A.18
    19 weeks Z3A.19
    20 weeks Z3A.20
    21 weeks Z3A.21
    22 weeks Z3A.22
    23 weeks Z3A.23
    24 weeks Z3A.24
    25 weeks Z3A.25
    26 weeks Z3A.26
    27 weeks Z3A.27
    28 weeks Z3A.28
    29 weeks Z3A.29
    30 weeks Z3A.30
    31 weeks Z3A.31
    32 weeks Z3A.32
    33 weeks Z3A.33
    34 weeks Z3A.34
    35 weeks Z3A.35
    36 weeks Z3A.36

▶ New   ⇒ Revised   ~~deleted~~ Deleted   • Use Additional Character(s)

Pregnancy *(Continued)*
 weeks of gestation *(Continued)*
  37 weeks Z3A.37
  38 weeks Z3A.38
  39 weeks Z3A.39
  40 weeks Z3A.40
  41 weeks Z3A.41
  42 weeks Z3A.42
  greater than 42 weeks Z3A.49
  less than 8 weeks Z3A.01
  not specified Z3A.00
Preiser's disease —*see* Osteonecrosis,
  secondary, due to, trauma, metacarpus
Pre-kwashiorkor —*see* Malnutrition, severe
Preleukemia (syndrome) D46.9
Preluxation, hip, congenital Q65.6
Premature —*see also* condition
 adrenarche E27.0
 aging E34.8
 beats I49.40
  atrial I49.1
  auricular I49.1
  supraventricular I49.1
 birth NEC —*see* Preterm, newborn
 closure, foramen ovale Q21.8
 contraction
  atrial I49.1
  atrioventricular I49.49
  auricular I49.1
  auriculoventricular I49.2
  heart (extrasystole) I49.49
  junctional I49.2
  ventricular I49.3
 delivery —*see also* Pregnancy, complicated by,
  preterm labor O60.10
 ejaculation F52.4
 infant NEC —*see* Preterm, newborn
  light-for-dates —*see* Light for dates
 labor —*see* Pregnancy, complicated by,
  preterm labor
 lungs P28.0
 menopause E28.319
  asymptomatic E28.319
  symptomatic E28.310
 newborn
  extreme (less than 28 completed weeks) —
   see Immaturity, extreme
  less than 37 completed weeks —*see*
   Preterm, newborn
 puberty E30.1
 rupture membranes or amnion —*see*
  Pregnancy, complicated by, premature
  rupture of membranes
 senility E34.8
 thelarche E30.8
 ventricular systole I49.3
Prematurity NEC (less than 37 completed
  weeks) —*see* Preterm, newborn
 extreme (less than 28 completed weeks) —*see*
  Immaturity, extreme
Premenstrual
 dysphoric disorder (PMDD) F32.81
 tension (syndrome) N94.3
Premolarization, cuspids K00.2
Prenatal
 care, normal pregnancy —*see* Pregnancy,
  normal
 screening of mother —*see also* Encounter,
  antenatal Z36.9
 teeth K00.6
Preparatory care for subsequent treatment NEC
 for dialysis Z49.01
  peritoneal Z49.02
Prepartum —*see* condition
Preponderance, left or right ventricular I51.7
Prepuce —*see* condition
PRES (posterior reversible encephalopathy
  syndrome) I67.83
Presbycardia R54
Presbycusis, presbyacusia H91.1-●
➡ Presbyesophagus K22.89

Presbyophrenia F03
Presbyopia H52.4
Prescription of contraceptives (initial) Z30.019
 barrier Z30.018
 diaphragm Z30.018
 emergency (postcoital) Z30.012
 implantable subdermal Z30.017
 injectable Z30.013
 intrauterine contraceptive device Z30.014
 pills Z30.011
 postcoital (emergency) Z30.012
 repeat Z30.40
  barrier Z30.49
  diaphragm Z30.49
  implantable subdermal Z30.46
  injectable Z30.42
  pills Z30.41
  specified type NEC Z30.49
  transdermal patch hormonal Z30.45
  vaginal ring hormonal Z30.44
 specified type NEC Z30.018
  transdermal patch hormonal Z30.016
  vaginal ring hormonal Z30.015
Presence (of)
 ankle-joint implant (functional) (prosthesis)
  Z96.66-●
 aortocoronary (bypass) graft Z95.1
 arterial-venous shunt (dialysis) Z99.2
 artificial
  eye (globe) Z97.0
  heart (fully implantable) (mechanical)
   Z95.812
  valve Z95.2
  larynx Z96.3
  lens (intraocular) Z96.1
  limb (complete) (partial) Z97.1-●
   arm Z97.1-●
    bilateral Z97.15
   leg Z97.1-●
    bilateral Z97.16
 audiological implant (functional) Z96.29
 bladder implant (functional) Z96.0
 bone
  conduction hearing device Z96.29
  implant (functional) NEC Z96.7
  joint (prosthesis) —*see* Presence, joint
   implant
 cardiac
  defibrillator (functional) (with synchronous
   cardiac pacemaker)Z95.810
  implant or graft Z95.9
   specified type NEC Z95.818
  pacemaker Z95.0
  resynchronization therapy
   defibrillator Z95.810
   pacemaker Z95.0
 cerebrospinal fluid drainage device Z98.2
 cochlear implant (functional) Z96.21
 contact lens (es) Z97.3
 coronary artery graft or prosthesis Z95.5
 CRT-D (cardiac resynchronization therapy
  defibrillator) Z95.810
 CRT-P (cardiac resynchronization therapy
  pacemaker) Z95.0
 cardioverter-defibrillator (ICD) Z95.810
 CSF shunt Z98.2
 dental prosthesis device Z97.2
 dentures Z97.2
 device (external) NEC Z97.8
  cardiac NEC Z95.818
  heart assist Z95.811
  implanted (functional) Z96.9
   specified NEC Z96.89
  prosthetic Z97.8
 ear implant Z96.20
  cochlear implant Z96.21
  myringotomy tube Z96.22
  specified type NEC Z96.29
 elbow-joint implant (functional) (prosthesis)
  Z96.62-●
 endocrine implant (functional) NEC Z96.49

Presence *(Continued)*
 eustachian tube stent or device (functional)
  Z96.29
 external hearing-aid or device Z97.4
 finger-joint implant (functional) (prosthetic)
  Z96.69-●
 functional implant Z96.9
  specified NEC Z96.89
 graft
  cardiac NEC Z95.818
  vascular NEC Z95.828
 hearing-aid or device (external) Z97.4
  implant (bone) (cochlear) (functional) Z96.21
 heart assist device Z95.811
 heart valve implant (functional) Z95.2
  prosthetic Z95.2
  specified type NEC Z95.4
  xenogenic Z95.3
 hip-joint implant (functional) (prosthesis)
  Z96.64-●
➡ ICD (cardioverter-defibrillator) Z95.810
 implanted device (artificial) (functional)
  (prosthetic) Z96.9
  automatic cardiac defibrillator (with
   synchronous cardiac pacemaker)
   Z95.810
  cardiac pacemaker Z95.0
  cochlear Z96.21
  dental Z96.5
  heart Z95.812
  heart valve Z95.2
   prosthetic Z95.2
   specified NEC Z95.4
   xenogenic Z95.3
  insulin pump Z96.41
  intraocular lens Z96.1
  joint Z96.60
   ankle Z96.66-●
   elbow Z96.62-●
   finger Z96.69-●
   hip Z96.64-●
   knee Z96.65-●
   shoulder Z96.61-●
   specified NEC Z96.698
   wrist Z96.63-●
  larynx Z96.3
  myringotomy tube Z96.22
  otological Z96.20
   cochlear Z96.21
   eustachian stent Z96.29
   myringotomy Z96.22
   specified NEC Z96.29
   stapes Z96.29
  skin Z96.81
  skull plate Z96.7
  specified NEC Z96.89
  urogenital Z96.0
 insulin pump (functional) Z96.41
 intestinal bypass or anastomosis Z98.0
 intraocular lens (functional) Z96.1
 intrauterine contraceptive device (IUD) Z97.5
 intravascular implant (functional) (prosthetic)
  NEC Z95.9
  coronary artery Z95.5
  defibrillator (with synchronous cardiac
   pacemaker) Z95.810
  peripheral vessel (with angioplasty) Z95.820
 joint implant (prosthetic) (any) Z96.60
  ankle —*see* Presence, ankle joint implant
  elbow —*see* Presence, elbow joint implant
  finger —*see* Presence, finger joint implant
  hip —*see* Presence, hip joint implant
  knee —*see* Presence, knee joint implant
  shoulder —*see* Presence, shoulder joint
   implant
  specified joint NEC Z96.698
  wrist —*see* Presence, wrist joint implant
 knee-joint implant (functional) (prosthesis)
  Z96.65-●
 laryngeal implant (functional) Z96.3
 mandibular implant (dental) Z96.5

Presence *(Continued)*
  myringotomy tube(s) Z96.22
  neurostimulator (brain) (gastric) (peripheral
    nerve) (sacral nerve) (spinal cord) (vagus
    nerve) Z96.82
  orthopedic-joint implant (prosthetic) (any) —
    see Presence, joint implant
  otological implant (functional) Z96.29
  shoulder-joint implant (functional)
    (prosthesis) Z96.61-●
  skull-plate implant Z96.7
  spectacles Z97.3
  stapes implant (functional) Z96.29
  systemic lupus erythematosus [SLE] inhibitor
    D68.62
  tendon implant (functional) (graft) Z96.7
  tooth root(s) implant Z96.5
  ureteral stent Z96.0
  urethral stent Z96.0
  urogenital implant (functional) Z96.0
  vascular implant or device Z95.9
    access port device Z95.828
    specified type NEC Z95.828
  wrist-joint implant (functional) (prosthesis)
    Z96.63-●
Presenile —*see also* condition
  dementia F03
  premature aging E34.8
Presentation, fetal —*see* Delivery, complicated
  by, malposition
Prespondylolisthesis (congenital) Q76.2
Pressure
  area, skin —*see* Ulcer, pressure, by site
  brachial plexus G54.0
  brain G93.5
    injury at birth NEC P11.1
  cerebral —*see* Pressure, brain
  chest R07.89
  cone, tentorial G93.5
  hyposystolic —*see also* Hypotension
    incidental reading, without diagnosis of
      hypotension R03.1
  increased
    intracranial, benign G93.2
      injury at birth P11.0
    intraocular H40.05-●
  injury —*see* Ulcer, pressure, by site
  lumbosacral plexus G54.1
  mediastinum J98.59
  necrosis (chronic) —*see* Ulcer, pressure,
    by site
  parental, inappropriate (excessive) Z62.6
  sore (chronic) —*see* Ulcer, pressure, by site
  spinal cord G95.20
  ulcer (chronic) —*see* Ulcer, pressure, by site
  venous, increased I87.8
Pre-syncope R55
Preterm
  delivery (*see also* Pregnancy, complicated by,
    preterm labor) O60.10
  labor —*see* Pregnancy, complicated by,
    preterm labor
  newborn (infant) P07.30
    gestational age
      28 completed weeks (28 weeks, 0 days
        through 28 weeks, 6 days) P07.31
      29 completed weeks (29 weeks, 0 days
        through 29 weeks, 6 days) P07.32
      30 completed weeks (30 weeks, 0 days
        through 30 weeks, 6 days) P07.33
      31 completed weeks (31 weeks, 0 days
        through 31 weeks, 6 days) P07.34
      32 completed weeks (32 weeks, 0 days
        through 32 weeks, 6 days) P07.35
      33 completed weeks (33 weeks, 0 days
        through 33 weeks, 6 days) P07.36
      34 completed weeks (34 weeks, 0 days
        through 34 weeks, 6 days) P07.37
      35 completed weeks (35 weeks, 0 days
        through 35 weeks, 6 days) P07.38
      36 completed weeks (36 weeks, 0 days
        through 36 weeks, 6 days) P07.39

Previa
  placenta (total) (without hemorrhage)
    O44.0-●
    with hemorrhage O44.1-●
    complete O44.0-●
      with hemorrhage O44.1-●
    low —*see also* Delivery, complicated, by,
      placenta, low O44.4-●
      with hemorrhage O44.5-●
    marginal O44.2-●
      with hemorrhage O44.3-●
    partial O44.2-●
      with hemorrhage O44.3-●
  vasa O69.4
Priapism N48.30
  due to
    disease classified elsewhere N48.32
    drug N48.33
    specified cause NEC N48.39
    trauma N48.31
Prickling sensation (skin) R20.2
Prickly heat L74.0
Primary —*see* condition
Primigravida
  elderly, affecting management of pregnancy,
    labor and delivery (supervision only) —
    see Pregnancy, complicated by, elderly,
    primigravida
  older, affecting management of pregnancy,
    labor and delivery (supervision only) —
    see Pregnancy, complicated by, elderly,
    primigravida
  very young, affecting management
    of pregnancy, labor and delivery
    (supervision only) —*see* Pregnancy,
    complicated by, young mother,
    primigravida
Primipara
  elderly, affecting management of pregnancy,
    labor and delivery (supervision only) —
    see Pregnancy, complicated by, elderly,
    primigravida
  older, affecting management of pregnancy,
    labor and delivery (supervision only) —
    see Pregnancy, complicated by, elderly,
    primigravida
  very young, affecting management
    of pregnancy, labor and delivery
    (supervision only) —*see* Pregnancy,
    complicated by, young mother,
    primigravida
Primus varus (bilateral) Q66.21-●
PRIND (Prolonged reversible ischemic
  neurologic deficit) I63.9
Pringle's disease (tuberous sclerosis) Q85.1
Prinzmetal angina I20.1
Prizefighter ear —*see* Cauliflower ear
Problem (with) (related to)
  academic Z55.8
  acculturation Z60.3
  adjustment (to)
    change of job Z56.1
    life-cycle transition Z60.0
    pension Z60.0
    retirement Z60.0
  adopted child Z62.821
  alcoholism in family Z63.72
  atypical parenting situation Z62.9
  bankruptcy Z59.89
  behavioral (adult) F69
    drug seeking Z76.5
  birth of sibling affecting child Z62.898
  care (of)
    provider dependency Z74.9
      specified NEC Z74.8
    sick or handicapped person in family or
      household Z63.6
  child
    abuse (affecting the child) —*see*
      Maltreatment, child
    custody or support proceedings Z65.3

Problem *(Continued)*
  child *(Continued)*
    in care of non-parental family member
      Z62.21
    in foster care Z62.21
    in welfare custody Z62.21
    living in orphanage or group home Z62.22
  child-rearing Z62.9
    specified NEC Z62.898
  communication (developmental) F80.9
  conflict or discord (with)
    boss Z56.4
    classmates Z55.4
    counselor Z64.4
    employer Z56.4
    family Z63.9
      specified NEC Z63.8
    probation officer Z64.4
    social worker Z64.4
    teachers Z55.4
    workmates Z56.4
  conviction in legal proceedings Z65.0
    with imprisonment Z65.1
  counselor Z64.4
  creditors Z59.89
  digestive K92.9
  drug addict in family Z63.72
  ear —*see* Disorder, ear
  economic Z59.9
    affecting care Z59.9
    specified NEC Z59.89
  education Z55.9
    specified NEC Z55.8
  employment Z56.9
    change of job Z56.1
    discord Z56.4
    environment Z56.5
    sexual harassment Z56.81
    specified NEC Z56.89
    stress NEC Z56.6
    stressful schedule Z56.3
    threat of job loss Z56.2
    unemployment Z56.0
  enuresis, child F98.0
  eye H57.9
  failed examinations (school) Z55.2
  falling Z91.81
  family —*see also* Disruption, family Z63.9-●
    specified NEC Z63.8
  feeding (elderly) (infant) R63.39
    newborn P92.9
      breast P92.5
      overfeeding P92.4
      slow P92.2
      specified NEC P92.8
      underfeeding P92.3
    nonorganic F50.89
  finance Z59.9
    specified NEC Z59.89
  foreclosure on loan Z59.89
  foster child Z62.822
  frightening experience(s) in childhood
    Z62.898
  genital NEC
    female N94.9
    male N50.9
  health care Z75.9
    specified NEC Z75.8
  hearing —*see* Deafness
  homelessness Z59.00
  housing Z59.9
    inadequate Z59.1
    isolated Z59.89
    specified NEC Z59.89
  identity (of childhood) F93.8
  illegitimate pregnancy (unwanted) Z64.0
  illiteracy Z55.0
  impaired mobility Z74.09
  imprisonment or incarceration Z65.1
  inadequate teaching affecting education
    Z55.8

▶ New   ⇒ Revised   ~~deleted~~ Deleted   ● Use Additional Character(s)

Problem *(Continued)*
  inappropriate (excessive) parental pressure Z62.6
  influencing health status NEC Z78.9
  in-law Z63.1
  institutionalization, affecting child Z62.22
  intrafamilial communication Z63.8
  jealousy, child F93.8
  landlord Z59.2
  language (developmental) F80.9
  learning (developmental) F81.9
  legal Z65.3
    conviction without imprisonment Z65.0
    imprisonment Z65.1
    release from prison Z65.2
  life-management Z73.9
    specified NEC Z73.89
  life-style Z72.9
    gambling Z72.6
    high-risk sexual behavior (heterosexual) Z72.51
      bisexual Z72.53
      homosexual Z72.52
    inappropriate eating habits Z72.4
    self-damaging behavior NEC Z72.89
    specified NEC Z72.89
    tobacco use Z72.0
  literacy Z55.9
    low level Z55.0
    specified NEC Z55.8
  living alone Z60.2
  lodgers Z59.2
  loss of love relationship in childhood Z62.898
  marital Z63.0
    involving
      divorce Z63.5
      estrangement Z63.5
      gender identity F66
  mastication K08.89
  medical
    care, within family Z63.6
    facilities Z75.9
      specified NEC Z75.8
  mental F48.9
  multiparity Z64.1
  negative life events in childhood Z62.9
    altered pattern of family relationships Z62.898
    frightening experience Z62.898
    loss of
      love relationship Z62.898
      self-esteem Z62.898
    physical abuse (alleged) —*see* Maltreatment, child
    removal from home Z62.29
    specified event NEC Z62.898
  neighbor Z59.2
  neurological NEC R29.818
  new step-parent affecting child Z62.898
  none (feared complaint unfounded) Z71.1
  occupational NEC Z56.89
  parent-child —*see* Conflict, parent-child
  personal hygiene Z91.89
  personality F69
  phase-of-life transition, adjustment Z60.0
  presence of sick or disabled person
    in family or household Z63.79
    needing care Z63.6
  primary support group (family) Z63.9
    specified NEC Z63.8
  probation officer Z64.4
  psychiatric F99
  psychosexual (development) F66
  psychosocial Z65.9
    religious or spiritual Z65.8
    specified NEC Z65.8
  relationship Z63.9
    childhood F93.8
  release from prison Z65.2
    religious or spiritual Z65.8

Problem *(Continued)*
  removal from home affecting child Z62.29
  seeking and accepting known hazardous and harmful
    behavioral or psychological interventions Z65.8
    chemical, nutritional or physical interventions Z65.8
  sexual function (nonorganic) F52.9
  sight H54.7
  sleep disorder, child F51.9
  smell —*see* Disturbance, sensation, smell
  social
    environment Z60.9
      specified NEC Z60.8
    exclusion and rejection Z60.4
    worker Z64.4
  speech R47.9
    developmental F80.9
    specified NEC R47.89
  swallowing —*see* Dysphagia
  taste —*see* Disturbance, sensation, taste
  tic, child F95.0
  underachievement in school Z55.3
  unemployment Z56.0
    threatened Z56.2
  unwanted pregnancy Z64.0
  upbringing Z62.9
    specified NEC Z62.898
  urinary N39.9
  voice production R47.89
  work schedule (stressful) Z56.3
Procedure (surgical)
  converted
    arthroscopic to open Z53.33
    laparoscopic to open Z53.31
    specified procedure NEC to open Z53.39
    thoracoscopic to open Z53.32
  for purpose other than remedying health state Z41.9
    specified NEC Z41.8
  not done Z53.9
    because of
      administrative reasons Z53.8
      contraindication Z53.09
        smoking Z53.01
      patient's decision Z53.20
        for reasons of belief or group pressure Z53.1
        ⇒left against medical advice (AMA) Z53.29
      ▶left without being seen Z53.21
        specified reason NEC Z53.29
      specified reason NEC Z53.8
Procidentia (uteri) N81.3
Proctalgia K62.89
  fugax K59.4
  spasmodic K59.4
Proctitis K62.89
  amebic (acute) A06.0
  chlamydial A56.3
  gonococcal A54.6
  granulomatous —*see* Enteritis, regional, large intestine
  herpetic A60.1
  radiation K62.7
  tuberculous A18.32
  ulcerative (chronic) K51.20
    with
      complication K51.219
        abscess K51.214
        fistula K51.213
        obstruction K51.212
        rectal bleeding K51.211
        specified NEC K51.218
Proctocele
  female (without uterine prolapse) N81.6
    with uterine prolapse N81.2
      complete N81.3
  male K62.3

Proctocolitis
  ▶allergic K52.29
  ⇒food-induced eosinophilic K52.29
  ⇒food protein-induced K52.29
  ⇒milk protein-induced K52.29
  mucosal —*see* Rectosigmoiditis, ulcerative
Proctoptosis K62.3
Proctorrhagia K62.5
Proctosigmoiditis K63.89
  ulcerative (chronic) —*see* Rectosigmoiditis, ulcerative
Proctospasm K59.4
  psychogenic F45.8
Profichet's disease —*see* Disorder, soft tissue, specified type NEC
Progeria E34.8
Prognathism (mandibular) (maxillary) M26.19
Progonoma (melanotic) —*see* Neoplasm, benign, by site
Progressive —*see* condition
Prolactinoma
  specified site —*see* Neoplasm, benign, by site
  unspecified site D35.2
Prolapse, prolapsed
  anus, anal (canal) (sphincter) K62.2
  arm or hand O32.2
    causing obstructed labor O64.4
  bladder (mucosa) (sphincter) (acquired)
    congenital Q79.4
    female —*see* Cystocele
    male N32.89
  breast implant (prosthetic) T85.49
  cecostomy K94.09
  cecum K63.4
  cervix, cervical (hypertrophied) N81.2
    anterior lip, obstructing labor O65.5
    congenital Q51.828
    postpartal, old N81.2
    stump N81.85
  ciliary body (traumatic) —*see* Laceration, eye(ball), with prolapse or loss of intraocular tissue
  colon (pedunculated) K63.4
  colostomy K94.09
  disc (intervertebral) —*see* Displacement, intervertebral disc
  eye implant (orbital) T85.398
    lens (ocular) —*see* Complications, intraocular lens
  fallopian tube N83.4-•
  gastric (mucosa) K31.89
  genital, female N81.9
    specified NEC N81.89
  globe, nontraumatic —*see* Luxation, globe
  ileostomy bud K94.19
  intervertebral disc —*see* Displacement, intervertebral disc
  intestine (small) K63.4
  iris (traumatic) —*see* Laceration, eye(ball), with prolapse or loss of interocular tissue
    nontraumatic H21.89
  kidney N28.83
    congenital Q63.2
  laryngeal muscles or ventricle J38.7
  liver K76.89
  meatus urinarius N36.8
  mitral (valve) I34.1
  ocular lens implant —*see* Complications, intraocular lens
  organ or site, congenital NEC —*see* Malposition, congenital
  ovary N83.4-•
  pelvic floor, female N81.89
  perineum, female N81.89
  rectum (mucosa) (sphincter) K62.3
    due to trichuris trichuria B79
  spleen D73.89
  stomach K31.89
  umbilical cord
    complicating delivery O69.0

Prolapse, prolapsed (Continued)
  urachus, congenital Q64.4
  ureter N28.89
    with obstruction N13.5
      with infection N13.6
  ureterovesical orifice N28.89
  urethra (acquired) (infected) (mucosa)
      N36.8
    congenital Q64.71
  urinary meatus N36.8
    congenital Q64.72
  uterovaginal N81.4
    complete N81.3
    incomplete N81.2
  uterus (with prolapse of vagina) N81.4
    complete N81.3
    congenital Q51.818
    first degree N81.2
    in pregnancy or childbirth —see
        Pregnancy, complicated by,
        abnormal, uterus
    incomplete N81.2
    postpartal (old) N81.4
    second degree N81.2
    third degree N81.3
  uveal (traumatic) —see Laceration, eye(ball),
      with prolapse or loss of interocular
      tissue
  vagina (anterior) (wall) —see Cystocele
    with prolapse of uterus N81.4
      complete N81.3
      incomplete N81.2
    posterior wall N81.6
    posthysterectomy N99.3
  vitreous (humor) H43.0-•
    in wound —see Laceration, eye(ball),
        with prolapse or loss of interocular
        tissue
  womb —see Prolapse, uterus
Prolapsus, female N81.9
  specified NEC N81.89
Proliferation(s)
  primary cutaneous CD30-positive large T-cell
      C86.6
  prostate, atypical small acinar N42.32
Proliferative —see condition
Prolonged, prolongation (of)
  bleeding (time) (idiopathic) R79.1
  coagulation (time) R79.1
  gestation (over 42 completed weeks)
    mother O48.1
    newborn P08.22
  interval I44.0
  labor O63.9
    first stage O63.0
    second stage O63.1
  partial thromboplastin time (PTT) R79.1
  pregnancy (more than 42 weeks gestation)
      O48.1
  prothrombin time R79.1
  QT interval R94.31
  uterine contractions in labor O62.4
Prominence, prominent
  ischial spine or sacral promontory with
      disproportion (fetopelvic) O33.0
    causing obstructed labor O65.0
  auricle (congenital) (ear) Q17.5
  nose (congenital) acquired M95.0
Promiscuity —see High, risk, sexual behavior
Pronation
  ankle —see Deformity, limb, foot, specified
      NEC
  foot —see also Deformity, limb, foot, specified
      NEC
    congenital Q74.2
Prophylactic
  administration of
    antibiotics, long-term Z79.2
      short-term use - omit code

Prophylactic (Continued)
  antibiotics, long-term (Continued)
    drug —see also Long-term (current) drug
        therapy (use of) Z79.899-•
    medication Z79.899
  organ removal (for neoplasia management)
      Z40.00
    breast Z40.01
    fallopian tube(s) Z40.03
      with ovary(s) Z40.02
    ovary(s) Z40.02
    specified site NEC Z40.09
  surgery Z40.9
    for risk factors related to malignant
        neoplasm —see Prophylactic, organ
        removal
    specified NEC Z40.8
  vaccination Z23
Propionic acidemia E71.121
Proptosis (ocular) —see also Exophthalmos
  thyroid —see Hyperthyroidism, with goiter
Prosecution, anxiety concerning Z65.3
Prosopagnosia R48.3
Prostadynia N42.81
Prostate, prostatic —see condition
Prostatism —see Hyperplasia, prostate
Prostatitis (congestive) (suppurative) (with
    cystitis) N41.9
  acute N41.0
  cavitary N41.8
  chronic N41.1
  diverticular N41.8
  due to Trichomonas (vaginalis) A59.02
  fibrous N41.1
  gonococcal (acute) (chronic) A54.22
  granulomatous N41.4
  hypertrophic N41.1
  subacute N41.1
  trichomonal A59.02
  tuberculous A18.14
Prostatocystitis N41.3
Prostatorrhea N42.89
Prostatosis N42.82
Prostration R53.83
  heat —see also Heat, exhaustion
    anhydrotic T67.3
    due to
      salt (and water) depletion T67.4
      water depletion T67.3
  nervous F48.8
  senile R54
Protanomaly (anomalous trichromat) H53.54
Protanopia (complete) (incomplete) H53.54
Protection (against) (from) —see Prophylactic
Protein
  deficiency NEC —see Malnutrition
  malnutrition —see Malnutrition
  sickness —see also Reaction, serum T80.69
Proteinemia R77.9
Proteinosis
  alveolar (pulmonary) J84.01
  lipid or lipoid (of Urbach) E78.89
Proteinuria R80.9
  Bence Jones R80.3
  complicating pregnancy —see Proteinuria,
      gestational
  gestational
    complicating
      childbirth O12.14
      pregnancy O12.1-•
        with edema O12.2-•
      puerperium O12.15
  idiopathic R80.0
  isolated R80.0
    with glomerular lesion N06.9
      C3
        glomerulonephritis N06.A
        glomerulopathy N06.A
          with dense deposit disease
              N06.6
      dense deposit disease N06.6

Proteinuria (Continued)
  isolated (Continued)
    with glomerular lesion (Continued)
      diffuse
        crescentic glomerulonephritis N06.7
        endocapillary proliferative
            glomerulonephritis N06.4
        mesangiocapillary glomerulonephritis
            N06.5
      focal and segmental hyalinosis or
          sclerosis N06.1
      membranous (diffuse) N06.2
      mesangial proliferative (diffuse) N06.3
      minimal change N06.0
      specified pathology NEC N06.8
  orthostatic R80.2
    with glomerular lesion —see Proteinuria,
        isolated, with glomerular lesion
  persistent R80.1
    with glomerular lesion —see Proteinuria,
        isolated, with glomerular lesion
  postural R80.2
    with glomerular lesion —see Proteinuria,
        isolated, with glomerular lesion
  pre-eclamptic —see Pre-eclampsia
  puerperal O12.15
  specified type NEC R80.8
Proteolysis, pathologic D65
Proteus (mirabilis) (morganii), as cause of
    disease classified elsewhere B96.4
Prothrombin gene mutation D68.52
Protoporphyria, erythropoietic E80.0
Protozoal —see also condition
  disease B64
    specified NEC B60.8
Protrusion, protrusio
  acetabuli M24.7
  acetabulum (into pelvis) M24.7
  device, implant or graft —see also
      Complications, by site and type,
      mechanical T85.698
    arterial graft NEC —see Complication,
        cardiovascular device, mechanical,
        vascular
    breast (implant) T85.49
    catheter NEC T85.698
      cystostomy T83.090
      dialysis (renal) T82.49
        intraperitoneal T85.691
      infusion NEC T82.594
        spinal (epidural) (subdural) T85.690
      urinary —see also Complications,
          catheter, urinary T83.098
    electronic (electrode) (pulse generator)
        (stimulator)
      bone T84.390
      nervous system —see Complication,
          prosthetic device, mechanical,
          electronic nervous system
          stimulator
    fixation, internal (orthopedic) NEC —
        see Complication, fixation device,
        mechanical
    gastrointestinal —see Complications,
        prosthetic device, mechanical,
        gastrointestinal device
    genital NEC T83.498
      intrauterine contraceptive device T83.39
      penile prosthesis (cylinder) (implanted)
          (pump) (reservoir) T83.490
      testicular prosthesis T83.491
    heart NEC —see Complication,
        cardiovascular device, mechanical
    joint prosthesis —see Complications, joint
        prosthesis, mechanical, specified NEC,
        by site
    ocular NEC —see Complications, prosthetic
        device, mechanical, ocular device
    orthopedic NEC —see Complication,
        orthopedic, device, mechanical
    specified NEC T85.628

▶ New   ⇒ Revised   ~~deleted~~ Deleted   • Use Additional Character(s)

Protrusion, protrusio (Continued)
device, implant or graft (Continued)
urinary NEC —see also Complication,
genitourinary, device, urinary,
mechanical
graft T83.29
vascular NEC —see Complication,
cardiovascular device, mechanical
ventricular intracranial shunt T85.09
intervertebral disc —see Displacement,
intervertebral disc
joint prosthesis —see Complications, joint
prosthesis, mechanical, specified NEC,
by site
nucleus pulposus —see Displacement,
intervertebral disc
Prune belly (syndrome) Q79.4
Prurigo (ferox) (gravis) (Hebrae) (Hebra's)
(mitis) (simplex) L28.2
Besnier's L20.0
estivalis L56.4
nodularis L28.1
psychogenic F45.8
Pruritus, pruritic (essential) L29.9
ani, anus L29.0
psychogenic F45.8
anogenital L29.3
psychogenic F45.8
due to onchocerca volvulus B73.1
gravidarum —see Pregnancy, complicated by,
specified pregnancy-related condition
NEC
hiemalis L29.8
neurogenic (any site) F45.8
perianal L29.0
psychogenic (any site) F45.8
scroti, scrotum L29.1
psychogenic F45.8
senile, senilis L29.8
specified NEC L29.8
psychogenic F45.8
Trichomonas A59.9
vulva, vulvae L29.2
psychogenic F45.8
Pseudarthrosis, pseudoarthrosis (bone) —see
Nonunion, fracture
clavicle, congenital Q74.0
joint, following fusion or arthrodesis M96.0
Pseudoaneurysm —see Aneurysm
Pseudoangina (pectoris) —see Angina
Pseudoangioma I81
Pseudoarteriosus Q28.8
Pseudoarthrosis —see Pseudarthrosis
Pseudobulbar affect (PBA) F48.2
Pseudochromhidrosis L67.8
Pseudocirrhosis, liver, pericardial I31.1
Pseudocowpox B08.03
Pseudocoxalgia M91.3-●
Pseudocroup J38.5
Pseudo-Cushing's syndrome, alcohol-induced
E24.4
Pseudocyesis F45.8
Pseudocyst
lung J98.4
pancreas K86.3
retina —see Cyst, retina
Pseudoelephantiasis neuroarthritica Q82.0
Pseudoexfoliation, capsule (lens) —see
Cataract, specified NEC
Pseudofolliculitis barbae L73.1
Pseudoglioma H44.89
Pseudohemophilia (Bernuth's) (hereditary)
(type B) D68.0
Type A D69.8
vascular D69.8
Pseudohermaphroditism Q56.3
adrenal E25.8
female Q56.2
with adrenocortical disorder E25.8
without adrenocortical disorder
Q56.2

Pseudohermaphroditism (Continued)
female (Continued)
adrenal (congenital) E25.0
unspecified E25.9
male Q56.1
with
adrenocortical disorder E25.8
androgen resistance E34.51
cleft scrotum Q56.1
feminizing testis E34.51
5-alpha-reductase deficiency E29.1
without gonadal disorder Q56.1
adrenal E25.8
unspecified E25.9
Pseudo-Hurler's polydystrophy E77.0
Pseudohydrocephalus G93.2
Pseudohypertrophic muscular dystrophy
(Erb's) G71.02
Pseudohypertrophy, muscle G71.09
Pseudohypoparathyroidism E20.1
Pseudoinsomnia F51.03
Pseudoleukemia, infantile D64.89
Pseudomembranous —see condition
Pseudomeningocele (cerebral) (infective) (post-
traumatic) G96.198
postprocedural (spinal) G97.82
Pseudomenses (newborn) P54.6
Pseudomenstruation (newborn) P54.6
Pseudomonas
aeruginosa, as cause of disease classified
elsewhere B96.5
mallei infection A24.0
as cause of disease classified elsewhere
B96.5
pseudomallei, as cause of disease classified
elsewhere B96.5
Pseudomyotonia G71.19
Pseudomyxoma peritonei C78.6
Pseudoneuritis, optic (nerve) (disc) (papilla),
congenital Q14.2
Pseudo-obstruction intestine (acute) (chronic)
(idiopathic) (intermittent secondary)
(primary) K59.89
colonic K59.81
Pseudopapilledema H47.33-●
congenital Q14.2
Pseudoparalysis
arm or leg R29.818
atonic, congenital P94.2
Pseudopelade L66.0
Pseudophakia Z96.1
Pseudopolyarthritis, rhizomelic M35.3
Pseudopolycythemia D75.1
Pseudopseudohypoparathyroidism E20.1
Pseudopterygium H11.81-●
Pseudoptosis (eyelid) —see Blepharochalasis
Pseudopuberty, precocious
female heterosexual E25.8
male isosexual E25.8
Pseudorickets (renal) N25.0
Pseudorubella B08.20
Pseudosclerema, newborn P83.88
Pseudosclerosis (brain)
Jakob's —see Creutzfeldt-Jakob disease or
syndrome
of Westphal (Strüümpell) E83.01
spastic —see Creutzfeldt-Jakob disease or
syndrome
Pseudotetanus —see Convulsions
Pseudotetany R29.0
hysterical F44.5
Pseudotruncus arteriosus Q25.49
Pseudotuberculosis A28.2
enterocolitis A04.8
pasteurella (infection) A28.0
Pseudotumor G93.2
cerebri G93.2
orbital H05.11-●
Pseudoxanthoma elasticum Q82.8
Psilosis (sprue) (tropical) K90.1
nontropical K90.0

Psittacosis A70
Psoitis M60.88
Psoriasis L40.9
arthropathic L40.50
arthritis mutilans L40.52
distal interphalangeal L40.51
juvenile L40.54
other specified L40.59
spondylitis L40.53
buccal K13.29
flexural L40.8
guttate L40.4
mouth K13.29
nummular L40.0
plaque L40.0
psychogenic F54
pustular (generalized) L40.1
palmaris et plantaris L40.3
specified NEC L40.8
vulgaris L40.0
Psychasthenia F48.8
Psychiatric disorder or problem F99
Psychogenic —see also condition
factors associated with physical conditions
F54
Psychological and behavioral factors affecting
medical condition F59
Psychoneurosis, psychoneurotic —see also
Neurosis
anxiety (state) F41.1
depersonalization F48.1
hypochondriacal F45.21
hysteria F44.9
neurasthenic F48.8
personality NEC F60.89
Psychopathy, psychopathic
affectionless F94.2
autistic F84.5
constitution, post-traumatic F07.81
personality —see Disorder, personality
sexual —see Deviation, sexual
state F60.2
Psychosexual identity disorder of childhood
F64.2
Psychosis, psychotic F29
acute (transient) F23
hysterical F44.9
affective —see Disorder, mood
alcoholic F10.959
with
abuse F10.159
anxiety disorder F10.980
with
abuse F10.180
dependence F10.280
delirium tremens F10.231
delusions F10.950
with
abuse F10.150
dependence F10.250
dementia F10.97
with dependence F10.27
dependence F10.259
hallucinosis F10.951
with
abuse F10.151
dependence F10.251
mood disorder F10.94
with
abuse F10.14
dependence F10.24
paranoia F10.950
with
abuse F10.150
dependence F10.250
persisting amnesia F10.96
with dependence F10.26
amnestic confabulatory F10.96
with dependence F10.26
delirium tremens F10.231
Korsakoff's, Korsakov's, Korsakow's F10.26

Psychosis, psychotic (*Continued*)
  alcoholic (*Continued*)
    paranoid type F10.950
      with
        abuse F10.150
        dependence F10.250
  anergastic —*see* Psychosis, organic
  arteriosclerotic (simple type) (uncomplicated)
      F01.50
    with behavioral disturbance F01.51
  childhood F84.0
    atypical F84.8
  climacteric —*see* Psychosis, involutional
  confusional F29
    acute or subacute F05
    reactive F23
  cycloid F23
  depressive —*see* Disorder, depressive
  disintegrative (childhood) F84.3
  drug-induced —*see* F11-F19 with .x59
    paranoid and hallucinatory states —*see*
        F11-F19 with .x50 or .x51
  due to or associated with
    addiction, drug —*see* F11-F19 with .X59
    dependence
      alcohol F10.259
      drug —*see* F11-F19 with .x59
    epilepsy F06.8
    Huntington's chorea F06.8
    ischemia, cerebrovascular (generalized)
        F06.8
    multiple sclerosis F06.8
    physical disease F06.8
    presenile dementia F03
    senile dementia F03
    vascular disease (arteriosclerotic) (cerebral)
        F01.50
      with behavioral disturbance F01.51
  epileptic F06.8
  episode F23
    due to or associated with physical
        condition F06.8
  exhaustive F43.0
  hallucinatory, chronic F28
  hypomanic F30.8
  hysterical (acute) F44.9
  induced F24
  infantile F84.0
    atypical F84.8
  infective (acute) (subacute) F05
  involutional F28
    depressive —*see* Disorder, depressive
    melancholic —*see* Disorder, depressive
    paranoid (state) F22
  Korsakoff's, Korsakov's, Korsakow's
      (nonalcoholic) F04
    alcoholic F10.96
      in dependence F10.26
    induced by other psychoactive
        substance —*see* categories F11-F19
        with .x5x
  mania, manic (single episode) F30.2
    recurrent type F31.89
  manic-depressive —*see* Disorder, bipolar
  menopausal —*see* Psychosis, involutional
  mixed schizophrenic and affective F25.8
  multi-infarct (cerebrovascular) F01.50
    with behavioral disturbance F01.51
  nonorganic F29
    specified NEC F28
  organic F09
    due to or associated with
      arteriosclerosis (cerebral) —*see*
          Psychosis, arteriosclerotic
      cerebrovascular disease,
          arteriosclerotic —*see* Psychosis,
          arteriosclerotic
      childbirth —*see* Psychosis, puerperal
      Creutzfeldt-Jakob disease or
          syndrome —*see* Creutzfeldt-Jakob
          disease or syndrome

Psychosis, psychotic (*Continued*)
  organic (*Continued*)
    due to or associated with (*Continued*)
      dependence, alcohol F10.259
      disease
        alcoholic liver F10.259
        brain, arteriosclerotic —*see* Psychosis,
            arteriosclerotic
        cerebrovascular F01.50
          with behavioral disturbance
              F01.51
        Creutzfeldt-Jakob —*see* Creutzfeldt-
            Jakob disease or syndrome
        endocrine or metabolic F06.8
          acute or subacute F05
        liver, alcoholic F10.259
      epilepsy transient (acute) F05
      infection
        brain (intracranial) F06.8
          acute or subacute F05
      intoxication
        alcoholic (acute) F10.259
        drug F11-F19 with .x59
      ischemia, cerebrovascular
          (generalized) —*see* Psychosis,
          arteriosclerotic
      puerperium —*see* Psychosis, puerperal
      trauma, brain (birth) (from electric
          current) (surgical) F06.8
        acute or subacute F05
    infective F06.8
      acute or subacute F05
    post-traumatic F06.8
      acute or subacute F05
  paranoiac F22
  paranoid (climacteric) (involutional)
      (menopausal) F22
    psychogenic (acute) F23
    schizophrenic F20.0
    senile F03
  postpartum F53.1
  presbyophrenic (type) F03
  presenile F03
  psychogenic (paranoid) F23
    depressive F32.3
  puerperal F53.1
    specified type —*see* Psychosis, by type
  reactive (brief) (transient) (emotional stress)
      (psychological trauma) F23
    depressive F32.3
      recurrent F33.3
    excitative type F30.8
  schizoaffective F25.9
    depressive type F25.1
    manic type F25.0
  schizophrenia, schizophrenic —*see*
      Schizophrenia
  schizophrenia-like, in epilepsy F06.2
  schizophreniform F20.81
    affective type F25.9
    brief F23
    confusional type F23
    mixed type F25.0
  senile NEC F03
    depressed or paranoid type F03
    simple deterioration F03
    specified type — code to condition
  shared F24
  situational (reactive) F23
  symbiotic (childhood) F84.3
  symptomatic F09
Psychosomatic —*see* Disorder,
    psychosomatic
Psychosyndrome, organic F07.9
Psychotic episode due to or associated with
    physical condition F06.8
Pterygium (eye) H11.00-●
  amyloid H11.01-●
  central H11.02-●
  colli Q18.3
  double H11.03-●

Psychosis, psychotic (*Continued*)
  peripheral
    progressive H11.05-●
    stationary H11.04-●
  recurrent H11.06-●
Ptilosis (eyelid) —*see* Madarosis
Ptomaine (poisoning) —*see* Poisoning, food
Ptosis —*see also* Blepharoptosis
  adiposa (false) —*see* Blepharoptosis
  breast N64.81
  brow H57.81-●
  cecum K63.4
  colon K63.4
  congenital (eyelid) Q10.0
    specified site NEC —*see* Anomaly, by site
  eyebrow H57.81-●
  eyelid —*see* Blepharoptosis
    congenital Q10.0
  gastric K31.89
  intestine K63.4
  kidney N28.83
  liver K76.89
  renal N28.83
  splanchnic K63.4
  spleen D73.89
  stomach K31.89
  viscera K63.4
PTP D69.51
Ptyalism (periodic) K11.7
  hysterical F45.8
  pregnancy —*see* Pregnancy, complicated by,
      specified pregnancy-related condition
      NEC
  psychogenic F45.8
Ptyalolithiasis K11.5
Pubarche, precocious E30.1
Pubertas praecox E30.1
Puberty (development state) Z00.3
  bleeding (excessive) N92.2
  delayed E30.0
  precocious (constitutional) (cryptogenic)
      (idiopathic) E30.1
    central E22.8
    due to
      ovarian hyperfunction E28.1
        estrogen E28.0
      testicular hyperfunction E29.0
  premature E30.1
    due to
      adrenal cortical hyperfunction E25.8
      pineal tumor E34.8
      pituitary (anterior) hyperfunction E22.8
Puckering, macula —*see* Degeneration, macula,
    puckering
Pudenda, pudendum —*see* condition
Puente's disease (simple glandular cheilitis)
    K13.0
Puerperal, puerperium (complicated by,
    complications)
  abnormal glucose (tolerance test) O99.815
  abscess
    areola O91.02
      associated with lactation O91.03
    Bartholin's gland O86.19
    breast O91.12
      associated with lactation O91.13
    cervix (uteri) O86.11
    genital organ NEC O86.19
    kidney O86.21
    mammary O91.12
      associated with lactation O91.13
    nipple O91.02
      associated with lactation O91.03
    peritoneum O85
    subareola O91.12
      associated with lactation O91.13
    urinary tract —*see* Puerperal, infection,
        urinary
    uterus O86.12
    vagina (wall) O86.13
    vaginorectal O86.13
    vulvovaginal gland O86.13

Puerperal, puerperium *(Continued)*
  adnexitis O86.19
  afibrinogenemia, or other coagulation defect
      O72.3
  albuminuria (acute) (subacute) —*see*
      Proteinuria, gestational
  alcohol use O99.315
  anemia O90.81
    pre-existing (pre-pregnancy) O99.03
  anesthetic death O89.8
  apoplexy O99.43
  bariatric surgery status O99.845
  blood disorder NEC O99.13
  blood dyscrasia O72.3
  cardiomyopathy O90.3
  cerebrovascular disorder (conditions in
      I60-I69) O99.43
  cervicitis O86.11
  circulatory system disorder O99.43
  coagulopathy (any) O99.13
    with hemorrhage O72.3
  complications O90.9
    specified NEC O90.89
  convulsions —*see* Eclampsia
  cystitis O86.22
  cystopyelitis O86.29
  delirium NEC F05
  diabetes O24.93
    gestational —*see* Puerperal, gestational
        diabetes
    pre-existing O24.33
      specified NEC O24.83
      type 1 O24.03
      type 2 O24.13
  digestive system disorder O99.63
  disease O90.9
    breast NEC O92.29
    cerebrovascular (acute) O99.43
    nonobstetric NEC O99.893
    tubo-ovarian O86.19
    Valsuani's O99.03
  disorder O90.9
    biliary tract O26.63
    lactation O92.70
    liver O26.63
    nonobstetric NEC O99.893
  disruption
    cesarean wound O90.0
    episiotomy wound O90.1
    perineal laceration wound O90.1
  drug use O99.325
  eclampsia (with pre-existing hypertension)
      O15.2
  embolism (pulmonary) (blood clot) —*see*
      Embolism, obstetric, puerperal
  endocrine, nutritional or metabolic disease
      NEC O99.285
  endophlebitis —*see* Puerperal, phlebitis
  endotrachelitis O86.11
  failure
    lactation (complete) O92.3
      partial O92.4
    renal, acute O90.4
  fever (of unknown origin) O86.4
    septic O85
  fissure, nipple O92.12
    associated with lactation O92.13
  fistula
    breast (due to mastitis) O91.12
      associated with lactation O91.13
    nipple O91.02
      associated with lactation O91.03
  galactophoritis O91.22
    associated with lactation O91.23
  galactorrhea O92.6
  gastric banding status O99.845
  gastric bypass status O99.845
  gastrointestinal disease NEC O99.63
  gestational
    diabetes O24.439
      diet controlled O24.430
      insulin (and diet) controlled O24.434

Puerperal, puerperium *(Continued)*
  gestational *(Continued)*
    diabetes *(Continued)*
      oral drug controlled (antidiabetic)
          (hypoglycemic) O24.435
    edema O12.05
      with proteinuria O12.25
    proteinuria O12.15
  gonorrhea O98.23
  hematoma, subdural O99.43
  hemiplegia, cerebral O99.355-●
    due to cerebrovascular disorder O99.43
  hemorrhage O72.1
    brain O99.43
    bulbar O99.43
    cerebellar O99.43
    cerebral O99.43
    cortical O99.43
    delayed or secondary O72.2
    extradural O99.43
    internal capsule O99.43
    intracranial O99.43
    intrapontine O99.43
    meningeal O99.43
    pontine O99.43
    retained placenta O72.0
    subarachnoid O99.43
    subcortical O99.43
    subdural O99.43
    third stage O72.0
    uterine, delayed O72.2
    ventricular O99.43
  hemorrhoids O87.2
  hepatorenal syndrome O90.4
  hypertension —*see* Hypertension,
      complicating, puerperium
  hypertrophy, breast O92.29
  induration breast (fibrous) O92.29
  infection O86.4
    cervix O86.11
    generalized O85
    genital tract NEC O86.19
      obstetric surgical wound O86.09
    kidney (bacillus coli) O86.21
    maternal O98.93
      carrier state NEC O99.835
      gonorrhea O98.23
      human immunodeficiency virus (HIV)
          O98.73
      protozoal O98.63
      sexually transmitted NEC O98.33
      specified NEC O98.83
      streptococcus group B (GBS) carrier state
          O99.825
      syphilis O98.13
      tuberculosis O98.03
      viral hepatitis O98.43
      viral NEC O98.53
    nipple O91.02
      associated with lactation O91.03
    peritoneum O85
    renal O86.21
    specified NEC O86.89
    urinary (asymptomatic) (tract) NEC O86.20
      bladder O86.22
      kidney O86.21
      specified site NEC O86.29
      urethra O86.22
    vagina O86.13
    vein —*see* Puerperal, phlebitis
  ischemia, cerebral O99.43
  lymphangitis O86.89
    breast O91.22
      associated with lactation O91.23
  malignancy O9A.13
  malnutrition O25.3
  mammillitis O91.02
    associated with lactation O91.03
  mammitis O91.22
    associated with lactation O91.23
  mania F30.8

Puerperal, puerperium *(Continued)*
  mastitis O91.22
    associated with lactation O91.23
    purulent O91.12
      associated with lactation O91.13
  melancholia —*see* Disorder, depressive
  mental disorder NEC O99.345
  metroperitonitis O85
  metrorrhagia —*see* Hemorrhage,
      postpartum
  metrosalpingitis O86.19
  metrovaginitis O86.13
  milk leg O87.1
  monoplegia, cerebral O99.43
  mood disturbance O90.6
  necrosis, liver (acute) (subacute)
      (conditions in subcategory K72.0) O26.63
    with renal failure O90.4
  nervous system disorder O99.355
  neuritis O90.89
  obesity (pre-existing prior to pregnancy)
      O99.215
  obesity surgery status O99.845
  occlusion, precerebral artery O99.43
  paralysis
    bladder (sphincter) O90.89
    cerebral O99.43
  paralytic stroke O99.43
  parametritis O85
  paravaginitis O86.13
  pelviperitonitis O85
  perimetritis O86.12
  perimetrosalpingitis O86.19
  perinephritis O86.21
  periphlebitis —*see* Puerperal phlebitis
  peritoneal infection O85
  peritonitis (pelvic) O85
  perivaginitis O86.13
  phlebitis O87.0
    deep O87.1
    pelvic O87.1
    superficial O87.0
  phlebothrombosis, deep O87.1
  phlegmasia alba dolens O87.1
  placental polyp O90.89
  pneumonia, embolic —*see* Embolism,
      obstetric, puerperal
  pre-eclampsia —*see* Pre-eclampsia
  psychosis F53.1
  pyelitis O86.21
  pyelocystitis O86.29
  pyelonephritis O86.21
  pyelonephrosis O86.21
  pyemia O85
  pyocystitis O86.29
  pyohemia O85
  pyometra O86.12
  pyonephritis O86.21
  pyosalpingitis O86.19
  pyrexia (of unknown origin) O86.4
  renal
    disease NEC O90.89
    failure O90.4
  respiratory disease NEC O99.53
  retention
    decidua —*see* Retention, decidua
    placenta O72.0
    secundines —*see* Retention,
        secundines
  retracted nipple O92.02
  salpingo-ovaritis O86.19
  salpingoperitonitis O85
  secondary perineal tear O90.1
  sepsis O85
  sepsis (pelvic) O85
  septic thrombophlebitis O86.81
  skin disorder NEC O99.73
  specified condition NEC O99.893
  stroke O99.43
  subinvolution (uterus) O90.89
  subluxation of symphysis (pubis) O26.73

Puerperal, puerperium *(Continued)*
  suppuration —*see* Puerperal, abscess
  tetanus A34
  thelitis O91.02
    associated with lactation O91.03
  thrombocytopenia O72.3
  thrombophlebitis (superficial) O87.0
    deep O87.1
    pelvic O87.1
    septic O86.81
  thrombosis (venous) —*see* Thrombosis, puerperal
  thyroiditis O90.5
  toxemia (eclamptic) (pre-eclamptic) (with convulsions) O15.2
  trauma, non-obstetric O9A.23
    caused by abuse (physical) (suspected) O9A.33
      confirmed O9A.33
      psychological (suspected) O9A.53
        confirmed O9A.53
      sexual (suspected) O9A.43
        confirmed O9A.43
  uremia (due to renal failure) O90.4
  urethritis O86.22
  vaginitis O86.13
  varicose veins (legs) O87.4
    vulva or perineum O87.8
  venous O87.9
  vulvitis O86.19
  vulvovaginitis O86.13
  white leg O87.1
Puerperium —*see* Puerperal
Pulmolithiasis J98.4
Pulmonary —*see* condition
Pulpitis (acute) (anachoretic) (chronic) (hyperplastic) (putrescent) (suppurative) (ulcerative) K04.01
  irreversible K04.02
  reversible K04.01
Pulpless tooth K04.99
Pulse
  alternating R00.8
  bigeminal R00.8
  fast R00.0
  feeble, rapid due to shock following injury T79.4
  rapid R00.0
  weak R09.89
Pulsus alternans or trigeminus R00.8
Punch drunk F07.81
Punctum lacrimale occlusion —*see* Obstruction, lacrimal
Puncture
  abdomen, abdominal
    wall S31.139
      with
        foreign body S31.149
        penetration into peritoneal cavity S31.639
          with foreign body S31.649
      epigastric region S31.132
        with
          foreign body S31.142
          penetration into peritoneal cavity S31.632
            with foreign body S31.642
      left
        lower quadrant S31.134
          with
            foreign body S31.144
            penetration into peritoneal cavity S31.634
              with foreign body S31.644
        upper quadrant S31.131
          with
            foreign body S31.141
            penetration into peritoneal cavity S31.631
              with foreign body S31.641

Puncture *(Continued)*
  abdomen, abdominal *(Continued)*
    wall *(Continued)*
      periumbilic region S31.135
        with
          foreign body S31.145
          penetration into peritoneal cavity S31.635
            with foreign body S31.645
      right
        lower quadrant S31.133
          with
            foreign body S31.143
            penetration into peritoneal cavity S31.633
              with foreign body S31.643
        upper quadrant S31.130
          with
            foreign body S31.140
            penetration into peritoneal cavity S31.630
              with foreign body S31.640
  accidental, complicating surgery —*see* Complication, accidental puncture or laceration
  alveolar (process) —*see* Puncture, oral cavity
  ankle S91.039
    with
      foreign body S91.049
    left S91.032
      with
        foreign body S91.042
    right S91.031
      with
        foreign body S91.041
  anus S31.833
    with foreign body S31.834
  arm (upper) S41.139
    with foreign body S41.149
    left S41.132
      with foreign body S41.142
    lower —*see* Puncture, forearm
    right S41.131
      with foreign body S41.141
  auditory canal (external) (meatus) —*see* Puncture, ear
  auricle, ear —*see* Puncture, ear
  axilla —*see* Puncture, arm
  back —*see also* Puncture, thorax, back
    lower S31.030
      with
        foreign body S31.040
          with penetration into retroperitoneal space S31.041
        penetration into retroperitoneal space S31.031
  bladder (traumatic) S37.29
    nontraumatic N32.89
  breast S21.039
    with foreign body S21.049
    left S21.032
      with foreign body S21.042
    right S21.031
      with foreign body S21.041
  buttock S31.803
    with foreign body S31.804
    left S31.823
      with foreign body S31.824
    right S31.813
      with foreign body S31.814
  by
    device, implant or graft —*see* Complications, by site and type, mechanical
    foreign body left accidentally in operative wound T81.539
    instrument (any) during a procedure, accidental —*see* Puncture, accidental complicating surgery
  calf —*see* Puncture, leg
  canaliculus lacrimalis —*see* Puncture, eyelid

Puncture *(Continued)*
  canthus, eye —*see* Puncture, eyelid
  cervical esophagus S11.23
    with foreign body S11.24
  cheek (external) S01.439
    with foreign body S01.449
    internal —*see* Puncture, oral cavity
    left S01.432
      with foreign body S01.442
    right S01.431
      with foreign body S01.441
  chest wall —*see* Puncture, thorax
  chin —*see* Puncture, head, specified site NEC
  clitoris —*see* Puncture, vulva
  costal region —*see* Puncture, thorax
  digit(s)
    foot —*see* Puncture, toe
    hand —*see* Puncture, finger
  ear (canal) (external) S01.339
    with foreign body S01.349
    drum S09.2-●
    left S01.332
      with foreign body S01.342
    right S01.331
      with foreign body S01.341
  elbow S51.039
    with
      foreign body S51.049
    left S51.032
      with
        foreign body S51.042
    right S51.031
      with
        foreign body S51.041
  epididymis —*see* Puncture, testis
  epigastric region —*see* Puncture, abdomen, wall, epigastric
  epiglottis S11.83
    with foreign body S11.84
  esophagus
    cervical S11.23
      with foreign body S11.24
    thoracic S27.818
  eyeball S05.6-●
    with foreign body S05.5-●
  eyebrow —*see* Puncture, eyelid
  eyelid S01.13-●
    with foreign body S01.14-●
    left S01.132
      with foreign body S01.142
    right S01.131
      with foreign body S01.141
  face NEC —*see* Puncture, head, specified site NEC
  finger(s) S61.239
    with
      damage to nail S61.339
        with
          foreign body S61.349
      foreign body S61.249
    index S61.238
      with
        damage to nail S61.338
          with
            foreign body S61.348
        foreign body S61.248
      left S61.231
        with
          damage to nail S61.331
            with
              foreign body S61.341
          foreign body S61.241
      right S61.230
        with
          damage to nail S61.330
            with
              foreign body S61.340
          foreign body S61.240
    little S61.238
      with
        damage to nail S61.338

▶ New   ⇒ Revised   ~~deleted~~ Deleted   ● Use Additional Character(s)

Puncture (Continued)
  finger (Continued)
    with (Continued)
      with (Continued)
        damage to nail (Continued)
          with
            foreign body S61.348
          foreign body S61.248
      left S61.237
        with
          damage to nail S61.337
            with
              foreign body S61.347
          foreign body S61.247
      right S61.236
        with
          damage to nail S61.336
            with
              foreign body S61.346
          foreign body S61.246
    middle S61.238
      with
        damage to nail S61.338
          with
            foreign body S61.348
        foreign body S61.248
      left S61.233
        with
          damage to nail S61.333
            with
              foreign body S61.343
          foreign body S61.243
      right S61.232
        with
          damage to nail S61.332
            with
              foreign body S61.342
          foreign body S61.242
    ring S61.238
      with
        damage to nail S61.338
          with
            foreign body S61.348
        foreign body S61.248
      left S61.235
        with
          damage to nail S61.335
            with
              foreign body S61.345
          foreign body S61.245
      right S61.234
        with
          damage to nail S61.334
            with
              foreign body S61.344
          foreign body S61.244
  flank S31.139
    with foreign body S31.149
  foot (except toe(s) alone) S91.339
    with foreign body S91.349
    left S91.332
      with foreign body S91.342
    right S91.331
      with foreign body S91.341
    toe —see Puncture, toe
  forearm S51.839
    with
      foreign body S51.849
    elbow only —see Puncture, elbow
    left S51.832
      with
        foreign body S51.842
    right S51.831
      with
        foreign body S51.841
  forehead —see Puncture, head, specified site NEC
  genital organs, external
    female S31.532
      with foreign body S31.542
      vagina —see Puncture, vagina
      vulva —see Puncture, vulva

Puncture (Continued)
  genital organs, external (Continued)
    male S31.531
      with foreign body S31.541
      penis —see Puncture, penis
      scrotum —see Puncture, scrotum
      testis —see Puncture, testis
  groin —see Puncture, abdomen, wall
  gum —see Puncture, oral cavity
  hand S61.439
    with
      foreign body S61.449
    finger —see Puncture, finger
    left S61.432
      with
        foreign body S61.442
    right S61.431
      with
        foreign body S61.441
    thumb —see Puncture, thumb
  head S01.93
    with foreign body S01.94
    cheek —see Puncture, cheek
    ear —see Puncture, ear
    eyelid —see Puncture, eyelid
    lip —see Puncture, oral cavity
    nose —see Puncture, nose
    oral cavity —see Puncture, oral cavity
    scalp S01.03
      with foreign body S01.04
    specified site NEC S01.83
      with foreign body S01.84
    temporomandibular area —see Puncture, cheek
  heart S26.99
    with hemopericardium S26.09
    without hemopericardium S26.19
  heel —see Puncture, foot
  hip S71.039
    with foreign body S71.049
    left S71.032
      with foreign body S71.042
    right S71.031
      with foreign body S71.041
  hymen —see Puncture, vagina
  hypochondrium —see Puncture, abdomen, wall
  hypogastric region —see Puncture, abdomen, wall
  inguinal region —see Puncture, abdomen, wall
  instep —see Puncture, foot
  internal organs —see Injury, by site
  interscapular region —see Puncture, thorax, back
  intestine
    large
      colon S36.599
        ascending S36.590
        descending S36.592
        sigmoid S36.593
        specified site NEC S36.598
        transverse S36.591
      rectum S36.69
    small S36.499
      duodenum S36.490
      specified site NEC S36.498
  intra-abdominal organ S36.99
    gallbladder S36.128
    intestine —see Puncture, intestine
    liver S36.118
    pancreas —see Puncture, pancreas
    peritoneum S36.81
    specified site NEC S36.898
    spleen S36.09
    stomach S36.39
  jaw —see Puncture, head, specified site NEC
  knee S81.039
    with foreign body S81.049
    left S81.032
      with foreign body S81.042

Puncture (Continued)
  knee (Continued)
    right S81.031
      with foreign body S81.041
  labium (majus) (minus) —see Puncture, vulva
  lacrimal duct —see Puncture, eyelid
  larynx S11.013
    with foreign body S11.014
  leg (lower) S81.839
    with foreign body S81.849
    foot —see Puncture, foot
    knee —see Puncture, knee
    left S81.832
      with foreign body S81.842
    right S81.831
      with foreign body S81.841
    upper —see Puncture, thigh
  lip S01.531
    with foreign body S01.541
  loin —see Puncture, abdomen, wall
  lower back —see Puncture, back, lower
  lumbar region —see Puncture, back, lower
  malar region —see Puncture, head, specified site NEC
  mammary —see Puncture, breast
  mastoid region —see Puncture, head, specified site NEC
  mouth —see Puncture, oral cavity
  nail
    finger —see Puncture, finger, with damage to nail
    toe —see Puncture, toe, with damage to nail
  nasal (septum) (sinus) —see Puncture, nose
  nasopharynx —see Puncture, head, specified site NEC
  neck S11.93
    with foreign body S11.94
    involving
      cervical esophagus —see Puncture, cervical esophagus
      larynx —see Puncture, larynx
      pharynx —see Puncture, pharynx
      thyroid gland —see Puncture, thyroid gland
      trachea —see Puncture, trachea
    specified site NEC S11.83
      with foreign body S11.84
  nose (septum) (sinus) S01.23
    with foreign body S01.24
  ocular —see Puncture, eyeball - oral cavity S01.532
    with foreign body S01.542
  orbit S05.4-●
  palate —see Puncture, oral cavity
  palm —see Puncture, hand
  pancreas S36.299
    body S36.291
    head S36.290
    tail S36.292
  pelvis —see Puncture, back, lower
  penis S31.23
    with foreign body S31.24
  perineum
    female S31.43
      with foreign body S31.44
    male S31.139
      with foreign body S31.149
  periocular area (with or without lacrimal passages) —see Puncture, eyelid
  phalanges
    finger —see Puncture, finger
    toe —see Puncture, toe
  pharynx S11.23
    with foreign body S11.24
  pinna —see Puncture, ear
  popliteal space —see Puncture, knee
  prepuce —see Puncture, penis
  pubic region S31.139
    with foreign body S31.149

Puncture *(Continued)*
  pudendum —*see* Puncture, genital organs,
    external
  rectovaginal septum —*see* Puncture,
    vagina
  sacral region —*see* Puncture, back,
    lower
  sacroiliac region —*see* Puncture, back,
    lower
  salivary gland —*see* Puncture, oral
    cavity
  scalp S01.03
    with foreign body S01.04
  scapular region —*see* Puncture,
    shoulder
  scrotum S31.33
    with foreign body S31.34
  shin —*see* Puncture, leg
  shoulder S41.039
    with foreign body S41.049
    left S41.032
      with foreign body S41.042
    right S41.031
      with foreign body S41.041
  spermatic cord —*see* Puncture, testis
  sternal region —*see* Puncture, thorax, front
  submaxillary region —*see* Puncture, head,
    specified site NEC
  submental region —*see* Puncture, head,
    specified site NEC
  subungual
    finger(s) —*see* Puncture, finger, with
      damage to nail
    toe —*see* Puncture, toe, with damage to
      nail
  supraclavicular fossa —*see* Puncture, neck,
    specified site NEC
  temple, temporal region —*see* Puncture, head,
    specified site NEC
  temporomandibular area —*see* Puncture,
    cheek
  testis S31.33
    with foreign body S31.34
  thigh S71.139
    with foreign body S71.149
    left S71.132
      with foreign body S71.142
    right S71.131
      with foreign body S71.141
  thorax, thoracic (wall) S21.93
    with foreign body S21.94
    back S21.23-●
      with
        foreign body S21.24-●
          with penetration S21.44
        penetration S21.43
    breast —*see* Puncture, breast
    front S21.13-●
      with
        foreign body S21.14-●
          with penetration S21.34
        penetration S21.33
  throat —*see* Puncture, neck
  thumb S61.039
    with
      damage to nail S61.139
        with
          foreign body S61.149
      foreign body S61.049
    left S61.032
      with
        damage to nail S61.132
          with
            foreign body S61.142
        foreign body S61.042
    right S61.031
      with
        damage to nail S61.131
          with
            foreign body S61.141
        foreign body S61.041

Puncture *(Continued)*
  thyroid gland S11.13
    with foreign body S11.14
  toe(s) S91.139
    with
      damage to nail S91.239
        with
          foreign body S91.249
      foreign body S91.149
    great S91.133
      with
        damage to nail S91.233
          with
            foreign body S91.243
        foreign body S91.143
      left S91.132
        with
          damage to nail S91.232
            with
              foreign body S91.242
          foreign body S91.142
      right S91.131
        with
          damage to nail S91.231
            with
              foreign body S91.241
          foreign body S91.141
    lesser S91.136
      with
        damage to nail S91.236
          with
            foreign body S91.246
        foreign body S91.146
      left S91.135
        with
          damage to nail S91.235
            with
              foreign body S91.245
        foreign body S91.145
      right S91.134
        with
          damage to nail S91.234
            with
              foreign body S91.244
        foreign body S91.144
  tongue —*see* Puncture, oral cavity
  trachea S11.023
    with foreign body S11.024
  tunica vaginalis —*see* Puncture, testis
  tympanum, tympanic membrane
    S09.2-●
  umbilical region S31.135
    with foreign body S31.145
  uvula —*see* Puncture, oral cavity
  vagina S31.43
    with foreign body S31.44
  vocal cords S11.033
    with foreign body S11.034
  vulva S31.43
    with foreign body S31.44
  wrist S61.539
    with
      foreign body S61.549
    left S61.532
      with
        foreign body S61.542
    right S61.531
      with
        foreign body S61.541
PUO (pyrexia of unknown origin) R50.9
Pupillary membrane (persistent) Q13.89
Pupillotonia —*see* Anomaly, pupil, function,
  tonic pupil
Purpura D69.2
  abdominal D69.0
  allergic D69.0
  anaphylactoid D69.0
  annularis telangiectodes L81.7
  arthritic D69.0
  autoerythrocyte sensitization D69.2
  autoimmune D69.0

Purpura *(Continued)*
  bacterial D69.0
  Bateman's (senile) D69.2
  capillary fragility (hereditary) (idiopathic)
    D69.8
  cryoglobulinemic D89.1
  Devil's pinches D69.2
  fibrinolytic —*see* Fibrinolysis
  fulminans, fulminous D65
  gangrenous D65
  hemorrhagic, hemorrhagica D69.3
    not due to thrombocytopenia D69.0
  Henoch (-Schönlein) (allergic) D69.0
  hypergammaglobulinemic (benign)
    (Waldenström's) D89.0
  idiopathic (thrombocytopenic) D69.3
    nonthrombocytopenic D69.0
  immune thrombocytopenic D69.3
  infectious D69.0
  malignant D69.0
  neonatorum P54.5
  nervosa D69.0
  newborn P54.5
  nonthrombocytopenic D69.2
    hemorrhagic D69.0
    idiopathic D69.0
  nonthrombopenic D69.2
  peliosis rheumatica D69.0
  posttransfusion (post-transfusion) (from
    (fresh) whole blood or blood products)
    D69.51
  primary D69.49
  red cell membrane sensitivity D69.2
  rheumatica D69.0
  Schönlein (-Henoch) (allergic) D69.0
  scorbutic E54 *[D77]*
  senile D69.2
  simplex D69.2
  symptomatica D69.0
  telangiectasia annularis L81.7
  thrombocytopenic D69.49
    congenital D69.42
    hemorrhagic D69.3
    hereditary D69.42
    idiopathic D69.3
    immune D69.3
    neonatal, transitory P61.0
  ➧thrombotic M31.19
  thrombohemolytic —*see* Fibrinolysis
  thrombolytic —*see* Fibrinolysis
  thrombopenic D69.49
  ➧thrombotic, thrombocytopenic
    M31.19
  toxic D69.0
  vascular D69.0
  visceral symptoms D69.0
Purpuric spots R23.3
Purulent —*see* condition
Pus
  in
    stool R19.5
    urine N39.0
  tube (rupture) —*see* Salpingo-oophoritis
Pustular rash L08.0
Pustule (nonmalignant) L08.9
  malignant A22.0
Pustulosis palmaris et plantaris
  L40.3
Putnam (-Dana) disease or syndrome —*see*
  Degeneration, combined
Putrescent pulp (dental) K04.1
Pyarthritis, pyarthrosis —*see* Arthritis,
  pyogenic or pyemic
  tuberculous —*see* Tuberculosis, joint
Pyelectasis —*see* Hydronephrosis
Pyelitis (congenital) (uremic) —*see also*
  Pyelonephritis
  with
    calculus —*see* category N20
      with hydronephrosis N13.6
    contracted kidney N11.9

▶ New   ➧ Revised   ~~deleted~~ Deleted   ● Use Additional Character(s)

Pyelitis *(Continued)*
  acute N10
  chronic N11.9
    with calculus —*see* category N20
      with hydronephrosis N13.6
  cystica N28.84
  puerperal (postpartum) O86.21
  tuberculous A18.11
Pyelocystitis —*see* Pyelonephritis
Pyelonephritis —*see also* Nephritis,
    tubulo-interstitial
  with
    calculus —*see* category N20
      with hydronephrosis N13.6
    contracted kidney N11.9
  acute N10
  calculus —*see* category N20
    with hydronephrosis N13.6
  chronic N11.9
    with calculus —*see* category N20
      with hydronephrosis N13.6
    associated with ureteral obstruction or
      stricture N11.1
    nonobstructive N11.8
      with reflux (vesicoureteral) N11.0
    obstructive N11.1
    specified NEC N11.8
  in (due to)
    brucellosis A23.9 *[N16]*
    cryoglobulinemia (mixed) D89.1 *[N16]*
    cystinosis E72.04
    diphtheria A36.84
    glycogen storage disease E74.09 *[N16]*
    leukemia NEC C95.9-• *[N16]*
    lymphoma NEC C85.90 *[N16]*
    multiple myeloma C90.0-• *[N16]*
    obstruction N11.1
    Salmonella infection A02.25
    sarcoidosis D86.84
    sepsis A41.9 *[N16]*
    Sjögren's disease M35.04
    toxoplasmosis B58.83
    transplant rejection T86.91 *[N16]*
    Wilson's disease E83.01 *[N16]*
  nonobstructive N12
    with reflux (vesicoureteral) N11.0
    chronic N11.8
  syphilitic A52.75

Pyelonephrosis (obstructive) N11.1
  chronic N11.9
Pyelophlebitis I80.8
Pyeloureteritis cystica N28.85
Pyemia, pyemic (fever) (infection) (purulent) —
    see also Sepsis
  joint —*see* Arthritis, pyogenic or pyemic
  liver K75.1
  pneumococcal A40.3
  portal K75.1
  postvaccinal T88.0
  puerperal, postpartum, childbirth O85
  specified organism NEC A41.89
  tuberculous —*see* Tuberculosis, miliary
Pygopagus Q89.4
Pyknoepilepsy (idiopathic) —*see* Pyknolepsy
Pyknolepsy G40.A09
  intractable G40.A19
    with status epilepticus G40.A11
    without status epilepticus G40.A19
  not intractable G40.A09
    with status epilepticus G40.A01
    without status epilepticus G40.A09
Pylephlebitis K75.1
Pyle's syndrome Q78.5
Pylethrombophlebitis K75.1
Pylethrombosis K75.1
Pyloritis K29.90
  with bleeding K29.91
Pylorospasm (reflex) NEC K31.3
  congenital or infantile Q40.0
  neurotic F45.8
  newborn Q40.0
  psychogenic F45.8
Pylorus, pyloric —*see* condition
Pyoarthrosis —*see* Arthritis, pyogenic or
    pyemic
Pyocele
  mastoid —*see* Mastoiditis, acute
  sinus (accessory) —*see* Sinusitis
  turbinate (bone) J32.9
  urethra —*see also* Urethritis N34.0
Pyocolpos —*see* Vaginitis
Pyocystitis N30.80
  with hematuria N30.81
Pyoderma, pyodermia L08.0
  gangrenosum L88
  newborn P39.4

Pyoderma, pyodermia *(Continued)*
  phagedenic L88
  vegetans L08.81
Pyodermatitis L08.0
  vegetans L08.81
Pyogenic —*see* condition
Pyohydronephrosis N13.6
Pyometra, pyometrium, pyometritis —*see*
    Endometritis
Pyomyositis (tropical) —*see* Myositis,
    infective
Pyonephritis N12
Pyonephrosis N13.6
  tuberculous A18.11
Pyo-oophoritis —*see* Salpingo-oophoritis
Pyo-ovarium —*see* Salpingo-oophoritis
Pyopericarditis, pyopericardium
    I30.1
Pyophlebitis —*see* Phlebitis
Pyopneumopericardium I30.1
Pyopneumothorax (infective) J86.9
  with fistula J86.0
  tuberculous NEC A15.6
Pyosalpinx, pyosalpingitis —*see also*
    Salpingo-oophoritis
Pyothorax J86.9
  with fistula J86.0
  tuberculous NEC A15.6
Pyoureter N28.89
  tuberculous A18.11
Pyramidopallidonigral syndrome
    G20
Pyrexia (of unknown origin) R50.9
  atmospheric T67.01
  during labor NEC O75.2
  heat T67.01
  newborn P81.9
    environmentally-induced P81.0
  persistent R50.9
  puerperal O86.4
Pyroglobulinemia NEC E88.09
Pyromania F63.1
Pyrosis R12
Pyuria (bacterial) R82.81

Q

Q fever A78
　with pneumonia A78
Quadricuspid aortic valve Q23.8
Quadrilateral fever A78
Quadriparesis —*see* Quadriplegia
　meaning muscle weakness M62.81
Quadriplegia G82.50-●
　complete
　　C1-C4 level G82.51
　　C5-C7 level G82.53
　congenital (cerebral) (spinal) G80.8
　　spastic G80.0

Quadriplegia (*Continued*)
　embolic (current episode) I63.4-●
　functional R53.2
　incomplete
　　C1-C4 level G82.52
　　C5-C7 level G82.54
　thrombotic (current episode) I63.3-●
　traumatic — code to injury with seventh
　　character S
　　current episode —*see* Injury, spinal (cord),
　　　cervical
Quadruplet, pregnancy —*see* Pregnancy,
　quadruplet
Quarrelsomeness F60.3

Queensland fever A77.3
Quervain's disease M65.4
　thyroid E06.1
Queyrat's erythroplasia D07.4
　penis D07.4
　specified site —*see* Neoplasm, skin,
　　in situ
　unspecified site D07.4
Quincke's disease or edema T78.3
　hereditary D84.1
Quinsy (gangrenous) J36
Quintan fever A79.0
Quintuplet, pregnancy —*see* Pregnancy,
　quintuplet

R

Rabbit fever —*see* Tularemia
Rabies A82.9
   contact Z20.3
   exposure to Z20.3
   inoculation reaction —*see* Complications,
      vaccination
   sylvatic A82.0
   urban A82.1
Rachischisis —*see* Spina bifida
Rachitic —*see also* condition
   deformities of spine (late effect) (sequelae)
      E64.3
   pelvis (late effect) (sequelae) E64.3
      with disproportion (fetopelvic) O33.0
         causing obstructed labor O65.0
Rachitis, rachitism (acute) (tarda) —*see also*
   Rickets
   renalis N25.0
   sequelae E64.3
Radial nerve —*see* condition
Radiation
   burn —*see* Burn
   effects NOS T66
   sickness NOS T66
   therapy, encounter for Z51.0
Radiculitis (pressure) (vertebrogenic) —*see*
   Radiculopathy
Radiculomyelitis —*see also* Encephalitis
   toxic, due to
      Clostridium tetani A35
      Corynebacterium diphtheriae A36.82
Radiculopathy M54.10
   cervical region M54.12
   cervicothoracic region M54.13
   due to
      disc disorder
         C3 M50.11
         C4 M50.11
         C5 M50.121
         C6 M50.122
         C7 M50.123
         C8 M50.13
      displacement of intervertebral disc —*see*
         Disorder, disc, with, radiculopathy
   leg M54.1-●
   lumbar region M54.16
   lumbosacral region M54.17
   occipito-atlanto-axial region M54.11
   postherpetic B02.29
   sacrococcygeal region M54.18
   syphilitic A52.11
   thoracic region (with visceral pain)
      M54.14
   thoracolumbar region M54.15
Radiodermal burns (acute, chronic, or
   occupational) —*see* Burn
Radiodermatitis L58.9
   acute L58.0
   chronic L58.1
Radiotherapy session Z51.0
RAEB (refractory anemia with excess blasts)
   D46.2-●
Rage, meaning rabies —*see* Rabies
Ragpicker's disease A22.1
Ragsorter's disease A22.1
Raillietiniasis B71.8
Railroad neurosis F48.8
Railway spine F48.8
Raised —*see also* Elevated
   antibody titer R76.0
Rake teeth, tooth M26.39
Rales R09.89
Ramifying renal pelvis Q63.8
Ramsay-Hunt disease or syndrome —*see also*
   Hunt's disease B02.21
   meaning dyssynergia cerebellaris myoclonica
      G11.19
Ranula K11.6
   congenital Q38.4

Rape
   adult
      confirmed T74.21
      suspected T76.21
   alleged, observation or examination, ruled out
      adult Z04.41
      child Z04.42
   child
      confirmed T74.22
      suspected T76.22
Rapid
   feeble pulse, due to shock, following injury
      T79.4
   heart (beat) R00.0
      psychogenic F45.8
   second stage (delivery) O62.3
   time-zone change syndrome G47.25
Rarefaction, bone —*see* Disorder, bone, density
   and structure, specified NEC
Rash (toxic) R21
   canker A38.9
   diaper L22
   drug (internal use) L27.0
      contact —*see also* Dermatitis, due to, drugs,
         external L25.1
   following immunization T88.1
   food —*see* Dermatitis, due to, food
   heat L74.0
   napkin (psoriasiform) L22
   nettle —*see* Urticaria
   pustular L08.0
   rose R21
      epidemic B06.9
   scarlet A38.9
   serum —*see also* Reaction, serum T80.69
   wandering tongue K14.1
Rasmussen aneurysm —*see* Tuberculosis,
   pulmonary
Rasmussen encephalitis G04.81
Rat-bite fever A25.9
   due to Streptobacillus moniliformis A25.1
   spirochetal (morsus muris) A25.0
Rathke's pouch tumor D44.3
Raymond (-Céstan) syndrome I65.8
Raynaud's disease, phenomenon or syndrome
   (secondary) I73.00
   with gangrene (symmetric) I73.01
RDS (newborn) (type I) P22.0
   type II P22.1
Reaction —*see also* Disorder
   adaptation —*see* Disorder, adjustment
   adjustment (anxiety) (conduct disorder)
      (depressiveness) (distress) —*see*
      Disorder, adjustment
      with
         mutism, elective (child) (adolescent) F94.0
   adverse
      food (any) (ingested) NEC T78.1
         anaphylactic —*see* Shock, anaphylactic,
            due to food
   anaphylactoid —*see* Shock, anaphylactic
   affective —*see* Disorder, mood
   allergic —*see* Allergy
   anaphylactic —*see* Shock, anaphylactic
   anesthesia —*see* Anesthesia, complication
   antitoxin (prophylactic) (therapeutic) —*see*
      Complications, vaccination
   anxiety F41.1
   Arthus —*see* Arthus' phenomenon
   asthenic F48.8
   combat and operational stress F43.0
   compulsive F42.8
   conversion F44.9
   crisis, acute F43.0
   deoxyribonuclease (DNA) (DNase)
      hypersensitivity D69.2
   depressive (single episode) F32.9
      affective (single episode) F31.4
         recurrent episode F33.9
      neurotic F34.1
      psychoneurotic F34.1

Reaction (*Continued*)
   depressive (*Continued*)
      psychotic F32.3
      recurrent —*see* Disorder, depressive,
         recurrent
   dissociative F44.9
   drug NEC T88.7
      addictive —*see* Dependence, drug
         transmitted via placenta or breast
            milk —*see* Absorption, drug,
            addictive, through placenta
      allergic —*see* Allergy, drug
      lichenoid L43.2
      newborn P93.8
         gray baby syndrome P93.0
      overdose or poisoning (by accident) —*see*
         Table of Drugs and Chemicals, by
         drug, poisoning
      photoallergic L56.1
      phototoxic L56.0
      withdrawal —*see* Dependence, by drug,
         with, withdrawal
         infant of dependent mother P96.1
         newborn P96.1
      wrong substance given or taken (by
         accident) —*see* Table of Drugs and
         Chemicals, by drug, poisoning
   fear F40.9
      child (abnormal) F93.8
   febrile nonhemolytic transfusion (FNHTR)
      R50.84
   fluid loss, cerebrospinal G97.1
   foreign
      body NEC —*see* Granuloma, foreign body
         in operative wound (inadvertently
           left) —*see* Foreign body, accidentally
           left during a procedure
      substance accidentally left during a
         procedure (chemical) (powder) (talc)
         T81.60
         aseptic peritonitis T81.61
         body or object (instrument) (sponge)
           (swab) —*see* Foreign body,
           accidentally left during a
           procedure
         specified reaction NEC T81.69
   grief —*see* Disorder, adjustment
   Herxheimer's R68.89
   hyperkinetic —*see* Hyperkinesia
   hypochondriacal F45.20
   hypoglycemic, due to insulin E16.0
      with coma (diabetic) —*see* Diabetes, coma
         nondiabetic E15
      therapeutic misadventure —*see*
         subcategory T38.3
   hypomanic F30.8
   hysterical F44.9
   immunization —*see* Complications, vaccination
   incompatibility
      ABO blood group (infusion) (transfusion) —
         see Complication(s), transfusion,
         incompatibility reaction, ABO
      delayed serologic T80.39
      minor blood group (Duffy) (E) (K) (Kell)
         (Kidd) (Lewis) (M) (N) (P) (S)
         T80.89
      Rh (factor) (infusion) (transfusion) —
         see Complication(s), transfusion,
         incompatibility reaction, Rh (factor)
   inflammatory —*see* Infection
   infusion —*see* Complications, infusion
   inoculation (immune serum) —*see*
      Complications, vaccination
   insulin T38.3-●
   involutional psychotic —*see* Disorder,
      depressive
   leukemoid D72.823
      basophilic D72.823
      lymphocytic D72.823
      monocytic D72.823
      myelocytic D72.823
      neutrophilic D72.823

Reaction *(Continued)*
  LSD (acute)
    due to drug abuse —*see* Abuse, drug,
      hallucinogen
    due to drug dependence —*see* Dependence,
      drug, hallucinogen
  lumbar puncture G97.1
  manic-depressive —*see* Disorder, bipolar
  neurasthenic F48.8
  neurogenic —*see* Neurosis
  neurotic F48.9
  neurotic-depressive F34.1
  nitritoid —*see* Crisis, nitritoid - obsessive-
    compulsive F42
  nonspecific
    to
      cell mediated immunity measurement
        of gamma interferon antigen
        response without active
        tuberculosis R76.12
      QuantiFERON-TB test (QFT) without
        active tuberculosis R76.12
      tuberculin test —*see also* Reaction,
        tuberculin skin test R76.11
  obsessive-compulsive F42.8
  organic, acute or subacute —*see* Delirium
  paranoid (acute) F23
    chronic F22
    senile F03
  passive dependency F60.7
  phobic F40.9
  post-traumatic stress, uncomplicated Z73.3
  psychogenic F99
  psychoneurotic —*see also* Neurosis
    compulsive F42.8
    depersonalization F48.1
    depressive F34.1
    hypochondriacal F45.20
    neurasthenic F48.8
    obsessive F42.8
  psychophysiologic —*see* Disorder,
    somatoform
  psychosomatic —*see* Disorder, somatoform
  psychotic —*see* Psychosis
  scarlet fever toxin —*see* Complications,
    vaccination
  schizophrenic F23
    acute (brief) (undifferentiated) F23
    latent F21
    undifferentiated (acute) (brief) F23
  serological for syphilis —*see* Serology for
    syphilis
  serum T80.69
    anaphylactic (immediate) —*see also* Shock,
      anaphylactic T80.59
    specified reaction NEC
      due to
        administration of blood and blood
          products T80.61
        immunization T80.62
        serum specified NEC T80.69
        vaccination T80.62
  situational —*see* Disorder, adjustment
  somatization —*see* Disorder, somatoform
  spinal puncture G97.1
    dural G97.1
  stress (severe) F43.9
    acute (agitation) ("daze") (disorientation)
      (disturbance of consciousness) (flight
      reaction) (fugue) F43.0
    specified NEC F43.8
  surgical procedure —*see* Complications,
    surgical procedure
  tetanus antitoxin —*see* Complications,
    vaccination
  toxic, to local anesthesia T81.59
    in labor and delivery O74.4
    in pregnancy O29.3X-•
    postpartum, puerperal O89.3
  toxin-antitoxin —*see* Complications,
    vaccination

Reaction *(Continued)*
  transfusion (blood) (bone marrow)
    (lymphocytes) (allergic) —*see*
    Complications, transfusion
  tuberculin skin test, abnormal R76.11
  vaccination (any) —*see* Complications,
    vaccination
  withdrawing, child or adolescent F93.8
Reactive airway disease —*see* Asthma
Reactive depression —*see* Reaction, depressive
Rearrangement
  chromosomal
    balanced (in) Q95.9
      abnormal individual (autosomal) Q95.2
        non-sex (autosomal) chromosomes
          Q95.2
        sex/non-sex chromosomes Q95.3
      specified NEC Q95.8
Recalcitrant patient —*see* Noncompliance
Recanalization, thrombus —*see* Thrombosis
Recession, receding
  chamber angle (eye) H21.55-•
  chin M26.09
  gingival (postinfective) (postoperative)
    generalized K06.020
      minimal K06.021
      moderate K06.022
      severe K06.023
    localized K06.010
      minimal K06.011
      moderate K06.012
      severe K06.013
Recklinghausen's disease Q85.01
  bones E21.0
Reclus' disease (cystic) —*see* Mastopathy, cystic
Recrudescent typhus (fever) A75.1
Recruitment, auditory H93.21-•
Rectalgia K62.89
Rectitis K62.89
Rectocele
  female (without uterine prolapse) N81.6
    with uterine prolapse N81.4
      incomplete N81.2
  in pregnancy —*see* Pregnancy, complicated
    by, abnormal, pelvic organs or tissues
    NEC
  male K62.3
Rectosigmoid junction —*see* condition
Rectosigmoiditis K63.89
  ulcerative (chronic) K51.30
    with
      complication K51.319
        abscess K51.314
        fistula K51.313
        obstruction K51.312
        rectal bleeding K51.311
        specified NEC K51.318
Rectourethral —*see* condition
Rectovaginal —*see* condition
Rectovesical —*see* condition
Rectum, rectal —*see* condition
Recurrent —*see* condition
  pregnancy loss —*see* Loss (of), pregnancy,
    recurrent
Red bugs B88.0
Red-cedar lung or pneumonitis J67.8
Red tide —*see also* Table of Drugs and
  Chemicals T65.82-•
Reduced
  mobility Z74.09
  ventilatory or vital capacity R94.2
Redundant, redundancy
  anus (congenital) Q43.8
  clitoris N90.89
  colon (congenital) Q43.8
  foreskin (congenital) N47.8
  intestine (congenital) Q43.8
  labia N90.69
  organ or site, congenital NEC —*see* Accessory
  panniculus (abdominal) E65
  prepuce (congenital) N47.8

Redundant, redundancy *(Continued)*
  pylorus K31.89
  rectum (congenital) Q43.8
  scrotum N50.89
  sigmoid (congenital) Q43.8
  skin L98.7
    and subcutaneous tissue L98.7
    of face L57.4
      eyelids —*see* Blepharochalasis
  stomach K31.89
Reduplication —*see* Duplication
Reflex R29.2
  hyperactive gag J39.2
  pupillary, abnormal —*see* Anomaly, pupil,
    function
  vasoconstriction I73.9
  vasovagal R55
Reflux K21.9
  acid K21.9
  esophageal K21.9
    with esophagitis (without bleeding) K21.00
      with bleeding K21.01
    newborn P78.83
  gastroesophageal K21.9
    with esophagitis (without bleeding) K21.00
      with bleeding K21.01
  mitral —*see* Insufficiency, mitral
  ureteral —*see* Reflux, vesicoureteral
  vesicoureteral (with scarring) N13.70
    with
      nephropathy N13.729
        with hydroureter N13.739
          bilateral N13.732
          unilateral N13.731
        without hydroureter N13.729
          bilateral N13.722
          unilateral N13.721
      bilateral N13.722
      unilateral N13.721
      pyelonephritis (chronic) N11.0
    without nephropathy N13.71
    congenital Q62.7
Reforming, artificial openings —*see* Attention
  to, artificial, opening
Refractive error —*see* Disorder, refraction
Refsum's disease or syndrome G60.1
Refusal of
  food, psychogenic F50.89
  treatment (because of) Z53.20
  ➠ left against medical advice (AMA) Z53.29
  ▶ left without being seen Z53.21
    patient's decision NEC Z53.29
    reasons of belief or group pressure Z53.1
Regional —*see* condition
Regurgitation R11.10
  aortic (valve) —*see* Insufficiency, aortic
  food —*see also* Vomiting
    with reswallowing —*see* Rumination
    newborn P92.1
  gastric contents —*see* Vomiting
  heart —*see* Endocarditis
  mitral (valve) —*see* Insufficiency, mitral
    congenital Q23.3
  myocardial —*see* Endocarditis
  pulmonary (valve) (heart) I37.1
    congenital Q22.2
    syphilitic A52.03
  tricuspid —*see* Insufficiency, tricuspid
  valve, valvular —*see* Endocarditis
    congenital Q24.8
  vesicoureteral —*see* Reflux, vesicoureteral
Reichmann's disease or syndrome K31.89
Reifenstein syndrome E34.52
Reinsertion
  implantable subdermal contraceptive Z30.46
  intrauterine contraceptive device Z30.433
Reiter's disease, syndrome, or urethritis
  M02.30
  ankle M02.37-•
  elbow M02.32-•
  foot joint M02.37-•
  hand joint M02.34-•

▶ New   ➠ Revised   ~~deleted~~ Deleted   • Use Additional Character(s)

Reiter's disease, syndrome, or urethritis
    (Continued)
  hip M02.35-●
  knee M02.36-●
  multiple site M02.39
  shoulder M02.31-●
  vertebra M02.38
  wrist M02.33-●
Rejection
  food, psychogenic F50.89
  transplant T86.91
    bone T86.830
      marrow T86.01
    cornea T86.840-●
    heart T86.21
      with lung(s) T86.31
    intestine T86.850
    kidney T86.11
    liver T86.41
    lung(s) T86.810
      with heart T86.31
    organ (immune or nonimmune cause)
      T86.91
    pancreas T86.890
    skin (allograft) (autograft) T86.820
    specified NEC T86.890
    stem cell (peripheral blood) (umbilical
      cord) T86.5
Relapsing fever A68.9
  Carter's (Asiatic) A68.1
  Dutton's (West African) A68.1
  Koch's A68.9
  louse-borne (epidemic) A68.0
  Novy's (American) A68.1
  Obermeyers's (European) A68.0
  Spirillum A68.9
  tick-borne (endemic) A68.1
Relationship
  occlusal
    open anterior M26.220
    open posterior M26.221
Relaxation
  anus (sphincter) K62.89
    psychogenic F45.8
  arch (foot) —see also Deformity, limb, flat foot
  back ligaments —see Instability, joint, spine
  bladder (sphincter) N31.2
  cardioesophageal K21.9
  cervix —see Incompetency, cervix
  diaphragm J98.6
  joint (capsule) (ligament) (paralytic) —see
    Flail, joint
    congenital NEC Q74.8
  lumbosacral (joint) —see subcategory M53.2
  pelvic floor N81.89
  perineum N81.89
  posture R29.3
  rectum (sphincter) K62.89
  sacroiliac (joint) —see subcategory M53.2
  scrotum N50.89
  urethra (sphincter) N36.44
  vesical N31.2
Release from prison, anxiety concerning Z65.2
Remains
  canal of Cloquet Q14.0
  capsule (opaque) Q14.8
Remittent fever (malarial) B54
Remnant
  canal of Cloquet Q14.0
  capsule (opaque) Q14.8
  cervix, cervical stump (acquired)
    (postoperative) N88.8
  cystic duct, postcholecystectomy K91.5
  fingernail L60.8
    congenital Q84.6
  meniscus, knee —see Derangement, knee,
    meniscus, specified NEC
  thyroglossal duct Q89.2
  tonsil J35.8
    infected (chronic) J35.01
  urachus Q64.4

Removal (from) (of)
  artificial
    arm Z44.00-●
      complete Z44.01-●
      partial Z44.02-●
    eye Z44.2-●
    leg Z44.10-●
      complete Z44.11-●
      partial Z44.12-●
  breast implant Z45.81
  cardiac pulse generator (battery) (end-of-life)
    Z45.010
  catheter (urinary) (indwelling) Z46.6
    from artificial opening —see Attention to,
      artificial, opening
    non-vascular Z46.82
    vascular NEC Z45.2
  device Z46.9
    contraceptive Z30.432
      implantable subdermal Z30.46
    implanted NEC Z45.89
    specified NEC Z46.89
  drains Z48.03
  dressing (nonsurgical) Z48.00
    surgical Z48.01
  external
    fixation device — code to fracture with
      seventh character D
    prosthesis, prosthetic device Z44.9
      breast Z44.3-●
      specified NEC Z44.8
  home in childhood (to foster home or
    institution) Z62.29
  ileostomy Z43.2
  insulin pump Z46.81
  myringotomy device (stent) (tube) Z45.82
  nervous system device NEC Z46.2
    brain neuropacemaker Z46.2
    visual substitution device Z46.2
      implanted Z45.31
  non-vascular catheter Z46.82
  organ, prophylactic (for neoplasia
    management) —see Prophylactic, organ
    removal
  orthodontic device Z46.4
  staples Z48.02
  stent
    ureteral Z46.6
  suture Z48.02
  urinary device Z46.6
  vascular access device or catheter Z45.2
Ren
  arcuatus Q63.1
  mobile, mobilis N28.89
    congenital Q63.8
  unguliformis Q63.1
Renal —see condition
Rendu-Osler-Weber disease or syndrome I78.0
Reninoma D41.0-●
Renon-Delille syndrome E23.3
Reovirus, as cause of disease classified
    elsewhere B97.5
Repeated falls NEC R29.6
Replaced chromosome by dicentric ring Q93.2
Replacement by artificial or mechanical device
    or prosthesis of
  bladder Z96.0
  blood vessel NEC Z95.828
  bone NEC Z96.7
  cochlea Z96.21
  coronary artery Z95.5
  eustachian tube Z96.29
  eye globe Z97.0
  heart Z95.812
    valve Z95.2
      prosthetic Z95.2
      specified NEC Z95.4
      xenogenic Z95.3
  intestine Z96.89
  joint Z96.60
    hip —see Presence, hip joint implant
    knee —see Presence, knee joint implant
    specified site NEC Z96.698

Replacement by artificial or mechanical device
    or prosthesis of (Continued)
  larynx Z96.3
  lens Z96.1
  limb(s) —see Presence, artificial, limb
  mandible NEC (for tooth root implant(s)) Z96.5
  organ NEC Z96.89
  peripheral vessel NEC Z95.828
  stapes Z96.29
  teeth Z97.2
  tendon Z96.7
  tissue NEC Z96.89
  tooth root(s) Z96.5
  vessel NEC Z95.828
    coronary (artery) Z95.5
Request for expert evidence Z04.89
Reserve, decreased or low
  cardiac —see Disease, heart
  kidney N28.89
▶Residing
▶in place not meant for human habitation
    (abandoned building) (car) (park)
    (sidewalk) Z59.02
▶on the street Z59.02
Residual —see also condition
  ovary syndrome N99.83
  state, schizophrenic F20.5
  urine R39.198
Resistance, resistant (to)
  activated protein C D68.51
  complicating pregnancy O26.89
  insulin E88.81
  organism(s)
    to
      drug Z16.30
        aminoglycosides Z16.29
        amoxicillin Z16.11
        ampicillin Z16.11
        antibiotic(s) Z16.20
          multiple Z16.24
          specified NEC Z16.29
        antifungal Z16.32
        antimicrobial (single) Z16.30
          multiple Z16.35
          specified NEC Z16.39
        antimycobacterial (single) Z16.341
          multiple Z16.342
        antiparasitic Z16.31
        antiviral Z16.33
        beta lactam antibiotics Z16.10
          specified NEC Z16.19
        cephalosporins Z16.19
        extended beta lactamase (ESBL) Z16.12
        fluoroquinolones Z16.23
        macrolides Z16.29
        methicillin —see MRSA
        multiple drugs (MDRO)
          antibiotics Z16.24
          antimicrobial Z16.35
          antimycobacterials Z16.342
        penicillins Z16.11
        quinine (and related compounds)
          Z16.31
        quinolones Z16.23
        sulfonamides Z16.29
        tetracyclines Z16.29
        tuberculostatics (single) Z16.341
          multiple Z16.342
        vancomycin Z16.21
          related antibiotics Z16.22
  thyroid hormone E07.89
Resorption
  dental (roots) K03.3
    alveoli M26.79
  teeth (external) (internal) (pathological)
    (roots) K03.3
Respiration
  Cheyne-Stokes R06.3
  decreased due to shock, following injury T79.4
  disorder of, psychogenic F45.8
  insufficient, or poor R06.89
    newborn P28.5

Respiration(Continued)
painful R07.1
sighing, psychogenic F45.8
Respiratory —see also condition
distress syndrome (newborn) (type I) P22.0
type II P22.1
syncytial virus, as cause of disease classified
elsewhere (see also Virus, respiratory
syncytial (RSV)) B97.4
Respite care Z75.5
Response (drug)
photoallergic L56.1
phototoxic L56.0
Restenosis
stent
vascular
end stent
adjacent to stent —see Arteriosclerosis

within the stent
coronary T82.855
peripheral T82.856
in stent
coronary vessel T82.855
peripheral vessel T82.856
Restless legs (syndrome) G25.81
Restlessness R45.1
Restoration (of)
dental
aesthetically inadequate or displeasing
K08.56
defective K08.50
specified NEC K08.59
failure of marginal integrity K08.51
failure of periodontal anatomical intergrity
K08.54
organ continuity from previous sterilization
(tuboplasty) (vasoplasty) Z31.0
aftercare Z31.42
tooth (existing)
contours biologically incompatible with
oral health K08.54
open margins K08.51
overhanging K08.52
poor aesthetic K08.56
poor gingival margins K08.51
unsatisfactory, of tooth K08.50
specified NEC K08.59
Restorative material (dental)
allergy to K08.55
fractured K08.539
with loss of material K08.531
without loss of material K08.530
unrepairable overhanging of K08.52
Restriction of housing space Z59.1
Rests, ovarian, in fallopian tube Q50.6
Restzustand (schizophrenic) F20.5
Retained —see also Retention
cholelithiasis following cholecystectomy K91.86
foreign body fragments (type of) Z18.9
acrylics Z18.2
animal quill(s) or spines Z18.31
cement Z18.83
concrete Z18.83
crystalline Z18.83
depleted isotope Z18.09
depleted uranium Z18.01
diethylhexyl phthalates Z18.2
glass Z18.81
isocyanate Z18.2
magnetic metal Z18.11
metal Z18.10
nonmagnetic metal Z18.12
nontherapeutic radioactive Z18.09
organic NEC Z18.39
plastic Z18.2
quill(s) (animal) Z18.31
radioactive (nontherapeutic) NEC Z18.09
specified NEC Z18.89
spine(s) (animal) Z18.31
stone Z18.83
tooth (teeth) Z18.32
wood Z18.33

Retained (Continued)
fragments (type of) Z18.9
acrylics Z18.2
animal quill(s) or spines Z18.31
cement Z18.83
fragments (type of) (Continued)
concrete Z18.83
crystalline Z18.83
depleted isotope Z18.09
depleted uranium Z18.01
diethylhexyl phthalates Z18.2
glass Z18.81
isocyanate Z18.2
magnetic metal Z18.11
metal Z18.10
nonmagnectic metal Z18.12
nontherapeutic radioactive Z18.09
organic NEC Z18.39
plastic Z18.2
quill(s) (animal) Z18.31
radioactive (nontherapeutic) NEC Z18.09
specified NEC Z18.89
spine(s) (animal) Z18.31
stone Z18.83
tooth (teeth) Z18.32
wood Z18.33
gallstones, following cholecystectomy K91.86
Retardation
development, developmental, specific —see
Disorder, developmental
endochondral bone growth —see Disorder,
bone, development or growth
growth R62.50
due to malnutrition E45
mental —see Disability, intellectual
motor function, specific F82
physical (child) R62.52
due to malnutrition E45
reading (specific) F81.0
spelling (specific) (without reading disorder)
F81.81
Retching —see Vomiting
Retention —see also Retained
bladder —see Retention, urine
carbon dioxide E87.2
cholelithiasis following cholecystectomy K91.86
cyst —see Cyst
dead
fetus (at or near term) (mother) O36.4
early fetal death O02.1
ovum O02.0
decidua (fragments) (following delivery)
(with hemorrhage) O72.2
without hemorrhage O73.1
deciduous tooth K00.6
dental root K08.3
fecal —see Constipation
fetus
dead O36.4
early O02.1
fluid R60.9
foreign body —see also Foreign body, retained
current trauma - code as Foreign body, by
site or type
gallstones, following cholecystectomy K91.86
gastric K31.89
intrauterine contraceptive device, in
pregnancy —see Pregnancy, complicated
by, retention, intrauterine device
membranes (complicating delivery) (with
hemorrhage) O72.2
with abortion —see Abortion, by type
without hemorrhage O73.1
meniscus —see Derangement, meniscus
menses N94.89
milk (puerperal, postpartum) O92.79
nitrogen, extrarenal R39.2
ovary syndrome N99.83
placenta (total) (with hemorrhage) O72.0
without hemorrhage O73.0
portions or fragments (with hemorrhage)
O72.2
without hemorrhage O73.1

Retention (Continued)
products of conception
early pregnancy (dead fetus) O02.1
following
delivery (with hemorrhage) O72.2
without hemorrhage O73.1
secundines (following delivery) (with
hemorrhage) O72.0
without hemorrhage O73.0
complicating puerperium (delayed
hemorrhage) O72.2
partial O72.2
without hemorrhage O73.1
smegma, clitoris N90.89
urine R33.9
drug-induced R33.0
due to hyperplasia (hypertrophy) of
prostate —see Hyperplasia, prostate
organic R33.8
drug-induced R33.0
psychogenic F45.8
specified NEC R33.8
water (in tissues) —see Edema
Reticular erythematous mucinosis L98.5
Reticulation, dust —see Pneumoconiosis
Reticulocytosis R70.1
Reticuloendotheliosis
acute infantile C96.0
leukemic C91.4-●
nonlipid C96.0
Reticulohistiocytoma (giant-cell) D76.3
Reticuloid, actinic L57.1
Reticulosis (skin)
acute of infancy C96.0
hemophagocytic, familial D76.1
histiocytic medullary C96.A
lipomelanotic I89.8
malignant (midline) C86.0
polymorphic C86.0
Sézary —see Sézary disease
Retina, retinal —see also condition
dark area D49.81
Retinitis —see also Inflammation, chorioretinal
albuminurica N18.9 [H32]
diabetic —see Diabetes, retinitis
disciformis —see Degeneration, macula
focal —see Inflammation, chorioretinal, focal
gravidarum —see Pregnancy, complicated by,
specified pregnancy-related condition
NEC
juxtapapillaris —see Inflammation,
chorioretinal, focal, juxtapapillary
luetic —see Retinitis, syphilitic
pigmentosa H35.52
proliferans —see Disorder, globe,
degenerative, specified type NEC
proliferating —see Disorder, globe,
degenerative, specified type NEC
renal N18.9 [H32]
syphilitic (early) (secondary) A51.43
central, recurrent A52.71
congenital (early) A50.01 [H32]
late A52.71
tuberculous A18.53
Retinoblastoma C69.2-●
differentiated C69.2-●
undifferentiated C69.2-●
Retinochoroiditis —see also Inflammation,
chorioretinal
disseminated —see Inflammation,
chorioretinal, disseminated
syphilitic A52.71
focal —see Inflammation, chorioretinal
juxtapapillaris —see Inflammation,
chorioretinal, focal, juxtapapillary
Retinopathy (background) H35.00
arteriosclerotic I70.8 [H35.0-●]
atherosclerotic I70.8 [H35.0-●]
central serous —see Chorioretinopathy,
central serous
Coats H35.02-●

▶ New   ⇒ Revised   ~~deleted~~ Deleted   ● Use Additional Character(s)

Retinopathy (Continued)
diabetic —see Diabetes, retinopathy
exudative H35.02-●
hypertensive H35.03-●
in (due to)
diabetes —see Diabetes, retinopathy
sickle-cell disorders D57.- ● [H36]
of prematurity H35.10-●
stage 0 H35.11-●
stage 1 H35.12-●
stage 2 H35.13-●
stage 3 H35.14-●
stage 4 H35.15-●
stage 5 H35.16-●
pigmentary, congenital —see Dystrophy,
retina
proliferative NEC H35.2-●
diabetic —see Diabetes, retinopathy,
proliferative
sickle-cell D57.- ● [H36]
solar H31.02-●
Retinoschisis H33.10-●
congenital Q14.1
specified type NEC H33.19-●
Retortamoniasis A07.8
Retractile testis Q55.22
Retraction
cervix —see Retroversion, uterus
drum (membrane) —see Disorder, tympanic
membrane, specified NEC
finger —see Deformity, finger
lid H02.539
left H02.536
lower H02.535
upper H02.534
right H02.533
lower H02.532
upper H02.531
lung J98.4
mediastinum J98.59
nipple N64.53
associated with
lactation O92.03
pregnancy O92.01-●
puerperium O92.02
congenital Q83.8
palmar fascia M72.0
pleura —see Pleurisy
ring, uterus (Bandl's) (pathological)
O62.4
sternum (congenital) Q76.7
acquired M95.4
uterus —see Retroversion, uterus
valve (heart) —see Endocarditis
Retrobulbar —see condition
Retrocecal —see condition
Retrocession —see Retroversion
Retrodisplacement —see Retroversion
Retroflection, retroflexion —see Retroversion
Retrognathia, retrognathism (mandibular)
(maxillary) M26.19
Retrograde menstruation N92.5
Retroperineal —see condition
Retroperitoneal —see condition
Retroperitonitis K68.9
Retropharyngeal —see condition
Retroplacental —see condition
Retroposition —see Retroversion
Retroprosthetic membrane T85.398
Retrosternal thyroid (congenital)
Q89.2
Retroversion, retroverted
cervix —see Retroversion, uterus
female NEC —see Retroversion, uterus
iris H21.89
testis (congenital) Q55.29
uterus (acquired) (acute) (any degree)
(asymptomatic) (cervix) (postinfectional)
(postpartal, old) N85.4
congenital Q51.818
in pregnancy O34.53-●

Retrovirus, as cause of disease classified
elsewhere B97.30
human
immunodeficiency, type 2 (HIV 2) B97.35
T-cell lymphotropic
type I (HTLV-I) B97.33
type II (HTLV-II) B97.34
lentivirus B97.31
oncovirus B97.32
specified NEC B97.39
Retrusion, premaxilla (developmental) M26.09
Rett's disease or syndrome F84.2
Reverse peristalsis R19.2
Reye's syndrome G93.7
Rh (factor)
hemolytic disease (newborn) P55.0
incompatibility, immunization or sensitization
affecting management of pregnancy NEC
O36.09-●
anti-D antibody O36.01-●
newborn P55.0
transfusion reaction —see Complication(s),
transfusion, incompatibility reaction,
Rh (factor)
negative mother affecting newborn P55.0
titer elevated —see Complication(s),
transfusion, incompatibility reaction, Rh
(factor)
transfusion reaction —see Complication(s),
transfusion, incompatibility reaction, Rh
(factor)
Rhabdomyolysis (idiopathic) NEC M62.82
traumatic T79.6
Rhabdomyoma —see also Neoplasm, connective
tissue, benign
adult —see Neoplasm, connective tissue, benign
fetal —see Neoplasm, connective tissue, benign
glycogenic —see Neoplasm, connective tissue,
benign
Rhabdomyosarcoma (any type) —see
Neoplasm, connective tissue, malignant
Rhabdosarcoma —see Rhabdomyosarcoma
Rhesus (factor) incompatibility —see Rh,
incompatibility
Rheumatic (acute) (subacute)
adherent pericardium I09.2
chronic I09.89
coronary arteritis I01.8
degeneration, myocardium I09.0
fever (acute) —see Fever, rheumatic
heart —see Disease, heart, rheumatic
myocardial degeneration —see Degeneration,
myocardium
myocarditis (chronic) (inactive) (with chorea)
I09.0
with chorea (acute) (rheumatic)
(Sydenham's) I02.0
active or acute I01.2
pancarditis, acute I01.8
with chorea (acute (rheumatic)
Sydenham's) I02.0
pericarditis (active) (acute) (with effusion)
(with pneumonia) I01.0
with chorea (acute) (rheumatic)
(Sydenham's) I02.0
chronic or inactive I09.2
pneumonia I00 [J17]
torticollis M43.6
typhoid fever A01.09
Rheumatism (articular) (neuralgic)
(nonarticular) M79.0
gout —see Arthritis, rheumatoid
intercostal, meaning Tietze's disease M94.0
palindromic (any site) M12.30
ankle M12.37-●
elbow M12.32-●
foot joint M12.37-●
hand joint M12.34-●
hip M12.35-●
knee M12.36-●
multiple site M12.39

Rheumatism (Continued)
palindromic (Continued)
shoulder M12.31-●
specified joint NEC M12.38
vertebrae M12.38
wrist M12.33-●
sciatic M54.4-●
Rheumatoid —see also condition
arthritis —see also Arthritis, rheumatoid
with involvement of organs NEC M05.60
ankle M05.67-●
elbow M05.62-●
foot joint M05.67-●
hand joint M05.64-●
hip M05.65-●
knee M05.66-●
multiple site M05.69
shoulder M05.61-●
vertebra —see Spondylitis, ankylosing
wrist M05.63-●
seronegative —see Arthritis, rheumatoid,
seronegative
seropositive —see Arthritis, rheumatoid,
seropositive
carditis M05.30
ankle M05.37-●
elbow M05.32-●
foot joint M05.37-●
hand joint M05.34-●
hip M05.35-●
knee M05.36-●
multiple site M05.39
shoulder M05.31-●
vertebra —see Spondylitis, ankylosing
wrist M05.33-●
endocarditis —see Rheumatoid, carditis
lung (disease) M05.10
ankle M05.17-●
elbow M05.12-●
foot joint M05.17-●
hand joint M05.14-●
hip M05.15-●
knee M05.16-●
multiple site M05.19
shoulder M05.11-●
vertebra —see Spondylitis, ankylosing
wrist M05.13-●
myocarditis —see Rheumatoid, carditis
myopathy M05.40
ankle M05.47-●
elbow M05.42-●
foot joint M05.47-●
hand joint M05.44-●
hip M05.45-●
knee M05.46-●
multiple site M05.49
shoulder M05.41-●
vertebra —see Spondylitis, ankylosing
wrist M05.43-●
pericarditis —see Rheumatoid, carditis
polyarthritis —see Arthritis, rheumatoid
polyneuropathy M05.50
ankle M05.57-●
elbow M05.52-●
foot joint M05.57-●
hand joint M05.54-●
hip M05.55-●
knee M05.56-●
multiple site M05.59
shoulder M05.51-●
vertebra —see Spondylitis, ankylosing
wrist M05.53-●
vasculitis M05.20
ankle M05.27-●
elbow M05.22-●
foot joint M05.27-●
hand joint M05.24-●
hip M05.25-●
knee M05.26-●
multiple site M05.29
shoulder M05.21-●
vertebra —see Spondylitis, ankylosing
wrist M05.23-●

Rhinitis (atrophic) (catarrhal) (chronic)
  (croupous) (fibrinous) (granulomatous)
  (hyperplastic) (hypertrophic)
  (membranous) (obstructive) (purulent)
  (suppurative) (ulcerative) J31.0
  with
    sore throat —see Nasopharyngitis
  acute J00
  allergic J30.9
    with asthma J45.909
      with
        exacerbation (acute) J45.901
        status asthmaticus J45.902
    due to
      food J30.5
      pollen J30.1
    nonseasonal J30.89
    perennial J30.89
    seasonal NEC J30.2
    specified NEC J30.89
  infective J00
  pneumococcal J00
  syphilitic A52.73
    congenital A50.05 [J99]
  tuberculous A15.8
  vasomotor J30.0
Rhinoantritis (chronic) —see Sinusitis,
  maxillary
Rhinodacryolith —see Dacryolith
Rhinolith (nasal sinus) J34.89
Rhinomegaly J34.89
Rhinopharyngitis (acute) (subacute) —see also
  Nasopharyngitis
  chronic J31.1
  destructive ulcerating A66.5
  mutilans A66.5
Rhinophyma L71.1
Rhinorrhea J34.89
  cerebrospinal (fluid) G96.01
    postoperative G96.08
    specified NEC G96.08
    spontaneous G96.01
    traumatic G96.08
  paroxysmal —see Rhinitis, allergic
  spasmodic —see Rhinitis, allergic
Rhinosalpingitis —see Salpingitis, eustachian
Rhinoscleroma A48.8
Rhinosporidiosis B48.1
Rhinovirus infection NEC B34.8
Rhizomelic chondrodysplasia punctata E71.540
Rhythm
  atrioventricular nodal I49.8
  disorder I49.9
    coronary sinus I49.8
    ectopic I49.8
    nodal I49.8
  escape I49.9
  heart, abnormal I49.9
  idioventricular I44.2
  nodal I49.8
  sleep, inversion G47.2-•
    nonorganic origin —see Disorder, sleep,
      circadian rhythm, psychogenic
Rhytidosis facialis L98.8
Rib —see also condition
  cervical Q76.5
Riboflavin deficiency E53.0
Rice bodies —see also Loose, body, joint
  knee M23.4-•
Richter syndrome —see Leukemia, chronic
  lymphocytic, B-cell type
Richter's hernia —see Hernia, abdomen, with
  obstruction
Ricinism —see Poisoning, food, noxious, plant
Rickets (active) (acute) (adolescent) (chest wall)
  (congenital) (current) (infantile) (intestinal)
  E55.0
  adult —see Osteomalacia
  celiac K90.0
  hypophosphatemic with nephrotic-glycosuric
    dwarfism E72.09

Rickets (Continued)
  inactive E64.3
  kidney N25.0
  renal N25.0
  sequelae, any E64.3
  vitamin-D-resistant E83.31 [M90.80]
Rickettsia 364D/R. philipii (Pacific Coast tick
  fever) A77.8
Rickettsial disease A79.9
  specified type NEC A79.89
Rickettsialpox (Rickettsia akari) A79.1
Rickettsiosis A79.9
  due to
    Ehrlichia sennetsu A79.81
    Neorickettsia sennetsu A79.81
    Rickettsia akari (rickettsialpox) A79.1
  specified type NEC A79.89
  tick-borne A77.9
  vesicular A79.1
Rider's bone —see Ossification, muscle,
  specified NEC
Ridge, alveolus —see also condition
  flabby K06.8
Ridged ear, congenital Q17.3
Riedel's
  lobe, liver Q44.7
  struma, thyroiditis or disease E06.5
Rieger's anomaly or syndrome Q13.81
Riehl's melanosis L81.4
Rietti-Greppi-Micheli anemia D56.9
Rieux's hernia —see Hernia, abdomen, specified
  site NEC
Riga (-Fede) disease K14.0
Riggs' disease —see Periodontitis
Right aortic arch Q25.47
Right middle lobe syndrome J98.11
Rigid, rigidity —see also condition
  abdominal R19.30
    with severe abdominal pain R10.0
    epigastric R19.36
    generalized R19.37
    left lower quadrant R19.34
    left upper quadrant R19.32
    periumbilic R19.35
    right lower quadrant R19.33
    right upper quadrant R19.31
  articular, multiple, congenital Q68.8
  cervix (uteri) in pregnancy —see Pregnancy,
    complicated by, abnormal, cervix
  hymen (acquired) (congenital) N89.6
  nuchal R29.1
  pelvic floor in pregnancy —see Pregnancy,
    complicated by, abnormal, pelvic organs
    or tissues NEC
  perineum or vulva in pregnancy —see
    Pregnancy, complicated by, abnormal,
    vulva
  spine —see Dorsopathy, specified NEC
  vagina in pregnancy —see Pregnancy,
    complicated by, abnormal, vagina
Rigors R68.89
  with fever R50.9
Riley-Day syndrome G90.1
RIND (reversible ischemic neurologic deficit)
  I63.9
Ring(s)
  aorta (vascular) Q25.45
  Bandl's O62.4
  contraction, complicating delivery O62.4
  esophageal, lower (muscular) K22.2
  Fleischer's (cornea) H18.04-•
  hymenal, tight (acquired) (congenital)
    N89.6
  Kayser-Fleischer (cornea) H18.04-•
  retraction, uterus, pathological O62.4
  Schatzki's (esophagus) (lower) K22.2
    congenital Q39.3
  Soemmerring's —see Cataract, secondary
  vascular (congenital) Q25.8
    aorta Q25.45
Ringed hair (congenital) Q84.1

Ringworm B35.9
  beard B35.0
  black dot B35.0
  body B35.4
  Burmese B35.5
  corporeal B35.4
  foot B35.3
  groin B35.6
  hand B35.2
  honeycomb B35.0
  nails B35.1
  perianal (area) B35.6
  scalp B35.0
  specified NEC B35.8
  Tokelau B35.5
Rise, venous pressure I87.8
Rising, PSA following treatment for malignant
  neoplasm of prostate R97.21
Risk
  for
    dental caries Z91.849
      high Z91.843
      low Z91.841
      moderate Z91.842
    ▶homelessness, imminent Z59.811
  suicidal
    ⇒meaning personal history of attempted
      suicide Z91.51
    meaning suicidal ideation —see Ideation,
      suicidal
Ritter's disease L00
Rivalry, sibling Z62.891
Rivalta's disease A42.2
River blindness B73.01
Robert's pelvis Q74.2
  with disproportion (fetopelvic) O33.0
    causing obstructed labor O65.0
Robin (-Pierre) syndrome Q87.0
Robinow-Silvermann-Smith syndrome Q87.19
Robinson's (hidrotic) ectodermal dysplasia or
  syndrome Q82.4
Robles' disease B73.01
Rocky Mountain (spotted) fever A77.0
Roetheln —see Rubella
Roger's disease Q21.0
Rokitansky-Aschoff sinuses (gallbladder) K82.8
Rolando's fracture (displaced) S62.22-•
  nondisplaced S62.22-•
Romano-Ward (prolonged QT interval)
  syndrome I45.81
Romberg's disease or syndrome G51.8
Roof, mouth —see condition
Rosacea L71.9
  acne L71.9
  keratitis L71.8
  specified NEC L71.8
Rosary, rachitic E55.0
Rose
  cold J30.1
  fever J30.1
  rash R21
    epidemic B06.9
Rosenbach's erysipeloid A26.0
Rosenthal's disease or syndrome D68.1
Roseola B09
  infantum B08.20
    due to human herpesvirus 6 B08.21
    due to human herpesvirus 7 B08.22
Ross River disease or fever B33.1
Rossbach's disease K31.89
  psychogenic F45.8
Rostan's asthma (cardiac) —see Failure,
  ventricular, left
Rotation
  anomalous, incomplete or insufficient,
    intestine Q43.3
  cecum (congenital) Q43.3
  colon (congenital) Q43.3
  spine, incomplete or insufficient —see
    Dorsopathy, deforming, specified NEC
  tooth, teeth, fully erupted M26.35
  vertebra, incomplete or insufficient —see
    Dorsopathy, deforming, specified NEC

▶ New   ⇒ Revised   ~~deleted~~ Deleted   • Use Additional Character(s)

Rotes Quérol disease or syndrome —*see* Hyperostosis, ankylosing
Roth (-Bernhardt) disease or syndrome —*see* Meralgia paraesthetica
Rothmund (-Thomson) syndrome Q82.8
Rotor's disease or syndrome E80.6
Round
  back (with wedging of vertebrae) —*see* Kyphosis
  sequelae (late effect) of rickets E64.3
  worms (large) (infestation) NEC B82.0
    Ascariasis —*see also* Ascariasis B77.9
Roussy-Lévy syndrome G60.0
Rubella (German measles) B06.9
  complication NEC B06.09
    neurological B06.00
  congenital P35.0
  contact Z20.4
  exposure to Z20.4
  maternal
    care for (suspected) damage to fetus O35.3
    manifest rubella in infant P35.0
    suspected damage to fetus affecting management of pregnancy O35.3
  specified complications NEC B06.89
Rubeola (meaning measles) —*see* Measles
  meaning rubella —*see* Rubella
Rubeosis, iris —*see* Disorder, iris, vascular
Rubinstein-Taybi syndrome Q87.2
Rudimentary (congenital) —*see also* Agenesis
  arm —*see* Defect, reduction, upper limb
  bone Q79.9
  cervix uteri Q51.828
  eye Q11.2
  lobule of ear Q17.3
  patella Q74.1
  respiratory organs in thoracopagus Q89.4
  tracheal bronchus Q32.4
  uterus Q51.818
    in male Q56.1
  vagina Q52.0
Ruled out condition —*see* Observation, suspected
Rumination R11.10
  with nausea R11.2
  disorder of infancy F98.21
  neurotic F42.8
  newborn P92.1
  obsessional F42.8
  psychogenic F42.8
Runeberg's disease D51.0
Runny nose R09.89
Rupia (syphilitic) A51.39
  congenital A50.06
  tertiary A52.79
Rupture, ruptured
  abscess (spontaneous) - code by site under Abscess
  aneurysm —*see* Aneurysm
  anus (sphincter) —*see* Laceration, anus
  aorta, aortic I71.8
    abdominal I71.3
    arch I71.1
    ascending I71.1
    descending I71.8
      abdominal I71.3
      thoracic I71.1
    syphilitic A52.01
    thoracoabdominal I71.5
    thorax, thoracic I71.1
    transverse I71.1
    traumatic —*see* Injury, aorta, laceration, major
    valve or cusp —*see also* Endocarditis, aortic I35.8
  appendix (with peritonitis) (*see also* Appendicitis) K35.32
    with localized peritonitis (*see also* Appendicitis) K35.32
  arteriovenous fistula, brain —*see* Fistula, arteriovenous, brain, ruptured

Rupture, ruptured (*Continued*)
  artery I77.2
    brain —*see* Hemorrhage, intracranial, intracerebral
    coronary —*see* Infarct, myocardium
    heart —*see* Infarct, myocardium
    pulmonary I28.8
    traumatic (complication) —*see* Injury, blood vessel
  bile duct (common) (hepatic) K83.2
    cystic K82.2
  bladder (sphincter) (nontraumatic) (spontaneous) N32.89
    following ectopic or molar pregnancy O08.6
    obstetrical trauma O71.5
    traumatic S37.29
  blood vessel —*see also* Hemorrhage
    brain —*see* Hemorrhage, intracranial, intracerebral
    heart —*see* Infarct, myocardium
    traumatic (complication) —*see* Injury, blood vessel, laceration, major, by site
  bone —*see* Fracture
  bowel (nontraumatic) K63.1
  brain
    aneurysm (congenital) —*see also* Hemorrhage, intracranial, subarachnoid
      syphilitic A52.05
    hemorrhagic —*see* Hemorrhage, intracranial, intracerebral
  capillaries I78.8
  cardiac (auricle) (ventricle) (wall) I23.3
    with hemopericardium I23.0
    infectional I40.9
    traumatic —*see* Injury, heart
  cartilage (articular) (current) —*see also* Sprain
    knee S83.3-•
    semilunar —*see* Tear, meniscus
  cecum (with peritonitis) K65.0
    with peritoneal abscess K35.33
    traumatic S36.598
  celiac artery, traumatic —*see* Injury, blood vessel, celiac artery, laceration, major
  cerebral aneurysm (congenital) (*see* Hemorrhage, intracranial, subarachnoid)
  cervix (uteri)
    with ectopic or molar pregnancy O08.6
    following ectopic or molar pregnancy O08.6
    obstetrical trauma O71.3
    traumatic S37.69
  chordae tendineae NEC I51.1
    concurrent with acute myocardial infarction —*see* Infarct, myocardium
    following acute myocardial infarction (current complication) I23.4
  choroid (direct) (indirect) (traumatic) H31.32-•
  circle of Willis I60.6
  colon (nontraumatic) K63.1
    traumatic —*see* Injury, intestine, large
  cornea (traumatic) —*see* Injury, eye, laceration
  coronary (artery) (thrombotic) —*see* Infarct, myocardium
  corpus luteum (infected) (ovary) N83.1-•
  cyst —*see* Cyst
  cystic duct K82.2
  Descemet's membrane —*see* Change, corneal membrane, Descemet's, rupture
    traumatic —*see* Injury, eye, laceration
  diaphragm, traumatic —*see* Injury, intrathoracic, diaphragm
  disc —*see* Rupture, intervertebral disc
  diverticulum (intestine) K57.80
    with bleeding K57.81
    bladder N32.3
    large intestine K57.20
      with
        bleeding K57.21
        small intestine K57.40
          with bleeding K57.41

Rupture, ruptured (*Continued*)
  diverticulum (*Continued*)
    small intestine K57.00
      with
        bleeding K57.01
        large intestine K57.40
          with bleeding K57.41
  duodenal stump K31.89
  ear drum (nontraumatic) —*see also* Perforation, tympanum
    traumatic S09.2-•
    due to blast injury —*see* Injury, blast, ear
  esophagus K22.3
  eye (without prolapse or loss of intraocular tissue) —*see* Injury, eye, laceration
  fallopian tube NEC (nonobstetric) (nontraumatic) N83.8
    due to pregnancy O00.10-•
    with intrauterine pregnancy O00.11-•
  fontanel P13.1
  gallbladder K82.2
    traumatic S36.128
  gastric —*see also* Rupture, stomach
    vessel K92.2
  globe (eye) (traumatic) —*see* Injury, eye, laceration
  graafian follicle (hematoma) N83.0-•
  heart —*see* Rupture, cardiac
  hymen (nontraumatic) (nonintentional) N89.8
  internal organ, traumatic —*see* Injury, by site
  intervertebral disc —*see* Displacement, intervertebral disc
    traumatic —*see* Rupture, traumatic, intervertebral disc
  intestine NEC (nontraumatic) K63.1
    traumatic —*see* Injury, intestine
  iris —*see also* Abnormality, pupillary
    traumatic —*see* Injury, eye, laceration
  joint capsule, traumatic —*see* Sprain
  kidney (traumatic) S37.06-•
    birth injury P15.8
    nontraumatic N28.89
  lacrimal duct (traumatic) —*see* Injury, eye, specified site NEC
  lens (cataract) (traumatic) —*see* Cataract, traumatic
  ligament, traumatic —*see* Rupture, traumatic, ligament, by site
  liver S36.116
    birth injury P15.0
  lymphatic vessel I89.8
  marginal sinus (placental) (with hemorrhage) —*see* Hemorrhage, antepartum, specified cause NEC
  membrana tympani (nontraumatic) —*see* Perforation, tympanum
  membranes (spontaneous)
    artificial
      delayed delivery following O75.5
    delayed delivery following —*see* Pregnancy, complicated by, premature rupture of membranes
  meningeal artery I60.8
  meniscus (knee) —*see also* Tear, meniscus
    old —*see* Derangement, meniscus
    site other than knee - code as Sprain
  mesenteric artery, traumatic —*see* Injury, mesenteric, artery, laceration, major
  mesentery (nontraumatic) K66.8
    traumatic —*see* Injury, intra-abdominal, specified, site NEC
  mitral (valve) I34.8
  muscle (traumatic) —*see also* Strain
    diastasis —*see* Diastasis, muscle
    nontraumatic M62.10
      ankle M62.17-•
      foot M62.17-•
      forearm M62.13-•
      hand M62.14-•
      lower leg M62.16-•
      pelvic region M62.15-•

Rupture, ruptured *(Continued)*
  muscle *(Continued)*
    nontraumatic *(Continued)*
      shoulder region M62.11-●
      specified site NEC M62.18
      thigh M62.15-●
      upper arm M62.12-●
    traumatic —*see* Strain, by site
  musculotendinous junction NEC,
    nontraumatic —*see* Rupture, tendon,
    spontaneous
  mycotic aneurysm causing cerebral
    hemorrhage —*see* Hemorrhage,
    intracranial, subarachnoid
  myocardium, myocardial —*see* Rupture,
    cardiac
    traumatic —*see* Injury, heart
  nontraumatic, meaning hernia —*see* Hernia
  obstructed —*see* Hernia, by site, obstructed
  operation wound —*see* Disruption, wound,
    operation
  ovary, ovarian N83.8
    corpus luteum cyst N83.1-●
    follicle (graafian) N83.0-●
  oviduct (nonobstetric) (nontraumatic)
    N83.8
    due to pregnancy O00.10-●
      with intrauterine pregnancy
        O00.11-●
  pancreas (nontraumatic) K86.89
    traumatic S36.299
  papillary muscle NEC I51.2
    following acute myocardial infarction
      (current complication) I23.5
  pelvic
    floor, complicating delivery O70.1
    organ NEC, obstetrical trauma O71.5
  perineum (nonobstetric) (nontraumatic)
    N90.89
    complicating delivery —*see* Delivery,
      complicated, by, laceration, anus
      (sphincter)
  postoperative wound —*see* Disruption,
    wound, operation
  prostate (traumatic) S37.828
  pulmonary
    artery I28.8
    valve (heart) I37.8
    vein I28.8
    vessel I28.8
  pus tube —*see* Salpingitis
  pyosalpinx —*see* Salpingitis
  rectum (nontraumatic) K63.1
    traumatic S36.69
  retina, retinal (traumatic) (without
    detachment) —*see also* Break, retina
    with detachment —*see* Detachment,
      retina, with retinal, break
  rotator cuff (nontraumatic) M75.10-●
    complete M75.12-●
    incomplete M75.11-●
  sclera —*see* Injury, eye, laceration
  sigmoid (nontraumatic) K63.1
    traumatic S36.593
  spinal cord —*see also* Injury, spinal cord, by
    region
    due to injury at birth P11.5
    newborn (birth injury) P11.5
  spleen (traumatic) S36.09
    birth injury P15.1
    congenital (birth injury) P15.1
    due to P. vivax malaria B51.0
    nontraumatic D73.5
    spontaneous D73.5
  splenic vein R58
    traumatic —*see* Injury, blood vessel,
      splenic vein
  stomach (nontraumatic) (spontaneous)
    K31.89
    traumatic S36.39

Rupture, ruptured *(Continued)*
  supraspinatus (complete) (incomplete)
    (nontraumatic) —*see* Tear, rotator cuff
  symphysis pubis
    obstetric O71.6
    traumatic S33.4
  synovium (cyst) M66.10
    ankle M66.17-●
    elbow M66.12-●
    finger M66.14-●
    foot M66.17-●
    forearm M66.13-●
    hand M66.14-●
    pelvic region M66.15-●
    shoulder region M66.11-●
    specified site NEC M66.18
    thigh M66.15-●
    toe M66.17-●
    upper arm M66.12-●
    wrist M66.13-●
  tendon (traumatic) —*see* Strain
    nontraumatic (spontaneous) M66.9
      ankle M66.87-●
      extensor M66.20
        ankle M66.27-●
        foot M66.27-●
        forearm M66.23-●
        hand M66.24-●
        lower leg M66.26-●
        multiple sites M66.29
        pelvic region M66.25-●
        shoulder region M66.21-●
        specified site NEC M66.28
        thigh M66.25-●
        upper arm M66.22-●
      flexor M66.30
        ankle M66.37-●
        foot M66.37-●
        forearm M66.33-●
        hand M66.34-●
        lower leg M66.36-●
        multiple sites M66.39
        pelvic region M66.35-●
        shoulder region M66.31-●
        specified site NEC M66.38
        thigh M66.35-●
        upper arm M66.32-●
      foot M66.87-●
      forearm M66.83-●
      hand M66.84-●
      lower leg M66.86-●
      multiple sites M66.89
      pelvic region M66.85-●
      shoulder region M66.81-●
      specified
        site NEC M66.88
        tendon M66.80
      thigh M66.85-●
      upper arm M66.82-●
  thoracic duct I89.8
  tonsil J35.8
  traumatic
    aorta —*see* Injury, aorta, laceration, major
    diaphragm —*see* Injury, intrathoracic,
      diaphragm
    external site —*see* Wound, open, by site
    eye —*see* Injury, eye, laceration
    internal organ —*see* Injury, by site
    intervertebral disc
      cervical S13.0
      lumbar S33.0
      thoracic S23.0
    kidney S37.06-●
    ligament —*see also* Sprain
      ankle —*see* Sprain, ankle
      carpus —*see* Rupture, traumatic,
        ligament, wrist
      collateral (hand) —*see* Rupture,
        traumatic, ligament, finger,
        collateral

Rupture, ruptured *(Continued)*
  traumatic *(Continued)*
    ligament *(Continued)*
      finger (metacarpophalangeal)
        (interphalangeal) S63.40-●
        collateral S63.41-●
          index S63.41-●
          little S63.41-●
          middle S63.41-●
          ring S63.41-●
        index S63.40-●
        little S63.40-●
        middle S63.40-●
        palmar S63.42-●
          index S63.42-●
          little S63.42-●
          middle S63.42-●
          ring S63.42-●
        ring S63.40-●
        specified site NEC S63.499
          index S63.49-●
          little S63.49-●
          middle S63.49-●
          ring S63.49-●
        volar plate S63.43-●
          index S63.43-●
          little S63.43-●
          middle S63.43-●
          ring S63.43-●
      foot —*see* Sprain, foot
      radial collateral S53.2-●
      radiocarpal —*see* Rupture, traumatic,
        ligament, wrist, radiocarpal
      ulnar collateral S53.3-●
      ulnocarpal —*see* Rupture, traumatic,
        ligament, wrist, ulnocarpal
      wrist S63.30-●
        collateral S63.31-●
        radiocarpal S63.32-●
        specified site NEC S63.39-●
        ulnocarpal (palmar) S63.33-●
    liver S36.116
    membrana tympani —*see* Rupture, ear
      drum, traumatic
    muscle or tendon —*see* Strain
    myocardium —*see* Injury, heart
    pancreas S36.299
    rectum S36.69
    sigmoid S36.593
    spleen S36.09
    stomach S36.39
    symphysis pubis S33.4
    tympanum, tympanic (membrane) —*see*
      Rupture, ear drum, traumatic
    ureter S37.19
    uterus S37.69
    vagina —*see* Injury, vagina
    vena cava —*see* Injury, vena cava,
      laceration, major
  tricuspid (heart) (valve) I07.8
  tube, tubal (nonobstetric) (nontraumatic)
    N83.8
    abscess —*see* Salpingitis
    due to pregnancy O00.10-●
      with intrauterine pregnancy O00.11-●
  tympanum, tympanic (membrane)
    (nontraumatic) —*see also* Perforation,
    tympanic membrane H72.9-●
    traumatic —*see* Rupture, ear drum,
      traumatic
  umbilical cord, complicating delivery
    O69.89
  ureter (traumatic) S37.19
    nontraumatic N28.89
  urethra (nontraumatic) N36.8
    with ectopic or molar pregnancy O08.6
    following ectopic or molar pregnancy
      O08.6
    obstetrical trauma O71.5
    traumatic S37.39

Rupture, ruptured *(Continued)*
  uterosacral ligament (nonobstetric)
    (nontraumatic) N83.8
  uterus (traumatic) S37.69
    before labor O71.0-●
    during or after labor O71.1
    nonpuerperal, nontraumatic N85.8
    pregnant (during labor) O71.1
      before labor O71.0-●
  vagina —*see* Injury, vagina
  valve, valvular (heart) —*see* Endocarditis
  varicose vein —*see* Varix

Rupture, ruptured *(Continued)*
  varix —*see* Varix
  vena cava R58
    traumatic —*see* Injury, vena cava,
      laceration, major
  vesical (urinary) N32.89
  vessel (blood) R58
    pulmonary I28.8
    traumatic —*see* Injury, blood vessel
  viscus R19.8
  vulva complicating delivery O70.0

Russell-Silver syndrome Q87.19
Russian spring-summer type encephalitis
  A84.0
Rust's disease (tuberculous cervical spondylitis)
  A18.01
Ruvalcaba-Myhre-Smith syndrome E71.440
Rytand-Lipsitch syndrome I44.2

S

Saber, sabre shin or tibia (syphilitic) A50.56
[M90.8-●]
Sac lacrimal —see condition
Saccharomyces infection B37.9
Saccharopinuria E72.3
Saccular —see condition
Sacculation
aorta (nonsyphilitic) —see Aneurysm, aorta
bladder N32.3
intralaryngeal (congenital) (ventricular)
Q31.3
larynx (congenital) (ventricular) Q31.3
organ or site, congenital —see Distortion
pregnant uterus —see Pregnancy, complicated
by, abnormal, uterus
ureter N28.89
urethra N36.1
vesical N32.3
Sachs' amaurotic familial idiocy or disease
E75.02
Sachs-Tay disease E75.02
Sacks-Libman disease M32.11
Sacralgia M53.3
Sacralization Q76.49
Sacrodynia M53.3
Sacroiliac joint —see condition
Sacroiliitis NEC M46.1
Sacrum —see condition
Saddle
back —see Lordosis
embolus
abdominal aorta I74.01
pulmonary artery I26.92
with acute cor pulmonale I26.02
injury — code to condition
nose M95.0
due to syphilis A50.57
Sadism (sexual) F65.52
Sadness, postpartal O90.6
Sadomasochism F65.50
Saemisch's ulcer (cornea) —see Ulcer, cornea,
central
Sagging
skin and subcutaneous tissue (following
bariatric surgery weight loss) (following
dietary weight loss) L98.7
Sahib disease B55.0
Sailors' skin L57.8
Saint
Anthony's fire —see Erysipelas
triad —see Hernia, diaphragm
Vitus' dance —see Chorea, Sydenham's
Salaam
attack(s) —see Epilepsy, spasms
tic R25.8
Salicylism
abuse F55.8
overdose or wrong substance given —see
Table of Drugs and Chemicals, by drug,
poisoning
Salivary duct or gland —see condition
Salivation, excessive K11.7
Salmonella —see Infection, Salmonella
Salmonellosis A02.0
Salpingitis (catarrhal) (fallopian tube) (nodular)
(pseudofollicular) (purulent) (septic)
N70.91
with oophoritis N70.93
acute N70.01
with oophoritis N70.03
chlamydial A56.11
chronic N70.11
with oophoritis N70.13
complicating abortion —see Abortion, by
type, complicated by, salpingitis
ear —see Salpingitis, eustachian
eustachian (tube) H68.00-●
acute H68.01-●
chronic H68.02-●

Salpingitis (Continued)
follicularis N70.11
with oophoritis N70.13
gonococcal (acute) (chronic) A54.24
interstitial, chronic N70.11
with oophoritis N70.13
isthmica nodosa N70.11
with oophoritis N70.13
specific (gonococcal) (acute) (chronic) A54.24
tuberculous (acute) (chronic) A18.17
venereal (gonococcal) (acute) (chronic) A54.24
Salpingocele N83.4-●
Salpingo-oophoritis (catarrhal) (purulent)
(ruptured) (septic) (suppurative) N70.93
acute N70.03
with ectopic or molar pregnancy O08.0
following ectopic or molar pregnancy
O08.0
gonococcal A54.24
chronic N70.13
following ectopic or molar pregnancy O08.0
gonococcal (acute) (chronic) A54.24
puerperal O86.19
specific (gonococcal) (acute) (chronic) A54.24
subacute N70.03
tuberculous (acute) (chronic) A18.17
venereal (gonococcal) (acute) (chronic) A54.24
Salpingo-ovaritis —see Salpingo-oophoritis
Salpingoperitonitis —see Salpingo-oophoritis
Salzmann's nodular dystrophy —see
Degeneration, cornea, nodular
Sampson's cyst or tumor N80.1
San Joaquin (Valley) fever B38.0
Sandblaster's asthma, lung or pneumoconiosis
J62.8
Sander's disease (paranoia) F22
Sandfly fever A93.1
Sandhoff's disease E75.01
Sanfilippo (Type B) (Type C) (Type D)
syndrome E76.22
Sanger-Brown ataxia G11.2
Sao Paulo fever or typhus A77.0
Saponification, mesenteric K65.8
Sarcocele (benign)
syphilitic A52.76
congenital A50.59
Sarcocystosis A07.8
Sarcoepiplocele —see Hernia
Sarcoepiplomphalocele Q79.2
Sarcoid —see also Sarcoidosis
arthropathy D86.86
Boeck's D86.9
Darier-Roussy D86.3
iridocyclitis D86.83
meningitis D86.81
myocarditis D86.85
myositis D86.87
pyelonephritis D86.84
Spiegler-Fendt L08.89
Sarcoidosis D86.9
with
cranial nerve palsies D86.82
hepatic granuloma D86.89
polyarthritis D86.86
tubulo-interstitial nephropathy D86.84
combined sites NEC D86.89
lung D86.0
and lymph nodes D86.2
lymph nodes D86.1
and lung D86.2
meninges D86.81
skin D86.3
specified type NEC D86.89
Sarcoma (of) —see also Neoplasm, connective
tissue, malignant
alveolar soft part —see Neoplasm, connective
tissue, malignant
ameloblastic C41.1
upper jaw (bone) C41.0
botryoid —see Neoplasm, connective tissue,
malignant

Sarcoma (Continued)
botryoides —see Neoplasm, connective tissue,
malignant
cerebellar C71.6
circumscribed (arachnoidal) C71.6
circumscribed (arachnoidal) cerebellar
C71.6
clear cell —see also Neoplasm, connective
tissue, malignant
kidney C64.-●
dendritic cells (accessory cells) C96.4
embryonal —see Neoplasm, connective tissue,
malignant
endometrial (stromal) C54.1
isthmus C54.0
epithelioid (cell) —see Neoplasm, connective
tissue, malignant
Ewing's —see Neoplasm, bone, malignant
follicular dendritic cell C96.4
germinoblastic (diffuse) —see Lymphoma,
diffuse, large cell
follicular —see Lymphoma, follicular,
specified NEC
giant cell (except of bone) —see also
Neoplasm, connective tissue, malignant
bone —see Neoplasm, bone, malignant
glomoid —see Neoplasm, connective tissue,
malignant
granulocytic C92.3-●
hemangioendothelial —see Neoplasm,
connective tissue, malignant
hemorrhagic, multiple —see Sarcoma,
Kaposi's
histiocytic C96.A
Hodgkin —see Lymphoma, Hodgkin
immunoblastic (diffuse) —see Lymphoma,
diffuse large cell
interdigitating dendritic cell C96.4
Kaposi's
colon C46.4
connective tissue C46.1
gastrointestinal organ C46.4
lung C46.5-●
lymph node(s) C46.3
palate (hard) (soft) C46.2
rectum C46.4
skin C46.0
specified site NEC C46.7
stomach C46.4
unspecified site C46.9
Kupffer cell C22.3
Langerhans cell C96.4
leptomeningeal —see Neoplasm, meninges,
malignant
liver NEC C22.4
lymphangioendothelial —see Neoplasm,
connective tissue, malignant
lymphoblastic —see Lymphoma,
lymphoblastic (diffuse)
lymphocytic —see Lymphoma, small cell
B-cell
mast cell C96.22
melanotic —see Melanoma
meningeal —see Neoplasm, meninges,
malignant
meningothelial —see Neoplasm, meninges,
malignant
mesenchymal —see also Neoplasm,
connective tissue, malignant
mixed —see Neoplasm, connective tissue,
malignant
mesothelial —see Mesothelioma
monstrocellular
specified site —see Neoplasm, malignant,
by site
unspecified site C71.9
myeloid C92.3-●
neurogenic —see Neoplasm, nerve,
malignant
odontogenic C41.1
upper jaw (bone) C41.0

▶ New   ➡ Revised   ~~deleted~~ Deleted   ● Use Additional Character(s)

Sarcoma (Continued)
  osteoblastic —see Neoplasm, bone, malignant
  osteogenic —see also Neoplasm, bone, malignant
    juxtacortical —see Neoplasm, bone, malignant
    periosteal —see Neoplasm, bone, malignant
  periosteal —see also Neoplasm, bone, malignant
    osteogenic —see Neoplasm, bone, malignant
  pleomorphic cell —see Neoplasm, connective tissue, malignant
  reticulum cell (diffuse) —see Lymphoma, diffuse large cell
    nodular —see Lymphoma, follicular
    pleomorphic cell type —see Lymphoma, diffuse large cell
  rhabdoid —see Neoplasm, malignant, by site
  round cell —see Neoplasm, connective tissue, malignant
  small cell —see Neoplasm, connective tissue, malignant
  soft tissue —see Neoplasm, connective tissue, malignant
  spindle cell —see Neoplasm, connective tissue, malignant
  stromal (endometrial) C54.1
    isthmus C54.0
  synovial —see also Neoplasm, connective tissue, malignant
    biphasic —see Neoplasm, connective tissue, malignant
    epithelioid cell —see Neoplasm, connective tissue, malignant
    spindle cell —see Neoplasm, connective tissue, malignant
Sarcomatosis
  meningeal —see Neoplasm, meninges, malignant
  specified site NEC —see Neoplasm, connective tissue, malignant
  unspecified site C80.1
Sarcopenia (age-related) M62.84
Sarcosinemia E72.59
Sarcosporidiosis (intestinal) A07.8
▶SARS-CoV-2 —see also COVID-19
  ▶sequelae (post acute) U09.9
Satiety, early R68.81
Saturnine —see condition
Saturnism
  overdose or wrong substance given or taken —see Table of Drugs and Chemicals, by drug, poisoning
Satyriasis F52.8
Sauriasis —see Ichthyosis
SBE (subacute bacterial endocarditis) I33.0
Scabies (any site) B86
Scabs R23.4
Scaglietti-Dagnini syndrome E22.0
Scald —see Burn
Scalenus anticus (anterior) syndrome G54.0
Scales R23.4
Scaling, skin R23.4
Scalp —see condition
Scapegoating affecting child Z62.3
Scaphocephaly Q75.0
Scapulalgia M89.8X1
Scapulohumeral myopathy G71.02
Scar, scarring —see also Cicatrix L90.5
  adherent L90.5
  atrophic L90.5
  cervix
    in pregnancy or childbirth —see Pregnancy, complicated by, abnormal cervix
  cheloid L91.0
  chorioretinal H31.00-•
    posterior pole macula H31.01-•
    postsurgical H59.81-•
    solar retinopathy H31.02-•
    specified type NEC H31.09-•

Scar, scarring (Continued)
  choroid —see Scar, chorioretinal
  conjunctiva H11.24-•
  cornea H17.9
    xerophthalmic —see also Opacity, cornea vitamin A deficiency E50.6
  defect (isthmocele) O34.22
  duodenum, obstructive K31.5
  hypertrophic L91.0
  keloid L91.0
  labia N90.89
  lung (base) J98.4
  macula —see Scar, chorioretinal, posterior pole
  muscle M62.89
  myocardium, myocardial I25.2
  painful L90.5
  posterior pole (eye) —see Scar, chorioretinal, posterior pole
  retina —see Scar, chorioretinal
  trachea J39.8
  transmural uterine, in pregnancy O34.29
  uterus N85.8
    in pregnancy O34.29
  vagina N89.8
    postoperative N99.2
  vulva N90.89
Scarabiasis B88.2
Scarlatina (anginosa) (maligna) A38.9
  myocarditis (acute) A38.1
    old —see Myocarditis
  otitis media A38.0
  ulcerosa A38.8
Scarlet fever (albuminuria) (angina) A38.9
Schamberg's disease (progressive pigmentary dermatosis) L81.7
Schatzki's ring (acquired) (esophagus) (lower) K22.2
  congenital Q39.3
Schaufenster krankheit I20.8
Schaumann's
  benign lymphogranulomatosis D86.1
  disease or syndrome —see Sarcoidosis
Scheie's syndrome E76.03
Schenck's disease B42.1
Scheuermann's disease or osteochondrosis — see Osteochondrosis, juvenile, spine
Schilder (-Flatau) disease G37.0
Schilling-type monocytic leukemia C93.0-•
Schimmelbusch's disease, cystic mastitis, or hyperplasia —see Mastopathy, cystic
Schistosoma infestation —see Infestation, Schistosoma
Schistosomiasis B65.9
  with muscle disorder B65.9 [M63.80]
    ankle B65.9 [M63.87-•]
    foot B65.9 [M63.87-•]
    forearm B65.9 [M63.83-•]
    hand B65.9 [M63.84-•]
    lower leg B65.9 [M63.86-•]
    multiple sites B65.9 [M63.89]
    pelvic region B65.9 [M63.85-•]
    shoulder region B65.9 [M63.81-•]
    specified site NEC B65.9 [M63.88]
    thigh B65.9 [M63.85-•]
    upper arm B65.9 [M63.82-•]
  Asiatic B65.2
  bladder B65.0
  chestermani B65.8
  colon B65.1
  cutaneous B65.3
  due to
    S. haematobium B65.0
    S. japonicum B65.2
    S. mansoni B65.1
    S. mattheii B65.8
  Eastern B65.2
  genitourinary tract B65.0
  intestinal B65.1
  lung NEC B65.9 [J99]
    pneumonia B65.9 [J17]
  Manson's (intestinal) B65.1

Schistosomiasis (Continued)
  oriental B65.2
  pulmonary NEC B65.9 [J99]
    pneumonia B65.9
  Schistosoma
    haematobium B65.0
    japonicum B65.2
    mansoni B65.1
  specified type NEC B65.8
  urinary B65.0
  vesical B65.0
Schizencephaly Q04.6
Schizoaffective psychosis F25.9
Schizodontia K00.2
Schizoid personality F60.1
Schizophrenia, schizophrenic F20.9
  acute (brief) (undifferentiated) F23
  atypical (form) F20.3
  borderline F21
  catalepsy F20.2
  catatonic (type) (excited) (withdrawn) F20.2
  cenesthopathic, cenesthesiopathic F20.89
  childhood type F84.5
  chronic undifferentiated F20.9
  cyclic F25.0
  disorganized (type) F20.1
  flexibilitas cerea F20.2
  hebephrenic (type) F20.1
  incipient F21
  latent F21
  negative type F20.5
  paranoid (type) F20.0
  paraphrenic F20.0
  post-psychotic depression F32.89
  prepsychotic F21
  prodromal F21
  pseudoneurotic F21
  pseudopsychopathic F21
  reaction F23
  residual (state) (type) F20.5
  restzustand F20.5
  schizoaffective (type) —see Psychosis, schizoaffective
  simple (type) F20.89
  simplex F20.89
  specified type NEC F20.89
  spectrum and other psychotic disorder F29
    specified NEC F28
  stupor F20.2
  syndrome of childhood F84.5
  undifferentiated (type) F20.3
    chronic F20.5
Schizothymia (persistent) F60.1
Schlatter-Osgood disease or osteochondrosis M92.52-•
Schlatter's tibia —see Osteochondrosis, juvenile, tibia
Schmidt's syndrome (polyglandular, autoimmune) E31.0
Schmincke's carcinoma or tumor —see Neoplasm, nasopharynx, malignant
Schmitz (-Stutzer) dysentery A03.0
Schmorl's disease or nodes
  lumbar region M51.46
  lumbosacral region M51.47
  sacrococcygeal region M53.3
  thoracic region M51.44
  thoracolumbar region M51.45
Schneiderian
  papilloma —see Neoplasm, nasopharynx benign
    specified site —see Neoplasm, benign, by site
    unspecified site D14.0
    specified site —see Neoplasm, malignant, by site
    unspecified site C30.0
Scholte's syndrome (malignant carcinoid) E34.0
Scholz (-Bielchowsky-Henneberg) disease or syndrome E75.25
Schönlein (-Henoch) disease or purpura (primary) (rheumatic) D69.0

Schottmuller's disease A01.4
Schroeder's syndrome (endocrine
    hypertensive) E27.0
Schüller-Christian disease or syndrome C96.5
Schultze's type acroparesthesia, simple I73.89
Schultz's disease or syndrome —see
    Agranulocytosis
Schwalbe-Ziehen-Oppenheim disease G24.1
Schwannoma —see also Neoplasm, nerve,
    benign
    malignant —see also Neoplasm, nerve,
        malignant
        with rhabdomyoblastic differentiation —
            see Neoplasm, nerve, malignant
    melanocytic —see Neoplasm, nerve, benign
    pigmented —see Neoplasm, nerve, benign
Schwannomatosis Q85.03
Schwartz (-Jampel) syndrome G71.13
Schwartz-Bartter syndrome E22.2
Schweniger-Buzzi anetoderma L90.1
Sciatic —see condition
▶ Sciatica (infective) M54.3
    with lumbago M54.4-●
        due to intervertebral disc disorder —see
            Disorder, disc, with, radiculopathy
        due to displacement of intervertebral disc
            (with lumbago) —see Disorder, disc,
            with, radiculopathy
    wallet M54.3-●
Scimitar syndrome Q26.8
Sclera —see condition
Sclerectasia H15.84-●
Scleredema
    adultorum —see Sclerosis, systemic
    Buschke's —see Sclerosis, systemic
    newborn P83.0
Sclerema (adiposum) (edematosum)
    (neonatorum) (newborn) P83.0
    adultorum —see Sclerosis, systemic
Scleriasis —see Scleroderma
Scleritis H15.00-●
    with corneal involvement H15.04-●
    anterior H15.01-●
    brawny H15.02-●
    in (due to) zoster B02.34
    posterior H15.03-●
    specified type NEC H15.09-●
    syphilitic A52.71
    tuberculous (nodular) A18.51
Sclerochoroiditis H31.8
Scleroconjunctivitis —see Scleritis
Sclerocystic ovary syndrome E28.2
Sclerodactyly, sclerodactylia L94.3
Scleroderma, sclerodermia (acrosclerotic)
    (diffuse) (generalized) (progressive)
    (pulmonary) —see also Sclerosis, systemic
    M34.9-●
    circumscribed L94.0
    linear L94.1
    localized L94.0
    newborn P83.88
    systemic M34.9
Sclerokeratitis H16.8
    tuberculous A18.52
Scleroma nasi A48.8
Scleromalacia (perforans) H15.05-●
Scleromyxedema L98.5
Sclérose en plaques G35
Sclerosis, sclerotic
    adrenal (gland) E27.8
    Alzheimer's —see Disease, Alzheimer's
    amyotrophic (lateral) G12.21
    aorta, aortic I70.0
        valve —see Endocarditis, aortic
    artery, arterial, arteriolar, arteriovascular —
        see Arteriosclerosis
    ascending multiple G35
    brain (generalized) (lobular) G37.9
        artery, arterial I67.2
        diffuse G37.0
        disseminated G35

Sclerosis, sclerotic (Continued)
    brain (Continued)
        insular G35
        Krabbe's E75.23
        miliary G35
        multiple G35
        presenile (Alzheimer's) —see Disease,
            Alzheimer's, early onset
        senile (arteriosclerotic) I67.2
        stem, multiple G35
        tuberous Q85.1
    bulbar, multiple G35
    bundle of His I44.39
    cardiac —see Disease, heart, ischemic,
        atherosclerotic
    cardiorenal —see Hypertension, cardiorenal
    cardiovascular —see also Disease,
        cardiovascular
        renal —see Hypertension, cardiorenal
    cerebellar —see Sclerosis, brain
    cerebral —see Sclerosis, brain
    cerebrospinal (disseminated) (multiple) G35
    cerebrovascular I67.2
    choroid —see Degeneration, choroid
    combined (spinal cord) —see also
        Degeneration, combined
        multiple G35
    concentric (Balo) G37.5
    cornea —see Opacity, cornea
    coronary (artery) I25.10
        with angina pectoris —see Arteriosclerosis,
            coronary (artery),
    corpus cavernosum
        female N90.89
        male N48.6
    diffuse (brain) (spinal cord) G37.0
    disseminated G35
    dorsal G35
    dorsolateral (spinal cord) —see Degeneration,
        combined
    endometrium N85.5
    extrapyramidal G25.9
    eye, nuclear (senile) —see Cataract, senile,
        nuclear
    focal and segmental (glomerular) —see also
        N00-N07 with fourth character .1 N05.1
    Friedreich's (spinal cord) G11.11
    funicular (spermatic cord) N50.89
    general (vascular) —see Arteriosclerosis
    gland (lymphatic) I89.8
    hepatic K74.1
        alcoholic K70.2
    hereditary
        cerebellar G11.9
        spinal (Friedreich's ataxia) G11.11
    hippocampal G93.81
    insular G35
    kidney —see Sclerosis, renal
    larynx J38.7
    lateral (amyotrophic) (descending) (spinal)
        G12.21
        primary G12.23
    lens, senile nuclear —see Cataract, senile,
        nuclear
    liver K74.1
        with fibrosis K74.2
            alcoholic K70.2
        alcoholic K70.2
        cardiac K76.1
    lung —see Fibrosis, lung
    mastoid —see Mastoiditis, chronic
    mesial temporal G93.81
    mitral I05.8
    Mönckeberg's (medial) —see Arteriosclerosis,
        extremities
    multiple (brain stem) (cerebral) (generalized)
        (spinal cord) G35
    myocardium, myocardial —see Disease, heart,
        ischemic, atherosclerotic
    nuclear (senile), eye —see Cataract, senile,
        nuclear

Sclerosis, sclerotic (Continued)
    ovary N83.8
    pancreas K86.89
    penis N48.6
    peripheral arteries —see Arteriosclerosis,
        extremities
    plaques G35
    pluriglandular E31.8
    polyglandular E31.8
    posterolateral (spinal cord) —see
        Degeneration, combined
    presenile (Alzheimer's) —see Disease,
        Alzheimer's, early onset
    primary, lateral G12.23
    progressive, systemic M34.0
    pulmonary —see Fibrosis, lung
        artery I27.0
        valve (heart) —see Endocarditis, pulmonary
    renal N26.9
        with
            cystine storage disease E72.09
            hypertensive heart disease (conditions in
                I11) —see Hypertension, cardiorenal
            arteriolar (hyaline) (hyperplastic) —see
                Hypertension, kidney
    retina (senile) (vascular) H35.00
    senile (vascular) —see Arteriosclerosis
    spinal (cord) (progressive) G95.89
        ascending G61.0
        combined —see also Degeneration,
            combined
            multiple G35
            syphilitic A52.11
        disseminated G35
        dorsolateral —see Degeneration, combined
        hereditary (Friedreich's) (mixed form)
            G11.11
        lateral (amyotrophic) G12.21
            progressive G12.23
        multiple G35
        posterior (syphilitic) A52.11
    stomach K31.89
    subendocardial, congenital I42.4
    systemic M34.9
        with
            lung involvement M34.81
            myopathy M34.82
            polyneuropathy M34.83
        drug-induced M34.2
        due to chemicals NEC M34.2
        progressive M34.0
        specified NEC M34.89
    temporal (mesial) G93.81
    tricuspid (heart) (valve) I07.8
    tuberous (brain) Q85.1
    tympanic membrane —see Disorder,
        tympanic membrane, specified NEC
    valve, valvular (heart) —see Endocarditis
    vascular —see Arteriosclerosis
    vein I87.8
Scoliosis (acquired) (postural) M41.9
    adolescent (idiopathic) —see Scoliosis,
        idiopathic, adolescent
    congenital Q67.5
        due to bony malformation Q76.3
        failure of segmentation (hemivertebra)
            Q76.3
        hemivertebra fusion Q76.3
        postural Q67.5
    degenerative M41.8-●
    idiopathic M41.20
        adolescent M41.129
            cervical region M41.122
            cervicothoracic region M41.123
            lumbar region M41.126
            lumbosacral region M41.127
            thoracic region M41.124
            thoracolumbar region
                M41.125
        cervical region M41.22
        cervicothoracic region M41.23

Scoliosis *(Continued)*
  idiopathic, *(Continued)*
    infantile M41.00
      cervical region M41.02
      cervicothoracic region M41.03
      lumbar region M41.06
      lumbosacral region M41.07
      sacrococcygeal region M41.08
      thoracic region M41.04
      thoracolumbar region M41.05
    juvenile M41.119
      cervical region M41.112
      cervicothoracic region M41.113
      lumbar region M41.116
      lumbosacral region M41.117
      thoracic region M41.114
      thoracolumbar region M41.115
    lumbar region M41.26
    lumbosacral region M41.27
    thoracic region M41.24
    thoracolumbar region M41.25
  infantile —*see* Scoliosis, idiopathic, infantile
  neuromuscular M41.40
    cervical region M41.42
    cervicothoracic region M41.43
    lumbar region M41.46
    lumbosacral region M41.47
    occipito-atlanto-axial region M41.41
    thoracic region M41.44
    thoracolumbar region M41.45
  paralytic —*see* Scoliosis, neuromuscular
  postradiation therapy M96.5
  rachitic (late effect or sequelae) E64.3 *[M49.80]*
    cervical region E64.3 *[M49.82]*
    cervicothoracic region E64.3 *[M49.83]*
    lumbar region E64.3 *[M49.86]*
    lumbosacral region E64.3 *[M49.87]*
    multiple sites E64.3 *[M49.89]*
    occipito-atlanto-axial region E64.3 *[M49.81]*
    sacrococcygeal region E64.3 *[M49.88]*
    thoracic region E64.3 *[M49.84]*
    thoracolumbar region E64.3 *[M49.85]*
  sciatic M54.4-●
  secondary (to) NEC M41.50
    cerebral palsy, Friedreich's ataxia,
      poliomyelitis, neuromuscular
      disorders —*see* Scoliosis,
      neuromuscular
    cervical region M41.52
    cervicothoracic region M41.53
    lumbar region M41.56
    lumbosacral region M41.57
    thoracic region M41.54
    thoracolumbar region M41.55
  specified form NEC M41.80
    cervical region M41.82
    cervicothoracic region M41.83
    lumbar region M41.86
    lumbosacral region M41.87
    thoracic region M41.84
    thoracolumbar region M41.85
  thoracogenic M41.30
    thoracic region M41.34
    thoracolumbar region M41.35
  tuberculous A18.01
Scoliotic pelvis
  with disproportion (fetopelvic) O33.0
    causing obstructed labor O65.0
Scorbutus, scorbutic —*see also* Scurvy
  anemia D53.2
Score, NIHSS (National Institutes of Health
  Stroke Scale) R29.7-●
Scotoma (arcuate) (Bjerrum) (central) (ring) —
  see also Defect, visual field, localized, scotoma
  scintillating H53.19
Scratch —*see* Abrasion
Scratchy throat R09.89
Screening (for) Z13.9
  alcoholism Z13.33
  anemia Z13.0
  anomaly, congenital Z13.89

Screening *(Continued)*
  antenatal, of mother —*see also* Encounter,
    antenatal Z36.9
  arterial hypertension Z13.6
  arthropod-borne viral disease NEC Z11.59
  autism Z13.41
  bacteriuria, asymptomatic Z13.89
    specified NEC Z13.39
  behavioral disorder Z13.30
  brain injury, traumatic Z13.850
  bronchitis, chronic Z13.83
  brucellosis Z11.2
  cardiovascular disorder Z13.6
  cataract Z13.5
  chlamydial diseases Z11.8
  cholera Z11.0
  chromosomal abnormalities (nonprocreative)
    NEC Z13.79
  colonoscopy Z12.11
  congenital
    dislocation of hip Z13.89
    eye disorder Z13.5
    malformation or deformation Z13.89
  contamination NEC Z13.88
  coronavirus (disease) (novel) 2019 Z11.52
  COVID-19 Z11.52
  cystic fibrosis Z13.228
  dengue fever Z11.59
  dental disorder Z13.84
  depression (adult) (adolescent) (child) Z13.31
    maternal Z13.32
    perinatal Z13.32
  developmental
    delays Z13.40
      global (milestones) Z13.42
      specified NEC Z13.49
    handicap Z13.42
      in early childhood Z13.42
  diabetes mellitus Z13.1
  diphtheria Z11.2
  disability, intellectual Z13.39
  disease or disorder Z13.9
    bacterial NEC Z11.2
      intestinal infectious Z11.0
      respiratory tuberculosis Z11.1
    behavioral Z13.30
      specified NEC Z13.39
    developmental delays Z13.40
      global (milestones) Z13.42
      specified NEC Z13.49
    mental health and behavioral Z13.30
      specified NEC Z13.39
    blood or blood-forming organ Z13.0
    cardiovascular Z13.6
    Chagas' Z11.6
    chlamydial Z11.8
    coronavirus (novel) 2019 Z11.52
    COVID-19 Z11.52
    dental Z13.89
    digestive tract NEC Z13.818
      lower GI Z13.811
      upper GI Z13.810
    ear Z13.5
    endocrine Z13.29
    eye Z13.5
    genitourinary Z13.89
    heart Z13.6
    human immunodeficiency virus (HIV)
      infection Z11.4
    immunity Z13.0
    infection
      intestinal Z11.0
        specified NEC Z11.6
      infectious Z11.9
    metabolic Z13.228
    neurological Z13.89
    nutritional Z13.21
      metabolic Z13.228
        lipoid disorders Z13.220
    protozoal Z11.6
      intestinal Z11.0

Screening *(Continued)*
  disease or disorder *(Continued)*
    respiratory Z13.83
    rheumatic Z13.828
    rickettsial Z11.8
    sexually-transmitted NEC Z11.3
      human immunodeficiency virus (HIV)
        Z11.4
    sickle-cell (trait) Z13.0
    skin Z13.89
    specified NEC Z13.89
    spirochetal Z11.8
    thyroid Z13.29
    vascular Z13.6
    venereal Z11.3
    viral NEC Z11.59
      coronavirus (disease) (novel) 2019
        Z11.52
      COVID-19 Z11.52
      human immunodeficiency virus (HIV)
        Z11.4
      intestinal Z11.0
      SARS-CoV-2 Z11.52
  elevated titer Z13.89
  emphysema Z13.83
  encephalitis, viral (mosquito- or tick-borne)
    Z11.59
  exposure to contaminants (toxic) Z13.88
  fever
    dengue Z11.59
    hemorrhagic Z11.59
    yellow Z11.59
  filariasis Z11.6
  galactosemia Z13.228
  gastrointestinal condition Z13.818
  genetic (nonprocreative)- for procreative
    management —*see* Testing, genetic, for
    procreative management
    disease carrier status (nonprocreative)
      Z13.71
    specified NEC (nonprocreative) Z13.79
  genitourinary condition Z13.89
  glaucoma Z13.5
  gonorrhea Z11.3
  gout Z13.89
  helminthiasis (intestinal) Z11.6
  hematopoietic malignancy Z12.89
  hemoglobinopathies NEC Z13.0
  hemorrhagic fever Z11.59
  Hodgkin disease Z12.89
  human immunodeficiency virus (HIV) Z11.4
  human papillomavirus Z11.51
  hypertension Z13.6
  infant or child (over 28 days old) Z00.129
    with abnormal findings Z00.121
  immunity disorders Z13.0
  infection
    mycotic Z11.8
    parasitic Z11.8
  ingestion of radioactive substance Z13.88
  intellectual disability Z13.39
  intestinal
    helminthiasis Z11.6
    infectious disease Z11.0
  leishmaniasis Z11.6
  leprosy Z11.2
  leptospirosis Z11.8
  leukemia Z12.89
  lymphoma Z12.89
  malaria Z11.6
  malnutrition Z13.29
    metabolic Z13.228
    nutritional Z13.21
  measles Z11.59
  mental health disorder Z13.30
    specified NEC Z13.39
  metabolic errors, inborn Z13.228
  multiphasic Z13.89
  musculoskeletal disorder Z13.828
    osteoporosis Z13.820
  mycoses Z11.8

Screening *(Continued)*
  myocardial infarction (acute) Z13.6
  neoplasm (malignant) (of) Z12.9
    bladder Z12.6
    blood Z12.89
    breast Z12.39
      routine mammogram Z12.31
    cervix Z12.4
    colon Z12.11
    genitourinary organs NEC Z12.79
      bladder Z12.6
      cervix Z12.4
      ovary Z12.73
      prostate Z12.5
      testis Z12.71
      vagina Z12.72
    hematopoietic system Z12.89
    intestinal tract Z12.10
      colon Z12.11
      rectum Z12.12
      small intestine Z12.13
    lung Z12.2
    lymph (glands) Z12.89
    nervous system Z12.82
    oral cavity Z12.81
    prostate Z12.5
    rectum Z12.12
    respiratory organs Z12.2
    skin Z12.83
    small intestine Z12.13
    specified site NEC Z12.89
    stomach Z12.0
  nephropathy Z13.89
  nervous system disorders NEC Z13.858
  neurological condition Z13.89
  osteoporosis Z13.820
  parasitic infestation Z11.9
    specified NEC Z11.8
  phenylketonuria Z13.228
  plague Z11.2
  poisoning (chemical) (heavy metal) Z13.88
  poliomyelitis Z11.59
  postnatal, chromosomal abnormalities Z13.89
  prenatal, of mother —*see also* Encounter,
      antenatal Z36.9
  protozoal disease Z11.6
    intestinal Z11.0
  pulmonary tuberculosis Z11.1
  radiation exposure Z13.88
  respiratory condition Z13.83
  respiratory tuberculosis Z11.1
  rheumatoid arthritis Z13.828
  rubella Z11.59
  SARS-CoV-2 Z11.52
  schistosomiasis Z11.6
  sexually-transmitted disease NEC Z11.3
    human immunodeficiency virus (HIV) Z11.4
  sickle-cell disease or trait Z13.0
  skin condition Z13.89
  sleeping sickness Z11.6
  special Z13.9
    specified NEC Z13.89
  syphilis Z11.3
  tetanus Z11.2
  trachoma Z11.8
  traumatic brain injury Z13.850
  trypanosomiasis Z11.6
  tuberculosis, respiratory Z11.1
    active Z11.1
    latent Z11.7
  venereal disease Z11.3
  viral encephalitis (mosquito- or tick-borne)
      Z11.59
  whooping cough Z11.2
  worms, intestinal Z11.6
  yaws Z11.8
  yellow fever Z11.59
Scrofula, scrofulosis (tuberculosis of cervical
    lymph glands) A18.2
Scrofulide (primary) (tuberculous) A18.4
Scrofuloderma, scrofulodermia (any site)
    (primary) A18.4

Scrofulosus lichen (primary) (tuberculous) A18.4
Scrofulous —*see* condition
Scrotal tongue K14.5
Scrotum —*see* condition
Scurvy, scorbutic E54
  anemia D53.2
  gum E54
  infantile E54
  rickets E55.0 *[M90.80]*
Sealpox B08.62
Seasickness T75.3
Seatworm (infection) (infestation) B80
Sebaceous —*see also* condition
  cyst —*see* Cyst, sebaceous
Seborrhea, seborrheic L21.9
  capillitii R23.8
  capitis L21.0
  dermatitis L21.9
    infantile L21.1
  eczema L21.9
    infantile L21.1
  sicca L21.0
Seckel's syndrome Q87.19
Seclusion, pupil —*see* Membrane, pupillary
Second hand tobacco smoke exposure (acute)
    (chronic) Z77.22
  in the perinatal period P96.81
Secondary
  dentin (in pulp) K04.3
  neoplasm, secondaries —*see* Table of
    Neoplasms, secondary
Secretion
  antidiuretic hormone, inappropriate E22.2
  catecholamine, by pheochromocytoma E27.5
  hormone
    antidiuretic, inappropriate (syndrome)
        E22.2
    by
      carcinoid tumor E34.0
      pheochromocytoma E27.5
    ectopic NEC E34.2
  urinary
    excessive R35.89
    suppression R34
Section
  nerve, traumatic —*see* Injury, nerve
Sedative, hypnotic, or anxiolytic-induced
  anxiety disorder F13.980
  bipolar and related disorder F13.94
  delirium F13.921
  depressive disorder F13.94
  major neurocognitive disorder F13.97
  mild neurocognitive disorder F13.988
  psychotic disorder F13.959
  sexual dysfunction F13.981
  sleep disorder F13.982
Segmentation, incomplete (congenital) —*see
  also* Fusion
  bone NEC Q78.8
  lumbosacral (joint) (vertebra) Q76.49
Seitelberger's syndrome (infantile neuraxonal
    dystrophy) G31.89
Seizure(s) —*see also* Convulsions R56.9
  absence G40.A-•
  akinetic —*see* Epilepsy, generalized, specified
      NEC
  atonic —*see* Epilepsy, generalized, specified
      NEC
  autonomic (hysterical) F44.5
  convulsive —*see* Convulsions
  cortical (focal) (motor) —*see* Epilepsy,
      localization-related, symptomatic, with
      simple partial seizures
  disorder —*see also* Epilepsy G40.909
  due to stroke —*see* Sequelae (of), disease,
      cerebrovascular, by type, specified NEC
  epileptic —*see* Epilepsy
  febrile (simple) R56.00
    with status epilepticus G40.901
    complex (atypical) (complicated) R56.01
      with status epilepticus G40.901

Seizure *(Continued)*
  grand mal G40.409
    intractable G40.419
      with status epilepticus G40.411
      without status epilepticus G40.419
    not intractable G40.409
      with status epilepticus G40.401
      without status epilepticus G40.409
  heart —*see* Disease, heart
  hysterical F44.5
  intractable G40.919
    with status epilepticus G40.911
  Jacksonian (focal) (motor type) (sensory
      type) —*see* Epilepsy, localization-related,
      symptomatic, with simple partial seizures
  newborn P90
  nonspecific epileptic
    atonic —*see* Epilepsy, generalized, specified
        NEC
    clonic —*see* Epilepsy, generalized, specified
        NEC
    myoclonic —*see* Epilepsy, generalized,
        specified NEC
    tonic —*see* Epilepsy, generalized, specified
        NEC
    tonic-clonic —*see* Epilepsy, generalized,
        specified NEC
  partial, developing into secondarily
      generalized seizures
    complex —*see* Epilepsy, localization-
        related, symptomatic, with complex
        partial seizures
    simple —*see* Epilepsy, localization-related,
        symptomatic, with simple partial
        seizures
  petit mal G40.A-•
  intractable G40.A1-•
    with status epilepticus G40.A11
    without status epilepticus G40.A19
  not intractable G40.A0 -•
    with status epilepticus G40.A01
    without status epilepticus G40.A01
  post traumatic R56.1
  recurrent G40.909
  specified NEC G40.89
  uncinate —*see* Epilepsy, localization-related,
      symptomatic, with complex partial
      seizures
Selenium deficiency, dietary E59
Self-damaging behavior (life-style) Z72.89
Self-harm (attempted)
  history (personal)
    in family Z81.8
    nonsuicidal Z91.52
    suicidal Z91.51
  nonsuicidal R45.88
Self-injury, nonsuicidal R45.88
  personal history Z91.52
Self-mutilation (attempted)
  history (personal)
    in family Z81.8
    nonsuicidal Z91.52
    suicidal Z91.51
  nonsuicidal R45.88
Self-poisoning
  history (personal)
    in family Z81.8
  observation following (alleged) attempt Z03.6
Semicoma R40.1
Seminal vesiculitis N49.0
Seminoma C62.9-•
  specified site —*see* Neoplasm, malignant, by
      site
Senear-Usher disease or syndrome L10.4
Senectus R54
Senescence (without mention of psychosis) R54
Senile, senility —*see also* condition R41.81
  with
    acute confusional state F05
    mental changes NOS F03
    psychosis NEC —*see* Psychosis, senile
  asthenia R54
  cervix (atrophic) N88.8

▶ New   ⇒ Revised   ~~deleted~~ Deleted   • Use Additional Character(s)

Septum, septate *(Continued)*
  vagina Q52.10
    in pregnancy —*see* Pregnancy, complicated
        by, abnormal vagina
      causing obstructed labor O65.5
    longitudinal Q52.129
      microperforate
        left side Q52.124
        right side Q52.123
      nonobstruction Q52.120
      obstructing Q52.129
        left side Q52.122
        right side Q52.121
    transverse Q52.11
Sequelae (of) —*see also* condition
  abscess, intracranial or intraspinal (conditions
      in G06) G09
  amputation — code to injury with seventh
      character S
  burn and corrosion — code to injury with
      seventh character S
  calcium deficiency E64.8
  cerebrovascular disease —*see* Sequelae,
      disease, cerebrovascular
  childbirth O94
  contusion — code to injury with seventh
      character S
  corrosion —*see* Sequelae, burn and corrosion
▶COVID-19 (post acute) U09.9
  crushing injury — code to injury with
      seventh character S
  disease
    cerebrovascular I69.90
      alteration of sensation I69.998
      aphasia I69.920
      apraxia I69.990
      ataxia I69.993
      cognitive deficits I69.91
      disturbance of vision I69.998
      dysarthria I69.922
      dysphagia I69.991
      dysphasia I69.921
      facial droop I69.992
      facial weakness I69.992
      fluency disorder I69.923
      hemiplegia I69.95-●
      hemorrhage
        intracerebral —*see* Sequelae,
            hemorrhage, intracerebral
        intracranial, nontraumatic NEC —
            see Sequelae, hemorrhage,
            intracranial, nontraumatic
        subarachnoid —*see* Sequelae,
            hemorrhage, subarachnoid
      language deficit I69.928
      monoplegia
        lower limb I69.94-●
        upper limb I69.93-●
      paralytic syndrome I69.96-●
      specified effect NEC I69.998
      specified type NEC I69.80
        alteration of sensation I69.898
        aphasia I69.820
        apraxia I69.890
        ataxia I69.893
        cognitive deficits I69.81
        disturbance of vision I69.898
        dysarthria I69.822
        dysphagia I69.891
        dysphasia I69.821
        facial droop I69.892
        facial weakness I69.892
        fluency disorder I69.823
        hemiplegia I69.85-●
        language deficit I69.828
        monoplegia
          lower limb I69.84-●
          upper limb I69.83-●
        paralytic syndrome I69.86-●
        specified effect NEC I69.898
      speech deficit I69.928
        speech deficit I69.828
    stroke NOS —*see* Sequelae, stroke NOS

Sequelae *(Continued)*
  dislocation — code to injury with seventh
      character S
  encephalitis or encephalomyelitis (conditions
      in G04) G09
    in infectious disease NEC B94.8
    viral B94.1
  external cause — code to injury with seventh
      character S
  foreign body entering natural orifice — code
      to injury with seventh character S
  fracture — code to injury with seventh
      character S
  frostbite — code to injury with seventh
      character S
  Hansen's disease B92
  hemorrhage
    intracerebral I69.10
      alteration of sensation I69.198
      aphasia I69.120
      apraxia I69.190
      ataxia I69.193
      cognitive deficits I69.11
      disturbance of vision I69.198
      dysarthria I69.122
      dysphagia I69.191
      dysphasia I69.121
      facial droop I69.192
      facial weakness I69.192
      fluency disorder I69.123
      hemiplegia I69.15-●
      language deficit NEC I69.128
      monoplegia
        lower limb I69.14-●
        upper limb I69.13-●
      paralytic syndrome I69.16-●
      specified effect NEC I69.198
      speech deficit NEC I69.128
    intracranial, nontraumatic NEC I69.20
      alteration of sensation I69.298
      aphasia I69.220
      apraxia I69.290
      ataxia I69.293
      cognitive deficits I69.21
      disturbance of vision I69.298
      dysarthria I69.222
      dysphagia I69.291
      dysphasia I69.221
      facial droop I69.292
      facial weakness I69.292
      fluency disorder I69.223
      hemiplegia I69.25-●
      language deficit NEC I69.228
      monoplegia
        lower limb I69.24-●
        upper limb I69.23-●
      paralytic syndrome I69.26-●
      specified effect NEC I69.298
      speech deficit NEC I69.228
    subarachnoid I69.00
      alteration of sensation I69.098
      aphasia I69.020
      apraxia I69.090
      ataxia I69.093
      cognitive deficits —*see* subcategory
          I69.01-●
      disturbance of vision I69.098
      dysarthria I69.022
      dysphagia I69.091
      dysphasia I69.021
      facial droop I69.092
      facial weakness I69.092
      fluency disorder I69.023
      hemiplegia I69.05-●
      language deficit NEC I69.028
      monoplegia
        lower limb I69.04-●
        upper limb I69.03-●
      paralytic syndrome I69.06-●
      specified effect NEC I69.098
      speech deficit NEC I69.028

Sequelae *(Continued)*
  hepatitis, viral B94.2
  hyperalimentation E68
  infarction
    cerebral I69.30
      alteration of sensation I69.398
      aphasia I69.320
      apraxia I69.390
      ataxia I69.393
      cognitive deficits I69.31
      disturbance of vision I69.398
      dysarthria I69.322
      dysphagia I69.391
      dysphasia I69.321
      facial droop I69.392
      facial weakness I69.392
      fluency disorder I69.323
      hemiplegia I69.35-●
      language deficit NEC I69.328
      monoplegia
        lower limb I69.34-●
        upper limb I69.33-●
      paralytic syndrome I69.36-●
      specified effect NEC I69.398
      speech deficit NEC I69.328
  infection, pyogenic, intracranial or intraspinal
      G09
  infectious disease B94.9
    specified NEC B94.8
  injury — code to injury with seventh
      character S
  leprosy B92
  meningitis
    bacterial (conditions in G00) G09
    other or unspecified cause (conditions in
        G03) G09
  muscle (and tendon) injury — code to injury
      with seventh character S
  myelitis —*see* Sequelae, encephalitis
  niacin deficiency E64.8
  nutritional deficiency E64.9
    specified NEC E64.8
  obstetrical condition O94
  parasitic disease B94.9
  phlebitis or thrombophlebitis of intracranial
      or intraspinal venous sinuses and veins
      (conditions in G08) G09
  poisoning — code to poisoning with seventh
      character S
    nonmedicinal substance —*see* Sequelae,
        toxic effect, nonmedicinal substance
  poliomyelitis (acute) B91
  pregnancy O94
  protein-energy malnutrition E64.0
  puerperium O94
  rickets E64.3
▶SARS-CoV-2 (post acute) U09.9
  selenium deficiency E64.8
  sprain and strain — code to injury with
      seventh character S
  stroke NOS I69.30
    alteration in sensation I69.398
    aphasia I69.320
    apraxia I69.390
    ataxia I69.393
    cognitive deficits I69.31
    disturbance of vision I69.398
    dysarthria I69.322
    dysphagia I69.391
    dysphasia I69.321
    facial droop I69.392
    facial weakness I69.392
    hemiplegia I69.35-●
    language deficit NEC I69.328
    monoplegia
      lower limb I69.34-●
      upper limb I69.33-●
    paralytic syndrome I69.36-●
    specified effect NEC I69.398
    speech deficit NEC I69.328
  tendon and muscle injury — code to injury
      with seventh character S

▶ New   ⇒ Revised   ~~deleted~~ Deleted   ● Use Additional Character(s)

Sequelae *(Continued)*
thiamine deficiency E64.8
trachoma B94.0
tuberculosis B90.9
bones and joints B90.2
central nervous system B90.0
genitourinary B90.1
pulmonary (respiratory) B90.9
specified organs NEC B90.8
viral
encephalitis B94.1
hepatitis B94.2
vitamin deficiency NEC E64.8
A E64.1
B E64.8
C E64.2
wound, open — code to injury with seventh
character S
Sequestration —*see also* Sequestrum
disc —*see* Displacement, intervertebral
disc
lung, congenital Q33.2
Sequestrum
bone —*see* Osteomyelitis, chronic
dental M27.2
jaw bone M27.2
orbit —*see* Osteomyelitis, orbit
sinus (accessory) (nasal) —*see* Sinusitis
Sequoiosis lung or pneumonitis J67.8
Serology for syphilis
doubtful
with signs or symptoms - code by site and
stage under Syphilis
follow-up of latent syphilis —*see* Syphilis,
latent
negative, with signs or symptoms — code by
site and stage under Syphilis
positive A53.0
with signs or symptoms - code by site and
stage under Syphilis
reactivated A53.0
Seroma —*see also* Hematoma
postprocedural —*see* Complication,
postprocedural, seroma
traumatic, secondary and recurrent
T79.2
Seropurulent —*see* condition
Serositis, multiple K65.8
pericardial I31.1
peritoneal K65.8
Serous —*see* condition
Sertoli cell
adenoma
specified site —*see* Neoplasm, benign, by
site
unspecified site
female D27.9
male D29.20
carcinoma
specified site —*see* Neoplasm, malignant,
by site
unspecified site (male) C62.9-●
female C56.9
tumor
with lipid storage
specified site —*see* Neoplasm, benign,
by site
unspecified site
female D27.9
male D29.20
specified site —*see* Neoplasm, benign, by
site
unspecified site
female D27.9
male D29.20
Sertoli-Leydig cell tumor —*see* Neoplasm,
benign, by site
specified site —*see* Neoplasm, benign, by site
unspecified site
female D27.9
male D29.20

Serum
allergy, allergic reaction —*see also* Reaction,
serum T80.69
shock —*see also* Shock, anaphylactic T80.59
arthritis —*see also* Reaction, serum T80.69
complication or reaction NEC —*see also*
Reaction, serum T80.69
disease NEC —*see also* Reaction, serum T80.69
hepatitis —*see also* Hepatitis, viral, type B
carrier (suspected) of B18.1
intoxication —*see also* Reaction, serum T80.69
neuritis —*see also* Reaction, serum T80.69
neuropathy G61.1
poisoning NEC —*see also* Reaction, serum
T80.69
rash NEC —*see also* Reaction, serum T80.69
reaction NEC —*see also* Reaction, serum
T80.69
sickness NEC —*see also* Reaction, serum
T80.69
urticaria —*see also* Reaction, serum T80.69
Sesamoiditis M25.8-●
Sever's disease or osteochondrosis —*see*
Osteochondrosis, juvenile, tarsus
Severe sepsis R65.20
with septic shock R65.21
Sex
chromosome mosaics Q97.8
lines with various numbers of
X chromosomes Q97.2
education Z70.8
reassignment surgery status Z87.890
Sextuplet pregnancy —*see* Pregnancy,
sextuplet
Sexual
function, disorder of (psychogenic) F52.9
immaturity (female) (male) E30.0
impotence (psychogenic) organic origin
NEC —*see* Dysfunction, sexual, male
precocity (constitutional) (cryptogenic)
(female) (idiopathic) (male) E30.1
Sexuality, pathologic —*see* Deviation, sexual
Sézary disease C84.1-●
Shadow, lung R91.8
Shaking palsy or paralysis —*see* Parkinsonism
Shallowness, acetabulum —*see* Derangement,
joint, specified type NEC, hip
Shaver's disease J63.1
Sheath (tendon) —*see* condition
Sheathing, retinal vessels H35.01-●
Shedding
nail L60.8
premature, primary (deciduous) teeth
K00.6
Sheehan's disease or syndrome E23.0
Shelf, rectal K62.89
Shell teeth K00.5
Shellshock (current) F43.0
lasting state —*see* Disorder, post-traumatic
stress
Shield kidney Q63.1
Shift
auditory threshold (temporary) H93.24-●
mediastinal R93.89
Shifting sleep-work schedule (affecting sleep)
G47.26
Shiga (-Kruse) dysentery A03.0
Shiga's bacillus A03.0
Shigella (dysentery) —*see* Dysentery,
bacillary
Shigellosis A03.9
Group A A03.0
Group B A03.1
Group C A03.2
Group D A03.3
Shin splints S86.89
Shingles —*see* Herpes, zoster
Shipyard disease or eye B30.0
Shirodkar suture, in pregnancy —*see*
Pregnancy, complicated by, incompetent
cervix

Shock R57.9
with ectopic or molar pregnancy O08.3
adrenal (cortical) (Addisonian) E27.2
adverse food reaction (anaphylactic) —*see*
Shock, anaphylactic, due to food
allergic —*see* Shock, anaphylactic
anaphylactic T78.2
chemical —*see* Table of Drugs and
Chemicals
due to drug or medicinal substance
correct substance properly administered
T88.6
overdose or wrong substance given or
taken (by accident) —*see* Table of
Drugs and Chemicals, by drug,
poisoning
due to food (nonpoisonous) T78.00
additives T78.06
dairy products T78.07
eggs T78.08
fish T78.03
shellfish T78.02
fruit T78.04
milk T78.07
nuts T78.05
multiple types T78.05
peanuts T78.01
peanuts T78.01
seeds T78.05
specified type NEC T78.09
vegetable T78.04
following sting(s) —*see* Venom
immunization T80.52
serum T80.59
blood and blood products T80.51
immunization T80.52
specified NEC T80.59
vaccination T80.52
anaphylactoid —*see* Shock, anaphylactic
anesthetic
correct substance properly administered
T88.2
overdose or wrong substance given
or taken —*see* Table of Drugs and
Chemicals, by drug, poisoning
specified anesthetic —*see* Table of
Drugs and Chemicals, by drug,
poisoning
cardiogenic R57.0
chemical substance —*see* Table of Drugs and
Chemicals
complicating ectopic or molar pregnancy O08.3
culture —*see* Disorder, adjustment
drug
due to correct substance properly
administered T88.6
overdose or wrong substance given or
taken (by accident) —*see* Table of
Drugs and Chemicals, by drug,
poisoning
during or after labor and delivery O75.1
electric T75.4
(taser) T75.4
endotoxic R65.21
postprocedural (resulting from a procedure,
not elsewhere classified) T81.12
following
ectopic or molar pregnancy O08.3
injury (immediate) (delayed) T79.4
labor and delivery O75.1
food (anaphylactic) —*see* Shock, anaphylactic,
due to food
from electroshock gun (taser) T75.4
gram-negative R65.21
postprocedural (resulting from a procedure,
not elsewhere classified) T81.12
hematologic R57.8
hemorrhagic R57.8
surgery (intraoperative) (postoperative)
T81.19
trauma T79.4

Shock *(Continued)*
  hypovolemic R57.1
    surgical T81.19
    traumatic T79.4
  insulin E15
    therapeutic misadventure —*see*
      subcategory T38.3
  kidney N17.0
    traumatic (following crushing) T79.5
  lightning T75.01
  liver K72.00
  lung J80
  obstetric O75.1
    with ectopic or molar pregnancy O08.3
    following ectopic or molar pregnancy
      O08.3
  pleural (surgical) T81.19
    due to trauma T79.4
  postprocedural (postoperative) T81.10
    with ectopic or molar pregnancy O08.3
    cardiogenic T81.11
    endotoxic T81.12
    following ectopic or molar pregnancy
      O08.3
    gram-negative T81.12
    hypovolemic T81.19
    septic T81.12
    specified type NEC T81.19
  psychic F43.0
  septic (due to severe sepsis) R65.21
  specified NEC R57.8
  surgical T81.10
  taser gun (taser) T75.4
  therapeutic misadventure NEC T81.10
  thyroxin
    overdose or wrong substance given
      or taken —*see* Table of Drugs and
      Chemicals, by drug, poisoning
  toxic, syndrome A48.3
  transfusion —*see* Complications, transfusion
  traumatic (immediate) (delayed) T79.4
Shoemaker's chest M95.4
Short, shortening, shortness
  arm (acquired) —*see also* Deformity, limb,
    unequal length
    congenital Q71.81-●
      forearm —*see* Deformity, limb, unequal
        length
  bowel syndrome K91.2
  breath R06.02
  cervical (complicating pregnancy) O26.87-●
    non-gravid uterus N88.3
  common bile duct, congenital Q44.5
  cord (umbilical), complicating delivery O69.3
  cystic duct, congenital Q44.5
  esophagus (congenital) Q39.8
  femur (acquired) —*see* Deformity, limb,
    unequal length, femur
    congenital —*see* Defect, reduction, lower
      limb, longitudinal, femur
  frenum, frenulum, linguae (congenital) Q38.1
  hip (acquired) —*see also* Deformity, limb,
    unequal length
    congenital Q65.89
  leg (acquired) —*see also* Deformity, limb,
    unequal length
    congenital Q72.81-●
      lower leg —*see also* Deformity, limb,
        unequal length
  limbed stature, with immunodeficiency
    D82.2
  lower limb (acquired) —*see also* Deformity,
    limb, unequal length
    congenital Q72.81-●
  organ or site, congenital NEC —*see* Distortion
  palate, congenital Q38.5
  radius (acquired) —*see also* Deformity, limb,
    unequal length
    congenital —*see* Defect, reduction, upper
      limb, longitudinal, radius
  rib syndrome Q77.2

Short, shortening, shortness*(Continued)*
  stature (child) (hereditary) (idiopathic) NEC
    R62.52
    constitutional E34.3
    due to endocrine disorder E34.3
    Laron-type E34.3
Short, shortening, shortness *(Continued)*
  tendon —*see also* Contraction, tendon
    with contracture of joint —*see* Contraction,
      joint
      Achilles (acquired) M67.0-●
        congenital Q66.89
      congenital Q79.8
    thigh (acquired) —*see also* Deformity, limb,
      unequal length, femur
      congenital —*see* Defect, reduction, lower
        limb, longitudinal, femur
    tibialis anterior (tendon) —*see* Contraction,
      tendon
  umbilical cord
    complicating delivery O69.3
  upper limb, congenital —*see* Defect, reduction,
    upper limb, specified type NEC
  urethra N36.8
  uvula, congenital Q38.5
  vagina (congenital) Q52.4
Shortsightedness —*see* Myopia
Shoshin (acute fulminating beriberi) E51.11
Shoulder —*see* condition
Shovel-shaped incisors K00.2
Shower, thromboembolic —*see* Embolism
Shunt
  arterial-venous (dialysis) Z99.2
  arteriovenous, pulmonary (acquired) I28.0
    congenital Q25.72
  cerebral ventricle (communicating) in situ Z98.2
  surgical, prosthetic, with complications —*see*
    Complications, cardiovascular, device or
    implant Shutdown, renal N28.9
Shutdown, renal N28.9
Shy-Drager syndrome G90.3
Sialadenitis, sialadenosis (any gland) (chronic)
  (periodic) (suppurative) —*see* Sialoadenitis
Sialectasia K11.8
Sialidosis E77.1
Sialitis, silitis (any gland) (chronic)
  (suppurative) —*see* Sialoadenitis
Sialoadenitis (any gland) (periodic)
  (suppurative) K11.20
  acute K11.21
    recurrent K11.22
  chronic K11.23
Sialoadenopathy K11.9
Sialoangitis —*see* Sialoadenitis
Sialodochitis (fibrinosa) —*see* Sialoadenitis
Sialodocholithiasis K11.5
Sialolithiasis K11.5
Sialometaplasia, necrotizing K11.8
Sialorrhea —*see also* Ptyalism
  periodic —*see* Sialoadenitis
Sialosis K11.7
Siamese twin Q89.4
Sibling rivalry Z62.891
Sicard's syndrome G52.7
➡Sicca syndrome —*see* Syndrome, Sjogren
  ~~with~~
    ~~keratoconjunctivitis M35.01~~
    ~~lung involvement M35.02~~
    ~~myopathy M35.03~~
    ~~renal tubulo-interstitial disorders M35.04~~
    ~~specified organ involvement NEC M35.09~~
Sick R69
  or handicapped person in family Z63.79
    needing care at home Z63.6
  sinus (syndrome) I49.5
Sick-euthyroid syndrome E07.81
Sickle-cell
  anemia —*see* Disease, sickle-cell
  beta plus —*see* Disease, sickle-cell,
    thalassemia, beta plus
  beta zero —*see* Disease, sickle-cell,
    thalassemia, beta zero
  trait D57.3

Sicklemia —*see also* Disease, sickle-cell
  trait D57.3
Sickness
  air (travel) T75.3
  airplane T75.3
  alpine T70.29
  altitude T70.20
  Andes T70.29
  aviator's T70.29
  balloon T70.29
  car T75.3
  compressed air T70.3
  decompression T70.3
  green D50.8
  milk —*see* Poisoning, food, noxious
  motion T75.3
  mountain T70.29
    acute D75.1
  protein —*see also* Reaction, serum T80.69
  radiation T66
  roundabout (motion) T75.3
  sea T75.3
  serum NEC —*see also* Reaction, serum T80.69
  sleeping (African) B56.9
    by Trypanosoma B56.9
      brucei
        gambiense B56.0
        rhodesiense B56.1
      East African B56.1
      Gambian B56.0
      Rhodesian B56.1
      West African B56.0
  swing (motion) T75.3
  train (railway) (travel) T75.3
  travel (any vehicle) T75.3
Sideropenia —*see* Anemia, iron deficiency
Siderosilicosis J62.8
Siderosis (lung) J63.4
  brain G93.89
  eye (globe) —*see* Disorder, globe,
    degenerative, siderosis
Siemens' syndrome (ectodermal dysplasia) Q82.8
Sighing R06.89
  psychogenic F45.8
Sigmoid —*see also* condition
  flexure —*see* condition
  kidney Q63.1
Sigmoiditis —*see also* Enteritis K52.9
  infectious A09
  noninfectious K52.9
Silfversköld's syndrome Q78.9
Silicosiderosis J62.8
Silicosis, silicotic (simple) (complicated) J62.8
  with tuberculosis J65
Silicotuberculosis J65
Silo-fillers' disease J68.8
  bronchitis J68.0
  pneumonitis J68.0
  pulmonary edema J68.1
Silver's syndrome Q87.19
Simian malaria B53.1
Simmonds' cachexia or disease E23.0
Simons' disease or syndrome (progressive
  lipodystrophy) E88.1
Simple, simplex —*see* condition
Simulation, conscious (of illness) Z76.5
Simultanagnosia (asimultagnosia) R48.3
Sin Nombre virus disease (Hantavirus)
  (cardio)-pulmonary syndrome) B33.4
Sinding-Larsen disease or osteochondrosis —
  see Osteochondrosis, juvenile, patella
Singapore hemorrhagic fever A91
Singer's node or nodule J38.2
Single
  atrium Q21.2
  coronary artery Q24.5
  umbilical artery Q27.0
  ventricle Q20.4
Singultus R06.6
  epidemicus B33.0
Sinus —*see also* Fistula
  abdominal K63.89
  arrest I45.5

▶ New   ⮕ Revised   ~~deleted~~ Deleted   ● Use Additional Character(s)

Sinus *(Continued)*
  arrhythmia I49.8
  bradycardia R00.1
  branchial cleft (internal) (external) Q18.0
  coccygeal —*see* Sinus, pilonidal
  dental K04.6
  dermal (congenital) Q06.8
    with abscess Q06.8
    coccygeal, pilonidal —*see* Sinus, coccygeal
  infected, skin NEC L08.89
  marginal, ruptured or bleeding —*see*
    Hemorrhage, antepartum, specified
    cause NEC
  medial, face and neck Q18.8
  pause I45.5
  pericranii Q01.9
  pilonidal (infected) (rectum) L05.92
    with abscess L05.02
  preauricular Q18.1
  rectovaginal N82.3
  Rokitansky-Aschoff (gallbladder) K82.8
  sacrococcygeal (dermoid) (infected) —*see*
    Sinus, pilonidal
  tachycardia R00.0
    paroxysmal I47.1
  tarsi syndrome M25.57-●
  testis N50.89
  tract (postinfective) —*see* Fistula
  urachus Q64.4
Sinusitis (accessory) (chronic) (hyperplastic)
  (nasal) (nonpurulent) (purulent) J32.9
  acute J01.90
    ethmoidal J01.20
      recurrent J01.21
    frontal J01.10
      recurrent J01.11
    involving more than one sinus, other than
      pansinusitis J01.80
      recurrent J01.81
    maxillary J01.00
      recurrent J01.01
    pansinusitis J01.40
      recurrent J01.41
    recurrent J01.91
    specified NEC J01.80
      recurrent J01.81
    sphenoidal J01.30
      recurrent J01.31
  allergic —*see* Rhinitis, allergic
  due to high altitude T70.1
  ethmoidal J32.2
    acute J01.20
      recurrent J01.21
  frontal J32.1
    acute J01.10
      recurrent J01.11
  influenzal —*see* Influenza, with, respiratory
    manifestations NEC
  involving more than one sinus but not
    pansinusitis J32.8
    acute J01.80
      recurrent J01.81
  maxillary J32.0
    acute J01.00
      recurrent J01.01
  sphenoidal J32.3
    acute J01.30
      recurrent J01.31
  tuberculous, any sinus A15.8
Sinusitis-bronchiectasis-situs inversus
  (syndrome) (triad) Q89.3
Sipple's syndrome E31.22
Sirenomelia (syndrome) Q87.2
Siriasis T67.01
Sirkari's disease B55.0
Siti A65
Situation, psychiatric F99
Situational
  disturbance (transient) —*see* Disorder,
    adjustment
    acute F43.0

Situational *(Continued)*
  maladjustment —*see* Disorder, adjustment
  reaction —*see* Disorder, adjustment
    acute F43.0
Situs inversus or transversus (abdominalis)
  (thoracis) Q89.3
Sixth disease B08.20
  due to human herpesvirus 6 B08.21
  due to human herpesvirus 7 B08.22
Sjögren-Larsson syndrome Q87.19
⇒Sjögren's syndrome or disease —*see* Syndrome,
  Sjogren
Skeletal —*see* condition
Skene's gland —*see* condition
Skenitis —*see* Urethritis
Skerljevo A65
Skevas-Zerfus disease —*see* Toxicity, venom,
  marine animal, sea anemone
Skin —*see also* condition
  clammy R23.1
  donor —*see* Donor, skin
▶dry L85.3
  hidebound M35.9
Slate-dressers' or slate-miners' lung J62.8
Sleep
  apnea —*see* Apnea, sleep
  deprivation Z72.820
  disorder or disturbance G47.9
    child F51.9
    nonorganic origin F51.9
    specified NEC G47.8
  disturbance G47.9
    nonorganic origin F51.9
  drunkenness F51.9
  rhythm inversion G47.2-●
  terrors F51.4
  walking F51.3
    hysterical F44.89
Sleep hygiene
  abuse Z72.821
  inadequate Z72.821
  poor Z72.821
Sleeping sickness —*see* Sickness, sleeping
Sleeplessness —*see* Insomnia
  menopausal N95.11
Sleep-wake schedule disorder G47.20
Slim disease (in HIV infection) B20
Slipped, slipping
  epiphysis (traumatic) —*see also*
    Osteochondropathy, specified type
    NEC
    capital femoral (traumatic)
      acute (on chronic) S79.01-●
    current traumatic - code as Fracture,
      by site
    upper femoral (nontraumatic) M93.00-●
      acute M93.01-●
        on chronic M93.03-●
      chronic M93.02-●
  intervertebral disc —*see* Displacement,
    intervertebral disc
  ligature, umbilical P51.8
  patella —*see* Disorder, patella, derangement
    NEC
  rib M89.8X8
  sacroiliac joint —*see* subcategory M53.2
  tendon —*see* Disorder, tendon
  ulnar nerve, nontraumatic —*see* Lesion,
    nerve, ulnar
  vertebra NEC —*see* Spondylolisthesis
Slocumb's syndrome E27.0
Sloughing (multiple) (phagedena) (skin) —*see*
  also Gangrene
  abscess —*see* Abscess
  appendix K38.8
  fascia —*see* Disorder, soft tissue, specified
    type NEC
  scrotum N50.89
  tendon —*see* Disorder, tendon
  transplanted organ —*see* Rejection, transplant
  ulcer —*see* Ulcer, skin

Slow
  feeding, newborn P92.2
  flow syndrome, coronary I20.8
  heart(beat) R00.1
Slowing, urinary stream R39.198
Sluder's neuralgia (syndrome) G44.89
Slurred, slurring speech R47.81
Small (ness)
  for gestational age —*see* Small for dates
  introitus, vagina N89.6
  kidney (unknown cause) N27.9
    bilateral N27.1
    unilateral N27.0
  ovary (congenital) Q50.39
  pelvis
    with disproportion (fetopelvic) O33.1
      causing obstructed labor O65.1
  uterus N85.8
  white kidney N03.9
Small-and-light-for-dates —*see* Small for
  dates
Small-for-dates (infant) P05.10
  with weight of
    499 grams or less P05.11
    500-749 grams P05.12
    750-999 grams P05.13
    1000-1249 grams P05.14
    1250-1499 grams P05.15
    1500-1749 grams P05.16
    1750-1999 grams P05.17
    2000-2499 grams P05.18
    2500 grams and over P05.19
  specified NEC P05.19
Smallpox B03
Smearing, fecal R15.1
SMEI (severe myoclonic epilepsy in infancy)
  G40.83-●
Smith-Lemli-Opitz syndrome E78.72
Smith's fracture S52.54-●
Smoker —*see* Dependence, drug, nicotine
Smoker's
  bronchitis J41.0
  cough J41.0
  palate K13.24
  throat J31.2
  tongue K13.24
Smoking
  passive Z77.22
Smothering spells R06.81
Snaggle teeth, tooth M26.39
Snapping
  finger —*see* Trigger finger
  hip —*see* Derangement, joint, specified type
    NEC, hip
    involving the iliotiblial band M76.3-●
  knee —*see* Derangement, knee
    involving the iliotiblial band M76.3-●
Sneddon-Wilkinson disease or syndrome
  (sub-corneal pustular dermatosis)
  L13.1
Sneezing (intractable) R06.7
Sniffing
  cocaine
    abuse —*see* Abuse, drug, cocaine
    dependence —*see* Dependence, drug,
      cocaine
  gasoline
    abuse —*see* Abuse, drug, inhalant
    dependence —*see* Dependence, drug,
      inhalant
  glue (airplane)
    abuse —*see* Abuse, drug, inhalant
    drug dependence —*see* Dependence, drug,
      inhalant
Sniffles
  newborn P28.89
Snoring R06.83
Snow blindness —*see* Photokeratitis
Snuffles (non-syphilitic) R06.5
  newborn P28.89
  syphilitic (infant) A50.05 *[J99]*

Social
  exclusion Z60.4
    due to discrimination or persecution
      (perceived) Z60.5
  ▶migrant Z59.00
    acculturation difficulty Z60.3
  rejection Z60.4
    due to discrimination or persecution Z60.5
  role conflict NEC Z73.5
  skills inadequacy NEC Z73.4
  transplantation Z60.3
Sodoku A25.0
Soemmerring's ring —see Cataract, secondary
Soft —see also condition
  nails L60.3
Softening
  bone —see Osteomalacia
  brain (necrotic) (progressive) G93.89
    congenital Q04.8
    embolic I63.4-●
    hemorrhagic —see Hemorrhage,
      intracranial, intracerebral
    occlusive I63.5-●
    thrombotic I63.3-●
  cartilage M94.2-●
    patella M22.4-●
  cerebellar —see Softening, brain
  cerebral —see Softening, brain
  cerebrospinal —see Softening, brain
  myocardial, heart —see Degeneration,
    myocardial
  spinal cord G95.89
  stomach K31.89
Soldier's
  heart F45.8
  patches I31.0
Solitary
  cyst, kidney N28.1
  kidney, congenital Q60.0
Solvent abuse —see Abuse, drug, inhalant
  dependence —see Dependence, drug,
    inhalant
Somatization reaction, somatic reaction —see
  Disorder, somatoform
Somnambulism F51.3
  hysterical F44.89
Somnolence R40.0
  nonorganic origin F51.11
Sonne dysentery A03.3
Soor B37.0
Sore
  bed —see Ulcer, pressure, by site
  chiclero B55.1
  Delhi B55.1
  desert —see Ulcer, skin
  eye H57.1-●
  Lahore B55.1
  mouth K13.79
    canker K12.0
  muscle M79.10
  Naga —see Ulcer, skin
  of skin —see Ulcer, skin - oriental B55.1
  pressure —see Ulcer, pressure, by site
  skin L98.9
  soft A57
  throat (acute) —see also Pharyngitis
    with influenza, flu, or grippe —see
      Influenza, with, respiratory
      manifestations NEC
    chronic J31.2
    coxsackie (virus) B08.5
    diphtheritic A36.0
    herpesviral B00.2
    influenzal —see Influenza, with, respiratory
      manifestations NEC
    septic J02.0
    streptococcal (ulcerative) J02.0
    viral NEC J02.8
      coxsackie B08.5
  tropical —see Ulcer, skin
  veldt —see Ulcer, skin

Soto's syndrome (cerebral gigantism) Q87.3
South African cardiomyopathy syndrome I42.8
Southeast Asian hemorrhagic fever A91
Spacing
  abnormal, tooth, teeth, fully erupted M26.30
  excessive, tooth, fully erupted M26.32
Spade-like hand (congenital) Q68.1
Spading nail L60.8
  congenital Q84.6
Spanish collar N47.1
Sparganosis B70.1
Spasm(s), spastic, spasticity —see also condition
  R25.2
  accommodation —see Spasm, of
    accommodation
  ampulla of Vater K83.4
  anus, ani (sphincter) (reflex) K59.4
    psychogenic F45.8
  artery I73.9
    cerebral G45.9
  Bell's G51.3-●
  bladder (sphincter, external or internal)
    N32.89
    psychogenic F45.8
  bronchus, bronchiole J98.01
  cardia K22.0
  cardiac I20.1
  carpopedal —see Tetany
  cerebral (arteries) (vascular) G45.9
  cervix, complicating delivery O62.4
  ciliary body (of accommodation) —see Spasm,
    of accommodation
  colon —see also Irritable, bowel K58.9
    with diarrhea K58.0
    psychogenic F45.8
  common duct K83.8
  compulsive —see Tic
  conjugate H51.8
  coronary (artery) I20.1
  diaphragm (reflex) R06.6
    epidemic B33.0
    psychogenic F45.8
  duodenum K59.89
  epidemic diaphragmatic (transient) B33.0
  esophagus (diffuse) K22.4
    psychogenic F45.8
  facial G51.3-●
  fallopian tube N83.8
  gastrointestinal (tract) K31.89
    psychogenic F45.8
  glottis J38.5
    hysterical F44.4
    psychogenic F45.8
      conversion reaction F44.4
    reflex through recurrent laryngeal nerve
      J38.5
  habit —see Tic
  heart I20.1
  hemifacial (clonic) G51.3-●
  hourglass —see Contraction, hourglass
  hysterical F44.4
  infantile —see Epilepsy, spasms
  inferior oblique, eye H51.8
  intestinal —see also Syndrome, irritable bowel
    K58.9
    psychogenic F45.8
  larynx, laryngeal J38.5
    hysterical F44.4
    psychogenic F45.8
      conversion reaction F44.4
  levator palpebrae superioris —see Disorder,
    eyelid function
  muscle NEC M62.838
    back M62.830
  nerve, trigeminal G51.0
  nervous F45.8
  nodding F98.4
  occupational F48.8
  oculogyric H51.8
    psychogenic F45.8
  of accommodation H52.53-●

Spasm(s), spastic, spasticity (Continued)
  ophthalmic artery —see Occlusion, artery,
    retina
  perineal, female N94.89
  peroneo-extensor —see also Deformity, limb,
    flat foot
  pharynx (reflex) J39.2
    hysterical F45.8
    psychogenic F45.8
  psychogenic F45.8
  pylorus NEC K31.3
    adult hypertrophic K31.89
    congenital or infantile Q40.0
    psychogenic F45.8
  rectum (sphincter) K59.4
    psychogenic F45.8
  retinal (artery) —see Occlusion, artery, retina
  sigmoid —see also Syndrome, irritable bowel
    K58.9
    psychogenic F45.8
  sphincter of Oddi K83.4
  stomach K31.89
    neurotic F45.8
  throat J39.2
    hysterical F45.8
    psychogenic F45.8
  tic F95.9
    chronic F95.1
    transient of childhood F95.0
  tongue K14.8
  torsion (progressive) G24.1
  trigeminal nerve —see Neuralgia, trigeminal
  ureter N13.5
  urethra (sphincter) N35.919
  uterus N85.8
    complicating labor O62.4
  vagina N94.2
    psychogenic F52.5
  vascular I73.9
  vasomotor I73.9
  vein NEC I87.8
  viscera —see Pain, abdominal
Spasmodic —see condition
Spasmophilia —see Tetany
Spasmus nutans F98.4
Spastic, spasticity —see also Spasm
  child (cerebral) (congenital) (paralysis)
    G80.1
Speaker's throat R49.8
Specific, specified —see condition
Speech
  defect, disorder, disturbance, impediment —
    see Disorder, speech R47.9
    psychogenic, in childhood and adolescence
      F98.8
    slurring R47.81
    specified NEC R47.89
Spencer's disease A08.19
Spens' syndrome (syncope with heart block)
  I45.9
Sperm counts (fertility testing) Z31.41
  postvasectomy Z30.8
  reversal Z31.42
Spermatic cord —see condition
Spermatocele N43.40
  congenital Q55.4
  multiple N43.42
  single N43.41
Spermatocystitis N49.0
Spermatocytoma C62.9-●
  specified site —see Neoplasm, malignant, by
    site
Spermatorrhea N50.89
Sphacelus —see Gangrene
Sphenoidal —see condition
Sphenoiditis (chronic) —see Sinusitis,
  sphenoidal
Sphenopalatine ganglion neuralgia
  G90.09
Sphericity, increased, lens (congenital)
  Q12.4

Spherocytosis (congenital) (familial) (hereditary) D58.0
  hemoglobin disease D58.0
  sickle-cell (disease) D57.8-●
Spherophakia Q12.4
Sphincter —*see* condition
Sphincteritis, sphincter of Oddi —*see* Cholangitis
Sphingolipidosis E75.3
  specified NEC E75.29
Sphingomyelinosis E75.3
Spicule tooth K00.2
Spider
  bite —*see* Toxicity, venom, spider
    nonvenomous —*see* Bite, by site, superficial, insect
  fingers —*see* Syndrome, Marfan's
  nevus I78.1
  toes —*see* Syndrome, Marfan's
  vascular I78.1
Spiegler-Fendt
  benign lymphocytoma L98.8
  sarcoid L08.89
Spielmeyer-Vogt disease E75.4
Spina bifida (aperta) Q05.9
  with hydrocephalus NEC Q05.4
  cervical Q05.5
    with hydrocephalus Q05.0
  dorsal Q05.6
    with hydrocephalus Q05.1
  lumbar Q05.7
    with hydrocephalus Q05.2
  lumbosacral Q05.7
    with hydrocephalus Q05.2
  occulta Q76.0
  sacral Q05.8
    with hydrocephalus Q05.3
  thoracic Q05.6
    with hydrocephalus Q05.1
  thoracolumbar Q05.6
    with hydrocephalus Q05.1
Spindle, Krukenberg's —*see* Pigmentation, cornea, posterior
Spine, spinal —*see* condition
Spiradenoma (eccrine) —*see* Neoplasm, skin, benign
Spirillosis A25.0
Spirillum
  minus A25.0
  obermeieri infection A68.0
Spirochetal —*see* condition
Spirochetosis A69.9
  arthritic, arthritica A69.9
  bronchopulmonary A69.8
  icterohemorrhagic A27.0
  lung A69.8
Spirometrosis B70.1
Spitting blood —*see* Hemoptysis
Splanchnoptosis K63.4
Spleen, splenic —*see* condition
Splenectasis —*see* Splenomegaly
Splenitis (interstitial) (malignant) (nonspecific) D73.89
  malarial —*see also* Malaria B54 [D77]
  tuberculous A18.85
Splenocele D73.89
Splenomegaly, splenomegalia (Bengal) (cryptogenic) (idiopathic) (tropical) R16.1
  with hepatomegaly R16.2
  cirrhotic D73.2
  congenital Q89.09
  congestive, chronic D73.2
  Egyptian B65.1
  Gaucher's E75.22
  malarial —*see also* Malaria B54 [D77]
  neutropenic D73.81
  Niemann-Pick —*see* Niemann-Pick disease or syndrome
  siderotic D73.2
  syphilitic A52.79
    congenital (early) A50.08 [D77]

Splenopathy D73.9
Splenoptosis D73.89
Splenosis D73.89
Splinter —*see* Foreign body, superficial, by site
Split, splitting
  foot Q72.7-●
  hand Q71.6
  heart sounds R01.2
  lip, congenital —*see* Cleft, lip
  nails L60.3
  urinary stream R39.13
Spondylarthrosis —*see* Spondylosis
Spondylitis (chronic) —*see also* Spondylopathy, inflammatory
  ankylopoietica —*see* Spondylitis, ankylosing
  ankylosing (chronic) M45.9
    with lung involvement M45.9 [J99]
    cervical region M45.2
    cervicothoracic region M45.3
    juvenile M08.1
    lumbar region M45.6
    lumbosacral region M45.7
    multiple sites M45.0
    occipito-atlanto-axial region M45.1
    sacrococcygeal region M45.8
    thoracic region M45.4
    thoracolumbar region M45.5
  atrophic (ligamentous) —*see* Spondylitis, ankylosing
  deformans (chronic) —*see* Spondylosis
  gonococcal A54.41
  gouty —*see also* Gout, by type, vertebrae M10.08
  in (due to)
    brucellosis A23.9 [M49.80]
      cervical region A23.9 [M49.82]
      cervicothoracic region A23.9 [M49.83]
      lumbar region A23.9 [M49.86]
      lumbosacral region A23.9 [M49.87]
      multiple sites A23.9 [M49.89]
      occipito-atlanto-axial region A23.9 [M49.81]
      sacrococcygeal region A23.9 [M49.88]
      thoracic region A23.9 [M49.84]
      thoracolumbar region A23.9 [M49.85]
    enterobacteria —*see also* subcategory M49.8 A04.9
    tuberculosis A18.01
  infectious NEC —*see* Spondylopathy, infective
  juvenile ankylosing (chronic) M08.1
  Kümmell's —*see* Spondylopathy, traumatic
  Marie-Strümpell —*see* Spondylitis, ankylosing
  muscularis —*see* Spondylopathy, specified NEC
  psoriatic L40.53
  rheumatoid —*see* Spondylitis, ankylosing
  rhizomelica —*see* Spondylitis, ankylosing
  sacroiliac NEC M46.1
  senescent, senile —*see* Spondylosis
  traumatic (chronic) or post-traumatic —*see* Spondylopathy, traumatic
  tuberculous A18.01
  typhosa A01.05
Spondyloarthritis
  axial —*see also* Spondlyitis, ankylosing
  ⇛non-radiographic M45.A0
    ⇛cervical M45.A2
    ⇛cervicothoracic M45.A3
    ⇛lumbar M45.A6
    ⇛lumbosacral M45.A7
    ⇛multiple sites M45.AB
    ⇛occipito-atlanto-axial region M45.A1
    ⇛sacral and sacrococcygeal M45.A8
    ⇛thoracic M45.A4
    ⇛thoracolumbar M45.A5
Spondylolisthesis (acquired) (degenerative) M43.10
  with disproportion (fetopelvic) O33.0
    causing obstructed labor O65.0

Spondylolisthesis (*Continued*)
  cervical region M43.12
  cervicothoracic region M43.13
  congenital Q76.2
  lumbar region M43.16
  lumbosacral region M43.17
  multiple sites M43.19
  occipito-atlanto-axial region M43.11
  sacrococcygeal region M43.18
  thoracic region M43.14
  thoracolumbar region M43.15
  traumatic (old) M43.10
    acute
      fifth cervical (displaced) S12.430
        nondisplaced S12.431
        specified type NEC (displaced) S12.450
          nondisplaced S12.451
        type III S12.44
      fourth cervical (displaced) S12.330
        nondisplaced S12.331
        specified type NEC (displaced) S12.350
          nondisplaced S12.351
        type III S12.34
      second cervical (displaced) S12.130
        nondisplaced S12.131
        specified type NEC (displaced) S12.150
          nondisplaced S12.151
        type III S12.14
      seventh cervical (displaced) S12.630
        nondisplaced S12.631
        specified type NEC (displaced) S12.650
          nondisplaced S12.651
        type III S12.64
      sixth cervical (displaced) S12.530
        nondisplaced S12.531
        specified type NEC (displaced) S12.550
          nondisplaced S12.551
        type III S12.54
      third cervical (displaced) S12.230
        nondisplaced S12.231
        specified type NEC (displaced) S12.250
          nondisplaced S12.251
        type III S12.24
Spondylolysis (acquired) M43.00
  cervical region M43.02
  cervicothoracic region M43.03
  congenital Q76.2
  lumbar region M43.06
  lumbosacral region M43.07
    with disproportion (fetopelvic) O33.0
      causing obstructed labor O65.8
  multiple sites M43.09
  occipito-atlanto-axial region M43.01
  sacrococcygeal region M43.08
  thoracic region M43.04
  thoracolumbar region M43.05
Spondylopathy M48.9
  infective NEC M46.50
    cervical region M46.52
    cervicothoracic region M46.53
    lumbar region M46.56
    lumbosacral region M46.57
    multiple sites M46.59
    occipito-atlanto-axial region M46.51
    sacrococcygeal region M46.58
    thoracic region M46.54
    thoracolumbar region M46.55
  inflammatory M46.90
    cervical region M46.92
    cervicothoracic region M46.93
    lumbar region M46.96
    lumbosacral region M46.97
    multiple sites M46.99
    occipito-atlanto-axial region M46.91
    sacrococcygeal region M46.98

Spondylopathy *(Continued)*
  inflammatory *(Continued)*
    specified type NEC M46.80
      cervical region M46.82
      cervicothoracic region M46.83
      lumbar region M46.86
      lumbosacral region M46.87
      multiple sites M46.89
      occipito-atlanto-axial region M46.81
      sacrococcygeal region M46.88
      thoracic region M46.84
      thoracolumbar region M46.85
    thoracic region M46.94
    thoracolumbar region M46.95
  neuropathic, in
    syringomyelia and syringobulbia G95.0
    tabes dorsalis A52.11
  specified NEC —*see* subcategory M48.8
  traumatic M48.30
    cervical region M48.32
    cervicothoracic region M48.33
    lumbar region M48.36
    lumbosacral region M48.37
    occipito-atlanto-axial region M48.31
    sacrococcygeal region M48.38
    thoracic region M48.34
    thoracolumbar region M48.35
Spondylosis M47.9
  with
    disproportion (fetopelvic) O33.0
      causing obstructed labor O65.0
    myelopathy NEC M47.10
      cervical region M47.12
      cervicothoracic region M47.13
      lumbar region M47.16
      occipito-atlanto-axial region M47.11
      thoracic region M47.14
      thoracolumbar region M47.15
    radiculopathy M47.20
      cervical region M47.22
      cervicothoracic region M47.23
      lumbar region M47.26
      lumbosacral region M47.27
      occipito-atlanto-axial region M47.21
      sacrococcygeal region M47.28
      thoracic region M47.24
      thoracolumbar region M47.25
  without myelopathy or radiculopathy
    M47.819
    cervical region M47.812
    cervicothoracic region M47.813
    lumbar region M47.816
    lumbosacral region M47.817
    occipito-atlanto-axial region M47.811
    sacrococcygeal region M47.818
    thoracic region M47.814
    thoracolumbar region M47.815
  specified NEC M47.899
    cervical region M47.892
    cervicothoracic region M47.893
  ▶facet joint (*see also* Spondylosis) M47.819
    lumbar region M47.896
    lumbosacral region M47.897
    occipito-atlanto-axial region M47.891
    sacrococcygeal region M47.898
    thoracic region M47.894
    thoracolumbar region M47.895
  traumatic —*see* Spondylopathy, traumatic
Sponge
  inadvertently left in operation wound —*see*
    Foreign body, accidentally left during a
    procedure
  kidney (medullary) Q61.5
Sponge-diver's disease —*see* Toxicity, venom,
  marine animal, sea anemone
Spongioblastoma (any type) —*see* Neoplasm,
  malignant, by site
  specified site —*see* Neoplasm, malignant, by
    site
  unspecified site C71.9
Spongioneuroblastoma —*see* Neoplasm,
  malignant, by site

Spontaneous —*see also* condition
  fracture (cause unknown) —*see* Fracture,
    pathological
Spoon nail L60.3
  congenital Q84.6
Sporadic —*see* condition
Sporothrix schenckii infection —*see*
  Sporotrichosis
Sporotrichosis B42.9
  arthritis B42.82
  disseminated B42.7
  generalized B42.7
  lymphocutaneous (fixed) (progressive)
    B42.1
  pulmonary B42.0
  specified NEC B42.89
Spots, spotting (in) (of)
  Bitot's —*see also* Pigmentation, conjunctiva
    in the young child E50.1
    vitamin A deficiency E50.1
  café, au lait L81.3
  Cayenne pepper I78.1
  cotton wool, retina —*see* Occlusion, artery,
    retina
  de Morgan's (senile angiomas) I78.1
  Fuchs' black (myopic) —*see also* Myopia,
    degenerative H44.2-●
  intermenstrual (regular) N92.0
    irregular N92.1
  Koplik's B05.9
  liver L81.4
  pregnancy O26.85-●
  purpuric R23.3
  ruby I78.1
Spotted fever —*see* Fever, spotted A77.9
Sprain (joint) (ligament)
  acromioclavicular joint or ligament S43.5-●
  ankle S93.40-●
    calcaneofibular ligament S93.41-●
    deltoid ligament S93.42-●
    internal collateral ligament —*see* Sprain,
      ankle, specified ligament NEC
    specified ligament NEC S93.49-●
    talofibular ligament —*see* Sprain, ankle,
      specified ligament NEC
    tibiofibular ligament S93.43-●
  anterior longitudinal, cervical S13.4
  atlas, atlanto-axial, atlanto-occipital S13.4
  breast bone —*see* Sprain, sternum
  calcaneofibular —*see* Sprain, ankle
  carpal —*see* Sprain, wrist
  carpometacarpal —*see* Sprain, hand, specified
    site NEC
  cartilage
    costal S23.41
    semilunar (knee) —*see* Sprain, knee,
      specified site NEC
      with current tear —*see* Tear, meniscus
    thyroid region S13.5
    xiphoid —*see* Sprain, sternum
  cervical, cervicodorsal, cervicothoracic S13.4
  chondrosternal S23.421
  coracoclavicular S43.8-●
  coracohumeral S43.41-●
  coronary, knee —*see* Sprain, knee, specified
    site NEC
  costal cartilage S23.41
  cricoarytenoid articulation or ligament S13.5
  cricothyroid articulation S13.5
  cruciate, knee —*see* Sprain, knee, cruciate
  deltoid, ankle —*see* Sprain, ankle
  dorsal (spine) S23.3
  elbow S53.40-●
    radial collateral ligament S53.43-●
    radiohumeral S53.41-●
    rupture
      radial collateral ligament —*see* Rupture,
        traumatic, ligament, radial
        collateral
      ulnar collateral ligament —*see* Rupture,
        traumatic, ligament, ulnar collateral

Sprain *(Continued)*
  elbow *(Continued)*
    specified type NEC S53.49-●
    ulnar collateral ligament S53.44-●
    ulnohumeral S53.42-●
  femur, head —*see* Sprain, hip
  fibular collateral, knee —*see* Sprain, knee,
    collateral
  fibulocalcaneal —*see* Sprain, ankle
  finger(s) S63.61-●
    index S63.61-●
    interphalangeal (joint) S63.63-●
      index S63.63-●
      little S63.63-●
      middle S63.63-●
      ring S63.63-●
    little S63.61-●
    metacarpophalangeal (joint) S63.65-●
    middle S63.61-●
    ring S63.61-●
    specified site NEC S63.69-●
      index S63.69-●
      little S63.69-●
      middle S63.69-●
      ring S63.69-●
  foot S93.60-●
    specified ligament NEC S93.69-●
    tarsal ligament S93.61-●
    tarsometatarsal ligament S93.62-●
    toe —*see* Sprain, toe
  hand S63.9-●
    finger —*see* Sprain, finger
    specified site NEC —*see* subcategory
      S63.8
    thumb —*see* Sprain, thumb
  head S03.9
  hip S73.10-●
    iliofemoral ligament S73.11-●
    ischiocapsular (ligament) S73.12-●
    specified NEC S73.19-●
  iliofemoral —*see* Sprain, hip
  innominate
    acetabulum —*see* Sprain, hip
    sacral junction S33.6
  internal
    collateral, ankle —*see* Sprain, ankle
    semilunar cartilage —*see* Sprain, knee,
      specified site NEC
  interphalangeal
    finger —*see* Sprain, finger, interphalangeal
      (joint)
    toe —*see* Sprain, toe, interphalangeal joint
  ischiocapsular —*see* Sprain, hip
  ischiofemoral —*see* Sprain, hip
  jaw (articular disc) (cartilage) (meniscus)
    S03.4-●
    old M26.69
  knee S83.9-●
    collateral ligament S83.40-●
      lateral (fibular) S83.42-●
      medial (tibial) S83.41-●
    cruciate ligament S83.50-●
      anterior S83.51-●
      posterior S83.52-●
    lateral (fibular) collateral ligament S83.42-●
    medial (tibial) collateral ligament S83.41-●
    patellar ligament S76.11-●
    specified site NEC S83.8X-●
    superior tibiofibular joint (ligament)
      S83.6-●
  lateral collateral, knee —*see* Sprain, knee,
    collateral
  lumbar (spine) S33.5
  lumbosacral S33.9
  mandible (articular disc) S03.4-●
    old M26.69
  medial collateral, knee —*see* Sprain, knee,
    collateral
  meniscus
    jaw S03.4-●
      old M26.69

Sprain (Continued)

meniscus (Continued)

knee —see Sprain, knee, specified site NEC
with current tear —see Tear, meniscus
old —see Derangement, knee,
meniscus, due to old tear
mandible S03.4-●
old M26.69
metacarpal (distal) (proximal) —see Sprain,
hand, specified site NEC
metacarpophalangeal —see Sprain, finger,
metacarpophalangeal (joint)
metatarsophalangeal —see Sprain, toe,
metatarsophalangeal joint
midcarpal —see Sprain, hand, specified site
NEC
midtarsal —see Sprain, foot, specified site
NEC
neck S13.9
anterior longitudinal cervical ligament
S13.4
atlanto-axial joint S13.4
atlanto-occipital joint S13.4
cervical spine S13.4
cricoarytenoid ligament S13.5
cricothyroid ligament S13.5
specified site NEC S13.8
thyroid region (cartilage) S13.5
nose S03.8
orbicular, hip —see Sprain, hip
patella —see Sprain, knee, specified site
NEC
patellar ligament S76.11-●
pelvis NEC S33.8
phalanx
finger —see Sprain, finger
toe —see Sprain, toe
pubofemoral —see Sprain, hip
radiocarpal —see Sprain, wrist
radiohumeral —see Sprain, elbow
radius, collateral —see Rupture, traumatic,
ligament, radial collateral
rib (cage) S23.41
rotator cuff (capsule) S43.42-●
sacroiliac (region)
chronic or old —see subcategory M53.2
joint S33.6
scaphoid (hand) —see Sprain, hand, specified
site NEC
scapula (r) —see Sprain, shoulder girdle,
specified site NEC
semilunar cartilage (knee) —see Sprain, knee,
specified site NEC
with current tear —see Tear, meniscus
old —see Derangement, knee, meniscus,
due to old tear
shoulder joint S43.40-●
acromioclavicular joint (ligament) —see
Sprain, acromioclavicular joint
blade —see Sprain, shoulder, girdle,
specified site NEC
coracoclavicular joint (ligament) —see
Sprain, coracoclavicular joint
coracohumeral ligament —see Sprain,
coracohumeral joint
girdle S43.9-●
specified site NEC S43.8-●
rotator cuff —see Sprain, rotator cuff
specified site NEC S43.49-●
sternoclavicular joint (ligament) —see
Sprain, sternoclavicular joint
spine
cervical S13.4
lumbar S33.5
thoracic S23.3
sternoclavicular joint S43.6-●
sternum S23.429
chondrosternal joint S23.421
specified site NEC S23.428
sternoclavicular (joint) (ligament)
S23.420

Sprain (Continued)

symphysis
jaw S03.4-●
old M26.69
mandibular S03.4-●
old M26.69
talofibular —see Sprain, ankle
tarsal —see Sprain, foot, specified site NEC
tarsometatarsal —see Sprain, foot, specified
site NEC
temporomandibular S03.4-●
old M26.69
thorax S23.9
ribs S23.41
specified site NEC S23.8
spine S23.3
sternum —see Sprain, sternum
thumb S63.60-●
interphalangeal (joint) S63.62-●
metacarpophalangeal (joint) S63.64-●
specified site NEC S63.68-●
thyroid cartilage or region S13.5
tibia (proximal end) —see Sprain, knee,
specified site NEC
tibial collateral, knee —see Sprain, knee,
collateral
tibiofibular
distal —see Sprain, ankle
superior —see Sprain, knee, specified site
NEC
toe(s) S93.50-●
great S93.50-●
interphalangeal joint S93.51-●
great S93.51-●
lesser S93.51-●
lesser S93.50-●
metatarsophalangeal joint S93.52-●
great S93.52-●
lesser S93.52-●
ulna, collateral —see Rupture, traumatic,
ligament, ulnar collateral
ulnohumeral —see Sprain, elbow
wrist S63.50-●
carpal S63.51-●
radiocarpal S63.52-●
specified site NEC S63.59-●
xiphoid cartilage —see Sprain, sternum
Sprengel's deformity (congenital) Q74.0
Sprue (tropical) K90.1
celiac K90.0
idiopathic K90.49
meaning thrush B37.0
nontropical K90.0
Spur, bone —see also Enthesopathy
calcaneal M77.3-●
iliac crest M76.2-●
nose (septum) J34.89
Spurway's syndrome Q78.0
Sputum
abnormal (amount) (color) (odor) (purulent)
R09.3
blood-stained R04.2
excessive (cause unknown) R09.3
Squamous —see also condition
epithelium in
cervical canal (congenital) Q51.828
uterine mucosa (congenital) Q51.818
Squashed nose M95.0
congenital Q67.4
Squeeze, diver's T70.3
Squint —see also Strabismus
accommodative —see Strabismus, convergent
concomitant
SSADHD (succinic semialdehyde
dehydrogenase deficiency) E72.81
St. Hubert's disease A82.9
Stab —see also Laceration
internal organs —see Injury, by site
Stafne's cyst or cavity M27.0
Staggering gait R26.0
hysterical F44.4

Staghorn calculus —see Calculus, kidney
Stähli's line (cornea) (pigment) —see
Pigmentation, cornea, anterior
Stain, staining
meconium (newborn) P96.83
port wine Q82.5
tooth, teeth (hard tissues) (extrinsic) K03.6
due to
accretions K03.6
deposits (betel) (black) (green) (materia
alba) (orange) (soft) (tobacco) K03.6
metals (copper) (silver) K03.7
nicotine K03.6
pulpal bleeding K03.7
tobacco K03.6
intrinsic K00.8
Stammering —see also Disorder, fluency
F80.81
Standstill
auricular I45.5
cardiac —see Arrest, cardiac
sinoatrial I45.5
ventricular —see Arrest, cardiac
Stannosis J63.5
Stanton's disease —see Melioidosis
Staphylitis (acute) (catarrhal) (chronic)
(gangrenous) (membranous) (suppurative)
(ulcerative) K12.2
Staphylococcal scalded skin syndrome L00
Staphylococcemia A41.2
Staphylococcus, staphylococcal —see also
condition
as cause of disease classified elsewhere
B95.8
aureus (methicillin susceptible) (MSSA)
B95.61
methicillin resistant (MRSA) B95.62
specified NEC, as cause of disease classified
elsewhere B95.7
Staphyloma (sclera)
cornea H18.72-●
equatorial H15.81-●
localized (anterior) H15.82-●
posticum H15.83-●
ring H15.85-●
Stargardt's disease —see Dystrophy, retina
Starvation (inanition) (due to lack of food)
T73.0
edema —see Malnutrition, severe
Stasis
bile (noncalculous) K83.1
bronchus J98.09
with infection —see Bronchitis
cardiac —see Failure, heart, congestive
cecum K59.89
colon K59.89
dermatitis I87.2
with
varicose ulcer —see Varix, leg, with ulcer,
with inflammation
varicose veins —see Varix, leg, with,
inflammation
due to postthrombotic syndrome —see
Syndrome, postthrombotic
duodenal K31.5
eczema —see Varix, leg, with, inflammation
edema —see Hypertension, venous (chronic),
idiopathic
foot T69.0-●
ileocecal coil K59.89
ileum K59.89
intestinal K59.89
jejunum K59.89
kidney N19
liver (cirrhotic) K76.1
lymphatic I89.8
pneumonia J18.2
pulmonary —see Edema, lung
rectal K59.89
renal N19
tubular N17.0

Stasis (Continued)

ulcer —see Varix, leg, with, ulcer
  without varicose veins I87.2
urine —see Retention, urine
venous I87.8

State (of)

affective and paranoid, mixed, organic
  psychotic F06.8
agitated R45.1
  acute reaction to stress F43.0
anxiety (neurotic) F41.1
apprehension F41.1
burn-out Z73.0
climacteric, female Z78.0
  symptomatic N95.1
compulsive F42.8
  mixed with obsessional thoughts F42.2
confusional (psychogenic) F44.89
  acute —see also Delirium
    with
      arteriosclerotic dementia F01.50
        with behavioral disturbance F01.51
      senility or dementia F05
     alcoholic F10.231
    epileptic F05
    reactive (from emotional stress,
     psychological trauma) F44.89
    subacute —see Delirium
convulsive —see Convulsions
crisis F43.0
depressive F32.A
  neurotic F34.1
dissociative F44.9
emotional shock (stress) R45.7
hypercoagulation —see Hypercoagulable
locked-in G83.5
menopausal Z78.0
  symptomatic N95.1
neurotic F48.9
  with depersonalization F48.1
obsessional F42.8
oneiroid (schizophrenia-like) F23
organic
  hallucinatory (nonalcoholic) F06.0
  paranoid (-hallucinatory) F06.2
panic F41.0
paranoid F22
  climacteric F22
  involutional F22
  menopausal F22
  organic F06.2
  senile F03
  simple F22
persistent vegetative R40.3
phobic F40.9
postleukotomy F07.0
pregnant
  gestational carrier Z33.3
  incidental Z33.1
psychogenic, twilight F44.89
psychopathic (constitutional) F60.2
psychotic, organic —see also Psychosis,
  organic
  mixed paranoid and affective F06.8
  senile or presenile F03
  transient NEC F06.8
    with
     depression F06.31
     hallucinations F06.0
residual schizophrenic F20.5
restlessness R45.1
stress (emotional) R45.7
tension (mental) F48.9
  specified NEC F48.8
transient organic psychotic NEC F06.8
  depressive type F06.31
  hallucinatory type F06.0
twilight
  epileptic F05
  psychogenic F44.89
vegetative, persistent R40.3

State (Continued)

vital exhaustion Z73.0
withdrawal —see Withdrawal, state

Status (post) —see also Presence (of)

absence, epileptic —see Epilepsy, by type,
  with status epilepticus
administration of tPA (rtPA) in a different
  facility within the last 24 hours prior to
  admission to the current facility
  Z92.82
adrenalectomy (unilateral) (bilateral)
  E89.6
anastomosis Z98.0
anginosus I20.9
angioplasty (peripheral) Z98.62
  with implant Z95.820
  coronary artery Z98.61
    with implant Z95.5
aortocoronary bypass Z95.1
arthrodesis Z98.1
artificial opening (of) Z93.9
  gastrointestinal tract Z93.4
  specified NEC Z93.8
  urinary tract Z93.6
  vagina Z93.8
asthmaticus —see Asthma, by type, with
  status asthmaticus
awaiting organ transplant Z76.82
bariatric surgery Z98.84
bed confinement Z74.01
bleb, filtering (vitreous), after glaucoma
  surgery Z98.83
breast implant Z98.82
  removal Z98.86
cataract extraction Z98.4-●
cholecystectomy Z90.49
clitorectomy N90.811
  with excision of labia minora N90.812
colectomy (complete) (partial) Z90.49
colonization —see Carrier (suspected) of
colostomy Z93.3
convulsivus idiopathicus —see Epilepsy, by
  type, with status epilepticus
coronary artery angioplasty —see Status,
  angioplasty, coronary artery
coronary artery bypass graft Z95.1
cystectomy (urinary bladder) Z90.6
cystostomy Z93.50
  appendico-vesicostomy Z93.52
  cutaneous Z93.51
  specified NEC Z93.59
delinquent immunization Z28.3
dental Z98.818
  crown Z98.811
  fillings Z98.811
  restoration Z98.811
  sealant Z98.810
  specified NEC Z98.818
deployment (current) (military) Z56.82
dialysis (hemodialysis) (peritoneal) Z99.2
do not resuscitate (DNR) Z66
donor —see Donor
embedded fragments —see Retained, foreign
  body fragments (type of)
embedded splinter —see Retained, foreign
  body fragments (type of)
enterostomy Z93.4
epileptic, epilepticus —see also Epilepsy, by
  type, with status epilepticus G40.901
estrogen receptor
  negative Z17.1
  positive Z17.0
female genital cutting —see Female genital
  mutilation status
female genital mutilation —see Female genital
  mutilation status
filtering (vitreous) bleb after glaucoma
  surgery Z98.83
gastrectomy (complete) (partial) Z90.3
gastric banding Z98.84
gastric bypass for obesity Z98.84

Status (Continued)

gastrostomy Z93.1
human immunodeficiency virus (HIV)
  infection, asymptomatic Z21
hysterectomy (complete) (total) Z90.710
  partial (with remaining cervial stump)
    Z90.711
ileostomy Z93.2
implant
  breast Z98.82
infibulation N90.813
intestinal bypass Z98.0
jejunostomy Z93.4
lapsed immunization schedule Z28.3
laryngectomy Z90.02
lymphaticus E32.8
malignancy
  castrate resistant prostate Z19.2
  hormone resistant Z19.2
  hormone sensitive Z19.1
marmoratus G80.3
mastectomy (unilateral) (bilateral) Z90.1-●
military deployment status (current) Z56.82
  in theater or in support of military war,
    peacekeeping and humanitarian
    operations Z56.82
nephrectomy (unilateral) (bilateral) Z90.5
nephrostomy Z93.6
obesity surgery Z98.84
oophorectomy
  bilateral Z90.722
  unilateral Z90.721
organ replacement
  by artificial or mechanical device or
    prosthesis of
    artery Z95.828
    bladder Z96.0
    blood vessel Z95.828
    breast Z97.8
    eye globe Z97.0
    heart Z95.812
     valve Z95.2
    intestine Z97.8
    joint Z96.60
     hip —see Presence, hip joint implant
     knee —see Presence, knee joint
      implant
     specified site NEC Z96.698
    kidney Z97.8
    larynx Z96.3
    lens Z96.1
    limbs —see Presence, artificial, limb
    liver Z97.8
    lung Z97.8
    pancreas Z97.8
  by organ transplant (heterologous)
    (homologous) —see Transplant
pacemaker
  brain Z96.89
  cardiac Z95.0
  specified NEC Z96.89
pancreatectomy Z90.410
  complete Z90.410
  partial Z90.411
  total Z90.410
pneumonectomy (complete) (partial) Z90.2
pneumothorax, therapeutic Z98.3
postcommotio cerebri F07.81
postoperative (postprocedural) NEC
  Z98.890
  breast implant Z98.82
  dental Z98.818
    crown Z98.811
    fillings Z98.811
    restoration Z98.811
    sealant Z98.810
    specified NEC Z98.818
  pneumothorax, therapeutic Z98.3
  uterine scar Z98.891
postpartum (routine follow-up) Z39.2
  care immediately after delivery Z39.0

Status *(Continued)*
  postsurgical (postprocedural) NEC
    Z98.890
    pneumothorax, therapeutic Z98.3
  pregnancy, incidental Z33.1
  prosthesis coronary angioplasty Z95.5
  pseudophakia Z96.1
  renal dialysis (hemodialysis) (peritoneal) Z99.2
  retained foreign body —*see* Retained, foreign
    body fragments (type of)
  reversed jejunal transposition (for bypass
    Z98.0
  salpingo-oophorectomy
    bilateral Z90.722
    unilateral Z90.721
  sex reassignment surgery status Z87.890
  shunt
    arteriovenous (for dialysis) Z99.2
    cerebrospinal fluid Z98.2
    ventricular (communicating) (for drainage)
      Z98.2
  splenectomy Z90.81
  thymicolymphaticus E32.8
  thymicus E32.8
  thymolymphaticus E32.8
  thyroidectomy (hypothyroidism) E89.0
  tooth (teeth) extraction —*see also* Absence,
    teeth, acquired K08.409
  tPA (rtPA) administration in a different
    facility within the last 24 hours prior to
    admission to current facility Z92.82
  tracheostomy Z93.0
  transplant —*see* Transplant
    organ removed Z98.85
  tubal ligation Z98.51
  underimmunization Z28.3
  ureterostomy Z93.6
  urethrostomy Z93.6
  vagina, artificial Z93.8
  vasectomy Z98.52
  wheelchair confinement Z99.3
Stealing
  child problem F91.8
    in company with others Z72.810
  pathological (compulsive) F63.2
Steam burn —*see* Burn
Steatocystoma multiplex L72.2
Steatohepatitis (nonalcoholic) (NASH) K75.81
Steatoma L72.3
  eyelid (cystic) —*see* Dermatosis, eyelid
    infected —*see* Hordeolum
Steatorrhea (chronic) K90.9
  with lacteal obstruction K90.2
  idiopathic (adult) (infantile) K90.9
  pancreatic K90.3
  primary K90.0
  tropical K90.1
Steatosis E88.89
  heart —*see* Degeneration, myocardial
  kidney N28.89
  liver NEC K76.0
Steele-Richardson-Olszewski disease or
  syndrome G23.1
Steinbrocker's syndrome G90.8
Steinert's disease G71.11
Stein-Leventhal syndrome E28.2
Stein's syndrome E28.2
STEMI —*see also* Infarct, myocardium, ST
  elevation I21.3
Stenocardia I20.8
Stenocephaly Q75.8
Stenosis, stenotic (cicatricial) —*see also*
  Stricture
  ampulla of Vater K83.1
  anus, anal (canal) (sphincter) K62.4
    and rectum K62.4
    congenital Q42.3
      with fistula Q42.2
  aorta (ascending) (supraventricular)
    (congenital) Q25.1
    arteriosclerotic I70.0

Stenosis, stenotic *(Continued)*
  aorta *(Continued)*
    calcified I70.0
    supravalvular Q25.3
  aortic (valve) I35.0
    with insufficiency I35.2
    congenital Q23.0
    rheumatic I06.0
      with
        incompetency, insufficiency or
          regurgitation I06.2
          with mitral (valve) disease I08.0
            with tricuspid (valve) disease
              I08.3
        mitral (valve) disease I08.0
          with tricuspid (valve) disease
            I08.3
        tricuspid (valve) disease I08.2
          with mitral (valve) disease I08.3
    specified cause NEC I35.0
    syphilitic A52.03
  aqueduct of Sylvius (congenital) Q03.0
    with spina bifida —*see* Spina bifida,
      by site, with hydrocephalus
    acquired G91.1
  artery NEC —*see also* Arteriosclerosis I77.1
    celiac I77.4
    cerebral —*see* Occlusion, artery, cerebral
    extremities —*see* Arteriosclerosis,
      extremities
    precerebral —*see* Occlusion, artery,
      precerebral
    pulmonary (congenital) Q25.6
      acquired I28.8
    renal I70.1
    stent
      coronary T82.855
      peripheral T82.856
  bile duct (common) (hepatic) K83.1
    congenital Q44.3
  bladder-neck (acquired) N32.0
    congenital Q64.31
  brain G93.89
  bronchus J98.09
    congenital Q32.3
    syphilitic A52.72
  cardia (stomach) K22.2
    congenital Q39.3
  cardiovascular —*see* Disease, cardiovascular
  caudal M48.08
  cervix, cervical (canal) N88.2
    congenital Q51.828
    in pregnancy or childbirth —*see*
      Pregnancy, complicated by, abnormal
      cervix
  colon —*see also* Obstruction, intestine
    congenital Q42.9
    specified NEC Q42.8
  colostomy K94.03
  common (bile) duct K83.1
    congenital Q44.3
  coronary (artery) —*see* Disease, heart,
    ischemic, atherosclerotic
  cystic duct —*see* Obstruction, gallbladder
  due to presence of device, implant or
    graft —*see also* Complications, by site
    and type, specified NEC T85.858
    arterial graft NEC T82.858
    breast (implant) T85.858
    catheter T85.858
      dialysis (renal) T82.858
        intraperitoneal T85.858
      infusion NEC T82.858
        spinal (epidural) (subdural)
          T85.850
      urinary (indwelling) T83.85
    fixation, internal (orthopedic) NEC
      T84.85
    gastrointestinal (bile duct) (esophagus)
      T85.858
    genital NEC T83.85

Stenosis, stenotic *(Continued)*
  due to presence of device, implant or graft
    (Continued)
    heart NEC T82.857
    joint prosthesis T84.85
    ocular (corneal graft) (orbital implant)
      NEC T85.858
    orthopedic NEC T84.85
    specified NEC T85.858
    urinary NEC T83.85
    vascular NEC T82.858
    ventricular intracranial shunt
      T85.850
  duodenum K31.5
    congenital Q41.0
  ejaculatory duct NEC N50.89
  endocervical os —*see* Stenosis, cervix
  enterostomy K94.13
  esophagus K22.2
    congenital Q39.3
    syphilitic A52.79
      congenital A50.59 *[K23]*
  eustachian tube —*see* Obstruction, eustachian
    tube
  external ear canal (acquired) H61.30-•
    congenital Q16.1
    due to
      inflammation H61.32-•
      trauma H61.31-•
    postprocedural H95.81-•
    specified cause NEC H61.39-•
  gallbladder —*see* Obstruction, gallbladder
  glottis J38.6
  heart valve (see also Endocarditis) I38
  aortic —*see* Stenosis, aortic
    ▶congenital Q24.8
    mitral —*see* Stenosis, mitral
    pulmonary —*see* Stenosis, pulmonary,
      valve
    tricuspid —*see* Stenosis, tricuspid Q22.4
  hepatic duct K83.1
  hymen N89.6
  hypertrophic subaortic (idiopathic) I42.1
  ileum —*see also* Obstruction, intestine,
    specified NEC K56.699
    congenital Q41.2
  infundibulum cardia Q24.3
  intervertebral foramina —*see also* Lesion,
    biomechanical, specified NEC
    connective tissue M99.79
      abdomen M99.79
      cervical region M99.71
      cervicothoracic M99.71
      head region M99.70
      lumbar region M99.73
      lumbosacral M99.73
      occipitocervical M99.70
      sacral region M99.74
      sacrococcygeal M99.74
      sacroiliac M99.74
      specified NEC M99.79
      thoracic region M99.72
      thoracolumbar M99.72
    disc M99.79
      abdomen M99.79
      cervical region M99.71
      cervicothoracic M99.71
      head region M99.70
      lower extremity M99.76
      lumbar region M99.73
      lumbosacral M99.73
      occipitocervical M99.70
      pelvic M99.75
      rib cage M99.78
      sacral region M99.74
      sacrococcygeal M99.74
      sacroiliac M99.74
      specified NEC M99.79
      thoracic region M99.72
      thoracolumbar M99.72
      upper extremity M99.77

Stenosis, stenotic *(Continued)*
  intervertebral foramina *(Continued)*
    osseous M99.69
      abdomen M99.69
      cervical region M99.61
      cervicothoracic M99.61
      head region M99.60
      lower extremity M99.66
      lumbar region M99.63
      lumbosacral M99.63
      occipitocervical M99.60
      pelvic M99.65
      rib cage M99.68
      sacral region M99.64
      sacrococcygeal M99.64
      sacroiliac M99.64
      specified NEC M99.69
      thoracic region M99.62
      thoracolumbar M99.62
      upper extremity M99.67
    subluxation —*see* Stenosis, intervertebral
      foramina, osseous
  intestine —*see also* Obstruction, intestine
    congenital (small) Q41.9
      large Q42.9
        specified NEC Q42.8
      specified NEC Q41.8
  jejunum —*see also* Obstruction, intestine,
    specified NEC K56.699
    congenital Q41.1
  lacrimal (passage)
    canaliculi H04.54-●
    congenital Q10.5
    duct H04.55-●
    punctum H04.56-●
    sac H04.57-●
  lacrimonasal duct —*see* Stenosis, lacrimal,
    duct
    congenital Q10.5
  larynx J38.6
    congenital NEC Q31.8
      subglottic Q31.1
    syphilitic A52.73
      congenital A50.59 *[J99]*
  mitral (chronic) (inactive) (valve) I05.0
    with
      aortic valve disease I08.0
      incompetency, insufficiency or
        regurgitation I05.2
    active or acute I01.1
      with rheumatic or Sydenham's chorea
        I02.0
    congenital Q23.2
    specified cause, except rheumatic I34.2
    syphilitic A52.03
  myocardium, myocardial —*see also*
    Degeneration, myocardial
    hypertrophic subaortic (idiopathic) I42.1
  nares (anterior) (posterior) J34.89
    congenital Q30.0
  nasal duct —*see also* Stenosis, lacrimal, duct
    congenital Q10.5
  nasolacrimal duct —*see also* Stenosis, lacrimal,
    duct
    congenital Q10.5
  neural canal —*see also* Lesion, biomechanical,
    specified NEC
    connective tissue M99.49
      abdomen M99.49
      cervical region M99.41
      cervicothoracic M99.41
      head region M99.40
      lower extremity M99.46
      lumbar region M99.43
      lumbosacral M99.43
      occipitocervical M99.40
      pelvic M99.45
      rib cage M99.48
      sacral region M99.44
      sacrococcygeal M99.44
      sacroiliac M99.44

Stenosis, stenotic *(Continued)*
  neural canal *(Continued)*
    connective tissue *(Continued)*
      specified NEC M99.49
      thoracic region M99.42
      thoracolumbar M99.42
      upper extremity M99.47
    intervertebral disc M99.59
      abdomen M99.59
      cervical region M99.51
      cervicothoracic M99.51
      head region M99.50
      lower extremity M99.56
      lumbar region M99.53
      lumbosacral M99.53
      occipitocervical M99.50
      pelvic M99.55
      rib cage M99.58
      sacral region M99.54
      sacrococcygeal M99.54
      sacroiliac M99.54
      specified NEC M99.59
      thoracic region M99.52
      thoracolumbar M99.52
      upper extremity M99.57
    osseous M99.39
      abdomen M99.39
      cervical region M99.31
      cervicothoracic M99.31
      head region M99.30
      lower extremity M99.36
      lumbar region M99.33
      lumbosacral M99.33
      occipitocervical M99.30
      pelvic M99.35
      rib cage M99.38
      sacral region M99.34
      sacrococcygeal M99.34
      sacroiliac M99.34
      specified NEC M99.39
      thoracic region M99.32
      thoracolumbar M99.32
      upper extremity M99.37
    subluxation M99.29
      cervical region M99.21
      cervicothoracic M99.21
      head region M99.20
      lower extremity M99.26
      lumbar region M99.23
      lumbosacral M99.23
      occipitocervical M99.20
      pelvic M99.25
      rib cage M99.28
      sacral region M99.24
      sacrococcygeal M99.24
      sacroiliac M99.24
      specified NEC M99.29
      thoracic region M99.22
      thoracolumbar M99.22
      upper extremity M99.27
  organ or site, congenital NEC —*see* Atresia,
    by site
  papilla of Vater K83.1
  pulmonary (artery) (congenital) Q25.6
    with ventricular septal defect,
      transposition of aorta, and
      hypertrophy of right ventricle
      Q21.3
    acquired I28.8
    in tetralogy of Fallot Q21.3
    infundibular Q24.3
    subvalvular Q24.3
    supravalvular Q25.6
    valve I37.0
      with insufficiency I37.2
      congenital Q22.1
      rheumatic I09.89
        with aortic, mitral or tricuspid (valve)
          disease I08.8
    vein, acquired I28.8
    vessel NEC I28.8

Stenosis, stenotic *(Continued)*
  pulmonic (congenital) Q22.1
    infundibular Q24.3
    subvalvular Q24.3
  pylorus (hypertrophic) (acquired) K31.1
    adult K31.1
    congenital Q40.0
    infantile Q40.0
  rectum (sphincter) —*see* Stricture, rectum
  renal artery I70.1
    congenital Q27.1
  salivary duct (any) K11.8
  sphincter of Oddi K83.1
  spinal M48.00
    cervical region M48.02
    cervicothoracic region M48.03
    lumbar region (NOS) (without neurogenic
      claudication) M48.061
      with neurogenic claudication M48.062
    lumbosacral region M48.07
    occipito-atlanto-axial region M48.01
    sacrococcygeal region M48.08
    thoracic region M48.04
    thoracolumbar region M48.05
  stent
    vascular
      end stent
        adjacent to stent —*see* Arteriosclerosis
        within the stent
          coronary T82.855
          peripheral T82.856
      in stent
        coronary vessel T82.855
        peripheral vessel T82.856
  stomach, hourglass K31.2
  subaortic (congenital) Q24.4
    hypertrophic (idiopathic) I42.1
  subglottic J38.6
    congenital Q31.1
    postprocedural J95.5
  trachea J39.8
    congenital Q32.1
    syphilitic A52.73
    tuberculous NEC A15.5
  tracheostomy J95.03
  tricuspid (valve) I07.0
    with
      aortic (valve) disease I08.2
      incompetency, insufficiency or
        regurgitation I07.2
      with aortic (valve) disease I08.2
        with mitral (valve) disease I08.3
      mitral (valve) disease I08.1
        with aortic (valve) disease I08.3
    congenital Q22.4
    nonrheumatic I36.0
      with insufficiency I36.2
  tubal N97.1
  ureter —*see* Atresia, ureter
  ureteropelvic junction, congenital
    Q62.11
  ureterovesical orifice, congenital Q62.12
  urethra (valve) —*see also* Stricture, urethra
    congenital Q64.32
  urinary meatus, congenital Q64.33
  vagina N89.5
    congenital Q52.4
    in pregnancy —*see* Pregnancy, complicated
      by, abnormal vagina
    causing obstructed labor O65.5
  valve (cardiac) (heart) —*see also* Endocarditis
    I38
    congenital Q24.8
      aortic Q23.0
      mitral Q23.2
      pulmonary Q22.1
      tricuspid Q22.4
  vena cava (inferior) (superior) I87.1
    congenital Q26.0
  vesicourethral orifice Q64.31
  vulva N90.5

▶ New   ⇒ Revised   ~~deleted~~ Deleted   ● Use Additional Character(s)

Stent jail T82.897
Stercolith (impaction) K56.41
    appendix K38.1
Stercoraceous, stercoral ulcer K63.3
    anus or rectum K62.6
Stereotypies NEC F98.4
Sterility —see Infertility
Sterilization —see Encounter (for), sterilization
Sternalgia —see Angina
Sternopagus Q89.4
Sternum bifidum Q76.7
Steroid
    effects (adverse) (adrenocortical)
            (iatrogenic)
        cushingoid E24.2
            correct substance properly
                administered —see Table of Drugs
                and Chemicals, by drug, adverse
                effect
            overdose or wrong substance given
                or taken —see Table of Drugs and
                Chemicals, by drug, poisoning
        diabetes —see category E09
            correct substance properly
                administered —see Table of Drugs
                and Chemicals, by drug, adverse
                effect
            overdose or wrong substance given
                or taken —see Table of Drugs and
                Chemicals, by drug, poisoning
        fever R50.2
        insufficiency E27.3
            correct substance properly
                administered —see Table of Drugs
                and Chemicals, by drug, adverse
                effect
            overdose or wrong substance given
                or taken —see Table of Drugs and
                Chemicals, by drug, poisoning
    responder H40.04-●
Stevens-Johnson disease or syndrome L51.1
    toxic epidermal necrolysis overlap L51.3
Stewart-Morel syndrome M85.2
Sticker's disease B08.3
Sticky eye —see Conjunctivitis, acute,
    mucopurulent
Stieda's disease —see Bursitis, tibial collateral
Stiff neck —see Torticollis
Stiff-man syndrome G25.82
Stiffness, joint NEC M25.60-●
    ankle M25.67-●
    ankylosis —see Ankylosis, joint
    contracture —see Contraction, joint
    elbow M25.62-●
    foot M25.67-●
    hand M25.64-●
    hip M25.65-●
    knee M25.66-●
    shoulder M25.61-●
    specified site NEC M25.69
    wrist M25.63-●
Stigmata congenital syphilis A50.59
Stillbirth P95
Still-Felty syndrome —see Felty's syndrome
Still's disease or syndrome (juvenile) M08.20
    adult-onset M06.1
    ankle M08.27-●
    elbow M08.22-●
    foot joint M08.27-●
    hand joint M08.24-●
    hip M08.25-●
    knee M08.26-●
    multiple site M08.29
    shoulder M08.21-●
    specified site NEC M08.2A
    vertebra M08.28
    wrist M08.23-●
Stimulation, ovary E28.1
Sting (venomous) (with allergic or anaphylactic
    shock) —see Table of Drugs and Chemicals,
    by animal or substance, poisoning

Stippled epiphyses Q78.8
Stitch
    abscess T81.41
    burst (in operation wound) —see Disruption,
        wound, operation
Stokes-Adams disease or syndrome
    I45.9
Stokes' disease E05.00
    with thyroid storm E05.01
Stokvis (-Talma) disease D74.8
Stoma malfunction
    colostomy K94.03
    enterostomy K94.13
    gastrostomy K94.23
    ileostomy K94.13
    tracheostomy J95.03
Stomach —see condition
Stomatitis (denture) (ulcerative)
    K12.1
    angular K13.0
        due to dietary or vitamin deficiency
        E53.0
    aphthous K12.0
    bovine B08.61
    candidal B37.0
    catarrhal K12.1
    diphtheritic A36.89
    due to
        dietary deficiency E53.0
        thrush B37.0
        vitamin deficiency
            B group NEC E53.9
            B2 (riboflavin) E53.0
    epidemic B08.8
    epizootic B08.8
    follicular K12.1
    gangrenous A69.0
    Geotrichum B48.3
    herpesviral, herpetic B00.2
    herpetiformis K12.0
    malignant K12.1
    membranous acute K12.1
    monilial B37.0
    mycotic B37.0
    necrotizing ulcerative A69.0
    parasitic B37.0
    septic K12.1
    spirochetal A69.1
    suppurative (acute) K12.2
    ulceromembranous A69.1
    vesicular K12.1
        with exanthem (enteroviral)
            B08.4
        virus disease A93.8
    Vincent's A69.1
Stomatocytosis D58.8
Stomatomycosis B37.0
Stomatorrhagia K13.79
Stone(s) —see also Calculus
    bladder (diverticulum) N21.0
    cystine E72.09
    heart syndrome I50.1
    kidney N20.0
    prostate N42.0
    pulpal (dental) K04.2
    renal N20.0
    salivary gland or duct (any) K11.5
    urethra (impacted) N21.1
    urinary (duct) (impacted) (passage)
        N20.9
        bladder (diverticulum) N21.0
        lower tract N21.9
        specified NEC N21.8
    xanthine E79.8 [N22]
Stonecutter's lung J62.8
Stonemason's asthma, disease, lung or
        pneumoconiosis J62.8
Stoppage
    heart —see Arrest, cardiac
    urine —see Retention, urine
Storm, thyroid —see Thyrotoxicosis

Strabismus (congenital) (nonparalytic)
    H50.9
    concomitant H50.40
        convergent —see Strabismus, convergent
            concomitant
        divergent —see Strabismus, divergent
            concomitant
    convergent concomitant H50.00
        accommodative component H50.43
        alternating H50.05
            with
                A pattern H50.06
                specified nonconcomitances NEC
                    H50.08
                V pattern H50.07
        monocular H50.01-●
            with
                A pattern H50.02-●
                specified nonconcomitances NEC
                    H50.04-●
                V pattern H50.03-●
        intermittent H50.31-●
            alternating H50.32
    cyclotropia H50.41
    divergent concomitant H50.10
        alternating H50.15
            with
                A pattern H50.16
                specified noncomitances NEC
                    H50.18
                V pattern H50.17
        monocular H50.11-●
            with
                A pattern H50.12-●
                specified noncomitances NEC
                    H50.14-●
                V pattern H50.13-●
        intermittent H50.33-●
            alternating H50.34
    Duane's syndrome H50.81-●
    due to adhesions, scars H50.69
    heterophoria H50.50
        alternating H50.55
        cyclophoria H50.54
        esophoria H50.51
        exophoria H50.52
        vertical H50.53
    heterotropia H50.40
        intermittent H50.30
    hypertropia H50.2-●
    hypotropia —see Hypertropia
    latent H50.50
    mechanical H50.60
        Brown's sheath syndrome H50.61-●
        specified type NEC H50.69
    monofixation syndrome H50.42
    paralytic H49.9
        abducens nerve H49.2-●
        fourth nerve H49.1-●
        Kearns-Sayre syndrome H49.81-●
        ophthalmoplegia (external)
            progressive H49.4-●
                with pigmentary retinopathy H49.81-●
            total H49.3-●
        sixth nerve H49.2-●
        specified type NEC H49.88-●
        third nerve H49.0-●
        trochlear nerve H49.1-●
    specified type NEC H50.89
    vertical H50.2-●
Strain
    back S39.012
    cervical S16.1
    eye NEC —see Disturbance, vision, subjective
    heart —see Disease, heart
    low back S39.012
    mental NOS Z73.3
        work-related Z56.6
    muscle (tendon) —see Injury, muscle, by site,
        strain
    neck S16.1

Strain *(Continued)*
 physical NOS Z73.3
  work-related Z56.6
 postural —*see also* Disorder, soft tissue, due
   to use
 psychological NEC Z73.3
 tendon —*see* Injury, muscle, by site, strain
Straining, on urination R39.16
Strand, vitreous —*see* Opacity, vitreous,
  membranes and strands
Strangulation, strangulated —*see also*
  Asphyxia, traumatic
 appendix K38.8
 bladder-neck N32.0
 bowel or colon K56.2
 food or foreign body —*see* Foreign body, by
   site
 hemorrhoids —*see* Hemorrhoids, with
  complication
 hernia —*see also* Hernia, by site, with
  obstruction
  with gangrene —*see* Hernia, by site, with
    gangrene
 intestine (large) (small) K56.2
  with hernia —*see also* Hernia, by site, with
    obstruction
   with gangrene —*see* Hernia, by site, with
     gangrene
 mesentery K56.2
 mucus —*see* Asphyxia, mucus
 omentum K56.2
 organ or site, congenital NEC —*see* Atresia,
   by site
 ovary —*see* Torsion, ovary
 penis N48.89
  foreign body T19.4
 rupture —*see* Hernia, by site, with obstruction
 stomach due to hernia —*see also* Hernia, by
   site, with obstruction
  with gangrene —*see* Hernia, by site, with
    gangrene
 vesicourethral orifice N32.0
Strangury R30.0
Straw itch B88.0
Strawberry
 gallbladder K82.4
 mark Q82.5
 tongue (red) (white) K14.3
Streak(s)
 macula, angioid H35.33
 ovarian Q50.32
Strephosymbolia F81.0
 secondary to organic lesion R48.8
Streptobacillary fever A25.1
Streptobacillosis A25.1
Streptobacillus moniliformis A25.1
Streptococcus, streptococcal —*see also*
  condition
 as cause of disease classified elsewhere B95.5
 group
  A, as cause of disease classified elsewhere
    B95.0
  B, as cause of disease classified elsewhere
    B95.1
  D, as cause of disease classified elsewhere
    B95.2
 pneumoniae, as cause of disease classified
   elsewhere B95.3
 specified NEC, as cause of disease classified
   elsewhere B95.4
Streptomycosis B47.1
Streptotrichosis A48.8
Stress F43.9
 family —*see* Disruption, family
 fetal P84
  complicating pregnancy O77.9
   due to drug administration O77.1
 mental NEC Z73.3
  work-related Z56.6
 physical NEC Z73.3
  work-related Z56.6

Stress *(Continued)*
 polycythemia D75.1
 reaction —*see also* Reaction, stress F43.9
 work schedule Z56.3
Stretching, nerve —*see* Injury, nerve
Striae albicantes, atrophicae or distensae
  (cutis) L90.6
Stricture —*see also* Stenosis
 ampulla of Vater K83.1
 anus (sphincter) K62.4
  congenital Q42.3
   with fistula Q42.2
  infantile Q42.3
   with fistula Q42.2
 aorta (ascending) (congenital) Q25.1
  arteriosclerotic I70.0
  calcified I70.0
  supravalvular, congenital Q25.3
 aortic (valve) —*see* Stenosis, aortic
 aqueduct of Sylvius (congenital) Q03.0
  with spina bifida —*see* Spina bifida, by site,
    with hydrocephalus
  acquired G91.1
 artery I77.1
  basilar —*see* Occlusion, artery, basilar
  carotid —*see* Occlusion, artery, carotid
  celiac I77.4
  congenital (peripheral) Q27.8
   cerebral Q28.3
   coronary Q24.5
   digestive system Q27.8
   lower limb Q27.8
   retinal Q14.1
   specified site NEC Q27.8
   umbilical Q27.0
   upper limb Q27.8
  coronary —*see* Disease, heart, ischemic,
    atherosclerotic
   congenital Q24.5
  precerebral —*see* Occlusion, artery,
    precerebral
  pulmonary (congenital) Q25.6
   acquired I28.8
  renal I70.1
  vertebral —*see* Occlusion, artery, vertebral
 auditory canal (external) (congenital)
  acquired —*see* Stenosis, external ear canal
 bile duct (common) (hepatic) K83.1
  congenital Q44.3
  postoperative K91.89
 bladder N32.89
  neck N32.0
 bowel —*see* Obstruction, intestine
 brain G93.89
 bronchus J98.09
  congenital Q32.3
  syphilitic A52.72
 cardia (stomach) K22.2
  congenital Q39.3
 cardiac —*see also* Disease, heart
  orifice (stomach) K22.2
 cecum —*see* Obstruction, intestine
 cervix, cervical (canal) N88.2
  congenital Q51.828
  in pregnancy —*see* Pregnancy, complicated
    by, abnormal cervix
   causing obstructed labor O65.5
 colon —*see also* Obstruction, intestine
  congenital Q42.9
   specified NEC Q42.8
 colostomy K94.03
 common (bile) duct K83.1
 coronary (artery) —*see* Disease, heart,
   ischemic, atherosclerotic
 cystic duct —*see* Obstruction, gallbladder
 digestive organs NEC, congenital Q45.8
 duodenum K31.5
  congenital Q41.0
 ear canal (external) (congenital) Q16.1
  acquired —*see* Stricture, auditory canal,
    acquired

Stricture *(Continued)*
 ejaculatory duct N50.89
 enterostomy K94.13
 esophagus K22.2
  congenital Q39.3
  syphilitic A52.79
   congenital A50.59 [K23]
 eustachian tube —*see also* Obstruction,
   eustachian tube
  congenital Q17.8
 fallopian tube N97.1
  gonococcal A54.24
  tuberculous A18.17
 gallbladder —*see* Obstruction, gallbladder
 glottis J38.6
 heart —*see also* Disease, heart
  valve (see also Endocarditis) I38
   aortic Q23.0
   mitral Q23.2
   pulmonary Q22.1
   tricuspid Q22.4
 hepatic duct K83.1
 hourglass, of stomach K31.2
 hymen N89.6
 hypopharynx J39.2
 ileum —*see also* Obstruction, intestine,
   specified NEC K56.699
  congenital Q41.2
 intestine —*see also* Obstruction, intestine
  congenital (small) Q41.9
   large Q42.9
    specified NEC Q42.8
   specified NEC Q41.8
  ischemic K55.1
 jejunum —*see also* Obstruction, intestine,
   specified NEC K56.699
  congenital Q41.1
 lacrimal passages —*see also* Stenosis, lacrimal
  congenital Q10.5
 larynx J38.6
  congenital NEC Q31.8
   subglottic Q31.1
  syphilitic A52.73
   congenital A50.59 [J99]
 meatus
  ear (congenital) Q16.1
   acquired —*see* Stricture, auditory canal,
     acquired
  osseous (ear) (congenital) Q16.1
   acquired —*see* Stricture, auditory canal,
     acquired
  urinarius —*see also* Stricture, urethra
   congenital Q64.33
 mitral (valve) —*see* Stenosis, mitral
 myocardium, myocardial I51.5
  hypertrophic subaortic (idiopathic) I42.1
 nares (anterior) (posterior) J34.89
  congenital Q30.0
 nasal duct —*see also* Stenosis, lacrimal, duct
  congenital Q10.5
 nasolacrimal duct —*see also* Stenosis, lacrimal,
   duct
  congenital Q10.5
 nasopharynx J39.2
  syphilitic A52.73
 nose J34.89
  congenital Q30.0
 nostril (anterior) (posterior) J34.89
  congenital Q30.0
  syphilitic A52.73
   congenital A50.59 [J99]
 organ or site, congenital NEC —*see* Atresia,
   by site
 os uteri —*see* Stricture, cervix
 osseous meatus (ear) (congenital) Q16.1
  acquired —*see* Stricture, auditory canal,
    acquired
 oviduct —*see* Stricture, fallopian tube
 pelviureteric junction (congenital) Q62.11
  acquired, with hydronephrosis N13.0
 penis, by foreign body T19.4

▶ New ⇒ Revised ~~deleted~~ Deleted ● Use Additional Character(s)

Stricture *(Continued)*
  pharynx J39.2
  prostate N42.89
  pulmonary, pulmonic
    artery (congenital) Q25.6
      acquired I28.8
      noncongenital I28.8
    infundibulum (congenital) Q24.3
    valve I37.0
      congenital Q22.1
    vein, acquired I28.8
    vessel NEC I28.8
  punctum lacrimale —*see also* Stenosis,
      lacrimal, punctum
    congenital Q10.5
  pylorus (hypertrophic) K31.1
    adult K31.1
    congenital Q40.0
    infantile Q40.0
  rectosigmoid —*see also* Obstruction, intestine,
      specified NEC K56.699
  rectum (sphincter) K62.4
    congenital Q42.1
      with fistula Q42.0
    due to
      chlamydial lymphogranuloma A55
      irradiation K91.89
      lymphogranuloma venereum A55
    gonococcal A54.6
    inflammatory (chlamydial) A55
    syphilitic A52.74
    tuberculous A18.32
  renal artery I70.1
    congenital Q27.1
  salivary duct or gland (any) K11.8
  sigmoid (flexure) —*see* Obstruction, intestine
  spermatic cord N50.89
  stoma (following) (of)
    colostomy K94.03
    enterostomy K94.13
    gastrostomy K94.23
    ileostomy K94.13
    tracheostomy J95.03
  stomach K31.89
    congenital Q40.2
    hourglass K31.2
  subaortic Q24.4
    hypertrophic (acquired) (idiopathic) I42.1
  subglottic J38.6
  syphilitic NEC A52.79
  trachea J39.8
    congenital Q32.1
    syphilitic A52.73
    tuberculous NEC A15.5
  tracheostomy J95.03
  tricuspid (valve) —*see* Stenosis, tricuspid
  tunica vaginalis N50.89
  ureter (postoperative) N13.5
    with
      hydronephrosis N13.1
        with infection N13.6
      pyelonephritis (chronic) N11.1
    congenital —*see* Atresia, ureter
    tuberculous A18.11
  ureteropelvic junction (congenital) Q62.11
    acquired, with hydronephrosis N13.0
  ureterovesical orifice N13.5
    with infection N13.6
  urethra (organic) (spasmodic) (*see also*
      Stricture, urethra, male N35.919
    associated with schistosomiasis
      B65.0 [N37]
    congenital Q64.39
      valvular (posterior) Q64.2
    due to
      infection —*see* Stricture, urethra,
          postinfective
      trauma —*see* Stricture, urethra,
          post-traumatic
    female N35.92
    gonococcal, gonorrheal A54.01

Stricture *(Continued)*
  urethra (organic) (spasmodic) *(Continued)*
    infective NEC —*see* Stricture, urethra,
        postinfective
    late effect (sequelae) of injury —*see*
        Stricture, urethra, post-traumatic
    male N35.919
      anterior urethra N35.914
      bulbous urethra N35.912
      meatal N35.911
      membranous urethra N35.913
      overlapping sites N35.916
    postcatheterization —*see* Stricture, urethra,
        postprocedural
    postinfective NEC
      female N35.12
      male N35.119
        anterior urethra N35.114
        bulbous urethra N35.112
        meatal N35.111
        membranous urethra N35.113
        overlapping sites N35.116
    postobstetric N35.021
    postoperative —*see* Stricture, urethra,
        postprocedural
    postprocedural
      female N99.12
      male N99.114
        anterior bulbous urethra N99.113
        bulbous urethra N99.111
        fossa navicularis N99.115
        meatal N99.110
        membranous urethra N99.112
        overlapping sites N35.116
    post-traumatic
      female N35.028
        due to childbirth N35.021
      male N35.014
        anterior urethra N35.013
        bulbous urethra N35.011
        meatal N35.010
        membranous urethra N35.012
        overlapping sites N35.016
    sequela (late effect) of
      childbirth N35.021
      injury —*see* Stricture, urethra,
          post-traumatic
    specified cause NEC
      female N35.82
      male N35.819
        anterior urethra N35.814
        bulbous urethra N35.812
        meatal N35.811
        membranous urethra N35.813
        overlapping sites N35.816
    syphilitic A52.76
    traumatic —*see* Stricture, urethra,
        post-traumatic
    valvular (posterior), congenital Q64.2
  urinary meatus —*see* Stricture, urethra
  uterus, uterine (synechiae) N85.6
    os (external) (internal) —*see* Stricture,
        cervix
  vagina (outlet) —*see* Stenosis, vagina
  valve (cardiac) (heart) —*see also* Endocarditis
    congenital
      aortic Q23.0
      mitral Q23.2
      pulmonary Q22.1
      tricuspid Q22.4
  vas deferens N50.89
    congenital Q55.4
  vein I87.1
  vena cava (inferior) (superior) NEC I87.1
    congenital Q26.0
  vesicourethral orifice N32.0
    congenital Q64.31
  vulva (acquired) N90.5
Stridor R06.1
  congenital (larynx) P28.89
Stridulous —*see* condition

Stroke (apoplectic) (brain) (embolic) (ischemic)
    (paralytic) (thrombotic) I63.9
  cerebral, perinatal P91.82-●
  cryptogenic —*see also* infarction, cerebral
      I63.9
  epileptic —*see* Epilepsy
  heat T67.01
    exertional T67.02
    specified NEC T67.09
  in evolution I63.9
  intraoperative
    during cardiac surgery I97.810
    during other surgery I97.811
  ischemic, perinatal arterial P91.82-●
  lightning —*see* Lightning
  meaning
    cerebral hemorrhage — code to
        Hemorrhage, intracranial
    cerebral infarction — code to Infarction,
        cerebral
  neonatal P91.82-●
  postprocedural
    following cardiac surgery I97.820
    following other surgery I97.821
  sun T67.01
    specified NEC T67.09
  unspecified (NOS) I63.9
Stromatosis, endometrial D39.0
Strongyloidiasis, strongyloidosis B78.9
  cutaneous B78.1
  disseminated B78.7
  intestinal B78.0
Strophulus pruriginosus L28.2
Struck by lightning —*see* Lightning
Struma —*see also* Goiter
  Hashimoto E06.3
  lymphomatosa E06.3
  nodosa (simplex) E04.9
    endemic E01.2
      multinodular E01.1
    multinodular E04.2
      iodine-deficiency related E01.1
    toxic or with hyperthyroidism E05.20
      with thyroid storm E05.21
      multinodular E05.20
        with thyroid storm E05.21
      uninodular E05.10
        with thyroid storm E05.11
    toxicosa E05.20
      with thyroid storm E05.21
      multinodular E05.20
        with thyroid storm E05.21
      uninodular E05.10
        with thyroid storm E05.11
    uninodular E04.1
  ovarii D27.-●
  Riedel's E06.5
Strumipriva cachexia E03.4
Strümpell-Marie spine —*see* Spondylitis,
    ankylosing
Strümpell-Westphal pseudosclerosis E83.01
Stuart deficiency disease (factor X) D68.2
Stuart-Prower factor deficiency (factor X)
    D68.2
Student's elbow —*see* Bursitis, elbow,
    olecranon
Stump —*see* Amputation
Stunting, nutritional E45
Stupor (catatonic) R40.1
  depressive (single episode) F32.89
    recurrent episode F33.8
  dissociative F44.2
  manic F30.2
  manic-depressive F31.89
  psychogenic (anergic) F44.2
  reaction to exceptional stress (transient) F43.0
Sturge (-Weber) (-Dimitri) (-Kalischer) disease
    or syndrome Q85.8
Stuttering F80.81
  adult onset F98.5
  childhood onset F80.81

▶ New ⇒ Revised ~~deleted~~ Deleted ● Use Additional Character(s)

Stuttering (Continued)
   following cerebrovascular disease —
      see Disorder, fluency, following
      cerebrovascular disease
   in conditions classified elsewhere R47.82
Sty, stye (external) (internal) (meibomian)
      (zeisian) —see Hordeolum
Subacidity, gastric K31.89
   psychogenic F45.8
Subacute —see condition
Subarachnoid —see condition
Subcortical —see condition
Subcostal syndrome, nerve compression —see
      Mononeuropathy, upper limb, specified
      site NEC
Subcutaneous, subcuticular —see condition
Subdural —see condition
Subendocardium —see condition
Subependymoma
   specified site —see Neoplasm, uncertain
      behavior, by site
   unspecified site D43.2
Suberosis J67.3
Subglossitis —see Glossitis
Subhemophilia D66
Subinvolution
   breast (postlactational) (postpuerperal)
      N64.89
   puerperal O90.89
   uterus (chronic) (nonpuerperal) N85.3
      puerperal O90.89
Sublingual —see condition
Sublinguitis —see Sialoadenitis
Subluxatable hip Q65.6
Subluxation —see also Dislocation
   acromioclavicular S43.11-●
   ankle S93.0-●
   atlantoaxial, recurrent M43.4
      with myelopathy M43.3
   carpometacarpal (joint) NEC S63.05-●
      thumb S63.04-●
   complex, vertebral —see Complex,
      subluxation
   congenital —see also Malposition, congenital
      hip —see Dislocation, hip, congenital,
         partial
      joint (excluding hip)
         lower limb Q68.8
         shoulder Q68.8
         upper limb Q68.8
   elbow (traumatic) S53.10-●
      anterior S53.11-●
      lateral S53.14-●
      medial S53.13-●
      posterior S53.12-●
      specified type NEC S53.19-●
   finger S63.20-●
      index S63.20-●
      interphalangeal S63.22-●
         distal S63.24-●
            index S63.24-●
            little S63.24-●
            middle S63.24-●
            ring S63.24-●
         index S63.22-●
         little S63.22-●
         middle S63.22-●
         proximal S63.23-●
            index S63.23-●
            little S63.23-●
            middle S63.23-●
            ring S63.23-●
         ring S63.22-●
      little S63.20-●
      metacarpophalangeal S63.21-●
         index S63.21-●
         little S63.21-●
         middle S63.21-●
         ring S63.21-●
      middle S63.20-●
      ring S63.20-●

Subluxation (Continued)
   foot S93.30-●
      specified site NEC S93.33-●
      tarsal joint S93.31-●
      tarsometatarsal joint S93.32-●
      toe —see Subluxation, toe
   hip S73.00-●
      anterior S73.03-●
         obturator S73.02-●
      central S73.04-●
      posterior S73.01-●
   interphalangeal (joint)
      finger S63.22-●
         distal joint S63.24-●
            index S63.24-●
            little S63.24-●
            middle S63.24-●
            ring S63.24-●
         index S63.22-●
         little S63.22-●
         middle S63.22-●
         proximal joint S63.23-●
            index S63.23-●
            little S63.23-●
            middle S63.23-●
            ring S63.23-●
         ring S63.22-●
      thumb S63.12-●
      toe S93.13-●
         great S93.13-●
         lesser S93.13-●
   joint prosthesis —see Complications, joint
      prosthesis, mechanical, displacement,
      by site
   knee S83.10-●
      cap —see Subluxation, patella
      patella —see Subluxation, patella
      proximal tibia
         anteriorly S83.11-●
         laterally S83.14-●
         medially S83.13-●
         posteriorly S83.12-●
      specified type NEC S83.19-●
   lens —see Dislocation, lens, partial
   ligament, traumatic —see Sprain,
      by site
   metacarpal (bone)
      proximal end S63.06-●
   metacarpophalangeal (joint)
      finger S63.21-●
         index S63.21-●
         little S63.21-●
         middle S63.21-●
         ring S63.21-●
      thumb S63.11-●
   metatarsophalangeal joint S93.14-●
      great toe S93.14-●
      lesser toe S93.14-●
   midcarpal (joint) S63.03-●
   patella S83.00-●
      lateral S83.01-●
      recurrent (nontraumatic) —see
         Dislocation, patella, recurrent,
         incomplete
      specified type NEC S83.09-●
   pathological —see Dislocation,
      pathological
   radial head S53.00-●
      anterior S53.01-●
      nursemaid's elbow S53.03-●
      posterior S53.02-●
      specified type NEC S53.09-●
   radiocarpal (joint) S63.02-●
   radioulnar (joint)
      distal S63.01-●
      proximal —see Subluxation, elbow
   shoulder
      congenital Q68.8
      girdle S43.30-●
         scapula S43.31-●
         specified site NEC S43.39-●

Subluxation (Continued)
   shoulder (Continued)
      traumatic S43.00-●
         anterior S43.01-●
         inferior S43.03-●
         posterior S43.02-●
         specified type NEC S43.08-●
   sternoclavicular (joint) S43.20-●
      anterior S43.21-●
      posterior S43.22-●
   symphysis (pubis)
   thumb S63.103
      interphalangeal joint —see Subluxation,
         interphalangeal (joint), thumb
      metacarpophalangeal joint —see
         Subluxation, metacarpophalangeal
         (joint), thumb
   toe(s) S93.10-●
      great S93.10-●
         interphalangeal joint S93.13-●
         metatarsophalangeal joint S93.14-●
      interphalangeal joint S93.13-●
      lesser S93.10-●
         interphalangeal joint S93.13-●
         metatarsophalangeal joint S93.14-●
      metatarsophalangeal joint S93.149
   ulnohumeral joint —see Subluxation, elbow
   vertebral
      recurrent NEC —see subcategory M43.5
      traumatic
         cervical S13.100
            atlantoaxial joint S13.120
            atlantooccipital joint S13.110
            atloidooccipital joint S13.110
            joint between
               C0 and C1 S13.110
               C1 and C2 S13.120
               C2 and C3 S13.130
               C3 and C4 S13.140
               C4 and C5 S13.150
               C5 and C6 S13.160
               C6 and C7 S13.170
               C7 and T1 S13.180
            occipitoatloid joint S13.110
         lumbar S33.100
            joint between
               L1 and L2 S33.110
               L2 and L3 S33.120
               L3 and L4 S33.130
               L4 and L5 S33.140
         thoracic S23.100
            joint between
               T1 and T2 S23.110
               T2 and T3 S23.120
               T3 and T4 S23.122
               T4 and T5 S23.130
               T5 and T6 S23.132
               T6 and T7 S23.140
               T7 and T8 S23.142
               T8 and T9 S23.150
               T9 and T10 S23.152
               T10 and T11 S23.160
               T11 and T12 S23.162
               T12 and L1 S23.170
   ulna
      distal end S63.07-●
      proximal end —see Subluxation, elbow
   wrist (carpal bone) S63.00-●
      carpometacarpal joint —see Subluxation,
         carpometacarpal (joint)
      distal radioulnar joint —see Subluxation,
         radioulnar (joint), distal
      metacarpal bone, proximal —see Subluxation,
         metacarpal (bone), proximal end
      midcarpal —see Subluxation, midcarpal
         (joint)
      radiocarpal joint —see Subluxation,
         radiocarpal (joint)
      recurrent —see Dislocation, recurrent, wrist
      specified site NEC S63.09-●
      ulna —see Subluxation, ulna, distal end

▶ New   ⇒ Revised   ~~deleted~~ Deleted   ● Use Additional Character(s)

Submaxillary —see condition
Submersion (fatal) (nonfatal) T75.1
Submucous —see condition
Subnormal, subnormality
   accommodation (old age) H52.4
   mental —see Disability, intellectual
   temperature (accidental) T68
Subphrenic —see condition
Subscapular nerve —see condition
Subseptus uterus Q51.28
Subsiding appendicitis K36
Substance (other psychoactive) -induced
   anxiety disorder F19.980
   bipolar and related disorder F19.94
   delirium F19.921
   depressive disorder F19.94
   major neurocognitive disorder F19.97
   mild neurocognitive disorder F19.988
   obsessive-compulsive and related disorder
      F19.988
   psychotic disorder F19.959
   sexual dysfunction F19.981
   sleep disorder F19.982
Substernal thyroid E04.9
   congenital Q89.2
Substitution disorder F44.9
Subtentorial —see condition
Subthyroidism (acquired) —see also
      Hypothyroidism
   congenital E03.1
Succenturiate placenta O43.19-●
Sucking thumb, child (excessive) F98.8
Sudamen, sudamina L74.1
Sudanese kala-azar B55.0
Sudden
   hearing loss —see Deafness, sudden
   heart failure —see Failure, heart
Sudeck's atrophy, disease, or syndrome —see
      Algoneurodystrophy
Suffocation —see Asphyxia, traumatic
Sugar
   blood
      high (transient) R73.9
      low (transient) E16.2
   in urine R81
Suicide, suicidal (attempted) T14.91
   by poisoning —see Table of Drugs and
      Chemicals
   ⇒history of (personal) Z91.51
      in family Z81.8
   ideation —see Ideation, suicidal
   risk
      ⇒meaning personal history of attempted
         suicide Z91.51
      meaning suicidal ideation —see Ideation,
         suicidal
   tendencies
      ⇒meaning personal history of attempted
         suicide Z91.51
      meaning suicidal ideation —see Ideation,
         suicidal
   trauma —see nature of injury by site
Suipestifer infection —see Infection, salmonella
Sulfhemoglobinemia, sulphemoglobinemia
      (acquired) (with methemoglobinemia) D74.8
Sumatran mite fever A75.3
Summer —see condition
Sunburn L55.9
   due to
      tanning bed (acute) L56.8
         chronic L57.8
      ultraviolet radiation (acute) L56.8
         chronic L57.8
   first degree L55.0
   second degree L55.1
   third degree L55.2
SUNCT (short lasting unilateral neuralgiform
      headache with conjunctival injection and
      tearing) G44.059
   intractable G44.051
   not intractable G44.059

Sundowning F05
Sunken acetabulum —see Derangement, joint,
      specified type NEC, hip
Sunstroke T67.01
   specified NEC T67.09
Superfecundation —see Pregnancy, multiple
Superfetation —see Pregnancy, multiple
Superinvolution (uterus) N85.8
Supernumerary (congenital)
   aortic cusps Q23.8
   auditory ossicles Q16.3
   bone Q79.8
   breast Q83.1
   carpal bones Q74.0
   cusps, heart valve NEC Q24.8
      aortic Q23.8
      mitral Q23.2
      pulmonary Q22.3
   digit(s) Q69.9
   ear (lobule) Q17.0
   fallopian tube Q50.6
   finger Q69.0
   hymen Q52.4
   kidney Q63.0
   lacrimonasal duct Q10.6
   lobule (ear) Q17.0
   mitral cusps Q23.2
   muscle Q79.8
   nipple(s) Q83.3
   organ or site not listed —see Accessory
   ossicles, auditory Q16.3
   ovary Q50.31
   oviduct Q50.6
   pulmonary, pulmonic cusps Q22.3
   rib Q76.6
      cervical or first (syndrome) Q76.5
   roots (of teeth) K00.2
   spleen Q89.09
   tarsal bones Q74.2
   teeth K00.1
   testis Q55.29
   thumb Q69.1
   toe Q69.2
   uterus Q51.28
   vagina Q52.1
   vertebra Q76.49
Supervision (of)
   contraceptive —see Prescription,
      contraceptives
   dietary (for) Z71.3
      allergy (food) Z71.3
      colitis Z71.3
      diabetes mellitus Z71.3
      food allergy or intolerance Z71.3
      gastritis Z71.3
      hypercholesterolemia Z71.3
      hypoglycemia Z71.3
      intolerance (food) Z71.3
      obesity Z71.3
      specified NEC Z71.3
   healthy infant or child Z76.2
      foundling Z76.1
   high-risk pregnancy —see Pregnancy,
      complicated by, high, risk
   lactation Z39.1
   pregnancy —see Pregnancy, supervision of
Supplemental teeth K00.1
Suppression
   binocular vision H53.34
   lactation O92.5
   menstruation N94.89
   ovarian secretion E28.39
   renal N28.9
   urine, urinary secretion R34
Suppuration, suppurative —see also condition
   accessory sinus (chronic) —see Sinusitis
   adrenal gland
   antrum (chronic) —see Sinusitis, maxillary
   bladder —see Cystitis
   brain G06.0
      sequelae G09

Suppuration, suppurative (Continued)
   breast N61.1
      puerperal, postpartum or gestational —see
         Mastitis, obstetric, purulent
   dental periosteum M27.3
   ear (middle) —see also Otitis, media
      external NEC —see Otitis, externa, infective
      internal —see subcategory H83.0
   ethmoidal (chronic) (sinus) —see Sinusitis,
      ethmoidal
   fallopian tube —see Salpingo-oophoritis
   frontal (chronic) (sinus) —see Sinusitis, frontal
   gallbladder (acute) K81.0
   gum K05.20
      generalized —see Periodontitis, aggressive,
         generalized
      localized —see Periodontitis, aggressive,
         localized
   intracranial G06.0
   joint —see Arthritis, pyogenic or pyemic
   labyrinthine —see subcategory H83.0
   lung —see Abscess, lung
   mammary gland N61.1
      puerperal, postpartum O91.12
         associated with lactation O91.13
   maxilla, maxillary M27.2
      sinus (chronic) —see Sinusitis, maxillary
   muscle —see Myositis, infective
   nasal sinus (chronic) —see Sinusitis
   pancreas, acute —see also Pancreatitis, acute
      K85.80
   parotid gland —see Sialoadenitis
   pelvis, pelvic
      female —see Disease, pelvis, inflammatory
      male K65.0
   pericranial —see Osteomyelitis
   salivary duct or gland (any) —see
      Sialoadenitis
   sinus (accessory) (chronic) (nasal) —see
      Sinusitis
   sphenoidal sinus (chronic) —see Sinusitis,
      sphenoidal
   thymus (gland) E32.1
   thyroid (gland) E06.0
   tonsil —see Tonsillitis
   uterus —see Endometritis
Supraeruption of tooth (teeth) M26.34
Supraglottitis J04.30
   with obstruction J04.31
Suprarenal (gland) —see condition
Suprascapular nerve —see condition
Suprasellar —see condition
Surfer's knots or nodules S89.8-●
Surgical
   emphysema T81.82
   procedures, complication or misadventure —
      see Complications, surgical procedures
   shock T81.10
Surveillance (of) (for) —see also Observation
   alcohol abuse Z71.41
   contraceptive —see Prescription, contraceptives
   dietary Z71.3
   drug abuse Z71.51
Susceptibility to disease, genetic Z15.89
   malignant neoplasm Z15.09
      breast Z15.01
      endometrium Z15.04
      ovary Z15.02
      prostate Z15.03
      specified NEC Z15.09
   multiple endocrine neoplasia Z15.81
Suspected condition, ruled out —see also
      Observation, suspected
   amniotic cavity and membrane Z03.71
   cervical shortening Z03.75
   fetal anomaly Z03.73
   fetal growth Z03.74
   maternal and fetal conditions NEC Z03.79
   newborn —see also Observation, newborn,
      suspected condition ruled out Z05.9
   oligohydramnios Z03.71

Suspected condition, ruled out *(Continued)*
- placental problem Z03.72
- polyhydramnios Z03.71

Suspended uterus
- in pregnancy or childbirth —*see* Pregnancy, complicated by, abnormal uterus

Sutton's nevus D22.9

Suture
- burst (in operation wound) T81.31
  - external operation wound T81.31
  - internal operation wound T81.32
- inadvertently left in operation wound —*see* Foreign body, accidentally left during a procedure
- removal Z48.02

Swab inadvertently left in operation wound —*see* Foreign body, accidentally left during a procedure

Swallowed, swallowing
- difficulty —*see* Dysphagia
- foreign body —*see* Foreign body, alimentary tract

Swan-neck deformity (finger) —*see* Deformity, finger, swan-neck

Swearing, compulsive F42.8
- in Gilles de la Tourette's syndrome F95.2

Sweat, sweats
- fetid L75.0
- night R61

Sweating, excessive R61

Sweeley-Klionsky disease E75.21

Sweet's disease or dermatosis L98.2

Swelling (of) R60.9
- abdomen, abdominal (not referable to any particular organ) —*see* Mass, abdominal
- ankle —*see* Effusion, joint, ankle
- arm M79.89
  - forearm M79.89
- breast —*see also* Lump, breast N63.0
- Calabar B74.3
- cervical gland R59.0
- chest, localized R22.2
- ear H93.8-●
- extremity (lower) (upper) —*see* Disorder, soft tissue, specified type NEC
- finger M79.89
- foot M79.89
- glands R59.9
  - generalized R59.1
  - localized R59.0
- hand M79.89
- head (localized) R22.0
- inflammatory —*see* Inflammation
- intra-abdominal —*see* Mass, abdominal
- joint —*see* Effusion, joint
- leg M79.89
  - lower M79.89
- limb —*see* Disorder, soft tissue, specified type NEC
- localized (skin) R22.9
  - chest R22.2
  - head R22.0
  - limb
    - lower —*see* Mass, localized, limb, lower
    - upper —*see* Mass, localized, limb, upper
  - neck R22.1
  - trunk R22.2
- neck (localized) R22.1
- pelvic —*see* Mass, abdominal
- scrotum N50.89
- splenic —*see* Splenomegaly
- testis N50.89
- toe M79.89
- umbilical R19.09
- wandering, due to Gnathostoma (spinigerum) B83.1
- white —*see* Tuberculosis, arthritis

Swift (-Feer) disease
- overdose or wrong substance given or taken —*see* Table of Drugs and Chemicals, by drug, poisoning

Swimmer's
- cramp T75.1
- ear H60.33-●
- itch B65.3

Swimming in the head R42

Swollen —*see* Swelling

Swyer syndrome Q99.1

Sycosis L73.8
- barbae (not parasitic) L73.8
- contagiosa (mycotic) B35.0
- lupoides L73.8
- mycotic B35.0
- parasitic B35.0
- vulgaris L73.8

Sydenham's chorea —*see* Chorea, Sydenham's

Sylvatic yellow fever A95.0

Sylvest's disease B33.0

Symblepharon H11.23-●
- congenital Q10.3

Symond's syndrome G93.2

Sympathetic —*see* condition

Sympatheticotonia G90.8

Sympathicoblastoma
- specified site —*see* Neoplasm, malignant, by site
- unspecified site C74.90

Sympathogonioma —*see* Sympathicoblastoma

Symphalangy (fingers) (toes) Q70.9

Symptoms NEC R68.89
- breast NEC N64.59
- cold J00
- development NEC R63.8
- factitious, self-induced —*see* Disorder, factitious
- genital organs, female R10.2
- involving
  - abdomen NEC R19.8
  - appearance NEC R46.89
  - awareness R41.9
    - altered mental status R41.82
    - amnesia —*see* Amnesia
    - borderline intellectual functioning R41.83
    - coma —*see* Coma
    - disorientation R41.0
    - neurologic neglect syndrome R41.4
    - senile cognitive decline R41.81
    - specified symptom NEC R41.89
  - behavior NEC R46.89
  - cardiovascular system NEC R09.89
  - chest NEC R09.89
  - circulatory system NEC R09.89
  - cognitive functions R41.9
    - altered mental status R41.82
    - amnesia —*see* Amnesia
    - borderline intellectual functioning R41.83
    - coma —*see* Coma
    - disorientation R41.0
    - neurologic neglect syndrome R41.4
    - senile cognitive decline R41.81
    - specified symptom NEC R41.89
  - development NEC R62.50
  - digestive system NEC R19.8
  - emotional state NEC R45.89
    - emotional lability R45.86
  - food and fluid intake R63.8
  - general perceptions and sensations R44.9
    - specified NEC R44.8
  - musculoskeletal system R29.91
    - specified NEC R29.898
  - nervous system R29.90
    - specified NEC R29.818
  - pelvis NEC R19.8
  - respiratory system NEC R09.89
  - skin and integument R23.9
  - urinary system R39.9
- menopausal N95.1
- metabolism NEC R63.8

Symptoms NEC *(Continued)*
- neurotic F48.8
- of infancy R68.19
- pelvis NEC, female R10.2
- skin and integument NEC R23.9
- subcutaneous tissue NEC R23.9
- viral cold J00

Sympus Q74.2

Syncephalus Q89.4

Synchondrosis
- abnormal (congenital) Q78.8
- ischiopubic M91.0

Synchysis (scintillans) (senile) (vitreous body) H43.89

Syncope (near) (pre-) R55
- anginosa I20.8
- bradycardia R00.1
- cardiac R55
- carotid sinus G90.01
- due to spinal (lumbar) puncture G97.1
- heart R55
- heat T67.1
- ▶laryngeal R05.4
- psychogenic F48.8
- ▶tussive R05.8
- vasoconstriction R55
- vasodepressor R55
- vasomotor R55
- vasovagal R55

Syndactylism, syndactyly Q70.9
- complex (with synostosis)
  - fingers Q70.0-●
  - toes Q70.2-●
- simple (without synostosis)
  - fingers Q70.1-●
  - toes Q70.3-●

Syndrome —*see also* Disease
- 5q minus NOS D46.C
- 48,XXXX Q97.1
- 49,XXXXX Q97.1
- abdominal
  - acute R10.0
  - muscle deficiency Q79.4
- abnormal innervation H02.519
  - left H02.516
    - lower H02.515
    - upper H02.514
  - right H02.513
    - lower H02.512
    - upper H02.511
- abstinence, neonatal P96.1
- acid pulmonary aspiration, obstetric O74.0
- acquired immunodeficiency —*see* Human, immunodeficiency virus (HIV) disease
- acute abdominal R10.0
- acute respiratory distress (adult) (child) J80
  - idiopathic J84.114
- Adair-Dighton Q78.0
- Adams-Stokes (-Morgagni) I45.9
- adiposogenital E23.6
- adrenal
  - hemorrhage (meningococcal) A39.1
  - meningococcic A39.1
- adrenocortical —*see* Cushing's, syndrome
- adrenogenital E25.9
  - congenital, associated with enzyme deficiency E25.0
- afferent loop NEC K91.89
- Alagille's Q44.7
- alcohol withdrawal (without convulsions) —*see* Dependence, alcohol, with, withdrawal
- Alder's D72.0
- Aldrich (-Wiskott) D82.0
- alien hand R41.4
- Alport Q87.81
- alveolar hypoventilation E66.2
- alveolocapillary block J84.10
- amnesic, amnestic (confabulatory) (due to) —*see* Disorder, amnesic
- amyostatic (Wilson's disease) E83.01

▶ New　　⇒ Revised　　~~deleted~~ Deleted　　● Use Additional Character(s)

Syndrome *(Continued)*
  androgen insensitivity E34.50
    complete E34.51
    partial E34.52
  androgen resistance *(see also* Syndrome,
      androgen insensitivity) E34.50
  Angelman Q93.51
  anginal —*see* Angina
  ankyloglossia superior Q38.1
  anterior
    chest wall R07.89
    cord G83.82
    spinal artery G95.19
      compression M47.019
        cervical region M47.012
        cervicothoracic region M47.013
        lumbar region M47.016
        occipito-atlanto-axial region M47.011
        thoracic region M47.014
        thoracolumbar region M47.015
    tibial M76.81-●
  antibody deficiency D80.9
    agammaglobulinemic D80.1
      hereditary D80.0
    congenital D80.0
    hypogammaglobulinemic D80.1
      hereditary D80.0
  anticardiolipin (-antibody) D68.61
  antidepressant discontinuation T43.205
  antiphospholipid (-antibody) D68.61
  aortic
    arch M31.4
    bifurcation I74.09
  aortomesenteric duodenum occlusion K31.5
  apical ballooning (transient left ventricular)
      I51.81
  arcuate ligament I77.4
  argentaffin, argentaffinoma E34.0
  Arnold-Chiari —*see* Arnold-Chiari disease
  Arrillaga-Ayerza I27.0
  arterial tortuosity Q87.82
  arteriovenous steal T82.898-●
  Asherman's N85.6
  aspiration, of newborn —*see* Aspiration, by
      substance, with pneumonia
    meconium P24.01
  ataxia-telangiectasia G11.3
  auriculotemporal G50.8
  autoerythrocyte sensitization (Gardner-
      Diamond) D69.2
  autoimmune lymphoproliferative [ALPS]
      D89.82
  autoimmune polyglandular E31.0
  autoinflammatory M04.9
    specified type NEC M04.8
  autosomal —*see* Abnormal, autosomes
  Avellis' G46.8
  Ayerza (-Arrillaga) I27.0
  Babinski-Nageotte G83.89
  Bakwin-Krida Q78.5
  bare lymphocyte D81.6
  Barré-Guillain G61.0
  Barré-Liéou M53.0
  Barrett's —*see* Barrett's, esophagus
  Barsony-Polgar K22.4
  Barsony-Teschendorf K22.4
  Barth E78.71
  Bartter's E26.81
  basal cell nevus Q87.89
  Basedow's E05.00
    with thyroid storm E05.01
  basilar artery G45.0
  Batten-Steinert G71.11
  battered
    baby or child —*see* Maltreatment, child,
        physical abuse
    spouse —*see* Maltreatment, adult, physical
        abuse
  Beals Q87.40
  Beau's I51.5
  Beck's I65.8

Syndrome *(Continued)*
  Benedikt's G46.3
  Béquez César (-Steinbrinck-Chédiak-Higashi)
      D70.330
  Bernhardt-Roth —*see* Meralgia paresthetica
  Bernheim's —*see* Failure, heart, right
  big spleen D73.1
  bilateral polycystic ovarian E28.2
  Bing-Horton's —*see* Horton's headache
  Birt-Hogg-Dube syndrome Q87.89
  Björck (-Thorsen) E34.0
  black
    lung J60
    widow spider bite —*see* Toxicity, venom,
        spider, black widow
  Blackfan-Diamond D61.01
  Blau M04.8
  blind loop K90.2
    congenital Q43.8
    postsurgical K91.2
  blue sclera Q78.0
  blue toe I75.02-●
  Boder-Sedgewick G11.3
  Boerhaave's K22.3
  Borjeson Forssman Lehmann Q89.8
  Bouillaud's I01.9
  Bourneville (-Pringle) Q85.1
  Bouveret (-Hoffman) I47.9
  brachial plexus G54.0
  bradycardia-tachycardia I49.5
  brain (nonpsychotic) F09
    with psychosis, psychotic reaction F09
    acute or subacute —*see* Delirium
    congenital —*see* Disability, intellectual
    organic F09
      post-traumatic (nonpsychotic) F07.81
        psychotic F09
      personality change F07.0
      postcontusional F07.81
      post-traumatic, nonpsychotic F07.81
      psycho-organic F09
      psychotic F06.8
  brain stem stroke G46.3
  Brandt's (acrodermatitis enteropathica)
      E83.2
  broad ligament laceration N83.8
  Brock's J98.11
  bronze baby P83.88
  Brown-Sequard G83.81
  Brugada I49.8
  bubbly lung P27.0
  Buchem's M85.2
  Budd-Chiari I82.0
  bulbar (progressive) G12.22
  Bürger-Grütz E78.3
  Burke's K86.89
  Burnett's (milk-alkali) E83.52
  burning feet E53.9
  Bywaters' T79.5
  Call-Fleming I67.841
  carbohydrate-deficient glycoprotein (CDGS)
      E77.8
  carcinogenic thrombophlebitis I82.1
  carcinoid E34.0
  cardiac asthma I50.1
  cardiacos negros I27.0
  cardiofaciocutaneous Q87.89
  cardiopulmonary-obesity E66.2
  cardiorenal —*see* Hypertension, cardiorenal
  cardiorespiratory distress (idiopathic),
      newborn P22.0
  cardiovascular renal —*see* Hypertension,
      cardiorenal
  carotid
    artery (hemispheric) (internal)
        G45.1
    body G90.01
    sinus G90.01
  carpal tunnel G56.0-●
  Cassidy (-Scholte) E34.0
  cat-cry Q93.4

Syndrome *(Continued)*
  cat eye Q92.8
  cauda equina G83.4
  causalgia —*see* Causalgia
  celiac K90.0
    artery compression I77.4
    axis I77.4
  central pain G89.0
  cerebellar
    hereditary G11.9
    stroke G46.4
  cerebellomedullary malformation —*see* Spina
      bifida
  cerebral
    artery
      anterior G46.1
      middle G46.0
      posterior G46.2
    gigantism E22.0
  cervical (root) M53.1
    disc —*see* Disorder, disc, cervical, with
        neuritis
    fusion Q76.1
    posterior, sympathicus M53.0
    rib Q76.5
    sympathetic paralysis G90.2
  cervicobrachial (diffuse) M53.1
  cervicocranial M53.0
  cervicodorsal outlet G54.2
  cervicothoracic outlet G54.0
  Céstan (-Raymond) I65.8
  Charcot's (angina cruris) (intermittent
      claudication) I73.9
  Charcot-Weiss-Baker G90.09
  CHARGE Q89.8
  Chédiak-Higashi (-Steinbrinck) E70.330
  chest wall R07.1
  Chiari's (hepatic vein thrombosis) I82.0
  Chilaiditi's Q43.3
  child maltreatment —*see* Maltreatment,
      child
  chondrocostal junction M94.0
  chondroectodermal dysplasia Q77.6
  chromosome 4 short arm deletion Q93.3
  chromosome 5 short arm deletion Q93.4
  chronic
    infantile neurological, cutaneous and
        articular (CINCA) M04.2
    pain G89.4
    personality F68.8
  Churg-Strauss M30.1
  Clarke-Hadfield K86.89
  Clerambault's automatism G93.89
  Clouston's (hidrotic ectodermal dysplasia)
      Q82.4
  clumsiness, clumsy child F82
  cluster headache G44.009
    intractable G44.001
    not intractable G44.009
  Coffin-Lowry Q89.8
  cold injury (newborn) P80.0
  combined immunity deficiency D81.9
  compartment (deep) (posterior) (traumatic)
      T79.A0
    abdomen T79.A3
    lower extremity (hip, buttock, thigh, leg,
        foot, toes) T79.A2
    nontraumatic
      abdomen M79.A3
      lower extremity (hip, buttock, thigh, leg,
          foot, toes) M79.A2-●
      specified site NEC M79.A9
      upper extremity (shoulder, arm, forearm,
          wrist, hand, fingers) M79.A1-●
    postprocedural —*see* Syndrome
        compartment, nontraumatic
    specified site NEC T79.A9
    upper extremity (shoulder, arm, forearm,
        wrist, hand, fingers) T79.A1
  complex regional pain —*see* Syndrome, pain,
      complex regional

Syndrome (Continued)
compression T79.5
    anterior spinal —see Syndrome, anterior,
        spinal artery, compression
    cauda equina G83.4
    celiac artery I77.4
    vertebral artery M47.029
        cervical region M47.022
        occipito-atlanto-axial region M47.021
concussion F07.81
congenital
    affecting multiple systems NEC Q87.89
    central alveolar hypoventilation G47.35
    facial diplegia Q87.0
    muscular hypertrophy-cerebral
        Q87.89
    oculo-auriculovertebral Q87.0
    oculofacial diplegia (Moebius)
        Q87.0
    rubella (manifest) P35.0
congestion-fibrosis (pelvic), female
    N94.89
congestive dysmenorrhea N94.6
Conn's E26.01
connective tissue M35.9
    overlap NEC M35.1
conus medullaris G95.81
cord
    anterior G83.82
    posterior G83.83
coronary
    acute NEC I24.9
    insufficiency or intermediate I20.0
    slow flow I20.8
Costen's (complex) M26.69
costochondral junction M94.0
costoclavicular G54.0
costovertebral E22.0
Cowden Q85.8
craniovertebral M53.0
Creutzfeldt-Jakob —see Creutzfeldt-Jakob
    disease or syndrome
cri-du-chat Q93.4
crib death R99
cricopharyngeal —see Dysphagia
croup J05.0
CRPS I —see Syndrome, pain, complex
    regional I
crush T79.5
cubital tunnel —see Lesion, nerve, ulnar
Curschmann (-Batten) (-Steinert) G71.11
Cushing's E24.9
    alcohol-induced E24.4
    drug-induced E24.2
    due to
        alcohol
        drugs E24.2
        ectopic ACTH E24.3
        overproduction of pituitary ACTH
            E24.0
    overdose or wrong substance given
        or taken —see Table of Drugs and
        Chemicals, by drug, poisoning
    pituitary-dependent E24.0
    specified type NEC E24.8
cryopyrin-associated periodic M04.2
cryptophthalmos Q87.0
cystic duct stump K91.5
cytokine release D89.839
    grade 1 D89.831
    grade 2 D89.832
    grade 3 D89.833
    grade 4 D89.834
    grade 5 D89.835
Dana-Putnam D51.0
Danbolt (-Cross) (acrodermatitis
    enteropathica) E83.2
Dandy-Walker Q03.1
    with spina bifida Q07.01
Danlos' (see also Syndrome, Ehlers-Danlos)
    Q79.60

Syndrome (Continued)
defibrination —see also Fibrinolysis
    with
        antepartum hemorrhage —see
            Hemorrhage, antepartum, with
            coagulation defect
        intrapartum hemorrhage —see
            Hemorrhage, complicating,
            delivery
        newborn P60
        postpartum O72.3
Degos' I77.8
Déjérine-Roussy G89.0
delayed sleep phase G47.21
demyelinating G37.9
dependence —see F10-F19 with fourth
    character .2
depersonalization (-derealization) F48.1
De Quervain E34.51
de Toni-Fanconi (-Debré) E72.09
    with cystinosis E72.04
de Vivo syndrome E74.810
diabetes mellitus-hypertension-nephrosis —
    see Diabetes, nephrosis
diabetes mellitus in newborn infant P70.2
diabetes-nephrosis —see Diabetes, nephrosis
diabetic amyotrophy —see Diabetes,
    amyotrophy
dialysis associated steal T82.898-●
Diamond-Blackfan D61.01
Diamond-Gardener D69.2
DIC (diffuse or disseminated intravascular
    coagulopathy) D65
di George's D82.1
Dighton's Q78.0
disequilibrium E87.8
Döhle body-panmyelopathic D72.0
dorsolateral medullary G46.4
double athetosis G80.3
Down (see also Down syndrome) Q90.9
Dravet (intractable) G40.834
    with status epilepticus G40.833
    without status epilepticus G40.834
Dresbach's (elliptocytosis) D58.1
DRESS (drug rash with eosinophilia and
    systemic symptoms) D72.12
Dressler's (postmyocardial infarction) I24.1
    postcardiotomy I97.0
drug rash with eosinophilia and systemic
    symptoms (DRESS) D72.12
drug withdrawal, infant of dependent mother
    P96.1
dry eye H04.12-●
due to abnormality
    chromosomal Q99.9
        sex
            female phenotype Q97.9
            male phenotype Q98.9
        specified NEC Q99.8
dumping (postgastrectomy) K91.1
    nonsurgical K31.89
Dupré's (meningism) R29.1
dysmetabolic X E88.81
dyspraxia, developmental F82
Eagle-Barrett Q79.4
Eaton-Lambert —see Syndrome, Lambert-Eaton
Ebstein's Q22.5
ectopic ACTH E24.3
eczema-thrombocytopenia D82.0
Eddowes' Q78.0
effort (psychogenic) F45.8
Ehlers-Danlos Q79.60
    classical (cEDS) (classical EDS) Q79.61
    hypermobile (hEDS) (hypermobile EDS)
        Q79.62
    specified NEC Q79.69
    vascular (vascular EDS) (vEDS) Q79.63
Eisenmenger's I27.83
Ekman's Q78.0
electric feet E53.8
Ellis-van Creveld Q77.6

Syndrome (Continued)
empty nest Z60.0
endocrine-hypertensive E27.0
entrapment —see Neuropathy, entrapment
eosinophilia-myalgia M35.89
epileptic —see also Epilepsy, by type
    absence G40.A09
        intractable G40.A19
            with status epilepticus G40.A11
            without status epilepticus G40.A19
        not intractable G40.A09
            with status epilepticus G40.A01
            without status epilepticus G40.A09
Erdheim-Chester (ECD) E88.89
Erdheim's E22.0
erythrocyte fragmentation D59.4
Evans D69.41
exhaustion F48.8
extrapyramidal G25.9
    specified NEC G25.89
eye retraction —see Strabismus
eyelid-malar-mandible Q87.0
Faber's D50.9
facet M47.89-●
► facet joint (see also Spondylosis) M47.819
facial pain, paroxysmal G50.0
Fallot's Q21.3
familial cold autoinflammatory M04.2
familial eczema-thrombocytopenia (Wiskott-
    Aldrich) D82.0
Fanconi (-de Toni) (-Debré) E72.09
    with cystinosis E72.04
Fanconi's (anemia) (congenital pancytopenia)
    D61.09
fatigue
    chronic R53.82
    psychogenic F48.8
faulty bowel habit K59.39
Feil-Klippel (brevicollis) Q76.1
Felty's —see Felty's syndrome
fertile eunuch E23.0
fetal
    alcohol (dysmorphic) Q86.0
    hydantoin Q86.1
Fiedler's I40.1
first arch Q87.0
fish odor E72.89
Fisher's G61.0
Fitzhugh-Curtis
    due to
        Chlamydia trachomatis A74.81
        Neisseria gonorrhorea (gonococcal
            peritonitis) A54.85
Fitz's —see also Pancreatitis, acute K85.80
Flajani (-Basedow) E05.00
    with thyroid storm E05.01
flatback —see Flatback syndrome
floppy
    baby P94.2
    iris (intraoeprative) (IFIS) H21.81
    mitral valve I34.1
flush E34.0
Foix-Alajouanine G95.19
Fong's Q87.2
food protein-induced enterocolitis (FPIES)
    K52.21
foramen magnum G93.5
Foster-Kennedy H47.14-●
Foville's (peduncular) G46.3
fragile X Q99.2
Franceschetti Q75.4
Frey's
    auriculotemporal G50.8
    hyperhidrosis L74.52
Friderichsen-Waterhouse A39.1
Froin's G95.89
frontal lobe F07.0
Fukuhara E88.49
functional
    bowel K59.9
    prepubertal castrate E29.1
Gaisböck's D75.1

Syndrome *(Continued)*
  ganglion (basal ganglia brain) G25.9
    geniculi G51.1
  Gardner-Diamond D69.2
  gastroesophageal
    junction K22.0
    laceration-hemorrhage K22.6
  gastrojejunal loop obstruction K91.89
  Gee-Herter-Heubner K90.0
  Gelineau's G47.419
    with cataplexy G47.411
  genito-anorectal A55
  Gerstmann-Sträussler-Scheinker (GSS) A81.82
  Gianotti-Crosti L44.4
  giant platelet (Bernard-Soulier) D69.1
  Gilles de la Tourette's F95.2
  Glass Q87.89
  Gleich's D72.118
  goiter-deafness E07.1
  Goldberg Q89.8
  Goldberg-Maxwell E34.51
  Good's D83.8
  Gopalan' (burning feet) E53.8
  Gorlin's Q87.89
  Gougerot-Blum L81.7
  Gouley's I31.1
  Gower's R55
  gray or grey (newborn) P93.0
    platelet D69.1
  Gubler-Millard G46.3
  Guillain-Barré (-Strohl) G61.0
  gustatory sweating G50.8
  Hadfield-Clarke K86.89
  hair tourniquet —*see* Constriction, external,
    by site
  Hamman's J98.19
  hand-foot L27.1
  hand-shoulder G90.8
  hantavirus (cardio)-pulmonary (HPS) (HCPS)
    B33.4
  happy puppet Q93.51
  Harada's H30.81-•
  Hayem-Faber D50.9
  headache NEC G44.89
    complicated NEC G44.59
  Heberden's I20.8
  Hedinger's E34.0
  Hegglin's D72.0
  HELLP (hemolysis, elevated liver enzymes
    and low platelet count) O14.2-•
    complicating
      childbirth O14.24
        puerperium O14.25
  hemolytic-uremic D59.3
  hemophagocytic, infection-associated D76.2
  Henoch-Schönlein D69.0
  hepatic flexure K59.89
  hepatopulmonary K76.81
  hepatorenal K76.7
    following delivery O90.4
    postoperative or postprocedural K91.83
    postpartum, puerperal O90.4
  hepatourologic K76.7
▶ hereditary alpha tryptasemia D89.44
  Herter (-Gee) (nontropical sprue) K90.0
  Heubner-Herter K90.0
  Heyd's K76.7
  Hilger's G90.09
  histamine-like (fish poisoning) —*see*
    Poisoning, fish
  histiocytic D76.3
  histiocytosis NEC D76.3
  HIV infection, acute B20
  Hoffmann-Werdnig G12.0
  Hollander-Simons E88.1
  Hoppe-Goldflam G70.00
    with exacerbation (acute) G70.01
    in crisis G70.01
  Horner's G90.2
  hungry bone E83.81
  hunterian glossitis D51.0
  Hutchinson's triad A50.53

Syndrome *(Continued)*
  hyperabduction G54.0
  hyperammonemia-hyperornithinemia-
    homocitrullinemia E72.4
  hypereosinophilic (HES) D72.119
    idiopathic (IHES) D72.110
    lymphocytic variant (LHES) D72.111
  ▶ myeloid D72.118
    specified NEC D72.118
  hyperimmunoglobulin D M04.1
  hyperimmunoglobulin E (IgE) D82.4
  hyperkalemic E87.5
  hyperkinetic —*see* Hyperkinesia
  hypermobility M35.7
  hypernatremia E87.0
  hyperosmolarity E87.0
  hyperperfusion G97.82
  hypersplenic D73.1
  hypertransfusion, newborn P61.1
  hyperventilation F45.8
  hyperviscosity (of serum)
    polycythemic D75.1
    sclerothymic D58.8
  hypoglycemic (familial) (neonatal) E16.2
  hypokalemic E87.6
  hyponatremic E87.1
  hypopituitarism E23.0
  hypoplastic left-heart Q23.4
  hypopotassemia E87.6
  hyposmolality E87.1
  hypotension, maternal O26.5-•
  hypothenar hammer I73.89
  hypoventilation, obesity (OHS) E66.2
  ICF (intravascular coagulation-fibrinolysis) D65
  idiopathic
    cardiorespiratory distress, newborn P22.0
    nephrotic (infantile) N04.9
  iliotibial band M76.3-•
  immobility, immobilization (paraplegic) M62.3
  ▶ immune effector cell-associated neurotoxicity
    (ICANS) G92.00
    ▶ grade
      ▶ 1 G92.01
      ▶ 2 G92.02
      ▶ 3 G92.03
      ▶ 4 G92.04
      ▶ 5 G92.05
      ▶ unspecified G92.00
  immune reconstitution D89.3
  immune reconstitution inflammatory [IRIS]
    D89.3
  immunity deficiency, combined D81.9
  immunodeficiency
    acquired —*see* Human, immunodeficiency
      virus (HIV) disease
    combined D81.9
  impending coronary I20.0
  impingement, shoulder M75.4-•
  inappropriate secretion of antidiuretic
    hormone E22.2
  infant
    gestational diabetes P70.0
    of diabetic mother P70.1
  infantilism (pituitary) E23.0
  inferior vena cava I87.1
  inspissated bile (newborn) P59.1
  institutional (childhood) F94.2
  insufficient sleep F51.12
  intermediate coronary (artery) I20.0
  interspinous ligament —*see* Spondylopathy,
    specified NEC
  intestinal
    carcinoid E34.0
    knot K56.2
  intravascular coagulation-fibrinolysis (ICF)
    D65
  iodine-deficiency, congenital E00.9
    type
      mixed E00.2
      myxedematous E00.1
      neurological E00.0
  IRDS (idiopathic respiratory distress,
    newborn) P22.0

Syndrome *(Continued)*
  irritable
    bowel K58.9
      with
        constipation K58.1
        diarrhea K58.0
      mixed K58.2
      psychogenic F45.8
      specified NEC K58.8
    heart (psychogenic) F45.8
    weakness F48.8
  ischemic
    bowel (transient) K55.9
      chronic K55.1
      due to mesenteric artery insufficiency
        K55.1
    steal T82.898
  IVC (intravascular coagulopathy) D65
  Ivemark's Q89.01
  Jaccoud's —*see* Arthropathy, postrheumatic,
    chronic
  Jackson's G83.89
  Jakob-Creutzfeldt —*see* Creutzfeldt-Jakob
    disease or syndrome
  jaw-winking Q07.8
  Jervell-Lange-Nielsen I45.81
  jet lag G47.25
  Job's D71
  Joseph-Diamond-Blackfan D61.01
  jugular foramen G52.7
  Kabuki Q89.8
  Kanner's (autism) F84.0
  Kartagener's Q89.3
  Kelly's D50.1
  Kimmelstiel-Wilson —*see* Diabetes,specified
    type, with Kimmelstiel-Wilson disease
  Klein (e)-Levine G47.13
  Klippel-Feil (brevicollis) Q76.1
  Köhler-Pellegrini-Steida —*see* Bursitis, tibial
    collateral
  König's K59.89
  Korsakoff (-Wernicke) (nonalcoholic) F04
    alcoholic F10.26
  Kostmann's D70.0
  Krabbe's congenital muscle hypoplasia Q79.8
  labyrinthine —*see* subcategory H83.2
  lacunar NEC G46.7
  Lambert-Eaton G70.80
    in
      neoplastic disease G73.1
      specified disease NEC G70.81
  Landau-Kleffner —*see* Epilepsy, specified NEC
  Larsen's Q74.8
  lateral
    cutaneous nerve of thigh G57.1-•
    medullary G46.4
  Launois' E22.0
  lazy
    leukocyte D70.8
    posture M62.3
  Lemiere I80.8
  Lennox-Gastaut G40.812
    intractable G40.814
      with status epilepticus G40.813
      without status epilepticus G40.814
    not intractable G40.812
      with status epilepticus G40.811
      without status epilepticus G40.812
  lenticular, progressive E83.01
  Leopold-Levi's E05.90
  Lev's I44.2
  Li-Fraumeni Z15.01
  Lichtheim's D51.0
  Lightwood's N25.89
  Lignac (de Toni) (-Fanconi) (-Debré)
    E72.09
    with cystinosis E72.04
  Likoff's I20.8
  limbic epilepsy personality F07.0
  liver-kidney K76.7
  lobotomy F07.0
  Löffler's J82.89
  long arm 18 or 21 deletion Q93.89

Syndrome *(Continued)*
  long QT I45.81
  Louis-Barré G11.3
  low
    atmospheric pressure T70.29
  ➡back M54.50
    output (cardiac) I50.9
  lower radicular, newborn (birth injury) P14.8
  Luetscher's (dehydration) E86.0
  Lupus anticoagulant D68.62
  Lutembacher's Q21.1
  macrophage activation D76.1
    due to infection D76.2
  magnesium-deficiency R29.0
  Majeed M04.8
  Mal de Debarquement R42
  malabsorption K90.9
    postsurgical K91.2
  malformation, congenital, due to
    alcohol Q86.0
    exogenous cause NEC Q86.8
    hydantoin Q86.1
    warfarin Q86.2
  malignant
    carcinoid E34.0
    neuroleptic G21.0
  Mallory-Weiss K22.6
  mandibulofacial dysostosis Q75.4
  manic-depressive —*see* Disorder, bipolar
  maple-syrup-urine E71.0
  Marable's I77.4
  Marfan's Q87.40
    with
      cardiovascular manifestations Q87.418
        aortic dilation Q87.410
      ocular manifestations Q87.42
      skeletal manifestations Q87.43
  Marie's (acromegaly) E22.0
  mast cell activation —*see* Activation, mast cell
  maternal hypotension —*see* Syndrome,
    hypotension, maternal
  May (-Hegglin) D72.0
  McArdle (-Schmidt) (-Pearson) E74.04
  McQuarrie's E16.2
  meconium plug (newborn) P76.0
  median arcuate ligament I77.4
  Meekeren-Ehlers-Danlos Q79.6
  megavitamin-B6 E67.2
  Meige G24.4
  MELAS E88.41
  Mendelson's O74.0
  MERRF (myoclonic epilepsy associated with
    ragged-red fibers) E88.42
  mesenteric
    artery (superior) K55.1
    vascular insufficiency K55.1
  metabolic E88.81
  metastatic carcinoid E34.0
  micrognathia-glossoptosis Q87.0
  midbrain NEC G93.89
  middle lobe (lung) J98.19
  middle radicular G54.0
  migraine —*see also* Migraine G43.909- •
  Mikulicz' K11.8
  milk-alkali E83.52
  Millard-Gubler G46.3
  Miller-Dieker Q93.88
  Miller-Fisher G61.0
  Minkowski-Chauffard D58.0
  Mirizzi's K83.1
  MNGIE (Mitochondrial Neurogastrointestinal
    Encephalopathy) E88.49
  Möbius, ophthalmoplegic migraine —*see*
    Migraine, ophthalmoplegic
  monofixation H50.42
  Morel-Moore M85.2
  Morel-Morgagni M85.2
  Morgagni (-Morel) (-Stewart) M85.2
  Morgagni-Adams-Stokes I45.9
  Mounier-Kuhn Q32.4
    with bronchiectasis J47.9

Syndrome *(Continued)*
  Mounier-Kuhn *(Continued)*
    with bronchiectasis*(Continued)*
      with
        exacerbation (acute) J47.1
        lower respiratory infection J47.0
      acquired J98.09
        with bronchiectasis J47.9
          with
            exacerbation (acute) J47.1
            lower respiratory infection J47.0
  Muckle-Wells M04.2
  mucocutaneous lymph node (acute febrile)
    (MCLS) M30.3
  multiple endocrine neoplasia (MEN) —*see*
    Neoplasia, endocrine, multiple (MEN)
  multiple operations —*see* Disorder, factitious
  multisystem inflammatory (in adults) (in
    children) M35.81
  myasthenic G70.9
    in
      diabetes mellitus —*see* Diabetes,
        amyotrophy
      endocrine disease NEC E34.9 *[G73.3]*
      neoplastic disease —*see also* Neoplasm
        D49.9 *[G73.3]*
      thyrotoxicosis (hyperthyroidism) E05.90
        [G73.3]
        with thyroid storm E05.91 *[G73.3]*
  myelodysplastic D46.9
    with
      5q deletion D46.C
      isolated del (5q) chromosomal
        abnormality D46.C
      multilineage dysplasia D46.A
        with ringed sideroblasts D46.B
    lesions, low grade D46.20
    specified NEC D46.Z
  myeloid hypereosinophilic D72.118
  myelopathic pain G89.0
  myeloproliferative (chronic) D47.1
  myofascial pain M79.18
  Naffziger's G54.0
  nail patella Q87.2
  NARP (Neuropathy, Ataxia and Retinitis
    pigmentosa) E88.49
  neonatal abstinence P96.1
  nephritic —*see also* Nephritis
    with edema —*see* Nephrosis
    acute N00.9
    chronic N03.9
    rapidly progressive N01.9
  nephrotic (congenital) —*see also* Nephrosis
    N04.9
    with
      C3
        glomerulonephritis N04.A
        glomerulopathy N04.A
          with dense deposit disease N04.6
      dense deposit disease N04.6
      diffuse
        crescentic glomerulonephritis N04.7
        endocapillary proliferative
          glomerulonephritis N04.4
        membranous glomerulonephritis N04.2
        mesangial proliferative
          glomerulonephritis N04.3
        mesangiocapillary glomerulonephritis
          N04.5
      focal and segmental glomerular lesions
        N04.1
      minor glomerular abnormality N04.0
      specified morphological changes NEC
        N04.8
    diabetic —*see* Diabetes, nephrosis
  neurologic neglect R41.4
  Nezelof's D81.4
  Nonne-Milroy-Meige Q82.0
  Nothnagel's vasomotor acroparesthesia I73.89
  obesity hypoventilation (OHS) E66.2
  oculomotor H51.9
  Ogilvie K59.81

Syndrome *(Continued)*
  ophthalmoplegia-cerebellar ataxia —*see*
    Strabismus, paralytic, third nerve
  oral allergy T78.1
  oral-facial-digital Q87.0
  organic
    affective F06.30
    amnesic (not alcohol- or drug-induced) F04
    brain F09
    depressive F06.31
    hallucinosis F06.0
    personality F07.0
  Ormond's N13.5
  oro-facial-digital Q87.0
  os trigonum Q68.8
  Osler-Weber-Rendu I78.0
  osteoporosis-osteomalacia M83.8
  Osterreicher-Turner Q87.2
  otolith —*see* subcategory H81.8
  oto-palatal-digital Q87.0
  outlet (thoracic) G54.0
  ovary
    polycystic E28.2
    resistant E28.39
    sclerocystic E28.2
  Owren's D68.2
  Paget-Schroetter I82.890
  pain —*see also* Pain
    complex regional I G90.50
      lower limb G90.52- •
      specified site NEC G90.59
      upper limb G90.51- •
    complex regional II —*see* Causalgia
  painful
    bruising D69.2
    feet E53.8
    prostate N42.81
  paralysis agitans —*see* Parkinsonism
  paralytic G83.9
    specified NEC G83.89
  Parinaud's H51.0
  parkinsonian —*see* Parkinsonism
  Parkinson's —*see* Parkinsonism
  paroxysmal facial pain G50.0
  Parry's E05.00
    with thyroid storm E05.01
  Parsonage (-Aldren)-Turner G54.5
  patella clunk M25.86- •
  Paterson (-Brown) (-Kelly) D50.1
  pectoral girdle I77.89
  pectoralis minor I77.89
  pediatric autoimmune neuropsychiatric
    disorders associated with streptococcal
    infections (PANDAS) D89.89
  pediatric inflammatory multisystem M35.81
  Pelger-Huet D72.0
  pellagra-cerebellar ataxia-renal
    aminoaciduria E72.02
  pellagroid E52
  Pellegrini-Stieda —*see* Bursitis, tibial collateral
  pelvic congestion-fibrosis, female N94.89
  penta X Q97.1
  peptic ulcer —*see* Ulcer, peptic
  perabduction I77.89
  periodic fever M04.1
  periodic fever, aphthous stomatitis, pharyngitis,
    and adenopathy [PFAPA] M04.8
  periodic headache, in adults and children —
    see Headache, periodic syndromes in
    adults and children
  periurethral fibrosis N13.5
  phantom limb (without pain) G54.7
    with pain G54.6
  pharyngeal pouch D82.1
  Pick's —*see* Disease, Pick's
  Pickwickian E66.2
  PIE (pulmonary infiltration with
    eosinophilia) J82.89
  pigmentary pallidal degeneration
    (progressive) G23.0
  pineal E34.8
  pituitary E22.0

▶ New ⟹ Revised ~~deleted~~ Deleted • Use Additional Character(s)

Syndrome *(Continued)*
  placental transfusion —*see* Pregnancy,
    complicated by, placental transfusion
    syndromes
  plantar fascia M72.2
  plateau iris (post-iridectomy)
    (postprocedural) H21.82
  Plummer-Vinson D50.1
  pluricarential of infancy E40
  plurideficiency E40
  pluriglandular (compensatory) E31.8
    autoimmune E31.0
  pneumatic hammer T75.21
  polyangiitis overlap M30.8
  polycarential of infancy E40
  polyglandular E31.8
    autoimmune E31.0
  polysplenia Q89.09
  pontine NEC G93.89
  popliteal
    artery entrapment I77.89
    web Q87.89
  postcardiac injury
    postcardiotomy I97.0
    postmyocardial infarction I24.1
  postcardiotomy I97.0
  post chemoembolization — code to
    associated conditions
  postcholecystectomy K91.5
  postcommissurotomy I97.0
  postconcussional F07.81
  postcontusional F07.81
▶post-COVID (-19) U09.9
  postencephalitic F07.89
  post endometrial ablation N99.85
  posterior
    cervical sympathetic M53.0
    cord G83.83
    fossa compression G93.5
    reversible encephalopathy (PRES) I67.83
  postgastrectomy (dumping) K91.1
  postgastric surgery K91.1
  postinfarction I24.1
  postlaminectomy NEC M96.1
  postleukotomy F07.0
  postmastectomy lymphedema I97.2
  postmyocardial infarction I24.1
  postoperative NEC T81.9
    blind loop K90.2
  postpartum panhypopituitary (Sheehan) E23.0
  postpolio (myelitic) G14
  postthrombotic I87.009
    with
      inflammation I87.02-●
        with ulcer I87.03-●
      specified complication NEC I87.09-●
      ulcer I87.01-●
        with inflammation I87.03-●
    asymptomatic I87.00-●
  postvagotomy K91.1
  postvalvulotomy I97.0
  postviral NEC G93.3
    fatigue G93.3
  Potain's K31.0
  potassium intoxication E87.5
  Prader-Willi Q87.11
  Prader-Willi-like Q87.19
  precerebral artery (multiple) (bilateral) G45.2
  preinfarction I20.0
  preleukemic D46.9
  premature senility E34.8
  premenstrual dysphoric F32.81
  premenstrual tension N94.3
  Prinzmetal-Massumi R07.1
  prune belly Q79.4
  pseudocarpal tunnel (sublimis) —*see*
    Syndrome, carpal tunnel
  pseudoparalytica G70.00
    with exacerbation (acute) G70.01
    in crisis G70.01
  pseudo-Turner's Q87.19

Syndrome *(Continued)*
  psycho-organic (nonpsychotic severity) F07.9
    acute or subacute F05
    depressive type F06.31
    hallucinatory type F06.0
    nonpsychotic severity F07.0
    specified NEC F07.89
  pulmonary
    arteriosclerosis I27.0
    dysmaturity (Wilson-Mikity) P27.0
    hypoperfusion (idiopathic) P22.0
    renal (hemorrhagic) (Goodpasture's) M31.0
  pure
    motor lacunar G46.5
    sensory lacunar G46.6
  Putnam-Dana D51.0
  pyogenic arthritis, pyoderma gangrenosum,
    and acne [PAPA] M04.8
  pyramidopallidonigral G20
  pyriformis —*see* Lesion, nerve, sciatic
  QT interval prolongation I45.81
  radicular NEC —*see* Radiculopathy
    upper limbs, newborn (birth injury) P14.3
  rapid time-zone change G47.25
  Rasmussen G04.81
  Raymond (-Céstan) I65.8
  Raynaud's I73.00
    with gangrene I73.01
  RDS (respiratory distress syndrome,
    newborn) P22.0
  reactive airways dysfunction J68.3
  Refsum's G60.1
  Reifenstein E34.52
  renal glomerulohyalinosis-diabetic —*see*
    Diabetes, nephrosis
  Rendu-Osler-Weber I78.0
  residual ovary N99.83
  resistant ovary E28.39
  respiratory
    distress
      acute J80
        adult J80
        child J80
        idiopathic J84.114
      newborn (idiopathic) (type I) P22.0
        type II P22.1
  restless legs G25.81
  retinoblastoma (familial) C69.2
  retroperitoneal fibrosis N13.5
  retroviral seroconversion (acute) Z21
  Reye's G93.7
  Richter —*see* Leukemia, chronic lymphocytic,
    B-cell type
  Ridley's I50.1
  right
    heart, hypoplastic Q22.6
    ventricular obstruction —*see* Failure, heart,
      right
  Romano-Ward (prolonged QT interval) I45.81
  rotator cuff, shoulder —*see also* Tear, rotator
    cuff M75.10-●
  Rotes Quérol —*see* Hyperostosis, ankylosing
  Roth —*see* Meralgia paresthetica
  rubella (congenital) P35.0
  Ruvalcaba-Myhre-Smith E71.440
  Rytand-Lipsitch I44.2
  salt
    depletion E87.1
      due to heat NEC T67.8
        causing heat exhaustion or prostration
          T67.4
    low E87.1
  salt-losing N28.89
  SATB2-associated Q87.89
  Scaglietti-Dagnini E22.0
  scalenus anticus (anterior) G54.0
  scapulocostal —*see* Mononeuropathy, upper
    limb, specified site NEC
  scapuloperoneal G71.09
  schizophrenic, of childhood NEC F84.5
  Schnitzler D47.2
  Scholte's E34.0

Syndrome *(Continued)*
  Schroeder's E27.0
  Schüller-Christian C96.5
  Schwachman's —*see* Syndrome, Shwachman's
  Schwartz (-Jampel) G71.13
  Schwartz-Bartter E22.2
  scimitar Q26.8
  sclerocystic ovary E28.2
  Seitelberger's G31.89
  septicemic adrenal hemorrhage A39.1
  seroconversion, retroviral (acute) Z21
  serous meningitis G93.2
  severe acute respiratory (SARS) J12.81
  coronavirus 2 -*see also* COVID-19 U07.1
    pneumonia J12.82
  shaken infant T74.4
  shock (traumatic) T79.4
    kidney N17.0
      following crush injury T79.5
    toxic A48.3
  shock-lung J80
  Shone's — code to specific anomalies
  short
    bowel K91.2
    rib Q77.2
  shoulder-hand —*see* Algoneurodystrophy
  Shwachman's D70.4
▸sicca —*see* Syndrome, Sjögren
  sick
    cell E87.1
    sinus I49.5
  sick-euthyroid E07.81
  sideropenic D50.1
  Siemens' ectodermal dysplasia Q82.4
  Silfversköld's Q78.9
  Simons' E88.1
  sinus tarsi M25.57-●
  sinusitis-bronchiectasis-situs inversus Q89.3
  Sipple's E31.22
  sirenomelia Q87.2
▶Sjögren M35.00
  ▶with
    ▶central nervous system involvement
      M35.07
    ▶dental involvement M35.0C
    ▶gastrointestinal involvement M35.08
    ▶glomerular disease M35.0A
    ▶inflammatory arthritis M35.05
    ▶keratoconjunctivitis M35.01
    ▶lung involvement M35.02
    ▶myopathy M35.03
    ▶peripheral nervous system involvement
      M35.06
    ▶renal tubular acidosis M35.04
    ▶specified organ involvement, NEC
      M35.09
    ▶tubulo-interstitial nephropathy M35.04
    ▶vasculitis M35.0B
  Slocumb's E27.0
  slow flow, coronary I20.8
  Sluder's G44.89
  Smith-Magenis Q93.88
  Sneddon-Wilkinson L13.1
  Sotos' Q87.3
  South African cardiomyopathy I42.8
  spasmodic
    upward movement, eyes H51.8
    winking F95.8
  Spen's I45.9
  splenic
    agenesis Q89.01
    flexure K59.89
    neutropenia D73.81
  Spurway's Q78.0
  staphylococcal scalded skin L00
  steal
    arteriovenous T82.898-●
    ischemic T82.898-●
    subclavian G45.8
  Stein-Leventhal E28.2
  Stein's E28.2
  Stevens-Johnson syndrome L51.1
    toxic epidermal necrolysis overlap L51.3

Syndrome *(Continued)*
Stewart-Morel M85.2
Stickler Q89.8
stiff baby Q89.8
stiff man G25.82
Still-Felty —*see* Felty's syndrome
Stokes (-Adams) I45.9
stone heart I50.1
straight back, congenital Q76.49
subclavian steal G45.8
subcoracoid-pectoralis minor G54.0
subcostal nerve compression I77.89
subphrenic interposition Q43.3
superior
  cerebellar artery I63.89
  mesenteric artery K55.1
  semi-circular canal dehiscence H83.8X-●
  vena cava I87.1
supine hypotensive (maternal) —*see*
  Syndrome, hypotension, maternal
suprarenal cortical E27.0
supraspinatus —*see also* Tear, rotator cuff
  M75.10-●
Susac G93.49
swallowed blood P78.2
sweat retention L74.0
Swyer Q99.1
Symond's G93.2
sympathetic
  cervical paralysis G90.2
  pelvic, female N94.89
systemic inflammatory response (SIRS), of
  non-infectious origin (without organ
  dysfunction) R65.10
  with acute organ dysfunction R65.11
tachycardia-bradycardia I49.5
takotsubo I51.81
TAR (thrombocytopenia with absent radius)
  Q87.2
tarsal tunnel G57.5-●
teething K00.7
tegmental G93.89
telangiectasic-pigmentation-cataract Q82.8
temporal pyramidal apex —*see* Otitis, media,
  suppurative, acute
temporomandibular joint-pain-dysfunction
  M26.62-●
Terry's —*see also* Myopia, degenerative
  H44.2-●
testicular feminization —*see also* Syndrome,
  androgen insensitivity E34.51
thalamic pain (hyperesthetic) G89.0
thoracic outlet (compression) G54.0
Thorson-Björck E34.0
thrombocytopenia with absent radius (TAR)
  Q87.2
thyroid-adrenocortical insufficiency E31.0
tibial
  anterior M76.81-●
  posterior M76.82-●
Tietze's M94.0
time-zone (rapid) G47.25
Toni-Fanconi E72.09
  with cystinosis E72.04
Touraine's Q79.8
tourniquet —*see* Constriction, external, by site
toxic shock A48.3
transient left ventricular apical ballooning
  I51.81
traumatic vasospastic T75.22
Treacher Collins Q75.4
triple X, female Q97.0
trisomy Q92.9
  13 Q91.7
    meiotic nondisjunction Q91.4
    mitotic nondisjunction Q91.5
    mosaicism Q91.5
    translocation Q91.6
  18 Q91.3
    meiotic nondisjunction Q91.0
    mitotic nondisjunction Q91.1
    mosaicism Q91.1
    translocation Q91.2

Syndrome *(Continued)*
trisomy Q92.9
  20 (q)(p) Q92.8
  21 Q90.9
    meiotic nondisjunction Q90.0
    mitotic nondisjunction Q90.1
    mosaicism Q90.1
    translocation Q90.2
  22 Q92.8
tropical wet feet T69.0-●
Trousseau's I82.1
tumor lysis (following antineoplastic
  chemotherapy) (spontaneous) NEC E88.3
tumor necrosis factor receptor associated
  periodic (TRAPS) M04.1
Twiddler's (due to)
  automatic implantable defibrillator T82.198
  cardiac pacemaker T82.198
Unverricht (-Lundborg) —*see* Epilepsy,
  generalized, idiopathic
upward gaze H51.8
uremia, chronic —*see also* Disease, kidney,
  chronic N18.9
urethral N34.3
urethro-oculo-articular —*see* Reiter's disease
urohepatic K76.7
vago-hypoglossal G52.7
van Buchem's M85.2
van der Hoeve's Q78.0
vascular NEC in cerebrovascular disease G46.8
vasoconstriction, reversible cerebrovascular
  I67.841
vasomotor I73.9
vasospastic (traumatic) T75.22
vasovagal R55
VATER Q87.2
velo-cardio-facial Q93.81
vena cava (inferior) (superior) (obstruction)
  I87.1
vertebral
  artery G45.0
    compression —*see* Syndrome, anterior,
    spinal artery, compression
  steal G45.0
vertebro-basilar artery G45.0
➠vertebrogenic (pain) (*see also* Pain,
  vertebrogenic) M54.89
vertiginous —*see* Disorder, vestibular function
Vinson-Plummer D50.1
virus B34.9
visceral larva migrans B83.0
visual disorientation H53.8
vitamin B6 deficiency E53.1
vitreal corneal H59.01-●
vitreous (touch) H59.01-●
Vogt-Koyanagi H20.82-●
Volkmann's T79.6
von Schroetter's I82.890
von Willebrand (-Jürgen) D68.0
Waldenström-Kjellberg D50.1
Wallenberg's G46.3
water retention E87.79
Waterhouse (-Friderichsen) A39.1
Weber-Gubler G46.3
Weber-Leyden G46.3
Weber's G46.3
Wegener's M31.30
  with
    kidney involvement M31.31
    lung involvement M31.30
      with kidney involvement M31.31
Weingarten's (tropical eosinophilia) J82.89
Weiss-Baker G90.09
Werdnig-Hoffman G12.0
Werner's E31.21
Werner's E34.8
Wernicke-Korsakoff (nonalcoholic) F04
  alcoholic F10.26
West's —*see* Epilepsy, spasms
Westphal-Strümpell E83.01
wet
  feet (maceration) (tropical) T69.0-●
  lung, newborn P22.1

Syndrome *(Continued)*
whiplash S13.4
whistling face Q87.0
Wilkie's K55.1
Wilkinson-Sneddon L13.1
Willebrand (-Jürgens) D68.0
Williams Q93.82
Wilson's (hepatolenticular degeneration) E83.01
Wiskott-Aldrich D82.0
withdrawal —*see* Withdrawal, state
  drug
    infant of dependent mother P96.1
    therapeutic use, newborn P96.2
Woakes' (ethmoiditis) J33.1
Wright's (hyperabduction) G54.0
X I20.9
XXXX Q97.1
XXXXX Q97.1
XXXXY Q98.1
XXY Q98.0
Yao M04.8
yellow nail L60.5
Zahorsky's B08.5
Zellweger syndrome E71.510
Zellweger-like syndrome E71.541
Synechia (anterior) (iris) (posterior) (pupil) —
  see also Adhesions, iris
  intra-uterine (traumatic) N85.6
Synesthesia R20.8
Syngamiasis, syngamosis B83.3
Synodontia K00.2
Synorchidism, synorchism Q55.1
Synostosis (congenital) Q78.8
  astragalo-scaphoid Q74.2
  radioulnar Q74.0
Synovial sarcoma —*see* Neoplasm, connective
  tissue, malignant
Synovioma (malignant) —*see also* Neoplasm,
  connective tissue, malignant
  benign —*see* Neoplasm, connective tissue,
    benign
Synoviosarcoma —*see* Neoplasm, connective
  tissue, malignant
Synovitis —*see also* Tenosynovitis M65.9
  crepitant
    hand M70.0-●
    wrist M70.03-●
  gonococcal A54.49
  gouty —*see* Gout
  in (due to)
    crystals M65.8-●
    gonorrhea A54.49
    syphilis (late) A52.78
    use, overuse, pressure —*see* Disorder, soft
      tissue, due to use
  infective NEC —*see* Tenosynovitis, infective
    NEC
  specified NEC —*see* Tenosynovitis, specified
    type NEC
  syphilitic A52.78
    congenital (early) A50.02
  toxic —*see* Synovitis, transient
  transient M67.3-●
    ankle M67.37-●
    elbow M67.32-●
    foot joint M67.37-●
    hand joint M67.34-●
    hip M67.35-●
    knee M67.36-●
    multiple site M67.39
    pelvic region M67.35-●
    shoulder M67.31-●
    specified joint NEC M67.38
    wrist M67.33-●
  traumatic, current —*see* Sprain
  tuberculous —*see* Tuberculosis, synovitis
  villonodular (pigmented) M12.2-●
    ankle M12.27-●
    elbow M12.22-●
    foot joint M12.27-●
    hand joint M12.24-●
    hip M12.25-●
    knee M12.26-●

▶ New   ➠ Revised   ~~deleted~~ Deleted   ● Use Additional Character(s)

Synovitis(Continued)
  villonodular(Continued)
    multiple site M12.29
    pelvic region M12.25-●
    shoulder M12.21-●
    specified joint NEC M12.28
    vertebrae M12.28
    wrist M12.23-●
Syphilid A51.39
  congenital A50.06
  newborn A50.06
  tubercular (late) A52.79
Syphilis, syphilitic (acquired) A53.9
  abdomen (late) A52.79
  acoustic nerve A52.15
  adenopathy (secondary) A51.49
  adrenal (gland) (with cortical hypofunction)
      A52.79
  age under 2 years NOS —see also Syphilis,
      congenital, early
    acquired A51.9
  alopecia (secondary) A51.32
  anemia (late) A52.79 [D63.8]
  aneurysm (aorta) (ruptured) A52.01
    central nervous system A52.05
    congenital A50.54 [I79.0]
  anus (late) A52.74
    primary A51.1
    secondary A51.39
  aorta (arch) (abdominal) (thoracic) A52.02
    aneurysm A52.01
  aortic (insufficiency) (regurgitation)
      (stenosis)A52.03
    aneurysm A52.01
  arachnoid (adhesive) (cerebral) (spinal) A52.13
  asymptomatic —see Syphilis, latent
  ataxia (locomotor) A52.11
  atrophoderma maculatum A51.39
  auricular fibrillation A52.06
  bladder (late) A52.76
  bone A52.77
    secondary A51.46
  brain A52.17
  breast (late) A52.79
  bronchus (late) A52.72
  bubo (primary) A51.0
  bulbar palsy A52.19
  bursa (late) A52.78
  cardiac decompensation A52.06
  cardiovascular A52.00
  central nervous system (late) (recurrent)
      (relapse) (tertiary) A52.3
    with
      ataxia A52.11
      general paralysis A52.17
        juvenile A50.45
      paresis (general) A52.17
        juvenile A50.45
      tabes (dorsalis) A52.11
        juvenile A50.45
      taboparesis A52.17
        juvenile A50.45
    aneurysm A52.05
    congenital A50.40
    juvenile A50.40
    remission in (sustained) A52.3
    serology doubtful, negative, or positive A52.3
    specified nature or site NEC A52.19
    vascular A52.05
  cerebral A52.17
    meningovascular A52.13
    nerves (multiple palsies) A52.15
    sclerosis A52.17
    thrombosis A52.05
  cerebrospinal (tabetic type) A52.12
  cerebrovascular A52.05
  cervix (late) A52.76
  chancre (multiple) A51.0
    extragenital A51.2
    Rollet's A51.0
  Charcot's joint A52.16
  chorioretinitis A51.43
    congenital A50.01

Syphilis, syphilitic (Continued)
  chorioretinitis (Continued)
    late A52.71
    prenatal A50.01
  choroiditis —see Syphilitic chorioretinitis
  choroidoretinitis —see Syphilitic chorioretinitis
  ciliary body (secondary) A51.43
    late A52.71
  colon (late) A52.74
  combined spinal sclerosis A52.11
  condyloma (latum) A51.31
  congenital A50.9
    with
      paresis (general) A50.45
      tabes (dorsalis) A50.45
      taboparesis A50.45
    chorioretinitis, choroiditis A50.01 [H32]
    early, or less than 2 years after birth NEC
        A50.2
      with manifestations —see Syphilis,
          congenital, early, symptomatic
      latent (without manifestations) A50.1
        negative spinal fluid test A50.1
        serology positive A50.1
      symptomatic A50.09
        cutaneous A50.06
        mucocutaneous A50.07
        oculopathy A50.01
        osteochondropathy A50.02
        pharyngitis A50.03
        pneumonia A50.04
        rhinitis A50.05
        visceral A50.08
    interstitial keratitis A50.31
    juvenile neurosyphilis A50.45
    late, or 2 years or more after birth NEC A50.7
      chorioretinitis, choroiditis A50.32
      interstitial keratitis A50.31
      juvenile neurosyphilis A50.45
      latent (without manifestations) A50.6
        negative spinal fluid test A50.6
        serology positive A50.6
      symptomatic or with manifestations
          NEC A50.59
        arthropathy A50.55
        cardiovascular A50.54
        Clutton's joints A50.51
        Hutchinson's teeth A50.52
        Hutchinson's triad A50.53
        osteochondropathy A50.56
        saddle nose A50.57
  conjugal A53.9
    tabes A52.11
  conjunctiva (late) A52.71
  contact Z20.2
  cord bladder A52.19
  cornea, late A52.71
  coronary (artery) (sclerosis) A52.06
  coryza, congenital A50.05
  cranial nerve A52.15
    multiple palsies A52.15
  cutaneous —see Syphilis, skin
  dacryocystitis (late) A52.71
  degeneration, spinal cord A52.12
  dementia paralytica A52.17
    juvenilis A50.45
  destruction of bone A52.77
  dilatation, aorta A52.01
  due to blood transfusion A53.9
  dura mater A52.13
  ear A52.79
    inner A52.79
      nerve (eighth) A52.15
      neurorecurrence A52.15
  early A51.9
    cardiovascular A52.00
    central nervous system A52.3
    latent (without manifestations) (less than 2
        years after infection) A51.5
      negative spinal fluid test A51.5
      serological relapse after treatment A51.5
      serology positive A51.5
    relapse (treated, untreated) A51.9

Syphilis, syphilitic (Continued)
  early (Continued)
    skin A51.39
    symptomatic A51.9
      extragenital chancre A51.2
      primary, except extragenital chancre
          A51.0
      secondary —see also Syphilis, secondary
          A51.39
        relapse (treated, untreated) A51.49
    ulcer A51.39
  eighth nerve (neuritis) A52.15
  endemic A65
  endocarditis A52.03
    aortic A52.03
    pulmonary A52.03
  epididymis (late) A52.76
  epiglottis (late) A52.73
  epiphysitis (congenital) (early) A50.02
  episcleritis (late) A52.71
  esophagus A52.79
  eustachian tube A52.73
  exposure to Z20.2
  eye A52.71
  eyelid (late) (with gumma) A52.71
  fallopian tube (late) A52.76
  fracture A52.77
  gallbladder (late) A52.74
  gastric (polyposis) (late) A52.74
  general A53.9
    paralysis A52.17
      juvenile A50.45
  genital (primary) A51.0
  glaucoma A52.71
  gumma NEC A52.79
    cardiovascular system A52.00
    central nervous system A52.3
    congenital A50.59
  heart (block) (decompensation) (disease)
      (failure) A52.06 [I52]
    valve NEC A52.03
  hemianesthesia A52.19
  hemianopia A52.71
  hemiparesis A52.17
  hemiplegia A52.17
  hepatic artery A52.09
  hepatis A52.74
  hepatomegaly, congenital A50.08
  hereditaria tarda —see Syphilis, congenital,
      late
  hereditary —see Syphilis, congenital
  Hutchinson's teeth A50.52
  hyalitis A52.71
  inactive —see Syphilis, latent
  infantum —see Syphilis, congenital
  inherited —see Syphilis, congenital
  internal ear A52.79
  intestine (late) A52.74
  iris, iritis (secondary) A51.43
    late A52.71
  joint (late) A52.77
  keratitis (congenital) (interstitial) (late) A50.31
  kidney (late) A52.75
  lacrimal passages (late) A52.71
  larynx (late) A52.73
  late A52.9
    cardiovascular A52.00
    central nervous system A52.3
    kidney A52.75
    latent or 2 years or more after infection
        (without manifestations) A52.8
      negative spinal fluid test A52.8
      serology positive A52.8
    paresis A52.17
    specified site NEC A52.79
    symptomatic or with manifestations
        A52.79
    tabes A52.11
  latent A53.9
    with signs or symptoms - code by site and
        stage under Syphilis

Syphilis, syphilitic *(Continued)*
latent *(Continued)*
central nervous system A52.2
date of infection unspecified A53.0
early, or less than 2 years after infection
A51.5
follow-up of latent syphilis A53.0
date of infection unspecified A53.0
late, or 2 years or more after infection
A52.8
late, or 2 years or more after infection A52.8
positive serology (only finding) A53.0
date of infection unspecified A53.0
early, or less than 2 years after infection
A51.5
late, or 2 years or more after infection
A52.8
lens (late) A52.71
leukoderma A51.39
late A52.79
lienitis A52.79
lip A51.39
chancre (primary) A51.2
late A52.79
Lissauer's paralysis A52.17
liver A52.74
locomotor ataxia A52.11
lung A52.72
lymph gland (early) (secondary) A51.49
late A52.79
lymphadenitis (secondary) A51.49
macular atrophy of skin A51.39
striated A52.79
mediastinum (late) A52.73
meninges (adhesive) (brain) (spinal cord)
A52.13
meningitis A52.13
acute (secondary) A51.41
congenital A50.41
meningoencephalitis A52.14
meningovascular A52.13
congenital A50.41
mesarteritis A52.09
brain A52.04
middle ear A52.77
mitral stenosis A52.03
monoplegia A52.17
mouth (secondary) A51.39
late A52.79
mucocutaneous (secondary) A51.39
late A52.79
mucous
membrane (secondary) A51.39
late A52.79
patches A51.39
congenital A50.07
mulberry molars A50.52
muscle A52.78
myocardium A52.06
nasal sinus (late) A52.73
neonatorum —*see* Syphilis, congenital
nephrotic syndrome (secondary) A51.44
nerve palsy (any cranial nerve) A52.15
multiple A52.15
nervous system, central A52.3
neuritis A52.15
acoustic A52.15
neurorecidive of retina A52.19
neuroretinitis A52.19
newborn —*see* Syphilis, congenital
nodular superficial (late) A52.79
nonvenereal A65
nose (late) A52.73
saddle back deformity A50.57
occlusive arterial disease A52.09
oculopathy A52.71
ophthalmic (late) A52.71
optic nerve (atrophy) (neuritis) (papilla)
A52.15
orbit (late) A52.71

organic A53.9
osseous (late) A52.77
osteochondritis (congenital) (early) A50.02
[M90.80]
osteoporosis A52.77
ovary (late) A52.76
oviduct (late) A52.76
palate (late) A52.79
pancreas (late) A52.74
paralysis A52.17
general A52.17
juvenile A50.45
paresis (general) A52.17
juvenile A50.45
paresthesia A52.19
Parkinson's disease or syndrome A52.19
paroxysmal tachycardia A52.06
pemphigus (congenital) A50.06
penis (chancre) A51.0
late A52.76
pericardium A52.06
perichondritis, larynx (late) A52.73
periosteum (late) A52.77
congenital (early) A50.02 [M90.80]
early (secondary) A51.46
peripheral nerve A52.79
petrous bone (late) A52.77
pharynx (late) A52.73
secondary A51.39
pituitary (gland) A52.79
pleura (late) A52.73
pneumonia, white A50.04
pontine lesion A52.17
portal vein A52.09
primary A51.0
anal A51.1
and secondary —*see* Syphilis, secondary
central nervous system A52.3
extragenital chancre NEC A51.2
fingers A51.2
genital A51.0
lip A51.2
specified site NEC A51.2
tonsils A51.2
prostate (late) A52.76
ptosis (eyelid) A52.71
pulmonary (late) A52.72
artery A52.09
pyelonephritis (late) A52.75
recently acquired, symptomatic A51.9
rectum (late) A52.74
respiratory tract (late) A52.73
retina, late A52.71
retrobulbar neuritis A52.15
salpingitis A52.76
sclera (late) A52.71
sclerosis
cerebral A52.17
coronary A52.06
multiple A52.11
scotoma (central) A52.71
scrotum (late) A52.76
secondary (and primary) A51.49
adenopathy A51.49
anus A51.39
bone A51.46
chorioretinitis, choroiditis A51.43
hepatitis A51.45
liver A51.45
lymphadenitis A51.49
meningitis (acute) A51.41
mouth A51.39
mucous membranes A51.39
periosteum, periostitis A51.46
pharynx A51.39
relapse (treated, untreated) A51.49
skin A51.39
specified form NEC A51.49
tonsil A51.39

secondary *(Continued)*
ulcer A51.39
viscera NEC A51.49
vulva A51.39
seminal vesicle (late) A52.76
seronegative with signs or symptoms - code
by site and stage under Syphilis
seropositive
with signs or symptoms - code by site and
stage under Syphilis
follow-up of latent syphilis —*see* Syphilis,
latent
only finding —*see* Syphilis, latent
seventh nerve (paralysis) A52.15
sinus, sinusitis (late) A52.73
skeletal system A52.77
skin (with ulceration) (early) (secondary)
A51.39
late or tertiary A52.79
small intestine A52.74
spastic spinal paralysis A52.17
spermatic cord (late) A52.76
spinal (cord) A52.12
spleen A52.79
splenomegaly A52.79
spondylitis A52.77
staphyloma A52.71
stigmata (congenital) A50.59
stomach A52.74
synovium A52.78
tabes dorsalis (late) A52.11
juvenile A50.45
tabetic type A52.11
juvenile A50.45
taboparesis A52.17
juvenile A50.45
tachycardia A52.06
tendon (late) A52.78
tertiary A52.9
with symptoms NEC A52.79
cardiovascular A52.00
central nervous system A52.3
multiple NEC A52.79
specified site NEC A52.79
testis A52.76
thorax A52.73
throat A52.73
thymus (gland) (late) A52.79
thyroid (late) A52.79
tongue (late) A52.79
tonsil (lingual) (late) A52.73
primary A51.2
secondary A51.39
trachea (late) A52.73
tunica vaginalis (late) A52.76
ulcer (any site) (early) (secondary)
A51.39
late A52.79
perforating A52.79
foot A52.11
urethra (late) A52.76
urogenital (late) A52.76
uterus (late) A52.76
uveal tract (secondary) A51.43
late A52.71
uveitis (secondary) A51.43
late A52.71
uvula (late) (perforated) A52.79
vagina A51.0
late A52.76
valvulitis NEC A52.03
vascular A52.00
brain (cerebral) A52.05
ventriculi A52.74
vesicae urinariae (late) A52.76
viscera (abdominal) (late) A52.74
secondary A51.49
vitreous (opacities) (late) A52.71
hemorrhage A52.71

► New ⇒ Revised ~~deleted~~ Deleted • Use Additional Character(s)

Syphilis, syphilitic *(Continued)*
  vulva A51.0
    late A52.76
    secondary A51.39
Syphiloma A52.79
  cardiovascular system A52.00
  central nervous system A52.3
  circulatory system A52.00
  congenital A50.59
Syphilophobia F45.29
Syringadenoma —*see also* Neoplasm, skin, benign
  papillary —*see* Neoplasm, skin, benign

Syringobulbia G95.0
Syringocystadenoma —*see* Neoplasm, skin, benign
  papillary —*see* Neoplasm, skin, benign
Syringoma —*see also* Neoplasm, skin, benign
  chondroid —*see* Neoplasm, skin, benign
Syringomyelia G95.0
Syringomyelitis —*see* Encephalitis
Syringomyelocele —*see* Spina bifida
Syringopontia G95.0

System, systemic —*see also* condition
  disease, combined —*see* Degeneration, combined
  inflammatory response syndrome (SIRS) of non-infectious origin (without organ dysfunction) R65.10
    with acute organ dysfunction R65.11
  lupus erythematosus M32.9
    inhibitor present D68.62

S

T

Tabacism, tabacosis, tabagism —*see also*
    Poisoning, tobacco
    meaning dependence (without remission)
        F17.200
    with
        disorder F17.299
            in remission F17.211
            specified disorder NEC F17.298
            withdrawal F17.203
Tabardillo A75.9
    flea-borne A75.2
    louse-borne A75.0
Tabes, tabetic A52.10
    with
        central nervous system syphilis A52.10
        Charcot's joint A52.16
        cord bladder A52.19
        crisis, viscera (any) A52.19
        paralysis, general A52.17
        paresis (general) A52.17
        perforating ulcer (foot) A52.19
    arthropathy (Charcot) A52.16
    bladder A52.19
    bone A52.11
    cerebrospinal A52.12
    congenital A50.45
    conjugal A52.10
    dorsalis A52.11
        juvenile A50.49
    juvenile A50.49
    latent A52.19
    mesenterica A18.39
    paralysis, insane, general A52.17
    spasmodic A52.17
    syphilis (cerebrospinal) A52.12
Taboparalysis A52.17
Taboparesis (remission) A52.17
    juvenile A50.45
TAC (trigeminal autonomic cephalgia) NEC
        G44.099
    intractable G44.091
    not intractable G44.099
Tache noir S60.22-●
Tachyalimentation K91.2
Tachyarrhythmia, tachyrhythmia —*see*
        Tachycardia
Tachycardia R00.0
    atrial (paroxysmal) I47.1
    auricular I47.1
    AV nodal re-entry (re-entrant) I47.1
    junctional (paroxysmal) I47.1
    newborn P29.11
    nodal (paroxysmal) I47.1
    non-paroxysmal AV nodal I45.89
    paroxysmal (sustained) (nonsustained)
        I47.9
        with sinus bradycardia I49.5
        atrial (PAT) I47.1
        atrioventricular (AV) (re-entrant) I47.1
            psychogenic F54
        junctional I47.1
            ectopic I47.1
        nodal I47.1
        psychogenic (atrial) (supraventricular)
            (ventricular) F54
        supraventricular (sustained) I47.1
            psychogenic F54
        ventricular I47.2
            psychogenic F54
    psychogenic F45.8
    sick sinus I49.5
    sinoauricular NOS R00.0
        paroxysmal I47.1
    sinus [sinusal] NOS R00.0
        paroxysmal I47.1
    supraventricular I47.1
    ventricular (paroxysmal) (sustained) I47.2
        psychogenic F54
Tachygastria K31.89

Tachypnea R06.82
    hysterical F45.8
    newborn (idiopathic) (transitory) P22.1
    psychogenic F45.8
    transitory, of newborn P22.1
TACO (transfusion associated circulatory
        overload) E87.71
Taenia (infection) (infestation) B68.9
    diminuta B71.0
    echinococcal infestation B67.90
    mediocanellata B68.1
    nana B71.0
    saginata B68.1
    solium (intestinal form) B68.0
        larval form —*see* Cysticercosis
Taeniasis (intestine) —*see* Taenia
Tag (hypertrophied skin) (infected) L91.8
    adenoid J35.8
    anus K64.4
    hemorrhoidal K64.4
    hymen N89.8
    perineal N90.89
    preauricular Q17.0
    sentinel K64.4
    skin L91.8
        accessory (congenital) Q82.8
        anus K64.4
        congenital Q82.8
        preauricular Q17.0
    tonsil J35.8
    urethra, urethral N36.8
    vulva N90.89
Tahyna fever B33.8
Takahara's disease E80.3
Takayasu's disease or syndrome M31.4
Talaromycosis B48.4
Talcosis (pulmonary) J62.0
Talipes (congenital) Q66.89
    acquired, planus —*see* Deformity, limb, flat foot
    asymmetric Q66.89
    calcaneovalgus Q66.4-●
    calcaneovarus Q66.1-●
    calcaneus Q66.89
    cavus Q66.7-●
    equinovalgus Q66.6
    equinovarus Q66.0-●
    equinus Q66.89
    percavus Q66.7-●
    planovalgus Q66.6
    planus (acquired) (any degree) —*see also*
        Deformity, limb, flat foot
        congenital Q66.5-●
        due to rickets (sequelae) E64.3
    valgus Q66.6
    varus Q66.3-●
Tall stature, constitutional E34.4
Talma's disease M62.89
Talon noir S90.3-●
    hand S60.22-●
    heel S90.3-●
    toe S90.1-●
Tamponade, heart I31.4
Tanapox (virus disease) B08.71
Tangier disease E78.6
Tantrum, child problem F91.8
Tapeworm (infection) (infestation) —*see*
        Infestation, tapeworm
Tapia's syndrome G52.7
TAR (thrombocytopenia with absent radius)
        syndrome Q87.2
Tarral-Besnier disease L44.0
Tarsal tunnel syndrome —*see* Syndrome, tarsal
        tunnel
Tarsalgia —*see* Pain, limb, lower
Tarsitis (eyelid) H01.8
    syphilitic A52.71
    tuberculous A18.4
Tartar (teeth) (dental calculus) K03.6
Tattoo (mark) L81.8
Tauri's disease E74.09
Taurodontism K00.2

Taussig-Bing syndrome Q20.1
Taybi's syndrome Q87.2
Tay-Sachs amaurotic familial idiocy or disease
        E75.02
TBI (traumatic brain injury) S06.9
Teacher's node or nodule J38.2
Tear, torn (traumatic) —*see also* Laceration
    with abortion —*see* Abortion
    annular fibrosis M51.35
    anus, anal (sphincter) S31.831
        complicating delivery
            with third degree perineal laceration —
                see also Delivery, complicated, by,
                laceration, perineum, third degree
                O70.20
                with mucosa O70.3
            without third degree perineal laceration
                O70.4
        nontraumatic (healed) (old) K62.81
    articular cartilage, old —*see* Derangement,
        joint, articular cartilage, by site
    bladder
        with ectopic or molar pregnancy O08.6
        following ectopic or molar pregnancy
            O08.6
        obstetrical O71.5
        traumatic —*see* Injury, bladder
    bowel
        with ectopic or molar pregnancy O08.6
        following ectopic or molar pregnancy
            O08.6
        obstetrical trauma O71.5
    broad ligament
        with ectopic or molar pregnancy O08.6
        following ectopic or molar pregnancy O08.6
        obstetrical trauma O71.6
    bucket handle (knee) (meniscus) —*see* Tear,
        meniscus
    capsule, joint —*see* Sprain
    cartilage —*see also* Sprain
        articular, old —*see* Derangement, joint,
            articular cartilage, by site
    cervix
        with ectopic or molar pregnancy O08.6
        following ectopic or molar pregnancy
            O08.6
        obstetrical trauma (current) O71.3
        old N88.1
        traumatic —*see* Injury, uterus
    dural G97.41
        nontraumatic G96.11
    internal organ —*see* Injury, by site
    knee cartilage
        articular (current) S83.3-●
        old —*see* Derangement, knee, meniscus,
            due to old tear
    ligament —*see* Sprain
    meniscus (knee) (current injury) S83.209
        bucket-handle S83.20-●
        lateral
            bucket-handle S83.25-●
            complex S83.27-●
            peripheral S83.26-●
            specified type NEC S83.28-●
        medial
            bucket-handle S83.21-●
            complex S83.23-●
            peripheral S83.22-●
            specified type NEC S83.24-●
        old —*see* Derangement, knee, meniscus,
            due to old tear
        site other than knee - code as Sprain
        specified type NEC S83.20-●
    muscle —*see* Strain
    pelvic
        floor, complicating delivery O70.1
        organ NEC, obstetrical trauma O71.5
            with ectopic or molar pregnancy O08.6
            following ectopic or molar pregnancy
                O08.6
    perineal, secondary O90.1

▶ New   ⇒ Revised   ~~deleted~~ Deleted   ● Use Additional Character(s)

Tear, torn *(Continued)*
  periurethral tissue, obstetrical trauma O71.82
    with ectopic or molar pregnancy O08.6
    following ectopic or molar pregnancy
      O08.6
  rectovaginal septum —*see* Laceration, vagina
  retina, retinal (without detachment)
      (horseshoe) —*see also* Break, retina,
      horseshoe
    with detachment —*see* Detachment, retina,
      with retinal, break
  rotator cuff (nontraumatic) M75.10-●
    complete M75.12-●
    incomplete M75.11-●
    traumatic S46.01-●
      capsule S43.42-●
  semilunar cartilage, knee —*see* Tear, meniscus
  supraspinatus (complete) (incomplete)
      (nontraumatic) —*see also* Tear, rotator
      cuff M75.10-●
  tendon —*see* Strain
  tentorial, at birth P10.4
  umbilical cord
    complicating delivery O69.89
  urethra
    with ectopic or molar pregnancy O08.6
    following ectopic or molar pregnancy
      O08.6
    obstetrical trauma O71.5
  uterus —*see* Injury, uterus
  vagina —*see* Laceration, vagina
  vessel, from catheter —*see* Puncture,
      accidental complicating surgery
  vulva, complicating delivery O70.0
Tear-stone —*see* Dacryolith
Teeth —*see also* condition
  grinding
    psychogenic F45.8
    sleep related G47.63
Teething (syndrome) K00.7
Telangiectasia, telangiectasis (verrucous) I78.1
  ataxic (cerebellar) (Louis-Bar) G11.3
  familial I78.0
  hemorrhagic, hereditary (congenital) (senile)
      I78.0
  hereditary, hemorrhagic (congenital) (senile)
      I78.0
  juxtafoveal H35.07-●
  macular H35.07-●
  macularis eruptiva perstans D47.01
  parafoveal H35.07-●
  retinal (idiopathic) (juxtafoveal) (macular)
      (parafoveal) H35.07-●
  spider I78.1
Telephone scatologia F65.89
Telescoped bowel or intestine K56.1
  congenital Q43.8
Temperature
  body, high (of unknown origin) R50.9
  cold, trauma from T69.9
    newborn P80.0
    specified effect NEC T69.8
Temple —*see* condition
Temporal —*see* condition
Temporomandibular joint pain-dysfunction
    syndrome M26.62-●
Temporosphenoidal —*see* condition
Tendency
  bleeding —*see* Defect, coagulation
  suicide
    ⟫meaning personal history of attempted
      suicide Z91.51
    meaning suicidal ideation —*see* Ideation,
      suicidal
  to fall R29.6
Tenderness, abdominal R10.819
  epigastric R10.816
  generalized R10.817
  left lower quadrant R10.814
  left upper quadrant R10.812
  periumbilic R10.815

Tenderness, abdominal *(Continued)*
  rebound R10.829
    epigastric R10.826
    generalized R10.827
    left lower quadrant R10.824
    left upper quadrant R10.822
    periumbilic R10.825
    right lower quadrant R10.823
    right upper quadrant R10.821
  right lower quadrant R10.813
  right upper quadrant R10.811
Tendinitis, tendonitis —*see also* Enthesopathy
  Achilles M76.6-●
  adhesive —*see* Tenosynovitis, specified type
    NEC
    shoulder —*see* Capsulitis, adhesive
  bicipital M75.2-●
  calcific M65.2-●
    ankle M65.27-●
    foot M65.27-●
    forearm M65.23-●
    hand M65.24-●
    lower leg M65.26-●
    multiple sites M65.29
    pelvic region M65.25-●
    shoulder M75.3-●
    specified site NEC M65.28
    thigh M65.25-●
    upper arm M65.22-●
  due to use, overuse, pressure —*see also*
    Disorder, soft tissue, due to use
    specified NEC —*see* Disorder, soft tissue,
      due to use, specified NEC
  gluteal M76.0-●
  patellar M76.5-●
  peroneal M76.7-●
  psoas M76.1-●
  tibial (posterior) M76.82-●
    anterior M76.81-●
  trochanteric —*see* Bursitis, hip, trochanteric
Tendon —*see* condition
Tendosynovitis —*see* Tenosynovitis
Tenesmus (rectal) R19.8
  vesical R30.1
Tennis elbow —*see* Epicondylitis, lateral
Tenonitis —*see also* Tenosynovitis
  eye (capsule) H05.04-●
Tenontosynovitis —*see* Tenosynovitis
Tenontothecitis —*see* Tenosynovitis
Tenophyte —*see* Disorder, synovium, specified
    type NEC
Tenosynovitis —*see also* Synovitis M65.9
  adhesive —*see* Tenosynovitis, specified type
    NEC
    shoulder —*see* Capsulitis, adhesive
  bicipital (calcifying) —*see* Tendinitis,
    bicipital
  gonococcal A54.49
  in (due to)
    crystals M65.8-●
    gonorrhea A54.49
    syphilis (late) A52.78
    use, overuse, pressure —*see also* Disorder,
      soft tissue, due to use
      specified NEC —*see* Disorder, soft tissue,
        due to use, specified NEC
  infective NEC M65.1-●
    ankle M65.17-●
    foot M65.17-●
    forearm M65.13-●
    hand M65.14-●
    lower leg M65.16-●
    multiple sites M65.19
    pelvic region M65.15-●
    shoulder region M65.11-●
    specified site NEC M65.18
    thigh M65.15-●
    upper arm M65.12-●
  radial styloid M65.4
  shoulder region M65.81-●
    adhesive —*see* Capsulitis, adhesive

Tenosynovitis *(Continued)*
  specified type NEC M65.88-●
    ankle M65.87-●
    foot M65.87-●
    forearm M65.83-●
    hand M65.84-●
    lower leg M65.86-●
    multiple sites M65.89
    pelvic region M65.85-●
    shoulder region M65.81-●
    specified site NEC M65.88
    thigh M65.85-●
    upper arm M65.82-●
  tuberculous —*see* Tuberculosis, tenosynovitis
Tenovaginitis —*see* Tenosynovitis
Tension
  arterial, high —*see also* Hypertension
    without diagnosis of hypertension R03.0
  headache G44.209
    intractable G44.201
    not intractable G44.209
  nervous R45.0
  pneumothorax J93.0
  premenstrual N94.3
  state (mental) F48.9
Tentorium —*see* condition
Teratencephalus Q89.8
Teratism Q89.7
Teratoblastoma (malignant) —*see* Neoplasm,
    malignant, by site
Teratocarcinoma —*see also* Neoplasm,
    malignant, by site
  liver C22.7
Teratoma (solid) —*see also* Neoplasm, uncertain
    behavior, by site
  with embryonal carcinoma, mixed —*see*
    Neoplasm, malignant, by site
  with malignant transformation —*see*
    Neoplasm, malignant, by site
  adult (cystic) —*see* Neoplasm, benign, by site
  benign —*see* Neoplasm, benign, by site
  combined with choriocarcinoma —*see*
    Neoplasm, malignant, by site
  cystic (adult) —*see* Neoplasm, benign, by site
  differentiated —*see* Neoplasm, benign, by site
  embryonal —*see also* Neoplasm, malignant,
    by site
    liver C22.7
  immature —*see* Neoplasm, malignant, by site
  liver C22.7
    adult, benign, cystic, differentiated type or
      mature D13.4
  malignant —*see also* Neoplasm, malignant,
    by site
    anaplastic —*see* Neoplasm, malignant, by
      site
    intermediate —*see* Neoplasm, malignant,
      by site
    specified site —*see* Neoplasm,
      malignant, by site
    unspecified site C62.90
    undifferentiated —*see* Neoplasm,
      malignant, by site
  mature —*see* Neoplasm, uncertain behavior,
    by site
  malignant —*see* Neoplasm, by site,
    malignant, by site
  ovary D27.-●
    embryonal, immature or malignant C56-●
  solid —*see* Neoplasm, uncertain behavior,
    by site
  testis C62.9-●
    adult, benign, cystic, differentiated type or
      mature D29.2-●
    scrotal C62.1-●
    undescended C62.0-●
Termination
  anomalous —*see also* Malposition, congenital
    right pulmonary vein Q26.3
  pregnancy, elective Z33.2
Ternidens diminutus infestation B81.8
Ternidensiasis B81.8

Terror(s) night (child) F51.4
Terrorism, victim of Z65.4
Terry's syndrome —see also Myopia,
    degenerative H44.2-●
Tertiary —see condition
Test, tests, testing (for)
    adequacy (for dialysis)
        hemodialysis Z49.31
        peritoneal Z49.32
    blood pressure Z01.30
        abnormal reading —see Blood, pressure
    blood typing Z01.83
        Rh typing Z01.83
    ⇒blood-alcohol Z02.83
        positive —see Findings, abnormal, in blood
    ⇒blood-drug Z02.83
        positive —see Findings, abnormal, in blood
    cardiac pulse generator (battery) Z45.010
    fertility Z31.41
    genetic
        disease carrier status for procreative
            management
            female Z31.430
            male Z31.440
        male partner of patient with recurrent
            pregnancy loss Z31.441
        procreative management NEC
            female Z31.438
            male Z31.448
    hearing Z01.10
        with abnormal findings NEC Z01.118
        infant or child (over 28 days old) Z00.129
            with abnormal findings Z00.121
    HIV (human immunodeficiency virus)
        nonconclusive (in infants) R75
        positive Z21
        seropositive Z21
    immunity status Z01.84
    intelligence NEC Z01.89
    laboratory (as part of a general medical
        examination) Z00.00
        with abnormal finding Z00.01
        for medicolegal reason NEC Z04.89
    male partner of patient with recurrent
        pregnancy loss Z31.441
    Mantoux (for tuberculosis) Z11.1
        abnormal result R76.11
    pregnancy, positive first pregnancy —see
        Pregnancy, normal, first
    procreative Z31.49
        fertility Z31.41
    skin, diagnostic
        allergy Z01.82
            special screening examination —see
                Screening, by name of disease
        Mantoux Z11.1
        tuberculin Z11.1
    specified NEC Z01.89
    tuberculin Z11.1
        abnormal result R76.11
    vision Z01.00
        with abnormal findings Z01.01
        following failed vision screening Z01.020
            with abnormal findings Z01.021
        infant or child (over 28 days old) Z00.129
            with abnormal findings Z00.121
    Wassermann Z11.3
        positive —see Serology for syphilis, positive
Testicle, testicular, testis —see also condition
    feminization syndrome —see also Syndrome,
        androgen insensitivity E34.51
    migrans Q55.29
Tetanus, tetanic (cephalic) (convulsions) A35
    with
        abortion A34
        ectopic or molar pregnancy O08.0
    following ectopic or molar pregnancy O08.0
    inoculation reaction (due to serum) —see
        Complications, vaccination
    neonatorum A33
    obstetrical A34
    puerperal, postpartum, childbirth A34

Tetany (due to) R29.0
    alkalosis E87.3
    associated with rickets E55.0
    convulsions R29.0
        hysterical F44.5
    functional (hysterical) F44.5
    hyperkinetic R29.0
        hysterical F44.5
    hyperpnea R06.4
        hysterical F44.5
        psychogenic F45.8
    hyperventilation —see also Hyperventilation
        R06.4
        hysterical F44.5
    neonatal (without calcium or magnesium
        deficiency) P71.3
    parathyroid (gland) E20.9
    parathyroprival E89.2
    post- (para)thyroidectomy E89.2
    postoperative E89.2
    pseudotetany R29.0
    psychogenic (conversion reaction) F44.5
Tetralogy of Fallot Q21.3
Tetraplegia (chronic) —see also Quadriplegia
    G82.50-●
Thailand hemorrhagic fever A91
Thalassanemia —see Thalassemia
Thalassemia (anemia) (disease) D56.9
    with other hemoglobinopathy D56.8
    alpha (major) (severe) (triple gene defect)
        D56.0
        minor D56.3
        silent carrier D56.3
        trait D56.3
    beta (severe) D56.1
        homozygous D56.1
        major D56.1
        minor D56.3
        trait D56.3
    delta-beta (homozygous) D56.2
        minor D56.3
        trait D56.3
    dominant D56.8
    hemoglobin
        C D56.8
        E-beta D56.5
    intermedia D56.1
    major D56.1
    minor D56.3
    mixed D56.8
    sickle-cell —see Disease, sickle-cell,
        thalassemia
    specified type NEC D56.8
    trait D56.3
    variants D56.8
Thanatophoric dwarfism or short stature Q77.1
Thaysen-Gee disease (nontropical sprue) K90.0
Thaysen's disease K90.0
Thecoma D27-●
    luteinized D27-●
    malignant C56-●
Thelarche, premature E30.8
Thelaziasis B83.8
Thelitis N61.0
    puerperal, postpartum or gestational —see
        Infection, nipple
Therapeutic —see condition
Therapy
    drug, long-term (current) (prophylactic)
        agents affecting estrogen receptors and
            estrogen levels NEC Z79.818
        anastrozole (Arimidex) Z79.811
        antibiotics Z79.2
            short-term use - omit code
        anticoagulants Z79.01
        anti-inflammatory Z79.1
        antiplatelet Z79.02
        antithrombotics Z79.02
        aromatase inhibitors Z79.811
        aspirin Z79.82
        birth control pill or patch Z79.3

Therapy (Continued)
    drug, long-term (Continued)
        bisphosphonates Z79.83
        contraceptive, oral Z79.3
        drug, specified NEC Z79.899
        estrogen receptor downregulators
            Z79.818
        Evista Z79.810
        exemestane (Aromasin) Z79.811
        Fareston Z79.810
        fulvestrant (Faslodex) Z79.818
        gonadotropin-releasing hormone (GnRH)
            agonist Z79.818
        goserelin acetate (Zoladex) Z79.818
        hormone replacement Z79.890
        insulin Z79.4
        letrozole (Femara) Z79.811
        leuprolide acetate (leuprorelin) (Lupron)
            Z79.818
        megestrol acetate (Megace) Z79.818
        methadone
            for pain management Z79.891
            maintenance therapy F11.20
        Nolvadex Z79.810
        opiate analgesic Z79.891
        oral contraceptive Z79.3
        raloxifene (Evista) Z79.810
        selective estrogen receptor modulators
            (SERMs) Z79.810
        short term - omit code
        steroids
            inhaled Z79.51
            systemic Z79.52
        tamoxifen (Nolvadex) Z79.810
        toremifene (Fareston) Z79.810
Thermic —see condition
Thermography (abnormal) —see also Abnormal,
    diagnostic imaging R93.89
    breast R92.8
Thermoplegia T67.01
Thesaurismosis, glycogen —see Disease,
    glycogen storage
Thiamin deficiency E51.9
    specified NEC E51.8
Thiaminic deficiency with beriberi E51.11
Thibierge-Weissenbach syndrome —see
    Sclerosis, systemic
Thickening
    bone —see Hypertrophy, bone
    breast N64.59
    endometrium R93.89
    epidermal L85.9
        specified NEC L85.8
    hymen N89.6
    larynx J38.7
    nail L60.2
        congenital Q84.5
    periosteal —see Hypertrophy, bone
    pleura J92.9
        with asbestos J92.0
    skin R23.4
    subepiglottic J38.7
    tongue K14.8
    valve, heart —see Endocarditis
Thigh —see condition
Thinning vertebra —see Spondylopathy,
    specified NEC
Thirst, excessive R63.1
    due to deprivation of water T73.1
Thomsen disease G71.12
Thoracic —see also condition
    kidney Q63.2
    outlet syndrome G54.0
Thoracogastroschisis (congenital)
    Q79.8
Thoracopagus Q89.4
Thorax —see condition
Thorn's syndrome N28.89
Thorson-Björck syndrome E34.0
Threadworm (infection) (infestation)
    B80

Threatened
  abortion O20.0
    with subsequent abortion O03.9
  job loss, anxiety concerning Z56.2
  labor (without delivery) O47.9
    at or after 37 completed weeks of gestation O47.1
    before 37 completed weeks of gestation O47.0-•
  loss of job, anxiety concerning Z56.2
  miscarriage O20.0
  unemployment, anxiety concerning Z56.2
Three-day fever A93.1
Threshers' lung J67.0
Thrix annulata (congenital) Q84.1
Throat —see condition
Thrombasthenia (Glanzmann) (hemorrhagic) (hereditary) D69.1
Thromboangiitis I73.1
  obliterans (general) I73.1
    cerebral I67.89
    vessels
      brain I67.89
      spinal cord I67.89
Thromboarteritis —see Arteritis
Thromboasthenia (Glanzmann) (hemorrhagic) (hereditary) D69.1
Thrombocytasthenia (Glanzmann) D69.1
Thrombocythemia (hemorrhagic) (see also Thrombocytosis) D75.839
  essential D47.3
  idiopathic D47.3
  primary D47.3
Thrombocytopathy (dystrophic) (granulopenic) D69.1
Thrombocytopenia, thrombocytopenic D69.6
  with absent radius (TAR) Q87.2
  congenital D69.42
  dilutional D69.59
  due to
    drugs D69.59
    extracorporeal circulation of blood D69.59
    (massive)blood transfusion D69.59
    platelet alloimmunization D69.59
  essential D69.3
  heparin induced (HIT) D75.82
  hereditary D69.42
  idiopathic D69.3
  neonatal, transitory P61.0
    due to
      exchange transfusion P61.0
      idiopathic maternal thrombocytopenia P61.0
      isoimmunization P61.0
  primary NEC D69.49
    idiopathic D69.3
  puerperal, postpartum O72.3
  secondary D69.59
  transient neonatal P61.0
Thrombocytosis, essential D47.3
  primary D47.3
Thrombocytosis D75.839
  essential D47.3
  idiopathic D47.3
  primary D47.3
  reactive D75.838
  secondary D75.838
  specified NEC D75.838
Thromboembolism —see Embolism
Thrombopathy (Bernard-Soulier) D69.1
  constitutional D68.0
  Willebrand-Jurgens D68.0
Thrombopenia —see Thrombocytopenia
Thrombophilia D68.59
  primary NEC D68.59
  secondary NEC D68.69
  specified NEC D68.69
Thrombophlebitis I80.9
  antepartum O22.2-•
    deep O22.3-•
    superficial O22.2-•
  calf muscular vein (NOS) I80.25-•

Thrombophlebitis (Continued)
  cavernous (venous) sinus G08
    complicating pregnancy O22.5-•
    nonpyogenic I67.6
  cerebral (sinus) (vein) G08
    nonpyogenic I67.6
    sequelae G09
  due to implanted device —see Complications, by site and type, specified NEC
  during or resulting from a procedure NEC T81.72
  femoral vein (superficial) I80.1-•
  femoropopliteal vein I80.0-•
  gastrocnemial vein I80.25-•
  hepatic (vein) I80.8
  idiopathic, recurrent I82.1
  iliac vein (common) (external) (internal) I80.21-•
  iliofemoral I80.1-•
  intracranial venous sinus (any) G08
    nonpyogenic I67.6
    sequelae G09
  intraspinal venous sinuses and veins G08
    nonpyogenic G95.19
  lateral (venous) sinus G08
    nonpyogenic I67.6
  leg I80.3
    superficial I80.0-•
  longitudinal (venous) sinus G08
    nonpyogenic I67.6
  lower extremity I80.299
  migrans, migrating I82.1
  pelvic
    with ectopic or molar pregnancy O08.0
    following ectopic or molar pregnancy O08.0
    puerperal O87.1
  peroneal vein I80.24-•
  popliteal vein —see Phlebitis, leg, deep, popliteal
  portal (vein) K75.1
  postoperative T81.72
  pregnancy —see Thrombophlebitis, antepartum
  puerperal, postpartum, childbirth O87.0
    deep O87.1
    pelvic O87.1
    septic O86.81
    superficial O87.0
  saphenous (greater) (lesser) I80.0-•
  sinus (intracranial) G08
    nonpyogenic I67.6
  soleal vein I80.25-•
  specified site NEC I80.8
  tibial vein (anterior) (posterior) I80.23-•
Thrombosis, thrombotic (bland) (multiple) (progressive) (silent) (vessel) I82.90
  anal K64.5
  antepartum —see Thrombophlebitis, antepartum
  aorta, aortic I74.10
    abdominal I74.09
      saddle I74.01
    bifurcation I74.09
      saddle I74.01
    specified site NEC I74.19
    terminal I74.09
    thoracic I74.11
    valve —see Endocarditis, aortic
  apoplexy I63.3-•
  artery, arteries (postinfectional) I74.9
    auditory, internal —see Occlusion, artery, precerebral, specified NEC
    basilar —see Occlusion, artery, basilar
    carotid (common) (internal) —see Occlusion, artery, carotid
    cerebellar (anterior inferior) (posterior inferior) (superior) —see Occlusion, artery, cerebellar
    cerebral —see Occlusion, artery, cerebral
    choroidal (anterior) —see Occlusion, artery, precerebral, specified NEC
    communicating, posterior —see Occlusion, artery, precerebral, specified NEC

Thrombosis, thrombotic (Continued)
  artery, arteries (Continued)
    coronary —see also Infarct, myocardium
      not resulting in infarction I24.0
    hepatic I74.8
    hypophyseal —see Occlusion, artery, precerebral, specified NEC
    iliac I74.5
    limb I74.4
      lower I74.3
      upper I74.2
    meningeal, anterior or posterior —see Occlusion, artery, cerebral, specified NEC
    mesenteric (with gangrene) —see also Infarct, intestine K55.069
    ophthalmic —see Occlusion, artery, retina
    pontine —see Occlusion, artery, precerebral, specified NEC
    precerebral —see Occlusion, artery, precerebral
    pulmonary (iatrogenic) —see Embolism, pulmonary
    renal N28.0
    retinal —see Occlusion, artery, retina
    spinal, anterior or posterior G95.11
    traumatic NEC T14.8
    vertebral —see Occlusion, artery, vertebral
  atrium, auricular —see Infarct, myocardium
    following acute myocardial infarction (current complication) I23.6
    not resulting in infarction I51.3
    old I51.3
  basilar (artery) —see Occlusion, artery, basilar
  brain (artery) (stem) —see also Occlusion, artery, cerebral
    due to syphilis A52.05
    puerperal O99.43
    sinus —see Thrombosis, intracranial venous sinus
  capillary I78.8
  cardiac —see also Infarct, myocardium
    not resulting in infarction I51.3
    valve —see Endocarditis
    old I51.3
  carotid (artery) (common) (internal) —see Occlusion, artery, carotid
  cavernous (venous) sinus —see Thrombosis, intracranial venous sinus
  cerebellar artery (anterior inferior) (posterior inferior) (superior) I66.3
  cerebral (artery) —see Occlusion, artery, cerebral
  cerebrovenous sinus —see also Thrombosis, intracranial venous sinus
    puerperium O87.3
  chronic I82.91
  coronary (artery) (vein) —see also Infarct, myocardium
    not resulting in infarction I24.0
  corpus cavernosum N48.89
  cortical I66.9
  deep —see Embolism, vein, lower extremity
  due to device, implant or graft —see also Complications, by site and type, specified NEC T85.868
    arterial graft NEC T82.868
    breast (implant) T85.868
    catheter NEC T85.868
      dialysis (renal) T82.868
        intraperitoneal T85.868
      infusion NEC T82.868
        spinal (epidural) (subdural) T85.860
      urinary (indwelling) T83.86
    electronic (electrode) (pulse generator) (stimulator)
      bone T84.86
      cardiac T82.867
      nervous system (brain) (peripheral nerve) (spinal) T85.860
      urinary T83.86
    fixation, internal (orthopedic) NEC T84.86
    gastrointestinal (bile duct) (esophagus) T85.868

Thrombosis, thrombotic *(Continued)*
  due to device, implant or graft *(Continued)*
    genital NEC T83.86
    heart T82.867
    joint prosthesis T84.86
    ocular (corneal graft) (orbital implant)
      NEC T85.868
    orthopedic NEC T84.86
    specified NEC T85.868
    urinary NEC T83.86
    vascular NEC T82.868
    ventricular intracranial shunt T85.860
  during the puerperium —*see* Thrombosis,
    puerperal
  endocardial —*see also* Infarct, myocardium
    not resulting in infarction I51.3
  eye —*see* Occlusion, retina
  genital organ
    female NEC N94.89
      pregnancy —*see* Thrombophlebitis,
        antepartum
    male N50.1
  gestational —*see* Phlebopathy, gestational
  heart (chamber) —*see also* Infarct, myocardium
    not resulting in infarction I51.3
    old I51.3
  hepatic (vein) I82.0
    artery I74.8
  history (of) Z86.718
  intestine (with gangrene) —*see also* Infarct,
    intestine K55.069
  intracardiac NEC (apical) (atrial) (auricular)
    (ventricular) (old) I51.3
  intracranial (arterial) I66.9
    venous sinus (any) G08
      nonpyogenic origin I67.6
      puerperium O87.3
  intramural —*see also* Infarct, myocardium
    not resulting in infarction I51.3
    old I51.3
  intraspinal venous sinuses and veins G08
    nonpyogenic G95.19
  kidney (artery) N28.0
  lateral (venous) sinus —*see* Thrombosis,
    intracranial venous sinus
  leg —*see* Thrombosis, vein, lower extremity
    arterial I74.3
  liver (venous) I82.0
    artery I74.8
    portal vein I81
  longitudinal (venous) sinus —*see* Thrombosis,
    intracranial venous sinus
  lower limb —*see* Thrombosis, vein, lower
    extremity
  lung (iatrogenic) (postoperative) —*see*
    Embolism, pulmonary
  meninges (brain) (arterial) I66.8
  mesenteric (artery) (with gangrene) —*see also*
    Infarct, intestine K55.069
    vein (inferior) (superior) K55.0-•
  mitral I34.8
  mural —*see also* Infarct, myocardium
    due to syphilis A52.06
    not resulting in infarction I51.3
    old I51.3
  omentum (with gangrene) —*see also* Infarct,
    intestine K55.069
  ophthalmic —*see* Occlusion, retina
  pampiniform plexus (male) N50.1
  parietal —*see also* Infarct, myocardium
    not resulting in infarction I24.0
  penis, superficial vein N48.81
  perianal venous K64.5
  peripheral arteries I74.4
    upper I74.2
  personal history (of) Z86.718
  portal I81
    due to syphilis A52.09
  precerebral artery —*see* Occlusion, artery,
    precerebral
  puerperal, postpartum O87.0
    brain (artery) O99.43
      venous (sinus) O87.3

Thrombosis, thrombotic *(Continued)*
  puerperal, postpartum*(Continued)*
    cardiac O99.43
    cerebral (artery) O99.43
      venous (sinus) O87.3
    superficial O87.0
  pulmonary (artery) (iatrogenic)
    (postoperative) (vein) —*see* Embolism,
    pulmonary
  renal (artery) N28.0
    vein I82.3
  resulting from presence of device, implant or
    graft —*see* Complications, by site and
    type, specified NEC
  retina, retinal —*see* Occlusion, retina
  scrotum N50.1
  seminal vesicle N50.1
  sigmoid (venous) sinus —*see* Thrombosis,
    intracranial venous sinus
  sinus, intracranial (any) —*see* Thrombosis,
    intracranial venous sinus
  specified site NEC I82.890
    chronic I82.891
  spermatic cord N50.1
  spinal cord (arterial) G95.11
    due to syphilis A52.09
    pyogenic origin G06.1
  spleen, splenic D73.5
    artery I74.8
  testis N50.1
  traumatic NEC T14.8
  tricuspid I07.8
  tumor —*see* Neoplasm, by site
  tunica vaginalis N50.1
  umbilical cord (vessels), complicating
    delivery O69.5
  vas deferens N50.1
  vein (acute) I82.90
    antecubital I82.61-•
      chronic I82.71-•
    axillary I82.A1-•
      chronic I82.A2-•
    basilic I82.61-•
      chronic I82.71-•
    brachial I82.62-•
      chronic I82.72-•
    brachiocephalic (innominate) I82.290
      chronic I82.291
    cerebral, nonpyogenic I67.6
    cephalic I82.61-•
      chronic I82.71-•
    chronic I82.91
    deep (DVT) I82.40-•
      calf I82.4Z-•
        chronic I82.5Z-•
      lower leg I82.4Z-•
        chronic I82.5Z-•
      thigh I82.4Y-•
        chronic I82.5Y-•
      ➡upper leg I82.4Y-•
      ➡chronic I82.5Y-•
    femoral I82.41-•
      chronic I82.51-•
    iliac (iliofemoral) I82.42-•
      chronic I82.52-•
    innominate I82.290
      chronic I82.291
    internal jugular I82.C1-•
      chronic I82.C2-•
    lower extremity
      deep I82.40-•
        chronic I82.50-•
        specified NEC I82.49-•
          chronic NEC I82.59-•
      distal
        deep I82.4Z-•
      proximal
        deep I82.4Y-•
          chronic I82.5Y-•
      superficial I82.81-•
    perianal K64.5
    popliteal I82.43-•
      chronic I82.53-•

Thrombosis, thrombotic *(Continued)*
  vein *(Continued)*
    radial I82.62-•
      chronic I82.72-•
    renal I82.3
    saphenous (greater) (lesser) I82.81-•
    specified NEC I82.890
      chronic NEC I82.891
    subclavian I82.B1-•
      chronic I82.B2-•
    thoracic NEC I82.290
      chronic I82.291
    tibial I82.44-•
      chronic I82.54-•
    ulnar I82.62-•
      chronic I82.72-•
    upper extremity I82.60-•
      chronic I82.70-•
      deep I82.62-•
        chronic I82.72-•
      superficial I82.61-•
        chronic I82.71-•
  vena cava
    inferior I82.220
      chronic I82.221
    superior I82.210
      chronic I82.211
  venous, perianal K64.5
  ventricle —*see also* Infarct, myocardium
    following acute myocardial infarction
      (current complication) I23.6
    not resulting in infarction I24.0
    old I51.3
Thrombus —*see* Thrombosis
Thrush —*see also* Candidiasis
  newborn P37.5
  oral B37.0
  vaginal B37.3
Thumb —*see also* condition
  sucking (child problem) F98.8
Thymitis E32.8
Thymoma —*see also* Neoplasm, thymus, by type
  malignant C37
  metaplastic C37
  microscopic D15.0
  sclerosing C37
  type A C37
  type AB C37
  type B1 C37
  type B2 C37
  type B3 C37
Thymus, thymic (gland) —*see* condition
Thyrocele —*see* Goiter
Thyroglossal —*see also* condition
  cyst Q89.2
  duct, persistent Q89.2
Thyroid (gland) (body) —*see also* condition
  hormone resistance E07.89
  lingual Q89.2
  nodule (cystic) (nontoxic) (single) E04.1
Thyroiditis E06.9
  acute (nonsuppurative) (pyogenic)
    (suppurative) E06.0
  autoimmune E06.3
  chronic (nonspecific) (sclerosing) E06.5
    with thyrotoxicosis, transient E06.2
    fibrous E06.5
    lymphadenoid E06.3
    lymphocytic E06.3
    lymphoid E06.3
  de Quervain's E06.1
  drug-induced E06.4
  fibrous (chronic) E06.5
  giant-cell (follicular) E06.1
  granulomatous (de Quervain) (subacute) E06.1
  Hashimoto's (struma lymphomatosa) E06.3
  iatrogenic E06.4
  ligneous E06.5
  lymphocytic (chronic) E06.3
  lymphoid E06.3
  lymphomatous E06.3
  nonsuppurative E06.1
  postpartum, puerperal O90.5

▶ New   ➡ Revised   ~~deleted~~ Deleted   • Use Additional Character(s)

Thyroiditis *(Continued)*
  pseudotuberculous E06.1
  pyogenic E06.0
  radiation E06.4
  Riedel's E06.5
  subacute (granulomatous) E06.1
  suppurative E06.0
  tuberculous A18.81
  viral E06.1
  woody E06.5
Thyrolingual duct, persistent Q89.2
Thyromegaly E01.0
Thyrotoxic
  crisis —*see* Thyrotoxicosis
  heart disease or failure —*see also*
    Thyrotoxicosis E05.90 [*143*]
    with thyroid storm E05.91 [*143*]
  storm —*see* Thyrotoxicosis
Thyrotoxicosis (recurrent) E05.90
  with
    goiter (diffuse) E05.00
      with thyroid storm E05.01
      adenomatous uninodular E05.10
        with thyroid storm E05.11
      multinodular E05.20
        with thyroid storm E05.21
      nodular E05.20
        with thyroid storm E05.21
      uninodular E05.10
        with thyroid storm E05.11
    infiltrative
      dermopathy E05.00
        with thyroid storm E05.01
      ophthalmopathy E05.00
        with thyroid storm E05.01
    single thyroid nodule E05.10
      with thyroid storm E05.11
    thyroid storm E05.91
  due to
    ectopic thyroid nodule or tissue E05.30
      with thyroid storm E05.31
    ingestion of (excessive) thyroid material
      E05.40
      with thyroid storm E05.41
    overproduction of thyroid-stimulating
      hormone E05.80
      with thyroid storm E05.81
    specified cause NEC E05.80
      with thyroid storm E05.81
  factitia E05.40
    with thyroid storm E05.41
  heart —*see also* Failure, heart, high-output
    E05.90 [*143*]
    with thyroid storm —*see also* Failure, heart,
      high-output E05.91 [*143*]
    failure —*see also* Failure, heart, high-output
      E05.90 [*143*]
  neonatal (transient) P72.1
  transient with chronic thyroiditis E06.2
Tibia vara M92.51-●
Tic (disorder) F95.9
  breathing F95.8
  child problem F95.0
  compulsive F95.1
  de la Tourette F95.2
  degenerative (generalized) (localized) G25.69
    facial G25.69
  disorder
    chronic
      motor F95.1
      vocal F95.1
    combined vocal and multiple motor F95.2
    transient F95.0
  douloureux G50.0
    atypical G50.1
    postherpetic, postzoster B02.22
  drug-induced G25.61
  eyelid F95.8
  habit F95.9
    chronic F95.1
    transient of childhood F95.0
  lid, transient of childhood F95.0

Tic *(Continued)*
  motor-verbal F95.2
  occupational F48.8
  orbicularis F95.8
    transient of childhood F95.0
  organic origin G25.69
  postchoreic G25.69
  provisional F95.0
  psychogenic, compulsive F95.1
  salaam R25.8
  spasm (motor or vocal) F95.9
    chronic F95.1
    transient of childhood F95.0
  specified NEC F95.8
Tick-borne —*see* condition
Tietze's disease or syndrome M94.0
Tight, tightness
  anus K62.89
  chest R07.89
  fascia (lata) M62.89
  foreskin (congenital) N47.1
  hymen, hymenal ring N89.6
  introitus (acquired) (congenital) N89.6
  rectal sphincter K62.89
  tendon —*see* Short, tendon
  urethral sphincter N35.919
Tilting vertebra —*see* Dorsopathy, deforming,
  specified NEC
Timidity, child F93.8
Tin-miner's lung J63.5
Tinea (intersecta) (tarsi) B35.9
  amiantacea L44.8
  asbestina B35.0
  barbae B35.0
  beard B35.0
  black dot B35.0
  blanca B36.2
  capitis B35.0
  corporis B35.4
  cruris B35.6
  flava B36.0
  foot B35.3
  furfuracea B36.0
  imbricata (Tokelau) B35.5
  kerion B35.0
  manuum B35.2
  microsporic —*see* Dermatophytosis
  nigra B36.1
  nodosa —*see* Piedra
  pedis B35.3
  scalp B35.0
  specified NEC B35.8
  sycosis B35.0
  tonsurans B35.0
  trichophytic —*see* Dermatophytosis
  unguium B35.1
  versicolor B36.0
Tingling sensation (skin) R20.2
Tinnitus NOS H93.1-●
  audible H93.1-●
  aurium H93.1-●
  pulsatile H93.A-●
  subjective H93.1-●
Tipped tooth (teeth) M26.33
Tipping
  pelvis M95.5
    with disproportion (fetopelvic) O33.0
      causing obstructed labor O65.0
  tooth (teeth), fully erupted M26.33
Tiredness R53.83
Tissue —*see* condition
Tobacco (nicotine)
  abuse —*see* Tobacco, use
  dependence —*see* Dependence, drug, nicotine
  harmful use Z72.0
  heart —*see* Tobacco, toxic effect
  maternal use, affecting newborn P04.2
  toxic effect —*see* Table of Drugs and
    Chemicals, by substance, poisoning
    chewing tobacco —*see* Table of Drugs
      and Chemicals, by substance, poisoning

Tobacco *(Continued)*
  toxic effect *(Continued)*
    cigarettes —*see* Table of Drugs and
      Chemicals, by substance, poisoning
  use Z72.0
    complicating
      childbirth O99.334
      pregnancy O99.33-●
      puerperium O99.335
    counseling and surveillance Z71.6
    history Z87.891
  withdrawal state —*see also* Dependence,
    drug, nicotine F17.203
Tocopherol deficiency E56.0
Todd's
  cirrhosis K74.3
  paralysis (postepileptic) (transitory) G83.84
Toe —*see* condition
Toilet, artificial opening —*see* Attention to,
  artificial, opening
Tokelau (ringworm) B35.5
Tollwut —*see* Rabies
Tommaselli's disease R31.9
  correct substance properly administered —*see*
    Table of Drugs and Chemicals, by drug,
    adverse effect
  overdose or wrong substance given
    or taken —*see* Table of Drugs and
    Chemicals, by drug, poisoning
Tongue —*see also* condition
  tie Q38.1
Tonic pupil —*see* Anomaly, pupil, function,
  tonic pupil
Toni-Fanconi syndrome (cystinosis)
  E72.09
  with cystinosis E72.04
Tonsil —*see* condition
Tonsillitis (acute) (catarrhal) (croupous)
  (follicular) (gangrenous) (infective)
  (lacunar) (lingual) (malignant)
  (membranous) (parenchymatous)
  (phlegmonous) (pseudomembranous)
  (purulent) (septic) (subacute) (suppurative)
  (toxic) (ulcerative) (vesicular) (viral) J03.90
  chronic J35.01
    with adenoiditis J35.03
  diphtheritic A36.0
  hypertrophic J35.01
    with adenoiditis J35.03
  recurrent J03.91
  specified organism NEC J03.80
    recurrent J03.81
  staphylococcal J03.80
    recurrent J03.81
  streptococcal J03.00
    recurrent J03.01
  tuberculous A15.8
  Vincent's A69.1
Tooth, teeth —*see* condition
Toothache K08.89
Topagnosis R20.8
Tophi —*see* Gout, chronic
TORCH infection —*see* Infection, congenital
  without active infection P00.2
Torn —*see* Tear
Tornwaldt's cyst or disease J39.2
Torsion
  accessory tube —*see* Torsion, fallopian tube
  adnexa (female) —*see* Torsion, fallopian tube
  aorta, acquired I77.1
  appendix epididymis N44.04
  appendix testis N44.03
  bile duct (common) (hepatic) K83.8
    congenital Q44.5
  bowel, colon or intestine K56.2
  cervix —*see* Malposition, uterus
  cystic duct K82.8
  dystonia —*see* Dystonia, torsion
  epididymis (appendix) N44.04
  fallopian tube N83.52-●
    with ovary N83.53

Torsion *(Continued)*
gallbladder K82.8
  congenital Q44.1
hydatid of Morgagni
  female N83.52-●
  male N44.03
kidney (pedicle) (leading to infarction) N28.0
Meckel's diverticulum (congenital) Q43.0
  malignant —*see* Table of Neoplasms, small intestine, malignant
mesentery K56.2
omentum K56.2
organ or site, congenital NEC —*see* Anomaly, by site
ovary (pedicle) N83.51-●
  with fallopian tube N83.53
  congenital Q50.2
oviduct —*see* Torsion, fallopian tube
penis (acquired) N48.82
  congenital Q55.63
spasm —*see* Dystonia, torsion
spermatic cord N44.02
  extravaginal N44.01
  intravaginal N44.02
spleen D73.5
testis, testicle N44.00
  appendix N44.03
tibia —*see* Deformity, limb, specified type NEC, lower leg
uterus —*see* Malposition, uterus
Torticollis (intermittent) (spastic) M43.6
congenital (sternomastoid) Q68.0
due to birth injury P15.8
hysterical F44.4
ocular R29.891
psychogenic F45.8
  conversion reaction F44.4
rheumatic M43.6
rheumatoid M06.88
spasmodic G24.3
traumatic, current S13.4
Tortipelvis G24.1
Tortuous
aortic arch Q25.46
artery I77.1
organ or site, congenital NEC —*see* Distortion
retinal vessel, congenital Q14.1
ureter N13.8
urethra N36.8
vein —*see* Varix
Torture, victim of Z65.4
Torula, torular (histolytica) (infection) —*see* Cryptococcosis
Torulosis —*see* Cryptococcosis
Torus (mandibularis) (palatinus) M27.0
fracture —*see* Fracture, by site, torus
Touraine's syndrome Q79.8
Tourette's syndrome F95.2
Tourniquet syndrome —*see* Constriction, external, by site
Tower skull Q75.0
with exophthalmos Q87.0
Toxemia R68.89
bacterial —*see* Sepsis
burn —*see* Burn
eclamptic (with pre-existing hypertension) — *see* Eclampsia
erysipelatous —*see* Erysipelas
fatigue R68.89
food —*see* Poisoning, food
gastrointestinal K52.1
intestinal K52.1
kidney —*see* Uremia
malarial —*see* Malaria
myocardial —*see* Myocarditis, toxic
of pregnancy —*see* Pre-eclampsia
pre-eclamptic —*see* Pre-eclampsia
small intestine K52.1
staphylococcal, due to food A05.0
stasis R68.89

Toxemia *(Continued)*
uremic —*see* Uremia
urinary —*see* Uremia
Toxemica cerebropathia psychica (nonalcoholic) F04
alcoholic —*see* Alcohol, amnestic disorder
Toxic (poisoning) —*see also* condition T65.91
effect —*see* Table of Drugs and Chemicals, by substance, poisoning
shock syndrome A48.3
thyroid (gland) —*see* Thyrotoxicosis
Toxicemia —*see* Toxemia
Toxicity —*see* Table of Drugs and Chemicals, by substance, poisoning
fava bean D55.0
food, noxious —*see* Poisoning, food
from drug or nonmedicinal substance —*see* Table of Drugs and Chemicals, by drug
Toxicosis —*see also* Toxemia
capillary, hemorrhagic D69.0
Toxinfection, gastrointestinal K52.1
Toxocariasis B83.0
Toxoplasma, toxoplasmosis (acquired) B58.9
with
  hepatitis B58.1
  meningoencephalitis B58.2
  ocular involvement B58.00
  other organ involvement B58.89
  pneumonia, pneumonitis B58.3
congenital (acute) (subacute) (chronic) P37.1
maternal, manifest toxoplasmosis in infant (acute) (subacute) (chronic) P37.1
tPA (rtPA) administation in a different facility within the last 24 hours prior to admission to current facility Z92.82
Trabeculation, bladder N32.89
Trachea —*see* condition
Tracheitis (catarrhal) (infantile) (membranous) (plastic) (septal) (suppurative) (viral) J04.10
with
  bronchitis (15 years of age and above) J40
    acute or subacute —*see* Bronchitis, acute
    chronic J42
    tuberculous NEC A15.5
    under 15 years of age J20.9
  laryngitis (acute) J04.2
    chronic J37.1
    tuberculous NEC A15.5
acute J04.10
  with obstruction J04.11
chronic J42
  with
    bronchitis (chronic) J42
    laryngitis (chronic) J37.1
diphtheritic (membranous) A36.89
due to external agent —*see* Inflammation, respiratory, upper, due to
syphilitic A52.73
tuberculous A15.5
Trachelitis (nonvenereal) —*see* Cervicitis
Tracheobronchial —*see* condition
Tracheobronchitis (15 years of age and above) —*see also* Bronchitis
due to
  Bordetella bronchiseptica A37.80
    with pneumonia A37.81
  Francisella tularensis A21.8
Tracheobronchomegaly Q32.4
with bronchiectasis J47.9
  with
    exacerbation (acute) J47.1
    lower respiratory infection J47.0
acquired J98.09
  with bronchiectasis J47.9
    with
      exacerbation (acute) J47.1
      lower respiratory infection J47.0
Tracheobronchopneumonitis —*see* Pneumonia, broncho-●
Tracheocele (external) (internal) J39.8
congenital Q32.1

Tracheomalacia J39.8
congenital Q32.0
Tracheopharyngitis (acute) J06.9
chronic J42
due to external agent —*see* Inflammation, respiratory, upper, due to
Tracheostenosis J39.8
Tracheostomy
complication —*see* Complication, tracheostomy
status Z93.0
  attention to Z43.0
  malfunctioning J95.03
Trachoma, trachomatous A71.9
active (stage) A71.1
contraction of conjunctiva A71.1
dubium A71.0
healed or sequelae B94.0
initial (stage) A71.0
pannus A71.1
Türck's J37.0
Traction, vitreomacular H43.82-●
Train sickness T75.3
Trait(s)
Hb-S D57.3
hemoglobin
  abnormal NEC D58.2
    with thalassemia D56.3
  C —*see* Disease, hemoglobin C
  S (Hb-S) D57.3
Lepore D56.3
personality, accentuated Z73.1
sickle-cell D57.3
  with elliptocytosis or spherocytosis D57.3
type A personality Z73.1
Tramp Z59.00
Trance R41.89
hysterical F44.89
Transaminasemia R74.01
Transection
abdomen (partial) S38.3
aorta (incomplete) —*see also* Injury, aorta
  complete —*see* Injury, aorta, laceration, major
carotid artery (incomplete) —*see also* Injury, blood vessel, carotid, laceration
  complete —*see* Injury, blood vessel, carotid, laceration, major
celiac artery (incomplete) S35.211
  branch (incomplete) S35.291
    complete S35.292
  complete S35.212
innominate
  artery (incomplete) —*see also* Injury, blood vessel, thoracic, innominate, artery, laceration
    complete —*see* Injury, blood vessel, thoracic, innominate, artery, laceration, major
  vein (incomplete) —*see also* Injury, blood vessel, thoracic, innominate, vein, laceration
    complete —*see* Injury, blood vessel, thoracic, innominate, vein, laceration, major
jugular vein (external) (incomplete) —*see also* Injury, blood vessel, jugular vein, laceration
  complete —*see* Injury, blood vessel, jugular vein, laceration, major
  internal (incomplete) —*see also* Injury, blood vessel, jugular vein, internal, laceration
    complete —*see* Injury, blood vessel, jugular vein, internal, laceration, major
mesenteric artery (incomplete) —*see also* Injury, mesenteric, artery, laceration
  complete —*see* Injury, mesenteric artery, laceration, major

▶ New   ⇥ Revised   ~~deleted~~ Deleted   ● Use Additional Character(s)

Transection (Continued)
pulmonary vessel (incomplete) —see also
Injury, blood vessel, thoracic, pulmonary,
laceration
complete —see Injury, blood vessel,
thoracic, pulmonary, laceration, major
subclavian —see Transection, innominate
vena cava (incomplete) —see also Injury, vena
cava
complete —see Injury, vena cava,
laceration, major
vertebral artery (incomplete) —see also Injury,
blood vessel, vertebral, laceration
complete —see Injury, blood vessel,
vertebral, laceration, major
Transfusion
associated (red blood cell) hemochromatosis
E83.111
blood
ABO incompatible —see Complication(s),
transfusion, incompatibility reaction,
ABO
minor blood group (Duffy) (E) (K) (Kell)
(Kidd) (Lewis) (M) (N) (P) (S)
T80.89
reaction or complication —see
Complications, transfusion
fetomaternal (mother) —see Pregnancy,
complicated by, placenta, transfusion
syndrome
maternofetal (mother) —see Pregnancy,
complicated by, placenta, transfusion
syndrome
placental (syndrome) (mother) —see
Pregnancy, complicated by, placenta,
transfusion syndrome
reaction (adverse) —see Complications,
transfusion
related acute lung injury (TRALI) J95.84
twin-to-twin —see Pregnancy, complicated
by, placenta, transfusion syndrome, fetus
to fetus
Transient (meaning homeless) —see also
condition Z59.00
Translocation
balanced autosomal Q95.9
in normal individual Q95.0
chromosomes NEC Q99.8
balanced and insertion in normal
individual Q95.0
Down's syndrome Q90.2
trisomy
13 Q91.6
18 Q91.2
21 Q90.2
Translucency, iris —see Degeneration, iris
Transmission of chemical substances through
the placenta —see Absorption, chemical,
through placenta
Transparency, lung, unilateral J43.0
Transplant (ed) (status) Z94.9
awaiting organ Z76.82
bone Z94.6
marrow Z94.81
candidate Z76.82
complication —see Complication, transplant
cornea Z94.7
heart Z94.1
and lung(s) Z94.3
valve Z95.2
prosthetic Z95.2
specified NEC Z95.4
xenogenic Z95.3
intestine Z94.82
kidney Z94.0
liver Z94.4
lung(s) Z94.2
and heart Z94.3
organ (failure) (infection) (rejection)Z94.9
removal status Z98.85
pancreas Z94.83

Transplant (Continued)
skin Z94.5
social Z60.3
specified organ or tissue NEC Z94.89
stem cells Z94.84
tissue Z94.9
Transplants, ovarian, endometrial N80.1
Transposed —see Transposition
Transposition (congenital) —see also
Malposition, congenital
abdominal viscera Q89.3
aorta (dextra) Q20.3
appendix Q43.8
colon Q43.8
corrected Q20.5
great vessels (complete) (partial) Q20.3
heart Q24.0
with complete transposition of viscera
Q89.3
intestine (large) (small) Q43.8
reversed jejunal (for bypass) (status) Z98.0
scrotum Q55.23
stomach Q40.2
with general transposition of viscera Q89.3
tooth, teeth, fully erupted M26.30
vessels, great (complete) (partial) Q20.3
viscera (abdominal) (thoracic) Q89.3
Transsexualism F64.0
Transverse —see also condition
arrest (deep), in labor O64.0
lie (mother) O32.2
causing obstructed labor O64.8
Transvestism, transvestitism (dual-role)
F64.1
fetishistic F65.1
Trapped placenta (with hemorrhage) O72.0
without hemorrhage O73.0
TRAPS (tumor necrosis factor receptor
associated periodic syndrome) M04.1
Trauma, traumatism —see also Injury
acoustic —see subcategory H83.3
birth —see Birth, injury
complicating ectopic or molar pregnancy
O08.6
during delivery O71.9
following ectopic or molar pregnancy O08.6
obstetric O71.9
specified NEC O71.89
occlusal
primary K08.81
secondary K08.82
Traumatic —see also condition
brain injury S06.9
Treacher Collins syndrome Q75.4
Treitz's hernia —see Hernia, abdomen, specified
site NEC
Trematode infestation —see Infestation, fluke
Trematodiasis —see Infestation, fluke
Trembling paralysis —see Parkinsonism
Tremor(s) R25.1
drug induced G25.1
essential (benign) G25.0
familial G25.0
hereditary G25.0
hysterical F44.4
intention G25.2
medication induced postural G25.1
mercurial —see subcategory T56.1
Parkinson's —see Parkinsonism
psychogenic (conversion reaction) F44.4
senilis R54
specified type NEC G25.2
Trench
fever A79.0
foot —see Immersion, foot
mouth A69.1
Treponema pallidum infection —see Syphilis
Treponematosis
due to
T. pallidum —see Syphilis
T. pertenue —see Yaws

Triad
Hutchinson's (congenital syphilis) A50.53
Kartagener's Q89.3
Saint's —see Hernia, diaphragm
Trichiasis (eyelid) H02.059
with entropion —see Entropion
left H02.056
lower H02.055
upper H02.054
right H02.053
lower H02.052
upper H02.051
Trichinella spiralis (infection) (infestation) B75
Trichinellosis, trichiniasis, trichinelliasis,
trichinosis B75
with muscle disorder B75 [M63.80]
ankle B75 [M63.87-●]
foot B75 [M63.87-●]
forearm B75 [M63.83-●]
hand B75 [M63.84-●]
lower leg B75 [M63.86-●]
multiple sites B75 [M63.89]
pelvic region B75 [M63.85-●]
shoulder region B75 [M63.81-●]
specified site NEC B75 [M63.88]
thigh B75 [M63.85-●]
upper arm B75 [M63.82-●]
Trichobezoar T18.9
intestine T18.3
stomach T18.2
Trichocephaliasis, trichocephalosis B79
Trichocephalus infestation B79
Trichoclasis L67.8
Trichoepithelioma —see also Neoplasm, skin,
benign
malignant —see Neoplasm, skin, malignant
Trichofolliculoma —see Neoplasm, skin,
benign
Tricholemmoma —see Neoplasm, skin,
benign
Trichomoniasis A59.9
bladder A59.03
cervix A59.09
intestinal A07.8
prostate A59.02
seminal vesicles A59.09
specified site NEC A59.8
urethra A59.03
urogenitalis A59.00
vagina A59.01
vulva A59.01
Trichomycosis
axillaris A48.8
nodosa, nodularis B36.8
Trichonodosis L67.8
Trichophytid, trichophyton infection —see
Dermatophytosis
Trichophytobezoar T18.9
intestine T18.3
stomach T18.2
Trichophytosis —see Dermatophytosis
Trichoptilosis L67.8
Trichorrhexis (nodosa) (invaginata) L67.0
Trichosis axillaris A48.8
Trichosporosis nodosa B36.2
Trichostasis spinulosa (congenital) Q84.1
Trichostrongyliasis, trichostrongylosis (small
intestine) B81.2
Trichostrongylus infection B81.2
Trichotillomania F63.3
Trichromat, trichromatopsia, anomalous
(congenital) H53.55
Trichuriasis B79
Trichuris trichiura (infection) (infestation) (any
site) B79
Tricuspid (valve) —see condition
Trifid —see also Accessory
kidney (pelvis) Q63.8
tongue Q38.3
Trigeminal neuralgia —see Neuralgia,
trigeminal

Trigeminy R00.8
Trigger finger (acquired) M65.30
　congenital Q74.0
　index finger M65.32-●
　little finger M65.35-●
　middle finger M65.33-●
　ring finger M65.34-●
　thumb M65.31-●
Trigonitis (bladder) (chronic)
　(pseudomembranous) N30.30
　with hematuria N30.31
Trigonocephaly Q75.0
Trilocular heart —see Cor triloculare
Trimethylaminuria E72.52
Tripartite placenta O43.19-●
Triphalangeal thumb Q74.0
Triple —see also Accessory
　kidneys Q63.0
　uteri Q51.818
　X, female Q97.0
Triple I O41.12-●
Triplegia G83.89
　congenital G80.8
Triplet (newborn) —see also Newborn, triplet
　complicating pregnancy —see Pregnancy, triplet
Triplication —see Accessory
Triploidy Q92.7
Trismus R25.2
　neonatorum A33
　newborn A33
Trisomy (syndrome) Q92.9
　13 (partial) Q91.7
　　meiotic nondisjunction Q91.4
　　mitotic nondisjunction Q91.5
　　mosaicism Q91.5
　　translocation Q91.6
　18 (partial) Q91.3
　　meiotic nondisjunction Q91.0
　　mitotic nondisjunction Q91.1
　　mosaicism Q91.1
　　translocation Q91.2
　20 Q92.8
　21 (partial) Q90.9
　　meiotic nondisjunction Q90.0
　　mitotic nondisjunction Q90.1
　　mosaicism Q90.1
　　translocation Q90.2
　22 Q92.8
　autosomes Q92.9
　chromosome specified NEC Q92.8
　　partial Q92.2
　　　due to unbalanced translocation Q92.5
　　specified NEC Q92.8
　　whole (nonsex chromosome)
　　　meiotic nondisjunction Q92.0
　　　mitotic nondisjunction Q92.1
　　　mosaicism Q92.1
　due to
　　dicentrics —see Extra, marker
　　　chromosomes
　　extra rings —see Extra, marker
　　　chromosomes
　　isochromosomes —see Extra, marker
　　　chromosomes
　specified NEC Q92.8
　whole chromosome Q92.9
　　meiotic nondisjunction Q92.0
　　mitotic nondisjunction Q92.1
　　mosaicism Q92.1
　　partial Q92.9
　　specified NEC Q92.8
Tritanomaly, tritanopia H53.55
Trombiculosis, trombiculiasis, trombidiosis
　B88.0
Trophedema (congenital) (hereditary) Q82.0
Trophoblastic disease —see also Mole,
　hydatidiform O01.9
Tropholymphedema Q82.0
Trophoneurosis NEC G96.89
　disseminated M34.9
Tropical —see condition

Trouble —see also Disease
　heart —see Disease, heart
　kidney —see Disease, renal
　nervous R45.0
　sinus —see Sinusitis
Trousseau's syndrome (thrombophlebitis
　migrans) I82.1
Truancy, childhood
　from school Z72.810
Truncus
　arteriosus (persistent) Q20.0
　communis Q20.0
Trunk —see condition
Trypanosomiasis
　African B56.9
　　by Trypanosoma brucei
　　　gambiense B56.0
　　　rhodesiense B56.1
　American —see Chagas' disease
　Brazilian —see Chagas' disease
　by Trypanosoma
　　brucei gambiense B56.0
　　brucei rhodesiense B56.1
　　cruzi —see Chagas' disease
　gambiensis, Gambian B56.0
　rhodesiensis, Rhodesian B56.1
　South American —see Chagas' disease
　where
　　African trypanosomiasis is prevalent
　　　B56.9
　　Chagas' disease is prevalent B57.2
▶Tryptasemia, hereditary alpha D89.44
T-shaped incisors K00.2
Tsutsugamushi (disease) (fever) A75.3
Tube, tubal, tubular —see condition
Tubercle —see also Tuberculosis
　brain, solitary A17.81
　Darwin's Q17.8
　Ghon, primary infection A15.7
Tuberculid, tuberculide (indurating,
　subcutaneous) (lichenoid) (miliary)
　(papulonecrotic) (primary) (skin) A18.4
Tuberculoma —see also Tuberculosis
　brain A17.81
　meninges (cerebral) (spinal) A17.1
　spinal cord A17.81
Tuberculosis, tubercular, tuberculous
　(calcification) (calcified) (caseous)
　(chromogenic acid-fast bacilli)
　(degeneration) (fibrocaseous) (fistula)
　(interstitial) (isolated circumscribed
　lesions) (necrosis) (parenchymatous)
　(ulcerative) A15.9
　with pneumoconiosis (any condition in
　　J60-J64) J65
　abdomen (lymph gland) A18.39
　abscess (respiratory) A15.9
　　bone A18.03
　　　hip A18.02
　　　knee A18.02
　　　sacrum A18.01
　　　specified site NEC A18.03
　　　spinal A18.01
　　　vertebra A18.01
　　brain A17.81
　　breast A18.89
　　Cowper's gland A18.15
　　dura (mater) (cerebral) (spinal) A17.81
　　epidural (cerebral) (spinal) A17.81
　　female pelvis A18.17
　　frontal sinus A15.8
　　genital organs NEC A18.10
　　genitourinary A18.10
　　gland (lymphatic) —see Tuberculosis,
　　　lymph gland
　　hip A18.02
　　intestine A18.32
　　ischiorectal A18.32
　　joint NEC A18.02
　　　hip A18.02
　　　knee A18.02

Tuberculosis, tubercular, tuberculous
　(Continued)
　abscess (Continued)
　　joint NEC (Continued)
　　　specified NEC A18.02
　　　vertebral A18.01
　　kidney A18.11
　　knee A18.02
　　latent Z22.7
　　lumbar (spine) A18.01
　　lung —see Tuberculosis, pulmonary
　　meninges (cerebral) (spinal) A17.0
　　muscle A18.09
　　perianal (fistula) A18.32
　　perinephritic A18.11
　　perirectal A18.32
　　rectum A18.32
　　retropharyngeal A15.8
　　sacrum A18.01
　　scrofulous A18.2
　　scrotum A18.15
　　skin (primary) A18.4
　　spinal cord A17.81
　　spine or vertebra (column) A18.01
　　subdiaphragmatic A18.31
　　testis A18.15
　　urinary A18.13
　　uterus A18.17
　accessory sinus —see Tuberculosis, sinus
　Addison's disease A18.7
　adenitis —see Tuberculosis, lymph gland
　adenoids A15.8
　adenopathy —see Tuberculosis, lymph gland
　adherent pericardium A18.84
　adnexa (uteri) A18.17
　adrenal (capsule) (gland) A18.7
　alimentary canal A18.32
　anemia A18.89
　ankle (joint) (bone) A18.02
　anus A18.32
　apex, apical —see Tuberculosis, pulmonary
　appendicitis, appendix A18.32
　arachnoid A17.0
　artery, arteritis A18.89
　　cerebral A18.89
　arthritis (chronic) (synovial) A18.02
　　spine or vertebra (column) A18.01
　articular —see Tuberculosis, joint
　ascites A18.31
　asthma —see Tuberculosis, pulmonary
　axilla, axillary (gland) A18.2
　bladder A18.12
　bone A18.03
　　hip A18.02
　　knee A18.02
　　limb NEC A18.03
　　sacrum A18.01
　　spine or vertebral column A18.01
　bowel (miliary) A18.32
　brain A17.81
　breast A18.89
　broad ligament A18.17
　bronchi, bronchial, bronchus A15.5
　　ectasia, ectasis (bronchiectasis) —see
　　　Tuberculosis, pulmonary
　　fistula A15.5
　　　primary (progressive) A15.7
　　gland or node A15.4
　　　primary (progressive) A15.7
　　lymph gland or node A15.4
　　　primary (progressive) A15.7
　bronchiectasis —see Tuberculosis, pulmonary
　bronchitis A15.5
　bronchopleural A15.6
　bronchopneumonia, bronchopneumonic —see
　　Tuberculosis, pulmonary
　bronchorrhagia A15.5
　bronchotracheal A15.5
　bronze disease A18.7
　buccal cavity A18.83
　bulbourethral gland A18.15

▶ New　⇒ Revised　deleted Deleted　● Use Additional Character(s)

Tuberculosis, tubercular, tuberculous
(Continued)
bursa A18.09
cachexia A15.9
cardiomyopathy A18.84
caries —see Tuberculosis, bone
cartilage A18.02
    intervertebral A18.01
catarrhal —see Tuberculosis, respiratory
cecum A18.32
cellulitis (primary) A18.4
cerebellum A17.81
cerebral, cerebrum A17.81
cerebrospinal A17.81
    meninges A17.0
cervical (lymph gland or node) A18.2
cervicitis, cervix (uteri) A18.16
chest —see Tuberculosis, respiratory
chorioretinitis A18.53
choroid, choroiditis A18.53
ciliary body A18.54
colitis A18.32
collier's J65
colliquativa (primary) A18.4
colon A18.32
complex, primary A15.7
congenital P37.0
conjunctiva A18.59
connective tissue (systemic) A18.89
contact Z20.1
cornea (ulcer) A18.52
Cowper's gland A18.15
coxae A18.02
coxalgia A18.02
cul-de-sac of Douglas A18.17
curvature, spine A18.01
cutis (colliquativa) (primary) A18.4
cyst, ovary A18.18
cystitis A18.12
dactylitis A18.03
diarrhea A18.32
diffuse —see Tuberculosis, miliary
digestive tract A18.32
disseminated —see Tuberculosis, miliary
duodenum A18.32
dura (mater) (cerebral) (spinal) A17.0
    abscess (cerebral) (spinal) A17.81
dysentery A18.32
ear (inner) (middle) A18.6
    bone A18.03
    external (primary) A18.4
    skin (primary) A18.4
elbow A18.02
emphysema —see Tuberculosis, pulmonary
empyema A15.6
encephalitis A17.82
endarteritis A18.89
endocarditis A18.84
    aortic A18.84
    mitral A18.84
    pulmonary A18.84
    tricuspid A18.84
endocrine glands NEC A18.82
endometrium A18.17
enteric, enterica, enteritis A18.32
enterocolitis A18.32
epididymis, epididymitis A18.15
epidural abscess (cerebral) (spinal) A17.81
epiglottis A15.5
episcleritis A18.51
erythema (induratum) (nodosum) (primary)
    A18.4
esophagus A18.83
eustachian tube A18.6
exposure (to) Z20.1
exudative —see Tuberculosis, pulmonary
eye A18.50
eyelid (primary) (lupus) A18.4
fallopian tube (acute) (chronic) A18.17
fascia A18.09
fauces A15.8

Tuberculosis, tubercular, tuberculous
(Continued)
female pelvic inflammatory disease
    A18.17
finger A18.03
first infection A15.7
gallbladder A18.83
ganglion A18.09
gastritis A18.83
gastrocolic fistula A18.32
gastroenteritis A18.32
gastrointestinal tract A18.32
general, generalized —see Tuberculosis,
    miliary
genital organs A18.10
genitourinary A18.10
genu A18.02
glandula suprarenalis A18.7
glandular, general A18.2
glottis A15.5
grinder's J65
gum A18.83
hand A18.03
heart A18.84
hematogenous —see Tuberculosis, miliary
hemoptysis —see Tuberculosis, pulmonary
hemorrhage NEC —see Tuberculosis,
    pulmonary
hemothorax A15.6
hepatitis A18.83
hilar lymph nodes A15.4
    primary (progressive) A15.7
hip (joint) (disease) (bone) A18.02
hydropneumothorax A15.6
hydrothorax A15.6
hypoadrenalism A18.7
hypopharynx A15.8
ileocecal (hyperplastic) A18.32
ileocolitis A18.32
ileum A18.32
iliac spine (superior) A18.03
immunological findings only A15.7
indurativa (primary) A18.4
infantile A15.7
infection A15.9
    without clinical manifestations A15.7
infraclavicular gland A18.2
inguinal gland A18.2
inguinalis A18.2
intestine (any part) A18.32
iridocyclitis A18.54
iris, iritis A18.54
ischiorectal A18.32
jaw A18.03
jejunum A18.32
joint A18.02
    vertebral A18.01
keratitis (interstitial) A18.52
keratoconjunctivitis A18.52
kidney A18.11
knee (joint) A18.02
kyphosis, kyphoscoliosis A18.01
laryngitis A15.5
larynx A15.5
latent Z22.7
leptomeninges, leptomeningitis (cerebral)
    (spinal) A17.0
lichenoides (primary) A18.4
linguae A18.83
lip A18.83
liver A18.83
lordosis A18.01
lung —see Tuberculosis, pulmonary
lupus vulgaris A18.4
lymph gland or node (peripheral) A18.2
    abdomen A18.39
    bronchial A15.4
        primary (progressive) A15.7
    cervical A18.2
    hilar A15.4
        primary (progressive) A15.7

Tuberculosis, tubercular, tuberculous
(Continued)
lymph gland or node (Continued)
    intrathoracic A15.4
        primary (progressive) A15.7
    mediastinal A15.4
        primary (progressive) A15.7
    mesenteric A18.39
    retroperitoneal A18.39
    tracheobronchial A15.4
        primary (progressive) A15.7
lymphadenitis —see Tuberculosis, lymph
    gland
lymphangitis —see Tuberculosis, lymph
    gland
lymphatic (gland) (vessel) —see Tuberculosis,
    lymph gland
mammary gland A18.89
marasmus A15.9
mastoiditis A18.03
mediastinal lymph gland or node
    A15.4
    primary (progressive) A15.7
mediastinitis A15.8
    primary (progressive) A15.7
mediastinum A15.8
    primary (progressive) A15.7
medulla A17.81
melanosis, Addisonian A18.7
meninges, meningitis (basilar) (cerebral)
    (cerebrospinal) (spinal) A17.0
meningoencephalitis A17.82
mesentery, mesenteric (gland or node)
    A18.39
miliary A19.9
    acute A19.2
        multiple sites A19.1
        single specified site A19.0
    chronic A19.8
    specified NEC A19.8
millstone makers' J65
miner's J65
molder's J65
mouth A18.83
multiple A19.9
    acute A19.1
    chronic A19.8
muscle A18.09
myelitis A17.82
myocardium, myocarditis A18.84
nasal (passage) (sinus) A15.8
nasopharynx A15.8
neck gland A18.2
nephritis A18.11
nerve (mononeuropathy) A17.83
nervous system A17.9
nose (septum) A15.8
ocular A18.50
omentum A18.31
oophoritis (acute) (chronic) A18.17
optic (nerve trunk) (papilla) A18.59
orbit A18.59
orchitis A18.15
organ, specified NEC A18.89
osseous —see Tuberculosis, bone
osteitis —see Tuberculosis, bone
osteomyelitis —see Tuberculosis, bone
otitis media A18.6
ovary, ovaritis (acute) (chronic) A18.17
oviduct (acute) (chronic) A18.17
pachymeningitis A17.0
palate (soft) A18.83
pancreas A18.83
papulonecrotic (a) (primary) A18.4
parathyroid glands A18.82
paronychia (primary) A18.4
parotid gland or region A18.83
pelvis (bony) A18.03
penis A18.15
peribronchitis A15.5
pericardium, pericarditis A18.84

Tuberculosis, tubercular, tuberculous
(Continued)
perichondritis, larynx A15.5
periostitis —see Tuberculosis, bone
perirectal fistula A18.32
peritoneum NEC A18.31
peritonitis A18.31
pharynx, pharyngitis A15.8
phlyctenulosis (keratoconjunctivitis) A18.52
phthisis NEC —see Tuberculosis, pulmonary
pituitary gland A18.82
pleura, pleural, pleurisy, pleuritis (fibrinous)
(obliterative) (purulent) (simple plastic)
(with effusion) A15.6
primary (progressive) A15.7
pneumonia, pneumonic —see Tuberculosis,
pulmonary
pneumothorax (spontaneous) (tense
valvular) —see Tuberculosis, pulmonary
polyneuropathy A17.89
polyserositis A19.9
acute A19.1
chronic A19.8
potter's J65
prepuce A18.15
primary (complex) A15.7
proctitis A18.32
prostate, prostatitis A18.14
pulmonalis —see Tuberculosis, pulmonary
pulmonary (cavitated) (fibrotic) (infiltrative)
(nodular) A15.0
childhood type or first infection A15.7
primary (complex) A15.7
pyelitis A18.11
pyelonephritis A18.11
pyemia —see Tuberculosis, miliary
pyonephrosis A18.11
pyopneumothorax A15.6
pyothorax A15.6
rectum (fistula) (with abscess) A18.32
reinfection stage —see Tuberculosis,
pulmonary
renal A18.11
renis A18.11
respiratory A15.9
primary A15.7
specified site NEC A15.8
retina, retinitis A18.53
retroperitoneal (lymph gland or node)
A18.39
rheumatism NEC A18.09
rhinitis A15.8
sacroiliac (joint) A18.01
sacrum A18.01
salivary gland A18.83
salpingitis (acute) (chronic) A18.17
sandblaster's J65
sclera A18.51
scoliosis A18.01
scrofulous A18.2
scrotum A18.15
seminal tract or vesicle A18.15
senile A15.9
septic —see Tuberculosis, miliary
shoulder (joint) A18.02
blade A18.03
sigmoid A18.32
sinus (any nasal) A15.8
bone A18.03
epididymis A18.15
skeletal NEC A18.03
skin (any site) (primary) A18.4
small intestine A18.32
soft palate A18.83
spermatic cord A18.15
spine, spinal (column) A18.01
cord A17.81
medulla A17.81
membrane A17.0
meninges A17.0
spleen, splenitis A18.85

Tuberculosis, tubercular, tuberculous
(Continued)
spondylitis A18.01
sternoclavicular joint A18.02
stomach A18.83
stonemason's J65
subcutaneous tissue (cellular) (primary)
A18.4
subcutis (primary) A18.4
subdeltoid bursa A18.83
submaxillary (region) A18.83
supraclavicular gland A18.2
suprarenal (capsule) (gland) A18.7
swelling, joint —see also category M01 (see also
Tuberculosis, joint) A18.02
symphysis pubis A18.02
synovitis A18.09
articular A18.02
spine or vertebra A18.01
systemic —see Tuberculosis, miliary
tarsitis A18.4
tendon (sheath) —see Tuberculosis,
tenosynovitis
tenosynovitis A18.09
spine or vertebra A18.01
testis A18.15
throat A15.8
thymus gland A18.82
thyroid gland A18.81
tongue A18.83
tonsil, tonsillitis A15.8
trachea, tracheal A15.5
lymph gland or node A15.4
primary (progressive) A15.7
tracheobronchial A15.5
lymph gland or node A15.4
primary (progressive) A15.7
tubal (acute) (chronic) A18.17
tunica vaginalis A18.15
ulcer (skin) (primary) A18.4
bowel or intestine A18.32
specified NEC - code under Tuberculosis,
by site
unspecified site A15.9
ureter A18.11
urethra, urethral (gland) A18.13
urinary organ or tract A18.13
uterus A18.17
uveal tract A18.54
uvula A18.83
vagina A18.18
vas deferens A18.15
verruca, verrucosa (cutis) (primary) A18.4
vertebra (column) A18.01
vesiculitis A18.15
vulva A18.18
wrist (joint) A18.02
Tuberculum
Carabelli —see Note at K00.2
occlusal —see Note at K00.2
paramolare K00.2
Tuberosity, enitre maxillary M26.07
Tuberous sclerosis (brain) Q85.1
Tubo-ovarian —see condition
Tuboplasty, after previous sterilization
Z31.0
aftercare Z31.42
Tubotympanitis, catarrhal (chronic) —see Otitis,
media, nonsuppurative, chronic, serous
Tularemia A21.9
with
conjunctivitis A21.1
pneumonia A21.2
abdominal A21.3
bronchopneumonic A21.2
conjunctivitis A21.1
cryptogenic A21.3
enteric A21.3
gastrointestinal A21.3
generalized A21.7
ingestion A21.3

Tularemia (Continued)
intestinal A21.3
oculoglandular A21.1
ophthalmic A21.1
pneumonia (any), pneumonic A21.2
pulmonary A21.2
sepsis A21.7
specified NEC A21.8
typhoidal A21.7
ulceroglandular A21.0
Tularensis conjunctivitis A21.1
Tumefaction —see also Swelling
liver —see Hypertrophy, liver
Tumor —see also Neoplasm, unspecified
behavior, by site
acinar cell —see Neoplasm, uncertain
behavior, by site
acinic cell —see Neoplasm, uncertain
behavior, by site
adenocarcinoid —see Neoplasm, malignant,
by site
adenomatoid —see also Neoplasm, benign,
by site
odontogenic —see Cyst, calcifying
odontogenic
adnexal (skin) —see Neoplasm, skin, benign,
by site
adrenal
cortical (benign) D35.0-●
malignant C74.0-●
rest —see Neoplasm, benign, by site
alpha-cell
malignant
pancreas C25.4
specified site NEC —see Neoplasm,
malignant, by site
unspecified site C25.4
pancreas D13.7
specified site NEC —see Neoplasm, benign,
by site
unspecified site D13.7
aneurysmal —see Aneurysm
aortic body D44.7
malignant C75.5
Askin's —see Neoplasm, connective tissue,
malignant
basal cell —see also Neoplasm, skin, uncertain
behavior D48.5
Bednar —see Neoplasm, skin, malignant
benign (unclassified) —see Neoplasm, benign,
by site
beta-cell
malignant
pancreas C25.4
specified site NEC —see Neoplasm,
malignant, by site
unspecified site C25.4
pancreas D13.7
specified site NEC —see Neoplasm, benign,
by site
unspecified site D13.7
Brenner D27.9
borderline malignancy D39.1-●
malignant C56-●
proliferating D39.1
bronchial alveolar, intravascular D38.1
Brooke's —see Neoplasm, skin, benign
brown fat —see Lipoma
Burkitt —see Lymphoma, Burkitt
calcifying epithelial odontogenic —see Cyst,
calcifying odontogenic
carcinoid D3A.00
benign D3A.00
appendix D3A.020
ascending colon D3A.022
bronchus (lung) D3A.090
cecum D3A.021
colon D3A.029
descending colon D3A.024
duodenum D3A.010
foregut NOS D3A.094

Tumor (Continued)
  carcinoid (Continued)
    malignant (Continued)
      hindgut NOS D3A.096
      ileum D3A.012
      jejunum D3A.011
      kidney D3A.093
      large intestine D3A.029
      lung (bronchus) D3A.090
      midgut NOS D3A.095
      rectum D3A.026
      sigmoid colon D3A.025
      small intestine D3A.019
      specified NEC D3A.098
      stomach D3A.092
      thymus D3A.091
      transverse colon D3A.023
    malignant C7A.00
      appendix C7A.020
      ascending colon C7A.022
      bronchus (lung) C7A.090
      cecum C7A.021
      colon C7A.029
      descending colon C7A.024
      duodenum C7A.010
      foregut NOS C7A.094
      hindgut NOS C7A.096
      ileum C7A.012
      jejunum C7A.011
      kidney C7A.093
      large intestine C7A.029
      lung (bronchus) C7A.090
      midgut NOS C7A.095
      rectum C7A.026
      sigmoid colon C7A.025
      small intestine C7A.019
      specified NEC C7A.098
      stomach C7A.092
      thymus C7A.091
      transverse colon C7A.023
    mesentary metastasis C7B.04
    secondary C7B.00
      bone C7B.03
      distant lymph nodes C7B.01
      liver C7B.02
      peritoneum C7B.04
      specified NEC C7B.09
  carotid body D44.6
    malignant C75.4
  cells —see also Neoplasm, unspecified
    behavior, by site
    benign —see Neoplasm, benign,
      by site
    malignant —see Neoplasm, malignant,
      by site
    uncertain whether benign or malignant —
      see Neoplasm, uncertain behavior,
      by site
  cervix, in pregnancy or childbirth —see
    Pregnancy, complicated by, tumor,
    cervix
  chondromatous giant cell —see Neoplasm,
    bone, benign
  chromaffin —see also Neoplasm, benign, by
    site
    malignant —see Neoplasm, malignant, by
      site
  Cock's peculiar L72.3
  Codman's —see Neoplasm, bone, benign
  dentigerous, mixed —see Cyst, calcifying
    odontogenic
  dermoid —see Neoplasm, benign,
    by site
    with malignant transformation C56-●
  desmoid (extra-abdominal) —see also
    Neoplasm, connective tissue, uncertain
    behavior
    abdominal —see Neoplasm, connective
      tissue, uncertain behavior
  embolus —see Neoplasm, secondary,
    by site

Tumor (Continued)
  embryonal (mixed) —see also Neoplasm,
    uncertain behavior, by site
    liver C22.7
  endodermal sinus
    specified site —see Neoplasm, malignant,
      by site
    unspecified site
      female C56.-●
      male C62.90
  epithelial
    benign —see Neoplasm, benign,
      by site
    malignant —see Neoplasm, malignant,
      by site
  Ewing's —see Neoplasm, bone, malignant,
    by site
  fatty —see Lipoma
  fibroid —see Leiomyoma
  G cell
    malignant
      pancreas C25.4
      specified site NEC —see Neoplasm,
        malignant, by site
      unspecified site C25.4
    specified site —see Neoplasm, uncertain
      behavior, by site
    unspecified site D37.8
  germ cell —see also Neoplasm, malignant,
    by site
    mixed —see Neoplasm, malignant,
      by site
  ghost cell, odontogenic —see Cyst, calcifying
    odontogenic
  giant cell —see also Neoplasm, uncertain
    behavior, by site
    bone D48.0
      malignant —see Neoplasm, bone,
        malignant
    chondromatous —see Neoplasm, bone,
      benign
    malignant —see Neoplasm, malignant,
      by site
    soft parts —see Neoplasm, connective
      tissue, uncertain behavior
      malignant —see Neoplasm, connective
        tissue, malignant
  glomus D18.00
    intra-abdominal D18.03
    intracranial D18.02
    jugulare D44.7
      malignant C75.5
    skin D18.01
    specified site NEC D18.09
  gonadal stromal —see Neoplasm, uncertain
    behavior, by site
  granular cell —see also Neoplasm, connective
    tissue, benign
    malignant —see Neoplasm, connective
      tissue, malignant
  granulosa cell D39.1-●
    juvenile D39.1-●
    malignant C56-●
  granulosa cell-theca cell D39.1-●
    malignant C56-●
  Grawitz's C64-●
  hemorrhoidal —see Hemorrhoids
  hilar cell D27-●
  hilus cell D27-●
  Hurthle cell (benign) D34
    malignant C73
  hydatid —see Echinococcus
  hypernephroid —see also Neoplasm,
    uncertain behavior, by site
  interstitial cell —see also Neoplasm, uncertain
    behavior, by site
    benign —see Neoplasm, benign, by site
    malignant —see Neoplasm, malignant,
      by site
  intravascular bronchial alveolar
    D38.1

Tumor (Continued)
  islet cell —see Neoplasm, benign, by site
    malignant —see Neoplasm, malignant, by
      site
      pancreas C25.4
      specified site NEC —see Neoplasm,
        malignant, by site
      unspecified site C25.4
    pancreas D13.7
    specified site NEC —see Neoplasm, benign,
      by site
    unspecified site D13.7
  juxtaglomerular D41.0-●
  Klatskin's C24.0
  Krukenberg's C79.6-●
  Leydig cell —see Neoplasm, uncertain
    behavior, by site
    benign —see Neoplasm, benign, by site
      specified site —see Neoplasm, benign,
        by site
      unspecified site
        female D27.9
        male D29.20
    malignant —see Neoplasm, malignant, by
      site
      specified site —see Neoplasm,
        malignant, by site
      unspecified site
        female C56.9
        male C62.90
    specified site —see Neoplasm, uncertain
      behavior, by site
    unspecified site
      female D39.10
      male D40.10
  lipid cell, ovary D27-●
  lipoid cell, ovary D27-●
  malignant —see also Neoplasm, malignant, by
    site C80.1
    fusiform cell (type) C80.1
    giant cell (type) C80.1
    localized, plasma cell —see Plasmacytoma,
      solitary
    mixed NEC C80.1
    small cell (type) C80.1
    spindle cell (type) C80.1
    unclassified C80.1
  mast cell D47.09
  melanotic, neuroectodermal —see Neoplasm,
    benign, by site
  Merkel cell —see Carcinoma, Merkel cell
  mesenchymal
    malignant —see Neoplasm, connective
      tissue, malignant
    mixed —see Neoplasm, connective tissue,
      uncertain behavior
  mesodermal, mixed —see also Neoplasm,
    malignant, by site
    liver C22.4
  mesonephric —see also Neoplasm, uncertain
    behavior, by site
    malignant —see Neoplasm, malignant, by
      site
  metastatic
    from specified site —see Neoplasm,
      malignant, by site
    of specified site —see Neoplasm,
      malignant, by site
    to specified site —see Neoplasm, secondary,
      by site
  mixed NEC —see also Neoplasm, benign, by
    site
    malignant —see Neoplasm, malignant, by
      site
  mucinous of low malignant potential
    specified site —see Neoplasm, malignant,
      by site
    unspecified site C56.9
  mucocarcinoid
    specified site —see Neoplasm, malignant,
      by site
    unspecified site C18.1

Tumor (Continued)

mucoepidermoid —see Neoplasm, uncertain behavior, by site

Müllerian, mixed
  specified site —see Neoplasm, malignant, by site
  unspecified site C54.9

myoepithelial —see Neoplasm, benign, by site

neuroectodermal (peripheral) —see Neoplasm, malignant, by site
  primitive
    specified site —see Neoplasm, malignant, by site
    unspecified site C71.9

neuroendocrine D3A.8
  malignant poorly differentiated C7A.1
  secondary NEC C7B.8
  specified NEC C7A.8

neurogenic olfactory C30.0

nonencapsulated sclerosing C73

odontogenic (adenomatoid) (benign) (calcifying epithelial) (keratocystic) (squamous) —see Cyst, calcifying odontogenic
  malignant C41.1
    upper jaw (bone) C41.0

ovarian stromal D39.1-●

ovary, in pregnancy —see Pregnancy, complicated by

pacinian —see Neoplasm, skin, benign

Pancoast's —see Pancoast's syndrome

papillary —see also Papilloma
  cystic D37.9
  mucinous of low malignant potential C56-●
    specified site —see Neoplasm, malignant, by site
    unspecified site C56.9
  serous of low malignant potential
    specified site —see Neoplasm, malignant, by site
    unspecified site C56.9

pelvic, in pregnancy or childbirth —see Pregnancy, complicated by

phantom F45.8

phyllodes D48.6-●
  benign D24-●
  malignant —see Neoplasm, breast, malignant

Pindborg —see Cyst, calcifying odontogenic

placental site trophoblastic D39.2

plasma cell (malignant) (localized) —see Plasmacytoma, solitary

polyvesicular vitelline
  specified site —see Neoplasm, malignant, by site
  unspecified site
    female C56.9
    male C62.90

Pott's puffy —see Osteomyelitis, specified NEC

Rathke's pouch D44.3

retinal anlage —see Neoplasm, benign, by site

salivary gland type, mixed —see Neoplasm, salivary gland, benign
  malignant —see Neoplasm, salivary gland, malignant

Sampson's N80.1

Schmincke's —see Neoplasm, nasopharynx, malignant

sclerosing stromal D27-●

sebaceous —see Cyst, sebaceous

secondary —see Neoplasm, secondary, by site
  carcinoid C7B.00
    bone C7B.03
    distant lymph nodes C7B.01
    liver C7B.02
    peritoneum C7B.04
    specified NEC C7B.09
  neuroendocrine NEC C7B.8

Tumor (Continued)

serous of low malignant potential
  specified site —see Neoplasm, malignant, by site
  unspecified site C56.9

Sertoli cell —see Neoplasm, benign, by site
  with lipid storage
    specified site —see Neoplasm, benign, by site
    unspecified site
      female D27.9
      male D29.20
  specified site —see Neoplasm, benign, by site
  unspecified site
    female D27.9
    male D29.20

Sertoli-Leydig cell —see Neoplasm, benign, by site
  specified site —see Neoplasm, benign, by site
  unspecified site
    female D27.9
    male D29.20

sex cord(-stromal) —see Neoplasm, uncertain behavior, by site
  with annular tubules D39.1-●

skin appendage —see Neoplasm, skin, benign

smooth muscle —see Neoplasm, connective tissue, uncertain behavior

soft tissue
  benign —see Neoplasm, connective tissue, benign
  malignant —see Neoplasm, connective tissue, malignant

sternomastoid (congenital) Q68.0

stromal
  endometrial D39.0
  gastric D48.1
    benign D21.4
    malignant C16.9
    uncertain behavior D48.1
  gastrointestinal C49.A-●
    benign D21.4
    esophagus C49.A1
    large intestine C49.A4
    malignant C49.A0
      colon C49.A4
      duodenum C49.A3
      esophagus C49.A1
      ileum C49.A3
      jejunum C49.A3
      Meckel diverticulum C49.A3
      large intestine C49.A4
      omentum C49.A9
      peritoneum C49.A9
      rectum C49.A5
      small intestine C49.A3
      specified site NEC C49.A9
      stomach C49.A2
    rectum C49.A5
    small intestine C49.A3
    specified site NEC C49.A9
    stomach C49.A2
    uncertain behavior D48.1
  intestine
    benign D21.4
    malignant
      large C49.A4
      small C49.A3
    uncertain behavior D48.1
  ovarian D39.1-●
  stomach C49.A2
    benign D21.4
    malignant C49.A2
    uncertain behavior D48.1

sweat gland —see also Neoplasm, skin, uncertain behavior
  benign —see Neoplasm, skin, benign
  malignant —see Neoplasm, skin, malignant

Tumor (Continued)

syphilitic, brain A52.17

testicular D40.10

testicular stromal D40.1-●

theca cell D27.-●

theca cell-granulosa cell D39.1-●

Triton, malignant —see Neoplasm, nerve, malignant

trophoblastic, placental site D39.2

turban D23.4

uterus (body), in pregnancy or childbirth — see Pregnancy, complicated by, tumor, uterus

vagina, in pregnancy or childbirth —see Pregnancy, complicated by

varicose —see Varix

von Recklinghausen's —see Neurofibromatosis

vulva or perineum, in pregnancy or childbirth —see Pregnancy, complicated by
  causing obstructed labor O65.5

Warthin's —see Neoplasm, salivary gland, benign

Wilms' C64-●

yolk sac —see Neoplasm, malignant, by site
  specified site —see Neoplasm, malignant, by site
  unspecified site
    female C56.9
    male C62.90

Tumor lysis syndrome (following antineoplastic chemotherapy) (spontaneous) NEC E88.3

Tumorlet —see Neoplasm, uncertain behavior, by site

Tungiasis B88.1

Tunica vasculosa lentis Q12.2

Turban tumor D23.4

Türck's trachoma J37.0

Turner-Kieser syndrome Q87.2

Turner-like syndrome Q87.19

Turner's
  hypoplasia (tooth) K00.4
  syndrome Q96.9
    specified NEC Q96.8
  tooth K00.4

Turner-Ullrich syndrome Q96.9

Tussis convulsiva —see Whooping cough

Twiddler's syndrome (due to)
  automatic implantable defibrillator T82.198
  cardiac pacemaker T82.198

Twilight state
  epileptic F05
  psychogenic F44.89

Twin (newborn) —see also Newborn, twin
  conjoined Q89.4
  pregnancy —see Pregnancy, twin

Twinning, teeth K00.2

Twist, twisted
  bowel, colon or intestine K56.2
  hair (congenital) Q84.1
  mesentery K56.2
  omentum K56.2
  organ or site, congenital NEC —see Anomaly, by site
  ovarian pedicle —see Torsion, ovary

Twitching R25.3

Tylosis (acquired) L84
  buccalis K13.29
  linguae K13.29
  palmaris et plantaris (congenital) (inherited) Q82.8
  acquired L85.1

Tympanism R14.0

Tympanites (abdominal) (intestinal) R14.0

Tympanitis —see Myringitis

Tympanosclerosis —see subcategory H74.0

Tympanum —see condition

▶ New   ⇒ Revised   ~~deleted~~ Deleted   ● Use Additional Character(s)

Tympany
  abdomen R14.0
  chest R09.89
Type A behavior pattern Z73.1
Typhlitis —see Appendicitis
Typhoenteritis —see Typhoid
Typhoid (abortive) (ambulant) (any site)
    (clinical) (fever) (hemorrhagic) (infection)
    (intermittent) (malignant) (rheumatic)
    (Widal negative) A01.00
  with pneumonia A01.03
  abdominal A01.09
  arthritis A01.04
  carrier (suspected) of Z22.0
  cholecystitis (current) A01.09
  endocarditis A01.02
  heart involvement A01.02
  inoculation reaction —see Complications,
    vaccination
  meningitis A01.01
  mesenteric lymph nodes A01.09
  myocarditis A01.02
  Orientia Tsutsugamushi (scrub typhus) A75.3
  osteomyelitis A01.05
  perichondritis, larynx A01.09
  pneumonia A01.03

Typhoid (Continued)
  specified NEC A01.09
  spine A01.05
  ulcer (perforating) A01.09
Typhomalaria (fever) —see Malaria
Typhomania A01.00
Typhoperitonitis A01.09
Typhus (fever) A75.9
  abdominal, abdominalis —see Typhoid
  African tick A77.1
  amarillic A95.9
  brain A75.9 [G94]
  cerebral A75.9 [G94]
  classical A75.0
  due to Rickettsia
    prowazekii A75.0
      recrudescent A75.1
    tsutsugamushi A75.3
    typhi A75.2
  endemic (flea-borne) A75.2
  epidemic (louse-borne) A75.0
  exanthematic NEC A75.0
  exanthematicus SAI A75.0
    brillii SAI A75.1
    mexicanus SAI A75.2
    typhus murinus A75.2

Typhus (Continued)
  exanthematicus (Continued)
    flea-borne A75.2
    India tick A77.1
    Kenya (tick) A77.1
    louse-borne A75.0
    Mexican A75.2
    mite-borne A75.3
    murine A75.2
    North Asian tick-borne A77.2
    petechial A75.9
    Queensland tick A77.3
    rat A75.2
    recrudescent A75.1
    recurrens —see Fever, relapsing
    Sao Paulo A77.0
    scrub (China) (India) (Malaysia) (New
      Guinea) A75.3
    shop (of Malaysia) A75.2
    Siberian tick A77.2
    tick-borne A77.9
    tropical (mite-borne) A75.3
Tyrosinemia E70.21
  newborn, transitory P74.5
Tyrosinosis E70.21
Tyrosinuria E70.29

U

Uhl's anomaly or disease Q24.8
Ulcer, ulcerated, ulcerating, ulceration, ulcerative
- alveolar process M27.3
- amebic (intestine) A06.1
  - skin A06.7
- anastomotic —see Ulcer, gastrojejunal
- anorectal K62.6
- antral —see Ulcer, stomach
- anus (sphincter) (solitary) K62.6
- aorta —see Aneurysm
- aphthous (oral) (recurrent) K12.0
  - genital organ(s)
    - female N76.6
    - male N50.89
- artery I77.2
- atrophic —see Ulcer, skin
  - decubitus —see Ulcer, pressure, by site
- back L98.429
  - with
    - bone involvement without evidence of necrosis L98.426
    - bone necrosis L98.424
    - exposed fat layer L98.422
    - muscle involvement without evidence of necrosis L98.425
    - muscle necrosis L98.423
    - skin breakdown only L98.421
    - specified severity NEC L98.428
- Barrett's (esophagus) K22.10
  - with bleeding K22.11
- bile duct (common) (hepatic) K83.8
- bladder (solitary) (sphincter) NEC N32.89
  - bilharzial B65.9 [N33]
  - in schistosomiasis (bilharzial) B65.9 [N33]
  - submucosal —see Cystitis, interstitial
  - tuberculous A18.12
- bleeding K27.4
- bone —see Osteomyelitis, specified type NEC
- bowel —see Ulcer, intestine
- breast N61.1
- bronchus J98.09
- buccal (cavity) (traumatic) K12.1
- Buruli A31.1
- buttock L98.419
  - with
    - bone involvement without evidence of necrosis L98.416
    - bone necrosis L98.414
    - exposed fat layer L98.412
    - muscle involvement without evidence of necrosis L98.415
    - muscle necrosis L98.413
    - skin breakdown only L98.411
    - specified severity NEC L98.418
- cancerous —see Neoplasm, malignant, by site
- cardia K22.10
  - with bleeding K22.11
- cardioesophageal (peptic) K22.10
  - with bleeding K22.11
- cecum —see Ulcer, intestine
- cervix (uteri) (decubitus) (trophic) N86
  - with cervicitis N72
- chancroidal A57
- chiclero B55.1
- chronic (cause unknown) —see Ulcer, skin
- Cochin-China B55.1
- colon —see Ulcer, intestine
- conjunctiva H10.89
- cornea H16.00-●
  - with hypopyon H16.03-●
  - central H16.01-●
  - dendritic (herpes simplex) B00.52
  - marginal H16.04-●
  - Mooren's H16.05-●
  - mycotic H16.06-●
  - perforated H16.07-●
  - ring H16.02-●
  - tuberculous (phlyctenular) A18.52

Ulcer, ulcerated, ulcerating, ulceration, ulcerative (Continued)
- corpus cavernosum (chronic) N48.5
- crural —see Ulcer, lower limb
- Curling's —see Ulcer, peptic, acute
- Cushing's —see Ulcer, peptic, acute
- cystic duct K82.8
- cystitis (interstitial) —see Cystitis, interstitial
- decubitus —see Ulcer, pressure, by site
- dendritic, cornea (herpes simplex) B00.52
- diabetes, diabetic —see Diabetes, ulcer
- Dieulafoy's K25.0
- due to
  - infection NEC —see Ulcer, skin
  - radiation NEC L59.8
  - trophic disturbance (any region) —see Ulcer, skin
  - X-ray L58.1
- duodenum, duodenal (eroded) (peptic) K26.9
  - with
    - hemorrhage K26.4
      - and perforation K26.6
    - perforation K26.5
  - acute K26.3
    - with
      - hemorrhage K26.0
        - and perforation K26.2
      - perforation K26.1
  - chronic K26.7
    - with
      - hemorrhage K26.4
        - and perforation K26.6
      - perforation K26.5
- dysenteric A09
- elusive —see Cystitis, interstitial
- endocarditis (acute) (chronic) (subacute) I28.8
- epiglottis J38.7
- esophagus (peptic) K22.10
  - with bleeding K22.11
  - due to
    - aspirin K22.10
      - with bleeding K22.11
    - gastrointestinal reflux disease (without bleeding) K21.00
      - with bleeding K21.01
    - ingestion of chemical or medicament K22.10
      - with bleeding K22.11
  - fungal K22.10
    - with bleeding K22.11
  - infective K22.10
    - with bleeding K22.11
  - varicose —see Varix, esophagus
- eyelid (region) H01.8
- fauces J39.2
- Fenwick (-Hunner) (solitary) —see Cystitis, interstitial
- fistulous —see Ulcer, skin
- foot (indolent) (trophic) —see Ulcer, lower limb
- frambesial, initial A66.0
- frenum (tongue) K14.0
- gallbladder or duct K82.8
- gangrenous —see Gangrene
- gastric —see Ulcer, stomach
- gastrocolic —see Ulcer, gastrojejunal
- gastroduodenal —see Ulcer, peptic
- gastroesophageal —see Ulcer, stomach
- gastrointestinal —see Ulcer, gastrojejunal
- gastrojejunal (peptic) K28.9
  - with
    - hemorrhage K28.4
      - and perforation K28.6
    - perforation K28.5
  - acute K28.3
    - with
      - hemorrhage K28.0
        - and perforation K28.2
      - perforation K28.1

Ulcer, ulcerated, ulcerating, ulceration, ulcerative (Continued)
- gastrojejunal (Continued)
  - chronic K28.7
    - with
      - hemorrhage K28.4
        - and perforation K28.6
      - perforation K28.5
- gastrojejunocolic —see Ulcer, gastrojejunal
- gingiva K06.8
- gingivitis K05.10
  - nonplaque induced K05.11
  - plaque induced K05.10
- glottis J38.7
- granuloma of pudenda A58
- gum K06.8
- gumma, due to yaws A66.4
- heel —see Ulcer, lower limb
- hemorrhoid —see also Hemorrhoids, by degree K64.8
- Hunner's —see Cystitis, interstitial
- hypopharynx J39.2
- hypopyon (chronic) (subacute) —see Ulcer, cornea, with hypopyon
- hypostaticum —see Ulcer, varicose
- ileum —see Ulcer, intestine
- intestine, intestinal K63.3
  - with perforation K63.1
  - amebic A06.1
  - duodenal —see Ulcer, duodenum
  - granulocytopenic (with hemorrhage) —see Neutropenia
  - marginal —see Ulcer, gastrojejunal
  - perforating K63.1
    - newborn P78.0
  - primary, small intestine K63.3
  - rectum K62.6
  - stercoraceous, stercoral K63.3
  - tuberculous A18.32
  - typhoid (fever) —see Typhoid
  - varicose I86.8
- jejunum, jejunal —see Ulcer, gastrojejunal
- keratitis —see Ulcer, cornea
- knee —see Ulcer, lower limb
- labium (majus) (minus) N76.6
- laryngitis —see Laryngitis
- larynx (aphthous) (contact) J38.7
  - diphtheritic A36.2
- leg —see Ulcer, lower limb
- lip K13.0
- Lipschütz's N76.6
- lower limb (atrophic) (chronic) (neurogenic) (perforating) (pyogenic) (trophic) (tropical) L97.909
  - with
    - bone involvement without evidence of necrosis L97.906
    - bone necrosis L97.904
    - exposed fat layer L97.902
    - muscle involvement without evidence of necrosis L97.905
    - muscle necrosis L97.903
    - skin breakdown only L97.901
    - specified severity NEC L97.908
  - ankle L97.309
    - with
      - bone involvement without evidence of necrosis L97.306
      - bone necrosis L97.304
      - exposed fat layer L97.302
      - muscle involvement without evidence of necrosis L97.305
      - muscle necrosis L97.303
      - skin breakdown only L97.301
      - specified severity NEC L97.308
    - left L97.329
      - with
        - bone involvement without evidence of necrosis L97.326
        - bone necrosis L97.324
        - exposed fat layer L97.322

▶ New   ⇒ Revised   ~~deleted~~ Deleted   ● Use Additional Character(s)

► New ⟹ Revised ~~deleted~~ Deleted ● Use Additional Character(s)

Ulcer, ulcerated, ulcerating, ulceration, ulcerative *(Continued)*
lower limb *(Continued)*
right L97.919
with
bone involvement without evidence of necrosis L97.916
bone necrosis L97.914
exposed fat layer L97.912
muscle involvement without evidence of necrosis L97.915
muscle necrosis L97.913
skin breakdown only L97.911
specified severity NEC L97.918
thigh L97.109
with
bone involvement without evidence of necrosis L97.106
bone necrosis L97.104
exposed fat layer L97.102
muscle involvement without evidence of necrosis L97.105
muscle necrosis L97.103
skin breakdown only L97.101
specified severity NEC L97.108
left L97.129
with
bone involvement without evidence of necrosis L97.126
bone necrosis L97.124
exposed fat layer L97.122
muscle involvement without evidence of necrosis L97.125
muscle necrosis L97.123
skin breakdown only L97.121
specified severity NEC L97.128
right L97.119
with
bone involvement without evidence of necrosis L97.116
bone necrosis L97.114
exposed fat layer L97.112
muscle involvement without evidence of necrosis L97.115
muscle necrosis L97.113
skin breakdown only L97.111
specified severity NEC L97.118
toe L97.509
with
bone involvement without evidence of necrosis L97.506
bone necrosis L97.504
exposed fat layer L97.502
muscle involvement without evidence of necrosis L97.505
muscle necrosis L97.503
skin breakdown only L97.501
specified severity NEC L97.508
left L97.529
with
bone involvement without evidence of necrosis L97.526
bone necrosis L97.524
exposed fat layer L97.522
muscle involvement without evidence of necrosis L97.525
muscle necrosis L97.523
skin breakdown only L97.521
specified severity NEC L97.528
right L97.519
with
bone involvement without evidence of necrosis L97.516
bone necrosis L97.514
exposed fat layer L97.512
muscle involvement without evidence of necrosis L97.515
muscle necrosis L97.513
skin breakdown only L97.511
specified severity NEC L97.518

Ulcer, ulcerated, ulcerating, ulceration, ulcerative *(Continued)*
lower limb *(Continued)*
leprous A30.1
syphilitic A52.19
varicose —*see* Varix, leg, with, ulcer
luetic —*see* Ulcer, syphilitic
lung J98.4
tuberculous —*see* Tuberculosis, pulmonary
malignant —*see* Neoplasm, malignant, by site
marginal NEC —*see* Ulcer, gastrojejunal
meatus (urinarius) N34.2
Meckel's diverticulum Q43.0
malignant —*see* Table of Neoplasms, small intestine, malignant
Meleney's (chronic undermining) —*see* Ulcer, skin
Mooren's (cornea) —*see* Ulcer, cornea, Mooren's
mycobacterial (skin) A31.1
nasopharynx J39.2
neck, uterus N86
neurogenic NEC —*see* Ulcer, skin
nose, nasal (passage) (infective) (septum) J34.0
skin —*see* Ulcer, skin
spirochetal A69.8
varicose (bleeding) I86.8
oral mucosa (traumatic) K12.1
palate (soft) K12.1
penis (chronic) N48.5
peptic (site unspecified) K27.9
with
hemorrhage K27.4
and perforation K27.6
perforation K27.5
acute K27.3
with
hemorrhage K27.0
and perforation K27.2
perforation K27.1
chronic K27.7
with
hemorrhage K27.4
and perforation K27.6
perforation K27.5
esophagus K22.10
with bleeding K22.11
newborn P78.82
perforating K27.5
skin —*see* Ulcer, skin
peritonsillar J35.8
phagedenic (tropical) —*see* Ulcer, skin
pharynx J39.2
phlebitis —*see* Phlebitis
plaster —*see* Ulcer, pressure, by site
popliteal space —*see* Ulcer, lower limb
postpyloric —*see* Ulcer, duodenum
prepuce N47.7
prepyloric —*see* Ulcer, stomach
pressure (pressure area) L89.9-●
ankle L89.5-●
back L89.1-●
buttock L89.3-●
coccyx L89.15-●
contiguous site of back, buttock, hip L89.4-●
elbow L89.0-●
face L89.81-●
head L89.81-●
heel L89.6-●
hip L89.2-●
sacral region (tailbone) L89.15-●
specified site NEC L89.89-●
stage 1 (healing) (pre-ulcer skin changes limited to persistent focal edema)
ankle L89.5-●
back L89.1-●
buttock L89.3-●
coccyx L89.15-●
contiguous site of back, buttock, hip L89.4-●

Ulcer, ulcerated, ulcerating, ulceration, ulcerative *(Continued)*
pressure *(Continued)*
stage 1 *(Continued)*
elbow L89.0-●
face L89.81-●
head L89.81-●
heel L89.6-●
hip L89.2-●
sacral region (tailbone) L89.15-●
specified site NEC L89.89-●
stage 2 (healing) (abrasion, blister, partial thickness skin loss involving epidermis and/or dermis)
ankle L89.5-●
back L89.1-●
buttock L89.3-●
coccyx L89.15-●
contiguous site of back, buttock, hip L89.4-●
elbow L89.0-●
face L89.81-●
head L89.81-●
heel L89.6-●
hip L89.2-●
sacral region (tailbone) L89.15-●
specified site NEC L89.89-●
stage 3 (healing) (full thickness skin loss involving damage or necrosis of subcutaneous tissue)
ankle L89.5-●
back L89.1-●
buttock L89.3-●
coccyx L89.15-●
contiguous site of back, buttock, hip L89.4-●
elbow L89.0-●
face L89.81-●
head L89.81-●
heel L89.6-●
hip L89.2-●
sacral region (tailbone) L89.15-●
specified site NEC L89.89-●
stage 4 (healing) (necrosis of soft tissues through to underlying muscle, tendon, or bone)
ankle L89.5-●
back L89.1-●
buttock L89.3-●
coccyx L89.15-●
contiguous site of back, buttock, hip L89.4-●
elbow L89.0-●
face L89.81-●
head L89.81-●
heel L89.6-●
hip L89.2-●
sacral region (tailbone) L89.15-●
specified site NEC L89.89-●
unspecified stage
ankle L89.5-●
back L89.1-●
buttock L89.3-●
coccyx L89.15-●
contiguous site of back, buttock, hip L89.4-●
elbow L89.0-●
face L89.81-●
head L89.81-●
heel L89.6-●
hip L89.2-●
sacral region (tailbone) L89.15-●
specified site NEC L89.89-●
unstageable
ankle L89.5-●
back L89.1-●
buttock L89.3-●
coccyx L89.15-●
contiguous site of back, buttock, hip L89.4-●
elbow L89.0-●

▶ New   ⇒ Revised   ~~deleted~~ Deleted   ● Use Additional Character(s)

Ulcer, ulcerated, ulcerating, ulceration, ulcerative *(Continued)*
  pressure *(Continued)*
    unstageable *(Continued)*
      face L89.81-●
      head L89.81-●
      heel L89.6-●
      hip L89.2-●
      sacral region (tailbone) L89.15-●
      specified site NEC L89.89-●
  primary of intestine K63.3
    with perforation K63.1
  prostate N41.9
  pyloric —*see* Ulcer, stomach
  rectosigmoid K63.3
    with perforation K63.1
  rectum (sphincter) (solitary) K62.6
    stercoraceous, stercoral K62.6
  retina —*see* Inflammation, chorioretinal
  rodent —*see also* Neoplasm, skin, malignant
  sclera —*see* Scleritis
  scrofulous (tuberculous) A18.2
  scrotum N50.89
    tuberculous A18.15
    varicose I86.1
  seminal vesicle N50.89
  sigmoid —*see* Ulcer, intestine
  skin (atrophic) (chronic) (neurogenic) (non-healing) (perforating) (pyogenic) (trophic) (tropical) L98.499
    with gangrene —*see* Gangrene
    amebic A06.7
    back —*see* Ulcer, back
    buttock —*see* Ulcer, buttock
    decubitus —*see* Ulcer, pressure
    lower limb —*see* Ulcer, lower limb
    mycobacterial A31.1
    specified site NEC L98.499
      with
        bone involvement without evidence of necrosis L98.496
        bone necrosis L98.494
        exposed fat layer L98.492
        muscle involvement without evidence of necrosis L98.495
        muscle necrosis L98.493
        skin breakdown only L98.491
        specified severity NEC L98.498
    tuberculous (primary) A18.4
    varicose —*see* Ulcer, varicose
  sloughing —*see* Ulcer, skin
  solitary, anus or rectum (sphincter) K62.6
  sore throat J02.9
    streptococcal J02.0
  spermatic cord N50.89
  spine (tuberculous) A18.01
  stasis (venous) —*see* Varix, leg, with, ulcer
    without varicose veins I87.2
  stercoraceous, stercoral K63.3
    with perforation K63.1
    anus or rectum K62.6
  stoma, stomal —*see* Ulcer, gastrojejunal
  stomach (eroded) (peptic) (round) K25.9
    with
      hemorrhage K25.4
        and perforation K25.6
      perforation K25.5
    acute K25.3
      with
        hemorrhage K25.0
          and perforation K25.2
        perforation K25.1
    chronic K25.7
      with
        hemorrhage K25.4
          and perforation K25.6
        perforation K25.5
  stomal —*see* Ulcer, gastrojejunal
  stomatitis K12.1
  stress —*see* Ulcer, peptic

Ulcer, ulcerated, ulcerating, ulceration, ulcerative *(Continued)*
  strumous (tuberculous) A18.2
  submucosal, bladder —*see* Cystitis, interstitial
  syphilitic (any site) (early) (secondary) A51.39
    late A52.79
    perforating A52.79
      foot A52.11
  testis N50.89
  thigh —*see* Ulcer, lower limb
  throat J39.2
    diphtheritic A36.0
  toe —*see* Ulcer, lower limb
  tongue (traumatic) K14.0
  tonsil J35.8
    diphtheritic A36.0
  trachea J39.8
  trophic —*see* Ulcer, skin
  tropical —*see* Ulcer, skin
  tuberculous —*see* Tuberculosis, ulcer
  tunica vaginalis N50.89
  turbinate J34.89
  typhoid (perforating) —*see* Typhoid
  unspecified site —*see* Ulcer, skin
  urethra (meatus) —*see* Urethritis
  uterus N85.8
    cervix N86
      with cervicitis N72
    neck N86
      with cervicitis N72
  vagina N76.5
    in Behçet's disease M35.2 *[N77.0]*
    pessary N89.8
  valve, heart I33.0
  varicose (lower limb, any part) —*see also* Varix, leg, with, ulcer
    broad ligament I86.2
    esophagus —*see* Varix, esophagus
    inflamed or infected —*see* Varix, leg, with ulcer, with inflammation
    nasal septum I86.8
    perineum I86.3
    scrotum I86.1
    specified site NEC I86.8
    sublingual I86.0
    vulva I86.3
  vas deferens N50.89
  vulva (acute) (infectional) N76.6
    in (due to)
      Behçet's disease M35.2 *[N77.0]*
      herpesviral (herpes simplex) infection A60.04
      tuberculosis A18.18
  vulvobuccal, recurring N76.6
  X-ray L58.1
  yaws A66.4
Ulcerosa scarlatina A38.8
Ulcus —*see also* Ulcer
  cutis tuberculosum A18.4
  duodeni —*see* Ulcer, duodenum
  durum (syphilitic) A51.0
    extragenital A51.2
  gastrojejunale —*see* Ulcer, gastrojejunal
  hypostaticum —*see* Ulcer, varicose
  molle (cutis) (skin) A57
  serpens corneae —*see* Ulcer, cornea, central
  ventriculi —*see* Ulcer, stomach
Ulegyria Q04.8
Ulerythema
  ophryogenes, congenital Q84.2
  sycosiforme L73.8
Ullrich(-Bonnevie)(-Turner) syndrome —*see also* Turner's syndrome Q87.19
Ullrich-Feichtiger syndrome Q87.0
Ulnar —*see* condition
Ulorrhagia, ulorrhea K06.8
Umbilicus, umbilical —*see* condition
Unacceptable
  contours of tooth K08.54
  morphology of tooth K08.54

Unavailability (of)
  bed at medical facility Z75.1
  health service-related agencies Z75.4
  medical facilities (at) Z75.3
    due to
      investigation by social service agency Z75.2
      lack of services at home Z75.0
      remoteness from facility Z75.3
      waiting list Z75.1
    home Z75.0
    outpatient clinic Z75.3
  schooling Z55.1
  social service agencies Z75.4
Uncinaria americana infestation B76.1
Uncinariasis B76.9
Uncongenial work Z56.5
Unconscious (ness) —*see* Coma
Underachievement in school Z55.3
Underdevelopment —*see also* Undeveloped
  nose Q30.1
  sexual E30.0
Underdosing —*see also* Table of Drugs and Chemicals, categories T36-T50, with final character 6 Z91.14
  intentional NEC Z91.128
    due to financial hardship of patient Z91.120
  unintentional NEC Z91.138
    due to patient's age related debility Z91.130
Underfeeding, newborn P92.3
Underfill, endodontic M27.53
Underimmunization status Z28.3
Undernourishment —*see* Malnutrition
Undernutrition —*see* Malnutrition
Under observation —*see* Observation
Underweight R63.6
  for gestational age —*see* Light for dates
Underwood's disease P83.0
Undescended —*see also* Malposition, congenital
  cecum Q43.3
  colon Q43.3
  testicle —*see* Cryptorchid
Undeveloped, undevelopment —*see also* Hypoplasia
  brain (congenital) Q02
  cerebral (congenital) Q02
  heart Q24.8
  lung Q33.6
  testis E29.1
  uterus E30.0
Undiagnosed (disease) R69
Undulant fever —*see* Brucellosis
Unemployment, anxiety concerning Z56.0
  threatened Z56.2
Unequal length (acquired) (limb) —*see also* Deformity, limb, unequal length
  leg —*see also* Deformity, limb, unequal length
    congenital Q72.9-●
Unextracted dental root K08.3
Unguis incarnatus L60.0
Unhappiness R45.2
Unicornate uterus Q51.4
  in pregnancy or childbirth O34.00
Unilateral —*see also* condition
  development, breast N64.89
  organ or site, congenital NEC —*see* Agenesis, by site
Unilocular heart Q20.8
Union, abnormal —*see also* Fusion
  larynx and trachea Q34.8
Universal mesentery Q43.3
Unrepairable overhanging of dental restorative materials K08.52
Unsatisfactory
  restoration of tooth K08.50
    specified NEC K08.59
  sample of cytologic smear
    anus R85.615
    cervix R87.615
    vagina R87.625
  surroundings Z59.1
  work Z56.5

Unsoundness of mind —see Psychosis
Unstable
　back NEC —see Instability, joint, spine
　hip (congenital) Q65.6
　　acquired —see Derangement, joint,
　　　specified type NEC, hip
　joint —see Instability, joint
　　secondary to removal of joint prosthesis
　　　M96.89
　lie (mother) O32.0
　lumbosacral joint (congenital) —see
　　　subcategory M53.2
　sacroiliac —see subcategory M53.2
　spine NEC —see Instability, joint, spine
Unsteadiness on feet R26.81
Untruthfulness, child problem F91.8
Unverricht(-Lundborg) disease or epilepsy —
　　see Epilepsy, generalized, idiopathic
Unwanted pregnancy Z64.0
▶Unwanted
　▶multiple moves in the last 12 months
　　　Z59.81- ●
　▶pregnancy Z64.0
Upbringing, institutional Z62.22
　away from parents NEC Z62.29
　in care of non-parental family member Z62.21
　in foster care Z62.21
　in orphanage or group home Z62.22
　in welfare custody Z62.21
Upper respiratory —see condition
Upset
　gastric K30
　gastrointestinal K30
　　psychogenic F45.8
　intestinal (large) (small) K59.9
　　psychogenic F45.8
　menstruation N93.9
　mental F48.9
　stomach K30
　　psychogenic F45.8
Urachus —see also condition
　patent or persistent Q64.4
Urbach-Oppenheim disease (necrobiosis
　　lipoidica diabeticorum) —see E08-E13 with
　　.620
Urbach's lipoid proteinosis E78.89
Urbach-Wiethe disease E78.89
Urban yellow fever A95.1
Urea
　blood, high —see Uremia
　cycle metabolism disorder —see Disorder,
　　urea cycle metabolism
Uremia, uremic N19
　with
　　ectopic or molar pregnancy O08.4
　　polyneuropathy N18.9 [G63]
　chronic NOS —see also Disease, kidney,
　　chronic N18.9
　　due to hypertension —see Hypertensive,
　　　kidney
　complicating
　　ectopic or molar pregnancy O08.4
　congenital P96.0
　extrarenal R39.2
　following ectopic or molar pregnancy O08.4
　newborn P96.0
　prerenal R39.2
Ureter, ureteral —see condition
Ureteralgia N23
Ureterectasis —see Hydroureter
Ureteritis N28.89
　cystica N28.86
　due to calculus N20.1
　　with calculus, kidney N20.2
　　　with hydronephrosis N13.2
　gonococcal (acute) (chronic) A54.21
　nonspecific N28.89
Ureterocele N28.89
　congenital (orthotopic) Q62.31
　　ectopic Q62.32
Ureterolith, ureterolithiasis —see Calculus, ureter
Ureterostomy
　attention to Z43.6

status Z93.6
Urethra, urethral —see condition
Urethralgia R39.89
Urethritis (anterior) (posterior) N34.2
　calculous N21.1
　candidal B37.41
　chlamydial A56.01
　diplococcal (gonococcal) A54.01
　　with abscess (accessory gland)
　　　(periurethral) A54.1
　gonococcal A54.01
　　with abscess (accessory gland)
　　　(periurethral) A54.1
　nongonococcal N34.1
　　Reiter's —see Reiter's disease
　nonspecific N34.1
　nonvenereal N34.1
　postmenopausal N34.2
　puerperal O86.22
　Reiter's —see Reiter's disease
　specified NEC N34.2
　trichomonal or due to Trichomonas
　　　(vaginalis) A59.03
Urethrocele N81.0
　with
　　cystocele —see Cystocele
　　prolapse of uterus —see Prolapse, uterus
Urethrolithiasis (with colic or infection) N21.1
Urethrorectal —see condition
Urethrorrhagia N36.8
Urethrorrhea R36.9
Urethrostomy
　attention to Z43.6
　status Z93.6
Urethrotrigonitis —see Trigonitis
Urethrovaginal —see condition
Urgency
　fecal R15.2
　hypertensive —see Hypertension
　urinary N39.15
Urhidrosis, uridrosis L74.8
Uric acid in blood (increased) E79.0
Uricacidemia (asymptomatic) E79.0
Uricemia (asymptomatic) E79.0
Uricosuria R82.998
Urinary —see condition
Urination
　frequent R35.0
　painful R30.9
Urine
　blood in —see Hematuria
⇒discharge, excessive R35.89
　enuresis, nonorganic origin F98.0
　extravasation R39.0
　frequency R35.0
　incontinence R32
　　nonorganic origin F98.0
　intermittent stream R39.198
　pus in N39.0
　retention or stasis R33.9
　　organic R33.8
　　　drug-induced R33.0
　　psychogenic F45.8
　secretion
　　deficient R34
⇒　excessive R35.89
　　frequency R35.0
　stream
　　intermittent R39.198
　　slowing R39.198
　　splitting R39.13
　　weak R39.12
Urinemia —see Uremia
Urinoma, urethra N36.8
Uroarthritis, infectious (Reiter's) —see Reiter's
　　disease
Urodialysis R34
Urolithiasis —see Calculus, urinary
Uronephrosis —see Hydronephrosis
Uropathy N39.9
　obstructive N13.9

　specified NEC N13.8
Uropathy (Continued)
　reflux N13.9
　　specified NEC N13.8
　vesicoureteral reflux-associated —see Reflux,
　　vesicoureteral
Urosepsis — code to condition
Urticaria L50.9
　with angioneurotic edema T78.3
　　hereditary D84.1
　allergic L50.0
　cholinergic L50.5
　chronic L50.8
　cold, familial L50.2
　contact L50.6
　dermatographic L50.3
　due to
　　cold or heat L50.2
　　drugs L50.0
　　food L50.0
　　inhalants L50.0
　　plants L50.6
　　serum —see also Reaction, serum
　　　T80.69
　factitial L50.3
　familial cold M04.2
　giant T78.3
　　hereditary D84.1
　gigantea T78.3
　idiopathic L50.1
　larynx T78.3
　　hereditary D84.1
　neonatorum P83.88
　nonallergic L50.1
　papulosa (Hebra) L28.2
　pigmentosa D47.01
　　congenital Q82.2
　　of neonatal onset Q82.2
　　of newborn onset Q82.2
　recurrent periodic L50.8
　serum —see also Reaction, serum T80.69
　solar L56.3
　specified type NEC L50.8
　thermal (cold) (heat) L50.2
　vibratory L50.4
　xanthelasmoidea —see Urticaria pigmentosa
Use (of)
　alcohol Z72.89
　　with
　　　intoxication F10.929
　　　sleep disorder F10.982
　　　withdrawal F10.939
　　　　with
　　　　　perceptual disturbance F10.932
　　　　delirium F10.931
　　　　uncomplicated F10.930
　　harmful —see Abuse, alcohol
　amphetamines —see Use, stimulant NEC
　caffeine —see Use, stimulant NEC
　cannabis F12.90
　　with
　　　anxiety disorder F12.980
　　　intoxication F12.929
　　　　with
　　　　　delirium F12.921
　　　　　perceptual disturbance F12.922
　　　　uncomplicated F12.920
　　　other specified disorder F12.988
　　　psychosis F12.959
　　　　delusions F12.950
　　　　hallucinations F12.951
　　　unspecified disorder F12.99
　　　withdrawal F12.93
　cocaine F14.90
　　with
　　　anxiety disorder F14.980
　　　intoxication F14.929
　　　　with
　　　　　delirium F14.921
　　　　　perceptual disturbance F14.922
　　　　uncomplicated F14.920

other specified disorder F14.988
Use *(Continued)*
  cocaine *(Continued)*
    with *(Continued)*
      psychosis F14.959
        delusions F14.950
        hallucinations F14.951
      sexual dysfunction F14.981
      sleep disorder F14.982
      unspecified disorder F14.99
      withdrawal F14.93
    harmful —*see* Abuse, drug, cocaine
  drug(s) NEC F19.90
    with sleep disorder F19.982
    harmful —*see* Abuse, drug, by type
  hallucinogen NEC F16.90
    with
      anxiety disorder F16.980
      intoxication F16.929
        with
          delirium F16.921
        uncomplicated F16.920
      mood disorder F16.94
      other specified disorder F16.988
      perception disorder (flashbacks) F16.983
      psychosis F16.959
        delusions F16.950
        hallucinations F16.951
      unspecified disorder F16.99
    harmful —*see* Abuse, drug, hallucinogen
      NEC
  inhalants F18.90
    with
      anxiety disorder F18.980
      intoxication F18.929
        with delirium F18.921
        uncomplicated F18.920
      mood disorder F18.94
      other specified disorder F18.988
      persisting dementia F18.97
      psychosis F18.959
        delusions F18.950
        hallucinations F18.951
      unspecified disorder F18.99
    harmful —*see* Abuse, drug, inhalant
  methadone —*see* Use, opioid
  nonprescribed drugs F19.90
    harmful —*see* Abuse, non-psychoactive
      substance
  opioid F11.90
    with
      disorder F11.99
        mood F11.94
        sleep F11.982
        specified type NEC F11.988
      intoxication F11.929
        with
          delirium F11.921
          perceptual disturbance F11.922
        uncomplicated F11.920
      withdrawal F11.93

harmful —*see* Abuse, drug, opioid
Use *(Continued)*
  patent medicines F19.90
    harmful —*see* Abuse, non-psychoactive
      substance
  psychoactive drug NEC F19.90
    with
      anxiety disorder F19.980
      intoxication F19.929
        with
          delirium F19.921
          perceptual disturbance
            F19.922
        uncomplicated F19.920
      mood disorder F19.94
      other specified disorder F19.988
      persisting
        amnestic disorder F19.96
        dementia F19.97
      psychosis F19.959
        delusions F19.950
        hallucinations F19.951
      sexual dysfunction F19.981
      sleep disorder F19.982
      unspecified disorder F19.99
      withdrawal F19.939
        with
          delirium F19.931
          perceptual disturbance
            F19.932
        uncomplicated F19.930
    harmful —*see* Abuse, drug NEC,
      psychoactive NEC
  sedative, hypnotic, or anxiolytic
    F13.90
    with
      anxiety disorder F13.980
      intoxication F13.929
        with
          delirium F13.921
        uncomplicated F13.920
      other specified disorder F13.988
      persisting
        amnestic disorder F13.96
        dementia F13.97
      psychosis F13.959
        delusions F13.950
        hallucinations F13.951
      sexual dysfunction F13.981
      sleep disorder F13.982
      unspecified disorder F13.99
    harmful —*see* Abuse, drug, sedative,
      hypnotic, or anxiolytic
  stimulant NEC F15.90
    with
      anxiety disorder F15.980
      intoxication F15.929
        with
          delirium F15.921
          perceptual disturbance
            F15.922

uncomplicated F15.920
Use *(Continued)*
  stimulant NEC *(Continued)*
    with *(Continued)*
      mood disorder F15.94
      other specified disorder F15.988
      psychosis F15.959
        delusions F15.950
        hallucinations F15.951
      sexual dysfunction F15.981
      sleep disorder F15.982
      unspecified disorder F15.99
      withdrawal F15.93
    harmful —*see* Abuse, drug, stimulant
      NEC
  tobacco Z72.0
    with dependence —*see* Dependence,
      drug, nicotine
  volatile solvents —*see also* Use, inhalant
    F18.90
    harmful —*see* Abuse, drug, inhalant
Usher-Senear disease or syndrome L10.4
Uta B55.1
Uteromegaly N85.2
Uterovaginal —*see* condition
Uterovesical —*see* condition
Uveal —*see* condition
Uveitis (anterior) —*see also* Iridocyclitis
  acute —*see* Iridocyclitis, acute
  chronic —*see* Iridocyclitis, chronic
  due to toxoplasmosis (acquired) B58.09
    congenital P37.1
  granulomatous —*see* Iridocyclitis,
    chronic
  heterochromic —*see* Cyclitis, Fuchs'
    heterochromic
  lens-induced —*see* Iridocyclitis,
    lens-induced
  posterior —*see* Chorioretinitis
  sympathetic H44.13-●
  syphilitic (secondary) A51.43
    congenital (early) A50.01
    late A52.71
  tuberculous A18.54
Uveoencephalitis —*see* Inflammation,
  chorioretinal
Uveokeratitis —*see* Iridocyclitis
Uveoparotitis D86.89
Uvula —*see* condition
Uvulitis (acute) (catarrhal) (chronic)
  (membranous) (suppurative) (ulcerative)
  K12.2

V

Vaccination (prophylactic)
  complication or reaction —*see* Complications, vaccination
  delayed Z28.9
  encounter for Z23
  not done —*see* Immunization, not done, because (of)
Vaccinia (generalized) (localized) T88.1
  without vaccination B08.011
  congenital P35.8
Vacuum, in sinus (accessory) (nasal) J34.89
Vagabond, vagabondage Z59.00
Vagabond's disease B85.1
Vagina, vaginal —*see* condition
Vaginalitis (tunica) (testis) N49.1
Vaginismus (reflex) N94.2
  functional F52.5
  nonorganic F52.5
  psychogenic F52.5
  secondary N94.2
Vaginitis (acute) (circumscribed) (diffuse) (emphysematous) (nonvenereal) (ulcerative) N76.0
  with ectopic or molar pregnancy O08.0
  amebic A06.82
  atrophic, postmenopausal N95.2
  bacterial N76.0
  blennorrhagic (gonococcal) A54.02
  candidal B37.3
  chlamydial A56.02
  chronic N76.1
  due to Trichomonas (vaginalis) A59.01
  following ectopic or molar pregnancy O08.0
  gonococcal A54.02
    with abscess (accessory gland) (periurethral) A54.1
  granuloma A58
  in (due to)
    candidiasis B37.3
    herpesviral (herpes simplex) infection A60.04
    pinworm infection B80 [N77.1]
  monilial B37.3
  mycotic (candidal) B37.3
  postmenopausal atrophic N95.2
  puerperal (postpartum) O86.13
  senile (atrophic) N95.2
  subacute or chronic N76.1
  syphilitic (early) A51.0
    late A52.76
  trichomonal A59.01
  tuberculous A18.18
Vaginosis —*see* Vaginitis
Vagotonia G52.2
Vagrancy Z59.00
VAIN —*see* Neoplasia, intraepithelial, vagina
Vallecula —*see* condition
Valley fever B38.0
Valsuani's disease —*see* Anemia, obstetric
Valve, valvular (formation) —*see also* condition
  cerebral ventricle (communicating) in situ Z98.2
  cervix, internal os Q51.828
  congenital NEC —*see* Atresia, by site
  ureter (pelvic junction) (vesical orifice) Q62.39
  urethra (congenital) (posterior) Q64.2
Valvulitis (chronic) —*see* Endocarditis
Valvulopathy —*see* Endocarditis
Van Bogaert's leukoencephalopathy (sclerosing) (subacute) A81.1
Van Bogaert-Scherer-Epstein disease or syndrome E75.5
Van Buchem's syndrome M85.2
Van Creveld-von Gierke disease E74.01
Van der Hoeve (-de Kleyn) syndrome Q78.0
Van der Woude's syndrome Q38.0
Van Neck's disease or osteochondrosis M91.0
Vanishing lung J44.9

Vapor asphyxia or suffocation T59.9
  specified agent —*see* Table of Drugs and Chemicals
Variance, lethal ball, prosthetic heart valve T82.09
Variants, thalassemic D56.8
Variations in hair color L67.1
Varicella B01.9
  with
    complications NEC B01.89
    encephalitis B01.11
    encephalomyelitis B01.11
    meningitis B01.0
    myelitis B01.12
    pneumonia B01.2
  congenital P35.8
Varices —*see* Varix
Varicocele (scrotum) (thrombosed) I86.1
  ovary I86.2
  perineum I86.3
  spermatic cord (ulcerated) I86.1
Varicose
  aneurysm (ruptured) I77.0
  dermatitis —*see* Varix, leg, with, inflammation
  eczema —*see* Varix, leg, with, inflammation
  phlebitis —*see* Varix, with, inflammation
  tumor —*see* Varix
  ulcer (lower limb, any part) —*see also* Varix, leg, with, ulcer
    anus —*see also* Hemorrhoids K64.8
    esophagus —*see* Varix, esophagus
    inflamed or infected —*see* Varix, leg, with, ulcer, with inflammation
    nasal septum I86.8
    perineum I86.3
    scrotum I86.1
    specified site NEC I86.8
  vein —*see* Varix
  vessel —*see* Varix, leg
Varicosis, varicosities, varicosity —*see* Varix
Variola (major) (minor) B03
Varioloid B03
Varix (lower limb) I83.90
  with
    bleeding I83.899
    edema I83.899
    inflammation I83.10
      with ulcer (venous) I83.209
    pain I83.819
    rupture I83.899
    specified complication NEC I83.899
    stasis dermatitis I83.10
      with ulcer (venous) I83.209
    swelling I83.899
    ulcer I83.009
      with inflammation I83.209
  aneurysmal I77.0
  asymptomatic I83.9-●
  bladder I86.2
  broad ligament I86.2
  complicating
    childbirth (lower extremity) O87.4
      anus or rectum O87.2
      genital (vagina, vulva or perineum) O87.8
    pregnancy (lower extremity) O22.0-●
      anus or rectum O22.4-●
      genital (vagina, vulva or perineum) O22.1-●
    puerperium (lower extremity) O87.4
      anus or rectum O87.2
      genital (vagina, vulva, perineum) O87.8
  congenital (any site) Q27.8
  esophagus (idiopathic) (primary) (ulcerated) I85.00
    bleeding I85.01
    congenital Q27.8
    in (due to)
      alcoholic liver disease I85.10
        bleeding I85.11
      cirrhosis of liver I85.10
        bleeding I85.11

Varix (Continued)
  esophagus (Continued)
    in (Continued)
      portal hypertension I85.10
        bleeding I85.11
      schistosomiasis I85.10
        bleeding I85.11
      toxic liver disease I85.10
        bleeding I85.11
    secondary I85.10
      bleeding I85.11
  gastric I86.4
  inflamed or infected I83.10
    ulcerated I83.209
  labia (majora) I86.3
  leg (asymptomatic) I83.9-●
    with
      edema I83.899
      inflammation I83.10
        with ulcer —*see* Varix, leg, with, ulcer, with inflammation by site
      pain I83.819
      specified complication NEC I83.899
      swelling I83.899
      ulcer I83.0-●
        with inflammation I83.2-●
        ankle I83.003
          with inflammation I83.203
        calf I83.002
          with inflammation I83.202
        foot NEC I83.005
          with inflammation I83.205
        heel I83.004
          with inflammation I83.204
        lower leg NEC I83.008
          with inflammation I83.208
        midfoot I83.004
          with inflammation I83.204
        thigh I83.001
          with inflammation I83.201
    bilateral (asymptomatic) I83.93
      with
        edema I83.893
        pain I83.813
        specified complication NEC I83.893
        swelling I83.893
        ulcer I83.0-●
          with inflammation I83.209
    left (asymptomatic) I83.92
      with
        edema I83.892
        inflammation I83.12
          with ulcer —*see* Varix, leg, with, ulcer, with inflammation by site
        pain I83.812
        specified complication NEC I83.892
        swelling I83.892
        ulcer I83.029
          with inflammation I83.229
        ankle I83.023
          with inflammation I83.223
        calf I83.022
          with inflammation I83.222
        foot NEC I83.025
          with inflammation I83.225
        heel I83.024
          with inflammation I83.224
        lower leg NEC I83.028
          with inflammation I83.228
        midfoot I83.024
          with inflammation I83.224
        thigh I83.021
          with inflammation I83.221
    right (asymptomatic) I83.91
      with
        edema I83.891
        inflammation I83.11
          with ulcer —*see* Varix, leg, with, ulcer, with inflammation by site

▶ New   ⇒ Revised   ~~deleted~~ Deleted   ● Use Additional Character(s)

Varix (Continued)
  leg (Continued)
    right (Continued)
      with (Continued)
        pain I83.811
        specified complication NEC I83.891
        swelling I83.891
        ulcer I83.019
          with inflammation I83.219
          ankle I83.013
            with inflammation I83.213
          calf I83.012
            with inflammation I83.212
          foot NEC I83.015
            with inflammation I83.215
          heel I83.014
            with inflammation I83.214
          lower leg NEC I83.018
            with inflammation I83.218
          midfoot I83.014
            with inflammation I83.214
          thigh I83.011
            with inflammation I83.211
  nasal septum I86.8
  orbit I86.8
    congenital Q27.8
  ovary I86.2
  papillary I78.1
  pelvis I86.2
  perineum I86.3
  pharynx I86.8
  placenta O43.89-●
  renal papilla I86.8
  retina H35.09
  scrotum (ulcerated) I86.1
  sigmoid colon I86.8
  specified site NEC I86.8
  spinal (cord) (vessels) I86.8
  spleen, splenic (vein) (with phlebolith) I86.8
  stomach I86.4
  sublingual I86.0
  ulcerated I83.009
    inflamed or infected I83.209
  uterine ligament I86.2
  vagina I86.8
  vocal cord I86.8
  vulva I86.3
Vas deferens —see condition
Vas deferentitis N49.1
Vasa previa O69.4
  hemorrhage from, affecting newborn P50.0
Vascular —see also condition
  loop on optic papilla Q14.2
  spasm I73.9
  spider I78.1
Vascularization, cornea —see
    Neovascularization, cornea
Vasculitis I77.6
  allergic D69.0
  cryoglobulinemic D89.1
  disseminated I77.6
  hypocomplementemic M31.8
  kidney I77.89
▶ leukocytoclastic M31.0
  livedoid L95.0
  nodular L95.8
  retina H35.06-●
  rheumatic —see Fever, rheumatic
  rheumatoid —see Rheumatoid, vasculitis
  skin (limited to) L95.9
    specified NEC L95.8
  systemic M31.8
Vasculopathy, necrotizing M31.9
  cardiac allograft T86.290
  specified NEC M31.8
Vasitis (nodosa) N49.1
  tuberculous A18.15
Vasodilation I73.9
Vasomotor —see condition
Vasoplasty, after previous sterilization Z31.0
  aftercare Z31.42

Vasospasm (vasoconstriction) I73.9
  cerebral (cerebrovascular) (artery)
      I67.848
    reversible I67.841
  coronary I20.1
  nerve
    arm —see Mononeuropathy, upper limb
    brachial plexus G54.0
    cervical plexus G54.2
    leg —see Mononeuropathy, lower limb
  peripheral NOS I73.9
  retina (artery) —see Occlusion, artery,
      retina
Vasospastic —see condition
Vasovagal attack (paroxysmal) R55
  psychogenic F45.8
VATER syndrome Q87.2
Vater's ampulla —see condition
Vegetation, vegetative
  adenoid (nasal fossa) J35.8
  endocarditis (acute) (any valve) (subacute)
      I33.0
  heart (mycotic) (valve) I33.0
Veil
  Jackson's Q43.3
Vein, venous —see condition
Veldt sore —see Ulcer, skin
Velpeau's hernia —see Hernia, femoral
Venereal
  bubo A55
  disease A64
  granuloma inguinale A58
  lymphogranuloma (Durand-Nicolas-Favre)
      A55
Venofibrosis I87.8
Venom, venomous —see Table of Drugs and
    Chemicals, by animal or substance,
    poisoning
Venous —see condition
Ventilator lung, newborn P27.8
Ventral —see condition
Ventricle, ventricular —see also condition
  escape I49.3
  inversion Q20.5
Ventriculitis (cerebral) —see also Encephalitis
    G04.90
Ventriculostomy status Z98.2
Vernet's syndrome G52.7
Verneuil's disease (syphilitic bursitis) A52.78
Verruca (due to HPV) (filiformis) (simplex)
    (viral) (vulgaris) B07.9
  acuminata A63.0
  necrogenica (primary) (tuberculosa) A18.4
  plana B07.8
  plantaris B07.0
  seborrheica L82.1
    inflamed L82.0
  senile (seborrheic) L82.1
    inflamed L82.0
  tuberculosa (primary) A18.4
  venereal A63.0
Verrucosities —see Verruca
Verruga peruana, peruviana A44.1
Version
  cervix —see Malposition, uterus
  uterus (postinfectional) (postpartal, old) —see
    Malposition, uterus
Vertebra, vertebral —see condition
Vertical talus (congenital) Q66.80
  left foot Q66.82
  right foot Q66.81
Vertigo R42
  auditory —see Vertigo, aural
  aural H81.31-●
  benign paroxysmal (positional) H81.1-●
  central (origin) H81.4
  cerebral H81.4
  Dix and Hallpike (epidemic) —see Neuronitis,
    vestibular
  due to infrasound T75.23

Vertigo (Continued)
  epidemic A88.1
    Dix and Hallpike —see Neuronitis,
      vestibular
    Pedersen's —see Neuronitis, vestibular
    vestibular neuronitis —see Neuronitis,
      vestibular
  hysterical F44.89
  infrasound T75.23
  labyrinthine —see subcategory H81.0
⇒ laryngeal R05.4
  malignant positional H81.4
  Ménière's —see subcategory H81.40
  menopausal N95.11
  otogenic —see Vertigo, aural
  paroxysmal positional, benign —see Vertigo,
    benign paroxysmal
  Pedersen's (epidemic) —see Neuronitis,
    vestibular
  peripheral NEC H81.39-●
  positional
    benign paroxysmal —see Vertigo, benign
      paroxysmal
    malignant H81.4
Very-low-density-lipoprotein-type (VLDL)
    hyperlipoproteinemia E78.1
Vesania —see Psychosis
Vesical —see condition
Vesicle
  cutaneous R23.8
  seminal —see condition
  skin R23.8
Vesicocolic —see condition
Vesicoperineal —see condition
Vesicorectal —see condition
Vesicourethrorectal —see condition
Vesicovaginal —see condition
Vesicular —see condition
Vesiculitis (seminal) N49.0
  amebic A06.82
  gonorrheal (acute) (chronic) A54.23
  trichomonal A59.09
  tuberculous A18.15
Vestibulitis (ear) —see also subcategory H83.0
  nose (external) J34.89
  vulvar N94.810
Vestibulopathy, acute peripheral (recurrent) —
    see Neuronitis, vestibular
Vestige, vestigial —see also Persistence
  branchial Q18.0
  structures in vitreous Q14.0
Vibration
  adverse effects T75.20
    pneumatic hammer syndrome T75.21
    specified effect NEC T75.29
    vasospastic syndrome T75.22
    vertigo from infrasound T75.23
  exposure (occupational) Z57.7
  vertigo T75.23
Vibriosis A28.9
Victim (of)
  crime Z65.4
  disaster Z65.5
  terrorism Z65.4
  torture Z65.4
  war Z65.5
Vidal's disease L28.0
Villaret's syndrome G52.7
Villous —see condition
VIN —see Neoplasia, intraepithelial, vulva
Vincent's infection (angina) (gingivitis) A69.1
  stomatitis NEC A69.1
Vinson-Plummer syndrome D50.1
Violence, physical R45.6
Viosterol deficiency —see Deficiency, calciferol
Vipoma —see Neoplasm, malignant, by site
Viremia B34.9
Virilism (adrenal) E25.9
  congenital E25.0
Virilization (female) (suprarenal) E25.9
  congenital E25.0
  isosexual E28.2

Virulent bubo A57
Virus, viral —see also condition
  as cause of disease classified elsewhere
    B97.89
  ➡respiratory syncytial virus (RSV) —see Virus,
      infection, respiratory syncytial (RSV)
  cytomegalovirus B25.9
  human immunodeficiency (HIV) —see
      Human, immunodeficiency virus (HIV)
      disease
  infection —see Infection, virus
  respiratory syncytial (RSV)
    as cause of disease classified elsewhere
      B97.4
    bronchiolitis J21.0
    bronchitis J20.5
    bronchopneumonia J12.1
    otitis media H65-• [B97.4]
    pneumonia J12.1
    upper respiratory infection J06.9 [B97.4]
  specified NEC B34.8
  swine influenza (viruses that normally cause
      infections in pigs) —see also Influenza,
      due to, identified novel influenza A virus
      J09.X2
  West Nile (fever) A92.30
    with
      complications NEC A92.39
      cranial nerve disorders A92.32
      encephalitis A92.31
      encephalomyelitis A92.31
      neurologic manifestation NEC A92.32
      optic neuritis A92.32
      polyradiculitis A92.32
Viscera, visceral —see condition
Visceroptosis K63.4
Visible peristalsis R19.2
Vision, visual
  binocular, suppression H53.34
  blurred, blurring H53.8
    hysterical F44.6
  defect, defective NEC H54.7
  disorientation (syndrome) H53.8
  disturbance H53.9
    hysterical F44.6
  double H53.2
  examination Z01.00
    with abnormal findings Z01.01
    following failed vision screening Z01.020
      with abnormal findings Z01.021
  field, limitation (defect) —see Defect, visual
      field
  hallucinations R44.1
  halos H53.19
  loss —see Loss, vision
    sudden —see Disturbance, vision,
        subjective, loss, sudden
  low (both eyes) —see Low, vision
  perception, simultaneous without fusion
      H53.33
Vitality, lack or want of R53.83
  newborn P96.89
Vitamin deficiency —see Deficiency, vitamin

Vitelline duct, persistent Q43.0
Vitiligo L80
  eyelid H02.739
    left H02.736
      lower H02.735
      upper H02.734
    right H02.733
      lower H02.732
      upper H02.731
  pinta A67.2
  vulva N90.89
Vitreal corneal syndrome H59.01-•
Vitreoretinopathy, proliferative —see also
    Retinopathy, proliferative
  with retinal detachment —see Detachment,
      retina, traction
Vitreous —see also condition
  touch syndrome —see Complication,
      postprocedural, following cataract
      surgery
Vocal cord —see condition
Vogt-Koyanagi syndrome H20.82-•
Vogt's disease or syndrome G80.3
Vogt-Spielmeyer amaurotic idiocy or disease
    E75.4
Voice
  change R49.9
    specified NEC R49.8
  loss —see Aphonia
Volhynian fever A79.0
Volkmann's ischemic contracture or paralysis
    (complicating trauma) T79.6
Volvulus (bowel) (colon) (intestine) K56.2
  with perforation K56.2
  congenital Q43.8
  duodenum K31.5
  fallopian tube —see Torsion, fallopian tube
  oviduct —see Torsion, fallopian tube
  stomach (due to absence of gastrocolic
      ligament) K31.89
Vomiting R11.10
  with nausea R11.2
  without nausea R11.11
  asphyxia —see Foreign body, by site, causing
      asphyxia, gastric contents
  bilious (cause unknown) R11.14
    following gastro-intestinal surgery K91.0
    in newborn P92.01
  blood —see Hematemesis
  causing asphyxia, choking, or suffocation —
      see Foreign body, by site
  cyclical, in migraine G43.A0
    with refractory migraine G43.A1
    intractable G43.A1
    not intractable G43.A0
    psychogenic F50.89
    without refractory migraine G43.A0
  cyclical syndrome NOS (unrelated to
      migraine) R53.1
    persistent R11.15

Vomiting (Continued)
  fecal mater R11.13
  following gastrointestinal surgery K91.0
    psychogenic F50.89
  functional K31.89
  hysterical F50.89
  nervous F50.89
  neurotic F50.89
  newborn NEC P92.09
    bilious P92.01
  periodic R11.10
    psychogenic F50.89
  projectile R11.12
  psychogenic F50.89
  uremic —see Uremia
Vomito negro —see Fever, yellow
Von Bezold's abscess —see Mastoiditis, acute
Von Economo-Cruchet disease A85.8
Von Eulenburg's disease G71.19
Von Gierke's disease E74.01
Von Hippel (-Lindau) disease or syndrome
    Q85.8
Von Jaksch's anemia or disease D64.89
Von Recklinghausen
  disease (neurofibromatosis) Q85.01
    bones E21.0
Von Schroetter's syndrome I82.890
Von Willebrand (-Jurgens)(-Minot) disease or
    syndrome D68.0
Von Zumbusch's disease L40.1
Voyeurism F65.3
Vrolik's disease Q78.0
Vulva —see condition
Vulvismus N94.2
Vulvitis (acute) (allergic) (atrophic)
    (hypertrophic) (intertriginous) (senile)
    N76.2
  with ectopic or molar pregnancy O08.0
  adhesive, congenital Q52.79
  blennorrhagic (gonococcal) A54.02
  candidal B37.3
  chlamydial A56.02
  due to Haemophilus ducreyi A57
  following ectopic or molar pregnancy O08.0
  gonococcal A54.02
    with abscess (accessory gland)
        (periurethral) A54.1
  herpesviral A60.04
  leukoplakic N90.4
  monilial B37.3
  puerperal (postpartum) O86.19
  subacute or chronic N76.3
  syphilitic (early) A51.0
    late A52.76
  trichomonal A59.01
  tuberculous A18.18
Vulvodynia N94.819
  specified NEC N94.818
Vulvorectal —see condition
Vulvovaginitis (acute) —see Vaginitis

W

Waiting list, person on Z75.1
    for organ transplant Z76.82
    undergoing social agency investigation Z75.2
Waldenström
    hypergammaglobulinemia D89.0
    syndrome or macroglobulinemia C88.0
Waldenström-Kjellberg syndrome D50.1
Walking
    difficulty R26.2
        psychogenic F44.4
    sleep F51.3
        hysterical F44.89
Wall, abdominal —see condition
Wallenberg's disease or syndrome G46.3
Wallgren's disease I87.8
Wandering
    gallbladder, congenital Q44.1
    in diseases classified elsewhere Z91.83
    kidney, congenital Q63.8
    organ or site, congenital NEC —see
        Malposition, congenital, by site
    pacemaker (heart) I49.8
    spleen D73.89
War neurosis F48.8
Wart (due to HPV) (filiform) (infectious)
        (viral) B07.9
    anogenital region (venereal) A63.0
    common B07.8
    external genital organs (venereal)
        A63.0
    flat B07.8
    Hassal-Henle's (of cornea) H18.49
    Peruvian A44.1
    plantar B07.0
    prosector (tuberculous) A18.4
    seborrheic L82.1
        inflamed L82.0
    senile (seborrheic) L82.1
        inflamed L82.0
    tuberculous A18.4
    venereal A63.0
Warthin's tumor —see Neoplasm, salivary
        gland, benign
Wassilieff's disease A27.0
Wasting
    disease R64
        ➡due to malnutrition E43
        ▶with marasmus E41
    ➡extreme (due to malnutrition) E43
        ▶with marasmus E41
    muscle NEC —see Atrophy, muscle
Water
    clefts (senile cataract) —see Cataract, senile,
        incipient
    deprivation of T73.1
    intoxication E87.79
    itch B76.9
    lack of T73.1
        ▶safe drinking Z58.6
    loading E87.70
    on
        brain —see Hydrocephalus
        chest J94.8
    poisoning E87.79
Waterbrash R12
Waterhouse(-Friderichsen) syndrome or
        disease (meningococcal) A39.1
Water-losing nephritis N25.89
Watermelon stomach K31.819
    with hemorrhage K31.811
    without hemorrhage K31.819
Watsoniasis B66.8
Wax in ear —see Impaction, cerumen
Weak, weakening, weakness (generalized)
        R53.1
    arches (acquired) —see also Deformity, limb,
        flat foot
    bladder (sphincter) R32

Weak, weakening, weakness (Continued)
    facial R29.810
        following
            cerebrovascular disease I69.992
                cerebral infarction I69.392
                intracerebral hemorrhage I69.192
                nontraumatic intracranial hemorrhage
                    NEC I69.292
                specified disease NEC I69.892
                stroke I69.392
                subarachnoid hemorrhage I69.092
    foot (double) —see also Weak, arches
    heart, cardiac —see Failure, heart
    mind F70
    muscle M62.81
    myocardium —see Failure, heart
    newborn P96.89
    pelvic fundus N81.89
    pubocervical tissue N81.82
    rectovaginal tissue N81.83
    senile R54
    urinary stream R39.12
    valvular —see Endocarditis
Wear, worn (with normal or routine use)
    articular bearing surface of internal joint
        prosthesis —see Complications, joint
            prosthesis, mechanical, wear of articular
            bearing surfaces, by site
    device, implant or graft —see Complications,
        by site, mechanical complication
    tooth, teeth (approximal) (hard tissues)
        (interproximal) (occlusal) K03.0
Weather, weathered
    effects of
        cold T69.9
            specified effect NEC T69.8
        hot —see Heat
    skin L57.8
Weaver's syndrome Q87.3
Web, webbed (congenital)
    duodenal Q43.8
    esophagus Q39.4
    fingers Q70.1
    larynx (glottic) (subglottic) Q31.0
    neck (pterygium colli) Q18.3
    Paterson-Kelly D50.1
    popliteal syndrome Q87.89
    toes Q70.3
Weber-Christian disease M35.6
Weber-Cockayne syndrome (epidermolysis
        bullosa) Q81.8
Weber-Gubler syndrome G46.3
Weber-Leyden syndrome G46.3
Weber-Osler syndrome I78.0
Weber's paralysis or syndrome G46.3
Wedge-shaped or wedging vertebra —see
        Collapse, vertebra NEC
Wegener's granulomatosis or syndrome
        M31.30
    with
        kidney involvement M31.31
        lung involvement M31.30
            with kidney involvement M31.31
Wegner's disease A50.02
Weight
    1000-2499 grams at birth (low) —see Low,
        birthweight
    999 grams or less at birth (extremely low) —
        see Low, birthweight, extreme
    and length below 10th percentile for
        gestational age P05.1-●
    below but length above 10th percentile for
        gestational age P05.0-●
    gain (abnormal) (excessive) R63.5
        in pregnancy —see Pregnancy, complicated
            by, excessive weight gain
        low —see Pregnancy, complicated by,
            insufficient, weight gain
    loss (abnormal) (cause unknown) R63.4
Weightlessness (effect of) T75.82

Weil (l)-Marchesani syndrome Q87.19
Weil's disease A27.0
Weingarten's syndrome J82.89
Weir Mitchell's disease I73.81
Weiss-Baker syndrome G90.09
Wells' disease L98.3
Wen —see Cyst, sebaceous
Wenckebach's block or phenomenon I44.1
Werdnig-Hoffmann syndrome (muscular
        atrophy) G12.0
Werlhof's disease D69.3
Werner-His disease A79.0
Wermer's disease or syndrome E31.21
Werner's disease or syndrome E34.8
Wernicke-Korsakoff's syndrome or psychosis
        (alcoholic) F10.96
    with dependence F10.26
    drug-induced
        due to drug abuse —see Abuse, drug, by
            type, with amnestic disorder
        due to drug dependence —see
            Dependence, drug, by type, with
            amnestic disorder
    nonalcoholic F04
Wernicke-Posadas disease B38.9
Wernicke's
    developmental aphasia F80.2
    disease or syndrome E51.2
    encephalopathy E51.2
    polioencephalitis, superior E51.2
West African fever B50.8
Westphal-Strümpell syndrome E83.01
West's syndrome —see Epilepsy, spasms
Wet
    feet, tropical (maceration) (syndrome) —see
        Immersion, foot
    lung (syndrome), newborn P22.1
Wharton's duct —see condition
Wheal —see Urticaria
Wheezing R06.2
Whiplash injury S13.4
Whipple's disease —see also subcategory
        M14.8-● K90.81
Whipworm (disease) (infection) (infestation)
        B79
Whistling face Q87.0
White —see also condition
    kidney, small N03.9
    leg, puerperal, postpartum, childbirth O87.1
    mouth B37.0
    patches of mouth K13.29
    spot lesions, teeth
        chewing surface K02.51
        pit and fissure surface K02.51
        smooth surface K02.61
Whitehead L70.0
Whitlow —see also Cellulitis, digit
    with lymphangitis —see Lymphangitis, acute,
        digit
    herpesviral B00.89
Whitmore's disease or fever —see Melioidosis
Whooping cough A37.90
    with pneumonia A37.91
        due to Bordetella
            bronchiseptica A37.81
            parapertussis A37.11
            pertussis A37.01
            specified organism NEC A37.81
    due to
        Bordetella
            bronchiseptica A37.80
                with pneumonia A37.81
            parapertussis A37.10
                with pneumonia A37.11
            pertussis A37.00
                with pneumonia A37.01
            specified NEC A37.80
                with pneumonia A37.81
Wichman's asthma J38.5
Wide cranial sutures, newborn P96.3

► New   ⇒ Revised   ~~deleted~~ Deleted   ● Use Additional Character(s)

Wound, open *(Continued)*
esophagus (thoracic) S27.819
  cervical —*see* Wound, open, cervical esophagus
  laceration S27.813
  specified type NEC S27.818
eye —*see* Wound, open, ocular
eyeball —*see* Wound, open, ocular
eyebrow —*see* Wound, open, eyelid
eyelid S01.10-●
  bite —*see* Bite, eyelid
  laceration —*see* Laceration, eyelid
  puncture —*see* Puncture, eyelid
face NEC —*see* Wound, open, head, specified site NEC
finger(s) S61.209
  with
    amputation —*see* Amputation, traumatic, finger
    damage to nail S61.309
  bite —*see* Bite, finger
  index S61.208
    with
      damage to nail S61.308
    left S61.201
      with
        damage to nail S61.301
    right S61.200
      with
        damage to nail S61.300
    laceration —*see* Laceration, finger
  little S61.208
    with
      damage to nail S61.308
    left S61.207
      with damage to nail S61.307
    right S61.206
      with damage to nail S61.306
  middle S61.208
    with
      damage to nail S61.308
    left S61.203
      with damage to nail S61.303
    right S61.202
      with damage to nail S61.302
  puncture —*see* Puncture, finger
  ring S61.208
    with
      damage to nail S61.308
    left S61.205
      with damage to nail S61.305
    right S61.204
      with damage to nail S61.304
flank —*see* Wound, open, abdomen, wall
foot (except toe(s) alone) S91.30-●
  with amputation —*see* Amputation, traumatic, foot
  bite —*see* Bite, foot
  laceration —*see* Laceration, foot
  puncture —*see* Puncture, foot
  toe —*see* Wound, open, toe
forearm S51.80-●
  with
    amputation —*see* Amputation, traumatic, forearm
  bite —*see* Bite, forearm
  elbow only —*see* Wound, open, elbow
  laceration —*see* Laceration, forearm
  puncture —*see* Puncture, forearm
forehead —*see* Wound, open, head, specified site NEC
genital organs, external
  with amputation —*see* Amputation, traumatic, genital organs
  bite —*see* Bite, genital organ
  female S31.502
    vagina S31.40
    vulva S31.40
  laceration —*see* Laceration, genital organ

Wound, open *(Continued)*
  genital organs, external *(Continued)*
    male S31.501
      penis S31.20
      scrotum S31.30
      testes S31.30
    puncture —*see* Puncture, genital organ
globe (eye) —*see* Wound, open, ocular
groin —*see* Wound, open, abdomen, wall
gum —*see* Wound, open, oral cavity
hand S61.40-●
  with
    amputation —*see* Amputation, traumatic, hand
  bite —*see* Bite, hand
  finger(s) —*see* Wound, open, finger
  laceration —*see* Laceration, hand
  puncture —*see* Puncture, hand
  thumb —*see* Wound, open, thumb
head S01.90
  bite —*see* Bite, head
  cheek —*see* Wound, open, cheek
  ear —*see* Wound, open, ear
  eyelid —*see* Wound, open, eyelid
  laceration —*see* Laceration, head
  lip —*see* Wound, open, lip
  nose S01.20
  oral cavity —*see* Wound, open, oral cavity
  puncture —*see* Puncture, head
  scalp —*see* Wound, open, scalp
  specified site NEC S01.80
  temporomandibular area —*see* Wound, open, cheek
heel —*see* Wound, open, foot
hip S71.00-●
  with amputation —*see* Amputation, traumatic, hip
  bite —*see* Bite, hip
  laceration —*see* Laceration, hip
  puncture —*see* Puncture, hip
hymen S31.40
  bite —*see* Bite, vulva
  laceration —*see* Laceration, vagina
  puncture —*see* Puncture, vagina
hypochondrium S31.109
  bite —*see* Bite, hypochondrium
  laceration —*see* Laceration, hypochondrium
  puncture —*see* Puncture, hypochondrium
hypogastric region S31.109
  bite —*see* Bite, hypogastric region
  laceration —*see* Laceration, hypogastric region
  puncture —*see* Puncture, hypogastric region
iliac (region) —*see* Wound, open, inguinal region
inguinal region S31.109
  bite —*see* Bite, abdomen, wall, lower quadrant
  laceration —*see* Laceration, inguinal region
  puncture —*see* Puncture, inguinal region
instep —*see* Wound, open, foot
interscapular region —*see* Wound, open, thorax, back
intraocular —*see* Wound, open, ocular
iris —*see* Wound, open, ocular
jaw —*see* Wound, open, head, specified site NEC
knee S81.00-●
  bite —*see* Bite, knee
  laceration —*see* Laceration, knee
  puncture —*see* Puncture, knee
labium (majus) (minus) —*see* Wound, open, vulva
laceration —*see* Laceration, by site
lacrimal duct —*see* Wound, open, eyelid

Wound, open *(Continued)*
larynx S11.019
  bite —*see* Bite, larynx
  laceration —*see* Laceration, larynx
  puncture —*see* Puncture, larynx
left
  lower quadrant S31.104
    with penetration into peritoneal cavity S31.604
    bite —*see* Bite, abdomen, wall, left, lower quadrant
    laceration —*see* Laceration, abdomen, wall, left, lower quadrant
    puncture —*see* Puncture, abdomen, wall, left, lower quadrant
  upper quadrant S31.101
    with penetration into peritoneal cavity S31.601
    bite —*see* Bite, abdomen, wall, left, upper quadrant
    laceration —*see* Laceration, abdomen, wall, left, upper quadrant
    puncture —*see* Puncture, abdomen, wall, left, upper quadrant
leg (lower) S81.80-●
  with amputation —*see* Amputation, traumatic, leg
  ankle —*see* Wound, open, ankle
  bite —*see* Bite, leg
  foot —*see* Wound, open, foot
  knee —*see* Wound, open, knee
  laceration —*see* Laceration, leg
  puncture —*see* Puncture, leg
  toe —*see* Wound, open, toe
  upper —*see* Wound, open, thigh
lip S01.501
  bite —*see* Bite, lip
  laceration —*see* Laceration, lip
  puncture —*see* Puncture, lip
loin S31.109
  bite —*see* Bite, abdomen, wall
  laceration —*see* Laceration, loin
  puncture —*see* Puncture, loin
lower back —*see* Wound, open, back, lower
lumbar region —*see* Wound, open, back, lower
malar region —*see* Wound, open, head, specified site NEC
mammary —*see* Wound, open, breast
mastoid region —*see* Wound, open, head, specified site NEC
mouth —*see* Wound, open, oral cavity
nail
  finger —*see* Wound, open, finger, with damage to nail
  toe —*see* Wound, open, toe, with damage to nail
nape (neck) —*see* Wound, open, neck
nasal (septum) (sinus) —*see* Wound, open, nose
nasopharynx —*see* Wound, open, head, specified site NEC
neck S11.90
  bite —*see* Bite, neck
  involving
    cervical esophagus S11.20
    larynx —*see* Wound, open, larynx
    pharynx S11.20
    thyroid S11.10
    trachea (cervical) S11.029
      bite —*see* Bite, trachea
      laceration S11.021
        with foreign body S11.022
      puncture S11.023
        with foreign body S11.024
  laceration —*see* Laceration, neck
  puncture —*see* Puncture, neck
  specified site NEC S11.80
    specified type NEC S11.89

Wound, open *(Continued)*
  nose (septum) (sinus) S01.20
    with amputation —*see* Amputation,
      traumatic, nose
    bite —*see* Bite, nose
    laceration —*see* Laceration, nose
    puncture —*see* Puncture, nose
  ocular S05.90
    avulsion (traumatic enucleation) S05.7-•
    eyeball S05.6-•
      with foreign body S05.5-•
    eyelid —*see* Wound, open, eyelid
    laceration and rupture S05.3-•
      with prolapse or loss of intraocular
        tissue S05.2-•
    orbit (penetrating) (with or without foreign
      body) S05.4-•
    periocular area —*see* Wound, open, eyelid
    specified NEC S05.8X-•
  oral cavity S01.502
    bite S01.552
    laceration —*see* Laceration, oral cavity
    puncture —*see* Puncture, oral cavity
  orbit —*see* Wound, open, ocular, orbit
  palate —*see* Wound, open, oral cavity
  palm —*see* Wound, open, hand
  pelvis, pelvic —*see also* Wound, open, back,
    lower
    girdle —*see* Wound, open, hip
  penetrating —*see* Puncture, by site
  penis S31.20
    with amputation —*see* Amputation,
      traumatic, penis
    bite S31.25
    laceration —*see* Laceration, penis
    puncture —*see* Puncture, penis
  perineum
    bite —*see* Bite, perineum
    female S31.502
    laceration —*see* Laceration, perineum
    male S31.501
    puncture —*see* Puncture, perineum
  periocular area (with or without lacrimal
    passages) —*see* Wound, open, eyelid
  periumbilic region S31.105
    with penetration into peritoneal cavity
      S31.605
    bite —*see* Bite, abdomen, wall, periumbilic
      region
    laceration —*see* Laceration, abdomen, wall,
      periumbilic region
    puncture —*see* Puncture, abdomen, wall,
      periumbilic region
  phalanges
    finger —*see* Wound, open, finger
    toe —*see* Wound, open, toe
  pharynx S11.20
  pinna —*see* Wound, open, ear
  popliteal space —*see* Wound, open, knee
  prepuce —*see* Wound, open, penis
  pubic region —*see* Wound, open, back, lower
  pudendum —*see* Wound, open, genital
    organs, external
  puncture wound —*see* Puncture
  rectovaginal septum —*see* Wound, open,
    vagina
  right
    lower quadrant S31.103
      with penetration into peritoneal cavity
        S31.603
      bite —*see* Bite, abdomen, wall, right,
        lower quadrant
      laceration —*see* Laceration, abdomen,
        wall, right, lower quadrant
      puncture —*see* Puncture, abdomen, wall,
        right, lower quadrant
    upper quadrant S31.100
      with penetration into peritoneal cavity
        S31.600

Wound, open *(Continued)*
  right *(Continued)*
    upper quadrant *(Continued)*
      bite —*see* Bite, abdomen, wall, right,
        upper quadrant
      laceration —*see* Laceration, abdomen,
        wall, right, upper quadrant
      puncture —*see* Puncture, abdomen, wall,
        right, upper quadrant
  sacral region —*see* Wound, open, back, lower
  sacroiliac region —*see* Wound, open, back,
    lower
  salivary gland —*see* Wound, open, oral cavity
  scalp S01.00
    bite S01.05
    laceration —*see* Laceration, scalp
    puncture —*see* Puncture, scalp
  scalpel, newborn (birth injury) P15.8
  scapular region —*see* Wound, open, shoulder
  sclera —*see* Wound, open, ocular
  scrotum S31.30
    with amputation —*see* Amputation,
      traumatic, scrotum
    bite S31.35
    laceration —*see* Laceration, scrotum
    puncture —*see* Puncture, scrotum
  shin —*see* Wound, open, leg
  shoulder S41.00-•
    with amputation —*see* Amputation,
      traumatic, arm
    bite —*see* Bite, shoulder
    laceration —*see* Laceration, shoulder
    puncture —*see* Puncture, shoulder
  skin NOS T14.8
  spermatic cord —*see* Wound, open, testis
  sternal region —*see* Wound, open, thorax,
    front wall
  submaxillary region —*see* Wound, open,
    head, specified site NEC
  submental region —*see* Wound, open, head,
    specified site NEC
  subungual
    finger(s) —*see* Wound, open, finger
    toe(s) —*see* Wound, open, toe
  supraclavicular region —*see* Wound, open,
    neck, specified site NEC
  temple, temporal region —*see* Wound, open,
    head, specified site NEC
  temporomandibular area —*see* Wound, open,
    cheek
  testis S31.30
    with amputation —*see* Amputation,
      traumatic, testes
    bite S31.35
    laceration —*see* Laceration, testis
    puncture —*see* Puncture, testis
  thigh S71.10-•
    with amputation —*see* Amputation,
      traumatic, hip
    bite —*see* Bite, thigh
    laceration —*see* Laceration, thigh
    puncture —*see* Puncture, thigh
  thorax, thoracic (wall) S21.90
    back S21.20-•
      with penetration S21.40
    bite —*see* Bite, thorax
    breast —*see* Wound, open, breast
    front S21.10-•
      with penetration S21.30
    laceration —*see* Laceration, thorax
    puncture —*see* Puncture, thorax
  throat —*see* Wound, open, neck
  thumb S61.009
    with
      amputation —*see* Amputation,
        traumatic, thumb
      damage to nail S61.109
    bite —*see* Bite, thumb
    laceration —*see* Laceration, thumb

Wound, open *(Continued)*
  thumb *(Continued)*
    left S61.002
      with
        damage to nail S61.102
      puncture —*see* Puncture, thumb
    right S61.001
      with
        damage to nail S61.101
  thyroid (gland) —*see* Wound, open, neck,
    thyroid
  toe(s) S91.109
    with
      amputation —*see* Amputation,
        traumatic, toe
      damage to nail S91.209
    bite —*see* Bite, toe
    great S91.103
      with
        damage to nail S91.203
      left S91.102
        with
          damage to nail S91.202
      right S91.101
        with
          damage to nail S91.201
    laceration —*see* Laceration, toe
    lesser S91.106
      with
        damage to nail S91.206
      left S91.105
        with
          damage to nail S91.205
      right S91.104
        with
          damage to nail S91.204
    puncture —*see* Puncture, toe
  tongue —*see* Wound, open, oral cavity
  trachea (cervical region) —*see* Wound, open,
    neck, trachea
  tunica vaginalis —*see* Wound, open, testis
  tympanum, tympanic membrane S09.2-•
    laceration —*see* Laceration, ear, drum
    puncture —*see* Puncture, tympanum
  umbilical region —*see* Wound, open,
    abdomen, wall, periumbilic region
  uvula —*see* Wound, open, oral cavity
  vagina S31.40
    bite S31.45
    laceration —*see* Laceration, vagina
    puncture —*see* Puncture, vagina
  vitreous (humor) —*see* Wound, open, ocular
  vocal cord S11.039
    bite —*see* Bite, vocal cord
    laceration S11.031
      with foreign body S11.032
    puncture S11.033
      with foreign body S11.034
  vulva S31.40
    with amputation —*see* Amputation,
      traumatic, vulva
    bite S31.45
    laceration —*see* Laceration, vulva
    puncture —*see* Puncture, vulva
  wrist S61.50-•
    bite —*see* Bite, wrist
    laceration —*see* Laceration, wrist
    puncture —*see* Puncture, wrist
Wound, superficial —*see* Injury *(see also*
  specified injury type)
Wright's syndrome G54.0
Wrist —*see* condition
Wrong drug (by accident) (given in error) —
  see Table of Drugs and Chemicals, by
  drug, poisoning
Wry neck —*see* Torticollis
Wuchereria (bancrofti) infestation B74.0
Wuchereriasis B74.0
Wuchernde Struma Langhans C73

▶ New ⇒ Revised ~~deleted~~ Deleted • Use Additional Character(s)

X

Xanthelasma (eyelid) (palpebrarum) H02.60
 left H02.66
  lower H02.65
  upper H02.64
 right H02.63
  lower H02.62
  upper H02.61
Xanthelasmatosis (essential) E78.2
Xanthinuria, hereditary E79.8
Xanthoastrocytoma
 specified site —*see* Neoplasm, malignant, by
  site
 unspecified site C71.9
Xanthofibroma —*see* Neoplasm, connective
  tissue, benign
Xanthogranuloma D76.3
Xanthoma(s), xanthomatosis (primary)
  (familial) (hereditary) E75.5
 with
  hyperlipoproteinemia
   Type I E78.3
   Type III E78.2
   Type IV E78.1
   Type V E78.3
 bone (generalisata) C96.5
 cerebrotendinous E75.5
 cutaneotendinous E75.5

Xanthoma(s), xanthomatosis (*Continued*)
 disseminatum (skin) E78.2
 eruptive E78.2
 hypercholesterinemic E78.00
 hypercholesterolemic E78.00
 hyperlipidemic E78.5
 joint E75.5
 multiple (skin) E78.2
 tendon (sheath) E75.5
 tuberosum E78.2
 tuberous E78.2
 tubo-eruptive E78.2
 verrucous, oral mucosa K13.4
Xanthosis R23.8
Xenophobia F40.10
Xeroderma —*see also* Ichthyosis
 acquired L85.0
  eyelid H01.149
   left H01.146
    lower H01.145
    upper H01.144
   right H01.143
    lower H01.142
    upper H01.141
 pigmentosum Q82.1
 vitamin A deficiency E50.8
Xerophthalmia (vitamin A deficiency) E50.7
 unrelated to vitamin A deficiency —*see*
   Keratoconjunctivitis

Xerosis
 conjunctiva H11.14-●
  with Bitot's spots —*see also* Pigmentation,
   conjunctiva
   vitamin A deficiency E50.1
  vitamin A deficiency E50.0
 cornea H18.89-●
  with ulceration —*see* Ulcer, cornea
   vitamin A deficiency E50.3
  vitamin A deficiency E50.2
 ⇒cutis (dry skin) L85.3
 skin L85.3
Xerostomia K11.7
Xiphopagus Q89.4
XO syndrome Q96.9
X-ray (of)
 abnormal findings —*see* Abnormal,
   diagnostic imaging
 breast (mammogram) (routine) Z12.31
 chest
  routine (as part of a general medical
   examination) Z00.00
   with abnormal findings Z00.01
 routine (as part of a general medical
   examination) Z00.00
  with abnormal findings Z00.01
XXXXY syndrome Q98.1
XXY syndrome Q98.0

Y

Yaba pox virus disease B08.72
Yatapoxvirus B08.70
  specified NEC B08.79
Yawning R06.89
  psychogenic F45.8
Yaws A66.9
  bone lesions A66.6
  butter A66.1
  chancre A66.0
  cutaneous, less than five years after infection
      A66.2
  early (cutaneous) (macular) (maculopapular)
      (micropapular) (papular) A66.2
    frambeside A66.2
    skin lesions NEC A66.2
  eyelid A66.2
  ganglion A66.6
  gangosis, gangosa A66.5
  gumma, gummata A66.4
    bone A66.6
  gummatous
    frambeside A66.4
    osteitis A66.6
    periostitis A66.6
  hydrarthrosis —see also subcategory
      M14.8-● A66.6
  hyperkeratosis (early) (late) A66.3

Yaws (Continued)
  initial lesions A66.0
  joint lesions —see also subcategory
      M14.8-● A66.6
  juxta-articular nodules A66.7
  late nodular (ulcerated) A66.4
  latent (without clinical manifestations) (with
      positive serology) A66.8
  mother A66.0
  mucosal A66.7
  multiple papillomata A66.1
  nodular, late (ulcerated) A66.4
  osteitis A66.6
  papilloma, plantar or palmar A66.1
  periostitis (hypertrophic) A66.6
  specified NEC A66.7
  ulcers A66.4
  wet crab A66.1
Yeast infection —see also Candidiasis B37.9
Yellow
  atrophy (liver) —see Failure, hepatic
  fever —see Fever, yellow
  jack —see Fever, yellow
  jaundice —see Jaundice
  nail syndrome L60.5
Yersiniosis —see also Infection, Yersinia
  extraintestinal A28.2
  intestinal A04.6

Z

Zahorsky's syndrome (herpangina) B08.5
Zellweger's syndrome E71.510
Zenker's diverticulum (esophagus) K22.5
Ziehen-Oppenheim disease G24.1
Zieve's syndrome K70.0
Zika NOS A92.5
  congenital P35.4
Zinc
  deficiency, dietary E60
  metabolism disorder E83.2
Zollinger-Ellison syndrome E16.4
Zona —see Herpes, zoster
Zoophobia F40.218
Zoster (herpes) —see Herpes, zoster
Zygomycosis B46.9
  specified NEC B46.8
Zymotic —see condition

Y, Z

▶ New   ⇒ Revised   ~~deleted~~ Deleted   ● Use Additional Character(s)

ICD-10-CM
Table of Neoplasms

	Malignant Primary	Malignant Secondary	Ca in situ	Benign	Uncertain Behavior	Unspecified Behavior

The list below gives the code numbers for neoplasms by anatomical site. For each site there are six possible code numbers according to whether the neoplasm in question is malignant, benign, in situ, of uncertain behavior, or of unspecified nature. The description of the neoplasm will often indicate which of the six columns is appropriate; e.g., malignant melanoma of skin, benign fibroadenoma of breast, carcinoma in situ of cervix uteri.

Where such descriptors are not present, the remainder of the Index should be consulted where guidance is given to the appropriate column for each morphological (histological) variety listed; e.g., Mesonephroma — *see Neoplasm, malignant;* Embryoma — *see also Neoplasm, uncertain behavior;* Disease, Bowen's — *see Neoplasm, skin, in situ.* However, the guidance in the Index can be overridden if one of the descriptors mentioned above is present; e.g., malignant adenoma of colon is coded to C18.9 and not to D12.6 as the adjective "Malignant" overrides the Index entry 'Adenoma — *see also Neoplasm, benign.*'

Codes listed with a dash -, following the code have a required additional character for laterality. The Tablular must be reviewed for the complete code.

	Malignant Primary	Malignant Secondary	Ca in situ	Benign	Uncertain Behavior	Unspecified Behavior
Neoplasm, neoplastic	C80.1	C79.9	D09.9	D36.9	D48.9	D49.9
abdomen, abdominal	C76.2	C79.8-●	D09.8	D36.7	D48.7	D49.89
cavity	C76.2	C79.8-●	D09.8	D36.7	D48.7	D49.89
organ	C76.2	C79.8-●	D09.8	D36.7	D48.7	D49.89
viscera	C76.2	C79.8-●	D09.8	D36.7	D48.7	D49.89
wall — *see also Neoplasm, abdomen, wall, skin*	C44.509	C79.2-●	D04.5	D23.5	D48.5	D49.2
connective tissue	C49.4	C79.8-●	—	D21.4	D48.1	D49.2
skin	C44.509					
basal cell carcinoma	C44.519	—	—	—	—	—
specified type NEC	C44.599	—	—	—	—	—
squamous cell carcinoma	C44.529	—	—	—	—	—
abdominopelvic	C76.8	C79.8-●	—	D36.7	D48.7	D49.89
accessory sinus — *see Neoplasm, sinus*						
acoustic nerve	C72.4-●	C79.49	—	D33.3	D43.3	D49.7
adenoid (pharynx) (tissue)	C11.1	C79.89	D00.08	D10.6	D37.05	D49.0
adipose tissue — *see also Neoplasm, connective tissue*	C49.4	C79.89	—	D21.9	D48.1	D49.2
adnexa (uterine)	C57.4	C79.89	D07.39	D28.7	D39.8	D49.59
adrenal	C74.9-●	C79.7-●	D09.3	D35.0-●	D44.1-●	D49.7
capsule	C74.9-●	C79.7-●	D09.3	D35.0-●	D44.1-●	D49.7
cortex	C74.0-●	C79.7-●	D09.3	D35.0-●	D44.1-●	D49.7
gland	C74.9-●	C79.7-●	D09.3	D35.0-●	D44.1-●	D49.7
medulla	C74.1-●	C79.7-●	D09.3	D35.0-●	D44.1-●	D49.7
ala nasi (external) — *see also Neoplasm, skin, nose*	C44.301	C79.2	D04.39	D23.39	D48.5	D49.2

	Malignant Primary	Malignant Secondary	Ca in situ	Benign	Uncertain Behavior	Unspecified Behavior
alimentary canal or tract NEC	C26.9	C78.80	D01.9	D13.9	D37.9	D49.0
alveolar	C03.9	C79.89	D00.03	D10.39	D37.09	D49.0
mucosa	C03.9	C79.89	D00.03	D10.39	D37.09	D49.0
lower	C03.1	C79.89	D00.03	D10.39	D37.09	D49.0
upper	C03.0	C79.89	D00.03	D10.39	D37.09	D49.0
ridge or process	C41.1	C79.51	—	D16.5-●	D48.0	D49.2
carcinoma	C03.9	C79.8-●	—	—	—	—
lower	C03.1	C79.8-●	—	—	—	—
upper	C03.0	C79.8-●	—	—	—	—
lower	C41.1	C79.51	—	D16.5-●	D48.0	D49.2
mucosa	C03.9	C79.89	D00.03	D10.39	D37.09	D49.0
lower	C03.1	C79.89	D00.03	D10.39	D37.09	D49.0
upper	C03.0	C79.89	D00.03	D10.39	D37.09	D49.0
upper	C41.0	C79.51	—	D16.4-●	D48.0	D49.2
sulcus	C06.1	C79.89	D00.02	D10.39	D37.09	D49.0
alveolus	C03.9	C79.89	D00.03	D10.39	D37.09	D49.0
lower	C03.1	C79.89	D00.03	D10.39	D37.09	D49.0
upper	C03.0	C79.89	D00.03	D10.39	D37.09	D49.0
ampulla of Vater	C24.1	C78.89	D01.5	D13.5	D37.6	D49.0
ankle NEC	C76.5-●	C79.89	D04.7-●	D36.7	D48.7	D49.89
anorectum, anorectal (junction)	C21.8	C78.5	D01.3	D12.9	D37.8	D49.0
antecubital fossa or space	C76.4-●	C79.89	D04.6-●	D36.7	D48.7	D49.89
antrum (Highmore) (maxillary)	C31.0	C78.39	D02.3	D14.0	D38.5	D49.1
pyloric	C16.3	C78.89	D00.2	D13.1	D37.1	D49.0
tympanicum	C30.1	C78.39	D02.3	D14.0	D38.5	D49.1
anus, anal	C21.0	C78.5	D01.3	D12.9	D37.8	D49.0
canal	C21.1	C78.5	D01.3	D12.9	D37.8	D49.0
cloacogenic zone	C21.2	C78.5	D01.3	D12.9	D37.8	D49.0
margin — *see also Neoplasm, anus, skin*	C44.500	C79.2	D04.5	D23.5	D48.5	D49.2
overlapping lesion with rectosigmoid junction or rectum	C21.8	—	—	—	—	—
skin	C44.500	C79.2	D04.5	D23.5	D48.5	D49.2
basal cell carcinoma	C44.510	—	—	—	—	—
specified type NEC	C44.590	—	—	—	—	—
squamous cell carcinoma	C44.520	—	—	—	—	—
sphincter	C21.1	C78.5	D01.3	D12.9	D37.8	D49.0
aorta (thoracic)	C49.3	C79.89	—	D21.3	D48.1	D49.2
abdominal	C49.4	C79.89	—	D21.4	D48.1	D49.2
aortic body	C75.5	C79.89		D35.6	D44.7	D49.7
aponeurosis	C49.9	C79.89	—	D21.9	D48.1	D49.2
palmar	C49.1-●	C79.89	—	D21.1-●	D48.1	D49.2
plantar	C49.2-●	C79.89	—	D21.2-●	D48.1	D49.2

	Malignant Primary	Malignant Secondary	Ca in situ	Benign	Uncertain Behavior	Unspecified Behavior
appendix	C18.1	C78.5	D01.0	D12.1	D37.3	D49.0
arachnoid	C70.9	C79.49	—	D32.9	D42.9	D49.7
cerebral	C70.0	C79.32	—	D32.0	D42.0	D49.7
spinal	C70.1	C79.49	—	D32.1	D42.1	D49.7
areola	C50.0-●	C79.81	D05.-●	D24.-●	D48.6-●	D49.3
arm NEC	C76.4-●	C79.89	D04.6-●	D36.7	D48.7	D49.89
artery — see Neoplasm, connective tissue						
aryepiglottic fold	C13.1	C79.89	D00.08	D10.7	D37.05	D49.0
hypopharyngeal aspect	C13.1	C79.89	D00.08	D10.7	D37.05	D49.0
laryngeal aspect	C32.1	C78.39	D02.0	D14.1	D38.0	D49.1
marginal zone	C13.1	C79.89	D00.08	D10.7	D37.05	D49.0
arytenoid (cartilage)	C32.3	C78.39	D02.0	D14.1	D38.0	D49.1
fold — see Neoplasm, aryepiglottic						
associated with transplanted organ	C80.2	—	—	—	—	—
atlas	C41.2	C79.51	—	D16.6	D48.0	D49.2
atrium, cardiac	C38.0	C79.89	—	D15.1	D48.7	D49.89
auditory						
canal (external) (skin)	C44.20-●	C79.2	D04.2-●	D23.2-●	D48.5	D49.2
internal	C30.1	C78.39	D02.3	D14.0	D38.5	D49.1
nerve	C72.4-●	C79.49	—	D33.3	D43.3	D49.7
tube	C30.1	C78.39	D02.3	D14.0	D38.5	D49.1
opening	C11.2	C79.89	D00.08	D10.6	D37.05	D49.0
auricle, ear — see also Neoplasm, skin, ear	C44.20-●	C79.2	D04.2-●	D23.2-●	D48.5	D49.2
auricular canal (external) — see also Neoplasm, skin, ear	C44.20-●	C79.2	D04.2-●	D23.2-●	D48.5	D49.2
internal	C30.1	C78.39	D02.3	D14.0	D38.5	D49.2
autonomic nerve or nervous system NEC (see Neoplasm, nerve, peripheral)						
axilla, axillary	C76.1	C79.89	D09.8	D36.7	D48.7	D49.89
fold — see also Neoplasm, skin, trunk	C44.509	C79.2	D04.5	D23.5	D48.5	D49.2
back NEC	C76.8	C79.89	D04.5	D36.7	D48.7	D49.89
Bartholin's gland	C51.0	C79.82	D07.1	D28.0	D39.8	D49.59
basal ganglia	C71.0	C79.31	—	D33.0	D43.0	D49.6
basis pedunculi	C71.7	C79.31	—	D33.1	D43.1	D49.6
bile or biliary (tract)	C24.9	C78.89	D01.5	D13.5	D37.6	D49.0
canaliculi (biliferi) (intrahepatic)	C22.1	C78.7	D01.5	D13.4	D37.6	D49.0
canals, interlobular	C22.1	C78.89	D01.5	D13.4	D37.6	D49.0

	Malignant Primary	Malignant Secondary	Ca in situ	Benign	Uncertain Behavior	Unspecified Behavior
bile or biliary (Continued)						
duct or passage (common)						
(cystic) (extrahepatic)	C24.0	C78.89	D01.5	D13.5	D37.6	D49.0
interlobular	C22.1	C78.89	D01.5	D13.4	D37.6	D49.0
intrahepatic	C22.1	C78.7	D01.5	D13.4	D37.6	D49.0
and extrahepatic	C24.8	C78.89	D01.5	D13.5	D37.6	D49.0
bladder (urinary)	C67.9	C79.11	D09.0	D30.3	D41.4	D49.4
dome	C67.1	C79.11	D09.0	D30.3	D41.4	D49.4
neck	C67.5	C79.11	D09.0	D30.3	D41.4	D49.4
orifice	C67.9	C79.11	D09.0	D30.3	D41.4	D49.4
ureteric	C67.6	C79.11	D09.0	D30.3	D41.4	D49.4
urethral	C67.5	C79.11	D09.0	D30.3	D41.4	D49.4
overlapping lesion	C67.8	—	—	—	—	—
sphincter	C67.8	C79.11	D09.0	D30.3	D41.4	D49.4
trigone	C67.0	C79.11	D09.0	D30.3	D41.4	D49.4
urachus	C67.7	C79.11	D09.0	D30.3	D41.4	D49.4
wall	C67.9	C79.11	D09.0	D30.3	D41.4	D49.4
anterior	C67.3	C79.11	D09.0	D30.3	D41.4	D49.4
lateral	C67.2	C79.11	D09.0	D30.3	D41.4	D49.4
posterior	C67.4	C79.11	D09.0	D30.3	D41.4	D49.4
blood vessel — see Neoplasm, connective tissue						
bone (periosteum)	C41.9	C79.51	—	D16.9-●	D48.0	D49.2
acetabulum	C41.4	C79.51	—	D16.8-●	D48.0	D49.2
ankle	C40.3-●	C79.51	—	D16.3-●	—	—
arm NEC	C40.0-●	C79.51	—	D16.0-●		
astragalus	C40.3-●	C79.51	—	D16.3-●	—	—
atlas	C41.2	C79.51	—	D16.6-●	D48.0	D49.2
axis	C41.2	C79.51	—	D16.6-●	D48.0	D49.2
back NEC	C41.2	C79.51	—	D16.6-●	D48.0	D49.2
calcaneus	C40.3-●	C79.51	—	D16.3-●	—	—
calvarium	C41.0	C79.51	—	D16.4-●	D48.0	D49.2
carpus (any)	C40.1-●	C79.51	—	D16.1-●	—	—
cartilage NEC	C41.9	C79.51	—	D16.9-●	D48.0	D49.2
clavicle	C41.3	C79.51	—	D16.7-●	D48.0	D49.2
clivus	C41.0	C79.51	—	D16.4-●	D48.0	D49.2
coccygeal vertebra	C41.4	C79.51	—	D16.8-●	D48.0	D49.2
coccyx	C41.4	C79.51	—	D16.8-●	D48.0	D49.2
costal cartilage	C41.3	C79.51	—	D16.7-●	D48.0	D49.2
costovertebral joint	C41.3	C79.51	—	D16.7-●	D48.0	D49.2
cranial	C41.0	C79.51	—	D16.4-●	D48.0	D49.2
cuboid	C40.3-●	C79.51	—	D16.3-●	—	—
cuneiform	C41.9	C79.51	—	D16.9-●	D48.0	D49.2
elbow	C40.0-●	C79.51	—	D16.0-●		

◀ New ◀▌ Revised ~~deleted~~ Deleted ● Use Additional Character(s)

	Malignant Primary	Malignant Secondary	Ca in situ	Benign	Uncertain Behavior	Unspecified Behavior
bone *(Continued)*						
ethmoid (labyrinth)	C41.0	C79.51	—	D16.4-●	D48.0	D49.2
face	C41.0	C79.51	—	D16.4-●	D48.0	D49.2
femur (any part)	C40.2-●	C79.51	—	D16.2-●	—	—
fibula (any part)	C40.2-●	C79.51	—	D16.2-●	—	—
finger (any)	C40.1-●	C79.51	—	D16.1-●	—	—
foot	C40.3-●	C79.51	—	D16.3-●	—	—
forearm	C40.0-●	C79.51	—	D16.0-●	—	—
frontal	C41.0	C79.51	—	D16.4-●	D48.0	D49.2
hand	C40.1-●	C79.51	—	D16.1-●	—	—
heel	C40.3-●	C79.51	—	D16.3-●	—	—
hip	C41.4	C79.51	—	D16.8-●	D48.0	D49.2
humerus (any part)	C40.0-●	C79.51	—	D16.0-●	—	—
hyoid	C41.0	C79.51	—	D16.4-●	D48.0	D49.2
ilium	C41.4	C79.51	—	D16.8-●	D48.0	D49.2
innominate	C41.4	C79.51	—	D16.8-●	D48.0	D49.2
intervertebral cartilage or disc	C41.2	C79.51	—	D16.6-●	D48.0	D49.2
ischium	C41.4	C79.51	—	D16.8-●	D48.0	D49.2
jaw (lower)	C41.1	C79.51	—	D16.5-●	D48.0	D49.2
knee	C40.2-●	C79.51	—	D16.2-●	—	—
leg NEC	C40.2-●	C79.51	—	D16.2-●	—	—
limb NEC	C40.9-●	C79.51	—	D16.9-●	—	—
lower (long bones)	C40.2-●	C79.51	—	D16.2-●	—	—
short bones	C40.3-●	C79.51	—	D16.3-●	—	—
upper (long bones)	C40.0-●	C79.51	—	D16.0-●	—	—
short bones	C40.1-●	C79.51	—	D16.1-●	—	—
malar	C41.0	C79.51	—	D16.4-●	D48.0	D49.2
mandible	C41.1	C79.51	—	D16.5-●	D48.0	D49.2
marrow NEC (any bone)	C96.9	C79.52	—	—	D47.9	D49.89
mastoid	C41.0	C79.51	—	D16.4-●	D48.0	D49.2
maxilla, maxillary (superior)	C41.0	C79.51	—	D16.4-●	D48.0	D49.2
inferior	C41.1	C79.51	—	D16.5-●	D48.0	D49.2
metacarpus (any)	C40.1-●	C79.51	—	D16.1-●	—	—
metatarsus (any)	C40.3-●	C79.51	—	D16.3-●	—	—
overlapping sites	C40.8-●	—	—	—	—	—
navicular						
ankle	C40.3-●	C79.51	—	—	—	—
hand	C40.1-●	C79.51	—	—	—	—
nose, nasal	C41.0	C79.51	—	D16.4-●	D48.0	D49.2
occipital	C41.0	C79.51	—	D16.4-●	D48.0	D49.2
orbit	C41.0	C79.51	—	D16.4-●	D48.0	D49.2
parietal	C41.0	C79.51	—	D16.4-●	D48.0	D49.2
patella	C40.2-●	C79.51	—	—	—	—
pelvic	C41.4	C79.51	—	D16.8	D48.0	D49.2

	Malignant Primary	Malignant Secondary	Ca in situ	Benign	Uncertain Behavior	Unspecified Behavior
bone *(Continued)*						
phalanges						
foot	C40.3-●	C79.51	—	—	—	—
hand	C40.1-●	C79.51	—	—	—	—
pubic	C41.4	C79.51	—	D16.8	D48.0	D49.2
radius (any part)	C40.0-●	C79.51	—	D16.0-●	—	—
rib	C41.3	C79.51	—	D16.7	D48.0	D49.2
sacral vertebra	C41.4	C79.51	—	D16.8	D48.0	D49.2
sacrum	C41.4	C79.51	—	D16.8	D48.0	D49.2
scaphoid	—	—	—	—	—	—
of ankle	C40.3-●	C79.51	—	—	—	—
of hand	C40.1-●	C79.51	—	—	—	—
scapula (any part)	C40.0-●	C79.51	—	D16.0-●	—	—
sella turcica	C41.0	C79.51	—	D16.4-●	D48.0	D49.2
shoulder	C40.0-●	C79.51	—	D16.0-●	—	—
skull	C41.0	C79.51	—	D16.4-●	D48.0	D49.2
sphenoid	C41.0	C79.51	—	D16.4-●	D48.0	D49.2
spine, spinal (column)	C41.2	C79.51	—	D16.6	D48.0	D49.2
coccyx	C41.4	C79.51	—	D16.8	D48.0	D49.2
sacrum	C41.4	C79.51	—	D16.8	D48.0	D49.2
sternum	C41.3	C79.51	—	D16.7	D48.0	D49.2
tarsus (any)	C40.3-●	C79.51	—	—	—	—
temporal	C41.0	C79.51	—	D16.4-●	D48.0	D49.2
thumb	C40.1-●	C79.51	—	—	—	—
tibia (any part)	C40.2-●	C79.51	—	—	—	—
toe (any)	C40.3-●	C79.51	—	—	—	—
trapezium	C40.1-●	C79.51	—	—	—	—
trapezoid	C40.1-●	C79.51	—	—	—	—
turbinate	C41.0	C79.51	—	D16.4-●	D48.0	D49.2
ulna (any part)	C40.0-●	C79.51	—	D16.0-●	—	—
unciform	C40.1-●	C79.51	—	—	—	—
vertebra (column)	C41.2	C79.51	—	D16.6	D48.0	D49.2
coccyx	C41.4	C79.51	—	D16.8	D48.0	D49.2
sacrum	C41.4	C79.51	—	D16.8	D48.0	D49.2
vomer	C41.0	C79.51	—	D16.4-●	D48.0	D49.2
wrist	C40.1-●	C79.51	—	—	—	—
xiphoid process	C41.3	C79.51	—	D16.7	D48.0	D49.2
zygomatic	C41.0	C79.51	—	D16.4-●	D48.0	D49.2
book-leaf (mouth)	C06.89	C79.89	D00.00	D10.39	D37.09	D49.0
bowel — *see Neoplasm, intestine*						
brachial plexus	C47.1-●	C79.89	—	D36.12	D48.2	D49.2
brain NEC	C71.9	C79.31	—	D33.2	D43.2	D49.6
basal ganglia	C71.0	C79.31	—	D33.0	D43.0	D49.6
cerebellopontine angle	C71.6	C79.31	—	D33.1	D43.1	D49.6

◀ New　◀█ Revised　~~deleted~~ Deleted　● Use Additional Character(s)

TABLE OF NEOPLASMS

	Malignant Primary	Malignant Secondary	Ca in situ	Benign	Uncertain Behavior	Unspecified Behavior
brain NEC *(Continued)*						
cerebellum NOS	C71.6	C79.31	—	D33.1	D43.1	D49.6
cerebrum	C71.0	C79.31	—	D33.0	D43.0	D49.6
choroid plexus	C71.7	C79.31	—	D33.1	D43.1	D49.6
corpus callosum	C71.8	C79.31	—	D33.2	D43.2	D49.6
corpus striatum	C71.0	C79.31	—	D33.0	D43.0	D49.6
cortex (cerebral)	C71.0	C79.31	—	D33.0	D43.0	D49.6
frontal lobe	C71.1	C79.31	—	D33.0	D43.0	D49.6
globus pallidus	C71.0	C79.31	—	D33.0	D43.0	D49.6
hippocampus	C71.2	C79.31	—	D33.0	D43.0	D49.6
hypothalamus	C71.0	C79.31	—	D33.0	D43.0	D49.6
internal capsule	C71.0	C79.31	—	D33.0	D43.0	D49.6
medulla oblongata	C71.7	C79.31	—	D33.1	D43.1	D49.6
meninges	C70.0	C79.32	—	D32.0	D42.0	D49.7
midbrain	C71.7	C79.31	—	D33.1	D43.1	D49.6
occipital lobe	C71.4	C79.31	—	D33.0	D43.0	D49.6
overlapping lesion	C71.8	C79.31	—	—	—	—
parietal lobe	C71.3	C79.31	—	D33.0	D43.0	D49.6
peduncle	C71.7	C79.31	—	D33.1	D43.1	D49.6
pons	C71.7	C79.31	—	D33.1	D43.1	D49.6
stem	C71.7	C79.31	—	D33.1	D43.1	D49.6
tapetum	C71.8	C79.31	—	D33.2	D43.2	D49.6
temporal lobe	C71.2	C79.31	—	D33.0	D43.0	D49.6
thalamus	C71.0	C79.31	—	D33.0	D43.0	D49.6
uncus	C71.2	C79.31	—	D33.0	D43.0	D49.6
ventricle (floor)	C71.5	C79.31	—	D33.0	D43.0	D49.6
fourth	C71.7	C79.31	—	D33.1	D43.1	D49.6
branchial (cleft) (cyst) (vestiges)	C10.4	C79.89	D00.08	D10.5	D37.05	D49.0
breast (connective tissue)						
(glandular tissue) (soft parts)	C50.9-●	C79.81	D05.-●	D24.-●	D48.6-●	D49.3
areola	C50.0-●	C79.81	D05.-●	D24.-●	D48.6-●	D49.3
axillary tail	C50.6-●	C79.81	D05.-●	D24.-●	D48.6-●	D49.3
central portion	C50.1-●	C79.81	D05.-●	D24.-●	D48.6-●	D49.3
inner	C50.8-●	C79.81	D05.-●	D24.-●	D48.6-●	D49.3
lower	C50.8-●	C79.81	D05.-●	D24.-●	D48.6-●	D49.3
lower-inner quadrant	C50.3-●	C79.81	D05.-●	D24.-●	D48.6-●	D49.3
lower-outer quadrant	C50.5-●	C79.81	D05.-●	D24.-●	D48.6-●	D49.3
mastectomy site (skin) — *see also Neoplasm, breast, skin*	C44.501	C79.2	—	—	—	—
specified as breast tissue	C50.8-●	C79.81	—	—	—	—
midline	C50.8-●	C79.81	D05.-●	D24.-●	D48.6-●	D49.3
nipple	C50.0-●	C79.81	D05.-●	D24.-●	D48.6-●	D49.3
outer	C50.8-●	C79.81	D05.-●	D24.-●	D48.6-●	D49.3
overlapping lesion	C50.8-●	—	—	—	—	—

	Malignant Primary	Malignant Secondary	Ca in situ	Benign	Uncertain Behavior	Unspecified Behavior
breast *(Continued)*						
skin	C44.501	C79.2	D04.5	D23.5	D48.5	D49.2
basal cell carcinoma	C44.511	—	—	—	—	—
specified type NEC	C44.591	—	—	—	—	—
squamous cell carcinoma	C44.521	—	—	—	—	—
tail (axillary)	C50.6-●	C79.81	D05.-●	D24.-●	D48.6-●	D49.3
upper	C50.8-●	C79.81	D05.-●	D24.-●	D48.6-●	D49.3
upper-inner quadrant	C50.2-●	C79.81	D05.-●	D24.-●	D48.6-●	D49.3
upper-outer quadrant	C50.4-●	C79.81	D05.-●	D24.-●	D48.6-●	D49.3
broad ligament	C57.1	C79.82	D07.39	D28.2	D39.8	D49.59
bronchiogenic, bronchogenic (lung)	C34.9-●	C78.0-●	D02.2-●	D14.3-●	D38.1	D49.1
bronchiole	C34.9-●	C78.0-●	D02.2-●	D14.3-●	D38.1	D49.1
bronchus	C34.9-●	C78.0-●	D02.2-●	D14.3-●	D38.1	D49.1
carina	C34.0-●	C78.0-●	D02.2-●	D14.3-●	D38.1	D49.1
lower lobe of lung	C34.3-●	C78.0-●	D02.2-●	D14.3-●	D38.1	D49.1
main	C34.0-●	C78.0-●	D02.2-●	D14.3-●	D38.1	D49.1
middle lobe of lung	C34.2	C78.0-●	D02.21	D14.31	D38.1	D49.1
overlapping lesion	C34.8-●	—	—	—	—	—
upper lobe of lung	C34.1-●	C78.0-●	D02.2-●	D14.3-●	D38.1	D49.1
brow	C44.309	C79.2	D04.39	D23.39	D48.5	D49.2
basal cell carcinoma	C44.319	—	—	—	—	—
specified type NEC	C44.399	—	—	—	—	—
squamous cell carcinoma	C44.329	—	—	—	—	—
buccal (cavity)	C06.9	C79.89	D00.00	D10.39	D37.09	D49.0
commissure	C06.0	C79.89	D00.02	D10.39	D37.09	D49.0
groove (lower) (upper)	C06.1	C79.89	D00.02	D10.39	D37.09	D49.0
mucosa	C06.0	C79.89	D00.02	D10.39	D37.09	D49.0
sulcus (lower) (upper)	C06.1	C79.89	D00.02	D10.39	D37.09	D49.0
bulbourethral gland	C68.0	C79.19	D09.19	D30.4	D41.3	D49.59
bursa — *see Neoplasm, connective tissue*						
buttock NEC	C76.3	C79.89	D04.5	D36.7	D48.7	D49.89
calf	C76.5-●	C79.89	D04.7-●	D36.7	D48.7	D49.89
calvarium	C41.0	C79.51	—	D16.4-●	D48.0	D49.2
calyx, renal	C65.-●	C79.0-●	D09.19	D30.1-●	D41.1-●	D49.51-●
canal						
anal	C21.1	C78.5	D01.3	D12.9	D37.8	D49.0
auditory (external) — *see also Neoplasm, skin, ear*	C44.20-●	C79.2	D04.2-●	D23.2-●	D48.5	D49.2
auricular (external) — *see also Neoplasm, skin, ear*	C44.20-●	C79.2	D04.2-●	D23.2-●	D48.5	D49.2
canaliculi, biliary (biliferi) (intrahepatic)	C22.1	C78.7	D01.5	D13.4	D37.6	D49.0

◀ New   ◀ Revised   ~~deleted~~ Deleted   ● Use Additional Character(s)

	Malignant Primary	Malignant Secondary	Ca in situ	Benign	Uncertain Behavior	Unspecified Behavior
canthus (eye) (inner) (outer)	C44.10-●	C79.2	D04.1-●	D23.1-●	D48.5	D49.2
basal cell carcinoma	C44.11-●	—	—	—	—	—
sebaceous cell	C44.13-●	—	—	—	—	—
specified type NEC	C44.19-●	—	—	—	—	—
squamous cell carcinoma	C44.12-●	—	—	—	—	—
capillary — see Neoplasm, connective tissue						
caput coli	C18.0	C78.5	D01.0	D12.0	D37.4	D49.0
carcinoid — see Tumor, carcinoid						
cardia (gastric)	C16.0	C78.89	D00.2	D13.1	D37.1	D49.0
cardiac orifice (stomach)	C16.0	C78.89	D00.2	D13.1	D37.1	D49.0
cardio-esophageal junction	C16.0	C78.89	D00.2	D13.1	D37.1	D49.0
cardio-esophagus	C16.0	C78.89	D00.2	D13.1	D37.1	D49.0
carina (bronchus)	C34.0-●	C78.0-●	D02.2-●	D14.3-●	D38.1	D49.1
carotid (artery)	C49.0	C79.89	—	D21.0	D48.1	D49.2
body	C75.4	C79.89	—	D35.5	D44.6	D49.7
carpus (any bone)	C40.1-●	C79.51		D16.1-●	—	—
cartilage (articular) (joint) NEC — see also Neoplasm, bone	C41.9	C79.51	—	D16.9-●	D48.0	D49.2
arytenoid	C32.3	C78.39	D02.0	D14.1	D38.0	D49.1
auricular	C49.0	C79.89	—	D21.0	D48.1	D49.2
bronchi	C34.0-●	C78.39		D14.3-●	D38.1	D49.1
costal	C41.3	C79.51		D16.7	D48.0	D49.2
cricoid	C32.3	C78.39	D02.0	D14.1	D38.0	D49.1
cuneiform	C32.3	C78.39	D02.0	D14.1	D38.0	D49.1
ear (external)	C49.0	C79.89	—	D21.0	D48.1	D49.2
ensiform	C41.3	C79.51		D16.7	D48.0	D49.2
epiglottis	C32.1	C78.39	D02.0	D14.1	D38.0	D49.1
anterior surface	C10.1	C79.89	D00.08	D10.5	D37.05	D49.0
eyelid	C49.0	C79.89	—	D21.0	D48.1	D49.2
intervertebral	C41.2	C79.51	—	D16.6	D48.0	D49.2
larynx, laryngeal	C32.3	C78.39	D02.0	D14.1	D38.0	D49.1
nose, nasal	C30.0	C78.39	D02.3	D14.0	D38.5	D49.1
pinna	C49.0	C79.89	—	D21.0	D48.1	D49.2
rib	C41.3	C79.51		D16.7	D48.0	D49.2
semilunar (knee)	C40.2-●	C79.51	—	D16.2-●	D48.0	D49.2
thyroid	C32.3	C78.39	D02.0	D14.1	D38.0	D49.1
trachea	C33	C78.39	D02.1	D14.2	D38.1	D49.1
cauda equina	C72.1	C79.49	—	D33.4	D43.4	D49.7
cavity						
buccal	C06.9	C79.89	D00.00	D10.30	D37.09	D49.0
nasal	C30.0	C78.39	D02.3	D14.0	D38.5	D49.1
oral	C06.9	C79.89	D00.00	D10.30	D37.09	D49.0

	Malignant Primary	Malignant Secondary	Ca in situ	Benign	Uncertain Behavior	Unspecified Behavior
cavity (Continued)						
peritoneal	C48.2	C78.6	—	D20.1	D48.4	D49.0
tympanic	C30.1	C78.39	D02.3	D14.0	D38.5	D49.1
cecum	C18.0	C78.5	D01.0	D12.0	D37.4	D49.0
central nervous system	C72.9	C79.40				—
cerebellopontine (angle)	C71.6	C79.31		D33.1	D43.1	D49.6
cerebellum, cerebellar	C71.6	C79.31	—	D33.1	D43.1	D49.6
cerebrum, cerebra (cortex) (hemisphere) (white matter)	C71.0	C79.31	—	D33.0	D43.0	D49.6
meninges	C70.0	C79.32	—	D32.0	D42.0	D49.7
peduncle	C71.7	C79.31	—	D33.1	D43.1	D49.6
ventricle	C71.5	C79.31	—	D33.0	D43.0	D49.6
fourth	C71.7	C79.31	—	D33.1	D43.1	D49.6
cervical region	C76.0	C79.89	D09.8	D36.7	D48.7	D49.89
cervix (cervical) (uteri) (uterus)	C53.9	C79.82	D06.9	D26.0	D39.0	D49.59
canal	C53.0	C79.82	D06.0	D26.0	D39.0	D49.59
endocervix (canal) (gland)	C53.0	C79.82	D06.0	D26.0	D39.0	D49.59
exocervix	C53.1	C79.82	D06.1	D26.0	D39.0	D49.59
external os	C53.1	C79.82	D06.1	D26.0	D39.0	D49.59
internal os	C53.0	C79.82	D06.0	D26.0	D39.0	D49.59
nabothian gland	C53.0	C79.82	D06.0	D26.0	D39.0	D49.59
overlapping lesion	C53.8	—	—	—	—	—
squamocolumnar junction	C53.8	C79.82	D06.7	D26.0	D39.0	D49.59
stump	C53.8	C79.82	D06.7	D26.0	D39.0	D49.59
cheek	C76.0	C79.89	D09.8	D36.7	D48.7	D49.89
external	C44.309	C79.2	D04.39	D23.39	D48.5	D49.2
basal cell carcinoma	C44.319	—	—	—	—	—
specified type NEC	C44.399	—	—	—	—	—
squamous cell carcinoma	C44.329	—	—	—	—	—
inner aspect	C06.0	C79.89	D00.02	D10.39	D37.09	D49.0
internal	C06.0	C79.89	D00.02	D10.39	D37.09	D49.0
mucosa	C06.0	C79.89	D00.02	D10.39	D37.09	D49.0
chest (wall) NEC	C76.1	C79.89	D09.8	D36.7	D48.7	D49.89
chiasma opticum	C72.3-●	C79.49	—	D33.3	D43.3	D49.7
chin	C44.309	C79.2	D04.39	D23.39	D48.5	D49.2
basal cell carcinoma	C44.319	—	—	—	—	—
specified type NEC	C44.399	—	—	—	—	—
squamous cell carcinoma	C44.329	—	—	—	—	—
choana	C11.3	C79.89	D00.08	D10.6	D37.05	D49.0
cholangiole	C22.1	C78.89	D01.5	D13.4	D37.6	D49.0
choledochal duct	C24.0	C78.89	D01.5	D13.5	D37.6	D49.0
choroid	C69.3-●	C79.49	D09.2-●	D31.3-●	D48.7	D49.81
plexus	C71.5	C79.31	—	D33.0	D43.0	D49.6
ciliary body	C69.4-●	C79.49	D09.2-●	D31.4-●	D48.7	D49.89

TABLE OF NEOPLASMS

	Malignant Primary	Malignant Secondary	Ca in situ	Benign	Uncertain Behavior	Unspecified Behavior
clavicle	C41.3	C79.51	—	D16.7	D48.0	D49.2
clitoris	C51.2	C79.82	D07.1	D28.0	D39.8	D49.59
clivus	C41.0	C79.51	—	D16.4-•	D48.0	D49.2
cloacogenic zone	C21.2	C78.5	D01.3	D12.9	D37.8	D49.0
coccygeal						
body or glomus	C49.5	C79.89	—	D21.5	D48.1	D49.2
vertebra	C41.4	C79.51	—	D16.8	D48.0	D49.2
coccyx	C41.4	C79.51	—	D16.8	D48.0	D49.2
colon — *see also Neoplasm, intestine, large*	C18.9	C78.5	—	—	—	—
with rectum	C19	C78.5	D01.1	D12.7	D37.5	D49.0
column, spinal — *see Neoplasm, spine*						
columnella — *see also Neoplasm, skin, face*	C44.390	C79.2	D04.39	D23.39	D48.5	D49.2
commissure						
labial, lip	C00.6	C79.89	D00.01	D10.39	D37.01	D49.0
laryngeal	C32.0	C78.39	D02.0	D14.1	D38.0	D49.1
common (bile) duct	C24.0	C78.89	D01.5	D13.5	D37.6	D49.0
concha — *see also Neoplasm, skin, ear*	C44.20-•	C79.2	D04.2-•	D23.2-•	D48.5	D49.2
nose	C30.0	C78.39	D02.3	D14.0	D38.5	D49.1
conjunctiva	C69.0-•	C79.49	D09.2-•	D31.0-•	D48.7	D49.89
connective tissue NEC	C49.9	C79.89	—	D21.9	D48.1	D49.2

Note: For neoplasms of connective tissue (blood vessel, bursa, fascia, ligament, muscle, peripheral nerves, sympathetic and parasympathetic nerves and ganglia, synovia, tendon, etc.) or of morphological types that indicate connective tissue, code according to the list under "Neoplasm, connective tissue." For sites that do not appear in this list, code to neoplasm of that site; e.g., fibrosarcoma, pancreas (C25.9)

Note: Morphological types that indicate connective tissue appear in their proper place in the alphabetic index with the instruction "*see Neoplasm, connective tissue ....*"

	Malignant Primary	Malignant Secondary	Ca in situ	Benign	Uncertain Behavior	Unspecified Behavior
abdomen	C49.4	C79.89	—	D21.4	D48.1	D49.2
abdominal wall	C49.4	C79.89	—	D21.4	D48.1	D49.2
ankle	C49.2-•	C79.89	—	D21.2-•	D48.1	D49.2
antecubital fossa or space	C49.1-•	C79.89	—	D21.1-•	D48.1	D49.2
arm	C49.1-•	C79.89	—	D21.1-•	D48.1	D49.2
auricle (ear)	C49.0	C79.89	—	D21.0	D48.1	D49.2
axilla	C49.3	C79.89	—	D21.3	D48.1	D49.2
back	C49.6	C79.89	—	D21.6	D48.1	D49.2
breast — *see Neoplasm, breast*						
buttock	C49.5	C79.89	—	D21.5	D48.1	D49.2
calf	C49.2-•	C79.89	—	D21.2-•	D48.1	D49.2
cervical region	C49.0	C79.89	—	D21.0	D48.1	D49.2

	Malignant Primary	Malignant Secondary	Ca in situ	Benign	Uncertain Behavior	Unspecified Behavior
connective tissue NEC *(Continued)*						
cheek	C49.0	C79.89	—	D21.0	D48.1	D49.2
chest (wall)	C49.3	C79.89	—	D21.3	D48.1	D49.2
chin	C49.0	C79.89	—	D21.0	D48.1	D49.2
diaphragm	C49.3	C79.89	—	D21.3	D48.1	D49.2
ear (external)	C49.0	C79.89	—	D21.0	D48.1	D49.2
elbow	C49.1-•	C79.89	—	D21.1-•	D48.1	D49.2
extrarectal	C49.5	C79.89	—	D21.5	D48.1	D49.2
extremity	C49.9	C79.89	—	D21.9	D48.1	D49.2
lower	C49.2-•	C79.89	—	D21.2-•	D48.1	D49.2
upper	C49.1-•	C79.89	—	D21.1-•	D48.1	D49.2
eyelid	C49.0	C79.89	—	D21.0	D48.1	D49.2
face	C49.0	C79.89	—	D21.0	D48.1	D49.2
finger	C49.1-•	C79.89	—	D21.1-•	D48.1	D49.2
flank	C49.6	C79.89	—	D21.6	D48.1	D49.2
foot	C49.2-•	C79.89	—	D21.2-•	D48.1	D49.2
forearm	C49.1-•	C79.89	—	D21.1-•	D48.1	D49.2
forehead	C49.0	C79.89	—	D21.0	D48.1	D49.2
gastric	C49.4	C79.89	—	D21.4	D48.1	D49.2
gastrointestinal	C49.4	C79.89	—	D21.4	D48.1	D49.2
gluteal region	C49.5	C79.89	—	D21.5	D48.1	D49.2
great vessels NEC	C49.3	C79.89	—	D21.3	D48.1	D49.2
groin	C49.5	C79.89	—	D21.5	D48.1	D49.2
hand	C49.1-•	C79.89	—	D21.1-•	D48.1	D49.2
head	C49.0	C79.89	—	D21.0	D48.1	D49.2
heel	C49.2-•	C79.89	—	D21.2-•	D48.1	D49.2
hip	C49.2-•	C79.89	—	D21.2-•	D48.1	D49.2
hypochondrium	C49.4	C79.89	—	D21.4	D48.1	D49.2
iliopsoas muscle	C49.5	C79.89	—	D21.5	D48.1	D49.2
infraclavicular region	C49.3	C79.89	—	D21.3	D48.1	D49.2
inguinal (canal) (region)	C49.5	C79.89	—	D21.5	D48.1	D49.2
intestinal	C49.4	C79.89	—	D21.4	D48.1	D49.2
intrathoracic	C49.3	C79.89	—	D21.3	D48.1	D49.2
ischiorectal fossa	C49.5	C79.89	—	D21.5	D48.1	D49.2
jaw	C03.9	C79.89	D00.03	D10.39	D48.1	D49.0
knee	C49.2-•	C79.89	—	D21.2-•	D48.1	D49.2
leg	C49.2-•	C79.89	—	D21.2-•	D48.1	D49.2
limb NEC	C49.9	C79.89	—	D21.9	D48.1	D49.2
lower	C49.2-•	C79.89	—	D21.2-•	D48.1	D49.2
upper	C49.1-•	C79.89	—	D21.1-•	D48.1	D49.2
nates	C49.5	C79.89	—	D21.5	D48.1	D49.2
neck	C49.0	C79.89	—	D21.0	D48.1	D49.2
orbit	C69.6-•	C79.49	D09.2-•	D31.6-•	D48.1	D49.89
overlapping lesion	C49.8	—	—	—	—	—

◀ New   ◀ Revised   ~~deleted~~ Deleted   • Use Additional Character(s)

	Malignant Primary	Malignant Secondary	Ca in situ	Benign	Uncertain Behavior	Unspecified Behavior
connective tissue NEC *(Continued)*						
pararectal	C49.5	C79.89	—	D21.5	D48.1	D49.2
para-urethral	C49.5	C79.89	—	D21.5	D48.1	D49.2
paravaginal	C49.5	C79.89	—	D21.5	D48.1	D49.2
pelvis (floor)	C49.5	C79.89	—	D21.5	D48.1	D49.2
pelvo-abdominal	C49.8	C79.89	—	D21.6	D48.1	D49.2
perineum	C49.5	C79.89	—	D21.5	D48.1	D49.2
perirectal (tissue)	C49.5	C79.89	—	D21.5	D48.1	D49.2
periurethral (tissue)	C49.5	C79.89	—	D21.5	D48.1	D49.2
popliteal fossa or space	C49.2-●	C79.89		D21.2-●	D48.1	D49.2
presacral	C49.5	C79.89	—	D21.5	D48.1	D49.2
psoas muscle	C49.4	C79.89	—	D21.4	D48.1	D49.2
pterygoid fossa	C49.0	C79.89	—	D21.0	D48.1	D49.2
rectovaginal septum or wall	C49.5	C79.89	—	D21.5	D48.1	D49.2
rectovesical	C49.5	C79.89	—	D21.5	D48.1	D49.2
retroperitoneum	C48.0	C78.6	—	D20.0	D48.3	D49.0
sacrococcygeal region	C49.5	C79.89	—	D21.5	D48.1	D49.2
scalp	C49.0	C79.89	—	D21.0	D48.1	D49.2
scapular region	C49.3	C79.89	—	D21.3	D48.1	D49.2
shoulder	C49.1-●	C79.89	—	D21.1-●	D48.1	D49.2
skin (dermis) NEC — *see also* Neoplasm, skin, by site	C44.90	C79.2	D04.9	D23.9	D48.5	D49.2
stomach	C49.4	C79.89	—	D21.4	D48.1	D49.2
submental	C49.0	C79.89	—	D21.0	D48.1	D49.2
supraclavicular region	C49.0	C79.89	—	D21.0	D48.1	D49.2
temple	C49.0	C79.89	—	D21.0	D48.1	D49.2
temporal region	C49.0	C79.89	—	D21.0	D48.1	D49.2
thigh	C49.2-●	C79.89	—	D21.2-●	D48.1	D49.2
thoracic (duct) (wall)	C49.3	C79.89	—	D21.3	D48.1	D49.2
thorax	C49.3	C79.89	—	D21.3	D48.1	D49.2
thumb	C49.1-●	C79.89	—	D21.1-●	D48.1	D49.2
toe	C49.2-●	C79.89	—	D21.2-●	D48.1	D49.2
trunk	C49.6	C79.89	—	D21.6	D48.1	D49.2
umbilicus	C49.4	C79.89	—	D21.4	D48.1	D49.2
vesicorectal	C49.5	C79.89	—	D21.5	D48.1	D49.2
wrist	C49.1-●	C79.89	—	D21.1-●	D48.1	D49.2
conus medullaris	C72.0	C79.49	—	D33.4	D43.4	D49.7
cord (true) (vocal)	C32.0	C78.39	D02.0	D14.1	D38.0	D49.1
false	C32.1	C78.39	D02.0	D14.1	D38.0	D49.1
spermatic	C63.1-●	C79.82	D07.69	D29.8	D40.8	D49.59
spinal (cervical) (lumbar) (thoracic)	C72.0	C79.49	—	D33.4	D43.4	D49.7
cornea (limbus)	C69.1-●	C79.49	D09.2-●	D31.1-●	D48.7	D49.89
corpus						

	Malignant Primary	Malignant Secondary	Ca in situ	Benign	Uncertain Behavior	Unspecified Behavior
corpus *(Continued)*						
albicans	C56.-●	C79.6-●	D07.39	D27.-●	D39.1-●	D49.59
callosum, brain	C71.0	C79.31	—	D33.2	D43.2	D49.6
cavernosum	C60.2	C79.82	D07.4	D29.0	D40.8	D49.59
gastric	C16.2	C78.89	D00.2	D13.1	D37.1	D49.0
overlapping sites	C54.8	—	—	—	—	—
penis	C60.2	C79.82	D07.4	D29.0	D40.8	D49.59
striatum, cerebrum	C71.0	C79.31	—	D33.0	D43.0	D49.6
uteri	C54.9	C79.82	D07.0	D26.1	D39.0	D49.59
isthmus	C54.0	C79.82	D07.0	D26.1	D39.0	D49.59
cortex						
adrenal	C74.0-●	C79.7-●	D09.3	D35.0-●	D44.1-●	D49.7
cerebral	C71.0	C79.31	—	D33.0	D43.0	D49.6
costal cartilage	C41.3	C79.51	—	D16.7	D48.0	D49.2
costovertebral joint	C41.3	C79.51	—	D16.7	D48.0	D49.2
Cowper's gland	C68.0	C79.19	D09.19	D30.4	D41.3	D49.59
cranial (fossa, any)	C71.9	C79.31	—	D33.2	D43.2	D49.6
meninges	C70.0	C79.32	—	D32.0	D42.0	D49.7
nerve	C72.50	C79.49	—	D33.3	D43.3	D49.7
specified NEC	C72.59	C79.49	—	D33.3	D43.3	D49.7
craniobuccal pouch	C75.2	C79.89	D09.3	D35.2	D44.3	D49.7
craniopharyngeal (duct) (pouch)	C75.2	C79.89	D09.3	D35.3	D44.4	D49.7
cricoid	C13.0	C79.89	D00.08	D10.7	D37.05	D49.0
cartilage	C32.3	C78.39	D02.0	D14.1	D38.0	D49.1
cricopharynx	C13.0	C79.89	D00.08	D10.7	D37.05	D49.0
crypt of Morgagni	C21.8	C78.5	D01.3	D12.9	D37.8	D49.0
crystalline lens	C69.4-●	C79.49	D09.2-●	D31.4-●	D48.7	D49.89
cul-de-sac (Douglas')	C48.1	C78.6	—	D20.1	D48.4	D49.0
cuneiform cartilage	C32.3	C78.39	D02.0	D14.1	D38.0	D49.1
cutaneous — *see Neoplasm, skin*						
cutis — *see Neoplasm, skin*						
cystic (bile) duct (common)	C24.0	C78.89	D01.5	D13.5	D37.6	D49.0
dermis — *see Neoplasm, skin*						
diaphragm	C49.3	C79.89	—	D21.3	D48.1	D49.2
digestive organs, system, tube, or tract NEC	C26.9	C78.89	D01.9	D13.9	D37.9	D49.0
disc, intervertebral	C41.2	C79.51	—	D16.6	D48.0	D49.2
disease, generalized	C80.0	—	—	—	—	—
disseminated	C80.0	—	—	—	—	—
Douglas' cul-de-sac or pouch	C48.1	C78.6	—	D20.1	D48.4	D49.0
duodenojejunal junction	C17.8	C78.4	D01.49	D13.39	D37.2	D49.0
duodenum	C17.0	C78.4	D01.49	D13.2	D37.2	D49.0

TABLE OF NEOPLASMS

TABLE OF NEOPLASMS

	Malignant Primary	Malignant Secondary	Ca in situ	Benign	Uncertain Behavior	Unspecified Behavior
dura (cranial) (mater)	C70.9	C79.49	—	D32.9	D42.9	D49.7
cerebral	C70.0	C79.32		D32.0	D42.0	D49.7
spinal	C70.1	C79.49	—	D32.1	D42.1	D49.7
ear (external) — see also Neoplasm, skin, ear	C44.20-•	C79.2	D04.2-•	D23.2-•	D48.5	D49.2
auricle or auris — see also Neoplasm, skin, ear	C44.20-•	C79.2	D04.2-•	D23.2-•	D48.5	D49.2
canal, external — see also Neoplasm, skin, ear	C44.20-•	C79.2	D04.2-•	D23.2-•	D48.5	D49.2
cartilage	C49.0	C79.89	—	D21.0	D48.1	D49.2
external meatus — see also Neoplasm, skin, ear	C44.20-•	C79.2	D04.2-•	D23.2-•	D48.5	D49.2
inner	C30.1	C78.39	D02.3	D14.0	D38.5	D49.1
lobule — see also Neoplasm, skin, ear	C44.20-•	C79.2	D04.2-•	D23.2-•	D48.5	D49.2
middle	C30.1	C78.39	D02.3	D14.0	D38.5	D49.1
overlapping lesion with accessory sinuses	C31.8	—	—	—	—	—
skin	C44.20-•	C79.2	D04.2-•	D23.2-•	D48.5	D49.2
basal cell carcinoma	C44.21-•	—	—	—	—	—
specified type NEC	C44.29-•	—	—	—	—	—
squamous cell carcinoma	C44.22-•	—	—	—	—	—
earlobe	C44.20-•	C79.2	D04.2-•	D23.2-•	D48.5	D49.2
basal cell carcinoma	C44.21-•	—	—	—	—	—
specified type NEC	C44.29-•	—	—	—	—	—
squamous cell carcinoma	C44.22-•	—	—	—	—	—
ejaculatory duct	C63.7	C79.82	D07.69	D29.8	D40.8	D49.59
elbow NEC	C76.4-•	C79.89	D04.6-•	D36.7	D48.7	D49.89
endocardium	C38.0	C79.89	—	D15.1	D48.7	D49.89
endocervix (canal) (gland)	C53.0	C79.82	D06.0	D26.0	D39.0	D49.59
endocrine gland NEC	C75.9	C79.89	D09.3	D35.9	D44.9	D49.7
pluriglandular	C75.8	C79.89	D09.3	D35.7	D44.9	D49.7
endometrium (gland) (stroma)	C54.1	C79.82	D07.0	D26.1	D39.0	D49.59
ensiform cartilage	C41.3	C79.51		D16.7	D48.0	D49.2
enteric — see Neoplasm, intestine						
ependyma (brain)	C71.5	C79.31		D33.0	D43.0	D49.6
fourth ventricle	C71.7	C79.31		D33.1	D43.1	D49.6
epicardium	C38.0	C79.89		D15.1	D48.7	D49.89
epididymis	C63.0-•	C79.82	D07.69	D29.3-•	D40.8	D49.59
epidural	C72.9	C79.49		D33.9	D43.9	D49.7
epiglottis	C32.1	C78.39	D02.0	D14.1	D38.0	D49.1
anterior aspect or surface	C10.1	C79.89	D00.08	D10.5	D37.05	D49.0
cartilage	C32.3	C78.39	D02.0	D14.1	D38.0	D49.1
free border (margin)	C10.1	C79.89	D00.08	D10.5	D37.05	D49.0

	Malignant Primary	Malignant Secondary	Ca in situ	Benign	Uncertain Behavior	Unspecified Behavior
junctional region	C10.8	C79.89	D00.08	D10.5	D37.05	D49.0
posterior (laryngeal) surface	C32.1	C78.39	D02.0	D14.1	D38.0	D49.1
suprahyoid portion	C32.1	C78.39	D02.0	D14.1	D38.0	D49.1
esophagogastric junction	C16.0	C78.89	D00.2	D13.1	D37.1	D49.0
esophagus	C15.9	C78.89	D00.1	D13.0	D37.8	D49.0
abdominal	C15.5	C78.89	D00.1	D13.0	D37.8	D49.0
cervical	C15.3	C78.89	D00.1	D13.0	D37.8	D49.0
distal (third)	C15.5	C78.89	D00.1	D13.0	D37.8	D49.0
lower (third)	C15.5	C78.89	D00.1	D13.0	D37.8	D49.0
middle (third)	C15.4	C78.89	D00.1	D13.0	D37.8	D49.0
overlapping lesion	C15.8	—	—	—	—	—
proximal (third)	C15.3	C78.89	D00.1	D13.0	D37.8	D49.0
thoracic	C15.4	C78.89	D00.1	D13.0	D37.8	D49.0
upper (third)	C15.3	C78.89	D00.1	D13.0	D37.8	D49.0
ethmoid (sinus)	C31.1	C78.39	D02.3	D14.0	D38.5	D49.1
bone or labyrinth	C41.0	C79.51	—	D16.4-•	D48.0	D49.2
eustachian tube	C30.1	C78.39	D02.3	D14.0	D38.5	D49.1
exocervix	C53.1	C79.82	D06.1	D26.0	D39.0	D49.59
external						
meatus (ear) — see also Neoplasm, skin, ear	C44.20-•	C79.2	D04.2-•	D23.2-•	D48.5	D49.2
os, cervix uteri	C53.1	C79.82	D06.1	D26.0	D39.0	D49.59
extradural	C72.9	C79.49	—	D33.9	D43.9	D49.7
extrahepatic (bile) duct	C24.0	C78.89	D01.5	D13.5	D37.6	D49.0
overlapping lesion with gallbladder	C24.8	—	—	—	—	—
extraocular muscle	C69.6-•	C79.49	D09.2-•	D31.6-•	D48.7	D49.89
extrarectal	C76.3	C79.89	D09.8	D36.7	D48.7	D49.89
extremity	C76.8	C79.89	D04.8	D36.7	D48.7	D49.89
lower	C76.5-•	C79.89	D04.7-•	D36.7	D48.7	D49.89
upper	C76.4-•	C79.89	D04.6-•	D36.7	D48.7	D49.89
eye NEC	C69.9-•	C79.49	D09.2	D31.9	D48.7	D49.89
overlapping sites	C69.8	—	—	—	—	—
eyeball	C69.9-•	C79.49	D09.2-•	D31.9-•	D48.7	D49.89
eyebrow	C44.309	C79.2	D04.39	D23.39	D48.5	D49.2
basal cell carcinoma	C44.319	—	—	—	—	—
specified type NEC	C44.399	—	—	—	—	—
squamous cell carcinoma	C44.329	—	—	—	—	—
eyelid (lower) (skin) (upper)	C44.10-•	—	—	—	—	—
basal cell carcinoma	C44.11-•	—	—	—	—	—
cartilage	C49.0	C79.89		D21.0	D48.1	D49.2
sebaceous cell	C44.13-•	—	—	—	—	—
specified type NEC	C44.19-•	—	—	—	—	—
squamous cell carcinoma	C44.12-•	—	—	—	—	—

◄ New   ◄◄ Revised   ~~deleted~~ Deleted   • Use Additional Character(s)

TABLE OF NEOPLASMS

	Malignant Primary	Malignant Secondary	Ca in situ	Benign	Uncertain Behavior	Unspecified Behavior
face NEC	C76.0	C79.89	D04.39	D36.7	D48.7	D49.89
fallopian tube (accessory)	C57.0-●	C79.82	D07.39	D28.2	D39.8	D49.59
falx (cerebella) (cerebri)	C70.0	C79.32	—	D32.0	D42.0	D49.7
fascia — see also Neoplasm, connective tissue						
palmar	C49.1-●	C79.89	—	D21.1-●	D48.1	D49.2
plantar	C49.2-●	C79.89	—	D21.2-●	D48.1	D49.2
fatty tissue — see Neoplasm, connective tissue						
fauces, faucial NEC	C10.9	C79.89	D00.08	D10.5	D37.05	D49.0
pillars	C09.1	C79.89	D00.08	D10.5	D37.05	D49.0
tonsil	C09.9	C79.89	D00.08	D10.4	D37.05	D49.0
femur (any part)	C40.2-●	—	—	D16.2-●	—	—
fetal membrane	C58	C79.82	D07.0	D26.7	D39.2	D49.59
fibrous tissue — see Neoplasm, connective tissue						
fibula (any part)	C40.2-●	C79.51	—	D16.2-●	—	—
filum terminale	C72.0	C79.49	—	D33.4	D43.4	D49.7
finger NEC	C76.4-●	C79.89	D04.6-●	D36.7	D48.7	D49.89
flank NEC	C76.8	C79.89	D04.5	D36.7	D48.7	D49.89
follicle, nabothian	C53.0	C79.82	D06.0	D26.0	D39.0	D49.59
foot NEC	C76.5-●	C79.89	D04.7-●	D36.7	D48.7	D49.89
forearm NEC	C76.4-●	C79.89	D04.6-●	D36.7	D48.7	D49.89
forehead (skin)	C44.309	C79.2	D04.39	D23.39	D48.5	D49.2
basal cell carcinoma	C44.319	—	—	—	—	—
specified type NEC	C44.399	—	—	—	—	—
squamous cell carcinoma	C44.329	—	—	—	—	—
foreskin	C60.0	C79.82	D07.4	D29.0	D40.8	D49.59
fornix						
pharyngeal	C11.3	C79.89	D00.08	D10.6	D37.05	D49.0
vagina	C52	C79.82	D07.2	D28.1	D39.8	D49.59
fossa (of)						
anterior (cranial)	C71.9	C79.31	—	D33.2	D43.2	D49.6
cranial	C71.9	C79.31	—	D33.2	D43.2	D49.6
ischiorectal	C76.3	C79.89	D09.8	D36.7	D48.7	D49.89
middle (cranial)	C71.9	C79.31	—	D33.2	D43.2	D49.6
piriform	C12	C79.89	D00.08	D10.7	D37.05	D49.0
pituitary	C75.1	C79.89	D09.3	D35.2	D44.3	D49.7
posterior (cranial)	C71.9	C79.31	—	D33.2	D43.2	D49.6
pterygoid	C49.0	C79.89	—	D21.0	D48.1	D49.2
pyriform	C12	C79.89	D00.08	D10.7	D37.05	D49.0
Rosenmuller	C11.2	C79.89	D00.08	D10.6	D37.05	D49.0
tonsillar	C09.0	C79.89	D00.08	D10.5	D37.05	D49.0
fourchette	C51.9	C79.82	D07.1	D28.0	D39.8	D49.59

	Malignant Primary	Malignant Secondary	Ca in situ	Benign	Uncertain Behavior	Unspecified Behavior
frenulum						
labii — see Neoplasm, lip, internal						
linguae	C02.2	C79.89	D00.07	D10.1	D37.02	D49.0
frontal						
bone	C41.0	C79.51	—	D16.4-●	D48.0	D49.2
lobe, brain	C71.1	C79.31	—	D33.0	D43.0	D49.6
pole	C71.1	C79.31	—	D33.0	D43.0	D49.6
sinus	C31.2	C78.39	D02.3	D14.0	D38.5	D49.1
fundus						
stomach	C16.1	C78.89	D00.2	D13.1	D37.1	D49.0
uterus	C54.3	C79.82	D07.0	D26.1	D39.0	D49.59
gall duct (extrahepatic)	C24.0	C78.89	D01.5	D13.5	D37.6	D49.0
intrahepatic	C22.1	C78.7	D01.5	D13.4	D37.6	D49.0
gallbladder	C23	C78.89	D01.5	D13.5	D37.6	D49.0
overlapping lesion with extrahepatic bile ducts	C24.8	—	—	—	—	—
ganglia — see also Neoplasm, nerve, peripheral	C47.9	C79.89	—	D36.10	D48.2	D49.2
basal	C71.0	C79.31	—	D33.0	D43.0	D49.6
cranial nerve	C72.50	C79.49	—	D33.3	D43.3	D49.7
Gartner's duct	C52	C79.82	D07.2	D28.1	D39.8	D49.59
gastric — see Neoplasm, stomach						
gastrocolic	C26.9	C78.89	D01.9	D13.9	D37.9	D49.0
gastroesophageal junction	C16.0	C78.89	D00.2	D13.1	D37.1	D49.0
gastrointestinal (tract) NEC	C26.9	C78.89	D01.9	D13.9	D37.9	D49.0
generalized	C80.0	—	—	—	—	—
genital organ or tract						
female NEC	C57.9	C79.82	D07.30	D28.9	D39.9	D49.59
overlapping lesion	C57.8	—	—	—	—	—
specified site NEC	C57.7	C79.82	D07.39	D28.7	D39.8	D49.59
male NEC	C63.9	C79.82	D07.60	D29.9	D40.9	D49.59
overlapping lesion	C63.8	—	—	—	—	—
specified site NEC	C63.7	C79.82	D07.69	D29.8	D40.8	D49.59
genitourinary tract						
female	C57.9	C79.82	D07.30	D28.9	D39.9	D49.59
male	C63.9	C79.82	D07.60	D29.9	D40.9	D49.59
gingiva (alveolar) (marginal)	C03.9	C79.89	D00.03	D10.39	D37.09	D49.0
lower	C03.1	C79.89	D00.03	D10.39	D37.09	D49.0
mandibular	C03.1	C79.89	D00.03	D10.39	D37.09	D49.0
maxillary	C03.0	C79.89	D00.03	D10.39	D37.09	D49.0
upper	C03.0	C79.89	D00.03	D10.39	D37.09	D49.0

◀ New   ◀ Revised   ~~deleted~~ Deleted   ● Use Additional Character(s)   489

TABLE OF NEOPLASMS

	Malignant Primary	Malignant Secondary	Ca in situ	Benign	Uncertain Behavior	Unspecified Behavior
gland, glandular (lymphatic) (system) — see also Neoplasm, lymph gland						
endocrine NEC	C75.9	C79.89	D09.3	D35.9	D44.9	D49.7
salivary — see Neoplasm, salivary gland						
glans penis	C60.1	C79.82	D07.4	D29.0	D40.8	D49.59
globus pallidus	C71.0	C79.31	—	D33.0	D43.0	D49.6
glomus						
coccygeal	C49.5	C79.89	—	D21.5	D48.1	D49.2
jugularis	C75.5	C79.89	—	D35.6	D44.7	D49.7
glosso-epiglottic fold(s)	C10.1	C79.89	D00.08	D10.5	D37.05	D49.0
glossopalatine fold	C09.1	C79.89	D00.08	D10.5	D37.05	D49.0
glossopharyngeal sulcus	C09.0	C79.89	D00.08	D10.5	D37.05	D49.0
glottis	C32.0	C78.39	D02.0	D14.1	D38.0	D49.1
gluteal region	C76.3	C79.89	D04.5	D36.7	D48.7	D49.89
great vessels NEC	C49.3	C79.89	—	D21.3	D48.1	D49.2
groin NEC	C76.3	C79.89	D04.5	D36.7	D48.7	D49.89
gum	C03.9	C79.89	D00.03	D10.39	D37.09	D49.0
lower	C03.1	C79.89	D00.03	D10.39	D37.09	D49.0
upper	C03.0	C79.89	D00.03	D10.39	D37.09	D49.0
hand NEC	C76.4-●	C79.89	D04.6-●	D36.7	D48.7	D49.89
head NEC	C76.0	C79.89	D04.4	D36.7	D48.7	D49.89
heart	C38.0	C79.89	—	D15.1	D48.7	D49.89
heel NEC	C76.5-●	C79.89	D04.7-●	D36.7	D48.7	D49.89
helix — see also Neoplasm, skin, ear	C44.20-●	C79.2	D04.2-●	D23.2-●	D48.5	D49.2
hematopoietic, hemopoietic tissue NEC	C96.9	—	—	—	—	—
specified NEC	C96.Z	—	—	—	—	—
hemisphere, cerebral	C71.0	C79.31	—	D33.0	D43.0	D49.6
hemorrhoidal zone	C21.1	C78.5	D01.3	D12.9	D37.8	D49.0
hepatic — see also Index to disease, by histology	C22.9	C78.7	D01.5	D13.4	D37.6	D49.0
duct (bile)	C24.0	C78.89	D01.5	D13.5	D37.6	D49.0
flexure (colon)	C18.3	C78.5	D01.0	D12.3	D37.4	D49.0
primary	C22.8	C78.7	D01.5	D13.4	D37.6	D49.0
hepatobiliary	C24.9	C79.89	D01.5	D13.5	D37.6	D49.0
hepatoblastoma	C22.2	C78.7	D01.5	D13.4	D37.6	D49.0
hepatoma	C22.0	C78.7	D01.5	D13.4	D37.6	D49.0
hilus of lung	C34.0-●	C78.0-●	D02.2-●	D14.3-●	D38.1	D49.1
hip NEC	C76.5-●	C79.89	D04.7-●	D36.7	D48.7	D49.89
hippocampus, brain	C71.2	C79.31	—	D33.0	D43.0	D49.6
humerus (any part)	C40.0-●	C79.51	—	D16.0-●	—	—
hymen	C52	C79.82	D07.2	D28.1	D39.8	D49.59
hypopharynx, hypopharyngeal NEC	C13.9	C79.89	D00.08	D10.7	D37.05	D49.0
overlapping lesion	C13.8	—	—	—	—	—
postcricoid region	C13.0	C79.89	D00.08	D10.7	D37.05	D49.0
posterior wall	C13.2	C79.89	D00.08	D10.7	D37.05	D49.0
pyriform fossa (sinus)	C12	C79.89	D00.08	D10.7	D37.05	D49.0
hypophysis	C75.1	C79.89	D09.3	D35.2	D44.3	D49.7
hypothalamus	C71.0	C79.31	—	D33.0	D43.0	D49.6
ileocecum, ileocecal (coil) (junction) (valve)	C18.0	C78.5	D01.0	D12.0	D37.4	D49.0
ileum	C17.2	C78.4	D01.49	D13.39	D37.2	D49.0
ilium	C41.4	C79.51	—	D16.8	D48.0	D49.2
immunoproliferative NEC	C88.9	—	—	—	—	—
infraclavicular (region)	C76.1	C79.89	D04.5	D36.7	D48.7	D49.89
inguinal (region)	C76.3	C79.89	D04.5	D36.7	D48.7	D49.89
insula	C71.0	C79.31	—	D33.0	D43.0	D49.6
insular tissue (pancreas)	C25.4	C78.89	D01.7	D13.7	D37.8	D49.0
brain	C71.0	C79.31	—	D33.0	D43.0	D49.6
interarytenoid fold	C13.1	C79.89	D00.08	D10.7	D37.05	D49.0
hypopharyngeal aspect	C13.1	C79.89	D00.08	D10.7	D37.05	D49.0
laryngeal aspect	C32.1	C78.39	D02.0	D14.1	D38.0	D49.1
marginal zone	C13.1	C79.89	D00.08	D10.7	D37.05	D49.0
interdental papillae	C03.9	C79.89	D00.03	D10.39	D37.09	D49.0
lower	C03.1	C79.89	D00.03	D10.39	D37.09	D49.0
upper	C03.0	C79.89	D00.03	D10.39	D37.09	D49.0
internal						
capsule	C71.0	C79.31	—	D33.0	D43.0	D49.6
os (cervix)	C53.0	C79.82	D06.0	D26.0	D39.0	D49.59
intervertebral cartilage or disc	C41.2	C79.51	—	D16.6	D48.0	D49.2
intestine, intestinal	C26.0	C78.80	D01.40	D13.9	D37.8	D49.0
large	C18.9	C78.5	D01.0	D12.6	D37.4	D49.0
appendix	C18.1	C78.5	D01.0	D12.1	D37.3	D49.0
caput coli	C18.0	C78.5	D01.0	D12.0	D37.4	D49.0
cecum	C18.0	C78.5	D01.0	D12.0	D37.4	D49.0
colon	C18.9	C78.5	D01.0	D12.6	D37.4	D49.0
and rectum	C19	C78.5	D01.1	D12.7	D37.5	D49.0
ascending	C18.2	C78.5	D01.0	D12.2	D37.4	D49.0
caput	C18.0	C78.5	D01.0	D12.0	D37.4	D49.0
descending	C18.6	C78.5	D01.0	D12.4	D37.4	D49.0
distal	C18.6	C78.5	D01.0	D12.4	D37.4	D49.0
left	C18.6	C78.5	D01.0	D12.4	D37.4	D49.0
overlapping lesion	C18.8	—	—	—	—	—
pelvic	C18.7	C78.5	D01.0	D12.5	D37.4	D49.0
right	C18.2	C78.5	D01.0	D12.2	D37.4	D49.0

◀ New   ◀◀ Revised   ~~deleted~~ Deleted   ● Use Additional Character(s)

	Malignant Primary	Malignant Secondary	Ca in situ	Benign	Uncertain Behavior	Unspecified Behavior
intestine, intestinal *(Continued)*						
large *(Continued)*						
colon *(Continued)*						
sigmoid (flexure)	C18.7	C78.5	D01.0	D12.5	D37.4	D49.0
transverse	C18.4	C78.5	D01.0	D12.3	D37.4	D49.0
hepatic flexure	C18.3	C78.5	D01.0	D12.3	D37.4	D49.0
ileocecum, ileocecal (coil) (valve)	C18.0	C78.5	D01.0	D12.0	D37.4	D49.0
overlapping lesion	C18.8	—	—	—	—	—
sigmoid flexure (lower) (upper)	C18.7	C78.5	D01.0	D12.5	D37.4	D49.0
splenic flexure	C18.5	C78.5	D01.0	D12.3	D37.4	D49.0
small	C17.9	C78.4	D01.40	D13.30	D37.2	D49.0
duodenum	C17.0	C78.4	D01.49	D13.2	D37.2	D49.0
ileum	C17.2	C78.4	D01.49	D13.39	D37.2	D49.0
jejunum	C17.1	C78.4	D01.49	D13.39	D37.2	D49.0
overlapping lesion	C17.8	—	—	—	—	—
tract NEC	C26.0	C78.89	D01.40	D13.9	D37.8	D49.0
intra-abdominal	C76.2	C79.89	D09.8	D36.7	D48.7	D49.89
intracranial NEC	C71.9	C79.31	—	D33.2	D43.2	D49.6
intrahepatic (bile) duct	C22.1	C78.7	D01.5	D13.4	D37.6	D49.0
intraocular	C69.9-●	C79.49	D09.2-●	D31.9-●	D48.7	D49.89
intraorbital	C69.6-●	C79.49	D09.2-●	D31.6-●	D48.7	D49.89
intrasellar	C75.1	C79.89	D09.3	D35.2	D44.3	D49.7
intrathoracic (cavity) (organs)	C76.1	C79.89	D09.8	D15.9	D48.7	D49.89
specified NEC	C76.1	C79.89	D09.8	D15.7	—	—
iris	C69.4-●	C79.49	D09.2-●	D31.4-●	D48.7	D49.89
ischiorectal (fossa)	C76.3	C79.89	D09.8	D36.7	D48.7	D49.89
ischium	C41.4	C79.51	—	D16.8	D48.0	D49.2
island of Reil	C71.0	C79.31	—	D33.0	D43.0	D49.6
islands or islets of Langerhans	C25.4	C78.89	D01.7	D13.7	D37.8	D49.0
isthmus uteri	C54.0	C79.82	D07.0	D26.1	D39.0	D49.59
jaw	C76.0	C79.89	D09.8	D36.7	D48.7	D49.89
bone	C41.1	C79.51	—	D16.5-●	D48.0	D49.2
lower	C41.1	C79.51	—	D16.5-●	—	—
upper	C41.0	C79.51	—	D16.4-●	—	—
carcinoma (any type) (lower) (upper)	C76.0	C79.89	—	—	—	—
skin — *see also Neoplasm, skin, face*	C44.309	C79.2	D04.39	D23.39	D48.5	D49.2
soft tissues	C03.9	C79.89	D00.03	D10.39	D37.09	D49.0
lower	C03.1	C79.89	D00.03	D10.39	D37.09	D49.0
upper	C03.0	C79.89	D00.03	D10.39	D37.09	D49.0
jejunum	C17.1	C78.4	D01.49	D13.39	D37.2	D49.0

	Malignant Primary	Malignant Secondary	Ca in situ	Benign	Uncertain Behavior	Unspecified Behavior
joint NEC — *see also Neoplasm, bone*	C41.9	C79.51	—	D16.9-●	D48.0	D49.2
acromioclavicular	C40.0-●	C79.51	—	D16.0-●	—	—
bursa or synovial membrane — *see Neoplasm, connective tissue*						
costovertebral	C41.3	C79.51	—	D16.7	D48.0	D49.2
sternocostal	C41.3	C79.51	—	D16.7	D48.0	D49.2
temporomandibular	C41.1	C79.51	—	D16.5-●	D48.0	D49.2
junction						
anorectal	C21.8	C78.5	D01.3	D12.9	D37.8	D49.0
cardioesophageal	C16.0	C78.89	D00.2	D13.1	D37.1	D49.0
esophagogastric	C16.0	C78.89	D00.2	D13.1	D37.1	D49.0
gastroesophageal	C16.0	C78.89	D00.2	D13.1	D37.1	D49.0
hard and soft palate	C05.9	C79.89	D00.00	D10.39	D37.09	D49.0
ileocecal	C18.0	C78.5	D01.0	D12.0	D37.4	D49.0
pelvirectal	C19	C78.5	D01.1	D12.7	D37.5	D49.0
pelviureteric	C65.-●	C79.0-●	D09.19	D30.1-●	D41.1-●	D49.59
rectosigmoid	C19	C78.5	D01.1	D12.7	D37.5	D49.0
squamocolumnar, of cervix	C53.8	C79.82	D06.7	D26.0	D39.0	D49.59
Kaposi's sarcoma — *see Kaposi's, sarcoma*						
kidney (parenchymal)	C64.-●	C79.0-●	D09.19	D30.0-●	D41.0-●	D49.51-●
calyx	C65.-●	C79.0-●	D09.19	D30.1-●	D41.1-●	D49.51-●
hilus	C65.-●	C79.0-●	D09.19	D30.1-●	D41.1-●	D49.51-●
pelvis	C65.-●	C79.0-●	D09.19	D30.1-●	D41.1-●	D49.51-●
knee NEC	C76.5-●	C79.89	D04.7-●	D36.7	D48.7	D49.89
labia (skin)	C51.9	C79.82	D07.1	D28.0	D39.8	D49.59
majora	C51.0	C79.82	D07.1	D28.0	D39.8	D49.59
minora	C51.1	C79.82	D07.1	D28.0	D39.8	D49.59
labial — *see also Neoplasm, lip*	C00.9	C79.89	D00.01	D10.0	D37.01	D49.0
sulcus (lower) (upper)	C06.1	C79.89	D00.02	D10.39	D37.09	D49.0
labium (skin)	C51.9	C79.82	D07.1	D28.0	D39.8	D49.59
majus	C51.0	C79.82	D07.1	D28.0	D39.8	D49.59
minus	C51.1	C79.82	D07.1	D28.0	D39.8	D49.59
lacrimal						
canaliculi	C69.5-●	C79.49	D09.2-●	D31.5-●	D48.7	D49.89
duct (nasal)	C69.5-●	C79.49	D09.2-●	D31.5-●	D48.7	D49.89
gland	C69.5-●	C79.49	D09.2-●	D31.5-●	D48.7	D49.89
punctum	C69.5-●	C79.49	D09.2-●	D31.5-●	D48.7	D49.89
sac	C69.5-●	C79.49	D09.2-●	D31.5-●	D48.7	D49.89
Langerhans, islands or islets	C25.4	C78.89	D01.7	D13.7	D37.8	D49.0
laryngopharynx	C13.9	C79.89	D00.08	D10.7	D37.05	D49.0

◀ New ◀ Revised ~~deleted~~ Deleted ● Use Additional Character(s)

TABLE OF NEOPLASMS

	Malignant Primary	Malignant Secondary	Ca in situ	Benign	Uncertain Behavior	Unspecified Behavior
larynx, laryngeal NEC	C32.9	C78.39	D02.0	D14.1	D38.0	D49.1
aryepiglottic fold	C32.1	C78.39	D02.0	D14.1	D38.0	D49.1
cartilage (arytenoid) (cricoid) (cuneiform) (thyroid)	C32.3	C78.39	D02.0	D14.1	D38.0	D49.1
commissure (anterior) (posterior)	C32.0	C78.39	D02.0	D14.1	D38.0	D49.1
extrinsic NEC	C32.1	C78.39	D02.0	D14.1	D38.0	D49.1
meaning hypopharynx	C13.9	C79.89	D00.08	D10.7	D37.05	D49.0
interarytenoid fold	C32.1	C78.39	D02.0	D14.1	D38.0	D49.1
intrinsic	C32.0	C78.39	D02.0	D14.1	D38.0	D49.1
overlapping lesion	C32.8	—	—	—	—	—
ventricular band	C32.1	C78.39	D02.0	D14.1	D38.0	D49.1
leg NEC	C76.5-•	C79.89	D04.7-•	D36.7	D48.7	D49.89
lens, crystalline	C69.4-•	C79.49	D09.2-•	D31.4-•	D48.7	D49.89
lid (lower) (upper)	C44.10-•	C79.2	D04.1-•	D23.1-•	D48.5	D49.2
basal cell carcinoma	C44.11-•	—	—	—	—	—
sebaceous cell	C44.13-•	—	—	—	—	—
specified type NEC	C44.19-•	—	—	—	—	—
squamous cell carcinoma	C44.12-•	—	—	—	—	—
ligament — *see also Neoplasm, connective tissue*						
broad	C57.1	C79.82	D07.39	D28.2	D39.8	D49.59
Mackenrodt's	C57.7	C79.82	D07.39	D28.7	D39.8	D49.59
non-uterine — *see Neoplasm, connective tissue*						
round	C57.2	C79.82	—	D28.2	D39.8	D49.59
sacro-uterine	C57.3	C79.82	—	D28.2	D39.8	D49.59
uterine	C57.3	C79.82	—	D28.2	D39.8	D49.59
utero-ovarian	C57.7	C79.82	D07.39	D28.2	D39.8	D49.59
uterosacral	C57.3	C79.82	—	D28.2	D39.8	D49.59
limb	C76.8	C79.89	D04.8	D36.7	D48.7	D49.89
lower	C76.5-•	C79.89	D04.7-•	D36.7	D48.7	D49.89
upper	C76.4-•	C79.89	D04.6-•	D36.7	D48.7	D49.89
limbus of cornea	C69.1-•	C79.49	D09.2-•	D31.1-•	D48.7	D49.89
lingual NEC — *see also Neoplasm, tongue*	C02.9	C79.89	D00.07	D10.1	D37.02	D49.0
lingula, lung	C34.1-•	C78.0-•	D02.2-•	D14.3-•	D38.1	D49.1
lip	C00.9	C79.89	D00.01	D10.0	D37.01	D49.0
buccal aspect — *see Neoplasm, lip, internal*						
commissure	C00.6	C79.89	D00.01	D10.0	D37.01	D49.0
external	C00.2	C79.89	D00.01	D10.0	D37.01	D49.0
lower	C00.1	C79.89	D00.01	D10.0	D37.01	D49.0
upper	C00.0	C79.89	D00.01	D10.0	D37.01	D49.0
frenulum — *see Neoplasm, lip, internal*						

	Malignant Primary	Malignant Secondary	Ca in situ	Benign	Uncertain Behavior	Unspecified Behavior
lip *(Continued)*						
inner aspect — *see Neoplasm, lip, internal*						
internal	C00.5	C79.89	D00.01	D10.0	D37.01	D49.0
lower	C00.4	C79.89	D00.01	D10.0	D37.01	D49.0
upper	C00.3	C79.89	D00.01	D10.0	D37.01	D49.0
lipstick area	C00.2	C79.89	D00.01	D10.0	D37.01	D49.0
lower	C00.1	C79.89	D00.01	D10.0	D37.01	D49.0
upper	C00.0	C79.89	D00.01	D10.0	D37.01	D49.0
lower	C00.1	C79.89	D00.01	D10.0	D37.01	D49.0
internal	C00.4	C79.89	D00.01	D10.0	D37.01	D49.0
mucosa — *see Neoplasm, lip, internal*						
oral aspect — *see Neoplasm, lip, internal*						
overlapping lesion	C00.8	—	—	—	—	—
with oral cavity or pharynx	C14.8	—	—	—	—	—
skin (commissure) (lower) (upper)	C44.00	C79.2	D04.0	D23.0	D48.5	D49.2
basal cell carcinoma	C44.01	—	—	—	—	—
specified type NEC	C44.09	—	—	—	—	—
squamous cell carcinoma	C44.02	—	—	—	—	—
upper	C00.0	C79.89	D00.01	D10.0	D37.01	D49.0
internal	C00.3	C79.89	D00.01	D10.0	D37.01	D49.0
vermilion border	C00.2	C79.89	D00.01	D10.0	D37.01	D49.0
lower	C00.1	C79.89	D00.01	D10.0	D37.01	D49.0
upper	C00.0	C79.89	D00.01	D10.0	D37.01	D49.0
lipomatous — *see Lipoma, by site*						
liver — *see also Index to disease, by histology*	C22.9	C78.7	D01.5	D13.4	D37.6	D49.0
primary	C22.8	C78.7	D01.5	D13.4	D37.6	D49.0
lumbosacral plexus	C47.5	C79.89	—	D36.16	D48.2	D49.2
lung	C34.9-•	C78.0-•	D02.2-•	D14.3-•	D38.1	D49.1
azygos lobe	C34.1-•	C78.0-•	D02.2-•	D14.3-•	D38.1	D49.1
carina	C34.0-•	C78.0-•	D02.2-•	D14.3-•	D38.1	D49.1
hilus	C34.0-•	C78.0-•	D02.2-•	D14.3-•	D38.1	D49.1
linqula	C34.1-•	C78.0-•	D02.2-•	D14.3-•	D38.1	D49.1
lobe NEC	C34.9-•	C78.0-•	D02.2-•	D14.3-•	D38.1	D49.1
lower lobe	C34.3-•	C78.0-•	D02.2-•	D14.3-•	D38.1	D49.1
main bronchus	C34.0-•	C78.0-•	D02.2-•	D14.3-•	D38.1	D49.1
mesothelioma — *see Mesothelioma*						
middle lobe	C34.2	C78.0-•	D02.21	D14.31	D38.1	D49.1
overlapping lesion	C34.8-•	—	—	—	—	—
upper lobe	C34.1-•	C78.0-•	D02.2-•	D14.3-•	D38.1	D49.1

◀ New ◀ Revised ~~deleted~~ Deleted • Use Additional Character(s)

	Malignant Primary	Malignant Secondary	Ca in situ	Benign	Uncertain Behavior	Unspecified Behavior
lymph, lymphatic channel NEC	C49.9	C79.89	—	D21.9	D48.1	D49.2
gland (secondary)	—	C77.9	—	D36.0	D48.7	D49.89
abdominal	—	C77.2	—	D36.0	D48.7	D49.89
aortic	—	C77.2	—	D36.0	D48.7	D49.89
arm	—	C77.3	—	D36.0	D48.7	D49.89
auricular (anterior) (posterior)	—	C77.0	—	D36.0	D48.7	D49.89
axilla, axillary	—	C77.3	—	D36.0	D48.7	D49.89
brachial	—	C77.3	—	D36.0	D48.7	D49.89
bronchial	—	C77.1	—	D36.0	D48.7	D49.89
bronchopulmonary	—	C77.1	—	D36.0	D48.7	D49.89
celiac	—	C77.2	—	D36.0	D48.7	D49.89
cervical	—	C77.0	—	D36.0	D48.7	D49.89
cervicofacial	—	C77.0	—	D36.0	D48.7	D49.89
Cloquet	—	C77.4	—	D36.0	D48.7	D49.89
colic	—	C77.2	—	D36.0	D48.7	D49.89
common duct	—	C77.2	—	D36.0	D48.7	D49.89
cubital	—	C77.3	—	D36.0	D48.7	D49.89
diaphragmatic	—	C77.1	—	D36.0	D48.7	D49.89
epigastric, inferior	—	C77.1	—	D36.0	D48.7	D49.89
epitrochlear	—	C77.3	—	D36.0	D48.7	D49.89
esophageal	—	C77.1	—	D36.0	D48.7	D49.89
face	—	C77.0	—	D36.0	D48.7	D49.89
femoral	—	C77.4	—	D36.0	D48.7	D49.89
gastric	—	C77.2	—	D36.0	D48.7	D49.89
groin	—	C77.4	—	D36.0	D48.7	D49.89
head	—	C77.0	—	D36.0	D48.7	D49.89
hepatic	—	C77.2	—	D36.0	D48.7	D49.89
hilar (pulmonary)	—	C77.1	—	D36.0	D48.7	D49.89
splenic	—	C77.2	—	D36.0	D48.7	D49.89
hypogastric	—	C77.5	—	D36.0	D48.7	D49.89
ileocolic	—	C77.2	—	D36.0	D48.7	D49.89
iliac	—	C77.5	—	D36.0	D48.7	D49.89
infraclavicular	—	C77.3	—	D36.0	D48.7	D49.89
inguina, inguinal	—	C77.4	—	D36.0	D48.7	D49.89
innominate	—	C77.1	—	D36.0	D48.7	D49.89
intercostal	—	C77.1	—	D36.0	D48.7	D49.89
intestinal	—	C77.2	—	D36.0	D48.7	D49.89
intrabdominal	—	C77.2	—	D36.0	D48.7	D49.89
intrapelvic	—	C77.5	—	D36.0	D48.7	D49.89
intrathoracic	—	C77.1	—	D36.0	D48.7	D49.89
jugular	—	C77.0	—	D36.0	D48.7	D49.89
leg	—	C77.4	—	D36.0	D48.7	D49.89
limb						
lower	—	C77.4	—	D36.0	D48.7	D49.89
upper	—	C77.3	—	D36.0	D48.7	D49.89

	Malignant Primary	Malignant Secondary	Ca in situ	Benign	Uncertain Behavior	Unspecified Behavior
lymph, lymphatic channel NEC (Continued)						
gland (Continued)						
lower limb	—	C77.4	—	D36.0	D48.7	D49.89
lumbar	—	C77.2	—	D36.0	D48.7	D49.89
mandibular	—	C77.0	—	D36.0	D48.7	D49.89
mediastinal	—	C77.1	—	D36.0	D48.7	D49.89
mesenteric (inferior) (superior)	—	C77.2	—	D36.0	D48.7	D49.89
midcolic	—	C77.2	—	D36.0	D48.7	D49.89
multiple sites in categories C77.0 - C77.5	—	C77.8	—	D36.0	D48.7	D49.89
neck	—	C77.0	—	D36.0	D48.7	D49.89
obturator	—	C77.5	—	D36.0	D48.7	D49.89
occipital	—	C77.0	—	D36.0	D48.7	D49.89
pancreatic	—	C77.2	—	D36.0	D48.7	D49.89
para-aortic	—	C77.2	—	D36.0	D48.7	D49.89
paracervical	—	C77.5	—	D36.0	D48.7	D49.89
parametrial	—	C77.5	—	D36.0	D48.7	D49.89
parasternal	—	C77.1	—	D36.0	D48.7	D49.89
parotid	—	C77.0	—	D36.0	D48.7	D49.89
pectoral	—	C77.3	—	D36.0	D48.7	D49.89
pelvic	—	C77.5	—	D36.0	D48.7	D49.89
peri-aortic	—	C77.2	—	D36.0	D48.7	D49.89
peripancreatic	—	C77.2	—	D36.0	D48.7	D49.89
popliteal	—	C77.4	—	D36.0	D48.7	D49.89
porta hepatis	—	C77.2	—	D36.0	D48.7	D49.89
portal	—	C77.2	—	D36.0	D48.7	D49.89
preauricular	—	C77.0	—	D36.0	D48.7	D49.89
prelaryngeal	—	C77.0	—	D36.0	D48.7	D49.89
presymphysial	—	C77.5	—	D36.0	D48.7	D49.89
pretracheal	—	C77.0	—	D36.0	D48.7	D49.89
primary (any site) NEC	C96.9	—	—	—	—	—
pulmonary (hiler)	—	C77.1	—	D36.0	D48.7	D49.89
pyloric	—	C77.2	—	D36.0	D48.7	D49.89
retroperitoneal	—	C77.2	—	D36.0	D48.7	D49.89
retropharyngeal	—	C77.0	—	D36.0	D48.7	D49.89
Rosenmuller's	—	C77.4	—	D36.0	D48.7	D49.89
sacral	—	C77.5	—	D36.0	D48.7	D49.89
scalene	—	C77.0	—	D36.0	D48.7	D49.89
site NEC	—	C77.9	—	D36.0	D48.7	D49.89
splenic (hilar)	—	C77.2	—	D36.0	D48.7	D49.89
subclavicular	—	C77.3	—	D36.0	D48.7	D49.89
subinguinal	—	C77.4	—	D36.0	D48.7	D49.89

TABLE OF NEOPLASMS

TABLE OF NEOPLASMS

	Malignant Primary	Malignant Secondary	Ca in situ	Benign	Uncertain Behavior	Unspecified Behavior
lymph, lymphatic channel NEC *(Continued)*						
gland *(Continued)*						
sublingual	—	C77.0	—	D36.0	D48.7	D49.89
submandibular	—	C77.0	—	D36.0	D48.7	D49.89
submaxillary	—	C77.0	—	D36.0	D48.7	D49.89
submental	—	C77.0	—	D36.0	D48.7	D49.89
subscapular	—	C77.3	—	D36.0	D48.7	D49.89
supraclavicular	—	C77.0	—	D36.0	D48.7	D49.89
thoracic	—	C77.1	—	D36.0	D48.7	D49.89
tibial	—	C77.4	—	D36.0	D48.7	D49.89
tracheal	—	C77.1	—	D36.0	D48.7	D49.89
tracheobronchial	—	C77.1	—	D36.0	D48.7	D49.89
upper limb	—	C77.3	—	D36.0	D48.7	D49.89
Virchow's	—	C77.0	—	D36.0	D48.7	D49.89
node — *see also Neoplasm, lymph gland*						
primary NEC	C96.9	—	—	—	—	—
vessel — *see also Neoplasm, connective tissue*	C49.9	C79.89	—	D21.9	D48.1	D49.2
Mackenrodt's ligament	C57.7	C79.82	D07.39	D28.7	D39.8	D49.59
malar	C41.0	C79.51	—	D16.4-●	D48.0	D49.2
region — *see Neoplasm, cheek*						
mammary gland — *see Neoplasm, breast*						
mandible	C41.1	C79.51	—	D16.5-●	D48.0	D49.2
alveolar						
mucosa (carcinoma)	C03.1	C79.89	D00.03	D10.39	D37.09	D49.0
ridge or process	C41.1	C79.51	—	D16.5-●	D48.0	D49.2
marrow (bone) NEC	C96.9	C79.52	—	—	D47.9	D49.89
mastectomy site (skin) — *see also Neoplasm, breast, skin*	C44.501	C79.2	—	—	—	—
specified as breast tissue	C50.8-●	C79.81	—	—	—	—
mastoid (air cells) (antrum) (cavity)	C30.1	C78.39	D02.3	D14.0	D38.5	D49.1
bone or process	C41.0	C79.51	—	D16.4-●	D48.0	D49.2
maxilla, maxillary (superior)	C41.0	C79.51	—	D16.4-●	D48.0	D49.2
alveolar						
mucosa	C03.0	C79.89	D00.03	D10.39	D37.09	D49.0
ridge or process (carcinoma)	C41.0	C79.51	—	D16.4-●	D48.0	D49.2
antrum	C31.0	C78.39	D02.3	D14.0	D38.5	D49.1
carcinoma	C03.0	C79.51	—	—	—	—
inferior — *see Neoplasm, mandible*						
sinus	C31.0	C78.39	D02.3	D14.0	D38.5	D49.1
meatus external (ear) — *see also Neoplasm, skin, ear*	C44.20-●	C79.2	D04.2-●	D23.2-●	D48.5	D49.2
Meckel diverticulum, malignant	C17.3	C78.4	D01.49	D13.39	D37.2	D49.0
mediastinum, mediastinal	C38.3	C78.1	—	D15.2	D38.3	D49.89
anterior	C38.1	C78.1	—	D15.2	D38.3	D49.89
posterior	C38.2	C78.1	—	D15.2	D38.3	D49.89
medulla						
adrenal	C74.1-●	C79.7-●	D09.3	D35.0-●	D44.1-●	D49.7
oblongata	C71.7	C79.31	—	D33.1	D43.1	D49.6
meibomian gland	C44.10-●	C79.2	D04.1-●	D23.1-●	D48.5	D49.2
basal cell carcinoma	C44.11-●	—	—	—	—	—
sebaceous cell	C44.13-●	—	—	—	—	—
specified type NEC	C44.19-●	—	—	—	—	—
squamous cell carcinoma	C44.12-●	—	—	—	—	—
melanoma — *see Melanoma*						
meninges	C70.9	C79.49	—	D32.9	D42.9	D49.7
brain	C70.0	C79.32	—	D32.0	D42.0	D49.7
cerebral	C70.0	C79.32	—	D32.0	D42.0	D49.7
crainial	C70.0	C79.32	—	D32.0	D42.0	D49.7
intracranial	C70.0	C79.32	—	D32.0	D42.0	D49.7
spinal (cord)	C70.1	C79.49	—	D32.1	D42.1	D49.7
meniscus, knee joint (lateral) (medial)	C40.2-●	C79.51	—	D16.2-●	D48.0	D49.2
Merkel cell — *see Carcinoma, Merkel cell*						
mesentery, mesenteric	C48.1	C78.6	—	D20.1	D48.4	D49.0
mesoappendix	C48.1	C78.6	—	D20.1	D48.4	D49.0
mesocolon	C48.1	C78.6	—	D20.1	D48.4	D49.0
mesopharynx — *see Neoplasm, oropharynx*						
mesosalpinx	C57.1	C79.82	D07.39	D28.2	D39.8	D49.59
mesothelial tissue — *see Mesothelioma*						
mesothelioma — *see Mesothelioma*						
mesovarium	C57.1	C79.82	D07.39	D28.2	D39.8	D49.59
metacarpus (any bone)	C40.1-●	C79.51	—	D16.1-●	—	—
metastatic NEC — *see also Neoplasm, by site, secondary*	—	C79.9	—	—	—	—
metatarsus (any bone)	C40.3-●	C79.51	—	D16.3-●	—	—
midbrain	C71.7	C79.31	—	D33.1	D43.1	D49.6
milk duct — *see Neoplasm, breast*						
mons						
pubis	C51.9	C79.82	D07.1	D28.0	D39.8	D49.59
veneris	C51.9	C79.82	D07.1	D28.0	D39.8	D49.59

TABLE OF NEOPLASMS

◀ New ◀◀ Revised ~~deleted~~ Deleted ● Use Additional Character(s)

	Malignant Primary	Malignant Secondary	Ca in situ	Benign	Uncertain Behavior	Unspecified Behavior
motor tract	C72.9	C79.49	—	D33.9	D43.9	D49.7
brain	C71.9	C79.31	—	D33.2	D43.2	D49.6
cauda equina	C72.1	C79.49	—	D33.4	D43.4	D49.7
spinal	C72.0	C79.49	—	D33.4	D43.4	D49.7
mouth	C06.9	C79.89	D00.00	D10.30	D37.09	D49.0
book-leaf	C06.89	C79.89	—	—	—	—
floor	C04.9	C79.89	D00.06	D10.2	D37.09	D49.0
anterior portion	C04.0	C79.89	D00.06	D10.2	D37.09	D49.0
lateral portion	C04.1	C79.89	D00.06	D10.2	D37.09	D49.0
overlapping lesion	C04.8					
overlapping NEC	C06.80	—	—	—	—	—
roof	C05.9	C79.89	D00.00	D10.39	D37.09	D49.0
specified part NEC	C06.89	C79.89	D00.00	D10.39	D37.09	D49.0
vestibule	C06.1	C79.89	D00.00	D10.39	D37.09	D49.0
mucosa						
alveolar (ridge or process)	C03.9	C79.89	D00.03	D10.39	D37.09	D49.0
lower	C03.1	C79.89	D00.03	D10.39	D37.09	D49.0
upper	C03.0	C79.89	D00.03	D10.39	D37.09	D49.0
buccal	C06.0	C79.89	D00.02	D10.39	D37.09	D49.0
cheek	C06.0	C79.89	D00.02	D10.39	D37.09	D49.0
lip — see Neoplasm, lip, internal						
nasal	C30.0	C78.39	D02.3	D14.0	D38.5	D49.1
oral	C06.0	C79.89	D00.02	D10.39	D37.09	D49.0
Mullerian duct						
female	C57.7	C79.82	D07.39	D28.7	D39.8	D49.59
male	C63.7	C79.82	D07.69	D29.8	D40.8	D49.59
muscle — see also Neoplasm, connective tissue						
extraocular	C69.6-●	C79.49	D09.2-●	D31.6-●	D48.7	D49.89
myocardium	C38.0	C79.89	—	D15.1	D48.7	D49.89
myometrium	C54.2	C79.82	D07.0	D26.1	D39.0	D49.59
myopericardium	C38.0	C79.89	—	D15.1	D48.7	D49.89
nabothian gland (follicle)	C53.0	C79.82	D06.0	D26.0	D39.0	D49.59
nail — see also Neoplasm, skin, limb	C44.90	C79.2	D04.9	D23.9	D48.5	D49.2
finger — see also Neoplasm, skin, limb, upper	C44.60-●	C79.2	D04.6-●	D23.6-●	D48.5	D49.2
toe — see also Neoplasm, skin, limb, lower	C44.70-●	C79.2	D04.7-●	D23.7-●	D48.5	D49.2
nares, naris (anterior) (posterior)	C30.0	C78.39	D02.3	D14.0	D38.5	D49.1
nasal — see Neoplasm, nose						
nasolabial groove — see also Neoplasm, skin, face	C44.309	C79.2	D04.39	D23.39	D48.5	D49.2
nasolacrimal duct	C69.5-●	C79.49	D09.2-●	D31.5-●	D48.7	D49.89

	Malignant Primary	Malignant Secondary	Ca in situ	Benign	Uncertain Behavior	Unspecified Behavior
nasopharynx, nasopharyngeal	C11.9	C79.89	D00.08	D10.6	D37.05	D49.0
floor	C11.3	C79.89	D00.08	D10.6	D37.05	D49.0
overlapping lesion	C11.8	—	—	—	—	—
roof	C11.0	C79.89	D00.08	D10.6	D37.05	D49.0
wall	C11.9	C79.89	D00.08	D10.6	D37.05	D49.0
anterior	C11.3	C79.89	D00.08	D10.6	D37.05	D49.0
lateral	C11.2	C79.89	D00.08	D10.6	D37.05	D49.0
posterior	C11.1	C79.89	D00.08	D10.6	D37.05	D49.0
superior	C11.0	C79.89	D00.08	D10.6	D37.05	D49.0
nates — see also Neoplasm, skin, trunk	C44.509	C79.2	D04.5	D23.5	D48.5	D49.2
neck NEC	C76.0	C79.89	D09.8	D36.7	D48.7	D49.89
skin	C44.40	—	—	—	—	—
basal cell carcinoma	C44.41					
specified type NEC	C44.49	—	—	—	—	—
squamous cell carcinoma	C44.42	—	—	—	—	—
nerve (ganglion)	C47.9	C79.89	—	D36.10	D48.2	D49.2
abducens	C72.59	C79.49	—	D33.3	D43.3	D49.7
accessory (spinal)	C72.59	C79.49	—	D33.3	D43.3	D49.7
acoustic	C72.4-●	C79.49	—	D33.3	D43.3	D49.7
auditory	C72.4-●	C79.49	—	D33.3	D43.3	D49.7
autonomic NEC — see also Neoplasm, nerve, peripheral	C47.9	C79.89	—	D36.10	D48.2	D49.2
brachial	C47.1-●	C79.89	—	D36.12	D48.2	D49.2
cranial	C72.50	C79.49	—	D33.3	D43.3	D49.7
specified NEC	C72.59	C79.49	—	D33.3	D43.3	D49.7
facial	C72.59	C79.49	—	D33.3	D43.3	D49.7
femoral	C47.2-●	C79.89	—	D36.13	D48.2	D49.2
ganglion NEC — see also Neoplasm, nerve, peripheral	C47.9	C79.89	—	D36.10	D48.2	D49.2
glossopharyngeal	C72.59	C79.49	—	D33.3	D43.3	D49.7
hypoglossal	C72.59	C79.49	—	D33.3	D43.3	D49.7
intercostal	C47.3	C79.89	—	D36.14	D48.2	D49.2
lumbar	C47.6	C79.89	—	D36.17	D48.2	D49.2
median	C47.1-●	C79.89	—	D36.12	D48.2	D49.2
obturator	C47.2-●	C79.89	—	D36.13	D48.2	D49.2
oculomotor	C72.59	C79.49	—	D33.3	D43.3	D49.7
olfactory	C47.2-●	C79.49	—	D33.3	D43.3	D49.7
optic	C72.3-●	C79.49	—	D33.3	D43.3	D49.7
parasympathetic NEC	C47.9	C79.89	—	D36.10	D48.2	D49.2
peripheral NEC	C47.9	C79.89	—	D36.10	D48.2	D49.2
abdomen	C47.4	C79.89	—	D36.15	D48.2	D49.2
abdominal wall	C47.4	C79.89	—	D36.15	D48.2	D49.2

TABLE OF NEOPLASMS

TABLE OF NEOPLASMS

nerve (Continued)	Malignant Primary	Malignant Secondary	Ca in situ	Benign	Uncertain Behavior	Unspecified Behavior
peripheral NEC (Continued)						
ankle	C47.2-●	C79.89	—	D36.13	D48.2	D49.2
antecubital fossa or space	C47.1-●	C79.89	—	D36.12	D48.2	D49.2
arm	C47.1-●	C79.89	—	D36.12	D48.2	D49.2
auricle (ear)	C47.0	C79.89	—	D36.11	D48.2	D49.2
axilla	C47.3	C79.89	—	D36.12	D48.2	D49.2
back	C47.6	C79.89	—	D36.17	D48.2	D49.2
buttock	C47.5	C79.89	—	D36.16	D48.2	D49.2
calf	C47.2-●	C79.89	—	D36.13	D48.2	D49.2
cervical region	C47.0	C79.89	—	D36.11	D48.2	D49.2
cheek	C47.0	C79.89	—	D36.11	D48.2	D49.2
chest (wall)	C47.3	C79.89	—	D36.14	D48.2	D49.2
chin	C47.0	C79.89	—	D36.11	D48.2	D49.2
ear (external)	C47.0	C79.89	—	D36.11	D48.2	D49.2
elbow	C47.1-●	C79.89	—	D36.12	D48.2	D49.2
extrarectal	C47.5	C79.89	—	D36.16	D48.2	D49.2
extremity	C47.9	C79.89	—	D36.10	D48.2	D49.2
lower	C47.2-●	C79.89	—	D36.13	D48.2	D49.2
upper	C47.1-●	C79.89	—	D36.12	D48.2	D49.2
eyelid	C47.0	C79.89	—	D36.11	D48.2	D49.2
face	C47.0	C79.89	—	D36.11	D48.2	D49.2
finger	C47.1-●	C79.89	—	D36.12	D48.2	D49.2
flank	C47.6	C79.89	—	D36.17	D48.2	D49.2
foot	C47.2-●	C79.89	—	D36.13	D48.2	D49.2
forearm	C47.1-●	C79.89	—	D36.12	D48.2	D49.2
forehead	C47.0	C79.89	—	D36.11	D48.2	D49.2
gluteal region	C47.5	C79.89	—	D36.16	D48.2	D49.2
groin	C47.5	C79.89	—	D36.16	D48.2	D49.2
hand	C47.1-●	C79.89	—	D36.12	D48.2	D49.2
head	C47.0	C79.89	—	D36.11	D48.2	D49.2
heel	C47.2-●	C79.89	—	D36.13	D48.2	D49.2
hip	C47.2-●	C79.89	—	D36.13	D48.2	D49.2
infraclavicular region	C47.3	C79.89	—	D36.14	D48.2	D49.2
inguinal (canal) (region)	C47.5	C79.89	—	D36.16	D48.2	D49.2
intrathoracic	C47.3	C79.89	—	D36.14	D48.2	D49.2
ischiorectal fossa	C47.5	C79.89	—	D36.16	D48.2	D49.2
knee	C47.2-●	C79.89	—	D36.13	D48.2	D49.2
leg	C47.2-●	C79.89	—	D36.13	D48.2	D49.2
limb NEC	C47.9	C79.89	—	D36.10	D48.2	D49.2
lower	C47.2-●	C79.89	—	D36.13	D48.2	D49.2
upper	C47.1-●	C79.89	—	D36.12	D48.2	D49.2
nates	C47.5	C79.89	—	D36.16	D48.2	D49.2
neck	C47.0	C79.89	—	D36.11	D48.2	D49.2

nerve (Continued)	Malignant Primary	Malignant Secondary	Ca in situ	Benign	Uncertain Behavior	Unspecified Behavior
peripheral NEC (Continued)						
orbit	C69.6-●	C79.49	—	D31.6-●	D48.7	D49.2
pararectal	C47.5	C79.89	—	D36.16	D48.2	D49.2
paraurethral	C47.5	C79.89	—	D36.16	D48.2	D49.2
paravaginal	C47.5	C79.89	—	D36.16	D48.2	D49.2
pelvis (floor)	C47.5	C79.89	—	D36.16	D48.2	D49.2
pelvoabdominal	C47.8	C79.89	—	D36.17	D48.2	D49.2
perineum	C47.5	C79.89	—	D36.16	D48.2	D49.2
perirectal (tissue)	C47.5	C79.89	—	D36.16	D48.2	D49.2
periurethral (tissue)	C47.5	C79.89	—	D36.16	D48.2	D49.2
popliteal fossa or space	C47.2-●	C79.89	—	D36.13	D48.2	D49.2
presacral	C47.5	C79.89	—	D36.16	D48.2	D49.2
pterygoid fossa	C47.0	C79.89	—	D36.11	D48.2	D49.2
rectovaginal septum or wall	C47.5	C79.89	—	D36.16	D48.2	D49.2
rectovesical	C47.5	C79.89	—	D36.16	D48.2	D49.2
sacrococcygeal region	C47.5	C79.89	—	D36.16	D48.2	D49.2
scalp	C47.0	C79.89	—	D36.11	D48.2	D49.2
scapular region	C47.3	C79.89	—	D36.14	D48.2	D49.2
shoulder	C47.1-●	C79.89	—	D36.12	D48.2	D49.2
submental	C47.0	C79.89	—	D36.11	D48.2	D49.2
supraclavicular region	C47.0	C79.89	—	D36.11	D48.2	D49.2
temple	C47.0	C79.89	—	D36.11	D48.2	D49.2
temporal region	C47.0	C79.89	—	D36.11	D48.2	D49.2
thigh	C47.2-●	C79.89	—	D36.13	D48.2	D49.2
thoracic (duct) (wall)	C47.3	C79.89	—	D36.14	D48.2	D49.2
thorax	C47.3	C79.89	—	D36.14	D48.2	D49.2
thumb	C47.1-●	C79.89	—	D36.12	D48.2	D49.2
toe	C47.2-●	C79.89	—	D36.13	D48.2	D49.2
trunk	C47.6	C79.89	—	D36.17	D48.2	D49.2
umbilicus	C47.4	C79.89	—	D36.15	D48.2	D49.2
vesicorectal	C47.5	C79.89	—	D36.16	D48.2	D49.2
wrist	C47.1-●	C79.89	—	D36.12	D48.2	D49.2
radial	C47.1-●	C79.89	—	D36.12	D48.2	D49.2
sacral	C47.5	C79.89	—	D36.16	D48.2	D49.2
sciatic	C47.2-●	C79.89	—	D36.13	D48.2	D49.2
spinal NEC	C47.9	C79.89	—	D36.10	D48.2	D49.2
accessory	C72.59	C79.49	—	D33.3	D43.3	D49.7
sympathetic NEC — see also Neoplasm, nerve, peripheral	C47.9	C79.89	—	D36.10	D48.2	D49.2
trigeminal	C72.59	C79.49	—	D33.3	D43.3	D49.7
trochlear	C72.59	C79.49	—	D33.3	D43.3	D49.7
ulnar	C47.1-●	C79.89	—	D36.12	D48.2	D49.2
vagus	C72.59	C79.49	—	D33.3	D43.3	D49.7

◄ New   ◀ Revised   ~~deleted~~ Deleted   ● Use Additional Character(s)

	Malignant Primary	Malignant Secondary	Ca in situ	Benign	Uncertain Behavior	Unspecified Behavior
nervous system (central)	C72.9	C79.40	—	D33.9	D43.9	D49.7
autonomic — see Neoplasm, nerve, peripheral						
parasympathetic — see Neoplasm, nerve, peripheral						
specified site NEC	—	C79.49	—	D33.7	D43.8	—
sympathetic — see Neoplasm, nerve, peripheral						
nevus — see Nevus						
nipple	C50.0-●	C79.81	D05.-	D24.-●	—	—
nose, nasal	C76.0	C79.89	D09.8	D36.7	D48.7	D49.89
ala (external) (nasi) — see also Neoplasm, nose, skin	C44.301	C79.2	D04.39	D23.39	D48.5	D49.2
bone	C41.0	C79.51	—	D16.4-●	D48.0	D49.2
cartilage	C30.0	C78.39	D02.3	D14.0	D38.5	D49.1
cavity	C30.0	C78.39	D02.3	D14.0	D38.5	D49.1
choana	C11.3	C79.89	D00.08	D10.6	D37.05	D49.0
external (skin) — see also Neoplasm, nose, skin	C44.301	C79.2	D04.39	D23.39	D48.5	D49.2
fossa	C30.0	C78.39	D02.3	D14.0	D38.5	D49.1
internal	C30.0	C78.39	D02.3	D14.0	D38.5	D49.1
mucosa	C30.0	C78.39	D02.3	D14.0	D38.5	D49.1
septum	C30.0	C78.39	D02.3	D14.0	D38.5	D49.1
posterior margin	C11.3	C79.89	D00.08	D10.6	D37.05	D49.0
sinus — see Neoplasm, sinus						
skin	C44.301	C79.2	D04.39	D23.39	D48.5	D49.2
basal cell carcinoma	C44.311	—	—	—	—	—
specified type NEC	C44.391	—	—	—	—	—
squamous cell carcinoma	C44.321	—	—	—	—	—
turbinate (mucosa)	C30.0	C78.39	D02.3	D14.0	D38.5	D49.1
bone	C41.0	C79.51	—	D16.4-●	D48.0	D49.2
vestibule	C30.0	C78.39	D02.3	D14.0	D38.5	D49.1
nostril	C30.0	C78.39	D02.3	D14.0	D38.5	D49.1
nucleus pulposus	C41.2	C79.51	—	D16.6	D48.0	D49.2
occipital						
bone	C41.0	C79.51	—	D16.4-●	D48.0	D49.2
lobe or pole, brain	C71.4	C79.31		D33.0	D43.0	D49.6
odontogenic — see Neoplasm, jaw bone						
olfactory nerve or bulb	C72.2-●	C79.49	—	D33.3	D43.3	D49.7
olive (brain)	C71.7	C79.31	—	D33.1	D43.1	D49.6
omentum	C48.1	C78.6	—	D20.1	D48.4	D49.0
operculum (brain)	C71.0	C79.31		D33.0	D43.0	D49.6
optic nerve, chiasm, or tract	C72.3-●	C79.49	—	D33.3	D43.3	D49.7

	Malignant Primary	Malignant Secondary	Ca in situ	Benign	Uncertain Behavior	Unspecified Behavior
oral (cavity)	C06.9	C79.89	D00.00	D10.30	D37.09	D49.0
ill-defined	C14.8	C79.89	D00.00	D10.30	D37.09	D49.0
mucosa	C06.0	C79.89	D00.02	D10.39	D37.09	D49.0
orbit	C69.6-●	C79.49	D09.2-●	D31.6-●	D48.7	D49.89
autonomic nerve	C69.6-●	C79.49	—	D31.6-●	D48.7	D49.2
bone	C41.0	C79.51	—	D16.4-●	D48.0	D49.2
eye	C69.6-●	C79.49	D09.2-●	D31.6-●	D48.7	D49.89
peripheral nerves	C69.6-●	C79.49	—	D31.6-●	D48.7	D49.2
soft parts	C69.6-●	C79.49	D09.2-●	D31.6-●	D48.7	D49.89
organ of Zuckerkandl	C75.5	C79.89	—	D35.6	D44.7	D49.7
oropharynx	C10.9	C79.89	D00.08	D10.5	D37.05	D49.0
branchial cleft (vestige)	C10.4	C79.89	D00.08	D10.5	D37.05	D49.0
junctional region	C10.8	C79.89	D00.08	D10.5	D37.05	D49.0
lateral wall	C10.2	C79.89	D00.08	D10.5	D37.05	D49.0
overlapping lesion	C10.8	—	—	—	—	—
pillars or fauces	C09.1	C79.89	D00.08	D10.5	D37.05	D49.0
posterior wall	C10.3	C79.89	D00.08	D10.5	D37.05	D49.0
vallecula	C10.0	C79.89	D00.08	D10.5	D37.05	D49.0
os						
external	C53.1	C79.82	D06.1	D26.0	D39.0	D49.59
internal	C53.0	C79.82	D06.0	D26.0	D39.0	D49.59
ovary	C56.-●	C79.6-●	D07.39	D27.-●	D39.1-●	D49.59
oviduct	C57.0-●	C79.82	D07.39	D28.2	D39.8	D49.59
palate	C05.9	C79.89	D00.00	D10.39	D37.09	D49.0
hard	C05.0	C79.89	D00.05	D10.39	D37.09	D49.0
junction of hard and soft palate	C05.9	C79.89	D00.00	D10.39	D37.09	D49.0
overlapping lesions	C05.8	—	—	—	—	—
soft	C05.1	C79.89	D00.04	D10.39	D37.09	D49.0
nasopharyngeal surface	C11.3	C79.89	D00.08	D10.6	D37.05	D49.0
posterior surface	C11.3	C79.89	D00.08	D10.6	D37.05	D49.0
superior surface	C11.3	C79.89	D00.08	D10.6	D37.05	D49.0
palatoglossal arch	C09.1	C79.89	D00.00	D10.5	D37.09	D49.0
palatopharyngeal arch	C09.1	C79.89	D00.00	D10.5	D37.09	D49.0
pallium	C71.0	C79.31	—	D33.0	D43.0	D49.6
palpebra	C44.10-●	C79.2	D04.1-●	D23.1-●	D48.5	D49.2
basal cell carcinoma	C44.11-●	—	—	—	—	—
sebaceous cell	C44.13-●	—	—	—	—	—
specified type NEC	C44.19-●	—	—	—	—	—
squamous cell carcinoma	C44.12-●	—	—	—	—	—
pancreas	C25.9	C78.89	D01.7	D13.6	D37.8	D49.0
body	C25.1	C78.89	D01.7	D13.6	D37.8	D49.0
duct (of Santorini) (of Wirsung)	C25.3	C78.89	D01.7	D13.6	D37.8	D49.0
ectopic tissue	C25.7	C78.89	—	D13.6	D37.8	D49.0
head	C25.0	C78.89	D01.7	D13.6	D37.8	D49.0

◀ New ◀▮ Revised ~~deleted~~ Deleted ● Use Additional Character(s)

TABLE OF NEOPLASMS

	Malignant Primary	Malignant Secondary	Ca in situ	Benign	Uncertain Behavior	Unspecified Behavior
pancreas *(Continued)*						
islet cells	C25.4	C78.89	D01.7	D13.7	D37.8	D49.0
neck	C25.7	C78.89	D01.7	D13.6	D37.8	D49.0
overlapping lesion	C25.8	—				
tail	C25.2	C78.89	D01.7	D13.6	D37.8	D49.0
para-aortic body	C75.5	C79.89	—	D35.6	D44.7	D49.7
paraganglion NEC	C75.5	C79.89	—	D35.6	D44.7	D49.7
parametrium	C57.3	C79.82		D28.2	D39.8	D49.59
paranephric	C48.0	C78.6		D20.0	D48.3	D49.0
pararectal	C76.3	C79.89		D36.7	D48.7	D49.89
parasagittal (region)	C76.0	C79.89	D09.8	D36.7	D48.7	D49.89
parasellar	C72.9	C79.49		D33.9	D43.8	D49.7
parathyroid (gland)	C75.0	C79.89	D09.3	D35.1	D44.2	D49.7
paraurethral	C76.3	C79.89		D36.7	D48.7	D49.89
gland	C68.1	C79.19	D09.19	D30.8	D41.8	D49.59
paravaginal	C76.3	C79.89		D36.7	D48.7	D49.89
parenchyma, kidney	C64.-●	C79.0-●	D09.19	D30.0-●	D41.0-●	D49.51-●
parietal						
bone	C41.0	C79.51	—	D16.4-●	D48.0	D49.2
lobe, brain	C71.3	C79.31		D33.0	D43.0	D49.6
paroophoron	C57.1	C79.82	D07.39	D28.2	D39.8	D49.59
parotid (duct) (gland)	C07	C79.89	D00.00	D11.0	D37.030	D49.0
parovarium	C57.1	C79.82	D07.39	D28.2	D39.8	D49.59
patella	C40.20	C79.51		—	—	—
peduncle, cerebral	C71.7	C79.31	—	D33.1	D43.1	D49.6
pelvirectal junction	C19	C78.5	D01.1	D12.7	D37.5	D49.0
pelvis, pelvic	C76.3	C79.89	D09.8	D36.7	D48.7	D49.89
bone	C41.4	C79.51	—	D16.8	D48.0	D49.2
floor	C76.3	C79.89	D09.8	D36.7	D48.7	D49.89
renal	C65.-●	C79.0-●	D09.19	D30.1-●	D41.1-●	D49.51-●
viscera	C76.3	C79.89	D09.8	D36.7	D48.7	D49.89
wall	C76.3	C79.89	D09.8	D36.7	D48.7	D49.89
pelvo-abdominal	C76.8	C79.89	D09.8	D36.7	D48.7	D49.89
penis	C60.9	C79.82	D07.4	D29.0	D40.8	D49.59
body	C60.2	C79.82	D07.4	D29.0	D40.8	D49.59
corpus (cavernosum)	C60.2	C79.82	D07.4	D29.0	D40.8	D49.59
glans	C60.1	C79.82	D07.4	D29.0	D40.8	D49.59
overlapping sites	C60.8	—		—	—	—
skin NEC	C60.9	C79.82	D07.4	D29.0	D40.8	D49.59
periadrenal (tissue)	C48.0	C78.6		D20.0	D48.3	D49.0
perianal (skin) — *see also Neoplasm, anus, skin*	C44.500	C79.2	D04.5	D23.5	D48.5	D49.2
pericardium	C38.0	C79.89	—	D15.1	D48.7	D49.89
perinephric	C48.0	C78.6	—	D20.0	D48.3	D49.0
perineum	C76.3	C79.89	D09.8	D36.7	D48.7	D49.89
periodontal tissue NEC	C03.9	C79.89	D00.03	D10.39	D37.09	D49.0
periosteum — *see Neoplasm, bone*						
peripancreatic	C48.0	C78.6	—	D20.0	D48.3	D49.0
peripheral nerve NEC	C47.9	C79.89	—	D36.10	D48.2	D49.2
perirectal (tissue)	C76.3	C79.89		D36.7	D48.7	D49.89
perirenal (tissue)	C48.0	C78.6		D20.0	D48.3	D49.0
peritoneum, peritoneal (cavity)	C48.2	C78.6	—	D20.1	D48.4	D49.0
benign mesothelial tissue — *see Mesothelioma, benign*						
overlapping lesion	C48.8	—		—	—	—
with digestive organs	C26.9	—		—	—	—
parietal	C48.1	C78.6		D20.1	D48.4	D49.0
pelvic	C48.1	C78.6		D20.1	D48.4	D49.0
specified part NEC	C48.1	C78.6	—	D20.1	D48.4	D49.0
peritonsillar (tissue)	C76.0	C79.89	D09.8	D36.7	D48.7	D49.89
periurethral tissue	C76.3	C79.89		D36.7	D48.7	D49.89
phalanges						
foot	C40.3-●	C79.51		D16.3-●	—	—
hand	C40.1-●	C79.51		D16.1-●	—	—
pharynx, pharyngeal	C14.0	C79.89	D00.08	D10.9	D37.05	D49.0
bursa	C11.1	C79.89	D00.08	D10.6	D37.05	D49.0
fornix	C11.3	C79.89	D00.08	D10.6	D37.05	D49.0
recess	C11.2	C79.89	D00.08	D10.6	D37.05	D49.0
region	C14.0	C79.89	D00.08	D10.9	D37.05	D49.0
tonsil	C11.1	C79.89	D00.08	D10.6	D37.05	D49.0
wall (lateral) (posterior)	C14.0	C79.89	D00.08	D10.9	D37.05	D49.0
pia mater	C70.9	C79.40	—	D32.9	D42.9	D49.7
cerebral	C70.0	C79.32		D32.0	D42.0	D49.7
cranial	C70.0	C79.32	—	D32.0	D42.0	D49.7
spinal	C70.1	C79.49		D32.1	D42.1	D49.7
pillars of fauces	C09.1	C79.89	D00.08	D10.5	D37.05	D49.0
pineal (body) (gland)	C75.3	C79.89	D09.3	D35.4	D44.5	D49.7
pinna (ear) NEC — *see also Neoplasm, skin, ear*	C44.20-●	C79.2	D04.2-●	D23.2-●	D48.5	D49.2
piriform fossa or sinus	C12	C79.89	D00.08	D10.7	D37.05	D49.0
pituitary (body) (fossa) (gland) (lobe)	C75.1	C79.89	D09.3	D35.2	D44.3	D49.7
placenta	C58	C79.82	D07.0	D26.7	D39.2	D49.59
pleura, pleural (cavity)	C38.4	C78.2	—	D19.0	D38.2	D49.1
overlapping lesion with heart or mediastinum	C38.8	—		—	—	—
parietal	C38.4	C78.2		D19.0	D38.2	D49.1
visceral	C38.4	C78.2		D19.0	D38.2	D49.1

◀ New   ◀◀ Revised   ~~deleted~~ Deleted   ● Use Additional Character(s)

	Malignant Primary	Malignant Secondary	Ca in situ	Benign	Uncertain Behavior	Unspecified Behavior
plexus						
brachial	C47.1-●	C79.89	—	D36.12	D48.2	D49.2
cervical	C47.0	C79.89	—	D36.11	D48.2	D49.2
choroid	C71.5	C79.31	—	D33.0	D43.0	D49.6
lumbosacral	C47.5	C79.89	—	D36.16	D48.2	D49.2
sacral	C47.5	C79.89	—	D36.16	D48.2	D49.2
pluriendocrine	C75.8	C79.89	D09.3	D35.7	D44.9	D49.7
pole						
frontal	C71.1	C79.31	—	D33.0	D43.0	D49.6
occipital	C71.4	C79.31	—	D33.0	D43.0	D49.6
pons (varolii)	C71.7	C79.31	—	D33.1	D43.1	D49.6
popliteal fossa or space	C76.5-●	C79.89	D04.7-●	D36.7	D48.7	D49.89
postcricoid (region)	C13.0	C79.89	D00.08	D10.7	D37.05	D49.0
posterior fossa (cranial)	C71.9	C79.31	—	D33.2	D43.2	D49.6
postnasal space	C11.9	C79.89	D00.08	D10.6	D37.05	D49.0
prepuce	C60.0	C79.82	D07.4	D29.0	D40.8	D49.59
prepylorus	C16.4	C78.89	D00.2	D13.1	D37.1	D49.0
presacral (region)	C76.3	C79.89	—	D36.7	D48.7	D49.89
prostate (gland)	C61	C79.82	D07.5	D29.1	D40.0	D49.59
utricle	C68.0	C79.19	D09.19	D30.4	D41.3	D49.59
pterygoid fossa	C49.0	C79.89	—	D21.0	D48.1	D49.2
pubic bone	C41.4	C79.51	—	D16.8	D48.0	D49.2
pudenda, pudendum (female)	C51.9	C79.82	D07.1	D28.0	D39.8	D49.59
pulmonary — see also Neoplasm, lung	C34.9-●	C78.0-●	D02.2-●	D14.3-●	D38.1	D49.1
putamen	C71.0	C79.31	—	D33.0	D43.0	D49.6
pyloric						
antrum	C16.3	C78.89	D00.2	D13.1	D37.1	D49.0
canal	C16.4	C78.89	D00.2	D13.1	D37.1	D49.0
pylorus	C16.4	C78.89	D00.2	D13.1	D37.1	D49.0
pyramid (brain)	C71.7	C79.31	—	D33.1	D43.1	D49.6
pyriform fossa or sinus	C12	C79.89	D00.08	D10.7	D37.05	D49.0
radius (any part)	C40.0-●	C79.51	—	D16.0-●	—	—
Rathke's pouch	C75.1	C79.89	D09.3	D35.2	D44.3	D49.7
rectosigmoid (junction)	C19	C78.5	D01.1	D12.7	D37.5	D49.0
overlapping lesion with anus or rectum	C21.8	—	—	—	—	—
rectouterine pouch	C48.1	C78.6	—	D20.1	D48.4	D49.0
rectovaginal septum or wall	C76.3	C79.89	D09.8	D36.7	D48.7	D49.89
rectovesical septum	C76.3	C79.89	D09.8	D36.7	D48.7	D49.89
rectum (ampulla)	C20	C78.5	D01.2	D12.8	D37.5	D49.0
and colon	C19	C78.5	D01.1	D12.7	D37.5	D49.0
overlapping lesion with anus or rectosigmoid junction	C21.8	—	—	—	—	—

	Malignant Primary	Malignant Secondary	Ca in situ	Benign	Uncertain Behavior	Unspecified Behavior
renal	C64.-●	C79.0-●	D09.19	D30.0-●	D41.0-●	D49.51-●
calyx	C65.-●	C79.0-●	D09.19	D30.1-●	D41.1-●	D49.51-●
hilus	C65.-●	C79.0-●	D09.19	D30.1-●	D41.1-●	D49.51-●
parenchyma	C64.-●	C79.0-●	D09.19	D30.0-●	D41.0-●	D49.51-●
pelvis	C65.-●	C79.0-●	D09.19	D30.1-●	D41.1-●	D49.51-●
respiratory						
organs or system NEC	C39.9	C78.30	D02.4	D14.4	D38.6	D49.1
tract NEC	C39.9	C78.30	D02.4	D14.4	D38.5	D49.1
upper	C39.0	C78.30	D02.4	D14.4	D38.5	D49.1
retina	C69.2-●	C79.49	D09.2-●	D31.2-●	D48.7	D49.81
retrobulbar	C69.6-●	C79.49	—	D31.6-●	D48.7	D49.89
retrocecal	C48.0	C78.6	—	D20.0	D48.3	D49.0
retromolar (area) (triangle) (trigone)	C06.2	C79.89	D00.00	D10.39	D37.09	D49.0
retro-orbital	C76.0	C79.89	D09.8	D36.7	D48.7	D49.89
retroperitoneal (space) (tissue)	C48.0	C78.6	—	D20.0	D48.3	D49.0
retroperitoneum	C48.0	C78.6	—	D20.0	D48.3	D49.0
retropharyngeal	C14.0	C79.89	D00.08	D10.9	D37.05	D49.0
retrovesical (septum)	C76.3	C79.89	D09.8	D36.7	D48.7	D49.89
rhinencephalon	C71.0	C79.31	—	D33.0	D43.0	D49.6
rib	C41.3	C79.51	—	D16.7	D48.0	D49.2
Rosenmuller's fossa	C11.2	C79.89	D00.08	D10.6	D37.05	D49.0
round ligament	C57.2	C79.82	—	D28.2	D39.8	D49.59
sacrococcyx, sacrococcygeal	C41.4	C79.51	—	D16.8	D48.0	D49.2
region	C76.3	C79.89	D09.8	D36.7	D48.7	D49.89
sacrouterine ligament	C57.3	C79.82	—	D28.2	D39.8	D49.59
sacrum, sacral (vertebra)	C41.4	C79.51	—	D16.8	D48.0	D49.2
salivary gland or duct (major)	C08.9	C79.89	D00.00	D11.9	D37.039	D49.0
minor NEC	C06.9	C79.89	D00.00	D10.39	D37.04	D49.0
overlapping lesion	C08.9	—	—	—	—	—
parotid	C07	C79.89	D00.00	D11.0	D37.030	D49.0
pluriglandular	C08.9	C79.89	D00.00	D11.9	D37.039	D49.0
sublingual	C08.1	C79.89	D00.00	D11.7	D37.031	D49.0
submandibular	C08.0	C79.89	D00.00	D11.7	D37.032	D49.0
submaxillary	C08.0	C79.89	D00.00	D11.7	D37.032	D49.0
salpinx (uterine)	C57.0-●	C79.82	D07.39	D28.2	D39.8	D49.59
Santorini's duct	C25.3	C78.89	D01.7	D13.6	D37.8	D49.0
scalp	C44.40	C79.2	D04.4	D23.4	D48.5	D49.2
basal cell carcinoma	C44.41	—	—	—	—	—
specified type NEC	C44.49	—	—	—	—	—
squamous cell carcinoma	C44.42	—	—	—	—	—
scapula (any part)	C40.0-●	C79.51	—	D16.0-●	—	—
scapular region	C76.1	C79.89	D09.8	D36.7	D48.7	D49.89

TABLE OF NEOPLASMS

	Malignant Primary	Malignant Secondary	Ca in situ	Benign	Uncertain Behavior	Unspecified Behavior
scar NEC — see also Neoplasm, skin, by site	C44.90	C79.2	D04.9	D23.9	D48.5	D49.2
sciatic nerve	C47.2-●	C79.89	—	D36.13	D48.2	D49.2
sclera	C69.4-●	C79.49	D09.2-●	D31.4-●	D48.7	D49.89
scrotum (skin)	C63.2	C79.82	D07.61	D29.4	D40.8	D49.59
sebaceous gland — see Neoplasm, skin						
sella turcica	C75.1	C79.89	D09.3	D35.2	D44.3	D49.7
bone	C41.0	C79.51	—	D16.4-●	D48.0	D49.2
semilunar cartilage (knee)	C40.2-●	C79.51	—	D16.2-●	D48.0	D49.2
seminal vesicle	C63.7	C79.82	D07.69	D29.8	D40.8	D49.59
septum						
nasal	C30.0	C78.39	D02.3	D14.0	D38.5	D49.1
posterior margin	C11.3	C79.89	D00.08	D10.6	D37.05	D49.0
rectovaginal	C76.3	C79.89	D09.8	D36.7	D48.7	D49.89
rectovesical	C76.3	C79.89	D09.8	D36.7	D48.7	D49.89
urethrovaginal	C57.9	C79.82	D07.30	D28.9	D39.9	D49.59
vesicovaginal	C57.9	C79.82	D07.30	D28.9	D39.9	D49.59
shoulder NEC	C76.4-●	C79.89	D04.6-●	D36.7	D48.7	D49.89
sigmoid flexure (lower) (upper)	C18.7	C78.5	D01.0	D12.5	D37.4	D49.0
sinus (accessory)	C31.9	C78.39	D02.3	D14.0	D38.5	D49.1
bone (any)	C41.0	C79.51	—	D16.4-●	D48.0	D49.2
ethmoidal	C31.1	C78.39	D02.3	D14.0	D38.5	D49.1
frontal	C31.2	C78.39	D02.3	D14.0	D38.5	D49.1
maxillary	C31.0	C78.39	D02.3	D14.0	D38.5	D49.1
nasal, paranasal NEC	C31.9	C78.39	D02.3	D14.0	D38.5	D49.1
overlapping lesion	C31.8	—	—	—	—	—
pyriform	C12	C79.89	D00.08	D10.7	D37.05	D49.0
sphenoid	C31.3	C78.39	D02.3	D14.0	D38.5	D49.1
skeleton, skeletal NEC	C41.9	C79.51	—	D16.9-●	D48.0	D49.2
Skene's gland	C68.1	C79.19	D09.19	D30.8	D41.8	D49.59
skin NOS	C44.90	C79.2	D04.9	D23.9	D48.5	D49.2
abdominal wall	C44.509	C79.2	D04.5	D23.5	D48.5	D49.2
basal cell carcinoma	C44.519	—	—	—	—	—
specified type NEC	C44.599	—	—	—	—	—
squamous cell carcinoma	C44.529	—	—	—	—	—
ala nasi — see also Neoplasm, nose, skin	C44.301	C79.2	D04.39	D23.39	D48.5	D49.2
ankle — see also Neoplasm, skin, limb, lower	C44.70-●	C79.2	D04.7-●	D23.7-●	D48.5	D49.2
antecubital space — see also Neoplasm, skin, limb, upper	C44.60-●	C79.2	D04.6-●	D23.6-●	D48.5	D49.2
skin NOS (Continued)						
anus	C44.500	C79.2	D04.5	D23.5	D48.5	D49.2
basal cell carcinoma	C44.510	—	—	—	—	—
specified type NEC	C44.590	—	—	—	—	—
squamous cell carcinoma	C44.520	—	—	—	—	—
arm — see also Neoplasm, skin, limb, upper	C44.60-●	C79.2	D04.6-●	D23.6-●	D48.5	D49.2
auditory canal (external) — see also Neoplasm, skin, ear	C44.20-●	C79.2	D04.2-●	D23.2-●	D48.5	D49.2
auricle (ear) — see also Neoplasm, skin, ear	C44.20-●	C79.2	D04.2-●	D23.2-●	D48.5	D49.2
auricular canal (external) — see also Neoplasm, skin, ear	C44.20-●	C79.2	D04.2-●	D23.2-●	D48.5	D49.2
axilla, axillary fold — see also Neoplasm, skin, trunk	C44.509	C79.2	D04.5	D23.5	D48.5	D49.2
back — see also Neoplasm, skin, trunk	C44.509	C79.2	D04.5	D23.5	D48.5	D49.2
basal cell carcinoma	C44.91					
breast	C44.501	C79.2	D04.5	D23.5	D48.5	D49.2
basal cell carcinoma	C44.511	—	—	—	—	—
specified type NEC	C44.591	—	—	—	—	—
squamous cell carcinoma	C44.521	—	—	—	—	—
brow — see also Neoplasm, skin, face	C44.309	C79.2	D04.39	D23.39	D48.5	D49.2
buttock — see also Neoplasm, skin, trunk	C44.509	C79.2	D04.5	D23.5	D48.5	D49.2
calf — see also Neoplasm, skin, limb, lower	C44.70-●	C79.2	D04.7-●	D23.7-●	D48.5	D49.2
canthus (eye) (inner) (outer)	C44.10-●	C79.2	D04.1-●	D23.1-●	D48.5	D49.2
basal cell carcinoma	C44.11-●	—	—	—	—	—
sebaceous cell	C44.13-●	—	—	—	—	—
specified type NEC	C44.19-●	—	—	—	—	—
squamous cell carcinoma	C44.12-●	—	—	—	—	—
cervical region — see also Neoplasm, skin, neck	C44.40	C79.2	D04.4	D23.4	D48.5	D49.2
cheek (external) — see also Neoplasm, skin, face	C44.309	C79.2	D04.39	D23.39	D48.5	D49.2
chest (wall) — see also Neoplasm, skin, trunk	C44.509	C79.2	D04.5	D23.5	D48.5	D49.2
chin — see also Neoplasm, skin, face	C44.309	C79.2	D04.39	D23.39	D48.5	D49.2
clavicular area — see also Neoplasm, skin, trunk	C44.509	C79.2	D04.5	D23.5	D48.5	D49.2
clitoris	C51.2	C79.82	D07.1	D28.0	D39.8	D49.59

skin NOS (Continued)

	Malignant Primary	Malignant Secondary	Ca in situ	Benign	Uncertain Behavior	Unspecified Behavior
columnella — see also Neoplasm, skin, face	C44.309	C79.2	D04.39	D23.39	D48.5	D49.2
concha — see also Neoplasm, skin, ear	C44.20-●	C79.2	D04.2-●	D23.2-●	D48.5	D49.2
ear (external)	C44.20-●	C79.2	D04.2-●	D23.2-●	D48.5	D49.2
basal cell carcinoma	C44.21-●	—	—	—	—	—
specified type NEC	C44.29-●	—	—	—	—	—
squamous cell carcinoma	C44.22-●	—	—	—	—	—
elbow — see also Neoplasm, skin, limb, upper	C44.60-●	C79.2	D04.6-●	D23.6-●	D48.5	D49.2
eyebrow — see also skin, face	C44.309	C79.2	D04.39	D23.39	D48.5	D49.2
eyelid	C44.10-●	C79.2	D04.1-●	D23.1-●	D48.5	D49.2
basal cell carcinoma	C44.11-●	—	—	—	—	—
sebaceous cell	C44.13-●	—	—	—	—	—
specified type NEC	C44.19-●	—	—	—	—	—
squamous cell carcinoma	C44.12-●	—	—	—	—	—
face NOS	C44.300	C79.2	D04.30	D23.30	D48.5	D49.2
basal cell carcinoma	C44.310	—	—	—	—	—
specified type NEC	C44.390	—	—	—	—	—
squamous cell carcinoma	C44.320	—	—	—	—	—
female genital organs (external)	C51.9	C79.82	D07.1	D28.0	D39.8	D49.59
clitoris	C51.2	C79.82	D07.1	D28.0	D39.8	D49.59
labium NEC	C51.9	C79.82	D07.1	D28.0	D39.8	D49.59
majus	C51.0	C79.82	D07.1	D28.0	D39.8	D49.59
minus	C51.1	C79.82	D07.1	D28.0	D39.8	D49.59
pudendum	C51.9	C79.82	D07.1	D28.0	D39.8	D49.59
vulva	C51.9	C79.82	D07.1	D28.0	D39.8	D49.59
finger — see also Neoplasm, skin, limb, upper	C44.60-●	C79.2	D04.6-●	D23.6-●	D48.5	D49.2
flank — see also Neoplasm, skin, trunk	C44.509	C79.2	D04.5	D23.5	D48.5	D49.2
foot — see also Neoplasm, skin, limb, lower	C44.70-●	C79.2	D04.7-●	D23.7-●	D48.5	D49.2
forearm — see also Neoplasm, skin, limb, upper	C44.60-●	C79.2	D04.6-●	D23.6-●	D48.5	D49.2
forehead — see also Neoplasm, skin, face	C44.309	C79.2	D04.39	D23.39	D48.5	D49.2
glabella — see also Neoplasm, skin, face	C44.309	C79.2	D04.39	D23.39	D48.5	D49.2
gluteal region — see also Neoplasm, skin, trunk	C44.509	C79.2	D04.5	D23.5	D48.5	D49.2
groin — see also Neoplasm, skin, trunk	C44.509	C79.2	D04.5	D23.5	D48.5	D49.2

skin NOS (Continued)

	Malignant Primary	Malignant Secondary	Ca in situ	Benign	Uncertain Behavior	Unspecified Behavior
hand — see also Neoplasm, skin, limb, upper	C44.60-●	C79.2	D04.6-●	D23.6-●	D48.5	D49.2
head NEC — see also Neoplasm, skin, scalp	C44.40	C79.2	D04.4	D23.4	D48.5	D49.2
heel — see also Neoplasm, skin, limb, lower	C44.70-●	C79.2	D04.7-●	D23.7-●	D48.5	D49.2
helix — see also Neoplasm, skin, ear	C44.20-●	C79.2	D04.2-●	D23.2-●	D48.5	D49.2
hip — see also Neoplasm, skin, limb, lower	C44.70-●	C79.2	D04.7-●	D23.7-●	D48.5	D49.2
infraclavicular region — see also Neoplasm, skin, trunk	C44.509	C79.2	D04.5	D23.5	D48.5	D49.2
inguinal region — see also Neoplasm, skin, trunk	C44.509	C79.2	D04.5	D23.5	D48.5	D49.2
jaw — see also Neoplasm, skin, face	C44.309	C79.2	D04.39	D23.39	D48.5	D49.2
Kaposi's sarcoma — see Kaposi's, sarcoma, skin						
knee — see also Neoplasm, skin, limb, lower	C44.70-●	C79.2	D04.7-●	D23.7-●	D48.5	D49.2
labia						
majora	C51.0	C79.82	D07.1	D28.0	D39.8	D49.59
minora	C51.1	C79.82	D07.1	D28.0	D39.8	D49.59
leg — see also Neoplasm, skin, limb, lower	C44.70-●	C79.2	D04.7-●	D23.7-●	D48.5	D49.2
lid (lower) (upper)	C44.10-●	C79.2	D04.1-●	D23.1-●	D48.5	D49.2
basal cell carcinoma	C44.11-●	—	—	—	—	—
sebaceous cell	C44.13-●	—	—	—	—	—
specified type NEC	C44.19-●	—	—	—	—	—
squamous cell carcinoma	C44.12-●	—	—	—	—	—
limb NEC	C44.90	C79.2	D04.9	D23.9	D48.5	D49.2
basal cell carcinoma	C44.91					
lower	C44.70-●	C79.2	D04.7-●	D23.7-●	D48.5	D49.2
basal cell carcinoma	C44.71-●	—	—	—	—	—
specified type NEC	C44.79-●	—	—	—	—	—
squamous cell carcinoma	C44.72-●	—	—	—	—	—
upper	C44.60-●	C79.2	D04.6-●	D23.6-●	D48.5	D49.2
basal cell carcinoma	C44.61-●	—	—	—	—	—
specified type NEC	C44.69-●	—	—	—	—	—
squamous cell carcinoma	C44.62-●	—	—	—	—	—
lip (lower) (upper)	C44.00	C79.2	D04.0	D23.0	D48.5	D49.2
basal cell carcinoma	C44.01	—	—	—	—	—
specified type NEC	C44.09	—	—	—	—	—
squamous cell carcinoma	C44.02	—	—	—	—	—

◄ New ◄ Revised ~~deleted~~ Deleted ● Use Additional Character(s)

TABLE OF NEOPLASMS

skin NOS (Continued)	Malignant Primary	Malignant Secondary	Ca in situ	Benign	Uncertain Behavior	Unspecified Behavior
male genital organs	C63.9	C79.82	D07.60	D29.9	D40.8	D49.59
penis	C60.9	C79.82	D07.4	D29.0	D40.8	D49.59
prepuce	C60.0	C79.82	D07.4	D29.0	D40.8	D49.59
scrotum	C63.2	C79.82	D07.61	D29.4	D40.8	D49.59
mastectomy site (skin) — see also Neoplasm, skin, breast	C44.501	C79.2	—			
specified as breast tissue	C50.8-●	C79.81	—			
meatus, acoustic (external) — see also Neoplasm, skin, ear	C44.20-●	C79.2	D04.2-●	D23.2-●	D48.5	D49.2
melanotic — see Melanoma						
Merkel cell — see Carcinoma, Merkel cell						
nates — see also Neoplasm, skin, trunk	C44.509	C79.2	D04.5	D23.5	D48.5	D49.2
neck	C44.40	C79.2	D04.4	D23.4	D48.5	D49.2
basal cell carcinoma	C44.41	—	—	—	—	—
specified type NEC	C44.49	—	—	—	—	—
squamous cell carcinoma	C44.42	—	—	—	—	—
nevus — see Nevus, skin						
nose (external) — see also Neoplasm, nose, skin	C44.301	C79.2	D04.39	D23.39	D48.5	D49.2
overlapping lesion	C44.80	—	—	—	—	—
basal cell carcinoma	C44.81	—	—	—	—	—
specified type NEC	C44.89	—	—	—	—	—
squamous cell carcinoma	C44.82	—	—	—	—	—
palm — see also Neoplasm, skin, limb, upper	C44.60-●	C79.2	D04.6-●	D23.6-●	D48.5	D49.2
palpebra	C44.10-●	C79.2	D04.1-●	D23.1-●	D48.5	D49.2
basal cell carcinoma	C44.11-●	—	—	—	—	—
sebaceous cell	C44.13-●	—	—	—	—	—
specified type NEC	C44.19-●	—	—	—	—	—
squamous cell carcinoma	C44.12-●	—	—	—	—	—
penis NEC	C60.9	C79.82	D07.4	D29.0	D40.8	D49.59
perianal — see also Neoplasm, skin, anus	C44.500	C79.2	D04.5	D23.5	D48.5	D49.2
perineum — see also Neoplasm, skin, anus	C44.500	C79.2	D04.5	D23.5	D48.5	D49.2
pinna — see also Neoplasm, skin, ear	C44.20-●	C79.2	D04.2-●	D23.2-●	D48.5	D49.2
plantar — see also Neoplasm, skin, limb, lower	C44.70-●	C79.2	D04.7-●	D23.7-●	D48.5	D49.2
popliteal fossa or space — see also Neoplasm, skin, limb, lower	C44.70-●	C79.2	D04.7-●	D23.7-●	D48.5	D49.2

skin NOS (Continued)	Malignant Primary	Malignant Secondary	Ca in situ	Benign	Uncertain Behavior	Unspecified Behavior
prepuce	C60.0	C79.82	D07.4	D29.0	D40.8	D49.59
pubes — see also Neoplasm, skin, trunk	C44.509	C79.2	D04.5	D23.5	D48.5	D49.2
sacrococcygeal region — see also Neoplasm, skin, trunk	C44.509	C79.2	D04.5	D23.5	D48.5	D49.2
scalp	C44.40	C79.2	D04.4	D23.4	D48.5	D49.2
basal cell carcinoma	C44.41	—	—	—	—	—
specified type NEC	C44.49	—	—	—	—	—
squamous cell carcinoma	C44.42	—	—	—	—	—
scapular region — see also Neoplasm, skin, trunk	C44.509	C79.2	D04.5	D23.5	D48.5	D49.2
scrotum	C63.2	C79.82	D07.61	D29.4	D40.8	D49.59
shoulder — see also Neoplasm, skin, limb, upper	C44.60-●	C79.2	D04.6-●	D23.6-●	D48.5	D49.2
sole (foot) — see also Neoplasm, skin, limb, lower	C44.70-●	C79.2	D04.7-●	D23.7-●	D48.5	D49.2
specified sites NEC	C44.80	C79.2	D04.8	D23.9	D48.5	D49.2
basal cell carcinoma	C44.81	—	—	—	—	—
specified type NEC	C44.89	—	—	—	—	—
squamous cell carcinoma	C44.82	—	—	—	—	—
specified type NEC	C44.99	—	—	—	—	—
squamous cell carcinoma	C44.92	—	—	—	—	—
submammary fold — see also Neoplasm, skin, trunk	C44.509	C79.2	D04.5	D23.5	D48.5	D49.2
supraclavicular region — see also Neoplasm, skin, neck	C44.40	C79.2	D04.4	D23.4	D48.5	D49.2
temple — see also Neoplasm, skin, face	C44.309	C79.2	D04.39	D23.39	D48.5	D49.2
thigh — see also Neoplasm, skin, limb, lower	C44.70-●	C79.2	D04.7-●	D23.7-●	D48.5	D49.2
thoracic wall — see also Neoplasm, skin, trunk	C44.509	C79.2	D04.5	D23.5	D48.5	D49.2
thumb — see also Neoplasm, skin, limb, upper	C44.60-●	C79.2	D04.6-●	D23.6-●	D48.5	D49.2
toe — see also Neoplasm, skin, limb, lower	C44.70-●	C79.2	D04.7-●	D23.7-●	D48.5	D49.2
tragus — see also Neoplasm, skin, ear	C44.20-●	C79.2	D04.2-●	D23.2-●	D48.5	D49.2
trunk	C44.509	C79.2	D04.5	D23.5	D48.5	D49.2
basal cell carcinoma	C44.519	—	—	—	—	—
specified type NEC	C44.599	—	—	—	—	—
squamous cell carcinoma	C44.529	—	—	—	—	—
umbilicus — see also Neoplasm, skin, trunk	C44.509	C79.2	D04.5	D23.5	D48.5	D49.2

◀ New   ◀ Revised   ~~deleted~~ Deleted   ● Use Additional Character(s)

	Malignant Primary	Malignant Secondary	Ca in situ	Benign	Uncertain Behavior	Unspecified Behavior
skin NOS *(Continued)*						
vulva	C51.9	C79.82	D07.1	D28.0	D39.8	D49.59
overlapping lesion	C51.8	—	—	—	—	—
wrist — *see also Neoplasm, skin, limb, upper*	C44.60-●	C79.2	D04.6-●	D23.6-●	D48.5	D49.2
skull	C41.0	C79.51	—	D16.4-●	D48.0	D49.2
soft parts or tissues — *see Neoplasm, connective tissue*						
specified site NEC	C76.8	C79.89	D09.8	D36.7	D48.7	D49.89
spermatic cord	C63.1-●	C79.82	D07.69	D29.8	D40.8	D49.59
sphenoid	C31.3	C78.39	D02.3	D14.0	D38.5	D49.1
bone	C41.0	C79.51	—	D16.4-●	D48.0	D49.2
sinus	C31.3	C78.39	D02.3	D14.0	D38.5	D49.1
sphincter						
anal	C21.1	C78.5	D01.3	D12.9	D37.8	D49.0
of Oddi	C24.0	C78.89	D01.5	D13.5	D37.6	D49.0
spine, spinal (column)	C41.2	C79.51	—	D16.6	D48.0	D49.2
bulb	C71.7	C79.31	—	D33.1	D43.1	D49.6
coccyx	C41.4	C79.51	—	D16.8	D48.0	D49.2
cord (cervical) (lumbar) (sacral) (thoracic)	C72.0	C79.49	—	D33.4	D43.4	D49.7
dura mater	C70.1	C79.49	—	D32.1	D42.1	D49.7
lumbosacral	C41.2	C79.51	—	D16.6	D48.0	D49.2
marrow NEC	C96.9	C79.52	—	—	D47.9	D49.89
membrane	C70.1	C79.49	—	D32.1	D42.1	D49.7
meninges	C70.1	C79.49	—	D32.1	D42.1	D49.7
nerve (root)	C47.9	C79.89	—	D36.10	D48.2	D49.2
pia mater	C70.1	C79.49	—	D32.1	D42.1	D49.7
root	C47.9	C79.89	—	D36.10	D48.2	D49.2
sacrum	C41.4	C79.51	—	D16.8	D48.0	D49.2
spleen, splenic NEC	C26.1	C78.89	D01.7	D13.9	D37.8	D49.0
flexure (colon)	C18.5	C78.5	D01.0	D12.3	D37.4	D49.0
stem, brain	C71.7	C79.31	—	D33.1	D43.1	D49.6
Stensen's duct	C07	C79.89	D00.00	D11.0	D37.030	D49.0
sternum	C41.3	C79.51	—	D16.7	D48.0	D49.2
stomach	C16.9	C78.89	D00.2	D13.1	D37.1	D49.0
antrum (pyloric)	C16.3	C78.89	D00.2	D13.1	D37.1	D49.0
body	C16.2	C78.89	D00.2	D13.1	D37.1	D49.0
cardia	C16.0	C78.89	D00.2	D13.1	D37.1	D49.0
cardiac orifice	C16.0	C78.89	D00.2	D13.1	D37.1	D49.0
corpus	C16.2	C78.89	D00.2	D13.1	D37.1	D49.0
fundus	C16.1	C78.89	D00.2	D13.1	D37.1	D49.0
greater curvature NEC	C16.6	C78.89	D00.2	D13.1	D37.1	D49.0
lesser curvature NEC	C16.5	C78.89	D00.2	D13.1	D37.1	D49.0

	Malignant Primary	Malignant Secondary	Ca in situ	Benign	Uncertain Behavior	Unspecified Behavior
stomach *(Continued)*						
overlapping lesion	C16.8	—	—	—	—	—
prepylorus	C16.4	C78.89	D00.2	D13.1	D37.1	D49.0
pylorus	C16.4	C78.89	D00.2	D13.1	D37.1	D49.0
wall NEC	C16.9	C78.89	D00.2	D13.1	D37.1	D49.0
anterior NEC	C16.8	C78.89	D00.2	D13.1	D37.1	D49.0
posterior NEC	C16.8	C78.89	D00.2	D13.1	D37.1	D49.0
stroma, endometrial	C54.1	C79.82	D07.0	D26.1	D39.0	D49.59
stump, cervical	C53.8	C79.82	D06.7	D26.0	D39.0	D49.59
subcutaneous (nodule) (tissue) NEC — *see Neoplasm, connective tissue*						
subdural	C70.9	C79.32	—	D32.9	D42.9	D49.7
subglottis, subglottic	C32.2	C78.39	D02.0	D14.1	D38.0	D49.1
sublingual	C04.9	C79.89	D00.06	D10.2	D37.09	D49.0
gland or duct	C08.1	C79.89	D00.00	D11.7	D37.031	D49.0
submandibular gland	C08.0	C79.89	D00.00	D11.7	D37.032	D49.0
submaxillary gland or duct	C08.0	C79.89	D00.00	D11.7	D37.032	D49.0
submental	C76.0	C79.89	D09.8	D36.7	D48.7	D49.89
subpleural	C34.9-●	C78.0-●	D02.2-●	D14.3-●	D38.1	D49.1
substernal	C38.1	C78.1	—	D15.2	D38.3	D49.89
sudoriferous, sudoriparous gland, site unspecified	C44.90	C79.2	D04.9	D23.9	D48.5	D49.2
specified site — *see Neoplasm, skin*						
supraclavicular region	C76.0	C79.89	D09.8	D36.7	D48.7	D49.89
supraglottis	C32.1	C78.39	D02.0	D14.1	D38.0	D49.1
suprarenal	C74.9-●	C79.7-●	D09.3	D35.0-●	D44.1-●	D49.7
capsule	C74.9-●	C79.7-●	D09.3	D35.0-●	D44.1-●	D49.7
cortex	C74.0-●	C79.7-●	D09.3	D35.0-●	D44.1-●	D49.7
gland	C74.9-●	C79.7-●	D09.3	D35.0-●	D44.1-●	D49.7
medulla	C74.1-●	C79.7-●	D09.3	D35.0-●	D44.1-●	D49.7
suprasellar (region)	C71.9	C79.31	—	D33.2	D43.2	D49.6
supratentorial (brain) NEC	C71.0	C79.31	—	D33.0	D43.0	D49.6
sweat gland (apocrine) (eccrine), site unspecified	C44.90	C79.2	D04.9	D23.9	D48.5	D49.2
specified site — *see Neoplasm, skin*						
sympathetic nerve or nervous system NEC	C47.9	C79.89	—	D36.10	D48.2	D49.2
symphysis pubis	C41.4	C79.51	—	D16.8	D48.0	D49.2
synovial membrane — *see Neoplasm, connective tissue*						
tapetum, brain	C71.8	C79.31	—	D33.2	D43.2	D49.6

TABLE OF NEOPLASMS

TABLE OF NEOPLASMS

	Malignant Primary	Malignant Secondary	Ca in situ	Benign	Uncertain Behavior	Unspecified Behavior
tarsus (any bone)	C40.3-•	C79.51	—	D16.3-•	—	—
temple (skin) — see also Neoplasm, skin, face	C44.309	C79.2	D04.39	D23.39	D48.5	D49.2
temporal						
bone	C41.0	C79.51	—	D16.4-•	D48.0	D49.2
lobe or pole	C71.2	C79.31	—	D33.0	D43.0	D49.6
region	C76.0	C79.89	D09.8	D36.7	D48.7	D49.89
skin — see also Neoplasm, skin, face	C44.309	C79.2	D04.39	D23.39	D48.5	D49.2
tendon (sheath) — see Neoplasm, connective tissue						
tentorium (cerebelli)	C70.0	C79.32	—	D32.0	D42.0	D49.7
testis, testes	C62.9-•	C79.82	D07.69	D29.2-•	D40.1-•	D49.59
descended	C62.1-•	C79.82	D07.69	D29.2-•	D40.1-•	D49.59
ectopic	C62.0-•	C79.82	D07.69	D29.2-•	D40.1-•	D49.59
retained	C62.0-•	C79.82	D07.69	D29.2-•	D40.1-•	D49.59
scrotal	C62.1-•	C79.82	D07.69	D29.2-•	D40.1-•	D49.59
undescended	C62.0-•	C79.82	D07.69	D29.2-•	D40.1-•	D49.59
unspecified whether descended or undescended	C62.9-•	C79.82	D07.69	D29.2-•	D40.1-•	D49.59
thalamus	C71.0	C79.31	—	D33.0	D43.0	D49.6
thigh NEC	C76.5-•	C79.89	D04.7-•	D36.7	D48.7	D49.89
thorax, thoracic (cavity) (organs NEC)	C76.1	C79.89	D09.8	D36.7	D48.7	D49.89
duct	C49.3	C79.89	—	D21.3	D48.1	D49.2
wall NEC	C76.1	C79.89	D09.8	D36.7	D48.7	D49.89
throat	C14.0	C79.89	D00.08	D10.9	D37.05	D49.0
thumb NEC	C76.4-•	C79.89	D04.6-•	D36.7	D48.7	D49.89
thymus (gland)	C37	C79.89	D09.3	D15.0	D38.4	D49.89
thyroglossal duct	C73	C79.89	D09.3	D34	D44.0	D49.7
thyroid (gland)	C73	C79.89	D09.3	D34	D44.0	D49.7
cartilage	C32.3	C78.39	D02.0	D14.1	D38.0	D49.1
tibia (any part)	C40.2-•	C79.51	—	D16.2-•	—	—
toe NEC	C76.5-•	C79.89	D04.7-•	D36.7	D48.7	D49.89
tongue	C02.9	C79.89	D00.07	D10.1	D37.02	D49.0
anterior (two-thirds) NEC	C02.3	C79.89	D00.07	D10.1	D37.02	D49.0
dorsal surface	C02.0	C79.89	D00.07	D10.1	D37.02	D49.0
ventral surface	C02.2	C79.89	D00.07	D10.1	D37.02	D49.0
base (dorsal surface)	C01	C79.89	D00.07	D10.1	D37.02	D49.0
border (lateral)	C02.1	C79.89	D00.07	D10.1	D37.02	D49.0
dorsal surface NEC	C02.0	C79.89	D00.07	D10.1	D37.02	D49.0
fixed part NEC	C01	C79.89	D00.07	D10.1	D37.02	D49.0
foreamen cecum	C02.0	C79.89	D00.07	D10.1	D37.02	D49.0
frenulum linguae	C02.2	C79.89	D00.07	D10.1	D37.02	D49.0

	Malignant Primary	Malignant Secondary	Ca in situ	Benign	Uncertain Behavior	Unspecified Behavior
tongue (Continued)						
junctional zone	C02.8	C79.89	D00.07	D10.1	D37.02	D49.0
margin (lateral)	C02.1	C79.89	D00.07	D10.1	D37.02	D49.0
midline NEC	C02.0	C79.89	D00.07	D10.1	D37.02	D49.0
mobile part NEC	C02.3	C79.89	D00.07	D10.1	D37.02	D49.0
overlapping lesion	C02.8	—	—	—	—	—
posterior (third)	C01	C79.89	D00.07	D10.1	D37.02	D49.0
root	C01	C79.89	D00.07	D10.1	D37.02	D49.0
surface (dorsal)	C02.0	C79.89	D00.07	D10.1	D37.02	D49.0
base	C01	C79.89	D00.07	D10.1	D37.02	D49.0
ventral	C02.2	C79.89	D00.07	D10.1	D37.02	D49.0
tip	C02.1	C79.89	D00.07	D10.1	D37.02	D49.0
tonsil	C02.4	C79.89	D00.07	D10.1	D37.02	D49.0
tonsil	C09.9	C79.89	D00.08	D10.4	D37.05	D49.0
fauces, faucial	C09.9	C79.89	D00.08	D10.4	D37.05	D49.0
lingual	C02.4	C79.89	D00.07	D10.1	D37.02	D49.0
overlapping sites	C09.8	—	—	—	—	—
palatine	C09.9	C79.89	D00.08	D10.4	D37.05	D49.0
pharyngeal	C11.1	C79.89	D00.08	D10.6	D37.05	D49.0
pillar (anterior) (posterior)	C09.1	C79.89	D00.08	D10.5	D37.05	D49.0
tonsillar fossa	C09.0	C79.89	D00.08	D10.5	D37.05	D49.0
tooth socket NEC	C03.9	C79.89	D00.03	D10.39	D37.09	D49.0
trachea (cartilage) (mucosa)	C33	C78.39	D02.1	D14.2	D38.1	D49.1
overlapping lesion with bronchus or lung	C34.8-•	—	—	—	—	—
tracheobronchial	C34.8-•	C78.39	D02.1	D14.2	D38.1	D49.1
overlapping lesion with lung	C34.8-•	—	—	—	—	—
tragus — see also Neoplasm, skin, ear	C44.20-•	C79.2	D04.2-•	D23.2-•	D48.5	D49.2
trunk NEC	C76.8	C79.89	D04.5	D36.7	D48.7	D49.89
tubo-ovarian	C57.8	C79.82	D07.39	D28.7	D39.8	D49.59
tunica vaginalis	C63.7	C79.82	D07.69	D29.8	D40.8	D49.59
turbinate (bone)	C41.0	C79.51	—	D16.4-•	D48.0	D49.2
nasal	C30.0	C78.39	D02.3	D14.0	D38.5	D49.1
tympanic cavity	C30.1	C78.39	D02.3	D14.0	D38.5	D49.1
ulna (any part)	C40.0-•	C79.51	—	D16.0-•	—	—
umbilicus, umbilical — see also Neoplasm, skin, trunk	C44.509	C79.2	D04.5	D23.5	D48.5	D49.2
uncus, brain	C71.2	C79.31	—	D33.0	D43.0	D49.6
unknown site or unspecified	C80.1	C79.9	D09.9	D36.9	D48.9	D49.9
urachus	C67.7	C79.11	D09.0	D30.3	D41.4	D49.4
ureter, ureteral	C66.-•	C79.19	D09.19	D30.2-•	D41.2-•	D49.59
orifice (bladder)	C67.6	C79.11	D09.0	D30.3	D41.4	D49.4
ureter-bladder (junction)	C67.6	C79.11	D09.0	D30.3	D41.4	D49.4

◀ New   ◀ Revised   ~~deleted~~ Deleted   • Use Additional Character(s)

	Malignant Primary	Malignant Secondary	Ca in situ	Benign	Uncertain Behavior	Unspecified Behavior
urethra, urethral (gland)	C68.0	C79.19	D09.19	D30.4	D41.3	D49.59
orifice, internal	C67.5	C79.11	D09.0	D30.3	D41.4	D49.4
urethrovaginal (septum)	C57.9	C79.82	D07.30	D28.9	D39.8	D49.59
urinary organ or system	C68.9	C79.10	D09.10	D30.9	D41.9	D49.59
bladder — *see Neoplasm, bladder*						
overlapping lesion	C68.8	—	—	—	—	—
specified sites NEC	C68.8	C79.19	D09.19	D30.8	D41.8	D49.59
utero-ovarian	C57.8	C79.82	D07.39	D28.7	D39.8	D49.59
ligament	C57.1	C79.82	D07.39	D28.2	D39.8	D49.59
uterosacral ligament	C57.3	C79.82	—	D28.2	D39.8	D49.59
uterus, uteri, uterine	C55	C79.82	D07.0	D26.9	D39.0	D49.59
adnexa NEC	C57.4	C79.82	D07.39	D28.7	D39.8	D49.59
body	C54.9	C79.82	D07.0	D26.1	D39.0	D49.59
cervix	C53.9	C79.82	D06.9	D26.0	D39.0	D49.59
cornu	C54.9	C79.82	D07.0	D26.1	D39.0	D49.59
corpus	C54.9	C79.82	D07.0	D26.1	D39.0	D49.59
endocervix (canal) (gland)	C53.0	C79.82	D06.0	D26.0	D39.0	D49.59
endometrium	C54.1	C79.82	D07.0	D26.1	D39.0	D49.59
exocervix	C53.1	C79.82	D06.1	D26.0	D39.0	D49.59
external os	C53.1	C79.82	D06.1	D26.0	D39.0	D49.59
fundus	C54.3	C79.82	D07.0	D26.1	D39.0	D49.59
internal os	C53.0	C79.82	D06.0	D26.0	D39.0	D49.59
isthmus	C54.0	C79.82	D07.0	D26.1	D39.0	D49.59
ligament	C57.3	C79.82	—	D28.2	D39.8	D49.59
broad	C57.1	C79.82	D07.39	D28.2	D39.8	D49.59
round	C57.2	C79.82	—	D28.2	D39.8	D49.59
lower segment	C54.0	C79.82	D07.0	D26.1	D39.0	D49.59
myometrium	C54.2	C79.82	D07.0	D26.1	D39.0	D49.59
overlapping sites	C54.8	—	—	—	—	—
squamocolumnar junction	C53.8	C79.82	D06.7	D26.0	D39.0	D49.59
tube	C57.0-•	C79.82	D07.39	D28.2	D39.8	D49.59
utricle, prostatic	C68.0	C79.19	D09.19	D30.4	D41.3	D49.59
uveal tract	C69.4-•	C79.49	D09.2-•	D31.4-•	D48.7	D49.89
uvula	C05.2	C79.89	D00.04	D10.39	D37.09	D49.0
vagina, vaginal (fornix) (vault) (wall)	C52	C79.82	D07.2	D28.1	D39.8	D49.59
vaginovesical	C57.9	C79.82	D07.30	D28.9	D39.9	D49.59
septum	C57.9	C79.82	D07.30	D28.9	D39.9	D49.59
vallecula (epiglottis)	C10.0	C79.89	D00.08	D10.5	D37.05	D49.0
vas deferens	C63.1-•	C79.82	D07.69	D29.8	D40.8	D49.59
vascular — *see Neoplasm, connective tissue*						

	Malignant Primary	Malignant Secondary	Ca in situ	Benign	Uncertain Behavior	Unspecified Behavior
Vater's ampulla	C24.1	C78.89	D01.5	D13.5	D37.6	D49.0
vein, venous — *see Neoplasm, connective tissue*						
vena cava (abdominal) (inferior)	C49.4	C79.89	—	D21.4	D48.1	D49.2
superior	C49.3	C79.89	—	D21.3	D48.1	D49.2
ventricle (cerebral) (floor) (lateral) (third)	C71.5	C79.31	—	D33.0	D43.0	D49.6
cardiac (left) (right)	C38.0	C79.89	—	D15.1	D48.7	D49.89
fourth	C71.7	C79.31	—	D33.1	D43.1	D49.6
ventricular band of larynx	C32.1	C78.39	D02.0	D14.1	D38.0	D49.1
ventriculus — *see Neoplasm, stomach*						
vermillion border — *see Neoplasm, lip*						
vermis, cerebellum	C71.6	C79.31	—	D33.1	D43.1	D49.6
vertebra (column)	C41.2	C79.51	—	D16.6	D48.0	D49.2
coccyx	C41.4	C79.51	—	D16.8-•	D48.0	D49.2
marrow NEC	C96.9	C79.52	—	—	D47.9	D49.89
sacrum	C41.4	C79.51	—	D16.8-•	D48.0	D49.2
vesical — *see Neoplasm, bladder*						
vesicle, seminal	C63.7	C79.82	D07.69	D29.8	D40.8	D49.59
vesicocervical tissue	C57.9	C79.82	D07.30	D28.9	D39.9	D49.59
vesicorectal	C76.3	C79.82	D09.8	D36.7	D48.7	D49.89
vesicovaginal	C57.9	C79.82	D07.30	D28.9	D39.9	D49.59
septum	C57.9	C79.82	D07.30	D28.9	D39.8	D49.59
vessel (blood) — *see Neoplasm, connective tissue*						
vestibular gland, greater	C51.0	C79.82	D07.1	D28.0	D39.8	D49.59
vestibule						
mouth	C06.1	C79.89	D00.00	D10.39	D37.09	D49.0
nose	C30.0	C78.39	D02.3	D14.0	D38.5	D49.1
Virchow's gland	C77.0	C77.0	—	D36.0	D48.7	D49.89
viscera NEC	C76.8	C79.89	D09.8	D36.7	D48.7	D49.89
vocal cords (true)	C32.0	C78.39	D02.0	D14.1	D38.0	D49.1
false	C32.1	C78.39	D02.0	D14.1	D38.0	D49.1
vomer	C41.0	C79.51	—	D16.4-•	D48.0	D49.2
vulva	C51.9	C79.82	D07.1	D28.0	D39.8	D49.59
vulvovaginal gland	C51.0	C79.82	D07.1	D28.0	D39.8	D49.59
Waldeyer's ring	C14.2	C79.89	D00.08	D10.9	D37.05	D49.0
Wharton's duct	C08.0	C79.89	D00.00	D11.7	D37.032	D49.0
white matter (central) (cerebral)	C71.0	C79.31	—	D33.0	D43.0	D49.6
windpipe	C33	C78.39	D02.1	D14.2	D38.1	D49.1

◀ New   ◀ Revised   ~~deleted~~ Deleted   • Use Additional Character(s)

	Malignant Primary	Malignant Secondary	Ca in situ	Benign	Uncertain Behavior	Unspecified Behavior
Wirsung's duct	C25.3	C78.89	D01.7	D13.6	D37.8	D49.0
wolffian (body) (duct)						
female	C57.7	C79.82	D07.39	D28.7	D39.8	D49.59
male	C63.7	C79.82	D07.69	D29.8	D40.8	D49.59

	Malignant Primary	Malignant Secondary	Ca in situ	Benign	Uncertain Behavior	Unspecified Behavior
womb — *see Neoplasm, uterus*						
wrist NEC	C76.4-●	C79.89	D04.6-●	D36.7	D48.7	D49.89
xiphoid process	C41.3	C79.51	—	D16.7	D48.0	D49.2
Zuckerkandl organ	C75.5	C79.89	—	D35.6	D44.7	D49.7

◀ New   ◀ Revised   ~~deleted~~ Deleted   ● Use Additional Character(s)

TABLE OF NEOPLASMS

ICD-10-CM
Table of Drugs and Chemicals

TOD

ICD-10-CM
Table of Drugs and Chemicals

Substance	Poisoning, Accidental (Unintentional)	Poisoning, Intentional Self-Harm	Poisoning, Assault	Poisoning, Undetermined	Adverse Effect	Underdosing
#						
1-propanol	T51.3X1	T51.3X2	T51.3X3	T51.3X4	—	—
2-propanol	T51.2X1	T51.2X2	T51.2X3	T51.2X4	—	—
2,4-D (dichlorophen-oxyacetic acid)	T60.3X1	T60.3X2	T60.3X3	T60.3X4	—	—
2,4-toluene diisocyanate	T65.0X1	T65.0X2	T65.0X3	T65.0X4	—	—
2,4,5-T (trichloro-phenoxyacetic acid)	T60.1X1	T60.1X2	T60.1X3	T60.1X4	—	—
3,4-methylenedioxy-methamphetamine	T43.641	T43.642	T43.643	T43.644	—	—
14-hydroxydihydro-morphinone	T40.2X1	T40.2X2	T40.2X3	T40.2X4	T40.2X5	T40.2X6
A						
ABOB	T37.5X1	T37.5X2	T37.5X3	T37.5X4	T37.5X5	T37.5X6
Abrine	T62.2X1	T62.2X2	T62.2X3	T62.2X4	—	—
Abrus (seed)	T62.2X1	T62.2X2	T62.2X3	T62.2X4	—	—
Absinthe	T51.0X1	T51.0X2	T51.0X3	T51.0X4	—	—
beverage	T51.0X1	T51.0X2	T51.0X3	T51.0X4	—	—
Acaricide	T60.8X1	T60.8X2	T60.8X3	T60.8X4	—	—
Acebutolol	T44.7X1	T44.7X2	T44.7X3	T44.7X4	T44.7X5	T44.7X6
Acecarbromal	T42.6X1	T42.6X2	T42.6X3	T42.6X4	T42.6X5	T42.6X6
Aceclidine	T44.1X1	T44.1X2	T44.1X3	T44.1X4	T44.1X5	T44.1X6
Acedapsone	T37.0X1	T37.0X2	T37.0X3	T37.0X4	T37.0X5	T37.0X6
Acefylline piperazine	T48.6X1	T48.6X2	T48.6X3	T48.6X4	T48.6X5	T48.6X6
Acemorphan	T40.2X1	T40.2X2	T40.2X3	T40.2X4	T40.2X5	T40.2X6
Acenocoumarin	T45.511	T45.512	T45.513	T45.514	T45.515	T45.516
Acenocoumarol	T45.511	T45.512	T45.513	T45.514	T45.515	T45.516
Acepifylline	T48.6X1	T48.6X2	T48.6X3	T48.6X4	T48.6X5	T48.6X6
Acepromazine	T43.3X1	T43.3X2	T43.3X3	T43.3X4	T43.3X5	T43.3X6
Acesulfamethoxypyridazine	T37.0X1	T37.0X2	T37.0X3	T37.0X4	T37.0X5	T37.0X6
Acetal	T52.8X1	T52.8X2	T52.8X3	T52.8X4	—	—
Acetaldehyde (vapor)	T52.8X1	T52.8X2	T52.8X3	T52.8X4	—	—
liquid	T65.891	T65.892	T65.893	T65.894	—	—
P-Acetamidophenol	T39.1X1	T39.1X2	T39.1X3	T39.1X4	T39.1X5	T39.1X6
Acetaminophen	T39.1X1	T39.1X2	T39.1X3	T39.1X4	T39.1X5	T39.1X6
Acetaminosalol	T39.1X1	T39.1X2	T39.1X3	T39.1X4	T39.1X5	T39.1X6
Acetanilide	T39.1X1	T39.1X2	T39.1X3	T39.1X4	T39.1X5	T39.1X6
Acetarsol	T37.3X1	T37.3X2	T37.3X3	T37.3X4	T37.3X5	T37.3X6
Acetazolamide	T50.2X1	T50.2X2	T50.2X3	T50.2X4	T50.2X5	T50.2X6
Acetiamine	T45.2X1	T45.2X2	T45.2X3	T45.2X4	T45.2X5	T45.2X6
Acetic						
acid	T54.2X1	T54.2X2	T54.2X3	T54.2X4	—	—
with sodium acetate (ointment)	T49.3X1	T49.3X2	T49.3X3	T49.3X4	T49.3X5	T49.3X6

Substance	Poisoning, Accidental (Unintentional)	Poisoning, Intentional Self-Harm	Poisoning, Assault	Poisoning, Undetermined	Adverse Effect	Underdosing
Acetic *(Continued)*						
acid *(Continued)*						
ester (solvent) (vapor)	T52.8X1	T52.8X2	T52.8X3	T52.8X4	—	—
irrigating solution	T50.3X1	T50.3X2	T50.3X3	T50.3X4	T50.3X5	T50.3X6
medicinal (lotion)	T49.2X1	T49.2X2	T49.2X3	T49.2X4	T49.2X5	T49.2X6
anhydride	T65.891	T65.892	T65.893	T65.894		
ether (vapor)	T52.8X1	T52.8X2	T52.8X3	T52.8X4		
Acetohexamide	T38.3X1	T38.3X2	T38.3X3	T38.3X4	T38.3X5	T38.3X6
Acetohydroxamic acid	T50.991	T50.992	T50.993	T50.994	T50.995	T50.996
Acetomenaphthone	T45.7X1	T45.7X2	T45.7X3	T45.7X4	T45.7X5	T45.7X6
Acetomorphine	T40.1X1	T40.1X2	T40.1X3	T40.1X4	—	—
Acetone (oils)	T52.4X1	T52.4X2	T52.4X3	T52.4X4		
chlorinated	T52.4X1	T52.4X2	T52.4X3	T52.4X4		
vapor	T52.4X1	T52.4X2	T52.4X3	T52.4X4		
Acetonitrile	T52.8X1	T52.8X2	T52.8X3	T52.8X4		
Acetophenazine	T43.3X1	T43.3X2	T43.3X3	T43.3X4	T43.3X5	T43.3X6
Acetophenetedin	T39.1X1	T39.1X2	T39.1X3	T39.1X4	T39.1X5	T39.1X6
Acetophenone	T52.4X1	T52.4X2	T52.4X3	T52.4X4		
Acetorphine	T40.2X1	T40.2X2	T40.2X3	T40.2X4		
Acetosulfone (sodium)	T37.1X1	T37.1X2	T37.1X3	T37.1X4	T37.1X5	T37.1X6
Acetrizoate (sodium)	T50.8X1	T50.8X2	T50.8X3	T50.8X4	T50.8X5	T50.8X6
Acetylcarbromal	T42.6X1	T42.6X2	T42.6X3	T42.6X4	T42.6X5	T42.6X6
Acetrizoic acid	T50.8X1	T50.8X2	T50.8X3	T50.8X4	T50.8X5	T50.8X6
Acetyl						
bromide	T53.6X1	T53.6X2	T53.6X3	T53.6X4		
chloride	T53.6X1	T53.6X2	T53.6X3	T53.6X4	—	—
Acetylcholine						
chloride	T44.1X1	T44.1X2	T44.1X3	T44.1X4	T44.1X5	T44.1X6
derivative	T44.1X1	T44.1X2	T44.1X3	T44.1X4	T44.1X5	T44.1X6
Acetylcysteine	T48.4X1	T48.4X2	T48.4X3	T48.4X4	T48.4X5	T48.4X6
Acetyldigitoxin	T46.0X1	T46.0X2	T46.0X3	T46.0X4	T46.0X5	T46.0X6
Acetyldigoxin	T46.0X1	T46.0X2	T46.0X3	T46.0X4	T46.0X5	T46.0X6
Acetyldihydrocodeine	T40.2X1	T40.2X2	T40.2X3	T40.2X4	—	—
Acetyldihydrocodeinone	T40.2X1	T40.2X2	T40.2X3	T40.2X4	—	—
Acetylene (gas)	T59.891	T59.892	T59.893	T59.894	—	—
dichloride	T53.6X1	T53.6X2	T53.6X3	T53.6X4	—	—
incomplete combustion of	T58.11	T58.12	T58.13	T58.14		
industrial	T59.891	T59.892	T59.893	T59.894		
tetrachloride	T53.6X1	T53.6X2	T53.6X3	T53.6X4	—	—
vapor	T53.6X1	T53.6X2	T53.6X3	T53.6X4		
Acetylphenylhydrazine	T39.8X1	T39.8X2	T39.8X3	T39.8X4	T39.8X5	T39.8X6
Acetylpheneturide	T42.6X1	T42.6X2	T42.6X3	T42.6X4	T42.6X5	T42.6X6

◄ New ◄ Revised ~~deleted~~ Deleted

TABLE OF DRUGS AND CHEMICALS

Substance	External Cause (T-Code)					
	Poisoning, Accidental (Unintentional)	Poisoning, Intentional Self-Harm	Poisoning, Assault	Poisoning, Undetermined	Adverse Effect	Underdosing
Acetylsalicylic acid (salts)	T39.011	T39.012	T39.013	T39.014	T39.015	T39.016
enteric coated	T39.011	T39.012	T39.013	T39.014	T39.015	T39.016
Acetylsulfamethoxypyridazine	T37.0X1	T37.0X2	T37.0X3	T37.0X4	T37.0X5	T37.0X6
Achromycin	T36.4X1	T36.4X2	T36.4X3	T36.4X4	T36.4X5	T36.4X6
ophthalmic preparation	T49.5X1	T49.5X2	T49.5X3	T49.5X4	T49.5X5	T49.5X6
topical NEC	T49.0X1	T49.0X2	T49.0X3	T49.0X4	T49.0X5	T49.0X6
Aciclovir	T37.5X1	T37.5X2	T37.5X3	T37.5X4	T37.5X5	T37.5X6
Acid (corrosive) NEC	T54.2X1	T54.2X2	T54.2X3	T54.2X4	—	—
Acidifying agent NEC	T50.901	T50.902	T50.903	T50.904	T50.905	T50.906
Acipimox	T46.6X1	T46.6X2	T46.6X3	T46.6X4	T46.6X5	T46.6X6
Acitretin	T50.991	T50.992	T50.993	T50.994	T50.995	T50.996
Aclarubicin	T45.1X1	T45.1X2	T45.1X3	T45.1X4	T45.1X5	T45.1X6
Aclatonium napadisilate	T48.1X1	T48.1X2	T48.1X3	T48.1X4	T48.1X5	T48.1X6
Aconite (wild)	T46.991	T46.992	T46.993	T46.994	T46.995	T46.996
Aconitine	T46.991	T46.992	T46.993	T46.994	T46.995	T46.996
Aconitum ferox	T46.991	T46.992	T46.993	T46.994	T46.995	T46.996
Acridine	T65.6X1	T65.6X2	T65.6X3	T65.6X4	—	—
vapor	T59.891	T59.892	T59.893	T59.894	—	—
Acriflavine	T37.91	T37.92	T37.93	T37.94	T37.95	T37.96
Acriflavinium chloride	T49.0X1	T49.0X2	T49.0X3	T49.0X4	T49.0X5	T49.0X6
Acrinol	T49.0X1	T49.0X2	T49.0X3	T49.0X4	T49.0X5	T49.0X6
Acrisorcin	T49.0X1	T49.0X2	T49.0X3	T49.0X4	T49.0X5	T49.0X6
Acrivastine	T45.0X1	T45.0X2	T45.0X3	T45.0X4	T45.0X5	T45.0X6
Acrolein (gas)	T59.891	T59.892	T59.893	T59.894	—	—
liquid	T54.1X1	T54.1X2	T54.1X3	T54.1X4	—	—
Acrylamide	T65.891	T65.892	T65.893	T65.894	—	—
Acrylic resin	T49.3X1	T49.3X2	T49.3X3	T49.3X4	T49.3X5	T49.3X6
Acrylonitrile	T65.891	T65.892	T65.893	T65.894	—	—
Actaea spicata	T62.2X1	T62.2X2	T62.2X3	T62.2X4	—	—
berry	T62.1X1	T62.1X2	T62.1X3	T62.1X4	—	—
Acterol	T37.3X1	T37.3X2	T37.3X3	T37.3X4	T37.3X5	T37.3X6
ACTH	T38.811	T38.812	T38.813	T38.814	T38.815	T38.816
Actinomycin C	T45.1X1	T45.1X2	T45.1X3	T45.1X4	T45.1X5	T45.1X6
Actinomycin D	T45.1X1	T45.1X2	T45.1X3	T45.1X4	T45.1X5	T45.1X6
Activated charcoal — see also Charcoal, medicinal	T47.6X1	T47.6X2	T47.6X3	T47.6X4	T47.6X5	T47.6X6
Acyclovir	T37.5X1	T37.5X2	T37.5X3	T37.5X4	T37.5X5	T37.5X6
Adenine	T45.2X1	T45.2X2	T45.2X3	T45.2X4	T45.2X5	T45.2X6
arabinoside	T37.5X1	T37.5X2	T37.5X3	T37.5X4	T37.5X5	T37.5X6
Adenosine (phosphate)	T46.2X1	T46.2X2	T46.2X3	T46.2X4	T46.2X5	T46.2X6
ADH	T38.891	T38.892	T38.893	T38.894	T38.895	T38.896
Adhesive NEC	T65.891	T65.892	T65.893	T65.894	—	—

Substance	External Cause (T-Code)					
	Poisoning, Accidental (Unintentional)	Poisoning, Intentional Self-Harm	Poisoning, Assault	Poisoning, Undetermined	Adverse Effect	Underdosing
Adicillin	T36.0X1	T36.0X2	T36.0X3	T36.0X4	T36.0X5	T36.0X6
Adiphenine	T44.3X1	T44.3X2	T44.3X3	T44.3X4	T44.3X5	T44.3X6
Adipiodone	T50.8X1	T50.8X2	T50.8X3	T50.8X4	T50.8X5	T50.8X6
Adjunct, pharmaceutical	T50.901	T50.902	T50.903	T50.904	T50.905	T50.906
Adrenal (extract, cortex or medulla) (glucocorticoids) (hormones) (mineralo corticoids)	T38.0X1	T38.0X2	T38.0X3	T38.0X4	T38.0X5	T38.0X6
ENT agent	T49.6X1	T49.6X2	T49.6X3	T49.6X4	T49.6X5	T49.6X6
ophthalmic preparation	T49.5X1	T49.5X2	T49.5X3	T49.5X4	T49.5X5	T49.5X6
topical NEC	T49.0X1	T49.0X2	T49.0X3	T49.0X4	T49.0X5	T49.0X6
Adrenaline	T44.5X1	T44.5X2	T44.5X3	T44.5X4	T44.5X5	T44.5X6
Adrenalin — see Adrenaline						
Adrenergic NEC	T44.901	T44.902	T44.903	T44.904	T44.905	T44.906
blocking agent NEC	T44.8X1	T44.8X2	T44.8X3	T44.8X4	T44.8X5	T44.8X6
beta, heart	T44.7X1	T44.7X2	T44.7X3	T44.7X4	T44.7X5	T44.7X6
specified NEC	T44.991	T44.992	T44.993	T44.994	T44.995	T44.996
Adrenochrome						
(mono) semicarbazone	T46.991	T46.992	T46.993	T46.994	T46.995	T46.996
derivative	T46.991	T46.992	T46.993	T46.994	T46.995	T46.996
Adrenocorticotrophic hormone	T38.811	T38.812	T38.813	T38.814	T38.815	T38.816
Adrenocorticotrophin	T38.811	T38.812	T38.813	T38.814	T38.815	T38.816
Adriamycin	T45.1X1	T45.1X2	T45.1X3	T45.1X4	T45.1X5	T45.1X6
Aerosol spray NEC	T65.91	T65.92	T65.93	T65.94	—	—
Aerosporin	T36.8X1	T36.8X2	T36.8X3	T36.8X4	T36.8X5	T36.8X6
ENT agent	T49.6X1	T49.6X2	T49.6X3	T49.6X4	T49.6X5	T49.6X6
ophthalmic preparation	T49.5X1	T49.5X2	T49.5X3	T49.5X4	T49.5X5	T49.5X6
topical NEC	T49.0X1	T49.0X2	T49.0X3	T49.0X4	T49.0X5	T49.0X6
Aethusa cynapium	T62.2X1	T62.2X2	T62.2X3	T62.2X4	—	—
Afghanistan black	T40.711	T40.712	T40.713	T40.714	T40.715	T40.716
Aflatoxin	T64.01	T64.02	T64.03	T64.04	—	—
Afloqualone	T42.8X1	T42.8X2	T42.8X3	T42.8X4	T42.8X5	T42.8X6
African boxwood	T62.2X1	T62.2X2	T62.2X3	T62.2X4	—	—
Agar	T47.4X1	T47.4X2	T47.4X3	T47.4X4	T47.4X5	T47.4X6
Agonist						
predominantly						
alpha-adrenoreceptor	T44.4X1	T44.4X2	T44.4X3	T44.4X4	T44.4X5	T44.4X6
beta-adrenoreceptor	T44.5X1	T44.5X2	T44.5X3	T44.5X4	T44.5X5	T44.5X6
Agricultural agent NEC	T65.91	T65.92	T65.93	T65.94	—	—
Agrypnal	T42.3X1	T42.3X2	T42.3X3	T42.3X4	T42.3X5	T42.3X6
AHLG	T50.Z11	T50.Z12	T50.Z13	T50.Z14	T50.Z15	T50.Z16
Air contaminant(s), source/type NOS	T65.91	T65.92	T65.93	T65.94	—	—

◀ New   ◀ Revised   ~~deleted~~ Deleted

Substance	Poisoning, Accidental (Unintentional)	Poisoning, Intentional Self-Harm	Poisoning, Assault	Poisoning, Undetermined	Adverse Effect	Underdosing
Ajmaline	T46.2X1	T46.2X2	T46.2X3	T46.2X4	T46.2X5	T46.2X6
Akritoin	T37.8X1	T37.8X2	T37.8X3	T37.8X4	T37.8X5	T37.8X6
Akee	T62.1X1	T62.1X2	T62.1X3	T62.1X4	—	—
Akrinol	T49.0X1	T49.0X2	T49.0X3	T49.0X4	T49.0X5	T49.0X6
Alacepril	T46.4X1	T46.4X2	T46.4X3	T46.4X4	T46.4X5	T46.4X6
Alantolactone	T37.4X1	T37.4X2	T37.4X3	T37.4X4	T37.4X5	T37.4X6
Albamycin	T36.8X1	T36.8X2	T36.8X3	T36.8X4	T36.8X5	T36.8X6
Albendazole	T37.4X1	T37.4X2	T37.4X3	T37.4X4	T37.4X5	T37.4X6
Albumin						
bovine	T45.8X1	T45.8X2	T45.8X3	T45.8X4	T45.8X5	T45.8X6
human serum	T45.8X1	T45.8X2	T45.8X3	T45.8X4	T45.8X5	T45.8X6
salt-poor	T45.8X1	T45.8X2	T45.8X3	T45.8X4	T45.8X5	T45.8X6
normal human serum	T45.8X1	T45.8X2	T45.8X3	T45.8X4	T45.8X5	T45.8X6
Albuterol	T48.6X1	T48.6X2	T48.6X3	T48.6X4	T48.6X5	T48.6X6
Albutoin	T42.0X1	T42.0X2	T42.0X3	T42.0X4	T42.0X5	T42.0X6
Alclometasone	T49.0X1	T49.0X2	T49.0X3	T49.0X4	T49.0X5	T49.0X6
Alcohol	T51.91	T51.92	T51.93	T51.94	—	—
absolute	T51.0X1	T51.0X2	T51.0X3	T51.0X4		
beverage	T51.0X1	T51.0X2	T51.0X3	T51.0X4	—	—
allyl	T51.8X1	T51.8X2	T51.8X3	T51.8X4		
amyl	T51.3X1	T51.3X2	T51.3X3	T51.3X4		
antifreeze	T51.1X1	T51.1X2	T51.1X3	T51.1X4		
beverage	T51.0X1	T51.0X2	T51.0X3	T51.0X4		
butyl	T51.3X1	T51.3X2	T51.3X3	T51.3X4		
dehydrated	T51.0X1	T51.0X2	T51.0X3	T51.0X4		
beverage	T51.0X1	T51.0X2	T51.0X3	T51.0X4	—	—
denatured	T51.0X1	T51.0X2	T51.0X3	T51.0X4		
deterrent NEC	T50.6X1	T50.6X2	T50.6X3	T50.6X4	T50.6X5	T50.6X6
diagnostic (gastric function)	T50.8X1	T50.8X2	T50.8X3	T50.8X4	T50.8X5	T50.8X6
ethyl	T51.0X1	T51.0X2	T51.0X3	T51.0X4		
beverage	T51.0X1	T51.0X2	T51.0X3	T51.0X4	—	—
grain	T51.0X1	T51.0X2	T51.0X3	T51.0X4		
beverage	T51.0X1	T51.0X2	T51.0X3	T51.0X4	—	—
industrial	T51.0X1	T51.0X2	T51.0X3	T51.0X4		
isopropyl	T51.2X1	T51.2X2	T51.2X3	T51.2X4		
methyl	T51.1X1	T51.1X2	T51.1X3	T51.1X4		
preparation for consumption	T51.0X1	T51.0X2	T51.0X3	T51.0X4	—	—
propyl	T51.3X1	T51.3X2	T51.3X3	T51.3X4		
secondary	T51.2X1	T51.2X2	T51.2X3	T51.2X4		
radiator	T51.1X1	T51.1X2	T51.1X3	T51.1X4		
rubbing	T51.2X1	T51.2X2	T51.2X3	T51.2X4		
specified type NEC	T51.8X1	T51.8X2	T51.8X3	T51.8X4	—	—

Substance	Poisoning, Accidental (Unintentional)	Poisoning, Intentional Self-Harm	Poisoning, Assault	Poisoning, Undetermined	Adverse Effect	Underdosing
Alcohol *(Continued)*						
surgical	T51.0X1	T51.0X2	T51.0X3	T51.0X4	—	—
vapor (from any type of Alcohol)	T59.891	T59.892	T59.893	T59.894	—	—
wood	T51.1X1	T51.1X2	T51.1X3	T51.1X4		—
Alcuronium (chloride)	T48.1X1	T48.1X2	T48.1X3	T48.1X4	T48.1X5	T48.1X6
Aldactone	T50.0X1	T50.0X2	T50.0X3	T50.0X4	T50.0X5	T50.0X6
Aldesulfone sodium	T37.1X1	T37.1X2	T37.1X3	T37.1X4	T37.1X5	T37.1X6
Aldicarb	T60.0X1	T60.0X2	T60.0X3	T60.0X4	—	—
Aldomet	T46.5X1	T46.5X2	T46.5X3	T46.5X4	T46.5X5	T46.5X6
Aldosterone	T50.0X1	T50.0X2	T50.0X3	T50.0X4	T50.0X5	T50.0X6
Aldrin (dust)	T60.1X1	T60.1X2	T60.1X3	T60.1X4	—	—
Aleve — *see* Naproxen						
Alexitol sodium	T47.1X1	T47.1X2	T47.1X3	T47.1X4	T47.1X5	T47.1X6
Alfacalcidol	T45.2X1	T45.2X2	T45.2X3	T45.2X4	T45.2X5	T45.2X6
Alfadolone	T41.1X1	T41.1X2	T41.1X3	T41.1X4	T41.1X5	T41.1X6
Alfaxalone	T41.1X1	T41.1X2	T41.1X3	T41.1X4	T41.1X5	T41.1X6
Alfentanil	T40.411	T40.412	T40.413	T40.414	T40.415	T40.416
Alfuzosin (hydrochloride)	T44.8X1	T44.8X2	T44.8X3	T44.8X4	T44.8X5	T44.8X6
Algae (harmful) (toxin)	T65.821	T65.822	T65.823	T65.824	—	—
Algeldrate	T47.1X1	T47.1X2	T47.1X3	T47.1X4	T47.1X5	T47.1X6
Algin	T47.8X1	T47.8X2	T47.8X3	T47.8X4	T47.8X5	T47.8X6
Alglucerase	T45.3X1	T45.3X2	T45.3X3	T45.3X4	T45.3X5	T45.3X6
Alidase	T45.3X1	T45.3X2	T45.3X3	T45.3X4	T45.3X5	T45.3X6
Alimemazine	T43.3X1	T43.3X2	T43.3X3	T43.3X4	T43.3X5	T43.3X6
Aliphatic thiocyanates	T65.0X1	T65.0X2	T65.0X3	T65.0X4	—	—
Alizapride	T45.0X1	T45.0X2	T45.0X3	T45.0X4	T45.0X5	T45.0X6
Alkali (caustic)	T54.3X1	T54.3X2	T54.3X3	T54.3X4	—	—
Alkalizing agent NEC	T50.901	T50.902	T50.903	T50.904	T50.905	T50.906
Alkaline antiseptic solution (aromatic)	T49.6X1	T49.6X2	T49.6X3	T49.6X4	T49.6X5	T49.6X6
Alkalinizing agents (medicinal)	T50.901	T50.902	T50.903	T50.904	T50.905	T50.906
Alka-seltzer	T39.011	T39.012	T39.013	T39.014	T39.015	T39.016
Alkavervir	T46.5X1	T46.5X2	T46.5X3	T46.5X4	T46.5X5	T46.5X6
Alkonium (bromide)	T49.0X1	T49.0X2	T49.0X3	T49.0X4	T49.0X5	T49.0X6
Alkylating drug NEC	T45.1X1	T45.1X2	T45.1X3	T45.1X4	T45.1X5	T45.1X6
antimyeloproliferative	T45.1X1	T45.1X2	T45.1X3	T45.1X4	T45.1X5	T45.1X6
lymphatic	T45.1X1	T45.1X2	T45.1X3	T45.1X4	T45.1X5	T45.1X6
Alkylisocyanate	T65.0X1	T65.0X2	T65.0X3	T65.0X4	—	—
Allantoin	T49.411	T49.412	T49.413	T49.414	T49.415	T49.416
Allegron	T43.0X1	T43.0X2	T43.0X3	T43.0X4	T43.0X5	T43.0X6
Allethrin	T49.0X1	T49.0X2	T49.0X3	T49.0X4	T49.0X5	T49.0X6
Allobarbital	T42.3X1	T42.3X2	T42.3X3	T42.3X4	T42.3X5	T42.3X6

◀ New   ◀ Revised   ~~deleted~~ Deleted

TABLE OF DRUGS AND CHEMICALS

	External Cause (T-Code)					
Substance	Poisoning, Accidental (Unintentional)	Poisoning, Intentional Self-Harm	Poisoning, Assault	Poisoning, Undetermined	Adverse Effect	Underdosing
Allopurinol	T50.4X1	T50.4X2	T50.4X3	T50.4X4	T50.4X5	T50.4X6
Allyl						
alcohol	T51.8X1	T51.8X2	T51.8X3	T51.8X4	—	—
disulfide	T46.6X1	T46.6X2	T46.6X3	T46.6X4	T46.6X5	T46.6X6
Allylestrenol	T38.5X1	T38.5X2	T38.5X3	T38.5X4	T38.5X5	T38.5X6
Allylisopropylacetylurea	T42.6X1	T42.6X2	T42.6X3	T42.6X4	T42.6X5	T42.6X6
Allylisopropylmalonylurea	T42.3X1	T42.3X2	T42.3X3	T42.3X4	T42.3X5	T42.3X6
Allylthiourea	T49.3X1	T49.3X2	T49.3X3	T49.3X4	T49.3X5	T49.3X6
Allyltribromide	T42.6X1	T42.6X2	T42.6X3	T42.6X4	T42.6X5	T42.6X6
Allypropymal	T42.3X1	T42.3X2	T42.3X3	T42.3X4	T42.3X5	T42.3X6
Almagate	T47.1X1	T47.1X2	T47.1X3	T47.1X4	T47.1X5	T47.1X6
Almasilate	T47.1X1	T47.1X2	T47.1X3	T47.1X4	T47.1X5	T47.1X6
Almitrine	T50.7X1	T50.7X2	T50.7X3	T50.7X4	T50.7X5	T50.7X6
Aloes	T47.2X1	T47.2X2	T47.2X3	T47.2X4	T47.2X5	T47.2X6
Aloglutamol	T47.1X1	T47.1X2	T47.1X3	T47.1X4	T47.1X5	T47.1X6
Aloin	T47.2X1	T47.2X2	T47.2X3	T47.2X4	T47.2X5	T47.2X6
Aloxidone	T42.2X1	T42.2X2	T42.2X3	T42.2X4	T42.2X5	T42.2X6
Alpha						
acetyldigoxin	T46.0X1	T46.0X2	T46.0X3	T46.0X4	T46.0X5	T46.0X6
adrenergic blocking drug	T44.6X1	T44.6X2	T44.6X3	T44.6X4	T44.6X5	T44.6X6
amylase	T45.3X1	T45.3X2	T45.3X3	T45.3X4	T45.3X5	T45.3X6
tocoferol (acetate)	T45.2X1	T45.2X2	T45.2X3	T45.2X4	T45.2X5	T45.2X6
tocopherol	T45.2X1	T45.2X2	T45.2X3	T45.2X4	T45.2X5	T45.2X6
Alphadolone	T41.1X1	T41.1X2	T41.1X3	T41.1X4	T41.1X5	T41.1X6
Alphaprodine	T40.491	T40.492	T40.493	T40.494	T40.495	T40.496
Alphaxalone	T41.1X1	T41.1X2	T41.1X3	T41.1X4	T41.1X5	T41.1X6
Alprazolam	T42.4X1	T42.4X2	T42.4X3	T42.4X4	T42.4X5	T42.4X6
Alprenolol	T44.7X1	T44.7X2	T44.7X3	T44.7X4	T44.7X5	T44.7X6
Alprostadil	T46.7X1	T46.7X2	T46.7X3	T46.7X4	T46.7X5	T46.7X6
Alsactide	T38.811	T38.812	T38.813	T38.814	T38.815	T38.816
Alseroxylon	T46.5X1	T46.5X2	T46.5X3	T46.5X4	T46.5X5	T46.5X6
Alteplase	T45.611	T45.612	T45.613	T45.614	T45.615	T45.616
Altizide	T50.2X1	T50.2X2	T50.2X3	T50.2X4	T50.2X5	T50.2X6
Altretamine	T45.1X1	T45.1X2	T45.1X3	T45.1X4	T45.1X5	T45.1X6
Alum (medicinal)	T49.4X1	T49.4X2	T49.4X3	T49.4X4	T49.4X5	T49.4X6
nonmedicinal (ammonium) (potassium)	T56.891	T56.892	T56.893	T56.894	—	—
Aluminium, aluminum						
acetate	T49.2X1	T49.2X2	T49.2X3	T49.2X4	T49.2X5	T49.2X6
solution	T49.0X1	T49.0X2	T49.0X3	T49.0X4	T49.0X5	T49.0X6
aspirin	T39.011	T39.012	T39.013	T39.014	T39.015	T39.016
bis (acetylsalicylate)	T39.011	T39.012	T39.013	T39.014	T39.015	T39.016

	External Cause (T-Code)					
Substance	Poisoning, Accidental (Unintentional)	Poisoning, Intentional Self-Harm	Poisoning, Assault	Poisoning, Undetermined	Adverse Effect	Underdosing
Aluminium, aluminum (Continued)						
carbonate (gel, basic)	T47.1X1	T47.1X2	T47.1X3	T47.1X4	T47.1X5	T47.1X6
chlorhydroxide-complex	T47.1X1	T47.1X2	T47.1X3	T47.1X4	T47.1X5	T47.1X6
chloride	T49.2X1	T49.2X2	T49.2X3	T49.2X4	T49.2X5	T49.2X6
clofibrate	T46.6X1	T46.6X2	T46.6X3	T46.6X4	T46.6X5	T46.6X6
diacetate	T49.2X1	T49.2X2	T49.2X3	T49.2X4	T49.2X5	T49.2X6
glycinate	T47.1X1	T47.1X2	T47.1X3	T47.1X4	T47.1X5	T47.1X6
hydroxide (gel)	T47.1X1	T47.1X2	T47.1X3	T47.1X4	T47.1X5	T47.1X6
hydroxide-magnesium carb. gel	T47.1X1	T47.1X2	T47.1X3	T47.1X4	T47.1X5	T47.1X6
magnesium silicate	T47.1X1	T47.1X2	T47.1X3	T47.1X4	T47.1X5	T47.1X6
nicotinate	T46.7X1	T46.7X2	T46.7X3	T46.7X4	T46.7X5	T46.7X6
ointment (surgical) (topical)	T49.3X1	T49.3X2	T49.3X3	T49.3X4	T49.3X5	T49.3X6
phosphate	T47.1X1	T47.1X2	T47.1X3	T47.1X4	T47.1X5	T47.1X6
salicylate	T39.091	T39.092	T39.093	T39.094	T39.095	T39.096
silicate	T47.1X1	T47.1X2	T47.1X3	T47.1X4	T47.1X5	T47.1X6
sodium silicate	T47.1X1	T47.1X2	T47.1X3	T47.1X4	T47.1X5	T47.1X6
subacetate	T49.2X1	T49.2X2	T49.2X3	T49.2X4	T49.2X5	T49.2X6
sulfate	T49.0X1	T49.0X2	T49.0X3	T49.0X4	T49.0X5	T49.0X6
tannate	T47.6X1	T47.6X2	T47.6X3	T47.6X4	T47.6X5	T47.6X6
topical NEC	T49.3X1	T49.3X2	T49.3X3	T49.3X4	T49.3X5	T49.3X6
Alurate	T42.3X1	T42.3X2	T42.3X3	T42.3X4	T42.3X5	T42.3X6
Alverine	T44.3X1	T44.3X2	T44.3X3	T44.3X4	T44.3X5	T44.3X6
Alvodine	T40.2X1	T40.2X2	T40.2X3	T40.2X4	T40.2X5	T40.2X6
Amanita phalloides	T62.0X1	T62.0X2	T62.0X3	T62.0X4	—	—
Amanitine	T62.0X1	T62.0X2	T62.0X3	T62.0X4	—	—
Amantadine	T42.8X1	T42.8X2	T42.8X3	T42.8X4	T42.8X5	T42.8X6
Ambazone	T49.6X1	T49.6X2	T49.6X3	T49.6X4	T49.6X5	T49.6X6
Ambenonium (chloride)	T44.0X1	T44.0X2	T44.0X3	T44.0X4	T44.0X5	T44.0X6
Ambroxol	T48.4X1	T48.4X2	T48.4X3	T48.4X4	T48.4X5	T48.4X6
Ambuphylline	T48.6X1	T48.6X2	T48.6X3	T48.6X4	T48.6X5	T48.6X6
Ambutonium bromide	T44.3X1	T44.3X2	T44.3X3	T44.3X4	T44.3X5	T44.3X6
Amcinonide	T49.0X1	T49.0X2	T49.0X3	T49.0X4	T49.0X5	T49.0X6
Amdinocilline	T36.0X1	T36.0X2	T36.0X3	T36.0X4	T36.0X5	T36.0X6
Ametazole	T50.8X1	T50.8X2	T50.8X3	T50.8X4	T50.8X5	T50.8X6
Amethocaine	T41.3X1	T41.3X2	T41.3X3	T41.3X4	T41.3X5	T41.3X6
regional	T41.3X1	T41.3X2	T41.3X3	T41.3X4	T41.3X5	T41.3X6
spinal	T41.3X1	T41.3X2	T41.3X3	T41.3X4	T41.3X5	T41.3X6
Amethopterin	T45.1X1	T45.1X2	T45.1X3	T45.1X4	T45.1X5	T45.1X6
Amezinium metilsulfate	T44.991	T44.992	T44.993	T44.994	T44.995	T44.996
Amfebutamone	T43.291	T43.292	T43.293	T43.294	T43.295	T43.296
Amfepramone	T50.5X1	T50.5X2	T50.5X3	T50.5X4	T50.5X5	T50.5X6

◀ New ◀◀ Revised ~~deleted~~ Deleted

Substance	External Cause (T-Code)					
	Poisoning, Accidental (Unintentional)	Poisoning, Intentional Self-Harm	Poisoning, Assault	Poisoning, Undetermined	Adverse Effect	Underdosing
Amfetamine	T43.621	T43.622	T43.623	T43.624	T43.625	T43.626
Amfetaminil	T43.621	T43.622	T43.623	T43.624	T43.625	T43.626
Amfomycin	T36.8X1	T36.8X2	T36.8X3	T36.8X4	T36.8X5	T36.8X6
Amidefrine mesilate	T48.5X1	T48.5X2	T48.5X3	T48.5X4	T48.5X5	T48.5X6
Amidone	T40.3X1	T40.3X2	T40.3X3	T40.3X4	T40.3X5	T40.3X6
Amidopyrine	T39.2X1	T39.2X2	T39.2X3	T39.2X4	T39.2X5	T39.2X6
Amidotrizoate	T50.8X1	T50.8X2	T50.8X3	T50.8X4	T50.8X5	T50.8X6
Amiflamine	T43.1X1	T43.1X2	T43.1X3	T43.1X4	T43.1X5	T43.1X6
Amikacin	T36.5X1	T36.5X2	T36.5X3	T36.5X4	T36.5X5	T36.5X6
Amikhelline	T46.3X1	T46.3X2	T46.3X3	T46.3X4	T46.3X5	T46.3X6
Amiloride	T50.2X1	T50.2X2	T50.2X3	T50.2X4	T50.2X5	T50.2X6
Aminacrine	T49.0X1	T49.0X2	T49.0X3	T49.0X4	T49.0X5	T49.0X6
Amineptine	T43.011	T43.012	T43.013	T43.014	T43.015	T43.016
Aminitrozole	T37.3X1	T37.3X2	T37.3X3	T37.3X4	T37.3X5	T37.3X6
Aminoacetic acid (derivatives)	T50.3X1	T50.3X2	T50.3X3	T50.3X4	T50.3X5	T50.3X6
Amino acids	T50.3X1	T50.3X2	T50.3X3	T50.3X4	T50.3X5	T50.3X6
Aminoacridine	T49.0X1	T49.0X2	T49.0X3	T49.0X4	T49.0X5	T49.0X6
Aminobenzoic acid (-p)	T49.3X1	T49.3X2	T49.3X3	T49.3X4	T49.3X5	T49.3X6
4-Aminobutyric acid	T43.8X1	T43.8X2	T43.8X3	T43.8X4	T43.8X5	T43.8X6
Aminocaproic acid	T45.621	T45.622	T45.623	T45.624	T45.625	T45.626
Aminofenazone	T39.2X1	T39.2X2	T39.2X3	T39.2X4	T39.2X5	T39.2X6
Aminoethylisothiourium	T45.8X1	T45.8X2	T45.8X3	T45.8X4	T45.8X5	T45.8X6
Aminoglutethimide	T45.1X1	T45.1X2	T45.1X3	T45.1X4	T45.1X5	T45.1X6
Aminohippuric acid	T50.8X1	T50.8X2	T50.8X3	T50.8X4	T50.8X5	T50.8X6
Aminomethylbenzoic acid	T45.691	T45.692	T45.693	T45.694	T45.695	T45.696
Aminometradine	T50.2X1	T50.2X2	T50.2X3	T50.2X4	T50.2X5	T50.2X6
Aminopentamide	T44.3X1	T44.3X2	T44.3X3	T44.3X4	T44.3X5	T44.3X6
Aminophenazone	T39.2X1	T39.2X2	T39.2X3	T39.2X4	T39.2X5	T39.2X6
Aminophenol	T54.0X1	T54.0X2	T54.0X3	T54.0X4	—	—
4-Aminophenol derivatives	T39.1X1	T39.1X2	T39.1X3	T39.1X4	T39.1X5	T39.1X6
Aminophenylpyridone	T43.591	T43.592	T43.593	T43.594	T43.595	T43.596
Aminophylline	T48.6X1	T48.6X2	T48.6X3	T48.6X4	T48.6X5	T48.6X6
Aminopterin sodium	T45.1X1	T45.1X2	T45.1X3	T45.1X4	T45.1X5	T45.1X6
Aminopyrine	T39.2X1	T39.2X2	T39.2X3	T39.2X4	T39.2X5	T39.2X6
8-Aminoquinoline drugs	T37.2X1	T37.2X2	T37.2X3	T37.2X4	T37.2X5	T37.2X6
Aminorex	T50.5X1	T50.5X2	T50.5X3	T50.5X4	T50.5X5	T50.5X6
Aminosalicylic acid	T37.1X1	T37.1X2	T37.1X3	T37.1X4	T37.1X5	T37.1X6
Aminosalylum	T37.1X1	T37.1X2	T37.1X3	T37.1X4	T37.1X5	T37.1X6
Amiodarone	T46.2X1	T46.2X2	T46.2X3	T46.2X4	T46.2X5	T46.2X6
Amiphenazole	T50.7X1	T50.7X2	T50.7X3	T50.7X4	T50.7X5	T50.7X6
Amiquinsin	T46.5X1	T46.5X2	T46.5X3	T46.5X4	T46.5X5	T46.5X6
Amisometradine	T50.2X1	T50.2X2	T50.2X3	T50.2X4	T50.2X5	T50.2X6

Substance	External Cause (T-Code)					
	Poisoning, Accidental (Unintentional)	Poisoning, Intentional Self-Harm	Poisoning, Assault	Poisoning, Undetermined	Adverse Effect	Underdosing
Amisulpride	T43.591	T43.592	T43.593	T43.594	T43.595	T43.596
Amitriptyline	T43.021	T43.022	T43.023	T43.024	T43.025	T43.026
Amitriptylinoxide	T43.021	T43.022	T43.023	T43.024	T43.025	T43.026
Amlexanox	T48.6X1	T48.6X2	T48.6X3	T48.6X4	T48.6X5	T48.6X6
Ammonia (fumes) (gas) (vapor)	T59.891	T59.892	T59.893	T59.894	—	—
aromatic spirit	T48.991	T48.992	T48.993	T48.994	T48.995	T48.996
liquid (household)	T54.3X1	T54.3X2	T54.3X3	T54.3X4	—	—
Ammoniated mercury	T49.0X1	T49.0X2	T49.0X3	T49.0X4	T49.0X5	T49.0X6
Ammonium						
acid tartrate	T49.5X1	T49.5X2	T49.5X3	T49.5X4	T49.5X5	T49.5X6
bromide	T42.6X1	T42.6X2	T42.6X3	T42.6X4	T42.6X5	T42.6X6
carbonate	T54.3X1	T54.3X2	T54.3X3	T54.3X4	—	—
chloride	T50.991	T50.992	T50.993	T50.994	T50.995	T50.996
expectorant	T48.4X1	T48.4X2	T48.4X3	T48.4X4	T48.4X5	T48.4X6
compounds (household) NEC	T54.3X1	T54.3X2	T54.3X3	T54.3X4	—	—
fumes (any usage)	T59.891	T59.892	T59.893	T59.894	—	—
industrial	T54.3X1	T54.3X2	T54.3X3	T54.3X4	—	—
ichthyosulronate	T49.4X1	T49.4X2	T49.4X3	T49.4X4	T49.4X5	T49.4X6
mandelate	T37.91	T37.92	T37.93	T37.94	T37.95	T37.96
sulfamate	T60.3X1	T60.3X2	T60.3X3	T60.3X4	—	—
sulfonate resin	T47.8X1	T47.8X2	T47.8X3	T47.8X4	T47.8X5	T47.8X6
Amobarbital (sodium)	T42.3X1	T42.3X2	T42.3X3	T42.3X4	T42.3X5	T42.3X6
Amodiaquine	T37.2X1	T37.2X2	T37.2X3	T37.2X4	T37.2X5	T37.2X6
Amopyroquin(e)	T37.2X1	T37.2X2	T37.2X3	T37.2X4	T37.2X5	T37.2X6
Amoxapine	T43.011	T43.012	T43.013	T43.014	T43.015	T43.016
Amoxicillin	T36.0X1	T36.0X2	T36.0X3	T36.0X4	T36.0X5	T36.0X6
Amperozide	T43.591	T43.592	T43.593	T43.594	T43.595	T43.596
Amphenidone	T43.591	T43.592	T43.593	T43.594	T43.595	T43.596
Amphetamine NEC	T43.621	T43.622	T43.623	T43.624	T43.625	T43.626
Amphomycin	T36.8X1	T36.8X2	T36.8X3	T36.8X4	T36.8X5	T36.8X6
Amphotalide	T37.4X1	T37.4X2	T37.4X3	T37.4X4	T37.4X5	T37.4X6
Amphotericin B	T36.7X1	T36.7X2	T36.7X3	T36.7X4	T36.7X5	T36.7X6
topical	T49.0X1	T49.0X2	T49.0X3	T49.0X4	T49.0X5	T49.0X6
Ampicillin	T36.0X1	T36.0X2	T36.0X3	T36.0X4	T36.0X5	T36.0X6
Amprotropine	T44.3X1	T44.3X2	T44.3X3	T44.3X4	T44.3X5	T44.3X6
Amsacrine	T45.1X1	T45.1X2	T45.1X3	T45.1X4	T45.1X5	T45.1X6
Amygdaline	T62.2X1	T62.2X2	T62.2X3	T62.2X4	—	—
Amyl						
acetate	T52.8X1	T52.8X2	T52.8X3	T52.8X4	—	—
vapor	T59.891	T59.892	T59.893	T59.894	—	—
alcohol	T51.3X1	T51.3X2	T51.3X3	T51.3X4	—	—
chloride	T53.6X1	T53.6X2	T53.6X3	T53.6X4	—	—

◀ New ◀ Revised ~~deleted~~ Deleted

	External Cause (T-Code)					
Substance	Poisoning, Accidental (Unintentional)	Poisoning, Intentional Self-Harm	Poisoning, Assault	Poisoning, Undetermined	Adverse Effect	Underdosing
Amyl *(Continued)*						
formate	T52.8X1	T52.8X2	T52.8X3	T52.8X4	—	—
nitrite	T46.3X1	T46.3X2	T46.3X3	T46.3X4	T46.3X5	T46.3X6
propionate	T65.891	T65.892	T65.893	T65.894	—	—
Amylase	T47.5X1	T47.5X2	T47.5X3	T47.5X4	T47.5X5	T47.5X6
Amyleine, regional	T41.3X1	T41.3X2	T41.3X3	T41.3X4	T41.3X5	T41.3X6
Amylene						
dichloride	T53.6X1	T53.6X2	T53.6X3	T53.6X4	—	—
hydrate	T51.3X1	T51.3X2	T51.3X3	T51.3X4	—	—
Amylmetacresol	T49.6X1	T49.6X2	T49.6X3	T49.6X4	T49.6X5	T49.6X6
Amylobarbitone	T42.3X1	T42.3X2	T42.3X3	T42.3X4	T42.3X5	T42.3X6
Amylocaine, regional	T41.3X1	T41.3X2	T41.3X3	T41.3X4	T41.3X5	T41.3X6
infiltration (subcutaneous)	T41.3X1	T41.3X2	T41.3X3	T41.3X4	T41.3X5	T41.3X6
nerve block (peripheral) (plexus)	T41.3X1	T41.3X2	T41.3X3	T41.3X4	T41.3X5	T41.3X6
spinal	T41.3X1	T41.3X2	T41.3X3	T41.3X4	T41.3X5	T41.3X6
topical (surface)	T41.3X1	T41.3X2	T41.3X3	T41.3X4	T41.3X5	T41.3X6
Amylopectin	T47.6X1	T47.6X2	T47.6X3	T47.6X4	T47.6X5	T47.6X6
Amytal (sodium)	T42.3X1	T42.3X2	T42.3X3	T42.3X4	T42.3X5	T42.3X6
Anabolic steroid	T38.7X1	T38.7X2	T38.7X3	T38.7X4	T38.7X5	T38.7X6
Analeptic NEC	T50.7X1	T50.7X2	T50.7X3	T50.7X4	T50.7X5	T50.7X6
Analgesic	T39.91	T39.92	T39.93	T39.94	T39.95	T39.96
anti-inflammatory NEC	T39.91	T39.92	T39.93	T39.94	T39.95	T39.96
propionic acid derivative	T39.311	T39.312	T39.313	T39.314	T39.315	T39.316
antirheumatic NEC	T39.4X1	T39.4X2	T39.4X3	T39.4X4	T39.4X5	T39.4X6
aromatic NEC	T39.1X1	T39.1X2	T39.1X3	T39.1X4	T39.1X5	T39.1X6
narcotic NEC	T40.601	T40.602	T40.603	T40.604	T40.605	T40.606
combination	T40.601	T40.602	T40.603	T40.604	T40.605	T40.606
obstetric	T40.601	T40.602	T40.603	T40.604	T40.605	T40.606
non-narcotic NEC	T39.91	T39.92	T39.93	T39.94	T39.95	T39.96
combination	T39.91	T39.92	T39.93	T39.94	T39.95	T39.96
pyrazole	T39.2X1	T39.2X2	T39.2X3	T39.2X4	T39.2X5	T39.2X6
specified NEC	T39.8X1	T39.8X2	T39.8X3	T39.8X4	T39.8X5	T39.8X6
Analgin	T39.2X1	T39.2X2	T39.2X3	T39.2X4	T39.2X5	T39.2X6
Anamirta cocculus	T62.1X1	T62.1X2	T62.1X3	T62.1X4	—	—
Ancillin	T36.0X1	T36.0X2	T36.0X3	T36.0X4	T36.0X5	T36.0X6
Ancrod	T45.691	T45.692	T45.693	T45.694	T45.695	T45.696
Androgen	T38.7X1	T38.7X2	T38.7X3	T38.7X4	T38.7X5	T38.7X6
Androgen-estrogen mixture	T38.7X1	T38.7X2	T38.7X3	T38.7X4	T38.7X5	T38.7X6
Androstalone	T38.7X1	T38.7X2	T38.7X3	T38.7X4	T38.7X5	T38.7X6
Androstanolone	T38.7X1	T38.7X2	T38.7X3	T38.7X4	T38.7X5	T38.7X6
Androsterone	T38.7X1	T38.7X2	T38.7X3	T38.7X4	T38.7X5	T38.7X6

	External Cause (T-Code)					
Substance	Poisoning, Accidental (Unintentional)	Poisoning, Intentional Self-Harm	Poisoning, Assault	Poisoning, Undetermined	Adverse Effect	Underdosing
Anemone pulsatilla	T62.2X1	T62.2X2	T62.2X3	T62.2X4	—	—
Anesthesia						
caudal	T41.3X1	T41.3X2	T41.3X3	T41.3X4	T41.3X5	T41.3X6
endotracheal	T41.0X1	T41.0X2	T41.0X3	T41.0X4	T41.0X5	T41.0X6
epidural	T41.3X1	T41.3X2	T41.3X3	T41.3X4	T41.3X5	T41.3X6
inhalation	T41.0X1	T41.0X2	T41.0X3	T41.0X4	T41.0X5	T41.0X6
local	T41.3X1	T41.3X2	T41.3X3	T41.3X4	T41.3X5	T41.3X6
mucosal	T41.3X1	T41.3X2	T41.3X3	T41.3X4	T41.3X5	T41.3X6
muscle relaxation	T48.1X1	T48.1X2	T48.1X3	T48.1X4	T48.1X5	T48.1X6
nerve blocking	T41.3X1	T41.3X2	T41.3X3	T41.3X4	T41.3X5	T41.3X6
plexus blocking	T41.3X1	T41.3X2	T41.3X3	T41.3X4	T41.3X5	T41.3X6
potentiated	T41.201	T41.202	T41.203	T41.204	T41.205	T41.206
rectal	T41.201	T41.202	T41.203	T41.204	T41.205	T41.206
general	T41.201	T41.202	T41.203	T41.204	T41.205	T41.206
local	T41.3X1	T41.3X2	T41.3X3	T41.3X4	T41.3X5	T41.3X6
regional	T41.3X1	T41.3X2	T41.3X3	T41.3X4	T41.3X5	T41.3X6
surface	T41.3X1	T41.3X2	T41.3X3	T41.3X4	T41.3X5	T41.3X6
Anesthetic NEC—*see also* Anesthesia	T41.41	T41.42	T41.43	T41.44	T41.45	T41.46
with muscle relaxant	T41.201	T41.202	T41.203	T41.204	T41.205	T41.206
general	T41.201	T41.202	T41.203	T41.204	T41.205	T41.206
local	T41.3X1	T41.3X2	T41.3X3	T41.3X4	T41.3X5	T41.3X6
gaseous NEC	T41.0X1	T41.0X2	T41.0X3	T41.0X4	T41.0X5	T41.0X6
general NEC	T41.201	T41.202	T41.203	T41.204	T41.205	T41.206
halogenated hydrocarbon derivatives NEC	T41.0X1	T41.0X2	T41.0X3	T41.0X4	T41.0X5	T41.0X6
infiltration NEC	T41.3X1	T41.3X2	T41.3X3	T41.3X4	T41.3X5	T41.3X6
intravenous NEC	T41.1X1	T41.1X2	T41.1X3	T41.1X4	T41.1X5	T41.1X6
local NEC	T41.3X1	T41.3X2	T41.3X3	T41.3X4	T41.3X5	T41.3X6
rectal	T41.201	T41.202	T41.203	T41.204	T41.205	T41.206
general	T41.201	T41.202	T41.203	T41.204	T41.205	T41.206
local	T41.3X1	T41.3X2	T41.3X3	T41.3X4	T41.3X5	T41.3X6
regional NEC	T41.3X1	T41.3X2	T41.3X3	T41.3X4	T41.3X5	T41.3X6
spinal NEC	T41.3X1	T41.3X2	T41.3X3	T41.3X4	T41.3X5	T41.3X6
thiobarbiturate	T41.1X1	T41.1X2	T41.1X3	T41.1X4	T41.1X5	T41.1X6
topical	T41.3X1	T41.3X2	T41.3X3	T41.3X4	T41.3X5	T41.3X6
Aneurine	T45.2X1	T45.2X2	T45.2X3	T45.2X4	T45.2X5	T45.2X6
Angio-Conray	T50.8X1	T50.8X2	T50.8X3	T50.8X4	T50.8X5	T50.8X6
Angiotensin	T44.5X1	T44.5X2	T44.5X3	T44.5X4	T44.5X5	T44.5X6
Angiotensinamide	T44.991	T44.992	T44.993	T44.994	T44.995	T44.996
Anhydrohydroxy-progesterone	T38.5X1	T38.5X2	T38.5X3	T38.5X4	T38.5X5	T38.5X6
Anhydron	T50.2X1	T50.2X2	T50.2X3	T50.2X4	T50.2X5	T50.2X6
Anileridine	T40.491	T40.492	T40.493	T40.494	T40.495	T40.496

◀ New ◀ Revised ~~deleted~~ Deleted

	External Cause (T-Code)					
Substance	Poisoning, Accidental (Unintentional)	Poisoning, Intentional Self-Harm	Poisoning, Assault	Poisoning, Undetermined	Adverse Effect	Underdosing
Aniline (dye) (liquid)	T65.3X1	T65.3X2	T65.3X3	T65.3X4	—	—
analgesic	T39.1X1	T39.1X2	T39.1X3	T39.1X4	T39.1X5	T39.1X6
derivatives, therapeutic NEC	T39.1X1	T39.1X2	T39.1X3	T39.1X4	T39.1X5	T39.1X6
vapor	T65.3X1	T65.3X2	T65.3X3	T65.3X4	—	—
Anise oil	T47.5X1	T47.5X2	T47.5X3	T47.5X4	T47.5X5	T47.5X6
Aniscoropine	T44.3X1	T44.3X2	T44.3X3	T44.3X4	T44.3X5	T44.3X6
Anisidine	T65.3X1	T65.3X2	T65.3X3	T65.3X4	—	—
Anisindione	T45.511	T45.512	T45.513	T45.514	T45.515	T45.516
Anisotropine methyl-bromide	T44.3X1	T44.3X2	T44.3X3	T44.3X4	T44.3X5	T44.3X6
Anistreplase	T45.611	T45.612	T45.613	T45.614	T45.615	T45.616
Anorexiant (central)	T50.5X1	T50.5X2	T50.5X3	T50.5X4	T50.5X5	T50.5X6
Anorexic agents	T50.5X1	T50.5X2	T50.5X3	T50.5X4	T50.5X5	T50.5X6
Ansamycin	T36.6X1	T36.6X2	T36.6X3	T36.6X4	T36.6X5	T36.6X6
Ant (bite) (sting)	T63.421	T63.422	T63.423	T63.424	—	—
Antabuse	T50.6X1	T50.6X2	T50.6X3	T50.6X4	T50.6X5	T50.6X6
Ant poison — see Insecticide						
Antacid NEC	T47.1X1	T47.1X2	T47.1X3	T47.1X4	T47.1X5	T47.1X6
Antagonist						
Aldosterone	T50.0X1	T50.0X2	T50.0X3	T50.0X4	T50.0X5	T50.0X6
alpha-adrenoreceptor	T44.6X1	T44.6X2	T44.6X3	T44.6X4	T44.6X5	T44.6X6
anticoagulant	T45.7X1	T45.7X2	T45.7X3	T45.7X4	T45.7X5	T45.7X6
beta-adrenoreceptor	T44.7X1	T44.7X2	T44.7X3	T44.7X4	T44.7X5	T44.7X6
extrapyramidal NEC	T44.3X1	T44.3X2	T44.3X3	T44.3X4	T44.3X5	T44.3X6
folic acid	T45.1X1	T45.1X2	T45.1X3	T45.1X4	T45.1X5	T45.1X6
H2 receptor	T47.0X1	T47.0X2	T47.0X3	T47.0X4	T47.0X5	T47.0X6
heavy metal	T45.8X1	T45.8X2	T45.8X3	T45.8X4	T45.8X5	T45.8X6
narcotic analgesic	T50.7X1	T50.7X2	T50.7X3	T50.7X4	T50.7X5	T50.7X6
opiate	T50.7X1	T50.7X2	T50.7X3	T50.7X4	T50.7X5	T50.7X6
pyrimidine	T45.1X1	T45.1X2	T45.1X3	T45.1X4	T45.1X5	T45.1X6
serotonin	T46.5X1	T46.5X2	T46.5X3	T46.5X4	T46.5X5	T46.5X6
Antazolin(e)	T45.0X1	T45.0X2	T45.0X3	T45.0X4	T45.0X5	T45.0X6
Anterior pituitary hormone NEC	T38.811	T38.812	T38.813	T38.814	T38.815	T38.816
Anthelmintic NEC	T37.4X1	T37.4X2	T37.4X3	T37.4X4	T37.4X5	T37.4X6
Anthiolimine	T37.4X1	T37.4X2	T37.4X3	T37.4X4	T37.4X5	T37.4X6
Anthralin	T49.4X1	T49.4X2	T49.4X3	T49.4X4	T49.4X5	T49.4X6
Anthramycin	T45.1X1	T45.1X2	T45.1X3	T45.1X4	T45.1X5	T45.1X6
Antiadrenergic NEC	T44.8X1	T44.8X2	T44.8X3	T44.8X4	T44.8X5	T44.8X6
Antiallergic NEC	T45.0X1	T45.0X2	T45.0X3	T45.0X4	T45.0X5	T45.0X6
Anti-anemic (drug) (preparation)	T45.8X1	T45.8X2	T45.8X3	T45.8X4	T45.8X5	T45.8X6
Antiandrogen NEC	T38.6X1	T38.6X2	T38.6X3	T38.6X4	T38.6X5	T38.6X6
Antianxiety drug NEC	T43.501	T43.502	T43.503	T43.504	T43.505	T43.506
Antiaris toxicaria	T65.891	T65.892	T65.893	T65.894	—	—

	External Cause (T-Code)					
Substance	Poisoning, Accidental (Unintentional)	Poisoning, Intentional Self-Harm	Poisoning, Assault	Poisoning, Undetermined	Adverse Effect	Underdosing
Antiarteriosclerotic drug	T46.6X1	T46.6X2	T46.6X3	T46.6X4	T46.6X5	T46.6X6
Antiasthmatic drug NEC	T48.6X1	T48.6X2	T48.6X3	T48.6X4	T48.6X5	T48.6X6
Antibiotic NEC	T36.91	T36.92	T36.93	T36.94	T36.95	T36.96
aminoglycoside	T36.5X1	T36.5X2	T36.5X3	T36.5X4	T36.5X5	T36.5X6
anticancer	T45.1X1	T45.1X2	T45.1X3	T45.1X4	T45.1X5	T45.1X6
antifungal	T36.7X1	T36.7X2	T36.7X3	T36.7X4	T36.7X5	T36.7X6
antimycobacterial	T36.5X1	T36.5X2	T36.5X3	T36.5X4	T36.5X5	T36.5X6
antineoplastic	T45.1X1	T45.1X2	T45.1X3	T45.1X4	T45.1X5	T45.1X6
cephalosporin (group)	T36.1X1	T36.1X2	T36.1X3	T36.1X4	T36.1X5	T36.1X6
chloramphenicol (group)	T36.2X1	T36.2X2	T36.2X3	T36.2X4	T36.2X5	T36.2X6
ENT	T49.6X1	T49.6X2	T49.6X3	T49.6X4	T49.6X5	T49.6X6
eye	T49.5X1	T49.5X2	T49.5X3	T49.5X4	T49.5X5	T49.5X6
fungicidal (local)	T49.0X1	T49.0X2	T49.0X3	T49.0X4	T49.0X5	T49.0X6
intestinal	T36.8X1	T36.8X2	T36.8X3	T36.8X4	T36.8X5	T36.8X6
b-lactam NEC	T36.1X1	T36.1X2	T36.1X3	T36.1X4	T36.1X5	T36.1X6
local	T49.0X1	T49.0X2	T49.0X3	T49.0X4	T49.0X5	T49.0X6
macrolides	T36.3X1	T36.3X2	T36.3X3	T36.3X4	T36.3X5	T36.3X6
polypeptide	T36.8X1	T36.8X2	T36.8X3	T36.8X4	T36.8X5	T36.8X6
specified NEC	T36.8X1	T36.8X2	T36.8X3	T36.8X4	T36.8X5	T36.8X6
tetracycline (group)	T36.4X1	T36.4X2	T36.4X3	T36.4X4	T36.4X5	T36.4X6
throat	T49.6X1	T49.6X2	T49.6X3	T49.6X4	T49.6X5	T49.6X6
Anticancer agents NEC	T45.1X1	T45.1X2	T45.1X3	T45.1X4	T45.1X5	T45.1X6
Anticholesterolemic drug NEC	T46.6X1	T46.6X2	T46.6X3	T46.6X4	T46.6X5	T46.6X6
Anticholinergic NEC	T44.3X1	T44.3X2	T44.3X3	T44.3X4	T44.3X5	T44.3X6
Anticholinesterase	T44.0X1	T44.0X2	T44.0X3	T44.0X4	T44.0X5	T44.0X6
organophosphorus	T44.0X1	T44.0X2	T44.0X3	T44.0X4	T44.0X5	T44.0X6
insecticide	T60.0X1	T60.0X2	T60.0X3	T60.0X4	—	—
nerve gas	T59.891	T59.892	T59.893	T59.894	—	—
reversible	T44.0X1	T44.0X2	T44.0X3	T44.0X4	T44.0X5	T44.0X6
ophthalmological	T49.5X1	T49.5X2	T49.5X3	T49.5X4	T49.5X5	T49.5X6
Anticoagulant NEC	T45.511	T45.512	T45.513	T45.514	T45.515	T45.516
Antagonist	T45.7X1	T45.7X2	T45.7X3	T45.7X4	T45.7X5	T45.7X6
Anti-common-cold drug NEC	T48.5X1	T48.5X2	T48.5X3	T48.5X4	T48.5X5	T48.5X6
Anticonvulsant	T42.71	T42.72	T42.73	T42.74	T42.75	T42.76
barbiturate	T42.3X1	T42.3X2	T42.3X3	T42.3X4	T42.3X5	T42.3X6
combination (with barbiturate)	T42.3X1	T42.3X2	T42.3X3	T42.3X4	T42.3X5	T42.3X6
hydantoin	T42.0X1	T42.0X2	T42.0X3	T42.0X4	T42.0X5	T42.0X6
hypnotic NEC	T42.6X1	T42.6X2	T42.6X3	T42.6X4	T42.6X5	T42.6X6
oxazolidinedione	T42.2X1	T42.2X2	T42.2X3	T42.2X4	T42.2X5	T42.2X6
pyrimidinedione	T42.6X1	T42.6X2	T42.6X3	T42.6X4	T42.6X5	T42.6X6
specified NEC	T42.6X1	T42.6X2	T42.6X3	T42.6X4	T42.6X5	T42.6X6
succinimide	T42.2X1	T42.2X2	T42.2X3	T42.2X4	T42.2X5	T42.2X6

◀ New ◀ Revised ~~deleted~~ Deleted

TABLE OF DRUGS AND CHEMICALS

Substance	Poisoning, Accidental (Unintentional)	Poisoning, Intentional Self-Harm	Poisoning, Assault	Poisoning, Undetermined	Adverse Effect	Underdosing
Anti-D immunoglobulin (human)	T50.Z11	T50.Z12	T50.Z13	T50.Z14	T50.Z15	T50.Z16
Antidepressant NEC	T43.201	T43.202	T43.203	T43.204	T43.205	T43.206
monoamine oxidase inhibitor	T43.1X1	T43.1X2	T43.1X3	T43.1X4	T43.1X5	T43.1X6
selective serotonin norepinephrine reuptake inhibitor	T43.211	T43.212	T43.213	T43.214	T43.215	T43.216
selective serotonin reuptake inhibitor	T43.221	T43.222	T43.223	T43.224	T43.225	T43.226
specified NEC	T43.291	T43.292	T43.293	T43.294	T43.295	T43.296
tetracyclic	T43.021	T43.022	T43.023	T43.024	T43.025	T43.026
triazolopyridine	T43.221	T43.222	T43.223	T43.224	T43.225	T43.226
tricyclic	T43.011	T43.012	T43.013	T43.014	T43.015	T43.016
Antidiabetic NEC	T38.3X1	T38.3X2	T38.3X3	T38.3X4	T38.3X5	T38.3X6
biguanide	T38.3X1	T38.3X2	T38.3X3	T38.3X4	T38.3X5	T38.3X6
and sulfonyl combined	T38.3X1	T38.3X2	T38.3X3	T38.3X4	T38.3X5	T38.3X6
combined	T38.3X1	T38.3X2	T38.3X3	T38.3X4	T38.3X5	T38.3X6
sulfonylurea	T38.3X1	T38.3X2	T38.3X3	T38.3X4	T38.3X5	T38.3X6
Antidiarrheal drug NEC	T47.6X1	T47.6X2	T47.6X3	T47.6X4	T47.6X5	T47.6X6
absorbent	T47.6X1	T47.6X2	T47.6X3	T47.6X4	T47.6X5	T47.6X6
Antidiphtheria serum	T50.Z11	T50.Z12	T50.Z13	T50.Z14	T50.Z15	T50.Z16
Antidiuretic hormone	T38.891	T38.892	T38.893	T38.894	T38.895	T38.896
Antidote NEC	T50.6X1	T50.6X2	T50.6X3	T50.6X4	T50.6X5	T50.6X6
heavy metal	T45.8X1	T45.8X2	T45.8X3	T45.8X4	T45.8X5	T45.8X6
Antidysrhythmic NEC	T46.2X1	T46.2X2	T46.2X3	T46.2X4	T46.2X5	T46.2X6
Antiemetic drug	T45.0X1	T45.0X2	T45.0X3	T45.0X4	T45.0X5	T45.0X6
Antiepilepsy agent	T42.71	T42.72	T42.73	T42.74	T42.75	T42.76
combination	T42.5X1	T42.5X2	T42.5X3	T42.5X4	T42.5X5	T42.5X6
mixed	T42.5X1	T42.5X2	T42.5X3	T42.5X4	T42.5X5	T42.5X6
specified, NEC	T42.6X1	T42.6X2	T42.6X3	T42.6X4	T42.6X5	T42.6X6
Antiestrogen NEC	T38.6X1	T38.6X2	T38.6X3	T38.6X4	T38.6X5	T38.6X6
Antifertility pill	T38.4X1	T38.4X2	T38.4X3	T38.4X4	T38.4X5	T38.4X6
Antifibrinolytic drug	T45.621	T45.622	T45.623	T45.624	T45.625	T45.626
Antifilarial drug	T37.4X1	T37.4X2	T37.4X3	T37.4X4	T37.4X5	T37.4X6
Antiflatulent	T47.5X1	T47.5X2	T47.5X3	T47.5X4	T47.5X5	T47.5X6
Antifreeze	T65.91	T65.92	T65.93	T65.94	—	—
alcohol	T51.1X1	T51.1X2	T51.1X3	T51.1X4	—	—
ethylene glycol	T51.8X1	T51.8X2	T51.8X3	T51.8X4	—	—
Antifungal						
antibiotic (systemic)	T36.7X1	T36.7X2	T36.7X3	T36.7X4	T36.7X5	T36.7X6
anti-infective NEC	T37.91	T37.92	T37.93	T37.94	T37.95	T37.96
disinfectant, local	T49.0X1	T49.0X2	T49.0X3	T49.0X4	T49.0X5	T49.0X6
nonmedicinal (spray)	T60.3X1	T60.3X2	T60.3X3	T60.3X4		
topical	T49.0X1	T49.0X2	T49.0X3	T49.0X4	T49.0X5	T49.0X6

Substance	Poisoning, Accidental (Unintentional)	Poisoning, Intentional Self-Harm	Poisoning, Assault	Poisoning, Undetermined	Adverse Effect	Underdosing
Anti-gastric-secretion drug NEC	T47.1X1	T47.1X2	T47.1X3	T47.1X4	T47.1X5	T47.1X6
Antigonadotrophin NEC	T38.6X1	T38.6X2	T38.6X3	T38.6X4	T38.6X5	T38.6X6
Antihallucinogen	T43.501	T43.502	T43.503	T43.504	T43.505	T43.506
Antihelmintics	T37.4X1	T37.4X2	T37.4X3	T37.4X4	T37.4X5	T37.4X6
Antihemophilic						
factor	T45.8X1	T45.8X2	T45.8X3	T45.8X4	T45.8X5	T45.8X6
fraction	T45.8X1	T45.8X2	T45.8X3	T45.8X4	T45.8X5	T45.8X6
globulin concentrate	T45.7X1	T45.7X2	T45.7X3	T45.7X4	T45.7X5	T45.7X6
human plasma	T45.8X1	T45.8X2	T45.8X3	T45.8X4	T45.8X5	T45.8X6
plasma, dried	T45.7X1	T45.7X2	T45.7X3	T45.7X4	T45.7X5	T45.7X6
Antihemorrhoidal preparation	T49.2X1	T49.2X2	T49.2X3	T49.2X4	T49.2X5	T49.2X6
Antiheparin drug	T45.7X1	T45.7X2	T45.7X3	T45.7X4	T45.7X5	T45.7X6
Antihistamine	T45.0X1	T45.0X2	T45.0X3	T45.0X4	T45.0X5	T45.0X6
Antihookworm drug	T37.4X1	T37.4X2	T37.4X3	T37.4X4	T37.4X5	T37.4X6
Anti-human lymphocytic globulin	T50.Z11	T50.Z12	T50.Z13	T50.Z14	T50.Z15	T50.Z16
Antihyperlipidemic drug	T46.6X1	T46.6X2	T46.6X3	T46.6X4	T46.6X5	T46.6X6
Antihypertensive drug NEC	T46.5X1	T46.5X2	T46.5X3	T46.5X4	T46.5X5	T46.5X6
Anti-infective NEC	T37.91	T37.92	T37.93	T37.94	T37.95	T37.96
anthelmintic	T37.4X1	T37.4X2	T37.4X3	T37.4X4	T37.4X5	T37.4X6
antibiotics	T36.91	T36.92	T36.93	T36.94	T36.95	T36.96
specified NEC	T36.8X1	T36.8X2	T36.8X3	T36.8X4	T36.8X5	T36.8X6
antimalarial	T37.2X1	T37.2X2	T37.2X3	T37.2X4	T37.2X5	T37.2X6
antimycobacterial NEC	T37.1X1	T37.1X2	T37.1X3	T37.1X4	T37.1X5	T37.1X6
antibiotics	T36.5X1	T36.5X2	T36.5X3	T36.5X4	T36.5X5	T36.5X6
antiprotozoal NEC	T37.3X1	T37.3X2	T37.3X3	T37.3X4	T37.3X5	T37.3X6
blood	T37.2X1	T37.2X2	T37.2X3	T37.2X4	T37.2X5	T37.2X6
antiviral	T37.5X1	T37.5X2	T37.5X3	T37.5X4	T37.5X5	T37.5X6
arsenical	T37.8X1	T37.8X2	T37.8X3	T37.8X4	T37.8X5	T37.8X6
bismuth, local	T49.0X1	T49.0X2	T49.0X3	T49.0X4	T49.0X5	T49.0X6
ENT	T49.6X1	T49.6X2	T49.6X3	T49.6X4	T49.6X5	T49.6X6
eye NEC	T49.5X1	T49.5X2	T49.5X3	T49.5X4	T49.5X5	T49.5X6
heavy metals NEC	T37.8X1	T37.8X2	T37.8X3	T37.8X4	T37.8X5	T37.8X6
local NEC	T49.0X1	T49.0X2	T49.0X3	T49.0X4	T49.0X5	T49.0X6
specified NEC	T49.0X1	T49.0X2	T49.0X3	T49.0X4	T49.0X5	T49.0X6
mixed	T37.91	T37.92	T37.93	T37.94	T37.95	T37.96
ophthalmic preparation	T49.5X1	T49.5X2	T49.5X3	T49.5X4	T49.5X5	T49.5X6
topical NEC	T49.0X1	T49.0X2	T49.0X3	T49.0X4	T49.0X5	T49.0X6
Anti-inflammatory drug NEC	T49.0X1	T49.0X2	T49.0X3	T49.0X4	T49.0X5	T49.0X6
local	T49.0X1	T49.0X2	T49.0X3	T49.0X4	T49.0X5	T49.0X6
nonsteroidal NEC	T39.391	T39.392	T39.393	T39.394	T39.395	T39.396
propionic acid derivative	T39.311	T39.312	T39.313	T39.314	T39.315	T39.316
specified NEC	T39.391	T39.392	T39.393	T39.394	T39.395	T39.396

◄ New   ◄ Revised   ~~deleted~~ Deleted

Substance	Poisoning, Accidental (Unintentional)	Poisoning, Intentional Self-Harm	Poisoning, Assault	Poisoning, Undetermined	Adverse Effect	Underdosing
Antikaluretic	T50.3X1	T50.3X2	T50.3X3	T50.3X4	T50.3X5	T50.3X6
Antiknock (tetraethyl lead)	T56.0X1	T56.0X2	T56.0X3	T56.0X4	—	—
Antilipemic drug NEC	T46.6X1	T46.6X2	T46.6X3	T46.6X4	T46.6X5	T46.6X6
Antimalarial	T37.2X1	T37.2X2	T37.2X3	T37.2X4	T37.2X5	T37.2X6
prophylactic NEC	T37.2X1	T37.2X2	T37.2X3	T37.2X4	T37.2X5	T37.2X6
pyrimidine derivative	T37.2X1	T37.2X2	T37.2X3	T37.2X4	T37.2X5	T37.2X6
Antimetabolite	T45.1X1	T45.1X2	T45.1X3	T45.1X4	T45.1X5	T45.1X6
Antimitotic agent	T45.1X1	T45.1X2	T45.1X3	T45.1X4	T45.1X5	T45.1X6
Antimony (compounds) (vapor) NEC	T56.891	T56.892	T56.893	T56.894	—	—
anti-infectives	T37.8X1	T37.8X2	T37.8X3	T37.8X4	T37.8X5	T37.8X6
dimercaptosuccinate	T37.3X1	T37.3X2	T37.3X3	T37.3X4	T37.3X5	T37.3X6
hydride	T56.891	T56.892	T56.893	T56.894	—	—
pesticide (vapor)	T60.8X1	T60.8X2	T60.8X3	T60.8X4	—	—
potassium (sodium) tartrate	T37.8X1	T37.8X2	T37.8X3	T37.8X4	T37.8X5	T37.8X6
sodium dimercaptosuccinate	T37.3X1	T37.3X2	T37.3X3	T37.3X4	T37.3X5	T37.3X6
tartrated	T37.8X1	T37.8X2	T37.8X3	T37.8X4	T37.8X5	T37.8X6
Antimuscarinic NEC	T44.3X1	T44.3X2	T44.3X3	T44.3X4	T44.3X5	T44.3X6
Antimycobacterial drug NEC	T37.1X1	T37.1X2	T37.1X3	T37.1X4	T37.1X5	T37.1X6
antibiotics	T36.5X1	T36.5X2	T36.5X3	T36.5X4	T36.5X5	T36.5X6
combination	T37.1X1	T37.1X2	T37.1X3	T37.1X4	T37.1X5	T37.1X6
Antinausea drug	T45.0X1	T45.0X2	T45.0X3	T45.0X4	T45.0X5	T45.0X6
Antinematode drug	T37.4X1	T37.4X2	T37.4X3	T37.4X4	T37.4X5	T37.4X6
Antineoplastic NEC	T45.1X1	T45.1X2	T45.1X3	T45.1X4	T45.1X5	T45.1X6
alkaloidal	T45.1X1	T45.1X2	T45.1X3	T45.1X4	T45.1X5	T45.1X6
antibiotics	T45.1X1	T45.1X2	T45.1X3	T45.1X4	T45.1X5	T45.1X6
combination	T45.1X1	T45.1X2	T45.1X3	T45.1X4	T45.1X5	T45.1X6
estrogen	T38.5X1	T38.5X2	T38.5X3	T38.5X4	T38.5X5	T38.5X6
steroid	T38.7X1	T38.7X2	T38.7X3	T38.7X4	T38.7X5	T38.7X6
Antiparasitic drug (systemic)	T37.91	T37.92	T37.93	T37.94	T37.95	T37.96
local	T49.0X1	T49.0X2	T49.0X3	T49.0X4	T49.0X5	T49.0X6
specified NEC	T37.8X1	T37.8X2	T37.8X3	T37.8X4	T37.8X5	T37.8X6
Antiparkinsonism drug NEC	T42.8X1	T42.8X2	T42.8X3	T42.8X4	T42.8X5	T42.8X6
Antiperspirant NEC	T49.2X1	T49.2X2	T49.2X3	T49.2X4	T49.2X5	T49.2X6
Antiphlogistic NEC	T39.4X1	T39.4X2	T39.4X3	T39.4X4	T39.4X5	T39.4X6
Antiplatyhelmintic drug	T37.4X1	T37.4X2	T37.4X3	T37.4X4	T37.4X5	T37.4X6
Antiprotozoal drug NEC	T37.3X1	T37.3X2	T37.3X3	T37.3X4	T37.3X5	T37.3X6
blood	T37.2X1	T37.2X2	T37.2X3	T37.2X4	T37.2X5	T37.2X6
local	T49.0X1	T49.0X2	T49.0X3	T49.0X4	T49.0X5	T49.0X6
Antipruritic drug NEC	T49.1X1	T49.1X2	T49.1X3	T49.1X4	T49.1X5	T49.1X6
Antipsychotic drug	T43.501	T43.502	T43.503	T43.504	T43.505	T43.506
specified NEC	T43.591	T43.592	T43.593	T43.594	T43.595	T43.596

Substance	Poisoning, Accidental (Unintentional)	Poisoning, Intentional Self-Harm	Poisoning, Assault	Poisoning, Undetermined	Adverse Effect	Underdosing
Antipyretic	T39.91	T39.92	T39.93	T39.94	T39.95	T39.96
specified NEC	T39.8X1	T39.8X2	T39.8X3	T39.8X4	T39.8X5	T39.8X6
Antipyrine	T39.2X1	T39.2X2	T39.2X3	T39.2X4	T39.2X5	T39.2X6
Antirabies hyperimmune serum	T50.Z11	T50.Z12	T50.Z13	T50.Z14	T50.Z15	T50.Z16
Antirheumatic NEC	T39.4X1	T39.4X2	T39.4X3	T39.4X4	T39.4X5	T39.4X6
Antirigidity drug NEC	T42.8X1	T42.8X2	T42.8X3	T42.8X4	T42.8X5	T42.8X6
Antischistosomal drug	T37.4X1	T37.4X2	T37.4X3	T37.4X4	T37.4X5	T37.4X6
Antiscorpion sera	T50.Z11	T50.Z12	T50.Z13	T50.Z14	T50.Z15	T50.Z16
Antiseborrheics	T49.4X1	T49.4X2	T49.4X3	T49.4X4	T49.4X5	T49.4X6
Antiseptics (external) (medicinal)	T49.0X1	T49.0X2	T49.0X3	T49.0X4	T49.0X5	T49.0X6
Antistine	T45.0X1	T45.0X2	T45.0X3	T45.0X4	T45.0X5	T45.0X6
Antitapeworm drug	T37.4X1	T37.4X2	T37.4X3	T37.4X4	T37.4X5	T37.4X6
Antitetanus immunoglobulin	T50.Z11	T50.Z12	T50.Z13	T50.Z14	T50.Z15	T50.Z16
Antithrombotic	T45.521	T45.522	T45.523	T45.524	T45.525	T45.526
Antithyroid drug NEC	T38.2X1	T38.2X2	T38.2X3	T38.2X4	T38.2X5	T38.2X6
Antitoxin	T50.Z11	T50.Z12	T50.Z13	T50.Z14	T50.Z15	T50.Z16
diphtheria	T50.Z11	T50.Z12	T50.Z13	T50.Z14	T50.Z15	T50.Z16
gas gangrene	T50.Z11	T50.Z12	T50.Z13	T50.Z14	T50.Z15	T50.Z16
tetanus	T50.Z11	T50.Z12	T50.Z13	T50.Z14	T50.Z15	T50.Z16
Antitoxin, any	T50.901	T50.902	T50.903	T50.904	T50.905	T50.906
Antitrichomonal drug	T37.3X1	T37.3X2	T37.3X3	T37.3X4	T37.3X5	T37.3X6
Antituberculars	T37.1X1	T37.1X2	T37.1X3	T37.1X4	T37.1X5	T37.1X6
antibiotics	T36.5X1	T36.5X2	T36.5X3	T36.5X4	T36.5X5	T36.5X6
Antitussive NEC	T48.3X1	T48.3X2	T48.3X3	T48.3X4	T48.3X5	T48.3X6
codeine mixture	T40.2X1	T40.2X2	T40.2X3	T40.2X4	T40.2X5	T40.2X6
opiate	T40.2X1	T40.2X2	T40.2X3	T40.2X4	T40.2X5	T40.2X6
Antivaricose drug	T46.8X1	T46.8X2	T46.8X3	T46.8X4	T46.8X5	T46.8X6
Antivenin, antivenom (sera)	T50.Z11	T50.Z12	T50.Z13	T50.Z14	T50.Z15	T50.Z16
crotaline	T50.Z11	T50.Z12	T50.Z13	T50.Z14	T50.Z15	T50.Z16
spider bite	T50.Z11	T50.Z12	T50.Z13	T50.Z14	T50.Z15	T50.Z16
Antivertigo drug	T45.0X1	T45.0X2	T45.0X3	T45.0X4	T45.0X5	T45.0X6
Antiviral drug NEC	T37.5X1	T37.5X2	T37.5X3	T37.5X4	T37.5X5	T37.5X6
eye	T49.5X1	T49.5X2	T49.5X3	T49.5X4	T49.5X5	T49.5X6
Antiwhipworm drug	T37.4X1	T37.4X2	T37.4X3	T37.4X4	T37.4X5	T37.4X6
Ant poisons — see Pesticides						
Antrol — see also by specific chemical substance	T60.91	T60.92	T60.93	T60.94	—	—
fungicide	T60.91	T60.92	T60.93	T60.94	—	—
ANTU (alpha naphthylthiourea)	T60.4X1	T60.4X2	T60.4X3	T60.4X4	—	—
Apalcillin	T36.0X1	T36.0X2	T36.0X3	T36.0X4	T36.0X5	T36.0X6
APC	T48.5X1	T48.5X2	T48.5X3	T48.5X4	T48.5X5	T48.5X6
Aplonidine	T44.4X1	T44.4X2	T44.4X3	T44.4X4	T44.4X5	T44.4X6
Apomorphine	T47.7X1	T47.7X2	T47.7X3	T47.7X4	T47.7X5	T47.7X6

◄ New ◄ Revised ~~deleted~~ Deleted

TABLE OF DRUGS AND CHEMICALS

Substance	Poisoning, Accidental (Unintentional)	Poisoning, Intentional Self-Harm	Poisoning, Assault	Poisoning, Undetermined	Adverse Effect	Underdosing
Appetite depressants, central	T50.5X1	T50.5X2	T50.5X3	T50.5X4	T50.5X5	T50.5X6
Apraclonidine (hydrochloride)	T44.4X1	T44.4X2	T44.4X3	T44.4X4	T44.4X5	T44.4X6
Apresoline	T46.5X1	T46.5X2	T46.5X3	T46.5X4	T46.5X5	T46.5X6
Aprindine	T46.2X1	T46.2X2	T46.2X3	T46.2X4	T46.2X5	T46.2X6
Aprobarbital	T42.3X1	T42.3X2	T42.3X3	T42.3X4	T42.3X5	T42.3X6
Apronalide	T42.6X1	T42.6X2	T42.6X3	T42.6X4	T42.6X5	T42.6X6
Aprotinin	T45.621	T45.622	T45.623	T45.624	T45.625	T45.626
Aptocaine	T41.3X1	T41.3X2	T41.3X3	T41.3X4	T41.3X5	T41.3X6
Aqua fortis	T54.2X1	T54.2X2	T54.2X3	T54.2X4	—	—
Ara-A	T37.5X1	T37.5X2	T37.5X3	T37.5X4	T37.5X5	T37.5X6
Ara-C	T45.1X1	T45.1X2	T45.1X3	T45.1X4	T45.1X5	T45.1X6
Arachis oil	T49.3X1	T49.3X2	T49.3X3	T49.3X4	T49.3X5	T49.3X6
cathartic	T47.4X1	T47.4X2	T47.4X3	T47.4X4	T47.4X5	T47.4X6
Aralen	T37.2X1	T37.2X2	T37.2X3	T37.2X4	T37.2X5	T37.2X6
Arecoline	T44.1X1	T44.1X2	T44.1X3	T44.1X4	T44.1X5	T44.1X6
Arginine	T50.991	T50.992	T50.993	T50.994	T50.995	T50.996
glutamate	T50.991	T50.992	T50.993	T50.994	T50.995	T50.996
Argyrol	T49.0X1	T49.0X2	T49.0X3	T49.0X4	T49.0X5	T49.0X6
ENT agent	T49.6X1	T49.6X2	T49.6X3	T49.6X4	T49.6X5	T49.6X6
ophthalmic preparation	T49.5X1	T49.5X2	T49.5X3	T49.5X4	T49.5X5	T49.5X6
Aristocort	T38.0X1	T38.0X2	T38.0X3	T38.0X4	T38.0X5	T38.0X6
ENT agent	T49.6X1	T49.6X2	T49.6X3	T49.6X4	T49.6X5	T49.6X6
ophthalmic preparation	T49.5X1	T49.5X2	T49.5X3	T49.5X4	T49.5X5	T49.5X6
topical NEC	T49.0X1	T49.0X2	T49.0X3	T49.0X4	T49.0X5	T49.0X6
Aromatics, corrosive	T54.1X1	T54.1X2	T54.1X3	T54.1X4	—	—
disinfectants	T54.1X1	T54.1X2	T54.1X3	T54.1X4	—	—
Arsenate of lead	T57.0X1	T57.0X2	T57.0X3	T57.0X4	—	—
herbicide	T57.0X1	T57.0X2	T57.0X3	T57.0X4	—	—
Arsenic, arsenicals (compounds) (dust) (vapor) NEC	T57.0X1	T57.0X2	T57.0X3	T57.0X4	—	—
anti-infectives	T37.8X1	T37.8X2	T37.8X3	T37.8X4	T37.8X5	T37.8X6
pesticide (dust) (fumes)	T57.0X1	T57.0X2	T57.0X3	T57.0X4	—	—
Arsine (gas)	T57.0X1	T57.0X2	T57.0X3	T57.0X4	—	—
Arsphenamine (silver)	T37.8X1	T37.8X2	T37.8X3	T37.8X4	T37.8X5	T37.8X6
Arsthinol	T37.3X1	T37.3X2	T37.3X3	T37.3X4	T37.3X5	T37.3X6
Artane	T44.3X1	T44.3X2	T44.3X3	T44.3X4	T44.3X5	T44.3X6
Arthropod (venomous) NEC	T63.481	T63.482	T63.483	T63.484	—	—
Articaine	T41.3X1	T41.3X2	T41.3X3	T41.3X4	T41.3X5	T41.3X6
Asbestos	T57.8X1	T57.8X2	T57.8X3	T57.8X4	—	—
Ascaridole	T37.4X1	T37.4X2	T37.4X3	T37.4X4	T37.4X5	T37.4X6
Ascorbic acid	T45.2X1	T45.2X2	T45.2X3	T45.2X4	T45.2X5	T45.2X6
Asiaticoside	T49.0X1	T49.0X2	T49.0X3	T49.0X4	T49.0X5	T49.0X6

Substance	Poisoning, Accidental (Unintentional)	Poisoning, Intentional Self-Harm	Poisoning, Assault	Poisoning, Undetermined	Adverse Effect	Underdosing
Asparaginase	T45.1X1	T45.1X2	T45.1X3	T45.1X4	T45.1X5	T45.1X6
Aspidium (oleoresin)	T37.4X1	T37.4X2	T37.4X3	T37.4X4	T37.4X5	T37.4X6
Aspirin (aluminum) (soluble)	T39.011	T39.012	T39.013	T39.014	T39.015	T39.016
Aspoxicillin	T36.0X1	T36.0X2	T36.0X3	T36.0X4	T36.0X5	T36.0X6
Astemizole	T45.0X1	T45.0X2	T45.0X3	T45.0X4	T45.0X5	T45.0X6
Astringent (local)	T49.2X1	T49.2X2	T49.2X3	T49.2X4	T49.2X5	T49.2X6
specified NEC	T49.2X1	T49.2X2	T49.2X3	T49.2X4	T49.2X5	T49.2X6
Astromicin	T36.5X1	T36.5X2	T36.5X3	T36.5X4	T36.5X5	T36.5X6
Ataractic drug NEC	T43.501	T43.502	T43.503	T43.504	T43.505	T43.506
Atenolol	T44.7X1	T44.7X2	T44.7X3	T44.7X4	T44.7X5	T44.7X6
Atonia drug, intestinal	T47.4X1	T47.4X2	T47.4X3	T47.4X4	T47.4X5	T47.4X6
Atophan	T50.4X1	T50.4X2	T50.4X3	T50.4X4	T50.4X5	T50.4X6
Atracurium besilate	T48.1X1	T48.1X2	T48.1X3	T48.1X4	T48.1X5	T48.1X6
Atropine	T44.3X1	T44.3X2	T44.3X3	T44.3X4	T44.3X5	T44.3X6
derivative	T44.3X1	T44.3X2	T44.3X3	T44.3X4	T44.3X5	T44.3X6
methonitrate	T44.3X1	T44.3X2	T44.3X3	T44.3X4	T44.3X5	T44.3X6
Attapulgite	T47.6X1	T47.6X2	T47.6X3	T47.6X4	T47.6X5	T47.6X6
Attenuvax	T50.991	T50.992	T50.993	T50.994	T50.995	T50.996
Auramine	T65.891	T65.892	T65.893	T65.894	—	—
dye	T65.6X1	T65.6X2	T65.6X3	T65.6X4	—	—
fungicide	T60.3X1	T60.3X2	T60.3X3	T60.3X4	—	—
Auranofin	T39.4X1	T39.4X2	T39.4X3	T39.4X4	T39.4X5	T39.4X6
Aurantiin	T46.991	T46.992	T46.993	T46.994	T46.995	T46.996
Aureomycin	T36.4X1	T36.4X2	T36.4X3	T36.4X4	T36.4X5	T36.4X6
ophthalmic preparation	T49.5X1	T49.5X2	T49.5X3	T49.5X4	T49.5X5	T49.5X6
topical NEC	T49.0X1	T49.0X2	T49.0X3	T49.0X4	T49.0X5	T49.0X6
Aurothioglucose	T39.4X1	T39.4X2	T39.4X3	T39.4X4	T39.4X5	T39.4X6
Aurothioglycanide	T39.4X1	T39.4X2	T39.4X3	T39.4X4	T39.4X5	T39.4X6
Aurothiomalate sodium	T39.4X1	T39.4X2	T39.4X3	T39.4X4	T39.4X5	T39.4X6
Aurotioprol	T39.4X1	T39.4X2	T39.4X3	T39.4X4	T39.4X5	T39.4X6
Automobile fuel	T52.0X1	T52.0X2	T52.0X3	T52.0X4	—	—
Autonomic nervous system agent NEC	T44.901	T44.902	T44.903	T44.904	T44.905	T44.906
Avlosulfon	T37.1X1	T37.1X2	T37.1X3	T37.1X4	T37.1X5	T37.1X6
Avomine	T42.6X1	T42.6X2	T42.6X3	T42.6X4	T42.6X5	T42.6X6
Axerophthol	T45.2X1	T45.2X2	T45.2X3	T45.2X4	T45.2X5	T45.2X6
Azacitidine	T45.1X1	T45.1X2	T45.1X3	T45.1X4	T45.1X5	T45.1X6
Azacyclonol	T43.591	T43.592	T43.593	T43.594	T43.595	T43.596
Azadirachta	T60.2X1	T60.2X2	T60.2X3	T60.2X4	—	—
Azanidazole	T37.3X1	T37.3X2	T37.3X3	T37.3X4	T37.3X5	T37.3X6
Azapetine	T46.7X1	T46.7X2	T46.7X3	T46.7X4	T46.7X5	T46.7X6
Azapropazone	T39.2X1	T39.2X2	T39.2X3	T39.2X4	T39.2X5	T39.2X6

◀ New ◀ Revised ~~deleted~~ Deleted

Substance	Poisoning, Accidental (Unintentional)	Poisoning, Intentional Self-Harm	Poisoning, Assault	Poisoning, Undetermined	Adverse Effect	Underdosing
Azaribine	T45.1X1	T45.1X2	T45.1X3	T45.1X4	T45.1X5	T45.1X6
Azaserine	T45.1X1	T45.1X2	T45.1X3	T45.1X4	T45.1X5	T45.1X6
Azatadine	T45.0X1	T45.0X2	T45.0X3	T45.0X4	T45.0X5	T45.0X6
Azatepa	T45.1X1	T45.1X2	T45.1X3	T45.1X4	T45.1X5	T45.1X6
Azathioprine	T45.1X1	T45.1X2	T45.1X3	T45.1X4	T45.1X5	T45.1X6
Azelaic acid	T49.0X1	T49.0X2	T49.0X3	T49.0X4	T49.0X5	T49.0X6
Azelastine	T45.0X1	T45.0X2	T45.0X3	T45.0X4	T45.0X5	T45.0X6
Azidocillin	T36.0X1	T36.0X2	T36.0X3	T36.0X4	T36.0X5	T36.0X6
Azidothymidine	T37.5X1	T37.5X2	T37.5X3	T37.5X4	T37.5X5	T37.5X6
Azinphos (ethyl) (methyl)	T60.0X1	T60.0X2	T60.0X3	T60.0X4	—	—
Aziridine (chelating)	T54.1X1	T54.1X2	T54.1X3	T54.1X4	—	—
Azithromycin	T36.3X1	T36.3X2	T36.3X3	T36.3X4	T36.3X5	T36.3X6
Azlocillin	T36.01	T36.02	T36.03	T36.04	T36.05	T36.06
Azobenzene smoke	T65.3X1	T65.3X2	T65.3X3	T65.3X4	—	—
acaricide	T60.8X1	T60.8X2	T60.8X3	T60.8X4	—	—
Azosulfamide	T37.0X1	T37.0X2	T37.0X3	T37.0X4	T37.0X5	T37.0X6
AZT	T37.5X1	T37.5X2	T37.5X3	T37.5X4	T37.5X5	T37.5X6
Aztreonam	T36.1X1	T36.1X2	T36.1X3	T36.1X4	T36.1X5	T36.1X6
Azulfidine	T37.0X1	T37.0X2	T37.0X3	T37.0X4	T37.0X5	T37.0X6
Azuresin	T50.8X1	T50.8X2	T50.8X3	T50.8X4	T50.8X5	T50.8X6
B						
Bacampicillin	T36.0X1	T36.0X2	T36.0X3	T36.0X4	T36.0X5	T36.0X6
Bacillus						
lactobacillus	T47.8X1	T47.8X2	T47.8X3	T47.8X4	T47.8X5	T47.8X6
subtilis	T47.6X1	T47.6X2	T47.6X3	T47.6X4	T47.6X5	T47.6X6
Bacimycin	T49.0X1	T49.0X2	T49.0X3	T49.0X4	T49.0X5	T49.0X6
ophthalmic preparation	T49.5X1	T49.5X2	T49.5X3	T49.5X4	T49.5X5	T49.5X6
Bacitracin zinc	T49.0X1	T49.0X2	T49.0X3	T49.0X4	T49.0X5	T49.0X6
with neomycin	T49.0X1	T49.0X2	T49.0X3	T49.0X4	T49.0X5	T49.0X6
ENT agent	T49.6X1	T49.6X2	T49.6X3	T49.6X4	T49.6X5	T49.6X6
ophthalmic preparation	T49.5X1	T49.5X2	T49.5X3	T49.5X4	T49.5X5	T49.5X6
topical NEC	T49.0X1	T49.0X2	T49.0X3	T49.0X4	T49.0X5	T49.0X6
Baclofen	T42.8X1	T42.8X2	T42.8X3	T42.8X4	T42.8X5	T42.8X6
Baking soda	T50.991	T50.992	T50.993	T50.994	T50.995	T50.996
BAL	T45.8X1	T45.8X2	T45.8X3	T45.8X4	T45.8X5	T45.8X6
Bambuterol	T48.6X1	T48.6X2	T48.6X3	T48.6X4	T48.6X5	T48.6X6
Bamethan (sulfate)	T46.7X1	T46.7X2	T46.7X3	T46.7X4	T46.7X5	T46.7X6
Bamifylline	T48.6X1	T48.6X2	T48.6X3	T48.6X4	T48.6X5	T48.6X6
Bamipine	T45.0X1	T45.0X2	T45.0X3	T45.0X4	T45.0X5	T45.0X6
Baneberry — see Actaea spicata						
Banewort — see Belladonna						

Substance	Poisoning, Accidental (Unintentional)	Poisoning, Intentional Self-Harm	Poisoning, Assault	Poisoning, Undetermined	Adverse Effect	Underdosing
Barbenyl	T42.3X1	T42.3X2	T42.3X3	T42.3X4	T42.3X5	T42.3X6
Barbexaclone	T42.6X1	T42.6X2	T42.6X3	T42.6X4	T42.6X5	T42.6X6
Barbital	T42.3X1	T42.3X2	T42.3X3	T42.3X4	T42.3X5	T42.3X6
sodium	T42.3X1	T42.3X2	T42.3X3	T42.3X4	T42.3X5	T42.3X6
Barbitone	T42.3X1	T42.3X2	T42.3X3	T42.3X4	T42.3X5	T42.3X6
Barbiturate NEC	T42.3X1	T42.3X2	T42.3X3	T42.3X4	T42.3X5	T42.3X6
with tranquilizer	T42.3X1	T42.3X2	T42.3X3	T42.3X4	T42.3X5	T42.3X6
anesthetic (intravenous)	T41.1X1	T41.1X2	T41.1X3	T41.1X4	T41.1X5	T41.1X6
Barium (carbonate) (chloride) (sulfite)	T57.8X1	T57.8X2	T57.8X3	T57.8X4	—	—
diagnostic agent	T50.8X1	T50.8X2	T50.8X3	T50.8X4	T50.8X5	T50.8X6
pesticide	T60.4X1	T60.4X2	T60.4X3	T60.4X4	—	—
rodenticide	T60.4X1	T60.4X2	T60.4X3	T60.4X4	—	—
sulfate (medicinal)	T50.8X1	T50.8X2	T50.8X3	T50.8X4	T50.8X5	T50.8X6
Barrier cream	T49.3X1	T49.3X2	T49.3X3	T49.3X4	T49.3X5	T49.3X6
Basic fuchsin	T49.0X1	T49.0X2	T49.0X3	T49.0X4	T49.0X5	T49.0X6
Battery acid or fluid	T54.2X1	T54.2X2	T54.2X3	T54.2X4	—	—
Bay rum	T51.8X1	T51.8X2	T51.8X3	T51.8X4	—	—
BCG (vaccine)	T50.A91	T50.A92	T50.A93	T50.A94	T50.A95	T50.A96
BCNU	T45.1X1	T45.1X2	T45.1X3	T45.1X4	T45.1X5	T45.1X6
Bearsfoot	T62.2X1	T62.2X2	T62.2X3	T62.2X4	—	—
Beclamide	T42.6X1	T42.6X2	T42.6X3	T42.6X4	T42.6X5	T42.6X6
Beclomethasone	T44.5X1	T44.5X2	T44.5X3	T44.5X4	T44.5X5	T44.5X6
Bee (sting) (venom)	T63.441	T63.442	T63.443	T63.444	—	—
Befunolol	T49.5X1	T49.5X2	T49.5X3	T49.5X4	T49.5X5	T49.5X6
Bekanamycin	T36.5X1	T36.5X2	T36.5X3	T36.5X4	T36.5X5	T36.5X6
Belladonna — see also Nightshade						
alkaloids	T44.3X1	T44.3X2	T44.3X3	T44.3X4	T44.3X5	T44.3X6
extract	T44.3X1	T44.3X2	T44.3X3	T44.3X4	T44.3X5	T44.3X6
herb	T44.3X1	T44.3X2	T44.3X3	T44.3X4	T44.3X5	T44.3X6
Bemegride	T50.7X1	T50.7X2	T50.7X3	T50.7X4	T50.7X5	T50.7X6
Benactyzine	T44.3X1	T44.3X2	T44.3X3	T44.3X4	T44.3X5	T44.3X6
Benadryl	T45.0X1	T45.0X2	T45.0X3	T45.0X4	T45.0X5	T45.0X6
Benaprizine	T44.3X1	T44.3X2	T44.3X3	T44.3X4	T44.3X5	T44.3X6
Benazepril	T46.4X1	T46.4X2	T46.4X3	T46.4X4	T46.4X5	T46.4X6
Bencyclane	T46.7X1	T46.7X2	T46.7X3	T46.7X4	T46.7X5	T46.7X6
Bendazol	T46.3X1	T46.3X2	T46.3X3	T46.3X4	T46.3X5	T46.3X6
Bendrofluazide	T50.2X1	T50.2X2	T50.2X3	T50.2X4	T50.2X5	T50.2X6
Bendroflumethiazide	T50.2X1	T50.2X2	T50.2X3	T50.2X4	T50.2X5	T50.2X6
Benemid	T50.4X1	T50.4X2	T50.4X3	T50.4X4	T50.4X5	T50.4X6
Benethamine penicillin	T36.0X1	T36.0X2	T36.0X3	T36.0X4	T36.0X5	T36.0X6
Benisone	T49.0X1	T49.0X2	T49.0X3	T49.0X4	T49.0X5	T49.0X6

TABLE OF DRUGS AND CHEMICALS

Substance	External Cause (T-Code)					
	Poisoning, Accidental (Unintentional)	Poisoning, Intentional Self-Harm	Poisoning, Assault	Poisoning, Undetermined	Adverse Effect	Underdosing
Benexate	T47.1X1	T47.1X2	T47.1X3	T47.1X4	T47.1X5	T47.1X6
Benfluorex	T46.6X1	T46.6X2	T46.6X3	T46.6X4	T46.6X5	T46.6X6
Benfotiamine	T45.2X1	T45.2X2	T45.2X4	T45.2X4	T45.2X5	T45.2X6
Benomyl	T60.0X1	T60.0X2	T60.0X3	T60.0X4	—	—
Benoquin	T49.8X1	T49.8X2	T49.8X3	T49.8X4	T49.8X5	T49.8X6
Benoxinate	T41.3X1	T41.3X2	T41.3X3	T41.3X4	T41.3X5	T41.3X6
Benperidol	T43.4X1	T43.4X2	T43.4X3	T43.4X4	T43.4X5	T43.4X6
Benproperine	T48.3X1	T48.3X2	T48.3X3	T48.3X4	T48.3X5	T48.3X6
Benserazide	T42.8X1	T42.8X2	T42.8X3	T42.8X4	T42.8X5	T42.8X6
Bentazepam	T42.4X1	T42.4X2	T42.4X3	T42.4X4	T42.4X5	T42.4X6
Bentiromide	T50.8X1	T50.8X2	T50.8X3	T50.8X4	T50.8X5	T50.8X6
Bentonite	T49.3X1	T49.3X2	T49.3X3	T49.3X4	T49.3X5	T49.3X6
Benzalbutyramide	T46.6X1	T46.6X2	T46.6X3	T46.6X4	T46.6X5	T46.6X6
Benzalkonium (chloride)	T49.0X1	T49.0X2	T49.0X3	T49.0X4	T49.0X5	T49.0X6
ophthalmic preparation	T49.5X1	T49.5X2	T49.5X3	T49.5X4	T49.5X5	T49.5X6
Benzamine	T41.3X1	T41.3X2	T41.3X3	T41.3X4	T41.3X5	T41.3X6
lactate	T49.1X1	T49.1X2	T49.1X3	T49.1X4	T49.1X5	T49.1X6
Benzamidosalicylate (calcium)	T37.1X1	T37.1X2	T37.1X3	T37.1X4	T37.1X5	T37.1X6
Benzamphetamine	T50.5X1	T50.5X2	T50.5X3	T50.5X4	T50.5X5	T50.5X6
Benzapril hydrochloride	T46.5X1	T46.5X2	T46.5X3	T46.5X4	T46.5X5	T46.5X6
Benzathine benzylpenicillin	T36.0X1	T36.0X2	T36.0X3	T36.0X4	T36.0X5	T36.0X6
Benzathine penicillin	T36.0X1	T36.0X2	T36.0X3	T36.0X4	T36.0X5	T36.0X6
Benzatropine	T42.8X1	T42.8X2	T42.8X3	T42.8X4	T42.8X5	T42.8X6
Benzbromarone	T50.4X1	T50.4X2	T50.4X3	T50.4X4	T50.4X5	T50.4X6
Benzcarbimine	T45.1X1	T45.1X2	T45.1X3	T45.1X4	T45.1X5	T45.1X6
Benzedrex	T44.991	T44.992	T44.993	T44.994	T44.995	T44.996
Benzedrine (amphetamine)	T43.621	T43.622	T43.623	T43.624	T43.625	T43.626
Benzenamine	T65.3X1	T65.3X2	T65.3X3	T65.3X4	—	—
Benzene	T52.1X1	T52.1X2	T52.1X3	T52.1X4	—	—
homologues (acetyl) (dimethyl) (methyl) (solvent)	T52.2X1	T52.2X2	T52.2X3	T52.2X4		
Benzethonium (chloride)	T49.0X1	T49.0X2	T49.0X3	T49.0X4	T49.0X5	T49.0X6
Benzfetamine	T50.5X1	T50.5X2	T50.5X3	T50.5X4	T50.5X5	T50.5X6
Benzhexol	T44.3X1	T44.3X2	T44.3X3	T44.3X4	T44.3X5	T44.3X6
Benzhydramine (chloride)	T45.0X1	T45.0X2	T45.0X3	T45.0X4	T45.0X5	T45.0X6
Benzidine	T65.891	T65.892	T65.893	T65.894	—	—
Benzilonium bromide	T44.3X1	T44.3X2	T44.3X3	T44.3X4	T44.3X5	T44.3X6
Benzimidazole	T60.3X1	T60.3X2	T60.3X3	T60.3X4	—	—
Benzin(e) — see Ligroin						
Benziodarone	T46.3X1	T46.3X2	T46.3X3	T46.3X4	T46.3X5	T46.3X6
Benznidazole	T37.3X1	T37.3X2	T37.3X3	T37.3X4	T37.3X5	T37.3X6
Benzocaine	T41.3X1	T41.3X2	T41.3X3	T41.3X4	T41.3X5	T41.3X6

Substance	External Cause (T-Code)					
	Poisoning, Accidental (Unintentional)	Poisoning, Intentional Self-Harm	Poisoning, Assault	Poisoning, Undetermined	Adverse Effect	Underdosing
Benzoctamine	T43.0X1	T43.0X2	T43.0X3	T43.0X4	T43.0X5	T43.0X6
Benzodiapin	T42.4X1	T42.4X2	T42.4X3	T42.4X4	T42.4X5	T42.4X6
Benzodiazepine NEC	T42.4X1	T42.4X2	T42.4X3	T42.4X4	T42.4X5	T42.4X6
Benzoic acid	T49.0X1	T49.0X2	T49.0X3	T49.0X4	T49.0X5	T49.0X6
with salicylic acid	T49.0X1	T49.0X2	T49.0X3	T49.0X4	T49.0X5	T49.0X6
Benzoin (tincture)	T48.5X1	T48.5X2	T48.5X3	T48.5X4	T48.5X5	T48.5X6
Benzol (benzene)	T52.1X1	T52.1X2	T52.1X3	T52.1X4	—	—
vapor	T52.0X1	T52.0X2	T52.0X3	T52.0X4	—	—
Benzomorphan	T40.2X1	T40.2X2	T40.2X3	T40.2X4	T40.2X5	T40.2X6
Benzonatate	T48.3X1	T48.3X2	T48.3X3	T48.3X4	T48.3X5	T48.3X6
Benzophenones	T49.3X1	T49.3X2	T49.3X3	T49.3X4	T49.3X5	T49.3X6
Benzopyrone	T46.991	T46.992	T46.993	T46.994	T46.995	T46.996
Benzothiadiazides	T50.2X1	T50.2X2	T50.2X3	T50.2X4	T50.2X5	T50.2X6
Benzoxonium chloride	T49.0X1	T49.0X2	T49.0X3	T49.0X4	T49.0X5	T49.0X6
Benzoyl peroxide	T49.0X1	T49.0X2	T49.0X3	T49.0X4	T49.0X5	T49.0X6
Benzoylpas calcium	T37.1X1	T37.1X2	T37.1X3	T37.1X4	T37.1X5	T37.1X6
Benzperidin	T43.591	T43.592	T43.593	T43.594	T43.595	T43.596
Benzperidol	T43.591	T43.592	T43.593	T43.594	T43.595	T43.596
Benzphetamine	T50.5X1	T50.5X2	T50.5X3	T50.5X4	T50.5X5	T50.5X6
Benzpyrinium bromide	T44.1X1	T44.1X2	T44.1X3	T44.1X4	T44.1X5	T44.1X6
Benzquinamide	T45.0X1	T45.0X2	T45.0X3	T45.0X4	T45.0X5	T45.0X6
Benzthiazide	T50.2X1	T50.2X2	T50.2X3	T50.2X4	T50.2X5	T50.2X6
Benztropine						
anticholinergic	T44.3X1	T44.3X2	T44.3X3	T44.3X4	T44.3X5	T44.3X6
antiparkinson	T42.8X1	T42.8X2	T42.8X3	T42.8X4	T42.8X5	T42.8X6
Benzydamine	T49.0X1	T49.0X2	T49.0X3	T49.0X4	T49.0X5	T49.0X6
Benzyl						
acetate	T52.8X1	T52.8X2	T52.8X3	T52.8X4	—	—
alcohol	T49.0X1	T49.0X2	T49.0X3	T49.0X4	T49.0X5	T49.0X6
benzoate	T49.0X1	T49.0X2	T49.0X3	T49.0X4	T49.0X5	T49.0X6
Benzoic acid	T49.0X1	T49.0X2	T49.0X3	T49.0X4	T49.0X5	T49.0X6
morphine	T40.2X1	T40.2X2	T40.2X3	T40.2X4	—	—
nicotinate	T46.6X1	T46.6X2	T46.6X3	T46.6X4	T46.6X5	T46.6X6
penicillin	T36.0X1	T36.0X2	T36.0X3	T36.0X4	T36.0X5	T36.0X6
Benzylhydrochlorthia-zide	T50.2X1	T50.2X2	T50.2X3	T50.2X4	T50.2X5	T50.2X6
Benzylpenicillin	T36.0X1	T36.0X2	T36.0X3	T36.0X4	T36.0X5	T36.0X6
Benzylthiouracil	T38.2X1	T38.2X2	T38.2X3	T38.2X4	T38.2X5	T38.2X6
Bephenium hydroxy-naphthoate	T37.4X1	T37.4X2	T37.4X3	T37.4X4	T37.4X5	T37.4X6
Bepridil	T46.1X1	T46.1X2	T46.1X3	T46.1X4	T46.1X5	T46.1X6
Bergamot oil	T65.891	T65.892	T65.893	T65.894	—	—
Bergapten	T50.991	T50.992	T50.993	T50.994	T50.995	T50.996
Berries, poisonous	T62.1X1	T62.1X2	T62.1X3	T62.1X4		

◀ New   ◀ Revised   ~~deleted~~ Deleted

Substance	Poisoning, Accidental (Unintentional)	Poisoning, Intentional Self-Harm	Poisoning, Assault	Poisoning, Undetermined	Adverse Effect	Underdosing
Beryllium (compounds)	T56.7X1	T56.7X2	T56.7X3	T56.7X4	—	—
b-acetyldigoxin	T46.0X1	T46.0X2	T46.0X3	T46.0X4	T46.0X5	T46.0X6
beta adrenergic blocking agent, heart	T44.7X1	T44.7X2	T44.7X3	T44.7X4	T44.7X5	T44.7X6
b-benzalbutyramide	T46.6X1	T46.6X2	T46.6X3	T46.6X4	T46.6X5	T46.6X6
Betacarotene	T45.2X1	T45.2X2	T45.2X3	T45.2X4	T45.2X5	T45.2X6
b-eucaine	T49.1X1	T49.1X2	T49.1X3	T49.1X4	T49.1X5	T49.1X6
Beta-Chlor	T42.6X1	T42.6X2	T42.6X3	T42.6X4	T42.6X5	T42.6X6
b-galactosidase	T47.5X1	T47.5X2	T47.5X3	T47.5X4	T47.5X5	T47.5X6
Betahistine	T46.7X1	T46.7X2	T46.7X3	T46.7X4	T46.7X5	T46.7X6
Betaine	T47.5X1	T47.5X2	T47.5X3	T47.5X4	T47.5X5	T47.5X6
Betamethasone	T49.0X1	T49.0X2	T49.0X3	T49.0X4	T49.0X5	T49.0X6
topical	T49.0X1	T49.0X2	T49.0X3	T49.0X4	T49.0X5	T49.0X6
Betamicin	T36.8X1	T36.8X2	T36.8X3	T36.8X4	T36.8X5	T36.8X6
Betanidine	T46.5X1	T46.5X2	T46.5X3	T46.5X4	T46.5X5	T46.5X6
b-sitosterol(s)	T46.6X1	T46.6X2	T46.6X3	T46.6X4	T46.6X5	T46.6X6
Betaxolol	T44.7X1	T44.7X2	T44.7X3	T44.7X4	T44.7X5	T44.7X6
Betazole	T50.8X1	T50.8X2	T50.8X3	T50.8X4	T50.8X5	T50.8X6
Bethanechol	T44.1X1	T44.1X2	T44.1X3	T44.1X4	T44.1X5	T44.1X6
chloride	T44.1X1	T44.1X2	T44.1X3	T44.1X4	T44.1X5	T44.1X6
Bethanidine	T46.5X1	T46.5X2	T46.5X3	T46.5X4	T46.5X5	T46.5X6
Betoxycaine	T41.3X1	T41.3X2	T41.3X3	T41.3X4	T41.3X5	T41.3X6
Betula oil	T49.3X1	T49.3X2	T49.3X3	T49.3X4	T49.3X5	T49.3X6
Bevantolol	T44.7X1	T44.7X2	T44.7X3	T44.7X4	T44.7X5	T44.7X6
Bevonium metilsulfate	T44.3X1	T44.3X2	T44.3X3	T44.3X4	T44.3X5	T44.3X6
Bezafibrate	T46.6X1	T46.6X2	T46.6X3	T46.6X4	T46.6X5	T46.6X6
Bezitramide	T40.491	T40.492	T40.493	T40.494	T40.495	T40.496
BHA	T50.991	T50.992	T50.993	T50.994	T50.995	T50.996
Bhang	T40.711	T40.712	T40.713	T40.714	T40.715	T40.716
BHC (medicinal)	T49.0X1	T49.0X2	T49.0X3	T49.0X4	T49.0X5	T49.0X6
nonmedicinal (vapor)	T53.6X1	T53.6X2	T53.6X3	T53.6X4	—	—
Bialamicol	T37.3X1	T37.3X2	T37.3X3	T37.3X4	T37.3X5	T37.3X6
Bibenzonium bromide	T48.3X1	T48.3X2	T48.3X3	T48.3X4	T48.3X5	T48.3X6
Bibrocathol	T49.5X1	T49.5X2	T49.5X3	T49.5X4	T49.5X5	T49.5X6
Bichloride of mercury — see Mercury, chloride						
Bichromates (calcium) (potassium) (sodium) (crystals)	T57.8X1	T57.8X2	T57.8X3	T57.8X4	—	—
fumes	T56.2X1	T56.2X2	T56.2X3	T56.2X4	—	—
Biclotymol	T49.6X1	T49.6X2	T49.6X3	T49.6X4	T49.6X5	T49.6X6
Bicuculline	T50.7X1	T50.7X2	T50.7X3	T50.7X4	T50.7X5	T50.7X6
Bifemelane	T43.291	T43.292	T43.293	T43.294	T43.295	T43.296
Biguanide derivatives, oral	T38.3X1	T38.3X2	T38.3X3	T38.3X4	T38.3X5	T38.3X6

Substance	Poisoning, Accidental (Unintentional)	Poisoning, Intentional Self-Harm	Poisoning, Assault	Poisoning, Undetermined	Adverse Effect	Underdosing
Biligrafin	T50.8X1	T50.8X2	T50.8X3	T50.8X4	T50.8X5	T50.8X6
Bile salts	T47.5X1	T47.5X2	T47.5X3	T47.5X4	T47.5X5	T47.5X6
Bilopaque	T50.8X1	T50.8X2	T50.8X3	T50.8X4	T50.8X5	T50.8X6
Binifibrate	T46.6X1	T46.6X2	T46.6X3	T46.6X4	T46.6X5	T46.6X6
Binitrobenzol	T65.3X1	T65.3X2	T65.3X3	T65.3X4	—	—
Bioflavonoid(s)	T46.991	T46.992	T46.993	T46.994	T46.995	T46.996
Biological substance NEC	T50.901	T50.902	T50.903	T50.904	T50.905	T50.906
Biotin	T45.2X1	T45.2X2	T45.2X3	T45.2X4	T45.2X5	T45.2X6
Biperiden	T44.3X1	T44.3X2	T44.3X3	T44.3X4	T44.3X5	T44.3X6
Bisacodyl	T47.2X1	T47.2X2	T47.2X3	T47.2X4	T47.2X5	T47.2X6
Bisbentiamine	T45.2X1	T45.2X2	T45.2X3	T45.2X4	T45.2X5	T45.2X6
Bisbutiamine	T45.2X1	T45.2X2	T45.2X3	T45.2X4	T45.2X5	T45.2X6
Bisdequalinium (salts) (diacetate)	T49.6X1	T49.6X2	T49.6X3	T49.6X4	T49.6X5	T49.6X6
Bishydroxycoumarin	T45.511	T45.512	T45.513	T45.514	T45.515	T45.516
Bismarsen	T37.8X1	T37.8X2	T37.8X3	T37.8X4	T37.8X5	T37.8X6
Bismuth salts	T47.6X1	T47.6X2	T47.6X3	T47.6X4	T47.6X5	T47.6X6
aluminate	T47.1X1	T47.1X2	T47.1X3	T47.1X4	T47.1X5	T47.1X6
anti-infectives	T37.8X1	T37.8X2	T37.8X3	T37.8X4	T37.8X5	T37.8X6
formic iodide	T49.0X1	T49.0X2	T49.0X3	T49.0X4	T49.0X5	T49.0X6
glycolylarsenate	T49.0X1	T49.0X2	T49.0X3	T49.0X4	T49.0X5	T49.0X6
nonmedicinal (compounds) NEC	T65.91	T65.92	T65.93	T65.94	—	—
subcarbonate	T47.6X1	T47.6X2	T47.6X3	T47.6X4	T47.6X5	T47.6X6
subsalicylate	T37.8X1	T37.8X2	T37.8X3	T37.8X4	T37.8X5	T37.8X6
sulfarsphenamine	T37.8X1	T37.8X2	T37.8X3	T37.8X4	T37.8X5	T37.8X6
Bisoprolol	T44.7X1	T44.7X2	T44.7X3	T44.7X4	T44.7X5	T44.7X6
Bisoxatin	T47.2X1	T47.2X2	T47.2X3	T47.2X4	T47.2X5	T47.2X6
Bisulepin (hydrochloride)	T45.0X1	T45.0X2	T45.0X3	T45.0X4	T45.0X5	T45.0X6
Bithionol	T37.8X1	T37.8X2	T37.8X3	T37.8X4	T37.8X5	T37.8X6
anthelminthic	T37.4X1	T37.4X2	T37.4X3	T37.4X4	T37.4X5	T37.4X6
Bitolterol	T48.6X1	T48.6X2	T48.6X3	T48.6X4	T48.6X5	T48.6X6
Bitoscanate	T37.4X1	T37.4X2	T37.4X3	T37.4X4	T37.4X5	T37.4X6
Bitter almond oil	T62.8X1	T62.8X2	T62.8X3	T62.8X4	—	—
Bittersweet	T62.2X1	T62.2X2	T62.2X3	T62.2X4	—	—
Black						
flag	T60.91	T60.92	T60.93	T60.94	—	—
henbane	T62.2X1	T62.2X2	T62.2X3	T62.2X4	—	—
leaf (40)	T60.91	T60.92	T60.93	T60.94	—	—
widow spider (bite)	T63.311	T63.312	T63.313	T63.314	—	—
antivenin	T50.Z11	T50.Z12	T50.Z13	T50.Z14	T50.Z15	T50.Z16
Blast furnace gas (carbon monoxide from)	T58.8X1	T58.8X2	T58.8X3	T58.8X4	—	—
Bleach	T54.91	T54.92	T54.93	T54.94	—	—

◀ New ◀▮ Revised ~~deleted~~ Deleted

521

TABLE OF DRUGS AND CHEMICALS

	External Cause (T-Code)					
Substance	Poisoning, Accidental (Unintentional)	Poisoning, Intentional Self-Harm	Poisoning, Assault	Poisoning, Undetermined	Adverse Effect	Underdosing
Bleaching agent (medicinal)	T49.4X1	T49.4X2	T49.4X3	T49.4X4	T49.4X5	T49.4X6
Bleomycin	T45.1X1	T45.1X2	T45.1X3	T45.1X4	T45.1X5	T45.1X6
Blockain	T41.3X1	T41.3X2	T41.3X3	T41.3X4	T41.3X5	T41.3X6
infiltration (subcutaneous)	T41.3X1	T41.3X2	T41.3X3	T41.3X4	T41.3X5	T41.3X6
nerve block (peripheral) (plexus)	T41.3X1	T41.3X2	T41.3X3	T41.3X4	T41.3X5	T41.3X6
topical (surface)	T41.3X1	T41.3X2	T41.3X3	T41.3X4	T41.3X5	T41.3X6
Blockers, calcium channel	T46.1X1	T46.1X2	T46.1X3	T46.1X4	T46.1X5	T46.1X6
Blood (derivatives) (natural) (plasma) (whole)	T45.8X1	T45.8X2	T45.8X3	T45.8X4	T45.8X5	T45.8X6
dried	T45.8X1	T45.8X2	T45.8X3	T45.8X4	T45.8X5	T45.8X6
drug affecting NEC	T45.91	T45.92	T45.93	T45.94	T45.95	T45.96
expander NEC	T45.8X1	T45.8X2	T45.8X3	T45.8X4	T45.8X5	T45.8X6
fraction NEC	T45.8X1	T45.8X2	T45.8X3	T45.8X4	T45.8X5	T45.8X6
substitute (macromolecular)	T45.8X1	T45.8X2	T45.8X3	T45.8X4	T45.8X5	T45.8X6
Blue velvet	T40.2X1	T40.2X2	T40.2X3	T40.2X4	—	—
Bone meal	T62.8X1	T62.8X2	T62.8X3	T62.8X4	—	—
Bonine	T45.0X1	T45.0X2	T45.0X3	T45.0X4	T45.0X5	T45.0X6
Bopindolol	T44.7X1	T44.7X2	T44.7X3	T44.7X4	T44.7X5	T44.7X6
Boracic acid	T49.0X1	T49.0X2	T49.0X3	T49.0X4	T49.0X5	T49.0X6
ENT agent	T49.6X1	T49.6X2	T49.6X3	T49.6X4	T49.6X5	T49.6X6
ophthalmic preparation	T49.5X1	T49.5X2	T49.5X3	T49.5X4	T49.5X5	T49.5X6
Borane complex	T57.8X1	T57.8X2	T57.8X3	T57.8X4	—	—
Borate(s)	T57.8X1	T57.8X2	T57.8X3	T57.8X4	—	—
buffer	T50.991	T50.992	T50.993	T50.994	T50.995	T50.996
cleanser	T54.91	T54.92	T54.93	T54.94	—	—
sodium	T57.8X1	T57.8X2	T57.8X3	T57.8X4	—	—
Borax (cleanser)	T54.91	T54.92	T54.93	T54.94	—	—
Bordeaux mixture	T60.3X1	T60.3X2	T60.3X3	T60.3X4	—	—
Boric acid	T49.0X1	T49.0X2	T49.0X3	T49.0X4	T49.0X5	T49.0X6
ENT agent	T49.6X1	T49.6X2	T49.6X3	T49.6X4	T49.6X5	T49.6X6
ophthalmic preparation	T49.5X1	T49.5X2	T49.5X3	T49.5X4	T49.5X5	T49.5X6
Bornaprine	T44.3X1	T44.3X2	T44.3X3	T44.3X4	T44.3X5	T44.3X6
Boron	T57.8X1	T57.8X2	T57.8X3	T57.8X4	—	—
hydride NEC	T57.8X1	T57.8X2	T57.8X3	T57.8X4	—	—
fumes or gas	T57.8X1	T57.8X2	T57.8X3	T57.8X4	—	—
trifluoride	T59.891	T59.892	T59.893	T59.894	—	—
Botox	T48.291	T48.292	T48.293	T48.294	T48.295	T48.296
Botulinus anti-toxin (type A, B)	T50.Z11	T50.Z12	T50.Z13	T50.Z14	T50.Z15	T50.Z16
Brake fluid vapor	T59.891	T59.892	T59.893	T59.894	—	—
Brallobarbital	T42.3X1	T42.3X2	T42.3X3	T42.3X4	T42.3X5	T42.3X6
Bran (wheat)	T47.4X1	T47.4X2	T47.4X3	T47.4X4	T47.4X5	T47.4X6
Brass (fumes)	T56.891	T56.892	T56.893	T56.894	—	—

	External Cause (T-Code)					
Substance	Poisoning, Accidental (Unintentional)	Poisoning, Intentional Self-Harm	Poisoning, Assault	Poisoning, Undetermined	Adverse Effect	Underdosing
Brasso	T52.0X1	T52.0X2	T52.0X3	T52.0X4	—	—
Bretylium tosilate	T46.2X1	T46.2X2	T46.2X3	T46.2X4	T46.2X5	T46.2X6
Brevital (sodium)	T41.1X1	T41.1X2	T41.1X3	T41.1X4	T41.1X5	T41.1X6
Brinase	T45.3X1	T45.3X2	T45.3X3	T45.3X4	T45.3X5	T45.3X6
British antilewisite	T45.8X1	T45.8X2	T45.8X3	T45.8X4	T45.8X5	T45.8X6
Brodifacoum	T60.4X1	T60.4X2	T60.4X3	T60.4X4	—	—
Bromal (hydrate)	T42.6X1	T42.6X2	T42.6X3	T42.6X4	T42.6X5	T42.6X6
Bromazepam	T42.4X1	T42.4X2	T42.4X3	T42.4X4	T42.4X5	T42.4X6
Bromazine	T45.0X1	T45.0X2	T45.0X3	T45.0X4	T45.0X5	T45.0X6
Brombenzylcyanide	T59.3X1	T59.3X2	T59.3X3	T59.3X4	—	—
Bromelains	T45.3X1	T45.3X2	T45.3X3	T45.3X4	T45.3X5	T45.3X6
Bromethalin	T60.4X1	T60.4X2	T60.4X3	T60.4X4	—	—
Bromhexine	T48.4X1	T48.4X2	T48.4X3	T48.4X4	T48.4X5	T48.4X6
Bromide salts	T42.6X1	T42.6X2	T42.6X3	T42.6X4	T42.6X5	T42.6X6
Bromindione	T45.511	T45.512	T45.513	T45.514	T45.515	T45.516
Bromine						
compounds (medicinal)	T42.6X1	T42.6X2	T42.6X3	T42.6X4	T42.6X5	T42.6X6
sedative	T42.6X1	T42.6X2	T42.6X3	T42.6X4	T42.6X5	T42.6X6
vapor	T59.891	T59.892	T59.893	T59.894	—	—
Bromisovalum	T42.6X1	T42.6X2	T42.6X3	T42.6X4	T42.6X5	T42.6X6
Bromisoval	T42.6X1	T42.6X2	T42.6X3	T42.6X4	T42.6X5	T42.6X6
Bromobenzylcyanide	T59.3X1	T59.3X2	T59.3X3	T59.3X4	—	—
Bromochlorosalicylani-lide	T49.0X1	T49.0X2	T49.0X3	T49.0X4	T49.0X5	T49.0X6
Bromocriptine	T42.8X1	T42.8X2	T42.8X3	T42.8X4	T42.8X5	T42.8X6
Bromodiphenhydramine	T45.0X1	T45.0X2	T45.0X3	T45.0X4	T45.0X5	T45.0X6
Bromoform	T42.6X1	T42.6X2	T42.6X3	T42.6X4	T42.6X5	T42.6X6
Bromophenol blue reagent	T50.991	T50.992	T50.993	T50.994	T50.995	T50.996
Bromopride	T47.8X1	T47.8X2	T47.8X3	T47.8X4	T47.8X5	T47.8X6
Bromosalicylchloranitide	T49.0X1	T49.0X2	T49.0X3	T49.0X4	T49.0X5	T49.0X6
Bromosalicylhydroxamic acid	T37.1X1	T37.1X2	T37.1X3	T37.1X4	T37.1X5	T37.1X6
Bromo-seltzer	T39.1X1	T39.1X2	T39.1X3	T39.1X4	T39.1X5	T39.1X6
Bromoxynil	T60.3X1	T60.3X2	T60.3X3	T60.3X4	—	—
Bromperidol	T43.4X1	T43.4X2	T43.4X3	T43.4X4	T43.4X5	T43.4X6
Brompheniramine	T45.0X1	T45.0X2	T45.0X3	T45.0X4	T45.0X5	T45.0X6
Bromsulfophthalein	T50.8X1	T50.8X2	T50.8X3	T50.8X4	T50.8X5	T50.8X6
Bromural	T42.6X1	T42.6X2	T42.6X3	T42.6X4	T42.6X5	T42.6X6
Bromvaletone	T42.6X1	T42.6X2	T42.6X3	T42.6X4	T42.6X5	T42.6X6
Bronchodilator NEC	T48.6X1	T48.6X2	T48.6X3	T48.6X4	T48.6X5	T48.6X6
Brotizolam	T42.4X1	T42.4X2	T42.4X3	T42.4X4	T42.4X5	T42.4X6
Brovincamine	T46.7X1	T46.7X2	T46.7X3	T46.7X4	T46.7X5	T46.7X6
Brown spider (bite) (venom)	T63.391	T63.392	T63.393	T63.394	—	—

◀ New　◀ Revised　~~deleted~~ Deleted

Substance	External Cause (T-Code)					
	Poisoning, Accidental (Unintentional)	Poisoning, Intentional Self-Harm	Poisoning, Assault	Poisoning, Undetermined	Adverse Effect	Underdosing
Brown recluse spider (bite) (venom)	T63.331	T63.332	T63.333	T63.334	—	—
Broxaterol	T48.6X1	T48.6X2	T48.6X3	T48.6X4	T48.6X5	T48.6X6
Broxuridine	T45.1X1	T45.1X2	T45.1X3	T45.1X4	T45.1X5	T45.1X6
Broxyquinoline	T37.8X1	T37.8X2	T37.8X3	T37.8X4	T37.8X5	T37.8X6
Bruceine	T48.291	T48.292	T48.293	T48.294	T48.295	T48.296
Brucia	T62.2X1	T62.2X2	T62.2X3	T62.2X4	—	—
Brucine	T65.1X1	T65.1X2	T65.1X3	T65.1X4	—	—
Brunswick green — see Copper						
Bruten — see Ibuprofen						
Bryonia	T47.2X1	T47.2X2	T47.2X3	T47.2X4	T47.2X5	T47.2X6
Buclizine	T45.0X1	T45.0X2	T45.0X3	T45.0X4	T45.0X5	T45.0X6
Buclosamide	T49.0X1	T49.0X2	T49.0X3	T49.0X4	T49.0X5	T49.0X6
Budesonide	T44.5X1	T44.5X2	T44.5X3	T44.5X4	T44.5X5	T44.5X6
Budralazine	T46.5X1	T46.5X2	T46.5X3	T46.5X4	T46.5X5	T46.5X6
Bufferin	T39.011	T39.012	T39.013	T39.014	T39.015	T39.016
Buflomedil	T46.7X1	T46.7X2	T46.7X3	T46.7X4	T46.7X5	T46.7X6
Buformin	T38.3X1	T38.3X2	T38.3X3	T38.3X4	T38.3X5	T38.3X6
Bufotenine	T40.991	T40.992	T40.993	T40.994	—	—
Bufrolin	T48.6X1	T48.6X2	T48.6X3	T48.6X4	T48.6X5	T48.6X6
Bufylline	T48.6X1	T48.6X2	T48.6X3	T48.6X4	T48.6X5	T48.6X6
Bulk filler	T50.5X1	T50.5X2	T50.5X3	T50.5X4	T50.5X5	T50.5X6
cathartic	T47.4X1	T47.4X2	T47.4X3	T47.4X4	T47.4X5	T47.4X6
Bumetanide	T50.1X1	T50.1X2	T50.1X3	T50.1X4	T50.1X5	T50.1X6
Bunaftine	T46.2X1	T46.2X2	T46.2X3	T46.2X4	T46.2X5	T46.2X6
Bunamiodyl	T50.8X1	T50.8X2	T50.8X3	T50.8X4	T50.8X5	T50.8X6
Bunazosin	T44.6X1	T44.6X2	T44.6X3	T44.6X4	T44.6X5	T44.6X6
Bunitrolol	T44.7X1	T44.7X2	T44.7X3	T44.7X4	T44.7X5	T44.7X6
Buphenine	T46.7X1	T46.7X2	T46.7X3	T46.7X4	T46.7X5	T46.7X6
Bupivacaine	T41.3X1	T41.3X2	T41.3X3	T41.3X4	T41.3X5	T41.3X6
infiltration (subcutaneous)	T41.3X1	T41.3X2	T41.3X3	T41.3X4	T41.3X5	T41.3X6
nerve block (peripheral) (plexus)	T41.3X1	T41.3X2	T41.3X3	T41.3X4	T41.3X5	T41.3X6
spinal	T41.3X1	T41.3X2	T41.3X3	T41.3X4	T41.3X5	T41.3X6
Bupranolol	T44.7X1	T44.7X2	T44.7X3	T44.7X4	T44.7X5	T44.7X6
Buprenorphine	T40.491	T40.492	T40.493	T40.494	T40.495	T40.496
Bupropion	T43.291	T43.292	T43.293	T43.294	T43.295	T43.296
Burimamide	T47.1X1	T47.1X2	T47.1X3	T47.1X4	T47.1X5	T47.1X6
Buserelin	T38.891	T38.892	T38.893	T38.894	T38.895	T38.896
Buspirone	T43.591	T43.592	T43.593	T43.594	T43.595	T43.596
Busulfan, busulphan	T45.1X1	T45.1X2	T45.1X3	T45.1X4	T45.1X5	T45.1X6
Butabarbital (sodium)	T42.3X1	T42.3X2	T42.3X3	T42.3X4	T42.3X5	T42.3X6
Butabarbitone	T42.3X1	T42.3X2	T42.3X3	T42.3X4	T42.3X5	T42.3X6

Substance	External Cause (T-Code)					
	Poisoning, Accidental (Unintentional)	Poisoning, Intentional Self-Harm	Poisoning, Assault	Poisoning, Undetermined	Adverse Effect	Underdosing
Butabarpal	T42.3X1	T42.3X2	T42.3X3	T42.3X4	T42.3X5	T42.3X6
Butacaine	T41.3X1	T41.3X2	T41.3X3	T41.3X4	T41.3X5	T41.3X6
Butalamine	T46.7X1	T46.7X2	T46.7X3	T46.7X4	T46.7X5	T46.7X6
Butalbital	T42.3X1	T42.3X2	T42.3X3	T42.3X4	T42.3X5	T42.3X6
Butallylonal	T42.3X1	T42.3X2	T42.3X3	T42.3X4	T42.3X5	T42.3X6
Butamben	T41.3X1	T41.3X2	T41.3X3	T41.3X4	T41.3X5	T41.3X6
Butamirate	T48.3X1	T48.3X2	T48.3X3	T48.3X4	T48.3X5	T48.3X6
Butane (distributed in mobile container)	T59.891	T59.892	T59.893	T59.894	—	—
distributed through pipes	T59.891	T59.892	T59.893	T59.894	—	—
incomplete combustion	T58.11	T58.12	T58.13	T58.14	—	—
Butanilicaine	T41.3X1	T41.3X2	T41.3X3	T41.3X4	T41.3X5	T41.3X6
Butanol	T51.3X1	T51.3X2	T51.3X3	T51.3X4		
Butanone, 2-butanone	T52.4X1	T52.4X2	T52.4X3	T52.4X4	—	—
Butantrone	T49.4X1	T49.4X2	T49.4X3	T49.4X4	T49.4X5	T49.4X6
Butaperazine	T43.3X1	T43.3X2	T43.3X3	T43.3X4	T43.3X5	T43.3X6
Butazolidin	T39.2X1	T39.2X2	T39.2X3	T39.2X4	T39.2X5	T39.2X6
Butetamate	T48.6X1	T48.6X2	T48.6X3	T48.6X4	T48.6X5	T48.6X6
Butethal	T42.3X1	T42.3X2	T42.3X3	T42.3X4	T42.3X5	T42.3X6
Butethamate	T44.3X1	T44.3X2	T44.3X3	T44.3X4	T44.3X5	T44.3X6
Buthalitone (sodium)	T41.1X1	T41.1X2	T41.1X3	T41.1X4	T41.1X5	T41.1X6
Butisol (sodium)	T42.3X1	T42.3X2	T42.3X3	T42.3X4	T42.3X5	T42.3X6
Butizide	T50.2X1	T50.2X2	T50.2X3	T50.2X4	T50.2X5	T50.2X6
Butobarbital	T42.3X1	T42.3X2	T42.3X3	T42.3X4	T42.3X5	T42.3X6
sodium	T42.3X1	T42.3X2	T42.3X3	T42.3X4	T42.3X5	T42.3X6
Butobarbitone	T42.3X1	T42.3X2	T42.3X3	T42.3X4	T42.3X5	T42.3X6
Butoconazole (nitrate)	T49.0X1	T49.0X2	T49.0X3	T49.0X4	T49.0X5	T49.0X6
Butorphanol	T40.491	T40.492	T40.493	T40.494	T40.495	T40.496
Butriptyline	T43.011	T43.012	T43.013	T43.014	T43.015	T43.016
Butropium bromide	T44.3X1	T44.3X2	T44.3X3	T44.3X4	T44.3X5	T44.3X6
Buttercups	T62.2X1	T62.2X2	T62.2X3	T62.2X4	—	—
Butter of antimony — see Antimony						
Butyl						
acetate (secondary)	T52.8X1	T52.8X2	T52.8X3	T52.8X4	—	—
alcohol	T51.3X1	T51.3X2	T51.3X3	T51.3X4	—	—
aminobenzoate	T41.3X1	T41.3X2	T41.3X3	T41.3X4	T41.3X5	T41.3X6
butyrate	T52.8X1	T52.8X2	T52.8X3	T52.8X4	—	—
carbinol	T51.3X1	T51.3X2	T51.3X3	T51.3X4	—	—
carbitol	T52.3X1	T52.3X2	T52.3X3	T52.3X4	—	—
cellosolve	T52.3X1	T52.3X2	T52.3X3	T52.3X4	—	—
chloral (hydrate)	T42.6X1	T42.6X2	T42.6X3	T42.6X4	T42.6X5	T42.6X6
formate	T52.8X1	T52.8X2	T52.8X3	T52.8X4	—	—

Substance	Poisoning, Accidental (Unintentional)	Poisoning, Intentional Self-Harm	Poisoning, Assault	Poisoning, Undetermined	Adverse Effect	Underdosing
Butyl *(Continued)*						
lactate	T52.8X1	T52.8X2	T52.8X3	T52.8X4	—	—
propionate	T52.8X1	T52.8X2	T52.8X3	T52.8X4	—	—
scopolamine bromide	T44.3X1	T44.3X2	T44.3X3	T44.3X4	T44.3X5	T44.3X6
thiobarbital sodium	T41.1X1	T41.1X2	T41.1X3	T41.1X4	T41.1X5	T41.1X6
Butylated hydroxy-anisole	T50.991	T50.992	T50.993	T50.994	T50.995	T50.996
Butylchloral hydrate	T42.6X1	T42.6X2	T42.6X3	T42.6X4	T42.6X5	T42.6X6
Butyltoluene	T52.2X1	T52.2X2	T52.2X3	T52.2X4	—	—
Butyn	T41.3X1	T41.3X2	T41.3X3	T41.3X4	T41.3X5	T41.3X6
Butyrophenone (-based tranquilizers)	T43.4X1	T43.4X2	T43.4X3	T43.4X4	T43.4X5	T43.4X6

C

Substance	Poisoning, Accidental (Unintentional)	Poisoning, Intentional Self-Harm	Poisoning, Assault	Poisoning, Undetermined	Adverse Effect	Underdosing
Cabergoline	T42.8X1	T42.8X2	T42.8X3	T42.8X4	T42.8X5	T42.8X6
Cacodyl, cacodylic acid	T57.0X1	T57.0X2	T57.0X3	T57.0X4	—	—
Cactinomycin	T45.1X1	T45.1X2	T45.1X3	T45.1X4	T45.1X5	T45.1X6
Cade oil	T49.4X1	T49.4X2	T49.4X3	T49.4X4	T49.4X5	T49.4X6
Cadexomer iodine	T49.0X1	T49.0X2	T49.0X3	T49.0X4	T49.0X5	T49.0X6
Cadmium (chloride) (fumes) (oxide)	T56.3X1	T56.3X2	T56.3X3	T56.3X4	—	—
sulfide (medicinal) NEC	T49.4X1	T49.4X2	T49.4X3	T49.4X4	T49.4X5	T49.4X6
Cadralazine	T46.5X1	T46.5X2	T46.5X3	T46.5X4	T46.5X5	T46.5X6
Caffeine	T43.611	T43.612	T43.613	T43.614	T43.615	T43.616
Calabar bean	T62.2X1	T62.2X2	T62.2X3	T62.2X4	—	—
Caladium seguinum	T62.2X1	T62.2X2	T62.2X3	T62.2X4	—	—
Calamine (lotion)	T49.3X1	T49.3X2	T49.3X3	T49.3X4	T49.3X5	T49.3X6
Calcifediol	T45.2X1	T45.2X2	T45.2X3	T45.2X4	T45.2X5	T45.2X6
Calciferol	T45.2X1	T45.2X2	T45.2X3	T45.2X4	T45.2X5	T45.2X6
Calcitonin	T50.991	T50.992	T50.993	T50.994	T50.995	T50.996
Calcitriol	T45.2X1	T45.2X2	T45.2X3	T45.2X4	T45.2X5	T45.2X6
Calcium	T50.3X1	T50.3X2	T50.3X3	T50.3X4	T50.3X5	T50.3X6
actylsalicylate	T39.011	T39.012	T39.013	T39.014	T39.015	T39.016
benzamidosalicylate	T37.1X1	T37.1X2	T37.1X3	T37.1X4	T37.1X5	T37.1X6
bromide	T42.6X1	T42.6X2	T42.6X3	T42.6X4	T42.6X5	T42.6X6
bromolactobionate	T42.6X1	T42.6X2	T42.6X3	T42.6X4	T42.6X5	T42.6X6
carbaspirin	T39.011	T39.012	T39.013	T39.014	T39.015	T39.016
carbimide	T50.6X1	T50.6X2	T50.6X3	T50.6X4	T50.6X5	T50.6X6
carbonate	T47.1X1	T47.1X2	T47.1X3	T47.1X4	T47.1X5	T47.1X6
chloride	T50.991	T50.992	T50.993	T50.994	T50.995	T50.996
anhydrous	T50.991	T50.992	T50.993	T50.994	T50.995	T50.996
cyanide	T57.8X1	T57.8X2	T57.8X3	T57.8X4	—	—
dioctyl sulfosuccinate	T47.4X1	T47.4X2	T47.4X3	T47.4X4	T47.4X5	T47.4X6
disodium edathamil	T45.8X1	T45.8X2	T45.8X3	T45.8X4	T45.8X5	T45.8X6

Substance	Poisoning, Accidental (Unintentional)	Poisoning, Intentional Self-Harm	Poisoning, Assault	Poisoning, Undetermined	Adverse Effect	Underdosing
Calcium *(Continued)*						
disodium edetate	T45.8X1	T45.8X2	T45.8X3	T45.8X4	T45.8X5	T45.8X6
dobesilate	T46.991	T46.992	T46.993	T46.994	T46.995	T46.996
EDTA	T45.8X1	T45.8X2	T45.8X3	T45.8X4	T45.8X5	T45.8X6
ferrous citrate	T45.4X1	T45.4X2	T45.4X3	T45.4X4	T45.4X5	T45.4X6
folinate	T45.8X1	T45.8X2	T45.8X3	T45.8X4	T45.8X5	T45.8X6
glubionate	T50.3X1	T50.3X2	T50.3X3	T50.3X4	T50.3X5	T50.3X6
gluconate	T50.3X1	T50.3X2	T50.3X3	T50.3X4	T50.3X5	T50.3X6
gluconogalactogluconate	T50.3X1	T50.3X2	T50.3X3	T50.3X4	T50.3X5	T50.3X6
hydrate, hydroxide	T54.3X1	T54.3X2	T54.3X3	T54.3X4	—	—
hypochlorite	T54.3X1	T54.3X2	T54.3X3	T54.3X4	—	—
iodide	T48.4X1	T48.4X2	T48.4X3	T48.4X4	T48.4X5	T48.4X6
ipodate	T50.8X1	T50.8X2	T50.8X3	T50.8X4	T50.8X5	T50.8X6
lactate	T50.3X1	T50.3X2	T50.3X3	T50.3X4	T50.3X5	T50.3X6
leucovorin	T45.8X1	T45.8X2	T45.8X3	T45.8X4	T45.8X5	T45.8X6
mandelate	T37.91	T37.92	T37.93	T37.94	T37.95	T37.96
oxide	T54.3X1	T54.3X2	T54.3X3	T54.3X4	—	—
pantothenate	T45.2X1	T45.2X2	T45.2X3	T45.2X4	T45.2X5	T45.2X6
phosphate	T50.3X1	T50.3X2	T50.3X3	T50.3X4	T50.3X5	T50.3X6
salicylate	T39.091	T39.092	T39.093	T39.094	T39.095	T39.096
salts	T50.3X1	T50.3X2	T50.3X3	T50.3X4	T50.3X5	T50.3X6
Calculus-dissolving drug	T50.991	T50.992	T50.993	T50.994	T50.995	T50.996
Calomel	T49.0X1	T49.0X2	T49.0X3	T49.0X4	T49.0X5	T49.0X6
Caloric agent	T50.3X1	T50.3X2	T50.3X3	T50.3X4	T50.3X5	T50.3X6
Calusterone	T38.7X1	T38.7X2	T38.7X3	T38.7X4	T38.7X5	T38.7X6
Camazepam	T42.4X1	T42.4X2	T42.4X3	T42.4X4	T42.4X5	T42.4X6
Camomile	T49.0X1	T49.0X2	T49.0X3	T49.0X4	T49.0X5	T49.0X6
Camoquin	T37.2X1	T37.2X2	T37.2X3	T37.2X4	T37.2X5	T37.2X6
Camphor						
insecticide	T60.2X1	T60.2X2	T60.2X3	T60.2X4	—	—
medicinal	T49.8X1	T49.8X2	T49.8X3	T49.8X4	T49.8X5	T49.8X6
Camylofin	T44.3X1	T44.3X2	T44.3X3	T44.3X4	T44.3X5	T44.3X6
Cancer chemotherapy drug regimen	T45.1X1	T45.1X2	T45.1X3	T45.1X4	T45.1X5	T45.1X6
Candeptin	T49.0X1	T49.0X2	T49.0X3	T49.0X4	T49.0X5	T49.0X6
Candicidin	T49.0X1	T49.0X2	T49.0X3	T49.0X4	T49.0X5	T49.0X6
Cannabinoids, synthetic	T40.721	T40.722	T40.723	T40.724	T40.725	T40.726
Cannabinol	T40.711	T40.712	T40.713	T40.714	T40.715	T40.716
Cannabis (derivatives)	T40.711	T40.712	T40.713	T40.714	T40.715	T40.716
Canned heat	T51.1X1	T51.1X2	T51.1X3	T51.1X4	—	—
Canrenoic acid	T50.0X1	T50.0X2	T50.0X3	T50.0X4	T50.0X5	T50.0X6
Canrenone	T50.0X1	T50.0X2	T50.0X3	T50.0X4	T50.0X5	T50.0X6

TABLE OF DRUGS AND CHEMICALS

◀ New ◀ Revised ~~deleted~~ Deleted

Substance	External Cause (T-Code)					
	Poisoning, Accidental (Unintentional)	Poisoning, Intentional Self-Harm	Poisoning, Assault	Poisoning, Undetermined	Adverse Effect	Underdosing
Cantharides, cantharidin, cantharis	T49.8X1	T49.8X2	T49.8X3	T49.8X4	T49.8X5	T49.8X6
Canthaxanthin	T50.991	T50.992	T50.993	T50.994	T50.995	T50.996
Capillary-active drug NEC	T46.901	T46.902	T46.903	T46.904	T46.905	T46.906
Capreomycin	T36.8X1	T36.8X2	T36.8X3	T36.8X4	T36.8X5	T36.8X6
Capsicum	T49.4X1	T49.4X2	T49.4X3	T49.4X4	T49.4X5	T49.4X6
Captafol	T60.3X1	T60.3X2	T60.3X3	T60.3X4	—	—
Captan	T60.3X1	T60.3X2	T60.3X3	T60.3X4	—	—
Captodiame, captodiamine	T43.591	T43.592	T43.593	T43.594	T43.595	T43.596
Captopril	T46.4X1	T46.4X2	T46.4X3	T46.4X4	T46.4X5	T46.4X6
Caramiphen	T44.3X1	T44.3X2	T44.3X3	T44.3X4	T44.3X5	T44.3X6
Carazolol	T44.7X1	T44.7X2	T44.7X3	T44.7X4	T44.7X5	T44.7X6
Carbachol	T44.1X1	T44.1X2	T44.1X3	T44.1X4	T44.1X5	T44.1X6
Carbacrylamine (resin)	T50.3X1	T50.3X2	T50.3X3	T50.3X4	T50.3X5	T50.3X6
Carbamate (insecticide)	T60.0X1	T60.0X2	T60.0X3	T60.0X4	—	—
Carbamate (sedative)	T42.6X1	T42.6X2	T42.6X3	T42.6X4	T42.6X5	T42.6X6
herbicide	T60.0X1	T60.0X2	T60.0X3	T60.0X4	—	—
insecticide	T60.0X1	T60.0X2	T60.0X3	T60.0X4	—	—
Carbamazepine	T42.1X1	T42.1X2	T42.1X3	T42.1X4	T42.1X5	T42.1X6
Carbamide	T47.3X1	T47.3X2	T47.3X3	T47.3X4	T47.3X5	T47.3X6
peroxide	T49.0X1	T49.0X2	T49.0X3	T49.0X4	T49.0X5	T49.0X6
topical	T49.8X1	T49.8X2	T49.8X3	T49.8X4	T49.8X5	T49.8X6
Carbamylcholine chloride	T44.1X1	T44.1X2	T44.1X3	T44.1X4	T44.1X5	T44.1X6
Carbaril	T60.0X1	T60.0X2	T60.0X3	T60.0X4	—	—
Carbarsone	T37.3X1	T37.3X2	T37.3X3	T37.3X4	T37.3X5	T37.3X6
Carbaryl	T60.0X1	T60.0X2	T60.0X3	T60.0X4	—	—
Carbaspirin	T39.011	T39.012	T39.013	T39.014	T39.015	T39.016
Carbazochrome (salicylate) (sodium sulfonate)	T49.4X1	T49.4X2	T49.4X3	T49.4X4	T49.4X5	T49.4X6
Carbenicillin	T36.0X1	T36.0X2	T36.0X3	T36.0X4	T36.0X5	T36.0X6
Carbenoxolone	T47.1X1	T47.1X2	T47.1X3	T47.1X4	T47.1X5	T47.1X6
Carbetapentane	T48.3X1	T48.3X2	T48.3X3	T48.3X4	T48.3X5	T48.3X6
Carbethyl salicylate	T39.091	T39.092	T39.093	T39.094	T39.095	T39.096
Carbidopa (with levodopa)	T42.8X1	T42.8X2	T42.8X3	T42.8X4	T42.8X5	T42.8X6
Carbimazole	T38.2X1	T38.2X2	T38.2X3	T38.2X4	T38.2X5	T38.2X6
Carbinol	T51.1X1	T51.1X2	T51.1X3	T51.1X4	—	—
Carbinoxamine	T45.0X1	T45.0X2	T45.0X3	T45.0X4	T45.0X5	T45.0X6
Carbiphene	T39.8X1	T39.8X2	T39.8X3	T39.8X4	T39.8X5	T39.8X6
Carbitol	T52.3X1	T52.3X2	T52.3X3	T52.3X4	—	—
Carbocaine	T41.3X1	T41.3X2	T41.3X3	T41.3X4	T41.3X5	T41.3X6
infiltration (subcutaneous)	T41.3X1	T41.3X2	T41.3X3	T41.3X4	T41.3X5	T41.3X6
nerve block (peripheral) (plexus)	T41.3X1	T41.3X2	T41.3X3	T41.3X4	T41.3X5	T41.3X6
topical (surface)	T41.3X1	T41.3X2	T41.3X3	T41.3X4	T41.3X5	T41.3X6

Substance	External Cause (T-Code)					
	Poisoning, Accidental (Unintentional)	Poisoning, Intentional Self-Harm	Poisoning, Assault	Poisoning, Undetermined	Adverse Effect	Underdosing
Carbo medicinalis	T47.6X1	T47.6X2	T47.6X3	T47.6X4	T47.6X5	T47.6X6
Carbomycin	T36.8X1	T36.8X2	T36.8X3	T36.8X4	T36.8X5	T36.8X6
Carbocisteine	T48.4X1	T48.4X2	T48.4X3	T48.4X4	T48.4X5	T48.4X6
Carbocromen	T46.3X1	T46.3X2	T46.3X3	T46.3X4	T46.3X5	T46.3X6
Carbol fuchsin	T49.0X1	T49.0X2	T49.0X3	T49.0X4	T49.0X5	T49.0X6
Carbolic acid — see also Phenol	T54.0X1	T54.0X2	T54.0X3	T54.0X4	—	—
Carbolonium (bromide)	T48.1X1	T48.1X2	T48.1X3	T48.1X4	T48.1X5	T48.1X6
Carbon						
bisulfide (liquid)	T65.4X1	T65.4X2	T65.4X3	T65.4X4	—	—
vapor	T65.4X1	T65.4X2	T65.4X3	T65.4X4	—	—
dioxide (gas)	T59.7X1	T59.7X2	T59.7X3	T59.7X4	—	—
medicinal	T41.5X1	T41.5X2	T41.5X3	T41.5X4	T41.5X5	T41.5X6
nonmedicinal	T59.7X1	T59.7X2	T59.7X3	T59.7X4	—	—
snow	T49.4X1	T49.4X2	T49.4X3	T49.4X4	T49.4X5	T49.4X6
disulfide (liquid)	T65.4X1	T65.4X2	T65.4X3	T65.4X4	—	—
vapor	T65.4X1	T65.4X2	T65.4X3	T65.4X4	—	—
monoxide (from incomplete combustion)	T58.91	T58.92	T58.93	T58.94	—	—
blast furnace gas	T58.8X1	T58.8X2	T58.8X3	T58.8X4	—	—
butane (distributed in mobile container)	T58.11	T58.12	T58.13	T58.14	—	—
distributed through pipes	T58.11	T58.12	T58.13	T58.14	—	—
charcoal fumes	T58.2X1	T58.2X2	T58.2X3	T58.2X4	—	—
coal	T58.2X1	T58.2X2	T58.2X3	T58.2X4	—	—
coke (in domestic stoves, fireplaces)	T58.2X1	T58.2X2	T58.2X3	T58.2X4	—	—
gas (piped)	T58.11	T58.12	T58.13	T58.14	—	—
solid (in domestic stoves, fireplaces)	T58.2X1	T58.2X2	T58.2X3	T58.2X4	—	—
exhaust gas (motor) not in transit	T58.01	T58.02	T58.03	T58.04	—	—
combustion engine, any not in watercraft	T58.01	T58.02	T58.03	T58.04	—	—
farm tractor, not in transit	T58.01	T58.02	T58.03	T58.04	—	—
gas engine	T58.01	T58.02	T58.03	T58.04	—	—
motor pump	T58.01	T58.02	T58.03	T58.04	—	—
motor vehicle, not in transit	T58.01	T58.02	T58.03	T58.04	—	—
fuel (in domestic use)	T58.2X1	T58.2X2	T58.2X3	T58.2X4	—	—
gas (piped)	T58.11	T58.12	T58.13	T58.14	—	—
in mobile container	T58.11	T58.12	T58.13	T58.14	—	—
utility	T58.11	T58.12	T58.13	T58.14	—	—
in mobile container	T58.11	T58.12	T58.13	T58.14	—	—
piped (natural)	T58.11	T58.12	T58.13	T58.14	—	—

◄ New ◄ Revised ~~deleted~~ Deleted

Substance	Poisoning, Accidental (Unintentional)	Poisoning, Intentional Self-Harm	Poisoning, Assault	Poisoning, Undetermined	Adverse Effect	Underdosing
Carbon *(Continued)*						
monoxide *(Continued)*						
illuminating gas	T58.11	T58.12	T58.13	T58.14	—	—
industrial fuels or gases, any	T58.8X1	T58.8X2	T58.8X3	T58.8X4	—	—
kerosene (in domestic stoves, fireplaces)	T58.2X1	T58.2X2	T58.2X3	T58.2X4	—	—
kiln gas or vapor	T58.8X1	T58.8X2	T58.8X3	T58.8X4	—	—
motor exhaust gas, not in transit	T58.01	T58.02	T58.03	T58.04	—	—
piped gas (manufactured) (natural)	T58.11	T58.12	T58.13	T58.14	—	—
producer gas	T58.8X1	T58.8X2	T58.8X3	T58.8X4	—	—
propane (distributed in mobile container)	T58.11	T58.12	T58.13	T58.14	—	—
distributed through pipes	T58.11	T58.12	T58.13	T58.14	—	—
specified source NEC	T58.8X1	T58.8X2	T58.8X3	T58.8X4	—	—
stove gas	T58.11	T58.12	T58.13	T58.14	—	—
piped	T58.11	T58.12	T58.13	T58.14	—	—
utility gas	T58.11	T58.12	T58.13	T58.14	—	—
piped	T58.11	T58.12	T58.13	T58.14	—	—
water gas	T58.11	T58.12	T58.13	T58.14	—	—
wood (in domestic stoves, fireplaces)	T58.2X1	T58.2X2	T58.2X3	T58.2X4	—	—
tetrachloride (vapor) NEC	T53.0X1	T53.0X2	T53.0X3	T53.0X4	—	—
liquid (cleansing agent) NEC	T53.0X1	T53.0X2	T53.0X3	T53.0X4	—	—
solvent	T53.0X1	T53.0X2	T53.0X3	T53.0X4	—	—
Carbonic acid gas	T59.7X1	T59.7X2	T59.7X3	T59.7X4	—	—
anhydrase inhibitor NEC	T50.2X1	T50.2X2	T50.2X3	T50.2X4	T50.2X5	T50.2X6
Carbophenothion	T60.0X1	T60.0X2	T60.0X3	T60.0X4	—	—
Carboplatin	T45.1X1	T45.1X2	T45.1X3	T45.1X4	T45.1X5	T45.1X6
Carboprost	T48.0X1	T48.0X2	T48.0X3	T48.0X4	T48.0X5	T48.0X6
Carboquone	T45.1X1	T45.1X2	T45.1X3	T45.1X4	T45.1X5	T45.1X6
Carbowax	T49.3X1	T49.3X2	T49.3X3	T49.3X4	T49.3X5	T49.3X6
Carboxymethyl-cellulose	T47.4X1	T47.4X2	T47.4X3	T47.4X4	T47.4X5	T47.4X6
S-Carboxymethyl-cysteine	T48.4X1	T48.4X2	T48.4X3	T48.4X4	T48.4X5	T48.4X6
Carbrital	T42.3X1	T42.3X2	T42.3X3	T42.3X4	T42.3X5	T42.3X6
Carbromal	T42.6X1	T42.6X2	T42.6X3	T42.6X4	T42.6X5	T42.6X6
Carbutamide	T38.3X1	T38.3X2	T38.3X3	T38.3X4	T38.3X5	T38.3X6
Carbuterol	T48.6X1	T48.6X2	T48.6X3	T48.6X4	T48.6X5	T48.6X6
Cardiac						
depressants	T46.2X1	T46.2X2	T46.2X3	T46.2X4	T46.2X5	T46.2X6
rhythm regulator	T46.2X1	T46.2X2	T46.2X3	T46.2X4	T46.2X5	T46.2X6
specified NEC	T46.2X1	T46.2X2	T46.2X3	T46.2X4	T46.2X5	T46.2X6

Substance	Poisoning, Accidental (Unintentional)	Poisoning, Intentional Self-Harm	Poisoning, Assault	Poisoning, Undetermined	Adverse Effect	Underdosing
Cardiografin	T50.8X1	T50.8X2	T50.8X3	T50.8X4	T50.8X5	T50.8X6
Cardio-green	T50.8X1	T50.8X2	T50.8X3	T50.8X4	T50.8X5	T50.8X6
Cardiotonic (glycoside) NEC	T46.0X1	T46.0X2	T46.0X3	T46.0X4	T46.0X5	T46.0X6
Cardiovascular drug NEC	T46.901	T46.902	T46.903	T46.904	T46.905	T46.906
Cardrase	T50.2X1	T50.2X2	T50.2X3	T50.2X4	T50.2X5	T50.2X6
Carfusin	T49.0X1	T49.0X2	T49.0X3	T49.0X4	T49.0X5	T49.0X6
Carfecillin	T36.0X1	T36.0X2	T36.0X3	T36.0X4	T36.0X5	T36.0X6
Carfenazine	T43.3X1	T43.3X2	T43.3X3	T43.3X4	T43.3X5	T43.3X6
Carindacillin	T36.0X1	T36.0X2	T36.0X3	T36.0X4	T36.0X5	T36.0X6
Carisoprodol	T42.8X1	T42.8X2	T42.8X3	T42.8X4	T42.8X5	T42.8X6
Carmellose	T47.4X1	T47.4X2	T47.4X3	T47.4X4	T47.4X5	T47.4X6
Carminative	T47.5X1	T47.5X2	T47.5X3	T47.5X4	T47.5X5	T47.5X6
Carmofur	T45.1X1	T45.1X2	T45.1X3	T45.1X4	T45.1X5	T45.1X6
Carmustine	T45.1X1	T45.1X2	T45.1X3	T45.1X4	T45.1X5	T45.1X6
Carotene	T45.2X1	T45.2X2	T45.2X3	T45.2X4	T45.2X5	T45.2X6
Carphenazine	T43.3X1	T43.3X2	T43.3X3	T43.3X4	T43.3X5	T43.3X6
Carpipramine	T42.4X1	T42.4X2	T42.4X3	T42.4X4	T42.4X5	T42.4X6
Carprofen	T39.311	T39.312	T39.313	T39.314	T39.315	T39.316
Carpronium chloride	T44.3X1	T44.3X2	T44.3X3	T44.3X4	T44.3X5	T44.3X6
Carrageenan	T47.8X1	T47.8X2	T47.8X3	T47.8X4	T47.8X5	T47.8X6
Carteolol	T44.7X1	T44.7X2	T44.7X3	T44.7X4	T44.7X5	T44.7X6
Carter's Little Pills	T47.2X1	T47.2X2	T47.2X3	T47.2X4	T47.2X5	T47.2X6
Cascara (sagrada)	T47.2X1	T47.2X2	T47.2X3	T47.2X4	T47.2X5	T47.2X6
Cassava	T62.2X1	T62.2X2	T62.2X3	T62.2X4	—	—
Castellani's paint	T49.0X1	T49.0X2	T49.0X3	T49.0X4	T49.0X5	T49.0X6
Castor						
bean	T62.2X1	T62.2X2	T62.2X3	T62.2X4	—	—
oil	T47.2X1	T47.2X2	T47.2X3	T47.2X4	T47.2X5	T47.2X6
Catalase	T45.3X1	T45.3X2	T45.3X3	T45.3X4	T45.3X5	T45.3X6
Caterpillar (sting)	T63.431	T63.432	T63.433	T63.434	—	—
Catha (edulis) (tea)	T43.691	T43.692	T43.693	T43.694	—	—
Cathartic NEC	T47.4X1	T47.4X2	T47.4X3	T47.4X4	T47.4X5	T47.4X6
anthracene derivative	T47.2X1	T47.2X2	T47.2X3	T47.2X4	T47.2X5	T47.2X6
bulk	T47.4X1	T47.4X2	T47.4X3	T47.4X4	T47.4X5	T47.4X6
contact	T47.2X1	T47.2X2	T47.2X3	T47.2X4	T47.2X5	T47.2X6
emollient NEC	T47.4X1	T47.4X2	T47.4X3	T47.4X4	T47.4X5	T47.4X6
irritant NEC	T47.2X1	T47.2X2	T47.2X3	T47.2X4	T47.2X5	T47.2X6
mucilage	T47.4X1	T47.4X2	T47.4X3	T47.4X4	T47.4X5	T47.4X6
saline	T47.3X1	T47.3X2	T47.3X3	T47.3X4	T47.3X5	T47.3X6
vegetable	T47.2X1	T47.2X2	T47.2X3	T47.2X4	T47.2X5	T47.2X6
Cathine	T50.5X1	T50.5X2	T50.5X3	T50.5X4	T50.5X5	T50.5X6
Cathomycin	T36.8X1	T36.8X2	T36.8X3	T36.8X4	T36.8X5	T36.8X6

◀ New   ◀ Revised   ~~deleted~~ Deleted

Substance	External Cause (T-Code)					
	Poisoning, Accidental (Unintentional)	Poisoning, Intentional Self-Harm	Poisoning, Assault	Poisoning, Undetermined	Adverse Effect	Underdosing
Cation exchange resin	T50.3X1	T50.3X2	T50.3X3	T50.3X4	T50.3X5	T50.3X6
Caustic(s) NEC	T54.91	T54.92	T54.93	T54.94	—	—
alkali	T54.3X1	T54.3X2	T54.3X3	T54.3X4	—	—
hydroxide	T54.3X1	T54.3X2	T54.3X3	T54.3X4	—	—
potash	T54.3X1	T54.3X2	T54.3X3	T54.3X4	—	—
soda	T54.3X1	T54.3X2	T54.3X3	T54.3X4	—	—
specified NEC	T54.91	T54.92	T54.93	T54.94	—	—
Ceepryn	T49.0X1	T49.0X2	T49.0X3	T49.0X4	T49.0X5	T49.0X6
ENT agent	T49.6X1	T49.6X2	T49.6X3	T49.6X4	T49.6X5	T49.6X6
lozenges	T49.6X1	T49.6X2	T49.6X3	T49.6X4	T49.6X5	T49.6X6
Cefacetrile	T36.1X1	T36.1X2	T36.1X3	T36.1X4	T36.1X5	T36.1X6
Cefaclor	T36.1X1	T36.1X2	T36.1X3	T36.1X4	T36.1X5	T36.1X6
Cefadroxil	T36.1X1	T36.1X2	T36.1X3	T36.1X4	T36.1X5	T36.1X6
Cefalexin	T36.1X1	T36.1X2	T36.1X3	T36.1X4	T36.1X5	T36.1X6
Cefaloglycin	T36.1X1	T36.1X2	T36.1X3	T36.1X4	T36.1X5	T36.1X6
Cefaloridine	T36.1X1	T36.1X2	T36.1X3	T36.1X4	T36.1X5	T36.1X6
Cefalosporins	T36.1X1	T36.1X2	T36.1X3	T36.1X4	T36.1X5	T36.1X6
Cefalotin	T36.1X1	T36.1X2	T36.1X3	T36.1X4	T36.1X5	T36.1X6
Cefamandole	T36.1X1	T36.1X2	T36.1X3	T36.1X4	T36.1X5	T36.1X6
Cefamycin antibiotic	T36.1X1	T36.1X2	T36.1X3	T36.1X4	T36.1X5	T36.1X6
Cefapirin	T36.1X1	T36.1X2	T36.1X3	T36.1X4	T36.1X5	T36.1X6
Cefatrizine	T36.1X1	T36.1X2	T36.1X3	T36.1X4	T36.1X5	T36.1X6
Cefazedone	T36.1X1	T36.1X2	T36.1X3	T36.1X4	T36.1X5	T36.1X6
Cefazolin	T36.1X1	T36.1X2	T36.1X3	T36.1X4	T36.1X5	T36.1X6
Cefbuperazone	T36.1X1	T36.1X2	T36.1X3	T36.1X4	T36.1X5	T36.1X6
Cefetamet	T36.1X1	T36.1X2	T36.1X3	T36.1X4	T36.1X5	T36.1X6
Cefixime	T36.1X1	T36.1X2	T36.1X3	T36.1X4	T36.1X5	T36.1X6
Cefmenoxime	T36.1X1	T36.1X2	T36.1X3	T36.1X4	T36.1X5	T36.1X6
Cefmetazole	T36.1X1	T36.1X2	T36.1X3	T36.1X4	T36.1X5	T36.1X6
Cefminox	T36.1X1	T36.1X2	T36.1X3	T36.1X4	T36.1X5	T36.1X6
Cefonicid	T36.1X1	T36.1X2	T36.1X3	T36.1X4	T36.1X5	T36.1X6
Cefoperazone	T36.1X1	T36.1X2	T36.1X3	T36.1X4	T36.1X5	T36.1X6
Ceforanide	T36.1X1	T36.1X2	T36.1X3	T36.1X4	T36.1X5	T36.1X6
Cefotaxime	T36.1X1	T36.1X2	T36.1X3	T36.1X4	T36.1X5	T36.1X6
Cefotetan	T36.1X1	T36.1X2	T36.1X3	T36.1X4	T36.1X5	T36.1X6
Cefotiam	T36.1X1	T36.1X2	T36.1X3	T36.1X4	T36.1X5	T36.1X6
Cefoxitin	T36.1X1	T36.1X2	T36.1X3	T36.1X4	T36.1X5	T36.1X6
Cefpimizole	T36.1X1	T36.1X2	T36.1X3	T36.1X4	T36.1X5	T36.1X6
Cefpiramide	T36.1X1	T36.1X2	T36.1X3	T36.1X4	T36.1X5	T36.1X6
Cefradine	T36.1X1	T36.1X2	T36.1X3	T36.1X4	T36.1X5	T36.1X6
Cefroxadine	T36.1X1	T36.1X2	T36.1X3	T36.1X4	T36.1X5	T36.1X6
Cefsulodin	T36.1X1	T36.1X2	T36.1X3	T36.1X4	T36.1X5	T36.1X6

Substance	External Cause (T-Code)					
	Poisoning, Accidental (Unintentional)	Poisoning, Intentional Self-Harm	Poisoning, Assault	Poisoning, Undetermined	Adverse Effect	Underdosing
Ceftazidime	T36.1X1	T36.1X2	T36.1X3	T36.1X4	T36.1X5	T36.1X6
Cefteram	T36.1X1	T36.1X2	T36.1X3	T36.1X4	T36.1X5	T36.1X6
Ceftezole	T36.1X1	T36.1X2	T36.1X3	T36.1X4	T36.1X5	T36.1X6
Ceftizoxime	T36.1X1	T36.1X2	T36.1X3	T36.1X4	T36.1X5	T36.1X6
Ceftriaxone	T36.1X1	T36.1X2	T36.1X3	T36.1X4	T36.1X5	T36.1X6
Cefuroxime	T36.1X1	T36.1X2	T36.1X3	T36.1X4	T36.1X5	T36.1X6
Cefuzonam	T36.1X1	T36.1X2	T36.1X3	T36.1X4	T36.1X5	T36.1X6
Celestone	T38.0X1	T38.0X2	T38.0X3	T38.0X4	T38.0X5	T38.0X6
topical	T49.0X1	T49.0X2	T49.0X3	T49.0X4	T49.0X5	T49.0X6
Celiprolol	T44.7X1	T44.7X2	T44.7X3	T44.7X4	T44.7X5	T44.7X6
Cellosolve	T52.91	T52.92	T52.93	T52.94	—	—
Cell stimulants and proliferants	T49.8X1	T49.8X2	T49.8X3	T49.8X4	T49.8X5	T49.8X6
Cellulose						
cathartic	T47.4X1	T47.4X2	T47.4X3	T47.4X4	T47.4X5	T47.4X6
hydroxyethyl	T47.4X1	T47.4X2	T47.4X3	T47.4X4	T47.4X5	T47.4X6
nitrates (topical)	T49.3X1	T49.3X2	T49.3X3	T49.3X4	T49.3X5	T49.3X6
oxidized	T49.4X1	T49.4X2	T49.4X3	T49.4X4	T49.4X5	T49.4X6
Centipede (bite)	T63.411	T63.412	T63.413	T63.414	—	—
Central nervous system						
depressants	T42.71	T42.72	T42.73	T42.74	T42.75	T42.76
anesthetic (general) NEC	T41.201	T41.202	T41.203	T41.204	T41.205	T41.206
gases NEC	T41.0X1	T41.0X2	T41.0X3	T41.0X4	T41.0X5	T41.0X6
intravenous	T41.1X1	T41.1X2	T41.1X3	T41.1X4	T41.1X5	T41.1X6
barbiturates	T42.3X1	T42.3X2	T42.3X3	T42.3X4	T42.3X5	T42.3X6
benzodiazepines	T42.4X1	T42.4X2	T42.4X3	T42.4X4	T42.4X5	T42.4X6
bromides	T42.6X1	T42.6X2	T42.6X3	T42.6X4	T42.6X5	T42.6X6
cannabis sativa	T40.711	T40.712	T40.713	T40.714	T40.715	T40.716
chloral hydrate	T42.6X1	T42.6X2	T42.6X3	T42.6X4	T42.6X5	T42.6X6
ethanol	T51.0X1	T51.0X2	T51.0X3	T51.0X4	—	—
hallucinogenics	T40.901	T40.902	T40.903	T40.904	T40.905	T40.906
hypnotics	T42.71	T42.72	T42.73	T42.74	T42.75	T42.76
specified NEC	T42.6X1	T42.6X2	T42.6X3	T42.6X4	T42.6X5	T42.6X6
muscle relaxants	T42.8X1	T42.8X2	T42.8X3	T42.8X4	T42.8X5	T42.8X6
paraldehyde	T42.6X1	T42.6X2	T42.6X3	T42.6X4	T42.6X5	T42.6X6
sedatives; sedative-hypnotics	T42.71	T42.72	T42.73	T42.74	T42.75	T42.76
mixed NEC	T42.6X1	T42.6X2	T42.6X3	T42.6X4	T42.6X5	T42.6X6
specified NEC	T42.6X1	T42.6X2	T42.6X3	T42.6X4	T42.6X5	T42.6X6
muscle-tone depressants	T42.8X1	T42.8X2	T42.8X3	T42.8X4	T42.8X5	T42.8X6
stimulants	T43.601	T43.602	T43.603	T43.604	T43.605	T43.606
amphetamines	T43.621	T43.622	T43.623	T43.624	T43.625	T43.626
analeptics	T50.7X1	T50.7X2	T50.7X3	T50.7X4	T50.7X5	T50.7X6

◀ New ◀ Revised ~~deleted~~ Deleted

	External Cause (T-Code)					
Substance	Poisoning, Accidental (Unintentional)	Poisoning, Intentional Self-Harm	Poisoning, Assault	Poisoning, Undetermined	Adverse Effect	Underdosing
Central nervous system (*Continued*)						
stimulants (*Continued*)						
antidepressants	T43.201	T43.202	T43.203	T43.204	T43.205	T43.206
opiate antagonists	T50.7X1	T50.7X2	T50.7X3	T50.7X4	T50.7X5	T50.7X6
specified NEC	T43.691	T43.692	T43.693	T43.694	T43.695	T43.696
Cephalexin	T36.1X1	T36.1X2	T36.1X3	T36.1X4	T36.1X5	T36.1X6
Cephaloglycin	T36.1X1	T36.1X2	T36.1X3	T36.1X4	T36.1X5	T36.1X6
Cephaloridine	T36.1X1	T36.1X2	T36.1X3	T36.1X4	T36.1X5	T36.1X6
Cephalosporins	T36.1X1	T36.1X2	T36.1X3	T36.1X4	T36.1X5	T36.1X6
N (adicillin)	T36.0X1	T36.0X2	T36.0X3	T36.0X4	T36.0X5	T36.0X6
Cephalothin	T36.1X1	T36.1X2	T36.1X3	T36.1X4	T36.1X5	T36.1X6
Cephalotin	T36.1X1	T36.1X2	T36.1X3	T36.1X4	T36.1X5	T36.1X6
Cephradine	T36.1X1	T36.1X2	T36.1X3	T36.1X4	T36.1X5	T36.1X6
Cerbera (odallam)	T62.2X1	T62.2X2	T62.2X3	T62.2X4	—	—
Cerberin	T46.0X1	T46.0X2	T46.0X3	T46.0X4	T46.0X5	T46.0X6
Cerebral stimulants	T43.601	T43.602	T43.603	T43.604	T43.605	T43.606
psychotherapeutic	T43.601	T43.602	T43.603	T43.604	T43.605	T43.606
specified NEC	T43.691	T43.692	T43.693	T43.694	T43.695	T43.696
Cerium oxalate	T45.0X1	T45.0X2	T45.0X3	T45.0X4	T45.0X5	T45.0X6
Cerous oxalate	T45.0X1	T45.0X2	T45.0X3	T45.0X4	T45.0X5	T45.0X6
Ceruletide	T50.8X1	T50.8X2	T50.8X3	T50.8X4	T50.8X5	T50.8X6
Cetalkonium (chloride)	T49.0X1	T49.0X2	T49.0X3	T49.0X4	T49.0X5	T49.0X6
Cethexonium chloride	T49.0X1	T49.0X2	T49.0X3	T49.0X4	T49.0X5	T49.0X6
Cetiedil	T46.7X1	T46.7X2	T46.7X3	T46.7X4	T46.7X5	T46.7X6
Cetirizine	T45.0X1	T45.0X2	T45.0X3	T45.0X4	T45.0X5	T45.0X6
Cetomacrogol	T50.991	T50.992	T50.993	T50.994	T50.995	T50.996
Cetotiamine	T45.2X1	T45.2X2	T45.2X3	T45.2X4	T45.2X5	T45.2X6
Cetoxime	T45.0X1	T45.0X2	T45.0X3	T45.0X4	T45.0X5	T45.0X6
Cetraxate	T47.1X1	T47.1X2	T47.1X3	T47.1X4	T47.1X5	T47.1X6
Cetrimide	T49.0X1	T49.0X2	T49.0X3	T49.0X4	T49.0X5	T49.0X6
Cetrimonium (bromide)	T49.0X1	T49.0X2	T49.0X3	T49.0X4	T49.0X5	T49.0X6
Cetylpyridinium chloride	T49.0X1	T49.0X2	T49.0X3	T49.0X4	T49.0X5	T49.0X6
ENT agent	T49.6X1	T49.6X2	T49.6X3	T49.6X4	T49.6X5	T49.6X6
lozenges	T49.6X1	T49.6X2	T49.6X3	T49.6X4	T49.6X5	T49.6X6
Cevadillasee Sabadilla						
Cevitamic acid	T45.2X1	T45.2X2	T45.2X3	T45.2X4	T45.2X5	T45.2X6
Chalk, precipitated	T47.1X1	T47.1X2	T47.1X3	T47.1X4	T47.1X5	T47.1X6
Chamomile	T49.0X1	T49.0X2	T49.0X3	T49.0X4	T49.0X5	T49.0X6
Ch'an su	T46.0X1	T46.0X2	T46.0X3	T46.0X4	T46.0X5	T46.0X6
Charcoal	T47.6X1	T47.6X2	T47.6X3	T47.6X4	T47.6X5	T47.6X6
activated — *see also Charcoal, medicinal*	T47.6X1	T47.6X2	T47.6X3	T47.6X4	T47.6X5	T47.6X6

	External Cause (T-Code)					
Substance	Poisoning, Accidental (Unintentional)	Poisoning, Intentional Self-Harm	Poisoning, Assault	Poisoning, Undetermined	Adverse Effect	Underdosing
Charcoal (*Continued*)						
fumes (Carbon monoxide)	T58.2X1	T58.2X2	T58.2X3	T58.2X4	—	—
industrial	T58.8X1	T58.8X2	T58.8X3	T58.8X4	—	—
medicinal (activated)	T47.6X1	T47.6X2	T47.6X3	T47.6X4	T47.6X5	T47.6X6
antidiarrheal	T47.6X1	T47.6X2	T47.6X3	T47.6X4	T47.6X5	T47.6X6
poison control	T47.8X1	T47.8X2	T47.8X3	T47.8X4	T47.8X5	T47.8X6
specified use other than for diarrhea	T47.8X1	T47.8X2	T47.8X3	T47.8X4	T47.8X5	T47.8X6
topical	T49.8X1	T49.8X2	T49.8X3	T49.8X4	T49.8X5	T49.8X6
Chaulmosulfone	T37.1X1	T37.1X2	T37.1X3	T37.1X4	T37.1X5	T37.1X6
Chelating agent NEC	T50.6X1	T50.6X2	T50.6X3	T50.6X4	T50.6X5	T50.6X6
Chelidonium majus	T62.2X1	T62.2X2	T62.2X3	T62.2X4	—	—
Chemical substance NEC	T65.91	T65.92	T65.93	T65.94	—	—
Chenodeoxycholic acid	T47.5X1	T47.5X2	T47.5X3	T47.5X4	T47.5X5	T47.5X6
Chenodiol	T47.5X1	T47.5X2	T47.5X3	T47.5X4	T47.5X5	T47.5X6
Chenopodium	T37.4X1	T37.4X2	T37.4X3	T37.4X4	T37.4X5	T37.4X6
Cherry laurel	T62.2X1	T62.2X2	T62.2X3	T62.2X4	—	—
Chinidin(e)	T46.2X1	T46.2X2	T46.2X3	T46.2X4	T46.2X5	T46.2X6
Chiniofon	T37.8X1	T37.8X2	T37.8X3	T37.8X4	T37.8X5	T37.8X6
Chlophedianol	T48.3X1	T48.3X2	T48.3X3	T48.3X4	T48.3X5	T48.3X6
Chloral	T42.6X1	T42.6X2	T42.6X3	T42.6X4	T42.6X5	T42.6X6
derivative	T42.6X1	T42.6X2	T42.6X3	T42.6X4	T42.6X5	T42.6X6
hydrate	T42.6X1	T42.6X2	T42.6X3	T42.6X4	T42.6X5	T42.6X6
Chloralamide	T42.6X1	T42.6X2	T42.6X3	T42.6X4	T42.6X5	T42.6X6
Chloralodol	T42.6X1	T42.6X2	T42.6X3	T42.6X4	T42.6X5	T42.6X6
Chloralose	T60.4X1	T60.4X2	T60.4X3	T60.4X4	—	—
Chlorambucil	T45.1X1	T45.1X2	T45.1X3	T45.1X4	T45.1X5	T45.1X6
Chloramine	T57.8X1	T57.8X2	T57.8X3	T57.8X4	—	—
T	T49.0X1	T49.0X2	T49.0X3	T49.0X4	T49.0X5	T49.0X6
topical	T49.0X1	T49.0X2	T49.0X3	T49.0X4	T49.0X5	T49.0X6
Chloramphenicol	T36.2X1	T36.2X2	T36.2X3	T36.2X4	T36.2X5	T36.2X6
ENT agent	T49.6X1	T49.6X2	T49.6X3	T49.6X4	T49.6X5	T49.6X6
ophthalmic preparation	T49.5X1	T49.5X2	T49.5X3	T49.5X4	T49.5X5	T49.5X6
topical NEC	T49.0X1	T49.0X2	T49.0X3	T49.0X4	T49.0X5	T49.0X6
Chlorate (potassium) (sodium) NEC	T60.3X1	T60.3X2	T60.3X3	T60.3X4	—	—
herbicide	T60.3X1	T60.3X2	T60.3X3	T60.3X4	—	—
Chlorazanil	T50.2X1	T50.2X2	T50.2X3	T50.2X4	T50.2X5	T50.2X6
Chlorbenzene, chlorbenzol	T53.7X1	T53.7X2	T53.7X3	T53.7X4	—	—
Chlorbenzoxamine	T44.3X1	T44.3X2	T44.3X3	T44.3X4	T44.3X5	T44.3X6
Chlorbutol	T42.6X1	T42.6X2	T42.6X3	T42.6X4	T42.6X5	T42.6X6
Chlorcyclizine	T45.0X1	T45.0X2	T45.0X3	T45.0X4	T45.0X5	T45.0X6

◀ New   ◀ Revised   ~~deleted~~ Deleted

Substance	External Cause (T-Code) Poisoning, Accidental (Unintentional)	Poisoning, Intentional Self-Harm	Poisoning, Assault	Poisoning, Undetermined	Adverse Effect	Underdosing
Chlordan(e) (dust)	T60.1X1	T60.1X2	T60.1X3	T60.1X4	—	—
Chlordantoin	T49.0X1	T49.0X2	T49.0X3	T49.0X4	T49.0X5	T49.0X6
Chlordiazepoxide	T42.4X1	T42.4X2	T42.4X3	T42.4X4	T42.4X5	T42.4X6
Chlordiethyl benzamide	T49.3X1	T49.3X2	T49.3X3	T49.3X4	T49.3X5	T49.3X6
Chloresium	T49.8X1	T49.8X2	T49.8X3	T49.8X4	T49.8X5	T49.8X6
Chlorethiazol	T42.6X1	T42.6X2	T42.6X3	T42.6X4	T42.6X5	T42.6X6
Chlorethyl — see Ethyl chloride						
Chloretone	T42.6X1	T42.6X2	T42.6X3	T42.6X4	T42.6X5	T42.6X6
Chlorex	T53.6X1	T53.6X2	T53.6X3	T53.6X4	—	—
insecticide	T60.1X1	T60.1X2	T60.1X3	T60.1X4	—	—
Chlorfenvinphos	T60.0X1	T60.0X2	T60.0X3	T60.0X4	—	—
Chlorhexadol	T42.6X1	T42.6X2	T42.6X3	T42.6X4	T42.6X5	T42.6X6
Chlorhexamide	T45.1X1	T45.1X2	T45.1X3	T45.1X4	T45.1X5	T45.1X6
Chlorhexidine	T49.0X1	T49.0X2	T49.0X3	T49.0X4	T49.0X5	T49.0X6
Chlorhydroxyquinolin	T49.0X1	T49.0X2	T49.0X3	T49.0X4	T49.0X5	T49.0X6
Chloride of lime (bleach)	T54.3X1	T54.3X2	T54.3X3	T54.3X4	—	—
Chlorimipramine	T43.011	T43.012	T43.013	T43.014	T43.015	T43.016
Chlorinated						
camphene	T53.6X1	T53.6X2	T53.6X3	T53.6X4	—	—
diphenyl	T53.7X1	T53.7X2	T53.7X3	T53.7X4	—	—
hydrocarbons NEC	T53.91	T53.92	T53.93	T53.94	—	—
solvents	T53.91	T53.92	T53.93	T53.94	—	—
lime (bleach)	T54.3X1	T54.3X2	T54.3X3	T54.3X4	—	—
and boric acid solution	T49.0X1	T49.0X2	T49.0X3	T49.0X4	T49.0X5	T49.0X6
naphthalene (insecticide)	T60.1X1	T60.1X2	T60.1X3	T60.1X4	—	—
industrial (non-pesticide)	T53.7X1	T53.7X2	T53.7X3	T53.7X4	—	—
pesticide NEC	T60.8X1	T60.8X2	T60.8X3	T60.8X4	—	—
soda — see also Sodium hypochlorite						
solution	T49.0X1	T49.0X2	T49.0X3	T49.0X4	T49.0X5	T49.0X6
Chlorine (fumes) (gas)	T59.4X1	T59.4X2	T59.4X3	T59.4X4	—	—
bleach	T54.3X1	T54.3X2	T54.3X3	T54.3X4	—	—
compound gas NEC	T59.4X1	T59.4X2	T59.4X3	T59.4X4	—	—
disinfectant	T59.4X1	T59.4X2	T59.4X3	T59.4X4	—	—
releasing agents NEC	T59.4X1	T59.4X2	T59.4X3	T59.4X4	—	—
Chlorisondamine chloride	T46.991	T46.992	T46.993	T46.994	T46.995	T46.996
Chlormadinone	T38.5X1	T38.5X2	T38.5X3	T38.5X4	T38.5X5	T38.5X6
Chlormephos	T60.0X1	T60.0X2	T60.0X3	T60.0X4	—	—
Chlormerodrin	T50.2X1	T50.2X2	T50.2X3	T50.2X4	T50.2X5	T50.2X6
Chlormethiazole	T42.6X1	T42.6X2	T42.6X3	T42.6X4	T42.6X5	T42.6X6
Chlormethine	T45.1X1	T45.1X2	T45.1X3	T45.1X4	T45.1X5	T45.1X6
Chlormethylenecycline	T36.4X1	T36.4X2	T36.4X3	T36.4X4	T36.4X5	T36.4X6

Substance	External Cause (T-Code) Poisoning, Accidental (Unintentional)	Poisoning, Intentional Self-Harm	Poisoning, Assault	Poisoning, Undetermined	Adverse Effect	Underdosing
Chlormezanone	T42.6X1	T42.6X2	T42.6X3	T42.6X4	T42.6X5	T42.6X6
Chloroacetic acid	T60.3X1	T60.3X2	T60.3X3	T60.3X4	—	—
Chloroacetone	T59.3X1	T59.3X2	T59.3X3	T59.3X4	—	—
Chloroacetophenone	T59.3X1	T59.3X2	T59.3X3	T59.3X4	—	—
Chloroaniline	T53.7X1	T53.7X2	T53.7X3	T53.7X4	—	—
Chlorobenzene, chlorobenzol	T53.7X1	T53.7X2	T53.7X3	T53.7X4	—	—
Chlorobromomethane (fire extinguisher)	T53.6X1	T53.6X2	T53.6X3	T53.6X4	—	—
Chlorobutanol	T49.0X1	T49.0X2	T49.0X3	T49.0X4	T49.0X5	T49.0X6
Chlorocresol	T49.0X1	T49.0X2	T49.0X3	T49.0X4	T49.0X5	T49.0X6
Chlorodehydro-methyltestosterone	T38.7X1	T38.7X2	T38.7X3	T38.7X4	T38.7X5	T38.7X6
Chlorodinitrobenzene	T53.7X1	T53.7X2	T53.7X3	T53.7X4	—	—
dust or vapor	T53.7X1	T53.7X2	T53.7X3	T53.7X4	—	—
Chlorodiphenyl	T53.7X1	T53.7X2	T53.7X3	T53.7X4	—	—
Chloroethane — see Ethyl chloride						
Chloroethylene	T53.6X1	T53.6X2	T53.6X3	T53.6X4	—	—
Chlorofluorocarbons	T53.5X1	T53.5X2	T53.5X3	T53.5X4	—	—
Chloroform (fumes) (vapor)	T53.1X1	T53.1X2	T53.1X3	T53.1X4	—	—
anesthetic	T41.0X1	T41.0X2	T41.0X3	T41.0X4	T41.0X5	T41.0X6
solvent	T53.1X1	T53.1X2	T53.1X3	T53.1X4	—	—
water, concentrated	T41.0X1	T41.0X2	T41.0X3	T41.0X4	T41.0X5	T41.0X6
Chloroguanide	T37.2X1	T37.2X2	T37.2X3	T37.2X4	T37.2X5	T37.2X6
Chloromycetin	T36.2X1	T36.2X2	T36.2X3	T36.2X4	T36.2X5	T36.2X6
ENT agent	T49.6X1	T49.6X2	T49.6X3	T49.6X4	T49.6X5	T49.6X6
ophthalmic preparation	T49.5X1	T49.5X2	T49.5X3	T49.5X4	T49.5X5	T49.5X6
otic solution	T49.6X1	T49.6X2	T49.6X3	T49.6X4	T49.6X5	T49.6X6
topical NEC	T49.0X1	T49.0X2	T49.0X3	T49.0X4	T49.0X5	T49.0X6
Chloronitrobenzene	T53.7X1	T53.7X2	T53.7X3	T53.7X4	—	—
dust or vapor	T53.7X1	T53.7X2	T53.7X3	T53.7X4	—	—
Chlorophacinone	T60.4X1	T60.4X2	T60.4X3	T60.4X4	—	—
Chlorophenol	T53.7X1	T53.7X2	T53.7X3	T53.7X4	—	—
Chlorophenothane	T60.1X1	T60.1X2	T60.1X3	T60.1X4	—	—
Chlorophyll	T50.991	T50.992	T50.993	T50.994	T50.995	T50.996
Chloropicrin (fumes)	T53.6X1	T53.6X2	T53.6X3	T53.6X4	—	—
fumigant	T60.8X1	T60.8X2	T60.8X3	T60.8X4	—	—
fungicide	T60.3X1	T60.3X2	T60.3X3	T60.3X4	—	—
pesticide	T60.8X1	T60.8X2	T60.8X3	T60.8X4	—	—
Chloroprocaine	T41.3X1	T41.3X2	T41.3X3	T41.3X4	T41.3X5	T41.3X6
infiltration (subcutaneous)	T41.3X1	T41.3X2	T41.3X3	T41.3X4	T41.3X5	T41.3X6
nerve block (peripheral) (plexus)	T41.3X1	T41.3X2	T41.3X3	T41.3X4	T41.3X5	T41.3X6
spinal	T41.3X1	T41.3X2	T41.3X3	T41.3X4	T41.3X5	T41.3X6

◄ New   ◄ Revised   deleted Deleted

TABLE OF DRUGS AND CHEMICALS

TABLE OF DRUGS AND CHEMICALS

Substance	External Cause (T-Code)					
	Poisoning, Accidental (Unintentional)	Poisoning, Intentional Self-Harm	Poisoning, Assault	Poisoning, Undetermined	Adverse Effect	Underdosing
Chloroptic	T49.5X1	T49.5X2	T49.5X3	T49.5X4	T49.5X5	T49.5X6
Chloropurine	T45.1X1	T45.1X2	T45.1X3	T45.1X4	T45.1X5	T45.1X6
Chloropyramine	T45.0X1	T45.0X2	T45.0X3	T45.0X4	T45.0X5	T45.0X6
Chloropyrifos	T60.0X1	T60.0X2	T60.0X3	T60.0X4	—	—
Chloropyrilene	T45.0X1	T45.0X2	T45.0X3	T45.0X4	T45.0X5	T45.0X6
Chloroquine	T37.2X1	T37.2X2	T37.2X3	T37.2X4	T37.2X5	T37.2X6
Chlorothalonil	T60.3X1	T60.3X2	T60.3X3	T60.3X4	—	—
Chlorothen	T45.0X1	T45.0X2	T45.0X3	T45.0X4	T45.0X5	T45.0X6
Chlorothiazide	T50.2X1	T50.2X2	T50.2X3	T50.2X4	T50.2X5	T50.2X6
Chlorothymol	T49.4X1	T49.4X2	T49.4X3	T49.4X4	T49.4X5	T49.4X6
Chlorotrianisene	T38.5X1	T38.5X2	T38.5X3	T38.5X4	T38.5X5	T38.5X6
Chlorovinyldichloro-arsine, not in war	T57.0X1	T57.0X2	T57.0X3	T57.0X4	—	—
Chloroxine	T49.4X1	T49.4X2	T49.4X3	T49.4X4	T49.4X5	T49.4X6
Chloroxylenol	T49.0X1	T49.0X2	T49.0X3	T49.0X4	T49.0X5	T49.0X6
Chlorphenamine	T45.0X1	T45.0X2	T45.0X3	T45.0X4	T45.0X5	T45.0X6
Chlorphenesin	T42.8X1	T42.8X2	T42.8X3	T42.8X4	T42.8X5	T42.8X6
topical (antifungal)	T49.0X1	T49.0X2	T49.0X3	T49.0X4	T49.0X5	T49.0X6
Chlorpheniramine	T45.0X1	T45.0X2	T45.0X3	T45.0X4	T45.0X5	T45.0X6
Chlorphenoxamine	T45.0X1	T45.0X2	T45.0X3	T45.0X4	T45.0X5	T45.0X6
Chlorphentermine	T50.5X1	T50.5X2	T50.5X3	T50.5X4	T50.5X5	T50.5X6
Chlorprocaine — see Chloroprocaine						
Chlorproguanil	T37.2X1	T37.2X2	T37.2X3	T37.2X4	T37.2X5	T37.2X6
Chlorpromazine	T43.3X1	T43.3X2	T43.3X3	T43.3X4	T43.3X5	T43.3X6
Chlorpropamide	T38.3X1	T38.3X2	T38.3X3	T38.3X4	T38.3X5	T38.3X6
Chlorprothixene	T43.4X1	T43.4X2	T43.4X3	T43.4X4	T43.4X5	T43.4X6
Chlorquinaldol	T49.0X1	T49.0X2	T49.0X3	T49.0X4	T49.0X5	T49.0X6
Chlorquinol	T49.0X1	T49.0X2	T49.0X3	T49.0X4	T49.0X5	T49.0X6
Chlortalidone	T50.2X1	T50.2X2	T50.2X3	T50.2X4	T50.2X5	T50.2X6
Chlortetracycline	T36.4X1	T36.4X2	T36.4X3	T36.4X4	T36.4X5	T36.4X6
Chlorthalidone	T50.2X1	T50.2X2	T50.2X3	T50.2X4	T50.2X5	T50.2X6
Chlorthiophos	T60.0X1	T60.0X2	T60.0X3	T60.0X4	—	—
Chlorotrianisene	T38.5X1	T38.5X2	T38.5X3	T38.5X4	T38.5X5	T38.5X6
Chlor-Trimeton	T45.0X1	T45.0X2	T45.0X3	T45.0X4	T45.0X5	T45.0X6
Chlorthion	T60.0X1	T60.0X2	T60.0X3	T60.0X4	—	—
Chlorzoxazone	T42.8X1	T42.8X2	T42.8X3	T42.8X4	T42.8X5	T42.8X6
Choke damp	T59.7X1	T59.7X2	T59.7X3	T59.7X4	—	—
Cholagogues	T47.5X1	T47.5X2	T47.5X3	T47.5X4	T47.5X5	T47.5X6
Cholebrine	T50.8X1	T50.8X2	T50.8X3	T50.8X4	T50.8X5	T50.8X6
Cholecalciferol	T45.2X1	T45.2X2	T45.2X3	T45.2X4	T45.2X5	T45.2X6
Cholecystokinin	T50.8X1	T50.8X2	T50.8X3	T50.8X4	T50.8X5	T50.8X6
Cholera vaccine	T50.A91	T50.A92	T50.A93	T50.A94	T50.A95	T50.A96

Substance	External Cause (T-Code)					
	Poisoning, Accidental (Unintentional)	Poisoning, Intentional Self-Harm	Poisoning, Assault	Poisoning, Undetermined	Adverse Effect	Underdosing
Choleretic	T47.5X1	T47.5X2	T47.5X3	T47.5X4	T47.5X5	T47.5X6
Cholesterol-lowering agents	T46.6X1	T46.6X2	T46.6X3	T46.6X4	T46.6X5	T46.6X6
Cholestyramine (resin)	T46.6X1	T46.6X2	T46.6X3	T46.6X4	T46.6X5	T46.6X6
Cholic acid	T47.5X1	T47.5X2	T47.5X3	T47.5X4	T47.5X5	T47.5X6
Choline	T48.6X1	T48.6X2	T48.6X3	T48.6X4	T48.6X5	T48.6X6
chloride	T50.991	T50.992	T50.993	T50.994	T50.995	T50.996
dihydrogen citrate	T50.991	T50.992	T50.993	T50.994	T50.995	T50.996
salicylate	T39.091	T39.092	T39.093	T39.094	T39.095	T39.096
theophyllinate	T48.6X1	T48.6X2	T48.6X3	T48.6X4	T48.6X5	T48.6X6
Cholinergic (drug) NEC	T44.1X1	T44.1X2	T44.1X3	T44.1X4	T44.1X5	T44.1X6
muscle tone enhancer	T44.1X1	T44.1X2	T44.1X3	T44.1X4	T44.1X5	T44.1X6
organophosphorus	T44.0X1	T44.0X2	T44.0X3	T44.0X4	T44.0X5	T44.0X6
insecticide	T60.0X1	T60.0X2	T60.0X3	T60.0X4	—	—
nerve gas	T59.891	T59.892	T59.893	T59.894		
trimethyl ammonium propanediol	T44.1X1	T44.1X2	T44.1X3	T44.1X4	T44.1X5	T44.1X6
Cholinesterase reactivator	T50.6X1	T50.6X2	T50.6X3	T50.6X4	T50.6X5	T50.6X6
Cholografin	T50.8X1	T50.8X2	T50.8X3	T50.8X4	T50.8X5	T50.8X6
Chorionic gonadotropin	T38.891	T38.892	T38.893	T38.894	T38.895	T38.896
Chromate	T56.2X1	T56.2X2	T56.2X3	T56.2X4	—	—
dust or mist	T56.2X1	T56.2X2	T56.2X3	T56.2X4	—	—
lead — see also Lead	T56.0X1	T56.0X2	T56.0X3	T56.0X4	—	—
paint	T56.0X1	T56.0X2	T56.0X3	T56.0X4		
Chromic						
acid	T56.2X1	T56.2X2	T56.2X3	T56.2X4	—	—
dust or mist	T56.2X1	T56.2X2	T56.2X3	T56.2X4	—	—
phosphate 32P	T45.1X1	T45.1X2	T45.1X3	T45.1X4	T45.1X5	T45.1X6
Chromium	T56.2X1	T56.2X2	T56.2X3	T56.2X4		
compounds — see Chromate						
sesquioxide	T50.8X1	T50.8X2	T50.8X3	T50.8X4	T50.8X5	T50.8X6
Chromomycin A3	T45.1X1	T45.1X2	T45.1X3	T45.1X4	T45.1X5	T45.1X6
Chromonar	T46.3X1	T46.3X2	T46.3X3	T46.3X4	T46.3X5	T46.3X6
Chromyl chloride	T56.2X1	T56.2X2	T56.2X3	T56.2X4	—	—
Chrysarobin	T49.4X1	T49.4X2	T49.4X3	T49.4X4	T49.4X5	T49.4X6
Chrysazin	T47.2X1	T47.2X2	T47.2X3	T47.2X4	T47.2X5	T47.2X6
Chymar	T45.3X1	T45.3X2	T45.3X3	T45.3X4	T45.3X5	T45.3X6
ophthalmic preparation	T49.5X1	T49.5X2	T49.5X3	T49.5X4	T49.5X5	T49.5X6
Chymopapain	T45.3X1	T45.3X2	T45.3X3	T45.3X4	T45.3X5	T45.3X6
Chymotrypsin	T45.3X1	T45.3X2	T45.3X3	T45.3X4	T45.3X5	T45.3X6
ophthalmic preparation	T49.5X1	T49.5X2	T49.5X3	T49.5X4	T49.5X5	T49.5X6
Cianidanol	T50.991	T50.992	T50.993	T50.994	T50.995	T50.996
Cianopramine	T43.011	T43.012	T43.013	T43.014	T43.015	T43.016
Cibenzoline	T46.2X1	T46.2X2	T46.2X3	T46.2X4	T46.2X5	T46.2X6

◄ New ◄ Revised ~~deleted~~ Deleted

TABLE OF DRUGS AND CHEMICALS

Substance	Poisoning, Accidental (Unintentional)	Poisoning, Intentional Self-Harm	Poisoning, Assault	Poisoning, Undetermined	Adverse Effect	Underdosing
Ciclacillin	T36.0X1	T36.0X2	T36.0X3	T36.0X4	T36.0X5	T36.0X6
Ciclobarbital — *see Hexobarbital*						
Ciclonicate	T46.7X1	T46.7X2	T46.7X3	T46.7X4	T46.7X5	T46.7X6
Ciclopirox (olamine)	T49.0X1	T49.0X2	T49.0X3	T49.0X4	T49.0X5	T49.0X6
Ciclosporin	T45.1X1	T45.1X2	T45.1X3	T45.1X4	T45.1X5	T45.1X6
Cicuta maculata or virosa	T62.2X1	T62.2X2	T62.2X3	T62.2X4	—	—
Cicutoxin	T62.2X1	T62.2X2	T62.2X3	T62.2X4	—	—
Cigarette lighter fluid	T52.0X1	T52.0X2	T52.0X3	T52.0X4	—	—
Cigarettes (tobacco)	T65.221	T65.222	T65.223	T65.224		
Ciguatoxin	T61.01	T61.02	T61.03	T61.04	—	—
Cilazapril	T46.4X1	T46.4X2	T46.4X3	T46.4X4	T46.4X5	T46.4X6
Cimetidine	T47.0X1	T47.0X2	T47.0X3	T47.0X4	T47.0X5	T47.0X6
Cimetropium bromide	T44.3X1	T44.3X2	T44.3X3	T44.3X4	T44.3X5	T44.3X6
Cinchocaine	T41.3X1	T41.3X2	T41.3X3	T41.3X4	T41.3X5	T41.3X6
topical (surface)	T41.3X1	T41.3X2	T41.3X3	T41.3X4	T41.3X5	T41.3X6
Cinchona	T37.2X1	T37.2X2	T37.2X3	T37.2X4	T37.2X5	T37.2X6
Cinchonine alkaloids	T37.2X1	T37.2X2	T37.2X3	T37.2X4	T37.2X5	T37.2X6
Cinchophen	T50.4X1	T50.4X2	T50.4X3	T50.4X4	T50.4X5	T50.4X6
Cinepazide	T46.7X1	T46.7X2	T46.7X3	T46.7X4	T46.7X5	T46.7X6
Cinnamedrine	T48.5X1	T48.5X2	T48.5X3	T48.5X4	T48.5X5	T48.5X6
Cinnarizine	T45.0X1	T45.0X2	T45.0X3	T45.0X4	T45.0X5	T45.0X6
Cinoxacin	T37.8X1	T37.8X2	T37.8X3	T37.8X4	T37.8X5	T37.8X6
Ciprofibrate	T46.6X1	T46.6X2	T46.6X3	T46.6X4	T46.6X5	T46.6X6
Ciprofloxacin	T36.8X1	T36.8X2	T36.8X3	T36.8X4	T36.8X5	T36.8X6
Cisapride	T47.8X1	T47.8X2	T47.8X3	T47.8X4	T47.8X5	T47.8X6
Cisplatin	T45.1X1	T45.1X2	T45.1X3	T45.1X4	T45.1X5	T45.1X6
Citalopram	T43.221	T43.222	T43.223	T43.224	T43.225	T43.226
Citanest	T41.3X1	T41.3X2	T41.3X3	T41.3X4	T41.3X5	T41.3X6
infiltration (subcutaneous)	T41.3X1	T41.3X2	T41.3X3	T41.3X4	T41.3X5	T41.3X6
nerve block (peripheral) (plexus)	T41.3X1	T41.3X2	T41.3X3	T41.3X4	T41.3X5	T41.3X6
Citric acid	T47.5X1	T47.5X2	T47.5X3	T47.5X4	T47.5X5	T47.5X6
Citrovorum (factor)	T45.8X1	T45.8X2	T45.8X3	T45.8X4	T45.8X5	T45.8X6
Claviceps purpurea	T62.2X1	T62.2X2	T62.2X3	T62.2X4	—	—
Clavulanic acid	T36.1X1	T36.1X2	T36.1X3	T36.1X4	T36.1X5	T36.1X6
Cleaner, cleansing agent, type not specified	T65.891	T65.892	T65.893	T65.894		
of paint or varnish	T52.91	T52.92	T52.93	T52.94		
specified type NEC	T65.891	T65.892	T65.893	T65.894	—	—
Clebopride	T47.8X1	T47.8X2	T47.8X3	T47.8X4	T47.8X5	T47.8X6
Clefamide	T37.3X1	T37.3X2	T37.3X3	T37.3X4	T37.3X5	T37.3X6
Clemastine	T45.0X1	T45.0X2	T45.0X3	T45.0X4	T45.0X5	T45.0X6
Clematis vitalba	T62.2X1	T62.2X2	T62.2X3	T62.2X4	—	—

Substance	Poisoning, Accidental (Unintentional)	Poisoning, Intentional Self-Harm	Poisoning, Assault	Poisoning, Undetermined	Adverse Effect	Underdosing
Clemizole	T45.0X1	T45.0X2	T45.0X3	T45.0X4	T45.0X5	T45.0X6
penicillin	T36.0X1	T36.0X2	T36.0X3	T36.0X4	T36.0X5	T36.0X6
Clenbuterol	T48.6X1	T48.6X2	T48.6X3	T48.6X4	T48.6X5	T48.6X6
Clidinium bromide	T44.3X1	T44.3X2	T44.3X3	T44.3X4	T44.3X5	T44.3X6
Clindamycin	T36.8X1	T36.8X2	T36.8X3	T36.8X4	T36.8X5	T36.8X6
Clinofibrate	T46.6X1	T46.6X2	T46.6X3	T46.6X4	T46.6X5	T46.6X6
Clioquinol	T37.8X1	T37.8X2	T37.8X3	T37.8X4	T37.8X5	T37.8X6
Cliradon	T40.2X1	T40.2X2	T40.2X3	T40.2X4	—	—
Clobazam	T42.4X1	T42.4X2	T42.4X3	T42.4X4	T42.4X5	T42.4X6
Clobenzorex	T50.5X1	T50.5X2	T50.5X3	T50.5X4	T50.5X5	T50.5X6
Clobetasol	T49.0X1	T49.0X2	T49.0X3	T49.0X4	T49.0X5	T49.0X6
Clobetasone	T49.0X1	T49.0X2	T49.0X3	T49.0X4	T49.0X5	T49.0X6
Clobutinol	T48.3X1	T48.3X2	T48.3X3	T48.3X4	T48.3X5	T48.3X6
Clocapramine	T43.0X1	T43.0X2	T43.0X3	T43.0X4	T43.0X5	T43.0X6
Clocortolone	T38.0X1	T38.0X2	T38.0X3	T38.0X4	T38.0X5	T38.0X6
Clodantoin	T49.0X1	T49.0X2	T49.0X3	T49.0X4	T49.0X5	T49.0X6
Clodronic acid	T50.991	T50.992	T50.993	T50.994	T50.995	T50.996
Clofazimine	T37.1X1	T37.1X2	T37.1X3	T37.1X4	T37.1X5	T37.1X6
Clofedanol	T48.3X1	T48.3X2	T48.3X3	T48.3X4	T48.3X5	T48.3X6
Clofenamide	T50.2X1	T50.2X2	T50.2X3	T50.2X4	T50.2X5	T50.2X6
Clofenotane	T49.0X1	T49.0X2	T49.0X3	T49.0X4	T49.0X5	T49.0X6
Clofezone	T39.2X1	T39.2X2	T39.2X3	T39.2X4	T39.2X5	T39.2X6
Clofibrate	T46.6X1	T46.6X2	T46.6X3	T46.6X4	T46.6X5	T46.6X6
Clofibride	T46.6X1	T46.6X2	T46.6X3	T46.6X4	T46.6X5	T46.6X6
Cloforex	T50.5X1	T50.5X2	T50.5X3	T50.5X4	T50.5X5	T50.5X6
Clomacran	T43.0X1	T43.0X2	T43.0X3	T43.0X4	T43.0X5	T43.0X6
Clomethiazole	T42.6X1	T42.6X2	T42.6X3	T42.6X4	T42.6X5	T42.6X6
Clometocillin	T36.0X1	T36.0X2	T36.0X3	T36.0X4	T36.0X5	T36.0X6
Clomifene	T38.5X1	T38.5X2	T38.5X3	T38.5X4	T38.5X5	T38.5X6
Clomiphene	T38.5X1	T38.5X2	T38.5X3	T38.5X4	T38.5X5	T38.5X6
Clomipramine	T43.011	T43.012	T43.013	T43.014	T43.015	T43.016
Clomocycline	T36.4X1	T36.4X2	T36.4X3	T36.4X4	T36.4X5	T36.4X6
Clonazepam	T42.4X1	T42.4X2	T42.4X3	T42.4X4	T42.4X5	T42.4X6
Clonidine	T46.5X1	T46.5X2	T46.5X3	T46.5X4	T46.5X5	T46.5X6
Clonixin	T39.8X1	T39.8X2	T39.8X3	T39.8X4	T39.8X5	T39.8X6
Clopamide	T50.2X1	T50.2X2	T50.2X3	T50.2X4	T50.2X5	T50.2X6
Clopenthixol	T43.4X1	T43.4X2	T43.4X3	T43.4X4	T43.4X5	T43.4X6
Cloperastine	T48.3X1	T48.3X2	T48.3X3	T48.3X4	T48.3X5	T48.3X6
Clophedianol	T48.3X1	T48.3X2	T48.3X3	T48.3X4	T48.3X5	T48.3X6
Cloponone	T36.2X1	T36.2X2	T36.2X3	T36.2X4	T36.2X5	T36.2X6
Cloprednol	T38.0X1	T38.0X2	T38.0X3	T38.0X4	T38.0X5	T38.0X6
Cloral betaine	T42.6X1	T42.6X2	T42.6X3	T42.6X4	T42.6X5	T42.6X6

TABLE OF DRUGS AND CHEMICALS

	External Cause (T-Code)					
Substance	Poisoning, Accidental (Unintentional)	Poisoning, Intentional Self-Harm	Poisoning, Assault	Poisoning, Undetermined	Adverse Effect	Underdosing
Cloramfenicol	T36.2X1	T36.2X2	T36.2X3	T36.2X4	T36.2X5	T36.2X6
Clorazepate (dipotassium)	T42.4X1	T42.4X2	T42.4X3	T42.4X4	T42.4X5	T42.4X6
Clorexolone	T50.2X1	T50.2X2	T50.2X3	T50.2X4	T50.2X5	T50.2X6
Clorox (bleach)	T54.91	T54.92	T54.93	T54.94	—	—
Clorfenamine	T45.0X1	T45.0X2	T45.0X3	T45.0X4	T45.0X5	T45.0X6
Clorgiline	T43.1X1	T43.1X2	T43.1X3	T43.1X4	T43.1X5	T43.1X6
Clorotepine	T44.3X1	T44.3X2	T44.3X3	T44.3X4	T44.3X5	T44.3X6
Clorprenaline	T48.6X1	T48.6X2	T48.6X3	T48.6X4	T48.6X5	T48.6X6
Clortermine	T50.5X1	T50.5X2	T50.5X3	T50.5X4	T50.5X5	T50.5X6
Clotiapine	T43.591	T43.592	T43.593	T43.594	T43.595	T43.596
Clotiazepam	T42.4X1	T42.4X2	T42.4X3	T42.4X4	T42.4X5	T42.4X6
Clotibric acid	T46.6X1	T46.6X2	T46.6X3	T46.6X4	T46.6X5	T46.6X6
Clotrimazole	T49.0X1	T49.0X2	T49.0X3	T49.0X4	T49.0X5	T49.0X6
Cloxacillin	T36.0X1	T36.0X2	T36.0X3	T36.0X4	T36.0X5	T36.0X6
Cloxazolam	T42.4X1	T42.4X2	T42.4X3	T42.4X4	T42.4X5	T42.4X6
Cloxiquine	T49.0X1	T49.0X2	T49.0X3	T49.0X4	T49.0X5	T49.0X6
Clozapine	T42.4X1	T42.4X2	T42.4X3	T42.4X4	T42.4X5	T42.4X6
Coagulant NEC	T45.7X1	T45.7X2	T45.7X3	T45.7X4	T45.7X5	T45.7X6
Coal (carbon monoxide from) — see also Carbon, monoxide, coal	T58.2X1	T58.2X2	T58.2X3	T58.2X4	—	—
oil — see Kerosene						
tar	T49.1X1	T49.1X2	T49.1X3	T49.1X4	T49.1X5	T49.1X6
fumes	T59.891	T59.892	T59.893	T59.894	—	—
medicinal (ointment)	T49.4X1	T49.4X2	T49.4X3	T49.4X4	T49.4X5	T49.4X6
analgesics NEC	T39.2X1	T39.2X2	T39.2X3	T39.2X4	T39.2X5	T39.2X6
naphtha (solvent)	T52.0X1	T52.0X2	T52.0X3	T52.0X4		
Cobalamine	T45.2X1	T45.2X2	T45.2X3	T45.2X4	T45.2X5	T45.2X6
Cobalt (nonmedicinal) (fumes) (industrial)	T56.891	T56.892	T56.893	T56.894		
medicinal (trace) (chloride)	T45.8X1	T45.8X2	T45.8X3	T45.8X4	T45.8X5	T45.8X6
Cobra (venom)	T63.041	T63.042	T63.043	T63.044		
Coca (leaf)	T40.5X1	T40.5X2	T40.5X3	T40.5X4	T40.5X5	T40.5X6
Cocaine	T40.5X1	T40.5X2	T40.5X3	T40.5X4	T40.5X5	T40.5X6
topical anesthetic	T41.3X1	T41.3X2	T41.3X3	T41.3X4	T41.3X5	T41.3X6
Cocarboxylase	T45.3X1	T45.3X2	T45.3X3	T45.3X4	T45.3X5	T45.3X6
Coccidioidin	T50.8X1	T50.8X2	T50.8X3	T50.8X4	T50.8X5	T50.8X6
Cocculus indicus	T62.1X1	T62.1X2	T62.1X3	T62.1X4		
Cochineal	T65.6X1	T65.6X2	T65.6X3	T65.6X4		
medicinal products	T50.991	T50.992	T50.993	T50.994	T50.995	T50.996
Codeine	T40.2X1	T40.2X2	T40.2X3	T40.2X4	T40.2X5	T40.2X6
Cod-liver oil	T45.2X1	T45.2X2	T45.2X3	T45.2X4	T45.2X5	T45.2X6

	External Cause (T-Code)					
Substance	Poisoning, Accidental (Unintentional)	Poisoning, Intentional Self-Harm	Poisoning, Assault	Poisoning, Undetermined	Adverse Effect	Underdosing
Coenzyme A	T50.991	T50.992	T50.993	T50.994	T50.995	T50.996
Coffee	T62.8X1	T62.8X2	T62.8X3	T62.8X4	—	—
Cogalactoisomerase	T50.991	T50.992	T50.993	T50.994	T50.995	T50.996
Cogentin	T44.3X1	T44.3X2	T44.3X3	T44.3X4	T44.3X5	T44.3X6
Coke fumes or gas (carbon monoxide)	T58.2X1	T58.2X2	T58.2X3	T58.2X4	—	—
industrial use	T58.8X1	T58.8X2	T58.8X3	T58.8X4	—	—
Colace	T47.4X1	T47.4X2	T47.4X3	T47.4X4	T47.4X5	T47.4X6
Colaspase	T45.1X1	T45.1X2	T45.1X3	T45.1X4	T45.1X5	T45.1X6
Colchicine	T50.4X1	T50.4X2	T50.4X3	T50.4X4	T50.4X5	T50.4X6
Colchicum	T62.2X1	T62.2X2	T62.2X3	T62.2X4	—	—
Cold cream	T49.3X1	T49.3X2	T49.3X3	T49.3X4	T49.3X5	T49.3X6
Colecalciferol	T45.2X1	T45.2X2	T45.2X3	T45.2X4	T45.2X5	T45.2X6
Colestipol	T46.6X1	T46.6X2	T46.6X3	T46.6X4	T46.6X5	T46.6X6
Colestyramine	T46.6X1	T46.6X2	T46.6X3	T46.6X4	T46.6X5	T46.6X6
Colimycin	T36.8X1	T36.8X2	T36.8X3	T36.8X4	T36.8X5	T36.8X6
Colistimethate	T36.8X1	T36.8X2	T36.8X3	T36.8X4	T36.8X5	T36.8X6
Colistin	T36.8X1	T36.8X2	T36.8X3	T36.8X4	T36.8X5	T36.8X6
sulfate (eye preparation)	T49.5X1	T49.5X2	T49.5X3	T49.5X4	T49.5X5	T49.5X6
Collagen	T50.991	T50.992	T50.993	T50.994	T50.995	T50.996
Collagenase	T49.4X1	T49.4X2	T49.4X3	T49.4X4	T49.4X5	T49.4X6
Collodion	T49.3X1	T49.3X2	T49.3X3	T49.3X4	T49.3X5	T49.3X6
Colocynth	T47.2X1	T47.2X2	T47.2X3	T47.2X4	T47.2X5	T47.2X6
Colophony adhesive	T49.3X1	T49.3X2	T49.3X3	T49.3X4	T49.3X5	T49.3X6
Colorant — see also Dye	T50.991	T50.992	T50.993	T50.994	T50.995	T50.996
Coloring matter — see Dye(s)						
Combustion gas (after combustion) — see Carbon, monoxide						
prior to combustion	T59.891	T59.892	T59.893	T59.894	—	—
Compazine	T43.3X1	T43.3X2	T43.3X3	T43.3X4	T43.3X5	T43.3X6
Compound						
42 (warfarin)	T60.4X1	T60.4X2	T60.4X3	T60.4X4	—	—
269 (endrin)	T60.1X1	T60.1X2	T60.1X3	T60.1X4	—	—
497 (dieldrin)	T60.1X1	T60.1X2	T60.1X3	T60.1X4	—	—
1080 (sodium fluoroacetate)	T60.4X1	T60.4X2	T60.4X3	T60.4X4	—	—
3422 (parathion)	T60.0X1	T60.0X2	T60.0X3	T60.0X4	—	—
3911 (phorate)	T60.0X1	T60.0X2	T60.0X3	T60.0X4	—	—
3956 (toxaphene)	T60.1X1	T60.1X2	T60.1X3	T60.1X4	—	—
4049 (malathion)	T60.0X1	T60.0X2	T60.0X3	T60.0X4	—	—
4069 (malathion)	T60.0X1	T60.0X2	T60.0X3	T60.0X4	—	—
4124 (dicapthon)	T60.0X1	T60.0X2	T60.0X3	T60.0X4	—	—

◀ New ◀ Revised ~~deleted~~ Deleted

Substance	Poisoning, Accidental (Unintentional)	Poisoning, Intentional Self-Harm	Poisoning, Assault	Poisoning, Undetermined	Adverse Effect	Underdosing
Compound *(Continued)*						
E (cortisone)	T38.0X1	T38.0X2	T38.0X3	T38.0X4	T38.0X5	T38.0X6
F (hydrocortisone)	T38.0X1	T38.0X2	T38.0X3	T38.0X4	T38.0X5	T38.0X6
Congener, anabolic	T38.7X1	T38.7X2	T38.7X3	T38.7X4	T38.7X5	T38.7X6
Congo red	T50.8X1	T50.8X2	T50.8X3	T50.8X4	T50.8X5	T50.8X6
Coniine, conine	T62.2X1	T62.2X2	T62.2X3	T62.2X4	—	—
Conium (maculatum)	T62.2X1	T62.2X2	T62.2X3	T62.2X4	—	—
Conjugated estrogenic substances	T38.5X1	T38.5X2	T38.5X3	T38.5X4	T38.5X5	T38.5X6
Contac	T48.5X1	T48.5X2	T48.5X3	T48.5X4	T48.5X5	T48.5X6
Contact lens solution	T49.5X1	T49.5X2	T49.5X3	T49.5X4	T49.5X5	T49.5X6
Contraceptive (oral)	T38.4X1	T38.4X2	T38.4X3	T38.4X4	T38.4X5	T38.4X6
vaginal	T49.8X1	T49.8X2	T49.8X3	T49.8X4	T49.8X5	T49.8X6
Contrast medium, radiography	T50.8X1	T50.8X2	T50.8X3	T50.8X4	T50.8X5	T50.8X6
Convallaria glycosides	T46.0X1	T46.0X2	T46.0X3	T46.0X4	T46.0X5	T46.0X6
Convallaria majalis	T62.2X1	T62.2X2	T62.2X3	T62.2X4	—	—
berry	T62.1X1	T62.1X2	T62.1X3	T62.1X4	—	—
Copper (dust) (fumes) (nonmedicinal) NEC	T56.4X1	T56.4X2	T56.4X3	T56.4X4	—	—
arsenate, arsenite	T57.0X1	T57.0X2	T57.0X3	T57.0X4	—	—
insecticide	T60.2X1	T60.2X2	T60.2X3	T60.2X4	—	—
emetic	T47.7X1	T47.7X2	T47.7X3	T47.7X4	T47.7X5	T47.7X6
fungicide	T60.3X1	T60.3X2	T60.3X3	T60.3X4	—	—
gluconate	T49.0X1	T49.0X2	T49.0X3	T49.0X4	T49.0X5	T49.0X6
insecticide	T60.2X1	T60.2X2	T60.2X3	T60.2X4	—	—
medicinal (trace)	T45.8X1	T45.8X2	T45.8X3	T45.8X4	T45.8X5	T45.8X6
oleate	T49.0X1	T49.0X2	T49.0X3	T49.0X4	T49.0X5	T49.0X6
sulfate	T56.4X1	T56.4X2	T56.4X3	T56.4X4	—	—
cupric	T56.4X1	T56.4X2	T56.4X3	T56.4X4	—	—
fungicide	T60.3X1	T60.3X2	T60.3X3	T60.3X4	—	—
medicinal						
ear	T49.6X1	T49.6X2	T49.6X3	T49.6X4	T49.6X5	T49.6X6
emetic	T47.7X1	T47.7X2	T47.7X3	T47.7X4	T47.7X5	T47.7X6
eye	T49.5X1	T49.5X2	T49.5X3	T49.5X4	T49.5X5	T49.5X6
cuprous	T56.4X1	T56.4X2	T56.4X3	T56.4X4	—	—
fungicide	T60.3X1	T60.3X2	T60.3X3	T60.3X4	—	—
medicinal						
ear	T49.6X1	T49.6X2	T49.6X3	T49.6X4	T49.6X5	T49.6X6
emetic	T47.7X1	T47.7X2	T47.7X3	T47.7X4	T47.7X5	T47.7X6
eye	T49.5X1	T49.5X2	T49.5X3	T49.5X4	T49.5X5	T49.5X6
Copperhead snake (bite) (venom)	T63.061	T63.062	T63.063	T63.064	—	—
Coral (sting)	T63.691	T63.692	T63.693	T63.694	—	—
snake (bite) (venom)	T63.021	T63.022	T63.023	T63.024	—	—
Corbadrine	T49.6X1	T49.6X2	T49.6X3	T49.6X4	T49.6X5	T49.6X6
Cordran	T49.0X1	T49.0X2	T49.0X3	T49.0X4	T49.0X5	T49.0X6
Cordite	T65.891	T65.892	T65.893	T65.894	—	—
vapor	T59.891	T59.892	T59.893	T59.894	—	—
Corn cures	T49.4X1	T49.4X2	T49.4X3	T49.4X4	T49.4X5	T49.4X6
Cornhusker's lotion	T49.3X1	T49.3X2	T49.3X3	T49.3X4	T49.3X5	T49.3X6
Corn starch	T49.3X1	T49.3X2	T49.3X3	T49.3X4	T49.3X5	T49.3X6
Coronary vasodilator NEC	T46.3X1	T46.3X2	T46.3X3	T46.3X4	T46.3X5	T46.3X6
Corrosive NEC	T54.91	T54.92	T54.93	T54.94		
acid NEC	T54.2X1	T54.2X2	T54.2X3	T54.2X4	—	—
aromatics	T54.1X1	T54.1X2	T54.1X3	T54.1X4	—	—
disinfectant	T54.1X1	T54.1X2	T54.1X3	T54.1X4	—	—
fumes NEC	T54.91	T54.92	T54.93	T54.94	—	—
specified NEC	T54.91	T54.92	T54.93	T54.94	—	—
sublimate	T56.1X1	T56.1X2	T56.1X3	T56.1X4	—	—
Cortate	T38.0X1	T38.0X2	T38.0X3	T38.0X4	T38.0X5	T38.0X6
Cort-Dome	T38.0X1	T38.0X2	T38.0X3	T38.0X4	T38.0X5	T38.0X6
ENT agent	T49.6X1	T49.6X2	T49.6X3	T49.6X4	T49.6X5	T49.6X6
ophthalmic preparation	T49.5X1	T49.5X2	T49.5X3	T49.5X4	T49.5X5	T49.5X6
topical NEC	T49.0X1	T49.0X2	T49.0X3	T49.0X4	T49.0X5	T49.0X6
Cortef	T38.0X1	T38.0X2	T38.0X3	T38.0X4	T38.0X5	T38.0X6
ENT agent	T49.6X1	T49.6X2	T49.6X3	T49.6X4	T49.6X5	T49.6X6
ophthalmic preparation	T49.5X1	T49.5X2	T49.5X3	T49.5X4	T49.5X5	T49.5X6
topical NEC	T49.0X1	T49.0X2	T49.0X3	T49.0X4	T49.0X5	T49.0X6
Corticosteroid	T38.0X1	T38.0X2	T38.0X3	T38.0X4	T38.0X5	T38.0X6
ENT agent	T49.6X1	T49.6X2	T49.6X3	T49.6X4	T49.6X5	T49.6X6
mineral	T50.0X1	T50.0X2	T50.0X3	T50.0X4	T50.0X5	T50.0X6
ophthalmic	T49.5X1	T49.5X2	T49.5X3	T49.5X4	T49.5X5	T49.5X6
topical NEC	T49.0X1	T49.0X2	T49.0X3	T49.0X4	T49.0X5	T49.0X6
Corticotropin	T38.811	T38.812	T38.813	T38.814	T38.815	T38.816
Cortisol	T49.0X1	T49.0X2	T49.0X3	T49.0X4	T49.0X5	T49.0X6
ENT agent	T49.6X1	T49.6X2	T49.6X3	T49.6X4	T49.6X5	T49.6X6
ophthalmic preparation	T49.5X1	T49.5X2	T49.5X3	T49.5X4	T49.5X5	T49.5X6
topical NEC	T49.0X1	T49.0X2	T49.0X3	T49.0X4	T49.0X5	T49.0X6
Cortisone (acetate)	T38.0X1	T38.0X2	T38.0X3	T38.0X4	T38.0X5	T38.0X6
ENT agent	T49.6X1	T49.6X2	T49.6X3	T49.6X4	T49.6X5	T49.6X6
ophthalmic preparation	T49.5X1	T49.5X2	T49.5X3	T49.5X4	T49.5X5	T49.5X6
topical NEC	T49.0X1	T49.0X2	T49.0X3	T49.0X4	T49.0X5	T49.0X6
Cortivazol	T38.0X1	T38.0X2	T38.0X3	T38.0X4	T38.0X5	T38.0X6
Cortogen	T38.0X1	T38.0X2	T38.0X3	T38.0X4	T38.0X5	T38.0X6
ENT agent	T49.6X1	T49.6X2	T49.6X3	T49.6X4	T49.6X5	T49.6X6
ophthalmic preparation	T49.5X1	T49.5X2	T49.5X3	T49.5X4	T49.5X5	T49.5X6

◀ New   ◀ Revised   ~~deleted~~ Deleted

Substance	External Cause (T-Code) Poisoning, Accidental (Unintentional)	Poisoning, Intentional Self-Harm	Poisoning, Assault	Poisoning, Undetermined	Adverse Effect	Underdosing
Cortone	T38.0X1	T38.0X2	T38.0X3	T38.0X4	T38.0X5	T38.0X6
ENT agent	T49.6X1	T49.6X2	T49.6X3	T49.6X4	T49.6X5	T49.6X6
ophthalmic preparation	T49.5X1	T49.5X2	T49.5X3	T49.5X4	T49.5X5	T49.5X6
Cortril	T38.0X1	T38.0X2	T38.0X3	T38.0X4	T38.0X5	T38.0X6
ENT agent	T49.6X1	T49.6X2	T49.6X3	T49.6X4	T49.6X5	T49.6X6
ophthalmic preparation	T49.5X1	T49.5X2	T49.5X3	T49.5X4	T49.5X5	T49.5X6
topical NEC	T49.0X1	T49.0X2	T49.0X3	T49.0X4	T49.0X5	T49.0X6
Corynebacterium parvum	T45.1X1	T45.1X2	T45.1X3	T45.1X4	T45.1X5	T45.1X6
Cosmetic preparation	T49.8X1	T49.8X2	T49.8X3	T49.8X4	T49.8X5	T49.8X6
Cosmetics	T49.8X1	T49.8X2	T49.8X3	T49.8X4	T49.8X5	T49.8X6
Cosyntropin	T38.811	T38.812	T38.813	T38.814	T38.815	T38.816
Cotarnine	T45.7X1	T45.7X2	T45.7X3	T45.7X4	T45.7X5	T45.7X6
Co-trimoxazole	T36.8X1	T36.8X2	T36.8X3	T36.8X4	T36.8X5	T36.8X6
Cottonseed oil	T49.3X1	T49.3X2	T49.3X3	T49.3X4	T49.3X5	T49.3X6
Cough mixture (syrup)	T48.4X1	T48.4X2	T48.4X3	T48.4X4	T48.4X5	T48.4X6
containing opiates	T40.2X1	T40.2X2	T40.2X3	T40.2X4	T40.2X5	T40.2X6
expectorants	T48.4X1	T48.4X2	T48.4X3	T48.4X4	T48.4X5	T48.4X6
Coumadin	T45.511	T45.512	T45.513	T45.514	T45.515	T45.516
rodenticide	T60.4X1	T60.4X2	T60.4X3	T60.4X4	—	—
Coumaphos	T60.0X1	T60.0X2	T60.0X3	T60.0X4	—	—
Coumarin	T45.511	T45.512	T45.513	T45.514	T45.515	T45.516
Coumetarol	T45.511	T45.512	T45.513	T45.514	T45.515	T45.516
Cowbane	T62.2X1	T62.2X2	T62.2X3	T62.2X4	—	—
Cozyme	T45.2X1	T45.2X2	T45.2X3	T45.2X4	T45.2X5	T45.2X6
Crack	T40.5X1	T40.5X2	T40.5X3	T40.5X4	—	—
Crataegus extract	T46.0X1	T46.0X2	T46.0X3	T46.0X4	T46.0X5	T46.0X6
Creolin	T54.1X1	T54.1X2	T54.1X3	T54.1X4		
disinfectant	T54.1X1	T54.1X2	T54.1X3	T54.1X4	—	—
Creosol (compound)	T49.0X1	T49.0X2	T49.0X3	T49.0X4	T49.0X5	T49.0X6
Creosote (coal tar) (beechwood)	T49.0X1	T49.0X2	T49.0X3	T49.0X4	T49.0X5	T49.0X6
medicinal (expectorant)	T48.4X1	T48.4X2	T48.4X3	T48.4X4	T48.4X5	T48.4X6
syrup	T48.4X1	T48.4X2	T48.4X3	T48.4X4	T48.4X5	T48.4X6
Cresol(s)	T49.0X1	T49.0X2	T49.0X3	T49.0X4	T49.0X5	T49.0X6
and soap solution	T49.0X1	T49.0X2	T49.0X3	T49.0X4	T49.0X5	T49.0X6
Cresyl acetate	T49.0X1	T49.0X2	T49.0X3	T49.0X4	T49.0X5	T49.0X6
Cresylic acid	T49.0X1	T49.0X2	T49.0X3	T49.0X4	T49.0X5	T49.0X6
Crimidine	T60.4X1	T60.4X2	T60.4X3	T60.4X4	—	—
Croconazole	T37.8X1	T37.8X2	T37.8X3	T37.8X4	T37.8X5	T37.8X6
Cromoglicic acid	T48.6X1	T48.6X2	T48.6X3	T48.6X4	T48.6X5	T48.6X6
Cromolyn	T48.6X1	T48.6X2	T48.6X3	T48.6X4	T48.6X5	T48.6X6
Cromonar	T46.3X1	T46.3X2	T46.3X3	T46.3X4	T46.3X5	T46.3X6

Substance	External Cause (T-Code) Poisoning, Accidental (Unintentional)	Poisoning, Intentional Self-Harm	Poisoning, Assault	Poisoning, Undetermined	Adverse Effect	Underdosing
Cropropamide	T39.8X1	T39.8X2	T39.8X3	T39.8X4	T39.8X5	T39.8X6
with crotethamide	T50.7X1	T50.7X2	T50.7X3	T50.7X4	T50.7X5	T50.7X6
Crotamiton	T49.0X1	T49.0X2	T49.0X3	T49.0X4	T49.0X5	T49.0X6
Crotethamide	T39.8X1	T39.8X2	T39.8X3	T39.8X4	T39.8X5	T39.8X6
with cropropamide	T50.7X1	T50.7X2	T50.7X3	T50.7X4	T50.7X5	T50.7X6
Croton (oil)	T47.2X1	T47.2X2	T47.2X3	T47.2X4	T47.2X5	T47.2X6
chloral	T42.6X1	T42.6X2	T42.6X3	T42.6X4	T42.6X5	T42.6X6
Crude oil	T52.0X1	T52.0X2	T52.0X3	T52.0X4	—	—
Cryogenine	T39.8X1	T39.8X2	T39.8X3	T39.8X4	T39.8X5	T39.8X6
Cryolite (vapor)	T60.1X1	T60.1X2	T60.1X3	T60.1X4	—	—
insecticide	T60.1X1	T60.1X2	T60.1X3	T60.1X4	—	—
Cryptenamine (tannates)	T46.5X1	T46.5X2	T46.5X3	T46.5X4	T46.5X5	T46.5X6
Crystal violet	T49.0X1	T49.0X2	T49.0X3	T49.0X4	T49.0X5	T49.0X6
Cuckoopint	T62.2X1	T62.2X2	T62.2X3	T62.2X4	—	—
Cumetharol	T45.511	T45.512	T45.513	T45.514	T45.515	T45.516
Cupric						
acetate	T60.3X1	T60.3X2	T60.3X3	T60.3X4		
acetoarsenite	T57.0X1	T57.0X2	T57.0X3	T57.0X4		
arsenate	T57.0X1	T57.0X2	T57.0X3	T57.0X4		
gluconate	T49.0X1	T49.0X2	T49.0X3	T49.0X4	T49.0X5	T49.0X6
oleate	T49.0X1	T49.0X2	T49.0X3	T49.0X4	T49.0X5	T49.0X6
sulfate	T56.4X1	T56.4X2	T56.4X3	T56.4X4		
Cuprous sulfate—see also Copper sulfate	T56.4X1	T56.4X2	T56.4X3	T56.4X4		
Curare, curarine	T48.1X1	T48.1X2	T48.1X3	T48.1X4	T48.1X5	T48.1X6
Cyamemazine	T43.3X1	T43.3X2	T43.3X3	T43.3X4	T43.3X5	T43.3X6
Cyamopsis tetragono-loba	T46.6X1	T46.6X2	T46.6X3	T46.6X4	T46.6X5	T46.6X6
Cyanacetyl hydrazide	T37.1X1	T37.1X2	T37.1X3	T37.1X4	T37.1X5	T37.1X6
Cyanic acid (gas)	T59.891	T59.892	T59.893	T59.894	—	—
Cyanide(s) (compounds) (potassium) (sodium) NEC	T65.0X1	T65.0X2	T65.0X3	T65.0X4	—	—
dust or gas (inhalation) NEC	T57.3X1	T57.3X2	T57.3X3	T57.3X4		
fumigant	T65.0X1	T65.0X2	T65.0X3	T65.0X4		
hydrogen	T57.3X1	T57.3X2	T57.3X3	T57.3X4		
mercuric—see Mercury						
pesticide (dust) (fumes)	T65.0X1	T65.0X2	T65.0X3	T65.0X4		
Cyanoacrylate adhesive	T49.3X1	T49.3X2	T49.3X3	T49.3X4	T49.3X5	T49.3X6
Cyanocobalamin	T45.8X1	T45.8X2	T45.8X3	T45.8X4	T45.8X5	T45.8X6
Cyanogen (chloride) (gas) NEC	T59.891	T59.892	T59.893	T59.894	—	—
Cyclacillin	T36.0X1	T36.0X2	T36.0X3	T36.0X4	T36.0X5	T36.0X6
Cyclaine	T41.3X1	T41.3X2	T41.3X3	T41.3X4	T41.3X5	T41.3X6
Cyclamate	T50.991	T50.992	T50.993	T50.994	T50.995	T50.996

◄ New ◄ Revised ~~deleted~~ Deleted

	External Cause (T-Code)					
Substance	Poisoning, Accidental (Unintentional)	Poisoning, Intentional Self-Harm	Poisoning, Assault	Poisoning, Undetermined	Adverse Effect	Underdosing
Cyclamen europaeum	T62.2X1	T62.2X2	T62.2X3	T62.2X4	—	—
Cyclandelate	T46.7X1	T46.7X2	T46.7X3	T46.7X4	T46.7X5	T46.7X6
Cyclazocine	T50.7X1	T50.7X2	T50.7X3	T50.7X4	T50.7X5	T50.7X6
Cyclizine	T45.0X1	T45.0X2	T45.0X3	T45.0X4	T45.0X5	T45.0X6
Cyclobarbital	T42.3X1	T42.3X2	T42.3X3	T42.3X4	T42.3X5	T42.3X6
Cyclobarbitone	T42.3X1	T42.3X2	T42.3X3	T42.3X4	T42.3X5	T42.3X6
Cyclobenzaprine	T48.1X1	T48.1X2	T48.1X3	T48.1X4	T48.1X5	T48.1X6
Cyclodrine	T44.3X1	T44.3X2	T44.3X3	T44.3X4	T44.3X5	T44.3X6
Cycloguanil embonate	T37.2X1	T37.2X2	T37.2X3	T37.2X4	T37.2X5	T37.2X6
Cycloheptadiene	T43.291	T43.292	T43.293	T43.294	T43.295	T43.296
Cyclohexane	T52.8X1	T52.8X2	T52.8X3	T52.8X4	—	—
Cyclohexanol	T51.8X1	T51.8X2	T51.8X3	T51.8X4	—	—
Cyclohexanone	T52.4X1	T52.4X2	T52.4X3	T52.4X4	—	—
Cycloheximide	T60.3X1	T60.3X2	T60.3X3	T60.3X4	—	—
Cyclohexyl acetate	T52.8X1	T52.8X2	T52.8X3	T52.8X4	—	—
Cycloleucin	T45.1X1	T45.1X2	T45.1X3	T45.1X4	T45.1X5	T45.1X6
Cyclomethycaine	T41.3X1	T41.3X2	T41.3X3	T41.3X4	T41.3X5	T41.3X6
Cyclopentamine	T44.4X1	T44.4X2	T44.4X3	T44.4X4	T44.4X5	T44.4X6
Cyclopenthiazide	T50.2X1	T50.2X2	T50.2X3	T50.2X4	T50.2X5	T50.2X6
Cyclopentolate	T44.3X1	T44.3X2	T44.3X3	T44.3X4	T44.3X5	T44.3X6
Cyclophosphamide	T45.1X1	T45.1X2	T45.1X3	T45.1X4	T45.1X5	T45.1X6
Cycloplegic drug	T49.5X1	T49.5X2	T49.5X3	T49.5X4	T49.5X5	T49.5X6
Cyclopropane	T41.291	T41.292	T41.293	T41.294	T41.295	T41.296
Cyclopyrabital	T39.8X1	T39.8X2	T39.8X3	T39.8X4	T39.8X5	T39.8X6
Cycloserine	T37.1X1	T37.1X2	T37.1X3	T37.1X4	T37.1X5	T37.1X6
Cyclosporin	T45.1X1	T45.1X2	T45.1X3	T45.1X4	T45.1X5	T45.1X6
Cyclothiazide	T50.2X1	T50.2X2	T50.2X3	T50.2X4	T50.2X5	T50.2X6
Cycrimine	T44.3X1	T44.3X2	T44.3X3	T44.3X4	T44.3X5	T44.3X6
Cyhalothrin	T60.1X1	T60.1X2	T60.1X3	T60.1X4	—	—
Cymarin	T46.0X1	T46.0X2	T46.0X3	T46.0X4	T46.0X5	T46.0X6
Cypermethrin	T60.1X1	T60.1X2	T60.1X3	T60.1X4	—	—
Cyphenothrin	T60.2X1	T60.2X2	T60.2X3	T60.2X4	—	—
Cyproheptadine	T45.0X1	T45.0X2	T45.0X3	T45.0X4	T45.0X5	T45.0X6
Cyprolidol	T43.291	T43.292	T43.293	T43.294	T43.295	T43.296
Cyproterone	T38.6X1	T38.6X2	T38.6X3	T38.6X4	T38.6X5	T38.6X6
Cysteamine	T50.6X1	T50.6X2	T50.6X3	T50.6X4	T50.6X5	T50.6X6
Cytarabine	T45.1X1	T45.1X2	T45.1X3	T45.1X4	T45.1X5	T45.1X6
Cytisus						
laburnum	T62.2X1	T62.2X2	T62.2X3	T62.2X4	—	—
scoparius	T62.2X1	T62.2X2	T62.2X3	T62.2X4	—	—
Cytochrome C	T47.5X1	T47.5X2	T47.5X3	T47.5X4	T47.5X5	T47.5X6
Cytomel	T38.1X1	T38.1X2	T38.1X3	T38.1X4	T38.1X5	T38.1X6

	External Cause (T-Code)					
Substance	Poisoning, Accidental (Unintentional)	Poisoning, Intentional Self-Harm	Poisoning, Assault	Poisoning, Undetermined	Adverse Effect	Underdosing
Cytosine arabinoside	T45.1X1	T45.1X2	T45.1X3	T45.1X4	T45.1X5	T45.1X6
Cytoxan	T45.1X1	T45.1X2	T45.1X3	T45.1X4	T45.1X5	T45.1X6
Cytozyme	T45.7X1	T45.7X2	T45.7X3	T45.7X4	T45.7X5	T45.7X6
2,4-D	T60.3X1	T60.3X2	T60.3X3	T60.3X4	—	—
			D			
Dacarbazine	T45.1X1	T45.1X2	T45.1X3	T45.1X4	T45.1X5	T45.1X6
Dactinomycin	T45.1X1	T45.1X2	T45.1X3	T45.1X4	T45.1X5	T45.1X6
DADPS	T37.1X1	T37.1X2	T37.1X3	T37.1X4	T37.1X5	T37.1X6
Dakin's solution	T49.0X1	T49.0X2	T49.0X3	T49.0X4	T49.0X5	T49.0X6
Dalapon (sodium)	T60.3X1	T60.3X2	T60.3X3	T60.3X4	—	—
Dalmane	T42.4X1	T42.4X2	T42.4X3	T42.4X4	T42.4X5	T42.4X6
Danazol	T38.6X1	T38.6X2	T38.6X3	T38.6X4	T38.6X5	T38.6X6
Danilone	T45.511	T45.512	T45.513	T45.514	T45.515	T45.516
Danthron	T47.2X1	T47.2X2	T47.2X3	T47.2X4	T47.2X5	T47.2X6
Dantrolene	T42.8X1	T42.8X2	T42.8X3	T42.8X4	T42.8X5	T42.8X6
Dantron	T47.2X1	T47.2X2	T47.2X3	T47.2X4	T47.2X5	T47.2X6
Daphne (gnidium) (mezereum)	T62.2X1	T62.2X2	T62.2X3	T62.2X4	—	—
berry	T62.1X1	T62.1X2	T62.1X3	T62.1X4	—	—
Dapsone	T37.1X1	T37.1X2	T37.1X3	T37.1X4	T37.1X5	T37.1X6
Daraprim	T37.2X1	T37.2X2	T37.2X3	T37.2X4	T37.2X5	T37.2X6
Darnel	T62.2X1	T62.2X2	T62.2X3	T62.2X4	—	—
Darvon	T39.8X1	T39.8X2	T39.8X3	T39.8X4	T39.8X5	T39.8X6
Daunomycin	T45.1X1	T45.1X2	T45.1X3	T45.1X4	T45.1X5	T45.1X6
Daunorubicin	T45.1X1	T45.1X2	T45.1X3	T45.1X4	T45.1X5	T45.1X6
DBI	T38.3X1	T38.3X2	T38.3X3	T38.3X4	T38.3X5	T38.3X6
D-Con	T60.91	T60.92	T60.93	T60.94	—	—
insecticide	T60.2X1	T60.2X2	T60.2X3	T60.2X4	—	—
rodenticide	T60.4X1	T60.4X2	T60.4X3	T60.4X4	—	—
DDAVP	T38.891	T38.892	T38.893	T38.894	T38.895	T38.896
DDE (bis(chlorophenyl)-dichloroethylene)	T60.2X1	T60.2X2	T60.2X3	T60.2X4	—	—
DDS	T37.1X1	T37.1X2	T37.1X3	T37.1X4	T37.1X5	T37.1X6
DDT (dust)	T60.1X1	T60.1X2	T60.1X3	T60.1X4	—	—
Deadly nightshade— *see also* Belladonna	T62.2X1	T62.2X2	T62.2X3	T62.2X4	—	—
berry	T62.1X1	T62.1X2	T62.1X3	T62.1X4	—	—
Deamino-D-arginine vasopressin	T38.891	T38.892	T38.893	T38.894	T38.895	T38.896
Deanol (aceglumate)	T50.991	T50.992	T50.993	T50.994	T50.995	T50.996
Debrisoquine	T46.5X1	T46.5X2	T46.5X3	T46.5X4	T46.5X5	T46.5X6
Decaborane	T57.8X1	T57.8X2	T57.8X3	T57.8X4	—	—
fumes	T59.891	T59.892	T59.893	T59.894	—	—

◀ New   ◀ Revised   ~~deleted~~ Deleted

TABLE OF DRUGS AND CHEMICALS

Substance	External Cause (T-Code)					
	Poisoning, Accidental (Unintentional)	Poisoning, Intentional Self-Harm	Poisoning, Assault	Poisoning, Undetermined	Adverse Effect	Underdosing
Decadron	T38.0X1	T38.0X2	T38.0X3	T38.0X4	T38.0X5	T38.0X6
ENT agent	T49.6X1	T49.6X2	T49.6X3	T49.6X4	T49.6X5	T49.6X6
ophthalmic preparation	T49.5X1	T49.5X2	T49.5X3	T49.5X4	T49.5X5	T49.5X6
topical NEC	T49.0X1	T49.0X2	T49.0X3	T49.0X4	T49.0X5	T49.0X6
Decahydronaphthalene	T52.8X1	T52.8X2	T52.8X3	T52.8X4	—	—
Decalin	T52.8X1	T52.8X2	T52.8X3	T52.8X4	—	—
Decamethonium (bromide)	T48.1X1	T48.1X2	T48.1X3	T48.1X4	T48.1X5	T48.1X6
Decholin	T47.5X1	T47.5X2	T47.5X3	T47.5X4	T47.5X5	T47.5X6
Declomycin	T36.4X1	T36.4X2	T36.4X3	T36.4X4	T36.4X5	T36.4X6
Decongestant, nasal (mucosa)	T48.5X1	T48.5X2	T48.5X3	T48.5X4	T48.5X5	T48.5X6
combination	T48.5X1	T48.5X2	T48.5X3	T48.5X4	T48.5X5	T48.5X6
Deet	T60.8X1	T60.8X2	T60.8X3	T60.8X4	—	—
Deferoxamine	T45.8X1	T45.8X2	T45.8X3	T45.8X4	T45.8X5	T45.8X6
Deflazacort	T38.0X1	T38.0X2	T38.0X3	T38.0X4	T38.0X5	T38.0X6
Deglycyrrhizinized extract of licorice	T48.4X1	T48.4X2	T48.4X3	T48.4X4	T48.4X5	T48.4X6
Dehydrocholic acid	T47.5X1	T47.5X2	T47.5X3	T47.5X4	T47.5X5	T47.5X6
Dehydroemetine	T37.3X1	T37.3X2	T37.3X3	T37.3X4	T37.3X5	T37.3X6
Dekalin	T52.8X1	T52.8X2	T52.8X3	T52.8X4	—	—
Delalutin	T38.5X1	T38.5X2	T38.5X3	T38.5X4	T38.5X5	T38.5X6
Delphinium	T62.2X1	T62.2X2	T62.2X3	T62.2X4	—	—
Deltasone	T38.0X1	T38.0X2	T38.0X3	T38.0X4	T38.0X5	T38.0X6
Deltra	T38.0X1	T38.0X2	T38.0X3	T38.0X4	T38.0X5	T38.0X6
Delvinal	T42.3X1	T42.3X2	T42.3X3	T42.3X4	T42.3X5	T42.3X6
Delorazepam	T42.4X1	T42.4X2	T42.4X3	T42.4X4	T42.4X5	T42.4X6
Deltamethrin	T60.1X1	T60.1X2	T60.1X3	T60.1X4	—	—
Demecarium (bromide)	T49.5X1	T49.5X2	T49.5X3	T49.5X4	T49.5X5	T49.5X6
Demeclocycline	T36.4X1	T36.4X2	T36.4X3	T36.4X4	T36.4X5	T36.4X6
Demecolcine	T45.1X1	T45.1X2	T45.1X3	T45.1X4	T45.1X5	T45.1X6
Demegestone	T38.5X1	T38.5X2	T38.5X3	T38.5X4	T38.5X5	T38.5X6
Demelanizing agents	T49.8X1	T49.8X2	T49.8X3	T49.8X4	T49.8X5	T49.8X6
Demephion -O and -S	T60.0X1	T60.0X2	T60.0X3	T60.0X4	—	—
Demerol	T40.2X1	T40.2X2	T40.2X3	T40.2X4	T40.2X5	T40.2X6
Demethylchlortetracycline	T36.4X1	T36.4X2	T36.4X3	T36.4X4	T36.4X5	T36.4X6
Demethyltetracycline	T36.4X1	T36.4X2	T36.4X3	T36.4X4	T36.4X5	T36.4X6
Demeton -O and -S	T60.0X1	T60.0X2	T60.0X3	T60.0X4	—	—
Demulcent (external)	T49.3X1	T49.3X2	T49.3X3	T49.3X4	T49.3X5	T49.3X6
specified NEC	T49.3X1	T49.3X2	T49.3X3	T49.3X4	T49.3X5	T49.3X6
Demulen	T38.4X1	T38.4X2	T38.4X3	T38.4X4	T38.4X5	T38.4X6
Denatured alcohol	T51.0X1	T51.0X2	T51.0X3	T51.0X4	—	—
Dendrid	T49.5X1	T49.5X2	T49.5X3	T49.5X4	T49.5X5	T49.5X6
Dental drug, topical application NEC	T49.7X1	T49.7X2	T49.7X3	T49.7X4	T49.7X5	T49.7X6

Substance	External Cause (T-Code)					
	Poisoning, Accidental (Unintentional)	Poisoning, Intentional Self-Harm	Poisoning, Assault	Poisoning, Undetermined	Adverse Effect	Underdosing
Dentifrice	T49.7X1	T49.7X2	T49.7X3	T49.7X4	T49.7X5	T49.7X6
Deodorant spray (feminine hygiene)	T49.8X1	T49.8X2	T49.8X3	T49.8X4	T49.8X5	T49.8X6
Deoxycortone	T50.0X1	T50.0X2	T50.0X3	T50.0X4	T50.0X5	T50.0X6
2-Deoxy-5-fluorouridine	T45.1X1	T45.1X2	T45.1X3	T45.1X4	T45.1X5	T45.1X6
5-Deoxy-5-fluorouridine	T45.1X1	T45.1X2	T45.1X3	T45.1X4	T45.1X5	T45.1X6
Deoxyribonuclease (pancreatic)	T45.3X1	T45.3X2	T45.3X3	T45.3X4	T45.3X5	T45.3X6
Depilatory	T49.4X1	T49.4X2	T49.4X3	T49.4X4	T49.4X5	T49.4X6
Deprenalin	T42.8X1	T42.8X2	T42.8X3	T42.8X4	T42.8X5	T42.8X6
Deprenyl	T42.8X1	T42.8X2	T42.8X3	T42.8X4	T42.8X5	T42.8X6
Depressant, appetite	T50.5X1	T50.5X2	T50.5X3	T50.5X4	T50.5X5	T50.5X6
Depressant						
appetite, central	T50.5X1	T50.5X2	T50.5X3	T50.5X4	T50.5X5	T50.5X6
cardiac	T46.2X1	T46.2X2	T46.2X3	T46.2X4	T46.2X5	T46.2X6
central nervous system (anesthetic) — see also Central nervous system, depressants	T42.71	T42.72	T42.73	T42.74	T42.75	T42.76
general anesthetic	T41.201	T41.202	T41.203	T41.204	T41.205	T41.206
muscle tone	T42.8X1	T42.8X2	T42.8X3	T42.8X4	T42.8X5	T42.8X6
muscle tone, central	T42.8X1	T42.8X2	T42.8X3	T42.8X4	T42.8X5	T42.8X6
psychotherapeutic	T43.501	T43.502	T43.503	T43.504	T43.505	T43.506
Deptropine	T45.0X1	T45.0X2	T45.0X3	T45.0X4	T45.0X5	T45.0X6
Dequalinium (chloride)	T49.0X1	T49.0X2	T49.0X3	T49.0X4	T49.0X5	T49.0X6
Derris root	T60.2X1	T60.2X2	T60.2X3	T60.2X4	—	—
Deserpidine	T43.011	T43.012	T43.013	T43.014	T43.015	T43.016
Desferrioxamine	T45.8X1	T45.8X2	T45.8X3	T45.8X4	T45.8X5	T45.8X6
Desipramine	T43.0X1	T43.0X2	T43.0X3	T43.0X4	T43.0X5	T43.0X6
Deslanoside	T46.0X1	T46.0X2	T46.0X3	T46.0X4	T46.0X5	T46.0X6
Desloughing agent	T49.4X1	T49.4X2	T49.4X3	T49.4X4	T49.4X5	T49.4X6
Desmethylimipramine	T43.011	T43.012	T43.013	T43.014	T43.015	T43.016
Desmopressin	T38.891	T38.892	T38.893	T38.894	T38.895	T38.896
Desocodeine	T40.2X1	T40.2X2	T40.2X3	T40.2X4	T40.2X5	T40.2X6
Desogestrel	T38.5X1	T38.5X2	T38.5X3	T38.5X4	T38.5X5	T38.5X6
Desomorphine	T40.2X1	T40.2X2	T40.2X3	T40.2X4	—	—
Desonide	T49.0X1	T49.0X2	T49.0X3	T49.0X4	T49.0X5	T49.0X6
Desoximetasone	T49.0X1	T49.0X2	T49.0X3	T49.0X4	T49.0X5	T49.0X6
Desoxycorticosteroid	T50.0X1	T50.0X2	T50.0X3	T50.0X4	T50.0X5	T50.0X6
Desoxycortone	T50.0X1	T50.0X2	T50.0X3	T50.0X4	T50.0X5	T50.0X6
Desoxyephedrine	T43.621	T43.622	T43.623	T43.624	T43.625	T43.626
Detaxtran	T46.6X1	T46.6X2	T46.6X3	T46.6X4	T46.6X5	T46.6X6
Detergent	T49.2X1	T49.2X2	T49.2X3	T49.2X4	T49.2X5	T49.2X6
external medication	T49.2X1	T49.2X2	T49.2X3	T49.2X4	T49.2X5	T49.2X6
local	T49.2X1	T49.2X2	T49.2X3	T49.2X4	T49.2X5	T49.2X6

◄ New   ◄ Revised   ~~deleted~~ Deleted

Substance	External Cause (T-Code)					
	Poisoning, Accidental (Unintentional)	Poisoning, Intentional Self-Harm	Poisoning, Assault	Poisoning, Undetermined	Adverse Effect	Underdosing
Detergent (Continued)						
medicinal	T49.2X1	T49.2X2	T49.2X3	T49.2X4	T49.2X5	T49.2X6
nonmedicinal	T55.1X1	T55.1X2	T55.1X3	T55.1X4	—	—
specified NEC	T55.1X1	T55.1X2	T55.1X3	T55.1X4	T55.1X5	T55.1X6
Deterrent, alcohol	T50.6X1	T50.6X2	T50.6X3	T50.6X4	T50.6X5	T50.6X6
Detoxifying agent	T50.6X1	T50.6X2	T50.6X3	T50.6X4	T50.6X5	T50.6X6
Detrothyronine	T38.1X1	T38.1X2	T38.1X3	T38.1X4	T38.1X5	T38.1X6
Dettol (external medication)	T49.0X1	T49.0X2	T49.0X3	T49.0X4	T49.0X5	T49.0X6
Dexamethasone	T38.0X1	T38.0X2	T38.0X3	T38.0X4	T38.0X5	T38.0X6
ENT agent	T49.6X1	T49.6X2	T49.6X3	T49.6X4	T49.6X5	T49.6X6
ophthalmic preparation	T49.5X1	T49.5X2	T49.5X3	T49.5X4	T49.5X5	T49.5X6
topical NEC	T49.0X1	T49.0X2	T49.0X3	T49.0X4	T49.0X5	T49.0X6
Dexamfetamine	T43.621	T43.622	T43.623	T43.624	T43.625	T43.626
Dexamphetamine	T43.621	T43.622	T43.623	T43.624	T43.625	T43.626
Dexbrompheniramine	T45.0X1	T45.0X2	T45.0X3	T45.0X4	T45.0X5	T45.0X6
Dexchlorpheniramine	T45.0X1	T45.0X2	T45.0X3	T45.0X4	T45.0X5	T45.0X6
Dexedrine	T43.621	T43.622	T43.623	T43.624	T43.625	T43.626
Dexetimide	T44.3X1	T44.3X2	T44.3X3	T44.3X4	T44.3X5	T44.3X6
Dexfenfluramine	T50.5X1	T50.5X2	T50.5X3	T50.5X4	T50.5X5	T50.5X6
Dexpanthenol	T45.2X1	T45.2X2	T45.2X3	T45.2X4	T45.2X5	T45.2X6
Dextran (40) (70) (150)	T45.8X1	T45.8X2	T45.8X3	T45.8X4	T45.8X5	T45.8X6
Dextriferron	T45.4X1	T45.4X2	T45.4X3	T45.4X4	T45.4X5	T45.4X6
Dextroamphetamine	T43.621	T43.622	T43.623	T43.624	T43.625	T43.626
Dextro calcium pantothenate	T45.2X1	T45.2X2	T45.2X3	T45.2X4	T45.2X5	T45.2X6
Dextromethorphan	T48.3X1	T48.3X2	T48.3X3	T48.3X4	T48.3X5	T48.3X6
Dextromoramide	T40.491	T40.492	T40.493	T40.494	—	—
topical	T49.8X1	T49.8X2	T49.8X3	T49.8X4	T49.8X5	T49.8X6
Dextro pantothenyl alcohol	T45.2X1	T45.2X2	T45.2X3	T45.2X4	T45.2X5	T45.2X6
Dextropropoxyphene	T40.491	T40.492	T40.493	T40.494	T40.495	T40.496
Dextrorphan	T40.2X1	T40.2X2	T40.2X3	T40.2X4	T40.2X5	T40.2X6
Dextrose	T50.3X1	T50.3X2	T50.3X3	T50.3X4	T50.3X5	T50.3X6
concentrated solution, intravenous	T46.8X1	T46.8X2	T46.8X3	T46.8X4	T46.8X5	T46.8X6
Dextrothyroxin	T38.1X1	T38.1X2	T38.1X3	T38.1X4	T38.1X5	T38.1X6
Dextrothyroxine sodium	T38.1X1	T38.1X2	T38.1X3	T38.1X4	T38.1X5	T38.1X6
DFP	T44.0X1	T44.0X2	T44.0X3	T44.0X4	T44.0X5	T44.0X6
DHE	T37.3X1	T37.3X2	T37.3X3	T37.3X4	T37.3X5	T37.3X6
45	T46.5X1	T46.5X2	T46.5X3	T46.5X4	T46.5X5	T46.5X6
Diabinese	T38.3X1	T38.3X2	T38.3X3	T38.3X4	T38.3X5	T38.3X6
Diacetone alcohol	T52.4X1	T52.4X2	T52.4X3	T52.4X4	—	—
Diacetyl monoxime	T50.991	T50.992	T50.993	T50.994	—	—
Diacetylmorphine	T40.1X1	T40.1X2	T40.1X3	T40.1X4	—	—

Substance	External Cause (T-Code)					
	Poisoning, Accidental (Unintentional)	Poisoning, Intentional Self-Harm	Poisoning, Assault	Poisoning, Undetermined	Adverse Effect	Underdosing
Diachylon plaster	T49.4X1	T49.4X2	T49.4X3	T49.4X4	T49.4X5	T49.4X6
Diaethylstilboestrolum	T38.5X1	T38.5X2	T38.5X3	T38.5X4	T38.5X5	T38.5X6
Diagnostic agent NEC	T50.8X1	T50.8X2	T50.8X3	T50.8X4	T50.8X5	T50.8X6
Dial (soap)	T49.2X1	T49.2X2	T49.2X3	T49.2X4	T49.2X5	T49.2X6
sedative	T42.3X1	T42.3X2	T42.3X3	T42.3X4	T42.3X5	T42.3X6
Dialkyl carbonate	T52.91	T52.92	T52.93	T52.94	—	—
Diallylbarbituric acid	T42.3X1	T42.3X2	T42.3X3	T42.3X4	T42.3X5	T42.3X6
Diallymal	T42.3X1	T42.3X2	T42.3X3	T42.3X4	T42.3X5	T42.3X6
Dialysis solution (intraperitoneal)	T50.3X1	T50.3X2	T50.3X3	T50.3X4	T50.3X5	T50.3X6
Diaminodiphenylsulfone	T37.1X1	T37.1X2	T37.1X3	T37.1X4	T37.1X5	T37.1X6
Diamorphine	T40.1X1	T40.1X2	T40.1X3	T40.1X4	—	—
Diamox	T50.2X1	T50.2X2	T50.2X3	T50.2X4	T50.2X5	T50.2X6
Diamthazole	T49.0X1	T49.0X2	T49.0X3	T49.0X4	T49.0X5	T49.0X6
Dianthone	T47.2X1	T47.2X2	T47.2X3	T47.2X4	T47.2X5	T47.2X6
Diaphenylsulfone	T37.0X1	T37.0X2	T37.0X3	T37.0X4	T37.0X5	T37.0X6
Diasone (sodium)	T37.1X1	T37.1X2	T37.1X3	T37.1X4	T37.1X5	T37.1X6
Diastase	T47.5X1	T47.5X2	T47.5X3	T47.5X4	T47.5X5	T47.5X6
Diatrizoate	T50.8X1	T50.8X2	T50.8X3	T50.8X4	T50.8X5	T50.8X6
Diazepam	T42.4X1	T42.4X2	T42.4X3	T42.4X4	T42.4X5	T42.4X6
Diazinon	T60.0X1	T60.0X2	T60.0X3	T60.0X4	—	—
Diazomethane (gas)	T59.891	T59.892	T59.893	T59.894	—	—
Diazoxide	T46.5X1	T46.5X2	T46.5X3	T46.5X4	T46.5X5	T46.5X6
Dibekacin	T36.5X1	T36.5X2	T36.5X3	T36.5X4	T36.5X5	T36.5X6
Dibenamine	T44.6X1	T44.6X2	T44.6X3	T44.6X4	T44.6X5	T44.6X6
Dibenzepin	T43.011	T43.012	T43.013	T43.014	T43.015	T43.016
Dibenzheptropine	T45.0X1	T45.0X2	T45.0X3	T45.0X4	T45.0X5	T45.0X6
Dibenzyline	T44.6X1	T44.6X2	T44.6X3	T44.6X4	T44.6X5	T44.6X6
Diborane (gas)	T59.891	T59.892	T59.893	T59.894	—	—
Dibromochloropropane	T60.8X1	T60.8X2	T60.8X3	T60.8X4	—	—
Dibromodulcitol	T45.1X1	T45.1X2	T45.1X3	T45.1X4	T45.1X5	T45.1X6
Dibromoethane	T53.6X1	T53.6X2	T53.6X3	T53.6X4	—	—
Dibromomannitol	T45.1X1	T45.1X2	T45.1X3	T45.1X4	T45.1X5	T45.1X6
Dibromopropamidine isethionate	T49.0X1	T49.0X2	T49.0X3	T49.0X4	T49.0X5	T49.0X6
Dibrompropamidine	T49.0X1	T49.0X2	T49.0X3	T49.0X4	T49.0X5	T49.0X6
Dibucaine	T41.3X1	T41.3X2	T41.3X3	T41.3X4	T41.3X5	T41.3X6
topical (surface)	T41.3X1	T41.3X2	T41.3X3	T41.3X4	T41.3X5	T41.3X6
Dibunate sodium	T48.3X1	T48.3X2	T48.3X3	T48.3X4	T48.3X5	T48.3X6
Dibutoline sulfate	T44.3X1	T44.3X2	T44.3X3	T44.3X4	T44.3X5	T44.3X6
Dicamba	T60.3X1	T60.3X2	T60.3X3	T60.3X4	—	—
Dicapthon	T60.0X1	T60.0X2	T60.0X3	T60.0X4	—	—
Dichlobenil	T60.3X1	T60.3X2	T60.3X3	T60.3X4	—	—
Dichlone	T60.3X1	T60.3X2	T60.3X3	T60.3X4	—	—

◀ New ◀ Revised ~~deleted~~ Deleted

TABLE OF DRUGS AND CHEMICALS

Substance	External Cause (T-Code)					
	Poisoning, Accidental (Unintentional)	Poisoning, Intentional Self-Harm	Poisoning, Assault	Poisoning, Undetermined	Adverse Effect	Underdosing
Dichloralphenozone	T42.6X1	T42.6X2	T42.6X3	T42.6X4	T42.6X5	T42.6X6
Dichlorbenzidine	T65.3X1	T65.3X2	T65.3X3	T65.3X4	—	—
Dichlorhydrin	T52.8X1	T52.8X2	T52.8X3	T52.8X4	—	—
Dichlorhydroxyquinoline	T37.8X1	T37.8X2	T37.8X3	T37.8X4	T37.8X5	T37.8X6
Dichlorobenzene	T53.7X1	T53.7X2	T53.7X3	T53.7X4	—	—
Dichlorobenzyl alcohol	T49.6X1	T49.6X2	T49.6X3	T49.6X4	T49.6X5	T49.6X6
Dichlorodifluoromethane	T53.5X1	T53.5X2	T53.5X3	T53.5X4	—	—
Dichloroethane	T52.8X1	T52.8X2	T52.8X3	T52.8X4	—	—
Sym-Dichloroethyl ether	T53.6X1	T53.6X2	T53.6X3	T53.6X4	—	—
Dichloroethyl sulfide, not in war	T59.891	T59.892	T59.893	T59.894		
Dichloroethylene	T53.6X1	T53.6X2	T53.6X3	T53.6X4	—	—
Dichloroformoxine, not in war	T59.891	T59.892	T59.893	T59.894		
Dichlorohydrin, alpha-dichlorohydrin	T52.8X1	T52.8X2	T52.8X3	T52.8X4		
Dichloromethane (solvent)	T53.4X1	T53.4X2	T53.4X3	T53.4X4	—	—
vapor	T53.4X1	T53.4X2	T53.4X3	T53.4X4	—	—
Dichloronaphthoquinone	T60.3X1	T60.3X2	T60.3X3	T60.3X4		
Dichlorophen	T37.4X1	T37.4X2	T37.4X3	T37.4X4	T37.4X5	T37.4X6
2,4-Dichlorophenoxy-acetic acid	T60.3X1	T60.3X2	T60.3X3	T60.3X4		
Dichloropropene	T60.3X1	T60.3X2	T60.3X3	T60.3X4		
Dichloropropionic acid	T60.3X1	T60.3X2	T60.3X3	T60.3X4	—	—
Dichlorphenamide	T50.2X1	T50.2X2	T50.2X3	T50.2X4	T50.2X5	T50.2X6
Dichlorvos	T60.0X1	T60.0X2	T60.0X3	T60.0X4		
Diclofenac	T39.391	T39.392	T39.393	T39.394	T39.395	T39.396
Diclofenamide	T50.2X1	T50.2X2	T50.2X3	T50.2X4	T50.2X5	T50.2X6
Diclofensine	T43.291	T43.292	T43.293	T43.294	T43.295	T43.296
Diclonixine	T39.8X1	T39.8X2	T39.8X3	T39.8X4	T39.8X5	T39.8X6
Dicloxacillin	T36.0X1	T36.0X2	T36.0X3	T36.0X4	T36.0X5	T36.0X6
Dicophane	T49.0X1	T49.0X2	T49.0X3	T49.0X4	T49.0X5	T49.0X6
Dicoumarol, dicoumarin, dicumarol	T45.511	T45.512	T45.513	T45.514	T45.515	T45.516
Dicrotophos	T60.0X1	T60.0X2	T60.0X3	T60.0X4	—	—
Dicyanogen (gas)	T65.0X1	T65.0X2	T65.0X3	T65.0X4	—	—
Dicyclomine	T44.3X1	T44.3X2	T44.3X3	T44.3X4	T44.3X5	T44.3X6
Dicycloverine	T44.3X1	T44.3X2	T44.3X3	T44.3X4	T44.3X5	T44.3X6
Dideoxycytidine	T37.5X1	T37.5X2	T37.5X3	T37.5X4	T37.5X5	T37.5X6
Dideoxyinosine	T37.5X1	T37.5X2	T37.5X3	T37.5X4	T37.5X5	T37.5X6
Dieldrin (vapor)	T60.1X1	T60.1X2	T60.1X3	T60.1X4	—	—
Diemal	T42.3X1	T42.3X2	T42.3X3	T42.3X4	T42.3X5	T42.3X6
Dienestrol	T38.5X1	T38.5X2	T38.5X3	T38.5X4	T38.5X5	T38.5X6
Dienoestrol	T38.5X1	T38.5X2	T38.5X3	T38.5X4	T38.5X5	T38.5X6
Dietetic drug NEC	T50.901	T50.902	T50.903	T50.904	T50.905	T50.906
Diethazine	T42.8X1	T42.8X2	T42.8X3	T42.8X4	T42.8X5	T42.8X6

Substance	External Cause (T-Code)					
	Poisoning, Accidental (Unintentional)	Poisoning, Intentional Self-Harm	Poisoning, Assault	Poisoning, Undetermined	Adverse Effect	Underdosing
Diethyl						
barbituric acid	T42.3X1	T42.3X2	T42.3X3	T42.3X4	T42.3X5	T42.3X6
carbamazine	T37.4X1	T37.4X2	T37.4X3	T37.4X4	T37.4X5	T37.4X6
carbinol	T51.3X1	T51.3X2	T51.3X3	T51.3X4	—	—
carbonate	T52.8X1	T52.8X2	T52.8X3	T52.8X4	—	—
ether (vapor) — see also Ether	T41.0X1	T41.0X2	T41.0X3	T41.0X4	T41.0X5	T41.0X6
oxide	T52.8X1	T52.8X2	T52.8X3	T52.8X4	—	—
propion	T50.5X1	T50.5X2	T50.5X3	T50.5X4	T50.5X5	T50.5X6
stilbestrol	T38.5X1	T38.5X2	T38.5X3	T38.5X4	T38.5X5	T38.5X6
toluamide (nonmedicinal)	T60.8X1	T60.8X2	T60.8X3	T60.8X4	—	—
medicinal	T49.3X1	T49.3X2	T49.3X3	T49.3X4	T49.3X5	T49.3X6
Diethylcarbamazine	T37.4X1	T37.4X2	T37.4X3	T37.4X4	T37.4X5	T37.4X6
Diethylene						
dioxide	T52.8X1	T52.8X2	T52.8X3	T52.8X4	—	—
glycol (monoacetate) (monobutyl ether) (monoethyl ether)	T52.3X1	T52.3X2	T52.3X3	T52.3X4	—	—
Diethylhexylphthalate	T65.891	T65.892	T65.893	T65.894	—	—
Diethylpropion	T50.5X1	T50.5X2	T50.5X3	T50.5X4	T50.5X5	T50.5X6
Diethylstilbestrol	T38.5X1	T38.5X2	T38.5X3	T38.5X4	T38.5X5	T38.5X6
Diethylstilboestrol	T38.5X1	T38.5X2	T38.5X3	T38.5X4	T38.5X5	T38.5X6
Diethylsulfone-diethylmethane	T42.6X1	T42.6X2	T42.6X3	T42.6X4	T42.6X5	T42.6X6
Diethyltoluamide	T49.0X1	T49.0X2	T49.0X3	T49.0X4	T49.0X5	T49.0X6
Diethyltryptamine (DET)	T40.991	T40.992	T40.993	T40.994	—	—
Difebarbamate	T42.3X1	T42.3X2	T42.3X3	T42.3X4	T42.3X5	T42.3X6
Difencloxazine	T40.2X1	T40.2X2	T40.2X3	T40.2X4	T40.2X5	T40.2X6
Difenidol	T45.0X1	T45.0X2	T45.0X3	T45.0X4	T45.0X5	T45.0X6
Difenoxin	T47.6X1	T47.6X2	T47.6X3	T47.6X4	T47.6X5	T47.6X6
Difetarsone	T37.3X1	T37.3X2	T37.3X3	T37.3X4	T37.3X5	T37.3X6
Diffusin	T45.3X1	T45.3X2	T45.3X3	T45.3X4	T45.3X5	T45.3X6
Diflorasone	T49.0X1	T49.0X2	T49.0X3	T49.0X4	T49.0X5	T49.0X6
Diflubenzuron	T60.1X1	T60.1X2	T60.1X3	T60.1X4	—	—
Diflos	T44.0X1	T44.0X2	T44.0X3	T44.0X4	T44.0X5	T44.0X6
Diflucortolone	T49.0X1	T49.0X2	T49.0X3	T49.0X4	T49.0X5	T49.0X6
Diflunisal	T39.091	T39.092	T39.093	T39.094	T39.095	T39.096
Difluoromethyldopa	T42.8X1	T42.8X2	T42.8X3	T42.8X4	T42.8X5	T42.8X6
Difluorophate	T44.0X1	T44.0X2	T44.0X3	T44.0X4	T44.0X5	T44.0X6
Digestant NEC	T47.5X1	T47.5X2	T47.5X3	T47.5X4	T47.5X5	T47.5X6
Digitalin(e)	T46.0X1	T46.0X2	T46.0X3	T46.0X4	T46.0X5	T46.0X6
Digitalis (leaf) (glycoside)	T46.0X1	T46.0X2	T46.0X3	T46.0X4	T46.0X5	T46.0X6
lanata	T46.0X1	T46.0X2	T46.0X3	T46.0X4	T46.0X5	T46.0X6
purpurea	T46.0X1	T46.0X2	T46.0X3	T46.0X4	T46.0X5	T46.0X6
Digitoxin	T46.0X1	T46.0X2	T46.0X3	T46.0X4	T46.0X5	T46.0X6

◀ New   ◀ Revised   ~~deleted~~ Deleted

Substance	External Cause (T-Code)					
	Poisoning, Accidental (Unintentional)	Poisoning, Intentional Self-Harm	Poisoning, Assault	Poisoning, Undetermined	Adverse Effect	Underdosing
Digitoxose	T46.0X1	T46.0X2	T46.0X3	T46.0X4	T46.0X5	T46.0X6
Digoxin	T46.0X1	T46.0X2	T46.0X3	T46.0X4	T46.0X5	T46.0X6
Digoxine	T46.0X1	T46.0X2	T46.0X3	T46.0X4	T46.0X5	T46.0X6
Dihydralazine	T46.5X1	T46.5X2	T46.5X3	T46.5X4	T46.5X5	T46.5X6
Dihydrazine	T46.5X1	T46.5X2	T46.5X3	T46.5X4	T46.5X5	T46.5X6
Dihydrocodeinone	T40.2X1	T40.2X2	T40.2X3	T40.2X4	T40.2X5	T40.2X6
Dihydroergocornine	T46.7X1	T46.7X2	T46.7X3	T46.7X4	T46.7X5	T46.7X6
Dihydroergocristine (mesilate)	T46.7X1	T46.7X2	T46.7X3	T46.7X4	T46.7X5	T46.7X6
Dihydroergokryptine	T46.7X1	T46.7X2	T46.7X3	T46.7X4	T46.7X5	T46.7X6
Dihydroergotamine	T46.5X1	T46.5X2	T46.5X3	T46.5X4	T46.5X5	T46.5X6
Dihydroergotoxine	T46.7X1	T46.7X2	T46.7X3	T46.7X4	T46.7X5	T46.7X6
mesilate	T46.7X1	T46.7X2	T46.7X3	T46.7X4	T46.7X5	T46.7X6
Dihydrohydroxycodein-one	T40.2X1	T40.2X2	T40.2X3	T40.2X4	T40.2X5	T40.2X6
Dihydrohydroxymorphinone	T40.2X1	T40.2X2	T40.2X3	T40.2X4	T40.2X5	T40.2X6
Dihydroisocodeine	T40.2X1	T40.2X2	T40.2X3	T40.2X4	T40.2X5	T40.2X6
Dihydromorphine	T40.2X1	T40.2X2	T40.2X3	T40.2X4	—	—
Dihydromorphinone	T40.2X1	T40.2X2	T40.2X3	T40.2X4	T40.2X5	T40.2X6
Dihydrostreptomycin	T36.5X1	T36.5X2	T36.5X3	T36.5X4	T36.5X5	T36.5X6
Dihydrotachysterol	T45.2X1	T45.2X2	T45.2X3	T45.2X4	T45.2X5	T45.2X6
Dihydroxyaluminum aminoacetate	T47.1X1	T47.1X2	T47.1X3	T47.1X4	T47.1X5	T47.1X6
Dihydroxyaluminum sodium carbonate	T47.1X1	T47.1X2	T47.1X3	T47.1X4	T47.1X5	T47.1X6
Dihydroxyanthraquinone	T47.2X1	T47.2X2	T47.2X3	T47.2X4	T47.2X5	T47.2X6
Dihydroxycodeinone	T40.2X1	T40.2X2	T40.2X3	T40.2X4	T40.2X5	T40.2X6
Dihydroxypropyl theophylline	T50.2X1	T50.2X2	T50.2X3	T50.2X4	T50.2X5	T50.2X6
Diiodohydroxyquin	T37.8X1	T37.8X2	T37.8X3	T37.8X4	T37.8X5	T37.8X6
topical	T49.0X1	T49.0X2	T49.0X3	T49.0X4	T49.0X5	T49.0X6
Diiodohydroxyquinoline	T37.8X1	T37.8X2	T37.8X3	T37.8X4	T37.8X5	T37.8X6
Diiodotyrosine	T38.2X1	T38.2X2	T38.2X3	T38.2X4	T38.2X5	T38.2X6
Diisopromine	T44.3X1	T44.3X2	T44.3X3	T44.3X4	T44.3X5	T44.3X6
Diisopropylamine	T46.3X1	T46.3X2	T46.3X3	T46.3X4	T46.3X5	T46.3X6
Diisopropylfluorophosphonate	T44.0X1	T44.0X2	T44.0X3	T44.0X4	T44.0X5	T44.0X6
Dilantin	T42.0X1	T42.0X2	T42.0X3	T42.0X4	T42.0X5	T42.0X6
Dilaudid	T40.2X1	T40.2X2	T40.2X3	T40.2X4	T40.2X5	T40.2X6
Dilazep	T46.3X1	T46.3X2	T46.3X3	T46.3X4	T46.3X5	T46.3X6
Dill	T47.5X1	T47.5X2	T47.5X3	T47.5X4	T47.5X5	T47.5X6
Diloxanide	T37.3X1	T37.3X2	T37.3X3	T37.3X4	T37.3X5	T37.3X6
Diltiazem	T46.1X1	T46.1X2	T46.1X3	T46.1X4	T46.1X5	T46.1X6
Dimazole	T49.0X1	T49.0X2	T49.0X3	T49.0X4	T49.0X5	T49.0X6
Dimefline	T50.7X1	T50.7X2	T50.7X3	T50.7X4	T50.7X5	T50.7X6
Dimefox	T60.0X1	T60.0X2	T60.0X3	T60.0X4	—	—

Substance	External Cause (T-Code)					
	Poisoning, Accidental (Unintentional)	Poisoning, Intentional Self-Harm	Poisoning, Assault	Poisoning, Undetermined	Adverse Effect	Underdosing
Dimemorfan	T48.3X1	T48.3X2	T48.3X3	T48.3X4	T48.3X5	T48.3X6
Dimenhydrinate	T45.0X1	T45.0X2	T45.0X3	T45.0X4	T45.0X5	T45.0X6
Dimercaprol (British anti-lewisite)	T45.8X1	T45.8X2	T45.8X3	T45.8X4	T45.8X5	T45.8X6
Dimercaptopropanol	T45.8X1	T45.8X2	T45.8X3	T45.8X4	T45.8X5	T45.8X6
Dimestrol	T38.5X1	T38.5X2	T38.5X3	T38.5X4	T38.5X5	T38.5X6
Dimetane	T45.0X1	T45.0X2	T45.0X3	T45.0X4	T45.0X5	T45.0X6
Dimethicone	T47.1X1	T47.1X2	T47.1X3	T47.1X4	T47.1X5	T47.1X6
Dimethindene	T45.0X1	T45.0X2	T45.0X3	T45.0X4	T45.0X5	T45.0X6
Dimethisoquin	T49.1X1	T49.1X2	T49.1X3	T49.1X4	T49.1X5	T49.1X6
Dimethisterone	T38.5X1	T38.5X2	T38.5X3	T38.5X4	T38.5X5	T38.5X6
Dimethoate	T60.0X1	T60.0X2	T60.0X3	T60.0X4	—	—
Dimethocaine	T41.3X1	T41.3X2	T41.3X3	T41.3X4	T41.3X5	T41.3X6
Dimethoxanate	T48.3X1	T48.3X2	T48.3X3	T48.3X4	T48.3X5	T48.3X6
Dimethyl						
arsine, arsinic acid	T57.0X1	T57.0X2	T57.0X3	T57.0X4	—	—
carbinol	T51.2X1	T51.2X2	T51.2X3	T51.2X4	—	—
carbonate	T52.8X1	T52.8X2	T52.8X3	T52.8X4	—	—
diguanide	T38.3X1	T38.3X2	T38.3X3	T38.3X4	T38.3X5	T38.3X6
ketone	T52.4X1	T52.4X2	T52.4X3	T52.4X4	—	—
vapor	T52.4X1	T52.4X2	T52.4X3	T52.4X4	—	—
meperidine	T40.2X1	T40.2X2	T40.2X3	T40.2X4	T40.2X5	T40.2X6
parathion	T60.0X1	T60.0X2	T60.0X3	T60.0X4	—	—
phthlate	T49.3X1	T49.3X2	T49.3X3	T49.3X4	T49.3X5	T49.3X6
polysiloxane	T47.8X1	T47.8X2	T47.8X3	T47.8X4	T47.8X5	T47.8X6
sulfate (fumes)	T59.891	T59.892	T59.893	T59.894	—	—
liquid	T65.891	T65.892	T65.893	T65.894	—	—
sulfoxide (nonmedicinal)	T52.8X1	T52.8X2	T52.8X3	T52.8X4	—	—
medicinal	T49.4X1	T49.4X2	T49.4X3	T49.4X4	T49.4X5	T49.4X6
tryptamine	T40.991	T40.992	T40.993	T40.994		
tubocurarine	T48.1X1	T48.1X2	T48.1X3	T48.1X4	T48.1X5	T48.1X6
Dimethylamine sulfate	T49.4X1	T49.4X2	T49.4X3	T49.4X4	T49.4X5	T49.4X6
Dimethylformamide	T52.8X1	T52.8X2	T52.8X3	T52.8X4		
Dimethyltubocurarinium chloride	T48.1X1	T48.1X2	T48.1X3	T48.1X4	T48.1X5	T48.1X6
Dimeticone	T47.1X1	T47.1X2	T47.1X3	T47.1X4	T47.1X5	T47.1X6
Dimetilan	T60.0X1	T60.0X2	T60.0X3	T60.0X4	—	—
Dimetindene	T45.0X1	T45.0X2	T45.0X3	T45.0X4	T45.0X5	T45.0X6
Dimetotiazine	T43.3X1	T43.3X2	T43.3X3	T43.3X4	T43.3X5	T43.3X6
Dimorpholamine	T50.7X1	T50.7X2	T50.7X3	T50.7X4	T50.7X5	T50.7X6
Dimoxyline	T46.3X1	T46.3X2	T46.3X3	T46.3X4	T46.3X5	T46.3X6
Dinitrobenzene	T65.3X1	T65.3X2	T65.3X3	T65.3X4	—	—
vapor	T59.891	T59.892	T59.893	T59.894	—	—

◀ New ◀ Revised ~~deleted~~ Deleted

Substance	External Cause (T-Code)					
	Poisoning, Accidental (Unintentional)	Poisoning, Intentional Self-Harm	Poisoning, Assault	Poisoning, Undetermined	Adverse Effect	Underdosing
Dinitrobenzol	T65.3X1	T65.3X2	T65.3X3	T65.3X4	—	—
vapor	T59.891	T59.892	T59.893	T59.894	—	—
Dinitrobutylphenol	T65.3X1	T65.3X2	T65.3X3	T65.3X4	—	—
Dinitro (-ortho-)cresol (pesticide) (spray)	T65.3X1	T65.3X2	T65.3X3	T65.3X4	—	—
Dinitrocyclohexylphenol	T65.3X1	T65.3X2	T65.3X3	T65.3X4	—	—
Dinitrophenol	T65.3X1	T65.3X2	T65.3X3	T65.3X4	—	—
Dinoprost	T48.0X1	T48.0X2	T48.0X3	T48.0X4	T48.0X5	T48.0X6
Dinoprostone	T48.0X1	T48.0X2	T48.0X3	T48.0X4	T48.0X5	T48.0X6
Dinoseb	T60.3X1	T60.3X2	T60.3X3	T60.3X4		
Dioctyl sulfosuccinate (calcium) (sodium)	T47.4X1	T47.4X2	T47.4X3	T47.4X4	T47.4X5	T47.4X6
Diodone	T50.8X1	T50.8X2	T50.8X3	T50.8X4	T50.8X5	T50.8X6
Diodoquin	T37.8X1	T37.8X2	T37.8X3	T37.8X4	T37.8X5	T37.8X6
Dionin	T40.2X1	T40.2X2	T40.2X3	T40.2X4	T40.2X5	T40.2X6
Diosmin	T46.991	T46.992	T46.993	T46.994	T46.995	T46.996
Dioxane	T52.8X1	T52.8X2	T52.8X3	T52.8X4	—	—
Dioxathion	T60.0X1	T60.0X2	T60.0X3	T60.0X4	—	—
Dioxin	T53.7X1	T53.7X2	T53.7X3	T53.7X4	—	—
Dioxopromethazine	T43.3X1	T43.3X2	T43.3X3	T43.3X4	T43.3X5	T43.3X6
Dioxyline	T46.3X1	T46.3X2	T46.3X3	T46.3X4	T46.3X5	T46.3X6
Dipentene	T52.8X1	T52.8X2	T52.8X3	T52.8X4	—	—
Diperodon	T41.3X1	T41.3X2	T41.3X3	T41.3X4	T41.3X5	T41.3X6
Diphacinone	T60.4X1	T60.4X2	T60.4X3	T60.4X4	—	—
Diphemanil	T44.3X1	T44.3X2	T44.3X3	T44.3X4	T44.3X5	T44.3X6
metilsulfate	T44.3X1	T44.3X2	T44.3X3	T44.3X4	T44.3X5	T44.3X6
Diphenadione	T45.511	T45.512	T45.513	T45.514	T45.515	T45.516
rodenticide	T60.4X1	T60.4X2	T60.4X3	T60.4X4	—	—
Diphenhydramine	T45.0X1	T45.0X2	T45.0X3	T45.0X4	T45.0X5	T45.0X6
Diphenidol	T45.0X1	T45.0X2	T45.0X3	T45.0X4	T45.0X5	T45.0X6
Diphenoxylate	T47.6X1	T47.6X2	T47.6X3	T47.6X4	T47.6X5	T47.6X6
Diphenylamine	T65.3X1	T65.3X2	T65.3X3	T65.3X4	—	—
Diphenylbutazone	T39.2X1	T39.2X2	T39.2X3	T39.2X4	T39.2X5	T39.2X6
Diphenylchloroarsine, not in war	T57.0X1	T57.0X2	T57.0X3	T57.0X4	—	—
Diphenylhydantoin	T42.0X1	T42.0X2	T42.0X3	T42.0X4	T42.0X5	T42.0X6
Diphenylmethane dye	T52.1X1	T52.1X2	T52.1X3	T52.1X4	—	—
Diphenylpyraline	T45.0X1	T45.0X2	T45.0X3	T45.0X4	T45.0X5	T45.0X6
Diphtheria						
antitoxin	T50.Z11	T50.Z12	T50.Z13	T50.Z14	T50.Z15	T50.Z16
toxoid	T50.A91	T50.A92	T50.A93	T50.A94	T50.A95	T50.A96
with tetanus toxoid	T50.A21	T50.A22	T50.A23	T50.A24	T50.A25	T50.A26
with pertussis component	T50.A11	T50.A12	T50.A13	T50.A14	T50.A15	T50.A16

Substance	External Cause (T-Code)					
	Poisoning, Accidental (Unintentional)	Poisoning, Intentional Self-Harm	Poisoning, Assault	Poisoning, Undetermined	Adverse Effect	Underdosing
Diphtheria (Continued)						
vaccine (combination)	T50.A91	T50.A92	T50.A93	T50.A94	T50.A95	T50.A96
combination						
including pertussis	T50.A11	T50.A12	T50.A13	T50.A14	T50.A15	T50.A16
without pertussis	T50.A21	T50.A22	T50.A23	T50.A24	T50.A25	T50.A26
Diphylline	T50.2X1	T50.2X2	T50.2X3	T50.2X4	T50.2X5	T50.2X6
Dipipanone	T40.491	T40.492	T40.493	T40.494	—	—
Dipivefrine	T49.5X1	T49.5X2	T49.5X3	T49.5X4	T49.5X5	T49.5X6
Diplovax	T50.B91	T50.B92	T50.B93	T50.B94	T50.B95	T50.B96
Diprophylline	T50.2X1	T50.2X2	T50.2X3	T50.2X4	T50.2X5	T50.2X6
Dipropyline	T48.291	T48.292	T48.293	T48.294	T48.295	T48.296
Dipyridamole	T46.3X1	T46.3X2	T46.3X3	T46.3X4	T46.3X5	T46.3X6
Dipyrone	T39.2X1	T39.2X2	T39.2X3	T39.2X4	T39.2X5	T39.2X6
Diquat (dibromide)	T60.3X1	T60.3X2	T60.3X3	T60.3X4	—	—
Disinfectant	T65.891	T65.892	T65.893	T65.894	—	—
alkaline	T54.3X1	T54.3X2	T54.3X3	T54.3X4	—	—
aromatic	T54.1X1	T54.1X2	T54.1X3	T54.1X4	—	—
intestinal	T37.8X1	T37.8X2	T37.8X3	T37.8X4	T37.8X5	T37.8X6
Disipal	T42.8X1	T42.8X2	T42.8X3	T42.8X4	T42.8X5	T42.8X6
Disodium edetate	T50.6X1	T50.6X2	T50.6X3	T50.6X4	T50.6X5	T50.6X6
Disoprofol	T41.291	T41.292	T41.293	T41.294	T41.295	T41.296
Disopyramide	T46.2X1	T46.2X2	T46.2X3	T46.2X4	T46.2X5	T46.2X6
Distigmine (bromide)	T44.0X1	T44.0X2	T44.0X3	T44.0X4	T44.0X5	T44.0X6
Disulfamide	T50.2X1	T50.2X2	T50.2X3	T50.2X4	T50.2X5	T50.2X6
Disulfanilamide	T37.0X1	T37.0X2	T37.0X3	T37.0X4	T37.0X5	T37.0X6
Disulfiram	T50.6X1	T50.6X2	T50.6X3	T50.6X4	T50.6X5	T50.6X6
Disulfoton	T60.0X1	T60.0X2	T60.0X3	T60.0X4	—	—
Dithiazanine iodide	T37.4X1	T37.4X2	T37.4X3	T37.4X4	T37.4X5	T37.4X6
Dithiocarbamate	T60.0X1	T60.0X2	T60.0X3	T60.0X4	—	—
Dithranol	T49.4X1	T49.4X2	T49.4X3	T49.4X4	T49.4X5	T49.4X6
Diucardin	T50.2X1	T50.2X2	T50.2X3	T50.2X4	T50.2X5	T50.2X6
Diupres	T50.2X1	T50.2X2	T50.2X3	T50.2X4	T50.2X5	T50.2X6
Diuretic NEC	T50.2X1	T50.2X2	T50.2X3	T50.2X4	T50.2X5	T50.2X6
benzothiadiazine	T50.2X1	T50.2X2	T50.2X3	T50.2X4	T50.2X5	T50.2X6
carbonic acid anhydrase inhibitors	T50.2X1	T50.2X2	T50.2X3	T50.2X4	T50.2X5	T50.2X6
furfuryl NEC	T50.2X1	T50.2X2	T50.2X3	T50.2X4	T50.2X5	T50.2X6
loop (high-ceiling)	T50.1X1	T50.1X2	T50.1X3	T50.1X4	T50.1X5	T50.1X6
mercurial NEC	T50.2X1	T50.2X2	T50.2X3	T50.2X4	T50.2X5	T50.2X6
osmotic	T50.2X1	T50.2X2	T50.2X3	T50.2X4	T50.2X5	T50.2X6
purine NEC	T50.2X1	T50.2X2	T50.2X3	T50.2X4	T50.2X5	T50.2X6
saluretic NEC	T50.2X1	T50.2X2	T50.2X3	T50.2X4	T50.2X5	T50.2X6

◄ New   ◄ Revised   ~~deleted~~ Deleted

Substance	Poisoning, Accidental (Unintentional)	Poisoning, Intentional Self-Harm	Poisoning, Assault	Poisoning, Undetermined	Adverse Effect	Underdosing
Diuretic NEC *(Continued)*						
sulfonamide	T50.2X1	T50.2X2	T50.2X3	T50.2X4	T50.2X5	T50.2X6
thiazide NEC	T50.2X1	T50.2X2	T50.2X3	T50.2X4	T50.2X5	T50.2X6
xanthine	T50.2X1	T50.2X2	T50.2X3	T50.2X4	T50.2X5	T50.2X6
Diurgin	T50.2X1	T50.2X2	T50.2X3	T50.2X4	T50.2X5	T50.2X6
Diuril	T50.2X1	T50.2X2	T50.2X3	T50.2X4	T50.2X5	T50.2X6
Diuron	T60.3X1	T60.3X2	T60.3X3	T60.3X4	—	—
Divalproex	T42.6X1	T42.6X2	T42.6X3	T42.6X4	T42.6X5	T42.6X6
Divinyl ether	T41.0X1	T41.0X2	T41.0X3	T41.0X4	T41.0X5	T41.0X6
Dixanthogen	T49.0X1	T49.0X2	T49.0X3	T49.0X4	T49.0X5	T49.0X6
Dixyrazine	T43.3X1	T43.3X2	T43.3X3	T43.3X4	T43.3X5	T43.3X6
D-lysergic acid diethylamide	T40.8X1	T40.8X2	T40.8X3	T40.8X4	—	—
DMCT	T36.4X1	T36.4X2	T36.4X3	T36.4X4	T36.4X5	T36.4X6
DMSO — *see Dimethyl sulfoxide*						
DNBP	T60.3X1	T60.3X2	T60.3X3	T60.3X4		
DNOC	T65.3X1	T65.3X2	T65.3X3	T65.3X4	—	—
DOCA	T38.0X1	T38.0X2	T38.0X3	T38.0X4	T38.0X5	T38.0X6
Dobutamine	T44.5X1	T44.5X2	T44.5X3	T44.5X4	T44.5X5	T44.5X6
Docusate sodium	T47.4X1	T47.4X2	T47.4X3	T47.4X4	T47.4X5	T47.4X6
Dodicin	T49.0X1	T49.0X2	T49.0X3	T49.0X4	T49.0X5	T49.0X6
Dofamium chloride	T49.0X1	T49.0X2	T49.0X3	T49.0X4	T49.0X5	T49.0X6
Dolophine	T40.3X1	T40.3X2	T40.3X3	T40.3X4	T40.3X5	T40.3X6
Doloxene	T39.8X1	T39.8X2	T39.8X3	T39.8X4	T39.8X5	T39.8X6
Domestic gas (after combustion) — *see Gas, utility*						
prior to combustion	T59.891	T59.892	T59.893	T59.894	—	—
Domiodol	T48.4X1	T48.4X2	T48.4X3	T48.4X4	T48.4X5	T48.4X6
Domiphen (bromide)	T49.0X1	T49.0X2	T49.0X3	T49.0X4	T49.0X5	T49.0X6
Domperidone	T45.0X1	T45.0X2	T45.0X3	T45.0X4	T45.0X5	T45.0X6
Dopa	T42.8X1	T42.8X2	T42.8X3	T42.8X4	T42.8X5	T42.8X6
Dopamine	T44.991	T44.992	T44.993	T44.994	T44.995	T44.996
Doriden	T42.6X1	T42.6X2	T42.6X3	T42.6X4	T42.6X5	T42.6X6
Dormiral	T42.3X1	T42.3X2	T42.3X3	T42.3X4	T42.3X5	T42.3X6
Dormison	T42.6X1	T42.6X2	T42.6X3	T42.6X4	T42.6X5	T42.6X6
Dornase	T48.4X1	T48.4X2	T48.4X3	T48.4X4	T48.4X5	T48.4X6
Dorsacaine	T41.3X1	T41.3X2	T41.3X3	T41.3X4	T41.3X5	T41.3X6
Dosulepin	T43.011	T43.012	T43.013	T43.014	T43.015	T43.016
Dothiepin	T43.011	T43.012	T43.013	T43.014	T43.015	T43.016
Doxantrazole	T48.6X1	T48.6X2	T48.6X3	T48.6X4	T48.6X5	T48.6X6
Doxapram	T50.7X1	T50.7X2	T50.7X3	T50.7X4	T50.7X5	T50.7X6
Doxazosin	T44.6X1	T44.6X2	T44.6X3	T44.6X4	T44.6X5	T44.6X6
Doxepin	T43.011	T43.012	T43.013	T43.014	T43.015	T43.016

Substance	Poisoning, Accidental (Unintentional)	Poisoning, Intentional Self-Harm	Poisoning, Assault	Poisoning, Undetermined	Adverse Effect	Underdosing
Doxifluridine	T45.1X1	T45.1X2	T45.1X3	T45.1X4	T45.1X5	T45.1X6
Doxorubicin	T45.1X1	T45.1X2	T45.1X3	T45.1X4	T45.1X5	T45.1X6
Doxycycline	T36.4X1	T36.4X2	T36.4X3	T36.4X4	T36.4X5	T36.4X6
Doxylamine	T45.0X1	T45.0X2	T45.0X3	T45.0X4	T45.0X5	T45.0X6
Dramamine	T45.0X1	T45.0X2	T45.0X3	T45.0X4	T45.0X5	T45.0X6
Drano (drain cleaner)	T54.3X1	T54.3X2	T54.3X3	T54.3X4	—	—
Dressing, live pulp	T49.7X1	T49.7X2	T49.7X3	T49.7X4	T49.7X5	T49.7X6
Drocode	T40.2X1	T40.2X2	T40.2X3	T40.2X4	T40.2X5	T40.2X6
Dromoran	T40.2X1	T40.2X2	T40.2X3	T40.2X4	T40.2X5	T40.2X6
Dromostanolone	T38.7X1	T38.7X2	T38.7X3	T38.7X4	T38.7X5	T38.7X6
Dronabinol	T40.711	T40.712	T40.713	T40.714	T40.715	T40.716 ◄
Droperidol	T43.591	T43.592	T43.593	T43.594	T43.595	T43.596
Dropropizine	T48.3X1	T48.3X2	T48.3X3	T48.3X4	T48.3X5	T48.3X6
Drostanolone	T38.7X1	T38.7X2	T38.7X3	T38.7X4	T38.7X5	T38.7X6
Drotaverine	T44.3X1	T44.3X2	T44.3X3	T44.3X4	T44.3X5	T44.3X6
Drotrecogin alfa	T45.511	T45.512	T45.513	T45.514	T45.515	T45.516
Drug NEC	T50.901	T50.902	T50.903	T50.904	T50.905	T50.906
specified NEC	T50.991	T50.992	T50.993	T50.994	T50.995	T50.996
DTIC	T45.1X1	T45.1X2	T45.1X3	T45.1X4	T45.1X5	T45.1X6
Duboisine	T44.3X1	T44.3X2	T44.3X3	T44.3X4	T44.3X5	T44.3X6
Dulcolax	T47.2X1	T47.2X2	T47.2X3	T47.2X4	T47.2X5	T47.2X6
Duponol (C) (EP)	T49.2X1	T49.2X2	T49.2X3	T49.2X4	T49.2X5	T49.2X6
Durabolin	T38.7X1	T38.7X2	T38.7X3	T38.7X4	T38.7X5	T38.7X6
Dyclone	T41.3X1	T41.3X2	T41.3X3	T41.3X4	T41.3X5	T41.3X6
Dyclonine	T41.3X1	T41.3X2	T41.3X3	T41.3X4	T41.3X5	T41.3X6
Dydrogesterone	T38.5X1	T38.5X2	T38.5X3	T38.5X4	T38.5X5	T38.5X6
Dye NEC	T65.6X1	T65.6X2	T65.6X3	T65.6X4	—	—
antiseptic	T49.0X1	T49.0X2	T49.0X3	T49.0X4	T49.0X5	T49.0X6
diagnostic agents	T50.8X1	T50.8X2	T50.8X3	T50.8X4	T50.8X5	T50.8X6
pharmaceutical NEC	T50.901	T50.902	T50.903	T50.904	T50.905	T50.906
Dyflos	T44.0X1	T44.0X2	T44.0X3	T44.0X4	T44.0X5	T44.0X6
Dymelor	T38.3X1	T38.3X2	T38.3X3	T38.3X4	T38.3X5	T38.3X6
Dynamite	T65.3X1	T65.3X2	T65.3X3	T65.3X4	—	—
fumes	T59.891	T59.892	T59.893	T59.894	—	—
Dyphylline	T44.3X1	T44.3X2	T44.3X3	T44.3X4	T44.3X5	T44.3X6
E						
Ear drug NEC	T49.6X1	T49.6X2	T49.6X3	T49.6X4	T49.6X5	T49.6X6
Ear preparations	T49.6X1	T49.6X2	T49.6X3	T49.6X4	T49.6X5	T49.6X6
Econazole	T49.0X1	T49.0X2	T49.0X3	T49.0X4	T49.0X5	T49.0X6
Ecothiopate iodide	T49.5X1	T49.5X2	T49.5X3	T49.5X4	T49.5X5	T49.5X6
Echothiophate, echothiopate, ecothiopate	T49.5X1	T49.5X2	T49.5X3	T49.5X4	T49.5X5	T49.5X6

◄ New　◄ Revised　~~deleted~~ Deleted

TABLE OF DRUGS AND CHEMICALS

Substance	Poisoning, Accidental (Unintentional)	Poisoning, Intentional Self-Harm	Poisoning, Assault	Poisoning, Undetermined	Adverse Effect	Underdosing
Ecstasy	T43.641	T43.642	T43.643	T43.644	—	—
Ectylurea	T42.6X1	T42.6X2	T42.6X3	T42.6X4	T42.6X5	T42.6X6
Edathamil disodium	T45.8X1	T45.8X2	T45.8X3	T45.8X4	T45.8X5	T45.8X6
Edecrin	T50.1X1	T50.1X2	T50.1X3	T50.1X4	T50.1X5	T50.1X6
Edetate, disodium (calcium)	T45.8X1	T45.8X2	T45.8X3	T45.8X4	T45.8X5	T45.8X6
Edoxudine	T49.5X1	T49.5X2	T49.5X3	T49.5X4	T49.5X5	T49.5X6
Edrophonium	T44.0X1	T44.0X2	T44.0X3	T44.0X4	T44.0X5	T44.0X6
chloride	T44.0X1	T44.0X2	T44.0X3	T44.0X4	T44.0X5	T44.0X6
EDTA	T50.6X1	T50.6X2	T50.6X3	T50.6X4	T50.6X5	T50.6X6
Eflornithine	T37.2X1	T37.2X2	T37.2X3	T37.2X4	T37.2X5	T37.2X6
Efloxate	T46.3X1	T46.3X2	T46.3X3	T46.3X4	T46.3X5	T46.3X6
Elase	T49.8X1	T49.8X2	T49.8X3	T49.8X4	T49.8X5	T49.8X6
Elastase	T47.5X1	T47.5X2	T47.5X3	T47.5X4	T47.5X5	T47.5X6
Elaterium	T47.2X1	T47.2X2	T47.2X3	T47.2X4	T47.2X5	T47.2X6
Elcatonin	T50.991	T50.992	T50.993	T50.994	T50.995	T50.996
Elder	T62.2X1	T62.2X2	T62.2X3	T62.2X4	—	—
berry (unripe)	T62.1X1	T62.1X2	T62.1X3	T62.1X4	—	—
Electrolyte balance drug	T50.3X1	T50.3X2	T50.3X3	T50.3X4	T50.3X5	T50.3X6
Electrolytes NEC	T50.3X1	T50.3X2	T50.3X3	T50.3X4	T50.3X5	T50.3X6
Electrolytic agent NEC	T50.3X1	T50.3X2	T50.3X3	T50.3X4	T50.3X5	T50.3X6
Elemental diet	T50.901	T50.902	T50.903	T50.904	T50.905	T50.906
Elliptinium acetate	T45.1X1	T45.1X2	T45.1X3	T45.1X4	T45.1X5	T45.1X6
Embramine	T45.0X1	T45.0X2	T45.0X3	T45.0X4	T45.0X5	T45.0X6
Emepronium (salts)	T44.3X1	T44.3X2	T44.3X3	T44.3X4	T44.3X5	T44.3X6
bromide	T44.3X1	T44.3X2	T44.3X3	T44.3X4	T44.3X5	T44.3X6
Emetic NEC	T47.7X1	T47.7X2	T47.7X3	T47.7X4	T47.7X5	T47.7X6
Emetine	T37.3X1	T37.3X2	T37.3X3	T37.3X4	T37.3X5	T37.3X6
Emollient NEC	T49.3X1	T49.3X2	T49.3X3	T49.3X4	T49.3X5	T49.3X6
Emorfazone	T39.8X1	T39.8X2	T39.8X3	T39.8X4	T39.8X5	T39.8X6
Emylcamate	T43.591	T43.592	T43.593	T43.594	T43.595	T43.596
Enalapril	T46.4X1	T46.4X2	T46.4X3	T46.4X4	T46.4X5	T46.4X6
Enalaprilat	T46.4X1	T46.4X2	T46.4X3	T46.4X4	T46.4X5	T46.4X6
Encainide	T46.2X1	T46.2X2	T46.2X3	T46.2X4	T46.2X5	T46.2X6
Endocaine	T41.3X1	T41.3X2	T41.3X3	T41.3X4	T41.3X5	T41.3X6
Endosulfan	T60.2X1	T60.2X2	T60.2X3	T60.2X4	—	—
Endothall	T60.3X1	T60.3X2	T60.3X3	T60.3X4	—	—
Endralazine	T46.5X1	T46.5X2	T46.5X3	T46.5X4	T46.5X5	T46.5X6
Endrin	T60.1X1	T60.1X2	T60.1X3	T60.1X4	—	—
Enflurane	T41.0X1	T41.0X2	T41.0X3	T41.0X4	T41.0X5	T41.0X6
Enhexymal	T42.3X1	T42.3X2	T42.3X3	T42.3X4	T42.3X5	T42.3X6
Enocitabine	T45.1X1	T45.1X2	T45.1X3	T45.1X4	T45.1X5	T45.1X6
Enovid	T38.4X1	T38.4X2	T38.4X3	T38.4X4	T38.4X5	T38.4X6

Substance	Poisoning, Accidental (Unintentional)	Poisoning, Intentional Self-Harm	Poisoning, Assault	Poisoning, Undetermined	Adverse Effect	Underdosing
Enoxacin	T36.8X1	T36.8X2	T36.8X3	T36.8X4	T36.8X5	T36.8X6
Enoxaparin (sodium)	T45.511	T45.512	T45.513	T45.514	T45.515	T45.516
Enpiprazole	T43.591	T43.592	T43.593	T43.594	T43.595	T43.596
Enprofylline	T48.6X1	T48.6X2	T48.6X3	T48.6X4	T48.6X5	T48.6X6
Enprostil	T47.1X1	T47.1X2	T47.1X3	T47.1X4	T47.1X5	T47.1X6
ENT preparations (anti-infectives)	T49.6X1	T49.6X2	T49.6X3	T49.6X4	T49.6X5	T49.6X6
Enviomycin	T36.8X1	T36.8X2	T36.8X3	T36.8X4	T36.8X5	T36.8X6
Enzodase	T45.3X1	T45.3X2	T45.3X3	T45.3X4	T45.3X5	T45.3X6
Enzyme NEC	T45.3X1	T45.3X2	T45.3X3	T45.3X4	T45.3X5	T45.3X6
depolymerizing	T49.8X1	T49.8X2	T49.8X3	T49.8X4	T49.8X5	T49.8X6
fibrolytic	T45.3X1	T45.3X2	T45.3X3	T45.3X4	T45.3X5	T45.3X6
gastric	T47.5X1	T47.5X2	T47.5X3	T47.5X4	T47.5X5	T47.5X6
intestinal	T47.5X1	T47.5X2	T47.5X3	T47.5X4	T47.5X5	T47.5X6
local action	T49.4X1	T49.4X2	T49.4X3	T49.4X4	T49.4X5	T49.4X6
proteolytic	T49.4X1	T49.4X2	T49.4X3	T49.4X4	T49.4X5	T49.4X6
thrombolytic	T45.3X1	T45.3X2	T45.3X3	T45.3X4	T45.3X5	T45.3X6
EPAB	T41.3X1	T41.3X2	T41.3X3	T41.3X4	T41.3X5	T41.3X6
Epanutin	T42.0X1	T42.0X2	T42.0X3	T42.0X4	T42.0X5	T42.0X6
Ephedra	T44.991	T44.992	T44.993	T44.994	T44.995	T44.996
Ephedrine	T44.991	T44.992	T44.993	T44.994	T44.995	T44.996
Epichlorhydrin, epichlorohydrin	T52.8X1	T52.8X2	T52.8X3	T52.8X4	—	—
Epicillin	T36.0X1	T36.0X2	T36.0X3	T36.0X4	T36.0X5	T36.0X6
Epiestriol	T38.5X1	T38.5X2	T38.5X3	T38.5X4	T38.5X5	T38.5X6
Epilim — see Sodium valproate						
Epimestrol	T38.5X1	T38.5X2	T38.5X3	T38.5X4	T38.5X5	T38.5X6
Epinephrine	T44.5X1	T44.5X2	T44.5X3	T44.5X4	T44.5X5	T44.5X6
Epirubicin	T45.1X1	T45.1X2	T45.1X3	T45.1X4	T45.1X5	T45.1X6
Epitiostanol	T38.7X1	T38.7X2	T38.7X3	T38.7X4	T38.7X5	T38.7X6
Epitizide	T50.2X1	T50.2X2	T50.2X3	T50.2X4	T50.2X5	T50.2X6
EPN	T60.0X1	T60.0X2	T60.0X3	T60.0X4	—	—
EPO	T45.8X1	T45.8X2	T45.8X3	T45.8X4	T45.8X5	T45.8X6
Epoetin alpha	T45.8X1	T45.8X2	T45.8X3	T45.8X4	T45.8X5	T45.8X6
Epomediol	T50.991	T50.992	T50.993	T50.994	T50.995	T50.996
Epoprostenol	T45.521	T45.522	T45.523	T45.524	T45.525	T45.526
Epoxy resin	T65.891	T65.892	T65.893	T65.894	—	—
Eprazinone	T48.4X1	T48.4X2	T48.4X3	T48.4X4	T48.4X5	T48.4X6
Epsilon amino-caproic acid	T45.621	T45.622	T45.623	T45.624	T45.625	T45.626
Epsom salt	T47.3X1	T47.3X2	T47.3X3	T47.3X4	T47.3X5	T47.3X6
Eptazocine	T40.491	T40.492	T40.493	T40.494	T40.495	T40.496
Equanil	T43.591	T43.592	T43.593	T43.594	T43.595	T43.596
Equisetum	T62.2X1	T62.2X2	T62.2X3	T62.2X4	—	—
diuretic	T50.2X1	T50.2X2	T50.2X3	T50.2X4	T50.2X5	T50.2X6

◀ New ◀ Revised ~~deleted~~ Deleted

Substance	External Cause (T-Code)					
	Poisoning, Accidental (Unintentional)	Poisoning, Intentional Self-Harm	Poisoning, Assault	Poisoning, Undetermined	Adverse Effect	Underdosing
Ergobasine	T48.0X1	T48.0X2	T48.0X3	T48.0X4	T48.0X5	T48.0X6
Ergocalciferol	T45.2X1	T45.2X2	T45.2X3	T45.2X4	T45.2X5	T45.2X6
Ergoloid mesylates	T46.7X1	T46.7X2	T46.7X3	T46.7X4	T46.7X5	T46.7X6
Ergometrine	T48.0X1	T48.0X2	T48.0X3	T48.0X4	T48.0X5	T48.0X6
Ergonovine	T48.0X1	T48.0X2	T48.0X3	T48.0X4	T48.0X5	T48.0X6
Ergot NEC	T64.81	T64.82	T64.83	T64.84	—	—
derivative	T48.0X1	T48.0X2	T48.0X3	T48.0X4	T48.0X5	T48.0X6
medicinal (alkaloids)	T48.0X1	T48.0X2	T48.0X3	T48.0X4	T48.0X5	T48.0X6
prepared	T48.0X1	T48.0X2	T48.0X3	T48.0X4	T48.0X5	T48.0X6
Ergotamine	T46.5X1	T46.5X2	T46.5X3	T46.5X4	T46.5X5	T46.5X6
Ergotocine	T48.0X1	T48.0X2	T48.0X3	T48.0X4	T48.0X5	T48.0X6
Ergotrate	T48.0X1	T48.0X2	T48.0X3	T48.0X4	T48.0X5	T48.0X6
Eritrityl tetranitrate	T46.3X1	T46.3X2	T46.3X3	T46.3X4	T46.3X5	T46.3X6
Erythrityl tetranitrate	T46.3X1	T46.3X2	T46.3X3	T46.3X4	T46.3X5	T46.3X6
Erythrol tetranitrate	T46.3X1	T46.3X2	T46.3X3	T46.3X4	T46.3X5	T46.3X6
Erythromycin (salts)	T36.3X1	T36.3X2	T36.3X3	T36.3X4	T36.3X5	T36.3X6
ophthalmic preparation	T49.5X1	T49.5X2	T49.5X3	T49.5X4	T49.5X5	T49.5X6
topical NEC	T49.0X1	T49.0X2	T49.0X3	T49.0X4	T49.0X5	T49.0X6
Erythropoietin	T45.8X1	T45.8X2	T45.8X3	T45.8X4	T45.8X5	T45.8X6
human	T45.8X1	T45.8X2	T45.8X3	T45.8X4	T45.8X5	T45.8X6
Escin	T46.991	T46.992	T46.993	T46.994	T46.995	T46.996
Esculin	T45.2X1	T45.2X2	T45.2X3	T45.2X4	T45.2X5	T45.2X6
Esculoside	T45.2X1	T45.2X2	T45.2X3	T45.2X4	T45.2X5	T45.2X6
ESDT (ether-soluble tar distillate)	T49.1X1	T49.1X2	T49.1X3	T49.1X4	T49.1X5	T49.1X6
Eserine	T49.5X1	T49.5X2	T49.5X3	T49.5X4	T49.5X5	T49.5X6
Esflurbiprofen	T39.311	T39.312	T39.313	T39.314	T39.315	T39.316
Eskabarb	T42.3X1	T42.3X2	T42.3X3	T42.3X4	T42.3X5	T42.3X6
Eskalith	T43.8X1	T43.8X2	T43.8X3	T43.8X4	T43.8X5	T43.8X6
Esmolol	T44.7X1	T44.7X2	T44.7X3	T44.7X4	T44.7X5	T44.7X6
Estanozolol	T38.7X1	T38.7X2	T38.7X3	T38.7X4	T38.7X5	T38.7X6
Estazolam	T42.4X1	T42.4X2	T42.4X3	T42.4X4	T42.4X5	T42.4X6
Estradiol	T38.5X1	T38.5X2	T38.5X3	T38.5X4	T38.5X5	T38.5X6
with testosterone	T38.7X1	T38.7X2	T38.7X3	T38.7X4	T38.7X5	T38.7X6
benzoate	T38.5X1	T38.5X2	T38.5X3	T38.5X4	T38.5X5	T38.5X6
Estramustine	T45.1X1	T45.1X2	T45.1X3	T45.1X4	T45.1X5	T45.1X6
Estriol	T38.5X1	T38.5X2	T38.5X3	T38.5X4	T38.5X5	T38.5X6
Estrogen	T38.5X1	T38.5X2	T38.5X3	T38.5X4	T38.5X5	T38.5X6
with progesterone	T38.5X1	T38.5X2	T38.5X3	T38.5X4	T38.5X5	T38.5X6
conjugated	T38.5X1	T38.5X2	T38.5X3	T38.5X4	T38.5X5	T38.5X6
Estrone	T38.5X1	T38.5X2	T38.5X3	T38.5X4	T38.5X5	T38.5X6
Estropipate	T38.5X1	T38.5X2	T38.5X3	T38.5X4	T38.5X5	T38.5X6

Substance	External Cause (T-Code)					
	Poisoning, Accidental (Unintentional)	Poisoning, Intentional Self-Harm	Poisoning, Assault	Poisoning, Undetermined	Adverse Effect	Underdosing
Etacrynate sodium	T50.1X1	T50.1X2	T50.1X3	T50.1X4	T50.1X5	T50.1X6
Etacrynic acid	T50.1X1	T50.1X2	T50.1X3	T50.1X4	T50.1X5	T50.1X6
Etafedrine	T48.6X1	T48.6X2	T48.6X3	T48.6X4	T48.6X5	T48.6X6
Etafenone	T46.3X1	T46.3X2	T46.3X3	T46.3X4	T46.3X5	T46.3X6
Etambutol	T37.1X1	T37.1X2	T37.1X3	T37.1X4	T37.1X5	T37.1X6
Etamiphyllin	T48.6X1	T48.6X2	T48.6X3	T48.6X4	T48.6X5	T48.6X6
Etamivan	T50.7X1	T50.7X2	T50.7X3	T50.7X4	T50.7X5	T50.7X6
Etamsylate	T45.7X1	T45.7X2	T45.7X3	T45.7X4	T45.7X5	T45.7X6
Etebenecid	T50.4X1	T50.4X2	T50.4X3	T50.4X4	T50.4X5	T50.4X6
Ethacridine	T49.0X1	T49.0X2	T49.0X3	T49.0X4	T49.0X5	T49.0X6
Ethacrynic acid	T50.1X1	T50.1X2	T50.1X3	T50.1X4	T50.1X5	T50.1X6
Ethadione	T42.2X1	T42.2X2	T42.2X3	T42.2X4	T42.2X5	T42.2X6
Ethambutol	T37.1X1	T37.1X2	T37.1X3	T37.1X4	T37.1X5	T37.1X6
Ethamide	T50.2X1	T50.2X2	T50.2X3	T50.2X4	T50.2X5	T50.2X6
Ethamivan	T50.7X1	T50.7X2	T50.7X3	T50.7X4	T50.7X5	T50.7X6
Ethamsylate	T45.7X1	T45.7X2	T45.7X3	T45.7X4	T45.7X5	T45.7X6
Ethanol	T51.0X1	T51.0X2	T51.0X3	T51.0X4	—	—
beverage	T51.0X1	T51.0X2	T51.0X3	T51.0X4	—	—
Ethanolamine oleate	T46.8X1	T46.8X2	T46.8X3	T46.8X4	T46.8X5	T46.8X6
Ethaverine	T44.3X1	T44.3X2	T44.3X3	T44.3X4	T44.3X5	T44.3X6
Ethchlorvynol	T42.6X1	T42.6X2	T42.6X3	T42.6X4	T42.6X5	T42.6X6
Ethebenecid	T50.4X1	T50.4X2	T50.4X3	T50.4X4	T50.4X5	T50.4X6
Ether (vapor)	T41.0X1	T41.0X2	T41.0X3	T41.0X4	T41.0X5	T41.0X6
anesthetic	T41.0X1	T41.0X2	T41.0X3	T41.0X4	T41.0X5	T41.0X6
divinyl	T41.0X1	T41.0X2	T41.0X3	T41.0X4	T41.0X5	T41.0X6
ethyl (medicinal)	T41.0X1	T41.0X2	T41.0X3	T41.0X4	T41.0X5	T41.0X6
nonmedicinal	T52.8X1	T52.8X2	T52.8X3	T52.8X4	—	—
petroleum — see Ligroin						
solvent	T52.8X1	T52.8X2	T52.8X3	T52.8X4	—	—
Ethiazide	T50.2X1	T50.2X2	T50.2X3	T50.2X4	T50.2X5	T50.2X6
Ethidium chloride (vapor)	T59.891	T59.892	T59.893	T59.894	—	—
Ethinamate	T42.6X1	T42.6X2	T42.6X3	T42.6X4	T42.6X5	T42.6X6
Ethinylestradiol, ethinyloestradiol	T38.5X1	T38.5X2	T38.5X3	T38.5X4	T38.5X5	T38.5X6
with						
levonorgestrel	T38.4X1	T38.4X2	T38.4X3	T38.4X4	T38.4X5	T38.4X6
norethisterone	T38.4X1	T38.4X2	T38.4X3	T38.4X4	T38.4X5	T38.4X6
Ethiodized oil (131 I)	T50.8X1	T50.8X2	T50.8X3	T50.8X4	T50.8X5	T50.8X6
Ethion	T60.0X1	T60.0X2	T60.0X3	T60.0X4	—	—
Ethionamide	T37.1X1	T37.1X2	T37.1X3	T37.1X4	T37.1X5	T37.1X6
Ethioniamide	T37.1X1	T37.1X2	T37.1X3	T37.1X4	T37.1X5	T37.1X6
Ethisterone	T38.5X1	T38.5X2	T38.5X3	T38.5X4	T38.5X5	T38.5X6
Ethobral	T42.3X1	T42.3X2	T42.3X3	T42.3X4	T42.3X5	T42.3X6

Substance	External Cause (T-Code)					
	Poisoning, Accidental (Unintentional)	Poisoning, Intentional Self-Harm	Poisoning, Assault	Poisoning, Undetermined	Adverse Effect	Underdosing
Ethocaine (infiltration) (topical)	T41.3X1	T41.3X2	T41.3X3	T41.3X4	T41.3X5	T41.3X6
nerve block (peripheral) (plexus)	T41.3X1	T41.3X2	T41.3X3	T41.3X4	T41.3X5	T41.3X6
spinal	T41.3X1	T41.3X2	T41.3X3	T41.3X4	T41.3X5	T41.3X6
Ethoheptazine	T40.491	T40.492	T40.493	T40.494	T40.495	T40.496
Ethopropazine	T44.3X1	T44.3X2	T44.3X3	T44.3X4	T44.3X5	T44.3X6
Ethosuximide	T42.2X1	T42.2X2	T42.2X3	T42.2X4	T42.2X5	T42.2X6
Ethotoin	T42.0X1	T42.0X2	T42.0X3	T42.0X4	T42.0X5	T42.0X6
Ethoxazene	T37.91	T37.92	T37.93	T37.94	T37.95	T37.96
Ethoxazorutoside	T46.991	T46.992	T46.993	T46.994	T46.995	T46.996
2-Ethoxyethanol	T52.3X1	T52.3X2	T52.3X3	T52.3X4	—	—
Ethoxzolamide	T50.2X1	T50.2X2	T50.2X3	T50.2X4	T50.2X5	T50.2X6
Ethyl						
acetate	T52.8X1	T52.8X2	T52.8X3	T52.8X4	—	—
alcohol	T51.0X1	T51.0X2	T51.0X3	T51.0X4	—	—
beverage	T51.0X1	T51.0X2	T51.0X3	T51.0X4	—	—
aldehyde (vapor)	T59.891	T59.892	T59.893	T59.894	—	—
liquid	T52.8X1	T52.8X2	T52.8X3	T52.8X4	—	—
aminobenzoate	T41.3X1	T41.3X2	T41.3X3	T41.3X4	T41.3X5	T41.3X6
aminophenothiazine	T43.3X1	T43.3X2	T43.3X3	T43.3X4	T43.3X5	T43.3X6
benzoate	T52.8X1	T52.8X2	T52.8X3	T52.8X4	—	—
biscoumacetate	T45.511	T45.512	T45.513	T45.514	T45.515	T45.516
bromide (anesthetic)	T41.0X1	T41.0X2	T41.0X3	T41.0X4	T41.0X5	T41.0X6
carbamate	T45.1X1	T45.1X2	T45.1X3	T45.1X4	T45.1X5	T45.1X6
carbinol	T51.3X1	T51.3X2	T51.3X3	T51.3X4	—	—
carbonate	T52.8X1	T52.8X2	T52.8X3	T52.8X4	—	—
chaulmoograte	T37.1X1	T37.1X2	T37.1X3	T37.1X4	T37.1X5	T37.1X6
chloride (anesthetic)	T41.0X1	T41.0X2	T41.0X3	T41.0X4	T41.0X5	T41.0X6
anesthetic (local)	T41.3X1	T41.3X2	T41.3X3	T41.3X4	T41.3X5	T41.3X6
inhaled	T41.0X1	T41.0X2	T41.0X3	T41.0X4	T41.0X5	T41.0X6
local	T49.4X1	T49.4X2	T49.4X3	T49.4X4	T49.4X5	T49.4X6
solvent	T53.6X1	T53.6X2	T53.6X3	T53.6X4	—	—
dibunate	T48.3X1	T48.3X2	T48.3X3	T48.3X4	T48.3X5	T48.3X6
dichloroarsine (vapor)	T57.0X1	T57.0X2	T57.0X3	T57.0X4	—	—
estranol	T38.7X1	T38.7X2	T38.7X3	T38.7X4	T38.7X5	T38.7X6
ether — see also Ether	T52.8X1	T52.8X2	T52.8X3	T52.8X4	—	—
formate NEC (solvent)	T52.0X1	T52.0X2	T52.0X3	T52.0X4	—	—
fumarate	T49.4X1	T49.4X2	T49.4X3	T49.4X4	T49.4X5	T49.4X6
hydroxyisobutyrate NEC (solvent)	T52.8X1	T52.8X2	T52.8X3	T52.8X4	—	—
iodoacetate	T59.3X1	T59.3X2	T59.3X3	T59.3X4	—	—
lactate NEC (solvent)	T52.8X1	T52.8X2	T52.8X3	T52.8X4	—	—
loflazepate	T42.4X1	T42.4X2	T42.4X3	T42.4X4	T42.4X5	T42.4X6

Substance	External Cause (T-Code)					
	Poisoning, Accidental (Unintentional)	Poisoning, Intentional Self-Harm	Poisoning, Assault	Poisoning, Undetermined	Adverse Effect	Underdosing
Ethyl (Continued)						
mercuric chloride	T56.1X1	T56.1X2	T56.1X3	T56.1X4	—	—
methylcarbinol	T51.8X1	T51.8X2	T51.8X3	T51.8X4	—	—
morphine	T40.2X1	T40.2X2	T40.2X3	T40.2X4	T40.2X5	T40.2X6
noradrenaline	T48.6X1	T48.6X2	T48.6X3	T48.6X4	T48.6X5	T48.6X6
oxybutyrate NEC (solvent)	T52.8X1	T52.8X2	T52.8X3	T52.8X4	—	—
Ethylene (gas)	T59.891	T59.892	T59.893	T59.894	—	—
anesthetic (general)	T41.0X1	T41.0X2	T41.0X3	T41.0X4	T41.0X5	T41.0X6
chlorohydrin	T52.8X1	T52.8X2	T52.8X3	T52.8X4	—	—
vapor	T53.6X1	T53.6X2	T53.6X3	T53.6X4	—	—
dichloride	T52.8X1	T52.8X2	T52.8X3	T52.8X4	—	—
vapor	T53.6X1	T53.6X2	T53.6X3	T53.6X4	—	—
dinitrate	T52.3X1	T52.3X2	T52.3X3	T52.3X4	—	—
glycol(s)	T52.8X1	T52.8X2	T52.8X3	T52.8X4	—	—
dinitrate	T52.3X1	T52.3X2	T52.3X3	T52.3X4	—	—
monobutyl ether	T52.3X1	T52.3X2	T52.3X3	T52.3X4	—	—
imine	T54.1X1	T54.1X2	T54.1X3	T54.1X4	—	—
oxide (fumigant) (nonmedicinal)	T59.891	T59.892	T59.893	T59.894	—	—
medicinal	T49.0X1	T49.0X2	T49.0X3	T49.0X4	T49.0X5	T49.0X6
Ethylenediamine theophylline	T48.6X1	T48.6X2	T48.6X3	T48.6X4	T48.6X5	T48.6X6
Ethylenediaminetetra-acetic acid	T50.6X1	T50.6X2	T50.6X3	T50.6X4	T50.6X5	T50.6X6
Ethylenedinitrilotetra-acetate	T50.6X1	T50.6X2	T50.6X3	T50.6X4	T50.6X5	T50.6X6
Ethylestrenol	T38.7X1	T38.7X2	T38.7X3	T38.7X4	T38.7X5	T38.7X6
Ethylhydroxycellulose	T47.4X1	T47.4X2	T47.4X3	T47.4X4	T47.4X5	T47.4X6
Ethylidene						
chloride NEC	T53.6X1	T53.6X2	T53.6X3	T53.6X4	—	—
diacetate	T60.3X1	T60.3X2	T60.3X3	T60.3X4	—	—
dicoumarin	T45.511	T45.512	T45.513	T45.514	T45.515	T45.516
dicoumarol	T45.511	T45.512	T45.513	T45.514	T45.515	T45.516
diethyl ether	T52.0X1	T52.0X2	T52.0X3	T52.0X4	—	—
Ethylmorphine	T40.2X1	T40.2X2	T40.2X3	T40.2X4	T40.2X5	T40.2X6
Ethylnorepinephrine	T48.6X1	T48.6X2	T48.6X3	T48.6X4	T48.6X5	T48.6X6
Ethylparachlorophen-oxyisobutyrate	T46.6X1	T46.6X2	T46.6X3	T46.6X4	T46.6X5	T46.6X6
Ethynodiol	T38.4X1	T38.4X2	T38.4X3	T38.4X4	T38.4X5	T38.4X6
with mestranol diacetate	T38.4X1	T38.4X2	T38.4X3	T38.4X4	T38.4X5	T38.4X6
Etidocaine	T41.3X1	T41.3X2	T41.3X3	T41.3X4	T41.3X5	T41.3X6
infiltration (subcutaneous)	T41.3X1	T41.3X2	T41.3X3	T41.3X4	T41.3X5	T41.3X6
nerve (peripheral) (plexus)	T41.3X1	T41.3X2	T41.3X3	T41.3X4	T41.3X5	T41.3X6
Etidronate	T50.991	T50.992	T50.993	T50.994	T50.995	T50.996
Etidronic acid (disodium salt)	T50.991	T50.992	T50.993	T50.994	T50.995	T50.996
Etifoxine	T42.6X1	T42.6X2	T42.6X3	T42.6X4	T42.6X5	T42.6X6

◀ New ◀ Revised deleted Deleted

Substance	Poisoning, Accidental (Unintentional)	Poisoning, Intentional Self-Harm	Poisoning, Assault	Poisoning, Undetermined	Adverse Effect	Underdosing
Etilefrine	T44.4X1	T44.4X2	T44.4X3	T44.4X4	T44.4X5	T44.4X6
Etilfen	T42.3X1	T42.3X2	T42.3X3	T42.3X4	T42.3X5	T42.3X6
Etinodiol	T38.4X1	T38.4X2	T38.4X3	T38.4X4	T38.4X5	T38.4X6
Etiroxate	T46.6X1	T46.6X2	T46.6X3	T46.6X4	T46.6X5	T46.6X6
Etizolam	T42.4X1	T42.4X2	T42.4X3	T42.4X4	T42.4X5	T42.4X6
Etodolac	T39.391	T39.392	T39.393	T39.394	T39.395	T39.396
Etofamide	T37.3X1	T37.3X2	T37.3X3	T37.3X4	T37.3X5	T37.3X6
Etofibrate	T46.6X1	T46.6X2	T46.6X3	T46.6X4	T46.6X5	T46.6X6
Etofylline	T46.7X1	T46.7X2	T46.7X3	T46.7X4	T46.7X5	T46.7X6
clofibrate	T46.6X1	T46.6X2	T46.6X3	T46.6X4	T46.6X5	T46.6X6
Etoglucid	T45.1X1	T45.1X2	T45.1X3	T45.1X4	T45.1X5	T45.1X6
Etomidate	T41.1X1	T41.1X2	T41.1X3	T41.1X4	T41.1X5	T41.1X6
Etomide	T39.8X1	T39.8X2	T39.8X3	T39.8X4	T39.8X5	T39.8X6
Etomidoline	T44.3X1	T44.3X2	T44.3X3	T44.3X4	T44.3X5	T44.3X6
Etoposide	T45.1X1	T45.1X2	T45.1X3	T45.1X4	T45.1X5	T45.1X6
Etorphine	T40.2X1	T40.2X2	T40.2X3	T40.2X4	T40.2X5	T40.2X6
Etoval	T42.3X1	T42.3X2	T42.3X3	T42.3X4	T42.3X5	T42.3X6
Etozolin	T50.1X1	T50.1X2	T50.1X3	T50.1X4	T50.1X5	T50.1X6
Etretinate	T50.991	T50.992	T50.993	T50.994	T50.995	T50.996
Etryptamine	T43.691	T43.692	T43.693	T43.694	T43.695	T43.696
Etybenzatropine	T44.3X1	T44.3X2	T44.3X3	T44.3X4	T44.3X5	T44.3X6
Etynodiol	T38.4X1	T38.4X2	T38.4X3	T38.4X4	T38.4X5	T38.4X6
Eucaine	T41.3X1	T41.3X2	T41.3X3	T41.3X4	T41.3X5	T41.3X6
Eucalyptus oil	T49.7X1	T49.7X2	T49.7X3	T49.7X4	T49.7X5	T49.7X6
Eucatropine	T49.5X1	T49.5X2	T49.5X3	T49.5X4	T49.5X5	T49.5X6
Eucodal	T40.2X1	T40.2X2	T40.2X3	T40.2X4	T40.2X5	T40.2X6
Euneryl	T42.3X1	T42.3X2	T42.3X3	T42.3X4	T42.3X5	T42.3X6
Euphthalmine	T44.3X1	T44.3X2	T44.3X3	T44.3X4	T44.3X5	T44.3X6
Eurax	T49.0X1	T49.0X2	T49.0X3	T49.0X4	T49.0X5	T49.0X6
Euresol	T49.4X1	T49.4X2	T49.4X3	T49.4X4	T49.4X5	T49.4X6
Euthroid	T38.1X1	T38.1X2	T38.1X3	T38.1X4	T38.1X5	T38.1X6
Evans blue	T50.8X1	T50.8X2	T50.8X3	T50.8X4	T50.8X5	T50.8X6
Evipal	T42.3X1	T42.3X2	T42.3X3	T42.3X4	T42.3X5	T42.3X6
sodium	T41.1X1	T41.1X2	T41.1X3	T41.1X4	T41.1X5	T41.1X6
Evipan	T42.3X1	T42.3X2	T42.3X3	T42.3X4	T42.3X5	T42.3X6
sodium	T41.1X1	T41.1X2	T41.1X3	T41.1X4	T41.1X5	T41.1X6
Exalamide	T49.0X1	T49.0X2	T49.0X3	T49.0X4	T49.0X5	T49.0X6
Exalgin	T39.1X1	T39.1X2	T39.1X3	T39.1X4	T39.1X5	T39.1X6
Excipients, pharmaceutical	T50.901	T50.902	T50.903	T50.904	T50.905	T50.906
Exhaust gas (engine) (motor vehicle)	T58.01	T58.02	T58.03	T58.04	—	—
Ex-Lax (phenolphthalein)	T47.2X1	T47.2X2	T47.2X3	T47.2X4	T47.2X5	T47.2X6
Expectorant NEC	T48.4X1	T48.4X2	T48.4X3	T48.4X4	T48.4X5	T48.4X6

Substance	Poisoning, Accidental (Unintentional)	Poisoning, Intentional Self-Harm	Poisoning, Assault	Poisoning, Undetermined	Adverse Effect	Underdosing
Extended insulin zinc suspension	T38.3X1	T38.3X2	T38.3X3	T38.3X4	T38.3X5	T38.3X6
External medications (skin) (mucous membrane)	T49.91	T49.92	T49.93	T49.94	T49.95	T49.96
dental agent	T49.7X1	T49.7X2	T49.7X3	T49.7X4	T49.7X5	T49.7X6
ENT agent	T49.6X1	T49.6X2	T49.6X3	T49.6X4	T49.6X5	T49.6X6
ophthalmic preparation	T49.5X1	T49.5X2	T49.5X3	T49.5X4	T49.5X5	T49.5X6
specified NEC	T49.8X1	T49.8X2	T49.8X3	T49.8X4	T49.8X5	T49.8X6
Extrapyramidal antagonist NEC	T44.3X1	T44.3X2	T44.3X3	T44.3X4	T44.3X5	T44.3X6
Eye agents (anti-infective)	T49.5X1	T49.5X2	T49.5X3	T49.5X4	T49.5X5	T49.5X6
Eye drug NEC	T49.5X1	T49.5X2	T49.5X3	T49.5X4	T49.5X5	T49.5X6
F						
FAC (fluorouracil + doxorubicin + cyclophosphamide)	T45.1X1	T45.1X2	T45.1X3	T45.1X4	T45.1X5	T45.1X6
Factor						
I (fibrinogen)	T45.8X1	T45.8X2	T45.8X3	T45.8X4	T45.8X5	T45.8X6
III (thromboplastin)	T45.8X1	T45.8X2	T45.8X3	T45.8X4	T45.8X5	T45.8X6
VIII (antihemophilic Factor) (Concentrate)	T45.8X1	T45.8X2	T45.8X3	T45.8X4	T45.8X5	T45.8X6
IX complex	T45.7X1	T45.7X2	T45.7X3	T45.7X4	T45.7X5	T45.7X6
human	T45.8X1	T45.8X2	T45.8X3	T45.8X4	T45.8X5	T45.8X6
Famotidine	T47.0X1	T47.0X2	T47.0X3	T47.0X4	T47.0X5	T47.0X6
Fat suspension, intravenous	T50.991	T50.992	T50.993	T50.994	T50.995	T50.996
Fazadinium bromide	T48.1X1	T48.1X2	T48.1X3	T48.1X4	T48.1X5	T48.1X6
Febarbamate	T42.3X1	T42.3X2	T42.3X3	T42.3X4	T42.3X5	T42.3X6
Fecal softener	T47.4X1	T47.4X2	T47.4X3	T47.4X4	T47.4X5	T47.4X6
Fedrilate	T48.3X1	T48.3X2	T48.3X3	T48.3X4	T48.3X5	T48.3X6
Felodipine	T46.1X1	T46.1X2	T46.1X3	T46.1X4	T46.1X5	T46.1X6
Felypressin	T38.891	T38.892	T38.893	T38.894	T38.895	T38.896
Femoxetine	T43.221	T43.222	T43.223	T43.224	T43.225	T43.226
Fenalcomine	T46.3X1	T46.3X2	T46.3X3	T46.3X4	T46.3X5	T46.3X6
Fenamisal	T37.1X1	T37.1X2	T37.1X3	T37.1X4	T37.1X5	T37.1X6
Fenazone	T39.2X1	T39.2X2	T39.2X3	T39.2X4	T39.2X5	T39.2X6
Fenbendazole	T37.4X1	T37.4X2	T37.4X3	T37.4X4	T37.4X5	T37.4X6
Fenbutrazate	T50.5X1	T50.5X2	T50.5X3	T50.5X4	T50.5X5	T50.5X6
Fencamfamine	T43.691	T43.692	T43.693	T43.694	T43.695	T43.696
Fendiline	T46.1X1	T46.1X2	T46.1X3	T46.1X4	T46.1X5	T46.1X6
Fenetylline	T43.691	T43.692	T43.693	T43.694	T43.695	T43.696
Fenflumizole	T39.391	T39.392	T39.393	T39.394	T39.395	T39.396
Fenfluramine	T50.5X1	T50.5X2	T50.5X3	T50.5X4	T50.5X5	T50.5X6
Fenobarbital	T42.3X1	T42.3X2	T42.3X3	T42.3X4	T42.3X5	T42.3X6
Fenofibrate	T46.6X1	T46.6X2	T46.6X3	T46.6X4	T46.6X5	T46.6X6
Fenoprofen	T39.311	T39.312	T39.313	T39.314	T39.315	T39.316
Fenoterol	T48.6X1	T48.6X2	T48.6X3	T48.6X4	T48.6X5	T48.6X6

◀ New   ◀ Revised   ~~deleted~~ Deleted

Substance	Poisoning, Accidental (Unintentional)	Poisoning, Intentional Self-Harm	Poisoning, Assault	Poisoning, Undetermined	Adverse Effect	Underdosing
Fenoverine	T44.3X1	T44.3X2	T44.3X3	T44.3X4	T44.3X5	T44.3X6
Fenoxazoline	T48.5X1	T48.5X2	T48.5X3	T48.5X4	T48.5X5	T48.5X6
Fenproporex	T50.5X1	T50.5X2	T50.5X3	T50.5X4	T50.5X5	T50.5X6
Fenquizone	T50.2X1	T50.2X2	T50.2X3	T50.2X4	T50.2X5	T50.2X6
Fentanyl (analogs)	T40.411	T40.412	T40.413	T40.414	T40.415	T40.416
Fentazin	T43.3X1	T43.3X2	T43.3X3	T43.3X4	T43.3X5	T43.3X6
Fenthion	T60.0X1	T60.0X2	T60.0X3	T60.0X4	—	—
Fenticlor	T49.0X1	T49.0X2	T49.0X3	T49.0X4	T49.0X5	T49.0X6
Fenylbutazone	T39.2X1	T39.2X2	T39.2X3	T39.2X4	T39.2X5	T39.2X6
Feprazone	T39.2X1	T39.2X2	T39.2X3	T39.2X4	T39.2X5	T39.2X6
Fer de lance (bite) (venom)	T63.061	T63.062	T63.063	T63.064	—	—
Ferric — see also Iron						
chloride	T45.4X1	T45.4X2	T45.4X3	T45.4X4	T45.4X5	T45.4X6
citrate	T45.4X1	T45.4X2	T45.4X3	T45.4X4	T45.4X5	T45.4X6
hydroxide						
colloidal	T45.4X1	T45.4X2	T45.4X3	T45.4X4	T45.4X5	T45.4X6
polymaltose	T45.4X1	T45.4X2	T45.4X3	T45.4X4	T45.4X5	T45.4X6
pyrophosphate	T45.4X1	T45.4X2	T45.4X3	T45.4X4	T45.4X5	T45.4X6
Ferritin	T45.4X1	T45.4X2	T45.4X3	T45.4X4	T45.4X5	T45.4X6
Ferrocholinate	T45.4X1	T45.4X2	T45.4X3	T45.4X4	T45.4X5	T45.4X6
Ferrodextrane	T45.4X1	T45.4X2	T45.4X3	T45.4X4	T45.4X5	T45.4X6
Ferropolimaler	T45.4X1	T45.4X2	T45.4X3	T45.4X4	T45.4X5	T45.4X6
Ferrous — see also Iron						
phosphate	T45.4X1	T45.4X2	T45.4X3	T45.4X4	T45.4X5	T45.4X6
salt	T45.4X1	T45.4X2	T45.4X3	T45.4X4	T45.4X5	T45.4X6
with folic acid	T45.4X1	T45.4X2	T45.4X3	T45.4X4	T45.4X5	T45.4X6
Ferrous fumarate, gluconate, lactate, salt NEC, sulfate (medicinal)	T45.4X1	T45.4X2	T45.4X3	T45.4X4	T45.4X5	T45.4X6
Ferrovanadium (fumes)	T59.891	T59.892	T59.893	T59.894	—	—
Ferrum — see Iron						
Fertilizers NEC	T65.891	T65.892	T65.893	T65.894	—	—
with herbicide mixture	T60.3X1	T60.3X2	T60.3X3	T60.3X4	—	—
Fetoxilate	T47.6X1	T47.6X2	T47.6X3	T47.6X4	T47.6X5	T47.6X6
Fiber, dietary	T47.4X1	T47.4X2	T47.4X3	T47.4X4	T47.4X5	T47.4X6
Fibrinogen (human)	T45.8X1	T45.8X2	T45.8X3	T45.8X4	T45.8X5	T45.8X6
Fibrinolysin (human)	T45.691	T45.692	T45.693	T45.694	T45.695	T45.696
Fibrinolysis						
affecting drug	T45.601	T45.602	T45.603	T45.604	T45.605	T45.606
inhibitor NEC	T45.621	T45.622	T45.623	T45.624	T45.625	T45.626
Fibrinolytic drug	T45.611	T45.612	T45.613	T45.614	T45.615	T45.616
Filix mas	T37.4X1	T37.4X2	T37.4X3	T37.4X4	T37.4X5	T37.4X6
Filtering cream	T49.3X1	T49.3X2	T49.3X3	T49.3X4	T49.3X5	T49.3X6

Substance	Poisoning, Accidental (Unintentional)	Poisoning, Intentional Self-Harm	Poisoning, Assault	Poisoning, Undetermined	Adverse Effect	Underdosing
Fiorinal	T39.011	T39.012	T39.013	T39.014	T39.015	T39.016
Firedamp	T59.891	T59.892	T59.893	T59.894	—	—
Fish, noxious, nonbacterial	T61.91	T61.92	T61.93	T61.94	—	—
ciguatera	T61.01	T61.02	T61.03	T61.04	—	—
scombroid	T61.11	T61.12	T61.13	T61.14	—	—
shell	T61.781	T61.782	T61.783	T61.784	—	—
specified NEC	T61.771	T61.772	T61.773	T61.774	—	—
Flagyl	T37.3X1	T37.3X2	T37.3X3	T37.3X4	T37.3X5	T37.3X6
Flavine adenine dinucleotide	T45.2X1	T45.2X2	T45.2X3	T45.2X4	T45.2X5	T45.2X6
Flavodic acid	T46.991	T46.992	T46.993	T46.994	T46.995	T46.996
Flavoxate	T44.3X1	T44.3X2	T44.3X3	T44.3X4	T44.3X5	T44.3X6
Flaxedil	T48.1X1	T48.1X2	T48.1X3	T48.1X4	T48.1X5	T48.1X6
Flaxseed (medicinal)	T49.3X1	T49.3X2	T49.3X3	T49.3X4	T49.3X5	T49.3X6
Flecainide	T46.2X1	T46.2X2	T46.2X3	T46.2X4	T46.2X5	T46.2X6
Fleroxacin	T36.8X1	T36.8X2	T36.8X3	T36.8X4	T36.8X5	T36.8X6
Floctafenine	T39.8X1	T39.8X2	T39.8X3	T39.8X4	T39.8X5	T39.8X6
Flomax	T44.6X1	T44.6X2	T44.6X3	T44.6X4	T44.6X5	T44.6X6
Flomoxef	T36.1X1	T36.1X2	T36.1X3	T36.1X4	T36.1X5	T36.1X6
Flopropione	T44.3X1	T44.3X2	T44.3X3	T44.3X4	T44.3X5	T44.3X6
Florantyrone	T47.5X1	T47.5X2	T47.5X3	T47.5X4	T47.5X5	T47.5X6
Floraquin	T37.8X1	T37.8X2	T37.8X3	T37.8X4	T37.8X5	T37.8X6
Florinef	T38.0X1	T38.0X2	T38.0X3	T38.0X4	T38.0X5	T38.0X6
ENT agent	T49.6X1	T49.6X2	T49.6X3	T49.6X4	T49.6X5	T49.6X6
ophthalmic preparation	T49.5X1	T49.5X2	T49.5X3	T49.5X4	T49.5X5	T49.5X6
topical NEC	T49.0X1	T49.0X2	T49.0X3	T49.0X4	T49.0X5	T49.0X6
Flowers of sulfur	T49.4X1	T49.4X2	T49.4X3	T49.4X4	T49.4X5	T49.4X6
Floxuridine	T45.1X1	T45.1X2	T45.1X3	T45.1X4	T45.1X5	T45.1X6
Fluanisone	T43.4X1	T43.4X2	T43.4X3	T43.4X4	T43.4X5	T43.4X6
Flubendazole	T37.4X1	T37.4X2	T37.4X3	T37.4X4	T37.4X5	T37.4X6
Fluclorolone acetonide	T49.0X1	T49.0X2	T49.0X3	T49.0X4	T49.0X5	T49.0X6
Flucloxacillin	T36.0X1	T36.0X2	T36.0X3	T36.0X4	T36.0X5	T36.0X6
Fluconazole	T37.8X1	T37.8X2	T37.8X3	T37.8X4	T37.8X5	T37.8X6
Flucytosine	T37.8X1	T37.8X2	T37.8X3	T37.8X4	T37.8X5	T37.8X6
Fludeoxyglucose (18F)	T50.8X1	T50.8X2	T50.8X3	T50.8X4	T50.8X5	T50.8X6
Fludiazepam	T42.4X1	T42.4X2	T42.4X3	T42.4X4	T42.4X5	T42.4X6
Fludrocortisone	T50.0X1	T50.0X2	T50.0X3	T50.0X4	T50.0X5	T50.0X6
ENT agent	T49.6X1	T49.6X2	T49.6X3	T49.6X4	T49.6X5	T49.6X6
ophthalmic preparation	T49.5X1	T49.5X2	T49.5X3	T49.5X4	T49.5X5	T49.5X6
topical NEC	T49.0X1	T49.0X2	T49.0X3	T49.0X4	T49.0X5	T49.0X6
Fludroxycortide	T49.0X1	T49.0X2	T49.0X3	T49.0X4	T49.0X5	T49.0X6
Flufenamic acid	T39.391	T39.392	T39.393	T39.394	T39.395	T39.396
Fluindione	T45.511	T45.512	T45.513	T45.514	T45.515	T45.516

◀ New   ◀ Revised   ~~deleted~~ Deleted

Substance	Poisoning, Accidental (Unintentional)	Poisoning, Intentional Self-Harm	Poisoning, Assault	Poisoning, Undetermined	Adverse Effect	Underdosing
Flumequine	T37.8X1	T37.8X2	T37.8X3	T37.8X4	T37.8X5	T37.8X6
Flumethasone	T49.0X1	T49.0X2	T49.0X3	T49.0X4	T49.0X5	T49.0X6
Flumethiazide	T50.2X1	T50.2X2	T50.2X3	T50.2X4	T50.2X5	T50.2X6
Flumidin	T37.5X1	T37.5X2	T37.5X3	T37.5X4	T37.5X5	T37.5X6
Flunarizine	T46.7X1	T46.7X2	T46.7X3	T46.7X4	T46.7X5	T46.7X6
Flunidazole	T37.8X1	T37.8X2	T37.8X3	T37.8X4	T37.8X5	T37.8X6
Flunisolide	T48.6X1	T48.6X2	T48.6X3	T48.6X4	T48.6X5	T48.6X6
Flunitrazepam	T42.4X1	T42.4X2	T42.4X3	T42.4X4	T42.4X5	T42.4X6
Fluocinolone (acetonide)	T49.0X1	T49.0X2	T49.0X3	T49.0X4	T49.0X5	T49.0X6
Fluocinonide	T49.0X1	T49.0X2	T49.0X3	T49.0X4	T49.0X5	T49.0X6
Fluocortin (butyl)	T49.0X1	T49.0X2	T49.0X3	T49.0X4	T49.0X5	T49.0X6
Fluocortolone	T49.0X1	T49.0X2	T49.0X3	T49.0X4	T49.0X5	T49.0X6
Fluohydrocortisone	T38.0X1	T38.0X2	T38.0X3	T38.0X4	T38.0X5	T38.0X6
ENT agent	T49.6X1	T49.6X2	T49.6X3	T49.6X4	T49.6X5	T49.6X6
ophthalmic preparation	T49.5X1	T49.5X2	T49.5X3	T49.5X4	T49.5X5	T49.5X6
topical NEC	T49.0X1	T49.0X2	T49.0X3	T49.0X4	T49.0X5	T49.0X6
Fluonid	T49.0X1	T49.0X2	T49.0X3	T49.0X4	T49.0X5	T49.0X6
Fluopromazine	T43.3X1	T43.3X2	T43.3X3	T43.3X4	T43.3X5	T43.3X6
Fluoroacetate	T60.8X1	T60.8X2	T60.8X3	T60.8X4	—	—
Fluorescein	T50.8X1	T50.8X2	T50.8X3	T50.8X4	T50.8X5	T50.8X6
Fluorhydrocortisone	T50.0X1	T50.0X2	T50.0X3	T50.0X4	T50.0X5	T50.0X6
Fluoride (nonmedicinal) (pesticide) (sodium) NEC	T60.8X1	T60.8X2	T60.8X3	T60.8X4		
hydrogen — see Hydrofluoric acid						
medicinal NEC	T50.991	T50.992	T50.993	T50.994	T50.995	T50.996
dental use	T49.7X1	T49.7X2	T49.7X3	T49.7X4	T49.7X5	T49.7X6
not pesticide NEC	T54.91	T54.92	T54.93	T54.94	—	—
stannous	T49.7X1	T49.7X2	T49.7X3	T49.7X4	T49.7X5	T49.7X6
Fluorinated corticosteroids	T38.0X1	T38.0X2	T38.0X3	T38.0X4	T38.0X5	T38.0X6
Fluorine (gas)	T59.5X1	T59.5X2	T59.5X3	T59.5X4	—	—
salt — see Fluoride(s)						
Fluoristan	T49.7X1	T49.7X2	T49.7X3	T49.7X4	T49.7X5	T49.7X6
Fluormetholone	T49.0X1	T49.0X2	T49.0X3	T49.0X4	T49.0X5	T49.0X6
Fluoroacetate	T60.8X1	T60.8X2	T60.8X3	T60.8X4	—	—
Fluorocarbon monomer	T53.6X1	T53.6X2	T53.6X3	T53.6X4	—	—
Fluorocytosine	T37.8X1	T37.8X2	T37.8X3	T37.8X4	T37.8X5	T37.8X6
Fluorodeoxyuridine	T45.1X1	T45.1X2	T45.1X3	T45.1X4	T45.1X5	T45.1X6
Fluorometholone	T49.0X1	T49.0X2	T49.0X3	T49.0X4	T49.0X5	T49.0X6
ophthalmic preparation	T49.5X1	T49.5X2	T49.5X3	T49.5X4	T49.5X5	T49.5X6
Fluorophosphate insecticide	T60.0X1	T60.0X2	T60.0X3	T60.0X4	—	—
Fluorosol	T46.3X1	T46.3X2	T46.3X3	T46.3X4	T46.3X5	T46.3X6
Fluorouracil	T45.1X1	T45.1X2	T45.1X3	T45.1X4	T45.1X5	T45.1X6

Substance	Poisoning, Accidental (Unintentional)	Poisoning, Intentional Self-Harm	Poisoning, Assault	Poisoning, Undetermined	Adverse Effect	Underdosing
Fluorphenylalanine	T49.5X1	T49.5X2	T49.5X3	T49.5X4	T49.5X5	T49.5X6
Fluothane	T41.0X1	T41.0X2	T41.0X3	T41.0X4	T41.0X5	T41.0X6
Fluoxetine	T43.221	T43.222	T43.223	T43.224	T43.225	T43.226
Fluoxymesterone	T38.7X1	T38.7X2	T38.7X3	T38.7X4	T38.7X5	T38.7X6
Flupenthixol	T43.4X1	T43.4X2	T43.4X3	T43.4X4	T43.4X5	T43.4X6
Flupentixol	T43.4X1	T43.4X2	T43.4X3	T43.4X4	T43.4X5	T43.4X6
Fluphenazine	T43.3X1	T43.3X2	T43.3X3	T43.3X4	T43.3X5	T43.3X6
Fluprednidene	T49.0X1	T49.0X2	T49.0X3	T49.0X4	T49.0X5	T49.0X6
Fluprednisolone	T38.0X1	T38.0X2	T38.0X3	T38.0X4	T38.0X5	T38.0X6
Fluradoline	T39.8X1	T39.8X2	T39.8X3	T39.8X4	T39.8X5	T39.8X6
Flurandrenolide	T49.0X1	T49.0X2	T49.0X3	T49.0X4	T49.0X5	T49.0X6
Flurandrenolone	T49.0X1	T49.0X2	T49.0X3	T49.0X4	T49.0X5	T49.0X6
Flurazepam	T42.4X1	T42.4X2	T42.4X3	T42.4X4	T42.4X5	T42.4X6
Flurbiprofen	T39.311	T39.312	T39.313	T39.314	T39.315	T39.316
Flurobate	T49.0X1	T49.0X2	T49.0X3	T49.0X4	T49.0X5	T49.0X6
Flurotyl	T43.291	T43.292	T43.293	T43.294	T43.295	T43.296
Fluroxene	T41.0X1	T41.0X2	T41.0X3	T41.0X4	T41.0X5	T41.0X6
Fluspirilene	T43.591	T43.592	T43.593	T43.594	T43.595	T43.596
Flutamide	T38.6X1	T38.6X2	T38.6X3	T38.6X4	T38.6X5	T38.6X6
Flutazolam	T42.4X1	T42.4X2	T42.4X3	T42.4X4	T42.4X5	T42.4X6
Fluticasone propionate	T38.0X1	T38.0X2	T38.0X3	T38.0X4	T38.0X5	T38.0X6
Flutoprazepam	T42.4X1	T42.4X2	T42.4X3	T42.4X4	T42.4X5	T42.4X6
Flutropium bromide	T48.6X1	T48.6X2	T48.6X3	T48.6X4	T48.6X5	T48.6X6
Fluvoxamine	T43.221	T43.222	T43.223	T43.224	T43.225	T43.226
Folacin	T45.8X1	T45.8X2	T45.8X3	T45.8X4	T45.8X5	T45.8X6
Folic acid	T45.8X1	T45.8X2	T45.8X3	T45.8X4	T45.8X5	T45.8X6
with ferrous salt	T45.2X1	T45.2X2	T45.2X3	T45.2X4	T45.2X5	T45.2X6
antagonist	T45.1X1	T45.1X2	T45.1X3	T45.1X4	T45.1X5	T45.1X6
Folinic acid	T45.8X1	T45.8X2	T45.8X3	T45.8X4	T45.8X5	T45.8X6
Folium stramoniae	T48.6X1	T48.6X2	T48.6X3	T48.6X4	T48.6X5	T48.6X6
Follicle-stimulating hormone, human	T38.811	T38.812	T38.813	T38.814	T38.815	T38.816
Folpet	T60.3X1	T60.3X2	T60.3X3	T60.3X4	—	—
Fominoben	T48.3X1	T48.3X2	T48.3X3	T48.3X4	T48.3X5	T48.3X6
Food, foodstuffs, noxious, nonbacterial, NEC	T62.91	T62.92	T62.93	T62.94	—	—
berries	T62.1X1	T62.1X2	T62.1X3	T62.1X4	—	—
fish — see also Fish	T61.91	T61.92	T61.93	T61.94	—	—
mushrooms	T62.0X1	T62.0X2	T62.0X3	T62.0X4	—	—
plants	T62.2X1	T62.2X2	T62.2X3	T62.2X4	—	—
seafood	T61.91	T61.92	T61.93	T61.94	—	—
specified NEC	T61.8X1	T61.8X2	T61.8X3	T61.8X4	—	—
seeds	T62.2X1	T62.2X2	T62.2X3	T62.2X4	—	—

◀ New　◀ Revised　~~deleted~~ Deleted

TABLE OF DRUGS AND CHEMICALS

Substance	External Cause (T-Code)					
	Poisoning, Accidental (Unintentional)	Poisoning, Intentional Self-Harm	Poisoning, Assault	Poisoning, Undetermined	Adverse Effect	Underdosing
Food, foodstuffs, noxious, nonbacterial, NEC *(Continued)*						
shellfish	T61.781	T61.782	T61.783	T61.784	—	—
specified NEC	T62.8X1	T62.8X2	T62.8X3	T62.8X4	—	—
Fool's parsley	T62.2X1	T62.2X2	T62.2X3	T62.2X4	—	—
Formaldehyde (solution), gas or vapor	T59.2X1	T59.2X2	T59.2X3	T59.2X4	—	—
fungicide	T60.3X1	T60.3X2	T60.3X3	T60.3X4	—	—
Formalin	T59.2X1	T59.2X2	T59.2X3	T59.2X4	—	—
fungicide	T60.3X1	T60.3X2	T60.3X3	T60.3X4	—	—
vapor	T59.2X1	T59.2X2	T59.2X3	T59.2X4	—	—
Formic acid	T54.2X1	T54.2X2	T54.2X3	T54.2X4	—	—
vapor	T59.891	T59.892	T59.893	T59.894	—	—
Foscarnet sodium	T37.5X1	T37.5X2	T37.5X3	T37.5X4	T37.5X5	T37.5X6
Fosfestrol	T38.5X1	T38.5X2	T38.5X3	T38.5X4	T38.5X5	T38.5X6
Fosfomycin	T36.8X1	T36.8X2	T36.8X3	T36.8X4	T36.8X5	T36.8X6
Fosfonet sodium	T37.5X1	T37.5X2	T37.5X3	T37.5X4	T37.5X5	T37.5X6
Fosinopril	T46.4X1	T46.4X2	T46.4X3	T46.4X4	T46.4X5	T46.4X6
sodium	T46.4X1	T46.4X2	T46.4X3	T46.4X4	T46.4X5	T46.4X6
Fowler's solution	T57.0X1	T57.0X2	T57.0X3	T57.0X4	—	—
Foxglove	T62.2X1	T62.2X2	T62.2X3	T62.2X4	—	—
Framycetin	T36.5X1	T36.5X2	T36.5X3	T36.5X4	T36.5X5	T36.5X6
Frangula	T47.2X1	T47.2X2	T47.2X3	T47.2X4	T47.2X5	T47.2X6
extract	T47.2X1	T47.2X2	T47.2X3	T47.2X4	T47.2X5	T47.2X6
Frei antigen	T50.8X1	T50.8X2	T50.8X3	T50.8X4	T50.8X5	T50.8X6
Freon	T53.5X1	T53.5X2	T53.5X3	T53.5X4	—	—
Fructose	T50.3X1	T50.3X2	T50.3X3	T50.3X4	T50.3X5	T50.3X6
Frusemide	T50.1X1	T50.1X2	T50.1X3	T50.1X4	T50.1X5	T50.1X6
FSH	T38.811	T38.812	T38.813	T38.814	T38.815	T38.816
Ftorafur	T45.1X1	T45.1X2	T45.1X3	T45.1X4	T45.1X5	T45.1X6
Fuel						
automobile	T52.0X1	T52.0X2	T52.0X3	T52.0X4	—	—
exhaust gas, not in transit	T58.01	T58.02	T58.03	T58.04	—	—
vapor NEC	T52.0X1	T52.0X2	T52.0X3	T52.0X4	—	—
gas (domestic use) — *see also Carbon, monoxide, fuel, utility*	T59.891	T59.892	T59.893	T59.894	—	—
utility	T59.891	T59.892	T59.893	T59.894	—	—
in mobile container	T59.891	T59.892	T59.893	T59.894	—	—
incomplete combustion of — *see Carbon, monoxide, fuel, utility*						
piped (natural)	T59.891	T59.892	T59.893	T59.894	—	—
industrial, incomplete combustion	T58.8X1	T58.8X2	T58.8X3	T58.8X4	—	—

Substance	External Cause (T-Code)					
	Poisoning, Accidental (Unintentional)	Poisoning, Intentional Self-Harm	Poisoning, Assault	Poisoning, Undetermined	Adverse Effect	Underdosing
Fugillin	T36.8X1	T36.8X2	T36.8X3	T36.8X4	T36.8X5	T36.8X6
Fulminate of mercury	T56.1X1	T56.1X2	T56.1X3	T56.1X4	—	—
Fulvicin	T36.7X1	T36.7X2	T36.7X3	T36.7X4	T36.7X5	T36.7X6
Fumadil	T36.8X1	T36.8X2	T36.8X3	T36.8X4	T36.8X5	T36.8X6
Fumagillin	T36.8X1	T36.8X2	T36.8X3	T36.8X4	T36.8X5	T36.8X6
Fumaric acid	T49.4X1	T49.4X2	T49.4X3	T49.4X4	T49.4X5	T49.4X6
Fumes (from)	T59.91	T59.92	T59.93	T59.94	—	—
carbon monoxide — *see Carbon, monoxide*						
charcoal (domestic use) — *see Charcoal, fumes*						
chloroform — *see Chloroform*						
coke (in domestic stoves, fireplaces) — *see Coke, fumes*						
corrosive NEC	T54.91	T54.92	T54.93	T54.94	—	—
ether — *see Ether*						
freons	T53.5X1	T53.5X2	T53.5X3	T53.5X4	—	—
hydrocarbons	T59.891	T59.892	T59.893	T59.894	—	—
petroleum (liquefied)	T59.891	T59.892	T59.893	T59.894	—	—
distributed through pipes (pure or mixed with air)	T59.891	T59.892	T59.893	T59.894	—	—
lead — *see Lead*						
metal — *see Metals, or the specified metal*						
nitrogen dioxide	T59.0X1	T59.0X2	T59.0X3	T59.0X4	—	—
pesticides — *see Pesticides*						
petroleum (liquefied)	T59.891	T59.892	T59.893	T59.894	—	—
distributed through pipes (pure or mixed with air)	T59.891	T59.892	T59.893	T59.894	—	—
polyester	T59.891	T59.892	T59.893	T59.894	—	—
specified source NEC — *see also substance specified*	T59.891	T59.892	T59.893	T59.894	—	—
sulfur dioxide	T59.1X1	T59.1X2	T59.1X3	T59.1X4	—	—
Fumigant NEC	T60.91	T60.92	T60.93	T60.94	—	—
Fungi, noxious, used as food	T62.0X1	T62.0X2	T62.0X3	T62.0X4	—	—
Fungicide NEC (nonmedicinal)	T60.3X1	T60.3X2	T60.3X3	T60.3X4	—	—
Fungizone	T36.7X1	T36.7X2	T36.7X3	T36.7X4	T36.7X5	T36.7X6
topical	T49.0X1	T49.0X2	T49.0X3	T49.0X4	T49.0X5	T49.0X6
Furacin	T49.0X1	T49.0X2	T49.0X3	T49.0X4	T49.0X5	T49.0X6
Furadantin	T37.91	T37.92	T37.93	T37.94	T37.95	T37.96
Furazolidone	T37.8X1	T37.8X2	T37.8X3	T37.8X4	T37.8X5	T37.8X6
Furazolium chloride	T49.0X1	T49.0X2	T49.0X3	T49.0X4	T49.0X5	T49.0X6
Furfural	T52.8X1	T52.8X2	T52.8X3	T52.8X4	—	—

◀ New   ◀ Revised   ~~deleted~~ Deleted

Substance	Poisoning, Accidental (Unintentional)	Poisoning, Intentional Self-Harm	Poisoning, Assault	Poisoning, Undetermined	Adverse Effect	Underdosing
Furnace (coal burning) (domestic), gas from industrial	T58.2X1	T58.2X2	T58.2X3	T58.2X4	—	—
industrial	T58.8X1	T58.8X2	T58.8X3	T58.8X4	—	—
Furniture polish	T65.891	T65.892	T65.893	T65.894	—	—
Furosemide	T50.1X1	T50.1X2	T50.1X3	T50.1X4	T50.1X5	T50.1X6
Furoxone	T37.91	T37.92	T37.93	T37.94	T37.95	T37.96
Fursultiamine	T45.2X1	T45.2X2	T45.2X3	T45.2X4	T45.2X5	T45.2X6
Fusafungine	T36.8X1	T36.8X2	T36.8X3	T36.8X4	T36.8X5	T36.8X6
Fusel oil (any) (amyl) (butyl) (propyl), vapor	T51.3X1	T51.3X2	T51.3X3	T51.3X4	—	—
Fusidate (ethanolamine) (sodium)	T36.8X1	T36.8X2	T36.8X3	T36.8X4	T36.8X5	T36.8X6
Fusidic acid	T36.8X1	T36.8X2	T36.8X3	T36.8X4	T36.8X5	T36.8X6
Fytic acid, nonasodium	T50.6X1	T50.6X2	T50.6X3	T50.6X4	T50.6X5	T50.6X6
G						
GABA	T43.8X1	T43.8X2	T43.8X3	T43.8X4	T43.8X5	T43.8X6
Gadopentetic acid	T50.8X1	T50.8X2	T50.8X3	T50.8X4	T50.8X5	T50.8X6
Galactose	T50.3X1	T50.3X2	T50.3X3	T50.3X4	T50.3X5	T50.3X6
b-Galactosidase	T47.5X1	T47.5X2	T47.5X3	T47.5X4	T47.5X5	T47.5X6
Galantamine	T44.0X1	T44.0X2	T44.0X3	T44.0X4	T44.0X5	T44.0X6
Gallamine (triethiodide)	T48.1X1	T48.1X2	T48.1X3	T48.1X4	T48.1X5	T48.1X6
Gallium citrate	T50.991	T50.992	T50.993	T50.994	T50.995	T50.996
Gallopamil	T46.1X1	T46.1X2	T46.1X3	T46.1X4	T46.1X5	T46.1X6
Gamboge	T47.2X1	T47.2X2	T47.2X3	T47.2X4	T47.2X5	T47.2X6
Gamimune	T50.Z11	T50.Z12	T50.Z13	T50.Z14	T50.Z15	T50.Z16
Gamma-aminobutyric acid	T43.8X1	T43.8X2	T43.8X3	T43.8X4	T43.8X5	T43.8X6
Gamma-benzene hexachloride (medicinal)	T49.0X1	T49.0X2	T49.0X3	T49.0X4	T49.0X5	T49.0X6
nonmedicinal, vapor	T53.6X1	T53.6X2	T53.6X3	T53.6X4	—	—
Gamma-BHC (medicinal) — see also Gamma-benzene hexachloride	T49.0X1	T49.0X2	T49.0X3	T49.0X4	T49.0X5	T49.0X6
Gamma globulin	T50.Z11	T50.Z12	T50.Z13	T50.Z14	T50.Z15	T50.Z16
Gamulin	T50.Z11	T50.Z12	T50.Z13	T50.Z14	T50.Z15	T50.Z16
Ganciclovir (sodium)	T37.5X1	T37.5X2	T37.5X3	T37.5X4	T37.5X5	T37.5X6
Ganglionic blocking drug NEC	T44.2X1	T44.2X2	T44.2X3	T44.2X4	T44.2X5	T44.2X6
specified NEC	T44.2X1	T44.2X2	T44.2X3	T44.2X4	T44.2X5	T44.2X6
Ganja	T40.711	T40.712	T40.713	T40.714	T40.715	T40.716
Garamycin	T36.5X1	T36.5X2	T36.5X3	T36.5X4	T36.5X5	T36.5X6
ophthalmic preparation	T49.5X1	T49.5X2	T49.5X3	T49.5X4	T49.5X5	T49.5X6
topical NEC	T49.0X1	T49.0X2	T49.0X3	T49.0X4	T49.0X5	T49.0X6
Gardenal	T42.3X1	T42.3X2	T42.3X3	T42.3X4	T42.3X5	T42.3X6
Gardepanyl	T42.3X1	T42.3X2	T42.3X3	T42.3X4	T42.3X5	T42.3X6

Substance	Poisoning, Accidental (Unintentional)	Poisoning, Intentional Self-Harm	Poisoning, Assault	Poisoning, Undetermined	Adverse Effect	Underdosing
Gas NEC	T59.91	T59.92	T59.93	T59.94	—	—
acetylene	T59.891	T59.892	T59.893	T59.894	—	—
incomplete combustion of	T58.11	T58.12	T58.13	T58.14		
air contaminants, source or type not specified	T59.91	T59.92	T59.93	T59.94	—	—
anesthetic	T41.0X1	T41.0X2	T41.0X3	T41.0X4	T41.0X5	T41.0X6
blast furnace	T58.8X1	T58.8X2	T58.8X3	T58.8X4	—	—
butane — see Butane						
carbon monoxide — see Carbon, monoxide						
chlorine	T59.4X1	T59.4X2	T59.4X3	T59.4X4	—	—
coal	T58.2X1	T58.2X2	T58.2X3	T58.2X4	—	—
cyanide	T57.3X1	T57.3X2	T57.3X3	T57.3X4	—	—
dicyanogen	T65.0X1	T65.0X2	T65.0X3	T65.0X4	—	—
domestic — see Domestic gas	T57.91	T57.92	T57.93	T57.94	—	—
exhaust	T57.91	T57.92	T57.93	T57.94	—	—
from utility (for cooking, heating, or lighting) (after combustion) — see Carbon, monoxide, fuel, utility						
prior to combustion	T59.891	T59.892	T59.893	T59.894	—	—
from wood or coal-burning stove or fireplace	T57.91	T57.92	T57.93	T57.94	—	—
fuel (domestic use) (after combustion) — see also Carbon, monoxide, fuel	T57.91	T57.92	T57.93	T57.94	—	—
industrial use	T58.8X1	T58.8X2	T58.8X3	T58.8X4	—	—
prior to combustion	T59.891	T59.892	T59.893	T59.894	—	—
utility	T59.891	T59.892	T59.893	T59.894	—	—
in mobile container	T59.891	T59.892	T59.893	T59.894	—	—
incomplete combustion of — see Carbon, monoxide, fuel, utility						
piped (natural)	T59.891	T59.892	T59.893	T59.894	—	—
garage	T58.01	T58.02	T58.03	T58.04		
hydrocarbon NEC	T59.891	T59.892	T59.893	T59.894	—	—
incomplete combustion of — see Carbon, monoxide, fuel, utility						
liquefied — see Butane						
piped	T59.891	T59.892	T59.893	T59.894	—	—
hydrocyanic acid	T65.0X1	T65.0X2	T65.0X3	T65.0X4	—	—

TABLE OF DRUGS AND CHEMICALS

TABLE OF DRUGS AND CHEMICALS

Substance	Poisoning, Accidental (Unintentional)	Poisoning, Intentional Self-Harm	Poisoning, Assault	Poisoning, Undetermined	Adverse Effect	Underdosing
Gas NEC (Continued)						
illuminating (after combustion)	T58.11	T58.12	T58.13	T58.14	—	—
prior to combustion	T59.891	T59.892	T59.893	T59.894	—	—
incomplete combustion, any — see Carbon, monoxide						
kiln	T58.8X1	T58.8X2	T58.8X3	T58.8X4	—	—
lacrimogenic	T59.3X1	T59.3X2	T59.3X3	T59.3X4	—	—
liquefied petroleum — see Butane						
marsh	T59.891	T59.892	T59.893	T59.894	—	—
motor exhaust, not in transit	T58.01	T58.02	T58.03	T58.04	—	—
mustard, not in war	T59.891	T59.892	T59.893	T59.894	—	—
natural	T59.891	T59.892	T59.893	T59.894	—	—
nerve, not in war	T59.91	T59.92	T59.93	T59.94	—	—
oil	T52.0X1	T52.0X2	T52.0X3	T52.0X4	—	—
petroleum (liquefied) (distributed in mobile containers)	T59.891	T59.892	T59.893	T59.894	—	—
piped (pure or mixed with air)	T59.891	T59.892	T59.893	T59.894	—	—
piped (manufactured) (natural) NEC	T59.891	T59.892	T59.893	T59.894	—	—
producer	T58.8X1	T58.8X2	T58.8X3	T58.8X4	—	—
propane — see Propane						
refrigerant (chlorofluoro-carbon)	T53.5X1	T53.5X2	T53.5X3	T53.5X4	—	—
not chlorofluoro-carbon	T59.891	T59.892	T59.893	T59.894	—	—
sewer	T59.91	T59.92	T59.93	T59.94	—	—
specified source NEC	T59.91	T59.92	T59.93	T59.94	—	—
stove (after combustion)	T58.11	T58.12	T58.13	T58.14	—	—
tear	T59.3X1	T59.3X2	T59.3X3	T59.3X4	—	—
therapeutic	T41.5X1	T41.5X2	T41.5X3	T41.5X4	T41.5X5	T41.5X6
utility (for cooking, heating, or lighting) (piped) NEC	T59.891	T59.892	T59.893	T59.894	—	—
in mobile container	T59.891	T59.892	T59.893	T59.894	—	—
incomplete combustion of — see Carbon, monoxide, fuel, utilty						
piped (natural)	T59.891	T59.892	T59.893	T59.894	—	—
water	T58.11	T58.12	T58.13	T58.14	—	—
incomplete combustion of — see Carbon, monoxide, fuel, utility						

Substance	Poisoning, Accidental (Unintentional)	Poisoning, Intentional Self-Harm	Poisoning, Assault	Poisoning, Undetermined	Adverse Effect	Underdosing
Gaseous substance — see Gas						
Gasoline	T52.0X1	T52.0X2	T52.0X3	T52.0X4	—	—
vapor	T52.0X1	T52.0X2	T52.0X3	T52.0X4	—	—
Gastric enzymes	T47.5X1	T47.5X2	T47.5X3	T47.5X4	T47.5X5	T47.5X6
Gastrografin	T50.8X1	T50.8X2	T50.8X3	T50.8X4	T50.8X5	T50.8X6
Gastrointestinal drug	T47.91	T47.92	T47.93	T47.94	T47.95	T47.96
biological	T47.8X1	T47.8X2	T47.8X3	T47.8X4	T47.8X5	T47.8X6
specified NEC	T47.8X1	T47.8X2	T47.8X3	T47.8X4	T47.8X5	T47.8X6
Gaultheria procumbens	T62.2X1	T62.2X2	T62.2X3	T62.2X4	—	—
Gelatin (intravenous)	T45.8X1	T45.8X2	T45.8X3	T45.8X4	T45.8X5	T45.8X6
absorbable (sponge)	T45.7X1	T45.7X2	T45.7X3	T45.7X4	T45.7X5	T45.7X6
Gefarnate	T44.3X1	T44.3X2	T44.3X3	T44.3X4	T44.3X5	T44.3X6
Gelfilm	T49.8X1	T49.8X2	T49.8X3	T49.8X4	T49.8X5	T49.8X6
Gelfoam	T45.7X1	T45.7X2	T45.7X3	T45.7X4	T45.7X5	T45.7X6
Gelsemine	T50.991	T50.992	T50.993	T50.994	T50.995	T50.996
Gelsemium (sempervirens)	T62.2X1	T62.2X2	T62.2X3	T62.2X4	—	—
Gemeprost	T48.0X1	T48.0X2	T48.0X3	T48.0X4	T48.0X5	T48.0X6
Gemfibrozil	T46.6X1	T46.6X2	T46.6X3	T46.6X4	T46.6X5	T46.6X6
Gemonil	T42.3X1	T42.3X2	T42.3X3	T42.3X4	T42.3X5	T42.3X6
Gentamicin	T36.5X1	T36.5X2	T36.5X3	T36.5X4	T36.5X5	T36.5X6
ophthalmic preparation	T49.5X1	T49.5X2	T49.5X3	T49.5X4	T49.5X5	T49.5X6
topical NEC	T49.0X1	T49.0X2	T49.0X3	T49.0X4	T49.0X5	T49.0X6
Gentian	T47.5X1	T47.5X2	T47.5X3	T47.5X4	T47.5X5	T47.5X6
violet	T49.0X1	T49.0X2	T49.0X3	T49.0X4	T49.0X5	T49.0X6
Gepefrine	T44.4X1	T44.4X2	T44.4X3	T44.4X4	T44.4X5	T44.4X6
Gestonorone caproate	T38.5X1	T38.5X2	T38.5X3	T38.5X4	T38.5X5	T38.5X6
Gexane	T49.0X1	T49.0X2	T49.0X3	T49.0X4	T49.0X5	T49.0X6
Gila monster (venom)	T63.111	T63.112	T63.113	T63.114	—	—
Ginger	T47.5X1	T47.5X2	T47.5X3	T47.5X4	T47.5X5	T47.5X6
Jamaica — see Jamaica, ginger						
Gitalin	T46.0X1	T46.0X2	T46.0X3	T46.0X4	T46.0X5	T46.0X6
amorphous	T46.0X1	T46.0X2	T46.0X3	T46.0X4	T46.0X5	T46.0X6
Gitaloxin	T46.0X1	T46.0X2	T46.0X3	T46.0X4	T46.0X5	T46.0X6
Gitoxin	T46.0X1	T46.0X2	T46.0X3	T46.0X4	T46.0X5	T46.0X6
Glafenine	T39.8X1	T39.8X2	T39.8X3	T39.8X4	T39.8X5	T39.8X6
Glandular extract (medicinal) NEC	T50.Z91	T50.Z92	T50.Z93	T50.Z94	T50.Z95	T50.Z96
Glaucarubin	T37.3X1	T37.3X2	T37.3X3	T37.3X4	T37.3X5	T37.3X6
Glibenclamide	T38.3X1	T38.3X2	T38.3X3	T38.3X4	T38.3X5	T38.3X6
Glibornuride	T38.3X1	T38.3X2	T38.3X3	T38.3X4	T38.3X5	T38.3X6
Gliclazide	T38.3X1	T38.3X2	T38.3X3	T38.3X4	T38.3X5	T38.3X6
Glimidine	T38.3X1	T38.3X2	T38.3X3	T38.3X4	T38.3X5	T38.3X6

◀ New ◀ Revised ~~deleted~~ Deleted

Substance	Poisoning, Accidental (Unintentional)	Poisoning, Intentional Self-Harm	Poisoning, Assault	Poisoning, Undetermined	Adverse Effect	Underdosing
Glipizide	T38.3X1	T38.3X2	T38.3X3	T38.3X4	T38.3X5	T38.3X6
Gliquidone	T38.3X1	T38.3X2	T38.3X3	T38.3X4	T38.3X5	T38.3X6
Glisolamide	T38.3X1	T38.3X2	T38.3X3	T38.3X4	T38.3X5	T38.3X6
Glisoxepide	T38.3X1	T38.3X2	T38.3X3	T38.3X4	T38.3X5	T38.3X6
Globin zinc insulin	T38.3X1	T38.3X2	T38.3X3	T38.3X4	T38.3X5	T38.3X6
Globulin						
antilymphocytic	T50.Z11	T50.Z12	T50.Z13	T50.Z14	T50.Z15	T50.Z16
antirhesus	T50.Z11	T50.Z12	T50.Z13	T50.Z14	T50.Z15	T50.Z16
antivenin	T50.Z11	T50.Z12	T50.Z13	T50.Z14	T50.Z15	T50.Z16
antiviral	T50.Z11	T50.Z12	T50.Z13	T50.Z14	T50.Z15	T50.Z16
Glucagon	T38.3X1	T38.3X2	T38.3X3	T38.3X4	T38.3X5	T38.3X6
Glucocorticoids	T38.0X1	T38.0X2	T38.0X3	T38.0X4	T38.0X5	T38.0X6
Glucocorticosteroid	T38.0X1	T38.0X2	T38.0X3	T38.0X4	T38.0X5	T38.0X6
Gluconic acid	T50.991	T50.992	T50.993	T50.994	T50.995	T50.996
Glucosamine sulfate	T39.4X1	T39.4X2	T39.4X3	T39.4X4	T39.4X5	T39.4X6
Glucose	T50.3X1	T50.3X2	T50.3X3	T50.3X4	T50.3X5	T50.3X6
with sodium chloride	T50.3X1	T50.3X2	T50.3X3	T50.3X4	T50.3X5	T50.3X6
Glucosulfone sodium	T37.1X1	T37.1X2	T37.1X3	T37.1X4	T37.1X5	T37.1X6
Glucurolactone	T47.8X1	T47.8X2	T47.8X3	T47.8X4	T47.8X5	T47.8X6
Glue NEC	T52.8X1	T52.8X2	T52.8X3	T52.8X4	—	—
Glutamic acid	T47.5X1	T47.5X2	T47.5X3	T47.5X4	T47.5X5	T47.5X6
Glutaral (medicinal)	T49.0X1	T49.0X2	T49.0X3	T49.0X4	T49.0X5	T49.0X6
nonmedicinal	T65.891	T65.892	T65.893	T65.894	—	—
Glutaraldehyde (nonmedicinal)	T65.891	T65.892	T65.893	T65.894	—	—
medicinal	T49.0X1	T49.0X2	T49.0X3	T49.0X4	T49.0X5	T49.0X6
Glutathione	T50.6X1	T50.6X2	T50.6X3	T50.6X4	T50.6X5	T50.6X6
Glutethimide	T42.6X1	T42.6X2	T42.6X3	T42.6X4	T42.6X5	T42.6X6
Glyburide	T38.3X1	T38.3X2	T38.3X3	T38.3X4	T38.3X5	T38.3X6
Glycerin	T47.4X1	T47.4X2	T47.4X3	T47.4X4	T47.4X5	T47.4X6
Glycerol	T47.4X1	T47.4X2	T47.4X3	T47.4X4	T47.4X5	T47.4X6
borax	T49.6X1	T49.6X2	T49.6X3	T49.6X4	T49.6X5	T49.6X6
intravenous	T50.3X1	T50.3X2	T50.3X3	T50.3X4	T50.3X5	T50.3X6
iodinated	T48.4X1	T48.4X2	T48.4X3	T48.4X4	T48.4X5	T48.4X6
Glycerophosphate	T50.991	T50.992	T50.993	T50.994	T50.995	T50.996
Glyceryl						
gualacolate	T48.4X1	T48.4X2	T48.4X3	T48.4X4	T48.4X5	T48.4X6
nitrate	T46.3X1	T46.3X2	T46.3X3	T46.3X4	T46.3X5	T46.3X6
triacetate (topical)	T49.0X1	T49.0X2	T49.0X3	T49.0X4	T49.0X5	T49.0X6
trinitrate	T46.3X1	T46.3X2	T46.3X3	T46.3X4	T46.3X5	T46.3X6
Glycine	T50.3X1	T50.3X2	T50.3X3	T50.3X4	T50.3X5	T50.3X6
Glyclopyramide	T38.3X1	T38.3X2	T38.3X3	T38.3X4	T38.3X5	T38.3X6
Glycobiarsol	T37.3X1	T37.3X2	T37.3X3	T37.3X4	T37.3X5	T37.3X6

Substance	Poisoning, Accidental (Unintentional)	Poisoning, Intentional Self-Harm	Poisoning, Assault	Poisoning, Undetermined	Adverse Effect	Underdosing
Glycols (ether)	T52.3X1	T52.3X2	T52.3X3	T52.3X4	—	—
Glyconiazide	T37.1X1	T37.1X2	T37.1X3	T37.1X4	T37.1X5	T37.1X6
Glycopyrrolate	T44.3X1	T44.3X2	T44.3X3	T44.3X4	T44.3X5	T44.3X6
Glycopyrronium	T44.3X1	T44.3X2	T44.3X3	T44.3X4	T44.3X5	T44.3X6
bromide	T44.3X1	T44.3X2	T44.3X3	T44.3X4	T44.3X5	T44.3X6
Glycoside, cardiac (stimulant)	T46.0X1	T46.0X2	T46.0X3	T46.0X4	T46.0X5	T46.0X6
Glycyclamide	T38.3X1	T38.3X2	T38.3X3	T38.3X4	T38.3X5	T38.3X6
Glycyrrhiza extract	T48.4X1	T48.4X2	T48.4X3	T48.4X4	T48.4X5	T48.4X6
Glycyrrhizic acid	T48.4X1	T48.4X2	T48.4X3	T48.4X4	T48.4X5	T48.4X6
Glycyrrhizinate potassium	T48.4X1	T48.4X2	T48.4X3	T48.4X4	T48.4X5	T48.4X6
Glymidine sodium	T38.3X1	T38.3X2	T38.3X3	T38.3X4	T38.3X5	T38.3X6
Glyphosate	T60.3X1	T60.3X2	T60.3X3	T60.3X4	—	—
Glyphylline	T48.6X1	T48.6X2	T48.6X3	T48.6X4	T48.6X5	T48.6X6
Gold						
colloidal (I98Au)	T45.1X1	T45.1X2	T45.1X3	T45.1X4	T45.1X5	T45.1X6
salts	T39.4X1	T39.4X2	T39.4X3	T39.4X4	T39.4X5	T39.4X6
Golden sulfide of antimony	T56.891	T56.892	T56.893	T56.894	—	—
Goldylocks	T62.2X1	T62.2X2	T62.2X3	T62.2X4	—	—
Gonadal tissue extract	T38.901	T38.902	T38.903	T38.904	T38.905	T38.906
female	T38.5X1	T38.5X2	T38.5X3	T38.5X4	T38.5X5	T38.5X6
male	T38.7X1	T38.7X2	T38.7X3	T38.7X4	T38.7X5	T38.7X6
Gonadorelin	T38.891	T38.892	T38.893	T38.894	T38.895	T38.896
Gonadotropin	T38.891	T38.892	T38.893	T38.894	T38.895	T38.896
chorionic	T38.891	T38.892	T38.893	T38.894	T38.895	T38.896
pituitary	T38.811	T38.812	T38.813	T38.814	T38.815	T38.816
Goserelin	T45.1X1	T45.1X2	T45.1X3	T45.1X4	T45.1X5	T45.1X6
Grain alcohol	T51.0X1	T51.0X2	T51.0X3	T51.0X4	—	—
Gramicidin	T49.0X1	T49.0X2	T49.0X3	T49.0X4	T49.0X5	T49.0X6
Granisetron	T45.0X1	T45.0X2	T45.0X3	T45.0X4	T45.0X5	T45.0X6
Gratiola officinalis	T62.2X1	T62.2X2	T62.2X3	T62.2X4	—	—
Grease	T65.891	T65.892	T65.893	T65.894	—	—
Green hellebore	T62.2X1	T62.2X2	T62.2X3	T62.2X4	—	—
Green soap	T49.2X1	T49.2X2	T49.2X3	T49.2X4	T49.2X5	T49.2X6
Grifulvin	T36.7X1	T36.7X2	T36.7X3	T36.7X4	T36.7X5	T36.7X6
Griseofulvin	T36.7X1	T36.7X2	T36.7X3	T36.7X4	T36.7X5	T36.7X6
Growth hormone	T38.811	T38.812	T38.813	T38.814	T38.815	T38.816
Guaiacol derivatives	T48.4X1	T48.4X2	T48.4X3	T48.4X4	T48.4X5	T48.4X6
Guaiac reagent	T50.991	T50.992	T50.993	T50.994	T50.995	T50.996
Guaifenesin	T48.4X1	T48.4X2	T48.4X3	T48.4X4	T48.4X5	T48.4X6
Guaimesal	T48.4X1	T48.4X2	T48.4X3	T48.4X4	T48.4X5	T48.4X6
Guaiphenesin	T48.4X1	T48.4X2	T48.4X3	T48.4X4	T48.4X5	T48.4X6
Guamecycline	T36.4X1	T36.4X2	T36.4X3	T36.4X4	T36.4X5	T36.4X6

◀ New   ◀ Revised   ~~deleted~~ Deleted

TABLE OF DRUGS AND CHEMICALS

TABLE OF DRUGS AND CHEMICALS

Substance	Poisoning, Accidental (Unintentional)	Poisoning, Intentional Self-Harm	Poisoning, Assault	Poisoning, Undetermined	Adverse Effect	Underdosing
Guanabenz	T46.5X1	T46.5X2	T46.5X3	T46.5X4	T46.5X5	T46.5X6
Guanacline	T46.5X1	T46.5X2	T46.5X3	T46.5X4	T46.5X5	T46.5X6
Guanadrel	T46.5X1	T46.5X2	T46.5X3	T46.5X4	T46.5X5	T46.5X6
Guanatol	T37.2X1	T37.2X2	T37.2X3	T37.2X4	T37.2X5	T37.2X6
Guanethidine	T46.5X1	T46.5X2	T46.5X3	T46.5X4	T46.5X5	T46.5X6
Guanfacine	T46.5X1	T46.5X2	T46.5X3	T46.5X4	T46.5X5	T46.5X6
Guano	T65.891	T65.892	T65.893	T65.894	—	—
Guanochlor	T46.5X1	T46.5X2	T46.5X3	T46.5X4	T46.5X5	T46.5X6
Guanoclor	T46.5X1	T46.5X2	T46.5X3	T46.5X4	T46.5X5	T46.5X6
Guanoctine	T46.5X1	T46.5X2	T46.5X3	T46.5X4	T46.5X5	T46.5X6
Guanoxabenz	T46.5X1	T46.5X2	T46.5X3	T46.5X4	T46.5X5	T46.5X6
Guanoxan	T46.5X1	T46.5X2	T46.5X3	T46.5X4	T46.5X5	T46.5X6
Guar gum (medicinal)	T46.6X1	T46.6X2	T46.6X3	T46.6X4	T46.6X5	T46.6X6
H						
Hachimycin	T36.7X1	T36.7X2	T36.7X3	T36.7X4	T36.7X5	T36.7X6
Hair						
dye	T49.4X1	T49.4X2	T49.4X3	T49.4X4	T49.4X5	T49.4X6
preparation NEC	T49.4X1	T49.4X2	T49.4X3	T49.4X4	T49.4X5	T49.4X6
Halazepam	T42.4X1	T42.4X2	T42.4X3	T42.4X4	T42.4X5	T42.4X6
Halcinolone	T49.0X1	T49.0X2	T49.0X3	T49.0X4	T49.0X5	T49.0X6
Halcinonide	T49.0X1	T49.0X2	T49.0X3	T49.0X4	T49.0X5	T49.0X6
Halethazole	T49.0X1	T49.0X2	T49.0X3	T49.0X4	T49.0X5	T49.0X6
Hallucinogen NOS	T40.901	T40.902	T40.903	T40.904	T40.905	T40.906
specified NEC	T40.991	T40.992	T40.993	T40.994	T40.995	T40.996
Halofantrine	T37.2X1	T37.2X2	T37.2X3	T37.2X4	T37.2X5	T37.2X6
Halofenate	T46.6X1	T46.6X2	T46.6X3	T46.6X4	T46.6X5	T46.6X6
Halometasone	T49.0X1	T49.0X2	T49.0X3	T49.0X4	T49.0X5	T49.0X6
Haloperidol	T43.4X1	T43.4X2	T43.4X3	T43.4X4	T43.4X5	T43.4X6
Haloprogin	T49.0X1	T49.0X2	T49.0X3	T49.0X4	T49.0X5	T49.0X6
Halotex	T49.0X1	T49.0X2	T49.0X3	T49.0X4	T49.0X5	T49.0X6
Halothane	T41.0X1	T41.0X2	T41.0X3	T41.0X4	T41.0X5	T41.0X6
Haloxazolam	T42.4X1	T42.4X2	T42.4X3	T42.4X4	T42.4X5	T42.4X6
Halquinols	T49.0X1	T49.0X2	T49.0X3	T49.0X4	T49.0X5	T49.0X6
Hamamelis	T49.2X1	T49.2X2	T49.2X3	T49.2X4	T49.2X5	T49.2X6
Haptendextran	T45.8X1	T45.8X2	T45.8X3	T45.8X4	T45.8X5	T45.8X6
Harmonyl	T46.5X1	T46.5X2	T46.5X3	T46.5X4	T46.5X5	T46.5X6
Hartmann's solution	T50.3X1	T50.3X2	T50.3X3	T50.3X4	T50.3X5	T50.3X6
Hashish	T40.711	T40.712	T40.713	T40.714	T40.715	T40.716
Hawaiian Woodrose seeds	T40.991	T40.992	T40.993	T40.994	—	—
HCB	T60.3X1	T60.3X2	T60.3X3	T60.3X4	—	—
HCH	T53.6X1	T53.6X2	T53.6X3	T53.6X4	—	—
medicinal	T49.0X1	T49.0X2	T49.0X3	T49.0X4	T49.0X5	T49.0X6

Substance	Poisoning, Accidental (Unintentional)	Poisoning, Intentional Self-Harm	Poisoning, Assault	Poisoning, Undetermined	Adverse Effect	Underdosing
HCN	T57.3X1	T57.3X2	T57.3X3	T57.3X4	—	—
Headache cures, drugs, powders NEC	T50.901	T50.902	T50.903	T50.904	T50.905	T50.906
Heavenly Blue (morning glory)	T40.991	T40.992	T40.993	T40.994	—	—
Heavy metal antidote	T45.8X1	T45.8X2	T45.8X3	T45.8X4	T45.8X5	T45.8X6
Hedaquinium	T49.0X1	T49.0X2	T49.0X3	T49.0X4	T49.0X5	T49.0X6
Hedge hyssop	T62.2X1	T62.2X2	T62.2X3	T62.2X4	—	—
Heet	T49.8X1	T49.8X2	T49.8X3	T49.8X4	T49.8X5	T49.8X6
Helium	T48.991	T48.992	T48.993	T48.994	T48.995	T48.996
Helenin	T37.4X1	T37.4X2	T37.4X3	T37.4X4	T37.4X5	T37.4X6
Hellebore (black) (green) (white)	T62.2X1	T62.2X2	T62.2X3	T62.2X4	—	—
Helium (nonmedicinal) NEC	T59.891	T59.892	T59.893	T59.894	—	—
medicinal	T48.991	T48.992	T48.993	T48.994	T48.995	T48.996
Hematin	T45.8X1	T45.8X2	T45.8X3	T45.8X4	T45.8X5	T45.8X6
Hematinic preparation	T45.8X1	T45.8X2	T45.8X3	T45.8X4	T45.8X5	T45.8X6
Hemlock	T62.2X1	T62.2X2	T62.2X3	T62.2X4	—	—
Hemostatic	T45.621	T45.622	T45.623	T45.624	T45.625	T45.626
drug, systemic	T45.621	T45.622	T45.623	T45.624	T45.625	T45.626
Hemostyptic	T49.4X1	T49.4X2	T49.4X3	T49.4X4	T49.4X5	T49.4X6
Henbane	T62.2X1	T62.2X2	T62.2X3	T62.2X4	—	—
Heparin (sodium)	T45.511	T45.512	T45.513	T45.514	T45.515	T45.516
action reverser	T45.7X1	T45.7X2	T45.7X3	T45.7X4	T45.7X5	T45.7X6
Heparin-fraction	T45.511	T45.512	T45.513	T45.514	T45.515	T45.516
Heparinoid (systemic)	T45.511	T45.512	T45.513	T45.514	T45.515	T45.516
Hepatic secretion stimulant	T47.8X1	T47.8X2	T47.8X3	T47.8X4	T47.8X5	T47.8X6
Hepatitis B						
immune globulin	T50.Z11	T50.Z12	T50.Z13	T50.Z14	T50.Z15	T50.Z16
vaccine	T50.B91	T50.B92	T50.B93	T50.B94	T50.B95	T50.B96
Hepronicate	T46.7X1	T46.7X2	T46.7X3	T46.7X4	T46.7X5	T46.7X6
Heptabarb	T42.3X1	T42.3X2	T42.3X3	T42.3X4	T42.3X5	T42.3X6
Heptabarbitone	T42.3X1	T42.3X2	T42.3X3	T42.3X4	T42.3X5	T42.3X6
Heptabarbital	T42.3X1	T42.3X2	T42.3X3	T42.3X4	T42.3X5	T42.3X6
Heptachlor	T60.1X1	T60.1X2	T60.1X3	T60.1X4	—	—
Heptalgin	T40.2X1	T40.2X2	T40.2X3	T40.2X4	T40.2X5	T40.2X6
Heptaminol	T46.3X1	T46.3X2	T46.3X3	T46.3X4	T46.3X5	T46.3X6
Herbicide NEC	T60.3X1	T60.3X2	T60.3X3	T60.3X4	—	—
Heroin	T40.1X1	T40.1X2	T40.1X3	T40.1X4	—	—
Herplex	T49.5X1	T49.5X2	T49.5X3	T49.5X4	T49.5X5	T49.5X6
HES	T45.8X1	T45.8X2	T45.8X3	T45.8X4	T45.8X5	T45.8X6
Hesperidin	T46.991	T46.992	T46.993	T46.994	T46.995	T46.996
Hetacillin	T36.0X1	T36.0X2	T36.0X3	T36.0X4	T36.0X5	T36.0X6

◄ New   ◄ Revised   deleted Deleted

Substance	Poisoning, Accidental (Unintentional)	Poisoning, Intentional Self-Harm	Poisoning, Assault	Poisoning, Undetermined	Adverse Effect	Underdosing
Hetastarch	T45.8X1	T45.8X2	T45.8X3	T45.8X4	T45.8X5	T45.8X6
HETP	T60.0X1	T60.0X2	T60.0X3	T60.0X4	—	—
Hexachlorobenzene (vapor)	T60.3X1	T60.3X2	T60.3X3	T60.3X4	—	—
Hexachlorocyclohexane	T53.6X1	T53.6X2	T53.6X3	T53.6X4	—	—
Hexachlorophene	T49.0X1	T49.0X2	T49.0X3	T49.0X4	T49.0X5	T49.0X6
Hexadiline	T46.3X1	T46.3X2	T46.3X3	T46.3X4	T46.3X5	T46.3X6
Hexadimethrine (bromide)	T45.7X1	T45.7X2	T45.7X3	T45.7X4	T45.7X5	T45.7X6
Hexadylamine	T46.3X1	T46.3X2	T46.3X3	T46.3X4	T46.3X5	T46.3X6
Hexaethyl tetraphosphate	T60.0X1	T60.0X2	T60.0X3	T60.0X4	—	—
Hexafluorenium bromide	T48.1X1	T48.1X2	T48.1X3	T48.1X4	T48.1X5	T48.1X6
Hexafluorodiethyl ether	T43.291	T43.292	T43.293	T43.294	T43.295	T43.296
Hexafluronium (bromide)	T48.1X1	T48.1X2	T48.1X3	T48.1X4	T48.1X5	T48.1X6
Hexahydrobenzol	T52.8X1	T52.8X2	T52.8X3	T52.8X4	—	—
Hexahydrocresol(s)	T51.8X1	T51.8X2	T51.8X3	T51.8X4	—	—
arsenide	T57.0X1	T57.0X2	T57.0X3	T57.0X4	—	—
arseniurated	T57.0X1	T57.0X2	T57.0X3	T57.0X4	—	—
cyanide	T57.3X1	T57.3X2	T57.3X3	T57.3X4	—	—
gas	T59.891	T59.892	T59.893	T59.894	—	—
Fluoride (liquid)	T57.8X1	T57.8X2	T57.8X3	T57.8X4	—	—
vapor	T59.891	T59.892	T59.893	T59.894	—	—
phophorated	T60.0X1	T60.0X2	T60.0X3	T60.0X4	—	—
sulfate	T57.8X1	T57.8X2	T57.8X3	T57.8X4	—	—
sulfide (gas)	T59.6X1	T59.6X2	T59.6X3	T59.6X4	—	—
arseniurated	T57.0X1	T57.0X2	T57.0X3	T57.0X4	—	—
sulfurated	T57.8X1	T57.8X2	T57.8X3	T57.8X4	—	—
Hexahydrophenol	T51.8X1	T51.8X2	T51.8X3	T51.8X4	—	—
Hexa-germ	T49.2X1	T49.2X2	T49.2X3	T49.2X4	T49.2X5	T49.2X6
Hexalen	T51.8X1	T51.8X2	T51.8X3	T51.8X4	—	—
Hexamethonium bromide	T44.2X1	T44.2X2	T44.2X3	T44.2X4	T44.2X5	T44.2X6
Hexamethylene	T52.8X1	T52.8X2	T52.8X3	T52.8X4	—	—
Hexamethylmelamine	T45.1X1	T45.1X2	T45.1X3	T45.1X4	T45.1X5	T45.1X6
Hexamidine	T49.0X1	T49.0X2	T49.0X3	T49.0X4	T49.0X5	T49.0X6
Hexamine (mandelate)	T37.8X1	T37.8X2	T37.8X3	T37.8X4	T37.8X5	T37.8X6
Hexanone, 2-hexanone	T52.4X1	T52.4X2	T52.4X3	T52.4X4	—	—
Hexanuorenium	T48.1X1	T48.1X2	T48.1X3	T48.1X4	T48.1X5	T48.1X6
Hexapropymate	T42.6X1	T42.6X2	T42.6X3	T42.6X4	T42.6X5	T42.6X6
Hexasonium iodide	T44.3X1	T44.3X2	T44.3X3	T44.3X4	T44.3X5	T44.3X6
Hexcarbacholine bromide	T48.1X1	T48.1X2	T48.1X3	T48.1X4	T48.1X5	T48.1X6
Hexemal	T42.3X1	T42.3X2	T42.3X3	T42.3X4	T42.3X5	T42.3X6
Hexestrol	T38.5X1	T38.5X2	T38.5X3	T38.5X4	T38.5X5	T38.5X6
Hexethal (sodium)	T42.3X1	T42.3X2	T42.3X3	T42.3X4	T42.3X5	T42.3X6
Hexetidine	T37.8X1	T37.8X2	T37.8X3	T37.8X4	T37.8X5	T37.8X6

Substance	Poisoning, Accidental (Unintentional)	Poisoning, Intentional Self-Harm	Poisoning, Assault	Poisoning, Undetermined	Adverse Effect	Underdosing
Hexobarbital	T42.3X1	T42.3X2	T42.3X3	T42.3X4	T42.3X5	T42.3X6
rectal	T41.291	T41.292	T41.293	T41.294	T41.295	T41.296
sodium	T41.1X1	T41.1X2	T41.1X3	T41.1X4	T41.1X5	T41.1X6
Hexobendine	T46.3X1	T46.3X2	T46.3X3	T46.3X4	T46.3X5	T46.3X6
Hexocyclium	T44.3X1	T44.3X2	T44.3X3	T44.3X4	T44.3X5	T44.3X6
metilsulfate	T44.3X1	T44.3X2	T44.3X3	T44.3X4	T44.3X5	T44.3X6
Hexoestrol	T38.5X1	T38.5X2	T38.5X3	T38.5X4	T38.5X5	T38.5X6
Hexone	T52.4X1	T52.4X2	T52.4X3	T52.4X4	—	—
Hexoprenaline	T48.6X1	T48.6X2	T48.6X3	T48.6X4	T48.6X5	T48.6X6
Hexylcaine	T41.3X1	T41.3X2	T41.3X3	T41.3X4	T41.3X5	T41.3X6
Hexylresorcinol	T52.2X1	T52.2X2	T52.2X3	T52.2X4	—	—
HGH (human growth hormone)	T38.811	T38.812	T38.813	T38.814	T38.815	T38.816
Hinkle's pills	T47.2X1	T47.2X2	T47.2X3	T47.2X4	T47.2X5	T47.2X6
Histalog	T50.8X1	T50.8X2	T50.8X3	T50.8X4	T50.8X5	T50.8X6
Histamine (phosphate)	T50.8X1	T50.8X2	T50.8X3	T50.8X4	T50.8X5	T50.8X6
Histoplasmin	T50.8X1	T50.8X2	T50.8X3	T50.8X4	T50.8X5	T50.8X6
Holly berries	T62.2X1	T62.2X2	T62.2X3	T62.2X4	—	—
Homatropine	T44.3X1	T44.3X2	T44.3X3	T44.3X4	T44.3X5	T44.3X6
methylbromide	T44.3X1	T44.3X2	T44.3X3	T44.3X4	T44.3X5	T44.3X6
Homochlorcyclizine	T45.0X1	T45.0X2	T45.0X3	T45.0X4	T45.0X5	T45.0X6
Homosalate	T49.3X1	T49.3X2	T49.3X3	T49.3X4	T49.3X5	T49.3X6
Homo-tet	T50.Z11	T50.Z12	T50.Z13	T50.Z14	T50.Z15	T50.Z16
Hormone	T38.801	T38.802	T38.803	T38.804	T38.805	T38.806
adrenal cortical steroids	T38.0X1	T38.0X2	T38.0X3	T38.0X4	T38.0X5	T38.0X6
androgenic	T38.7X1	T38.7X2	T38.7X3	T38.7X4	T38.7X5	T38.7X6
anterior pituitary NEC	T38.811	T38.812	T38.813	T38.814	T38.815	T38.816
antidiabetic agents	T38.3X1	T38.3X2	T38.3X3	T38.3X4	T38.3X5	T38.3X6
antidiuretic	T38.891	T38.892	T38.893	T38.894	T38.895	T38.896
cancer therapy	T45.1X1	T45.1X2	T45.1X3	T45.1X4	T45.1X5	T45.1X6
follicle stimulating	T38.811	T38.812	T38.813	T38.814	T38.815	T38.816
gonadotropic	T38.891	T38.892	T38.893	T38.894	T38.895	T38.896
pituitary	T38.811	T38.812	T38.813	T38.814	T38.815	T38.816
growth	T38.811	T38.812	T38.813	T38.814	T38.815	T38.816
luteinizing	T38.811	T38.812	T38.813	T38.814	T38.815	T38.816
ovarian	T38.5X1	T38.5X2	T38.5X3	T38.5X4	T38.5X5	T38.5X6
oxytocic	T48.0X1	T48.0X2	T48.0X3	T48.0X4	T48.0X5	T48.0X6
parathyroid (derivatives)	T50.991	T50.992	T50.993	T50.994	T50.995	T50.996
pituitary (posterior) NEC	T38.891	T38.892	T38.893	T38.894	T38.895	T38.896
anterior	T38.811	T38.812	T38.813	T38.814	T38.815	T38.816
specified, NEC	T38.891	T38.892	T38.893	T38.894	T38.895	T38.896
thyroid	T38.1X1	T38.1X2	T38.1X3	T38.1X4	T38.1X5	T38.1X6
Hornet (sting)	T63.451	T63.452	T63.453	T63.454	—	—

◀ New ◀ Revised ~~deleted~~ Deleted

	External Cause (T-Code)					
Substance	Poisoning, Accidental (Unintentional)	Poisoning, Intentional Self-Harm	Poisoning, Assault	Poisoning, Undetermined	Adverse Effect	Underdosing
Horse anti-human lymphocytic serum	T50.Z11	T50.Z12	T50.Z13	T50.Z14	T50.Z15	T50.Z16
Horticulture agent NEC	T65.91	T65.92	T65.93	T65.94	—	—
with pesticide	T60.91	T60.92	T60.93	T60.94	—	—
Human						
albumin	T45.8X1	T45.8X2	T45.8X3	T45.8X4	T45.8X5	T45.8X6
growth hormone (HGH)	T38.811	T38.812	T38.813	T38.814	T38.815	T38.816
immune serum	T50.Z11	T50.Z12	T50.Z13	T50.Z14	T50.Z15	T50.Z16
Hyaluronidase	T45.3X1	T45.3X2	T45.3X3	T45.3X4	T45.3X5	T45.3X6
Hyazyme	T45.3X1	T45.3X2	T45.3X3	T45.3X4	T45.3X5	T45.3X6
Hycodan	T40.2X1	T40.2X2	T40.2X3	T40.2X4	T40.2X5	T40.2X6
Hydantoin derivative NEC	T42.0X1	T42.0X2	T42.0X3	T42.0X4	T42.0X5	T42.0X6
Hydeltra	T38.0X1	T38.0X2	T38.0X3	T38.0X4	T38.0X5	T38.0X6
Hydergine	T44.6X1	T44.6X2	T44.6X3	T44.6X4	T44.6X5	T44.6X6
Hydrabamine penicillin	T36.0X1	T36.0X2	T36.0X3	T36.0X4	T36.0X5	T36.0X6
Hydralazine	T46.5X1	T46.5X2	T46.5X3	T46.5X4	T46.5X5	T46.5X6
Hydrargaphen	T49.0X1	T49.0X2	T49.0X3	T49.0X4	T49.0X5	T49.0X6
Hydrargyri amino-chloridum	T49.0X1	T49.0X2	T49.0X3	T49.0X4	T49.0X5	T49.0X6
Hydrastine	T48.291	T48.292	T48.293	T48.294	T48.295	T48.296
Hydrazine	T54.1X1	T54.1X2	T54.1X3	T54.1X4	—	—
monoamine oxidase inhibitors	T43.1X1	T43.1X2	T43.1X3	T43.1X4	T43.1X5	T43.1X6
Hydrazoic acid, azides	T54.2X1	T54.2X2	T54.2X3	T54.2X4	—	—
Hydriodic acid	T48.4X1	T48.4X2	T48.4X3	T48.4X4	T48.4X5	T48.4X6
Hydrocarbon gas	T59.891	T59.892	T59.893	T59.894		
incomplete combustion of — see Carbon, monoxide, fuel, utility						
liquefied (mobile container)	T59.891	T59.892	T59.893	T59.894	—	—
piped (natural)	T59.891	T59.892	T59.893	T59.894	—	—
Hydrochloric acid (liquid)	T54.2X1	T54.2X2	T54.2X3	T54.2X4	—	—
medicinal (digestant)	T47.5X1	T47.5X2	T47.5X3	T47.5X4	T47.5X5	T47.5X6
vapor	T59.891	T59.892	T59.893	T59.894	—	—
Hydrochlorothiazide	T50.2X1	T50.2X2	T50.2X3	T50.2X4	T50.2X5	T50.2X6
Hydrocodone	T40.2X1	T40.2X2	T40.2X3	T40.2X4	T40.2X5	T40.2X6
Hydrocortisone (derivatives)	T38.0X1	T38.0X2	T38.0X3	T38.0X4	T38.0X5	T38.0X6
aceponate	T49.0X1	T49.0X2	T49.0X3	T49.0X4	T49.0X5	T49.0X6
ENT agent	T49.6X1	T49.6X2	T49.6X3	T49.6X4	T49.6X5	T49.6X6
ophthalmic preparation	T49.5X1	T49.5X2	T49.5X3	T49.5X4	T49.5X5	T49.5X6
topical NEC	T49.0X1	T49.0X2	T49.0X3	T49.0X4	T49.0X5	T49.0X6
Hydrocortone	T38.0X1	T38.0X2	T38.0X3	T38.0X4	T38.0X5	T38.0X6
ENT agent	T49.6X1	T49.6X2	T49.6X3	T49.6X4	T49.6X5	T49.6X6
ophthalmic preparation	T49.5X1	T49.5X2	T49.5X3	T49.5X4	T49.5X5	T49.5X6
topical NEC	T49.0X1	T49.0X2	T49.0X3	T49.0X4	T49.0X5	T49.0X6

	External Cause (T-Code)					
Substance	Poisoning, Accidental (Unintentional)	Poisoning, Intentional Self-Harm	Poisoning, Assault	Poisoning, Undetermined	Adverse Effect	Underdosing
Hydrocyanic acid (liquid)	T57.3X1	T57.3X2	T57.3X3	T57.3X4	—	—
gas	T65.0X1	T65.0X2	T65.0X3	T65.0X4	—	—
Hydroflumethiazide	T50.2X1	T50.2X2	T50.2X3	T50.2X4	T50.2X5	T50.2X6
Hydrofluoric acid (liquid)	T54.2X1	T54.2X2	T54.2X3	T54.2X4	—	—
vapor	T59.891	T59.892	T59.893	T59.894	—	—
Hydrogen	T59.891	T59.892	T59.893	T59.894	—	—
arsenide	T57.0X1	T57.0X2	T57.0X3	T57.0X4	—	—
arseniureted	T57.0X1	T57.0X2	T57.0X3	T57.0X4	—	—
chloride	T57.8X1	T57.8X2	T57.8X3	T57.8X4	—	—
cyanide (salts)	T57.3X1	T57.3X2	T57.3X3	T57.3X4	—	—
gas	T57.3X1	T57.3X2	T57.3X3	T57.3X4	—	—
Fluoride	T59.5X1	T59.5X2	T59.5X3	T59.5X4	—	—
vapor	T59.5X1	T59.5X2	T59.5X3	T59.5X4	—	—
peroxide	T49.0X1	T49.0X2	T49.0X3	T49.0X4	T49.0X5	T49.0X6
phosphureted	T57.1X1	T57.1X2	T57.1X3	T57.1X4	—	—
sulfide	T59.6X1	T59.6X2	T59.6X3	T59.6X4	—	—
arseniureted	T57.0X1	T57.0X2	T57.0X3	T57.0X4	—	—
sulfureted	T59.6X1	T59.6X2	T59.6X3	T59.6X4	—	—
Hydromethylpyridine	T46.7X1	T46.7X2	T46.7X3	T46.7X4	T46.7X5	T46.7X6
Hydromorphinol	T40.2X1	T40.2X2	T40.2X3	T40.2X4		
Hydromorphinone	T40.2X1	T40.2X2	T40.2X3	T40.2X4	T40.2X5	T40.2X6
Hydromorphone	T40.2X1	T40.2X2	T40.2X3	T40.2X4	T40.2X5	T40.2X6
Hydromox	T50.2X1	T50.2X2	T50.2X3	T50.2X4	T50.2X5	T50.2X6
Hydrophilic lotion	T49.3X1	T49.3X2	T49.3X3	T49.3X4	T49.3X5	T49.3X6
Hydroquinidine	T46.2X1	T46.2X2	T46.2X3	T46.2X4	T46.2X5	T46.2X6
Hydroquinone	T52.2X1	T52.2X2	T52.2X3	T52.2X4		
vapor	T59.891	T59.892	T59.893	T59.894	—	—
Hydrosulfuric acid (gas)	T59.6X1	T59.6X2	T59.6X3	T59.6X4	—	—
Hydrotalcite	T47.1X1	T47.1X2	T47.1X3	T47.1X4	T47.1X5	T47.1X6
Hydrous wool fat	T49.3X1	T49.3X2	T49.3X3	T49.3X4	T49.3X5	T49.3X6
Hydroxide, caustic	T54.3X1	T54.3X2	T54.3X3	T54.3X4		
Hydroxocobalamin	T45.8X1	T45.8X2	T45.8X3	T45.8X4	T45.8X5	T45.8X6
Hydroxyamphetamine	T49.5X1	T49.5X2	T49.5X3	T49.5X4	T49.5X5	T49.5X6
Hydroxycarbamide	T45.1X1	T45.1X2	T45.1X3	T45.1X4	T45.1X5	T45.1X6
Hydroxychloroquine	T37.8X1	T37.8X2	T37.8X3	T37.8X4	T37.8X5	T37.8X6
Hydroxydihydrocodeinone	T40.2X1	T40.2X2	T40.2X3	T40.2X4	T40.2X5	T40.2X6
Hydroxyestrone	T38.5X1	T38.5X2	T38.5X3	T38.5X4	T38.5X5	T38.5X6
Hydroxyethyl starch	T45.8X1	T45.8X2	T45.8X3	T45.8X4	T45.8X5	T45.8X6
Hydroxymethylpentanone	T52.4X1	T52.4X2	T52.4X3	T52.4X4	—	—
Hydroxyphenamate	T43.591	T43.592	T43.593	T43.594	T43.595	T43.596
Hydroxyphenylbutazone	T39.2X1	T39.2X2	T39.2X3	T39.2X4	T39.2X5	T39.2X6

◀ New ◀ Revised ~~deleted~~ Deleted

Substance	Poisoning, Accidental (Unintentional)	Poisoning, Intentional Self-Harm	Poisoning, Assault	Poisoning, Undetermined	Adverse Effect	Underdosing
Hydroxyprogesterone	T38.5X1	T38.5X2	T38.5X3	T38.5X4	T38.5X5	T38.5X6
caproate	T38.5X1	T38.5X2	T38.5X3	T38.5X4	T38.5X5	T38.5X6
Hydroxyquinoline (derivatives) NEC	T37.8X1	T37.8X2	T37.8X3	T37.8X4	T37.8X5	T37.8X6
Hydroxystilbamidine	T37.3X1	T37.3X2	T37.3X3	T37.3X4	T37.3X5	T37.3X6
Hydroxytoluene (nonmedicinal)	T54.0X1	T54.0X2	T54.0X3	T54.0X4	—	—
medicinal	T49.0X1	T49.0X2	T49.0X3	T49.0X4	T49.0X5	T49.0X6
Hydroxyurea	T45.1X1	T45.1X2	T45.1X3	T45.1X4	T45.1X5	T45.1X6
Hydroxyzine	T43.591	T43.592	T43.593	T43.594	T43.595	T43.596
Hyoscine	T44.3X1	T44.3X2	T44.3X3	T44.3X4	T44.3X5	T44.3X6
Hyoscyamine	T44.3X1	T44.3X2	T44.3X3	T44.3X4	T44.3X5	T44.3X6
Hyoscyamus	T44.3X1	T44.3X2	T44.3X3	T44.3X4	T44.3X5	T44.3X6
dry extract	T44.3X1	T44.3X2	T44.3X3	T44.3X4	T44.3X5	T44.3X6
Hypaque	T50.8X1	T50.8X2	T50.8X3	T50.8X4	T50.8X5	T50.8X6
Hypertussis	T50.Z11	T50.Z12	T50.Z13	T50.Z14	T50.Z15	T50.Z16
Hypnotic	T42.71	T42.72	T42.73	T42.74	T42.75	T42.76
anticonvulsant	T42.71	T42.72	T42.73	T42.74	T42.75	T42.76
specified NEC	T42.6X1	T42.6X2	T42.6X3	T42.6X4	T42.6X5	T42.6X6
Hypochlorite	T49.0X1	T49.0X2	T49.0X3	T49.0X4	T49.0X5	T49.0X6
Hypophysis, posterior	T38.891	T38.892	T38.893	T38.894	T38.895	T38.896
Hypotensive NEC	T46.5X1	T46.5X2	T46.5X3	T46.5X4	T46.5X5	T46.5X6
Hypromellose	T49.5X1	T49.5X2	T49.5X3	T49.5X4	T49.5X5	T49.5X6

I

Substance	Poisoning, Accidental (Unintentional)	Poisoning, Intentional Self-Harm	Poisoning, Assault	Poisoning, Undetermined	Adverse Effect	Underdosing
Ibacitabine	T37.5X1	T37.5X2	T37.5X3	T37.5X4	T37.5X5	T37.5X6
Ibopamine	T44.991	T44.992	T44.993	T44.994	T44.995	T44.996
Ibufenac	T39.311	T39.312	T39.313	T39.314	T39.315	T39.316
Ibuprofen	T39.311	T39.312	T39.313	T39.314	T39.315	T39.316
Ibuproxam	T39.311	T39.312	T39.313	T39.314	T39.315	T39.316
Ibuterol	T48.6X1	T48.6X2	T48.6X3	T48.6X4	T48.6X5	T48.6X6
Ichthammol	T49.0X1	T49.0X2	T49.0X3	T49.0X4	T49.0X5	T49.0X6
Ichthyol	T49.4X1	T49.4X2	T49.4X3	T49.4X4	T49.4X5	T49.4X6
Idarubicin	T45.1X1	T45.1X2	T45.1X3	T45.1X4	T45.1X5	T45.1X6
Idrocilamide	T42.8X1	T42.8X2	T42.8X3	T42.8X4	T42.8X5	T42.8X6
Ifenprodil	T46.7X1	T46.7X2	T46.7X3	T46.7X4	T46.7X5	T46.7X6
Ifosfamide	T45.1X1	T45.1X2	T45.1X3	T45.1X4	T45.1X5	T45.1X6
Iletin	T38.3X1	T38.3X2	T38.3X3	T38.3X4	T38.3X5	T38.3X6
Ilex	T62.2X1	T62.2X2	T62.2X3	T62.2X4	—	—
Illuminating gas (after combustion)	T58.11	T58.12	T58.13	T58.14	—	—
prior to combustion	T59.891	T59.892	T59.893	T59.894	—	—
Ilopan	T45.2X1	T45.2X2	T45.2X3	T45.2X4	T45.2X5	T45.2X6
Iloprost	T46.7X1	T46.7X2	T46.7X3	T46.7X4	T46.7X5	T46.7X6

Substance	Poisoning, Accidental (Unintentional)	Poisoning, Intentional Self-Harm	Poisoning, Assault	Poisoning, Undetermined	Adverse Effect	Underdosing
Ilotycin	T36.3X1	T36.3X2	T36.3X3	T36.3X4	T36.3X5	T36.3X6
ophthalmic preparation	T49.5X1	T49.5X2	T49.5X3	T49.5X4	T49.5X5	T49.5X6
topical NEC	T49.0X1	T49.0X2	T49.0X3	T49.0X4	T49.0X5	T49.0X6
Imidazole-4-carboxamide	T45.1X1	T45.1X2	T45.1X3	T45.1X4	T45.1X5	T45.1X6
Imipenem	T36.0X1	T36.0X2	T36.0X3	T36.0X4	T36.0X5	T36.0X6
Imipramine	T43.011	T43.012	T43.013	T43.014	T43.015	T43.016
Iminostilbene	T42.1X1	T42.1X2	T42.1X3	T42.1X4	T42.1X5	T42.1X6
Immu-G	T50.Z11	T50.Z12	T50.Z13	T50.Z14	T50.Z15	T50.Z16
Immuglobin	T50.Z11	T50.Z12	T50.Z13	T50.Z14	T50.Z15	T50.Z16
Immune						
globulin	T50.Z11	T50.Z12	T50.Z13	T50.Z14	T50.Z15	T50.Z16
serum globulin	T50.Z11	T50.Z12	T50.Z13	T50.Z14	T50.Z15	T50.Z16
Immunoglobin human (intravenous) (normal)	T50.Z11	T50.Z12	T50.Z13	T50.Z14	T50.Z15	T50.Z16
unmodified	T50.Z11	T50.Z12	T50.Z13	T50.Z14	T50.Z15	T50.Z16
Immunosuppressive drug	T45.1X1	T45.1X2	T45.1X3	T45.1X4	T45.1X5	T45.1X6
Immu-tetanus	T50.Z11	T50.Z12	T50.Z13	T50.Z14	T50.Z15	T50.Z16
Indalpine	T43.221	T43.222	T43.223	T43.224	T43.225	T43.226
Indanazoline	T48.5X1	T48.5X2	T48.5X3	T48.5X4	T48.5X5	T48.5X6
Indandione (derivatives)	T45.511	T45.512	T45.513	T45.514	T45.515	T45.516
Indapamide	T46.5X1	T46.5X2	T46.5X3	T46.5X4	T46.5X5	T46.5X6
Indendione (derivatives)	T45.511	T45.512	T45.513	T45.514	T45.515	T45.516
Indenolol	T44.7X1	T44.7X2	T44.7X3	T44.7X4	T44.7X5	T44.7X6
Inderal	T44.7X1	T44.7X2	T44.7X3	T44.7X4	T44.7X5	T44.7X6
Indian						
hemp	T40.711	T40.712	T40.713	T40.714	T40.715	T40.716
tobacco	T62.2X1	T62.2X2	T62.2X3	T62.2X4	—	—
Indigo carmine	T50.8X1	T50.8X2	T50.8X3	T50.8X4	T50.8X5	T50.8X6
Indobufen	T45.521	T45.522	T45.523	T45.524	T45.525	T45.526
Indocin	T39.2X1	T39.2X2	T39.2X3	T39.2X4	T39.2X5	T39.2X6
Indocyanine green	T50.8X1	T50.8X2	T50.8X3	T50.8X4	T50.8X5	T50.8X6
Indometacin	T39.391	T39.392	T39.393	T39.394	T39.395	T39.396
Indomethacin	T39.391	T39.392	T39.393	T39.394	T39.395	T39.396
farnesil	T39.4X1	T39.4X2	T39.4X3	T39.4X4	T39.4X5	T39.4X6
Indoramin	T44.6X1	T44.6X2	T44.6X3	T44.6X4	T44.6X5	T44.6X6
Industrial						
alcohol	T51.0X1	T51.0X2	T51.0X3	T51.0X4	—	—
fumes	T59.891	T59.892	T59.893	T59.894	—	—
solvents (fumes) (vapors)	T52.91	T52.92	T52.93	T52.94	—	—
Influenza vaccine	T50.B91	T50.B92	T50.B93	T50.B94	T50.B95	T50.B96
Ingested substance NEC	T65.91	T65.92	T65.93	T65.94	—	—
INH	T37.1X1	T37.1X2	T37.1X3	T37.1X4	T37.1X5	T37.1X6

TABLE OF DRUGS AND CHEMICALS

TABLE OF DRUGS AND CHEMICALS (left margin, vertical)

Substance	External Cause (T-Code) Poisoning, Accidental (Unintentional)	Poisoning, Intentional Self-Harm	Poisoning, Assault	Poisoning, Undetermined	Adverse Effect	Underdosing
Inhalation, gas (noxious) — see Gas						
Inhibitor						
angiotensin-converting enzyme	T46.4X1	T46.4X2	T46.4X3	T46.4X4	T46.4X5	T46.4X6
carbonic anhydrase	T50.2X1	T50.2X2	T50.2X3	T50.2X4	T50.2X5	T50.2X6
fibrinolysis	T45.621	T45.622	T45.623	T45.624	T45.625	T45.626
monoamine oxidase NEC	T43.1X1	T43.1X2	T43.1X3	T43.1X4	T43.1X5	T43.1X6
hydrazine	T43.1X1	T43.1X2	T43.1X3	T43.1X4	T43.1X5	T43.1X6
postsynaptic	T43.8X1	T43.8X2	T43.8X3	T43.8X4	T43.8X5	T43.8X6
prothrombin synthesis	T45.511	T45.512	T45.513	T45.514	T45.515	T45.516
Ink	T65.891	T65.892	T65.893	T65.894	—	—
Inorganic substance NEC	T57.91	T57.92	T57.93	T57.94	—	—
Inosine pranobex	T37.5X1	T37.5X2	T37.5X3	T37.5X4	T37.5X5	T37.5X6
Inositol	T50.991	T50.992	T50.993	T50.994	T50.995	T50.996
nicotinate	T46.7X1	T46.7X2	T46.7X3	T46.7X4	T46.7X5	T46.7X6
Inproquone	T45.1X1	T45.1X2	T45.1X3	T45.1X4	T45.1X5	T45.1X6
Insect (sting), venomous	T63.481	T63.482	T63.483	T63.484	—	—
ant	T63.421	T63.422	T63.423	T63.424	—	—
bee	T63.441	T63.442	T63.443	T63.444	—	—
caterpillar	T63.431	T63.432	T63.433	T63.434	—	—
hornet	T63.451	T63.452	T63.453	T63.454	—	—
wasp	T63.461	T63.462	T63.463	T63.464	—	—
Insecticide NEC	T60.91	T60.92	T60.93	T60.94	—	—
carbamate	T60.0X1	T60.0X2	T60.0X3	T60.0X4	—	—
chlorinated	T60.1X1	T60.1X2	T60.1X3	T60.1X4	—	—
mixed	T60.91	T60.92	T60.93	T60.94	—	—
organochlorine	T60.1X1	T60.1X2	T60.1X3	T60.1X4	—	—
organophosphorus	T60.0X1	T60.0X2	T60.0X3	T60.0X4	—	—
Insular tissue extract	T38.3X1	T38.3X2	T38.3X3	T38.3X4	T38.3X5	T38.3X6
Insulin (amorphous) (globin) (isophane) (Lente) (NPH) (Semilente) (Ultralente)	T38.3X1	T38.3X2	T38.3X3	T38.3X4	T38.3X5	T38.3X6
defalan	T38.3X1	T38.3X2	T38.3X3	T38.3X4	T38.3X5	T38.3X6
human	T38.3X1	T38.3X2	T38.3X3	T38.3X4	T38.3X5	T38.3X6
injection, soluble	T38.3X1	T38.3X2	T38.3X3	T38.3X4	T38.3X5	T38.3X6
biphasic	T38.3X1	T38.3X2	T38.3X3	T38.3X4	T38.3X5	T38.3X6
intermediate acting	T38.3X1	T38.3X2	T38.3X3	T38.3X4	T38.3X5	T38.3X6
protamine zinc	T38.3X1	T38.3X2	T38.3X3	T38.3X4	T38.3X5	T38.3X6
slow acting	T38.3X1	T38.3X2	T38.3X3	T38.3X4	T38.3X5	T38.3X6
zinc						
protamine injection	T38.3X1	T38.3X2	T38.3X3	T38.3X4	T38.3X5	T38.3X6
suspension (amorphous) (crystalline)	T38.3X1	T38.3X2	T38.3X3	T38.3X4	T38.3X5	T38.3X6

Substance	External Cause (T-Code) Poisoning, Accidental (Unintentional)	Poisoning, Intentional Self-Harm	Poisoning, Assault	Poisoning, Undetermined	Adverse Effect	Underdosing
Interferon (alpha) (beta) (gamma)	T37.5X1	T37.5X2	T37.5X3	T37.5X4	T37.5X5	T37.5X6
Intestinal motility control drug	T47.6X1	T47.6X2	T47.6X3	T47.6X4	T47.6X5	T47.6X6
biological	T47.8X1	T47.8X2	T47.8X3	T47.8X4	T47.8X5	T47.8X6
Intranarcon	T41.1X1	T41.1X2	T41.1X3	T41.1X4	T41.1X5	T41.1X6
Intravenous						
amino acids	T50.991	T50.992	T50.993	T50.994	T50.995	T50.996
fat suspension	T50.991	T50.992	T50.993	T50.994	T50.995	T50.996
Inulin	T50.8X1	T50.8X2	T50.8X3	T50.8X4	T50.8X5	T50.8X6
Invert sugar	T50.3X1	T50.3X2	T50.3X3	T50.3X4	T50.3X5	T50.3X6
Inza — see Naproxen						
Iobenzamic acid	T50.8X1	T50.8X2	T50.8X3	T50.8X4	T50.8X5	T50.8X6
Iocarmic acid	T50.8X1	T50.8X2	T50.8X3	T50.8X4	T50.8X5	T50.8X6
Iocetamic acid	T50.8X1	T50.8X2	T50.8X3	T50.8X4	T50.8X5	T50.8X6
Iodamide	T50.8X1	T50.8X2	T50.8X3	T50.8X4	T50.8X5	T50.8X6
Iodide NEC — see also Iodine	T49.0X1	T49.0X2	T49.0X3	T49.0X4	T49.0X5	T49.0X6
mercury (ointment)	T49.0X1	T49.0X2	T49.0X3	T49.0X4	T49.0X5	T49.0X6
methylate	T49.0X1	T49.0X2	T49.0X3	T49.0X4	T49.0X5	T49.0X6
potassium (expectorant) NEC	T48.4X1	T48.4X2	T48.4X3	T48.4X4	T48.4X5	T48.4X6
Iodinated						
contrast medium	T50.8X1	T50.8X2	T50.8X3	T50.8X4	T50.8X5	T50.8X6
glycerol	T48.4X1	T48.4X2	T48.4X3	T48.4X4	T48.4X5	T48.4X6
human serum albumin (131I)	T50.8X1	T50.8X2	T50.8X3	T50.8X4	T50.8X5	T50.8X6
Iodine (antiseptic, external) (tincture) NEC	T49.0X1	T49.0X2	T49.0X3	T49.0X4	T49.0X5	T49.0X6
125 — see also Radiation sickness, and Exposure to radioactivce isotopes	T50.8X1	T50.8X2	T50.8X3	T50.8X4	T50.8X5	T50.8X6
therapeutic	T50.991	T50.992	T50.993	T50.994	T50.995	T50.996
131 — see also Radiation sickness, and Exposure to radioactivce isotopes	T50.8X1	T50.8X2	T50.8X3	T50.8X4	T50.8X5	T50.8X6
therapeutic	T38.2X1	T38.2X2	T38.2X3	T38.2X4	T38.2X5	T38.2X6
diagnostic	T50.8X1	T50.8X2	T50.8X3	T50.8X4	T50.8X5	T50.8X6
for thyroid conditions (antithyroid)	T38.2X1	T38.2X2	T38.2X3	T38.2X4	T38.2X5	T38.2X6
solution	T49.0X1	T49.0X2	T49.0X3	T49.0X4	T49.0X5	T49.0X6
vapor	T59.891	T59.892	T59.893	T59.894	—	—
Iodipamide	T50.8X1	T50.8X2	T50.8X3	T50.8X4	T50.8X5	T50.8X6
Iodized (poppy seed) oil	T50.8X1	T50.8X2	T50.8X3	T50.8X4	T50.8X5	T50.8X6
Iodobismitol	T37.8X1	T37.8X2	T37.8X3	T37.8X4	T37.8X5	T37.8X6
Iodochlorhydroxyquin	T37.8X1	T37.8X2	T37.8X3	T37.8X4	T37.8X5	T37.8X6
topical	T49.0X1	T49.0X2	T49.0X3	T49.0X4	T49.0X5	T49.0X6
Iodochlorhydroxyquino-line	T37.8X1	T37.8X2	T37.8X3	T37.8X4	T37.8X5	T37.8X6
Iodocholesterol (131I)	T50.8X1	T50.8X2	T50.8X3	T50.8X4	T50.8X5	T50.8X6

◀ New   ◀ Revised   ~~deleted~~ Deleted

	External Cause (T-Code)					
Substance	Poisoning, Accidental (Unintentional)	Poisoning, Intentional Self-Harm	Poisoning, Assault	Poisoning, Undetermined	Adverse Effect	Underdosing
Iodoform	T49.0X1	T49.0X2	T49.0X3	T49.0X4	T49.0X5	T49.0X6
Iodohippuric acid	T50.8X1	T50.8X2	T50.8X3	T50.8X4	T50.8X5	T50.8X6
Iodopanoic acid	T50.8X1	T50.8X2	T50.8X3	T50.8X4	T50.8X5	T50.8X6
Iodophthalein (sodium)	T50.8X1	T50.8X2	T50.8X3	T50.8X4	T50.8X5	T50.8X6
Iodopyracet	T50.8X1	T50.8X2	T50.8X3	T50.8X4	T50.8X5	T50.8X6
Iodoquinol	T37.8X1	T37.8X2	T37.8X3	T37.8X4	T37.8X5	T37.8X6
Iodoxamic acid	T50.8X1	T50.8X2	T50.8X3	T50.8X4	T50.8X5	T50.8X6
Iofendylate	T50.8X1	T50.8X2	T50.8X3	T50.8X4	T50.8X5	T50.8X6
Ioglycamic acid	T50.8X1	T50.8X2	T50.8X3	T50.8X4	T50.8X5	T50.8X6
Iohexol	T50.8X1	T50.8X2	T50.8X3	T50.8X4	T50.8X5	T50.8X6
Ion exchange resin						
anion	T47.8X1	T47.8X2	T47.8X3	T47.8X4	T47.8X5	T47.8X6
cation	T50.3X1	T50.3X2	T50.3X3	T50.3X4	T50.3X5	T50.3X6
cholestyramine	T46.6X1	T46.6X2	T46.6X3	T46.6X4	T46.6X5	T46.6X6
intestinal	T47.8X1	T47.8X2	T47.8X3	T47.8X4	T47.8X5	T47.8X6
Iopamidol	T50.8X1	T50.8X2	T50.8X3	T50.8X4	T50.8X5	T50.8X6
Iopanoic acid	T50.8X1	T50.8X2	T50.8X3	T50.8X4	T50.8X5	T50.8X6
Iophenoic acid	T50.8X1	T50.8X2	T50.8X3	T50.8X4	T50.8X5	T50.8X6
Iopodate, sodium	T50.8X1	T50.8X2	T50.8X3	T50.8X4	T50.8X5	T50.8X6
Iopodic acid	T50.8X1	T50.8X2	T50.8X3	T50.8X4	T50.8X5	T50.8X6
Iopromide	T50.8X1	T50.8X2	T50.8X3	T50.8X4	T50.8X5	T50.8X6
Iopydol	T50.8X1	T50.8X2	T50.8X3	T50.8X4	T50.8X5	T50.8X6
Iotalamic acid	T50.8X1	T50.8X2	T50.8X3	T50.8X4	T50.8X5	T50.8X6
Iothalamate	T50.8X1	T50.8X2	T50.8X3	T50.8X4	T50.8X5	T50.8X6
Iothiouracil	T38.2X1	T38.2X2	T38.2X3	T38.2X4	T38.2X5	T38.2X6
Iotrol	T50.8X1	T50.8X2	T50.8X3	T50.8X4	T50.8X5	T50.8X6
Iotrolan	T50.8X1	T50.8X2	T50.8X3	T50.8X4	T50.8X5	T50.8X6
Iotroxate	T50.8X1	T50.8X2	T50.8X3	T50.8X4	T50.8X5	T50.8X6
Iotroxic acid	T50.8X1	T50.8X2	T50.8X3	T50.8X4	T50.8X5	T50.8X6
Ioversol	T50.8X1	T50.8X2	T50.8X3	T50.8X4	T50.8X5	T50.8X6
Ioxaglate	T50.8X1	T50.8X2	T50.8X3	T50.8X4	T50.8X5	T50.8X6
Ioxaglic acid	T50.8X1	T50.8X2	T50.8X3	T50.8X4	T50.8X5	T50.8X6
Ioxitalamic acid	T50.8X1	T50.8X2	T50.8X3	T50.8X4	T50.8X5	T50.8X6
Ipecac	T47.7X1	T47.7X2	T47.7X3	T47.7X4	T47.7X5	T47.7X6
Ipecacuanha	T48.4X1	T48.4X2	T48.4X3	T48.4X4	T48.4X5	T48.4X6
Ipodate, calcium	T50.8X1	T50.8X2	T50.8X3	T50.8X4	T50.8X5	T50.8X6
Ipral	T42.3X1	T42.3X2	T42.3X3	T42.3X4	T42.3X5	T42.3X6
Ipratropium (bromide)	T48.6X1	T48.6X2	T48.6X3	T48.6X4	T48.6X5	T48.6X6
Ipriflavone	T46.3X1	T46.3X2	T46.3X3	T46.3X4	T46.3X5	T46.3X6
Iprindole	T43.011	T43.012	T43.013	T43.014	T43.015	T43.016
Iproclozide	T43.1X1	T43.1X2	T43.1X3	T43.1X4	T43.1X5	T43.1X6
Iprofenin	T50.8X1	T50.8X2	T50.8X3	T50.8X4	T50.8X5	T50.8X6

	External Cause (T-Code)					
Substance	Poisoning, Accidental (Unintentional)	Poisoning, Intentional Self-Harm	Poisoning, Assault	Poisoning, Undetermined	Adverse Effect	Underdosing
Iproheptine	T49.2X1	T49.2X2	T49.2X3	T49.2X4	T49.2X5	T49.2X6
Iproniazid	T43.1X1	T43.1X2	T43.1X3	T43.1X4	T43.1X5	T43.1X6
Iproplatin	T45.1X1	T45.1X2	T45.1X3	T45.1X4	T45.1X5	T45.1X6
Iproveratril	T46.1X1	T46.1X2	T46.1X3	T46.1X4	T46.1X5	T46.1X6
Iron (compounds) (medicinal) NEC	T45.4X1	T45.4X2	T45.4X3	T45.4X4	T45.4X5	T45.4X6
ammonium	T45.4X1	T45.4X2	T45.4X3	T45.4X4	T45.4X5	T45.4X6
dextran injection	T45.4X1	T45.4X2	T45.4X3	T45.4X4	T45.4X5	T45.4X6
nonmedicinal	T56.891	T56.892	T56.893	T56.894	—	—
salts	T45.4X1	T45.4X2	T45.4X3	T45.4X4	T45.4X5	T45.4X6
sorbitex	T45.4X1	T45.4X2	T45.4X3	T45.4X4	T45.4X5	T45.4X6
sorbitol citric acid complex	T45.4X1	T45.4X2	T45.4X3	T45.4X4	T45.4X5	T45.4X6
Irrigating fluid (vaginal)	T49.8X1	T49.8X2	T49.8X3	T49.8X4	T49.8X5	T49.8X6
eye	T49.5X1	T49.5X2	T49.5X3	T49.5X4	T49.5X5	T49.5X6
Isepamicin	T36.5X1	T36.5X2	T36.5X3	T36.5X4	T36.5X5	T36.5X6
Isoaminile (citrate)	T48.3X1	T48.3X2	T48.3X3	T48.3X4	T48.3X5	T48.3X6
Isoamyl nitrite	T46.3X1	T46.3X2	T46.3X3	T46.3X4	T46.3X5	T46.3X6
Isobenzan	T60.1X1	T60.1X2	T60.1X3	T60.1X4	—	—
Isobutyl acetate	T52.8X1	T52.8X2	T52.8X3	T52.8X4	—	—
Isocarboxazid	T43.1X1	T43.1X2	T43.1X3	T43.1X4	T43.1X5	T43.1X6
Isoconazole	T49.0X1	T49.0X2	T49.0X3	T49.0X4	T49.0X5	T49.0X6
Isocyanate	T65.0X1	T65.0X2	T65.0X3	T65.0X4	—	—
Isoephedrine	T44.991	T44.992	T44.993	T44.994	T44.995	T44.996
Isoetarine	T48.6X1	T48.6X2	T48.6X3	T48.6X4	T48.6X5	T48.6X6
Isoethadione	T42.2X1	T42.2X2	T42.2X3	T42.2X4	T42.2X5	T42.2X6
Isoetharine	T44.5X1	T44.5X2	T44.5X3	T44.5X4	T44.5X5	T44.5X6
Isoflurane	T41.0X1	T41.0X2	T41.0X3	T41.0X4	T41.0X5	T41.0X6
Isoflurophate	T44.0X1	T44.0X2	T44.0X3	T44.0X4	T44.0X5	T44.0X6
Isomaltose, ferric complex	T45.4X1	T45.4X2	T45.4X3	T45.4X4	T45.4X5	T45.4X6
Isometheptene	T44.3X1	T44.3X2	T44.3X3	T44.3X4	T44.3X5	T44.3X6
Isoniazid	T37.1X1	T37.1X2	T37.1X3	T37.1X4	T37.1X5	T37.1X6
with						
rifampicin	T36.6X1	T36.6X2	T36.6X3	T36.6X4	T36.6X5	T36.6X6
thioacetazone	T37.1X1	T37.1X2	T37.1X3	T37.1X4	T37.1X5	T37.1X6
Isonicotinic acid hydrazide	T37.1X1	T37.1X2	T37.1X3	T37.1X4	T37.1X5	T37.1X6
Isonipecaine	T40.491	T40.492	T40.493	T40.494	T40.495	T40.496
Isopentaquine	T37.2X1	T37.2X2	T37.2X3	T37.2X4	T37.2X5	T37.2X6
Isophane insulin	T38.3X1	T38.3X2	T38.3X3	T38.3X4	T38.3X5	T38.3X6
Isophorone	T65.891	T65.892	T65.893	T65.894	—	—
Isophosphamide	T45.1X1	T45.1X2	T45.1X3	T45.1X4	T45.1X5	T45.1X6
Isopregnenone	T38.5X1	T38.5X2	T38.5X3	T38.5X4	T38.5X5	T38.5X6
Isoprenaline	T48.6X1	T48.6X2	T48.6X3	T48.6X4	T48.6X5	T48.6X6
Isopromethazine	T43.3X1	T43.3X2	T43.3X3	T43.3X4	T43.3X5	T43.3X6

◀ New   ◀▌ Revised   ~~deleted~~ Deleted

Substance	Poisoning, Accidental (Unintentional)	Poisoning, Intentional Self-Harm	Poisoning, Assault	Poisoning, Undetermined	Adverse Effect	Underdosing
External Cause (T-Code)						
Isopropamide	T44.3X1	T44.3X2	T44.3X3	T44.3X4	T44.3X5	T44.3X6
iodide	T44.3X1	T44.3X2	T44.3X3	T44.3X4	T44.3X5	T44.3X6
Isopropanol	T51.2X1	T51.2X2	T51.2X3	T51.2X4	—	—
Isopropyl						
acetate	T52.8X1	T52.8X2	T52.8X3	T52.8X4	—	—
alcohol	T51.2X1	T51.2X2	T51.2X3	T51.2X4	—	—
medicinal	T49.4X1	T49.4X2	T49.4X3	T49.4X4	T49.4X5	T49.4X6
ether	T52.8X1	T52.8X2	T52.8X3	T52.8X4	—	—
Isopropylaminophena-zone	T39.2X1	T39.2X2	T39.2X3	T39.2X4	T39.2X5	T39.2X6
Isoproterenol	T48.6X1	T48.6X2	T48.6X3	T48.6X4	T48.6X5	T48.6X6
Isosorbide dinitrate	T46.3X1	T46.3X2	T46.3X3	T46.3X4	T46.3X5	T46.3X6
Isothipendyl	T45.0X1	T45.0X2	T45.0X3	T45.0X4	T45.0X5	T45.0X6
Isotretinoin	T50.991	T50.992	T50.993	T50.994	T50.995	T50.996
Isoxazolyl penicillin	T36.0X1	T36.0X2	T36.0X3	T36.0X4	T36.0X5	T36.0X6
Isoxicam	T39.391	T39.392	T39.393	T39.394	T39.395	T39.396
Isoxsuprine	T46.7X1	T46.7X2	T46.7X3	T46.7X4	T46.7X5	T46.7X6
Ispagula	T47.4X1	T47.4X2	T47.4X3	T47.4X4	T47.4X5	T47.4X6
husk	T47.4X1	T47.4X2	T47.4X3	T47.4X4	T47.4X5	T47.4X6
Isradipine	T46.1X1	T46.1X2	T46.1X3	T46.1X4	T46.1X5	T46.1X6
I-thyroxine sodium	T38.1X1	T38.1X2	T38.1X3	T38.1X4	T38.1X5	T38.1X6
Itraconazole	T37.8X1	T37.8X2	T37.8X3	T37.8X4	T37.8X5	T37.8X6
Itramin tosilate	T46.3X1	T46.3X2	T46.3X3	T46.3X4	T46.3X5	T46.3X6
Ivermectin	T37.4X1	T37.4X2	T37.4X3	T37.4X4	T37.4X5	T37.4X6
Izoniazid	T37.1X1	T37.1X2	T37.1X3	T37.1X4	T37.1X5	T37.1X6
with thioacetazone	T37.1X1	T37.1X2	T37.1X3	T37.1X4	T37.1X5	T37.1X6
J						
Jalap	T47.2X1	T47.2X2	T47.2X3	T47.2X4	T47.2X5	T47.2X6
Jamaica						
dogwood (bark)	T39.8X1	T39.8X2	T39.8X3	T39.8X4	T39.8X5	T39.8X6
ginger	T65.891	T65.892	T65.893	T65.894	—	—
root	T62.2X1	T62.2X2	T62.2X3	T62.2X4	—	—
Jatropha	T62.2X1	T62.2X2	T62.2X3	T62.2X4	—	—
curcas	T62.2X1	T62.2X2	T62.2X3	T62.2X4	—	—
Jectofer	T45.4X1	T45.4X2	T45.4X3	T45.4X4	T45.4X5	T45.4X6
Jellyfish (sting)	T63.621	T63.622	T63.623	T63.624	—	—
Jequirity (bean)	T62.2X1	T62.2X2	T62.2X3	T62.2X4	—	—
Jimson weed (stramonium)	T62.2X1	T62.2X2	T62.2X3	T62.2X4	—	—
seeds	T62.2X1	T62.2X2	T62.2X3	T62.2X4	—	—
Josamycin	T36.3X1	T36.3X2	T36.3X3	T36.3X4	T36.3X5	T36.3X6
Juniper tar	T49.1X1	T49.1X2	T49.1X3	T49.1X4	T49.1X5	T49.1X6

Substance	Poisoning, Accidental (Unintentional)	Poisoning, Intentional Self-Harm	Poisoning, Assault	Poisoning, Undetermined	Adverse Effect	Underdosing
External Cause (T-Code)						
K						
Kallidinogenase	T46.7X1	T46.7X2	T46.7X3	T46.7X4	T46.7X5	T46.7X6
Kallikrein	T46.7X1	T46.7X2	T46.7X3	T46.7X4	T46.7X5	T46.7X6
Kanamycin	T36.5X1	T36.5X2	T36.5X3	T36.5X4	T36.5X5	T36.5X6
Kantrex	T36.5X1	T36.5X2	T36.5X3	T36.5X4	T36.5X5	T36.5X6
Kaolin	T47.6X1	T47.6X2	T47.6X3	T47.6X4	T47.6X5	T47.6X6
light	T47.6X1	T47.6X2	T47.6X3	T47.6X4	T47.6X5	T47.6X6
Karaya (gum)	T47.4X1	T47.4X2	T47.4X3	T47.4X4	T47.4X5	T47.4X6
Kebuzone	T39.2X1	T39.2X2	T39.2X3	T39.2X4	T39.2X5	T39.2X6
Kelevan	T60.1X1	T60.1X2	T60.1X3	T60.1X4	—	—
Kemithal	T41.1X1	T41.1X2	T41.1X3	T41.1X4	T41.1X5	T41.1X6
Kenacort	T38.0X1	T38.0X2	T38.0X3	T38.0X4	T38.0X5	T38.0X6
Keratolytic drug NEC	T49.4X1	T49.4X2	T49.4X3	T49.4X4	T49.4X5	T49.4X6
anthracene	T49.4X1	T49.4X2	T49.4X3	T49.4X4	T49.4X5	T49.4X6
Keratoplastic NEC	T49.4X1	T49.4X2	T49.4X3	T49.4X4	T49.4X5	T49.4X6
Kerosene, kerosine (fuel) (solvent) NEC	T52.0X1	T52.0X2	T52.0X3	T52.0X4	—	—
insecticide	T52.0X1	T52.0X2	T52.0X3	T52.0X4	—	—
vapor	T52.0X1	T52.0X2	T52.0X3	T52.0X4	—	—
Ketamine	T41.291	T41.292	T41.293	T41.294	T41.295	T41.296
Ketazolam	T42.4X1	T42.4X2	T42.4X3	T42.4X4	T42.4X5	T42.4X6
Ketazon	T39.2X1	T39.2X2	T39.2X3	T39.2X4	T39.2X5	T39.2X6
Ketobemidone	T40.491	T40.492	T40.493	T40.494	—	—
Ketoconazole	T49.0X1	T49.0X2	T49.0X3	T49.0X4	T49.0X5	T49.0X6
Ketols	T52.4X1	T52.4X2	T52.4X3	T52.4X4	—	—
Ketone oils	T52.4X1	T52.4X2	T52.4X3	T52.4X4	—	—
Ketoprofen	T39.311	T39.312	T39.313	T39.314	T39.315	T39.316
Ketorolac	T39.8X1	T39.8X2	T39.8X3	T39.8X4	T39.8X5	T39.8X6
Ketotifen	T45.0X1	T45.0X2	T45.0X3	T45.0X4	T45.0X5	T45.0X6
Khat	T43.691	T43.692	T43.693	T43.694	—	—
Khellin	T46.3X1	T46.3X2	T46.3X3	T46.3X4	T46.3X5	T46.3X6
Khelloside	T46.3X1	T46.3X2	T46.3X3	T46.3X4	T46.3X5	T46.3X6
Kiln gas or vapor (carbon monoxide)	T58.8X1	T58.8X2	T58.8X3	T58.8X4	—	—
Kitasamycin	T36.3X1	T36.3X2	T36.3X3	T36.3X4	T36.3X5	T36.3X6
Konsyl	T47.4X1	T47.4X2	T47.4X3	T47.4X4	T47.4X5	T47.4X6
Kosam seed	T62.2X1	T62.2X2	T62.2X3	T62.2X4	—	—
Krait (venom)	T63.091	T63.092	T63.093	T63.094	—	—
Kwell (insecticide)	T60.1X1	T60.1X2	T60.1X3	T60.1X4	—	—
anti-infective (topical)	T49.0X1	T49.0X2	T49.0X3	T49.0X4	T49.0X5	T49.0X6

◀ New ◀ Revised ~~deleted~~ Deleted

Substance	Poisoning, Accidental (Unintentional)	Poisoning, Intentional Self-Harm	Poisoning, Assault	Poisoning, Undetermined	Adverse Effect	Underdosing
L						
Labetalol	T44.8X1	T44.8X2	T44.8X3	T44.8X4	T44.8X5	T44.8X6
Laburnum (seeds)	T62.2X1	T62.2X2	T62.2X3	T62.2X4	—	—
leaves	T62.2X1	T62.2X2	T62.2X3	T62.2X4	—	—
Lachesine	T49.5X1	T49.5X2	T49.5X3	T49.5X4	T49.5X5	T49.5X6
Lacidipine	T46.5X1	T46.5X2	T46.5X3	T46.5X4	T46.5X5	T46.5X6
Lacquer	T65.6X1	T65.6X2	T65.6X3	T65.6X4	—	—
Lacrimogenic gas	T59.3X1	T59.3X2	T59.3X3	T59.3X4	—	—
Lactated potassic saline	T50.3X1	T50.3X2	T50.3X3	T50.3X4	T50.3X5	T50.3X6
Lactic acid	T49.8X1	T49.8X2	T49.8X3	T49.8X4	T49.8X5	T49.8X6
Lactobacillus						
acidophilus	T47.6X1	T47.6X2	T47.6X3	T47.6X4	T47.6X5	T47.6X6
compound	T47.6X1	T47.6X2	T47.6X3	T47.6X4	T47.6X5	T47.6X6
bifidus, lyophilized	T47.6X1	T47.6X2	T47.6X3	T47.6X4	T47.6X5	T47.6X6
bulgaricus	T47.6X1	T47.6X2	T47.6X3	T47.6X4	T47.6X5	T47.6X6
sporogenes	T47.6X1	T47.6X2	T47.6X3	T47.6X4	T47.6X5	T47.6X6
Lactoflavin	T45.2X1	T45.2X2	T45.2X3	T45.2X4	T45.2X5	T45.2X6
Lactose (as excipient)	T50.901	T50.902	T50.903	T50.904	T50.905	T50.906
Lactuca (virosa) (extract)	T42.6X1	T42.6X2	T42.6X3	T42.6X4	T42.6X5	T42.6X6
Lactucarium	T42.6X1	T42.6X2	T42.6X3	T42.6X4	T42.6X5	T42.6X6
Lactulose	T47.3X1	T47.3X2	T47.3X3	T47.3X4	T47.3X5	T47.3X6
Laevo — see Levo-						
Lanatosides	T46.0X1	T46.0X2	T46.0X3	T46.0X4	T46.0X5	T46.0X6
Lanolin	T49.3X1	T49.3X2	T49.3X3	T49.3X4	T49.3X5	T49.3X6
Largactil	T43.3X1	T43.3X2	T43.3X3	T43.3X4	T43.3X5	T43.3X6
Larkspur	T62.2X1	T62.2X2	T62.2X3	T62.2X4	—	—
Laroxyl	T43.011	T43.012	T43.013	T43.014	T43.015	T43.016
Lassar's paste	T49.4X1	T49.4X2	T49.4X3	T49.4X4	T49.4X5	T49.4X6
Lasix	T50.1X1	T50.1X2	T50.1X3	T50.1X4	T50.1X5	T50.1X6
Latamoxef	T36.1X1	T36.1X2	T36.1X3	T36.1X4	T36.1X5	T36.1X6
Latex	T65.811	T65.812	T65.813	T65.814	—	—
Lathyrus (seed)	T62.2X1	T62.2X2	T62.2X3	T62.2X4	—	—
Laudanum	T40.0X1	T40.0X2	T40.0X3	T40.0X4	T40.0X5	T40.0X6
Laudexium	T48.1X1	T48.1X2	T48.1X3	T48.1X4	T48.1X5	T48.1X6
Laughing gas	T41.0X1	T41.0X2	T41.0X3	T41.0X4	T41.0X5	T41.0X6
Laurel, black or cherry	T62.2X1	T62.2X2	T62.2X3	T62.2X4	—	—
Laurolinium	T49.0X1	T49.0X2	T49.0X3	T49.0X4	T49.0X5	T49.0X6
Lauryl sulfoacetate	T49.2X1	T49.2X2	T49.2X3	T49.2X4	T49.2X5	T49.2X6

Substance	Poisoning, Accidental (Unintentional)	Poisoning, Intentional Self-Harm	Poisoning, Assault	Poisoning, Undetermined	Adverse Effect	Underdosing
Laxative NEC	T47.4X1	T47.4X2	T47.4X3	T47.4X4	T47.4X5	T47.4X6
osmotic	T47.3X1	T47.3X2	T47.3X3	T47.3X4	T47.3X5	T47.3X6
saline	T47.3X1	T47.3X2	T47.3X3	T47.3X4	T47.3X5	T47.3X6
stimulant	T47.2X1	T47.2X2	T47.2X3	T47.2X4	T47.2X5	T47.2X6
L-dopa	T42.8X1	T42.8X2	T42.8X3	T42.8X4	T42.8X5	T42.8X6
Lead (dust) (fumes) (vapor) NEC	T56.0X1	T56.0X2	T56.0X3	T56.0X4	—	—
acetate	T49.2X1	T49.2X2	T49.2X3	T49.2X4	T49.2X5	T49.2X6
alkyl (fuel additive)	T56.0X1	T56.0X2	T56.0X3	T56.0X4	—	—
anti-infectives	T37.8X1	T37.8X2	T37.8X3	T37.8X4	T37.8X5	T37.8X6
antiknock compound (tetraethyl)	T56.0X1	T56.0X2	T56.0X3	T56.0X4	—	—
arsenate, arsenite (dust) (herbicide) (insecticide) (vapor)	T57.0X1	T57.0X2	T57.0X3	T57.0X4	—	—
carbonate	T56.0X1	T56.0X2	T56.0X3	T56.0X4	—	—
paint	T56.0X1	T56.0X2	T56.0X3	T56.0X4	—	—
chromate	T56.0X1	T56.0X2	T56.0X3	T56.0X4	—	—
paint	T56.0X1	T56.0X2	T56.0X3	T56.0X4	—	—
dioxide	T56.0X1	T56.0X2	T56.0X3	T56.0X4	—	—
inorganic	T56.0X1	T56.0X2	T56.0X3	T56.0X4	—	—
iodide	T56.0X1	T56.0X2	T56.0X3	T56.0X4	—	—
pigment (paint)	T56.0X1	T56.0X2	T56.0X3	T56.0X4	—	—
monoxide (dust)	T56.0X1	T56.0X2	T56.0X3	T56.0X4	—	—
paint	T56.0X1	T56.0X2	T56.0X3	T56.0X4	—	—
organic	T56.0X1	T56.0X2	T56.0X3	T56.0X4	—	—
oxide	T56.0X1	T56.0X2	T56.0X3	T56.0X4	—	—
paint	T56.0X1	T56.0X2	T56.0X3	T56.0X4	—	—
paint	T56.0X1	T56.0X2	T56.0X3	T56.0X4	—	—
salts	T56.0X1	T56.0X2	T56.0X3	T56.0X4	—	—
specified compound NEC	T56.0X1	T56.0X2	T56.0X3	T56.0X4	—	—
tetra-ethyl	T56.0X1	T56.0X2	T56.0X3	T56.0X4	—	—
Lebanese red	T40.711	T40.712	T40.713	T40.714	T40.715	T40.716
Lefetamine	T39.8X1	T39.8X2	T39.8X3	T39.8X4	T39.8X5	T39.8X6
Lenperone	T43.4X1	T43.4X2	T43.4X3	T43.4X4	T43.4X5	T43.4X6
Lente lietin (insulin)	T38.3X1	T38.3X2	T38.3X3	T38.3X4	T38.3X5	T38.3X6
Leptazol	T50.7X1	T50.7X2	T50.7X3	T50.7X4	T50.7X5	T50.7X6
Leptophos	T60.0X1	T60.0X2	T60.0X3	T60.0X4	—	—
Leritine	T40.2X1	T40.2X2	T40.2X3	T40.2X4	T40.2X5	T40.2X6
Letosteine	T48.4X1	T48.4X2	T48.4X3	T48.4X4	T48.4X5	T48.4X6
Letter	T38.1X1	T38.1X2	T38.1X3	T38.1X4	T38.1X5	T38.1X6
Lettuce opium	T42.6X1	T42.6X2	T42.6X3	T42.6X4	T42.6X5	T42.6X6
Leucinocaine	T41.3X1	T41.3X2	T41.3X3	T41.3X4	T41.3X5	T41.3X6

◀ New   ◀ Revised   deleted Deleted

	External Cause (T-Code)					
Substance	Poisoning, Accidental (Unintentional)	Poisoning, Intentional Self-Harm	Poisoning, Assault	Poisoning, Undetermined	Adverse Effect	Underdosing
Leucocianidol	T46.991	T46.992	T46.993	T46.994	T46.995	T46.996
Leucovorin (factor)	T45.8X1	T45.8X2	T45.8X3	T45.8X4	T45.8X5	T45.8X6
Leukeran	T45.1X1	T45.1X2	T45.1X3	T45.1X4	T45.1X5	T45.1X6
Leuprolide	T38.891	T38.892	T38.893	T38.894	T38.895	T38.896
Levalbuterol	T48.6X1	T48.6X2	T48.6X3	T48.6X4	T48.6X5	T48.6X6
Levallorphan	T50.7X1	T50.7X2	T50.7X3	T50.7X4	T50.7X5	T50.7X6
Levamisole	T37.4X1	T37.4X2	T37.4X3	T37.4X4	T37.4X5	T37.4X6
Levanil	T42.6X1	T42.6X2	T42.6X3	T42.6X4	T42.6X5	T42.6X6
Levarterenol	T44.4X1	T44.4X2	T44.4X3	T44.4X4	T44.4X5	T44.4X6
Levdropropizine	T48.3X1	T48.3X2	T48.3X3	T48.3X4	T48.3X5	T48.3X6
Levobunolol	T49.5X1	T49.5X2	T49.5X3	T49.5X4	T49.5X5	T49.5X6
Levocabastine (hydrochloride)	T45.0X1	T45.0X2	T45.0X3	T45.0X4	T45.0X5	T45.0X6
Levocarnitine	T50.991	T50.992	T50.993	T50.994	T50.995	T50.996
Levodopa	T42.8X1	T42.8X2	T42.8X3	T42.8X4	T42.8X5	T42.8X6
with carbidopa	T42.8X1	T42.8X2	T42.8X3	T42.8X4	T42.8X5	T42.8X6
Levo-dromoran	T40.2X1	T40.2X2	T40.2X3	T40.2X4	T40.2X5	T40.2X6
Levoglutamide	T50.991	T50.992	T50.993	T50.994	T50.995	T50.996
Levoid	T38.1X1	T38.1X2	T38.1X3	T38.1X4	T38.1X5	T38.1X6
Levo-iso-methadone	T40.3X1	T40.3X2	T40.3X3	T40.3X4	T40.3X5	T40.3X6
Levomepromazine	T43.3X1	T43.3X2	T43.3X3	T43.3X4	T43.3X5	T43.3X6
Levonordefrin	T49.6X1	T49.6X2	T49.6X3	T49.6X4	T49.6X5	T49.6X6
Levonorgestrel	T38.4X1	T38.4X2	T38.4X3	T38.4X4	T38.4X5	T38.4X6
with ethinylestradiol	T38.5X1	T38.5X2	T38.5X3	T38.5X4	T38.5X5	T38.5X6
Levopromazine	T43.3X1	T43.3X2	T43.3X3	T43.3X4	T43.3X5	T43.3X6
Levoprome	T42.6X1	T42.6X2	T42.6X3	T42.6X4	T42.6X5	T42.6X6
Levopropoxyphene	T40.491	T40.492	T40.493	T40.494	T40.495	T40.496
Levopropylhexedrine	T50.5X1	T50.5X2	T50.5X3	T50.5X4	T50.5X5	T50.5X6
Levoproxyphylline	T48.6X1	T48.6X2	T48.6X3	T48.6X4	T48.6X5	T48.6X6
Levorphanol	T40.491	T40.492	T40.493	T40.494	T40.495	T40.496
Levothyroxine	T38.1X1	T38.1X2	T38.1X3	T38.1X4	T38.1X5	T38.1X6
sodium	T38.1X1	T38.1X2	T38.1X3	T38.1X4	T38.1X5	T38.1X6
Levsin	T44.3X1	T44.3X2	T44.3X3	T44.3X4	T44.3X5	T44.3X6
Levulose	T50.3X1	T50.3X2	T50.3X3	T50.3X4	T50.3X5	T50.3X6
Lewisite (gas), not in war	T57.0X1	T57.0X2	T57.0X3	T57.0X4	—	—
Librium	T42.4X1	T42.4X2	T42.4X3	T42.4X4	T42.4X5	T42.4X6
Lidex	T49.0X1	T49.0X2	T49.0X3	T49.0X4	T49.0X5	T49.0X6
Lidocaine	T41.3X1	T41.3X2	T41.3X3	T41.3X4	T41.3X5	T41.3X6
regional	T41.3X1	T41.3X2	T41.3X3	T41.3X4	T41.3X5	T41.3X6
spinal	T41.3X1	T41.3X2	T41.3X3	T41.3X4	T41.3X5	T41.3X6
Lidofenin	T50.8X1	T50.8X2	T50.8X3	T50.8X4	T50.8X5	T50.8X6
Lidoflazine	T46.1X1	T46.1X2	T46.1X3	T46.1X4	T46.1X5	T46.1X6
Lighter fluid	T52.0X1	T52.0X2	T52.0X3	T52.0X4	—	—

	External Cause (T-Code)					
Substance	Poisoning, Accidental (Unintentional)	Poisoning, Intentional Self-Harm	Poisoning, Assault	Poisoning, Undetermined	Adverse Effect	Underdosing
Lignin hemicellulose	T47.6X1	T47.6X2	T47.6X3	T47.6X4	T47.6X5	T47.6X6
Lignocaine	T41.3X1	T41.3X2	T41.3X3	T41.3X4	T41.3X5	T41.3X6
regional	T41.3X1	T41.3X2	T41.3X3	T41.3X4	T41.3X5	T41.3X6
spinal	T41.3X1	T41.3X2	T41.3X3	T41.3X4	T41.3X5	T41.3X6
Ligroin(e) (solvent)	T52.0X1	T52.0X2	T52.0X3	T52.0X4	—	—
vapor	T59.891	T59.892	T59.893	T59.894	—	—
Ligustrum vulgare	T62.2X1	T62.2X2	T62.2X3	T62.2X4	—	—
Lily of the valley	T62.2X1	T62.2X2	T62.2X3	T62.2X4	—	—
Lime (chloride)	T54.3X1	T54.3X2	T54.3X3	T54.3X4	—	—
Limonene	T52.8X1	T52.8X2	T52.8X3	T52.8X4	—	—
Lincomycin	T36.8X1	T36.8X2	T36.8X3	T36.8X4	T36.8X5	T36.8X6
Lindane (insecticide) (nonmedicinal) (vapor)	T53.6X1	T53.6X2	T53.6X3	T53.6X4	—	—
medicinal	T49.0X1	T49.0X2	T49.0X3	T49.0X4	T49.0X5	T49.0X6
Liniments NEC	T49.91	T49.92	T49.93	T49.94	T49.95	T49.96
Linoleic acid	T46.6X1	T46.6X2	T46.6X3	T46.6X4	T46.6X5	T46.6X6
Linolenic acid	T46.6X1	T46.6X2	T46.6X3	T46.6X4	T46.6X5	T46.6X6
Linseed	T47.4X1	T47.4X2	T47.4X3	T47.4X4	T47.4X5	T47.4X6
Liothyronine	T38.1X1	T38.1X2	T38.1X3	T38.1X4	T38.1X5	T38.1X6
Liotrix	T38.1X1	T38.1X2	T38.1X3	T38.1X4	T38.1X5	T38.1X6
Lipancreatin	T47.5X1	T47.5X2	T47.5X3	T47.5X4	T47.5X5	T47.5X6
Lipo-alprostadil	T46.7X1	T46.7X2	T46.7X3	T46.7X4	T46.7X5	T46.7X6
Lipo-Lutin	T38.5X1	T38.5X2	T38.5X3	T38.5X4	T38.5X5	T38.5X6
Lipotropic drug NEC	T50.901	T50.902	T50.903	T50.904	T50.905	T50.906
Liquefied petroleum gases	T59.891	T59.892	T59.893	T59.894	—	—
piped (pure or mixed with air)	T59.891	T59.892	T59.893	T59.894	—	—
Liquid						
paraffin	T47.4X1	T47.4X2	T47.4X3	T47.4X4	T47.4X5	T47.4X6
petrolatum	T47.4X1	T47.4X2	T47.4X3	T47.4X4	T47.4X5	T47.4X6
topical	T49.3X1	T49.3X2	T49.3X3	T49.3X4	T49.3X5	T49.3X6
specified NEC	T65.891	T65.892	T65.893	T65.894	—	—
substance	T65.91	T65.92	T65.93	T65.94	—	—
Liquor creosolis compositus	T65.891	T65.892	T65.893	T65.894	—	—
Liquorice	T48.4X1	T48.4X2	T48.4X3	T48.4X4	T48.4X5	T48.4X6
extract	T47.8X1	T47.8X2	T47.8X3	T47.8X4	T47.8X5	T47.8X6
Lirugen	T50.991	T50.992	T50.993	T50.994	T50.995	T50.996
Lisinopril	T46.4X1	T46.4X2	T46.4X3	T46.4X4	T46.4X5	T46.4X6
Lisuride	T42.8X1	T42.8X2	T42.8X3	T42.8X4	T42.8X5	T42.8X6
Lithane	T43.8X1	T43.8X2	T43.8X3	T43.8X4	T43.8X5	T43.8X6
Lithium	T56.891	T56.892	T56.893	T56.894	—	—
gluconate	T43.591	T43.592	T43.593	T43.594	T43.595	T43.596
salts (carbonate)	T43.591	T43.592	T43.593	T43.594	T43.595	T43.596

◀ New   ◀ Revised   ~~deleted~~ Deleted

Substance	External Cause (T-Code)					
	Poisoning, Accidental (Unintentional)	Poisoning, Intentional Self-Harm	Poisoning, Assault	Poisoning, Undetermined	Adverse Effect	Underdosing
Lithonate	T43.8X1	T43.8X2	T43.8X3	T43.8X4	T43.8X5	T43.8X6
Liver						
extract	T45.8X1	T45.8X2	T45.8X3	T45.8X4	T45.8X5	T45.8X6
for parenteral use	T45.8X1	T45.8X2	T45.8X3	T45.8X4	T45.8X5	T45.8X6
fraction 1	T45.8X1	T45.8X2	T45.8X3	T45.8X4	T45.8X5	T45.8X6
hydrolysate	T45.8X1	T45.8X2	T45.8X3	T45.8X4	T45.8X5	T45.8X6
Lizard (bite) (venom)	T63.121	T63.122	T63.123	T63.124	—	—
LMD	T45.8X1	T45.8X2	T45.8X3	T45.8X4	T45.8X5	T45.8X6
Lobelia	T62.2X1	T62.2X2	T62.2X3	T62.2X4		
Lobeline	T50.7X1	T50.7X2	T50.7X3	T50.7X4	T50.7X5	T50.7X6
Local action drug NEC	T49.8X1	T49.8X2	T49.8X3	T49.8X4	T49.8X5	T49.8X6
Locorten	T49.0X1	T49.0X2	T49.0X3	T49.0X4	T49.0X5	T49.0X6
Lofepramine	T43.011	T43.012	T43.013	T43.014	T43.015	T43.016
Lolium temulentum	T62.2X1	T62.2X2	T62.2X3	T62.2X4	—	—
Lomotil	T47.6X1	T47.6X2	T47.6X3	T47.6X4	T47.6X5	T47.6X6
Lomustine	T45.1X1	T45.1X2	T45.1X3	T45.1X4	T45.1X5	T45.1X6
Lonidamine	T45.1X1	T45.1X2	T45.1X3	T45.1X4	T45.1X5	T45.1X6
Loperamide	T47.6X1	T47.6X2	T47.6X3	T47.6X4	T47.6X5	T47.6X6
Loprazolam	T42.4X1	T42.4X2	T42.4X3	T42.4X4	T42.4X5	T42.4X6
Lorajmine	T46.2X1	T46.2X2	T46.2X3	T46.2X4	T46.2X5	T46.2X6
Loratidine	T45.0X1	T45.0X2	T45.0X3	T45.0X4	T45.0X5	T45.0X6
Lorazepam	T42.4X1	T42.4X2	T42.4X3	T42.4X4	T42.4X5	T42.4X6
Lorcainide	T46.2X1	T46.2X2	T46.2X3	T46.2X4	T46.2X5	T46.2X6
Lormetazepam	T42.4X1	T42.4X2	T42.4X3	T42.4X4	T42.4X5	T42.4X6
Lotions NEC	T49.91	T49.92	T49.93	T49.94	T49.95	T49.96
Lotusate	T42.3X1	T42.3X2	T42.3X3	T42.3X4	T42.3X5	T42.3X6
Lovastatin	T46.6X1	T46.6X2	T46.6X3	T46.6X4	T46.6X5	T46.6X6
Loxapine	T43.591	T43.592	T43.593	T43.594	T43.595	T43.596
Lowila	T49.2X1	T49.2X2	T49.2X3	T49.2X4	T49.2X5	T49.2X6
Lozenges (throat)	T49.6X1	T49.6X2	T49.6X3	T49.6X4	T49.6X5	T49.6X6
LSD	T40.8X1	T40.8X2	T40.8X3	T40.8X4	—	—
L-Tryptophan — see Amino acid						
Lubricant, eye	T49.5X1	T49.5X2	T49.5X3	T49.5X4	T49.5X5	T49.5X6
Lubricating oil NEC	T52.0X1	T52.0X2	T52.0X3	T52.0X4	—	—
Lucanthone	T37.4X1	T37.4X2	T37.4X3	T37.4X4	T37.4X5	T37.4X6
Luminal	T42.3X1	T42.3X2	T42.3X3	T42.3X4	T42.3X5	T42.3X6
Lung irritant (gas) NEC	T59.91	T59.92	T59.93	T59.94	—	—
Luteinizing hormone	T38.811	T38.812	T38.813	T38.814	T38.815	T38.816
Lutocylol	T38.5X1	T38.5X2	T38.5X3	T38.5X4	T38.5X5	T38.5X6
Lutromone	T38.5X1	T38.5X2	T38.5X3	T38.5X4	T38.5X5	T38.5X6
Lututrin	T48.291	T48.292	T48.293	T48.294	T48.295	T48.296
Lye (Concentrated)	T54.3X1	T54.3X2	T54.3X3	T54.3X4	—	—

Substance	External Cause (T-Code)					
	Poisoning, Accidental (Unintentional)	Poisoning, Intentional Self-Harm	Poisoning, Assault	Poisoning, Undetermined	Adverse Effect	Underdosing
Lygranum (skin test)	T50.8X1	T50.8X2	T50.8X3	T50.8X4	T50.8X5	T50.8X6
Lymecycline	T36.4X1	T36.4X2	T36.4X3	T36.4X4	T36.4X5	T36.4X6
Lymphogranuloma venereum antigen	T50.8X1	T50.8X2	T50.8X3	T50.8X4	T50.8X5	T50.8X6
Lynestrenol	T38.4X1	T38.4X2	T38.4X3	T38.4X4	T38.4X5	T38.4X6
Lypressin	T38.891	T38.892	T38.893	T38.894	T38.895	T38.896
Lyovac Sodium Edecrin	T50.1X1	T50.1X2	T50.1X3	T50.1X4	T50.1X5	T50.1X6
Lysergic acid diethylamide	T40.8X1	T40.8X2	T40.8X3	T40.8X4	—	—
Lysergide	T40.8X1	T40.8X2	T40.8X3	T40.8X4	—	—
Lysine vasopressin	T38.891	T38.892	T38.893	T38.894	T38.895	T38.896
Lysol	T54.1X1	T54.1X2	T54.1X3	T54.1X4	—	—
Lysozyme	T49.0X1	T49.0X2	T49.0X3	T49.0X4	T49.0X5	T49.0X6
Lytta (vitatta)	T49.8X1	T49.8X2	T49.8X3	T49.8X4	T49.8X5	T49.8X6
M						
Mace	T59.3X1	T59.3X2	T59.3X3	T59.3X4	—	—
Macrogol	T50.991	T50.992	T50.993	T50.994	T50.995	T50.996
Macrolide						
anabolic drug	T38.7X1	T38.7X2	T38.7X3	T38.7X4	T38.7X5	T38.7X6
antibiotic	T36.3X1	T36.3X2	T36.3X3	T36.3X4	T36.3X5	T36.3X6
Mafenide	T49.0X1	T49.0X2	T49.0X3	T49.0X4	T49.0X5	T49.0X6
Magaldrate	T47.1X1	T47.1X2	T47.1X3	T47.1X4	T47.1X5	T47.1X6
Magic mushroom	T40.991	T40.992	T40.993	T40.994		
Magnamycin	T36.8X1	T36.8X2	T36.8X3	T36.8X4	T36.8X5	T36.8X6
Magnesia magma	T47.1X1	T47.1X2	T47.1X3	T47.1X4	T47.1X5	T47.1X6
Magnesium NEC	T56.891	T56.892	T56.893	T56.894	—	—
carbonate	T47.1X1	T47.1X2	T47.1X3	T47.1X4	T47.1X5	T47.1X6
citrate	T47.4X1	T47.4X2	T47.4X3	T47.4X4	T47.4X5	T47.4X6
hydroxide	T47.1X1	T47.1X2	T47.1X3	T47.1X4	T47.1X5	T47.1X6
oxide	T47.1X1	T47.1X2	T47.1X3	T47.1X4	T47.1X5	T47.1X6
peroxide	T49.0X1	T49.0X2	T49.0X3	T49.0X4	T49.0X5	T49.0X6
salicylate	T39.091	T39.092	T39.093	T39.094	T39.095	T39.096
silicofluoride	T50.3X1	T50.3X2	T50.3X3	T50.3X4	T50.3X5	T50.3X6
sulfate	T47.4X1	T47.4X2	T47.4X3	T47.4X4	T47.4X5	T47.4X6
thiosulfate	T45.0X1	T45.0X2	T45.0X3	T45.0X4	T45.0X5	T45.0X6
trisilicate	T47.1X1	T47.1X2	T47.1X3	T47.1X4	T47.1X5	T47.1X6
Malathion (medicinal)	T49.0X1	T49.0X2	T49.0X3	T49.0X4	T49.0X5	T49.0X6
insecticide	T60.0X1	T60.0X2	T60.0X3	T60.0X4	—	—
Male fern extract	T37.4X1	T37.4X2	T37.4X3	T37.4X4	T37.4X5	T37.4X6
M-AMSA	T45.1X1	T45.1X2	T45.1X3	T45.1X4	T45.1X5	T45.1X6
Mandelic acid	T37.8X1	T37.8X2	T37.8X3	T37.8X4	T37.8X5	T37.8X6
Manganese (dioxide) (salts)	T57.2X1	T57.2X2	T57.2X3	T57.2X4	—	—
medicinal	T50.991	T50.992	T50.993	T50.994	T50.995	T50.996

◀ New   ◀ Revised   ~~deleted~~ Deleted

TABLE OF DRUGS AND CHEMICALS

Substance	External Cause (T-Code)					
	Poisoning, Accidental (Unintentional)	Poisoning, Intentional Self-Harm	Poisoning, Assault	Poisoning, Undetermined	Adverse Effect	Underdosing
Mannitol	T47.3X1	T47.3X2	T47.3X3	T47.3X4	T47.3X5	T47.3X6
hexanitrate	T46.3X1	T46.3X2	T46.3X3	T46.3X4	T46.3X5	T46.3X6
Mannomustine	T45.1X1	T45.1X2	T45.1X3	T45.1X4	T45.1X5	T45.1X6
MAO inhibitors	T43.1X1	T43.1X2	T43.1X3	T43.1X4	T43.1X5	T43.1X6
Mapharsen	T37.8X1	T37.8X2	T37.8X3	T37.8X4	T37.8X5	T37.8X6
Maphenide	T49.0X1	T49.0X2	T49.0X3	T49.0X4	T49.0X5	T49.0X6
Maprotiline	T43.021	T43.022	T43.023	T43.024	T43.025	T43.026
Marcaine	T41.3X1	T41.3X2	T41.3X3	T41.3X4	T41.3X5	T41.3X6
infiltration (subcutaneous)	T41.3X1	T41.3X2	T41.3X3	T41.3X4	T41.3X5	T41.3X6
nerve block (peripheral) (plexus)	T41.3X1	T41.3X2	T41.3X3	T41.3X4	T41.3X5	T41.3X6
Marezine	T45.0X1	T45.0X2	T45.0X3	T45.0X4	T45.0X5	T45.0X6
Marihuana	T40.711	T40.712	T40.713	T40.714	T40.715	T40.716
Marijuana	T40.711	T40.712	T40.713	T40.714	T40.715	T40.716
Marine (sting)	T63.691	T63.692	T63.693	T63.694	—	—
animals (sting)	T63.691	T63.692	T63.693	T63.694	—	—
plants (sting)	T63.711	T63.712	T63.713	T63.714	—	—
Marplan	T43.1X1	T43.1X2	T43.1X3	T43.1X4	T43.1X5	T43.1X6
Marsh gas	T59.891	T59.892	T59.893	T59.894	—	—
Marsilid	T43.1X1	T43.1X2	T43.1X3	T43.1X4	T43.1X5	T43.1X6
Matulane	T45.1X1	T45.1X2	T45.1X3	T45.1X4	T45.1X5	T45.1X6
Mazindol	T50.5X1	T50.5X2	T50.5X3	T50.5X4	T50.5X5	T50.5X6
MCPA	T60.3X1	T60.3X2	T60.3X3	T60.3X4	—	—
MDMA	T43.641	T43.642	T43.643	T43.644	—	—
Meadow saffron	T62.2X1	T62.2X2	T62.2X3	T62.2X4	—	—
Measles virus vaccine (attenuated)	T50.B91	T50.B92	T50.B93	T50.B94	T50.B95	T50.B96
Meat, noxious	T62.8X1	T62.8X2	T62.8X3	T62.8X4	—	—
Meballymal	T42.3X1	T42.3X2	T42.3X3	T42.3X4	T42.3X5	T42.3X6
Mebanazine	T43.1X1	T43.1X2	T43.1X3	T43.1X4	T43.1X5	T43.1X6
Mebaral	T42.3X1	T42.3X2	T42.3X3	T42.3X4	T42.3X5	T42.3X6
Mebendazole	T37.4X1	T37.4X2	T37.4X3	T37.4X4	T37.4X5	T37.4X6
Mebeverine	T44.3X1	T44.3X2	T44.3X3	T44.3X4	T44.3X5	T44.3X6
Mebhydrolin	T45.0X1	T45.0X2	T45.0X3	T45.0X4	T45.0X5	T45.0X6
Mebumal	T42.3X1	T42.3X2	T42.3X3	T42.3X4	T42.3X5	T42.3X6
Mebutamate	T43.591	T43.592	T43.593	T43.594	T43.595	T43.596
Mecamylamine	T44.2X1	T44.2X2	T44.2X3	T44.2X4	T44.2X5	T44.2X6
Mechlorethamine	T45.1X1	T45.1X2	T45.1X3	T45.1X4	T45.1X5	T45.1X6
Mecillinam	T36.0X1	T36.0X2	T36.0X3	T36.0X4	T36.0X5	T36.0X6
Meclizine (hydrochloride)	T45.0X1	T45.0X2	T45.0X3	T45.0X4	T45.0X5	T45.0X6
Meclocycline	T36.4X1	T36.4X2	T36.4X3	T36.4X4	T36.4X5	T36.4X6
Meclofenamate	T39.391	T39.392	T39.393	T39.394	T39.395	T39.396
Meclofenamic acid	T39.391	T39.392	T39.393	T39.394	T39.395	T39.396

Substance	External Cause (T-Code)					
	Poisoning, Accidental (Unintentional)	Poisoning, Intentional Self-Harm	Poisoning, Assault	Poisoning, Undetermined	Adverse Effect	Underdosing
Meclofenoxate	T43.691	T43.692	T43.693	T43.694	T43.695	T43.696
Meclozine	T45.0X1	T45.0X2	T45.0X3	T45.0X4	T45.0X5	T45.0X6
Mecobalamin	T45.8X1	T45.8X2	T45.8X3	T45.8X4	T45.8X5	T45.8X6
Mecoprop	T60.3X1	T60.3X2	T60.3X3	T60.3X4	—	—
Mecrilate	T49.3X1	T49.3X2	T49.3X3	T49.3X4	T49.3X5	T49.3X6
Mecysteine	T48.4X1	T48.4X2	T48.4X3	T48.4X4	T48.4X5	T48.4X6
Medazepam	T42.4X1	T42.4X2	T42.4X3	T42.4X4	T42.4X5	T42.4X6
Medicament NEC	T50.901	T50.902	T50.903	T50.904	T50.905	T50.906
Medinal	T42.3X1	T42.3X2	T42.3X3	T42.3X4	T42.3X5	T42.3X6
Medomin	T42.3X1	T42.3X2	T42.3X3	T42.3X4	T42.3X5	T42.3X6
Medrogestone	T38.5X1	T38.5X2	T38.5X3	T38.5X4	T38.5X5	T38.5X6
Medroxalol	T44.8X1	T44.8X2	T44.8X3	T44.8X4	T44.8X5	T44.8X6
Medroxyprogesterone acetate (depot)	T38.5X1	T38.5X2	T38.5X3	T38.5X4	T38.5X5	T38.5X6
Medrysone	T49.0X1	T49.0X2	T49.0X3	T49.0X4	T49.0X5	T49.0X6
Mefenamic acid	T39.391	T39.392	T39.393	T39.394	T39.395	T39.396
Mefenorex	T50.5X1	T50.5X2	T50.5X3	T50.5X4	T50.5X5	T50.5X6
Mefloquine	T37.2X1	T37.2X2	T37.2X3	T37.2X4	T37.2X5	T37.2X6
Mefruside	T50.2X1	T50.2X2	T50.2X3	T50.2X4	T50.2X5	T50.2X6
Megahallucinogen	T40.901	T40.902	T40.903	T40.904	T40.905	T40.906
Megestrol	T38.5X1	T38.5X2	T38.5X3	T38.5X4	T38.5X5	T38.5X6
Meglumine						
antimoniate	T37.8X1	T37.8X2	T37.8X3	T37.8X4	T37.8X5	T37.8X6
diatrizoate	T50.8X1	T50.8X2	T50.8X3	T50.8X4	T50.8X5	T50.8X6
iodipamide	T50.8X1	T50.8X2	T50.8X3	T50.8X4	T50.8X5	T50.8X6
iotroxate	T50.8X1	T50.8X2	T50.8X3	T50.8X4	T50.8X5	T50.8X6
MEK (methyl ethyl ketone)	T52.4X1	T52.4X2	T52.4X3	T52.4X4	—	—
Meladrazine	T44.3X1	T44.3X2	T44.3X3	T44.3X4	T44.3X5	T44.3X6
Meladinin	T49.3X1	T49.3X2	T49.3X3	T49.3X4	T49.3X5	T49.3X6
Melaleuca alternifolia oil	T49.0X1	T49.0X2	T49.0X3	T49.0X4	T49.0X5	T49.0X6
Melanizing agents	T49.3X1	T49.3X2	T49.3X3	T49.3X4	T49.3X5	T49.3X6
Melanocyte-stimulating hormone	T38.891	T38.892	T38.893	T38.894	T38.895	T38.896
Melarsonyl potassium	T37.3X1	T37.3X2	T37.3X3	T37.3X4	T37.3X5	T37.3X6
Melarsoprol	T37.3X1	T37.3X2	T37.3X3	T37.3X4	T37.3X5	T37.3X6
Melia azedarach	T62.2X1	T62.2X2	T62.2X3	T62.2X4	—	—
Melitracen	T43.011	T43.012	T43.013	T43.014	T43.015	T43.016
Mellaril	T43.3X1	T43.3X2	T43.3X3	T43.3X4	T43.3X5	T43.3X6
Meloxine	T49.3X1	T49.3X2	T49.3X3	T49.3X4	T49.3X5	T49.3X6
Melperone	T43.4X1	T43.4X2	T43.4X3	T43.4X4	T43.4X5	T43.4X6
Melphalan	T45.1X1	T45.1X2	T45.1X3	T45.1X4	T45.1X5	T45.1X6
Memantine	T43.8X1	T43.8X2	T43.8X3	T43.8X4	T43.8X5	T43.8X6

◀ New ◀ Revised ~~deleted~~ Deleted

	External Cause (T-Code)					
Substance	Poisoning, Accidental (Unintentional)	Poisoning, Intentional Self-Harm	Poisoning, Assault	Poisoning, Undetermined	Adverse Effect	Underdosing
Menadiol	T45.7X1	T45.7X2	T45.7X3	T45.7X4	T45.7X5	T45.7X6
sodium sulfate	T45.7X1	T45.7X2	T45.7X3	T45.7X4	T45.7X5	T45.7X6
Menadione	T45.7X1	T45.7X2	T45.7X3	T45.7X4	T45.7X5	T45.7X6
sodium bisulfite	T45.7X1	T45.7X2	T45.7X3	T45.7X4	T45.7X5	T45.7X6
Menaphthone	T45.7X1	T45.7X2	T45.7X3	T45.7X4	T45.7X5	T45.7X6
Menaquinone	T45.7X1	T45.7X2	T45.7X3	T45.7X4	T45.7X5	T45.7X6
Menatetrenone	T45.7X1	T45.7X2	T45.7X3	T45.7X4	T45.7X5	T45.7X6
Meningococcal vaccine	T50.A91	T50.A92	T50.A93	T50.A94	T50.A95	T50.A96
Menningovax (-AC) (-C)	T50.A91	T50.A92	T50.A93	T50.A94	T50.A95	T50.A96
Menotropins	T38.811	T38.812	T38.813	T38.814	T38.815	T38.816
Menthol	T48.5X1	T48.5X2	T48.5X3	T48.5X4	T48.5X5	T48.5X6
Mepacrine	T37.2X1	T37.2X2	T37.2X3	T37.2X4	T37.2X5	T37.2X6
Meparfynol	T42.6X1	T42.6X2	T42.6X3	T42.6X4	T42.6X5	T42.6X6
Mepartricin	T36.7X1	T36.7X2	T36.7X3	T36.7X4	T36.7X5	T36.7X6
Mepazine	T43.3X1	T43.3X2	T43.3X3	T43.3X4	T43.3X5	T43.3X6
Mepenzolate	T44.3X1	T44.3X2	T44.3X3	T44.3X4	T44.3X5	T44.3X6
bromide	T44.3X1	T44.3X2	T44.3X3	T44.3X4	T44.3X5	T44.3X6
Meperidine	T40.491	T40.492	T40.493	T40.494	T40.495	T40.496
Mephebarbital	T42.3X1	T42.3X2	T42.3X3	T42.3X4	T42.3X5	T42.3X6
Mephenamin(e)	T42.8X1	T42.8X2	T42.8X3	T42.8X4	T42.8X5	T42.8X6
Mephenesin	T42.8X1	T42.8X2	T42.8X3	T42.8X4	T42.8X5	T42.8X6
Mephenhydramine	T45.0X1	T45.0X2	T45.0X3	T45.0X4	T45.0X5	T45.0X6
Mephenoxalone	T42.8X1	T42.8X2	T42.8X3	T42.8X4	T42.8X5	T42.8X6
Mephentermine	T44.991	T44.992	T44.993	T44.994	T44.995	T44.996
Mephenytoin	T42.0X1	T42.0X2	T42.0X3	T42.0X4	T42.0X5	T42.0X6
with phenobarbital	T42.3X1	T42.3X2	T42.3X3	T42.3X4	T42.3X5	T42.3X6
Mephobarbital	T42.3X1	T42.3X2	T42.3X3	T42.3X4	T42.3X5	T42.3X6
Mephosfolan	T60.0X1	T60.0X2	T60.0X3	T60.0X4	—	—
Mepindolol	T44.7X1	T44.7X2	T44.7X3	T44.7X4	T44.7X5	T44.7X6
Mepiperphenidol	T44.3X1	T44.3X2	T44.3X3	T44.3X4	T44.3X5	T44.3X6
Mepitiostane	T38.7X1	T38.7X2	T38.7X3	T38.7X4	T38.7X5	T38.7X6
Mepivacaine	T41.3X1	T41.3X2	T41.3X3	T41.3X4	T41.3X5	T41.3X6
epidural	T41.3X1	T41.3X2	T41.3X3	T41.3X4	T41.3X5	T41.3X6
Meprednisone	T38.0X1	T38.0X2	T38.0X3	T38.0X4	T38.0X5	T38.0X6
Meprobam	T43.591	T43.592	T43.593	T43.594	T43.595	T43.596
Meprobamate	T43.591	T43.592	T43.593	T43.594	T43.595	T43.596
Meproscillarin	T46.0X1	T46.0X2	T46.0X3	T46.0X4	T46.0X5	T46.0X6
Meprylcaine	T41.3X1	T41.3X2	T41.3X3	T41.3X4	T41.3X5	T41.3X6
Meptazinol	T39.8X1	T39.8X2	T39.8X3	T39.8X4	T39.8X5	T39.8X6
Mepyramine	T45.0X1	T45.0X2	T45.0X3	T45.0X4	T45.0X5	T45.0X6
Mequitazine	T43.3X1	T43.3X2	T43.3X3	T43.3X4	T43.3X5	T43.3X6
Meralluride	T50.2X1	T50.2X2	T50.2X3	T50.2X4	T50.2X5	T50.2X6

	External Cause (T-Code)					
Substance	Poisoning, Accidental (Unintentional)	Poisoning, Intentional Self-Harm	Poisoning, Assault	Poisoning, Undetermined	Adverse Effect	Underdosing
Merbaphen	T50.2X1	T50.2X2	T50.2X3	T50.2X4	T50.2X5	T50.2X6
Merbromin	T49.0X1	T49.0X2	T49.0X3	T49.0X4	T49.0X5	T49.0X6
Mercaptobenzothiazole salts	T49.0X1	T49.0X2	T49.0X3	T49.0X4	T49.0X5	T49.0X6
Mercaptomerin	T50.2X1	T50.2X2	T50.2X3	T50.2X4	T50.2X5	T50.2X6
Mercaptopurine	T45.1X1	T45.1X2	T45.1X3	T45.1X4	T45.1X5	T45.1X6
Mercumatilin	T50.2X1	T50.2X2	T50.2X3	T50.2X4	T50.2X5	T50.2X6
Mercuramide	T50.2X1	T50.2X2	T50.2X3	T50.2X4	T50.2X5	T50.2X6
Mercurochrome	T49.0X1	T49.0X2	T49.0X3	T49.0X4	T49.0X5	T49.0X6
Mercurophylline	T50.2X1	T50.2X2	T50.2X3	T50.2X4	T50.2X5	T50.2X6
Mercury, mercurial, mercuric, mercurous (compounds) (cyanide) (fumes) (nonmedicinal) (vapor) NEC	T56.1X1	T56.1X2	T56.1X3	T56.1X4	—	—
ammoniated	T49.0X1	T49.0X2	T49.0X3	T49.0X4	T49.0X5	T49.0X6
anti-infective						
local	T49.0X1	T49.0X2	T49.0X3	T49.0X4	T49.0X5	T49.0X6
systemic	T37.8X1	T37.8X2	T37.8X3	T37.8X4	T37.8X5	T37.8X6
topical	T49.0X1	T49.0X2	T49.0X3	T49.0X4	T49.0X5	T49.0X6
chloride (ammoniated)	T49.0X1	T49.0X2	T49.0X3	T49.0X4	T49.0X5	T49.0X6
fungicide	T56.1X1	T56.1X2	T56.1X3	T56.1X4	—	—
diuretic NEC	T50.2X1	T50.2X2	T50.2X3	T50.2X4	T50.2X5	T50.2X6
fungicide	T56.1X1	T56.1X2	T56.1X3	T56.1X4	—	—
organic (fungicide)	T56.1X1	T56.1X2	T56.1X3	T56.1X4	—	—
oxide, yellow	T49.0X1	T49.0X2	T49.0X3	T49.0X4	T49.0X5	T49.0X6
Mersalyl	T50.2X1	T50.2X2	T50.2X3	T50.2X4	T50.2X5	T50.2X6
Merthiolate	T49.0X1	T49.0X2	T49.0X3	T49.0X4	T49.0X5	T49.0X6
ophthalmic preparation	T49.5X1	T49.5X2	T49.5X3	T49.5X4	T49.5X5	T49.5X6
Meruvax	T50.B91	T50.B92	T50.B93	T50.B94	T50.B95	T50.B96
Mesalazine	T47.8X1	T47.8X2	T47.8X3	T47.8X4	T47.8X5	T47.8X6
Mescal buttons	T40.991	T40.992	T40.993	T40.994	—	—
Mescaline	T40.991	T40.992	T40.993	T40.994	—	—
Mesna	T48.4X1	T48.4X2	T48.4X3	T48.4X4	T48.4X5	T48.4X6
Mesoglycan	T46.6X1	T46.6X2	T46.6X3	T46.6X4	T46.6X5	T46.6X6
Mesoridazine	T43.3X1	T43.3X2	T43.3X3	T43.3X4	T43.3X5	T43.3X6
Mestanolone	T38.7X1	T38.7X2	T38.7X3	T38.7X4	T38.7X5	T38.7X6
Mesterolone	T38.7X1	T38.7X2	T38.7X3	T38.7X4	T38.7X5	T38.7X6
Mestranol	T38.5X1	T38.5X2	T38.5X3	T38.5X4	T38.5X5	T38.5X6
Mesulergine	T42.8X1	T42.8X2	T42.8X3	T42.8X4	T42.8X5	T42.8X6
Mesulfen	T49.0X1	T49.0X2	T49.0X3	T49.0X4	T49.0X5	T49.0X6
Mesuximide	T42.2X1	T42.2X2	T42.2X3	T42.2X4	T42.2X5	T42.2X6
Metabutethamine	T41.3X1	T41.3X2	T41.3X3	T41.3X4	T41.3X5	T41.3X6
Metactesylacetate	T49.0X1	T49.0X2	T49.0X3	T49.0X4	T49.0X5	T49.0X6

◀ New ◀|| Revised ~~deleted~~ Deleted

TABLE OF DRUGS AND CHEMICALS

	External Cause (T-Code)					
Substance	Poisoning, Accidental (Unintentional)	Poisoning, Intentional Self-Harm	Poisoning, Assault	Poisoning, Undetermined	Adverse Effect	Underdosing
Metacycline	T36.4X1	T36.4X2	T36.4X3	T36.4X4	T36.4X5	T36.4X6
Metaldehyde (snail killer) NEC	T60.8X1	T60.8X2	T60.8X3	T60.8X4	—	—
Metals (heavy) (nonmedicinal)	T56.91	T56.92	T56.93	T56.94	—	—
dust, fumes, or vapor NEC	T56.91	T56.92	T56.93	T56.94	—	—
light NEC	T56.91	T56.92	T56.93	T56.94	—	—
dust, fumes, or vapor NEC	T56.91	T56.92	T56.93	T56.94	—	—
specified NEC	T56.891	T56.892	T56.893	T56.894	—	—
thallium	T56.811	T56.812	T56.813	T56.814	—	—
Metamfetamine	T43.621	T43.622	T43.623	T43.624	T43.625	T43.626
Metamizole sodium	T39.2X1	T39.2X2	T39.2X3	T39.2X4	T39.2X5	T39.2X6
Metampicillin	T36.0X1	T36.0X2	T36.0X3	T36.0X4	T36.0X5	T36.0X6
Metamucil	T47.4X1	T47.4X2	T47.4X3	T47.4X4	T47.4X5	T47.4X6
Metaphen	T49.0X1	T49.0X2	T49.0X3	T49.0X4	T49.0X5	T49.0X6
Metandienone	T38.7X1	T38.7X2	T38.7X3	T38.7X4	T38.7X5	T38.7X6
Metandrostenolone	T38.7X1	T38.7X2	T38.7X3	T38.7X4	T38.7X5	T38.7X6
Metaphos	T60.0X1	T60.0X2	T60.0X3	T60.0X4	—	—
Metapramine	T43.011	T43.012	T43.013	T43.014	T43.015	T43.016
Metaproterenol	T48.291	T48.292	T48.293	T48.294	T48.295	T48.296
Metaraminol	T44.4X1	T44.4X2	T44.4X3	T44.4X4	T44.4X5	T44.4X6
Metaxalone	T42.8X1	T42.8X2	T42.8X3	T42.8X4	T42.8X5	T42.8X6
Metenolone	T38.7X1	T38.7X2	T38.7X3	T38.7X4	T38.7X5	T38.7X6
Metergoline	T42.8X1	T42.8X2	T42.8X3	T42.8X4	T42.8X5	T42.8X6
Metescufylline	T46.991	T46.992	T46.993	T46.994	T46.995	T46.996
Metetoin	T42.0X1	T42.0X2	T42.0X3	T42.0X4	T42.0X5	T42.0X6
Metformin	T38.3X1	T38.3X2	T38.3X3	T38.3X4	T38.3X5	T38.3X6
Methacholine	T44.1X1	T44.1X2	T44.1X3	T44.1X4	T44.1X5	T44.1X6
Methacycline	T36.4X1	T36.4X2	T36.4X3	T36.4X4	T36.4X5	T36.4X6
Methadone	T40.3X1	T40.3X2	T40.3X3	T40.3X4	T40.3X5	T40.3X6
Methallenestril	T38.5X1	T38.5X2	T38.5X3	T38.5X4	T38.5X5	T38.5X6
Methallenoestril	T38.5X1	T38.5X2	T38.5X3	T38.5X4	T38.5X5	T38.5X6
Methamphetamine	T43.621	T43.622	T43.623	T43.624	T43.625	T43.626
Methampyrone	T39.2X1	T39.2X2	T39.2X3	T39.2X4	T39.2X5	T39.2X6
Methandienone	T38.7X1	T38.7X2	T38.7X3	T38.7X4	T38.7X5	T38.7X6
Methandriol	T38.7X1	T38.7X2	T38.7X3	T38.7X4	T38.7X5	T38.7X6
Methandrostenolone	T38.7X1	T38.7X2	T38.7X3	T38.7X4	T38.7X5	T38.7X6
Methane	T59.891	T59.892	T59.893	T59.894	—	—
Methanethiol	T59.891	T59.892	T59.893	T59.894	—	—
Methaniazide	T37.1X1	T37.1X2	T37.1X3	T37.1X4	T37.1X5	T37.1X6
Methanol (vapor)	T51.1X1	T51.1X2	T51.1X3	T51.1X4	—	—
Methantheline	T44.3X1	T44.3X2	T44.3X3	T44.3X4	T44.3X5	T44.3X6
Methanthelinium bromide	T44.3X1	T44.3X2	T44.3X3	T44.3X4	T44.3X5	T44.3X6
Methaphenilene	T45.0X1	T45.0X2	T45.0X3	T45.0X4	T45.0X5	T45.0X6

	External Cause (T-Code)					
Substance	Poisoning, Accidental (Unintentional)	Poisoning, Intentional Self-Harm	Poisoning, Assault	Poisoning, Undetermined	Adverse Effect	Underdosing
Methapyrilene	T45.0X1	T45.0X2	T45.0X3	T45.0X4	T45.0X5	T45.0X6
Methaqualone (compound)	T42.6X1	T42.6X2	T42.6X3	T42.6X4	T42.6X5	T42.6X6
Metharbital	T42.3X1	T42.3X2	T42.3X3	T42.3X4	T42.3X5	T42.3X6
Methazolamide	T50.2X1	T50.2X2	T50.2X3	T50.2X4	T50.2X5	T50.2X6
Methdilazine	T43.3X1	T43.3X2	T43.3X3	T43.3X4	T43.3X5	T43.3X6
Methedrine	T43.621	T43.622	T43.623	T43.624	T43.625	T43.626
Methenamine (mandelate)	T37.8X1	T37.8X2	T37.8X3	T37.8X4	T37.8X5	T37.8X6
Methenolone	T38.7X1	T38.7X2	T38.7X3	T38.7X4	T38.7X5	T38.7X6
Methergine	T48.0X1	T48.0X2	T48.0X3	T48.0X4	T48.0X5	T48.0X6
Methetoin	T42.0X1	T42.0X2	T42.0X3	T42.0X4	T42.0X5	T42.0X6
Methiacil	T38.2X1	T38.2X2	T38.2X3	T38.2X4	T38.2X5	T38.2X6
Methicillin	T36.0X1	T36.0X2	T36.0X3	T36.0X4	T36.0X5	T36.0X6
Methimazole	T38.2X1	T38.2X2	T38.2X3	T38.2X4	T38.2X5	T38.2X6
Methiodal sodium	T50.8X1	T50.8X2	T50.8X3	T50.8X4	T50.8X5	T50.8X6
Methionine	T50.991	T50.992	T50.993	T50.994	T50.995	T50.996
Methisazone	T37.5X1	T37.5X2	T37.5X3	T37.5X4	T37.5X5	T37.5X6
Methisoprinol	T37.5X1	T37.5X2	T37.5X3	T37.5X4	T37.5X5	T37.5X6
Methitural	T42.3X1	T42.3X2	T42.3X3	T42.3X4	T42.3X5	T42.3X6
Methixene	T44.3X1	T44.3X2	T44.3X3	T44.3X4	T44.3X5	T44.3X6
Methobarbital, methobarbitone	T42.3X1	T42.3X2	T42.3X3	T42.3X4	T42.3X5	T42.3X6
Methocarbamol	T42.8X1	T42.8X2	T42.8X3	T42.8X4	T42.8X5	T42.8X6
skeletal muscle relaxant	T48.1X1	T48.1X2	T48.1X3	T48.1X4	T48.1X5	T48.1X6
Methohexital	T41.1X1	T41.1X2	T41.1X3	T41.1X4	T41.1X5	T41.1X6
Methohexitone	T41.1X1	T41.1X2	T41.1X3	T41.1X4	T41.1X5	T41.1X6
Methoin	T42.0X1	T42.0X2	T42.0X3	T42.0X4	T42.0X5	T42.0X6
Methopholine	T39.8X1	T39.8X2	T39.8X3	T39.8X4	T39.8X5	T39.8X6
Methopromazine	T43.3X1	T43.3X2	T43.3X3	T43.3X4	T43.3X5	T43.3X6
Methorate	T48.3X1	T48.3X2	T48.3X3	T48.3X4	T48.3X5	T48.3X6
Methoserpidine	T46.5X1	T46.5X2	T46.5X3	T46.5X4	T46.5X5	T46.5X6
Methotrexate	T45.1X1	T45.1X2	T45.1X3	T45.1X4	T45.1X5	T45.1X6
Methotrimeprazine	T43.3X1	T43.3X2	T43.3X3	T43.3X4	T43.3X5	T43.3X6
Methoxa-Dome	T49.3X1	T49.3X2	T49.3X3	T49.3X4	T49.3X5	T49.3X6
Methoxamine	T44.4X1	T44.4X2	T44.4X3	T44.4X4	T44.4X5	T44.4X6
Methoxsalen	T50.991	T50.992	T50.993	T50.994	T50.995	T50.996
Methoxyaniline	T65.3X1	T65.3X2	T65.3X3	T65.3X4	—	—
Methoxybenzyl penicillin	T36.0X1	T36.0X2	T36.0X3	T36.0X4	T36.0X5	T36.0X6
Methoxychlor	T53.7X1	T53.7X2	T53.7X3	T53.7X4	—	—
Methoxy-DDT	T53.7X1	T53.7X2	T53.7X3	T53.7X4	—	—
2-Methoxyethanol	T52.3X1	T52.3X2	T52.3X3	T52.3X4	—	—
Methoxyflurane	T41.0X1	T41.0X2	T41.0X3	T41.0X4	T41.0X5	T41.0X6
Methoxyphenamine	T48.6X1	T48.6X2	T48.6X3	T48.6X4	T48.6X5	T48.6X6
Methoxypromazine	T43.3X1	T43.3X2	T43.3X3	T43.3X4	T43.3X5	T43.3X6

◀ New   ◀ Revised   ~~deleted~~ Deleted

Substance	External Cause (T-Code)					
	Poisoning, Accidental (Unintentional)	Poisoning, Intentional Self-Harm	Poisoning, Assault	Poisoning, Undetermined	Adverse Effect	Underdosing
5-Methoxypsoralen (5-MOP)	T50.991	T50.992	T50.993	T50.994	T50.995	T50.996
8-Methoxypsoralen (8-MOP)	T50.991	T50.992	T50.993	T50.994	T50.995	T50.996
Methscopolamine bromide	T44.3X1	T44.3X2	T44.3X3	T44.3X4	T44.3X5	T44.3X6
Methsuximide	T42.2X1	T42.2X2	T42.2X3	T42.2X4	T42.2X5	T42.2X6
Methylclothiazide	T50.2X1	T50.2X2	T50.2X3	T50.2X4	T50.2X5	T50.2X6
Methyl						
acetate	T52.4X1	T52.4X2	T52.4X3	T52.4X4	—	—
acetone	T52.4X1	T52.4X2	T52.4X3	T52.4X4	—	—
acrylate	T65.891	T65.892	T65.893	T65.894	—	—
alcohol	T51.1X1	T51.1X2	T51.1X3	T51.1X4	—	—
aminophenol	T65.3X1	T65.3X2	T65.3X3	T65.3X4	—	—
amphetamine	T43.621	T43.622	T43.623	T43.624	T43.625	T43.626
androstanolone	T38.7X1	T38.7X2	T38.7X3	T38.7X4	T38.7X5	T38.7X6
atropine	T44.3X1	T44.3X2	T44.3X3	T44.3X4	T44.3X5	T44.3X6
benzene	T52.2X1	T52.2X2	T52.2X3	T52.2X4	—	—
benzoate	T52.8X1	T52.8X2	T52.8X3	T52.8X4	—	—
benzol	T52.2X1	T52.2X2	T52.2X3	T52.2X4	—	—
bromide (gas)	T59.891	T59.892	T59.893	T59.894	—	—
fumigant	T60.8X1	T60.8X2	T60.8X3	T60.8X4	—	—
butanol	T51.3X1	T51.3X2	T51.3X3	T51.3X4	—	—
carbinol	T51.1X1	T51.1X2	T51.1X3	T51.1X4	—	—
carbonate	T52.8X1	T52.8X2	T52.8X3	T52.8X4	—	—
CCNU	T45.1X1	T45.1X2	T45.1X3	T45.1X4	T45.1X5	T45.1X6
cellosolve	T52.91	T52.92	T52.93	T52.94	—	—
cellulose	T47.4X1	T47.4X2	T47.4X3	T47.4X4	T47.4X5	T47.4X6
chloride (gas)	T59.891	T59.892	T59.893	T59.894	—	—
chloroformate	T59.3X1	T59.3X2	T59.3X3	T59.3X4	—	—
cyclohexane	T52.8X1	T52.8X2	T52.8X3	T52.8X4	—	—
cyclohexanol	T51.8X1	T51.8X2	T51.8X3	T51.8X4	—	—
cyclohexanone	T52.8X1	T52.8X2	T52.8X3	T52.8X4	—	—
cyclohexyl acetate	T52.8X1	T52.8X2	T52.8X3	T52.8X4	—	—
demeton	T60.0X1	T60.0X2	T60.0X3	T60.0X4	—	—
dihydromorphinone	T40.2X1	T40.2X2	T40.2X3	T40.2X4	T40.2X5	T40.2X6
ergometrine	T48.0X1	T48.0X2	T48.0X3	T48.0X4	T48.0X5	T48.0X6
ergonovine	T48.0X1	T48.0X2	T48.0X3	T48.0X4	T48.0X5	T48.0X6
ethyl ketone	T52.4X1	T52.4X2	T52.4X3	T52.4X4	—	—
glucamine antimonate	T37.8X1	T37.8X2	T37.8X3	T37.8X4	T37.8X5	T37.8X6
hydrazine	T65.891	T65.892	T65.893	T65.894	—	—
iodide	T65.891	T65.892	T65.893	T65.894	—	—
isobutyl ketone	T52.4X1	T52.4X2	T52.4X3	T52.4X4	—	—
isothiocyanate	T60.3X1	T60.3X2	T60.3X3	T60.3X4	—	—
mercaptan	T59.891	T59.892	T59.893	T59.894	—	—

Substance	External Cause (T-Code)					
	Poisoning, Accidental (Unintentional)	Poisoning, Intentional Self-Harm	Poisoning, Assault	Poisoning, Undetermined	Adverse Effect	Underdosing
Methyl (Continued)						
morphine NEC	T40.2X1	T40.2X2	T40.2X3	T40.2X4	T40.2X5	T40.2X6
nicotinate	T49.4X1	T49.4X2	T49.4X3	T49.4X4	T49.4X5	T49.4X6
paraben	T49.0X1	T49.0X2	T49.0X3	T49.0X4	T49.0X5	T49.0X6
parafynol	T42.6X1	T42.6X2	T42.6X3	T42.6X4	T42.6X5	T42.6X6
parathion	T60.0X1	T60.0X2	T60.0X3	T60.0X4	—	—
peridol	T43.4X1	T43.4X2	T43.4X3	T43.4X4	T43.4X5	T43.4X6
phenidate	T43.631	T43.632	T43.633	T43.634	T43.635	T43.636
prednisolone	T38.0X1	T38.0X2	T38.0X3	T38.0X4	T38.0X5	T38.0X6
ENT agent	T49.6X1	T49.6X2	T49.6X3	T49.6X4	T49.6X5	T49.6X6
ophthalmic preparation	T49.5X1	T49.5X2	T49.5X3	T49.5X4	T49.5X5	T49.5X6
topical NEC	T49.0X1	T49.0X2	T49.0X3	T49.0X4	T49.0X5	T49.0X6
propylcarbinol	T51.3X1	T51.3X2	T51.3X3	T51.3X4	—	—
rosaniline NEC	T49.0X1	T49.0X2	T49.0X3	T49.0X4	T49.0X5	T49.0X6
salicylate	T49.2X1	T49.2X2	T49.2X3	T49.2X4	T49.2X5	T49.2X6
sulfate (fumes)	T59.891	T59.892	T59.893	T59.894	—	—
liquid	T52.8X1	T52.8X2	T52.8X3	T52.8X4	—	—
sulfonal	T42.6X1	T42.6X2	T42.6X3	T42.6X4	T42.6X5	T42.6X6
testosterone	T38.7X1	T38.7X2	T38.7X3	T38.7X4	T38.7X5	T38.7X6
thiouracil	T38.2X1	T38.2X2	T38.2X3	T38.2X4	T38.2X5	T38.2X6
Methylamphetamine	T43.621	T43.622	T43.623	T43.624	T43.625	T43.626
Methylated spirit	T51.1X1	T51.1X2	T51.1X3	T51.1X4	—	—
Methylatropine nitrate	T44.3X1	T44.3X2	T44.3X3	T44.3X4	T44.3X5	T44.3X6
Methylbenactyzium bromide	T44.3X1	T44.3X2	T44.3X3	T44.3X4	T44.3X5	T44.3X6
Methylbenzethonium chloride	T49.0X1	T49.0X2	T49.0X3	T49.0X4	T49.0X5	T49.0X6
Methylcellulose	T47.4X1	T47.4X2	T47.4X3	T47.4X4	T47.4X5	T47.4X6
laxative	T47.4X1	T47.4X2	T47.4X3	T47.4X4	T47.4X5	T47.4X6
Methylchlorophenoxy-acetic acid	T60.3X1	T60.3X2	T60.3X3	T60.3X4	—	—
Methyldopa	T46.5X1	T46.5X2	T46.5X3	T46.5X4	T46.5X5	T46.5X6
Methyldopate	T46.5X1	T46.5X2	T46.5X3	T46.5X4	T46.5X5	T46.5X6
Methylene						
blue	T50.6X1	T50.6X2	T50.6X3	T50.6X4	T50.6X5	T50.6X6
chloride or dichloride (solvent) NEC	T53.4X1	T53.4X2	T53.4X3	T53.4X4	—	—
Methylenedioxyamphet-amine	T43.621	T43.622	T43.623	T43.624	T43.625	T43.626
Methylenedioxymethamphetamine	T43.641	T43.642	T43.643	T43.644	—	—
Methylergometrine	T48.0X1	T48.0X2	T48.0X3	T48.0X4	T48.0X5	T48.0X6
Methylergonovine	T48.0X1	T48.0X2	T48.0X3	T48.0X4	T48.0X5	T48.0X6
Methylestrenolone	T38.5X1	T38.5X2	T38.5X3	T38.5X4	T38.5X5	T38.5X6
Methylethyl cellulose	T50.991	T50.992	T50.993	T50.994	T50.995	T50.996
Methylhexabital	T42.3X1	T42.3X2	T42.3X3	T42.3X4	T42.3X5	T42.3X6
Methylmorphine	T40.2X1	T40.2X2	T40.2X3	T40.2X4	T40.2X5	T40.2X6

◀ New   ◀◀ Revised   ~~deleted~~ Deleted

TABLE OF DRUGS AND CHEMICALS

Substance	External Cause (T-Code)					
	Poisoning, Accidental (Unintentional)	Poisoning, Intentional Self-Harm	Poisoning, Assault	Poisoning, Undetermined	Adverse Effect	Underdosing
Methylparaben (ophthalmic)	T49.5X1	T49.5X2	T49.5X3	T49.5X4	T49.5X5	T49.5X6
Methylparafynol	T42.6X1	T42.6X2	T42.6X3	T42.6X4	T42.6X5	T42.6X6
Methylpentynol, methylpenthynol	T42.6X1	T42.6X2	T42.6X3	T42.6X4	T42.6X5	T42.6X6
Methylphenidate	T43.631	T43.632	T43.633	T43.634	T43.635	T43.636
Methylphenobarbital	T42.3X1	T42.3X2	T42.3X3	T42.3X4	T42.3X5	T42.3X6
Methylpolysiloxane	T47.1X1	T47.1X2	T47.1X3	T47.1X4	T47.1X5	T47.1X6
Methylprednisolone — see Methyl, prednisolone						
Methylrosaniline	T49.0X1	T49.0X2	T49.0X3	T49.0X4	T49.0X5	T49.0X6
Methylrosanilinium chloride	T49.0X1	T49.0X2	T49.0X3	T49.0X4	T49.0X5	T49.0X6
Methyltestosterone	T38.7X1	T38.7X2	T38.7X3	T38.7X4	T38.7X5	T38.7X6
Methylthionine chloride	T50.6X1	T50.6X2	T50.6X3	T50.6X4	T50.6X5	T50.6X6
Methylthioninium chloride	T50.6X1	T50.6X2	T50.6X3	T50.6X4	T50.6X5	T50.6X6
Methylthiouracil	T38.2X1	T38.2X2	T38.2X3	T38.2X4	T38.2X5	T38.2X6
Methyprylon	T42.6X1	T42.6X2	T42.6X3	T42.6X4	T42.6X5	T42.6X6
Methysergide	T46.5X1	T46.5X2	T46.5X3	T46.5X4	T46.5X5	T46.5X6
Metiamide	T47.1X1	T47.1X2	T47.1X3	T47.1X4	T47.1X5	T47.1X6
Meticillin	T36.0X1	T36.0X2	T36.0X3	T36.0X4	T36.0X5	T36.0X6
Meticrane	T50.2X1	T50.2X2	T50.2X3	T50.2X4	T50.2X5	T50.2X6
Metildigoxin	T46.0X1	T46.0X2	T46.0X3	T46.0X4	T46.0X5	T46.0X6
Metipranolol	T49.5X1	T49.5X2	T49.5X3	T49.5X4	T49.5X5	T49.5X6
Metirosine	T46.5X1	T46.5X2	T46.5X3	T46.5X4	T46.5X5	T46.5X6
Metisazone	T37.5X1	T37.5X2	T37.5X3	T37.5X4	T37.5X5	T37.5X6
Metixene	T44.3X1	T44.3X2	T44.3X3	T44.3X4	T44.3X5	T44.3X6
Metizoline	T48.5X1	T48.5X2	T48.5X3	T48.5X4	T48.5X5	T48.5X6
Metoclopramide	T45.0X1	T45.0X2	T45.0X3	T45.0X4	T45.0X5	T45.0X6
Metofenazate	T43.3X1	T43.3X2	T43.3X3	T43.3X4	T43.3X5	T43.3X6
Metofoline	T39.8X1	T39.8X2	T39.8X3	T39.8X4	T39.8X5	T39.8X6
Metolazone	T50.2X1	T50.2X2	T50.2X3	T50.2X4	T50.2X5	T50.2X6
Metopon	T40.2X1	T40.2X2	T40.2X3	T40.2X4	T40.2X5	T40.2X6
Metoprine	T45.1X1	T45.1X2	T45.1X3	T45.1X4	T45.1X5	T45.1X6
Metoprolol	T44.7X1	T44.7X2	T44.7X3	T44.7X4	T44.7X5	T44.7X6
Metrifonate	T60.0X1	T60.0X2	T60.0X3	T60.0X4	—	—
Metrizamide	T50.8X1	T50.8X2	T50.8X3	T50.8X4	T50.8X5	T50.8X6
Metrizoic acid	T50.8X1	T50.8X2	T50.8X3	T50.8X4	T50.8X5	T50.8X6
Metronidazole	T37.8X1	T37.8X2	T37.8X3	T37.8X4	T37.8X5	T37.8X6
Metycaine	T41.3X1	T41.3X2	T41.3X3	T41.3X4	T41.3X5	T41.3X6
infiltration (subcutaneous)	T41.3X1	T41.3X2	T41.3X3	T41.3X4	T41.3X5	T41.3X6
nerve block (peripheral) (plexus)	T41.3X1	T41.3X2	T41.3X3	T41.3X4	T41.3X5	T41.3X6
topical (surface)	T41.3X1	T41.3X2	T41.3X3	T41.3X4	T41.3X5	T41.3X6
Metyrapone	T50.8X1	T50.8X2	T50.8X3	T50.8X4	T50.8X5	T50.8X6
Mevinphos	T60.0X1	T60.0X2	T60.0X3	T60.0X4	—	—

Substance	External Cause (T-Code)					
	Poisoning, Accidental (Unintentional)	Poisoning, Intentional Self-Harm	Poisoning, Assault	Poisoning, Undetermined	Adverse Effect	Underdosing
Mexazolam	T42.4X1	T42.4X2	T42.4X3	T42.4X4	T42.4X5	T42.4X6
Mexenone	T49.3X1	T49.3X2	T49.3X3	T49.3X4	T49.3X5	T49.3X6
Mexiletine	T46.2X1	T46.2X2	T46.2X3	T46.2X4	T46.2X5	T46.2X6
Mezereon	T62.2X1	T62.2X2	T62.2X3	T62.2X4	—	—
berries	T62.1X1	T62.1X2	T62.1X3	T62.1X4	—	—
Mezlocillin	T36.0X1	T36.0X2	T36.0X3	T36.0X4	T36.0X5	T36.0X6
Mianserin	T43.021	T43.022	T43.023	T43.024	T43.025	T43.026
Micatin	T49.0X1	T49.0X2	T49.0X3	T49.0X4	T49.0X5	T49.0X6
Miconazole	T49.0X1	T49.0X2	T49.0X3	T49.0X4	T49.0X5	T49.0X6
Micronomicin	T36.5X1	T36.5X2	T36.5X3	T36.5X4	T36.5X5	T36.5X6
Midazolam	T42.4X1	T42.4X2	T42.4X3	T42.4X4	T42.4X5	T42.4X6
Midecamycin	T36.3X1	T36.3X2	T36.3X3	T36.3X4	T36.3X5	T36.3X6
Mifepristone	T38.6X1	T38.6X2	T38.6X3	T38.6X4	T38.6X5	T38.6X6
Milk of magnesia	T47.1X1	T47.1X2	T47.1X3	T47.1X4	T47.1X5	T47.1X6
Millipede (tropical) (venomous)	T63.411	T63.412	T63.413	T63.414	—	—
Miltown	T43.591	T43.592	T43.593	T43.594	T43.595	T43.596
Milverine	T44.3X1	T44.3X2	T44.3X3	T44.3X4	T44.3X5	T44.3X6
Minaprine	T43.291	T43.292	T43.293	T43.294	T43.295	T43.296
Minaxolone	T41.291	T41.292	T41.293	T41.294	T41.295	T41.296
Mineral						
acids	T54.2X1	T54.2X2	T54.2X3	T54.2X4	—	—
oil (laxative) (medicinal)	T47.4X1	T47.4X2	T47.4X3	T47.4X4	T47.4X5	T47.4X6
emulsion	T47.2X1	T47.2X2	T47.2X3	T47.2X4	T47.2X5	T47.2X6
nonmedicinal	T52.0X1	T52.0X2	T52.0X3	T52.0X4	—	—
topical	T49.3X1	T49.3X2	T49.3X3	T49.3X4	T49.3X5	T49.3X6
salt NEC	T50.3X1	T50.3X2	T50.3X3	T50.3X4	T50.3X5	T50.3X6
spirits	T52.0X1	T52.0X2	T52.0X3	T52.0X4	—	—
Mineralocorticosteroid	T50.0X1	T50.0X2	T50.0X3	T50.0X4	T50.0X5	T50.0X6
Minocycline	T36.4X1	T36.4X2	T36.4X3	T36.4X4	T36.4X5	T36.4X6
Minoxidil	T46.7X1	T46.7X2	T46.7X3	T46.7X4	T46.7X5	T46.7X6
Miokamycin	T36.3X1	T36.3X2	T36.3X3	T36.3X4	T36.3X5	T36.3X6
Miotic drug	T49.5X1	T49.5X2	T49.5X3	T49.5X4	T49.5X5	T49.5X6
Mipafox	T60.0X1	T60.0X2	T60.0X3	T60.0X4	—	—
Mirex	T60.1X1	T60.1X2	T60.1X3	T60.1X4	—	—
Mirtazapine	T43.021	T43.022	T43.023	T43.024	T43.025	T43.026
Misonidazole	T37.3X1	T37.3X2	T37.3X3	T37.3X4	T37.3X5	T37.3X6
Misoprostol	T47.1X1	T47.1X2	T47.1X3	T47.1X4	T47.1X5	T47.1X6
Mithramycin	T45.1X1	T45.1X2	T45.1X3	T45.1X4	T45.1X5	T45.1X6
Mitobronitol	T45.1X1	T45.1X2	T45.1X3	T45.1X4	T45.1X5	T45.1X6
Mitoguazone	T45.1X1	T45.1X2	T45.1X3	T45.1X4	T45.1X5	T45.1X6
Mitolactol	T45.1X1	T45.1X2	T45.1X3	T45.1X4	T45.1X5	T45.1X6
Mitomycin	T45.1X1	T45.1X2	T45.1X3	T45.1X4	T45.1X5	T45.1X6

◀ New ◀ Revised ~~deleted~~ Deleted

Substance	Poisoning, Accidental (Unintentional)	Poisoning, Intentional Self-Harm	Poisoning, Assault	Poisoning, Undetermined	Adverse Effect	Underdosing
Mitopodozide	T45.1X1	T45.1X2	T45.1X3	T45.1X4	T45.1X5	T45.1X6
Mitotane	T45.1X1	T45.1X2	T45.1X3	T45.1X4	T45.1X5	T45.1X6
Mitoxantrone	T45.1X1	T45.1X2	T45.1X3	T45.1X4	T45.1X5	T45.1X6
Mivacurium chloride	T48.1X1	T48.1X2	T48.1X3	T48.1X4	T48.1X5	T48.1X6
Miyari bacteria	T47.6X1	T47.6X2	T47.6X3	T47.6X4	T47.6X5	T47.6X6
Moclobemide	T43.1X1	T43.1X2	T43.1X3	T43.1X4	T43.1X5	T43.1X6
Moderil	T46.5X1	T46.5X2	T46.5X3	T46.5X4	T46.5X5	T46.5X6
Mofebutazone	T39.2X1	T39.2X2	T39.2X3	T39.2X4	T39.2X5	T39.2X6
Mogadon — *see Nitrazepam*						
Molindone	T43.591	T43.592	T43.593	T43.594	T43.595	T43.596
Molsidomine	T46.3X1	T46.3X2	T46.3X3	T46.3X4	T46.3X5	T46.3X6
Mometasone	T49.0X1	T49.0X2	T49.0X3	T49.0X4	T49.0X5	T49.0X6
Monistat	T49.0X1	T49.0X2	T49.0X3	T49.0X4	T49.0X5	T49.0X6
Monkshood	T62.2X1	T62.2X2	T62.2X3	T62.2X4	—	—
Monoamine oxidase inhibitor NEC	T43.1X1	T43.1X2	T43.1X3	T43.1X4	T43.1X5	T43.1X6
hydrazine	T43.1X1	T43.1X2	T43.1X3	T43.1X4	T43.1X5	T43.1X6
Monobenzone	T49.4X1	T49.4X2	T49.4X3	T49.4X4	T49.4X5	T49.4X6
Monochloroacetic acid	T60.3X1	T60.3X2	T60.3X3	T60.3X4		
Monochlorobenzene	T53.7X1	T53.7X2	T53.7X3	T53.7X4	—	—
Monoethanolamine	T46.8X1	T46.8X2	T46.8X3	T46.8X4	T46.8X5	T46.8X6
oleate	T46.8X1	T46.8X2	T46.8X3	T46.8X4	T46.8X5	T46.8X6
Monooctanoin	T50.991	T50.992	T50.993	T50.994	T50.995	T50.996
Monophenylbutazone	T39.2X1	T39.2X2	T39.2X3	T39.2X4	T39.2X5	T39.2X6
Monosodium glutamate	T65.891	T65.892	T65.893	T65.894	—	—
Monosulfiram	T49.0X1	T49.0X2	T49.0X3	T49.0X4	T49.0X5	T49.0X6
Monoxide, carbon — *see Carbon, monoxide*	T57.91	T57.92	T57.93	T57.94	—	—
Monoxidine hydrochloride	T46.1X1	T46.1X2	T46.1X3	T46.1X4	T46.1X5	T46.1X6
Monuron	T60.3X1	T60.3X2	T60.3X3	T60.3X4	—	—
Moperone	T43.4X1	T43.4X2	T43.4X3	T43.4X4	T43.4X5	T43.4X6
Mopidamol	T45.1X1	T45.1X2	T45.1X3	T45.1X4	T45.1X5	T45.1X6
MOPP (mechlorethamine + vincristine + prednisone + procarbazine)	T45.1X1	T45.1X2	T45.1X3	T45.1X4	T45.1X5	T45.1X6
Morfin	T40.2X1	T40.2X2	T40.2X3	T40.2X4	T40.2X5	T40.2X6
Morinamide	T37.1X1	T37.1X2	T37.1X3	T37.1X4	T37.1X5	T37.1X6
Morning glory seeds	T40.991	T40.992	T40.993	T40.994	—	—
Moroxydine	T37.5X1	T37.5X2	T37.5X3	T37.5X4	T37.5X5	T37.5X6
Morphazinamide	T37.1X1	T37.1X2	T37.1X3	T37.1X4	T37.1X5	T37.1X6
Morphine	T40.2X1	T40.2X2	T40.2X3	T40.2X4	T40.2X5	T40.2X6
antagonist	T50.7X1	T50.7X2	T50.7X3	T50.7X4	T50.7X5	T50.7X6
Morpholinylethylmorphine	T40.2X1	T40.2X2	T40.2X3	T40.2X4	—	—
Morsuximide	T42.2X1	T42.2X2	T42.2X3	T42.2X4	T42.2X5	T42.2X6

Substance	Poisoning, Accidental (Unintentional)	Poisoning, Intentional Self-Harm	Poisoning, Assault	Poisoning, Undetermined	Adverse Effect	Underdosing
Mosapramine	T43.591	T43.592	T43.593	T43.594	T43.595	T43.596
Moth balls — *see also Pesticides*	T60.2X1	T60.2X2	T60.2X3	T60.2X4	—	—
naphthalene	T60.2X1	T60.2X2	T60.2X3	T60.2X4		
paradichlorobenzene	T60.1X1	T60.1X2	T60.1X3	T60.1X4		
Motor exhaust gas	T58.01	T58.02	T58.03	T58.04		
Mouthwash (antiseptic) (zinc chloride)	T49.6X1	T49.6X2	T49.6X3	T49.6X4	T49.6X5	T49.6X6
Moxastine	T45.0X1	T45.0X2	T45.0X3	T45.0X4	T45.0X5	T45.0X6
Moxaverine	T44.3X1	T44.3X2	T44.3X3	T44.3X4	T44.3X5	T44.3X6
Moxifensine	T43.291	T43.292	T43.293	T43.294	T43.295	T43.296
Moxisylyte	T46.7X1	T46.7X2	T46.7X3	T46.7X4	T46.7X5	T46.7X6
Mucilage, plant	T47.4X1	T47.4X2	T47.4X3	T47.4X4	T47.4X5	T47.4X6
Mucolytic drug	T48.4X1	T48.4X2	T48.4X3	T48.4X4	T48.4X5	T48.4X6
Mucomyst	T48.4X1	T48.4X2	T48.4X3	T48.4X4	T48.4X5	T48.4X6
Mucous membrane agents (external)	T49.91	T49.92	T49.93	T49.94	T49.95	T49.96
specified NEC	T49.8X1	T49.8X2	T49.8X3	T49.8X4	T49.8X5	T49.8X6
Multiple unspecified drugs, medicaments and biological substances	T50.911	T50.912	T50.913	T50.914	T50.915	T50.916
Mumps						
immune globulin (human)	T50.Z11	T50.Z12	T50.Z13	T50.Z14	T50.Z15	T50.Z16
skin test antigen	T50.8X1	T50.8X2	T50.8X3	T50.8X4	T50.8X5	T50.8X6
vaccine	T50.B91	T50.B92	T50.B93	T50.B94	T50.B95	T50.B96
Mumpsvax	T50.B91	T50.B92	T50.B93	T50.B94	T50.B95	T50.B96
Mupirocin	T49.0X1	T49.0X2	T49.0X3	T49.0X4	T49.0X5	T49.0X6
Muriatic acid — *see Hydrochloric acid*						
Muromonab-CD3	T45.1X1	T45.1X2	T45.1X3	T45.1X4	T45.1X5	T45.1X6
Muscle relaxant — *see Relaxant, muscle*						
Muscle-action drug NEC	T48.201	T48.202	T48.203	T48.204	T48.205	T48.206
Muscle affecting agents NEC	T48.201	T48.202	T48.203	T48.204	T48.205	T48.206
oxytocic	T48.0X1	T48.0X2	T48.0X3	T48.0X4	T48.0X5	T48.0X6
relaxants	T48.201	T48.202	T48.203	T48.204	T48.205	T48.206
central nervous system	T42.8X1	T42.8X2	T42.8X3	T42.8X4	T42.8X5	T42.8X6
skeletal	T48.1X1	T48.1X2	T48.1X3	T48.1X4	T48.1X5	T48.1X6
smooth	T44.3X1	T44.3X2	T44.3X3	T44.3X4	T44.3X5	T44.3X6
Muscle-tone depressant, central NEC	T42.8X1	T42.8X2	T42.8X3	T42.8X4	T42.8X5	T42.8X6
specified NEC	T42.8X1	T42.8X2	T42.8X3	T42.8X4	T42.8X5	T42.8X6
Mushroom, noxious	T62.0X1	T62.0X2	T62.0X3	T62.0X4	—	—
Mussel, noxious	T61.781	T61.782	T61.783	T61.784		

◀ New ◀ Revised ~~deleted~~ Deleted

TABLE OF DRUGS AND CHEMICALS

TABLE OF DRUGS AND CHEMICALS

Substance	External Cause (T-Code)					
	Poisoning, Accidental (Unintentional)	Poisoning, Intentional Self-Harm	Poisoning, Assault	Poisoning, Undetermined	Adverse Effect	Underdosing
Mustard (emetic)	T47.7X1	T47.7X2	T47.7X3	T47.7X4	T47.7X5	T47.7X6
black	T47.7X1	T47.7X2	T47.7X3	T47.7X4	T47.7X5	T47.7X6
gas, not in war	T59.91	T59.92	T59.93	T59.94	—	—
nitrogen	T45.1X1	T45.1X2	T45.1X3	T45.1X4	T45.1X5	T45.1X6
Mustine	T45.1X1	T45.1X2	T45.1X3	T45.1X4	T45.1X5	T45.1X6
M-vac	T45.1X1	T45.1X2	T45.1X3	T45.1X4	T45.1X5	T45.1X6
Mycifradin	T36.5X1	T36.5X2	T36.5X3	T36.5X4	T36.5X5	T36.5X6
topical	T49.0X1	T49.0X2	T49.0X3	T49.0X4	T49.0X5	T49.0X6
Mycitracin	T36.8X1	T36.8X2	T36.8X3	T36.8X4	T36.8X5	T36.8X6
ophthalmic preparation	T49.5X1	T49.5X2	T49.5X3	T49.5X4	T49.5X5	T49.5X6
Mycostatin	T36.7X1	T36.7X2	T36.7X3	T36.7X4	T36.7X5	T36.7X6
topical	T49.0X1	T49.0X2	T49.0X3	T49.0X4	T49.0X5	T49.0X6
Mycotoxins	T64.81	T64.82	T64.83	T64.84	—	—
aflatoxin	T64.01	T64.02	T64.03	T64.04	—	—
specified NEC	T64.81	T64.82	T64.83	T64.84	—	—
Mydriacyl	T44.3X1	T44.3X2	T44.3X3	T44.3X4	T44.3X5	T44.3X6
Mydriatic drug	T49.5X1	T49.5X2	T49.5X3	T49.5X4	T49.5X5	T49.5X6
Myelobromal	T45.1X1	T45.1X2	T45.1X3	T45.1X4	T45.1X5	T45.1X6
Myleran	T45.1X1	T45.1X2	T45.1X3	T45.1X4	T45.1X5	T45.1X6
Myochrysin(e)	T39.2X1	T39.2X2	T39.2X3	T39.2X4	T39.2X5	T39.2X6
Myoneural blocking agents	T48.1X1	T48.1X2	T48.1X3	T48.1X4	T48.1X5	T48.1X6
Myralact	T49.0X1	T49.0X2	T49.0X3	T49.0X4	T49.0X5	T49.0X6
Myristica fragrans	T62.2X1	T62.2X2	T62.2X3	T62.2X4	—	—
Myristicin	T65.891	T65.892	T65.893	T65.894	—	—
Mysoline	T42.3X1	T42.3X2	T42.3X3	T42.3X4	T42.3X5	T42.3X6
N						
Nabilone	T40.711	T40.712	T40.713	T40.714	T40.715	T40.716
Nabumetone	T39.391	T39.392	T39.393	T39.394	T39.395	T39.396
Nadolol	T44.7X1	T44.7X2	T44.7X3	T44.7X4	T44.7X5	T44.7X6
Nafcillin	T36.0X1	T36.0X2	T36.0X3	T36.0X4	T36.0X5	T36.0X6
Nafoxidine	T38.6X1	T38.6X2	T38.6X3	T38.6X4	T38.6X5	T38.6X6
Naftazone	T46.991	T46.992	T46.993	T46.994	T46.995	T46.996
Naftidrofuryl (oxalate)	T46.7X1	T46.7X2	T46.7X3	T46.7X4	T46.7X5	T46.7X6
Naftifine	T49.0X1	T49.0X2	T49.0X3	T49.0X4	T49.0X5	T49.0X6
Nail polish remover	T52.91	T52.92	T52.93	T52.94	—	—
Nalbuphine	T40.491	T40.492	T40.493	T40.494	T40.495	T40.496
Naled	T60.0X1	T60.0X2	T60.0X3	T60.0X4	—	—
Nalidixic acid	T37.8X1	T37.8X2	T37.8X3	T37.8X4	T37.8X5	T37.8X6
Nalorphine	T50.7X1	T50.7X2	T50.7X3	T50.7X4	T50.7X5	T50.7X6
Naloxone	T50.7X1	T50.7X2	T50.7X3	T50.7X4	T50.7X5	T50.7X6
Naltrexone	T50.7X1	T50.7X2	T50.7X3	T50.7X4	T50.7X5	T50.7X6
Namenda	T43.8X1	T43.8X2	T43.8X3	T43.8X4	T43.8X5	T43.8X6

Substance	External Cause (T-Code)					
	Poisoning, Accidental (Unintentional)	Poisoning, Intentional Self-Harm	Poisoning, Assault	Poisoning, Undetermined	Adverse Effect	Underdosing
Nandrolone	T38.7X1	T38.7X2	T38.7X3	T38.7X4	T38.7X5	T38.7X6
Naphazoline	T48.5X1	T48.5X2	T48.5X3	T48.5X4	T48.5X5	T48.5X6
Naphtha (painters') (petroleum)	T52.0X1	T52.0X2	T52.0X3	T52.0X4	—	—
solvent	T52.0X1	T52.0X2	T52.0X3	T52.0X4	—	—
vapor	T52.0X1	T52.0X2	T52.0X3	T52.0X4	—	—
Naphthalene (non-chlorinated)	T60.2X1	T60.2X2	T60.2X3	T60.2X4	—	—
chlorinated	T60.1X1	T60.1X2	T60.1X3	T60.1X4	—	—
vapor	T60.1X1	T60.1X2	T60.1X3	T60.1X4	—	—
insecticide or moth repellent	T60.2X1	T60.2X2	T60.2X3	T60.2X4	—	—
chlorinated	T60.1X1	T60.1X2	T60.1X3	T60.1X4	—	—
vapor	T60.2X1	T60.2X2	T60.2X3	T60.2X4	—	—
chlorinated	T60.1X1	T60.1X2	T60.1X3	T60.1X4	—	—
Naphthol	T65.891	T65.892	T65.893	T65.894	—	—
Naphthylamine	T65.891	T65.892	T65.893	T65.894	—	—
Naphthylthiourea (ANTU)	T60.4X1	T60.4X2	T60.4X3	T60.4X4	—	—
Naprosyn — see Naproxen						
Naproxen	T39.311	T39.312	T39.313	T39.314	T39.315	T39.316
Narcotic (drug)	T40.601	T40.602	T40.603	T40.604	T40.605	T40.606
analgesic NEC	T40.601	T40.602	T40.603	T40.604	T40.605	T40.606
antagonist	T50.7X1	T50.7X2	T50.7X3	T50.7X4	T50.7X5	T50.7X6
specified NEC	T40.691	T40.692	T40.693	T40.694	T40.695	T40.696
synthetic	T40.491	T40.492	T40.493	T40.494	T40.495	T40.496
Narcotine	T48.3X1	T48.3X2	T48.3X3	T48.3X4	T48.3X5	T48.3X6
Nardil	T43.1X1	T43.1X2	T43.1X3	T43.1X4	T43.1X5	T43.1X6
Nasal drug NEC	T49.6X1	T49.6X2	T49.6X3	T49.6X4	T49.6X5	T49.6X6
Natamycin	T49.0X1	T49.0X2	T49.0X3	T49.0X4	T49.0X5	T49.0X6
Natrium cyanide — see Cyanide(s)						
Natural gas	T59.891	T59.892	T59.893	T59.894	—	—
incomplete combustion	T57.91	T57.92	T57.93	T57.94	—	—
Natural						
blood (product)	T45.8X1	T45.8X2	T45.8X3	T45.8X4	T45.8X5	T45.8X6
gas (piped)	T59.891	T59.892	T59.893	T59.894	—	—
incomplete combustion	T58.11	T58.12	T58.13	T58.14	—	—
Nealbarbital	T42.3X1	T42.3X2	T42.3X3	T42.3X4	T42.3X5	T42.3X6
Nectadon	T48.3X1	T48.3X2	T48.3X3	T48.3X4	T48.3X5	T48.3X6
Nedocromil	T48.6X1	T48.6X2	T48.6X3	T48.6X4	T48.6X5	T48.6X6
Nefopam	T39.8X1	T39.8X2	T39.8X3	T39.8X4	T39.8X5	T39.8X6
Nematocyst (sting)	T63.691	T63.692	T63.693	T63.694	—	—
Nembutal	T42.3X1	T42.3X2	T42.3X3	T42.3X4	T42.3X5	T42.3X6
Nemonapride	T43.591	T43.592	T43.593	T43.594	T43.595	T43.596
Neoarsphenamine	T37.8X1	T37.8X2	T37.8X3	T37.8X4	T37.8X5	T37.8X6

◀ New　◀ Revised　~~deleted~~ Deleted

Substance	External Cause (T-Code) Poisoning, Accidental (Unintentional)	Poisoning, Intentional Self-Harm	Poisoning, Assault	Poisoning, Undetermined	Adverse Effect	Underdosing
Neocinchophen	T50.4X1	T50.4X2	T50.4X3	T50.4X4	T50.4X5	T50.4X6
Neomycin (derivatives)	T36.5X1	T36.5X2	T36.5X3	T36.5X4	T36.5X5	T36.5X6
with						
bacitracin	T49.0X1	T49.0X2	T49.0X3	T49.0X4	T49.0X5	T49.0X6
neostigmine	T44.0X1	T44.0X2	T44.0X3	T44.0X4	T44.0X5	T44.0X6
ENT agent	T49.6X1	T49.6X2	T49.6X3	T49.6X4	T49.6X5	T49.6X6
ophthalmic preparation	T49.5X1	T49.5X2	T49.5X3	T49.5X4	T49.5X5	T49.5X6
topical NEC	T49.0X1	T49.0X2	T49.0X3	T49.0X4	T49.0X5	T49.0X6
Neonal	T42.3X1	T42.3X2	T42.3X3	T42.3X4	T42.3X5	T42.3X6
Neoprontosil	T37.0X1	T37.0X2	T37.0X3	T37.0X4	T37.0X5	T37.0X6
Neosalvarsan	T37.8X1	T37.8X2	T37.8X3	T37.8X4	T37.8X5	T37.8X6
Neosilversalvarsan	T37.8X1	T37.8X2	T37.8X3	T37.8X4	T37.8X5	T37.8X6
Neosporin	T36.8X1	T36.8X2	T36.8X3	T36.8X4	T36.8X5	T36.8X6
ENT agent	T49.6X1	T49.6X2	T49.6X3	T49.6X4	T49.6X5	T49.6X6
opthalmic preparation	T49.5X1	T49.5X2	T49.5X3	T49.5X4	T49.5X5	T49.5X6
topical NEC	T49.0X1	T49.0X2	T49.0X3	T49.0X4	T49.0X5	T49.0X6
Neostigmine bromide	T44.0X1	T44.0X2	T44.0X3	T44.0X4	T44.0X5	T44.0X6
Neraval	T42.3X1	T42.3X2	T42.3X3	T42.3X4	T42.3X5	T42.3X6
Neravan	T42.3X1	T42.3X2	T42.3X3	T42.3X4	T42.3X5	T42.3X6
Nerium oleander	T62.2X1	T62.2X2	T62.2X3	T62.2X4	—	—
Nerve gas, not in war	T59.91	T59.92	T59.93	T59.94	—	—
Nesacaine	T41.3X1	T41.3X2	T41.3X3	T41.3X4	T41.3X5	T41.3X6
infiltration (subcutaneous)	T41.3X1	T41.3X2	T41.3X3	T41.3X4	T41.3X5	T41.3X6
nerve block (peripheral) (plexus)	T41.3X1	T41.3X2	T41.3X3	T41.3X4	T41.3X5	T41.3X6
Netilmicin	T36.5X1	T36.5X2	T36.5X3	T36.5X4	T36.5X5	T36.5X6
Neurobarb	T42.3X1	T42.3X2	T42.3X3	T42.3X4	T42.3X5	T42.3X6
Neuroleptic drug NEC	T43.501	T43.502	T43.503	T43.504	T43.505	T43.506
Neuromuscular blocking drug	T48.1X1	T48.1X2	T48.1X3	T48.1X4	T48.1X5	T48.1X6
Neutral insulin injection	T38.3X1	T38.3X2	T38.3X3	T38.3X4	T38.3X5	T38.3X6
Neutral spirits	T51.0X1	T51.0X2	T51.0X3	T51.0X4	—	—
beverage	T51.0X1	T51.0X2	T51.0X3	T51.0X4	—	—
Niacin	T46.7X1	T46.7X2	T46.7X3	T46.7X4	T46.7X5	T46.7X6
Niacinamide	T45.2X1	T45.2X2	T45.2X3	T45.2X4	T45.2X5	T45.2X6
Nialamide	T43.1X1	T43.1X2	T43.1X3	T43.1X4	T43.1X5	T43.1X6
Niaprazine	T42.6X1	T42.6X2	T42.6X3	T42.6X4	T42.6X5	T42.6X6
Nicametate	T46.7X1	T46.7X2	T46.7X3	T46.7X4	T46.7X5	T46.7X6
Nicardipine	T46.1X1	T46.1X2	T46.1X3	T46.1X4	T46.1X5	T46.1X6
Nicergoline	T46.7X1	T46.7X2	T46.7X3	T46.7X4	T46.7X5	T46.7X6
Nickel (carbonyl) (tetra-carbonyl) (fumes) (vapor)	T56.891	T56.892	T56.893	T56.894	—	—

Substance	External Cause (T-Code) Poisoning, Accidental (Unintentional)	Poisoning, Intentional Self-Harm	Poisoning, Assault	Poisoning, Undetermined	Adverse Effect	Underdosing
Nickelocene	T56.891	T56.892	T56.893	T56.894	—	—
Niclosamide	T37.4X1	T37.4X2	T37.4X3	T37.4X4	T37.4X5	T37.4X6
Nicofuranose	T46.7X1	T46.7X2	T46.7X3	T46.7X4	T46.7X5	T46.7X6
Nicomorphine	T40.2X1	T40.2X2	T40.2X3	T40.2X4	—	—
Nicorandil	T46.3X1	T46.3X2	T46.3X3	T46.3X4	T46.3X5	T46.3X6
Nicotiana (plant)	T62.2X1	T62.2X2	T62.2X3	T62.2X4	—	—
Nicotinamide	T45.2X1	T45.2X2	T45.2X3	T45.2X4	T45.2X5	T45.2X6
Nicotine (insecticide) (spray) (sulfate) NEC	T60.2X1	T60.2X2	T60.2X3	T60.2X4	—	—
from tobacco	T65.291	T65.292	T65.293	T65.294	—	—
cigarettes	T65.221	T65.222	T65.223	T65.224	—	—
not insecticide	T65.291	T65.292	T65.293	T65.294	—	—
Nicotinic acid	T46.7X1	T46.7X2	T46.7X3	T46.7X4	T46.7X5	T46.7X6
Nicotinyl alcohol	T46.7X1	T46.7X2	T46.7X3	T46.7X4	T46.7X5	T46.7X6
Nicoumalone	T45.511	T45.512	T45.513	T45.514	T45.515	T45.516
Nifedipine	T46.1X1	T46.1X2	T46.1X3	T46.1X4	T46.1X5	T46.1X6
Nifenazone	T39.2X1	T39.2X2	T39.2X3	T39.2X4	T39.2X5	T39.2X6
Nifuraldezone	T37.91	T37.92	T37.93	T37.94	T37.95	T37.96
Nifuratel	T37.8X1	T37.8X2	T37.8X3	T37.8X4	T37.8X5	T37.8X6
Nifurtimox	T37.3X1	T37.3X2	T37.3X3	T37.3X4	T37.3X5	T37.3X6
Nifurtoinol	T37.8X1	T37.8X2	T37.8X3	T37.8X4	T37.8X5	T37.8X6
Nightshade, deadly (solanum) — see also Belladonna	T62.2X1	T62.2X2	T62.2X3	T62.2X4	—	—
berry	T62.1X1	T62.1X2	T62.1X3	T62.1X4	—	—
Nikethamide	T50.7X1	T50.7X2	T50.7X3	T50.7X4	T50.7X5	T50.7X6
Nilstat	T36.7X1	T36.7X2	T36.7X3	T36.7X4	T36.7X5	T36.7X6
topical	T49.0X1	T49.0X2	T49.0X3	T49.0X4	T49.0X5	T49.0X6
Nilutamide	T38.6X1	T38.6X2	T38.6X3	T38.6X4	T38.6X5	T38.6X6
Nimesulide	T39.391	T39.392	T39.393	T39.394	T39.395	T39.396
Nimetazepam	T42.4X1	T42.4X2	T42.4X3	T42.4X4	T42.4X5	T42.4X6
Nimodipine	T46.1X1	T46.1X2	T46.1X3	T46.1X4	T46.1X5	T46.1X6
Nimorazole	T37.3X1	T37.3X2	T37.3X3	T37.3X4	T37.3X5	T37.3X6
Nimustine	T45.1X1	T45.1X2	T45.1X3	T45.1X4	T45.1X5	T45.1X6
Niridazole	T37.4X1	T37.4X2	T37.4X3	T37.4X4	T37.4X5	T37.4X6
Nisentil	T40.2X1	T40.2X2	T40.2X3	T40.2X4	T40.2X5	T40.2X6
Nisoldipine	T46.1X1	T46.1X2	T46.1X3	T46.1X4	T46.1X5	T46.1X6
Nitramine	T65.3X1	T65.3X2	T65.3X3	T65.3X4	—	—
Nitrate, organic	T46.3X1	T46.3X2	T46.3X3	T46.3X4	T46.3X5	T46.3X6
Nitrazepam	T42.4X1	T42.4X2	T42.4X3	T42.4X4	T42.4X5	T42.4X6
Nitrefazole	T50.6X1	T50.6X2	T50.6X3	T50.6X4	T50.6X5	T50.6X6
Nitrendipine	T46.1X1	T46.1X2	T46.1X3	T46.1X4	T46.1X5	T46.1X6

◀ New ◀ Revised ~~deleted~~ Deleted

Substance	Poisoning, Accidental (Unintentional)	Poisoning, Intentional Self-Harm	Poisoning, Assault	Poisoning, Undetermined	Adverse Effect	Underdosing
Nitric						
acid (liquid)	T54.2X1	T54.2X2	T54.2X3	T54.2X4	—	—
vapor	T59.891	T59.892	T59.893	T59.894	—	—
oxide (gas)	T59.0X1	T59.0X2	T59.0X3	T59.0X4	—	—
Nitrimidazine	T37.3X1	T37.3X2	T37.3X3	T37.3X4	T37.3X5	T37.3X6
Nitrite, amyl (medicinal) (vapor)	T46.3X1	T46.3X2	T46.3X3	T46.3X4	T46.3X5	T46.3X6
Nitroaniline	T65.3X1	T65.3X2	T65.3X3	T65.3X4	—	—
vapor	T59.891	T59.892	T59.893	T59.894	—	—
Nitrobenzene, nitrobenzol	T65.3X1	T65.3X2	T65.3X3	T65.3X4	—	—
vapor	T65.3X1	T65.3X2	T65.3X3	T65.3X4	—	—
Nitrocellulose	T65.891	T65.892	T65.893	T65.894	—	—
lacquer	T65.891	T65.892	T65.893	T65.894	—	—
Nitrodiphenyl	T65.3X1	T65.3X2	T65.3X3	T65.3X4	—	—
Nitrofural	T49.0X1	T49.0X2	T49.0X3	T49.0X4	T49.0X5	T49.0X6
Nitrofurantoin	T37.8X1	T37.8X2	T37.8X3	T37.8X4	T37.8X5	T37.8X6
Nitrofurazone	T49.0X1	T49.0X2	T49.0X3	T49.0X4	T49.0X5	T49.0X6
Nitrogen	T59.0X1	T59.0X2	T59.0X3	T59.0X4	—	—
mustard	T45.1X1	T45.1X2	T45.1X3	T45.1X4	T45.1X5	T45.1X6
Nitroglycerin, nitro-glycerol (medicinal)	T46.3X1	T46.3X2	T46.3X3	T46.3X4	T46.3X5	T46.3X6
nonmedicinal	T65.5X1	T65.5X2	T65.5X3	T65.5X4	—	—
fumes	T65.5X1	T65.5X2	T65.5X3	T65.5X4	—	—
Nitroglycol	T52.3X1	T52.3X2	T52.3X3	T52.3X4	—	—
Nitrohydrochloric acid	T54.2X1	T54.2X2	T54.2X3	T54.2X4	—	—
Nitromersol	T49.0X1	T49.0X2	T49.0X3	T49.0X4	T49.0X5	T49.0X6
Nitronaphthalene	T65.891	T65.892	T65.893	T65.894	—	—
Nitrophenol	T54.0X1	T54.0X2	T54.0X3	T54.0X4	—	—
Nitropropane	T52.8X1	T52.8X2	T52.8X3	T52.8X4	—	—
Nitroprusside	T46.5X1	T46.5X2	T46.5X3	T46.5X4	T46.5X5	T46.5X6
Nitrosodimethylamine	T65.3X1	T65.3X2	T65.3X3	T65.3X4	—	—
Nitrothiazol	T37.4X1	T37.4X2	T37.4X3	T37.4X4	T37.4X5	T37.4X6
Nitrotoluene, nitrotoluol	T65.3X1	T65.3X2	T65.3X3	T65.3X4	—	—
vapor	T65.3X1	T65.3X2	T65.3X3	T65.3X4	—	—
Nitrous						
acid (liquid)	T54.2X1	T54.2X2	T54.2X3	T54.2X4	—	—
fumes	T59.891	T59.892	T59.893	T59.894	—	—
ether spirit	T46.3X1	T46.3X2	T46.3X3	T46.3X4	T46.3X5	T46.3X6
oxide	T41.0X1	T41.0X2	T41.0X3	T41.0X4	T41.0X5	T41.0X6
Nitroxoline	T37.8X1	T37.8X2	T37.8X3	T37.8X4	T37.8X5	T37.8X6
Nitrozone	T49.0X1	T49.0X2	T49.0X3	T49.0X4	T49.0X5	T49.0X6
Nizatidine	T47.0X1	T47.0X2	T47.0X3	T47.0X4	T47.0X5	T47.0X6

Substance	Poisoning, Accidental (Unintentional)	Poisoning, Intentional Self-Harm	Poisoning, Assault	Poisoning, Undetermined	Adverse Effect	Underdosing
Nizofenone	T43.8X1	T43.8X2	T43.8X3	T43.8X4	T43.8X5	T43.8X6
Noctec	T42.6X1	T42.6X2	T42.6X3	T42.6X4	T42.6X5	T42.6X6
Noludar	T42.6X1	T42.6X2	T42.6X3	T42.6X4	T42.6X5	T42.6X6
Noptil	T42.3X1	T42.3X2	T42.3X3	T42.3X4	T42.3X5	T42.3X6
Nomegestrol	T38.5X1	T38.5X2	T38.5X3	T38.5X4	T38.5X5	T38.5X6
Nomifensine	T43.291	T43.292	T43.293	T43.294	T43.295	T43.296
Nonoxinol	T49.8X1	T49.8X2	T49.8X3	T49.8X4	T49.8X5	T49.8X6
Nonylphenoxy (polyethoxy-ethanol)	T49.8X1	T49.8X2	T49.8X3	T49.8X4	T49.8X5	T49.8X6
Noptil	T42.3X1	T42.3X2	T42.3X3	T42.3X4	T42.3X5	T42.3X6
Noradrenaline	T44.4X1	T44.4X2	T44.4X3	T44.4X4	T44.4X5	T44.4X6
Noramidopyrine	T39.2X1	T39.2X2	T39.2X3	T39.2X4	T39.2X5	T39.2X6
methanesulfonate sodium	T39.2X1	T39.2X2	T39.2X3	T39.2X4	T39.2X5	T39.2X6
Norbormide	T60.4X1	T60.4X2	T60.4X3	T60.4X4	—	—
Nordazepam	T42.4X1	T42.4X2	T42.4X3	T42.4X4	T42.4X5	T42.4X6
Norepinephrine	T44.4X1	T44.4X2	T44.4X3	T44.4X4	T44.4X5	T44.4X6
Norethandrolone	T38.7X1	T38.7X2	T38.7X3	T38.7X4	T38.7X5	T38.7X6
Norethindrone	T38.4X1	T38.4X2	T38.4X3	T38.4X4	T38.4X5	T38.4X6
Norethisterone (acetate) (enantate)	T38.4X1	T38.4X2	T38.4X3	T38.4X4	T38.4X5	T38.4X6
with ethinylestradiol	T38.5X1	T38.5X2	T38.5X3	T38.5X4	T38.5X5	T38.5X6
Noretynodrel	T38.5X1	T38.5X2	T38.5X3	T38.5X4	T38.5X5	T38.5X6
Norfenefrine	T44.4X1	T44.4X2	T44.4X3	T44.4X4	T44.4X5	T44.4X6
Norfloxacin	T36.8X1	T36.8X2	T36.8X3	T36.8X4	T36.8X5	T36.8X6
Norgestrel	T38.4X1	T38.4X2	T38.4X3	T38.4X4	T38.4X5	T38.4X6
Norgestrienone	T38.4X1	T38.4X2	T38.4X3	T38.4X4	T38.4X5	T38.4X6
Norlestrin	T38.4X1	T38.4X2	T38.4X3	T38.4X4	T38.4X5	T38.4X6
Norlutin	T38.4X1	T38.4X2	T38.4X3	T38.4X4	T38.4X5	T38.4X6
Normal serum albumin (human), salt-poor	T45.8X1	T45.8X2	T45.8X3	T45.8X4	T45.8X5	T45.8X6
Normethandrone	T38.5X1	T38.5X2	T38.5X3	T38.5X4	T38.5X5	T38.5X6
Normison — see Benzodiazepines						
Normorphine	T40.2X1	T40.2X2	T40.2X3	T40.2X4	—	—
Norpseudoephedrine	T50.5X1	T50.5X2	T50.5X3	T50.5X4	T50.5X5	T50.5X6
Nortestosterone (furanpropionate)	T38.7X1	T38.7X2	T38.7X3	T38.7X4	T38.7X5	T38.7X6
Nortriptyline	T43.011	T43.012	T43.013	T43.014	T43.015	T43.016
Noscapine	T48.3X1	T48.3X2	T48.3X3	T48.3X4	T48.3X5	T48.3X6
Nose preparations	T49.6X1	T49.6X2	T49.6X3	T49.6X4	T49.6X5	T49.6X6
Novobiocin	T36.5X1	T36.5X2	T36.5X3	T36.5X4	T36.5X5	T36.5X6
Novocain (infiltration) (topical)	T41.3X1	T41.3X2	T41.3X3	T41.3X4	T41.3X5	T41.3X6
nerve block (peripheral) (plexus)	T41.3X1	T41.3X2	T41.3X3	T41.3X4	T41.3X5	T41.3X6
spinal	T41.3X1	T41.3X2	T41.3X3	T41.3X4	T41.3X5	T41.3X6

◀ New   ◀ Revised   ~~deleted~~ Deleted

Substance	Poisoning, Accidental (Unintentional)	Poisoning, Intentional Self-Harm	Poisoning, Assault	Poisoning, Undetermined	Adverse Effect	Underdosing
Noxious foodstuff	T62.91	T62.92	T62.93	T62.94	—	—
specified NEC	T62.8X1	T62.8X2	T62.8X3	T62.8X4	—	—
Noxiptiline	T43.011	T43.012	T43.013	T43.014	T43.015	T43.016
Noxytiolin	T49.0X1	T49.0X2	T49.0X3	T49.0X4	T49.0X5	T49.0X6
NPH Iletin (insulin)	T38.3X1	T38.3X2	T38.3X3	T38.3X4	T38.3X5	T38.3X6
Numorphan	T40.2X1	T40.2X2	T40.2X3	T40.2X4	T40.2X5	T40.2X6
Nunol	T42.3X1	T42.3X2	T42.3X3	T42.3X4	T42.3X5	T42.3X6
Nupercaine (spinal anesthetic)	T41.3X1	T41.3X2	T41.3X3	T41.3X4	T41.3X5	T41.3X6
topical (surface)	T41.3X1	T41.3X2	T41.3X3	T41.3X4	T41.3X5	T41.3X6
Nutmeg oil (liniment)	T49.3X1	T49.3X2	T49.3X3	T49.3X4	T49.3X5	T49.3X6
Nutritional supplement	T50.901	T50.902	T50.903	T50.904	T50.905	T50.906
Nux vomica	T65.1X1	T65.1X2	T65.1X3	T65.1X4	—	—
Nydrazid	T37.1X1	T37.1X2	T37.1X3	T37.1X4	T37.1X5	T37.1X6
Nylidrin	T46.7X1	T46.7X2	T46.7X3	T46.7X4	T46.7X5	T46.7X6
Nystatin	T36.7X1	T36.7X2	T36.7X3	T36.7X4	T36.7X5	T36.7X6
topical	T49.0X1	T49.0X2	T49.0X3	T49.0X4	T49.0X5	T49.0X6
Nytol	T45.0X1	T45.0X2	T45.0X3	T45.0X4	T45.0X5	T45.0X6

○

Substance	Poisoning, Accidental (Unintentional)	Poisoning, Intentional Self-Harm	Poisoning, Assault	Poisoning, Undetermined	Adverse Effect	Underdosing
Obidoxime chloride	T50.6X1	T50.6X2	T50.6X3	T50.6X4	T50.6X5	T50.6X6
Octafonium (chloride)	T49.3X1	T49.3X2	T49.3X3	T49.3X4	T49.3X5	T49.3X6
Octamethyl pyrophos-phoramide	T60.0X1	T60.0X2	T60.0X3	T60.0X4	—	—
Octanoin	T50.991	T50.992	T50.993	T50.994	T50.995	T50.996
Octatropine methyl-bromide	T44.3X1	T44.3X2	T44.3X3	T44.3X4	T44.3X5	T44.3X6
Octotiamine	T45.2X1	T45.2X2	T45.2X3	T45.2X4	T45.2X5	T45.2X6
Octoxinol (9)	T49.8X1	T49.8X2	T49.8X3	T49.8X4	T49.8X5	T49.8X6
Octreotide	T38.991	T38.992	T38.993	T38.994	T38.995	T38.996
Octyl nitrite	T46.3X1	T46.3X2	T46.3X3	T46.3X4	T46.3X5	T46.3X6
Oestradiol	T38.5X1	T38.5X2	T38.5X3	T38.5X4	T38.5X5	T38.5X6
Oestriol	T38.5X1	T38.5X2	T38.5X3	T38.5X4	T38.5X5	T38.5X6
Oestrogen	T38.5X1	T38.5X2	T38.5X3	T38.5X4	T38.5X5	T38.5X6
Oestrone	T38.5X1	T38.5X2	T38.5X3	T38.5X4	T38.5X5	T38.5X6
Ofloxacin	T36.8X1	T36.8X2	T36.8X3	T36.8X4	T36.8X5	T36.8X6
Oil (of)	T65.891	T65.892	T65.893	T65.894	—	—
bitter almond	T62.8X1	T62.8X2	T62.8X3	T62.8X4	—	—
cloves	T49.7X1	T49.7X2	T49.7X3	T49.7X4	T49.7X5	T49.7X6
colors	T65.6X1	T65.6X2	T65.6X3	T65.6X4	—	—
fumes	T59.891	T59.892	T59.893	T59.894	—	—
lubricating	T52.0X1	T52.0X2	T52.0X3	T52.0X4	—	—
Niobe	T52.8X1	T52.8X2	T52.8X3	T52.8X4	—	—

Substance	Poisoning, Accidental (Unintentional)	Poisoning, Intentional Self-Harm	Poisoning, Assault	Poisoning, Undetermined	Adverse Effect	Underdosing
Oil (of) *(Continued)*						
vitriol (liquid)	T54.2X1	T54.2X2	T54.2X3	T54.2X4	—	—
fumes	T54.2X1	T54.2X2	T54.2X3	T54.2X4	—	—
wintergreen (bitter) NEC	T49.3X1	T49.3X2	T49.3X3	T49.3X4	T49.3X5	T49.3X6
Oily preparation (for skin)	T49.3X1	T49.3X2	T49.3X3	T49.3X4	T49.3X5	T49.3X6
Ointment NEC	T49.3X1	T49.3X2	T49.3X3	T49.3X4	T49.3X5	T49.3X6
Olanzapine	T43.591	T43.592	T43.593	T43.594	T43.595	T43.596
Oleander	T62.2X1	T62.2X2	T62.2X3	T62.2X4	—	—
Oleandomycin	T36.3X1	T36.3X2	T36.3X3	T36.3X4	T36.3X5	T36.3X6
Oleandrin	T46.0X1	T46.0X2	T46.0X3	T46.0X4	T46.0X5	T46.0X6
Oleic acid	T46.6X1	T46.6X2	T46.6X3	T46.6X4	T46.6X5	T46.6X6
Oleovitamin A	T45.2X1	T45.2X2	T45.2X3	T45.2X4	T45.2X5	T45.2X6
Oleum ricini	T47.2X1	T47.2X2	T47.2X3	T47.2X4	T47.2X5	T47.2X6
Olive oil (medicinal) NEC	T47.4X1	T47.4X2	T47.4X3	T47.4X4	T47.4X5	T47.4X6
Olivomycin	T45.1X1	T45.1X2	T45.1X3	T45.1X4	T45.1X5	T45.1X6
Olsalazine	T47.8X1	T47.8X2	T47.8X3	T47.8X4	T47.8X5	T47.8X6
Omeprazole	T47.1X1	T47.1X2	T47.1X3	T47.1X4	T47.1X5	T47.1X6
OMPA	T60.0X1	T60.0X2	T60.0X3	T60.0X4	—	—
Ondansetron	T45.0X1	T45.0X2	T45.0X3	T45.0X4	T45.0X5	T45.0X6
Oncovin	T45.1X1	T45.1X2	T45.1X3	T45.1X4	T45.1X5	T45.1X6
Ophthaine	T41.3X1	T41.3X2	T41.3X3	T41.3X4	T41.3X5	T41.3X6
Ophthetic	T41.3X1	T41.3X2	T41.3X3	T41.3X4	T41.3X5	T41.3X6
Opiate NEC	T40.601	T40.602	T40.603	T40.604	T40.605	T40.606
antagonists	T50.7X1	T50.7X2	T50.7X3	T50.7X4	T50.7X5	T50.7X6
Opioid NEC	T40.2X1	T40.2X2	T40.2X3	T40.2X4	T40.2X5	T40.2X6
Opipramol	T43.011	T43.012	T43.013	T43.014	T43.015	T43.016
Opium alkaloids (total)	T40.0X1	T40.0X2	T40.0X3	T40.0X4	T40.0X5	T40.0X6
standardized powdered	T40.0X1	T40.0X2	T40.0X3	T40.0X4	T40.0X5	T40.0X6
tincture (camphorated)	T40.0X1	T40.0X2	T40.0X3	T40.0X4	T40.0X5	T40.0X6
Oracon	T38.4X1	T38.4X2	T38.4X3	T38.4X4	T38.4X5	T38.4X6
Oragrafin	T50.8X1	T50.8X2	T50.8X3	T50.8X4	T50.8X5	T50.8X6
Oral contraceptives	T38.4X1	T38.4X2	T38.4X3	T38.4X4	T38.4X5	T38.4X6
Oral rehydration salts	T50.3X1	T50.3X2	T50.3X3	T50.3X4	T50.3X5	T50.3X6
Orazamide	T50.991	T50.992	T50.993	T50.994	T50.995	T50.996
Orciprenaline	T48.291	T48.292	T48.293	T48.294	T48.295	T48.296
Organidin	T48.4X1	T48.4X2	T48.4X3	T48.4X4	T48.4X5	T48.4X6
Organonitrate NEC	T46.3X1	T46.3X2	T46.3X3	T46.3X4	T46.3X5	T46.3X6
Organophosphates	T60.0X1	T60.0X2	T60.0X3	T60.0X4	—	—
Orimune	T50.B91	T50.B92	T50.B93	T50.B94	T50.B95	T50.B96
Orinase	T38.3X1	T38.3X2	T38.3X3	T38.3X4	T38.3X5	T38.3X6
Ormeloxifene	T38.6X1	T38.6X2	T38.6X3	T38.6X4	T38.6X5	T38.6X6

◀ New ◀ Revised ~~deleted~~ Deleted

Substance	External Cause (T-Code)					
	Poisoning, Accidental (Unintentional)	Poisoning, Intentional Self-Harm	Poisoning, Assault	Poisoning, Undetermined	Adverse Effect	Underdosing
Ornidazole	T37.3X1	T37.3X2	T37.3X3	T37.3X4	T37.3X5	T37.3X6
Ornithine aspartate	T50.991	T50.992	T50.993	T50.994	T50.995	T50.996
Ornoprostil	T47.1X1	T47.1X2	T47.1X3	T47.1X4	T47.1X5	T47.1X6
Orphenadrine (hydrochloride)	T42.8X1	T42.8X2	T42.8X3	T42.8X4	T42.8X5	T42.8X6
Ortal (sodium)	T42.3X1	T42.3X2	T42.3X3	T42.3X4	T42.3X5	T42.3X6
Orthoboric acid	T49.0X1	T49.0X2	T49.0X3	T49.0X4	T49.0X5	T49.0X6
ENT agent	T49.6X1	T49.6X2	T49.6X3	T49.6X4	T49.6X5	T49.6X6
ophthalmic preparation	T49.5X1	T49.5X2	T49.5X3	T49.5X4	T49.5X5	T49.5X6
Orthocaine	T41.3X1	T41.3X2	T41.3X3	T41.3X4	T41.3X5	T41.3X6
Orthodichlorobenzene	T53.7X1	T53.7X2	T53.7X3	T53.7X4	—	—
Ortho-Novum	T38.4X1	T38.4X2	T38.4X3	T38.4X4	T38.4X5	T38.4X6
Orthotolidine (reagent)	T54.2X1	T54.2X2	T54.2X3	T54.2X4	—	—
Osmic acid (liquid)	T54.2X1	T54.2X2	T54.2X3	T54.2X4	—	—
fumes	T54.2X1	T54.2X2	T54.2X3	T54.2X4	—	—
Osmotic diuretics	T50.2X1	T50.2X2	T50.2X3	T50.2X4	T50.2X5	T50.2X6
Otilonium bromide	T44.3X1	T44.3X2	T44.3X3	T44.3X4	T44.3X5	T44.3X6
Otorhinolaryngological drug NEC	T49.6X1	T49.6X2	T49.6X3	T49.6X4	T49.6X5	T49.6X6
Ouabain(e)	T46.0X1	T46.0X2	T46.0X3	T46.0X4	T46.0X5	T46.0X6
Ovarian						
hormone	T38.5X1	T38.5X2	T38.5X3	T38.5X4	T38.5X5	T38.5X6
stimulant	T38.5X1	T38.5X2	T38.5X3	T38.5X4	T38.5X5	T38.5X6
Ovral	T38.4X1	T38.4X2	T38.4X3	T38.4X4	T38.4X5	T38.4X6
Ovulen	T38.4X1	T38.4X2	T38.4X3	T38.4X4	T38.4X5	T38.4X6
Oxacillin	T36.0X1	T36.0X2	T36.0X3	T36.0X4	T36.0X5	T36.0X6
Oxalic acid	T54.2X1	T54.2X2	T54.2X3	T54.2X4	—	—
ammonium salt	T50.991	T50.992	T50.993	T50.994	T50.995	T50.996
Oxamniquine	T37.4X1	T37.4X2	T37.4X3	T37.4X4	T37.4X5	T37.4X6
Oxanamide	T43.591	T43.592	T43.593	T43.594	T43.595	T43.596
Oxandrolone	T38.7X1	T38.7X2	T38.7X3	T38.7X4	T38.7X5	T38.7X6
Oxantel	T37.4X1	T37.4X2	T37.4X3	T37.4X4	T37.4X5	T37.4X6
Oxapium iodide	T44.3X1	T44.3X2	T44.3X3	T44.3X4	T44.3X5	T44.3X6
Oxaprotiline	T43.021	T43.022	T43.023	T43.024	T43.025	T43.026
Oxaprozin	T39.311	T39.312	T39.313	T39.314	T39.315	T39.316
Oxatomide	T45.0X1	T45.0X2	T45.0X3	T45.0X4	T45.0X5	T45.0X6
Oxazepam	T42.4X1	T42.4X2	T42.4X3	T42.4X4	T42.4X5	T42.4X6
Oxazimedrine	T50.5X1	T50.5X2	T50.5X3	T50.5X4	T50.5X5	T50.5X6
Oxazolam	T42.4X1	T42.4X2	T42.4X3	T42.4X4	T42.4X5	T42.4X6
Oxazolidine derivatives	T42.2X1	T42.2X2	T42.2X3	T42.2X4	T42.2X5	T42.2X6
Oxazolidinedione (derivative)	T42.2X1	T42.2X2	T42.2X3	T42.2X4	T42.2X5	T42.2X6
Ox bile extract	T47.5X1	T47.5X2	T47.5X3	T47.5X4	T47.5X5	T47.5X6
Oxcarbazepine	T42.1X1	T42.1X2	T42.1X3	T42.1X4	T42.1X5	T42.1X6
Oxedrine	T44.4X1	T44.4X2	T44.4X3	T44.4X4	T44.4X5	T44.4X6

Substance	External Cause (T-Code)					
	Poisoning, Accidental (Unintentional)	Poisoning, Intentional Self-Harm	Poisoning, Assault	Poisoning, Undetermined	Adverse Effect	Underdosing
Oxeladin (citrate)	T48.3X1	T48.3X2	T48.3X3	T48.3X4	T48.3X5	T48.3X6
Oxendolone	T38.5X1	T38.5X2	T38.5X3	T38.5X4	T38.5X5	T38.5X6
Oxetacaine	T41.3X1	T41.3X2	T41.3X3	T41.3X4	T41.3X5	T41.3X6
Oxethazine	T41.3X1	T41.3X2	T41.3X3	T41.3X4	T41.3X5	T41.3X6
Oxetorone	T39.8X1	T39.8X2	T39.8X3	T39.8X4	T39.8X5	T39.8X6
Oxiconazole	T49.0X1	T49.0X2	T49.0X3	T49.0X4	T49.0X5	T49.0X6
Oxidizing agent NEC	T54.91	T54.92	T54.93	T54.94	—	—
Oxipurinol	T50.4X1	T50.4X2	T50.4X3	T50.4X4	T50.4X5	T50.4X6
Oxitriptan	T43.291	T43.292	T43.293	T43.294	T43.295	T43.296
Oxitropium bromide	T48.6X1	T48.6X2	T48.6X3	T48.6X4	T48.6X5	T48.6X6
Oxodipine	T46.1X1	T46.1X2	T46.1X3	T46.1X4	T46.1X5	T46.1X6
Oxolamine	T48.3X1	T48.3X2	T48.3X3	T48.3X4	T48.3X5	T48.3X6
Oxolinic acid	T37.8X1	T37.8X2	T37.8X3	T37.8X4	T37.8X5	T37.8X6
Oxomemazine	T43.3X1	T43.3X2	T43.3X3	T43.3X4	T43.3X5	T43.3X6
Oxophenarsine	T37.3X1	T37.3X2	T37.3X3	T37.3X4	T37.3X5	T37.3X6
Oxprenolol	T44.7X1	T44.7X2	T44.7X3	T44.7X4	T44.7X5	T44.7X6
Oxsoralen	T49.3X1	T49.3X2	T49.3X3	T49.3X4	T49.3X5	T49.3X6
Oxtriphylline	T48.6X1	T48.6X2	T48.6X3	T48.6X4	T48.6X5	T48.6X6
Oxybate sodium	T41.291	T41.292	T41.293	T41.294	T41.295	T41.296
Oxybuprocaine	T41.3X1	T41.3X2	T41.3X3	T41.3X4	T41.3X5	T41.3X6
Oxybutynin	T44.3X1	T44.3X2	T44.3X3	T44.3X4	T44.3X5	T44.3X6
Oxychlorosene	T49.0X1	T49.0X2	T49.0X3	T49.0X4	T49.0X5	T49.0X6
Oxycodone	T40.2X1	T40.2X2	T40.2X3	T40.2X4	T40.2X5	T40.2X6
Oxyfedrine	T46.3X1	T46.3X2	T46.3X3	T46.3X4	T46.3X5	T46.3X6
Oxygen	T41.5X1	T41.5X2	T41.5X3	T41.5X4	T41.5X5	T41.5X6
Oxylone	T49.0X1	T49.0X2	T49.0X3	T49.0X4	T49.0X5	T49.0X6
ophthalmic preparation	T49.5X1	T49.5X2	T49.5X3	T49.5X4	T49.5X5	T49.5X6
Oxymesterone	T38.7X1	T38.7X2	T38.7X3	T38.7X4	T38.7X5	T38.7X6
Oxymetazoline	T48.5X1	T48.5X2	T48.5X3	T48.5X4	T48.5X5	T48.5X6
Oxymetholone	T38.7X1	T38.7X2	T38.7X3	T38.7X4	T38.7X5	T38.7X6
Oxymorphone	T40.2X1	T40.2X2	T40.2X3	T40.2X4	T40.2X5	T40.2X6
Oxypertine	T43.591	T43.592	T43.593	T43.594	T43.595	T43.596
Oxyphenbutazone	T39.2X1	T39.2X2	T39.2X3	T39.2X4	T39.2X5	T39.2X6
Oxyphencyclimine	T44.3X1	T44.3X2	T44.3X3	T44.3X4	T44.3X5	T44.3X6
Oxyphenisatine	T47.2X1	T47.2X2	T47.2X3	T47.2X4	T47.2X5	T47.2X6
Oxyphenonium bromide	T44.3X1	T44.3X2	T44.3X3	T44.3X4	T44.3X5	T44.3X6
Oxypolygelatin	T45.8X1	T45.8X2	T45.8X3	T45.8X4	T45.8X5	T45.8X6
Oxyquinoline (derivatives)	T37.8X1	T37.8X2	T37.8X3	T37.8X4	T37.8X5	T37.8X6
Oxytetracycline	T36.4X1	T36.4X2	T36.4X3	T36.4X4	T36.4X5	T36.4X6
Oxytocic drug NEC	T48.0X1	T48.0X2	T48.0X3	T48.0X4	T48.0X5	T48.0X6
Oxytocin (synthetic)	T48.0X1	T48.0X2	T48.0X3	T48.0X4	T48.0X5	T48.0X6
Ozone	T59.891	T59.892	T59.893	T59.894	—	—

◀ New　◀ Revised　deleted Deleted

Substance	Poisoning, Accidental (Unintentional)	Poisoning, Intentional Self-Harm	Poisoning, Assault	Poisoning, Undetermined	Adverse Effect	Underdosing
P						
PABA	T49.3X1	T49.3X2	T49.3X3	T49.3X4	T49.3X5	T49.3X6
Packed red cells	T45.8X1	T45.8X2	T45.8X3	T45.8X4	T45.8X5	T45.8X6
Padimate	T49.3X1	T49.3X2	T49.3X3	T49.3X4	T49.3X5	T49.3X6
Paint NEC	T65.6X1	T65.6X2	T65.6X3	T65.6X4	—	—
cleaner	T52.91	T52.92	T52.93	T52.94	—	—
fumes NEC	T59.891	T59.892	T59.893	T59.894	—	—
lead (fumes)	T56.0X1	T56.0X2	T56.0X3	T56.0X4	—	—
solvent NEC	T52.8X1	T52.8X2	T52.8X3	T52.8X4	—	—
stripper	T52.8X1	T52.8X2	T52.8X3	T52.8X4	—	—
Palfium	T40.2X1	T40.2X2	T40.2X3	T40.2X4	—	—
Palm kernel oil	T50.991	T50.992	T50.993	T50.994	T50.995	T50.996
Paludrine	T37.2X1	T37.2X2	T37.2X3	T37.2X4	T37.2X5	T37.2X6
PAM (pralidoxime)	T50.6X1	T50.6X2	T50.6X3	T50.6X4	T50.6X5	T50.6X6
Pamaquine (naphthoute)	T37.2X1	T37.2X2	T37.2X3	T37.2X4	T37.2X5	T37.2X6
Panadol	T39.1X1	T39.1X2	T39.1X3	T39.1X4	T39.1X5	T39.1X6
Pancreatic						
digestive secretion stimulant	T47.8X1	T47.8X2	T47.8X3	T47.8X4	T47.8X5	T47.8X6
dornase	T45.3X1	T45.3X2	T45.3X3	T45.3X4	T45.3X5	T45.3X6
Pancreatin	T47.5X1	T47.5X2	T47.5X3	T47.5X4	T47.5X5	T47.5X6
Pancrelipase	T47.5X1	T47.5X2	T47.5X3	T47.5X4	T47.5X5	T47.5X6
Pancuronium (bromide)	T48.1X1	T48.1X2	T48.1X3	T48.1X4	T48.1X5	T48.1X6
Pangamic acid	T45.2X1	T45.2X2	T45.2X3	T45.2X4	T45.2X5	T45.2X6
Panthenol	T45.2X1	T45.2X2	T45.2X3	T45.2X4	T45.2X5	T45.2X6
topical	T49.8X1	T49.8X2	T49.8X3	T49.8X4	T49.8X5	T49.8X6
Pantopon	T40.0X1	T40.0X2	T40.0X3	T40.0X4	T40.0X5	T40.0X6
Pantothenic acid	T45.2X1	T45.2X2	T45.2X3	T45.2X4	T45.2X5	T45.2X6
Panwarfin	T45.511	T45.512	T45.513	T45.514	T45.515	T45.516
Papain	T47.5X1	T47.5X2	T47.5X3	T47.5X4	T47.5X5	T47.5X6
digestant	T47.5X1	T47.5X2	T47.5X3	T47.5X4	T47.5X5	T47.5X6
Papaveretum	T40.0X1	T40.0X2	T40.0X3	T40.0X4	T40.0X5	T40.0X6
Papaverine	T44.3X1	T44.3X2	T44.3X3	T44.3X4	T44.3X5	T44.3X6
Para-acetamidophenol	T39.1X1	T39.1X2	T39.1X3	T39.1X4	T39.1X5	T39.1X6
Para-aminobenzoic acid	T49.3X1	T49.3X2	T49.3X3	T49.3X4	T49.3X5	T49.3X6
Para-aminophenol derivatives	T39.1X1	T39.1X2	T39.1X3	T39.1X4	T39.1X5	T39.1X6
Para-aminosalicylic acid	T37.1X1	T37.1X2	T37.1X3	T37.1X4	T37.1X5	T37.1X6
Paracetaldehyde	T42.6X1	T42.6X2	T42.6X3	T42.6X4	T42.6X5	T42.6X6
Paracetamol	T39.1X1	T39.1X2	T39.1X3	T39.1X4	T39.1X5	T39.1X6
Parachlorophenol (camphorated)	T49.0X1	T49.0X2	T49.0X3	T49.0X4	T49.0X5	T49.0X6
Paracodin	T40.2X1	T40.2X2	T40.2X3	T40.2X4	T40.2X5	T40.2X6
Paradione	T42.2X1	T42.2X2	T42.2X3	T42.2X4	T42.2X5	T42.2X6

Substance	Poisoning, Accidental (Unintentional)	Poisoning, Intentional Self-Harm	Poisoning, Assault	Poisoning, Undetermined	Adverse Effect	Underdosing
Paraffin(s) (wax)	T52.0X1	T52.0X2	T52.0X3	T52.0X4	—	—
liquid (medicinal)	T47.4X1	T47.4X2	T47.4X3	T47.4X4	T47.4X5	T47.4X6
nonmedicinal	T52.0X1	T52.0X2	T52.0X3	T52.0X4	—	—
Paraformaldehyde	T60.3X1	T60.3X2	T60.3X3	T60.3X4	—	—
Paraldehyde	T42.6X1	T42.6X2	T42.6X3	T42.6X4	T42.6X5	T42.6X6
Paramethadione	T42.2X1	T42.2X2	T42.2X3	T42.2X4	T42.2X5	T42.2X6
Paramethasone	T38.0X1	T38.0X2	T38.0X3	T38.0X4	T38.0X5	T38.0X6
acetate	T49.0X1	T49.0X2	T49.0X3	T49.0X4	T49.0X5	T49.0X6
Paraoxon	T60.0X1	T60.0X2	T60.0X3	T60.0X4	—	—
Paraquat	T60.3X1	T60.3X2	T60.3X3	T60.3X4	—	—
Parasympatholytic NEC	T44.3X1	T44.3X2	T44.3X3	T44.3X4	T44.3X5	T44.3X6
Parasympathomimetic drug NEC	T44.1X1	T44.1X2	T44.1X3	T44.1X4	T44.1X5	T44.1X6
Parathion	T60.0X1	T60.0X2	T60.0X3	T60.0X4	—	—
Parathormone	T50.991	T50.992	T50.993	T50.994	T50.995	T50.996
Parathyroid extract	T50.991	T50.992	T50.993	T50.994	T50.995	T50.996
Paratyphoid vaccine	T50.A91	T50.A92	T50.A93	T50.A94	T50.A95	T50.A96
Paredrine	T44.4X1	T44.4X2	T44.4X3	T44.4X4	T44.4X5	T44.4X6
Paregoric	T40.0X1	T40.0X2	T40.0X3	T40.0X4	T40.0X5	T40.0X6
Pargyline	T46.5X1	T46.5X2	T46.5X3	T46.5X4	T46.5X5	T46.5X6
Paris green	T57.0X1	T57.0X2	T57.0X3	T57.0X4	—	—
insecticide	T57.0X1	T57.0X2	T57.0X3	T57.0X4	—	—
Parnate	T43.1X1	T43.1X2	T43.1X3	T43.1X4	T43.1X5	T43.1X6
Paromomycin	T36.5X1	T36.5X2	T36.5X3	T36.5X4	T36.5X5	T36.5X6
Paroxypropione	T45.1X1	T45.1X2	T45.1X3	T45.1X4	T45.1X5	T45.1X6
Parzone	T40.2X1	T40.2X2	T40.2X3	T40.2X4	T40.2X5	T40.2X6
PAS	T37.1X1	T37.1X2	T37.1X3	T37.1X4	T37.1X5	T37.1X6
Pasiniazid	T37.1X1	T37.1X2	T37.1X3	T37.1X4	T37.1X5	T37.1X6
PBB (polybrominated biphenyls)	T65.891	T65.892	T65.893	T65.894	—	—
PCB	T65.891	T65.892	T65.893	T65.894	—	—
PCP						
meaning pentachlorophenol	T60.1X1	T60.1X2	T60.1X3	T60.1X4	—	—
fungicide	T60.3X1	T60.3X2	T60.3X3	T60.3X4	—	—
herbicide	T60.3X1	T60.3X2	T60.3X3	T60.3X4	—	—
insecticide	T60.1X1	T60.1X2	T60.1X3	T60.1X4	—	—
meaning phencyclidine	T40.991	T40.992	T40.993	T40.994	—	—
Peach kernel oil (emulsion)	T47.4X1	T47.4X2	T47.4X3	T47.4X4	T47.4X5	T47.4X6
Peanut oil (emulsion) NEC	T47.4X1	T47.4X2	T47.4X3	T47.4X4	T47.4X5	T47.4X6
topical	T49.3X1	T49.3X2	T49.3X3	T49.3X4	T49.3X5	T49.3X6
Pearly Gates (morning glory seeds)	T40.991	T40.992	T40.993	T40.994	—	—
Pecazine	T43.3X1	T43.3X2	T43.3X3	T43.3X4	T43.3X5	T43.3X6
Pectin	T47.6X1	T47.6X2	T47.6X3	T47.6X4	T47.6X5	T47.6X6

TABLE OF DRUGS AND CHEMICALS

	External Cause (T-Code)					
Substance	Poisoning, Accidental (Unintentional)	Poisoning, Intentional Self-Harm	Poisoning, Assault	Poisoning, Undetermined	Adverse Effect	Underdosing
Pefloxacin	T37.8X1	T37.8X2	T37.8X3	T37.8X4	T37.8X5	T37.8X6
Pegademase, bovine	T50.Z91	T50.Z92	T50.Z93	T50.Z94	T50.Z95	T50.Z96
Pelletierine tannate	T37.4X1	T37.4X2	T37.4X3	T37.4X4	T37.4X5	T37.4X6
Pemirolast (potassium)	T48.6X1	T48.6X2	T48.6X3	T48.6X4	T48.6X5	T48.6X6
Pemoline	T50.7X1	T50.7X2	T50.7X3	T50.7X4	T50.7X5	T50.7X6
Pempidine	T44.2X1	T44.2X2	T44.2X3	T44.2X4	T44.2X5	T44.2X6
Penamecillin	T36.0X1	T36.0X2	T36.0X3	T36.0X4	T36.0X5	T36.0X6
Penbutolol	T44.7X1	T44.7X2	T44.7X3	T44.7X4	T44.7X5	T44.7X6
Penethamate	T36.0X1	T36.0X2	T36.0X3	T36.0X4	T36.0X5	T36.0X6
Penfluridol	T43.591	T43.592	T43.593	T43.594	T43.595	T43.596
Penflutizide	T50.2X1	T50.2X2	T50.2X3	T50.2X4	T50.2X5	T50.2X6
Pengitoxin	T46.0X1	T46.0X2	T46.0X3	T46.0X4	T46.0X5	T46.0X6
Penicillamine	T50.6X1	T50.6X2	T50.6X3	T50.6X4	T50.6X5	T50.6X6
Penicillin (any)	T36.0X1	T36.0X2	T36.0X3	T36.0X4	T36.0X5	T36.0X6
Penicillinase	T45.3X1	T45.3X2	T45.3X3	T45.3X4	T45.3X5	T45.3X6
Penicilloyl polylysine	T50.8X1	T50.8X2	T50.8X3	T50.8X4	T50.8X5	T50.8X6
Penimepicycline	T36.4X1	T36.4X2	T36.4X3	T36.4X4	T36.4X5	T36.4X6
Pentachloroethane	T53.6X1	T53.6X2	T53.6X3	T53.6X4	—	—
Pentachloronaphthalene	T53.7X1	T53.7X2	T53.7X3	T53.7X4	—	—
Pentachlorophenol (pesticide)	T60.1X1	T60.1X2	T60.1X3	T60.1X4	—	—
fungicide	T60.3X1	T60.3X2	T60.3X3	T60.3X4	—	—
herbicide	T60.3X1	T60.3X2	T60.3X3	T60.3X4	—	—
insecticide	T60.1X1	T60.1X2	T60.1X3	T60.1X4	—	—
Pentaerythritol tetranitrate	T46.3X1	T46.3X2	T46.3X3	T46.3X4	T46.3X5	T46.3X6
Pentaerythritol	T46.3X1	T46.3X2	T46.3X3	T46.3X4	T46.3X5	T46.3X6
chloral	T42.6X1	T42.6X2	T42.6X3	T42.6X4	T42.6X5	T42.6X6
tetranitrate NEC	T46.3X1	T46.3X2	T46.3X3	T46.3X4	T46.3X5	T46.3X6
Pentagastrin	T50.8X1	T50.8X2	T50.8X3	T50.8X4	T50.8X5	T50.8X6
Pentalin	T53.6X1	T53.6X2	T53.6X3	T53.6X4	—	—
Pentamethonium bromide	T44.2X1	T44.2X2	T44.2X3	T44.2X4	T44.2X5	T44.2X6
Pentamidine	T37.3X1	T37.3X2	T37.3X3	T37.3X4	T37.3X5	T37.3X6
Pentanol	T51.3X1	T51.3X2	T51.3X3	T51.3X4	—	—
Pentapyrrolinium (bitartrate)	T44.2X1	T44.2X2	T44.2X3	T44.2X4	T44.2X5	T44.2X6
Pentaquine	T37.2X1	T37.2X2	T37.2X3	T37.2X4	T37.2X5	T37.2X6
Pentazocine	T40.491	T40.492	T40.493	T40.494	T40.495	T40.496
Pentetrazole	T50.7X1	T50.7X2	T50.7X3	T50.7X4	T50.7X5	T50.7X6
Penthienate bromide	T44.3X1	T44.3X2	T44.3X3	T44.3X4	T44.3X5	T44.3X6
Pentifylline	T46.7X1	T46.7X2	T46.7X3	T46.7X4	T46.7X5	T46.7X6
Pentobarbital	T42.3X1	T42.3X2	T42.3X3	T42.3X4	T42.3X5	T42.3X6
sodium	T42.3X1	T42.3X2	T42.3X3	T42.3X4	T42.3X5	T42.3X6
Pentobarbitone	T42.3X1	T42.3X2	T42.3X3	T42.3X4	T42.3X5	T42.3X6
Pentolonium tartrate	T44.2X1	T44.2X2	T44.2X3	T44.2X4	T44.2X5	T44.2X6

	External Cause (T-Code)					
Substance	Poisoning, Accidental (Unintentional)	Poisoning, Intentional Self-Harm	Poisoning, Assault	Poisoning, Undetermined	Adverse Effect	Underdosing
Pentosan polysulfate (sodium)	T39.8X1	T39.8X2	T39.8X3	T39.8X4	T39.8X5	T39.8X6
Pentostatin	T45.1X1	T45.1X2	T45.1X3	T45.1X4	T45.1X5	T45.1X6
Pentothal	T41.1X1	T41.1X2	T41.1X3	T41.1X4	T41.1X5	T41.1X6
Pentoxifylline	T46.7X1	T46.7X2	T46.7X3	T46.7X4	T46.7X5	T46.7X6
Pentoxyverine	T48.3X1	T48.3X2	T48.3X3	T48.3X4	T48.3X5	T48.3X6
Pentrinat	T46.3X1	T46.3X2	T46.3X3	T46.3X4	T46.3X5	T46.3X6
Pentylenetetrazole	T50.7X1	T50.7X2	T50.7X3	T50.7X4	T50.7X5	T50.7X6
Pentylsalicylamide	T37.1X1	T37.1X2	T37.1X3	T37.1X4	T37.1X5	T37.1X6
Pentymal	T42.3X1	T42.3X2	T42.3X3	T42.3X4	T42.3X5	T42.3X6
Peplomycin	T45.1X1	T45.1X2	T45.1X3	T45.1X4	T45.1X5	T45.1X6
Peppermint (oil)	T47.5X1	T47.5X2	T47.5X3	T47.5X4	T47.5X5	T47.5X6
Pepsin	T47.5X1	T47.5X2	T47.5X3	T47.5X4	T47.5X5	T47.5X6
digestant	T47.5X1	T47.5X2	T47.5X3	T47.5X4	T47.5X5	T47.5X6
Pepstatin	T47.1X1	T47.1X2	T47.1X3	T47.1X4	T47.1X5	T47.1X6
Peptavlon	T50.8X1	T50.8X2	T50.8X3	T50.8X4	T50.8X5	T50.8X6
Perazine	T43.3X1	T43.3X2	T43.3X3	T43.3X4	T43.3X5	T43.3X6
Percaine (spinal)	T41.3X1	T41.3X2	T41.3X3	T41.3X4	T41.3X5	T41.3X6
topical (surface)	T41.3X1	T41.3X2	T41.3X3	T41.3X4	T41.3X5	T41.3X6
Perchloroethylene	T53.3X1	T53.3X2	T53.3X3	T53.3X4	—	—
medicinal	T37.4X1	T37.4X2	T37.4X3	T37.4X4	T37.4X5	T37.4X6
vapor	T53.3X1	T53.3X2	T53.3X3	T53.3X4	—	—
Percodan	T40.2X1	T40.2X2	T40.2X3	T40.2X4	T40.2X5	T40.2X6
Percogesic — see also Acetaminophen	T45.0X1	T45.0X2	T45.0X3	T45.0X4	T45.0X5	T45.0X6
Percorten	T38.0X1	T38.0X2	T38.0X3	T38.0X4	T38.0X5	T38.0X6
Pergolide	T42.8X1	T42.8X2	T42.8X3	T42.8X4	T42.8X5	T42.8X6
Pergonal	T38.811	T38.812	T38.813	T38.814	T38.815	T38.816
Perhexilene	T46.3X1	T46.3X2	T46.3X3	T46.3X4	T46.3X5	T46.3X6
Perhexiline (maleate)	T46.3X1	T46.3X2	T46.3X3	T46.3X4	T46.3X5	T46.3X6
Periactin	T45.0X1	T45.0X2	T45.0X3	T45.0X4	T45.0X5	T45.0X6
Periciazine	T43.3X1	T43.3X2	T43.3X3	T43.3X4	T43.3X5	T43.3X6
Periclor	T42.6X1	T42.6X2	T42.6X3	T42.6X4	T42.6X5	T42.6X6
Perindopril	T46.4X1	T46.4X2	T46.4X3	T46.4X4	T46.4X5	T46.4X6
Perisoxal	T39.8X1	T39.8X2	T39.8X3	T39.8X4	T39.8X5	T39.8X6
Peritrate	T46.3X1	T46.3X2	T46.3X3	T46.3X4	T46.3X5	T46.3X6
Peritoneal dialysis solution	T50.3X1	T50.3X2	T50.3X3	T50.3X4	T50.3X5	T50.3X6
Perlapine	T42.4X1	T42.4X2	T42.4X3	T42.4X4	T42.4X5	T42.4X6
Permanganate	T65.891	T65.892	T65.893	T65.894	—	—
Permethrin	T60.1X1	T60.1X2	T60.1X3	T60.1X4	—	—
Pernocton	T42.3X1	T42.3X2	T42.3X3	T42.3X4	T42.3X5	T42.3X6
Pernoston	T42.3X1	T42.3X2	T42.3X3	T42.3X4	T42.3X5	T42.3X6
Peronine	T40.2X1	T40.2X2	T40.2X3	T40.2X4	—	—
Perphenazine	T43.3X1	T43.3X2	T43.3X3	T43.3X4	T43.3X5	T43.3X6

◀ New   ◀ Revised   ~~deleted~~ Deleted

Substance	Poisoning, Accidental (Unintentional)	Poisoning, Intentional Self-Harm	Poisoning, Assault	Poisoning, Undetermined	Adverse Effect	Underdosing
Pertofrane	T43.011	T43.012	T43.013	T43.014	T43.015	T43.016
Pertussis						
immune serum (human)	T50.Z11	T50.Z12	T50.Z13	T50.Z14	T50.Z15	T50.Z16
vaccine (with diphtheria toxoid) (with tetanus toxoid)	T50.A11	T50.A12	T50.A13	T50.A14	T50.A15	T50.A16
Peruvian balsam	T49.0X1	T49.0X2	T49.0X3	T49.0X4	T49.0X5	T49.0X6
Peruvoside	T46.0X1	T46.0X2	T46.0X3	T46.0X4	T46.0X5	T46.0X6
Pesticide (dust) (fumes) (vapor) NEC	T60.91	T60.92	T60.93	T60.94	—	—
arsenic	T57.0X1	T57.0X2	T57.0X3	T57.0X4	—	—
chlorinated	T60.1X1	T60.1X2	T60.1X3	T60.1X4	—	—
cyanide	T65.0X1	T65.0X2	T65.0X3	T65.0X4	—	—
kerosene	T52.0X1	T52.0X2	T52.0X3	T52.0X4	—	—
mixture (of compounds)	T60.91	T60.92	T60.93	T60.94	—	—
naphthalene	T60.2X1	T60.2X2	T60.2X3	T60.2X4	—	—
organochlorine (compounds)	T60.1X1	T60.1X2	T60.1X3	T60.1X4	—	—
petroleum (distillate) (products) NEC	T60.8X1	T60.8X2	T60.8X3	T60.8X4	—	—
specified ingredient NEC	T60.8X1	T60.8X2	T60.8X3	T60.8X4	—	—
strychnine	T65.1X1	T65.1X2	T65.1X3	T65.1X4	—	—
thallium	T60.4X1	T60.4X2	T60.4X3	T60.4X4	—	—
Pethidine	T40.491	T40.492	T40.493	T40.494	T40.495	T40.496
Petrichloral	T42.6X1	T42.6X2	T42.6X3	T42.6X4	T42.6X5	T42.6X6
Petrol	T52.0X1	T52.0X2	T52.0X3	T52.0X4	—	—
vapor	T52.0X1	T52.0X2	T52.0X3	T52.0X4	—	—
Petrolatum	T49.3X1	T49.3X2	T49.3X3	T49.3X4	T49.3X5	T49.3X6
hydrophilic	T49.3X1	T49.3X2	T49.3X3	T49.3X4	T49.3X5	T49.3X6
liquid	T47.4X1	T47.4X2	T47.4X3	T47.4X4	T47.4X5	T47.4X6
topical	T49.3X1	T49.3X2	T49.3X3	T49.3X4	T49.3X5	T49.3X6
nonmedicinal	T52.0X1	T52.0X2	T52.0X3	T52.0X4	—	—
red veterinary	T49.3X1	T49.3X2	T49.3X3	T49.3X4	T49.3X5	T49.3X6
white	T49.3X1	T49.3X2	T49.3X3	T49.3X4	T49.3X5	T49.3X6
Petroleum (products) NEC	T52.0X1	T52.0X2	T52.0X3	T52.0X4	—	—
benzine(s) — see Ligroin						
ether — see Ligroin						
jelly — see Petrolatum						
naphtha — see Ligroin						
pesticide	T60.8X1	T60.8X2	T60.8X3	T60.8X4	—	—
solids	T52.0X1	T52.0X2	T52.0X3	T52.0X4	—	—
solvents	T52.0X1	T52.0X2	T52.0X3	T52.0X4	—	—
vapor	T52.0X1	T52.0X2	T52.0X3	T52.0X4	—	—
Peyote	T40.991	T40.992	T40.993	T40.994	—	—
Phanodorm, phanodorn	T42.3X1	T42.3X2	T42.3X3	T42.3X4	T42.3X5	T42.3X6

Substance	Poisoning, Accidental (Unintentional)	Poisoning, Intentional Self-Harm	Poisoning, Assault	Poisoning, Undetermined	Adverse Effect	Underdosing
Phanquinone	T37.3X1	T37.3X2	T37.3X3	T37.3X4	T37.3X5	T37.3X6
Phanquone	T37.3X1	T37.3X2	T37.3X3	T37.3X4	T37.3X5	T37.3X6
Pharmaceutical						
adjunct NEC	T50.901	T50.902	T50.903	T50.904	T50.905	T50.906
excipient NEC	T50.901	T50.902	T50.903	T50.904	T50.905	T50.906
sweetener	T50.901	T50.902	T50.903	T50.904	T50.905	T50.906
viscous agent	T50.901	T50.902	T50.903	T50.904	T50.905	T50.906
Phemitone	T42.3X1	T42.3X2	T42.3X3	T42.3X4	T42.3X5	T42.3X6
Phenacaine	T41.3X1	T41.3X2	T41.3X3	T41.3X4	T41.3X5	T41.3X6
Phenacemide	T42.6X1	T42.6X2	T42.6X3	T42.6X4	T42.6X5	T42.6X6
Phenacetin	T39.1X1	T39.1X2	T39.1X3	T39.1X4	T39.1X5	T39.1X6
Phenadoxone	T40.2X1	T40.2X2	T40.2X3	T40.2X4	—	—
Phenaglycodol	T43.591	T43.592	T43.593	T43.594	T43.595	T43.596
Phenantoin	T42.0X1	T42.0X2	T42.0X3	T42.0X4	T42.0X5	T42.0X6
Phenaphthazine reagent	T50.991	T50.992	T50.993	T50.994	T50.995	T50.996
Phenazocine	T40.491	T40.492	T40.493	T40.494	T40.495	T40.496
Phenazone	T39.2X1	T39.2X2	T39.2X3	T39.2X4	T39.2X5	T39.2X6
Phenazopyridine	T39.8X1	T39.8X2	T39.8X3	T39.8X4	T39.8X5	T39.8X6
Phenbenicillin	T36.0X1	T36.0X2	T36.0X3	T36.0X4	T36.0X5	T36.0X6
Phenbutrazate	T50.5X1	T50.5X2	T50.5X3	T50.5X4	T50.5X5	T50.5X6
Phencyclidine	T40.991	T40.992	T40.993	T40.994	T40.995	T40.996
Phendimetrazine	T50.5X1	T50.5X2	T50.5X3	T50.5X4	T50.5X5	T50.5X6
Phenelzine	T43.1X1	T43.1X2	T43.1X3	T43.1X4	T43.1X5	T43.1X6
Phenemal	T42.3X1	T42.3X2	T42.3X3	T42.3X4	T42.3X5	T42.3X6
Phenergan	T42.6X1	T42.6X2	T42.6X3	T42.6X4	T42.6X5	T42.6X6
Pheneticillin	T36.0X1	T36.0X2	T36.0X3	T36.0X4	T36.0X5	T36.0X6
Pheneturide	T42.6X1	T42.6X2	T42.6X3	T42.6X4	T42.6X5	T42.6X6
Phenformin	T38.3X1	T38.3X2	T38.3X3	T38.3X4	T38.3X5	T38.3X6
Phenglutarimide	T44.3X1	T44.3X2	T44.3X3	T44.3X4	T44.3X5	T44.3X6
Phenicarbazide	T39.8X1	T39.8X2	T39.8X3	T39.8X4	T39.8X5	T39.8X6
Phenindamine	T45.0X1	T45.0X2	T45.0X3	T45.0X4	T45.0X5	T45.0X6
Phenindione	T45.511	T45.512	T45.513	T45.514	T45.515	T45.516
Pheniprazine	T43.1X1	T43.1X2	T43.1X3	T43.1X4	T43.1X5	T43.1X6
Pheniramine	T45.0X1	T45.0X2	T45.0X3	T45.0X4	T45.0X5	T45.0X6
Phenisatin	T47.2X1	T47.2X2	T47.2X3	T47.2X4	T47.2X5	T47.2X6
Phenmetrazine	T50.5X1	T50.5X2	T50.5X3	T50.5X4	T50.5X5	T50.5X6
Phenobal	T42.3X1	T42.3X2	T42.3X3	T42.3X4	T42.3X5	T42.3X6
Phenobarbital	T42.3X1	T42.3X2	T42.3X3	T42.3X4	T42.3X5	T42.3X6
with						
mephenytoin	T42.3X1	T42.3X2	T42.3X3	T42.3X4	T42.3X5	T42.3X6
phenytoin	T42.3X1	T42.3X2	T42.3X3	T42.3X4	T42.3X5	T42.3X6
sodium	T42.3X1	T42.3X2	T42.3X3	T42.3X4	T42.3X5	T42.3X6

◀ New ◀ Revised ~~deleted~~ Deleted

Substance	External Cause (T-Code) Poisoning, Accidental (Unintentional)	Poisoning, Intentional Self-Harm	Poisoning, Assault	Poisoning, Undetermined	Adverse Effect	Underdosing
Phenobarbitone	T42.3X1	T42.3X2	T42.3X3	T42.3X4	T42.3X5	T42.3X6
Phenobutiodil	T50.8X1	T50.8X2	T50.8X3	T50.8X4	T50.8X5	T50.8X6
Phenoctide	T49.0X1	T49.0X2	T49.0X3	T49.0X4	T49.0X5	T49.0X6
Phenol	T49.0X1	T49.0X2	T49.0X3	T49.0X4	T49.0X5	T49.0X6
disinfectant	T54.0X1	T54.0X2	T54.0X3	T54.0X4	—	—
in oil injection	T46.8X1	T46.8X2	T46.8X3	T46.8X4	T46.8X5	T46.8X6
medicinal	T49.1X1	T49.1X2	T49.1X3	T49.1X4	T49.1X5	T49.1X6
nonmedicinal NEC	T54.0X1	T54.0X2	T54.0X3	T54.0X4	—	—
pesticide	T60.8X1	T60.8X2	T60.8X3	T60.8X4		
red	T50.8X1	T50.8X2	T50.8X3	T50.8X4	T50.8X5	T50.8X6
Phenolic preparation	T49.1X1	T49.1X2	T49.1X3	T49.1X4	T49.1X5	T49.1X6
Phenolphthalein	T47.2X1	T47.2X2	T47.2X3	T47.2X4	T47.2X5	T47.2X6
Phenolsulfonphthalein	T50.8X1	T50.8X2	T50.8X3	T50.8X4	T50.8X5	T50.8X6
Phenomorphan	T40.2X1	T40.2X2	T40.2X3	T40.2X4		
Phenonyl	T42.3X1	T42.3X2	T42.3X3	T42.3X4	T42.3X5	T42.3X6
Phenoperidine	T40.491	T40.492	T40.493	T40.494	—	—
Phenopyrazone	T46.991	T46.992	T46.993	T46.994	T46.995	T46.996
Phenoquin	T50.4X1	T50.4X2	T50.4X3	T50.4X4	T50.4X5	T50.4X6
Phenothiazine (psychotropic) NEC	T43.3X1	T43.3X2	T43.3X3	T43.3X4	T43.3X5	T43.3X6
insecticide	T60.2X1	T60.2X2	T60.2X3	T60.2X4	—	—
Phenothrin	T49.0X1	T49.0X2	T49.0X3	T49.0X4	T49.0X5	T49.0X6
Phenoxybenzamine	T46.7X1	T46.7X2	T46.7X3	T46.7X4	T46.7X5	T46.7X6
Phenoxyethanol	T49.0X1	T49.0X2	T49.0X3	T49.0X4	T49.0X5	T49.0X6
Phenoxymethyl penicillin	T36.0X1	T36.0X2	T36.0X3	T36.0X4	T36.0X5	T36.0X6
Phenprobamate	T42.8X1	T42.8X2	T42.8X3	T42.8X4	T42.8X5	T42.8X6
Phenprocoumon	T45.511	T45.512	T45.513	T45.514	T45.515	T45.516
Phensuximide	T42.2X1	T42.2X2	T42.2X3	T42.2X4	T42.2X5	T42.2X6
Phentermine	T50.5X1	T50.5X2	T50.5X3	T50.5X4	T50.5X5	T50.5X6
Phenthicillin	T36.0X1	T36.0X2	T36.0X3	T36.0X4	T36.0X5	T36.0X6
Phentolamine	T46.7X1	T46.7X2	T46.7X3	T46.7X4	T46.7X5	T46.7X6
Phenyl						
butazone	T39.2X1	T39.2X2	T39.2X3	T39.2X4	T39.2X5	T39.2X6
enediamine	T65.3X1	T65.3X2	T65.3X3	T65.3X4	—	—
hydrazine	T65.3X1	T65.3X2	T65.3X3	T65.3X4	—	—
antineoplastic	T45.1X1	T45.1X2	T45.1X3	T45.1X4	T45.1X5	T45.1X6
mercuric compounds — see Mercury						
salicylate	T49.3X1	T49.3X2	T49.3X3	T49.3X4	T49.3X5	T49.3X6
Phenylalanine mustard	T45.1X1	T45.1X2	T45.1X3	T45.1X4	T45.1X5	T45.1X6
Phenylbutazone	T39.2X1	T39.2X2	T39.2X3	T39.2X4	T39.2X5	T39.2X6
Phenylenediamine	T65.3X1	T65.3X2	T65.3X3	T65.3X4		
Phenylephrine	T44.4X1	T44.4X2	T44.4X3	T44.4X4	T44.4X5	T44.4X6

Substance	External Cause (T-Code) Poisoning, Accidental (Unintentional)	Poisoning, Intentional Self-Harm	Poisoning, Assault	Poisoning, Undetermined	Adverse Effect	Underdosing
Phenylethylbiguanide	T38.3X1	T38.3X2	T38.3X3	T38.3X4	T38.3X5	T38.3X6
Phenylmercuric						
acetate	T49.0X1	T49.0X2	T49.0X3	T49.0X4	T49.0X5	T49.0X6
borate	T49.0X1	T49.0X2	T49.0X3	T49.0X4	T49.0X5	T49.0X6
nitrate	T49.0X1	T49.0X2	T49.0X3	T49.0X4	T49.0X5	T49.0X6
Phenylmethylbarbitone	T42.3X1	T42.3X2	T42.3X3	T42.3X4	T42.3X5	T42.3X6
Phenylpropanol	T47.5X1	T47.5X2	T47.5X3	T47.5X4	T47.5X5	T47.5X6
Phenylpropanolamine	T44.991	T44.992	T44.993	T44.994	T44.995	T44.996
Phenylsulfthion	T60.0X1	T60.0X2	T60.0X3	T60.0X4	—	—
Phenyltoloxamine	T45.0X1	T45.0X2	T45.0X3	T45.0X4	T45.0X5	T45.0X6
Phenyramidol, phenyramidon	T39.8X1	T39.8X2	T39.8X3	T39.8X4	T39.8X5	T39.8X6
Phenytoin	T42.0X1	T42.0X2	T42.0X3	T42.0X4	T42.0X5	T42.0X6
with Phenobarbital	T42.3X1	T42.3X2	T42.3X3	T42.3X4	T42.3X5	T42.3X6
pHisoHex	T49.2X1	T49.2X2	T49.2X3	T49.2X4	T49.2X5	T49.2X6
Pholcodine	T48.3X1	T48.3X2	T48.3X3	T48.3X4	T48.3X5	T48.3X6
Pholedrine	T46.991	T46.992	T46.993	T46.994	T46.995	T46.996
Phorate	T60.0X1	T60.0X2	T60.0X3	T60.0X4	—	—
Phosdrin	T60.0X1	T60.0X2	T60.0X3	T60.0X4	—	—
Phosfolan	T60.0X1	T60.0X2	T60.0X3	T60.0X4	—	—
Phosgene (gas)	T59.891	T59.892	T59.893	T59.894		
Phosphamidon	T60.0X1	T60.0X2	T60.0X3	T60.0X4	—	—
Phosphate	T65.891	T65.892	T65.893	T65.894	—	—
laxative	T47.4X1	T47.4X2	T47.4X3	T47.4X4	T47.4X5	T47.4X6
organic	T60.0X1	T60.0X2	T60.0X3	T60.0X4	—	—
solvent	T52.91	T52.92	T52.93	T52.94	—	—
tricresyl	T65.891	T65.892	T65.893	T65.894	—	—
Phosphine	T57.1X1	T57.1X2	T57.1X3	T57.1X4		
fumigant	T57.1X1	T57.1X2	T57.1X3	T57.1X4	—	—
Phospholine	T49.5X1	T49.5X2	T49.5X3	T49.5X4	T49.5X5	T49.5X6
Phosphoric acid	T54.2X1	T54.2X2	T54.2X3	T54.2X4	—	—
Phosphorus (compound) NEC	T57.1X1	T57.1X2	T57.1X3	T57.1X4	—	—
pesticide	T60.0X1	T60.0X2	T60.0X3	T60.0X4	—	—
Phthalates	T65.891	T65.892	T65.893	T65.894	—	—
Phthalic anhydride	T65.891	T65.892	T65.893	T65.894	—	—
Phthalimidoglutarimide	T42.6X1	T42.6X2	T42.6X3	T42.6X4	T42.6X5	T42.6X6
Phthalylsulfathiazole	T37.0X1	T37.0X2	T37.0X3	T37.0X4	T37.0X5	T37.0X6
Phylloquinone	T45.7X1	T45.7X2	T45.7X3	T45.7X4	T45.7X5	T45.7X6
Physeptone	T40.3X1	T40.3X2	T40.3X3	T40.3X4	T40.3X5	T40.3X6
Physostigma venenosum	T62.2X1	T62.2X2	T62.2X3	T62.2X4	—	—
Physostigmine	T49.5X1	T49.5X2	T49.5X3	T49.5X4	T49.5X5	T49.5X6
Phytolacca decandra	T62.2X1	T62.2X2	T62.2X3	T62.2X4	—	—
berries	T62.1X1	T62.1X2	T62.1X3	T62.1X4	—	—

◀ New ◀ Revised ~~deleted~~ Deleted

Substance	Poisoning, Accidental (Unintentional)	Poisoning, Intentional Self-Harm	Poisoning, Assault	Poisoning, Undetermined	Adverse Effect	Underdosing
Phytomenadione	T45.7X1	T45.7X2	T45.7X3	T45.7X4	T45.7X5	T45.7X6
Phytonadione	T45.7X1	T45.7X2	T45.7X3	T45.7X4	T45.7X5	T45.7X6
Picoperine	T48.3X1	T48.3X2	T48.3X3	T48.3X4	T48.3X5	T48.3X6
Picosulfate (sodium)	T47.2X1	T47.2X2	T47.2X3	T47.2X4	T47.2X5	T47.2X6
Picric (acid)	T54.2X1	T54.2X2	T54.2X3	T54.2X4	—	—
Picrotoxin	T50.7X1	T50.7X2	T50.7X3	T50.7X4	T50.7X5	T50.7X6
Piketoprofen	T49.0X1	T49.0X2	T49.0X3	T49.0X4	T49.0X5	T49.0X6
Pilocarpine	T44.1X1	T44.1X2	T44.1X3	T44.1X4	T44.1X5	T44.1X6
Pilocarpus (jaborandi) extract	T44.1X1	T44.1X2	T44.1X3	T44.1X4	T44.1X5	T44.1X6
Pilsicainide (hydrochloride)	T46.2X1	T46.2X2	T46.2X3	T46.2X4	T46.2X5	T46.2X6
Pimaricin	T36.7X1	T36.7X2	T36.7X3	T36.7X4	T36.7X5	T36.7X6
Pimeclone	T50.7X1	T50.7X2	T50.7X3	T50.7X4	T50.7X5	T50.7X6
Pimelic ketone	T52.8X1	T52.8X2	T52.8X3	T52.8X4	—	—
Pimethixene	T45.0X1	T45.0X2	T45.0X3	T45.0X4	T45.0X5	T45.0X6
Piminodine	T40.2X1	T40.2X2	T40.2X3	T40.2X4	T40.2X5	T40.2X6
Pimozide	T43.591	T43.592	T43.593	T43.594	T43.595	T43.596
Pinacidil	T46.5X1	T46.5X2	T46.5X3	T46.5X4	T46.5X5	T46.5X6
Pinaverium bromide	T44.3X1	T44.3X2	T44.3X3	T44.3X4	T44.3X5	T44.3X6
Pinazepam	T42.4X1	T42.4X2	T42.4X3	T42.4X4	T42.4X5	T42.4X6
Pindolol	T44.7X1	T44.7X2	T44.7X3	T44.7X4	T44.7X5	T44.7X6
Pindone	T60.4X1	T60.4X2	T60.4X3	T60.4X4	—	—
Pine oil (disinfectant)	T65.891	T65.892	T65.893	T65.894	—	—
Pinkroot	T37.4X1	T37.4X2	T37.4X3	T37.4X4	T37.4X5	T37.4X6
Pipadone	T40.2X1	T40.2X2	T40.2X3	T40.2X4	—	—
Pipamazine	T45.0X1	T45.0X2	T45.0X3	T45.0X4	T45.0X5	T45.0X6
Pipamperone	T43.4X1	T43.4X2	T43.4X3	T43.4X4	T43.4X5	T43.4X6
Pipazetate	T48.3X1	T48.3X2	T48.3X3	T48.3X4	T48.3X5	T48.3X6
Pipemidic acid	T37.8X1	T37.8X2	T37.8X3	T37.8X4	T37.8X5	T37.8X6
Pipenzolate bromide	T44.3X1	T44.3X2	T44.3X3	T44.3X4	T44.3X5	T44.3X6
Piperacetazine	T43.3X1	T43.3X2	T43.3X3	T43.3X4	T43.3X5	T43.3X6
Piperacillin	T36.0X1	T36.0X2	T36.0X3	T36.0X4	T36.0X5	T36.0X6
Piperazine	T37.4X1	T37.4X2	T37.4X3	T37.4X4	T37.4X5	T37.4X6
estrone sulfate	T38.5X1	T38.5X2	T38.5X3	T38.5X4	T38.5X5	T38.5X6
Piper cubeba	T62.2X1	T62.2X2	T62.2X3	T62.2X4	—	—
Piperidione	T48.3X1	T48.3X2	T48.3X3	T48.3X4	—	—
Piperidolate	T44.3X1	T44.3X2	T44.3X3	T44.3X4	T44.3X5	T44.3X6
Piperocaine	T41.3X1	T41.3X2	T41.3X3	T41.3X4	T41.3X5	T41.3X6
infiltration (subcutaneous)	T41.3X1	T41.3X2	T41.3X3	T41.3X4	T41.3X5	T41.3X6
nerve block (peripheral) (plexus)	T41.3X1	T41.3X2	T41.3X3	T41.3X4	T41.3X5	T41.3X6
topical (surface)	T41.3X1	T41.3X2	T41.3X3	T41.3X4	T41.3X5	T41.3X6
Piperonyl butoxide	T60.8X1	T60.8X2	T60.8X3	T60.8X4	—	—
Pipethanate	T44.3X1	T44.3X2	T44.3X3	T44.3X4	T44.3X5	T44.3X6

Substance	Poisoning, Accidental (Unintentional)	Poisoning, Intentional Self-Harm	Poisoning, Assault	Poisoning, Undetermined	Adverse Effect	Underdosing
Pipobroman	T45.1X1	T45.1X2	T45.1X3	T45.1X4	T45.1X5	T45.1X6
Pipofezine	T43.0X1	T43.0X2	T43.0X3	T43.0X4	T43.0X5	T43.0X6
Pipotiazine	T43.3X1	T43.3X2	T43.3X3	T43.3X4	T43.3X5	T43.3X6
Pipoxizine	T45.0X1	T45.0X2	T45.0X3	T45.0X4	T45.0X5	T45.0X6
Pipradrol	T43.691	T43.692	T43.693	T43.694	T43.695	T43.696
Piprinhydrinate	T45.0X1	T45.0X2	T45.0X3	T45.0X4	T45.0X5	T45.0X6
Pirarubicin	T45.1X1	T45.1X2	T45.1X3	T45.1X4	T45.1X5	T45.1X6
Pirazinamide	T37.1X1	T37.1X2	T37.1X3	T37.1X4	T37.1X5	T37.1X6
Pirbuterol	T48.6X1	T48.6X2	T48.6X3	T48.6X4	T48.6X5	T48.6X6
Pirenzepine	T47.1X1	T47.1X2	T47.1X3	T47.1X4	T47.1X5	T47.1X6
Piretanide	T50.1X1	T50.1X2	T50.1X3	T50.1X4	T50.1X5	T50.1X6
Piribedil	T42.8X1	T42.8X2	T42.8X3	T42.8X4	T42.8X5	T42.8X6
Piridoxilate	T46.3X1	T46.3X2	T46.3X3	T46.3X4	T46.3X5	T46.3X6
Piritramide	T40.491	T40.492	T40.493	T40.494	—	—
Pirlindole	T43.0X1	T43.0X2	T43.0X3	T43.0X4	T43.0X5	T43.0X6
Piromidic acid	T37.8X1	T37.8X2	T37.8X3	T37.8X4	T37.8X5	T37.8X6
Piroxicam	T39.391	T39.392	T39.393	T39.394	T39.395	T39.396
beta-cyclodextrin complex	T39.8X1	T39.8X2	T39.8X3	T39.8X4	T39.8X5	T39.8X6
Pirozadil	T46.6X1	T46.6X2	T46.6X3	T46.6X4	T46.6X5	T46.6X6
Piscidia (bark) (erythrina)	T39.8X1	T39.8X2	T39.8X3	T39.8X4	T39.8X5	T39.8X6
Pitch	T65.891	T65.892	T65.893	T65.894	—	—
Pitkin's solution	T41.3X1	T41.3X2	T41.3X3	T41.3X4	T41.3X5	T41.3X6
Pitocin	T48.0X1	T48.0X2	T48.0X3	T48.0X4	T48.0X5	T48.0X6
Pitressin (tannate)	T38.891	T38.892	T38.893	T38.894	T38.895	T38.896
Pituitary extracts (posterior)	T38.891	T38.892	T38.893	T38.894	T38.895	T38.896
anterior	T38.811	T38.812	T38.813	T38.814	T38.815	T38.816
Pituitrin	T38.891	T38.892	T38.893	T38.894	T38.895	T38.896
Pivampicillin	T36.0X1	T36.0X2	T36.0X3	T36.0X4	T36.0X5	T36.0X6
Pivmecillinam	T36.0X1	T36.0X2	T36.0X3	T36.0X4	T36.0X5	T36.0X6
Placental hormone	T38.891	T38.892	T38.893	T38.894	T38.895	T38.896
Placidyl	T42.6X1	T42.6X2	T42.6X3	T42.6X4	T42.6X5	T42.6X6
Plague vaccine	T50.A91	T50.A92	T50.A93	T50.A94	T50.A95	T50.A96
Plant						
food or fertilizer NEC	T65.891	T65.892	T65.893	T65.894	—	—
containing herbicide	T60.3X1	T60.3X2	T60.3X3	T60.3X4	—	—
noxious, used as food	T62.2X1	T62.2X2	T62.2X3	T62.2X4	—	—
berries	T62.1X1	T62.1X2	T62.1X3	T62.1X4	—	—
seeds	T62.2X1	T62.2X2	T62.2X3	T62.2X4	—	—
specified type NEC	T62.2X1	T62.2X2	T62.2X3	T62.2X4	—	—
Plasma	T45.8X1	T45.8X2	T45.8X3	T45.8X4	T45.8X5	T45.8X6
expander NEC	T45.8X1	T45.8X2	T45.8X3	T45.8X4	T45.8X5	T45.8X6
protein fraction (human)	T45.8X1	T45.8X2	T45.8X3	T45.8X4	T45.8X5	T45.8X6

◀ New   ◀ Revised   ~~deleted~~ Deleted

Substance	Poisoning, Accidental (Unintentional)	Poisoning, Intentional Self-Harm	Poisoning, Assault	Poisoning, Undetermined	Adverse Effect	Underdosing
Plasmanate	T45.8X1	T45.8X2	T45.8X3	T45.8X4	T45.8X5	T45.8X6
Plasminogen (tissue) activator	T45.611	T45.612	T45.613	T45.614	T45.615	T45.616
Plaster dressing	T49.3X1	T49.3X2	T49.3X3	T49.3X4	T49.3X5	T49.3X6
Plastic dressing	T49.3X1	T49.3X2	T49.3X3	T49.3X4	T49.3X5	T49.3X6
Plegicil	T43.3X1	T43.3X2	T43.3X3	T43.3X4	T43.3X5	T43.3X6
Plicamycin	T45.1X1	T45.1X2	T45.1X3	T45.1X4	T45.1X5	T45.1X6
Podophyllotoxin	T49.8X1	T49.8X2	T49.8X3	T49.8X4	T49.8X5	T49.8X6
Podophyllum (resin)	T49.4X1	T49.4X2	T49.4X3	T49.4X4	T49.4X5	T49.4X6
Poison NEC	T65.91	T65.92	T65.93	T65.94	—	—
Poisonous berries	T62.1X1	T62.1X2	T62.1X3	T62.1X4	—	—
Pokeweed (any part)	T62.2X1	T62.2X2	T62.2X3	T62.2X4	—	—
Poldine metilsulfate	T44.3X1	T44.3X2	T44.3X3	T44.3X4	T44.3X5	T44.3X6
Polidexide (sulfate)	T46.6X1	T46.6X2	T46.6X3	T46.6X4	T46.6X5	T46.6X6
Polidocanol	T46.8X1	T46.8X2	T46.8X3	T46.8X4	T46.8X5	T46.8X6
Poliomyelitis vaccine	T50.B91	T50.B92	T50.B93	T50.B94	T50.B95	T50.B96
Polish (car) (floor) (furniture) (metal) (porcelain) (silver)	T65.891	T65.892	T65.893	T65.894	—	—
abrasive	T65.891	T65.892	T65.893	T65.894	—	—
porcelain	T65.891	T65.892	T65.893	T65.894	—	—
Poloxalkol	T47.4X1	T47.4X2	T47.4X3	T47.4X4	T47.4X5	T47.4X6
Poloxamer	T47.4X1	T47.4X2	T47.4X3	T47.4X4	T47.4X5	T47.4X6
Polyaminostyrene resins	T50.3X1	T50.3X2	T50.3X3	T50.3X4	T50.3X5	T50.3X6
Polycarbophil	T47.4X1	T47.4X2	T47.4X3	T47.4X4	T47.4X5	T47.4X6
Polychlorinated biphenyl	T65.891	T65.892	T65.893	T65.894	—	—
Polycycline	T36.4X1	T36.4X2	T36.4X3	T36.4X4	T36.4X5	T36.4X6
Polyester fumes	T59.891	T59.892	T59.893	T59.894	—	—
Polyester resin hardener	T52.91	T52.92	T52.93	T52.94	—	—
fumes	T59.891	T59.892	T59.893	T59.894	—	—
Polyestradiol phosphate	T38.5X1	T38.5X2	T38.5X3	T38.5X4	T38.5X5	T38.5X6
Polyethanolamine alkyl sulfate	T49.2X1	T49.2X2	T49.2X3	T49.2X4	T49.2X5	T49.2X6
Polyethylene adhesive	T49.3X1	T49.3X2	T49.3X3	T49.3X4	T49.3X5	T49.3X6
Polyferose	T45.4X1	T45.4X2	T45.4X3	T45.4X4	T45.4X5	T45.4X6
Polygeline	T45.8X1	T45.8X2	T45.8X3	T45.8X4	T45.8X5	T45.8X6
Polymyxin	T36.8X1	T36.8X2	T36.8X3	T36.8X4	T36.8X5	T36.8X6
B	T36.8X1	T36.8X2	T36.8X3	T36.8X4	T36.8X5	T36.8X6
ENT agent	T49.6X1	T49.6X2	T49.6X3	T49.6X4	T49.6X5	T49.6X6
ophthalmic preparation	T49.5X1	T49.5X2	T49.5X3	T49.5X4	T49.5X5	T49.5X6
topical NEC	T49.0X1	T49.0X2	T49.0X3	T49.0X4	T49.0X5	T49.0X6
E sulfate (eye preparation)	T49.5X1	T49.5X2	T49.5X3	T49.5X4	T49.5X5	T49.5X6
Polynoxylin	T49.0X1	T49.0X2	T49.0X3	T49.0X4	T49.0X5	T49.0X6
Polyoestradiol phosphate	T38.5X1	T38.5X2	T38.5X3	T38.5X4	T38.5X5	T38.5X6
Polyoxymethyleneurea	T49.0X1	T49.0X2	T49.0X3	T49.0X4	T49.0X5	T49.0X6

Substance	Poisoning, Accidental (Unintentional)	Poisoning, Intentional Self-Harm	Poisoning, Assault	Poisoning, Undetermined	Adverse Effect	Underdosing
Polysilane	T47.8X1	T47.8X2	T47.8X3	T47.8X4	T47.8X5	T47.8X6
Polytetrafluoroethylene (inhaled)	T59.891	T59.892	T59.893	T59.894	—	—
Polythiazide	T50.2X1	T50.2X2	T50.2X3	T50.2X4	T50.2X5	T50.2X6
Polyvidone	T45.8X1	T45.8X2	T45.8X3	T45.8X4	T45.8X5	T45.8X6
Polyvinylpyrrolidone	T45.8X1	T45.8X2	T45.8X3	T45.8X4	T45.8X5	T45.8X6
Pontocaine (hydrochloride) (infiltration) (topical)	T41.3X1	T41.3X2	T41.3X3	T41.3X4	T41.3X5	T41.3X6
nerve block (peripheral) (plexus)	T41.3X1	T41.3X2	T41.3X3	T41.3X4	T41.3X5	T41.3X6
spinal	T41.3X1	T41.3X2	T41.3X3	T41.3X4	T41.3X5	T41.3X6
Porfiromycin	T45.1X1	T45.1X2	T45.1X3	T45.1X4	T45.1X5	T45.1X6
Posterior pituitary hormone NEC	T38.891	T38.892	T38.893	T38.894	T38.895	T38.896
Pot	T40.711	T40.712	T40.713	T40.714	T40.715	T40.716
Potash (caustic)	T54.3X1	T54.3X2	T54.3X3	T54.3X4	—	—
Potassic saline injection (lactated)	T50.3X1	T50.3X2	T50.3X3	T50.3X4	T50.3X5	T50.3X6
Potassium (salts) NEC	T50.3X1	T50.3X2	T50.3X3	T50.3X4	T50.3X5	T50.3X6
aminobenzoate	T45.8X1	T45.8X2	T45.8X3	T45.8X4	T45.8X5	T45.8X6
aminosalicylate	T37.1X1	T37.1X2	T37.1X3	T37.1X4	T37.1X5	T37.1X6
antimony 'tartrate'	T37.8X1	T37.8X2	T37.8X3	T37.8X4	T37.8X5	T37.8X6
arsenite (solution)	T57.0X1	T57.0X2	T57.0X3	T57.0X4	—	—
bichromate	T56.2X1	T56.2X2	T56.2X3	T56.2X4	—	—
bisulfate	T47.3X1	T47.3X2	T47.3X3	T47.3X4	T47.3X5	T47.3X6
bromide	T42.6X1	T42.6X2	T42.6X3	T42.6X4	T42.6X5	T42.6X6
canrenoate	T50.0X1	T50.0X2	T50.0X3	T50.0X4	T50.0X5	T50.0X6
carbonate	T54.3X1	T54.3X2	T54.3X3	T54.3X4	—	—
chlorate NEC	T65.891	T65.892	T65.893	T65.894	—	—
chloride	T50.3X1	T50.3X2	T50.3X3	T50.3X4	T50.3X5	T50.3X6
citrate	T50.991	T50.992	T50.993	T50.994	T50.995	T50.996
cyanide	T65.0X1	T65.0X2	T65.0X3	T65.0X4	—	—
ferric hexacyanoferrate (medicinal)	T50.6X1	T50.6X2	T50.6X3	T50.6X4	T50.6X5	T50.6X6
nonmedicinal	T65.891	T65.892	T65.893	T65.894	—	—
Fluoride	T57.8X1	T57.8X2	T57.8X3	T57.8X4	—	—
glucaldrate	T47.1X1	T47.1X2	T47.1X3	T47.1X4	T47.1X5	T47.1X6
hydroxide	T54.3X1	T54.3X2	T54.3X3	T54.3X4	—	—
iodate	T49.0X1	T49.0X2	T49.0X3	T49.0X4	T49.0X5	T49.0X6
iodide	T48.4X1	T48.4X2	T48.4X3	T48.4X4	T48.4X5	T48.4X6
nitrate	T57.8X1	T57.8X2	T57.8X3	T57.8X4	—	—
oxalate	T65.891	T65.892	T65.893	T65.894	—	—
perchlorate (nonmedicinal) NEC	T65.891	T65.892	T65.893	T65.894	—	—
antithyroid	T38.2X1	T38.2X2	T38.2X3	T38.2X4	T38.2X5	T38.2X6
medicinal	T38.2X1	T38.2X2	T38.2X3	T38.2X4	T38.2X5	T38.2X6

◀ New ◀ Revised ~~deleted~~ Deleted

Substance	External Cause (T-Code)					
	Poisoning, Accidental (Unintentional)	Poisoning, Intentional Self-Harm	Poisoning, Assault	Poisoning, Undetermined	Adverse Effect	Underdosing
Permanganate (nonmedicinal)	T65.891	T65.892	T65.893	T65.894	—	—
medicinal	T49.0X1	T49.0X2	T49.0X3	T49.0X4	T49.0X5	T49.0X6
sulfate	T47.2X1	T47.2X2	T47.2X3	T47.2X4	T47.2X5	T47.2X6
Potassium-removing resin	T50.3X1	T50.3X2	T50.3X3	T50.3X4	T50.3X5	T50.3X6
Potassium-retaining drug	T50.3X1	T50.3X2	T50.3X3	T50.3X4	T50.3X5	T50.3X6
Povidone	T45.8X1	T45.8X2	T45.8X3	T45.8X4	T45.8X5	T45.8X6
iodine	T49.0X1	T49.0X2	T49.0X3	T49.0X4	T49.0X5	T49.0X6
Practolol	T44.7X1	T44.7X2	T44.7X3	T44.7X4	T44.7X5	T44.7X6
Prajmalium bitartrate	T46.2X1	T46.2X2	T46.2X3	T46.2X4	T46.2X5	T46.2X6
Pralidoxime (iodide)	T50.6X1	T50.6X2	T50.6X3	T50.6X4	T50.6X5	T50.6X6
chloride	T50.6X1	T50.6X2	T50.6X3	T50.6X4	T50.6X5	T50.6X6
Pramiverine	T44.3X1	T44.3X2	T44.3X3	T44.3X4	T44.3X5	T44.3X6
Pramocaine	T49.1X1	T49.1X2	T49.1X3	T49.1X4	T49.1X5	T49.1X6
Pramoxine	T49.1X1	T49.1X2	T49.1X3	T49.1X4	T49.1X5	T49.1X6
Prasterone	T38.7X1	T38.7X2	T38.7X3	T38.7X4	T38.7X5	T38.7X6
Pravastatin	T46.6X1	T46.6X2	T46.6X3	T46.6X4	T46.6X5	T46.6X6
Prazepam	T42.4X1	T42.4X2	T42.4X3	T42.4X4	T42.4X5	T42.4X6
Praziquantel	T37.4X1	T37.4X2	T37.4X3	T37.4X4	T37.4X5	T37.4X6
Prazitone	T43.291	T43.292	T43.293	T43.294	T43.295	T43.296
Prazosin	T44.6X1	T44.6X2	T44.6X3	T44.6X4	T44.6X5	T44.6X6
Prednicarbate	T49.0X1	T49.0X2	T49.0X3	T49.0X4	T49.0X5	T49.0X6
Prednimustine	T45.1X1	T45.1X2	T45.1X3	T45.1X4	T45.1X5	T45.1X6
Prednisolone	T38.0X1	T38.0X2	T38.0X3	T38.0X4	T38.0X5	T38.0X6
ENT agent	T49.6X1	T49.6X2	T49.6X3	T49.6X4	T49.6X5	T49.6X6
ophthalmic preparation	T49.5X1	T49.5X2	T49.5X3	T49.5X4	T49.5X5	T49.5X6
steaglate	T49.0X1	T49.0X2	T49.0X3	T49.0X4	T49.0X5	T49.0X6
topical NEC	T49.0X1	T49.0X2	T49.0X3	T49.0X4	T49.0X5	T49.0X6
Prednisone	T38.0X1	T38.0X2	T38.0X3	T38.0X4	T38.0X5	T38.0X6
Prednylidene	T38.0X1	T38.0X2	T38.0X3	T38.0X4	T38.0X5	T38.0X6
Pregnandiol	T38.5X1	T38.5X2	T38.5X3	T38.5X4	T38.5X5	T38.5X6
Pregneninolone	T38.5X1	T38.5X2	T38.5X3	T38.5X4	T38.5X5	T38.5X6
Preludin	T43.691	T43.692	T43.693	T43.694	T43.695	T43.696
Premarin	T38.5X1	T38.5X2	T38.5X3	T38.5X4	T38.5X5	T38.5X6
Premedication anesthetic	T41.201	T41.202	T41.203	T41.204	T41.205	T41.206
Prenalterol	T44.5X1	T44.5X2	T44.5X3	T44.5X4	T44.5X5	T44.5X6
Prenoxdiazine	T48.3X1	T48.3X2	T48.3X3	T48.3X4	T48.3X5	T48.3X6
Prenylamine	T46.3X1	T46.3X2	T46.3X3	T46.3X4	T46.3X5	T46.3X6
Preparation, local	T49.4X1	T49.4X2	T49.4X3	T49.4X4	T49.4X5	T49.4X6
Preparation H	T49.8X1	T49.8X2	T49.8X3	T49.8X4	T49.8X5	T49.8X6
Preservative (nonmedicinal)	T65.891	T65.892	T65.893	T65.894	—	—
medicinal	T50.901	T50.902	T50.903	T50.904	T50.905	T50.906
wood	T60.91	T60.92	T60.93	T60.94	—	—

Substance	External Cause (T-Code)					
	Poisoning, Accidental (Unintentional)	Poisoning, Intentional Self-Harm	Poisoning, Assault	Poisoning, Undetermined	Adverse Effect	Underdosing
Prethcamide	T50.7X1	T50.7X2	T50.7X3	T50.7X4	T50.7X5	T50.7X6
Pride of China	T62.2X1	T62.2X2	T62.2X3	T62.2X4	—	—
Pridinol	T44.3X1	T44.3X2	T44.3X3	T44.3X4	T44.3X5	T44.3X6
Prifinium bromide	T44.3X1	T44.3X2	T44.3X3	T44.3X4	T44.3X5	T44.3X6
Prilocaine	T41.3X1	T41.3X2	T41.3X3	T41.3X4	T41.3X5	T41.3X6
infiltration (subcutaneous)	T41.3X1	T41.3X2	T41.3X3	T41.3X4	T41.3X5	T41.3X6
nerve block (peripheral) (plexus)	T41.3X1	T41.3X2	T41.3X3	T41.3X4	T41.3X5	T41.3X6
regional	T41.3X1	T41.3X2	T41.3X3	T41.3X4	T41.3X5	T41.3X6
Primaquine	T37.2X1	T37.2X2	T37.2X3	T37.2X4	T37.2X5	T37.2X6
Primidone	T42.6X1	T42.6X2	T42.6X3	T42.6X4	T42.6X5	T42.6X6
Primula (veris)	T62.2X1	T62.2X2	T62.2X3	T62.2X4	—	—
Prinadol	T40.2X1	T40.2X2	T40.2X3	T40.2X4	T40.2X5	T40.2X6
Priscol, Priscoline	T44.6X1	T44.6X2	T44.6X3	T44.6X4	T44.6X5	T44.6X6
Pristinamycin	T36.3X1	T36.3X2	T36.3X3	T36.3X4	T36.3X5	T36.3X6
Privet	T62.2X1	T62.2X2	T62.2X3	T62.2X4	—	—
berries	T62.1X1	T62.1X2	T62.1X3	T62.1X4	—	—
Privine	T44.4X1	T44.4X2	T44.4X3	T44.4X4	T44.4X5	T44.4X6
Pro-Banthine	T44.3X1	T44.3X2	T44.3X3	T44.3X4	T44.3X5	T44.3X6
Probarbital	T42.3X1	T42.3X2	T42.3X3	T42.3X4	T42.3X5	T42.3X6
Probenecid	T50.4X1	T50.4X2	T50.4X3	T50.4X4	T50.4X5	T50.4X6
Probucol	T46.6X1	T46.6X2	T46.6X3	T46.6X4	T46.6X5	T46.6X6
Procainamide	T46.2X1	T46.2X2	T46.2X3	T46.2X4	T46.2X5	T46.2X6
Procaine	T41.3X1	T41.3X2	T41.3X3	T41.3X4	T41.3X5	T41.3X6
benzylpenicillin	T36.0X1	T36.0X2	T36.0X3	T36.0X4	T36.0X5	T36.0X6
nerve block (peripheral) (plexus)	T41.3X1	T41.3X2	T41.3X3	T41.3X4	T41.3X5	T41.3X6
penicillin G	T36.0X1	T36.0X2	T36.0X3	T36.0X4	T36.0X5	T36.0X6
regional	T41.3X1	T41.3X2	T41.3X3	T41.3X4	T41.3X5	T41.3X6
spinal	T41.3X1	T41.3X2	T41.3X3	T41.3X4	T41.3X5	T41.3X6
Procalmidol	T43.591	T43.592	T43.593	T43.594	T43.595	T43.596
Procarbazine	T45.1X1	T45.1X2	T45.1X3	T45.1X4	T45.1X5	T45.1X6
Procaterol	T44.5X1	T44.5X2	T44.5X3	T44.5X4	T44.5X5	T44.5X6
Prochlorperazine	T43.3X1	T43.3X2	T43.3X3	T43.3X4	T43.3X5	T43.3X6
Procyclidine	T44.3X1	T44.3X2	T44.3X3	T44.3X4	T44.3X5	T44.3X6
Producer gas	T58.8X1	T58.8X2	T58.8X3	T58.8X4	—	—
Profadol	T40.491	T40.492	T40.493	T40.494	T40.495	T40.496
Profenamine	T44.3X1	T44.3X2	T44.3X3	T44.3X4	T44.3X5	T44.3X6
Profenil	T44.3X1	T44.3X2	T44.3X3	T44.3X4	T44.3X5	T44.3X6
Proflavine	T49.0X1	T49.0X2	T49.0X3	T49.0X4	T49.0X5	T49.0X6
Progabide	T42.6X1	T42.6X2	T42.6X3	T42.6X4	T42.6X5	T42.6X6
Progestin	T38.5X1	T38.5X2	T38.5X3	T38.5X4	T38.5X5	T38.5X6
oral contraceptive	T38.4X1	T38.4X2	T38.4X3	T38.4X4	T38.4X5	T38.4X6

TABLE OF DRUGS AND CHEMICALS

Substance	Poisoning, Accidental (Unintentional)	Poisoning, Intentional Self-Harm	Poisoning, Assault	Poisoning, Undetermined	Adverse Effect	Underdosing
Progesterone	T38.5X1	T38.5X2	T38.5X3	T38.5X4	T38.5X5	T38.5X6
Progestogen NEC	T38.5X1	T38.5X2	T38.5X3	T38.5X4	T38.5X5	T38.5X6
Progestone	T38.5X1	T38.5X2	T38.5X3	T38.5X4	T38.5X5	T38.5X6
Proglumide	T47.1X1	T47.1X2	T47.1X3	T47.1X4	T47.1X5	T47.1X6
Proguanil	T37.2X1	T37.2X2	T37.2X3	T37.2X4	T37.2X5	T37.2X6
Prolactin	T38.811	T38.812	T38.813	T38.814	T38.815	T38.816
Prolintane	T43.691	T43.692	T43.693	T43.694	T43.695	T43.696
Proloid	T38.1X1	T38.1X2	T38.1X3	T38.1X4	T38.1X5	T38.1X6
Proluton	T38.5X1	T38.5X2	T38.5X3	T38.5X4	T38.5X5	T38.5X6
Promacetin	T37.1X1	T37.1X2	T37.1X3	T37.1X4	T37.1X5	T37.1X6
Promazine	T43.3X1	T43.3X2	T43.3X3	T43.3X4	T43.3X5	T43.3X6
Promedol	T40.2X1	T40.2X2	T40.2X3	T40.2X4	—	—
Promegestone	T38.5X1	T38.5X2	T38.5X3	T38.5X4	T38.5X5	T38.5X6
Promethazine (teoclate)	T43.3X1	T43.3X2	T43.3X3	T43.3X4	T43.3X5	T43.3X6
Promin	T37.1X1	T37.1X2	T37.1X3	T37.1X4	T37.1X5	T37.1X6
Pronase	T45.3X1	T45.3X2	T45.3X3	T45.3X4	T45.3X5	T45.3X6
Pronestyl (hydrochloride)	T46.2X1	T46.2X2	T46.2X3	T46.2X4	T46.2X5	T46.2X6
Pronetalol	T44.7X1	T44.7X2	T44.7X3	T44.7X4	T44.7X5	T44.7X6
Prontosil	T37.0X1	T37.0X2	T37.0X3	T37.0X4	T37.0X5	T37.0X6
Propachlor	T60.3X1	T60.3X2	T60.3X3	T60.3X4	—	—
Propafenone	T46.2X1	T46.2X2	T46.2X3	T46.2X4	T46.2X5	T46.2X6
Propallylonal	T42.3X1	T42.3X2	T42.3X3	T42.3X4	T42.3X5	T42.3X6
Propamidine	T49.0X1	T49.0X2	T49.0X3	T49.0X4	T49.0X5	T49.0X6
Propane (distributed in mobile container)	T59.891	T59.892	T59.893	T59.894	—	—
distributed through pipes	T59.891	T59.892	T59.893	T59.894	—	—
incomplete combustion	T57.11	T57.12	T57.13	T57.14	—	—
Propanidid	T41.291	T41.292	T41.293	T41.294	T41.295	T41.296
Propanil	T60.3X1	T60.3X2	T60.3X3	T60.3X4	—	—
1-Propanol	T51.3X1	T51.3X2	T51.3X3	T51.3X4	—	—
2-Propanol	T51.2X1	T51.2X2	T51.2X3	T51.2X4	—	—
Propantheline	T44.3X1	T44.3X2	T44.3X3	T44.3X4	T44.3X5	T44.3X6
bromide	T44.3X1	T44.3X2	T44.3X3	T44.3X4	T44.3X5	T44.3X6
Proparacaine	T41.3X1	T41.3X2	T41.3X3	T41.3X4	T41.3X5	T41.3X6
Propatylnitrate	T46.3X1	T46.3X2	T46.3X3	T46.3X4	T46.3X5	T46.3X6
Propicillin	T36.0X1	T36.0X2	T36.0X3	T36.0X4	T36.0X5	T36.0X6
Propiolactone	T49.0X1	T49.0X2	T49.0X3	T49.0X4	T49.0X5	T49.0X6
Propiomazine	T45.0X1	T45.0X2	T45.0X3	T45.0X4	T45.0X5	T45.0X6
Propionaldehyde (medicinal)	T42.6X1	T42.6X2	T42.6X3	T42.6X4	T42.6X5	T42.6X6
Propionate (calcium) (sodium)	T49.0X1	T49.0X2	T49.0X3	T49.0X4	T49.0X5	T49.0X6
Propion gel	T49.0X1	T49.0X2	T49.0X3	T49.0X4	T49.0X5	T49.0X6

Substance	Poisoning, Accidental (Unintentional)	Poisoning, Intentional Self-Harm	Poisoning, Assault	Poisoning, Undetermined	Adverse Effect	Underdosing
Propitocaine	T41.3X1	T41.3X2	T41.3X3	T41.3X4	T41.3X5	T41.3X6
infiltration (subcutaneous)	T41.3X1	T41.3X2	T41.3X3	T41.3X4	T41.3X5	T41.3X6
nerve block (peripheral) (plexus)	T41.3X1	T41.3X2	T41.3X3	T41.3X4	T41.3X5	T41.3X6
Propofol	T41.291	T41.292	T41.293	T41.294	T41.295	T41.296
Propoxur	T60.0X1	T60.0X2	T60.0X3	T60.0X4	—	—
Propoxycaine	T41.3X1	T41.3X2	T41.3X3	T41.3X4	T41.3X5	T41.3X6
infiltration (subcutaneous)	T41.3X1	T41.3X2	T41.3X3	T41.3X4	T41.3X5	T41.3X6
nerve block (peripheral) (plexus)	T41.3X1	T41.3X2	T41.3X3	T41.3X4	T41.3X5	T41.3X6
topical (surface)	T41.3X1	T41.3X2	T41.3X3	T41.3X4	T41.3X5	T41.3X6
Propoxyphene	T40.491	T40.492	T40.493	T40.494	T40.495	T40.496
Propranolol	T44.7X1	T44.7X2	T44.7X3	T44.7X4	T44.7X5	T44.7X6
Propyl						
alcohol	T51.3X1	T51.3X2	T51.3X3	T51.3X4	—	—
carbinol	T51.3X1	T51.3X2	T51.3X3	T51.3X4	—	—
hexadrine	T44.4X1	T44.4X2	T44.4X3	T44.4X4	T44.4X5	T44.4X6
iodone	T50.8X1	T50.8X2	T50.8X3	T50.8X4	T50.8X5	T50.8X6
thiouracil	T38.2X1	T38.2X2	T38.2X3	T38.2X4	T38.2X5	T38.2X6
Propylaminophenothiazine	T43.3X1	T43.3X2	T43.3X3	T43.3X4	T43.3X5	T43.3X6
Propylene	T59.891	T59.892	T59.893	T59.894	—	—
Propylhexedrine	T48.5X1	T48.5X2	T48.5X3	T48.5X4	T48.5X5	T48.5X6
Propyliodone	T50.8X1	T50.8X2	T50.8X3	T50.8X4	T50.8X5	T50.8X6
Propylthiouracil	T38.2X1	T38.2X2	T38.2X3	T38.2X4	T38.2X5	T38.2X6
Propylparaben (ophthalmic)	T49.5X1	T49.5X2	T49.5X3	T49.5X4	T49.5X5	T49.5X6
Propyphenazone	T39.2X1	T39.2X2	T39.2X3	T39.2X4	T39.2X5	T39.2X6
Proquazone	T39.391	T39.392	T39.393	T39.394	T39.395	T39.396
Proscillaridin	T46.0X1	T46.0X2	T46.0X3	T46.0X4	T46.0X5	T46.0X6
Prostacyclin	T45.521	T45.522	T45.523	T45.524	T45.525	T45.526
Prostaglandin (I2)	T45.521	T45.522	T45.523	T45.524	T45.525	T45.526
E1	T46.7X1	T46.7X2	T46.7X3	T46.7X4	T46.7X5	T46.7X6
E2	T48.0X1	T48.0X2	T48.0X3	T48.0X4	T48.0X5	T48.0X6
F2 alpha	T48.0X1	T48.0X2	T48.0X3	T48.0X4	T48.0X5	T48.0X6
Prostigmin	T44.0X1	T44.0X2	T44.0X3	T44.0X4	T44.0X5	T44.0X6
Prosultiamine	T45.2X1	T45.2X2	T45.2X3	T45.2X4	T45.2X5	T45.2X6
Protamine sulfate	T45.7X1	T45.7X2	T45.7X3	T45.7X4	T45.7X5	T45.7X6
zinc insulin	T38.3X1	T38.3X2	T38.3X3	T38.3X4	T38.3X5	T38.3X6
Protease	T47.5X1	T47.5X2	T47.5X3	T47.5X4	T47.5X5	T47.5X6
Protectant, skin NEC	T49.3X1	T49.3X2	T49.3X3	T49.3X4	T49.3X5	T49.3X6
Protein hydrolysate	T50.991	T50.992	T50.993	T50.994	T50.995	T50.996
Prothiaden — see Dothiepin hydrochloride						
Prothionamide	T37.1X1	T37.1X2	T37.1X3	T37.1X4	T37.1X5	T37.1X6

◀ New ◀ Revised ~~deleted~~ Deleted

	External Cause (T-Code)					
Substance	Poisoning, Accidental (Unintentional)	Poisoning, Intentional Self-Harm	Poisoning, Assault	Poisoning, Undetermined	Adverse Effect	Underdosing
Prothipendyl	T43.591	T43.592	T43.593	T43.594	T43.595	T43.596
Prothoate	T60.0X1	T60.0X2	T60.0X3	T60.0X4	—	—
Prothrombin						
activator	T45.7X1	T45.7X2	T45.7X3	T45.7X4	T45.7X5	T45.7X6
synthesis inhibitor	T45.511	T45.512	T45.513	T45.514	T45.515	T45.516
Protionamide	T37.1X1	T37.1X2	T37.1X3	T37.1X4	T37.1X5	T37.1X6
Protirelin	T38.891	T38.892	T38.893	T38.894	T38.895	T38.896
Protokylol	T48.6X1	T48.6X2	T48.6X3	T48.6X4	T48.6X5	T48.6X6
Protopam	T50.6X1	T50.6X2	T50.6X3	T50.6X4	T50.6X5	T50.6X6
Protoveratrine(s) (A) (B)	T46.5X1	T46.5X2	T46.5X3	T46.5X4	T46.5X5	T46.5X6
Protriptyline	T43.011	T43.012	T43.013	T43.014	T43.015	T43.016
Provera	T38.5X1	T38.5X2	T38.5X3	T38.5X4	T38.5X5	T38.5X6
Provitamin A	T45.2X1	T45.2X2	T45.2X3	T45.2X4	T45.2X5	T45.2X6
Proxibarbal	T42.3X1	T42.3X2	T42.3X3	T42.3X4	T42.3X5	T42.3X6
Proxymetacaine	T41.3X1	T41.3X2	T41.3X3	T41.3X4	T41.3X5	T41.3X6
Proxyphylline	T48.6X1	T48.6X2	T48.6X3	T48.6X4	T48.6X5	T48.6X6
Prozac — see Fluoxetine hydrochloride						
Prunus						
laurocerasus	T62.2X1	T62.2X2	T62.2X3	T62.2X4	—	—
virginiana	T62.2X1	T62.2X2	T62.2X3	T62.2X4	—	—
Prussian blue						
commercial	T65.891	T65.892	T65.893	T65.894	—	—
therapeutic	T50.6X1	T50.6X2	T50.6X3	T50.6X4	T50.6X5	T50.6X6
Prussic acid	T65.0X1	T65.0X2	T65.0X3	T65.0X4	—	—
vapor	T57.3X1	T57.3X2	T57.3X3	T57.3X4	—	—
Pseudoephedrine	T44.991	T44.992	T44.993	T44.994	T44.995	T44.996
Psilocin	T40.991	T40.992	T40.993	T40.994	—	—
Psilocybin	T40.991	T40.992	T40.993	T40.994	—	—
Psilocybine	T40.991	T40.992	T40.993	T40.994	—	—
Psoralene (nonmedicinal)	T65.891	T65.892	T65.893	T65.894	—	—
Psoralens (medicinal)	T50.991	T50.992	T50.993	T50.994	T50.995	T50.996
PSP (phenolsulfonphthalein)	T50.8X1	T50.8X2	T50.8X3	T50.8X4	T50.8X5	T50.8X6
Psychodysleptic drug NOS	T40.901	T40.902	T40.903	T40.904	T40.905	T40.906
specified NEC	T40.991	T40.992	T40.993	T40.994	T40.995	T40.996
Psychostimulant	T43.601	T43.602	T43.603	T43.604	T43.605	T43.606
amphetamine	T43.621	T43.622	T43.623	T43.624	T43.625	T43.626
caffeine	T43.611	T43.612	T43.613	T43.614	T43.615	T43.616
methylphenidate	T43.631	T43.632	T43.633	T43.634	T43.635	T43.636
specified NEC	T43.691	T43.692	T43.693	T43.694	T43.695	T43.696
Psychotherapeutic drug NEC	T43.91	T43.92	T43.93	T43.94	T43.95	T43.96
antidepressants — see also Antidepressant	T43.201	T43.202	T43.203	T43.204	T43.205	T43.206

	External Cause (T-Code)					
Substance	Poisoning, Accidental (Unintentional)	Poisoning, Intentional Self-Harm	Poisoning, Assault	Poisoning, Undetermined	Adverse Effect	Underdosing
Psychotherapeutic drug NEC (Continued)						
specified NEC	T43.8X1	T43.8X2	T43.8X3	T43.8X4	T43.8X5	T43.8X6
tranquilizers NEC	T43.501	T43.502	T43.503	T43.504	T43.505	T43.506
Psychotomimetic agents	T40.901	T40.902	T40.903	T40.904	T40.905	T40.906
Psychotropic drug NEC	T43.91	T43.92	T43.93	T43.94	T43.95	T43.96
specified NEC	T43.8X1	T43.8X2	T43.8X3	T43.8X4	T43.8X5	T43.8X6
Psyllium hydrophilic mucilloid	T47.4X1	T47.4X2	T47.4X3	T47.4X4	T47.4X5	T47.4X6
Pteroylglutamic acid	T45.8X1	T45.8X2	T45.8X3	T45.8X4	T45.8X5	T45.8X6
Pteroyltriglutamate	T45.1X1	T45.1X2	T45.1X3	T45.1X4	T45.1X5	T45.1X6
PTFE — see Polytetrafluoroethylene						
Pulp						
devitalizing paste	T49.7X1	T49.7X2	T49.7X3	T49.7X4	T49.7X5	T49.7X6
dressing	T49.7X1	T49.7X2	T49.7X3	T49.7X4	T49.7X5	T49.7X6
Pulsatilla	T62.2X1	T62.2X2	T62.2X3	T62.2X4	—	—
Pumpkin seed extract	T37.4X1	T37.4X2	T37.4X3	T37.4X4	T37.4X5	T37.4X6
Purex (bleach)	T54.91	T54.92	T54.93	T54.94		
Purgative NEC — see also Cathartic	T47.4X1	T47.4X2	T47.4X3	T47.4X4	T47.4X5	T47.4X6
Purine analogue (antineoplastic)	T45.1X1	T45.1X2	T45.1X3	T45.1X4	T45.1X5	T45.1X6
Purine diuretics	T50.2X1	T50.2X2	T50.2X3	T50.2X4	T50.2X5	T50.2X6
Purinethol	T45.1X1	T45.1X2	T45.1X3	T45.1X4	T45.1X5	T45.1X6
PVP	T45.8X1	T45.8X2	T45.8X3	T45.8X4	T45.8X5	T45.8X6
Pyrabital	T39.8X1	T39.8X2	T39.8X3	T39.8X4	T39.8X5	T39.8X6
Pyramidon	T39.2X1	T39.2X2	T39.2X3	T39.2X4	T39.2X5	T39.2X6
Pyrantel	T37.4X1	T37.4X2	T37.4X3	T37.4X4	T37.4X5	T37.4X6
Pyrathiazine	T45.0X1	T45.0X2	T45.0X3	T45.0X4	T45.0X5	T45.0X6
Pyrazinamide	T37.1X1	T37.1X2	T37.1X3	T37.1X4	T37.1X5	T37.1X6
Pyrazinoic acid (amide)	T37.1X1	T37.1X2	T37.1X3	T37.1X4	T37.1X5	T37.1X6
Pyrazole (derivatives)	T39.2X1	T39.2X2	T39.2X3	T39.2X4	T39.2X5	T39.2X6
Pyrazolone analgesic NEC	T39.2X1	T39.2X2	T39.2X3	T39.2X4	T39.2X5	T39.2X6
Pyrethrin, pyrethrum (nonmedicinal)	T60.2X1	T60.2X2	T60.2X3	T60.2X4	—	—
Pyrethrum extract	T49.0X1	T49.0X2	T49.0X3	T49.0X4	T49.0X5	T49.0X6
Pyribenzamine	T45.0X1	T45.0X2	T45.0X3	T45.0X4	T45.0X5	T45.0X6
Pyridine	T52.8X1	T52.8X2	T52.8X3	T52.8X4	—	—
aldoxime methiodide	T50.6X1	T50.6X2	T50.6X3	T50.6X4	T50.6X5	T50.6X6
aldoxime methyl chloride	T50.6X1	T50.6X2	T50.6X3	T50.6X4	T50.6X5	T50.6X6
vapor	T59.891	T59.892	T59.893	T59.894	—	—
Pyridium	T39.8X1	T39.8X2	T39.8X3	T39.8X4	T39.8X5	T39.8X6
Pyridostigmine bromide	T44.0X1	T44.0X2	T44.0X3	T44.0X4	T44.0X5	T44.0X6
Pyridoxal phosphate	T45.2X1	T45.2X2	T45.2X3	T45.2X4	T45.2X5	T45.2X6

◀ New　◀ Revised　~~deleted~~ Deleted

TABLE OF DRUGS AND CHEMICALS

Substance	External Cause (T-Code)					
	Poisoning, Accidental (Unintentional)	Poisoning, Intentional Self-Harm	Poisoning, Assault	Poisoning, Undetermined	Adverse Effect	Underdosing
Pyridoxine	T45.2X1	T45.2X2	T45.2X3	T45.2X4	T45.2X5	T45.2X6
Pyrilamine	T45.0X1	T45.0X2	T45.0X3	T45.0X4	T45.0X5	T45.0X6
Pyrimethamine	T37.2X1	T37.2X2	T37.2X3	T37.2X4	T37.2X5	T37.2X6
with sulfadoxine	T37.2X1	T37.2X2	T37.2X3	T37.2X4	T37.2X5	T37.2X6
Pyrimidine antagonist	T45.1X1	T45.1X2	T45.1X3	T45.1X4	T45.1X5	T45.1X6
Pyriminil	T60.4X1	T60.4X2	T60.4X3	T60.4X4	—	—
Pyrithione zinc	T49.4X1	T49.4X2	T49.4X3	T49.4X4	T49.4X5	T49.4X6
Pyrithyldione	T42.6X1	T42.6X2	T42.6X3	T42.6X4	T42.6X5	T42.6X6
Pyrogallic acid	T49.0X1	T49.0X2	T49.0X3	T49.0X4	T49.0X5	T49.0X6
Pyrogallol	T49.0X1	T49.0X2	T49.0X3	T49.0X4	T49.0X5	T49.0X6
Pyroxylin	T49.3X1	T49.3X2	T49.3X3	T49.3X4	T49.3X5	T49.3X6
Pyrrobutamine	T45.0X1	T45.0X2	T45.0X3	T45.0X4	T45.0X5	T45.0X6
Pyrrolizidine alkaloids	T62.8X1	T62.8X2	T62.8X3	T62.8X4	—	—
Pyrvinium chloride	T37.4X1	T37.4X2	T37.4X3	T37.4X4	T37.4X5	T37.4X6
PZI	T38.3X1	T38.3X2	T38.3X3	T38.3X4	T38.3X5	T38.3X6
Q						
Quaalude	T42.6X1	T42.6X2	T42.6X3	T42.6X4	T42.6X5	T42.6X6
Quarternary ammonium						
anti-infective	T49.0X1	T49.0X2	T49.0X3	T49.0X4	T49.0X5	T49.0X6
ganglion blocking	T44.2X1	T44.2X2	T44.2X3	T44.2X4	T44.2X5	T44.2X6
parasympatholytic	T44.3X1	T44.3X2	T44.3X3	T44.3X4	T44.3X5	T44.3X6
Quazepam	T42.4X1	T42.4X2	T42.4X3	T42.4X4	T42.4X5	T42.4X6
Quicklime	T54.3X1	T54.3X2	T54.3X3	T54.3X4	—	—
Quillaja extract	T48.4X1	T48.4X2	T48.4X3	T48.4X4	T48.4X5	T48.4X6
Quinacrine	T37.2X1	T37.2X2	T37.2X3	T37.2X4	T37.2X5	T37.2X6
Quinaglute	T46.2X1	T46.2X2	T46.2X3	T46.2X4	T46.2X5	T46.2X6
Quinalbarbital	T42.3X1	T42.3X2	T42.3X3	T42.3X4	T42.3X5	T42.3X6
Quinalbarbitone sodium	T42.3X1	T42.3X2	T42.3X3	T42.3X4	T42.3X5	T42.3X6
Quinalphos	T60.0X1	T60.0X2	T60.0X3	T60.0X4	—	—
Quinapril	T46.4X1	T46.4X2	T46.4X3	T46.4X4	T46.4X5	T46.4X6
Quinestradiol	T38.5X1	T38.5X2	T38.5X3	T38.5X4	T38.5X5	T38.5X6
Quinestradol	T38.5X1	T38.5X2	T38.5X3	T38.5X4	T38.5X5	T38.5X6
Quinestrol	T38.5X1	T38.5X2	T38.5X3	T38.5X4	T38.5X5	T38.5X6
Quinethazone	T50.2X1	T50.2X2	T50.2X3	T50.2X4	T50.2X5	T50.2X6
Quingestanol	T38.4X1	T38.4X2	T38.4X3	T38.4X4	T38.4X5	T38.4X6
Quinidine	T46.2X1	T46.2X2	T46.2X3	T46.2X4	T46.2X5	T46.2X6
Quinine	T37.2X1	T37.2X2	T37.2X3	T37.2X4	T37.2X5	T37.2X6
Quiniobine	T37.8X1	T37.8X2	T37.8X3	T37.8X4	T37.8X5	T37.8X6
Quinisocaine	T49.1X1	T49.1X2	T49.1X3	T49.1X4	T49.1X5	T49.1X6
Quinocide	T37.2X1	T37.2X2	T37.2X3	T37.2X4	T37.2X5	T37.2X6
Quinoline (derivatives) NEC	T37.8X1	T37.8X2	T37.8X3	T37.8X4	T37.8X5	T37.8X6

Substance	External Cause (T-Code)					
	Poisoning, Accidental (Unintentional)	Poisoning, Intentional Self-Harm	Poisoning, Assault	Poisoning, Undetermined	Adverse Effect	Underdosing
Quinupramine	T43.011	T43.012	T43.013	T43.014	T43.015	T43.016
Quotane	T41.3X1	T41.3X2	T41.3X3	T41.3X4	T41.3X5	T41.3X6
R						
Rabies						
immune globulin (human)	T50.Z11	T50.Z12	T50.Z13	T50.Z14	T50.Z15	T50.Z16
vaccine	T50.B91	T50.B92	T50.B93	T50.B94	T50.B95	T50.B96
Racemoramide	T40.2X1	T40.2X2	T40.2X3	T40.2X4	—	—
Racemorphan	T40.2X1	T40.2X2	T40.2X3	T40.2X4	T40.2X5	T40.2X6
Racepinefrin	T44.5X1	T44.5X2	T44.5X3	T44.5X4	T44.5X5	T44.5X6
Raclopride	T43.591	T43.592	T43.593	T43.594	T43.595	T43.596
Radiator alcohol	T51.1X1	T51.1X2	T51.1X3	T51.1X4	—	—
Radioactive drug NEC	T50.8X1	T50.8X2	T50.8X3	T50.8X4	T50.8X5	T50.8X6
Radio-opaque (drugs) (materials)	T50.8X1	T50.8X2	T50.8X3	T50.8X4	T50.8X5	T50.8X6
Ramifenazone	T39.2X1	T39.2X2	T39.2X3	T39.2X4	T39.2X5	T39.2X6
Ramipril	T46.4X1	T46.4X2	T46.4X3	T46.4X4	T46.4X5	T46.4X6
Ranitidine	T47.0X1	T47.0X2	T47.0X3	T47.0X4	T47.0X5	T47.0X6
Ranunculus	T62.2X1	T62.2X2	T62.2X3	T62.2X4	—	—
Rat poison NEC	T60.4X1	T60.4X2	T60.4X3	T60.4X4	—	—
Rattlesnake (venom)	T63.011	T63.012	T63.013	T63.014	—	—
Raubasine	T46.7X1	T46.7X2	T46.7X3	T46.7X4	T46.7X5	T46.7X6
Raudixin	T46.5X1	T46.5X2	T46.5X3	T46.5X4	T46.5X5	T46.5X6
Rautensin	T46.5X1	T46.5X2	T46.5X3	T46.5X4	T46.5X5	T46.5X6
Rautina	T46.5X1	T46.5X2	T46.5X3	T46.5X4	T46.5X5	T46.5X6
Rautotal	T46.5X1	T46.5X2	T46.5X3	T46.5X4	T46.5X5	T46.5X6
Rauwiloid	T46.5X1	T46.5X2	T46.5X3	T46.5X4	T46.5X5	T46.5X6
Rauwoldin	T46.5X1	T46.5X2	T46.5X3	T46.5X4	T46.5X5	T46.5X6
Rauwolfia (alkaloids)	T46.5X1	T46.5X2	T46.5X3	T46.5X4	T46.5X5	T46.5X6
Razoxane	T45.1X1	T45.1X2	T45.1X3	T45.1X4	T45.1X5	T45.1X6
Realgar	T57.0X1	T57.0X2	T57.0X3	T57.0X4	—	—
Recombinant (R) — see specific protein						
Red blood cells, packed	T45.8X1	T45.8X2	T45.8X3	T45.8X4	T45.8X5	T45.8X6
Red squill (scilliroside)	T60.4X1	T60.4X2	T60.4X3	T60.4X4	—	—
Reducing agent, industrial NEC	T65.891	T65.892	T65.893	T65.894	—	—
Refrigerant gas (chlorofluoro-carbon)	T53.5X1	T53.5X2	T53.5X3	T53.5X4	—	—
not chlorofluoro-carbon	T59.891	T59.892	T59.893	T59.894	—	—
Regroton	T50.2X1	T50.2X2	T50.2X3	T50.2X4	T50.2X5	T50.2X6
Rehydration salts (oral)	T50.3X1	T50.3X2	T50.3X3	T50.3X4	T50.3X5	T50.3X6
Rela	T42.8X1	T42.8X2	T42.8X3	T42.8X4	T42.8X5	T42.8X6

◀ New   ◀ Revised   ~~deleted~~ Deleted

| | External Cause (T-Code) | | | | | |
Substance	Poisoning, Accidental (Unintentional)	Poisoning, Intentional Self-Harm	Poisoning, Assault	Poisoning, Undetermined	Adverse Effect	Underdosing
Relaxant, muscle						
anesthetic	T48.1X1	T48.1X2	T48.1X3	T48.1X4	T48.1X5	T48.1X6
central nervous system	T42.8X1	T42.8X2	T42.8X3	T42.8X4	T42.8X5	T42.8X6
skeletal NEC	T48.1X1	T48.1X2	T48.1X3	T48.1X4	T48.1X5	T48.1X6
smooth NEC	T44.3X1	T44.3X2	T44.3X3	T44.3X4	T44.3X5	T44.3X6
Remoxipride	T43.591	T43.592	T43.593	T43.594	T43.595	T43.596
Renese	T50.2X1	T50.2X2	T50.2X3	T50.2X4	T50.2X5	T50.2X6
Renografin	T50.8X1	T50.8X2	T50.8X3	T50.8X4	T50.8X5	T50.8X6
Replacement solution	T50.3X1	T50.3X2	T50.3X3	T50.3X4	T50.3X5	T50.3X6
Reproterol	T48.6X1	T48.6X2	T48.6X3	T48.6X4	T48.6X5	T48.6X6
Rescinnamine	T46.5X1	T46.5X2	T46.5X3	T46.5X4	T46.5X5	T46.5X6
Reserpin(e)	T46.5X1	T46.5X2	T46.5X3	T46.5X4	T46.5X5	T46.5X6
Resorcin, resorcinol (nonmedicinal)	T65.891	T65.892	T65.893	T65.894	—	—
medicinal	T49.4X1	T49.4X2	T49.4X3	T49.4X4	T49.4X5	T49.4X6
Respaire	T48.4X1	T48.4X2	T48.4X3	T48.4X4	T48.4X5	T48.4X6
Respiratory drug NEC	T48.901	T48.902	T48.903	T48.904	T48.905	T48.906
antiasthmatic NEC	T48.6X1	T48.6X2	T48.6X3	T48.6X4	T48.6X5	T48.6X6
anti-common-cold NEC	T48.5X1	T48.5X2	T48.5X3	T48.5X4	T48.5X5	T48.5X6
expectorant NEC	T48.4X1	T48.4X2	T48.4X3	T48.4X4	T48.4X5	T48.4X6
stimulant	T48.901	T48.902	T48.903	T48.904	T48.905	T48.906
Retinoic acid	T49.0X1	T49.0X2	T49.0X3	T49.0X4	T49.0X5	T49.0X6
Retinol	T45.2X1	T45.2X2	T45.2X3	T45.2X4	T45.2X5	T45.2X6
Rh (D) immune globulin (human)	T50.Z11	T50.Z12	T50.Z13	T50.Z14	T50.Z15	T50.Z16
Rhodine	T39.011	T39.012	T39.013	T39.014	T39.015	T39.016
RhoGAM	T50.Z11	T50.Z12	T50.Z13	T50.Z14	T50.Z15	T50.Z16
Rhubarb						
dry extract	T47.2X1	T47.2X2	T47.2X3	T47.2X4	T47.2X5	T47.2X6
tincture, compound	T47.2X1	T47.2X2	T47.2X3	T47.2X4	T47.2X5	T47.2X6
Ribavirin	T37.5X1	T37.5X2	T37.5X3	T37.5X4	T37.5X5	T37.5X6
Riboflavin	T45.2X1	T45.2X2	T45.2X3	T45.2X4	T45.2X5	T45.2X6
Ribostamycin	T36.5X1	T36.5X2	T36.5X3	T36.5X4	T36.5X5	T36.5X6
Ricin	T62.2X1	T62.2X2	T62.2X3	T62.2X4	—	—
Ricinus communis	T62.2X1	T62.2X2	T62.2X3	T62.2X4	—	—
Rickettsial vaccine NEC	T50.A91	T50.A92	T50.A93	T50.A94	T50.A95	T50.A96
Rifabutin	T36.6X1	T36.6X2	T36.6X3	T36.6X4	T36.6X5	T36.6X6
Rifamide	T36.6X1	T36.6X2	T36.6X3	T36.6X4	T36.6X5	T36.6X6
Rifampicin	T36.6X1	T36.6X2	T36.6X3	T36.6X4	T36.6X5	T36.6X6
with isoniazid	T37.1X1	T37.1X2	T37.1X3	T37.1X4	T37.1X5	T37.1X6
Rifampin	T36.6X1	T36.6X2	T36.6X3	T36.6X4	T36.6X5	T36.6X6
Rifamycin	T36.6X1	T36.6X2	T36.6X3	T36.6X4	T36.6X5	T36.6X6
Rifaximin	T36.6X1	T36.6X2	T36.6X3	T36.6X4	T36.6X5	T36.6X6

| | External Cause (T-Code) | | | | | |
Substance	Poisoning, Accidental (Unintentional)	Poisoning, Intentional Self-Harm	Poisoning, Assault	Poisoning, Undetermined	Adverse Effect	Underdosing
Rimantadine	T37.5X1	T37.5X2	T37.5X3	T37.5X4	T37.5X5	T37.5X6
Rimazolium metilsulfate	T39.8X1	T39.8X2	T39.8X3	T39.8X4	T39.8X5	T39.8X6
Rimifon	T37.1X1	T37.1X2	T37.1X3	T37.1X4	T37.1X5	T37.1X6
Rimiterol	T48.6X1	T48.6X2	T48.6X3	T48.6X4	T48.6X5	T48.6X6
Ringer (lactate) solution	T50.3X1	T50.3X2	T50.3X3	T50.3X4	T50.3X5	T50.3X6
Ristocetin	T36.8X1	T36.8X2	T36.8X3	T36.8X4	T36.8X5	T36.8X6
Ritalin	T43.631	T43.632	T43.633	T43.634	T43.635	T43.636
Ritodrine	T44.5X1	T44.5X2	T44.5X3	T44.5X4	T44.5X5	T44.5X6
Roach killer — see Insecticide						
Rociverine	T44.3X1	T44.3X2	T44.3X3	T44.3X4	T44.3X5	T44.3X6
Rocky Mountain spotted fever vaccine	T50.A91	T50.A92	T50.A93	T50.A94	T50.A95	T50.A96
Rodenticide NEC	T60.4X1	T60.4X2	T60.4X3	T60.4X4	—	—
Rohypnol	T42.4X1	T42.4X2	T42.4X3	T42.4X4	T42.4X5	T42.4X6
Rokitamycin	T36.3X1	T36.3X2	T36.3X3	T36.3X4	T36.3X5	T36.3X6
Rolaids	T47.1X1	T47.1X2	T47.1X3	T47.1X4	T47.1X5	T47.1X6
Rolitetracycline	T36.4X1	T36.4X2	T36.4X3	T36.4X4	T36.4X5	T36.4X6
Romilar	T48.3X1	T48.3X2	T48.3X3	T48.3X4	T48.3X5	T48.3X6
Ronifibrate	T46.6X1	T46.6X2	T46.6X3	T46.6X4	T46.6X5	T46.6X6
Rosaprostol	T47.1X1	T47.1X2	T47.1X3	T47.1X4	T47.1X5	T47.1X6
Rose bengal sodium (131I)	T50.8X1	T50.8X2	T50.8X3	T50.8X4	T50.8X5	T50.8X6
Rose water ointment	T49.3X1	T49.3X2	T49.3X3	T49.3X4	T49.3X5	T49.3X6
Rosoxacin	T37.8X1	T37.8X2	T37.8X3	T37.8X4	T37.8X5	T37.8X6
Rotenone	T60.2X1	T60.2X2	T60.2X3	T60.2X4	—	—
Rotoxamine	T45.0X1	T45.0X2	T45.0X3	T45.0X4	T45.0X5	T45.0X6
Rough-on-rats	T60.4X1	T60.4X2	T60.4X3	T60.4X4	—	—
Roxatidine	T47.0X1	T47.0X2	T47.0X3	T47.0X4	T47.0X5	T47.0X6
Roxithromycin	T36.3X1	T36.3X2	T36.3X3	T36.3X4	T36.3X5	T36.3X6
Rt-PA	T45.611	T45.612	T45.613	T45.614	T45.615	T45.616
Rubbing alcohol	T51.2X1	T51.2X2	T51.2X3	T51.2X4	—	—
Rubefacient	T49.4X1	T49.4X2	T49.4X3	T49.4X4	T49.4X5	T49.4X6
Rubella vaccine	T50.B91	T50.B92	T50.B93	T50.B94	T50.B95	T50.B96
Rubelogen	T50.B91	T50.B92	T50.B93	T50.B94	T50.B95	T50.B96
Rubeovax	T50.991	T50.992	T50.993	T50.994	T50.995	T50.996
Rubidium chloride Rb82	T50.8X1	T50.8X2	T50.8X3	T50.8X4	T50.8X5	T50.8X6
Rubidomycin	T45.1X1	T45.1X2	T45.1X3	T45.1X4	T45.1X5	T45.1X6
Rue	T62.2X1	T62.2X2	T62.2X3	T62.2X4	—	—
Rufocromomycin	T45.1X1	T45.1X2	T45.1X3	T45.1X4	T45.1X5	T45.1X6
Russel's viper venin	T45.7X1	T45.7X2	T45.7X3	T45.7X4	T45.7X5	T45.7X6
Ruta (graveolens)	T62.2X1	T62.2X2	T62.2X3	T62.2X4	—	—
Rutinum	T46.991	T46.992	T46.993	T46.994	T46.995	T46.996
Rutoside	T46.991	T46.992	T46.993	T46.994	T46.995	T46.996

TABLE OF DRUGS AND CHEMICALS

TABLE OF DRUGS AND CHEMICALS

	External Cause (T-Code)					
Substance	Poisoning, Accidental (Unintentional)	Poisoning, Intentional Self-Harm	Poisoning, Assault	Poisoning, Undetermined	Adverse Effect	Underdosing
S						
Sabadilla (plant)	T62.2X1	T62.2X2	T62.2X3	T62.2X4	—	—
pesticide	T60.2X1	T60.2X2	T60.2X3	T60.2X4	—	—
Saccharated iron oxide	T45.8X1	T45.8X2	T45.8X3	T45.8X4	T45.8X5	T45.8X6
Saccharin	T50.901	T50.902	T50.903	T50.904	T50.905	T50.906
Saccharomyces boulardii	T47.6X1	T47.6X2	T47.6X3	T47.6X4	T47.6X5	T47.6X6
Safflower oil	T46.6X1	T46.6X2	T46.6X3	T46.6X4	T46.6X5	T46.6X6
Safrazine	T43.1X1	T43.1X2	T43.1X3	T43.1X4	T43.1X5	T43.1X6
Salazosulfapyridine	T37.0X1	T37.0X2	T37.0X3	T37.0X4	T37.0X5	T37.0X6
Salbutamol	T48.6X1	T48.6X2	T48.6X3	T48.6X4	T48.6X5	T48.6X6
Salicylamide	T39.091	T39.092	T39.093	T39.094	T39.095	T39.096
Salicylate NEC	T39.091	T39.092	T39.093	T39.094	T39.095	T39.096
methyl	T49.3X1	T49.3X2	T49.3X3	T49.3X4	T49.3X5	T49.3X6
theobromine calcium	T50.2X1	T50.2X2	T50.2X3	T50.2X4	T50.2X5	T50.2X6
Salicylazosulfapyridine	T37.0X1	T37.0X2	T37.0X3	T37.0X4	T37.0X5	T37.0X6
Salicylhydroxamic acid	T49.0X1	T49.0X2	T49.0X3	T49.0X4	T49.0X5	T49.0X6
Salicylic acid	T49.4X1	T49.4X2	T49.4X3	T49.4X4	T49.4X5	T49.4X6
with benzoic acid	T49.4X1	T49.4X2	T49.4X3	T49.4X4	T49.4X5	T49.4X6
congeners	T39.091	T39.092	T39.093	T39.094	T39.095	T39.096
derivative	T39.091	T39.092	T39.093	T39.094	T39.095	T39.096
salts	T39.091	T39.092	T39.093	T39.094	T39.095	T39.096
Salinazid	T37.1X1	T37.1X2	T37.1X3	T37.1X4	T37.1X5	T37.1X6
Salmeterol	T48.6X1	T48.6X2	T48.6X3	T48.6X4	T48.6X5	T48.6X6
Salol	T49.3X1	T49.3X2	T49.3X3	T49.3X4	T49.3X5	T49.3X6
Salsalate	T39.091	T39.092	T39.093	T39.094	T39.095	T39.096
Salt substitute	T50.901	T50.902	T50.903	T50.904	T50.905	T50.906
Salt-replacing drug	T50.901	T50.902	T50.903	T50.904	T50.905	T50.906
Salt-retaining mineralocorticoid	T50.0X1	T50.0X2	T50.0X3	T50.0X4	T50.0X5	T50.0X6
Saluretic NEC	T50.2X1	T50.2X2	T50.2X3	T50.2X4	T50.2X5	T50.2X6
Saluron	T50.2X1	T50.2X2	T50.2X3	T50.2X4	T50.2X5	T50.2X6
Salvarsan 606 (neosilver) (silver)	T37.8X1	T37.8X2	T37.8X3	T37.8X4	T37.8X5	T37.8X6
Sambucus canadensis	T62.2X1	T62.2X2	T62.2X3	T62.2X4	—	—
berry	T62.1X1	T62.1X2	T62.1X3	T62.1X4	—	—
Sandril	T46.5X1	T46.5X2	T46.5X3	T46.5X4	T46.5X5	T46.5X6
Sanguinaria canadensis	T62.2X1	T62.2X2	T62.2X3	T62.2X4	—	—
Saniflush (cleaner)	T54.2X1	T54.2X2	T54.2X3	T54.2X4	—	—
Santonin	T37.4X1	T37.4X2	T37.4X3	T37.4X4	T37.4X5	T37.4X6
Santyl	T49.8X1	T49.8X2	T49.8X3	T49.8X4	T49.8X5	T49.8X6
Saralasin	T46.5X1	T46.5X2	T46.5X3	T46.5X4	T46.5X5	T46.5X6
Sarcolysin	T45.1X1	T45.1X2	T45.1X3	T45.1X4	T45.1X5	T45.1X6
Sarkomycin	T45.1X1	T45.1X2	T45.1X3	T45.1X4	T45.1X5	T45.1X6
Saroten	T43.011	T43.012	T43.013	T43.014	T43.015	T43.016

	External Cause (T-Code)					
Substance	Poisoning, Accidental (Unintentional)	Poisoning, Intentional Self-Harm	Poisoning, Assault	Poisoning, Undetermined	Adverse Effect	Underdosing
Saturnine — see Lead						
Savin (oil)	T49.4X1	T49.4X2	T49.4X3	T49.4X4	T49.4X5	T49.4X6
Scammony	T47.2X1	T47.2X2	T47.2X3	T47.2X4	T47.2X5	T47.2X6
Scarlet red	T49.8X1	T49.8X2	T49.8X3	T49.8X4	T49.8X5	T49.8X6
Scheele's green	T57.0X1	T57.0X2	T57.0X3	T57.0X4	—	—
insecticide	T57.0X1	T57.0X2	T57.0X3	T57.0X4	—	—
Schizontozide (blood) (tissue)	T37.2X1	T37.2X2	T37.2X3	T37.2X4	T37.2X5	T37.2X6
Schradan	T60.0X1	T60.0X2	T60.0X3	T60.0X4	—	—
Schweinfurth green	T57.0X1	T57.0X2	T57.0X3	T57.0X4	—	—
insecticide	T57.0X1	T57.0X2	T57.0X3	T57.0X4	—	—
Scilla, rat poison	T60.4X1	T60.4X2	T60.4X3	T60.4X4	—	—
Scillaren	T60.4X1	T60.4X2	T60.4X3	T60.4X4	—	—
Sclerosing agent	T46.8X1	T46.8X2	T46.8X3	T46.8X4	T46.8X5	T46.8X6
Scombrotoxin	T61.11	T61.12	T61.13	T61.14		
Scopolamine	T44.3X1	T44.3X2	T44.3X3	T44.3X4	T44.3X5	T44.3X6
Scopolia extract	T44.3X1	T44.3X2	T44.3X3	T44.3X4	T44.3X5	T44.3X6
Scouring powder	T65.891	T65.892	T65.893	T65.894		
Sea						
anemone (sting)	T63.631	T63.632	T63.633	T63.634	—	—
cucumber (sting)	T63.691	T63.692	T63.693	T63.694	—	—
snake (bite) (venom)	T63.091	T63.092	T63.093	T63.094	—	—
urchin spine (puncture)	T63.691	T63.692	T63.693	T63.694	—	—
Seafood	T61.91	T61.92	T61.93	T61.94		
specified NEC	T61.8X1	T61.8X2	T61.8X3	T61.8X4		
Secbutabarbital	T42.3X1	T42.3X2	T42.3X3	T42.3X4	T42.3X5	T42.3X6
Secbutabarbitone	T42.3X1	T42.3X2	T42.3X3	T42.3X4	T42.3X5	T42.3X6
Secnidazole	T37.3X1	T37.3X2	T37.3X3	T37.3X4	T37.3X5	T37.3X6
Secobarbital	T42.3X1	T42.3X2	T42.3X3	T42.3X4	T42.3X5	T42.3X6
Seconal	T42.3X1	T42.3X2	T42.3X3	T42.3X4	T42.3X5	T42.3X6
Secretin	T50.8X1	T50.8X2	T50.8X3	T50.8X4	T50.8X5	T50.8X6
Sedative NEC	T42.71	T42.72	T42.73	T42.74	T42.75	T42.76
mixed NEC	T42.6X1	T42.6X2	T42.6X3	T42.6X4	T42.6X5	T42.6X6
Sedormid	T42.6X1	T42.6X2	T42.6X3	T42.6X4	T42.6X5	T42.6X6
Seed disinfectant or dressing	T60.8X1	T60.8X2	T60.8X3	T60.8X4	—	—
Seeds (poisonous)	T62.2X1	T62.2X2	T62.2X3	T62.2X4	—	—
Selegiline	T42.8X1	T42.8X2	T42.8X3	T42.8X4	T42.8X5	T42.8X6
Selenium NEC	T56.891	T56.892	T56.893	T56.894	—	—
disulfide or sulfide	T49.4X1	T49.4X2	T49.4X3	T49.4X4	T49.4X5	T49.4X6
fumes	T59.891	T59.892	T59.893	T59.894	—	—
sulfide	T49.4X1	T49.4X2	T49.4X3	T49.4X4	T49.4X5	T49.4X6
Selenomethionine (75Se)	T50.8X1	T50.8X2	T50.8X3	T50.8X4	T50.8X5	T50.8X6
Selsun	T49.4X1	T49.4X2	T49.4X3	T49.4X4	T49.4X5	T49.4X6

◀ New ◀ Revised ~~deleted~~ Deleted

	External Cause (T-Code)					
Substance	Poisoning, Accidental (Unintentional)	Poisoning, Intentional Self-Harm	Poisoning, Assault	Poisoning, Undetermined	Adverse Effect	Underdosing
Semustine	T45.1X1	T45.1X2	T45.1X3	T45.1X4	T45.1X5	T45.1X6
Senega syrup	T48.4X1	T48.4X2	T48.4X3	T48.4X4	T48.4X5	T48.4X6
Senna	T47.2X1	T47.2X2	T47.2X3	T47.2X4	T47.2X5	T47.2X6
Sennoside A+B	T47.2X1	T47.2X2	T47.2X3	T47.2X4	T47.2X5	T47.2X6
Septisol	T49.2X1	T49.2X2	T49.2X3	T49.2X4	T49.2X5	T49.2X6
Seractide	T38.811	T38.812	T38.813	T38.814	T38.815	T38.816
Serax	T42.4X1	T42.4X2	T42.4X3	T42.4X4	T42.4X5	T42.4X6
Serenesil	T42.6X1	T42.6X2	T42.6X3	T42.6X4	T42.6X5	T42.6X6
Serenium (hydrochloride)	T37.91	T37.92	T37.93	T37.94	T37.95	T37.96
Serepax — see Oxazepam						
Sermorelin	T38.891	T38.892	T38.893	T38.894	T38.895	T38.896
Sernyl	T41.1X1	T41.1X2	T41.1X3	T41.1X4	T41.1X5	T41.1X6
Serotonin	T50.991	T50.992	T50.993	T50.994	T50.995	T50.996
Serpasil	T46.5X1	T46.5X2	T46.5X3	T46.5X4	T46.5X5	T46.5X6
Serrapeptase	T45.3X1	T45.3X2	T45.3X3	T45.3X4	T45.3X5	T45.3X6
Serum						
antibotulinus	T50.Z11	T50.Z12	T50.Z13	T50.Z14	T50.Z15	T50.Z16
anticytotoxic	T50.Z11	T50.Z12	T50.Z13	T50.Z14	T50.Z15	T50.Z16
antidiphtheria	T50.Z11	T50.Z12	T50.Z13	T50.Z14	T50.Z15	T50.Z16
antimeningococcus	T50.Z11	T50.Z12	T50.Z13	T50.Z14	T50.Z15	T50.Z16
anti-Rh	T50.Z11	T50.Z12	T50.Z13	T50.Z14	T50.Z15	T50.Z16
anti-snake-bite	T50.Z11	T50.Z12	T50.Z13	T50.Z14	T50.Z15	T50.Z16
antitetanic	T50.Z11	T50.Z12	T50.Z13	T50.Z14	T50.Z15	T50.Z16
antitoxic	T50.Z11	T50.Z12	T50.Z13	T50.Z14	T50.Z15	T50.Z16
complement (inhibitor)	T45.8X1	T45.8X2	T45.8X3	T45.8X4	T45.8X5	T45.8X6
convalescent	T50.Z11	T50.Z12	T50.Z13	T50.Z14	T50.Z15	T50.Z16
hemolytic complement	T45.8X1	T45.8X2	T45.8X3	T45.8X4	T45.8X5	T45.8X6
immune (human)	T50.Z11	T50.Z12	T50.Z13	T50.Z14	T50.Z15	T50.Z16
protective NEC	T50.Z11	T50.Z12	T50.Z13	T50.Z14	T50.Z15	T50.Z16
Setastine	T45.0X1	T45.0X2	T45.0X3	T45.0X4	T45.0X5	T45.0X6
Setoperone	T43.591	T43.592	T43.593	T43.594	T43.595	T43.596
Sewer gas	T59.91	T59.92	T59.93	T59.94	—	—
Shampoo	T55.0X1	T55.0X2	T55.0X3	T55.0X4	—	—
Shellfish, noxious, nonbacterial	T61.781	T61.782	T61.783	T61.784	—	—
Sildenafil	T46.7X1	T46.7X2	T46.7X3	T46.7X4	T46.7X5	T46.7X6
Silibinin	T50.991	T50.992	T50.993	T50.994	T50.995	T50.996
Silicone NEC	T65.891	T65.892	T65.893	T65.894	—	—
medicinal	T49.3X1	T49.3X2	T49.3X3	T49.3X4	T49.3X5	T49.3X6
Silvadene	T49.0X1	T49.0X2	T49.0X3	T49.0X4	T49.0X5	T49.0X6
Silver	T49.0X1	T49.0X2	T49.0X3	T49.0X4	T49.0X5	T49.0X6
anti-infectives	T49.0X1	T49.0X2	T49.0X3	T49.0X4	T49.0X5	T49.0X6
arsphenamine	T37.8X1	T37.8X2	T37.8X3	T37.8X4	T37.8X5	T37.8X6

	External Cause (T-Code)					
Substance	Poisoning, Accidental (Unintentional)	Poisoning, Intentional Self-Harm	Poisoning, Assault	Poisoning, Undetermined	Adverse Effect	Underdosing
Silver *(Continued)*						
colloidal	T49.0X1	T49.0X2	T49.0X3	T49.0X4	T49.0X5	T49.0X6
nitrate	T49.0X1	T49.0X2	T49.0X3	T49.0X4	T49.0X5	T49.0X6
ophthalmic preparation	T49.5X1	T49.5X2	T49.5X3	T49.5X4	T49.5X5	T49.5X6
toughened (keratolytic)	T49.4X1	T49.4X2	T49.4X3	T49.4X4	T49.4X5	T49.4X6
nonmedicinal (dust)	T56.891	T56.892	T56.893	T56.894	—	—
protein	T49.5X1	T49.5X2	T49.5X3	T49.5X4	T49.5X5	T49.5X6
salvarsan	T37.8X1	T37.8X2	T37.8X3	T37.8X4	T37.8X5	T37.8X6
sulfadiazine	T49.4X1	T49.4X2	T49.4X3	T49.4X4	T49.4X5	T49.4X6
Silymarin	T50.991	T50.992	T50.993	T50.994	T50.995	T50.996
Simaldrate	T47.1X1	T47.1X2	T47.1X3	T47.1X4	T47.1X5	T47.1X6
Simazine	T60.3X1	T60.3X2	T60.3X3	T60.3X4	—	—
Simethicone	T47.1X1	T47.1X2	T47.1X3	T47.1X4	T47.1X5	T47.1X6
Simfibrate	T46.6X1	T46.6X2	T46.6X3	T46.6X4	T46.6X5	T46.6X6
Simvastatin	T46.6X1	T46.6X2	T46.6X3	T46.6X4	T46.6X5	T46.6X6
Sincalide	T50.8X1	T50.8X2	T50.8X3	T50.8X4	T50.8X5	T50.8X6
Sinequan	T43.011	T43.012	T43.013	T43.014	T43.015	T43.016
Singoserp	T46.5X1	T46.5X2	T46.5X3	T46.5X4	T46.5X5	T46.5X6
Sintrom	T45.511	T45.512	T45.513	T45.514	T45.515	T45.516
Sisomicin	T36.5X1	T36.5X2	T36.5X3	T36.5X4	T36.5X5	T36.5X6
Sitosterols	T46.6X1	T46.6X2	T46.6X3	T46.6X4	T46.6X5	T46.6X6
Skeletal muscle relaxants	T48.1X1	T48.1X2	T48.1X3	T48.1X4	T48.1X5	T48.1X6
Skin						
agents (external)	T49.91	T49.92	T49.93	T49.94	T49.95	T49.96
specified NEC	T49.8X1	T49.8X2	T49.8X3	T49.8X4	T49.8X5	T49.8X6
test antigen	T50.8X1	T50.8X2	T50.8X3	T50.8X4	T50.8X5	T50.8X6
Sleep-eze	T45.0X1	T45.0X2	T45.0X3	T45.0X4	T45.0X5	T45.0X6
Sleeping draught, pill	T42.71	T42.72	T42.73	T42.74	T42.75	T42.76
Smallpox vaccine	T50.B11	T50.B12	T50.B13	T50.B14	T50.B15	T50.B16
Smelter fumes NEC	T56.91	T56.92	T56.93	T56.94	—	—
Smog	T59.1X1	T59.1X2	T59.1X3	T59.1X4	—	—
Smoke NEC	T59.811	T59.812	T59.813	T59.814	—	—
Smooth muscle relaxant	T44.3X1	T44.3X2	T44.3X3	T44.3X4	T44.3X5	T44.3X6
Snail killer NEC	T60.8X1	T60.8X2	T60.8X3	T60.8X4	—	—
Snake venom or bite	T63.001	T63.002	T63.003	T63.004	—	—
hemocoagulase	T45.7X1	T45.7X2	T45.7X3	T45.7X4	T45.7X5	T45.7X6
Snuff	T65.211	T65.212	T65.213	T65.214	—	—
Soap (powder) (product)	T55.0X1	T55.0X2	T55.0X3	T55.0X4	—	—
enema	T47.4X1	T47.4X2	T47.4X3	T47.4X4	T47.4X5	T47.4X6
medicinal, soft	T49.2X1	T49.2X2	T49.2X3	T49.2X4	T49.2X5	T49.2X6
superfatted	T49.2X1	T49.2X2	T49.2X3	T49.2X4	T49.2X5	T49.2X6
Sobrerol	T48.4X1	T48.4X2	T48.4X3	T48.4X4	T48.4X5	T48.4X6

◄ New   ◀ Revised   ~~deleted~~ Deleted

Substance	Poisoning, Accidental (Unintentional)	Poisoning, Intentional Self-Harm	Poisoning, Assault	Poisoning, Undetermined	Adverse Effect	Underdosing
Soda (caustic)	T54.3X1	T54.3X2	T54.3X3	T54.3X4	—	—
bicarb	T47.1X1	T47.1X2	T47.1X3	T47.1X4	T47.1X5	T47.1X6
chlorinated — *see Sodium, hypochlorite*						
Sodium						
acetosulfone	T37.1X1	T37.1X2	T37.1X3	T37.1X4	T37.1X5	T37.1X6
acetrizoate	T50.8X1	T50.8X2	T50.8X3	T50.8X4	T50.8X5	T50.8X6
acid phosphate	T50.3X1	T50.3X2	T50.3X3	T50.3X4	T50.3X5	T50.3X6
alginate	T47.8X1	T47.8X2	T47.8X3	T47.8X4	T47.8X5	T47.8X6
amidotrizoate	T50.8X1	T50.8X2	T50.8X3	T50.8X4	T50.8X5	T50.8X6
aminopterin	T45.1X1	T45.1X2	T45.1X3	T45.1X4	T45.1X5	T45.1X6
amylosulfate	T47.8X1	T47.8X2	T47.8X3	T47.8X4	T47.8X5	T47.8X6
amytal	T42.3X1	T42.3X2	T42.3X3	T42.3X4	T42.3X5	T42.3X6
antimony gluconate	T37.3X1	T37.3X2	T37.3X3	T37.3X4	T37.3X5	T37.3X6
arsenate	T57.0X1	T57.0X2	T57.0X3	T57.0X4	—	—
aurothiomalate	T39.4X1	T39.4X2	T39.4X3	T39.4X4	T39.4X5	T39.4X6
aurothiosulfate	T39.4X1	T39.4X2	T39.4X3	T39.4X4	T39.4X5	T39.4X6
barbiturate	T42.3X1	T42.3X2	T42.3X3	T42.3X4	T42.3X5	T42.3X6
basic phosphate	T47.4X1	T47.4X2	T47.4X3	T47.4X4	T47.4X5	T47.4X6
bicarbonate	T47.1X1	T47.1X2	T47.1X3	T47.1X4	T47.1X5	T47.1X6
bichromate	T57.8X1	T57.8X2	T57.8X3	T57.8X4	—	—
biphosphate	T50.3X1	T50.3X2	T50.3X3	T50.3X4	T50.3X5	T50.3X6
bisulfate	T65.891	T65.892	T65.893	T65.894	—	—
borate						
cleanser	T57.8X1	T57.8X2	T57.8X3	T57.8X4	—	—
eye	T49.5X1	T49.5X2	T49.5X3	T49.5X4	T49.5X5	T49.5X6
therapeutic	T49.8X1	T49.8X2	T49.8X3	T49.8X4	T49.8X5	T49.8X6
bromide	T42.6X1	T42.6X2	T42.6X3	T42.6X4	T42.6X5	T42.6X6
cacodylate (nonmedicinal) NEC	T50.8X1	T50.8X2	T50.8X3	T50.8X4	T50.8X5	T50.8X6
anti-infective	T37.8X1	T37.8X2	T37.8X3	T37.8X4	T37.8X5	T37.8X6
herbicide	T60.3X1	T60.3X2	T60.3X3	T60.3X4	—	—
calcium edetate	T45.8X1	T45.8X2	T45.8X3	T45.8X4	T45.8X5	T45.8X6
carbonate NEC	T54.3X1	T54.3X2	T54.3X3	T54.3X4	—	—
chlorate NEC	T65.891	T65.892	T65.893	T65.894	—	—
herbicide	T54.91	T54.92	T54.93	T54.94	—	—
chloride	T50.3X1	T50.3X2	T50.3X3	T50.3X4	T50.3X5	T50.3X6
with glucose	T50.3X1	T50.3X2	T50.3X3	T50.3X4	T50.3X5	T50.3X6
chromate	T65.891	T65.892	T65.893	T65.894	—	—
citrate	T50.991	T50.992	T50.993	T50.994	T50.995	T50.996
cromoglicate	T48.6X1	T48.6X2	T48.6X3	T48.6X4	T48.6X5	T48.6X6
cyanide	T65.0X1	T65.0X2	T65.0X3	T65.0X4	—	—
cyclamate	T50.3X1	T50.3X2	T50.3X3	T50.3X4	T50.3X5	T50.3X6

Substance	Poisoning, Accidental (Unintentional)	Poisoning, Intentional Self-Harm	Poisoning, Assault	Poisoning, Undetermined	Adverse Effect	Underdosing
Sodium *(Continued)*						
dehydrocholate	T45.8X1	T45.8X2	T45.8X3	T45.8X4	T45.8X5	T45.8X6
diatrizoate	T50.8X1	T50.8X2	T50.8X3	T50.8X4	T50.8X5	T50.8X6
dibunate	T48.4X1	T48.4X2	T48.4X3	T48.4X4	T48.4X5	T48.4X6
dioctyl sulfosuccinate	T47.4X1	T47.4X2	T47.4X3	T47.4X4	T47.4X5	T47.4X6
dipantoyl ferrate	T45.8X1	T45.8X2	T45.8X3	T45.8X4	T45.8X5	T45.8X6
edetate	T45.8X1	T45.8X2	T45.8X3	T45.8X4	T45.8X5	T45.8X6
ethacrynate	T50.1X1	T50.1X2	T50.1X3	T50.1X4	T50.1X5	T50.1X6
feredetate	T45.8X1	T45.8X2	T45.8X3	T45.8X4	T45.8X5	T45.8X6
Fluoride — *see Fluoride*						
fluoroacetate (dust) (pesticide)	T60.4X1	T60.4X2	T60.4X3	T60.4X4	—	—
free salt	T50.3X1	T50.3X2	T50.3X3	T50.3X4	T50.3X5	T50.3X6
fusidate	T36.8X1	T36.8X2	T36.8X3	T36.8X4	T36.8X5	T36.8X6
glucaldrate	T47.1X1	T47.1X2	T47.1X3	T47.1X4	T47.1X5	T47.1X6
glucosulfone	T37.1X1	T37.1X2	T37.1X3	T37.1X4	T37.1X5	T37.1X6
glutamate	T45.8X1	T45.8X2	T45.8X3	T45.8X4	T45.8X5	T45.8X6
hydrogen carbonate	T50.3X1	T50.3X2	T50.3X3	T50.3X4	T50.3X5	T50.3X6
hydroxide	T54.3X1	T54.3X2	T54.3X3	T54.3X4	—	—
hypochlorite (bleach) NEC	T54.3X1	T54.3X2	T54.3X3	T54.3X4	—	—
disinfectant	T54.3X1	T54.3X2	T54.3X3	T54.3X4	—	—
medicinal (anti-infective) (external)	T49.0X1	T49.0X2	T49.0X3	T49.0X4	T49.0X5	T49.0X6
vapor	T54.3X1	T54.3X2	T54.3X3	T54.3X4	—	—
hyposulfite	T49.0X1	T49.0X2	T49.0X3	T49.0X4	T49.0X5	T49.0X6
indigotin disulfonate	T50.8X1	T50.8X2	T50.8X3	T50.8X4	T50.8X5	T50.8X6
iodide	T50.991	T50.992	T50.993	T50.994	T50.995	T50.996
I-131	T50.8X1	T50.8X2	T50.8X3	T50.8X4	T50.8X5	T50.8X6
therapeutic	T38.2X1	T38.2X2	T38.2X3	T38.2X4	T38.2X5	T38.2X6
iodohippurate (131I)	T50.8X1	T50.8X2	T50.8X3	T50.8X4	T50.8X5	T50.8X6
iopodate	T50.8X1	T50.8X2	T50.8X3	T50.8X4	T50.8X5	T50.8X6
iothalamate	T50.8X1	T50.8X2	T50.8X3	T50.8X4	T50.8X5	T50.8X6
iron edetate	T45.4X1	T45.4X2	T45.4X3	T45.4X4	T45.4X5	T45.4X6
lactate (compound solution)	T45.8X1	T45.8X2	T45.8X3	T45.8X4	T45.8X5	T45.8X6
lauryl (sulfate)	T49.2X1	T49.2X2	T49.2X3	T49.2X4	T49.2X5	T49.2X6
(L)-triiodothyronine	T38.1X1	T38.1X2	T38.1X3	T38.1X4	T38.1X5	T38.1X6
magnesium citrate	T50.991	T50.992	T50.993	T50.994	T50.995	T50.996
mersalate	T50.2X1	T50.2X2	T50.2X3	T50.2X4	T50.2X5	T50.2X6
metasilicate	T65.891	T65.892	T65.893	T65.894	—	—
metrizoate	T50.8X1	T50.8X2	T50.8X3	T50.8X4	T50.8X5	T50.8X6
monofluoroacetate (pesticide)	T60.1X1	T60.1X2	T60.1X3	T60.1X4	—	—
morrhuate	T46.8X1	T46.8X2	T46.8X3	T46.8X4	T46.8X5	T46.8X6
nafcillin	T36.0X1	T36.0X2	T36.0X3	T36.0X4	T36.0X5	T36.0X6

◀ New ◀ Revised ~~deleted~~ Deleted

Substance	External Cause (T-Code)					
	Poisoning, Accidental (Unintentional)	Poisoning, Intentional Self-Harm	Poisoning, Assault	Poisoning, Undetermined	Adverse Effect	Underdosing
Sodium *(Continued)*						
nitrate (oxidizing agent)	T65.891	T65.892	T65.893	T65.894	—	—
nitrite	T50.6X1	T50.6X2	T50.6X3	T50.6X4	T50.6X5	T50.6X6
nitroferricyanide	T46.5X1	T46.5X2	T46.5X3	T46.5X4	T46.5X5	T46.5X6
nitroprusside	T46.5X1	T46.5X2	T46.5X3	T46.5X4	T46.5X5	T46.5X6
oxalate	T65.891	T65.892	T65.893	T65.894		
oxide/peroxide	T65.891	T65.892	T65.893	T65.894	—	—
oxybate	T41.291	T41.292	T41.293	T41.294	T41.295	T41.296
para-aminohippurate	T50.8X1	T50.8X2	T50.8X3	T50.8X4	T50.8X5	T50.8X6
perborate (nonmedicinal) NEC	T65.891	T65.892	T65.893	T65.894	—	—
medicinal	T49.0X1	T49.0X2	T49.0X3	T49.0X4	T49.0X5	T49.0X6
soap	T55.0X1	T55.0X2	T55.0X3	T55.0X4	—	—
percarbonate — *see Sodium, perborate*						
pertechnetate Tc99m	T50.8X1	T50.8X2	T50.8X3	T50.8X4	T50.8X5	T50.8X6
phosphate						
cellulose	T45.8X1	T45.8X2	T45.8X3	T45.8X4	T45.8X5	T45.8X6
dibasic	T47.2X1	T47.2X2	T47.2X3	T47.2X4	T47.2X5	T47.2X6
monobasic	T47.2X1	T47.2X2	T47.2X3	T47.2X4	T47.2X5	T47.2X6
phytate	T50.6X1	T50.6X2	T50.6X3	T50.6X4	T50.6X5	T50.6X6
picosulfate	T47.2X1	T47.2X2	T47.2X3	T47.2X4	T47.2X5	T47.2X6
polyhydroxyaluminium monocarbonate	T47.1X1	T47.1X2	T47.1X3	T47.1X4	T47.1X5	T47.1X6
polystyrene sulfonate	T50.3X1	T50.3X2	T50.3X3	T50.3X4	T50.3X5	T50.3X6
propionate	T49.0X1	T49.0X2	T49.0X3	T49.0X4	T49.0X5	T49.0X6
propyl hydroxybenzoate	T50.991	T50.992	T50.993	T50.994	T50.995	T50.996
psylliate	T46.8X1	T46.8X2	T46.8X3	T46.8X4	T46.8X5	T46.8X6
removing resins	T50.3X1	T50.3X2	T50.3X3	T50.3X4	T50.3X5	T50.3X6
salicylate	T39.091	T39.092	T39.093	T39.094	T39.095	T39.096
salt NEC	T50.3X1	T50.3X2	T50.3X3	T50.3X4	T50.3X5	T50.3X6
selenate	T60.2X1	T60.2X2	T60.2X3	T60.2X4	—	—
stibogluconate	T37.3X1	T37.3X2	T37.3X3	T37.3X4	T37.3X5	T37.3X6
sulfate	T47.4X1	T47.4X2	T47.4X3	T47.4X4	T47.4X5	T47.4X6
sulfoxone	T37.1X1	T37.1X2	T37.1X3	T37.1X4	T37.1X5	T37.1X6
tetradecyl sulfate	T46.8X1	T46.8X2	T46.8X3	T46.8X4	T46.8X5	T46.8X6
thiopental	T41.1X1	T41.1X2	T41.1X3	T41.1X4	T41.1X5	T41.1X6
thiosalicylate	T39.091	T39.092	T39.093	T39.094	T39.095	T39.096
thiosulfate	T50.6X1	T50.6X2	T50.6X3	T50.6X4	T50.6X5	T50.6X6
tolbutamide	T38.3X1	T38.3X2	T38.3X3	T38.3X4	T38.3X5	T38.3X6
l-triiodothyronine	T38.1X1	T38.1X2	T38.1X3	T38.1X4	T38.1X5	T38.1X6
tyropanoate	T50.8X1	T50.8X2	T50.8X3	T50.8X4	T50.8X5	T50.8X6
valproate	T42.6X1	T42.6X2	T42.6X3	T42.6X4	T42.6X5	T42.6X6
versenate	T50.6X1	T50.6X2	T50.6X3	T50.6X4	T50.6X5	T50.6X6

Substance	External Cause (T-Code)					
	Poisoning, Accidental (Unintentional)	Poisoning, Intentional Self-Harm	Poisoning, Assault	Poisoning, Undetermined	Adverse Effect	Underdosing
Sodium-free salt	T50.901	T50.902	T50.903	T50.904	T50.905	T50.906
Sodium-removing resin	T50.3X1	T50.3X2	T50.3X3	T50.3X4	T50.3X5	T50.3X6
Soft soap	T55.0X1	T55.0X2	T55.0X3	T55.0X4	—	—
Solanine	T62.2X1	T62.2X2	T62.2X3	T62.2X4	—	—
berries	T62.1X1	T62.1X2	T62.1X3	T62.1X4	—	—
Solanum dulcamara	T62.2X1	T62.2X2	T62.2X3	T62.2X4	—	—
berries	T62.1X1	T62.1X2	T62.1X3	T62.1X4	—	—
Solapsone	T37.1X1	T37.1X2	T37.1X3	T37.1X4	T37.1X5	T37.1X6
Solar lotion	T49.3X1	T49.3X2	T49.3X3	T49.3X4	T49.3X5	T49.3X6
Solasulfone	T37.1X1	T37.1X2	T37.1X3	T37.1X4	T37.1X5	T37.1X6
Soldering fluid	T65.891	T65.892	T65.893	T65.894		
Solid substance	T65.91	T65.92	T65.93	T65.94		
specified NEC	T65.891	T65.892	T65.893	T65.894	—	—
Solvent, industrial NEC	T52.91	T52.92	T52.93	T52.94		
naphtha	T52.0X1	T52.0X2	T52.0X3	T52.0X4	—	—
petroleum	T52.0X1	T52.0X2	T52.0X3	T52.0X4	—	—
specified NEC	T52.8X1	T52.8X2	T52.8X3	T52.8X4	—	—
Soma	T42.8X1	T42.8X2	T42.8X3	T42.8X4	T42.8X5	T42.8X6
Somatorelin	T38.891	T38.892	T38.893	T38.894	T38.895	T38.896
Somatostatin	T38.991	T38.992	T38.993	T38.994	T38.995	T38.996
Somatotropin	T38.811	T38.812	T38.813	T38.814	T38.815	T38.816
Somatrem	T38.811	T38.812	T38.813	T38.814	T38.815	T38.816
Somatropin	T38.811	T38.812	T38.813	T38.814	T38.815	T38.816
Sominex	T45.0X1	T45.0X2	T45.0X3	T45.0X4	T45.0X5	T45.0X6
Somnos	T42.6X1	T42.6X2	T42.6X3	T42.6X4	T42.6X5	T42.6X6
Somonal	T42.3X1	T42.3X2	T42.3X3	T42.3X4	T42.3X5	T42.3X6
Soneryl	T42.3X1	T42.3X2	T42.3X3	T42.3X4	T42.3X5	T42.3X6
Soothing syrup	T50.901	T50.902	T50.903	T50.904	T50.905	T50.906
Sopor	T42.6X1	T42.6X2	T42.6X3	T42.6X4	T42.6X5	T42.6X6
Soporific	T42.71	T42.72	T42.73	T42.74	T42.75	T42.76
Soporific drug	T42.71	T42.72	T42.73	T42.74	T42.75	T42.76
specified type NEC	T42.6X1	T42.6X2	T42.6X3	T42.6X4	T42.6X5	T42.6X6
Sorbide nitrate	T46.3X1	T46.3X2	T46.3X3	T46.3X4	T46.3X5	T46.3X6
Sorbitol	T47.4X1	T47.4X2	T47.4X3	T47.4X4	T47.4X5	T47.4X6
Sotalol	T44.7X1	T44.7X2	T44.7X3	T44.7X4	T44.7X5	T44.7X6
Sotradecol	T46.8X1	T46.8X2	T46.8X3	T46.8X4	T46.8X5	T46.8X6
Soysterol	T46.6X1	T46.6X2	T46.6X3	T46.6X4	T46.6X5	T46.6X6
Spacoline	T44.3X1	T44.3X2	T44.3X3	T44.3X4	T44.3X5	T44.3X6
Spanish fly	T49.8X1	T49.8X2	T49.8X3	T49.8X4	T49.8X5	T49.8X6
Sparine	T43.3X1	T43.3X2	T43.3X3	T43.3X4	T43.3X5	T43.3X6
Sparteine	T48.0X1	T48.0X2	T48.0X3	T48.0X4	T48.0X5	T48.0X6

◀ New ◀ Revised ~~deleted~~ Deleted

Substance	Poisoning, Accidental (Unintentional)	Poisoning, Intentional Self-Harm	Poisoning, Assault	Poisoning, Undetermined	Adverse Effect	Underdosing
Spasmolytic						
anticholinergics	T44.3X1	T44.3X2	T44.3X3	T44.3X4	T44.3X5	T44.3X6
autonomic	T44.3X1	T44.3X2	T44.3X3	T44.3X4	T44.3X5	T44.3X6
bronchial NEC	T48.6X1	T48.6X2	T48.6X3	T48.6X4	T48.6X5	T48.6X6
quaternary ammonium	T44.3X1	T44.3X2	T44.3X3	T44.3X4	T44.3X5	T44.3X6
skeletal muscle NEC	T48.1X1	T48.1X2	T48.1X3	T48.1X4	T48.1X5	T48.1X6
Spectinomycin	T36.5X1	T36.5X2	T36.5X3	T36.5X4	T36.5X5	T36.5X6
Speed	T43.621	T43.622	T43.623	T43.624	T43.625	T43.626
Spermicide	T49.8X1	T49.8X2	T49.8X3	T49.8X4	T49.8X5	T49.8X6
Spider (bite) (venom)	T63.391	T63.392	T63.393	T63.394	—	—
antivenin	T50.Z11	T50.Z12	T50.Z13	T50.Z14	T50.Z15	T50.Z16
Spigelia (root)	T37.4X1	T37.4X2	T37.4X3	T37.4X4	T37.4X5	T37.4X6
Spindle inactivator	T50.4X1	T50.4X2	T50.4X3	T50.4X4	T50.4X5	T50.4X6
Spiperone	T43.4X1	T43.4X2	T43.4X3	T43.4X4	T43.4X5	T43.4X6
Spiramycin	T36.3X1	T36.3X2	T36.3X3	T36.3X4	T36.3X5	T36.3X6
Spirapril	T46.4X1	T46.4X2	T46.4X3	T46.4X4	T46.4X5	T46.4X6
Spirilene	T43.591	T43.592	T43.593	T43.594	T43.595	T43.596
Spirit(s) (neutral) NEC	T51.0X1	T51.0X2	T51.0X3	T51.0X4	—	—
beverage	T51.0X1	T51.0X2	T51.0X3	T51.0X4	—	—
industrial	T51.0X1	T51.0X2	T51.0X3	T51.0X4	—	—
mineral	T52.0X1	T52.0X2	T52.0X3	T52.0X4	—	—
of salt — see Hydrochloric acid						
surgical	T51.0X1	T51.0X2	T51.0X3	T51.0X4	—	—
Spironolactone	T50.0X1	T50.0X2	T50.0X3	T50.0X4	T50.0X5	T50.0X6
Spiroperidol	T43.4X1	T43.4X2	T43.4X3	T43.4X4	T43.4X5	T43.4X6
Sponge, absorbable (gelatin)	T45.7X1	T45.7X2	T45.7X3	T45.7X4	T45.7X5	T45.7X6
Sporostacin	T49.0X1	T49.0X2	T49.0X3	T49.0X4	T49.0X5	T49.0X6
Spray (aerosol)	T65.91	T65.92	T65.93	T65.94	—	—
cosmetic	T65.891	T65.892	T65.893	T65.894	—	—
medicinal NEC	T50.901	T50.902	T50.903	T50.904	T50.905	T50.906
pesticides — see Pesticides						
specified content — see specific substance						
Spurge flax	T62.2X1	T62.2X2	T62.2X3	T62.2X4	—	—
Spurges	T62.2X1	T62.2X2	T62.2X3	T62.2X4	—	—
Sputum viscosity-lowering drug	T48.4X1	T48.4X2	T48.4X3	T48.4X4	T48.4X5	T48.4X6
Squill	T46.0X1	T46.0X2	T46.0X3	T46.0X4	T46.0X5	T46.0X6
rat poison	T60.4X1	T60.4X2	T60.4X3	T60.4X4	—	—
Squirting cucumber (cathartic)	T47.2X1	T47.2X2	T47.2X3	T47.2X4	T47.2X5	T47.2X6
Stains	T65.6X1	T65.6X2	T65.6X3	T65.6X4	—	—
Stannous fluoride	T49.7X1	T49.7X2	T49.7X3	T49.7X4	T49.7X5	T49.7X6
Stanolone	T38.7X1	T38.7X2	T38.7X3	T38.7X4	T38.7X5	T38.7X6

Substance	Poisoning, Accidental (Unintentional)	Poisoning, Intentional Self-Harm	Poisoning, Assault	Poisoning, Undetermined	Adverse Effect	Underdosing
Stanozolol	T38.7X1	T38.7X2	T38.7X3	T38.7X4	T38.7X5	T38.7X6
Staphisagria or stavesacre (pediculicide)	T49.0X1	T49.0X2	T49.0X3	T49.0X4	T49.0X5	T49.0X6
Starch	T50.901	T50.902	T50.903	T50.904	T50.905	T50.906
Stelazine	T43.3X1	T43.3X2	T43.3X3	T43.3X4	T43.3X5	T43.3X6
Stemetil	T43.3X1	T43.3X2	T43.3X3	T43.3X4	T43.3X5	T43.3X6
Stepronin	T48.4X1	T48.4X2	T48.4X3	T48.4X4	T48.4X5	T48.4X6
Sterculia	T47.4X1	T47.4X2	T47.4X3	T47.4X4	T47.4X5	T47.4X6
Sternutator gas	T59.891	T59.892	T59.893	T59.894	—	—
Steroid	T38.0X1	T38.0X2	T38.0X3	T38.0X4	T38.0X5	T38.0X6
anabolic	T38.7X1	T38.7X2	T38.7X3	T38.7X4	T38.7X5	T38.7X6
androgenic	T38.7X1	T38.7X2	T38.7X3	T38.7X4	T38.7X5	T38.7X6
antineoplastic, hormone	T38.7X1	T38.7X2	T38.7X3	T38.7X4	T38.7X5	T38.7X6
estrogen	T38.5X1	T38.5X2	T38.5X3	T38.5X4	T38.5X5	T38.5X6
ENT agent	T49.6X1	T49.6X2	T49.6X3	T49.6X4	T49.6X5	T49.6X6
ophthalmic preparation	T49.5X1	T49.5X2	T49.5X3	T49.5X4	T49.5X5	T49.5X6
topical NEC	T49.0X1	T49.0X2	T49.0X3	T49.0X4	T49.0X5	T49.0X6
Stibine	T56.891	T56.892	T56.893	T56.894	—	—
Stibogluconate	T37.3X1	T37.3X2	T37.3X3	T37.3X4	T37.3X5	T37.3X6
Stibophen	T37.4X1	T37.4X2	T37.4X3	T37.4X4	T37.4X5	T37.4X6
Stilbamidine (isetionate)	T37.3X1	T37.3X2	T37.3X3	T37.3X4	T37.3X5	T37.3X6
Stilbestrol	T38.5X1	T38.5X2	T38.5X3	T38.5X4	T38.5X5	T38.5X6
Stilboestrol	T38.5X1	T38.5X2	T38.5X3	T38.5X4	T38.5X5	T38.5X6
Stimulant						
central nervous system — see also Psychostimulant	T43.601	T43.602	T43.603	T43.604	T43.605	T43.606
analeptics	T50.7X1	T50.7X2	T50.7X3	T50.7X4	T50.7X5	T50.7X6
opiate antagonist	T50.7X1	T50.7X2	T50.7X3	T50.7X4	T50.7X5	T50.7X6
psychotherapeutic NEC — see also Psychotherapeutic drug	T43.601	T43.602	T43.603	T43.604	T43.605	T43.606
specified NEC	T43.691	T43.692	T43.693	T43.694	T43.695	T43.696
respiratory	T48.901	T48.902	T48.903	T48.904	T48.905	T48.906
Stone-dissolving drug	T50.901	T50.902	T50.903	T50.904	T50.905	T50.906
Storage battery (cells) (acid)	T54.2X1	T54.2X2	T54.2X3	T54.2X4	—	—
Stovaine	T41.3X1	T41.3X2	T41.3X3	T41.3X4	T41.3X5	T41.3X6
infiltration (subcutaneous)	T41.3X1	T41.3X2	T41.3X3	T41.3X4	T41.3X5	T41.3X6
nerve block (peripheral) (plexus)	T41.3X1	T41.3X2	T41.3X3	T41.3X4	T41.3X5	T41.3X6
spinal	T41.3X1	T41.3X2	T41.3X3	T41.3X4	T41.3X5	T41.3X6
topical (surface)	T41.3X1	T41.3X2	T41.3X3	T41.3X4	T41.3X5	T41.3X6
Stovarsal	T37.8X1	T37.8X2	T37.8X3	T37.8X4	T37.8X5	T37.8X6
Stove gas — see Gas, stove	T57.91	T57.92	T57.93	T57.94	—	—

◀ New ◀ Revised ~~deleted~~ Deleted

Substance	Poisoning, Accidental (Unintentional)	Poisoning, Intentional Self-Harm	Poisoning, Assault	Poisoning, Undetermined	Adverse Effect	Underdosing
	External Cause (T-Code)					
Stoxil	T49.5X1	T49.5X2	T49.5X3	T49.5X4	T49.5X5	T49.5X6
Stramonium	T48.6X1	T48.6X2	T48.6X3	T48.6X4	T48.6X5	T48.6X6
natural state	T62.2X1	T62.2X2	T62.2X3	T62.2X4	—	—
Streptodornase	T45.3X1	T45.3X2	T45.3X3	T45.3X4	T45.3X5	T45.3X6
Streptoduocin	T36.5X1	T36.5X2	T36.5X3	T36.5X4	T36.5X5	T36.5X6
Streptokinase	T45.611	T45.612	T45.613	T45.614	T45.615	T45.616
Streptomycin (derivative)	T36.5X1	T36.5X2	T36.5X3	T36.5X4	T36.5X5	T36.5X6
Streptonivicin	T36.5X1	T36.5X2	T36.5X3	T36.5X4	T36.5X5	T36.5X6
Streptovarycin	T36.5X1	T36.5X2	T36.5X3	T36.5X4	T36.5X5	T36.5X6
Streptozocin	T45.1X1	T45.1X2	T45.1X3	T45.1X4	T45.1X5	T45.1X6
Streptozotocin	T45.1X1	T45.1X2	T45.1X3	T45.1X4	T45.1X5	T45.1X6
Stripper (paint) (solvent)	T52.8X1	T52.8X2	T52.8X3	T52.8X4	—	—
Strobane	T60.1X1	T60.1X2	T60.1X3	T60.1X4	—	—
Strofantina	T46.0X1	T46.0X2	T46.0X3	T46.0X4	T46.0X5	T46.0X6
Strophanthin (g) (k)	T46.0X1	T46.0X2	T46.0X3	T46.0X4	T46.0X5	T46.0X6
Strophanthus	T46.0X1	T46.0X2	T46.0X3	T46.0X4	T46.0X5	T46.0X6
Strophantin	T46.0X1	T46.0X2	T46.0X3	T46.0X4	T46.0X5	T46.0X6
Strophantin-g	T46.0X1	T46.0X2	T46.0X3	T46.0X4	T46.0X5	T46.0X6
Strychnine (nonmedicinal) (pesticide) (salts)	T65.1X1	T65.1X2	T65.1X3	T65.1X4	—	—
medicinal	T48.291	T48.292	T48.293	T48.294	T48.295	T48.296
Strychnos (ignatii) — see Strychnine						
Styramate	T42.8X1	T42.8X2	T42.8X3	T42.8X4	T42.8X5	T42.8X6
Styrene	T65.891	T65.892	T65.893	T65.894	—	—
Succinimide, antiepileptic or anticonvulsant	T42.2X1	T42.2X2	T42.2X3	T42.2X4	T42.2X5	T42.2X6
mercuric — see Mercury						
Succinylcholine	T48.1X1	T48.1X2	T48.1X3	T48.1X4	T48.1X5	T48.1X6
Succinylsulfathiazole	T37.0X1	T37.0X2	T37.0X3	T37.0X4	T37.0X5	T37.0X6
Sucralfate	T47.1X1	T47.1X2	T47.1X3	T47.1X4	T47.1X5	T47.1X6
Sucrose	T50.3X1	T50.3X2	T50.3X3	T50.3X4	T50.3X5	T50.3X6
Sufentanil	T40.411	T40.412	T40.413	T40.414	T40.415	T40.416
Sulbactam	T36.0X1	T36.0X2	T36.0X3	T36.0X4	T36.0X5	T36.0X6
Sulbenicillin	T36.0X1	T36.0X2	T36.0X3	T36.0X4	T36.0X5	T36.0X6
Sulbentine	T49.0X1	T49.0X2	T49.0X3	T49.0X4	T49.0X5	T49.0X6
Sulfacetamide	T49.0X1	T49.0X2	T49.0X3	T49.0X4	T49.0X5	T49.0X6
ophthalmic preparation	T49.5X1	T49.5X2	T49.5X3	T49.5X4	T49.5X5	T49.5X6
Sulfachlorpyridazine	T37.0X1	T37.0X2	T37.0X3	T37.0X4	T37.0X5	T37.0X6
Sulfacitine	T37.0X1	T37.0X2	T37.0X3	T37.0X4	T37.0X5	T37.0X6
Sulfadiasulfone sodium	T37.0X1	T37.0X2	T37.0X3	T37.0X4	T37.0X5	T37.0X6
Sulfadiazine	T37.0X1	T37.0X2	T37.0X3	T37.0X4	T37.0X5	T37.0X6
silver (topical)	T49.0X1	T49.0X2	T49.0X3	T49.0X4	T49.0X5	T49.0X6

Substance	Poisoning, Accidental (Unintentional)	Poisoning, Intentional Self-Harm	Poisoning, Assault	Poisoning, Undetermined	Adverse Effect	Underdosing
	External Cause (T-Code)					
Sulfadimethoxine	T37.0X1	T37.0X2	T37.0X3	T37.0X4	T37.0X5	T37.0X6
Sulfadimidine	T37.0X1	T37.0X2	T37.0X3	T37.0X4	T37.0X5	T37.0X6
Sulfadoxine	T37.0X1	T37.0X2	T37.0X3	T37.0X4	T37.0X5	T37.0X6
with pyrimethamine	T37.2X1	T37.2X2	T37.2X3	T37.2X4	T37.2X5	T37.2X6
Sulfaethidole	T37.0X1	T37.0X2	T37.0X3	T37.0X4	T37.0X5	T37.0X6
Sulfafurazole	T37.0X1	T37.0X2	T37.0X3	T37.0X4	T37.0X5	T37.0X6
Sulfaguanidine	T37.0X1	T37.0X2	T37.0X3	T37.0X4	T37.0X5	T37.0X6
Sulfalene	T37.0X1	T37.0X2	T37.0X3	T37.0X4	T37.0X5	T37.0X6
Sulfaloxate	T37.0X1	T37.0X2	T37.0X3	T37.0X4	T37.0X5	T37.0X6
Sulfaloxic acid	T37.0X1	T37.0X2	T37.0X3	T37.0X4	T37.0X5	T37.0X6
Sulfamazone	T39.2X1	T39.2X2	T39.2X3	T39.2X4	T39.2X5	T39.2X6
Sulfamerazine	T37.0X1	T37.0X2	T37.0X3	T37.0X4	T37.0X5	T37.0X6
Sulfameter	T37.0X1	T37.0X2	T37.0X3	T37.0X4	T37.0X5	T37.0X6
Sulfamethazine	T37.0X1	T37.0X2	T37.0X3	T37.0X4	T37.0X5	T37.0X6
Sulfamethizole	T37.0X1	T37.0X2	T37.0X3	T37.0X4	T37.0X5	T37.0X6
Sulfamethoxazole	T37.0X1	T37.0X2	T37.0X3	T37.0X4	T37.0X5	T37.0X6
with trimethoprim	T36.8X1	T36.8X2	T36.8X3	T36.8X4	T36.8X5	T36.8X6
Sulfamethoxydiazine	T37.0X1	T37.0X2	T37.0X3	T37.0X4	T37.0X5	T37.0X6
Sulfamethoxypyridazine	T37.0X1	T37.0X2	T37.0X3	T37.0X4	T37.0X5	T37.0X6
Sulfamethylthiazole	T37.0X1	T37.0X2	T37.0X3	T37.0X4	T37.0X5	T37.0X6
Sulfametoxydiazine	T37.0X1	T37.0X2	T37.0X3	T37.0X4	T37.0X5	T37.0X6
Sulfamidopyrine	T39.2X1	T39.2X2	T39.2X3	T39.2X4	T39.2X5	T39.2X6
Sulfamonomethoxine	T37.0X1	T37.0X2	T37.0X3	T37.0X4	T37.0X5	T37.0X6
Sulfamoxole	T37.0X1	T37.0X2	T37.0X3	T37.0X4	T37.0X5	T37.0X6
Sulfamylon	T49.0X1	T49.0X2	T49.0X3	T49.0X4	T49.0X5	T49.0X6
Sulfan blue (diagnostic dye)	T50.8X1	T50.8X2	T50.8X3	T50.8X4	T50.8X5	T50.8X6
Sulfanilamide	T37.0X1	T37.0X2	T37.0X3	T37.0X4	T37.0X5	T37.0X6
Sulfanilylguanidine	T37.0X1	T37.0X2	T37.0X3	T37.0X4	T37.0X5	T37.0X6
Sulfaperin	T37.0X1	T37.0X2	T37.0X3	T37.0X4	T37.0X5	T37.0X6
Sulfaphenazole	T37.0X1	T37.0X2	T37.0X3	T37.0X4	T37.0X5	T37.0X6
Sulfaphenylthiazole	T37.0X1	T37.0X2	T37.0X3	T37.0X4	T37.0X5	T37.0X6
Sulfaproxyline	T37.0X1	T37.0X2	T37.0X3	T37.0X4	T37.0X5	T37.0X6
Sulfapyridine	T37.0X1	T37.0X2	T37.0X3	T37.0X4	T37.0X5	T37.0X6
Sulfapyrimidine	T37.0X1	T37.0X2	T37.0X3	T37.0X4	T37.0X5	T37.0X6
Sulfarsphenamine	T37.8X1	T37.8X2	T37.8X3	T37.8X4	T37.8X5	T37.8X6
Sulfasalazine	T37.0X1	T37.0X2	T37.0X3	T37.0X4	T37.0X5	T37.0X6
Sulfasuxidine	T37.0X1	T37.0X2	T37.0X3	T37.0X4	T37.0X5	T37.0X6
Sulfasymazine	T37.0X1	T37.0X2	T37.0X3	T37.0X4	T37.0X5	T37.0X6
Sulfated amylopectin	T47.8X1	T47.8X2	T47.8X3	T47.8X4	T47.8X5	T47.8X6
Sulfathiazole	T37.0X1	T37.0X2	T37.0X3	T37.0X4	T37.0X5	T37.0X6
Sulfatostearate	T49.2X1	T49.2X2	T49.2X3	T49.2X4	T49.2X5	T49.2X6
Sulfinpyrazone	T50.4X1	T50.4X2	T50.4X3	T50.4X4	T50.4X5	T50.4X6

◀ New   ◀ Revised   deleted Deleted

TABLE OF DRUGS AND CHEMICALS

Substance	Poisoning, Accidental (Unintentional)	Poisoning, Intentional Self-Harm	Poisoning, Assault	Poisoning, Undetermined	Adverse Effect	Underdosing
Sulfiram	T49.0X1	T49.0X2	T49.0X3	T49.0X4	T49.0X5	T49.0X6
Sulfisomidine	T37.0X1	T37.0X2	T37.0X3	T37.0X4	T37.0X5	T37.0X6
Sulfisoxazole	T37.0X1	T37.0X2	T37.0X3	T37.0X4	T37.0X5	T37.0X6
ophthalmic preparation	T49.5X1	T49.5X2	T49.5X3	T49.5X4	T49.5X5	T49.5X6
Sulfobromophthalein (sodium)	T50.8X1	T50.8X2	T50.8X3	T50.8X4	T50.8X5	T50.8X6
Sulfobromphthalein	T50.8X1	T50.8X2	T50.8X3	T50.8X4	T50.8X5	T50.8X6
Sulfogaiacol	T48.4X1	T48.4X2	T48.4X3	T48.4X4	T48.4X5	T48.4X6
Sulfomyxin	T36.8X1	T36.8X2	T36.8X3	T36.8X4	T36.8X5	T36.8X6
Sulfonal	T42.6X1	T42.6X2	T42.6X3	T42.6X4	T42.6X5	T42.6X6
Sulfonamide NEC	T37.0X1	T37.0X2	T37.0X3	T37.0X4	T37.0X5	T37.0X6
eye	T49.5X1	T49.5X2	T49.5X3	T49.5X4	T49.5X5	T49.5X6
Sulfonazide	T37.1X1	T37.1X2	T37.1X3	T37.1X4	T37.1X5	T37.1X6
Sulfones	T37.1X1	T37.1X2	T37.1X3	T37.1X4	T37.1X5	T37.1X6
Sulfonethylmethane	T42.6X1	T42.6X2	T42.6X3	T42.6X4	T42.6X5	T42.6X6
Sulfonmethane	T42.6X1	T42.6X2	T42.6X3	T42.6X4	T42.6X5	T42.6X6
Sulfonphthal, sulfonphthol	T50.8X1	T50.8X2	T50.8X3	T50.8X4	T50.8X5	T50.8X6
Sulfonylurea derivatives, oral	T38.3X1	T38.3X2	T38.3X3	T38.3X4	T38.3X5	T38.3X6
Sulforidazine	T43.3X1	T43.3X2	T43.3X3	T43.3X4	T43.3X5	T43.3X6
Sulfoxone	T37.1X1	T37.1X2	T37.1X3	T37.1X4	T37.1X5	T37.1X6
Sulfur, sulfurated, sulfuric, sulfurous, sulfuryl (compounds NEC) (medicinal)	T49.4X1	T49.4X2	T49.4X3	T49.4X4	T49.4X5	T49.4X6
acid	T54.2X1	T54.2X2	T54.2X3	T54.2X4	—	—
dioxide (gas)	T59.1X1	T59.1X2	T59.1X3	T59.1X4	—	—
ether — see Ether(s)						
hydrogen	T59.6X1	T59.6X2	T59.6X3	T59.6X4	—	—
medicinal (keratolytic) (ointment) NEC	T49.4X1	T49.4X2	T49.4X3	T49.4X4	T49.4X5	T49.4X6
ointment	T49.0X1	T49.0X2	T49.0X3	T49.0X4	T49.0X5	T49.0X6
pesticide (vapor)	T60.91	T60.92	T60.93	T60.94	—	—
vapor NEC	T59.891	T59.892	T59.893	T59.894	—	—
Sulfuric acid	T54.2X1	T54.2X2	T54.2X3	T54.2X4	—	—
Sulglicotide	T47.1X1	T47.1X2	T47.1X3	T47.1X4	T47.1X5	T47.1X6
Sulindac	T39.391	T39.392	T39.393	T39.394	T39.395	T39.396
Sulisatin	T47.2X1	T47.2X2	T47.2X3	T47.2X4	T47.2X5	T47.2X6
Sulisobenzone	T49.3X1	T49.3X2	T49.3X3	T49.3X4	T49.3X5	T49.3X6
Sulkowitch's reagent	T50.8X1	T50.8X2	T50.8X3	T50.8X4	T50.8X5	T50.8X6
Sulmetozine	T44.3X1	T44.3X2	T44.3X3	T44.3X4	T44.3X5	T44.3X6
Suloctidil	T46.7X1	T46.7X2	T46.7X3	T46.7X4	T46.7X5	T46.7X6
Sulph — see also Sulf-						
Sulphadiazine	T37.0X1	T37.0X2	T37.0X3	T37.0X4	T37.0X5	T37.0X6
Sulphadimethoxine	T37.0X1	T37.0X2	T37.0X3	T37.0X4	T37.0X5	T37.0X6

Substance	Poisoning, Accidental (Unintentional)	Poisoning, Intentional Self-Harm	Poisoning, Assault	Poisoning, Undetermined	Adverse Effect	Underdosing
Sulphadimidine	T37.0X1	T37.0X2	T37.0X3	T37.0X4	T37.0X5	T37.0X6
Sulphadione	T37.1X1	T37.1X2	T37.1X3	T37.1X4	T37.1X5	T37.1X6
Sulphafurazole	T37.0X1	T37.0X2	T37.0X3	T37.0X4	T37.0X5	T37.0X6
Sulphamethizole	T37.0X1	T37.0X2	T37.0X3	T37.0X4	T37.0X5	T37.0X6
Sulphamethoxazole	T37.0X1	T37.0X2	T37.0X3	T37.0X4	T37.0X5	T37.0X6
Sulphan blue	T50.8X1	T50.8X2	T50.8X3	T50.8X4	T50.8X5	T50.8X6
Sulphaphenazole	T37.0X1	T37.0X2	T37.0X3	T37.0X4	T37.0X5	T37.0X6
Sulphapyridine	T37.0X1	T37.0X2	T37.0X3	T37.0X4	T37.0X5	T37.0X6
Sulphasalazine	T37.0X1	T37.0X2	T37.0X3	T37.0X4	T37.0X5	T37.0X6
Sulphinpyrazone	T50.4X1	T50.4X2	T50.4X3	T50.4X4	T50.4X5	T50.4X6
Sulpiride	T43.591	T43.592	T43.593	T43.594	T43.595	T43.596
Sulprostone	T48.0X1	T48.0X2	T48.0X3	T48.0X4	T48.0X5	T48.0X6
Sulpyrine	T39.2X1	T39.2X2	T39.2X3	T39.2X4	T39.2X5	T39.2X6
Sultamicillin	T36.0X1	T36.0X2	T36.0X3	T36.0X4	T36.0X5	T36.0X6
Sulthiame	T42.6X1	T42.6X2	T42.6X3	T42.6X4	T42.6X5	T42.6X6
Sultiame	T42.6X1	T42.6X2	T42.6X3	T42.6X4	T42.6X5	T42.6X6
Sultopride	T43.591	T43.592	T43.593	T43.594	T43.595	T43.596
Sumatriptan	T39.8X1	T39.8X2	T39.8X3	T39.8X4	T39.8X5	T39.8X6
Sunflower seed oil	T46.6X1	T46.6X2	T46.6X3	T46.6X4	T46.6X5	T46.6X6
Superinone	T48.4X1	T48.4X2	T48.4X3	T48.4X4	T48.4X5	T48.4X6
Suprofen	T39.311	T39.312	T39.313	T39.314	T39.315	T39.316
Suramin (sodium)	T37.4X1	T37.4X2	T37.4X3	T37.4X4	T37.4X5	T37.4X6
Surfacaine	T41.3X1	T41.3X2	T41.3X3	T41.3X4	T41.3X5	T41.3X6
Surital	T41.1X1	T41.1X2	T41.1X3	T41.1X4	T41.1X5	T41.1X6
Sutilains	T45.3X1	T45.3X2	T45.3X3	T45.3X4	T45.3X5	T45.3X6
Suxamethonium (chloride)	T48.1X1	T48.1X2	T48.1X3	T48.1X4	T48.1X5	T48.1X6
Suxethonium (chloride)	T48.1X1	T48.1X2	T48.1X3	T48.1X4	T48.1X5	T48.1X6
Suxibuzone	T39.2X1	T39.2X2	T39.2X3	T39.2X4	T39.2X5	T39.2X6
Sweet oil (birch)	T49.3X1	T49.3X2	T49.3X3	T49.3X4	T49.3X5	T49.3X6
Sweet niter spirit	T46.3X1	T46.3X2	T46.3X3	T46.3X4	T46.3X5	T46.3X6
Sweetener	T50.901	T50.902	T50.903	T50.904	T50.905	T50.906
Sym-dichloroethyl ether	T53.6X1	T53.6X2	T53.6X3	T53.6X4	—	—
Sympatholytic NEC	T44.8X1	T44.8X2	T44.8X3	T44.8X4	T44.8X5	T44.8X6
haloalkylamine	T44.8X1	T44.8X2	T44.8X3	T44.8X4	T44.8X5	T44.8X6
Sympathomimetic NEC	T44.901	T44.902	T44.903	T44.904	T44.905	T44.906
anti-common-cold	T48.5X1	T48.5X2	T48.5X3	T48.5X4	T48.5X5	T48.5X6
bronchodilator	T48.6X1	T48.6X2	T48.6X3	T48.6X4	T48.6X5	T48.6X6
specified NEC	T44.991	T44.992	T44.993	T44.994	T44.995	T44.996
Synagis	T50.B91	T50.B92	T50.B93	T50.B94	T50.B95	T50.B96
Synalar	T49.0X1	T49.0X2	T49.0X3	T49.0X4	T49.0X5	T49.0X6
Synthetic cannabinoids	T40.721	T40.722	T40.723	T40.724	T40.725	T40.726
Synthroid	T38.1X1	T38.1X2	T38.1X3	T38.1X4	T38.1X5	T38.1X6

◀ New   ◀ Revised   ~~deleted~~ Deleted

Substance	Poisoning, Accidental (Unintentional)	Poisoning, Intentional Self-Harm	Poisoning, Assault	Poisoning, Undetermined	Adverse Effect	Underdosing
Syntocinon	T48.0X1	T48.0X2	T48.0X3	T48.0X4	T48.0X5	T48.0X6
Syrosingopine	T46.5X1	T46.5X2	T46.5X3	T46.5X4	T46.5X5	T46.5X6
Systemic drug	T45.91	T45.92	T45.93	T45.94	T45.95	T45.96
specified NEC	T45.8X1	T45.8X2	T45.8X3	T45.8X4	T45.8X5	T45.8X6
2,4,5-T	T60.3X1	T60.3X2	T60.3X3	T60.3X4	—	—

T

Substance	Poisoning, Accidental (Unintentional)	Poisoning, Intentional Self-Harm	Poisoning, Assault	Poisoning, Undetermined	Adverse Effect	Underdosing
Tablets — see also specified substance	T50.901	T50.902	T50.903	T50.904	T50.905	T50.906
Tace	T38.5X1	T38.5X2	T38.5X3	T38.5X4	T38.5X5	T38.5X6
Tacrine	T44.0X1	T44.0X2	T44.0X3	T44.0X4	T44.0X5	T44.0X6
Tadalafil	T46.7X1	T46.7X2	T46.7X3	T46.7X4	T46.7X5	T46.7X6
Talampicillin	T36.0X1	T36.0X2	T36.0X3	T36.0X4	T36.0X5	T36.0X6
Talbutal	T42.3X1	T42.3X2	T42.3X3	T42.3X4	T42.3X5	T42.3X6
Talc powder	T49.3X1	T49.3X2	T49.3X3	T49.3X4	T49.3X5	T49.3X6
Talcum	T49.3X1	T49.3X2	T49.3X3	T49.3X4	T49.3X5	T49.3X6
Taleranol	T38.6X1	T38.6X2	T38.6X3	T38.6X4	T38.6X5	T38.6X6
Tamoxifen	T38.6X1	T38.6X2	T38.6X3	T38.6X4	T38.6X5	T38.6X6
Tamsulosin	T44.6X1	T44.6X2	T44.6X3	T44.6X4	T44.6X5	T44.6X6
Tandearil, tanderil	T39.2X1	T39.2X2	T39.2X3	T39.2X4	T39.2X5	T39.2X6
Tannic acid	T49.2X1	T49.2X2	T49.2X3	T49.2X4	T49.2X5	T49.2X6
medicinal (astringent)	T49.2X1	T49.2X2	T49.2X3	T49.2X4	T49.2X5	T49.2X6
Tannin — see Tannic acid						
Tansy	T62.2X1	T62.2X2	T62.2X3	T62.2X4	—	—
TAO	T36.3X1	T36.3X2	T36.3X3	T36.3X4	T36.3X5	T36.3X6
Tapazole	T38.2X1	T38.2X2	T38.2X3	T38.2X4	T38.2X5	T38.2X6
Tar NEC	T52.0X1	T52.0X2	T52.0X3	T52.0X4		
camphor	T60.1X1	T60.1X2	T60.1X3	T60.1X4		
distillate	T49.1X1	T49.1X2	T49.1X3	T49.1X4	T49.1X5	T49.1X6
fumes	T59.891	T59.892	T59.893	T59.894	—	—
medicinal	T49.1X1	T49.1X2	T49.1X3	T49.1X4	T49.1X5	T49.1X6
ointment	T49.1X1	T49.1X2	T49.1X3	T49.1X4	T49.1X5	T49.1X6
Taractan	T43.591	T43.592	T43.593	T43.594	T43.595	T43.596
Tarantula (venomous)	T63.321	T63.322	T63.323	T63.324		
Tartar emetic	T37.8X1	T37.8X2	T37.8X3	T37.8X4	T37.8X5	T37.8X6
Tartaric acid	T65.891	T65.892	T65.893	T65.894	—	—
Tartrated antimony (anti-infective)	T37.8X1	T37.8X2	T37.8X3	T37.8X4	T37.8X5	T37.8X6
Tartrate, laxative	T47.4X1	T47.4X2	T47.4X3	T47.4X4	T47.4X5	T47.4X6
Tauromustine	T45.1X1	T45.1X2	T45.1X3	T45.1X4	T45.1X5	T45.1X6
TCA — see Trichloroacetic acid						
TCDD	T53.7X1	T53.7X2	T53.7X3	T53.7X4	—	—
TDI (vapor)	T65.0X1	T65.0X2	T65.0X3	T65.0X4	—	—

Substance	Poisoning, Accidental (Unintentional)	Poisoning, Intentional Self-Harm	Poisoning, Assault	Poisoning, Undetermined	Adverse Effect	Underdosing
Tear						
gas	T59.3X1	T59.3X2	T59.3X3	T59.3X4	—	—
solution	T49.5X1	T49.5X2	T49.5X3	T49.5X4	T49.5X5	T49.5X6
Teclothiazide	T50.2X1	T50.2X2	T50.2X3	T50.2X4	T50.2X5	T50.2X6
Teclozan	T37.3X1	T37.3X2	T37.3X3	T37.3X4	T37.3X5	T37.3X6
Tegafur	T45.1X1	T45.1X2	T45.1X3	T45.1X4	T45.1X5	T45.1X6
Tegretol	T42.1X1	T42.1X2	T42.1X3	T42.1X4	T42.1X5	T42.1X6
Teicoplanin	T36.8X1	T36.8X2	T36.8X3	T36.8X4	T36.8X5	T36.8X6
Telepaque	T50.8X1	T50.8X2	T50.8X3	T50.8X4	T50.8X5	T50.8X6
Tellurium	T56.891	T56.892	T56.893	T56.894	—	—
fumes	T56.891	T56.892	T56.893	T56.894	—	—
TEM	T45.1X1	T45.1X2	T45.1X3	T45.1X4	T45.1X5	T45.1X6
Temazepam	T42.4X1	T42.4X2	T42.4X3	T42.4X4	T42.4X5	T42.4X6
Temocillin	T36.0X1	T36.0X2	T36.0X3	T36.0X4	T36.0X5	T36.0X6
Tenamfetamine	T43.621	T43.622	T43.623	T43.624	T43.625	T43.626
Teniposide	T45.1X1	T45.1X2	T45.1X3	T45.1X4	T45.1X5	T45.1X6
Tenitramine	T46.3X1	T46.3X2	T46.3X3	T46.3X4	T46.3X5	T46.3X6
Tenoglicin	T48.4X1	T48.4X2	T48.4X3	T48.4X4	T48.4X5	T48.4X6
Tenonitrozole	T37.3X1	T37.3X2	T37.3X3	T37.3X4	T37.3X5	T37.3X6
Tenoxicam	T39.391	T39.392	T39.393	T39.394	T39.395	T39.396
TEPA	T45.1X1	T45.1X2	T45.1X3	T45.1X4	T45.1X5	T45.1X6
TEPP	T60.0X1	T60.0X2	T60.0X3	T60.0X4	—	—
Teprotide	T46.5X1	T46.5X2	T46.5X3	T46.5X4	T46.5X5	T46.5X6
Terazosin	T44.6X1	T44.6X2	T44.6X3	T44.6X4	T44.6X5	T44.6X6
Terbufos	T60.0X1	T60.0X2	T60.0X3	T60.0X4	—	—
Terbutaline	T48.6X1	T48.6X2	T48.6X3	T48.6X4	T48.6X5	T48.6X6
Terconazole	T49.0X1	T49.0X2	T49.0X3	T49.0X4	T49.0X5	T49.0X6
Terfenadine	T45.0X1	T45.0X2	T45.0X3	T45.0X4	T45.0X5	T45.0X6
Teriparatide (acetate)	T50.991	T50.992	T50.993	T50.994	T50.995	T50.996
Terizidone	T37.1X1	T37.1X2	T37.1X3	T37.1X4	T37.1X5	T37.1X6
Terlipressin	T38.891	T38.892	T38.893	T38.894	T38.895	T38.896
Terodiline	T46.3X1	T46.3X2	T46.3X3	T46.3X4	T46.3X5	T46.3X6
Teroxalene	T37.4X1	T37.4X2	T37.4X3	T37.4X4	T37.4X5	T37.4X6
Terpin(cis) hydrate	T48.4X1	T48.4X2	T48.4X3	T48.4X4	T48.4X5	T48.4X6
Terramycin	T36.4X1	T36.4X2	T36.4X3	T36.4X4	T36.4X5	T36.4X6
Tertatolol	T44.7X1	T44.7X2	T44.7X3	T44.7X4	T44.7X5	T44.7X6
Tessalon	T48.3X1	T48.3X2	T48.3X3	T48.3X4	T48.3X5	T48.3X6
Testolactone	T38.7X1	T38.7X2	T38.7X3	T38.7X4	T38.7X5	T38.7X6
Testosterone	T38.7X1	T38.7X2	T38.7X3	T38.7X4	T38.7X5	T38.7X6
Tetanus toxoid or vaccine	T50.A91	T50.A92	T50.A93	T50.A94	T50.A95	T50.A96
antitoxin	T50.Z11	T50.Z12	T50.Z13	T50.Z14	T50.Z15	T50.Z16
immune globulin (human)	T50.Z11	T50.Z12	T50.Z13	T50.Z14	T50.Z15	T50.Z16

Substance	Poisoning, Accidental (Unintentional)	Poisoning, Intentional Self-Harm	Poisoning, Assault	Poisoning, Undetermined	Adverse Effect	Underdosing
Tetanus toxoid or vaccine *(Continued)*						
toxoid	T50.A91	T50.A92	T50.A93	T50.A94	T50.A95	T50.A96
with diphtheria toxoid	T50.A21	T50.A22	T50.A23	T50.A24	T50.A25	T50.A26
with pertussis	T50.A11	T50.A12	T50.A13	T50.A14	T50.A15	T50.A16
Tetrabenazine	T43.591	T43.592	T43.593	T43.594	T43.595	T43.596
Tetracaine	T41.3X1	T41.3X2	T41.3X3	T41.3X4	T41.3X5	T41.3X6
nerve block (peripheral) (plexus)	T41.3X1	T41.3X2	T41.3X3	T41.3X4	T41.3X5	T41.3X6
regional	T41.3X1	T41.3X2	T41.3X3	T41.3X4	T41.3X5	T41.3X6
spinal	T41.3X1	T41.3X2	T41.3X3	T41.3X4	T41.3X5	T41.3X6
Tetrachlorethylene — *see* Tetrachloroethylene						
Tetrachlormethiazide	T50.2X1	T50.2X2	T50.2X3	T50.2X4	T50.2X5	T50.2X6
2,3,7,8-Tetrachlorodibenzo-p-dioxin	T53.7X1	T53.7X2	T53.7X3	T53.7X4	—	—
Tetrachloroethane	T53.6X1	T53.6X2	T53.6X3	T53.6X4	—	—
vapor	T53.6X1	T53.6X2	T53.6X3	T53.6X4	—	—
paint or varnish	T53.6X1	T53.6X2	T53.6X3	T53.6X4	—	—
Tetrachloroethylene (liquid)	T53.3X1	T53.3X2	T53.3X3	T53.3X4	—	—
medicinal	T37.4X1	T37.4X2	T37.4X3	T37.4X4	T37.4X5	T37.4X6
vapor	T53.3X1	T53.3X2	T53.3X3	T53.3X4	—	—
Tetrachloromethane — *see* Carbon tetrachloride						
Tetracosactide	T38.811	T38.812	T38.813	T38.814	T38.815	T38.816
Tetracosactrin	T38.811	T38.812	T38.813	T38.814	T38.815	T38.816
Tetracycline	T36.4X1	T36.4X2	T36.4X3	T36.4X4	T36.4X5	T36.4X6
ophthalmic preparation	T49.5X1	T49.5X2	T49.5X3	T49.5X4	T49.5X5	T49.5X6
topical NEC	T49.0X1	T49.0X2	T49.0X3	T49.0X4	T49.0X5	T49.0X6
Tetradifon	T60.8X1	T60.8X2	T60.8X3	T60.8X4	—	—
Tetradotoxin	T61.771	T61.772	T61.773	T61.774	—	—
Tetraethyl						
lead	T56.0X1	T56.0X2	T56.0X3	T56.0X4	—	—
pyrophosphate	T60.0X1	T60.0X2	T60.0X3	T60.0X4	—	—
Tetraethylammonium chloride	T44.2X1	T44.2X2	T44.2X3	T44.2X4	T44.2X5	T44.2X6
Tetraethylthiuram disulfide	T50.6X1	T50.6X2	T50.6X3	T50.6X4	T50.6X5	T50.6X6
Tetrahydroaminoacridine	T44.0X1	T44.0X2	T44.0X3	T44.0X4	T44.0X5	T44.0X6
Tetrahydrocannabinol	T40.711	T40.712	T40.713	T40.714	T40.715	T40.716
Tetrahydrofuran	T52.8X1	T52.8X2	T52.8X3	T52.8X4	—	—
Tetrahydronaphthalene	T52.8X1	T52.8X2	T52.8X3	T52.8X4	—	—
Tetrahydrozoline	T49.5X1	T49.5X2	T49.5X3	T49.5X4	T49.5X5	T49.5X6
Tetralin	T52.8X1	T52.8X2	T52.8X3	T52.8X4	—	—
Tetramethrin	T60.2X1	T60.2X2	T60.2X3	T60.2X4	—	—

Substance	Poisoning, Accidental (Unintentional)	Poisoning, Intentional Self-Harm	Poisoning, Assault	Poisoning, Undetermined	Adverse Effect	Underdosing
Tetramethylthiuram (disulfide) NEC	T60.3X1	T60.3X2	T60.3X3	T60.3X4	—	—
medicinal	T49.0X1	T49.0X2	T49.0X3	T49.0X4	T49.0X5	T49.0X6
Tetramisole	T37.4X1	T37.4X2	T37.4X3	T37.4X4	T37.4X5	T37.4X6
Tetranicotinoyl fructose	T46.7X1	T46.7X2	T46.7X3	T46.7X4	T46.7X5	T46.7X6
Tetronal	T42.6X1	T42.6X2	T42.6X3	T42.6X4	T42.6X5	T42.6X6
Tetrazepam	T42.4X1	T42.4X2	T42.4X3	T42.4X4	T42.4X5	T42.4X6
Tetryl	T65.3X1	T65.3X2	T65.3X3	T65.3X4	—	—
Tetrylammonium chloride	T44.2X1	T44.2X2	T44.2X3	T44.2X4	T44.2X5	T44.2X6
Tetryzoline	T49.5X1	T49.5X2	T49.5X3	T49.5X4	T49.5X5	T49.5X6
Thalidomide	T45.1X1	T45.1X2	T45.1X3	T45.1X4	T45.1X5	T45.1X6
Thallium (compounds) (dust) NEC	T56.811	T56.812	T56.813	T56.814	—	—
pesticide	T60.4X1	T60.4X2	T60.4X3	T60.4X4	—	—
THC	T40.711	T40.712	T40.713	T40.714	T40.715	T40.716
Thebacon	T48.3X1	T48.3X2	T48.3X3	T48.3X4	T48.3X5	T48.3X6
Thebaine	T40.2X1	T40.2X2	T40.2X3	T40.2X4	T40.2X5	T40.2X6
Thenoic acid	T49.6X1	T49.6X2	T49.6X3	T49.6X4	T49.6X5	T49.6X6
Thenyldiamine	T45.0X1	T45.0X2	T45.0X3	T45.0X4	T45.0X5	T45.0X6
Theobromine (calcium salicylate)	T48.6X1	T48.6X2	T48.6X3	T48.6X4	T48.6X5	T48.6X6
sodium salicylate	T48.6X1	T48.6X2	T48.6X3	T48.6X4	T48.6X5	T48.6X6
Theophyllamine	T48.6X1	T48.6X2	T48.6X3	T48.6X4	T48.6X5	T48.6X6
Theophylline	T48.6X1	T48.6X2	T48.6X3	T48.6X4	T48.6X5	T48.6X6
aminobenzoic acid	T48.6X1	T48.6X2	T48.6X3	T48.6X4	T48.6X5	T48.6X6
ethylenediamine	T48.6X1	T48.6X2	T48.6X3	T48.6X4	T48.6X5	T48.6X6
piperazine p-amino-benzoate	T48.6X1	T48.6X2	T48.6X3	T48.6X4	T48.6X5	T48.6X6
Thiabendazole	T37.4X1	T37.4X2	T37.4X3	T37.4X4	T37.4X5	T37.4X6
Thialbarbital	T41.1X1	T41.1X2	T41.1X3	T41.1X4	T41.1X5	T41.1X6
Thiamazole	T38.2X1	T38.2X2	T38.2X3	T38.2X4	T38.2X5	T38.2X6
Thiambutosine	T37.1X1	T37.1X2	T37.1X3	T37.1X4	T37.1X5	T37.1X6
Thiamine	T45.2X1	T45.2X2	T45.2X3	T45.2X4	T45.2X5	T45.2X6
Thiamphenicol	T36.2X1	T36.2X2	T36.2X3	T36.2X4	T36.2X5	T36.2X6
Thiamylal	T41.1X1	T41.1X2	T41.1X3	T41.1X4	T41.1X5	T41.1X6
sodium	T41.1X1	T41.1X2	T41.1X3	T41.1X4	T41.1X5	T41.1X6
Thiazesim	T43.291	T43.292	T43.293	T43.294	T43.295	T43.296
Thiazides (diuretics)	T50.2X1	T50.2X2	T50.2X3	T50.2X4	T50.2X5	T50.2X6
Thiazinamium metilsulfate	T43.3X1	T43.3X2	T43.3X3	T43.3X4	T43.3X5	T43.3X6
Thiethylperazine	T43.3X1	T43.3X2	T43.3X3	T43.3X4	T43.3X5	T43.3X6
Thimerosal	T49.0X1	T49.0X2	T49.0X3	T49.0X4	T49.0X5	T49.0X6
ophthalmic preparation	T49.5X1	T49.5X2	T49.5X3	T49.5X4	T49.5X5	T49.5X6
Thioacetazone	T37.1X1	T37.1X2	T37.1X3	T37.1X4	T37.1X5	T37.1X6
with isoniazid	T37.1X1	T37.1X2	T37.1X3	T37.1X4	T37.1X5	T37.1X6
Thiobarbital sodium	T41.1X1	T41.1X2	T41.1X3	T41.1X4	T41.1X5	T41.1X6

◀ New   ◀◀ Revised   ~~deleted~~ Deleted

Substance	Poisoning, Accidental (Unintentional)	Poisoning, Intentional Self-Harm	Poisoning, Assault	Poisoning, Undetermined	Adverse Effect	Underdosing
Thiobarbiturate anesthetic	T41.1X1	T41.1X2	T41.1X3	T41.1X4	T41.1X5	T41.1X6
Thiobismol	T37.8X1	T37.8X2	T37.8X3	T37.8X4	T37.8X5	T37.8X6
Thiobutabarbital sodium	T41.1X1	T41.1X2	T41.1X3	T41.1X4	T41.1X5	T41.1X6
Thiocarbamate (insecticide)	T60.0X1	T60.0X2	T60.0X3	T60.0X4	—	—
Thiocarbamide	T38.2X1	T38.2X2	T38.2X3	T38.2X4	T38.2X5	T38.2X6
Thiocarbarsone	T37.8X1	T37.8X2	T37.8X3	T37.8X4	T37.8X5	T37.8X6
Thiocarlide	T37.1X1	T37.1X2	T37.1X3	T37.1X4	T37.1X5	T37.1X6
Thioctamide	T50.991	T50.992	T50.993	T50.994	T50.995	T50.996
Thioctic acid	T50.991	T50.992	T50.993	T50.994	T50.995	T50.996
Thiofos	T60.0X1	T60.0X2	T60.0X3	T60.0X4	—	—
Thioglycolate	T49.4X1	T49.4X2	T49.4X3	T49.4X4	T49.4X5	T49.4X6
Thioglycolic acid	T65.891	T65.892	T65.893	T65.894	—	—
Thioguanine	T45.1X1	T45.1X2	T45.1X3	T45.1X4	T45.1X5	T45.1X6
Thiomercaptomerin	T50.2X1	T50.2X2	T50.2X3	T50.2X4	T50.2X5	T50.2X6
Thiomerin	T50.2X1	T50.2X2	T50.2X3	T50.2X4	T50.2X5	T50.2X6
Thiomersal	T49.0X1	T49.0X2	T49.0X3	T49.0X4	T49.0X5	T49.0X6
Thionazin	T60.0X1	T60.0X2	T60.0X3	T60.0X4	—	—
Thiopental (sodium)	T41.1X1	T41.1X2	T41.1X3	T41.1X4	T41.1X5	T41.1X6
Thiopentone (sodium)	T41.1X1	T41.1X2	T41.1X3	T41.1X4	T41.1X5	T41.1X6
Thiopropazate	T43.3X1	T43.3X2	T43.3X3	T43.3X4	T43.3X5	T43.3X6
Thioproperazine	T43.3X1	T43.3X2	T43.3X3	T43.3X4	T43.3X5	T43.3X6
Thioridazine	T43.3X1	T43.3X2	T43.3X3	T43.3X4	T43.3X5	T43.3X6
Thiosinamine	T49.3X1	T49.3X2	T49.3X3	T49.3X4	T49.3X5	T49.3X6
Thiotepa	T45.1X1	T45.1X2	T45.1X3	T45.1X4	T45.1X5	T45.1X6
Thiothixene	T43.4X1	T43.4X2	T43.4X3	T43.4X4	T43.4X5	T43.4X6
Thiouracil (benzyl) (methyl) (propyl)	T38.2X1	T38.2X2	T38.2X3	T38.2X4	T38.2X5	T38.2X6
Thiourea	T38.2X1	T38.2X2	T38.2X3	T38.2X4	T38.2X5	T38.2X6
Thiphenamil	T44.3X1	T44.3X2	T44.3X3	T44.3X4	T44.3X5	T44.3X6
Thiram	T60.3X1	T60.3X2	T60.3X3	T60.3X4	—	—
medicinal	T49.2X1	T49.2X2	T49.2X3	T49.2X4	T49.2X5	T49.2X6
Thonzylamine (systemic)	T45.0X1	T45.0X2	T45.0X3	T45.0X4	T45.0X5	T45.0X6
mucosal decongestant	T48.5X1	T48.5X2	T48.5X3	T48.5X4	T48.5X5	T48.5X6
Thorazine	T43.3X1	T43.3X2	T43.3X3	T43.3X4	T43.3X5	T43.3X6
Thorium dioxide suspension	T50.8X1	T50.8X2	T50.8X3	T50.8X4	T50.8X5	T50.8X6
Thornapple	T62.2X1	T62.2X2	T62.2X3	T62.2X4	—	—
Throat drug NEC	T49.6X1	T49.6X2	T49.6X3	T49.6X4	T49.6X5	T49.6X6
Thrombin	T45.7X1	T45.7X2	T45.7X3	T45.7X4	T45.7X5	T45.7X6
Thrombolysin	T45.611	T45.612	T45.613	T45.614	T45.615	T45.616
Thromboplastin	T45.7X1	T45.7X2	T45.7X3	T45.7X4	T45.7X5	T45.7X6
Thurfyl nicotinate	T46.7X1	T46.7X2	T46.7X3	T46.7X4	T46.7X5	T46.7X6
Thymol	T49.0X1	T49.0X2	T49.0X3	T49.0X4	T49.0X5	T49.0X6

Substance	Poisoning, Accidental (Unintentional)	Poisoning, Intentional Self-Harm	Poisoning, Assault	Poisoning, Undetermined	Adverse Effect	Underdosing
Thymopentin	T37.5X1	T37.5X2	T37.5X3	T37.5X4	T37.5X5	T37.5X6
Thymoxamine	T46.7X1	T46.7X2	T46.7X3	T46.7X4	T46.7X5	T46.7X6
Thymus extract	T38.891	T38.892	T38.893	T38.894	T38.895	T38.896
Thyreotrophic hormone	T38.811	T38.812	T38.813	T38.814	T38.815	T38.816
Thyroglobulin	T38.1X1	T38.1X2	T38.1X3	T38.1X4	T38.1X5	T38.1X6
Thyroid (hormone)	T38.1X1	T38.1X2	T38.1X3	T38.1X4	T38.1X5	T38.1X6
Thyrolar	T38.1X1	T38.1X2	T38.1X3	T38.1X4	T38.1X5	T38.1X6
Thyrotrophin	T38.811	T38.812	T38.813	T38.814	T38.815	T38.816
Thyrotropic hormone	T38.811	T38.812	T38.813	T38.814	T38.815	T38.816
Thyroxine	T38.1X1	T38.1X2	T38.1X3	T38.1X4	T38.1X5	T38.1X6
Tiabendazole	T37.4X1	T37.4X2	T37.4X3	T37.4X4	T37.4X5	T37.4X6
Tiamizide	T50.2X1	T50.2X2	T50.2X3	T50.2X4	T50.2X5	T50.2X6
Tianeptine	T43.291	T43.292	T43.293	T43.294	T43.295	T43.296
Tiapamil	T46.1X1	T46.1X2	T46.1X3	T46.1X4	T46.1X5	T46.1X6
Tiapride	T43.591	T43.592	T43.593	T43.594	T43.595	T43.596
Tiaprofenic acid	T39.311	T39.312	T39.313	T39.314	T39.315	T39.316
Tiaramide	T39.8X1	T39.8X2	T39.8X3	T39.8X4	T39.8X5	T39.8X6
Ticarcillin	T36.0X1	T36.0X2	T36.0X3	T36.0X4	T36.0X5	T36.0X6
Ticlatone	T49.0X1	T49.0X2	T49.0X3	T49.0X4	T49.0X5	T49.0X6
Ticlopidine	T45.521	T45.522	T45.523	T45.524	T45.525	T45.526
Ticrynafen	T50.1X1	T50.1X2	T50.1X3	T50.1X4	T50.1X5	T50.1X6
Tidiacic	T50.991	T50.992	T50.993	T50.994	T50.995	T50.996
Tiemonium	T44.3X1	T44.3X2	T44.3X3	T44.3X4	T44.3X5	T44.3X6
iodide	T44.3X1	T44.3X2	T44.3X3	T44.3X4	T44.3X5	T44.3X6
Tienilic acid	T50.1X1	T50.1X2	T50.1X3	T50.1X4	T50.1X5	T50.1X6
Tifenamil	T44.3X1	T44.3X2	T44.3X3	T44.3X4	T44.3X5	T44.3X6
Tigan	T45.0X1	T45.0X2	T45.0X3	T45.0X4	T45.0X5	T45.0X6
Tigloidine	T44.3X1	T44.3X2	T44.3X3	T44.3X4	T44.3X5	T44.3X6
Tilactase	T47.5X1	T47.5X2	T47.5X3	T47.5X4	T47.5X5	T47.5X6
Tiletamine	T41.291	T41.292	T41.293	T41.294	T41.295	T41.296
Tilidine	T40.441	T40.442	T40.443	T40.444	—	—
Timepidium bromide	T44.3X1	T44.3X2	T44.3X3	T44.3X4	T44.3X5	T44.3X6
Timiperone	T43.4X1	T43.4X2	T43.4X3	T43.4X4	T43.4X5	T43.4X6
Timolol	T44.7X1	T44.7X2	T44.7X3	T44.7X4	T44.7X5	T44.7X6
Tin (chloride) (dust) (oxide) NEC	T56.6X1	T56.6X2	T56.6X3	T56.6X4	—	—
anti-infectives	T37.8X1	T37.8X2	T37.8X3	T37.8X4	T37.8X5	T37.8X6
Tincture, iodine — see Iodine						
Tindal	T43.3X1	T43.3X2	T43.3X3	T43.3X4	T43.3X5	T43.3X6
Tinidazole	T37.3X1	T37.3X2	T37.3X3	T37.3X4	T37.3X5	T37.3X6
Tinoridine	T39.8X1	T39.8X2	T39.8X3	T39.8X4	T39.8X5	T39.8X6
Tiocarlide	T37.1X1	T37.1X2	T37.1X3	T37.1X4	T37.1X5	T37.1X6
Tioclomarol	T45.511	T45.512	T45.513	T45.514	T45.515	T45.516

◀ New   ◀ Revised   ~~deleted~~ Deleted

TABLE OF DRUGS AND CHEMICALS

TABLE OF DRUGS AND CHEMICALS

Substance	Poisoning, Accidental (Unintentional)	Poisoning, Intentional Self-Harm	Poisoning, Assault	Poisoning, Undetermined	Adverse Effect	Underdosing
Tioconazole	T49.0X1	T49.0X2	T49.0X3	T49.0X4	T49.0X5	T49.0X6
Tioguanine	T45.1X1	T45.1X2	T45.1X3	T45.1X4	T45.1X5	T45.1X6
Tiopronin	T50.991	T50.992	T50.993	T50.994	T50.995	T50.996
Tiotixene	T43.4X1	T43.4X2	T43.4X3	T43.4X4	T43.4X5	T43.4X6
Tioxolone	T49.4X1	T49.4X2	T49.4X3	T49.4X4	T49.4X5	T49.4X6
Tipepidine	T48.3X1	T48.3X2	T48.3X3	T48.3X4	T48.3X5	T48.3X6
Tiquizium bromide	T44.3X1	T44.3X2	T44.3X3	T44.3X4	T44.3X5	T44.3X6
Tiratricol	T38.1X1	T38.1X2	T38.1X3	T38.1X4	T38.1X5	T38.1X6
Tisopurine	T50.4X1	T50.4X2	T50.4X3	T50.4X4	T50.4X5	T50.4X6
Titanium (compounds) (vapor)	T56.891	T56.892	T56.893	T56.894	—	—
dioxide	T49.3X1	T49.3X2	T49.3X3	T49.3X4	T49.3X5	T49.3X6
ointment	T49.3X1	T49.3X2	T49.3X3	T49.3X4	T49.3X5	T49.3X6
oxide	T49.3X1	T49.3X2	T49.3X3	T49.3X4	T49.3X5	T49.3X6
tetrachloride	T56.891	T56.892	T56.893	T56.894	—	—
Titanocene	T56.891	T56.892	T56.893	T56.894	—	—
Titroid	T38.1X1	T38.1X2	T38.1X3	T38.1X4	T38.1X5	T38.1X6
Tizanidine	T42.8X1	T42.8X2	T42.8X3	T42.8X4	T42.8X5	T42.8X6
TMTD	T60.3X1	T60.3X2	T60.3X3	T60.3X4		
TNT (fumes)	T65.3X1	T65.3X2	T65.3X3	T65.3X4	—	—
Toadstool	T62.0X1	T62.0X2	T62.0X3	T62.0X4		
Tobacco NEC	T65.291	T65.292	T65.293	T65.294		
cigarettes	T65.221	T65.222	T65.223	T65.224		
Indian	T62.2X1	T62.2X2	T62.2X3	T62.2X4	—	—
smoke, second-hand	T65.221	T65.222	T65.223	T65.224	—	—
Tobramycin	T36.5X1	T36.5X2	T36.5X3	T36.5X4	T36.5X5	T36.5X6
Tocainide	T46.2X1	T46.2X2	T46.2X3	T46.2X4	T46.2X5	T46.2X6
Tocoferol	T45.2X1	T45.2X2	T45.2X3	T45.2X4	T45.2X5	T45.2X6
Tocopherol	T45.2X1	T45.2X2	T45.2X3	T45.2X4	T45.2X5	T45.2X6
acetate	T45.2X1	T45.2X2	T45.2X3	T45.2X4	T45.2X5	T45.2X6
Tocosamine	T48.0X1	T48.0X2	T48.0X3	T48.0X4	T48.0X5	T48.0X6
Todralazine	T46.5X1	T46.5X2	T46.5X3	T46.5X4	T46.5X5	T46.5X6
Tofisopam	T42.4X1	T42.4X2	T42.4X3	T42.4X4	T42.4X5	T42.4X6
Tofranil	T43.011	T43.012	T43.013	T43.014	T43.015	T43.016
Toilet deodorizer	T65.891	T65.892	T65.893	T65.894	—	—
Tolamolol	T44.7X1	T44.7X2	T44.7X3	T44.7X4	T44.7X5	T44.7X6
Tolazamide	T38.3X1	T38.3X2	T38.3X3	T38.3X4	T38.3X5	T38.3X6
Tolazoline	T46.7X1	T46.7X2	T46.7X3	T46.7X4	T46.7X5	T46.7X6
Tolbutamide (sodium)	T38.3X1	T38.3X2	T38.3X3	T38.3X4	T38.3X5	T38.3X6
Tolciclate	T49.0X1	T49.0X2	T49.0X3	T49.0X4	T49.0X5	T49.0X6
Tolmetin	T39.391	T39.392	T39.393	T39.394	T39.395	T39.396
Tolnaftate	T49.0X1	T49.0X2	T49.0X3	T49.0X4	T49.0X5	T49.0X6
Tolonidine	T46.5X1	T46.5X2	T46.5X3	T46.5X4	T46.5X5	T46.5X6

Substance	Poisoning, Accidental (Unintentional)	Poisoning, Intentional Self-Harm	Poisoning, Assault	Poisoning, Undetermined	Adverse Effect	Underdosing
Toloxatone	T42.6X1	T42.6X2	T42.6X3	T42.6X4	T42.6X5	T42.6X6
Tolperisone	T44.3X1	T44.3X2	T44.3X3	T44.3X4	T44.3X5	T44.3X6
Tolserol	T42.8X1	T42.8X2	T42.8X3	T42.8X4	T42.8X5	T42.8X6
Toluene (liquid)	T52.2X1	T52.2X2	T52.2X3	T52.2X4	—	—
diisocyanate	T65.0X1	T65.0X2	T65.0X3	T65.0X4	—	—
Toluidine	T65.891	T65.892	T65.893	T65.894	—	—
vapor	T59.891	T59.892	T59.893	T59.894	—	—
Toluol (liquid)	T52.2X1	T52.2X2	T52.2X3	T52.2X4	—	—
vapor	T52.2X1	T52.2X2	T52.2X3	T52.2X4	—	—
Toluylenediamine	T65.3X1	T65.3X2	T65.3X3	T65.3X4	—	—
Tolylene-2,4-diisocyanate	T65.0X1	T65.0X2	T65.0X3	T65.0X4	—	—
Tonic NEC	T50.901	T50.902	T50.903	T50.904	T50.905	T50.906
Topical action drug NEC	T49.91	T49.92	T49.93	T49.94	T49.95	T49.96
ear, nose or throat	T49.6X1	T49.6X2	T49.6X3	T49.6X4	T49.6X5	T49.6X6
eye	T49.5X1	T49.5X2	T49.5X3	T49.5X4	T49.5X5	T49.5X6
skin	T49.91	T49.92	T49.93	T49.94	T49.95	T49.96
specified NEC	T49.8X1	T49.8X2	T49.8X3	T49.8X4	T49.8X5	T49.8X6
Toquizine	T44.3X1	T44.3X2	T44.3X3	T44.3X4	T44.3X5	T44.3X6
Toremifene	T38.6X1	T38.6X2	T38.6X3	T38.6X4	T38.6X5	T38.6X6
Tosylchloramide sodium	T49.8X1	T49.8X2	T49.8X3	T49.8X4	T49.8X5	T49.8X6
Toxaphene (dust) (spray)	T60.1X1	T60.1X2	T60.1X3	T60.1X4	—	—
Toxin, diphtheria (Schick Test)	T50.8X1	T50.8X2	T50.8X3	T50.8X4	T50.8X5	T50.8X6
Toxoid						
combined	T50.A21	T50.A22	T50.A23	T50.A24	T50.A25	T50.A26
diphtheria	T50.A91	T50.A92	T50.A93	T50.A94	T50.A95	T50.A96
tetanus	T50.A91	T50.A92	T50.A93	T50.A94	T50.A95	T50.A96
Trace element NEC	T45.8X1	T45.8X2	T45.8X3	T45.8X4	T45.8X5	T45.8X6
Tractor fuel NEC	T52.0X1	T52.0X2	T52.0X3	T52.0X4	—	—
Tragacanth	T50.991	T50.992	T50.993	T50.994	T50.995	T50.996
Tramadol	T40.421	T40.422	T40.423	T40.424	T40.425	T40.426
Tramazoline	T48.5X1	T48.5X2	T48.5X3	T48.5X4	T48.5X5	T48.5X6
Tranexamic acid	T45.621	T45.622	T45.623	T45.624	T45.625	T45.626
Tranilast	T45.0X1	T45.0X2	T45.0X3	T45.0X4	T45.0X5	T45.0X6
Tranquilizer NEC	T43.501	T43.502	T43.503	T43.504	T43.505	T43.506
with hypnotic or sedative	T42.6X1	T42.6X2	T42.6X3	T42.6X4	T42.6X5	T42.6X6
benzodiazepine NEC	T42.4X1	T42.4X2	T42.4X3	T42.4X4	T42.4X5	T42.4X6
butyrophenone NEC	T43.4X1	T43.4X2	T43.4X3	T43.4X4	T43.4X5	T43.4X6
carbamate	T43.591	T43.592	T43.593	T43.594	T43.595	T43.596
dimethylamine	T43.3X1	T43.3X2	T43.3X3	T43.3X4	T43.3X5	T43.3X6
ethylamine	T43.3X1	T43.3X2	T43.3X3	T43.3X4	T43.3X5	T43.3X6
hydroxyzine	T43.591	T43.592	T43.593	T43.594	T43.595	T43.596
major NEC	T43.501	T43.502	T43.503	T43.504	T43.505	T43.506

◀ New ◀ Revised ~~deleted~~ Deleted

Substance	Poisoning, Accidental (Unintentional)	Poisoning, Intentional Self-Harm	Poisoning, Assault	Poisoning, Undetermined	Adverse Effect	Underdosing
Tranquilizer NEC *(Continued)*						
penothiazine NEC	T43.3X1	T43.3X2	T43.3X3	T43.3X4	T43.3X5	T43.3X6
phenothiazine-based	T43.3X1	T43.3X2	T43.3X3	T43.3X4	T43.3X5	T43.3X6
piperazine NEC	T43.3X1	T43.3X2	T43.3X3	T43.3X4	T43.3X5	T43.3X6
piperidine	T43.3X1	T43.3X2	T43.3X3	T43.3X4	T43.3X5	T43.3X6
propylamine	T43.3X1	T43.3X2	T43.3X3	T43.3X4	T43.3X5	T43.3X6
specified NEC	T43.591	T43.592	T43.593	T43.594	T43.595	T43.596
thioxanthene NEC	T43.591	T43.592	T43.593	T43.594	T43.595	T43.596
Tranxene	T42.4X1	T42.4X2	T42.4X3	T42.4X4	T42.4X5	T42.4X6
Tranylcypromine	T43.1X1	T43.1X2	T43.1X3	T43.1X4	T43.1X5	T43.1X6
Trapidil	T46.3X1	T46.3X2	T46.3X3	T46.3X4	T46.3X5	T46.3X6
Trasentine	T44.3X1	T44.3X2	T44.3X3	T44.3X4	T44.3X5	T44.3X6
Travert	T50.3X1	T50.3X2	T50.3X3	T50.3X4	T50.3X5	T50.3X6
Trazodone	T43.211	T43.212	T43.213	T43.214	T43.215	T43.216
Trecator	T37.1X1	T37.1X2	T37.1X3	T37.1X4	T37.1X5	T37.1X6
Treosulfan	T45.1X1	T45.1X2	T45.1X3	T45.1X4	T45.1X5	T45.1X6
Tretamine	T45.1X1	T45.1X2	T45.1X3	T45.1X4	T45.1X5	T45.1X6
Tretinoin	T49.0X1	T49.0X2	T49.0X3	T49.0X4	T49.0X5	T49.0X6
Tretoquinol	T48.6X1	T48.6X2	T48.6X3	T48.6X4	T48.6X5	T48.6X6
Triacetin	T49.0X1	T49.0X2	T49.0X3	T49.0X4	T49.0X5	T49.0X6
Triacetoxyanthracene	T49.4X1	T49.4X2	T49.4X3	T49.4X4	T49.4X5	T49.4X6
Triacetyloleandomycin	T36.3X1	T36.3X2	T36.3X3	T36.3X4	T36.3X5	T36.3X6
Triamcinolone	T38.0X1	T38.0X2	T38.0X3	T38.0X4	T38.0X5	T38.0X6
ENT agent	T49.6X1	T49.6X2	T49.6X3	T49.6X4	T49.6X5	T49.6X6
hexacetonide	T49.0X1	T49.0X2	T49.0X3	T49.0X4	T49.0X5	T49.0X6
ophthalmic preparation	T49.5X1	T49.5X2	T49.5X3	T49.5X4	T49.5X5	T49.5X6
topical NEC	T49.0X1	T49.0X2	T49.0X3	T49.0X4	T49.0X5	T49.0X6
Triampyzine	T44.3X1	T44.3X2	T44.3X3	T44.3X4	T44.3X5	T44.3X6
Triamterene	T50.2X1	T50.2X2	T50.2X3	T50.2X4	T50.2X5	T50.2X6
Triazine (herbicide)	T60.3X1	T60.3X2	T60.3X3	T60.3X4	—	—
Triaziquone	T45.1X1	T45.1X2	T45.1X3	T45.1X4	T45.1X5	T45.1X6
Triazolam	T42.4X1	T42.4X2	T42.4X3	T42.4X4	T42.4X5	T42.4X6
Triazole (herbicide)	T60.3X1	T60.3X2	T60.3X3	T60.3X4	—	—
Tribenoside	T46.991	T46.992	T46.993	T46.994	T46.995	T46.996
Tribromacetaldehyde	T42.6X1	T42.6X2	T42.6X3	T42.6X4	T42.6X5	T42.6X6
Tribromoethanol, rectal	T41.291	T41.292	T41.293	T41.294	T41.295	T41.296
Tribromomethane	T42.6X1	T42.6X2	T42.6X3	T42.6X4	T42.6X5	T42.6X6
Trichlorethane	T53.2X1	T53.2X2	T53.2X3	T53.2X4	—	—
Trichlorethylene	T53.2X1	T53.2X2	T53.2X3	T53.2X4	—	—
Trichlorfon	T60.0X1	T60.0X2	T60.0X3	T60.0X4	—	—
Trichlormethiazide	T50.2X1	T50.2X2	T50.2X3	T50.2X4	T50.2X5	T50.2X6
Trichlormethine	T45.1X1	T45.1X2	T45.1X3	T45.1X4	T45.1X5	T45.1X6

Substance	Poisoning, Accidental (Unintentional)	Poisoning, Intentional Self-Harm	Poisoning, Assault	Poisoning, Undetermined	Adverse Effect	Underdosing
Trichloroacetic acid, Trichloracetic acid	T54.2X1	T54.2X2	T54.2X3	T54.2X4	—	—
medicinal	T49.4X1	T49.4X2	T49.4X3	T49.4X4	T49.4X5	T49.4X6
Trichloroethane	T53.2X1	T53.2X2	T53.2X3	T53.2X4	—	—
Trichloroethanol	T42.6X1	T42.6X2	T42.6X3	T42.6X4	T42.6X5	T42.6X6
Trichloroethylene (liquid) (vapor)	T53.2X1	T53.2X2	T53.2X3	T53.2X4	—	—
anesthetic (gas)	T41.0X1	T41.0X2	T41.0X3	T41.0X4	T41.0X5	T41.0X6
vapor NEC	T53.2X1	T53.2X2	T53.2X3	T53.2X4	—	—
Trichloroethyl phosphate	T42.6X1	T42.6X2	T42.6X3	T42.6X4	T42.6X5	T42.6X6
Trichlorofluoromethane NEC	T53.5X1	T53.5X2	T53.5X3	T53.5X4	—	—
Trichloronate	T60.0X1	T60.0X2	T60.0X3	T60.0X4	—	—
2,4,5-Trichlorophen-oxyacetic acid	T60.3X1	T60.3X2	T60.3X3	T60.3X4	—	—
Trichloropropane	T53.6X1	T53.6X2	T53.6X3	T53.6X4	—	—
Trichlorotriethylamine	T45.1X1	T45.1X2	T45.1X3	T45.1X4	T45.1X5	T45.1X6
Trichomonacides NEC	T37.3X1	T37.3X2	T37.3X3	T37.3X4	T37.3X5	T37.3X6
Trichomycin	T36.7X1	T36.7X2	T36.7X3	T36.7X4	T36.7X5	T36.7X6
Triclobisonium chloride	T49.0X1	T49.0X2	T49.0X3	T49.0X4	T49.0X5	T49.0X6
Triclocarban	T49.0X1	T49.0X2	T49.0X3	T49.0X4	T49.0X5	T49.0X6
Triclofos	T42.6X1	T42.6X2	T42.6X3	T42.6X4	T42.6X5	T42.6X6
Triclosan	T49.0X1	T49.0X2	T49.0X3	T49.0X4	T49.0X5	T49.0X6
Tricresyl phosphate	T65.891	T65.892	T65.893	T65.894	—	—
solvent	T52.91	T52.92	T52.93	T52.94	—	—
Tricyclamol chloride	T44.3X1	T44.3X2	T44.3X3	T44.3X4	T44.3X5	T44.3X6
Tridesilon	T49.0X1	T49.0X2	T49.0X3	T49.0X4	T49.0X5	T49.0X6
Tridihexethyl iodide	T44.3X1	T44.3X2	T44.3X3	T44.3X4	T44.3X5	T44.3X6
Tridione	T42.2X1	T42.2X2	T42.2X3	T42.2X4	T42.2X5	T42.2X6
Trientine	T45.8X1	T45.8X2	T45.8X3	T45.8X4	T45.8X5	T45.8X6
Triethanolamine NEC	T54.3X1	T54.3X2	T54.3X3	T54.3X4	—	—
detergent	T54.3X1	T54.3X2	T54.3X3	T54.3X4	—	—
trinitrate (biphosphate)	T46.3X1	T46.3X2	T46.3X3	T46.3X4	T46.3X5	T46.3X6
Triethanomelamine	T45.1X1	T45.1X2	T45.1X3	T45.1X4	T45.1X5	T45.1X6
Triethylenemelamine	T45.1X1	T45.1X2	T45.1X3	T45.1X4	T45.1X5	T45.1X6
Triethylenephosphoramide	T45.1X1	T45.1X2	T45.1X3	T45.1X4	T45.1X5	T45.1X6
Triethylenethiophosphoramide	T45.1X1	T45.1X2	T45.1X3	T45.1X4	T45.1X5	T45.1X6
Trifluoperazine	T43.3X1	T43.3X2	T43.3X3	T43.3X4	T43.3X5	T43.3X6
Trifluoroethyl vinyl ether	T41.0X1	T41.0X2	T41.0X3	T41.0X4	T41.0X5	T41.0X6
Trifluperidol	T43.4X1	T43.4X2	T43.4X3	T43.4X4	T43.4X5	T43.4X6
Triflupromazine	T43.3X1	T43.3X2	T43.3X3	T43.3X4	T43.3X5	T43.3X6
Trifluridine	T37.5X1	T37.5X2	T37.5X3	T37.5X4	T37.5X5	T37.5X6
Triflusal	T45.521	T45.522	T45.523	T45.524	T45.525	T45.526
Trihexyphenidyl	T44.3X1	T44.3X2	T44.3X3	T44.3X4	T44.3X5	T44.3X6
Triiodothyronine	T38.1X1	T38.1X2	T38.1X3	T38.1X4	T38.1X5	T38.1X6

TABLE OF DRUGS AND CHEMICALS

	External Cause (T-Code)					
Substance	Poisoning, Accidental (Unintentional)	Poisoning, Intentional Self-Harm	Poisoning, Assault	Poisoning, Undetermined	Adverse Effect	Underdosing
Trilene	T41.0X1	T41.0X2	T41.0X3	T41.0X4	T41.0X5	T41.0X6
Trilostane	T38.991	T38.992	T38.993	T38.994	T38.995	T38.996
Trimebutine	T44.3X1	T44.3X2	T44.3X3	T44.3X4	T44.3X5	T44.3X6
Trimecaine	T41.3X1	T41.3X2	T41.3X3	T41.3X4	T41.3X5	T41.3X6
Trimeprazine (tartrate)	T44.3X1	T44.3X2	T44.3X3	T44.3X4	T44.3X5	T44.3X6
Trimetaphan camsilate	T44.2X1	T44.2X2	T44.2X4	T44.2X4	T44.2X5	T44.2X6
Trimetazidine	T46.7X1	T46.7X2	T46.7X3	T46.7X4	T46.7X5	T46.7X6
Trimethadione	T42.2X1	T42.2X2	T42.2X3	T42.2X4	T42.2X5	T42.2X6
Trimethaphan	T44.2X1	T44.2X2	T44.2X3	T44.2X4	T44.2X5	T44.2X6
Trimethidinium	T44.2X1	T44.2X2	T44.2X3	T44.2X4	T44.2X5	T44.2X6
Trimethobenzamide	T45.0X1	T45.0X2	T45.0X3	T45.0X4	T45.0X5	T45.0X6
Trimethoprim	T37.8X1	T37.8X2	T37.8X3	T37.8X4	T37.8X5	T37.8X6
with sulfamethoxazole	T36.8X1	T36.8X2	T36.8X3	T36.8X4	T36.8X5	T36.8X6
Trimethylcarbinol	T51.3X1	T51.3X2	T51.3X3	T51.3X4	—	—
Trimethylpsoralen	T49.3X1	T49.3X2	T49.3X3	T49.3X4	T49.3X5	T49.3X6
Trimeton	T45.0X1	T45.0X2	T45.0X3	T45.0X4	T45.0X5	T45.0X6
Trimetrexate	T45.1X1	T45.1X2	T45.1X3	T45.1X4	T45.1X5	T45.1X6
Trimipramine	T43.011	T43.012	T43.013	T43.014	T43.015	T43.016
Trimustine	T45.1X1	T45.1X2	T45.1X3	T45.1X4	T45.1X5	T45.1X6
Trinitrine	T46.3X1	T46.3X2	T46.3X3	T46.3X4	T46.3X5	T46.3X6
Trinitrobenzol	T65.3X1	T65.3X2	T65.3X3	T65.3X4	—	—
Trinitrophenol	T65.3X1	T65.3X2	T65.3X3	T65.3X4	—	—
Trinitrotoluene (fumes)	T65.3X1	T65.3X2	T65.3X3	T65.3X4	—	—
Trional	T42.6X1	T42.6X2	T42.6X3	T42.6X4	T42.6X5	T42.6X6
Triorthocresyl phosphate	T65.891	T65.892	T65.893	T65.894	—	—
Trioxide of arsenic	T57.0X1	T57.0X2	T57.0X3	T57.0X4	—	—
Trioxysalen	T49.4X1	T49.4X2	T49.4X3	T49.4X4	T49.4X5	T49.4X6
Tripamide	T50.2X1	T50.2X2	T50.2X3	T50.2X4	T50.2X5	T50.2X6
Triparanol	T46.6X1	T46.6X2	T46.6X3	T46.6X4	T46.6X5	T46.6X6
Tripelennamine	T45.0X1	T45.0X2	T45.0X3	T45.0X4	T45.0X5	T45.0X6
Triperiden	T44.3X1	T44.3X2	T44.3X3	T44.3X4	T44.3X5	T44.3X6
Triperidol	T43.4X1	T43.4X2	T43.4X3	T43.4X4	T43.4X5	T43.4X6
Triphenylphosphate	T65.891	T65.892	T65.893	T65.894	—	—
Triple						
bromides	T42.6X1	T42.6X2	T42.6X3	T42.6X4	T42.6X5	T42.6X6
carbonate	T47.1X1	T47.1X2	T47.1X3	T47.1X4	T47.1X5	T47.1X6
vaccine						
DPT	T50.A11	T50.A12	T50.A13	T50.A14	T50.A15	T50.A16
including pertussis	T50.A11	T50.A12	T50.A13	T50.A14	T50.A15	T50.A16
MMR	T50.B91	T50.B92	—	—	—	—
Triprolidine	T45.0X1	T45.0X2	T45.0X3	T45.0X4	T45.0X5	T45.0X6
Trisodium hydrogen edetate	T50.6X1	T50.6X2	T50.6X3	T50.6X4	T50.6X5	T50.6X6

	External Cause (T-Code)					
Substance	Poisoning, Accidental (Unintentional)	Poisoning, Intentional Self-Harm	Poisoning, Assault	Poisoning, Undetermined	Adverse Effect	Underdosing
Trisoralen	T49.3X1	T49.3X2	T49.3X3	T49.3X4	T49.3X5	T49.3X6
Trisulfapyrimidines	T37.0X1	T37.0X2	T37.0X3	T37.0X4	T37.0X5	T37.0X6
Trithiozine	T44.3X1	T44.3X2	T44.3X3	T44.3X4	T44.3X5	T44.3X6
Tritiozine	T44.3X1	T44.3X2	T44.3X3	T44.3X4	T44.3X5	T44.3X6
Tritoqualine	T45.0X1	T45.0X2	T45.0X3	T45.0X4	T45.0X5	T45.0X6
Trofosfamide	T45.1X1	T45.1X2	T45.1X3	T45.1X4	T45.1X5	T45.1X6
Troleandomycin	T36.3X1	T36.3X2	T36.3X3	T36.3X4	T36.3X5	T36.3X6
Trolnitrate (phosphate)	T46.3X1	T46.3X2	T46.3X3	T46.3X4	T46.3X5	T46.3X6
Tromantadine	T37.5X1	T37.5X2	T37.5X3	T37.5X4	T37.5X5	T37.5X6
Trometamol	T50.2X1	T50.2X2	T50.2X3	T50.2X4	T50.2X5	T50.2X6
Tromethamine	T50.2X1	T50.2X2	T50.2X3	T50.2X4	T50.2X5	T50.2X6
Tronothane	T41.3X1	T41.3X2	T41.3X3	T41.3X4	T41.3X5	T41.3X6
Tropacine	T44.3X1	T44.3X2	T44.3X3	T44.3X4	T44.3X5	T44.3X6
Tropatepine	T44.3X1	T44.3X2	T44.3X3	T44.3X4	T44.3X5	T44.3X6
Tropicamide	T44.3X1	T44.3X2	T44.3X3	T44.3X4	T44.3X5	T44.3X6
Trospium chloride	T44.3X1	T44.3X2	T44.3X3	T44.3X4	T44.3X5	T44.3X6
Troxerutin	T46.991	T46.992	T46.993	T46.994	T46.995	T46.996
Troxidone	T42.2X1	T42.2X2	T42.2X3	T42.2X4	T42.2X5	T42.2X6
Tryparsamide	T37.3X1	T37.3X2	T37.3X3	T37.3X4	T37.3X5	T37.3X6
Trypsin	T45.3X1	T45.3X2	T45.3X3	T45.3X4	T45.3X5	T45.3X6
Tryptizol	T43.011	T43.012	T43.013	T43.014	T43.015	T43.016
TSH	T38.811	T38.812	T38.813	T38.814	T38.815	T38.816
Tuaminoheptane	T48.5X1	T48.5X2	T48.5X3	T48.5X4	T48.5X5	T48.5X6
Tuberculin, purified protein derivative (PPD)	T50.8X1	T50.8X2	T50.8X3	T50.8X4	T50.8X5	T50.8X6
Tubocurare	T48.1X1	T48.1X2	T48.1X3	T48.1X4	T48.1X5	T48.1X6
Tubocurarine (chloride)	T48.1X1	T48.1X2	T48.1X3	T48.1X4	T48.1X5	T48.1X6
Tulobuterol	T48.6X1	T48.6X2	T48.6X3	T48.6X4	T48.6X5	T48.6X6
Turpentine (spirits of)	T52.8X1	T52.8X2	T52.8X3	T52.8X4	—	—
vapor	T52.8X1	T52.8X2	T52.8X3	T52.8X4	—	—
Tybamate	T43.591	T43.592	T43.593	T43.594	T43.595	T43.596
Tyloxapol	T48.4X1	T48.4X2	T48.4X3	T48.4X4	T48.4X5	T48.4X6
Tymazoline	T48.5X1	T48.5X2	T48.5X3	T48.5X4	T48.5X5	T48.5X6
Typhoid-paratyphoid vaccine	T50.A91	T50.A92	T50.A93	T50.A94	T50.A95	T50.A96
Typhus vaccine	T50.A91	T50.A92	T50.A93	T50.A94	T50.A95	T50.A96
Tyropanoate	T50.8X1	T50.8X2	T50.8X3	T50.8X4	T50.8X5	T50.8X6
Tyrothricin	T49.6X1	T49.6X2	T49.6X3	T49.6X4	T49.6X5	T49.6X6
ENT agent	T49.6X1	T49.6X2	T49.6X3	T49.6X4	T49.6X5	T49.6X6
ophthalmic preparation	T49.5X1	T49.5X2	T49.5X3	T49.5X4	T49.5X5	T49.5X6
U						
Ufenamate	T39.391	T39.392	T39.393	T39.394	T39.395	T39.396
Ultraviolet light protectant	T49.3X1	T49.3X2	T49.3X3	T49.3X4	T49.3X5	T49.3X6

◄ New   ◄| Revised   ~~deleted~~ Deleted

Substance	External Cause (T-Code)					
	Poisoning, Accidental (Unintentional)	Poisoning, Intentional Self-Harm	Poisoning, Assault	Poisoning, Undetermined	Adverse Effect	Underdosing
Undecenoic acid	T49.0X1	T49.0X2	T49.0X3	T49.0X4	T49.0X5	T49.0X6
Undecoylium	T49.0X1	T49.0X2	T49.0X3	T49.0X4	T49.0X5	T49.0X6
Undecylenic acid (derivatives)	T49.0X1	T49.0X2	T49.0X3	T49.0X4	T49.0X5	T49.0X6
Unna's boot	T49.3X1	T49.3X2	T49.3X3	T49.3X4	T49.3X5	T49.3X6
Unsaturated fatty acid	T46.6X1	T46.6X2	T46.6X3	T46.6X4	T46.6X5	T46.6X6
Uracil mustard	T45.1X1	T45.1X2	T45.1X3	T45.1X4	T45.1X5	T45.1X6
Uramustine	T45.1X1	T45.1X2	T45.1X3	T45.1X4	T45.1X5	T45.1X6
Urapidil	T46.5X1	T46.5X2	T46.5X3	T46.5X4	T46.5X5	T46.5X6
Urari	T48.1X1	T48.1X2	T48.1X3	T48.1X4	T48.1X5	T48.1X6
Urate oxidase	T50.4X1	T50.4X2	T50.4X3	T50.4X4	T50.4X5	T50.4X6
Urea	T47.3X1	T47.3X2	T47.3X3	T47.3X4	T47.3X5	T47.3X6
peroxide	T49.0X1	T49.0X2	T49.0X3	T49.0X4	T49.0X5	T49.0X6
stibamine	T37.4X1	T37.4X2	T37.4X3	T37.4X4	T37.4X5	T37.4X6
topical	T49.8X1	T49.8X2	T49.8X3	T49.8X4	T49.8X5	T49.8X6
Urethane	T45.1X1	T45.1X2	T45.1X3	T45.1X4	T45.1X5	T45.1X6
Urginea (maritima) (scilla) — see Squill						
Uric acid metabolism drug NEC	T50.4X1	T50.4X2	T50.4X3	T50.4X4	T50.4X5	T50.4X6
Uricosuric agent	T50.4X1	T50.4X2	T50.4X3	T50.4X4	T50.4X5	T50.4X6
Urinary anti-infective	T37.8X1	T37.8X2	T37.8X3	T37.8X4	T37.8X5	T37.8X6
Urofollitropin	T38.811	T38.812	T38.813	T38.814	T38.815	T38.816
Urokinase	T45.611	T45.612	T45.613	T45.614	T45.615	T45.616
Urokon	T50.8X1	T50.8X2	T50.8X3	T50.8X4	T50.8X5	T50.8X6
Ursodeoxycholic acid	T50.991	T50.992	T50.993	T50.994	T50.995	T50.996
Ursodiol	T50.991	T50.992	T50.993	T50.994	T50.995	T50.996
Urtica	T62.2X1	T62.2X2	T62.2X3	T62.2X4	—	—
Utility gas — see Gas, utility						
V						
Vaccine NEC	T50.Z91	T50.Z92	T50.Z93	T50.Z94	T50.Z95	T50.Z96
antineoplastic	T50.Z91	T50.Z92	T50.Z93	T50.Z94	T50.Z95	T50.Z96
bacterial NEC	T50.A91	T50.A92	T50.A93	T50.A94	T50.A95	T50.A96
with						
other bacterial component	T50.A91	T50.A92	T50.A93	T50.A94	T50.A95	T50.A96
pertussis component	T50.A91	T50.A92	T50.A93	T50.A94	T50.A95	T50.A96
viral-rickettsial component	T50.A91	T50.A92	T50.A93	T50.A94	T50.A95	T50.A96
mixed NEC	T50.A91	T50.A92	T50.A93	T50.A94	T50.A95	T50.A96
BCG	T50.A91	T50.A92	T50.A93	T50.A94	T50.A95	T50.A96
cholera	T50.A91	T50.A92	T50.A93	T50.A94	T50.A95	T50.A96
diphtheria	T50.A91	T50.A92	T50.A93	T50.A94	T50.A95	T50.A96
with tetanus	T50.A21	T50.A22	T50.A23	T50.A24	T50.A25	T50.A26
and pertussis	T50.A11	T50.A12	T50.A13	T50.A14	T50.A15	T50.A16

Substance	External Cause (T-Code)					
	Poisoning, Accidental (Unintentional)	Poisoning, Intentional Self-Harm	Poisoning, Assault	Poisoning, Undetermined	Adverse Effect	Underdosing
Vaccine NEC *(Continued)*						
influenza	T50.B91	T50.B92	T50.B93	T50.B94	T50.B95	T50.B96
measles	T50.B91	T50.B92	T50.B93	T50.B94	T50.B95	T50.B96
with mumps and rubella	T50.B91	T50.B92	T50.B93	T50.B94	T50.B95	T50.B96
meningococcal	T50.A91	T50.A92	T50.A93	T50.A94	T50.A95	T50.A96
mumps	T50.B91	T50.B92	T50.B93	T50.B94	T50.B95	T50.B96
paratyphoid	T50.A91	T50.A92	T50.A93	T50.A94	T50.A95	T50.A96
pertussis	T50.A11	T50.A12	T50.A13	T50.A14	T50.A15	T50.A16
with diphtheria	T50.A11	T50.A12	T50.A13	T50.A14	T50.A15	T50.A16
and tetanus	T50.A11	T50.A12	T50.A13	T50.A14	T50.A15	T50.A16
plague	T50.A91	T50.A92	T50.A93	T50.A94	T50.A95	T50.A96
poliomyelitis	T50.B91	T50.B92	T50.B93	T50.B94	T50.B95	T50.B96
poliovirus	T50.B91	T50.B92	T50.B93	T50.B94	T50.B95	T50.B96
rabies	T50.B91	T50.B92	T50.B93	T50.B94	T50.B95	T50.B96
respiratory syncytial virus	T50.B91	T50.B92	T50.B93	T50.B94	T50.B95	T50.B96
rickettsial NEC	T50.A91	T50.A92	T50.A93	T50.A94	T50.A95	T50.A96
with						
bacterial component	T50.A21	T50.A22	T50.A23	T50.A24	T50.A25	T50.A26
Rocky Mountain spotted fever	T50.A91	T50.A92	T50.A93	T50.A94	T50.A95	T50.A96
rubella	T50.B91	T50.B92	T50.B93	T50.B94	T50.B95	T50.B96
sabin oral	T50.B91	T50.B92	T50.B93	T50.B94	T50.B95	T50.B96
smallpox	T50.B11	T50.B12	T50.B13	T50.B14	T50.B15	T50.B16
TAB	T50.A91	T50.A92	T50.A93	T50.A94	T50.A95	T50.A96
tetanus	T50.A91	T50.A92	T50.A93	T50.A94	T50.A95	T50.A96
typhoid	T50.A91	T50.A92	T50.A93	T50.A94	T50.A95	T50.A96
typhus	T50.A91	T50.A92	T50.A93	T50.A94	T50.A95	T50.A96
viral NEC	T50.B91	T50.B92	T50.B93	T50.B94	T50.B95	T50.B96
yellow fever	T50.B91	T50.B92	T50.B93	T50.B94	T50.B95	T50.B96
Vaccinia immune globulin	T50.Z11	T50.Z12	T50.Z13	T50.Z14	T50.Z15	T50.Z16
Vaginal contraceptives	T49.8X1	T49.8X2	T49.8X3	T49.8X4	T49.8X5	T49.8X6
Valerian						
root	T42.6X1	T42.6X2	T42.6X3	T42.6X4	T42.6X5	T42.6X6
tincture	T42.6X1	T42.6X2	T42.6X3	T42.6X4	T42.6X5	T42.6X6
Valethamate bromide	T44.3X1	T44.3X2	T44.3X3	T44.3X4	T44.3X5	T44.3X6
Valisone	T49.0X1	T49.0X2	T49.0X3	T49.0X4	T49.0X5	T49.0X6
Valium	T42.4X1	T42.4X2	T42.4X3	T42.4X4	T42.4X5	T42.4X6
Valmid	T42.6X1	T42.6X2	T42.6X3	T42.6X4	T42.6X5	T42.6X6
Valnoctamide	T42.6X1	T42.6X2	T42.6X3	T42.6X4	T42.6X5	T42.6X6
Valproate (sodium)	T42.6X1	T42.6X2	T42.6X3	T42.6X4	T42.6X5	T42.6X6
Valproic acid	T42.6X1	T42.6X2	T42.6X3	T42.6X4	T42.6X5	T42.6X6
Valpromide	T42.6X1	T42.6X2	T42.6X3	T42.6X4	T42.6X5	T42.6X6
Vanadium	T56.891	T56.892	T56.893	T56.894	—	—

◄ New   ◄═ Revised   ~~deleted~~ Deleted

TABLE OF DRUGS AND CHEMICALS

Substance	External Cause (T-Code)					
	Poisoning, Accidental (Unintentional)	Poisoning, Intentional Self-Harm	Poisoning, Assault	Poisoning, Undetermined	Adverse Effect	Underdosing
Vancomycin	T36.8X1	T36.8X2	T36.8X3	T36.8X4	T36.8X5	T36.8X6
Vapor — see also Gas	T59.91	T59.92	T59.93	T59.94	—	—
kiln (carbon monoxide)	T58.8X1	T58.8X2	T58.8X3	T58.8X4	—	—
lead — see Lead						
specified source NEC	T59.891	T59.892	T59.893	T59.894	—	—
Vardenafil	T46.7X1	T46.7X2	T46.7X3	T46.7X4	T46.7X5	T46.7X6
Varicose reduction drug	T46.8X1	T46.8X2	T46.8X3	T46.8X4	T46.8X5	T46.8X6
Varnish	T65.4X1	T65.4X2	T65.4X3	T65.4X4		
cleaner	T52.91	T52.92	T52.93	T52.94	—	—
Vaseline	T49.3X1	T49.3X2	T49.3X3	T49.3X4	T49.3X5	T49.3X6
Vasodilan	T46.7X1	T46.7X2	T46.7X3	T46.7X4	T46.7X5	T46.7X6
Vasodilator						
coronary NEC	T46.3X1	T46.3X2	T46.3X3	T46.3X4	T46.3X5	T46.3X6
peripheral NEC	T46.7X1	T46.7X2	T46.7X3	T46.7X4	T46.7X5	T46.7X6
Vasopressin	T38.891	T38.892	T38.893	T38.894	T38.895	T38.896
Vasopressor drugs	T38.891	T38.892	T38.893	T38.894	T38.895	T38.896
Vecuronium bromide	T48.1X1	T48.1X2	T48.1X3	T48.1X4	T48.1X5	T48.1X6
Vegetable extract, astringent	T49.2X1	T49.2X2	T49.2X3	T49.2X4	T49.2X5	T49.2X6
Venlafaxine	T43.211	T43.212	T43.213	T43.214	T43.215	T43.216
Venom, venomous (bite) (sting)	T63.91	T63.92	T63.93	T63.94	—	—
amphibian NEC	T63.831	T63.832	T63.833	T63.834	—	—
animal NEC	T63.891	T63.892	T63.893	T63.894	—	—
ant	T63.421	T63.422	T63.423	T63.424	—	—
arthropod NEC	T63.481	T63.482	T63.483	T63.484	—	—
bee	T63.441	T63.442	T63.443	T63.444	—	—
centipede	T63.411	T63.412	T63.413	T63.414	—	—
fish	T63.591	T63.592	T63.593	T63.594	—	—
frog	T63.811	T63.812	T63.813	T63.814	—	—
hornet	T63.451	T63.452	T63.453	T63.454	—	—
insect NEC	T63.481	T63.482	T63.483	T63.484	—	—
lizard	T63.121	T63.122	T63.123	T63.124	—	—
marine						
animals	T63.691	T63.692	T63.693	T63.694	—	—
bluebottle	T63.611	T63.612	T63.613	T63.614	—	—
jellyfish NEC	T63.621	T63.622	T63.623	T63.624	—	—
Portuguese Man-o-war	T63.611	T63.612	T63.613	T63.614	—	—
sea anemone	T63.631	T63.632	T63.633	T63.634	—	—
specified NEC	T63.691	T63.692	T63.693	T63.694	—	—
fish	T63.591	T63.592	T63.593	T63.594	—	—
plants	T63.711	T63.712	T63.713	T63.714	—	—
sting ray	T63.511	T63.512	T63.513	T63.514	—	—

Substance	External Cause (T-Code)					
	Poisoning, Accidental (Unintentional)	Poisoning, Intentional Self-Harm	Poisoning, Assault	Poisoning, Undetermined	Adverse Effect	Underdosing
Venom, venomous (Continued)						
millipede (tropical)	T63.411	T63.412	T63.413	T63.414	—	—
plant NEC	T63.791	T63.792	T63.793	T63.794	—	—
marine	T63.711	T63.712	T63.713	T63.714	—	—
reptile	T63.191	T63.192	T63.193	T63.194	—	—
gila monster	T63.111	T63.112	T63.113	T63.114	—	—
lizard NEC	T63.121	T63.122	T63.123	T63.124	—	—
scorpion	T63.2X1	T63.2X2	T63.2X3	T63.2X4	—	—
snake	T63.001	T63.002	T63.003	T63.004	—	—
African NEC	T63.081	T63.082	T63.083	T63.084	—	—
American (North) (South) NEC	T63.061	T63.062	T63.063	T63.064	—	—
Asian	T63.081	T63.082	T63.083	T63.084	—	—
Australian	T63.071	T63.072	T63.073	T63.074	—	—
cobra	T63.041	T63.042	T63.043	T63.044	—	—
coral snake	T63.021	T63.022	T63.023	T63.024	—	—
rattlesnake	T63.011	T63.012	T63.013	T63.014	—	—
specified NEC	T63.091	T63.092	T63.093	T63.094	—	—
taipan	T63.031	T63.032	T63.033	T63.034	—	—
specified NEC	T63.891	T63.892	T63.893	T63.894	—	—
spider	T63.301	T63.302	T63.303	T63.304	—	—
black widow	T63.311	T63.312	T63.313	T63.314	—	—
brown recluse	T63.331	T63.332	T63.333	T63.334	—	—
specified NEC	T63.391	T63.392	T63.393	T63.394	—	—
tarantula	T63.321	T63.322	T63.323	T63.324	—	—
sting ray	T63.511	T63.512	T63.513	T63.514	—	—
toad	T63.821	T63.822	T63.823	T63.824	—	—
wasp	T63.461	T63.462	T63.463	T63.464	—	—
Venous sclerosing drug NEC	T46.8X1	T46.8X2	T46.8X3	T46.8X4	T46.8X5	T46.8X6
Ventolin — see Albuterol						
Verapamil	T46.1X1	T46.1X2	T46.1X3	T46.1X4	T46.1X5	T46.1X6
Veramon	T42.3X1	T42.3X2	T42.3X3	T42.3X4	T42.3X5	T42.3X6
Veratrine	T46.5X1	T46.5X2	T46.5X3	T46.5X4	T46.5X5	T46.5X6
Veratrum						
album	T62.2X1	T62.2X2	T62.2X3	T62.2X4	—	—
alkaloids	T46.5X1	T46.5X2	T46.5X3	T46.5X4	T46.5X5	T46.5X6
viride	T62.2X1	T62.2X2	T62.2X3	T62.2X4	—	—
Verdigris	T60.3X1	T60.3X2	T60.3X3	T60.3X4	—	—
Veronal	T42.3X1	T42.3X2	T42.3X3	T42.3X4	T42.3X5	T42.3X6
Veroxil	T37.4X1	T37.4X2	T37.4X3	T37.4X4	T37.4X5	T37.4X6
Versenate	T50.6X1	T50.6X2	T50.6X3	T50.6X4	T50.6X5	T50.6X6

◄ New   ◄ Revised   ~~deleted~~ Deleted

Substance	Poisoning, Accidental (Unintentional)	Poisoning, Intentional Self-Harm	Poisoning, Assault	Poisoning, Undetermined	Adverse Effect	Underdosing
Versidyne	T39.8X1	T39.8X2	T39.8X3	T39.8X4	T39.8X5	T39.8X6
Vetrabutine	T48.0X1	T48.0X2	T48.0X3	T48.0X4	T48.0X5	T48.0X6
Vidarabine	T37.5X1	T37.5X2	T37.5X3	T37.5X4	T37.5X5	T37.5X6
Vienna						
green	T57.0X1	T57.0X2	T57.0X3	T57.0X4	—	—
insecticide	T60.2X1	T60.2X2	T60.2X3	T60.2X4		
red	T57.0X1	T57.0X2	T57.0X3	T57.0X4	—	—
pharmaceutical dye	T50.991	T50.992	T50.993	T50.994	T50.995	T50.996
Vigabatrin	T42.6X1	T42.6X2	T42.6X3	T42.6X4	T42.6X5	T42.6X6
Viloxazine	T43.291	T43.292	T43.293	T43.294	T43.295	T43.296
Viminol	T39.8X1	T39.8X2	T39.8X3	T39.8X4	T39.8X5	T39.8X6
Vinbarbital, vinbarbitone	T42.3X1	T42.3X2	T42.3X3	T42.3X4	T42.3X5	T42.3X6
Vinblastine	T45.1X1	T45.1X2	T45.1X3	T45.1X4	T45.1X5	T45.1X6
Vinburnine	T46.7X1	T46.7X2	T46.7X3	T46.7X4	T46.7X5	T46.7X6
Vincamine	T45.1X1	T45.1X2	T45.1X3	T45.1X4	T45.1X5	T45.1X6
Vincristine	T45.1X1	T45.1X2	T45.1X3	T45.1X4	T45.1X5	T45.1X6
Vindesine	T45.1X1	T45.1X2	T45.1X3	T45.1X4	T45.1X5	T45.1X6
Vinesthene, vinethene	T41.0X1	T41.0X2	T41.0X3	T41.0X4	T41.0X5	T41.0X6
Vinorelbine tartrate	T45.1X1	T45.1X2	T45.1X3	T45.1X4	T45.1X5	T45.1X6
Vinpocetine	T46.7X1	T46.7X2	T46.7X3	T46.7X4	T46.7X5	T46.7X6
Vinyl						
acetate	T65.891	T65.892	T65.893	T65.894	—	—
bital	T42.3X1	T42.3X2	T42.3X3	T42.3X4	T42.3X5	T42.3X6
bromide	T65.891	T65.892	T65.893	T65.894	—	—
chloride	T59.891	T59.892	T59.893	T59.894	—	—
ether	T41.0X1	T41.0X2	T41.0X3	T41.0X4	T41.0X5	T41.0X6
Vinylbital	T42.3X1	T42.3X2	T42.3X3	T42.3X4	T42.3X5	T42.3X6
Vinylidene chloride	T65.891	T65.892	T65.893	T65.894	—	—
Vioform	T37.8X1	T37.8X2	T37.8X3	T37.8X4	T37.8X5	T37.8X6
topical	T49.0X1	T49.0X2	T49.0X3	T49.0X4	T49.0X5	T49.0X6
Viomycin	T36.8X1	T36.8X2	T36.8X3	T36.8X4	T36.8X5	T36.8X6
Viosterol	T45.2X1	T45.2X2	T45.2X3	T45.2X4	T45.2X5	T45.2X6
Viper (venom)	T63.091	T63.092	T63.093	T63.094	—	—
Viprynium	T37.4X1	T37.4X2	T37.4X3	T37.4X4	T37.4X5	T37.4X6
Viquidil	T46.7X1	T46.7X2	T46.7X3	T46.7X4	T46.7X5	T46.7X6
Viral vaccine NEC	T50.B91	T50.B92	T50.B93	T50.B94	T50.B95	T50.B96
Virginiamycin	T36.8X1	T36.8X2	T36.8X3	T36.8X4	T36.8X5	T36.8X6
Virugon	T37.5X1	T37.5X2	T37.5X3	T37.5X4	T37.5X5	T37.5X6
Viscous agent	T50.901	T50.902	T50.903	T50.904	T50.905	T50.906
Visine	T49.5X1	T49.5X2	T49.5X3	T49.5X4	T49.5X5	T49.5X6
Visnadine	T46.3X1	T46.3X2	T46.3X3	T46.3X4	T46.3X5	T46.3X6

Substance	Poisoning, Accidental (Unintentional)	Poisoning, Intentional Self-Harm	Poisoning, Assault	Poisoning, Undetermined	Adverse Effect	Underdosing
Vitamin NEC	T45.2X1	T45.2X2	T45.2X3	T45.2X4	T45.2X5	T45.2X6
A	T45.2X1	T45.2X2	T45.2X3	T45.2X4	T45.2X5	T45.2X6
B NEC	T45.2X1	T45.2X2	T45.2X3	T45.2X4	T45.2X5	T45.2X6
nicotinic acid	T46.7X1	T46.7X2	T46.7X3	T46.7X4	T46.7X5	T46.7X6
B1	T45.2X1	T45.2X2	T45.2X3	T45.2X4	T45.2X5	T45.2X6
B2	T45.2X1	T45.2X2	T45.2X3	T45.2X4	T45.2X5	T45.2X6
B6	T45.2X1	T45.2X2	T45.2X3	T45.2X4	T45.2X5	T45.2X6
B12	T45.2X1	T45.2X2	T45.2X3	T45.2X4	T45.2X5	T45.2X6
B15	T45.2X1	T45.2X2	T45.2X3	T45.2X4	T45.2X5	T45.2X6
C	T45.2X1	T45.2X2	T45.2X3	T45.2X4	T45.2X5	T45.2X6
D	T45.2X1	T45.2X2	T45.2X3	T45.2X4	T45.2X5	T45.2X6
D2	T45.2X1	T45.2X2	T45.2X3	T45.2X4	T45.2X5	T45.2X6
D3	T45.2X1	T45.2X2	T45.2X3	T45.2X4	T45.2X5	T45.2X6
E	T45.2X1	T45.2X2	T45.2X3	T45.2X4	T45.2X5	T45.2X6
E acetate	T45.2X1	T45.2X2	T45.2X3	T45.2X4	T45.2X5	T45.2X6
hematopoietic	T45.8X1	T45.8X2	T45.8X3	T45.8X4	T45.8X5	T45.8X6
K NEC	T45.7X1	T45.7X2	T45.7X3	T45.7X4	T45.7X5	T45.7X6
K1	T45.7X1	T45.7X2	T45.7X3	T45.7X4	T45.7X5	T45.7X6
K2	T45.7X1	T45.7X2	T45.7X3	T45.7X4	T45.7X5	T45.7X6
PP	T45.2X1	T45.2X2	T45.2X3	T45.2X4	T45.2X5	T45.2X6
ulceroprotectant	T47.1X1	T47.1X2	T47.1X3	T47.1X4	T47.1X5	T47.1X6
Vleminckx's solution	T49.4X1	T49.4X2	T49.4X3	T49.4X4	T49.4X5	T49.4X6
Voltaren — *see Diclofenac sodium*						
W						
Warfarin	T45.511	T45.512	T45.513	T45.514	T45.515	T45.516
rodenticide	T60.4X1	T60.4X2	T60.4X3	T60.4X4	—	—
sodium	T45.511	T45.512	T45.513	T45.514	T45.515	T45.516
Wasp (sting)	T63.461	T63.462	T63.463	T63.464	—	—
Water						
balance drug	T50.3X1	T50.3X2	T50.3X3	T50.3X4	T50.3X5	T50.3X6
distilled	T50.3X1	T50.3X2	T50.3X3	T50.3X4	T50.3X5	T50.3X6
gas — *see Gas, water*						
incomplete combustion of — *see Carbon, monoxide, fuel, utility*						
hemlock	T62.2X1	T62.2X2	T62.2X3	T62.2X4	—	—
moccasin (venom)	T63.061	T63.062	T63.063	T63.064	—	—
purified	T50.3X1	T50.3X2	T50.3X3	T50.3X4	T50.3X5	T50.3X6
Wax (paraffin) (petroleum)	T52.0X1	T52.0X2	T52.0X3	T52.0X4	—	—
automobile	T65.891	T65.892	T65.893	T65.894	—	—
floor	T52.0X1	T52.0X2	T52.0X3	T52.0X4	—	—

◀ New   ◀ Revised   ~~deleted~~ Deleted

TABLE OF DRUGS AND CHEMICALS

Substance	Poisoning, Accidental (Unintentional)	Poisoning, Intentional Self-Harm	Poisoning, Assault	Poisoning, Undetermined	Adverse Effect	Underdosing
Weed killers NEC	T60.3X1	T60.3X2	T60.3X3	T60.3X4	—	—
Welldorm	T42.6X1	T42.6X2	T42.6X3	T42.6X4	T42.6X5	T42.6X6
White						
arsenic	T57.0X1	T57.0X2	T57.0X3	T57.0X4	—	—
helebore	T62.2X1	T62.2X2	T62.2X3	T62.2X4	—	—
lotion (keratolytic)	T49.4X1	T49.4X2	T49.4X3	T49.4X4	T49.4X5	T49.4X6
spirit	T52.0X1	T52.0X2	T52.0X3	T52.0X4	—	—
Whitewash	T65.891	T65.892	T65.893	T65.894	—	—
Whole blood (human)	T45.8X1	T45.8X2	T45.8X3	T45.8X4	T45.8X5	T45.8X6
Wild						
black cherry	T62.2X1	T62.2X2	T62.2X3	T62.2X4	—	—
poisonous plants NEC	T62.2X1	T62.2X2	T62.2X3	T62.2X4	—	—
Window cleaning fluid	T65.891	T65.892	T65.893	T65.894	—	—
Wintergreen (oil)	T49.3X1	T49.3X2	T49.3X3	T49.3X4	T49.3X5	T49.3X6
Wisterine	T62.2X1	T62.2X2	T62.2X3	T62.2X4	—	—
Witch hazel	T49.2X1	T49.2X2	T49.2X3	T49.2X4	T49.2X5	T49.2X6
Wood alcohol or spirit	T51.1X1	T51.1X2	T51.1X3	T51.1X4	—	—
Wool fat (hydrous)	T49.3X1	T49.3X2	T49.3X3	T49.3X4	T49.3X5	T49.3X6
Woorali	T48.1X1	T48.1X2	T48.1X3	T48.1X4	T48.1X5	T48.1X6
Wormseed, American	T37.4X1	T37.4X2	T37.4X3	T37.4X4	T37.4X5	T37.4X6
X						
Xamoterol	T44.5X1	T44.5X2	T44.5X3	T44.5X4	T44.5X5	T44.5X6
Xanthine diuretics	T50.2X1	T50.2X2	T50.2X3	T50.2X4	T50.2X5	T50.2X6
Xanthinol nicotinate	T46.7X1	T46.7X2	T46.7X3	T46.7X4	T46.7X5	T46.7X6
Xanthotoxin	T49.3X1	T49.3X2	T49.3X3	T49.3X4	T49.3X5	T49.3X6
Xantinol nicotinate	T46.7X1	T46.7X2	T46.7X3	T46.7X4	T46.7X5	T46.7X6
Xantocillin	T36.0X1	T36.0X2	T36.0X3	T36.0X4	T36.0X5	T36.0X6
Xenon (127Xe) (133Xe)	T50.8X1	T50.8X2	T50.8X3	T50.8X4	T50.8X5	T50.8X6
Xenysalate	T49.4X1	T49.4X2	T49.4X3	T49.4X4	T49.4X5	T49.4X6
Xibornol	T37.8X1	T37.8X2	T37.8X3	T37.8X4	T37.8X5	T37.8X6
Xigris	T45.511	T45.512	T45.513	T45.514	T45.515	T45.516
Xipamide	T50.2X1	T50.2X2	T50.2X3	T50.2X4	T50.2X5	T50.2X6
Xylene (vapor)	T52.2X1	T52.2X2	T52.2X3	T52.2X4	—	—
Xylocaine (infiltration) (topical)	T41.3X1	T41.3X2	T41.3X3	T41.3X4	T41.3X5	T41.3X6
nerve block (peripheral) (plexus)	T41.3X1	T41.3X2	T41.3X3	T41.3X4	T41.3X5	T41.3X6
spinal	T41.3X1	T41.3X2	T41.3X3	T41.3X4	T41.3X5	T41.3X6
Xylol (vapor)	T52.2X1	T52.2X2	T52.2X3	T52.2X4	—	—
Xylometazoline	T48.5X1	T48.5X2	T48.5X3	T48.5X4	T48.5X5	T48.5X6

Substance	Poisoning, Accidental (Unintentional)	Poisoning, Intentional Self-Harm	Poisoning, Assault	Poisoning, Undetermined	Adverse Effect	Underdosing
Y						
Yeast	T45.2X1	T45.2X2	T45.2X3	T45.2X4	T45.2X5	T45.2X6
dried	T45.2X1	T45.2X2	T45.2X3	T45.2X4	T45.2X5	T45.2X6
Yellow						
fever vaccine	T50.B91	T50.B92	T50.B93	T50.B94	T50.B95	T50.B96
jasmine	T62.2X1	T62.2X2	T62.2X3	T62.2X4	—	—
phenolphthalein	T47.2X1	T47.2X2	T47.2X3	T47.2X4	T47.2X5	T47.2X6
Yew	T62.2X1	T62.2X2	T62.2X3	T62.2X4	—	—
Yohimbic acid	T40.991	T40.992	T40.993	T40.994	T40.995	T40.996
Z						
Zactane	T39.8X1	T39.8X2	T39.8X3	T39.8X4	T39.8X5	T39.8X6
Zalcitabine	T37.5X1	T37.5X2	T37.5X3	T37.5X4	T37.5X5	T37.5X6
Zaroxolyn	T50.2X1	T50.2X2	T50.2X3	T50.2X4	T50.2X5	T50.2X6
Zephiran (topical)	T49.0X1	T49.0X2	T49.0X3	T49.0X4	T49.0X5	T49.0X6
ophthalmic preparation	T49.5X1	T49.5X2	T49.5X3	T49.5X4	T49.5X5	T49.5X6
Zeranol	T38.7X1	T38.7X2	T38.7X3	T38.7X4	T38.7X5	T38.7X6
Zerone	T51.1X1	T51.1X2	T51.1X3	T51.1X4	—	—
Zidovudine	T37.5X1	T37.5X2	T37.5X3	T37.5X4	T37.5X5	T37.5X6
Zimeldine	T43.221	T43.222	T43.223	T43.224	T43.225	T43.226
Zinc (compounds) (fumes) (vapor) NEC	T56.5X1	T56.5X2	T56.5X3	T56.5X4	—	—
anti-infectives	T49.0X1	T49.0X2	T49.0X3	T49.0X4	T49.0X5	T49.0X6
antivaricose	T46.8X1	T46.8X2	T46.8X3	T46.8X4	T46.8X5	T46.8X6
bacitracin	T49.0X1	T49.0X2	T49.0X3	T49.0X4	T49.0X5	T49.0X6
chloride (mouthwash)	T49.6X1	T49.6X2	T49.6X3	T49.6X4	T49.6X5	T49.6X6
chromate	T56.5X1	T56.5X2	T56.5X3	T56.5X4	—	—
gelatin	T49.3X1	T49.3X2	T49.3X3	T49.3X4	T49.3X5	T49.3X6
oxide	T49.3X1	T49.3X2	T49.3X3	T49.3X4	T49.3X5	T49.3X6
plaster	T49.3X1	T49.3X2	T49.3X3	T49.3X4	T49.3X5	T49.3X6
peroxide	T49.0X1	T49.0X2	T49.0X3	T49.0X4	T49.0X5	T49.0X6
pesticides	T56.5X1	T56.5X2	T56.5X3	T56.5X4	—	—
phosphide	T60.4X1	T60.4X2	T60.4X3	T60.4X4	—	—
pyrithionate	T49.4X1	T49.4X2	T49.4X3	T49.4X4	T49.4X5	T49.4X6
stearate	T49.3X1	T49.3X2	T49.3X3	T49.3X4	T49.3X5	T49.3X6
sulfate	T49.5X1	T49.5X2	T49.5X3	T49.5X4	T49.5X5	T49.5X6
ENT agent	T49.6X1	T49.6X2	T49.6X3	T49.6X4	T49.6X5	T49.6X6
ophthalmic solution	T49.5X1	T49.5X2	T49.5X3	T49.5X4	T49.5X5	T49.5X6
topical NEC	T49.0X1	T49.0X2	T49.0X3	T49.0X4	T49.0X5	T49.0X6
undecylenate	T49.0X1	T49.0X2	T49.0X3	T49.0X4	T49.0X5	T49.0X6

◀ New   ◀|| Revised   ~~deleted~~ Deleted

| Substance | External Cause (T-Code) | | | | | |
	Poisoning, Accidental (Unintentional)	Poisoning, Intentional Self-Harm	Poisoning, Assault	Poisoning, Undetermined	Adverse Effect	Underdosing
Zineb	T60.0X1	T60.0X2	T60.0X3	T60.0X4	—	—
Zinostatin	T45.1X1	T45.1X2	T45.1X3	T45.1X4	T45.1X5	T45.1X6
Zipeprol	T48.3X1	T48.3X2	T48.3X3	T48.3X4	T48.3X5	T48.3X6
Zofenopril	T46.4X1	T46.4X2	T46.4X3	T46.4X4	T46.4X5	T46.4X6
Zolpidem	T42.6X1	T42.6X2	T42.6X3	T42.6X4	T42.6X5	T42.6X6
Zomepirac	T39.391	T39.392	T39.393	T39.394	T39.395	T39.396
Zopiclone	T42.6X1	T42.6X2	T42.6X3	T42.6X4	T42.6X5	T42.6X6

| Substance | External Cause (T-Code) | | | | | |
	Poisoning, Accidental (Unintentional)	Poisoning, Intentional Self-Harm	Poisoning, Assault	Poisoning, Undetermined	Adverse Effect	Underdosing
Zorubicin	T45.1X1	T45.1X2	T45.1X3	T45.1X4	T45.1X5	T45.1X6
Zotepine	T43.591	T43.592	T43.593	T43.594	T43.595	T43.596
Zovant	T45.511	T45.512	T45.513	T45.514	T45.515	T45.516
Zoxazolamine	T42.8X1	T42.8X2	T42.8X3	T42.8X4	T42.8X5	T42.8X6
Zuclopenthixol	T43.4X1	T43.4X2	T43.4X3	T43.4X4	T43.4X5	T43.4X6
Zygadenus (venenosus)	T62.2X1	T62.2X2	T62.2X3	T62.2X4	—	—
Zyprexa	T43.591	T43.592	T43.593	T43.594	T43.595	T43.596

◀ New   ◀ Revised   ~~deleted~~ Deleted

TABLE OF DRUGS AND CHEMICALS

External Cause
of Injuries Index

ICD-10-CM EXTERNAL CAUSE OF INJURIES INDEX

A

Abandonment (causing exposure to weather conditions) (with intent to injure or kill) NEC X58

Abuse (adult) (child) (mental) (physical) (sexual) X58

Accident (to) X58
- aircraft (in transit) (powered) —see also Accident, transport, aircraft
  - due to, caused by cataclysm —see Forces of nature, by type
- animal-drawn vehicle —see Accident, transport, animal-drawn vehicle occupant
- animal-rider —see Accident, transport, animal-rider
- automobile —see Accident, transport, car occupant
- bare foot water skiier V94.4
- boat, boating —see also Accident, watercraft
  - striking swimmer
    - powered V94.11
    - unpowered V94.12
- bus —see Accident, transport, bus occupant
- cable car, not on rails V98.0
  - on rails —see Accident, transport, streetcar occupant
- car —see Accident, transport, car occupant
- caused by, due to
  - animal NEC W64
  - chain hoist W24.0
  - cold (excessive) —see Exposure, cold
  - corrosive liquid, substance —see Table of Drugs and Chemicals
  - cutting or piercing instrument —see Contact, with, by type of instrument
  - drive belt W24.0
  - electric
    - current —see Exposure, electric current
    - motor —see also Contact, with, by type of machine W31.3
    - current (of) W86.8
  - environmental factor NEC X58
  - explosive material —see Explosion
  - fire, flames —see Exposure, fire
  - firearm missile —see Discharge, firearm by type
  - heat (excessive) —see Heat
  - hot —see Contact, with, hot
  - ignition —see Ignition
  - lifting device W24.0
  - lightning —see subcategory T75.0
    - causing fire —see Exposure, fire
  - machine, machinery —see Contact, with, by type of machine
  - natural factor NEC X58
  - pulley (block) W24.0
  - radiation —see Radiation
  - steam X13.1
    - inhalation X13.0
    - pipe X16
  - thunderbolt —see subcategory T75.0
    - causing fire —see Exposure, fire
  - transmission device W24.1
- coach —see Accident, transport, bus occupant
- coal car —see Accident, transport, industrial vehicle occupant
- diving —see also Fall, into, water
  - with
    - drowning or submersion —see Drowning
- forklift —see Accident, transport, industrial vehicle occupant
- heavy transport vehicle NOS —see Accident, transport, truck occupant
- ice yacht V98.2

Accident (Continued)
- in
  - medical, surgical procedure
    - as, or due to misadventure —see Misadventure
    - causing an abnormal reaction or later complication without mention of misadventure —see also Complication of or following, by type of procedure Y84.9
- land yacht V98.1
- late effect of —see W00-X58 with 7th character S
- logging car —see Accident, transport, industrial vehicle occupant
- machine, machinery —see also Contact, with, by type of machine
  - on board watercraft V93.69
    - explosion —see Explosion, in, watercraft
    - fire —see Burn, on board watercraft
    - powered craft V93.63
      - ferry boat V93.61
      - fishing boat V93.62
      - jet ski V93.63
      - liner V93.61
      - merchant ship V93.60
      - passenger ship V93.61
      - sailboat V93.64
- mine tram —see Accident, transport, industrial vehicle occupant
- mobility scooter (motorized) —see Accident, transport, pedestrian, conveyance, specified type NEC
- motor scooter —see Accident, transport, motorcyclist
- motor vehicle NOS (traffic) —see also Accident, transport V89.2
  - nontraffic V89.0
  - three-wheeled NOS —see Accident, transport, three-wheeled motor vehicle occupant
- motorcycle NOS —see Accident, transport, motorcyclist
- nonmotor vehicle NOS (nontraffic) —see also Accident, transport V89.1
  - traffic NOS V89.3
- nontraffic (victim's mode of transport NOS) V88.9
  - collision (between) V88.7
    - bus and truck V88.5
    - car and:
      - bus V88.3
      - pickup V88.2
      - three-wheeled motor vehicle V88.0
      - train V88.6
      - truck V88.4
      - two-wheeled motor vehicle V88.0
      - van V88.2
    - specified vehicle NEC and:
      - three-wheeled motor vehicle V88.1
      - two-wheeled motor vehicle V88.1
  - known mode of transport —see Accident, transport, by type of vehicle
  - noncollision V88.8
- on board watercraft V93.89
  - powered craft V93.83
    - ferry boat V93.81
    - fishing boat V93.82
    - jet ski V93.83
    - liner V93.81
    - merchant ship V93.80
    - passenger ship V93.81
  - unpowered craft V93.88
    - canoe V93.85
    - inflatable V93.86
      - in tow
        - recreational V94.31
        - specified NEC V94.32
    - kayak V93.85

Accident (Continued)
- on board watercraft (Continued)
  - unpowered craft (Continued)
    - sailboat V93.84
    - surf-board V93.88
    - water skis V93.87
    - windsurfer V93.88
- parachutist V97.29
  - entangled in object V97.21
  - injured on landing V97.22
- pedal cycle —see Accident, transport, pedal cyclist
- pedestrian (on foot)
  - with
    - another pedestrian W51
      - with fall W03
        - due to ice or snow W00.0
      - on pedestrian conveyance NEC V00.09
    - rider of
      - hoverboard V00.038
      - Segway V00.038
      - standing
        - electric scooter V00.031
        - micro-mobility pedestrian conveyance NEC V00.038
      - roller skater (in-line) V00.01
      - skate boarder V00.02
    - transport vehicle —see Accident, transport
  - on pedestrian conveyance —see Accident, transport, pedestrian, conveyance
- pick-up truck or van —see Accident, transport, pickup truck occupant
- quarry truck —see Accident, transport, industrial vehicle occupant
- railway vehicle (any) (in motion) —see Accident, transport, railway vehicle occupant
  - due to cataclysm —see Forces of nature, by type
- scooter (non-motorized) —see Accident, transport, pedestrian, conveyance, scooter
- sequelae of —see W00-X58 with 7th character S
- skateboard —see Accident, transport, pedestrian, conveyance, skateboard
- ski (ing) —see Accident, transport, pedestrian, conveyance
  - lift V98.3
- specified cause NEC X58
- streetcar —see Accident, transport, streetcar occupant
- traffic (victim's mode of transport NOS) V87.9
  - collision (between) V87.7
    - bus and truck V87.5
    - car and:
      - bus V87.3
      - pickup V87.2
      - three-wheeled motor vehicle V87.0
      - train V87.6
      - truck V87.4
      - two-wheeled motor vehicle V87.0
      - van V87.2
    - specified vehicle NEC V86.39
      - and
        - three-wheeled motor vehicle V87.1
        - two-wheeled motor vehicle V87.1
    - driver V86.09
    - person on outside V86.29
    - passenger V86.19
    - while boarding or alighting V86.49
  - known mode of transport —see Accident, transport, by type of vehicle
  - noncollision V87.8

▶ New　⇒ Revised　~~deleted~~ Deleted　● Use Additional Character(s)

Accident *(Continued)*
 transport (involving injury to) V99
  18 wheeler —*see* Accident, transport, truck
   occupant
  agricultural vehicle occupant (nontraffic)
   V84.9
   driver V84.5
   hanger-on V84.7
   passenger V84.6
   traffic V84.3
    driver V84.0
    hanger-on V84.2
    passenger V84.1
   while boarding or alighting
    V84.4
  aircraft NEC V97.89
   military NEC V97.818
    with civilian aircraft V97.810
    civilian injured by V97.811
   occupant injured (in)
    nonpowered craft accident V96.9
     balloon V96.00
      collision V96.03
      crash V96.01
      explosion V96.05
      fire V96.04
      forced landing V96.02
      specified type NEC V96.09
     glider V96.20
      collision V96.23
      crash V96.21
      explosion V96.25
      fire V96.24
      forced landing V96.22
      specified type NEC V96.29
     hang glider V96.10
      collision V96.13
      crash V96.11
      explosion V96.15
      fire V96.14
      forced landing V96.12
      specified type NEC V96.19
     specified craft NEC V96.8
    powered craft accident V95.9
     fixed wing NEC
      commercial V95.30
       collision V95.33
       crash V95.31
       explosion V95.35
       fire V95.34
       forced landing V95.32
       specified type NEC V95.39
      private V95.20
       collision V95.23
       crash V95.21
       explosion V95.25
       fire V95.24
       forced landing V95.22
       specified type NEC V95.29
     glider V95.10
      collision V95.13
      crash V95.11
      explosion V95.15
      fire V95.14
      forced landing V95.12
      specified type NEC V95.19
     helicopter V95.00
      collision V95.03
      crash V95.01
      explosion V95.05
      fire V95.04
      forced landing V95.02
      specified type NEC V95.09
     spacecraft V95.40
      collision V95.43
      crash V95.41
      explosion V95.45
      fire V95.44
      forced landing V95.42
      specified type NEC V95.49
     specified craft NEC V95.8

Accident *(Continued)*
 transport *(Continued)*
  aircraft NEC *(Continued)*
   occupant injured *(Continued)*
     powered craft accident *(Continued)*
      ultralight V95.10
       collision V95.13
       crash V95.11
       explosion V95.15
       fire V95.14
       forced landing V95.12
       specified type NEC V95.19
     specified accident NEC V97.0
    while boarding or alighting V97.1
   person (injured by)
    falling from, in or on aircraft V97.0
    machinery on aircraft V97.89
    on ground with aircraft involvement
     V97.39
    rotating propeller V97.32
    struck by object falling from aircraft
     V97.31
    sucked into aircraft jet V97.33
    while boarding or alighting aircraft
     V97.1
  airport (battery-powered) passenger
   vehicle —*see* Accident, transport,
   industrial vehicle occupant
  all-terrain vehicle occupant (nontraffic)
   V86.95
   driver V86.55
   dune buggy —*see* Accident, transport,
    dune buggy occupant
   hanger-on V86.75
   passenger V86.65
   snowmobile —*see* Accident, transport,
    snowmobile occupant
   specified type NEC V86.99
    driver V86.59
    passenger V86.69
    person on outside V86.79
   traffic V86.35
    driver V86.05
    hanger-on V86.25
    passenger V86.15
   while boarding or alighting V86.45
  ambulance occupant (traffic) V86.31
   driver V86.01
   hanger-on V86.21
   nontraffic V86.91
    driver V86.51
    hanger-on V86.71
    passenger V86.61
   passenger V86.11
   while boarding or alighting V86.41
  animal-drawn vehicle occupant (in) V80.929
   collision (with)
    animal V80.12
     being ridden V80.711
    animal-drawn vehicle V80.721
    bus V80.42
    car V80.42
    fixed or stationary object V80.82
    military vehicle V80.920
    nonmotor vehicle V80.791
    pedal cycle V80.22
    pedestrian V80.12
    pickup V80.42
    railway train or vehicle V80.62
    specified motor vehicle NEC V80.52
    streetcar V80.731
    truck V80.42
    two-or three-wheeled motor vehicle
     V80.32
    van V80.42
   noncollision V80.02
   specified circumstance NEC V80. 928
  animal-rider V80.919
   collision (with)
    animal V80.11
     being ridden V80.710

Accident *(Continued)*
 transport *(Continued)*
  animal-rider *(Continued)*
   collision *(Continued)*
    animal-drawn vehicle V80.720
    bus V80.41
    car V80.41
    fixed or stationary object V80.81
    military vehicle V80.910
    nonmotor vehicle V80.790
    pedal cycle V80.21
    pedestrian V80.11
    pickup V80.41
    railway train or vehicle V80.61
    specified motor vehicle NEC V80.51
    streetcar V80.730
    truck V80.41
    two- or three-wheeled motor vehicle
     V80.31
    van V80.41
   noncollision V80.018
    specified as horse rider V80.010
   specified circumstance NEC V80.918
  armored car —*see* Accident, transport,
   truck occupant
  battery-powered truck (baggage) (mail) —
   see Accident, transport, industrial
   vehicle occupant
  bus occupant V79.9
   collision (with)
    animal (traffic) V70.9
     being ridden (traffic) V76.9
      nontraffic V76.3
       while boarding or alighting V76.4
     nontraffic V70.3
      while boarding or alighting V70.4
    animal-drawn vehicle (traffic) V76.9
     nontraffic V76.3
      while boarding or alighting V76.4
    bus (traffic) V74.9
     nontraffic V74.3
      while boarding or alighting V74.4
    car (traffic) V73.9
     nontraffic V73.3
      while boarding or alighting V73.4
    motor vehicle NOS (traffic) V79.60
     nontraffic V79.20
     specified type NEC (traffic) V79.69
      nontraffic V79.29
    pedal cycle (traffic) V71.9
     nontraffic V71.3
      while boarding or alighting V71.4
    pickup truck (traffic) V73.9
     nontraffic V73.3
      while boarding or alighting V73.4
    railway vehicle (traffic) V75.9
     nontraffic V75.3
      while boarding or alighting V75.4
    specified vehicle NEC (traffic) V76.9
     nontraffic V76.3
      while boarding or alighting V76.4
    stationary object (traffic) V77.9
     nontraffic V77.3
      while boarding or alighting V77.4
    streetcar (traffic) V76.9
     nontraffic V76.3
      while boarding or alighting V76.4
    three wheeled motor vehicle (traffic)
     V72.9
     nontraffic V72.3
      while boarding or alighting V72.4
    truck (traffic) V74.9
     nontraffic V74.3
      while boarding or alighting V74.4
    two wheeled motor vehicle (traffic)
     V72.9
     nontraffic V72.3
      while boarding or alighting V72.4
    van (traffic) V73.9
     nontraffic V73.3
      while boarding or alighting V73.4

Accident (Continued)
  transport (Continued)
    bus occupant (Continued)
      driver
        collision (with)
          animal (traffic) V70.5
            being ridden (traffic) V76.5
              nontraffic V76.0
            nontraffic V70.0
          animal-drawn vehicle (traffic) V76.5
            nontraffic V76.0
          bus (traffic) V74.5
            nontraffic V74.0
          car (traffic) V73.5
            nontraffic V73.0
          motor vehicle NOS (traffic) V79.40
            nontraffic V79.00
            specified type NEC (traffic) V79.49
              nontraffic V79.09
          pedal cycle (traffic) V71.5
            nontraffic V71.0
          pickup truck (traffic) V73.5
            nontraffic V73.0
          railway vehicle (traffic) V75.5
            nontraffic V75.0
          specified vehicle NEC (traffic) V76.5
            nontraffic V76.0
          stationary object (traffic) V77.5
            nontraffic V77.0
          streetcar (traffic) V76.5
            nontraffic V76.0
          three wheeled motor vehicle (traffic) V72.5
            nontraffic V72.0
          truck (traffic) V74.5
            nontraffic V74.0
          two wheeled motor vehicle (traffic) V72.5
            nontraffic V72.0
          van (traffic) V73.5
            nontraffic V73.0
        noncollision accident (traffic) V78.5
          nontraffic V78.0
      hanger-on
        collision (with)
          animal (traffic) V70.7
            being ridden (traffic) V76.7
              nontraffic V76.2
            nontraffic V70.2
          animal-drawn vehicle (traffic) V76.7
            nontraffic V76.2
          bus (traffic) V74.7
            nontraffic V74.2
          car (traffic) V73.7
            nontraffic V73.2
          pedal cycle (traffic) V71.7
            nontraffic V71.2
          pickup truck (traffic) V73.7
            nontraffic V73.2
          railway vehicle (traffic) V75.7
            nontraffic V75.2
          specified vehicle NEC (traffic) V76.7
            nontraffic V76.2
          stationary object (traffic) V77.7
            nontraffic V77.2
          streetcar (traffic) V76.7
            nontraffic V76.2
          three wheeled motor vehicle (traffic) V72.7
            nontraffic V72.2
          truck (traffic) V74.7
            nontraffic V74.2
          two wheeled motor vehicle (traffic) V72.7
            nontraffic V72.2
          van (traffic) V73.7
            nontraffic V73.2
        noncollision accident (traffic) V78.7
          nontraffic V78.2

Accident (Continued)
  transport (Continued)
    bus occupant (Continued)
      noncollision accident (traffic) V78.9
        nontraffic V78.3
        while boarding or alighting V78.4
      nontraffic V79.3
      passenger
        collision (with)
          animal (traffic) V70.6
            being ridden (traffic) V76.6
              nontraffic V76.1
            nontraffic V70.1
          animal-drawn vehicle (traffic) V76.6
            nontraffic V76.1
          bus (traffic) V74.6
            nontraffic V74.1
          car (traffic) V73.6
            nontraffic V73.1
          motor vehicle NOS (traffic) V79.50
            nontraffic V79.10
            specified type NEC (traffic) V79.59
              nontraffic V79.19
          pedal cycle (traffic) V71.6
            nontraffic V71.1
          pickup truck (traffic) V73.6
            nontraffic V73.1
          railway vehicle (traffic) V75.6
            nontraffic V75.1
          specified vehicle NEC (traffic) V76.6
            nontraffic V76.1
          stationary object (traffic) V77.6
            nontraffic V77.1
          streetcar (traffic) V76.6
            nontraffic V76.1
          three wheeled motor vehicle (traffic) V72.6
            nontraffic V72.1
          truck (traffic) V74.6
            nontraffic V74.1
          two wheeled motor vehicle (traffic) V72.6
            nontraffic V72.1
          van (traffic) V73.6
            nontraffic V73.1
        noncollision accident (traffic) V78.6
          nontraffic V78.1
      specified type NEC V79.88
      military vehicle V79.81
    cable car, not on rails V98.0
      on rails —see Accident, transport, streetcar occupant
    car occupant V49.9
      ambulance occupant —see Accident, transport, ambulance occupant
      collision (with)
        animal (traffic) V40.9
          being ridden (traffic) V46.9
            nontraffic V46.3
            while boarding or alighting V46.4
          nontraffic V40.3
          while boarding or alighting V40.4
        animal-drawn vehicle (traffic) V46.9
          nontraffic V46.3
          while boarding or alighting V46.4
        bus (traffic) V44.9
          nontraffic V44.3
          while boarding or alighting V44.4
        car (traffic) V43.92
          nontraffic V43.32
          while boarding or alighting V43.42
        motor vehicle NOS (traffic) V49.60
          nontraffic V49.20
          specified type NEC (traffic) V49.69
            nontraffic V49.29
        pedal cycle (traffic) V41.9
          nontraffic V41.3
          while boarding or alighting V41.4

Accident (Continued)
  transport (Continued)
    car occupant (Continued)
      collision (Continued)
        pickup truck (traffic) V43.93
          nontraffic V43.33
          while boarding or alighting V43.43
        railway vehicle (traffic) V45.9
          nontraffic V45.3
          while boarding or alighting V45.4
        specified vehicle NEC (traffic) V46.9
          nontraffic V46.3
          while boarding or alighting V46.4
        sport utility vehicle (traffic) V43.91
          nontraffic V43.31
          while boarding or alighting V43.41
        stationary object (traffic) V47.9
          nontraffic V47.3
          while boarding or alighting V47.4
        streetcar (traffic) V46.9
          nontraffic V46.3
          while boarding or alighting V46.4
        three wheeled motor vehicle (traffic) V42.9
          nontraffic V42.3
          while boarding or alighting V42.4
        truck (traffic) V44.9
          nontraffic V44.3
          while boarding or alighting V44.4
        two wheeled motor vehicle (traffic) V42.9
          nontraffic V42.3
          while boarding or alighting V42.4
        van (traffic) V43.94
          nontraffic V43.34
          while boarding or alighting V43.44
      driver
        collision (with)
          animal (traffic) V40.5
           being ridden (traffic) V46.5
            nontraffic V46.0
           nontraffic V40.0
          animal-drawn vehicle (traffic) V46.5
           nontraffic V46.0
          bus (traffic) V44.5
           nontraffic V44.0
          car (traffic) V43.52
           nontraffic V43.02
          motor vehicle NOS (traffic) V49.40
           nontraffic V49.00
           specified type NEC (traffic) V49.49
            nontraffic V49.09
          pedal cycle (traffic) V41.5
           nontraffic V41.0
          pickup truck (traffic) V43.53
           nontraffic V43.03
          railway vehicle (traffic) V45.5
           nontraffic V45.0
          specified vehicle NEC (traffic) V46.5
           nontraffic V46.0
          sport utility vehicle (traffic) V43.51
           nontraffic V43.01
          stationary object (traffic) V47.5
           nontraffic V47.0
          streetcar (traffic) V46.5
           nontraffic V46.0
          three wheeled motor vehicle (traffic) V42.5
           nontraffic V42.0
          truck (traffic) V44.5
           nontraffic V44.0
          two wheeled motor vehicle (traffic) V42.5
           nontraffic V42.0
          van (traffic) V43.54
           nontraffic V43.04
        noncollision accident (traffic) V48.5
          nontraffic V48.0

▶ New   ⇒ Revised   ~~deleted~~ Deleted   ● Use Additional Character(s)

Accident *(Continued)*
  transport *(Continued)*
    car occupant *(Continued)*
      hanger-on
        collision (with)
          animal (traffic) V40.7
            being ridden (traffic) V46.7
              nontraffic V46.2
            nontraffic V40.2
          animal-drawn vehicle (traffic) V46.7
            nontraffic V46.2
          bus (traffic) V44.7
            nontraffic V44.2
          car (traffic) V43.72
            nontraffic V43.22
          pedal cycle (traffic) V41.7
            nontraffic V41.2
          pickup truck (traffic) V43.73
            nontraffic V43.23
          railway vehicle (traffic) V45.7
            nontraffic V45.2
          specified vehicle NEC (traffic) V46.7
            nontraffic V46.2
          sport utility vehicle (traffic) V43.71
            nontraffic V43.21
          stationary object (traffic) V47.7
            nontraffic V47.2
          streetcar (traffic) V46.7
            nontraffic V46.2
          three wheeled motor vehicle (traffic) V42.7
            nontraffic V42.2
          truck (traffic) V44.7
            nontraffic V44.2
          two wheeled motor vehicle (traffic) V42.7
            nontraffic V42.2
          van (traffic) V43.74
            nontraffic V43.24
        noncollision accident (traffic) V48.7
          nontraffic V48.2
      noncollision accident (traffic) V48.9
        nontraffic V48.3
        while boarding or alighting V48.4
      nontraffic V49.3
      passenger
        collision (with)
          animal (traffic) V40.6
            being ridden (traffic) V46.6
              nontraffic V46.1
            nontraffic V40.1
          animal-drawn vehicle (traffic) V46.6
            nontraffic V46.1
          bus (traffic) V44.6
            nontraffic V44.1
          car (traffic) V43.62
            nontraffic V43.12
          motor vehicle NOS (traffic) V49.50
            nontraffic V49.10
            specified type NEC (traffic) V49.59
              nontraffic V49.19
          pedal cycle (traffic) V41.6
            nontraffic V41.1
          pickup truck (traffic) V43.63
            nontraffic V43.13
          railway vehicle (traffic) V45.6
            nontraffic V45.1
          specified vehicle NEC (traffic) V46.6
            nontraffic V46.1
          sport utility vehicle (traffic) V43.61
            nontraffic V43.11
          stationary object (traffic) V47.6
            nontraffic V47.1
          streetcar (traffic) V46.6
            nontraffic V46.1
          three wheeled motor vehicle (traffic) V42.6
            nontraffic V42.1
          truck (traffic) V44.6
            nontraffic V44.1

Accident *(Continued)*
  transport *(Continued)*
    car occupant *(Continued)*
      passenger *(Continued)*
        collision *(Continued)*
          two wheeled motor vehicle (traffic) V42.6
            nontraffic V42.1
          van (traffic) V43.64
            nontraffic V43.14
        noncollision accident (traffic) V48.6
          nontraffic V48.1
        specified type NEC V49.88
        military vehicle V49.81
      coal car —*see* Accident, transport, industrial vehicle occupant
      construction vehicle occupant (nontraffic) V85.9
        driver V85.5
        hanger-on V85.7
        passenger V85.6
        traffic V85.3
          driver V85.0
          hanger-on V85.2
          passenger V85.1
        while boarding or alighting V85.4
      dirt bike rider (nontraffic) V86.96
        driver V86.56
        hanger-on V86.76
        passenger V86.66
        traffic V86.36
          driver V86.06
          hanger-on V86.26
          passenger V86.16
        while boarding or alighting V86.46
      due to cataclysm —*see* Forces of nature, by type
      dune buggy occupant (nontraffic) V86.93
        driver V86.53
        hanger-on V86.73
        passenger V86.63
        traffic V86.33
          driver V86.03
          hanger-on V86.23
          passenger V86.13
        while boarding or alighting V86.43
      forklift —*see* Accident, transport, industrial vehicle occupant
      go cart —*see* Accident, transport, all-terrain vehicle occupant
      golf cart —*see* Accident, transport, all-terrain vehicle occupant
      heavy transport vehicle occupant — *see* Accident, transport, truck occupant
      hoverboard V00.848
      ice yacht V98.2
      industrial vehicle occupant (nontraffic) V83.9
        driver V83.5
        hanger-on V83.7
        passenger V83.6
        traffic V83.3
          driver V83.0
          hanger-on V83.2
          passenger V83.1
        while boarding or alighting V83.4
      interurban electric car —*see* Accident, transport, streetcar
      land yacht V98.1
      logging car —*see* Accident, transport, industrial vehicle occupant
      military vehicle occupant (traffic) V86.34
        driver V86.04
        hanger-on V86.24
        nontraffic V86.94
          driver V86.54
          hanger-on V86.74
          passenger V86.64
        passenger V86.14
        while boarding or alighting V86.44

Accident *(Continued)*
  transport *(Continued)*
    mine tram —*see* Accident, transport, industrial vehicle occupant
    motor vehicle NEC occupant (traffic) V89.2
    motorcoach —*see* Accident, transport, bus occupant
    motor/cross bike rider —*see also* Accident, transport, dirt bike rider V86.96
    motorcyclist V29.9
      collision (with)
        animal (traffic) V20.9
          being ridden (traffic) V26.9
            nontraffic V26.2
            while boarding or alighting V26.3
          nontraffic V20.2
          while boarding or alighting V20.3
        animal-drawn vehicle (traffic) V26.9
          nontraffic V26.2
          while boarding or alighting V26.3
        bus (traffic) V24.9
          nontraffic V24.2
          while boarding or alighting V24.3
        car (traffic) V23.9
          nontraffic V23.2
          while boarding or alighting V23.3
        motor vehicle NOS (traffic) V29.60
          nontraffic V29.20
          specified type NEC (traffic) V29.69
            nontraffic V29.29
        pedal cycle (traffic) V21.9
          nontraffic V21.2
          while boarding or alighting V21.3
        pickup truck (traffic) V23.9
          nontraffic V23.2
          while boarding or alighting V23.3
        railway vehicle (traffic) V25.9
          nontraffic V25.2
          while boarding or alighting V25.3
        specified vehicle NEC (traffic) V26.9
          nontraffic V26.2
          while boarding or alighting V26.3
        stationary object (traffic) V27.9
          nontraffic V27.2
          while boarding or alighting V27.3
        streetcar (traffic) V26.9
          nontraffic V26.2
          while boarding or alighting V26.3
        three wheeled motor vehicle (traffic) V22.9
          nontraffic V22.2
          while boarding or alighting V22.3
        truck (traffic) V24.9
          nontraffic V24.2
          while boarding or alighting V24.3
        two wheeled motor vehicle (traffic) V22.9
          nontraffic V22.2
          while boarding or alighting V22.3
        van (traffic) V23.9
          nontraffic V23.2
          while boarding or alighting V23.3
      driver
        collision (with)
          animal (traffic) V20.4
            being ridden (traffic) V26.4
              nontraffic V26.0
            nontraffic V20.0
          animal-drawn vehicle (traffic) V26.4
            nontraffic V26.0
          bus (traffic) V24.4
            nontraffic V24.0
          car (traffic) V23.4
            nontraffic V23.0
          motor vehicle NOS (traffic) V29.40
            nontraffic V29.00
            specified type NEC (traffic) V29.49
              nontraffic V29.09
          pedal cycle (traffic) V21.4
            nontraffic V21.0

Accident (Continued)
  transport (Continued)
    motorcyclist (Continued)
      driver (Continued)
        collision (Continued)
          pickup truck (traffic) V23.4
            nontraffic V23.0
          railway vehicle (traffic) V25.4
            nontraffic V25.0
          specified vehicle NEC (traffic) V26.4
            nontraffic V26.0
          stationary object (traffic) V27.4
            nontraffic V27.0
          streetcar (traffic) V26.4
            nontraffic V26.0
          three wheeled motor vehicle
              (traffic) V22.4
            nontraffic V22.0
          truck (traffic) V24.4
            nontraffic V24.0
          two wheeled motor vehicle (traffic)
              V22.4
            nontraffic V22.0
          van (traffic) V23.4
            nontraffic V23.0
        noncollision accident (traffic) V28.4
          nontraffic V28.0
      noncollision accident (traffic) V28.9
        nontraffic V28.2
        while boarding or alighting V28.3
      nontraffic V29.3
      passenger
        collision (with)
          animal (traffic) V20.5
            being ridden (traffic) V26.5
              nontraffic V26.1
            nontraffic V20.1
          animal-drawn vehicle (traffic) V26.5
            nontraffic V26.1
          bus (traffic) V24.5
            nontraffic V24.1
          car (traffic) V23.5
            nontraffic V23.1
          motor vehicle NOS (traffic) V29.50
            nontraffic V29.10
            specified type NEC (traffic)
                V29.59
              nontraffic V29.19
          pedal cycle (traffic) V21.5
            nontraffic V21.1
          pickup truck (traffic) V23.5
            nontraffic V23.1
          railway vehicle (traffic) V25.5
            nontraffic V25.1
          specified vehicle NEC (traffic) V26.5
            nontraffic V26.1
          stationary object (traffic) V27.5
            nontraffic V27.1
          streetcar (traffic) V26.5
            nontraffic V26.1
          three wheeled motor vehicle
              (traffic) V22.5
            nontraffic V22.1
          truck (traffic) V24.5
            nontraffic V24.1
          two wheeled motor vehicle (traffic)
              V22.5
            nontraffic V22.1
          van (traffic) V23.5
            nontraffic V23.1
        noncollision accident (traffic) V28.5
          nontraffic V28.1
      specified type NEC V29.88
      military vehicle V29.81
    occupant (of)
      aircraft (powered) V95.9
        fixed wing
          commercial —see Accident,
              transport, aircraft, occupant,
              powered, fixed wing,
              commercial

Accident (Continued)
  transport (Continued)
    occupant (Continued)
      aircraft (Continued)
        fixed wing (Continued)
          private —see Accident, transport,
              aircraft, occupant, powered,
              fixed wing, private
        nonpowered V96.9
        specified NEC V95.8
      airport battery-powered vehicle —see
          Accident, transport, industrial
          vehicle occupant
      all-terrain vehicle (ATV) —see Accident,
          transport, all-terrain vehicle
          occupant
      animal-drawn vehicle —see Accident,
          transport, animal-drawn vehicle
          occupant
      automobile —see Accident, transport, car
          occupant
      balloon V96.00
      battery-powered vehicle —see Accident,
          transport, industrial vehicle
          occupant
      bicycle —see Accident, transport, pedal
          cyclist
        motorized —see Accident, transport,
            motorcycle rider
      boat NEC —see Accident, watercraft
      bulldozer —see Accident, transport,
          construction vehicle occupant
      bus —see Accident, transport, bus
          occupant
      cable car (on rails) —see also Accident,
          transport, streetcar occupant
        not on rails V98.0
      car —see also Accident, transport, car
          occupant
        cable (on rails) —see also Accident,
            transport, streetcar occupant
          not on rails V98.0
      coach —see Accident, transport, bus
          occupant
      coal-car —see Accident, transport,
          industrial vehicle occupant
      digger —see Accident, transport,
          construction vehicle occupant
      dump truck —see Accident, transport,
          construction vehicle occupant
      earth-leveler —see Accident, transport,
          construction vehicle occupant
      farm machinery (self-propelled) —see
          Accident, transport, agricultural
          vehicle occupant
      forklift —see Accident, transport,
          industrial vehicle occupant
      glider (unpowered) V96.20
        hang V96.10
        powered (microlight) (ultralight) —see
            Accident, transport, aircraft,
            occupant, powered, glider
      glider (unpowered) NEC V96.20
      hang-glider V96.10
      harvester —see Accident, transport,
          agricultural vehicle occupant
      heavy (transport) vehicle —see Accident,
          transport, truck occupant
      helicopter —see Accident, transport,
          aircraft, occupant, helicopter
      ice-yacht V98.2
      kite (carrying person) V96.8
      land-yacht V98.1
      logging car —see Accident, transport,
          industrial vehicle occupant
      mechanical shovel —see Accident,
          transport, construction vehicle
          occupant
      microlight —see Accident, transport,
          aircraft, occupant, powered,
          glider

Accident (Continued)
  transport (Continued)
    occupant (Continued)
      minibus —see Accident, transport,
          pickup truck occupant
      minivan —see Accident, transport,
          pickup truck occupant
      moped —see Accident, transport,
          motorcycle
      motor scooter —see Accident, transport,
          motorcycle
      motorcycle (with sidecar) —see Accident,
          transport, motorcycle
      off-road motor-vehicle —see also
          Accident, transport, all-terrain
          vehicle occupant V86.99
      pedal cycle —see also Accident,
          transport, pedal cyclist
      pick-up (truck) —see Accident, transport,
          pickup truck occupant
      railway (train) (vehicle) (subterranean)
          (elevated) —see Accident, transport,
          railway vehicle occupant
      rickshaw —see Accident, transport,
          pedal cycle
        pedal driven —see Accident, transport,
            pedal cyclist
      road-roller —see Accident, transport,
          construction vehicle occupant
      ship NOS V94.9
      ski-lift (chair) (gondola) V98.3
      snowmobile —see Accident, transport,
          snowmobile occupant
      spacecraft, spaceship —see Accident,
          transport, aircraft, occupant,
          spacecraft
      sport utility vehicle —see Accident,
          transport, pickup truck occupant
      streetcar (interurban) (operating on
          public street or highway) —see
          Accident, transport, streetcar
          occupant
      SUV —see Accident, transport, pickup
          truck occupant
      téléférique V98.0
      three-wheeled vehicle (motorized) —see
          also Accident, transport, three-
          wheeled motor vehicle occupant
        nonmotorized —see Accident,
            transport, pedal cycle
      tractor (farm) (and trailer) —see
          Accident, transport, agricultural
          vehicle occupant
      train —see Accident, transport, railway
          vehicle occupant
      tram —see Accident, transport, streetcar
          occupant
        in mine or quarry —see Accident,
            transport, industrial vehicle
            occupant
      tricycle —see Accident, transport, pedal
          cycle
        motorized —see Accident, transport,
            three-wheeled motor vehicle
      trolley —see Accident, transport,
          streetcar occupant
        in mine or quarry —see Accident,
            transport, industrial vehicle
            occupant
      tub, in mine or quarry —see Accident,
          transport, industrial vehicle
          occupant
      ultralight —see Accident, transport,
          aircraft, occupant, powered, glider
      van —see Accident, transport, van
          occupant
      vehicle NEC V89.9
        heavy transport —see Accident,
            transport, truck occupant
        motor (traffic) NEC V89.2
          nontraffic NEC V89.0

▶ New   ⇒ Revised   ~~deleted~~ Deleted   ● Use Additional Character(s)

Accident (Continued)
 transport (Continued)
  pedestrian (Continued)
   conveyance (Continued)
    flat-bottomed NEC (Continued)
     collision (Continued)
      vehicle (Continued)
       motor
        nontraffic V09.00
        traffic V09.20
      fall V00.381
      nontraffic V09.1
       involving motor vehicle NEC
        V09.00
      snow
       board —see Accident, transport,
        pedestrian, conveyance,
        snow board
       ski —see Accident, transport,
        pedestrian, conveyance, skis
        (snow)
      traffic V09.3
       involving motor vehicle NEC
        V09.20
    gliding type NEC V00.288
     collision (with) V09.9
      animal being ridden or animal
       drawn vehicle V06.99
       nontraffic V06.09
       traffic V06.19
      bus or heavy transport
       V04.99
       nontraffic V04.09
       traffic V04.19
      car V03.99
       nontraffic V03.09
       traffic V03.19
      pedal cycle V01.99
       nontraffic V01.09
       traffic V01.19
      pick-up truck or van V03.99
       nontraffic V03.09
       traffic V03.19
      railway (train) (vehicle) V05.99
       nontraffic V05.09
       traffic V05.19
      stationary object V00.282
      streetcar V06.99
       nontraffic V06.09
       traffic V06.19
      two- or three-wheeled motor
       vehicle V02.99
       nontraffic V02.09
       traffic V02.19
      vehicle V09.9
       animal-drawn V06.99
        nontraffic V06.09
        traffic V06.19
       motor
        nontraffic V09.00
        traffic V09.20
     fall V00.281
     heelies —see Accident, transport,
      pedestrian, conveyance,
      heelies
     hoverboard
      collision with
       animal being ridden or animal
        drawn vehicle V06.938
        nontraffic V06.038
        traffic V06.138
       bus or heavy transport
        V04.938
        nontraffic V04.038
        traffic V04.138
       car V03.938
        nontraffic V03.038
        traffic V03.138
       pedal cycle V01.938
        nontraffic V01.038
        traffic V01.138

Accident (Continued)
 transport (Continued)
  pedestrian (Continued)
   conveyance (Continued)
    gliding type NEC (Continued)
     hoverboard (Continued)
      collision with (Continued)
       pick-up or van V03.938
        nontraffic V03.038
        traffic V03.138
       railway (train) (vehicle) V05.938
        nontraffic V05.038
        traffic V05.138
       streetcar V06.938
        nontraffic V06.038
        traffic V06.138
       three-wheeled motor vehicle
        V02.938
        nontraffic V02.038
        traffic V02.138
       two-wheeled motor vehicle
        V02.938
        nontraffic V02.038
        traffic V02.138
       vehicle, nonmotor, specified
        NEC V06.938
        nontraffic V06.038
        traffic V06.138
      fall V00.848
     ice skate —see Accident, transport,
      pedestrian, conveyance, ice
      skate
     nontraffic V09.1
      involving motor vehicle NEC
       V09.00
     Segway
      collision with
       animal being ridden or animal
        drawn vehicle V06.938
        nontraffic V06.038
        traffic V06.138
       bus or heavy transport V04.938
        nontraffic V04.038
        traffic V04.138
       car V03.938
        nontraffic V03.038
        traffic V03.138
       pedal cycle V01.938
        nontraffic V01.038
        traffic V01.138
       pick-up or van V03.038
        nontraffic V01.038
        traffic V03.138
       railway (train) (vehicle) V05.938
        nontraffic V05.038
        traffic V05.138
       streetcar V06.938
        nontraffic V06.038
        traffic V06.138
       three-wheeled motor vehicle
        V02.938
        nontraffic V02.038
        traffic V02.138
       two-wheeled motor vehicle
        V02.938
        nontraffic V02.038
        traffic V02.138
       vehicle, nonmotor, specified
        NEC V06.938
        nontraffic V06.038
        traffic V06.138
      fall V00.848
     sled —see Accident, transport,
      pedestrian, conveyance, sled
    standing
     electric scooter
      collision with
       animal being ridden or
        animal drawn vehicle
        V06.931
        nontraffic V06.031
        traffic V06.131

Accident (Continued)
 transport (Continued)
  pedestrian (Continued)
   conveyance (Continued)
    gliding type NEC (Continued)
     standing (Continued)
      electric scooter (Continued)
       collision with (Continued)
        bus or heavy transport
         V04.931
         nontraffic V04.031
         traffic V04.131
        car V03.931
         nontraffic V03.031
         traffic V03.131
        pedal cycle V01.931
         nontraffic V01.031
         traffic V01.131
        pick-up or van V03.931
         nontraffic V03.031
         traffic V03.131
        railway (train) (vehicle)
         V05.931
         nontraffic V05.031
         traffic V05.131
        streetcar V06.931
         nontraffic V06.031
         traffic V06.131
        three-wheeled motor vehicle
         V02.931
         nontraffic V02.031
         traffic V02.131
        two-wheeled motor vehicle
         V02.931
         nontraffic V02.031
         traffic V02.131
        vehicle, nonmotor, specified
         NEC V06.931
         nontraffic V06.031
         traffic V06.131
       fall V00.841
      micro-mobility pedestrian
       conveyance
       collision with
        animal being ridden or
         animal drawn vehicle
         V06.938
         nontraffic V06.038
         traffic V06.138
        bus or heavy transport
         V04.938
         nontraffic V04.038
         traffic V04.138
        car V03.938
         nontraffic V03.038
         traffic V03.138
        pedal cycle V01.938
         nontraffic V01.038
         traffic V01.138
        pick-up or van V03.938
         nontraffic V03.038
         traffic V03.138
        railway (train) (vehicle)
         V05.938
         nontraffic V05.038
         traffic V05.138
        stationary object V00.842
        streetcar V06.938
         nontraffic V06.038
         traffic V06.138
        three-wheeled motor vehicle
         V02.938
         nontraffic V02.038
         traffic V02.138
        two-wheeled motor vehicle
         V02.938
         nontraffic V02.038
         traffic V02.138
        vehicle, nonmotor, specified
         NEC V06.938
         nontraffic V06.038
         traffic V06.138
       fall V00.848

▶ New   ⇒ Revised   ~~deleted~~ Deleted   ● Use Additional Character(s)

Accident *(Continued)*
 transport *(Continued)*
  pedestrian *(Continued)*
   conveyance *(Continued)*
    gliding type NEC *(Continued)*
     traffic V09.3
      involving motor vehicle NEC
       V09.20
      wheelies —*see* Accident,
       transport, pedestrian,
       conveyance, heelies
    heelies V00.158
     colliding with stationary object
      V00.152
     fall V00.151
    ice skates V00.218
     collision (with) V09.9
      animal being ridden or animal
       drawn vehicle V06.99
        nontraffic V06.09
        traffic V06.19
      bus or heavy transport V04.99
       nontraffic V04.09
       traffic V04.19
      car V03.99
       nontraffic V03.09
       traffic V03.19
      pedal cycle V01.99
       nontraffic V01.09
       traffic V01.19
      pick-up truck or van V03.99
       nontraffic V03.09
       traffic V03.19
      railway (train) (vehicle)
       V05.99
        nontraffic V05.09
        traffic V05.19
      stationary object V00.212
      streetcar V06.99
       nontraffic V06.09
       traffic V06.19
      two- or three-wheeled motor
       vehicle V02.99
        nontraffic V02.09
        traffic V02.19
      vehicle V09.9
       animal-drawn V06.99
        nontraffic V06.09
        traffic V06.19
       motor
        nontraffic V09.00
        traffic V09.20
     fall V00.211
     nontraffic V09.1
      involving motor vehicle NEC
       V09.00
     traffic V09.3
      involving motor vehicle NEC
       V09.20
    motorized mobility scooter
     V00.838
     collision with stationary object
      V00.832
     fall from V00.831
     nontraffic V09.1
      involving motor vehicle
       V09.00
       military V09.01
       specified type NEC V09.09
    roller skates (non in-line) V00.128
     collision (with) V09.9
      animal being ridden or animal
       drawn vehicle V06.91
        nontraffic V06.01
        traffic V06.11
      bus or heavy transport V04.91
       nontraffic V04.01
       traffic V04.11
      car V03.91
       nontraffic V03.01
       traffic V03.11

Accident *(Continued)*
 transport *(Continued)*
  pedestrian *(Continued)*
   conveyance *(Continued)*
    roller skates *(Continued)*
     collision *(Continued)*
      pedal cycle V01.91
       nontraffic V01.01
       traffic V01.11
      pick-up truck or van
       V03.91
       nontraffic V03.01
       traffic V03.11
      railway (train) (vehicle)
       V05.91
       nontraffic V05.01
       traffic V05.11
      stationary object V00.122
      streetcar V06.91
       nontraffic V06.01
       traffic V06.11
      two- or three-wheeled motor
       vehicle V02.91
        nontraffic V02.01
        traffic V02.11
      vehicle V09.9
       animal-drawn V06.91
        nontraffic V06.01
        traffic V06.11
       motor
        nontraffic V09.00
        traffic V09.20
     fall V00.121
     in-line V00.118
      collision —*see also* Accident,
       transport, pedestrian,
       conveyance occupant, roller
       skates, collision
       with stationary object
        V00.112
      fall V00.111
      nontraffic V09.1
       involving motor vehicle NEC
        V09.00
      traffic V09.3
       involving motor vehicle NEC
        V09.20
    rolling shoes V00.158
     colliding with stationary object
      V00.152
     fall V00.151
    rolling type NEC V00.188
     collision (with) V09.9
      animal being ridden or animal
       drawn vehicle V06.99
        nontraffic V06.09
        traffic V06.19
      bus or heavy transport V04.99
       nontraffic V04.09
       traffic V04.19
      car V03.99
       nontraffic V03.09
       traffic V03.19
      pedal cycle V01.99
       nontraffic V01.09
       traffic V01.19
      pick-up truck or van V03.99
       nontraffic V03.09
       traffic V03.19
      railway (train) (vehicle)
       V05.99
       nontraffic V05.09
       traffic V05.19
      stationary object V00.182
      streetcar V06.99
       nontraffic V06.09
       traffic V06.19
      two- or three-wheeled motor
       vehicle V02.99
        nontraffic V02.09
        traffic V02.19

Accident *(Continued)*
 transport *(Continued)*
  pedestrian *(Continued)*
   conveyance *(Continued)*
    rolling type NEC *(Continued)*
     collision *(Continued)*
      vehicle V09.9
       animal-drawn V06.99
        nontraffic V06.09
        traffic V06.19
       motor
        nontraffic V09.00
        traffic V09.20
     fall V00.181
     in-line roller skate —*see* Accident,
      transport, pedestrian,
      conveyance, roller skate,
      in-line
     nontraffic V09.1
      involving motor vehicle NEC
       V09.00
     roller skate —*see* Accident,
      transport, pedestrian,
      conveyance, roller skate
     scooter (non-motorized) —
      see Accident, transport,
      pedestrian, conveyance,
      scooter
     skateboard —*see* Accident,
      transport, pedestrian,
      conveyance, skateboard
     traffic V09.3
      involving motor vehicle NEC
       V09.20
    scooter (non-motorized) V00.148
     collision (with) V09.9
      animal being ridden or
       animal drawn vehicle
       V06.99
        nontraffic V06.09
        traffic V06.19
      bus or heavy transport
       V04.99
       nontraffic V04.09
       traffic V04.19
      car V03.99
       nontraffic V03.09
       traffic V03.19
      pedal cycle V01.99
       nontraffic V01.09
       traffic V01.19
      pick-up truck or van
       V03.99
       nontraffic V03.09
       traffic V03.19
      railway (train) (vehicle)
       V05.99
       nontraffic V05.09
       traffic V05.19
      stationary object V00.142
      streetcar V06.99
       nontraffic V06.09
       traffic V06.19
      two- or three-wheeled motor
       vehicle V02.99
        nontraffic V02.09
        traffic V02.19
      vehicle V09.9
       animal-drawn V06.99
        nontraffic V06.09
        traffic V06.19
       motor
        nontraffic V09.00
        traffic V09.20
     fall V00.141
     nontraffic V09.1
      involving motor vehicle NEC
       V09.00
     traffic V09.3
      involving motor vehicle NEC
       V09.20

A

Accident *(Continued)*
  transport *(Continued)*
    pedestrian *(Continued)*
      conveyance *(Continued)*
        skate board V00.138
          collision (with) V09.9
            animal being ridden or animal
                drawn vehicle V06.92
              nontraffic V06.02
              traffic V06.12
            bus or heavy transport
                V04.92
              nontraffic V04.02
              traffic V04.12
            car V03.92
              nontraffic V03.02
              traffic V03.12
            pedal cycle V01.92
              nontraffic V01.02
              traffic V01.12
            pick-up truck or van V03.92
              nontraffic V03.02
              traffic V03.12
            railway (train) (vehicle) V05.92
              nontraffic V05.02
              traffic V05.12
            stationary object V00.132
            streetcar V06.92
              nontraffic V06.02
              traffic V06.12
            two- or three-wheeled motor
                vehicle V02.92
              nontraffic V02.02
              traffic V02.12
            vehicle V09.9
              animal-drawn V06.92
                nontraffic V06.02
                traffic V06.12
              motor
                nontraffic V09.00
                traffic V09.20
          fall V00.131
          nontraffic V09.1
            involving motor vehicle NEC
                V09.00
          traffic V09.3
            involving motor vehicle NEC
                V09.20
        skis (snow) V00.328
          collision (with) V09.9
            animal being ridden or animal
                drawn vehicle V06.99
              nontraffic V06.09
              traffic V06.19
            bus or heavy transport V04.99
              nontraffic V04.09
              traffic V04.19
            car V03.99
              nontraffic V03.09
              traffic V03.19
            pedal cycle V01.99
              nontraffic V01.09
              traffic V01.19
            pick-up truck or van V03.99
              nontraffic V03.09
              traffic V03.19
            railway (train) (vehicle) V05.99
              nontraffic V05.09
              traffic V05.19
            stationary object V00.322
            streetcar V06.99
              nontraffic V06.09
              traffic V06.19
            two- or three-wheeled motor
                vehicle V02.99
              nontraffic V02.09
              traffic V02.19
            vehicle V09.9
              animal-drawn V06.99
                nontraffic V06.09
                traffic V06.19

Accident *(Continued)*
  transport *(Continued)*
    pedestrian *(Continued)*
      conveyance *(Continued)*
        sled *(Continued)*
          collision *(Continued)*
            vehicle *(Continued)*
              motor
                nontraffic V09.00
                traffic V09.20
          fall V00.321
          nontraffic V09.1
            involving motor vehicle NEC
                V09.00
          traffic V09.3
            involving motor vehicle NEC
                V09.20
        sled V00.228
          collision (with) V09.9
            animal being ridden or animal
                drawn vehicle V06.99
              nontraffic V06.09
              traffic V06.19
            bus or heavy transport V04.99
              nontraffic V04.09
              traffic V04.19
            car V03.99
              nontraffic V03.09
              traffic V03.19
            pedal cycle V01.99
              nontraffic V01.09
              traffic V01.19
            pick-up truck or van V03.99
              nontraffic V03.09
              traffic V03.19
            railway (train) (vehicle) V05.99
              nontraffic V05.09
              traffic V05.19
            stationary object V00.222
            streetcar V06.99
              nontraffic V06.09
              traffic V06.19
            two- or three-wheeled motor
                vehicle V02.99
              nontraffic V02.09
              traffic V02.19
            vehicle V09.9
              animal-drawn V06.99
                nontraffic V06.09
                traffic V06.19
              motor
                nontraffic V09.00
                traffic V09.20
          fall V00.221
          nontraffic V09.1
            involving motor vehicle NEC
                V09.00
          traffic V09.3
            involving motor vehicle NEC
                V09.20
        snow board V00.318
          collision (with) V09.9
            animal being ridden or animal
                drawn vehicle V06.99
              nontraffic V06.09
              traffic V06.19
            bus or heavy transport V04.99
              nontraffic V04.09
              traffic V04.19
            car V03.99
              nontraffic V03.09
              traffic V03.19
            pedal cycle V01.99
              nontraffic V01.09
              traffic V01.19
            pick-up truck or van V03.99
              nontraffic V03.09
              traffic V03.19
            railway (train) (vehicle) V05.99
              nontraffic V05.09
              traffic V05.19

Accident *(Continued)*
  transport *(Continued)*
    pedestrian *(Continued)*
      conveyance *(Continued)*
        snow board *(Continued)*
          collision *(Continued)*
            stationary object V00.312
            streetcar V06.99
              nontraffic V06.09
              traffic V06.19
            two- or three-wheeled motor
                vehicle V02.99
              nontraffic V02.09
              traffic V02.19
            vehicle V09.9
              animal-drawn V06.99
                nontraffic V06.09
                traffic V06.19
              motor
                nontraffic V09.00
                traffic V09.20
          fall V00.311
          nontraffic V09.1
            involving motor vehicle NEC
                V09.00
          traffic V09.3
            involving motor vehicle NEC
                V09.20
        specified type NEC V00.898
          collision (with) V09.9
            animal being ridden or animal
                drawn vehicle V06.99
              nontraffic V06.09
              traffic V06.19
            bus or heavy transport V04.99
              nontraffic V04.09
              traffic V04.19
            car V03.99
              nontraffic V03.09
              traffic V03.19
            pedal cycle V01.99
              nontraffic V01.09
              traffic V01.19
            pick-up truck or van V03.99
              nontraffic V03.09
              traffic V03.19
            railway (train) (vehicle) V05.99
              nontraffic V05.09
              traffic V05.19
            stationary object V00.892
            streetcar V06.99
              nontraffic V06.09
              traffic V06.19
            two- or three-wheeled motor
                vehicle V02.99
              nontraffic V02.09
              traffic V02.19
            vehicle V09.9
              animal-drawn V06.99
                nontraffic V06.09
                traffic V06.19
              motor
                nontraffic V09.00
                traffic V09.20
          fall V00.891
          nontraffic V09.1
            involving motor vehicle NEC
                V09.00
          traffic V09.3
            involving motor vehicle NEC
                V09.20
        traffic V09.3
          involving motor vehicle V09.20
            military V09.21
            specified type NEC V09.29
        wheelchair (powered) V00.818
          collision (with) V09.9
            animal being ridden or animal
                drawn vehicle V06.99
              nontraffic V06.09
              traffic V06.19

▶ New   ⇒ Revised   ~~deleted~~ Deleted   ● Use Additional Character(s)

Accident *(Continued)*
  transport *(Continued)*
    pedestrian *(Continued)*
      conveyance *(Continued)*
        wheelchair *(Continued)*
          collision *(Continued)*
            bus or heavy transport V04.99
              nontraffic V04.09
              traffic V04.19
            car V03.99
              nontraffic V03.09
              traffic V03.19
            pedal cycle V01.99
              nontraffic V01.09
              traffic V01.19
            pick-up truck or van V03.99
              nontraffic V03.09
              traffic V03.19
            railway (train) (vehicle) V05.99
              nontraffic V05.09
              traffic V05.19
            stationary object V00.812
            streetcar V06.99
              nontraffic V06.09
              traffic V06.19
            two- or three-wheeled motor
              vehicle V02.99
              nontraffic V02.09
              traffic V02.19
            vehicle V09.9
              animal-drawn V06.99
                nontraffic V06.09
                traffic V06.19
              motor
                nontraffic V09.00
                traffic V09.20
        fall V00.811
        nontraffic V09.1
          involving motor vehicle NEC
            V09.00
        traffic V09.3
          involving motor vehicle NEC
            V09.20
      wheeled shoe V00.158
        colliding with stationary object
          V00.152
        fall V00.151
      on foot —*see also* Accident, pedestrian
      collision (with)
        animal being ridden or animal
          drawn vehicle V06.90
          nontraffic V06.00
          traffic V06.10
        bus or heavy transport V04.90
          nontraffic V04.00
          traffic V04.10
        car V03.90
          nontraffic V03.00
          traffic V03.10
        pedal cycle V01.90
          nontraffic V01.00
          traffic V01.10
        pick-up truck or van V03.90
          nontraffic V03.00
          traffic V03.10
        railway (train) (vehicle) V05.90
          nontraffic V05.00
          traffic V05.10
        streetcar V06.90
          nontraffic V06.00
          traffic V06.10
        two- or three-wheeled motor
          vehicle V02.90
          nontraffic V02.00
          traffic V02.10
        vehicle V09.9
          animal-drawn V06.90
            nontraffic V06.00
            traffic V06.10
          motor
            nontraffic V09.00
            traffic V09.20

Accident *(Continued)*
  transport *(Continued)*
    pedestrian *(Continued)*
      on foot *(Continued)*
        nontraffic V09.1
          involving motor vehicle V09.00
            military V09.01
            specified type NEC V09.09
        traffic V09.3
          involving motor vehicle V09.20
            military V09.21
            specified type NEC V09.29
    person NEC (unknown way or
      transportation) V99
      collision (between)
        bus (with)
          heavy transport vehicle (traffic)
            V87.5
            nontraffic V88.5
        car (with)
          nontraffic V88.5
          bus (traffic) V87.3
            nontraffic V88.3
          heavy transport vehicle (traffic)
            V87.4
            nontraffic V88.4
          pick-up truck or van (traffic)
            V87.2
            nontraffic V88.2
          train or railway vehicle (traffic)
            V87.6
            nontraffic V88.6
          two- or three-wheeled motor
            vehicle (traffic) V87.0
            nontraffic V88.0
        motor vehicle (traffic) NEC V87.7
          nontraffic V88.7
        two- or three-wheeled vehicle (with)
          (traffic)
          motor vehicle NEC V87.1
            nontraffic V88.1
      nonmotor vehicle (collision)
        (noncollision) (traffic) V87.9
        nontraffic V88.9
    pickup truck occupant V59.9
      collision (with)
        animal (traffic) V50.9
          being ridden (traffic) V56.9
            nontraffic V56.3
            while boarding or alighting
              V56.4
          nontraffic V50.3
          while boarding or alighting V50.4
        animal-drawn vehicle (traffic) V56.9
          nontraffic V56.3
          while boarding or alighting V56.4
        bus (traffic) V54.9
          nontraffic V54.3
          while boarding or alighting V54.4
        car (traffic) V53.9
          nontraffic V53.3
          while boarding or alighting V53.4
        motor vehicle NOS (traffic) V59.60
          nontraffic V59.20
          specified type NEC (traffic) V59.69
            nontraffic V59.29
        pedal cycle (traffic) V51.9
          nontraffic V51.3
          while boarding or alighting V51.4
        pickup truck (traffic) V53.9
          nontraffic V53.3
          while boarding or alighting V53.4
        railway vehicle (traffic) V55.9
          nontraffic V55.3
          while boarding or alighting V55.4
        specified vehicle NEC (traffic) V56.9
          nontraffic V56.3
          while boarding or alighting V56.4
        stationary object (traffic) V57.9
          nontraffic V57.3
          while boarding or alighting V57.4

Accident *(Continued)*
  transport *(Continued)*
    pickup truck occupant *(Continued)*
      collision (with) *(Continued)*
        streetcar (traffic) V56.9
          nontraffic V56.3
          while boarding or alighting V56.4
        three wheeled motor vehicle (traffic)
          V52.9
          nontraffic V52.3
          while boarding or alighting V52.4
        truck (traffic) V54.9
          nontraffic V54.3
          while boarding or alighting V54.4
        two wheeled motor vehicle (traffic)
          V52.9
          nontraffic V52.3
          while boarding or alighting V52.4
        van (traffic) V53.9
          nontraffic V53.3
          while boarding or alighting V53.4
    driver
      collision (with)
        animal (traffic) V50.5
          being ridden (traffic) V56.5
            nontraffic V56.0
          nontraffic V50.0
        animal-drawn vehicle (traffic)
          V56.5
          nontraffic V56.0
        bus (traffic) V54.5
          nontraffic V54.0
        car (traffic) V53.5
          nontraffic V53.0
        motor vehicle NOS (traffic) V59.40
          nontraffic V59.00
          specified type NEC (traffic)
            V59.49
            nontraffic V59.09
        pedal cycle (traffic) V51.5
          nontraffic V51.0
        pickup truck (traffic) V53.5
          nontraffic V53.0
        railway vehicle (traffic) V55.5
          nontraffic V55.0
        specified vehicle NEC (traffic) V56.5
          nontraffic V56.0
        stationary object (traffic) V57.5
          nontraffic V57.0
        streetcar (traffic) V56.5
          nontraffic V56.0
        three wheeled motor vehicle
          (traffic) V52.5
          nontraffic V52.0
        truck (traffic) V54.5
          nontraffic V54.0
        two wheeled motor vehicle (traffic)
          V52.5
          nontraffic V52.0
        van (traffic) V53.5
          nontraffic V53.0
      noncollision accident (traffic) V58.5
        nontraffic V58.0
    hanger-on
      collision (with)
        animal (traffic) V50.7
          being ridden (traffic) V56.7
            nontraffic V56.2
          nontraffic V50.2
        animal-drawn vehicle (traffic) V56.7
          nontraffic V56.2
        bus (traffic) V54.7
          nontraffic V54.2
        car (traffic) V53.7
          nontraffic V53.2
        pedal cycle (traffic) V51.7
          nontraffic V51.2
        pickup truck (traffic) V53.7
          nontraffic V53.2
        railway vehicle (traffic) V55.7
          nontraffic V55.2

Accident *(Continued)*
transport *(Continued)*
pickup truck occupant *(Continued)*
hanger-on *(Continued)*
collision *(Continued)*
specified vehicle NEC (traffic) V56.7
nontraffic V56.2
stationary object (traffic) V57.7
nontraffic V57.2
streetcar (traffic) V56.7
nontraffic V56.2
three wheeled motor vehicle
(traffic) V52.7
nontraffic V52.2
truck (traffic) V54.7
nontraffic V54.2
two wheeled motor vehicle (traffic)
V52.7
nontraffic V52.2
van (traffic) V53.7
nontraffic V53.2
noncollision accident (traffic) V58.7
nontraffic V58.2
noncollision accident (traffic) V58.9
nontraffic V58.3
while boarding or alighting V58.4
nontraffic V59.3
passenger
collision (with)
animal (traffic) V50.6
being ridden (traffic) V56.6
nontraffic V56.1
nontraffic V50.1
animal-drawn vehicle (traffic) V56.6
nontraffic V56.1
bus (traffic) V54.6
nontraffic V54.1
car (traffic) V53.6
nontraffic V53.1
motor vehicle NOS (traffic) V59.50
nontraffic V59.10
specified type NEC (traffic) V59.59
nontraffic V59.19
pedal cycle (traffic) V51.6
nontraffic V51.1
pickup truck (traffic) V53.6
nontraffic V53.1
railway vehicle (traffic) V55.6
nontraffic V55.1
specified vehicle NEC (traffic) V56.6
nontraffic V56.1
stationary object (traffic) V57.6
nontraffic V57.1
streetcar (traffic) V56.6
nontraffic V56.1
three wheeled motor vehicle
(traffic) V52.6
nontraffic V52.1
truck (traffic) V54.6
nontraffic V54.1
two wheeled motor vehicle (traffic)
V52.6
nontraffic V52.1
van (traffic) V53.6
nontraffic V53.1
noncollision accident (traffic) V58.6
nontraffic V58.1
specified type NEC V59.88
military vehicle V59.81
quarry truck —*see* Accident, transport,
industrial vehicle occupant
race car —*see* Accident, transport, motor
vehicle NEC occupant
railway vehicle occupant V81.9
collision (with) V81.3
motor vehicle (non-military) (traffic)
V81.1
military V81.83
nontraffic V81.0
rolling stock V81.2
specified object NEC V81.3

Accident *(Continued)*
transport *(Continued)*
railway vehicle occupant *(Continued)*
during derailment V81.7
with antecedent collision —*see*
Accident, transport, railway
vehicle occupant, collision
explosion V81.81
fall (in railway vehicle) V81.5
during derailment V81.7
with antecedent collision —*see*
Accident, transport, railway
vehicle occupant, collision
from railway vehicle V81.6
during derailment V81.7
with antecedent collision —*see*
Accident, transport,
railway vehicle occupant,
collision
while boarding or alighting V81.4
fire V81.81
object falling onto train V81.82
specified type NEC V81.89
while boarding or alighting V81.4
Segway V00.848
ski lift V98.3
snowmobile occupant (nontraffic) V86.92
driver V86.52
hanger-on V86.72
passenger V86.62
traffic V86.32
driver V86.02
hanger-on V86.22
passenger V86.12
while boarding or alighting V86.42
specified NEC V98.8
sport utility vehicle occupant —*see also*
Accident, transport, pickup truck
occupant
streetcar occupant V82.9
collision (with) V82.3
motor vehicle (traffic) V82.1
nontraffic V82.0
rolling stock V82.2
during derailment V82.7
with antecedent collision —*see*
Accident, transport, streetcar
occupant, collision
fall (in streetcar) V82.5
during derailment V82.7
with antecedent collision —*see*
Accident, transport, streetcar
occupant, collision
from streetcar V82.6
during derailment V82.7
with antecedent collision —*see*
Accident, transport, streetcar
occupant, collision
while boarding or alighting
V82.4
while boarding or alighting V82.4
specified type NEC V82.8
while boarding or alighting V82.4
three-wheeled motor vehicle occupant
V39.9
collision (with)
animal (traffic) V30.9
being ridden (traffic) V36.9
nontraffic V36.3
while boarding or alighting V36.4
nontraffic V30.3
while boarding or alighting V30.4
animal-drawn vehicle (traffic) V36.9
nontraffic V36.3
while boarding or alighting V36.4
bus (traffic) V34.9
nontraffic V34.3
while boarding or alighting V34.4
car (traffic) V33.9
nontraffic V33.3
while boarding or alighting V33.4

Accident *(Continued)*
transport *(Continued)*
three-wheeled motor vehicle occupant
(Continued)
collision *(Continued)*
motor vehicle NOS (traffic) V39.60
nontraffic V39.20
specified type NEC (traffic)
V39.69
nontraffic V39.29
pedal cycle (traffic) V31.9
nontraffic V31.3
while boarding or alighting
V31.4
pickup truck (traffic) V33.9
nontraffic V33.3
while boarding or alighting
V33.4
railway vehicle (traffic) V35.9
nontraffic V35.3
while boarding or alighting
V35.4
specified vehicle NEC (traffic) V36.9
nontraffic V36.3
while boarding or alighting V36.4
stationary object (traffic) V37.9
nontraffic V37.3
while boarding or alighting V37.4
streetcar (traffic) V36.9
nontraffic V36.3
while boarding or alighting V36.4
three wheeled motor vehicle (traffic)
V32.9
nontraffic V32.3
while boarding or alighting V32.4
truck (traffic) V34.9
nontraffic V34.3
while boarding or alighting V34.4
two wheeled motor vehicle (traffic)
V32.9
nontraffic V32.3
while boarding or alighting V32.4
van (traffic) V33.9
nontraffic V33.3
while boarding or alighting V33.4
driver
collision (with)
animal (traffic) V30.5
being ridden (traffic) V36.5
nontraffic V36.0
nontraffic V30.0
animal-drawn vehicle (traffic) V36.5
nontraffic V36.0
bus (traffic) V34.5
nontraffic V34.0
car (traffic) V33.5
nontraffic V33.0
motor vehicle NOS (traffic)
V39.40
nontraffic V39.00
specified type NEC (traffic)
V39.49
nontraffic V39.09
pedal cycle (traffic) V31.5
nontraffic V31.0
pickup truck (traffic) V33.5
nontraffic V33.0
railway vehicle (traffic) V35.5
nontraffic V35.0
specified vehicle NEC (traffic)
V36.5
nontraffic V36.0
stationary object (traffic) V37.5
nontraffic V37.0
streetcar (traffic) V36.5
nontraffic V36.0
three wheeled motor vehicle
(traffic) V32.5
nontraffic V32.0
truck (traffic) V34.5
nontraffic V34.0

▶ New ⟾ Revised ~~deleted~~ Deleted ● Use Additional Character(s)

Accident *(Continued)*
 transport *(Continued)*
  three-wheeled motor vehicle occupant
   (Continued)
   driver *(Continued)*
    collision *(Continued)*
     two wheeled motor vehicle (traffic)
      V32.5
      nontraffic V32.0
     van (traffic) V33.5
      nontraffic V33.0
    noncollision accident (traffic) V38.5
     nontraffic V38.0
   hanger-on
    collision (with)
     animal (traffic) V30.7
      being ridden (traffic) V36.7
       nontraffic V36.2
      nontraffic V30.2
     animal-drawn vehicle (traffic) V36.7
      nontraffic V36.2
     bus (traffic) V34.7
      nontraffic V34.2
     car (traffic) V33.7
      nontraffic V33.2
     pedal cycle (traffic) V31.7
      nontraffic V31.2
     pickup truck (traffic) V33.7
      nontraffic V33.2
     railway vehicle (traffic) V35.7
      nontraffic V35.2
     specified vehicle NEC (traffic) V36.7
      nontraffic V36.2
     stationary object (traffic) V37.7
      nontraffic V37.2
     streetcar (traffic) V36.7
      nontraffic V36.2
     three wheeled motor vehicle
      (traffic) V32.7
      nontraffic V32.2
     truck (traffic) V34.7
      nontraffic V34.2
     two wheeled motor vehicle (traffic)
      V32.7
      nontraffic V32.2
     van (traffic) V33.7
      nontraffic V33.2
    noncollision accident (traffic) V38.7
     nontraffic V38.2
   noncollision accident (traffic) V38.9
    nontraffic V38.3
    while boarding or alighting V38.4
   nontraffic V39.3
   passenger
    collision (with)
     animal (traffic) V30.6
      being ridden (traffic) V36.6
       nontraffic V36.1
      nontraffic V30.1
     animal-drawn vehicle (traffic) V36.6
      nontraffic V36.1
     bus (traffic) V34.6
      nontraffic V34.1
     car (traffic) V33.6
      nontraffic V33.1
     motor vehicle NOS (traffic) V39.50
      nontraffic V39.10
      specified type NEC (traffic)
       V39.59
       nontraffic V39.19
     pedal cycle (traffic) V31.6
      nontraffic V31.1
     pickup truck (traffic) V33.6
      nontraffic V33.1
     railway vehicle (traffic) V35.6
      nontraffic V35.1
     specified vehicle NEC (traffic)
      V36.6
      nontraffic V36.1
     stationary object (traffic) V37.6
      nontraffic V37.1

Accident *(Continued)*
 transport *(Continued)*
  three-wheeled motor vehicle occupant
   (Continued)
   passenger *(Continued)*
    collision *(Continued)*
     streetcar (traffic) V36.6
      nontraffic V36.1
     three wheeled motor vehicle
      (traffic) V32.6
      nontraffic V32.1
     truck (traffic) V34.6
      nontraffic V34.1
     two wheeled motor vehicle (traffic)
      V32.6
      nontraffic V32.1
     van (traffic) V33.6
      nontraffic V33.1
    noncollision accident (traffic)
     V38.6
     nontraffic V38.1
   specified type NEC V39.89
    military vehicle V39.81
  tractor (farm) (and trailer) —*see* Accident,
   transport, agricultural vehicle
   occupant
  tram —*see* Accident, transport, streetcar
   in mine or quarry —*see* Accident,
    transport, industrial vehicle
    occupant
  trolley —*see* Accident, transport, streetcar
   in mine or quarry —*see* Accident,
    transport, industrial vehicle
    occupant
  truck (heavy) occupant V69.9
   collision (with)
    animal (traffic) V60.9
     being ridden (traffic) V66.9
      nontraffic V66.3
      while boarding or alighting
       V66.4
     nontraffic V60.3
     while boarding or alighting V60.4
    animal-drawn vehicle (traffic) V66.9
     nontraffic V66.3
     while boarding or alighting V66.4
    bus (traffic) V64.9
     nontraffic V64.3
     while boarding or alighting V64.4
    car (traffic) V63.9
     nontraffic V63.3
     while boarding or alighting V63.4
    motor vehicle NOS (traffic) V69.60
     nontraffic V69.20
     specified type NEC (traffic) V69.69
      nontraffic V69.29
    pedal cycle (traffic) V61.9
     nontraffic V61.3
     while boarding or alighting V61.4
    pickup truck (traffic) V63.9
     nontraffic V63.3
     while boarding or alighting V63.4
    railway vehicle (traffic) V65.9
     nontraffic V65.3
     while boarding or alighting V65.4
    specified vehicle NEC (traffic) V66.9
     nontraffic V66.3
     while boarding or alighting V66.4
    stationary object (traffic) V67.9
     nontraffic V67.3
     while boarding or alighting V67.4
    streetcar (traffic) V66.9
     nontraffic V66.3
     while boarding or alighting V66.4
    three wheeled motor vehicle (traffic)
     V62.9
     nontraffic V62.3
     while boarding or alighting V62.4
    truck (traffic) V64.9
     nontraffic V64.3
     while boarding or alighting V64.4

Accident *(Continued)*
 transport *(Continued)*
  truck occupant *(Continued)*
   collision *(Continued)*
    two wheeled motor vehicle (traffic)
     V62.9
     nontraffic V62.3
     while boarding or alighting V62.4
    van (traffic) V63.9
     nontraffic V63.3
     while boarding or alighting V63.4
   driver
    collision (with)
     animal (traffic) V60.5
      being ridden (traffic) V66.5
       nontraffic V66.0
      nontraffic V60.0
     animal-drawn vehicle (traffic) V66.5
      nontraffic V66.0
     bus (traffic) V64.5
      nontraffic V64.0
     car (traffic) V63.5
      nontraffic V63.0
     motor vehicle NOS (traffic) V69.40
      nontraffic V69.00
      specified type NEC (traffic)
       V69.49
       nontraffic V69.09
     pedal cycle (traffic) V61.5
      nontraffic V61.0
     pickup truck (traffic) V63.5
      nontraffic V63.0
     railway vehicle (traffic) V65.5
      nontraffic V65.0
     specified vehicle NEC (traffic) V66.5
      nontraffic V66.0
     stationary object (traffic) V67.5
      nontraffic V67.0
     streetcar (traffic) V66.5
      nontraffic V66.0
     three wheeled motor vehicle
      (traffic) V62.5
      nontraffic V62.0
     truck (traffic) V64.5
      nontraffic V64.0
     two wheeled motor vehicle (traffic)
      V62.5
      nontraffic V62.0
     van (traffic) V63.5
      nontraffic V63.0
    noncollision accident (traffic) V68.5
     nontraffic V68.0
   dump —*see* Accident, transport,
    construction vehicle occupant
   hanger-on
    collision (with)
     animal (traffic) V60.7
      being ridden (traffic) V66.7
       nontraffic V66.2
      nontraffic V60.2
     animal-drawn vehicle (traffic) V66.7
      nontraffic V66.2
     bus (traffic) V64.7
      nontraffic V64.2
     car (traffic) V63.7
      nontraffic V63.2
     pedal cycle (traffic) V61.7
      nontraffic V61.2
     pickup truck (traffic) V63.7
      nontraffic V63.2
     railway vehicle (traffic) V65.7
      nontraffic V65.2
     specified vehicle NEC (traffic) V66.7
      nontraffic V66.2
     stationary object (traffic) V67.7
      nontraffic V67.2
     streetcar (traffic) V66.7
      nontraffic V66.2
     three wheeled motor vehicle
      (traffic) V62.7
      nontraffic V62.2

Accident (Continued)
  transport (Continued)
    truck occupant (Continued)
      hanger-on (Continued)
        collision (Continued)
          truck (traffic) V64.7
            nontraffic V64.2
          two wheeled motor vehicle (traffic) V62.7
            nontraffic V62.2
          van (traffic) V63.7
            nontraffic V63.2
        noncollision accident (traffic) V68.7
          nontraffic V68.2
      noncollision accident (traffic) V68.9
        nontraffic V68.3
        while boarding or alighting V68.4
      nontraffic V69.3
      passenger
        collision (with)
          animal (traffic) V60.6
            being ridden (traffic) V66.6
              nontraffic V66.1
            nontraffic V60.1
          animal-drawn vehicle (traffic) V66.6
            nontraffic V66.1
          bus (traffic) V64.6
            nontraffic V64.1
          car (traffic) V63.6
            nontraffic V63.1
          motor vehicle NOS (traffic) V69.50
            nontraffic V69.10
            specified type NEC (traffic) V69.59
              nontraffic V69.19
          pedal cycle (traffic) V61.6
            nontraffic V61.1
          pickup truck (traffic) V63.6
            nontraffic V63.1
          railway vehicle (traffic) V65.6
            nontraffic V65.1
          specified vehicle NEC (traffic) V66.6
            nontraffic V66.1
          stationary object (traffic) V67.6
            nontraffic V67.1
          streetcar (traffic) V66.6
            nontraffic V66.1
          three wheeled motor vehicle (traffic) V62.6
            nontraffic V62.1
          truck (traffic) V64.6
            nontraffic V64.1
          two wheeled motor vehicle (traffic) V62.6
            nontraffic V62.1
          van (traffic) V63.6
            nontraffic V63.1
        noncollision accident (traffic) V68.6
          nontraffic V68.1
      pickup —see Accident, transport, pickup truck occupant
      specified type NEC V69.88
        military vehicle V69.81
    van occupant V59.9
      collision (with)
        animal (traffic) V50.9
          being ridden (traffic) V56.9
            nontraffic V56.3
              while boarding or alighting V56.4
          nontraffic V50.3
          while boarding or alighting V50.4
        animal-drawn vehicle (traffic) V56.9
          nontraffic V56.3
          while boarding or alighting V56.4
        bus (traffic) V54.9
          nontraffic V54.3
          while boarding or alighting V54.4
        car (traffic) V53.9
          nontraffic V53.3
          while boarding or alighting V53.4

Accident (Continued)
  transport (Continued)
    van occupant (Continued)
      collision (Continued)
        motor vehicle NOS (traffic) V59.60
          nontraffic V59.20
          specified type NEC (traffic) V59.69
            nontraffic V59.29
        pedal cycle (traffic) V51.9
          nontraffic V51.3
          while boarding or alighting V51.4
        pickup truck (traffic) V53.9
          nontraffic V53.3
          while boarding or alighting V53.4
        railway vehicle (traffic) V55.9
          nontraffic V55.3
          while boarding or alighting V55.4
        specified vehicle NEC (traffic) V56.9
          nontraffic V56.3
          while boarding or alighting V56.4
        stationary object (traffic) V57.9
          nontraffic V57.3
          while boarding or alighting V57.4
        streetcar (traffic) V56.9
          nontraffic V56.3
          while boarding or alighting V56.4
        three wheeled motor vehicle (traffic) V52.9
          nontraffic V52.3
          while boarding or alighting V52.4
        truck (traffic) V54.9
          nontraffic V54.3
          while boarding or alighting V54.4
        two wheeled motor vehicle (traffic) V52.9
          nontraffic V52.3
          while boarding or alighting V52.4
        van (traffic) V53.9
          nontraffic V53.3
          while boarding or alighting V53.4
      driver
        collision (with)
          animal (traffic) V50.5
            being ridden (traffic) V56.5
              nontraffic V56.0
            nontraffic V50.0
          animal-drawn vehicle (traffic) V56.5
            nontraffic V56.0
          bus (traffic) V54.5
            nontraffic V54.0
          car (traffic) V53.5
            nontraffic V53.0
          motor vehicle NOS (traffic) V59.40
            nontraffic V59.00
            specified type NEC (traffic) V59.49
              nontraffic V59.09
          pedal cycle (traffic) V51.5
            nontraffic V51.0
          pickup truck (traffic) V53.5
            nontraffic V53.0
          railway vehicle (traffic) V55.5
            nontraffic V55.0
          specified vehicle NEC (traffic) V56.5
            nontraffic V56.0
          stationary object (traffic) V57.5
            nontraffic V57.0
          streetcar (traffic) V56.5
            nontraffic V56.0
          three wheeled motor vehicle (traffic) V52.5
            nontraffic V52.0
          truck (traffic) V54.5
            nontraffic V54.0
          two wheeled motor vehicle (traffic) V52.5
            nontraffic V52.0
          van (traffic) V53.5
            nontraffic V53.0
        noncollision accident (traffic) V58.5
          nontraffic V58.0

Accident (Continued)
  transport (Continued)
    van occupant (Continued)
      hanger-on
        collision (with)
          animal (traffic) V50.7
            being ridden (traffic) V56.7
              nontraffic V56.2
            nontraffic V50.2
          animal-drawn vehicle (traffic) V56.7
            nontraffic V56.2
          bus (traffic) V54.7
            nontraffic V54.2
          car (traffic) V53.7
            nontraffic V53.2
          pedal cycle (traffic) V51.7
            nontraffic V51.2
          pickup truck (traffic) V53.7
            nontraffic V53.2
          railway vehicle (traffic) V55.7
            nontraffic V55.2
          specified vehicle NEC (traffic) V56.7
            nontraffic V56.2
          stationary object (traffic) V57.7
            nontraffic V57.2
          streetcar (traffic) V56.7
            nontraffic V56.2
          three wheeled motor vehicle (traffic) V52.7
            nontraffic V52.2
          truck (traffic) V54.7
            nontraffic V54.2
          two wheeled motor vehicle (traffic) V52.7
            nontraffic V52.2
          van (traffic) V53.7
            nontraffic V53.2
        noncollision accident (traffic) V58.7
          nontraffic V58.2
      noncollision accident (traffic) V58.9
        nontraffic V58.3
        while boarding or alighting V58.4
      nontraffic V59.3
      passenger
        collision (with)
          animal (traffic) V50.6
            being ridden (traffic) V56.6
              nontraffic V56.1
            nontraffic V50.1
          animal-drawn vehicle (traffic) V56.6
            nontraffic V56.1
          bus (traffic) V54.6
            nontraffic V54.1
          car (traffic) V53.6
            nontraffic V53.1
          motor vehicle NOS (traffic) V59.50
            nontraffic V59.10
            specified type NEC (traffic) V59.59
              nontraffic V59.19
          pedal cycle (traffic) V51.6
            nontraffic V51.1
          pickup truck (traffic) V53.6
            nontraffic V53.1
          railway vehicle (traffic) V55.6
            nontraffic V55.1
          specified vehicle NEC (traffic) V56.6
            nontraffic V56.1
          stationary object (traffic) V57.6
            nontraffic V57.1
          streetcar (traffic) V56.6
            nontraffic V56.1
          three wheeled motor vehicle (traffic) V52.6
            nontraffic V52.1
          truck (traffic) V54.6
            nontraffic V54.1
          two wheeled motor vehicle (traffic) V52.6
            nontraffic V52.1
          van (traffic) V53.6
            nontraffic V53.1

▶ New   ⇒ Revised   ~~deleted~~ Deleted   ● Use Additional Character(s)

Accident *(Continued)*
  transport *(Continued)*
    van occupant *(Continued)*
      passenger *(Continued)*
        noncollision accident (traffic) V58.6
        nontraffic V58.1
      specified type NEC V59.88
      military vehicle V59.81
    watercraft occupant —*see* Accident,
      watercraft
  vehicle NEC V89.9
    animal-drawn NEC —*see* Accident,
      transport, animal-drawn vehicle
      occupant
    special
      agricultural —*see* Accident, transport,
        agricultural vehicle occupant
      construction —*see* Accident, transport,
        construction vehicle occupant
      industrial —*see* Accident, transport,
        industrial vehicle occupant
      three-wheeled NEC (motorized) —*see*
        Accident, transport, three-wheeled
        motor vehicle occupant
  watercraft V94.9
    causing
      drowning —*see* Drowning, due to,
        accident to, watercraft
      injury NEC V91.89
        crushed between craft and object
          V91.19
          powered craft V91.13
            ferry boat V91.11
            fishing boat V91.12
            jet ski V91.13
            liner V91.11
            merchant ship V91.10
            passenger ship V91.11
          unpowered craft V91.18
            canoe V91.15
            inflatable V91.16
            kayak V91.15
            sailboat V91.14
            surf-board V91.18
            windsurfer V91.18
        fall on board V91.29
          powered craft V91.23
            ferry boat V91.21
            fishing boat V91.22
            jet ski V91.23
            liner V91.21
            merchant ship V91.20
            passenger ship V91.21
          unpowered craft
            canoe V91.25
            inflatable V91.26
            kayak V91.25
            sailboat V91.24
        fire on board causing burn V91.09
          powered craft V91.03
            ferry boat V91.01
            fishing boat V91.02
            jet ski V91.03
            liner V91.01
            merchant ship V91.00
            passenger ship V91.01
          unpowered craft V91.08
            canoe V91.05
            inflatable V91.06
            kayak V91.05
            sailboat V91.04
            surf-board V91.08
            water skis V91.07
            windsurfer V91.08
        hit by falling object V91.39
          powered craft V91.33
            ferry boat V91.31
            fishing boat V91.32
            jet skis V91.33
            liner V91.31
            merchant ship V91.30
            passenger ship V91.31

Accident *(Continued)*
  watercraft *(Continued)*
    causing *(Continued)*
      injury NEC *(Continued)*
        hit by falling object *(Continued)*
          unpowered craft V91.38
            canoe V91.35
            inflatable V91.36
            kayak V91.35
            sailboat V91.34
            surf-board V91.38
            water skis V91.37
            windsurfer V91.38
        specified type NEC V91.89
          powered craft V91.83
            ferry boat V91.81
            fishing boat V91.82
            jet ski V91.83
            liner V91.81
            merchant ship V91.80
            passenger ship V91.81
          unpowered craft V91.88
            canoe V91.85
            inflatable V91.86
            kayak V91.85
            sailboat V91.84
            surf-board V91.88
            water skis V91.87
            windsurfer V91.88
      due to, caused by cataclysm —*see* Forces of
        nature, by type
      military NEC V94.818
        with civilian watercraft V94.810
        civilian in water injured by V94.811
      nonpowered, struck by
        nonpowered vessel V94.22
        powered vessel V94.21
      specified type NEC V94.89
      striking swimmer
        powered V94.11
        unpowered V94.12
Acid throwing (assault) Y08.89
Activity (involving) (of victim at time of event)
  Y93.9
  aerobic and step exercise (class) Y93.A3
  alpine skiing Y93.23
  animal care NEC Y93.K9
  arts and handcrafts NEC Y93.D9
  athletics NEC Y93.79
  athletics played as a team or group NEC
    Y93.69
  athletics played individually NEC Y93.59
  baking Y93.G3
  ballet Y93.41
  barbells Y93.B3
  BASE (Building, Antenna, Span, Earth)
    jumping Y93.33
  baseball Y93.64
  basketball Y93.67
  bathing (personal) Y93.E1
  beach volleyball Y93.68
  bike riding Y93.55
  blackout game Y93.85
  boogie boarding Y93.18
  bowling Y93.54
  boxing Y93.71
  brass instrument playing Y93.J4
  building construction Y93.H3
  bungee jumping Y93.34
  calisthenics Y93.A2
  canoeing (in calm and turbulent water) Y93.16
  capture the flag Y93.6A
  cardiorespiratory exercise NEC Y93.A9
  caregiving (providing) NEC Y93.F9
    bathing Y93.F1
    lifting Y93.F2
  cellular
    communication device Y93.C2
    telephone Y93.C2
  challenge course Y93.A5
  cheerleading Y93.45

Activity *(Continued)*
  choking game Y93.85
  circuit training Y93.A4
  cleaning
    floor Y93.E5
  climbing NEC Y93.39
    mountain Y93.31
    rock Y93.31
    wall Y93.31
  clothing care and maintenance NEC Y93.E9
  combatives Y93.75
  computer
    keyboarding Y93.C1
    technology NEC Y93.C9
  confidence course Y93.A5
  construction (building) Y93.H3
  cooking and baking Y93.G3
  cool down exercises Y93.A2
  cricket Y93.69
  crocheting Y93.D1
  cross country skiing Y93.24
  dancing (all types) Y93.41
  digging
    dirt Y93.H1
  dirt digging Y93.H1
  dishwashing Y93.G1
  diving (platform) (springboard) Y93.12
    underwater Y93.15
  dodge ball Y93.6A
  downhill skiing Y93.23
  drum playing Y93.J2
  dumbbells Y93.B3
  electronic
    devices NEC Y93.C9
      hand held interactive Y93.C2
    game playing (using) (with)
      interactive device Y93.C2
      keyboard or other stationary device
        Y93.C1
  elliptical machine Y93.A1
  exercise(s)
    machines ((primarily) for)
      cardiorespiratory conditioning Y93.A1
      muscle strengthening Y93.B1
    muscle strengthening (non-machine) NEC
      Y93.B9
  external motion NEC Y93.I9
    rollercoaster Y93.I1
  fainting game Y93.85
  field hockey Y93.65
  figure skating (pairs) (singles) Y93.21
  flag football Y93.62
  floor mopping and cleaning Y93.E5
  food preparation and clean up Y93.G1
  football (American) NOS Y93.61
    flag Y93.62
    tackle Y93.61
    touch Y93.62
  four square Y93.6A
  free weights Y93.B3
  frisbee (ultimate) Y93.74
  furniture
    building Y93.D3
    finishing Y93.D3
    repair Y93.D3
  game playing (electronic)
    using interactive device Y93.C2
    using keyboard or other stationary device
      Y93.C1
  gardening Y93.H2
  golf Y93.53
  grass drills Y93.A6
  grilling and smoking food Y93.G2
  grooming and shearing an animal Y93.K3
  guerilla drills Y93.A6
  gymnastics (rhythmic) Y93.43
  hand held interactive electronic device Y93.C2
  handball Y93.73
  handcrafts NEC Y93.D9
  hang gliding Y93.35
  hiking (on level or elevated terrain) Y93.01

▶ New   ⇒ Revised   ~~deleted~~ Deleted   ● Use Additional Character(s)

Activity (Continued)
hockey (ice) Y93.22
   field Y93.65
horseback riding Y93.52
household (interior) maintenance NEC Y93.
   E9
ice NEC Y93.29
   dancing Y93.21
   hockey Y93.22
   skating Y93.21
inline roller skating Y93.51
ironing Y93.E4
judo Y93.75
jumping (off) NEC Y93.39
   BASE (Building, Antenna, Span, Earth)
     Y93.33
   bungee Y93.34
   jacks Y93.A2
   rope Y93.56
jumping jacks Y93.A2
jumping rope Y93.56
karate Y93.75
kayaking (in calm and turbulent water) Y93.16
keyboarding (computer) Y93.C1
kickball Y93.6A
knitting Y93.D1
lacrosse Y93.65
land maintenance NEC Y93.H9
landscaping Y93.H2
laundry Y93.E2
machines (exercise)
   primarily for cardiorespiratory
     conditioning Y93.A1
   primarily for muscle strengthening Y93.B1
maintenance
   exterior building NEC Y93.H9
   household (interior) NEC Y93.E9
   land Y93.H9
   property Y93.H9
marching (on level or elevated terrain) Y93.01
martial arts Y93.75
microwave oven Y93.G3
milking an animal Y93.K2
mopping (floor) Y93.E5
mountain climbing Y93.31
muscle strengthening
   exercises (non-machine) NEC Y93.B9
   machines Y93.B1
musical keyboard (electronic) playing Y93.J1
nordic skiing Y93.24
obstacle course Y93.A5
oven (microwave) Y93.G3
packing up and unpacking in moving to a
   new residence Y93.E6
parasailing Y93.19
pass out game Y93.85
percussion instrument playing NEC Y93.J2
personal
   bathing and showering Y93.E1
   hygiene NEC Y93.E8
   showering Y93.E1
physical games generally associated with
   school recess, summer camp and
   children Y93.6A
physical training NEC Y93.A9
piano playing Y93.J1
pilates Y93.B4
platform diving Y93.12
playing musical instrument
   brass instrument Y93.J4
   drum Y93.J2
   musical keyboard (electronic) Y93.J1
   percussion instrument NEC Y93.J2
   piano Y93.J1
   string instrument Y93.J3
   winds instrument Y93.J4
property maintenance
   exterior NEC Y93.H9
   interior NEC Y93.E9
pruning (garden and lawn) Y93.H2

Activity (Continued)
pull-ups Y93.B2
push-ups Y93.B2
racquetball Y93.73
rafting (in calm and turbulent water) Y93.16
raking (leaves) Y93.H1
rappelling Y93.32
refereeing a sports activity Y93.81
residential relocation Y93.E6
rhythmic gymnastics Y93.43
rhythmic movement NEC Y93.49
riding
   horseback Y93.52
   rollercoaster Y93.I1
rock climbing Y93.31
roller skating (inline) Y93.51
rollercoaster riding Y93.I1
rough housing and horseplay Y93.83
rowing (in calm and turbulent water)
   Y93.16
rugby Y93.63
SCUBA diving Y93.15
sewing Y93.D2
shoveling Y93.H1
   dirt Y93.H1
   snow Y93.H1
showering (personal) Y93.E1
sit-ups Y93.B2
skateboarding Y93.51
skating (ice) Y93.21
   roller Y93.51
skiing (alpine) (downhill) Y93.23
   cross country Y93.24
   nordic Y93.24
   water Y93.17
sledding (snow) Y93.23
sleeping (sleep) Y93.84
smoking and grilling food Y93.G2
snorkeling Y93.15
snow NEC Y93.29
   boarding Y93.23
   shoveling Y93.H1
   sledding Y93.23
   tubing Y93.23
soccer Y93.66
softball Y93.64
specified NEC Y93.89
spectator at an event Y93.82
sports NEC Y93.79
   sports played as a team or group NEC
     Y93.69
   sports played individually NEC Y93.59
springboard diving Y93.12
squash Y93.73
stationary bike Y93.A1
step (stepping) exercise (class) Y93.A3
stepper machine Y93.A1
stove Y93.G3
string instrument playing Y93.J3
surfing Y93.18
   wind Y93.18
swimming Y93.11
tackle football Y93.61
tap dancing Y93.41
tennis Y93.73
tobogganing Y93.23
touch football Y93.62
track and field events (non-running) Y93.57
   running Y93.02
trampoline Y93.44
treadmill Y93.A1
trimming shrubs Y93.H2
tubing (in calm and turbulent water) Y93.16
   snow Y93.23
ultimate frisbee Y93.74
underwater diving Y93.15
unpacking in moving to a new residence
   Y93.E6
use of stove, oven and microwave oven Y93.
   G3

Activity (Continued)
vacuuming Y93.E3
volleyball (beach) (court) Y93.68
wake boarding Y93.17
walking (on level or elevated terrain)
   Y93.01
   an animal Y93.K1
walking an animal Y93.K1
wall climbing Y93.31
warm up and cool down exercises Y93.A2
water NEC Y93.19
   aerobics Y93.14
   craft NEC Y93.19
   exercise Y93.14
   polo Y93.13
   skiing Y93.17
   sliding Y93.18
   survival training and testing Y93.19
weeding (garden and lawn) Y93.H2
wind instrument playing Y93.J4
windsurfing Y93.18
wrestling Y93.72
yoga Y93.42
Adverse effect of drugs —*see* Table of Drugs
   and Chemicals
Aerosinusitis —*see* Air, pressure
After-effect, late —*see* Sequelae
Air
   blast in war operations —*see* War operations,
     air blast
   pressure
     change, rapid
       during
         ascent W94.29
           while (in) (surfacing from)
             aircraft W94.23
             deep water diving W94.21
             underground W94.22
         descent W94.39
           in
             aircraft W94.31
             water W94.32
     high, prolonged W94.0
     low, prolonged W94.12
       due to residence or long visit at high
         altitude W94.11
Alpine sickness W94.11
Altitude sickness W94.11
Anaphylactic shock, anaphylaxis —*see* Table of
   Drugs and Chemicals
Andes disease W94.11
Arachnidism, arachnoidism X58
Arson (with intent to injure or kill) X97
Asphyxia, asphyxiation
   by
     food (bone) (seed) —*see* categories T17
       and T18
     gas —*see also* Table of Drugs and
       Chemicals
       legal
         execution —*see* Legal, intervention,
           gas
         intervention —*see* Legal, intervention,
           gas
   from
     fire —*see also* Exposure, fire
       in war operations —*see* War operations,
         fire
     ignition —*see* Ignition
     vomitus T17.81
   in war operations —*see* War operations,
     restriction of airway
Aspiration
   food (any type) (into respiratory tract) (with
     asphyxia, obstruction respiratory tract,
     suffocation) —*see* categories T17 and T18
   foreign body —*see* Foreign body, aspiration
   vomitus (with asphyxia, obstruction
     respiratory tract, suffocation) T17.81
Assassination (attempt) —*see* Assault

▶ New   ⟹ Revised   ~~deleted~~ Deleted   ● Use Additional Character(s)

Assault (homicidal) (by) (in) Y09
  arson X97
  bite (of human being) Y04.1
  bodily force Y04.8
    bite Y04.1
    bumping into Y04.2
    sexual —*see* subcategories T74.0, T76.0
    unarmed fight Y04.0
  bomb X96.9
    antipersonnel X96.0
    fertilizer X96.3
    gasoline X96.1
    letter X96.2
    petrol X96.1
    pipe X96.3
    specified NEC X96.8
  brawl (hand) (fists) (foot) (unarmed)
      Y04.0
  burning, burns (by fire) NEC X97
    acid Y08.89
    caustic, corrosive substance Y08.89
    chemical from swallowing caustic,
        corrosive substance —*see* Table of
        Drugs and Chemicals
    cigarette(s) X97
    hot object X98.9
      fluid NEC X98.2
      household appliance X98.3
      specified NEC X98.8
      steam X98.0
      tap water X98.1
      vapors X98.0
    scalding —*see* Assault, burning
    steam X98.0
    vitriol Y08.89
  caustic, corrosive substance (gas) Y08.89
  crashing of
    aircraft Y08.81
    motor vehicle Y03.8
      pushed in front of Y02.0
      run over Y03.0
      specified NEC Y03.8
  cutting or piercing instrument X99.9
    dagger X99.2
    glass X99.0

Assault *(Continued)*
  cutting or piercing instrument *(Continued)*
    knife X99.1
    specified NEC X99.8
    sword X99.2
  dagger X99.2
  drowning (in) X92.9
    bathtub X92.0
    natural water X92.3
    specified NEC X92.8
    swimming pool X92.1
      following fall X92.2
  dynamite X96.8
  explosive(s) (material) X96.9
  fight (hand) (fists) (foot) (unarmed)
      Y04.0
    with weapon —*see* Assault, by type of
        weapon
  fire X97
  firearm X95.9
    airgun X95.01
    handgun X93
    hunting rifle X94.1
    larger X94.9
      specified NEC X94.8
    machine gun X94.2
    shotgun X94.0
    specified NEC X95.8
  from high place Y01
  gunshot (wound) NEC —*see* Assault, firearm,
      by type
  incendiary device X97
  injury Y09
    to child due to criminal abortion attempt
        NEC Y08.89
  knife X99.1
  late effect of —*see* X92-Y08 with 7th
      character S
  placing before moving object NEC
      Y02.8
    motor vehicle Y02.0
  poisoning —*see* categories T36-T65 with 7th
      character S
  puncture, any part of body —*see* Assault,
      cutting or piercing instrument

Assault *(Continued)*
  pushing
    before moving object NEC Y02.8
      motor vehicle Y02.0
      subway train Y02.1
      train Y02.1
  rape T74.2-●
  scalding —*see* Assault, burning
  sequelae of —*see* X92-Y08 with 7th character S
  sexual (by bodily force) T74.2-●
  shooting —*see* Assault, firearm
  specified means NEC Y08.89
  stab, any part of body —*see* Assault, cutting
      or piercing instrument
  steam X98.0
  striking against
    other person Y04.2
    sports equipment Y08.09
      baseball bat Y08.02
      hockey stick Y08.01
  struck by
    sports equipment Y08.09
      baseball bat Y08.02
      hockey stick Y08.01
  submersion —*see* Assault, drowning
  violence Y09
  weapon Y09
    blunt Y00
    cutting or piercing —*see* Assault, cutting or
        piercing instrument
    firearm —*see* Assault, firearm
  wound Y09
    cutting —*see* Assault, cutting or piercing
        instrument
    gunshot —*see* Assault, firearm
    knife X99.1
    piercing —*see* Assault, cutting or piercing
        instrument
    puncture —*see* Assault, cutting or piercing
        instrument
    stab —*see* Assault, cutting or piercing
        instrument
Attack by mammals NEC W55.89
Avalanche —*see* Landslide
Aviator's disease —*see* Air, pressure

B

Barotitis, barodontalgia, barosinusitis,
   barotrauma (otitic) (sinus) —see Air,
   pressure
Battered (baby) (child) (person) (syndrome)
   X58
Bayonet wound W26.1
   in
      legal intervention —see Legal,
         intervention, sharp object,
         bayonet
      war operations —see War operations,
         combat
   stated as undetermined whether accidental or
      intentional Y28.8
   suicide (attempt) X78.2
Bean in nose —see categories T17 and T18
Bed set on fire NEC —see Exposure, fire,
   uncontrolled, building, bed
Beheading (by guillotine)
   homicide X99.9
   legal execution —see Legal, intervention
Bending, injury in (prolonged) (static) X50.1
Bends —see Air, pressure, change
Bite, bitten by
   alligator W58.01
   arthropod (nonvenomous) NEC W57
   bull W55.21
   cat W55.01
   cow W55.21
   crocodile W58.11
   dog W54.0
   goat W55.31
   hoof stock NEC W55.31
   horse W55.11
   human being (accidentally) W50.3
      with intent to injure or kill Y04.1
      as, or caused by, a crowd or human
         stampede (with fall) W52
      assault Y04.1
      homicide (attempt) Y04.1
      in
         fight Y04.1
   insect (nonvenomous) W57
   lizard (nonvenomous) W59.01
   mammal NEC W55.81
      marine W56.31
   marine animal (nonvenomous) W56.81
   millipede W57
   moray eel W56.51
   mouse W53.01
   person(s) (accidentally) W50.3
      with intent to injure or kill Y04.1
      as, or caused by, a crowd or human
         stampede (with fall) W52
      assault Y04.1
      homicide (attempt) Y04.1
      in
         fight Y04.1
   pig W55.41
   raccoon W55.51
   rat W53.11
   reptile W59.81
      lizard W59.01
      snake W59.11
      turtle W59.21
      terrestrial W59.81
   rodent W53.81
      mouse W53.01
      rat W53.11
      specified NEC W53.81
      squirrel W53.21
   shark W56.41
   sheep W55.31
   snake (nonvenomous) W59.11
   spider (nonvenomous) W57
   squirrel W53.21
Blast (air) in war operations —see War
   operations, blast
Blizzard X37.2

Blood alcohol level Y90.9
   20-39mg/100ml Y90.1
   40-59mg/100ml Y90.2
   60-79mg/100ml Y90.3
   80-99mg/100ml Y90.4
   100-119mg/100ml Y90.5
   120-199mg/100ml Y90.6
   200-239mg/100ml Y90.7
   less than 20mg/100ml Y90.0
   presence in blood, level not specified
      Y90.9
Blow X58
   by law-enforcing agent, police (on duty) —see
      Legal, intervention, manhandling
      blunt object —see Legal, intervention, blunt
         object
Blowing up —see Explosion
Brawl (hand) (fists) (foot) Y04.0
Breakage (accidental) (part of)
   ladder (causing fall) W11
   scaffolding (causing fall) W12
Broken
   glass, contact with —see Contact, with, glass
   power line (causing electric shock) W85
Bumping against, into (accidentally)
   object NEC W22.8
      with fall —see Fall, due to, bumping
         against, object
      caused by crowd or human stampede
         (with fall) W52
      sports equipment W21.9
   person(s) W51
      with fall W03
         due to ice or snow W00.0
      assault Y04.2
      caused by, a crowd or human stampede
         (with fall) W52
      homicide (attempt) Y04.2
   sports equipment W21.9
Burn, burned, burning (accidental) (by) (from)
   (on)
   acid NEC —see Table of Drugs and
      Chemicals
   bed linen —see Exposure, fire, uncontrolled,
      in building, bed
   blowtorch X08.8
      with ignition of clothing NEC X06.2
         nightwear X05
   bonfire, campfire (controlled) —see also
      Exposure, fire, controlled, not in
      building
      uncontrolled —see Exposure, fire,
         uncontrolled, not in building
   candle X08.8
      with ignition of clothing NEC X06.2
         nightwear X05
   caustic liquid, substance (external) (internal)
      NEC —see Table of Drugs and
      Chemicals
   chemical (external) (internal) —see also Table
      of Drugs and Chemicals
      in war operations —see War operations, fire
   cigar(s) or cigarette(s) X08.8
      with ignition of clothing NEC X06.2
         nightwear X05
   clothes, clothing NEC (from controlled fire)
      X06.2
      with conflagration —see Exposure, fire,
         uncontrolled, building
      not in building or structure —see
         Exposure, fire, uncontrolled, not in
         building
   cooker (hot) X15.8
      stated as undetermined whether accidental
         or intentional Y27.3
      suicide (attempt) X77.3
   electric blanket X16
   engine (hot) X17
   fire, flames —see Exposure, fire
   flare, Very pistol —see Discharge, firearm
      NEC

Burn, burned, burning (Continued)
   heat
      from appliance (electrical) (household)
         X15.8
         cooker X15.8
         hotplate X15.2
         kettle X15.8
         light bulb X15.8
         saucepan X15.3
         skillet X15.3
         stated as undetermined whether
            accidental or intentional Y27.3
         stove X15.0
         suicide (attempt) X77.3
         toaster X15.1
      in local application or packing during
         medical or surgical procedure
         Y63.5
   heating
      appliance, radiator or pipe X16
   homicide (attempt) —see Assault, burning
   hot
      air X14.1
      cooker X15.8
      drink X10.0
      engine X17
      fat X10.2
      fluid NEC X12
      food X10.1
      gases X14.1
      heating appliance X16
      household appliance NEC X15.8
      kettle X15.8
      liquid NEC X12
      machinery X17
      metal (molten) (liquid) NEC X18
      object (not producing fire or flames) NEC
         X19
      oil (cooking) X10.2
      pipe(s) X16
      radiator X16
      saucepan (glass) (metal) X15.3
      stove (kitchen) X15.0
      substance NEC X19
         caustic or corrosive NEC —see Table of
            Drugs and Chemicals
      toaster X15.1
      tool X17
      vapor X13.1
      water (tap) —see Contact, with, hot, tap
         water
   hotplate X15.2
      suicide (attempt) X77.3
   ignition —see Ignition
   in war operations —see War operations, fire
   inflicted by other person X97
      by hot objects, hot vapor, and steam —see
         Assault, burning, hot object
   internal, from swallowed caustic, corrosive
      liquid, substance —see Table of Drugs
      and Chemicals
   iron (hot) X15.8
      stated as undetermined whether accidental
         or intentional Y27.3
      suicide (attempt) X77.3
   kettle (hot) X15.8
      stated as undetermined whether accidental
         or intentional Y27.3
      suicide (attempt) X77.3
   lamp (flame) X08.8
      with ignition of clothing NEC X06.2
         nightwear X05
   lighter (cigar) (cigarette) X08.8
      with ignition of clothing NEC X06.2
         nightwear X05
   lightning —see subcategory T75.0
      causing fire —see Exposure, fire
   liquid (boiling) (hot) NEC X12
      stated as undetermined whether accidental
         or intentional Y27.2
      suicide (attempt) X77.2

▶ New   ➡ Revised   ~~deleted~~ Deleted   ● Use Additional Character(s)

Burn, burned, burning *(Continued)*
  local application of externally applied
    substance in medical or surgical care
    Y63.5
  machinery (hot) X17
  matches X08.8
    with ignition of clothing NEC X06.2
      nightwear X05
  mattress —*see* Exposure, fire, uncontrolled,
    building, bed
  medicament, externally applied Y63.5
  metal (hot) (liquid) (molten) NEC X18
  nightwear (nightclothes, nightdress, gown,
    pajamas, robe) X05
  object (hot) NEC X19
  on board watercraft
    due to
      accident to watercraft V91.09
        powered craft V91.03
          ferry boat V91.01
          fishing boat V91.02
          jet ski V91.03
          liner V91.01
          merchant ship V91.00
          passenger ship V91.01
        unpowered craft V91.08
          canoe V91.05
          inflatable V91.06
          kayak V91.05
          sailboat V91.04
          surf-board V91.08
          water skis V91.07
          windsurfer V91.08
      fire on board V93.09
        ferry boat V93.01
        fishing boat V93.02
        jet ski V93.03
        liner V93.01
        merchant ship V93.00
        passenger ship V93.01
        powered craft NEC V93.03
        sailboat V93.04

Burn, burned, burning *(Continued)*
  on board watercraft *(Continued)*
    due to *(Continued)*
      specified heat source NEC on board
        V93.19
        ferry boat V93.11
        fishing boat V93.12
        jet ski V93.13
        liner V93.11
        merchant ship V93.10
        passenger ship V93.11
        powered craft NEC V93.13
        sailboat V93.14
  pipe (hot) X16
    smoking X08.8
      with ignition of clothing NEC X06.2
        nightwear X05
  powder —*see* Powder burn
  radiator (hot) X16
  saucepan (hot) (glass) (metal) X15.3
    stated as undetermined whether
      accidental or intentional
      Y27.3
    suicide (attempt) X77.3
  self-inflicted X76
    stated as undetermined whether
      accidental or intentional
      Y26
  stated as undetermined whether
    accidental or intentional Y27.0
  steam X13.1
    pipe X16
      stated as undetermined whether
        accidental or intentional
        Y27.8
    stated as undetermined whether
      accidental or intentional Y27.0
    suicide (attempt) X77.0
  stove (hot) (kitchen) X15.0
    stated as undetermined whether
      accidental or intentional Y27.3
    suicide (attempt) X77.3

Burn, burned, burning *(Continued)*
  substance (hot) NEC X19
    boiling X12
      stated as undetermined whether
        accidental or intentional Y27.2
      suicide (attempt) X77.2
    molten (metal) X18
  suicide (attempt) NEC X76
    hot
      household appliance X77.3
      object X77.9
  stated as undetermined whether accidental or
    intentional Y27.0
  therapeutic misadventure
    heat in local application or packing during
      medical or surgical procedure Y63.5
    overdose of radiation Y63.2
  toaster (hot) X15.1
    stated as undetermined whether accidental
      or intentional Y27.3
    suicide (attempt) X77.3
  tool (hot) X17
  torch, welding X08.8
    with ignition of clothing NEC X06.2
      nightwear X05
  trash fire (controlled) —*see* Exposure, fire,
    controlled, not in building
    uncontrolled —*see* Exposure, fire,
      uncontrolled, not in building
  vapor (hot) X13.1
    stated as undetermined whether accidental
      or intentional Y27.0
    suicide (attempt) X77.0
  Very pistol —*see* Discharge, firearm NEC
Butted by animal W55.82
  bull W55.22
  cow W55.22
  goat W55.32
  horse W55.12
  pig W55.42
  sheep W55.32

C

Caisson disease—*see* Air, pressure, change
Campfire (exposure to) (controlled)—*see also* Exposure, fire, controlled, not in building
  uncontrolled—*see* Exposure, fire, uncontrolled, not in building
Capital punishment (any means)—*see* Legal, intervention
Car sickness T75.3
Casualty (not due to war) NEC X58
  war—*see* War operations
Cat
  bite W55.01
  scratch W55.03
Cataclysm, cataclysmic (any injury) NEC—*see* Forces of nature
Catching fire—*see* Exposure, fire
Caught
  between
    folding object W23.0
    objects (moving) (stationary and moving) W23.0
      and machinery—*see* Contact, with, by type of machine
    stationary W23.1
    sliding door and door frame W23.0
  by, in
    machinery (moving parts of)—*see* Contact, with, by type of machine
    washing-machine wringer W23.0
  under packing crate (due to losing grip) W23.1
Cave-in caused by cataclysmic earth surface movement or eruption—*see* Landslide
Change(s) in air pressure—*see* Air, pressure, change
Choked, choking (on) (any object except food or vomitus)
  food (bone) (seed)—*see* categories T17 and T18
  vomitus T17.81-●
Civil insurrection—*see* War operations
Cloudburst (any injury) X37.8
Cold, exposure to (accidental) (excessive) (extreme) (natural) (place) NEC—*see* Exposure, cold
Collapse
  building W20.1
    burning (uncontrolled fire) X00.2
  dam or man-made structure (causing earth movement) X36.0
  machinery—*see* Contact, with, by type of machine
  structure W20.1
    burning (uncontrolled fire) X00.2
Collision (accidental) NEC—*see also* Accident, transport V89.9
  pedestrian W51
    with fall W03
      due to ice or snow W00.0
      involving pedestrian conveyance—*see* Accident, transport, pedestrian, conveyance
    and
      crowd or human stampede (with fall) W52
      object W22.8
        with fall—*see* Fall, due to, bumping against, object
      person(s)—*see* Collision, pedestrian
  transport vehicle NEC V89.9
    and
      avalanche, fallen or not moving—*see* Accident, transport
        falling or moving—*see* Landslide
      landslide, fallen or not moving—*see* Accident, transport
        falling or moving—*see* Landslide

Collision NEC *(Continued)*
  transport vehicle NEC *(Continued)*
    due to cataclysm—*see* Forces of nature, by type
    intentional, purposeful suicide (attempt)—*see* Suicide, collision
Combustion, spontaneous—*see* Ignition
Complication (delayed) of or following (medical or surgical procedure) Y84.9
  with misadventure—*see* Misadventure
  amputation of limb(s) Y83.5
  anastomosis (arteriovenous) (blood vessel) (gastrojejunal) (tendon) (natural or artificial material) Y83.2
  aspiration (of fluid) Y84.4
    tissue Y84.8
  biopsy Y84.8
  blood
    sampling Y84.7
    transfusion
      procedure Y84.8
  bypass Y83.2
  catheterization (urinary) Y84.6
    cardiac Y84.0
  colostomy Y83.3
  cystostomy Y83.3
  dialysis (kidney) Y84.1
  drug—*see* Table of Drugs and Chemicals
  due to misadventure—*see* Misadventure
  duodenostomy Y83.3
  electroshock therapy Y84.3
  external stoma, creation of Y83.3
  formation of external stoma Y83.3
  gastrostomy Y83.3
  graft Y83.2
  hypothermia (medically-induced) Y84.8
  implant, implantation (of)
    artificial
      internal device (cardiac pacemaker) (electrodes in brain) (heart valve prosthesis) (orthopedic) Y83.1
      material or tissue (for anastomosis or bypass) Y83.2
        with creation of external stoma Y83.3
    natural tissues (for anastomosis or bypass) Y83.2
      with creation of external stoma Y83.3
  infusion
    procedure Y84.8
  injection—*see* Table of Drugs and Chemicals
    procedure Y84.8
  insertion of gastric or duodenal sound Y84.5
  insulin-shock therapy Y84.3
  paracentesis (abdominal) (thoracic) (aspirative) Y84.4
  procedures other than surgical operation—*see* Complication of or following, by type of procedure
  radiological procedure or therapy Y84.2
  removal of organ (partial) (total) NEC Y83.6
  sampling
    blood Y84.7
    fluid NEC Y84.4
    tissue Y84.8
  shock therapy Y84.3
  surgical operation NEC—*see also* Complication of or following, by type of operation Y83.9
    reconstructive NEC Y83.4
      with
        anastomosis, bypass or graft Y83.2
        formation of external stoma Y83.3
    specified NEC Y83.8
  transfusion—*see also* Table of Drugs and Chemicals
    procedure Y84.8
  transplant, transplantation (heart) (kidney) (liver) (whole organ, any) Y83.0
    partial organ Y83.4
  ureterostomy Y83.3

Complication of or following *(Continued)*
  vaccination—*see also* Table of Drugs and Chemicals
    procedure Y84.8
Compression
  divers' squeeze—*see* Air, pressure, change
  trachea by
    food (lodged in esophagus)—*see* categories T17 and T18
    vomitus (lodged in esophagus) T17.81-●
Conflagration—*see* Exposure, fire, uncontrolled
Constriction (external)
  hair W49.01
  jewelry W49.04
  ring W49.04
  rubber band W49.03
  specified item NEC W49.09
  string W49.02
  thread W49.02
Contact (accidental)
  with
    abrasive wheel (metalworking) W31.1
    alligator W58.09
      bite W58.01
      crushing W58.03
      strike W58.02
    amphibian W62.9
      frog W62.0
      toad W62.1
    animal (nonvenomous) NEC W64
      marine W56.89
        bite W56.81
        dolphin—*see* Contact, with, dolphin
        fish NEC—*see* Contact, with, fish
        mammal—*see* Contact, with, mammal, marine
        orca—*see* Contact, with, orca
        sea lion—*see* Contact, with, sea lion
        shark—*see* Contact, with, shark
        strike W56.82
    animate mechanical force NEC W64
    arrow W21.89
      not thrown, projected or falling W45.8
    arthropods (nonvenomous) W57
    axe W27.0
    band-saw (industrial) W31.2
    bayonet—*see* Bayonet wound
    bee(s) X58
    bench-saw (industrial) W31.2
    bird W61.99
      bite W61.91
      chicken—*see* Contact, with, chicken
      duck—*see* Contact, with, duck
      goose—*see* Contact, with, goose
      macaw—*see* Contact, with, macaw
      parrot—*see* Contact, with, parrot
      psittacine—*see* Contact, with, psittacine
      strike W61.92
      turkey—*see* Contact, with, turkey
    blender W29.0
    boiling water X12
      stated as undetermined whether accidental or intentional Y27.2
      suicide (attempt) X77.2
    bore, earth-drilling or mining (land) (seabed) W31.0
    buffalo—*see* Contact, with, hoof stock NEC
    bull W55.29
      bite W55.21
      gored W55.22
      strike W55.22
    bumper cars W31.81
    camel—*see* Contact, with, hoof stock NEC
    can
      lid W26.8
      opener W27.4
        powered W29.0
    cat W55.09
      bite W55.01
      scratch W55.03
    caterpillar (venomous) X58

▶ New   ➡ Revised   ~~deleted~~ Deleted   ● Use Additional Character(s)

Contact *(Continued)*
  with *(Continued)*
    centipede (venomous) X58
    chain
      hoist W24.Ø
        agricultural operations W30.89
      saw W29.3
    chicken W61.39
      peck W61.33
      strike W61.32
    chisel W27.Ø
    circular saw W31.2
    cobra X58
    combine (harvester) W30.Ø
    conveyer belt W24.1
    cooker (hot) X15.8
      stated as undetermined whether
        accidental or intentional Y27.3
      suicide (attempt) X77.3
    coral X58
    cotton gin W31.82
    cow W55.29
      bite W55.21
      strike W55.22
    crane W24.Ø
      agricultural operations W30.89
    crocodile W58.19
      bite W58.11
      crushing W58.13
      strike W58.12
    dagger W26.1
      stated as undetermined whether
        accidental or intentional Y28.2
      suicide (attempt) X78.2
    dairy equipment W31.82
    dart W21.89
      not thrown, projected or falling W45.8
    deer —*see* Contact, with, hoof stock
      NEC
    derrick W24.Ø
      agricultural operations W30.89
        hay W30.2
    dog W54.8
      bite W54.Ø
      strike W54.1
    dolphin W56.Ø9
      bite W56.Ø1
      strike W56.Ø2
    donkey —*see* Contact, with, hoof stock
      NEC
    drill (powered) W29.8
      earth (land) (seabed) W31.Ø
      nonpowered W27.8
    drive belt W24.Ø
      agricultural operations W30.89
    dry ice —*see* Exposure, cold, man-made
    dryer (clothes) (powered) (spin) W29.2
    duck W61.69
      bite W61.61
      strike W61.62
    earth(-)
      drilling machine (industrial) W31.Ø
      scraping machine in stationary use
        W31.83
    edge of stiff paper W26.2
    electric
      beater W29.Ø
      blanket X16
      fan W29.2
        commercial W31.82
      knife W29.1
      mixer W29.Ø
    elevator (building) W24.Ø
      agricultural operations W30.89
        grain W30.3
    engine(s), hot NEC X17
    excavating machine W31.Ø
    farm machine W30.9
    feces —*see* Contact, with, by type of
      animal
    fer de lance X58

Contact *(Continued)*
  with *(Continued)*
    fish W56.59
      bite W56.51
      shark —*see* Contact, with, shark
      strike W56.52
    flying horses W31.81
    forging (metalworking) machine
      W31.1
    fork W27.4
    forklift (truck) W24.Ø
      agricultural operations W30.89
    frog W62.Ø
    garden
      cultivator (powered) W29.3
        riding W30.89
      fork W27.1
    gas turbine W31.3
    Gila monster X58
    giraffe —*see* Contact, with, hoof stock
      NEC
    glass (sharp) (broken) W25
      with subsequent fall W18.Ø2
      assault X99.Ø
      due to fall —*see* Fall, by type
      stated as undetermined whether
        accidental or intentional Y28. Ø
      suicide (attempt) X78.Ø
    goat W55.39
      bite W55.31
      strike W55.32
    goose W61.59
      bite W61.51
      strike W61.52
    hand
      saw W27.Ø
      tool (not powered) NEC W27.8
        powered W29.8
    harvester W30.Ø
    hay-derrick W30.2
    heat NEC X19
      from appliance (electrical)
        (household) —*see* Contact, with,
        hot, household appliance
      heating appliance X16
    heating
      appliance (hot) X16
      pad (electric) X16
    hedge-trimmer (powered) W29.3
    hoe W27.1
    hoist (chain) (shaft) NEC W24.Ø
      agricultural W30.89
    hoof stock NEC W55.39
      bite W55.31
      strike W55.32
    hornet(s) X58
    horse W55.19
      bite W55.11
      strike W55.12
    hot
      air X14.1
        inhalation X14.Ø
      cooker X15.8
      drinks X10.Ø
      engine X17
      fats X10.2
      fluids NEC X12
        assault X98.2
        suicide (attempt) X77.2
        undetermined whether accidental or
          intentional Y27.2
      food X10.1
      gases X14.1
        inhalation X14.Ø
      heating appliance X16
      household appliance X15.8
        assault X98.3
        cooker X15.8
        hotplate X15.2
        kettle X15.8
        light bulb X15.8

Contact *(Continued)*
  with *(Continued)*
    hot *(Continued)*
      household appliance *(Continued)*
        object NEC X19
          assault X98.8
          stated as undetermined whether
            accidental or intentional Y27.9
          suicide (attempt) X77.8
        saucepan X15.3
        skillet X15.3
        stated as undetermined whether
          accidental or intentional Y27.3
        stove X15.Ø
        suicide (attempt) X77.3
        toaster X15.1
      kettle X15.8
      light bulb X15.8
      liquid NEC —*see also* Burn X12
        drinks X10.Ø
        stated as undetermined whether
          accidental or intentional Y27.2
        suicide (attempt) X77.2
        tap water X11.8
          stated as undetermined whether
            accidental or intentional Y27.1
          suicide (attempt) X77.1
      machinery X17
      metal (molten) (liquid) NEC X18
      object (not producing fire or flames)
        NEC X19
      oil (cooking) X10.2
      pipe X16
      plate X15.2
      radiator X16
      saucepan (glass) (metal) X15.3
      skillet X15.3
      stove (kitchen) X15.Ø
      substance NEC X19
      tap-water X11.8
        assault X98.1
        heated on stove X12
          stated as undetermined whether
            accidental or intentional Y27.2
          suicide (attempt) X77.2
        in bathtub X11.Ø
        running X11.1
        stated as undetermined whether
          accidental or intentional Y27.1
        suicide (attempt) X77.1
      toaster X15.1
      tool X17
      vapors X13.1
        inhalation X13.Ø
      water (tap) X11.8
        boiling X12
          stated as undetermined whether
            accidental or intentional Y27.2
          suicide (attempt) X77.2
        heated on stove X12
          stated as undetermined whether
            accidental or intentional Y27.2
          suicide (attempt) X77.2
        in bathtub X11.Ø
        running X11.1
        stated as undetermined whether
          accidental or intentional Y27.1
        suicide (attempt) X77.1
    hotplate X15.2
    ice-pick W27.4
    insect (nonvenomous) NEC W57
    kettle (hot) X15.8
    knife W26.Ø
      assault X99.1
      electric W29.1
      stated as undetermined whether
        accidental or intentional Y28.1
      suicide (attempt) X78.1
    lathe (metalworking) W31.1
      turnings W45.8
      woodworking W31.2

Contact *(Continued)*
  with *(Continued)*
    lawnmower (powered) (ridden) W28
      causing electrocution W86.8
        suicide (attempt) X83.1
      unpowered W27.1
    lift, lifting (devices) W24.0
      agricultural operations W30.89
      shaft W24.0
    liquefied gas —*see* Exposure, cold,
      man-made
    liquid air, hydrogen, nitrogen —*see*
      Exposure, cold, man-made
    lizard (nonvenomous) W59.09
      bite W59.01
      strike W59.02
    llama —*see* Contact, with, hoof stock NEC
    macaw W61.19
      bite W61.11
      strike W61.12
    machine, machinery W31.9
      abrasive wheel W31.1
      agricultural including animal-powered
        W30.9
        combine harvester W30.0
        grain storage elevator W30.3
        hay derrick W30.2
        power take-off device W30.1
        reaper W30.0
        specified NEC W30.89
        thresher W30.0
        transport vehicle, stationary W30.81
      band saw W31.2
      bench saw W31.2
      circular saw W31.2
      commercial NEC W31.82
      drilling, metal (industrial) W31.1
      earth-drilling W31.0
      earthmoving or scraping W31.89
      excavating W31.89
      forging machine W31.1
      gas turbine W31.3
      hot X17
      internal combustion engine W31.3
      land drill W31.0
      lathe W31.1
      lifting (devices) W24.0
      metal drill W31.1
      metalworking (industrial) W31.1
      milling, metal W31.1
      mining W31.0
      molding W31.2
      overhead plane W31.2
      power press, metal W31.1
      prime mover W31.3
      printing W31.89
      radial saw W31.2
      recreational W31.81
      roller-coaster W31.81
      rolling mill, metal W31.1
      sander W31.2
      seabed drill W31.0
      shaft
        hoist W31.0
        lift W31.0
      specified NEC W31.89
      spinning W31.89
      steam engine W31.3
      transmission W24.1
      undercutter W31.0
      water driven turbine W31.3
      weaving W31.89
      woodworking or forming (industrial)
        W31.2
    mammal (feces) (urine) W55.89
      bull —*see* Contact, with, bull
      cat —*see* Contact, with, cat
      cow —*see* Contact, with, cow
      goat —*see* Contact, with, goat
      hoof stock —*see* Contact, with, hoof
        stock

Contact *(Continued)*
  with *(Continued)*
    mammal *(Continued)*
      horse —*see* Contact, with, horse
      marine W56.39
        dolphin —*see* Contact, with, dolphin
        orca —*see* Contact, with, orca
        sea lion —*see* Contact, with, sea lion
        specified NEC W56.39
          bite W56.31
          strike W56.32
      pig —*see* Contact, with, pig
      raccoon —*see* Contact, with, raccoon
      rodent —*see* Contact, with, rodent
      sheep —*see* Contact, with, sheep
      specified NEC W55.89
        bite W55.81
        strike W55.82
    marine
      animal W56.89
        bite W56.81
        dolphin —*see* Contact, with, dolphin
        fish NEC —*see* Contact, with, fish
        mammal —*see* Contact, with,
          mammal, marine
        orca —*see* Contact, with, orca
        sea lion —*see* Contact, with, sea lion
        shark —*see* Contact, with, shark
        strike W56.82
    meat
      grinder (domestic) W29.0
        industrial W31.82
        nonpowered W27.4
      slicer (domestic) W29.0
        industrial W31.82
    merry go round W31.81
    metal, (hot) (liquid) (molten) NEC X18
    millipede W57
    nail W45.0
      gun W29.4
    needle (sewing) W27.3
      hypodermic W46.0
        contaminated W46.1
    object (blunt) NEC
      hot NEC X19
      legal intervention —*see* Legal,
        intervention, blunt object
      sharp NEC W45.8
        inflicted by other person NEC W45.8
          stated as
            intentional homicide (attempt) —
              see Assault, cutting or
              piercing instrument
        legal intervention —*see* Legal,
          intervention, sharp object
        self-inflicted X78.9
    orca W56.29
      bite W56.21
      strike W56.22
    overhead plane W31.2
    paper (as sharp object) W26.2
    paper-cutter W27.5
    parrot W61.09
      bite W61.01
      strike W61.02
    pig W55.49
      bite W55.41
      strike W55.42
    pipe, hot X16
    pitchfork W27.1
    plane (metal) (wood) W27.0
      overhead W27.0
    plant thorns, spines, sharp leaves or other
      mechanisms W60
    powered
      garden cultivator W29.3
      household appliance, implement, or
        machine W29.8
      saw (industrial) W31.2
        hand W29.8
    printing machine W31.89

Contact *(Continued)*
  with *(Continued)*
    psittacine bird W61.29
      bite W61.21
      macaw —*see* Contact, with, macaw
      parrot —*see* Contact, with, parrot
      strike W61.22
    pulley (block) (transmission) W24.0
      agricultural operations W30.89
    raccoon W55.59
      bite W55.51
      strike W55.52
    radial-saw (industrial) W31.2
    radiator (hot) X16
    rake W27.1
    rattlesnake X58
    reaper W30.0
    reptile W59.89
      lizard —*see* Contact, with, lizard
      snake —*see* Contact, with, snake
      specified NEC W59.89
        bite W59.81
        crushing W59.83
        strike W59.82
      turtle —*see* Contact, with, turtle
    rivet gun (powered) W29.4
    road scraper —*see* Accident, transport,
      construction vehicle
    rodent (feces) (urine) W53.89
      bite W53.81
      mouse W53.09
        bite W53.01
      rat W53.19
        bite W53.11
      specified NEC W53.89
        bite W53.81
      squirrel W53.29
        bite W53.21
    roller coaster W31.81
    rope NEC W24.0
      agricultural operations W30.89
    saliva —*see* Contact, with, by type of
      animal
    sander W29.8
      industrial W31.2
    saucepan (hot) (glass) (metal) X15.3
    saw W27.0
      band (industrial) W31.2
      bench (industrial) W31.2
      chain W29.3
      hand W27.0
    sawing machine, metal W31.1
    scissors W27.2
    scorpion X58
    screwdriver W27.0
      powered W29.8
    sea
      anemone, cucumber or urchin (spine)
        X58
      lion W56.19
        bite W56.11
        strike W56.12
    serpent —*see* Contact, with, snake, by type
    sewing-machine (electric) (powered) W29.2
      not powered W27.8
    shaft (hoist) (lift) (transmission) NEC W24.0
      agricultural W30.89
    shark W56.49
      bite W56.41
      strike W56.42
    sharp object(s) W26.9
      specified NEC W26.8
    shears (hand) W27.2
      powered (industrial) W31.1
        domestic W29.2
    sheep W55.39
      bite W55.31
      strike W55.32
    shovel W27.8
      steam —*see* Accident, transport,
        construction vehicle

Contact *(Continued)*
  with *(Continued)*
    snake (nonvenomous) W59.19
      bite W59.11
      crushing W59.13
      strike W59.12
    spade W27.1
    spider (venomous) X58
    spin-drier W29.2
    spinning machine W31.89
    splinter W45.8
    sports equipment W21.9
    staple gun (powered) W29.8
    steam X13.1
      engine W31.3
      inhalation X13.0
      pipe X16
      shovel W31.89
    stove (hot) (kitchen) X15.0
    substance, hot NEC X19
      molten (metal) X18
    sword W26.1
      assault X99.2
      stated as undetermined whether
        accidental or intentional
        Y28.2
      suicide (attempt) X78.2
    tarantula X58
    thresher W30.0
    tin can lid W26.8
    toad W62.1
    toaster (hot) X15.1
    tool W27.8
      hand (not powered) W27.8
        auger W27.0
        axe W27.0
        can opener W27.4
        chisel W27.0
        fork W27.4
        garden W27.1
        handsaw W27.0
        hoe W27.1
        ice-pick W27.4
        kitchen utensil W27.4
        manual
          lawn mower W27.1
          sewing machine W27.8
        meat grinder W27.4
        needle (sewing) W27.3
          hypodermic W46.0
            contaminated W46.1
        paper cutter W27.5
        pitchfork W27.1
        rake W27.1
        scissors W27.2
        screwdriver W27.0
        specified NEC W27.8
        workbench W27.0
      hot X17
      powered W29.8
        blender W29.0
          commercial W31.82
        can opener W29.0
          commercial W31.82
        chainsaw W29.3
        clothes dryer W29.2
          commercial W31.82
        dishwasher W29.2
          commercial W31.82
        edger W29.3
        electric fan W29.2
          commercial W31.82
        electric knife W29.1
        food processor W29.0
          commercial W31.82
        garbage disposal W29.0
          commercial W31.82

Contact *(Continued)*
  with *(Continued)*
    tool *(Continued)*
      powered *(Continued)*
        garden tool W29.3
        hedge trimmer W29.3
        ice maker W29.0
          commercial W31.82
        kitchen appliance W29.0
          commercial W31.82
        lawn mower W28
        meat grinder W29.0
          commercial W31.82
        mixer W29.0
          commercial W31.82
        rototiller W29.3
        sewing machine W29.2
          commercial W31.82
        washing machine W29.2
          commercial W31.82
    transmission device (belt, cable, chain,
      gear, pinion, shaft) W24.1
      agricultural operations W30.89
    turbine (gas) (water-driven) W31.3
    turkey W61.49
      peck W61.43
      strike W61.42
    turtle (nonvenomous) W59.29
      bite W59.21
      strike W59.22
      terrestrial W59.89
        bite W59.81
        crushing W59.83
        strike W59.82
    under-cutter W31.0
    urine —*see* Contact, with, by type of animal
    vehicle
      agricultural use (transport) —*see*
        Accident, transport, agricultural
        vehicle
        not on public highway W30.81
      industrial use (transport) —*see*
        Accident, transport, industrial
        vehicle
        not on public highway W31.83
      off-road use (transport) —*see* Accident,
        transport, all-terrain or off-road
        vehicle
        not on public highway W31.83
      special construction use (transport) —*see*
        Accident, transport, construction
        vehicle
        not on public highway W31.83
    venomous
      animal X58
      arthropods X58
      lizard X58
      marine animal NEC X58
      marine plant NEC X58
      millipedes (tropical) X58
      plant(s) X58
      snake X58
      spider X58
      viper X58
    washing-machine (powered) W29.2
    wasp X58
    weaving-machine W31.89
    winch W24.0
      agricultural operations W30.89
    wire NEC W24.0
      agricultural operations W30.89
    wood slivers W45.8
    yellow jacket X58
    zebra —*see* Contact, with, hoof stock NEC
  pressure X50.9
  stress X50.9
Coup de soleil X32

Crash
  aircraft (in transit) (powered) V95.9
    balloon V96.01
    fixed wing NEC (private) V95.21
      commercial V95.31
    glider V96.21
      hang V96.11
      powered V95.11
    helicopter V95.01
    in war operations —*see* War operations,
      destruction of aircraft
    microlight V95.11
    nonpowered V96.9
      specified NEC V96.8
    powered NEC V95.8
    stated as
      homicide (attempt) Y08.81
      suicide (attempt) X83.0
    ultralight V95.11
  spacecraft V95.41
  transport vehicle NEC —*see also* Accident,
    transport V89.9
    homicide (attempt) Y03.8
    motor NEC (traffic) V89.2
      homicide (attempt) Y03.8
      suicide (attempt) —*see* Suicide, collision
Cruelty (mental) (physical) (sexual) X58
Crushed (accidentally) X58
  between objects (moving) (stationary and
    moving) W23.0
    stationary W23.1
  by
    alligator W58.03
    avalanche NEC —*see* Landslide
    cave-in W20.0
      caused by cataclysmic earth surface
        movement —*see* Landslide
    crocodile W58.13
    crowd or human stampede W52
    falling
      aircraft V97.39
        in war operations —*see* War
          operations, destruction of aircraft
      earth, material W20.0
        caused by cataclysmic earth surface
          movement —*see* Landslide
      object NEC W20.8
    landslide NEC —*see* Landslide
    lizard (nonvenomous) W59.09
    machinery —*see* Contact, with, by type of
      machine
    reptile NEC W59.89
    snake (nonvenomous) W59.13
  in
    machinery —*see* Contact, with, by type of
      machine
Cut, cutting (any part of body) (accidental) —
  see also Contact, with, by object or machine
  during medical or surgical treatment as
    misadventure —*see* Index to Diseases
    and Injuries, Complications
  homicide (attempt) —*see* Assault, cutting or
    piercing instrument
  inflicted by other person —*see* Assault,
    cutting or piercing instrument
  legal
    execution —*see* Legal, intervention
    intervention —*see* Legal, intervention,
      sharp object
  machine NEC —*see also* Contact, with, by
    type of machine W31.9
  self-inflicted —*see* Suicide, cutting or piercing
    instrument
  suicide (attempt) —*see* Suicide, cutting or
    piercing instrument
Cyclone (any injury) X37.1

D

Decapitation (accidental circumstances)
NEC X58
homicide X99.9
legal execution —*see* Legal, intervention
Dehydration from lack of water X58
Deprivation X58
Derailment (accidental)
railway (rolling stock) (train) (vehicle)
(without antecedent collision) V81.7
with antecedent collision —*see* Accident,
transport, railway vehicle occupant
streetcar (without antecedent collision) V82.7
with antecedent collision —*see* Accident,
transport, streetcar occupant
Descent
parachute (voluntary) (without accident to
aircraft) V97.29
due to accident to aircraft —*see* Accident,
transport, aircraft
Desertion X58
Destitution X58
Disability, late effect or sequela of injury —*see*
Sequelae
Discharge (accidental)
airgun W34.010
assault X95.01
homicide (attempt) X95.01
stated as undetermined whether accidental
or intentional Y24.0
suicide (attempt) X74.01
BB gun —*see* Discharge, airgun
firearm (accidental) W34.00
assault X95.9
handgun (pistol) (revolver) W32.0
assault X93
homicide (attempt) X93
legal intervention —*see* Legal,
intervention, firearm, handgun
stated as undetermined whether
accidental or intentional Y22
suicide (attempt) X72
homicide (attempt) X95.9
hunting rifle W33.02
assault X94.1
homicide (attempt) X94.1
legal intervention
injuring
bystander Y35.032
law enforcement personnel Y35.031
suspect Y35.033
unspecified person Y35.039
stated as undetermined whether
accidental or intentional Y23.1
suicide (attempt) X73.1
larger W33.00
assault X94.9
homicide (attempt) X94.9
hunting rifle —*see* Discharge, firearm,
hunting rifle
legal intervention —*see* Legal,
intervention, firearm by type of
firearm
machine gun —*see* Discharge, firearm,
machine gun
shotgun —*see* Discharge, firearm,
shotgun
specified NEC W33.09
assault X94.8
homicide (attempt) X94.8
legal intervention
injuring
bystander Y35.092
law enforcement personnel
Y35.091
suspect Y35.093
unspecified person Y35.099
stated as undetermined whether
accidental or intentional Y23.8
suicide (attempt) X73.8

Discharge (Continued)
firearm (Continued)
larger (Continued)
stated as undetermined whether
accidental or intentional Y23.9
suicide (attempt) X73.9
legal intervention
injuring
bystander Y35.002
law enforcement personnel Y35.001
suspect Y35.03
unspecified person Y35.009
using rubber bullet
injuring
bystander Y35.042
law enforcement personnel Y35.041
suspect Y35.043
unspecified person Y35.049
machine gun W33.03
assault X94.2
homicide (attempt) X94.2
legal intervention —*see* Legal,
intervention, firearm, machine gun
stated as undetermined whether
accidental or intentional Y23.3
suicide (attempt) X73.2
pellet gun —*see* Discharge, airgun
shotgun W33.01
assault X94.0
homicide (attempt) X94.0
legal intervention —*see* Legal,
intervention, firearm, specified NEC
stated as undetermined whether
accidental or intentional Y23.0
suicide (attempt) X73.0
specified NEC W34.09
assault X95.8
homicide (attempt) X95.8
legal intervention —*see* Legal,
intervention, firearm, specified NEC
stated as undetermined whether
accidental or intentional Y24.8
suicide (attempt) X74.8
stated as undetermined whether accidental
or intentional Y24.9
suicide (attempt) X74.9
Very pistol W34.09
assault X95.8
homicide (attempt) X95.8
stated as undetermined whether
accidental or intentional Y24.8
suicide (attempt) X74.8
firework(s) W39
stated as undetermined whether accidental
or intentional Y25
gas-operated gun NEC W34.018
airgun —*see* Discharge, airgun
assault X95.09
homicide (attempt) X95.09
paintball gun —*see* Discharge, paintball gun
stated as undetermined whether accidental
or intentional Y24.8
suicide (attempt) X74.09
gun NEC —*see also* Discharge, firearm NEC
air —*see* Discharge, airgun
BB —*see* Discharge, airgun
for single hand use —*see* Discharge,
firearm, handgun
hand —*see* Discharge, firearm, handgun
machine —*see* Discharge, firearm, machine
gun
other specified —*see* Discharge, firearm
NEC
paintball —*see* Discharge, paintball gun
pellet —*see* Discharge, airgun
handgun —*see* Discharge, firearm, handgun
machine gun —*see* Discharge, firearm,
machine gun
paintball gun W34.011
assault X95.02
homicide (attempt) X95.02

Discharge (Continued)
paintball gun (Continued)
stated as undetermined whether accidental
or intentional Y24.8
suicide (attempt) X74.02
pistol —*see* Discharge, firearm, handgun
flare —*see* Discharge, firearm, Very pistol
pellet —*see* Discharge, airgun
Very —*see* Discharge, firearm, Very pistol
revolver —*see* Discharge, firearm, handgun
rifle (hunting) —*see* Discharge, firearm,
hunting rifle
shotgun —*see* Discharge, firearm, shotgun
spring-operated gun NEC W34.018
assault X95.09
homicide (attempt) X95.09
stated as undetermined whether accidental
or intentional Y24.8
suicide (attempt) X74.09
Disease
Andes W94.11
aviator's —*see* Air, pressure
range W94.11
Diver's disease, palsy, paralysis, squeeze —*see*
Air, pressure
Diving (into water) —*see* Accident, diving
Dog bite W54.0
Dragged by transport vehicle NEC —*see also*
Accident, transport V09.9
Drinking poison (accidental) —*see* Table of
Drugs and Chemicals
Dropped (accidentally) while being carried or
supported by other person W04
Drowning (accidental) W74
assault X92.9
due to
accident (to)
machinery —*see* Contact, with, by type
of machine
watercraft V90.89
burning V90.29
powered V90.23
fishing boat V90.22
jet ski V90.23
merchant ship V90.20
passenger ship V90.21
unpowered V90.28
canoe V90.25
inflatable V90.26
kayak V90.25
sailboat V90.24
water skis V90.27
crushed V90.39
powered V90.33
fishing boat V90.32
jet ski V90.33
merchant ship V90.30
passenger ship V90.31
unpowered V90.38
canoe V90.35
inflatable V90.36
kayak V90.35
sailboat V90.34
water skis V90.37
overturning V90.09
powered V90.03
fishing boat V90.02
jet ski V90.03
merchant ship V90.00
passenger ship V90.01
unpowered V90.08
canoe V90.05
inflatable V90.06
kayak V90.05
sailboat V90.04
sinking V90.19
powered V90.13
fishing boat V90.12
jet ski V90.13
merchant ship V90.10
passenger ship V90.11

▶ New   ⇒ Revised   ~~deleted~~ Deleted   ● Use Additional Character(s)

E

Earth (surface) movement NEC —see Forces of
   nature, earth movement
Earth falling (on) W20.0
   caused by cataclysmic earth surface
      movement or eruption —see Landslide
Earthquake (any injury) X34
Effect(s) (adverse) of
   air pressure (any) —see Air, pressure
   cold, excessive (exposure to) —see Exposure,
      cold
   heat (excessive) —see Heat
   hot place (weather) —see Heat
   insolation X30
   late —see Sequelae
   motion —see Motion
   nuclear explosion or weapon in war
      operations —see War operations, nuclear
      weapon
   radiation —see Radiation
   travel —see Travel
Electric shock (accidental) (by) (in) —see
   Exposure, electric current
Electrocution (accidental) —see Exposure,
   electric current
Endotracheal tube wrongly placed during
   anesthetic procedure Y65.3
Entanglement
   in
      bed linen, causing suffocation —see
         category T71
      wheel of pedal cycle V19.88
Entry of foreign body or material —see Foreign
   body
Environmental pollution related condition —
   see Z57
Execution, legal (any method) —see Legal,
   intervention
Exhaustion
   cold —see Exposure, cold
   due to excessive exertion —see also
      Overexertion X50.9
   heat —see Heat
Explosion (accidental) (of) (with secondary fire)
   W40.9
   acetylene W40.1
   aerosol can W36.1
   air tank (compressed) (in machinery) W36.2
   aircraft (in transit) (powered) NEC V95.9
      balloon V96.05
      fixed wing NEC (private) V95.25
         commercial V95.35
      glider V96.25
         hang V96.15
         powered V95.15
      helicopter V95.05
      in war operations —see War operations,
         destruction of aircraft
      microlight V95.15
      nonpowered V96.9
         specified NEC V96.8
      powered NEC V95.8
      stated as
         homicide (attempt) Y03.8
         suicide (attempt) X83.0
      ultralight V95.15
   anesthetic gas in operating room W40.1
   antipersonnel bomb W40.8
      assault X96.0
      homicide (attempt) X96.0
      suicide (attempt) X75
   assault X96.9
   bicycle tire W37.0
   blasting (cap) (materials) W40.0
   boiler (machinery), not on transport vehicle
      W35
      on watercraft —see Explosion, in,
         watercraft
   butane W40.1
   caused by other person X96.9
   coal gas W40.1

Explosion (Continued)
   detonator W40.0
   dump (munitions) W40.8
   dynamite W40.0
      in
         assault X96.8
         homicide (attempt) X96.8
         legal intervention
            injuring
               bystander Y35.112
               law enforcement personnel Y35.111
               suspect Y35.113
               unspecified person Y35.119
         suicide (attempt) X75
   explosive (material) W40.9
      gas W40.1
      in blasting operation W40.0
      specified NEC W40.8
         in
            assault X96.8
            homicide (attempt) X96.8
            legal intervention
               injuring
                  bystander Y35.192
                  law enforcement personnel
                    Y35.191
                  suspect Y35.193
                  unspecified person Y35.199
            suicide (attempt) X75
   factory (munitions) W40.8
   fertilizer bomb W40.8
      assault X96.3
      homicide (attempt) X96.3
      suicide (attempt) X75
   fire-damp W40.1
   firearm (parts) NEC W34.19
      airgun W34.110
      BB gun W34.110
      gas, air or spring-operated gun NEC W34.118
      handgun W32.1
      hunting rifle W33.12
      larger firearm W33.10
         specified NEC W33.19
      machine gun W33.13
      paintball gun W34.111
      pellet gun W34.110
      shotgun W33.11
      Very pistol [flare] W34.19
   fireworks W39
   gas (coal) (explosive) W40.1
      cylinder W36.9
         aerosol can W36.1
         air tank W36.2
         pressurized W36.3
         specified NEC W36.8
   gasoline (fumes) (tank) not in moving motor
      vehicle W40.1
      bomb W40.8
         assault X96.1
         homicide (attempt) X96.1
         suicide (attempt) X75
      in motor vehicle —see Accident, transport,
         by type of vehicle
   grain store W40.8
   grenade W40.8
      in
         assault X96.8
         homicide (attempt) X96.8
         legal intervention
            injuring
               bystander Y35.192
               law enforcement personnel Y35.191
               suspect Y35.193
               unspecified person Y35.199
         suicide (attempt) X75
   handgun (parts) —see Explosion, firearm,
      handgun (parts)
   homicide (attempt) X96.9
      antipersonnel bomb —see Explosion,
         antipersonnel bomb
      fertilizer bomb —see Explosion, fertilizer
         bomb

Explosion (Continued)
   homicide (Continued)
      gasoline bomb —see Explosion, gasoline
         bomb
      letter bomb —see Explosion, letter bomb
      pipe bomb —see Explosion, pipe bomb
      specified NEC X96.8
   hose, pressurized W37.8
   hot water heater, tank (in machinery) W35
      on watercraft —see Explosion, in, watercraft
   in, on
      dump W40.8
      factory W40.8
      mine (of explosive gases) NEC W40.1
      watercraft V93.59
         powered craft V93.53
            ferry boat V93.51
            fishing boat V93.52
            jet ski V93.53
            liner V93.51
            merchant ship V93.50
            passenger ship V93.51
            sailboat V93.54
   letter bomb W40.8
      assault X96.2
      homicide (attempt) X96.2
      suicide (attempt) X75
   machinery —see also Contact, with, by type
      of machine
      on board watercraft —see Explosion, in,
         watercraft
      pressure vessel —see Explosion, by type
         of vessel
   methane W40.1
   mine W40.1
   missile NEC W40.8
   mortar bomb W40.8
      in
         assault X96.8
         homicide (attempt) X96.8
         legal intervention
            injuring
               bystander Y35.192
               law enforcement personnel Y35.191
               suspect Y35.193
               unspecified person Y35.199
         suicide (attempt) X75
   munitions (dump) (factory) W40.8
   pipe, pressurized W37.8
      bomb W40.8
         assault X96.4
         homicide (attempt) X96.4
         suicide (attempt) X75
   pressure, pressurized
      cooker W38
      gas tank (in machinery) W36.3
      hose W37.8
      pipe W37.8
      specified device NEC W38
      tire W37.8
         bicycle W37.0
      vessel (in machinery) W38
   propane W40.1
   self-inflicted X75
   shell (artillery) NEC W40.8
      during war operations —see War
         operations, explosion
      in
         legal intervention
            injuring
               bystander Y35.122
               law enforcement personnel Y35.121
               suspect Y35.123
               unspecified person Y35.129
      war —see War operations, explosion
   spacecraft V95.45
   stated as undetermined whether accidental or
      intentional Y25
   steam or water lines (in machinery) W37.8
   stove W40.9
   suicide (attempt) X75

▶ New   ⇒ Revised   ~~deleted~~ Deleted   • Use Additional Character(s)

Explosion *(Continued)*
  tire, pressurized W37.8
    bicycle W37.Ø
  undetermined whether accidental or
    intentional Y25
  vehicle tire NEC W37.8
    bicycle W37.Ø
  war operations —*see* War operations,
    explosion
Exposure (to) X58
  air pressure change —*see* Air, pressure
  cold (accidental) (excessive) (extreme)
    (natural) (place) X31
    assault YØ8.89
    due to
      man-made conditions W93.8
        dry ice (contact) W93.Ø1
          inhalation W93.Ø2
        liquid air (contact) (hydrogen)
          (nitrogen) W93.11
          inhalation W93.12
        refrigeration unit (deep freeze)
          W93.2
    suicide (attempt) X83.2
    weather (conditions) X31
    homicide (attempt) YØ8.89
    self-inflicted X83.2
  due to abandonment or neglect X58
  electric current W86.8
    appliance (faulty) W86.8
      domestic W86.Ø
    caused by other person YØ8.89
    conductor (faulty) W86.1
    control apparatus (faulty) W86.1
    electric power generating plant,
      distribution station W86.1
    electroshock gun —*see* Exposure, electric
      current, taser
    high-voltage cable W85
    homicide (attempt) YØ8.89
    legal execution —*see* Legal, intervention,
      specified means NEC
    lightning —*see* subcategory T75.Ø
    live rail W86.8
    misadventure in medical or surgical
      procedure in electroshock therapy
      Y63.4
    motor (electric) (faulty) W86.8
      domestic W86.Ø
    self-inflicted X83.1
    specified NEC W86.8
      domestic W86.Ø
    stun gun —*see* Exposure, electric current,
      taser
    suicide (attempt) X83.1
    taser W86.8
      assault YØ8.89
      legal intervention —*see* category Y35
      self-harm (intentional) X83.8
      undetermined intent Y33
    third rail W86.8
    transformer (faulty) W86.1
    transmission lines W85
  environmental tobacco smoke X58
  excessive
    cold —*see* Exposure, cold
    heat (natural) NEC X30
      man-made W92
  factor(s) NOS X58
    environmental NEC X58
      man-made NEC W99
      natural NEC —*see* Forces of nature
    specified NEC X58
  fire, flames (accidental) XØ8.8
    assault X97
    campfire —*see* Exposure, fire, controlled,
      not in building
    controlled (in)
      with ignition (of) clothing —*see also*
        Ignition, clothes XØ6.2
        nightwear XØ5

Exposure *(Continued)*
  fire, flames *(Continued)*
    controlled *(Continued)*
      bonfire —*see* Exposure, fire, controlled,
        not in building
      brazier (in building or structure) —*see
        also* Exposure, fire, controlled,
        building
        not in building or structure —*see*
          Exposure, fire, controlled, not in
          building
      building or structure XØ2.Ø
        with
          fall from building XØ2.3
          from building XØ2.5
          injury due to building collapse
            XØ2.2
          smoke inhalation XØ2.1
        hit by object from building XØ2.4
        specified mode of injury NEC XØ2.8
      fireplace, furnace or stove —*see*
        Exposure, fire, controlled, building
      not in building or structure XØ3.Ø
        with
          fall XØ3.3
          smoke inhalation XØ3.1
        hit by object XØ3.4
        specified mode of injury NEC XØ3.8
      trash —*see* Exposure, fire, controlled, not
        in building
    fireplace —*see* Exposure, fire, controlled,
      building
    fittings or furniture (in building or
      structure) (uncontrolled) —*see*
      Exposure, fire, uncontrolled, building
    forest (uncontrolled) —*see* Exposure, fire,
      uncontrolled, not in building
    grass (uncontrolled) —*see* Exposure, fire,
      uncontrolled, not in building
    hay (uncontrolled) —*see* Exposure, fire,
      uncontrolled, not in building
    homicide (attempt) X97
    ignition of highly flammable material XØ4
    in, of, on, starting in
      machinery —*see* Contact, with, by type
        of machine
      motor vehicle (in motion) —*see also*
        Accident, transport, occupant by
        type of vehicle V87.8
        with collision —*see* Collision
      railway rolling stock, train, vehicle
        V81.81
        with collision —*see* Accident,
          transport, railway vehicle
          occupant
      street car (in motion) V82.8
        with collision —*see* Accident,
          transport, streetcar occupant
      transport vehicle NEC —*see also*
        Accident, transport
        with collision —*see* Collision
      war operations —*see also* War operations,
        fire
        from nuclear explosion —*see* War
          operations, nuclear weapons
      watercraft (in transit) (not in transit)
        V91.Ø9
        localized —*see* Burn, on board
          watercraft, due to, fire on board
        powered craft V91.Ø3
          ferry boat V91.Ø1
          fishing boat V91.Ø2
          jet skis V91.Ø3
          liner V91.Ø1
          merchant ship V91.ØØ
          passenger ship V91.Ø1
        unpowered craft V91.Ø8
          canoe V91.Ø5
          inflatable V91.Ø6
          kayak V91.Ø5
          sailboat V91.Ø4

Exposure *(Continued)*
  fire, flames *(Continued)*
    in, of, on, starting in *(Continued)*
      watercraft *(Continued)*
        unpowered craft *(Continued)*
          surf-board V91.Ø8
          waterskis V91.Ø7
          windsurfer V91.Ø8
    lumber (uncontrolled) —*see* Exposure, fire,
      uncontrolled, not in building
    mine (uncontrolled) —*see* Exposure, fire,
      uncontrolled, not in building
    prairie (uncontrolled) —*see* Exposure, fire,
      uncontrolled, not in building
    resulting from
      explosion —*see* Explosion
      lightning XØ8.8
    self-inflicted X76
    specified NEC XØ8.8
    started by other person X97
    stated as undetermined whether accidental
      or intentional Y26
    stove —*see* Exposure, fire, controlled,
      building
    suicide (attempt) X76
    tunnel (uncontrolled) —*see* Exposure, fire,
      uncontrolled, not in building
    uncontrolled
      in building or structure XØØ.Ø
        with
          fall from building XØØ.3
          injury due to building collapse
            XØØ.2
          jump from building XØØ.5
          smoke inhalation XØØ.1
        bed XØ8.ØØ
          due to
            cigarette XØ8.Ø1
            specified material NEC XØ8.Ø9
        furniture NEC XØ8.2Ø
          due to
            cigarette XØ8.21
            specified material NEC XØ8.29
        hit by object from building XØØ.4
        sofa XØ8.1Ø
          due to
            cigarette XØ8.11
            specified material NEC
              XØ8.19
        specified mode of injury NEC
          XØØ.8
      not in building or structure (any)
        XØ1.Ø
        with
          fall XØ1.3
          smoke inhalation XØ1.1
        hit by object XØ1.4
        specified mode of injury NEC
          XØ1.8
    undetermined whether accidental or
      intentional Y26
  forces of nature NEC —*see* Forces of nature
  G-forces (abnormal) W49.9
  gravitational forces (abnormal) W49.9
  heat (natural) NEC —*see* Heat
  high-pressure jet (hydraulic) (pneumatic)
    W49.9
  hydraulic jet W49.9
  inanimate mechanical force W49.9
  jet, high-pressure (hydraulic) (pneumatic)
    W49.9
  lightning —*see* subcategory T75.Ø
    causing fire —*see* Exposure, fire
  mechanical forces NEC W49.9
    animate NEC W64
    inanimate NEC W49.9
  noise W42.9
    supersonic W42.Ø
  noxious substance —*see* Table of Drugs and
    Chemicals
  pneumatic jet W49.9

Exposure (*Continued*)
   prolonged in deep-freeze unit or refrigerator W93.2
   radiation —*see* Radiation
   smoke —*see also* Exposure, fire
     tobacco, second hand Z77.22
   specified factors NEC X58
   sunlight X32
     man-made (sun lamp) W89.8
       tanning bed W89.1
   supersonic waves W42.0
   transmission line(s), electric W85
   vibration W49.9

Exposure (*Continued*)
   waves
     infrasound W49.9
     sound W42.9
     supersonic W42.0
   weather NEC —*see* Forces of nature
External cause status Y99.9
   child assisting in compensated work for family Y99.8
   civilian activity done for financial or other compensation Y99.0
   civilian activity done for income or pay Y99.0

External cause status (*Continued*)
   family member assisting in compensated work for other family member Y99.8
   hobby not done for income Y99.8
   leisure activity Y99.8
   military activity Y99.1
   off-duty activity of military personnel Y99.8
   recreation or sport not for income or while a student Y99.8
   specified NEC Y99.8
   student activity Y99.8
   volunteer activity Y99.2

▶ New   ⟹ Revised   ~~deleted~~ Deleted   ● Use Additional Character(s)

F

Factors, supplemental
  alcohol
    blood level
      less than 20mg/100ml Y90.0
      presence in blood, level not specified
        Y90.9
      20-39mg/100ml Y90.1
      40-59mg/100ml Y90.2
      60-79mg/100ml Y90.3
      80-99mg/100ml Y90.4
      100-119mg/100ml Y90.5
      120-199mg/100ml Y90.6
      200-239mg/100ml Y90.7
      240mg/100ml or more Y90.8
    presence in blood, but level not specified
      Y90.9
  environmental-pollution-related condition —
    see Z57
  nosocomial condition Y95
  work-related condition Y99.0
Failure
  in suture or ligature during surgical
    procedure Y65.2
  mechanical, of instrument or apparatus
    (any) (during any medical or surgical
    procedure) Y65.8
  sterile precautions (during medical and
    surgical care) —see Misadventure,
    failure, sterile precautions, by type of
    procedure
  to
    introduce tube or instrument Y65.4
    endotracheal tube during anesthesia Y65.3
    make curve (transport vehicle) NEC —see
      Accident, transport
    remove tube or instrument Y65.4
Fall, falling (accidental) W19
  building W20.1
    burning (uncontrolled fire) X00.3
  down
    embankment W17.81
    escalator W10.0
    hill W17.81
    ladder W11
    ramp W10.2
    stairs, steps W10.9
  due to
    bumping against
      object W18.00
        sharp glass W18.02
        specified NEC W18.09
        sports equipment W18.01
      person W03
        due to ice or snow W00.0
        on pedestrian conveyance —see
          Accident, transport, pedestrian,
          conveyance
    collision with another person W03
      due to ice or snow W00.0
      involving pedestrian conveyance —see
        Accident, transport, pedestrian,
        conveyance
    grocery cart tipping over W17.82
    ice or snow W00.9
      from one level to another W00.2
        on stairs or steps W00.1
      involving pedestrian conveyance —see
        Accident, transport, pedestrian,
        conveyance
      on same level W00.0
    slipping (on moving sidewalk) W01.0
      with subsequent striking against object
        W01.10
        furniture W01.190
        sharp object W01.119
          glass W01.110
          power tool or machine W01.111
          specified NEC W01.118
        specified NEC W01.198

Fall, falling (Continued)
  due to (Continued)
    striking against
      object W18.00
        sharp glass W18.02
        specified NEC W18.09
        sports equipment W18.01
      person W03
        due to ice or snow W00.0
        on pedestrian conveyance —see
          Accident, transport, pedestrian,
          conveyance
  earth (with asphyxia or suffocation (by
    pressure)) —see Earth, falling
  from, off, out of
    aircraft NEC (with accident to aircraft
      NEC) V97.0
      while boarding or alighting V97.1
    balcony W13.0
    bed W06
    boat, ship, watercraft NEC (with drowning
      or submersion) —see Drowning, due
      to, fall overboard
      with hitting bottom or object V94.0
    bridge W13.1
    building W13.9
      burning (uncontrolled fire) X00.3
    cavity W17.2
    chair W07
    cherry picker W17.89
    cliff W15
    dock W17.4
    embankment W17.81
    escalator W10.0
    flagpole W13.8
    furniture NEC W08
    grocery cart W17.82
    haystack W17.89
    high place NEC W17.89
      stated as undetermined whether
        accidental or intentional Y30
    hole W17.2
    incline W10.2
    ladder W11
    lifting device W17.89
    machine, machinery —see also Contact,
      with, by type of machine
      not in operation W17.89
    manhole W17.1
    mobile elevated work platform [MEWP]
      W17.89
    motorized mobility scooter W05.2
    one level to another NEC W17.89
      intentional, purposeful, suicide
        (attempt) X80
      stated as undetermined whether
        accidental or intentional Y30
    pit W17.2
    playground equipment W09.8
      jungle gym W09.2
      slide W09.0
      swing W09.1
    quarry W17.89
    railing W13.9
    ramp W10.2
    roof W13.2
    scaffolding W12
    scooter (nonmotorized) W05.1
      motorized mobility W05.2
    sky lift W17.89
    stairs, steps W10.9
      curb W10.1
      due to ice or snow W00.1
      escalator W10.0
      incline W10.2
      ramp W10.2
      sidewalk curb W10.1
      specified NEC W10.8
    Standing
      electric scooter V00.841
      micro-mobility pedestrian conveyance
        V00.848

Fall, falling (Continued)
  from, off, out of (Continued)
    stepladder W11
    storm drain W17.1
    streetcar NEC V82.6
      with antecedent collision —see
        Accident, transport, streetcar
        occupant
      while boarding or alighting V82.4
    structure NEC W13.8
      burning (uncontrolled fire) X00.3
    table W08
    toilet W18.11
      with subsequent striking against object
        W18.12
    train NEC V81.6
      during derailment (without antecedent
        collision) V81.7
      with antecedent collision —see
        Accident, transport, railway
        vehicle occupant
      while boarding or alighting V81.4
    transport vehicle after collision —see
      Accident, transport, by type of
      vehicle, collision
    tree W14
    vehicle (in motion) NEC —see also
      Accident, transport V89.9
      motor NEC —see also Accident,
        transport, occupant, by type of
        vehicle V87.8
      stationary W17.89
        while boarding or alighting —see
          Accident, transport, by type of
          vehicle, while boarding or
          alighting
    viaduct W13.8
    wall W13.8
    watercraft —see also Drowning, due to, fall
      overboard
      with hitting bottom or object V94.0
    well W17.0
    wheelchair, non-moving W05.0
      powered —see Accident, transport,
        pedestrian, conveyance occupant,
        specified type NEC
    window W13.4
  in, on
    aircraft NEC V97.0
      with accident to aircraft V97.0
      while boarding or alighting V97.1
    bathtub (empty) W18.2
      filled W16.212
        causing drowning W16.211
    escalator W10.0
    incline W10.2
    ladder W11
    machine, machinery —see Contact, with,
      by type of machine
    object, edged, pointed or sharp (with
      cut) —see Fall, by type
    playground equipment W09.8
      jungle gym W09.2
      slide W09.0
      swing W09.1
    ramp W10.2
    scaffolding W12
    shower W18.2
      causing drowning W16.211
    staircase, stairs, steps W10.9
      curb W10.1
      due to ice or snow W00.1
      escalator W10.0
      incline W10.2
      specified NEC W10.8
    streetcar (without antecedent collision)
      V82.5
      with antecedent collision —see
        Accident, transport, streetcar
        occupant
      while boarding or alighting V82.4

Fall, falling *(Continued)*
  in, on *(Continued)*
    train (without antecedent collision) V81.5
      with antecedent collision —*see* Accident,
          transport, railway vehicle occupant
      during derailment (without antecedent
          collision) V81.7
        with antecedent collision —*see*
            Accident, transport, railway
            vehicle occupant
      while boarding or alighting V81.4
    transport vehicle after collision —*see*
        Accident, transport, by type of
        vehicle, collision
    watercraft V93.39
      due to
        accident to craft V91.29
          powered craft V91.23
            ferry boat V91.21
            fishing boat V91.22
            jet ski V91.23
            liner V91.21
            merchant ship V91.20
            passenger ship V91.21
          unpowered craft
            canoe V91.25
            inflatable V91.26
            kayak V91.25
            sailboat V91.24
        powered craft V93.33
          ferry boat V93.31
          fishing boat V93.32
          jet ski V93.33
          liner V93.31
          merchant ship V93.30
          passenger ship V93.31
        unpowered craft V93.38
          canoe V93.35
          inflatable V93.36
          kayak V93.35
          sailboat V93.34
          surf-board V93.38
          windsurfer V93.38
  into
    cavity W17.2
    dock W17.4
    fire —*see* Exposure, fire, by type
    haystack W17.89
    hole W17.2
    manhole W17.1
    moving part of machinery —*see* Contact,
        with, by type of machine
    ocean —*see* Fall, into, water
    opening in surface NEC W17.89
    pit W17.2
    pond —*see* Fall, into, water
    quarry W17.89
    river —*see* Fall, into, water
    shaft W17.89
    storm drain W17.1
    stream —*see* Fall, into, water
    swimming pool —*see also* Fall, into, water,
        in, swimming pool
      empty W17.3
    tank W17.89
    water W16.42
      causing drowning W16.41
      from watercraft —*see* Drowning, due to,
          fall overboard
      hitting diving board W21.4
      in
        bathtub W16.212
          causing drowning W16.211
        bucket W16.222
          causing drowning W16.221
        natural body of water W16.112
          causing drowning W16.111
          striking
            bottom W16.122
              causing drowning
                  W16.121

Fall, falling *(Continued)*
  into *(Continued)*
    water *(Continued)*
      in *(Continued)*
        natural body of water *(Continued)*
          striking *(Continued)*
            side W16.132
              causing drowning W16.131
        specified water NEC W16.312
          causing drowning W16.311
          striking
            bottom W16.322
              causing drowning W16.321
            wall W16.332
              causing drowning W16.331
        swimming pool W16.012
          causing drowning W16.011
          striking
            bottom W16.022
              causing drowning W16.021
            wall W16.032
              causing drowning W16.031
        utility bucket W16.222
          causing drowning W16.221
    well W17.0
  involving
    bed W06
    chair W07
    furniture NEC W08
    glass —*see* Fall, by type
    playground equipment W09.8
      jungle gym W09.2
      slide W09.0
      swing W09.1
    roller blades —*see* Accident, transport,
        pedestrian, conveyance
    skateboard(s) —*see* Accident, transport,
        pedestrian, conveyance
    skates (ice) (in line) (roller) —*see*
        Accident, transport, pedestrian,
        conveyance
    skis —*see* Accident, transport, pedestrian,
        conveyance
    table W08
    wheelchair, non-moving W05.0
      powered —*see* Accident, transport,
          pedestrian, conveyance, specified
          type NEC
  object —*see* Struck by, object, falling
  off
    toilet W18.11
      with subsequent striking against object
          W18.12
  on same level W18.30
    due to
      specified NEC W18.39
      stepping on an object W18.31
  out of
    bed W06
    building NEC W13.8
    chair W07
    furniture NEC W08
    wheelchair, non-moving W05.0
      powered —*see* Accident, transport,
          pedestrian, conveyance, specified
          type NEC
    window W13.4
  over
    animal W01.0
    cliff W15
    embankment W17.81
    small object W01.0
  rock W20.8
  same level W18.30
    from
      being crushed, pushed, or stepped on
          by a crowd or human stampede
          W52
      collision, pushing, shoving, by or with
          other person W03
      slipping, stumbling, tripping W01.0

Fall, falling *(Continued)*
  same level *(Continued)*
    involving ice or snow W00.0
      involving skates (ice) (roller),
          skateboard, skis —*see* Accident,
          transport, pedestrian, conveyance
  snowslide (avalanche) —*see* Landslide
  stone W20.8
  structure W20.1
    burning (uncontrolled fire) X00.3
  through
    bridge W13.1
    floor W13.3
    roof W13.2
    wall W13.8
    window W13.4
  timber W20.8
  tree (caused by lightning) W20.8
  while being carried or supported by other
      person(s) W04
Fallen on by
  animal (not being ridden) NEC W55.89
Felo-de-se —*see* Suicide
Fight (hand) (fists) (foot) —*see* Assault, fight
Fire (accidental) —*see* Exposure, fire
Firearm discharge —*see* Discharge, firearm
Fireball effects from nuclear explosion in war
    operations —*see* War operations, nuclear
    weapons
Fireworks (explosion) W39
Flash burns from explosion —*see* Explosion
Flood (any injury) (caused by) X38
  collapse of man-made structure causing earth
      movement X36.0
  tidal wave —*see* Forces of nature, tidal wave
Food (any type) in
  air passages (with asphyxia, obstruction, or
      suffocation) —*see* categories T17 and T18
  alimentary tract causing asphyxia (due to
      compression of trachea) —*see* categories
      T17 and T18
Forces of nature X39.8
  avalanche X36.1
    causing transport accident —*see* Accident,
        transport, by type of vehicle
  blizzard X37.2
  cataclysmic storm X37.9
    with flood X38
    blizzard X37.2
    cloudburst X37.8
    cyclone X37.1
    dust storm X37.3
    hurricane X37.0
    specified storm NEC X37.8
    storm surge X37.0
    tornado X37.1
    twister X37.1
    typhoon X37.0
  cloudburst X37.8
  cold (natural) X31
  cyclone X37.1
  dam collapse causing earth movement X36.0
  dust storm X37.3
  earth movement X36.1
    caused by dam or structure collapse X36.0
    earthquake X34
  earthquake X34
  flood (caused by) X38
    dam collapse X36.0
    tidal wave —*see* Forces of nature, tidal
        wave
  heat (natural) X30
  hurricane X37.0
  landslide X36.1
    causing transport accident —*see* Accident,
        transport, by type of vehicle
  lightning —*see* subcategory T75.0
    causing fire —*see* Exposure, fire
  mudslide X36.1
    causing transport accident —*see* Accident,
        transport, by type of vehicle

▶ New   ⇒ Revised   ~~deleted~~ Deleted   ● Use Additional Character(s)

Forces of nature (Continued)
radiation (natural) X39.08
radon X39.01
radon X39.01
specified force NEC X39.8
storm surge X37.0
structure collapse causing
earth movement
X36.0
sunlight X32
tidal wave X37.41
due to
earthquake X37.41
landslide X37.43
storm X37.42
volcanic eruption X37.41
tornado X37.1

Forces of nature (Continued)
tsunami X37.41
twister X37.1
typhoon X37.0
volcanic eruption X35
Foreign body
aspiration —see Index to Diseases and
Injuries, Foreign body, respitory
tract
embedded in skin W45
entering through skin W45.8
can lid W26.2
nail W45.0
paper W26.2
specified NEC 45.8
splinter W45.8

Forest fire (exposure to) —see Exposure, fire,
uncontrolled, not in building
Found injured X58
from exposure (to) —see Exposure
on
highway, road(way), street V89.9
railway right of way V81.9
Fracture (circumstances unknown or
unspecified) X58
due to specified cause NEC X58
Freezing —see Exposure, cold
Frostbite X31
due to man-made conditions —see Exposure,
cold, man-made
Frozen —see Exposure, cold

G

Gored by bull W55.22
Gunshot wound W34.00

H

Hailstones, injured by X39.8
Hanged herself or himself —see Hanging,
self-inflicted
Hanging (accidental) —see also category T71
legal execution —see Legal, intervention,
specified means NEC
Heat (effects of) (excessive) X30
due to
man-made conditions W92
on board watercraft V93.29
fishing boat V93.22
merchant ship V93.20
passenger ship V93.21
sailboat V93.24
specified powered craft NEC V93.23
weather (conditions) X30

Heat (Continued)
from
electric heating apparatus causing
burning X16
nuclear explosion in war operations —
see War operations, nuclear
weapons
inappropriate in local application or
packing in medical or surgical
procedure Y63.5
Hemorrhage
delayed following medical or surgical
treatment without mention of
misadventure —see Index to Diseases
and Injuries, Complication(s)
during medical or surgical treatment as
misadventure —see Index to Diseases
and Injuries, Complication(s)

High
altitude (effects) —see Air, pressure, low
level of radioactivity, effects —see Radiation
pressure (effects) —see Air, pressure, high
temperature, effects —see Heat
Hit, hitting (accidental) by —see Struck by
Hitting against —see Striking against
Homicide (attempt) (justifiable) —see Assault
Hot
place, effects —see also Heat
weather, effects X30
House fire (uncontrolled) —see Exposure, fire,
uncontrolled, building
Humidity, causing problem X39.8
Hunger X58
Hurricane (any injury) X37.0
Hypobarism, hypobaropathy —see Air,
pressure, low

F, G, & H

I

Ictus
caloris —*see also* Heat
solaris X30
Ignition (accidental) —*see also* Exposure, fire
    X08.8
  anesthetic gas in operating room W40.1
  apparel X06.2
    from highly flammable material X04
    nightwear X05
  bed linen (sheets) (spreads) (pillows)
    (mattress) —*see* Exposure, fire,
    uncontrolled, building, bed
  benzine X04
  clothes, clothing NEC (from controlled fire)
    X06.2
    from
      highly flammable material X04
  ether X04
    in operating room W40.1
  explosive material —*see* Explosion
  gasoline X04
  jewelry (plastic) (any) X06.0
  kerosene X04
  material
    explosive —*see* Explosion
    highly flammable with secondary
      explosion X04
  nightwear X05
  paraffin X04
  petrol X04
Immersion (accidental) —*see also* Drowning
  hand or foot due to cold (excessive) X31
Implantation of quills of porcupine W55.89
Inanition (from) (hunger) X58
  thirst X58.8
Inappropriate operation performed
  correct operation on wrong side or body part
    (wrong side) (wrong site) Y65.53
  operation intended for another patient done
    on wrong patient Y65.52
  wrong operation performed on correct
    patient Y65.51
Inattention after, at birth (homicidal intent)
  (infanticidal intent) X58
Incident, adverse
  device
    anesthesiology Y70.8
      accessory Y70.2
      diagnostic Y70.0
      miscellaneous Y70.8
      monitoring Y70.0
      prosthetic Y70.2
      rehabilitative Y70.1
      surgical Y70.3
      therapeutic Y70.1
    cardiovascular Y71.8
      accessory Y71.2
      diagnostic Y71.0
      miscellaneous Y71.8
      monitoring Y71.0
      prosthetic Y71.2
      rehabilitative Y71.1
      surgical Y71.3
      therapeutic Y71.1
    gastroenterology Y73.8
      accessory Y73.2
      diagnostic Y73.0
      miscellaneous Y73.8
      monitoring Y73.0
      prosthetic Y73.2
      rehabilitative Y73.1
      surgical Y73.3
      therapeutic Y73.1
    general
      hospital Y74.8
        accessory Y74.2
        diagnostic Y74.0
        miscellaneous Y74.8
        monitoring Y74.0

Incident, adverse *(Continued)*
  device *(Continued)*
    general *(Continued)*
      hospital *(Continued)*
        prosthetic Y74.2
        rehabilitative Y74.1
        surgical Y74.3
        therapeutic Y74.1
      surgical Y81.8
        accessory Y81.2
        diagnostic Y81.0
        miscellaneous Y81.8
        monitoring Y81.0
        prosthetic Y81.2
        rehabilitative Y81.1
        surgical Y81.3
        therapeutic Y81.1
    gynecological Y76.8
      accessory Y76.2
      diagnostic Y76.0
      miscellaneous Y76.8
      monitoring Y76.0
      prosthetic Y76.2
      rehabilitative Y76.1
      surgical Y76.3
      therapeutic Y76.1
    medical Y82.9
      specified type NEC Y82.8
    neurological Y75.8
      accessory Y75.2
      diagnostic Y75.0
      miscellaneous Y75.8
      monitoring Y75.0
      prosthetic Y75.2
      rehabilitative Y75.1
      surgical Y75.3
      therapeutic Y75.1
    obstetrical Y76.8
      accessory Y76.2
      diagnostic Y76.0
      miscellaneous Y76.8
      monitoring Y76.0
      prosthetic Y76.2
      rehabilitative Y76.1
      surgical Y76.3
      therapeutic Y76.1
    ophthalmic Y77.8
      accessory Y77.2
      contact lens (rigid gas permeable)
        (soft) (hydrophilic)) Y77.11
      diagnostic Y77.0
      miscellaneous Y77.8
      monitoring Y77.0
      prosthetic Y77.2
      rehabilitative Y77.19
      surgical Y77.3
      therapeutic Y77.19
    orthopedic Y79.8
      accessory Y79.2
      diagnostic Y79.0
      miscellaneous Y79.8
      monitoring Y79.0
      prosthetic Y79.2
      rehabilitative Y79.1
      surgical Y79.3
      therapeutic Y79.1
    otorhinolaryngological Y72.8
      accessory Y72.2
      diagnostic Y72.0
      miscellaneous Y72.8
      monitoring Y72.0
      prosthetic Y72.2
      rehabilitative Y72.1
      surgical Y72.3
      therapeutic Y72.1
    personal use Y74.8
      accessory Y74.2
      diagnostic Y74.0
      miscellaneous Y74.8
      monitoring Y74.0
      prosthetic Y74.2

Incident, adverse *(Continued)*
  device *(Continued)*
    personal use *(Continued)*
      rehabilitative Y74.1
      surgical Y74.3
      therapeutic Y74.1
    physical medicine Y80.8
      accessory Y80.2
      diagnostic Y80.0
      miscellaneous Y80.8
      monitoring Y80.0
      prosthetic Y80.2
      rehabilitative Y80.1
      surgical Y80.3
      therapeutic Y80.1
    plastic surgical Y81.8
      accessory Y81.2
      diagnostic Y81.0
      miscellaneous Y81.8
      monitoring Y81.0
      prosthetic Y81.2
      rehabilitative Y81.1
      surgical Y81.3
      therapeutic Y81.1
    radiological Y78.8
      accessory Y78.2
      diagnostic Y78.0
      miscellaneous Y78.8
      monitoring Y78.0
      prosthetic Y78.2
      rehabilitative Y78.1
      surgical Y78.3
      therapeutic Y78.1
    urology Y73.8
      accessory Y73.2
      diagnostic Y73.0
      miscellaneous Y73.8
      monitoring Y73.0
      prosthetic Y73.2
      rehabilitative Y73.1
      surgical Y73.3
      therapeutic Y73.1
Incineration (accidental) —*see* Exposure, fire
Infanticide —*see* Assault
Infrasound waves (causing injury) W49.9
Ingestion
  foreign body (causing injury) (with
    obstruction) —*see* Foreign body,
    alimentary canal
  poisonous
    plant(s) X58
    substance NEC —*see* Table of Drugs and
      Chemicals
Inhalation
  excessively cold substance, man-made —*see*
    Exposure, cold, man-made
  food (any type) (into respiratory tract) (with
    asphyxia, obstruction respiratory tract,
    suffocation) —*see* categories T17 and T18
  foreign body —*see* Foreign body, aspiration
  gastric contents (with asphyxia, obstruction
    respiratory passage, suffocation) T17.81-●
  hot air or gases X14.0
  liquid air, hydrogen, nitrogen W93.12
    suicide (attempt) X83.2
  steam X13.0
    assault X98.0
    stated as undetermined whether accidental
      or intentional Y27.0
    suicide (attempt) X77.0
  toxic gas —*see* Table of Drugs and
    Chemicals
  vomitus (with asphyxia, obstruction
    respiratory passage, suffocation) T17.81-●
Injury, injured (accidental(ly)) NOS X58
  by, caused by, from
    assault —*see* Assault
    law-enforcing agent, police, in course
      of legal intervention —*see* Legal
      intervention
    suicide (attempt) X83.8

▶ New   ⇒ Revised   ~~deleted~~ Deleted   ● Use Additional Character(s)

Injury, injured NOS (Continued)
  due to, in
    civil insurrection —see War
      operations
    fight —see also Assault, fight
      Y04.0
    war operations —see War
      operations
  homicide —see also Assault Y09
  inflicted (by)
    in course of arrest (attempted), suppression
      of disturbance, maintenance of order,
      by law-enforcing agents —see Legal
      intervention

Injury, injured NOS (Continued)
  inflicted (Continued)
    other person
      stated as
        accidental X58
        intentional, homicide (attempt) —see
          Assault
        undetermined whether accidental or
          intentional Y33
    purposely (inflicted) by other person(s) —see
      Assault
    self-inflicted X83.8
      stated as accidental X58
    specified cause NEC X58

Injury, injured NOS (Continued)
  undetermined whether accidental or
    intentional Y33
Insolation, effects X30
Insufficient nourishment X58
Interruption of respiration (by)
  food (lodged in esophagus) —see categories
    T17 and T18
  vomitus (lodged in esophagus) T17.81-•
Intervention, legal —see Legal intervention
Intoxication
  drug —see Table of Drugs and Chemicals
  poison —see Table of Drugs and
    Chemicals

J

Jammed (accidentally)
  between objects (moving) (stationary and
    moving) W23.0
  stationary W23.1
Jumped, jumping
  before moving object NEC X81.8
    motor vehicle X81.0
    subway train X81.1
    train X81.1
    undetermined whether accidental or
      intentional Y31
  from
    boat (into water) voluntarily,
      without accident (to or on boat)
      W16.712
      with
        accident to or on boat —see Accident,
          watercraft
        drowning or submersion W16.711
          suicide (attempt) X71.3

Jumped, jumping (Continued)
  from (Continued)
    boat voluntarily, without accident
      (Continued)
      striking bottom W16.722
        causing drowning W16.721
    building —see also Jumped, from,
      high place W13.9
      burning (uncontrolled fire)
        X00.5
    high place NEC W17.89
      suicide (attempt) X80
      undetermined whether accidental or
        intentional Y30
    structure —see also Jumped, from, high
      place W13.9
      burning (uncontrolled fire)
        X00.5
  into water W16.92
    causing drowning W16.91
    from, off watercraft —see Jumped, from,
      boat

Jumped, jumping (Continued)
  into water (Continued)
    in
      natural body W16.612
        causing drowning W16.611
        striking bottom W16.622
          causing drowning W16.621
      specified place NEC W16.812
        causing drowning W16.811
        striking
          bottom W16.822
            causing drowning W16.821
          wall W16.832
            causing drowning W16.831
      swimming pool W16.512
        causing drowning W16.511
        striking
          bottom W16.522
            causing drowning W16.521
          wall W16.532
            causing drowning W16.531
    suicide (attempt) X71.3

K

Kicked by
  animal NEC W55.82
  person(s) (accidentally) W50.1
    with intent to injure or kill Y04.0
    as, or caused by, a crowd or human
      stampede (with fall) W52
    assault Y04.0
    homicide (attempt) Y04.0
    in
      fight Y04.0
      legal intervention
        injuring
          bystander Y35.812
          law enforcement personnel
            Y35.811
          suspect Y35.813
          unspecified person Y35.819

Kicking
  against
    object W22.8
      sports equipment W21.9
      stationary W22.09
        sports equipment W21.89
    person —see Striking against, person
      sports equipment W21.9
  carpet stretcher with knee X50.3
Killed, killing (accidentally) NOS —see also
  Injury X58
  in
    action —see War operations
    brawl, fight (hand) (fists) (foot) Y04.0
      by weapon —see also Assault
        cutting, piercing —see Assault, cutting
          or piercing instrument
        firearm —see Discharge, firearm, by
          type, homicide

Killed, killing NOS (Continued)
  self
    stated as
      accident NOS X58
      suicide —see Suicide
      undetermined whether accidental or
        intentional Y33
Kneeling (prolonged) (static) X50.1
Knocked down (accidentally) (by) NOS X58
  animal (not being ridden) NEC —see also
    Struck by, by type of animal
  crowd or human stampede W52
  person W51
    in brawl, fight Y04.0
  transport vehicle NEC —see also Accident,
    transport V09.9

L

Laceration NEC —see Injury
Lack of
  care (helpless person) (infant) (newborn) X58
  food except as result of abandonment or
    neglect X58
    due to abandonment or neglect X58
  water except as result of transport accident
    X58
    due to transport accident —see Accident,
      transport, by type
  helpless person, infant, newborn X58
Landslide (falling on transport vehicle) X36.1
  caused by collapse of man-made structure
    X36.0
Late effect —see Sequelae
Legal
  execution (any method) —see Legal,
    intervention
  intervention (by)
    baton —see Legal, intervention, blunt
      object, baton
    bayonet —see Legal, intervention, sharp
      object, bayonet
    blow —see Legal, intervention,
      manhandling
    blunt object
      baton
        injuring
          bystander Y35.312
          law enforcement personnel Y35.311
          suspect Y35.313
          unspecified person Y35.319
        injuring
          bystander Y35.302
          law enforcement personnel Y35.301
          suspect Y35.303
          unspecified person Y35.309
        specified NEC
          injuring
            bystander Y35.392
            law enforcement personnel Y35.391
            suspect Y35.393
            unspecified person Y35.399
        stave
          injuring
            bystander Y35.392
            law enforcement personnel Y35.391
            suspect Y35.393
            unspecified person Y35.399
    bomb —see Legal, intervention, explosive
    conducted energy device
      injuring
        bystander Y35.832
        law enforcement personnel Y35.831
        suspect Y35.833
        unspecified person Y35.839
    cutting or piercing instrument —see Legal,
      intervention, sharp object
    dynamite —see Legal, intervention,
      explosive, dynamite
    electroshock device (taser)
      injuring
        bystander Y35.832
        law enforcement personnel Y35.831
        suspect Y35.833
        unspecified person Y35.839
    explosive(s)
      dynamite
        injuring
          bystander Y35.112
          law enforcement personnel Y35.111
          suspect Y35.113
          unspecified person Y35.119
      grenade
        injuring
          bystander Y35.192
          law enforcement personnel Y35.191
          suspect Y35.193
          unspecified person Y35.199

Legal (Continued)
  intervention (Continued)
    explosive (Continued)
      injuring
        bystander Y35.102
        law enforcement personnel Y35.101
        suspect Y35.103
        unspecified person Y35.109
      mortar bomb
        injuring
          bystander Y35.192
          law enforcement personnel Y35.191
          suspect Y35.193
          unspecified person Y35.199
      shell
        injuring
          bystander Y35.122
          law enforcement personnel Y35.121
          suspect Y35.123
          unspecified person Y35.129
      specified NEC
        injuring
          bystander Y35.192
          law enforcement personnel Y35.191
          suspect Y35.193
          unspecified person Y35.199
    firearm(s) (discharge)
      handgun
        injuring
          bystander Y35.022
          law enforcement personnel Y35.021
          suspect Y35.023
          unspecified person Y35.029
      injuring
        bystander Y35.002
        law enforcement personnel Y35.001
        suspect Y35.003
        unspecified person Y35.009
      machine gun
        injuring
          bystander Y35.012
          law enforcement personnel Y35.011
          suspect Y35.013
          unspecified person Y35.019
      rifle pellet
        injuring
          bystander Y35.032
          law enforcement personnel Y35.031
          suspect Y35.033
          unspecified person Y35.039
      rubber bullet
        injuring
          bystander Y35.042
          law enforcement personnel Y35.041
          suspect Y35.043
          unspecified person Y35.049
      shotgun —see Legal, intervention,
        firearm, specified NEC
      specified NEC
        injuring
          bystander Y35.092
          law enforcement personnel Y35.091
          suspect Y35.093
          unspecified person Y35.099
    gas (asphyxiation) (poisoning)
      injuring
        bystander Y35.202
        law enforcement personnel Y35.201
        suspect Y35.203
        unspecified person Y35.209
      specified NEC
        injuring
          bystander Y35.292
          law enforcement personnel Y35.291
          suspect Y35.293
          unspecified person Y35.299
      tear gas
        injuring
          bystander Y35.212
          law enforcement personnel Y35.211
          suspect Y35.213
          unspecified person Y35.219

Legal (Continued)
  intervention (Continued)
    grenade —see Legal, intervention,
      explosive, grenade
    injuring
      bystander Y35.92
      law enforcement personnel Y35.91
      suspect Y35.93
      unspecified person Y35.99
    late effect (of) —see with 7th character S
      Y35
    manhandling
      injuring
        bystander Y35.812
        law enforcement personnel Y35.811
        suspect Y35.813
        unspecified person Y35.819
    sequelae (of) —see with 7th character S Y35
    sharp objects
      bayonet
        injuring
          bystander Y35.412
          law enforcement personnel
            Y35.411
          suspect Y35.413
          unspecified person Y35.419
      injuring
        bystander Y35.402
        law enforcement personnel Y35.401
        suspect Y35.403
        unspecified person Y35.409
      specified NEC
        injuring
          bystander Y35.492
          law enforcement personnel Y35.491
          suspect Y35.493
          unspecified person Y35.499
    specified means NEC
      injuring
        bystander Y35.892
        law enforcement personnel Y35.891
        suspect Y35.893
        ▶unspecified person Y35.899
    stabbing —see Legal, intervention, sharp
      object
    stave —see Legal, intervention, blunt
      object, stave
    stun gun
      injuring
        bystander Y35.832
        law enforcement personnel Y35.831
        suspect Y35.833
        unspecified person Y35.839
    taser
      injuring
        bystander Y35.832
        law enforcement personnel Y35.831
        suspect Y35.833
        unspecified person Y35.839
    tear gas —see Legal, intervention, gas, tear
      gas
    truncheon —see Legal, intervention, blunt
      object, stave
Lifting —see also Overexertion
  heavy objects X50.0
  weights X50.0
Lightning (shock) (stroke) (struck by) —see
    subcategory T75.0
  causing fire —see Exposure, fire
Loss of control (transport vehicle) NEC —see
    Accident, transport
Lost at sea NOS —see Drowning, due to, fall
    overboard
Low
  pressure (effects) —see Air, pressure, low
  temperature (effects) —see Exposure, cold
Lying before train, vehicle or other moving
    object X81.8
  subway train X81.1
  train X81.1
  undetermined whether accidental or
    intentional Y31
Lynching —see Assault

▶ New   ⇒ Revised   ~~deleted~~ Deleted   ● Use Additional Character(s)

M

Malfunction (mechanism or component) (of)
 firearm
  airgun W34.10
  BB gun W34.110
  gas, air or spring-operated gun NEC
   W34.118
  handgun W32.1
  hunting rifle W33.12
  larger firearm W33.10
   specified NEC W33.19
  machine gun W33.13
  paintball gun W34.111
  pellet gun W34.110
  shotgun W33.11
  specified NEC W34.19
  Very pistol [flare] W34.19
 handgun —see Malfunction, firearm,
  handgun
Maltreatment —see Perpetrator
Mangled (accidentally) NOS X58
Manhandling (in brawl, fight) Y04.0
 legal intervention —see Legal, intervention,
  manhandling
Manslaughter (nonaccidental) —see Assault
Mauled by animal NEC W55.89
Medical procedure, complication of
  (delayed or as an abnormal reaction
  without mention of misadventure) —see
  Complication of or following, by specified
  type of procedure
 due to or as a result of misadventure —see
  Misadventure
Melting (due to fire) —see also Exposure, fire
 apparel NEC X06.3
 clothes, clothing NEC X06.3
  nightwear X05
 fittings or furniture (burning building)
  (uncontrolled fire) X00.8
 nightwear X05
 plastic jewelry X06.1
Mental cruelty X58
Military operations (injuries to military and
  civilians occuring during peacetime on
  military property and during routine
  military exercises and operations) (by)
  (from) (involving) Y37.90-●
 air blast Y37.20-●
 aircraft
  destruction —see Military operations,
   destruction of aircraft
  airway restriction —see Military operations,
   restriction of airways
  asphyxiation —see Military operations,
   restriction of airways
 biological weapons Y37.6X-●
 blast Y37.20-●
 blast fragments Y37.20-●
 blast wave Y37.20-●
 blast wind Y37.20-●
 bomb Y37.20-●
  dirty Y37.50-●
  gasoline Y37.31-●
  incendiary Y37.31-●
  petrol Y37.31-●
 bullet Y37.43-●
  incendiary Y37.32-●
  rubber Y37.41-●
 chemical weapons Y37.7X-●
 combat
  hand to hand (unarmed) combat
   Y37.44-●
  using blunt or piercing object Y37.45-●
 conflagration —see Military operations, fire
 conventional warfare NEC Y37.49-●
 depth-charge Y37.01-●
 destruction of aircraft Y37.10-●
  due to
   air to air missile Y37.11-●
   collision with other aircraft Y37.12-●

Military operations (Continued)
 destruction of aircraft (Continued)
  due to (Continued)
   detonation (accidental) of onboard
    munitions and explosives Y37.14-●
   enemy fire or explosives Y37.11-●
   explosive placed on aircraft Y37.11-●
   onboard fire Y37.13-●
   rocket propelled grenade [RPG] Y37.11-●
   small arms fire Y37.11-●
   surface to air missile Y37.11-●
  specified NEC Y37.19-●
 detonation (accidental) of
  onboard marine weapons Y37.05-●
  own munitions or munitions launch device
   Y37.24-
 dirty bomb Y37.50-●
 explosion (of) Y37.20-●
  aerial bomb Y37.21-●
  bomb NOS —see also Military operations,
   bomb(s) Y37.20-●
  fragments Y37.20-●
  grenade Y37.29-●
  guided missile Y37.22-●
  improvised explosive device [IED]
   (person-borne) (roadside) (vehicle-
   borne) Y37.23-●
  land mine Y37.29-●
  marine mine (at sea) (in harbor) Y37.02-●
  marine weapon Y37.00-●
   specified NEC Y37.09-●
  own munitions or munitions launch device
   (accidental) Y37.24-●
  sea-based artillery shell Y37.03-●
  specified NEC Y37.29-●
  torpedo Y37.04-●
 fire Y37.30-●
  specified NEC Y37.39-●
 firearms
  discharge Y37.43-●
  pellets Y37.42-●
 flamethrower Y37.33-●
 fragments (from) (of)
  improvised explosive device [IED]
   (person-borne) (roadside) (vehicle-
   borne) Y37.26-●
  munitions Y37.25-●
  specified NEC Y37.29-●
  weapons Y37.27-●
 friendly fire Y37.92-●
 hand to hand (unarmed) combat Y37.44-●
 hot substances —see Military operations, fire
 incendiary bullet Y37.32-●
 nuclear weapon (effects of) Y37.50-●
  acute radiation exposure Y37.54-●
  blast pressure Y37.51-●
  direct blast Y37.51-●
  direct heat Y37.53-●
  fallout exposure Y37.54-●
  fireball Y37.53-●
  indirect blast (struck or crushed by blast
   debris) (being thrown by blast)
   Y37.52-●
  ionizing radiation (immediate exposure)
   Y37.54-●
  nuclear radiation Y37.54-●
  radiation
   ionizing (immediate exposure) Y37.54-●
   nuclear Y37.54-●
   thermal Y37.53-●
  secondary effects Y37.54-●
  specified NEC Y37.59-●
  thermal radiation Y37.53-●
 restriction of air (airway)
  intentional Y37.46-●
  unintentional Y37.47-●
 rubber bullets Y37.41-●
 shrapnel NOS Y37.29-●
 suffocation —see Military operations,
  restriction of airways
 unconventional warfare NEC Y37.7X-●

Military operations (Continued)
 underwater blast NOS Y37.00-●
 warfare
  conventional NEC Y37.49-●
  unconventional NEC Y37.7X-●
 weapon of mass destruction [WMD]
  Y37.91-●
 weapons
  biological weapons Y37.6X-●
  chemical Y37.7X-●
  nuclear (effects of) Y37.50-●
   acute radiation exposure Y37.54-●
   blast pressure Y37.51-●
   direct blast Y37.51-●
   direct heat Y37.53-●
   fallout exposure Y37.54-●
   fireball Y37.53-●
   radiation
    ionizing (immediate exposure)
     Y37.54-●
    nuclear Y37.54-●
    thermal Y37.53-●
   secondary effects Y37.54-●
   specified NEC Y37.59-●
  of mass destruction [WMD] Y37.91-●
Misadventure(s) to patient(s) during surgical
  or medical care Y69
 contaminated medical or biological substance
  (blood, drug, fluid) Y64.9
  administered (by) NEC Y64.9
   immunization Y64.1
   infusion Y64.0
   injection Y64.1
   specified means NEC Y64.8
   transfusion Y64.0
   vaccination Y64.1
 excessive amount of blood or other fluid
  during transfusion or infusion Y63.0
 failure
  in dosage Y63.9
   electroshock therapy Y63.4
   inappropriate temperature (too hot or
    too cold) in local application and
    packing Y63.5
   infusion
    excessive amount of fluid Y63.0
    incorrect dilution of fluid Y63.1
   insulin-shock therapy Y63.4
   nonadministration of necessary drug or
    biological substance Y63.6
   overdose —see Table of Drugs and
    Chemicals
   radiation, in therapy Y63.2
  radiation
   overdose Y63.2
  specified procedure NEC Y63.8
  transfusion
   excessive amount of blood Y63.0
 mechanical, of instrument or apparatus
  (any) (during any procedure) Y65.8
 sterile precautions (during procedure)
  Y62.9
  aspiration of fluid or tissue (by puncture
   or catheterization, except heart)
   Y62.6
  biopsy (except needle aspiration)
   Y62.8
   needle (aspirating) Y62.6
  blood sampling Y62.6
  catheterization Y62.6
   heart Y62.5
  dialysis (kidney) Y62.2
  endoscopic examination Y62.4
  enema Y62.8
  immunization Y62.3
  infusion Y62.1
  injection Y62.3
  needle biopsy Y62.6
  paracentesis (abdominal) (thoracic)
   Y62.6
  perfusion Y62.2

M

Misadventure(s) to patient(s) during surgical or medical care *(Continued)*
  failure *(Continued)*
    sterile precautions *(Continued)*
      puncture (lumbar) Y62.6
      removal of catheter or packing Y62.8
      specified procedure NEC Y62.8
      surgical operation Y62.0
      transfusion Y62.1
      vaccination Y62.3
    suture or ligature during surgical procedure Y65.2
    to introduce or to remove tube or instrument —*see* Failure, to
  hemorrhage —*see* Index to Diseases and Injuries, Complication(s)
  inadvertent exposure of patient to radiation Y63.3
  inappropriate
    operation performed —*see* Inappropriate operation performed
    temperature (too hot or too cold) in local application or packing Y63.5

Misadventure(s) to patient(s) during surgical or medical care *(Continued)*
  infusion —*see also* Misadventure, by type, infusion Y69
    excessive amount of fluid Y63.0
    incorrect dilution of fluid Y63.1
    wrong fluid Y65.1
  mismatched blood in transfusion Y65.0
  nonadministration of necessary drug or biological substance Y63.6
  overdose —*see* Table of Drugs and Chemicals
    radiation (in therapy) Y63.2
  perforation —*see* Index to Diseases and Injuries, Complication(s)
  performance of inappropriate operation —*see* Inappropriate operation performed
  puncture —*see* Index to Diseases and Injuries, Complication(s)
  specified type NEC Y65.8
    failure
      suture or ligature during surgical operation Y65.2
      to introduce or to remove tube or instrument —*see* Failure, to
    infusion of wrong fluid Y65.1

Misadventure(s) to patient(s) during surgical or medical care *(Continued)*
  specified type NEC *(Continued)*
    performance of inappropriate operation —*see* Inappropriate operation performed
    transfusion of mismatched blood Y65.0
    wrong
      fluid in infusion Y65.1
      placement of endotracheal tube during anesthetic procedure Y65.3
  transfusion —*see* Misadventure, by type, transfusion
    excessive amount of blood Y63.0
    mismatched blood Y65.0
  wrong
    drug given in error —*see* Table of Drugs and Chemicals
    fluid in infusion Y65.1
    placement of endotracheal tube during anesthetic procedure Y65.3
Mismatched blood in transfusion Y65.0
Motion sickness T75.3
Mountain sickness W94.11
Mudslide (of cataclysmic nature) —*see* Landslide
Murder (attempt) —*see* Assault

N

Nail
  contact with W45.0
    gun W29.4
  embedded in skin W45.0
Neglect (criminal) (homicidal intent) X58

Noise (causing injury) (pollution) W42.9
  supersonic W42.0
Nonadministration (of)
  drug or biological substance (necessary) Y63.6
  surgical and medical care Y66
Nosocomial condition Y95

O

Object
  falling
    from, in, on, hitting
      machinery —*see* Contact, with, by type of machine
  set in motion by
    accidental explosion or rupture of pressure vessel W38
    firearm —*see* Discharge, firearm, by type
    machine (ry) —*see* Contact, with, by type of machine
Overdose (drug) —*see* Table of Drugs and Chemicals
  radiation Y63.2

Overexertion X50.9
  from
    prolonged static or awkward postures X50.1
    repetitive movements X50.3
    specified strenuous movements or postures NEC X50.9
    strenuous movement or load X50.0
Overexposure (accidental) (to)
  cold —*see also* Exposure, cold X31
    due to man-made conditions —*see* Exposure, cold, man-made
  heat —*see also* Heat X30
  radiation —*see* Radiation
  radioactivity W88.0
  sun (sunburn) X32

Overexposure *(Continued)*
  weather NEC —*see* Forces of nature
  wind NEC —*see* Forces of nature
Overheated —*see* Heat
Overturning (accidental)
  machinery —*see* Contact, with, by type of machine
  transport vehicle NEC —*see also* Accident, transport V89.9
  watercraft (causing drowning, submersion) —*see also* Drowning, due to, accident to, watercraft, overturning
    causing injury except drowning or submersion —*see* Accident, watercraft, causing, injury NEC

▶ New   ⇒ Revised   ~~deleted~~ Deleted   • Use Additional Character(s)

M, N, & O

P

Parachute descent (voluntary) (without
　accident to aircraft) V97.29
　due to accident to aircraft —see Accident,
　　transport, aircraft
Pecked by bird W61.99
Perforation during medical or surgical
　treatment as misadventure —see Index to
　Diseases and Injuries, Complication(s)
Perpetrator, perpetration, of assault,
　maltreatment and neglect (by) Y07.9
　boyfriend Y07.03
　brother Y07.410
　　stepbrother Y07.435
　coach Y07.53
　cousin
　　female Y07.491
　　male Y07.490
　daycare provider Y07.519
　　at-home
　　　adult care Y07.512
　　　childcare Y07.510
　　care center
　　　adult care Y07.513
　　　childcare Y07.511
　family member NEC Y07.499
　father Y07.11
　　adoptive Y07.13
　　foster Y07.420
　　stepfather Y07.430
　foster father Y07.420
　foster mother Y07.421
　girl friend Y07.04
　healthcare provider Y07.529
　　mental health Y07.521
　　specified NEC Y07.528
　husband Y07.01
　instructor Y07.53
　mother Y07.12
　　adoptive Y07.14
　　foster Y07.421
　　stepmother Y07.433
　nonfamily member Y07.50
　　specified NEC Y07.59
　nurse Y07.528
　occupational therapist Y07.528
　partner of parent
　　female Y07.434
　　male Y07.432
　physical therapist Y07.528
　sister Y07.411
　speech therapist Y07.528
　stepbrother Y07.435
　stepfather Y07.430
　stepmother Y07.433
　stepsister Y07.436
　teacher Y07.53
　wife Y07.02
Piercing —see Contact, with, by type of object
　or machine
Pinched
　between objects (moving) (stationary and
　　moving) W23.0
　　stationary W23.1
Pinned under machine (ry) —see Contact, with,
　by type of machine
Place of occurrence Y92.9
　abandoned house Y92.89
　airplane Y92.813
　airport Y92.520
　ambulatory health services establishment
　　NEC Y92.538
　ambulatory surgery center Y92.530
　amusement park Y92.831
　apartment (co-op) —see Place of occurrence,
　　residence, apartment
　assembly hall Y92.29
　bank Y92.510
　barn Y92.71
　baseball field Y92.320

Place of occurrence (Continued)
　basketball court Y92.310
　beach Y92.832
　boarding house —see Place of occurrence,
　　residence, boarding house
　boat Y92.814
　bowling alley Y92.39
　bridge Y92.89
　building under construction Y92.61
　bus Y92.811
　　station Y92.521
　cafe Y92.511
　campsite Y92.833
　campus —see Place of occurrence, school
　canal Y92.89
　car Y92.810
　casino Y92.59
　children's home —see Place of occurrence,
　　residence, institutional, orphanage
　church Y92.22
　cinema Y92.26
　clubhouse Y92.29
　coal pit Y92.64
　college (community) Y92.214
　condominium —see Place of occurrence,
　　residence, apartment
　construction area —see Place of occurrence,
　　industrial and construction area
　convalescent home —see Place of occurrence,
　　residence, institutional, nursing home
　court-house Y92.240
　cricket ground Y92.328
　cultural building Y92.258
　　art gallery Y92.250
　　museum Y92.251
　　music hall Y92.252
　　opera house Y92.253
　　specified NEC Y92.258
　　theater Y92.254
　dancehall Y92.252
　day nursery Y92.210
　dentist office Y92.531
　derelict house Y92.89
　desert Y92.820
　dock NOS Y92.89
　dockyard Y92.62
　doctor's office Y92.531
　dormitory —see Place of occurrence,
　　residence, institutional, school dormitory
　dry dock Y92.62
　factory (building) (premises) Y92.63
　farm (land under cultivation) (outbuildings)
　　Y92.79
　　barn Y92.71
　　chicken coop Y92.72
　　field Y92.73
　　hen house Y92.72
　　house —see Place of occurrence, residence,
　　　house
　　orchard Y92.74
　　specified NEC Y92.79
　football field Y92.321
　forest Y92.821
　freeway Y92.411
　gallery Y92.250
　garage (commercial) Y92.59
　　boarding house Y92.044
　　military base Y92.135
　　mobile home Y92.025
　　nursing home Y92.124
　　orphanage Y92.114
　　private house Y92.015
　　reform school Y92.155
　gas station Y92.524
　gasworks Y92.69
　golf course Y92.39
　gravel pit Y92.64
　grocery Y92.512
　gymnasium Y92.39
　handball court Y92.318
　harbor Y92.89

Place of occurrence (Continued)
　harness racing course Y92.39
　healthcare provider office Y92.531
　highway (interstate) Y92.411
　hill Y92.828
　hockey rink Y92.330
　home —see Place of occurrence, residence
　hospice —see Place of occurrence, residence,
　　institutional, nursing home
　hospital Y92.239
　　cafeteria Y92.233
　　corridor Y92.232
　　operating room Y92.234
　　patient
　　　bathroom Y92.231
　　　room Y92.230
　　specified NEC Y92.238
　hotel Y92.59
　house —see also Place of occurrence, residence
　　abandoned Y92.89
　　under construction Y92.61
　industrial and construction area (yard)
　　Y92.69
　　building under construction Y92.61
　　dock Y92.62
　　dry dock Y92.62
　　factory Y92.63
　　gasworks Y92.69
　　mine Y92.64
　　oil rig Y92.65
　　pit Y92.64
　　power station Y92.69
　　shipyard Y92.62
　　specified NEC Y92.69
　　tunnel under construction Y92.69
　　workshop Y92.69
　kindergarten Y92.211
　lacrosse field Y92.328
　lake Y92.828
　library Y92.241
　mall Y92.59
　market Y92.512
　marsh Y92.828
　military
　　base —see Place of occurrence, residence,
　　　institutional, military base
　　training ground Y92.84
　mine Y92.64
　mosque Y92.22
　motel Y92.59
　motorway (interstate) Y92.411
　mountain Y92.828
　movie-house Y92.26
　museum Y92.251
　music-hall Y92.252
　not applicable Y92.9
　nuclear power station Y92.69
　nursing home —see Place of occurrence,
　　residence, institutional, nursing home
　office building Y92.59
　offshore installation Y92.65
　oil rig Y92.65
　old people's home —see Place of occurrence,
　　residence, institutional, specified NEC
　opera-house Y92.253
　orphanage —see Place of occurrence,
　　residence, institutional, orphanage
　outpatient surgery center Y92.530
　park (public) Y92.830
　　amusement Y92.831
　parking garage Y92.89
　　lot Y92.481
　pavement Y92.480
　physician office Y92.531
　polo field Y92.328
　pond Y92.828
　post office Y92.242
　power station Y92.69
　prairie Y92.828
　prison —see Place of occurrence, residence,
　　institutional, prison

Place of occurrence (Continued)
  public
    administration building Y92.248
      city hall Y92.243
      courthouse Y92.240
      library Y92.241
      post office Y92.242
      specified NEC Y92.248
    building NEC Y92.29
    hall Y92.29
    place NOS Y92.89
  race course Y92.39
  radio station Y92.59
  railway line (bridge) Y92.85
  ranch (outbuildings) —see Place of
      occurrence, farm
  recreation area Y92.838
    amusement park Y92.831
    beach Y92.832
    campsite Y92.833
    park (public) Y92.830
    seashore Y92.832
    specified NEC Y92.838
  reform school —see Place of occurrence,
      residence, institutional, reform school
  religious institution Y92.22
  residence (non-institutional) (private) Y92.009
    apartment Y92.039
      bathroom Y92.031
      bedroom Y92.032
      kitchen Y92.030
      specified NEC Y92.038
    bathroom Y92.002
    bedroom Y92.003
    boarding house Y92.049
      bathroom Y92.041
      bedroom Y92.042
      driveway Y92.043
      garage Y92.044
      garden Y92.046
      kitchen Y92.040
      specified NEC Y92.048
      swimming pool Y92.045
      yard Y92.046
    dining room Y92.001
    garden Y92.007
    home Y92.009
    house, single family Y92.019
      bathroom Y92.012
      bedroom Y92.013
      dining room Y92.011
      driveway Y92.014
      garage Y92.015
      garden Y92.017
      kitchen Y92.010
      specified NEC Y92.018
      swimming pool Y92.016
      yard Y92.017
    institutional Y92.10
      children's home —see Place of
          occurrence, residence, institutional,
          orphanage
      hospice —see Place of occurrence,
          residence, institutional, nursing
          home
      military base Y92.139
        barracks Y92.133
        garage Y92.135
        garden Y92.137
        kitchen Y92.130
        mess hall Y92.131
        specified NEC Y92.138
        swimming pool Y92.136
        yard Y92.137
      nursing home Y92.129
        bathroom Y92.121
        bedroom Y92.122
        driveway Y92.123
        garage Y92.124
        garden Y92.126
        kitchen Y92.120

Place of occurrence (Continued)
  residence (Continued)
    institutional (Continued)
      nursing home (Continued)
        specified NEC Y92.128
        swimming pool Y92.125
        yard Y92.126
      orphanage Y92.119
        bathroom Y92.111
        bedroom Y92.112
        driveway Y92.113
        garage Y92.114
        garden Y92.116
        kitchen Y92.110
        specified NEC Y92.118
        swimming pool Y92.115
        yard Y92.116
      prison Y92.149
        bathroom Y92.142
        cell Y92.143
        courtyard Y92.147
        dining room Y92.141
        kitchen Y92.140
        specified NEC Y92.148
        swimming pool Y92.146
      reform school Y92.159
        bathroom Y92.152
        bedroom Y92.153
        dining room Y92.151
        driveway Y92.154
        garage Y92.155
        garden Y92.157
        kitchen Y92.150
        specified NEC Y92.158
        swimming pool Y92.156
        yard Y92.157
      school dormitory Y92.169
        bathroom Y92.162
        bedroom Y92.163
        dining room Y92.161
        kitchen Y92.160
        specified NEC Y92.168
      specified NEC Y92.199
        bathroom Y92.192
        bedroom Y92.193
        dining room Y92.191
        driveway Y92.194
        garage Y92.195
        garden Y92.197
        kitchen Y92.190
        specified NEC Y92.198
        swimming pool Y92.196
        yard Y92.197
    kitchen Y92.000
    mobile home Y92.029
      bathroom Y92.022
      bedroom Y92.023
      dining room Y92.021
      driveway Y92.024
      garage Y92.025
      garden Y92.027
      kitchen Y92.020
      specified NEC Y92.028
      swimming pool Y92.026
      yard Y92.027
    specified place in residence NEC Y92.008
    specified residence type NEC Y92.099
      bathroom Y92.091
      bedroom Y92.092
      driveway Y92.093
      garage Y92.094
      garden Y92.096
      kitchen Y92.090
      specified NEC Y92.098
      swimming pool Y92.095
      yard Y92.096
  restaurant Y92.511
  riding school Y92.39
  river Y92.828
  road Y92.410
  rodeo ring Y92.39

Place of occurrence (Continued)
  rugby field Y92.328
  same day surgery center Y92.530
  sand pit Y92.64
  school (private) (public) (state) Y92.219
    college Y92.214
    daycare center Y92.210
    elementary school Y92.211
    high school Y92.213
    kindergarten Y92.211
    middle school Y92.212
    specified NEC Y92.218
    trace school Y92.215
    university Y92.214
    vocational school Y92.215
  sea (shore) Y92.832
  senior citizen center Y92.29
  service area
    airport Y92.520
    bus station Y92.521
    gas station Y92.524
    highway rest stop Y92.523
    railway station Y92.522
  shipyard Y92.62
  shop(commercial) Y92.513
  sidewalk Y92.480
  silo Y92.79
  skating rink (roller) Y92.331
    ice Y92.330
  slaughter house Y92.86
  soccer field Y92.322
  specified place NEC Y92.89
  sports area Y92.39
    athletic
      court Y92.318
        basketball Y92.310
        specified NEC Y92.318
        squash Y92.311
        tennis Y92.312
      field Y92.328
        baseball Y92.320
        cricket ground Y92.328
        football Y92.321
        hockey Y92.328
        soccer Y92.322
        specified NEC Y92.328
    golf course Y92.39
    gymnasium Y92.39
    riding school Y92.39
    skating rink (roller) Y92.331
      ice Y92.330
    stadium Y92.39
    swimming pool Y92.34
  squash court Y92.311
  stadium Y92.39
  steeplechasing course Y92.39
  store Y92.512
  stream Y92.828
  street and highway Y92.410
    bike path Y92.482
    freeway Y92.411
    highway ramp Y92.415
    interstate highway Y92.411
    local residential or business street
        Y92.414
    motorway Y92.411
    parking lot Y92.481
    parkway Y92.412
    sidewalk Y92.480
    specified NEC Y92.488
    state road Y92.413
  subway car Y92.816
  supermarket Y92.512
  swamp Y92.828
  swimming pool (public) Y92.34
    private (at) Y92.095
      boarding house Y92.045
      military base Y92.136
      mobile home Y92.026
      nursing home Y92.125
      orphanage Y92.115

▶ New   ⇛ Revised   ~~deleted~~ Deleted   ● Use Additional Character(s)

Place of occurrence (Continued)
swimming pool (Continued)
  private (Continued)
    prison Y92.146
    reform school Y92.156
    single family residence
      Y92.016
synagogue Y92.22
television station Y92.59
tennis court Y92.312
theater Y92.254
trade area Y92.59
  bank Y92.510
  cafe Y92.511
  casino Y92.59
  garage Y92.59
  hotel Y92.59
  market Y92.512
  office building Y92.59
  radio station Y92.59
  restaurant Y92.511
  shop Y92.513
  shopping mall Y92.59
  store Y92.512
  supermarket Y92.512
  television station Y92.59
  warehouse Y92.59
trailer park, residential —see Place of
  occurrence, residence, mobile
  home
trailer site NOS Y92.89
train Y92.815
  station Y92.522
truck Y92.812
tunnel under construction Y92. 69
university Y92.214
urgent (health) care center Y92.532
vehicle (transport) Y92.818
  airplane Y92.813
  boat Y92.814
  bus Y92.811
  car Y92.810
  specified NEC Y92.818
  subway car Y92.816
  train Y92.815
  truck Y92.812
warehouse Y92.59
water reservoir Y92.89
wilderness area Y92.828
  desert Y92.820
  forest Y92.821
  marsh Y92.828
  mountain Y92.828
  prairie Y92.828
  specified NEC Y92.828
  swamp Y92.828
workshop Y92.69
yard, private Y92.096
  boarding house Y92.046
  mobile home Y92.027
  single family house Y92.017

Place of occurrence (Continued)
youth center Y92.29
zoo (zoological garden) Y92.834
Plumbism —see Table of Drugs and Chemicals,
  lead
Poisoning (accidental) (by) —see also Table of
  Drugs and Chemicals
by plant, thorns, spines, sharp leaves or other
  mechanisms NEC X58
carbon monoxide
  generated by
    motor vehicle —see Accident, transport
    watercraft (in transit) (not in transit)
      V93.89
      ferry boat V93.81
      fishing boat V93.82
      jet skis V93.83
      liner V93.81
      merchant ship V93.80
      passenger ship V93.81
      powered craft NEC V93.83
caused by injection of poisons into skin by
  plant thorns, spines, sharp leaves X58
marine or sea plants (venomous) X58
exhaust gas
  generated by
    motor vehicle —see Accident, transport
    watercraft (in transit) (not in transit)
      V93.89
      ferry boat V93.81
      fishing boat V93.82
      jet skis V93.83
      liner V93.81
      merchant ship V93.80
      passenger ship V93.81
      powered craft NEC V93.83
fumes or smoke due to
  explosion —see also Explosion W40.9
  fire —see Exposure, fire
  ignition —see Ignition
gas
  in legal intervention —see Legal,
    intervention, gas
  legal execution —see Legal, intervention,
    gas
in war operations —see War operations
legal
  execution —see Legal, intervention, gas
  intervention
    by gas —see Legal, intervention, gas
    other specified means —see Legal,
      intervention, specified means
      NEC
Powder burn (by) (from)
airgun W34.110
BB gun W34.110
firearm NEC W34.19
gas, air or spring-operated gun NEC
  W34.118
handgun W32.1
hunting rifle W33.12

Powder burn (Continued)
larger firearm W33.10
  specified NEC W33.19
machine gun W33.13
paintball gun W34.111
pellet gun W34.110
shotgun W33.11
Very pistol [flare] W34.19
Premature cessation (of) surgical and medical
  care Y66
Privation (food) (water) X58
Procedure (operation)
correct, on wrong side or body part (wrong
  side) (wrong site) Y65.53
intended for another patient done on wrong
  patient Y65.52
performed on patient not scheduled for
  surgery Y65.52
performed on wrong patient Y65.52
wrong, performed on correct patient Y65.51
Prolonged
sitting in transport vehicle —see Travel, by
  type of vehicle
stay in
  high altitude as cause of anoxia,
    barodontalgia, barotitis or hypoxia
    W94.11
  weightless environment X52
Pulling, excessive —see also Overexertion
  X50.9
Puncture, puncturing —see also Contact, with,
  by type of object or machine
by
  plant thorns, spines, sharp leaves or other
    mechanisms NEC W60
during medical or surgical treatment as
  misadventure —see Index to Diseases
  and Injuries, Complication(s)
Pushed, pushing (accidental) (injury in)
by other person(s) (accidental) W51
  with fall W03
    due to ice or snow W00.0
  as, or caused by, a crowd or human
    stampede (with fall) W52
  before moving object NEC Y02.8
    motor vehicle Y02.0
    subway train Y02.1
    train Y02.1
  from
    high place NEC
      in accidental circumstances W17.89
      stated as
        intentional, homicide (attempt) Y01
        undetermined whether accidental
          or intentional Y30
    transport vehicle NEC —see also
      Accident, transport V89.9
      stated as
        intentional, homicide (attempt)
          Y08.89
    overexertion X50.9

P

R

Radiation (exposure to)
  arc lamps W89.0
  atomic power plant (malfunction) NEC
      W88.1
  complication of or abnormal reaction to
      medical radiotherapy Y84.2
  electromagnetic, ionizing W88.0
  gamma rays W88.1
  in
    war operations (from or following
        nuclear explosion) —see also War
        operations
  inadvertent exposure of patient (receiving
      test or therapy) Y63.3
  infrared (heaters and lamps) W90.1
    excessive heat from W92
  ionized, ionizing (particles, artificially
      accelerated)
    radioisotopes W88.1
    specified NEC W88.8
    x-rays W88.0
  isotopes, radioactive —see Radiation,
      radioactive isotopes
  laser(s) W90.2
    in war operations —see War operations
    misadventure in medical care Y63.2
  light sources (man-made visible and
      ultraviolet) W89.9
    natural X32
    specified NEC W89.8
    tanning bed W89.1
    welding light W89.0
  man-made visible light W89.9
    specified NEC W89.8
    tanning bed W89.1
    welding light W89.0
  microwave W90.8
  misadventure in medical or surgical
      procedure Y63.2

Radiation (Continued)
  natural NEC X39.08
    radon X39.01
  overdose (in medical or surgical procedure)
      Y63.2
  radar W90.0
  radioactive isotopes (any) W88.1
    atomic power plant malfunction W88.1
    misadventure in medical or surgical
        treatment Y63.2
  radiofrequency W90.0
  radium NEC W88.1
  sun X32
  ultraviolet (light) (man-made) W89.9
    natural X32
    specified NEC W89.8
    tanning bed W89.1
    welding light W89.0
  welding arc, torch, or light W89.0
    excessive heat from W92
  x-rays (hard) (soft) W88.0
Range disease W94.11
Rape (attempted) T74.2-●
Rat bite W53.11
Reaching (prolonged) (static) X50.1
Reaction, abnormal to medical procedure —see
    also Complication of or following, by type
    of procedure Y84.9
  with misadventure —see Misadventure
  biologicals —see Table of Drugs and
      Chemicals
  drugs —see Table of Drugs and Chemicals
  vaccine —see Table of Drugs and
      Chemicals
Recoil
  airgun W34.110
  BB gun W34.110
  firearm NEC W34.19
  gas, air or spring-operated gun NEC W34.118

Recoil (Continued)
  handgun W32.1
  hunting rifle W33.12
  larger firearm W33.10
    specified NEC W33.19
  machine gun W33.13
  paintball gun W34.111
  pellet W34.110
  shotgun W33.11
  Very pistol [flare] W34.19
Reduction in
  atmospheric pressure —see Air, pressure,
      change
Rock falling on or hitting (accidentally)
    (person) W20.8
  in cave-in W20.0
Run over (accidentally) (by)
  animal (not being ridden) NEC W55.89
  machinery —see Contact, with, by specified
      type of machine
  transport vehicle NEC —see also Accident,
      transport V09.9
    intentional homicide (attempt) Y03.0
    motor NEC V09.20
      intentional homicide (attempt) Y03.0
Running
  before moving object X81.8
    motor vehicle X81.0
Running off, away
  animal (being ridden) —see also Accident,
      transport V80.918
    not being ridden W55.89
  animal-drawn vehicle NEC —see also
      Accident, transport V80.928
  highway, road(way), street
    transport vehicle NEC —see also Accident,
        transport V89.9
Rupture pressurized devices —see Explosion,
    by type of device

▶ New   ⇒ Revised   ~~deleted~~ Deleted   ● Use Additional Character(s)

S

Saturnism —see Table of Drugs and Chemicals, lead
Scald, scalding (accidental) (by) (from) (in) X19
air (hot) X14.1
gases (hot) X14.1
homicide (attempt) —see Assault, burning, hot object
inflicted by other person
stated as intentional, homicide (attempt) —see Assault, burning, hot object
liquid (boiling) (hot) NEC X12
stated as undetermined whether accidental or intentional Y27.2
suicide (attempt) X77.2
local application of externally applied substance in medical or surgical care Y63.5
metal (molten) (liquid) (hot) NEC X18
self-inflicted X77.9
stated as undetermined whether accidental or intentional Y27.8
steam X13.1
assault X98.0
stated as undetermined whether accidental or intentional Y27.0
suicide (attempt) X77.0
suicide (attempt) X77.9
vapor (hot) X13.1
assault X98.0
stated as undetermined whether accidental or intentional Y27.0
suicide (attempt) X77.0
Scratched by
cat W55.03
person(s) (accidentally) W50.4
with intent to injure or kill Y04.0
as, or caused by, a crowd or human stampede (with fall) W52
assault Y04.0
homicide (attempt) Y04.0
in
fight Y04.0
legal intervention
injuring
bystander Y35.892
law enforcement personnel Y35.891
suspect Y35.893
▶unspecified person Y35.899
Seasickness T75.3
Self-harm NEC —see also External cause by type, undetermined whether accidental or intentional
intentional —see Suicide
poisoning NEC —see Table of drugs and biologicals, accident
Self-inflicted (injury) NEC —see also External cause by type, undetermined whether accidental or intentional
intentional —see Suicide
poisoning NEC —see Table of drugs and biologicals, accident
Sequelae (of)
accident NEC —see W00-X58 with 7th character S
assault (homicidal) (any means) —see X92-Y08 with 7th character S
homicide, attempt (any means) —see X92-Y08 with 7th character S
injury undetermined whether accidentally or purposely inflicted —see Y21-Y33 with 7th character S
intentional self-harm (classifiable to X71-X83) —see X71-X83 with 7th character S
legal intervention (see with 7th character S Y35)
motor vehicle accident —see V00-V99 with 7th character S
suicide, attempt (any means) —see X71-X83 with 7th character S

Sequelae (Continued)
transport accident —see V00-V99 with 7th character S
war operations —see War operations
Shock
electric —see Exposure, electric current
from electric appliance (any) (faulty) W86.8
domestic W86.0
suicide (attempt) X83.1
Shooting, shot (accidental (ly)) —see also Discharge, firearm, by type
herself or himself —see Discharge, firearm by type, self-inflicted
homicide (attempt) —see Discharge, firearm by type, homicide
in war operations —see War operations
inflicted by other person —see Discharge, firearm by type, homicide
accidental —see Discharge, firearm, by type of firearm
legal
execution —see Legal, intervention, firearm
intervention —see Legal, intervention, firearm
self-inflicted —see Discharge, firearm by type, suicide
accidental —see Discharge, firearm, by type of firearm
suicide (attempt) —see Discharge, firearm by type, suicide
Shoving (accidentally) by other person —see Pushed, by other person
Sickness
alpine W94.11
motion —see Motion
mountain W94.11
Sinking (accidental)
watercraft (causing drowning, submersion) —see also Drowning, due to, accident to, watercraft, sinking
causing injury except drowning or submersion —see Accident, watercraft, causing, injury NEC
Siriasis X32
Sitting (prolonged) (static) X50.1
Slashed wrists —see Cut, self-inflicted
Slipping (accidental) (on same level) (with fall) W01.0
without fall W18.40
due to
specified NEC W18.49
stepping from one level to another W18.43
stepping into hole or opening W18.42
stepping on object W18.41
on
ice W00.0
with skates —see Accident, transport, pedestrian, conveyance
mud W01.0
oil W01.0
snow W00.0
with skis —see Accident, transport, pedestrian, conveyance
surface (slippery) (wet) NEC W01.0
Sliver, wood, contact with W45.8
Smoldering (due to fire) —see Exposure, fire
Sodomy (attempted) by force T74.2-●
Sound waves (causing injury) W42.9
supersonic W42.0
Splinter, contact with W45.8
Stab, stabbing —see Cut
Standing (prolonged) (static) X50.1
Starvation X58
Status of external cause Y99.9
child assisting in compensated work for family Y99.8
civilian activity done for financial or other compensation Y99.0
civilian activity done for income or pay Y99.0

Status of external cause (Continued)
family member assisting in compensated work for other family member Y99.8
hobby not done for income Y99.8
leisure activity Y99.8
military activity Y99.1
off-duty activity of military personnel Y99.8
recreation or sport not for income or while a student Y99.8
specified NEC Y99.8
student activity Y99.8
volunteer activity Y99.2
Stepped on
by
animal (not being ridden) NEC W55.89
crowd or human stampede W52
person W50.0
Stepping on
object W22.8
with fall W18.31
sports equipment W21.9
stationary W22.09
sports equipment W21.89
person W51
by crowd or human stampede W52
sports equipment W21.9
Sting
arthropod, nonvenomous W57
insect, nonvenomous W57
Storm (cataclysmic) —see Forces of nature, cataclysmic storm
Straining, excessive —see also Overexertion X50.9
Strangling —see Strangulation
Strangulation (accidental) —see category T71
Strenuous movements —see also Overexertion X50.9
Striking against
airbag (automobile) W22.10
driver side W22.11
front passenger side W22.12
specified NEC W22.19
bottom when
diving or jumping into water (in) W16.822
causing drowning W16.821
from boat W16.722
causing drowning W16.721
natural body W16.622
causing drowning W16.821
swimming pool W16.522
causing drowning W16.521
falling into water (in) W16.322
causing drowning W16.321
fountain —see Striking against, bottom when, falling into water, specified NEC
natural body W16.122
causing drowning W16.121
reservoir —see Striking against, bottom when, falling into water, specified NEC
specified NEC W16.322
causing drowning W16.321
swimming pool W16.022
causing drowning W16.021
diving board (swimming-pool) W21.4
object W22.8
with
drowning or submersion —see Drowning
fall —see Fall, due to, bumping against, object
caused by crowd or human stampede (with fall) W52
furniture W22.03
lamppost W22.02
sports equipment W21.9
stationary W22.09
sports equipment W21.89
wall W22.01

Striking against (Continued)
  person(s) W51
    with fall W03
      due to ice or snow W00.0
    as, or caused by, a crowd or human
      stampede (with fall) W52
    assault Y04.2
    homicide (attempt) Y04.2
  sports equipment W21.9
  wall (when) W22.01
    diving or jumping into water (in) W16.832
      causing drowning W16.831
        swimming pool W16.532
          causing drowning W16.531
    falling into water (in) W16.332
      causing drowning W16.331
      fountain —see Striking against, wall
        when, falling into water, specified
        NEC
      natural body W16.132
        causing drowning W16.131
      reservoir —see Striking against, wall
        when, falling into water, specified
        NEC
      specified NEC W16.332
        causing drowning W16.331
      swimming pool W16.032
        causing drowning W16.031
    swimming pool (when) W22.042
      causing drowning W22.041
      diving or jumping into water W16.532
        causing drowning W16.531
      falling into water W16.032
        causing drowning W16.031
Struck (accidentally) **by**
  airbag (automobile) W22.10
    driver side W22.11
    front passenger side W22.12
    specified NEC W22.19
  alligator W58.02
  animal (not being ridden) NEC W55.89
  avalanche —see Landslide
  ball (hit) (thrown) W21.00
    assault Y08.09
    baseball W21.03
    basketball W21.05
    football W21.01
    golf ball W21.04
    football W21.01
    soccer W21.02
    softball W21.07
    specified NEC W21.09
    volleyball W21.06
  bat or racquet
    baseball bat W21.11
      assault Y08.02
    golf club W21.13
      assault Y08.09
    specified NEC W21.19
      assault Y08.09
    tennis racquet W21.12
      assault Y08.09
  bullet —see also Discharge, firearm by type
    in war operations —see War operations
  crocodile W58.12
  dog W54.1
  flare, Very pistol —see Discharge, firearm
    NEC
  hailstones X39.8
  hockey (ice)
    field
      puck W21.221
      stick W21.211
    puck W21.220
    stick W21.210
      assault Y08.01
  landslide —see Landslide
  law-enforcement agent (on duty) —see Legal,
    intervention, manhandling
    with blunt object —see Legal, intervention,
      blunt object

Struck by (Continued)
  lightning —see subcategory T75.0
    causing fire —see Exposure, fire
  machine —see Contact, with, by type of
    machine
  mammal NEC W55.89
    marine W56.32
  marine animal W56.82
  missile
    firearm —see Discharge, firearm by type
    in war operations —see War operations,
      missile
  object W22.8
    blunt W22.8
      assault Y00
      suicide (attempt) X79
      undetermined whether accidental or
        intentional Y29
    falling W20.8
      from, in, on
        building W20.1
          burning (uncontrolled fire) X00.4
        cataclysmic
          earth surface movement NEC —see
            Landslide
          storm —see Forces of nature,
            cataclysmic storm
        cave-in W20.0
        earthquake X34
        machine (in operation) —see Contact,
          with, by type of machine
        structure W20.1
          burning X00.4
        transport vehicle (in motion) —see
          Accident, transport, by type of
          vehicle
        watercraft V93.49
          due to
            accident to craft V91.39
              powered craft V91.33
                ferry boat V91.31
                fishing boat V91.32
                jet ski V91.33
                liner V91.31
                merchant ship V91.30
                passenger ship V91.31
              unpowered craft V91.38
                canoe V91.35
                inflatable V91.36
                kayak V91.35
                sailboat V91.34
                surf-board V91.38
                windsurfer V91.38
            powered craft V93.43
              ferry boat V93.41
              fishing boat V93.42
              jet ski V93.43
              liner V93.41
              merchant ship V93.40
              passenger ship V93.41
            unpowered craft V93.48
              sailboat V93.44
              surf-board V93.48
              windsurfer V93.48
    moving NEC W20.8
    projected W20.8
      assault Y00
      in sports W21.9
        assault Y08.09
        ball W21.00
          baseball W21.03
          basketball W21.05
          football W21.01
          golf ball W21.04
          soccer W21.02
          softball W21.07
          specified NEC W21.09
          volleyball W21.06
        bat or racquet
          baseball bat W21.11
            assault Y08.02

Struck by (Continued)
  object (Continued)
    projected (Continued)
      in sports (Continued)
        bat or racquet (Continued)
          golf club W21.13
            assault Y08.09-●
          specified NEC W21.19
            assault Y08.09
          tennis racquet W21.12
            assault Y08.09
        hockey (ice)
          field
            puck W21.221
            stick W21.211
          puck W21.220
          stick W21.210
            assault Y08.01
        specified NEC W21.89
    set in motion by explosion —see Explosion
    thrown W20.8
      assault Y00
      in sports W21.9
        assault Y08.09
        ball W21.00
          baseball W21.03
          basketball W21.05
          football W21.01
          golf ball W21.04
          soccer W21.02
          soft ball W21.07
          specified NEC W21.09
          volleyball W21.06
        bat or racquet
          baseball bat W21.11
            assault Y08.02
          golf club W21.13
            assault Y08.09
          specified NEC W21.19
            assault Y08.09
          tennis racquet W21.12
            assault Y08.09
        hockey (ice)
          field
            puck W21.221
            stick W21.211
          puck W21.220
          stick W21.210
            assault Y08.01
        specified NEC W21.89
  other person(s) W50.0
    with
      blunt object W22.8
        intentional, homicide (attempt) Y00
        sports equipment W21.9
        undetermined whether accidental or
          intentional Y29
      fall W03
        due to ice or snow W00.0
      as, or caused by, a crowd or human
        stampede (with fall) W52
      assault Y04.2
      homicide (attempt) Y04.2
    in legal intervention
      injuring
        bystander Y35.812
        law enforcement personnel Y35.811
        suspect Y35.813
        unspecified person Y35.819
    sports equipment W21.9
  police (on duty) —see Legal, intervention,
    manhandling
    with blunt object —see Legal, intervention,
      blunt object
  sports equipment W21.9
    assault Y08.09
    ball W21.00
      baseball W21.03
      basketball W21.05
      football W21.01
      golf ball W21.04
      soccer W21.02

▶ New   ⇒ Revised   ~~deleted~~ Deleted   ● Use Additional Character(s)

Struck by *(Continued)*
  sports equipment *(Continued)*
    ball *(Continued)*
      soft ball W21.07
      specified NEC W21.09
      volleyball W21.06
    bat or racquet
      baseball bat W21.11
        assault Y08.02
      golf club W21.13
        assault Y08.09
      specified NEC W21.19
      tennis racquet W21.12
        assault Y08.09
    cleats (shoe) W21.31
    foot wear NEC W21.39
    football helmet W21.81
    hockey (ice)
      field
        puck W21.221
        stick W21.211
      puck W21.220
      stick W21.210
        assault Y08.01
    skate blades W21.32
    specified NEC W21.89
      assault Y08.09
  thunderbolt *—see* subcategory
    T75.0
    causing fire *—see* Exposure, fire
  transport vehicle NEC *—see also* Accident,
    transport V09.9
    intentional, homicide (attempt) Y03.0
    motor NEC *—see also* Accident, transport
      V09.20
      homicide Y03.0
  vehicle (transport) NEC *—see* Accident,
    transport, by type of vehicle
    stationary (falling from jack,
      hydraulic lift, ramp)
      W20.8
Stumbling
  without fall W18.40
    due to
      specified NEC W18.49
      stepping from one level to another
        W18.43
      stepping into hole or opening W18.42
      stepping on object W18.41
  over
    animal NEC W01.0
      with fall W18.09
    carpet, rug or (small) object W22.8
      with fall W18.09
    person W51
      with fall W03
        due to ice or snow W00.0

Submersion (accidental) *—see* Drowning
Suffocation (accidental) (by external means)
  (by pressure) (mechanical) *—see also*
    category T71
  due to, by
    avalanche *—see* Landslide
    explosion *—see* Explosion
    fire *—see* Exposure, fire
    food, any type (aspiration) (ingestion)
      (inhalation) *—see* categories T17 and
      T18
    ignition *—see* Ignition
    landslide *—see* Landslide
    machine (ry) *—see* Contact, with, by type
      of machine
    vomitus (aspiration) (inhalation)
      T17.81-●
  in
    burning building X00.8
Suicide, suicidal (attempted) (by) X83.8
  blunt object X79
  burning, burns X76
    hot object X77.9
      fluid NEC X77.2
      household appliance X77.3
      specified NEC X77.8
      steam X77.0
      tap water X77.1
      vapors X77.0
  caustic substance *—see* Table of Drugs and
    Chemicals
  cold, extreme X83.2
  collision of motor vehicle with
    motor vehicle X82.0
    specified NEC X82.8
    train X82.1
    tree X82.2
  crashing of aircraft X83.0
  cut (any part of body) X78.9
  cutting or piercing instrument X78.9
    dagger X78.2
    glass X78.0
    knife X78.1
    specified NEC X78.8
    sword X78.2
  drowning (in) X71.9
    bathtub X71.0
    natural water X71.3
    specified NEC X71.8
    swimming pool X71.1
      following fall X71.2
  electrocution X83.1
  explosive(s) (material) X75
  fire, flames X76
  firearm X74.9
    airgun X74.01
    handgun X72

Suicide, suicidal *(Continued)*
  firearm *(Continued)*
    hunting rifle X73.1
    larger X73.9
      specified NEC X73.8
    machine gun X73.2
    shotgun X73.0
    specified NEC X74.8
  hanging X83.8
  hot object *—see* Suicide, burning, hot object
  jumping
    before moving object X81.8
      motor vehicle X81.0
      subway train X81.1
      train X81.1
    from high place X80
  late effect of attempt *—see* X71-X83 with 7th
    character S
  lying before moving object, train, vehicle X81.8
  poisoning *—see* Table of Drugs and
    Chemicals
  puncture (any part of body) *—see* Suicide,
    cutting or piercing instrument
  scald *—see* Suicide, burning, hot object
  sequelae of attempt *—see* X71-X83 with 7th
    character S
  sharp object (any) *—see* Suicide, cutting or
    piercing instrument
  shooting *—see* Suicide, firearm
  specified means NEC X83.8
  stab (any part of body) *—see* Suicide, cutting
    or piercing instrument
  steam, hot vapors X77.0
  strangulation X83.8
  submersion *—see* Suicide, drowning
  suffocation X83.8
  wound NEC X83.8
Sunstroke X32
Supersonic waves (causing injury) W42.0
Surgical procedure, complication of (delayed
  or as an abnormal reaction without
  mention of misadventure) *—see also*
  Complication of or following, by type of
  procedure
  due to or as a result of misadventure *—see*
    Misadventure
Swallowed, swallowing
  foreign body *—see* Foreign body, alimentary
    canal
  poison *—see* Table of Drugs and Chemicals
  substance
    caustic or corrosive *—see* Table of Drugs
      and Chemicals
    poisonous *—see* Table of Drugs and
      Chemicals

S

T

Tackle in sport W03
Terrorism (involving) Y38.80
  biological weapons Y38.6X-●
  chemical weapons Y38.7X-●
  conflagration Y38.3X-●
  drowning and submersion Y38.89-●
  explosion Y38.2X-●
    destruction of aircraft Y38.1X-●
    marine weapons Y38.0X-●
  fire Y38.3X-●
  firearms Y38.4X-●
  hot substances Y38.3X-●
  lasers Y38.89-●
  nuclear weapons Y38.5X-●
  piercing or stabbing instruments
    Y38.89-●
  secondary effects Y38.9X-●
  specified method NEC Y38.89-●
  suicide bomber Y38.81-●
Thirst X58
Threat to breathing
  aspiration —see Aspiration
  due to cave-in, falling earth or substance
    NEC —see category T71
Thrown (accidentally)
  against part (any) of or object in transport
    vehicle (in motion) NEC —see also
    Accident, transport

Thrown (Continued)
  from
    high place, homicide (attempt) Y01
    machinery —see Contact, with, by type of
      machine
    transport vehicle NEC —see also Accident,
      transport V89.9
  off —see Thrown, from
Thunderbolt —see subcategory T75.0
  causing fire —see Exposure, fire
Tidal wave (any injury) NEC —see Forces of
  nature, tidal wave
Took
  overdose (drug) —see Table of Drugs and
    Chemicals
  poison —see Table of Drugs and
    Chemicals
Tornado (any injury) X37.1
Torrential rain (any injury) X37.8
Torture X58
Trampled by animal NEC W55.89
Trapped (accidentally)
  between objects (moving) (stationary and
    moving) —see Caught
  by part (any) of
    motorcycle V29.88
    pedal cycle V19.88
    transport vehicle NEC —see also Accident,
      transport V89.9
Travel (effects) (sickness) T75.3

Tree falling on or hitting (accidentally)
  (person) W20.8
Tripping
  without fall W18.40
    due to
      specified NEC W18.49
      stepping from one level to another
        W18.43
      stepping into hole or opening
        W18.42
      stepping on object W18.41
    over
      animal W01.0
        with fall W01.0
      carpet, rug or (small) object W22.8
        with fall W18.09
      person W51
        with fall W03
          due to ice or snow W00.0
Twisted by person(s) (accidentally) W50.2
  with intent to injure or kill Y04.0
  as, or caused by, a crowd or human stampede
    (with fall) W52
  assault Y04.0
  homicide (attempt) Y04.0
  in
    fight Y04.0
    legal intervention —see Legal, intervention,
      manhandling
Twisting (prolonged) (static) X50.1

U

Underdosing of necessary drugs, medicaments
  or biological substances Y63.6
Undetermined intent (contact)
  (exposure)
  automobile collision Y32
  blunt object Y29
  drowning (submersion) (in) Y21.9
    bathtub Y21.0
      after fall Y21.1
    natural water (lake) (ocean) (pond) (river)
      (stream) Y21.4
    specified place NEC Y21.8
    swimming pool Y21.2
      after fall Y21.3
  explosive material Y25
  fall, jump or push from high place Y30
  falling, lying or running before moving object
    Y31
  fire Y26

Undetermined intent (Continued)
  firearm discharge Y24.9
    airgun (BB) (pellet) Y24.0
    handgun (pistol) (revolver)
      Y22
    hunting rifle Y23.1
    larger Y23.9
      hunting rifle Y23.1
      machine gun Y23.3
      military Y23.2
      shotgun Y23.0
      specified type NEC Y23.8
    machine gun Y23.3
    military Y23.2
    shotgun Y23.0
    specified type NEC Y24.8
    Very pistol Y24.8
  hot object Y27.9
    fluid NEC Y27.2
    household appliance Y27.3
    specified object NEC Y27.8

Undetermined intent (Continued)
  hot object (Continued)
    steam Y27.0
    tap water Y27.1
    vapor Y27.0
  jump, fall or push from high place Y30
  lying, falling or running before moving object
    Y31
  motor vehicle crash Y32
  push, fall or jump from high place Y30
  running, falling or lying before moving object
    Y31
  sharp object Y28.9
    dagger Y28.2
    glass Y28.0
    knife Y28.1
    specified object NEC Y28.8
    sword Y28.2
  smoke Y26
  specified event NEC Y33
Use of hand as hammer X50.3

V

Vibration (causing injury) W49.9
Victim (of)
  avalanche —see Landslide
  earth movements NEC —see Forces of nature,
    earth movement
  earthquake X34

Victim (Continued)
  flood —see Flood
  landslide —see Landslide
  lightning —see subcategory T75.0
    causing fire —see Exposure, fire
  storm (cataclysmic) NEC —see Forces of
    nature, cataclysmic storm
  volcanic eruption X35

Volcanic eruption (any injury) X35
Vomitus, gastric contents in air passages (with
  asphyxia, obstruction or
  suffocation) T17.81-●

▶ New   ⏩ Revised   ~~deleted~~ Deleted   ● Use Additional Character(s)

W

Walked into stationary object (any) W22.09
  furniture W22.03
  lamppost W22.02
  wall W22.01
War operations (injuries to military personnel
    and civilians during war, civil insurrection
    and peacekeeping missions) (by) (from)
    (involving) Y36.90-●
  after cessation of hostilities Y36.89-●
    explosion (of)
      bomb placed during war operations
        Y36.82-●
      mine placed during war operations
        Y36.81-●
    specified NEC Y36.88-●
  air blast Y36.20-●
  aircraft
    destruction —see War operations,
      destruction of aircraft
  airway restriction —see War operations,
    restriction of airways
  asphyxiation —see War operations, restriction
    of airways
  biological weapons Y36.6X-●
  blast Y36.20-●
  blast fragments Y36.20-●
  blast wave Y36.20-●
  blast wind Y36.20-●
  bomb Y36.20-●
    dirty Y36.50-●
    gasoline Y36.31-●
    incendiary Y36.31-●
    petrol Y36.31-●
  bullet Y36.43-●
    incendiary Y36.32-●
    rubber Y36.41-●
  chemical weapons Y36.7X-●
  combat
    hand to hand (unarmed) combat Y36.44-●
    using blunt or piercing object Y36.45-●
  conflagration —see War operations, fire
  conventional warfare NEC Y36.49-●
  depth-charge Y36.01-●
  destruction of aircraft Y36.10-●
    due to
      air to air missile Y36.11-●
      collision with other aircraft Y36.12-●
      detonation (accidental) of onboard
        munitions and explosives Y36.14-●
      enemy fire or explosives Y36.11-●
      explosive placed on aircraft Y36.11-●
      onboard fire Y36.13-●
      rocket propelled grenade [RPG] Y36.11-●
      small arms fire Y36.11-●
      surface to air missile Y36.11-●
    specified NEC Y36.19-●
  detonation (accidental) of
    onboard marine weapons Y36.05-●
    own munitions or munitions launch device
      Y36.24-●

War operations (Continued)
  dirty bomb Y36.50-●
  explosion (of) Y36.20-●
    aerial bomb Y36.21-●
    after cessation of hostilities
      bomb placed during war operations
        Y36.82-●
      mine placed during war operations
        Y36.81-●
    bomb NOS —see also War operations,
      bomb(s) Y36.20-●
    fragments Y36.20-●
    grenade Y36.29-●
    guided missile Y36.22-●
    improvised explosive device [IED]
      (person-borne) (roadside)
      (vehicle-borne) Y36.23-●
    land mine Y36.29-●
    marine mine (at sea) (in harbor)
      Y36.02-●
    marine weapon Y36.00-●
      specified NEC Y36.09-●
    own munitions or munitions launch
      device (accidental) Y36.24-●
    sea-based artillery shell Y36.03-●
    specified NEC Y36.29-●
    torpedo Y36.04-●
  fire Y36.30-●
    specified NEC Y36.39-●
  firearms
    discharge Y36.43-●
    pellets Y36.42-●
  flamethrower Y36.33-●
  fragments (from) (of)
    improvised explosive device [IED]
      (person-borne) (roadside)
      (vehicle-borne) Y36.26-●
    munitions Y36.25-●
    specified NEC Y36.29-●
    weapons Y36.27-●
  friendly fire Y36.92
  hand to hand (unarmed) combat
    Y36.44-●
  hot substances —see War operations,
    fire
  incendiary bullet Y36.32-●
  nuclear weapon (effects of) Y36.50-●
    acute radiation exposure Y36.54-●
    blast pressure Y36.51-●
    direct blast Y36.51-●
    direct heat Y36.53-●
    fallout exposure Y36.54-●
    fireball Y36.53-●
    indirect blast (struck or crushed by blast
      debris) (being thrown by blast)
      Y36.52-●
    ionizing radiation (immediate exposure)
      Y36.54-●
    nuclear radiation Y36.54-●
    radiation
      ionizing (immediate exposure)
        Y36.54-●

War operations (Continued)
  nuclear weapon (Continued)
    radiation (Continued)
      nuclear Y36.54-●
      thermal Y36.53-●
    secondary NEC Y36.54-●
    specified NEC Y36.59-●
    thermal radiation Y36.53-●
  restriction of air (airway)
    intentional Y36.46-●
    unintentional Y36.47-●
  rubber bullets Y36.41-●
  shrapnel NOS Y36.29-●
  suffocation —see War operations, restriction
    of airways
  unconventional warfare NEC Y36.7X-●
  underwater blast NOS Y36.00-●
  warfare
    conventional NEC Y36.49-●
    unconventional NEC Y36.7X-●
  weapon of mass destruction [WMD] Y36.91
  weapons
    biological weapons Y36.6X-●
    chemical Y36.7X-●
    nuclear (effects of) Y36.50-●
      acute radiation exposure Y36.54-●
      blast pressure Y36.51-●
      direct blast Y36.51-●
      direct heat Y36.53-●
      fallout exposure Y36.54-●
      fireball Y36.53-●
      radiation
        ionizing (immediate exposure)
          Y36.54-●
        nuclear Y36.54-●
        thermal Y36.53-●
      secondary effects Y36.54-●
      specified NEC Y36.59-●
    of mass destruction [WMD] Y36.91-●
Washed
  away by flood —see Flood
  off road by storm (transport vehicle) —see
    Forces of nature, cataclysmic storm
Weather exposure NEC —see Forces of nature
Weightlessness (causing injury) (effects of) (in
    spacecraft, real or simulated) X52
Work related condition Y99.0
Wound (accidental) NEC —see also Injury X58
  battle —see also War operations Y36.90
  gunshot —see Discharge, firearm by type
Wreck transport vehicle NEC —see also
    Accident, transport V89.9
Wrong
  device implanted into correct surgical site
    Y65.51
  fluid in infusion Y65.1
  patient, procedure performed on Y65.52
  procedure (operation) on correct patient
    Y65.51

PART III

ICD-1O-CM Tabular List of Diseases and Injuries

CHAPTER 1

CERTAIN INFECTIOUS AND PARASITIC DISEASES (A00-B99)

OGCR Chapter-Specific Coding Guidelines

1. **Chapter 1: Certain Infectious and Parasitic Diseases (A00-B99)**

   a. **Human Immunodeficiency Virus (HIV) Infections**

   1) **Code only confirmed cases**

   Code only confirmed cases of HIV infection/illness. This is an exception to the hospital inpatient guideline Section II, H.

   In this context, "confirmation" does not require documentation of positive serology or culture for HIV; the provider's diagnostic statement that the patient is HIV positive, or has an HIV-related illness is sufficient.

   2) **Selection and sequencing of HIV codes**

   (a) **Patient admitted for HIV-related condition**

   If a patient is admitted for an HIV-related condition, the principal diagnosis should be B20, Human immunodeficiency virus [HIV] disease followed by additional diagnosis codes for all reported HIV-related conditions.

   (b) **Patient with HIV disease admitted for unrelated condition**

   If a patient with HIV disease is admitted for an unrelated condition (such as a traumatic injury), the code for the unrelated condition (e.g., the nature of injury code) should be the principal diagnosis. Other diagnoses would be B20 followed by additional diagnosis codes for all reported HIV-related conditions.

   (c) **Whether the patient is newly diagnosed**

   Whether the patient is newly diagnosed or has had previous admissions/encounters for HIV conditions is irrelevant to the sequencing decision.

   (d) **Asymptomatic human immunodeficiency virus**

   Z21, Asymptomatic human immunodeficiency virus [HIV] infection status, is to be applied when the patient without any documentation of symptoms is listed as being "HIV positive," "known HIV," "HIV test positive," or similar terminology. Do not use this code if the term "AIDS" is used or if the patient is treated for any HIV-related illness or is described as having any condition(s) resulting from his/her HIV positive status; use B20 in these cases.

   (e) **Patients with inconclusive HIV serology**

   Patients with inconclusive HIV serology, but no definitive diagnosis or manifestations of the illness, may be assigned code R75, Inconclusive laboratory evidence of human immunodeficiency virus [HIV].

   (f) **Previously diagnosed HIV-related illness**

   Patients with any known prior diagnosis of an HIV-related illness should be coded to B20. Once a patient has developed an HIV-related illness, the patient should always be assigned code B20 on every subsequent admission/encounter. Patients previously diagnosed with any HIV illness (B20) should never be assigned to R75 or Z21, Asymptomatic human immunodeficiency virus [HIV] infection status.

   (g) **HIV Infection in Pregnancy, Childbirth and the Puerperium**

   During pregnancy, childbirth or the puerperium, a patient admitted (or presenting for a health care encounter) because of an HIV-related illness should receive a principal diagnosis code of O98.7-, Human immunodeficiency [HIV] disease complicating pregnancy, childbirth and the puerperium, followed by B20 and the code(s) for the HIV-related illness(es). Codes from Chapter 15 always take sequencing priority.

   Patients with asymptomatic HIV infection status admitted (or presenting for a health care encounter) during pregnancy, childbirth, or the puerperium should receive codes of O98.7- and Z21.

   (h) **Encounters for testing for HIV**

   If a patient is being seen to determine his/her HIV status, use code Z11.4, Encounter for screening for human immunodeficiency virus [HIV]. Use additional codes for any associated high-risk behavior.

   If a patient with signs or symptoms is being seen for HIV testing, code the signs and symptoms. An additional counseling code Z71.7, Human immunodeficiency virus [HIV] counseling, may be used if counseling is provided during the encounter for the test.

   When a patient returns to be informed of his/her HIV test results and the test result is negative, use code Z71.7, Human immunodeficiency virus [HIV] counseling.

If the results are positive, see previous guidelines and assign codes as appropriate.

   b. **Infectious agents as the cause of diseases classified to other chapters**

   Certain infections are classified in chapters other than Chapter 1 and no organism is identified as part of the infection code. In these instances, it is necessary to use an additional code from Chapter 1 to identify the organism. A code from category B95, Streptococcus, Staphylococcus, and Enterococcus as the cause of diseases classified to other chapters, B96, Other bacterial agents as the cause of diseases classified to other chapters, or B97, Viral agents as the cause of diseases classified to other chapters, is to be used as an additional code to identify the organism. An instructional note will be found at the infection code advising that an additional organism code is required.

   c. **Infections resistant to antibiotics**

   Many bacterial infections are resistant to current antibiotics. It is necessary to identify all infections documented as antibiotic resistant. Assign a code from category Z16, Resistance to antimicrobial drugs, following the infection code only if the infection code does not identify drug resistance.

   d. **Sepsis, Severe Sepsis, and Septic Shock**

   1) **Coding of Sepsis and Severe Sepsis**

   (a) **Sepsis**

   For a diagnosis of sepsis, assign the appropriate code for the underlying systemic infection. If the type of infection or causal organism is not further specified, assign code A41.9, Sepsis, unspecified organism.

   A code from subcategory R65.2, Severe sepsis, should not be assigned unless severe sepsis or an associated acute organ dysfunction is documented.

   (i) Negative or inconclusive blood cultures and sepsis

   Negative or inconclusive blood cultures do not preclude a diagnosis of sepsis in patients with clinical evidence of the condition, however, the provider should be queried.

   (ii) Urosepsis

   The term urosepsis is a nonspecific term. It is not to be considered synonymous with sepsis. It has no default code in the Alphabetic Index. Should a provider use this term, he/she must be queried for clarification.

   (iii) Sepsis with organ dysfunction

   If a patient has sepsis and associated acute organ dysfunction or multiple organ dysfunction (MOD), follow the instructions for coding severe sepsis.

   (iv) Acute organ dysfunction that is not clearly associated with the sepsis

   If a patient has sepsis and an acute organ dysfunction, but the medical record documentation indicates that the acute organ dysfunction is related to a medical condition other than the sepsis, do not assign a code from subcategory R65.2, Severe sepsis. An acute organ dysfunction must be associated with the sepsis in order to assign the severe sepsis code. If the documentation is not clear as to whether an acute organ dysfunction is related to the sepsis or another medical condition, query the provider.

   (b) **Severe sepsis**

   The coding of severe sepsis requires a minimum of 2 codes: first a code for the underlying systemic infection, followed by a code from subcategory R65.2, Severe sepsis. If the causal organism is not documented, assign code A41.9, Sepsis, unspecified organism, for the infection. Additional code(s) for the associated acute organ dysfunction are also required.

   Due to the complex nature of severe sepsis, some cases may require querying the provider prior to assignment of the codes.

   2) **Septic shock**

   (a) Septic shock generally refers to circulatory failure associated with severe sepsis, and therefore, it represents a type of acute organ dysfunction.

   For all cases of septic shock, the code for the systemic infection should be sequenced first, followed by code R65.21, Severe sepsis with septic shock or code T81.12, Postprocedural septic shock.

Any additional codes for the other acute organ dysfunctions should also be assigned. As noted in the sequencing instructions in the Tabular List, the code for septic shock cannot be assigned as a principal diagnosis.

3) Sequencing of severe sepsis

If severe sepsis is present on admission, and meets the definition of principal diagnosis, the underlying systemic infection should be assigned as principal diagnosis followed by the appropriate code from subcategory R65.2 as required by the sequencing rules in the Tabular List. A code from subcategory R65.2 can never be assigned as a principal diagnosis.

When severe sepsis develops during an encounter (it was not present on admission) the underlying systemic infection and the appropriate code from subcategory R65.2 should be assigned as secondary diagnoses.

Severe sepsis may be present on admission but the diagnosis may not be confirmed until sometime after admission. If the documentation is not clear whether severe sepsis was present on admission, the provider should be queried.

4) Sepsis and severe sepsis with a localized infection

If the reason for admission is both sepsis or severe sepsis and a localized infection, such as pneumonia or cellulitis, a code(s) for the underlying systemic infection should be assigned first and the code for the localized infection should be assigned as a secondary diagnosis. If the patient has severe sepsis, a code from subcategory R65.2 should also be assigned as a secondary diagnosis. If the patient is admitted with a localized infection, such as pneumonia, and sepsis/severe sepsis doesn't develop until after admission, the localized infection should be assigned first, followed by the appropriate sepsis/severe sepsis codes.

5) Sepsis due to a postprocedural infection

(a) Documentation of causal relationship

As with all postprocedural complications, code assignment is based on the provider's documentation of the relationship between the infection and the procedure.

(b) Sepsis due to a postprocedural infection

For infections following a procedure, a code from T81.40, to T81.43, Infection following a procedure, or O86.00 to O86.03, Infection of obstetric surgical wound, that identifies the site of the infection should be coded first, if known. Assign an additional code for sepsis following a procedure (T81.44) or sepsis following an obstetrical procedure (O86.04). Use an additional code to identify the infectious agent. If the patient has severe sepsis the appropriate code from subcategory R65.2 should also be assigned with the additional code(s) for any acute organ dysfunction.

For infections following infusion, transfusion, therapeutic injection, or immunization, a code from subcategory T80.2, Infections following infusion, transfusion, and therapeutic injection, or code T88.0-, Infection following immunization, should be coded first, followed by the code for the specific infection. If the patient has severe sepsis, the appropriate code from subcategory R65.2 should also be assigned, with the additional codes(s) for any acute organ dysfunction.

(c) Postprocedural infection and postprocedural septic shock

If a postprocedural infection has resulted in postprocedural septic shock, assign the codes indicated above for sepsis due to a postprocedural infection, followed by code T81.12-, Postprocedural septic shock. Do not assign code R65.21, Severe sepsis with septic shock. Additional code(s) should be assigned for any acute organ dysfunction.

6) Sepsis and severe sepsis associated with a noninfectious process (condition)

In some cases a noninfectious process (condition), such as trauma, may lead to an infection which can result in sepsis or severe sepsis. If sepsis or severe sepsis is documented as associated with a noninfectious condition, such as a burn or serious injury, and this condition meets the definition for principal diagnosis, the code for the noninfectious condition should be sequenced first, followed by the code for the resulting infection. If severe sepsis is present, a code from subcategory R65.2 should also be assigned with any associated organ dysfunction(s) codes. It is not necessary to assign a code from subcategory R65.1, Systemic inflammatory response syndrome (SIRS) of noninfectious origin, for these cases.

If the infection meets the definition of principal diagnosis it should be sequenced before the noninfectious condition. When both the associated noninfectious condition and the infection meet the definition of principal diagnosis either may be assigned as principal diagnosis.

Only one code from category R65, Symptoms and signs specifically associated with systemic inflammation and infection, should be assigned. Therefore, when a noninfectious condition leads to an infection resulting in severe sepsis, assign the appropriate code from subcategory R65.2, Severe sepsis. Do not additionally assign a code from subcategory R65.1, Systemic inflammatory response syndrome (SIRS) of noninfectious origin.
See Section I.C.18. SIRS due to non-infectious process

7) Sepsis and septic shock complicating abortion, pregnancy, childbirth, and the puerperium

See Section I.C.15. Sepsis and septic shock complicating abortion, pregnancy, childbirth and the puerperium

8) Newborn sepsis

See Section I.C.16. f. Bacterial sepsis of Newborn

e. Methicillin Resistant Staphylococcus aureus (MRSA) Conditions

1) Selection and sequencing of MRSA codes

(a) Combination codes for MRSA infection

When a patient is diagnosed with an infection that is due to methicillin resistant *Staphylococcus aureus* (MRSA), and that infection has a combination code that includes the causal organism (e.g., sepsis, pneumonia) assign the appropriate combination code for the condition (e.g., code A41.02, Sepsis due to Methicillin resistant Staphylococcus aureus or code J15.212, Pneumonia due to Methicillin resistant Staphylococcus aureus). Do not assign code B95.62, Methicillin resistant Staphylococcus aureus infection as the cause of diseases classified elsewhere, as an additional code because the combination code includes the type of infection and the MRSA organism. Do not assign a code from subcategory Z16.11, Resistance to penicillins, as an additional diagnosis.
See Section C.1. for instructions on coding and sequencing of sepsis and severe sepsis.

(b) Other codes for MRSA infection

When there is documentation of a current infection (e.g., wound infection, stitch abscess, urinary tract infection) due to MRSA, and that infection does not have a combination code that includes the causal organism, assign the appropriate code to identify the condition along with code B95.62, Methicillin resistant Staphylococcus aureus infection as the cause of diseases classified elsewhere for the MRSA infection. Do not assign a code from subcategory Z16.11, Resistance to penicillins.

(c) Methicillin susceptible Staphylococcus aureus (MSSA) and MRSA colonization

The condition or state of being colonized or carrying MSSA or MRSA is called colonization or carriage, while an individual person is described as being colonized or being a carrier. Colonization means that MSSA or MSRA is present on or in the body without necessarily causing illness. A positive MRSA colonization test might be documented by the provider as "MRSA screen positive" or "MRSA nasal swab positive".

Assign code Z22.322, Carrier or suspected carrier of Methicillin resistant Staphylococcus aureus, for patients documented as having MRSA colonization. Assign code Z22.321, Carrier or suspected carrier of Methicillin susceptible Staphylococcus aureus, for patient documented as having MSSA colonization. Colonization is not necessarily indicative of a disease process or as the cause of a specific condition the patient may have unless documented as such by the provider.

(d) MRSA colonization and infection

If a patient is documented as having both MRSA colonization and infection during a hospital admission, code Z22.322, Carrier or suspected carrier of Methicillin resistant Staphylococcus aureus, and a code for the MRSA infection may both be assigned.

f. Zika virus infections

1) Code only confirmed cases

Code only a confirmed diagnosis of Zika virus (A92.5, Zika virus disease) as documented by the provider. This is an exception to the hospital inpatient guideline Section II, H.

In this context, "confirmation" does not require documentation of the type of test performed; the physician's diagnostic statement that the condition is confirmed is sufficient. This code should be assigned regardless of the stated mode of transmission.

If the provider documents "suspected", "possible" or "probable" Zika, do not assign code A92.5. Assign a code(s) explaining the reason for encounter (such as fever, rash, or joint pain) or Z20.821, Contact with and (suspected) exposure to Zika virus.

CHAPTER 1

CERTAIN INFECTIOUS AND PARASITIC DISEASES (A00-B99)

Includes   diseases generally recognized as communicable or transmissible

Use additional code to identify resistance to antimicrobial drugs (Z16.-)

Excludes1   certain localized infections - see body system-related chapters

Excludes2   carrier or suspected carrier of infectious disease (Z22.-)

infectious and parasitic diseases complicating pregnancy, childbirth and the puerperium (O98.-)

infectious and parasitic diseases specific to the perinatal period (P35-P39)

influenza and other acute respiratory infections (J00-J22)

This chapter contains the following blocks:

A00-A09	Intestinal infectious diseases
A15-A19	Tuberculosis
A20-A28	Certain zoonotic bacterial diseases
A30-A49	Other bacterial diseases
A50-A64	Infections with a predominantly sexual mode of transmission
A65-A69	Other spirochetal diseases
A70-A74	Other diseases caused by chlamydiae
A75-A79	Rickettsioses
A80-A89	Viral and prion infections of the central nervous system
A90-A99	Arthropod-borne viral fevers and viral hemorrhagic fevers
B00-B09	Viral infections characterized by skin and mucous membrane lesions
B10	Other human herpesviruses
B15-B19	Viral hepatitis
B20	Human immunodeficiency virus [HIV] disease
B25-B34	Other viral diseases
B35-B49	Mycoses
B50-B64	Protozoal diseases
B65-B83	Helminthiases
B85-B89	Pediculosis, acariasis and other infestations
B90-B94	Sequelae of infectious and parasitic diseases
B95-B97	Bacterial and viral infectious agents
B99	Other infectious diseases

INTESTINAL INFECTIOUS DISEASES (A00-A09)

● **A00   Cholera**
A serious, often deadly, infectious disease of the small intestine

A00.0   Cholera due to Vibrio cholerae 01, biovar cholerae
Classical cholera

A00.1   Cholera due to Vibrio cholerae 01, biovar eltor
Cholera eltor

A00.9   Cholera, unspecified

● **A01   Typhoid and paratyphoid fevers**
Caused by Salmonella typhi and Salmonella paratyphi A, B, and C bacteria

● **A01.0   Typhoid fever**
Infection due to Salmonella typhi

     A01.00   Typhoid fever, unspecified

     A01.01   Typhoid meningitis

     A01.02   Typhoid fever with heart involvement
         Typhoid endocarditis
         Typhoid myocarditis

     A01.03   Typhoid pneumonia 🐾

     A01.04   Typhoid arthritis 🐾

     A01.05   Typhoid osteomyelitis 🐾

     A01.09   Typhoid fever with other complications

A01.1   Paratyphoid fever A

A01.2   Paratyphoid fever B

A01.3   Paratyphoid fever C

A01.4   Paratyphoid fever, unspecified
Infection due to Salmonella paratyphi NOS

● **A02   Other salmonella infections**
Includes   infection or foodborne intoxication due to any Salmonella species other than S. typhi and S. paratyphi

A02.0   Salmonella enteritis
Salmonellosis

A02.1   Salmonella sepsis 🐾

● **A02.2   Localized salmonella infections**

     A02.20   Localized salmonella infection, unspecified
         Specified in the documentation as localized, but unspecified as to type

     A02.21   Salmonella meningitis
         Specified as localized in the meninges

     A02.22   Salmonella pneumonia 🐾
         Specified as localized in the lungs

     A02.23   Salmonella arthritis 🐾
         Specified as localized in the joints

     A02.24   Salmonella osteomyelitis 🐾
         Specified as localized in bone

     A02.25   Salmonella pyelonephritis
         Salmonella tubulo-interstitial nephropathy

     A02.29   Salmonella with other localized infection
         Specified as localized (because it is still under localized heading) but does not assign into any of the above codes

A02.8   Other specified salmonella infections
Any specified salmonella infection which does NOT assign into any of the above codes (not specified as localized)

A02.9   Salmonella infection, unspecified
Unspecified in the documentation as to specific type of salmonella

● **A03   Shigellosis**
An infectious disease caused by bacteria (Shigella)

A03.0   Shigellosis due to Shigella dysenteriae
Group A shigellosis [Shiga-Kruse dysentery]

A03.1   Shigellosis due to Shigella flexneri
Group B shigellosis

A03.2   Shigellosis due to Shigella boydii
Group C shigellosis

A03.3   Shigellosis due to Shigella sonnei
Group D shigellosis

A03.8   Other shigellosis

A03.9   Shigellosis, unspecified
Bacillary dysentery NOS

Item 1-1   Salmonella is a bacterium that lives in the intestines of fowl and mammals and can spread to humans through improper food preparation and cooking. Salmonellosis is an infection with the bacterium. Symptoms include diarrhea, fever, and abdominal cramps 12 to 72 hours after infection. The illness usually lasts 4 to 7 days, and most persons recover without treatment. The diarrhea may be so severe that the patient needs to be hospitalized. Patients with immunocompromised systems in chronic, ill health are more likely to have the infection invade their bloodstream with life-threatening results. For example, patients with sickle cell disease are more prone to salmonella osteomyelitis than others.

▶ New   ⏵ Revised   ~~deleted~~ Deleted   Excludes 1   Excludes 2   Includes   Use additional   Code first   Code also   Key words

OGCR Official Guidelines   X Assign placeholder X   ● Use Additional Character(s)   ▶ Manifestation Code   🐾 Hierarchical Condition Category   **Coding Clinic**

Figure 1-1   Electron micrograph of escherichia coli (E. coli) expressing P fimbriae. (Getty Image)

Item 1-2   *Escherichia coli [E. coli]* is a Gram-negative bacterium found in the intestinal tracts of humans and animals and is usually nonpathogenic. Pathogenic strains can cause diarrhea or pyogenic (pus-producing) infections. Can be a threat to food safety.

● **A04**   **Other bacterial intestinal infections**

     Excludes1   bacterial foodborne intoxications, NEC (A05.-)
                   tuberculous enteritis (A18.32)

     A04.0   **Enteropathogenic Escherichia coli infection**
             Pertaining to or producing intestinal disease

     A04.1   **Enterotoxigenic Escherichia coli infection**
             Producing or containing intestinal toxin

     A04.2   **Enteroinvasive Escherichia coli infection**
             Capable of penetrating and spreading through intestinal mucosal epithelium

     A04.3   **Enterohemorrhagic Escherichia coli infection**
             Causing bloody diarrhea, resulting from microorganisms

     A04.4   **Other intestinal Escherichia coli infections**
             Escherichia coli enteritis NOS

     A04.5   **Campylobacter enteritis**
             Spiral shaped bacterium

     A04.6   **Enteritis due to Yersinia enterocolitica**

             Excludes1   extraintestinal yersiniosis (A28.2)

             Transmitted by infected food/water and person-to-person contact, affecting intestinal tract

●   **A04.7**   **Enterocolitis due to Clostridium difficile**
             Foodborne intoxication by Clostridium difficile
             Pseudomembraneous colitis
             Marked by fibrinous deposit (false membrane) with enmeshed necrotic cells

         A04.71   **Enterocolitis due to Clostridium difficile, recurrent**
                   Coding Clinic: 2020, Q1, P18

         A04.72   **Enterocolitis due to Clostridium difficile, not specified as recurrent**

     A04.8   **Other specified bacterial intestinal infections**

     A04.9   **Bacterial intestinal infection, unspecified**
             Bacterial enteritis NOS

● **A05**   **Other bacterial foodborne intoxications, not elsewhere classified**

     Excludes1   Clostridium difficile foodborne intoxication and infection (A04.7-)
                   Escherichia coli infection (A04.0-A04.4)
                   listeriosis (A32.-)
                   salmonella foodborne intoxication and infection (A02.-)
                   toxic effect of noxious foodstuffs (T61-T62)

     A05.0   **Foodborne staphylococcal intoxication**

     A05.1   **Botulism food poisoning**
             Botulism NOS
             Classical foodborne intoxication due to Clostridium botulinum

             Excludes1   infant botulism (A48.51)
                        wound botulism (A48.52)

     A05.2   **Foodborne Clostridium perfringens [Clostridium welchii] intoxication**
             Type A causes gas gangrene and necrotizing colitis; major cause of food poisoning in humans
             Enteritis necroticans
             Pig-bel

     A05.3   **Foodborne Vibrio parahaemolyticus intoxication**
             Organism that survives only in high salt environment (halophilic), major cause of gastroenteritis due to consumption of raw or improperly cooked fish/seafood

     A05.4   **Foodborne Bacillus cereus intoxication**
             Spore-forming species commonly found in soil, causes food poisoning from formation of intestinal toxins in contaminated foods

     A05.5   **Foodborne Vibrio vulnificus intoxication**
             Species that survives in high salt environment (halophilic) with infection by eating raw seafood causes septicemia and cellulitis

     A05.8   **Other specified bacterial foodborne intoxications**

     A05.9   **Bacterial foodborne intoxication, unspecified**

● **A06**   **Amebiasis**
     An intestinal illness caused by the microscopic parasite Entamoeba histolytica

     Includes   infection due to Entamoeba histolytica

     Excludes1   other protozoal intestinal diseases (A07.-)

     Excludes2   acanthamebiasis (B60.1-)
                   Naegleriasis (B60.2)

     A06.0   **Acute amebic dysentery**
             Acute amebiasis
             Intestinal amebiasis NOS

     A06.1   **Chronic intestinal amebiasis**

     A06.2   **Amebic nondysenteric colitis**
             Pertaining to single cell microorganism

     A06.3   **Ameboma of intestine**
             Tumorlike mass produced by localized inflammation often in intestine
             Ameboma NOS

     A06.4   **Amebic liver abscess**
             Hepatic amebiasis

     A06.5   **Amebic lung abscess** 🔍
             Amebic abscess of lung (and liver)

     A06.6   **Amebic brain abscess**
             Amebic abscess of brain (and liver) (and lung)

     A06.7   **Cutaneous amebiasis**

●   **A06.8**   **Amebic infection of other sites**

         A06.81   **Amebic cystitis**

         A06.82   **Other amebic genitourinary infections**
                   Amebic balanitis
                   Amebic vesiculitis
                   Amebic vulvovaginitis

         A06.89   **Other amebic infections**
                   Amebic appendicitis
                   Amebic splenic abscess

     A06.9   **Amebiasis, unspecified**

● **A07   Other protozoal intestinal diseases**

A07.0   Balantidiasis
Balantidial dysentery
Infection by protozoa that may cause diarrhea and dysentery, with ulceration of colonic mucous membranes

A07.1   Giardiasis [lambliasis]
Common infection in small intestine spread by contaminated food, water, or direct person-to-person contact

A07.2   Cryptosporidiosis
Human infection with protozoa usually seen as self-limited diarrhea in those who work with cattle

A07.3   Isosporiasis
Human intestinal disease caused by protozoa
Infection due to Isospora belli and Isospora hominis
Intestinal coccidiosis
Isosporosis

A07.4   Cyclosporiasis
Infection by protozoa with most common species infecting humans being C cayetanensis

A07.8   Other specified protozoal intestinal diseases
Intestinal microsporidiosis
Intestinal trichomoniasis
Sarcocystosis
Sarcosporidiosis

A07.9   Protozoal intestinal disease, unspecified
Flagellate diarrhea
Protozoal colitis
Protozoal diarrhea
Protozoal dysentery

● **A08   Viral and other specified intestinal infections**
Excludes1   influenza with involvement of gastrointestinal tract (J09.X3, J10.2, J11.2)

A08.0   Rotaviral enteritis

● **A08.1   Acute gastroenteropathy due to Norwalk agent and other small round viruses**

A08.11   Acute gastroenteropathy due to Norwalk agent
Acute gastroenteropathy due to Norovirus
Acute gastroenteropathy due to Norwalk-like agent

A08.19   Acute gastroenteropathy due to other small round viruses
Acute gastroenteropathy due to small round virus [SRV] NOS

A08.2   Adenoviral enteritis

● **A08.3   Other viral enteritis**
A08.31   Calicivirus enteritis
A08.32   Astrovirus enteritis
A08.39   Other viral enteritis
Coxsackie virus enteritis
Echovirus enteritis
Enterovirus enteritis NEC
Torovirus enteritis

A08.4   Viral intestinal infection, unspecified
Viral enteritis NOS
Viral gastroenteritis NOS
Viral gastroenteropathy NOS
Coding Clinic: 2016, Q3, P12

A08.8   Other specified intestinal infections

A09   Infectious gastroenteritis and colitis, unspecified
Infectious colitis NOS
Infectious enteritis NOS
Infectious gastroenteritis NOS
Excludes1   colitis NOS (K52.9)
diarrhea NOS (R19.7)
enteritis NOS (K52.9)
gastroenteritis NOS (K52.9)
noninfective gastroenteritis and colitis, unspecified (K52.9)

Figure 1-2   Far advanced bilateral pulmonary tuberculosis before and after 8 months of treatment with streptomycin, PAS, and isoniazid. (Getty Image)

Item 1–3 Tuberculosis is a common and deadly infectious disease caused by the *Mycobacterium tuberculosis* organism. The first tuberculosis infection is called the **primary infection** and most commonly attacks the lungs but can affect the central nervous system, lymphatic system, circulatory system, genitourinary system, bones, joints, and even the skin. A **Ghon** lesion is the **initial lesion.** A **secondary lesion** occurs when the tubercle bacilli are carried to other areas.

Item 1–4 Although it primarily affects the lungs, the bacteria *Mycobacterium tuberculosis* can travel from the pulmonary circulation to virtually any organ in the body, much as a cancer metastasizes to a secondary site. If the immune system becomes compromised by age or disease, what would otherwise be a self-limiting primary tuberculosis in the lungs will develop in other organs. These are known as extrapulmonary sites.

TUBERCULOSIS (A15-A19)

Includes   infections due to Mycobacterium tuberculosis and Mycobacterium bovis
Excludes1   congenital tuberculosis (P37.0)
nonspecific reaction to test for tuberculosis without active tuberculosis (R76.1-)
pneumoconiosis associated with tuberculosis, any type in A15 (J65)
positive PPD (R76.11)
positive tuberculin skin test without active tuberculosis (R76.11)
sequelae of tuberculosis (B90.-)
silicotuberculosis (J65)

● **A15   Respiratory tuberculosis**

A15.0   Tuberculosis of lung
Tuberculous bronchiectasis
Chronic dilatation of bronchi
Tuberculous fibrosis of lung
Tuberculous pneumonia
Tuberculous pneumothorax

A15.4   Tuberculosis of intrathoracic lymph nodes
Tuberculosis of hilar lymph nodes
Tuberculosis of mediastinal lymph nodes
Tuberculosis of tracheobronchial lymph nodes
Excludes1   tuberculosis specified as primary (A15.7)

A15.5   Tuberculosis of larynx, trachea and bronchus
Tuberculosis of bronchus
Tuberculosis of glottis
Tuberculosis of larynx
Tuberculosis of trachea

A15.6   Tuberculous pleurisy
Tuberculosis of pleura
Tuberculous empyema
Excludes1   primary respiratory tuberculosis (A15.7)

A15.7   Primary respiratory tuberculosis

A15.8   Other respiratory tuberculosis
Mediastinal tuberculosis
Nasopharyngeal tuberculosis
Tuberculosis of nose
Tuberculosis of sinus [any nasal]

A15.9   Respiratory tuberculosis unspecified

● **A17**   **Tuberculosis of nervous system**

   A17.0   **Tuberculous meningitis**
   Tuberculosis of meninges (cerebral) (spinal)
   Tuberculous leptomeningitis
   > **Excludes1**   tuberculous meningoencephalitis
   >   (A17.82)

   A17.1   **Meningeal tuberculoma**
   Tuberculoma of meninges (cerebral) (spinal)
   > **Excludes2**   tuberculoma of brain and spinal cord
   >   (A17.81)

   ● **A17.8**   **Other tuberculosis of nervous system**

      A17.81   **Tuberculoma of brain and spinal cord**
      Tuberculous abscess of brain and spinal cord

      A17.82   **Tuberculous meningoencephalitis**
      *Inflammation of brain and meninges; AKA
      cerebromeningitis and encephalomeningitis*
      Tuberculous myelitis

      A17.83   **Tuberculous neuritis**
      Tuberculous mononeuropathy

      A17.89   **Other tuberculosis of nervous system**
      Tuberculous polyneuropathy

   A17.9   **Tuberculosis of nervous system, unspecified**

● **A18**   **Tuberculosis of other organs**

   ● **A18.0**   **Tuberculosis of bones and joints**

      A18.01   **Tuberculosis of spine**
      Pott's disease or curvature of spine
      Tuberculous arthritis
      Tuberculous osteomyelitis of spine
      Tuberculous spondylitis

      A18.02   **Tuberculous arthritis of other joints**
      Tuberculosis of hip (joint)
      Tuberculosis of knee (joint)

      A18.03   **Tuberculosis of other bones**
      Tuberculous mastoiditis
      Tuberculous osteomyelitis

      A18.09   **Other musculoskeletal tuberculosis**
      Tuberculous myositis
      Tuberculous synovitis
      Tuberculous tenosynovitis

   ● **A18.1**   **Tuberculosis of genitourinary system**

      A18.10   **Tuberculosis of genitourinary system, unspecified**

      A18.11   **Tuberculosis of kidney and ureter**

      A18.12   **Tuberculosis of bladder**

      A18.13   **Tuberculosis of other urinary organs**
      Tuberculous urethritis

      A18.14   **Tuberculosis of prostate** ♂   A

      A18.15   **Tuberculosis of other male genital organs** ♂

      A18.16   **Tuberculosis of cervix** ♀

      A18.17   **Tuberculous female pelvic inflammatory disease** ♀
      Tuberculous endometritis
      Tuberculous oophoritis and salpingitis
      *Oophoritis = inflammation of ovary
      Salpingitis = inflammation of fallopian tube*

      A18.18   **Tuberculosis of other female genital organs** ♀
      Tuberculous ulceration of vulva

   A18.2   **Tuberculous peripheral lymphadenopathy**
   Tuberculous adenitis
   > **Excludes2**   tuberculosis of bronchial and mediastinal
   >   lymph nodes (A15.4)
   >   tuberculosis of mesenteric and
   >   retroperitoneal lymph nodes
   >   (A18.39)
   >   tuberculous tracheobronchial adenopathy
   >   (A15.4)

● **A18.3**   **Tuberculosis of intestines, peritoneum and mesenteric glands**

   A18.31   **Tuberculous peritonitis**
   Tuberculous ascites

   A18.32   **Tuberculous enteritis**
   Tuberculosis of anus and rectum
   Tuberculosis of intestine (large) (small)

   A18.39   **Retroperitoneal tuberculosis**
   Tuberculosis of mesenteric glands
   Tuberculosis of retroperitoneal (lymph glands)

A18.4   **Tuberculosis of skin and subcutaneous tissue**
   Erythema induratum, tuberculous
   Lupus excedens
   Lupus vulgaris NOS
   Lupus vulgaris of eyelid
   *Cutaneous tuberculosis characterized by reddish brown
   plaque on skin surrounded by papules and nodules*
   Scrofuloderma
   *Type of cutaneous tuberculosis, with direct extension of
   tuberculosis into skin from underlying structures;
   AKA tuberculosis colliquativa*
   Tuberculosis of external ear
   > **Excludes2**   lupus erythematosus (L93.-)
   >   systemic lupus erythematosus (M32.-)

● **A18.5**   **Tuberculosis of eye**
   > **Excludes2**   lupus vulgaris of eyelid (A18.4)

   A18.50   **Tuberculosis of eye, unspecified**

   A18.51   **Tuberculous episcleritis**
   Inflammation of episclera and adjacent tissues

   A18.52   **Tuberculous keratitis**
   Tuberculous interstitial keratitis
   Tuberculous keratoconjunctivitis (interstitial)
   (phlyctenular)
   Inflammation of cornea and conjunctiva

   A18.53   **Tuberculous chorioretinitis**
   *Inflammation of choroid and retina;
   retinochoroiditis*

   A18.54   **Tuberculous iridocyclitis**
   Inflammation of iris and ciliary body

   A18.59   **Other tuberculosis of eye**
   Tuberculous conjunctivitis

A18.6   **Tuberculosis of (inner) (middle) ear**
   Tuberculous otitis media
   > **Excludes2**   tuberculosis of external ear (A18.4)
   >   tuberculous mastoiditis (A18.03)

A18.7   **Tuberculosis of adrenal glands**
   Tuberculous Addison's disease

● **A18.8**   **Tuberculosis of other specified organs**

   A18.81   **Tuberculosis of thyroid gland**

   A18.82   **Tuberculosis of other endocrine glands**
   Tuberculosis of pituitary gland
   Tuberculosis of thymus gland

   A18.83   **Tuberculosis of digestive tract organs, not elsewhere classified**
   > **Excludes1**   tuberculosis of intestine (A18.32)

   A18.84   **Tuberculosis of heart**
   Tuberculous cardiomyopathy
   Tuberculous endocarditis
   Tuberculous myocarditis
   Tuberculous pericarditis

   A18.85   **Tuberculosis of spleen**

   A18.89   **Tuberculosis of other sites**
   Tuberculosis of muscle
   Tuberculous cerebral arteritis

CHAPTER 1 (A00–B99)

Item 1–5 Miliary tuberculosis can be a life-threatening condition. If a tuberculous lesion enters a blood vessel, immense dissemination of tuberculous organisms can occur if the immune system is weak. High-risk populations—children under 4 years of age, the elderly, or the immunocompromised—are particularly prone to this type of infection. The lesions will have a millet seedlike appearance on chest x-ray. Bronchial washings and biopsy may aid in diagnosis.

● A19 Miliary tuberculosis

> **Includes** disseminated tuberculosis
> generalized tuberculosis
> tuberculous polyserositis

A19.0 Acute miliary tuberculosis of a single specified site

A19.1 Acute miliary tuberculosis of multiple sites

A19.2 Acute miliary tuberculosis, unspecified

A19.8 Other miliary tuberculosis

A19.9 Miliary tuberculosis, unspecified

CERTAIN ZOONOTIC BACTERIAL DISEASES (A20-A28)

● A20 Plague

> *Infectious disease caused by a Yersinia pestis bacterium, transmitted by a rodent flea bite or handling of infected animal*

> **Includes** infection due to Yersinia pestis

A20.0 Bubonic plague

A20.1 Cellulocutaneous plague
> *Skin and subcutaneous tissue plague*

A20.2 Pneumonic plague 🦠

A20.3 Plague meningitis

A20.7 Septicemic plague 🦠

A20.8 Other forms of plague
> Abortive plague
> Asymptomatic plague
> Pestis minor
> > *Systemic bacterial disease*

A20.9 Plague, unspecified

● A21 Tularemia

> *Caused by Francisella tularensis bacterium found in rodents, rabbits, and hares and transmitted to humans by contact with infected animal tissues or by ticks, biting flies, or mosquitoes*

> **Includes** deer-fly fever
> infection due to Francisella tularensis
> rabbit fever

Coding Clinic: 2016, Q4, P25

A21.0 Ulceroglandular tularemia
> *Most common form of tularemia in humans is painful, swollen, erythematous papule at point of inoculation that ruptures to form shallow ulcer*

A21.1 Oculoglandular tularemia
> *Primary site of entry is conjunctival sac, results in granulomatous corneal lesions*
> Ophthalmic tularemia

A21.2 Pulmonary tularemia 🦠

A21.3 Gastrointestinal tularemia
> Abdominal tularemia

A21.7 Generalized tularemia

A21.8 Other forms of tularemia

A21.9 Tularemia, unspecified

● A22 Anthrax

> *An acute infectious disease caused by the spore-forming Bacillus anthracis; occurs in humans exposed to infected animals or tissue from infected animals*

> **Includes** infection due to Bacillus anthracis

A22.0 Cutaneous anthrax
> Malignant carbuncle
> Malignant pustule

A22.1 Pulmonary anthrax 🦠
> Inhalation anthrax
> Ragpicker's disease
> Woolsorter's disease

A22.2 Gastrointestinal anthrax

A22.7 Anthrax sepsis 🦠
> *Infectious bacterial disease*

A22.8 Other forms of anthrax
> Anthrax meningitis

A22.9 Anthrax, unspecified

● A23 Brucellosis

> **Includes** Malta fever
> Mediterranean fever
> undulant fever

A23.0 Brucellosis due to Brucella melitensis
> *Resulting in flu-like symptoms that may lead to chronic symptoms that include recurrent fevers, joint pain, and fatigue*

A23.1 Brucellosis due to Brucella abortus
> *Most common cause of brucellosis in humans; AKA Bang bacillus*

A23.2 Brucellosis due to Brucella suis
> *Species found primarily in pigs, rabbits, and reindeer*

A23.3 Brucellosis due to Brucella canis
> *Species that causes respiratory tract infection in humans*

A23.8 Other brucellosis

A23.9 Brucellosis, unspecified

● A24 Glanders and melioidosis

> *Infection, usually of rodents, which spreads to other animals and humans, caused by Burkholderia pseudomallei through break in skin contaminated with infested soil or water*

A24.0 Glanders
> Infection due to Pseudomonas mallei
> Malleus

A24.1 Acute and fulminating melioidosis
> Melioidosis pneumonia
> Melioidosis sepsis

A24.2 Subacute and chronic melioidosis

A24.3 Other melioidosis

A24.9 Melioidosis, unspecified
> Infection due to Pseudomonas pseudomallei NOS
> Whitmore's disease

Item 1–6 Brucellosis: An infectious disease caused by the bacterium Brucella. Humans are infected by contact with contaminated animals or animal products. In humans brucellosis symptoms that are similar to the flu include fever, sweats, headaches, back pains, and physical weakness. Severe infections of the central nervous system or lining of the heart may occur. Brucellosis can also cause chronic symptoms that include recurrent fevers, joint pain, and fatigue.

▶ New ⟹ Revised ~~deleted~~ Deleted | Excludes 1 | Excludes 2 | Includes | Use additional | Code first | Code also | Key words

OGCR Official Guidelines X Assign placeholder X ● Use Additional Character(s) ▶ Manifestation Code 🦠 Hierarchical Condition Category **Coding Clinic**

● **A25 Rat-bite fevers**
RBF, infectious disease caused by Streptobacillus moniliformis or Spirillum minus.

  A25.0 Spirillosis
Any disease condition caused by spirilla
Sodoku

  A25.1 Streptobacillosis
Acute, febrile human illness caused by bacteria transmitted by rats in most cases, passed from rodent to human via rodent's urine or mucous secretions; AKA rat fever
Epidemic arthritic erythema
Haverhill fever
Streptobacillary rat-bite fever

  A25.9 Rat-bite fever, unspecified

● **A26 Erysipeloid**
Infection with Erysipelothrix rhusiopathiae, occurring often as occupational disease resulting from handling infected fish, shellfish, meat, or poultry

  A26.0 Cutaneous erysipeloid
Erythema migrans

  A26.7 Erysipelothrix sepsis 🐾

  A26.8 Other forms of erysipeloid

  A26.9 Erysipeloid, unspecified

● **A27 Leptospirosis**
Occurs most commonly in the tropics

  A27.0 Leptospirosis icterohemorrhagica
Leptospiral or spirochetal jaundice (hemorrhagic)
Weil's disease

  ● **A27.8 Other forms of leptospirosis**

    A27.81 Aseptic meningitis in leptospirosis

    A27.89 Other forms of leptospirosis

  A27.9 Leptospirosis, unspecified

● **A28 Other zoonotic bacterial diseases, not elsewhere classified**

  A28.0 Pasteurellosis
Infection of humans or other animals by species of Pasteurella

  A28.1 Cat-scratch disease
Cat-scratch fever

  A28.2 Extraintestinal yersiniosis
Infection from Yersinia enterocolitica; AKA enteric yersiniosis, intestinal yersiniosis, Yersinia enteritis

    Excludes1   enteritis due to Yersinia enterocolitica (A04.6)
                plague (A20.-)

  A28.8 Other specified zoonotic bacterial diseases, not elsewhere classified

  A28.9 Zoonotic bacterial disease, unspecified

OTHER BACTERIAL DISEASES (A30-A49)

● **A30 Leprosy [Hansen's disease]**
Chronic infectious disease attacking the skin, peripheral nerves, and mucous membranes

  Includes   infection due to Mycobacterium leprae

  Excludes1 sequelae of leprosy (B92)

  A30.0 Indeterminate leprosy
I leprosy

  A30.1 Tuberculoid leprosy
TT leprosy

  A30.2 Borderline tuberculoid leprosy
BT leprosy

  A30.3 Borderline leprosy
BB leprosy

  A30.4 Borderline lepromatous leprosy
BL leprosy

  A30.5 Lepromatous leprosy
LL leprosy

  A30.8 Other forms of leprosy

  A30.9 Leprosy, unspecified

● **A31 Infection due to other mycobacteria**

  Excludes2 leprosy (A30.-)
              tuberculosis (A15-A19)

  A31.0 Pulmonary mycobacterial infection 🐾
Infection due to Mycobacterium avium
Infection due to Mycobacterium intracellulare [Battey bacillus]
Infection due to Mycobacterium kansasii

  A31.1 Cutaneous mycobacterial infection
Buruli ulcer
Infection due to Mycobacterium marinum
Infection due to Mycobacterium ulcerans

  A31.2 Disseminated mycobacterium avium-intracellulare complex (DMAC) 🐾
MAC sepsis

  A31.8 Other mycobacterial infections

  A31.9 Mycobacterial infection, unspecified
Atypical mycobacterial infection NOS
Mycobacteriosis NOS

● **A32 Listeriosis**
Infection caused by Listeria monocytogenes

  Includes   listerial foodborne infection

  Excludes1 neonatal (disseminated) listeriosis (P37.2)

  A32.0 Cutaneous listeriosis

  ● **A32.1 Listerial meningitis and meningoencephalitis**

    A32.11 Listerial meningitis

    A32.12 Listerial meningoencephalitis

  A32.7 Listerial sepsis 🐾

  ● **A32.8 Other forms of listeriosis**

    A32.81 Oculoglandular listeriosis
Primary infection site is conjunctival sac, which if untreated may result in perforation of cornea and optic atrophy

    A32.82 Listerial endocarditis
Exudative and proliferative inflammatory condition of endocardium caused by listeria bacteria

    A32.89 Other forms of listeriosis
Listerial cerebral arteritis

  A32.9 Listeriosis, unspecified

A33 Tetanus neonatorum   N
Neonate = newborn

A34 Obstetrical tetanus ♀   M

A35 Other tetanus
Tetanus NOS

  Excludes1 tetanus neonatorum (A33)
             obstetrical tetanus (A34)

● **A36 Diphtheria**

  A36.0 Pharyngeal diphtheria
Diphtheritic membranous angina
Tonsillar diphtheria

  A36.1 Nasopharyngeal diphtheria

  A36.2 Laryngeal diphtheria
Diphtheritic laryngotracheitis

  A36.3 Cutaneous diphtheria

    Excludes2 erythrasma (L08.1)

Item 1-7 Diphtheria: A highly contagious bacterial disease that results in the formation of an adherent membrane in the throat that may lead to suffocation. In its most poisonous form, it attacks the heart and lungs. It is spread by direct physical contact or breathing the aerosolized secretions of infected individuals. The exact location is specified in the codes.

CHAPTER 1 (A00-B99)

CHAPTER 1 (A00-B99)

● **A36.8 Other diphtheria**

    A36.81 Diphtheritic cardiomyopathy
        Diphtheritic myocarditis

    A36.82 Diphtheritic radiculomyelitis

    A36.83 Diphtheritic polyneuritis

    A36.84 Diphtheritic tubulo-interstitial nephropathy

    A36.85 Diphtheritic cystitis

    A36.86 Diphtheritic conjunctivitis

    A36.89 Other diphtheritic complications
        Diphtheritic peritonitis

  A36.9 Diphtheria, unspecified

● **A37 Whooping cough**
    Pertussis is a highly contagious disease caused by the bacterium
    Bordetella pertussis and results in a whooping sounding cough.

  ● **A37.0 Whooping cough due to Bordetella pertussis**

    A37.00 Whooping cough due to Bordetella pertussis without pneumonia
      ▶Paroxysmal cough due to Bordetella pertussis without pneumonia

    A37.01 Whooping cough due to Bordetella pertussis with pneumonia
      ▶Paroxysmal cough due to Bordetella pertussis without pneumonia

  ● **A37.1 Whooping cough due to Bordetella parapertussis**

    A37.10 Whooping cough due to Bordetella parapertussis without pneumonia

    A37.11 Whooping cough due to Bordetella parapertussis with pneumonia

  ● **A37.8 Whooping cough due to other Bordetella species**

    A37.80 Whooping cough due to other Bordetella species without pneumonia

    A37.81 Whooping cough due to other Bordetella species with pneumonia

  ● **A37.9 Whooping cough, unspecified species**

    A37.90 Whooping cough, unspecified species without pneumonia

    A37.91 Whooping cough, unspecified species with pneumonia

● **A38 Scarlet fever**
    Most commonly caused by the bacteria Streptococcus pneumoniae and Neisseria meningitides

    Includes scarlatina
    Excludes2 streptococcal sore throat (J02.0)

  A38.0 Scarlet fever with otitis media

  A38.1 Scarlet fever with myocarditis

  A38.8 Scarlet fever with other complications

  A38.9 Scarlet fever, uncomplicated
    Scarlet fever, NOS

● **A39 Meningococcal infection**
    Most commonly caused by the bacteria Streptococcus pneumoniae and Neisseria meningitides

  A39.0 Meningococcal meningitis

  A39.1 Waterhouse-Friderichsen syndrome
    Fulminating complication of meningococcemia
    Meningococcal hemorrhagic adrenalitis
    Meningococcic adrenal syndrome

  A39.2 Acute meningococcemia

  A39.3 Chronic meningococcemia

  A39.4 Meningococcemia, unspecified

  ● **A39.5 Meningococcal heart disease**

    A39.50 Meningococcal carditis, unspecified

    A39.51 Meningococcal endocarditis

    A39.52 Meningococcal myocarditis

    A39.53 Meningococcal pericarditis

● **A39.8 Other meningococcal infections**

    A39.81 Meningococcal encephalitis

    A39.82 Meningococcal retrobulbar neuritis
      Optic neuritis in portion of optic nerve posterior to eyeball; AKA postocular optic neuritis

    A39.83 Meningococcal arthritis

    A39.84 Postmeningococcal arthritis

    A39.89 Other meningococcal infections
      Meningococcal conjunctivitis

  A39.9 Meningococcal infection, unspecified
    Meningococcal disease NOS

● **A40 Streptococcal sepsis**
    Code first
      postprocedural streptococcal sepsis (T81.44)
      streptococcal sepsis during labor (O75.3)
      streptococcal sepsis following abortion or ectopic or molar pregnancy (O03-O07, O08.0)
      streptococcal sepsis following immunization (T88.0)
      streptococcal sepsis following infusion, transfusion or therapeutic injection (T80.2-)

    Excludes1 neonatal (P36.0-P36.1)
        puerperal sepsis (O85)
        sepsis due to Streptococcus, group D (A41.81)

  A40.0 Sepsis due to streptococcus, group A

  A40.1 Sepsis due to streptococcus, group B
    Coding Clinic: 2019, Q1, P14

  A40.3 Sepsis due to Streptococcus pneumoniae
    Pneumococcal sepsis

  A40.8 Other streptococcal sepsis

  A40.9 Streptococcal sepsis, unspecified

● **A41 Other sepsis**
    Code first
      postprocedural sepsis (T81.44)
      sepsis during labor (O75.3)
      sepsis following abortion, ectopic or molar pregnancy (O03-O07, O08.0)
      sepsis following immunization (T88.0)
      sepsis following infusion, transfusion or therapeutic injection (T80.2-)

    Excludes1 bacteremia NOS (R78.81)
        neonatal (P36.-)
        puerperal sepsis (O85)
        streptococcal sepsis (A40.-)

    Excludes2 sepsis (due to) (in) actinomycotic (A42.7)
        sepsis (due to) (in) anthrax (A22.7)
        sepsis (due to) (in) candidal (B37.7)
        sepsis (due to) (in) Erysipelothrix (A26.7)
        sepsis (due to) (in) extraintestinal yersiniosis (A28.2)
        sepsis (due to) (in) gonococcal (A54.86)
        sepsis (due to) (in) herpesviral (B00.7)
        sepsis (due to) (in) listerial (A32.7)
        sepsis (due to) (in) melioidosis (A24.1)
        sepsis (due to) (in) meningococcal (A39.2-A39.4)
        sepsis (due to) (in) plague (A20.7)
        sepsis (due to) (in) tularemia (A21.7)
        toxic shock syndrome (A48.3)
    Coding Clinic: 2016, Q1, P39

  ● **A41.0 Sepsis due to Staphylococcus aureus**

    A41.01 Sepsis due to Methicillin susceptible Staphylococcus aureus
      MSSA sepsis
      Staphylococcus aureus sepsis NOS

    A41.02 Sepsis due to Methicillin resistant Staphylococcus aureus

▶ New ▥ Revised ~~deleted~~ Deleted Excludes 1 Excludes 2 Includes Use additional Code first Code also Key words

OGCR Official Guidelines X Assign placeholder X ● Use Additional Character(s) ▶ Manifestation Code Hierarchical Condition Category **Coding Clinic**

Item 1–8 **Gas gangrene** is a necrotizing subcutaneous infection that will cause tissue death. Patients with poor circulation (e.g., diabetes, peripheral nephropathy) will have low oxygen content in their tissues (hypoxia), which allows the Clostridium bacteria to flourish. Gas gangrene often occurs at the site of a surgical wound or trauma. Onset is sudden and dramatic. Treatment can include debridement, amputation, and/or hyperbaric oxygen treatments.

A41.1   **Sepsis due to other specified staphylococcus** 🦠
        Coagulase negative staphylococcus sepsis

A41.2   **Sepsis due to unspecified staphylococcus** 🦠

A41.3   **Sepsis due to Hemophilus influenzae** 🦠

A41.4   **Sepsis due to anaerobes** 🦠
        Excludes1   gas gangrene (A48.0)

● A41.5   **Sepsis due to other Gram-negative organisms**
        A41.50   **Gram-negative sepsis, unspecified** 🦠
                 Gram-negative sepsis NOS
        A41.51   **Sepsis due to Escherichia coli [E. coli]** 🦠
                 Coding Clinic: 2018, Q1, P16
        A41.52   **Sepsis due to Pseudomonas** 🦠
                 Pseudomonas aeroginosa
        A41.53   **Sepsis due to Serratia** 🦠
        A41.59   **Other Gram-negative sepsis** 🦠
                 Coding Clinic: 2019, Q1, P13

● A41.8   **Other specified sepsis**
        A41.81   **Sepsis due to Enterococcus** 🦠
        A41.89   **Other specified sepsis** 🦠
                 Coding Clinic: 2021, Q1, P33; 2016, Q3, P8-14

A41.9   **Sepsis, unspecified organism** 🦠
        Septicemia NOS
        Coding Clinic: 2018, Q4, P18

● A42   **Actinomycosis**
        Excludes1   actinomycetoma (B47.1)
        A42.0   **Pulmonary actinomycosis** 🦠
        A42.1   **Abdominal actinomycosis**
        A42.2   **Cervicofacial actinomycosis**
        A42.7   **Actinomycotic sepsis** 🦠
      ● A42.8   **Other forms of actinomycosis**
                A42.81   **Actinomycotic meningitis**
                A42.82   **Actinomycotic encephalitis**
                A42.89   **Other forms of actinomycosis**
        A42.9   **Actinomycosis, unspecified**

● A43   **Nocardiosis**
        A43.0   **Pulmonary nocardiosis** 🦠
        A43.1   **Cutaneous nocardiosis**
        A43.8   **Other forms of nocardiosis**
        A43.9   **Nocardiosis, unspecified**

● A44   **Bartonellosis**
        A44.0   **Systemic bartonellosis**
                Oroya fever
        A44.1   **Cutaneous and mucocutaneous bartonellosis**
                Verruga peruana
        A44.8   **Other forms of bartonellosis**
        A44.9   **Bartonellosis, unspecified**

  A46   **Erysipelas**
        Excludes1   postpartum or puerperal erysipelas (O86.89)

● A48   **Other bacterial diseases, not elsewhere classified**
        Excludes1   actinomycetoma (B47.1)
        A48.0   **Gas gangrene** 🦠
                Clostridial cellulitis
                Clostridial myonecrosis
                Coding Clinic: 2017, Q4, P102

A48.1   **Legionnaires' disease** 🦠
A48.2   **Nonpneumonic Legionnaires' disease [Pontiac fever]**
A48.3   **Toxic shock syndrome** 🦠
        Use additional code to identify the organism (B95, B96)
        Excludes1   endotoxic shock NOS (R57.8)
                        sepsis NOS (A41.9)

A48.4   **Brazilian purpuric fever**
        Systemic Hemophilus aegyptius infection

● A48.5   **Other specified botulism**
        Non-foodborne intoxication due to toxins of
          Clostridium botulinum [C. botulinum]
        Excludes1   food poisoning due to toxins of
                        Clostridium botulinum (A05.1)
        A48.51   **Infant botulism**   P
        A48.52   **Wound botulism**
                 Non-foodborne botulism NOS
                 Use additional code for associated wound

A48.8   **Other specified bacterial diseases**

● A49   **Bacterial infection of unspecified site**
        Excludes1   bacterial agents as the cause of diseases classified
                        elsewhere (B95-B96)
                        chlamydial infection NOS (A74.9)
                        meningococcal infection NOS (A39.9)
                        rickettsial infection NOS (A79.9)
                        spirochetal infection NOS (A69.9)
      ● A49.0   **Staphylococcal infection, unspecified site**
                A49.01   **Methicillin susceptible Staphylococcus aureus
                         infection, unspecified site**
                         Methicillin susceptible Staphylococcus aureus
                           (MSSA) infection
                         Staphylococcus aureus infection NOS
                A49.02   **Methicillin resistant Staphylococcus aureus
                         infection, unspecified site**
                         Methicillin resistant Staphylococcus aureus
                           (MRSA) infection
        A49.1   **Streptococcal infection, unspecified site**
        A49.2   **Hemophilus influenzae infection, unspecified site**
                 Any of seven bacterium of genus Haemophilus
        A49.3   **Mycoplasma infection, unspecified site**
                 *Bacterium of class Mollicutes, unusual group of bacteria
                 distinguished by absence of cell wall*
        A49.8   **Other bacterial infections of unspecified site**
        A49.9   **Bacterial infection, unspecified**
                 Excludes1   bacteremia NOS (R78.81)

INFECTIONS WITH A PREDOMINANTLY SEXUAL MODE OF TRANSMISSION (A50-A64)

        Excludes1   human immunodeficiency virus [HIV] disease
                        (B20)
                        nonspecific and nongonococcal urethritis (N34.1)
                        Reiter's disease (M02.3-)

● A50   **Congenital syphilis**
      ● A50.0   **Early congenital syphilis, symptomatic**
                Any congenital syphilitic condition specified as early or
                  manifest less than two years after birth
                A50.01   **Early congenital syphilitic oculopathy**
                A50.02   **Early congenital syphilitic osteochondropathy**
                A50.03   **Early congenital syphilitic pharyngitis**
                         Early congenital syphilitic laryngitis
                A50.04   **Early congenital syphilitic pneumonia**
                A50.05   **Early congenital syphilitic rhinitis**
                A50.06   **Early cutaneous congenital syphilis**
                A50.07   **Early mucocutaneous congenital syphilis**
                A50.08   **Early visceral congenital syphilis**
                A50.09   **Other early congenital syphilis, symptomatic**

CHAPTER 1 (A00-B99)

Figure 1-3 Chancre of primary syphilis. (From James WD, Berger TG, Elston DM: Andrews' Diseases of the Skin: Clinical Dermatology, Philadelphia, Saunders Elsevier, 2006)

Item 1–9 Syphilis, also known as lues, is the most serious of the venereal diseases caused by *Treponema pallidum*. The **primary** stage is characterized by an ulceration known as **chancre,** which usually appears on the genitals but can also develop on the anus, lips, tonsils, breasts, or fingers. Syphilis is easy to cure in its early stages. A single intramuscular injection of penicillin will usually cure a person who has had syphilis for less than a year.

The **secondary** stage is characterized by a rash that can affect any area of the body. **Latent** syphilis is divided into **early,** which is diagnosed within two years of infection, and **late,** which is diagnosed two years or more after infection. Additional doses of penicillin or another antibiotic are needed to treat someone who has had syphilis for longer than a year. For those allergic to penicillin, there are other antibiotic treatments. **Congenital** syphilis is also labeled **early** or **late** based on the time of diagnosis.

A50.1   **Early congenital syphilis, latent**
Congenital syphilis without clinical manifestations, with positive serological reaction and negative spinal fluid test, less than two years after birth

A50.2   **Early congenital syphilis, unspecified**
Congenital syphilis NOS less than two years after birth

● A50.3   **Late congenital syphilitic oculopathy**
Excludes1   Hutchinson's triad (A50.53)

A50.30   **Late congenital syphilitic oculopathy, unspecified**

A50.31   **Late congenital syphilitic interstitial keratitis**

A50.32   **Late congenital syphilitic chorioretinitis**

A50.39   **Other late congenital syphilitic oculopathy**

● A50.4   **Late congenital neurosyphilis [juvenile neurosyphilis]**
Use additional code to identify any associated mental disorder
Excludes1   Hutchinson's triad (A50.53)

A50.40   **Late congenital neurosyphilis, unspecified**
Juvenile neurosyphilis NOS

A50.41   **Late congenital syphilitic meningitis**

A50.42   **Late congenital syphilitic encephalitis**

A50.43   **Late congenital syphilitic polyneuropathy**

A50.44   **Late congenital syphilitic optic nerve atrophy**

A50.45   **Juvenile general paresis**
Dementia paralytica juvenilis
Juvenile tabetoparetic neurosyphilis

A50.49   **Other late congenital neurosyphilis**
Juvenile tabes dorsalis

● A50.5   **Other late congenital syphilis, symptomatic**
Any congenital syphilitic condition specified as late or manifest two years or more after birth

A50.51   **Clutton's joints**

A50.52   **Hutchinson's teeth**

A50.53   **Hutchinson's triad**

A50.54   **Late congenital cardiovascular syphilis**

A50.55   **Late congenital syphilitic arthropathy** 🅗

A50.56   **Late congenital syphilitic osteochondropathy**

A50.57   **Syphilitic saddle nose**

A50.59   **Other late congenital syphilis, symptomatic**

A50.6   **Late congenital syphilis, latent**
Congenital syphilis without clinical manifestations, with positive serological reaction and negative spinal fluid test, two years or more after birth.

A50.7   **Late congenital syphilis, unspecified**
Congenital syphilis NOS two years or more after birth.

A50.9   **Congenital syphilis, unspecified**

● A51   **Early syphilis**
A51.0   **Primary genital syphilis**
Syphilitic chancre NOS

A51.1   **Primary anal syphilis**

A51.2   **Primary syphilis of other sites**

● A51.3   **Secondary syphilis of skin and mucous membranes**

A51.31   **Condyloma latum**

A51.32   **Syphilitic alopecia**

A51.39   **Other secondary syphilis of skin**
Syphilitic leukoderma
Syphilitic mucous patch
Excludes1   late syphilitic leukoderma (A52.79)

● A51.4   **Other secondary syphilis**

A51.41   **Secondary syphilitic meningitis**

A51.42   **Secondary syphilitic female pelvic disease** ♀

A51.43   **Secondary syphilitic oculopathy**
Secondary syphilitic chorioretinitis
Secondary syphilitic iridocyclitis, iritis
Secondary syphilitic uveitis

A51.44   **Secondary syphilitic nephritis**

A51.45   **Secondary syphilitic hepatitis**

A51.46   **Secondary syphilitic osteopathy**

A51.49   **Other secondary syphilitic conditions**
Secondary syphilitic lymphadenopathy
Secondary syphilitic myositis

A51.5   **Early syphilis, latent**
Syphilis (acquired) without clinical manifestations, with positive serological reaction and negative spinal fluid test, less than two years after infection.

A51.9   **Early syphilis, unspecified**

● A52   **Late syphilis**
● A52.0   **Cardiovascular and cerebrovascular syphilis**

A52.00   **Cardiovascular syphilis, unspecified**

A52.01   **Syphilitic aneurysm of aorta**

A52.02   **Syphilitic aortitis**

A52.03   **Syphilitic endocarditis**
Syphilitic aortic valve incompetence or stenosis
Syphilitic mitral valve stenosis
Syphilitic pulmonary valve regurgitation

A52.04   **Syphilitic cerebral arteritis**

A52.05   **Other cerebrovascular syphilis**
Syphilitic cerebral aneurysm (ruptured) (non-ruptured)
Syphilitic cerebral thrombosis

A52.06   **Other syphilitic heart involvement**
Syphilitic coronary artery disease
Syphilitic myocarditis
Syphilitic pericarditis

A52.09   **Other cardiovascular syphilis**

● A52.1   **Symptomatic neurosyphilis**

A52.10   **Symptomatic neurosyphilis, unspecified**

A52.11   **Tabes dorsalis**
Cognitive decline with progressive degeneration of posterior columns, roots, and ganglia of spinal cord, occur 15-20 years after initial infection of syphilis; AKA Duchenne disease
Locomotor ataxia (progressive)
Tabetic neurosyphilis

A52.12   **Other cerebrospinal syphilis**

A52.13   **Late syphilitic meningitis**

A52.14   **Late syphilitic encephalitis**

A52.15   **Late syphilitic neuropathy**
Late syphilitic acoustic neuritis
Late syphilitic optic (nerve) atrophy
Late syphilitic polyneuropathy
Late syphilitic retrobulbar neuritis

▶ New   ⟹ Revised   d̶e̶l̶e̶t̶e̶d̶ Deleted   Excludes 1   Excludes 2   Includes   Use additional   Code first   Code also   Key words
OGCR Official Guidelines   X Assign placeholder X   ● Use Additional Character(s)   ▶ Manifestation Code   🅗 Hierarchical Condition Category   **Coding Clinic**

A52.16　Charcôt's arthropathy (tabetic)
Progressive musculoskeletal condition characterized by joint dislocation, fractures, and deformities, results in progressive destruction of bone and soft tissue of weight-bearing joints

A52.17　General paresis
Chronic meningoencephalitis results in loss of cortical function, or progressive dementia and generalized paralysis, occurring 10-20 years after initial infection of syphilis; AKA Bayle disease, dementia paralytica, paralytic dementiaparetic neurosyphilis, syphilitic meningoencephalitis
Dementia paralytica

A52.19　Other symptomatic neurosyphilis
Syphilitic parkinsonism

A52.2　Asymptomatic neurosyphilis

A52.3　Neurosyphilis, unspecified
Gumma (syphilitic)
Destructive lesions of syphilis
Syphilis (late)
Syphiloma
Coding Clinic: 2021, Q2, P6

A52.7　Other symptomatic late syphilis

A52.71　Late syphilitic oculopathy
Late syphilitic chorioretinitis
Late syphilitic episcleritis

A52.72　Syphilis of lung and bronchus

A52.73　Symptomatic late syphilis of other respiratory organs

A52.74　Syphilis of liver and other viscera
Late syphilitic peritonitis

A52.75　Syphilis of kidney and ureter
Syphilitic glomerular disease

A52.76　Other genitourinary symptomatic late syphilis ♀
Late syphilitic female pelvic inflammatory disease

A52.77　Syphilis of bone and joint

A52.78　Syphilis of other musculoskeletal tissue
Late syphilitic bursitis
Syphilis [stage unspecified] of bursa
Syphilis [stage unspecified] of muscle
Syphilis [stage unspecified] of synovium
Syphilis [stage unspecified] of tendon

A52.79　Other symptomatic late syphilis
Late syphilitic leukoderma
Syphilis of adrenal gland
Syphilis of pituitary gland
Syphilis of thyroid gland
Syphilitic splenomegaly
Excludes1　syphilitic leukoderma (secondary) (A51.39)

A52.8　Late syphilis, latent
Syphilis (acquired) without clinical manifestations, with positive serological reaction and negative spinal fluid test, two years or more after infection

A52.9　Late syphilis, unspecified

A53　Other and unspecified syphilis

A53.0　Latent syphilis, unspecified as early or late
Latent syphilis NOS
Positive serological reaction for syphilis

A53.9　Syphilis, unspecified
Infection due to Treponema pallidum NOS
Syphilis (acquired) NOS
Excludes1　syphilis NOS under two years of age (A50.2)

Item 1-10 An STD (sexually transmitted disease) caused by **Neisseria gonorrhoeae** that flourishes in the warm, moist areas of the reproductive tract. Untreated gonorrhea spreads to other parts of the body, causing inflammation of the testes or prostate or pelvic inflammatory disease (PID).

A54　Gonococcal infection

A54.0　Gonococcal infection of lower genitourinary tract without periurethral or accessory gland abscess
Excludes1　gonococcal infection with genitourinary gland abscess (A54.1)
gonococcal infection with periurethral abscess (A54.1)

A54.00　Gonococcal infection of lower genitourinary tract, unspecified

A54.01　Gonococcal cystitis and urethritis, unspecified

A54.02　Gonococcal vulvovaginitis, unspecified ♀

A54.03　Gonococcal cervicitis, unspecified ♀

A54.09　Other gonococcal infection of lower genitourinary tract

A54.1　Gonococcal infection of lower genitourinary tract with periurethral and accessory gland abscess
Gonococcal Bartholin's gland abscess

A54.2　Gonococcal pelviperitonitis and other gonococcal genitourinary infection

A54.21　Gonococcal infection of kidney and ureter

A54.22　Gonococcal prostatitis ♂

A54.23　Gonococcal infection of other male genital organs ♂
Gonococcal epididymitis
Gonococcal orchitis

A54.24　Gonococcal female pelvic inflammatory disease ♀
Gonococcal pelviperitonitis
Excludes1　gonococcal peritonitis (A54.85)

A54.29　Other gonococcal genitourinary infections

A54.3　Gonococcal infection of eye

A54.30　Gonococcal infection of eye, unspecified

A54.31　Gonococcal conjunctivitis
Form of bacterial conjunctivitis contracted by newborns during delivery; AKA neonatal conjunctivitis
Ophthalmia neonatorum due to gonococcus

A54.32　Gonococcal iridocyclitis
Inflammation of iris and of ciliary body due to gonococcal infection

A54.33　Gonococcal keratitis
Inflammation of cornea due to gonococcal infection; AKA keratoconjunctivitis, keratopathy

A54.39　Other gonococcal eye infection
Gonococcal endophthalmia

A54.4　Gonococcal infection of musculoskeletal system

A54.40　Gonococcal infection of musculoskeletal system, unspecified 🔗

A54.41　Gonococcal spondylopathy 🔗
Disorder of vertebrae due to gonococcal infection; AKA rachiopathy

A54.42　Gonococcal arthritis 🔗
Excludes2　gonococcal infection of spine (A54.41)

A54.43　Gonococcal osteomyelitis 🔗
Excludes2　gonococcal infection of spine (A54.41)

A54.49　Gonococcal infection of other musculoskeletal tissue 🔗
Gonococcal bursitis
Gonococcal myositis
Gonococcal synovitis
Gonococcal tenosynovitis

A54.5   Gonococcal pharyngitis

A54.6   Gonococcal infection of anus and rectum

● A54.8   Other gonococcal infections

     A54.81   Gonococcal meningitis

     A54.82   Gonococcal brain abscess

     A54.83   Gonococcal heart infection
            Gonococcal endocarditis
            Gonococcal myocarditis
            Gonococcal pericarditis

     A54.84   Gonococcal pneumonia ⬥

     A54.85   Gonococcal peritonitis ⬥

         Excludes1   gonococcal pelviperitonitis (A54.24)

     A54.86   Gonococcal sepsis ⬥

     A54.89   Other gonococcal infections
            Gonococcal keratoderma
            Gonococcal lymphadenitis

A54.9   Gonococcal infection, unspecified

A55   Chlamydial lymphogranuloma (venereum)
     Climatic or tropical bubo
     Durand-Nicolas-Favre disease
     Esthiomene
     Lymphogranuloma inguinale

● A56   Other sexually transmitted chlamydial diseases

     Includes   sexually transmitted diseases due to Chlamydia trachomatis

     Excludes1   neonatal chlamydial conjunctivitis (P39.1)
            neonatal chlamydial pneumonia (P23.1)

     Excludes2   chlamydial lymphogranuloma (A55)
            conditions classified to A74.-

 ● A56.0   Chlamydial infection of lower genitourinary tract

     A56.00   Chlamydial infection of lower genitourinary tract, unspecified

     A56.01   Chlamydial cystitis and urethritis

     A56.02   Chlamydial vulvovaginitis ♀

     A56.09   Other chlamydial infection of lower genitourinary tract
            Chlamydial cervicitis

 ● A56.1   Chlamydial infection of pelviperitoneum and other genitourinary organs

     A56.11   Chlamydial female pelvic inflammatory disease ♀

     A56.19   Other chlamydial genitourinary infection
            Chlamydial epididymitis
            Chlamydial orchitis

   A56.2   Chlamydial infection of genitourinary tract, unspecified

   A56.3   Chlamydial infection of anus and rectum

   A56.4   Chlamydial infection of pharynx

   A56.8   Sexually transmitted chlamydial infection of other sites

A57   Chancroid
     Ulcus molle
     Sexually transmitted infection caused by bacteria, Haemophilus ducreyi

A58   Granuloma inguinale
     Chronic, progressive, ulcerative granulomatous disease
     Donovanosis

● A59   Trichomoniasis

     Excludes2   intestinal trichomoniasis (A07.8)

     A common STD caused by a parasite, Trichomonas vaginalis

 ● A59.0   Urogenital trichomoniasis

     A59.00   Urogenital trichomoniasis, unspecified
            Fluor (vaginalis) due to Trichomonas
            Leukorrhea (vaginalis) due to Trichomonas

     A59.01   Trichomonal vulvovaginitis ♀

     A59.02   Trichomonal prostatitis ♂

     A59.03   Trichomonal cystitis and urethritis

     A59.09   Other urogenital trichomoniasis
            Common sexually transmitted disease (STD) caused by single-celled protozoan parasite; AKA trich
            Trichomonas cervicitis

   A59.8   Trichomoniasis of other sites

   A59.9   Trichomoniasis, unspecified

● A60   Anogenital herpesviral [herpes simplex] infections

 ● A60.0   Herpesviral infection of genitalia and urogenital tract

     A60.00   Herpesviral infection of urogenital system, unspecified

     A60.01   Herpesviral infection of penis ♂

     A60.02   Herpesviral infection of other male genital organs ♂

     A60.03   Herpesviral cervicitis ♀

     A60.04   Herpesviral vulvovaginitis ♀
            Herpesviral [herpes simplex] ulceration
            Herpesviral [herpes simplex] vaginitis
            Herpesviral [herpes simplex] vulvitis

     A60.09   Herpesviral infection of other urogenital tract
            Coding Clinic: 2020, Q1, P20

   A60.1   Herpesviral infection of perianal skin and rectum

   A60.9   Anogenital herpesviral infection, unspecified

● A63   Other predominantly sexually transmitted diseases, not elsewhere classified

     Excludes2   molluscum contagiosum (B08.1)
            papilloma of cervix (D26.0)

   A63.0   Anogenital (venereal) warts
     Anogenital warts due to (human) papillomavirus [HPV]
     Condyloma acuminatum

   A63.8   Other specified predominantly sexually transmitted diseases

A64   Unspecified sexually transmitted disease

OTHER SPIROCHETAL DISEASES (A65-A69)

     Excludes2   leptospirosis (A27.-)
            syphilis (A50-A53)

A65   Nonvenereal syphilis
     Bejel
     Endemic syphilis
     Njovera

● A66   Yaws
     Endemic, infectious, tropical disease caused by spirochete, spread by direct contact; AKA frambesia, framboesia, frambesia tropica

     Includes   bouba
            frambesia (tropica)
            pian

   A66.0   Initial lesions of yaws
     Chancre of yaws
     Frambesia, initial or primary
     Initial frambesial ulcer
     Mother yaw

   A66.1   Multiple papillomata and wet crab yaws
     Frambesioma
     Pianoma
     Plantar or palmar papilloma of yaws

   A66.2   Other early skin lesions of yaws
     Cutaneous yaws, less than five years after infection
     Early yaws (cutaneous)(macular)(maculopapular) (micropapular)(papular)
     Frambeside of early yaws

▶ New   ⇒ Revised   ~~deleted~~ Deleted   Excludes 1   Excludes 2   Includes   Use additional   Code first   Code also   Key words

OGCR Official Guidelines   X Assign placeholder X   ● Use Additional Character(s)   ▷ Manifestation Code   ⬥ Hierarchical Condition Category   **Coding Clinic**

A66.3 Hyperkeratosis of yaws
Hypertrophy of stratum corneum of skin in which there are small, hard, verrucous scales
Ghoul hand
Hyperkeratosis, palmar or plantar (early) (late) due to yaws
Worm-eaten soles

A66.4 Gummata and ulcers of yaws
Small, rubbery granuloma with necrotic center and inflamed characteristic of advanced stage of syphilis; AKA syphiloma
Gummatous frambeside
Nodular late yaws (ulcerated)

A66.5 Gangosa
Manifestation of yaws that develops in the soft palate and spreads eroding bone, cartilage, and soft tissue
Rhinopharyngitis mutilans

A66.6 Bone and joint lesions of yaws 🪲
Yaws ganglion
Yaws goundou
Yaws gumma, bone
Yaws gummatous osteitis or periostitis
Yaws hydrarthrosis
Yaws osteitis
Yaws periostitis (hypertrophic)

A66.7 Other manifestations of yaws
Juxta-articular nodules of yaws
Mucosal yaws

A66.8 Latent yaws
Yaws without clinical manifestations, with positive serology

A66.9 Yaws, unspecified

● **A67 Pinta [carate]**
Group of nonvenereal diseases caused by Treponema species

A67.0 Primary lesions of pinta
Chancre (primary) of pinta
Papule (primary) of pinta

A67.1 Intermediate lesions of pinta
Erythematous plaques of pinta
Hyperchromic lesions of pinta
Hyperkeratosis of pinta
Pintids

A67.2 Late lesions of pinta
Achromic skin lesions of pinta
Cicatricial skin lesions of pinta
Dyschromic skin lesions of pinta

A67.3 Mixed lesions of pinta
Achromic with hyperchromic skin lesions of pinta [carate]

A67.9 Pinta, unspecified

● **A68 Relapsing fevers**
Includes   recurrent fever
Excludes2 Lyme disease (A69.2-)

A68.0 Louse-borne relapsing fever
Relapsing fever due to Borrelia recurrentis

A68.1 Tick-borne relapsing fever
Relapsing fever due to any Borrelia species other than Borrelia recurrentis

A68.9 Relapsing fever, unspecified

Item 1-11 Cancrum oris, also known as **noma** or **gangrenous stomatitis,** begins as an ulcer of the gingiva and results in a progressive gangrenous process.

● **A69 Other spirochetal infections**

A69.0 Necrotizing ulcerative stomatitis
Cancrum oris
Fusospirochetal gangrene
Noma
Stomatitis gangrenosa

A69.1 Other Vincent's infections
Fusospirochetal pharyngitis
Necrotizing ulcerative (acute) gingivitis
Necrotizing ulcerative (acute) gingivostomatitis
Spirochetal stomatitis
Trench mouth
Vincent's angina
Vincent's gingivitis

● **A69.2 Lyme disease**
Erythema chronicum migrans due to Borrelia burgdorferi

A69.20 Lyme disease, unspecified

A69.21 Meningitis due to Lyme disease

A69.22 Other neurologic disorders in Lyme disease
Cranial neuritis
Meningoencephalitis
Polyneuropathy

A69.23 Arthritis due to Lyme disease 🪲

A69.29 Other conditions associated with Lyme disease
Myopericarditis due to Lyme disease
Coding Clinic: 2016, Q3, P12

A69.8 Other specified spirochetal infections

A69.9 Spirochetal infection, unspecified

OTHER DISEASES CAUSED BY CHLAMYDIAE (A70-A74)

Excludes1 sexually transmitted chlamydial diseases (A55-A56)

A70 Chlamydia psittaci infections
Ornithosis
Parrot fever
Psittacosis

● **A71 Trachoma**
Excludes1 sequelae of trachoma (B94.0)

A71.0 Initial stage of trachoma
Trachoma dubium

A71.1 Active stage of trachoma
Granular conjunctivitis (trachomatous)
Trachomatous follicular conjunctivitis
Trachomatous pannus

A71.9 Trachoma, unspecified

● **A74 Other diseases caused by chlamydiae**
Excludes1 neonatal chlamydial conjunctivitis (P39.1)
neonatal chlamydial pneumonia (P23.1)
Reiter's disease (M02.3-)
sexually transmitted chlamydial diseases (A55-A56)

Excludes2 chlamydial pneumonia (J16.0)

A74.0 Chlamydial conjunctivitis
Paratrachoma

● **A74.8 Other chlamydial diseases**

A74.81 Chlamydial peritonitis

A74.89 Other chlamydial diseases

A74.9 Chlamydial infection, unspecified
Chlamydiosis NOS

CHAPTER 1 (A00-B99)

Item 1–12 **Rickettsioses** are diseases spread from ticks, lice, fleas, or mites to humans.

Typhus is spread to humans chiefly by the fleas of rats.

Endemic identifies a disease as being present in low numbers of humans at all times, whereas **epidemic** identifies a disease as being present in high numbers of humans at a specific time. Morbidity (death) is higher in epidemic diseases.

Brill's disease, also known as **Brill-Zinsser disease,** is spread from human to human by body lice and also from the lice of flying squirrels. **Scrub typhus** is spread in the same ways as Brill's disease.

Malaria is spread to humans by mosquitoes.

RICKETTSIOSES (A75-A79)

● **A75　Typhus fever**
　　Excludes1　rickettsiosis due to Ehrlichia sennetsu (A79.81)

　　A75.0　Epidemic louse-borne typhus fever due to Rickettsia prowazekii
　　　　Organisms transmitted between humans via louse
　　　　Classical typhus (fever)
　　　　Epidemic (louse-borne) typhus

　　A75.1　Recrudescent typhus [Brill's disease]
　　　　Brill-Zinsser disease

　　A75.2　Typhus fever due to Rickettsia typhi
　　　　Murine (flea-borne) typhus

　　A75.3　Typhus fever due to Rickettsia tsutsugamushi
　　　　Scrub (mite-borne) typhus
　　　　Tsutsugamushi fever
　　　　Typhus fever due to Orientia Tsutsugamushi (scrub typhus)

　　A75.9　Typhus fever, unspecified
　　　　Typhus (fever) NOS

● **A77　Spotted fever [tick-borne rickettsioses]**

　　A77.0　Spotted fever due to Rickettsia rickettsii
　　　　Rocky Mountain spotted fever
　　　　Sao Paulo fever

　　A77.1　Spotted fever due to Rickettsia conorii
　　　　African tick typhus
　　　　Boutonneuse fever
　　　　India tick typhus
　　　　Kenya tick typhus
　　　　Marseilles fever
　　　　Mediterranean tick fever

　　A77.2　Spotted fever due to Rickettsia siberica
　　　　North Asian tick fever
　　　　Siberian tick typhus

　　A77.3　Spotted fever due to Rickettsia australis
　　　　Queensland tick typhus

　● **A77.4　Ehrlichiosis**
　　　　Type of tick-borne fever caused by bacteria infection
　　　　Excludes1　~~Rickettsiosis due to Ehrlichia sennetsu (A79.81)~~
　　　　　▶anaplasmosis [A. phagocytophilum] (A79.82)
　　　　　▶rickettsiosis due to Ehrlichia sennetsu (A79.81)
　　　　A77.40　Ehrlichiosis, unspecified
　　　　A77.41　Ehrlichiosis chafeensis [E. chafeensis]
　　　　A77.49　Other ehrlichiosis
　　　　　　Ehrlichiosis due to E. ewingii
　　　　　　Ehrlichiosis due to E. muris euclairensis

　　A77.8　Other spotted fevers
　　　　Rickettsia 364D/R. philipii (Pacific Coast tick fever)
　　　　Spotted fever due to Rickettsia africae (African tick bite fever)
　　　　Spotted fever due to Rickettsia parkeri]

　　A77.9　Spotted fever, unspecified
　　　　Tick-borne typhus NOS

A78　Q fever
　　Infection due to Coxiella burnetii
　　Nine Mile fever
　　Quadrilateral fever

● **A79　Other rickettsioses**

　　A79.0　Trench fever
　　　　Quintan fever
　　　　Wolhynian fever

　　A79.1　Rickettsialpox due to Rickettsia akari
　　　　Kew Garden fever
　　　　Vesicular rickettsiosis

　● **A79.8　Other specified rickettsioses**
　　　　A79.81　Rickettsiosis due to Ehrlichia sennetsu
　　　　　　Rickettsiosis due to Neorickettsia sennetsu
　　　　▶**A79.82　Anaplasmosis [A. phagocytophilum]**
　　　　　　▶Transfusion transmitted A. phagocytophilum
　　　　A79.89　Other specified rickettsioses

　　A79.9　Rickettsiosis, unspecified
　　　　Rickettsial infection NOS

VIRAL AND PRION INFECTIONS OF THE CENTRAL NERVOUS SYSTEM (A80-A89)

　　Excludes1　postpolio syndrome (G14)
　　　　　　sequelae of poliomyelitis (B91)
　　　　　　sequelae of viral encephalitis (B94.1)

● **A80　Acute poliomyelitis**
　　▶**Excludes1**　acute flaccid myelitis (G04.82)
　　A80.0　Acute paralytic poliomyelitis, vaccine-associated
　　A80.1　Acute paralytic poliomyelitis, wild virus, imported
　　A80.2　Acute paralytic poliomyelitis, wild virus, indigenous
　● **A80.3　Acute paralytic poliomyelitis, other and unspecified**
　　　　A80.30　Acute paralytic poliomyelitis, unspecified
　　　　A80.39　Other acute paralytic poliomyelitis
　　A80.4　Acute nonparalytic poliomyelitis
　　A80.9　Acute poliomyelitis, unspecified

● **A81　Atypical virus infections of central nervous system**
　　Includes　diseases of the central nervous system caused by prions
　　Use additional code to identify:
　　　dementia with behavioral disturbance (F02.81)
　　　dementia without behavioral disturbance (F02.80)
　● **A81.0　Creutzfeldt-Jakob disease**
　　　　A81.00　Creutzfeldt-Jakob disease, unspecified
　　　　　　Jakob-Creutzfeldt disease, unspecified
　　　　A81.01　Variant Creutzfeldt-Jakob disease
　　　　　　vCJD
　　　　A81.09　Other Creutzfeldt-Jakob disease
　　　　　　CJD
　　　　　　Familial Creutzfeldt-Jakob disease
　　　　　　Iatrogenic Creutzfeldt-Jakob disease
　　　　　　Sporadic Creutzfeldt-Jakob disease
　　　　　　Subacute spongiform encephalopathy (with dementia)
　　A81.1　Subacute sclerosing panencephalitis
　　　　Type of viral encephalitis that causes parenchymatous lesions in gray and white matter of brain
　　　　Dawson's inclusion body encephalitis
　　　　Van Bogaert's sclerosing leukoencephalopathy
　　A81.2　Progressive multifocal leukoencephalopathy
　　　　Group of diseases affecting white matter of brain
　　　　Multifocal leukoencephalopathy NOS

Item 1-13　Acute Poliomyelitis: Also called infantile paralysis and is caused by the poliovirus, which enters the body orally and infects the intestinal wall and then enters the blood stream and central nervous system, causing muscle weakness and paralysis. This disease has been nearly eradicated with the polio vaccine.

▶ New　　⇒ Revised　　~~deleted~~ Deleted　　Excludes 1　　Excludes 2　　Includes　　Use additional　　Code first　　Code also　　Key words

OGCR Official Guidelines　　X Assign placeholder X　　● Use Additional Character(s)　　▶ Manifestation Code　　🅗 Hierarchical Condition Category　　**Coding Clinic**

● A81.8 **Other atypical virus infections of central nervous system**

　　A81.81 **Kuru**

　　A81.82 **Gerstmann-Sträussler-Scheinker syndrome**
　　　　　　GSS syndrome

　　A81.83 **Fatal familial insomnia**
　　　　　　FFI

　　A81.89 **Other atypical virus infections of central nervous system**

● A81.9 **Atypical virus infection of central nervous system, unspecified**
　　　　Prion diseases of the central nervous system NOS

● **A82 Rabies**
　　Viral disease affecting the central nervous system and transmitted from infected mammals to man

　A82.0 **Sylvatic rabies**

　A82.1 **Urban rabies**

　A82.9 **Rabies, unspecified**

● **A83 Mosquito-borne viral encephalitis**
　　Inflammation of the brain caused most commonly by Herpes Simplex virus

　　Includes   mosquito-borne viral meningoencephalitis
　　Excludes2   Venezuelan equine encephalitis (A92.2)
　　　　　　　　West Nile fever (A92.3-)
　　　　　　　　West Nile virus (A92.3-)

　A83.0 **Japanese encephalitis**

　A83.1 **Western equine encephalitis**

　A83.2 **Eastern equine encephalitis**

　A83.3 **St. Louis encephalitis**

　A83.4 **Australian encephalitis**
　　　　Kunjin virus disease

　A83.5 **California encephalitis**
　　　　California meningoencephalitis
　　　　La Crosse encephalitis

　A83.6 **Rocio virus disease**
　　　　Mosquito-borne virus

　A83.8 **Other mosquito-borne viral encephalitis**

　A83.9 **Mosquito-borne viral encephalitis, unspecified**

● **A84 Tick-borne viral encephalitis**
　　Includes   tick-borne viral meningoencephalitis

　A84.0 **Far Eastern tick-borne encephalitis [Russian spring-summer encephalitis]**

　A84.1 **Central European tick-borne encephalitis**

　A84.8 **Other tick-borne viral encephalitis**

　　A84.81 **Powassan virus disease**

　　A84.89 **Other tick-borne viral encephalitis**
　　　　　　Louping ill
　　　　　　Code first, if applicable, transfusion related infection (T80.22-)

　A84.9 **Tick-borne viral encephalitis, unspecified**

● **A85 Other viral encephalitis, not elsewhere classified**

　　Includes   specified viral encephalomyelitis NEC
　　　　　　　　specified viral meningoencephalitis NEC
　　Excludes1   benign myalgic encephalomyelitis (G93.3)
　　　　　　　　encephalitis due to cytomegalovirus (B25.8)
　　　　　　　　encephalitis due to herpesvirus NEC (B10.0-)
　　　　　　　　encephalitis due to herpesvirus [herpes simplex] (B00.4)
　　　　　　　　encephalitis due to measles virus (B05.0)
　　　　　　　　encephalitis due to mumps virus (B26.2)
　　　　　　　　encephalitis due to poliomyelitis virus (A80.-)
　　　　　　　　encephalitis due to zoster (B02.0)
　　　　　　　　lymphocytic choriomeningitis (A87.2)

　A85.0 **Enteroviral encephalitis**
　　　　Enteroviral encephalomyelitis

　A85.1 **Adenoviral encephalitis**
　　　　Adenoviral meningoencephalitis

　A85.2 **Arthropod-borne viral encephalitis, unspecified**
　　　　Excludes1   West nile virus with encephalitis (A92.31)

　A85.8 **Other specified viral encephalitis**
　　　　Encephalitis lethargica
　　　　Von Economo-Cruchet disease

● **A86 Unspecified viral encephalitis**
　　Viral encephalomyelitis NOS
　　Viral meningoencephalitis NOS

● **A87 Viral meningitis**
　　Excludes1   meningitis due to herpesvirus [herpes simplex] (B00.3)
　　　　　　　　meningitis due to measles virus (B05.1)
　　　　　　　　meningitis due to mumps virus (B26.1)
　　　　　　　　meningitis due to poliomyelitis virus (A80.-)
　　　　　　　　meningitis due to zoster (B02.1)

　A87.0 **Enteroviral meningitis**
　　　　Group of common viruses responsible for the majority of viral meningitis
　　　　Coxsackievirus meningitis
　　　　Echovirus meningitis

　A87.1 **Adenoviral meningitis**

　A87.2 **Lymphocytic choriomeningitis**
　　　　Lymphocytic meningoencephalitis

　A87.8 **Other viral meningitis**

　A87.9 **Viral meningitis, unspecified**

● **A88 Other viral infections of central nervous system, not elsewhere classified**
　　Excludes1   viral encephalitis NOS (A86)
　　　　　　　　viral meningitis NOS (A87.9)

　A88.0 **Enteroviral exanthematous fever [Boston exanthem]**
　　　　Infectious skin eruption

　A88.1 **Epidemic vertigo**

　A88.8 **Other specified viral infections of central nervous system**

　A89 **Unspecified viral infection of central nervous system**

OGCR Section I. C.1.f.

Certain Infectious and Parasitic Diseases (A00-B99)

Zika virus infections

Code only confirmed cases

Code only a confirmed diagnosis of Zika virus (A92.5, Zika virus disease) as documented by the provider. This is an exception to the hospital inpatient guideline Section II, H.

In this context, "confirmation" does not require documentation of the type of test performed; the physician's diagnostic statement that the condition is confirmed is sufficient. This code should be assigned regardless of the stated mode of transmission.

If the provider documents "suspected", "possible" or "probable" Zika, do not assign code A92.5. Assign a code(s) explaining the reason for encounter (such as fever, rash, or joint pain) or Z20.828, Contact with and (suspected) exposure to other viral communicable diseases.

Item 1-14 Encephalitis is an inflammation of the brain most often caused by a virus but may also be caused by a bacteria and most commonly transmitted by a mosquito. **Myelitis** is an inflammation of the spinal cord that may disrupt CNS function. Untreated myelitis may rapidly lead to permanent damage to the spinal cord. **Encephalomyelitis** is a general term for an inflammation of the brain and spinal cord.

CHAPTER 1 (A00-B99)

CHAPTER 1 (A00-B99)

ARTHROPOD-BORNE VIRAL FEVERS AND VIRAL HEMORRHAGIC FEVERS (A90-A99)

A90   Dengue fever [classical dengue]
Acute, self-limited disease, characterized by fever, prostration, severe muscle pains, headache, rash, lymphadenopathy, and leukopenia, caused by dengue virus; AKA breakbone, dandy

     Excludes1   dengue hemorrhagic fever (A91)

     Coding Clinic: 2016, Q3, P13

A91   Dengue hemorrhagic fever
Serious follow-up to regular dengue, with symptoms of hemorrhage

● **A92   Other mosquito-borne viral fevers**

     Excludes1   Ross River disease (B33.1)

   A92.0   Chikungunya virus disease
Transmitted by mosquitoes
Chikungunya (hemorrhagic) fever

   A92.1   O'nyong-nyong fever
Acute, nonfatal febrile disease transmitted by mosquitoes, which clinically resembles dengue and chikungunya

   A92.2   Venezuelan equine fever
Venezuelan equine encephalitis
Venezuelan equine encephalomyelitis virus disease

  ● **A92.3   West Nile virus infection**
West Nile fever

      A92.30   West Nile virus infection, unspecified
West Nile fever NOS
West Nile fever without complications
West Nile virus NOS

      A92.31   West Nile virus infection with encephalitis
West Nile encephalitis
West Nile encephalomyelitis
Coding Clinic: 2016, Q3, P13

      A92.32   West Nile virus infection with other neurologic manifestation
Use additional code to specify the neurologic manifestation

      A92.39   West Nile virus infection with other complications
Use additional code to specify the other conditions

   A92.4   Rift Valley fever

   A92.5   Zika virus disease
Zika virus fever
Zika virus infection
Zika NOS

     Excludes1   congenital Zika virus disease (P35.4)

     Coding Clinic: 2016, Q4, P4-7, 121

   A92.8   Other specified mosquito-borne viral fevers

   A92.9   Mosquito-borne viral fever, unspecified

● **A93   Other arthropod-borne viral fevers, not elsewhere classified**

   A93.0   Oropouche virus disease
Tropical viral infection
Oropouche fever

   A93.1   Sandfly fever
Pappataci fever
Phlebotomus fever

   A93.2   Colorado tick fever

   A93.8   Other specified arthropod-borne viral fevers
Piry virus disease
Vesicular stomatitis virus disease [Indiana fever]

A94   Unspecified arthropod-borne viral fever
Arboviral fever NOS
Arbovirus infection NOS

● **A95   Yellow fever**
Acute infectious disease transmitted by mosquitoes

   A95.0   Sylvatic yellow fever
Jungle yellow fever

   A95.1   Urban yellow fever

   A95.9   Yellow fever, unspecified

● **A96   Arenaviral hemorrhagic fever**
Virus that causes various hemorrhagic fevers

   A96.0   Junin hemorrhagic fever
Argentinian hemorrhagic fever

   A96.1   Machupo hemorrhagic fever
Transmitted by contact with infected rodents
Bolivian hemorrhagic fever

   A96.2   Lassa fever
Acute type of hemorrhagic fever caused by contact with disease carrying mouse or person

   A96.8   Other arenaviral hemorrhagic fevers

   A96.9   Arenaviral hemorrhagic fever, unspecified

● **A98   Other viral hemorrhagic fevers, not elsewhere classified**

     Excludes1   chikungunya hemorrhagic fever (A92.0)
dengue hemorrhagic fever (A91)

   A98.0   Crimean-Congo hemorrhagic fever
Virus transmitted by ticks and contact with blood, secretions, or fluids from infected humans or animals
Central Asian hemorrhagic fever

   A98.1   Omsk hemorrhagic fever
Transmitted to humans by bites of infected ticks or contact with infected muskrats

   A98.2   Kyasanur Forest disease
Transmitted via infected monkeys, voles, ticks

   A98.3   Marburg virus disease
Rare, acute, often fatal type of hemorrhagic fever

   A98.4   Ebola virus disease

   A98.5   Hemorrhagic fever with renal syndrome
Epidemic hemorrhagic fever
Korean hemorrhagic fever
Russian hemorrhagic fever
Hantaan virus disease
Hantavirus disease with renal manifestations
Nephropathia epidemica
Songo fever

     Excludes1   hantavirus (cardio)-pulmonary syndrome (B33.4)

   A98.8   Other specified viral hemorrhagic fevers

A99   Unspecified viral hemorrhagic fever

VIRAL INFECTIONS CHARACTERIZED BY SKIN AND MUCOUS MEMBRANE LESIONS (B00-B09)

● **B00   Herpesviral [herpes simplex] infections**

     Excludes1   congenital herpesviral infections (P35.2)
     Excludes2   anogenital herpesviral infection (A60.-)
gammaherpesviral mononucleosis (B27.0-)
herpangina (B08.5)

   B00.0   Eczema herpeticum
Cutaneous eruption caused by herpes simplex virus (HSV) type 1, HSV-2, coxsackievirus A16, or vaccinia virus
Kaposi's varicelliform eruption

   B00.1   Herpesviral vesicular dermatitis
Vesicle formation; characteristics include formation of blisters and scabs on feet and legs
Herpes simplex facialis
Herpes simplex labialis
Herpes simplex otitis externa
Vesicular dermatitis of ear
Vesicular dermatitis of lip

Figure 1-4 Primary herpes simplex in and around the mouth. The infection is usually acquired from siblings or parents and is readily transmitted to other direct contacts. (Getty Image)

Item 1-15   Herpes is a viral disease for which there is no cure. There are two types of the herpes simplex virus: **Type I** causes **cold sores** or **fever blisters,** and **Type II** causes **genital herpes.** The virus can be spread from a sore on the lips to the genitals or from the genitals to the lips.

▶ New   ⇒ Revised   ~~deleted~~ Deleted   Excludes 1   Excludes 2   Includes   Use additional   Code first   Code also   Key words

   OGCR Official Guidelines   X Assign placeholder X   ● Use Additional Character(s)   ▶ Manifestation Code   🐾 Hierarchical Condition Category   **Coding Clinic**

B00.2   Herpesviral gingivostomatitis and pharyngotonsillitis
Inflammation involving both gingivae and oral mucosa
Herpesviral pharyngitis
Inflammation of pharynx and tonsils; AKA tonsillopharyngitis

B00.3   Herpesviral meningitis

B00.4   Herpesviral encephalitis
Herpesviral meningoencephalitis
Simian B disease

> **Excludes1**   herpesviral encephalitis due to herpesvirus 6 and 7 (B10.01, B10.09)
> non-simplex herpesviral encephalitis (B10.0-)

● **B00.5   Herpesviral ocular disease**

　B00.50   Herpesviral ocular disease, unspecified

　B00.51   Herpesviral iridocyclitis
　Herpesviral iritis
　Herpesviral uveitis, anterior

　B00.52   Herpesviral keratitis
　Herpesviral keratoconjunctivitis

　B00.53   Herpesviral conjunctivitis

　B00.59   Other herpesviral disease of eye
　Herpesviral dermatitis of eyelid

B00.7   Disseminated herpesviral disease
Herpesviral sepsis

● **B00.8   Other forms of herpesviral infections**

　B00.81   Herpesviral hepatitis

　B00.82   Herpes simplex myelitis

　B00.89   Other herpesviral infection
　Herpesviral whitlow

B00.9   Herpesviral infection, unspecified
Herpes simplex infection NOS

● **B01   Varicella [chickenpox]**
Very contagious disease caused by the varicella zoster virus that results in an itchy outbreak of skin blisters (varicella). The same virus causes shingles (zoster).

B01.0   Varicella meningitis

● **B01.1   Varicella encephalitis, myelitis and encephalomyelitis**
Postchickenpox encephalitis, myelitis and encephalomyelitis

　B01.11   Varicella encephalitis and encephalomyelitis
　Postchickenpox encephalitis and encephalomyelitis

　B01.12   Varicella myelitis
　Postchickenpox myelitis

B01.2   Varicella pneumonia

● **B01.8   Varicella with other complications**

　B01.81   Varicella keratitis

　B01.89   Other varicella complications

B01.9   Varicella without complication
Varicella NOS

● **B02   Zoster [herpes zoster]**

> **Includes**   shingles
> zona

B02.0   Zoster encephalitis
Zoster meningoencephalitis

B02.1   Zoster meningitis

● **B02.2   Zoster with other nervous system involvement**
Coding Clinic: 2019, Q1, P18

　B02.21   Postherpetic geniculate ganglionitis

　B02.22   Postherpetic trigeminal neuralgia

　B02.23   Postherpetic polyneuropathy

Item 1-16 Zoster: Also known as ***shingles*** and is caused by the same virus as chickenpox. After exposure, the virus lies dormant in nerve tissue and is activated by factors including aging, stress, suppression of the immune system, and certain medication. It begins as a unilateral rash that leads to blisters and sores on the skin. It may involve the nerve pathways of the eye, forehead, nose, and eyelids and may be very painful with long-term systemic effects.

Figure 1-5 Photograph of eyelids with marginal blepharitis. (From Hoyt CS, Taylor D: Pediatric Ophthalmology and Strabismus, London, Elsevier Saunders, 2005)

Item 1–17 Blepharitis is a common condition in which the eyelid is swollen and yellow scaling and conjunctivitis develop. Usually the hair on the scalp and brow is involved.

　B02.24   Postherpetic myelitis
　Herpes zoster myelitis

　B02.29   Other postherpetic nervous system involvement
　Postherpetic radiculopathy

● **B02.3   Zoster ocular disease**

　B02.30   Zoster ocular disease, unspecified

　B02.31   Zoster conjunctivitis

　B02.32   Zoster iridocyclitis

　B02.33   Zoster keratitis
　Herpes zoster keratoconjunctivitis

　B02.34   Zoster scleritis

　B02.39   Other herpes zoster eye disease
　Zoster blepharitis

B02.7   Disseminated zoster

B02.8   Zoster with other complications
Herpes zoster otitis externa

B02.9   Zoster without complications
Zoster NOS

B03   Smallpox

> **Note:** In 1980 the 33rd World Health Assembly declared that smallpox had been eradicated. The classification is maintained for surveillance purposes.

B04   Monkeypox
Disease occurring in captive monkeys and other mammals that may be transmitted to humans, clinically similar to smallpox

● **B05   Measles**

> **Includes**   morbilli
> **Excludes1**   subacute sclerosing panencephalitis (A81.1)

B05.0   Measles complicated by encephalitis
Postmeasles encephalitis

B05.1   Measles complicated by meningitis
Postmeasles meningitis

B05.2   Measles complicated by pneumonia
Postmeasles pneumonia

B05.3   Measles complicated by otitis media
Postmeasles otitis media

B05.4   Measles with intestinal complications

● **B05.8   Measles with other complications**

　B05.81   Measles keratitis and keratoconjunctivitis

　B05.89   Other measles complications

B05.9   Measles without complication
Measles NOS

● **B06   Rubella [German measles]**

> **Excludes1**   congenital rubella (P35.0)

● **B06.0   Rubella with neurological complications**

　B06.00   Rubella with neurological complication, unspecified

　B06.01   Rubella encephalitis
　Rubella meningoencephalitis

　B06.02   Rubella meningitis

　B06.09   Other neurological complications of rubella

● **B06.8   Rubella with other complications**

　B06.81   Rubella pneumonia

　B06.82   Rubella arthritis

　B06.89   Other rubella complications

B06.9   Rubella without complication
Rubella NOS

● **B07   Viral warts**

     Includes   verruca simplex
                    verruca vulgaris
                    viral warts due to human papillomavirus

     Excludes2   anogenital (venereal) warts (A63.0)
                     papilloma of bladder (D41.4)
                     papilloma of cervix (D26.0)
                     papilloma larynx (D14.1)

   B07.0   Plantar wart
         Verruca plantaris

   B07.8   Other viral warts
         Common wart
         Flat wart
         Verruca plana

   B07.9   Viral wart, unspecified

● **B08   Other viral infections characterized by skin and mucous membrane lesions, not elsewhere classified**

     Excludes1   vesicular stomatitis virus disease (A93.8)

 ● **B08.0   Other orthopoxvirus infections**

       Excludes2   monkeypox (B04)

     ● **B08.01   Cowpox and vaccinia not from vaccine**

         B08.010   Cowpox

         B08.011   Vaccinia not from vaccine

              Excludes1   vaccinia (from
                           vaccination)
                           (generalized) (T88.1)

     B08.02   Orf virus disease
           Contagious pustular dermatitis
           Ecthyma contagiosum

     B08.03   Pseudocowpox [milker's node]

     B08.04   Paravaccinia, unspecified

     B08.09   Other orthopoxvirus infections
           Orthopoxvirus infection NOS

   B08.1   Molluscum contagiosum
       Various skin diseases characterized by soft, rounded, cutaneous lesions

 ● **B08.2   Exanthema subitum [sixth disease] Roseola infantum**
       Acute, short-lived high fever in infants and young children followed by a rash mainly on the trunk, caused by human herpesvirus 6

     B08.20   Exanthema subitum [sixth disease], unspecified Roseola infantum, unspecified   P

     B08.21   Exanthema subitum [sixth disease] due to human herpesvirus 6 Roseola infantum due to human herpesvirus 6   P
            Virus results in sudden rash; infection results in lifelong persistence

     B08.22   Exanthema subitum [sixth disease] due to human herpesvirus 7 Roseola infantum due to human herpesvirus 7   P

   B08.3   Erythema infectiosum [fifth disease]
       Moderately contagious, epidemic disease in children caused by B19 virus; onset of rash that begins as redness of cheeks, later there is rash on trunk and limbs; when this fades, there may be central clearing that leaves lacelike pattern

   B08.4   Enteroviral vesicular stomatitis with exanthem
       Hand, foot and mouth disease
       Check your documentation—this code is HAND, foot, and mouth disease. Code B08.8 is foot and mouth disease.

   B08.5   Enteroviral vesicular pharyngitis
       Herpangina

 ● **B08.6   Parapoxvirus infections**

     B08.60   Parapoxvirus infection, unspecified

     B08.61   Bovine stomatitis

     B08.62   Sealpox

     B08.69   Other parapoxvirus infections

 ● **B08.7   Yatapoxvirus infections**

     B08.70   Yatapoxvirus infection, unspecified

     B08.71   Tanapox virus disease

     B08.72   Yaba pox virus disease
           Yaba monkey tumor disease

     B08.79   Other yatapoxvirus infections

   B08.8   Other specified viral infections characterized by skin and mucous membrane lesions
       Enteroviral lymphonodular pharyngitis
       Foot-and-mouth disease
         Check your documentation. Code B08.4 is for HAND, foot, and mouth disease.
       Poxvirus NEC

B09   Unspecified viral infection characterized by skin and mucous membrane lesions
       Viral enanthema NOS
       Viral exanthema NOS

OTHER HUMAN HERPESVIRUSES (B10)

● **B10   Other human herpesviruses**

     Excludes2   cytomegalovirus (B25.9)
                  Epstein-Barr virus (B27.0-)
                  herpes NOS (B00.9)
                  herpes simplex (B00.-)
                  herpes zoster (B02.-)
                  human herpesvirus NOS (B00.-)
                  human herpesvirus 1 and 2 (B00.-)
                  human herpesvirus 3 (B01.-, B02.-)
                  human herpesvirus 4 (B27.0-)
                  human herpesvirus 5 (B25.-)
                  varicella (B01.-)
                  zoster (B02.-)

 ● **B10.0   Other human herpesvirus encephalitis**

       Excludes2   herpes encephalitis NOS (B00.4)
                    herpes simplex encephalitis (B00.4)
                    human herpesvirus encephalitis (B00.4)
                    simian B herpes virus encephalitis (B00.4)

     B10.01   Human herpesvirus 6 encephalitis
           Sudden rash or roseola

     B10.09   Other human herpesvirus encephalitis
           Human herpesvirus 7 encephalitis
           Virus closely related to human herpesvirus 6, but not known to cause any disease

 ● **B10.8   Other human herpesvirus infection**

     B10.81   Human herpesvirus 6 infection
           Causative agent of exanthema subitum that results in sudden rash

     B10.82   Human herpesvirus 7 infection
           Closely related to human herpesvirus 6, but not known cause any disease

     B10.89   Other human herpesvirus infection
           Human herpesvirus 8 infection
           May be the cause of Kaposi sarcoma, a malignant tumor
           Kaposi's sarcoma-associated herpesvirus infection

Figure 1-6   Hepatitis B viral infection. **A.** Liver parenchyma showing hepatocytes with diffuse granular cytoplasm, so-called ground glass hepatocytes (H&E). **B.** Immunoperoxidase stains from the same case, showing cytoplasmic inclusions of viral particles. (From Kumar: Robbins and Cotran: Pathologic Basis of Disease, ed 8, Saunders, An Imprint of Elsevier, 2009)

CHAPTER 1 (A00-B99)

▶ New   ⇒ Revised   ~~deleted~~ Deleted   Excludes 1   Excludes 2   Includes   Use additional   Code first   Code also   Key words

OGCR Official Guidelines   X Assign placeholder X   ● Use Additional Character(s)   ▶ Manifestation Code   🏷 Hierarchical Condition Category   **Coding Clinic**

Item 1–18 Hepatitis A (HAV) was formerly called epidemic, infectious, short-incubation, or acute catarrhal jaundice hepatitis. The primary transmission mode is the oral–fecal route. **Hepatitis B (HBV)** was formerly called long-incubation period, serum, or homologous serum hepatitis. Transmission modes are through blood from infected persons and from body fluids of infected mother to neonate. **Hepatitis C (HCV),** caused by the hepatitis C virus, is primarily transfusion associated. **Hepatitis D (HDV),** also called delta hepatitis, is caused by the hepatitis D virus in patients formerly or currently infected with hepatitis B. **Hepatitis E (HEV)** is also called enterically transmitted non-A, non-B hepatitis. The primary transmission mode is the oral–fecal route, usually through contaminated water.

VIRAL HEPATITIS (B15-B19)

Excludes1	sequelae of viral hepatitis (B94.2)
Excludes2	cytomegaloviral hepatitis (B25.1)
	herpesviral [herpes simplex] hepatitis (B00.81)

● **B15   Acute hepatitis A**
  B15.0   Hepatitis A with hepatic coma
  B15.9   Hepatitis A without hepatic coma
      Hepatitis A (acute) (viral) NOS

● **B16   Acute hepatitis B**
  B16.0   Acute hepatitis B with delta-agent with hepatic coma
  B16.1   Acute hepatitis B with delta-agent without hepatic coma
  B16.2   Acute hepatitis B without delta-agent with hepatic coma
  B16.9   Acute hepatitis B without delta-agent and without hepatic coma
      Hepatitis B (acute) (viral) NOS
      Coding Clinic: 2016, Q3, P13

● **B17   Other acute viral hepatitis**
  B17.0   Acute delta-(super) infection of hepatitis B carrier
  ● **B17.1   Acute hepatitis C**
      B17.10   Acute hepatitis C without hepatic coma
          Acute hepatitis C NOS
      B17.11   Acute hepatitis C with hepatic coma
  B17.2   Acute hepatitis E
  B17.8   Other specified acute viral hepatitis
      Hepatitis non-A non-B (acute) (viral) NEC
  B17.9   Acute viral hepatitis, unspecified
      Acute hepatitis NOS
      Acute infectious hepatitis NOS

● **B18   Chronic viral hepatitis**
Includes	Carrier of viral hepatitis
  B18.0   Chronic viral hepatitis B with delta-agent 🔊
  B18.1   Chronic viral hepatitis B without delta-agent 🔊
      Carrier of viral hepatitis B
      Chronic (viral) hepatitis B
  B18.2   Chronic viral hepatitis C 🔊
      Carrier of viral hepatitis C
      Coding Clinic: 2018, Q1, P4; 2017, Q1, P41
  B18.8   Other chronic viral hepatitis 🔊
      Carrier of other viral hepatitis
  B18.9   Chronic viral hepatitis, unspecified 🔊
      Carrier of unspecified viral hepatitis

● **B19   Unspecified viral hepatitis**
  B19.0   Unspecified viral hepatitis with hepatic coma
  ● **B19.1   Unspecified viral hepatitis B**
      B19.10   Unspecified viral hepatitis B without hepatic coma
          Unspecified viral hepatitis B NOS
      B19.11   Unspecified viral hepatitis B with hepatic coma
  ● **B19.2   Unspecified viral hepatitis C**
      B19.20   Unspecified viral hepatitis C without hepatic coma
          Viral hepatitis C NOS
      B19.21   Unspecified viral hepatitis C with hepatic coma
  B19.9   Unspecified viral hepatitis without hepatic coma
      Viral hepatitis NOS

Figure 1-7 Kaposi's sarcoma. There are large confluent hyperpigmented patch-stage lesions with lymphedema. (From Kanski, JJ: Clinical Diagnosis in Ophthalmology, London, Elsevier Mosby, 2006)

Item 1–19 AIDS (acquired immune deficiency syndrome) is caused by **HIV** (human immunodeficiency virus). HIV affects certain white blood cells (T-4 lymphocytes) and destroys the ability of the cells to fight infections, making patients susceptible to a host of infectious diseases (e.g., ***Pneumocystis carinii pneumonia [PCP], Kaposi's sarcoma,*** and ***lymphoma***). ***AIDS-related complex (ARC)*** is an early stage of AIDS in which tests for HIV are positive but the symptoms are mild.

OGCR Section I. C.1.a.

Certain Infectious and Parasitic Diseases (A00-B99)
a. Human Immunodeficiency Virus (HIV) Infections
  1) Code only confirmed cases
      Code only confirmed cases of HIV infection illness. This is an exception to the hospital inpatient guideline Section II, H.
      In this context, "confirmation" does not require documentation of positive serology or culture for HIV; the provider's diagnostic statement that the patient is HIV positive or has an HIV-related illness is sufficient.

HUMAN IMMUNODEFICIENCY VIRUS [HIV] DISEASE (B20)

B20   Human immunodeficiency virus [HIV] disease 🔊
Includes	acquired immune deficiency syndrome [AIDS]
	AIDS-related complex [ARC]
	HIV infection, symptomatic

  Code first Human immunodeficiency virus [HIV] disease complicating pregnancy, childbirth and the puerperium, if applicable (O98.7-)

  Use additional code(s) to identify all manifestations of HIV infection

Excludes1	asymptomatic human immunodeficiency virus [HIV] infection status (Z21)
	exposure to HIV virus (Z20.6)
	inconclusive serologic evidence of HIV (R75)

  Coding Clinic: 2021, Q2, P6; 2019, Q1, P9-11

OTHER VIRAL DISEASES (B25-B34)

● **B25   Cytomegaloviral disease**
  AKA: HCMV or Human Herpesvirus 5 (HHV-5)
Excludes1	congenital cytomegalovirus infection (P35.1)
	cytomegaloviral mononucleosis (B27.1-)

  B25.0   Cytomegaloviral pneumonitis 🔊
  B25.1   Cytomegaloviral hepatitis 🔊
  B25.2   Cytomegaloviral pancreatitis 🔊
  B25.8   Other cytomegaloviral diseases 🔊
      Cytomegaloviral encephalitis
  B25.9   Cytomegaloviral disease, unspecified 🔊

● **B26   Mumps**
Includes	epidemic parotitis
	infectious parotitis
  Acute, contagious, viral disease
  B26.0   Mumps orchitis ♂
  B26.1   Mumps meningitis
  B26.2   Mumps encephalitis
  B26.3   Mumps pancreatitis

● B26.8 Mumps with other complications
    B26.81   Mumps hepatitis
    B26.82   Mumps myocarditis
    B26.83   Mumps nephritis
    B26.84   Mumps polyneuropathy
    B26.85   Mumps arthritis 🪙
    B26.89   Other mumps complications
  B26.9 Mumps without complication
           Mumps NOS
           Mumps parotitis NOS

● B27 Infectious mononucleosis
       Includes   glandular fever
                      monocytic angina
                      Pfeiffer's disease
● B27.0 Gammaherpesviral mononucleosis
         AKA: Pfeiffer's disease, infective mononucleosis
         Mononucleosis due to Epstein-Barr virus
    B27.00   Gammaherpesviral mononucleosis without
              complication
              Infective mononucleosis
    B27.01   Gammaherpesviral mononucleosis with
              polyneuropathy
    B27.02   Gammaherpesviral mononucleosis with
              meningitis
    B27.09   Gammaherpesviral mononucleosis with other
              complications
              Hepatomegaly in gammaherpesviral
                mononucleosis
● B27.1 Cytomegaloviral mononucleosis
         Infectious disease resembling infectious mononucleosis
    B27.10   Cytomegaloviral mononucleosis without
              complications
    B27.11   Cytomegaloviral mononucleosis with
              polyneuropathy
    B27.12   Cytomegaloviral mononucleosis with
              meningitis
    B27.19   Cytomegaloviral mononucleosis with other
              complication
              Hepatomegaly in cytomegaloviral
                mononucleosis
● B27.8 Other infectious mononucleosis
    B27.80   Other infectious mononucleosis without
              complication
    B27.81   Other infectious mononucleosis with
              polyneuropathy
    B27.82   Other infectious mononucleosis with
              meningitis
    B27.89   Other infectious mononucleosis with other
              complication
              Hepatomegaly in other infectious
                mononucleosis
● B27.9 Infectious mononucleosis, unspecified
    B27.90   Infectious mononucleosis, unspecified without
              complication
    B27.91   Infectious mononucleosis, unspecified with
              polyneuropathy
    B27.92   Infectious mononucleosis, unspecified with
              meningitis
    B27.99   Infectious mononucleosis, unspecified with
              other complication
              Hepatomegaly in unspecified infectious
                mononucleosis

● B30 Viral conjunctivitis
       Excludes1   herpesviral [herpes simplex] ocular disease
                       (B00.5)
                       ocular zoster (B02.3)
    B30.0   Keratoconjunctivitis due to adenovirus
             Epidemic keratoconjunctivitis
             Shipyard eye
    B30.1   Conjunctivitis due to adenovirus
             Acute adenoviral follicular conjunctivitis
             Swimming-pool conjunctivitis
    B30.2   Viral pharyngoconjunctivitis
    B30.3   Acute epidemic hemorrhagic conjunctivitis (enteroviral)
             Conjunctivitis due to coxsackievirus 24
             Conjunctivitis due to enterovirus 70
             Hemorrhagic conjunctivitis (acute)(epidemic)
    B30.8   Other viral conjunctivitis
             Newcastle conjunctivitis
    B30.9   Viral conjunctivitis, unspecified

● B33 Other viral diseases, not elsewhere classified
    B33.0   Epidemic myalgia
             Acute infectious disease, caused by group A coxsackie viruses
             or other enteroviruses with symptoms that include
             sudden pain in chest or upper abdomen with fever
             Bornholm disease
    B33.1   Ross River disease
             Epidemic polyarthritis and exanthema
             Ross River fever
● B33.2   Viral carditis
             Coxsackie (virus) carditis
    B33.20   Viral carditis, unspecified
    B33.21   Viral endocarditis
    B33.22   Viral myocarditis
    B33.23   Viral pericarditis
    B33.24   Viral cardiomyopathy 🪙
    B33.3   Retrovirus infections, not elsewhere classified
             Retrovirus infection NOS
    B33.4   Hantavirus (cardio)-pulmonary syndrome [HPS] [HCPS]
             Hantavirus disease with pulmonary manifestations
             Sin nombre virus disease
             Use additional code to identify any associated acute
                kidney failure (N17.9)
             Excludes1   hantavirus disease with renal
                             manifestations (A98.5)
                             hemorrhagic fever with renal
                             manifestations (A98.5)
    B33.8   Other specified viral diseases
             Excludes1   anogenital human papillomavirus
                             infection (A63.0)
                             viral warts due to human papillomavirus
                             infection (B07)

● B34 Viral infection of unspecified site
       Excludes1   anogenital human papillomavirus infection
                       (A63.0)
                       cytomegaloviral disease NOS (B25.9)
                       herpesvirus [herpes simplex] infection NOS
                       (B00.9)
                       retrovirus infection NOS (B33.3)
                       viral agents as the cause of diseases classified
                       elsewhere (B97.-)
                       viral warts due to human papillomavirus
                       infection (B07)
    B34.0   Adenovirus infection, unspecified
    B34.1   Enterovirus infection, unspecified
             Intestinal tract infection
             Coxsackievirus infection NOS
             Echovirus infection NOS
    B34.2   Coronavirus infection, unspecified
             Excludes1   COVID-19 (U07.1)
                             pneumonia due to SARS-associated
                             coronavirus (J12.81)

B34.3   Parvovirus infection, unspecified
B34.4   Papovavirus infection, unspecified
B34.8   Other viral infections of unspecified site
B34.9   Viral infection, unspecified
     Viremia NOS
     Coding Clinic: 2016, Q3, P10

MYCOSES (B35-B49)

Excludes2	hypersensitivity pneumonitis due to organic dust (J67.-)
	mycosis fungoides (C84.0-)

● **B35   Dermatophytosis**
    AKA tinea or ringworm

Includes	favus
	infections due to species of Epidermophyton, Micro-sporum and Trichophyton
	tinea, any type except those in B36.-

B35.0   **Tinea barbae and tinea capitis**
    Beard ringworm
    Kerion
    Scalp ringworm
    Sycosis, mycotic

B35.1   **Tinea unguium**
    White patches or pits on surface or edges of nails, followed by infection under nail plate
    Dermatophytic onychia
    Dermatophytosis of nail
    Onychomycosis
    Ringworm of nails

B35.2   **Tinea manuum**
    Tinea of hands
    Dermatophytosis of hand
    Hand ringworm

B35.3   **Tinea pedis**
    Tinea affecting feet
    Athlete's foot
    Dermatophytosis of foot
    Foot ringworm

B35.4   **Tinea corporis**
    Infecting skin areas other than hands
    Ringworm of the body

B35.5   **Tinea imbricata**
    Chronic tropical tinea corporis; AKA Oriental ringworm, tinea inguinalis, tinea cruris
    Tokelau

B35.6   **Tinea cruris**
    In groin or perineal area, spreading to adjacent regions; AKA jock itch, eczema marginatum, ringworm of groin, or tinea inguinalis
    Dhobi itch
    Groin ringworm
    Jock itch

B35.8   **Other dermatophytoses**
    Disseminated dermatophytosis
    Granulomatous dermatophytosis

B35.9   **Dermatophytosis, unspecified**
    Ringworm NOS

● **B36   Other superficial mycoses**
B36.0   **Pityriasis versicolor**
    Common, chronic, symptomless disorder that includes macular patches of various sizes and shapes; AKA liver spots
    Tinea flava
    Tinea versicolor

B36.1   **Tinea nigra**
    Minor fungal infection, with dark lesions, usually on skin of hands
    Keratomycosis nigricans palmaris
    Microsporosis nigra
    Pityriasis nigra

Figure 1-8 Oral candidiasis (thrush). (From James WD, Berger T, Elston D: Andrews' Diseases of the Skin: Clinical Dermatology, 11e, Saunders, 2011)

Item 1–20 Candidiasis, also called oidiomycosis or moniliasis, is a fungal infection. It most often appears on moist cutaneous areas of the body but can also be responsible for a variety of systemic infections such as endocarditis, meningitis, arthritis, and myositis. Antifungal medications cure most yeast infections.

B36.2   **White piedra**
    White to light brown nodules on hair of beard, axilla, or groin; AKA trichosporosis
    Tinea blanca

B36.3   **Black piedra**
    Characterized by small black or brown nodules on shafts of scalp hair

B36.8   **Other specified superficial mycoses**
B36.9   **Superficial mycosis, unspecified**

● **B37   Candidiasis**

Includes	candidosis
	moniliasis

Excludes1	neonatal candidiasis (P37.5)

B37.0   **Candidal stomatitis**
    Oral thrush

B37.1   **Pulmonary candidiasis** 🔗
    Candidal bronchitis
    Candidal pneumonia

B37.2   **Candidiasis of skin and nail**
    Candidal onychia
    Candidal paronychia

Excludes2	diaper dermatitis (L22)

B37.3   **Candidiasis of vulva and vagina** ♀
    Candidal vulvovaginitis
    Monilial vulvovaginitis
    Vaginal thrush

● **B37.4   Candidiasis of other urogenital sites**
    B37.41   **Candidal cystitis and urethritis**
    B37.42   **Candidal balanitis** ♂
        Male condition only
    B37.49   **Other urogenital candidiasis**
        Candidal pyelonephritis

B37.5   **Candidal meningitis**
B37.6   **Candidal endocarditis**
B37.7   **Candidal sepsis** 🔗
    Disseminated candidiasis systemic candidiasis

● **B37.8   Candidiasis of other sites**
    B37.81   **Candidal esophagitis** 🔗
    B37.82   **Candidal enteritis**
        Candidal proctitis
    B37.83   **Candidal cheilitis**
        Inflammation affecting lip
    B37.84   **Candidal otitis externa**
        Inflammation of external auditory canal
    B37.89   **Other sites of candidiasis**
        Infection manifested by invasive candidiasis
        Candidal osteomyelitis

B37.9   **Candidiasis, unspecified**
    Thrush NOS

CHAPTER 1 (A00-B99)

Item 1–21 Bird and bat droppings that fall into the soil give rise to a fungus that can spread airborne spores. When inhaled into the lungs, these spores divide and multiply into lesions. Histoplasmosis capsulatum takes three forms: primary (lodged in the lungs only), chronic (resembles TB), and disseminated (infection has moved to other organs). This is an opportunistic infection in immunosuppressed patients.

● **B38   Coccidioidomycosis**
   Fungal disease; AKA coccidioidosis, coccidioidal granuloma, Posadas, or Posadas-Wernicke disease

   B38.0   Acute pulmonary coccidioidomycosis 🦠
   B38.1   Chronic pulmonary coccidioidomycosis 🦠
   B38.2   Pulmonary coccidioidomycosis, unspecified 🦠
   B38.3   Cutaneous coccidioidomycosis
   B38.4   Coccidioidomycosis meningitis
   B38.7   Disseminated coccidioidomycosis
            Generalized coccidioidomycosis
   ● B38.8   Other forms of coccidioidomycosis
            B38.81   Prostatic coccidioidomycosis ♂
            B38.89   Other forms of coccidioidomycosis
   B38.9   Coccidioidomycosis, unspecified

● **B39   Histoplasmosis**
   Infection resulting from inhalation or ingestion of spores; AKA Darling disease

   Code first associated AIDS (B20)

   Use additional code for any associated manifestations, such as:
            endocarditis (I39)
            meningitis (G02)
            pericarditis (I32)
            retinitis (H32)

   B39.0   Acute pulmonary histoplasmosis capsulati 🦠
   B39.1   Chronic pulmonary histoplasmosis capsulati 🦠
   B39.2   Pulmonary histoplasmosis capsulati, unspecified 🦠
   B39.3   Disseminated histoplasmosis capsulati
            Generalized histoplasmosis capsulati
   B39.4   Histoplasmosis capsulati, unspecified
            American histoplasmosis
   B39.5   Histoplasmosis duboisii
            African histoplasmosis
   B39.9   Histoplasmosis, unspecified

● **B40   Blastomycosis**
   Rare and potentially fatal infection caused by inhaling fungus found in moist soil in temperate climates.

   Excludes1   Brazilian blastomycosis (B41.-)
                  keloidal blastomycosis (B48.0)
   B40.0   Acute pulmonary blastomycosis 🦠
   B40.1   Chronic pulmonary blastomycosis 🦠
   B40.2   Pulmonary blastomycosis, unspecified 🦠
   B40.3   Cutaneous blastomycosis
   B40.7   Disseminated blastomycosis
            Generalized blastomycosis
   ● B40.8   Other forms of blastomycosis
            B40.81   Blastomycotic meningoencephalitis
                     Meningomyelitis due to blastomycosis
            B40.89   Other forms of blastomycosis
   B40.9   Blastomycosis, unspecified

● **B41   Paracoccidioidomycosis**
   Fungal infection usually chronic that begins in lungs, spreads to mucocutaneous areas which may extend to skin, tonsils, gastrointestinal lymphatics, liver, and spleen; AKA Almeida or Lutz-Splendore-Almeida disease, Brazilian or South American blastomycosis, or paracoccidioidal granuloma

   Includes   Brazilian blastomycosis
                  Lutz' disease
   B41.0   Pulmonary paracoccidioidomycosis 🦠
   B41.7   Disseminated paracoccidioidomycosis
            Generalized paracoccidioidomycosis

   B41.8   Other forms of paracoccidioidomycosis
   B41.9   Paracoccidioidomycosis, unspecified

● **B42   Sporotrichosis**
   Chronic fungal infection with nodular lesions
   B42.0   Pulmonary sporotrichosis
   B42.1   Lymphocutaneous sporotrichosis
   B42.7   Disseminated sporotrichosis
            Generalized sporotrichosis
   ● B42.8   Other forms of sporotrichosis
            B42.81   Cerebral sporotrichosis
                     Meningitis due to sporotrichosis
            B42.82   Sporotrichosis arthritis 🦠
            B42.89   Other forms of sporotrichosis
   B42.9   Sporotrichosis, unspecified

● **B43   Chromomycosis and pheomycotic abscess**
   Chronic fungal infection of skin, initiated at site of puncture affecting lower limb or foot (mossy foot)
   B43.0   Cutaneous chromomycosis
            Dermatitis verrucosa
   B43.1   Pheomycotic brain abscess
            Cerebral chromomycosis
   B43.2   Subcutaneous pheomycotic abscess and cyst
   B43.8   Other forms of chromomycosis
   B43.9   Chromomycosis, unspecified

● **B44   Aspergillosis**
   Infection marked by inflammatory lesions in skin, ear, orbit, nasal sinuses, lungs, and occasionally bones and meninges
   Includes   aspergilloma
   B44.0   Invasive pulmonary aspergillosis 🦠
   B44.1   Other pulmonary aspergillosis 🦠
   B44.2   Tonsillar aspergillosis 🦠
   B44.7   Disseminated aspergillosis 🦠
            Generalized aspergillosis
   ● B44.8   Other forms of aspergillosis
            B44.81   Allergic bronchopulmonary aspergillosis 🦠
            B44.89   Other forms of aspergillosis 🦠
   B44.9   Aspergillosis, unspecified 🦠

● **B45   Cryptococcosis**
   Infection in the immunocompromised and fatal if left untreated; AKA torulosis, Buschke, or Busse-Buschke disease
   B45.0   Pulmonary cryptococcosis 🦠
   B45.1   Cerebral cryptococcosis 🦠
            Cryptococcal meningitis
            Cryptococcosis meningocerebralis
   B45.2   Cutaneous cryptococcosis 🦠
   B45.3   Osseous cryptococcosis 🦠
   B45.7   Disseminated cryptococcosis 🦠
            Generalized cryptococcosis
   B45.8   Other forms of cryptococcosis 🦠
   B45.9   Cryptococcosis, unspecified 🦠

● **B46   Zygomycosis**
   Fungal infections including subcutaneous lesions and infection of sinuses, brain, or lungs
   B46.0   Pulmonary mucormycosis 🦠
            Fungal infection affecting lung
   B46.1   Rhinocerebral mucormycosis 🦠
   B46.2   Gastrointestinal mucormycosis 🦠
   B46.3   Cutaneous mucormycosis 🦠
            Subcutaneous mucormycosis
   B46.4   Disseminated mucormycosis 🦠
            Generalized mucormycosis
   B46.5   Mucormycosis, unspecified 🦠
   B46.8   Other zygomycoses
            Entomophthoromycosis
   B46.9   Zygomycosis, unspecified 🦠
            Phycomycosis NOS

▶ New   ⇒ Revised   ~~deleted~~ Deleted   Excludes 1   Excludes 2   Includes   Use additional   Code first   Code also   Key words

OGCR Official Guidelines   X Assign placeholder X   ● Use Additional Character(s)   ⟩ Manifestation Code   🦠 Hierarchical Condition Category   **Coding Clinic**

● **B47** **Mycetoma**
Slow progressive, destructive fungal infection of cutaneous and subcutaneous tissues, fascia, and bone, primarily seen in foot (Madura foot) or leg

    B47.0 **Eumycetoma**
        Madura foot, mycotic Maduromycosis

    B47.1 **Actinomycetoma**

    B47.9 **Mycetoma, unspecified**
        Madura foot NOS

● **B48** **Other mycoses, not elsewhere classified**

    B48.0 **Lobomycosis**
        Infection with symptoms of red, smooth, hard cutaneous nodules resembling keloids
        Keloidal blastomycosis
        Lobo's disease

    B48.1 **Rhinosporidiosis**
        Chronic, localized granulomatous fungal infection, affecting mucocutaneous tissues, usually of nose characterized by polyps, papillomas, and wartlike lesions

    B48.2 **Allescheriasis**
        Fungal infection
        Infection due to Pseudallescheria boydii
        Excludes1   eumycetoma (B47.0)

    B48.3 **Geotrichosis**
        Fungal infection usually of bronchi, lungs, mouth, or intestinal tract
        Geotrichum stomatitis

    B48.4 **Penicillosis** 🔖
        Fungal infection
        Talaromycosis

    B48.8 **Other specified mycoses** 🔖
        Adiaspiromycosis
        Infection of tissue and organs by Alternaria
        Infection of tissue and organs by Drechslera
        Infection of tissue and organs by Fusarium
        Infection of tissue and organs by saprophytic fungi NEC

  B49 **Unspecified mycosis**
        Fungemia NOS

PROTOZOAL DISEASES (B50-B64)

    Excludes1   amebiasis (A06.-)
            other protozoal intestinal diseases (A07.-)

● **B50** **Plasmodium falciparum malaria**
Severe form of malaria that can be fatal

    Includes   mixed infections of Plasmodium falciparum with any other Plasmodium species

    B50.0 **Plasmodium falciparum malaria with cerebral complications**
        Cerebral malaria NOS

    B50.8 **Other severe and complicated Plasmodium falciparum malaria**
        Severe or complicated Plasmodium falciparum malaria NOS

    B50.9 **Plasmodium falciparum malaria, unspecified**

● **B51** **Plasmodium vivax malaria**

    Includes   mixed infections of Plasmodium vivax with other Plasmodium species, except Plasmodium falciparum

    Excludes1   plasmodium vivax with Plasmodium falciparum (B50.-)

    B51.0 **Plasmodium vivax malaria with rupture of spleen**

    B51.8 **Plasmodium vivax malaria with other complications**

    B51.9 **Plasmodium vivax malaria without complication**
        Plasmodium vivax malaria NOS

● **B52** **Plasmodium malariae malaria**
Causes fever that recurs at approximately three-day intervals (quartan fever), longer than two-day (tertian) intervals of other malarial parasites

    Includes   mixed infections of Plasmodium malariae with other Plasmodium species, except Plasmodium falciparum and Plasmodium vivax

    Excludes1   plasmodium falciparum (B50.-)
            plasmodium vivax (B51.-)

    B52.0 **Plasmodium malariae malaria with nephropathy**

    B52.8 **Plasmodium malariae malaria with other complications**

    B52.9 **Plasmodium malariae malaria without complication**
        Plasmodium malariae malaria NOS

● **B53** **Other specified malaria**

    B53.0 **Plasmodium ovale malaria**
        Least diagnosed type of malaria spread by female mosquitoes of rare species
        Excludes1   plasmodium ovale with Plasmodium falciparum (B50.-)
                 plasmodium ovale with Plasmodium malariae (B52.-)
                 plasmodium ovale with Plasmodium vivax (B51.-)

    B53.1 **Malaria due to simian plasmodia**
        Malaria-like disease (parasite infection)
        Excludes1   malaria due to simian plasmodia with Plasmodium falciparum (B50.-)
                 malaria due to simian plasmodia with Plasmodium malariae (B52.-)
                 malaria due to simian plasmodia with Plasmodium ovale (B53.0)
                 malaria due to simian plasmodia with Plasmodium vivax (B51.-)

    B53.8 **Other malaria, not elsewhere classified**

  B54 **Unspecified malaria**

● **B55** **Leishmaniasis**
Protozoal infection

    B55.0 **Visceral leishmaniasis**
        Kala-azar
        Post-kala-azar dermal leishmaniasis

    B55.1 **Cutaneous leishmaniasis**

    B55.2 **Mucocutaneous leishmaniasis**

    B55.9 **Leishmaniasis, unspecified**

● **B56** **African trypanosomiasis**
Human African trypanosomiasis (HAT) is transmitted by fly bites

    B56.0 **Gambiense trypanosomiasis**
        Infection due to Trypanosoma brucei gambiense
        West African sleeping sickness

    B56.1 **Rhodesiense trypanosomiasis**
        East African sleeping sickness
        Infection due to Trypanosoma brucei rhodesiense

    B56.9 **African trypanosomiasis, unspecified**
        Sleeping sickness NOS

● **B57** **Chagas' disease**
Tropical parasitic disease

    Includes   American trypanosomiasis
            infection due to Trypanosoma cruzi

    B57.0 **Acute Chagas' disease with heart involvement**
        Acute Chagas' disease with myocarditis

    B57.1 **Acute Chagas' disease without heart involvement**
        Acute Chagas' disease NOS

    B57.2 **Chagas' disease (chronic) with heart involvement**
        American trypanosomiasis NOS
        Chagas' disease (chronic) NOS
        Chagas' disease (chronic) with myocarditis
        Trypanosomiasis NOS

CHAPTER 1 (A00-B99)

CHAPTER 1 (A00-B99)

- **B57.3 Chagas' disease (chronic) with digestive system involvement**
  - B57.30 Chagas' disease with digestive system involvement, unspecified
  - B57.31 Megaesophagus in Chagas' disease
  - B57.32 Megacolon in Chagas' disease
  - B57.39 Other digestive system involvement in Chagas' disease

- **B57.4 Chagas' disease (chronic) with nervous system involvement**
  - B57.40 Chagas' disease with nervous system involvement, unspecified
  - B57.41 Meningitis in Chagas' disease
  - B57.42 Meningoencephalitis in Chagas' disease
  - B57.49 Other nervous system involvement in Chagas' disease

- B57.5 Chagas' disease (chronic) with other organ involvement

- **B58 Toxoplasmosis**
  Infection by protozoon transmitted in cysts in feces of cats
  | **Includes** | infection due to Toxoplasma gondii |
  | **Excludes1** | congenital toxoplasmosis (P37.1) |
  - **B58.0 Toxoplasma oculopathy**
    - B58.00 Toxoplasma oculopathy, unspecified
    - B58.01 Toxoplasma chorioretinitis
    - B58.09 Other toxoplasma oculopathy
      Toxoplasma uveitis
  - B58.1 Toxoplasma hepatitis
  - B58.2 Toxoplasma meningoencephalitis 🝢
  - B58.3 Pulmonary toxoplasmosis 🝢
  - **B58.8 Toxoplasmosis with other organ involvement**
    - B58.81 Toxoplasma myocarditis
    - B58.82 Toxoplasma myositis
    - B58.83 Toxoplasma tubulo-interstitial nephropathy
      Toxoplasma pyelonephritis
    - B58.89 Toxoplasmosis with other organ involvement
  - B58.9 Toxoplasmosis, unspecified

- B59 **Pneumocystosis** 🝢
  Caused by fungus
  Pneumonia due to Pneumocystis carinii
  Pneumonia due to Pneumocystis jiroveci

- **B60 Other protozoal diseases, not elsewhere classified**
Excludes1	cryptosporidiosis (A07.2)
	intestinal microsporidiosis (A07.8)
	isosporiasis (A07.3)
  - **B60.0 Babesiosis**
    Tickborne disease caused by microscopic organisms
    - B60.00 Babesiosis, unspecified
      Babesiosis due to unspecified Babesia species
      Piroplasmosis, unspecified
    - B60.01 Babesiosis due to Babesia microti
      Infection due to B. microti
    - B60.02 Babesiosis due to Babesia duncani
      Infection due to B. duncani and B. duncani-type species
    - B60.03 Babesiosis due to Babesia divergens
      Babesiosis due to Babesia MO-1
      Infection due to B. divergens and B. divergens-like strains
    - B60.09 Other babesiosis
      Babesiosis due to Babesia KO-1
      Babesiosis due to Babesia venatorum
      Infection due to other Babesia species
      Infection due to other protozoa of the order Piroplasmida
      Other piroplasmosis

Item 1–22 Toxoplasmosis is caused by the protozoa **Toxoplasma gondii,** of which the house cat can be a host. Human infection occurs when contact is made with materials containing the pathogen, such as feces, contaminated soil, or ingestion of infected lamb, goat; or pork. Of the infected, very few have symptoms because a healthy person's immune system keeps the parasite from causing illness. When the immune system is compromised, symptoms may occur. Clinical symptoms include flu-like symptoms, but the disease progresses to include the eyes and the brain in babies.

- **B60.1 Acanthamebiasis**
  - B60.10 Acanthamebiasis, unspecified
  - B60.11 Meningoencephalitis due to Acanthamoeba (culbertsoni)
  - B60.12 Conjunctivitis due to Acanthamoeba
  - B60.13 Keratoconjunctivitis due to Acanthamoeba
  - B60.19 Other acanthamebic disease
- B60.2 Naegleriasis
  Infection with microscopic organisms
  Primary amebic meningoencephalitis
- B60.8 Other specified protozoal diseases
  Microsporidiosis

- B64 **Unspecified protozoal disease**

HELMINTHIASES (B65-B83)
Diseases or infestations caused by parasitic worms

- **B65 Schistosomiasis [bilharziasis]**
  Infection with flukes (flat parasitic worms)
  | **Includes** | snail fever |
  - B65.0 Schistosomiasis due to Schistosoma haematobium [urinary schistosomiasis]
  - B65.1 Schistosomiasis due to Schistosoma mansoni [intestinal schistosomiasis]
  - B65.2 Schistosomiasis due to Schistosoma japonicum
    Asiatic schistosomiasis
  - B65.3 Cercarial dermatitis
    Swimmer's itch
  - B65.8 Other schistosomiasis
    Infection due to Schistosoma intercalatum
    Infection due to Schistosoma mattheei
    Infection due to Schistosoma mekongi
  - B65.9 Schistosomiasis, unspecified
- **B66 Other fluke infections**
  Trematode (parasitic worms)
  - B66.0 Opisthorchiasis
    Infection due to cat liver fluke
    Infection due to Opisthorchis (felineus)(viverrini)
  - B66.1 Clonorchiasis
    Chinese liver fluke disease
    Infection due to Clonorchis sinensis
    Oriental liver fluke disease
  - B66.2 Dicroceliasis
    Liver fluke
    Infection due to Dicrocoelium dendriticum
    Lancet fluke infection
  - B66.3 Fascioliasis
    Infection due to Fasciola gigantica
    Infection due to Fasciola hepatica
    Infection due to Fasciola indica
    Sheep liver fluke disease
  - B66.4 Paragonimiasis 🝢
    Infection due to Paragonimus species
    Lung fluke disease
    Pulmonary distomiasis
  - B66.5 Fasciolopsiasis
    Largest intestinal fluke in humans
    Infection due to Fasciolopsis buski
    Intestinal distomiasis

▶ New   ⇒ Revised   ~~deleted~~ Deleted   Excludes 1   Excludes 2   Includes   Use additional   Code first   Code also   Key words

OGCR Official Guidelines   X Assign placeholder X   ● Use Additional Character(s)   ▶ Manifestation Code   🝢 Hierarchical Condition Category   **Coding Clinic**

Item 1-23 Echinococcosis: Also known as hydatid disease; is caused by Echinococcus granulosus, E. multilocularis, and E. vogeli tapeworms; and is contracted from infected food. Found in southern South America, the Mediterranean, the Middle East, central Asia, and Africa and uncommon in the United States but has been reported in California, New Mexico, Arizona and Utah. The disease is treated with medication over a long course, as it is resistive.

B66.8 **Other specified fluke infections**
Echinostomiasis
Heterophyiasis
Metagonimiasis
Nanophyetiasis
Watsoniasis

B66.9 **Fluke infection, unspecified**

● **B67** **Echinococcosis**
Larval forms of tapeworms usually of liver or lungs
Includes hydatidosis

B67.0 **Echinococcus granulosus infection of liver**

B67.1 **Echinococcus granulosus infection of lung** 🔊

B67.2 **Echinococcus granulosus infection of bone**

● **B67.3** **Echinococcus granulosus infection, other and multiple sites**

B67.31 **Echinococcus granulosus infection, thyroid gland**

B67.32 **Echinococcus granulosus infection, multiple sites**

B67.39 **Echinococcus granulosus infection, other sites**

B67.4 **Echinococcus granulosus infection, unspecified**
Dog tapeworm (infection)

B67.5 **Echinococcus multilocularis infection of liver**

● **B67.6** **Echinococcus multilocularis infection, other and multiple sites**

B67.61 **Echinococcus multilocularis infection, multiple sites**

B67.69 **Echinococcus multilocularis infection, other sites**

B67.7 **Echinococcus multilocularis infection, unspecified**

B67.8 **Echinococcosis, unspecified, of liver**

● **B67.9** **Echinococcosis, other and unspecified**

B67.90 **Echinococcosis, unspecified**
Echinococcosis NOS

B67.99 **Other echinococcosis**

● **B68** **Taeniasis**
Intestinal tapeworm (cestode) infection from raw or undercooked meat of infected animal
Excludes1 cysticercosis (B69.-)

B68.0 **Taenia solium taeniasis**
Pork tapeworm (infection)

B68.1 **Taenia saginata taeniasis**
Beef tapeworm (infection)
Infection due to adult tapeworm Taenia saginata

B68.9 **Taeniasis, unspecified**

● **B69** **Cysticercosis**
Systemic illness caused by the larvae of pork tapeworm
Includes cysticerciasis infection due to larval form of Taenia solium

B69.0 **Cysticercosis of central nervous system**

B69.1 **Cysticercosis of eye**

● **B69.8** **Cysticercosis of other sites**

B69.81 **Myositis in cysticercosis**

B69.89 **Cysticercosis of other sites**

B69.9 **Cysticercosis, unspecified**

● **B70** **Diphyllobothriasis and sparganosis**
Infection with tapeworms seen most often from inadequately cooked fish

B70.0 **Diphyllobothriasis**
Diphyllobothrium (adult) (latum) (pacificum) infection
Fish tapeworm (infection)
Excludes2 larval diphyllobothriasis (B70.1)

B70.1 **Sparganosis**
Infection with migrating tapeworm larvae, which invade subcutaneous tissues, causing inflammation and fibrosis that resembles cellulitis
Infection due to Sparganum (mansoni) (proliferum)
Infection due to Spirometra larva
Larval diphyllobothriasis
Spirometrosis

● **B71** **Other cestode infections**

B71.0 **Hymenolepiasis**
Intestinal infestation with tapeworms
Dwarf tapeworm infection
Rat tapeworm (infection)

B71.1 **Dipylidiasis**
Infection with tapeworm common to dogs and cats and seen in children having close contact with infected pets

B71.8 **Other specified cestode infections**
Infection by the larval stage of a tapeworm, usually through fruit or vegetables
Coenurosis

B71.9 **Cestode infection, unspecified**
Tapeworm (infection) NOS

B72 **Dracunculiasis**
Infection with roundworms
Includes guinea worm infection
infection due to Dracunculus medinensis

● **B73** **Onchocerciasis**
Infection with parasitic worm
Includes onchocerca volvulus infection
onchocercosis
river blindness

● **B73.0** **Onchocerciasis with eye disease**

B73.00 **Onchocerciasis with eye involvement, unspecified**

B73.01 **Onchocerciasis with endophthalmitis**

B73.02 **Onchocerciasis with glaucoma**

B73.09 **Onchocerciasis with other eye involvement**
Infestation of eyelid due to onchocerciasis

B73.1 **Onchocerciasis without eye disease**

● **B74** **Filariasis**
Infestation with slender threadlike worms
➡ **Excludes2** onchocerciasis (B73)
tropical (pulmonary) eosinophilia NOS (J82.89)

B74.0 **Filariasis due to Wuchereria bancrofti**
Bancroftian elephantiasis
Bancroftian filariasis

B74.1 **Filariasis due to Brugia malayi**

B74.2 **Filariasis due to Brugia timori**

B74.3 **Loiasis**
Infection with round worms growing in subcutaneous connective tissue
Calabar swelling
Eyeworm disease of Africa
Loa loa infection

B74.4 **Mansonelliasis**
Infection with filarial parasite
Infection due to Mansonella ozzardi
Infection due to Mansonella perstans
Infection due to Mansonella streptocerca

B74.8 **Other filariases**
Dirofilariasis

B74.9 **Filariasis, unspecified**

CHAPTER 1 (A00-B99)

B75   Trichinellosis
*Infestation with parasitic roundworms ingested in undercooked
contaminated meat*
> **Includes**   infection due to Trichinella species trichiniasis

● B76   Hookworm diseases
*Occurs in hot, humid parts of world where larvae are soil borne, enter
digestive tract through skin of feet/legs or in contaminated food/
water; AKA ground itch*
> **Includes**   uncinariasis

    B76.0   Ancylostomiasis
        Infection due to Ancylostoma species

    B76.1   Necatoriasis
        Infection due to Necator americanus

    B76.8   Other hookworm diseases

    B76.9   Hookworm disease, unspecified
        Cutaneous larva migrans NOS

● B77   Ascariasis
Infection by roundworm in small intestine
> **Includes**   ascaridiasis
> roundworm infection

    B77.0   Ascariasis with intestinal complications

    ● B77.8   Ascariasis with other complications

        B77.81   Ascariasis pneumonia

        B77.89   Ascariasis with other complications

    B77.9   Ascariasis, unspecified

● B78   Strongyloidiasis
Infection with adult female roundworms
> **Excludes1**   trichostrongyliasis (B81.2)

    B78.0   Intestinal strongyloidiasis

    B78.1   Cutaneous strongyloidiasis

    B78.7   Disseminated strongyloidiasis

    B78.9   Strongyloidiasis, unspecified

B79   Trichuriasis
Intestinal infection with roundworms
> **Includes**   trichocephaliasis
> whipworm (disease)(infection)

B80   Enterobiasis
Intestinal infection with pinworms
> **Includes**   oxyuriasis
> pinworm infection
> threadworm infection

● B81   Other intestinal helminthiases, not elsewhere classified
Diseases or infestations caused by parasitic worms
> **Excludes1**   angiostrongyliasis due to:
> Angiostrongylus cantonensis (B83.2)
> Parastrongylus cantonensis (B83.2)

    B81.0   Anisakiasis
        *Roundworm infection via contaminated undercooked infected
fish or marine mammals*
        Infection due to Anisakis larva

    B81.1   Intestinal capillariasis
        Infestation with of parasites (nematodes)
        Capillariasis NOS
        Infection due to Capillaria philippinensis
> > **Excludes2**   hepatic capillariasis (B83.8)

    B81.2   Trichostrongyliasis

    B81.3   Intestinal angiostrongyliasis
        Angiostrongyliasis due to:
        Angiostrongylus costaricensis (B83.2)
        Parastrongylus costaricensis (B83.2)

    B81.4   Mixed intestinal helminthiases
        Infection due to intestinal helminths classified to more
than one of the categories B65.0-B81.3 and B81.8
        Mixed helminthiasis NOS

    B81.8   Other specified intestinal helminthiases
        Infection due to Oesophagostomum species
[esophagostomiasis]
        Infection due to Ternidens diminutus [ternidensiasis]

● B82   Unspecified intestinal parasitism

    B82.0   Intestinal helminthiasis, unspecified
        Infected with worms

    B82.9   Intestinal parasitism, unspecified

● B83   Other helminthiases
Caused by parasitic worms
> **Excludes1**   capillariasis NOS (B81.1)
> **Excludes2**   intestinal capillariasis (B81.1)

    B83.0   Visceral larva migrans
        Prolonged migration of nematode larvae
        Toxocariasis

    B83.1   Gnathostomiasis
        *Infection with nematode occurring from ingested undercooked
fish contaminated with larvae; larvae migrate to
subcutaneous tissue or deeper tissues, results are
abscesses*
        Wandering swelling

    B83.2   Angiostrongyliasis due to Parastrongylus cantonensis
        *Nematode infection caused by eating contaminated raw
snails, slugs, or paratenic hosts such as prawns or
crabs; larval worms migrate to central nervous system
resulting in eosinophilic meningitis*
        Eosinophilic meningoencephalitis due to
Parastrongylus cantonensis
> > **Excludes2**   intestinal angiostrongyliasis (B81.3)

    B83.3   Syngamiasis
        *Infestation with gapeworm from turkey, pheasant, guinea fowl,
goose, and wild birds*
        Syngamosis

    B83.4   Internal hirudiniasis
        Infestation by leeches
> > **Excludes2**   external hirudiniasis (B88.3)

    B83.8   Other specified helminthiases
        Parasitic worm infestation
        Acanthocephaliasis
        Gongylonemiasis
        Hepatic capillariasis
        Metastrongyliasis
        Thelaziasis

    B83.9   Helminthiasis, unspecified
        Worms NOS
> > **Excludes1**   intestinal helminthiasis NOS (B82.0)

PEDICULOSIS, ACARIASIS AND OTHER INFESTATIONS (B85-B89)

● B85   Pediculosis and phthiriasis
Infestation of lice

    B85.0   Pediculosis due to Pediculus humanus capitis
        Head-louse infestation

    B85.1   Pediculosis due to Pediculus humanus corporis
        Body-louse infestation

    B85.2   Pediculosis, unspecified

    B85.3   Phthiriasis
        Crab or pubic lice
        Infestation by crab-louse
        Infestation by Phthirus pubis

    B85.4   Mixed pediculosis and phthiriasis
        Infestation classifiable to more than one of the
categories B85.0-B85.3

B86   Scabies
Contagious dermatitis caused by mites
Sarcoptic itch

- B87 **Myiasis**
  Infestation by fly maggots
  | Includes | infestation by larva of flies |
  - B87.0 **Cutaneous myiasis**
    Creeping myiasis
  - B87.1 **Wound myiasis**
    Traumatic myiasis
  - B87.2 **Ocular myiasis**
  - B87.3 **Nasopharyngeal myiasis**
    Laryngeal myiasis
  - B87.4 **Aural myiasis**
  - B87.8 **Myiasis of other sites**
    - B87.81 **Genitourinary myiasis**
    - B87.82 **Intestinal myiasis**
    - B87.89 **Myiasis of other sites**
  - B87.9 **Myiasis, unspecified**

- B88 **Other infestations**
  - B88.0 **Other acariasis**
    Acarine dermatitis
    Dermatitis due to Demodex species
    Dermatitis due to Dermanyssus gallinae
    Dermatitis due to Liponyssoides sanguineus
    Trombiculosis
    | Excludes2 | scabies (B86) |
  - B88.1 **Tungiasis [sandflea infestation]**
    Inflammatory skin disease caused by infestation of fleas
  - B88.2 **Other arthropod infestations**
    Scarabiasis
  - B88.3 **External hirudiniasis**
    Leech infestation NOS
    | Excludes2 | internal hirudiniasis (B83.4) |
  - B88.8 **Other specified infestations**
    Infection of topical fresh water fish parasite
    Ichthyoparasitism due to Vandellia cirrhosa
    Linguatulosis
    Porocephaliasis
  - B88.9 **Infestation, unspecified**
    Infestation (skin) NOS
    Infestation by mites NOS
    Skin parasites NOS

- B89 **Unspecified parasitic disease**

SEQUELAE OF INFECTIOUS AND PARASITIC DISEASES (B90-B94)

Note: Categories B90-B94 are to be used to indicate conditions in categories A00-B89 as the cause of sequelae, which are themselves classified elsewhere. The 'sequelae' include conditions specified as such; they also include residuals of diseases classifiable to the above categories if there is evidence that the disease itself is no longer present. Codes from these categories are not to be used for chronic infections. Code chronic current infections to active infectious disease as appropriate.

Code first condition resulting from (sequela) the infectious or parasitic disease

- B90 **Sequelae of tuberculosis**
  Condition resulting from tuberculosis
  - B90.0 **Sequelae of central nervous system tuberculosis**
  - B90.1 **Sequelae of genitourinary tuberculosis**
  - B90.2 **Sequelae of tuberculosis of bones and joints**
  - B90.8 **Sequelae of tuberculosis of other organs**
    | Excludes2 | sequelae of respiratory tuberculosis (B90.9) |
  - B90.9 **Sequelae of respiratory and unspecified tuberculosis**
    Sequelae of tuberculosis NOS

- B91 **Sequelae of poliomyelitis**
  | Excludes1 | postpolio syndrome (G14) |

- B92 **Sequelae of leprosy**

- B94 **Sequelae of other and unspecified infectious and parasitic diseases**
  - B94.0 **Sequelae of trachoma**
  - B94.1 **Sequelae of viral encephalitis**
  - B94.2 **Sequelae of viral hepatitis**
  - B94.8 **Sequelae of other specified infectious and parasitic diseases**
    Coding Clinic: 2021, Q1, P34,37,41,44,46,48
  - B94.9 **Sequelae of unspecified infectious and parasitic disease**
    ▶ **Excludes2** post COVID-19 condition (U09.9)
    Coding Clinic: 2017, Q4, P109

OGCR Section I.C.1.b.

Certain infectious and parasitic diseases
Infectious agents as the cause of diseases classified to other chapters
Certain infections are classified in chapters other than Chapter 1 and no organism is identified as part of the infection code. In these instances, it is necessary to use an additional code from Chapter 1 to identify the organism. A code from category B95, Streptococcus, Staphylococcus, and Enterococcus as the cause of diseases classified to other chapters, B96, Other bacterial agents as the cause of diseases classified to other chapters, or B97, Viral agents as the cause of diseases classified to other chapters, is to be used as an additional code to identify the organism. An instructional note will be found at the infection code advising that an additional organism code is required.

BACTERIAL AND VIRAL INFECTIOUS AGENTS (B95-B97)

Note: These categories are provided for use as supplementary or additional codes to identify the infectious agent(s) in diseases classified elsewhere.
Code the disease first, then the bacterium. Do not report codes from B95-B97 for sepsis.

- B95 **Streptococcus, Staphylococcus, and Enterococcus as the cause of diseases classified elsewhere**
  - B95.0 **Streptococcus, group A, as the cause of diseases classified elsewhere**
  - B95.1 **Streptococcus, group B, as the cause of diseases classified elsewhere**
    Coding Clinic: 2020, Q1, P10; 2019, Q2, P9-10; 2018, Q4, P23
  - B95.2 **Enterococcus as the cause of diseases classified elsewhere**
  - B95.3 **Streptococcus pneumoniae as the cause of diseases classified elsewhere**
  - B95.4 **Other streptococcus as the cause of diseases classified elsewhere**
  - B95.5 **Unspecified streptococcus as the cause of diseases classified elsewhere**
  - B95.6 **Staphylococcus aureus as the cause of diseases classified elsewhere**
    - B95.61 **Methicillin susceptible Staphylococcus aureus infection as the cause of diseases classified elsewhere**
      Methicillin susceptible Staphylococcus aureus (MSSA) infection as the cause of diseases classified elsewhere
      Staphylococcus aureus infection NOS as the cause of diseases classified elsewhere
    - B95.62 **Methicillin resistant Staphylococcus aureus infection as the cause of diseases classified elsewhere**
      Methicillin resistant staphylococcus aureus (MRSA) infection as the cause of diseases classified elsewhere
      Coding Clinic: 2016, Q1, P13
  - B95.7 **Other staphylococcus as the cause of diseases classified elsewhere**
  - B95.8 **Unspecified staphylococcus as the cause of diseases classified elsewhere**

CHAPTER 1 (A00-B99)

CHAPTER 1 (A00-B99)

● **B96** **Other bacterial agents as the cause of diseases classified elsewhere**

　B96.0 **Mycoplasma pneumoniae [M. pneumoniae] as the cause of diseases classified elsewhere**
　　　Pleuro-pneumonia-like-organism [PPLO]

　B96.1 **Klebsiella pneumoniae [K. pneumoniae] as the cause of diseases classified elsewhere**

● **B96.2** **Escherichia coli [E. coli] as the cause of diseases classified elsewhere**

　　B96.20 **Unspecified Escherichia coli [E. coli] as the cause of diseases classified elsewhere**
　　　　Escherichia coli [E. coli] NOS
　　　　Coding Clinic: 2018, Q4, P34; 2018, Q1, P16

　　B96.21 **Shiga toxin-producing Escherichia coli [E. coli] [STEC] O157 as the cause of diseases classified elsewhere**
　　　　E. coli O157:H- (nonmotile) with confirmation of Shiga toxin
　　　　E. coli O157 with confirmation of Shiga toxin when H antigen is unknown, or is not H7
　　　　O157:H7 Escherichia coli [E.coli] with or without confirmation of Shiga toxin-production
　　　　Shiga toxin-producing Escherichia coli [E.coli] O157:H7 with or without confirmation of Shiga toxin-production
　　　　STEC O157:H7 with or without confirmation of Shiga toxin-production

　　B96.22 **Other specified Shiga toxin-producing Escherichia coli [E. coli] [STEC] as the cause of diseases classified elsewhere**
　　　　Non-O157 Shiga toxin-producing Escherichia coli [E.coli]
　　　　Non-O157 Shiga toxin-producing Escherichia coli [E.coli] with known O group

　　B96.23 **Unspecified Shiga toxin-producing Escherichia coli [E. coli] [STEC] as the cause of diseases classified elsewhere**
　　　　Shiga toxin-producing Escherichia coli [E. coli] with unspecified O group
　　　　STEC NOS

　　B96.29 **Other Escherichia coli [E. coli] as the cause of diseases classified elsewhere**
　　　　Non-Shiga toxin-producing E. coli

　B96.3 **Hemophilus influenzae [H. influenzae] as the cause of diseases classified elsewhere**

　B96.4 **Proteus (mirabilis) (morganii) as the cause of diseases classified elsewhere**

　B96.5 **Pseudomonas (aeruginosa) (mallei) (pseudomallei) as the cause of diseases classified elsewhere**
　　　Coding Clinic: 2015, Q1, P18

　B96.6 **Bacteroides fragilis [B. fragilis] as the cause of diseases classified elsewhere**

　B96.7 **Clostridium perfringens [C. perfringens] as the cause of diseases classified elsewhere**

● **B96.8** **Other specified bacterial agents as the cause of diseases classified elsewhere**

　　B96.81 **Helicobacter pylori [H. pylori] as the cause of diseases classified elsewhere**

　　B96.82 **Vibrio vulnificus as the cause of diseases classified elsewhere**

　　B96.89 **Other specified bacterial agents as the cause of diseases classified elsewhere**

● **B97** **Viral agents as the cause of diseases classified elsewhere**

　B97.0 **Adenovirus as the cause of diseases classified elsewhere**

● **B97.1** **Enterovirus as the cause of diseases classified elsewhere**

　　B97.10 **Unspecified enterovirus as the cause of diseases classified elsewhere**

　　B97.11 **Coxsackievirus as the cause of diseases classified elsewhere**

　　B97.12 **Echovirus as the cause of diseases classified elsewhere**

　　B97.19 **Other enterovirus as the cause of diseases classified elsewhere**

● **B97.2** **Coronavirus as the cause of diseases classified elsewhere**

　　B97.21 **SARS-associated coronavirus as the cause of diseases classified elsewhere**
　　　　Excludes1　pneumonia due to SARS-associated coronavirus (J12.81)

　　B97.29 **Other coronavirus as the cause of diseases classified elsewhere**

Item 1–24 **Retrovirus** develops by copying its RNA, genetic materials, into the DNA, which then produces new virus particles. It is from the Retroviridae virus family. **Human T-cell lymphotropic virus, Type I (HTLV-I),** is also called human T-cell leukemia virus, Type I, and is a retrovirus thought to cause T-cell leukemia/lymphoma. **Human T-cell lymphotropic virus, Type II (HTLV-II),** is also called human T-cell leukemia virus, Type II, and is a retrovirus associated with hematologic disorders.

　HIV-2 is one of the serotypes of HIV and is usually confined to West Africa, whereas **HIV-1** is found worldwide.

● **B97.3** **Retrovirus as the cause of diseases classified elsewhere**
　　　Excludes1　human immunodeficiency virus [HIV] disease (B20)

　　B97.30 **Unspecified retrovirus as the cause of diseases classified elsewhere**

　　B97.31 **Lentivirus as the cause of diseases classified elsewhere**

　　B97.32 **Oncovirus as the cause of diseases classified elsewhere**

　　B97.33 **Human T-cell lymphotrophic virus, type I [HTLV-I] as the cause of diseases classified elsewhere**

　　B97.34 **Human T-cell lymphotrophic virus, type II [HTLV-II] as the cause of diseases classified elsewhere**

　　B97.35 **Human immunodeficiency virus, type 2 [HIV 2] as the cause of diseases classified elsewhere** 🐾

　　B97.39 **Other retrovirus as the cause of diseases classified elsewhere**

　B97.4 **Respiratory syncytial virus as the cause of diseases classified elsewhere**
　　　RSV as the cause of diseases classified elsewhere
　　　Code first related disorders, such as:
　　　　otitis media (H65.-)
　　　　upper respiratory infection (J06.9)
　　　Excludes1　acute bronchiolitis due to respiratory syncytial virus (RSV) (J21.0)
　　　　　acute bronchitis due to respiratory syncytial virus (RSV) (J20.5)
　　　　　respiratory syncytial virus (RSV) pneumonia (J12.1)

　B97.5 **Reovirus as the cause of diseases classified elsewhere**

　B97.6 **Parvovirus as the cause of diseases classified elsewhere**

　B97.7 **Papillomavirus as the cause of diseases classified elsewhere**

● **B97.8** **Other viral agents as the cause of diseases classified elsewhere**

　　B97.81 **Human metapneumovirus as the cause of diseases classified elsewhere**

　　B97.89 **Other viral agents as the cause of diseases classified elsewhere**
　　　　Coding Clinic: 2016, Q3, P8-10, 14

OTHER INFECTIOUS DISEASES (B99)

● **B99** **Other and unspecified infectious diseases**

　B99.8 **Other infectious disease**

　B99.9 **Unspecified infectious disease**

▶ New　　➡ Revised　　~~deleted~~ Deleted　　Excludes 1　　Excludes 2　　Includes　　Use additional　　Code first　　Code also　　Key words

OGCR Official Guidelines　　X Assign placeholder X　　● Use Additional Character(s)　　▶ Manifestation Code　　🐾 Hierarchical Condition Category　　**Coding Clinic**

CHAPTER 2

NEOPLASMS (C00-D49)

OGCR Chapter-Specific Coding Guidelines

2. Chapter 2: Neoplasms (C00-D49)
General guidelines
Chapter 2 of the ICD-10-CM contains the codes for most benign and all malignant neoplasms. Certain benign neoplasms, such as prostatic adenomas, may be found in the specific body system chapters. To properly code a neoplasm it is necessary to determine from the record if the neoplasm is benign, in-situ, malignant, or of uncertain histologic behavior. If malignant, any secondary (metastatic) sites should also be determined.

Primary malignant neoplasms overlapping site boundaries
A primary malignant neoplasm that overlaps two or more contiguous (next to each other) sites should be classified to the subcategory/code .8 ('overlapping lesion'), unless the combination is specifically indexed elsewhere. For multiple neoplasms of the same site that are not contiguous such as tumors in different quadrants of the same breast, codes for each site should be assigned.

Malignant neoplasm of ectopic tissue
Malignant neoplasms of ectopic tissue are to be coded to the site of origin mentioned, e.g., ectopic pancreatic malignant neoplasms involving the stomach are coded to malignant neoplasm of pancreas, unspecified (C25.9).

The neoplasm table in the Alphabetic Index should be referenced first. However, if the histological term is documented, that term should be referenced first, rather than going immediately to the Neoplasm Table, in order to determine which column in the Neoplasm Table is appropriate. For example, if the documentation indicates "adenoma," refer to the term in the Alphabetic Index to review the entries under this term and the instructional note to "see also neoplasm, by site, benign." The table provides the proper code based on the type of neoplasm and the site. It is important to select the proper column in the table that corresponds to the type of neoplasm. The Tabular List should then be referenced to verify that the correct code has been selected from the table and that a more specific site code does not exist.

See Section I.C.21. Factors influencing health status and contact with health services, Status, for information regarding Z15.0, codes for genetic susceptibility to cancer.

a. Treatment directed at the malignancy
If the treatment is directed at the malignancy, designate the malignancy as the principal diagnosis.

The only exception to this guideline is if a patient admission/encounter is solely for the administration of chemotherapy, immunotherapy or external beam radiation therapy, assign the appropriate Z51.— code as the first-listed or principal diagnosis, and the diagnosis or problem for which the service is being performed as a secondary diagnosis.

b. Treatment of secondary site
When a patient is admitted because of a primary neoplasm with metastasis and treatment is directed toward the secondary site only, the secondary neoplasm is designated as the principal diagnosis even though the primary malignancy is still present.

c. Coding and sequencing of complications
Coding and sequencing of complications associated with the malignancies or with the therapy thereof are subject to the following guidelines:

1) Anemia associated with malignancy
When admission/encounter is for management of an anemia associated with the malignancy, and the treatment is only for anemia, the appropriate code for the malignancy is sequenced as the principal or first-listed diagnosis followed by the appropriate code for the anemia (such as code D63.0, Anemia in neoplastic disease).

2) Anemia associated with chemotherapy, immunotherapy and radiation therapy
When the admission/encounter is for management of an anemia associated with an adverse effect of the administration of chemotherapy or immunotherapy and the only treatment is for the anemia, the anemia code is sequenced first followed by the appropriate codes for the neoplasm and the adverse effect (T45.1X5, Adverse effect of antineoplastic and immunosuppressive drugs).

When the admission/encounter is for management of an anemia associated with an adverse effect of radiotherapy, the anemia code should be sequenced first, followed by the appropriate neoplasm code and code Y84.2, Radiological procedure and radiotherapy as the cause of abnormal reaction of the patient, or of later complication, without mention of misadventure at the time of the procedure.

3) Management of dehydration due to the malignancy
When the admission/encounter is for management of dehydration due to the malignancy and only the dehydration is being treated (intravenous rehydration), the dehydration is sequenced first, followed by the code(s) for the malignancy.

4) Treatment of a complication resulting from a surgical procedure
When the admission/encounter is for treatment of a complication resulting from a surgical procedure, designate the complication as the principal or first-listed diagnosis if treatment is directed at resolving the complication.

d. Primary malignancy previously excised
When a primary malignancy has been previously excised or eradicated from its site and there is no further treatment directed to that site and there is no evidence of any existing primary malignancy at that site, a code from category Z85, Personal history of malignant neoplasm, should be used to indicate the former site of the malignancy. Any mention of extension, invasion, or metastasis to another site is coded as a secondary malignant neoplasm to that site. The secondary site may be the principal or first-listed with the Z85 code used as a secondary code.

e. Admissions/Encounters involving chemotherapy, immunotherapy and radiation therapy

1) Episode of care involves surgical removal of neoplasm
When an episode of care involves the surgical removal of a neoplasm, primary or secondary site, followed by adjunct chemotherapy or radiation treatment during the same episode of care, the code for the neoplasm should be assigned as principal or first-listed diagnosis.

2) Patient admission/encounter solely for administration of chemotherapy, immunotherapy and radiation therapy
If a patient admission/encounter is solely for the administration of chemotherapy, immunotherapy or external beam radiation therapy assign code Z51.0, Encounter for antineoplastic radiation therapy, or Z51.11, Encounter for antineoplastic chemotherapy, or Z51.12, Encounter for antineoplastic immunotherapy as the first-listed or principal diagnosis. If a patient receives more than one of these therapies during the same admission more than one of these codes may be assigned, in any sequence.

The malignancy for which the therapy is being administered should be assigned as a secondary diagnosis.

If a patient admission/encounter is for the insertion or implantation of radioactive elements (e.g., brachytherapy) the appropriate code for the malignancy is sequenced as the principal or first-listed diagnosis. Code Z51.0 should not be assigned.

3) Patient admitted for radiation therapy, chemotherapy or immunotherapy and develops complications
When a patient is admitted for the purpose of external beam radiotherapy, immunotherapy or chemotherapy and develops complications such as uncontrolled nausea and vomiting or dehydration, the principal or first-listed diagnosis is Z51.0, Encounter for antineoplastic radiation therapy, or Z51.11, Encounter for antineoplastic chemotherapy, or Z51.12, Encounter for antineoplastic immunotherapy followed by any codes for the complications.

When a patient is admitted for the purpose of insertion or implantation of radioactive elements (e.g., brachytherapy) and develops complications such as uncontrolled nausea and vomiting or dehydration, the principal or first-listed diagnosis is the appropriate code for the malignancy followed by any codes for the complications.

f. Admission/encounter to determine extent of malignancy
When the reason for admission/encounter is to determine the extent of the malignancy, or for a procedure such as paracentesis

or thoracentesis, the primary malignancy or appropriate metastatic site is designated as the principal or first-listed diagnosis, even though chemotherapy or radiotherapy is administered.

g. Symptoms, signs, and abnormal findings listed in Chapter 18 associated with neoplasms

Symptoms, signs, and ill-defined conditions listed in Chapter 18 characteristic of, or associated with, an existing primary or secondary site malignancy cannot be used to replace the malignancy as principal or first-listed diagnosis, regardless of the number of admissions or encounters for treatment and care of the neoplasm.

See Section I.C.21. Factors influencing health status and contact with health services, Encounter for prophylactic organ removal.

h. Admission/encounter for pain control/management

See Section I.C.6. for information on coding admission/encounter for pain control/management.

i. Malignancy in two or more noncontiguous sites

A patient may have more than one malignant tumor in the same organ. These tumors may represent different primaries or metastatic disease, depending on the site. Should the documentation be unclear, the provider should be queried as to the status of each tumor so that the correct codes can be assigned.

j. Disseminated malignant neoplasm, unspecified

Code C80.0, Disseminated malignant neoplasm, unspecified, is for use only in those cases where the patient has advanced metastatic disease and no known primary or secondary sites are specified. It should not be used in place of assigning codes for the primary site and all known secondary sites.

k. Malignant neoplasm without specification of site

Code C80.1, Malignant (primary) neoplasm, unspecified, equates to Cancer, unspecified. This code should only be used when no determination can be made as to the primary site of a malignancy. This code should rarely be used in the inpatient setting.

l. Sequencing of neoplasm codes

1) Encounter for treatment of primary malignancy

If the reason for the encounter is for treatment of a primary malignancy, assign the malignancy as the principal/first-listed diagnosis. The primary site is to be sequenced first, followed by any metastatic sites.

2) Encounter for treatment of secondary malignancy

When an encounter is for a primary malignancy with metastasis and treatment is directed toward the metastatic (secondary) site(s) only, the metastatic site(s) is designated as the principal/first-listed diagnosis. The primary malignancy is coded as an additional code.

3) Malignant neoplasm in a pregnant patient

When a pregnant woman has a malignant neoplasm, a code from subcategory O9A.1-, Malignant neoplasm complicating pregnancy, childbirth, and the puerperium, should be sequenced first, followed by the appropriate code from Chapter 2 to indicate the type of neoplasm.

4) Encounter for complication associated with a neoplasm

When an encounter is for management of a complication associated with a neoplasm, such as dehydration, and the treatment is only for the complication, the complication is coded first, followed by the appropriate code(s) for the neoplasm.

The exception to this guideline is anemia. When the admission/encounter is for management of an anemia associated with the malignancy, and the treatment is only for anemia, the appropriate code for the malignancy is sequenced as the principal or first-listed diagnosis followed by code D63.0, Anemia in neoplastic disease.

5) Complication from surgical procedure for treatment of a neoplasm

When an encounter is for treatment of a complication resulting from a surgical procedure performed for the treatment of the neoplasm, designate the complication as the principal/first-listed diagnosis. See guideline regarding the coding of a current malignancy versus personal history to determine if the code for the neoplasm should also be assigned.

6) Pathologic fracture due to a neoplasm

When an encounter is for a pathological fracture due to a neoplasm, and the focus of treatment is the fracture, a code from subcategory M84.5, Pathological fracture in neoplastic disease, should be sequenced first, followed by the code for the neoplasm.

If the focus of treatment is the neoplasm with an associated pathological fracture, the neoplasm code should be sequenced first, followed by a code from M84.5 for the pathological fracture.

m. Current malignancy versus personal history of malignancy

When a primary malignancy has been excised but further treatment, such as an additional surgery for the malignancy, radiation therapy or chemotherapy is directed to that site, the primary malignancy code should be used until treatment is completed.

When a primary malignancy has been previously excised or eradicated from its site, there is no further treatment (of the malignancy) directed to that site, and there is no evidence of any existing primary malignancy at that site, a code from category Z85, Personal history of malignant neoplasm, should be used to indicate the former site of the malignancy.

Subcategories Z85.0–Z85.7 should only be assigned for the former site of a primary malignancy, not the site of a secondary malignancy. Codes from subcategory Z85.8-, may be assigned for the former site(s) of either a primary or secondary malignancy included in this subcategory.

See Section I.C.21. Factors influencing health status and contact with health services, History (of)

n. Leukemia, Multiple Myeloma, and Malignant Plasma Cell Neoplasms in remission versus personal history

The categories for leukemia, and category C90, Multiple myeloma and malignant plasma cell neoplasms, have codes indicating whether or not the leukemia has achieved remission. There are also codes Z85.6, Personal history of leukemia, and Z85.79, Personal history of other malignant neoplasms of lymphoid, hematopoietic and related tissues. If the documentation is unclear, as to whether the leukemia has achieved remission, the provider should be queried.

See Section I.C.21. Factors influencing health status and contact with health services, History (of)

o. Aftercare following surgery for neoplasm

See Section I.C.21. Factors influencing health status and contact with health services, Aftercare

p. Follow-up care for completed treatment of a malignancy

See Section I.C.21. Factors influencing health status and contact with health services, Follow-up

q. Prophylactic organ removal for prevention of malignancy

See Section I.C. 21, Factors influencing health status and contact with health services, Prophylactic organ removal

r. Malignant neoplasm associated with transplanted organ

A malignant neoplasm of a transplanted organ should be coded as a transplant complication. Assign first the appropriate code from category T86.-, Complications of transplanted organs and tissue, followed by code C80.2, Malignant neoplasm associated with transplanted organ. Use an additional code for the specific malignancy.

Item 2-1 Neoplasm: Neo = new, plasm = growth, development, formation. This new growth (mass, tumor) can be malignant or benign, which is confirmed by the pathology report. Do not assign a code to a neoplasm until you review the pathology report. Certain CPT codes will specify benign or malignant lesion, so be certain the diagnosis code supports the procedure code.

CHAPTER 2

NEOPLASMS (C00-D49)

This chapter contains the following blocks:

C00-C14	Malignant neoplasms of lip, oral cavity and pharynx
C15-C26	Malignant neoplasms of digestive organs
C30-C39	Malignant neoplasms of respiratory and intrathoracic organs
C40-C41	Malignant neoplasms of bone and articular cartilage
C43-C44	Melanoma and other malignant neoplasms of skin
C45-C49	Malignant neoplasms of mesothelial and soft tissue
C50	Malignant neoplasms of breast
C51-C58	Malignant neoplasms of female genital organs
C60-C63	Malignant neoplasms of male genital organs
C64-C68	Malignant neoplasms of urinary tract
C69-C72	Malignant neoplasms of eye, brain and other parts of central nervous system
C73-C75	Malignant neoplasms of thyroid and other endocrine glands
C7A	Malignant neuroendocrine tumors
C7B	Secondary neuroendocrine tumors
C76-C80	Malignant neoplasms of ill-defined, other secondary and unspecified sites
C81-C96	Malignant neoplasms of lymphoid, hematopoietic and related tissue
D00-D09	In situ neoplasms
D10-D36	Benign neoplasms, except benign neuroendocrine tumors
D3A	Benign neuroendocrine tumors
D37-D48	Neoplasms of uncertain behavior, polycythemia vera and myelodysplastic syndromes
D49	Neoplasms of unspecified behavior

Notes: Functional activity

All neoplasms are classified in this chapter, whether they are functionally active or not. An additional code from Chapter 4 may be used, to identify functional activity associated with any neoplasm.

Morphology [Histology]

Chapter 2 classifies neoplasms primarily by site (topography), with broad groupings for behavior, malignant, in situ, benign, etc. The Table of Neoplasms should be used to identify the correct topography code. In a few cases, such as for malignant melanoma and certain neuroendocrine tumors, the morphology (histologic type) is included in the category and codes.

Primary malignant neoplasms overlapping site boundaries

A primary malignant neoplasm that overlaps two or more contiguous (next to each other) sites should be classified to the subcategory/code .8 ("overlapping lesion"), unless the combination is specifically indexed elsewhere. For multiple neoplasms of the same site that are not contiguous, such as tumors in different quadrants of the same breast, codes for each site should be assigned.

Malignant neoplasm of ectopic tissue

Malignant neoplasms of ectopic tissue are to be coded to the site mentioned, e.g., ectopic pancreatic malignant neoplasms are coded to pancreas, unspecified (C25.9).

MALIGNANT NEOPLASMS (C00-C96)

MALIGNANT NEOPLASMS, STATED OR PRESUMED TO BE PRIMARY (OF SPECIFIED SITES), AND CERTAIN SPECIFIED HISTOLOGIES, EXCEPT NEUROENDOCRINE, AND OF LYMPHOID, HEMATOPOIETIC AND RELATED TISSUE (C00-C75)

MALIGNANT NEOPLASMS OF LIP, ORAL CAVITY AND PHARYNX (C00-C14)

● C00   **Malignant neoplasm of lip**

Use additional code to identify:
  alcohol abuse and dependence (F10.-)
  history of tobacco dependence (Z87.891)
  tobacco dependence (F17.-)
  tobacco use (Z72.0)

Excludes1   malignant melanoma of lip (C43.0)
  Merkel cell carcinoma of lip (C4A.0)
  other and unspecified malignant neoplasm of skin of lip (C44.0-)

C00.0   **Malignant neoplasm of external upper lip**
  Malignant neoplasm of lipstick area of upper lip
  Malignant neoplasm of upper lip NOS
  Malignant neoplasm of vermilion border of upper lip

C00.1   **Malignant neoplasm of external lower lip**
  Malignant neoplasm of lower lip NOS
  Malignant neoplasm of lipstick area of lower lip
  Malignant neoplasm of vermilion border of lower lip

C00.2   **Malignant neoplasm of external lip, unspecified**
  Malignant neoplasm of vermilion border of lip NOS

C00.3   **Malignant neoplasm of upper lip, inner aspect**
  Malignant neoplasm of buccal aspect of upper lip
  Malignant neoplasm of frenulum of upper lip
  Malignant neoplasm of mucosa of upper lip
  Malignant neoplasm of oral aspect of upper lip

C00.4   **Malignant neoplasm of lower lip, inner aspect**
  Malignant neoplasm of buccal aspect of lower lip
  Malignant neoplasm of frenulum of lower lip
  Malignant neoplasm of mucosa of lower lip
  Malignant neoplasm of oral aspect of lower lip

C00.5   **Malignant neoplasm of lip, unspecified, inner aspect**
  Malignant neoplasm of buccal aspect of lip, unspecified
  Malignant neoplasm of frenulum of lip, unspecified
  Malignant neoplasm of mucosa of lip, unspecified
  Malignant neoplasm of oral aspect of lip, unspecified

C00.6   **Malignant neoplasm of commissure of lip, unspecified**
  Commissure: Site of union of corresponding parts

C00.8   **Malignant neoplasm of overlapping sites of lip**

C00.9   **Malignant neoplasm of lip, unspecified**

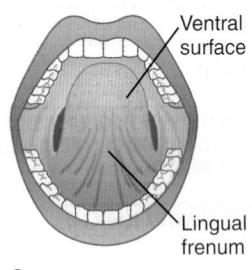

Transitional or vermilion surfaces

Lips are connected to
A   the gums by frenulum

B

- Hard palate
- Soft palate
- Vestibule
- Uvula
- Tonsil
- Dorsal surface (anterior two-thirds of tongue)

Ventral surface

Lingual frenum

C

Figure 2-1 Anatomical structures of the mouth and lips. **A.** Transitional or vermilion borders. Lips are connected to the gums by frenulum. **B.** Dorsal surface. **C.** Ventral surface.

CHAPTER 2 (C00-D49)

C01   Malignant neoplasm of base of tongue 🏷
     Malignant neoplasm of dorsal surface of base of tongue
     Malignant neoplasm of fixed part of tongue NOS
     Malignant neoplasm of posterior third of tongue

     Use additional code to identify:
       alcohol abuse and dependence (F10.-)
       history of tobacco dependence (Z87.891)
       tobacco dependence (F17.-)
       tobacco use (Z72.0)

● **C02**   Malignant neoplasm of other and unspecified parts of tongue
     Use additional code to identify:
       alcohol abuse and dependence (F10.-)
       history of tobacco dependence (Z87.891)
       tobacco dependence (F17.-)
       tobacco use (Z72.0)

    C02.0   Malignant neoplasm of dorsal surface of tongue 🏷
       Malignant neoplasm of anterior two-thirds of tongue, dorsal surface

       Excludes2   malignant neoplasm of dorsal surface of base of tongue (C01)

    C02.1   Malignant neoplasm of border of tongue 🏷
       Malignant neoplasm of tip of tongue

    C02.2   Malignant neoplasm of ventral surface of tongue 🏷
       Malignant neoplasm of anterior two-thirds of tongue, ventral surface
       Malignant neoplasm of frenulum linguae

    C02.3   Malignant neoplasm of anterior two-thirds of tongue, part unspecified 🏷
       Malignant neoplasm of middle third of tongue NOS
       Malignant neoplasm of mobile part of tongue NOS

    C02.4   Malignant neoplasm of lingual tonsil 🏷
       Lingual tonsil: Aggregation of lymph follicles at root of tongue

       Excludes2   malignant neoplasm of tonsil NOS (C09.9)

    C02.8   Malignant neoplasm of overlapping sites of tongue 🏷
       Malignant neoplasm of two or more contiguous sites of tongue

    C02.9   Malignant neoplasm of tongue, unspecified 🏷

● **C03**   Malignant neoplasm of gum
    Includes   malignant neoplasm of alveolar (ridge) mucosa
       malignant neoplasm of gingiva

    Use additional code to identify:
       alcohol abuse and dependence (F10.-)
       history of tobacco dependence (Z87.891)
       tobacco dependence (F17.-)
       tobacco use (Z72.0)

    Excludes2   malignant odontogenic neoplasms (C41.0-C41.1)

    C03.0   Malignant neoplasm of upper gum 🏷
    C03.1   Malignant neoplasm of lower gum 🏷
    C03.9   Malignant neoplasm of gum, unspecified 🏷

● **C04**   Malignant neoplasm of floor of mouth
    Use additional code to identify:
       alcohol abuse and dependence (F10.-)
       history of tobacco dependence (Z87.891)
       tobacco dependence (F17.-)
       tobacco use (Z72.0)

    C04.0   Malignant neoplasm of anterior floor of mouth 🏷
       Malignant neoplasm of anterior to the premolar-canine junction

    C04.1   Malignant neoplasm of lateral floor of mouth 🏷
    C04.8   Malignant neoplasm of overlapping sites of floor of mouth 🏷
    C04.9   Malignant neoplasm of floor of mouth, unspecified 🏷

● **C05**   Malignant neoplasm of palate
    Use additional code to identify:
       alcohol abuse and dependence (F10.-)
       history of tobacco dependence (Z87.891)
       tobacco dependence (F17.-)
       tobacco use (Z72.0)

    Excludes1   Kaposi's sarcoma of palate (C46.2)

    C05.0   Malignant neoplasm of hard palate 🏷
    C05.1   Malignant neoplasm of soft palate 🏷

       Excludes2   malignant neoplasm of nasopharyngeal surface of soft palate (C11.3)

    C05.2   Malignant neoplasm of uvula 🏷
    C05.8   Malignant neoplasm of overlapping sites of palate 🏷
    C05.9   Malignant neoplasm of palate, unspecified 🏷
       Malignant neoplasm of roof of mouth

● **C06**   Malignant neoplasm of other and unspecified parts of mouth
    Use additional code to identify:
       alcohol abuse and dependence (F10.-)
       history of tobacco dependence (Z87.891)
       tobacco dependence (F17.-)
       tobacco use (Z72.0)

    C06.0   Malignant neoplasm of cheek mucosa 🏷
       Malignant neoplasm of buccal mucosa NOS
       Malignant neoplasm of internal cheek

    C06.1   Malignant neoplasm of vestibule of mouth 🏷
       Malignant neoplasm of buccal sulcus (upper) (lower)
       Malignant neoplasm of labial sulcus (upper) (lower)

    C06.2   Malignant neoplasm of retromolar area 🏷
●   **C06.8**   Malignant neoplasm of overlapping sites of other and unspecified parts of mouth

       C06.80   Malignant neoplasm of overlapping sites of unspecified parts of mouth 🏷

       C06.89   Malignant neoplasm of overlapping sites of other parts of mouth 🏷
          'book leaf' neoplasm [ventral surface of tongue and floor of mouth]

    C06.9   Malignant neoplasm of mouth, unspecified 🏷
       Malignant neoplasm of minor salivary gland, unspecified site
       Malignant neoplasm of oral cavity NOS

▶ New   ⇒ Revised   ~~deleted~~ Deleted   Excludes 1   Excludes 2   Includes   Use additional   Code first   Code also   Key words
OGCR Official Guidelines   X Assign placeholder X   ● Use Additional Character(s)   ▶ Manifestation Code   🏷 Hierarchical Condition Category   **Coding Clinic**

Parotid gland
Sublingual gland
Submandibular gland

Figure 2-2 Major salivary glands.

C07   Malignant neoplasm of parotid gland 🦠
Use additional code to identify:
alcohol abuse and dependence (F10.-)
exposure to environmental tobacco smoke (Z77.22)
exposure to tobacco smoke in the perinatal period (P96.81)
history of tobacco dependence (Z87.891)
occupational exposure to environmental tobacco smoke (Z57.31)
tobacco dependence (F17.-)
tobacco use (Z72.0)

● **C08   Malignant neoplasm of other and unspecified major salivary glands**
    Includes   malignant neoplasm of salivary ducts
Use additional code to identify:
alcohol abuse and dependence (F10.-)
exposure to environmental tobacco smoke (Z77.22)
exposure to tobacco smoke in the perinatal period (P96.81)
history of tobacco dependence (Z87.891)
occupational exposure to environmental tobacco smoke (Z57.31)
tobacco dependence (F17.-)
tobacco use (Z72.0)
    Excludes1   malignant neoplasms of specified minor salivary glands which are classified according to their anatomical location
    Excludes2   malignant neoplasms of minor salivary glands NOS (C06.9)
malignant neoplasm of parotid gland (C07)

C08.0   Malignant neoplasm of submandibular gland 🦠
Malignant neoplasm of submaxillary gland

C08.1   Malignant neoplasm of sublingual gland 🦠

C08.9   Malignant neoplasm of major salivary gland, unspecified 🦠
Malignant neoplasm of salivary gland (major) NOS

★ **(See Plate 28 of the Anatomy Illustrations.)**

● **C09   Malignant neoplasm of tonsil**
Use additional code to identify:
alcohol abuse and dependence (F10.-)
exposure to environmental tobacco smoke (Z77.22)
exposure to tobacco smoke in the perinatal period (P96.81)
history of tobacco dependence (Z87.891)
occupational exposure to environmental tobacco smoke (Z57.31)
tobacco dependence (F17.-)
tobacco use (Z72.0)
    Excludes2   malignant neoplasm of lingual tonsil (C02.4)
malignant neoplasm of pharyngeal tonsil (C11.1)

C09.0   Malignant neoplasm of tonsillar fossa 🦠
Surface of palatine (two masses of lymphatic tissue on sides of throat) tonsils

C09.1   Malignant neoplasm of tonsillar pillar (anterior) (posterior) 🦠
Extension from palatine (two masses of lymphatic tissue on sides of throat) tonsils

C09.8   Malignant neoplasm of overlapping sites of tonsil 🦠

C09.9   Malignant neoplasm of tonsil, unspecified 🦠
Malignant neoplasm of tonsil NOS
Malignant neoplasm of faucial tonsils
Malignant neoplasm of palatine tonsils

● **C10   Malignant neoplasm of oropharynx**
Area of throat at back of mouth
Use additional code to identify:
alcohol abuse and dependence (F10.-)
exposure to environmental tobacco smoke (Z77.22)
exposure to tobacco smoke in the perinatal period (P96.81)
history of tobacco dependence (Z87.891)
occupational exposure to environmental tobacco smoke (Z57.31)
tobacco dependence (F17.-)
tobacco use (Z72.0)
    Excludes2   malignant neoplasm of tonsil (C09.-)

C10.0   Malignant neoplasm of vallecula 🦠
Vallecula, depression or furrow

C10.1   Malignant neoplasm of anterior surface of epiglottis 🦠
Malignant neoplasm of epiglottis, free border [margin]
Malignant neoplasm of glossoepiglottic fold(s)
    Excludes2   malignant neoplasm of epiglottis (suprahyoid portion) NOS (C32.1)

C10.2   Malignant neoplasm of lateral wall of oropharynx 🦠

C10.3   Malignant neoplasm of posterior wall of oropharynx 🦠

C10.4   Malignant neoplasm of branchial cleft 🦠
Congenital slitlike openings formed between branchial arches pharyngeal groove
Malignant neoplasm of branchial cyst [site of neoplasm]

C10.8   Malignant neoplasm of overlapping sites of oropharynx 🦠
Malignant neoplasm of junctional region of oropharynx

C10.9   Malignant neoplasm of oropharynx, unspecified 🦠

● **C11   Malignant neoplasm of nasopharynx**
Use additional code to identify:
exposure to environmental tobacco smoke (Z77.22)
exposure to tobacco smoke in the perinatal period (P96.81)
history of tobacco dependence (Z87.891)
occupational exposure to environmental tobacco smoke (Z57.31)
tobacco dependence (F17.-)
tobacco use (Z72.0)

C11.0   Malignant neoplasm of superior wall of nasopharynx 🦠
Part of pharynx that lies above soft palate
Malignant neoplasm of roof of nasopharynx

C11.1   Malignant neoplasm of posterior wall of nasopharynx 🦠
Malignant neoplasm of adenoid
Malignant neoplasm of pharyngeal tonsil

C11.2   Malignant neoplasm of lateral wall of nasopharynx 🦠
Malignant neoplasm of fossa of Rosenmüller
Malignant neoplasm of opening of auditory tube
Malignant neoplasm of pharyngeal recess

C11.3   Malignant neoplasm of anterior wall of nasopharynx 🦠
Malignant neoplasm of floor of nasopharynx
Malignant neoplasm of nasopharyngeal (anterior) (posterior) surface of soft palate
Malignant neoplasm of posterior margin of nasal choana
Malignant neoplasm of posterior margin of nasal septum

C11.8   Malignant neoplasm of overlapping sites of nasopharynx 🦠

C11.9   Malignant neoplasm of nasopharynx, unspecified 🦠
Malignant neoplasm of nasopharyngeal wall NOS

C12   Malignant neoplasm of pyriform sinus 🦠
Malignant neoplasm of pyriform fossa
Use additional code to identify:
exposure to environmental tobacco smoke (Z77.22)
exposure to tobacco smoke in the perinatal period (P96.81)
history of tobacco dependence (Z87.891)
occupational exposure to environmental tobacco smoke (Z57.31)
tobacco dependence (F17.-)
tobacco use (Z72.0)

CHAPTER 2 (C00-D49)

● **C13**   **Malignant neoplasm of hypopharynx**
Use additional code to identify:
exposure to environmental tobacco smoke (Z77.22)
exposure to tobacco smoke in the perinatal period (P96.81)
history of tobacco dependence (Z87.891)
occupational exposure to environmental tobacco smoke
(Z57.31)
tobacco dependence (F17.-)
tobacco use (Z72.0)
Excludes2   malignant neoplasm of pyriform sinus (C12)

C13.0   **Malignant neoplasm of postcricoid region** 🔗
Behind the cricoid cartilage of neck

C13.1   **Malignant neoplasm of aryepiglottic fold, hypopharyngeal aspect** 🔗
Arytenoepiglottic fold, triangular opening between side of epiglottis and apex of arytenoid cartilage
Malignant neoplasm of aryepiglottic fold, marginal zone
Malignant neoplasm of aryepiglottic fold NOS
Malignant neoplasm of interarytenoid fold, marginal zone
Malignant neoplasm of interarytenoid fold NOS
Excludes2   malignant neoplasm of aryepiglottic fold or interarytenoid fold, laryngeal aspect (C32.1)

C13.2   **Malignant neoplasm of posterior wall of hypopharynx** 🔗

C13.8   **Malignant neoplasm of overlapping sites of hypopharynx** 🔗

C13.9   **Malignant neoplasm of hypopharynx, unspecified** 🔗
Malignant neoplasm of hypopharyngeal wall NOS

● **C14**   **Malignant neoplasm of other and ill-defined sites in the lip, oral cavity and pharynx**
Use additional code to identify:
alcohol abuse and dependence (F10.-)
exposure to environmental tobacco smoke (Z77.22)
exposure to tobacco smoke in the perinatal period (P96.81)
history of tobacco dependence (Z87.891)
occupational exposure to environmental tobacco smoke
(Z57.31)
tobacco dependence (F17.-)
tobacco use (Z72.0)
Excludes1   malignant neoplasm of oral cavity NOS (C06.9)

C14.0   **Malignant neoplasm of pharynx, unspecified** 🔗

C14.2   **Malignant neoplasm of Waldeyer's ring** 🔗

C14.8   **Malignant neoplasm of overlapping sites of lip, oral cavity and pharynx** 🔗
Primary malignant neoplasm of two or more contiguous sites of lip, oral cavity and pharynx
Excludes1   'book leaf' neoplasm [ventral surface of tongue and floor of mouth] (C06.89)

MALIGNANT NEOPLASM OF DIGESTIVE ORGANS (C15-C26)

Excludes1   Kaposi's sarcoma of gastrointestinal sites (C46.4)
Excludes2   gastrointestinal stromal tumors (C49.A-)

● **C15**   **Malignant neoplasms of esophagus**
Use additional code to identify:
alcohol abuse and dependence (F10.-)

C15.3   **Malignant neoplasm of upper third of esophagus** 🔗

C15.4   **Malignant neoplasm of middle third of esophagus** 🔗

C15.5   **Malignant neoplasm of lower third of esophagus** 🔗
Excludes1   malignant neoplasm of cardio-esophageal junction (C16.0)

C15.8   **Malignant neoplasm of overlapping sites of esophagus** 🔗

C15.9   **Malignant neoplasm of esophagus, unspecified** 🔗

● **C16**   **Malignant neoplasm of stomach**
Use additional code to identify:
alcohol abuse and dependence (F10.-)
Excludes2   malignant carcinoid tumor of the stomach (C7A.092)

C16.0   **Malignant neoplasm of cardia** 🔗
Malignant neoplasm of cardiac orifice
Malignant neoplasm of cardio-esophageal junction
Malignant neoplasm of esophagus and stomach
Malignant neoplasm of gastro-esophageal junction

C16.1   **Malignant neoplasm of fundus of stomach** 🔗

C16.2   **Malignant neoplasm of body of stomach** 🔗

C16.3   **Malignant neoplasm of pyloric antrum** 🔗
Malignant neoplasm of gastric antrum

C16.4   **Malignant neoplasm of pylorus** 🔗
Malignant neoplasm of prepylorus
Malignant neoplasm of pyloric canal

C16.5   **Malignant neoplasm of lesser curvature of stomach, unspecified** 🔗
Malignant neoplasm of lesser curvature of stomach, not classifiable to C16.1-C16.4

C16.6   **Malignant neoplasm of greater curvature of stomach, unspecified** 🔗
Malignant neoplasm of greater curvature of stomach, not classifiable to C16.0-C16.4

C16.8   **Malignant neoplasm of overlapping sites of stomach** 🔗

C16.9   **Malignant neoplasm of stomach, unspecified** 🔗
Gastric cancer NOS

Figure 2-3   The esophagus is the muscular tube that connects the pharynx and the stomach. The 10 inch (25 cm) long esophagus is divided into three parts: **cervical, thoracic,** and **abdominal.**

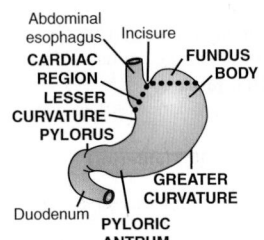

Figure 2-4   Parts of the stomach.

Item 2–2   The esophagus opens into the stomach through the **cardiac orifice,** also called the **cardioesophageal junction.** The **cardia** is adjacent to the cardiac orifice. The stomach widens into the **greater** and **lesser curvatures.** The **pyloric antrum** precedes the **pylorus,** which opens to the duodenum.

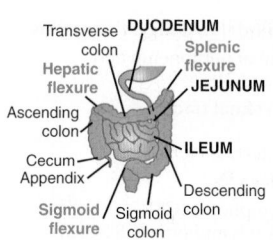

Transverse
colon **DUODENUM**
Hepatic   **Splenic**
flexure   **flexure**
Ascending   **JEJUNUM**
colon
Cecum   → **ILEUM**
Appendix
     Descending
Sigmoid / Sigmoid   colon
flexure   colon

Figure 2-5   Small intestine and colon.

● **C17   Malignant neoplasm of small intestine**

     Excludes1   malignant carcinoid tumor of the small intestine (C7A.01)

   C17.0   Malignant neoplasm of duodenum 🔍
     First or proximal portion of small intestine, extending from pylorus to jejunum

   C17.1   Malignant neoplasm of jejunum 🔍
     Second section of small intestine, extending from duodenum to ileum

   C17.2   Malignant neoplasm of ileum 🔍
     Distal and longest portion of small intestine, extending from jejunum to cecum

     Excludes1   malignant neoplasm of ileocecal valve (C18.0)

   C17.3   Meckel's diverticulum, malignant 🔍
     Appendage of ileum

     Excludes1   Meckel's diverticulum, congenital (Q43.0)

   C17.8   Malignant neoplasm of overlapping sites of small intestine 🔍

   C17.9   Malignant neoplasm of small intestine, unspecified 🔍

● **C18   Malignant neoplasm of colon**

     Excludes1   malignant carcinoid tumors of the colon (C7A.02)

   C18.0   Malignant neoplasm of cecum 🔍
     First section of large intestine
     Malignant neoplasm of ileocecal valve

   C18.1   Malignant neoplasm of appendix 🔍
     Blind ended tube connected to the cecum; AKA vermiform appendix

   C18.2   Malignant neoplasm of ascending colon 🔍
     Ascending colon is between cecum and right colic flexure

   C18.3   Malignant neoplasm of hepatic flexure 🔍
     A flexure is a bending in a structure or organ. Note the three flexures illustrated in Figure 2–5.

   C18.4   Malignant neoplasm of transverse colon 🔍
     Portion of colon that runs transversely across upper part of abdomen, between right and left colic flexures

   C18.5   Malignant neoplasm of splenic flexure 🔍
     Bend at junction of transverse and descending colon

   C18.6   Malignant neoplasm of descending colon 🔍
     Portion between left colic flexure and sigmoid colon at pelvic brim; AKA iliac colon

   C18.7   Malignant neoplasm of sigmoid colon 🔍
     S-shaped part of colon extending from pelvic brim to third segment of sacrum
     Malignant neoplasm of sigmoid (flexure)

     Excludes1   malignant neoplasm of rectosigmoid junction (C19)

   C18.8   Malignant neoplasm of overlapping sites of colon 🔍

   C18.9   Malignant neoplasm of colon, unspecified 🔍
     Malignant neoplasm of large intestine NOS

C19   Malignant neoplasm of rectosigmoid junction 🔍
     Malignant neoplasm of colon with rectum
     Malignant neoplasm of rectosigmoid (colon)

     Excludes1   malignant carcinoid tumors of the colon (C7A.02-)

C20   Malignant neoplasm of rectum 🔍
     Malignant neoplasm of rectal ampulla

     Excludes1   malignant carcinoid tumor of the rectum (C7A.026)

● **C21   Malignant neoplasm of anus and anal canal**

     Excludes2   malignant carcinoid tumors of the colon (C7A.02-)
         malignant melanoma of anal margin (C43.51)
         malignant melanoma of anal skin (C43.51)
         malignant melanoma of perianal skin (C43.51)
         other and unspecified malignant neoplasm of anal margin (C44.500, C44.510, C44.520, C44.590)
         other and unspecified malignant neoplasm of anal skin (C44.500, C44.510, C44.520, C44.590)
         other and unspecified malignant neoplasm of perianal skin (C44.500, C44.510, C44.520, C44.590)

   C21.0   Malignant neoplasm of anus, unspecified 🔍

   C21.1   Malignant neoplasm of anal canal 🔍
     Terminal part of large intestine
     Malignant neoplasm of anal sphincter

   C21.2   Malignant neoplasm of cloacogenic zone 🔍

   C21.8   Malignant neoplasm of overlapping sites of rectum, anus and anal canal 🔍
     Malignant neoplasm of anorectal junction
     Malignant neoplasm of anorectum
     Primary malignant neoplasm of two or more contiguous sites of rectum, anus and anal canal

● **C22   Malignant neoplasm of liver and intrahepatic bile ducts**
     Intrahepatic: Within liver

     Use additional code to identify:
         alcohol abuse and dependence (F10.-)
         hepatitis B (B16.-, B18.0-B18.1) hepatitis C (B17.1-, B18.2)

     Excludes1   malignant neoplasm of biliary tract NOS (C24.9)
         secondary malignant neoplasm of liver and intrahepatic bile duct (C78.7)

   C22.0   Liver cell carcinoma 🔍
     Hepatocellular carcinoma
     Hepatoma

   C22.1   Intrahepatic bile duct carcinoma 🔍
     Cholangiocarcinoma
     Adenocarcinoma (cancer that originates in glandular tissue) arising from epithelium of intrahepatic bile ducts

     Excludes1   malignant neoplasm of hepatic duct (C24.0)

   C22.2   Hepatoblastoma 🔍
     Malignant intrahepatic tumor

   C22.3   Angiosarcoma of liver 🔍
     Kupffer cell sarcoma

   C22.4   Other sarcomas of liver 🔍

   C22.7   Other specified carcinomas of liver 🔍

   C22.8   Malignant neoplasm of liver, primary, unspecified as to type 🔍

   C22.9   Malignant neoplasm of liver, not specified as primary or secondary 🔍

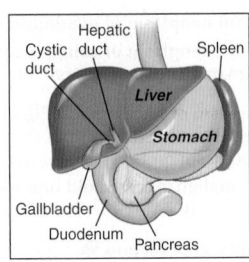

Figure 2-6 Diagram of liver, gallbladder, hepatic duct, pancreas, and spleen. (From Thibodeau and Patton: Anatomy and Physiology, ed 7, Mosby, 2010)

C23 Malignant neoplasm of gallbladder 🐾

● C24 Malignant neoplasm of other and unspecified parts of biliary tract
     Excludes1 malignant neoplasm of intrahepatic bile duct (C22.1)

    C24.0 Malignant neoplasm of extrahepatic bile duct 🐾
        Extrahepatic = outside the liver
        Malignant neoplasm of biliary duct or passage NOS
        Malignant neoplasm of common bile duct
        Malignant neoplasm of cystic duct
        Malignant neoplasm of hepatic duct

    C24.1 Malignant neoplasm of ampulla of Vater 🐾
        Union of pancreatic duct and common bile duct

    C24.8 Malignant neoplasm of overlapping sites of biliary tract 🐾
        Malignant neoplasm involving both intrahepatic and extrahepatic bile ducts
        Primary malignant neoplasm of two or more contiguous sites of biliary tract

    C24.9 Malignant neoplasm of biliary tract, unspecified 🐾

● C25 Malignant neoplasm of pancreas
    Check documentation for specific site.
    ➡ Code also if applicable exocrine pancreatic insufficiency (K86.81)
    Use additional code to identify:
        alcohol abuse and dependence (F10.-)

    C25.0 Malignant neoplasm of head of pancreas 🐾
    C25.1 Malignant neoplasm of body of pancreas 🐾
        Coding Clinic: 2018, Q4, P40
    C25.2 Malignant neoplasm of tail of pancreas 🐾
    C25.3 Malignant neoplasm of pancreatic duct 🐾
    C25.4 Malignant neoplasm of endocrine pancreas 🐾
        Malignant neoplasm of islets of Langerhans
        That part of the pancreas that acts as endocrine gland and consists of islets of Langerhans
        Use additional code to identify any functional activity.
    C25.7 Malignant neoplasm of other parts of pancreas 🐾
        Malignant neoplasm of neck of pancreas
    C25.8 Malignant neoplasm of overlapping sites of pancreas 🐾
    C25.9 Malignant neoplasm of pancreas, unspecified 🐾

Item 2-3 **Islets** of Langerhans (endocrine producing cells comprising 1% to 2% of the pancreatic mass) make and secrete hormones that regulate the body's production of insulin, glucagon, and stomach acid. Breakdown of the insulin-producing cells can cause diabetes mellitus. Islet cell tumors can be benign or malignant and include glucagonomas, insulinomas, gastrinomas, and neuroendocrine tumor. The neoplasm table must be consulted for the correct neoplasm code.

Figure 2-7 Paranasal sinuses. (From Buck CJ: Step-by-Step Medical Coding, ed 2016, St. Louis, Elsevier, 2016)

● C26 Malignant neoplasm of other and ill-defined digestive organs
     Excludes1 malignant neoplasm of peritoneum and retroperitoneum (C48.-)

    C26.0 Malignant neoplasm of intestinal tract, part unspecified 🐾
        Malignant neoplasm of intestine NOS

    C26.1 Malignant neoplasm of spleen 🐾
        Excludes1 Hodgkin lymphoma (C81.-)
                 non-Hodgkin lymphoma (C82-C85)

    C26.9 Malignant neoplasm of ill-defined sites within the digestive system 🐾
        Malignant neoplasm of alimentary canal or tract NOS
        Malignant neoplasm of gastrointestinal tract NOS
        Excludes1 malignant neoplasm of abdominal NOS (C76.2)
                 malignant neoplasm of intra-abdominal NOS (C76.2)

MALIGNANT NEOPLASMS OF RESPIRATORY AND INTRATHORACIC ORGANS (C30-C39)

    Includes malignant neoplasm of middle ear
    Excludes1 mesothelioma (C45.-)

● C30 Malignant neoplasm of nasal cavity and middle ear
    C30.0 Malignant neoplasm of nasal cavity 🐾
        Malignant neoplasm of cartilage of nose
        Malignant neoplasm of nasal concha
        Malignant neoplasm of internal nose
        Malignant neoplasm of septum of nose
        Malignant neoplasm of vestibule of nose
        Anterior part of nasal cavity
        Excludes1 malignant neoplasm of nasal bone (C41.0)
                 malignant neoplasm of nose NOS (C76.0)
                 malignant neoplasm of olfactory bulb (C72.2-)
                 malignant neoplasm of posterior margin of nasal septum and choana (C11.3)
                 malignant melanoma of skin of nose (C43.31)
           ➡ malignant neoplasm of turbinates (C41.0)
                 other and unspecified malignant neoplasm of skin of nose (C44.301, C44.311, C44.321, C44.391)

    C30.1 Malignant neoplasm of middle ear 🐾
        Malignant neoplasm of antrum tympanicum
        Boney cavity or chamber
        Malignant neoplasm of auditory tube
        Malignant neoplasm of eustachian tube
        Malignant neoplasm of inner ear
        Malignant neoplasm of mastoid air cells
        Malignant neoplasm of tympanic cavity
        Excludes1 malignant neoplasm of auricular canal (external) (C43.2-, C44.2-)
                 malignant neoplasm of bone of ear (meatus) (C41.0)
                 malignant neoplasm of cartilage of ear (C49.0)
                 malignant melanoma of skin of (external) ear (C43.2-)
                 other and unspecified malignant neoplasm of skin of (external) ear (C44.2-)

● C31 Malignant neoplasm of accessory sinuses
    Paired sinuses in bones of face
    C31.0 Malignant neoplasm of maxillary sinus 🐾
        Malignant neoplasm of antrum (Highmore) (maxillary)
    C31.1 Malignant neoplasm of ethmoidal sinus 🐾
    C31.2 Malignant neoplasm of frontal sinus 🐾
    C31.3 Malignant neoplasm of sphenoid sinus 🐾
    C31.8 Malignant neoplasm of overlapping sites of accessory sinuses 🐾
    C31.9 Malignant neoplasm of accessory sinus, unspecified 🐾

▶ New   ➡ Revised   ~~deleted~~ Deleted   Excludes 1   Excludes 2   Includes   Use additional   Code first   Code also   Key words

OGCR Official Guidelines   X Assign placeholder X   ● Use Additional Character(s)   ▸ Manifestation Code   🐾 Hierarchical Condition Category   **Coding Clinic**

● **C32**   **Malignant neoplasm of larynx**

     Use additional code to identify:
        alcohol abuse and dependence (F10.-)
        exposure to environmental tobacco smoke (Z77.22)
        exposure to tobacco smoke in the perinatal period (P96.81)
        history of tobacco dependence (Z87.891)
        occupational exposure to environmental tobacco smoke
          (Z57.31)
        tobacco dependence (F17.-)
        tobacco use (Z72.0)

   C32.0   **Malignant neoplasm of glottis** 🔎
       Vocal apparatus of larynx, consisting of true vocal cords (plicae vocales) and opening between them (rima glottidis)
       Malignant neoplasm of intrinsic larynx
       Malignant neoplasm of laryngeal commissure (anterior) (posterior)
       Malignant neoplasm of vocal cord (true) NOS
         True vocal cords ("lower vocal folds") produce vocalization when air from the lungs passes between them. Check your documentation. Code C32.1 is for malignant neoplasm of the false vocal cords.

   C32.1   **Malignant neoplasm of supraglottis** 🔎
       Area of pharynx above glottis
       Malignant neoplasm of aryepiglottic fold or interarytenoid fold, laryngeal aspect
       Malignant neoplasm of epiglottis (suprahyoid portion) NOS
       Malignant neoplasm of extrinsic larynx
       Malignant neoplasm of false vocal cord
         False vocal cords ("upper vocal folds") are not involved in vocalization. Check your documentation. Code C32.0 is for true vocal cords.
       Malignant neoplasm of posterior (laryngeal) surface of epiglottis
       Malignant neoplasm of ventricular bands

     Excludes2   malignant neoplasm of anterior surface of epiglottis (C10.1)
          malignant neoplasm of aryepiglottic fold or interarytenoid fold, hypopharyngeal aspect (C13.1)
          malignant neoplasm of aryepiglottic fold or interarytenoid fold, marginal zone (C13.1)
          malignant neoplasm of aryepiglottic fold or interarytenoid fold NOS (C13.1)

   C32.2   **Malignant neoplasm of subglottis** 🔎
       Lowest part of larynx from just below vocal cords down to top of trachea

   C32.3   **Malignant neoplasm of laryngeal cartilage** 🔎
       Cartilages of larynx, including cricoid, thyroid, and epiglottic, and two each of arytenoid, corniculate, and cuneiform

   C32.8   **Malignant neoplasm of overlapping sites of larynx** 🔎

   C32.9   **Malignant neoplasm of larynx, unspecified** 🔎

● **C33**   **Malignant neoplasm of trachea** 🔎

     Use additional code to identify:
        exposure to environmental tobacco smoke (Z77.22)
        exposure to tobacco smoke in the perinatal period (P96.81)
        history of tobacco dependence (Z87.891)
        occupational exposure to environmental tobacco smoke
          (Z57.31)
        tobacco dependence (F17.-)
        tobacco use (Z72.0)

● **C34**   **Malignant neoplasm of bronchus and lung**

     Use additional code to identify:
        exposure to environmental tobacco smoke (Z77.22)
        exposure to tobacco smoke in the perinatal period (P96.81)
        history of tobacco dependence (Z87.891)
        occupational exposure to environmental tobacco smoke
          (Z57.31)
        tobacco dependence (F17.-)
        tobacco use (Z72.0)

     Excludes1   Kaposi's sarcoma of lung (C46.5-)
          malignant carcinoid tumor of the bronchus and lung (C7A.090)

   ● **C34.0**   **Malignant neoplasm of main bronchus**
       Malignant neoplasm of carina
         Ridgelike structure
       Malignant neoplasm of hilus (of lung)
         Anatomic depression or pit

     C34.00   **Malignant neoplasm of unspecified main bronchus** 🔎

     C34.01   **Malignant neoplasm of right main bronchus** 🔎

     C34.02   **Malignant neoplasm of left main bronchus** 🔎

   ● **C34.1**   **Malignant neoplasm of upper lobe, bronchus or lung**

     C34.10   **Malignant neoplasm of unspecified bronchus or lung** 🔎

     C34.11   **Malignant neoplasm of upper lobe, right bronchus or lung** 🔎

     C34.12   **Malignant neoplasm of upper lobe, left bronchus or lung** 🔎

   C34.2   **Malignant neoplasm of middle lobe, bronchus or lung** 🔎

   ● **C34.3**   **Malignant neoplasm of lower lobe, bronchus or lung**

     C34.30   **Malignant neoplasm of lower lobe, unspecified bronchus or lung** 🔎

     C34.31   **Malignant neoplasm of lower lobe, right bronchus or lung** 🔎

     C34.32   **Malignant neoplasm of lower lobe, left bronchus or lung** 🔎

   ● **C34.8**   **Malignant neoplasm of overlapping sites of bronchus and lung**

     C34.80   **Malignant neoplasm of overlapping sites of unspecified bronchus and lung** 🔎

     C34.81   **Malignant neoplasm of overlapping sites of right bronchus and lung** 🔎

     C34.82   **Malignant neoplasm of overlapping sites of left bronchus and lung** 🔎

   ● **C34.9**   **Malignant neoplasm of unspecified part of bronchus or lung**

     C34.90   **Malignant neoplasm of unspecified part of unspecified bronchus or lung** 🔎
         Lung cancer NOS

     C34.91   **Malignant neoplasm of unspecified part of right bronchus or lung** 🔎

     C34.92   **Malignant neoplasm of unspecified part of left bronchus or lung** 🔎

  C37   **Malignant neoplasm of thymus** 🔎

     Excludes1   malignant carcinoid tumor of the thymus (C7A.091)

CHAPTER 2 (C00–D49)

● C38 Malignant neoplasm of heart, mediastinum and pleura
       Excludes1 mesothelioma (C45.-)

   C38.0 Malignant neoplasm of heart 🦠
          Malignant neoplasm of pericardium
          Excludes1 malignant neoplasm of great vessels
                         (C49.3)

   C38.1 Malignant neoplasm of anterior mediastinum 🦠

   C38.2 Malignant neoplasm of posterior mediastinum 🦠

   C38.3 Malignant neoplasm of mediastinum,
          part unspecified 🦠

   C38.4 Malignant neoplasm of pleura 🦠

   C38.8 Malignant neoplasm of overlapping sites of heart,
          mediastinum and pleura 🦠
          *Pleura are comprised of serous membrane that lines the
          thoracic cavity (parietal) and covers the lungs (visceral).*

● C39 Malignant neoplasm of other and ill-defined sites in the
       respiratory system and intrathoracic organs
       Intrathoracic: within thorax/chest
       Use additional code to identify:
          exposure to environmental tobacco smoke (Z77.22)
          exposure to tobacco smoke in the perinatal period (P96.81)
          history of tobacco dependence (Z87.891)
          occupational exposure to environmental tobacco smoke
             (Z57.31)
          tobacco dependence (F17.-)
          tobacco use (Z72.0)
       Excludes1 intrathoracic malignant neoplasm NOS (C76.1)
                      thoracic malignant neoplasm NOS (C76.1)

   C39.0 Malignant neoplasm of upper respiratory tract,
          part unspecified 🦠

   C39.9 Malignant neoplasm of lower respiratory tract,
          part unspecified 🦠
          Malignant neoplasm of respiratory tract NOS

MALIGNANT NEOPLASMS OF BONE AND ARTICULAR CARTILAGE (C40-C41)

       Includes   malignant neoplasm of cartilage (articular) (joint)
                       malignant neoplasm of periosteum
       Excludes1   malignant neoplasm of bone marrow NOS (C96.9)
                       malignant neoplasm of synovia (C49.-)

● C40 Malignant neoplasm of bone and articular cartilage of limbs
       Use additional code to identify major osseous defect, if
       applicable (M89.7-)

 ● C40.0 Malignant neoplasm of scapula and long bones of upper
          limb
       C40.00 Malignant neoplasm of scapula and long bones
               of unspecified upper limb 🦠
       C40.01 Malignant neoplasm of scapula and long bones
               of right upper limb 🦠
       C40.02 Malignant neoplasm of scapula and long bones
               of left upper limb 🦠

 ● C40.1 Malignant neoplasm of short bones of upper limb
       C40.10 Malignant neoplasm of short bones
               of unspecified upper limb 🦠
       C40.11 Malignant neoplasm of short bones of right
               upper limb 🦠
       C40.12 Malignant neoplasm of short bones of left
               upper limb 🦠

 ● C40.2 Malignant neoplasm of long bones of lower limb
       C40.20 Malignant neoplasm of long bones
               of unspecified lower limb 🦠
       C40.21 Malignant neoplasm of long bones of right
               lower limb 🦠
       C40.22 Malignant neoplasm of long bones of left lower
               limb 🦠

Figure 2-8 Diagram of skeleton of trunk and limbs with bones labeled.
(From Thibodeau and Patton: Anatomy and Physiology, ed 7, Mosby,
2010)

 ● C40.3 Malignant neoplasm of short bones of lower limb
       C40.30 Malignant neoplasm of short bones
               of unspecified lower limb 🦠
       C40.31 Malignant neoplasm of short bones of right
               lower limb 🦠
       C40.32 Malignant neoplasm of short bones of left
               lower limb 🦠

 ● C40.8 Malignant neoplasm of overlapping sites of bone and
          articular cartilage of limb
       C40.80 Malignant neoplasm of overlapping sites of
               bone and articular cartilage of unspecified
               limb 🦠
       C40.81 Malignant neoplasm of overlapping sites of
               bone and articular cartilage of right limb 🦠
       C40.82 Malignant neoplasm of overlapping sites of
               bone and articular cartilage of left limb 🦠

 ● C40.9 Malignant neoplasm of unspecified bones and articular
          cartilage of limb
       C40.90 Malignant neoplasm of unspecified bones and
               articular cartilage of unspecified limb 🦠
       C40.91 Malignant neoplasm of unspecified bones and
               articular cartilage of right limb 🦠
       C40.92 Malignant neoplasm of unspecified bones and
               articular cartilage of left limb 🦠

● C41 Malignant neoplasm of bone and articular cartilage of other and
       unspecified sites
       Excludes1   malignant neoplasm of bones of limbs (C40.-)
                       malignant neoplasm of cartilage of ear (C49.0)
                       malignant neoplasm of cartilage of eyelid (C49.0)
                       malignant neoplasm of cartilage of larynx (C32.3)
                       malignant neoplasm of cartilage of limbs (C40.-)
                       malignant neoplasm of cartilage of nose (C30.0)

   C41.0 Malignant neoplasm of bones of skull and face 🦠
          Malignant neoplasm of maxilla (superior)
          Malignant neoplasm of orbital bone
          Excludes2   carcinoma, any type except intraosseous
                          or odontogenic of:
                             maxillary sinus (C31.0)
                             upper jaw (C03.0)
                          malignant neoplasm of jaw bone (lower)
                             (C41.1)

▶ New   ⟾ Revised   ~~deleted~~ Deleted   Excludes 1   Excludes 2   Includes   Use additional   Code first   Code also   Key words

OGCR Official Guidelines   X Assign placeholder X   ● Use Additional Character(s)   ▷ Manifestation Code   🦠 Hierarchical Condition Category   **Coding Clinic**

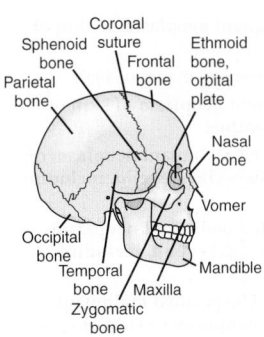

Figure 2-9 Bones of the skull.

Figure 2-10 Malignant melanoma of skin. (Getty Image)

Item 2–4 Malignant melanoma is a serious form of skin cancer that affects the melanocytes (pigment-forming cells) and is caused by ultraviolet (UV) rays from the sun that damage skin. It is most commonly seen in the 40- to 60-year-olds with fair skin, blue or green eyes, and red or blond hair who sunburn easily.

Melanoma can spread very rapidly and is the most deadly form of skin cancer. It is less common than other types of skin cancer. The rate of melanoma is increasing and currently is the leading cause of death from skin disease.

C41.1 Malignant neoplasm of mandible 🔖
    Malignant neoplasm of inferior maxilla
    Malignant neoplasm of lower jaw bone
    Excludes2 carcinoma, any type except intraosseous
            or odontogenic of:
            jaw NOS (C03.9)
            lower (C03.1)
            malignant neoplasm of upper jaw bone
            (C41.0)

C41.2 Malignant neoplasm of vertebral column 🔖
    Excludes1 malignant neoplasm of sacrum and
            coccyx (C41.4)

C41.3 Malignant neoplasm of ribs, sternum and clavicle 🔖

C41.4 Malignant neoplasm of pelvic bones, sacrum and coccyx 🔖

C41.9 Malignant neoplasm of bone and articular cartilage, unspecified 🔖

MELANOMA AND OTHER MALIGNANT NEOPLASMS OF SKIN (C43-C44)

● **C43** Malignant melanoma of skin
    Excludes1 melanoma in situ (D03.-)
    Excludes2 malignant melanoma of skin of genital organs
            (C51-C52, C60.-, C63.-)
            Merkel cell carcinoma (C4A.-)
            sites other than skin-code to malignant neoplasm
            of the site

C43.0 Malignant melanoma of lip 🔖
    Excludes1 malignant neoplasm of vermilion border
            of lip (C00.0-C00.2)

● **C43.1** Malignant melanoma of eyelid, including canthus
    Canthus: Either corner of eye where upper and lower eyelids
    meet
    C43.10 Malignant melanoma of unspecified eyelid,
            including canthus 🔖
    ● **C43.11** Malignant melanoma of right eyelid, including
            canthus 🔖
        C43.111 Malignant melanoma of right upper
                 eyelid, including canthus 🔖
        C43.112 Malignant melanoma of right lower
                 eyelid, including canthus 🔖
    ● **C43.12** Malignant melanoma of left eyelid, including
            canthus 🔖
        C43.121 Malignant melanoma of left upper
                 eyelid, including canthus 🔖
        C43.122 Malignant melanoma of left lower
                 eyelid, including canthus 🔖

● **C43.2** Malignant melanoma of ear and external auricular canal
    C43.20 Malignant melanoma of unspecified ear and
            external auricular canal 🔖
    C43.21 Malignant melanoma of right ear and external
            auricular canal 🔖
    C43.22 Malignant melanoma of left ear and external
            auricular canal 🔖

● **C43.3** Malignant melanoma of other and unspecified parts of face
    C43.30 Malignant melanoma of unspecified part of
            face 🔖
    C43.31 Malignant melanoma of nose 🔖
    C43.39 Malignant melanoma of other parts of face 🔖

C43.4 Malignant melanoma of scalp and neck 🔖

● **C43.5** Malignant melanoma of trunk
    Excludes2 malignant neoplasm of anus NOS (C21.0)
            malignant neoplasm of scrotum (C63.2)
    C43.51 Malignant melanoma of anal skin 🔖
        Malignant melanoma of anal margin
        Malignant melanoma of perianal skin
    C43.52 Malignant melanoma of skin of breast 🔖
    C43.59 Malignant melanoma of other part of trunk 🔖

● **C43.6** Malignant melanoma of upper limb, including shoulder
    C43.60 Malignant melanoma of upper limb, including
            shoulder, unspecified side 🔖
    C43.61 Malignant melanoma of right upper limb,
            including shoulder 🔖
    C43.62 Malignant melanoma of left upper limb,
            including shoulder 🔖

● **C43.7** Malignant melanoma of lower limb, including hip
    C43.70 Malignant melanoma of unspecified lower
            limb, including hip 🔖
    C43.71 Malignant melanoma of right lower limb,
            including hip 🔖
    C43.72 Malignant melanoma of left lower limb,
            including hip 🔖

C43.8 Malignant melanoma of overlapping sites of skin 🔖

C43.9 Malignant melanoma of skin, unspecified 🔖
    Malignant melanoma of unspecified site of skin
    Melanoma (malignant) NOS

● **C4A** Merkel cell carcinoma
    C4A.0 Merkel cell carcinoma of lip 🔖
        Excludes1 malignant neoplasm of vermilion border
                of lip (C00.0-C00.2)

  ● **C4A.1** Merkel cell carcinoma of eyelid, including canthus
      C4A.10 Merkel cell carcinoma of unspecified eyelid,
              including canthus 🔖
      ● **C4A.11** Merkel cell carcinoma of right eyelid, including
             canthus 🔖
         C4A.111 Merkel cell carcinoma of right upper
                  eyelid, including canthus 🔖
         C4A.112 Merkel cell carcinoma of right lower
                  eyelid, including canthus 🔖
      ● **C4A.12** Merkel cell carcinoma of left eyelid, including
             canthus 🔖
         C4A.121 Merkel cell carcinoma of left upper
                  eyelid, including canthus 🔖
         C4A.122 Merkel cell carcinoma of left lower
                  eyelid, including canthus 🔖

CHAPTER 2 (C00-D49)

● **C4A.2** Merkel cell carcinoma of ear and external auricular canal

　　C4A.20 Merkel cell carcinoma of unspecified ear and external auricular canal 🐾

　　C4A.21 Merkel cell carcinoma of right ear and external auricular canal 🐾

　　C4A.22 Merkel cell carcinoma of left ear and external auricular canal 🐾

● **C4A.3** Merkel cell carcinoma of other and unspecified parts of face

　　C4A.30 Merkel cell carcinoma of unspecified part of face 🐾

　　C4A.31 Merkel cell carcinoma of nose 🐾

　　C4A.39 Merkel cell carcinoma of other parts of face 🐾

● **C4A.4** Merkel cell carcinoma of scalp and neck 🐾

● **C4A.5** Merkel cell carcinoma of trunk

　　Excludes2　malignant neoplasm of anus NOS (C21.0)
　　　　　　　　malignant neoplasm of scrotum (C63.2)

　　C4A.51 Merkel cell carcinoma of anal skin 🐾
　　　　　Merkel cell carcinoma of anal margin
　　　　　Merkel cell carcinoma of perianal skin

　　C4A.52 Merkel cell carcinoma of skin of breast 🐾

　　C4A.59 Merkel cell carcinoma of other part of trunk 🐾

● **C4A.6** Merkel cell carcinoma of upper limb, including shoulder

　　C4A.60 Merkel cell carcinoma of unspecified upper limb, including shoulder 🐾

　　C4A.61 Merkel cell carcinoma of right upper limb, including shoulder 🐾

　　C4A.62 Merkel cell carcinoma of left upper limb, including shoulder 🐾

● **C4A.7** Merkel cell carcinoma of lower limb, including hip

　　C4A.70 Merkel cell carcinoma of unspecified lower limb, including hip 🐾

　　C4A.71 Merkel cell carcinoma of right lower limb, including hip 🐾

　　C4A.72 Merkel cell carcinoma of left lower limb, including hip 🐾

● **C4A.8** Merkel cell carcinoma of overlapping sites 🐾

● **C4A.9** Merkel cell carcinoma, unspecified 🐾
　　　　Merkel cell carcinoma of unspecified site
　　　　Merkel cell carcinoma NOS

● **C44** Other and unspecified malignant neoplasm of skin

　　Includes　malignant neoplasm of sebaceous glands
　　　　　　　malignant neoplasm of sweat glands

　　Excludes1　Kaposi's sarcoma of skin (C46.0)
　　　　　　　malignant melanoma of skin (C43.-)
　　　　　　　malignant neoplasm of skin of genital organs
　　　　　　　　　(C51-C52, C60.-, C63.2)
　　　　　　　Merkel cell carcinoma (C4A.-)

● **C44.0** Other and unspecified malignant neoplasm of skin of lip

　　Excludes1　malignant neoplasm of lip (C00.-)

　　C44.00 Unspecified malignant neoplasm of skin of lip

　　C44.01 Basal cell carcinoma of skin of lip

　　C44.02 Squamous cell carcinoma of skin of lip

　　C44.09 Other specified malignant neoplasm of skin of lip

● **C44.1** Other and unspecified malignant neoplasm of skin of eyelid, including canthus

　　Excludes1　connective tissue of eyelid (C49.0)

● **C44.10** Unspecified malignant neoplasm of skin of eyelid, including canthus

　　C44.101 Unspecified malignant neoplasm of skin of unspecified eyelid, including canthus

● **C44.102** Unspecified malignant neoplasm of skin of right eyelid, including canthus

　　　C44.1021 Unspecified malignant neoplasm of skin of right upper eyelid, including canthus

　　　C44.1022 Unspecified malignant neoplasm of skin of right lower eyelid, including canthus

● **C44.109** Unspecified malignant neoplasm of skin of left eyelid, including canthus

　　　C44.1091 Unspecified malignant neoplasm of skin of left upper eyelid, including canthus

　　　C44.1092 Unspecified malignant neoplasm of skin of left lower eyelid, including canthus

● **C44.11** Basal cell carcinoma of skin of eyelid, including canthus

　　C44.111 Basal cell carcinoma of skin of unspecified eyelid, including canthus

● **C44.112** Basal cell carcinoma of skin of right eyelid, including canthus

　　　C44.1121 Basal cell carcinoma of skin of right upper eyelid, including canthus

　　　C44.1122 Basal cell carcinoma of skin of right lower eyelid, including canthus

● **C44.119** Basal cell carcinoma of skin of left eyelid, including canthus

　　　C44.1191 Basal cell carcinoma of skin of left upper eyelid, including canthus

　　　C44.1192 Basal cell carcinoma of skin of left lower eyelid, including canthus

● **C44.12** Squamous cell carcinoma of skin of eyelid, including canthus

　　C44.121 Squamous cell carcinoma of skin of unspecified eyelid, including canthus

● **C44.122** Squamous cell carcinoma of skin of right eyelid, including canthus

　　　C44.1221 Squamous cell carcinoma of skin of right upper eyelid, including canthus

　　　C44.1222 Squamous cell carcinoma of skin of right lower eyelid, including canthus

● **C44.129** Squamous cell carcinoma of skin of left eyelid, including canthus

　　　C44.1291 Squamous cell carcinoma of skin of left upper eyelid, including canthus

　　　C44.1292 Squamous cell carcinoma of skin of left lower eyelid, including canthus

● C44.13   Sebaceous cell carcinoma of skin of eyelid, including canthus

    C44.131   Sebaceous cell carcinoma of skin of unspecified eyelid, including canthus

●   C44.132   Sebaceous cell carcinoma of skin of right eyelid, including canthus

      C44.1321   Sebaceous cell carcinoma of skin of right upper eyelid, including canthus

      C44.1322   Sebaceous cell carcinoma of skin of right lower eyelid, including canthus

●   C44.139   Sebaceous cell carcinoma of skin of left eyelid, including canthus

      C44.1391   Sebaceous cell carcinoma of skin of left upper eyelid, including canthus

      C44.1392   Sebaceous cell carcinoma of skin of left lower eyelid, including canthus

● C44.19   Other specified malignant neoplasm of skin of eyelid, including canthus

    C44.191   Other specified malignant neoplasm of skin of unspecified eyelid, including canthus

●   C44.192   Other specified malignant neoplasm of skin of right eyelid, including canthus

      C44.1921   Other specified malignant neoplasm of skin of right upper eyelid, including canthus

      C44.1922   Other specified malignant neoplasm of skin of right lower eyelid, including canthus

●   C44.199   Other specified malignant neoplasm of skin of left eyelid, including canthus

      C44.1991   Other specified malignant neoplasm of skin of left upper eyelid, including canthus

      C44.1992   Other specified malignant neoplasm of skin of left lower eyelid, including canthus

● C44.2   Other and unspecified malignant neoplasm of skin of ear and external auricular canal

    Excludes1   connective tissue of ear (C49.0)

● C44.20   Unspecified malignant neoplasm of skin of ear and external auricular canal

    C44.201   Unspecified malignant neoplasm of skin of unspecified ear and external auricular canal

    C44.202   Unspecified malignant neoplasm of skin of right ear and external auricular canal

    C44.209   Unspecified malignant neoplasm of skin of left ear and external auricular canal

● C44.21   Basal cell carcinoma of skin of ear and external auricular canal

    C44.211   Basal cell carcinoma of skin of unspecified ear and external auricular canal

    C44.212   Basal cell carcinoma of skin of right ear and external auricular canal

    C44.219   Basal cell carcinoma of skin of left ear and external auricular canal

● C44.22   Squamous cell carcinoma of skin of ear and external auricular canal

    C44.221   Squamous cell carcinoma of skin of unspecified ear and external auricular canal

    C44.222   Squamous cell carcinoma of skin of right ear and external auricular canal

    C44.229   Squamous cell carcinoma of skin of left ear and external auricular canal

● C44.29   Other specified malignant neoplasm of skin of ear and external auricular canal

    C44.291   Other specified malignant neoplasm of skin of unspecified ear and external auricular canal

    C44.292   Other specified malignant neoplasm of skin of right ear and external auricular canal

    C44.299   Other specified malignant neoplasm of skin of left ear and external auricular canal

● C44.3   Other and unspecified malignant neoplasm of skin of other and unspecified parts of face

● C44.30   Unspecified malignant neoplasm of skin of other and unspecified parts of face

    C44.300   Unspecified malignant neoplasm of skin of unspecified part of face

    C44.301   Unspecified malignant neoplasm of skin of nose

    C44.309   Unspecified malignant neoplasm of skin of other parts of face

● C44.31   Basal cell carcinoma of skin of other and unspecified parts of face

    C44.310   Basal cell carcinoma of skin of unspecified parts of face

    C44.311   Basal cell carcinoma of skin of nose

    C44.319   Basal cell carcinoma of skin of other parts of face
       Coding Clinic: 2017, Q1, P4

● C44.32   Squamous cell carcinoma of skin of other and unspecified parts of face

    C44.320   Squamous cell carcinoma of skin of unspecified parts of face

    C44.321   Squamous cell carcinoma of skin of nose

    C44.329   Squamous cell carcinoma of skin of other parts of face

● C44.39   Other specified malignant neoplasm of skin of other and unspecified parts of face

    C44.390   Other specified malignant neoplasm of skin of unspecified parts of face

    C44.391   Other specified malignant neoplasm of skin of nose

    C44.399   Other specified malignant neoplasm of skin of other parts of face

● C44.4   Other and unspecified malignant neoplasm of skin of scalp and neck

    C44.40   Unspecified malignant neoplasm of skin of scalp and neck

    C44.41   Basal cell carcinoma of skin of scalp and neck

    C44.42   Squamous cell carcinoma of skin of scalp and neck

    C44.49   Other specified malignant neoplasm of skin of scalp and neck

CHAPTER 2 (C00–D49)

CHAPTER 2 (C00-D49)

● C44.5   **Other and unspecified malignant neoplasm of skin of trunk**

     Excludes1   anus NOS (C21.0)
                          scrotum (C63.2)

   ● C44.50   **Unspecified malignant neoplasm of skin of trunk**

      C44.500   Unspecified malignant neoplasm of **anal skin**

           Unspecified malignant neoplasm of anal margin
           Unspecified malignant neoplasm of perianal skin

      C44.501   Unspecified malignant neoplasm of **skin of breast**

      C44.509   Unspecified malignant neoplasm of skin of **other part** of trunk

   ● C44.51   **Basal cell carcinoma** of skin of trunk

      C44.510   Basal cell carcinoma of **anal skin**
           Basal cell carcinoma of anal margin
           Basal cell carcinoma of perianal skin

      C44.511   Basal cell carcinoma of skin of **breast**

      C44.519   Basal cell carcinoma of skin of **other** part of trunk

   ● C44.52   **Squamous cell carcinoma** of skin of trunk

      C44.520   Squamous cell carcinoma of **anal skin**
           Squamous cell carcinoma of anal margin
           Squamous cell carcinoma of perianal skin

      C44.521   Squamous cell carcinoma of **skin of breast**

      C44.529   Squamous cell carcinoma of skin of **other part** of trunk

   ● C44.59   **Other** specified malignant neoplasm of skin of trunk

      C44.590   Other specified malignant neoplasm of **anal skin**
           Other specified malignant neoplasm of anal margin
           Other specified malignant neoplasm of perianal skin

      C44.591   Other specified malignant neoplasm of **skin of breast**

      C44.599   Other specified malignant neoplasm of skin of **other part** of trunk

● C44.6   **Other and unspecified malignant neoplasm of skin of upper limb, including shoulder**

   ● C44.60   **Unspecified** malignant neoplasm of skin of upper limb, including shoulder

      C44.601   Unspecified malignant neoplasm of skin of **unspecified** upper limb, including shoulder

      C44.602   Unspecified malignant neoplasm of skin of **right** upper limb, including shoulder

      C44.609   Unspecified malignant neoplasm of skin of **left** upper limb, including shoulder

   ● C44.61   **Basal cell carcinoma** of skin of upper limb, including shoulder

      C44.611   Basal cell carcinoma of skin of **unspecified** upper limb, including shoulder

      C44.612   Basal cell carcinoma of skin of **right** upper limb, including shoulder

      C44.619   Basal cell carcinoma of skin of **left** upper limb, including shoulder

   ● C44.62   **Squamous cell carcinoma** of skin of upper limb, including shoulder

      C44.621   Squamous cell carcinoma of skin of **unspecified** upper limb, including shoulder

      C44.622   Squamous cell carcinoma of skin of **right** upper limb, including shoulder

      C44.629   Squamous cell carcinoma of skin of **left** upper limb, including shoulder

   ● C44.69   **Other specified** malignant neoplasm of skin of upper limb, including shoulder

      C44.691   Other specified malignant neoplasm of skin of **unspecified** upper limb, including shoulder

      C44.692   Other specified malignant neoplasm of skin of **right** upper limb, including shoulder

      C44.699   Other specified malignant neoplasm of skin of **left** upper limb, including shoulder

● C44.7   **Other and unspecified malignant neoplasm of skin of lower limb, including hip**

   ● C44.70   **Unspecified** malignant neoplasm of skin of lower limb, including hip

      C44.701   Unspecified malignant neoplasm of skin of **unspecified** lower limb, including hip

      C44.702   Unspecified malignant neoplasm of skin of **right** lower limb, including hip

      C44.709   Unspecified malignant neoplasm of skin of **left** lower limb, including hip

   ● C44.71   **Basal cell carcinoma** of skin of lower limb, including hip

      C44.711   Basal cell carcinoma of skin of **unspecified** lower limb, including hip

      C44.712   Basal cell carcinoma of skin of **right** lower limb, including hip

      C44.719   Basal cell carcinoma of skin of **left** lower limb, including hip

   ● C44.72   **Squamous cell carcinoma** of skin of lower limb, including hip

      C44.721   Squamous cell carcinoma of skin of **unspecified** lower limb, including hip

      C44.722   Squamous cell carcinoma of skin of **right** lower limb, including hip

      C44.729   Squamous cell carcinoma of skin of **left** lower limb, including hip

   ● C44.79   **Other specified** malignant neoplasm of skin of lower limb, including hip

      C44.791   Other specified malignant neoplasm of skin of **unspecified** lower limb, including hip

      C44.792   Other specified malignant neoplasm of skin of **right** lower limb, including hip

      C44.799   Other specified malignant neoplasm of skin of **left** lower limb, including hip

● C44.8   **Other and unspecified malignant neoplasm of overlapping sites of skin**

      C44.80   **Unspecified** malignant neoplasm of overlapping sites of skin

      C44.81   **Basal cell carcinoma** of overlapping sites of skin

      C44.82   **Squamous cell carcinoma** of overlapping sites of skin

      C44.89   **Other** specified malignant neoplasm of overlapping sites of skin

▶ New   ⟹ Revised   ~~deleted~~ Deleted   Excludes 1   Excludes 2   Includes   Use additional   Code first   Code also   Key words

OGCR Official Guidelines   X Assign placeholder X   ● Use Additional Character(s)   ▶ Manifestation Code   🐱 Hierarchical Condition Category   **Coding Clinic**

● C44.9   **Other and unspecified malignant neoplasm of skin, unspecified**

      C44.90   **Unspecified malignant neoplasm of skin, unspecified**
                   Malignant neoplasm of unspecified site of skin

      C44.91   **Basal cell carcinoma of skin, unspecified**

      C44.92   **Squamous cell carcinoma of skin, unspecified**

      C44.99   **Other specified malignant neoplasm of skin, unspecified**

MALIGNANT NEOPLASMS OF MESOTHELIAL AND SOFT TISSUE (C45-C49)

● C45   **Mesothelioma**
      Malignant cells develop in protective lining that covers internal organs (mesothelium) caused by exposure to asbestos

      C45.0   **Mesothelioma of pleura**
                   Excludes1   other malignant neoplasm of pleura (C38.4)
                   Coding Clinic: 2017, Q2, P11

      C45.1   **Mesothelioma of peritoneum**
                   Mesothelioma of cul-de-sac
                   Mesothelioma of mesentery
                   Mesothelioma of mesocolon
                   Mesothelioma of omentum
                   Mesothelioma of peritoneum (parietal) (pelvic)
                   Excludes1   other malignant neoplasm of soft tissue of peritoneum (C48.-)

      C45.2   **Mesothelioma of pericardium**
                   Excludes1   other malignant neoplasm of pericardium (C38.0)

      C45.7   **Mesothelioma of other sites**

      C45.9   **Mesothelioma, unspecified**

● C46   **Kaposi's sarcoma**
      Code first any human immunodeficiency virus [HIV] disease (B20)

      C46.0   **Kaposi's sarcoma of skin**

      C46.1   **Kaposi's sarcoma of soft tissue**
                   Kaposi's sarcoma of blood vessel
                   Kaposi's sarcoma of connective tissue
                   Kaposi's sarcoma of fascia
                   Kaposi's sarcoma of ligament
                   Kaposi's sarcoma of lymphatic(s) NEC
                   Kaposi's sarcoma of muscle
                   Excludes2   Kaposi's sarcoma of lymph glands and nodes (C46.3)

      C46.2   **Kaposi's sarcoma of palate**

      C46.3   **Kaposi's sarcoma of lymph nodes**

      C46.4   **Kaposi's sarcoma of gastrointestinal sites**

  ● C46.5   **Kaposi's sarcoma of lung**

      C46.50   **Kaposi's sarcoma of unspecified lung**

      C46.51   **Kaposi's sarcoma of right lung**

      C46.52   **Kaposi's sarcoma of left lung**

      C46.7   **Kaposi's sarcoma of other sites**

      C46.9   **Kaposi's sarcoma, unspecified**
                   Kaposi's sarcoma of unspecified site

Figure 2-11 Kaposi's sarcoma. There are large confluent hyperpigmented patch-stage lesions with lymphedema. (From Goldman L, Ausiello D, Arend W, Armitage J, Clemmons D, Drazen J, Griggs R, et al: Cecil Medicine: Expert Consult, 23e, Saunders, 2007)

● C47   **Malignant neoplasm of peripheral nerves and autonomic nervous system**

      Includes   malignant neoplasm of sympathetic and parasympathetic nerves and ganglia

      Excludes1   Kaposi's sarcoma of soft tissue (C46.1)

      C47.0   **Malignant neoplasm of peripheral nerves of head, face and neck**
                   Excludes1   malignant neoplasm of peripheral nerves of orbit (C69.6-)

  ● C47.1   **Malignant neoplasm of peripheral nerves of upper limb, including shoulder**

      C47.10   **Malignant neoplasm of peripheral nerves of unspecified upper limb, including shoulder**

      C47.11   **Malignant neoplasm of peripheral nerves of right upper limb, including shoulder**

      C47.12   **Malignant neoplasm of peripheral nerves of left upper limb, including shoulder**

  ● C47.2   **Malignant neoplasm of peripheral nerves of lower limb, including hip**

      C47.20   **Malignant neoplasm of peripheral nerves of unspecified lower limb, including hip**

      C47.21   **Malignant neoplasm of peripheral nerves of right lower limb, including hip**

      C47.22   **Malignant neoplasm of peripheral nerves of left lower limb, including hip**

      C47.3   **Malignant neoplasm of peripheral nerves of thorax**

      C47.4   **Malignant neoplasm of peripheral nerves of abdomen**

      C47.5   **Malignant neoplasm of peripheral nerves of pelvis**

      C47.6   **Malignant neoplasm of peripheral nerves of trunk, unspecified**
                   Malignant neoplasm of peripheral nerves of unspecified part of trunk

      C47.8   **Malignant neoplasm of overlapping sites of peripheral nerves and autonomic nervous system**

      C47.9   **Malignant neoplasm of peripheral nerves and autonomic nervous system, unspecified**
                   Malignant neoplasm of unspecified site of peripheral nerves and autonomic nervous system

● C48   **Malignant neoplasm of retroperitoneum and peritoneum**
      Excludes1   Kaposi's sarcoma of connective tissue (C46.1)
                   mesothelioma (C45.-)

      C48.0   **Malignant neoplasm of retroperitoneum**
                   Behind/outside of peritoneum

      C48.1   **Malignant neoplasm of specified parts of peritoneum**
                   Serous membrane lining abdominopelvic walls and covering viscera
                   Malignant neoplasm of cul-de-sac
                   Malignant neoplasm of mesentery
                   Malignant neoplasm of mesocolon
                   Malignant neoplasm of omentum
                   Malignant neoplasm of parietal peritoneum
                   Malignant neoplasm of pelvic peritoneum

      C48.2   **Malignant neoplasm of peritoneum, unspecified**

      C48.8   **Malignant neoplasm of overlapping sites of retroperitoneum and peritoneum**

CHAPTER 2 (C00-D49)

Item 2–5   Kaposi's sarcoma is a cancer that causes patches of abnormal tissue to grow under the skin; in the lining of the mouth, nose, and throat; or in other organs, often beginning and spreading to other organs. Patients who have had organ transplants or patients with AIDS are at high risk for this malignancy.

● C49 Malignant neoplasm of other connective and soft tissue

Includes	malignant neoplasm of blood vessel
	malignant neoplasm of bursa
	malignant neoplasm of cartilage
	malignant neoplasm of fascia
	malignant neoplasm of fat
	malignant neoplasm of ligament, except uterine
	malignant neoplasm of lymphatic vessel
	malignant neoplasm of muscle
	malignant neoplasm of synovia
	malignant neoplasm of tendon (sheath)

Excludes1	malignant neoplasm of cartilage (of):
	articular (C40-C41)
	larynx (C32.3)
	nose (C30.0)
	malignant neoplasm of connective tissue of breast (C50.-)

Excludes2	Kaposi's sarcoma of soft tissue (C46.1)
	malignant neoplasm of heart (C38.0)
	malignant neoplasm of peripheral nerves and autonomic nervous system (C47.-)
	malignant neoplasm of peritoneum (C48.2)
	malignant neoplasm of retroperitoneum (C48.0)
	malignant neoplasm of uterine ligament (C57.3)
	mesothelioma (C45.-)

C49.0 Malignant neoplasm of connective and soft tissue of head, face and neck 🐾
    Malignant neoplasm of connective tissue of ear
    Malignant neoplasm of connective tissue of eyelid

    Excludes1   connective tissue of orbit (C69.6-)

● C49.1 Malignant neoplasm of connective and soft tissue of upper limb, including shoulder

    C49.10 Malignant neoplasm of connective and soft tissue of unspecified upper limb, including shoulder 🐾

    C49.11 Malignant neoplasm of connective and soft tissue of right upper limb, including shoulder 🐾

    C49.12 Malignant neoplasm of connective and soft tissue of left upper limb, including shoulder 🐾

● C49.2 Malignant neoplasm of connective and soft tissue of lower limb, including hip

    C49.20 Malignant neoplasm of connective and soft tissue of unspecified lower limb, including hip 🐾

    C49.21 Malignant neoplasm of connective and soft tissue of right lower limb, including hip 🐾

    C49.22 Malignant neoplasm of connective and soft tissue of left lower limb, including hip 🐾

C49.3 Malignant neoplasm of connective and soft tissue of thorax 🐾
    Malignant neoplasm of axilla
    Malignant neoplasm of diaphragm
    Malignant neoplasm of great vessels

    Excludes1   malignant neoplasm of breast (C50.-)
         malignant neoplasm of heart (C38.0)
         malignant neoplasm of mediastinum (C38.1-C38.3)
         malignant neoplasm of thymus (C37)
    Coding Clinic: 2015, Q3, P19

C49.4 Malignant neoplasm of connective and soft tissue of abdomen 🐾
    Malignant neoplasm of abdominal wall
    Malignant neoplasm of hypochondrium
    Coding Clinic: 2019, Q4, P44

C49.5 Malignant neoplasm of connective and soft tissue of pelvis 🐾
    Malignant neoplasm of buttock
    Malignant neoplasm of groin
    Malignant neoplasm of perineum

C49.6 Malignant neoplasm of connective and soft tissue of trunk, unspecified 🐾
    Malignant neoplasm of back NOS

C49.8 Malignant neoplasm of overlapping sites of connective and soft tissue 🐾
    Primary malignant neoplasm of two or more contiguous sites of connective and soft tissue

C49.9 Malignant neoplasm of connective and soft tissue, unspecified 🐾

● C49.A Gastrointestinal stromal tumor
    Coding Clinic: 2016, Q4, P8

    C49.A0 Gastrointestinal stromal tumor, unspecified site 🐾

    C49.A1 Gastrointestinal stromal tumor of esophagus 🐾

    C49.A2 Gastrointestinal stromal tumor of stomach 🐾

    C49.A3 Gastrointestinal stromal tumor of small intestine 🐾

    C49.A4 Gastrointestinal stromal tumor of large intestine 🐾

    C49.A5 Gastrointestinal stromal tumor of rectum 🐾

    C49.A9 Gastrointestinal stromal tumor of other sites 🐾

MALIGNANT NEOPLASMS OF BREAST (C50)

● C50 Malignant neoplasm of breast

Includes	connective tissue of breast
	Paget's disease of breast
	Paget's disease of nipple
	Intraductal carcinoma of breast characterized by eczema-like inflammatory skin changes

Use additional code to identify estrogen receptor status (Z17.0, Z17.1)

Excludes1	skin of breast (C44.501, C44.511, C44.521, C44.591)

● C50.0 Malignant neoplasm of nipple and areola

    ● C50.01 Malignant neoplasm of nipple and areola, female

        C50.011 Malignant neoplasm of nipple and areola, right female breast ♀ 🐾

        C50.012 Malignant neoplasm of nipple and areola, left female breast ♀ 🐾

        C50.019 Malignant neoplasm of nipple and areola, unspecified female breast ♀ 🐾

    ● C50.02 Malignant neoplasm of nipple and areola, male

        C50.021 Malignant neoplasm of nipple and areola, right male breast ♂ 🐾

        C50.022 Malignant neoplasm of nipple and areola, left male breast ♂ 🐾

        C50.029 Malignant neoplasm of nipple and areola, unspecified male breast ♂ 🐾

● C50.1 Malignant neoplasm of central portion of breast

    ● C50.11 Malignant neoplasm of central portion of breast, female

        C50.111 Malignant neoplasm of central portion of right female breast ♀ 🐾

        C50.112 Malignant neoplasm of central portion of left female breast ♀ 🐾

        C50.119 Malignant neoplasm of central portion of unspecified female breast ♀ 🐾

    ● C50.12 Malignant neoplasm of central portion of breast, male

        C50.121 Malignant neoplasm of central portion of right male breast ♂ 🐾

        C50.122 Malignant neoplasm of central portion of left male breast ♂ 🐾

        C50.129 Malignant neoplasm of central portion of unspecified male breast ♂ 🐾

AXILLARY TAIL
UPPER-INNER
UPPER-OUTER
Nipple and areola
Central portion
LOWER-OUTER
LOWER-INNER

Figure 2-12 Female breast quadrants and axillary tail.

● **C50.2** Malignant neoplasm of upper-inner quadrant of breast
  ● **C50.21** Malignant neoplasm of upper-inner quadrant of breast, female
    C50.211 Malignant neoplasm of upper-inner quadrant of right female breast ♀ 🐾
    C50.212 Malignant neoplasm of upper-inner quadrant of left female breast ♀ 🐾
    C50.219 Malignant neoplasm of upper-inner quadrant of unspecified female breast ♀ 🐾
  ● **C50.22** Malignant neoplasm of upper-inner quadrant of breast, male
    C50.221 Malignant neoplasm of upper-inner quadrant of right male breast ♂ 🐾
    C50.222 Malignant neoplasm of upper-inner quadrant of left male breast ♂ 🐾
    C50.229 Malignant neoplasm of upper-inner quadrant of unspecified male breast ♂ 🐾
● **C50.3** Malignant neoplasm of lower-inner quadrant of breast
  ● **C50.31** Malignant neoplasm of lower-inner quadrant of breast, female
    C50.311 Malignant neoplasm of lower-inner quadrant of right female breast ♀ 🐾
    C50.312 Malignant neoplasm of lower-inner quadrant of left female breast ♀ 🐾
    C50.319 Malignant neoplasm of lower-inner quadrant of unspecified female breast ♀ 🐾
  ● **C50.32** Malignant neoplasm of lower-inner quadrant of breast, male
    C50.321 Malignant neoplasm of lower-inner quadrant of right male breast ♂ 🐾
    C50.322 Malignant neoplasm of lower-inner quadrant of left male breast ♂ 🐾
    C50.329 Malignant neoplasm of lower-inner quadrant of unspecified male breast ♂ 🐾
● **C50.4** Malignant neoplasm of upper-outer quadrant of breast
  ● **C50.41** Malignant neoplasm of upper-outer quadrant of breast, female
    C50.411 Malignant neoplasm of upper-outer quadrant of right female breast ♀ 🐾
    C50.412 Malignant neoplasm of upper-outer quadrant of left female breast ♀ 🐾
    C50.419 Malignant neoplasm of upper-outer quadrant of unspecified female breast ♀ 🐾
  ● **C50.42** Malignant neoplasm of upper-outer quadrant of breast, male
    C50.421 Malignant neoplasm of upper-outer quadrant of right male breast ♂ 🐾
    C50.422 Malignant neoplasm of upper-outer quadrant of left male breast ♂ 🐾
    C50.429 Malignant neoplasm of upper-outer quadrant of unspecified male breast ♂ 🐾

● **C50.5** Malignant neoplasm of lower-outer quadrant of breast
  ● **C50.51** Malignant neoplasm of lower-outer quadrant of breast, female
    C50.511 Malignant neoplasm of lower-outer quadrant of right female breast ♀ 🐾
    C50.512 Malignant neoplasm of lower-outer quadrant of left female breast ♀ 🐾
    C50.519 Malignant neoplasm of lower-outer quadrant of unspecified female breast ♀ 🐾
  ● **C50.52** Malignant neoplasm of lower-outer quadrant of breast, male
    C50.521 Malignant neoplasm of lower-outer quadrant of right male breast ♂ 🐾
    C50.522 Malignant neoplasm of lower-outer quadrant of left male breast ♂ 🐾
    C50.529 Malignant neoplasm of lower-outer quadrant of unspecified male breast ♂ 🐾
● **C50.6** Malignant neoplasm of axillary tail of breast
  ● **C50.61** Malignant neoplasm of axillary tail of breast, female
    C50.611 Malignant neoplasm of axillary tail of right female breast ♀ 🐾
    C50.612 Malignant neoplasm of axillary tail of left female breast ♀ 🐾
    C50.619 Malignant neoplasm of axillary tail of unspecified female breast ♀ 🐾
  ● **C50.62** Malignant neoplasm of axillary tail of breast, male
    C50.621 Malignant neoplasm of axillary tail of right male breast ♂ 🐾
    C50.622 Malignant neoplasm of axillary tail of left male breast ♂ 🐾
    C50.629 Malignant neoplasm of axillary tail of unspecified male breast ♂ 🐾
● **C50.8** Malignant neoplasm of overlapping sites of breast
  ● **C50.81** Malignant neoplasm of overlapping sites of breast, female
    C50.811 Malignant neoplasm of overlapping sites of right female breast ♀ 🐾
    C50.812 Malignant neoplasm of overlapping sites of left female breast ♀ 🐾
    C50.819 Malignant neoplasm of overlapping sites of unspecified female breast ♀ 🐾
  ● **C50.82** Malignant neoplasm of overlapping sites of breast, male
    C50.821 Malignant neoplasm of overlapping sites of right male breast ♂ 🐾
    C50.822 Malignant neoplasm of overlapping sites of left male breast ♂ 🐾
    C50.829 Malignant neoplasm of overlapping sites of unspecified male breast ♂ 🐾
● **C50.9** Malignant neoplasm of breast of unspecified site
  ● **C50.91** Malignant neoplasm of breast of unspecified site, female
    C50.911 Malignant neoplasm of unspecified site of right female breast ♀ 🐾
    C50.912 Malignant neoplasm of unspecified site of left female breast ♀ 🐾
    C50.919 Malignant neoplasm of unspecified site of unspecified female breast ♀ 🐾
  ● **C50.92** Malignant neoplasm of breast of unspecified site, male
    C50.921 Malignant neoplasm of unspecified site of right male breast ♂ 🐾
    C50.922 Malignant neoplasm of unspecified site of left male breast ♂ 🐾
    C50.929 Malignant neoplasm of unspecified site of unspecified male breast ♂ 🐾

CHAPTER 2 (C00-D49)

CHAPTER 2 (C00-D49)

MALIGNANT NEOPLASMS OF FEMALE GENITAL ORGANS (C51-C58)

Includes   malignant neoplasm of skin of female genital organs

- **C51**   **Malignant neoplasm of vulva**

    Excludes1   carcinoma in situ of vulva (D07.1)

    C51.0   **Malignant neoplasm of labium majus ♀ 🐾**
    Outer folds of skin external female genitalia
    Malignant neoplasm of Bartholin's [greater vestibular] gland

    C51.1   **Malignant neoplasm of labium minus ♀ 🐾**
    Two inner folds surrounding vulva in female genitalia

    C51.2   **Malignant neoplasm of clitoris ♀ 🐾**

    C51.8   **Malignant neoplasm of overlapping sites of vulva ♀ 🐾**

    C51.9   **Malignant neoplasm of vulva, unspecified ♀ 🐾**
    Malignant neoplasm of external female genitalia NOS
    Malignant neoplasm of pudendum

- **C52**   **Malignant neoplasm of vagina ♀ 🐾**

    Excludes1   carcinoma in situ of vagina (D07.2)

- **C53**   **Malignant neoplasm of cervix uteri**

    Excludes1   carcinoma in situ of cervix uteri (D06.-)

    C53.0   **Malignant neoplasm of endocervix ♀ 🐾**
    Inside the cervix

    C53.1   **Malignant neoplasm of exocervix ♀ 🐾**
    Outside the cervix

    C53.8   **Malignant neoplasm of overlapping sites of cervix uteri ♀ 🐾**

    C53.9   **Malignant neoplasm of cervix uteri, unspecified ♀ 🐾**
    Coding Clinic: 2017, Q4, P103

- **C54**   **Malignant neoplasm of corpus uteri**

    C54.0   **Malignant neoplasm of isthmus uteri ♀ 🐾**
    Constricted part of uterus between cervix and body
    Malignant neoplasm of lower uterine segment

    C54.1   **Malignant neoplasm of endometrium ♀ 🐾**
    Lining of uterus

    C54.2   **Malignant neoplasm of myometrium ♀ 🐾**
    Middle layer of uterine wall consisting of smooth muscle supporting stromal and vascular tissue

    C54.3   **Malignant neoplasm of fundus uteri ♀ 🐾**
    Top rounded portion of uterus

    C54.8   **Malignant neoplasm of overlapping sites of corpus uteri ♀ 🐾**
    Main body of uterus

    C54.9   **Malignant neoplasm of corpus uteri, unspecified ♀ 🐾**

- **C55**   **Malignant neoplasm of uterus, part unspecified ♀ 🐾**

- **C56**   **Malignant neoplasm of ovary**
    Use additional code to identify any functional activity

    C56.1   **Malignant neoplasm of right ovary ♀ 🐾**
    C56.2   **Malignant neoplasm of left ovary ♀ 🐾**
    ▶**C56.3**   **Malignant neoplasm of bilateral ovaries**
    C56.9   **Malignant neoplasm of unspecified ovary ♀ 🐾**

- **C57**   **Malignant neoplasm of other and unspecified female genital organs**

    - **C57.0**   **Malignant neoplasm of fallopian tube**
        Malignant neoplasm of oviduct
        Malignant neoplasm of uterine tube

        C57.00   **Malignant neoplasm of unspecified fallopian tube ♀ 🐾**

        C57.01   **Malignant neoplasm of right fallopian tube ♀ 🐾**

        C57.02   **Malignant neoplasm of left fallopian tube ♀ 🐾**

    - **C57.1**   **Malignant neoplasm of broad ligament**

        C57.10   **Malignant neoplasm of unspecified broad ligament ♀ 🐾**

        C57.11   **Malignant neoplasm of right broad ligament ♀ 🐾**

        C57.12   **Malignant neoplasm of left broad ligament ♀ 🐾**

    - **C57.2**   **Malignant neoplasm of round ligament**

        C57.20   **Malignant neoplasm of unspecified round ligament ♀ 🐾**

        C57.21   **Malignant neoplasm of right round ligament ♀ 🐾**

        C57.22   **Malignant neoplasm of left round ligament ♀ 🐾**

    C57.3   **Malignant neoplasm of parametrium ♀ 🐾**
    Malignant neoplasm of uterine ligament NOS

    C57.4   **Malignant neoplasm of uterine adnexa, unspecified ♀ 🐾**

    C57.7   **Malignant neoplasm of other specified female genital organs ♀ 🐾**
    Malignant neoplasm of wolffian body or duct

    C57.8   **Malignant neoplasm of overlapping sites of female genital organs ♀ 🐾**
    Primary malignant neoplasm of two or more contiguous sites of the female genital organs whose point of origin cannot be determined
    Primary tubo-ovarian malignant neoplasm whose point of origin cannot be determined
    Primary utero-ovarian malignant neoplasm whose point of origin cannot be determined

    C57.9   **Malignant neoplasm of female genital organ, unspecified ♀ 🐾**
    Malignant neoplasm of female genitourinary tract NOS

- C58   **Malignant neoplasm of placenta ♀ 🐾**   M

    Includes   choriocarcinoma NOS
    chorionepithelioma NOS

    Excludes1   chorioadenoma (destruens) (D39.2)
    hydatidiform mole NOS (O01.9)
    invasive hydatidiform mole (D39.2)
    male choriocarcinoma NOS (C62.9-)
    malignant hydatidiform mole (D39.2)

MALIGNANT NEOPLASMS OF MALE GENITAL ORGANS (C60-C63)

Includes   malignant neoplasm of skin of male genital organs

- **C60**   **Malignant neoplasm of penis**

    C60.0   **Malignant neoplasm of prepuce ♂ 🐾**
    Malignant neoplasm of foreskin

    C60.1   **Malignant neoplasm of glans penis ♂ 🐾**

    C60.2   **Malignant neoplasm of body of penis ♂ 🐾**
    Malignant neoplasm of corpus cavernosum

    C60.8   **Malignant neoplasm of overlapping sites of penis ♂ 🐾**

    C60.9   **Malignant neoplasm of penis, unspecified ♂ 🐾**
    Malignant neoplasm of skin of penis NOS

- C61   **Malignant neoplasm of prostate ♂ 🐾**
    Use additional code to identify:
    hormone sensitivity status (Z19.1-Z19.2)
    rising PSA following treatment for malignant neoplasm of prostate (R97.21)

    Excludes1   malignant neoplasm of seminal vesicle (C63.7)

Figure 2-13   Cervix uteri.

▶ New   ⇒ Revised   ~~deleted~~ Deleted   Excludes 1   Excludes 2   Includes   Use additional   Code first   Code also   Key words

OGCR Official Guidelines   X Assign placeholder X   ● Use Additional Character(s)   ▶ Manifestation Code   🐾 Hierarchical Condition Category   **Coding Clinic**

Figure 2-14 Penis and other male genital organs.

● C62   Malignant neoplasm of testis
　　　　Use additional code to identify any functional activity.

　● C62.0   Malignant neoplasm of undescended testis
　　　　　　Malignant neoplasm of ectopic testis
　　　　　　Malignant neoplasm of retained testis

　　　C62.00   Malignant neoplasm of unspecified
　　　　　　　　undescended testis ♂ 🐾

　　　C62.01   Malignant neoplasm of undescended right
　　　　　　　　testis ♂ 🐾

　　　C62.02   Malignant neoplasm of undescended left
　　　　　　　　testis ♂ 🐾

　● C62.1   Malignant neoplasm of descended testis
　　　　　　Malignant neoplasm of scrotal testis

　　　C62.10   Malignant neoplasm of unspecified descended
　　　　　　　　testis, unspecified side ♂ 🐾

　　　C62.11   Malignant neoplasm of descended right
　　　　　　　　testis ♂ 🐾

　　　C62.12   Malignant neoplasm of descended left
　　　　　　　　testis ♂ 🐾

　● C62.9   Malignant neoplasm of testis, unspecified whether
　　　　　　descended or undescended

　　　C62.90   Malignant neoplasm of unspecified
　　　　　　　　testis, unspecified whether descended or
　　　　　　　　undescended ♂ 🐾
　　　　　　　　　Malignant neoplasm of testis NOS

　　　C62.91   Malignant neoplasm of right testis, unspecified
　　　　　　　　whether descended or undescended ♂ 🐾

　　　C62.92   Malignant neoplasm of left testis, unspecified
　　　　　　　　whether descended or undescended ♂ 🐾

● C63   Malignant neoplasm of other and unspecified male genital organs

　● C63.0   Malignant neoplasm of epididymis

　　　C63.00   Malignant neoplasm of unspecified
　　　　　　　　epididymis ♂ 🐾

　　　C63.01   Malignant neoplasm of right epididymis ♂ 🐾

　　　C63.02   Malignant neoplasm of left epididymis ♂ 🐾

　● C63.1   Malignant neoplasm of spermatic cord

　　　C63.10   Malignant neoplasm of unspecified spermatic
　　　　　　　　cord ♂ 🐾

　　　C63.11   Malignant neoplasm of right spermatic cord ♂ 🐾

　　　C63.12   Malignant neoplasm of left spermatic cord ♂ 🐾

　● C63.2   Malignant neoplasm of scrotum ♂ 🐾
　　　　　　Malignant neoplasm of skin of scrotum

　● C63.7   Malignant neoplasm of other specified male genital
　　　　　　organs ♂ 🐾
　　　　　　Malignant neoplasm of seminal vesicle
　　　　　　Malignant neoplasm of tunica vaginalis

　● C63.8   Malignant neoplasm of overlapping sites of male genital
　　　　　　organs ♂ 🐾
　　　　　　Primary malignant neoplasm of two or more
　　　　　　　contiguous sites of male genital organs whose
　　　　　　　point of origin cannot be determined

　● C63.9   Malignant neoplasm of male genital
　　　　　　organ, unspecified ♂ 🐾
　　　　　　Malignant neoplasm of male genitourinary tract NOS

MALIGNANT NEOPLASMS OF URINARY TRACT (C64-C68)

● C64   Malignant neoplasm of kidney, except renal pelvis
　　　Excludes1   malignant carcinoid tumor of the kidney
　　　　　　　　　　(C7A.093)
　　　　　　　　malignant neoplasm of renal calyces (C65.-)
　　　　　　　　malignant neoplasm of renal pelvis (C65.-)

　　C64.1   Malignant neoplasm of right kidney, except renal
　　　　　　pelvis 🐾

　　C64.2   Malignant neoplasm of left kidney, except renal
　　　　　　pelvis 🐾

　　C64.9   Malignant neoplasm of unspecified kidney, except renal
　　　　　　pelvis 🐾

● C65   Malignant neoplasm of renal pelvis
　　　Includes   malignant neoplasm of pelviureteric junction
　　　　　　　　malignant neoplasm of renal calyces

　　C65.1   Malignant neoplasm of right renal pelvis 🐾

　　C65.2   Malignant neoplasm of left renal pelvis 🐾

　　C65.9   Malignant neoplasm of unspecified renal pelvis 🐾

● C66   Malignant neoplasm of ureter
　　　Excludes1   malignant neoplasm of ureteric orifice of bladder
　　　　　　　　(C67.6)

　　C66.1   Malignant neoplasm of right ureter 🐾

　　C66.2   Malignant neoplasm of left ureter 🐾

　　C66.9   Malignant neoplasm of unspecified ureter 🐾

● C67   Malignant neoplasm of bladder

　　C67.0   Malignant neoplasm of trigone of bladder 🐾
　　　　　　Triangular area formed by three openings in the floor of
　　　　　　urinary bladder

　　C67.1   Malignant neoplasm of dome of bladder 🐾
　　　　　　Vaulted roof

　　C67.2   Malignant neoplasm of lateral wall of bladder 🐾
　　　　　　Side walls

　　C67.3   Malignant neoplasm of anterior wall of bladder 🐾
　　　　　　Front wall

　　C67.4   Malignant neoplasm of posterior wall of bladder 🐾
　　　　　　Back wall

　　C67.5   Malignant neoplasm of bladder neck 🐾
　　　　　　Joining of bladder and urethra
　　　　　　Malignant neoplasm of internal urethral orifice

　　C67.6   Malignant neoplasm of ureteric orifice 🐾
　　　　　　Opening from bladder to ureters

　　C67.7   Malignant neoplasm of urachus 🐾
　　　　　　Embryonic canal that connects the urinary bladder with the
　　　　　　structure that forms the umbilical cord (allantois)

　　C67.8   Malignant neoplasm of overlapping sites of bladder 🐾

　　C67.9   Malignant neoplasm of bladder, unspecified 🐾
　　　　　　Coding Clinic: 2017, Q1, P6; 2016, Q1, P19

● C68   Malignant neoplasm of other and unspecified urinary organs
　　　Excludes1   malignant neoplasm of female genitourinary tract
　　　　　　　　NOS (C57.9)
　　　　　　　　malignant neoplasm of male genitourinary tract
　　　　　　　　NOS (C63.9)

　　C68.0   Malignant neoplasm of urethra 🐾
　　　　　　Excludes1   malignant neoplasm of urethral orifice of
　　　　　　　　　　　bladder (C67.5)

　　C68.1   Malignant neoplasm of paraurethral glands 🐾
　　　　　　Group of glands of female urethra drained by paraurethral
　　　　　　ducts; AKA Skene glands, female prostate

　　C68.8   Malignant neoplasm of overlapping sites of urinary
　　　　　　organs 🐾
　　　　　　Primary malignant neoplasm of two or more
　　　　　　　contiguous sites of urinary organs whose point of
　　　　　　　origin cannot be determined

　　C68.9   Malignant neoplasm of urinary organ, unspecified 🐾
　　　　　　Malignant neoplasm of urinary system NOS

CHAPTER 2 (C00-D49)

MALIGNANT NEOPLASMS OF EYE, BRAIN AND OTHER PARTS OF CENTRAL NERVOUS SYSTEM (C69-C72)

● C69 **Malignant neoplasm of eye and adnexa**
    Excludes1 malignant neoplasm of connective tissue of eyelid (C49.0)
                 malignant neoplasm of eyelid (skin) (C43.1-, C44.1-)
                 malignant neoplasm of optic nerve (C72.3-)

● C69.0 **Malignant neoplasm of conjunctiva**
    C69.00 Malignant neoplasm of unspecified conjunctiva
    C69.01 Malignant neoplasm of right conjunctiva
    C69.02 Malignant neoplasm of left conjunctiva

● C69.1 **Malignant neoplasm of cornea**
    C69.10 Malignant neoplasm of unspecified cornea
    C69.11 Malignant neoplasm of right cornea
    C69.12 Malignant neoplasm of left cornea

● C69.2 **Malignant neoplasm of retina**
    Excludes1 dark area on retina (D49.81)
             neoplasm of unspecified behavior of retina and choroid (D49.81)
             retinal freckle (D49.81)
    C69.20 Malignant neoplasm of unspecified retina
    C69.21 Malignant neoplasm of right retina
    C69.22 Malignant neoplasm of left retina

● C69.3 **Malignant neoplasm of choroid**
    C69.30 Malignant neoplasm of unspecified choroid
    C69.31 Malignant neoplasm of right choroid
    C69.32 Malignant neoplasm of left choroid

● C69.4 **Malignant neoplasm of ciliary body**
    C69.40 Malignant neoplasm of unspecified ciliary body
    C69.41 Malignant neoplasm of right ciliary body
    C69.42 Malignant neoplasm of left ciliary body

● C69.5 **Malignant neoplasm of lacrimal gland and duct**
    Malignant neoplasm of lacrimal sac
    Malignant neoplasm of nasolacrimal duct
    C69.50 Malignant neoplasm of unspecified lacrimal gland and duct
    C69.51 Malignant neoplasm of right lacrimal gland and duct
    C69.52 Malignant neoplasm of left lacrimal gland and duct

● C69.6 **Malignant neoplasm of orbit**
    Malignant neoplasm of connective tissue of orbit
    Malignant neoplasm of extraocular muscle
    Malignant neoplasm of peripheral nerves of orbit
    Malignant neoplasm of retrobulbar tissue
    Malignant neoplasm of retro-ocular tissue
    Excludes1 malignant neoplasm of orbital bone (C41.0)
    C69.60 Malignant neoplasm of unspecified orbit
    C69.61 Malignant neoplasm of right orbit
    C69.62 Malignant neoplasm of left orbit

● C69.8 **Malignant neoplasm of overlapping sites of eye and adnexa**
    C69.80 Malignant neoplasm of overlapping sites of unspecified eye and adnexa
    C69.81 Malignant neoplasm of overlapping sites of right eye and adnexa
    C69.82 Malignant neoplasm of overlapping sites of left eye and adnexa

● C69.9 **Malignant neoplasm of unspecified site of eye**
    Malignant neoplasm of eyeball
    C69.90 Malignant neoplasm of unspecified site of unspecified eye
    C69.91 Malignant neoplasm of unspecified site of right eye
    C69.92 Malignant neoplasm of unspecified site of left eye

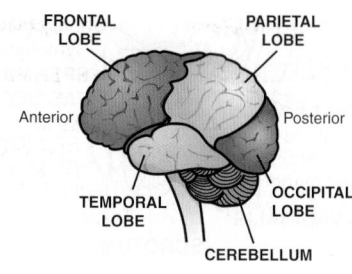

Figure 2-15 The brain.

● C70 **Malignant neoplasm of meninges**
    C70.0 Malignant neoplasm of cerebral meninges
    C70.1 Malignant neoplasm of spinal meninges
    C70.9 Malignant neoplasm of meninges, unspecified

● C71 **Malignant neoplasm of brain**
    Excludes1 malignant neoplasm of cranial nerves (C72.2-C72.5)
             retrobulbar malignant neoplasm (C69.6-)
    C71.0 Malignant neoplasm of cerebrum, except lobes and ventricles
        Malignant neoplasm of supratentorial NOS
    C71.1 Malignant neoplasm of frontal lobe
    C71.2 Malignant neoplasm of temporal lobe
    C71.3 Malignant neoplasm of parietal lobe
    C71.4 Malignant neoplasm of occipital lobe
    C71.5 Malignant neoplasm of cerebral ventricle
        Excludes1 malignant neoplasm of fourth cerebral ventricle (C71.7)
    C71.6 Malignant neoplasm of cerebellum
    C71.7 Malignant neoplasm of brain stem
        Malignant neoplasm of fourth cerebral ventricle
        Infratentorial malignant neoplasm NOS
    C71.8 Malignant neoplasm of overlapping sites of brain
    C71.9 Malignant neoplasm of brain, unspecified

● C72 **Malignant neoplasm of spinal cord, cranial nerves and other parts of central nervous system**
    Excludes1 malignant neoplasm of meninges (C70.-)
             malignant neoplasm of peripheral nerves and autonomic nervous system (C47.-)
    C72.0 Malignant neoplasm of spinal cord
    C72.1 Malignant neoplasm of cauda equina
        Lower end of spinal column
    ● C72.2 Malignant neoplasm of olfactory nerve
        Malignant neoplasm of olfactory bulb
        C72.20 Malignant neoplasm of unspecified olfactory nerve
        C72.21 Malignant neoplasm of right olfactory nerve
        C72.22 Malignant neoplasm of left olfactory nerve
    ● C72.3 Malignant neoplasm of optic nerve
        C72.30 Malignant neoplasm of unspecified optic nerve
        C72.31 Malignant neoplasm of right optic nerve
        C72.32 Malignant neoplasm of left optic nerve
    ● C72.4 Malignant neoplasm of acoustic nerve
        C72.40 Malignant neoplasm of unspecified acoustic nerve
        C72.41 Malignant neoplasm of right acoustic nerve
        C72.42 Malignant neoplasm of left acoustic nerve

▶ New   ⇒ Revised   ~~deleted~~ Deleted   Excludes 1   Excludes 2   Includes   Use additional   Code first   Code also   Key words
OGCR Official Guidelines   X Assign placeholder X   ● Use Additional Character(s)   ▶ Manifestation Code   🐾 Hierarchical Condition Category   **Coding Clinic**

● **C72.5** Malignant neoplasm of other and unspecified cranial nerves

  C72.50 Malignant neoplasm of unspecified cranial nerve 🦠

    Malignant neoplasm of cranial nerve NOS

  C72.59 Malignant neoplasm of other cranial nerves 🦠

C72.9 Malignant neoplasm of central nervous system, unspecified 🦠

    Malignant neoplasm of unspecified site of central nervous system

    Malignant neoplasm of nervous system NOS

MALIGNANT NEOPLASMS OF THYROID AND OTHER ENDOCRINE GLANDS (C73-C75)

C73 Malignant neoplasm of thyroid gland 🦠

    Use additional code to identify any functional activity

● **C74** Malignant neoplasm of adrenal gland

  ● **C74.0** Malignant neoplasm of cortex of adrenal gland

    C74.00 Malignant neoplasm of cortex of unspecified adrenal gland 🦠

    C74.01 Malignant neoplasm of cortex of right adrenal gland 🦠

    C74.02 Malignant neoplasm of cortex of left adrenal gland 🦠

  ● **C74.1** Malignant neoplasm of medulla of adrenal gland

    Pair of glands situated on top of or above each kidney ("suprarenal")

    C74.10 Malignant neoplasm of medulla of unspecified adrenal gland 🦠

    C74.11 Malignant neoplasm of medulla of right adrenal gland 🦠

    C74.12 Malignant neoplasm of medulla of left adrenal gland 🦠

  ● **C74.9** Malignant neoplasm of unspecified part of adrenal gland

    C74.90 Malignant neoplasm of unspecified part of unspecified adrenal gland 🦠

    C74.91 Malignant neoplasm of unspecified part of right adrenal gland 🦠

    C74.92 Malignant neoplasm of unspecified part of left adrenal gland 🦠

● **C75** Malignant neoplasm of other endocrine glands and related structures

  Excludes1 malignant carcinoid tumors (C7A.0-)
    malignant neoplasm of adrenal gland (C74.-)
    malignant neoplasm of endocrine pancreas (C25.4)
    malignant neoplasm of islets of Langerhans (C25.4)
    malignant neoplasm of ovary (C56.-)
    malignant neoplasm of testis (C62.-)
    malignant neoplasm of thymus (C37)
    malignant neoplasm of thyroid gland (C73)
    malignant neuroendocrine tumors (C7A.-)

  C75.0 Malignant neoplasm of parathyroid gland 🦠

  C75.1 Malignant neoplasm of pituitary gland 🦠

  C75.2 Malignant neoplasm of craniopharyngeal duct 🦠

  C75.3 Malignant neoplasm of pineal gland 🦠

  C75.4 Malignant neoplasm of carotid body 🦠

  C75.5 Malignant neoplasm of aortic body and other paraganglia 🦠

  C75.8 Malignant neoplasm with pluriglandular involvement, unspecified 🦠

  C75.9 Malignant neoplasm of endocrine gland, unspecified 🦠

MALIGNANT NEUROENDOCRINE TUMORS (C7A)

● **C7A** Malignant neuroendocrine tumors

    Code also any associated multiple endocrine neoplasia [MEN] syndromes (E31.2-)

    Use additional code to identify any associated endocrine syndrome, such as:
    carcinoid syndrome (E34.0)

    Excludes2 malignant pancreatic islet cell tumors (C25.4)
      Merkel cell carcinoma (C4A.-)

  ● **C7A.0** Malignant carcinoid tumors

    C7A.00 Malignant carcinoid tumor of unspecified site 🦠

    ● **C7A.01** Malignant carcinoid tumors of the small intestine

      C7A.010 Malignant carcinoid tumor of the duodenum 🦠

      C7A.011 Malignant carcinoid tumor of the jejunum 🦠

      C7A.012 Malignant carcinoid tumor of the ileum 🦠

      C7A.019 Malignant carcinoid tumor of the small intestine, unspecified portion 🦠

    ● **C7A.02** Malignant carcinoid tumors of the appendix, large intestine, and rectum

      C7A.020 Malignant carcinoid tumor of the appendix 🦠

      C7A.021 Malignant carcinoid tumor of the cecum 🦠

      C7A.022 Malignant carcinoid tumor of the ascending colon 🦠

      C7A.023 Malignant carcinoid tumor of the transverse colon 🦠

      C7A.024 Malignant carcinoid tumor of the descending colon 🦠

      C7A.025 Malignant carcinoid tumor of the sigmoid colon 🦠

      C7A.026 Malignant carcinoid tumor of the rectum 🦠

      C7A.029 Malignant carcinoid tumor of the large intestine, unspecified portion 🦠

        Malignant carcinoid tumor of the colon NOS

    ● **C7A.09** Malignant carcinoid tumors of other sites

      C7A.090 Malignant carcinoid tumor of the bronchus and lung 🦠

      C7A.091 Malignant carcinoid tumor of the thymus 🦠

      C7A.092 Malignant carcinoid tumor of the stomach 🦠

      C7A.093 Malignant carcinoid tumor of the kidney 🦠

      C7A.094 Malignant carcinoid tumor of the foregut, unspecified 🦠

      C7A.095 Malignant carcinoid tumor of the midgut, unspecified 🦠

      C7A.096 Malignant carcinoid tumor of the hindgut, unspecified 🦠

      C7A.098 Malignant carcinoid tumors of other sites 🦠

  C7A.1 Malignant poorly differentiated neuroendocrine tumors 🦠

    Malignant poorly differentiated neuroendocrine tumor NOS

    Malignant poorly differentiated neuroendocrine carcinoma, any site

    High grade neuroendocrine carcinoma, any site

  C7A.8 Other malignant neuroendocrine tumors 🦠

    Secondary neuroendocrine tumors (C7B)

    Coding Clinic: 2019, Q3, P7

N Newborn Age: 0   **P** Pediatric Age: 0–17   **M** Maternity DX: 9–64   **A** Adult Age: 15–124   ♀ Females Only   ♂ Males Only

CHAPTER 2 (C00-D49)

699

CHAPTER 2 (C00-D49)

SECONDARY NEUROENDOCRINE TUMORS (C7B)

● **C7B Secondary neuroendocrine tumors**
Use additional code to identify any functional activity

 ● **C7B.0 Secondary carcinoid tumors**
 C7B.00 Secondary carcinoid tumors, unspecified site 🐾
 C7B.01 Secondary carcinoid tumors of distant lymph nodes 🐾
 C7B.02 Secondary carcinoid tumors of liver 🐾
 C7B.03 Secondary carcinoid tumors of bone 🐾
 C7B.04 Secondary carcinoid tumors of peritoneum 🐾
 Mesentary metastasis of carcinoid tumor
 C7B.09 Secondary carcinoid tumors of other sites 🐾
 C7B.1 Secondary Merkel cell carcinoma 🐾
 Merkel cell carcinoma nodal presentation
 Merkel cell carcinoma visceral metastatic presentation
 C7B.8 Other secondary neuroendocrine tumors 🐾
 Coding Clinic: 2019, Q3, P7

MALIGNANT NEOPLASMS OF ILL-DEFINED, OTHER SECONDARY AND UNSPECIFIED SITES (C76-C80)

● **C76 Malignant neoplasm of other and ill-defined sites**
 Excludes1 malignant neoplasm of female genitourinary tract NOS (C57.9)
 malignant neoplasm of male genitourinary tract NOS (C63.9)
 malignant neoplasm of lymphoid, hematopoietic and related tissue (C81-C96)
 malignant neoplasm of skin (C44.-)
 malignant neoplasm of unspecified site NOS (C80.1)

 C76.0 Malignant neoplasm of head, face and neck 🐾
 Malignant neoplasm of cheek NOS
 Malignant neoplasm of nose NOS
 C76.1 Malignant neoplasm of thorax 🐾
 Intrathoracic malignant neoplasm NOS
 Malignant neoplasm of axilla NOS
 Thoracic malignant neoplasm NOS
 C76.2 Malignant neoplasm of abdomen 🐾
 C76.3 Malignant neoplasm of pelvis 🐾
 Malignant neoplasm of groin NOS
 Malignant neoplasm of sites overlapping systems within the pelvis
 Rectovaginal (septum) malignant neoplasm
 Between rectum and vagina
 Rectovesical (septum) malignant neoplasm
 Between rectum and urinary bladder; AKA vesicorectal
 ● **C76.4 Malignant neoplasm of upper limb**
 C76.40 Malignant neoplasm of unspecified upper limb 🐾
 C76.41 Malignant neoplasm of right upper limb 🐾
 C76.42 Malignant neoplasm of left upper limb 🐾
 ● **C76.5 Malignant neoplasm of lower limb**
 C76.50 Malignant neoplasm of unspecified lower limb 🐾
 C76.51 Malignant neoplasm of right lower limb 🐾
 C76.52 Malignant neoplasm of left lower limb 🐾
 C76.8 Malignant neoplasm of other specified ill-defined sites 🐾
 Malignant neoplasm of overlapping ill-defined sites

● **C77 Secondary and unspecified malignant neoplasm of lymph nodes**
 Excludes1 malignant neoplasm of lymph nodes, specified as primary (C81-C86, C88, C96.-)
 mesentary metastasis of carcinoid tumor (C7B.04)
 secondary carcinoid tumors of distant lymph nodes (C7B.01)

 C77.0 Secondary and unspecified malignant neoplasm of lymph nodes of head, face and neck 🐾
 Secondary and unspecified malignant neoplasm of supraclavicular lymph nodes

 C77.1 Secondary and unspecified malignant neoplasm of intrathoracic lymph nodes 🐾
 C77.2 Secondary and unspecified malignant neoplasm of intra-abdominal lymph nodes 🐾
 C77.3 Secondary and unspecified malignant neoplasm of axilla and upper limb lymph nodes 🐾
 Secondary and unspecified malignant neoplasm of pectoral lymph nodes
 C77.4 Secondary and unspecified malignant neoplasm of inguinal and lower limb lymph nodes 🐾
 C77.5 Secondary and unspecified malignant neoplasm of intrapelvic lymph nodes 🐾
 C77.8 Secondary and unspecified malignant neoplasm of lymph nodes of multiple regions 🐾
 C77.9 Secondary and unspecified malignant neoplasm of lymph node, unspecified 🐾

● **C78 Secondary malignant neoplasm of respiratory and digestive organs**
 Excludes1 secondary carcinoid tumors of liver (C7B.02)
 secondary carcinoid tumors of peritoneum (C7B.04)
 Excludes2 lymph node metastases (C77.0)
 ● **C78.0 Secondary malignant neoplasm of lung**
 C78.00 Secondary malignant neoplasm of unspecified lung 🐾
 C78.01 Secondary malignant neoplasm of right lung 🐾
 C78.02 Secondary malignant neoplasm of left lung 🐾
 C78.1 Secondary malignant neoplasm of mediastinum 🐾
 Thoracic cavity between pleural cavities
 C78.2 Secondary malignant neoplasm of pleura 🐾
 Serous membrane covering lungs and lining thoracic cavity
 ● **C78.3 Secondary malignant neoplasm of other and unspecified respiratory organs**
 C78.30 Secondary malignant neoplasm of unspecified respiratory organ 🐾
 C78.39 Secondary malignant neoplasm of other respiratory organs 🐾
 C78.4 Secondary malignant neoplasm of small intestine 🐾
 C78.5 Secondary malignant neoplasm of large intestine and rectum 🐾
 C78.6 Secondary malignant neoplasm of retroperitoneum and peritoneum 🐾
 Coding Clinic: 2017, Q2, P12
 C78.7 Secondary malignant neoplasm of liver and intrahepatic bile duct 🐾
 ● **C78.8 Secondary malignant neoplasm of other and unspecified digestive organs**
 C78.80 Secondary malignant neoplasm of unspecified digestive organ 🐾
 C78.89 Secondary malignant neoplasm of other digestive organs 🐾
 Code also exocrine pancreatic insufficiency (K86.81)

● **C79 Secondary malignant neoplasm of other and unspecified sites**
 Excludes1 secondary carcinoid tumors (C7B.-)
 secondary neuroendocrine tumors (C7B.-)
 ● **C79.0 Secondary malignant neoplasm of kidney and renal pelvis**
 C79.00 Secondary malignant neoplasm of unspecified kidney and renal pelvis 🐾
 C79.01 Secondary malignant neoplasm of right kidney and renal pelvis 🐾
 C79.02 Secondary malignant neoplasm of left kidney and renal pelvis 🐾

Item 2-6 The adrenal glands are a pair of glands situated on top of or above each kidney ("suprarenal") and chiefly responsible for regulating the stress response through the synthesis of corticosteroids and catecholamines, including cortisol and adrenaline.

▶ New ⟹ Revised ~~deleted~~ Deleted Excludes 1 Excludes 2 Includes Use additional Code first Code also Key words
OGCR Official Guidelines X Assign placeholder X ● Use Additional Character(s) ▌ Manifestation Code 🐾 Hierarchical Condition Category **Coding Clinic**

- C79.1   Secondary malignant neoplasm of bladder and other and unspecified urinary organs
  - C79.10   Secondary malignant neoplasm of unspecified urinary organs 🐾
  - C79.11   Secondary malignant neoplasm of bladder 🐾
    - **Excludes2**   lymph node metastases (C77.0)
  - C79.19   Secondary malignant neoplasm of other urinary organs 🐾
  - C79.2   Secondary malignant neoplasm of skin 🐾
    - **Excludes1**   secondary Merkel cell carcinoma (C7B.1)
- C79.3   Secondary malignant neoplasm of brain and cerebral meninges
  - C79.31   Secondary malignant neoplasm of brain 🐾
  - C79.32   Secondary malignant neoplasm of cerebral meninges 🐾
    Coding Clinic: 2020, Q1, P13
- C79.4   Secondary malignant neoplasm of other and unspecified parts of nervous system
  - C79.40   Secondary malignant neoplasm of unspecified part of nervous system 🐾
  - C79.49   Secondary malignant neoplasm of other parts of nervous system 🐾
- C79.5   Secondary malignant neoplasm of bone and bone marrow
  - **Excludes1**   secondary carcinoid tumors of bone (C7B.03)
  - C79.51   Secondary malignant neoplasm of bone 🐾
  - C79.52   Secondary malignant neoplasm of bone marrow 🐾
- C79.6   Secondary malignant neoplasm of ovary
  - C79.60   Secondary malignant neoplasm of unspecified ovary ♀ 🐾
  - C79.61   Secondary malignant neoplasm of right ovary ♀ 🐾
  - C79.62   Secondary malignant neoplasm of left ovary ♀ 🐾
  - ▶C79.63   Secondary malignant neoplasm of bilateral ovaries
- C79.7   Secondary malignant neoplasm of adrenal gland
  - C79.70   Secondary malignant neoplasm of unspecified adrenal gland 🐾
  - C79.71   Secondary malignant neoplasm of right adrenal gland 🐾
  - C79.72   Secondary malignant neoplasm of left adrenal gland 🐾
- C79.8   Secondary malignant neoplasm of other specified sites
  - C79.81   Secondary malignant neoplasm of breast 🐾
  - C79.82   Secondary malignant neoplasm of genital organs 🐾
  - C79.89   Secondary malignant neoplasm of other specified sites 🐾
    Coding Clinic: 2017, Q2, P11
  - C79.9   Secondary malignant neoplasm of unspecified site 🐾
    Metastatic cancer NOS
    Metastatic disease NOS
    - **Excludes1**   carcinomatosis NOS (C80.0)
      generalized cancer NOS (C80.0)
      malignant (primary) neoplasm of unspecified site (C80.1)

OGCR Section I.C.2.j and k

Disseminated malignant neoplasm, unspecified

j. Code C80.0, Disseminated malignant neoplasm, unspecified, is for use only in those cases where the patient has advanced metastatic disease and no known primary or secondary sites are specified. It should not be used in place of assigning codes for the primary site and all known secondary sites.

Malignant neoplasm without specification of site

k. Code C80.1, Malignant (primary) neoplasm, unspecified, equates to Cancer, unspecified. This code should only be used when no determination can be made as to the primary site of a malignancy. This code should rarely be used in the inpatient setting.

- C80   Malignant neoplasm without specification of site
  - **Excludes1**   malignant carcinoid tumor of unspecified site (C7A.00)
    malignant neoplasm of specified multiple sites-code to each site
  - C80.0   Disseminated malignant neoplasm, unspecified 🐾
    Carcinomatosis NOS
    Generalized cancer, unspecified site (primary) (secondary)
    Generalized malignancy, unspecified site (primary) (secondary)
  - C80.1   Malignant (primary) neoplasm, unspecified 🐾
    Cancer NOS
    Cancer unspecified site (primary)
    Carcinoma unspecified site (primary)
    Malignancy unspecified site (primary)
    - **Excludes1**   secondary malignant neoplasm of unspecified site (C79.9)
  - C80.2   Malignant neoplasm associated with transplanted organ 🐾
    Code first complication of transplanted organ (T86.-)
    Use additional code to identify the specific malignancy

★ **(See Plate 1 of the Anatomy Illustrations.)**

MALIGNANT NEOPLASMS OF LYMPHOID, HEMATOPOIETIC AND RELATED TISSUE (C81-C96)

- **Excludes2**   Kaposi's sarcoma of lymph nodes (C46.3)
  secondary and unspecified neoplasm of lymph nodes (C77.-)
  secondary neoplasm of bone marrow (C79.52)
  secondary neoplasm of spleen (C78.89)

- C81   Hodgkin lymphoma
  Form of malignant lymphoma with four types, nodular sclerosis, mixed cellularity, lymphocyte depleted, and lymphocyte predominant
  - **Excludes1**   personal history of Hodgkin lymphoma (Z85.71)
  - C81.0   Nodular lymphocyte predominant Hodgkin lymphoma
    Least aggressive, least common, typically no symptoms
    Lymphocytic-histiocytic predominance Hodgkin's disease
    - C81.00   Nodular lymphocyte predominant Hodgkin lymphoma, unspecified site 🐾
    - C81.01   Nodular lymphocyte predominant Hodgkin lymphoma, lymph nodes of head, face, and neck 🐾
    - C81.02   Nodular lymphocyte predominant Hodgkin lymphoma, intrathoracic lymph nodes 🐾
    - C81.03   Nodular lymphocyte predominant Hodgkin lymphoma, intra-abdominal lymph nodes 🐾
    - C81.04   Nodular lymphocyte predominant Hodgkin lymphoma, lymph nodes of axilla and upper limb 🐾
    - C81.05   Nodular lymphocyte predominant Hodgkin lymphoma, lymph nodes of inguinal region and lower limb 🐾
    - C81.06   Nodular lymphocyte predominant Hodgkin lymphoma, intrapelvic lymph nodes 🐾
    - C81.07   Nodular lymphocyte predominant Hodgkin lymphoma, spleen 🐾
    - C81.08   Nodular lymphocyte predominant Hodgkin lymphoma, lymph nodes of multiple sites 🐾
    - C81.09   Nodular lymphocyte predominant Hodgkin lymphoma, extranodal and solid organ sites 🐾

CHAPTER 2 (C00-D49)

● **C81.1**   Nodular sclerosis Hodgkin lymphoma
     Nodular sclerosis classical Hodgkin lymphoma
     Moderately aggressive; most common in young adults

     C81.10   Nodular sclerosis Hodgkin lymphoma, unspecified site 🐾

     C81.11   Nodular sclerosis Hodgkin lymphoma, lymph nodes of head, face, and neck 🐾

     C81.12   Nodular sclerosis Hodgkin lymphoma, intrathoracic lymph nodes 🐾

     C81.13   Nodular sclerosis Hodgkin lymphoma, intra-abdominal lymph nodes 🐾

     C81.14   Nodular sclerosis Hodgkin lymphoma, lymph nodes of axilla and upper limb 🐾

     C81.15   Nodular sclerosis Hodgkin lymphoma, lymph nodes of inguinal region and lower limb 🐾

     C81.16   Nodular sclerosis Hodgkin lymphoma, intrapelvic lymph nodes 🐾

     C81.17   Nodular sclerosis Hodgkin lymphoma, spleen 🐾

     C81.18   Nodular sclerosis Hodgkin lymphoma, lymph nodes of multiple sites 🐾

     C81.19   Nodular sclerosis Hodgkin lymphoma, extranodal and solid organ sites 🐾

● **C81.2**   Mixed cellularity Hodgkin lymphoma
     Mixed cellularity classical Hodgkin lymphoma
     A type of Hodgkin's that is moderately aggressive with mixed cell types

     C81.20   Mixed cellularity Hodgkin lymphoma, unspecified site 🐾

     C81.21   Mixed cellularity Hodgkin lymphoma, lymph nodes of head, face, and neck 🐾

     C81.22   Mixed cellularity Hodgkin lymphoma, intrathoracic lymph nodes 🐾

     C81.23   Mixed cellularity Hodgkin lymphoma, intra-abdominal lymph nodes 🐾

     C81.24   Mixed cellularity Hodgkin lymphoma, lymph nodes of axilla and upper limb 🐾

     C81.25   Mixed cellularity Hodgkin lymphoma, lymph nodes of inguinal region and lower limb 🐾

     C81.26   Mixed cellularity Hodgkin lymphoma, intrapelvic lymph nodes 🐾

     C81.27   Mixed cellularity Hodgkin lymphoma, spleen 🐾

     C81.28   Mixed cellularity Hodgkin lymphoma, lymph nodes of multiple sites 🐾

     C81.29   Mixed cellularity Hodgkin lymphoma, extranodal and solid organ sites 🐾

● **C81.3**   Lymphocyte depleted Hodgkin lymphoma
     Lymphocyte depleted classical Hodgkin lymphoma
     Most aggressive type with poor prognosis

     C81.30   Lymphocyte depleted Hodgkin lymphoma, unspecified site 🐾

     C81.31   Lymphocyte depleted Hodgkin lymphoma, lymph nodes of head, face, and neck 🐾

     C81.32   Lymphocyte depleted Hodgkin lymphoma, intrathoracic lymph nodes 🐾

     C81.33   Lymphocyte depleted Hodgkin lymphoma, intra-abdominal lymph nodes 🐾

     C81.34   Lymphocyte depleted Hodgkin lymphoma, lymph nodes of axilla and upper limb 🐾

     C81.35   Lymphocyte depleted Hodgkin lymphoma, lymph nodes of inguinal region and lower limb 🐾

     C81.36   Lymphocyte depleted Hodgkin lymphoma, intrapelvic lymph nodes 🐾

     C81.37   Lymphocyte depleted Hodgkin lymphoma, spleen 🐾

     C81.38   Lymphocyte depleted Hodgkin lymphoma, lymph nodes of multiple sites 🐾

     C81.39   Lymphocyte depleted Hodgkin lymphoma, extranodal and solid organ sites 🐾

● **C81.4**   Lymphocyte-rich Hodgkin lymphoma
     Lymphocyte-rich classical Hodgkin lymphoma
     Excludes1   nodular lymphocyte predominant Hodgkin lymphoma (C81.0-)

     C81.40   Lymphocyte-rich Hodgkin lymphoma, unspecified site 🐾

     C81.41   Lymphocyte-rich Hodgkin lymphoma, lymph nodes of head, face, and neck 🐾

     C81.42   Lymphocyte-rich Hodgkin lymphoma, intrathoracic lymph nodes 🐾

     C81.43   Lymphocyte-rich Hodgkin lymphoma, intra-abdominal lymph nodes 🐾

     C81.44   Lymphocyte-rich Hodgkin lymphoma, lymph nodes of axilla and upper limb 🐾

     C81.45   Lymphocyte-rich Hodgkin lymphoma, lymph nodes of inguinal region and lower limb 🐾

     C81.46   Lymphocyte-rich Hodgkin lymphoma, intrapelvic lymph nodes 🐾

     C81.47   Lymphocyte-rich Hodgkin lymphoma, spleen 🐾

     C81.48   Lymphocyte-rich Hodgkin lymphoma, lymph nodes of multiple sites 🐾

     C81.49   Lymphocyte-rich Hodgkin lymphoma, extranodal and solid organ sites 🐾

● **C81.7**   Other Hodgkin lymphoma
     Classical Hodgkin lymphoma NOS
     Other classical Hodgkin lymphoma

     C81.70   Other Hodgkin lymphoma, unspecified site 🐾

     C81.71   Other Hodgkin lymphoma, lymph nodes of head, face, and neck 🐾

     C81.72   Other Hodgkin lymphoma, intrathoracic lymph nodes 🐾

     C81.73   Other Hodgkin lymphoma, intra-abdominal lymph nodes 🐾

     C81.74   Other Hodgkin lymphoma, lymph nodes of axilla and upper limb 🐾

     C81.75   Other Hodgkin lymphoma, lymph nodes of inguinal region and lower limb 🐾

     C81.76   Other Hodgkin lymphoma, intrapelvic lymph nodes 🐾

     C81.77   Other Hodgkin lymphoma, spleen 🐾

     C81.78   Other Hodgkin lymphoma, lymph nodes of multiple sites 🐾

     C81.79   Other Hodgkin lymphoma, extranodal and solid organ sites 🐾

● **C81.9**   Hodgkin lymphoma, unspecified

     C81.90   Hodgkin lymphoma, unspecified, unspecified site 🐾

     C81.91   Hodgkin lymphoma, unspecified, lymph nodes of head, face, and neck 🐾

     C81.92   Hodgkin lymphoma, unspecified, intrathoracic lymph nodes 🐾

     C81.93   Hodgkin lymphoma, unspecified, intra-abdominal lymph nodes 🐾

     C81.94   Hodgkin lymphoma, unspecified, lymph nodes of axilla and upper limb 🐾

     C81.95   Hodgkin lymphoma, unspecified, lymph nodes of inguinal region and lower limb 🐾

     C81.96   Hodgkin lymphoma, unspecified, intrapelvic lymph nodes 🐾

     C81.97   Hodgkin lymphoma, unspecified, spleen 🐾

     C81.98   Hodgkin lymphoma, unspecified, lymph nodes of multiple sites 🐾

     C81.99   Hodgkin lymphoma, unspecified, extranodal and solid organ sites 🐾

CHAPTER 2 (C00-D49)

▶ New   ⇒ Revised   ~~deleted~~ Deleted   Excludes 1   Excludes 2   Includes   Use additional   Code first   Code also   Key words
OGCR Official Guidelines   X Assign placeholder X   ● Use Additional Character(s)   ▷ Manifestation Code   🐾 Hierarchical Condition Category   **Coding Clinic**

● **C82**   Follicular lymphoma
     Group of malignant lymphomas
     Includes   follicular lymphoma with or without diffuse areas
     Excludes1   mature T/NK-cell lymphomas (C84.-)
                 personal history of non-Hodgkin lymphoma (Z85.72)

● **C82.0**   Follicular lymphoma grade I
     C82.00   Follicular lymphoma grade I, unspecified site 🦠
     C82.01   Follicular lymphoma grade I, lymph nodes of head, face, and neck 🦠
     C82.02   Follicular lymphoma grade I, intrathoracic lymph nodes 🦠
     C82.03   Follicular lymphoma grade I, intra-abdominal lymph nodes 🦠
     C82.04   Follicular lymphoma grade I, lymph nodes of axilla and upper limb 🦠
     C82.05   Follicular lymphoma grade I, lymph nodes of inguinal region and lower limb 🦠
     C82.06   Follicular lymphoma grade I, intrapelvic lymph nodes 🦠
     C82.07   Follicular lymphoma grade I, spleen 🦠
     C82.08   Follicular lymphoma grade I, lymph nodes of multiple sites 🦠
     C82.09   Follicular lymphoma grade I, extranodal and solid organ sites 🦠

● **C82.1**   Follicular lymphoma grade II
     C82.10   Follicular lymphoma grade II, unspecified site 🦠
     C82.11   Follicular lymphoma grade II, lymph nodes of head, face, and neck 🦠
     C82.12   Follicular lymphoma grade II, intrathoracic lymph nodes 🦠
     C82.13   Follicular lymphoma grade II, intra-abdominal lymph nodes 🦠
     C82.14   Follicular lymphoma grade II, lymph nodes of axilla and upper limb 🦠
     C82.15   Follicular lymphoma grade II, lymph nodes of inguinal region and lower limb 🦠
     C82.16   Follicular lymphoma grade II, intrapelvic lymph nodes 🦠
     C82.17   Follicular lymphoma grade II, spleen 🦠
     C82.18   Follicular lymphoma grade II, lymph nodes of multiple sites 🦠
     C82.19   Follicular lymphoma grade II, extranodal and solid organ sites 🦠

● **C82.2**   Follicular lymphoma grade III, unspecified
     C82.20   Follicular lymphoma grade III, unspecified, unspecified site 🦠
     C82.21   Follicular lymphoma grade III, unspecified, lymph nodes of head, face, and neck 🦠
     C82.22   Follicular lymphoma grade III, unspecified, intrathoracic lymph nodes 🦠
     C82.23   Follicular lymphoma grade III, unspecified, intra-abdominal lymph nodes 🦠
     C82.24   Follicular lymphoma grade III, unspecified, lymph nodes of axilla and upper limb 🦠
     C82.25   Follicular lymphoma grade III, unspecified, lymph nodes of inguinal region and lower limb 🦠
     C82.26   Follicular lymphoma grade III, unspecified, intrapelvic lymph nodes 🦠
     C82.27   Follicular lymphoma grade III, unspecified, spleen 🦠
     C82.28   Follicular lymphoma grade III, unspecified, lymph nodes of multiple sites 🦠
     C82.29   Follicular lymphoma grade III, unspecified, extranodal and solid organ sites 🦠

● **C82.3**   Follicular lymphoma grade IIIa
     C82.30   Follicular lymphoma grade IIIa, unspecified site 🦠
     C82.31   Follicular lymphoma grade IIIa, lymph nodes of head, face, and neck 🦠
     C82.32   Follicular lymphoma grade IIIa, intrathoracic lymph nodes 🦠
     C82.33   Follicular lymphoma grade IIIa, intra-abdominal lymph nodes 🦠
     C82.34   Follicular lymphoma grade IIIa, lymph nodes of axilla and upper limb 🦠
     C82.35   Follicular lymphoma grade IIIa, lymph nodes of inguinal region and lower limb 🦠
     C82.36   Follicular lymphoma grade IIIa, intrapelvic lymph nodes 🦠
     C82.37   Follicular lymphoma grade IIIa, spleen 🦠
     C82.38   Follicular lymphoma grade IIIa, lymph nodes of multiple sites 🦠
     C82.39   Follicular lymphoma grade IIIa, extranodal and solid organ sites 🦠

● **C82.4**   Follicular lymphoma grade IIIb
     C82.40   Follicular lymphoma grade IIIb, unspecified site 🦠
     C82.41   Follicular lymphoma grade IIIb, lymph nodes of head, face, and neck 🦠
     C82.42   Follicular lymphoma grade IIIb, intrathoracic lymph nodes 🦠
     C82.43   Follicular lymphoma grade IIIb, intra-abdominal lymph nodes 🦠
     C82.44   Follicular lymphoma grade IIIb, lymph nodes of axilla and upper limb 🦠
     C82.45   Follicular lymphoma grade IIIb, lymph nodes of inguinal region and lower limb 🦠
     C82.46   Follicular lymphoma grade IIIb, intrapelvic lymph nodes 🦠
     C82.47   Follicular lymphoma grade IIIb, spleen 🦠
     C82.48   Follicular lymphoma grade IIIb, lymph nodes of multiple sites 🦠
     C82.49   Follicular lymphoma grade IIIb, extranodal and solid organ sites 🦠

● **C82.5**   Diffuse follicle center lymphoma
     C82.50   Diffuse follicle center lymphoma, unspecified site 🦠
     C82.51   Diffuse follicle center lymphoma, lymph nodes of head, face, and neck 🦠
     C82.52   Diffuse follicle center lymphoma, intrathoracic lymph nodes 🦠
     C82.53   Diffuse follicle center lymphoma, intra-abdominal lymph nodes 🦠
     C82.54   Diffuse follicle center lymphoma, lymph nodes of axilla and upper limb 🦠
     C82.55   Diffuse follicle center lymphoma, lymph nodes of inguinal region and lower limb 🦠
     C82.56   Diffuse follicle center lymphoma, intrapelvic lymph nodes 🦠
     C82.57   Diffuse follicle center lymphoma, spleen 🦠
     C82.58   Diffuse follicle center lymphoma, lymph nodes of multiple sites 🦠
     C82.59   Diffuse follicle center lymphoma, extranodal and solid organ sites 🦠

● **C82.6**   Cutaneous follicle center lymphoma
     C82.60   Cutaneous follicle center lymphoma, unspecified site 🦠
     C82.61   Cutaneous follicle center lymphoma, lymph nodes of head, face, and neck 🦠
     C82.62   Cutaneous follicle center lymphoma, intrathoracic lymph nodes 🦠
     C82.63   Cutaneous follicle center lymphoma, intra-abdominal lymph nodes 🦠

CHAPTER 2 (C00-D49)

C82.64   Cutaneous follicle center lymphoma, lymph nodes of axilla and upper limb 🐾

C82.65   Cutaneous follicle center lymphoma, lymph nodes of inguinal region and lower limb 🐾

C82.66   Cutaneous follicle center lymphoma, intrapelvic lymph nodes 🐾

C82.67   Cutaneous follicle center lymphoma, spleen 🐾

C82.68   Cutaneous follicle center lymphoma, lymph nodes of multiple sites 🐾

C82.69   Cutaneous follicle center lymphoma, extranodal and solid organ sites 🐾

● C82.8   Other types of follicular lymphoma

C82.80   Other types of follicular lymphoma, unspecified site 🐾

C82.81   Other types of follicular lymphoma, lymph nodes of head, face, and neck 🐾

C82.82   Other types of follicular lymphoma, intrathoracic lymph nodes 🐾

C82.83   Other types of follicular lymphoma, intra-abdominal lymph nodes 🐾

C82.84   Other types of follicular lymphoma, lymph nodes of axilla and upper limb 🐾

C82.85   Other types of follicular lymphoma, lymph nodes of inguinal region and lower limb 🐾

C82.86   Other types of follicular lymphoma, intrapelvic lymph nodes 🐾

C82.87   Other types of follicular lymphoma, spleen 🐾

C82.88   Other types of follicular lymphoma, lymph nodes of multiple sites 🐾

C82.89   Other types of follicular lymphoma, extranodal and solid organ sites 🐾

● C82.9   Follicular lymphoma, unspecified

C82.90   Follicular lymphoma, unspecified, unspecified site 🐾

C82.91   Follicular lymphoma, unspecified, lymph nodes of head, face, and neck 🐾

C82.92   Follicular lymphoma, unspecified, intrathoracic lymph nodes 🐾

C82.93   Follicular lymphoma, unspecified, intra-abdominal lymph nodes 🐾

C82.94   Follicular lymphoma, unspecified, lymph nodes of axilla and upper limb 🐾

C82.95   Follicular lymphoma, unspecified, lymph nodes of inguinal region and lower limb 🐾

C82.96   Follicular lymphoma, unspecified, intrapelvic lymph nodes 🐾

C82.97   Follicular lymphoma, unspecified, spleen 🐾

C82.98   Follicular lymphoma, unspecified, lymph nodes of multiple sites 🐾

C82.99   Follicular lymphoma, unspecified, extranodal and solid organ sites 🐾

● C83   Non-follicular lymphoma

    Excludes1   personal history of non-Hodgkin lymphoma (Z85.72)

● C83.0   Small cell B-cell lymphoma

    Lymphoplasmacytic lymphoma
    Nodal marginal zone lymphoma
    Non-leukemic variant of B-CLL
    Splenic marginal zone lymphoma

    Excludes1   chronic lymphocytic leukemia (C91.1)
                mature T/NK-cell lymphomas (C84.-)
                Waldenström macroglobulinemia (C88.0)

C83.00   Small cell B-cell lymphoma, unspecified site 🐾

C83.01   Small cell B-cell lymphoma, lymph nodes of head, face, and neck 🐾

C83.02   Small cell B-cell lymphoma, intrathoracic lymph nodes 🐾

C83.03   Small cell B-cell lymphoma, intra-abdominal lymph nodes 🐾

C83.04   Small cell B-cell lymphoma, lymph nodes of axilla and upper limb 🐾

C83.05   Small cell B-cell lymphoma, lymph nodes of inguinal region and lower limb 🐾

C83.06   Small cell B-cell lymphoma, intrapelvic lymph nodes 🐾

C83.07   Small cell B-cell lymphoma, spleen 🐾

C83.08   Small cell B-cell lymphoma, lymph nodes of multiple sites 🐾

C83.09   Small cell B-cell lymphoma, extranodal and solid organ sites 🐾

● C83.1   Mantle cell lymphoma

    Centrocytic lymphoma
    Malignant lymphomatous polyposis

C83.10   Mantle cell lymphoma, unspecified site 🐾

C83.11   Mantle cell lymphoma, lymph nodes of head, face, and neck 🐾

C83.12   Mantle cell lymphoma, intrathoracic lymph nodes 🐾

C83.13   Mantle cell lymphoma, intra-abdominal lymph nodes 🐾

C83.14   Mantle cell lymphoma, lymph nodes of axilla and upper limb 🐾

C83.15   Mantle cell lymphoma, lymph nodes of inguinal region and lower limb 🐾

C83.16   Mantle cell lymphoma, intrapelvic lymph nodes 🐾

C83.17   Mantle cell lymphoma, spleen 🐾

C83.18   Mantle cell lymphoma, lymph nodes of multiple sites 🐾

C83.19   Mantle cell lymphoma, extranodal and solid organ sites 🐾

● C83.3   Diffuse large B-cell lymphoma

    Anaplastic diffuse large B-cell lymphoma
    CD30-positive diffuse large B-cell lymphoma
    Centroblastic diffuse large B-cell lymphoma
    Diffuse large B-cell lymphoma, subtype not specified
    Immunoblastic diffuse large B-cell lymphoma
    Plasmablastic diffuse large B-cell lymphoma
    Diffuse large B-cell lymphoma, subtype not specified
    T-cell rich diffuse large B-cell lymphoma

    Excludes1   mediastinal (thymic) large B-cell lymphoma (C85.2-)
                mature T/NK-cell lymphomas (C84.-)

C83.30   Diffuse large B-cell lymphoma, unspecified site 🐾

C83.31   Diffuse large B-cell lymphoma, lymph nodes of head, face, and neck 🐾

C83.32   Diffuse large B-cell lymphoma, intrathoracic lymph nodes 🐾

C83.33   Diffuse large B-cell lymphoma, intra-abdominal lymph nodes 🐾

C83.34   Diffuse large B-cell lymphoma, lymph nodes of axilla and upper limb 🐾

C83.35   Diffuse large B-cell lymphoma, lymph nodes of inguinal region and lower limb 🐾

C83.36   Diffuse large B-cell lymphoma, intrapelvic lymph nodes 🐾

C83.37   Diffuse large B-cell lymphoma, spleen 🐾

C83.38   Diffuse large B-cell lymphoma, lymph nodes of multiple sites 🐾

C83.39   Diffuse large B-cell lymphoma, extranodal and solid organ sites 🐾

● **C83.5** **Lymphoblastic (diffuse) lymphoma**
Highly malignant type of non-Hodgkin lymphoma with diffuse infiltration
B-precursor lymphoma
Lymphoblastic B-cell lymphoma
Lymphoblastic lymphoma NOS
Lymphoblastic T-cell lymphoma
T-precursor lymphoma

C83.50 Lymphoblastic (diffuse) lymphoma, unspecified site 🦠

C83.51 Lymphoblastic (diffuse) lymphoma, lymph nodes of head, face, and neck 🦠

C83.52 Lymphoblastic (diffuse) lymphoma, intrathoracic lymph nodes 🦠

C83.53 Lymphoblastic (diffuse) lymphoma, intra-abdominal lymph nodes 🦠

C83.54 Lymphoblastic (diffuse) lymphoma, lymph nodes of axilla and upper limb 🦠

C83.55 Lymphoblastic (diffuse) lymphoma, lymph nodes of inguinal region and lower limb 🦠

C83.56 Lymphoblastic (diffuse) lymphoma, intrapelvic lymph nodes 🦠

C83.57 Lymphoblastic (diffuse) lymphoma, spleen 🦠

C83.58 Lymphoblastic (diffuse) lymphoma, lymph nodes of multiple sites 🦠

C83.59 Lymphoblastic (diffuse) lymphoma, extranodal and solid organ sites 🦠

● **C83.7** **Burkitt lymphoma**
Form of small cell lymphoma
Atypical Burkitt lymphoma
Burkitt-like lymphoma

    Excludes1 mature B-cell leukemia Burkitt type (C91.A-)

C83.70 Burkitt lymphoma, unspecified site 🦠

C83.71 Burkitt lymphoma, lymph nodes of head, face, and neck 🦠

C83.72 Burkitt lymphoma, intrathoracic lymph nodes 🦠

C83.73 Burkitt lymphoma, intra-abdominal lymph nodes 🦠

C83.74 Burkitt lymphoma, lymph nodes of axilla and upper limb 🦠

C83.75 Burkitt lymphoma, lymph nodes of inguinal region and lower limb 🦠

C83.76 Burkitt lymphoma, intrapelvic lymph nodes 🦠

C83.77 Burkitt lymphoma, spleen 🦠

C83.78 Burkitt lymphoma, lymph nodes of multiple sites 🦠

C83.79 Burkitt lymphoma, extranodal and solid organ sites 🦠

● **C83.8** **Other non-follicular lymphoma**
Intravascular large B-cell lymphoma
Lymphoid granulomatosis
Primary effusion B-cell lymphoma

    Excludes1 mediastinal (thymic) large B-cell lymphoma (C85.2-)
            T-cell rich B-cell lymphoma (C83.3-)

C83.80 Other non-follicular lymphoma, unspecified site 🦠

C83.81 Other non-follicular lymphoma, lymph nodes of head, face, and neck 🦠

C83.82 Other non-follicular lymphoma, intrathoracic lymph nodes 🦠

C83.83 Other non-follicular lymphoma, intra-abdominal lymph nodes 🦠

C83.84 Other non-follicular lymphoma, lymph nodes of axilla and upper limb 🦠

C83.85 Other non-follicular lymphoma, lymph nodes of inguinal region and lower limb 🦠

C83.86 Other non-follicular lymphoma, intrapelvic lymph nodes 🦠

C83.87 Other non-follicular lymphoma, spleen 🦠

C83.88 Other non-follicular lymphoma, lymph nodes of multiple sites 🦠

C83.89 Other non-follicular lymphoma, extranodal and solid organ sites 🦠

● **C83.9** **Non-follicular (diffuse) lymphoma, unspecified**

C83.90 Non-follicular (diffuse) lymphoma, unspecified, unspecified site 🦠

C83.91 Non-follicular (diffuse) lymphoma, unspecified, lymph nodes of head, face, and neck 🦠

C83.92 Non-follicular (diffuse) lymphoma, unspecified, intrathoracic lymph nodes 🦠

C83.93 Non-follicular (diffuse) lymphoma, unspecified, intra-abdominal lymph nodes 🦠

C83.94 Non-follicular (diffuse) lymphoma, unspecified, lymph nodes of axilla and upper limb 🦠

C83.95 Non-follicular (diffuse) lymphoma, unspecified, lymph nodes of inguinal region and lower limb 🦠

C83.96 Non-follicular (diffuse) lymphoma, unspecified, intrapelvic lymph nodes 🦠

C83.97 Non-follicular (diffuse) lymphoma, unspecified, spleen 🦠

C83.98 Non-follicular (diffuse) lymphoma, unspecified, lymph nodes of multiple sites 🦠

C83.99 Non-follicular (diffuse) lymphoma, unspecified, extranodal and solid organ sites 🦠

● **C84** **Mature T/NK-cell lymphomas**

    Excludes1 personal history of non-Hodgkin lymphoma (Z85.72)

● **C84.0** **Mycosis fungoides**
Chronic or rapidly progressive form of cutaneous T-cell lymphoma; AKA granuloma fungoides

    Excludes1 peripheral T-cell lymphoma, not classified (C84.4-)

C84.00 Mycosis fungoides, unspecified site 🦠

C84.01 Mycosis fungoides, lymph nodes of head, face, and neck 🦠

C84.02 Mycosis fungoides, intrathoracic lymph nodes 🦠

C84.03 Mycosis fungoides, intra-abdominal lymph nodes 🦠

C84.04 Mycosis fungoides, lymph nodes of axilla and upper limb 🦠

C84.05 Mycosis fungoides, lymph nodes of inguinal region and lower limb 🦠

C84.06 Mycosis fungoides, intrapelvic lymph nodes 🦠

C84.07 Mycosis fungoides, spleen 🦠

C84.08 Mycosis fungoides, lymph nodes of multiple sites 🦠

C84.09 Mycosis fungoides, extranodal and solid organ sites 🦠

● **C84.1** **Sézary disease**
Type of cutaneous lymphoma affecting T-cells

C84.10 Sézary disease, unspecified site 🦠

C84.11 Sézary disease, lymph nodes of head, face, and neck 🦠

C84.12 Sézary disease, intrathoracic lymph nodes 🦠

C84.13 Sézary disease, intra-abdominal lymph nodes 🦠

C84.14 Sézary disease, lymph nodes of axilla and upper limb 🦠

C84.15 Sézary disease, lymph nodes of inguinal region and lower limb 🦠

C84.16 Sézary disease, intrapelvic lymph nodes 🦠

C84.17 Sézary disease, spleen 🦠

C84.18 Sézary disease, lymph nodes of multiple sites 🦠

C84.19 Sézary disease, extranodal and solid organ sites 🦠

CHAPTER 2 (C00-D49)

● C84.4 **Peripheral T-cell lymphoma, not classified**
           Diverse group of blood carcinomas originating from T-cells,
           requiring aggressive chemotherapy
           Lennert's lymphoma
           Lymphoepithelioid lymphoma
           Mature T-cell lymphoma, not elsewhere classified

   C84.40 Peripheral T-cell lymphoma, not
           classified, unspecified site 🐾

   C84.41 Peripheral T-cell lymphoma, not classified,
           lymph nodes of head, face, and neck 🐾

   C84.42 Peripheral T-cell lymphoma, not classified,
           intrathoracic lymph nodes 🐾

   C84.43 Peripheral T-cell lymphoma, not classified,
           intra-abdominal lymph nodes 🐾

   C84.44 Peripheral T-cell lymphoma, not classified,
           lymph nodes of axilla and upper limb 🐾

   C84.45 Peripheral T-cell lymphoma, not classified,
           lymph nodes of inguinal region and lower
           limb 🐾

   C84.46 Peripheral T-cell lymphoma, not classified,
           intrapelvic lymph nodes 🐾

   C84.47 Peripheral T-cell lymphoma, not classified,
           spleen 🐾

   C84.48 Peripheral T-cell lymphoma, not classified,
           lymph nodes of multiple sites 🐾

   C84.49 Peripheral T-cell lymphoma, not classified,
           extranodal and solid organ sites 🐾

● C84.6 **Anaplastic large cell lymphoma, ALK-positive**
           Anaplastic large cell lymphoma, CD30-positive

   C84.60 Anaplastic large cell lymphoma, ALK-
           positive, unspecified site 🐾

   C84.61 Anaplastic large cell lymphoma, ALK-positive,
           lymph nodes of head, face, and neck 🐾

   C84.62 Anaplastic large cell lymphoma, ALK-positive,
           intrathoracic lymph nodes 🐾

   C84.63 Anaplastic large cell lymphoma, ALK-positive,
           intra-abdominal lymph nodes 🐾

   C84.64 Anaplastic large cell lymphoma, ALK-positive,
           lymph nodes of axilla and upper limb 🐾

   C84.65 Anaplastic large cell lymphoma, ALK-positive,
           lymph nodes of inguinal region and lower
           limb 🐾

   C84.66 Anaplastic large cell lymphoma, ALK-positive,
           intrapelvic lymph nodes 🐾

   C84.67 Anaplastic large cell lymphoma, ALK-positive,
           spleen 🐾

   C84.68 Anaplastic large cell lymphoma, ALK-positive,
           lymph nodes of multiple sites 🐾

   C84.69 Anaplastic large cell lymphoma, ALK-positive,
           extranodal and solid organ sites 🐾

● C84.7 **Anaplastic large cell lymphoma, ALK-negative**

   Excludes1   primary cutaneous CD30-positive T-cell
                   proliferations (C86.6-)

   C84.70 Anaplastic large cell lymphoma, ALK-
           negative, unspecified site 🐾

   C84.71 Anaplastic large cell lymphoma, ALK-negative,
           lymph nodes of head, face, and neck 🐾

   C84.72 Anaplastic large cell lymphoma, ALK-negative,
           intrathoracic lymph nodes 🐾

   C84.73 Anaplastic large cell lymphoma, ALK-negative,
           intra-abdominal lymph nodes 🐾

   C84.74 Anaplastic large cell lymphoma, ALK-negative,
           lymph nodes of axilla and upper limb 🐾

   C84.75 Anaplastic large cell lymphoma, ALK-negative,
           lymph nodes of inguinal region and lower
           limb 🐾

   C84.76 Anaplastic large cell lymphoma, ALK-negative,
           intrapelvic lymph nodes 🐾

   C84.77 Anaplastic large cell lymphoma, ALK-negative,
           spleen 🐾

Item 2–7 Lymphosarcoma, also known as malignant lymphoma, is a
cancer of the lymph system exhibiting abnormal cells encompassing an entire
lymph node creating a diffuse pattern without any definite organization. Diffuse
pattern lymphoma has a more unfavorable survival outlook than those with a
follicular or nodular pattern. Reticulosarcoma is the most common aggressive
form of non-Hodgkin lymphoma.

   C84.78 Anaplastic large cell lymphoma, ALK-negative,
           lymph nodes of multiple sites 🐾

   C84.79 Anaplastic large cell lymphoma, ALK-negative,
           extranodal and solid organ sites 🐾

▶ C84.7A Anaplastic large cell lymphoma, ALK-negative,
           breast
           ▶Breast implant associated anaplastic large cell
             lymphoma (BIA-ALCL)
       ▶Use additional code to identify:
             ▶breast implant status (Z98.82)
             ▶personal history of breast implant removal
               (Z98.86)

● C84.A **Cutaneous T-cell lymphoma, unspecified**

   C84.A0 Cutaneous T-cell lymphoma, unspecified,
           unspecified site 🐾

   C84.A1 Cutaneous T-cell lymphoma, unspecified lymph
           nodes of head, face, and neck 🐾

   C84.A2 Cutaneous T-cell lymphoma, unspecified,
           intrathoracic lymph nodes 🐾

   C84.A3 Cutaneous T-cell lymphoma, unspecified,
           intra-abdominal lymph nodes 🐾

   C84.A4 Cutaneous T-cell lymphoma, unspecified,
           lymph nodes of axilla and upper limb 🐾

   C84.A5 Cutaneous T-cell lymphoma, unspecified,
           lymph nodes of inguinal region and lower
           limb 🐾

   C84.A6 Cutaneous T-cell lymphoma, unspecified,
           intrapelvic lymph nodes 🐾

   C84.A7 Cutaneous T-cell lymphoma, unspecified,
           spleen 🐾
           ▶Coding Clinic: 2021, Q2, P7

   C84.A8 Cutaneous T-cell lymphoma, unspecified,
           lymph nodes of multiple sites 🐾
           ▶Coding Clinic: 2021, Q2, P7

   C84.A9 Cutaneous T-cell lymphoma, unspecified,
           extranodal and solid organ sites 🐾

● C84.Z **Other mature T/NK-cell lymphomas**

   Note: If T-cell lineage or involvement is mentioned in
           conjunction with a specific lymphoma, code to the
           more specific description.

   Excludes1   angioimmunoblastic T-cell lymphoma
                   (C86.5)
                   blastic NK-cell lymphoma (C86.4)
                   enteropathy-type T-cell lymphoma (C86.2)
                   extranodal NK-cell lymphoma, nasal type
                   (C86.0)
                   hepatosplenic T-cell lymphoma (C86.1)
                   primary cutaneous CD30-positive T-cell
                   proliferations (C86.6)
                   subcutaneous panniculitis-like T-cell
                   lymphoma (C86.3)
                   T-cell leukemia (C91.1-)

   C84.Z0 Other mature T/NK-cell
           lymphomas, unspecified site 🐾

   C84.Z1 Other mature T/NK-cell lymphomas, lymph
           nodes of head, face, and neck 🐾

   C84.Z2 Other mature T/NK-cell lymphomas,
           intrathoracic lymph nodes 🐾

   C84.Z3 Other mature T/NK-cell lymphomas, intra-
           abdominal lymph nodes 🐾

   C84.Z4 Other mature T/NK-cell lymphomas, lymph
           nodes of axilla and upper limb 🐾

   C84.Z5 Other mature T/NK-cell lymphomas, lymph
           nodes of inguinal region and lower limb 🐾

   C84.Z6 Other mature T/NK-cell lymphomas,
           intrapelvic lymph nodes 🐾

▶ New   ⇒ Revised   ~~deleted~~ Deleted   Excludes 1   Excludes 2   Includes   Use additional   Code first   Code also   Key words

OGCR Official Guidelines   X Assign placeholder X   ● Use Additional Character(s)   ▷ Manifestation Code   🐾 Hierarchical Condition Category   **Coding Clinic**

C84.Z7 Other mature T/NK-cell lymphomas, spleen 🐾

C84.Z8 Other mature T/NK-cell lymphomas, lymph nodes of multiple sites 🐾

C84.Z9 Other mature T/NK-cell lymphomas, extranodal and solid organ sites 🐾

● C84.9 Mature T/NK-cell lymphomas, unspecified
NK/T cell lymphoma NOS

> **Excludes1**   mature T-cell lymphoma, not elsewhere classified (C84.4-)

C84.90 Mature T/NK-cell lymphomas, unspecified, unspecified site 🐾

C84.91 Mature T/NK-cell lymphomas, unspecified, lymph nodes of head, face, and neck 🐾

C84.92 Mature T/NK-cell lymphomas, unspecified, intrathoracic lymph nodes 🐾

C84.93 Mature T/NK-cell lymphomas, unspecified, intra-abdominal lymph nodes 🐾

C84.94 Mature T/NK-cell lymphomas, unspecified, lymph nodes of axilla and upper limb 🐾

C84.95 Mature T/NK-cell lymphomas, unspecified, lymph nodes of inguinal region and lower limb 🐾

C84.96 Mature T/NK-cell lymphomas, unspecified, intrapelvic lymph nodes 🐾

C84.97 Mature T/NK-cell lymphomas, unspecified, spleen 🐾

C84.98 Mature T/NK-cell lymphomas, unspecified, lymph nodes of multiple sites 🐾

C84.99 Mature T/NK-cell lymphomas, unspecified, extranodal and solid organ sites 🐾

● C85 Other specified and unspecified types of non-Hodgkin lymphoma

> **Excludes1**   other specified types of T/NK-cell lymphoma (C86.-)
> personal history of non-Hodgkin lymphoma (Z85.72)

● C85.1 Unspecified B-cell lymphoma

> **Note:** If B-cell lineage or involvement is mentioned in conjunction with a specific lymphoma, code to the more specific description.

C85.10 Unspecified B-cell lymphoma, unspecified site 🐾

C85.11 Unspecified B-cell lymphoma, lymph nodes of head, face, and neck 🐾

C85.12 Unspecified B-cell lymphoma, intrathoracic lymph nodes 🐾

C85.13 Unspecified B-cell lymphoma, intra-abdominal lymph nodes 🐾

C85.14 Unspecified B-cell lymphoma, lymph nodes of axilla and upper limb 🐾

C85.15 Unspecified B-cell lymphoma, lymph nodes of inguinal region and lower limb 🐾

C85.16 Unspecified B-cell lymphoma, intrapelvic lymph nodes 🐾

C85.17 Unspecified B-cell lymphoma, spleen 🐾

C85.18 Unspecified B-cell lymphoma, lymph nodes of multiple sites 🐾

C85.19 Unspecified B-cell lymphoma, extranodal and solid organ sites 🐾

● C85.2 Mediastinal (thymic) large B-cell lymphoma

C85.20 Mediastinal (thymic) large B-cell lymphoma, unspecified site 🐾

C85.21 Mediastinal (thymic) large B-cell lymphoma, lymph nodes of head, face, and neck 🐾

C85.22 Mediastinal (thymic) large B-cell lymphoma, intrathoracic lymph nodes 🐾

C85.23 Mediastinal (thymic) large B-cell lymphoma, intra-abdominal lymph nodes 🐾

C85.24 Mediastinal (thymic) large B-cell lymphoma, lymph nodes of axilla and upper limb 🐾

C85.25 Mediastinal (thymic) large B-cell lymphoma, lymph nodes of inguinal region and lower limb 🐾

C85.26 Mediastinal (thymic) large B-cell lymphoma, intrapelvic lymph nodes 🐾

C85.27 Mediastinal (thymic) large B-cell lymphoma, spleen 🐾

C85.28 Mediastinal (thymic) large B-cell lymphoma, lymph nodes of multiple sites 🐾

C85.29 Mediastinal (thymic) large B-cell lymphoma, extranodal and solid organ sites 🐾

● C85.8 Other specified types of non-Hodgkin lymphoma

C85.80 Other specified types of non-Hodgkin lymphoma, unspecified site 🐾

C85.81 Other specified types of non-Hodgkin lymphoma, lymph nodes of head, face, and neck 🐾

C85.82 Other specified types of non-Hodgkin lymphoma, intrathoracic lymph nodes 🐾

C85.83 Other specified types of non-Hodgkin lymphoma, intra-abdominal lymph nodes 🐾

C85.84 Other specified types of non-Hodgkin lymphoma, lymph nodes of axilla and upper limb 🐾

C85.85 Other specified types of non-Hodgkin lymphoma, lymph nodes of inguinal region and lower limb 🐾

C85.86 Other specified types of non-Hodgkin lymphoma, intrapelvic lymph nodes 🐾

C85.87 Other specified types of non-Hodgkin lymphoma, spleen 🐾

C85.88 Other specified types of non-Hodgkin lymphoma, lymph nodes of multiple sites 🐾

C85.89 Other specified types of non-Hodgkin lymphoma, extranodal and solid organ sites 🐾

● C85.9 Non-Hodgkin lymphoma, unspecified
Lymphoma NOS
Malignant lymphoma NOS
Non-Hodgkin lymphoma NOS

C85.90 Non-Hodgkin lymphoma, unspecified, unspecified site 🐾

C85.91 Non-Hodgkin lymphoma, unspecified, lymph nodes of head, face, and neck 🐾

C85.92 Non-Hodgkin lymphoma, unspecified, intrathoracic lymph nodes 🐾

C85.93 Non-Hodgkin lymphoma, unspecified, intra-abdominal lymph nodes 🐾

C85.94 Non-Hodgkin lymphoma, unspecified, lymph nodes of axilla and upper limb 🐾

C85.95 Non-Hodgkin lymphoma, unspecified, lymph nodes of inguinal region and lower limb 🐾

C85.96 Non-Hodgkin lymphoma, unspecified, intrapelvic lymph nodes 🐾

C85.97 Non-Hodgkin lymphoma, unspecified, spleen 🐾

C85.98 Non-Hodgkin lymphoma, unspecified, lymph nodes of multiple sites 🐾

C85.99 Non-Hodgkin lymphoma, unspecified, extranodal and solid organ sites 🐾

CHAPTER 2 (C00-D49)

● **C86**   **Other specified types of T/NK-cell lymphoma**

     Excludes1   anaplastic large cell lymphoma, ALK negative
                 (C84.7-)
               anaplastic large cell lymphoma, ALK positive
                 (C84.6-)
               mature T/NK-cell lymphomas (C84.-)
               other specified types of non-Hodgkin lymphoma
                 (C85.8-)

   C86.0   **Extranodal NK/T-cell lymphoma, nasal type** 🐾

   C86.1   **Hepatosplenic T-cell lymphoma** 🐾
           Alpha-beta and gamma delta types

   C86.2   **Enteropathy-type (intestinal) T-cell lymphoma** 🐾
           Enteropathy associated T-cell lymphoma

   C86.3   **Subcutaneous panniculitis-like T-cell lymphoma** 🐾

   C86.4   **Blastic NK-cell lymphoma** 🐾
           Blastic plasmacytoid dendritic cell neoplasm (BPDCN)

   C86.5   **Angioimmunoblastic T-cell lymphoma** 🐾
           Angioimmunoblastic lymphadenopathy with
              dysproteinemia (AILD)

   C86.6   **Primary cutaneous CD30-positive T-cell proliferations** 🐾
           Lymphomatoid papulosis
           Primary cutaneous anaplastic large cell lymphoma
           Primary cutaneous CD30-positive large T-cell lymphoma

● **C88**   **Malignant immunoproliferative diseases and certain other B-cell lymphomas**
     Diseases involving immune system

     Excludes1   B-cell lymphoma, unspecified (C85.1-)
               personal history of other malignant neoplasms of
                 lymphoid, hematopoietic and related tissues
                 (Z85.79)

   C88.0   **Waldenström's macroglobulinemia** 🐾
           Lymphoplasmacytic lymphoma with IgM-production
           Macroglobulinemia (idiopathic) (primary)

     Excludes1   small cell B-cell lymphoma (C83.0)

   C88.2   **Heavy chain disease** 🐾
           Franklin disease
           Gamma heavy chain disease
           Mu heavy chain disease

   C88.3   **Immunoproliferative small intestinal disease** 🐾
           Alpha heavy chain disease
           Mediterranean lymphoma

   C88.4   **Extranodal marginal zone B-cell lymphoma of mucosa-associated lymphoid tissue [MALT-lymphoma]** 🐾
           Lymphoma of skin-associated lymphoid tissue [SALT-lymphoma]
           Lymphoma of bronchial-associated lymphoid tissue [BALT-lymphoma]

     Excludes1   high malignant (diffuse large B-cell)
               lymphoma (C83.3-)

   C88.8   **Other malignant immunoproliferative diseases** 🐾

   C88.9   **Malignant immunoproliferative disease, unspecified** 🐾
           Immunoproliferative disease NOS

● **C90**   **Multiple myeloma and malignant plasma cell neoplasms**

     Excludes1   personal history of other malignant neoplasms of
               lymphoid, hematopoietic and related tissues
               (Z85.79)

   ● **C90.0**   **Multiple myeloma**
           Kahler's disease
           Medullary plasmacytoma
           Myelomatosis
           Plasma cell myeloma

     Excludes1   solitary myeloma (C90.3-)
               solitary plasmacytoma (C90.3-)

     C90.00   **Multiple myeloma** not having achieved remission 🐾
            Multiple myeloma with failed remission
            Multiple myeloma NOS

     C90.01   **Multiple myeloma** in remission 🐾

     C90.02   **Multiple myeloma** in relapse 🐾

Item 2–8   **Multiple myeloma** is a cancer of a plasma cell (a type of white blood cell) and is an incurable but treatable disease. Immunoproliferative neoplasm is a term for diseases (mostly cancers) in which the immune system cells proliferate.

   ● **C90.1**   **Plasma cell leukemia**
           Rare type of acute leukemia
           Plasmacytic leukemia
           Coding Clinic: 2019, Q2, P30

     C90.10   **Plasma cell leukemia** not having achieved remission 🐾
            Plasma cell leukemia with failed remission
            Plasma cell leukemia NOS
            Coding Clinic: 2019, Q2, P30

     C90.11   **Plasma cell leukemia** in remission 🐾

     C90.12   **Plasma cell leukemia** in relapse 🐾

   ● **C90.2**   **Extramedullary plasmacytoma**
           Malignant monoclonal plasma cell tumor growing in soft tissue; AKA plasma cell dyscrasias

     C90.20   **Extramedullary plasmacytoma** not having achieved remission 🐾
            Extramedullary plasmacytoma with failed remission
            Extramedullary plasmacytoma NOS

     C90.21   **Extramedullary plasmacytoma** in remission 🐾

     C90.22   **Extramedullary plasmacytoma** in relapse 🐾

   ● **C90.3**   **Solitary plasmacytoma**
           Localized malignant plasma cell tumor NOS
           Plasmacytoma NOS
           Solitary myeloma

     C90.30   **Solitary plasmacytoma** not having achieved remission 🐾
            Solitary plasmacytoma with failed remission
            Solitary plasmacytoma NOS

     C90.31   **Solitary plasmacytoma** in remission 🐾

     C90.32   **Solitary plasmacytoma** in relapse 🐾

● **C91**   **Lymphoid leukemia**
     Type of leukemia affecting circulating cells of lymphoid origin

     Excludes1   personal history of leukemia (Z85.6)

   ● **C91.0**   **Acute lymphoblastic leukemia [ALL]**
           Note: Codes in subcategory C91.0 should only be used
                for T-cell and B-cell precursor leukemia

     C91.00   **Acute lymphoblastic leukemia** not having achieved remission 🐾
            Acute lymphoblastic leukemia with failed remission
            Acute lymphoblastic leukemia NOS

     C91.01   **Acute lymphoblastic leukemia,** in remission 🐾

     C91.02   **Acute lymphoblastic leukemia,** in relapse 🐾

   ● **C91.1**   **Chronic lymphocytic leukemia of** B-cell type
           Lymphoplasmacytic leukemia
           Richter syndrome

     Excludes1   lymphoplasmacytic lymphoma (C83.0-)

     C91.10   **Chronic lymphocytic leukemia of B-cell type** not having achieved remission 🐾
            Chronic lymphocytic leukemia of B-cell type with failed remission
            Chronic lymphocytic leukemia of B-cell type NOS

     C91.11   **Chronic lymphocytic leukemia of B-cell type** in remission 🐾

     C91.12   **Chronic lymphocytic leukemia of B-cell type** in relapse 🐾

Item 2–9   Leukemia is a cancer (acute or chronic) of the blood-forming tissues of the bone marrow. Blood cells all start out as stem cells. They mature and become red cells, white cells, or platelets. There are three main types of leukocytes (white cells that fight infection): monocytes, lymphocytes, and granulocytes. **Acute monocytic leukemia** (AML) affects monocytes. **Acute lymphoid leukemia** (ALL) affects lymphocytes, and **acute myeloid leukemia** (AML) affects cells that typically develop into white blood cells (not lymphocytes), though it may develop in other blood cells.

▶ New   ⇒ Revised   ~~deleted~~ Deleted   Excludes 1   Excludes 2   Includes   Use additional   Code first   Code also   Key words

OGCR Official Guidelines   **X** Assign placeholder X   ● Use Additional Character(s)   ▶ Manifestation Code   🐾 Hierarchical Condition Category   **Coding Clinic**

● **C91.3 Prolymphocytic leukemia of B-cell type**
     Chronic leukemia with symptoms of large number of circulating lymphocytes

     C91.30 Prolymphocytic leukemia of B-cell type not having achieved remission 🔍
         Prolymphocytic leukemia of B-cell type with failed remission
         Prolymphocytic leukemia of B-cell type NOS

     C91.31 Prolymphocytic leukemia of B-cell type, in remission 🔍

     C91.32 Prolymphocytic leukemia of B-cell type, in relapse 🔍

● **C91.4 Hairy cell leukemia**
     Chronic leukemia with splenomegaly and excessive number of abnormal large mononuclear cells covered by hairlike villi
     Leukemic reticuloendotheliosis

     C91.40 Hairy cell leukemia not having achieved remission 🔍
         Hairy cell leukemia with failed remission
         Hairy cell leukemia NOS

     C91.41 Hairy cell leukemia, in remission 🔍

     C91.42 Hairy cell leukemia, in relapse 🔍

● **C91.5 Adult T-cell lymphoma/leukemia (HTLV-1-associated)**
     Acute variant of adult T-cell lymphoma/leukemia (HTLV-1-associated)
     Chronic variant of adult T-cell lymphoma/leukemia (HTLV-1-associated)
     Lymphomatoid variant of adult T-cell lymphoma/leukemia (HTLV-1-associated)
     Smouldering variant of adult T-cell lymphoma/leukemia (HTLV-1-associated)

     C91.50 Adult T-cell lymphoma/leukemia (HTLV-1-associated) not having achieved remission 🔍   A
         Adult T-cell lymphoma/leukemia (HTLV-1-associated) with failed remission
         Adult T-cell lymphoma/leukemia (HTLV-1-associated) NOS

     C91.51 Adult T-cell lymphoma/leukemia (HTLV-1-associated), in remission 🔍   A

     C91.52 Adult T-cell lymphoma/leukemia (HTLV-1-associated), in relapse 🔍   A

● **C91.6 Prolymphocytic leukemia of T-cell type**

     C91.60 Prolymphocytic leukemia of T-cell type not having achieved remission 🔍
         Prolymphocytic leukemia of T-cell type with failed remission
         Prolymphocytic leukemia of T-cell type NOS

     C91.61 Prolymphocytic leukemia of T-cell type, in remission 🔍

     C91.62 Prolymphocytic leukemia of T-cell type, in relapse 🔍

● **C91.A Mature B-cell leukemia Burkitt-type**

     Excludes1   Burkitt lymphoma (C83.7-)

     C91.A0 Mature B-cell leukemia Burkitt-type not having achieved remission 🔍
         Mature B-cell leukemia Burkitt-type with failed remission
         Mature B-cell leukemia Burkitt-type NOS

     C91.A1 Mature B-cell leukemia Burkitt-type, in remission 🔍

     C91.A2 Mature B-cell leukemia Burkitt-type, in relapse 🔍

● **C91.Z Other lymphoid leukemia**
     T-cell large granular lymphocytic leukemia (associated with rheumatoid arthritis)

     C91.Z0 Other lymphoid leukemia not having achieved remission 🔍
         Other lymphoid leukemia with failed remission
         Other lymphoid leukemia NOS
         Coding Clinic: 2019, Q2, P25

     C91.Z1 Other lymphoid leukemia, in remission 🔍
     C91.Z2 Other lymphoid leukemia, in relapse 🔍

● **C91.9 Lymphoid leukemia, unspecified**

     C91.90 Lymphoid leukemia, unspecified not having achieved remission 🔍
         Lymphoid leukemia with failed remission
         Lymphoid leukemia NOS

     C91.91 Lymphoid leukemia, unspecified, in remission 🔍

     C91.92 Lymphoid leukemia, unspecified, in relapse 🔍

● **C92 Myeloid leukemia**

     Includes   granulocytic leukemia
                 myelogenous leukemia

     Excludes1   personal history of leukemia (Z85.6)
     Coding Clinic: 2019, Q1, P16

● **C92.0 Acute myeloblastic leukemia**
     Acute myeloblastic leukemia, minimal differentiation
     Acute myeloblastic leukemia (with maturation)
     Acute myeloblastic leukemia 1/ETO
     Acute myeloblastic leukemia M0
     Acute myeloblastic leukemia M1
     Acute myeloblastic leukemia M2
     Acute myeloblastic leukemia with t(8;21)
     Acute myeloblastic leukemia (without a FAB classification) NOS
     Refractory anemia with excess blasts in transformation [RAEB T]

     Excludes1   acute exacerbation of chronic myeloid leukemia (C92.10)
                 refractory anemia with excess of blasts not in transformation (D46.2-)

     Coding Clinic: 2018, Q4, P87

     C92.00 Acute myeloblastic leukemia, not having achieved remission 🔍
         Acute myeloblastic leukemia with failed remission
         Acute myeloblastic leukemia NOS

     C92.01 Acute myeloblastic leukemia, in remission 🔍
     C92.02 Acute myeloblastic leukemia, in relapse 🔍

● **C92.1 Chronic myeloid leukemia, BCR/ABL-positive**
     Chronic myelogenous leukemia, Philadelphia chromosome (Ph1) positive
     Chronic myelogenous leukemia, t(9;22) (q34;q11)
     Chronic myelogenous leukemia with crisis of blast cells

     Excludes1   atypical chronic myeloid leukemia BCR/ABL-negative (C92.2-)
                 chronic myelomonocytic leukemia (C93.1-)
                 chronic myeloproliferative disease (D47.1)

     C92.10 Chronic myeloid leukemia, BCR/ABL-positive, not having achieved remission 🔍
         Chronic myeloid leukemia, BCR/ABL-positive with failed remission
         Chronic myeloid leukemia, BCR/ABL-positive NOS
         Coding Clinic: 2017, Q1, P7

     C92.11 Chronic myeloid leukemia, BCR/ABL-positive, in remission 🔍

     C92.12 Chronic myeloid leukemia, BCR/ABL-positive, in relapse 🔍

● **C92.2 Atypical chronic myeloid leukemia, BCR/ABL-negative**

     C92.20 Atypical chronic myeloid leukemia, BCR/ABL-negative, not having achieved remission 🔍
         Atypical chronic myeloid leukemia, BCR/ABL-negative with failed remission
         Atypical chronic myeloid leukemia, BCR/ABL-negative NOS

     C92.21 Atypical chronic myeloid leukemia, BCR/ABL-negative, in remission 🔍

     C92.22 Atypical chronic myeloid leukemia, BCR/ABL-negative, in relapse 🔍

CHAPTER 2 (C00-D49)

CHAPTER 2 (C00–D49)

● **C92.3   Myeloid sarcoma**
     A malignant tumor of immature myeloid cells
     Chloroma
     Granulocytic sarcoma

     C92.30   Myeloid sarcoma, not having achieved remission 🦌
          Myeloid sarcoma with failed remission
          Myeloid sarcoma NOS

     C92.31   Myeloid sarcoma, in remission 🦌

     C92.32   Myeloid sarcoma, in relapse 🦌

● **C92.4   Acute promyelocytic leukemia**
     AML M3
     AML Me with t(15;17) and variants

     C92.40   Acute promyelocytic leukemia, not having achieved remission 🦌
          Acute promyelocytic leukemia with failed remission
          Acute promyelocytic leukemia NOS

     C92.41   Acute promyelocytic leukemia, in remission 🦌

     C92.42   Acute promyelocytic leukemia, in relapse 🦌

● **C92.5   Acute myelomonocytic leukemia**
     AML M4
     AML M4 Eo with inv(16) or t(16;16)

     C92.50   Acute myelomonocytic leukemia, not having achieved remission 🦌
          Acute myelomonocytic leukemia with failed remission
          Acute myelomonocytic leukemia NOS

     C92.51   Acute myelomonocytic leukemia, in remission 🦌

     C92.52   Acute myelomonocytic leukemia, in relapse 🦌

● **C92.6   Acute myeloid leukemia with 11q23-abnormality**
     Acute myeloid leukemia with variation of MLL-gene

     C92.60   Acute myeloid leukemia with 11q23-abnormality not having achieved remission 🦌
          Acute myeloid leukemia with 11q23-abnormality with failed remission
          Acute myeloid leukemia with 11q23-abnormality NOS

     C92.61   Acute myeloid leukemia with 11q23-abnormality in remission 🦌

     C92.62   Acute myeloid leukemia with 11q23-abnormality in relapse 🦌

● **C92.A   Acute myeloid leukemia with multilineage dysplasia**
     Acute myeloid leukemia with dysplasia of remaining hematopoesis and/or myelodysplastic disease in its history

     C92.A0   Acute myeloid leukemia with multilineage dysplasia, not having achieved remission 🦌
          Acute myeloid leukemia with multilineage dysplasia with failed remission
          Acute myeloid leukemia with multilineage dysplasia NOS

     C92.A1   Acute myeloid leukemia with multilineage dysplasia, in remission 🦌

     C92.A2   Acute myeloid leukemia with multilineage dysplasia, in relapse 🦌

● **C92.Z   Other myeloid leukemia**

     C92.Z0   Other myeloid leukemia not having achieved remission 🦌
          Myeloid leukemia NEC with failed remission
          Myeloid leukemia NEC

     C92.Z1   Other myeloid leukemia, in remission 🦌

     C92.Z2   Other myeloid leukemia, in relapse 🦌

● **C92.9   Myeloid leukemia, unspecified**

     C92.90   Myeloid leukemia, unspecified, not having achieved remission 🦌
          Myeloid leukemia, unspecified with failed remission
          Myeloid leukemia, unspecified NOS

     C92.91   Myeloid leukemia, unspecified in remission 🦌

     C92.92   Myeloid leukemia, unspecified in relapse 🦌

● **C93   Monocytic leukemia**

     Includes   monocytoid leukemia

     Excludes1   personal history of leukemia (Z85.6)

● **C93.0   Acute monoblastic/monocytic leukemia**
     AML M5
     AML M5a
     AML M5b

     C93.00   Acute monoblastic/monocytic leukemia, not having achieved remission 🦌
          Acute monoblastic/monocytic leukemia with failed remission
          Acute monoblastic/monocytic leukemia NOS

     C93.01   Acute monoblastic/monocytic leukemia, in remission 🦌

     C93.02   Acute monoblastic/monocytic leukemia, in relapse 🦌

● **C93.1   Chronic myelomonocytic leukemia**
     Chronic monocytic leukemia
     CMML-1
     CMML-2
     CMML with eosinophilia
     Code also, if applicable, eosinophilia (D72.18)

     C93.10   Chronic myelomonocytic leukemia not having achieved remission 🦌
          Chronic myelomonocytic leukemia with failed remission
          Chronic myelomonocytic leukemia NOS

     C93.11   Chronic myelomonocytic leukemia, in remission 🦌

     C93.12   Chronic myelomonocytic leukemia, in relapse 🦌

● **C93.3   Juvenile myelomonocytic leukemia**

     C93.30   Juvenile myelomonocytic leukemia, not having achieved remission 🦌   P
          Juvenile myelomonocytic leukemia with failed remission
          Juvenile myelomonocytic leukemia NOS

     C93.31   Juvenile myelomonocytic leukemia, in remission 🦌   P

     C93.32   Juvenile myelomonocytic leukemia, in relapse 🦌   P

● **C93.Z   Other monocytic leukemia**

     C93.Z0   Other monocytic leukemia, not having achieved remission 🦌
          Other monocytic leukemia NOS

     C93.Z1   Other monocytic leukemia, in remission 🦌

     C93.Z2   Other monocytic leukemia, in relapse 🦌

● **C93.9   Monocytic leukemia, unspecified**

     C93.90   Monocytic leukemia, unspecified, not having achieved remission 🦌
          Monocytic leukemia, unspecified with failed remission
          Monocytic leukemia, unspecified NOS

     C93.91   Monocytic leukemia, unspecified in remission 🦌

     C93.92   Monocytic leukemia, unspecified in relapse 🦌

● **C94   Other leukemias of specified cell type**

     Excludes1   leukemic reticuloendotheliosis (C91.4-)
                 myelodysplastic syndromes (D46.-)
                 personal history of leukemia (Z85.6)
                 plasma cell leukemia (C90.1-)

● **C94.0   Acute erythroid leukemia**
     Acute myeloid leukemia M6(a)(b)
     Erythroleukemia

     C94.00   Acute erythroid leukemia, not having achieved remission 🦌
          Acute erythroid leukemia with failed remission
          Acute erythroid leukemia NOS

     C94.01   Acute erythroid leukemia, in remission 🦌

     C94.02   Acute erythroid leukemia, in relapse 🦌

▶ New   ⇒ Revised   ~~deleted~~ Deleted   Excludes 1   Excludes 2   Includes   Use additional   Code first   Code also   Key words

OGCR Official Guidelines   **X** Assign placeholder X   ● Use Additional Character(s)   ▶ Manifestation Code   🦌 Hierarchical Condition Category   **Coding Clinic**

● **C94.2 Acute megakaryoblastic leukemia**
  Acute myeloid leukemia M7
  Acute megakaryocytic leukemia

  C94.20 Acute megakaryoblastic leukemia not having achieved remission 🐾
    Acute megakaryoblastic leukemia with failed remission
    Acute megakaryoblastic leukemia NOS

  C94.21 Acute megakaryoblastic leukemia, in remission 🐾

  C94.22 Acute megakaryoblastic leukemia, in relapse 🐾

● **C94.3 Mast cell leukemia**

  C94.30 Mast cell leukemia not having achieved remission 🐾
    Mast cell leukemia with failed remission
    Mast cell leukemia NOS

  C94.31 Mast cell leukemia, in remission 🐾

  C94.32 Mast cell leukemia, in relapse 🐾

● **C94.4 Acute panmyelosis with myelofibrosis**
  Acute myelofibrosis

  Excludes1 myelofibrosis NOS (D75.81)
      secondary myelofibrosis NOS (D75.81)

  C94.40 Acute panmyelosis with myelofibrosis not having achieved remission 🐾
    Acute myelofibrosis NOS
    Acute panmyelosis with myelofibrosis with failed remission
    Acute panmyelosis NOS

  C94.41 Acute panmyelosis with myelofibrosis, in remission 🐾

  C94.42 Acute panmyelosis with myelofibrosis, in relapse 🐾

● **C94.6 Myelodysplastic disease, not classified** 🐾
  Myeloproliferative disease, not classified

● **C94.8 Other specified leukemias**
  Aggressive NK-cell leukemia
  Acute basophilic leukemia

  C94.80 Other specified leukemias not having achieved remission 🐾
    Other specified leukemia with failed remission
    Other specified leukemias NOS

  C94.81 Other specified leukemias, in remission 🐾

  C94.82 Other specified leukemias, in relapse 🐾

● **C95 Leukemia of unspecified cell type**

  Excludes1 personal history of leukemia (Z85.6)

● **C95.0 Acute leukemia of unspecified cell type**
  Acute bilineal leukemia
  Acute mixed lineage leukemia
  Biphenotypic acute leukemia
  Stem cell leukemia of unclear lineage

  Excludes1 acute exacerbation of unspecified chronic leukemia (C95.10)

  C95.00 Acute leukemia of unspecified cell type not having achieved remission 🐾
    Acute leukemia of unspecified cell type with failed remission
    Acute leukemia NOS

  C95.01 Acute leukemia of unspecified cell type, in remission 🐾

  C95.02 Acute leukemia of unspecified cell type, in relapse 🐾

● **C95.1 Chronic leukemia of unspecified cell type**

  C95.10 Chronic leukemia of unspecified cell type not having achieved remission 🐾
    Chronic leukemia of unspecified cell type with failed remission
    Chronic leukemia NOS

  C95.11 Chronic leukemia of unspecified cell type, in remission 🐾

  C95.12 Chronic leukemia of unspecified cell type, in relapse 🐾

● **C95.9 Leukemia, unspecified**

  C95.90 Leukemia, unspecified not having achieved remission 🐾
    Leukemia, unspecified with failed remission
    Leukemia NOS

  C95.91 Leukemia, unspecified, in remission 🐾

  C95.92 Leukemia, unspecified, in relapse 🐾

● **C96 Other and unspecified malignant neoplasms of lymphoid, hematopoietic and related tissue**

  Excludes1 personal history of other malignant neoplasms of lymphoid, hematopoietic and related tissues (Z85.79)

  C96.0 Multifocal and multisystemic (disseminated) Langerhans-cell histiocytosis 🐾
    Histiocytosis X, multisystemic
    Letterer-Siwe disease

    Excludes1 adult pulmonary Langerhans cell histiocytosis (J84.82)
      multifocal and unisystemic Langerhans-cell histiocytosis (C96.5)
      unifocal Langerhans-cell histiocytosis (C96.6)

  C96.2 Malignant mast cell neoplasm

    Excludes1 indolent mastocytosis (D47.02)
      mast cell leukemia (C94.30)
      mastocytosis (congenital) (cutaneous) (Q82.2)

  C96.20 Malignant mast cell neoplasm, unspecified 🐾

  C96.21 Aggressive systemic mastocytosis 🐾

  C96.22 Mast cell sarcoma 🐾

  C96.29 Other malignant mast cell neoplasm 🐾

  C96.4 Sarcoma of dendritic cells (accessory cells) 🐾
    Follicular dendritic cell sarcoma
    Interdigitating dendritic cell sarcoma
    Langerhans cell sarcoma

  C96.5 Multifocal and unisystemic Langerhans-cell histiocytosis 🐾
    Hand-Schüller-Christian disease
    Histiocytosis X, multifocal

    Excludes1 multifocal and multisystemic (disseminated) Langerhans-cell histiocytosis (C96.0)
      unifocal Langerhans-cell histiocytosis (C96.6)

  C96.6 Unifocal Langerhans-cell histiocytosis 🐾
    Eosinophilic granuloma
    Histiocytosis X, unifocal
    Histiocytosis X NOS
    Langerhans-cell histiocytosis NOS

    Excludes1 multifocal and multisysemic (disseminated) Langerhans-cell histiocytosis (C96.0)
      multifocal and unisystemic Langerhans-cell histiocytosis (C96.5)

  C96.A Histiocytic sarcoma 🐾
    Malignant histiocytosis

  C96.Z Other specified malignant neoplasms of lymphoid, hematopoietic and related tissue 🐾

  C96.9 Malignant neoplasm of lymphoid, hematopoietic and related tissue, unspecified 🐾

CHAPTER 2 (C00-D49)

CHAPTER 2 (C00-D49)

IN SITU NEOPLASMS (D00-D09)

In situ is carcinoma involving cells in localized tissues that has not spread to nearby tissues

> **Includes**   Bowen's disease
>   erythroplasia
>   grade III intraepithelial neoplasia
>   Queyrat's erythroplasia

● **D00** **Carcinoma in situ of oral cavity, esophagus and stomach**
> **Excludes1**   melanoma in situ (D03.-)

● **D00.0** **Carcinoma in situ of lip, oral cavity and pharynx**
> Use additional code to identify:
> exposure to environmental tobacco smoke (Z77.22)
> exposure to tobacco smoke in the perinatal period (P96.81)
> history of tobacco dependence (Z87.891)
> occupational exposure to environmental tobacco smoke (Z57.31)
> tobacco dependence (F17.-)
> tobacco use (Z72.0)
>
> > **Excludes1**   carcinoma in situ of aryepiglottic fold or interarytenoid fold, laryngeal aspect (D02.0)
> > carcinoma in situ of epiglottis NOS (D02.0)
> > carcinoma in situ of epiglottis suprahyoid portion (D02.0)
> > carcinoma in situ of skin of lip (D03.0, D04.0)

     D00.00 Carcinoma in situ of oral cavity, unspecified site

     D00.01 Carcinoma in situ of labial mucosa and vermilion border

     D00.02 Carcinoma in situ of buccal mucosa

     D00.03 Carcinoma in situ of gingiva and edentulous alveolar ridge

     D00.04 Carcinoma in situ of soft palate

     D00.05 Carcinoma in situ of hard palate

     D00.06 Carcinoma in situ of floor of mouth

     D00.07 Carcinoma in situ of tongue

     D00.08 Carcinoma in situ of pharynx
> Carcinoma in situ of aryepiglottic fold NOS
> Carcinoma in situ of hypopharyngeal aspect of aryepiglottic fold
> Carcinoma in situ of marginal zone of aryepiglottic fold

   D00.1 Carcinoma in situ of esophagus

   D00.2 Carcinoma in situ of stomach

● **D01** **Carcinoma in situ of other and unspecified digestive organs**
> **Excludes1**   melanoma in situ (D03.-)

   D01.0 Carcinoma in situ of colon
> > **Excludes1**   carcinoma in situ of rectosigmoid junction (D01.1)

   D01.1 Carcinoma in situ of rectosigmoid junction

   D01.2 Carcinoma in situ of rectum

   D01.3 Carcinoma in situ of anus and anal canal
> Anal intraepithelial neoplasia III [AIN III]
> Severe dysplasia of anus
> > **Excludes1**   anal intraepithelial neoplasia I and II [AIN I and AIN II] (K62.82)
> > carcinoma in situ of anal margin (D04.5)
> > carcinoma in situ of anal skin (D04.5)
> > carcinoma in situ of perianal skin (D04.5)

● **D01.4** Carcinoma in situ of other and unspecified parts of intestine
> > **Excludes1**   carcinoma in situ of ampulla of Vater (D01.5)

     D01.40 Carcinoma in situ of unspecified part of intestine

     D01.49 Carcinoma in situ of other parts of intestine

   D01.5 Carcinoma in situ of liver, gallbladder and bile ducts
> Carcinoma in situ of ampulla of Vater

   D01.7 Carcinoma in situ of other specified digestive organs
> Carcinoma in situ of pancreas

   D01.9 Carcinoma in situ of digestive organ, unspecified

● **D02** **Carcinoma in situ of middle ear and respiratory system**
> Use additional code to identify:
> exposure to environmental tobacco smoke (Z77.22)
> exposure to tobacco smoke in the perinatal period (P96.81)
> history of tobacco dependence (Z87.891)
> occupational exposure to environmental tobacco smoke (Z57.31)
> tobacco dependence (F17.-)
> tobacco use (Z72.0)
> > **Excludes1**   melanoma in situ (D03.-)

   D02.0 Carcinoma in situ of larynx
> Carcinoma in situ of aryepiglottic fold or interarytenoid fold, laryngeal aspect
> Carcinoma in situ of epiglottis (suprahyoid portion)
> > **Excludes1**   carcinoma in situ of aryepiglottic fold or interarytenoid fold NOS (D00.08)
> > carcinoma in situ of hypopharyngeal aspect (D00.08)
> > carcinoma in situ of marginal zone (D00.08)

   D02.1 Carcinoma in situ of trachea

● **D02.2** Carcinoma in situ of bronchus and lung

     D02.20 Carcinoma in situ of unspecified bronchus and lung

     D02.21 Carcinoma in situ of right bronchus and lung

     D02.22 Carcinoma in situ of left bronchus and lung

   D02.3 Carcinoma in situ of other parts of respiratory system
> Carcinoma in situ of accessory sinuses
> Carcinoma in situ of middle ear
> Carcinoma in situ of nasal cavities
> > **Excludes1**   carcinoma in situ of ear (external) (skin) (D04.2-)
> > carcinoma in situ of nose NOS (D09.8)
> > carcinoma in situ of skin of nose (D04.3)

   D02.4 Carcinoma in situ of respiratory system, unspecified

● **D03** **Melanoma in situ**

   D03.0 Melanoma in situ of lip 🐾

● **D03.1** Melanoma in situ of eyelid, including canthus

     D03.10 Melanoma in situ of unspecified eyelid, including canthus 🐾

     ● **D03.11** Melanoma in situ of right eyelid, including canthus 🐾

         D03.111 Melanoma in situ of right upper eyelid, including canthus 🐾

         D03.112 Melanoma in situ of right lower eyelid, including canthus 🐾

     ● **D03.12** Melanoma in situ of left eyelid, including canthus 🐾

         D03.121 Melanoma in situ of left upper eyelid, including canthus 🐾

         D03.122 Melanoma in situ of left lower eyelid, including canthus 🐾

● **D03.2** Melanoma in situ of ear and external auricular canal

     D03.20 Melanoma in situ of unspecified ear and external auricular canal 🐾

     D03.21 Melanoma in situ of right ear and external auricular canal 🐾

     D03.22 Melanoma in situ of left ear and external auricular canal 🐾

● **D03.3** Melanoma in situ of other and unspecified parts of face

     D03.30 Melanoma in situ of unspecified part of face 🐾

     D03.39 Melanoma in situ of other parts of face 🐾

   D03.4 Melanoma in situ of scalp and neck 🐾

● D03.5   Melanoma in situ of trunk
     D03.51   Melanoma in situ of anal skin 🐾
         Melanoma in situ of anal margin
         Melanoma in situ of perianal skin
     D03.52   Melanoma in situ of breast (skin) (soft tissue)🐾
     D03.59   Melanoma in situ of other part of trunk 🐾

● D03.6   Melanoma in situ of upper limb, including shoulder
     D03.60   Melanoma in situ of unspecified upper limb, including shoulder 🐾
     D03.61   Melanoma in situ of right upper limb, including shoulder 🐾
     D03.62   Melanoma in situ of left upper limb, including shoulder 🐾

● D03.7   Melanoma in situ of lower limb, including hip
     D03.70   Melanoma in situ of unspecified lower limb, including hip 🐾
     D03.71   Melanoma in situ of right lower limb, including hip 🐾
     D03.72   Melanoma in situ of left lower limb, including hip 🐾

   D03.8   Melanoma in situ of other sites 🐾
         Melanoma in situ of scrotum
     Excludes1   carcinoma in situ of scrotum (D07.61)

   D03.9   Melanoma in situ, unspecified 🐾

● D04   Carcinoma in situ of skin
     Excludes1   erythroplasia of Queyrat (penis) NOS (D07.4)
         melanoma in situ (D03.-)

   D04.0   Carcinoma in situ of skin of lip
     Excludes2   carcinoma in situ of vermilion border of lip (D00.01)

● D04.1   Carcinoma in situ of skin of eyelid, including canthus
     D04.10   Carcinoma in situ of skin of unspecified eyelid, including canthus
     ● D04.11   Carcinoma in situ of skin of right eyelid, including canthus
         D04.111   Carcinoma in situ of skin of right upper eyelid, including canthus
         D04.112   Carcinoma in situ of skin of right lower eyelid, including canthus
     ● D04.12   Carcinoma in situ of skin of left eyelid, including canthus
         D04.121   Carcinoma in situ of skin of left upper eyelid, including canthus
         D04.122   Carcinoma in situ of skin of left lower eyelid, including canthus

● D04.2   Carcinoma in situ of skin of ear and external auricular canal
     D04.20   Carcinoma in situ of skin of unspecified ear and external auricular canal
     D04.21   Carcinoma in situ of skin of right ear and external auricular canal
     D04.22   Carcinoma in situ of skin of left ear and external auricular canal

● D04.3   Carcinoma in situ of skin of other and unspecified parts of face
     D04.30   Carcinoma in situ of skin of unspecified part of face
     D04.39   Carcinoma in situ of skin of other parts of face

   D04.4   Carcinoma in situ of skin of scalp and neck

   D04.5   Carcinoma in situ of skin of trunk
         Carcinoma in situ of anal margin
         Carcinoma in situ of anal skin
         Carcinoma in situ of perianal skin
         Carcinoma in situ of skin of breast
     Excludes1   carcinoma in situ of anus NOS (D01.3)
         carcinoma in situ of scrotum (D07.61)
         carcinoma in situ of skin of genital organs (D07.-)

● D04.6   Carcinoma in situ of skin of upper limb, including shoulder
     D04.60   Carcinoma in situ of skin of unspecified upper limb, including shoulder
     D04.61   Carcinoma in situ of skin of right upper limb, including shoulder
     D04.62   Carcinoma in situ of skin of left upper limb, including shoulder

● D04.7   Carcinoma in situ of skin of lower limb, including hip
     D04.70   Carcinoma in situ of skin of unspecified lower limb, including hip
     D04.71   Carcinoma in situ of skin of right lower limb, including hip
     D04.72   Carcinoma in situ of skin of left lower limb, including hip

   D04.8   Carcinoma in situ of skin of other sites

   D04.9   Carcinoma in situ of skin, unspecified

● D05   Carcinoma in situ of breast
     Excludes1   carcinoma in situ of skin of breast (D04.5)
         melanoma in situ of breast (skin) (D03.5)
         Paget's disease of breast or nipple (C50.-)

● D05.0   Lobular carcinoma in situ of breast
     D05.00   Lobular carcinoma in situ of unspecified breast
     D05.01   Lobular carcinoma in situ of right breast
     D05.02   Lobular carcinoma in situ of left breast

● D05.1   Intraductal carcinoma in situ of breast
     D05.10   Intraductal carcinoma in situ of unspecified breast
     D05.11   Intraductal carcinoma in situ of right breast
     D05.12   Intraductal carcinoma in situ of left breast

● D05.8   Other specified type of carcinoma in situ of breast
     D05.80   Other specified type of carcinoma in situ of unspecified breast
     D05.81   Other specified type of carcinoma in situ of right breast
     D05.82   Other specified type of carcinoma in situ of left breast

● D05.9   Unspecified type of carcinoma in situ of breast
     D05.90   Unspecified type of carcinoma in situ of unspecified breast
     D05.91   Unspecified type of carcinoma in situ of right breast
     D05.92   Unspecified type of carcinoma in situ of left breast

● D06   Carcinoma in situ of cervix uteri
     Includes   cervical adenocarcinoma in situ
         cervical intraepithelial glandular neoplasia
         cervical intraepithelial neoplasia III [CIN III]
         severe dysplasia of cervix uteri
     Excludes1   cervical intraepithelial neoplasia II [CIN II] (N87.1)
         cytologic evidence of malignancy of cervix without histologic confirmation (R87.614)
         high grade squamous intraepithelial lesion (HGSIL) of cervix (R87.613)
         melanoma in situ of cervix (D03.5)
         moderate cervical dysplasia (N87.1)

   D06.0   Carcinoma in situ of endocervix ♀
   D06.1   Carcinoma in situ of exocervix ♀
   D06.7   Carcinoma in situ of other parts of cervix ♀
   D06.9   Carcinoma in situ of cervix, unspecified ♀

CHAPTER 2 (C00–D49)

● **D07**   **Carcinoma in situ of other and unspecified genital organs**

      Excludes1   melanoma in situ of trunk (D03.5)

    D07.0   Carcinoma in situ of endometrium ♀

    D07.1   Carcinoma in situ of vulva ♀
         Severe dysplasia of vulva
         Vulvar intraepithelial neoplasia III [VIN III]

         Excludes1   moderate dysplasia of vulva (N90.1)
                    vulvar intraepithelial neoplasia II [VIN II] (N90.1)

    D07.2   Carcinoma in situ of vagina ♀
         Severe dysplasia of vagina
         Vaginal intraepithelial neoplasia III [VIN III]

         Excludes1   moderate dysplasia of vagina (N89.1)
                    vaginal intraepithelial neoplasia II [VIN II] (N89.1)

● **D07.3**   Carcinoma in situ of other and unspecified female genital organs

       D07.30   Carcinoma in situ of unspecified female genital organs ♀

       D07.39   Carcinoma in situ of other female genital organs ♀

    D07.4   Carcinoma in situ of penis ♂
         Erythroplasia of Queyrat NOS

    D07.5   Carcinoma in situ of prostate ♂
         Prostatic intraepithelial neoplasia III (PIN III)
         Severe dysplasia of prostate

         Excludes1   dysplasia (mild) (moderate) of prostate (N42.3-)
                    prostatic intraepithelial neoplasia II [PIN II] (N42.3-)

● **D07.6**   Carcinoma in situ of other and unspecified male genital organs

       D07.60   Carcinoma in situ of unspecified male genital organs ♂

       D07.61   Carcinoma in situ of scrotum ♂

       D07.69   Carcinoma in situ of other male genital organs ♂

● **D09**   **Carcinoma in situ of other and unspecified sites**

      Excludes1   melanoma in situ (D03.-)

    D09.0   Carcinoma in situ of bladder

● **D09.1**   Carcinoma in situ of other and unspecified urinary organs

       D09.10   Carcinoma in situ of unspecified urinary organ

       D09.19   Carcinoma in situ of other urinary organs

● **D09.2**   Carcinoma in situ of eye

       Excludes1   carcinoma in situ of skin of eyelid (D04.1-)

       D09.20   Carcinoma in situ of unspecified eye

       D09.21   Carcinoma in situ of right eye

       D09.22   Carcinoma in situ of left eye

    D09.3   Carcinoma in situ of thyroid and other endocrine glands

       Excludes1   carcinoma in situ of endocrine pancreas (D01.7)
                 carcinoma in situ of ovary (D07.39)
                 carcinoma in situ of testis (D07.69)

    D09.8   Carcinoma in situ of other specified sites

    D09.9   Carcinoma in situ, unspecified

Figure 2-16   The esophagus is the muscular tube that connects the pharynx and the stomach. The 10 inch (25 cm) long esophagus is divided into three parts: **cervical, thoracic,** and **abdominal.**

BENIGN NEOPLASMS, EXCEPT BENIGN NEUROENDOCRINE TUMORS (D10-D36)

● **D10**   **Benign neoplasm of mouth and pharynx**

    D10.0   Benign neoplasm of lip
         Benign neoplasm of lip (frenulum) (inner aspect) (mucosa) (vermilion border)

         Excludes1   benign neoplasm of skin of lip (D22.0, D23.0)

    D10.1   Benign neoplasm of tongue
         Benign neoplasm of lingual tonsil

    D10.2   Benign neoplasm of floor of mouth

● **D10.3**   Benign neoplasm of other and unspecified parts of mouth

       D10.30   Benign neoplasm of unspecified part of mouth

       D10.39   Benign neoplasm of other parts of mouth
           Benign neoplasm of minor salivary gland NOS

           Excludes1   benign odontogenic neoplasms (D16.4-D16.5)
                    benign neoplasm of mucosa of lip (D10.0)
                    benign neoplasm of nasopharyngeal surface of soft palate (D10.6)

    D10.4   Benign neoplasm of tonsil
         Benign neoplasm of tonsil (faucial) (palatine)

         Excludes1   benign neoplasm of lingual tonsil (D10.1)
                  benign neoplasm of pharyngeal tonsil (D10.6)
                  benign neoplasm of tonsillar fossa (D10.5)
                  benign neoplasm of tonsillar pillars (D10.5)

    D10.5   Benign neoplasm of other parts of oropharynx
         Division of pharynx lying between soft palate and upper edge of epiglottis
         Benign neoplasm of epiglottis, anterior aspect
         Benign neoplasm of tonsillar fossa
         Benign neoplasm of tonsillar pillars
         Benign neoplasm of vallecula

         Excludes1   benign neoplasm of epiglottis NOS (D14.1)
                  benign neoplasm of epiglottis, suprahyoid portion (D14.1)

    D10.6   Benign neoplasm of nasopharynx
         Segment of pharynx that lies above soft palate
         Benign neoplasm of pharyngeal tonsil
         Benign neoplasm of posterior margin of septum and choanae

▶ New   ➠ Revised   ~~deleted~~ Deleted   Excludes 1   Excludes 2   Includes   Use additional   Code first   Code also   Key words

OGCR Official Guidelines   **X** Assign placeholder X   ● Use Additional Character(s)   ▶ Manifestation Code   Hierarchical Condition Category   **Coding Clinic**

D10.7   Benign neoplasm of hypopharynx
Segment of pharynx that lies below upper edge of epiglottis and opens into larynx and esophagus

D10.9   Benign neoplasm of pharynx, unspecified

● **D11**   Benign neoplasm of major salivary glands
     Excludes1   benign neoplasms of specified minor salivary glands which are classified according to their anatomical location
                 benign neoplasms of minor salivary glands NOS (D10.39)

D11.0   Benign neoplasm of parotid gland

D11.7   Benign neoplasm of other major salivary glands
Benign neoplasm of sublingual salivary gland
Benign neoplasm of submandibular salivary gland

D11.9   Benign neoplasm of major salivary gland, unspecified

● **D12**   Benign neoplasm of colon, rectum, anus and anal canal
     Excludes1   benign carcinoid tumors of the large intestine, and rectum (D3A.02-)
                 polyp of colon NOS (K63.5)
     Coding Clinic: 2017, Q1, P15; 2015, Q2, P14

D12.0   Benign neoplasm of cecum
Benign neoplasm of ileocecal valve

D12.1   Benign neoplasm of appendix
     Excludes1   benign carcinoid tumor of the appendix (D3A.020)

D12.2   Benign neoplasm of ascending colon
     Coding Clinic: 2018, Q2, P14; 2017, Q1, P15

D12.3   Benign neoplasm of transverse colon
Benign neoplasm of hepatic flexure
Benign neoplasm of splenic flexure
Flexure is a bending in a structure or organ. Note the three flexures illustrated in Figure 2–17. Hepatic = liver, sigmoid = colon, splenic = spleen.
     Coding Clinic: 2017, Q1, P16

D12.4   Benign neoplasm of descending colon
     Coding Clinic: 2015, Q2, P14

D12.5   Benign neoplasm of sigmoid colon

D12.6   Benign neoplasm of colon, unspecified
Adenomatosis of colon
Benign neoplasm of large intestine NOS
Polyposis (hereditary) of colon
     Excludes1   inflammatory polyp of colon (K51.4-)
     Coding Clinic: 2017, Q1, P8-9

D12.7   Benign neoplasm of rectosigmoid junction
Angle where sigmoid colon becomes rectum

D12.8   Benign neoplasm of rectum
     Excludes1   benign carcinoid tumor of the rectum (D3A.026)
     Coding Clinic: 2018, Q1, P7

D12.9   Benign neoplasm of anus and anal canal
Benign neoplasm of anus NOS
     Excludes1   benign neoplasm of anal margin (D22.5, D23.5)
                 benign neoplasm of anal skin (D22.5, D23.5)
                 benign neoplasm of perianal skin (D22.5, D23.5)

● **D13**   Benign neoplasm of other and ill-defined parts of digestive system
     Excludes1   benign stromal tumors of digestive system (D21.4)

D13.0   Benign neoplasm of esophagus

D13.1   Benign neoplasm of stomach
     Excludes1   benign carcinoid tumor of the stomach (D3A.092)

D13.2   Benign neoplasm of duodenum
     Excludes1   benign carcinoid tumor of the duodenum (D3A.010)

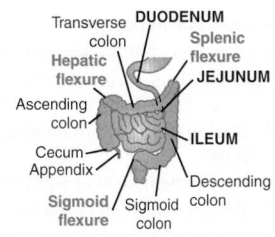

Figure 2-17   Small intestine and colon.

● **D13.3**   Benign neoplasm of other and unspecified parts of small intestine
     Excludes1   benign carcinoid tumors of the small intestine (D3A.01-)
                 benign neoplasm of ileocecal valve (D12.0)

D13.30   Benign neoplasm of unspecified part of small intestine

D13.39   Benign neoplasm of other parts of small intestine

D13.4   Benign neoplasm of liver
Benign neoplasm of intrahepatic bile ducts

D13.5   Benign neoplasm of extrahepatic bile ducts
Extensions of common hepatic bile duct (tube that collects bile from liver)

D13.6   Benign neoplasm of pancreas
     Excludes1   benign neoplasm of endocrine pancreas (D13.7)

D13.7   Benign neoplasm of endocrine pancreas
Pancreatic islets: Cells scattered throughout pancreas
Islet cell tumor
Benign neoplasm of islets of Langerhans
Use additional code to identify any functional activity.

D13.9   Benign neoplasm of ill-defined sites within the digestive system
Benign neoplasm of digestive system NOS
Benign neoplasm of intestine NOS
Benign neoplasm of spleen

● **D14**   Benign neoplasm of middle ear and respiratory system

D14.0   Benign neoplasm of middle ear, nasal cavity and accessory sinuses
Benign neoplasm of cartilage of nose
     Excludes1   benign neoplasm of auricular canal (external) (D22.2-, D23.2-)
                 benign neoplasm of bone of ear (D16.4)
                 benign neoplasm of bone of nose (D16.4)
                 benign neoplasm of cartilage of ear (D21.0)
                 benign neoplasm of ear (external) (skin) (D22.2-, D23.2-)
                 benign neoplasm of nose NOS (D36.7)
                 benign neoplasm of skin of nose (D22.39, D23.39)
                 benign neoplasm of olfactory bulb (D33.3)
                 benign neoplasm of posterior margin of septum and choanae (D10.6)
                 polyp of accessory sinus (J33.8)
                 polyp of ear (middle) (H74.4)
                 polyp of nasal (cavity) (J33.-)

D14.1   Benign neoplasm of larynx
Adenomatous polyp of larynx
Benign neoplasm of epiglottis (suprahyoid portion)
Horseshoe-shaped bone in anterior midline of neck between chin and thyroid cartilage
     Excludes1   benign neoplasm of epiglottis, anterior aspect (D10.5)
                 polyp (nonadenomatous) of vocal cord or larynx (J38.1)

D14.2 Benign neoplasm of trachea

● **D14.3** Benign neoplasm of bronchus and lung

  Excludes1 benign carcinoid tumor of the bronchus and lung (D3A.090)

  D14.30 Benign neoplasm of unspecified bronchus and lung

  D14.31 Benign neoplasm of right bronchus and lung

  D14.32 Benign neoplasm of left bronchus and lung

D14.4 Benign neoplasm of respiratory system, unspecified

● **D15** Benign neoplasm of other and unspecified intrathoracic organs

  Excludes1 benign neoplasm of mesothelial tissue (D19.-)

  D15.0 Benign neoplasm of thymus

    Excludes1 benign carcinoid tumor of the thymus (D3A.091)

  D15.1 Benign neoplasm of heart

    Excludes1 benign neoplasm of great vessels (D21.3)

  D15.2 Benign neoplasm of mediastinum

  D15.7 Benign neoplasm of other specified intrathoracic organs

  D15.9 Benign neoplasm of intrathoracic organ, unspecified

● **D16** Benign neoplasm of bone and articular cartilage

  Excludes1 benign neoplasm of connective tissue of ear (D21.0)

    benign neoplasm of connective tissue of eyelid (D21.0)

    benign neoplasm of connective tissue of larynx (D14.1)

    benign neoplasm of connective tissue of nose (D14.0)

    benign neoplasm of synovia (D21.-)

  ● **D16.0** Benign neoplasm of scapula and long bones of upper limb

    D16.00 Benign neoplasm of scapula and long bones of unspecified upper limb

    D16.01 Benign neoplasm of scapula and long bones of right upper limb

    D16.02 Benign neoplasm of scapula and long bones of left upper limb

  ● **D16.1** Benign neoplasm of short bones of upper limb

    D16.10 Benign neoplasm of short bones of unspecified upper limb

    D16.11 Benign neoplasm of short bones of right upper limb

    D16.12 Benign neoplasm of short bones of left upper limb

  ● **D16.2** Benign neoplasm of long bones of lower limb

    D16.20 Benign neoplasm of long bones of unspecified lower limb

    D16.21 Benign neoplasm of long bones of right lower limb

    D16.22 Benign neoplasm of long bones of left lower limb

  ● **D16.3** Benign neoplasm of short bones of lower limb

    D16.30 Benign neoplasm of short bones of unspecified lower limb

    D16.31 Benign neoplasm of short bones of right lower limb

    D16.32 Benign neoplasm of short bones of left lower limb

  D16.4 Benign neoplasm of bones of skull and face

    Benign neoplasm of maxilla (superior)
    Benign neoplasm of orbital bone
    Cavity or socket of skull in which eye and its appendages are located
    Keratocyst of maxilla
    Keratocystic odontogenic tumor of maxilla

    Excludes2 benign neoplasm of lower jaw bone (D16.5)

D16.5 Benign neoplasm of lower jaw bone

  Keratocyst of mandible
  Keratocystic odontogenic tumor of mandible

D16.6 Benign neoplasm of vertebral column

  Excludes1 benign neoplasm of sacrum and coccyx (D16.8)

D16.7 Benign neoplasm of ribs, sternum and clavicle

D16.8 Benign neoplasm of pelvic bones, sacrum and coccyx

D16.9 Benign neoplasm of bone and articular cartilage, unspecified

● **D17** Benign lipomatous neoplasm

  Slow-growing benign tumors (rubbery masses) of mature fat cells enclosed in a thin fibrous capsule

  D17.0 Benign lipomatous neoplasm of skin and subcutaneous tissue of head, face and neck

  D17.1 Benign lipomatous neoplasm of skin and subcutaneous tissue of trunk

  ● **D17.2** Benign lipomatous neoplasm of skin and subcutaneous tissue of limb

    D17.20 Benign lipomatous neoplasm of skin and subcutaneous tissue of unspecified limb

    D17.21 Benign lipomatous neoplasm of skin and subcutaneous tissue of right arm

    D17.22 Benign lipomatous neoplasm of skin and subcutaneous tissue of left arm

    D17.23 Benign lipomatous neoplasm of skin and subcutaneous tissue of right leg

    D17.24 Benign lipomatous neoplasm of skin and subcutaneous tissue of left leg

  ● **D17.3** Benign lipomatous neoplasm of skin and subcutaneous tissue of other and unspecified sites

    D17.30 Benign lipomatous neoplasm of skin and subcutaneous tissue of unspecified sites

    D17.39 Benign lipomatous neoplasm of skin and subcutaneous tissue of other sites

  D17.4 Benign lipomatous neoplasm of intrathoracic organs

  D17.5 Benign lipomatous neoplasm of intra-abdominal organs

    Excludes1 benign lipomatous neoplasm of peritoneum and retroperitoneum (D17.79)

  D17.6 Benign lipomatous neoplasm of spermatic cord ♂

  ● **D17.7** Benign lipomatous neoplasm of other sites

    D17.71 Benign lipomatous neoplasm of kidney

    D17.72 Benign lipomatous neoplasm of other genitourinary organ

    D17.79 Benign lipomatous neoplasm of other sites
      Benign lipomatous neoplasm of peritoneum
      Benign lipomatous neoplasm of retroperitoneum

  D17.9 Benign lipomatous neoplasm, unspecified
    Lipoma NOS

● **D18** Hemangioma and lymphangioma, any site

  Excludes1 benign neoplasm of glomus jugulare (D35.6)
    blue or pigmented nevus (D22.-)
    nevus NOS (D22.-)
    vascular nevus (Q82.5)

  ● **D18.0** Hemangioma

    Common type of vascular malformation
    Angioma NOS
    Cavernous nevus

    D18.00 Hemangioma unspecified site

    D18.01 Hemangioma of skin and subcutaneous tissue

    D18.02 Hemangioma of intracranial structures 🐾

    D18.03 Hemangioma of intra-abdominal structures

    D18.09 Hemangioma of other sites

  D18.1 Lymphangioma, any site
    Coding Clinic: 2018, Q2, P13

CHAPTER 2 (C00-D49)

Figure 2-18   Hemangioma of skin and subcutaneous tissue. (Getty Image)

Item 2-10   Hemangiomas are abnormally dense collections of dilated capillaries that occur on the skin or in internal organs. Hemangiomas are both deep and superficial and undergo a rapid growth phase when the size increases rapidly, followed by a rest phase, in which the tumor changes very little, followed by an involutional phase in which the tumor begins to and can disappear altogether. **Lymphangiomas** or cystic hygroma are benign collections of overgrown lymph vessels and, although rare, may occur anywhere but most commonly on the head and neck of children and infants. Visceral organs, lungs, and gastrointestinal tract may also be involved.

● **D19   Benign neoplasm of mesothelial tissue**
     Mesothelial tissue is the membrane lining several body cavities

     D19.0   Benign neoplasm of mesothelial tissue of pleura

     D19.1   Benign neoplasm of mesothelial tissue of peritoneum

     D19.7   Benign neoplasm of mesothelial tissue of other sites

     D19.9   Benign neoplasm of mesothelial tissue, unspecified
         Benign mesothelioma NOS

● **D20   Benign neoplasm of soft tissue of retroperitoneum and peritoneum**
     Excludes1   benign lipomatous neoplasm of peritoneum and retroperitoneum (D17.79)
                 benign neoplasm of mesothelial tissue (D19.-)

     D20.0   Benign neoplasm of soft tissue of retroperitoneum

     D20.1   Benign neoplasm of soft tissue of peritoneum

● **D21   Other benign neoplasms of connective and other soft tissue**
     Includes   benign neoplasm of blood vessel
                benign neoplasm of bursa
                benign neoplasm of cartilage
                benign neoplasm of fascia
                benign neoplasm of fat
                benign neoplasm of ligament, except uterine
                benign neoplasm of lymphatic channel
                benign neoplasm of muscle
                benign neoplasm of synovia
                benign neoplasm of tendon (sheath)
                benign stromal tumors

     Excludes1   benign neoplasm of articular cartilage (D16.-)
                 benign neoplasm of cartilage of larynx (D14.1)
                 benign neoplasm of cartilage of nose (D14.0)
                 benign neoplasm of connective tissue of breast (D24.-)
                 benign neoplasm of peripheral nerves and autonomic nervous system (D36.1-)
                 benign neoplasm of peritoneum (D20.1)
                 benign neoplasm of retroperitoneum (D20.0)
                 benign neoplasm of uterine ligament, any (D28.2)
                 benign neoplasm of vascular tissue (D18.-)
                 hemangioma (D18.0-)
                 lipomatous neoplasm (D17.-)
                 lymphangioma (D18.1)
                 uterine leiomyoma (D25.-)

     D21.0   Benign neoplasm of connective and other soft tissue of head, face and neck
         Benign neoplasm of connective tissue of ear
         Benign neoplasm of connective tissue of eyelid
         Excludes1   benign neoplasm of connective tissue of orbit (D31.6-)

● **D21.1   Benign neoplasm of connective and other soft tissue of upper limb, including shoulder**

     D21.10   Benign neoplasm of connective and other soft tissue of unspecified upper limb, including shoulder

     D21.11   Benign neoplasm of connective and other soft tissue of right upper limb, including shoulder

     D21.12   Benign neoplasm of connective and other soft tissue of left upper limb, including shoulder

● **D21.2   Benign neoplasm of connective and other soft tissue of lower limb, including hip**

     D21.20   Benign neoplasm of connective and other soft tissue of unspecified lower limb, including hip

     D21.21   Benign neoplasm of connective and other soft tissue of right lower limb, including hip

     D21.22   Benign neoplasm of connective and other soft tissue of left lower limb, including hip

     D21.3   Benign neoplasm of connective and other soft tissue of thorax
         Benign neoplasm of axilla
         Benign neoplasm of diaphragm
         Benign neoplasm of great vessels
         Excludes1   benign neoplasm of heart (D15.1)
                 benign neoplasm of mediastinum (D15.2)
                 benign neoplasm of thymus (D15.0)

     D21.4   Benign neoplasm of connective and other soft tissue of abdomen
         Benign stromal tumors of abdomen

     D21.5   Benign neoplasm of connective and other soft tissue of pelvis
         Excludes1   benign neoplasm of any uterine ligament (D28.2)
                 uterine leiomyoma (D25.-)

     D21.6   Benign neoplasm of connective and other soft tissue of trunk, unspecified
         Benign neoplasm of connective and other soft tissue of back NOS

     D21.9   Benign neoplasm of connective and other soft tissue, unspecified

● **D22   Melanocytic nevi**
     Includes   atypical nevus
                blue hairy pigmented nevus
                nevus NOS

     D22.0   Melanocytic nevi of lip
         Skin lesions composed of nests of nevus cells with macules/ papules

● **D22.1   Melanocytic nevi of eyelid, including canthus**

     D22.10   Melanocytic nevi of unspecified eyelid, including canthus

●   **D22.11   Melanocytic nevi of right eyelid, including canthus**

         D22.111   Melanocytic nevi of right upper eyelid, including canthus

         D22.112   Melanocytic nevi of right lower eyelid, including canthus

●   **D22.12   Melanocytic nevi of left eyelid, including canthus**

         D22.121   Melanocytic nevi of left upper eyelid, including canthus

         D22.122   Melanocytic nevi of left lower eyelid, including canthus

● **D22.2   Melanocytic nevi of ear and external auricular canal**

     D22.20   Melanocytic nevi of unspecified ear and external auricular canal

     D22.21   Melanocytic nevi of right ear and external auricular canal

     D22.22   Melanocytic nevi of left ear and external auricular canal

CHAPTER 2 (C00-D49)

● **D22.3** Melanocytic nevi of other and unspecified parts of face
     D22.30 Melanocytic nevi of unspecified part of face
     D22.39 Melanocytic nevi of other parts of face
   D22.4 Melanocytic nevi of scalp and neck
   D22.5 Melanocytic nevi of trunk
     Melanocytic nevi of anal margin
     Melanocytic nevi of anal skin
     Melanocytic nevi of perianal skin
     Melanocytic nevi of skin of breast
● **D22.6** Melanocytic nevi of upper limb, including shoulder
     D22.60 Melanocytic nevi of unspecified upper limb, including shoulder
     D22.61 Melanocytic nevi of right upper limb, including shoulder
     D22.62 Melanocytic nevi of left upper limb, including shoulder
● **D22.7** Melanocytic nevi of lower limb, including hip
     D22.70 Melanocytic nevi of unspecified lower limb, including hip
     D22.71 Melanocytic nevi of right lower limb, including hip
     D22.72 Melanocytic nevi of left lower limb, including hip
   D22.9 Melanocytic nevi, unspecified

● **D23** Other benign neoplasms of skin
     Includes   benign neoplasm of hair follicles
               benign neoplasm of sebaceous glands
               benign neoplasm of sweat glands
     Excludes1   benign lipomatous neoplasms of skin (D17.0-D17.3)
     Excludes2   melanocytic nevi (D22.-)
   D23.0 Other benign neoplasm of skin of lip
     Excludes1   benign neoplasm of vermilion border of lip (D10.0)
● **D23.1** Other benign neoplasm of skin of eyelid, including canthus
     D23.10 Other benign neoplasm of skin unspecified of eyelid, including canthus
     ● **D23.11** Other benign neoplasm of skin of right eyelid, including canthus
         D23.111 Other benign neoplasm of skin of right upper eyelid, including canthus
         D23.112 Other benign neoplasm of skin of right lower eyelid, including canthus
     ● **D23.12** Other benign neoplasm of skin of left eyelid, including canthus
         D23.121 Other benign neoplasm of skin of left upper eyelid, including canthus
         D23.122 Other benign neoplasm of skin of left lower eyelid, including canthus
● **D23.2** Other benign neoplasm of skin of ear and external auricular canal
     D23.20 Other benign neoplasm of skin of unspecified ear and external auricular canal
     D23.21 Other benign neoplasm of skin of right ear and external auricular canal
     D23.22 Other benign neoplasm of skin of left ear and external auricular canal
● **D23.3** Other benign neoplasm of skin of other and unspecified parts of face
     D23.30 Other benign neoplasm of skin of unspecified part of face
     D23.39 Other benign neoplasm of skin of other parts of face
   D23.4 Other benign neoplasm of skin of scalp and neck

● **D23.5** Other benign neoplasm of skin of trunk
     Other benign neoplasm of anal margin
     Other benign neoplasm of anal skin
     Other benign neoplasm of perianal skin
     Other benign neoplasm of skin of breast
     Excludes1   benign neoplasm of anus NOS (D12.9)
● **D23.6** Other benign neoplasm of skin of upper limb, including shoulder
     D23.60 Other benign neoplasm of skin of unspecified upper limb, including shoulder
     D23.61 Other benign neoplasm of skin of right upper limb, including shoulder
     D23.62 Other benign neoplasm of skin of left upper limb, including shoulder
● **D23.7** Other benign neoplasm of skin of lower limb, including hip
     D23.70 Other benign neoplasm of skin of unspecified lower limb, including hip
     D23.71 Other benign neoplasm of skin of right lower limb, including hip
     D23.72 Other benign neoplasm of skin of left lower limb, including hip
   D23.9 Other benign neoplasm of skin, unspecified

● **D24** Benign neoplasm of breast
     Includes   benign neoplasm of connective tissue of breast
               benign neoplasm of soft parts of breast
               fibroadenoma of breast
     Excludes2   adenofibrosis of breast (N60.2)
               benign cyst of breast (N60.-)
               benign mammary dysplasia (N60.-)
               benign neoplasm of skin of breast (D22.5, D23.5)
               fibrocystic disease of breast (N60.-)
   D24.1 Benign neoplasm of right breast
     Coding Clinic: 2017, Q1, P5
   D24.2 Benign neoplasm of left breast
   D24.9 Benign neoplasm of unspecified breast

● **D25** Leiomyoma of uterus
     Benign tumors or nodules of the uterine wall
     Includes   uterine fibroid
               uterine fibromyoma
               uterine myoma
   D25.0 Submucous leiomyoma of uterus ♀
   D25.1 Intramural leiomyoma of uterus ♀
     Interstitial leiomyoma of uterus
   D25.2 Subserosal leiomyoma of uterus ♀
     Subperitoneal leiomyoma of uterus
   D25.9 Leiomyoma of uterus, unspecified ♀

● **D26** Other benign neoplasms of uterus
   D26.0 Other benign neoplasm of cervix uteri ♀
   D26.1 Other benign neoplasm of corpus uteri ♀
   D26.7 Other benign neoplasm of other parts of uterus ♀
   D26.9 Other benign neoplasm of uterus, unspecified ♀

● **D27** Benign neoplasm of ovary
     Use additional code to identify any functional activity.
     Excludes2   corpus albicans cyst (N83.2-)
               corpus luteum cyst (N83.1-)
               endometrial cyst (N80.1)
               follicular (atretic) cyst (N83.0-)
               graafian follicle cyst (N83.0-)
               ovarian cyst NEC (N83.2-)
               ovarian retention cyst (N83.2-)
   D27.0 Benign neoplasm of right ovary ♀
   D27.1 Benign neoplasm of left ovary ♀
   D27.9 Benign neoplasm of unspecified ovary ♀
     Ovarian teratoma

▶ New   ⇒ Revised   ~~deleted~~ Deleted   Excludes 1   Excludes 2   Includes   Use additional   Code first   Code also   Key words
OGCR Official Guidelines   X Assign placeholder X   ● Use Additional Character(s)   ▷ Manifestation Code   Hierarchical Condition Category   **Coding Clinic**

Item 2–11 Teratoma: terat = monster, oma = mass, tumor. Alternate terms: dermoid cyst of the ovary, ovarian teratoma. Teratomas are neoplasms and arise from germ cells (ovaries in female and testes in male) and can be benign or malignant. Teratomas have been known to contain hair, nails, and teeth, giving them a bizarre ("monster") appearance.

● **D28 Benign neoplasm of other and unspecified female genital organs**

  Includes   adenomatous polyp
         benign neoplasm of skin of female genital organs
         benign teratoma

  Excludes1 epoophoron cyst (Q50.5)
         fimbrial cyst (Q50.4)
         Gartner's duct cyst (Q52.4)
         parovarian cyst (Q50.5)

  D28.0 Benign neoplasm of vulva ♀

  D28.1 Benign neoplasm of vagina ♀

  D28.2 Benign neoplasm of uterine tubes and ligaments ♀
      Benign neoplasm of fallopian tube
      Benign neoplasm of uterine ligament (broad) (round)

  D28.7 Benign neoplasm of other specified female genital organs ♀

  D28.9 Benign neoplasm of female genital organ, unspecified ♀

● **D29 Benign neoplasm of male genital organs**

  Includes   benign neoplasm of skin of male genital organs

  D29.0 Benign neoplasm of penis ♂

  D29.1 Benign neoplasm of prostate ♂
      Excludes1 enlarged prostate (N40.-)

  ● D29.2 Benign neoplasm of testis
       Use additional code to identify any functional activity.

    D29.20 Benign neoplasm of unspecified testis ♂

    D29.21 Benign neoplasm of right testis ♂

    D29.22 Benign neoplasm of left testis ♂

  ● D29.3 Benign neoplasm of epididymis

    D29.30 Benign neoplasm of unspecified epididymis ♂

    D29.31 Benign neoplasm of right epididymis ♂

    D29.32 Benign neoplasm of left epididymis ♂

  D29.4 Benign neoplasm of scrotum ♂
      Benign neoplasm of skin of scrotum

  D29.8 Benign neoplasm of other specified male genital organs ♂
      Benign neoplasm of seminal vesicle
      Benign neoplasm of spermatic cord
      Benign neoplasm of tunica vaginalis

  D29.9 Benign neoplasm of male genital organ, unspecified ♂

● **D30 Benign neoplasm of urinary organs**

  ● D30.0 Benign neoplasm of kidney
      Excludes1 benign carcinoid tumor of the kidney (D3A.093)
             benign neoplasm of renal calyces (D30.1-)
             benign neoplasm of renal pelvis (D30.1-)

    D30.00 Benign neoplasm of unspecified kidney

    D30.01 Benign neoplasm of right kidney

    D30.02 Benign neoplasm of left kidney

  ● D30.1 Benign neoplasm of renal pelvis

    D30.10 Benign neoplasm of unspecified renal pelvis

    D30.11 Benign neoplasm of right renal pelvis

    D30.12 Benign neoplasm of left renal pelvis

  ● D30.2 Benign neoplasm of ureter
      Excludes1 benign neoplasm of ureteric orifice of bladder (D30.3)

    D30.20 Benign neoplasm of unspecified ureter

    D30.21 Benign neoplasm of right ureter

    D30.22 Benign neoplasm of left ureter

  D30.3 Benign neoplasm of bladder
      Benign neoplasm of ureteric orifice of bladder
      Benign neoplasm of urethral orifice of bladder

  D30.4 Benign neoplasm of urethra
      Excludes1 benign neoplasm of urethral orifice of bladder (D30.3)

  D30.8 Benign neoplasm of other specified urinary organs
      Benign neoplasm of paraurethral glands

  D30.9 Benign neoplasm of urinary organ, unspecified
      Benign neoplasm of urinary system NOS

● **D31 Benign neoplasm of eye and adnexa**
    Excludes1 benign neoplasm of connective tissue of eyelid (D21.0)
           benign neoplasm of optic nerve (D33.3)
           benign neoplasm of skin of eyelid (D22.1-, D23.1-)

  ● D31.0 Benign neoplasm of conjunctiva

    D31.00 Benign neoplasm of unspecified conjunctiva

    D31.01 Benign neoplasm of right conjunctiva

    D31.02 Benign neoplasm of left conjunctiva

  ● D31.1 Benign neoplasm of cornea

    D31.10 Benign neoplasm of unspecified cornea

    D31.11 Benign neoplasm of right cornea

    D31.12 Benign neoplasm of left cornea

  ● D31.2 Benign neoplasm of retina
      Excludes1 dark area on retina (D49.81)
             hemangioma of retina (D49.81)
             neoplasm of unspecified behavior of retina and choroid (D49.81)
             retinal freckle (D49.81)

    D31.20 Benign neoplasm of unspecified retina

    D31.21 Benign neoplasm of right retina

    D31.22 Benign neoplasm of left retina

  ● D31.3 Benign neoplasm of choroid

    D31.30 Benign neoplasm of unspecified choroid

    D31.31 Benign neoplasm of right choroid

    D31.32 Benign neoplasm of left choroid

  ● D31.4 Benign neoplasm of ciliary body

    D31.40 Benign neoplasm of unspecified ciliary body

    D31.41 Benign neoplasm of right ciliary body

    D31.42 Benign neoplasm of left ciliary body

  ● D31.5 Benign neoplasm of lacrimal gland and duct
      Benign neoplasm of lacrimal sac
      Benign neoplasm of nasolacrimal duct

    D31.50 Benign neoplasm of unspecified lacrimal gland and duct

    D31.51 Benign neoplasm of right lacrimal gland and duct

    D31.52 Benign neoplasm of left lacrimal gland and duct

  ● D31.6 Benign neoplasm of unspecified site of orbit
      Benign neoplasm of connective tissue of orbit
      Benign neoplasm of extraocular muscle
      Benign neoplasm of peripheral nerves of orbit
      Benign neoplasm of retrobulbar tissue
      Benign neoplasm of retro-ocular tissue
      Excludes1 benign neoplasm of orbital bone (D16.4)

    D31.60 Benign neoplasm of unspecified site of unspecified orbit

    D31.61 Benign neoplasm of unspecified site of right orbit

    D31.62 Benign neoplasm of unspecified site of left orbit

  ● D31.9 Benign neoplasm of unspecified part of eye
      Benign neoplasm of eyeball

    D31.90 Benign neoplasm of unspecified part of unspecified eye

    D31.91 Benign neoplasm of unspecified part of right eye

    D31.92 Benign neoplasm of unspecified part of left eye

CHAPTER 2 (C00–D49)

CHAPTER 2 (C00-D49)

● D32   **Benign neoplasm of** meninges
    D32.0   **Benign neoplasm of** cerebral meninges 🝖
    D32.1   **Benign neoplasm of** spinal meninges 🝖
    D32.9   **Benign neoplasm of meninges,** unspecified 🝖
        Meningioma NOS

● D33   **Benign neoplasm of** brain and other parts of central nervous system
    Excludes1   angioma (D18.0-)
        benign neoplasm of meninges (D32.-)
        benign neoplasm of peripheral nerves and autonomic nervous system (D36.1-)
        hemangioma (D18.0-)
        neurofibromatosis (Q85.0-)
        retro-ocular benign neoplasm (D31.6-)
    D33.0   **Benign neoplasm of** brain, supratentorial 🝖
        Benign neoplasm of cerebral ventricle
        Benign neoplasm of cerebrum
        Benign neoplasm of frontal lobe
        Benign neoplasm of occipital lobe
        Benign neoplasm of parietal lobe
        Benign neoplasm of temporal lobe
        Excludes1   benign neoplasm of fourth ventricle (D33.1)
    D33.1   **Benign neoplasm of** brain, infratentorial 🝖
        Benign neoplasm of brain stem
        Benign neoplasm of cerebellum
        Benign neoplasm of fourth ventricle
    D33.2   **Benign neoplasm of** brain, unspecified 🝖
    D33.3   **Benign neoplasm of** cranial nerves 🝖
        Benign neoplasm of olfactory bulb
    D33.4   **Benign neoplasm of** spinal cord 🝖
    D33.7   **Benign neoplasm of** other specified parts of central nervous system 🝖
    D33.9   **Benign neoplasm of central nervous system,** unspecified 🝖
        Benign neoplasm of nervous system (central) NOS

D34   **Benign neoplasm of** thyroid gland
    Use additional code to identify any functional activity.

● D35   **Benign neoplasm of** other and unspecified endocrine glands
    Use additional code to identify any functional activity.
    Excludes1   benign neoplasm of endocrine pancreas (D13.7)
        benign neoplasm of ovary (D27.-)
        benign neoplasm of testis (D29.2-)
        benign neoplasm of thymus (D15.0)
 ● D35.0   **Benign neoplasm of** adrenal gland
     D35.00   **Benign neoplasm of** unspecified adrenal gland
     D35.01   **Benign neoplasm of** right adrenal gland
     D35.02   **Benign neoplasm of** left adrenal gland
    D35.1   **Benign neoplasm of** parathyroid gland
    D35.2   **Benign neoplasm of** pituitary gland 🝖
    D35.3   **Benign neoplasm of** craniopharyngeal duct 🝖
    D35.4   **Benign neoplasm of** pineal gland 🝖
    D35.5   **Benign neoplasm of** carotid body
    D35.6   **Benign neoplasm of** aortic body and other paraganglia
        Benign tumor of glomus jugulare
    D35.7   **Benign neoplasm of** other specified endocrine glands
    D35.9   **Benign neoplasm of endocrine gland,** unspecified
        Benign neoplasm of unspecified endocrine gland

● D36   **Benign neoplasm of** other and unspecified sites
    D36.0   **Benign neoplasm of** lymph nodes
        Excludes1   lymphangioma (D18.1)
 ● D36.1   **Benign neoplasm of** peripheral nerves and autonomic nervous system
        Excludes1   benign neoplasm of peripheral nerves of orbit (D31.6-)
          neurofibromatosis (Q85.0-)
     D36.10   **Benign neoplasm of peripheral nerves and autonomic nervous system,** unspecified
     D36.11   **Benign neoplasm of peripheral nerves and autonomic nervous system of** face, head, and neck
     D36.12   **Benign neoplasm of peripheral nerves and autonomic nervous system,** upper limb, including shoulder
     D36.13   **Benign neoplasm of peripheral nerves and autonomic nervous system of** lower limb, including hip
     D36.14   **Benign neoplasm of peripheral nerves and autonomic nervous system of** thorax
     D36.15   **Benign neoplasm of peripheral nerves and autonomic nervous system of** abdomen
     D36.16   **Benign neoplasm of peripheral nerves and autonomic nervous system of** pelvis
     D36.17   **Benign neoplasm of peripheral nerves and autonomic nervous system of** trunk, unspecified
    D36.7   **Benign neoplasm of** other specified sites
        Benign neoplasm of nose NOS
        Benign neoplasm of back NOS
    D36.9   **Benign neoplasm,** unspecified site

BENIGN NEUROENDOCRINE TUMORS (D3A)

● D3A   **Benign neuroendocrine tumors**
    Code also any associated multiple endocrine neoplasia [MEN] syndromes (E31.2-)
    Use additional code to identify any associated endocrine syndrome, such as:
    carcinoid syndrome (E34.0)
    Excludes2   benign pancreatic islet cell tumors (D13.7)
 ● D3A.0   **Benign** carcinoid tumors
     D3A.00   **Benign carcinoid tumor of** unspecified site
        Carcinoid tumor NOS
  ● D3A.01   **Benign carcinoid tumors of the** small intestine
      D3A.010   **Benign carcinoid tumor of the** duodenum
      D3A.011   **Benign carcinoid tumor of the** jejunum
      D3A.012   **Benign carcinoid tumor of the** ileum
      D3A.019   **Benign carcinoid tumor of the small intestine,** unspecified portion
  ● D3A.02   **Benign carcinoid tumors of the** appendix, large intestine, and rectum
      D3A.020   **Benign carcinoid tumor of the** appendix
      D3A.021   **Benign carcinoid tumor of the** cecum
      D3A.022   **Benign carcinoid tumor of the** ascending colon
      D3A.023   **Benign carcinoid tumor of the** transverse colon
      D3A.024   **Benign carcinoid tumor of the** descending colon
      D3A.025   **Benign carcinoid tumor of the** sigmoid colon
      D3A.026   **Benign carcinoid tumor of the** rectum
      D3A.029   **Benign carcinoid tumor of the large intestine,** unspecified portion
        Benign carcinoid tumor of the colon NOS

▶ New   ⇒ Revised   ~~deleted~~ Deleted   Excludes 1   Excludes 2   Includes   Use additional   Code first   Code also   Key words
OGCR Official Guidelines   X Assign placeholder X   ● Use Additional Character(s)   ▮ Manifestation Code   🝖 Hierarchical Condition Category   **Coding Clinic**

● **D3A.09** **Benign carcinoid tumors of other sites**

    D3A.090 Benign carcinoid tumor of the bronchus and lung

    D3A.091 Benign carcinoid tumor of the thymus

    D3A.092 Benign carcinoid tumor of the stomach

    D3A.093 Benign carcinoid tumor of the kidney

    D3A.094 Benign carcinoid tumor of the foregut, unspecified

    D3A.095 Benign carcinoid tumor of the midgut, unspecified

    D3A.096 Benign carcinoid tumor of the hindgut, unspecified

    D3A.098 Benign carcinoid tumors of other sites

D3A.8 **Other benign neuroendocrine tumors**
    Neuroendocrine tumor NOS

NEOPLASMS OF UNCERTAIN BEHAVIOR, POLYCYTHEMIA VERA AND MYELODYSPLASTIC SYNDROMES (D37-D48)

Note: Categories D37-D44, and D48 classify by site neoplasms of uncertain behavior, i.e., histologic confirmation whether the neoplasm is malignant or benign cannot be made.

    Excludes1   neoplasms of unspecified behavior (D49.-)

● **D37** **Neoplasm of uncertain behavior of oral cavity and digestive organs**

    Excludes1   stromal tumors of uncertain behavior of digestive system (D48.1)

● **D37.0** **Neoplasm of uncertain behavior of lip, oral cavity and pharynx**

    Excludes1   neoplasm of uncertain behavior of aryepiglottic fold or interarytenoid fold, laryngeal aspect (D38.0)
          neoplasm of uncertain behavior of epiglottis NOS (D38.0)
          neoplasm of uncertain behavior of skin of lip (D48.5)
          neoplasm of uncertain behavior of suprahyoid portion of epiglottis (D38.0)

    D37.01 **Neoplasm of uncertain behavior of lip**
        Neoplasm of uncertain behavior of vermilion border of lip

    D37.02 **Neoplasm of uncertain behavior of tongue**

●   **D37.03** **Neoplasm of uncertain behavior of the major salivary glands**

        D37.030 Neoplasm of uncertain behavior of the parotid salivary glands

        D37.031 Neoplasm of uncertain behavior of the sublingual salivary glands

        D37.032 Neoplasm of uncertain behavior of the submandibular salivary glands

        D37.039 Neoplasm of uncertain behavior of the major salivary glands, unspecified

    D37.04 **Neoplasm of uncertain behavior of the minor salivary glands**
        Neoplasm of uncertain behavior of submucosal salivary glands of lip
        Neoplasm of uncertain behavior of submucosal salivary glands of cheek
        Neoplasm of uncertain behavior of submucosal salivary glands of hard palate
        Neoplasm of uncertain behavior of submucosal salivary glands of soft palate

    D37.05 **Neoplasm of uncertain behavior of pharynx**
        Neoplasm of uncertain behavior of aryepiglottic fold of pharynx NOS
        Neoplasm of uncertain behavior of hypopharyngeal aspect of aryepiglottic fold of pharynx
        Neoplasm of uncertain behavior of marginal zone of aryepiglottic fold of pharynx

    D37.09 **Neoplasm of uncertain behavior of other specified sites of the oral cavity**

D37.1 **Neoplasm of uncertain behavior of stomach**

D37.2 **Neoplasm of uncertain behavior of small intestine**

D37.3 **Neoplasm of uncertain behavior of appendix**

D37.4 **Neoplasm of uncertain behavior of colon**

D37.5 **Neoplasm of uncertain behavior of rectum**
    Neoplasm of uncertain behavior of rectosigmoid junction
    Rectosigmoid junction: Angle where sigmoid colon becomes rectum

D37.6 **Neoplasm of uncertain behavior of liver, gallbladder and bile ducts**
    Neoplasm of uncertain behavior of ampulla of Vater
    Ampulla of Vater: Enlarged segment of ducts from liver and pancreas at entry point to small intestine

D37.8 **Neoplasm of uncertain behavior of other specified digestive organs**
    Neoplasm of uncertain behavior of anal canal
    Neoplasm of uncertain behavior of anal sphincter
    Neoplasm of uncertain behavior of anus NOS
    Neoplasm of uncertain behavior of esophagus
    Neoplasm of uncertain behavior of intestine NOS
    Neoplasm of uncertain behavior of pancreas

    Excludes1   neoplasm of uncertain behavior of anal margin (D48.5)
          neoplasm of uncertain behavior of anal skin (D48.5)
          neoplasm of uncertain behavior of perianal skin (D48.5)

D37.9 **Neoplasm of uncertain behavior of digestive organ, unspecified**

Figure 2-19 Major salivary glands.

Parotid gland
Sublingual gland
Submandibular gland

CHAPTER 2 (C00-D49)

CHAPTER 2 (C00-D49)

● **D38** **Neoplasm of uncertain behavior of middle ear and respiratory and intrathoracic organs**

  Excludes1   neoplasm of uncertain behavior of heart (D48.7)

  D38.0 **Neoplasm of uncertain behavior of larynx**
      Neoplasm of uncertain behavior of aryepiglottic fold or interarytenoid fold, laryngeal aspect
      Neoplasm of uncertain behavior of epiglottis (suprahyoid portion)

      Excludes1   neoplasm of uncertain behavior of aryepiglottic fold or interarytenoid fold NOS (D37.05)
          neoplasm of uncertain behavior of hypopharyngeal aspect of aryepiglottic fold (D37.05)
          neoplasm of uncertain behavior of marginal zone of aryepiglottic fold (D37.05)

  D38.1 **Neoplasm of uncertain behavior of trachea, bronchus and lung**

  D38.2 **Neoplasm of uncertain behavior of pleura**

  D38.3 **Neoplasm of uncertain behavior of mediastinum**

  D38.4 **Neoplasm of uncertain behavior of thymus**

  D38.5 **Neoplasm of uncertain behavior of other respiratory organs**
      Neoplasm of uncertain behavior of accessory sinuses
      Neoplasm of uncertain behavior of cartilage of nose
      Neoplasm of uncertain behavior of middle ear
      Neoplasm of uncertain behavior of nasal cavities

      Excludes1   neoplasm of uncertain behavior of ear (external) (skin) (D48.5)
          neoplasm of uncertain behavior of nose NOS (D48.7)
          neoplasm of uncertain behavior of skin of nose (D48.5)

  D38.6 **Neoplasm of uncertain behavior of respiratory organ, unspecified**

● **D39** **Neoplasm of uncertain behavior of female genital organs**

  D39.0 **Neoplasm of uncertain behavior of uterus** ♀

● **D39.1** **Neoplasm of uncertain behavior of ovary**
      Use additional code to identify any functional activity.

    D39.10 **Neoplasm of uncertain behavior of unspecified ovary** ♀

    D39.11 **Neoplasm of uncertain behavior of right ovary** ♀

    D39.12 **Neoplasm of uncertain behavior of left ovary** ♀

  D39.2 **Neoplasm of uncertain behavior of placenta** ♀ M
      Chorioadenoma destruens
      Invasive hydatidiform mole
      Malignant hydatidiform mole

      Excludes1   hydatidiform mole NOS (O01.9)

  D39.8 **Neoplasm of uncertain behavior of other specified female genital organs** ♀
      Neoplasm of uncertain behavior of skin of female genital organs

  D39.9 **Neoplasm of uncertain behavior of female genital organ, unspecified** ♀

● **D40** **Neoplasm of uncertain behavior of male genital organs**

  D40.0 **Neoplasm of uncertain behavior of prostate** ♂

● **D40.1** **Neoplasm of uncertain behavior of testis**

    D40.10 **Neoplasm of uncertain behavior of unspecified testis** ♂

    D40.11 **Neoplasm of uncertain behavior of right testis** ♂

    D40.12 **Neoplasm of uncertain behavior of left testis** ♂

  D40.8 **Neoplasm of uncertain behavior of other specified male genital organs** ♂
      Neoplasm of uncertain behavior of skin of male genital organs

  D40.9 **Neoplasm of uncertain behavior of male genital organ, unspecified** ♂

● **D41** **Neoplasm of uncertain behavior of urinary organs**

● **D41.0** **Neoplasm of uncertain behavior of kidney**

      Excludes1   neoplasm of uncertain behavior of renal pelvis (D41.1-)

    D41.00 **Neoplasm of uncertain behavior of unspecified kidney**

    D41.01 **Neoplasm of uncertain behavior of right kidney**

    D41.02 **Neoplasm of uncertain behavior of left kidney**

● **D41.1** **Neoplasm of uncertain behavior of renal pelvis**

    D41.10 **Neoplasm of uncertain behavior of unspecified renal pelvis**

    D41.11 **Neoplasm of uncertain behavior of right renal pelvis**

    D41.12 **Neoplasm of uncertain behavior of left renal pelvis**

● **D41.2** **Neoplasm of uncertain behavior of ureter**

    D41.20 **Neoplasm of uncertain behavior of unspecified ureter**

    D41.21 **Neoplasm of uncertain behavior of right ureter**

    D41.22 **Neoplasm of uncertain behavior of left ureter**

  D41.3 **Neoplasm of uncertain behavior of urethra**

  D41.4 **Neoplasm of uncertain behavior of bladder**

  D41.8 **Neoplasm of uncertain behavior of other specified urinary organs**

  D41.9 **Neoplasm of uncertain behavior of unspecified urinary organ**

● **D42** **Neoplasm of uncertain behavior of meninges**

  D42.0 **Neoplasm of uncertain behavior of cerebral meninges** 🐾

  D42.1 **Neoplasm of uncertain behavior of spinal meninges** 🐾

  D42.9 **Neoplasm of uncertain behavior of meninges, unspecified** 🐾

● **D43** **Neoplasm of uncertain behavior of brain and central nervous system**

  Excludes1   neoplasm of uncertain behavior of peripheral nerves and autonomic nervous system (D48.2)

  D43.0 **Neoplasm of uncertain behavior of brain, supratentorial** 🐾
      Superior to tentorium of cerebellum
      Neoplasm of uncertain behavior of cerebral ventricle
      Neoplasm of uncertain behavior of cerebrum
      Neoplasm of uncertain behavior of frontal lobe
      Neoplasm of uncertain behavior of occipital lobe
      Neoplasm of uncertain behavior of parietal lobe
      Neoplasm of uncertain behavior of temporal lobe

      Excludes1   neoplasm of uncertain behavior of fourth ventricle (D43.1)

  D43.1 **Neoplasm of uncertain behavior of brain, infratentorial** 🐾
      Beneath the tentorium of cerebellum
      Neoplasm of uncertain behavior of brain stem
      Neoplasm of uncertain behavior of cerebellum
      Neoplasm of uncertain behavior of fourth ventricle

  D43.2 **Neoplasm of uncertain behavior of brain, unspecified** 🐾

  D43.3 **Neoplasm of uncertain behavior of cranial nerves** 🐾

  D43.4 **Neoplasm of uncertain behavior of spinal cord** 🐾

  D43.8 **Neoplasm of uncertain behavior of other specified parts of central nervous system** 🐾

  D43.9 **Neoplasm of uncertain behavior of central nervous system, unspecified** 🐾
      Neoplasm of uncertain behavior of nervous system (central) NOS

▶ New   ⇒ Revised   ~~deleted~~ Deleted   Excludes 1   Excludes 2   Includes   Use additional   Code first   Code also   Key words
OGCR Official Guidelines   X Assign placeholder X   ● Use Additional Character(s)   ▌ Manifestation Code   🐾 Hierarchical Condition Category   **Coding Clinic**

● **D44**   **Neoplasm of uncertain behavior of endocrine glands**

     Excludes1   multiple endocrine adenomatosis (E31.2-)
              multiple endocrine neoplasia (E31.2-)
              neoplasm of uncertain behavior of endocrine
                 pancreas (D37.8)
              neoplasm of uncertain behavior of ovary (D39.1-)
              neoplasm of uncertain behavior of testis (D40.1-)
              neoplasm of uncertain behavior of thymus
                 (D38.4)

     D44.0   Neoplasm of uncertain behavior of thyroid gland

●   **D44.1**   Neoplasm of uncertain behavior of adrenal gland
         Use additional code to identify any functional activity.

         D44.10   Neoplasm of uncertain behavior of unspecified adrenal gland

         D44.11   Neoplasm of uncertain behavior of right adrenal gland

         D44.12   Neoplasm of uncertain behavior of left adrenal gland

     D44.2   Neoplasm of uncertain behavior of parathyroid gland

     D44.3   Neoplasm of uncertain behavior of pituitary gland
         Use additional code to identify any functional activity.

     D44.4   Neoplasm of uncertain behavior of craniopharyngeal duct

     D44.5   Neoplasm of uncertain behavior of pineal gland

     D44.6   Neoplasm of uncertain behavior of carotid body

     D44.7   Neoplasm of uncertain behavior of aortic body and other paraganglia
         Coding Clinic: 2016, Q4, P26

     D44.9   Neoplasm of uncertain behavior of unspecified endocrine gland

● **D45**   **Polycythemia vera**

     Excludes1   familial polycythemia (D75.0)
              secondary polycythemia (D75.1)
     Primary polycythemia. Secondary polycythemia is D75.1. Check your documentation. Polycythemia is caused by too many red blood cells, which increase the thickness of blood (viscosity). This can cause engorgement of the spleen (splenomegaly) with extra RBCs and potential clot formation.

● **D46**   **Myelodysplastic syndromes**

     Use additional code for adverse effect, if applicable, to identify drug (T36-T50 with fifth or sixth character 5)

     Excludes2   drug-induced aplastic anemia (D61.1)

     D46.0   Refractory anemia without ring sideroblasts, so stated
         Refractory anemia without sideroblasts, without excess of blasts

     D46.1   Refractory anemia with ring sideroblasts RARS

●   **D46.2**   Refractory anemia with excess of blasts [RAEB]
         Form of myelodysplasia with increased immature white blood cells (blasts) in bone marrow

         D46.20   Refractory anemia with excess of blasts, unspecified RAEB NOS

         D46.21   Refractory anemia with excess of blasts 1 RAEB 1
             Bone marrow disease which results in insufficient RBCs (anemia) in which level of blasts is less than 10%

         D46.22   Refractory anemia with excess of blasts 2 RAEB 2
             Bone marrow disease manifested by insufficient numbers of RBCs (anemia) with level of blasts 10-20%

     D46.A   Refractory cytopenia with multilineage dysplasia

     D46.B   Refractory cytopenia with multilineage dysplasia and ring sideroblasts
         RCMD RS

     D46.C   Myelodysplastic syndrome with isolated del(5q) chromosomal abnormality
         Myelodysplastic syndrome with 5q deletion
         5q minus syndrome NOS

     D46.4   Refractory anemia, unspecified

     D46.Z   Other myelodysplastic syndromes
         Excludes1   chronic myelomonocytic leukemia (C93.1-)

     D46.9   Myelodysplastic syndrome, unspecified
         Myelodysplasia NOS

● **D47**   **Other neoplasms of uncertain behavior of lymphoid, hematopoietic and related tissue**

●   **D47.0**   Mast cell neoplasms of uncertain behavior

         Excludes1   congenital cutaneous mastocytosis (Q82.2)
                histiocytic neoplasms of uncertain behavior (D47.Z9)
                malignant mast cell neoplasm (C96.2-)

         D47.01   Cutaneous mastocytosis
             Diffuse cutaneous mastocytosis
             Maculopapular cutaneous mastocytosis
             Solitary mastocytoma
             Telangiectasia macularis eruptiva perstans
             Urticaria pigmentosa
             Excludes1   congenital (diffuse) (maculopapular) cutaneous mastocytosis (Q82.2)
                      congenital urticaria pigmentosa (Q82.2)
                      extracutaneous mastocytoma (D47.09)

         D47.02   Systemic mastocytosis
             Indolent systemic mastocytosis
             Isolated bone marrow mastocytosis
             Smoldering systemic mastocytosis
             Systemic mastocytosis, with an associated hematological non-mast cell lineage disease (SM-AHNMD)
             Code also if applicable, any associated hematological non-mast cell lineage disease, such as:
               acute myeloid leukemia (C92.6-, C92.A-)
               chronic myelomonocytic leukemia (C93.1-)
               essential thrombocytosis (D47.3)
               hypereosinophilic syndrome (D72.1)
               myelodysplastic syndrome (D46.9)
               myeloproliferative syndrome (D47.1)
               non-Hodgkin lymphoma (C82-C85)
               plasma cell myeloma (C90.0-)
               polycythemia vera (D45)
             Excludes1   aggressive systemic mastocytosis (C96.21)
                      mast cell leukemia (C94.3-)

         D47.09   Other mast cell neoplasms of uncertain behavior
             Extracutaneous mastocytoma
             Mast cell tumor NOS
             Mastocytoma NOS
             Mastocytosis NOS

     D47.1   Chronic myeloproliferative disease
         Chronic neutrophilic leukemia
         Myeloproliferative disease, unspecified
         Excludes1   atypical chronic myeloid leukemia BCR/ABL-negative (C92.2-)
                chronic myeloid leukemia BCR/ABL-positive (C92.1-)
                myelofibrosis NOS (D75.81)
                myelophthisic anemia (D61.82)
                myelophthisis (D61.82)
                secondary myelofibrosis NOS (D75.81)

D47.2 Monoclonal gammopathy
Monoclonal gammopathy of undetermined significance [MGUS]

D47.3 Essential (hemorrhagic) thrombocythemia 🐾
Essential thrombocytosis
Idiopathic hemorrhagic thrombocythemia
▶Primary thrombocytosis
Excludes2 reactive thrombocytosis (D75.838)
▶secondary thrombocytosis (D75.838)
▶thrombocythemia NOS (D75.839)
▶thrombocytosis NOS (D75.839)

D47.4 Osteomyelofibrosis 🐾
Chronic idiopathic myelofibrosis
Myelofibrosis (idiopathic) (with myeloid metaplasia)
Myelosclerosis (megakaryocytic) with myeloid metaplasia
Secondary myelofibrosis in myeloproliferative disease
Excludes1 acute myelofibrosis (C94.4-)

● **D47.Z Other specified neoplasms of uncertain behavior of lymphoid, hematopoietic and related tissue**

D47.Z1 Post-transplant lymphoproliferative disorder (PTLD) 🐾
Code first complications of transplanted organs and tissue (T86.-)

D47.Z2 Castleman disease 🐾
➡Code also if applicable, human herpesvirus 8 infection (B10.89)
Excludes2 Kaposi's sarcoma (C46.-)
Coding Clinic: 2016, Q4, P8

D47.Z9 Other specified neoplasms of uncertain behavior of lymphoid, hematopoietic and related tissue 🐾
Histiocytic tumors of uncertain behavior

D47.9 Neoplasm of uncertain behavior of lymphoid, hematopoietic and related tissue, unspecified 🐾
Lymphoproliferative disease NOS

● **D48 Neoplasm of uncertain behavior of other and unspecified sites**
Excludes1 neurofibromatosis (nonmalignant) (Q85.0-)

D48.0 Neoplasm of uncertain behavior of bone and articular cartilage
Excludes1 neoplasm of uncertain behavior of cartilage of ear (D48.1)
neoplasm of uncertain behavior of cartilage of larynx (D38.0)
neoplasm of uncertain behavior of cartilage of nose (D38.5)
neoplasm of uncertain behavior of connective tissue of eyelid (D48.1)
neoplasm of uncertain behavior of synovia (D48.1)

D48.1 Neoplasm of uncertain behavior of connective and other soft tissue
Neoplasm of uncertain behavior of connective tissue of ear
Neoplasm of uncertain behavior of connective tissue of eyelid
Stromal tumors of uncertain behavior of digestive system
Excludes1 neoplasm of uncertain behavior of articular cartilage (D48.0)
neoplasm of uncertain behavior of cartilage of larynx (D38.0)
neoplasm of uncertain behavior of cartilage of nose (D38.5)
neoplasm of uncertain behavior of connective tissue of breast (D48.6-)

D48.2 Neoplasm of uncertain behavior of peripheral nerves and autonomic nervous system
Excludes1 neoplasm of uncertain behavior of peripheral nerves of orbit (D48.7)

D48.3 Neoplasm of uncertain behavior of retroperitoneum

D48.4 Neoplasm of uncertain behavior of peritoneum

D48.5 Neoplasm of uncertain behavior of skin
Neoplasm of uncertain behavior of anal margin
Neoplasm of uncertain behavior of anal skin
Neoplasm of uncertain behavior of perianal skin
Neoplasm of uncertain behavior of skin of breast
Excludes1 neoplasm of uncertain behavior of anus NOS (D37.8)
neoplasm of uncertain behavior of skin of genital organs (D39.8, D40.8)
neoplasm of uncertain behavior of vermilion border of lip (D37.0)

● **D48.6 Neoplasm of uncertain behavior of breast**
Neoplasm of uncertain behavior of connective tissue of breast
Cystosarcoma phyllodes
Excludes1 neoplasm of uncertain behavior of skin of breast (D48.5)

D48.60 Neoplasm of uncertain behavior of unspecified breast

D48.61 Neoplasm of uncertain behavior of right breast

D48.62 Neoplasm of uncertain behavior of left breast

D48.7 Neoplasm of uncertain behavior of other specified sites
Neoplasm of uncertain behavior of eye
Neoplasm of uncertain behavior of heart
Neoplasm of uncertain behavior of peripheral nerves of orbit
Excludes1 neoplasm of uncertain behavior of connective tissue (D48.1)
neoplasm of uncertain behavior of skin of eyelid (D48.5)

D48.9 Neoplasm of uncertain behavior, unspecified

● **D49 Neoplasms of unspecified behavior**
Note: Category D49 classifies by site neoplasms of unspecified morphology and behavior. The term "mass," unless otherwise stated, is not to be regarded as a neoplastic growth.
Includes 'growth' NOS
neoplasm NOS
new growth NOS
tumor NOS
Excludes1 neoplasms of uncertain behavior (D37-D44, D48)

D49.0 Neoplasm of unspecified behavior of digestive system
Excludes1 neoplasm of unspecified behavior of margin of anus (D49.2)
neoplasm of unspecified behavior of perianal skin (D49.2)
neoplasm of unspecified behavior of skin of anus (D49.2)

D49.1 Neoplasm of unspecified behavior of respiratory system

D49.2 Neoplasm of unspecified behavior of bone, soft tissue, and skin
Excludes1 neoplasm of unspecified behavior of anal canal (D49.0)
neoplasm of unspecified behavior of anus NOS (D49.0)
neoplasm of unspecified behavior of bone marrow (D49.89)
neoplasm of unspecified behavior of cartilage of larynx (D49.1)
neoplasm of unspecified behavior of cartilage of nose (D49.1)
neoplasm of unspecified behavior of connective tissue of breast (D49.3)
neoplasm of unspecified behavior of skin of genital organs (D49.59)
neoplasm of unspecified behavior of vermilion border of lip (D49.0)

CHAPTER 2 (C00-D49)

D49.3 Neoplasm of unspecified behavior of breast
> **Excludes1** neoplasm of unspecified behavior of skin of breast (D49.2)

D49.4 Neoplasm of unspecified behavior of bladder

● D49.5 Neoplasm of unspecified behavior of other genitourinary organs

  ● D49.51 Neoplasm of unspecified behavior of kidney

    D49.511 Neoplasm of unspecified behavior of right kidney
      Coding Clinic: 2016, Q4, P9

    D49.512 Neoplasm of unspecified behavior of left kidney
      Coding Clinic: 2016, Q4, P9

    D49.519 Neoplasm of unspecified behavior of unspecified kidney
      Coding Clinic: 2016, Q4, P9

  D49.59 Neoplasm of unspecified behavior of other genitourinary organ
    Coding Clinic: 2016, Q4, P9

D49.6 Neoplasm of unspecified behavior of brain 🔗
> **Excludes1** neoplasm of unspecified behavior of cerebral meninges (D49.7)
> neoplasm of unspecified behavior of cranial nerves (D49.7)

D49.7 Neoplasm of unspecified behavior of endocrine glands and other parts of nervous system
> **Excludes1** neoplasm of unspecified behavior of peripheral, sympathetic, and parasympathetic nerves and ganglia (D49.2)

● D49.8 Neoplasm of unspecified behavior of other specified sites
> **Excludes1** neoplasm of unspecified behavior of eyelid (skin) (D49.2)
> neoplasm of unspecified behavior of eyelid cartilage (D49.2)
> neoplasm of unspecified behavior of great vessels (D49.2)
> neoplasm of unspecified behavior of optic nerve (D49.7)

  D49.81 Neoplasm of unspecified behavior of retina and choroid
    Dark area on retina
    Retinal freckle

  D49.89 Neoplasm of unspecified behavior of other specified sites

D49.9 Neoplasm of unspecified behavior of unspecified site

CHAPTER 3 (D50-D89)

OGCR Chapter-Specific Coding Guidelines

3. Chapter 3: Disease of the blood and blood-forming organs and certain disorders involving the immune mechanism (D50-D89)
Reserved for future guideline expansion

CHAPTER 3

DISEASES OF THE BLOOD AND BLOOD-FORMING ORGANS AND CERTAIN DISORDERS INVOLVING THE IMMUNE MECHANISM (D50-D89)

Excludes2 autoimmune disease (systemic) NOS (M35.9)
certain conditions originating in the perinatal period (P00-P96)
complications of pregnancy, childbirth and the puerperium (O00-O9A)
congenital malformations, deformations and chromosomal abnormalities (Q00-Q99)
endocrine, nutritional and metabolic diseases (E00-E88)
human immunodeficiency virus [HIV] disease (B20)
injury, poisoning and certain other consequences of external causes (S00-T88)
neoplasms (C00-D49)
symptoms, signs and abnormal clinical and laboratory findings, not elsewhere classified (R00-R94)

This chapter contains the following blocks:

D50-D53	Nutritional anemias
D55-D59	Hemolytic anemias
D60-D64	Aplastic and other anemias and other bone marrow failure syndromes
D65-D69	Coagulation defects, purpura and other hemorrhagic conditions
D70-D77	Other disorders of blood and blood-forming organs
D78	Intraoperative and postprocedural complications of the spleen
D80-D89	Certain disorders involving the immune mechanism

NUTRITIONAL ANEMIAS (D50-D53)

● **D50 Iron deficiency anemia**
A disease characterized by a decrease in the number of red cells (hemoglobin) in the blood.

Includes asiderotic anemia
hypochromic anemia

D50.0 Iron deficiency anemia secondary to blood loss (chronic)
Posthemorrhagic anemia (chronic)

Excludes1 acute posthemorrhagic anemia (D62)
congenital anemia from fetal blood loss (P61.3)

Coding Clinic: 2019, Q3, P17

D50.1 Sideropenic dysphagia
Weblike growth of membranes in throat that makes swallowing difficult
Kelly-Paterson syndrome
Plummer-Vinson syndrome

D50.8 Other iron deficiency anemias
Iron deficiency anemia due to inadequate dietary iron intake

D50.9 Iron deficiency anemia, unspecified

● **D51 Vitamin B12 deficiency anemia**
Excludes1 vitamin B12 deficiency (E53.8)

D51.0 Vitamin B12 deficiency anemia due to intrinsic factor deficiency
Addison anemia
Biermer anemia
Pernicious (congenital) anemia
Congenital intrinsic factor deficiency

D51.1 Vitamin B12 deficiency anemia due to selective vitamin B12 malabsorption with proteinuria
Imerslund (Gräsbeck) syndrome
Megaloblastic hereditary anemia

D51.2 Transcobalamin II deficiency

D51.3 Other dietary vitamin B12 deficiency anemia
Vegan anemia

D51.8 Other vitamin B12 deficiency anemias

D51.9 Vitamin B12 deficiency anemia, unspecified

● **D52 Folate deficiency anemia**
Excludes1 folate deficiency without anemia (E53.8)

D52.0 Dietary folate deficiency anemia
Nutritional megaloblastic anemia

D52.1 Drug-induced folate deficiency anemia
Use additional code for adverse effect, if applicable, to identify drug (T36-T50 with fifth or sixth character 5)

D52.8 Other folate deficiency anemias

D52.9 Folate deficiency anemia, unspecified
Folic acid deficiency anemia NOS

● **D53 Other nutritional anemias**
Includes megaloblastic anemia unresponsive to vitamin B12 or folate therapy

D53.0 Protein deficiency anemia
Amino-acid deficiency anemia
Orotaciduric anemia
Excludes1 Lesch-Nyhan syndrome (E79.1)

D53.1 Other megaloblastic anemias, not elsewhere classified
Megaloblastic anemia NOS
Excludes1 Di Guglielmo's disease (C94.0)

D53.2 Scorbutic anemia
Anemia resulting from deficiency of ascorbic acid (vitamin C)
Excludes1 scurvy (E54)

D53.8 Other specified nutritional anemias
Anemia associated with deficiency of copper
Anemia associated with deficiency of molybdenum
Anemia associated with deficiency of zinc
Excludes1 nutritional deficiencies without anemia, such as:
copper deficiency NOS (E61.0)
molybdenum deficiency NOS (E61.5)
zinc deficiency NOS (E60)

D53.9 Nutritional anemia, unspecified
Simple chronic anemia
Excludes1 anemia NOS (D64.9)
Coding Clinic: 2018, Q4, P88

HEMOLYTIC ANEMIAS (D55-D59)

● **D55 Anemia due to enzyme disorders**
Excludes1 drug-induced enzyme deficiency anemia (D59.2)

D55.0 Anemia due to glucose-6-phosphate dehydrogenase [G6PD] deficiency 🅒🅒
Favism
G6PD deficiency anemia
Excludes1 glucose-6-phosphate dehydrogenase (G6PD) deficiency without anemia (D75.A)

D55.1 Anemia due to other disorders of glutathione metabolism 🅒🅒
Anemia (due to) enzyme deficiencies, except G6PD, related to the hexose monophosphate [HMP] shunt pathway
Anemia (due to) hemolytic nonspherocytic (hereditary), type I

▶ New   ▮▶ Revised   ~~deleted~~ Deleted   Excludes 1   Excludes 2   Includes   Use additional   Code first   Code also   Key words

OGCR Official Guidelines   X Assign placeholder X   ● Use Additional Character(s)   ▸ Manifestation Code   🅒🅒 Hierarchical Condition Category   **Coding Clinic**

- **D55.2 Anemia due to disorders of glycolytic enzymes** 🔎
  - ~~Hemolytic nonspherocytic (hereditary) anemia, type II~~
  - ~~Hexokinase deficiency anemia~~
  - ~~Pyruvate kinase [PK] deficiency anemia~~
  - ~~Triose-phosphate isomerase deficiency anemia~~
  - ▶ **D55.21 Anemia due to pyruvate kinase deficiency**
    - ▶ PK deficiency anemia
    - ▶ Pyruvate kinase deficiency anemia
  - ▶ **D55.29 Anemia due to other disorders of glycolytic enzymes**
    - ▶ Hexokinase deficiency anemia
    - ▶ Triose-phosphate isomerase deficiency anemia
    - **Excludes1** disorders of glycolysis not associated with anemia (E74.81-)
- **D55.3 Anemia due to disorders of nucleotide metabolism** 🔎
- **D55.8 Other anemias due to enzyme disorders** 🔎
- **D55.9 Anemia due to enzyme disorder, unspecified** 🔎

- **D56 Thalassemia**
  - *Hereditary disorders characterized by low production of hemoglobin or excessive destruction of red blood cells*
  - **Excludes1** sickle-cell thalassemia (D57.4-)
  - **D56.0 Alpha thalassemia** 🔎
    - Alpha thalassemia major
    - Hemoglobin H Constant Spring
    - Hemoglobin H disease
    - Hydrops fetalis due to alpha thalassemia
    - Severe alpha thalassemia
    - Triple gene defect alpha thalassemia
    - Use additional code, if applicable, for hydrops fetalis due to alpha thalassemia (P56.99)
    - **Excludes1** alpha thalassemia trait or minor (D56.3)
      - asymptomatic alpha thalassemia (D56.3)
      - hydrops fetalis due to isoimmunization (P56.0)
      - hydrops fetalis not due to immune hemolysis (P83.2)
  - **D56.1 Beta thalassemia** 🔎
    - Beta thalassemia major
    - Cooley's anemia
    - Homozygous beta thalassemia
    - Severe beta thalassemia
    - Thalassemia intermedia
    - Thalassemia major
    - **Excludes1** beta thalassemia minor (D56.3)
      - beta thalassemia trait (D56.3)
      - delta-beta thalassemia (D56.2)
      - hemoglobin E-beta thalassemia (D56.5)
      - sickle-cell beta thalassemia (D57.4-)
  - **D56.2 Delta-beta thalassemia** 🔎
    - Homozygous delta-beta thalassemia
    - **Excludes1** delta-beta thalassemia minor (D56.3)
      - delta-beta thalassemia trait (D56.3)
  - **D56.3 Thalassemia minor**
    - *Genetic disorders that have in common defective production of hemoglobin*
    - Alpha thalassemia minor
    - Alpha thalassemia silent carrier
    - Alpha thalassemia trait
    - Beta thalassemia minor
    - Beta thalassemia trait
    - Delta-beta thalassemia minor
    - Delta-beta thalassemia trait
    - Thalassemia trait NOS
    - **Excludes1** alpha thalassemia (D56.0)
      - beta thalassemia (D56.1)
      - delta-beta thalassemia (D56.2)
      - hemoglobin E-beta thalassemia (D56.5)
      - sickle-cell trait (D57.3)
  - **D56.4 Hereditary persistence of fetal hemoglobin [HPFH]** 🔎
    - *Persistent production of hemoglobin*

- **D56.5 Hemoglobin E-beta thalassemia** 🔎
  - **Excludes1** beta thalassemia (D56.1)
    - beta thalassemia minor (D56.3)
    - beta thalassemia trait (D56.3)
    - delta-beta thalassemia (D56.2)
    - delta-beta thalassemia trait (D56.3)
    - hemoglobin E disease (D58.2)
    - other hemoglobinopathies (D58.2)
    - sickle-cell beta thalassemia (D57.4-)
- **D56.8 Other thalassemias** 🔎
  - Dominant thalassemia
  - Hemoglobin C thalassemia
  - Mixed thalassemia
  - Thalassemia with other hemoglobinopathy
  - **Excludes1** hemoglobin C disease (D58.2)
    - hemoglobin E disease (D58.2)
    - other hemoglobinopathies (D58.2)
    - sickle cell anemia (D57.-)
    - sickle-cell thalassemia (D57.4)
- **D56.9 Thalassemia, unspecified**
  - Mediterranean anemia (with other hemoglobinopathy)

- **D57 Sickle-cell disorders**
  - *Inherited disease in which red blood cells, normally disc-shaped, become crescent shaped*
  - Use additional code for any associated fever (R50.81)
  - **Excludes1** other hemoglobinopathies (D58.-)
  - **D57.0 Hb-SS disease with crisis**
    - Sickle-cell disease with crisis
    - Hb-SS disease with vasoocclusive pain
    - **D57.00 Hb-SS disease with crisis, unspecified** 🔎
      - Hb-SS disease with (painful) crisis NOS
      - Hb-SS disease with vasoocclusive pain NOS
    - **D57.01 Hb-SS disease with acute chest syndrome** 🔎
    - **D57.02 Hb-SS disease with splenic sequestration** 🔎
    - **D57.03 Hb-SS disease with cerebral vascular involvement**
      - Code also, if applicable, cerebral infarction (I63.-)
    - **D57.09 Hb-SS disease with crisis with other specified complication**
      - Use additional code to identify complications, such as:
        - cholelithiasis (K80.-)
        - priapism (N48.32)
  - **D57.1 Sickle-cell disease without crisis Hb-SS disease without crisis** 🔎
    - Sickle-cell anemia NOS
    - Sickle-cell disease NOS
    - Sickle-cell disorder NOS
  - **D57.2 Sickle-cell/Hb-C disease**
    - Hb-SC disease
    - Hb-S/Hb-C disease
    - **D57.20 Sickle-cell/Hb-C disease without crisis** 🔎
    - **D57.21 Sickle-cell/Hb-C disease with crisis**
      - **D57.211 Sickle-cell/Hb-C disease with acute chest syndrome** 🔎
      - **D57.212 Sickle-cell/Hb-C disease with splenic sequestration** 🔎
      - **D57.213 Sickle-cell/Hb-C disease with cerebral vascular involvement**
        - Code also, if applicable, cerebral infarction (I63.-)
      - **D57.218 Sickle-cell/Hb-C disease with crisis with other specified complication**
        - Use additional code to identify complications, such as:
          - cholelithiasis (K80.-)
          - priapism (N48.32)
      - **D57.219 Sickle-cell/Hb-C disease with crisis, unspecified** 🔎
        - Sickle-cell/Hb-C disease with crisis NOS
        - Sickle-cell/Hb-C disease with vasoocclusive pain NOS

CHAPTER 3 (D50-D89)

D57.3 **Sickle-cell trait** 🐾
    Hb-S trait
    Heterozygous hemoglobin S

● **D57.4** **Sickle-cell thalassemia**
    Sickle-cell beta thalassemia
    Thalassemia Hb-S disease

  D57.40 **Sickle-cell thalassemia without crisis** 🐾
    Microdrepanocytosis
    Sickle-cell thalassemia NOS

  ● **D57.41** **Sickle-cell thalassemia, unspecified, with crisis**
    Sickle-cell "crisis" is precipitated when abnormally crescent-shaped red blood cells form clots and interrupt blood flow to major organs, causing severe pain and organ damage.
    Sickle-cell thalassemia with (painful) crisis NOS
    Sickle-cell thalassemia with vasoocclusive pain NOS

    D57.411 **Sickle-cell thalassemia, unspecified, with acute chest syndrome** 🐾

    D57.412 **Sickle-cell thalassemia with, unspecified, splenic sequestration** 🐾

    D57.413 **Sickle-cell thalassemia, unspecified, with cerebral vascular involvement**
      Code also, if applicable cerebral infarction (I63.-)

    D57.418 **Sickle-cell thalassemia, unspecified, with crisis with other specified complication**
      Use additional code to identify complications, such as:
        cholelithiasis (K80.-)
        priapism (N48.32)

    D57.419 **Sickle-cell thalassemia with, unspecified, crisis** 🐾
      Sickle-cell thalassemia with (painful) crisis NOS
      ➡Sickle-cell thalassemia with vasoocclusive pain NOS

  D57.42 **Sickle-cell thalassemia beta zero without crisis**
    HbS-beta zero without crisis
    Sickle-cell beta zero without crisis

  ● **D57.43** **Sickle-cell thalassemia beta zero with crisis**
    HbS-beta zero with crisis
    Sickle-cell beta zero with crisis

    D57.431 **Sickle-cell thalassemia beta zero with acute chest syndrome**
      HbS-beta zero with acute chest syndrome
      Sickle-cell beta zero with acute chest syndrome

    D57.432 **Sickle-cell thalassemia beta zero with splenic sequestration**
      HbS-beta zero with splenic sequestration
      Sickle-cell beta zero with splenic sequestration

    D57.433 **Sickle-cell thalassemia beta zero with cerebral vascular involvement**
      HbS-beta zero with cerebral vascular involvement
      Sickle-cell beta zero with cerebral vascular involvement
      Code also, if applicable cerebral infarction (I63.-)

    D57.438 **Sickle-cell thalassemia beta zero with crisis with other specified complication**
      HbS-beta zero with other specified complication
      Sickle-cell beta zero with other specified complication
      Use additional code to identify complications, such as:
        cholelithiasis (K80.-)
        priapism (N48.32)

    D57.439 **Sickle-cell thalassemia beta zero with crisis, unspecified**
      HbS-beta zero with other specified complication
      Sickle-cell beta zero with crisis unspecified
      Sickle-cell thalassemia beta zero with (painful) crisis NOS
      ➡Sickle-cell thalassemia beta zero with vasoocclusive pain NOS

  D57.44 **Sickle-cell thalassemia beta plus without crisis**
    HbS-beta plus without crisis
    Sickle-cell beta plus without crisis

  ● **D57.45** **Sickle-cell thalassemia beta plus with crisis**
    HbS-beta plus with crisis
    Sickle-cell beta plus with crisis

    D57.451 **Sickle-cell thalassemia beta plus with acute chest syndrome**
      HbS-beta plus with acute chest syndrome
      Sickle-cell beta plus with acute chest syndrome

    D57.452 **Sickle-cell thalassemia beta plus with splenic sequestration**
      HbS-beta plus with splenic sequestration
      Sickle-cell beta plus with splenic sequestration

    D57.453 **Sickle-cell thalassemia beta plus with cerebral vascular involvement**
      HbS-beta plus with cerebral vascular involvement
      Sickle-cell beta plus with cerebral vascular involvement
      Code also, if applicable cerebral infarction (I63.-)

    D57.458 **Sickle-cell thalassemia beta plus with crisis with other specified complication**
      HbS-beta plus with crisis with other specified complication
      Sickle-cell beta plus with crisis with other specified complication
      Use additional code to identify complications, such as:
        cholelithiasis (K80.-)
        priapism (N48.32)

    D57.459 **Sickle-cell thalassemia beta plus with crisis, unspecified**
      HbS-beta plus with crisis with unspecified complication
      Sickle-cell beta plus with crisis with unspecified complication
      Sickle-cell thalassemia beta plus with (painful) crisis NOS
      ➡Sickle-cell thalassemia beta plus with vasoocclusive pain NOS

● **D57.8** **Other sickle-cell disorders**
    Hb-SD disease
    Hb-SE disease

  D57.80 **Other sickle-cell disorders without crisis** 🐾

  ● **D57.81** **Other sickle-cell disorders with crisis**

    D57.811 **Other sickle-cell disorders with acute chest syndrome** 🐾

    D57.812 **Other sickle-cell disorders with splenic sequestration** 🐾

    D57.813 **Other sickle-cell disorders with cerebral vascular involvement**
      Code also, if applicable: cerebral infarction (I63.-)

▶ New   ➡ Revised   ~~deleted~~ Deleted   Excludes 1   Excludes 2   Includes   Use additional   Code first   Code also   Key words
OGCR Official Guidelines   X Assign placeholder X   ● Use Additional Character(s)   ▷ Manifestation Code   🐾 Hierarchical Condition Category   **Coding Clinic**

D57.818   Other sickle-cell disorders with crisis with other specified complication

> Use additional code to identify complications, such as:
> cholelithiasis (K80.-)
> priapism (N48.32)

D57.819   Other sickle-cell disorders with crisis, unspecified 🦤
> Other sickle-cell disorders with crisis NOS
> Other sickle-cell disorders with vasoocclusive pain NOS

● **D58**   Other hereditary hemolytic anemias
Genetic condition in which bone marrow is unable to compensate for premature destruction of red blood cells

> **Excludes1**   hemolytic anemia of the newborn (P55.-)

D58.0   Hereditary spherocytosis 🦤
Presence of spherocytes (spherically shaped red blood cells)
> Acholuric (familial) jaundice
> Congenital (spherocytic) hemolytic icterus
> Minkowski-Chauffard syndrome

D58.1   Hereditary elliptocytosis 🦤
Presence of large numbers of elliptocytes in blood
> Elliptocytosis (congenital)
> Ovalocytosis (congenital) (hereditary)

D58.2   Other hemoglobinopathies 🦤
> Abnormal hemoglobin NOS
> Congenital Heinz body anemia
> Hb-C disease
> Hb-D disease
> Hb-E disease
> Hemoglobinopathy NOS
> Unstable hemoglobin hemolytic disease
>
> > **Excludes1**   familial polycythemia (D75.0)
> > Hb-M disease (D74.0)
> > hemoglobin E-beta thalassemia (D56.5)
> > hereditary persistence of fetal hemoglobin [HPFH] (D56.4)
> > high-altitude polycythemia (D75.1)
> > methemoglobinemia (D74.-)
> > other hemoglobinopathies with thalassemia (D56.8)

D58.8   Other specified hereditary hemolytic anemias 🦤
> Stomatocytosis

D58.9   Hereditary hemolytic anemia, unspecified 🦤

● **D59**   Acquired hemolytic anemia

D59.0   Drug-induced autoimmune hemolytic anemia 🦤
> Use additional code for adverse effect, if applicable, to identify drug (T36-T50 with fifth or sixth character 5)

D59.1   Other autoimmune hemolytic anemias 🦤
> **Excludes2**   Evans syndrome (D69.41)
> hemolytic disease of newborn (P55.-)
> paroxysmal cold hemoglobinuria (D59.6)

D59.10   Autoimmune hemolytic anemia, unspecified

D59.11   Warm autoimmune hemolytic anemia
> Warm type (primary) (secondary) (symptomatic) autoimmune hemolytic anemia
> Warm type autoimmune hemolytic disease

D59.12   Cold autoimmune hemolytic anemia
> Chronic cold hemagglutinin disease
> Cold agglutinin disease
> Cold agglutinin hemoglobinuria
> Cold type (primary) (secondary) (symptomatic) autoimmune hemolytic anemia
> Cold type autoimmune hemolytic disease

D59.13   Mixed type autoimmune hemolytic anemia
> Mixed type autoimmune hemolytic disease
> Mixed type, cold and warm, (primary) (secondary) (symptomatic) autoimmune hemolyticanemia

D59.19   Other autoimmune hemolytic anemia

D59.2   Drug-induced nonautoimmune hemolytic anemia 🦤
> Drug-induced enzyme deficiency anemia
> Use additional code for adverse effect, if applicable, to identify drug (T36-T50 with fifth or sixth character 5)

D59.3   Hemolytic-uremic syndrome 🦤
> Use additional code to identify associated:
> E. coli infection (B96.2-)
> Pneumococcal pneumonia (J13)
> Shigella dysenteriae (A03.9)

D59.4   Other nonautoimmune hemolytic anemias 🦤
> Mechanical hemolytic anemia
> Microangiopathic hemolytic anemia
> Toxic hemolytic anemia

D59.5   Paroxysmal nocturnal hemoglobinuria [Marchiafava-Micheli] 🦤
> **Excludes1**   hemoglobinuria NOS (R82.3)

D59.6   Hemoglobinuria due to hemolysis from other external causes 🦤
> Hemoglobinuria from exertion
> March hemoglobinuria
> Paroxysmal cold hemoglobinuria
> Use additional code (Chapter 20) to identify external cause
>
> > **Excludes1**   hemoglobinuria NOS (R82.3)

D59.8   Other acquired hemolytic anemias 🦤

D59.9   Acquired hemolytic anemia, unspecified 🦤
> Idiopathic hemolytic anemia, chronic

APLASTIC AND OTHER ANEMIAS AND OTHER BONE MARROW FAILURE SYNDROMES (D60-D64)

● **D60**   Acquired pure red cell aplasia [erythroblastopenia]
Deficiency of erythroblasts
> **Includes**   red cell aplasia (acquired) (adult) (with thymoma)
> **Excludes1**   congenital red cell aplasia (D61.01)

D60.0   Chronic acquired pure red cell aplasia 🦤
Lack of development of blood cell

D60.1   Transient acquired pure red cell aplasia 🦤

D60.8   Other acquired pure red cell aplasias 🦤

D60.9   Acquired pure red cell aplasia, unspecified 🦤

● **D61**   Other aplastic anemias and other bone marrow failure syndromes
> **Excludes2**   neutropenia (D70.-)

● **D61.0**   Constitutional aplastic anemia
Condition where bone marrow is unable to produce blood cells

D61.01   Constitutional (pure) red blood cell aplasia 🦤
> Blackfan-Diamond syndrome
> Congenital (pure) red cell aplasia
> Familial hypoplastic anemia
> Primary (pure) red cell aplasia
> Red cell (pure) aplasia of infants
>
> > **Excludes1**   acquired red cell aplasia (D60.9)

D61.09   Other constitutional aplastic anemia 🦤
> Fanconi's anemia
> Pancytopenia with malformations

D61.1   Drug-induced aplastic anemia 🦤
> Use additional code for adverse effect, if applicable, to identify drug (T36-T50 with fifth or sixth character 5)

D61.2   Aplastic anemia due to other external agents 🦤
> *Code first*, if applicable, toxic effects of substances chiefly nonmedicinal as to source (T51-T65)

D61.3   Idiopathic aplastic anemia 🦤

● **D61.8 Other specified aplastic anemias and other bone marrow failure syndromes**

  ● **D61.81 Pancytopenia**

  Marked deficiency of all the blood elements: Red blood cells (erythrocytes), white blood cells (leukocytes), and platelets (thrombocytes). Check laboratory results.

  Excludes1 pancytopenia (due to) (with) aplastic anemia (D61.9)

  pancytopenia (due to) (with) bone marrow infiltration (D61.82)

  pancytopenia (due to) (with) congenital (pure) red cell aplasia (D61.01)

  pancytopenia (due to) (with) hairy cell leukemia (C91.4-)

  pancytopenia (due to) (with) human immunodeficiency virus disease (B20.-)

  pancytopenia (due to) (with) leukoerythroblastic anemia (D61.82)

  pancytopenia (due to) (with) myeloproliferative disease (D47.1)

  Excludes2 pancytopenia (due to) (with) myelodysplastic syndromes (D46.-)

  D61.810 Antineoplastic chemotherapy induced pancytopenia 🐾

  Excludes2 aplastic anemia due to antineoplastic chemotherapy (D61.1)

  D61.811 Other drug-induced pancytopenia 🐾

  Excludes2 aplastic anemia due to drugs (D61.1)

  D61.818 Other pancytopenia 🐾
  Coding Clinic: 2019, Q1, P16

  D61.82 Myelophthisis 🐾
  Leukoerythroblastic anemia
  Myelophthisic anemia
  Panmyelophthisis

  Code also the underlying disorder, such as:
  malignant neoplasm of breast (C50.-)
  tuberculosis (A15.-)

  Excludes1 idiopathic myelofibrosis (D47.1)
  myelofibrosis NOS (D75.81)
  myelofibrosis with myeloid metaplasia (D47.4)
  primary myelofibrosis (D47.1)
  secondary myelofibrosis (D75.81)

  D61.89 Other specified aplastic anemias and other bone marrow failure syndromes 🐾

● **D61.9 Aplastic anemia, unspecified** 🐾
  Hypoplastic anemia NOS
  Medullary hypoplasia

D62 Acute posthemorrhagic anemia

  Excludes1 anemia due to chronic blood loss (D50.0)
  blood loss anemia NOS (D50.0)
  congenital anemia from fetal blood loss (P61.3)
  Coding Clinic: 2019, Q3, P13,17

● **D63 Anemia in chronic diseases classified elsewhere**

  ▷ **D63.0 Anemia in neoplastic disease**
  Code first neoplasm (C00-D49)

  Excludes1 aplastic anemia due to antineoplastic chemotherapy (D61.1)

  Excludes2 anemia due to antineoplastic chemotherapy (D64.81)

  ▷ **D63.1 Anemia in chronic kidney disease**
  Erythropoietin resistant anemia (EPO resistant anemia)
  Code first underlying chronic kidney disease (CKD) (N18.-)

  ▷ **D63.8 Anemia in other chronic diseases classified elsewhere**
  Code first underlying disease, such as:
  diphyllobothriasis (B70.0)
  hookworm disease (B76.0-B76.9)
  hypothyroidism (E00.0-E03.9)
  malaria (B50.0-B54)
  symptomatic late syphilis (A52.79)
  tuberculosis (A18.89)

● **D64 Other anemias**

  Excludes1 refractory anemia (D46.-)
  refractory anemia with excess blasts in transformation [RAEB T] (C92.0-)

  D64.0 Hereditary sideroblastic anemia 🐾
  Abnormal production RBCs (erythrocytes)
  Sex-linked hypochromic sideroblastic anemia

  ▷ **D64.1 Secondary sideroblastic anemia due to disease** 🐾
  Code first underlying disease

  D64.2 Secondary sideroblastic anemia due to drugs and toxins 🐾
  Code first poisoning due to drug or toxin, if applicable (T36-T65 with fifth or sixth character 1-4 or 6)

  Use additional code for adverse effect, if applicable, to identify drug (T36-T50 with fifth or sixth character 5)

  D64.3 Other sideroblastic anemias 🐾
  Sideroblastic anemia NOS
  Pyridoxine-responsive sideroblastic anemia NEC

  D64.4 Congenital dyserythropoietic anemia
  Any of several rare hereditary anemias, mostly types of macrocytic anemia
  Dyshematopoietic anemia (congenital)

  Excludes1 Blackfan-Diamond syndrome (D61.01)
  Di Guglielmo's disease (C94.0)

● **D64.8 Other specified anemias**

  D64.81 Anemia due to antineoplastic chemotherapy
  Antineoplastic chemotherapy induced anemia

  ~~Excludes1~~ ~~aplastic anemia due to antineoplastic chemotherapy (D61.1)~~

  ▶ aplastic anemia due to antineoplastic chemotherapy (D61.1)

  Excludes2 anemia in neoplastic disease (D63.0)

  D64.89 Other specified anemias
  Infantile pseudoleukemia

  D64.9 Anemia, unspecified
  Coding Clinic: 2018, Q4, P88; 2017, Q1, P7

▶ New   ⟹ Revised   ~~deleted~~ Deleted   Excludes 1   Excludes 2   Includes   Use additional   Code first   Code also   Key words

730   OGCR Official Guidelines   X Assign placeholder X   ● Use Additional Character(s)   ▷ Manifestation Code   🐾 Hierarchical Condition Category   Coding Clinic

COAGULATION DEFECTS, PURPURA AND OTHER HEMORRHAGIC CONDITIONS (D65-D69)

D65   Disseminated intravascular coagulation [defibrination syndrome] 🦠
Blood clots form and consume all coagulation proteins and platelets and disrupt normal coagulation, resulting in abnormal bleeding
Afibrinogenemia, acquired
Consumption coagulopathy
Diffuse or disseminated intravascular coagulation [DIC]
Fibrinolytic hemorrhage, acquired
Fibrinolytic purpura
Purpura fulminans

> **Excludes1**   disseminated intravascular coagulation (complicating):
> abortion or ectopic or molar pregnancy (O00-O07, O08.1)
> in newborn (P60)
> pregnancy, childbirth and the puerperium (O45.0, O46.0, O67.0, O72.3)

Coding Clinic: 2021, Q1, P39; 2019, Q2, P25

D66   Hereditary factor VIII deficiency 🦠
Inherited coagulation disorder carried by females but most often affecting males
Classical hemophilia
Deficiency factor VIII (with functional defect)
Hemophilia NOS
Hemophilia A

> **Excludes1**   factor VIII deficiency with vascular defect (D68.0)

D67   Hereditary factor IX deficiency 🦠
Christmas disease
Factor IX deficiency (with functional defect)
Hemophilia B
Plasma thromboplastin component [PTC] deficiency

● D68   Other coagulation defects

> **Excludes1**   abnormal coagulation profile (R79.1)
> coagulation defects complicating abortion or ectopic or molar pregnancy (O00-O07, O08.1)
> coagulation defects complicating pregnancy, childbirth and the puerperium (O45.0, O46.0, O67.0, O72.3)

Coding Clinic: 2016, Q1, P14

D68.0   Von Willebrand's disease 🦠
Congenital bleeding disorder
Angiohemophilia
Factor VIII deficiency with vascular defect
Vascular hemophilia

> **Excludes1**   capillary fragility (hereditary) (D69.8)
> factor VIII deficiency NOS (D66)
> factor VIII deficiency with functional defect (D66)

D68.1   Hereditary factor XI deficiency 🦠
Deficiency of blood coagulation resulting in systemic blood-clotting defect
Hemophilia C
Plasma thromboplastin antecedent [PTA] deficiency
Rosenthal's disease

D68.2   Hereditary deficiency of other clotting factors 🦠
Blood clotting disorders caused by hereditary deficiencies of one or more clotting factors
AC globulin deficiency
Congenital afibrinogenemia
Deficiency of factor I [fibrinogen]
Deficiency of factor II [prothrombin]
Deficiency of factor V [labile]
Deficiency of factor VII [stable]
Deficiency of factor X [Stuart-Prower]
Deficiency of factor XII [Hageman]
Deficiency of factor XIII [fibrin stabilizing]
Dysfibrinogenemia (congenital)
Hypoproconvertinemia
Owren's disease
Proaccelerin deficiency

● D68.3   Hemorrhagic disorder due to circulating anticoagulants
Blood clotting disorders caused by anticoagulants (warfarin and heparin)

● D68.31   Hemorrhagic disorder due to intrinsic circulating anticoagulants, antibodies, or inhibitors

D68.311   Acquired hemophilia 🦠
Autoimmune hemophilia
Autoimmune inhibitors to clotting factors
Secondary hemophilia

D68.312   Antiphospholipid antibody with hemorrhagic disorder 🦠
Lupus anticoagulant (LAC) with hemorrhagic disorder
Systemic lupus erythematosus [SLE] inhibitor with hemorrhagic disorder

> **Excludes1**   antiphospholipid antibody, finding without diagnosis (R76.0)
> antiphospholipid antibody syndrome (D68.61)
> antiphospholipid antibody with hypercoagulable state (D68.61)
> lupus anticoagulant (LAC) finding without diagnosis (R76.0)
> lupus anticoagulant (LAC) with hypercoagulable state (D68.62)
> systemic lupus erythematosus [SLE] inhibitor finding without diagnosis (R76.0)
> systemic lupus erythematosus [SLE] inhibitor with hypercoagulable state (D68.62)

D68.318   Other hemorrhagic disorder due to intrinsic circulating anticoagulants, antibodies, or inhibitors 🦠
Antithromboplastinemia
Antithromboplastinogenemia
Hemorrhagic disorder due to intrinsic increase in antithrombin
Hemorrhagic disorder due to intrinsic increase in anti-VIIIa
Hemorrhagic disorder due to intrinsic increase in anti-IXa
Hemorrhagic disorder due to intrinsic increase in anti-XIa

CHAPTER 3 (D50–D89)

D68.32 **Hemorrhagic disorder due to extrinsic circulating anticoagulants** 🅗
- Drug-induced hemorrhagic disorder
- Hemorrhagic disorder due to increase in anti-IIa
- Hemorrhagic disorder due to increase in anti-Xa
- Hyperheparinemia
  - Use additional code for adverse effect, if applicable, to identify drug (T45.515, T45.525)
  - *Coding Clinic: 2021, Q1, P5; 2016, Q1, P14-15*

D68.4 **Acquired coagulation factor deficiency** 🅗
- Deficiency of coagulation factor due to liver disease
- Deficiency of coagulation factor due to vitamin K deficiency
  - **Excludes1**   vitamin K deficiency of newborn (P53)

● **D68.5** **Primary thrombophilia**
AKA idiopathic thrombocytopenia, may be acquired or congenital and is a common cause of coagulation disorders.
- Primary hypercoagulable states
  - **Excludes1**   antiphospholipid syndrome (D68.61)
    - lupus anticoagulant (D68.62)
    - secondary activated protein C resistance (D68.69)
    - secondary antiphospholipid antibody syndrome (D68.69)
    - secondary lupus anticoagulant with hypercoagulable state (D68.69)
    - secondary systemic lupus erythematosus [SLE] inhibitor with hypercoagulable state (D68.69)
    - systemic lupus erythematosus [SLE] inhibitor finding without diagnosis (R76.0)
    - systemic lupus erythematosus [SLE] inhibitor with hemorrhagic disorder (D68.312)
    - ➡ thrombotic thrombocytopenic purpura (M31.19)

D68.51 **Activated protein C resistance** 🅗
- Factor V Leiden mutation

D68.52 **Prothrombin gene mutation** 🅗

D68.59 **Other primary thrombophilia** 🅗
- Antithrombin III deficiency
- Hypercoagulable state NOS
- Primary hypercoagulable state NEC
- Primary thrombophilia NEC
- Protein C deficiency
- Protein S deficiency
- Thrombophilia NOS
  - ▶ *Coding Clinic: 2021, Q2, P8-9*

● **D68.6** **Other thrombophilia**
- Other hypercoagulable states
  - **Excludes1**   diffuse or disseminated intravascular coagulation [DIC] (D65)
    - heparin induced thrombocytopenia (HIT) (D75.82)
    - hyperhomocysteinemia (E72.11)

D68.61 **Antiphospholipid syndrome** 🅗
- Anticardiolipin syndrome
- Antiphospholipid antibody syndrome
  - **Excludes1**   anti-phospholipid antibody, finding without diagnosis (R76.0)
    - anti-phospholipid antibody with hemorrhagic disorder (D68.312)
    - lupus anticoagulant syndrome (D68.62)

D68.62 **Lupus anticoagulant syndrome** 🅗
- Lupus anticoagulant
- Presence of systemic lupus erythematosus [SLE] inhibitor
  - **Excludes1**   anticardiolipin syndrome (D68.61)
    - antiphospholipid syndrome (D68.61)
    - lupus anticoagulant (LAC) finding without diagnosis (R76.0)
    - lupus anticoagulant (LAC) with hemorrhagic disorder (D68.312)

D68.69 **Other thrombophilia** 🅗
- Hypercoagulable states NEC
- Secondary hypercoagulable state NOS
  - ▶ *Coding Clinic: 2021, Q2, P8*

D68.8 **Other specified coagulation defects** 🅗
- **Excludes1**   hemorrhagic disease of newborn (P53)
- *Coding Clinic: 2021, Q1, P39-40*

D68.9 **Coagulation defect, unspecified** 🅗

● **D69** **Purpura and other hemorrhagic conditions**
Group of conditions characterized by small hemorrhages in skin, mucous membranes, or serosal surfaces
- **Excludes1**   benign hypergammaglobulinemic purpura (D89.0)
  - cryoglobulinemic purpura (D89.1)
  - essential (hemorrhagic) thrombocythemia (D47.3)
  - hemorrhagic thrombocythemia (D47.3)
  - purpura fulminans (D65)
  - ➡ thrombotic thrombocytopenic purpura (M31.19)
  - Waldenström hypergammaglobulinemic purpura (D89.0)

D69.0 **Allergic purpura** 🅗
- Allergic vasculitis
- Nonthrombocytopenic hemorrhagic purpura
- Nonthrombocytopenic idiopathic purpura
- Purpura anaphylactoid
- Purpura Henoch(-Schönlein)
- Purpura rheumatica
- Vascular purpura
  - **Excludes1**   thrombocytopenic hemorrhagic purpura (D69.3)

D69.1 **Qualitative platelet defects** 🅗
- Bernard-Soulier [giant platelet] syndrome
- Glanzmann's disease
- Grey platelet syndrome
- Thromboasthenia (hemorrhagic) (hereditary)
- Thrombocytopathy
  - **Excludes1**   von Willebrand's disease (D68.0)

D69.2 **Other nonthrombocytopenic purpura** 🅗
- Purpura NOS
- Purpura simplex
- Senile purpura

D69.3 **Immune thrombocytopenic purpura** 🅗
- Hemorrhagic (thrombocytopenic) purpura
- Idiopathic thrombocytopenic purpura
- Tidal platelet dysgenesis

● **D69.4** **Other primary thrombocytopenia**
- **Excludes1**   transient neonatal thrombocytopenia (P61.0)
  - Wiskott-Aldrich syndrome (D82.0)

D69.41 **Evans syndrome** 🅗
Acquired hemolytic anemia and thrombocytopenia

▶ New   ➡ Revised   ~~deleted~~ Deleted   Excludes 1   Excludes 2   Includes   Use additional   Code first   Code also   Key words
OGCR Official Guidelines   X Assign placeholder X   ● Use Additional Character(s)   ▶ Manifestation Code   🅗 Hierarchical Condition Category   Coding Clinic

D69.42   **Congenital and hereditary thrombocytopenia purpura** 🔗
  Congenital thrombocytopenia
  Hereditary thrombocytopenia
  Code first congenital or hereditary disorder,
    such as:
      thrombocytopenia with absent radius (TAR
      syndrome) (Q87.2)

D69.49   **Other primary thrombocytopenia** 🔗
  Megakaryocytic hypoplasia
  Primary thrombocytopenia NOS

● **D69.5**   **Secondary thrombocytopenia**
  Acquired reduction of number of platelets required for blood
    clotting

Excludes1	heparin induced thrombocytopenia (HIT) (D75.82)
	transient thrombocytopenia of newborn (P61.0)

D69.51   **Posttransfusion purpura**
  Posttransfusion purpura from whole blood
  (fresh) or blood products PTP

D69.59   **Other secondary thrombocytopenia**

D69.6   **Thrombocytopenia, unspecified** 🔗

D69.8   **Other specified hemorrhagic conditions** 🔗
  Capillary fragility (hereditary)
  Vascular pseudohemophilia

D69.9   **Hemorrhagic condition, unspecified** 🔗

OTHER DISORDERS OF BLOOD AND BLOOD-FORMING ORGANS (D70-D77)

● **D70**   **Neutropenia**
  Decrease in number of neutrophils (type of white blood cell)

Includes	agranulocytosis
	decreased absolute neurophile count (ANC)

  Use additional code for any associated:
    fever (R50.81)
    mucositis (J34.81, K12.3-, K92.81, N76.81)

Excludes1	neutropenic splenomegaly (D73.81)
	transient neonatal neutropenia (P61.5)

D70.0   **Congenital agranulocytosis** 🔗
  Reduced numbers of neutrophils (type of white blood cell)
  Congenital neutropenia
  Infantile genetic agranulocytosis
  Kostmann's disease

D70.1   **Agranulocytosis secondary to cancer chemotherapy** 🔗
  Decreased numbers of granulocytes (type of white blood cell)
  Code also *underlying neoplasm*
  Use additional code for adverse effect, if applicable, to
    identify drug (T45.1X5)

D70.2   **Other drug-induced agranulocytosis** 🔗
  Use additional code for adverse effect, if applicable,
    to identify drug (T36-T50 with fifth or sixth
    character 5)

D70.3   **Neutropenia due to infection** 🔗

D70.4   **Cyclic neutropenia** 🔗
  Chronic neutropenia (low number of type of white blood cell)
  Cyclic hematopoiesis
  Periodic neutropenia

D70.8   **Other neutropenia** 🔗

D70.9   **Neutropenia, unspecified** 🔗
  Coding Clinic: 2019, Q2, P25

D71   **Functional disorders of polymorphonuclear neutrophils** 🔗
  Polymorphonuclear: varying shapes of nucleus; AKA PMNs
  Cell membrane receptor complex [CR3] defect
  Chronic (childhood) granulomatous disease
  Congenital dysphagocytosis
  Progressive septic granulomatosis

● **D72**   **Other disorders of white blood cells**

Excludes1	basophilia (D72.824)
	immunity disorders (D80-D89)
	neutropenia (D70)
	preleukemia (syndrome) (D46.9)

D72.0   **Genetic anomalies of leukocytes** 🔗
  Alder (granulation) (granulocyte) anomaly
  Alder syndrome
  Hereditary leukocytic hypersegmentation
  Hereditary leukocytic hyposegmentation
  Hereditary leukomelanopathy
  May-Hegglin (granulation) (granulocyte) anomaly
  May-Hegglin syndrome
  Pelger-Huët (granulation) (granulocyte) anomaly
  Pelger-Huët syndrome

Excludes1	Chédiak (-Steinbrinck)-Higashi syndrome (E70.330)

● **D72.1**   **Eosinophilia**
  Formation and accumulation of high number of white cells in
    blood/tissue

➡ **Excludes2**	Löffler's syndrome (J82.89)
	➡ pulmonary eosinophilia (J82.-)

D72.10   **Eosinophilia, unspecified**

● **D72.11**   **Hypereosinophilic syndrome [HES]**

  D72.110   **Idiopathic hypereosinophilic syndrome [IHES]**

  D72.111   **Lymphocytic Variant Hypereosinophilic Syndrome [LHES]**
    Lymphocyte variant
      hypereosinophilia
    Code also, if applicable, any
      associated lymphocytic
      neoplastic disorder

  D72.118   **Other hypereosinophilic syndrome**
    Episodic angioedema with
      eosinophilia
    Gleich's syndrome

  D72.119   **Hypereosinophilic syndrome [HES], unspecified**

  D72.12   **Drug rash with eosinophilia and systemic symptoms syndrome**
    DRESS syndrome
    Use additional code for adverse effect, if
      applicable, to identify drug (T36-T50 with
      fifth or sixth character 5)

  D72.18   *Eosinophilia in diseases classified elsewhere*
    Code first underlying disease, such as:
      chronic myelomonocytic leukemia (C93.1-)

  D72.19   **Other eosinophilia**
    Familial eosinophilia
    Hereditary eosinophilia

● **D72.8**   **Other specified disorders of white blood cells**

Excludes1	leukemia (C91-C95)

● **D72.81**   **Decreased white blood cell count**

Excludes1	neutropenia (D70.-)

  D72.810   **Lymphocytopenia**
    Decreased lymphocytes
    Reduction in number of lympho cytes
      in blood

  D72.818   **Other decreased white blood cell count**
    Basophilic leukopenia
    Eosinophilic leukopenia
    Monocytopenia
    Other decreased leukocytes
    Plasmacytopenia

  D72.819   **Decreased white blood cell count, unspecified**
    Decreased leukocytes, unspecified
    Leukocytopenia, unspecified
    Leukopenia

Excludes1	malignant leukopenia (D70.9)

CHAPTER 3 (D50-D89)

● **D72.82   Elevated white blood cell count**
> Excludes1   eosinophilia (D72.1)

     D72.820   Lymphocytosis (symptomatic)
        Elevated lymphocytes
        Excess of normal lymphocytes

     D72.821   Monocytosis (symptomatic)
> Excludes1   infectious mononucleosis (B27.-)

     D72.822   Plasmacytosis
        Presence of excess plasma cells

     D72.823   Leukemoid reaction
        Basophilic leukemoid reaction
        Leukemoid reaction NOS
        Lymphocytic leukemoid reaction
        Monocytic leukemoid reaction
        Myelocytic leukemoid reaction
        Neutrophilic leukemoid reaction

     D72.824   Basophilia
        Increase of basophils in blood

     D72.825   Bandemia
        Bandemia without diagnosis of specific infection
        Excess number of band cells (immature white blood cells) released by bone marrow
> Excludes1   confirmed infection -code to infection
> leukemia (C91.-, C92.-, C93.-, C94.-, C95.-)

     D72.828   Other elevated white blood cell count

     D72.829   Elevated white blood cell count, unspecified
        Elevated leukocytes, unspecified
        Leukocytosis, unspecified

   D72.89   Other specified disorders of white blood cells
     Abnormality of white blood cells NEC

   D72.9   Disorder of white blood cells, unspecified
     Abnormal leukocyte differential NOS

● **D73   Diseases of spleen**

   D73.0   Hyposplenism
     Diminished functioning of spleen
     Atrophy of spleen
> Excludes1   asplenia (congenital) (Q89.01)
> postsurgical absence of spleen (Z90.81)

   D73.1   Hypersplenism
     Accelerated function of spleen
> Excludes1   neutropenic splenomegaly (D73.81)
> primary splenic neutropenia (D73.81)
> splenitis, splenomegaly in late syphilis (A52.79)
> splenitis, splenomegaly in tuberculosis (A18.85)
> splenomegaly NOS (R16.1)
> splenomegaly congenital (Q89.0)

   D73.2   Chronic congestive splenomegaly
     Enlargement of spleen

   D73.3   Abscess of spleen

   D73.4   Cyst of spleen

   D73.5   Infarction of spleen
     Splenic rupture, nontraumatic
     Torsion of spleen
> Excludes1   rupture of spleen due to Plasmodium vivax malaria (B51.0)
> traumatic rupture of spleen (S36.03-)

● **D73.8   Other diseases of spleen**

   D73.81   Neutropenic splenomegaly
     Werner-Schultz disease
     Enlarged spleen responding to inadequate number of neutrophils

   D73.89   Other diseases of spleen
     Fibrosis of spleen NOS
     Perisplenitis
     Splenitis NOS

   D73.9   Disease of spleen, unspecified

● **D74   Methemoglobinemia**
   Excessive methemoglobin (form of hemoglobin)

   D74.0   Congenital methemoglobinemia
     Congenital NADH-methemoglobin reductase deficiency
     Hemoglobin-M [Hb-M] disease
     Methemoglobinemia, hereditary

   D74.8   Other methemoglobinemias
     Acquired methemoglobinemia (with sulfhemoglobinemia)
     Toxic methemoglobinemia

   D74.9   Methemoglobinemia, unspecified

● **D75   Other and unspecified diseases of blood and blood-forming organs**
> Excludes2   acute lymphadenitis (L04.-)
> chronic lymphadenitis (I88.1)
> enlarged lymph nodes (R59.-)
> hypergammaglobulinemia NOS (D89.2)
> lymphadenitis NOS (I88.9)
> mesenteric lymphadenitis (acute) (chronic) (I88.0)

   D75.A   Glucose-6-phosphate dehydrogenase (G6PD) deficiency without anemia
> Excludes1   glucose-6-phosphate dehydrogenase (G6PD) deficiency with anemia (D55.0)

   D75.0   Familial erythrocytosis
     Genetic mutation of gene that results in increased circulating RBCs
     Benign polycythemia
     Familial polycythemia
> Excludes1   hereditary ovalocytosis (D58.1)

   D75.1   Secondary polycythemia
     Increase in total red cell mass
     Acquired polycythemia
     Emotional polycythemia
     Erythrocytosis NOS
     Hypoxemic polycythemia
     Nephrogenous polycythemia
     Polycythemia due to erythropoietin
     Polycythemia due to fall in plasma volume
     Polycythemia due to high altitude
     Polycythemia due to stress
     Polycythemia NOS
     Relative polycythemia
> Excludes1   polycythemia neonatorum (P61.1)
> polycythemia vera (D45)

▶ New   ⫸ Revised   ~~deleted~~ Deleted   Excludes 1   Excludes 2   Includes   Use additional   Code first   Code also   Key words
OGCR Official Guidelines   X Assign placeholder X   ● Use Additional Character(s)   ▌ Manifestation Code   Hierarchical Condition Category   **Coding Clinic**

- **D75.8**   **Other specified diseases of blood and blood-forming organs**
  - ▸ *D75.81*   *Myelofibrosis* 🔁
    Replacing bone marrow by fibrous tissue
    Myelofibrosis NOS
    Secondary myelofibrosis NOS
    Code first the underlying disorder, such as:
        malignant neoplasm of breast (C50.-)
    Use additional code, if applicable, for associated therapy-related myelodysplastic syndrome (D46.-)
    Use additional code for adverse effect, if applicable, to identify drug (T45.1X5)
    - **Excludes1**   acute myelofibrosis (C94.4-)
      idiopathic myelofibrosis (D47.1)
      leukoerythroblastic anemia (D61.82)
      myelofibrosis with myeloid metaplasia (D47.4)
      myelophthisic anemia (D61.82)
      myelophthisis (D61.82)
      primary myelofibrosis (D47.1)
  - **D75.82**   **Heparin induced thrombocytopenia (HIT)** 🔁
  - ▸● **D75.83 Thrombocytosis**
    - ▸**Excludes2**   essential thrombocythemia (D47.3)
    - ▸**D75.838 Other thrombocytosis**
      - ▸Reactive thrombocytosis
      - ▸Secondary thrombocytosis
      - ▸Code also, underlying condition, if known and applicable
    - ▸**D75.839 Thrombocytosis, unspecified**
      - ▸Thrombocythemia NOS
      - ▸Thrombocytosis NOS
  - **D75.89**   **Other specified diseases of blood and blood-forming organs**
  - **D75.9**   **Disease of blood and blood-forming organs, unspecified**
- ● **D76**   **Other specified diseases with participation of lymphoreticular and reticulohistiocytic tissue**
  - **Excludes1**   (Abt-) Letterer-Siwe disease (C96.0)
    eosinophilic granuloma (C96.6)
    Hand-Schüller-Christian disease (C96.5)
    histiocytic medullary reticulosis (C96.9)
    histiocytic sarcoma (C96.A)
    histiocytosis X, multifocal (C96.5)
    histiocytosis X, unifocal (C96.6)
    Langerhans-cell histiocytosis, multifocal (C96.5)
    Langerhans-cell histiocytosis NOS (C96.6)
    Langerhans-cell histiocytosis, unifocal (C96.6)
    leukemic reticuloendotheliosis (C91.4-)
    lipomelanotic reticulosis (I89.8)
    malignant histiocytosis (C96.A)
    malignant reticulosis (C86.0)
    nonlipid reticuloendotheliosis (C96.0)
  - **D76.1**   **Hemophagocytic lymphohistiocytosis** 🔁
    Familial hemophagocytic reticulosis
    Histiocytoses of mononuclear phagocytes
  - **D76.2**   **Hemophagocytic syndrome, infection-associated** 🔁
    Use additional code to identify infectious agent or disease.
  - **D76.3**   **Other histiocytosis syndromes** 🔁
    Reticulohistiocytoma (giant-cell)
    Sinus histiocytosis with massive lymphadenopathy
    Xanthogranuloma

- ▸ **D77**   *Other disorders of blood and blood-forming organs in diseases classified elsewhere*
  Code first underlying disease, such as:
      amyloidosis (E85.-)
      congenital early syphilis (A50.0)
      echinococcosis (B67.0-B67.9)
      malaria (B50.0-B54)
      schistosomiasis [bilharziasis] (B65.0-B65.9)
      vitamin C deficiency (E54)
  - **Excludes1**   rupture of spleen due to Plasmodium vivax malaria (B51.0)
    splenitis, splenomegaly in late syphilis (A52.79)
    splenitis, splenomegaly in tuberculosis (A18.85)

INTRAOPERATIVE AND POSTPROCEDURAL COMPLICATIONS OF THE SPLEEN (D78)

- ● **D78**   **Intraoperative and postprocedural complications of the spleen**
  Coding Clinic: 2016, Q4, P9
  - ● **D78.0**   **Intraoperative hemorrhage and hematoma of the spleen complicating a procedure**
    - **Excludes1**   intraoperative hemorrhage and hematoma of the spleen due to accidental puncture or laceration during a procedure (D78.1-)
    - **D78.01**   Intraoperative hemorrhage and hematoma of the spleen complicating a procedure on the spleen
    - **D78.02**   Intraoperative hemorrhage and hematoma of the spleen complicating other procedure
  - ● **D78.1**   **Accidental puncture and laceration of the spleen during a procedure**
    - **D78.11**   Accidental puncture and laceration of the spleen during a procedure on the spleen
    - **D78.12**   Accidental puncture and laceration of the spleen during other procedure
  - ● **D78.2**   **Postprocedural hemorrhage of the spleen following a procedure**
    - **D78.21**   Postprocedural hemorrhage of the spleen following a procedure on the spleen
    - **D78.22**   Postprocedural hemorrhage of the spleen following other procedure
  - ● **D78.3**   **Postprocedural hematoma and seroma of the spleen following a procedure**
    - **D78.31**   Postprocedural hematoma of the spleen following a procedure on the spleen
    - **D78.32**   Postprocedural hematoma of the spleen following other procedure
    - **D78.33**   Postprocedural seroma of the spleen following a procedure on the spleen
    - **D78.34**   Postprocedural seroma of the spleen following other procedure
  - ● **D78.8**   **Other intraoperative and postprocedural complications of the spleen**
    Use additional code, if applicable, to further specify disorder
    - **D78.81**   Other intraoperative complications of the spleen
    - **D78.89**   Other postprocedural complications of the spleen

---

CERTAIN DISORDERS INVOLVING THE IMMUNE MECHANISM (D80-D89)

Includes	defects in the complement system
	immunodeficiency disorders, except human
	immunodeficiency virus [HIV] disease
	sarcoidosis

Excludes1	autoimmune disease (systemic) NOS (M35.9)
	functional disorders of polymorphonuclear
	neutrophils (D71)
	human immunodeficiency virus [HIV] disease (B20)

● **D80   Immunodeficiency with predominantly antibody defects**

D80.0   Hereditary hypogammaglobulinemia 🐾
Autosomal recessive agammaglobulinemia (Swiss type)
X-linked agammaglobulinemia [Bruton] (with growth hormone deficiency)

D80.1   Nonfamilial hypogammaglobulinemia 🐾
Abnormally low levels of all classes of immunoglobulins
Agammaglobulinemia with immunoglobulin-bearing B-lymphocytes
Common variable agammaglobulinemia [CVAgamma]
Hypogammaglobulinemia NOS

D80.2   Selective deficiency of immunoglobulin A [IgA] 🐾

D80.3   Selective deficiency of immunoglobulin G [IgG] subclasses 🐾

D80.4   Selective deficiency of immunoglobulin M [IgM] 🐾

D80.5   Immunodeficiency with increased immunoglobulin M [IgM] 🐾

D80.6   Antibody deficiency with near-normal immunoglobulins or with hyperimmunoglobulinemia 🐾
Abnormally high levels of immunoglobulins in serum

D80.7   Transient hypogammaglobulinemia of infancy 🐾

D80.8   Other immunodeficiencies with predominantly antibody defects
Kappa light chain deficiency

D80.9   Immunodeficiency with predominantly antibody defects, unspecified 🐾

● **D81   Combined immunodeficiencies**

Excludes1	autosomal recessive agammaglobulinemia
	(Swiss type) (D80.0)

D81.0   Severe combined immunodeficiency [SCID] with reticular dysgenesis 🐾

D81.1   Severe combined immunodeficiency [SCID] with low T- and B-cell numbers 🐾

D81.2   Severe combined immunodeficiency [SCID] with low or normal B-cell numbers 🐾

● **D81.3   Adenosine deaminase [ADA] deficiency** 🐾

D81.30   Adenosine deaminase deficiency, unspecified
ADA deficiency NOS

D81.31   Severe combined immunodeficiency due to adenosine deaminase deficiency
ADA deficiency with SCID
Adenosine deaminase [ADA] deficiency with severe combined immunodeficiency

D81.32   Adenosine deaminase 2 deficiency
ADA2 deficiency
Adenosine deaminase deficiency type 2
Code also, if applicable, any associated manifestations, such as:
polyarteritis nodosa (M30.0)
stroke (I63.-)

D81.39   Other adenosine deaminase deficiency
Adenosine deaminase [ADA] deficiency type 1, NOS
Adenosine deaminase [ADA] deficiency type 1, without SCID
Adenosine deaminase [ADA] deficiency type 1, without severe combined immunodeficiency
Partial ADA deficiency (type 1)
Partial adenosine deaminase deficiency (type 1)

D81.4   Nezelof's syndrome 🐾

D81.5   Purine nucleoside phosphorylase [PNP] deficiency 🐾

D81.6   Major histocompatibility complex class I deficiency 🐾
Bare lymphocyte syndrome

D81.7   Major histocompatibility complex class II deficiency 🐾

● **D81.8   Other combined immunodeficiencies**

● **D81.81   Biotin-dependent carboxylase deficiency**
Multiple carboxylase deficiency

Excludes1	biotin-dependent carboxylase
	deficiency due to dietary
	deficiency of biotin (E53.8)

D81.810   Biotinidase deficiency

D81.818   Other biotin-dependent carboxylase deficiency
Holocarboxylase synthetase deficiency
Other multiple carboxylase deficiency

D81.819   Biotin-dependent carboxylase deficiency, unspecified
Multiple carboxylase deficiency, unspecified

D81.89   Other combined immunodeficiencies 🐾

D81.9   Combined immunodeficiency, unspecified 🐾
Severe combined immunodeficiency disorder [SCID] NOS

● **D82   Immunodeficiency associated with other major defects**

Excludes1	ataxia telangiectasia [Louis-Bar] (G11.3)

D82.0   Wiskott-Aldrich syndrome 🐾
X-linked immunodeficiency
Immunodeficiency with thrombocytopenia and eczema

D82.1   Di George's syndrome 🐾
Congenital disorder with defective development of third and fourth pharyngeal pouches
Pharyngeal pouch syndrome
Thymic alymphoplasia
Thymic aplasia or hypoplasia with immunodeficiency
Coding Clinic: 2019, Q3, P14

D82.2   Immunodeficiency with short-limbed stature 🐾

D82.3   Immunodeficiency following hereditary defective response to Epstein-Barr virus 🐾
X-linked lymphoproliferative disease

D82.4   Hyperimmunoglobulin E [IgE] syndrome 🐾
Suspected genetic defect that produces high levels of antibody immunoglobulin (IgE) that causes skin and lung infections and eczema

D82.8   Immunodeficiency associated with other specified major defects 🐾

D82.9   Immunodeficiency associated with major defect, unspecified 🐾

● **D83   Common variable immunodeficiency**

D83.0   Common variable immunodeficiency with predominant abnormalities of B-cell numbers and function 🐾

D83.1   Common variable immunodeficiency with predominant immunoregulatory T-cell disorders 🐾

D83.2   Common variable immunodeficiency with autoantibodies to B- or T-cells 🐾

D83.8   Other common variable immunodeficiencies 🐾

D83.9   Common variable immunodeficiency, unspecified 🐾

● **D84   Other immunodeficiencies**

D84.0   Lymphocyte function antigen-1 [LFA-1] defect 🐾

● **D84.1   Defects in the complement system** 🐾
C1 esterase inhibitor [C1-INH] deficiency

CHAPTER 3 (D50-D89)

▶ New	⇒ Revised	~~deleted~~ Deleted	Excludes 1	Excludes 2	Includes	Use additional	Code first	Code also	Key words

OGCR Official Guidelines   X Assign placeholder X   ● Use Additional Character(s)   ▷ Manifestation Code   🐾 Hierarchical Condition Category   **Coding Clinic**

D84.8   **Other specified immunodeficiencies** 🖐

> D84.81   *Immunodeficiency due to conditions classified elsewhere*

> > *Code first* underlying condition, such as:
> > chromosomal abnormalities (Q90-Q99)
> > diabetes mellitus (E08-E13)
> > malignant neoplasms (C00-C96)

> > **Excludes1**   *certain disorders involving the immune mechanism (D80-D83, D84.0, D84.1, D84.9)*
> > *human immunodeficiency virus [HIV] disease (B20)*

● D84.82   **Immunodeficiency due to drugs and external causes**

    D84.821   **Immunodeficiency due to drugs**

      Immunodeficiency due to (current or past) medication

      Use additional code for adverse effect if applicable, to identify adverse effect of drug (T36-T50 with fifth or six character 5)

      Use additional code, if applicable, for associated long term (current) drug therapy drug or medication such as:
      long term (current) drug therapy systemic steroids (Z79.52)
      other long term (current) drug therapy (Z79.899)

    D84.822   **Immunodeficiency due to external causes**

      Code also, if applicable, radiological procedure and radiotherapy (Y84.2)

      Use additional code for external cause such as:
      exposure to ionizing radiation (W88)

    D84.89   **Other immunodeficiencies**

D84.9   **Immunodeficiency, unspecified** 🖐
    Immunocompromised NOS
    Immunodeficient NOS
    Immunosuppressed NOS]

● D86   **Sarcoidosis**

D86.0   **Sarcoidosis of lung** 🖐

D86.1   **Sarcoidosis of lymph nodes**

D86.2   **Sarcoidosis of lung with sarcoidosis of lymph nodes** 🖐

D86.3   **Sarcoidosis of skin**

● D86.8   **Sarcoidosis of other sites**

    D86.81   **Sarcoid meningitis**

    D86.82   **Multiple cranial nerve palsies in sarcoidosis** 🖐

    D86.83   **Sarcoid iridocyclitis**
      Rare large tumor with irregular surface of iris

    D86.84   **Sarcoid pyelonephritis**
      Systemic disease of unknown etiology characterized by chronic granulomatous inflammation with tissue destruction of pelvis kidney
      Tubulo-interstitial nephropathy in sarcoidosis

    D86.85   **Sarcoid myocarditis**

    D86.86   **Sarcoid arthropathy**
      Polyarthritis in sarcoidosis

    D86.87   **Sarcoid myositis**
      Granumloma of muscle

    D86.89   **Sarcoidosis of other sites**
      Hepatic granuloma
      Uveoparotid fever [Heerfordt]

D86.9   **Sarcoidosis, unspecified**

Item 3-1 Sarcoidosis: A symptom of an inflammation producing tiny lumps of cells (granulomas) in various organs, most commonly the lungs and lymph nodes, that affect organ function. Cause is unknown occurring primarily in 20- to 40-year-olds, African-American, especially women, and those of Asian, German, Irish, Scandinavian, and Puerto Rican heritage.

● D89   **Other disorders involving the immune mechanism, not elsewhere classified**

    Excludes1   hyperglobulinemia NOS (R77.1)
      monoclonal gammopathy (of undetermined significance) (D47.2)

    Excludes2   transplant failure and rejection (T86.-)

D89.0   **Polyclonal hypergammaglobulinemia**
    Benign hypergammaglobulinemic purpura
    Polyclonal gammopathy NOS

D89.1   **Cryoglobulinemia** 🖐
    Cryoglobulin (proteins) in blood that precipitate temperatures below 98.6° F; usually symptomatic of underlying disease
    Cryoglobulinemic purpura
    Cryoglobulinemic vasculitis
    Essential cryoglobulinemia
    Idiopathic cryoglobulinemia
    Mixed cryoglobulinemia
    Primary cryoglobulinemia
    Secondary cryoglobulinemia

D89.2   **Hypergammaglobulinemia, unspecified**

D89.3   **Immune reconstitution syndrome** 🖐
    Immune reconstitution inflammatory syndrome [IRIS]

    Use additional code for adverse effect, if applicable, to identify drug (T36-T50 with fifth or sixth character 5)

● D89.4   **Mast cell activation syndrome and related disorders**

    Excludes1   aggressive systemic mastocytosis (C96.21)
      congenital cutaneous mastocytosis (Q82.2)
      (non-congenital) cutaneous mastocytosis (D47.01)
      (indolent) systemic mastocytosis (D47.02)
      malignant mast cell neoplasm (C96.2-)
      malignant mastocytoma (C96.29)
      mast cell leukemia (C94.3-)
      mast cell sarcoma (C96.22)
      mastocytoma NOS (D47.09)
      other mast cell neoplasms of uncertain behavior (D47.09)
      systemic mastocytosis associated with a clonal hematologic non-mast cell lineage disease (SM-AHNMD) (D47.02)

    Coding Clinic: 2016, Q4, P11

    D89.40   **Mast cell activation, unspecified** 🖐
      Mast cell activation disorder, unspecified
      Mast cell activation syndrome, NOS

    D89.41   **Monoclonal mast cell activation syndrome** 🖐
      Coding Clinic: 2016, Q4, P11

    D89.42   **Idiopathic mast cell activation syndrome** 🖐
      Coding Clinic: 2016, Q4, P11

> D89.44   **Hereditary alpha tryptasemia**
> > Use additional code, if applicable, for:
> > > allergy status, other than to drugs and biological substances (Z91.0-)
> > > personal history of anaphylaxis (Z87.892)

    D89.43   **Secondary mast cell activation** 🖐
      Secondary mast cell activation syndrome
      Code also underlying etiology, if known
      Coding Clinic: 2016, Q4, P11

    D89.49   **Other mast cell activation disorder** 🖐
      Other mast cell activation syndrome
      Coding Clinic: 2016, Q4, P11

CHAPTER 3 (D50-D89)

● **D89.8** **Other specified disorders involving the immune mechanism, not elsewhere classified**

● **D89.81** **Graft-versus-host disease**

Code first underlying cause, such as:
  complications of transplanted organs and
    tissue (T86.-)
  complications of blood transfusion (T80.89)

Use additional code to identify associated
  manifestations, such as:
  desquamative dermatitis (L30.8)
  diarrhea (R19.7)
  elevated bilirubin (R17)
  hair loss (L65.9)

D89.810 **Acute** graft-versus-host disease ℞

D89.811 **Chronic** graft-versus-host disease ℞

D89.812 **Acute on chronic** graft-versus-host
disease ℞

D89.813 **Graft-versus-host disease,
unspecified** ℞

D89.82 **Autoimmune lymphoproliferative syndrome
[ALPS]** ℞

● **D89.83** **Cytokine release syndrome**

Code first underlying cause, such as:
  complications following infusion,
    transfusion and therapeutic injection
    (T80.89-)
  complications of transplanted organs and
    tissue (T86.-)

Use additional code to identify associated
  manifestations

D89.831 **Cytokine release syndrome, grade 1**

D89.832 **Cytokine release syndrome, grade 2**

D89.833 **Cytokine release syndrome,
grade 3**

D89.834 **Cytokine release syndrome,
grade 4**

D89.835 **Cytokine release syndrome,
grade 5**

D89.839 **Cytokine release syndrome, grade
unspecified**

D89.89 **Other specified disorders involving the
immune mechanism, not elsewhere classified** ℞

Excludes1 human immunodeficiency virus
disease (B20)

Coding Clinic: 2017, Q4, P109

D89.9 **Disorder involving the immune
mechanism, unspecified** ℞

Immune disease NOS

Coding Clinic: 2015, Q3, P22

▶ New   ⇒ Revised   ~~deleted~~ Deleted   Excludes 1   Excludes 2   Includes   Use additional   Code first   Code also   Key words

OGCR Official Guidelines   X Assign placeholder X   ● Use Additional Character(s)   ▶ Manifestation Code   ℞ Hierarchical Condition Category   **Coding Clinic**

CHAPTER 4

ENDOCRINE, NUTRITIONAL AND METABOLIC DISEASES (E00-E89)

OGCR Chapter-Specific Coding Guidelines

4. **Chapter 4: Endocrine, Nutritional, and Metabolic Diseases (E00-E89)**

a. **Diabetes mellitus**

The diabetes mellitus codes are combination codes that include the type of diabetes mellitus, the body system affected, and the complications affecting that body system. As many codes within a particular category as are necessary to describe all of the complications of the disease may be used. They should be sequenced based on the reason for a particular encounter. Assign as many codes from categories E08 – E13 as needed to identify all of the associated conditions that the patient has.

1) **Type of diabetes**

The age of a patient is not the sole determining factor, though most type 1 diabetics develop the condition before reaching puberty. For this reason type 1 diabetes mellitus is also referred to as juvenile diabetes.

2) **Type of diabetes mellitus not documented**

If the type of diabetes mellitus is not documented in the medical record the default is E11.-, Type 2 diabetes mellitus.

3) **Diabetes mellitus and the use of insulin oral hypoglycemics**

If the documentation in a medical record does not indicate the type of diabetes but does indicate that the patient uses insulin, code E11, Type 2 diabetes mellitus, should be assigned. An additional code should be assigned from category Z79 to identify the long-term (current) use of insulin or oral hypoglycemic drugs. If the patient is treated with both oral medications and insulin, only the code for long-term (current) use of insulin should be assigned. Code Z79.4 should not be assigned if insulin is given temporarily to bring a type 2 patient's blood sugar under control during an encounter.

4) **Diabetes mellitus in pregnancy and gestational diabetes**

See Section I.C.15. Diabetes mellitus in pregnancy.
See Section I.C.15. Gestational (pregnancy induced) diabetes

5) **Complications due to insulin pump malfunction**

(a) **Underdose of insulin due to insulin pump failure**

An underdose of insulin due to an insulin pump failure should be assigned to a code from subcategory T85.6, Mechanical complication of other specified internal and external prosthetic devices, implants and grafts, that specifies the type of pump malfunction, as the principal or first-listed code, followed by code T38.3X6-, Underdosing of insulin and oral hypoglycemic [antidiabetic] drugs. Additional codes for the type of diabetes mellitus and any associated complications due to the underdosing should also be assigned.

(b) **Overdose of insulin due to insulin pump failure**

The principal or first-listed code for an encounter due to an insulin pump malfunction resulting in an overdose of insulin, should also be T85.6-, Mechanical complication of other specified internal and external prosthetic devices, implants and grafts, followed by code T38.3X1-, Poisoning by insulin and oral hypoglycemic [antidiabetic] drugs, accidental (unintentional).

6) **Secondary diabetes mellitus**

Codes under categories E08, Diabetes mellitus due to underlying condition, E09, Drug or chemical induced diabetes mellitus and E13, Other specified diabetes mellitus, identify complications/ manifestations associated with secondary diabetes mellitus. Secondary diabetes is always caused by another condition or event (e.g., cystic fibrosis, malignant neoplasm of pancreas, pancreatectomy, adverse effect of drug, or poisoning).

(a) **Secondary diabetes mellitus and the use of insulin or hypoglycemic drugs**

For patients with secondary diabetes mellitus who routinely use insulin or oral hypoglycemic drugs, an additional code from category Z79 should be assigned to identify the long-term (current) use of insulin or oral hypoglycemic drugs. If the patient is treated with both oral medications and insulin, only the code for long-term (current) use of insulin should be assigned. Code Z79.4 should not be assigned if insulin is given temporarily to bring a type 2 patient's blood sugar under control during an encounter.

(b) **Assigning and sequencing secondary diabetes codes and its causes**

The sequencing of the secondary diabetes codes in relationship to codes for the cause of the diabetes is based on the Tabular List instructions for categories E08, E09 and E13.

(i) **Secondary diabetes mellitus due to pancreatectomy** For postpancreatectomy diabetes mellitus (lack of insulin due to the surgical removal of all or part of the pancreas), assign code E89.1, Postprocedural hypoinsulinemia. Assign a code from category E13 and a code from subcategory Z90.41-, Acquired absence of pancreas, as additional codes.

(ii) **Secondary diabetes due to drugs** Secondary diabetes may be caused by an adverse effect of correctly administered medications, poisoning or sequela of poisoning.

See Section I.C.19.e for coding of adverse effects and poisoning, and Section I.C.20 for external cause code reporting.

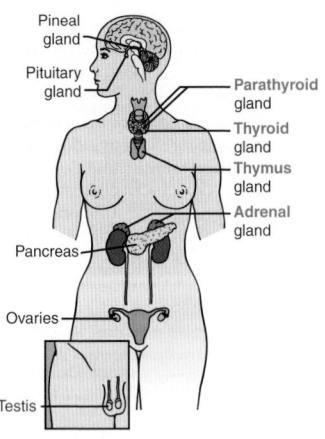

Figure 4-1 The endocrine system. (From Buck CJ: Step-by-Step Medical Coding, ed 2016, St. Louis, Elsevier, 2016)

CHAPTER 4

ENDOCRINE, NUTRITIONAL AND METABOLIC DISEASES (E00-E89)

All neoplasms, whether functionally active or not, are classified in Chapter 2. Appropriate codes in this chapter (i.e., E05.8, E07.0, E16-E31, E34.-) may be used as additional codes to indicate either functional activity by neoplasms and ectopic endocrine tissue or hyperfunction and hypofunction of endocrine glands associated with neoplasms and other conditions classified elsewhere.

Excludes1   transitory endocrine and metabolic disorders specific to newborn (P70-P74)

This chapter contains the following blocks:

E00-E07	Disorders of thyroid gland
E08-E13	Diabetes mellitus
E15-E16	Other disorders of glucose regulation and pancreatic internal secretion
E20-E35	Disorders of other endocrine glands
E36	Intraoperative complications of endocrine system
E40-E46	Malnutrition
E50-E64	Other nutritional deficiencies
E65-E68	Overweight, obesity and other hyperalimentation
E70-E88	Metabolic disorders
E89	Postprocedural endocrine and metabolic complications and disorders, not elsewhere classified

DISORDERS OF THYROID GLAND (E00-E07)

● **E00**   **Congenital iodine-deficiency syndrome**

Use additional code (F70-F79) to identify associated intellectual disabilities.

Excludes1   subclinical iodine-deficiency hypothyroidism (E02)

E00.0   **Congenital iodine-deficiency syndrome, neurological type**
Endemic cretinism, neurological type

E00.1   **Congenital iodine-deficiency syndrome, myxedematous type**
Dry, waxy type of swelling (nonpitting edema) with abnormal deposits of mucin in skin (mucinosis) and other tissues
Endemic hypothyroid cretinism
Endemic cretinism, myxedematous type

E00.2   **Congenital iodine-deficiency syndrome, mixed type**
Endemic cretinism, mixed type

E00.9   **Congenital iodine-deficiency syndrome, unspecified**
Congenital iodine-deficiency hypothyroidism NOS
Endemic cretinism NOS

Figure 4-2   Goiter is an enlargement of the thyroid gland.

Item 4-1   Simple goiter indicates no nodules are present. The most common type of goiter is a **diffuse colloidal,** also called a **nontoxic** or **endemic** goiter.

● **E01**   **Iodine-deficiency related thyroid disorders and allied conditions**

Excludes1   congenital iodine-deficiency syndrome (E00.-)
subclinical iodine-deficiency hypothyroidism (E02)

E01.0   **Iodine-deficiency related diffuse (endemic) goiter**
Thyroid gland is enlarged

E01.1   **Iodine-deficiency related multinodular (endemic) goiter**
Iodine-deficiency related nodular goiter

E01.2   **Iodine-deficiency related (endemic) goiter, unspecified**
Endemic goiter NOS

E01.8   **Other iodine-deficiency related thyroid disorders and allied conditions**
Acquired iodine-deficiency hypothyroidism NOS

E02   **Subclinical iodine-deficiency hypothyroidism**
Coding Clinic: 2021, Q1, P8-9

● **E03**   **Other hypothyroidism**

Excludes1   iodine-deficiency related hypothyroidism (E00-E02)
postprocedural hypothyroidism (E89.0)

E03.0   **Congenital hypothyroidism with diffuse goiter**
Congenital parenchymatous goiter (nontoxic)
Congenital goiter (nontoxic) NOS

Excludes1   transitory congenital goiter with normal function (P72.0)

E03.1   **Congenital hypothyroidism without goiter**
Aplasia of thyroid (with myxedema)
Congenital atrophy of thyroid
Congenital hypothyroidism NOS

E03.2   **Hypothyroidism due to medicaments and other exogenous substances**
Code first poisoning due to drug or toxin, if applicable (T36-T65 with fifth or sixth character 1-4 or 6)
Use additional code for adverse effect, if applicable, to identify drug (T36-T50 with fifth or sixth character 5)

E03.3   **Postinfectious hypothyroidism**

E03.4   **Atrophy of thyroid (acquired)**
Excludes1   congenital atrophy of thyroid (E03.1)

E03.5   **Myxedema coma** 🐾
Often fatal complication of long-term hypothyroidism

E03.8   **Other specified hypothyroidism**

E03.9   **Hypothyroidism, unspecified**
Myxedema NOS
Coding Clinic: 2021, Q1, P9

Item 4-2   Hypothyroidism is a condition in which there are insufficient levels of thyroxine. **Cretinism** is congenital hypothyroidism, which can result in mental and physical retardation.

▶ New   ⇒ Revised   ~~deleted~~ Deleted   Excludes 1   Excludes 2   Includes   Use additional   Code first   Code also   Key words
OGCR Official Guidelines   X Assign placeholder X   ● Use Additional Character(s)   ▶ Manifestation Code   🐾 Hierarchical Condition Category   **Coding Clinic**

● **E04   Other nontoxic goiter**

Excludes1   congenital goiter (NOS) (diffuse)
(parenchymatous) (E03.0)
iodine-deficiency related goiter (E00-E02)

E04.0   Nontoxic diffuse goiter
Thyroid gland is enlarged
Diffuse (colloid) nontoxic goiter
Simple nontoxic goiter

E04.1   Nontoxic single thyroid nodule
Colloid nodule (cystic) (thyroid)
Nontoxic uninodular goiter
Thyroid (cystic) nodule NOS

E04.2   Nontoxic multinodular goiter
Enlarged thyroid gland with multiple nodules
Cystic goiter NOS
Multinodular (cystic) goiter NOS

E04.8   Other specified nontoxic goiter

E04.9   Nontoxic goiter, unspecified
Goiter NOS
Nodular goiter (nontoxic) NOS

● **E05   Thyrotoxicosis [hyperthyroidism]**
Enlarged thyroid gland with multiple nodules

Excludes1   chronic thyroiditis with transient thyrotoxicosis
(E06.2)
neonatal thyrotoxicosis (P72.1)

● **E05.0   Thyrotoxicosis with diffuse goiter**
Exophthalmic or toxic goiter NOS
Graves' disease
Toxic diffuse goiter

**E05.00   Thyrotoxicosis with diffuse goiter without
thyrotoxic crisis or storm**

**E05.01   Thyrotoxicosis with diffuse goiter with
thyrotoxic crisis or storm**

● **E05.1   Thyrotoxicosis with toxic single thyroid nodule**
Thyrotoxicosis with toxic uninodular goiter

**E05.10   Thyrotoxicosis with toxic single thyroid nodule
without thyrotoxic crisis or storm**

**E05.11   Thyrotoxicosis with toxic single thyroid nodule
with thyrotoxic crisis or storm**

● **E05.2   Thyrotoxicosis with toxic multinodular goiter**
Toxic nodular goiter NOS

**E05.20   Thyrotoxicosis with toxic multinodular goiter
without thyrotoxic crisis or storm**

**E05.21   Thyrotoxicosis with toxic multinodular goiter
with thyrotoxic crisis or storm**

● **E05.3   Thyrotoxicosis from ectopic thyroid tissue**

**E05.30   Thyrotoxicosis from ectopic thyroid tissue
without thyrotoxic crisis or storm**

**E05.31   Thyrotoxicosis from ectopic thyroid tissue with
thyrotoxic crisis or storm**

● **E05.4   Thyrotoxicosis factitia**

**E05.40   Thyrotoxicosis factitia without thyrotoxic crisis
or storm**

**E05.41   Thyrotoxicosis factitia with thyrotoxic crisis or
storm**

● **E05.8   Other thyrotoxicosis**
Overproduction of thyroid-stimulating hormone

**E05.80   Other thyrotoxicosis without thyrotoxic crisis or
storm**

**E05.81   Other thyrotoxicosis with thyrotoxic crisis or
storm**

● **E05.9   Thyrotoxicosis, unspecified**
Hyperthyroidism NOS

**E05.90   Thyrotoxicosis, unspecified without thyrotoxic
crisis or storm**

**E05.91   Thyrotoxicosis, unspecified with thyrotoxic
crisis or storm**

● **E06   Thyroiditis**
*An inflammation of the thyroid gland which results in an inability to
convert iodine into thyroid hormone*

Excludes1   postpartum thyroiditis (O90.5)

E06.0   Acute thyroiditis
Abscess of thyroid
Pyogenic thyroiditis
Suppurative thyroiditis
Use additional code (B95-B97) to identify infectious
agent.

E06.1   Subacute thyroiditis
*Inflammation of thyroid gland following viral upper
respiratory infection*
de Quervain thyroiditis
Giant-cell thyroiditis
Granulomatous thyroiditis
Nonsuppurative thyroiditis
Viral thyroiditis

Excludes1   autoimmune thyroiditis (E06.3)

E06.2   Chronic thyroiditis with transient thyrotoxicosis
*Chronic inflammation of thyroid gland with intermittent
overproduction of thyroid hormone*

Excludes1   autoimmune thyroiditis (E06.3)

E06.3   Autoimmune thyroiditis
Hashimoto's thyroiditis
Hashitoxicosis (transient)
Lymphadenoid goiter
Lymphocytic thyroiditis
Struma lymphomatosa

E06.4   Drug-induced thyroiditis
Use additional code for adverse effect, if applicable,
to identify drug (T36-T50 with fifth or sixth
character 5)

E06.5   Other chronic thyroiditis
Chronic fibrous thyroiditis
Chronic thyroiditis NOS
Ligneous thyroiditis
Riedel thyroiditis

E06.9   Thyroiditis, unspecified

● **E07   Other disorders of thyroid**

E07.0   Hypersecretion of calcitonin
C-cell hyperplasia of thyroid
Hypersecretion of thyrocalcitonin

E07.1   Dyshormogenetic goiter
*Group of several types of goiter resulting from enzyme defects
in hormone synthesis*
Familial dyshormogenetic goiter
Pendred's syndrome

Excludes1   transitory congenital goiter with normal
function (P72.0)

● **E07.8   Other specified disorders of thyroid**

E07.81   Sick-euthyroid syndrome
Euthyroid sick-syndrome

E07.89   Other specified disorders of thyroid
Abnormality of thyroid-binding globulin
Hemorrhage of thyroid
Infarction of thyroid

E07.9   Disorder of thyroid, unspecified

Figure 4-3 Graves' disease. In Graves'
disease, exophthalmos often looks more
pronounced than it actually is because of the
extreme lid retraction that may occur. This
patient, for instance, had minimal proptosis
of the left eye but marked lid retraction. (From
Lissauer T, Clayden G, and Craft A: Illustrated
Textbook of Paediatrics, Edinburgh, Mosby,
2015)

Item 4–3 Thyrotoxicosis is a condition caused by excessive amounts
of the thyroid hormone thyroxine production or hyperthyroidism. **Graves'
disease is associated with hyperthyroidism** (known as **Basedow's
disease** in Europe).

CHAPTER 4 (E00-E89)

OGCR Section I.C.4.a.

Diabetes mellitus

The diabetes mellitus codes are combination codes that include the type of diabetes mellitus, body system affected, and the complications affecting that body system. As many codes within a particular category as are necessary to describe all of the complications of the disease may be used. They should be sequenced based on the reason for a particular visit. Assign as many codes from categories E08–E13 as needed to identify all of the associated conditions that the patient has.

DIABETES MELLITUS (E08-E13)

A metabolic disease that results in persistent hyperglycemia
Coding Clinic: 2016, Q4, P142

● **E08   Diabetes mellitus due to underlying condition**

Code first the underlying condition, such as:
congenital rubella (P35.0)
Cushing's syndrome (E24.-)
cystic fibrosis (E84.-)
malignant neoplasm (C00-C96)
malnutrition (E40-E46)
pancreatitis and other diseases of the pancreas (K85-K86.-)

Use additional code to identify control using:
insulin (Z79.4)
oral antidiabetic drugs (Z79.84)
oral hypoglycemic drugs (Z79.84)

Excludes1   drug or chemical induced diabetes mellitus (E09.-)
gestational diabetes (O24.4-)
neonatal diabetes mellitus (P70.2)
postpancreatectomy diabetes mellitus (E13.-)
postprocedural diabetes mellitus (E13.-)
secondary diabetes mellitus NEC (E13.-)
type 1 diabetes mellitus (E10.-)
type 2 diabetes mellitus (E11.-)

● **E08.0   Diabetes mellitus due to underlying condition with hyperosmolarity**

▷ *E08.00   Diabetes mellitus due to underlying condition with hyperosmolarity without nonketotic hyperglycemic-hyperosmolar coma (NKHHC)* 🖥

▷ *E08.01   Diabetes mellitus due to underlying condition with hyperosmolarity with coma* 🖥

● **E08.1   Diabetes mellitus due to underlying condition with ketoacidosis**

▷ *E08.10   Diabetes mellitus due to underlying condition with ketoacidosis without coma* 🖥

▷ *E08.11   Diabetes mellitus due to underlying condition with ketoacidosis with coma* 🖥

● **E08.2   Diabetes mellitus due to underlying condition with kidney complications**

▷ *E08.21   Diabetes mellitus due to underlying condition with diabetic nephropathy* 🖥
Diabetes mellitus due to underlying condition with intercapillary glomerulosclerosis
Diabetes mellitus due to underlying condition with intracapillary glomerulonephrosis
Diabetes mellitus due to underlying condition with Kimmelstiel-Wilson disease

▷ *E08.22   Diabetes mellitus due to underlying condition with diabetic chronic kidney disease* 🖥
Use additional code to identify stage of chronic kidney disease (N18.1-N18.6)

▷ *E08.29   Diabetes mellitus due to underlying condition with other diabetic kidney complication* 🖥
Renal tubular degeneration in diabetes mellitus due to underlying condition

● **E08.3   Diabetes mellitus due to underlying condition with ophthalmic complications**
Changes in blood vessels of retina in which blood vessels swell and leak fluid into retinal surface.
Coding Clinic: 2016, Q4, P11

● **E08.31   Diabetes mellitus due to underlying condition with unspecified diabetic retinopathy**

▷ *E08.311   Diabetes mellitus due to underlying condition with unspecified diabetic retinopathy with macular edema* 🖥

▷ *E08.319   Diabetes mellitus due to underlying condition with unspecified diabetic retinopathy without macular edema* 🖥

● **E08.32   Diabetes mellitus due to underlying condition with mild nonproliferative diabetic retinopathy**
Diabetes mellitus due to underlying condition with nonproliferative diabetic retinopathy NOS

One of the following 7th characters is to be assigned to codes in subcategory E08.32 to designate laterality of the disease:

1	right eye
2	left eye
3	bilateral
9	unspecified eye

●▷ *E08.321   Diabetes mellitus due to underlying condition with mild nonproliferative diabetic retinopathy with macular edema* 🖥

●▷ *E08.329   Diabetes mellitus due to underlying condition with mild nonproliferative diabetic retinopathy without macular edema* 🖥

● **E08.33   Diabetes mellitus due to underlying condition with moderate nonproliferative diabetic retinopathy**

One of the following 7th characters is to be assigned to codes in subcategory E08.33 to designate laterality of the disease:

1	right eye
2	left eye
3	bilateral
9	unspecified eye

●▷ *E08.331   Diabetes mellitus due to underlying condition with moderate nonproliferative diabetic retinopathy with macular edema* 🖥

●▷ *E08.339   Diabetes mellitus due to underlying condition with moderate nonproliferative diabetic retinopathy without macular edema* 🖥

● **E08.34   Diabetes mellitus due to underlying condition with severe nonproliferative diabetic retinopathy**

One of the following 7th characters is to be assigned to codes in subcategory E08.34 to designate laterality of the disease:

1	right eye
2	left eye
3	bilateral
9	unspecified eye

●▷ *E08.341   Diabetes mellitus due to underlying condition with severe nonproliferative diabetic retinopathy with macular edema* 🖥

●▷ *E08.349   Diabetes mellitus due to underlying condition with severe nonproliferative diabetic retinopathy without macular edema* 🖥

▶ New   ⇒ Revised   ~~deleted~~ Deleted   Excludes 1   Excludes 2   Includes   Use additional   Code first   Code also   Key words
OGCR Official Guidelines   X Assign placeholder X   ● Use Additional Character(s)   ▷ Manifestation Code   🖥 Hierarchical Condition Category   **Coding Clinic**

● **E08.35**   **Diabetes mellitus due to underlying condition with proliferative diabetic retinopathy**

One of the following 7th characters is to be assigned to codes in subcategory E08.35 to designate laterality of the disease:

1	right eye
2	left eye
3	bilateral
9	unspecified eye

● ▶ *E08.351*   *Diabetes mellitus due to underlying condition with proliferative diabetic retinopathy with macular edema* 🔍

● ▶ *E08.352*   *Diabetes mellitus due to underlying condition with proliferative diabetic retinopathy with traction retinal detachment involving the macula* 🔍

● ▶ *E08.353*   *Diabetes mellitus due to underlying condition with proliferative diabetic retinopathy with traction retinal detachment not involving the macula* 🔍

● ▶ *E08.354*   *Diabetes mellitus due to underlying condition with proliferative diabetic retinopathy with combined traction retinal detachment and rhegmatogenous retinal detachment* 🔍

● ▶ *E08.355*   *Diabetes mellitus due to underlying condition with stable proliferative diabetic retinopathy* 🔍

● ▶ *E08.359*   *Diabetes mellitus due to underlying condition with proliferative diabetic retinopathy without macular edema* 🔍

▶ *E08.36*   *Diabetes mellitus due to underlying condition with diabetic cataract* 🔍

X ● ▶ *E08.37*   *Diabetes mellitus due to underlying condition with diabetic macular edema, resolved following treatment* 🔍

One of the following 7th characters is to be assigned to code E08.37 to designate laterality of the disease:

1	right eye
2	left eye
3	bilateral
9	unspecified eye

▶ *E08.39*   *Diabetes mellitus due to underlying condition with other diabetic ophthalmic complication* 🔍

Use additional code to identify manifestation, such as:
     diabetic glaucoma (H40-H42)

● **E08.4**   **Diabetes mellitus due to underlying condition with neurological complications**

▶ *E08.40*   *Diabetes mellitus due to underlying condition with diabetic neuropathy, unspecified* 🔍

▶ *E08.41*   *Diabetes mellitus due to underlying condition with diabetic mononeuropathy* 🔍

▶ *E08.42*   *Diabetes mellitus due to underlying condition with diabetic polyneuropathy* 🔍
     Diabetes mellitus due to underlying condition with diabetic neuralgia

▶ *E08.43*   *Diabetes mellitus due to underlying condition with diabetic autonomic (poly)neuropathy* 🔍
     Diabetes mellitus due to underlying condition with diabetic gastroparesis

▶ *E08.44*   *Diabetes mellitus due to underlying condition with diabetic amyotrophy* 🔍

▶ *E08.49*   *Diabetes mellitus due to underlying condition with other diabetic neurological complication* 🔍

● **E08.5**   **Diabetes mellitus due to underlying condition with circulatory complications**

▶ *E08.51*   *Diabetes mellitus due to underlying condition with diabetic peripheral angiopathy without gangrene* 🔍

▶ *E08.52*   *Diabetes mellitus due to underlying condition with diabetic peripheral angiopathy with gangrene* 🔍
     Diabetes mellitus due to underlying condition with diabetic gangrene

▶ *E08.59*   *Diabetes mellitus due to underlying condition with other circulatory complications* 🔍

● **E08.6**   **Diabetes mellitus due to underlying condition with other specified complications**

● **E08.61**   **Diabetes mellitus due to underlying condition with diabetic arthropathy**

▶ *E08.610*   *Diabetes mellitus due to underlying condition with diabetic neuropathic arthropathy* 🔍
     Diabetes mellitus due to underlying condition with Charcôt's joints

▶ *E08.618*   *Diabetes mellitus due to underlying condition with other diabetic arthropathy* 🔍

● **E08.62**   **Diabetes mellitus due to underlying condition with skin complications**

▶ *E08.620*   *Diabetes mellitus due to underlying condition with diabetic dermatitis* 🔍
     Diabetes mellitus due to underlying condition with diabetic necrobiosis lipoidica

▶ *E08.621*   *Diabetes mellitus due to underlying condition with foot ulcer* 🔍
     Use additional code to identify site of ulcer (L97.4-, L97.5-)

▶ *E08.622*   *Diabetes mellitus due to underlying condition with other skin ulcer* 🔍
     Use additional code to identify site of ulcer (L97.1-L97.9, L98.41-L98.49)

▶ *E08.628*   *Diabetes mellitus due to underlying condition with other skin complications* 🔍

● **E08.63**   **Diabetes mellitus due to underlying condition with oral complications**

▶ *E08.630*   *Diabetes mellitus due to underlying condition with periodontal disease* 🔍

▶ *E08.638*   *Diabetes mellitus due to underlying condition with other oral complications* 🔍

● **E08.64**   **Diabetes mellitus due to underlying condition with hypoglycemia**

▶ *E08.641*   *Diabetes mellitus due to underlying condition with hypoglycemia with coma* 🔍

▶ *E08.649*   *Diabetes mellitus due to underlying condition with hypoglycemia without coma* 🔍

▶ *E08.65*   *Diabetes mellitus due to underlying condition with hyperglycemia* 🔍

▶ *E08.69*   *Diabetes mellitus due to underlying condition with other specified complication* 🔍
     Use additional code to identify complication

▶ *E08.8*   *Diabetes mellitus due to underlying condition with unspecified complications* 🔍

▶ *E08.9*   *Diabetes mellitus due to underlying condition without complications* 🔍

● **E09**   **Drug or chemical induced diabetes mellitus**

Code first poisoning due to drug or toxin, if applicable (T36-T65 with fifth or sixth character 1-4 or 6)

Use additional code for adverse effect, if applicable, to identify drug (T36-T50 with fifth or sixth character 5)

Use additional code to identify control using:
     insulin (Z79.4)
     oral antidiabetic drugs (Z79.84)
     oral hypoglycemic drugs (Z79.84)

     Excludes1   diabetes mellitus due to underlying condition (E08.-)
               gestational diabetes (O24.4-)
               neonatal diabetes mellitus (P70.2)
               postpancreatectomy diabetes mellitus (E13.-)
               postprocedural diabetes mellitus (E13.-)
               secondary diabetes mellitus NEC (E13.-)
               type 1 diabetes mellitus (E10.-)
               type 2 diabetes mellitus (E11.-)

● **E09.0**   **Drug or chemical induced diabetes mellitus with hyperosmolarity**

     E09.00   Drug or chemical induced diabetes mellitus with hyperosmolarity **without nonketotic hyperglycemic-hyperosmolar coma (NKHHC)** 🐾

     E09.01   Drug or chemical induced diabetes mellitus with hyperosmolarity **with coma** 🐾

● **E09.1**   **Drug or chemical induced diabetes mellitus with ketoacidosis**

     E09.10   Drug or chemical induced diabetes mellitus with ketoacidosis **without coma** 🐾

     E09.11   Drug or chemical induced diabetes mellitus with ketoacidosis **with coma** 🐾

● **E09.2**   **Drug or chemical induced diabetes mellitus with kidney complications**

     E09.21   Drug or chemical induced diabetes mellitus with diabetic **nephropathy** 🐾
           Drug or chemical induced diabetes mellitus with intercapillary glomerulosclerosis
           Drug or chemical induced diabetes mellitus with intracapillary glomerulonephrosis
           Drug or chemical induced diabetes mellitus with Kimmelstiel-Wilson disease

     E09.22   Drug or chemical induced diabetes mellitus with diabetic **chronic kidney disease** 🐾
           Use additional code to identify stage of chronic kidney disease (N18.1-N18.6)

     E09.29   Drug or chemical induced diabetes mellitus with **other diabetic kidney complication** 🐾
           Drug or chemical induced diabetes mellitus with renal tubular degeneration

● **E09.3**   **Drug or chemical induced diabetes mellitus with ophthalmic complications**
     Coding Clinic: 2016, Q4, P11

     ● **E09.31**   Drug or chemical induced diabetes mellitus with **unspecified** diabetic retinopathy

         E09.311   Drug or chemical induced diabetes mellitus with unspecified diabetic retinopathy **with macular edema** 🐾

         E09.319   Drug or chemical induced diabetes mellitus with unspecified diabetic retinopathy **without macular edema** 🐾

● **E09.32**   **Drug or chemical induced diabetes mellitus with mild nonproliferative diabetic retinopathy**
     Drug or chemical induced diabetes mellitus with nonproliferative diabetic retinopathy NOS

     One of the following 7th characters is to be assigned to codes in subcategory E09.32 to designate laterality of the disease:

1	right eye
2	left eye
3	bilateral
9	unspecified eye

     ● **E09.321**   Drug or chemical induced diabetes mellitus with mild nonproliferative diabetic retinopathy **with macular edema** 🐾

     ● **E09.329**   Drug or chemical induced diabetes mellitus with mild nonproliferative diabetic retinopathy **without macular edema** 🐾

● **E09.33**   **Drug or chemical induced diabetes mellitus with moderate nonproliferative diabetic retinopathy**

     One of the following 7th characters is to be assigned to codes in subcategory E09.33 to designate laterality of the disease:

1	right eye
2	left eye
3	bilateral
9	unspecified eye

     ● **E09.331**   Drug or chemical induced diabetes mellitus with moderate nonproliferative diabetic retinopathy **with macular edema** 🐾

     ● **E09.339**   Drug or chemical induced diabetes mellitus with moderate nonproliferative diabetic retinopathy **without macular edema** 🐾

● **E09.34**   **Drug or chemical induced diabetes mellitus with severe nonproliferative diabetic retinopathy**

     One of the following 7th characters is to be assigned to codes in subcategory E09.34 to designate laterality of the disease:

1	right eye
2	left eye
3	bilateral
9	unspecified eye

     ● **E09.341**   Drug or chemical induced diabetes mellitus with severe nonproliferative diabetic retinopathy **with macular edema** 🐾

     ● **E09.349**   Drug or chemical induced diabetes mellitus with severe nonproliferative diabetic retinopathy **without macular edema** 🐾

▶ New   ➡ Revised   ~~deleted~~ Deleted   Excludes 1   Excludes 2   Includes   Use additional   Code first   Code also   Key words

OGCR Official Guidelines   X Assign placeholder X   ● Use Additional Character(s)   ▶ Manifestation Code   🐾 Hierarchical Condition Category   Coding Clinic

● E09.35   **Drug or chemical induced diabetes mellitus with proliferative diabetic retinopathy**

One of the following 7th characters is to be assigned to codes in subcategory E09.35 to designate laterality of the disease:

1	right eye
2	left eye
3	bilateral
9	unspecified eye

● E09.351   Drug or chemical induced diabetes mellitus with proliferative diabetic retinopathy with macular edema 🦟

● E09.352   Drug or chemical induced diabetes mellitus with proliferative diabetic retinopathy with traction retinal 🦟 detachment involving the macula

● E09.353   Drug or chemical induced diabetes mellitus with proliferative diabetic retinopathy with traction retinal detachment not involving the macula 🦟

● E09.354   Drug or chemical induced diabetes mellitus with proliferative diabetic retinopathy with combined traction retinal detachment and rhegmatogenous retinal detachment 🦟

● E09.355   Drug or chemical induced diabetes mellitus with stable proliferative diabetic retinopathy 🦟

● E09.359   Drug or chemical induced diabetes mellitus with proliferative diabetic retinopathy without macular edema 🦟

E09.36   Drug or chemical induced diabetes mellitus with diabetic cataract 🦟

X ● E09.37   **Drug or chemical induced diabetes mellitus with diabetic macular edema, resolved following treatment** 🦟

One of the following 7th characters is to be assigned to code E09.37 to designate laterality of the disease:

1	right eye
2	left eye
3	bilateral
9	unspecified eye

E09.39   Drug or chemical induced diabetes mellitus with other diabetic ophthalmic complication 🦟

Use additional code to identify manifestation, such as:
diabetic glaucoma (H40-H42)

● E09.4   **Drug or chemical induced diabetes mellitus with neurological complications**

E09.40   Drug or chemical induced diabetes mellitus with neurological complications with diabetic neuropathy, unspecified 🦟

E09.41   Drug or chemical induced diabetes mellitus with neurological complications with diabetic mononeuropathy 🦟

E09.42   Drug or chemical induced diabetes mellitus with neurological complications with diabetic polyneuropathy 🦟
Drug or chemical induced diabetes mellitus with diabetic neuralgia

E09.43   Drug or chemical induced diabetes mellitus with neurological complications with diabetic autonomic (poly)neuropathy 🦟
Drug or chemical induced diabetes mellitus with diabetic gastroparesis

E09.44   Drug or chemical induced diabetes mellitus with neurological complications with diabetic amyotrophy 🦟

E09.49   Drug or chemical induced diabetes mellitus with neurological complications with other diabetic neurological complication 🦟

● E09.5   **Drug or chemical induced diabetes mellitus with circulatory complications**

E09.51   Drug or chemical induced diabetes mellitus with diabetic peripheral angiopathy without gangrene 🦟

E09.52   Drug or chemical induced diabetes mellitus with diabetic peripheral angiopathy with gangrene 🦟
Drug or chemical induced diabetes mellitus with diabetic gangrene

E09.59   Drug or chemical induced diabetes mellitus with other circulatory complications 🦟

● E09.6   **Drug or chemical induced diabetes mellitus with other specified complications**

● E09.61   Drug or chemical induced diabetes mellitus with diabetic arthropathy

E09.610   Drug or chemical induced diabetes mellitus with diabetic neuropathic arthropathy 🦟
Drug or chemical induced diabetes mellitus with Charcôt's joints
Progressive degeneration of weight-bearing joint

E09.618   Drug or chemical induced diabetes mellitus with other diabetic arthropathy 🦟

● E09.62   Drug or chemical induced diabetes mellitus with skin complications

E09.620   Drug or chemical induced diabetes mellitus with diabetic dermatitis 🦟
Drug or chemical induced diabetes mellitus with diabetic necrobiosis lipoidica
Necrotizing skin condition

E09.621   Drug or chemical induced diabetes mellitus with foot ulcer 🦟
Use additional code to identify site of ulcer (L97.4-, L97.5-)

E09.622   Drug or chemical induced diabetes mellitus with other skin ulcer 🦟
Use additional code to identify site of ulcer (L97.1-L97.9, L98.41-L98.49)

E09.628   Drug or chemical induced diabetes mellitus with other skin complications 🦟

● E09.63   Drug or chemical induced diabetes mellitus with oral complications

E09.630   Drug or chemical induced diabetes mellitus with periodontal disease 🦟

E09.638   Drug or chemical induced diabetes mellitus with other oral complications 🦟

● E09.64   Drug or chemical induced diabetes mellitus with hypoglycemia

E09.641   Drug or chemical induced diabetes mellitus with hypoglycemia with coma 🦟

E09.649   Drug or chemical induced diabetes mellitus with hypoglycemia without coma 🦟

E09.65   Drug or chemical induced diabetes mellitus with hyperglycemia 🦟

E09.69   Drug or chemical induced diabetes mellitus with other specified complication 🦟
Use additional code to identify complication

E09.8   Drug or chemical induced diabetes mellitus with unspecified complications 🦟

E09.9   Drug or chemical induced diabetes mellitus without complications 🦟

CHAPTER 4 (E00-E89)

● **E10**   **Type 1 diabetes mellitus**

    Includes   brittle diabetes (mellitus)
                     diabetes (mellitus) due to autoimmune process
                     diabetes (mellitus) due to immune mediated
                         pancreatic islet beta-cell destruction
                     idiopathic diabetes (mellitus)
                     juvenile onset diabetes (mellitus)
                     ketosis-prone diabetes (mellitus)

    Excludes1   diabetes mellitus due to underlying condition
                         (E08.-)
                     drug or chemical induced diabetes mellitus
                         (E09.-)
                     gestational diabetes (O24.4-)
                     hyperglycemia NOS (R73.9)
                     neonatal diabetes mellitus (P70.2)
                     postpancreatectomy diabetes mellitus (E13.-)
                     postprocedural diabetes mellitus (E13.-)
                     secondary diabetes mellitus NEC (E13.-)
                     type 2 diabetes mellitus (E11.-)

● **E10.1**   **Type 1 diabetes mellitus with ketoacidosis**
        Acidosis accompanied by accumulation of ketone bodies
          (ketosis) in body tissues and fluids

    E10.10   **Type 1 diabetes mellitus with ketoacidosis
             without coma** 🦠
             Coding Clinic: 2013, Q3, P20

    E10.11   **Type 1 diabetes mellitus with ketoacidosis with
             coma** 🦠

● **E10.2**   **Type 1 diabetes mellitus with kidney complications**

    E10.21   **Type 1 diabetes mellitus with diabetic
             nephropathy** 🦠
             Type 1 diabetes mellitus with intercapillary
                glomerulosclerosis
             Type 1 diabetes mellitus with intracapillary
                glomerulonephrosis
             Type 1 diabetes mellitus with Kimmelstiel-
                Wilson disease

    E10.22   **Type 1 diabetes mellitus with diabetic chronic
             kidney disease** 🦠
             Use additional code to identify stage of chronic
                kidney disease (N18.1-N18.6)

    E10.29   **Type 1 diabetes mellitus with other diabetic
             kidney complication** 🦠
             Type 1 diabetes mellitus with renal tubular
                degeneration
             Coding Clinic: 2016, Q1, P13

● **E10.3**   **Type 1 diabetes mellitus with ophthalmic complications**
        Coding Clinic: 2016, Q4, P11

  ● **E10.31**   **Type 1 diabetes mellitus with unspecified
             diabetic retinopathy**

       E10.311   **Type 1 diabetes mellitus
                with unspecified diabetic retinopathy
                with macular edema** 🦠

       E10.319   **Type 1 diabetes mellitus
                with unspecified diabetic retinopathy
                without macular edema** 🦠

  ● **E10.32**   **Type 1 diabetes mellitus with mild
             nonproliferative diabetic retinopathy**
             Type 1 diabetes mellitus with nonproliferative
                diabetic retinopathy NOS

             One of the following 7th characters is to be
                assigned to codes in subcategory E10.32 to
                designate laterality of the disease:

1	right eye
2	left eye
3	bilateral
9	unspecified eye

     ● **E10.321**   **Type 1 diabetes mellitus with mild
                nonproliferative diabetic retinopathy
                with macular edema** 🦠

     ● **E10.329**   **Type 1 diabetes mellitus with mild
                nonproliferative diabetic retinopathy
                without macular edema** 🦠

● **E10.33**   **Type 1 diabetes mellitus with moderate
         nonproliferative diabetic retinopathy**

         One of the following 7th characters is to be
             assigned to codes in subcategory E10.33 to
             designate laterality of the disease:

1	right eye
2	left eye
3	bilateral
9	unspecified eye

  ● **E10.331**   **Type 1 diabetes mellitus with
             moderate nonproliferative diabetic
             retinopathy with macular edema** 🦠

  ● **E10.339**   **Type 1 diabetes mellitus with
             moderate nonproliferative diabetic
             retinopathy without macular
             edema** 🦠

● **E10.34**   **Type 1 diabetes mellitus with severe
         nonproliferative diabetic retinopathy**

         One of the following 7th characters is to be
             assigned to codes in subcategory E10.34 to
             designate laterality of the disease:

1	right eye
2	left eye
3	bilateral
9	unspecified eye

  ● **E10.341**   **Type 1 diabetes mellitus with severe
             nonproliferative diabetic retinopathy
             with macular edema** 🦠

  ● **E10.349**   **Type 1 diabetes mellitus with severe
             nonproliferative diabetic retinopathy
             without macular edema** 🦠

● **E10.35**   **Type 1 diabetes mellitus with proliferative
         diabetic retinopathy**

         One of the following 7th characters is to be
             assigned to codes in subcategory E10.35 to
             designate laterality of the disease:

1	right eye
2	left eye
3	bilateral
9	unspecified eye

  ● **E10.351**   **Type 1 diabetes mellitus with
             proliferative diabetic retinopathy
             with macular edema** 🦠

  ● **E10.352**   **Type 1 diabetes mellitus with
             proliferative diabetic retinopathy
             with traction retinal detachment
             involving the macula** 🦠

  ● **E10.353**   **Type 1 diabetes mellitus with
             proliferative diabetic retinopathy
             with traction retinal detachment not
             involving the macula** 🦠

  ● **E10.354**   **Type 1 diabetes mellitus with
             proliferative diabetic retinopathy
             with combined traction retinal
             detachment and rhegmatogenous
             retinal detachment** 🦠

  ● **E10.355**   **Type 1 diabetes mellitus with stable
             proliferative diabetic retinopathy** 🦠

  ● **E10.359**   **Type 1 diabetes mellitus with
             proliferative diabetic retinopathy
             without macular edema** 🦠

▶ New   ➠ Revised   ~~deleted~~ Deleted   Excludes 1   Excludes 2   Includes   Use additional   Code first   Code also   Key words

OGCR Official Guidelines   X Assign placeholder X   ● Use Additional Character(s)   ▸ Manifestation Code   🦠 Hierarchical Condition Category   **Coding Clinic**

E10.36   Type 1 diabetes mellitus with diabetic cataract 🗝

X ⬤ E10.37   Type 1 diabetes mellitus with diabetic macular edema, resolved following treatment 🗝

     One of the following 7th characters is to be assigned to code E10.37 to designate laterality of the disease:

1	right eye
2	left eye
3	bilateral
9	unspecified eye

E10.39   Type 1 diabetes mellitus with other diabetic ophthalmic complication 🗝

     Use additional code to identify manifestation, such as:
     diabetic glaucoma (H40-H42)

⬤ E10.4   Type 1 diabetes mellitus with neurological complications

E10.40   Type 1 diabetes mellitus with diabetic neuropathy, unspecified 🗝

E10.41   Type 1 diabetes mellitus with diabetic mononeuropathy 🗝

E10.42   Type 1 diabetes mellitus with diabetic polyneuropathy 🗝
     Type 1 diabetes mellitus with diabetic neuralgia

E10.43   Type 1 diabetes mellitus with diabetic autonomic (poly)neuropathy 🗝
     Type 1 diabetes mellitus with diabetic gastroparesis

E10.44   Type 1 diabetes mellitus with diabetic amyotrophy 🗝

E10.49   Type 1 diabetes mellitus with other diabetic neurological complication 🗝

⬤ E10.5   Type 1 diabetes mellitus with circulatory complications

E10.51   Type 1 diabetes mellitus with diabetic peripheral angiopathy without gangrene 🗝

E10.52   Type 1 diabetes mellitus with diabetic peripheral angiopathy with gangrene 🗝
     Type 1 diabetes mellitus with diabetic gangrene

E10.59   Type 1 diabetes mellitus with other circulatory complications 🗝

⬤ E10.6   Type 1 diabetes mellitus with other specified complications

⬤ E10.61   Type 1 diabetes mellitus with diabetic arthropathy

E10.610   Type 1 diabetes mellitus with diabetic neuropathic arthropathy 🗝
     Type 1 diabetes mellitus with Charcôt's joints

E10.618   Type 1 diabetes mellitus with other diabetic arthropathy 🗝

⬤ E10.62   Type 1 diabetes mellitus with skin complications

E10.620   Type 1 diabetes mellitus with diabetic dermatitis 🗝
     Type 1 diabetes mellitus with diabetic necrobiosis lipoidica

E10.621   Type 1 diabetes mellitus with foot ulcer 🗝
     Use additional code to identify site of ulcer (L97.4-, L97.5-)

E10.622   Type 1 diabetes mellitus with other skin ulcer 🗝
     Use additional code to identify site of ulcer (L97.1-L97.9, L98.41-L98.49)

E10.628   Type 1 diabetes mellitus with other skin complications 🗝

⬤ E10.63   Type 1 diabetes mellitus with oral complications

E10.630   Type 1 diabetes mellitus with periodontal disease 🗝

E10.638   Type 1 diabetes mellitus with other oral complications 🗝

⬤ E10.64   Type 1 diabetes mellitus with hypoglycemia

E10.641   Type 1 diabetes mellitus with hypoglycemia with coma 🗝

E10.649   Type 1 diabetes mellitus with hypoglycemia without coma 🗝
     Coding Clinic: 2016, Q1, P13

E10.65   Type 1 diabetes mellitus with hyperglycemia 🗝
     Coding Clinic: 2013, Q3, P20

E10.69   Type 1 diabetes mellitus with other specified complication 🗝
     Use additional code to identify complication

E10.8   Type 1 diabetes mellitus with unspecified complications 🗝

E10.9   Type 1 diabetes mellitus without complications 🗝

⬤ E11   **Type 2 diabetes mellitus**

     Includes   diabetes (mellitus) due to insulin secretory defect
          diabetes NOS
          insulin resistant diabetes (mellitus)

     Use additional code to identify control using:
     insulin (Z79.4)
     oral antidiabetic drugs (Z79.84)
     oral hypoglycemic drugs (Z79.84)

     Excludes1   diabetes mellitus due to underlying condition (E08.-)
          drug or chemical induced diabetes mellitus (E09.-)
          gestational diabetes (O24.4-)
          neonatal diabetes mellitus (P70.2)
          postpancreatectomy diabetes mellitus (E13.-)
          postprocedural diabetes mellitus (E13.-)
          secondary diabetes mellitus NEC (E13.-)
          type 1 diabetes mellitus (E10.-)

     Coding Clinic: 2020, Q1, P12; 2016, Q4, P121, Q2, P10

⬤ E11.0   Type 2 diabetes mellitus with hyperosmolarity

E11.00   Type 2 diabetes mellitus with hyperosmolarity without nonketotic hyperglycemic-hyperosmolar coma (NKHHC) 🗝

E11.01   Type 2 diabetes mellitus with hyperosmolarity with coma 🗝

⬤ E11.1   Type 2 diabetes mellitus with ketoacidosis

E11.10   Type 2 diabetes mellitus with ketoacidosis without coma 🗝
     Coding Clinic: 2017, Q4, P6

E11.11   Type 2 diabetes mellitus with ketoacidosis with coma 🗝

⬤ E11.2   Type 2 diabetes mellitus with kidney complications

E11.21   Type 2 diabetes mellitus with diabetic nephropathy 🗝
     Type 2 diabetes mellitus with intercapillary glomerulosclerosis
     Type 2 diabetes mellitus with intracapillary glomerulonephrosis
     Type 2 diabetes mellitus with Kimmelstiel-Wilson disease
     Coding Clinic: 2019, Q3, P3

E11.22   Type 2 diabetes mellitus with diabetic chronic kidney disease 🗝
     Use additional code to identify stage of chronic kidney disease (N18.1-N18.6)
     Coding Clinic: 2019, Q3, P3; 2018, Q4, P88; 2016, Q2, P36, Q1, P13

E11.29   Type 2 diabetes mellitus with other diabetic kidney complication 🗝
     Type 2 diabetes mellitus with renal tubular degeneration

CHAPTER 4 (E00-E89)

CHAPTER 4 (E00-E89)

● E11.3   Type 2 diabetes mellitus with ophthalmic complications
          Coding Clinic: 2016, Q4, P11

  ● E11.31   Type 2 diabetes mellitus with unspecified diabetic retinopathy

     E11.311   Type 2 diabetes mellitus with unspecified diabetic retinopathy with macular edema 🦠

     E11.319   Type 2 diabetes mellitus with unspecified diabetic retinopathy without macular edema 🦠
               Coding Clinic: 2013, Q3, P20

  ● E11.32   Type 2 diabetes mellitus with mild nonproliferative diabetic retinopathy
             Type 2 diabetes mellitus with nonproliferative diabetic retinopathy NOS

             One of the following 7th characters is to be assigned to codes in subcategory E11.32 to designate laterality of the disease:

1	right eye
2	left eye
3	bilateral
9	unspecified eye

     ● E11.321   Type 2 diabetes mellitus with mild nonproliferative diabetic retinopathy with macular edema 🦠

     ● E11.329   Type 2 diabetes mellitus with mild nonproliferative diabetic retinopathy without macular edema 🦠

  ● E11.33   Type 2 diabetes mellitus with moderate nonproliferative diabetic retinopathy

             One of the following 7th characters is to be assigned to codes in subcategory E11.33 to designate laterality of the disease:

1	right eye
2	left eye
3	bilateral
9	unspecified eye

     ● E11.331   Type 2 diabetes mellitus with moderate nonproliferative diabetic retinopathy with macular edema 🦠

     ● E11.339   Type 2 diabetes mellitus with moderate nonproliferative diabetic retinopathy without macular edema 🦠

  ● E11.34   Type 2 diabetes mellitus with severe nonproliferative diabetic retinopathy

             One of the following 7th characters is to be assigned to codes in subcategory E11.34 to designate laterality of the disease:

1	right eye
2	left eye
3	bilateral
9	unspecified eye

     ● E11.341   Type 2 diabetes mellitus with severe nonproliferative diabetic retinopathy with macular edema 🦠

     ● E11.349   Type 2 diabetes mellitus with severe nonproliferative diabetic retinopathy without macular edema 🦠

● E11.35   Type 2 diabetes mellitus with proliferative diabetic retinopathy

           One of the following 7th characters is to be assigned to codes in subcategory E11.35 to designate laterality of the disease:

1	right eye
2	left eye
3	bilateral
9	unspecified eye

  ● E11.351   Type 2 diabetes mellitus with proliferative diabetic retinopathy with macular edema 🦠

  ● E11.352   Type 2 diabetes mellitus with proliferative diabetic retinopathy with traction retinal detachment involving the macula 🦠

  ● E11.353   Type 2 diabetes mellitus with proliferative diabetic retinopathy with traction retinal detachment not involving the macula 🦠

  ● E11.354   Type 2 diabetes mellitus with proliferative diabetic retinopathy with combined traction retinal detachment and rhegmatogenous retinal detachment 🦠

  ● E11.355   Type 2 diabetes mellitus with stable proliferative diabetic retinopathy 🦠

  ● E11.359   Type 2 diabetes mellitus with proliferative diabetic retinopathy without macular edema 🦠

  E11.36   Type 2 diabetes mellitus with diabetic cataract 🦠
           Coding Clinic: 2019, Q2, P30-31; 2016, Q2, P36

X ● E11.37   Type 2 diabetes mellitus with diabetic macular edema, resolved following treatment 🦠

           One of the following 7th characters is to be assigned to code E11.37 to designate laterality of the disease:

1	right eye
2	left eye
3	bilateral
9	unspecified eye

  E11.39   Type 2 diabetes mellitus with other diabetic ophthalmic complication 🦠
           Use additional code to identify manifestation, such as:
           diabetic glaucoma (H40-H42)

● E11.4   Type 2 diabetes mellitus with neurological complications

  E11.40   Type 2 diabetes mellitus with diabetic neuropathy, unspecified 🦠

  E11.41   Type 2 diabetes mellitus with diabetic mononeuropathy 🦠

  E11.42   Type 2 diabetes mellitus with diabetic polyneuropathy 🦠
           Type 2 diabetes mellitus with diabetic neuralgia
           Coding Clinic: 2020, Q1, P12; 2016, Q1, P13

  E11.43   Type 2 diabetes mellitus with diabetic autonomic (poly)neuropathy 🦠
           Type 2 diabetes mellitus with diabetic gastroparesis
           Coding Clinic: 2016, Q2, P36

  E11.44   Type 2 diabetes mellitus with diabetic amyotrophy 🦠
           Coding Clinic: 2016, Q2, P36

  E11.49   Type 2 diabetes mellitus with other diabetic neurological complication 🦠

▶ New   ⇒ Revised   ~~deleted~~ Deleted   Excludes 1   Excludes 2   Includes   Use additional   Code first   Code also   Key words
OGCR Official Guidelines   X Assign placeholder X   ● Use Additional Character(s)   ⟩ Manifestation Code   🦠 Hierarchical Condition Category   Coding Clinic

- ● E11.5   Type 2 diabetes mellitus with circulatory complications
  - E11.51   Type 2 diabetes mellitus with diabetic peripheral angiopathy without gangrene 🔖
  - E11.52   Type 2 diabetes mellitus with diabetic peripheral angiopathy with gangrene 🔖
    - Type 2 diabetes mellitus with diabetic gangrene
    - Coding Clinic: 2017, Q4, P102
  - E11.59   Type 2 diabetes mellitus with other circulatory complications 🔖
- ● E11.6   Type 2 diabetes mellitus with other specified complications
  - ● E11.61   Type 2 diabetes mellitus with diabetic arthropathy
    - E11.610   Type 2 diabetes mellitus with diabetic neuropathic arthropathy 🔖
      - Type 2 diabetes mellitus with Charcôt's joints
      - Coding Clinic: 2016, Q2, P36
    - E11.618   Type 2 diabetes mellitus with other diabetic arthropathy 🔖
      - Coding Clinic: 2018, Q2, P7; 2016, Q2, P36
  - ● E11.62   Type 2 diabetes mellitus with skin complications
    - E11.620   Type 2 diabetes mellitus with diabetic dermatitis 🔖
      - Type 2 diabetes mellitus with diabetic necrobiosis lipoidica
    - E11.621   Type 2 diabetes mellitus with foot ulcer 🔖
      - Use additional code to identify site of ulcer (L97.4-, L97.5-)
      - Coding Clinic: 2020, Q1, P12; 2016, Q1, P12
    - E11.622   Type 2 diabetes mellitus with other skin ulcer 🔖
      - Use additional code to identify site of ulcer (L97.1-L97.9, L98.41-L98.49)
      - Coding Clinic: 2021, Q1, P8; 2017, Q4, P17
    - E11.628   Type 2 diabetes mellitus with other skin complications 🔖
  - ● E11.63   Type 2 diabetes mellitus with oral complications
    - E11.630   Type 2 diabetes mellitus with periodontal disease 🔖
    - E11.638   Type 2 diabetes mellitus with other oral complications 🔖
  - ● E11.64   Type 2 diabetes mellitus with hypoglycemia
    - E11.641   Type 2 diabetes mellitus with hypoglycemia with coma 🔖
    - E11.649   Type 2 diabetes mellitus with hypoglycemia without coma 🔖
      - Coding Clinic: 2016, Q3, P42; 2015, Q3, P21
  - E11.65   Type 2 diabetes mellitus with hyperglycemia 🔖
    - Coding Clinic: 2013, Q3, P20
  - E11.69   Type 2 diabetes mellitus with other specified complication 🔖
    - Use additional code to identify complication
    - Coding Clinic: 2020, Q1, P12; 2016, Q4, P142
- E11.8   Type 2 diabetes mellitus with unspecified complications 🔖
- E11.9   Type 2 diabetes mellitus without complications 🔖
  - Coding Clinic: 2016, Q4, P142, Q2, P36

- ● E13   Other specified diabetes mellitus
  - **Includes**   diabetes mellitus due to genetic defects of beta-cell function
    - diabetes mellitus due to genetic defects in insulin action
    - postpancreatectomy diabetes mellitus
    - postprocedural diabetes mellitus
    - secondary diabetes mellitus NEC
  - Use additional code to identify control using:
    - insulin (Z79.4)
    - oral antidiabetic drugs (Z79.84)
    - oral hypoglycemic drugs (Z79.84)
  - **Excludes1**   diabetes (mellitus) due to autoimmune process (E10.-)
    - diabetes (mellitus) due to immune mediated pancreatic islet beta-cell destruction (E10.-)
    - diabetes mellitus due to underlying condition (E08.-)
    - drug or chemical induced diabetes mellitus (E09.-)
    - gestational diabetes (O24.4-)
    - neonatal diabetes mellitus (P70.2)
    - type 1 diabetes mellitus (E10.-)
  - ● E13.0   Other specified diabetes mellitus with hyperosmolarity
    - E13.00   Other specified diabetes mellitus with hyperosmolarity without nonketotic hyperglycemic-hyperosmolar coma (NKHHC) 🔖
      - **Excludes2**   type 2 diabetes mellitus (E11.-)
    - E13.01   Other specified diabetes mellitus with hyperosmolarity with coma 🔖
  - ● E13.1   Other specified diabetes mellitus with ketoacidosis
    - E13.10   Other specified diabetes mellitus with ketoacidosis without coma 🔖
      - Coding Clinic: 2016, Q2, P10; 2013, Q1, P26
    - E13.11   Other specified diabetes mellitus with ketoacidosis with coma 🔖
  - ● E13.2   Other specified diabetes mellitus with kidney complications
    - E13.21   Other specified diabetes mellitus with diabetic nephropathy 🔖
      - Other specified diabetes mellitus with intercapillary glomerulosclerosis
      - Other specified diabetes mellitus with intracapillary glomerulonephrosis
      - Other specified diabetes mellitus with Kimmelstiel-Wilson disease
    - E13.22   Other specified diabetes mellitus with diabetic chronic kidney disease 🔖
      - Use additional code to identify stage of chronic kidney disease (N18.1-N18.6)
    - E13.29   Other specified diabetes mellitus with other diabetic kidney complication 🔖
      - Other specified diabetes mellitus with renal tubular degeneration
  - ● E13.3   Other specified diabetes mellitus with ophthalmic complications
    - Coding Clinic: 2016, Q4, P11
    - ● E13.31   Other specified diabetes mellitus with unspecified diabetic retinopathy
      - E13.311   Other specified diabetes mellitus with unspecified diabetic retinopathy with macular edema 🔖
      - E13.319   Other specified diabetes mellitus with unspecified diabetic retinopathy without macular edema 🔖

● **E13.32**   Other specified diabetes mellitus with mild nonproliferative diabetic retinopathy

Other specified diabetes mellitus with nonproliferative diabetic retinopathy NOS

One of the following 7th characters is to be assigned to codes in subcategory E13.32 to designate laterality of the disease:

1	right eye
2	left eye
3	bilateral
9	unspecified eye

● **E13.321**   Other specified diabetes mellitus with mild nonproliferative diabetic retinopathy with macular edema ⬡

● **E13.329**   Other specified diabetes mellitus with mild nonproliferative diabetic retinopathy without macular edema ⬡

● **E13.33**   Other specified diabetes mellitus with moderate nonproliferative diabetic retinopathy

One of the following 7th characters is to be assigned to codes in subcategory E13.33 to designate laterality of the disease:

1	right eye
2	left eye
3	bilateral
9	unspecified eye

● **E13.331**   Other specified diabetes mellitus with moderate nonproliferative diabetic retinopathy with macular edema ⬡

● **E13.339**   Other specified diabetes mellitus with moderate nonproliferative diabetic retinopathy without macular edema ⬡

● **E13.34**   Other specified diabetes mellitus with severe nonproliferative diabetic retinopathy

One of the following 7th characters is to be assigned to codes in subcategory E13.34 to designate laterality of the disease:

1	right eye
2	left eye
3	bilateral
9	unspecified eye

● **E13.341**   Other specified diabetes mellitus with severe nonproliferative diabetic retinopathy with macular edema ⬡

● **E13.349**   Other specified diabetes mellitus with severe nonproliferative diabetic retinopathy without macular edema ⬡

● **E13.35**   Other specified diabetes mellitus with proliferative diabetic retinopathy

One of the following 7th characters is to be assigned to codes in subcategory E13.35 to designate laterality of the disease:

1	right eye
2	left eye
3	bilateral
9	unspecified eye

● **E13.351**   Other specified diabetes mellitus with proliferative diabetic retinopathy with macular edema ⬡

● **E13.352**   Other specified diabetes mellitus with proliferative diabetic retinopathy with traction retinal detachment involving the macula ⬡

● **E13.353**   Other specified diabetes mellitus with proliferative diabetic retinopathy with traction retinal detachment not involving the macula ⬡

● **E13.354**   Other specified diabetes mellitus with proliferative diabetic retinopathy with combined traction retinal detachment and rhegmatogenous retinal detachment ⬡

● **E13.355**   Other specified diabetes mellitus with stable proliferative diabetic retinopathy ⬡

● **E13.359**   Other specified diabetes mellitus with proliferative diabetic retinopathy without macular edema ⬡

E13.36   Other specified diabetes mellitus with diabetic cataract ⬡

X ● **E13.37**   Other specified diabetes mellitus with diabetic macular edema, resolved following treatment ⬡

One of the following 7th characters is to be assigned to code E13.37 to designate laterality of the disease:

1	right eye
2	left eye
3	bilateral
9	unspecified eye

E13.39   Other specified diabetes mellitus with other diabetic ophthalmic complication ⬡

Use additional code to identify manifestation, such as:
diabetic glaucoma (H40-H42)

● **E13.4**   **Other specified diabetes mellitus with neurological complications**

E13.40   Other specified diabetes mellitus with diabetic neuropathy, unspecified ⬡

E13.41   Other specified diabetes mellitus with diabetic mononeuropathy ⬡

E13.42   Other specified diabetes mellitus with diabetic polyneuropathy ⬡

Other specified diabetes mellitus with diabetic neuralgia

E13.43   Other specified diabetes mellitus with diabetic autonomic (poly)neuropathy ⬡

Other specified diabetes mellitus with diabetic gastroparesis

E13.44   Other specified diabetes mellitus with diabetic amyotrophy ⬡

E13.49   Other specified diabetes mellitus with other diabetic neurological complication ⬡

● **E13.5**   **Other specified diabetes mellitus with circulatory complications**

E13.51   Other specified diabetes mellitus with diabetic peripheral angiopathy without gangrene ⬡

E13.52   Other specified diabetes mellitus with diabetic peripheral angiopathy with gangrene ⬡

Other specified diabetes mellitus with diabetic gangrene

E13.59   Other specified diabetes mellitus with other circulatory complications ⬡

● **E13.6**   **Other specified diabetes mellitus with other specified complications**

● **E13.61**   Other specified diabetes mellitus with diabetic arthropathy

E13.610   Other specified diabetes mellitus with diabetic neuropathic arthropathy ⬡

Other specified diabetes mellitus with Charcôt's joints

E13.618   Other specified diabetes mellitus with other diabetic arthropathy ⬡

▶ New   ⟫ Revised   ~~deleted~~ Deleted   Excludes 1   Excludes 2   Includes   Use additional   Code first   Code also   Key words

OGCR Official Guidelines   X Assign placeholder X   ● Use Additional Character(s)   ▷ Manifestation Code   ⬡ Hierarchical Condition Category   **Coding Clinic**

● **E13.62** Other specified diabetes mellitus with skin complications

    E13.620 Other specified diabetes mellitus with diabetic dermatitis

        Other specified diabetes mellitus with diabetic necrobiosis lipoidica

    E13.621 Other specified diabetes mellitus with foot ulcer

        Use additional code to identify site of ulcer (L97.4-, L97.5-)

    E13.622 Other specified diabetes mellitus with other skin ulcer

        Use additional code to identify site of ulcer (L97.1-L97.9, L98.41-L98.49)

    E13.628 Other specified diabetes mellitus with other skin complications

● **E13.63** Other specified diabetes mellitus with oral complications

    E13.630 Other specified diabetes mellitus with periodontal disease

    E13.638 Other specified diabetes mellitus with other oral complications

● **E13.64** Other specified diabetes mellitus with hypoglycemia

    E13.641 Other specified diabetes mellitus with hypoglycemia with coma

    E13.649 Other specified diabetes mellitus with hypoglycemia without coma

    E13.65 Other specified diabetes mellitus with hyperglycemia

    E13.69 Other specified diabetes mellitus with other specified complication

        Use additional code to identify complication

E13.8 Other specified diabetes mellitus with unspecified complications

E13.9 Other specified diabetes mellitus without complications

OTHER DISORDERS OF GLUCOSE REGULATION AND PANCREATIC INTERNAL SECRETION (E15-E16)

E15 Nondiabetic hypoglycemic coma

    Includes drug-induced insulin coma in nondiabetic hyperinsulinism with hypoglycemic coma hypoglycemic coma NOS

● **E16** Other disorders of pancreatic internal secretion

    E16.0 Drug-induced hypoglycemia without coma

        Excludes1 diabetes with hypoglycemia without coma (E09.649)

        Use additional code for adverse effect, if applicable, to identify drug (T36-T50 with fifth or sixth character 5)

    E16.1 Other hypoglycemia

        Functional hyperinsulinism

        Functional nonhyperinsulinemic hypoglycemia

        Hyperinsulinism NOS

        Hyperplasia of pancreatic islet beta cells NOS

        Excludes1 diabetes with hypoglycemia (E08.649, E10.649, E11.649, E13.649) hypoglycemia in infant of diabetic mother (P70.1) neonatal hypoglycemia (P70.4)

    E16.2 Hypoglycemia, unspecified

        Excludes1 diabetes with hypoglycemia (E08.649, E10.649, E11.649, E13.649)

        Coding Clinic: 2016, Q3, P42

    E16.3 Increased secretion of glucagon

        Hyperplasia of pancreatic endocrine cells with glucagon excess

    E16.4 Increased secretion of gastrin

        Hypergastrinemia

        Hyperplasia of pancreatic endocrine cells with gastrin excess

        Zollinger-Ellison syndrome

    E16.8 Other specified disorders of pancreatic internal secretion

        Increased secretion from endocrine pancreas of growth hormone-releasing hormone

        Increased secretion from endocrine pancreas of pancreatic polypeptide

        Increased secretion from endocrine pancreas of somatostatin

        Increased secretion from endocrine pancreas of vasoactive-intestinal polypeptide

    E16.9 Disorder of pancreatic internal secretion, unspecified

        Islet-cell hyperplasia NOS

        Pancreatic endocrine cell hyperplasia NOS

DISORDERS OF OTHER ENDOCRINE GLANDS (E20-E35)

    Excludes1 galactorrhea (N64.3)
        gynecomastia (N62)

● **E20** Hypoparathyroidism

    Greatly reduced function of parathyroid glands; AKA parathyroid insufficiency

    Excludes1 Di George's syndrome (D82.1)
        postprocedural hypoparathyroidism (E89.2)
        tetany NOS (R29.0)
        transitory neonatal hypoparathyroidism (P71.4)

    E20.0 Idiopathic hypoparathyroidism

        Rare condition, unknown cause; short dwarf-like with round face

    E20.1 Pseudohypoparathyroidism

        Hereditary condition resembling hypoparathyroidism, but caused by inability to respond to parathyroid hormone

    E20.8 Other hypoparathyroidism

    E20.9 Hypoparathyroidism, unspecified

        Parathyroid tetany

● **E21** Hyperparathyroidism and other disorders of parathyroid gland

    Excludes1 adult osteomalacia (M83.-)
        ectopic hyperparathyroidism (E34.2)
        ~~familial hypocalciuric hypercalcemia (E83.52)~~
        hungry bone syndrome (E83.81)
        infantile and juvenile osteomalacia (E55.0)

    ▶ **Excludes2** familial hypocalciuric hypercalcemia (E83.52)

    E21.0 Primary hyperparathyroidism

        Hyperplasia of parathyroid

        Osteitis fibrosa cystica generalisata [von Recklinghausen's disease of bone]

    E21.1 Secondary hyperparathyroidism, not elsewhere classified

        Excludes1 secondary hyperparathyroidism of renal origin (N25.81)

    E21.2 Other hyperparathyroidism

        Tertiary hyperparathyroidism

        Excludes1 familial hypocalciuric hypercalcemia (E83.52)

    E21.3 Hyperparathyroidism, unspecified

    E21.4 Other specified disorders of parathyroid gland

    E21.5 Disorder of parathyroid gland, unspecified

Item 4–4 Hyperparathyroidism is an overactive parathyroid gland that secretes excessive parathormone, causing increased levels of circulating calcium. This results in a loss of calcium in the bone (osteoporosis).

    Hypoparathyroidism is an underactive parathyroid gland that results in decreased levels of circulating calcium. The primary manifestation is **tetany,** a continuous muscle spasm.

Figure 4-4 Tetany caused by hypoparathyroidism.

CHAPTER 4 (E00-E89)

Item 4–5 Hyperadrenalism is overactivity of the adrenal cortex, which secretes corticosteroid hormones. Excessive glucocorticoid hormone results in hyperglycemia **(Cushing's syndrome),** and excessive aldosterone results in **Conn's syndrome. Adrenogenital syndrome** is the result of excessive secretion of androgens, male hormones, which stimulates premature sexual development. **Hypoadrenalism, Addison's disease,** is a condition in which the adrenal glands atrophy.

Figure 4-5 Centripetal and generalized obesity and dorsal kyphosis in a woman with Cushing's disease. (From Salvo SG: Mosby's Pathology for Massage Therapists, St. Louis, MO: Mosby/Elsevier, 2009)

● **E22   Hyperfunction of pituitary gland**
  Excludes1   Cushing's syndrome (E24.-)
                   Nelson's syndrome (E24.1)
                   overproduction of ACTH not associated with
                       Cushing's disease (E27.0)
                   overproduction of pituitary ACTH (E24.0)
                   overproduction of thyroid-stimulating hormone
                       (E05.8-)

  E22.0   Acromegaly and pituitary gigantism 🐾
          Chronic disease caused by hypersecretion of growth hormone
          Overproduction of growth hormone
          Excludes1   constitutional gigantism (E34.4)
                           constitutional tall stature (E34.4)
                           increased secretion from endocrine
                               pancreas of growth hormone-
                               releasing hormone (E16.8)

  E22.1   Hyperprolactinemia 🐾
          Increased levels of prolactin
          Use additional code for adverse effect, if applicable,
              to identify drug (T36-T50 with fifth or sixth
              character 5)

  **E22.2   Syndrome of inappropriate secretion of antidiuretic
             hormone** 🐾

  E22.8   Other hyperfunction of pituitary gland 🐾
          Central precocious puberty

  E22.9   Hyperfunction of pituitary gland, unspecified 🐾

● **E23   Hypofunction and other disorders of the pituitary gland**
  Includes   the listed conditions whether the disorder is in
                  the pituitary or the hypothalamus
  Excludes1   postprocedural hypopituitarism (E89.3)

  E23.0   Hypopituitarism 🐾
          Fertile eunuch syndrome
          Hypogonadotropic hypogonadism
          Idiopathic growth hormone deficiency
          Isolated deficiency of gonadotropin
          Isolated deficiency of growth hormone
          Isolated deficiency of pituitary hormone
          Kallmann's syndrome
          Lorain-Levi short stature
          Necrosis of pituitary gland (postpartum)
          Panhypopituitarism
          Pituitary cachexia
          Pituitary insufficiency NOS
          Pituitary short stature
          Sheehan's syndrome
          Simmonds' disease

  E23.1   Drug-induced hypopituitarism 🐾
          Use additional code for adverse effect, if applicable,
              to identify drug (T36-T50 with fifth or sixth
              character 5)

  E23.2   Diabetes insipidus 🐾
          Excludes1   nephrogenic diabetes insipidus (N25.1)

  E23.3   Hypothalamic dysfunction, not elsewhere classified 🐾
          Excludes1   Prader-Willi syndrome (Q87.11)
                           Russell-Silver syndrome (Q87.19)

  E23.6   Other disorders of pituitary gland 🐾
          Abscess of pituitary
          Adiposogenital dystrophy

  E23.7   Disorder of pituitary gland, unspecified 🐾

● **E24   Cushing's syndrome**
  Excludes1   congenital adrenal hyperplasia (E25.0)

  E24.0   Pituitary-dependent Cushing's disease 🐾
          Overproduction of pituitary ACTH
          Pituitary-dependent hypercorticalism

  E24.1   Nelson's syndrome 🐾

  E24.2   Drug-induced Cushing's syndrome 🐾
          Use additional code for adverse effect, if applicable,
              to identify drug (T36-T50 with fifth or sixth
              character 5)

  E24.3   Ectopic ACTH syndrome 🐾
  E24.4   Alcohol-induced pseudo-Cushing's syndrome 🐾
  E24.8   Other Cushing's syndrome 🐾
  E24.9   Cushing's syndrome, unspecified 🐾

● **E25   Adrenogenital disorders**
  Disorder of production of steroid hormone in adrenal gland
  Includes   adrenogenital syndromes, virilizing or
                  feminizing, whether acquired or due to
                  adrenal hyperplasia consequent on inborn
                  enzyme defects in hormone synthesis
                  female adrenal pseudohermaphroditism
                  female heterosexual precocious pseudopuberty
                  male isosexual precocious pseudopuberty
                  male macrogenitosomia praecox
                  male sexual precocity with adrenal hyperplasia
                  male virilization (female)
  Excludes1   indeterminate sex and pseudohermaphroditism
                  (Q56)
                  chromosomal abnormalities (Q90-Q99)

  **E25.0   Congenital adrenogenital disorders associated with
             enzyme deficiency** 🐾
          Congenital adrenal hyperplasia
          21-Hydroxylase deficiency
          Salt-losing congenital adrenal hyperplasia

  E25.8   Other adrenogenital disorders 🐾
          Idiopathic adrenogenital disorder
          Use additional code for adverse effect, if applicable,
              to identify drug (T36-T50 with fifth or sixth
              character 5)

  E25.9   Adrenogenital disorder, unspecified 🐾
          Adrenogenital syndrome NOS

● **E26   Hyperaldosteronism**
  *Abnormality of electrolyte metabolism caused by excessive secretion
   of aldosterone*

  ● **E26.0   Primary hyperaldosteronism**
      E26.01   Conn's syndrome 🐾
              Code also adrenal adenoma (D35.0-)

      E26.02   Glucocorticoid-remediable aldosteronism 🐾
              Familial aldosteronism type I

      E26.09   Other primary hyperaldosteronism 🐾
              Primary aldosteronism due to adrenal
                  hyperplasia (bilateral)

  E26.1   Secondary hyperaldosteronism 🐾
  ● **E26.8   Other hyperaldosteronism** 🐾
      E26.81   Bartter's syndrome 🐾
      E26.89   Other hyperaldosteronism 🐾

  E26.9   Hyperaldosteronism, unspecified 🐾
          Aldosteronism NOS
          Hyperaldosteronism NOS

● **E27   Other disorders of adrenal gland**
  E27.0   Other adrenocortical overactivity 🐾
          Overproduction of ACTH, not associated with
              Cushing's disease
          Premature adrenarche
          Excludes1   Cushing's syndrome (E24.-)

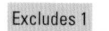

▶ New   ➡ Revised   ~~deleted~~ Deleted   Excludes 1   Excludes 2   Includes   Use additional   Code first   Code also   Key words

OGCR Official Guidelines   X Assign placeholder X   ● Use Additional Character(s)   ▶ Manifestation Code   🐾 Hierarchical Condition Category   **Coding Clinic**

E27.1   **Primary adrenocortical insufficiency** 🕮
     Addison's disease
     Autoimmune adrenalitis
     Excludes1   Addison only phenotype
                adrenoleukodystrophy (E71.528)
                amyloidosis (E85.-)
                tuberculous Addison's disease (A18.7)
                Waterhouse-Friderichsen syndrome
                  (A39.1)

E27.2   **Addisonian crisis** 🕮
     Acute onset of adrenocortical insufficiency
     Adrenal crisis
     Adrenocortical crisis

E27.3   **Drug-induced adrenocortical insufficiency** 🕮
     Use additional code for adverse effect, if applicable,
        to identify drug (T36-T50 with fifth or sixth
        character 5)

● **E27.4**   **Other and unspecified adrenocortical insufficiency**
     Excludes1   adrenoleukodystrophy [Addison-
                Schilder] (E71.528)
                Waterhouse-Friderichsen syndrome
                  (A39.1)

     E27.40   **Unspecified adrenocortical insufficiency** 🕮
           Adrenocortical insufficiency NOS
           Hypoaldosteronism

     E27.49   **Other adrenocortical insufficiency** 🕮
           Adrenal hemorrhage
           Adrenal infarction

E27.5   **Adrenomedullary hyperfunction** 🕮
     Adrenomedullary hyperplasia
     Catecholamine hypersecretion

E27.8   **Other specified disorders of adrenal gland** 🕮
     Abnormality of cortisol-binding globulin

E27.9   **Disorder of adrenal gland, unspecified** 🕮

● **E28**   **Ovarian dysfunction**
     Excludes1   isolated gonadotropin deficiency (E23.0)
                postprocedural ovarian failure (E89.4-)

E28.0   **Estrogen excess** ♀
     Use additional code for adverse effect, if applicable,
        to identify drug (T36-T50 with fifth or
        sixth character 5)

E28.1   **Androgen excess** ♀
     Hypersecretion of ovarian androgens
     Use additional code for adverse effect, if applicable,
        to identify drug (T36-T50 with fifth or
        sixth character 5)

E28.2   **Polycystic ovarian syndrome** ♀
     Sclerocystic ovary syndrome
     Stein-Leventhal syndrome

● **E28.3**   **Primary ovarian failure**
     Excludes1   pure gonadal dysgenesis (Q99.1)
                Turner's syndrome (Q96.-)

     ● **E28.31**   **Premature menopause**
         E28.310   **Symptomatic premature
                 menopause** ♀   A
                 Symptoms such as flushing,
                   sleeplessness, headache, lack of
                   concentration, associated with
                   premature menopause

         E28.319   **Asymptomatic premature
                 menopause** ♀   A
                 Premature menopause NOS

     E28.39   **Other primary ovarian failure** ♀
           Decreased estrogen
           Resistant ovary syndrome

E28.8   **Other ovarian dysfunction** ♀
     Ovarian hyperfunction NOS
     Excludes1   postprocedural ovarian failure (E89.4-)

E28.9   **Ovarian dysfunction, unspecified** ♀

● **E29**   **Testicular dysfunction**
     Excludes1   androgen insensitivity syndrome (E34.5-)
                azoospermia or oligospermia NOS (N46.0-N46.1)
                isolated gonadotropin deficiency (E23.0)
                Klinefelter's syndrome (Q98.0-Q98.1, Q98.4)

E29.0   **Testicular hyperfunction** ♂
     Hypersecretion of testicular hormones

E29.1   **Testicular hypofunction** ♂
     Defective biosynthesis of testicular androgen NOS
     5-delta-Reductase deficiency (with male
        pseudohermaphroditism)
     Testicular hypogonadism NOS
     Use additional code for adverse effect, if applicable,
        to identify drug (T36-T50 with fifth or sixth
        character 5)
     Excludes1   postprocedural testicular hypofunction
                (E89.5)

E29.8   **Other testicular dysfunction** ♂

E29.9   **Testicular dysfunction, unspecified** ♂

● **E30**   **Disorders of puberty, not elsewhere classified**
     E30.0   **Delayed puberty**
         Constitutional delay of puberty
         Delayed sexual development

     E30.1   **Precocious puberty**   P
         Sexual maturation at earlier age than normal, or before age
         8 in girls and 9 in boys, usually hormonal; AKA sexual
         precocity or pubertas praecox
         Precocious menstruation
         Excludes1   Albright (-McCune) (-Sternberg)
                  syndrome (Q78.1)
                  central precocious puberty (E22.8)
                  congenital adrenal hyperplasia (E25.0)
                  female heterosexual precocious
                    pseudopuberty (E25.-)
                  male isosexual precocious pseudopuberty
                    (E25.-)

     E30.8   **Other disorders of puberty**   P
         Premature thelarche

     E30.9   **Disorder of puberty, unspecified**

● **E31**   **Polyglandular dysfunction**
     Excludes1   ataxia telangiectasia [Louis-Bar] (G11.3)
                dystrophia myotonica [Steinert] (G71.11)
                pseudohypoparathyroidism (E20.1)

     E31.0   **Autoimmune polyglandular failure** 🕮
         Schmidt's syndrome

     E31.1   **Polyglandular hyperfunction** 🕮
         Excludes1   multiple endocrine adenomatosis (E31.2-)
                  multiple endocrine neoplasia (E31.2-)

     ● **E31.2**   **Multiple endocrine neoplasia [MEN] syndromes**
         Adenomatous hyperplasia and malignant tumors in
         endocrine glands
         Multiple endocrine adenomatosis
         Code also any associated malignancies and other
           conditions associated with the syndromes

         E31.20   **Multiple endocrine neoplasia [MEN]
                 syndrome, unspecified** 🕮
                 Multiple endocrine adenomatosis NOS
                 Multiple endocrine neoplasia [MEN]
                   syndrome NOS

         E31.21   **Multiple endocrine neoplasia [MEN] type I** 🕮
                 Wermer's syndrome

         E31.22   **Multiple endocrine neoplasia [MEN] type
                 IIA** 🕮
                 Sipple's syndrome

         E31.23   **Multiple endocrine neoplasia [MEN] type
                 IIB** 🕮

     E31.8   **Other polyglandular dysfunction** 🕮

     E31.9   **Polyglandular dysfunction, unspecified** 🕮

N   Newborn Age: 0   **P**   Pediatric Age: 0–17   **M**   Maternity DX: 9–64   **A**   Adult Age: 15–124   ♀   Females Only   ♂   Males Only

● **E32   Diseases of thymus**
    Excludes1   aplasia or hypoplasia of thymus with
          immunodeficiency (D82.1)
          myasthenia gravis (G70.0)

    E32.0   Persistent hyperplasia of thymus 🔖
        Hypertrophy of thymus

    E32.1   Abscess of thymus 🔖

    E32.8   Other diseases of thymus 🔖
        Excludes1   aplasia or hypoplasia with
            immunodeficiency (D82.1)
            thymoma (D15.0)

    E32.9   Disease of thymus, unspecified 🔖

● **E34   Other endocrine disorders**
    Excludes1   pseudohypoparathyroidism (E20.1)

    E34.0   Carcinoid syndrome 🔖
        Note: May be used as an additional code to identify
          functional activity associated with a carcinoid
          tumor.

    E34.1   Other hypersecretion of intestinal hormones

    E34.2   Ectopic hormone secretion, not elsewhere classified
        Excludes1   ectopic ACTH syndrome (E24.3)

    E34.3   Short stature due to endocrine disorder
        Constitutional short stature
        Laron-type short stature
        Excludes1   achondroplastic short stature (Q77.4)
            hypochondroplastic short stature (Q77.4)
            nutritional short stature (E45)
            pituitary short stature (E23.0)
            progeria (E34.8)
            renal short stature (N25.0)
            Russell-Silver syndrome (Q87.19)
            short-limbed stature with
              immunodeficiency (D82.2)
            short stature in specific dysmorphic
              syndromes - code to syndrome - see
              Alphabetical Index
            short stature NOS (R62.52)

    E34.4   Constitutional tall stature 🔖
        Constitutional gigantism

●   **E34.5   Androgen insensitivity syndrome**
        E34.50   Androgen insensitivity syndrome, unspecified
           Androgen insensitivity NOS

        E34.51   Complete androgen insensitivity syndrome
           Complete androgen insensitivity
           de Quervain syndrome
           Goldberg-Maxwell syndrome

        E34.52   Partial androgen insensitivity syndrome
           Partial androgen insensitivity
           Reifenstein syndrome

    E34.8   Other specified endocrine disorders
        Pineal gland dysfunction
        Progeria
        Excludes2   pseudohypoparathyroidism (E20.1)

    E34.9   Endocrine disorder, unspecified
        Endocrine disturbance NOS
        Hormone disturbance NOS

▷ *E35   Disorders of endocrine glands in diseases classified elsewhere*
    Code first underlying disease, such as:
        late congenital syphilis of thymus gland [Dubois disease]
          (A50.5)
    Use additional code, if applicable, to identify:
        sequelae of tuberculosis of other organs (B90.8)
    Excludes1   Echinococcus granulosus infection of thyroid
            gland (B67.3)
            meningococcal hemorrhagic adrenalitis (A39.1)
            syphilis of endocrine gland (A52.79)
            tuberculosis of adrenal gland, except calcification
              (A18.7)
            tuberculosis of endocrine gland NEC (A18.82)
            tuberculosis of thyroid gland (A18.81)
            Waterhouse-Friderichsen syndrome (A39.1)

INTRAOPERATIVE COMPLICATIONS OF ENDOCRINE SYSTEM (E36)

● **E36   Intraoperative complications of endocrine system**
    Excludes2   postprocedural endocrine and metabolic
            complications and disorders, not elsewhere
            classified (E89.-)

●   **E36.0   Intraoperative hemorrhage and hematoma of an
        endocrine system organ or structure complicating a
        procedure**
        Excludes1   intraoperative hemorrhage and
            hematoma of an endocrine system
            organ or structure due to accidental
            puncture or laceration during a
            procedure (E36.1-)

        **E36.01   Intraoperative hemorrhage and hematoma
           of an endocrine system organ or structure
           complicating an endocrine system procedure**
           Coding Clinic: 2020, Q1, P19

        **E36.02   Intraoperative hemorrhage and hematoma
           of an endocrine system organ or structure
           complicating other procedure**

●   **E36.1   Accidental puncture and laceration of an endocrine
        system organ or structure during a procedure**
        **E36.11   Accidental puncture and laceration of an
           endocrine system organ or structure during an
           endocrine system procedure**

        **E36.12   Accidental puncture and laceration of an
           endocrine system organ or structure during
           other procedure**

    E36.8   Other intraoperative complications of endocrine system
        Use additional code, if applicable, to further specify
        disorder

MALNUTRITION (E40-E46)

    Excludes1   intestinal malabsorption (K90.-)
            sequelae of protein-calorie malnutrition (E64.0)
    Excludes2   nutritional anemias (D50-D53)
            starvation (T73.0)

E40   Kwashiorkor 🔖
    Malnutrition produced by severe protein deficiency
    Severe malnutrition with nutritional edema with
        dyspigmentation of skin and hair
    Excludes1   marasmic kwashiorkor (E42)
    Coding Clinic: 22017, Q3, P25

E41   Nutritional marasmus 🔖
    Severe malnutrition with marasmus
    Excludes1   marasmic kwashiorkor (E42)
    Coding Clinic: 2017, Q3, P24-25

E42   Marasmic kwashiorkor 🔖
    Severe protein malnutrition
    Intermediate form severe protein-calorie malnutrition
    Severe protein-calorie malnutrition with signs of both
        kwashiorkor and marasmus
    Coding Clinic: 2017, Q3, P25

E43   Unspecified severe protein-calorie malnutrition 🔖
    Starvation edema
    Coding Clinic: 2020, Q1, P5-6; 2017, Q4, P108-109; 2017, Q3, P25

● **E44   Protein-calorie malnutrition of moderate and mild degree**
    E44.0   Moderate protein-calorie malnutrition 🔖
    E44.1   Mild protein-calorie malnutrition 🔖

**E45   Retarded development following protein-calorie
malnutrition** 🔖
    Nutritional short stature
    Nutritional stunting
    Physical retardation due to malnutrition

E46 Unspecified protein-calorie malnutrition
　　　Malnutrition NOS
　　　Protein-calorie imbalance NOS
　　　Excludes1 nutritional deficiency NOS (E63.9)
　　　Coding Clinic: 2017, Q3, P25

OTHER NUTRITIONAL DEFICIENCIES (E50-E64)

　　　Excludes2 nutritional anemias (D50-D53)

● **E50 Vitamin A deficiency**
　　　Excludes1 sequelae of vitamin A deficiency (E64.1)
　　E50.0 Vitamin A deficiency with conjunctival xerosis
　　E50.1 Vitamin A deficiency with Bitot's spot and conjunctival xerosis
　　　　Bitot's spot in the young child
　　E50.2 Vitamin A deficiency with corneal xerosis
　　E50.3 Vitamin A deficiency with corneal ulceration and xerosis
　　E50.4 Vitamin A deficiency with keratomalacia
　　　　Eye disorder that results in dry cornea caused by vitamin A deficiency
　　E50.5 Vitamin A deficiency with night blindness
　　E50.6 Vitamin A deficiency with xerophthalmic scars of cornea
　　　　Abnormal dryness and thickening of conjunctiva and cornea due to vitamin A deficiency
　　E50.7 Other ocular manifestations of vitamin A deficiency
　　　　Xerophthalmia NOS
　　E50.8 Other manifestations of vitamin A deficiency
　　　　Follicular keratosis
　　　　Xeroderma
　　E50.9 Vitamin A deficiency, unspecified
　　　　Hypovitaminosis A NOS

● **E51 Thiamine deficiency**
　　　Excludes1 sequelae of thiamine deficiency (E64.8)
　● **E51.1 Beriberi**
　　　E51.11 Dry beriberi
　　　　　Thiamine deficiency with nervous system manifestation most often caused by excessive alcohol consumption
　　　　　Beriberi NOS
　　　　　Beriberi with polyneuropathy
　　　E51.12 Wet beriberi
　　　　　Thiamine deficiency with cardiovascular manifestation most often caused by excessive alcohol consumption
　　　　　Beriberi with cardiovascular manifestations
　　　　　Cardiovascular beriberi
　　　　　Shoshin disease
　　E51.2 Wernicke's encephalopathy
　　　　Acute disease of brain due to thiamine deficiency most often associated with excessive alcohol consumption
　　E51.8 Other manifestations of thiamine deficiency
　　E51.9 Thiamine deficiency, unspecified

　 E52 Niacin deficiency [pellagra]
　　　Niacin (-tryptophan) deficiency
　　　Nicotinamide deficiency
　　　Pellagra (alcoholic)
　　　Excludes1 sequelae of niacin deficiency (E64.8)

Item 4–6 Bitot's spots are the result of a buildup of keratin debris found on the superficial surface the conjunctiva; oval, triangular, or irregular in shape; and a sign of vitamin A deficiency and associated with night blindness. The disease may progress to **keratomalacia,** which can result in eventual prolapse of the iris and loss of the lens.

Figure 4-6 Bitot's spot on the conjunctiva.

Figure 4-7 The sharply demarcated, characteristic scaling dermatitis of pellagra. (From James WD, Berger TG, Elston DM: Andrews' Diseases of the Skin: Clinical Dermatology, Philadelphia, Saunders Elsevier, 2006)

Item 4–7 Pellagra is associated with a deficiency of niacin and its precursor, **tryptophan.** Characteristics of the condition include diarrhea, dermatitis on exposed skin surfaces, dementia, and death. It is prevalent in developing countries where nutrition is inadequate. **Beriberi** is associated with thiamine deficiency.

● **E53 Deficiency of other B group vitamins**
　　　Excludes1 sequelae of vitamin B deficiency (E64.8)
　　E53.0 Riboflavin deficiency
　　　　Ariboflavinosis
　　　　Vitamin B2 deficiency
　　E53.1 Pyridoxine deficiency
　　　　Vitamin B6 deficiency
　　　　Excludes1 pyridoxine-responsive sideroblastic anemia (D64.3)
　　E53.8 Deficiency of other specified B group vitamins
　　　　Biotin deficiency
　　　　Cyanocobalamin deficiency
　　　　Folate deficiency
　　　　Folic acid deficiency
　　　　Pantothenic acid deficiency
　　　　Vitamin B12 deficiency
　　　　Excludes1 folate deficiency anemia (D52.-)
　　　　　　　　　vitamin B12 deficiency anemia (D51.-)
　　E53.9 Vitamin B deficiency, unspecified

　 E54 Ascorbic acid deficiency
　　　Deficiency of vitamin C
　　　Scurvy
　　　Excludes1 scorbutic anemia (D53.2)
　　　　　　　sequelae of vitamin C deficiency (E64.2)

● **E55 Vitamin D deficiency**
　　　Excludes1 adult osteomalacia (M83.-)
　　　　　　　osteoporosis (M80.-)
　　　　　　　sequelae of rickets (E64.3)
　　E55.0 Rickets, active
　　　　Infantile osteomalacia
　　　　Juvenile osteomalacia
　　　　Softening of bone
　　　　Excludes1 celiac rickets (K90.0)
　　　　　　　Crohn's rickets (K50.-)
　　　　　　　hereditary vitamin D-dependent rickets (E83.32)
　　　　　　　inactive rickets (E64.3)
　　　　　　　renal rickets (N25.0)
　　　　　　　sequelae of rickets (E64.3)
　　　　　　　vitamin D-resistant rickets (E83.31)
　　E55.9 Vitamin D deficiency, unspecified
　　　　Avitaminosis D

● **E56 Other vitamin deficiencies**
　　　Excludes1 sequelae of other vitamin deficiencies (E64.8)
　　E56.0 Deficiency of vitamin E
　　E56.1 Deficiency of vitamin K
　　　　Excludes1 deficiency of coagulation factor due to vitamin K deficiency (D68.4)
　　　　　　　vitamin K deficiency of newborn (P53)
　　E56.8 Deficiency of other vitamins
　　E56.9 Vitamin deficiency, unspecified

CHAPTER 4 (E00-E89)

CHAPTER 4 (E00-E89)

E58   **Dietary calcium deficiency**
> **Excludes1**   disorders of calcium metabolism (E83.5-)
> sequelae of calcium deficiency (E64.8)

E59   **Dietary selenium deficiency**
> Keshan disease
> **Excludes1**   sequelae of selenium deficiency (E64.8)

E60   **Dietary zinc deficiency**

E61   **Deficiency of other nutrient elements**
> Use additional code for adverse effect, if applicable, to identify drug (T36-T50 with fifth or sixth character 5)
> **Excludes1**   disorders of mineral metabolism (E83.-)
> iodine deficiency related thyroid disorders (E00-E02)
> sequelae of malnutrition and other nutritional deficiencies (E64.-)

E61.0   **Copper deficiency**
E61.1   **Iron deficiency**
> **Excludes1**   iron deficiency anemia (D50.-)

E61.2   **Magnesium deficiency**
E61.3   **Manganese deficiency**
E61.4   **Chromium deficiency**
E61.5   **Molybdenum deficiency**
E61.6   **Vanadium deficiency**
E61.7   **Deficiency of multiple nutrient elements**
E61.8   **Deficiency of other specified nutrient elements**
E61.9   **Deficiency of nutrient element, unspecified**

E63   **Other nutritional deficiencies**
> **Excludes1**
> **Excludes2**   dehydration (E86.0)
> failure to thrive, adult (R62.7)
> failure to thrive, child (R62.51)
> feeding problems in newborn (P92.-)
> sequelae of malnutrition and other nutritional deficiencies (E64.-)

E63.0   **Essential fatty acid [EFA] deficiency**
E63.1   **Imbalance of constituents of food intake**
E63.8   **Other specified nutritional deficiencies**
E63.9   **Nutritional deficiency, unspecified**

E64   **Sequelae of malnutrition and other nutritional deficiencies**
> *Pathological condition resulting from disease, injury, or other trauma*
> **Note:** This category is to be used to indicate conditions in categories E43, E44, E46, E50-E63 as the cause of sequelae, which are themselves classified elsewhere. The "sequelae" include conditions specified as such; they also include the late effects of diseases classifiable to the above categories if the disease itself is no longer present
> *Code first condition resulting from (sequela) of malnutrition and other nutritional deficiencies*

E64.0   **Sequelae of protein-calorie malnutrition** 🦠
> **Excludes2**   retarded development following protein-calorie malnutrition (E45)

E64.1   **Sequelae of vitamin A deficiency**
E64.2   **Sequelae of vitamin C deficiency**
E64.3   **Sequelae of rickets**
E64.8   **Sequelae of other nutritional deficiencies**
E64.9   **Sequelae of unspecified nutritional deficiency**

OVERWEIGHT, OBESITY AND OTHER HYPERALIMENTATION (E65-E68)

E65   **Localized adiposity**
> Fat pad

E66   **Overweight and obesity**
> *Code first obesity complicating pregnancy, childbirth and the puerperium, if applicable (O99.21-)*
> Use additional code to identify body mass index (BMI), if known (Z68.-)
> **Excludes1**   adiposogenital dystrophy (E23.6)
> lipomatosis NOS (E88.2)
> lipomatosis dolorosa [Dercum] (E88.2)
> Prader-Willi syndrome (Q87.11)
> Coding Clinic: 2018, Q4, P80

E66.0   **Obesity due to excess calories**
> **E66.01**   **Morbid (severe) obesity due to excess calories** 🦠
> > **Excludes1**   morbid (severe) obesity with alveolar hypoventilation (E66.2)
> > Coding Clinic: 2018, Q4, P79
> **E66.09**   **Other obesity due to excess calories**

E66.1   **Drug-induced obesity**
> Use additional code for adverse effect, if applicable, to identify drug (T36-T50 with fifth or sixth character 5)

E66.2   **Morbid (severe) obesity with alveolar hypoventilation** 🦠
> *Uncommon condition of unknown cause leading to inadequate ventilation in lungs, even though lungs and airways are normal*
> Obesity hypoventilation syndrome (OHS)
> Pickwickian syndrome

E66.3   **Overweight**
E66.8   **Other obesity**
E66.9   **Obesity, unspecified**
> Obesity NOS
> Coding Clinic: 2021, Q2, P10-11

E67   **Other hyperalimentation**
> *Ingestion of more than optimal amount of nutrients*
> **Excludes1**   hyperalimentation NOS (R63.2)
> sequelae of hyperalimentation (E68)

E67.0   **Hypervitaminosis A**
E67.1   **Hypercarotenemia**
E67.2   **Megavitamin-B6 syndrome**
E67.3   **Hypervitaminosis D**
E67.8   **Other specified hyperalimentation**

E68   **Sequelae of hyperalimentation**
> *Code first condition resulting from (sequela) of hyperalimentation*

METABOLIC DISORDERS (E70-E88)

> **Excludes1**   androgen insensitivity syndrome (E34.5-)
> congenital adrenal hyperplasia (E25.0)
> Ehlers-Danlos syndromes (Q79.6-)
> hemolytic anemias attributable to enzyme disorders (D55.-)
> Marfan's syndrome (Q87.4)
> 5-alpha-reductase deficiency (E29.1)
> **Excludes2**   Ehlers-Danlos syndromes (Q79.6-)

E70   **Disorders of aromatic amino-acid metabolism**
> **E70.0**   **Classical phenylketonuria** 🦠
> > *Inherited disorder that increases to harmful levels amino acid phenylalanine*
> **E70.1**   **Other hyperphenylalaninemias** 🦠

● **E70.2**   **Disorders of tyrosine metabolism**
     Excludes1   transitory tyrosinemia of newborn (P74.5)
     E70.20   **Disorder of tyrosine metabolism, unspecified**
         Tyrosine: Nonessential amino acid occurring in most proteins
     E70.21   **Tyrosinemia** 🔎
         Congenital amino acid metabolism
         Hypertyrosinemia
     E70.29   **Other disorders of tyrosine metabolism** 🔎
         Alkaptonuria
         Ochronosis

● **E70.3**   **Albinism**
     Congenital condition of reduced or absent pigment in eyes, skin, and hair
     E70.30   **Albinism, unspecified** 🔎
    ● **E70.31**   **Ocular albinism**
         E70.310   **X-linked ocular albinism** 🔎
         E70.311   **Autosomal recessive ocular albinism** 🔎
         E70.318   **Other ocular albinism** 🔎
         E70.319   **Ocular albinism, unspecified** 🔎
    ● **E70.32**   **Oculocutaneous albinism**
         Partial or total lack of melanin pigment in eyes
         Excludes1   Chediak-Higashi syndrome (E70.330)
                 Hermansky-Pudlak syndrome (E70.331)
         E70.320   **Tyrosinase negative oculocutaneous albinism** 🔎
             Albinism I
             Oculocutaneous albinism ty-neg
         E70.321   **Tyrosinase positive oculocutaneous albinism** 🔎
             Albinism II
             Oculocutaneous albinism ty-pos
         E70.328   **Other oculocutaneous albinism** 🔎
             Cross syndrome
         E70.329   **Oculocutaneous albinism, unspecified** 🔎
    ● **E70.33**   **Albinism with hematologic abnormality**
         E70.330   **Chediak-Higashi syndrome** 🔎
         E70.331   **Hermansky-Pudlak syndrome** 🔎
         E70.338   **Other albinism with hematologic abnormality** 🔎
         E70.339   **Albinism with hematologic abnormality, unspecified** 🔎
     E70.39   **Other specified albinism** 🔎
         Piebaldism

● **E70.4**   **Disorders of histidine metabolism**
     E70.40   **Disorders of histidine metabolism, unspecified** 🔎
     E70.41   **Histidinemia** 🔎
     E70.49   **Other disorders of histidine metabolism** 🔎

   E70.5   **Disorders of tryptophan metabolism** 🔎

● **E70.8**   **Other disorders of aromatic amino-acid metabolism** 🔎
     E70.81   **Aromatic L-amino acid decarboxylase deficiency**
         AADC deficiency
     E70.89   **Other disorders of aromatic amino-acid metabolism**

   E70.9   **Disorder of aromatic amino-acid metabolism, unspecified** 🔎

● **E71**   **Disorders of branched-chain amino-acid metabolism and fatty-acid metabolism**
   E71.0   **Maple-syrup-urine disease** 🔎
     Due to defect in amino acid catabolism, causing severe ketoacidosis with smell of maple syrup in urine and on body
    ● **E71.1**   **Other disorders of branched-chain amino-acid metabolism**
     ● **E71.11**   **Branched-chain organic acidurias**
         E71.110   **Isovaleric acidemia** 🔎
         E71.111   **3-methylglutaconic aciduria** 🔎
         E71.118   **Other branched-chain organic acidurias** 🔎
     ● **E71.12**   **Disorders of propionate metabolism**
         E71.120   **Methylmalonic acidemia** 🔎
         E71.121   **Propionic acidemia** 🔎
         E71.128   **Other disorders of propionate metabolism** 🔎
     E71.19   **Other disorders of branched-chain amino-acid metabolism** 🔎
         Hyperleucine-isoleucinemia
         Hypervalinemia
   E71.2   **Disorder of branched-chain amino-acid metabolism, unspecified** 🔎
    ● **E71.3**   **Disorders of fatty-acid metabolism**
     Excludes1   peroxisomal disorders (E71.5)
               Refsum's disease (G60.1)
               Schilder's disease (G37.0)
     Excludes2   carnitine deficiency due to inborn error of metabolism (E71.42)
     E71.30   **Disorder of fatty-acid metabolism, unspecified**
    ● **E71.31**   **Disorders of fatty-acid oxidation**
         E71.310   **Long chain/very long chain acyl CoA dehydrogenase deficiency** 🔎
             LCAD
             VLCAD
         E71.311   **Medium chain acyl CoA dehydrogenase deficiency** 🔎
             MCAD
         E71.312   **Short chain acyl CoA dehydrogenase deficiency** 🔎
             SCAD
         E71.313   **Glutaric aciduria type II** 🔎
             Glutaric aciduria type II A
             Glutaric aciduria type II B
             Glutaric aciduria type II C
             Excludes1   glutaric aciduria (type 1) NOS (E72.3)
         E71.314   **Muscle carnitine palmitoyltransferase deficiency** 🔎
         E71.318   **Other disorders of fatty-acid oxidation** 🔎
     E71.32   **Disorders of ketone metabolism** 🔎
     E71.39   **Other disorders of fatty-acid metabolism** 🔎
    ● **E71.4**   **Disorders of carnitine metabolism**
     Excludes1   muscle carnitine palmitoyltransferase deficiency (E71.314)
     E71.40   **Disorder of carnitine metabolism, unspecified** 🔎
     E71.41   **Primary carnitine deficiency** 🔎
     E71.42   **Carnitine deficiency due to inborn errors of metabolism** 🔎
         Code also associated inborn error or metabolism
     E71.43   **Iatrogenic carnitine deficiency** 🔎
         Iatrogenic: Outcomes from activity of physicians
         Carnitine deficiency due to hemodialysis
         Carnitine deficiency due to Valproic acid therapy

CHAPTER 4 (E00–E89)

● E71.44 Other secondary carnitine deficiency
    E71.440 Ruvalcaba-Myhre-Smith syndrome 🐾
    E71.448 Other secondary carnitine deficiency 🐾

● E71.5 Peroxisomal disorders
    Class of conditions which lead to disorders of lipid metabolism
    Excludes1 Schilder's disease (G37.0)

    E71.50 Peroxisomal disorder, unspecified 🐾
● E71.51 Disorders of peroxisome biogenesis
    Group 1 peroxisomal disorders
    Excludes1 Refsum's disease (G60.1)
    E71.510 Zellweger syndrome 🐾
    E71.511 Neonatal adrenoleukodystrophy 🐾
        Excludes1 X-linked adrenoleuko-
                       dystrophy
                       (E71.42-)
    E71.518 Other disorders of peroxisome biogenesis 🐾
● E71.52 X-linked adrenoleukodystrophy
    E71.520 Childhood cerebral X-linked adrenoleukodystrophy 🐾
    E71.521 Adolescent X-linked adrenoleukodystrophy 🐾
    E71.522 Adrenomyeloneuropathy 🐾
    E71.528 Other X-linked adrenoleukodystrophy 🐾
        Addison only phenotype adrenoleukodystrophy
        Addison-Schilder adrenoleukodystrophy
    E71.529 X-linked adrenoleukodystrophy, unspecified type 🐾
    E71.53 Other group 2 peroxisomal disorders 🐾
● E71.54 Other peroxisomal disorders
    E71.540 Rhizomelic chondrodysplasia punctata 🐾
        Rare, severe, inherited disorder with limb shortening, bone and cartilage abnormalities, abnormal facial appearance, severe mental retardation, psychomotor retardation, and cataracts
        Excludes1 chondrodysplasia punctata NOS (Q77.3)
    E71.541 Zellweger-like syndrome 🐾
    E71.542 Other group 3 peroxisomal disorders 🐾
    E71.548 Other peroxisomal disorders 🐾

● E72 Other disorders of amino-acid metabolism
    Excludes1 disorders of:
        aromatic amino-acid metabolism (E70.-)
        branched-chain amino-acid metabolism (E71.0-E71.2)
        fatty-acid metabolism (E71.3)
        purine and pyrimidine metabolism (E79.-)
        gout (M1A.-, M10.-)
● E72.0 Disorders of amino-acid transport
    Excludes1 disorders of tryptophan metabolism (E70.5)
    E72.00 Disorders of amino-acid transport, unspecified 🐾
    E72.01 Cystinuria 🐾
        Hereditary aminoaciduria due to impairment of renal transport with predominant symptom of urinary cystine calculi
    E72.02 Hartnup's disease 🐾
        Inborn error of metabolism

E72.03 Lowe's syndrome 🐾
    X-linked disorder with rickets, hydrophthalmia, congenital glaucoma, cataracts, mental retardation, and renal tubule dysfunction
    Use additional code for associated glaucoma (H42)
E72.04 Cystinosis 🐾
    Genetic disease with excessive depostits of amino acid cystine in cells
    Fanconi (-de Toni) (-Debré) syndrome with cystinosis
    Excludes1 Fanconi (-de Toni) (-Debré) syndrome without cystinosis (E72.09)
E72.09 Other disorders of amino-acid transport 🐾
    Fanconi (-de Toni) (-Debré) syndrome, unspecified
● E72.1 Disorders of sulfur-bearing amino-acid metabolism
    Excludes1 cystinosis (E72.04)
                   cystinuria (E72.01)
                   transcobalamin II deficiency (D51.2)
    E72.10 Disorders of sulfur-bearing amino-acid metabolism, unspecified 🐾
    E72.11 Homocystinuria 🐾
        Cystathionine synthase deficiency
    E72.12 Methylenetetrahydrofolate reductase deficiency 🐾
    E72.19 Other disorders of sulfur-bearing amino-acid metabolism 🐾
        Cystathioninuria
        Methioninemia
        Sulfite oxidase deficiency
● E72.2 Disorders of urea cycle metabolism
    Excludes1 disorders of ornithine metabolism (E72.4)
    E72.20 Disorder of urea cycle metabolism, unspecified 🐾
        Hyperammonemia
        Elevated levels of ammonia
        Excludes1 hyperammonemia-hyperornithinemia-homocitrullinemia syndrome E72.4
                       transient hyperammonemia of newborn (P74.6)
    E72.21 Argininemia 🐾
        Disorder in which deficiency of enzyme arginase causes build-up of arginine and ammonia in blood
    E72.22 Arginosuccinic aciduria 🐾
        Gene disorder of urea cycle resulting accumulation of ammonia
    E72.23 Citrullinemia 🐾
        Urea cycle disorder that causes ammonia and other toxic substances to accumulate in blood
    E72.29 Other disorders of urea cycle metabolism 🐾
E72.3 Disorders of lysine and hydroxylysine metabolism 🐾
    Glutaric aciduria NOS
    Glutaric aciduria (type I)
    Hydroxylysinemia
    Hyperlysinemia
    Excludes1 glutaric aciduria type II (E71.313)
                   Refsum's disease (G60.1)
                   Zellweger syndrome (E71.510)
E72.4 Disorders of ornithine metabolism 🐾
    Hyperammonemia-Hyperornithinemia-Homocitrullinemia syndrome
    Ornithinemia (types I, II)
    Ornithine transcarbamylase deficiency
    Excludes1 hereditary choroidal dystrophy (H31.2-)

▶ New ➥ Revised ~~deleted~~ Deleted Excludes 1 Excludes 2 Includes Use additional Code first Code also Key words
OGCR Official Guidelines **X** Assign placeholder X ● Use Additional Character(s) ▶ Manifestation Code 🐾 Hierarchical Condition Category **Coding Clinic**

● **E72.5   Disorders of glycine metabolism**
     E72.50   Disorder of glycine metabolism, unspecified 🦴
     E72.51   Non-ketotic hyperglycinemia 🦴
     E72.52   Trimethylaminuria 🦴
     E72.53   Primary hyperoxaluria 🦴
            Oxalosis
            Oxaluria
     E72.59   Other disorders of glycine metabolism 🦴
            D-glycericacidemia
            Hyperhydroxyprolinemia
            Hyperprolinemia (types I, II)
            Sarcosinemia

● **E72.8   Other specified disorders of amino-acid metabolism 🦴**
     E72.81   Disorders of gamma aminobutyric acid metabolism 🦴
            4-hydroxybutyric aciduria
            Disorders of GABA metabolism
            GABA metabolic defect
            GABA transaminase deficiency
            GABA-T deficiency
            Gamma-hydroxybutyric aciduria
            SSADHD
            Succinic semialdehyde dehydrogenase deficiency
     E72.89   Other specified disorders of amino-acid metabolism 🦴
            Disorders of beta-amino-acid metabolism
            Disorders of gamma-glutamyl cycle
     E72.9   Disorder of amino-acid metabolism, unspecified 🦴

● **E73   Lactose intolerance**
     Intolerance for lactose, due to inherited deficiency of lactase activity in intestinal mucosa
     E73.0   Congenital lactase deficiency
     E73.1   Secondary lactase deficiency
     E73.8   Other lactose intolerance
     E73.9   Lactose intolerance, unspecified

● **E74   Other disorders of carbohydrate metabolism**
     Excludes1   diabetes mellitus (E08-E13)
            hypoglycemia NOS (E16.2)
            increased secretion of glucagon (E16.3)
            mucopolysaccharidosis (E76.0-E76.3)
   ● **E74.0   Glycogen storage disease**
     E74.00   Glycogen storage disease, unspecified 🦴
     E74.01   von Gierke's disease 🦴
            Type I glycogen storage disease
     E74.02   Pompe disease 🦴
            Cardiac glycogenosis
            Type II glycogen storage disease
     E74.03   Cori disease 🦴
            Forbes' disease
            Type III glycogen storage disease
     E74.04   McArdle disease 🦴
            Type V glycogen storage disease
     E74.09   Other glycogen storage disease 🦴
            Andersen disease
            Hers disease
            Tauri disease
            Glycogen storage disease, types 0, IV, VI-XI
            Liver phosphorylase deficiency
            Muscle phosphofructokinase deficiency
   ● **E74.1   Disorders of fructose metabolism**
     Excludes1   muscle phosphofructokinase deficiency (E74.09)
     E74.10   Disorder of fructose metabolism, unspecified
     E74.11   Essential fructosuria
            Fructokinase deficiency
     E74.12   Hereditary fructose intolerance
            Fructosemia
     E74.19   Other disorders of fructose metabolism
            Fructose-1, 6-diphosphatase deficiency

● **E74.2   Disorders of galactose metabolism**
     E74.20   Disorders of galactose metabolism, unspecified 🦴
     E74.21   Galactosemia
            Genetic disorders resulting from defective simple sugar (galactose) metabolism
     E74.29   Other disorders of galactose metabolism 🦴
            Galactokinase deficiency
● **E74.3   Other disorders of intestinal carbohydrate absorption**
     Excludes2   lactose intolerance (E73.-)
     E74.31   Sucrase-isomaltase deficiency
            Deficiency in metabolism in intestinal mucosa results in malabsorption of sucrose and starch
     E74.39   Other disorders of intestinal carbohydrate absorption
            Disorder of intestinal carbohydrate absorption NOS
            Glucose-galactose malabsorption
            Sucrase deficiency
● **E74.4   Disorders of pyruvate metabolism and gluconeogenesis 🦴**
     Deficiency of phosphoenolpyruvate carboxykinase
     Deficiency of pyruvate carboxylase
     Deficiency of pyruvate dehydrogenase
     Excludes1   disorders of pyruvate metabolism and gluconeogenesis with anemia (D55.-)
            Leigh's syndrome (G31.82)
● **E74.8   Other specified disorders of carbohydrate metabolism 🦴**
   ● **E74.81   Disorders of glucose transport, not elsewhere classified**
       E74.810   Glucose transporter protein type 1 deficiency
            De Vivo syndrome
            Glucose transport defect, blood-brain barrier
            GLUT1 deficiency
            GLUT1 deficiency syndrome 1, infantile onset
            GLUT1 deficiency syndrome 2, childhood onset
       E74.818   Other disorders of glucose transport
            (Familial) renal glycosuria
       E74.819   Disorders of glucose transport, unspecified
     E74.89   Other specified disorders of carbohydrate metabolism
            Essential pentosuria
     E74.9   Disorder of carbohydrate metabolism, unspecified 🦴
● **E75   Disorders of sphingolipid metabolism and other lipid storage disorders**
     Excludes1   mucolipidosis, types I-III (E77.0-E77.1)
            Refsum's disease (G60.1)
   ● **E75.0   GM2 gangliosidosis**
     Rare metabolic disorder that causes destruction of nerve cells of brain and spinal cord
     E75.00   GM2 gangliosidosis, unspecified
     E75.01   Sandhoff disease
     E75.02   Tay-Sachs disease
     E75.09   Other GM2 gangliosidosis
            Adult GM2 gangliosidosis
            Juvenile GM2 gangliosidosis
   ● **E75.1   Other and unspecified gangliosidosis**
     E75.10   Unspecified gangliosidosis
            Gangliosidosis NOS
     E75.11   Mucolipidosis IV
            Disorder with symptoms of psychomotor retardation and severe visual impairment
     E75.19   Other gangliosidosis
            GM1 gangliosidosis
            GM3 gangliosidosis

CHAPTER 4 (E00-E89)

Item 4–8 Leukodystrophy is characterized by degeneration and/or failure of the myelin formation of the central nervous system and sometimes of the peripheral nervous system. The disease is inherited and progressive.

● **E75.2 Other sphingolipidosis**
Lysosomal (a particle in a cytoplasm cell that contains digestive enzymes) storage diseases with symptoms of abnormal storage of amino acids

    Excludes1   adrenoleukodystrophy [Addison-Schilder] (E71.528)

    E75.21 Fabry (-Anderson) disease 🔢

    E75.22 Gaucher disease 🔢

    E75.23 Krabbe disease

● **E75.24 Niemann-Pick disease**
     ▶Acid sphingomyelinase deficiency (ASMD)

      E75.240 Niemann-Pick disease type A 🔢
       ▶Acid sphingomyelinase deficiency type A (ASMD type A)
       ▶Infantile neurovisceral acid sphingomyelinase deficiency

      E75.241 Niemann-Pick disease type B 🔢
       ▶Acid sphingomyelinase deficiency type B (ASMD type B)
       ▶Chronic visceral acid sphingomyelinase deficiency

      E75.242 Niemann-Pick disease type C 🔢

      E75.243 Niemann-Pick disease type D 🔢

   ▶ **E75.244 Niemann-Pick disease type A/B**
       ▶Acid sphingomyelinase deficiency type A/B (ASMD type A/B)
       ▶Chronic neurovisceral acid sphingomyelinase deficiency

      E75.248 Other Niemann-Pick disease 🔢

      E75.249 Niemann-Pick disease, unspecified 🔢
       ▶Acid sphingomyelinase deficiency (ASMD) NOS

    E75.25 Metachromatic leukodystrophy

    E75.26 Sulfatase deficiency
      Multiple sulfatase deficiency (MSD)

    E75.29 Other sphingolipidosis
      Farber's syndrome
      Sulfatide lipidosis

   E75.3 Sphingolipidosis, unspecified 🔢

   E75.4 Neuronal ceroid lipofuscinosis
      Batten disease
      Bielschowsky-Jansky disease
      Kufs disease
      Spielmeyer-Vogt disease

   E75.5 Other lipid storage disorders
      Cerebrotendinous cholesterosis [van Bogaert-Scherer-Epstein]
      Wolman's disease

   E75.6 Lipid storage disorder, unspecified

● **E76 Disorders of glycosaminoglycan metabolism**

● **E76.0 Mucopolysaccharidosis, type I**
Inborn metabolic disorder of enzymes that break down carbohydrates

    E76.01 Hurler's syndrome 🔢

    E76.02 Hurler-Scheie syndrome 🔢

    E76.03 Scheie's syndrome 🔢

   E76.1 Mucopolysaccharidosis, type II 🔢
Inborn metabolic disorder of enzymes that break down carbohydrates occurs in 2-4 year old males
      Hunter's syndrome

● **E76.2 Other mucopolysaccharidoses**

● **E76.21 Morquio mucopolysaccharidoses**

      E76.210 Morquio A mucopolysaccharidoses 🔢
        Classic Morquio syndrome
        Morquio syndrome A
        Mucopolysaccharidosis, type IVA

      E76.211 Morquio B mucopolysaccharidoses 🔢
        Morquio-like mucopolysaccharidoses
        Morquio-like syndrome
        Morquio syndrome B
        Mucopolysaccharidosis, type IVB

      E76.219 Morquio mucopolysaccharidoses, unspecified 🔢
        Morquio syndrome
        Mucopolysaccharidosis, type IV

    E76.22 Sanfilippo mucopolysaccharidoses 🔢
      Mucopolysaccharidosis, type III (A) (B) (C) (D)
      Sanfilippo A syndrome
      Sanfilippo B syndrome
      Sanfilippo C syndrome
      Sanfilippo D syndrome

    E76.29 Other mucopolysaccharidoses 🔢
      beta-Glucuronidase deficiency
      Maroteaux-Lamy (mild) (severe) syndrome
      Mucopolysaccharidosis, types VI, VII

   E76.3 Mucopolysaccharidosis, unspecified 🔢

   E76.8 Other disorders of glucosaminoglycan metabolism 🔢

   E76.9 Glucosaminoglycan metabolism disorder, unspecified 🔢

● **E77 Disorders of glycoprotein metabolism**

   E77.0 Defects in post-translational modification of lysosomal enzymes 🔢
      Mucolipidosis II [I-cell disease]
      Mucolipidosis III [pseudo-Hurler polydystrophy]

   E77.1 Defects in glycoprotein degradation 🔢
      Aspartylglucosaminuria
      Fucosidosis
      Mannosidosis
      Sialidosis [mucolipidosis I]

   E77.8 Other disorders of glycoprotein metabolism 🔢

   E77.9 Disorder of glycoprotein metabolism, unspecified 🔢

● **E78 Disorders of lipoprotein metabolism and other lipidemias**
    Excludes1   sphingolipidosis (E75.0-E75.3)

● **E78.0 Pure hypercholesterolemia**
    Coding Clinic: 2016, Q4, P13

      E78.00 Pure hypercholesterolemia, unspecified
        Fredrickson's hyperlipoproteinemia, type IIa
        Hyperbetalipoproteinemia
        Low-density-lipoprotein-type [LDL] hyperlipoproteinemia
        (Pure) hypercholesterolemia NOS
        Coding Clinic: 2016, Q4, P13

      E78.01 Familial hypercholesterolemia
        Coding Clinic: 2016, Q4, P13

   E78.1 Pure hyperglyceridemia
      Elevated fasting triglycerides
      Endogenous hyperglyceridemia
      Fredrickson's hyperlipoproteinemia, type IV
      Hyperlipidemia, group B
      Hyperprebetalipoproteinemia
      Very-low-density-lipoprotein-type [VLDL] hyperlipoproteinemia

   E78.2 Mixed hyperlipidemia
      Broad- or floating-betalipoproteinemia
      Combined hyperlipidemia NOS
      Elevated cholesterol with elevated triglycerides NEC
      Fredrickson's hyperlipoproteinemia, type IIb or III
      Hyperbetalipoproteinemia with prebetalipoproteinemia
      Hypercholesteremia with endogenous hyperglyceridemia
      Hyperlipidemia, group C
      Tubo-eruptive xanthoma
      Xanthoma tuberosum

    Excludes1   cerebrotendinous cholesterosis [van Bogaert-Scherer-Epstein] (E75.5)
         familial combined hyperlipidemia (E78.49)

   E78.3 Hyperchylomicronemia
      Chylomicron retention disease
      Fredrickson's hyperlipoproteinemia, type I or V
      Hyperlipidemia, group D
      Mixed hyperglyceridemia

CHAPTER 4 (E00-E89)

● **E78.4**   **Other hyperlipidemia**

     E78.41   **Elevated Lipoprotein(a)**
          Elevated Lp(a)

     E78.49   **Other hyperlipidemia**
          Familial combined hyperlipidemia

E78.5   **Hyperlipidemia, unspecified**

E78.6   **Lipoprotein deficiency**
     Abetalipoproteinemia
     Depressed HDL cholesterol
     High-density lipoprotein deficiency
     Hypoalphalipoproteinemia
     Hypobetalipoproteinemia (familial)
     Lecithin cholesterol acyltransferase deficiency
     Tangier disease

● **E78.7**   **Disorders of bile acid and cholesterol metabolism**
     Excludes1   Niemann-Pick disease type C (E75.242)

     E78.70   **Disorder of bile acid and cholesterol metabolism, unspecified**

     E78.71   **Barth syndrome**

     E78.72   **Smith-Lemli-Opitz syndrome**

     E78.79   **Other disorders of bile acid and cholesterol metabolism**

● **E78.8**   **Other disorders of lipoprotein metabolism**

     E78.81   **Lipoid dermatoarthritis**

     E78.89   **Other lipoprotein metabolism disorders**

E78.9   **Disorder of lipoprotein metabolism, unspecified**

● **E79**   **Disorders of purine and pyrimidine metabolism**
Purines, along with pyrimidines, signal RNA and DNA production
     Excludes1   Ataxia-telangiectasia (Q87.19)
          Bloom's syndrome (Q82.8)
          Cockayne's syndrome (Q87.19)
          calculus of kidney (N20.0)
          combined immunodeficiency disorders (D81.-)
          Fanconi's anemia (D61.09)
          gout (M1A.-, M10.-)
          orotaciduric anemia (D53.0)
          progeria (E34.8)
          Werner's syndrome (E34.8)
          xeroderma pigmentosum (Q82.1)

E79.0   **Hyperuricemia without signs of inflammatory arthritis and tophaceous disease**
     Asymptomatic hyperuricemia

E79.1   **Lesch-Nyhan syndrome** 🔊
     HGPRT deficiency

E79.2   **Myoadenylate deaminase deficiency** 🔊

E79.8   **Other disorders of purine and pyrimidine metabolism** 🔊
     Hereditary xanthinuria

E79.9   **Disorder of purine and pyrimidine metabolism, unspecified** 🔊

● **E80**   **Disorders of porphyrin and bilirubin metabolism**
Group of chemical compounds in RBCs that combine with iron to form heme
     Includes   defects of catalase and peroxidase

E80.0   **Hereditary erythropoietic porphyria** 🔊
     Congenital erythropoietic porphyria
     Erythropoietic protoporphyria

E80.1   **Porphyria cutanea tarda** 🔊

● **E80.2**   **Other and unspecified porphyria**

     E80.20   **Unspecified porphyria** 🔊
          Porphyria NOS

     E80.21   **Acute intermittent (hepatic) porphyria** 🔊

     E80.29   **Other porphyria** 🔊
          Hereditary coproporphyria

E80.3   **Defects of catalase and peroxidase** 🔊
     Acatalasia [Takahara]

E80.4   **Gilbert syndrome**

E80.5   **Crigler-Najjar syndrome**

E80.6   **Other disorders of bilirubin metabolism**
     Dubin-Johnson syndrome
     Rotor's syndrome

E80.7   **Disorder of bilirubin metabolism, unspecified**

● **E83**   **Disorders of mineral metabolism**
     Excludes1   dietary mineral deficiency (E58-E61)
          parathyroid disorders (E20-E21)
          vitamin D deficiency (E55.-)

● **E83.0**   **Disorders of copper metabolism**

     E83.00   **Disorder of copper metabolism, unspecified**

     E83.01   **Wilson's disease**
          Code also associated Kayser Fleischer ring (H18.04-)

     E83.09   **Other disorders of copper metabolism**
          Menkes' (kinky hair) (steely hair) disease

● **E83.1**   **Disorders of iron metabolism**
     Excludes1   iron deficiency anemia (D50.-)
          sideroblastic anemia (D64.0-D64.3)

     E83.10   **Disorder of iron metabolism, unspecified**

     ● **E83.11**   **Hemochromatosis**
          Excludes1   GALD (P78.84)
              Gestational alloimmune liver disease (P78.84)
              Neonatal hemochromatosis (P78.84)

         E83.110   **Hereditary hemochromatosis** 🔊
              Bronzed diabetes
              Pigmentary cirrhosis (of liver)
              Primary (hereditary) hemochromatosis

         E83.111   **Hemochromatosis due to repeated red blood cell transfusions**
              Iron overload due to repeated red blood cell transfusions
              Transfusion (red blood cell) associated hemochromatosis

         E83.118   **Other hemochromatosis**

         E83.119   **Hemochromatosis, unspecified**

     E83.19   **Other disorders of iron metabolism**
          Use additional code, if applicable, for idiopathic pulmonary hemosiderosis (J84.03)

E83.2   **Disorders of zinc metabolism**
     Acrodermatitis enteropathica

● **E83.3**   **Disorders of phosphorus metabolism and phosphatases**
     Excludes1   adult osteomalacia (M83.-)
          osteoporosis (M80.-)

     E83.30   **Disorder of phosphorus metabolism, unspecified**

     E83.31   **Familial hypophosphatemia**
          Vitamin D-resistant osteomalacia
          Vitamin D-resistant rickets
          Excludes1   vitamin D-deficiency rickets (E55.0)

     E83.32   **Hereditary vitamin D-dependent rickets (type 1) (type 2)**
          25-hydroxyvitamin D 1-alpha-hydroxylase deficiency
          Pseudovitamin D deficiency
          Vitamin D receptor defect

     E83.39   **Other disorders of phosphorus metabolism**
          Acid phosphatase deficiency
          Hypophosphatasia

● **E83.4**   **Disorders of magnesium metabolism**

     E83.40   **Disorders of magnesium metabolism, unspecified**

     E83.41   **Hypermagnesemia**
          Coding Clinic: 2016, Q4, P55

     E83.42   **Hypomagnesemia**

     E83.49   **Other disorders of magnesium metabolism**

N Newborn Age: 0   **P** Pediatric Age: 0–17   **M** Maternity DX: 9–64   **A** Adult Age: 15–124   ♀ Females Only   ♂ Males Only

CHAPTER 4 (E00-E89)

761

CHAPTER 4 (E00-E89)

● **E83.5 Disorders of calcium metabolism**
    Excludes1 chondrocalcinosis (M11.1-M11.2)
                   hungry bone syndrome (E83.81)
                   hyperparathyroidism (E21.0-E21.3)

    E83.50 **Unspecified disorder of calcium metabolism**

    E83.51 **Hypocalcemia**

    E83.52 **Hypercalcemia**
          Familial hypocalciuric hypercalcemia

    E83.59 **Other disorders of calcium metabolism**
          Idiopathic hypercalciuria

● **E83.8 Other disorders of mineral metabolism**
    E83.81 **Hungry bone syndrome**
    E83.89 **Other disorders of mineral metabolism**

  E83.9 **Disorder of mineral metabolism, unspecified**

● **E84 Cystic fibrosis**
    Includes mucoviscidosis

  Code also exocrine pancreatic insufficiency (K86.81)

  E84.0 **Cystic fibrosis with pulmonary manifestations** 🐾
         Use additional code to identify any infectious organism
            present, such as:
            Pseudomonas (B96.5)
            Coding Clinic: 2021, Q1, P24

● **E84.1 Cystic fibrosis with intestinal manifestations**
    E84.11 **Meconium ileus in cystic fibrosis** 🐾   N
         Excludes1 meconium ileus not due to cystic
                    fibrosis (P76.0)

    E84.19 **Cystic fibrosis with other intestinal
           manifestations** 🐾
          Distal intestinal obstruction syndrome

  E84.8 **Cystic fibrosis with other manifestations** 🐾

  E84.9 **Cystic fibrosis, unspecified** 🐾

● **E85 Amyloidosis**
    *A disorder resulting from the abnormal deposition of a particular
    protein (amyloid) into tissues of the body*

    Excludes2 Alzheimer's disease (G30.0-)

  E85.0 **Non-neuropathic heredofamilial amyloidosis** 🐾
        Hereditary amyloid nephropathy

        Code also associated disorders, such as:
          autoinflammatory syndromes (M04.-)

        Excludes2 Transthyretin-related (ATTR) familial
                 amyloid cardiomyopathy (E85.4)

  E85.1 **Neuropathic heredofamilial amyloidosis** 🐾
        Amyloid polyneuropathy (Portuguese)
        Transthyretin-related (ATTR) familial amyloid
          polyneuropathy
        Coding Clinic: 2012, Q4, P100

  E85.2 **Heredofamilial amyloidosis, unspecified** 🐾

  E85.3 **Secondary systemic amyloidosis** 🐾
        Hemodialysis-associated amyloidosis

  E85.4 **Organ-limited amyloidosis** 🐾
        Localized amyloidosis
        Transthyretin-related (ATTR) familial amyloid
          cardiomyopathy

● **E85.8 Other amyloidosis**
    E85.81 **Light chain (AL) amyloidosis** 🐾

    E85.82 **Wild-type transthyretin-related (ATTR)
          amyloidosis** 🐾
          Senile systemic amyloidosis (SSA)

    E85.89 **Other amyloidosis** 🐾

  E85.9 **Amyloidosis, unspecified** 🐾

Item 4–9 Circulating fluid volume is regulated by the amount of water and sodium ingested, excreted by the kidneys into the urine, and lost through the gastrointestinal tract, lungs, and skin. To maintain blood volume within a normal range, the kidneys regulate the amount of water and sodium lost into the urine. Too much **(fluid overload)** or too little fluid volume **(volume depletion)** will affect blood pressure. Severe cases of vomiting, diarrhea, bleeding, and burns (fluid loss through exposed burn surface area) can contribute to fluid loss. Internal body environment must maintain a precise balance (homeostasis) between too much fluid and too little fluid. This complex balancing mechanism is critical to good health.

● **E86 Volume depletion**
    Excludes1 dehydration of newborn (P74.1)
               postprocedural hypovolemic shock (T81.19)
               traumatic hypovolemic shock (T79.4)

    Excludes2 hypovolemic shock NOS (R57.1)

  Use additional code(s) for any associated disorders of
     electrolyte and acid-base balance (E87.-)
  Coding Clinic: 2019, Q2, P7

  E86.0 **Dehydration**
        Excessive loss of body water
        Coding Clinic: 2019, Q2, P7-8

  E86.1 **Hypovolemia**
        Diminished volume of circulating blood
        Depletion of volume of plasma

  E86.9 **Volume depletion, unspecified**
        Coding Clinic: 2019, Q2, P7-8

● **E87 Other disorders of fluid, electrolyte and acid-base balance**
    Excludes1 diabetes insipidus (E23.2)
            electrolyte imbalance associated with
               hyperemesis gravidarum (O21.1)
            electrolyte imbalance following ectopic or molar
               pregnancy (O08.5)
            familial periodic paralysis (G72.3)

  E87.0 **Hyperosmolality and hypernatremia**
        Sodium [Na] excess
        Sodium [Na] overload
        Coding Clinic: 2018, Q2, P6

  E87.1 **Hypo-osmolality and hyponatremia**
        Sodium [Na] deficiency

       Excludes1 syndrome of inappropriate secretion of
                 antidiuretic hormone (E22.2)
        Coding Clinic: 2018, Q2, P6

  E87.2 **Acidosis**
        Acidosis NOS
        Lactic acidosis
        Metabolic acidosis
        Respiratory acidosis

    ⇒ **Excludes1** diabetic acidosis - see categories E08-E10,
                 E11, E13 with ketoacidosis

  E87.3 **Alkalosis**
        Alkalosis NOS
        Metabolic alkalosis
        Respiratory alkalosis

  E87.4 **Mixed disorder of acid-base balance**

  E87.5 **Hyperkalemia**
        Potassium [K] excess
        Potassium [K] overload

  E87.6 **Hypokalemia**
        Potassium [K] deficiency

▶ New   ⇒ Revised   ~~deleted~~ Deleted   Excludes 1   Excludes 2   Includes   Use additional   Code first   Code also   Key words

OGCR Official Guidelines   X Assign placeholder X   ● Use Additional Character(s)   ▷ Manifestation Code   🐾 Hierarchical Condition Category   **Coding Clinic**

● **E87.7**   **Fluid overload**

> **Excludes1**   edema NOS (R60.9)
> fluid retention (R60.9)

E87.70   **Fluid overload, unspecified**

E87.71   **Transfusion associated circulatory overload**
Fluid overload due to transfusion (blood) (blood components) TACO

E87.79   **Other fluid overload**

E87.8   **Other disorders of electrolyte and fluid balance, not elsewhere classified**
Electrolyte imbalance NOS
Hyperchloremia
Hypochloremia

● **E88**   **Other and unspecified metabolic disorders**
Use additional codes for associated conditions

> **Excludes1**   histiocytosis X (chronic) (C96.6)

● **E88.0**   **Disorders of plasma-protein metabolism, not elsewhere classified**

> **Excludes1**   monoclonal gammopathy (of undetermined significance) (D47.2)
> polyclonal hypergammaglobulinemia (D89.0)
> Waldenström macroglobulinemia (C88.0)

> **Excludes2**   disorder of lipoprotein metabolism (E78.-)

E88.01   **Alpha-1-antitrypsin deficiency AAT deficiency** 🔖

E88.02   **Plasminogen deficiency**
Dysplasminogenemia
Hypoplasminogenemia
Type 1 plasminogen deficiency
Type 2 plasminogen deficiency

> Code also, if applicable, ligneous conjunctivitis (H10.51)

> Use additional code for associated findings, such as:
> hydrocephalus (G91.4)
> otitis media (H67.-)
> respiratory disorder related to plasminogen deficiency (J99)

E88.09   **Other disorders of plasma-protein metabolism, not elsewhere classified**
Bisalbuminemia

E88.1   **Lipodystrophy, not elsewhere classified**
Defective fat metabolism resulting in absence of subcutaneous fat
Lipodystrophy NOS

> **Excludes1**   Whipple's disease (K90.81)

E88.2   **Lipomatosis, not elsewhere classified**
Abnormal tumorlike accumulations of fat in tissue
Lipomatosis NOS
Lipomatosis (Check) dolorosa [Dercum]

E88.3   **Tumor lysis syndrome**
Tumor lysis syndrome (spontaneous)
Tumor lysis syndrome following antineoplastic drug chemotherapy

> Use additional code for adverse effect, if applicable, to identify drug (T45.1X5)
> **Coding Clinic: 2019, Q2, P25**

● **E88.4**   **Mitochondrial metabolism disorders**
Congenital disorder of metabolism

> **Excludes1**   disorders of pyruvate metabolism (E74.4)
> Kearns-Sayre syndrome (H49.81)
> Leber's disease (H47.22)
> Leigh's encephalopathy (G31.82)
> Mitochondrial myopathy, NEC (G71.3)
> Reye's syndrome (G93.7)

E88.40   **Mitochondrial metabolism disorder, unspecified** 🔖

E88.41   **MELAS syndrome** 🔖
Mitochondrial myopathy, encephalopathy, lactic acidosis and stroke-like episodes

E88.42   **MERRF syndrome** 🔖
Myoclonic epilepsy associated with ragged-red fibers

> Code also progressive myoclonic epilepsy (G40.3-)

E88.49   **Other mitochondrial metabolism disorders** 🔖

● **E88.8**   **Other specified metabolic disorders**

E88.81   **Metabolic syndrome**
Dysmetabolic syndrome X

> Use additional codes for associated manifestations, such as:
> obesity (E66.-)

E88.89   **Other specified metabolic disorders** 🔖
Launois-Bensaude adenolipomatosis

> **Excludes1**   adult pulmonary Langerhans cell histiocytosis (J84.82)

E88.9   **Metabolic disorder, unspecified**

POSTPROCEDURAL ENDOCRINE AND METABOLIC COMPLICATIONS AND DISORDERS, NOT ELSEWHERE CLASSIFIED (E89)

● **E89**   **Postprocedural endocrine and metabolic complications and disorders, not elsewhere classified**

> **Excludes2**   intraoperative complications of endocrine system organ or structure (E36.0-, E36.1-, E36.8)

E89.0   **Postprocedural hypothyroidism**
Postirradiation hypothyroidism
Postsurgical hypothyroidism

E89.1   **Postprocedural hypoinsulinemia**
Postpancreatectomy hyperglycemia
Postsurgical hypoinsulinemia

> Use additional code, if applicable, to identify:
> acquired absence of pancreas (Z90.41-)
> diabetes mellitus (postpancreatectomy) (postprocedural) (E13.-)
> insulin use (Z79.4)

> **Excludes1**   transient postprocedural hyperglycemia (R73.9)
> transient postprocedural hypoglycemia (E16.2)

E89.2   **Postprocedural hypoparathyroidism** 🔖
Parathyroprival tetany

E89.3   **Postprocedural hypopituitarism** 🔖
Postirradiation hypopituitarism

● **E89.4**   **Postprocedural ovarian failure**

E89.40   **Asymptomatic postprocedural ovarian failure** ♀
Postprocedural ovarian failure NOS

E89.41   **Symptomatic postprocedural ovarian failure** ♀
Symptoms such as flushing, sleeplessness, headache, lack of concentration, associated with postprocedural menopause

CHAPTER 4 (E00–E89)

E89.5   Postprocedural testicular hypofunction ♂

E89.6   Postprocedural adrenocortical (-medullary) hypofunction 🐾

● E89.8   Other postprocedural endocrine and metabolic complications and disorders
       Coding Clinic: 2016, Q4, P9

     ● E89.81   Postprocedural hemorrhage of an endocrine system organ or structure following a procedure

         E89.810   Postprocedural hemorrhage of an endocrine system organ or structure following an endocrine system procedure

         E89.811   Postprocedural hemorrhage of an endocrine system organ or structure following other procedure

   ● E89.82   Postprocedural hematoma and seroma of an endocrine system organ or structure

         E89.820   Postprocedural hematoma of an endocrine system organ or structure following an endocrine system procedure

         E89.821   Postprocedural hematoma of an endocrine system organ or structure following other procedure

         E89.822   Postprocedural seroma of an endocrine system organ or structure following an endocrine system procedure

         E89.823   Postprocedural seroma of an endocrine system organ or structure following other procedure

   E89.89   Other postprocedural endocrine and metabolic complications and disorders

       Use additional code, if applicable, to further specify disorder

CHAPTER 5

MENTAL, BEHAVIORAL AND NEURODEVELOPMENTAL DISORDERS (F01-F99)

OGCR Chapter-Specific Coding Guidelines

5. Chapter 5: Mental, Behavioral and Neurodevelopmental disorders (F01 – F99)

a. Pain disorders related to psychological factors

Assign code F45.41, for pain that is exclusively related to psychological disorders. As indicated by the Excludes 1 note under category G89, a code from category G89 should not be assigned with code F45.41

Code F45.42, Pain disorders with related psychological factors, should be used with a code from category G89, Pain, not elsewhere classified, if there is documentation of a psychological component for a patient with acute or chronic pain.

See Section I.C.6. Pain

b. Mental and behavioral disorders due to psychoactive substance use

1) In Remission

Selection of codes for "in remission" for categories F10-F19, Mental and behavioral disorders due to psychoactive substance use (categories F10-F19 with -11, -.21) requires the provider's clinical judgment. The appropriate codes for "in remission" are assigned only on the basis of provider documentation (as defined in the Official Guidelines for Coding and Reporting), unless otherwise instructed by the classification.

Mild substance use disorders in early or sustained remission are classified to the appropriate codes for substance abuse in remission, and moderate or severe substance use disorders in early or sustained remission are classified to the appropriate codes for substance dependence in remission.

2) Psychoactive Substance Use, Abuse and Dependence

When the provider documentation refers to use, abuse and dependence of the same substance (e.g., alcohol, opioid, cannabis, etc.), only one code should be assigned to identify the pattern of use based on the following hierarchy:

- If both use and abuse are documented, assign only the code for abuse
- If both abuse and dependence are documented, assign only the code for dependence
- If use, abuse and dependence are all documented, assign only the code for dependence
- If both use and dependence are documented, assign only the code for dependence

3) Psychoactive Substance Use, Unspecified

As with all other unspecified diagnoses, the codes for unspecified psychoactive substance use disorders (F10.9-, F11.9-, F12.9-, F13.9-, F14.9-, F15.9-, F16.9-, F19.9-, F19.9-) should only be assigned based on provider documentation and when they meet the definition of a reportable diagnosis (see Section III, Reporting Additional Diagnoses). These codes are to be used only when the psychoactive substance use is associated with a physical, mental or behavioral disorder, and such a relationship is documented by the provider.

c. Factitious Disorder

Factitious disorder imposed on self or Munchausen's syndrome is a disorder in which a person falsely reports or causes his or her own physical or psychological signs or symptoms. For patients with documented factitious disorder on self or Munchausen's syndrome, assign the appropriate code from subcategory F68.1-, Factitious disorder imposed on self.

Munchausen's syndrome by proxy (MSBP) is a disorder in which a caregiver (perpetrator) falsely reports or causes an illness or injury in another person (victim) under his or her care, such as a child, an elderly adult, or a person who has a disability. The condition is also referred to as "factitious disorder imposed on another" or "factitious disorder by proxy." The perpetrator, not the victim, receives this diagnosis. Assign code F68.A, Factitious disorder imposed on another, to the perpetrator's record. For the victim of a patient suffering from MSBP, assign the appropriate code from categories T74, Adult and child abuse, neglect and other maltreatment, confirmed, or T76, Adult and child abuse, neglect and other maltreatment, suspected.

See Section I.C.19.f. Adult and child abuse, neglect and other maltreatment

CHAPTER 5

MENTAL, BEHAVIORAL AND NEURODEVELOPMENTAL DISORDERS (F01-F99)

Includes	disorders of psychological development
Excludes2	symptoms, signs and abnormal clinical laboratory findings, not elsewhere classified (R00-R99)

This chapter contains the following blocks:

F01-F09	Mental disorders due to known physiological conditions
F10-F19	Mental and behavioral disorders due to psychoactive substance use
F20-F29	Schizophrenia, schizotypal, delusional, and other non-mood psychotic disorders
F30-F39	Mood [affective] disorders
F40-F48	Anxiety, dissociative, stress-related, somatoform and other nonpsychotic mental disorders
F50-F59	Behavioral syndromes associated with physiological disturbances and physical factors
F60-F69	Disorders of adult personality and behavior
F70-F79	Intellectual disabilities
F80-F89	Pervasive and specific developmental disorders
F90-F98	Behavioral and emotional disorders with onset usually occurring in childhood and adolescence
F99	Unspecified mental disorder

MENTAL DISORDERS DUE TO KNOWN PHYSIOLOGICAL CONDITIONS (F01-F09)

This block comprises a range of mental disorders grouped together on the basis of their having in common a demonstrable etiology in cerebral disease, brain injury, or other insult leading to cerebral dysfunction. The dysfunction may be primary, as in diseases, injuries, and insults that affect the brain directly and selectively; or secondary, as in systemic diseases and disorders that attack the brain only as one of the multiple organs or systems of the body that are involved.

● **F01**   **Vascular dementia**

Vascular dementia as a result of infarction of the brain due to vascular disease, including hypertensive cerebrovascular disease.

Includes	arteriosclerotic dementia

Code first the underlying physiological condition or sequelae of cerebrovascular disease.

● **F01.5**   **Vascular dementia**

F01.50   **Vascular dementia without behavioral disturbance**   A

Major neurocognitive disorder without behavioral disturbance

Coding Clinic: 2021, Q2, P4

F01.51   **Vascular dementia with behavioral disturbance**   A

Major neurocognitive disorder due to vascular disease, with behavioral disturbance

Major neurocognitive disorder with aggressive behavior

Major neurocognitive disorder with combative behavior

Major neurocognitive disorder with violent behavior

Vascular dementia with aggressive behavior

Vascular dementia with combative behavior

Vascular dementia with violent behavior

Use additional code, if applicable, to identify wandering in vascular dementia (Z91.83)

CHAPTER 5 (F01-F99)

● **F02** **Dementia in other diseases classified elsewhere**

Code first the underlying physiological condition, such as:
Alzheimer's (G30.-)
cerebral lipidosis (E75.4)
Creutzfeldt-Jakob disease (A81.0-)
dementia with Lewy bodies (G31.83)
dementia with Parkinsonism (G31.83)
epilepsy and recurrent seizures (G40.-)
frontotemporal dementia (G31.09)
hepatolenticular degeneration (E83.0)
human immunodeficiency virus [HIV] disease (B20)
Huntington's disease (G10)
hypercalcemia (E83.52)
hypothyroidism, acquired (E00-E03.-)
intoxications (T36-T65)
Jakob-Creutzfeldt disease (A81.0-)
multiple sclerosis (G35)
neurosyphilis (A52.17)
niacin deficiency [pellagra] (E52)
Parkinson's disease (G20)
Pick's disease (G31.01)
polyarteritis nodosa (M30.0)
prion disease (A81.9)
systemic lupus erythematosus (M32.-)
traumatic brain injury (S06.-)
trypanosomiasis (B56.-, B57.-)
vitamin B deficiency (E53.8)

Includes Major neurocognitive disorder in other diseases classified elsewhere

Excludes2 dementia in alcohol and psychoactive substance disorders (F10-F19, with .17, .27, .97)
vascular dementia (F01.5-)
Coding Clinic: 2016, Q4, P141

● **F02.8** **Dementia in other diseases classified elsewhere**

▸ **F02.80** *Dementia in other diseases classified elsewhere without behavioral disturbance*
Dementia in other diseases classified elsewhere NOS
Major neurocognitive disorder in other diseases classified elsewhere
Coding Clinic: 2017, Q1, P43; 2016, Q2, P6

▸ **F02.81** *Dementia in other diseases classified elsewhere with behavioral disturbance*
Dementia in other diseases classified elsewhere with aggressive behavior
Dementia in other diseases classified elsewhere with combative behavior
Dementia in other diseases classified elsewhere with violent behavior
Major neurocognitive disorder in other diseases classified elsewhere with aggressive behavior
Major neurocognitive disorder in other diseases classified elsewhere with combative behavior
Major neurocognitive disorder in other diseases classified elsewhere with violent behavior
Use additional code, if applicable, to identify wandering in dementia in conditions classified elsewhere (Z91.83)
Coding Clinic: 2017, Q2, P8, Q1, P43

Item 5-1 Psychosis was a term formerly applied to any mental disorder but is now restricted to disturbances of a great magnitude in which there is a personality disintegration and loss of contact with reality.

● **F03** **Unspecified dementia**
Presenile dementia NOS
Presenile psychosis NOS
Primary degenerative dementia NOS
Senile dementia NOS
Senile dementia depressed or paranoid type
Senile psychosis NOS

Excludes1 senility NOS (R41.81)
Excludes2 mild memory disturbance due to known physiological condition (F06.8)
senile dementia with delirium or acute confusional state (F05)

● **F03.9** **Unspecified dementia**
F03.90 **Unspecified dementia without behavioral disturbance**   A
Dementia NOS
Coding Clinic: 2021, Q2, P4; 2012, Q4, P92

F03.91 **Unspecified dementia with behavioral disturbance**   A
Unspecified dementia with aggressive behavior
Unspecified dementia with combative behavior
Unspecified dementia with violent behavior
Use additional code, if applicable, to identify wandering in unspecified dementia (Z91.83)

F04 **Amnestic disorder due to known physiological condition**
Korsakov's psychosis or syndrome, nonalcoholic
Code first the underlying physiological condition
Excludes1 amnesia NOS (R41.3)
anterograde amnesia (R41.1)
dissociative amnesia (F44.0)
retrograde amnesia (R41.2)
Excludes2 alcohol-induced or unspecified Korsakov's syndrome (F10.26, F10.96)
Korsakov's syndrome induced by other psychoactive substances (F13.26, F13.96, F19.16, F19.26, F19.96)

F05 **Delirium due to known physiological condition**
Acute or subacute brain syndrome
Acute or subacute confusional state (nonalcoholic)
Acute or subacute infective psychosis
Acute or subacute organic reaction
Acute or subacute psycho-organic syndrome
Delirium of mixed etiology
Delirium superimposed on dementia
Sundowning
Code first the underlying physiological condition
Excludes1 delirium NOS (R41.0)
Excludes2 delirium tremens alcohol-induced or unspecified (F10.231, F10.921)
Coding Clinic: 2019, Q2, P34

● **F06** **Other mental disorders due to known physiological condition**
Includes mental disorders due to endocrine disorder
mental disorders due to exogenous hormone
mental disorders due to exogenous toxic substance
mental disorders due to primary cerebral disease
mental disorders due to somatic illness
mental disorders due to systemic disease affecting the brain
Code first the underlying physiological condition
Excludes1 unspecified dementia (F03)
Excludes2 delirium due to known physiological condition (F05)
dementia as classified in F01-F02
other mental disorders associated with alcohol and other psychoactive substances (F10-F19)

F06.0   **Psychotic disorder with hallucinations due to known physiological condition**
    Organic hallucinatory state (nonalcoholic)
    Excludes2   hallucinations and perceptual disturbance induced by alcohol and other psychoactive substances (F10-F19 with .151, .251, .951)
       schizophrenia (F20.-)

F06.1   **Catatonic disorder due to known physiological condition**
    Catatonia associated with another mental disorder
    Catatonia NOS
    Excludes1   catatonic stupor (R40.1)
       stupor NOS (R40.1)
    Excludes2   catatonic schizophrenia (F20.2)
       dissociative stupor (F44.2)

F06.2   **Psychotic disorder with delusions due to known physiological condition**
    Paranoid and paranoid-hallucinatory organic states
    Schizophrenia-like psychosis in epilepsy
    Excludes2   alcohol and drug-induced psychotic disorder (F10-F19 with .150, .250, .950)
       brief psychotic disorder (F23)
       delusional disorder (F22)
       schizophrenia (F20.-)

F06.3   **Mood disorder due to known physiological condition**
    Excludes2   mood disorders due to alcohol and other psychoactive substances (F10-F19 with .14, .24, .94)
       mood disorders, not due to known physiological condition or unspecified (F30-F39)

F06.30   **Mood disorder due to known physiological condition, unspecified**

F06.31   **Mood disorder due to known physiological condition with depressive features**
    Depressive disorder due to known physiological condition, with depressive features

F06.32   **Mood disorder due to known physiological condition with major depressive-like episode**
    Depressive disorder due to known physiological condition, with major depressive-like episode

F06.33   **Mood disorder due to known physiological condition with manic features**
    Bipolar and related disorder due to a known physiological condition, with manic features
    Bipolar and related disorder due to known physiological condition, with manic- or hypomanic-like episodes

F06.34   **Mood disorder due to known physiological condition with mixed features**
    Bipolar and related disorder due to known physiological condition, with mixed features
    Depressive disorder due to known physiological condition, with mixed features

F06.4   **Anxiety disorder due to known physiological condition**
    Excludes2   anxiety disorders due to alcohol and other psychoactive substances (F10-F19 with .180, .280, .980)
       anxiety disorders, not due to known physiological condition or unspecified (F40.-, F41.-)

F06.8   **Other specified mental disorders due to known physiological condition**
    Epileptic psychosis NOS
    Obsessive-compulsive and related disorder due to a known physiological condition
    Organic dissociative disorder
    Organic emotionally labile [asthenic] disorder

F07   **Personality and behavioral disorders due to known physiological condition**
    Code first the underlying physiological condition

F07.0   **Personality change due to known physiological condition**
    ◦ Frontal lobe syndrome
    Limbic epilepsy personality syndrome
    Lobotomy syndrome
    Organic personality disorder
    Organic pseudopsychopathic personality
    Organic pseudoretarded personality
    Postleucotomy syndrome
    Code first underlying physiological condition
    Excludes1   mild cognitive impairment (G31.84)
       postconcussional syndrome (F07.81)
       postencephalitic syndrome (F07.89)
       signs and symptoms involving emotional state (R45.-)
    Excludes2   specific personality disorder (F60.-)

F07.8   **Other personality and behavioral disorders due to known physiological condition**

F07.81   **Postconcussional syndrome**
    Postcontusional syndrome (encephalopathy)
    Post-traumatic brain syndrome, nonpsychotic
    Use additional code to identify associated post-traumatic headache, if applicable (G44.3-)
    Excludes1   current concussion (brain) (S06.0-)
       postencephalitic syndrome (F07.89)

F07.89   **Other personality and behavioral disorders due to known physiological condition**
    Postencephalitic syndrome
    Damage to temporal brain lobes with memory loss and abnormal behavior
    Right hemispheric organic affective disorder

F07.9   **Unspecified personality and behavioral disorder due to known physiological condition**
    Organic psychosyndrome
    Due to exposure to organic solvents

F09   **Unspecified mental disorder due to known physiological condition**
    Mental disorder NOS due to known physiological condition
    Organic brain syndrome NOS
    Organic mental disorder NOS
    Organic psychosis NOS
    Symptomatic psychosis NOS
    Code first the underlying physiological condition
    Excludes1   psychosis NOS (F29)

MENTAL AND BEHAVIORAL DISORDERS DUE TO PSYCHOACTIVE SUBSTANCE USE (F10-F19)

F10   **Alcohol related disorders**
    Use additional code for blood alcohol level, if applicable (Y90.-)
    Coding Clinic: 2019, Q3, P8

F10.1   **Alcohol abuse**
    Excludes1   alcohol dependence (F10.2-)
       alcohol use, unspecified (F10.9-)

F10.10   **Alcohol abuse, uncomplicated**
    Alcohol use disorder, mild

F10.11   **Alcohol abuse, in remission**
    Alcohol use disorder, mild, in early remission
    Alcohol use disorder, mild, in sustained remission

F10.12   **Alcohol abuse with intoxication**

F10.120   **Alcohol abuse with intoxication, uncomplicated** 🔗

F10.121   **Alcohol abuse with intoxication, delirium** 🔗

F10.129   **Alcohol abuse with intoxication, unspecified** 🔗

● F10.13 **Alcohol abuse, with withdrawal**
 F10.130 Alcohol abuse with withdrawal, uncomplicated
 F10.131 Alcohol abuse with withdrawal delirium
 F10.132 Alcohol abuse with withdrawal with perceptual disturbance
 F10.139 Alcohol abuse with withdrawal, unspecified
 F10.14 **Alcohol abuse with alcohol-induced mood disorder** 🐾
  Alcohol use disorder, mild, with alcohol-induced bipolar or related disorder
  Alcohol use disorder, mild, with alcohol-induced depressive disorder
● F10.15 **Alcohol abuse with alcohol-induced psychotic disorder**
 F10.150 Alcohol abuse with alcohol-induced psychotic disorder with delusions 🐾
 F10.151 Alcohol abuse with alcohol-induced psychotic disorder with hallucinations 🐾
 F10.159 Alcohol abuse with alcohol-induced psychotic disorder, unspecified 🐾
● F10.18 **Alcohol abuse with other alcohol-induced disorders**
 F10.180 Alcohol abuse with alcohol-induced anxiety disorder 🐾
 F10.181 Alcohol abuse with alcohol-induced sexual dysfunction 🐾
 F10.182 Alcohol abuse with alcohol-induced sleep disorder 🐾
 F10.188 Alcohol abuse with other alcohol-induced disorder 🐾
 F10.19 Alcohol abuse with unspecified alcohol-induced disorder 🐾
● F10.2 **Alcohol dependence**
 Excludes1 alcohol abuse (F10.1-)
  alcohol use, unspecified (F10.9-)
 Excludes2 toxic effect of alcohol (T51.0-)
 Coding Clinic: 2019, Q3, P8
 F10.20 **Alcohol dependence, uncomplicated** 🐾
  Alcohol use disorder, moderate
  Alcohol use disorder, severe
  Coding Clinic: 2020, Q1, P9
 F10.21 **Alcohol dependence, in remission** 🐾
  Alcohol use disorder, moderate, in early remission
  Alcohol use disorder, moderate, in sustained remission
  Alcohol use disorder, severe, in early remission
  Alcohol use disorder, severe, in sustained remission
● F10.22 **Alcohol dependence with intoxication**
  Acute drunkenness (in alcoholism)
  Excludes2 alcohol dependence with withdrawal (F10.23-)
 F10.220 Alcohol dependence with intoxication, uncomplicated 🐾
 F10.221 Alcohol dependence with intoxication delirium 🐾
 F10.229 Alcohol dependence with intoxication, unspecified 🐾
● F10.23 **Alcohol dependence with withdrawal**
 Excludes2 alcohol dependence with intoxication (F10.22-)
 F10.230 Alcohol dependence with withdrawal, uncomplicated 🐾
 F10.231 Alcohol dependence with withdrawal delirium 🐾

 F10.232 Alcohol dependence with withdrawal with perceptual disturbance 🐾
 F10.239 Alcohol dependence with withdrawal, unspecified 🐾
  Coding Clinic: 2015, Q2, P15
 F10.24 **Alcohol dependence with alcohol-induced mood disorder** 🐾
  Alcohol use disorder, moderate, with alcohol-induced bipolar or related disorder
  Alcohol use disorder, moderate, with alcohol-induced depressive disorder
  Alcohol use disorder, severe, with alcohol-induced bipolar or related disorder
  Alcohol use disorder, severe, with alcohol-induced depressive disorder
● F10.25 **Alcohol dependence with alcohol-induced psychotic disorder**
 F10.250 Alcohol dependence with alcohol-induced psychotic disorder with delusions 🐾
 F10.251 Alcohol dependence with alcohol-induced psychotic disorder with hallucinations 🐾
 F10.259 Alcohol dependence with alcohol-induced psychotic disorder, unspecified 🐾
 F10.26 **Alcohol dependence with alcohol-induced persisting amnestic disorder** 🐾
  Alcohol use disorder, moderate, with alcohol-induced major neurocognitive disorder, amnestic-confabulatory type
  Alcohol use disorder, severe, with alcohol-induced major neurocognitive disorder, amnestic-confabulatory type
 F10.27 **Alcohol dependence with alcohol-induced persisting dementia** 🐾
  Alcohol use disorder, moderate, with alcohol-induced major neurocognitive disorder, nonamnestic-confabulatory type
  Alcohol use disorder, severe, with alcohol-induced major neurocognitive disorder, nonamnestic-confabulatory type
● F10.28 **Alcohol dependence with other alcohol-induced disorders**
 F10.280 Alcohol dependence with alcohol-induced anxiety disorder 🐾
 F10.281 Alcohol dependence with alcohol-induced sexual dysfunction 🐾
 F10.282 Alcohol dependence with alcohol-induced sleep disorder 🐾
 F10.288 Alcohol dependence with other alcohol-induced disorder 🐾
  Alcohol use disorder, moderate, with alcohol-induced mild neurocognitive disorder
  Alcohol use disorder, severe, with alcohol-induced mild neurocognitive disorder
  Coding Clinic: 2020, Q1, P9
 F10.29 Alcohol dependence with unspecified alcohol-induced disorder 🐾
● F10.9 **Alcohol use, unspecified**
 Excludes1 alcohol abuse (F10.1-)
  alcohol dependence (F10.2-)
● F10.92 **Alcohol use, unspecified with intoxication**
 F10.920 Alcohol use, unspecified with intoxication, uncomplicated 🐾
 F10.921 Alcohol use, unspecified with intoxication delirium 🐾
 F10.929 Alcohol use, unspecified with intoxication, unspecified 🐾

▶ New ⇒ Revised ~~deleted~~ Deleted Excludes 1 Excludes 2 Includes Use additional Code first Code also Key words
OGCR Official Guidelines X Assign placeholder X ● Use Additional Character(s) ▶ Manifestation Code 🐾 Hierarchical Condition Category **Coding Clinic**

CHAPTER 5 (F01-F99)

● F10.93   Alcohol use, unspecified with withdrawal

    F10.930   Alcohol use, unspecified with withdrawal, uncomplicated

    F10.931   Alcohol use, unspecified with withdrawal delirium

    F10.932   Alcohol use, unspecified with withdrawal with perceptual disturbance

    F10.939   Alcohol use, unspecified with withdrawal, unspecified

   F10.94   Alcohol use, unspecified with alcohol-induced mood disorder 🦠

      Alcohol-induced bipolar or related disorder, without use disorder

      Alcohol-induced depressive disorder, without use disorder

● F10.95   Alcohol use, unspecified with alcohol-induced psychotic disorder

    F10.950   Alcohol use, unspecified with alcohol-induced psychotic disorder with delusions 🦠

    F10.951   Alcohol use, unspecified with alcohol-induced psychotic disorder with hallucinations 🦠

    F10.959   Alcohol use, unspecified with alcohol-induced psychotic disorder, unspecified 🦠

      Alcohol-induced psychotic disorder without use disorder

   F10.96   Alcohol use, unspecified with alcohol-induced persisting amnestic disorder 🦠

      Alcohol-induced major neurocognitive disorder, amnestic-confabulatory type, without use disorder

   F10.97   Alcohol use, unspecified with alcohol-induced persisting dementia 🦠

      Alcohol-induced major neurocognitive disorder, nonamnestic-confabulatory type, without use disorder

● F10.98   Alcohol use, unspecified with other alcohol-induced disorders

    F10.980   Alcohol use, unspecified with alcohol-induced anxiety disorder 🦠

      Alcohol-induced anxiety disorder, without use disorder

    F10.981   Alcohol use, unspecified with alcohol-induced sexual dysfunction 🦠

      Alcohol-induced sexual dysfunction, without use disorder

    F10.982   Alcohol use, unspecified with alcohol-induced sleep disorder 🦠

      Alcohol-induced sleep disorder, without use disorder

    F10.988   Alcohol use, unspecified with other alcohol-induced disorder 🦠

      Alcohol-induced mild neurocognitive disorder, without use disorder

      Coding Clinic: 2019, Q3, P8

   F10.99   Alcohol use, unspecified with unspecified alcohol-induced disorder 🦠

● F11   Opioid related disorders

● F11.1   Opioid abuse

     Excludes1   opioid dependence (F11.2-)
                opioid use, unspecified (F11.9-)

   F11.10   Opioid abuse, uncomplicated

      Opioid use disorder, mild

   F11.11   Opioid abuse, in remission

      Opioid use disorder, mild, in early remission

      Opioid use disorder, mild, in sustained remission

● F11.12   Opioid abuse with intoxication

    F11.120   Opioid abuse with intoxication, uncomplicated 🦠

    F11.121   Opioid abuse with intoxication delirium 🦠

    F11.122   Opioid abuse with intoxication with perceptual disturbance 🦠

    F11.129   Opioid abuse with intoxication, unspecified 🦠

   F11.13   Opioid abuse with withdrawal

   F11.14   Opioid abuse with opioid-induced mood disorder 🦠

      Opioid use disorder, mild, with opioid-induced depressive disorder

● F11.15   Opioid abuse with opioid-induced psychotic disorder

    F11.150   Opioid abuse with opioid-induced psychotic disorder with delusions 🦠

    F11.151   Opioid abuse with opioid-induced psychotic disorder with hallucinations 🦠

    F11.159   Opioid abuse with opioid-induced psychotic disorder, unspecified 🦠

● F11.18   Opioid abuse with other opioid-induced disorder

    F11.181   Opioid abuse with opioid-induced sexual dysfunction 🦠

    F11.182   Opioid abuse with opioid-induced sleep disorder 🦠

    F11.188   Opioid abuse with other opioid-induced disorder 🦠

   F11.19   Opioid abuse with unspecified opioid-induced disorder 🦠

● F11.2   Opioid dependence

     Excludes1   opioid abuse (F11.1-)
                opioid use, unspecified (F11.9-)

     Excludes2   opioid poisoning (T40.0—T40.2-)

   F11.20   Opioid dependence, uncomplicated 🦠

      Opioid use disorder, moderate

      Opioid use disorder, severe

   F11.21   Opioid dependence, in remission 🦠

      Opioid use disorder, moderate, in early remission

      Opioid use disorder, moderate, in sustained remission

      Opioid use disorder, severe, in early remission

      Opioid use disorder, severe, in sustained remission

● F11.22   Opioid dependence with intoxication

     Excludes1   opioid dependence with withdrawal (F11.23)

    F11.220   Opioid dependence with intoxication, uncomplicated 🦠

    F11.221   Opioid dependence with intoxication delirium 🦠

    F11.222   Opioid dependence with intoxication with perceptual disturbance 🦠

    F11.229   Opioid dependence with intoxication, unspecified 🦠

   F11.23   Opioid dependence with withdrawal 🦠

     Excludes1   opioid dependence with intoxication (F11.22-)

   F11.24   Opioid dependence with opioid-induced mood disorder 🦠

      Opioid use disorder, moderate, with opioid-induced depressive disorder

CHAPTER 5 (F01-F99)

CHAPTER 5 (F01-F99)

● F11.25   Opioid dependence with opioid-induced psychotic disorder
- F11.250   Opioid dependence with opioid-induced psychotic disorder with delusions 🦋
- F11.251   Opioid dependence with opioid-induced psychotic disorder with hallucinations 🦋
- F11.259   Opioid dependence with opioid-induced psychotic disorder, unspecified 🦋

● F11.28   Opioid dependence with other opioid-induced disorder
- F11.281   Opioid dependence with opioid-induced sexual dysfunction 🦋
- F11.282   Opioid dependence with opioid-induced sleep disorder 🦋
- F11.288   Opioid dependence with other opioid-induced disorder 🦋

   F11.29   Opioid dependence with unspecified opioid-induced disorder 🦋

● F11.9   Opioid use, unspecified

     Excludes1   opioid abuse (F11.1-)
                      opioid dependence (F11.2-)

   F11.90   Opioid use, unspecified, uncomplicated

● F11.92   Opioid use, unspecified with intoxication

     Excludes1   opioid use, unspecified with withdrawal (F11.93)
- F11.920   Opioid use, unspecified with intoxication, uncomplicated 🦋
- F11.921   Opioid use, unspecified with intoxication delirium 🦋
  Opioid-induced delirium
- F11.922   Opioid use, unspecified with intoxication with perceptual disturbance 🦋
- F11.929   Opioid use, unspecified with intoxication, unspecified 🦋

   F11.93   Opioid use, unspecified with withdrawal 🦋

     Excludes1   opioid use, unspecified with intoxication (F11.92-)

   F11.94   Opioid use, unspecified with opioid-induced mood disorder 🦋
  Opioid-induced depressive disorder, without use disorder

● F11.95   Opioid use, unspecified with opioid-induced psychotic disorder
- F11.950   Opioid use, unspecified with opioid-induced psychotic disorder with delusions 🦋
- F11.951   Opioid use, unspecified with opioid-induced psychotic disorder with hallucinations 🦋
- F11.959   Opioid use, unspecified with opioid-induced psychotic disorder, unspecified 🦋

● F11.98   Opioid use, unspecified with other specified opioid-induced disorder
- F11.981   Opioid use, unspecified with opioid-induced sexual dysfunction 🦋
  Opioid-induced sexual dysfunction, without use disorder
- F11.982   Opioid use, unspecified with opioid-induced sleep disorder 🦋
  Opioid-induced sleep disorder, without use disorder
- F11.988   Opioid use, unspecified with other opioid-induced disorder 🦋
  Opioid-induced anxiety disorder, without use disorder

   F11.99   Opioid use, unspecified with unspecified opioid-induced disorder 🦋

● F12   Cannabis related disorders

     Includes   marijuana

     Coding Clinic: 2020, Q1, P8

● F12.1   Cannabis abuse

     Excludes1   cannabis dependence (F12.2-)
                      cannabis use, unspecified (F12.9-)

   F12.10   Cannabis abuse, uncomplicated
  Cannabis use disorder, mild

   F12.11   Cannabis abuse, in remission
  Cannabis use disorder, mild, in early remission
  Cannabis use disorder, mild, in sustained remission

● F12.12   Cannabis abuse with intoxication
- F12.120   Cannabis abuse with intoxication, uncomplicated 🦋
- F12.121   Cannabis abuse with intoxication delirium 🦋
- F12.122   Cannabis abuse with intoxication with perceptual disturbance 🦋
- F12.129   Cannabis abuse with intoxication, unspecified 🦋

   F12.13   Cannabis abuse with withdrawal

● F12.15   Cannabis abuse with psychotic disorder
- F12.150   Cannabis abuse with psychotic disorder with delusions 🦋
- F12.151   Cannabis abuse with psychotic disorder with hallucinations 🦋
- F12.159   Cannabis abuse with psychotic disorder, unspecified 🦋

● F12.18   Cannabis abuse with other cannabis-induced disorder
- F12.180   Cannabis abuse with cannabis-induced anxiety disorder 🦋
- F12.188   Cannabis abuse with other cannabis-induced disorder 🦋
  Cannabis use disorder, mild, with cannabis-induced sleep disorder

   F12.19   Cannabis abuse with unspecified cannabis-induced disorder 🦋

● F12.2   Cannabis dependence

     Excludes1   cannabis abuse (F12.1-)
                      cannabis use, unspecified (F12.9-)

     Excludes2   cannabis poisoning (T40.7-)

   F12.20   Cannabis dependence, uncomplicated 🦋
  Cannabis use disorder, moderate
  Cannabis use disorder, severe

   F12.21   Cannabis dependence, in remission 🦋
  Cannabis use disorder, moderate, in early remission
  Cannabis use disorder, moderate, in sustained remission
  Cannabis use disorder, severe, in early remission
  Cannabis use disorder, severe, in sustained remission

● F12.22   Cannabis dependence with intoxication
- F12.220   Cannabis dependence with intoxication, uncomplicated 🦋
- F12.221   Cannabis dependence with intoxication delirium 🦋
- F12.222   Cannabis dependence with intoxication with perceptual disturbance 🦋
- F12.229   Cannabis dependence with intoxication, unspecified 🦋

   F12.23   Cannabis dependence with withdrawal 🦋

▶ New   ⇒ Revised   ~~deleted~~ Deleted   Excludes 1   Excludes 2   Includes   Use additional   Code first   Code also   Key words

OGCR Official Guidelines   **X** Assign placeholder X   ● Use Additional Character(s)   ▎ Manifestation Code   🦋 Hierarchical Condition Category   **Coding Clinic**

● F12.25　Cannabis dependence with psychotic disorder

　　　F12.250　Cannabis dependence with psychotic disorder with delusions 🐾

　　　F12.251　Cannabis dependence with psychotic disorder with hallucinations 🐾

　　　F12.259　Cannabis dependence with psychotic disorder, unspecified 🐾

● F12.28　Cannabis dependence with other cannabis-induced disorder

　　　F12.280　Cannabis dependence with cannabis-induced anxiety disorder 🐾

　　　F12.288　Cannabis dependence with other cannabis-induced disorder 🐾
　　　　　　Cannabis use disorder, moderate, with cannabis-induced sleep disorder
　　　　　　Cannabis use disorder, severe, with cannabis-induced sleep disorder

　　F12.29　Cannabis dependence with unspecified cannabis-induced disorder 🐾

● F12.9　Cannabis use, unspecified

　　Excludes1　cannabis abuse (F12.1-)
　　　　　　cannabis dependence (F12.2-)

　　F12.90　Cannabis use, unspecified, uncomplicated

● F12.92　Cannabis use, unspecified with intoxication

　　　F12.920　Cannabis use, unspecified with intoxication, uncomplicated 🐾

　　　F12.921　Cannabis use, unspecified with intoxication delirium 🐾

　　　F12.922　Cannabis use, unspecified with intoxication with perceptual disturbance 🐾

　　　F12.929　Cannabis use, unspecified with intoxication, unspecified 🐾

　　F12.93　Cannabis use, unspecified with withdrawal 🐾

● F12.95　Cannabis use, unspecified with psychotic disorder

　　　F12.950　Cannabis use, unspecified with psychotic disorder with delusions 🐾

　　　F12.951　Cannabis use, unspecified with psychotic disorder with hallucinations 🐾

　　　F12.959　Cannabis use, unspecified with psychotic disorder, unspecified 🐾
　　　　　　Cannabis-induced psychotic disorder, without use disorder

● F12.98　Cannabis use, unspecified with other cannabis-induced disorder

　　　F12.980　Cannabis use, unspecified with anxiety disorder 🐾
　　　　　　Cannabis-induced anxiety disorder, without use disorder

　　　F12.988　Cannabis use, unspecified with other cannabis-induced disorder 🐾
　　　　　　Cannabis-induced sleep disorder, without use disorder

　　F12.99　Cannabis use, unspecified with unspecified cannabis-induced disorder 🐾

● F13　Sedative, hypnotic, or anxiolytic related disorders

● F13.1　Sedative, hypnotic or anxiolytic-related abuse

　　Excludes1　sedative, hypnotic or anxiolytic-related dependence (F13.2-)
　　　　　　sedative, hypnotic, or anxiolytic use, unspecified (F13.9-)

　　F13.10　Sedative, hypnotic or anxiolytic abuse, uncomplicated
　　　　　　Sedative, hypnotic, or anxiolytic use disorder, mild

　　F13.11　Sedative, hypnotic or anxiolytic abuse, in remission
　　　　　　Sedative, hypnotic or anxiolytic use disorder, mild, in early remission
　　　　　　Sedative, hypnotic or anxiolytic use disorder, mild, in sustained remission

● F13.12　Sedative, hypnotic or anxiolytic abuse with intoxication

　　　F13.120　Sedative, hypnotic or anxiolytic abuse with intoxication, uncomplicated 🐾

　　　F13.121　Sedative, hypnotic or anxiolytic abuse with intoxication delirium 🐾

　　　F13.129　Sedative, hypnotic or anxiolytic abuse with intoxication, unspecified 🐾

● F13.13　Sedative, hypnotic or anxiolytic abuse with withdrawal

　　　F13.130　Sedative, hypnotic or anxiolytic abuse with withdrawal, uncomplicated

　　　F13.131　Sedative, hypnotic or anxiolytic abuse with withdrawal delirium

　　　F13.132　Sedative, hypnotic or anxiolytic abuse with withdrawal with perceptual disturbance

　　　F13.139　Sedative, hypnotic or anxiolytic abuse with withdrawal, unspecified

　　F13.14　Sedative, hypnotic or anxiolytic abuse with sedative, hypnotic or anxiolytic-induced mood disorder 🐾
　　　　　　Sedative, hypnotic, or anxiolytic use disorder, mild, with sedative, hypnotic, or anxiolytic-induced bipolar or related disorder
　　　　　　Sedative, hypnotic, or anxiolytic use disorder, mild, with sedative, hypnotic, or anxiolytic-induced depressive disorder

● F13.15　Sedative, hypnotic or anxiolytic abuse with sedative, hypnotic or anxiolytic-induced psychotic disorder

　　　F13.150　Sedative, hypnotic or anxiolytic abuse with sedative, hypnotic or anxiolytic-induced psychotic disorder with delusions 🐾

　　　F13.151　Sedative, hypnotic or anxiolytic abuse with sedative, hypnotic or anxiolytic-induced psychotic disorder with hallucinations 🐾

　　　F13.159　Sedative, hypnotic or anxiolytic abuse with sedative, hypnotic or anxiolytic-induced psychotic disorder, unspecified 🐾

● F13.18　Sedative, hypnotic or anxiolytic abuse with other sedative, hypnotic or anxiolytic-induced disorders

　　　F13.180　Sedative, hypnotic or anxiolytic abuse with sedative, hypnotic or anxiolytic-induced anxiety disorder 🐾

　　　F13.181　Sedative, hypnotic or anxiolytic abuse with sedative, hypnotic or anxiolytic-induced sexual dysfunction 🐾

　　　F13.182　Sedative, hypnotic or anxiolytic abuse with sedative, hypnotic or anxiolytic-induced sleep disorder 🐾

　　　F13.188　Sedative, hypnotic or anxiolytic abuse with other sedative, hypnotic or anxiolytic-induced disorder 🐾

　　F13.19　Sedative, hypnotic or anxiolytic abuse with unspecified sedative, hypnotic or anxiolytic-induced disorder 🐾

● F13.2　Sedative, hypnotic or anxiolytic-related dependence

N Newborn Age: 0　**P** Pediatric Age: 0–17　**M** Maternity DX: 9–64　**A** Adult Age: 15–124　♀ Females Only　♂ Males Only

771

Excludes1 sedative, hypnotic or anxiolytic-related
abuse (F13.1-)
sedative, hypnotic, or anxiolytic use,
unspecified (F13.9-)

Excludes2 sedative, hypnotic, or anxiolytic
poisoning (T42.-)

F13.20 Sedative, hypnotic or anxiolytic dependence,
uncomplicated

F13.21 Sedative, hypnotic or anxiolytic dependence, in
remission
Sedative, hypnotic or anxiolytic use disorder,
moderate, in early remission
Sedative, hypnotic or anxiolytic use disorder,
moderate, in sustained remission
Sedative, hypnotic or anxiolytic use disorder,
severe, in early remission
Sedative, hypnotic or anxiolytic use disorder,
severe, in sustained remission

● **F13.22** Sedative, hypnotic or anxiolytic dependence
with intoxication
Excludes1 sedative, hypnotic or anxiolytic
dependence with
withdrawal (F13.23-)

F13.220 Sedative, hypnotic or anxiolytic
dependence with intoxication,
uncomplicated

F13.221 Sedative, hypnotic or anxiolytic
dependence with intoxication
delirium

F13.229 Sedative, hypnotic or anxiolytic
dependence with
intoxication, unspecified

● **F13.23** Sedative, hypnotic or anxiolytic dependence
with withdrawal
Sedative, hypnotic, or anxiolytic use disorder,
moderate
Sedative, hypnotic, or anxiolytic use disorder,
severe
Excludes1 sedative, hypnotic or anxiolytic
dependence with
intoxication (F13.22-)

F13.230 Sedative, hypnotic or anxiolytic
dependence with withdrawal,
uncomplicated

F13.231 Sedative, hypnotic or anxiolytic
dependence with withdrawal
delirium

F13.232 Sedative, hypnotic or anxiolytic
dependence with withdrawal with
perceptual disturbance
Sedative, hypnotic, or anxiolytic
withdrawal with perceptual
disturbances

F13.239 Sedative, hypnotic or anxiolytic
dependence with
withdrawal, unspecified
Sedative, hypnotic, or anxiolytic
withdrawal without perceptual
disturbances

F13.24 Sedative, hypnotic or anxiolytic dependence
with sedative, hypnotic or anxiolytic-induced
mood disorder
Sedative, hypnotic, or anxiolytic use disorder,
moderate, with sedative, hypnotic, or
anxiolytic-induced bipolar or related
disorder
Sedative, hypnotic, or anxiolytic use disorder,
moderate, with sedative, hypnotic, or
anxiolytic-induced depressive disorder
Sedative, hypnotic, or anxiolytic use disorder,
severe, with sedative, hypnotic, or
anxiolytic-induced bipolar or related
disorder
Sedative, hypnotic, or anxiolytic use disorder,
severe, with sedative, hypnotic, or
anxiolytic-induced depressive disorder

● **F13.25** Sedative, hypnotic or anxiolytic dependence
with sedative, hypnotic or anxiolytic-induced
psychotic disorder
F13.250 Sedative, hypnotic or anxiolytic
dependence with sedative, hypnotic
or anxiolytic-induced psychotic
disorder with delusions

F13.251 Sedative, hypnotic or anxiolytic
dependence with sedative, hypnotic
or anxiolytic-induced psychotic
disorder with hallucinations

F13.259 Sedative, hypnotic or anxiolytic
dependence with sedative, hypnotic
or anxiolytic-induced psychotic
disorder, unspecified

F13.26 Sedative, hypnotic or anxiolytic dependence
with sedative, hypnotic or anxiolytic-induced
persisting amnestic disorder

F13.27 Sedative, hypnotic or anxiolytic dependence
with sedative, hypnotic or anxiolytic-induced
persisting dementia
Sedative, hypnotic, or anxiolytic use disorder,
moderate, with sedative, hypnotic, or
anxiolytic-induced major neurocognitive
disorder
Sedative, hypnotic, or anxiolytic use disorder,
severe, with sedative, hypnotic, or
anxiolytic-induced major neurocognitive
disorder

● **F13.28** Sedative, hypnotic or anxiolytic dependence
with other sedative, hypnotic or anxiolytic-
induced disorders
F13.280 Sedative, hypnotic or anxiolytic
dependence with sedative, hypnotic
or anxiolytic-induced anxiety
disorder

F13.281 Sedative, hypnotic or anxiolytic
dependence with sedative, hypnotic
or anxiolytic-induced sexual
dysfunction

F13.282 Sedative, hypnotic or anxiolytic
dependence with sedative, hypnotic
or anxiolytic-induced sleep
disorder

F13.288 Sedative, hypnotic or anxiolytic dependence with other sedative, hypnotic or anxiolytic-induced disorder 🔖
  Sedative, hypnotic, or anxiolytic use disorder, moderate, with sedative, hypnotic, or anxiolytic-induced mild neurocognitive disorder
  Sedative, hypnotic, or anxiolytic use disorder, severe, with sedative, hypnotic, or anxiolytic-induced mild neurocognitive disorder

F13.29 Sedative, hypnotic or anxiolytic dependence with unspecified sedative, hypnotic or anxiolytic-induced disorder 🔖

● F13.9 Sedative, hypnotic or anxiolytic-related use, unspecified
  Excludes1   sedative, hypnotic or anxiolytic-related abuse (F13.1-)
    sedative, hypnotic or anxiolytic-related dependence (F13.2-)

F13.90 Sedative, hypnotic, or anxiolytic use, unspecified, uncomplicated

● F13.92 Sedative, hypnotic or anxiolytic use, unspecified with intoxication
  Excludes1   sedative, hypnotic or anxiolytic use, unspecified with withdrawal (F13.93-)

F13.920 Sedative, hypnotic or anxiolytic use, unspecified with intoxication, uncomplicated 🔖

F13.921 Sedative, hypnotic or anxiolytic use, unspecified with intoxication delirium 🔖
  Sedative, hypnotic, or anxiolytic-induced delirium

F13.929 Sedative, hypnotic or anxiolytic use, unspecified with intoxication, unspecified 🔖

● F13.93 Sedative, hypnotic or anxiolytic use, unspecified with withdrawal
  Excludes1   sedative, hypnotic or anxiolytic use, unspecified with intoxication (F13.92-)

F13.930 Sedative, hypnotic or anxiolytic use, unspecified with withdrawal, uncomplicated 🔖

F13.931 Sedative, hypnotic or anxiolytic use, unspecified with withdrawal delirium 🔖

F13.932 Sedative, hypnotic or anxiolytic use, unspecified with withdrawal with perceptual disturbances 🔖

F13.939 Sedative, hypnotic or anxiolytic use, unspecified with withdrawal, unspecified 🔖

F13.94 Sedative, hypnotic or anxiolytic use, unspecified with sedative, hypnotic or anxiolytic-induced mood disorder 🔖
  Sedative, hypnotic, or anxiolytic-induced bipolar or related disorder, without use disorder
  Sedative, hypnotic, or anxiolytic-induced depressive disorder, without use disorder

● F13.95 Sedative, hypnotic or anxiolytic use, unspecified with sedative, hypnotic or anxiolytic-induced psychotic disorder

F13.950 Sedative, hypnotic or anxiolytic use, unspecified with sedative, hypnotic or anxiolytic-induced psychotic disorder with delusions 🔖

F13.951 Sedative, hypnotic or anxiolytic use, unspecified with sedative, hypnotic or anxiolytic-induced psychotic disorder with hallucinations 🔖

F13.959 Sedative, hypnotic or anxiolytic use, unspecified with sedative, hypnotic or anxiolytic-induced psychotic disorder, unspecified 🔖
  Sedative, hypnotic, or anxiolytic-induced psychotic disorder, without use disorder

F13.96 Sedative, hypnotic or anxiolytic use, unspecified with sedative, hypnotic or anxiolytic-induced persisting amnestic disorder 🔖

F13.97 Sedative, hypnotic or anxiolytic use, unspecified with sedative, hypnotic or anxiolytic-induced persisting dementia 🔖
  Sedative, hypnotic, or anxiolytic-induced major neurocognitive disorder, without use disorder

● F13.98 Sedative, hypnotic or anxiolytic use, unspecified with other sedative, hypnotic or anxiolytic-induced disorders

F13.980 Sedative, hypnotic or anxiolytic use, unspecified with sedative, hypnotic or anxiolytic-induced anxiety disorder 🔖
  Sedative, hypnotic, or anxiolytic-induced anxiety disorder, without use disorder

F13.981 Sedative, hypnotic or anxiolytic use, unspecified with sedative, hypnotic or anxiolytic-induced sexual dysfunction 🔖
  Sedative, hypnotic, or anxiolytic-induced sexual dysfunction disorder, without use disorder

F13.982 Sedative, hypnotic or anxiolytic use, unspecified with sedative, hypnotic or anxiolytic-induced sleep disorder 🔖
  Sedative, hypnotic, or anxiolytic-induced sleep disorder, without use disorder

F13.988 Sedative, hypnotic or anxiolytic use, unspecified with other sedative, hypnotic or anxiolytic-induced disorder 🔖
  Sedative, hypnotic, or anxiolytic-induced mild neurocognitive disorder

F13.99 Sedative, hypnotic or anxiolytic use, unspecified with unspecified sedative, hypnotic or anxiolytic-induced disorder 🔖

CHAPTER 5 (F01-F99)

● F14   Cocaine related disorders
      Excludes2   other stimulant-related disorders (F15.-)

● F14.1   Cocaine abuse
      Excludes1   cocaine dependence (F14.2-)
                   cocaine use, unspecified (F14.9-)

     F14.10   **Cocaine abuse, uncomplicated**
               Cocaine use disorder, mild

     F14.11   **Cocaine abuse, in remission**
               Cocaine use disorder, mild, in early remission
               Cocaine use disorder, mild, in sustained remission

    ● F14.12   **Cocaine abuse with intoxication**
        F14.120   **Cocaine abuse with intoxication, uncomplicated** 🝚
        F14.121   **Cocaine abuse with intoxication with delirium** 🝚
        F14.122   **Cocaine abuse with intoxication with perceptual disturbance** 🝚
        F14.129   **Cocaine abuse with intoxication, unspecified** 🝚

     F14.13   **Cocaine abuse, unspecified with withdrawal**

     F14.14   **Cocaine abuse with cocaine-induced mood disorder** 🝚
               Cocaine use disorder, mild, with cocaine-induced bipolar or related disorder
               Cocaine use disorder, mild, with cocaine-induced depressive disorder

    ● F14.15   **Cocaine abuse with cocaine-induced psychotic disorder**
        F14.150   **Cocaine abuse with cocaine-induced psychotic disorder with delusions** 🝚
        F14.151   **Cocaine abuse with cocaine-induced psychotic disorder with hallucinations** 🝚
        F14.159   **Cocaine abuse with cocaine-induced psychotic disorder, unspecified** 🝚

    ● F14.18   **Cocaine abuse with other cocaine-induced disorder**
        F14.180   **Cocaine abuse with cocaine-induced anxiety disorder** 🝚
        F14.181   **Cocaine abuse with cocaine-induced sexual dysfunction** 🝚
        F14.182   **Cocaine abuse with cocaine-induced sleep disorder** 🝚
        F14.188   **Cocaine abuse with other cocaine-induced disorder** 🝚
               Cocaine use disorder, mild, with cocaine-induced obsessive-compulsive or related disorder

     F14.19   **Cocaine abuse with unspecified cocaine-induced disorder** 🝚

● F14.2   Cocaine dependence
      Excludes1   cocaine abuse (F14.1-)
                   cocaine use, unspecified (F14.9-)
      Excludes2   cocaine poisoning (T40.5-)

     F14.20   **Cocaine dependence, uncomplicated** 🝚
               Cocaine use disorder, moderate
               Cocaine use disorder, severe

     F14.21   **Cocaine dependence, in remission** 🝚
               Cocaine use disorder, moderate, in early remission
               Cocaine use disorder, moderate, in sustained remission
               Cocaine use disorder, severe, in early remission
               Cocaine use disorder, severe, in sustained remission
               Coding Clinic: 2017, Q2, P27

● F14.22   Cocaine dependence with intoxication
      Excludes1   cocaine dependence with withdrawal (F14.23)

     F14.220   **Cocaine dependence with intoxication, uncomplicated** 🝚
     F14.221   **Cocaine dependence with intoxication delirium** 🝚
     F14.222   **Cocaine dependence with intoxication with perceptual disturbance** 🝚
     F14.229   **Cocaine dependence with intoxication, unspecified** 🝚

     F14.23   **Cocaine dependence with withdrawal** 🝚
      Excludes1   cocaine dependence with intoxication (F14.22-)

     F14.24   **Cocaine dependence with cocaine-induced mood disorder** 🝚
               Cocaine use disorder, moderate, with cocaine-induced bipolar or related disorder
               Cocaine use disorder, moderate, with cocaine-induced depressive disorder
               Cocaine use disorder, severe, with cocaine-induced bipolar or related disorder
               Cocaine use disorder, severe, with cocaine-induced depressive disorder

    ● F14.25   **Cocaine dependence with cocaine-induced psychotic disorder**
        F14.250   **Cocaine dependence with cocaine-induced psychotic disorder with delusions** 🝚
        F14.251   **Cocaine dependence with cocaine-induced psychotic disorder with hallucinations** 🝚
        F14.259   **Cocaine dependence with cocaine-induced psychotic disorder, unspecified** 🝚

    ● F14.28   **Cocaine dependence with other cocaine-induced disorder**
        F14.280   **Cocaine dependence with cocaine-induced anxiety disorder** 🝚
        F14.281   **Cocaine dependence with cocaine-induced sexual dysfunction** 🝚
        F14.282   **Cocaine dependence with cocaine-induced sleep disorder** 🝚
        F14.288   **Cocaine dependence with other cocaine-induced disorder** 🝚
               Cocaine use disorder, moderate, with cocaine-induced obsessive-compulsive or related disorder
               Cocaine use disorder, severe, with cocaine-induced obsessive-compulsive or related disorder

     F14.29   **Cocaine dependence with unspecified cocaine-induced disorder** 🝚

● F14.9   Cocaine use, unspecified
      Excludes1   cocaine abuse (F14.1-)
                   cocaine dependence (F14.2-)

     F14.90   **Cocaine use, unspecified, uncomplicated**
               Coding Clinic: 2018, Q2, P11

    ● F14.92   **Cocaine use, unspecified with intoxication**
        F14.920   **Cocaine use, unspecified with intoxication, uncomplicated** 🝚
        F14.921   **Cocaine use, unspecified with intoxication delirium** 🝚
        F14.922   **Cocaine use, unspecified with intoxication with perceptual disturbance** 🝚
        F14.929   **Cocaine use, unspecified with intoxication, unspecified** 🝚

► New   ⇒ Revised   ~~deleted~~ Deleted   Excludes 1   Excludes 2   Includes   Use additional   Code first   Code also   Key words
OGCR Official Guidelines   X Assign placeholder X   ● Use Additional Character(s)   ▌ Manifestation Code   🝚 Hierarchical Condition Category   **Coding Clinic**

F14.93   Cocaine use, unspecified with withdrawal

F14.94   Cocaine use, unspecified with cocaine-induced mood disorder 🔖
    Cocaine-induced bipolar or related disorder, without use disorder
    Cocaine-induced depressive disorder, without use disorder

● F14.95   Cocaine use, unspecified with cocaine-induced psychotic disorder

    F14.950   Cocaine use, unspecified with cocaine-induced psychotic disorder with delusions 🔖

    F14.951   Cocaine use, unspecified with cocaine-induced psychotic disorder with hallucinations 🔖

    F14.959   Cocaine use, unspecified with cocaine-induced psychotic disorder, unspecified 🔖
        Cocaine-induced psychotic disorder, without use disorder

● F14.98   Cocaine use, unspecified with other specified cocaine-induced disorder

    F14.980   Cocaine use, unspecified with cocaine-induced anxiety disorder 🔖
        Cocaine-induced anxiety disorder, without use disorder

    F14.981   Cocaine use, unspecified with cocaine-induced sexual dysfunction 🔖
        Cocaine-induced sexual dysfunction, without use disorder

    F14.982   Cocaine use, unspecified with cocaine-induced sleep disorder 🔖
        Cocaine-induced sleep disorder, without use disorder

    F14.988   Cocaine use, unspecified with other cocaine-induced disorder 🔖
        Cocaine-induced obsessive-compulsive or related disorder

F14.99   Cocaine use, unspecified with unspecified cocaine-induced disorder 🔖

● F15   Other stimulant related disorders

    Includes   amphetamine-related disorders
                  caffeine

    Excludes2   cocaine-related disorders (F14.-)

● F15.1   Other stimulant abuse

    Excludes1   other stimulant dependence (F15.2-)
                  other stimulant use, unspecified (F15.9-)

    F15.10   Other stimulant abuse, uncomplicated
        Amphetamine type substance use disorder, mild
        Other or unspecified stimulant use disorder, mild

    F15.11   Other stimulant abuse, in remission
        Amphetamine type substance use disorder, mild, in early remission
        Amphetamine type substance use disorder, mild, in sustained remission
        Other or unspecified stimulant use disorder, mild, in early remission
        Other or unspecified stimulant use disorder, mild, in sustained remission

● F15.12   Other stimulant abuse with intoxication

    F15.120   Other stimulant abuse with intoxication, uncomplicated 🔖

    F15.121   Other stimulant abuse with intoxication delirium 🔖

    F15.122   Other stimulant abuse with intoxication with perceptual disturbance 🔖
        Amphetamine or other stimulant use disorder, mild, with amphetamine or other stimulant intoxication, with perceptual disturbances

    F15.129   Other stimulant abuse with intoxication, unspecified 🔖
        Amphetamine or other stimulant use disorder, mild, with amphetamine or other stimulant intoxication, without perceptual disturbances

F15.13   Other stimulant abuse with withdrawal

F15.14   Other stimulant abuse with stimulant-induced mood disorder 🔖
    Amphetamine or other stimulant use disorder, mild, with amphetamine or other stimulant-induced bipolar or related disorder
    Amphetamine or other stimulant use disorder, mild, with amphetamine or other stimulant-induced depressive disorder

● F15.15   Other stimulant abuse with stimulant-induced psychotic disorder

    F15.150   Other stimulant abuse with stimulant-induced psychotic disorder with delusions 🔖

    F15.151   Other stimulant abuse with stimulant-induced psychotic disorder with hallucinations 🔖

    F15.159   Other stimulant abuse with stimulant-induced psychotic disorder, unspecified 🔖

● F15.18   Other stimulant abuse with other stimulant-induced disorder

    F15.180   Other stimulant abuse with stimulant-induced anxiety disorder 🔖

    F15.181   Other stimulant abuse with stimulant-induced sexual dysfunction 🔖

    F15.182   Other stimulant abuse with stimulant-induced sleep disorder 🔖

    F15.188   Other stimulant abuse with other stimulant-induced disorder 🔖
        Amphetamine or other stimulant use disorder, mild, with amphetamine or other stimulant-induced obsessive-compulsive or related disorder

F15.19   Other stimulant abuse with unspecified stimulant-induced disorder 🔖

● F15.2   Other stimulant dependence

    Excludes1   other stimulant abuse (F15.1-)
                  other stimulant use, unspecified (F15.9-)

    F15.20   Other stimulant dependence, uncomplicated 🔖
        Amphetamine type substance use disorder, moderate
        Amphetamine type substance use disorder, severe
        Other or unspecified stimulant use disorder, moderate
        Other or unspecified stimulant use disorder, severe

CHAPTER 5 (F01-F99)

CHAPTER 5 (F01-F99)

F15.21   Other stimulant dependence, in remission 🐾
    Amphetamine type substance use disorder, moderate, in early remission
    Amphetamine type substance use disorder, moderate, in sustained remission
    Amphetamine type substance use disorder, severe, in early remission
    Amphetamine type substance use disorder, severe, in sustained remission
    Other or unspecified stimulant use disorder, moderate, in early remission
    Other or unspecified stimulant use disorder, moderate, in sustained remission
    Other or unspecified stimulant use disorder, severe, in early remission
    Other or unspecified stimulant use disorder, severe, in sustained remission

● **F15.22**   Other stimulant dependence with intoxication

    Excludes1   other stimulant dependence with withdrawal (F15.23)

    F15.220   Other stimulant dependence with intoxication, uncomplicated 🐾

    F15.221   Other stimulant dependence with intoxication delirium 🐾

    F15.222   Other stimulant dependence with intoxication with perceptual disturbance 🐾
       Amphetamine or other stimulant use disorder, moderate, with amphetamine or other stimulant intoxication, with perceptual disturbances
       Amphetamine or other stimulant use disorder, severe, with amphetamine or other stimulant intoxication, with perceptual disturbances

    F15.229   Other stimulant dependence with intoxication, unspecified 🐾
       Amphetamine or other stimulant use disorder, moderate, with amphetamine or other stimulant intoxication, without perceptual disturbances
       Amphetamine or other stimulant use disorder, severe, with amphetamine or other stimulant intoxication, without perceptual disturbances

F15.23   Other stimulant dependence with withdrawal 🐾
    Amphetamine or other stimulant withdrawal

    Excludes1   other stimulant dependence with intoxication (F15.22-)

F15.24   Other stimulant dependence with stimulant-induced mood disorder 🐾
    Amphetamine or other stimulant use disorder, moderate, with amphetamine or other stimulant-induced bipolar or related disorder
    Amphetamine or other stimulant use disorder, moderate, with amphetamine or other stimulant-induced depressive disorder
    Amphetamine or other stimulant use disorder, severe, with amphetamine or other stimulant-induced bipolar or related disorder
    Amphetamine or other stimulant use disorder, severe, with amphetamine or other stimulant-induced depressive disorder

● **F15.25**   Other stimulant dependence with stimulant-induced psychotic disorder

    F15.250   Other stimulant dependence with stimulant-induced psychotic disorder with delusions 🐾

    F15.251   Other stimulant dependence with stimulant-induced psychotic disorder with hallucinations 🐾

    F15.259   Other stimulant dependence with stimulant-induced psychotic disorder, unspecified 🐾

● **F15.28**   Other stimulant dependence with other stimulant-induced disorder

    F15.280   Other stimulant dependence with stimulant-induced anxiety disorder 🐾

    F15.281   Other stimulant dependence with stimulant-induced sexual dysfunction 🐾

    F15.282   Other stimulant dependence with stimulant-induced sleep disorder 🐾

    F15.288   Other stimulant dependence with other stimulant-induced disorder 🐾
       Amphetamine or other stimulant use disorder, moderate, with amphetamine or other stimulant-induced obsessive-compulsive or related disorder
       Amphetamine or other stimulant use disorder, severe, with amphetamine or other stimulant-induced obsessive-compulsive or related disorder

F15.29   Other stimulant dependence with unspecified stimulant-induced disorder 🐾

● **F15.9**   Other stimulant use, unspecified

    Excludes1   other stimulant abuse (F15.1-)
                 other stimulant dependence (F15.2-)

    F15.90   Other stimulant use, unspecified, uncomplicated

●   **F15.92**   Other stimulant use, unspecified with intoxication

    Excludes1   other stimulant use, unspecified with withdrawal (F15.93)

    F15.920   Other stimulant use, unspecified with intoxication, uncomplicated 🐾

    F15.921   Other stimulant use, unspecified with intoxication delirium 🐾
       Amphetamine or other stimulant-induced delirium

    F15.922   Other stimulant use, unspecified with intoxication with perceptual disturbance 🐾

    F15.929   Other stimulant use, unspecified with intoxication, unspecified 🐾
       Caffeine intoxication

F15.93   Other stimulant use, unspecified with withdrawal 🐾
    Caffeine withdrawal

    Excludes1   other stimulant use, unspecified with intoxication (F15.92-)

F15.94   Other stimulant use, unspecified with stimulant-induced mood disorder 🐾
    Amphetamine or other stimulant-induced bipolar or related disorder, without use disorder
    Amphetamine or other stimulant-induced depressive disorder, without use disorder

▶ New   ⇒ Revised   ~~deleted~~ Deleted   Excludes 1   Excludes 2   Includes   Use additional   Code first   Code also   Key words
OGCR Official Guidelines   X Assign placeholder X   ● Use Additional Character(s)   ⫸ Manifestation Code   🐾 Hierarchical Condition Category   **Coding Clinic**

● **F15.95** **Other stimulant use, unspecified with stimulant-induced psychotic disorder**
    F15.950 **Other stimulant use, unspecified with stimulant-induced psychotic disorder with delusions** 🔍
    F15.951 **Other stimulant use, unspecified with stimulant-induced psychotic disorder with hallucinations** 🔍
    F15.959 **Other stimulant use, unspecified with stimulant-induced psychotic disorder, unspecified** 🔍
       Amphetamine or other stimulant-induced psychotic disorder, without use disorder

● **F15.98** **Other stimulant use, unspecified with other stimulant-induced disorder**
    F15.980 **Other stimulant use, unspecified with stimulant-induced anxiety disorder** 🔍
       Amphetamine or other stimulant-induced anxiety disorder, without use disorder
       Caffeine-induced anxiety disorder, without use disorder
    F15.981 **Other stimulant use, unspecified with stimulant-induced sexual dysfunction** 🔍
       Amphetamine or other stimulant-induced sexual dysfunction, without use disorder
    F15.982 **Other stimulant use, unspecified with stimulant-induced sleep disorder** 🔍
       Amphetamine or other stimulant-induced sleep disorder, without use disorder
       Caffeine-induced sleep disorder, without use disorder
    F15.988 **Other stimulant use, unspecified with other stimulant-induced disorder** 🔍
       Amphetamine or other stimulant-induced obsessive-compulsive or related disorder, without use disorder
   F15.99 **Other stimulant use, unspecified with unspecified stimulant-induced disorder** 🔍

● **F16** **Hallucinogen related disorders**
   Includes   ecstasy
                PCP
                phencyclidine

● **F16.1** **Hallucinogen abuse**
   Excludes1   hallucinogen dependence (F16.2-)
                hallucinogen use, unspecified (F16.9-)
   F16.10 **Hallucinogen abuse, uncomplicated**
       Other hallucinogen use disorder, mild
       Phencyclidine use disorder, mild
       Coding Clinic: 2018, Q4, P31
   F16.11 **Hallucinogen abuse, in remission**
       Other hallucinogen use disorder, mild, in early remission
       Other hallucinogen use disorder, mild, in sustained remission
       Phencyclidine use disorder, mild, in early remission
       Phencyclidine use disorder, mild, in sustained remission
● **F16.12** **Hallucinogen abuse with intoxication**
    F16.120 **Hallucinogen abuse with intoxication, uncomplicated** 🔍
    F16.121 **Hallucinogen abuse with intoxication with delirium** 🔍
    F16.122 **Hallucinogen abuse with intoxication with perceptual disturbance** 🔍
    F16.129 **Hallucinogen abuse with intoxication, unspecified** 🔍

F16.14 **Hallucinogen abuse with hallucinogen-induced mood disorder** 🔍
       Other hallucinogen use disorder, mild, with other hallucinogen-induced bipolar or related disorder
       Other hallucinogen use disorder, mild, with other hallucinogen-induced depressive disorder
       Phencyclidine use disorder, mild, with phencyclidine-induced bipolar or related disorder
       Phencyclidine use disorder, mild, with phencyclidine-induced depressive disorder
● **F16.15** **Hallucinogen abuse with hallucinogen-induced psychotic disorder**
    F16.150 **Hallucinogen abuse with hallucinogen-induced psychotic disorder with delusions** 🔍
    F16.151 **Hallucinogen abuse with hallucinogen-induced psychotic disorder with hallucinations** 🔍
    F16.159 **Hallucinogen abuse with hallucinogen-induced psychotic disorder, unspecified** 🔍
● **F16.18** **Hallucinogen abuse with other hallucinogen-induced disorder**
    F16.180 **Hallucinogen abuse with hallucinogen-induced anxiety disorder** 🔍
    F16.183 **Hallucinogen abuse with hallucinogen persisting perception disorder (flashbacks)** 🔍
    F16.188 **Hallucinogen abuse with other hallucinogen-induced disorder** 🔍
   F16.19 **Hallucinogen abuse with unspecified hallucinogen-induced disorder** 🔍
● **F16.2** **Hallucinogen dependence**
   Excludes1   hallucinogen abuse (F16.1-)
                hallucinogen use, unspecified (F16.9-)
   F16.20 **Hallucinogen dependence, uncomplicated** 🔍
       Other hallucinogen use disorder, moderate
       Other hallucinogen use disorder, severe
       Phencyclidine use disorder, moderate
       Phencyclidine use disorder, severe
   F16.21 **Hallucinogen dependence, in remission** 🔍
       Other hallucinogen use disorder, moderate, in early remission
       Other hallucinogen use disorder, moderate, in sustained remission
       Other hallucinogen use disorder, severe, in early remission
       Other hallucinogen use disorder, severe, in sustained remission
       Phencyclidine use disorder, moderate, in early remission
       Phencyclidine use disorder, moderate, in sustained remission
       Phencyclidine use disorder, severe, in early remission
       Phencyclidine use disorder, severe, in sustained remission
● **F16.22** **Hallucinogen dependence with intoxication**
    F16.220 **Hallucinogen dependence with intoxication, uncomplicated** 🔍
    F16.221 **Hallucinogen dependence with intoxication with delirium** 🔍
    F16.229 **Hallucinogen dependence with intoxication, unspecified** 🔍

CHAPTER 5 (FØ1-F99)

F16.24 **Hallucinogen dependence with hallucinogen-induced mood disorder** 🐷
Other hallucinogen use disorder, moderate, with other hallucinogen-induced bipolar or related disorder
Other hallucinogen use disorder, moderate, with other hallucinogen-induced depressive disorder
Other hallucinogen use disorder, severe, with other hallucinogen-induced bipolar or related disorder
Other hallucinogen use disorder, severe, with other hallucinogen-induced depressive disorder
Phencyclidine use disorder, moderate, with phencyclidine-induced bipolar or related disorder
Phencyclidine use disorder, moderate, with phencyclidine-induced depressive disorder
Phencyclidine use disorder, severe, with phencyclidine-induced bipolar or related disorder
Phencyclidine use disorder, severe, with phencyclidine-induced depressive disorder

● **F16.25** **Hallucinogen dependence with hallucinogen-induced psychotic disorder**
F16.250 Hallucinogen dependence with hallucinogen-induced psychotic disorder with delusions 🐷
F16.251 Hallucinogen dependence with hallucinogen-induced psychotic disorder with hallucinations 🐷
F16.259 Hallucinogen dependence with hallucinogen-induced psychotic disorder, unspecified 🐷

● **F16.28** **Hallucinogen dependence with other hallucinogen-induced disorder**
F16.280 Hallucinogen dependence with hallucinogen-induced anxiety disorder 🐷
F16.283 Hallucinogen dependence with hallucinogen persisting perception disorder (flashbacks) 🐷
F16.288 Hallucinogen dependence with other hallucinogen-induced disorder 🐷

F16.29 **Hallucinogen dependence with unspecified hallucinogen-induced disorder** 🐷

● **F16.9** **Hallucinogen use, unspecified**
Excludes1 hallucinogen abuse (F16.1-)
hallucinogen dependence (F16.2-)

F16.90 **Hallucinogen use, unspecified, uncomplicated**
● **F16.92** **Hallucinogen use, unspecified with intoxication**
F16.920 Hallucinogen use, unspecified with intoxication, uncomplicated 🐷
F16.921 Hallucinogen use, unspecified with intoxication with delirium 🐷
Other hallucinogen intoxication delirium
F16.929 Hallucinogen use, unspecified with intoxication, unspecified 🐷

F16.94 **Hallucinogen use, unspecified with hallucinogen-induced mood disorder** 🐷
Other hallucinogen-induced bipolar or related disorder, without use disorder
Other hallucinogen-induced depressive disorder, without use disorder
Phencyclidine-induced bipolar or related disorder, without use disorder
Phencyclidine-induced depressive disorder, without use disorder

● **F16.95** **Hallucinogen use, unspecified with hallucinogen-induced psychotic disorder**
F16.950 Hallucinogen use, unspecified with hallucinogen-induced psychotic disorder with delusions 🐷
F16.951 Hallucinogen use, unspecified with hallucinogen-induced psychotic disorder with hallucinations 🐷
F16.959 Hallucinogen use, unspecified with hallucinogen-induced psychotic disorder, unspecified 🐷
Other hallucinogen-induced psychotic disorder, without use disorder
Phencyclidine-induced psychotic disorder, without use disorder

● **F16.98** **Hallucinogen use, unspecified with other specified hallucinogen-induced disorder**
F16.980 Hallucinogen use, unspecified with hallucinogen-induced anxiety disorder 🐷
Other hallucinogen-induced anxiety disorder, without use disorder
Phencyclidine-induced anxiety disorder, without use disorder
F16.983 Hallucinogen use, unspecified with hallucinogen persisting perception disorder (flashbacks) 🐷
F16.988 Hallucinogen use, unspecified with other hallucinogen-induced disorder 🐷

F16.99 **Hallucinogen use, unspecified with unspecified hallucinogen-induced disorder** 🐷

● **F17** **Nicotine dependence**
Excludes1 history of tobacco dependence (Z87.891)
tobacco use NOS (Z72.0)
Excludes2 tobacco use (smoking) during pregnancy, childbirth and the puerperium (O99.33-)
toxic effect of nicotine (T65.2-)

● **F17.2** **Nicotine dependence**
● **F17.20** **Nicotine dependence, unspecified**
F17.200 Nicotine dependence, unspecified, uncomplicated
Tobacco use disorder, mild
Tobacco use disorder, moderate
Tobacco use disorder, severe
Coding Clinic: 2016, Q1, P37
F17.201 Nicotine dependence, unspecified, in remission
Tobacco use disorder, mild, in early remission
Tobacco use disorder, mild, in sustained remission
Tobacco use disorder, moderate, in early remission
Tobacco use disorder, moderate, in sustained remission
Tobacco use disorder, severe, in early remission
Tobacco use disorder, severe, in sustained remission
F17.203 Nicotine dependence unspecified, with withdrawal
Tobacco withdrawal
F17.208 Nicotine dependence, unspecified, with other nicotine-induced disorders
F17.209 Nicotine dependence, unspecified, with unspecified nicotine-induced disorders

● **F17.21** **Nicotine dependence, cigarettes**
F17.210 Nicotine dependence, cigarettes, uncomplicated
Coding Clinic: 2017, Q2, P28-29

▶ New ⏩ Revised ~~deleted~~ Deleted | Excludes 1 | Excludes 2 | Includes | Use additional | Code first | Code also | Key words
OGCR Official Guidelines X Assign placeholder X ● Use Additional Character(s) ▌ Manifestation Code 🐷 Hierarchical Condition Category **Coding Clinic**

F17.211   **Nicotine dependence, cigarettes, in
           remission**
               Tobacco use disorder, cigarettes,
                   mild, in early remission
               Tobacco use disorder, cigarettes,
                   mild, in sustained remission
               Tobacco use disorder, cigarettes,
                   moderate, in early remission
               Tobacco use disorder, cigarettes,
                   moderate, in sustained
                   remission
               Tobacco use disorder, cigarettes,
                   severe, in early remission
               Tobacco use disorder, cigarettes,
                   severe, in sustained remission
F17.213   **Nicotine dependence, cigarettes, with
           withdrawal**
F17.218   **Nicotine dependence, cigarettes, with
           other nicotine-induced disorders**
F17.219   **Nicotine dependence, cigarettes,
           with unspecified nicotine-induced
           disorders**

● F17.22   **Nicotine dependence, chewing tobacco**
F17.220   **Nicotine dependence, chewing
           tobacco, uncomplicated**
F17.221   **Nicotine dependence, chewing
           tobacco, in remission**
               Tobacco use disorder, chewing
                   tobacco, mild, in early
                   remission
               Tobacco use disorder, chewing
                   tobacco, mild, in sustained
                   remission
               Tobacco use disorder, chewing
                   tobacco, moderate, in early
                   remission
               Tobacco use disorder, chewing
                   tobacco, moderate, in sustained
                   remission
               Tobacco use disorder, chewing
                   tobacco, severe, in early
                   remission
               Tobacco use disorder, chewing
                   tobacco, severe, in sustained
                   remission
F17.223   **Nicotine dependence, chewing
           tobacco, with withdrawal**
F17.228   **Nicotine dependence, chewing
           tobacco, with other nicotine-induced
           disorders**
F17.229   **Nicotine dependence, chewing
           tobacco, with unspecified nicotine-
           induced disorders**

● F17.29   **Nicotine dependence, other tobacco product**
F17.290   **Nicotine dependence, other tobacco
           product, uncomplicated**
               Coding Clinic: 2017, Q2, P28-29
F17.291   **Nicotine dependence, other tobacco
           product, in remission**
               Tobacco use disorder, other tobacco
                   product, mild, in early
                   remission
               Tobacco use disorder, other tobacco
                   product, mild, in sustained
                   remission
               Tobacco use disorder, other tobacco
                   product, moderate, in early
                   remission
               Tobacco use disorder, other tobacco
                   product, moderate, in sustained
                   remission
               Tobacco use disorder, other tobacco
                   product, severe, in early
                   remission
               Tobacco use disorder, other tobacco
                   product, severe, in sustained
                   remission

F17.293   **Nicotine dependence, other tobacco
           product, with withdrawal**
F17.298   **Nicotine dependence, other tobacco
           product, with other nicotine-induced
           disorders**
F17.299   **Nicotine dependence, other tobacco
           product, with unspecified nicotine-
           induced disorders**

● F18   **Inhalant related disorders**
           Includes   volatile solvents
   ● F18.1   **Inhalant abuse**
           Excludes1   inhalant dependence (F18.2-)
                        inhalant use, unspecified (F18.9-)
       F18.10   **Inhalant abuse, uncomplicated**
                   Inhalant use disorder, mild
       F18.11   **Inhalant abuse, in remission**
                   Inhalant use disorder, mild, in early remission
                   Inhalant use disorder, mild, in sustained
                       remission
   ● F18.12   **Inhalant abuse with intoxication**
       F18.120   **Inhalant abuse with intoxication,
                   uncomplicated** 🔒
       F18.121   **Inhalant abuse with intoxication
                   delirium** 🔒
       F18.129   **Inhalant abuse with
                   intoxication, unspecified** 🔒
       F18.14   **Inhalant abuse with inhalant-induced mood
                   disorder** 🔒
                   Inhalant use disorder, mild, with inhalant-
                       induced depressive disorder
   ● F18.15   **Inhalant abuse with inhalant-induced psychotic
               disorder**
       F18.150   **Inhalant abuse with inhalant-induced
                   psychotic disorder with delusions** 🔒
       F18.151   **Inhalant abuse with inhalant-induced
                   psychotic disorder with
                   hallucinations** 🔒
       F18.159   **Inhalant abuse with inhalant-induced
                   psychotic disorder, unspecified** 🔒
       F18.17   **Inhalant abuse with inhalant-induced
                   dementia** 🔒
                   Inhalant use disorder, mild, with inhalant-
                       induced major neurocognitive disorder
   ● F18.18   **Inhalant abuse with other inhalant-induced
               disorders**
       F18.180   **Inhalant abuse with inhalant-induced
                   anxiety disorder** 🔒
       F18.188   **Inhalant abuse with other inhalant-
                   induced disorder** 🔒
                   Inhalant use disorder, mild,
                       with inhalant-induced mild
                       neurocognitive disorder
       F18.19   **Inhalant abuse with unspecified inhalant-
                   induced disorder** 🔒
   ● F18.2   **Inhalant dependence**
           Excludes1   inhalant abuse (F18.1-)
                        inhalant use, unspecified (F18.9-)
       F18.20   **Inhalant dependence, uncomplicated** 🔒
                   Inhalant use disorder, moderate
                   Inhalant use disorder, severe
       F18.21   **Inhalant dependence, in remission** 🔒
                   Inhalant use disorder, moderate, in early
                       remission
                   Inhalant use disorder, moderate, in sustained
                       remission
                   Inhalant use disorder, severe, in early
                       remission
                   Inhalant use disorder, severe, in sustained
                       remission

CHAPTER 5 (FØ1-F99)

CHAPTER 5 (F01-F99)

● **F18.22 Inhalant dependence with intoxication**

　　F18.220 Inhalant dependence with intoxication, uncomplicated 🦠

　　F18.221 Inhalant dependence with intoxication delirium 🦠

　　F18.229 Inhalant dependence with intoxication, unspecified 🦠

　F18.24 Inhalant dependence with inhalant-induced mood disorder 🦠
　　　Inhalant use disorder, moderate, with inhalant-induced depressive disorder
　　　Inhalant use disorder, severe, with inhalant-induced depressive disorder

● **F18.25 Inhalant dependence with inhalant-induced psychotic disorder**

　　F18.250 Inhalant dependence with inhalant-induced psychotic disorder with delusions 🦠

　　F18.251 Inhalant dependence with inhalant-induced psychotic disorder with hallucinations 🦠

　　F18.259 Inhalant dependence with inhalant-induced psychotic disorder, unspecified 🦠

　F18.27 Inhalant dependence with inhalant-induced dementia 🦠
　　　Inhalant use disorder, moderate, with inhalant-induced major neurocognitive disorder
　　　Inhalant use disorder, severe, with inhalant-induced major neurocognitive disorder

● **F18.28 Inhalant dependence with other inhalant-induced disorders**

　　F18.280 Inhalant dependence with inhalant-induced anxiety disorder 🦠

　　F18.288 Inhalant dependence with other inhalant-induced disorder 🦠
　　　　Inhalant use disorder, moderate, with inhalant-induced mild neurocognitive disorder
　　　　Inhalant use disorder, severe, with inhalant-induced mild neurocognitive disorder

　F18.29 Inhalant dependence with unspecified inhalant-induced disorder 🦠

● **F18.9 Inhalant use, unspecified**

　Excludes1 inhalant abuse (F18.1-)
　　　　　inhalant dependence (F18.2-)

　F18.90 Inhalant use, unspecified, uncomplicated

● **F18.92 Inhalant use, unspecified with intoxication**

　　F18.920 Inhalant use, unspecified with intoxication, uncomplicated 🦠

　　F18.921 Inhalant use, unspecified with intoxication with delirium 🦠

　　F18.929 Inhalant use, unspecified with intoxication, unspecified 🦠

　F18.94 Inhalant use, unspecified with inhalant-induced mood disorder 🦠
　　　Inhalant-induced depressive disorder

● **F18.95 Inhalant use, unspecified with inhalant-induced psychotic disorder**

　　F18.950 Inhalant use, unspecified with inhalant-induced psychotic disorder with delusions 🦠

　　F18.951 Inhalant use, unspecified with inhalant-induced psychotic disorder with hallucinations 🦠

　　F18.959 Inhalant use, unspecified with inhalant-induced psychotic disorder, unspecified 🦠

　F18.97 Inhalant use, unspecified with inhalant-induced persisting dementia 🦠
　　　Inhalant-induced major neurocognitive disorder

● **F18.98 Inhalant use, unspecified with other inhalant-induced disorders**

　　F18.980 Inhalant use, unspecified with inhalant-induced anxiety disorder 🦠

　　F18.988 Inhalant use, unspecified with other inhalant-induced disorder 🦠
　　　Inhalant-induced mild neurocognitive disorder

　F18.99 Inhalant use, unspecified with unspecified inhalant-induced disorder 🦠

● **F19 Other psychoactive substance related disorders**

　Includes polysubstance drug use (indiscriminate drug use)

● **F19.1 Other psychoactive substance abuse**

　Excludes1 other psychoactive substance dependence (F19.2-)
　　　　　other psychoactive substance use, unspecified (F19.9-)

　F19.10 Other psychoactive substance abuse, uncomplicated
　　　Other (or unknown) substance use disorder, mild

　F19.11 Other psychoactive substance abuse, in remission
　　　Other (or unknown) substance use disorder, mild, in early remission
　　　Other (or unknown) substance use disorder, mild, in sustained remission

● **F19.12 Other psychoactive substance abuse with intoxication**

　　F19.120 Other psychoactive substance abuse with intoxication, uncomplicated 🦠

　　F19.121 Other psychoactive substance abuse with intoxication delirium 🦠

　　F19.122 Other psychoactive substance abuse with intoxication with perceptual disturbances 🦠

　　F19.129 Other psychoactive substance abuse with intoxication, unspecified 🦠

● **F19.13 Other psychoactive substance abuse with withdrawal**

　　F19.130 Other psychoactive substance abuse with withdrawal, uncomplicated

　　F19.131 Other psychoactive substance abuse with withdrawal delirium

　　F19.132 Other psychoactive substance abuse with withdrawal with perceptual disturbance

　　F19.139 Other psychoactive substance abuse with withdrawal, unspecified

　F19.14 Other psychoactive substance abuse with psychoactive substance-induced mood disorder 🦠
　　　Other (or unknown) substance use disorder, mild, with other (or unknown) substance-induced bipolar or related disorder
　　　Other (or unknown) substance use disorder, mild, with other (or unknown) substance-induced depressive disorder

● **F19.15 Other psychoactive substance abuse with psychoactive substance-induced psychotic disorder**

　　F19.150 Other psychoactive substance abuse with psychoactive substance-induced psychotic disorder with delusions 🦠

　　F19.151 Other psychoactive substance abuse with psychoactive substance-induced psychotic disorder with hallucinations 🦠

　　F19.159 Other psychoactive substance abuse with psychoactive substance-induced psychotic disorder, unspecified 🦠

F19.16   Other psychoactive substance abuse with psychoactive substance-induced persisting amnestic disorder 🔖

F19.17   Other psychoactive substance abuse with psychoactive substance-induced persisting dementia 🔖
> Other (or unknown) substance use disorder, mild, with other (or unknown) substance-induced major neurocognitive disorder

● F19.18   Other psychoactive substance abuse with other psychoactive substance-induced disorders

     F19.180   Other psychoactive substance abuse with psychoactive substance-induced anxiety disorder 🔖

     F19.181   Other psychoactive substance abuse with psychoactive substance-induced sexual dysfunction 🔖

     F19.182   Other psychoactive substance abuse with psychoactive substance-induced sleep disorder 🔖

     F19.188   Other psychoactive substance abuse with other psychoactive substance-induced disorder 🔖
> Other (or unknown) substance use disorder, mild, with other (or unknown) substance-induced mild neurocognitive disorder
> Other (or unknown) substance use disorder, mild, with other (or unknown) substance-induced obsessive-compulsive or related disorder

F19.19   Other psychoactive substance abuse with unspecified psychoactive substance-induced disorder 🔖

● F19.2   Other psychoactive substance dependence

     Excludes1   other psychoactive substance abuse (F19.1-)
>   other psychoactive substance use, unspecified (F19.9-)

F19.20   Other psychoactive substance dependence, uncomplicated 🔖
> Other (or unknown) substance use disorder, moderate
> Other (or unknown) substance use disorder, severe

F19.21   Other psychoactive substance dependence, in remission 🔖
> Other (or unknown) substance use disorder, moderate, in early remission
> Other (or unknown) substance use disorder, moderate, in sustained remission
> Other (or unknown) substance use disorder, severe, in early remission
> Other (or unknown) substance use disorder, severe, in sustained remission

● F19.22   Other psychoactive substance dependence with intoxication

     Excludes1   other psychoactive substance dependence with withdrawal (F19.23-)

     F19.220   Other psychoactive substance dependence with intoxication, uncomplicated 🔖

     F19.221   Other psychoactive substance dependence with intoxication delirium 🔖

     F19.222   Other psychoactive substance dependence with intoxication with perceptual disturbance 🔖

     F19.229   Other psychoactive substance dependence with intoxication, unspecified 🔖

● F19.23   Other psychoactive substance dependence with withdrawal

     Excludes1   other psychoactive substance dependence with intoxication (F19.22-)

     F19.230   Other psychoactive substance dependence with withdrawal, uncomplicated 🔖

     F19.231   Other psychoactive substance dependence with withdrawal delirium 🔖

     F19.232   Other psychoactive substance dependence with withdrawal with perceptual disturbance 🔖

     F19.239   Other psychoactive substance dependence with withdrawal, unspecified 🔖

F19.24   Other psychoactive substance dependence with psychoactive substance-induced mood disorder 🔖
> Other (or unknown) substance use disorder, moderate, with other (or unknown) substance-induced bipolar or related disorder
> Other (or unknown) substance use disorder, moderate, with other (or unknown) substance-induced depressive disorder
> Other (or unknown) substance use disorder, severe, with other (or unknown) substance-induced bipolar or related disorder
> Other (or unknown) substance use disorder, severe, with other (or unknown) substance-induced depressive disorder

● F19.25   Other psychoactive substance dependence with psychoactive substance-induced psychotic disorder

     F19.250   Other psychoactive substance dependence with psychoactive substance-induced psychotic disorder with delusions 🔖

     F19.251   Other psychoactive substance dependence with psychoactive substance-induced psychotic disorder with hallucinations 🔖

     F19.259   Other psychoactive substance dependence with psychoactive substance-induced psychotic disorder, unspecified 🔖

F19.26   Other psychoactive substance dependence with psychoactive substance-induced persisting amnestic disorder 🔖

F19.27   Other psychoactive substance dependence with psychoactive substance-induced persisting dementia 🔖
> Other (or unknown) substance use disorder, moderate, with other (or unknown) substance-induced major neurocognitive disorder
> Other (or unknown) substance use disorder, severe, with other (or unknown) substance-induced major neurocognitive disorder

● F19.28   Other psychoactive substance dependence with other psychoactive substance-induced disorders

     F19.280   Other psychoactive substance dependence with psychoactive substance-induced anxiety disorder 🔖

     F19.281   Other psychoactive substance dependence with psychoactive substance-induced sexual dysfunction 🔖

     F19.282   Other psychoactive substance dependence with psychoactive substance-induced sleep disorder 🔖

F19.288 Other psychoactive substance dependence with other psychoactive substance-induced disorder 🐾
Other (or unknown) substance use disorder, moderate, with other (or unknown) substance-induced mild neurocognitive disorder
Other (or unknown) substance use disorder, severe, with other (or unknown) substance-induced mild neurocognitive disorder
Other (or unknown) substance use disorder, moderate, with other (or unknown) substance-induced obsessive-compulsive or related disorder
Other (or unknown) substance use disorder, severe, with other (or unknown) substance-induced obsessive-compulsive or related disorder

F19.29 Other psychoactive substance dependence with unspecified psychoactive substance-induced disorder 🐾

● **F19.9** Other psychoactive substance use, unspecified
Excludes1 other psychoactive substance abuse (F19.1-)
other psychoactive substance dependence (F19.2-)

F19.90 Other psychoactive substance use, unspecified, uncomplicated

● **F19.92** Other psychoactive substance use, unspecified with intoxication
Excludes1 other psychoactive substance use, unspecified with withdrawal (F19.93)

F19.920 Other psychoactive substance use, unspecified with intoxication, uncomplicated 🐾

F19.921 Other psychoactive substance use, unspecified with intoxication with delirium 🐾
Other (or unknown) substance-induced delirium

F19.922 Other psychoactive substance use, unspecified with intoxication with perceptual disturbance 🐾

F19.929 Other psychoactive substance use, unspecified with intoxication, unspecified 🐾

● **F19.93** Other psychoactive substance use, unspecified with withdrawal
Excludes1 other psychoactive substance use, unspecified with intoxication (F19.92-)

F19.930 Other psychoactive substance use, unspecified with withdrawal, uncomplicated 🐾

F19.931 Other psychoactive substance use, unspecified with withdrawal delirium 🐾

F19.932 Other psychoactive substance use, unspecified with withdrawal with perceptual disturbance 🐾

F19.939 Other psychoactive substance use, unspecified with withdrawal, unspecified 🐾

F19.94 Other psychoactive substance use, unspecified with psychoactive substance-induced mood disorder 🐾
Other (or unknown) substance-induced bipolar or related disorder, without use disorder
Other (or unknown) substance-induced depressive disorder, without use disorder

● **F19.95** Other psychoactive substance use, unspecified with psychoactive substance-induced psychotic disorder

F19.950 Other psychoactive substance use, unspecified with psychoactive substance-induced psychotic disorder with delusions 🐾

F19.951 Other psychoactive substance use, unspecified with psychoactive substance-induced psychotic disorder with hallucinations 🐾

F19.959 Other psychoactive substance use, unspecified with psychoactive substance-induced psychotic disorder, unspecified 🐾
Other or unknown substance-induced psychotic disorder, without use disorder

F19.96 Other psychoactive substance use, unspecified with psychoactive substance-induced persisting amnestic disorder 🐾

F19.97 Other psychoactive substance use, unspecified with psychoactive substance-induced persisting dementia 🐾
Other (or unknown) substance-induced major neurocognitive disorder, without use disorder

● **F19.98** Other psychoactive substance use, unspecified with other psychoactive substance-induced disorders

F19.980 Other psychoactive substance use, unspecified with psychoactive substance-induced anxiety disorder 🐾
Other (or unknown) substance-induced anxiety disorder, without use disorder

F19.981 Other psychoactive substance use, unspecified with psychoactive substance-induced sexual dysfunction 🐾
Other (or unknown) substance-induced sexual dysfunction, without use disorder

F19.982 Other psychoactive substance use, unspecified with psychoactive substance-induced sleep disorder 🐾
Other (or unknown) substance-induced sleep disorder, without use disorder

F19.988 Other psychoactive substance use, unspecified with other psychoactive substance-induced disorder 🐾
Other (or unknown) substance-induced mild neurocognitive disorder, without use disorder
Other (or unknown) substance-induced obsessive-compulsive or related disorder, without use disorder

F19.99 Other psychoactive substance use, unspecified with unspecified psychoactive substance-induced disorder 🐾

▶ New   ⇒ Revised   ~~deleted~~ Deleted   Excludes 1   Excludes 2   Includes   Use additional   Code first   Code also   Key words
OGCR Official Guidelines   X Assign placeholder X   ● Use Additional Character(s)   ▷ Manifestation Code   🐾 Hierarchical Condition Category   **Coding Clinic**

SCHIZOPHRENIA, SCHIZOTYPAL, DELUSIONAL, AND OTHER NON-MOOD PSYCHOTIC DISORDERS (F2Ø-F29)

● **F2Ø**   **Schizophrenia**

Personality disorders characterized by multiple mental and behavioral irregularities (may exhibit disorganized thinking, delusions, and auditory hallucinations)

> **Excludes1**   brief psychotic disorder (F23)
> cyclic schizophrenia (F25.Ø)
> mood [affective] disorders with psychotic symptoms (F3Ø.2, F31.2, F31.5, F31.64, F32.3, F33.3)
> schizoaffective disorder (F25.-)
> schizophrenic reaction NOS (F23)

> **Excludes2**   schizophrenic reaction in:
> alcoholism (F1Ø.15-, F1Ø.25-, F1Ø.95-)
> brain disease (FØ6.2)
> epilepsy (FØ6.2)
> psychoactive drug use (F11-F19 with .15, .25, .95)
> schizotypal disorder (F21)

Coding Clinic: 2019, Q2, P32

F2Ø.Ø   **Paranoid schizophrenia** 🔒

Paraphrenic schizophrenia

> **Excludes1**   involutional paranoid state (F22)
> paranoia (F22)

F2Ø.1   **Disorganized schizophrenia** 🔒

Hebephrenic schizophrenia
Hebephrenia

F2Ø.2   **Catatonic schizophrenia** 🔒

Schizophrenic catalepsy
Schizophrenic catatonia
Schizophrenic flexibilitas cerea

> **Excludes1**   catatonic stupor (R4Ø.1)

F2Ø.3   **Undifferentiated schizophrenia** 🔒

Atypical schizophrenia

> **Excludes1**   acute schizophrenia-like psychotic disorder (F23)

> **Excludes2**   post-schizophrenic depression (F32.89)

F2Ø.5   **Residual schizophrenia** 🔒

Restzustand (schizophrenic)
Schizophrenic residual state

● **F2Ø.8**   **Other schizophrenia**

F2Ø.81   **Schizophreniform disorder** 🔒

Schizophreniform psychosis NOS

F2Ø.89   **Other schizophrenia** 🔒

Cenesthopathic schizophrenia
Simple schizophrenia

F2Ø.9   **Schizophrenia, unspecified** 🔒

Coding Clinic: 2019, Q2, P32

F21   **Schizotypal disorder**

Personality disorder characterized by need for social isolation, odd behavior and thinking, and often unconventional beliefs

Borderline schizophrenia
Latent schizophrenia
Latent schizophrenic reaction
Prepsychotic schizophrenia
Prodromal schizophrenia
Pseudoneurotic schizophrenia
Pseudopsychopathic schizophrenia
Schizotypal personality disorder

> **Excludes2**   Asperger's syndrome (F84.5)
> schizoid personality disorder (F6Ø.1)

F22   **Delusional disorders** 🔒

Delusional dysmorphophobia
Involutional paranoid state
Paranoia
Paranoia querulans
Paranoid psychosis
Paranoid state
Paraphrenia (late)
Sensitiver Beziehungswahn

> **Excludes1**   mood [affective] disorders with psychotic symptoms (F3Ø.2, F31.2, F31.5, F31.64, F32.3, F33.3)
> paranoid schizophrenia (F2Ø.Ø)

> **Excludes2**   paranoid personality disorder (F6Ø.Ø)
> paranoid psychosis, psychogenic (F23)
> paranoid reaction (F23)

F23   **Brief psychotic disorder**

Paranoid reaction
Psychogenic paranoid psychosis

> **Excludes2**   mood [affective] disorders with psychotic symptoms (F3Ø.2, F31.2, F31.5, F31.64, F32.3, F33.3)

Coding Clinic: 2019, Q2, P32

F24   **Shared psychotic disorder** 🔒

Folie à deux
Induced paranoid disorder
Induced psychotic disorder

● **F25**   **Schizoaffective disorders**

Mental disorder exhibiting major depressive episode, manic episode, or mixed episode occurs with symptoms of schizophrenia, and mood disorder

> **Excludes1**   mood [affective] disorders with psychotic symptoms (F3Ø.2, F31.2, F31.5, F31.64, F32.3, F33.3)
> schizophrenia (F2Ø.-)

F25.Ø   **Schizoaffective disorder, bipolar type** 🔒

Cyclic schizophrenia
Schizoaffective disorder, manic type
Schizoaffective disorder, mixed type
Schizoaffective psychosis, bipolar type

F25.1   **Schizoaffective disorder, depressive type** 🔒

Schizoaffective psychosis, depressive type

F25.8   **Other schizoaffective disorders** 🔒

F25.9   **Schizoaffective disorder, unspecified** 🔒

Schizoaffective psychosis NOS

F28   **Other psychotic disorder not due to a substance or known physiological condition**

Chronic hallucinatory psychosis
Other specified schizophrenia spectrum and other psychotic disorder

F29   **Unspecified psychosis not due to a substance or known physiological condition**

Psychosis NOS
Unspecified schizophrenia spectrum and other psychotic disorder

> **Excludes1**   mental disorder NOS (F99)
> unspecified mental disorder due to known physiological condition (FØ9)

CHAPTER 5 (FØ1-F99)

MOOD [AFFECTIVE] DISORDERS (F30-F39)

● **F30   Manic episode**
Elevated, expansive, or irritable mood

| **Includes** | bipolar disorder, single manic episode |
| | mixed affective episode |

Excludes1	bipolar disorder (F31.-)
	major depressive disorder, single episode (F32.-)
	major depressive disorder, recurrent (F33.-)

● **F30.1   Manic episode without psychotic symptoms**

F30.10   Manic episode without psychotic symptoms, unspecified 🐾

F30.11   Manic episode without psychotic symptoms, mild 🐾

F30.12   Manic episode without psychotic symptoms, moderate 🐾

F30.13   Manic episode, severe, without psychotic symptoms 🐾

F30.2   Manic episode, severe with psychotic symptoms 🐾
Manic stupor
Mania with mood-congruent psychotic symptoms
Mania with mood-incongruent psychotic symptoms

F30.3   Manic episode in partial remission 🐾

F30.4   Manic episode in full remission 🐾

F30.8   Other manic episodes 🐾
Abnormality of mood resembling mania but less intense
Hypomania

F30.9   Manic episode, unspecified 🐾
Mania NOS

● **F31   Bipolar disorder**
Mood disorders with history of manic, mixed, or hypomanic episodes

Includes	bipolar I disorder
	bipolar type I disorder
	manic-depressive illness
	manic-depressive psychosis
	manic-depressive reaction

Excludes1	bipolar disorder, single manic episode (F30.-)
	major depressive disorder, single episode (F32.-)
	major depressive disorder, recurrent (F33.-)

| **Excludes2** | cyclothymia (F34.0) |

Coding Clinic: 2020, Q1, P23

F31.0   Bipolar disorder, current episode hypomanic 🐾

● **F31.1   Bipolar disorder, current episode manic without psychotic features**

F31.10   Bipolar disorder, current episode manic without psychotic features, unspecified 🐾

F31.11   Bipolar disorder, current episode manic without psychotic features, mild 🐾

F31.12   Bipolar disorder, current episode manic without psychotic features, moderate 🐾

F31.13   Bipolar disorder, current episode manic without psychotic features, severe 🐾

F31.2   Bipolar disorder, current episode manic severe with psychotic features 🐾
Bipolar disorder, current episode manic with mood-congruent psychotic symptoms
Bipolar disorder, current episode manic with mood-incongruent psychotic symptoms
Bipolar I disorder, current or most recent episode manic with psychotic features

● **F31.3   Bipolar disorder, current episode depressed, mild or moderate severity**

F31.30   Bipolar disorder, current episode depressed, mild or moderate severity, unspecified 🐾

F31.31   Bipolar disorder, current episode depressed, mild 🐾

F31.32   Bipolar disorder, current episode depressed, moderate 🐾

F31.4   Bipolar disorder, current episode depressed, severe, without psychotic features 🐾

F31.5   Bipolar disorder, current episode depressed, severe, with psychotic features 🐾
Bipolar disorder, current episode depressed with mood-incongruent psychotic symptoms
Bipolar disorder, current episode depressed with mood-congruent psychotic symptoms
Bipolar I disorder, current or most recent episode depressed, with psychotic features

● **F31.6   Bipolar disorder, current episode mixed**

F31.60   Bipolar disorder, current episode mixed, unspecified 🐾

F31.61   Bipolar disorder, current episode mixed, mild 🐾

F31.62   Bipolar disorder, current episode mixed, moderate 🐾

F31.63   Bipolar disorder, current episode mixed, severe, without psychotic features 🐾

F31.64   Bipolar disorder, current episode mixed, severe, with psychotic features 🐾
Bipolar disorder, current episode mixed with mood-congruent psychotic symptoms
Bipolar disorder, current episode mixed with mood-incongruent psychotic symptoms

● **F31.7   Bipolar disorder, currently in remission**

F31.70   Bipolar disorder, currently in remission, most recent episode unspecified 🐾

F31.71   Bipolar disorder, in partial remission, most recent episode hypomanic 🐾

F31.72   Bipolar disorder, in full remission, most recent episode hypomanic 🐾

F31.73   Bipolar disorder, in partial remission, most recent episode manic 🐾

F31.74   Bipolar disorder, in full remission, most recent episode manic 🐾

F31.75   Bipolar disorder, in partial remission, most recent episode depressed 🐾

F31.76   Bipolar disorder, in full remission, most recent episode depressed 🐾

F31.77   Bipolar disorder, in partial remission, most recent episode mixed 🐾

F31.78   Bipolar disorder, in full remission, most recent episode mixed 🐾

● **F31.8   Other bipolar disorders**

F31.81   Bipolar II disorder 🐾
Bipolar disorder, type 2

F31.89   Other bipolar disorder 🐾
Recurrent manic episodes NOS

F31.9   Bipolar disorder, unspecified 🐾
Manic depression
Coding Clinic: 2020, Q1, P23

➠● **F32   Depressive episode**

Includes	single episode of agitated depression
	single episode of depressive reaction
	single episode of major depression
	single episode of psychogenic depression
	single episode of reactive depression
	single episode of vital depression

Excludes1	bipolar disorder (F31.-)
	manic episode (F30.-)
	recurrent depressive disorder (F33.-)

| **Excludes2** | adjustment disorder (F43.2) |

F32.0   Major depressive disorder, single episode, mild 🐾

F32.1   Major depressive disorder, single episode, moderate 🐾

F32.2   Major depressive disorder, single episode, severe without psychotic features 🐾

▶ New   ➠ Revised   ~~deleted~~ Deleted | Excludes 1 | | Excludes 2 | | Includes | | Use additional | | Code first | | Code also | | Key words |

OGCR Official Guidelines   **X** Assign placeholder X   ● Use Additional Character(s)   ▶ Manifestation Code   🐾 Hierarchical Condition Category   **Coding Clinic**

F32.3   **Major depressive disorder, single episode, severe with psychotic features** 🐾
      Single episode of major depression with mood-congruent psychotic symptoms
      Single episode of major depression with mood-incongruent psychotic symptoms
      Single episode of major depression with psychotic symptoms
      Single episode of psychogenic depressive psychosis
      Single episode of psychotic depression
      Single episode of reactive depressive psychosis

F32.4   **Major depressive disorder, single episode, in partial remission** 🐾

F32.5   **Major depressive disorder, single episode, in full remission** 🐾

● **F32.8**   **Other depressive episodes**
     F32.81   **Premenstrual dysphoric disorder** ♀
         Excludes1   premenstrual tension syndrome (N94.3)
         Coding Clinic: 2016, Q4, P14

     F32.89   **Other specified depressive episodes**
         Atypical depression
         Post-schizophrenic depression
         Single episode of 'masked' depression NOS
         Coding Clinic: 2016, Q4, P14

F32.9   **Major depressive disorder, single episode, unspecified**
      ~~Depression NOS~~
      ~~Depressive disorder NOS~~
      Major depression NOS
      Coding Clinic: 2021, Q1, P10

▶ **F32.A**   **Depression, unspecified**
      ▶Depression NOS
      ▶Depressive disorder NOS

● **F33**   **Major depressive disorder, recurrent**
     Includes   recurrent episodes of depressive reaction
         recurrent episodes of endogenous depression
         recurrent episodes of major depression
         recurrent episodes of psychogenic depression
         recurrent episodes of reactive depression
         recurrent episodes of seasonal depressive disorder
         recurrent episodes of vital depression
     Excludes1   bipolar disorder (F31.-)
         manic episode (F30.-)
     Coding Clinic: 2020, Q1, P23

F33.0   **Major depressive disorder, recurrent, mild** 🐾
F33.1   **Major depressive disorder, recurrent, moderate** 🐾
F33.2   **Major depressive disorder, recurrent severe without psychotic features** 🐾
F33.3   **Major depressive disorder, recurrent, severe with psychotic symptoms** 🐾
      Endogenous depression with psychotic symptoms
      Major depressive disorder, recurrent, with psychotic features
      Recurrent severe episodes of major depression with mood-congruent psychotic symptoms
      Recurrent severe episodes of major depression with mood-incongruent psychotic symptoms
      Recurrent severe episodes of major depression with psychotic symptoms
      Recurrent severe episodes of psychogenic depressive psychosis
      Recurrent severe episodes of psychotic depression
      Recurrent severe episodes of reactive depressive psychosis

● **F33.4**   **Major depressive disorder, recurrent, in remission**
     F33.40   **Major depressive disorder, recurrent, in remission, unspecified** 🐾
     F33.41   **Major depressive disorder, recurrent, in partial remission** 🐾
     F33.42   **Major depressive disorder, recurrent, in full remission** 🐾

F33.8   **Other recurrent depressive disorders** 🐾
      Recurrent brief depressive episodes

F33.9   **Major depressive disorder, recurrent, unspecified** 🐾
      Monopolar depression NOS

Figure 5-1   PET scan of depressed individual's brain before and after recovery. (From Fortinash KM: Psychiatric Mental Health Nursing, ed 4, St. Louis, Mosby, 2008)

● **F34**   **Persistent mood [affective] disorders**
     F34.0   **Cyclothymic disorder**
         Affective personality disorder
         Cycloid personality
         Cyclothymia
         Cyclothymic personality

     F34.1   **Dysthymic disorder**
         Depressive neurosis
         Depressive personality disorder
         Dysthymia
         Neurotic depression
         Persistent anxiety depression
         Persistent depressive disorder
         Excludes2   anxiety depression (mild or not persistent) (F41.8)

● **F34.8**   **Other persistent mood [affective] disorders**
     F34.81   **Disruptive mood dysregulation disorder** 🐾
         Coding Clinic: 2016, Q4, P14
     F34.89   **Other specified persistent mood disorders** 🐾
         Coding Clinic: 2016, Q4, P14

     F34.9   **Persistent mood [affective] disorder, unspecified** 🐾

F39   **Unspecified mood [affective] disorder** 🐾
      Affective psychosis NOS

ANXIETY, DISSOCIATIVE, STRESS-RELATED, SOMATOFORM AND OTHER NONPSYCHOTIC MENTAL DISORDERS (F40-F48)

● **F40**   **Phobic anxiety disorders**
     Irrational fear with avoidance of the feared subject, activity, or situation even though the individual knows that the reaction is excessive

● **F40.0**   **Agoraphobia**
     Intense, irrational fear of open spaces
     F40.00   **Agoraphobia, unspecified**
     F40.01   **Agoraphobia with panic disorder**
         Panic disorder with agoraphobia
         Excludes1   panic disorder without agoraphobia (F41.0)
     F40.02   **Agoraphobia without panic disorder**

● **F40.1**   **Social phobias**
      Anthropophobia
      Social anxiety disorder
      Social anxiety disorder of childhood
      Social neurosis
     F40.10   **Social phobia, unspecified**
     F40.11   **Social phobia, generalized**

CHAPTER 5 (F01-F99)

● **F40.2**   Specific (isolated) phobias
     Excludes2   dysmorphophobia (nondelusional)
                     (F45.22)
                     nosophobia (F45.22)
    ● **F40.21**   Animal type phobia
        F40.210   Arachnophobia
                 Fear of spiders
        F40.218   Other animal type phobia
    ● **F40.22**   Natural environment type phobia
        F40.220   Fear of thunderstorms
        F40.228   Other natural environment type
                 phobia
    ● **F40.23**   Blood, injection, injury type phobia
        F40.230   Fear of blood
        F40.231   Fear of injections and transfusions
        F40.232   Fear of other medical care
        F40.233   Fear of injury
    ● **F40.24**   Situational type phobia
        F40.240   Claustrophobia
                 Fear of closed spaces
        F40.241   Acrophobia
                 Fear of heights
        F40.242   Fear of bridges
        F40.243   Fear of flying
        F40.248   Other situational type phobia
    ● **F40.29**   Other specified phobia
        F40.290   Androphobia
                 Fear of men
        F40.291   Gynephobia
                 Fear of women
        F40.298   Other specified phobia
   F40.8   Other phobic anxiety disorders
       Phobic anxiety disorder of childhood
   F40.9   Phobic anxiety disorder, unspecified
       Phobia NOS
       Phobic state NOS

● **F41**   Other anxiety disorders
     Excludes2   anxiety in:
                 acute stress reaction (F43.0)
                 transient adjustment reaction (F43.2)
                 neurasthenia (F48.8)
                 psychophysiologic disorders (F45.-)
                 separation anxiety (F93.0)
   F41.0   Panic disorder [episodic paroxysmal anxiety]
       Panic attack
       Panic state
       Excludes1   panic disorder with agoraphobia (F40.01)
   F41.1   Generalized anxiety disorder
       Anxiety neurosis
       Anxiety reaction
       Anxiety state
       Overanxious disorder
       Excludes2   neurasthenia (F48.8)
   F41.3   Other mixed anxiety disorders
   F41.8   Other specified anxiety disorders
       Anxiety depression (mild or not persistent)
       Anxiety hysteria
       Mixed anxiety and depressive disorder
       Coding Clinic: 2021, Q1, P11
   F41.9   Anxiety disorder, unspecified
       Anxiety NOS
       Coding Clinic: 2021, Q1, P11

● **F42**   Obsessive-compulsive disorder
     Anxiety disorder with recurrent obsessions or compulsions
     Excludes2   obsessive-compulsive personality (disorder)
                   (F60.5)
                   obsessive-compulsive symptoms occurring in
                       depression (F32-F33)
                   obsessive-compulsive symptoms occurring in
                       schizophrenia (F20.-)
   F42.2   Mixed obsessional thoughts and acts
       Coding Clinic: 2016, Q4, P15
   F42.3   Hoarding disorder
       Coding Clinic: 2016, Q4, P14-15
   F42.4   Excoriation (skin-picking) disorder
       Excludes1   factitial dermatitis (L98.1)
                 other specified behavioral and emotional
                       disorders with onset usually
                       occurring in early childhood and
                       adolescence (F98.8)
       Coding Clinic: 2016, Q4, P14-15
   F42.8   Other obsessive-compulsive disorder
       Anancastic neurosis
       Obsessive-compulsive neurosis
       Coding Clinic: 2016, Q4, P15
   F42.9   Obsessive-compulsive disorder, unspecified
       Coding Clinic: 2016, Q4, P15

● **F43**   Reaction to severe stress and adjustment disorders
   F43.0   Acute stress reaction
       Acute crisis reaction
       Acute reaction to stress
       Combat and operational stress reaction
       Combat fatigue
       Crisis state
       Psychic shock
   ● **F43.1**   Post-traumatic stress disorder (PTSD)
       Traumatic neurosis
      F43.10   Post-traumatic stress disorder, unspecified
      F43.11   Post-traumatic stress disorder, acute
      F43.12   Post-traumatic stress disorder, chronic
   ● **F43.2**   Adjustment disorders
       Culture shock
       Grief reaction
       Hospitalism in children
       Excludes2   separation anxiety disorder of childhood
                 (F93.0)
      F43.20   Adjustment disorder, unspecified
      F43.21   Adjustment disorder with depressed mood
      F43.22   Adjustment disorder with anxiety
      F43.23   Adjustment disorder with mixed anxiety and
               depressed mood
      F43.24   Adjustment disorder with disturbance of
               conduct
      F43.25   Adjustment disorder with mixed disturbance of
               emotions and conduct
      F43.29   Adjustment disorder with other symptoms
   F43.8   Other reactions to severe stress
       Other specified trauma and stressor-related disorder
   F43.9   Reaction to severe stress, unspecified
       Trauma and stressor-related disorder, NOS

CHAPTER 5 (F01-F99)

▶ New   ⇨ Revised   ~~deleted~~ Deleted   Excludes 1   Excludes 2   Includes   Use additional   Code first   Code also   Key words

OGCR Official Guidelines   **X** Assign placeholder X   ● Use Additional Character(s)   ▶ Manifestation Code   🝢 Hierarchical Condition Category   **Coding Clinic**

● **F44   Dissociative and conversion disorders**

> **Includes**   conversion hysteria
> conversion reaction
> hysteria
> hysterical psychosis

> **Excludes2**   malingering [conscious simulation] (Z76.5)

F44.0   Dissociative amnesia

Sudden loss of memory for personal information

> **Excludes1**   amnesia NOS (R41.3)
> anterograde amnesia (R41.1)
> dissociative amnesia with dissociative
> fugue (F44.1)
> retrograde amnesia (R41.2)

> **Excludes2**   alcohol or other psychoactive substance-
> induced amnestic disorder (F10, F13,
> F19 with .26, .96)
> amnestic disorder due to known
> physiological condition (F04)
> postictal amnesia in epilepsy (G40.-)

F44.1   Dissociative fugue

*Characterized by episode of sudden, unexpected travel with
amnesia for past and partial to total confusion about
identity or assumption of new identity*
Dissociative amnesia with dissociative fugue

> **Excludes2**   postictal fugue in epilepsy (G40.-)

F44.2   Dissociative stupor

*Profound diminution or absence of voluntary movement and
responsiveness to external stimuli*

> **Excludes1**   catatonic stupor (R40.1)
> stupor NOS (R40.1)

> **Excludes2**   catatonic disorder due to known
> physiological condition (F06.1)
> depressive stupor (F32, F33)
> manic stupor (F30, F31)

F44.4   Conversion disorder with motor symptom or deficit

Conversion disorder with abnormal movement
Conversion disorder with speech symptoms
Conversion disorder with swallowing symptoms
Conversion disorder with weakness/paralysis
Dissociative motor disorders
Psychogenic aphonia
Psychogenic dysphonia

F44.5   Conversion disorder with seizures or convulsions

Conversion disorder with attacks or seizures
Dissociative convulsions
Coding Clinic: 2019, Q1, P19

F44.6   Conversion disorder with sensory symptom or deficit

Conversion disorder with anesthesia or sensory loss
Conversion disorder with special sensory symptoms
Dissociative anesthesia and sensory loss
Psychogenic deafness

F44.7   Conversion disorder with mixed symptom presentation

● **F44.8   Other dissociative and conversion disorders**

F44.81   Dissociative identity disorder

Multiple personality disorder

F44.89   Other dissociative and conversion disorders

Ganser's syndrome
Psychogenic confusion
Psychogenic twilight state
Trance and possession disorders

F44.9   Dissociative and conversion disorder, unspecified

Dissociative disorder NOS

OGCR Section I.C.5.a.

> Pain disorders related to psychological factors
> Assign code F45.41, for pain that is exclusively related to psychological
> disorders. As indicated by the Excludes 1 note under category G89,
> a code from category G89 should not be assigned with code F45.41
> Code F45.42, Pain disorders with related psychological factors, should
> be used with a code from category G89, Pain, not elsewhere classified,
> if there is documentation of a psychological component for a patient
> with acute or chronic pain.
> *See Section I.C.6. Pain*

● **F45   Somatoform disorders**

*Mental disorders characterized by symptoms suggesting general
medical condition*

> **Excludes2**   dissociative and conversion disorders (F44.-)
> factitious disorders (F68.1-, F68.A)
> hair-plucking (F63.3)
> lalling (F80.0)
> lisping (F80.0)
> malingering [conscious simulation] (Z76.5)
> nail-biting (F98.8)
> psychological or behavioral factors associated
> with disorders or diseases classified
> elsewhere (F54)
> sexual dysfunction, not due to a substance or
> known physiological condition (F52.-)
> thumb-sucking (F98.8)
> tic disorders (in childhood and adolescence) (F95.-)
> Tourette's syndrome (F95.2)
> trichotillomania (F63.3)

F45.0   Somatization disorder

Briquet's disorder
Multiple psychosomatic disorder

F45.1   Undifferentiated somatoform disorder

Somatic symptom disorder
Undifferentiated psychosomatic disorder

● **F45.2   Hypochondriacal disorders**

*Persistent, unrealistic preoccupation with possibility of
having serious disease*

> **Excludes2**   delusional dysmorphophobia (F22)
> fixed delusions about bodily functions or
> shape (F22)

F45.20   Hypochondriacal disorder, unspecified

F45.21   Hypochondriasis

Hypochondriacal neurosis
Illness anxiety disorder

F45.22   Body dysmorphic disorder

Dysmorphophobia (nondelusional)
Nosophobia

F45.29   Other hypochondriacal disorders

● **F45.4   Pain disorders related to psychological factors**

> **Excludes1**   pain NOS (R52)

**F45.41   Pain disorder exclusively related to
psychological factors**

Somatoform pain disorder (persistent)

F45.42   Pain disorder with related psychological factors

Code also associated acute or chronic pain
(G89.-)

F45.8   Other somatoform disorders

Psychogenic dysmenorrhea
Psychogenic dysphagia, including 'globus hystericus'
Psychogenic pruritus
Psychogenic torticollis
Somatoform autonomic dysfunction
Teeth grinding

> **Excludes1**   sleep related teeth grinding (G47.63)

Coding Clinic: 2016, Q4, P118

F45.9   Somatoform disorder, unspecified

Psychosomatic disorder NOS

● **F48   Other nonpsychotic mental disorders**

F48.1   Depersonalization-derealization syndrome

F48.2   Pseudobulbar affect

Involuntary emotional expression disorder

Code first underlying cause, if known, such as:
amyotrophic lateral sclerosis (G12.21)
multiple sclerosis (G35)
sequelae of cerebrovascular disease (I69.-)
sequelae of traumatic intracranial injury (S06.-)

CHAPTER 5 (F01-F99)

F48.8   Other specified nonpsychotic mental disorders
Dhat syndrome
Neurasthenia
Occupational neurosis, including writer's cramp
Psychasthenia
Psychasthenic neurosis
Psychogenic syncope

F48.9   Nonpsychotic mental disorder, unspecified
Neurosis NOS

BEHAVIORAL SYNDROMES ASSOCIATED WITH PHYSIOLOGICAL DISTURBANCES AND PHYSICAL FACTORS (F50-F59)

● **F50**   Eating disorders
Excludes1   anorexia NOS (R63.0)
~~feeding difficulties (R63.3)~~
feeding problems of newborn (P92.-)
polyphagia (R63.2)
Excludes2 ► feeding difficulties (R63.3)
feeding disorder in infancy or childhood (F98.2-)

● **F50.0**   Anorexia nervosa
Excludes1   loss of appetite (R63.0)
psychogenic loss of appetite (F50.89)

F50.00   Anorexia nervosa, unspecified

F50.01   Anorexia nervosa, restricting type

F50.02   Anorexia nervosa, binge eating/purging type
Excludes1   bulimia nervosa (F50.2)

F50.2   Bulimia nervosa
Bulimia NOS
Hyperorexia nervosa
Excludes1   anorexia nervosa, binge eating/purging type (F50.02)

● **F50.8**   Other eating disorders
Excludes2   pica of infancy and childhood (F98.3)

F50.81   Binge eating disorder
Coding Clinic: 2016, Q4, P15

F50.82   Avoidant/restrictive food intake disorder

F50.89   Other specified eating disorder
Pica in adults
Psychogenic loss of appetite
Coding Clinic: 2016, Q4, P16

F50.9   Eating disorder, unspecified
Atypical anorexia nervosa
Atypical bulimia nervosa
Feeding or eating disorder, unspecified
Other specified feeding disorder

● **F51**   Sleep disorders not due to a substance or known physiological condition
Excludes2   organic sleep disorders (G47.-)

● **F51.0**   Insomnia not due to a substance or known physiological condition
Excludes2   alcohol related insomnia (F10.182, F10.282, F10.982)
drug-related insomnia (F11.182, F11.282, F11.982, F13.182, F13.282, F13.982, F14.182, F14.282, F14.982, F15.182, F15.282, F15.982, F19.182, F19.282, F19.982)
insomnia NOS (G47.0-)
insomnia due to known physiological condition (G47.0-)
organic insomnia (G47.0-)
sleep deprivation (Z72.820)

F51.01   Primary insomnia
Idiopathic insomnia

F51.02   Adjustment insomnia

F51.03   Paradoxical insomnia

F51.04   Psychophysiologic insomnia

F51.05   Insomnia due to other mental disorder
Code also associated mental disorder

F51.09   Other insomnia not due to a substance or known physiological condition

● **F51.1**   Hypersomnia not due to a substance or known physiological condition
Hypersomnia: Excessive sleeping/sleepiness
Excludes2   alcohol related hypersomnia (F10.182, F10.282, F10.982)
drug-related hypersomnia (F11.182, F11.282, F11.982, F13.182, F13.282, F13.982, F14.182, F14.282, F14.982, F15.182, F15.282, F15.982, F19.182, F19.282, F19.982)
hypersomnia NOS (G47.10)
hypersomnia due to known physiological condition (G47.10)
idiopathic hypersomnia (G47.11, G47.12)
narcolepsy (G47.4-)

F51.11   Primary hypersomnia

F51.12   Insufficient sleep syndrome
Excludes1   sleep deprivation (Z72.820)

F51.13   Hypersomnia due to other mental disorder
Code also associated mental disorder

F51.19   Other hypersomnia not due to a substance or known physiological condition

F51.3   Sleepwalking [somnambulism]
Non-rapid eye movement sleep arousal disorders, sleepwalking type

F51.4   Sleep terrors [night terrors]
Non-rapid eye movement sleep arousal disorders, sleep terror type

F51.5   Nightmare disorder
Dream anxiety disorder

F51.8   Other sleep disorders not due to a substance or known physiological condition

F51.9   Sleep disorder not due to a substance or known physiological condition, unspecified
Emotional sleep disorder NOS

● **F52**   Sexual dysfunction not due to a substance or known physiological condition
Excludes2   Dhat syndrome (F48.8)

F52.0   Hypoactive sexual desire disorder
Total loss of feeling of sexual pleasure
Lack or loss of sexual desire
Male hypoactive sexual desire disorder
Sexual anhedonia
Excludes1   decreased libido (R68.82)

F52.1   Sexual aversion disorder
Sexual aversion and lack of sexual enjoyment

● **F52.2**   Sexual arousal disorders
Failure of genital response

F52.21   Male erectile disorder ♂
Erectile disorder
Psychogenic impotence
Excludes1   impotence of organic origin (N52.-)
impotence NOS (N52.-)

F52.22   Female sexual arousal disorder ♀
Female sexual interest/arousal disorder

● **F52.3**   Orgasmic disorder
Inhibited orgasm
Psychogenic anorgasmy

F52.31   Female orgasmic disorder ♀

F52.32   Male orgasmic disorder ♂
Delayed ejaculation

F52.4   Premature ejaculation ♂

F52.5   **Vaginismus not due to a substance or known physiological condition** ♀
    Psychogenic vaginismus
    Excludes2   vaginismus (due to a known physiological condition) (N94.2)

F52.6   **Dyspareunia not due to a substance or known physiological condition**
    Dyspareunia: Difficult or painful sexual intercourse
    Genito-pelvic pain penetration disorder
    Psychogenic dyspareunia
    Excludes2   dyspareunia (due to a known physiological condition) (N94.1-)

F52.8   **Other sexual dysfunction not due to a substance or known physiological condition**
    Excessive sexual drive
    Nymphomania
    Satyriasis

F52.9   **Unspecified sexual dysfunction not due to a substance or known physiological condition**
    Sexual dysfunction NOS

● F53   **Mental and behavioral disorders associated with the puerperium, not elsewhere classified**
    Acute mental illness with sudden onset following childbirth with symptoms of affective psychosis, disorientation, and confusion are prevalent
    Excludes1   mood disorders with psychotic features (F30.2, F31.2, F31.5, F31.64, F32.3, F33.3)
       postpartum dysphoria (O90.6)
       psychosis in schizophrenia, schizotypal, delusional, and other psychotic disorders (F20-F29)

F53.0   **Postpartum depression** ♀   M
    Postnatal depression, NOS
    Postpartum depression, NOS
    Coding Clinic: 2018, Q4, P8

F53.1   **Puerperal psychosis** ♀   M
    Postpartum psychosis
    Puerperal psychosis, NOS
    Coding Clinic: 2018, Q4, P9

▷ F54   *Psychological and behavioral factors associated with disorders or diseases classified elsewhere*
    Psychological factors affecting physical conditions
    Code first the associated physical disorder, such as:
      asthma (J45.-)
      dermatitis (L23-L25)
      gastric ulcer (K25.-)
      mucous colitis (K58.-)
      ulcerative colitis (K51.-)
      urticaria (L50.-)
    Excludes2   tension-type headache (G44.2)

● F55   **Abuse of non-psychoactive substances**
    Excludes2   abuse of psychoactive substances (F10-F19)
   F55.0   **Abuse of antacids**
   F55.1   **Abuse of herbal or folk remedies**
   F55.2   **Abuse of laxatives**
   F55.3   **Abuse of steroids or hormones**
   F55.4   **Abuse of vitamins**
   F55.8   **Abuse of other non-psychoactive substances**

F59   **Unspecified behavioral syndromes associated with physiological disturbances and physical factors**
    Psychogenic physiological dysfunction NOS

DISORDERS OF ADULT PERSONALITY AND BEHAVIOR (F60-F69)

● F60   **Specific personality disorders**
    Long-term patterns of thoughts and behaviors causing serious problems with relationships and work

F60.0   **Paranoid personality disorder**
    Hostile, devious, and combative response to disappointments
    Expansive paranoid personality (disorder)
    Fanatic personality (disorder)
    Querulant personality (disorder)
    Paranoid personality (disorder)
    Sensitive paranoid personality (disorder)
    Excludes2   paranoia (F22)
       paranoia querulans (F22)
       paranoid psychosis (F22)
       paranoid schizophrenia (F20.0)
       paranoid state (F22)

F60.1   **Schizoid personality disorder**
    Detachment from social relationships with minimal emotional experiences and expressions
    Excludes2   Asperger's syndrome (F84.5)
       delusional disorder (F22)
       schizoid disorder of childhood (F84.5)
       schizophrenia (F20.-)
       schizotypal disorder (F21)

F60.2   **Antisocial personality disorder**
    Continuous and chronic antisocial behavior
    Amoral personality (disorder)
    Asocial personality (disorder)
    Dissocial personality disorder
    Psychopathic personality (disorder)
    Sociopathic personality (disorder)
    Excludes1   conduct disorders (F91.-)
    Excludes2   borderline personality disorder (F60.3)

F60.3   **Borderline personality disorder**
    Instability of mood, self-image or sense of self, and interpersonal relationships
    Aggressive personality (disorder)
    Emotionally unstable personality disorder
    Explosive personality (disorder)
    Excludes2   antisocial personality disorder (F60.2)

F60.4   **Histrionic personality disorder**
    Personality disorder with excessive emotional and attention-seeking behavior
    Hysterical personality (disorder)
    Psychoinfantile personality (disorder)

F60.5   **Obsessive-compulsive personality disorder**
    Anankastic personality (disorder)
    Compulsive personality (disorder)
    Obsessional personality (disorder)
    Excludes2   obsessive-compulsive disorder (F42.-)

F60.6   **Avoidant personality disorder**
    Anxious personality disorder

F60.7   **Dependent personality disorder**
    Asthenic personality (disorder)
    Inadequate personality (disorder)
    Passive personality (disorder)

● F60.8   **Other specific personality disorders**

   F60.81   **Narcissistic personality disorder**
      Vanity, conceit, egotism or indifference to plight of others

   F60.89   **Other specific personality disorders**
      Eccentric personality disorder
      'Haltlose' type personality disorder
      Immature personality disorder
      Passive-aggressive personality disorder
      Psychoneurotic personality disorder
      Self-defeating personality disorder

F60.9   **Personality disorder, unspecified**
    Character disorder NOS
    Character neurosis NOS
    Pathological personality NOS

CHAPTER 5 (F01-F99)

● **F63** **Impulse disorders**
    Excludes2   habitual excessive use of alcohol or psychoactive
                substances (F10-F19)
                impulse disorders involving sexual behavior (F65.-)

    F63.0 **Pathological gambling**
        Compulsive gambling
        Gambling disorder
        Excludes1 gambling and betting NOS (Z72.6)
        Excludes2 excessive gambling by manic patients
                    (F30, F31)
                    gambling in antisocial personality
                      disorder (F60.2)

    F63.1 **Pyromania**
        Pathological fire-setting
        Excludes2 fire-setting (by) (in):
                    adult with antisocial personality
                      disorder (F60.2)
                    alcohol or psychoactive substance
                      intoxication (F10-F19)
                    conduct disorders (F91.-)
                    mental disorders due to known
                      physiological condition (F01-F09)
                    schizophrenia (F20.-)

    F63.2 **Kleptomania**
        Pathological stealing
        Excludes1 shoplifting as the reason for observation
                    for suspected mental disorder
                    (Z03.8)
        Excludes2 depressive disorder with stealing
                    (F31-F33)
                    stealing due to underlying mental
                    condition-code to mental condition
                    stealing in mental disorders due to known
                    physiological condition (F01-F09)

    F63.3 **Trichotillomania**
        Hair plucking
        Excludes2 other stereotyped movement disorder
                    (F98.4)

  ● **F63.8** **Other impulse disorders**
        F63.81 **Intermittent explosive disorder**
        F63.89 **Other impulse disorders**

    F63.9 **Impulse disorder, unspecified**
        Impulse control disorder NOS

● **F64** **Gender identity disorders**
    F64.0 **Transsexualism**
        Gender identity disorder in adolescence and adulthood
        Gender dysphoria in adolescents and adults
        Coding Clinic: 2016, Q4, P16

    F64.1 **Dual role transvestism**
        Use additional code to identify sex reassignment status
            (Z87.890)
        Excludes1 gender identity disorder in childhood
                    (F64.2)
        Excludes2 fetishistic transvestism (F65.1)
        Coding Clinic: 2016, Q4, P16

    F64.2 **Gender identity disorder of childhood**   P
        Gender dysphoria in children
        Excludes1 gender identity disorder in adolescence
                    and adulthood (F64.0)
        Excludes2 sexual maturation disorder (F66)

    F64.8 **Other gender identity disorders**
        Other specified gender dysphoria

    F64.9 **Gender identity disorder, unspecified**
        Gender dysphoria, unspecified
        Gender-role disorder NOS

● **F65** **Paraphilias**
    F65.0 **Fetishism**
        Intense sexual urges and arousing fantasies using inanimate
           objects
        Fetishistic disorder

    F65.1 **Transvestic fetishism**
        Intense sexual urges, arousal, or orgasm associated with
           fantasized/actual cross-dressing
        Fetishistic transvestism
        Transvestic disorder

    F65.2 **Exhibitionism**
        Exhibitionistic disorder

    F65.3 **Voyeurism**
        Sexual urges or arousal involving real or fantasized
           observation of unsuspecting people who are naked,
           disrobing, or engaging in sexual activity
        Voyeuristic disorder

    F65.4 **Pedophilia**
        Pedophilic disorder

  ● **F65.5** **Sadomasochism**
        F65.50 **Sadomasochism, unspecified**
        F65.51 **Sexual masochism**
                Sexual masochism disorder
        F65.52 **Sexual sadism**
                Sexual sadism disorder

  ● **F65.8** **Other paraphilias**
        F65.81 **Frotteurism**
                Sexual arousal or orgasm is achieved by rubbing
                  up against another person (or fantasies of), in
                  crowded place with unsuspecting victim
                Frotteuristic disorder
        F65.89 **Other paraphilias**
                Necrophilia
                Other specified paraphilic disorder

    F65.9 **Paraphilia, unspecified**
        Paraphilic disorder, unspecified
        Sexual deviation NOS

  F66 **Other sexual disorders**
        Sexual maturation disorder
        Sexual relationship disorder

● **F68** **Other disorders of adult personality and behavior**
  ● **F68.1** **Factitious disorder imposed on self**
        Compensation neurosis
        Elaboration of physical symptoms for psychological
          reasons
        Hospital hopper syndrome
        Münchhausen's syndrome
        Peregrinating patient
        Excludes2 factitial dermatitis (L98.1)
                    person feigning illness (with obvious
                    motivation) (Z76.5)
        F68.10 **Factitious disorder imposed on self,**
                unspecified
        F68.11 **Factitious disorder imposed on self with**
                predominantly psychological signs and
                symptoms
        F68.12 **Factitious disorder imposed on self with**
                predominantly physical signs and symptoms
        F68.13 **Factitious disorder imposed on self with**
                combined psychological and physical signs and
                symptoms

    F68.8 **Other specified disorders of adult personality and behavior**

    F68.A **Factitious disorder imposed on another**
        Factitious disorder by proxy
        Münchausen's by proxy

  F69 **Unspecified disorder of adult personality and behavior**   A

▶ New   ⫸ Revised   ~~deleted~~ Deleted   Excludes 1   Excludes 2   Includes   Use additional   Code first   Code also   Key words
OGCR Official Guidelines   X Assign placeholder X   ● Use Additional Character(s)   ▷ Manifestation Code   🕪 Hierarchical Condition Category   **Coding Clinic**

INTELLECTUAL DISABILITIES (F70-F79)

Code first any associated physical or developmental disorders

Excludes1 borderline intellectual functioning, IQ above 70 to 84 (R41.83)

F70 **Mild intellectual disabilities**
IQ level 50-55 to approximately 70
Mild mental subnormality

F71 **Moderate intellectual disabilities**
IQ level 35-40 to 50-55
Moderate mental subnormality

F72 **Severe intellectual disabilities**
IQ 20-25 to 35-40
Severe mental subnormality

F73 **Profound intellectual disabilities**
IQ level below 20-25
Profound mental subnormality

● **F78** **Other intellectual disabilities**

▶● **F78.A** **Other genetic related intellectual disabilities**

▶ **F78.A1** **SYNGAP1-related intellectual disability**
▶ *Code also, if applicable, any associated:*
▶ autism spectrum disorder (F84.0)
▶ autistic disorder (F84.0)
▶ encephalopathy (G93.4-)
▶ epilepsy and recurrent seizures (G40.-)
▶ other pervasive developmental disorders (F84.8)
▶ pervasive developmental disorder, NOS (F84.9)

▶ **F78.A9** **Other genetic related intellectual disability**
Code also, if applicable, any associated disorders

F79 **Unspecified intellectual disabilities**
Mental deficiency NOS
Mental subnormality NOS

PERVASIVE AND SPECIFIC DEVELOPMENTAL DISORDERS (F80-F89)

● **F80** **Specific developmental disorders of speech and language**

F80.0 **Phonological disorder**
Communication disorder of unknown cause, characterized by failure to use age-appropriate sounds
Dyslalia
Functional speech articulation disorder
Lalling
Lisping
Phonological developmental disorder
Speech articulation developmental disorder
Speech-sound disorder

Excludes1 speech articulation impairment due to aphasia NOS (R47.01)
speech articulation impairment due to apraxia (R48.2)

Excludes2 speech articulation impairment due to hearing loss (F80.4)
speech articulation impairment due to intellectual disabilities (F70-F79)
speech articulation impairment with expressive language developmental disorder (F80.1)
speech articulation impairment with mixed receptive expressive language developmental disorder (F80.2)

F80.1 **Expressive language disorder**
Developmental dysphasia or aphasia, expressive type

Excludes1 mixed receptive-expressive language disorder (F80.2)
dysphasia and aphasia NOS (R47.-)

Excludes2 acquired aphasia with epilepsy [Landau-Kleffner] (G40.80-)
intellectual disabilities (F70-F79)
pervasive developmental disorders (F84.-)
selective mutism (F94.0)

F80.2 **Mixed receptive-expressive language disorder**
Developmental dysphasia or aphasia, receptive type
Developmental Wernicke's aphasia

Excludes1 central auditory processing disorder (H93.25)
dysphasia or aphasia NOS (R47.-)
expressive language disorder (F80.1)
expressive type dysphasia or aphasia (F80.1)
word deafness (H93.25)

Excludes2 acquired aphasia with epilepsy [Landau-Kleffner] (G40.80-)
intellectual disabilities (F70-F79)
pervasive developmental disorders (F84.-)
selective mutism (F94.0)

F80.4 **Speech and language development delay due to hearing loss**
Code also type of hearing loss (H90.-, H91.-)

● **F80.8** **Other developmental disorders of speech or language**

F80.81 **Childhood onset fluency disorder**
Cluttering NOS
Stuttering NOS

Excludes1 adult onset fluency disorder (F98.5)
fluency disorder in conditions classified elsewhere (R47.82)
fluency disorder (stuttering) following cerebrovascular disease (I69. with final characters -23)

F80.82 **Social pragmatic communication disorder**
Excludes1 Asperger's syndrome (F84.5)
autistic disorder (F84.0)
Coding Clinic: 2016, Q4, P16

F80.89 **Other developmental disorders of speech and language**
Coding Clinic: 2017, Q1, P27

F80.9 **Developmental disorder of speech and language, unspecified**
Communication disorder NOS
Language disorder NOS

● **F81** **Specific developmental disorders of scholastic skills**

F81.0 **Specific reading disorder**
'Backward reading'
Developmental dyslexia
Specific learning disorder, with impairment in reading
Specific reading retardation

Excludes1 alexia NOS (R48.0)
dyslexia NOS (R48.0)

F81.2 **Mathematics disorder**
Developmental acalculia
Developmental arithmetical disorder
Developmental Gerstmann's syndrome
Specific learning disorder, with impairment in mathematics

Excludes1 acalculia NOS (R48.8)

Excludes2 arithmetical difficulties associated with a reading disorder (F81.0)
arithmetical difficulties associated with a spelling disorder (F81.81)
arithmetical difficulties due to inadequate teaching (Z55.8)

● **F81.8** **Other developmental disorders of scholastic skills**

F81.81 **Disorder of written expression**
Specific learning disorder, with impairment in written expression
Specific spelling disorder

F81.89 **Other developmental disorders of scholastic skills**

F81.9   Developmental disorder of scholastic skills, unspecified
Knowledge acquisition disability NOS
Learning disability NOS
Learning disorder NOS

F82   Specific developmental disorder of motor function
Clumsy child syndrome
Developmental coordination disorder
Developmental dyspraxia

> **Excludes1**   abnormalities of gait and mobility (R26.-)
> lack of coordination (R27.-)

> **Excludes2**   lack of coordination secondary to intellectual disabilities (F70-F79)

F84   Pervasive developmental disorders
~~Use additional code to identify any associated medical condition and intellectual disabilities.~~

> ▶Code also any associated medical condition and intellectual disabilities

F84.0   Autistic disorder
Autism spectrum disorder
Infantile autism
Infantile psychosis
Kanner's syndrome

> **Excludes1**   Asperger's syndrome (F84.5)
> **Coding Clinic: 2017, Q1, P27**

F84.2   Rett's syndrome
Neurodevelopmental disorder

> **Excludes1**   Asperger's syndrome (F84.5)
> Autistic disorder (F84.0)
> other childhood disintegrative disorder (F84.3)

F84.3   Other childhood disintegrative disorder   P
Dementia infantilis
At least two years of normal development followed by significant loss of language abilities, social skills, bowel/bladder control, motor skills
Disintegrative psychosis
Heller's syndrome
At least two years of normal development followed by significant loss of language abilities, social skills, bowel/bladder control, motor skills
Symbiotic psychosis
Abnormal relationship to mothering figure, characterized by intense separation anxiety, severe regression, giving up of useful speech, and autism

Use additional code to identify any associated neurological condition.

> **Excludes1**   Asperger's syndrome (F84.5)
> Autistic disorder (F84.0)
> Rett's syndrome (F84.2)

F84.5   Asperger's syndrome
Developmental disorder
Asperger's disorder
Autistic psychopathy
Schizoid disorder of childhood

F84.8   Other pervasive developmental disorders
Overactive disorder associated with intellectual disabilities and stereotyped movements

F84.9   Pervasive developmental disorder, unspecified
Atypical autism

F88   Other disorders of psychological development
Developmental agnosia
Global developmental delay
Other specified neurodevelopmental disorder

F89   Unspecified disorder of psychological development
Developmental disorder NOS
Neurodevelopmental disorder NOS

BEHAVIORAL AND EMOTIONAL DISORDERS WITH ONSET USUALLY OCCURRING IN CHILDHOOD AND ADOLESCENCE (F90-F98)

Note: Codes within categories F90-F98 may be used regardless of the age of a patient. These disorders generally have onset within the childhood or adolescent years, but may continue throughout life or not be diagnosed until adulthood.

F90   Attention-deficit hyperactivity disorders
Attention deficit disorder with hyperactivity=ADHD

> **Includes**   attention deficit disorder with hyperactivity
> attention deficit syndrome with hyperactivity

> **Excludes2**   anxiety disorders (F40.-, F41.-)
> mood [affective] disorders (F30-F39)
> pervasive developmental disorders (F84.-)
> schizophrenia (F20.-)

F90.0   Attention-deficit hyperactivity disorder, predominantly inattentive type
Attention-deficit/hyperactivity disorder, predominantly inattentive presentation

F90.1   Attention-deficit hyperactivity disorder, predominantly hyperactive type
Attention-deficit/hyperactivity disorder, predominantly hyperactive impulsive presentation

F90.2   Attention-deficit hyperactivity disorder, combined type
Attention-deficit/hyperactivity disorder, combined presentation

F90.8   Attention-deficit hyperactivity disorder, other type

F90.9   Attention-deficit hyperactivity disorder, unspecified type
Attention-deficit hyperactivity disorder of childhood or adolescence NOS
Attention-deficit hyperactivity disorder NOS

F91   Conduct disorders
Childhood/adolescence disruptive behavior disorder

> **Excludes1**   antisocial behavior (Z72.81-)
> antisocial personality disorder (F60.2)

> **Excludes2**   conduct problems associated with attention-deficit hyperactivity disorder (F90.-)
> mood [affective] disorders (F30-F39)
> pervasive developmental disorders (F84.-)
> schizophrenia (F20.-)

F91.0   Conduct disorder confined to family context

F91.1   Conduct disorder, childhood-onset type
Unsocialized conduct disorder
Conduct disorder, solitary aggressive type
Unsocialized aggressive disorder

F91.2   Conduct disorder, adolescent-onset type
Socialized conduct disorder
Conduct disorder, group type

F91.3   Oppositional defiant disorder

F91.8   Other conduct disorders
Other specified conduct disorder
Other specified disruptive disorder

F91.9   Conduct disorder, unspecified
Behavioral disorder NOS
Conduct disorder NOS
Disruptive behavior disorder NOS
Disruptive disorder NOS

F93   Emotional disorders with onset specific to childhood

F93.0   Separation anxiety disorder of childhood

> **Excludes2**   mood [affective] disorders (F30-F39)
> nonpsychotic mental disorders (F40-F48)
> phobic anxiety disorder of childhood (F40.8)
> social phobia (F40.1)

F93.8   Other childhood emotional disorders
Identity disorder

> **Excludes2**   gender identity disorder of childhood (F64.2)

F93.9   Childhood emotional disorder, unspecified

▶ New   ➠ Revised   ~~deleted~~ Deleted   Excludes 1   Excludes 2   Includes   Use additional   Code first   Code also   Key words
OGCR Official Guidelines   X Assign placeholder X   ● Use Additional Character(s)   ▌ Manifestation Code   🝮 Hierarchical Condition Category   **Coding Clinic**

● **F94**   **Disorders of social functioning with onset specific to childhood and adolescence**

    F94.0   **Selective mutism**
         Elective mutism

         Excludes2   pervasive developmental disorders (F84.-)
                      schizophrenia (F20.-)
                      specific developmental disorders of speech and language (F80.-)
                      transient mutism as part of separation anxiety in young children (F93.0)

    F94.1   **Reactive attachment disorder of childhood**
         Use additional code to identify any associated failure to thrive or growth retardation

         Excludes1   disinhibited attachment disorder of childhood (F94.2)
                      normal variation in pattern of selective attachment

         Excludes2   Asperger's syndrome (F84.5)
                      maltreatment syndromes (T74.-)
                      sexual or physical abuse in childhood, resulting in psychosocial problems (Z62.81-)

    F94.2   **Disinhibited attachment disorder of childhood**
         Affectionless psychopathy
         Institutional syndrome

         Excludes1   reactive attachment disorder of childhood (F94.1)

         Excludes2   Asperger's syndrome (F84.5)
                      attention-deficit hyperactivity disorders (F90.-)
                      hospitalism in children (F43.2-)

    F94.8   **Other childhood disorders of social functioning**

    F94.9   **Childhood disorder of social functioning, unspecified**

● **F95**   **Tic disorder**
     Involuntary twitch

    F95.0   **Transient tic disorder**
         Provisional tic disorder

    F95.1   **Chronic motor or vocal tic disorder**

    F95.2   **Tourette's disorder**
         Combined vocal and multiple motor tic disorder [de la Tourette]
         Tourette's syndrome

    F95.8   **Other tic disorders**

    F95.9   **Tic disorder, unspecified**
         Tic NOS

● **F98**   **Other behavioral and emotional disorders with onset usually occurring in childhood and adolescence**

     Excludes2   breath-holding spells (R06.89)
                gender identity disorder of childhood (F64.2)
                Kleine-Levin syndrome (G47.13)
                obsessive-compulsive disorder (F42.3-)
                sleep disorders not due to a substance or known physiological condition (F51.-)

    F98.0   **Enuresis not due to a substance or known physiological condition**
         Enuresis: Urinary incontinence
         Enuresis (primary) (secondary) of nonorganic origin
         Functional enuresis
         Psychogenic enuresis
         Urinary incontinence of nonorganic origin

         Excludes1   enuresis NOS (R32)

    F98.1   **Encopresis not due to a substance or known physiological condition**
         Encopresis: Fecal incontinence
         Functional encopresis
         Incontinence of feces of nonorganic origin
         Psychogenic encopresis

         Use additional code to identify the cause of any coexisting constipation.

         Excludes1   encopresis NOS (R15.-)

● **F98.2**   **Other feeding disorders of infancy and childhood**
         ~~**Excludes1** feeding difficulties (R63.3)~~

         Excludes2   anorexia nervosa and other eating disorders (F50.-)
                 ▶ feeding difficulties (R63.3)
                 feeding problems of newborn (P92.-)
                 pica of infancy or childhood (F98.3)

    F98.21   **Rumination disorder of infancy**

    F98.29   **Other feeding disorders of infancy and early childhood**

    F98.3   **Pica of infancy and childhood**
         Craving and eating substances such as paint, clay, or dirt to replace a nutritional deficit in the body.

    F98.4   **Stereotyped movement disorders**
         Stereotype/habit disorder

         Excludes1   abnormal involuntary movements (R25.-)

         Excludes2   compulsions in obsessive-compulsive disorder (F42.-)
                 hair plucking (F63.3)
                 movement disorders of organic origin (G20-G25)
                 nail-biting (F98.8)
                 nose-picking (F98.8)
                 stereotypies that are part of a broader psychiatric condition (F01-F95)
                 thumb-sucking (F98.8)
                 tic disorders (F95.-)
                 trichotillomania (F63.3)

    F98.5   **Adult onset fluency disorder**

         Excludes1   childhood onset fluency disorder (F80.81)
                 dysphasia (R47.02)
                 fluency disorder in conditions classified elsewhere (R47.82)
                 fluency disorder (stuttering) following cerebrovascular disease (I69. with final characters -23)
                 tic disorders (F95.-)

    F98.8   **Other specified behavioral and emotional disorders with onset usually occurring in childhood and adolescence**
         Excessive masturbation
         Nail-biting
         Nose-picking
         Thumb-sucking

    F98.9   **Unspecified behavioral and emotional disorders with onset usually occurring in childhood and adolescence**

UNSPECIFIED MENTAL DISORDER (F99)

F99   **Mental disorder, not otherwise specified**
     Mental illness NOS

     Excludes1   unspecified mental disorder due to known physiological condition (F09)

Item 5-2 Enuresis: Bed wetting by children at night. Causes can be either psychological or medical (diabetes, urinary tract infections, or abnormalities). **Encopresis:** Overflow incontinence of bowels sometimes resulting from chronic constipation or fecal impaction. Check the documentation for additional diagnoses.

CHAPTER 6

DISEASES OF THE NERVOUS SYSTEM (G00-G99)

OGCR Chapter-Specific Coding Guidelines

6. **Chapter 6: Diseases of the Nervous System (G00-G99)**

   a. **Dominant/nondominant side**

   Codes from category G81, Hemiplegia and hemiparesis, and subcategories, G83.1, Monoplegia of lower limb, G83.2, Monoplegia of upper limb, and G83.3, Monoplegia, unspecified, identify whether the dominant or nondominant side is affected. Should the affected side be documented, but not specified as dominant or nondominant, and the classification system does not indicate a default, code selection is as follows:

   - For ambidextrous patients, the default should be dominant.
   - If the left side is affected, the default is nondominant.
   - If the right side is affected, the default is dominant.

   b. **Pain - Category G89**

   1) **General coding information**

   Codes in category G89, Pain, not elsewhere classified, may be used in conjunction with codes from other categories and chapters to provide more detail about acute or chronic pain and neoplasm-related pain, unless otherwise indicated below.

   If the pain is not specified as acute or chronic, post-thoracotomy, postprocedural, or neoplasm-related, do not assign codes from category G89.

   A code from category G89 should not be assigned if the underlying (definitive) diagnosis is known, unless the reason for the encounter is pain control/management and not management of the underlying condition.

   When an admission or encounter is for a procedure aimed at treating the underlying condition (e.g., spinal fusion, kyphoplasty), a code for the underlying condition (e.g., vertebral fracture, spinal stenosis) should be assigned as the principal diagnosis. No code from category G89 should be assigned.

   (a) **Category G89 Codes as Principal or First-Listed Diagnosis**

   Category G89 codes are acceptable as principal diagnosis or the first-listed code:

   - When pain control or pain management is the reason for the admission/encounter (e.g., a patient with displaced intervertebral disc, nerve impingement and severe back pain presents for injection of steroid into the spinal canal). The underlying cause of the pain should be reported as an additional diagnosis, if known.
   - When a patient is admitted for the insertion of a neurostimulator for pain control, assign the appropriate pain code as the principal or first-listed diagnosis. When an admission or encounter is for a procedure aimed at treating the underlying condition and a neurostimulator is inserted for pain control during the same admission/encounter, a code for the underlying condition should be assigned as the principal diagnosis and the appropriate pain code should be assigned as a secondary diagnosis.

   (b) **Use of Category G89 Codes in Conjunction with Site Specific Pain Codes**

   (i) **Assigning Category G89 and Site-Specific Pain Codes**

   Codes from category G89 may be used in conjunction with codes that identify the site of pain (including codes from Chapter 18) if the category G89 code provides additional information. For example, if the code describes the site of the pain, but does not fully describe whether the pain is acute or chronic, then both codes should be assigned.

   (ii) **Sequencing of Category G89 Codes with Site-Specific Pain Codes**

   The sequencing of category G89 codes with site-specific pain codes (including Chapter 18 codes), is dependent on the circumstances of the encounter/admission as follows:

   - If the encounter is for pain control or pain management, assign the code from category G89 followed by the code identifying the specific site of pain (e.g., encounter for pain management for acute neck pain from trauma is assigned code G89.11, Acute pain due to trauma, followed by code M54.2, Cervicalgia, to identify the site of pain).
   - If the encounter is for any other reason except pain control or pain management, and a related definitive diagnosis has not been established (confirmed) by the provider, assign the code for the specific site of pain first, followed by the appropriate code from category G89.

   2) **Pain due to devices, implants and grafts**
   See Section I.C.19. Pain due to medical devices

   3) **Postoperative Pain**

   The provider's documentation should be used to guide the coding of postoperative pain, as well as *Section III. Reporting Additional Diagnoses* and *Section IV. Diagnostic Coding and Reporting in the Outpatient Setting*.

   The default for post-thoracotomy and other postoperative pain not specified as acute or chronic is the code for the acute form.

   Routine or expected postoperative pain immediately after surgery should not be coded.

   (a) **Postoperative pain not associated with specific postoperative complication**

   Postoperative pain not associated with a specific postoperative complication is assigned to the appropriate postoperative pain code in category G89.

   (b) **Postoperative pain associated with specific postoperative complication**

   Postoperative pain associated with a specific postoperative complication (such as painful wire sutures) is assigned to the appropriate code(s) found in Chapter 19, Injury, poisoning, and certain other consequences of external causes. If appropriate, use additional code(s) from category G89 to identify acute or chronic pain (G89.18 or G89.28).

   4) **Chronic pain**

   Chronic pain is classified to subcategory G89.2. There is no time frame defining when pain becomes chronic pain. The provider's documentation should be used to guide use of these codes.

   5) **Neoplasm Related Pain**

   Code G89.3 is assigned to pain documented as being related, associated or due to cancer, primary or secondary malignancy, or tumor. This code is assigned regardless of whether the pain is acute or chronic.

   This code may be assigned as the principal or first-listed code when the stated reason for the admission/encounter is documented as pain control/pain management. The underlying neoplasm should be reported as an additional diagnosis.

   When the reason for the admission/encounter is management of the neoplasm and the pain associated with the neoplasm is also documented, code G89.3 may be assigned as an additional diagnosis. It is not necessary to assign an additional code for the site of the pain.

   See Section I.C.2 for instructions on the sequencing of neoplasms for all other stated reasons for the admission/encounter (except for pain control/pain management).

   6) **Chronic pain syndrome**

   Central pain syndrome (G89.0) and chronic pain syndrome (G89.4) are different than the term "chronic pain," and therefore codes should only be used when the provider has specifically documented this condition.

   See Section I.C.5. Pain disorders related to psychological factors

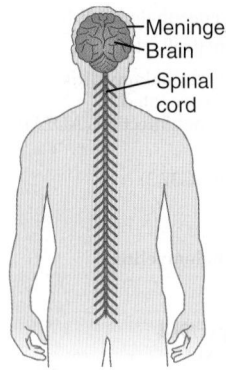

—Meninges
—Brain
—Spinal cord

Figure 6-1 The brain and spinal cord make up the central nervous system.

Item 6-1 The two major classifications of the nervous system are the peripheral nervous system and the central nervous system (CNS). The central nervous system is composed of the brain and the spinal cord. The peripheral nervous system is composed of the parasympathetic and sympathetic systems. **Encephalitis** is the swelling of the brain. **Meningitis** is swelling of the covering of the brain, the meninges. Types and causes of brain infections are:

Type	Cause
purulent	bacterial
aseptic/abacterial	viral
chronic meningitis	mycobacterial and fungal

CHAPTER 6

DISEASES OF THE NERVOUS SYSTEM (G00-G99)

Excludes2   certain conditions originating in the perinatal period (P04-P96)
certain infectious and parasitic diseases (A00-B99)
complications of pregnancy, childbirth and the puerperium (O00-O9A)
congenital malformations, deformations, and chromosomal abnormalities (Q00-Q99)
endocrine, nutritional and metabolic diseases (E00-E88)
injury, poisoning and certain other consequences of external causes (S00-T88)
neoplasms (C00-D49)
symptoms, signs and abnormal clinical and laboratory findings, not elsewhere classified (R00-R94)

This chapter contains the following blocks:

G00-G09	Inflammatory diseases of the central nervous system
G10-G14	Systemic atrophies primarily affecting the central nervous system
G20-G26	Extrapyramidal and movement disorders
G30-G32	Other degenerative diseases of the nervous system
G35-G37	Demyelinating diseases of the central nervous system
G40-G47	Episodic and paroxysmal disorders
G50-G59	Nerve, nerve root and plexus disorders
G60-G65	Polyneuropathies and other disorders of the peripheral nervous system
G70-G73	Diseases of myoneural junction and muscle
G80-G83	Cerebral palsy and other paralytic syndromes
G89-G99	Other disorders of the nervous system

INFLAMMATORY DISEASES OF THE CENTRAL NERVOUS SYSTEM (G00-G09)

● **G00**   **Bacterial meningitis, not elsewhere classified**
An infection of the cerebrospinal fluid surrounding the spinal cord and brain.

     Includes   bacterial arachnoiditis
bacterial leptomeningitis
bacterial meningitis
bacterial pachymeningitis

     Excludes1   bacterial meningoencephalitis (G04.2)
bacterial meningomyelitis (G04.2)

   G00.0   **Hemophilus meningitis**
Meningitis due to Hemophilus influenzae

   G00.1   **Pneumococcal meningitis**
Meningitis due to Streptococcal pneumoniae

   G00.2   **Streptococcal meningitis**
Use additional code to further identify organism (B95.0-B95.5)

   G00.3   **Staphylococcal meningitis**
Use additional code to further identify organism (B95.61-B95.8)

   G00.8   **Other bacterial meningitis**
Meningitis due to Escherichia coli
Meningitis due to Friedländer bacillus
Meningitis due to Klebsiella
Use additional code to further identify organism (B96.-)

   G00.9   **Bacterial meningitis, unspecified**
Meningitis due to gram-negative bacteria, unspecified
Purulent meningitis NOS
Pyogenic meningitis NOS
Suppurative meningitis NOS

▷ **G01**   *Meningitis in bacterial diseases classified elsewhere*
Code first underlying disease

     Excludes1   meningitis (in):
gonococcal (A54.81)
leptospirosis (A27.81)
listeriosis (A32.11)
Lyme disease (A69.21)
meningococcal (A39.0)
neurosyphilis (A52.13)
tuberculosis (A17.0)
meningoencephalitis and meningomyelitis in bacterial diseases classified elsewhere (G05)

▷ **G02**   *Meningitis in other infectious and parasitic diseases classified elsewhere*

     Code first underlying disease, such as:
African trypanosomiasis (B56.-)
poliovirus infection (A80.-)

     Excludes1   candidal meningitis (B37.5)
coccidioidomycosis meningitis (B38.4)
cryptococcal meningitis (B45.1)
herpesviral [herpes simplex] meningitis (B00.3)
infectious mononucleosis complicated by meningitis (B27.- with fourth character 2)
measles complicated by meningitis (B05.1)
meningoencephalitis and meningomyelitis in other infectious and parasitic diseases classified elsewhere (G05)
mumps meningitis (B26.1)
rubella meningitis (B06.02)
varicella [chickenpox] meningitis (B01.0)
zoster meningitis (B02.1)

● **G03** **Meningitis due to other and unspecified causes**
- **Includes** arachnoiditis NOS
  - leptomeningitis NOS
  - meningitis NOS
  - pachymeningitis NOS
- **Excludes1** meningoencephalitis (G04.-)
  - meningomyelitis (G04.-)

G03.0 **Nonpyogenic meningitis**
- Aseptic meningitis
- Nonbacterial meningitis

G03.1 **Chronic meningitis**

G03.2 **Benign recurrent** meningitis [Mollaret]

G03.8 **Meningitis due to other specified causes**

G03.9 **Meningitis, unspecified**
- Arachnoiditis (spinal) NOS

● **G04** **Encephalitis, myelitis and encephalomyelitis**
- **Includes** acute ascending myelitis
  - meningoencephalitis
  - meningomyelitis
- **Excludes1** encephalopathy NOS (G93.40)
  - other noninfectious acute disseminated encephalomyelitis (noninfectious ADEM) (G04.81)
- **Excludes2** acute transverse myelitis (G37.3-)
  - alcoholic encephalopathy (G31.2)
  - benign myalgic encephalomyelitis (G93.3)
  - multiple sclerosis (G35)
  - subacute necrotizing myelitis (G37.4)
  - ⇒ toxic encephalitis (G92.8)
  - ⇒ toxic encephalopathy (G92.8)

● **G04.0** **Acute disseminated encephalitis and encephalomyelitis (ADEM)**
- **Excludes1** acute necrotizing hemorrhagic encephalopathy (G04.3-)

G04.00 **Acute disseminated encephalitis and encephalomyelitis, unspecified**

▷ *G04.01* *Postinfectious acute disseminated encephalitis and encephalomyelitis (postinfectious ADEM)*
- **Excludes1** post chickenpox encephalitis (B01.1)
  - post measles encephalitis (B05.0)
  - post measles myelitis (B05.1)

G04.02 **Postimmunization acute disseminated encephalitis, myelitis and encephalomyelitis**
- Encephalitis, post immunization
- Encephalomyelitis, post immunization
- Use additional code to identify the vaccine (T50.A-, T50.B-, T50.Z-)

G04.1 **Tropical spastic paraplegia** 🐾

G04.2 **Bacterial meningoencephalitis and meningomyelitis, not elsewhere classified**

● **G04.3** **Acute necrotizing hemorrhagic encephalopathy**
- *Sudden and severe CNS disease with pathology of hemorrhages and necrosis of white matter*
- **Excludes1** acute disseminated encephalitis and encephalomyelitis (G04.0-)

G04.30 **Acute necrotizing hemorrhagic encephalopathy, unspecified**

G04.31 **Postinfectious acute necrotizing hemorrhagic encephalopathy**

G04.32 **Postimmunization acute necrotizing hemorrhagic encephalopathy**
- Use additional code to identify vaccine (T50.A-, T50.B-, T50.Z-)

G04.39 **Other acute necrotizing hemorrhagic encephalopathy**
- Code also underlying etiology, if applicable

● **G04.8** **Other encephalitis, myelitis and encephalomyelitis**
- Code also any associated seizure (G40.-, R56.9)

G04.81 **Other encephalitis and encephalomyelitis**
- Noninfectious acute disseminated encephalomyelitis (noninfectious ADEM)

▶ **G04.82** **Acute flaccid myelitis**
- ▶ **Excludes1** transverse myelitis (G37.3)

G04.89 **Other myelitis** 🐾
- Coding Clinic: 2020, Q1, P14

● **G04.9** **Encephalitis, myelitis and encephalomyelitis, unspecified**

G04.90 **Encephalitis and encephalomyelitis, unspecified**
- Ventriculitis (cerebral) NOS

G04.91 **Myelitis, unspecified** 🐾

● **G05** **Encephalitis, myelitis and encephalomyelitis in diseases classified elsewhere**
- *Code first underlying disease, such as:*
  - ▶ congenital toxoplasmosis encephalitis, myelitis and encephalomyelitis (P37.1)
  - ▶ cytomegaloviral encephalitis, myelitis and encephalomyelitis (B25.8)
  - ▶ encephalitis, myelitis and encephalomyelitis (in) systemic lupus erythematosus (M32.19)
  - ▶ eosinophilic meningoencephalitis (B83.2)
  - human immunodeficiency virus [HIV] disease (B20)
  - poliovirus (A80.-)
  - suppurative otitis media (H66.01-H66.4)
  - trichinellosis (B75)
- **Excludes1** adenoviral encephalitis, myelitis and encephalomyelitis (A85.1)
  - ~~congenital toxoplasmosis encephalitis, myelitis and encephalomyelitis (P37.1)~~
  - ~~cytomegaloviral encephalitis, myelitis and encephalomyelitis (B25.8)~~
  - encephalitis, myelitis and encephalomyelitis (in) measles (B05.0)
  - ~~encephalitis, myelitis and encephalomyelitis (in) systemic lupus erythematosus (M32.19)~~
  - enteroviral encephalitis, myelitis and encephalomyelitis (A85.0)
  - ~~eosinophilic meningoencephalitis (B83.2)~~
  - herpesviral [herpes simplex] encephalitis, myelitis and encephalomyelitis (B00.4)
  - listerial encephalitis, myelitis and encephalomyelitis (A32.12)
  - meningococcal encephalitis, myelitis and encephalomyelitis (A39.81)
  - mumps encephalitis, myelitis and encephalomyelitis (B26.2)
  - postchickenpox encephalitis, myelitis and encephalomyelitis (B01.1-)
  - rubella encephalitis, myelitis and encephalomyelitis (B06.01)
  - toxoplasmosis encephalitis, myelitis and encephalomyelitis (B58.2)
  - zoster encephalitis, myelitis and encephalomyelitis (B02.0)

▷ *G05.3* *Encephalitis and encephalomyelitis in diseases classified elsewhere*
- Meningoencephalitis in diseases classified elsewhere

▷ *G05.4* *Myelitis in diseases classified elsewhere* 🐾
- Meningomyelitis in diseases classified elsewhere

▶ New　　⇒ Revised　　~~deleted~~ Deleted　　Excludes 1　　Excludes 2　　Includes　　Use additional　　Code first　　Code also　　Key words

OGCR Official Guidelines　　X Assign placeholder X　　● Use Additional Character(s)　　▷ Manifestation Code　　🐾 Hierarchical Condition Category　　**Coding Clinic**

● **G06   Intracranial and intraspinal abscess and granuloma**
An accumulation of pus in either the brain or spinal cord
     Use additional code (B95-B97) to identify infectious agent.

     G06.0   Intracranial abscess and granuloma
         Brain [any part] abscess (embolic)
         Cerebellar abscess (embolic)
         Cerebral abscess (embolic)
         Intracranial epidural abscess or granuloma
         Intracranial extradural abscess or granuloma
         Intracranial subdural abscess or granuloma
         Otogenic abscess (embolic)
         Excludes1   tuberculous intracranial abscess and
                        granuloma (A17.81)

     G06.1   Intraspinal abscess and granuloma
         Abscess (embolic) of spinal cord [any part]
         Intraspinal epidural abscess or granuloma
         Intraspinal extradural abscess or granuloma
         Intraspinal subdural abscess or granuloma
         Excludes1   tuberculous intraspinal abscess and
                        granuloma (A17.81)

     G06.2   Extradural and subdural abscess, unspecified

▶ *G07   Intracranial and intraspinal abscess and granuloma in diseases
classified elsewhere*
     Code first underlying disease, such as:
         schistosomiasis granuloma of brain (B65.-)
     Excludes1   abscess of brain:
                amebic (A06.6)
                chromomycotic (B43.1)
                gonococcal (A54.82)
                tuberculous (A17.81)
                tuberculoma of meninges (A17.1)

G08   Intracranial and intraspinal phlebitis and thrombophlebitis
     Septic embolism of intracranial or intraspinal venous sinuses
         and veins
     Septic endophlebitis of intracranial or intraspinal venous
         sinuses and veins
     Septic phlebitis of intracranial or intraspinal venous sinuses
         and veins
     Septic thrombophlebitis of intracranial or intraspinal venous
         sinuses and veins
     Septic thrombosis of intracranial or intraspinal venous sinuses
         and veins
     Excludes1   intracranial phlebitis and thrombophlebitis
                complicating:
                  abortion, ectopic or molar pregnancy
                     (O00-O07, O08.7)
                  pregnancy, childbirth and the puerperium
                     (O22.5, O87.3)
                  nonpyogenic intracranial phlebitis and
                     thrombophlebitis (I67.6)
     Excludes2   intracranial phlebitis and thrombophlebitis
                complicating nonpyogenic intraspinal
                phlebitis and thrombophlebitis (G95.1)

G09   Sequelae of inflammatory diseases of central nervous system
     Note: Category G09 is to be used to indicate conditions
            whose primary classification is to G00-G08 as the cause of
            sequelae, themselves classifiable elsewhere. The 'sequelae'
            include conditions specified as residuals.
     *Code first condition resulting from (sequela) of inflammatory diseases
     of central nervous system*

SYSTEMIC ATROPHIES PRIMARILY AFFECTING
THE CENTRAL NERVOUS SYSTEM (G10-G14)

G10   Huntington's disease 🔖
     *Genetic disease with degeneration of cells of the nervous system,
         including brain*
     Huntington's chorea
     Huntington's dementia
     Code also dementia in other diseases classified elsewhere
         without behavioral disturbance (F02.80)

Item 6–2: Huntington's chorea is an inherited degenerative disorder of
the central nervous system and is characterized by ceaseless, jerky movements
and progressive cognitive and behavioral deterioration.

● **G11   Hereditary ataxia**
     Genetic neurological disorder affecting coordination
     Excludes2   cerebral palsy (G80.-)
                hereditary and idiopathic neuropathy (G60.-)
                metabolic disorders (E70-E88)

     G11.0   Congenital nonprogressive ataxia 🔖
●   **G11.1   Early-onset cerebellar ataxia** 🔖
         G11.10 Early-onset cerebellar ataxia, unspecified
         G11.11 Friedreich ataxia
              Autosomal recessive Friedreich ataxia
              Friedreich ataxia with retained reflexes
         G11.19 Other early-onset cerebellar ataxia
              Early-onset cerebellar ataxia with essential
                tremor
              Early-onset cerebellar ataxia with myoclonus
                [Hunt's ataxia]
              Early-onset cerebellar ataxia with retained
                tendon reflexes
              X-linked recessive spinocerebellar ataxia

     G11.2   Late-onset cerebellar ataxia 🔖   A
     G11.3   Cerebellar ataxia with defective DNA repair 🔖
         Ataxia telangiectasia [Louis-Bar]
         Excludes2   Cockayne's syndrome (Q87.19)
                    other disorders of purine and pyrimidine
                      metabolism (E79.-)
                    xeroderma pigmentosum (Q82.1)

     G11.4   Hereditary spastic paraplegia 🔖
     G11.8   Other hereditary ataxias 🔖
     G11.9   Hereditary ataxia, unspecified 🔖
         Hereditary cerebellar ataxia NOS
         Hereditary cerebellar degeneration
         Hereditary cerebellar disease
         Hereditary cerebellar syndrome

● **G12   Spinal muscular atrophy and related syndromes**
     **G12.0   Infantile spinal muscular atrophy, type I
             [Werdnig-Hoffman]** 🔖
     G12.1   Other inherited spinal muscular atrophy 🔖
         Adult form spinal muscular atrophy
         Childhood form, type II spinal muscular atrophy
         Distal spinal muscular atrophy
         Juvenile form, type III spinal muscular atrophy
             [Kugelberg-Welander]
         Progressive bulbar palsy of childhood [Fazio-Londe]
         Scapuloperoneal form spinal muscular atrophy
●   **G12.2   Motor neuron disease**
         *Progressive disease of motor neurons that carry impulses to
             muscles to move*
         G12.20   Motor neuron disease, unspecified 🔖
         G12.21   Amyotrophic lateral sclerosis 🔖   A
                Lou Gehrig's disease (ALS)
         G12.22   Progressive bulbar palsy 🔖
         G12.23   Primary lateral sclerosis 🔖
         G12.24   Familial motor neuron disease 🔖
         G12.25   Progressive spinal muscle atrophy 🔖
         G12.29   Other motor neuron disease 🔖
     **G12.8   Other spinal muscular atrophies and related
             syndromes** 🔖
     G12.9   Spinal muscular atrophy, unspecified 🔖

● **G13   Systemic atrophies primarily affecting central nervous system
in diseases classified elsewhere**
     ▶ *G13.0   Paraneoplastic neuromyopathy and neuropathy* 🔖
         Carcinomatous neuromyopathy
         Sensorial paraneoplastic neuropathy [Denny Brown]
         Code first underlying neoplasm (C00-D49)
     ▶ *G13.1   Other systemic atrophy primarily affecting central
             nervous system in neoplastic disease* 🔖
         Paraneoplastic limbic encephalopathy
         Code first underlying neoplasm (C00-D49)

▌ **G13.2** *Systemic atrophy primarily affecting the central nervous system in myxedema*
     Code first underlying disease, such as:
       hypothyroidism (E03.-)
       myxedematous congenital iodine deficiency (E00.1)

▌ **G13.8** *Systemic atrophy primarily affecting central nervous system in other diseases classified elsewhere*
     Code first underlying disease

G14   **Postpolio syndrome**
    Includes   Postpolio myelitic syndrome
    Excludes1   sequelae of poliomyelitis (B91)

EXTRAPYRAMIDAL AND MOVEMENT DISORDERS (G20-G26)

● **G20**   **Parkinson's disease** 🐾
    Progressive disease of the nervous system that affects muscle coordination
    Hemiparkinsonism
    Idiopathic Parkinsonism or Parkinson's disease
    Paralysis agitans
    Parkinsonism or Parkinson's disease NOS
    Primary Parkinsonism or Parkinson's disease
    Use additional code to identify:
      dementia with behavioral disturbance (F02.81)
      dementia without behavioral disturbance (F02.80)
    Excludes1   dementia with Parkinsonism (G31.83)
    Coding Clinic: 2017, Q2, P7-8; 2016, Q2, P7

● **G21**   **Secondary parkinsonism**
    Symptoms of Parkinson's caused by medicines, illness, or other nervous system disorder
    Excludes1   dementia with Parkinsonism (G31.83)
                 Huntington's disease (G10)
                  Shy-Drager syndrome (G90.3)
                  syphilitic Parkinsonism (A52.19)

   G21.0   **Malignant neuroleptic syndrome**
       Use additional code for adverse effect, if applicable, to identify drug (T43.3X5, T43.4X5, T43.505, T43.595)
       Excludes1   neuroleptic induced parkinsonism (G21.11)

 ● **G21.1**   **Other drug-induced secondary parkinsonism**
      G21.11   **Neuroleptic induced parkinsonism** 🐾
          Use additional code for adverse effect, if applicable, to identify drug (T43.3X5, T43.4X5, T43.505, T43.595)
          Excludes1   malignant neuroleptic syndrome (G21.0)

      G21.19   **Other drug induced secondary parkinsonism** 🐾
          Other medication-induced parkinsonism
          Use additional code for adverse effect, if applicable, to identify drug (T36-T50 with fifth or sixth character 5)

   G21.2   **Secondary parkinsonism due to other external agents** 🐾
       Code first (T51-T65) to identify external agent

   G21.3   **Postencephalitic parkinsonism** 🐾
   G21.4   **Vascular parkinsonism** 🐾
   G21.8   **Other secondary parkinsonism** 🐾
   G21.9   **Secondary parkinsonism, unspecified** 🐾

● **G23**   **Other degenerative diseases of basal ganglia**
    Excludes2   multi-system degeneration of the autonomic nervous system (G90.3)

   G23.0   **Hallervorden-Spatz disease** 🐾
       Pigmentary pallidal degeneration

   G23.1   **Progressive supranuclear ophthalmoplegia [Steele-Richardson-Olszewski]** 🐾
       Progressive supranuclear palsy

   G23.2   **Striatonigral degeneration** 🐾
   G23.8   **Other specified degenerative diseases of basal ganglia** 🐾
       Calcification of basal ganglia
   G23.9   **Degenerative disease of basal ganglia, unspecified** 🐾

● **G24**   **Dystonia**
    Involuntary movements
    Includes   dyskinesia
    Excludes2   athetoid cerebral palsy (G80.3)

 ● **G24.0**   **Drug induced dystonia**
       Use additional code for adverse effect, if applicable, to identify drug (T36-T50 with fifth or sixth character 5)

      G24.01   **Drug induced subacute dyskinesia**
          Drug induced blepharospasm
          Drug induced orofacial dyskinesia
          Neuroleptic induced tardive dyskinesia
          Tardive dyskinesia

      G24.02   **Drug induced acute dystonia**
          Acute dystonic reaction to drugs
          Neuroleptic induced acute dystonia

      G24.09   **Other drug induced dystonia**

   G24.1   **Genetic torsion dystonia**
       Dystonia deformans progressiva
       Dystonia musculorum deformans
       Familial torsion dystonia
       Idiopathic familial dystonia
       Idiopathic (torsion) dystonia NOS
       (Schwalbe-) Ziehen-Oppenheim disease

   G24.2   **Idiopathic nonfamilial dystonia**

   G24.3   **Spasmodic torticollis**
       Head tilts toward one side and chin is elevated and turned toward opposite side (wry neck)
       Excludes1   congenital torticollis (Q68.0)
                  hysterical torticollis (F44.4)
                  ocular torticollis (R29.891)
                  psychogenic torticollis (F45.8)
                  torticollis NOS (M43.6)
                  traumatic recurrent torticollis (S13.4)

   G24.4   **Idiopathic orofacial dystonia**
       Orofacial dyskinesia
       Excludes1   drug induced orofacial dyskinesia (G24.01)

   G24.5   **Blepharospasm**
       Tonic spasm of orbicularis oculi muscle, producing closure of eyelids
       Excludes1   drug induced blepharospasm (G24.01)

   G24.8   **Other dystonia**
       Acquired torsion dystonia NOS

   G24.9   **Dystonia, unspecified**
       Dyskinesia NOS

● **G25**   **Other extrapyramidal and movement disorders**
    Extrapyramidal: Other than pyramidal tracts
    Excludes2   sleep related movement disorders (G47.6-)

   G25.0   **Essential tremor**
       Familial tremor
       Excludes1   tremor NOS (R25.1)

   G25.1   **Drug-induced tremor**
       Use additional code for adverse effect, if applicable, to identify drug (T36-T50 with fifth or sixth character 5)

   G25.2   **Other specified forms of tremor**
       Intention tremor

   G25.3   **Myoclonus**
       Shocklike contractions muscle(s)
       Drug-induced myoclonus
       Palatal myoclonus
       Use additional code for adverse effect, if applicable, to identify drug (T36-T50 with fifth or sixth character 5)
       Excludes1   facial myokymia (G51.4)
                  myoclonic epilepsy (G40.-)

CHAPTER 6 (G00-G99)

▶ New   ⇒ Revised   ~~deleted~~ Deleted   Excludes 1   Excludes 2   Includes   Use additional   Code first   Code also   Key words

OGCR Official Guidelines   X Assign placeholder X   ● Use Additional Character(s)   ▌ Manifestation Code   🐾 Hierarchical Condition Category   **Coding Clinic**

G25.4   Drug-induced chorea

> Use additional code for adverse effect, if applicable, to identify drug (T36-T50 with fifth or sixth character 5)

G25.5   Other chorea

> *Continual, involuntary, jerky, movements*
> Chorea NOS

> > **Excludes1**   chorea NOS with heart involvement (I02.0)
> > Huntington's chorea (G10)
> > rheumatic chorea (I02.-)
> > Sydenham's chorea (I02.-)

G25.6   Drug induced tics and other tics of organic origin

    G25.61   Drug induced tics

> > Use additional code for adverse effect, if applicable, to identify drug (T36-T50 with fifth or sixth character 5)

    G25.69   Other tics of organic origin

> > > **Excludes1**   habit spasm (F95.9)
> > > tic NOS (F95.9)
> > > Tourette's syndrome (F95.2)

G25.7   Other and unspecified drug induced movement disorders

> Use additional code for adverse effect, if applicable, to identify drug (T36-T50 with fifth or sixth character 5)

    G25.70   Drug induced movement disorder, unspecified

    G25.71   Drug induced akathisia

> > Drug induced acathisia
> > Neuroleptic induced acute akathisia
> > Tardive akathisia

    G25.79   Other drug induced movement disorders

G25.8   Other specified extrapyramidal and movement disorders

    G25.81   Restless legs syndrome

    G25.82   Stiff-man syndrome

    G25.83   Benign shuddering attacks

    G25.89   Other specified extrapyramidal and movement disorders

G25.9   Extrapyramidal and movement disorder, unspecified

▶ *G26*   *Extrapyramidal and movement disorders in diseases classified elsewhere*

> *Code first underlying disease*

OTHER DEGENERATIVE DISEASES OF THE NERVOUS SYSTEM (G30-G32)

● **G30**   Alzheimer's disease

> *Progressive central neurodegenerative disorder*

> > **Includes**   Alzheimer's dementia senile and presenile forms

> Use additional code to identify:
>   delirium, if applicable (F05)
>   dementia with behavioral disturbance (F02.81)
>   dementia without behavioral disturbance (F02.80)

> > **Excludes1**   senile degeneration of brain NEC (G31.1)
> > senile dementia NOS (F03)
> > senility NOS (R41.81)

    G30.0   Alzheimer's disease with early onset

    G30.1   Alzheimer's disease with late onset   A

    G30.8   Other Alzheimer's disease

    G30.9   Alzheimer's disease, unspecified

> > **Coding Clinic: 2017, Q1, P43; 2016, Q2, P6; 2012, Q4, P95**

● **G31**   Other degenerative diseases of nervous system, not elsewhere classified

> For codes G31.0-G31.83, G31.85-G31.9, use additional code to identify:
>   dementia with behavioral disturbance (F02.81)
>   dementia without behavioral disturbance (F02.80)

> > **Excludes2**   Reye's syndrome (G93.7)

● **G31.0**   Frontotemporal dementia

    G31.01   Pick's disease

> > Primary progressive aphasia
> > Progressive isolated aphasia

    G31.09   Other frontotemporal dementia

> > Frontal dementia

G31.1   Senile degeneration of brain, not elsewhere classified

> > **Excludes1**   Alzheimer's disease (G30.-)
> > senility NOS (R41.81)

G31.2   Degeneration of nervous system due to alcohol

> Alcoholic cerebellar ataxia
> Alcoholic cerebellar degeneration
> Alcoholic cerebral degeneration
> Alcoholic encephalopathy
> Dysfunction of the autonomic nervous system due to alcohol

> *Code also* associated alcoholism (F10.-)

● **G31.8**   Other specified degenerative diseases of nervous system

    G31.81   Alpers' disease

> > *Rare neuronal degeneration of cerebral cortex disease of young children*
> > Grey-matter degeneration
> > **Coding Clinic: 2017, Q2, P7**

    G31.82   Leigh's disease

> > *Rare neurometabolic disorder that affects central nervous system*
> > Subacute necrotizing encephalopathy

    G31.83   Dementia with Lewy bodies

> > *Closely allied to Parkinson's Disease*
> > Dementia with Parkinsonism
> > Lewy body dementia
> > Lewy body disease
> > **Coding Clinic: 2017, Q2, P7; 2016, Q4, P141**

    G31.84   Mild cognitive impairment, so stated

> > Mild neurocognitive disorder

> > > **Excludes1**   age related cognitive decline (R41.81)
> > > altered mental status (R41.82)
> > > cerebral degeneration (G31.9)
> > > change in mental status (R41.82)
> > > cognitive deficits following (sequelae of) cerebral hemorrhage or infarction (I69.01-, I69.11-, I69.21-, I69.31-, I69.81-, I69.91-)
> > > cognitive impairment due to intracranial or head injury (S06.-)
> > > dementia (F01.-, F02.-, F03)
> > > mild memory disturbance (F06.8)
> > > neurologic neglect syndrome (R41.4)
> > > personality change, nonpsychotic (F68.8)

    G31.85   Corticobasal degeneration

    G31.89   Other specified degenerative diseases of nervous system

G31.9   Degenerative disease of nervous system, unspecified

● **G32**   Other degenerative disorders of nervous system in diseases classified elsewhere

▶ *G32.0*   *Subacute combined degeneration of spinal cord in diseases classified elsewhere* 🔾

> > Dana-Putnam syndrome
> > Sclerosis of spinal cord (combined) (dorsolateral) (posterolateral)

> > *Code first underlying disease, such as:*
> >   anemia (D51.9)
> >   dietary (D51.3)
> >   pernicious (D51.0)
> >   vitamin B12 deficiency (E53.8)

> > > **Excludes1**   syphilitic combined degeneration of spinal cord (A52.11)

CHAPTER 6 (G00-G99)

● G32.8   **Other specified degenerative disorders of nervous system in diseases classified elsewhere**
    Code first underlying disease, such as:
      amyloidosis cerebral degeneration (E85.-)
      cerebral degeneration (due to) hypothyroidism (E00.0-E03.9)
      cerebral degeneration (due to) neoplasm (C00-D49)
      cerebral degeneration (due to) vitamin B deficiency, except thiamine (E52-E53.-)

    Excludes1   superior hemorrhagic polioencephalitis [Wernicke's encephalopathy] (E51.2)

▷ G32.81   *Cerebellar ataxia in diseases classified elsewhere* 🔖
     Code first underlying disease, such as:
      celiac disease (with gluten ataxia) (K90.0)
      cerebellar ataxia (in) neoplastic disease (paraneoplastic cerebellar degeneration) (C00-D49)
      non-celiac gluten ataxia (M35.9)

     Excludes1   systemic atrophy primarily affecting the central nervous system in alcoholic cerebellar ataxia (G31.2)
           systemic atrophy primarily affecting the central nervous system in myxedema (G13.2)

▷ G32.89   *Other specified degenerative disorders of nervous system in diseases classified elsewhere*
     Degenerative encephalopathy in diseases classified elsewhere

DEMYELINATING DISEASES OF THE CENTRAL NERVOUS SYSTEM (G35-G37)

G35   **Multiple sclerosis** 🔖
   Destruction of central nervous system; four types: relapsing remitting, secondary progressive, primary progressive, and progressive relapsing
   Disseminated multiple sclerosis
   Generalized multiple sclerosis
   Multiple sclerosis NOS
   Multiple sclerosis of brain stem
   Multiple sclerosis of cord
   Coding Clinic: 2021, Q1, P7

● G36   **Other acute disseminated demyelination**
    Excludes1   postinfectious encephalitis and encephalomyelitis NOS (G04.01)

G36.0   **Neuromyelitis optica [Devic]** 🔖
    Inflammatory disorder in which immune system attacks optic nerves and spinal cord producing inflammation of optic nerve (optic neuritis) and spinal cord (myelitis)
    Demyelination in optic neuritis
    Excludes1   optic neuritis NOS (H46)

G36.1   **Acute and subacute hemorrhagic leukoencephalitis [Hurst]** 🔖

G36.8   **Other specified acute disseminated demyelination** 🔖

G36.9   **Acute disseminated demyelination, unspecified** 🔖

● G37   **Other demyelinating diseases of central nervous system**
   Destruction of central nervous system

G37.0   **Diffuse sclerosis of central nervous system** 🔖
    Periaxial encephalitis
    Schilder's disease
    Excludes1   X linked adrenoleukodystrophy (E71.52-)

Item 6–3   **Multiple sclerosis** (MS) is a nervous system disease affecting the brain and spinal cord by damaging the myelin sheath surrounding and protecting nerve cells. The damage slows down/blocks messages between the brain and body. Symptoms are visual disturbances, muscle weakness, coordination and balance issues, numbness, prickling, thinking and memory problems. The cause is unknown, though it is thought that it may be an autoimmune disease. It affects women more than men, between 20 and 40 years of age. MS can be mild, but it may cause the loss of ability to write, walk, and speak. There is no cure, but medication may slow or control symptoms.

G37.1   **Central demyelination of corpus callosum** 🔖

G37.2   **Central pontine myelinolysis** 🔖

G37.3   **Acute transverse myelitis in demyelinating disease of central nervous system** 🔖
    Acute transverse myelitis NOS
    Acute transverse myelopathy
   ▷ **Excludes1**   acute flaccid myelitis (G04.82)
           multiple sclerosis (G35)
           neuromyelitis optica [Devic] (G36.0)

G37.4   **Subacute necrotizing myelitis of central nervous system** 🔖

G37.5   **Concentric sclerosis [Baló] of central nervous system** 🔖

G37.8   **Other specified demyelinating diseases of central nervous system** 🔖

G37.9   **Demyelinating disease of central nervous system, unspecified** 🔖

EPISODIC AND PAROXYSMAL DISORDERS (G40-G47)

● G40   **Epilepsy and recurrent seizures**
   Note: The following terms are to be considered equivalent to intractable: pharmacoresistant (pharmacologically resistant), treatment resistant, refractory (medically) and poorly controlled

    Excludes1   conversion disorder with seizures (F44.5)
           convulsions NOS (R56.9)
           post traumatic seizures (R56.1)
           seizure (convulsive) NOS (R56.9)
           seizure of newborn (P90)

    Excludes2   hippocampal sclerosis (G93.81)
           mesial temporal sclerosis (G93.81)
           temporal sclerosis (G93.81)
           Todd's paralysis (G83.84)

● G40.0   **Localization-related (focal) (partial) idiopathic epilepsy and epileptic syndromes with seizures of localized onset**
    Benign childhood epilepsy with centrotemporal EEG spikes
    Childhood epilepsy with occipital EEG paroxysms
    Excludes1   adult onset localization-related epilepsy (G40.1-, G40.2-)

● G40.00   **Localization-related (focal) (partial) idiopathic epilepsy and epileptic syndromes with seizures of localized onset, not intractable**
    Localization-related (focal) (partial) idiopathic epilepsy and epileptic syndromes with seizures of localized onset without intractability

     G40.001   **Localization-related (focal) (partial) idiopathic epilepsy and epileptic syndromes with seizures of localized onset, not intractable, with status epilepticus** 🔖

     G40.009   **Localization-related (focal) (partial) idiopathic epilepsy and epileptic syndromes with seizures of localized onset, not intractable, without status epilepticus** 🔖
        Localization-related (focal) (partial) idiopathic epilepsy and epileptic syndromes with seizures of localized onset NOS

● G40.01   **Localization-related (focal) (partial) idiopathic epilepsy and epileptic syndromes with seizures of localized onset, intractable**

     G40.011   **Localization-related (focal) (partial) idiopathic epilepsy and epileptic syndromes with seizures of localized onset, intractable, with status epilepticus** 🔖

     G40.019   **Localization-related (focal) (partial) idiopathic epilepsy and epileptic syndromes with seizures of localized onset, intractable, without status epilepticus** 🔖

▶ New   ⇒ Revised   deleted Deleted   Excludes 1   Excludes 2   Includes   Use additional   Code first   Code also   Key words

OGCR Official Guidelines   X Assign placeholder X   ● Use Additional Character(s)   ▷ Manifestation Code   🔖 Hierarchical Condition Category   **Coding Clinic**

● **G40.1** **Localization-related (focal) (partial) symptomatic epilepsy and epileptic syndromes with simple partial seizures**

     Attacks without alteration of consciousness
     Epilepsia partialis continua [Kozhevnikof]
     Simple partial seizures developing into secondarily generalized seizures

  ● **G40.10** **Localization-related (focal) (partial) symptomatic epilepsy and epileptic syndromes with simple partial seizures, not intractable**

     Localization-related (focal) (partial) symptomatic epilepsy and epileptic syndromes with simple partial seizures without intractability

     G40.101 **Localization-related (focal) (partial) symptomatic epilepsy and epileptic syndromes with simple partial seizures, not intractable, with status epilepticus** 🕮

     G40.109 **Localization-related (focal) (partial) symptomatic epilepsy and epileptic syndromes with simple partial seizures, not intractable, without status epilepticus** 🕮

         Localization-related (focal) (partial) symptomatic epilepsy and epileptic syndromes with simple partial seizures NOS

  ● **G40.11** **Localization-related (focal) (partial) symptomatic epilepsy and epileptic syndromes with simple partial seizures, intractable**

     G40.111 **Localization-related (focal) (partial) symptomatic epilepsy and epileptic syndromes with simple partial seizures, intractable, with status epilepticus** 🕮

     G40.119 **Localization-related (focal) (partial) symptomatic epilepsy and epileptic syndromes with simple partial seizures, intractable, without status epilepticus** 🕮

● **G40.2** **Localization-related (focal) (partial) symptomatic epilepsy and epileptic syndromes with complex partial seizures**

     Attacks with alteration of consciousness, often with automatisms
     Complex partial seizures developing into secondarily generalized seizures

  ● **G40.20** **Localization-related (focal) (partial) symptomatic epilepsy and epileptic syndromes with complex partial seizures, not intractable**

     Localization-related (focal) (partial) symptomatic epilepsy and epileptic syndromes with complex partial seizures without intractability

     G40.201 **Localization-related (focal) (partial) symptomatic epilepsy and epileptic syndromes with complex partial seizures, not intractable, with status epilepticus** 🕮

     G40.209 **Localization-related (focal) (partial) symptomatic epilepsy and epileptic syndromes with complex partial seizures, not intractable, without status epilepticus** 🕮

         Localization-related (focal) (partial) symptomatic epilepsy and epileptic syndromes with complex partial seizures NOS

● **G40.21** **Localization-related (focal) (partial) symptomatic epilepsy and epileptic syndromes with complex partial seizures, intractable**

     G40.211 **Localization-related (focal) (partial) symptomatic epilepsy and epileptic syndromes with complex partial seizures, intractable, with status epilepticus** 🕮

     G40.219 **Localization-related (focal) (partial) symptomatic epilepsy and epileptic syndromes with complex partial seizures, intractable, without status epilepticus** 🕮

● **G40.3** **Generalized idiopathic epilepsy and epileptic syndromes**

     Code also MERRF syndrome, if applicable (E88.42)

  ● **G40.30** **Generalized idiopathic epilepsy and epileptic syndromes, not intractable**

     Generalized idiopathic epilepsy and epileptic syndromes without intractability

     G40.301 **Generalized idiopathic epilepsy and epileptic syndromes, not intractable, with status epilepticus** 🕮

     G40.309 **Generalized idiopathic epilepsy and epileptic syndromes, not intractable, without status epilepticus** 🕮

         Generalized idiopathic epilepsy and epileptic syndromes NOS

  ● **G40.31** **Generalized idiopathic epilepsy and epileptic syndromes, intractable**

     G40.311 **Generalized idiopathic epilepsy and epileptic syndromes, intractable, with status epilepticus** 🕮

     G40.319 **Generalized idiopathic epilepsy and epileptic syndromes, intractable, without status epilepticus** 🕮

● **G40.4** **Other generalized epilepsy and epileptic syndromes**

     Epilepsy with grand mal seizures on awakening
     Epilepsy with myoclonic absences
     Epilepsy with myoclonic-astatic seizures
     Grand mal seizure NOS
     Nonspecific atonic epileptic seizures
     Nonspecific clonic epileptic seizures
     Nonspecific myoclonic epileptic seizures
     Nonspecific tonic epileptic seizures
     Nonspecific tonic-clonic epileptic seizures
     Symptomatic early myoclonic encephalopathy

  ● **G40.40** **Other generalized epilepsy and epileptic syndromes, not intractable**

     Other generalized epilepsy and epileptic syndromes without intractability
     Other generalized epilepsy and epileptic syndromes NOS

     G40.401 **Other generalized epilepsy and epileptic syndromes, not intractable, with status epilepticus** 🕮

     G40.409 **Other generalized epilepsy and epileptic syndromes, not intractable, without status epilepticus** 🕮

  ● **G40.41** **Other generalized epilepsy and epileptic syndromes, intractable**

     G40.411 **Other generalized epilepsy and epileptic syndromes, intractable, with status epilepticus** 🕮

     G40.419 **Other generalized epilepsy and epileptic syndromes, intractable, without status epilepticus** 🕮

     G40.42 **Cyclin-Dependent Kinase-Like 5 Deficiency Disorder**

         CDKL5

         Use additional code, if known, to identify associated manifestations, such as:
          cortical blindness (H47.61-)
          global developmental delay (F88)

CHAPTER 6 (G00-G99)

● **G40.5 Epileptic seizures related to external causes**
     Epileptic seizures related to alcohol
     Epileptic seizures related to drugs
     Epileptic seizures related to hormonal changes
     Epileptic seizures related to sleep deprivation
     Epileptic seizures related to stress
     Code also, if applicable, associated epilepsy and
        recurrent seizures (G40.-)
     Use additional code for adverse effect, if applicable,
        to identify drug (T36-T50 with fifth or sixth
        character 5)

   ● **G40.50 Epileptic seizures related to external causes, not intractable**

       G40.501 Epileptic seizures related to external causes, not intractable, with status epilepticus 🔗

       G40.509 Epileptic seizures related to external causes, not intractable, without status epilepticus 🔗
          Epileptic seizures related to external causes, NOS

● **G40.8 Other epilepsy and recurrent seizures**
     Epilepsies and epileptic syndromes undetermined as to
        whether they are focal or generalized
     Landau-Kleffner syndrome

   ● **G40.80 Other epilepsy**

       G40.801 Other epilepsy, not intractable, with status epilepticus 🔗
          Other epilepsy without intractability with status epilepticus

       G40.802 Other epilepsy, not intractable, without status epilepticus 🔗
          Other epilepsy NOS
          Other epilepsy without intractability without status epilepticus

       G40.803 Other epilepsy, intractable, with status epilepticus 🔗

       G40.804 Other epilepsy, intractable, without status epilepticus 🔗

   ● **G40.81 Lennox-Gastaut syndrome**

       G40.811 Lennox-Gastaut syndrome, not intractable, with status epilepticus 🔗

       G40.812 Lennox-Gastaut syndrome, not intractable, without status epilepticus 🔗

       G40.813 Lennox-Gastaut syndrome, intractable, with status epilepticus 🔗

       G40.814 Lennox-Gastaut syndrome, intractable, without status epilepticus 🔗

   ● **G40.82 Epileptic spasms**
       Infantile spasms
       Salaam attacks
       West's syndrome

       G40.821 Epileptic spasms, not intractable, with status epilepticus 🔗

       G40.822 Epileptic spasms, not intractable, without status epilepticus 🔗

       G40.823 Epileptic spasms, intractable, with status epilepticus 🔗

       G40.824 Epileptic spasms, intractable, without status epilepticus 🔗

   ● **G40.83 Dravet syndrome**
       Polymorphic epilepsy in infancy (PMEI)
       Severe myoclonic epilepsy in infancy (SMEI)

       G40.833 Dravet syndrome, intractable, with status epilepticus

       G40.834 Dravet syndrome, intractable, without status epilepticus
          Dravet syndrome NOS

   G40.89 Other seizures 🔗
       Excludes1   post traumatic seizures (R56.1)
               recurrent seizures NOS (G40.909)
               seizure NOS (R56.9)

● **G40.9 Epilepsy, unspecified**

   ● **G40.90 Epilepsy, unspecified, not intractable**
       Epilepsy, unspecified, without intractability

       G40.901 Epilepsy, unspecified, not intractable, with status epilepticus 🔗

       G40.909 Epilepsy, unspecified, not intractable, without status epilepticus 🔗
          Epilepsy NOS
          Epileptic convulsions NOS
          Epileptic fits NOS
          Epileptic seizures NOS
          Recurrent seizures NOS
          Seizure disorder NOS
          Coding Clinic: 2021, Q2, P3

   ● **G40.91 Epilepsy, unspecified, intractable**
       Intractable seizure disorder NOS

       G40.911 Epilepsy, unspecified, intractable, with status epilepticus 🔗

       G40.919 Epilepsy, unspecified, intractable, without status epilepticus 🔗

● **G40.A Absence epileptic syndrome**
     Childhood absence epilepsy [pyknolepsy]
     Juvenile absence epilepsy
     Absence epileptic syndrome, NOS

   ● **G40.A0 Absence epileptic syndrome, not intractable**

       G40.A01 Absence epileptic syndrome, not intractable, with status epilepticus 🔗

       G40.A09 Absence epileptic syndrome, not intractable, without status epilepticus 🔗

   ● **G40.A1 Absence epileptic syndrome, intractable**

       G40.A11 Absence epileptic syndrome, intractable, with status epilepticus 🔗

       G40.A19 Absence epileptic syndrome, intractable, without status epilepticus 🔗

● **G40.B Juvenile myoclonic epilepsy [impulsive petit mal]**

   ● **G40.B0 Juvenile myoclonic epilepsy, not intractable**

       G40.B01 Juvenile myoclonic epilepsy, not intractable, with status epilepticus 🔗

       G40.B09 Juvenile myoclonic epilepsy, not intractable, without status epilepticus 🔗

   ● **G40.B1 Juvenile myoclonic epilepsy, intractable**

       G40.B11 Juvenile myoclonic epilepsy, intractable, with status epilepticus 🔗

       G40.B19 Juvenile myoclonic epilepsy, intractable, without status epilepticus 🔗

● **G43 Migraine**
     Note: The following terms are to be considered equivalent
        to intractable: pharmacoresistant (pharmacologically
        resistant), treatment resistant, refractory (medically) and
        poorly controlled
     Use additional code for adverse effect, if applicable, to identify
        drug (T36-T50 with fifth or sixth character 5)

     Excludes1   headache NOS (R51.9)
               lower half migraine (G44.00)

     Excludes2   headache syndromes (G44.-)

   ● **G43.0 Migraine without aura**
       Neurological disorder, generally recurring headaches without
          early symptom (aura)
       Common migraine

       Excludes1   chronic migraine without aura (G43.7-)

     ● **G43.00 Migraine without aura, not intractable**
         Neurological disorder, generally recurring
            headaches without early symptom (aura);
            resistant to cure, relief, or control
         Migraine without aura without mention of
            refractory migraine

▶ New   ⇒ Revised   ~~deleted~~ Deleted   Excludes 1   Excludes 2   Includes   Use additional   Code first   Code also   Key words
OGCR Official Guidelines   X Assign placeholder X   ● Use Additional Character(s)   ▷ Manifestation Code   🔗 Hierarchical Condition Category   **Coding Clinic**

        G43.001   Migraine without aura, not intractable, with status migrainosus

        G43.009   Migraine without aura, not intractable, without status migrainosus
                   Migraine without aura NOS

    ● **G43.01**   Migraine without aura, intractable
          Intractable migraine: Not easily cured or managed; relentless pain from a migraine
          Migraine without aura with refractory migraine

        G43.011   Migraine without aura, intractable, with status migrainosus

        G43.019   Migraine without aura, intractable, without status migrainosus

● **G43.1**   Migraine with aura
      Basilar migraine
      Classical migraine
      Migraine equivalents
      Migraine preceded or accompanied by transient focal neurological phenomena
      Migraine triggered seizures
      Migraine with acute-onset aura
      Migraine with aura without headache (migraine equivalents)
      Migraine with prolonged aura
      Migraine with typical aura
      Retinal migraine

      Code also any associated seizure (G40.-, R56.9)

      Excludes1   persistent migraine aura (G43.5-, G43.6-)

    ● **G43.10**   Migraine with aura, not intractable
          Migraine with aura without mention of refractory migraine

        G43.101   Migraine with aura, not intractable, with status migrainosus

        G43.109   Migraine with aura, not intractable, without status migrainosus
                  Migraine with aura NOS

    ● **G43.11**   Migraine with aura, intractable
          Migraine with aura with refractory migraine

        G43.111   Migraine with aura, intractable, with status migrainosus

        G43.119   Migraine with aura, intractable, without status migrainosus

● **G43.4**   Hemiplegic migraine
      Inherited migraine disorder causing temporary paralysis of one side of body followed by severe headache and nausea
      Familial migraine
      Sporadic migraine

    ● **G43.40**   Hemiplegic migraine, not intractable
          Hemiplegic migraine without refractory migraine

        G43.401   Hemiplegic migraine, not intractable, with status migrainosus

        G43.409   Hemiplegic migraine, not intractable, without status migrainosus
                  Hemiplegic migraine NOS

    ● **G43.41**   Hemiplegic migraine, intractable
          Hemiplegic migraine with refractory migraine

        G43.411   Hemiplegic migraine, intractable, with status migrainosus

        G43.419   Hemiplegic migraine, intractable, without status migrainosus

● **G43.5**   Persistent migraine aura without cerebral infarction

    ● **G43.50**   Persistent migraine aura without cerebral infarction, not intractable
          Persistent migraine aura without cerebral infarction, without refractory migraine

        G43.501   Persistent migraine aura without cerebral infarction, not intractable, with status migrainosus

        G43.509   Persistent migraine aura without cerebral infarction, not intractable, without status migrainosus
                  Persistent migraine aura NOS

    ● **G43.51**   Persistent migraine aura without cerebral infarction, intractable
          Persistent migraine aura without cerebral infarction, with refractory migraine

        G43.511   Persistent migraine aura without cerebral infarction, intractable, with status migrainosus

        G43.519   Persistent migraine aura without cerebral infarction, intractable, without status migrainosus

● **G43.6**   Persistent migraine aura with cerebral infarction
      Visual, motor, or psychic disturbances, paresthesias, and related neurologic abnormalities accompanying migraine

      Code also the type of cerebral infarction (I63.-)

    ● **G43.60**   Persistent migraine aura with cerebral infarction, not intractable
          Persistent migraine aura with cerebral infarction, without refractory migraine

        G43.601   Persistent migraine aura with cerebral infarction, not intractable, with status migrainosus

        G43.609   Persistent migraine aura with cerebral infarction, not intractable, without status migrainosus

    ● **G43.61**   Persistent migraine aura with cerebral infarction, intractable
          Persistent migraine aura with cerebral infarction, with refractory migraine

        G43.611   Persistent migraine aura with cerebral infarction, intractable, with status migrainosus

        G43.619   Persistent migraine aura with cerebral infarction, intractable, without status migrainosus

● **G43.7**   Chronic migraine without aura
      Transformed migraine

      Excludes1   migraine without aura (G43.0-)

    ● **G43.70**   Chronic migraine without aura, not intractable
          Chronic migraine without aura, without refractory migraine

        G43.701   Chronic migraine without aura, not intractable, with status migrainosus

        G43.709   Chronic migraine without aura, not intractable, without status migrainosus
                  Chronic migraine without aura NOS

    ● **G43.71**   Chronic migraine without aura, intractable
          Chronic migraine without aura, with refractory migraine

        G43.711   Chronic migraine without aura, intractable, with status migrainosus

        G43.719   Chronic migraine without aura, intractable, without status migrainosus

CHAPTER 6 (G00-G99)

Item 6–4   Migraine headache is described as an intense pulsing or throbbing pain in one area of the head. It can be accompanied by extreme sensitivity to light (photophobic) and sound and is three times more common in women than in men. Symptoms include nausea and vomiting. Research indicates migraine headaches are caused by inherited abnormalities in genes that control the activities of certain cell populations in the brain.

● G43.A   Cyclical vomiting
   Excludes1   cyclical vomiting syndrome unrelated to migraine (R11.15)

    G43.A0   Cyclical vomiting, in migraine, not intractable
        Cyclical vomiting, without refractory migraine

    G43.A1   Cyclical vomiting, in migraine, intractable
        Cyclical vomiting, with refractory migraine

● G43.B   Ophthalmoplegic migraine

    G43.B0   Ophthalmoplegic migraine, not intractable
        Ophthalmoplegic migraine, without refractory migraine

    G43.B1   Ophthalmoplegic migraine, intractable
        Ophthalmoplegic migraine, with refractory migraine

● G43.C   Periodic headache syndromes in child or adult

    G43.C0   Periodic headache syndromes in child or adult, not intractable
        Periodic headache syndromes in child or adult, without refractory migraine

    G43.C1   Periodic headache syndromes in child or adult, intractable
        Periodic headache syndromes in child or adult, with refractory migraine

● G43.D   Abdominal migraine

    G43.D0   Abdominal migraine, not intractable
        Abdominal migraine, without refractory migraine

    G43.D1   Abdominal migraine, intractable
        Abdominal migraine, with refractory migraine

● G43.8   Other migraine

   ● G43.80   Other migraine, not intractable
        Other migraine, without refractory migraine

      G43.801   Other migraine, not intractable, with status migrainosus

      G43.809   Other migraine, not intractable, without status migrainosus

   ● G43.81   Other migraine, intractable
        Other migraine, with refractory migraine

      G43.811   Other migraine, intractable, with status migrainosus

      G43.819   Other migraine, intractable, without status migrainosus

   ● G43.82   Menstrual migraine, not intractable
        Menstrual headache, not intractable
        Menstrual migraine, without refractory migraine
        Menstrually related migraine, not intractable
        Pre-menstrual headache, not intractable
        Pre-menstrual migraine, not intractable
        Pure menstrual migraine, not intractable
        Code also associated premenstrual tension syndrome (N94.3)

      G43.821   Menstrual migraine, not intractable, with status migrainosus ♀

      G43.829   Menstrual migraine, not intractable, without status migrainosus ♀
         Menstrual migraine NOS

   ● G43.83   Menstrual migraine, intractable
        Menstrual headache, intractable
        Menstrual migraine, with refractory migraine
        Menstrually related migraine, intractable
        Pre-menstrual headache, intractable
        Pre-menstrual migraine, intractable
        Pure menstrual migraine, intractable
        Code also associated premenstrual tension syndrome (N94.3)

      G43.831   Menstrual migraine, intractable, with status migrainosus ♀

      G43.839   Menstrual migraine, intractable, without status migrainosus ♀

● G43.9   Migraine, unspecified

   ● G43.90   Migraine, unspecified, not intractable
        Migraine, unspecified, without refractory migraine

      G43.901   Migraine, unspecified, not intractable, with status migrainosus
         Status migrainosus NOS

      G43.909   Migraine, unspecified, not intractable, without status migrainosus
         Migraine NOS

   ● G43.91   Migraine, unspecified, intractable
        Migraine, unspecified, with refractory migraine

      G43.911   Migraine, unspecified, intractable, with status migrainosus

      G43.919   Migraine, unspecified, intractable, without status migrainosus

● G44   Other headache syndromes
   Excludes1   headache NOS (R51.9)
   Excludes2   atypical facial pain (G50.1)
        headache due to lumbar puncture (G97.1)
        migraines (G43.-)
        trigeminal neuralgia (G50.0)

● G44.0   Cluster headaches and other trigeminal autonomic cephalgias (TAC)

   ● G44.00   Cluster headache syndrome, unspecified
        Ciliary neuralgia
        Cluster headache NOS
        Histamine cephalgia
        Lower half migraine
        Migrainous neuralgia

      G44.001   Cluster headache syndrome, unspecified, intractable

      G44.009   Cluster headache syndrome, unspecified, not intractable
         Cluster headache syndrome NOS

   ● G44.01   Episodic cluster headache

      G44.011   Episodic cluster headache, intractable

      G44.019   Episodic cluster headache, not intractable
         Episodic cluster headache NOS

   ● G44.02   Chronic cluster headache

      G44.021   Chronic cluster headache, intractable

      G44.029   Chronic cluster headache, not intractable
         Chronic cluster headache NOS

   ● G44.03   Episodic paroxysmal hemicrania
        Paroxysmal hemicrania NOS

      G44.031   Episodic paroxysmal hemicrania, intractable

      G44.039   Episodic paroxysmal hemicrania, not intractable
         Episodic paroxysmal hemicrania NOS

   ● G44.04   Chronic paroxysmal hemicrania
        Unilateral headache

      G44.041   Chronic paroxysmal hemicrania, intractable

      G44.049   Chronic paroxysmal hemicrania, not intractable
         Chronic paroxysmal hemicrania NOS

   ● G44.05   Short lasting unilateral neuralgiform headache with conjunctival injection and tearing (SUNCT)

      G44.051   Short lasting unilateral neuralgiform headache with conjunctival injection and tearing (SUNCT), intractable

G44.059 **Short lasting unilateral neuralgiform headache with conjunctival injection and tearing (SUNCT), not intractable**
Short lasting unilateral neuralgiform headache with conjunctival injection and tearing (SUNCT) NOS

● G44.09 **Other trigeminal autonomic cephalgias (TAC)**
Cluster headaches

G44.091 **Other trigeminal autonomic cephalgias (TAC), intractable**

G44.099 **Other trigeminal autonomic cephalgias (TAC), not intractable**

G44.1 **Vascular headache, not elsewhere classified**

Excludes2 cluster headache (G44.0)
complicated headache syndromes (G44.5-)
drug-induced headache (G44.4-)
migraine (G43.-)
other specified headache syndromes (G44.8-)
post-traumatic headache (G44.3-)
tension-type headache (G44.2-)

● G44.2 **Tension-type headache**

● G44.20 **Tension-type headache, unspecified**

G44.201 **Tension-type headache, unspecified, intractable**

G44.209 **Tension-type headache, unspecified, not intractable**
Tension headache NOS

● G44.21 **Episodic tension-type headache**

G44.211 **Episodic tension-type headache, intractable**

G44.219 **Episodic tension-type headache, not intractable**
Episodic tension-type headache NOS

● G44.22 **Chronic tension-type headache**

G44.221 **Chronic tension-type headache, intractable**

G44.229 **Chronic tension-type headache, not intractable**
Chronic tension-type headache NOS

● G44.3 **Post-traumatic headache**

● G44.30 **Post-traumatic headache, unspecified**

G44.301 **Post-traumatic headache, unspecified, intractable**

G44.309 **Post-traumatic headache, unspecified, not intractable**
Post-traumatic headache NOS

● G44.31 **Acute post-traumatic headache**

G44.311 **Acute post-traumatic headache, intractable**

G44.319 **Acute post-traumatic headache, not intractable**
Acute post-traumatic headache NOS

● G44.32 **Chronic post-traumatic headache**

G44.321 **Chronic post-traumatic headache, intractable**

G44.329 **Chronic post-traumatic headache, not intractable**
Chronic post-traumatic headache NOS

● G44.4 **Drug-induced headache, not elsewhere classified**
Medication overuse headache

Use additional code for adverse effect, if applicable, to identify drug (T36-T50 with fifth or sixth character 5)

G44.40 **Drug-induced headache, not elsewhere classified, not intractable**

G44.41 **Drug-induced headache, not elsewhere classified, intractable**

● G44.5 **Complicated headache syndromes**

G44.51 **Hemicrania continua**
Persistent unilateral headache

G44.52 **New daily persistent headache (NDPH)**

G44.53 **Primary thunderclap headache**

G44.59 **Other complicated headache syndrome**

● G44.8 **Other specified headache syndromes**

Excludes2 headache with orthostatic or positional component, not elsewhere classified (R51.0)

G44.81 **Hypnic headache**
Benign primary headaches

G44.82 **Headache associated with sexual activity**
Orgasmic headache
Preorgasmic headache

G44.83 **Primary cough headache**

G44.84 **Primary exertional headache**

G44.85 **Primary stabbing headache**

▶ G44.86 **Cervicogenic headache**
Code also associated cervical spinal condition, if known

G44.89 **Other headache syndrome**

● G45 **Transient cerebral ischemic attacks and related syndromes**

Excludes1 neonatal cerebral ischemia (P91.0)
transient retinal artery occlusion (H34.0-)

Coding Clinic: 2018, Q2, P9

G45.0 **Vertebro-basilar artery syndrome**

G45.1 **Carotid artery syndrome (hemispheric)**

G45.2 **Multiple and bilateral precerebral artery syndromes**

G45.3 **Amaurosis fugax**
Transient visual loss in one eye

G45.4 **Transient global amnesia**
Episode of short-term memory loss, nonrecurrent, lasting few hours

Excludes1 amnesia NOS (R41.3)

G45.8 **Other transient cerebral ischemic attacks and related syndromes**

G45.9 **Transient cerebral ischemic attack, unspecified**
Spasm of cerebral artery
TIA
Transient cerebral ischemia NOS

● G46 **Vascular syndromes of brain in cerebrovascular diseases**
Code first underlying cerebrovascular disease (I60-I69)

G46.0 **Middle cerebral artery syndrome**

G46.1 **Anterior cerebral artery syndrome**

G46.2 **Posterior cerebral artery syndrome**

G46.3 **Brain stem stroke syndrome**
Benedikt syndrome
Claude syndrome
Foville syndrome
Millard-Gubler syndrome
Wallenberg syndrome
Weber syndrome

G46.4 **Cerebellar stroke syndrome**

G46.5 **Pure motor lacunar syndrome**
Occlusion of single deep penetrating artery

G46.6 **Pure sensory lacunar syndrome**

G46.7 **Other lacunar syndromes**

G46.8 **Other vascular syndromes of brain in cerebrovascular diseases**

● G47 **Sleep disorders**

Excludes2 nightmares (F51.5)
nonorganic sleep disorders (F51.-)
sleep terrors (F51.4)
sleepwalking (F51.3)

CHAPTER 6 (G00-G99)

● **G47.0** **Insomnia**
> **Excludes2** alcohol related insomnia (F10.182, F10.282, F10.982)
> drug-related insomnia (F11.182, F11.282, F11.982, F13.182, F13.282, F13.982, F14.182, F14.282, F14.982, F15.182, F15.282, F15.982, F19.182, F19.282, F19.982)
> idiopathic insomnia (F51.01)
> insomnia due to a mental disorder (F51.05)
> insomnia not due to a substance or known physiological condition (F51.0-)
> nonorganic insomnia (F51.0-)
> primary insomnia (F51.01)
> sleep apnea (G47.3-)

    G47.00 **Insomnia, unspecified**
        Insomnia NOS

    G47.01 **Insomnia due to medical condition**
        Code also associated medical condition

    G47.09 **Other insomnia**

● **G47.1** **Hypersomnia**
> **Excludes2** alcohol-related hypersomnia (F10.182, F10.282, F10.982)
> drug-related hypersomnia (F11.182, F11.282, F11.982, F13.182, F13.282, F13.982, F14.182, F14.282, F14.982, F15.182, F15.282, F15.982, F19.182, F19.282, F19.982)
> hypersomnia due to a mental disorder (F51.13)
> hypersomnia not due to a substance or known physiological condition (F51.1-)
> primary hypersomnia (F51.11)
> sleep apnea (G47.3-)

    G47.10 **Hypersomnia, unspecified**
        Hypersomnia NOS

    G47.11 **Idiopathic hypersomnia with long sleep time**
        Idiopathic hypersomnia NOS

    G47.12 **Idiopathic hypersomnia without long sleep time**

    G47.13 **Recurrent hypersomnia**
        Kleine-Levin syndrome
        Menstrual related hypersomnia

    G47.14 **Hypersomnia due to medical condition**
        Code also associated medical condition

    G47.19 **Other hypersomnia**

● **G47.2** **Circadian rhythm sleep disorders**
    Disorders of the sleep wake schedule
    Inversion of nyctohemeral rhythm
    Inversion of sleep rhythm

    G47.20 **Circadian rhythm sleep disorder, unspecified type**
        Sleep wake schedule disorder NOS

    G47.21 **Circadian rhythm sleep disorder, delayed sleep phase type**
        Delayed sleep phase syndrome

    G47.22 **Circadian rhythm sleep disorder, advanced sleep phase type**

    G47.23 **Circadian rhythm sleep disorder, irregular sleep wake type**
        Irregular sleep-wake pattern

    G47.24 **Circadian rhythm sleep disorder, free running type**
        Circadian rhythm sleep disorder, non-24-hour sleep-wake type

    G47.25 **Circadian rhythm sleep disorder, jet lag type**

    G47.26 **Circadian rhythm sleep disorder, shift work type**

▸ **G47.27** *Circadian rhythm sleep disorder in conditions classified elsewhere*
> *Code first underlying condition*

    G47.29 **Other circadian rhythm sleep disorder**

● **G47.3** **Sleep apnea**
    Characterized by episodes in which breathing stops during sleep
    Code also any associated underlying condition
> **Excludes1** apnea NOS (R06.81)
> Cheyne-Stokes breathing (R06.3)
> pickwickian syndrome (E66.2)
> sleep apnea of newborn (P28.3)

    G47.30 **Sleep apnea, unspecified**
        Sleep apnea NOS

    G47.31 **Primary central sleep apnea**
        Idiopathic central sleep apnea

    G47.32 **High altitude periodic breathing**

    G47.33 **Obstructive sleep apnea (adult) (pediatric)**
        Obstructive sleep apnea hypopnea
> **Excludes1** obstructive sleep apnea of newborn (P28.3)

    G47.34 **Idiopathic sleep related nonobstructive alveolar hypoventilation**
        Sleep related hypoxia

    G47.35 **Congenital central alveolar hypoventilation syndrome**

▸ **G47.36** *Sleep related hypoventilation in conditions classified elsewhere*
        Sleep related hypoxemia in conditions classified elsewhere
> *Code first underlying condition*

▸ **G47.37** **Central** *sleep apnea in conditions classified elsewhere*
> *Code first underlying condition*

    G47.39 **Other sleep apnea**

● **G47.4** **Narcolepsy and cataplexy**
    *Cataplexy is a disorder evidenced by seizures including minor slacking of the facial muscles to complete collapse and often affects people who have **narcolepsy**, a disorder in which there is great difficulty remaining awake during the daytime.*

    ● **G47.41** **Narcolepsy**
        G47.411 **Narcolepsy with cataplexy**
        G47.419 **Narcolepsy without cataplexy**
            Narcolepsy NOS

    ● **G47.42** **Narcolepsy in conditions classified elsewhere**
> *Code first underlying condition*

     ▸ **G47.421** *Narcolepsy in conditions classified elsewhere **with** cataplexy*

     ▸ **G47.429** *Narcolepsy in conditions classified elsewhere **without** cataplexy*

● **G47.5** **Parasomnia**
> **Excludes1** alcohol induced parasomnia (F10.182, F10.282, F10.982)
> drug induced parasomnia (F11.182, F11.282, F11.982, F13.182, F13.282, F13.982, F14.182, F14.282, F14.982, F15.182, F15.282, F15.982, F19.182, F19.282, F19.982)
> parasomnia not due to a substance or known physiological condition (F51.8)

    G47.50 **Parasomnia, unspecified**
        Parasomnia NOS

    G47.51 **Confusional arousals**

    G47.52 **REM sleep behavior disorder**

    G47.53 **Recurrent isolated sleep paralysis**

▸ New   ⫸ Revised   ~~deleted~~ Deleted   Excludes 1   Excludes 2   Includes   Use additional   Code first   Code also   Key words
OGCR Official Guidelines   **X** Assign placeholder X   ● Use Additional Character(s)   ▸ Manifestation Code   🗪 Hierarchical Condition Category   **Coding Clinic**

▶ *G47.54*   *Parasomnia in conditions classified elsewhere*
     Code first underlying condition

G47.59   Other parasomnia

● G47.6   Sleep related movement disorders
     Excludes2   restless legs syndrome (G25.81)

G47.61   Periodic limb movement disorder

G47.62   Sleep related leg cramps

G47.63   Sleep related bruxism
     Excludes1   psychogenic bruxism (F45.8)
     Coding Clinic: 2016, Q4, P118

G47.69   Other sleep related movement disorders

G47.8   Other sleep disorders
     Other specified sleep-wake disorder

G47.9   Sleep disorder, unspecified
     Sleep disorder NOS
     Unspecified sleep-wake disorder

★ **(See Plate 6 of the Anatomy Illustrations.)**

NERVE, NERVE ROOT AND PLEXUS DISORDERS (G50-G59)

Excludes1   current traumatic nerve, nerve root and plexus
     disorders - see Injury, nerve by body region
     neuralgia NOS (M79.2)
     neuritis NOS (M79.2)
     peripheral neuritis in pregnancy (O26.82-)
     radiculitis NOS (M54.1-)

● G50   Disorders of trigeminal nerve
     Includes   disorders of 5th cranial nerve

G50.0   Trigeminal neuralgia
     Syndrome of paroxysmal facial pain
     Tic douloureux

G50.1   Atypical facial pain

G50.8   Other disorders of trigeminal nerve

G50.9   Disorder of trigeminal nerve, unspecified

● G51   Facial nerve disorders
     Includes   disorders of 7th cranial nerve

G51.0   Bell's palsy
     Facial palsy

G51.1   Geniculate ganglionitis
     Rare disorder with symptoms of severe pain deep in ear,
     spreading to ear canal, outer ear, mastoid or eye regions
     Excludes1   postherpetic geniculate ganglionitis
     (B02.21)

G51.2   Melkersson's syndrome
     Melkersson-Rosenthal syndrome

● G51.3   Clonic hemifacial spasm

G51.31   Clonic hemifacial spasm, right

G51.32   Clonic hemifacial spasm, left
     Coding Clinic: 2018, Q4, P10

G51.33   Clonic hemifacial spasm, bilateral

G51.39   Clonic hemifacial spasm, unspecified

G51.4   Facial myokymia
     Involuntary facial muscle movement

G51.8   Other disorders of facial nerve

G51.9   Disorder of facial nerve, unspecified

● G52   Disorders of other cranial nerves
     Excludes2   disorders of acoustic [8th] nerve (H93.3)
     disorders of optic [2nd] nerve (H46, H47.0)
     paralytic strabismus due to nerve palsy
     (H49.0-H49.2)

G52.0   Disorders of olfactory nerve
     Disorders of 1st cranial nerve

G52.1   Disorders of glossopharyngeal nerve
     Disorder of 9th cranial nerve
     Glossopharyngeal neuralgia

G52.2   Disorders of vagus nerve
     Disorders of pneumogastric [10th] nerve

G52.3   Disorders of hypoglossal nerve
     Disorders of 12th cranial nerve

G52.7   Disorders of multiple cranial nerves
     Polyneuritis cranialis

G52.8   Disorders of other specified cranial nerves

G52.9   Cranial nerve disorder, unspecified

▶ *G53*   *Cranial nerve disorders in diseases classified elsewhere*
     Code first underlying disease, such as:
     neoplasm (C00-D49)
     Excludes1   multiple cranial nerve palsy in sarcoidosis (D86.82)
     multiple cranial nerve palsy in syphilis (A52.15)
     postherpetic geniculate ganglionitis (B02.21)
     postherpetic trigeminal neuralgia (B02.22)

● G54   Nerve root and plexus disorders
     Raiculopathy (nerve root disorder) caused by pressure on nerve root,
     most common cause is herniation of intervertebral disk. Plexus
     disorders (plexopathies) are due to compression or injury.
     Excludes1   current traumatic nerve root and plexus disorders
     - see nerve injury by body region
     intervertebral disc disorders (M50-M51)
     neuralgia or neuritis NOS (M79.2)
     neuritis or radiculitis brachial NOS (M54.13)
     neuritis or radiculitis lumbar NOS (M54.16)
     neuritis or radiculitis lumbosacral NOS (M54.17)
     neuritis or radiculitis thoracic NOS (M54.14)
     radiculitis NOS (M54.10)
     radiculopathy NOS (M54.10)
     spondylosis (M47.-)

G54.0   Brachial plexus disorders
     Thoracic outlet syndrome

G54.1   Lumbosacral plexus disorders

G54.2   Cervical root disorders, not elsewhere classified

G54.3   Thoracic root disorders, not elsewhere classified

G54.4   Lumbosacral root disorders, not elsewhere classified

G54.5   Neuralgic amyotrophy
     Parsonage-Aldren-Turner syndrome
     Shoulder-girdle neuritis
     Excludes1   neuralgic amyotrophy in diabetes
     mellitus (E08-E13 with .44)

G54.6   Phantom limb syndrome with pain 🔗
     Sensations (cramping, itching) in a limb that no longer
     exists

G54.7   Phantom limb syndrome without pain 🔗
     Phantom limb syndrome NOS

G54.8   Other nerve root and plexus disorders

G54.9   Nerve root and plexus disorder, unspecified

Item 6–5 Trigeminal neuralgia, tic douloureux, is a pain syndrome diagnosed from the patient's history alone. The condition is characterized by pain and a brief facial spasm or tic. Pain is unilateral and follows the sensory distribution of cranial nerve V, typically radiating to the maxillary (V2) or mandibular (V3) area.

Item 6–6 The most common facial nerve disorder is **Bell's Palsy,** which occurs suddenly and results in facial drooping unilaterally. This disorder is the result of a reaction to a virus that causes the facial nerve in the ear to swell, resulting in pressure in the bony canal.

CHAPTER 6 (G00-G99)

▷ G55   Nerve root and plexus compressions in diseases classified
        elsewhere
        Code first underlying disease, such as:
            neoplasm (C00-D49)
        Excludes1   nerve root compression (due to) (in) ankylosing
                        spondylitis (M45.-)
                        nerve root compression (due to) (in)dorsopathies
                        (M53.-, M54.-)
                        nerve root compression (due to) (in)intervertebral
                        disc disorders (M50.1.-, M51.1.-)
                        nerve root compression (due to) (in)
                        spondylopathies (M46.-, M48.-)
                    ▶ nerve root compression (due to) (in) spondylosis
                        (M47.0-, M47.2.-)

★ **(See Plates 472 and 473 on pages 56 and 57.)**

● G56   Mononeuropathies of upper limb
        Excludes1   current traumatic nerve disorder - see nerve
                        injury by body region
    ● G56.0   Carpal tunnel syndrome
            G56.00   Carpal tunnel syndrome, unspecified upper
                     limb
            G56.01   Carpal tunnel syndrome, right upper limb
            G56.02   Carpal tunnel syndrome, left upper limb
            G56.03   Carpal tunnel syndrome, bilateral upper
                     limbs
                     Coding Clinic: 2016, Q4, P17
    ● G56.1   Other lesions of median nerve
            G56.10   Other lesions of median nerve, unspecified side
            G56.11   Other lesions of median nerve, right upper
                     limb
            G56.12   Other lesions of median nerve, left upper limb
            G56.13   Other lesions of median nerve, bilateral upper
                     limbs
                     Coding Clinic: 2016, Q4, P17
    ● G56.2   Lesion of ulnar nerve
            Tardy ulnar nerve palsy
            G56.20   Lesion of ulnar nerve, unspecified upper limb
            G56.21   Lesion of ulnar nerve, right upper limb
            G56.22   Lesion of ulnar nerve, left upper limb
            G56.23   Lesion of ulnar nerve, bilateral upper limbs
                     Coding Clinic: 2016, Q4, P17
    ● G56.3   Lesion of radial nerve
            G56.30   Lesion of radial nerve, unspecified upper limb
            G56.31   Lesion of radial nerve, right upper limb
            G56.32   Lesion of radial nerve, left upper limb
            G56.33   Lesion of radial nerve, bilateral upper limbs
                     Coding Clinic: 2016, Q4, P17
    ● G56.4   Causalgia of upper limb
            Intense burning pain and sensitivity to slight touch
            Complex regional pain syndrome II of upper limb
            Excludes1   complex regional pain syndrome I of
                            lower limb (G90.52-)
                            complex regional pain syndrome I of
                            upper limb (G90.51-)
                            complex regional pain syndrome II of
                            lower limb (G57.7-)
                            reflex sympathetic dystrophy of lower
                            limb (G90.52-)
                            reflex sympathetic dystrophy (G90.51-)
            G56.40   Causalgia of unspecified upper limb
            G56.41   Causalgia of right upper limb
            G56.42   Causalgia of left upper limb
            G56.43   Causalgia of bilateral upper limbs
                     Coding Clinic: 2016, Q4, P17

● G56.8   Other specified mononeuropathies of upper limb
        Disease of a single nerve
        Interdigital neuroma of upper limb
        G56.80   Other specified mononeuropathies
                 of unspecified upper limb
        G56.81   Other specified mononeuropathies of right
                 upper limb
        G56.82   Other specified mononeuropathies of left upper
                 limb
        G56.83   Other specified mononeuropathies of bilateral
                 upper limbs
                 Coding Clinic: 2016, Q4, P17
● G56.9   Unspecified mononeuropathy of upper limb
        Disease of a single nerve
        G56.90   Unspecified mononeuropathy of unspecified
                 upper limb
        G56.91   Unspecified mononeuropathy of right upper
                 limb
        G56.92   Unspecified mononeuropathy of left upper
                 limb
        G56.93   Unspecified mononeuropathy of bilateral upper
                 limbs
                 Coding Clinic: 2016, Q4, P17

● G57   Mononeuropathies of lower limb
        Excludes1   current traumatic nerve disorder - see nerve
                        injury by body region

★ **(See Plates 544 and 545 on pages 58 and 59.)**

    ● G57.0   Lesion of sciatic nerve
            Excludes1   sciatica NOS (M54.3-)
            Excludes2   sciatica attributed to intervertebral disc
                            disorder (M51.1.-)
            G57.00   Lesion of sciatic nerve, unspecified lower limb
            G57.01   Lesion of sciatic nerve, right lower limb
            G57.02   Lesion of sciatic nerve, left lower limb
            G57.03   Lesion of sciatic nerve, bilateral lower limbs
                     Coding Clinic: 2016, Q4, P1
    ● G57.1   Meralgia paresthetica
            Numbness or pain in outer thigh caused by injury to nerve
            Lateral cutaneous nerve of thigh syndrome
            G57.10   Meralgia paresthetica, unspecified lower limb
            G57.11   Meralgia paresthetica, right lower limb
            G57.12   Meralgia paresthetica, left lower limb
            G57.13   Meralgia paresthetica, bilateral lower limbs
                     Coding Clinic: 2016, Q4, P1
    ● G57.2   Lesion of femoral nerve
            G57.20   Lesion of femoral nerve, unspecified lower limb
            G57.21   Lesion of femoral nerve, right lower limb
            G57.22   Lesion of femoral nerve, left lower limb
            G57.23   Lesion of femoral nerve, bilateral lower limbs
                     Coding Clinic: 2016, Q4, P1
    ● G57.3   Lesion of lateral popliteal nerve
            Peroneal nerve palsy
            G57.30   Lesion of lateral popliteal nerve, unspecified
                     lower limb
            G57.31   Lesion of lateral popliteal nerve, right lower
                     limb
            G57.32   Lesion of lateral popliteal nerve, left lower limb
            G57.33   Lesion of lateral popliteal nerve, bilateral lower
                     limbs
                     Coding Clinic: 2016, Q4, P1
    ● G57.4   Lesion of medial popliteal nerve
            G57.40   Lesion of medial popliteal nerve, unspecified
                     lower limb
            G57.41   Lesion of medial popliteal nerve, right lower
                     limb

CHAPTER 6 (G00-G99)

▶ New   ⇒ Revised   ~~deleted~~ Deleted   Excludes 1   Excludes 2   Includes   Use additional   Code first   Code also   Key words

OGCR Official Guidelines   X Assign placeholder X   ● Use Additional Character(s)   ▷ Manifestation Code   🔑 Hierarchical Condition Category   Coding Clinic

G57.42   Lesion of medial popliteal nerve, left lower limb

G57.43   Lesion of medial popliteal nerve, bilateral lower limbs
     Coding Clinic: 2016, Q4, P1

● G57.5   Tarsal tunnel syndrome

G57.50   Tarsal tunnel syndrome, unspecified lower limb

G57.51   Tarsal tunnel syndrome, right lower limb

G57.52   Tarsal tunnel syndrome, left lower limb

G57.53   Tarsal tunnel syndrome, bilateral lower limbs
     Coding Clinic: 2016, Q4, P1

● G57.6   Lesion of plantar nerve
     Morton's metatarsalgia

G57.60   Lesion of plantar nerve, unspecified lower limb

G57.61   Lesion of plantar nerve, right lower limb

G57.62   Lesion of plantar nerve, left lower limb

G57.63   Lesion of plantar nerve, bilateral lower limbs
     Coding Clinic: 2016, Q4, P1

● G57.7   Causalgia of lower limb
     Complex regional pain syndrome II of lower limb

     Excludes1   complex regional pain syndrome I of lower limb (G90.52-)
               complex regional pain syndrome I of upper limb (G90.51-)
               complex regional pain syndrome II of upper limb (G56.4-)
               reflex sympathetic dystrophy of lower limb (G90.52-)
               reflex sympathetic dystrophy of upper limb (G90.51-)

G57.70   Causalgia of unspecified lower limb

G57.71   Causalgia of right lower limb

G57.72   Causalgia of left lower limb

G57.73   Causalgia of bilateral lower limbs
     Coding Clinic: 2016, Q4, P1

● G57.8   Other specified mononeuropathies of lower limb
     Interdigital neuroma of lower limb

G57.80   Other specified mononeuropathies of unspecified lower limb

G57.81   Other specified mononeuropathies of right lower limb

G57.82   Other specified mononeuropathies of left lower limb

G57.83   Other specified mononeuropathies of bilateral lower limbs
     Coding Clinic: 2016, Q4, P17

● G57.9   Unspecified mononeuropathy of lower limb

G57.90   Unspecified mononeuropathy of unspecified lower limb

G57.91   Unspecified mononeuropathy of right lower limb

G57.92   Unspecified mononeuropathy of left lower limb

G57.93   Unspecified mononeuropathy of bilateral lower limbs
     Coding Clinic: 2016, Q4, P17

● G58   Other mononeuropathies

G58.0   Intercostal neuropathy

G58.7   Mononeuritis multiplex

G58.8   Other specified mononeuropathies

G58.9   Mononeuropathy, unspecified

▷ G59   *Mononeuropathy in diseases classified elsewhere*

     Code first underlying disease

     Excludes1   diabetic mononeuropathy (E08-E13 with .41)
               syphilitic nerve paralysis (A52.19)
               syphilitic neuritis (A52.15)
               tuberculous mononeuropathy (A17.83)

POLYNEUROPATHIES AND OTHER DISORDERS OF THE PERIPHERAL NERVOUS SYSTEM (G60-G65)

     Excludes1   neuralgia NOS (M79.2)
               neuritis NOS (M79.2)
               peripheral neuritis in pregnancy (O26.82-)
               radiculitis NOS (M54.10)

● G60   Hereditary and idiopathic neuropathy

G60.0   Hereditary motor and sensory neuropathy
     Charcot-Marie-Tooth disease
     Déjerine-Sottas disease
     Hereditary motor and sensory neuropathy, types I-IV
     Hypertrophic neuropathy of infancy
     Peroneal muscular atrophy (axonal type) (hypertrophic type)
     Roussy-Lévy syndrome

G60.1   Refsum's disease
     Genetic disorder affecting fatty acid metabolism
     Infantile Refsum disease

G60.2   Neuropathy in association with hereditary ataxia

G60.3   Idiopathic progressive neuropathy

G60.8   Other hereditary and idiopathic neuropathies
     Dominantly inherited sensory neuropathy
     Morvan's disease
     Nelaton's syndrome
     Recessively inherited sensory neuropathy

G60.9   Hereditary and idiopathic neuropathy, unspecified

Figure 6-2 Actions of parasympathetic and sympathetic nerves. (From Chabner: The Language of Medicine, ed 9, St. Louis, Saunders, 2011)

Item 6-7 The **peripheral nervous system** consists of 31 pairs of spinal nerves, 12 pairs of cranial nerves, and the autonomic nerves, which are divided into the parasympathetic and sympathetic nerves. The cranial nerves are: olfactory (I), optic (II), oculomotor (III), trochlear (IV), trigeminal (V), abducens (VI), facial (VII), vestibulocochlear (VIII), glossopharyngeal (IX), vagus (X), accessory (XI), and hypoglossal (XII).

● G61   **Inflammatory polyneuropathy**
     G61.0   **Guillain-Barré syndrome** 🜲
         Autoimmune disease affecting peripheral nervous system
         Acute (post-)infective polyneuritis
         Miller Fisher Syndrome
     G61.1   **Serum neuropathy** 🜲
         Use additional code for adverse effect, if applicable, to identify serum (T50.-)
     ● G61.8   **Other inflammatory polyneuropathies**
         G61.81   **Chronic inflammatory demyelinating polyneuritis** 🜲
         G61.82   **Multifocal motor neuropathy** 🜲
            MMN
         G61.89   **Other inflammatory polyneuropathies** 🜲
     G61.9   **Inflammatory polyneuropathy, unspecified** 🜲

● G62   **Other and unspecified polyneuropathies**
     G62.0   **Drug-induced polyneuropathy** 🜲
         Use additional code for adverse effect, if applicable, to identify drug (T36-T50 with fifth or sixth character 5)
     G62.1   **Alcoholic polyneuropathy** 🜲
         Malfunction of many peripheral nerves throughout the body
         Coding Clinic: 2019, Q3, P8
     G62.2   **Polyneuropathy due to other toxic agents** 🜲
         Code first (T51-T65) to identify toxic agent
     ● G62.8   **Other specified polyneuropathies**
         G62.81   **Critical illness polyneuropathy** 🜲
            Acute motor neuropathy
         G62.82   **Radiation-induced polyneuropathy** 🜲
            Use additional external cause code (W88-W90, X39.0-) to identify cause
            Coding Clinic: 2016, Q4, P18
         G62.89   **Other specified polyneuropathies**
            Coding Clinic: 2016, Q2, P11
     G62.9   **Polyneuropathy, unspecified**
         Neuropathy NOS

▷ G63   *Polyneuropathy in diseases classified elsewhere* 🜲
     Code first underlying disease, such as:
         amyloidosis (E85.-)
         endocrine disease, except diabetes (E00-E07, E15-E16, E20-E34)
         metabolic diseases (E70-E88)
         neoplasm (C00-D49)
         nutritional deficiency (E40-E64)
     Excludes1   polyneuropathy (in):
         diabetes mellitus (E08-E13 with .42)
         diphtheria (A36.83)
         ~~infectious mononucleosis (B27.0-B27.9 with 1)~~
         ⇒ infectious mononucleosis complicated by polyneuropathy (B27.0-B27.9 with fifth character 1)
         Lyme disease (A69.22)
         mumps (B26.84)
         postherpetic (B02.23)
         rheumatoid arthritis (M05.5-)
         scleroderma (M34.83)
         systemic lupus erythematosus (M32.19)
     Coding Clinic: 2021, Q1, P7; 2012, Q4, P100

G64   **Other disorders of peripheral nervous system**
     Disorder of peripheral nervous system NOS

● G65   **Sequelae of inflammatory and toxic polyneuropathies**
     Code first condition resulting from (sequela) of inflammatory and toxic polyneuropathies
     G65.0   **Sequelae of Guillain-Barré syndrome** 🜲
     G65.1   **Sequelae of other inflammatory polyneuropathy** 🜲
     G65.2   **Sequelae of toxic polyneuropathy** 🜲

DISEASES OF MYONEURAL JUNCTION AND MUSCLE (G70-G73)

● G70   **Myasthenia gravis and other myoneural disorders**
     Excludes1   botulism (A05.1, A48.51-A48.52)
         transient neonatal myasthenia gravis (P94.0)
     ● G70.0   **Myasthenia gravis**
         Acquired and results in fatigable muscle weakness exacerbated by activity and improved with rest
         G70.00   **Myasthenia gravis without (acute) exacerbation** 🜲
            Myasthenia gravis NOS
         G70.01   **Myasthenia gravis with (acute) exacerbation** 🜲
            Myasthenia gravis in crisis
     G70.1   **Toxic myoneural disorders** 🜲
         Dysfunction at junction of muscle and motor nerve (myoneural junction)
         Code first (T51-T65) to identify toxic agent
     G70.2   **Congenital and developmental myasthenia** 🜲
     ● G70.8   **Other specified myoneural disorders**
         G70.80   **Lambert-Eaton syndrome, unspecified** 🜲
            Lambert-Eaton syndrome NOS
         ▷ G70.81   *Lambert-Eaton syndrome in disease classified elsewhere* 🜲
            Code first underlying disease
            Excludes1   Lambert-Eaton syndrome in neoplastic disease (G73.1)
         G70.89   **Other specified myoneural disorders** 🜲
     G70.9   **Myoneural disorder, unspecified** 🜲

● G71   **Primary disorders of muscles**
     Excludes2   arthrogryposis multiplex congenita (Q74.3)
         metabolic disorders (E70-E88)
         myositis (M60.-)
     ● G71.0   **Muscular dystrophy** 🜲
         G71.00   **Muscular dystrophy, unspecified** 🜲
         G71.01   **Duchenne or Becker muscular dystrophy** 🜲
            Autosomal recessive, childhood type, muscular dystrophy resembling Duchenne or Becker muscular dystrophy
            Benign [Becker] muscular dystrophy
            Severe [Duchenne] muscular dystrophy
         G71.02   **Facioscapulohumeral muscular dystrophy** 🜲
            Scapulohumeral muscular dystrophy
            Coding Clinic: 2018, Q4, P12
         G71.09   **Other specified muscular dystrophies** 🜲
            Benign scapuloperoneal muscular dystrophy with early contractures [Emery-Dreifuss]
            Congenital muscular dystrophy NOS
            Congenital muscular dystrophy with specific morphological abnormalities of the muscle fiber
            Distal muscular dystrophy
            Limb-girdle muscular dystrophy
            Ocular muscular dystrophy
            Oculopharyngeal muscular dystrophy
            Scapuloperoneal muscular dystrophy
     ● G71.1   **Myotonic disorders**
         Inherited disorder that affects muscles tone
         G71.11   **Myotonic muscular dystrophy** 🜲
            Dystrophia myotonica [Steinert]
            Myotonia atrophica
            Myotonic dystrophy
            Proximal myotonic myopathy (PROMM)
            Steinert disease

Item 6-8   Muscular dystrophies (MD) are a group of rare inherited muscle diseases. Voluntary muscles become progressively weaker. In the late stages of MD, fat and connective tissue replace muscle fibers. In some types of muscular dystrophy, heart muscles, other involuntary muscles, and other organs are affected. **Myopathies** is a general term for neuromuscular diseases in which the muscle fibers dysfunction for any one of many reasons, resulting in muscular weakness.

▶ New   ⇒ Revised   ~~deleted~~ Deleted   Excludes 1   Excludes 2   Includes   Use additional   Code first   Code also   Key words
OGCR Official Guidelines   X Assign placeholder X   ● Use Additional Character(s)   ▷ Manifestation Code   🜲 Hierarchical Condition Category   **Coding Clinic**

G71.12 **Myotonia congenita**
　　　　Acetazolamide responsive myotonia congenita
　　　　Dominant myotonia congenita [Thomsen disease]
　　　　Myotonia levior
　　　　Recessive myotonia congenita [Becker disease]

G71.13 **Myotonic chondrodystrophy**
　　　　Chondrodystrophic myotonia
　　　　Congenital myotonic chondrodystrophy
　　　　Schwartz-Jampel disease

G71.14 **Drug induced myotonia**
　　　　Use additional code for adverse effect, if applicable, to identify drug (T36-T50 with fifth or sixth character 5)

G71.19 **Other specified myotonic disorders**
　　　　Myotonia fluctuans
　　　　Myotonia permanens
　　　　Neuromyotonia [Isaacs]
　　　　Paramyotonia congenita (of von Eulenburg)
　　　　Pseudomyotonia
　　　　Symptomatic myotonia

G71.2 **Congenital myopathies** 🔆
　　Excludes2　arthrogryposis multiplex congenita (Q74.3)

➠ G71.20 **Congenital myopathy, unspecified**

G71.21 **Nemaline myopathy**

● G71.22 **Centronuclear myopathy**
　　　　G71.220 **X-linked myotubular myopathy**
　　　　　　　　Myotubular (centronuclear) myopathy
　　　　G71.228 **Other centronuclear myopathy**
　　　　　　　　Autosomal centronuclear myopathy
　　　　　　　　Autosomal dominant centronuclear myopathy
　　　　　　　　Autosomal recessive centronuclear myopathy
　　　　　　　　Centronuclear myopathy, NOS

G71.29 **Other congenital myopathy**
　　　　Central core disease
　　　　Minicore disease
　　　　Multicore disease
　　　　Multiminicore disease

G71.3 **Mitochondrial myopathy, not elsewhere classified**
　　　Myopathies associated with increased number of enlarged, often abnormal, mitochondria in muscle fibers
　　Excludes1　Kearns-Sayre syndrome (H49.81)
　　　　　　　　Leber's disease (H47.21)
　　　　　　　　Leigh's encephalopathy (G31.82)
　　　　　　　　mitochondrial metabolism disorders (E88.4.-)
　　　　　　　　Reye's syndrome (G93.7)

G71.8 **Other primary disorders of muscles**

G71.9 **Primary disorder of muscle, unspecified**
　　　　Hereditary myopathy NOS

● G72 **Other and unspecified myopathies**
　　Excludes1　arthrogryposis multiplex congenita (Q74.3)
　　　　　　　　dermatopolymyositis (M33.-)
　　　　　　　　ischemic infarction of muscle (M62.2-)
　　　　　　　　myositis (M60.-)
　　　　　　　　polymyositis (M33.2-)

G72.0 **Drug-induced myopathy**
　　　　Use additional code for adverse effect, if applicable, to identify drug (T36-T50 with fifth or sixth character 5)

G72.1 **Alcoholic myopathy**
　　　　Use additional code to identify alcoholism (F10.-)

G72.2 **Myopathy due to other toxic agents**
　　　Code first (T51-T65) to identify toxic agent

G72.3 **Periodic paralysis**
　　　　Familial periodic paralysis
　　　　Hyperkalemic periodic paralysis (familial)
　　　　Hypokalemic periodic paralysis (familial)
　　　　Myotonic periodic paralysis (familial)
　　　　Normokalemic paralysis (familial)
　　　　Potassium sensitive periodic paralysis
　　Excludes1　paramyotonia congenita (of von Eulenburg) (G71.19)

● G72.4 **Inflammatory and immune myopathies, not elsewhere classified**
　　　　G72.41 **Inclusion body myositis [IBM]**
　　　　G72.49 **Other inflammatory and immune myopathies, not elsewhere classified**
　　　　　　　　Inflammatory myopathy NOS

● G72.8 **Other specified myopathies**
　　　　G72.81 **Critical illness myopathy**
　　　　　　　　Acute necrotizing myopathy
　　　　　　　　Acute quadriplegic myopathy
　　　　　　　　Intensive care (ICU) myopathy
　　　　　　　　Myopathy of critical illness
　　　　G72.89 **Other specified myopathies**

G72.9 **Myopathy, unspecified**

● G73 **Disorders of myoneural junction and muscle in diseases classified elsewhere**

▌ *G73.1* **Lambert-Eaton syndrome in neoplastic disease** 🔆
　　　Rare autoimmune disorder affecting calcium channels of nerve-muscle (neuromuscular) junction
　　　Code first underlying neoplasm (C00-D49)
　　Excludes1　Lambert-Eaton syndrome not associated with neoplasm (G70.80-G70.81)

▌ *G73.3* **Myasthenic syndromes in other diseases classified elsewhere** 🔆
　　　Code first underlying disease, such as:
　　　　neoplasm (C00-D49)
　　　　thyrotoxicosis (E05.-)

▌ *G73.7* **Myopathy in diseases classified elsewhere**
　　　Code first underlying disease, such as:
　　　　hyperparathyroidism (E21.0, E21.3)
　　　　hypoparathyroidism (E20.-)
　　　　glycogen storage disease (E74.0)
　　　　lipid storage disorders (E75.-)
　　Excludes1　myopathy in:
　　　　　　　　rheumatoid arthritis (M05.32)
　　　　　　　　sarcoidosis (D86.87)
　　　　　　　　scleroderma (M34.82)
　　➠　　　　Sjögren syndrome (M35.03)
　　　　　　　　systemic lupus erythematosus (M32.19)

CEREBRAL PALSY AND OTHER PARALYTIC SYNDROMES (G80-G83)

● G80 **Cerebral palsy**
　　Excludes1　hereditary spastic paraplegia (G11.4)

G80.0 **Spastic quadriplegic cerebral palsy** 🔆
　　　　Congenital spastic paralysis (cerebral)

G80.1 **Spastic diplegic cerebral palsy** 🔆
　　　　Spastic cerebral palsy NOS

G80.2 **Spastic hemiplegic cerebral palsy** 🔆

G80.3 **Athetoid cerebral palsy** 🔆
　　　Result of damage to cerebellum or basal ganglia responsible for processing neuromuscular signals
　　　　Double athetosis (syndrome)
　　　　Dyskinetic cerebral palsy
　　　　Dystonic cerebral palsy
　　　　Vogt disease

G80.4 **Ataxic cerebral palsy** 🔆
　　　Poor muscle tone and coordination

G80.8 **Other cerebral palsy** 🔆
　　　　Mixed cerebral palsy syndromes

G80.9 **Cerebral palsy, unspecified** 🔆
　　　　Cerebral palsy NOS

CHAPTER 6 (G00-G99)

OGCR Section I.C.6.a.

Dominant/nondominant side

Codes from category G81, Hemiplegia and hemiparesis, and subcategories, G83.1, Monoplegia of lower limb, G83.2, Monoplegia of upper limb, and G83.3, Monoplegia, unspecified, identify whether the dominant and nondominant side is affected. Should the affected side be documented, but not specified as dominant or nondominant, and the classification system does not indicate a default, code selection is as follows:

- For ambidextrous patients, the default should be dominant.
- If the left side is affected, the default is nondominant.
- If the right side is affected, the default is dominant.

● **G81**   **Hemiplegia and hemiparesis**

    Note: This category is to be used only when hemiplegia (complete)(incomplete) is reported without further specification, or is stated to be old or longstanding but of unspecified cause. The category is also for use in multiple coding to identify these types of hemiplegia resulting from any cause.

    Excludes1   congenital cerebral palsy (G80.-)
              hemiplegia and hemiparesis due to sequela of cerebrovascular disease (I69.05-, I69.15-, I69.25-, I69.35-, I69.85-, I69.95-)

    Coding Clinic: 2012, Q4, P106

● **G81.0**   **Flaccid hemiplegia**

    Paralysis of half of body with loss of tone of muscles of paralyzed part and absence of tendon reflexes

    G81.00   Flaccid hemiplegia affecting unspecified side 🦠

    G81.01   Flaccid hemiplegia affecting right dominant side 🦠

    G81.02   Flaccid hemiplegia affecting left dominant side 🦠

    G81.03   Flaccid hemiplegia affecting right nondominant side 🦠

    G81.04   Flaccid hemiplegia affecting left nondominant side 🦠

● **G81.1**   **Spastic hemiplegia**

    Paralysis of half of body with spasticity of muscles of paralyzed part and increased tendon reflexes

    G81.10   Spastic hemiplegia affecting unspecified side 🦠

    G81.11   Spastic hemiplegia affecting right dominant side 🦠

    G81.12   Spastic hemiplegia affecting left dominant side 🦠

    G81.13   Spastic hemiplegia affecting right nondominant side 🦠

    G81.14   Spastic hemiplegia affecting left nondominant side 🦠

● **G81.9**   **Hemiplegia, unspecified**

    G81.90   Hemiplegia, unspecified affecting unspecified side 🦠

    G81.91   Hemiplegia, unspecified affecting right dominant side 🦠

    G81.92   Hemiplegia, unspecified affecting left dominant side 🦠

    G81.93   Hemiplegia, unspecified affecting right nondominant side 🦠

    G81.94   Hemiplegia, unspecified affecting left nondominant side 🦠

        Coding Clinic: 2015, Q1, P26

Item 6-9 Hemiplegia is complete paralysis of one side of the body—arm, leg, and trunk. **Hemiparesis** is a generalized weakness or incomplete paralysis of one side of the body. If most activities (eating, writing) are performed with the right hand, the right is the dominant side, and the left is the nondominant side. **Quadriplegia,** also called tetraplegia, is the complete paralysis of all four limbs. **Quadriparesis** is the incomplete paralysis of all four limbs. Nerve damage in C1–C4 is associated with lower limb paralysis, and C5–C7 damage is associated with upper limb paralysis. **Diplegia** is the paralysis of the upper limbs. **Monoplegia** is the complete paralysis of one limb.

● **G82**   **Paraplegia (paraparesis) and quadriplegia (quadriparesis)**

    Note: This category is to be used only when the listed conditions are reported without further specification, or are stated to be old or longstanding but of unspecified cause. The category is also for use in multiple coding to identify these conditions resulting from any cause.

    Excludes1   congenital cerebral palsy (G80.-)
              functional quadriplegia (R53.2)
              hysterical paralysis (F44.4)

● **G82.2**   **Paraplegia**

    Paralysis of both lower limbs NOS
    Paraparesis (lower) NOS
    Paraplegia (lower) NOS

    G82.20   Paraplegia, unspecified 🦠
            Coding Clinic: 2017, Q3, P3

    G82.21   Paraplegia, complete 🦠

    G82.22   Paraplegia, incomplete 🦠

● **G82.5**   **Quadriplegia**

    Paralysis of all limbs; AKA tetraplegia

    G82.50   Quadriplegia, unspecified 🦠

    G82.51   Quadriplegia, C1-C4 complete 🦠

    G82.52   Quadriplegia, C1-C4 incomplete 🦠

    G82.53   Quadriplegia, C5-C7 complete 🦠

    G82.54   Quadriplegia, C5-C7 incomplete 🦠

● **G83**   **Other paralytic syndromes**

    Note: This category is to be used only when the listed conditions are reported without further specification, or are stated to be old or longstanding but of unspecified cause. The category is also for use in multiple coding to identify these conditions resulting from any cause.

    Includes   paralysis (complete) (incomplete), except as in G80-G82

● **G83.0**   **Diplegia of upper limbs** 🦠

    Paralysis affecting limbs on both sides; AKA bilateral paralysis
    Diplegia (upper)
    Paralysis of both upper limbs

● **G83.1**   **Monoplegia of lower limb**

    Paralysis of limb on one side
    Paralysis of lower limb

    Excludes1   monoplegia of lower limbs due to sequela of cerebrovascular disease (I69.04-, I69.14-, I69.24-, I69.34-, I69.84-, I69.94-)

    Coding Clinic: 2012, Q4, P106

    G83.10   Monoplegia of lower limb affecting unspecified side 🦠

    G83.11   Monoplegia of lower limb affecting right dominant side 🦠

    G83.12   Monoplegia of lower limb affecting left dominant side 🦠

    G83.13   Monoplegia of lower limb affecting right nondominant side 🦠

    G83.14   Monoplegia of lower limb affecting left nondominant side 🦠

● **G83.2**   **Monoplegia of upper limb**

    Paralysis of upper limb

    Excludes1   monoplegia of upper limbs due to sequela of cerebrovascular disease (I69.03-, I69.13-, I69.23-, I69.33-, I69.83-, I69.93-)

    Coding Clinic: 2012, Q4, P106

    G83.20   Monoplegia of upper limb affecting unspecified side 🦠

    G83.21   Monoplegia of upper limb affecting right dominant side 🦠

    G83.22   Monoplegia of upper limb affecting left dominant side 🦠

    G83.23   Monoplegia of upper limb affecting right nondominant side 🦠

    G83.24   Monoplegia of upper limb affecting left nondominant side 🦠

▶ New   ⟫ Revised   ~~deleted~~ Deleted   Excludes 1   Excludes 2   Includes   Use additional   Code first   Code also   Key words

OGCR Official Guidelines   X Assign placeholder X   ● Use Additional Character(s)   ▶ Manifestation Code   🦠 Hierarchical Condition Category   **Coding Clinic**

● **G83.3**   **Monoplegia, unspecified**
     Coding Clinic: 2012, Q4, P106
     G83.30   Monoplegia, unspecified affecting unspecified side 🔖
     G83.31   Monoplegia, unspecified affecting right dominant side 🔖
     G83.32   Monoplegia, unspecified affecting left dominant side 🔖
     G83.33   Monoplegia, unspecified affecting right nondominant side 🔖
     G83.34   Monoplegia, unspecified affecting left nondominant side 🔖

G83.4   **Cauda equina syndrome** 🔖
     Aching pain due to compression of spinal nerve roots
     Neurogenic bladder due to cauda equina syndrome
     Excludes1   cord bladder NOS (G95.89)
                neurogenic bladder NOS (N31.9)

G83.5   **Locked-in state** 🔖
● **G83.8**   **Other specified paralytic syndromes**
     Excludes1   paralytic syndromes due to current spinal cord injury-code to spinal cord injury (S14, S24, S34)
     G83.81   Brown-Séquard syndrome 🔖
     G83.82   Anterior cord syndrome 🔖
     G83.83   Posterior cord syndrome 🔖
     G83.84   Todd's paralysis (postepileptic) 🔖
     G83.89   Other specified paralytic syndromes 🔖

G83.9   **Paralytic syndrome, unspecified** 🔖

OTHER DISORDERS OF THE NERVOUS SYSTEM (G89-G99)

● **G89**   **Pain, not elsewhere classified**
     Code also related psychological factors associated with pain (F45.42)
     Excludes1   generalized pain NOS (R52)
                pain disorders exclusively related to psychological factors (F45.41)
                pain NOS (R52)
     Excludes2   atypical face pain (G50.1)
                headache syndromes (G44.-)
                localized pain, unspecified type - code to pain by site, such as:
                     abdomen pain (R10.-)
                     back pain (M54.9)
                     breast pain (N64.4)
                     chest pain (R07.1-R07.9)
                     ear pain (H92.0-)
                     eye pain (H57.1)
                     headache (R51.9)
                     joint pain (M25.5-)
                     limb pain (M79.6-)
         ➡   lumbar region pain (M54.5-)
                     painful urination (R30.9)
                     pelvic and perineal pain (R10.2)
                     shoulder pain (M25.51-)
                     spine pain (M54.-)
                     throat pain (R07.0)
                     tongue pain (K14.6)
                     tooth pain (K08.8)
                 renal colic (N23)
                 migraines (G43.-)
                 myalgia (M79.1-)
                 pain from prosthetic devices, implants, and grafts (T82.84, T83.84, T84.84, T85.84-)
                 phantom limb syndrome with pain (G54.6)
                 vulvar vestibulitis (N94.810)
                 vulvodynia (N94.81-)

     G89.0   **Central pain syndrome**
         Neurological condition causing intractable pain resulting from damage to CNS
         Déjérine-Roussy syndrome
         Myelopathic pain syndrome
         Thalamic pain syndrome (hyperesthetic)

● **G89.1**   **Acute pain, not elsewhere classified**
     G89.11   Acute pain due to trauma
     G89.12   Acute post-thoracotomy pain
               Post-thoracotomy pain NOS
     G89.18   Other acute postprocedural pain
               Postoperative pain NOS
               Postprocedural pain NOS

● **G89.2**   **Chronic pain, not elsewhere classified**
     Excludes1   causalgia, lower limb (G57.7-)
                causalgia, upper limb (G56.4-)
                central pain syndrome (G89.0)
                chronic pain syndrome (G89.4)
                complex regional pain syndrome II, lower limb (G57.7-)
                complex regional pain syndrome II, upper limb (G56.4-)
                neoplasm related chronic pain (G89.3)
                reflex sympathetic dystrophy (G90.5-)
     G89.21   Chronic pain due to trauma
     G89.22   Chronic post-thoracotomy pain
     G89.28   Other chronic postprocedural pain
               Other chronic postoperative pain
     G89.29   Other chronic pain

G89.3   **Neoplasm related pain (acute) (chronic)**
     Cancer associated pain
     Pain due to malignancy (primary) (secondary)
     Tumor associated pain

G89.4   **Chronic pain syndrome**
     Chronic pain associated with significant psychosocial dysfunction

● **G90**   **Disorders of autonomic nervous system**
     Excludes1   dysfunction of the autonomic nervous system due to alcohol (G31.2)
   ● **G90.0**   **Idiopathic peripheral autonomic neuropathy**
     G90.01   Carotid sinus syncope
               Carotid sinus syndrome
     G90.09   Other idiopathic peripheral autonomic neuropathy
               Idiopathic peripheral autonomic neuropathy NOS

G90.1   **Familial dysautonomia [Riley-Day]** 🔖
     Inherited disorder that affects nerve function

G90.2   **Horner's syndrome**
     Due to damage of the sympathetic nervous system
     Bernard(-Horner) syndrome
     Cervical sympathetic dystrophy or paralysis

G90.3   **Multi-system degeneration of the autonomic nervous system** 🔖
     Neurogenic orthostatic hypotension [Shy-Drager]
     Excludes1   orthostatic hypotension NOS (I95.1)

G90.4   **Autonomic dysreflexia**
     Syndrome resulting from lesions of spinal cord
     Use additional code to identify the cause, such as:
         fecal impaction (K56.41)
         pressure ulcer (pressure area) (L89.-)
         urinary tract infection (N39.0)

● **G90.5**   **Complex regional pain syndrome I (CRPS I)**
     Reflex sympathetic dystrophy
     Excludes1   causalgia of lower limb (G57.7-)
                causalgia of upper limb (G56.4-)
                complex regional pain syndrome II of lower limb (G57.7-)
                complex regional pain syndrome II of upper limb (G56.4-)
     G90.50   Complex regional pain syndrome I, unspecified
   ● **G90.51**   Complex regional pain syndrome I of upper limb
         G90.511   Complex regional pain syndrome I of right upper limb
         G90.512   Complex regional pain syndrome I of left upper limb

CHAPTER 6 (G00-G99)

G90.513 Complex regional pain syndrome I of upper limb, **bilateral**

G90.519 Complex regional pain syndrome I of **unspecified** upper limb

● G90.52 Complex regional pain syndrome I of **lower** limb

G90.521 Complex regional pain syndrome I of **right** lower limb

G90.522 Complex regional pain syndrome I of **left** lower limb

G90.523 Complex regional pain syndrome I of lower limb, **bilateral**

G90.529 Complex regional pain syndrome I of **unspecified** lower limb

G90.59 Complex regional pain syndrome I of **other** specified site

G90.8 **Other disorders of autonomic nervous system**

G90.9 **Disorder of the autonomic nervous system, unspecified**

● **G91 Hydrocephalus**

Dilatation of cerebral ventricles, accompanied by accumulation of cerebrospinal fluid

Includes acquired hydrocephalus

Excludes1 Arnold-Chiari syndrome with hydrocephalus (Q07.-)
congenital hydrocephalus (Q03.-)
spina bifida with hydrocephalus (Q05.-)

G91.0 **Communicating hydrocephalus**
Secondary normal pressure hydrocephalus

G91.1 **Obstructive hydrocephalus**

G91.2 **(Idiopathic) normal pressure hydrocephalus**
Normal pressure hydrocephalus NOS

G91.3 **Post-traumatic hydrocephalus, unspecified**

▷ G91.4 *Hydrocephalus in diseases classified elsewhere*

Code first underlying condition, such as:
congenital syphilis (A50.4-)
neoplasm (C00-D49)
plasminogen deficiency (E88.02)

Excludes1 hydrocephalus due to congenital toxoplasmosis (P37.1)

G91.8 **Other hydrocephalus**

G91.9 **Hydrocephalus, unspecified**

G92 **Toxic encephalopathy**

▶● **G92.0 Immune effector cell-associated neurotoxicity syndrome**

▶*Code first* underlying cause such as:
▶complications of immune effector cellular therapy (T80.82)

▶Code also associated signs and symptoms, such as seizures and cerebral edema

▶Code also, if applicable:
▶cerebral edema (G93.6)
▶unspecified convulsions (R56.9)

▶ G92.00 Immune effector cell-associated neurotoxicity syndrome, grade unspecified
▶ICANS, grade unspecified

▶ G92.01 Immune effector cell-associated neurotoxicity syndrome, grade 1
▶ICANS, grade 1

▶ G92.02 Immune effector cell-associated neurotoxicity syndrome, grade 2
▶ICANS, grade 2

▶ G92.03 Immune effector cell-associated neurotoxicity syndrome, grade 3
▶ICANS, grade 3

▶ G92.04 Immune effector cell-associated neurotoxicity syndrome, grade 4
▶ICANS, grade 4

▶ G92.05 Immune effector cell-associated neurotoxicity syndrome, grade 5
▶ICANS, grade 5

▶ G92.8 **Other toxic encephalopathy**
▶Toxic encephalitis
▶Toxic metabolic encephalopathy

▶*Code first* poisoning due to drug or toxin, if applicable, (T36-T65 with fifth or sixth character 1-4 or 6)

▶Use Additional code for adverse effect, if applicable, to identify drug (T36-T50 with fifth or sixth character 5)

▶ G92.9 **Unspecified toxic encephalopathy**

▶*Code first* poisoning due to drug or toxin, if applicable, (T36-T65 with fifth or sixth character 1-4 or 6)

▶Use Additional code for adverse effect, if applicable, to identify drug (T36-T50 with fifth or sixth character 5)

Disorder or disease of brain caused by chemicals
~~Toxic encephalitis~~
~~Toxic metabolic encephalopathy~~

~~*Code first if applicable, drug induced (T36-T50) or use (T51-T65) to identify toxic agent*~~

Coding Clinic: 2021, Q1, P13; 2017, Q1, P39-40

● **G93 Other disorders of brain**

G93.0 **Cerebral cysts**
Arachnoid cyst
Porencephalic cyst, acquired

Excludes1 acquired periventricular cysts of newborn (P91.1)
congenital cerebral cysts (Q04.6)

G93.1 **Anoxic brain damage, not elsewhere classified** 🅗

Permanent brain damage by lack of oxygen perfusion through brain tissues.

Excludes1 cerebral anoxia due to anesthesia during labor and delivery (O74.3)
cerebral anoxia due to anesthesia during the puerperium (O89.2)
neonatal anoxia (P84)

G93.2 **Benign intracranial hypertension**
Pseudotumor

Excludes1 hypertensive encephalopathy (I67.4)
obstructive hydrocephalus (G91.1)

G93.3 **Postviral fatigue syndrome**
Benign myalgic encephalomyelitis

Excludes1 chronic fatigue syndrome NOS (R53.82)

● G93.4 **Other and unspecified encephalopathy**

Excludes1 alcoholic encephalopathy (G31.2)
encephalopathy in diseases classified elsewhere (G94)
hypertensive encephalopathy (I67.4)

⇒ **Excludes2** toxic (metabolic) encephalopathy (G92.8)

Coding Clinic: 2017, Q2, P9

G93.40 **Encephalopathy, unspecified**

G93.41 **Metabolic encephalopathy**
Septic encephalopathy
Coding Clinic: 2017, Q2, P8; 2016, Q3, P42; 2015, Q3, P21

G93.49 **Other encephalopathy**
Encephalopathy NEC
Coding Clinic: 2021, Q2, P3; 2018, Q4, P16; 2018, Q2, P22; 2017, Q2, P9

G93.5 **Compression of brain** 🅗
Arnold-Chiari type 1 compression of brain
Compression of brain (stem)
Herniation of brain (stem)

Excludes1 ~~diffuse traumatic compression of brain (S06.2-)~~
~~focal traumatic compression of brain (S06.3-)~~
▶traumatic compression of brain (S06.A-)

G93.6 **Cerebral edema** 🅗

Excludes1 cerebral edema due to birth injury (P11.0)
traumatic cerebral edema (S06.1-)

▶ New ⇒ Revised ~~deleted~~ Deleted Excludes 1 Excludes 2 Includes Use additional Code first Code also Key words

OGCR Official Guidelines X Assign placeholder X ● Use Additional Character(s) ▷ Manifestation Code 🅗 Hierarchical Condition Category **Coding Clinic**

G93.7   **Reye's syndrome**   P
Life-threatening neurological condition, usually follows viral illness

Code first (poisoning due to salicylates, if applicable (T39.0-, with sixth character 1-4)

Use additional code for adverse effect due to salicylates, if applicable (T39.0-, with sixth character 5)

● **G93.8**   **Other specified disorders of brain**

     G93.81   **Temporal sclerosis**
           Hippocampal sclerosis
           Mesial temporal sclerosis

     G93.82   **Brain death**

     G93.89   **Other specified disorders of brain**
           Postradiation encephalopathy
           Coding Clinic: 2019, Q3, P9; 2016, Q4, P7

G93.9   **Disorder of brain, unspecified**

▷ **G94**   *Other disorders of brain in diseases classified elsewhere*

     Code first underlying disease

     Excludes1   encephalopathy in congenital syphilis (A50.49)
           encephalopathy in influenza (J09.X9, J10.81, J11.81)
           encephalopathy in syphilis (A52.19)
           hydrocephalus in diseases classified elsewhere (G91.4)

     Coding Clinic: 2018, Q2, P22; 2017, Q2, P8

● **G95**   **Other and unspecified diseases of spinal cord**

     Excludes2   myelitis (G04.-)

G95.0   **Syringomyelia and syringobulbia** 🔖

● **G95.1**   **Vascular myelopathies**

     Excludes2   intraspinal phlebitis and thrombophlebitis, except non-pyogenic (G08)

     G95.11   **Acute infarction of spinal cord (embolic) (nonembolic)** 🔖
           Anoxia of spinal cord
           Arterial thrombosis of spinal cord

     G95.19   **Other vascular myelopathies** 🔖
           Edema of spinal cord
           Hematomyelia
           Nonpyogenic intraspinal phlebitis and thrombophlebitis
           Subacute necrotic myelopathy

● **G95.2**   **Other and unspecified cord compression**

     G95.20   **Unspecified cord compression** 🔖

     G95.29   **Other cord compression** 🔖

● **G95.8**   **Other specified diseases of spinal cord**

     Excludes1   neurogenic bladder NOS (N31.9)
           neurogenic bladder due to cauda equina syndrome (G83.4)
           neuromuscular dysfunction of bladder without spinal cord lesion (N31.-)

     G95.81   **Conus medullaris syndrome** 🔖
           Damage to gray matter and/or nerve roots in lower end of spinal cord

     G95.89   **Other specified diseases of spinal cord** 🔖
           Cord bladder NOS
           Drug-induced myelopathy
           Radiation-induced myelopathy
           Excludes1   myelopathy NOS (G95.9)

G95.9   **Disease of spinal cord, unspecified** 🔖
       Myelopathy NOS

● **G96**   **Other disorders of central nervous system**

● **G96.0**   **Cerebrospinal fluid leak**

     Code also if applicable:
       intracranial hypotension (G96.81-)

     Excludes1   cerebrospinal fluid leak from spinal puncture (G97.0)

     Coding Clinic: 2018, Q2, P13

G96.00   **Cerebrospinal fluid leak, unspecified**

       Code also if applicable:
         head injury (S00.- to S09.-)

G96.01   **Cranial cerebrospinal fluid leak, spontaneous**
       Otorrhea due to spontaneous cerebrospinal fluid CSF leak
       Rhinorrhea due to spontaneous cerebrospinal fluid CSF leak
       Spontaneous cerebrospinal fluid leak from skull base

G96.02   **Spinal cerebrospinal fluid leak, spontaneous**
       Spontaneous cerebrospinal fluid leak from spine

G96.08   **Other cranial cerebrospinal fluid leak**
       Postoperative cranial cerebrospinal fluid leak
       Traumatic cranial cerebrospinal fluid leak
       Code also if applicable:
         head injury (S00.- to S09.-)

G96.09   **Other spinal cerebrospinal fluid leak**
       Other spinal CSF leak
       Postoperative spinal cerebrospinal fluid leak
       Traumatic spinal cerebrospinal fluid leak
       Code also if applicable:
         head injury (S00.- to S09.-)

● **G96.1**   **Disorders of meninges, not elsewhere classified**

     G96.11   **Dural tear**
         Code also intracranial hypotension, if applicable (G96.81-)
         Excludes1   accidental puncture or laceration of dura during a procedure (G97.41)

     G96.12   **Meningeal adhesions (cerebral) (spinal)**

●   **G96.19**   **Other disorders of meninges, not elsewhere classified**

         G96.191   **Perineural cyst**
              Cervical nerve root cyst
              Lumbar nerve root cyst
              Sacral nerve root cyst
              Tarlov cyst
              Thoracic nerve root cyst

         G96.198   **Other disorders of meninges, not elsewhere classified**

● **G96.8**   **Other specified disorders of central nervous system**

●   **G96.81**   **Intracranial hypotension**

         Code also any associated diagnoses, such as:
         Brachial amyotrophy (G54.5)
         Cerebrospinal fluid leak from spine (G96.02)
         Cranial nerve disorders in diseases classified elsewhere (G53)
         Nerve root and compressions in diseases classified elsewhere (G55)
         Nonpyogenic thrombosis of intracranial venous system (I67.6)
         Nontraumatic intracerebral hemorrhage (I61.-)
         Nontraumatic subdural hemorrhage (I62.0-)
         Other and unspecified cord compression (G95.2-)
         Other secondary parkinsonism (G21.8)
         Reversible cerebrovascular vasoconstriction syndrome (I67.841)
         Spinal cord herniation (G95.89)
         Stroke (I63.-)
         Syringomyelia (G95.0)

         G96.810   **Intracranial hypotension, unspecified**

         G96.811   **Intracranial hypotension, spontaneous**

         G96.819   **Other intracranial hypotension**

     G96.89   **Other specified disorders of central nervous system**

G96.9   **Disorder of central nervous system, unspecified**

- **G97 Intraoperative and postprocedural complications and disorders of nervous system, not elsewhere classified**
  - **Excludes2**   intraoperative and postprocedural cerebrovascular infarction (I97.81-, I97.82-)
  - Coding Clinic: 2016, Q4, P9
  - **G97.0 Cerebrospinal fluid leak from spinal puncture**
    - Code also any associated diagnoses or complications, such as:
      - intracranial hypotension following a procedure (G97.83-G97.84)
  - **G97.1 Other reaction to spinal and lumbar puncture**
    - Headache due to lumbar puncture
    - Other reaction to spinal dural puncture
    - Code also, if applicable, any associated headache with orthostatic component (R51.0)
  - **G97.2 Intracranial hypotension following ventricular shunting**
    - Code also any associated diagnoses or complications
  - **G97.3 Intraoperative hemorrhage and hematoma of a nervous system organ or structure complicating a procedure**
    - **Excludes1**   intraoperative hemorrhage and hematoma of a nervous system organ or structure due to accidental puncture and laceration during a procedure (G97.4-)
    - **G97.31 Intraoperative hemorrhage and hematoma of a nervous system organ or structure complicating a nervous system procedure**
    - **G97.32 Intraoperative hemorrhage and hematoma of a nervous system organ or structure complicating other procedure**
  - **G97.4 Accidental puncture and laceration of a nervous system organ or structure during a procedure**
    - **G97.41 Accidental puncture or laceration of dura during a procedure**
      - Incidental (inadvertent) durotomy
      - Code also any associated diagnoses or complications
    - **G97.48 Accidental puncture and laceration of other nervous system organ or structure during a nervous system procedure**
    - **G97.49 Accidental puncture and laceration of other nervous system organ or structure during other procedure**
  - **G97.5 Postprocedural hemorrhage of a nervous system organ or structure following a procedure**
    - **G97.51 Postprocedural hemorrhage of a nervous system organ or structure following a nervous system procedure**
    - **G97.52 Postprocedural hemorrhage of a nervous system organ or structure following other procedure**
  - **G97.6 Postprocedural hematoma and seroma of a nervous system organ or structure following a procedure**
    - **G97.61 Postprocedural hematoma of a nervous system organ or structure following a nervous system procedure**
    - **G97.62 Postprocedural hematoma of a nervous system organ or structure following other procedure**
    - **G97.63 Postprocedural seroma of a nervous system organ or structure following a nervous system procedure**
    - **G97.64 Postprocedural seroma of a nervous system organ or structure following other procedure**

- **G97.8 Other intraoperative and postprocedural complications and disorders of nervous system**
  - Use additional code to further specify disorder
  - **G97.81 Other intraoperative complications of nervous system**
  - **G97.82 Other postprocedural complications and disorders of nervous system**
  - **G97.83 Intracranial hypotension following lumbar cerebrospinal fluid shunting**
    - Code also any associated diagnoses or complications
  - **G97.84 Intracranial hypotension following other procedure**
    - Code also, if applicable:
      - accidental puncture or laceration of dura during a procedure (G97.41)
      - cerebrospinal fluid leak from spinal puncture (G97.0)

- **G98 Other disorders of nervous system not elsewhere classified**
  - **Includes**   nervous system disorder NOS
  - **G98.0 Neurogenic arthritis, not elsewhere classified**
    - Nonsyphilitic neurogenic arthropathy NEC
    - Nonsyphilitic neurogenic spondylopathy NEC
    - **Excludes1**   spondylopathy (in):
      - syringomyelia and syringobulbia (G95.0)
      - tabes dorsalis (A52.11)
  - **G98.8 Other disorders of nervous system**
    - Nervous system disorder NOS

- **G99 Other disorders of nervous system in diseases classified elsewhere**
  - *G99.0 Autonomic neuropathy in diseases classified elsewhere*
    - Code first underlying disease, such as:
      - amyloidosis (E85.-)
      - gout (M1A.-, M10.-)
      - hyperthyroidism (E05.-)
    - **Excludes1**   diabetic autonomic neuropathy (E08-E13 with .43)
  - *G99.2 Myelopathy in diseases classified elsewhere* 🐾
    - Code first underlying disease, such as:
      - neoplasm (C00-D49)
    - **Excludes1**   myelopathy in:
      - intervertebral disease (M50.0-, M51.0-)
      - spondylosis (M47.0-, M47.1-)
  - *G99.8 Other specified disorders of nervous system in diseases classified elsewhere*
    - Code first underlying disorder, such as:
      - amyloidosis (E85.-)
      - avitaminosis (E56.9)
    - **Excludes1**   nervous system involvement in:
      - cysticercosis (B69.0)
      - rubella (B06.0-)
      - syphilis (A52.1-)

► New   ⇒ Revised   ~~deleted~~ Deleted   Excludes 1   Excludes 2   Includes   Use additional   Code first   Code also   Key words

816   OGCR Official Guidelines   X Assign placeholder X   ● Use Additional Character(s)   ▌ Manifestation Code   🐾 Hierarchical Condition Category   Coding Clinic

CHAPTER 7

DISEASES OF THE EYE AND ADNEXA
(H00-H59)

7. Chapter 7: Diseases of the Eye and Adnexa (H00-H59)

a. Glaucoma

1) Assigning Glaucoma Codes

Assign as many codes from category H40, Glaucoma, as needed to identify the type of glaucoma, the affected eye, and the glaucoma stage.

2) Bilateral glaucoma with same type and stage

When a patient has bilateral glaucoma and both eyes are documented as being the same type and stage, and there is a code for bilateral glaucoma, report only the code for the type of glaucoma, bilateral, with the seventh character for the stage.

When a patient has bilateral glaucoma and both eyes are documented as being the same type and stage, and the classification does not provide a code for bilateral glaucoma (i.e., subcategories H40.10, H40.11, and H40.20) report only one code for the type of glaucoma with the appropriate seventh character for the stage.

3) Bilateral glaucoma stage with different types or stages

When a patient has bilateral glaucoma and each eye is documented as having a different type or stage, and the classification distinguishes laterality, assign the appropriate code for each eye rather than the code for bilateral glaucoma.

When a patient has bilateral glaucoma and each eye is documented as having a different type, and the classification does not distinguish laterality (i.e., subcategories H40.10, H40.11 and H40.20), assign one code for each type of glaucoma with the appropriate seventh character for the stage.

When a patient has bilateral glaucoma and each eye is documented as having the same type, but different stage, and the classification does not distinguish laterality (i.e., subcategories H40.10, H40.11, and H40.20), assign a code for the type of glaucoma for each eye with the seventh character for the specific glaucoma stage documented for each eye.

4) Patient admitted with glaucoma and stage evolves during the admission

If a patient is admitted with glaucoma and the stage progresses during the admission, assign the code for highest stage documented.

5) Indeterminate stage glaucoma

Assignment of the seventh character "4" for "indeterminate stage" should be based on the clinical documentation. The seventh character "4" is used for glaucomas whose stage cannot be clinically determined. This seventh character should not be confused with the seventh character "0", unspecified, which should be assigned when there is no documentation regarding the stage of the glaucoma.

b. Blindness

If "blindness" or "low vision" of both eyes is documented but the visual impairment category is not documented, assign code H54.3, Unqualified visual loss, both eyes. If "blindness" or "low vision" in one eye is documented but the visual impairment category is not documented, assign a code from H54.6-, Unqualified visual loss, one eye. If "blindness" or "visual loss" is documented without any information about whether one or both eyes are affected, assign code H54.7, Unspecified visual loss.

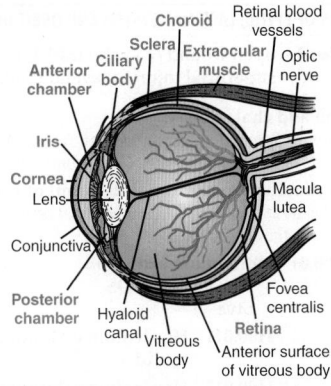

Figure 7-1 Eye and ocular adnexa. (From Buck CJ: Step-by-Step Medical Coding, ed 2016, St. Louis, Elsevier, 2016)

★**(See Plate 15 of the Anatomy Illustrations.)**

CHAPTER 7

DISEASES OF THE EYE AND ADNEXA
(H00-H59)

Note: Use an external cause code following the code for the eye condition, if applicable, to identify the cause of the eye condition

| Excludes2 | certain conditions originating in the perinatal period (P04-P96) |

Excludes2   certain conditions originating in the perinatal period (P04-P96)
certain infectious and parasitic diseases (A00-B99)
complications of pregnancy, childbirth and the puerperium (O00-O9A)
congenital malformations, deformations, and chromosomal abnormalities (Q00-Q99)
diabetes mellitus related eye conditions (E09.3-, E10.3-, E11.3-, E13.3-)
endocrine, nutritional and metabolic diseases (E00-E88)
injury (trauma) of eye and orbit (S05.-)
injury, poisoning and certain other consequences of external causes (S00-T88)
neoplasms (C00-D49)
symptoms, signs and abnormal clinical and laboratory findings, not elsewhere classified (R00-R94)
syphilis related eye disorders (A50.01, A50.3-, A51.43, A52.71)

This chapter contains the following blocks:

H00-H05	Disorders of eyelid, lacrimal system and orbit
H10-H11	Disorders of conjunctiva
H15-H22	Disorders of sclera, cornea, iris and ciliary body
H25-H28	Disorders of lens
H30-H36	Disorders of choroid and retina
H40-H42	Glaucoma
H43-H44	Disorders of vitreous body and globe
H46-H47	Disorders of optic nerve and visual pathways
H49-H52	Disorders of ocular muscles, binocular movement, accommodation and refraction
H53-H54	Visual disturbances and blindness
H55-H57	Other disorders of eye and adnexa
H59	Intraoperative and postprocedural complications and disorders of eye and adnexa, not elsewhere classified

DISORDERS OF EYELID, LACRIMAL SYSTEM AND ORBIT (H00-H05)

Excludes2   open wound of eyelid (S01.1-)
superficial injury of eyelid (S00.1-, S00.2-)

H00 Hordeolum and chalazion

Hordeolum: inflammatory staphylococcal infection of sebaceous glands of eyelids; AKA stye. Chalazion: eyelid mass

H00.0 Hordeolum (externum) (internum) of eyelid

Bacterial infection (staphylococcus) of the sebaceous gland of the eyelid (stye)

H00.01 Hordeolum externum

Hordeolum NOS
Stye

H00.011 Hordeolum externum right upper eyelid

H00.012 Hordeolum externum right lower eyelid

H00.013 Hordeolum externum right eye, unspecified eyelid

H00.014 Hordeolum externum left upper eyelid

H00.015 Hordeolum externum left lower eyelid

H00.016 Hordeolum externum left eye, unspecified eyelid

H00.019 Hordeolum externum unspecified eye, unspecified eyelid

H00.02 Hordeolum internum

Infection of meibomian gland

H00.021 Hordeolum internum right upper eyelid

H00.022 Hordeolum internum right lower eyelid

H00.023 Hordeolum internum right eye, unspecified eyelid

H00.024 Hordeolum internum left upper eyelid

H00.025 Hordeolum internum left lower eyelid

H00.026 Hordeolum internum left eye, unspecified eyelid

H00.029 Hordeolum internum unspecified eye, unspecified eyelid

H00.03 Abscess of eyelid

Furuncle of eyelid

H00.031 Abscess of right upper eyelid

H00.032 Abscess of right lower eyelid

H00.033 Abscess of eyelid right eye, unspecified eyelid

H00.034 Abscess of left upper eyelid

H00.035 Abscess of left lower eyelid

H00.036 Abscess of eyelid left eye, unspecified eyelid

H00.039 Abscess of eyelid unspecified eye, unspecified eyelid

H00.1 Chalazion

Often caused by accumulation of meibomian gland secretions resulting from a blockage of duct.

Meibomian (gland) cyst

Excludes2   infected meibomian gland (H00.02-)

H00.11 Chalazion right upper eyelid

H00.12 Chalazion right lower eyelid

H00.13 Chalazion right eye, unspecified eyelid

H00.14 Chalazion left upper eyelid

H00.15 Chalazion left lower eyelid

H00.16 Chalazion left eye, unspecified eyelid

H00.19 Chalazion unspecified eye, unspecified eyelid

H01 Other inflammation of eyelid

H01.0 Blepharitis

Inflammation of eyelids

Excludes1   blepharoconjunctivitis (H10.5-)

H01.00 Unspecified blepharitis

H01.001 Unspecified blepharitis right upper eyelid

H01.002 Unspecified blepharitis right lower eyelid

H01.003 Unspecified blepharitis right eye, unspecified eyelid

H01.004 Unspecified blepharitis left upper eyelid

H01.005 Unspecified blepharitis left lower eyelid

H01.006 Unspecified blepharitis left eye, unspecified eyelid

H01.009 Unspecified blepharitis unspecified eye, unspecified eyelid

H01.00A Unspecified blepharitis right eye, upper and lower eyelids

H01.00B Unspecified blepharitis left eye, upper and lower eyelids

H01.01 Ulcerative blepharitis

H01.011 Ulcerative blepharitis right upper eyelid

H01.012 Ulcerative blepharitis right lower eyelid

H01.013 Ulcerative blepharitis right eye, unspecified eyelid

H01.014 Ulcerative blepharitis left upper eyelid

H01.015 Ulcerative blepharitis left lower eyelid

H01.016 Ulcerative blepharitis left eye, unspecified eyelid

H01.019 Ulcerative blepharitis unspecified eye, unspecified eyelid

H01.01A Ulcerative blepharitis right eye, upper and lower eyelids

H01.01B Ulcerative blepharitis left eye, upper and lower eyelids

H01.02 Squamous blepharitis

H01.021 Squamous blepharitis right upper eyelid

H01.022 Squamous blepharitis right lower eyelid

H01.023 Squamous blepharitis right eye, unspecified eyelid

H01.024 Squamous blepharitis left upper eyelid

H01.025 Squamous blepharitis left lower eyelid

H01.026 Squamous blepharitis left eye, unspecified eyelid

H01.029 Squamous blepharitis unspecified eye, unspecified eyelid

H01.02A Squamous blepharitis right eye, upper and lower eyelids

H01.02B Squamous blepharitis left eye, upper and lower eyelids

H01.1 Noninfectious dermatoses of eyelid

H01.11 Allergic dermatitis of eyelid

Contact dermatitis of eyelid

H01.111 Allergic dermatitis of right upper eyelid

H01.112 Allergic dermatitis of right lower eyelid

H01.113 Allergic dermatitis of right eye, unspecified eyelid

▶ New   ▶ Revised   ~~deleted~~ Deleted   Excludes 1   Excludes 2   Includes   Use additional   Code first   Code also   Key words

OGCR Official Guidelines   X Assign placeholder X   ● Use Additional Character(s)   ▶ Manifestation Code   🝮 Hierarchical Condition Category   **Coding Clinic**

H01.114   Allergic dermatitis of left upper eyelid

H01.115   Allergic dermatitis of left lower eyelid

H01.116   Allergic dermatitis of left eye, unspecified eyelid

H01.119   Allergic dermatitis of unspecified eye, unspecified eyelid

● H01.12   Discoid lupus erythematosus of eyelid

H01.121   Discoid lupus erythematosus of right upper eyelid

H01.122   Discoid lupus erythematosus of right lower eyelid

H01.123   Discoid lupus erythematosus of right eye, unspecified eyelid

H01.124   Discoid lupus erythematosus of left upper eyelid

H01.125   Discoid lupus erythematosus of left lower eyelid

H01.126   Discoid lupus erythematosus of left eye, unspecified eyelid

H01.129   Discoid lupus erythematosus of unspecified eye, unspecified eyelid

● H01.13   Eczematous dermatitis of eyelid

H01.131   Eczematous dermatitis of right upper eyelid

H01.132   Eczematous dermatitis of right lower eyelid

H01.133   Eczematous dermatitis of right eye, unspecified eyelid

H01.134   Eczematous dermatitis of left upper eyelid

H01.135   Eczematous dermatitis of left lower eyelid

H01.136   Eczematous dermatitis of left eye, unspecified eyelid

H01.139   Eczematous dermatitis of unspecified eye, unspecified eyelid

● H01.14   Xeroderma of eyelid
Abnormally dry

H01.141   Xeroderma of right upper eyelid

H01.142   Xeroderma of right lower eyelid

H01.143   Xeroderma of right eye, unspecified eyelid

H01.144   Xeroderma of left upper eyelid

H01.145   Xeroderma of left lower eyelid

H01.146   Xeroderma of left eye, unspecified eyelid

H01.149   Xeroderma of unspecified eye, unspecified eyelid

H01.8   Other specified inflammations of eyelid

H01.9   Unspecified inflammation of eyelid
Inflammation of eyelid NOS

● H02   Other disorders of eyelid
Turning inward (inversion) of eyelid margin and ingrowing eyelashes

Excludes1   congenital malformations of eyelid (Q10.0-Q10.3)

● H02.0   Entropion and trichiasis of eyelid

● H02.00   Unspecified entropion of eyelid

H02.001   Unspecified entropion of right upper eyelid

H02.002   Unspecified entropion of right lower eyelid

H02.003   Unspecified entropion of right eye, unspecified eyelid

H02.004   Unspecified entropion of left upper eyelid

H02.005   Unspecified entropion of left lower eyelid

Figure 7-2 Right lower eyelid entropion. Note the inward rotation of the tarsal plate about the horizontal axis and the resultant contact between the mucocutaneous junction and ocular surface. (From Glynn M, Drake WM, Hutchison R: Hutchison's Clinical Methods: An Integrated Approach to Clinical Practice, Edinburgh, Saunders/Elsevier, 2012)

H02.006   Unspecified entropion of left eye, unspecified eyelid

H02.009   Unspecified entropion of unspecified eye, unspecified eyelid

● H02.01   Cicatricial entropion of eyelid
Scar

H02.011   Cicatricial entropion of right upper eyelid

H02.012   Cicatricial entropion of right lower eyelid

H02.013   Cicatricial entropion of right eye, unspecified eyelid

H02.014   Cicatricial entropion of left upper eyelid

H02.015   Cicatricial entropion of left lower eyelid

H02.016   Cicatricial entropion of left eye, unspecified eyelid

H02.019   Cicatricial entropion of unspecified eye, unspecified eyelid

● H02.02   Mechanical entropion of eyelid
Turning inward (inversion) of eyelid margin due to lack of support

H02.021   Mechanical entropion of right upper eyelid

H02.022   Mechanical entropion of right lower eyelid

H02.023   Mechanical entropion of right eye, unspecified eyelid

H02.024   Mechanical entropion of left upper eyelid

H02.025   Mechanical entropion of left lower eyelid

H02.026   Mechanical entropion of left eye, unspecified eyelid

H02.029   Mechanical entropion of unspecified eye, unspecified eyelid

● H02.03   Senile entropion of eyelid
Turning inward (inversion) of eyelid margin due to aging

H02.031   Senile entropion of right upper eyelid   A

H02.032   Senile entropion of right lower eyelid   A

H02.033   Senile entropion of right eye, unspecified eyelid   A

H02.034   Senile entropion of left upper eyelid A

H02.035   Senile entropion of left lower eyelid A

H02.036   Senile entropion of left eye, unspecified eyelid   A

H02.039   Senile entropion of unspecified eye, unspecified eyelid   A

● H02.04   Spastic entropion of eyelid
Turning inward (inversion) of eyelid margin caused by spasm of muscle

H02.041   Spastic entropion of right upper eyelid

H02.042   Spastic entropion of right lower eyelid

H02.043   Spastic entropion of right eye, unspecified eyelid

CHAPTER 7 (H00-H59)

CHAPTER 7 (H00-H59)

H02.044   Spastic entropion of left upper eyelid

H02.045   Spastic entropion of left lower eyelid

H02.046   Spastic entropion of left eye, unspecified eyelid

H02.049   Spastic entropion of unspecified eye, unspecified eyelid

● H02.05   Trichiasis without entropion
Ingrowing hairs of eyelashes

    H02.051   Trichiasis without entropion right upper eyelid

    H02.052   Trichiasis without entropion right lower eyelid

    H02.053   Trichiasis without entropion right eye, unspecified eyelid

    H02.054   Trichiasis without entropion left upper eyelid

    H02.055   Trichiasis without entropion left lower eyelid

    H02.056   Trichiasis without entropion left eye, unspecified eyelid

    H02.059   Trichiasis without entropion unspecified eye, unspecified eyelid

● H02.1   Ectropion of eyelid
Eversion (pulling away) of eyelid

  ● H02.10   Unspecified ectropion of eyelid

    H02.101   Unspecified ectropion of right upper eyelid

    H02.102   Unspecified ectropion of right lower eyelid

    H02.103   Unspecified ectropion of right eye, unspecified eyelid

    H02.104   Unspecified ectropion of left upper eyelid

    H02.105   Unspecified ectropion of left lower eyelid

    H02.106   Unspecified ectropion of left eye, unspecified eyelid

    H02.109   Unspecified ectropion of unspecified eye, unspecified eyelid

  ● H02.11   Cicatricial ectropion of eyelid
Pulling of eyelid down and away from eye due to scar or tightening

    H02.111   Cicatricial ectropion of right upper eyelid

    H02.112   Cicatricial ectropion of right lower eyelid

    H02.113   Cicatricial ectropion of right eye, unspecified eyelid

    H02.114   Cicatricial ectropion of left upper eyelid

    H02.115   Cicatricial ectropion of left lower eyelid

    H02.116   Cicatricial ectropion of left eye, unspecified eyelid

    H02.119   Cicatricial ectropion of unspecified eye, unspecified eyelid

  ● H02.12   Mechanical ectropion of eyelid
Eversion (pulling away) of eyelid due to lack of support

    H02.121   Mechanical ectropion of right upper eyelid

    H02.122   Mechanical ectropion of right lower eyelid

    H02.123   Mechanical ectropion of right eye, unspecified eyelid

    H02.124   Mechanical ectropion of left upper eyelid

    H02.125   Mechanical ectropion of left lower eyelid

    H02.126   Mechanical ectropion of left eye, unspecified eyelid

    H02.129   Mechanical ectropion of unspecified eye, unspecified eyelid

  ● H02.13   Senile ectropion of eyelid
Eversion (pulling away) of eyelid due to age

    H02.131   Senile ectropion of right upper eyelid   A

    H02.132   Senile ectropion of right lower eyelid

    H02.133   Senile ectropion of right eye, unspecified eyelid   A

    H02.134   Senile ectropion of left upper eyelid A

    H02.135   Senile ectropion of left lower eyelid A

    H02.136   Senile ectropion of left eye, unspecified eyelid   A

    H02.139   Senile ectropion of unspecified eye, unspecified eyelid   A

  ● H02.14   Spastic ectropion of eyelid
Eversion (pulling away) of eyelid due to tonic muscle spasm

    H02.141   Spastic ectropion of right upper eyelid

    H02.142   Spastic ectropion of right lower eyelid

    H02.143   Spastic ectropion of right eye, unspecified eyelid

    H02.144   Spastic ectropion of left upper eyelid

    H02.145   Spastic ectropion of left lower eyelid

    H02.146   Spastic ectropion of left eye, unspecified eyelid

    H02.149   Spastic ectropion of unspecified eye, unspecified eyelid

  ● H02.15   Paralytic ectropion of eyelid

    H02.151   Paralytic ectropion of right upper eyelid

    H02.152   Paralytic ectropion of right lower eyelid

    H02.153   Paralytic ectropion of right eye, unspecified eyelid

    H02.154   Paralytic ectropion of left upper eyelid

    H02.155   Paralytic ectropion of left lower eyelid

    H02.156   Paralytic ectropion of left eye, unspecified eyelid

    H02.159   Paralytic ectropion of unspecified eye, unspecified eyelid

● H02.2   Lagophthalmos
Condition in which eye cannot completely close

  ● H02.20   Unspecified lagophthalmos

    H02.201   Unspecified lagophthalmos right upper eyelid

    H02.202   Unspecified lagophthalmos right lower eyelid

    H02.203   Unspecified lagophthalmos right eye, unspecified eyelid

    H02.204   Unspecified lagophthalmos left upper eyelid

    H02.205   Unspecified lagophthalmos left lower eyelid

    H02.206   Unspecified lagophthalmos left eye, unspecified eyelid

    H02.209   Unspecified lagophthalmos unspecified eye, unspecified eyelid

    H02.20A   Unspecified lagophthalmos right eye, upper and lower eyelids

    H02.20B   Unspecified lagophthalmos left eye, upper and lower eyelids

    H02.20C   Unspecified lagophthalmos, bilateral, upper and lower eyelids

▶ New   ⇒ Revised   ~~deleted~~ Deleted   Excludes 1   Excludes 2   Includes   Use additional   Code first   Code also   Key words

OGCR Official Guidelines   X Assign placeholder X   ● Use Additional Character(s)   ▶ Manifestation Code   🏥 Hierarchical Condition Category   **Coding Clinic**

● H02.21   **Cicatricial** lagophthalmos
       Upper or lower eyelid does not close due to scar or tightening
   H02.211   Cicatricial lagophthalmos right upper eyelid
   H02.212   Cicatricial lagophthalmos right lower eyelid
   H02.213   Cicatricial lagophthalmos right eye, unspecified eyelid
   H02.214   Cicatricial lagophthalmos left upper eyelid
   H02.215   Cicatricial lagophthalmos left lower eyelid
   H02.216   Cicatricial lagophthalmos left eye, unspecified eyelid
   H02.219   Cicatricial lagophthalmos unspecified eye, unspecified eyelid
   H02.21A   Cicatricial lagophthalmos right eye, upper and lower eyelids
   H02.21B   Cicatricial lagophthalmos left eye, upper and lower eyelids
   H02.21C   Cicatricial lagophthalmos, bilateral, upper and lower eyelids

● H02.22   **Mechanical** lagophthalmos
       Inability to close lids due to structural disorder
   H02.221   Mechanical lagophthalmos right upper eyelid
   H02.222   Mechanical lagophthalmos right lower eyelid
   H02.223   Mechanical lagophthalmos right eye, unspecified eyelid
   H02.224   Mechanical lagophthalmos left upper eyelid
   H02.225   Mechanical lagophthalmos left lower eyelid
   H02.226   Mechanical lagophthalmos left eye, unspecified eyelid
   H02.229   Mechanical lagophthalmos unspecified eye, unspecified eyelid
   H02.22A   Mechanical lagophthalmos right eye, upper and lower eyelids
   H02.22B   Mechanical lagophthalmos left eye, upper and lower eyelids
   H02.22C   Mechanical lagophthalmos, bilateral, upper and lower eyelids

● H02.23   **Paralytic** lagophthalmos
       Eyelids do not close due to paralysis
   H02.231   Paralytic lagophthalmos right upper eyelid
   H02.232   Paralytic lagophthalmos right lower eyelid
   H02.233   Paralytic lagophthalmos right eye, unspecified eyelid
   H02.234   Paralytic lagophthalmos left upper eyelid
   H02.235   Paralytic lagophthalmos left lower eyelid
   H02.236   Paralytic lagophthalmos left eye, unspecified eyelid
   H02.239   Paralytic lagophthalmos unspecified eye, unspecified eyelid
   H02.23A   Paralytic lagophthalmos right eye, upper and lower eyelids
   H02.23B   Paralytic lagophthalmos left eye, upper and lower eyelids
   H02.23C   Paralytic lagophthalmos, bilateral, upper and lower eyelids

Figure 7-3   Ptosis of eyelid. (From Kanski JJ: Clinical Diagnosis in Ophthalmology, London, Elsevier Mosby, 2006)

Item 7-1   Ptosis of eyelid is drooping of the upper eyelid over the pupil when the eyes are fully opened resulting from nerve or muscle damage, which may require surgical correction.

★ **(See Plate 17 of the Anatomy Illustrations.)**
● H02.3   **Blepharochalasis**
       Relaxation of skin of eyelid, due to atrophy of intercellular tissue
       Pseudoptosis
   H02.30   Blepharochalasis unspecified eye, unspecified eyelid
   H02.31   Blepharochalasis right upper eyelid
   H02.32   Blepharochalasis right lower eyelid
   H02.33   Blepharochalasis right eye, unspecified eyelid
   H02.34   Blepharochalasis left upper eyelid
   H02.35   Blepharochalasis left lower eyelid
   H02.36   Blepharochalasis left eye, unspecified eyelid

● H02.4   **Ptosis of eyelid**
       Falling forward, drooping, sagging of eyelid
 ● H02.40   **Unspecified** ptosis of eyelid
   H02.401   Unspecified ptosis of right eyelid
   H02.402   Unspecified ptosis of left eyelid
   H02.403   Unspecified ptosis of bilateral eyelids
   H02.409   Unspecified ptosis of unspecified eyelid
 ● H02.41   **Mechanical** ptosis of eyelid
   H02.411   Mechanical ptosis of right eyelid
   H02.412   Mechanical ptosis of left eyelid
   H02.413   Mechanical ptosis of bilateral eyelids
   H02.419   Mechanical ptosis of unspecified eyelid
 ● H02.42   **Myogenic** ptosis of eyelid
   H02.421   Myogenic ptosis of right eyelid
   H02.422   Myogenic ptosis of left eyelid
   H02.423   Myogenic ptosis of bilateral eyelids
   H02.429   Myogenic ptosis of unspecified eyelid
 ● H02.43   **Paralytic** ptosis of eyelid
       Neurogenic ptosis of eyelid
   H02.431   Paralytic ptosis of right eyelid
   H02.432   Paralytic ptosis of left eyelid
   H02.433   Paralytic ptosis of bilateral eyelids
   H02.439   Paralytic ptosis unspecified eyelid
● H02.5   **Other disorders affecting eyelid function**
   Excludes2   blepharospasm (G24.5)
           organic tic (G25.69)
           psychogenic tic (F95.-)
 ● H02.51   **Abnormal innervation syndrome**
   H02.511   Abnormal innervation syndrome right upper eyelid
   H02.512   Abnormal innervation syndrome right lower eyelid
   H02.513   Abnormal innervation syndrome right eye, unspecified eyelid
   H02.514   Abnormal innervation syndrome left upper eyelid
   H02.515   Abnormal innervation syndrome left lower eyelid
   H02.516   Abnormal innervation syndrome left eye, unspecified eyelid
   H02.519   Abnormal innervation syndrome unspecified eye, unspecified eyelid

H02.52 Blepharophimosis
Drooping of eyelid with reduced lid size
Ankyloblepharon
H02.521 Blepharophimosis right upper eyelid
H02.522 Blepharophimosis right lower eyelid
H02.523 Blepharophimosis right eye, unspecified eyelid
H02.524 Blepharophimosis left upper eyelid
H02.525 Blepharophimosis left lower eyelid
H02.526 Blepharophimosis left eye, unspecified eyelid
H02.529 Blepharophimosis unspecified eye, unspecified lid

H02.53 Eyelid retraction
Eyelid lag
H02.531 Eyelid retraction right upper eyelid
H02.532 Eyelid retraction right lower eyelid
H02.533 Eyelid retraction right eye, unspecified eyelid
H02.534 Eyelid retraction left upper eyelid
H02.535 Eyelid retraction left lower eyelid
H02.536 Eyelid retraction left eye, unspecified eyelid
H02.539 Eyelid retraction unspecified eye, unspecified lid

H02.59 Other disorders affecting eyelid function
Deficient blink reflex
Sensory disorders

H02.6 Xanthelasma of eyelid
Yellow-to-orange patches or pimples clustered together on eyelid
H02.60 Xanthelasma of unspecified eye, unspecified eyelid
H02.61 Xanthelasma of right upper eyelid
H02.62 Xanthelasma of right lower eyelid
H02.63 Xanthelasma of right eye, unspecified eyelid
H02.64 Xanthelasma of left upper eyelid
H02.65 Xanthelasma of left lower eyelid
H02.66 Xanthelasma of left eye, unspecified eyelid

H02.7 Other and unspecified degenerative disorders of eyelid and periocular area
H02.70 Unspecified degenerative disorders of eyelid and periocular area
H02.71 Chloasma of eyelid and periocular area
Dyspigmentation of eyelid
Hyperpigmentation of eyelid
H02.711 Chloasma of right upper eyelid and periocular area
H02.712 Chloasma of right lower eyelid and periocular area
H02.713 Chloasma of right eye, unspecified eyelid and periocular area
H02.714 Chloasma of left upper eyelid and periocular area
H02.715 Chloasma of left lower eyelid and periocular area
H02.716 Chloasma of left eye, unspecified eyelid and periocular area
H02.719 Chloasma of unspecified eye, unspecified eyelid and periocular area
H02.72 Madarosis of eyelid and periocular area
Loss of eyelashes and/or eyebrows
Hypotrichosis of eyelid
H02.721 Madarosis of right upper eyelid and periocular area
H02.722 Madarosis of right lower eyelid and periocular area
H02.723 Madarosis of right eye, unspecified eyelid and periocular area

H02.724 Madarosis of left upper eyelid and periocular area
H02.725 Madarosis of left lower eyelid and periocular area
H02.726 Madarosis of left eye, unspecified eyelid and periocular area
H02.729 Madarosis of unspecified eye, unspecified eyelid and periocular area
H02.73 Vitiligo of eyelid and periocular area
Skin pigmentation disease characterized by white patches
Hypopigmentation of eyelid
H02.731 Vitiligo of right upper eyelid and periocular area
H02.732 Vitiligo of right lower eyelid and periocular area
H02.733 Vitiligo of right eye, unspecified eyelid and periocular area
H02.734 Vitiligo of left upper eyelid and periocular area
H02.735 Vitiligo of left lower eyelid and periocular area
H02.736 Vitiligo of left eye, unspecified eyelid and periocular area
H02.739 Vitiligo of unspecified eye, unspecified eyelid and periocular area
H02.79 Other degenerative disorders of eyelid and periocular area

H02.8 Other specified disorders of eyelid
H02.81 Retained foreign body in eyelid
Use additional code to identify the type of retained foreign body (Z18.-)
Excludes1 laceration of eyelid with foreign body (S01.12-)
retained intraocular foreign body (H44.6-, H44.7-)
superficial foreign body of eyelid and periocular area (S00.25-)
H02.811 Retained foreign body in right upper eyelid
H02.812 Retained foreign body in right lower eyelid
H02.813 Retained foreign body in right eye, unspecified eyelid
H02.814 Retained foreign body in left upper eyelid
H02.815 Retained foreign body in left lower eyelid
H02.816 Retained foreign body in left eye, unspecified eyelid
H02.819 Retained foreign body in unspecified eye, unspecified eyelid
H02.82 Cysts of eyelid
Sebaceous cyst of eyelid
H02.821 Cysts of right upper eyelid
H02.822 Cysts of right lower eyelid
H02.823 Cysts of right eye, unspecified eyelid
H02.824 Cysts of left upper eyelid
H02.825 Cysts of left lower eyelid
H02.826 Cysts of left eye, unspecified eyelid
H02.829 Cysts of unspecified eye, unspecified eyelid
H02.83 Dermatochalasis of eyelid
Skin is inelastic and hangs loosely in folds
H02.831 Dermatochalasis of right upper eyelid
H02.832 Dermatochalasis of right lower eyelid
H02.833 Dermatochalasis of right eye, unspecified eyelid
H02.834 Dermatochalasis of left upper eyelid

H02.835   Dermatochalasis of left lower eyelid

H02.836   Dermatochalasis of left eye, unspecified eyelid

H02.839   Dermatochalasis of unspecified eye, unspecified eyelid

● H02.84   Edema of eyelid
           Hyperemia of eyelid

H02.841   Edema of right upper eyelid

H02.842   Edema of right lower eyelid

H02.843   Edema of right eye, unspecified eyelid

H02.844   Edema of left upper eyelid

H02.845   Edema of left lower eyelid

H02.846   Edema of left eye, unspecified eyelid

H02.849   Edema of unspecified eye, unspecified eyelid

● H02.85   Elephantiasis of eyelid
           Massive secondary lymphedema with hypertrophy of skin and subcutaneous tissues (pachyderma)

H02.851   Elephantiasis of right upper eyelid

H02.852   Elephantiasis of right lower eyelid

H02.853   Elephantiasis of right eye, unspecified eyelid

H02.854   Elephantiasis of left upper eyelid

H02.855   Elephantiasis of left lower eyelid

H02.856   Elephantiasis of left eye, unspecified eyelid

H02.859   Elephantiasis of unspecified eye, unspecified eyelid

● H02.86   Hypertrichosis of eyelid
           Excessive growth of hair

H02.861   Hypertrichosis of right upper eyelid

H02.862   Hypertrichosis of right lower eyelid

H02.863   Hypertrichosis of right eye, unspecified eyelid

H02.864   Hypertrichosis of left upper eyelid

H02.865   Hypertrichosis of left lower eyelid

H02.866   Hypertrichosis of left eye, unspecified eyelid

H02.869   Hypertrichosis of unspecified eye, unspecified eyelid

● H02.87   Vascular anomalies of eyelid

H02.871   Vascular anomalies of right upper eyelid

H02.872   Vascular anomalies of right lower eyelid

H02.873   Vascular anomalies of right eye, unspecified eyelid

H02.874   Vascular anomalies of left upper eyelid

H02.875   Vascular anomalies of left lower eyelid

H02.876   Vascular anomalies of left eye, unspecified eyelid

H02.879   Vascular anomalies of unspecified eye, unspecified eyelid

● H02.88   Meibomian gland dysfunction of eyelid

H02.881   Meibomian gland dysfunction right upper eyelid

H02.882   Meibomian gland dysfunction right lower eyelid

H02.883   Meibomian gland dysfunction of right eye, unspecified eyelid

H02.884   Meibomian gland dysfunction left upper eyelid

H02.885   Meibomian gland dysfunction left lower eyelid

H02.886   Meibomian gland dysfunction of left eye, unspecified eyelid

H02.889   Meibomian gland dysfunction of unspecified eye, unspecified eyelid

H02.88A   Meibomian gland dysfunction right eye, upper and lower eyelids

H02.88B   Meibomian gland dysfunction left eye, upper and lower eyelids

H02.89   Other specified disorders of eyelid
           Hemorrhage of eyelid

H02.9   Unspecified disorder of eyelid
           Disorder of eyelid NOS

● H04   Disorders of lacrimal system
           Excludes1   congenital malformations of lacrimal system (Q10.4-Q10.6)

● H04.0   Dacryoadenitis
           Inflammation of lacrimal gland

● H04.00   Unspecified dacryoadenitis

H04.001   Unspecified dacryoadenitis, right lacrimal gland

H04.002   Unspecified dacryoadenitis, left lacrimal gland

H04.003   Unspecified dacryoadenitis, bilateral lacrimal glands

H04.009   Unspecified dacryoadenitis, unspecified lacrimal gland

● H04.01   Acute dacryoadenitis

H04.011   Acute dacryoadenitis, right lacrimal gland

H04.012   Acute dacryoadenitis, left lacrimal gland

H04.013   Acute dacryoadenitis, bilateral lacrimal glands

H04.019   Acute dacryoadenitis, unspecified lacrimal gland

★**(See Plate 19 of the Anatomy Illustrations.)**

● H04.02   Chronic dacryoadenitis

H04.021   Chronic dacryoadenitis, right lacrimal gland

H04.022   Chronic dacryoadenitis, left lacrimal gland

H04.023   Chronic dacryoadenitis, bilateral lacrimal gland

H04.029   Chronic dacryoadenitis, unspecified lacrimal gland

● H04.03   Chronic enlargement of lacrimal gland

H04.031   Chronic enlargement of right lacrimal gland

H04.032   Chronic enlargement of left lacrimal gland

H04.033   Chronic enlargement of bilateral lacrimal glands

H04.039   Chronic enlargement of unspecified lacrimal gland

● H04.1   Other disorders of lacrimal gland

● H04.11   Dacryops
           Watery eye or distention of lacrimal duct due to fluid

H04.111   Dacryops of right lacrimal gland

H04.112   Dacryops of left lacrimal gland

H04.113   Dacryops of bilateral lacrimal glands

H04.119   Dacryops of unspecified lacrimal gland

Figure 7-4   Lacrimal apparatus. (From Buck CJ: Step-by-Step Medical Coding, 2016, St. Louis, Elsevier, 2016)

CHAPTER 7 (H00-H59)

● **H04.12 Dry eye syndrome**
    Tear film insufficiency, NOS
    H04.121   Dry eye syndrome of right lacrimal gland
    H04.122   Dry eye syndrome of left lacrimal gland
    H04.123   Dry eye syndrome of bilateral lacrimal glands
    H04.129   Dry eye syndrome of unspecified lacrimal gland

● **H04.13 Lacrimal cyst**
    Lacrimal cystic degeneration
    H04.131   Lacrimal cyst right lacrimal gland
    H04.132   Lacrimal cyst left lacrimal gland
    H04.133   Lacrimal cyst bilateral lacrimal glands
    H04.139   Lacrimal cyst unspecified lacrimal gland

● **H04.14 Primary lacrimal gland atrophy**
    H04.141   Primary lacrimal gland atrophy, right lacrimal gland
    H04.142   Primary lacrimal gland atrophy, left lacrimal gland
    H04.143   Primary lacrimal gland atrophy, bilateral lacrimal glands
    H04.149   Primary lacrimal gland atrophy, unspecified lacrimal gland

● **H04.15 Secondary lacrimal gland atrophy**
    H04.151   Secondary lacrimal gland atrophy, right lacrimal gland
    H04.152   Secondary lacrimal gland atrophy, left lacrimal gland
    H04.153   Secondary lacrimal gland atrophy, bilateral lacrimal glands
    H04.159   Secondary lacrimal gland atrophy, unspecified lacrimal gland

● **H04.16 Lacrimal gland dislocation**
    H04.161   Lacrimal gland dislocation, right lacrimal gland
    H04.162   Lacrimal gland dislocation, left lacrimal gland
    H04.163   Lacrimal gland dislocation, bilateral lacrimal glands
    H04.169   Lacrimal gland dislocation, unspecified lacrimal gland

    H04.19 Other specified disorders of lacrimal gland

● **H04.2 Epiphora**
    Overflow of tears due to stricture of lacrimal passages; AKA lacrimation

● **H04.20 Unspecified epiphora**
    H04.201   Unspecified epiphora, right side
    H04.202   Unspecified epiphora, left side
    H04.203   Unspecified epiphora, bilateral
    H04.209   Unspecified epiphora, unspecified side

● **H04.21 Epiphora due to excess lacrimation**
    H04.211   Epiphora due to excess lacrimation, right lacrimal gland
    H04.212   Epiphora due to excess lacrimation, left lacrimal gland
    H04.213   Epiphora due to excess lacrimation, bilateral lacrimal glands
    H04.219   Epiphora due to excess lacrimation, unspecified lacrimal gland

● **H04.22 Epiphora due to insufficient drainage**
    H04.221   Epiphora due to insufficient drainage, right side
    H04.222   Epiphora due to insufficient drainage, left side
    H04.223   Epiphora due to insufficient drainage, bilateral
    H04.229   Epiphora due to insufficient drainage, unspecified side

● **H04.3 Acute and unspecified inflammation of lacrimal passages**
    Excludes1   neonatal dacryocystitis (P39.1)

● **H04.30 Unspecified dacryocystitis**
    H04.301   Unspecified dacryocystitis of right lacrimal passage
    H04.302   Unspecified dacryocystitis of left lacrimal passage
    H04.303   Unspecified dacryocystitis of bilateral lacrimal passages
    H04.309   Unspecified dacryocystitis of unspecified lacrimal passage

● **H04.31 Phlegmonous dacryocystitis**
    Cellulitis of lacrimal sac
    H04.311   Phlegmonous dacryocystitis of right lacrimal passage
    H04.312   Phlegmonous dacryocystitis of left lacrimal passage
    H04.313   Phlegmonous dacryocystitis of bilateral lacrimal passages
    H04.319   Phlegmonous dacryocystitis of unspecified lacrimal passage

● **H04.32 Acute dacryocystitis**
    Acute dacryopericystitis
    H04.321   Acute dacryocystitis of right lacrimal passage
    H04.322   Acute dacryocystitis of left lacrimal passage
    H04.323   Acute dacryocystitis of bilateral lacrimal passages
    H04.329   Acute dacryocystitis of unspecified lacrimal passage

● **H04.33 Acute lacrimal canaliculitis**
    H04.331   Acute lacrimal canaliculitis of right lacrimal passage
    H04.332   Acute lacrimal canaliculitis of left lacrimal passage
    H04.333   Acute lacrimal canaliculitis of bilateral lacrimal passages
    H04.339   Acute lacrimal canaliculitis of unspecified lacrimal passage

● **H04.4 Chronic inflammation of lacrimal passages**

● **H04.41 Chronic dacryocystitis**
    Inflammation of lacrimal sac
    H04.411   Chronic dacryocystitis of right lacrimal passage
    H04.412   Chronic dacryocystitis of left lacrimal passage
    H04.413   Chronic dacryocystitis of bilateral lacrimal passages
    H04.419   Chronic dacryocystitis of unspecified lacrimal passage

● **H04.42 Chronic lacrimal canaliculitis**
    Inflammation of lacrimal ducts
    H04.421   Chronic lacrimal canaliculitis of right lacrimal passage
    H04.422   Chronic lacrimal canaliculitis of left lacrimal passage
    H04.423   Chronic lacrimal canaliculitis of bilateral lacrimal passages
    H04.429   Chronic lacrimal canaliculitis of unspecified lacrimal passage

● **H04.43 Chronic lacrimal mucocele**
    Accumulation of mucous secretion
    H04.431   Chronic lacrimal mucocele of right lacrimal passage
    H04.432   Chronic lacrimal mucocele of left lacrimal passage
    H04.433   Chronic lacrimal mucocele of bilateral lacrimal passages
    H04.439   Chronic lacrimal mucocele of unspecified lacrimal passage

● **H04.5   Stenosis and insufficiency of lacrimal passages**
   ● **H04.51   Dacryolith**
      Concretion in lacrimal sac/duct; AKA lacrimal
      calculus
      H04.511   Dacryolith of right lacrimal passage
      H04.512   Dacryolith of left lacrimal passage
      H04.513   Dacryolith of bilateral lacrimal
              passages
      H04.519   Dacryolith of unspecified lacrimal
              passage
   ● **H04.52   Eversion of lacrimal punctum**
      Turning out of lacrimal drainage opening
      H04.521   Eversion of right lacrimal punctum
      H04.522   Eversion of left lacrimal punctum
      H04.523   Eversion of bilateral lacrimal
              punctum
      H04.529   Eversion of unspecified lacrimal
              punctum
   ● **H04.53   Neonatal obstruction of nasolacrimal duct**
      Excludes 1   congenital stenosis and stricture
              of lacrimal duct (Q10.5)
      H04.531   Neonatal obstruction of right
              nasolacrimal duct   N
      H04.532   Neonatal obstruction of left
              nasolacrimal duct   N
      H04.533   Neonatal obstruction of bilateral
              nasolacrimal duct   N
      H04.539   Neonatal obstruction of unspecified
              nasolacrimal duct   N
   ● **H04.54   Stenosis of lacrimal canaliculi**
      H04.541   Stenosis of right lacrimal canaliculi
      H04.542   Stenosis of left lacrimal canaliculi
      H04.543   Stenosis of bilateral lacrimal
              canaliculi
      H04.549   Stenosis of unspecified lacrimal
              canaliculi
   ● **H04.55   Acquired stenosis of nasolacrimal duct**
      H04.551   Acquired stenosis of right
              nasolacrimal duct
      H04.552   Acquired stenosis of left nasolacrimal
              duct
      H04.553   Acquired stenosis of bilateral
              nasolacrimal duct
      H04.559   Acquired stenosis of unspecified
              nasolacrimal duct
   ● **H04.56   Stenosis of lacrimal punctum**
      H04.561   Stenosis of right lacrimal punctum
      H04.562   Stenosis of left lacrimal punctum
      H04.563   Stenosis of bilateral lacrimal punctum
      H04.569   Stenosis of unspecified lacrimal
              punctum
   ● **H04.57   Stenosis of lacrimal sac**
      H04.571   Stenosis of right lacrimal sac
      H04.572   Stenosis of left lacrimal sac
      H04.573   Stenosis of bilateral lacrimal sac
      H04.579   Stenosis of unspecified lacrimal sac
● **H04.6   Other changes of lacrimal passages**
   ● **H04.61   Lacrimal fistula**
      H04.611   Lacrimal fistula right lacrimal passage
      H04.612   Lacrimal fistula left lacrimal passage
      H04.613   Lacrimal fistula bilateral lacrimal
              passages
      H04.619   Lacrimal fistula unspecified lacrimal
              passage
   H04.69   Other changes of lacrimal passages

● **H04.8   Other disorders of lacrimal system**
   ● **H04.81   Granuloma of lacrimal passages**
      Inflammatory response due to infectious or
      noninfectious agents
      H04.811   Granuloma of right lacrimal passage
      H04.812   Granuloma of left lacrimal passage
      H04.813   Granuloma of bilateral lacrimal
              passages
      H04.819   Granuloma of unspecified lacrimal
              passage
      H04.89   Other disorders of lacrimal system
   H04.9   Disorder of lacrimal system, unspecified
● **H05   Disorders of orbit**
      Excludes 1   congenital malformation of orbit (Q10.7)
   ● **H05.0   Acute inflammation of orbit**
      H05.00   Unspecified acute inflammation of orbit
      ● **H05.01   Cellulitis of orbit**
         Infection of soft tissue of orbit
         Abscess of orbit
         H05.011   Cellulitis of right orbit
         H05.012   Cellulitis of left orbit
         H05.013   Cellulitis of bilateral orbits
         H05.019   Cellulitis of unspecified orbit
      ● **H05.02   Osteomyelitis of orbit**
         Infection of boney orbit of eye
         H05.021   Osteomyelitis of right orbit
         H05.022   Osteomyelitis of left orbit
         H05.023   Osteomyelitis of bilateral orbits
         H05.029   Osteomyelitis of unspecified orbit
      ● **H05.03   Periostitis of orbit**
         Inflammation of periosteum (membrane covering
         bone surface)
         H05.031   Periostitis of right orbit
         H05.032   Periostitis of left orbit
         H05.033   Periostitis of bilateral orbits
         H05.039   Periostitis of unspecified orbit
      ● **H05.04   Tenonitis of orbit**
         Inflammation of tenon capsule (space enclosing
         fascia of Tenon between eyeball and fat of
         orbit)
         H05.041   Tenonitis of right orbit
         H05.042   Tenonitis of left orbit
         H05.043   Tenonitis of bilateral orbits
         H05.049   Tenonitis of unspecified orbit
   ● **H05.1   Chronic inflammatory disorders of orbit**
      H05.10   Unspecified chronic inflammatory disorders of
             orbit
      ● **H05.11   Granuloma of orbit**
         Pseudotumor (inflammatory) of orbit
         H05.111   Granuloma of right orbit
         H05.112   Granuloma of left orbit
         H05.113   Granuloma of bilateral orbits
         H05.119   Granuloma of unspecified orbit
      ● **H05.12   Orbital myositis**
         Inflammation of extraocular muscles of orbit
         H05.121   Orbital myositis, right orbit
         H05.122   Orbital myositis, left orbit
         H05.123   Orbital myositis, bilateral
         H05.129   Orbital myositis, unspecified orbit

Figure 7-5   Exophthalmos. (From Black JM, Hokanson JH: Medical-Surgical Nursing: Clinical Management for Positive Outcomes, St. Louis, Saunders Elsevier, 2009)

⬤ H05.2   **Exophthalmic conditions**
     Bulging eyes

H05.20   Unspecified exophthalmos

⬤ H05.21   Displacement (lateral) of globe

     H05.211   Displacement (lateral) of globe, right eye

     H05.212   Displacement (lateral) of globe, left eye

     H05.213   Displacement (lateral) of globe, bilateral

     H05.219   Displacement (lateral) of globe, unspecified eye

⬤ H05.22   Edema of orbit
     Orbital congestion

     H05.221   Edema of right orbit

     H05.222   Edema of left orbit

     H05.223   Edema of bilateral orbit

     H05.229   Edema of unspecified orbit

⬤ H05.23   Hemorrhage of orbit

     H05.231   Hemorrhage of right orbit

     H05.232   Hemorrhage of left orbit

     H05.233   Hemorrhage of bilateral orbit

     H05.239   Hemorrhage of unspecified orbit

⬤ H05.24   Constant exophthalmos
     Constant bulging eyes, often symptom of Graves disease

     H05.241   Constant exophthalmos, right eye

     H05.242   Constant exophthalmos, left eye

     H05.243   Constant exophthalmos, bilateral

     H05.249   Constant exophthalmos, unspecified eye

⬤ H05.25   Intermittent exophthalmos
     Intermittent bulging eye occurring with bending forward or sharp turning of head

     H05.251   Intermittent exophthalmos, right eye

     H05.252   Intermittent exophthalmos, left eye

     H05.253   Intermittent exophthalmos, bilateral

     H05.259   Intermittent exophthalmos, unspecified eye

⬤ H05.26   Pulsating exophthalmos
     Bulging eyes with pulsation and bruit, often due to aneurysm pushing eye forward

     H05.261   Pulsating exophthalmos, right eye

     H05.262   Pulsating exophthalmos, left eye

     H05.263   Pulsating exophthalmos, bilateral

     H05.269   Pulsating exophthalmos, unspecified eye

⬤ H05.3   **Deformity of orbit**
     Excludes1   congenital deformity of orbit (Q10.7)
             hypertelorism (Q75.2)

H05.30   Unspecified deformity of orbit

⬤ H05.31   Atrophy of orbit

     H05.311   Atrophy of right orbit

     H05.312   Atrophy of left orbit

     H05.313   Atrophy of bilateral orbit

     H05.319   Atrophy of unspecified orbit

⬤ H05.32   Deformity of orbit due to bone disease
     Code also associated bone disease

     H05.321   Deformity of right orbit due to bone disease

     H05.322   Deformity of left orbit due to bone disease

     H05.323   Deformity of bilateral orbits due to bone disease

     H05.329   Deformity of unspecified orbit due to bone disease

⬤ H05.33   Deformity of orbit due to trauma or surgery

     H05.331   Deformity of right orbit due to trauma or surgery

     H05.332   Deformity of left orbit due to trauma or surgery

     H05.333   Deformity of bilateral orbits due to trauma or surgery

     H05.339   Deformity of unspecified orbit due to trauma or surgery

⬤ H05.34   Enlargement of orbit

     H05.341   Enlargement of right orbit

     H05.342   Enlargement of left orbit

     H05.343   Enlargement of bilateral orbits

     H05.349   Enlargement of unspecified orbit

⬤ H05.35   Exostosis of orbit

     H05.351   Exostosis of right orbit

     H05.352   Exostosis of left orbit

     H05.353   Exostosis of bilateral orbits

     H05.359   Exostosis of unspecified orbit

⬤ H05.4   **Enophthalmos**
     Recessed eyeball into orbit

⬤ H05.40   Unspecified enophthalmos

     H05.401   Unspecified enophthalmos, right eye

     H05.402   Unspecified enophthalmos, left eye

     H05.403   Unspecified enophthalmos, bilateral

     H05.409   Unspecified enophthalmos, unspecified eye

⬤ H05.41   Enophthalmos due to atrophy of orbital tissue

     H05.411   Enophthalmos due to atrophy of orbital tissue, right eye

     H05.412   Enophthalmos due to atrophy of orbital tissue, left eye

     H05.413   Enophthalmos due to atrophy of orbital tissue, bilateral

     H05.419   Enophthalmos due to atrophy of orbital tissue, unspecified eye

⬤ H05.42   Enophthalmos due to trauma or surgery

     H05.421   Enophthalmos due to trauma or surgery, right eye

     H05.422   Enophthalmos due to trauma or surgery, left eye

     H05.423   Enophthalmos due to trauma or surgery, bilateral

     H05.429   Enophthalmos due to trauma or surgery, unspecified eye

● **H05.5**   **Retained (old) foreign body following penetrating wound of orbit**
     Retrobulbar foreign body
     Use additional code to identify the type of retained foreign body (Z18.-)
     Excludes1   current penetrating wound of orbit (S05.4-)
     Excludes2   retained foreign body of eyelid (H02.81-) retained intraocular foreign body (H44.6-, H44.7-)
     H05.50   Retained (old) foreign body following penetrating wound of unspecified orbit
     H05.51   Retained (old) foreign body following penetrating wound of right orbit
     H05.52   Retained (old) foreign body following penetrating wound of left orbit
     H05.53   Retained (old) foreign body following penetrating wound of bilateral orbits

● **H05.8**   Other disorders of orbit
   ● **H05.81**   Cyst of orbit
     Encephalocele of orbit
     H05.811   Cyst of right orbit
     H05.812   Cyst of left orbit
     H05.813   Cyst of bilateral orbits
     H05.819   Cyst of unspecified orbit
   ● **H05.82**   Myopathy of extraocular muscles
     Weakness of muscles of eye
     H05.821   Myopathy of extraocular muscles, right orbit
     H05.822   Myopathy of extraocular muscles, left orbit
     H05.823   Myopathy of extraocular muscles, bilateral
     H05.829   Myopathy of extraocular muscles, unspecified orbit
   H05.89   Other disorders of orbit
  H05.9   Unspecified disorder of orbit

DISORDERS OF CONJUNCTIVA (H10-H11)

★ **(See Plate 18 of the Anatomy Illustrations.)**

● **H10**   Conjunctivitis
   Inflammation of membrane of the inside of the eyelid or on surface of eye (conjunctiva)
   Excludes1   keratoconjunctivitis (H16.2-)
  ● **H10.0**   Mucopurulent conjunctivitis
   ● **H10.01**   Acute follicular conjunctivitis
     H10.011   Acute follicular conjunctivitis, right eye
     H10.012   Acute follicular conjunctivitis, left eye
     H10.013   Acute follicular conjunctivitis, bilateral
     H10.019   Acute follicular conjunctivitis, unspecified eye
   ● **H10.02**   Other mucopurulent conjunctivitis
     H10.021   Other mucopurulent conjunctivitis, right eye
     H10.022   Other mucopurulent conjunctivitis, left eye
     H10.023   Other mucopurulent conjunctivitis, bilateral
     H10.029   Other mucopurulent conjunctivitis, unspecified eye
  ● **H10.1**   Acute atopic conjunctivitis
   Acute papillary conjunctivitis
     H10.10   Acute atopic conjunctivitis, unspecified eye
     H10.11   Acute atopic conjunctivitis, right eye
     H10.12   Acute atopic conjunctivitis, left eye
     H10.13   Acute atopic conjunctivitis, bilateral

● **H10.2**   Other acute conjunctivitis
   ● **H10.21**   Acute toxic conjunctivitis
     Acute chemical conjunctivitis
     Code first (T51-T65) to identify chemical and intent
     Excludes1   burn and corrosion of eye and adnexa (T26.-)
     H10.211   Acute toxic conjunctivitis, right eye
     H10.212   Acute toxic conjunctivitis, left eye
     H10.213   Acute toxic conjunctivitis, bilateral
     H10.219   Acute toxic conjunctivitis, unspecified eye
   ● **H10.22**   Pseudomembranous conjunctivitis
     H10.221   Pseudomembranous conjunctivitis, right eye
     H10.222   Pseudomembranous conjunctivitis, left eye
     H10.223   Pseudomembranous conjunctivitis, bilateral
     H10.229   Pseudomembranous conjunctivitis, unspecified eye
   ● **H10.23**   Serous conjunctivitis, except viral
     Excludes1   viral conjunctivitis (B30.-)
     H10.231   Serous conjunctivitis, except viral, right eye
     H10.232   Serous conjunctivitis, except viral, left eye
     H10.233   Serous conjunctivitis, except viral, bilateral
     H10.239   Serous conjunctivitis, except viral, unspecified eye
  ● **H10.3**   Unspecified acute conjunctivitis
     Excludes1   ophthalmia neonatorum NOS (P39.1)
     H10.30   Unspecified acute conjunctivitis, unspecified eye
     H10.31   Unspecified acute conjunctivitis, right eye
     H10.32   Unspecified acute conjunctivitis, left eye
     H10.33   Unspecified acute conjunctivitis, bilateral
  ● **H10.4**   Chronic conjunctivitis
   ● **H10.40**   Unspecified chronic conjunctivitis
     H10.401   Unspecified chronic conjunctivitis, right eye
     H10.402   Unspecified chronic conjunctivitis, left eye
     H10.403   Unspecified chronic conjunctivitis, bilateral
     H10.409   Unspecified chronic conjunctivitis, unspecified eye
   ● **H10.41**   Chronic giant papillary conjunctivitis
     Inflammation of membrane of the inside of the eyelid or on surface of eye often associated with contact lens wear
     H10.411   Chronic giant papillary conjunctivitis, right eye
     H10.412   Chronic giant papillary conjunctivitis, left eye
     H10.413   Chronic giant papillary conjunctivitis, bilateral
     H10.419   Chronic giant papillary conjunctivitis, unspecified eye
   ● **H10.42**   Simple chronic conjunctivitis
     H10.421   Simple chronic conjunctivitis, right eye
     H10.422   Simple chronic conjunctivitis, left eye
     H10.423   Simple chronic conjunctivitis, bilateral
     H10.429   Simple chronic conjunctivitis, unspecified eye

CHAPTER 7 (H00-H59)

● H10.43   Chronic follicular conjunctivitis
> *Inflammation of membrane of the inside of the eyelid or on surface of eye due to topical medications or infection*

     H10.431   Chronic follicular conjunctivitis, right eye

     H10.432   Chronic follicular conjunctivitis, left eye

     H10.433   Chronic follicular conjunctivitis, bilateral

     H10.439   Chronic follicular conjunctivitis, unspecified eye

   H10.44   Vernal conjunctivitis
> *Affecting children, especially boys in which there are flattened papules with thick, gelatinous exudate on conjunctivae on inside of upper lid*

     Excludes1   vernal keratoconjunctivitis with limbar and corneal involvement (H16.26-)

   H10.45   Other chronic allergic conjunctivitis

● H10.5   Blepharoconjunctivitis
> *Inflammation of eyelids and conjunctiva*

 ● H10.50   Unspecified blepharoconjunctivitis

     H10.501   Unspecified blepharoconjunctivitis, right eye

     H10.502   Unspecified blepharoconjunctivitis, left eye

     H10.503   Unspecified blepharoconjunctivitis, bilateral

     H10.509   Unspecified blepharoconjunctivitis, unspecified eye

 ● H10.51   Ligneous conjunctivitis
> Code also underlying condition if known, such as:
> plasminogen deficiency (E88.02)

     H10.511   Ligneous conjunctivitis, right eye

     H10.512   Ligneous conjunctivitis, left eye

     H10.513   Ligneous conjunctivitis, bilateral

     H10.519   Ligneous conjunctivitis, unspecified eye

 ● H10.52   Angular blepharoconjunctivitis

     H10.521   Angular blepharoconjunctivitis, right eye

     H10.522   Angular blepharoconjunctivitis, left eye

     H10.523   Angular blepharoconjunctivitis, bilateral

     H10.529   Angular blepharoconjunctivitis, unspecified eye

 ● H10.53   Contact blepharoconjunctivitis

     H10.531   Contact blepharoconjunctivitis, right eye

     H10.532   Contact blepharoconjunctivitis, left eye

     H10.533   Contact blepharoconjunctivitis, bilateral

     H10.539   Contact blepharoconjunctivitis, unspecified eye

● H10.8   Other conjunctivitis

 ● H10.81   Pingueculitis
> *Inflammation of a yellow, raised thickening on the white of the eye associated with chronic dry eyes*

     Excludes1   pinguecula (H11.15-)

     H10.811   Pingueculitis, right eye

     H10.812   Pingueculitis, left eye

     H10.813   Pingueculitis, bilateral

     H10.819   Pingueculitis, unspecified eye

 ● H10.82   Rosacea conjunctivitis
> Code first underlying rosacea dermatitis (L71.-)

     H10.821   Rosacea conjunctivitis, right eye

     H10.822   Rosacea conjunctivitis, left eye

     H10.823   Rosacea conjunctivitis, bilateral
> **Coding Clinic: 2018, Q4, P15**

     H10.829   Rosacea conjunctivitis, unspecified eye

   H10.89   Other conjunctivitis

   H10.9   Unspecified conjunctivitis

● H11   Other disorders of conjunctiva
     Excludes1   keratoconjunctivitis (H16.2-)

 ● H11.0   Pterygium of eye
     Excludes1   pseudopterygium (H11.81-)

 ● H11.00   Unspecified pterygium of eye

     H11.001   Unspecified pterygium of right eye

     H11.002   Unspecified pterygium of left eye

     H11.003   Unspecified pterygium of eye, bilateral

     H11.009   Unspecified pterygium of unspecified eye

 ● H11.01   Amyloid pterygium

     H11.011   Amyloid pterygium of right eye

     H11.012   Amyloid pterygium of left eye

     H11.013   Amyloid pterygium of eye, bilateral

     H11.019   Amyloid pterygium of unspecified eye

 ● H11.02   Central pterygium of eye

     H11.021   Central pterygium of right eye

     H11.022   Central pterygium of left eye

     H11.023   Central pterygium of eye, bilateral

     H11.029   Central pterygium of unspecified eye

 ● H11.03   Double pterygium of eye

     H11.031   Double pterygium of right eye

     H11.032   Double pterygium of left eye

     H11.033   Double pterygium of eye, bilateral

     H11.039   Double pterygium of unspecified eye

 ● H11.04   Peripheral pterygium of eye, stationary

     H11.041   Peripheral pterygium, stationary, right eye

     H11.042   Peripheral pterygium, stationary, left eye

     H11.043   Peripheral pterygium, stationary, bilateral

     H11.049   Peripheral pterygium, stationary, unspecified eye

 ● H11.05   Peripheral pterygium of eye, progressive

     H11.051   Peripheral pterygium, progressive, right eye

     H11.052   Peripheral pterygium, progressive, left eye

     H11.053   Peripheral pterygium, progressive, bilateral

     H11.059   Peripheral pterygium, progressive, unspecified eye

 ● H11.06   Recurrent pterygium of eye

     H11.061   Recurrent pterygium of right eye

     H11.062   Recurrent pterygium of left eye

     H11.063   Recurrent pterygium of eye, bilateral

     H11.069   Recurrent pterygium of unspecified eye

Figure 7-6   Double pterygium. Note both nasal and temporal pterygia in a 57-year-old farmer. (From Brightbill FS, McDonnell PJ: Corneal Surgery: Theory, Technique and Tissue, S.l., Mosby Elsevier, 2009)

Item 7-2   **Pterygium** is Greek for batlike. The condition is characterized by a membrane that extends from the limbus to the center of the cornea and resembles a wing.

▶ New   ⇒ Revised   ~~deleted~~ Deleted   Excludes 1   Excludes 2   Includes   Use additional   Code first   Code also   Key words

OGCR Official Guidelines   X Assign placeholder X   ● Use Additional Character(s)   ▌ Manifestation Code   ⚙ Hierarchical Condition Category   **Coding Clinic**

● **H11.1**   **Conjunctival degenerations and deposits**
      Excludes2   pseudopterygium (H11.81)
    H11.10   Unspecified conjunctival degenerations
● H11.11   Conjunctival deposits
      H11.111   Conjunctival deposits, right eye
      H11.112   Conjunctival deposits, left eye
      H11.113   Conjunctival deposits, bilateral
      H11.119   Conjunctival deposits, unspecified eye
● H11.12   Conjunctival concretions
      White to yellow nodules within or beneath conjunctiva
      H11.121   Conjunctival concretions, right eye
      H11.122   Conjunctival concretions, left eye
      H11.123   Conjunctival concretions, bilateral
      H11.129   Conjunctival concretions, unspecified eye
● H11.13   Conjunctival pigmentations
      Conjunctival argyrosis [argyria]
      H11.131   Conjunctival pigmentations, right eye
      H11.132   Conjunctival pigmentations, left eye
      H11.133   Conjunctival pigmentations, bilateral
      H11.139   Conjunctival pigmentations, unspecified eye
● H11.14   Conjunctival xerosis, unspecified
      Excludes1   xerosis of conjunctiva due to vitamin A deficiency (E50.0, E50.1)
      H11.141   Conjunctival xerosis, unspecified, right eye
      H11.142   Conjunctival xerosis, unspecified, left eye
      H11.143   Conjunctival xerosis, unspecified, bilateral
      H11.149   Conjunctival xerosis, unspecified, unspecified eye
● H11.15   Pinguecula
      Yellowish spot near sclerocorneal junction, usually on nasal side; associated with aging
      Excludes1   pingueculitis (H10.81-)
      H11.151   Pinguecula, right eye
      H11.152   Pinguecula, left eye
      H11.153   Pinguecula, bilateral
      H11.159   Pinguecula, unspecified eye
● **H11.2**   **Conjunctival scars**
● H11.21   Conjunctival adhesions and strands (localized)
      H11.211   Conjunctival adhesions and strands (localized), right eye
      H11.212   Conjunctival adhesions and strands (localized), left eye
      H11.213   Conjunctival adhesions and strands (localized), bilateral
      H11.219   Conjunctival adhesions and strands (localized), unspecified eye
● H11.22   Conjunctival granuloma
      H11.221   Conjunctival granuloma, right eye
      H11.222   Conjunctival granuloma, left eye
      H11.223   Conjunctival granuloma, bilateral
      H11.229   Conjunctival granuloma, unspecified
● H11.23   Symblepharon
      Adhesion between tarsal conjunctiva and bulbar conjunctiva
      H11.231   Symblepharon, right eye
      H11.232   Symblepharon, left eye
      H11.233   Symblepharon, bilateral
      H11.239   Symblepharon, unspecified eye

● H11.24   Scarring of conjunctiva
      H11.241   Scarring of conjunctiva, right eye
      H11.242   Scarring of conjunctiva, left eye
      H11.243   Scarring of conjunctiva, bilateral
      H11.249   Scarring of conjunctiva, unspecified eye
● **H11.3**   **Conjunctival hemorrhage**
    Subconjunctival hemorrhage
    H11.30   Conjunctival hemorrhage, unspecified eye
    H11.31   Conjunctival hemorrhage, right eye
    H11.32   Conjunctival hemorrhage, left eye
    H11.33   Conjunctival hemorrhage, bilateral
● **H11.4**   **Other conjunctival vascular disorders and cysts**
● H11.41   Vascular abnormalities of conjunctiva
      Conjunctival aneurysm
      H11.411   Vascular abnormalities of conjunctiva, right eye
      H11.412   Vascular abnormalities of conjunctiva, left eye
      H11.413   Vascular abnormalities of conjunctiva, bilateral
      H11.419   Vascular abnormalities of conjunctiva, unspecified eye
● H11.42   Conjunctival edema
      H11.421   Conjunctival edema, right eye
      H11.422   Conjunctival edema, left eye
      H11.423   Conjunctival edema, bilateral
      H11.429   Conjunctival edema, unspecified eye
● H11.43   Conjunctival hyperemia
      H11.431   Conjunctival hyperemia, right eye
      H11.432   Conjunctival hyperemia, left eye
      H11.433   Conjunctival hyperemia, bilateral
      H11.439   Conjunctival hyperemia, unspecified eye
● H11.44   Conjunctival cysts
      H11.441   Conjunctival cysts, right eye
      H11.442   Conjunctival cysts, left eye
      H11.443   Conjunctival cysts, bilateral
      H11.449   Conjunctival cysts, unspecified eye
● **H11.8**   **Other specified disorders of conjunctiva**
● H11.81   Pseudopterygium of conjunctiva
      Conjunctival scar attached to cornea
      H11.811   Pseudopterygium of conjunctiva, right eye
      H11.812   Pseudopterygium of conjunctiva, left eye
      H11.813   Pseudopterygium of conjunctiva, bilateral
      H11.819   Pseudopterygium of conjunctiva, unspecified eye
● H11.82   Conjunctivochalasis
      Conjunctiva bulges over eyelid margin or covers lower punctum
      H11.821   Conjunctivochalasis, right eye
      H11.822   Conjunctivochalasis, left eye
      H11.823   Conjunctivochalasis, bilateral
      H11.829   Conjunctivochalasis, unspecified eye
    H11.89   Other specified disorders of conjunctiva
  H11.9   Unspecified disorder of conjunctiva

CHAPTER 7 (H00-H59)

DISORDERS OF SCLERA, CORNEA, IRIS AND CILIARY BODY (H15-H22)

● H15   Disorders of sclera
   ● H15.0   Scleritis
     Inflammation of the white (sclera and episclera) of the eye.
     ● H15.00   Unspecified scleritis
       H15.001   Unspecified scleritis, right eye
       H15.002   Unspecified scleritis, left eye
       H15.003   Unspecified scleritis, bilateral
       H15.009   Unspecified scleritis, unspecified eye
     ● H15.01   Anterior scleritis
       H15.011   Anterior scleritis, right eye
       H15.012   Anterior scleritis, left eye
       H15.013   Anterior scleritis, bilateral
       H15.019   Anterior scleritis, unspecified eye
     ● H15.02   Brawny scleritis
       Swelling around the cornea that is gelantinous in appearance
       H15.021   Brawny scleritis, right eye
       H15.022   Brawny scleritis, left eye
       H15.023   Brawny scleritis, bilateral
       H15.029   Brawny scleritis, unspecified eye
     ● H15.03   Posterior scleritis
       Sclerotenonitis
       H15.031   Posterior scleritis, right eye
       H15.032   Posterior scleritis, left eye
       H15.033   Posterior scleritis, bilateral
       H15.039   Posterior scleritis, unspecified eye
     ● H15.04   Scleritis with corneal involvement
       H15.041   Scleritis with corneal involvement, right eye
       H15.042   Scleritis with corneal involvement, left eye
       H15.043   Scleritis with corneal involvement, bilateral
       H15.049   Scleritis with corneal involvement, unspecified eye
     ● H15.05   Scleromalacia perforans
       Necrotic without inflammation; usually associated with rheumatoid arthritis
       H15.051   Scleromalacia perforans, right eye
       H15.052   Scleromalacia perforans, left eye
       H15.053   Scleromalacia perforans, bilateral
       H15.059   Scleromalacia perforans, unspecified eye
     ● H15.09   Other scleritis
       Scleral abscess
       H15.091   Other scleritis, right eye
       H15.092   Other scleritis, left eye
       H15.093   Other scleritis, bilateral
       H15.099   Other scleritis, unspecified eye
   ● H15.1   Episcleritis
     Inflammation of the white (sclera and episclera) of the eye.
     ● H15.10   Unspecified episcleritis
       H15.101   Unspecified episcleritis, right eye
       H15.102   Unspecified episcleritis, left eye
       H15.103   Unspecified episcleritis, bilateral
       H15.109   Unspecified episcleritis, unspecified eye
     ● H15.11   Episcleritis periodica fugax
       Transient, recurrent inflammation of portion of episclera (connective tissue on the surface of the sclera)
       H15.111   Episcleritis periodica fugax, right eye
       H15.112   Episcleritis periodica fugax, left eye
       H15.113   Episcleritis periodica fugax, bilateral
       H15.119   Episcleritis periodica fugax, unspecified eye

     ● H15.12   Nodular episcleritis
       Characterized by tender, localized, moveable nodule within inflamed area
       H15.121   Nodular episcleritis, right eye
       H15.122   Nodular episcleritis, left eye
       H15.123   Nodular episcleritis, bilateral
       H15.129   Nodular episcleritis, unspecified eye
   ● H15.8   Other disorders of sclera
     Excludes2   blue sclera (Q13.5)
       degenerative myopia (H44.2-)
     ● H15.81   Equatorial staphyloma
       H15.811   Equatorial staphyloma, right eye
       H15.812   Equatorial staphyloma, left eye
       H15.813   Equatorial staphyloma, bilateral
       H15.819   Equatorial staphyloma, unspecified eye
     ● H15.82   Localized anterior staphyloma
       H15.821   Localized anterior staphyloma, right eye
       H15.822   Localized anterior staphyloma, left eye
       H15.823   Localized anterior staphyloma, bilateral
       H15.829   Localized anterior staphyloma, unspecified eye
     ● H15.83   Staphyloma posticum
       H15.831   Staphyloma posticum, right eye
       H15.832   Staphyloma posticum, left eye
       H15.833   Staphyloma posticum, bilateral
       H15.839   Staphyloma posticum, unspecified eye
     ● H15.84   Scleral ectasia
       H15.841   Scleral ectasia, right eye
       H15.842   Scleral ectasia, left eye
       H15.843   Scleral ectasia, bilateral
       H15.849   Scleral ectasia, unspecified eye
     ● H15.85   Ring staphyloma
       H15.851   Ring staphyloma, right eye
       H15.852   Ring staphyloma, left eye
       H15.853   Ring staphyloma, bilateral
       H15.859   Ring staphyloma, unspecified eye
     H15.89   Other disorders of sclera
   H15.9   Unspecified disorder of sclera

● H16   Keratitis
   ● H16.0   Corneal ulcer
     ● H16.00   Unspecified corneal ulcer
       H16.001   Unspecified corneal ulcer, right eye
       H16.002   Unspecified corneal ulcer, left eye
       H16.003   Unspecified corneal ulcer, bilateral
       H16.009   Unspecified corneal ulcer, unspecified eye
     ● H16.01   Central corneal ulcer
       H16.011   Central corneal ulcer, right eye
       H16.012   Central corneal ulcer, left eye
       H16.013   Central corneal ulcer, bilateral
       H16.019   Central corneal ulcer, unspecified eye
     ● H16.02   Ring corneal ulcer
       H16.021   Ring corneal ulcer, right eye
       H16.022   Ring corneal ulcer, left eye
       H16.023   Ring corneal ulcer, bilateral
       H16.029   Ring corneal ulcer, unspecified eye
     ● H16.03   Corneal ulcer with hypopyon
       H16.031   Corneal ulcer with hypopyon, right eye
       H16.032   Corneal ulcer with hypopyon, left eye
       H16.033   Corneal ulcer with hypopyon, bilateral
       H16.039   Corneal ulcer with hypopyon, unspecified eye

▶ New   ⇒ Revised   ~~deleted~~ Deleted   Excludes 1   Excludes 2   Includes   Use additional   Code first   Code also   Key words

OGCR Official Guidelines   X Assign placeholder X   ● Use Additional Character(s)   ▶ Manifestation Code   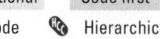 Hierarchical Condition Category   **Coding Clinic**

Marginal (catarrhal) ulcer   Ring ulcer   Central corneal ulcer   Rosacea ulcer   Mooren's (rodent) ulcer

Figure 7-7   Corneal ulcers: marginal, ring, central corneal, rosacea, and Mooren's.

Item 7-3   An infected ulcer is usually called a **serpiginous** or **hypopyon** ulcer, which is a pus sac in the anterior chamber of the eye. **Marginal** ulcers are usually asymptomatic, not primary, and are often superficial and simple. More severe marginal ulcers spread to form a ring ulcer. **Ring** ulcers can extend around the entire corneal periphery. **Central corneal** ulcers develop when there is an abrasion to the epithelium and an infection develops in the eroded area. The **pyocyaneal** ulcer is the most serious corneal infection, which, if left untreated, can lead to loss of the eye.

● H16.04   Marginal corneal ulcer
     H16.041   Marginal corneal ulcer, right eye
     H16.042   Marginal corneal ulcer, left eye
     H16.043   Marginal corneal ulcer, bilateral
     H16.049   Marginal corneal ulcer, unspecified eye

● H16.05   Mooren's corneal ulcer
     H16.051   Mooren's corneal ulcer, right eye
     H16.052   Mooren's corneal ulcer, left eye
     H16.053   Mooren's corneal ulcer, bilateral
     H16.059   Mooren's corneal ulcer, unspecified eye

● H16.06   Mycotic corneal ulcer
     H16.061   Mycotic corneal ulcer, right eye
     H16.062   Mycotic corneal ulcer, left eye
     H16.063   Mycotic corneal ulcer, bilateral
     H16.069   Mycotic corneal ulcer, unspecified eye

● H16.07   Perforated corneal ulcer
     H16.071   Perforated corneal ulcer, right eye
     H16.072   Perforated corneal ulcer, left eye
     H16.073   Perforated corneal ulcer, bilateral
     H16.079   Perforated corneal ulcer, unspecified eye

● H16.1   Other and unspecified superficial keratitis without conjunctivitis
  ● H16.10   Unspecified superficial keratitis
     H16.101   Unspecified superficial keratitis, right eye
     H16.102   Unspecified superficial keratitis, left eye
     H16.103   Unspecified superficial keratitis, bilateral
     H16.109   Unspecified superficial keratitis, unspecified eye

  ● H16.11   Macular keratitis
     Areolar keratitis
     Nummular keratitis
     Stellate keratitis
     Striate keratitis
     H16.111   Macular keratitis, right eye
     H16.112   Macular keratitis, left eye
     H16.113   Macular keratitis, bilateral
     H16.119   Macular keratitis, unspecified eye

  ● H16.12   Filamentary keratitis
     H16.121   Filamentary keratitis, right eye
     H16.122   Filamentary keratitis, left eye
     H16.123   Filamentary keratitis, bilateral
     H16.129   Filamentary keratitis, unspecified eye

● H16.13   Photokeratitis
     Snow blindness
     Welders' keratitis
     H16.131   Photokeratitis, right eye
     H16.132   Photokeratitis, left eye
     H16.133   Photokeratitis, bilateral
     H16.139   Photokeratitis, unspecified eye

● H16.14   Punctate keratitis
     H16.141   Punctate keratitis, right eye
     H16.142   Punctate keratitis, left eye
     H16.143   Punctate keratitis, bilateral
     H16.149   Punctate keratitis, unspecified eye

● H16.2   Keratoconjunctivitis
  ● H16.20   Unspecified keratoconjunctivitis
     Superficial keratitis with conjunctivitis NOS
     H16.201   Unspecified keratoconjunctivitis, right eye
     H16.202   Unspecified keratoconjunctivitis, left eye
     H16.203   Unspecified keratoconjunctivitis, bilateral
     H16.209   Unspecified keratoconjunctivitis, unspecified eye

  ● H16.21   Exposure keratoconjunctivitis
     H16.211   Exposure keratoconjunctivitis, right eye
     H16.212   Exposure keratoconjunctivitis, left eye
     H16.213   Exposure keratoconjunctivitis, bilateral
     H16.219   Exposure keratoconjunctivitis, unspecified eye

  ● H16.22   Keratoconjunctivitis sicca, not specified as Sjögren's
     Excludes1   Sjogren's syndrome (M35.01)
     H16.221   Keratoconjunctivitis sicca, not specified as Sjögren's, right eye
     H16.222   Keratoconjunctivitis sicca, not specified as Sjögren's, left eye
     H16.223   Keratoconjunctivitis sicca, not specified as Sjögren's, bilateral
     H16.229   Keratoconjunctivitis sicca, not specified as Sjögren's, unspecified eye

  ● H16.23   Neurotrophic keratoconjunctivitis
     H16.231   Neurotrophic keratoconjunctivitis, right eye
     H16.232   Neurotrophic keratoconjunctivitis, left eye
     H16.233   Neurotrophic keratoconjunctivitis, bilateral
     H16.239   Neurotrophic keratoconjunctivitis, unspecified eye

  ● H16.24   Ophthalmia nodosa
     H16.241   Ophthalmia nodosa, right eye
     H16.242   Ophthalmia nodosa, left eye
     H16.243   Ophthalmia nodosa, bilateral
     H16.249   Ophthalmia nodosa, unspecified eye

  ● H16.25   Phlyctenular keratoconjunctivitis
     H16.251   Phlyctenular keratoconjunctivitis, right eye
     H16.252   Phlyctenular keratoconjunctivitis, left eye
     H16.253   Phlyctenular keratoconjunctivitis, bilateral
     H16.259   Phlyctenular keratoconjunctivitis, unspecified eye

CHAPTER 7 (H00-H59)

● H16.26 **Vernal keratoconjunctivitis, with limbar and corneal involvement**
> **Excludes1** vernal conjunctivitis without limbar and corneal involvement (H10.44)

H16.261 Vernal keratoconjunctivitis, with limbar and corneal involvement, right eye
H16.262 Vernal keratoconjunctivitis, with limbar and corneal involvement, left eye
H16.263 Vernal keratoconjunctivitis, with limbar and corneal involvement, bilateral
H16.269 Vernal keratoconjunctivitis, with limbar and corneal involvement, unspecified eye

● H16.29 **Other keratoconjunctivitis**
H16.291 Other keratoconjunctivitis, right eye
H16.292 Other keratoconjunctivitis, left eye
H16.293 Other keratoconjunctivitis, bilateral
H16.299 Other keratoconjunctivitis, unspecified eye

● H16.3 **Interstitial and deep keratitis**
● H16.30 **Unspecified interstitial keratitis**
H16.301 Unspecified interstitial keratitis, right eye
H16.302 Unspecified interstitial keratitis, left eye
H16.303 Unspecified interstitial keratitis, bilateral
H16.309 Unspecified interstitial keratitis, unspecified eye

● H16.31 **Corneal abscess**
H16.311 Corneal abscess, right eye
H16.312 Corneal abscess, left eye
H16.313 Corneal abscess, bilateral
H16.319 Corneal abscess, unspecified eye

● H16.32 **Diffuse interstitial keratitis**
Cogan's syndrome
H16.321 Diffuse interstitial keratitis, right eye
H16.322 Diffuse interstitial keratitis, left eye
H16.323 Diffuse interstitial keratitis, bilateral
H16.329 Diffuse interstitial keratitis, unspecified eye

● H16.33 **Sclerosing keratitis**
H16.331 Sclerosing keratitis, right eye
H16.332 Sclerosing keratitis, left eye
H16.333 Sclerosing keratitis, bilateral
H16.339 Sclerosing keratitis, unspecified eye

● H16.39 **Other interstitial and deep keratitis**
H16.391 Other interstitial and deep keratitis, right eye
H16.392 Other interstitial and deep keratitis, left eye
H16.393 Other interstitial and deep keratitis, bilateral
H16.399 Other interstitial and deep keratitis, unspecified eye

● H16.4 **Corneal neovascularization**
● H16.40 **Unspecified corneal neovascularization**
H16.401 Unspecified corneal neovascularization, right eye
H16.402 Unspecified corneal neovascularization, left eye
H16.403 Unspecified corneal neovascularization, bilateral
H16.409 Unspecified corneal neovascularization, unspecified eye

● H16.41 **Ghost vessels (corneal)**
H16.411 Ghost vessels (corneal), right eye
H16.412 Ghost vessels (corneal), left eye
H16.413 Ghost vessels (corneal), bilateral
H16.419 Ghost vessels (corneal), unspecified eye

● H16.42 **Pannus (corneal)**
H16.421 Pannus (corneal), right eye
H16.422 Pannus (corneal), left eye
H16.423 Pannus (corneal), bilateral
H16.429 Pannus (corneal), unspecified eye

● H16.43 **Localized vascularization of cornea**
H16.431 Localized vascularization of cornea, right eye
H16.432 Localized vascularization of cornea, left eye
H16.433 Localized vascularization of cornea, bilateral
H16.439 Localized vascularization of cornea, unspecified eye

● H16.44 **Deep vascularization of cornea**
H16.441 Deep vascularization of cornea, right eye
H16.442 Deep vascularization of cornea, left eye
H16.443 Deep vascularization of cornea, bilateral
H16.449 Deep vascularization of cornea, unspecified eye

H16.8 **Other keratitis**
H16.9 **Unspecified keratitis**

● H17 **Corneal scars and opacities**
● H17.0 **Adherent leukoma**
H17.00 Adherent leukoma, unspecified eye
H17.01 Adherent leukoma, right eye
H17.02 Adherent leukoma, left eye
H17.03 Adherent leukoma, bilateral

● H17.1 **Central corneal opacity**
H17.10 Central corneal opacity, unspecified eye
H17.11 Central corneal opacity, right eye
H17.12 Central corneal opacity, left eye
H17.13 Central corneal opacity, bilateral

● H17.8 **Other corneal scars and opacities**
● H17.81 **Minor opacity of cornea**
Corneal nebula
H17.811 Minor opacity of cornea, right eye
H17.812 Minor opacity of cornea, left eye
H17.813 Minor opacity of cornea, bilateral
H17.819 Minor opacity of cornea, unspecified eye

● H17.82 **Peripheral opacity of cornea**
H17.821 Peripheral opacity of cornea, right eye
H17.822 Peripheral opacity of cornea, left eye
H17.823 Peripheral opacity of cornea, bilateral
H17.829 Peripheral opacity of cornea, unspecified eye

H17.89 Other corneal scars and opacities
H17.9 **Unspecified corneal scar and opacity**

● H18 **Other disorders of cornea**
● H18.0 **Corneal pigmentations and deposits**
● H18.00 **Unspecified corneal deposit**
H18.001 Unspecified corneal deposit, right eye
H18.002 Unspecified corneal deposit, left eye
H18.003 Unspecified corneal deposit, bilateral
H18.009 Unspecified corneal deposit, unspecified eye

● **H18.01 Anterior corneal pigmentations**
     Staehli's line

     H18.011   Anterior corneal pigmentations, right eye

     H18.012   Anterior corneal pigmentations, left eye

     H18.013   Anterior corneal pigmentations, bilateral

     H18.019   Anterior corneal pigmentations, unspecified eye

● **H18.02 Argentous corneal deposits**

     H18.021   Argentous corneal deposits, right eye

     H18.022   Argentous corneal deposits, left eye

     H18.023   Argentous corneal deposits, bilateral

     H18.029   Argentous corneal deposits, unspecified eye

● **H18.03 Corneal deposits in metabolic disorders**
     Code also associated metabolic disorder

     H18.031   Corneal deposits in metabolic disorders, right eye

     H18.032   Corneal deposits in metabolic disorders, left eye

     H18.033   Corneal deposits in metabolic disorders, bilateral

     H18.039   Corneal deposits in metabolic disorders, unspecified eye

● **H18.04 Kayser-Fleischer ring**
     Code also associated Wilson's disease (E83.01)

     H18.041   Kayser-Fleischer ring, right eye

     H18.042   Kayser-Fleischer ring, left eye

     H18.043   Kayser-Fleischer ring, bilateral

     H18.049   Kayser-Fleischer ring, unspecified eye

● **H18.05 Posterior corneal pigmentations**
     Krukenberg's spindle

     H18.051   Posterior corneal pigmentations, right eye

     H18.052   Posterior corneal pigmentations, left eye

     H18.053   Posterior corneal pigmentations, bilateral

     H18.059   Posterior corneal pigmentations, unspecified eye

● **H18.06 Stromal corneal pigmentations**
     Hematocornea

     H18.061   Stromal corneal pigmentations, right eye

     H18.062   Stromal corneal pigmentations, left eye

     H18.063   Stromal corneal pigmentations, bilateral

     H18.069   Stromal corneal pigmentations, unspecified eye

● **H18.1 Bullous keratopathy**

     H18.10   Bullous keratopathy, unspecified eye

     H18.11   Bullous keratopathy, right eye

     H18.12   Bullous keratopathy, left eye

     H18.13   Bullous keratopathy, bilateral

● **H18.2 Other and unspecified corneal edema**

     H18.20   Unspecified corneal edema

●   **H18.21 Corneal edema secondary to contact lens**

        Excludes2   other corneal disorders due to contact lens (H18.82-)

     H18.211   Corneal edema secondary to contact lens, right eye

     H18.212   Corneal edema secondary to contact lens, left eye

     H18.213   Corneal edema secondary to contact lens, bilateral

     H18.219   Corneal edema secondary to contact lens, unspecified eye

● **H18.22 Idiopathic corneal edema**

     H18.221   Idiopathic corneal edema, right eye

     H18.222   Idiopathic corneal edema, left eye

     H18.223   Idiopathic corneal edema, bilateral

     H18.229   Idiopathic corneal edema, unspecified eye

● **H18.23 Secondary corneal edema**

     H18.231   Secondary corneal edema, right eye

     H18.232   Secondary corneal edema, left eye

     H18.233   Secondary corneal edema, bilateral

     H18.239   Secondary corneal edema, unspecified eye

● **H18.3 Changes of corneal membranes**

     H18.30   Unspecified corneal membrane change

● **H18.31 Folds and rupture in Bowman's membrane**

     H18.311   Folds and rupture in Bowman's membrane, right eye

     H18.312   Folds and rupture in Bowman's membrane, left eye

     H18.313   Folds and rupture in Bowman's membrane, bilateral

     H18.319   Folds and rupture in Bowman's membrane, unspecified eye

● **H18.32 Folds in Descemet's membrane**

     H18.321   Folds in Descemet's membrane, right eye

     H18.322   Folds in Descemet's membrane, left eye

     H18.323   Folds in Descemet's membrane, bilateral

     H18.329   Folds in Descemet's membrane, unspecified eye

● **H18.33 Rupture in Descemet's membrane**

     H18.331   Rupture in Descemet's membrane, right eye

     H18.332   Rupture in Descemet's membrane, left eye

     H18.333   Rupture in Descemet's membrane, bilateral

     H18.339   Rupture in Descemet's membrane, unspecified eye

● **H18.4 Corneal degeneration**

     Excludes1   Mooren's ulcer (H16.0-)
                         recurrent erosion of cornea (H18.83-)

     H18.40   Unspecified corneal degeneration

● **H18.41 Arcus senilis**
     Senile corneal changes

     H18.411   Arcus senilis, right eye

     H18.412   Arcus senilis, left eye

     H18.413   Arcus senilis, bilateral

     H18.419   Arcus senilis, unspecified eye

● **H18.42 Band keratopathy**

     H18.421   Band keratopathy, right eye

     H18.422   Band keratopathy, left eye

     H18.423   Band keratopathy, bilateral

     H18.429   Band keratopathy, unspecified eye

     H18.43   Other calcerous corneal degeneration

● **H18.44 Keratomalacia**

     Excludes1   keratomalacia due to vitamin A deficiency (E50.4)

     H18.441   Keratomalacia, right eye

     H18.442   Keratomalacia, left eye

     H18.443   Keratomalacia, bilateral

     H18.449   Keratomalacia, unspecified eye

CHAPTER 7 (H00-H59)

CHAPTER 7 (H00-H59)

● H18.45   Nodular corneal degeneration
    H18.451   Nodular corneal degeneration, right eye
    H18.452   Nodular corneal degeneration, left eye
    H18.453   Nodular corneal degeneration, bilateral
    H18.459   Nodular corneal degeneration, unspecified eye

● H18.46   Peripheral corneal degeneration
    H18.461   Peripheral corneal degeneration, right eye
    H18.462   Peripheral corneal degeneration, left eye
    H18.463   Peripheral corneal degeneration, bilateral
    H18.469   Peripheral corneal degeneration, unspecified eye

   H18.49   Other corneal degeneration

● H18.5   Hereditary corneal dystrophies

● H18.50   Unspecified hereditary corneal dystrophies
    H18.501   Unspecified hereditary corneal dystrophies, right eye
    H18.502   Unspecified hereditary corneal dystrophies, left eye
    H18.503   Unspecified hereditary corneal dystrophies, bilateral
    H18.509   Unspecified hereditary corneal dystrophies, unspecified eye

● H18.51   Endothelial corneal dystrophy
     Fuchs' dystrophy
    H18.511   Endothelial corneal dystrophy, right eye
    H18.512   Endothelial corneal dystrophy, left eye
    H18.513   Endothelial corneal dystrophy, bilateral
    H18.519   Endothelial corneal dystrophy, unspecified eye

● H18.52   Epithelial (juvenile) corneal dystrophy
    H18.521   Epithelial (juvenile) corneal dystrophy, right eye
    H18.522   Epithelial (juvenile) corneal dystrophy, left eye
    H18.523   Epithelial (juvenile) corneal dystrophy, bilateral
    H18.529   Epithelial (juvenile) corneal dystrophy, unspecified eye

● H18.53   Granular corneal dystrophy
    H18.531   Granular corneal dystrophy, right eye
    H18.532   Granular corneal dystrophy, left eye
    H18.533   Granular corneal dystrophy, bilateral
    H18.539   Granular corneal dystrophy, unspecified eye

● H18.54   Lattice corneal dystrophy
    H18.541   Lattice corneal dystrophy, right eye
    H18.542   Lattice corneal dystrophy, left eye
    H18.543   Lattice corneal dystrophy, bilateral
    H18.549   Lattice corneal dystrophy, unspecified eye

● H18.55   Macular corneal dystrophy
    H18.551   Macular corneal dystrophy, right eye
    H18.552   Macular corneal dystrophy, left eye
    H18.553   Macular corneal dystrophy, bilateral
    H18.559   Macular corneal dystrophy, unspecified eye

● H18.59   Other hereditary corneal dystrophies
    H18.591   Other hereditary corneal dystrophies, right eye
    H18.592   Other hereditary corneal dystrophies, left eye
    H18.593   Other hereditary corneal dystrophies, bilateral
    H18.599   Other hereditary corneal dystrophies, unspecified eye

● H18.6   Keratoconus

● H18.60   Keratoconus, unspecified
    H18.601   Keratoconus, unspecified, right eye
    H18.602   Keratoconus, unspecified, left eye
    H18.603   Keratoconus, unspecified, bilateral
    H18.609   Keratoconus, unspecified, unspecified eye

● H18.61   Keratoconus, stable
    H18.611   Keratoconus, stable, right eye
    H18.612   Keratoconus, stable, left eye
    H18.613   Keratoconus, stable, bilateral
    H18.619   Keratoconus, stable, unspecified eye

● H18.62   Keratoconus, unstable
     Acute hydrops
    H18.621   Keratoconus, unstable, right eye
    H18.622   Keratoconus, unstable, left eye
    H18.623   Keratoconus, unstable, bilateral
    H18.629   Keratoconus, unstable, unspecified eye

● H18.7   Other and unspecified corneal deformities
    Excludes1   congenital malformations of cornea (Q13.3-Q13.4)

   H18.70   Unspecified corneal deformity

● H18.71   Corneal ectasia
    H18.711   Corneal ectasia, right eye
    H18.712   Corneal ectasia, left eye
    H18.713   Corneal ectasia, bilateral
    H18.719   Corneal ectasia, unspecified eye

● H18.72   Corneal staphyloma
    H18.721   Corneal staphyloma, right eye
    H18.722   Corneal staphyloma, left eye
    H18.723   Corneal staphyloma, bilateral
    H18.729   Corneal staphyloma, unspecified eye

● H18.73   Descemetocele
    H18.731   Descemetocele, right eye
    H18.732   Descemetocele, left eye
    H18.733   Descemetocele, bilateral
    H18.739   Descemetocele, unspecified eye

● H18.79   Other corneal deformities
    H18.791   Other corneal deformities, right eye
    H18.792   Other corneal deformities, left eye
    H18.793   Other corneal deformities, bilateral
    H18.799   Other corneal deformities, unspecified eye

Figure 7-8   Lateral view of the displacement of the cone apex in keratoconus. (From Yanoff: Ophthalmology, ed 3, Mosby, Inc., 2008)

Item 7-4 Keratoconus results in corneal degeneration that begins in childhood, gradually changes the cornea from a round to cone shape, decreasing visual acuity. Treatment includes contact lenses. In severe cases the need for corneal transplant may be the treatment of choice; however, newer technologies may use high-frequency radio energy to shrink the edges of the cornea, pulling the central area back to a more normal shape. It can help delay or avoid the need for a corneal transplantation.

▶ New   ➡ Revised   ~~deleted~~ Deleted   Excludes 1   Excludes 2   Includes   Use additional   Code first   Code also   Key words

OGCR Official Guidelines   X Assign placeholder X   ● Use Additional Character(s)   ▶ Manifestation Code   🔗 Hierarchical Condition Category   **Coding Clinic**

- ● H18.8   Other specified disorders of cornea
  - ● H18.81   Anesthesia and hypoesthesia of cornea
    - H18.811   Anesthesia and hypoesthesia of cornea, right eye
    - H18.812   Anesthesia and hypoesthesia of cornea, left eye
    - H18.813   Anesthesia and hypoesthesia of cornea, bilateral
    - H18.819   Anesthesia and hypoesthesia of cornea, unspecified eye
  - ● H18.82   Corneal disorder due to contact lens
    - **Excludes2**   corneal edema due to contact lens (H18.21-)
    - H18.821   Corneal disorder due to contact lens, right eye
    - H18.822   Corneal disorder due to contact lens, left eye
    - H18.823   Corneal disorder due to contact lens, bilateral
    - H18.829   Corneal disorder due to contact lens, unspecified eye
  - ● H18.83   Recurrent erosion of cornea
    - H18.831   Recurrent erosion of cornea, right eye
    - H18.832   Recurrent erosion of cornea, left eye
    - H18.833   Recurrent erosion of cornea, bilateral
    - H18.839   Recurrent erosion of cornea, unspecified eye
  - ● H18.89   Other specified disorders of cornea
    - H18.891   Other specified disorders of cornea, right eye
    - H18.892   Other specified disorders of cornea, left eye
    - H18.893   Other specified disorders of cornea, bilateral
    - H18.899   Other specified disorders of cornea, unspecified eye
- H18.9   Unspecified disorder of cornea

- ● H20   Iridocyclitis
  - ● H20.0   Acute and subacute iridocyclitis
    - Acute anterior uveitis
    - Acute cyclitis
    - Acute iritis
    - Subacute anterior uveitis
    - Subacute cyclitis
    - Subacute iritis
    - **Excludes1**   iridocyclitis, iritis, uveitis (due to) (in) diabetes mellitus (E08-E13 with .39)
      - iridocyclitis, iritis, uveitis (due to) (in) diphtheria (A36.89)
      - iridocyclitis, iritis, uveitis (due to) (in) gonococcal (A54.32)
      - iridocyclitis, iritis, uveitis (due to) (in) herpes (simplex) (B00.51)
      - iridocyclitis, iritis, uveitis (due to) (in) herpes zoster (B02.32)
      - iridocyclitis, iritis, uveitis (due to) (in) late congenital syphilis (A50.39)
      - iridocyclitis, iritis, uveitis (due to) (in) late syphilis (A52.71)
      - iridocyclitis, iritis, uveitis (due to) (in) sarcoidosis (D86.83)
      - iridocyclitis, iritis, uveitis (due to) (in) syphilis (A51.43)
      - iridocyclitis, iritis, uveitis (due to) (in) toxoplasmosis (B58.09)
      - iridocyclitis, iritis, uveitis (due to) (in) tuberculosis (A18.54)
    - H20.00   Unspecified acute and subacute iridocyclitis
    - ● H20.01   Primary iridocyclitis
      - H20.011   Primary iridocyclitis, right eye
      - H20.012   Primary iridocyclitis, left eye
      - H20.013   Primary iridocyclitis, bilateral
      - H20.019   Primary iridocyclitis, unspecified eye
    - ● H20.02   Recurrent acute iridocyclitis
      - H20.021   Recurrent acute iridocyclitis, right eye
      - H20.022   Recurrent acute iridocyclitis, left eye
      - H20.023   Recurrent acute iridocyclitis, bilateral
      - H20.029   Recurrent acute iridocyclitis, unspecified eye
    - ● H20.03   Secondary infectious iridocyclitis
      - H20.031   Secondary infectious iridocyclitis, right eye
      - H20.032   Secondary infectious iridocyclitis, left eye
      - H20.033   Secondary infectious iridocyclitis, bilateral
      - H20.039   Secondary infectious iridocyclitis, unspecified eye
    - ● H20.04   Secondary noninfectious iridocyclitis
      - H20.041   Secondary noninfectious iridocyclitis, right eye
      - H20.042   Secondary noninfectious iridocyclitis, left eye
      - H20.043   Secondary noninfectious iridocyclitis, bilateral
      - H20.049   Secondary noninfectious iridocyclitis, unspecified eye
    - ● H20.05   Hypopyon
      - H20.051   Hypopyon, right eye
      - H20.052   Hypopyon, left eye
      - H20.053   Hypopyon, bilateral
      - H20.059   Hypopyon, unspecified eye
  - ● H20.1   Chronic iridocyclitis
    - Use additional code for any associated cataract (H26.21-)
    - **Excludes2**   posterior cyclitis (H30.2-)
    - H20.10   Chronic iridocyclitis, unspecified eye
    - H20.11   Chronic iridocyclitis, right eye
    - H20.12   Chronic iridocyclitis, left eye
    - H20.13   Chronic iridocyclitis, bilateral
  - ● H20.2   Lens-induced iridocyclitis
    - H20.20   Lens-induced iridocyclitis, unspecified eye
    - H20.21   Lens-induced iridocyclitis, right eye
    - H20.22   Lens-induced iridocyclitis, left eye
    - H20.23   Lens-induced iridocyclitis, bilateral
  - ● H20.8   Other iridocyclitis
    - **Excludes2**   glaucomatocyclitis crises (H40.4-)
      - posterior cyclitis (H30.2-)
      - sympathetic uveitis (H44.13-)
    - ● H20.81   Fuchs' heterochromic cyclitis
      - H20.811   Fuchs' heterochromic cyclitis, right eye
      - H20.812   Fuchs' heterochromic cyclitis, left eye
      - H20.813   Fuchs' heterochromic cyclitis, bilateral
      - H20.819   Fuchs' heterochromic cyclitis, unspecified eye
    - ● H20.82   Vogt-Koyanagi syndrome
      - H20.821   Vogt-Koyanagi syndrome, right eye
      - H20.822   Vogt-Koyanagi syndrome, left eye
      - H20.823   Vogt-Koyanagi syndrome, bilateral
      - H20.829   Vogt-Koyanagi syndrome, unspecified eye
  - H20.9   Unspecified iridocyclitis
    - Uveitis NOS

CHAPTER 7 (H00-H59)

● H21　Other disorders of iris and ciliary body
　　Excludes2　sympathetic uveitis (H44.1-)
　● H21.0　Hyphema
　　　Excludes1　traumatic hyphema (S05.1-)
　　　H21.00　Hyphema, unspecified eye
　　　H21.01　Hyphema, right eye
　　　H21.02　Hyphema, left eye
　　　H21.03　Hyphema, bilateral
　● H21.1　Other vascular disorders of iris and ciliary body
　　　Neovascularization of iris or ciliary body
　　　Rubeosis iridis
　　　Rubeosis of iris
　　● H21.1X　Other vascular disorders of iris and ciliary body
　　　　H21.1X1　Other vascular disorders of iris and ciliary body, right eye
　　　　H21.1X2　Other vascular disorders of iris and ciliary body, left eye
　　　　H21.1X3　Other vascular disorders of iris and ciliary body, bilateral
　　　　H21.1X9　Other vascular disorders of iris and ciliary body, unspecified eye
　● H21.2　Degeneration of iris and ciliary body
　　● H21.21　Degeneration of chamber angle
　　　　H21.211　Degeneration of chamber angle, right eye
　　　　H21.212　Degeneration of chamber angle, left eye
　　　　H21.213　Degeneration of chamber angle, bilateral
　　　　H21.219　Degeneration of chamber angle, unspecified eye
　　● H21.22　Degeneration of ciliary body
　　　　H21.221　Degeneration of ciliary body, right eye
　　　　H21.222　Degeneration of ciliary body, left eye
　　　　H21.223　Degeneration of ciliary body, bilateral
　　　　H21.229　Degeneration of ciliary body, unspecified eye
　　● H21.23　Degeneration of iris (pigmentary)
　　　　Translucency of iris
　　　　H21.231　Degeneration of iris (pigmentary), right eye
　　　　H21.232　Degeneration of iris (pigmentary), left eye
　　　　H21.233　Degeneration of iris (pigmentary), bilateral
　　　　H21.239　Degeneration of iris (pigmentary), unspecified eye
　　● H21.24　Degeneration of pupillary margin
　　　　H21.241　Degeneration of pupillary margin, right eye
　　　　H21.242　Degeneration of pupillary margin, left eye
　　　　H21.243　Degeneration of pupillary margin, bilateral
　　　　H21.249　Degeneration of pupillary margin, unspecified eye
　　● H21.25　Iridoschisis
　　　　H21.251　Iridoschisis, right eye
　　　　H21.252　Iridoschisis, left eye
　　　　H21.253　Iridoschisis, bilateral
　　　　H21.259　Iridoschisis, unspecified eye
　　● H21.26　Iris atrophy (essential) (progressive)
　　　　H21.261　Iris atrophy (essential) (progressive), right eye

　　　　H21.262　Iris atrophy (essential) (progressive), left eye
　　　　H21.263　Iris atrophy (essential) (progressive), bilateral
　　　　H21.269　Iris atrophy (essential) (progressive), unspecified eye
　● H21.27　Miotic pupillary cyst
　　　　H21.271　Miotic pupillary cyst, right eye
　　　　H21.272　Miotic pupillary cyst, left eye
　　　　H21.273　Miotic pupillary cyst, bilateral
　　　　H21.279　Miotic pupillary cyst, unspecified eye
　　　H21.29　Other iris atrophy
　● H21.3　Cyst of iris, ciliary body and anterior chamber
　　　Excludes2　miotic pupillary cyst (H21.27-)
　　● H21.30　Idiopathic cysts of iris, ciliary body or anterior chamber
　　　　Cyst of iris, ciliary body or anterior chamber NOS
　　　　H21.301　Idiopathic cysts of iris, ciliary body or anterior chamber, right eye
　　　　H21.302　Idiopathic cysts of iris, ciliary body or anterior chamber, left eye
　　　　H21.303　Idiopathic cysts of iris, ciliary body or anterior chamber, bilateral
　　　　H21.309　Idiopathic cysts of iris, ciliary body or anterior chamber, unspecified eye
　　● H21.31　Exudative cysts of iris or anterior chamber
　　　　H21.311　Exudative cysts of iris or anterior chamber, right eye
　　　　H21.312　Exudative cysts of iris or anterior chamber, left eye
　　　　H21.313　Exudative cysts of iris or anterior chamber, bilateral
　　　　H21.319　Exudative cysts of iris or anterior chamber, unspecified eye
　　● H21.32　Implantation cysts of iris, ciliary body or anterior chamber
　　　　H21.321　Implantation cysts of iris, ciliary body or anterior chamber, right eye
　　　　H21.322　Implantation cysts of iris, ciliary body or anterior chamber, left eye
　　　　H21.323　Implantation cysts of iris, ciliary body or anterior chamber, bilateral
　　　　H21.329　Implantation cysts of iris, ciliary body or anterior chamber, unspecified eye
　　● H21.33　Parasitic cyst of iris, ciliary body or anterior chamber
　　　　H21.331　Parasitic cyst of iris, ciliary body or anterior chamber, right eye
　　　　H21.332　Parasitic cyst of iris, ciliary body or anterior chamber, left eye
　　　　H21.333　Parasitic cyst of iris, ciliary body or anterior chamber, bilateral
　　　　H21.339　Parasitic cyst of iris, ciliary body or anterior chamber, unspecified eye
　　● H21.34　Primary cyst of pars plana
　　　　H21.341　Primary cyst of pars plana, right eye
　　　　H21.342　Primary cyst of pars plana, left eye
　　　　H21.343　Primary cyst of pars plana, bilateral
　　　　H21.349　Primary cyst of pars plana, unspecified eye
　　● H21.35　Exudative cyst of pars plana
　　　　H21.351　Exudative cyst of pars plana, right eye
　　　　H21.352　Exudative cyst of pars plana, left eye
　　　　H21.353　Exudative cyst of pars plana, bilateral
　　　　H21.359　Exudative cyst of pars plana, unspecified eye

▶ New　⇒ Revised　deleted Deleted　Excludes 1　Excludes 2　Includes　Use additional　Code first　Code also　Key words
OGCR Official Guidelines　X Assign placeholder X　● Use Additional Character(s)　▶ Manifestation Code　🦶 Hierarchical Condition Category　**Coding Clinic**

● **H21.4   Pupillary membranes**
Iris bombé
Pupillary occlusion
Pupillary seclusion
> **Excludes1**   congenital pupillary membranes (Q13.8)

H21.40   Pupillary membranes, unspecified eye

H21.41   Pupillary membranes, right eye

H21.42   Pupillary membranes, left eye

H21.43   Pupillary membranes, bilateral

● **H21.5   Other and unspecified adhesions and disruptions of iris and ciliary body**
> **Excludes1**   corectopia (Q13.2)

● **H21.50   Unspecified adhesions of iris**
Synechia (iris) NOS

     H21.501   Unspecified adhesions of iris, right eye

     H21.502   Unspecified adhesions of iris, left eye

     H21.503   Unspecified adhesions of iris, bilateral

     H21.509   Unspecified adhesions of iris and ciliary body, unspecified eye

● **H21.51   Anterior synechiae (iris)**

     H21.511   Anterior synechiae (iris), right eye

     H21.512   Anterior synechiae (iris), left eye

     H21.513   Anterior synechiae (iris), bilateral

     H21.519   Anterior synechiae (iris), unspecified eye

● **H21.52   Goniosynechiae**

     H21.521   Goniosynechiae, right eye

     H21.522   Goniosynechiae, left eye

     H21.523   Goniosynechiae, bilateral

     H21.529   Goniosynechiae, unspecified eye

● **H21.53   Iridodialysis**

     H21.531   Iridodialysis, right eye

     H21.532   Iridodialysis, left eye

     H21.533   Iridodialysis, bilateral

     H21.539   Iridodialysis, unspecified eye

● **H21.54   Posterior synechiae (iris)**

     H21.541   Posterior synechiae (iris), right eye

     H21.542   Posterior synechiae (iris), left eye

     H21.543   Posterior synechiae (iris), bilateral

     H21.549   Posterior synechiae (iris), unspecified eye

● **H21.55   Recession of chamber angle**

     H21.551   Recession of chamber angle, right eye

     H21.552   Recession of chamber angle, left eye

     H21.553   Recession of chamber angle, bilateral

     H21.559   Recession of chamber angle, unspecified eye

● **H21.56   Pupillary abnormalities**
Deformed pupil
Ectopic pupil
Rupture of sphincter, pupil
> **Excludes1**   congenital deformity of pupil (Q13.2-)

     H21.561   Pupillary abnormality, right eye

     H21.562   Pupillary abnormality, left eye

     H21.563   Pupillary abnormality, bilateral

     H21.569   Pupillary abnormality, unspecified eye

● **H21.8   Other specified disorders of iris and ciliary body**

H21.81   Floppy iris syndrome
Intraoperative floppy iris syndrome (IFIS)
> Use additional code for adverse effect, if applicable, to identify drug (T36-T50 with fifth or sixth character 5)

H21.82   Plateau iris syndrome (post-iridectomy) (postprocedural)

H21.89   Other specified disorders of iris and ciliary body

H21.9   Unspecified disorder of iris and ciliary body

▌ **H22   *Disorders of iris and ciliary body in diseases classified elsewhere***
> *Code first* underlying disease, such as:
> gout (M1A.-, M10.-)
> leprosy (A30.-)
> parasitic disease (B89)

DISORDERS OF LENS (H25-H28)

● **H25   Age-related cataract**
Senile cataract
> **Excludes2**   capsular glaucoma with pseudoexfoliation of lens (H40.1-)

● **H25.0   Age-related incipient cataract**

● **H25.01   Cortical age-related cataract**

     H25.011   Cortical age-related cataract, right eye   A

     H25.012   Cortical age-related cataract, left eye   A

     H25.013   Cortical age-related cataract, bilateral   A

     H25.019   Cortical age-related cataract, unspecified eye   A

● **H25.03   Anterior subcapsular polar age-related cataract**

     H25.031   Anterior subcapsular polar age-related cataract, right eye   A

     H25.032   Anterior subcapsular polar age-related cataract, left eye   A

     H25.033   Anterior subcapsular polar age-related cataract, bilateral   A

     H25.039   Anterior subcapsular polar age-related cataract, unspecified eye   A

● **H25.04   Posterior subcapsular polar age-related cataract**

     H25.041   Posterior subcapsular polar age-related cataract, right eye   A

     H25.042   Posterior subcapsular polar age-related cataract, left eye   A

     H25.043   Posterior subcapsular polar age-related cataract, bilateral   A

     H25.049   Posterior subcapsular polar age-related cataract, unspecified eye   A

Figure 7-9   Age-related cataract.
Nuclear sclerosis and cortical lens opacities are present. (From Ignatavicius DD, Workman ML: *Medical-Surgical Nursing: Patient-Centered Collaborative Care*, St. Louis, MO, Saunders/Elsevier, 2010)

Item 7-5 Senile cataracts are linked to the aging process. The most common area for the formation of a cataract is the cortical area of the lens. **Polar cataracts** can be either anterior or posterior. **Anterior polar cataracts** are more common and are small, white, capsular cataracts located on the anterior portion of the lens. **Total cataracts,** also called **complete** or **mature,** cause an opacity of all fibers of the lens. **Hypermature** describes a mature cataract with a swollen, milky cortex that covers the entire lens. **Immature**, also called **incipient,** cataracts have a clear cortex and are only slightly opaque. Treatment for all cataracts is the removal of the lens.

CHAPTER 7 (H00-H59)

● **H25.09**   Other age-related incipient cataract
     Coronary age-related cataract
     Punctate age-related cataract
     Water clefts

     H25.091   Other age-related incipient cataract, right eye   A

     H25.092   Other age-related incipient cataract, left eye   A

     H25.093   Other age-related incipient cataract, bilateral   A

     H25.099   Other age-related incipient cataract, unspecified eye   A

● **H25.1**   Age-related nuclear cataract
     Cataracta brunescens
     Nuclear sclerosis cataract

     H25.10   Age-related nuclear cataract, unspecified eye   A

     H25.11   Age-related nuclear cataract, right eye   A
        Coding Clinic: 2019, Q2, P30

     H25.12   Age-related nuclear cataract, left eye   A
        Coding Clinic: 2016, Q1, P33

     H25.13   Age-related nuclear cataract, bilateral   A
        Coding Clinic: 2016, Q1, P32

● **H25.2**   Age-related cataract, morgagnian type
     Age-related hypermature cataract

     H25.20   Age-related cataract, morgagnian type, unspecified eye   A

     H25.21   Age-related cataract, morgagnian type, right eye   A

     H25.22   Age-related cataract, morgagnian type, left eye   A

     H25.23   Age-related cataract, morgagnian type, bilateral   A

● **H25.8**   Other age-related cataract

   ● **H25.81**   Combined forms of age-related cataract

     H25.811   Combined forms of age-related cataract, right eye   A

     H25.812   Combined forms of age-related cataract, left eye   A

     H25.813   Combined forms of age-related cataract, bilateral   A
        Coding Clinic: 2019, Q2, P30

     H25.819   Combined forms of age-related cataract, unspecified eye   A

     H25.89   Other age-related cataract   A

   H25.9   Unspecified age-related cataract   A

● **H26**   Other cataract

     Excludes1   congenital cataract (Q12.0)

   ● **H26.0**   Infantile and juvenile cataract

   ● **H26.00**   Unspecified infantile and juvenile cataract

     H26.001   Unspecified infantile and juvenile cataract, right eye   P

     H26.002   Unspecified infantile and juvenile cataract, left eye   P

     H26.003   Unspecified infantile and juvenile cataract, bilateral   P

     H26.009   Unspecified infantile and juvenile cataract, unspecified eye   P

   ● **H26.01**   Infantile and juvenile cortical, lamellar, or zonular cataract

     H26.011   Infantile and juvenile cortical, lamellar, or zonular cataract, right eye   P

     H26.012   Infantile and juvenile cortical, lamellar, or zonular cataract, left eye   P

     H26.013   Infantile and juvenile cortical, lamellar, or zonular cataract, bilateral   P

     H26.019   Infantile and juvenile cortical, lamellar, or zonular cataract, unspecified eye   P

● **H26.03**   Infantile and juvenile nuclear cataract

     H26.031   Infantile and juvenile nuclear cataract, right eye   P

     H26.032   Infantile and juvenile nuclear cataract, left eye   P

     H26.033   Infantile and juvenile nuclear cataract, bilateral   P

     H26.039   Infantile and juvenile nuclear cataract, unspecified eye   P

● **H26.04**   Anterior subcapsular polar infantile and juvenile cataract

     H26.041   Anterior subcapsular polar infantile and juvenile cataract, right eye   P

     H26.042   Anterior subcapsular polar infantile and juvenile cataract, left eye   P

     H26.043   Anterior subcapsular polar infantile and juvenile cataract, bilateral   P

     H26.049   Anterior subcapsular polar infantile and juvenile cataract, unspecified eye   P

● **H26.05**   Posterior subcapsular polar infantile and juvenile cataract

     H26.051   Posterior subcapsular polar infantile and juvenile cataract, right eye   P

     H26.052   Posterior subcapsular polar infantile and juvenile cataract, left eye   P

     H26.053   Posterior subcapsular polar infantile and juvenile cataract, bilateral   P

     H26.059   Posterior subcapsular polar infantile and juvenile cataract, unspecified eye   P

● **H26.06**   Combined forms of infantile and juvenile cataract

     H26.061   Combined forms of infantile and juvenile cataract, right eye   P

     H26.062   Combined forms of infantile and juvenile cataract, left eye   P

     H26.063   Combined forms of infantile and juvenile cataract bilateral   P

     H26.069   Combined forms of infantile and juvenile cataract, unspecified eye   P

     H26.09   Other infantile and juvenile cataract   P

● **H26.1**   Traumatic cataract
     Use additional code (Chapter 20) to identify external cause

   ● **H26.10**   Unspecified traumatic cataract

     H26.101   Unspecified traumatic cataract, right eye

     H26.102   Unspecified traumatic cataract, left eye

     H26.103   Unspecified traumatic cataract, bilateral

     H26.109   Unspecified traumatic cataract, unspecified eye

   ● **H26.11**   Localized traumatic opacities

     H26.111   Localized traumatic opacities, right eye

     H26.112   Localized traumatic opacities, left eye

     H26.113   Localized traumatic opacities, bilateral

     H26.119   Localized traumatic opacities, unspecified eye

   ● **H26.12**   Partially resolved traumatic cataract

     H26.121   Partially resolved traumatic cataract, right eye

     H26.122   Partially resolved traumatic cataract, left eye

     H26.123   Partially resolved traumatic cataract, bilateral

     H26.129   Partially resolved traumatic cataract, unspecified eye

---

▶ New   ⇒ Revised   ~~deleted~~ Deleted   Excludes 1   Excludes 2   Includes   Use additional   Code first   Code also   Key words

OGCR Official Guidelines   X Assign placeholder X   ● Use Additional Character(s)   ▶ Manifestation Code   ⊕ Hierarchical Condition Category   **Coding Clinic**

● H26.13   Total traumatic cataract
     H26.131   Total traumatic cataract, right eye
     H26.132   Total traumatic cataract, left eye
     H26.133   Total traumatic cataract, bilateral
     H26.139   Total traumatic cataract, unspecified eye

● H26.2   Complicated cataract
     H26.20   Unspecified complicated cataract
         Cataracta complicata NOS

● H26.21   Cataract with neovascularization
     Code also associated condition, such as:
     chronic iridocyclitis (H20.1-)
     H26.211   Cataract with neovascularization, right eye
     H26.212   Cataract with neovascularization, left eye
     H26.213   Cataract with neovascularization, bilateral
     H26.219   Cataract with neovascularization, unspecified eye

● H26.22   Cataract secondary to ocular disorders (degenerative) (inflammatory)
     Code also associated ocular disorder
     H26.221   Cataract secondary to ocular disorders (degenerative) (inflammatory), right eye
     H26.222   Cataract secondary to ocular disorders (degenerative) (inflammatory), left eye
     H26.223   Cataract secondary to ocular disorders (degenerative) (inflammatory), bilateral
     H26.229   Cataract secondary to ocular disorders (degenerative) (inflammatory), unspecified eye

● H26.23   Glaucomatous flecks (subcapsular)
     Code first underlying glaucoma (H40-H42)
     H26.231   Glaucomatous flecks (subcapsular), right eye
     H26.232   Glaucomatous flecks (subcapsular), left eye
     H26.233   Glaucomatous flecks (subcapsular), bilateral
     H26.239   Glaucomatous flecks (subcapsular), unspecified eye

● H26.3   Drug-induced cataract
     Toxic cataract
     Use additional code for adverse effect, if applicable, to identify drug (T36-T50 with fifth or sixth character 5)
     H26.30   Drug-induced cataract, unspecified eye
     H26.31   Drug-induced cataract, right eye
     H26.32   Drug-induced cataract, left eye
     H26.33   Drug-induced cataract, bilateral

● H26.4   Secondary cataract
     Coding Clinic: 2018, Q2, P14
     H26.40   Unspecified secondary cataract
   ● H26.41   Soemmering's ring
     H26.411   Soemmering's ring, right eye
     H26.412   Soemmering's ring, left eye
     H26.413   Soemmering's ring, bilateral
     H26.419   Soemmering's ring, unspecified eye

● H26.49   Other secondary cataract
     H26.491   Other secondary cataract, right eye
     H26.492   Other secondary cataract, left eye
         Coding Clinic: 2018, Q2, P13
     H26.493   Other secondary cataract, bilateral
     H26.499   Other secondary cataract, unspecified eye

H26.8   Other specified cataract
H26.9   Unspecified cataract

● H27   Other disorders of lens
     Excludes1   congenital lens malformations (Q12.-)
         mechanical complications of intraocular lens implant (T85.2)
         pseudophakia (Z96.1)

   ● H27.0   Aphakia
     Acquired absence of lens
     Acquired aphakia
     Aphakia due to trauma
     Excludes1   cataract extraction status (Z98.4-)
         congenital absence of lens (Q12.3)
         congenital aphakia (Q12.3)
     H27.00   Aphakia, unspecified eye
     H27.01   Aphakia, right eye
     H27.02   Aphakia, left eye
     H27.03   Aphakia, bilateral

   ● H27.1   Dislocation of lens
     H27.10   Unspecified dislocation of lens
   ● H27.11   Subluxation of lens
     H27.111   Subluxation of lens, right eye
     H27.112   Subluxation of lens, left eye
     H27.113   Subluxation of lens, bilateral
     H27.119   Subluxation of lens, unspecified eye
   ● H27.12   Anterior dislocation of lens
     H27.121   Anterior dislocation of lens, right eye
     H27.122   Anterior dislocation of lens, left eye
     H27.123   Anterior dislocation of lens, bilateral
     H27.129   Anterior dislocation of lens, unspecified eye
   ● H27.13   Posterior dislocation of lens
     H27.131   Posterior dislocation of lens, right eye
     H27.132   Posterior dislocation of lens, left eye
     H27.133   Posterior dislocation of lens, bilateral
     H27.139   Posterior dislocation of lens, unspecified eye

H27.8   Other specified disorders of lens
H27.9   Unspecified disorder of lens

▷ *H28*   *Cataract in diseases classified elsewhere*
     Code first underlying disease, such as:
     hypoparathyroidism (E20.-)
     myotonia (G71.1-)
     myxedema (E03.-)
     protein-calorie malnutrition (E40-E46)
     Excludes1   cataract in diabetes mellitus (E08.36, E09.36, E10.36, E11.36, E13.36)

CHAPTER 7 (H00-H59)

DISORDERS OF CHOROID AND RETINA (H30-H36)

⭐ **(See Plate 16 of the Anatomy Illustrations.)**

● H30   Chorioretinal inflammation
  ● H30.0   Focal chorioretinal inflammation
    Focal chorioretinitis
    Focal choroiditis
    Focal retinitis
    Focal retinochoroiditis
    ● H30.00   Unspecified focal chorioretinal inflammation
      Focal chorioretinitis NOS
      Focal choroiditis NOS
      Focal retinitis NOS
      Focal retinochoroiditis NOS
      H30.001   Unspecified focal chorioretinal inflammation, right eye
      H30.002   Unspecified focal chorioretinal inflammation, left eye
      H30.003   Unspecified focal chorioretinal inflammation, bilateral
      H30.009   Unspecified focal chorioretinal inflammation, unspecified eye
    ● H30.01   Focal chorioretinal inflammation, juxtapapillary
      H30.011   Focal chorioretinal inflammation, juxtapapillary, right eye
      H30.012   Focal chorioretinal inflammation, juxtapapillary, left eye
      H30.013   Focal chorioretinal inflammation, juxtapapillary, bilateral
      H30.019   Focal chorioretinal inflammation, juxtapapillary, unspecified eye
    ● H30.02   Focal chorioretinal inflammation of posterior pole
      H30.021   Focal chorioretinal inflammation of posterior pole, right eye
      H30.022   Focal chorioretinal inflammation of posterior pole, left eye
      H30.023   Focal chorioretinal inflammation of posterior pole, bilateral
      H30.029   Focal chorioretinal inflammation of posterior pole, unspecified eye
    ● H30.03   Focal chorioretinal inflammation, peripheral
      H30.031   Focal chorioretinal inflammation, peripheral, right eye
      H30.032   Focal chorioretinal inflammation, peripheral, left eye
      H30.033   Focal chorioretinal inflammation, peripheral, bilateral
      H30.039   Focal chorioretinal inflammation, peripheral, unspecified eye
    ● H30.04   Focal chorioretinal inflammation, macular or paramacular
      H30.041   Focal chorioretinal inflammation, macular or paramacular, right eye
      H30.042   Focal chorioretinal inflammation, macular or paramacular, left eye
      H30.043   Focal chorioretinal inflammation, macular or paramacular, bilateral
      H30.049   Focal chorioretinal inflammation, macular or paramacular, unspecified eye

● H30.1   Disseminated chorioretinal inflammation
    Disseminated chorioretinitis
    Disseminated choroiditis
    Disseminated retinitis
    Disseminated retinochoroiditis
    Excludes2   exudative retinopathy (H35.02-)
    ● H30.10   Unspecified disseminated chorioretinal inflammation
      Disseminated chorioretinitis NOS
      Disseminated choroiditis NOS
      Disseminated retinitis NOS
      Disseminated retinochoroiditis NOS
      H30.101   Unspecified disseminated chorioretinal inflammation, right eye
      H30.102   Unspecified disseminated chorioretinal inflammation, left eye
      H30.103   Unspecified disseminated chorioretinal inflammation, bilateral
      H30.109   Unspecified disseminated chorioretinal inflammation, unspecified eye
    ● H30.11   Disseminated chorioretinal inflammation of posterior pole
      H30.111   Disseminated chorioretinal inflammation of posterior pole, right eye
      H30.112   Disseminated chorioretinal inflammation of posterior pole, left eye
      H30.113   Disseminated chorioretinal inflammation of posterior pole, bilateral
      H30.119   Disseminated chorioretinal inflammation of posterior pole, unspecified eye
    ● H30.12   Disseminated chorioretinal inflammation, peripheral
      H30.121   Disseminated chorioretinal inflammation, peripheral right eye
      H30.122   Disseminated chorioretinal inflammation, peripheral, left eye
      H30.123   Disseminated chorioretinal inflammation, peripheral, bilateral
      H30.129   Disseminated chorioretinal inflammation, peripheral, unspecified eye
    ● H30.13   Disseminated chorioretinal inflammation, generalized
      H30.131   Disseminated chorioretinal inflammation, generalized, right eye
      H30.132   Disseminated chorioretinal inflammation, generalized, left eye
      H30.133   Disseminated chorioretinal inflammation, generalized, bilateral
      H30.139   Disseminated chorioretinal inflammation, generalized, unspecified eye
    ● H30.14   Acute posterior multifocal placoid pigment epitheliopathy
      H30.141   Acute posterior multifocal placoid pigment epitheliopathy, right eye
      H30.142   Acute posterior multifocal placoid pigment epitheliopathy, left eye
      H30.143   Acute posterior multifocal placoid pigment epitheliopathy, bilateral
      H30.149   Acute posterior multifocal placoid pigment epitheliopathy, unspecified eye

● **H30.2** Posterior cyclitis
     Pars planitis
     H30.20 Posterior cyclitis, unspecified eye
     H30.21 Posterior cyclitis, right eye
     H30.22 Posterior cyclitis, left eye
     H30.23 Posterior cyclitis, bilateral

● **H30.8** Other chorioretinal inflammations
   ● **H30.81** Harada's disease
       H30.811 Harada's disease, right eye
       H30.812 Harada's disease, left eye
       H30.813 Harada's disease, bilateral
       H30.819 Harada's disease, unspecified eye
   ● **H30.89** Other chorioretinal inflammations
       H30.891 Other chorioretinal inflammations, right eye
       H30.892 Other chorioretinal inflammations, left eye
       H30.893 Other chorioretinal inflammations, bilateral
       H30.899 Other chorioretinal inflammations, unspecified eye

● **H30.9** Unspecified chorioretinal inflammation
     Chorioretinitis NOS
     Choroiditis NOS
     Neuroretinitis NOS
     Retinitis NOS
     Retinochoroiditis NOS
     H30.90 Unspecified chorioretinal inflammation, unspecified eye
     H30.91 Unspecified chorioretinal inflammation, right eye
     H30.92 Unspecified chorioretinal inflammation, left eye
     H30.93 Unspecified chorioretinal inflammation, bilateral

● **H31** Other disorders of choroid
   ● **H31.0** Chorioretinal scars
       Excludes2   postsurgical chorioretinal scars (H59.81-)
     ● **H31.00** Unspecified chorioretinal scars
       H31.001 Unspecified chorioretinal scars, right eye
       H31.002 Unspecified chorioretinal scars, left eye
       H31.003 Unspecified chorioretinal scars, bilateral
       H31.009 Unspecified chorioretinal scars, unspecified eye
     ● **H31.01** Macula scars of posterior pole (postinflammatory) (post-traumatic)
         Excludes1   postprocedural chorioretinal scar (H59.81-)
       H31.011 Macula scars of posterior pole (postinflammatory) (post-traumatic), right eye
       H31.012 Macula scars of posterior pole (postinflammatory) (post-traumatic), left eye
       H31.013 Macula scars of posterior pole (postinflammatory) (post-traumatic), bilateral
       H31.019 Macula scars of posterior pole (postinflammatory) (post-traumatic), unspecified eye
     ● **H31.02** Solar retinopathy
       H31.021 Solar retinopathy, right eye
       H31.022 Solar retinopathy, left eye
       H31.023 Solar retinopathy, bilateral
       H31.029 Solar retinopathy, unspecified eye

   ● **H31.09** Other chorioretinal scars
       H31.091 Other chorioretinal scars, right eye
       H31.092 Other chorioretinal scars, left eye
       H31.093 Other chorioretinal scars, bilateral
       H31.099 Other chorioretinal scars, unspecified eye

● **H31.1** Choroidal degeneration
     Excludes2   angioid streaks of macula (H35.33)
   ● **H31.10** Unspecified choroidal degeneration
     Choroidal sclerosis NOS
       H31.101 Choroidal degeneration, unspecified, right eye
       H31.102 Choroidal degeneration, unspecified, left eye
       H31.103 Choroidal degeneration, unspecified, bilateral
       H31.109 Choroidal degeneration, unspecified, unspecified eye
   ● **H31.11** Age-related choroidal atrophy
       H31.111 Age-related choroidal atrophy, right eye   A
       H31.112 Age-related choroidal atrophy, left eye   A
       H31.113 Age-related choroidal atrophy, bilateral   A
       H31.119 Age-related choroidal atrophy, unspecified eye   A
   ● **H31.12** Diffuse secondary atrophy of choroid
       H31.121 Diffuse secondary atrophy of choroid, right eye
       H31.122 Diffuse secondary atrophy of choroid, left eye
       H31.123 Diffuse secondary atrophy of choroid, bilateral
       H31.129 Diffuse secondary atrophy of choroid, unspecified eye

● **H31.2** Hereditary choroidal dystrophy
     Excludes2   hyperornithinemia (E72.4)
                 ornithinemia (E72.4)
     H31.20 Hereditary choroidal dystrophy, unspecified
     H31.21 Choroideremia
     H31.22 Choroidal dystrophy (central areolar) (generalized) (peripapillary)
     H31.23 Gyrate atrophy, choroid
     H31.29 Other hereditary choroidal dystrophy

● **H31.3** Choroidal hemorrhage and rupture
   ● **H31.30** Unspecified choroidal hemorrhage
       H31.301 Unspecified choroidal hemorrhage, right eye
       H31.302 Unspecified choroidal hemorrhage, left eye
       H31.303 Unspecified choroidal hemorrhage, bilateral
       H31.309 Unspecified choroidal hemorrhage, unspecified eye
   ● **H31.31** Expulsive choroidal hemorrhage
       H31.311 Expulsive choroidal hemorrhage, right eye
       H31.312 Expulsive choroidal hemorrhage, left eye
       H31.313 Expulsive choroidal hemorrhage, bilateral
       H31.319 Expulsive choroidal hemorrhage, unspecified eye
   ● **H31.32** Choroidal rupture
       H31.321 Choroidal rupture, right eye
       H31.322 Choroidal rupture, left eye
       H31.323 Choroidal rupture, bilateral
       H31.329 Choroidal rupture, unspecified eye

CHAPTER 7 (H00-H59)

● H31.4 Choroidal detachment
 ● H31.40 Unspecified choroidal detachment
  H31.401 Unspecified choroidal detachment, right eye
  H31.402 Unspecified choroidal detachment, left eye
  H31.403 Unspecified choroidal detachment, bilateral
  H31.409 Unspecified choroidal detachment, unspecified eye
 ● H31.41 Hemorrhagic choroidal detachment
  H31.411 Hemorrhagic choroidal detachment, right eye
  H31.412 Hemorrhagic choroidal detachment, left eye
  H31.413 Hemorrhagic choroidal detachment, bilateral
  H31.419 Hemorrhagic choroidal detachment, unspecified eye
 ● H31.42 Serous choroidal detachment
  H31.421 Serous choroidal detachment, right eye
  H31.422 Serous choroidal detachment, left eye
  H31.423 Serous choroidal detachment, bilateral
  H31.429 Serous choroidal detachment, unspecified eye
 H31.8 Other specified disorders of choroid
 H31.9 Unspecified disorder of choroid

▷ H32 Chorioretinal disorders in diseases classified elsewhere
 Code first underlying disease, such as:
  congenital toxoplasmosis (P37.1)
  histoplasmosis (B39.-)
  leprosy (A30.-)
 Excludes1 chorioretinitis (in):
  toxoplasmosis (acquired) (B58.01)
  tuberculosis (A18.53)

● H33 Retinal detachments and breaks
 Excludes1 detachment of retinal pigment epithelium (H35.72-, H35.73-)
 ● H33.0 Retinal detachment with retinal break
  Rhegmatogenous retinal detachment
  Excludes1 serous retinal detachment (without retinal break) (H33.2-)
  ● H33.00 Unspecified retinal detachment with retinal break
   H33.001 Unspecified retinal detachment with retinal break, right eye
   H33.002 Unspecified retinal detachment with retinal break, left eye
   H33.003 Unspecified retinal detachment with retinal break, bilateral
   H33.009 Unspecified retinal detachment with retinal break, unspecified eye
  ● H33.01 Retinal detachment with single break
   H33.011 Retinal detachment with single break, right eye
   H33.012 Retinal detachment with single break, left eye
   H33.013 Retinal detachment with single break, bilateral
   H33.019 Retinal detachment with single break, unspecified eye

NON-RHEGMATOGENOUS RETINAL DETACHMENT

VITREOUS DETACHMENT

RHEGMATOGENOUS RETINAL DETACHMENT

Figure 7-10 Retinal detachment. (From Kumar: Robbins and Cotran: Pathologic Basis of Disease, ed 7, Saunders, 2005)

Item 7–6 Retinal detachments and defects are conditions of the eye in which the retina separates from the underlying tissue. Initial detachment may be localized, requiring rapid treatment (medical emergency) to avoid the entire retina from detaching, which leads to vision loss and blindness.

● H33.02 Retinal detachment with multiple breaks
 H33.021 Retinal detachment with multiple breaks, right eye
 H33.022 Retinal detachment with multiple breaks, left eye
 H33.023 Retinal detachment with multiple breaks, bilateral
 H33.029 Retinal detachment with multiple breaks, unspecified eye
● H33.03 Retinal detachment with giant retinal tear
 H33.031 Retinal detachment with giant retinal tear, right eye
 H33.032 Retinal detachment with giant retinal tear, left eye
 H33.033 Retinal detachment with giant retinal tear, bilateral
 H33.039 Retinal detachment with giant retinal tear, unspecified eye
● H33.04 Retinal detachment with retinal dialysis
 H33.041 Retinal detachment with retinal dialysis, right eye
 H33.042 Retinal detachment with retinal dialysis, left eye
 H33.043 Retinal detachment with retinal dialysis, bilateral
 H33.049 Retinal detachment with retinal dialysis, unspecified eye

● H33.05   Total retinal detachment
    H33.051   Total retinal detachment, right eye
    H33.052   Total retinal detachment, left eye
    H33.053   Total retinal detachment, bilateral
    H33.059   Total retinal detachment, unspecified eye
● H33.1   Retinoschisis and retinal cysts
    Excludes1   congenital retinoschisis (Q14.1)
         microcystoid degeneration of retina (H35.42-)
● H33.10   Unspecified retinoschisis
    H33.101   Unspecified retinoschisis, right eye
    H33.102   Unspecified retinoschisis, left eye
    H33.103   Unspecified retinoschisis, bilateral
    H33.109   Unspecified retinoschisis, unspecified eye
● H33.11   Cyst of ora serrata
    H33.111   Cyst of ora serrata, right eye
    H33.112   Cyst of ora serrata, left eye
    H33.113   Cyst of ora serrata, bilateral
    H33.119   Cyst of ora serrata, unspecified eye
● H33.12   Parasitic cyst of retina
    H33.121   Parasitic cyst of retina, right eye
    H33.122   Parasitic cyst of retina, left eye
    H33.123   Parasitic cyst of retina, bilateral
    H33.129   Parasitic cyst of retina, unspecified eye
● H33.19   Other retinoschisis and retinal cysts
    Pseudocyst of retina
    H33.191   Other retinoschisis and retinal cysts, right eye
    H33.192   Other retinoschisis and retinal cysts, left eye
    H33.193   Other retinoschisis and retinal cysts, bilateral
    H33.199   Other retinoschisis and retinal cysts, unspecified eye
● H33.2   Serous retinal detachment
    Retinal detachment NOS
    Retinal detachment without retinal break
    Excludes1   central serous chorioretinopathy (H35.71-)
    H33.20   Serous retinal detachment, unspecified eye
    H33.21   Serous retinal detachment, right eye
    H33.22   Serous retinal detachment, left eye
    H33.23   Serous retinal detachment, bilateral
● H33.3   Retinal breaks without detachment
    Excludes1   chorioretinal scars after surgery for detachment (H59.81-)
         peripheral retinal degeneration without break (H35.4-)
● H33.30   Unspecified retinal break
    H33.301   Unspecified retinal break, right eye
    H33.302   Unspecified retinal break, left eye
    H33.303   Unspecified retinal break, bilateral
    H33.309   Unspecified retinal break, unspecified eye
● H33.31   Horseshoe tear of retina without detachment
    Operculum of retina without detachment
    H33.311   Horseshoe tear of retina without detachment, right eye
    H33.312   Horseshoe tear of retina without detachment, left eye
    H33.313   Horseshoe tear of retina without detachment, bilateral
    H33.319   Horseshoe tear of retina without detachment, unspecified eye

● H33.32   Round hole of retina without detachment
    H33.321   Round hole, right eye
    H33.322   Round hole, left eye
    H33.323   Round hole, bilateral
    H33.329   Round hole, unspecified eye
● H33.33   Multiple defects of retina without detachment
    H33.331   Multiple defects of retina without detachment, right eye
    H33.332   Multiple defects of retina without detachment, left eye
    H33.333   Multiple defects of retina without detachment, bilateral
    H33.339   Multiple defects of retina without detachment, unspecified eye
● H33.4   Traction detachment of retina
    Proliferative vitreo-retinopathy with retinal detachment
    H33.40   Traction detachment of retina, unspecified eye
    H33.41   Traction detachment of retina, right eye
    H33.42   Traction detachment of retina, left eye
    H33.43   Traction detachment of retina, bilateral
   H33.8   Other retinal detachments
● H34   Retinal vascular occlusions
    Blockage in vessel of the retina
    Excludes1   amaurosis fugax (G45.3)
● H34.0   Transient retinal artery occlusion
    H34.00   Transient retinal artery occlusion, unspecified eye
    H34.01   Transient retinal artery occlusion, right eye
    H34.02   Transient retinal artery occlusion, left eye
    H34.03   Transient retinal artery occlusion, bilateral
● H34.1   Central retinal artery occlusion
    H34.10   Central retinal artery occlusion, unspecified eye
    H34.11   Central retinal artery occlusion, right eye
    H34.12   Central retinal artery occlusion, left eye
    H34.13   Central retinal artery occlusion, bilateral
● H34.2   Other retinal artery occlusions
● H34.21   Partial retinal artery occlusion
    Hollenhorst's plaque
    Retinal microembolism
    H34.211   Partial retinal artery occlusion, right eye
    H34.212   Partial retinal artery occlusion, left eye
    H34.213   Partial retinal artery occlusion, bilateral
    H34.219   Partial retinal artery occlusion, unspecified eye
● H34.23   Retinal artery branch occlusion
    H34.231   Retinal artery branch occlusion, right eye
    H34.232   Retinal artery branch occlusion, left eye
    H34.233   Retinal artery branch occlusion, bilateral
    H34.239   Retinal artery branch occlusion, unspecified eye

● **H34.8 Other retinal vascular occlusions**
Coding Clinic: 2016, Q4, P19

● **H34.81 Central retinal vein occlusion**

One of the following 7th characters is to be assigned to codes in subcategory H34.81 to designate the severity of the occlusion:

0	with macular edema
1	with retinal neovascularization
2	stable
	Old central retinal vein occlusion

● H34.811 Central retinal vein occlusion, right eye
● H34.812 Central retinal vein occlusion, left eye
● H34.813 Central retinal vein occlusion, bilateral
● H34.819 Central retinal vein occlusion, unspecified eye

● **H34.82 Venous engorgement**
Incipient retinal vein occlusion
Partial retinal vein occlusion
H34.821 Venous engorgement, right eye
H34.822 Venous engorgement, left eye
H34.823 Venous engorgement, bilateral
H34.829 Venous engorgement, unspecified eye

● **H34.83 Tributary (branch) retinal vein occlusion**

One of the following 7th characters is to be assigned to codes in subcategory H34.83 to designate the severity of the occlusion:

0	with macular edema
1	with retinal neovascularization
2	stable
	Old tributary (branch) retinal vein occlusion

● H34.831 Tributary (branch) retinal vein occlusion, right eye
● H34.832 Tributary (branch) retinal vein occlusion, left eye
● H34.833 Tributary (branch) retinal vein occlusion, bilateral
● H34.839 Tributary (branch) retinal vein occlusion, unspecified eye

H34.9 Unspecified retinal vascular occlusion

● **H35 Other retinal disorders**
Excludes2 diabetic retinal disorders (E08.311-E08.359, E09.311-E09.359, E10.311-E10.359, E11.311-E11.359, E13.311-E13.359)

● **H35.0 Background retinopathy and retinal vascular changes**
⟹ Code also any associated hypertension (I10)
OGCR Section I. C.9.a.5.

Hypertensive Retinopathy
Subcategory H35.0, Background retinopathy and retinal vascular changes, should be used with a code from category I10–I15, Hypertensive disease to include the systemic hypertension. The sequencing is based on the reason for the encounter.

H35.00 Unspecified background retinopathy
● H35.01 Changes in retinal vascular appearance
Retinal vascular sheathing
H35.011 Changes in retinal vascular appearance, right eye
H35.012 Changes in retinal vascular appearance, left eye

H35.013 Changes in retinal vascular appearance, bilateral
H35.019 Changes in retinal vascular appearance, unspecified eye

● **H35.02 Exudative retinopathy**
Coats retinopathy
H35.021 Exudative retinopathy, right eye
H35.022 Exudative retinopathy, left eye
H35.023 Exudative retinopathy, bilateral
H35.029 Exudative retinopathy, unspecified eye

● **H35.03 Hypertensive retinopathy**
H35.031 Hypertensive retinopathy, right eye
H35.032 Hypertensive retinopathy, left eye
H35.033 Hypertensive retinopathy, bilateral
H35.039 Hypertensive retinopathy, unspecified eye

● **H35.04 Retinal micro-aneurysms, unspecified**
H35.041 Retinal micro-aneurysms, unspecified, right eye
H35.042 Retinal micro-aneurysms, unspecified, left eye
H35.043 Retinal micro-aneurysms, unspecified, bilateral
H35.049 Retinal micro-aneurysms, unspecified, unspecified eye

● **H35.05 Retinal neovascularization, unspecified**
H35.051 Retinal neovascularization, unspecified, right eye
H35.052 Retinal neovascularization, unspecified, left eye
H35.053 Retinal neovascularization, unspecified, bilateral
H35.059 Retinal neovascularization, unspecified, unspecified eye

● **H35.06 Retinal vasculitis**
Eales disease
Retinal perivasculitis
H35.061 Retinal vasculitis, right eye
H35.062 Retinal vasculitis, left eye
H35.063 Retinal vasculitis, bilateral
H35.069 Retinal vasculitis, unspecified eye

● **H35.07 Retinal telangiectasis**
H35.071 Retinal telangiectasis, right eye
H35.072 Retinal telangiectasis, left eye
H35.073 Retinal telangiectasis, bilateral
H35.079 Retinal telangiectasis, unspecified eye

H35.09 Other intraretinal microvascular abnormalities
Retinal varices

● **H35.1 Retinopathy of prematurity**
● **H35.10 Retinopathy of prematurity, unspecified**
Retinopathy of prematurity NOS
H35.101 Retinopathy of prematurity, unspecified, right eye
H35.102 Retinopathy of prematurity, unspecified, left eye
H35.103 Retinopathy of prematurity, unspecified, bilateral
H35.109 Retinopathy of prematurity, unspecified, unspecified eye

● **H35.11 Retinopathy of prematurity, stage 0**
H35.111 Retinopathy of prematurity, stage 0, right eye
H35.112 Retinopathy of prematurity, stage 0, left eye
H35.113 Retinopathy of prematurity, stage 0, bilateral
H35.119 Retinopathy of prematurity, stage 0, unspecified eye

● H35.12   Retinopathy of prematurity, stage 1
  H35.121   Retinopathy of prematurity, stage 1, right eye
  H35.122   Retinopathy of prematurity, stage 1, left eye
  H35.123   Retinopathy of prematurity, stage 1, bilateral
  H35.129   Retinopathy of prematurity, stage 1, unspecified eye

● H35.13   Retinopathy of prematurity, stage 2
  H35.131   Retinopathy of prematurity, stage 2, right eye
  H35.132   Retinopathy of prematurity, stage 2, left eye
  H35.133   Retinopathy of prematurity, stage 2, bilateral
  H35.139   Retinopathy of prematurity, stage 2, unspecified eye

● H35.14   Retinopathy of prematurity, stage 3
  H35.141   Retinopathy of prematurity, stage 3, right eye
  H35.142   Retinopathy of prematurity, stage 3, left eye
  H35.143   Retinopathy of prematurity, stage 3, bilateral
  H35.149   Retinopathy of prematurity, stage 3, unspecified eye

● H35.15   Retinopathy of prematurity, stage 4
  H35.151   Retinopathy of prematurity, stage 4, right eye
  H35.152   Retinopathy of prematurity, stage 4, left eye
  H35.153   Retinopathy of prematurity, stage 4, bilateral
  H35.159   Retinopathy of prematurity, stage 4, unspecified eye

● H35.16   Retinopathy of prematurity, stage 5
  H35.161   Retinopathy of prematurity, stage 5, right eye
  H35.162   Retinopathy of prematurity, stage 5, left eye
  H35.163   Retinopathy of prematurity, stage 5, bilateral
  H35.169   Retinopathy of prematurity, stage 5, unspecified eye

● H35.17   Retrolental fibroplasia
  H35.171   Retrolental fibroplasia, right eye
  H35.172   Retrolental fibroplasia, left eye
  H35.173   Retrolental fibroplasia, bilateral
  H35.179   Retrolental fibroplasia, unspecified eye

● H35.2   Other non-diabetic proliferative retinopathy
  Proliferative vitreo-retinopathy

  Excludes1   proliferative vitreo-retinopathy with retinal detachment (H33.4-)

  H35.20   Other non-diabetic proliferative retinopathy, unspecified eye
  H35.21   Other non-diabetic proliferative retinopathy, right eye
  H35.22   Other non-diabetic proliferative retinopathy, left eye
  H35.23   Other non-diabetic proliferative retinopathy, bilateral

● H35.3   Degeneration of macula and posterior pole
  H35.30   Unspecified macular degeneration   A
    Age-related macular degeneration

● H35.31   Nonexudative age-related macular degeneration
    Atrophic age-related macular degeneration
    Dry age-related macular degeneration

    One of the following 7th characters is to be assigned to codes in subcategory H35.31 to designate the stage of the disease:

Ø	stage unspecified
1	early dry stage
2	intermediate dry stage
3	advanced atrophic without subfoveal involvement
	advanced dry stage
4	advanced atrophic with subfoveal involvement

  ● H35.311   Nonexudative age-related macular degeneration, right eye   A
      Coding Clinic: 2016, Q4, P20-21
  ● H35.312   Nonexudative age-related macular degeneration, left eye   A
      Coding Clinic: 2016, Q4, P20-21
  ● H35.313   Nonexudative age-related macular degeneration, bilateral   A
      Coding Clinic: 2016, Q4, P20
  ● H35.319   Nonexudative age-related macular degeneration, unspecified eye   A
      Coding Clinic: 2016, Q4, P20

● H35.32   Exudative age-related macular degeneration
    Wet age-related macular degeneration

    One of the following 7th characters is to be assigned to codes in subcategory H35.32 to designate the stage of the disease:

Ø	stage unspecified
1	with active choroidal neovascularization
2	with inactive choroidal neovascularization
	with involuted or regressed neovascularization
3	with inactive scar

    Coding Clinic: 2016, Q4, P20

  ● H35.321   Exudative age-related macular degeneration, right eye 🔲   A
  ● H35.322   Exudative age-related macular degeneration, left eye 🔲   A
  ● H35.323   Exudative age-related macular degeneration, bilateral 🔲   A
  ● H35.329   Exudative age-related macular degeneration, unspecified eye 🔲   A

  H35.33   Angioid streaks of macula

● H35.34   Macular cyst, hole, or pseudohole
  H35.341   Macular cyst, hole, or pseudohole, right eye
  H35.342   Macular cyst, hole, or pseudohole, left eye
  H35.343   Macular cyst, hole, or pseudohole, bilateral
  H35.349   Macular cyst, hole, or pseudohole, unspecified eye

Item 7–7 Macular degeneration is typically age-related, chronic, and is evidenced by deterioration of the macula (the part of the retina that provides for central field vision), resulting in blurred vision or a blind spot in the center of visual field while not affecting peripheral vision.

CHAPTER 7 (H00-H59)

● H35.35 Cystoid macular degeneration
    Excludes1   cystoid macular edema
                   following cataract surgery
                   (H59.03-)

  H35.351 Cystoid macular degeneration, right
         eye
  H35.352 Cystoid macular degeneration, left
         eye
  H35.353 Cystoid macular degeneration,
         bilateral
  H35.359 Cystoid macular degeneration,
         unspecified eye

● H35.36 Drusen (degenerative) of macula
  H35.361 Drusen (degenerative) of macula,
         right eye
         Coding Clinic: 2016, Q4, P21
  H35.362 Drusen (degenerative) of macula, left
         eye
         Coding Clinic: 2016, Q4, P21
  H35.363 Drusen (degenerative) of macula,
         bilateral
         Coding Clinic: 2017, Q1, P51
  H35.369 Drusen (degenerative) of macula,
         unspecified eye

● H35.37 Puckering of macula
  H35.371 Puckering of macula, right eye
  H35.372 Puckering of macula, left eye
  H35.373 Puckering of macula, bilateral
  H35.379 Puckering of macula, unspecified eye

● H35.38 Toxic maculopathy
    Code first poisoning due to drug or toxin, if
       applicable (T36-T65 with fifth or sixth
       character 1-4 or 6)
    Use additional code for adverse effect, if
       applicable, to identify drug (T36-T50
       with fifth or sixth character 5)
  H35.381 Toxic maculopathy, right eye
  H35.382 Toxic maculopathy, left eye
  H35.383 Toxic maculopathy, bilateral
  H35.389 Toxic maculopathy, unspecified eye

● H35.4 Peripheral retinal degeneration
    Excludes1   hereditary retinal degeneration
               (dystrophy) (H35.5-)
               peripheral retinal degeneration with
               retinal break (H33.3-)

  H35.40 Unspecified peripheral retinal degeneration
● H35.41 Lattice degeneration of retina
    Palisade degeneration of retina
  H35.411 Lattice degeneration of retina, right
         eye
  H35.412 Lattice degeneration of retina, left eye
  H35.413 Lattice degeneration of retina,
         bilateral
  H35.419 Lattice degeneration of retina,
         unspecified eye

● H35.42 Microcystoid degeneration of retina
  H35.421 Microcystoid degeneration of retina,
         right eye
  H35.422 Microcystoid degeneration of retina,
         left eye
  H35.423 Microcystoid degeneration of retina,
         bilateral
  H35.429 Microcystoid degeneration of retina,
         unspecified eye

● H35.43 Paving stone degeneration of retina
  H35.431 Paving stone degeneration of retina,
         right eye
  H35.432 Paving stone degeneration of retina,
         left eye

  H35.433 Paving stone degeneration of retina,
         bilateral
  H35.439 Paving stone degeneration of retina,
         unspecified eye

● H35.44 Age-related reticular degeneration of retina
  H35.441 Age-related reticular degeneration of
         retina, right eye   A
  H35.442 Age-related reticular degeneration of
         retina, left eye   A
  H35.443 Age-related reticular degeneration of
         retina, bilateral   A
  H35.449 Age-related reticular degeneration of
         retina, unspecified eye   A

● H35.45 Secondary pigmentary degeneration
  H35.451 Secondary pigmentary degeneration,
         right eye
  H35.452 Secondary pigmentary degeneration,
         left eye
  H35.453 Secondary pigmentary degeneration,
         bilateral
  H35.459 Secondary pigmentary degeneration,
         unspecified eye

● H35.46 Secondary vitreoretinal degeneration
  H35.461 Secondary vitreoretinal degeneration,
         right eye
  H35.462 Secondary vitreoretinal degeneration,
         left eye
  H35.463 Secondary vitreoretinal degeneration,
         bilateral
  H35.469 Secondary vitreoretinal degeneration,
         unspecified eye

● H35.5 Hereditary retinal dystrophy
    Excludes1   dystrophies primarily involving Bruch's
               membrane (H31.1-)

  H35.50 Unspecified hereditary retinal dystrophy
  H35.51 Vitreoretinal dystrophy
  H35.52 Pigmentary retinal dystrophy
    Albipunctate retinal dystrophy
    Retinitis pigmentosa
    Tapetoretinal dystrophy
  H35.53 Other dystrophies primarily involving the
    sensory retina
    Stargardt's disease
  H35.54 Dystrophies primarily involving the retinal
    pigment epithelium
    Vitelliform retinal dystrophy

● H35.6 Retinal hemorrhage
  H35.60 Retinal hemorrhage, unspecified eye
  H35.61 Retinal hemorrhage, right eye
  H35.62 Retinal hemorrhage, left eye
  H35.63 Retinal hemorrhage, bilateral

● H35.7 Separation of retinal layers
    Excludes1   retinal detachment (serous) (H33.2-)
               rhegmatogenous retinal detachment
               (H33.0-)

  H35.70 Unspecified separation of retinal layers
● H35.71 Central serous chorioretinopathy
  H35.711 Central serous chorioretinopathy,
         right eye
  H35.712 Central serous chorioretinopathy, left
         eye
  H35.713 Central serous chorioretinopathy,
         bilateral
  H35.719 Central serous chorioretinopathy,
         unspecified eye

CHAPTER 7 (H00-H59)

▶ New   ⇒ Revised   ~~deleted~~ Deleted   Excludes 1   Excludes 2   Includes   Use additional   Code first   Code also   Key words
OGCR Official Guidelines   X Assign placeholder X   ● Use Additional Character(s)   ▷ Manifestation Code   🐷 Hierarchical Condition Category   Coding Clinic

● **H35.72 Serous detachment of retinal pigment epithelium**

    H35.721 Serous detachment of retinal pigment epithelium, right eye

    H35.722 Serous detachment of retinal pigment epithelium, left eye

    H35.723 Serous detachment of retinal pigment epithelium, bilateral

    H35.729 Serous detachment of retinal pigment epithelium, unspecified eye

● **H35.73 Hemorrhagic detachment of retinal pigment epithelium**

    H35.731 Hemorrhagic detachment of retinal pigment epithelium, right eye

    H35.732 Hemorrhagic detachment of retinal pigment epithelium, left eye

    H35.733 Hemorrhagic detachment of retinal pigment epithelium, bilateral

    H35.739 Hemorrhagic detachment of retinal pigment epithelium, unspecified eye

● **H35.8 Other specified retinal disorders**

    Excludes2 retinal hemorrhage (H35.6-)

    H35.81 Retinal edema
        Retinal cotton wool spots

    H35.82 Retinal ischemia

    H35.89 Other specified retinal disorders

  H35.9 Unspecified retinal disorder

▷ *H36 Retinal disorders in diseases classified elsewhere*

    Code first underlying disease, such as:
      lipid storage disorders (E75.-)
      sickle-cell disorders (D57.-)

    Excludes1 arteriosclerotic retinopathy (H35.0-)
        diabetic retinopathy (E08.3-, E09.3-, E10.3-, E11.3-, E13.3-)

GLAUCOMA (H40-H42)

● **H40 Glaucoma**

    Intraocular pressure (IOP) that is too high results from too much aqueous humor and because of excess production or inadequate drainage, optic nerve damage and vision loss may occur.

    Excludes1 absolute glaucoma (H44.51-)
        congenital glaucoma (Q15.0)
        traumatic glaucoma due to birth injury (P15.3)

● **H40.0 Glaucoma suspect**

  ● **H40.00 Preglaucoma, unspecified**

    H40.001 Preglaucoma, unspecified, right eye

    H40.002 Preglaucoma, unspecified, left eye

    H40.003 Preglaucoma, unspecified, bilateral

    H40.009 Preglaucoma, unspecified, unspecified eye

  ● **H40.01 Open angle with borderline findings, low risk**
      Open angle, low risk

    H40.011 Open angle with borderline findings, low risk, right eye

    H40.012 Open angle with borderline findings, low risk, left eye

    H40.013 Open angle with borderline findings, low risk, bilateral

    H40.019 Open angle with borderline findings, low risk, unspecified eye

  ● **H40.02 Open angle with borderline findings, high risk**
      Open angle, high risk

    H40.021 Open angle with borderline findings, high risk, right eye

    H40.022 Open angle with borderline findings, high risk, left eye

    H40.023 Open angle with borderline findings, high risk, bilateral

    H40.029 Open angle with borderline findings, high risk, unspecified eye

● **H40.03 Anatomical narrow angle**
    Primary angle closure suspect

    H40.031 Anatomical narrow angle, right eye

    H40.032 Anatomical narrow angle, left eye

    H40.033 Anatomical narrow angle, bilateral

    H40.039 Anatomical narrow angle, unspecified eye

● **H40.04 Steroid responder**

    H40.041 Steroid responder, right eye

    H40.042 Steroid responder, left eye

    H40.043 Steroid responder, bilateral

    H40.049 Steroid responder, unspecified eye

● **H40.05 Ocular hypertension**

    H40.051 Ocular hypertension, right eye

    H40.052 Ocular hypertension, left eye

    H40.053 Ocular hypertension, bilateral

    H40.059 Ocular hypertension, unspecified eye

● **H40.06 Primary angle closure without glaucoma damage**

    H40.061 Primary angle closure without glaucoma damage, right eye

    H40.062 Primary angle closure without glaucoma damage, left eye

    H40.063 Primary angle closure without glaucoma damage, bilateral

    H40.069 Primary angle closure without glaucoma damage, unspecified eye

● **H40.1 Open-angle glaucoma**

  X ● **H40.10 Unspecified open-angle glaucoma**

    One of the following 7th characters is to be assigned to code H40.10 to designate the stage of glaucoma

0	stage unspecified
1	mild stage
2	moderate stage
3	severe stage
4	indeterminate stage

● **H40.11 Primary open-angle glaucoma**
    Chronic simple glaucoma

    One of the following 7th characters is to be assigned to each code in subcategory H40.11 to designate the stage of glaucoma

0	stage unspecified
1	mild stage
2	moderate stage
3	severe stage
4	indeterminate stage

    Coding Clinic: 2016, Q4, P22

  ● H40.111 Primary open-angle glaucoma, right eye
        Coding Clinic: 2019, Q2, P31

  ● H40.112 Primary open-angle glaucoma, left eye

  ● H40.113 Primary open-angle glaucoma, bilateral

  ● H40.119 Primary open-angle glaucoma, unspecified eye

● H40.12 Low-tension glaucoma

One of the following 7th characters is to be assigned to each code in subcategory H40.12 to designate the stage of glaucoma

0	stage unspecified
1	mild stage
2	moderate stage
3	severe stage
4	indeterminate stage

● H40.121 Low-tension glaucoma, right eye
● H40.122 Low-tension glaucoma, left eye
● H40.123 Low-tension glaucoma, bilateral
● H40.129 Low-tension glaucoma, unspecified eye

● H40.13 Pigmentary glaucoma

One of the following 7th characters is to be assigned to each code in subcategory H40.13 to designate the stage of glaucoma

0	stage unspecified
1	mild stage
2	moderate stage
3	severe stage
4	indeterminate stage

● H40.131 Pigmentary glaucoma, right eye
● H40.132 Pigmentary glaucoma, left eye
● H40.133 Pigmentary glaucoma, bilateral
● H40.139 Pigmentary glaucoma, unspecified eye

● H40.14 Capsular glaucoma with pseudoexfoliation of lens

One of the following 7th characters is to be assigned to each code in subcategory H40.14 to designate the stage of glaucoma

0	stage unspecified
1	mild stage
2	moderate stage
3	severe stage
4	indeterminate stage

● H40.141 Capsular glaucoma with pseudoexfoliation of lens, right eye
● H40.142 Capsular glaucoma with pseudoexfoliation of lens, left eye
● H40.143 Capsular glaucoma with pseudoexfoliation of lens, bilateral
● H40.149 Capsular glaucoma with pseudoexfoliation of lens, unspecified eye

● H40.15 Residual stage of open-angle glaucoma

H40.151 Residual stage of open-angle glaucoma, right eye
H40.152 Residual stage of open-angle glaucoma, left eye
H40.153 Residual stage of open-angle glaucoma, bilateral
H40.159 Residual stage of open-angle glaucoma, unspecified eye

● H40.2 Primary angle-closure glaucoma

Excludes1   aqueous misdirection (H40.83-)
malignant glaucoma (H40.83-)

X ● H40.20 Unspecified primary angle-closure glaucoma

One of the following 7th characters is to be assigned to code H40.20 to designate the stage of glaucoma

0	stage unspecified
1	mild stage
2	moderate stage
3	severe stage
4	indeterminate stage

● H40.21 Acute angle-closure glaucoma

Acute angle-closure glaucoma attack
Acute angle-closure glaucoma crisis

H40.211 Acute angle-closure glaucoma, right eye
H40.212 Acute angle-closure glaucoma, left eye
H40.213 Acute angle-closure glaucoma, bilateral
H40.219 Acute angle-closure glaucoma, unspecified eye

● H40.22 Chronic angle-closure glaucoma

Chronic primary angle closure glaucoma

One of the following 7th characters is to be assigned to each code in subcategory H40.22 to designate the stage of glaucoma

0	stage unspecified
1	mild stage
2	moderate stage
3	severe stage
4	indeterminate stage

● H40.221 Chronic angle-closure glaucoma, right eye
● H40.222 Chronic angle-closure glaucoma, left eye
● H40.223 Chronic angle-closure glaucoma, bilateral
● H40.229 Chronic angle-closure glaucoma, unspecified eye

● H40.23 Intermittent angle-closure glaucoma

H40.231 Intermittent angle-closure glaucoma, right eye
H40.232 Intermittent angle-closure glaucoma, left eye
H40.233 Intermittent angle-closure glaucoma, bilateral
H40.239 Intermittent angle-closure glaucoma, unspecified eye

● H40.24 Residual stage of angle-closure glaucoma

H40.241 Residual stage of angle-closure glaucoma, right eye
H40.242 Residual stage of angle-closure glaucoma, left eye
H40.243 Residual stage of angle-closure glaucoma, bilateral
H40.249 Residual stage of angle-closure glaucoma, unspecified eye

● **H40.3 Glaucoma secondary to eye trauma**
    Code also underlying condition
    One of the following 7th characters is to be assigned to each code in subcategory H40.3 to designate the stage of glaucoma

> Ø   stage unspecified
> 1   mild stage
> 2   moderate stage
> 3   severe stage
> 4   indeterminate stage

X ● **H40.30 Glaucoma secondary to eye trauma, unspecified eye**
X ● **H40.31 Glaucoma secondary to eye trauma, right eye**
X ● **H40.32 Glaucoma secondary to eye trauma, left eye**
X ● **H40.33 Glaucoma secondary to eye trauma, bilateral**

● **H40.4 Glaucoma secondary to eye inflammation**
    Code also underlying condition
    One of the following 7th characters is to be assigned to each code in subcategory H40.4 to designate the stage of glaucoma

> Ø   stage unspecified
> 1   mild stage
> 2   moderate stage
> 3   severe stage
> 4   indeterminate stage

X ● **H40.40 Glaucoma secondary to eye inflammation, unspecified eye**
X ● **H40.41 Glaucoma secondary to eye inflammation, right eye**
X ● **H40.42 Glaucoma secondary to eye inflammation, left eye**
X ● **H40.43 Glaucoma secondary to eye inflammation, bilateral**

● **H40.5 Glaucoma secondary to other eye disorders**
    Code also underlying eye disorder
    One of the following 7th characters is to be assigned to each code in subcategory H40.5 to designate the stage of glaucoma

> Ø   stage unspecified
> 1   mild stage
> 2   moderate stage
> 3   severe stage
> 4   indeterminate stage

X ● **H40.50 Glaucoma secondary to other eye disorders, unspecified eye**
X ● **H40.51 Glaucoma secondary to other eye disorders, right eye**
X ● **H40.52 Glaucoma secondary to other eye disorders, left eye**
X ● **H40.53 Glaucoma secondary to other eye disorders, bilateral**

● **H40.6 Glaucoma secondary to drugs**
    Use additional code for adverse effect, if applicable, to identify drug (T36-T50 with fifth or sixth character 5)
    One of the following 7th characters is to be assigned to each code in subcategory H40.6 to designate the stage of glaucoma

> Ø   stage unspecified
> 1   mild stage
> 2   moderate stage
> 3   severe stage
> 4   indeterminate stage

X ● **H40.60 Glaucoma secondary to drugs, unspecified eye**
X ● **H40.61 Glaucoma secondary to drugs, right eye**
X ● **H40.62 Glaucoma secondary to drugs, left eye**
X ● **H40.63 Glaucoma secondary to drugs, bilateral**

● **H40.8 Other glaucoma**
   ● **H40.81 Glaucoma with increased episcleral venous pressure**
      H40.811 Glaucoma with increased episcleral venous pressure, right eye
      H40.812 Glaucoma with increased episcleral venous pressure, left eye
      H40.813 Glaucoma with increased episcleral venous pressure, bilateral
      H40.819 Glaucoma with increased episcleral venous pressure, unspecified eye
   ● **H40.82 Hypersecretion glaucoma**
      H40.821 Hypersecretion glaucoma, right eye
      H40.822 Hypersecretion glaucoma, left eye
      H40.823 Hypersecretion glaucoma, bilateral
      H40.829 Hypersecretion glaucoma, unspecified eye
   ● **H40.83 Aqueous misdirection**
      Malignant glaucoma
      H40.831 Aqueous misdirection, right eye
      H40.832 Aqueous misdirection, left eye
      H40.833 Aqueous misdirection, bilateral
      H40.839 Aqueous misdirection, unspecified eye
      H40.89 Other specified glaucoma

   H40.9 Unspecified glaucoma

▸ **H42 Glaucoma in diseases classified elsewhere**
    Code first underlying condition, such as:
     amyloidosis (E85.-)
     aniridia (Q13.1)
     glaucoma (in) diabetes mellitus (E08.39, E09.39, E10.39, E11.39, E13.39)
     Lowe's syndrome (E72.03)
     Reiger's anomaly (Q13.81)
     specified metabolic disorder (E70-E88)

    Excludes1   glaucoma (in) onchocerciasis (B73.02)
               glaucoma (in) syphilis (A52.71)
               glaucoma (in) tuberculous (A18.59)

DISORDERS OF VITREOUS BODY AND GLOBE (H43-H44)

● **H43 Disorders of vitreous body**
   ● **H43.0 Vitreous prolapse**
     Excludes1   vitreous syndrome following cataract surgery (H59.0-)
               traumatic vitreous prolapse (S05.2-)
     H43.00 Vitreous prolapse, unspecified eye
     H43.01 Vitreous prolapse, right eye
     H43.02 Vitreous prolapse, left eye
     H43.03 Vitreous prolapse, bilateral

CHAPTER 7 (HØØ-H59)

● **H43.1 Vitreous hemorrhage**
  H43.10 Vitreous hemorrhage, unspecified eye 🔗
  H43.11 Vitreous hemorrhage, right eye 🔗
  H43.12 Vitreous hemorrhage, left eye 🔗
  H43.13 Vitreous hemorrhage, bilateral 🔗
● **H43.2 Crystalline deposits in vitreous body**
  H43.20 Crystalline deposits in vitreous body, unspecified eye
  H43.21 Crystalline deposits in vitreous body, right eye
  H43.22 Crystalline deposits in vitreous body, left eye
  H43.23 Crystalline deposits in vitreous body, bilateral
● **H43.3 Other vitreous opacities**
 ● H43.31 Vitreous membranes and strands
   H43.311 Vitreous membranes and strands, right eye
   H43.312 Vitreous membranes and strands, left eye
   H43.313 Vitreous membranes and strands, bilateral
   H43.319 Vitreous membranes and strands, unspecified eye
 ● H43.39 Other vitreous opacities
   Vitreous floaters
    Small clumps of cells that float in the vitreous of the eye, appearing as black specks or dots in the field of vision and common in the aging eye.
   H43.391 Other vitreous opacities, right eye
   H43.392 Other vitreous opacities, left eye
   H43.393 Other vitreous opacities, bilateral
   H43.399 Other vitreous opacities, unspecified eye
● **H43.8 Other disorders of vitreous body**
  Excludes1 proliferative vitreo-retinopathy with retinal detachment (H33.4)
  Excludes2 vitreous abscess (H44.02-)
 ● H43.81 Vitreous degeneration
   Vitreous detachment
   H43.811 Vitreous degeneration, right eye
   H43.812 Vitreous degeneration, left eye
   H43.813 Vitreous degeneration, bilateral
   H43.819 Vitreous degeneration, unspecified eye
 ● H43.82 Vitreomacular adhesion
   Vitreomacular traction
   H43.821 Vitreomacular adhesion, right eye A
   H43.822 Vitreomacular adhesion, left eye A
   H43.823 Vitreomacular adhesion, bilateral A
   H43.829 Vitreomacular adhesion, unspecified eye A
  H43.89 Other disorders of vitreous body
 H43.9 Unspecified disorder of vitreous body

● **H44 Disorders of globe**
  Includes disorders affecting multiple structures of eye
● **H44.0 Purulent endophthalmitis**
  Use additional code to identify organism
  Excludes1 bleb associated endophthalmitis (H59.4-)
 ● H44.00 Unspecified purulent endophthalmitis
   H44.001 Unspecified purulent endophthalmitis, right eye
   H44.002 Unspecified purulent endophthalmitis, left eye
   H44.003 Unspecified purulent endophthalmitis, bilateral
   H44.009 Unspecified purulent endophthalmitis, unspecified eye

 ● H44.01 Panophthalmitis (acute)
   H44.011 Panophthalmitis (acute), right eye
   H44.012 Panophthalmitis (acute), left eye
   H44.013 Panophthalmitis (acute), bilateral
   H44.019 Panophthalmitis (acute), unspecified eye
 ● H44.02 Vitreous abscess (chronic)
   H44.021 Vitreous abscess (chronic), right eye
   H44.022 Vitreous abscess (chronic), left eye
   H44.023 Vitreous abscess (chronic), bilateral
   H44.029 Vitreous abscess (chronic), unspecified eye
● **H44.1 Other endophthalmitis**
  Excludes1 bleb associated endophthalmitis (H59.4-)
  Excludes2 ophthalmia nodosa (H16.2-)
 ● H44.11 Panuveitis
   H44.111 Panuveitis, right eye
   H44.112 Panuveitis, left eye
   H44.113 Panuveitis, bilateral
   H44.119 Panuveitis, unspecified eye
 ● H44.12 Parasitic endophthalmitis, unspecified
   H44.121 Parasitic endophthalmitis, unspecified, right eye
   H44.122 Parasitic endophthalmitis, unspecified, left eye
   H44.123 Parasitic endophthalmitis, unspecified, bilateral
   H44.129 Parasitic endophthalmitis, unspecified, unspecified eye
 ● H44.13 Sympathetic uveitis
   H44.131 Sympathetic uveitis, right eye
   H44.132 Sympathetic uveitis, left eye
   H44.133 Sympathetic uveitis, bilateral
   H44.139 Sympathetic uveitis, unspecified eye
  H44.19 Other endophthalmitis
● **H44.2 Degenerative myopia**
  Malignant myopia
  H44.20 Degenerative myopia, unspecified eye
  H44.21 Degenerative myopia, right eye
  H44.22 Degenerative myopia, left eye
  H44.23 Degenerative myopia, bilateral
 ● H44.2A Degenerative myopia with choroidal neovascularization
   Use Additional code for any associated choroid disorders (H31.-)
   H44.2A1 Degenerative myopia with choroidal neovascularization, right eye
   H44.2A2 Degenerative myopia with choroidal neovascularization, left eye
   H44.2A3 Degenerative myopia with choroidal neovascularization, bilateral eye
   H44.2A9 Degenerative myopia with choroidal neovascularization, unspecified eye
 ● H44.2B Degenerative myopia with macular hole
   H44.2B1 Degenerative myopia with macular hole, right eye
   H44.2B2 Degenerative myopia with macular hole, left eye
   H44.2B3 Degenerative myopia with macular hole, bilateral eye
   H44.2B9 Degenerative myopia with macular hole, unspecified eye

- H44.2C Degenerative myopia with retinal detachment
  - Use Additional code to identify the retinal detachment (H33.-)
  - H44.2C1 Degenerative myopia with retinal detachment, right eye
  - H44.2C2 Degenerative myopia with retinal detachment, left eye
  - H44.2C3 Degenerative myopia with retinal detachment, bilateral eye
  - H44.2C9 Degenerative myopia with retinal detachment, unspecified eye
- H44.2D Degenerative myopia with foveoschisis
  - H44.2D1 Degenerative myopia with foveoschisis, right eye
  - H44.2D2 Degenerative myopia with foveoschisis, left eye
  - H44.2D3 Degenerative myopia with foveoschisis, bilateral eye
  - H44.2D9 Degenerative myopia with foveoschisis, unspecified eye
- H44.2E Degenerative myopia with other maculopathy
  - H44.2E1 Degenerative myopia with other maculopathy, right eye
  - H44.2E2 Degenerative myopia with other maculopathy, left eye
  - H44.2E3 Degenerative myopia with other maculopathy, bilateral eye
  - H44.2E9 Degenerative myopia with other maculopathy, unspecified eye
- H44.3 Other and unspecified degenerative disorders of globe
  - H44.30 Unspecified degenerative disorder of globe
  - H44.31 Chalcosis
    - H44.311 Chalcosis, right eye
    - H44.312 Chalcosis, left eye
    - H44.313 Chalcosis, bilateral
    - H44.319 Chalcosis, unspecified eye
  - H44.32 Siderosis of eye
    - H44.321 Siderosis of eye, right eye
    - H44.322 Siderosis of eye, left eye
    - H44.323 Siderosis of eye, bilateral
    - H44.329 Siderosis of eye, unspecified eye
  - H44.39 Other degenerative disorders of globe
    - H44.391 Other degenerative disorders of globe, right eye
    - H44.392 Other degenerative disorders of globe, left eye
    - H44.393 Other degenerative disorders of globe, bilateral
    - H44.399 Other degenerative disorders of globe, unspecified eye
- H44.4 Hypotony of eye
  - H44.40 Unspecified hypotony of eye
  - H44.41 Flat anterior chamber hypotony of eye
    - H44.411 Flat anterior chamber hypotony of right eye
    - H44.412 Flat anterior chamber hypotony of left eye
    - H44.413 Flat anterior chamber hypotony of eye, bilateral
    - H44.419 Flat anterior chamber hypotony of unspecified eye
  - H44.42 Hypotony of eye due to ocular fistula
    - H44.421 Hypotony of right eye due to ocular fistula
    - H44.422 Hypotony of left eye due to ocular fistula

- H44.423 Hypotony of eye due to ocular fistula, bilateral
- H44.429 Hypotony of unspecified eye due to ocular fistula
- H44.43 Hypotony of eye due to other ocular disorders
  - H44.431 Hypotony of eye due to other ocular disorders, right eye
  - H44.432 Hypotony of eye due to other ocular disorders, left eye
  - H44.433 Hypotony of eye due to other ocular disorders, bilateral
  - H44.439 Hypotony of eye due to other ocular disorders, unspecified eye
- H44.44 Primary hypotony of eye
  - H44.441 Primary hypotony of right eye
  - H44.442 Primary hypotony of left eye
  - H44.443 Primary hypotony of eye, bilateral
  - H44.449 Primary hypotony of unspecified eye
- H44.5 Degenerated conditions of globe
  - H44.50 Unspecified degenerated conditions of globe
  - H44.51 Absolute glaucoma
    - H44.511 Absolute glaucoma, right eye
    - H44.512 Absolute glaucoma, left eye
    - H44.513 Absolute glaucoma, bilateral
    - H44.519 Absolute glaucoma, unspecified eye
  - H44.52 Atrophy of globe
    - Phthisis bulbi
    - H44.521 Atrophy of globe, right eye
    - H44.522 Atrophy of globe, left eye
    - H44.523 Atrophy of globe, bilateral
    - H44.529 Atrophy of globe, unspecified eye
  - H44.53 Leucocoria
    - H44.531 Leucocoria, right eye
    - H44.532 Leucocoria, left eye
    - H44.533 Leucocoria, bilateral
    - H44.539 Leucocoria, unspecified eye
- H44.6 Retained (old) intraocular foreign body, magnetic
  - Use additional code to identify magnetic foreign body (Z18.11)
  - **Excludes1** current intraocular foreign body (S05.-)
  - **Excludes2** retained foreign body in eyelid (H02.81-)
    retained (old) foreign body following penetrating wound of orbit (H05.5-)
    retained (old) intraocular foreign body, nonmagnetic (H44.7-)
  - H44.60 Unspecified retained (old) intraocular foreign body, magnetic
    - H44.601 Unspecified retained (old) intraocular foreign body, magnetic, right eye
    - H44.602 Unspecified retained (old) intraocular foreign body, magnetic, left eye
    - H44.603 Unspecified retained (old) intraocular foreign body, magnetic, bilateral
    - H44.609 Unspecified retained (old) intraocular foreign body, magnetic, unspecified eye
  - H44.61 Retained (old) magnetic foreign body in anterior chamber
    - H44.611 Retained (old) magnetic foreign body in anterior chamber, right eye
    - H44.612 Retained (old) magnetic foreign body in anterior chamber, left eye
    - H44.613 Retained (old) magnetic foreign body in anterior chamber, bilateral
    - H44.619 Retained (old) magnetic foreign body in anterior chamber, unspecified eye

● H44.62   Retained (old) magnetic foreign body in iris or ciliary body

     H44.621   Retained (old) magnetic foreign body in iris or ciliary body, right eye

     H44.622   Retained (old) magnetic foreign body in iris or ciliary body, left eye

     H44.623   Retained (old) magnetic foreign body in iris or ciliary body, bilateral

     H44.629   Retained (old) magnetic foreign body in iris or ciliary body, unspecified eye

● H44.63   Retained (old) magnetic foreign body in lens

     H44.631   Retained (old) magnetic foreign body in lens, right eye

     H44.632   Retained (old) magnetic foreign body in lens, left eye

     H44.633   Retained (old) magnetic foreign body in lens, bilateral

     H44.639   Retained (old) magnetic foreign body in lens, unspecified eye

● H44.64   Retained (old) magnetic foreign body in posterior wall of globe

     H44.641   Retained (old) magnetic foreign body in posterior wall of globe, right eye

     H44.642   Retained (old) magnetic foreign body in posterior wall of globe, left eye

     H44.643   Retained (old) magnetic foreign body in posterior wall of globe, bilateral

     H44.649   Retained (old) magnetic foreign body in posterior wall of globe, unspecified eye

● H44.65   Retained (old) magnetic foreign body in vitreous body

     H44.651   Retained (old) magnetic foreign body in vitreous body, right eye

     H44.652   Retained (old) magnetic foreign body in vitreous body, left eye

     H44.653   Retained (old) magnetic foreign body in vitreous body, bilateral

     H44.659   Retained (old) magnetic foreign body in vitreous body, unspecified eye

● H44.69   Retained (old) intraocular foreign body, magnetic, in other or multiple sites

     H44.691   Retained (old) intraocular foreign body, magnetic, in other or multiple sites, right eye

     H44.692   Retained (old) intraocular foreign body, magnetic, in other or multiple sites, left eye

     H44.693   Retained (old) intraocular foreign body, magnetic, in other or multiple sites, bilateral

     H44.699   Retained (old) intraocular foreign body, magnetic, in other or multiple sites, unspecified eye

● H44.7   Retained (old) intraocular foreign body, nonmagnetic

Use additional code to identify nonmagnetic foreign body (Z18.01-Z18.10, Z18.12, Z18.2-Z18.9)

> **Excludes1**   current intraocular foreign body (S05.-)

> **Excludes2**   retained foreign body in eyelid (H02.81-)
> retained (old) foreign body following penetrating wound of orbit (H05.5-)
> retained (old) intraocular foreign body, magnetic (H44.6-)

● H44.70   Unspecified retained (old) intraocular foreign body, nonmagnetic

     H44.701   Unspecified retained (old) intraocular foreign body, nonmagnetic, right eye

     H44.702   Unspecified retained (old) intraocular foreign body, nonmagnetic, left eye

     H44.703   Unspecified retained (old) intraocular foreign body, nonmagnetic, bilateral

     H44.709   Unspecified retained (old) intraocular foreign body, nonmagnetic, unspecified eye

         Retained (old) intraocular foreign body NOS

● H44.71   Retained (nonmagnetic) (old) foreign body in anterior chamber

     H44.711   Retained (nonmagnetic) (old) foreign body in anterior chamber, right eye

     H44.712   Retained (nonmagnetic) (old) foreign body in anterior chamber, left eye

     H44.713   Retained (nonmagnetic) (old) foreign body in anterior chamber, bilateral

     H44.719   Retained (nonmagnetic) (old) foreign body in anterior chamber, unspecified eye

● H44.72   Retained (nonmagnetic) (old) foreign body in iris or ciliary body

     H44.721   Retained (nonmagnetic) (old) foreign body in iris or ciliary body, right eye

     H44.722   Retained (nonmagnetic) (old) foreign body in iris or ciliary body, left eye

     H44.723   Retained (nonmagnetic) (old) foreign body in iris or ciliary body, bilateral

     H44.729   Retained (nonmagnetic) (old) foreign body in iris or ciliary body, unspecified eye

● H44.73   Retained (nonmagnetic) (old) foreign body in lens

     H44.731   Retained (nonmagnetic) (old) foreign body in lens, right eye

     H44.732   Retained (nonmagnetic) (old) foreign body in lens, left eye

     H44.733   Retained (nonmagnetic) (old) foreign body in lens, bilateral

     H44.739   Retained (nonmagnetic) (old) foreign body in lens, unspecified eye

● H44.74   Retained (nonmagnetic) (old) foreign body in posterior wall of globe

     H44.741   Retained (nonmagnetic) (old) foreign body in posterior wall of globe, right eye

     H44.742   Retained (nonmagnetic) (old) foreign body in posterior wall of globe, left eye

     H44.743   Retained (nonmagnetic) (old) foreign body in posterior wall of globe, bilateral

     H44.749   Retained (nonmagnetic) (old) foreign body in posterior wall of globe, unspecified eye

● H44.75   Retained (nonmagnetic) (old) foreign body in vitreous body

     H44.751   Retained (nonmagnetic) (old) foreign body in vitreous body, right eye

     H44.752   Retained (nonmagnetic) (old) foreign body in vitreous body, left eye

     H44.753   Retained (nonmagnetic) (old) foreign body in vitreous body, bilateral

     H44.759   Retained (nonmagnetic) (old) foreign body in vitreous body, unspecified eye

● H44.79   Retained (old) intraocular foreign body, nonmagnetic, in other or multiple sites

     H44.791   Retained (old) intraocular foreign body, nonmagnetic, in other or multiple sites, right eye

     H44.792   Retained (old) intraocular foreign body, nonmagnetic, in other or multiple sites, left eye

     H44.793   Retained (old) intraocular foreign body, nonmagnetic, in other or multiple sites, bilateral

     H44.799   Retained (old) intraocular foreign body, nonmagnetic, in other or multiple sites, unspecified eye

● H44.8   Other disorders of globe

  ● H44.81   Hemophthalmos

     H44.811   Hemophthalmos, right eye

     H44.812   Hemophthalmos, left eye

     H44.813   Hemophthalmos, bilateral

     H44.819   Hemophthalmos, unspecified eye

  ● H44.82   Luxation of globe

     H44.821   Luxation of globe, right eye

     H44.822   Luxation of globe, left eye

     H44.823   Luxation of globe, bilateral

     H44.829   Luxation of globe, unspecified eye

     H44.89   Other disorders of globe

   H44.9   Unspecified disorder of globe

★ **(See Plate 7 of the Anatomy Illustrations.)**

DISORDERS OF OPTIC NERVE AND VISUAL PATHWAYS (H46-H47)

● H46   Optic neuritis

     Excludes2   ischemic optic neuropathy (H47.01-)
               neuromyelitis optica [Devic] (G36.0)

  ● H46.0   Optic papillitis

     H46.00   Optic papillitis, unspecified eye

     H46.01   Optic papillitis, right eye

     H46.02   Optic papillitis, left eye

     H46.03   Optic papillitis, bilateral

  ● H46.1   Retrobulbar neuritis

     Retrobulbar neuritis NOS

     Excludes1   syphilitic retrobulbar neuritis (A52.15)

     H46.10   Retrobulbar neuritis, unspecified eye

     H46.11   Retrobulbar neuritis, right eye

     H46.12   Retrobulbar neuritis, left eye

     H46.13   Retrobulbar neuritis, bilateral

   H46.2   Nutritional optic neuropathy

   H46.3   Toxic optic neuropathy

     Code first (T51-T65) to identify cause

   H46.8   Other optic neuritis

   H46.9   Unspecified optic neuritis

● H47   Other disorders of optic [2nd] nerve and visual pathways

  ● H47.0   Disorders of optic nerve, not elsewhere classified

    ● H47.01   Ischemic optic neuropathy

     H47.011   Ischemic optic neuropathy, right eye

     H47.012   Ischemic optic neuropathy, left eye

     H47.013   Ischemic optic neuropathy, bilateral

     H47.019   Ischemic optic neuropathy, unspecified eye

    ● H47.02   Hemorrhage in optic nerve sheath

     H47.021   Hemorrhage in optic nerve sheath, right eye

     H47.022   Hemorrhage in optic nerve sheath, left eye

     H47.023   Hemorrhage in optic nerve sheath, bilateral

     H47.029   Hemorrhage in optic nerve sheath, unspecified eye

    ● H47.03   Optic nerve hypoplasia

     H47.031   Optic nerve hypoplasia, right eye

     H47.032   Optic nerve hypoplasia, left eye

     H47.033   Optic nerve hypoplasia, bilateral

     H47.039   Optic nerve hypoplasia, unspecified eye

    ● H47.09   Other disorders of optic nerve, not elsewhere classified

       Compression of optic nerve

     H47.091   Other disorders of optic nerve, not elsewhere classified, right eye

     H47.092   Other disorders of optic nerve, not elsewhere classified, left eye

     H47.093   Other disorders of optic nerve, not elsewhere classified, bilateral

     H47.099   Other disorders of optic nerve, not elsewhere classified, unspecified eye

  ● H47.1   Papilledema

     H47.10   Unspecified papilledema

     H47.11   Papilledema associated with increased intracranial pressure

     H47.12   Papilledema associated with decreased ocular pressure

     H47.13   Papilledema associated with retinal disorder

    ● H47.14   Foster-Kennedy syndrome

     H47.141   Foster-Kennedy syndrome, right eye

     H47.142   Foster-Kennedy syndrome, left eye

     H47.143   Foster-Kennedy syndrome, bilateral

     H47.149   Foster-Kennedy syndrome, unspecified eye

  ● H47.2   Optic atrophy

     H47.20   Unspecified optic atrophy

    ● H47.21   Primary optic atrophy

     H47.211   Primary optic atrophy, right eye

     H47.212   Primary optic atrophy, left eye

     H47.213   Primary optic atrophy, bilateral

     H47.219   Primary optic atrophy, unspecified eye

     H47.22   Hereditary optic atrophy

       Leber's optic atrophy

Figure 7-11   Stages of papilledema according to the Frisén grading scale. **A,** Very eary papilledema (Frisén stage 1). **B,** Early papilledema (Frisén stage 2). **C,** Moderate papilledema (Frisén stage 3). **D,** Marked papilledema (Frisén stage 4). **E,** Severe papilledema. (From Youmans JR, Winn HR: Youmans Neurological Surgery, Philadelphia, PA, Elsevier/Saunders, 2011)

Item 7-8   Papilledema is swelling of the optic disc caused by increased intracranial pressure. It is most often bilateral and occurs quickly (hours) or over weeks of time. It is a common symptom of a brain tumor. The term should not be used to describe optic disc swelling with underlying infectious, infiltrative, or inflammatory etiologies.

CHAPTER 7 (H00-H59)

CHAPTER 7 (H00-H59)

● H47.23   Glaucomatous optic atrophy
     H47.231   Glaucomatous optic atrophy, right eye
     H47.232   Glaucomatous optic atrophy, left eye
     H47.233   Glaucomatous optic atrophy, bilateral
     H47.239   Glaucomatous optic atrophy, unspecified eye
● H47.29   Other optic atrophy
     Temporal pallor of optic disc
     H47.291   Other optic atrophy, right eye
     H47.292   Other optic atrophy, left eye
     H47.293   Other optic atrophy, bilateral
     H47.299   Other optic atrophy, unspecified eye
● H47.3   Other disorders of optic disc
   ● H47.31   Coloboma of optic disc
     H47.311   Coloboma of optic disc, right eye
     H47.312   Coloboma of optic disc, left eye
     H47.313   Coloboma of optic disc, bilateral
     H47.319   Coloboma of optic disc, unspecified eye
   ● H47.32   Drusen of optic disc
     H47.321   Drusen of optic disc, right eye
     H47.322   Drusen of optic disc, left eye
     H47.323   Drusen of optic disc, bilateral
     H47.329   Drusen of optic disc, unspecified eye
   ● H47.33   Pseudopapilledema of optic disc
     H47.331   Pseudopapilledema of optic disc, right eye
     H47.332   Pseudopapilledema of optic disc, left eye
     H47.333   Pseudopapilledema of optic disc, bilateral
     H47.339   Pseudopapilledema of optic disc, unspecified eye
   ● H47.39   Other disorders of optic disc
     H47.391   Other disorders of optic disc, right eye
     H47.392   Other disorders of optic disc, left eye
     H47.393   Other disorders of optic disc, bilateral
     H47.399   Other disorders of optic disc, unspecified eye
● H47.4   Disorders of optic chiasm
     Code also underlying condition
   H47.41   Disorders of optic chiasm in (due to) inflammatory disorders
   H47.42   Disorders of optic chiasm in (due to) neoplasm
   H47.43   Disorders of optic chiasm in (due to) vascular disorders
   H47.49   Disorders of optic chiasm in (due to) other disorders
● H47.5   Disorders of other visual pathways
     Disorders of optic tracts, geniculate nuclei and optic radiations
     Code also underlying condition
   ● H47.51   Disorders of visual pathways in (due to) inflammatory disorders
     H47.511   Disorders of visual pathways in (due to) inflammatory disorders, right side
     H47.512   Disorders of visual pathways in (due to) inflammatory disorders, left side
     H47.519   Disorders of visual pathways in (due to) inflammatory disorders, unspecified side

   ● H47.52   Disorders of visual pathways in (due to) neoplasm
     H47.521   Disorders of visual pathways in (due to) neoplasm, right side
     H47.522   Disorders of visual pathways in (due to) neoplasm, left side
     H47.529   Disorders of visual pathways in (due to) neoplasm, unspecified side
   ● H47.53   Disorders of visual pathways in (due to) vascular disorders
     H47.531   Disorders of visual pathways in (due to) vascular disorders, right side
     H47.532   Disorders of visual pathways in (due to) vascular disorders, left side
     H47.539   Disorders of visual pathways in (due to) vascular disorders, unspecified side
● H47.6   Disorders of visual cortex
     Code also underlying condition
     Excludes1   injury to visual cortex S04.04-
   ● H47.61   Cortical blindness
     H47.611   Cortical blindness, right side of brain
     H47.612   Cortical blindness, left side of brain
     H47.619   Cortical blindness, unspecified side of brain
   ● H47.62   Disorders of visual cortex in (due to) inflammatory disorders
     H47.621   Disorders of visual cortex in (due to) inflammatory disorders, right side of brain
     H47.622   Disorders of visual cortex in (due to) inflammatory disorders, left side of brain
     H47.629   Disorders of visual cortex in (due to) inflammatory disorders, unspecified side of brain
   ● H47.63   Disorders of visual cortex in (due to) neoplasm
     H47.631   Disorders of visual cortex in (due to) neoplasm, right side of brain
     H47.632   Disorders of visual cortex in (due to) neoplasm, left side of brain
     H47.639   Disorders of visual cortex in (due to) neoplasm, unspecified side of brain
   ● H47.64   Disorders of visual cortex in (due to) vascular disorders
     H47.641   Disorders of visual cortex in (due to) vascular disorders, right side of brain
     H47.642   Disorders of visual cortex in (due to) vascular disorders, left side of brain
     H47.649   Disorders of visual cortex in (due to) vascular disorders, unspecified side of brain
H47.9   Unspecified disorder of visual pathways

DISORDERS OF OCULAR MUSCLES, BINOCULAR MOVEMENT, ACCOMMODATION AND REFRACTION (H49-H52)

Excludes2   nystagmus and other irregular eye movements (H55)

● H49   Paralytic strabismus
   Excludes2   internal ophthalmoplegia (H52.51-)
     internuclear ophthalmoplegia (H51.2-)
     progressive supranuclear ophthalmoplegia (G23.1)
   ● H49.0   Third [oculomotor] nerve palsy
     H49.00   Third [oculomotor] nerve palsy, unspecified eye
     H49.01   Third [oculomotor] nerve palsy, right eye
     H49.02   Third [oculomotor] nerve palsy, left eye
     H49.03   Third [oculomotor] nerve palsy, bilateral

Item 7–9 Strabismus or esotropia (crossed eyes) is a condition of the extraocular eye muscles, resulting in an inability of the eyes to focus and also affects depth perception.

Figure 7-12 **A.** Image of strabismus. **B.** Exotropia. (**A** from Yanoff: Ophthalmology, ed 3, Mosby, Inc., 2008. **B** from Zitelli BJ, Davis HW, Pediatric Physical Diagnosis: Atlas of Pediatric Physical Diagnosis, Philadelphia, Elsevier Saunders, 2012)

●H49.1 Fourth [trochlear] nerve palsy
  H49.10 Fourth [trochlear] nerve palsy, unspecified eye
  H49.11 Fourth [trochlear] nerve palsy, right eye
  H49.12 Fourth [trochlear] nerve palsy, left eye
  H49.13 Fourth [trochlear] nerve palsy, bilateral
●H49.2 Sixth [abducent] nerve palsy
  H49.20 Sixth [abducent] nerve palsy, unspecified eye
  H49.21 Sixth [abducent] nerve palsy, right eye
  H49.22 Sixth [abducent] nerve palsy, left eye
  H49.23 Sixth [abducent] nerve palsy, bilateral
●H49.3 Total (external) ophthalmoplegia
  H49.30 Total (external) ophthalmoplegia, unspecified eye
  H49.31 Total (external) ophthalmoplegia, right eye
  H49.32 Total (external) ophthalmoplegia, left eye
  H49.33 Total (external) ophthalmoplegia, bilateral
●H49.4 Progressive external ophthalmoplegia
  Excludes1 Kearns-Sayre syndrome (H49.81-)
  H49.40 Progressive external ophthalmoplegia, unspecified eye
  H49.41 Progressive external ophthalmoplegia, right eye
  H49.42 Progressive external ophthalmoplegia, left eye
  H49.43 Progressive external ophthalmoplegia, bilateral
●H49.8 Other paralytic strabismus
  ●H49.81 Kearns-Sayre syndrome
    Progressive external ophthalmoplegia with pigmentary retinopathy
    Use additional code for other manifestation, such as:
    heart block (I45.9)
    H49.811 Kearns-Sayre syndrome, right eye
    H49.812 Kearns-Sayre syndrome, left eye
    H49.813 Kearns-Sayre syndrome, bilateral
    H49.819 Kearns-Sayre syndrome, unspecified eye
  ●H49.88 Other paralytic strabismus
    External ophthalmoplegia NOS
    H49.881 Other paralytic strabismus, right eye
    H49.882 Other paralytic strabismus, left eye
    H49.883 Other paralytic strabismus, bilateral
    H49.889 Other paralytic strabismus, unspecified eye
H49.9 Unspecified paralytic strabismus

●H50 Other strabismus
  ●H50.0 Esotropia
    Convergent concomitant strabismus
    Excludes1 intermittent esotropia (H50.31-, H50.32)
    H50.00 Unspecified esotropia
    ●H50.01 Monocular esotropia
      H50.011 Monocular esotropia, right eye
      H50.012 Monocular esotropia, left eye
    ●H50.02 Monocular esotropia with A pattern
      H50.021 Monocular esotropia with A pattern, right eye
      H50.022 Monocular esotropia with A pattern, left eye
    ●H50.03 Monocular esotropia with V pattern
      H50.031 Monocular esotropia with V pattern, right eye
      H50.032 Monocular esotropia with V pattern, left eye
    ●H50.04 Monocular esotropia with other noncomitancies
      H50.041 Monocular esotropia with other noncomitancies, right eye
      H50.042 Monocular esotropia with other noncomitancies, left eye
    H50.05 Alternating esotropia
    H50.06 Alternating esotropia with A pattern
    H50.07 Alternating esotropia with V pattern
    H50.08 Alternating esotropia with other noncomitancies
  ●H50.1 Exotropia
    Misalignment in which one eye deviates outward (away from nose) while the other fixates normally
    Divergent concomitant strabismus
    Excludes1 intermittent exotropia (H50.33-, H50.34)
    H50.10 Unspecified exotropia
    ●H50.11 Monocular exotropia
      H50.111 Monocular exotropia, right eye
      H50.112 Monocular exotropia, left eye
    ●H50.12 Monocular exotropia with A pattern
      H50.121 Monocular exotropia with A pattern, right eye
      H50.122 Monocular exotropia with A pattern, left eye
    ●H50.13 Monocular exotropia with V pattern
      H50.131 Monocular exotropia with V pattern, right eye
      H50.132 Monocular exotropia with V pattern, left eye
    ●H50.14 Monocular exotropia with other noncomitancies
      H50.141 Monocular exotropia with other noncomitancies, right eye
      H50.142 Monocular exotropia with other noncomitancies, left eye
    H50.15 Alternating exotropia
    H50.16 Alternating exotropia with A pattern
    H50.17 Alternating exotropia with V pattern
    H50.18 Alternating exotropia with other noncomitancies
  ●H50.2 Vertical strabismus
    Hypertropia
    H50.21 Vertical strabismus, right eye
    H50.22 Vertical strabismus, left eye

CHAPTER 7 (H00-H59)

● H50.3   Intermittent heterotropia
      Displacement of an organ or part of an organ from its normal position

    H50.30   Unspecified intermittent heterotropia
●   H50.31   Intermittent monocular esotropia
        H50.311   Intermittent monocular esotropia, right eye
        H50.312   Intermittent monocular esotropia, left eye
    H50.32   Intermittent alternating esotropia
●   H50.33   Intermittent monocular exotropia
        H50.331   Intermittent monocular exotropia, right eye
        H50.332   Intermittent monocular exotropia, left eye
    H50.34   Intermittent alternating exotropia
● H50.4   Other and unspecified heterotropia
    H50.40   Unspecified heterotropia
●   H50.41   Cyclotropia
        H50.411   Cyclotropia, right eye
        H50.412   Cyclotropia, left eye
    H50.42   Monofixation syndrome
    H50.43   Accommodative component in esotropia
● H50.5   Heterophoria
      One or both eyes wander away from the position where both eyes are looking together in the same direction

    H50.50   Unspecified heterophoria
    H50.51   Esophoria
        Eye deviates inward (toward the nose)
    H50.52   Exophoria
        Eye deviates outward (toward the ear)
    H50.53   Vertical heterophoria
    H50.54   Cyclophoria
    H50.55   Alternating heterophoria
● H50.6   Mechanical strabismus
    H50.60   Mechanical strabismus, unspecified
●   H50.61   Brown's sheath syndrome
        H50.611   Brown's sheath syndrome, right eye
        H50.612   Brown's sheath syndrome, left eye
    H50.69   Other mechanical strabismus
        Strabismus due to adhesions
        Traumatic limitation of duction of eye muscle
● H50.8   Other specified strabismus
●   H50.81   Duane's syndrome
        H50.811   Duane's syndrome, right eye
        H50.812   Duane's syndrome, left eye
    H50.89   Other specified strabismus
    H50.9   Unspecified strabismus

● H51   Other disorders of binocular movement
    H51.0   Palsy (spasm) of conjugate gaze
●   H51.1   Convergence insufficiency and excess
    H51.11   Convergence insufficiency
    H51.12   Convergence excess
●   H51.2   Internuclear ophthalmoplegia
    H51.20   Internuclear ophthalmoplegia, unspecified eye
    H51.21   Internuclear ophthalmoplegia, right eye
    H51.22   Internuclear ophthalmoplegia, left eye
    H51.23   Internuclear ophthalmoplegia, bilateral
    H51.8   Other specified disorders of binocular movement
    H51.9   Unspecified disorder of binocular movement

● H52   Disorders of refraction and accommodation
●   H52.0   Hypermetropia
    H52.00   Hypermetropia, unspecified eye
    H52.01   Hypermetropia, right eye
    H52.02   Hypermetropia, left eye
    H52.03   Hypermetropia, bilateral

Item 7–10   Disorders of refraction: **Hypermetropia,** or farsightedness, means focus at a distance is adequate but not on close objects. **Myopia** is near-sightedness or short-sightedness and means the focus on nearby objects is clear but distant objects appear blurred. **Astigmatism** is warping of the curvature of the cornea so light rays entering do not meet a single focal point, resulting in a distorted image. **Anisometropia** is unequal refractive power in which one eye may be myopic (near-sighted) and the other hyperopic (far-sighted). **Presbyopia** is the loss of focus on near objects, which occurs with age because the lens loses elasticity.

● H52.1   Myopia
    Excludes1   degenerative myopia (H44.2-)
    H52.10   Myopia, unspecified eye
    H52.11   Myopia, right eye
    H52.12   Myopia, left eye
    H52.13   Myopia, bilateral
● H52.2   Astigmatism
●   H52.20   Unspecified astigmatism
        H52.201   Unspecified astigmatism, right eye
        H52.202   Unspecified astigmatism, left eye
        H52.203   Unspecified astigmatism, bilateral
        H52.209   Unspecified astigmatism, unspecified eye
●   H52.21   Irregular astigmatism
        H52.211   Irregular astigmatism, right eye
        H52.212   Irregular astigmatism, left eye
        H52.213   Irregular astigmatism, bilateral
        H52.219   Irregular astigmatism, unspecified eye
●   H52.22   Regular astigmatism
        H52.221   Regular astigmatism, right eye
        H52.222   Regular astigmatism, left eye
        H52.223   Regular astigmatism, bilateral
        H52.229   Regular astigmatism, unspecified eye
● H52.3   Anisometropia and aniseikonia
    H52.31   Anisometropia
    H52.32   Aniseikonia
    H52.4   Presbyopia
●   H52.5   Disorders of accommodation
●   H52.51   Internal ophthalmoplegia (complete) (total)
        H52.511   Internal ophthalmoplegia (complete) (total), right eye
        H52.512   Internal ophthalmoplegia (complete) (total), left eye
        H52.513   Internal ophthalmoplegia (complete) (total), bilateral
        H52.519   Internal ophthalmoplegia (complete) (total), unspecified eye
●   H52.52   Paresis of accommodation
        H52.521   Paresis of accommodation, right eye
        H52.522   Paresis of accommodation, left eye
        H52.523   Paresis of accommodation, bilateral
        H52.529   Paresis of accommodation, unspecified eye
●   H52.53   Spasm of accommodation
        H52.531   Spasm of accommodation, right eye
        H52.532   Spasm of accommodation, left eye
        H52.533   Spasm of accommodation, bilateral
        H52.539   Spasm of accommodation, unspecified eye
    H52.6   Other disorders of refraction
    H52.7   Unspecified disorder of refraction

VISUAL DISTURBANCES AND BLINDNESS (H53-H54)

● H53   Visual disturbances
●   H53.0   Amblyopia ex anopsia
    Excludes1   amblyopia due to vitamin A deficiency (E50.5)

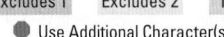

▶ New   ⯮ Revised   ~~deleted~~ Deleted   Excludes 1   Excludes 2   Includes   Use additional   Code first   Code also   Key words

OGCR Official Guidelines   X Assign placeholder X   ● Use Additional Character(s)   ▶ Manifestation Code   🐱 Hierarchical Condition Category   **Coding Clinic**

● **H53.00** Unspecified amblyopia
     H53.001   Unspecified amblyopia, right eye
     H53.002   Unspecified amblyopia, left eye
     H53.003   Unspecified amblyopia, bilateral
     H53.009   Unspecified amblyopia, unspecified eye

● **H53.01** Deprivation amblyopia
     H53.011   Deprivation amblyopia, right eye
     H53.012   Deprivation amblyopia, left eye
     H53.013   Deprivation amblyopia, bilateral
     H53.019   Deprivation amblyopia, unspecified eye

● **H53.02** Refractive amblyopia
     H53.021   Refractive amblyopia, right eye
     H53.022   Refractive amblyopia, left eye
     H53.023   Refractive amblyopia, bilateral
     H53.029   Refractive amblyopia, unspecified eye

● **H53.03** Strabismic amblyopia
     Excludes1   strabismus (H50.-)
     H53.031   Strabismic amblyopia, right eye
     H53.032   Strabismic amblyopia, left eye
     H53.033   Strabismic amblyopia, bilateral
     H53.039   Strabismic amblyopia, unspecified eye

● **H53.04** Amblyopia suspect
     Coding Clinic: 2016, Q4, P22
     H53.041   Amblyopia suspect, right eye
     H53.042   Amblyopia suspect, left eye
     H53.043   Amblyopia suspect, bilateral
     H53.049   Amblyopia suspect, unspecified eye

● **H53.1** Subjective visual disturbances
     Excludes1   subjective visual disturbances due to vitamin A deficiency (E50.5)
                 visual hallucinations (R44.1)
     H53.10   Unspecified subjective visual disturbances
     H53.11   Day blindness
            Hemeralopia
●   **H53.12** Transient visual loss
            Scintillating scotoma
     Excludes1   amaurosis fugax (G45.3-)
                  transient retinal artery occlusion (H34.0-)
     H53.121   Transient visual loss, right eye
     H53.122   Transient visual loss, left eye
     H53.123   Transient visual loss, bilateral
     H53.129   Transient visual loss, unspecified eye
●   **H53.13** Sudden visual loss
     H53.131   Sudden visual loss, right eye
     H53.132   Sudden visual loss, left eye
     H53.133   Sudden visual loss, bilateral
     H53.139   Sudden visual loss, unspecified eye
●   **H53.14** Visual discomfort
            Asthenopia
            Photophobia
     H53.141   Visual discomfort, right eye
     H53.142   Visual discomfort, left eye
     H53.143   Visual discomfort, bilateral
     H53.149   Visual discomfort, unspecified
     H53.15   Visual distortions of shape and size
            Metamorphopsia
     H53.16   Psychophysical visual disturbances
     H53.19   Other subjective visual disturbances
            Visual halos

H53.2 Diplopia
     Double vision

● **H53.3** Other and unspecified disorders of binocular vision
     H53.30   Unspecified disorder of binocular vision
     H53.31   Abnormal retinal correspondence
     H53.32   Fusion with defective stereopsis
     H53.33   Simultaneous visual perception without fusion
     H53.34   Suppression of binocular vision

● **H53.4** Visual field defects
     H53.40   Unspecified visual field defects
●   **H53.41** Scotoma involving central area
            Central scotoma
     H53.411   Scotoma involving central area, right eye
     H53.412   Scotoma involving central area, left eye
     H53.413   Scotoma involving central area, bilateral
     H53.419   Scotoma involving central area, unspecified eye
●   **H53.42** Scotoma of blind spot area
            Enlarged blind spot
     H53.421   Scotoma of blind spot area, right eye
     H53.422   Scotoma of blind spot area, left eye
     H53.423   Scotoma of blind spot area, bilateral
     H53.429   Scotoma of blind spot area, unspecified eye
●   **H53.43** Sector or arcuate defects
            Arcuate scotoma
            Bjerrum scotoma
     H53.431   Sector or arcuate defects, right eye
     H53.432   Sector or arcuate defects, left eye
     H53.433   Sector or arcuate defects, bilateral
     H53.439   Sector or arcuate defects, unspecified eye
●   **H53.45** Other localized visual field defect
            Peripheral visual field defect
            Ring scotoma NOS
            Scotoma NOS
     H53.451   Other localized visual field defect, right eye
     H53.452   Other localized visual field defect, left eye
     H53.453   Other localized visual field defect, bilateral
     H53.459   Other localized visual field defect, unspecified eye
●   **H53.46** Homonymous bilateral field defects
            Homonymous hemianopia
            Homonymous hemianopsia
            Quadrant anopia
            Quadrant anopsia
     H53.461   Homonymous bilateral field defects, right side
     H53.462   Homonymous bilateral field defects, left side
     H53.469   Homonymous bilateral field defects, unspecified side
            Homonymous bilateral field defects NOS
     H53.47   Heteronymous bilateral field defects
            Heteronymous hemianop(s)ia
●   **H53.48** Generalized contraction of visual field
     H53.481   Generalized contraction of visual field, right eye
     H53.482   Generalized contraction of visual field, left eye
     H53.483   Generalized contraction of visual field, bilateral
     H53.489   Generalized contraction of visual field, unspecified eye

CHAPTER 7 (H00-H59)

H53.5 **Color vision deficiencies**
  Color blindness
  Excludes2 day blindness (H53.11)

H53.50 **Unspecified color vision deficiencies**
  Color blindness NOS

H53.51 Achromatopsia

H53.52 Acquired color vision deficiency

H53.53 Deuteranomaly
  Deuteranopia

H53.54 Protanomaly
  Protanopia

H53.55 Tritanomaly
  Tritanopia

H53.59 Other color vision deficiencies

H53.6 **Night blindness**
  Excludes1 night blindness due to vitamin A
    deficiency (E50.5)

H53.60 **Unspecified night blindness**

H53.61 **Abnormal dark adaptation curve**

H53.62 **Acquired night blindness**

H53.63 **Congenital night blindness**

H53.69 **Other night blindness**

H53.7 Vision sensitivity deficiencies

H53.71 **Glare sensitivity**

H53.72 **Impaired contrast** sensitivity

H53.8 Other visual disturbances

H53.9 **Unspecified** visual disturbance

● H54 **Blindness and low vision**
  Note: For definition of visual impairment categories see table
    below.
  Code first any associated underlying cause of the blindness
  Excludes1 amaurosis fugax (G45.3)

●H54.0 **Blindness, both eyes**
  Visual impairment categories 3, 4, 5 in both eyes.

  ●H54.0X **Blindness, both eyes, different category levels**
    H54.0X3 **Blindness right eye, category 3**
      H54.0X33 Blindness right eye
        category 3, blindness left
        eye category 3
      H54.0X34 Blindness right eye
        category 3, blindness left
        eye category 4
      H54.0X35 Blindness right eye
        category 3, blindness left
        eye category 5

    ●H54.0X4 **Blindness right eye, category 4**
      H54.0X43 Blindness right eye
        category 4, blindness left
        eye category 3
      H54.0X44 Blindness right eye
        category 4, blindness left
        eye category 4
      H54.0X45 Blindness right eye
        category 4, blindness left
        eye category 5

    ●H54.0X5 **Blindness right eye, category 5**
      H54.0X53 Blindness right eye
        category 5, blindness left
        eye category 3
      H54.0X54 Blindness right eye
        category 5, blindness left
        eye category 4
      H54.0X55 Blindness right eye
        category 5, blindness left
        eye category 5

● H54.1 **Blindness, one eye, low vision other eye**
  Visual impairment categories 3, 4, 5 in one eye, with
    categories 1 or 2 in the other eye.

  H54.10 **Blindness, one eye, low vision other eye,
    unspecified eyes**

  ●H54.11 **Blindness, right eye, low vision left eye**
    ●H54.113 **Blindness right eye category 3, low
      vision left eye**
      H54.1131 **Blindness right eye
        category 3, low vision left
        eye category 1**
      H54.1132 **Blindness right eye
        category 3, low vision left
        eye category 2**

    ●H54.114 **Blindness right eye category 4, low
      vision left eye**
      H54.1141 **Blindness right eye
        category 4, low vision left
        eye category 1**
      H54.1142 **Blindness right eye
        category 4, low vision left
        eye category 2**

    ●H54.115 **Blindness right eye category 5, low
      vision left eye**
      H54.1151 **Blindness right eye
        category 5, low vision left
        eye category 1**
      H54.1152 **Blindness right eye
        category 5, low vision left
        eye category 2**

  ●H54.12 **Blindness, left eye, low vision right eye**
    ●H54.121 **Low vision right eye category 1,
      blindness left eye**
      H54.1213 **Low vision right eye
        category 1, blindness left
        eye category 3**
      H54.1214 **Low vision right eye
        category 1, blindness left
        eye category 4**
      H54.1215 **Low vision right eye
        category 1, blindness left
        eye category 5**

    ●H54.122 **Low vision right eye category 2,
      blindness left eye**
      H54.1223 **Low vision right eye
        category 2, blindness left
        eye category 3**
      H54.1224 **Low vision right eye
        category 2, blindness left
        eye category 4**
      H54.1225 **Low vision right eye
        category 2, blindness left
        eye category 5**

● H54.2 **Low vision, both eyes**
  Visual impairment categories 1 or 2 in both eyes.

  ●H54.2X **Low vision, both eyes, different category levels**
    ●H54.2X1 **Low vision, right eye, category 1**
      H54.2X11 **Low vision right eye
        category 1, low vision left
        eye category 1**
      H54.2X12 **Low vision right eye
        category 1, low vision left
        eye category 2**

    ●H54.2X2 **Low vision, right eye, category 2**
      H54.2X21 **Low vision right eye
        category 2, low vision left
        eye category 1**
      H54.2X22 **Low vision right eye
        category 2, low vision left
        eye category 2**

H54.3   Unqualified visual loss, both eyes
     Visual impairment category 9 in both eyes.

● H54.4   Blindness, one eye
     Visual impairment categories 3, 4, 5 in one eye [normal vision in other eye]

   H54.40   Blindness, one eye, unspecified eye

●   H54.41   Blindness, right eye, normal vision left eye

     ● H54.413   Blindness, right eye, category 3

         H54.413A   Blindness right eye category 3, normal vision left eye

     ● H54.414   Blindness, right eye, category 4

         H54.414A   Blindness right eye category 4, normal vision left eye

     ● H54.415   Blindness, right eye, category 5

         H54.415A   Blindness right eye category 5, normal vision left eye

●   H54.42   Blindness, left eye, normal vision right eye

     ● H54.42A   Blindness, left eye, category 3-5

         H54.42A3   Blindness left eye category 3, normal vision right eye

         H54.42A4   Blindness left eye category 4, normal vision right eye

         H54.42A5   Blindness left eye category 5, normal vision right eye

● H54.5   Low vision, one eye
     Visual impairment categories 1 or 2 in one eye [normal vision in other eye].

   H54.50   Low vision, one eye, unspecified eye

●   H54.51   Low vision, right eye, normal vision left eye

     ● H54.511   Low vision, right eye, category 1-2

         H54.511A   Low vision right eye category 1, normal vision left eye

         H54.512A   Low vision right eye category 2, normal vision left eye

●   H54.52   Low vision, left eye, normal vision right eye

     ● H54.52A   Low vision, left eye, category 1-2

         H54.52A1   Low vision left eye category 1, normal vision right eye

         H54.52A2   Low vision left eye category 2, normal vision right eye

● H54.6   Unqualified visual loss, one eye
     Visual impairment category 9 in one eye [normal vision in other eye].

   H54.60   Unqualified visual loss, one eye, unspecified

   H54.61   Unqualified visual loss, right eye, normal vision left eye

   H54.62   Unqualified visual loss, left eye, normal vision right eye

OGCR Section I.C.7.b.

Blindness

If "blindness" or "low vision" of both eyes is documented but the visual impairment category is not documented, assign code H54.3, Unqualified visual loss, both eyes. If "blindness" or "low vision" in one eye is documented but the visual impairment category is not documented, assign a code from H54.6-, Unqualified visual loss, one eye. If "blindness" or "visual loss" is documented without any information about whether one or both eyes are affected, assign code H54.7, Unspecified visual loss.

H54.7   Unspecified visual loss
     Visual impairment category 9 NOS

H54.8   Legal blindness, as defined in USA
     Blindness NOS according to USA definition

     Excludes1   legal blindness with specification of impairment level (H54.0-H54.7)

     Note: The table below gives a classification of severity of visual impairment recommended by a WHO Study Group on the Prevention of Blindness, Geneva, 6-10 November 1972.

         The term "low vision" in category H54 comprises categories 1 and 2 of the table, the term "blindness" categories 3, 4, and 5, and the term "unqualified visual loss" category 9.

         If the extent of the visual field is taken into account, patients with a field no greater than 10 but greater than 5 around central fixation should be placed in category 3 and patients with a field no greater than 5 around central fixation should be placed in category 4, even if the central acuity is not impaired.

(Document 508 compliance requires all cells in the following table to be filled.)

Category of visual impairment	Visual acuity with best possible correction	
	Maximum less than:	Minimum equal to or better than:
—	6/18	6/60
3/10 (0.3)	1/10 (0.1)	—
20/70	20/200	—
—	6/60	3/60
1/10 (0.1)	1/20 (0.05)	—
20/200	20/400	—
—	3/60	1/60 (finger counting at one meter)
1/20 (0.05)	1/50 (0.02)	—
20/400	5/300 (20/1200)	—
—	1/60 (finger counting at one meter)	Light perception
1/50 (0.02)	—	—
5/300	—	—
—	No light perception	—
—	Undetermined or unspecified	—

OTHER DISORDERS OF EYE AND ADNEXA (H55-H57)

● H55   Nystagmus and other irregular eye movements

   ● H55.0   Nystagmus
     Rapid, involuntary movements of the eyes in the horizontal or vertical direction

     H55.00   Unspecified nystagmus

     H55.01   Congenital nystagmus

     H55.02   Latent nystagmus

     H55.03   Visual deprivation nystagmus

     H55.04   Dissociated nystagmus

     H55.09   Other forms of nystagmus

   ● H55.8   Other irregular eye movements

     H55.81   Deficient saccadic eye movements

     H55.82   Deficient smooth pursuit eye movements

     H55.89   Other irregular eye movements

CHAPTER 7 (H00-H59)

● H57   Other disorders of eye and adnexa
   ● H57.0   Anomalies of pupillary function
     H57.00   Unspecified anomaly of pupillary function
     H57.01   Argyll Robertson pupil, atypical
       Excludes1   syphilitic Argyll Robertson pupil (A52.19)
     H57.02   Anisocoria
     H57.03   Miosis
     H57.04   Mydriasis
    ● H57.05   Tonic pupil
       H57.051   Tonic pupil, right eye
       H57.052   Tonic pupil, left eye
       H57.053   Tonic pupil, bilateral
       H57.059   Tonic pupil, unspecified eye
     H57.09   Other anomalies of pupillary function
   ● H57.1   Ocular pain
     H57.10   Ocular pain, unspecified eye
     H57.11   Ocular pain, right eye
     H57.12   Ocular pain, left eye
     H57.13   Ocular pain, bilateral
   ● H57.8   Other specified disorders of eye and adnexa
    ● H57.81   Brow ptosis
       H57.811   Brow ptosis, right
       H57.812   Brow ptosis, left
       H57.813   Brow ptosis, bilateral
       H57.819   Brow ptosis, unspecified
     H57.89   Other specified disorders of eye and adnexa
   H57.9   Unspecified disorder of eye and adnexa

INTRAOPERATIVE AND POSTPROCEDURAL COMPLICATIONS AND DISORDERS OF EYE AND ADNEXA, NOT ELSEWHERE CLASSIFIED (H59)

● H59   Intraoperative and postprocedural complications and disorders of eye and adnexa, not elsewhere classified
   Excludes1   mechanical complication of intraocular lens (T85.2)
       mechanical complication of other ocular prosthetic devices, implants and grafts (T85.3)
       pseudophakia (Z96.1)
       secondary cataracts (H26.4-)
   ● H59.0   Disorders of the eye following cataract surgery
    ● H59.01   Keratopathy (bullous aphakic) following cataract surgery
       Vitreal corneal syndrome
       Vitreous (touch) syndrome
       H59.011   Keratopathy (bullous aphakic) following cataract surgery, right eye
       H59.012   Keratopathy (bullous aphakic) following cataract surgery, left eye
       H59.013   Keratopathy (bullous aphakic) following cataract surgery, bilateral
       H59.019   Keratopathy (bullous aphakic) following cataract surgery, unspecified eye
    ● H59.02   Cataract (lens) fragments in eye following cataract surgery
       H59.021   Cataract (lens) fragments in eye following cataract surgery, right eye
       H59.022   Cataract (lens) fragments in eye following cataract surgery, left eye
       H59.023   Cataract (lens) fragments in eye following cataract surgery, bilateral
       H59.029   Cataract (lens) fragments in eye following cataract surgery, unspecified eye

    ● H59.03   Cystoid macular edema following cataract surgery
       H59.031   Cystoid macular edema following cataract surgery, right eye
       H59.032   Cystoid macular edema following cataract surgery, left eye
       H59.033   Cystoid macular edema following cataract surgery, bilateral
       H59.039   Cystoid macular edema following cataract surgery, unspecified eye
    ● H59.09   Other disorders of the eye following cataract surgery
       H59.091   Other disorders of the right eye following cataract surgery
       H59.092   Other disorders of the left eye following cataract surgery
       H59.093   Other disorders of the eye following cataract surgery, bilateral
       H59.099   Other disorders of unspecified eye following cataract surgery
   ● H59.1   Intraoperative hemorrhage and hematoma of eye and adnexa complicating a procedure
       Excludes1   intraoperative hemorrhage and hematoma of eye and adnexa due to accidental puncture or laceration during a procedure (H59.2-)
    ● H59.11   Intraoperative hemorrhage and hematoma of eye and adnexa complicating an ophthalmic procedure
       H59.111   Intraoperative hemorrhage and hematoma of right eye and adnexa complicating an ophthalmic procedure
       H59.112   Intraoperative hemorrhage and hematoma of left eye and adnexa complicating an ophthalmic procedure
       H59.113   Intraoperative hemorrhage and hematoma of eye and adnexa complicating an ophthalmic procedure, bilateral
       H59.119   Intraoperative hemorrhage and hematoma of unspecified eye and adnexa complicating an ophthalmic procedure
    ● H59.12   Intraoperative hemorrhage and hematoma of eye and adnexa complicating other procedure
       H59.121   Intraoperative hemorrhage and hematoma of right eye and adnexa complicating other procedure
       H59.122   Intraoperative hemorrhage and hematoma of left eye and adnexa complicating other procedure
       H59.123   Intraoperative hemorrhage and hematoma of eye and adnexa complicating other procedure, bilateral
       H59.129   Intraoperative hemorrhage and hematoma of unspecified eye and adnexa complicating other procedure
   ● H59.2   Accidental puncture and laceration of eye and adnexa during a procedure
    ● H59.21   Accidental puncture and laceration of eye and adnexa during an ophthalmic procedure
       H59.211   Accidental puncture and laceration of right eye and adnexa during an ophthalmic procedure
       H59.212   Accidental puncture and laceration of left eye and adnexa during an ophthalmic procedure

▶ New   ⇒ Revised   ~~deleted~~ Deleted   Excludes 1   Excludes 2   Includes   Use additional   Code first   Code also   Key words
OGCR Official Guidelines   X Assign placeholder X   ● Use Additional Character(s)   ▷ Manifestation Code   🐾 Hierarchical Condition Category   **Coding Clinic**

H59.213   Accidental puncture and laceration of eye and adnexa during an ophthalmic procedure, bilateral

H59.219   Accidental puncture and laceration of unspecified eye and adnexa during an ophthalmic procedure

● H59.22   Accidental puncture and laceration of eye and adnexa during other procedure

H59.221   Accidental puncture and laceration of right eye and adnexa during other procedure

H59.222   Accidental puncture and laceration of left eye and adnexa during other procedure

H59.223   Accidental puncture and laceration of eye and adnexa during other procedure, bilateral

H59.229   Accidental puncture and laceration of unspecified eye and adnexa during other procedure

● H59.3   Postprocedural hemorrhage, hematoma, and seroma of eye and adnexa following other procedure
Coding Clinic: 2016, Q4, P10

● H59.31   Postprocedural hemorrhage of eye and adnexa following an ophthalmic procedure

H59.311   Postprocedural hemorrhage of right eye and adnexa following an ophthalmic procedure

H59.312   Postprocedural hemorrhage of left eye and adnexa following an ophthalmic procedure

H59.313   Postprocedural hemorrhage of eye and adnexa following an ophthalmic procedure, bilateral

H59.319   Postprocedural hemorrhage of unspecified eye and adnexa following an ophthalmic procedure

● H59.32   Postprocedural hemorrhage of eye and adnexa following other procedure

H59.321   Postprocedural hemorrhage of right eye and adnexa following other procedure

H59.322   Postprocedural hemorrhage of left eye and adnexa following other procedure

H59.323   Postprocedural hemorrhage of eye and adnexa following other procedure, bilateral

H59.329   Postprocedural hemorrhage of unspecified eye and adnexa following other procedure

● H59.33   Postprocedural hematoma of eye and adnexa following an ophthalmic procedure

H59.331   Postprocedural hematoma of right eye and adnexa following an ophthalmic procedure

H59.332   Postprocedural hematoma of left eye and adnexa following an ophthalmic procedure

H59.333   Postprocedural hematoma of eye and adnexa following an ophthalmic procedure, bilateral

H59.339   Postprocedural hematoma of unspecified eye and adnexa following an ophthalmic procedure

● H59.34   Postprocedural hematoma of eye and adnexa following other procedure

H59.341   Postprocedural hematoma of right eye and adnexa following other procedure

H59.342   Postprocedural hematoma of left eye and adnexa following other procedure

H59.343   Postprocedural hematoma of eye and adnexa following other procedure, bilateral

H59.349   Postprocedural hematoma of unspecified eye and adnexa following other procedure

● H59.35   Postprocedural seroma of eye and adnexa following an ophthalmic procedure

H59.351   Postprocedural seroma of right eye and adnexa following an ophthalmic procedure

H59.352   Postprocedural seroma of left eye and adnexa following an ophthalmic procedure

H59.353   Postprocedural seroma of eye and adnexa following an ophthalmic procedure, bilateral

H59.359   Postprocedural seroma of unspecified eye and adnexa following an ophthalmic procedure

● H59.36   Postprocedural seroma of eye and adnexa following other procedure

H59.361   Postprocedural seroma of right eye and adnexa following other procedure

H59.362   Postprocedural seroma of left eye and adnexa following other procedure

H59.363   Postprocedural seroma of eye and adnexa following other procedure, bilateral

H59.369   Postprocedural seroma of unspecified eye and adnexa following other procedure

● H59.4   Inflammation (infection) of postprocedural bleb
Postprocedural blebitis

Excludes1   filtering (vitreous) bleb after glaucoma surgery status (Z98.83)

H59.40   Inflammation (infection) of postprocedural bleb, unspecified

H59.41   Inflammation (infection) of postprocedural bleb, stage 1

H59.42   Inflammation (infection) of postprocedural bleb, stage 2

H59.43   Inflammation (infection) of postprocedural bleb, stage 3
Bleb endophthalmitis

● H59.8   Other intraoperative and postprocedural complications and disorders of eye and adnexa, not elsewhere classified

● H59.81   Chorioretinal scars after surgery for detachment

H59.811   Chorioretinal scars after surgery for detachment, right eye

H59.812   Chorioretinal scars after surgery for detachment, left eye

H59.813   Chorioretinal scars after surgery for detachment, bilateral

H59.819   Chorioretinal scars after surgery for detachment, unspecified eye

H59.88   Other intraoperative complications of eye and adnexa, not elsewhere classified

H59.89   Other postprocedural complications and disorders of eye and adnexa, not elsewhere classified

CHAPTER 7 (H00-H59)

CHAPTER 8

DISEASES OF THE EAR AND MASTOID PROCESS (H60-H95)

OGCR Chapter-Specific Coding Guidelines

8. Chapter 8: Diseases of the Ear and Mastoid Process (H60-H95)
Reserved for future guideline expansion

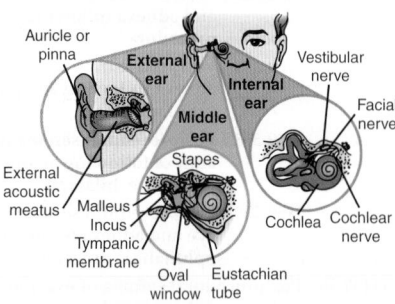

Figure 8-1 Auditory system. (From Buck CJ: Step-by-Step Medical Coding, ed 2016, St. Louis, Elsevier, 2016)

★ **(See Plate 20 of the Anatomy Illustrations.)**

CHAPTER 8

DISEASES OF THE EAR AND MASTOID PROCESS (H60-H95)

Note: Use an external cause code following the code for the ear condition, if applicable, to identify the cause of the ear condition

Excludes2 certain conditions originating in the perinatal period (P04-P96)
certain infectious and parasitic diseases (A00-B99)
complications of pregnancy, childbirth and the puerperium (O00-O9A)
congenital malformations, deformations and chromosomal abnormalities (Q00-Q99)
endocrine, nutritional and metabolic diseases (E00-E88)
injury, poisoning and certain other consequences of external causes (S00-T88)
neoplasms (C00-D49)
symptoms, signs and abnormal clinical and laboratory findings, not elsewhere classified (R00-R94)

This chapter contains the following blocks:

H60-H62	Diseases of external ear
H65-H75	Diseases of middle ear and mastoid
H80-H83	Diseases of inner ear
H90-H94	Other disorders of ear
H95	Intraoperative and postprocedural complications and disorders of ear and mastoid process, not elsewhere classified

DISEASES OF EXTERNAL EAR (H60-H62)

● H60 Otitis externa

● H60.0 Abscess of external ear
Boil of external ear
Carbuncle of auricle or external auditory canal
Furuncle of external ear

　H60.00 Abscess of external ear, unspecified ear
　H60.01 Abscess of right external ear
　H60.02 Abscess of left external ear
　H60.03 Abscess of external ear, bilateral

● H60.1 Cellulitis of external ear
Cellulitis of auricle
Cellulitis of external auditory canal

　H60.10 Cellulitis of external ear, unspecified ear
　H60.11 Cellulitis of right external ear
　H60.12 Cellulitis of left external ear
　H60.13 Cellulitis of external ear, bilateral

● H60.2 Malignant otitis externa

　H60.20 Malignant otitis externa, unspecified ear
　H60.21 Malignant otitis externa, right ear
　H60.22 Malignant otitis externa, left ear
　H60.23 Malignant otitis externa, bilateral

● H60.3 Other infective otitis externa

● H60.31 Diffuse otitis externa
　　H60.311 Diffuse otitis externa, right ear
　　H60.312 Diffuse otitis externa, left ear
　　H60.313 Diffuse otitis externa, bilateral
　　H60.319 Diffuse otitis externa, unspecified ear

● H60.32 Hemorrhagic otitis externa
　　H60.321 Hemorrhagic otitis externa, right ear
　　H60.322 Hemorrhagic otitis externa, left ear
　　H60.323 Hemorrhagic otitis externa, bilateral
　　H60.329 Hemorrhagic otitis externa, unspecified ear

● H60.33 Swimmer's ear
　　H60.331 Swimmer's ear, right ear
　　H60.332 Swimmer's ear, left ear
　　H60.333 Swimmer's ear, bilateral
　　H60.339 Swimmer's ear, unspecified ear

● H60.39 Other infective otitis externa
　　H60.391 Other infective otitis externa, right ear
　　H60.392 Other infective otitis externa, left ear
　　H60.393 Other infective otitis externa, bilateral
　　H60.399 Other infective otitis externa, unspecified ear

● H60.4 Cholesteatoma of external ear
Keratosis obturans of external ear (canal)

Excludes2 cholesteatoma of middle ear (H71.-)
recurrent cholesteatoma of postmastoidectomy cavity (H95.0-)

　H60.40 Cholesteatoma of external ear, unspecified ear
　H60.41 Cholesteatoma of right external ear
　H60.42 Cholesteatoma of left external ear
　H60.43 Cholesteatoma of external ear, bilateral

● H60.5 Acute noninfective otitis externa

● H60.50 Unspecified acute noninfective otitis externa
Acute otitis externa NOS
　　H60.501 Unspecified acute noninfective otitis externa, right ear
　　H60.502 Unspecified acute noninfective otitis externa, left ear
　　H60.503 Unspecified acute noninfective otitis externa, bilateral
　　H60.509 Unspecified acute noninfective otitis externa, unspecified ear

● H60.51 Acute actinic otitis externa
　　H60.511 Acute actinic otitis externa, right ear
　　H60.512 Acute actinic otitis externa, left ear
　　H60.513 Acute actinic otitis externa, bilateral
　　H60.519 Acute actinic otitis externa, unspecified ear

CHAPTER 8 (H60-H95)

● H60.52   Acute chemical otitis externa
     H60.521   Acute chemical otitis externa, right ear
     H60.522   Acute chemical otitis externa, left ear
     H60.523   Acute chemical otitis externa, bilateral
     H60.529   Acute chemical otitis externa, unspecified ear

● H60.53   Acute contact otitis externa
     H60.531   Acute contact otitis externa, right ear
     H60.532   Acute contact otitis externa, left ear
     H60.533   Acute contact otitis externa, bilateral
     H60.539   Acute contact otitis externa, unspecified ear

● H60.54   Acute eczematoid otitis externa
     H60.541   Acute eczematoid otitis externa, right ear
     H60.542   Acute eczematoid otitis externa, left ear
     H60.543   Acute eczematoid otitis externa, bilateral
     H60.549   Acute eczematoid otitis externa, unspecified ear

● H60.55   Acute reactive otitis externa
     H60.551   Acute reactive otitis externa, right ear
     H60.552   Acute reactive otitis externa, left ear
     H60.553   Acute reactive otitis externa, bilateral
     H60.559   Acute reactive otitis externa, unspecified ear

● H60.59   Other noninfective acute otitis externa
     H60.591   Other noninfective acute otitis externa, right ear
     H60.592   Other noninfective acute otitis externa, left ear
     H60.593   Other noninfective acute otitis externa, bilateral
     H60.599   Other noninfective acute otitis externa, unspecified ear

● H60.6   Unspecified chronic otitis externa
     H60.60   Unspecified chronic otitis externa, unspecified ear
     H60.61   Unspecified chronic otitis externa, right ear
     H60.62   Unspecified chronic otitis externa, left ear
     H60.63   Unspecified chronic otitis externa, bilateral

● H60.8   Other otitis externa
   ● H60.8X   Other otitis externa
     H60.8X1   Other otitis externa, right ear
     H60.8X2   Other otitis externa, left ear
     H60.8X3   Other otitis externa, bilateral
     H60.8X9   Other otitis externa, unspecified ear

● H60.9   Unspecified otitis externa
     H60.90   Unspecified otitis externa, unspecified ear
     H60.91   Unspecified otitis externa, right ear
     H60.92   Unspecified otitis externa, left ear
     H60.93   Unspecified otitis externa, bilateral

● H61   Other disorders of external ear
   ● H61.0   Chondritis and perichondritis of external ear
     Chondrodermatitis nodularis chronica helicis
     Perichondritis of auricle
     Perichondritis of pinna
     ● H61.00   Unspecified perichondritis of external ear
     H61.001   Unspecified perichondritis of right external ear
     H61.002   Unspecified perichondritis of left external ear
     H61.003   Unspecified perichondritis of external ear, bilateral
     H61.009   Unspecified perichondritis of external ear, unspecified ear

● H61.01   Acute perichondritis of external ear
     H61.011   Acute perichondritis of right external ear
     H61.012   Acute perichondritis of left external ear
     H61.013   Acute perichondritis of external ear, bilateral
     H61.019   Acute perichondritis of external ear, unspecified ear

● H61.02   Chronic perichondritis of external ear
     H61.021   Chronic perichondritis of right external ear
     H61.022   Chronic perichondritis of left external ear
     H61.023   Chronic perichondritis of external ear, bilateral
     H61.029   Chronic perichondritis of external ear, unspecified ear

● H61.03   Chondritis of external ear
     Chondritis of auricle
     Chondritis of pinna
     H61.031   Chondritis of right external ear
     H61.032   Chondritis of left external ear
        Coding Clinic: 2015, Q1, P18
     H61.033   Chondritis of external ear, bilateral
     H61.039   Chondritis of external ear, unspecified ear

● H61.1   Noninfective disorders of pinna
     Excludes2   cauliflower ear (M95.1-)
                gouty tophi of ear (M1A.-)

● H61.10   Unspecified noninfective disorders of pinna
     Disorder of pinna NOS
     H61.101   Unspecified noninfective disorders of pinna, right ear
     H61.102   Unspecified noninfective disorders of pinna, left ear
     H61.103   Unspecified noninfective disorders of pinna, bilateral
     H61.109   Unspecified noninfective disorders of pinna, unspecified ear

● H61.11   Acquired deformity of pinna
     Acquired deformity of auricle
     Excludes2   cauliflower ear (M95.1-)
     H61.111   Acquired deformity of pinna, right ear
     H61.112   Acquired deformity of pinna, left ear
     H61.113   Acquired deformity of pinna, bilateral
     H61.119   Acquired deformity of pinna, unspecified ear

● H61.12   Hematoma of pinna
     Hematoma of auricle
     H61.121   Hematoma of pinna, right ear
     H61.122   Hematoma of pinna, left ear
     H61.123   Hematoma of pinna, bilateral
     H61.129   Hematoma of pinna, unspecified ear

● H61.19   Other noninfective disorders of pinna
     H61.191   Noninfective disorders of pinna, right ear
     H61.192   Noninfective disorders of pinna, left ear
     H61.193   Noninfective disorders of pinna, bilateral
     H61.199   Noninfective disorders of pinna, unspecified ear

CHAPTER 8 (H60-H95)

● **H61.2 Impacted cerumen**
     Wax in ear
     H61.20 Impacted cerumen, unspecified ear
     H61.21 Impacted cerumen, right ear
     H61.22 Impacted cerumen, left ear
     H61.23 Impacted cerumen, bilateral

● **H61.3 Acquired stenosis of external ear canal**
     Collapse of external ear canal
     Excludes1 postprocedural stenosis of external ear canal (H95.81-)

     ● **H61.30 Acquired stenosis of external ear canal, unspecified**
         H61.301 Acquired stenosis of right external ear canal, unspecified
         H61.302 Acquired stenosis of left external ear canal, unspecified
         H61.303 Acquired stenosis of external ear canal, unspecified, bilateral
         H61.309 Acquired stenosis of external ear canal, unspecified, unspecified ear

     ● **H61.31 Acquired stenosis of external ear canal secondary to trauma**
         H61.311 Acquired stenosis of right external ear canal secondary to trauma
         H61.312 Acquired stenosis of left external ear canal secondary to trauma
         H61.313 Acquired stenosis of external ear canal secondary to trauma, bilateral
         H61.319 Acquired stenosis of external ear canal secondary to trauma, unspecified ear

     ● **H61.32 Acquired stenosis of external ear canal secondary to inflammation and infection**
         H61.321 Acquired stenosis of right external ear canal secondary to inflammation and infection
         H61.322 Acquired stenosis of left external ear canal secondary to inflammation and infection
         H61.323 Acquired stenosis of external ear canal secondary to inflammation and infection, bilateral
         H61.329 Acquired stenosis of external ear canal secondary to inflammation and infection, unspecified ear

     ● **H61.39 Other acquired stenosis of external ear canal**
         H61.391 Other acquired stenosis of right external ear canal
         H61.392 Other acquired stenosis of left external ear canal
         H61.393 Other acquired stenosis of external ear canal, bilateral
         H61.399 Other acquired stenosis of external ear canal, unspecified ear

● **H61.8 Other specified disorders of external ear**
     ● **H61.81 Exostosis of external canal**
         H61.811 Exostosis of right external canal
         H61.812 Exostosis of left external canal
         H61.813 Exostosis of external canal, bilateral
         H61.819 Exostosis of external canal, unspecified ear

     ● **H61.89 Other specified disorders of external ear**
         H61.891 Other specified disorders of right external ear
         H61.892 Other specified disorders of left external ear
         H61.893 Other specified disorders of external ear, bilateral
         H61.899 Other specified disorders of external ear, unspecified ear

● **H61.9 Disorder of external ear, unspecified**
     H61.90 Disorder of external ear, unspecified, unspecified ear
     H61.91 Disorder of right external ear, unspecified
     H61.92 Disorder of left external ear, unspecified
     H61.93 Disorder of external ear, unspecified, bilateral

● **H62 Disorders of external ear in diseases classified elsewhere**
     ● **H62.4 Otitis externa in other diseases classified elsewhere**
     Code first underlying disease, such as:
         erysipelas (A46)
         impetigo (L01.0)
     Excludes1 otitis externa (in):
         candidiasis (B37.84)
         herpes viral [herpes simplex] (B00.1)
         herpes zoster (B02.8)

     ▷ *H62.40 Otitis externa in other diseases classified elsewhere, unspecified ear*
     ▷ *H62.41 Otitis externa in other diseases classified elsewhere, right ear*
     ▷ *H62.42 Otitis externa in other diseases classified elsewhere, left ear*
     ▷ *H62.43 Otitis externa in other diseases classified elsewhere, bilateral*

     ● **H62.8 Other disorders of external ear in diseases classified elsewhere**
     Code first underlying disease, such as:
         gout (M1A.-, M10.-)

     ● **H62.8X Other disorders of external ear in diseases classified elsewhere**
     ▷ *H62.8X1 Other disorders of right external ear in diseases classified elsewhere*
     ▷ *H62.8X2 Other disorders of left external ear in diseases classified elsewhere*
     ▷ *H62.8X3 Other disorders of external ear in diseases classified elsewhere, bilateral*
     ▷ *H62.8X9 Other disorders of external ear in diseases classified elsewhere, unspecified ear*

DISEASES OF MIDDLE EAR AND MASTOID (H65-H75)

★ **(See Plate 21 of the Anatomy Illustrations.)**

● **H65 Nonsuppurative otitis media**
Bacterial or viral infection or inflammation of the middle ear; may result in fluid accumulation with pain and temporary hearing loss.

     Includes nonsuppurative otitis media with myringitis

     Use additional code for any associated perforated tympanic membrane (H72.-)
     Use additional code to identify:
         exposure to environmental tobacco smoke (Z77.22)
         exposure to tobacco smoke in the perinatal period (P96.81)
         history of tobacco dependence (Z87.891)
         infectious agent (B95-B97)
         occupational exposure to environmental tobacco smoke (Z57.31)
         tobacco dependence (F17.-)
         tobacco use (Z72.0)

● **H65.0 Acute serous otitis media**
     Acute and subacute secretory otitis
     H65.00 Acute serous otitis media, unspecified ear
     H65.01 Acute serous otitis media, right ear
     H65.02 Acute serous otitis media, left ear
     H65.03 Acute serous otitis media, bilateral
     H65.04 Acute serous otitis media, recurrent, right ear
     H65.05 Acute serous otitis media, recurrent, left ear
     H65.06 Acute serous otitis media, recurrent, bilateral
     H65.07 Acute serous otitis media, recurrent, unspecified ear

● **H65.1**   Other acute nonsuppurative otitis media

> **Excludes1**   otitic barotrauma (T70.0)
> otitis media (acute) NOS (H66.9)

   ● **H65.11**   Acute and subacute allergic otitis media (mucoid) (sanguinous) (serous)

     H65.111   Acute and subacute allergic otitis media (mucoid) (sanguinous) (serous), right ear

     H65.112   Acute and subacute allergic otitis media (mucoid) (sanguinous) (serous), left ear

     H65.113   Acute and subacute allergic otitis media (mucoid) (sanguinous) (serous), bilateral

     H65.114   Acute and subacute allergic otitis media (mucoid) (sanguinous) (serous), recurrent, right ear

     H65.115   Acute and subacute allergic otitis media (mucoid) (sanguinous) (serous), recurrent, left ear

     H65.116   Acute and subacute allergic otitis media (mucoid) (sanguinous) (serous), recurrent, bilateral

     H65.117   Acute and subacute allergic otitis media (mucoid) (sanguinous) (serous), recurrent, unspecified ear

     H65.119   Acute and subacute allergic otitis media (mucoid) (sanguinous) (serous), unspecified ear

   ● **H65.19**   Other acute nonsuppurative otitis media

> Acute and subacute mucoid otitis media
> Acute and subacute nonsuppurative otitis media NOS
> Acute and subacute sanguinous otitis media
> Acute and subacute seromucinous otitis media

     H65.191   Other acute nonsuppurative otitis media, right ear

     H65.192   Other acute nonsuppurative otitis media, left ear

     H65.193   Other acute nonsuppurative otitis media, bilateral

     H65.194   Other acute nonsuppurative otitis media, recurrent, right ear

     H65.195   Other acute nonsuppurative otitis media, recurrent, left ear

     H65.196   Other acute nonsuppurative otitis media, recurrent, bilateral

     H65.197   Other acute nonsuppurative otitis media recurrent, unspecified ear

     H65.199   Other acute nonsuppurative otitis media, unspecified ear

● **H65.2**   Chronic serous otitis media

> Chronic tubotympanal catarrh

   H65.20   Chronic serous otitis media, unspecified ear

   H65.21   Chronic serous otitis media, right ear

   H65.22   Chronic serous otitis media, left ear

   H65.23   Chronic serous otitis media, bilateral

● **H65.3**   Chronic mucoid otitis media

> Chronic mucinous otitis media
> Chronic secretory otitis media
> Chronic transudative otitis media
> Glue ear

> **Excludes1**   adhesive middle ear disease (H74.1)

   H65.30   Chronic mucoid otitis media, unspecified ear

   H65.31   Chronic mucoid otitis media, right ear

   H65.32   Chronic mucoid otitis media, left ear

   H65.33   Chronic mucoid otitis media, bilateral

● **H65.4**   Other chronic nonsuppurative otitis media

   ● **H65.41**   Chronic allergic otitis media

     H65.411   Chronic allergic otitis media, right ear

     H65.412   Chronic allergic otitis media, left ear

     H65.413   Chronic allergic otitis media, bilateral

     H65.419   Chronic allergic otitis media, unspecified ear

   ● **H65.49**   Other chronic nonsuppurative otitis media

> Chronic exudative otitis media
> Chronic nonsuppurative otitis media NOS
> Chronic otitis media with effusion (nonpurulent)
> Chronic seromucinous otitis media

     H65.491   Other chronic nonsuppurative otitis media, right ear

     H65.492   Other chronic nonsuppurative otitis media, left ear

     H65.493   Other chronic nonsuppurative otitis media, bilateral

     H65.499   Other chronic nonsuppurative otitis media, unspecified ear

● **H65.9**   Unspecified nonsuppurative otitis media

> Allergic otitis media NOS
> Catarrhal otitis media NOS
> Exudative otitis media NOS
> Mucoid otitis media NOS
> Otitis media with effusion (nonpurulent) NOS
> Secretory otitis media NOS
> Seromucinous otitis media NOS
> Serous otitis media NOS
> Transudative otitis media NOS

   H65.90   Unspecified nonsuppurative otitis media, unspecified ear

   H65.91   Unspecified nonsuppurative otitis media, right ear

   H65.92   Unspecified nonsuppurative otitis media, left ear

   H65.93   Unspecified nonsuppurative otitis media, bilateral

● **H66**   Suppurative and unspecified otitis media

> *Suppurative: Discharging pus*

> **Includes**   suppurative and unspecified otitis media with myringitis

> Use additional code to identify:
> exposure to environmental tobacco smoke (Z77.22)
> exposure to tobacco smoke in the perinatal period (P96.81)
> history of tobacco dependence (Z87.891)
> occupational exposure to environmental tobacco smoke (Z57.31)
> tobacco dependence (F17.-)
> tobacco use (Z72.0)

   ● **H66.0**   Acute suppurative otitis media

     ● **H66.00**   Acute suppurative otitis media without spontaneous rupture of ear drum

       H66.001   Acute suppurative otitis media without spontaneous rupture of ear drum, right ear
> Coding Clinic: 2016, Q1, P34

       H66.002   Acute suppurative otitis media without spontaneous rupture of ear drum, left ear

       H66.003   Acute suppurative otitis media without spontaneous rupture of ear drum, bilateral

       H66.004   Acute suppurative otitis media without spontaneous rupture of ear drum, recurrent, right ear

       H66.005   Acute suppurative otitis media without spontaneous rupture of ear drum, recurrent, left ear

       H66.006   Acute suppurative otitis media without spontaneous rupture of ear drum, recurrent, bilateral

       H66.007   Acute suppurative otitis media without spontaneous rupture of ear drum, recurrent, unspecified ear

       H66.009   Acute suppurative otitis media without spontaneous rupture of ear drum, unspecified ear

● H66.01   Acute suppurative otitis media with spontaneous rupture of ear drum

     H66.011   Acute suppurative otitis media with spontaneous rupture of ear drum, right ear

     H66.012   Acute suppurative otitis media with spontaneous rupture of ear drum, left ear

     H66.013   Acute suppurative otitis media with spontaneous rupture of ear drum, bilateral

     H66.014   Acute suppurative otitis media with spontaneous rupture of ear drum, recurrent, right ear

     H66.015   Acute suppurative otitis media with spontaneous rupture of ear drum, recurrent, left ear

     H66.016   Acute suppurative otitis media with spontaneous rupture of ear drum, recurrent, bilateral

     H66.017   Acute suppurative otitis media with spontaneous rupture of ear drum, recurrent, unspecified ear

     H66.019   Acute suppurative otitis media with spontaneous rupture of ear drum, unspecified ear

● H66.1   Chronic tubotympanic suppurative otitis media

     Benign chronic suppurative otitis media
     Chronic tubotympanic disease

     Use additional code for any associated perforated tympanic membrane (H72.-)

     H66.10   Chronic tubotympanic suppurative otitis media, unspecified

     H66.11   Chronic tubotympanic suppurative otitis media, right ear

     H66.12   Chronic tubotympanic suppurative otitis media, left ear

     H66.13   Chronic tubotympanic suppurative otitis media, bilateral

● H66.2   Chronic atticoantral suppurative otitis media

     Chronic atticoantral disease

     Use additional code for any associated perforated tympanic membrane (H72.-)

     H66.20   Chronic atticoantral suppurative otitis media, unspecified ear

     H66.21   Chronic atticoantral suppurative otitis media, right ear

     H66.22   Chronic atticoantral suppurative otitis media, left ear

     H66.23   Chronic atticoantral suppurative otitis media, bilateral

● H66.3   Other chronic suppurative otitis media

     Chronic suppurative otitis media NOS

     Use additional code for any associated perforated tympanic membrane (H72.-)

     Excludes1   tuberculous otitis media (A18.6)

● H66.3X   Other chronic suppurative otitis media

     H66.3X1   Other chronic suppurative otitis media, right ear

     H66.3X2   Other chronic suppurative otitis media, left ear

     H66.3X3   Other chronic suppurative otitis media, bilateral

     H66.3X9   Other chronic suppurative otitis media, unspecified ear

● H66.4   Suppurative otitis media, unspecified

     Purulent otitis media NOS

     Use additional code for any associated perforated tympanic membrane (H72.-)

     H66.40   Suppurative otitis media, unspecified, unspecified ear

     H66.41   Suppurative otitis media, unspecified, right ear

     H66.42   Suppurative otitis media, unspecified, left ear

     H66.43   Suppurative otitis media, unspecified, bilateral

● H66.9   Otitis media, unspecified

     Otitis media NOS
     Acute otitis media NOS
     Chronic otitis media NOS

     Use additional code for any associated perforated tympanic membrane (H72.-)

     H66.90   Otitis media, unspecified, unspecified ear

     H66.91   Otitis media, unspecified, right ear

     H66.92   Otitis media, unspecified, left ear

     H66.93   Otitis media, unspecified, bilateral

● H67   Otitis media in diseases classified elsewhere

     Code first underlying disease, such as:
     plasminogen deficiency (E88.02)
     viral disease NEC (B00-B34)

     Use additional code for any associated perforated tympanic membrane (H72.-)

     Excludes1   otitis media in:
         influenza (J09.X9, J10.83, J11.83)
         measles (B05.3)
         scarlet fever (A38.0)
         tuberculosis (A18.6)

▷ *H67.1*   *Otitis media in diseases classified elsewhere, right ear*

▷ *H67.2*   *Otitis media in diseases classified elsewhere, left ear*

▷ *H67.3*   *Otitis media in diseases classified elsewhere, bilateral*

▷ *H67.9*   *Otitis media in diseases classified elsewhere, unspecified ear*

● H68   Eustachian salpingitis and obstruction

   ● H68.0   Eustachian salpingitis

     ● H68.00   Unspecified Eustachian salpingitis

       H68.001   Unspecified Eustachian salpingitis, right ear

       H68.002   Unspecified Eustachian salpingitis, left ear

       H68.003   Unspecified Eustachian salpingitis, bilateral

       H68.009   Unspecified Eustachian salpingitis, unspecified ear

     ● H68.01   Acute Eustachian salpingitis

       H68.011   Acute Eustachian salpingitis, right ear

       H68.012   Acute Eustachian salpingitis, left ear

       H68.013   Acute Eustachian salpingitis, bilateral

       H68.019   Acute Eustachian salpingitis, unspecified ear

     ● H68.02   Chronic Eustachian salpingitis

       H68.021   Chronic Eustachian salpingitis, right ear

       H68.022   Chronic Eustachian salpingitis, left ear

       H68.023   Chronic Eustachian salpingitis, bilateral

       H68.029   Chronic Eustachian salpingitis, unspecified ear

CHAPTER 8 (H60-H95)

▶ New   ⇒ Revised   ~~deleted~~ Deleted   Excludes 1   Excludes 2   Includes   Use additional   Code first   Code also   Key words

OGCR Official Guidelines   X Assign placeholder X   ● Use Additional Character(s)   ▷ Manifestation Code   🏷 Hierarchical Condition Category   **Coding Clinic**

● **H68.1**   **Obstruction** of Eustachian tube
    Stenosis of Eustachian tube
    Stricture of Eustachian tube
   ● **H68.10**   **Unspecified** obstruction of Eustachian tube
     H68.101   Unspecified obstruction of Eustachian tube, **right** ear
     H68.102   Unspecified obstruction of Eustachian tube, **left** ear
     H68.103   Unspecified obstruction of Eustachian tube, **bilateral**
     H68.109   Unspecified obstruction of Eustachian tube, **unspecified** ear
   ● **H68.11**   **Osseous** obstruction of Eustachian tube
     H68.111   Osseous obstruction of Eustachian tube, **right** ear
     H68.112   Osseous obstruction of Eustachian tube, **left** ear
     H68.113   Osseous obstruction of Eustachian tube, **bilateral**
     H68.119   Osseous obstruction of Eustachian tube, **unspecified** ear
   ● **H68.12**   **Intrinsic cartilagenous** obstruction of Eustachian tube
     H68.121   Intrinsic cartilagenous obstruction of Eustachian tube, **right** ear
     H68.122   Intrinsic cartilagenous obstruction of Eustachian tube, **left** ear
     H68.123   Intrinsic cartilagenous obstruction of Eustachian tube, **bilateral**
     H68.129   Intrinsic cartilagenous obstruction of Eustachian tube, **unspecified** ear
   ● **H68.13**   **Extrinsic cartilagenous** obstruction of Eustachian tube
     Compression of Eustachian tube
     H68.131   Extrinsic cartilagenous obstruction of Eustachian tube, **right** ear
     H68.132   Extrinsic cartilagenous obstruction of Eustachian tube, **left** ear
     H68.133   Extrinsic cartilagenous obstruction of Eustachian tube, **bilateral**
     H68.139   Extrinsic cartilagenous obstruction of Eustachian tube, **unspecified** ear

● **H69**   **Other** and unspecified disorders of Eustachian tube
   ● **H69.0**   **Patulous** Eustachian tube
     H69.00   Patulous Eustachian tube, **unspecified** ear
     H69.01   Patulous Eustachian tube, **right** ear
     H69.02   Patulous Eustachian tube, **left** ear
     H69.03   Patulous Eustachian tube, **bilateral**
   ● **H69.8**   **Other specified** disorders of Eustachian tube
     H69.80   Other specified disorders of Eustachian tube, **unspecified** ear
     H69.81   Other specified disorders of Eustachian tube, **right** ear
     H69.82   Other specified disorders of Eustachian tube, **left** ear
     H69.83   Other specified disorders of Eustachian tube, **bilateral**
   ● **H69.9**   **Unspecified** Eustachian tube disorder
     H69.90   Unspecified Eustachian tube disorder, **unspecified** ear
     H69.91   Unspecified Eustachian tube disorder, **right** ear
     H69.92   Unspecified Eustachian tube disorder, **left** ear
     H69.93   Unspecified Eustachian tube disorder, **bilateral**

● **H70**   Mastoiditis and related conditions
   ● **H70.0**   **Acute** mastoiditis
     Abscess of mastoid
     Empyema of mastoid
   ● **H70.00**   Acute mastoiditis **without complications**
     H70.001   Acute mastoiditis without complications, **right** ear
     H70.002   Acute mastoiditis without complications, **left** ear
     H70.003   Acute mastoiditis without complications, **bilateral**
     H70.009   Acute mastoiditis without complications, **unspecified** ear
   ● **H70.01**   **Subperiosteal abscess** of mastoid
     H70.011   Subperiosteal abscess of mastoid, **right** ear
     H70.012   Subperiosteal abscess of mastoid, **left** ear
     H70.013   Subperiosteal abscess of mastoid, **bilateral**
     H70.019   Subperiosteal abscess of mastoid, **unspecified** ear
   ● **H70.09**   Acute mastoiditis with **other complications**
     H70.091   Acute mastoiditis with other complications, **right** ear
     H70.092   Acute mastoiditis with other complications, **left** ear
     H70.093   Acute mastoiditis with other complications, **bilateral**
     H70.099   Acute mastoiditis with other complications, **unspecified** ear
   ● **H70.1**   **Chronic** mastoiditis
     Caries of mastoid
     Fistula of mastoid
     Excludes1   tuberculous mastoiditis (A18.03)
     H70.10   Chronic mastoiditis, **unspecified** ear
     H70.11   Chronic mastoiditis, **right** ear
     H70.12   Chronic mastoiditis, **left** ear
     H70.13   Chronic mastoiditis, **bilateral**
   ● **H70.2**   **Petrositis**
     Inflammation of petrous bone
   ● **H70.20**   **Unspecified petrositis**
     H70.201   Unspecified petrositis, **right** ear
     H70.202   Unspecified petrositis, **left** ear
     H70.203   Unspecified petrositis, **bilateral**
     H70.209   Unspecified petrositis, **unspecified** ear
   ● **H70.21**   **Acute petrositis**
     H70.211   Acute petrositis, **right** ear
     H70.212   Acute petrositis, **left** ear
     H70.213   Acute petrositis, **bilateral**
     H70.219   Acute petrositis, **unspecified** ear
   ● **H70.22**   **Chronic petrositis**
     H70.221   Chronic petrositis, **right** ear
     H70.222   Chronic petrositis, **left** ear
     H70.223   Chronic petrositis, **bilateral**
     H70.229   Chronic petrositis, **unspecified** ear

CHAPTER 8 (H60-H95)

Item 8-1   **Mastoiditis** is an infection of the portion of the temporal bone of the skull that is behind the ear (mastoid process) caused by an untreated otitis media, leading to an infection of the surrounding structures which may include the brain.

● H70.8   Other mastoiditis and related conditions
    Excludes1   preauricular sinus and cyst (Q18.1)
       sinus, fistula, and cyst of branchial cleft (Q18.0)
   ● H70.81   Postauricular fistula
    H70.811   Postauricular fistula, right ear
    H70.812   Postauricular fistula, left ear
    H70.813   Postauricular fistula, bilateral
    H70.819   Postauricular fistula, unspecified ear
   ● H70.89   Other mastoiditis and related conditions
    H70.891   Other mastoiditis and related conditions, right ear
    H70.892   Other mastoiditis and related conditions, left ear
    H70.893   Other mastoiditis and related conditions, bilateral
    H70.899   Other mastoiditis and related conditions, unspecified ear
● H70.9   Unspecified mastoiditis
    H70.90   Unspecified mastoiditis, unspecified ear
    H70.91   Unspecified mastoiditis, right ear
    H70.92   Unspecified mastoiditis, left ear
    H70.93   Unspecified mastoiditis, bilateral

● H71   Cholesteatoma of middle ear
    Excludes2   cholesteatoma of external ear (H60.4-)
       recurrent cholesteatoma of postmastoidectomy cavity (H95.0-)
● H71.0   Cholesteatoma of attic
    H71.00   Cholesteatoma of attic, unspecified ear
    H71.01   Cholesteatoma of attic, right ear
    H71.02   Cholesteatoma of attic, left ear
    H71.03   Cholesteatoma of attic, bilateral
● H71.1   Cholesteatoma of tympanum
    H71.10   Cholesteatoma of tympanum, unspecified ear
    H71.11   Cholesteatoma of tympanum, right ear
    H71.12   Cholesteatoma of tympanum, left ear
    H71.13   Cholesteatoma of tympanum, bilateral
● H71.2   Cholesteatoma of mastoid
    H71.20   Cholesteatoma of mastoid, unspecified ear
    H71.21   Cholesteatoma of mastoid, right ear
    H71.22   Cholesteatoma of mastoid, left ear
    H71.23   Cholesteatoma of mastoid, bilateral
● H71.3   Diffuse cholesteatosis
    H71.30   Diffuse cholesteatosis, unspecified ear
    H71.31   Diffuse cholesteatosis, right ear
    H71.32   Diffuse cholesteatosis, left ear
    H71.33   Diffuse cholesteatosis, bilateral
● H71.9   Unspecified cholesteatoma
    H71.90   Unspecified cholesteatoma, unspecified ear
    H71.91   Unspecified cholesteatoma, right ear
    H71.92   Unspecified cholesteatoma, left ear
    H71.93   Unspecified cholesteatoma, bilateral

★ **(See Plate 22 of the Anatomy Illustrations.)**

● H72   Perforation of tympanic membrane
    Hole or rupture in ear drum
    Includes   persistent post-traumatic perforation of ear drum
       postinflammatory perforation of ear drum
    Code first any associated otitis media (H65.-, H66.1-, H66.2-, H66.3-, H66.4-, H66.9-, H67.-)
    Excludes1   acute suppurative otitis media with rupture of the tympanic membrane (H66.01-)
       traumatic rupture of ear drum (S09.2-)
● H72.0   Central perforation of tympanic membrane
    H72.00   Central perforation of tympanic membrane, unspecified ear
    H72.01   Central perforation of tympanic membrane, right ear
    H72.02   Central perforation of tympanic membrane, left ear
    H72.03   Central perforation of tympanic membrane, bilateral
● H72.1   Attic perforation of tympanic membrane
    Perforation of pars flaccida
    H72.10   Attic perforation of tympanic membrane, unspecified ear
    H72.11   Attic perforation of tympanic membrane, right ear
    H72.12   Attic perforation of tympanic membrane, left ear
    H72.13   Attic perforation of tympanic membrane, bilateral
● H72.2   Other marginal perforations of tympanic membrane
   ● H72.2X   Other marginal perforations of tympanic membrane
    H72.2X1   Other marginal perforations of tympanic membrane, right ear
    H72.2X2   Other marginal perforations of tympanic membrane, left ear
    H72.2X3   Other marginal perforations of tympanic membrane, bilateral
    H72.2X9   Other marginal perforations of tympanic membrane, unspecified ear
● H72.8   Other perforations of tympanic membrane
   ● H72.81   Multiple perforations of tympanic membrane
    H72.811   Multiple perforations of tympanic membrane, right ear
    H72.812   Multiple perforations of tympanic membrane, left ear
    H72.813   Multiple perforations of tympanic membrane, bilateral
    H72.819   Multiple perforations of tympanic membrane, unspecified ear
   ● H72.82   Total perforations of tympanic membrane
    H72.821   Total perforations of tympanic membrane, right ear
    H72.822   Total perforations of tympanic membrane, left ear
    H72.823   Total perforations of tympanic membrane, bilateral
    H72.829   Total perforations of tympanic membrane, unspecified ear
● H72.9   Unspecified perforation of tympanic membrane
    H72.90   Unspecified perforation of tympanic membrane, unspecified ear
    H72.91   Unspecified perforation of tympanic membrane, right ear
    H72.92   Unspecified perforation of tympanic membrane, left ear
    H72.93   Unspecified perforation of tympanic membrane, bilateral

CHAPTER 8 (H60-H95)

▶ New   ⇒ Revised   ~~deleted~~ Deleted   Excludes 1   Excludes 2   Includes   Use additional   Code first   Code also   Key words
OGCR Official Guidelines   X Assign placeholder X   ● Use Additional Character(s)   ▮ Manifestation Code   🖉 Hierarchical Condition Category   Coding Clinic

● H73   Other disorders of tympanic membrane
   ● H73.0   Acute myringitis
      Excludes1   acute myringitis with otitis media (H65, H66)
     ● H73.00   Unspecified acute myringitis
        Acute tympanitis NOS
       H73.001   Acute myringitis, right ear
       H73.002   Acute myringitis, left ear
       H73.003   Acute myringitis, bilateral
       H73.009   Acute myringitis, unspecified ear
     ● H73.01   Bullous myringitis
       H73.011   Bullous myringitis, right ear
       H73.012   Bullous myringitis, left ear
       H73.013   Bullous myringitis, bilateral
       H73.019   Bullous myringitis, unspecified ear
     ● H73.09   Other acute myringitis
       H73.091   Other acute myringitis, right ear
       H73.092   Other acute myringitis, left ear
       H73.093   Other acute myringitis, bilateral
       H73.099   Other acute myringitis, unspecified ear
   ● H73.1   Chronic myringitis
      Chronic tympanitis
      Excludes1   chronic myringitis with otitis media (H65, H66)
     H73.10   Chronic myringitis, unspecified ear
     H73.11   Chronic myringitis, right ear
     H73.12   Chronic myringitis, left ear
     H73.13   Chronic myringitis, bilateral
   ● H73.2   Unspecified myringitis
     H73.20   Unspecified myringitis, unspecified ear
     H73.21   Unspecified myringitis, right ear
     H73.22   Unspecified myringitis, left ear
     H73.23   Unspecified myringitis, bilateral
   ● H73.8   Other specified disorders of tympanic membrane
     ● H73.81   Atrophic flaccid tympanic membrane
       H73.811   Atrophic flaccid tympanic membrane, right ear
       H73.812   Atrophic flaccid tympanic membrane, left ear
       H73.813   Atrophic flaccid tympanic membrane, bilateral
       H73.819   Atrophic flaccid tympanic membrane, unspecified ear
     ● H73.82   Atrophic nonflaccid tympanic membrane
       H73.821   Atrophic nonflaccid tympanic membrane, right ear
       H73.822   Atrophic nonflaccid tympanic membrane, left ear
       H73.823   Atrophic nonflaccid tympanic membrane, bilateral
       H73.829   Atrophic nonflaccid tympanic membrane, unspecified ear
     ● H73.89   Other specified disorders of tympanic membrane
       H73.891   Other specified disorders of tympanic membrane, right ear
       H73.892   Other specified disorders of tympanic membrane, left ear
       H73.893   Other specified disorders of tympanic membrane, bilateral
       H73.899   Other specified disorders of tympanic membrane, unspecified ear

   ● H73.9   Unspecified disorder of tympanic membrane
     H73.90   Unspecified disorder of tympanic membrane, unspecified ear
     H73.91   Unspecified disorder of tympanic membrane, right ear
     H73.92   Unspecified disorder of tympanic membrane, left ear
     H73.93   Unspecified disorder of tympanic membrane, bilateral
● H74   Other disorders of middle ear mastoid
      Excludes2   mastoiditis (H70.-)
   ● H74.0   Tympanosclerosis
     H74.01   Tympanosclerosis, right ear
     H74.02   Tympanosclerosis, left ear
     H74.03   Tympanosclerosis, bilateral
     H74.09   Tympanosclerosis, unspecified ear
   ● H74.1   Adhesive middle ear disease
      Adhesive otitis
      Excludes1   glue ear (H65.3-)
     H74.11   Adhesive right middle ear disease
     H74.12   Adhesive left middle ear disease
     H74.13   Adhesive middle ear disease, bilateral
     H74.19   Adhesive middle ear disease, unspecified ear
   ● H74.2   Discontinuity and dislocation of ear ossicles
     H74.20   Discontinuity and dislocation of ear ossicles, unspecified ear
     H74.21   Discontinuity and dislocation of right ear ossicles
     H74.22   Discontinuity and dislocation of left ear ossicles
     H74.23   Discontinuity and dislocation of ear ossicles, bilateral
   ● H74.3   Other acquired abnormalities of ear ossicles
     ● H74.31   Ankylosis of ear ossicles
       H74.311   Ankylosis of ear ossicles, right ear
       H74.312   Ankylosis of ear ossicles, left ear
       H74.313   Ankylosis of ear ossicles, bilateral
       H74.319   Ankylosis of ear ossicles, unspecified ear
     ● H74.32   Partial loss of ear ossicles
       H74.321   Partial loss of ear ossicles, right ear
       H74.322   Partial loss of ear ossicles, left ear
       H74.323   Partial loss of ear ossicles, bilateral
       H74.329   Partial loss of ear ossicles, unspecified ear
     ● H74.39   Other acquired abnormalities of ear ossicles
       H74.391   Other acquired abnormalities of right ear ossicles
       H74.392   Other acquired abnormalities of left ear ossicles
       H74.393   Other acquired abnormalities of ear ossicles, bilateral
       H74.399   Other acquired abnormalities of ear ossicles, unspecified ear
   ● H74.4   Polyp of middle ear
     H74.40   Polyp of middle ear, unspecified ear
     H74.41   Polyp of right middle ear
     H74.42   Polyp of left middle ear
     H74.43   Polyp of middle ear, bilateral

● H74.8   Other specified disorders of middle ear and mastoid
   ● H74.8X   Other specified disorders of middle ear and mastoid
     H74.8X1   Other specified disorders of right middle ear and mastoid
     H74.8X2   Other specified disorders of left middle ear and mastoid
     H74.8X3   Other specified disorders of middle ear and mastoid, bilateral
     H74.8X9   Other specified disorders of middle ear and mastoid, unspecified ear
   ● H74.9   Unspecified disorder of middle ear and mastoid
     H74.90   Unspecified disorder of middle ear and mastoid, unspecified ear
     H74.91   Unspecified disorder of right middle ear and mastoid
     H74.92   Unspecified disorder of left middle ear and mastoid
     H74.93   Unspecified disorder of middle ear and mastoid, bilateral

● H75   Other disorders of middle ear and mastoid in diseases classified elsewhere
   Code first underlying disease
   ● H75.0   Mastoiditis in infectious and parasitic diseases classified elsewhere
     Excludes1   mastoiditis (in):
         syphilis (A52.77)
         tuberculosis (A18.03)
     ▷ *H75.00*   *Mastoiditis in infectious and parasitic diseases classified elsewhere, unspecified ear*
     ▷ *H75.01*   *Mastoiditis in infectious and parasitic diseases classified elsewhere, right ear*
     ▷ *H75.02*   *Mastoiditis in infectious and parasitic diseases classified elsewhere, left ear*
     ▷ *H75.03*   *Mastoiditis in infectious and parasitic diseases classified elsewhere, bilateral*
   ● H75.8   Other specified disorders of middle ear and mastoid in diseases classified elsewhere
     ▷ *H75.80*   *Other specified disorders of middle ear and mastoid in diseases classified elsewhere, unspecified ear*
     ▷ *H75.81*   *Other specified disorders of right middle ear and mastoid in diseases classified elsewhere*
     ▷ *H75.82*   *Other specified disorders of left middle ear and mastoid in diseases classified elsewhere*
     ▷ *H75.83*   *Other specified disorders of middle ear and mastoid in diseases classified elsewhere, bilateral*

DISEASES OF INNER EAR (H80-H83)

★ **(See Plate 23 of the Anatomy Illustrations.)**

● H80   Otosclerosis
   Inherited middle ear spongelike bone growth causing hearing loss
   Includes   Otospongiosis
   ● H80.0   Otosclerosis involving oval window, nonobliterative
     H80.00   Otosclerosis involving oval window, nonobliterative, unspecified ear
     H80.01   Otosclerosis involving oval window, nonobliterative, right ear
     H80.02   Otosclerosis involving oval window, nonobliterative, left ear
     H80.03   Otosclerosis involving oval window, nonobliterative, bilateral

● H80.1   Otosclerosis involving oval window, obliterative
   H80.10   Otosclerosis involving oval window, obliterative, unspecified ear
   H80.11   Otosclerosis involving oval window, obliterative, right ear
   H80.12   Otosclerosis involving oval window, obliterative, left ear
   H80.13   Otosclerosis involving oval window, obliterative, bilateral
● H80.2   Cochlear otosclerosis
   Otosclerosis involving otic capsule
   Otosclerosis involving round window
   H80.20   Cochlear otosclerosis, unspecified ear
   H80.21   Cochlear otosclerosis, right ear
   H80.22   Cochlear otosclerosis, left ear
   H80.23   Cochlear otosclerosis, bilateral
● H80.8   Other otosclerosis
   H80.80   Other otosclerosis, unspecified ear
   H80.81   Other otosclerosis, right ear
   H80.82   Other otosclerosis, left ear
   H80.83   Other otosclerosis, bilateral
● H80.9   Unspecified otosclerosis
   H80.90   Unspecified otosclerosis, unspecified ear
   H80.91   Unspecified otosclerosis, right ear
   H80.92   Unspecified otosclerosis, left ear
   H80.93   Unspecified otosclerosis, bilateral

● H81   Disorders of vestibular function
   Excludes1   epidemic vertigo (A88.1)
         vertigo NOS (R42)
   ● H81.0   Ménière's disease
     Vestibular disorder that produces recurring symptoms including severe and intermittent hearing loss including the feeling of ear pressure or pain
     Labyrinthine hydrops
     Ménière's syndrome or vertigo
     H81.01   Ménière's disease, right ear
     H81.02   Ménière's disease, left ear
     H81.03   Ménière's disease, bilateral
     H81.09   Ménière's disease, unspecified ear
   ● H81.1   Benign paroxysmal vertigo
     H81.10   Benign paroxysmal vertigo, unspecified ear
     H81.11   Benign paroxysmal vertigo, right ear
     H81.12   Benign paroxysmal vertigo, left ear
     H81.13   Benign paroxysmal vertigo, bilateral
   ● H81.2   Vestibular neuronitis
     H81.20   Vestibular neuronitis, unspecified ear
     H81.21   Vestibular neuronitis, right ear
     H81.22   Vestibular neuronitis, left ear
     H81.23   Vestibular neuronitis, bilateral
   ● H81.3   Other peripheral vertigo
     ● H81.31   Aural vertigo
       H81.311   Aural vertigo, right ear
       H81.312   Aural vertigo, left ear
       H81.313   Aural vertigo, bilateral
       H81.319   Aural vertigo, unspecified ear
     ● H81.39   Other peripheral vertigo
       Lermoyez' syndrome
       Otogenic vertigo
       Peripheral vertigo NOS
       H81.391   Other peripheral vertigo, right ear
       H81.392   Other peripheral vertigo, left ear
       H81.393   Other peripheral vertigo, bilateral
       H81.399   Other peripheral vertigo, unspecified ear
   H81.4   Vertigo of central origin
     Central positional nystagmus

▶ New   ⫸ Revised   ~~deleted~~ Deleted   Excludes 1   Excludes 2   Includes   Use additional   Code first   Code also   Key words
OGCR Official Guidelines   X Assign placeholder X   ● Use Additional Character(s)   ▷ Manifestation Code   🅗🅒🅒 Hierarchical Condition Category   **Coding Clinic**

● H81.8   Other disorders of vestibular function
   ● H81.8X   Other disorders of vestibular function
       H81.8X1   Other disorders of vestibular function, right ear
       H81.8X2   Other disorders of vestibular function, left ear
       H81.8X3   Other disorders of vestibular function, bilateral
       H81.8X9   Other disorders of vestibular function, unspecified ear

● H81.9   Unspecified disorder of vestibular function
       Vertiginous syndrome NOS
       H81.90   Unspecified disorder of vestibular function, unspecified ear
       H81.91   Unspecified disorder of vestibular function, right ear
       H81.92   Unspecified disorder of vestibular function, left ear
       H81.93   Unspecified disorder of vestibular function, bilateral

● H82   Vertiginous syndromes in diseases classified elsewhere
       Code first underlying disease
       Excludes1   epidemic vertigo (A88.1)
  ▷ *H82.1*   *Vertiginous syndromes in diseases classified elsewhere, right ear*
  ▷ *H82.2*   *Vertiginous syndromes in diseases classified elsewhere, left ear*
  ▷ *H82.3*   *Vertiginous syndromes in diseases classified elsewhere, bilateral*
  ▷ *H82.9*   *Vertiginous syndromes in diseases classified elsewhere, unspecified ear*

● H83   Other diseases of inner ear
   ● H83.0   Labyrinthitis
       Balance disorder that follows URI or head injury
       H83.01   Labyrinthitis, right ear
       H83.02   Labyrinthitis, left ear
       H83.03   Labyrinthitis, bilateral
       H83.09   Labyrinthitis, unspecified ear
   ● H83.1   Labyrinthine fistula
       H83.11   Labyrinthine fistula, right ear
       H83.12   Labyrinthine fistula, left ear
       H83.13   Labyrinthine fistula, bilateral
       H83.19   Labyrinthine fistula, unspecified ear
   ● H83.2   Labyrinthine dysfunction
       Labyrinthine hypersensitivity
       Labyrinthine hypofunction
       Labyrinthine loss of function
    ● H83.2X   Labyrinthine dysfunction
       H83.2X1   Labyrinthine dysfunction, right ear
       H83.2X2   Labyrinthine dysfunction, left ear
       H83.2X3   Labyrinthine dysfunction, bilateral
       H83.2X9   Labyrinthine dysfunction, unspecified ear
   ● H83.3   Noise effects on inner ear
       Acoustic trauma of inner ear
       Noise-induced hearing loss of inner ear
    ● H83.3X   Noise effects on inner ear
       H83.3X1   Noise effects on right inner ear
       H83.3X2   Noise effects on left inner ear
       H83.3X3   Noise effects on inner ear, bilateral
       H83.3X9   Noise effects on inner ear, unspecified ear

● H83.8   Other specified diseases of inner ear
   ● H83.8X   Other specified diseases of inner ear
       H83.8X1   Other specified diseases of right inner ear
       H83.8X2   Other specified diseases of left inner ear
       H83.8X3   Other specified diseases of inner ear, bilateral
       H83.8X9   Other specified diseases of inner ear, unspecified ear

● H83.9   Unspecified disease of inner ear
       H83.90   Unspecified disease of inner ear, unspecified ear
       H83.91   Unspecified disease of right inner ear
       H83.92   Unspecified disease of left inner ear
       H83.93   Unspecified disease of inner ear, bilateral

OTHER DISORDERS OF EAR (H90-H94)

● H90   Conductive and sensorineural hearing loss
       Excludes1   deaf nonspeaking NEC (H91.3)
                  deafness NOS (H91.9-)
                  hearing loss NOS (H91.9-)
                  noise-induced hearing loss (H83.3-)
                  ototoxic hearing loss (H91.0-)
                  sudden (idiopathic) hearing loss (H91.2-)
    H90.0   Conductive hearing loss, bilateral
   ● H90.1   Conductive hearing loss, unilateral with unrestricted hearing on the contralateral side
       H90.11   Conductive hearing loss, unilateral, right ear, with unrestricted hearing on the contralateral side
       H90.12   Conductive hearing loss, unilateral, left ear, with unrestricted hearing on the contralateral side
    H90.2   Conductive hearing loss, unspecified
       Conductive deafness NOS
    H90.3   Sensorineural hearing loss, bilateral
   ● H90.4   Sensorineural hearing loss, unilateral with unrestricted hearing on the contralateral side
       H90.41   Sensorineural hearing loss, unilateral, right ear, with unrestricted hearing on the contralateral side
       H90.42   Sensorineural hearing loss, unilateral, left ear, with unrestricted hearing on the contralateral side
    H90.5   Unspecified sensorineural hearing loss
       Central hearing loss NOS
       Congenital deafness NOS
       Neural hearing loss NOS
       Perceptive hearing loss NOS
       Sensorineural deafness NOS
       Sensory hearing loss NOS
       Excludes1   abnormal auditory perception (H93.2-)
                  psychogenic deafness (F44.6)
    H90.6   Mixed conductive and sensorineural hearing loss, bilateral
       Coding Clinic: 2015, Q2, P7
   ● H90.7   Mixed conductive and sensorineural hearing loss, unilateral with unrestricted hearing on the contralateral side
       H90.71   Mixed conductive and sensorineural hearing loss, unilateral, right ear, with unrestricted hearing on the contralateral side
       H90.72   Mixed conductive and sensorineural hearing loss, unilateral, left ear, with unrestricted hearing on the contralateral side
    H90.8   Mixed conductive and sensorineural hearing loss, unspecified

- H90.A **Conductive and sensorineural hearing loss with restricted hearing on the contralateral side**
  Coding Clinic: 2016, Q4, P23-24
  - H90.A1 **Conductive** hearing loss, **unilateral**, with restricted hearing on the contralateral side
    - H90.A11 Conductive hearing loss, unilateral, **right** ear with restricted hearing on the contralateral side
    - H90.A12 Conductive hearing loss, unilateral, **left** ear with restricted hearing on the contralateral side
      Coding Clinic: 2016, Q4, P25
  - H90.A2 **Sensorineural** hearing loss, **unilateral**, with restricted hearing on the contralateral side
    - H90.A21 Sensorineural hearing loss, unilateral, **right** ear, with restricted hearing on the contralateral side
    - H90.A22 Sensorineural hearing loss, unilateral, **left** ear, with restricted hearing on the contralateral side
  - H90.A3 **Mixed** conductive and sensorineural hearing loss, **unilateral** with restricted hearing on the contralateral side
    - H90.A31 Mixed conductive and sensorineural hearing loss, unilateral, **right** ear with restricted hearing on the contralateral side
    - H90.A32 Mixed conductive and sensorineural hearing loss, unilateral, **left** ear with restricted hearing on the contralateral side

- H91 **Other and unspecified hearing loss**
  - **Excludes1** abnormal auditory perception (H93.2-)
    hearing loss as classified in H90.-
    impacted cerumen (H61.2-)
    noise-induced hearing loss (H83.3-)
    psychogenic deafness (F44.6)
    transient ischemic deafness (H93.01-)
  - H91.0 **Ototoxic hearing loss**
    Code first poisoning due to drug or toxin, if applicable (T36-T65 with fifth or sixth character 1-4 or 6)
    Use additional code for adverse effect, if applicable, to identify drug (T36-T50 with fifth or sixth character 5)
    - H91.01 Ototoxic hearing loss, **right** ear
    - H91.02 Ototoxic hearing loss, **left** ear
    - H91.03 Ototoxic hearing loss, **bilateral**
    - H91.09 Ototoxic hearing loss, **unspecified** ear
  - H91.1 **Presbycusis**
    Presbyacusia
    - H91.10 Presbycusis, **unspecified** ear
    - H91.11 Presbycusis, **right** ear
    - H91.12 Presbycusis, **left** ear
    - H91.13 Presbycusis, **bilateral**
  - H91.2 **Sudden idiopathic hearing loss**
    Sudden hearing loss NOS
    - H91.20 Sudden idiopathic hearing loss, **unspecified** ear
    - H91.21 Sudden idiopathic hearing loss, **right** ear
    - H91.22 Sudden idiopathic hearing loss, **left** ear
    - H91.23 Sudden idiopathic hearing loss, **bilateral**
  - H91.3 Deaf nonspeaking, not elsewhere classified
  - H91.8 **Other specified hearing loss**
    - H91.8X **Other** specified hearing loss
      - H91.8X1 Other specified hearing loss, **right** ear
      - H91.8X2 Other specified hearing loss, **left** ear
      - H91.8X3 Other specified hearing loss, **bilateral**
      - H91.8X9 Other specified hearing loss, **unspecified** ear

- H91.9 **Unspecified** hearing loss
  Deafness NOS
  High frequency deafness
  Low frequency deafness
  - H91.90 Unspecified hearing loss, **unspecified** ear
  - H91.91 Unspecified hearing loss, **right** ear
  - H91.92 Unspecified hearing loss, **left** ear
  - H91.93 Unspecified hearing loss, **bilateral**

- H92 **Otalgia and effusion of ear**
  - H92.0 **Otalgia**
    - H92.01 Otalgia, **right** ear
    - H92.02 Otalgia, **left** ear
    - H92.03 Otalgia, **bilateral**
    - H92.09 Otalgia, **unspecified** ear
  - H92.1 **Otorrhea**
    Excludes1 leakage of cerebrospinal fluid through ear (G96.0)
    - H92.10 Otorrhea, **unspecified** ear
    - H92.11 Otorrhea, **right** ear
    - H92.12 Otorrhea, **left** ear
    - H92.13 Otorrhea, **bilateral**
  - H92.2 **Otorrhagia**
    Excludes1 traumatic otorrhagia - code to injury
    - H92.20 Otorrhagia, **unspecified** ear
    - H92.21 Otorrhagia, **right** ear
    - H92.22 Otorrhagia, **left** ear
    - H92.23 Otorrhagia, **bilateral**

- H93 **Other disorders of ear, not elsewhere classified**
  - H93.0 **Degenerative and vascular disorders of ear**
    Excludes1 presbycusis (H91.1)
    - H93.01 **Transient ischemic deafness**
      - H93.011 Transient ischemic deafness, **right** ear
      - H93.012 Transient ischemic deafness, **left** ear
      - H93.013 Transient ischemic deafness, **bilateral**
      - H93.019 Transient ischemic deafness, **unspecified** ear
    - H93.09 **Unspecified** degenerative and vascular disorders of ear
      - H93.091 Unspecified degenerative and vascular disorders of **right** ear
      - H93.092 Unspecified degenerative and vascular disorders of **left** ear
      - H93.093 Unspecified degenerative and vascular disorders of ear, **bilateral**
      - H93.099 Unspecified degenerative and vascular disorders of **unspecified** ear
  - H93.1 **Tinnitus**
    Perception of sound (ringing, buzzing, humming, whistling tunes, or singing)
    - H93.11 Tinnitus, **right** ear
    - H93.12 Tinnitus, **left** ear
    - H93.13 Tinnitus, **bilateral**
    - H93.19 Tinnitus, **unspecified** ear
  - H93.A **Pulsatile tinnitus**
    Coding Clinic: 2016, Q4, P25
    - H93.A1 Pulsatile tinnitus, **right** ear
      Coding Clinic: 2016, Q4, P26
    - H93.A2 Pulsatile tinnitus, **left** ear
    - H93.A3 Pulsatile tinnitus, **bilateral**
    - H93.A9 Pulsatile tinnitus, **unspecified** ear

▶ New ⇒ Revised ~~deleted~~ Deleted Excludes 1 Excludes 2 Includes Use additional Code first Code also Key words
OGCR Official Guidelines X Assign placeholder X ● Use Additional Character(s) ▸ Manifestation Code 🦘 Hierarchical Condition Category **Coding Clinic**

● **H93.2**   **Other abnormal auditory perceptions**
     Excludes2   auditory hallucinations (R44.0)

    ● **H93.21**   **Auditory recruitment**
       H93.211   Auditory recruitment, right ear
       H93.212   Auditory recruitment, left ear
       H93.213   Auditory recruitment, bilateral
       H93.219   Auditory recruitment, unspecified ear

    ● **H93.22**   **Diplacusis**
       H93.221   Diplacusis, right ear
       H93.222   Diplacusis, left ear
       H93.223   Diplacusis, bilateral
       H93.229   Diplacusis, unspecified ear

    ● **H93.23**   **Hyperacusis**
       H93.231   Hyperacusis, right ear
       H93.232   Hyperacusis, left ear
       H93.233   Hyperacusis, bilateral
       H93.239   Hyperacusis, unspecified ear

    ● **H93.24**   **Temporary auditory threshold shift**
       H93.241   Temporary auditory threshold shift, right ear
       H93.242   Temporary auditory threshold shift, left ear
       H93.243   Temporary auditory threshold shift, bilateral
       H93.249   Temporary auditory threshold shift, unspecified ear

    H93.25   **Central auditory processing disorder**
       Congenital auditory imperception
       Word deafness
       Excludes1   mixed receptive-expressive language disorder (F80.2)

    ● **H93.29**   **Other abnormal auditory perceptions**
       H93.291   Other abnormal auditory perceptions, right ear
       H93.292   Other abnormal auditory perceptions, left ear
       H93.293   Other abnormal auditory perceptions, bilateral
       H93.299   Other abnormal auditory perceptions, unspecified ear

● **H93.3**   **Disorders of acoustic nerve**
     Disorder of 8th cranial nerve
     Excludes1   acoustic neuroma (D33.3)
                syphilitic acoustic neuritis (A52.15)

    ● **H93.3X**   **Disorders of acoustic nerve**
       H93.3X1   Disorders of right acoustic nerve
       H93.3X2   Disorders of left acoustic nerve
       H93.3X3   Disorders of bilateral acoustic nerves
       H93.3X9   Disorders of unspecified acoustic nerve

● **H93.8**   **Other specified disorders of ear**
    ● **H93.8X**   **Other specified disorders of ear**
       H93.8X1   Other specified disorders of right ear
       H93.8X2   Other specified disorders of left ear
       H93.8X3   Other specified disorders of ear, bilateral
       H93.8X9   Other specified disorders of ear, unspecified ear

● **H93.9**   **Unspecified disorder of ear**
     H93.90   Unspecified disorder of ear, unspecified ear
     H93.91   Unspecified disorder of right ear
     H93.92   Unspecified disorder of left ear
     H93.93   Unspecified disorder of ear, bilateral

● **H94**   **Other disorders of ear in diseases classified elsewhere**
    ● **H94.0**   **Acoustic neuritis in infectious and parasitic diseases classified elsewhere**
       Code first underlying disease, such as:
       parasitic disease (B65-B89)
       Excludes1   acoustic neuritis (in):
                  herpes zoster (B02.29)
                  syphilis (A52.15)

      ▌ *H94.00*   *Acoustic neuritis in infectious and parasitic diseases classified elsewhere, unspecified ear*
      ▌ *H94.01*   *Acoustic neuritis in infectious and parasitic diseases classified elsewhere, right ear*
      ▌ *H94.02*   *Acoustic neuritis in infectious and parasitic diseases classified elsewhere, left ear*
      ▌ *H94.03*   *Acoustic neuritis in infectious and parasitic diseases classified elsewhere, bilateral*

    ● **H94.8**   **Other specified disorders of ear in diseases classified elsewhere**
       Code first underlying disease, such as:
       congenital syphilis (A50.0)
       Excludes1   aural myiasis (B87.4)
                  syphilitic labyrinthitis (A52.79)

      ▌ *H94.80*   *Other specified disorders of ear in diseases classified elsewhere, unspecified ear*
      ▌ *H94.81*   *Other specified disorders of right ear in diseases classified elsewhere*
      ▌ *H94.82*   *Other specified disorders of left ear in diseases classified elsewhere*
      ▌ *H94.83*   *Other specified disorders of ear in diseases classified elsewhere, bilateral*

INTRAOPERATIVE AND POSTPROCEDURAL COMPLICATIONS AND DISORDERS OF EAR AND MASTOID PROCESS, NOT ELSEWHERE CLASSIFIED (H95)

● **H95**   **Intraoperative and postprocedural complications and disorders of ear and mastoid process, not elsewhere classified**
     Coding Clinic: 2016, Q4, P10

    ● **H95.0**   **Recurrent cholesteatoma of postmastoidectomy cavity**
       H95.00   Recurrent cholesteatoma of postmastoidectomy cavity, unspecified ear
       H95.01   Recurrent cholesteatoma of postmastoidectomy cavity, right ear
       H95.02   Recurrent cholesteatoma of postmastoidectomy cavity, left ear
       H95.03   Recurrent cholesteatoma of postmastoidectomy cavity, bilateral ears

    ● **H95.1**   **Other disorders of ear and mastoid process following mastoidectomy**
      ● **H95.11**   **Chronic inflammation of postmastoidectomy cavity**
         H95.111   Chronic inflammation of postmastoidectomy cavity, right ear
         H95.112   Chronic inflammation of postmastoidectomy cavity, left ear
         H95.113   Chronic inflammation of postmastoidectomy cavity, bilateral ears
         H95.119   Chronic inflammation of postmastoidectomy cavity, unspecified ear

      ● **H95.12**   **Granulation of postmastoidectomy cavity**
         H95.121   Granulation of postmastoidectomy cavity, right ear
         H95.122   Granulation of postmastoidectomy cavity, left ear
         H95.123   Granulation of postmastoidectomy cavity, bilateral ears
         H95.129   Granulation of postmastoidectomy cavity, unspecified ear

CHAPTER 8 (H60-H95)

● H95.13   Mucosal cyst of postmastoidectomy cavity

     H95.131   Mucosal cyst of postmastoidectomy cavity, right ear

     H95.132   Mucosal cyst of postmastoidectomy cavity, left ear

     H95.133   Mucosal cyst of postmastoidectomy cavity, bilateral ears

     H95.139   Mucosal cyst of postmastoidectomy cavity, unspecified ear

● H95.19   Other disorders following mastoidectomy

     H95.191   Other disorders following mastoidectomy, right ear

     H95.192   Other disorders following mastoidectomy, left ear

     H95.193   Other disorders following mastoidectomy, bilateral ears

     H95.199   Other disorders following mastoidectomy, unspecified ear

● H95.2   Intraoperative hemorrhage and hematoma of ear and mastoid process complicating a procedure

     Excludes1   intraoperative hemorrhage and hematoma of ear and mastoid process due to accidental puncture or laceration during a procedure (H95.3-)

     H95.21   Intraoperative hemorrhage and hematoma of ear and mastoid process complicating a procedure on the ear and mastoid process

     H95.22   Intraoperative hemorrhage and hematoma of ear and mastoid process complicating other procedure

● H95.3   Accidental puncture and laceration of ear and mastoid process during a procedure

     H95.31   Accidental puncture and laceration of the ear and mastoid process during a procedure on the ear and mastoid process

     H95.32   Accidental puncture and laceration of the ear and mastoid process during other procedure

● H95.4   Postprocedural hemorrhage of ear and mastoid process following a procedure

     H95.41   Postprocedural hemorrhage of ear and mastoid process following a procedure on the ear and mastoid process

     H95.42   Postprocedural hemorrhage of ear and mastoid process following other procedure

● H95.5   Postprocedural hematoma and seroma of ear and mastoid process following a procedure

     H95.51   Postprocedural hematoma of ear and mastoid process following a procedure on the ear and mastoid process

     H95.52   Postprocedural hematoma of ear and mastoid process following other procedure

     H95.53   Postprocedural seroma of ear and mastoid process following a procedure on the ear and mastoid process

     H95.54   Postprocedural seroma of ear and mastoid process following other procedure

● H95.8   Other intraoperative and postprocedural complications and disorders of the ear and mastoid process, not elsewhere classified

     Excludes2   postprocedural complications and disorders following mastoidectomy (H95.Ø-, H95.1-)

● H95.81   Postprocedural stenosis of external ear canal

     H95.811   Postprocedural stenosis of right external ear canal

     H95.812   Postprocedural stenosis of left external ear canal

     H95.813   Postprocedural stenosis of external ear canal, bilateral

     H95.819   Postprocedural stenosis of unspecified external ear canal

     H95.88   Other intraoperative complications and disorders of the ear and mastoid process, not elsewhere classified

         Use additional code, if applicable, to further specify disorder

     H95.89   Other postprocedural complications and disorders of the ear and mastoid process, not elsewhere classified

         Use additional code, if applicable, to further specify disorder

CHAPTER 9

DISEASES OF THE CIRCULATORY SYSTEM (I00-I99)

OGCR Chapter-Specific Coding Guidelines

9. **Chapter 9: Diseases of the Circulatory System (I00-I99)**

a. **Hypertension**

The classification presumes a causal relationship between hypertension and heart involvement and between hypertension and kidney involvement, as the two conditions are linked by the term "with" in the Alphabetic Index. These conditions should be coded as related even in the absence of provider documentation explicitly linking them, unless the documentation clearly states the conditions are unrelated.

For hypertension and conditions not specifically linked by relational terms such as "with," "associated with" or "due to" in the classification, provider documentation must link the conditions in order to code them as related.

1) **Hypertension with Heart Disease**

Hypertension with heart conditions classified to I50.- or I51.4-I51.7, I51.89, I51.9, are assigned to, a code from category I11, Hypertensive heart disease. Use additional code(s) from category I50, Heart failure, to identify the type(s) of heart failure in those patients with heart failure.

The same heart conditions (I50.-, I51.4-I51.7, I51.89, I51.9) with hypertension, are coded separately if the provider has documented they are unrelated to the hypertension. Sequence according to the circumstances of the admission/encounter.

2) **Hypertensive Chronic Kidney Disease**

Assign codes from category I12, Hypertensive chronic kidney disease, when both hypertension and a condition classifiable to category N18, Chronic kidney disease (CKD), are present. CKD should not be coded as hypertension if the provider indicates the CKD is not related to the hypertension.

The appropriate code from category N18 should be used as a secondary code with a code from category I12 to identify the stage of chronic kidney disease.

See Section I.C.14. Chronic kidney disease.

If a patient has hypertensive chronic kidney disease and acute renal failure, an additional code for the acute renal failure is required.

3) **Hypertensive Heart and Chronic Kidney Disease**

Assign codes from combination category I13, Hypertensive heart and chronic kidney disease, when there is hypertension with both heart and kidney involvement. If heart failure is present, assign an additional code from category I50 to identify the type of heart failure.

The appropriate code from category N18, Chronic kidney disease, should be used as a secondary code with a code from category I13 to identify the stage of chronic kidney disease.

See Section I.C.14. Chronic kidney disease.

The codes in category I13, Hypertensive heart and chronic kidney disease, are combination codes that include hypertension, heart disease and chronic kidney disease. The Includes note at I13 specifies that the conditions included at I11 and I12 are included together in I13. If a patient has hypertension, heart disease and chronic kidney disease then a code from I13 should be used, not individual codes for hypertension, heart disease and chronic kidney disease, or codes from I11 or I12.

For patients with both acute renal failure and chronic kidney disease an additional code for acute renal failure is required.

4) **Hypertensive Cerebrovascular Disease**

For hypertensive cerebrovascular disease, first assign the appropriate code from categories I60-I69, followed by the appropriate hypertension code.

5) **Hypertensive Retinopathy**

Subcategory H35.0, Background retinopathy and retinal vascular changes, should be used with a code from category I10 – I15, Hypertensive disease to include the systemic hypertension. The sequencing is based on the reason for the encounter.

6) **Hypertension, Secondary**

Secondary hypertension is due to an underlying condition. Two codes are required: one to identify the underlying etiology and one from category I15 to identify the hypertension. Sequencing of codes is determined by the reason for admission/encounter.

7) **Hypertension, Transient**

Assign code R03.0, Elevated blood pressure reading without diagnosis of hypertension, unless patient has an established diagnosis of hypertension. Assign code O13.-, Gestational [pregnancy-induced] hypertension without significant proteinuria, or O14.-, Pre-eclampsia, for transient hypertension of pregnancy.

8) **Hypertension, Controlled**

This diagnostic statement usually refers to an existing state of hypertension under control by therapy. Assign the appropriate code from categories I10-I15, Hypertensive diseases.

9) **Hypertension, Uncontrolled**

Uncontrolled hypertension may refer to untreated hypertension or hypertension not responding to current therapeutic regimen. In either case, assign the appropriate code from categories I10-I15, Hypertensive diseases.

10) **Hypertensive Crisis**

Assign a code from category I16, Hypertensive crisis, for documented hypertensive urgency, hypertensive emergency or unspecified hypertensive crisis. Code also any identified hypertensive disease (I10-I15). The sequencing is based on the reason for the encounter.

11) **Pulmonary Hypertension**

Pulmonary hypertension is classified to category I27, Other pulmonary heart diseases. For secondary pulmonary hypertension (I27.1, I27.2-), code also any associated conditions or adverse effects of drugs or toxins. The sequencing is based on the reason for the encounter, except for adverse effects of drugs.

See Section I.C.19.e Adverse Effects, Poisoning, Underdosing and Toxic Effects.

b. **Atherosclerotic Coronary Artery Disease and Angina**

ICD-10-CM has combination codes for atherosclerotic heart disease with angina pectoris. The subcategories for these codes are I25.11, Atherosclerotic heart disease of native coronary artery with angina pectoris and I25.7, Atherosclerosis of coronary artery bypass graft(s) and coronary artery of transplanted heart with angina pectoris.

When using one of these combination codes it is not necessary to use an additional code for angina pectoris. A causal relationship can be assumed in a patient with both atherosclerosis and angina pectoris, unless the documentation indicates the angina is due to something other than the atherosclerosis.

If a patient with coronary artery disease is admitted due to an acute myocardial infarction (AMI), the AMI should be sequenced before the coronary artery disease.

See Section I.C.9. Acute myocardial infarction (AMI).

c. **Intraoperative and Postprocedural Cerebrovascular Accident**

Medical record documentation should clearly specify the cause-and-effect relationship between the medical intervention and the cerebrovascular accident in order to assign a code for intraoperative or postprocedural cerebrovascular accident.

Proper code assignment depends on whether it was an infarction or hemorrhage and whether it occurred intraoperatively or postoperatively. If it was a cerebral hemorrhage, code assignment depends on the type of procedure performed.

d. **Sequelae of Cerebrovascular Disease**

1) **Category I69, Sequelae of Cerebrovascular disease**

Category I69 is used to indicate conditions classifiable to categories I60-I67 as the causes of sequela (neurologic deficits), themselves classified elsewhere. These "late effects" include neurologic deficits that persist after initial onset of conditions classifiable to categories I60-I67. The neurologic deficits caused by cerebrovascular disease may be present from the onset or may arise at any time after the onset of the condition classifiable to categories I60-I67.

Codes from category I69, Sequelae of cerebrovascular disease, that specify hemiplegia, hemiparesis and monoplegia identify whether the dominant or nondominant side is affected. Should the affected side be documented, but not specified as dominant or nondominant, and the classification system does not indicate a default, code selection is as follows:

- For ambidextrous patients, the default should be dominant.
- If the left side is affected, the default is nondominant.
- If the right side is affected, the default is dominant.

2) **Codes from category I69 with codes from I60-I67**

Codes from category I69 may be assigned on a health care record with codes from I60-I67, if the patient has a current cerebrovascular disease and deficits from an old cerebrovascular disease.

    3)   Codes from category I69 and Personal history of transient ischemic attack (TIA) and cerebral infarction (Z86.73)

Codes from category I69 should not be assigned if the patient does not have neurologic deficits.

    See Section I.C.21. 4. History (of) for use of personal history codes.

  e. **Acute myocardial infarction (AMI)**

    1) **Type 1 ST elevation myocardial infarction (STEMI) and non-ST elevation myocardial infarction (NSTEMI)**

The ICD-10-CM codes for acute type 1 myocardial infarction (AMI) identify the site, such as anterolateral wall or true posterior wall. Subcategories I21.0-I21.2 and code I21.3 are used for type 1 ST elevation myocardial infarction (STEMI). Code I21.4, non-ST elevation (NSTEMI) myocardial infarction, is used for type 1 non-ST elevation myocardial infarction (NSTEMI) and nontransmural MIs.

    If a type 1 NSTEMI evolves to STEMI, assign the STEMI code. If a type 1 STEMI converts to NSTEMI due to thrombolytic therapy, it is still coded as STEMI.

    For encounters occurring while the myocardial infarction is equal to, or less than, four weeks old, including transfers to another acute setting or a postacute setting, and the myocardial infarction meets the definition for "other diagnoses" (see Section III, Reporting Additional Diagnoses), codes from category I21 may continue to be reported. For encounters after the 4-week time frame and the patient is still receiving care related to the myocardial infarction, the appropriate aftercare code should be assigned, rather than a code from category I21. For old or healed myocardial infarctions not requiring further care, code I25.2, Old myocardial infarction, may be assigned.

    2) **Acute myocardial infarction, unspecified**

Code I21.9, Acute myocardial infarction, unspecified, is the default for unspecified acute myocardial infarction or unspecified type. If only type 1 STEMI or transmural MI without the site is documented, assign code I21.3, ST elevation (STEMI) myocardial infarction of unspecified site.

    3) **AMI documented as nontransmural or subendocardial but site provided**

If an AMI is documented as nontransmural or subendocardial, but the site is provided, it is still coded as a subendocardial AMI.

    See Section I.C.21.3 for information on coding status post administration of tPA in a different facility within the last 24 hours.

    4) **Subsequent acute myocardial infarction**

A code from category I22, Subsequent ST elevation (STEMI) and non-ST elevation (NSTEMI) myocardial infarction, is to be used when a patient who has suffered a type 1 or unspecified AMI has a new AMI within the 4-week time frame of the initial AMI. A code from category I22 must be used in conjunction with a code from category I21. The sequencing of the I22 and I21 codes depends on the circumstances of the encounter.

    Do not assign code I22 for subsequent myocardial infarctions other than type 1 or unspecified. For subsequent type 2 AMI assign only code I21.A1. For subsequent type 4 or type 5 AMI, assign only code I21.A9.

    If a subsequent myocardial infarction of one type occurs within 4 weeks of a myocardial infarction of a different type, assign the appropriate codes from category I21 to identify each type. Do not assign a code from I22. Codes from category I22 should only be assigned if both the initial and subsequent myocardial infarctions are type 1 or unspecified.

    5) **Other Types of Myocardial Infarction**

The ICD-10-CM provides codes for different types of myocardial infarction. Type 1 myocardial infarctions are assigned to codes I21.0-I21.4 and I21.9.

    Type 2 myocardial infarction, and myocardial infarction due to demand ischemia or secondary to ischemic balance, is assigned to code I21.A1, Myocardial infarction type 2 with a code for the underlying cause. Do not assign code I24.8, Other forms of acute ischemic heart disease for the demand ischemia. Sequencing of type 2 AMI or the underlying cause is dependent on the circumstances of admission. When a type 2 AMI code is described as NSTEMI or STEMI, only assign code I21.A1. Codes I21.01-I21.4 should only be assigned for type 1 AMIs.

    Acute myocardial infarctions type 3, 4a, 4b, 4c, and 5 are assigned to code I21.A9, Other myocardial infarction type.

    The "Code also" and "Code first" notes should be followed related to complications, and for coding of postprocedural myocardial infarctions during or following cardiac surgery.

Figure 9-1   Cardiovascular valves.

Item 9–1 Rheumatic fever is the inflammation of the valve(s) of the heart, usually the mitral or aortic, which leads to valve damage. Rheumatic heart inflammations are usually **pericarditis** (sac surrounding heart), **endocarditis** (heart cavity), or **myocarditis** (heart muscle).

CHAPTER 9

DISEASES OF THE CIRCULATORY SYSTEM
(I00-I99)

  Excludes2   certain conditions originating in the perinatal period (P04-P96)

    certain infectious and parasitic diseases (A00-B99)

    complications of pregnancy, childbirth and the puerperium (O00-O9A)

    congenital malformations, deformations, and chromosomal abnormalities (Q00-Q99)

    endocrine, nutritional and metabolic diseases (E00-E88)

    injury, poisoning and certain other consequences of external causes (S00-T88)

    neoplasms (C00-D49)

    symptoms, signs and abnormal clinical and laboratory findings, not elsewhere classified (R00-R94)

    systemic connective tissue disorders (M30-M36)

    transient cerebral ischemic attacks and related syndromes (G45.-)

This chapter contains the following blocks:

I00-I02	Acute rheumatic fever
I05-I09	Chronic rheumatic heart diseases
I10-I16	Hypertensive diseases
I20-I25	Ischemic heart diseases
I26-I28	Pulmonary heart disease and diseases of pulmonary circulation
I30-I5A	Other forms of heart disease
I60-I69	Cerebrovascular diseases
I70-I79	Diseases of arteries, arterioles and capillaries
I80-I89	Diseases of veins, lymphatic vessels and lymph nodes, not elsewhere classified
I95-I99	Other and unspecified disorders of the circulatory system

---

ACUTE RHEUMATIC FEVER (I00-I02)

I00   **Rheumatic fever without heart involvement**

    Includes   arthritis, rheumatic, acute or subacute

    Excludes1   rheumatic fever with heart involvement (I01.0-I01.9)

● **I01**   **Rheumatic fever with heart involvement**

    Excludes1   chronic diseases of rheumatic origin (I05-I09) unless rheumatic fever is also present or there is evidence of reactivation or activity of the rheumatic process.

  I01.0   **Acute rheumatic pericarditis**

    Any condition in I00 with pericarditis

    Rheumatic pericarditis (acute)

    Excludes1   acute pericarditis not specified as rheumatic (I30.-)

  I01.1   **Acute rheumatic endocarditis**

    Any condition in I00 with endocarditis or valvulitis

    Acute rheumatic valvulitis

▶ New   ⇒ Revised   ~~deleted~~ Deleted   Excludes 1   Excludes 2   Includes   Use additional   Code first   Code also   Key words

OGCR Official Guidelines   X Assign placeholder X   ● Use Additional Character(s)   ▶ Manifestation Code   🔖 Hierarchical Condition Category   **Coding Clinic**

Item 9–2 Rheumatic chorea, also called Sydenham's, juvenile, minor, simple, or St. Vitus' dance, is a major symptom of rheumatic fever and is characterized by ceaseless, involuntary, jerky, purposeless movements.

I01.2 Acute rheumatic myocarditis
Any condition in I00 with myocarditis

I01.8 Other acute rheumatic heart disease
Any condition in I00 with other or multiple types of heart involvement
Acute rheumatic pancarditis

I01.9 Acute rheumatic heart disease, unspecified
Any condition in I00 with unspecified type of heart involvement
Rheumatic carditis, acute
Rheumatic heart disease, active or acute

● **I02 Rheumatic chorea**
Includes Sydenham's chorea
Excludes1 chorea NOS (G25.5)
Huntington's chorea (G10)

I02.0 Rheumatic chorea with heart involvement
Chorea NOS with heart involvement
Rheumatic chorea with heart involvement of any type classifiable under I01.-

I02.9 Rheumatic chorea without heart involvement
Rheumatic chorea NOS

CHRONIC RHEUMATIC HEART DISEASES (I05-I09)

● **I05 Rheumatic mitral valve diseases**
Includes conditions classifiable to both I05.0 and I05.2-I05.9, whether specified as rheumatic or not
Excludes1 mitral valve disease specified as nonrheumatic (I34.-)
mitral valve disease with aortic and/or tricuspid valve involvement (I08.-)

I05.0 Rheumatic mitral stenosis
Mitral (valve) obstruction (rheumatic)

I05.1 Rheumatic mitral insufficiency
Rheumatic mitral incompetence
Rheumatic mitral regurgitation
Excludes1 mitral insufficiency not specified as rheumatic (I34.0)

I05.2 Rheumatic mitral stenosis with insufficiency
Rheumatic mitral stenosis with incompetence or regurgitation

I05.8 Other rheumatic mitral valve diseases
Rheumatic mitral (valve) failure

I05.9 Rheumatic mitral valve disease, unspecified
Rheumatic mitral (valve) disorder (chronic) NOS

● **I06 Rheumatic aortic valve diseases**
Excludes1 aortic valve disease not specified as rheumatic (I35.-)
aortic valve disease with mitral and/or tricuspid valve involvement (I08.-)

I06.0 Rheumatic aortic stenosis
Rheumatic aortic (valve) obstruction

I06.1 Rheumatic aortic insufficiency
Rheumatic aortic incompetence
Rheumatic aortic regurgitation

I06.2 Rheumatic aortic stenosis with insufficiency
Rheumatic aortic stenosis with incompetence or regurgitation

★ **(See Plate 33 of the Anatomy Illustrations.)**

Item 9–3 Mitral stenosis is the narrowing of the mitral valve separating the left atrium from the left ventricle. **Mitral insufficiency** is the improper closure of the mitral valve, which may lead to enlargement (hypertrophy) of the left atrium.

Item 9–4 Aortic stenosis is the narrowing of the aortic valve located between the left ventricle and the aorta. **Aortic insufficiency** is the improper closure of the aortic valve, which may lead to enlargement (hypertrophy) of the left ventricle.

I06.8 Other rheumatic aortic valve diseases

I06.9 Rheumatic aortic valve disease, unspecified
Rheumatic aortic (valve) disease NOS

● **I07 Rheumatic tricuspid valve diseases**
Includes rheumatic tricuspid valve diseases specified as rheumatic or unspecified
Excludes1 tricuspid valve disease specified as nonrheumatic (I36.-)
tricuspid valve disease with aortic and/or mitral valve involvement (I08.-)

I07.0 Rheumatic tricuspid stenosis
Tricuspid (valve) stenosis (rheumatic)

I07.1 Rheumatic tricuspid insufficiency
Tricuspid (valve) insufficiency (rheumatic)

I07.2 Rheumatic tricuspid stenosis and insufficiency

I07.8 Other rheumatic tricuspid valve diseases

I07.9 Rheumatic tricuspid valve disease, unspecified
Rheumatic tricuspid valve disorder NOS

● **I08 Multiple valve diseases**
Includes multiple valve diseases specified as rheumatic or unspecified
Excludes1 endocarditis, valve unspecified (I38)
multiple valve disease specified as nonrheumatic (I34.-, I35.-, I36.-, I37.-, I38.-, Q22.-, Q23.-, Q24.8-)
rheumatic valve disease NOS (I09.1)
Coding Clinic: 2019, Q2, P5

I08.0 Rheumatic disorders of both mitral and aortic valves
Involvement of both mitral and aortic valves specified as rheumatic or unspecified
Coding Clinic: 2019, Q2, P5

I08.1 Rheumatic disorders of both mitral and tricuspid valves

I08.2 Rheumatic disorders of both aortic and tricuspid valves

I08.3 Combined rheumatic disorders of mitral, aortic and tricuspid valves

I08.8 Other rheumatic multiple valve diseases

I08.9 Rheumatic multiple valve disease, unspecified

● **I09 Other rheumatic heart diseases**
I09.0 Rheumatic myocarditis
Excludes1 myocarditis not specified as rheumatic (I51.4)

I09.1 Rheumatic diseases of endocardium, valve unspecified
Rheumatic endocarditis (chronic)
Rheumatic valvulitis (chronic)
Excludes1 endocarditis, valve unspecified (I38)

I09.2 Chronic rheumatic pericarditis
Adherent pericardium, rheumatic
Chronic rheumatic mediastinopericarditis
Chronic rheumatic myopericarditis
Excludes1 chronic pericarditis not specified as rheumatic (I31.-)

● **I09.8 Other specified rheumatic heart diseases**
I09.81 Rheumatic heart failure 🔗
Use additional code to identify type of heart failure (I50.-)

I09.89 Other specified rheumatic heart diseases
Rheumatic disease of pulmonary valve

I09.9 Rheumatic heart disease, unspecified
Rheumatic carditis
Excludes1 rheumatoid carditis (M05.31)

CHAPTER 9 (I00-I99)

Item 9–5 Hypertension is caused by high arterial blood pressure in the arteries. **Essential, primary,** or **idiopathic** hypertension occurs without identifiable organic cause. **Secondary** hypertension is that which has an organic cause. **Malignant** hypertension is severely elevated blood pressure. **Benign** hypertension is mildly elevated blood pressure.

HYPERTENSIVE DISEASES (I10-I16)

Use additional code to identify:
    exposure to environmental tobacco smoke (Z77.22)
    history of tobacco dependence (Z87.891)
    occupational exposure to environmental tobacco smoke (Z57.31)
    tobacco dependence (F17.-)
    tobacco use (Z72.0)

Excludes1   neonatal hypertension (P29.2)
           primary pulmonary hypertension (I27.0)

Excludes2   hypertensive disease complicating pregnancy, childbirth and the puerperium (O10-O11, O13-O16)

I10   **Essential (primary) hypertension**
     Includes   high blood pressure
              hypertension (arterial) (benign) (essential) (malignant) (primary) (systemic)

     Excludes1   hypertensive disease complicating pregnancy, childbirth and the puerperium (O10-O11, O13-O16)

     Excludes2   essential (primary) hypertension involving vessels of brain (I60-I69)
              essential (primary) hypertension involving vessels of eye (H35.0-)

● **I11**   **Hypertensive heart disease**
     Includes   any condition in I50.- or I51.4-I51.7, I51.89, I51.9 due to hypertension

   I11.0   **Hypertensive heart disease with heart failure** 🦠
        Hypertensive heart failure
        Use additional code to identify type of heart failure (I50.-)
        Coding Clinic: 2017, Q1, P47

   I11.9   **Hypertensive heart disease without heart failure**
        Hypertensive heart disease NOS

OGCR Section I.C.9.a.2.

Hypertensive Chronic Kidney Disease

Assign codes from category I12, Hypertensive chronic kidney disease, when both hypertension and a condition classifiable to category N18, Chronic kidney disease (CKD), are present. **CKD should not be coded as hypertensive if the physician has specifically documented a different cause.**

The appropriate code from category N18 should be used as a secondary code with a code from category I12 to identify the stage of chronic kidney disease.
See Section I.C.14. Chronic kidney disease.

If a patient has hypertensive chronic kidney disease and acute renal failure, an additional code for the acute renal failure is required.

● **I12**   **Hypertensive chronic kidney disease**
     Includes   any condition in N18 and N26 - due to hypertension
              arteriosclerosis of kidney
              arteriosclerotic nephritis (chronic) (interstitial)
              hypertensive nephropathy
              nephrosclerosis

     Excludes1   hypertension due to kidney disease (I15.0, I15.1)
              renovascular hypertension (I15.0)
              secondary hypertension (I15.-)

     Excludes2   acute kidney failure (N17.-)

     Coding Clinic: 2018, Q4, P89; 2016, Q4, P123

   I12.0   **Hypertensive chronic kidney disease with stage 5 chronic kidney disease or end stage renal disease** 🦠
        Use additional code to identify the stage of chronic kidney disease (N18.5, N18.6)
        Coding Clinic: 2016, Q3, P23

   I12.9   **Hypertensive chronic kidney disease with stage 1 through stage 4 chronic kidney disease, or unspecified chronic kidney disease**
        Hypertensive chronic kidney disease NOS
        Hypertensive renal disease NOS
        Use additional code to identify the stage of chronic kidney disease (N18.1-N18.4, N18.9)
        Coding Clinic: 2018, Q4, P88

OGCR Section I.c.9.a.3.

Hypertensive Heart and Chronic Kidney Disease

Assign codes from combination category I13, Hypertensive heart and chronic kidney disease, when **there is hypertension with both heart and kidney involvement.** If heart failure is present, assign an additional code from category I50 to identify the type of heart failure.

The appropriate code from category N18, Chronic kidney disease, should be used as a secondary code with a code from category I13 to identify the stage of chronic kidney disease.
See Section I.C.14. Chronic kidney disease.

The codes in category I13, Hypertensive heart and chronic kidney disease, are combination codes that include hypertension, heart disease and chronic kidney disease. The Includes note at I13 specifies that the conditions included at I11 and I12 are included together in I13. If a patient has hypertension, heart disease and chronic kidney disease then a code from I13 should be used, not individual codes for hypertension, heart disease and chronic kidney disease, or codes from I11 or I12.

For patients with both acute renal failure and chronic kidney disease an additional code for acute renal failure is required.

● **I13**   **Hypertensive heart and chronic kidney disease**
     Includes   any condition in I11.- with any condition in I12.-
              cardiorenal disease
              cardiovascular renal disease
     Coding Clinic: 2016, Q4, P123

   I13.0   **Hypertensive heart and chronic kidney disease with heart failure and stage 1 through stage 4 chronic kidney disease, or unspecified chronic kidney disease** 🦠
        Use additional code to identify type of heart failure (I50.-)
        Use additional code to identify stage of chronic kidney disease (N18.1-N18.4, N18.9)

● **I13.1**   **Hypertensive heart and chronic kidney disease without heart failure**

     I13.10   **Hypertensive heart and chronic kidney disease without heart failure, with stage 1 through stage 4 chronic kidney disease, or unspecified chronic kidney disease**
         Hypertensive heart disease and hypertensive chronic kidney disease NOS
         Use additional code to identify the stage of chronic kidney disease (N18.1-N18.4, N18.9)

     I13.11   **Hypertensive heart and chronic kidney disease without heart failure, with stage 5 chronic kidney disease, or end stage renal disease** 🦠
         Use additional code to identify the stage of chronic kidney disease (N18.5, N18.6)

   I13.2   **Hypertensive heart and chronic kidney disease with heart failure and with stage 5 chronic kidney disease, or end stage renal disease** 🦠
        Use additional code to identify type of heart failure (I50.-)
        Use additional code to identify the stage of chronic kidney disease (N18.5, N18.6)

▶ New   ⇨ Revised   ~~deleted~~ Deleted   Excludes 1   Excludes 2   Includes   Use additional   Code first   Code also   Key words

OGCR Official Guidelines   X Assign placeholder X   ● Use Additional Character(s)   ▷ Manifestation Code   🦠 Hierarchical Condition Category   **Coding Clinic**

OGCR Section I.9.a.6.

Hypertension, Secondary
Secondary hypertension is due to an underlying condition. Two codes are required: one to identify the underlying etiology and one from category I15 to identify the hypertension. Sequencing of codes is determined by the reason for admission/encounter.

● **I15**   **Secondary hypertension**
    Code also underlying condition
    Excludes1   postprocedural hypertension (I97.3)
    Excludes2   secondary hypertension involving vessels of
           · brain (I60-I69)
           secondary hypertension involving vessels of eye
             (H35.0-)

   I15.0   **Renovascular hypertension**

   I15.1   **Hypertension secondary to other renal disorders**
         Coding Clinic: 2016, Q3, P23

   I15.2   **Hypertension secondary to endocrine disorders**

   I15.8   **Other secondary hypertension**

   I15.9   **Secondary hypertension, unspecified**

● **I16**   **Hypertensive crisis**
    Code also any identified hypertensive disease (I10-I15)
    Coding Clinic: 2016, Q4, P26-27, 123

   I16.0   **Hypertensive urgency**

   I16.1   **Hypertensive emergency**

   I16.9   **Hypertensive crisis, unspecified**

ISCHEMIC HEART DISEASES (I20-I25)

~~Use additional code to identify presence of hypertension (I10-I16)~~

▶ Code also the presence of hypertension (I10-I16)

● **I20**   **Angina pectoris**
    Chest pain/discomfort due to lack of oxygen to the heart muscle.
    Principal symptom of myocardial infarction.
    Use additional code to identify:
      exposure to environmental tobacco smoke (Z77.22)
      history of tobacco dependence (Z87.891)
      occupational exposure to environmental tobacco smoke
        (Z57.31)
      tobacco dependence (F17.-)
      tobacco use (Z72.0)
    Excludes1   angina pectoris with atherosclerotic heart disease
          of native coronary arteries (I25.1-)
          atherosclerosis of coronary artery bypass graft(s)
            and coronary artery of transplanted heart
            with angina pectoris (I25.7-)
          postinfarction angina (I23.7)

   I20.0   **Unstable angina** 🔗
      Accelerated angina
      Crescendo angina
      De novo effort angina
      Intermediate coronary syndrome
      Preinfarction syndrome
      Worsening effort angina

   I20.1   **Angina pectoris with documented spasm** 🔗
      Angiospastic angina
      Prinzmetal angina
      Spasm-induced angina
      Variant angina

   I20.8   **Other forms of angina pectoris** 🔗
      Angina equivalent
      Angina of effort
      Coronary slow flow syndrome
      Stable angina
      Stenocardia
      Use additional code(s) for symptoms associated with
        angina equivalent

   I20.9   **Angina pectoris, unspecified** 🔗
      Angina NOS
      Anginal syndrome
      Cardiac angina
      Ischemic chest pain

● **I21**   **Acute myocardial infarction**
    Includes   cardiac infarction
           coronary (artery) embolism
           coronary (artery) occlusion
           coronary (artery) rupture
           coronary (artery) thrombosis
           infarction of heart, myocardium, or ventricle
           myocardial infarction specified as acute or with a
             stated duration of 4 weeks (28 days) or less
             from onset
    Use additional code, if applicable, to identify:
      exposure to environmental tobacco smoke (Z77.22)
      history of tobacco dependence (Z87.891)
      occupational exposure to environmental tobacco smoke
        (Z57.31)
      status post administration of tPA (rtPA) in a different facility
        within the last 24 hours prior to admission to current
        facility (Z92.82)
      tobacco dependence (F17.-)
      tobacco use (Z72.0)
    Excludes2   old myocardial infarction (I25.2)
          postmyocardial infarction syndrome (I24.1)
          subsequent type 1 myocardial infarction (I22.-)
    Coding Clinic: 2016, Q4, P140; 2013, Q1, P25-26; 2012, Q4, P103

   ● **I21.0**   **ST elevation (STEMI) myocardial infarction of anterior
        wall**
        Type 1 ST elevation myocardial infarction of anterior
          wall
        Coding Clinic: 2013, Q1, P26

     I21.01   **ST elevation (STEMI) myocardial infarction
          involving left main coronary artery** 🔗

     I21.02   **ST elevation (STEMI) myocardial infarction
          involving left anterior descending coronary
          artery** 🔗
            ST elevation (STEMI) myocardial infarction
              involving diagonal coronary artery
          Coding Clinic: 2013, Q1, P26

     I21.09   **ST elevation (STEMI) myocardial infarction
          involving other coronary artery of anterior
          wall** 🔗
            Acute transmural myocardial infarction of
              anterior wall
            Anteroapical transmural (Q wave) infarction
              (acute)
            Anterolateral transmural (Q wave) infarction
              (acute)
            Anteroseptal transmural (Q wave) infarction
              (acute)
            Transmural (Q wave) infarction (acute) (of)
              anterior (wall) NOS
          Coding Clinic: 2012, Q4, P102, 104

   ● **I21.1**   **ST elevation (STEMI) myocardial infarction of inferior
        wall**
        Type 1 ST elevation myocardial infarction of inferior
          wall
        Coding Clinic: 2013, Q1, P26

     I21.11   **ST elevation (STEMI) myocardial infarction
          involving right coronary artery** 🔗
            Inferoposterior transmural (Q wave) infarction
              (acute)

     I21.19   **ST elevation (STEMI) myocardial infarction
          involving other coronary artery of inferior
          wall** 🔗
            Acute transmural myocardial infarction of
              inferior wall
            Inferolateral transmural (Q wave) infarction
              (acute)
            Transmural (Q wave) infarction (acute) (of)
              diaphragmatic wall
            Transmural (Q wave) infarction (acute) (of)
              inferior (wall) NOS
        Excludes2   ST elevation (STEMI)
              myocardial infarction involving
              left circumflex coronary
              artery (I21.21)

        Coding Clinic: 2012, Q4, P97

CHAPTER 9 (I00-I99)

● **I21.2   ST elevation (STEMI) myocardial infarction of other sites**
  Type 1 ST elevation myocardial infarction of other sites
  Coding Clinic: 2013, Q1, P26

  I21.21   ST elevation (STEMI) myocardial infarction involving left circumflex coronary artery 🅗
    ST elevation (STEMI) myocardial infarction involving oblique marginal coronary artery

  I21.29   ST elevation (STEMI) myocardial infarction involving other sites 🅗
    Acute transmural myocardial infarction of other sites
    Apical-lateral transmural (Q wave) infarction (acute)
    Basal-lateral transmural (Q wave) infarction (acute)
    High lateral transmural (Q wave) infarction (acute)
    Lateral (wall) NOS transmural (Q wave) infarction (acute)
    Posterior (true) transmural (Q wave) infarction (acute)
    Posterobasal transmural (Q wave) infarction (acute)
    Posterolateral transmural (Q wave) infarction (acute)
    Posteroseptal transmural (Q wave) infarction (acute)
    Septal transmural (Q wave) infarction (acute) NOS

OGCR Section I.c.9.e.2.

Acute myocardial infarction, unspecified
Code I21.9, Acute myocardial infarction, unspecified, is the default for unspecified acute myocardial infarction or unspecified type. If only type 1 STEMI or transmural MI without the site is documented, assign I21.3, ST elevation (STEMI) myocardial infarction of unspecified site.

I21.3   ST elevation (STEMI) myocardial infarction of unspecified site 🅗
  Acute transmural myocardial infarction of unspecified site
  Transmural (Q wave) myocardial infarction NOS
  Type 1 ST elevation myocardial infarction of unspecified site
  Coding Clinic: 2013, Q1, P26

I21.4   Non-ST elevation (NSTEMI) myocardial infarction 🅗
  Acute subendocardial myocardial infarction
  Non-Q wave myocardial infarction NOS
  Nontransmural myocardial infarction NOS
  Type 1 non-ST elevation myocardial infarction
  Coding Clinic: 2017, Q1, P44; 2015, Q2, P16; 2013, Q1, P26

I21.9   Acute myocardial infarction, unspecified 🅗
  Myocardial infarction (acute) NOS

● **I21.A   Other type of myocardial infarction**

  I21.A1   Myocardial infarction type 2 🅗
    Myocardial infarction due to demand ischemia
    Myocardial infarction secondary to ischemic imbalance
    Code first the underlying cause, such as:
    anemia (D50.0-D64.9)
    chronic obstructive pulmonary disease (J44.-)
    paroxysmal tachycardia (I47.0-I47.9)
    shock (R57.0-R57.9)
    Coding Clinic: 2017, Q4, P13-14

  I21.A9   Other myocardial infarction type 🅗
    Myocardial infarction associated with revascularization procedure
    Myocardial infarction type 3
    Myocardial infarction type 4a
    Myocardial infarction type 4b
    Myocardial infarction type 4c
    Myocardial infarction type 5

    Code first, if applicable, postprocedural myocardial infarction following cardiac surgery (I97.190), or postprocedural myocardial infarction during cardiac surgery (I97.790)
    Code also complication, if known and applicable, such as:
    (acute) stent occlusion (T82.897-)
    (acute) stent stenosis (T82.857-)
    (acute) stent thrombosis (T82.865-)
    cardiac arrest due to underlying cardiac condition (I46.2)
    complication of percutaneous coronary intervention (PCI) (I97.89)
    occlusion of coronary artery bypass graft (T82.218-)
    Coding Clinic: 2019, Q2, P32-33

● **I22   Subsequent ST elevation (STEMI) and non-ST elevation (NSTEMI) myocardial infarction**

  Includes   acute myocardial infarction occurring within four weeks (28 days) of a previous acute myocardial infarction, regardless of site
    cardiac infarction
    coronary (artery) embolism
    coronary (artery) occlusion
    coronary (artery) rupture
    coronary (artery) thrombosis
    infarction of heart, myocardium, or ventricle
    recurrent myocardial infarction
    reinfarction of myocardium
    rupture of heart, myocardium, or ventricle
    subsequent type 1 myocardial infarction

  Excludes1   subsequent myocardial infarction, type 2 (I21.A1)
    subsequent myocardial infarction of other type (type 3) (type 4) (type 5) (I21.A9)

  Use additional code, if applicable, to identify:
    exposure to environmental tobacco smoke (Z77.22)
    history of tobacco dependence (Z87.891)
    occupational exposure to environmental tobacco smoke (Z57.31)
    status post administration of tPA (rtPA) in a different facility within the last 24 hours prior to admission to current facility (Z92.82)
    tobacco dependence (F17.-)
    tobacco use (Z72.0)
    Coding Clinic: 2017, Q4, P14; 2013, Q1, P25; 2012, Q4, P103

  I22.0   Subsequent ST elevation (STEMI) myocardial infarction of anterior wall 🅗
    Subsequent acute transmural myocardial infarction of anterior wall
    Subsequent transmural (Q wave) infarction (acute)(of) anterior (wall) NOS
    Subsequent anteroapical transmural (Q wave) infarction (acute)
    Subsequent anterolateral transmural (Q wave) infarction (acute)
    Subsequent anteroseptal transmural (Q wave) infarction (acute)

  I22.1   Subsequent ST elevation (STEMI) myocardial infarction of inferior wall 🅗
    Subsequent acute transmural myocardial infarction of inferior wall
    Subsequent transmural (Q wave) infarction (acute)(of) diaphragmatic wall
    Subsequent transmural (Q wave) infarction (acute)(of) inferior (wall) NOS
    Subsequent inferolateral transmural (Q wave) infarction (acute)
    Subsequent inferoposterior transmural (Q wave) infarction (acute)
    Coding Clinic: 2012, Q4, P97, 102, 104

▶ New   ⮞ Revised   ~~deleted~~ Deleted   Excludes 1   Excludes 2   Includes   Use additional   Code first   Code also   Key words
OGCR Official Guidelines   X Assign placeholder X   ● Use Additional Character(s)   ▌ Manifestation Code   🅗 Hierarchical Condition Category   **Coding Clinic**

I22.2   **Subsequent non-ST elevation (NSTEMI) myocardial infarction** 🦠
- Subsequent acute subendocardial myocardial infarction
- Subsequent non-Q wave myocardial infarction NOS
- Subsequent nontransmural myocardial infarction NOS

I22.8   **Subsequent ST elevation (STEMI) myocardial infarction of other sites** 🦠
- Subsequent acute transmural myocardial infarction of other sites
- Subsequent apical-lateral transmural (Q wave) myocardial infarction (acute)
- Subsequent basal-lateral transmural (Q wave) myocardial infarction (acute)
- Subsequent high lateral transmural (Q wave) myocardial infarction (acute)
- Subsequent transmural (Q wave) myocardial infarction (acute)(of) lateral (wall) NOS
- Subsequent posterior (true) transmural (Q wave) myocardial infarction (acute)
- Subsequent posterobasal transmural (Q wave) myocardial infarction (acute)
- Subsequent posterolateral transmural (Q wave) myocardial infarction (acute)
- Subsequent posteroseptal transmural (Q wave) myocardial infarction (acute)
- Subsequent septal NOS transmural (Q wave) myocardial infarction (acute)

I22.9   **Subsequent ST elevation (STEMI) myocardial infarction of unspecified site**
- Subsequent acute myocardial infarction of unspecified site
- Subsequent myocardial infarction (acute) NOS

● **I23**   **Certain current complications following ST elevation (STEMI) and non-ST elevation (NSTEMI) myocardial infarction (within the 28 day period)**
    Coding Clinic: 2017, Q2, P11

I23.0   **Hemopericardium as current complication following acute myocardial infarction** 🦠   A

    Excludes1   hemopericardium not specified as current complication following acute myocardial infarction (I31.2)

I23.1   **Atrial septal defect as current complication following acute myocardial infarction** 🦠   A

    Excludes1   acquired atrial septal defect not specified as current complication following acute myocardial infarction (I51.0)

I23.2   **Ventricular septal defect as current complication following acute myocardial infarction** 🦠   A

    Excludes1   acquired ventricular septal defect not specified as current complication following acute myocardial infarction (I51.0)

I23.3   **Rupture of cardiac wall without hemopericardium as current complication following acute myocardial infarction** 🦠   A
    Coding Clinic: 2017, Q2, P11

I23.4   **Rupture of chordae tendineae as current complication following acute myocardial infarction** 🦠

    Excludes1   rupture of chordae tendineae not specified as current complication following acute myocardial infarction (I51.1)

I23.5   **Rupture of papillary muscle as current complication following acute myocardial infarction** 🦠

    Excludes1   rupture of papillary muscle not specified as current complication following acute myocardial infarction (I51.2)

I23.6   **Thrombosis of atrium, auricular appendage, and ventricle as current complications following acute myocardial infarction** 🦠   A

    Excludes1   thrombosis of atrium, auricular appendage, and ventricle not specified as current complication following acute myocardial infarction (I51.3)

I23.7   **Postinfarction angina** 🦠   A
    Coding Clinic: 2015, Q2, P16-17

I23.8   **Other current complications following acute myocardial infarction** 🦠   A

● **I24**   **Other acute ischemic heart diseases**

    Excludes1   angina pectoris (I20.-)
                  transient myocardial ischemia in newborn (P29.4)

▶   **Excludes2**   non-ischemic myocardial injury (I5A)

I24.0   **Acute coronary thrombosis not resulting in myocardial infarction** 🦠
- Acute coronary (artery) (vein) embolism not resulting in myocardial infarction
- Acute coronary (artery) (vein) occlusion not resulting in myocardial infarction
- Acute coronary (artery) (vein) thromboembolism not resulting in myocardial infarction

    Excludes1   atherosclerotic heart disease (I25.1-)
    Coding Clinic: 2013, Q1, P24

I24.1   **Dressler's syndrome** 🦠
- Postmyocardial infarction syndrome

    Excludes1   postinfarction angina (I23.7)

I24.8   **Other forms of acute ischemic heart disease** 🦠

    Excludes1   myocardial infarction due to demand ischemia (I21.A1)

    Coding Clinic: 2017, Q4, P13

I24.9   **Acute ischemic heart disease, unspecified** 🦠

    Excludes1   ischemic heart disease (chronic) NOS (I25.9)

● **I25**   **Chronic ischemic heart disease**

▶   **Excludes2**   non-ischemic myocardial injury (I5A)

    Use additional code to identify:
- chronic total occlusion of coronary artery (I25.82)
- exposure to environmental tobacco smoke (Z77.22)
- history of tobacco dependence (Z87.891)
- occupational exposure to environmental tobacco smoke (Z57.31)
- tobacco dependence (F17.-)
- tobacco use (Z72.0)

★ **(See Plates 218 and 219 on pages 74 and 75.)**

● **I25.1**   **Atherosclerotic heart disease of native coronary artery**
    Disease in which fatty deposits form on the walls of arteries
- Atherosclerotic cardiovascular disease
- Coronary (artery) atheroma
- Coronary (artery) atherosclerosis
- Coronary (artery) disease
- Coronary (artery) sclerosis

    Use additional code, if applicable, to identify:
- coronary atherosclerosis due to calcified coronary lesion (I25.84)
- coronary atherosclerosis due to lipid rich plaque (I25.83)

    Excludes2   atheroembolism (I75.-)
                  atherosclerosis of coronary artery bypass graft(s) and transplanted heart (I25.7-)

    I25.10   **Atherosclerotic heart disease of native coronary artery without angina pectoris**   A
       Atherosclerotic heart disease NOS
       Coding Clinic: 2015, Q2, P17; 2012, Q4, P92

Item 9–6   Classification is based on the location of the atherosclerosis. **"Of native coronary artery"** indicates the atherosclerosis is within an original heart artery. **"Of autologous vein bypass graft"** indicates that the atherosclerosis is within a vein graft that was taken from within the patient. **"Of nonautologous biological bypass graft"** indicates the atherosclerosis is within a vessel grafted from other than the patient. **"Of artery bypass graft"** indicates the atherosclerosis is within an artery that was grafted from within the patient.

Figure 9-2 Atherosclerotic plaque.

Atherosclerotic
plaque
(atheromas)

OGCR See Section I.9.b.

Atherosclerotic Coronary Artery Disease and Angina

ICD-10-CM has combination codes for atherosclerotic heart disease
with angina pectoris. The subcategories for these codes are I25.11,
Atherosclerotic heart disease of native coronary artery with angina
pectoris and I25.7, Atherosclerosis of coronary artery bypass graft(s)
and coronary artery of transplanted heart with angina pectoris.

When using one of these combination codes it is not necessary to use
an additional code for angina pectoris. A causal relationship can be
assumed in a patient with both atherosclerosis and angina pectoris,
unless the documentation indicates the angina is due to something
other than the atherosclerosis.

If a patient with coronary artery disease is admitted due to an acute
myocardial infarction (AMI), the AMI should be sequenced before the
coronary artery disease.

See Section I.C.9. Acute myocardial infarction (AMI).

● **I25.11** **Atherosclerotic heart disease of native coronary
               artery with angina pectoris**

   I25.110 **Atherosclerotic heart disease of native
                         coronary artery with unstable angina
                         pectoris** 🐾   A

      Excludes1 unstable angina
                                              without
                                              atherosclerotic
                                              heart disease
                                              (I20.0)

   I25.111 **Atherosclerotic heart disease of native
                         coronary artery with angina pectoris
                         with documented spasm** 🐾   A

      Excludes1 angina pectoris with
                                              documented
                                              spasm without
                                              atherosclerotic
                                              heart disease
                                              (I20.1)

   I25.118 **Atherosclerotic heart disease of native
                         coronary artery with other forms of
                         angina pectoris** 🐾   A

      Excludes1 other forms of angina
                                              pectoris without
                                              atherosclerotic
                                              heart disease
                                              (I20.8)

      Coding Clinic: 2015, Q2, P16-17

   I25.119 **Atherosclerotic heart disease of native
                         coronary artery with unspecified
                         angina pectoris** 🐾   A

      Atherosclerotic heart disease with
                         angina NOS
                         Atherosclerotic heart disease with
                         ischemic chest pain

      Excludes1 unspecified angina
                                              pectoris without
                                              atherosclerotic
                                              heart disease
                                              (I20.9)

  I25.2 **Old myocardial infarction**
      Healed myocardial infarction
      Past myocardial infarction diagnosed by ECG or
                         other investigation, but currently presenting no
                         symptoms

  I25.3 **Aneurysm of heart**
      Mural aneurysm
      Ventricular aneurysm

● **I25.4** **Coronary artery aneurysm and dissection**

   I25.41 **Coronary artery aneurysm**
      Coronary arteriovenous fistula, acquired

      Excludes1 congenital coronary (artery)
                                              aneurysm (Q24.5)

   I25.42 **Coronary artery dissection**

  I25.5 **Ischemic cardiomyopathy**

      Excludes2 coronary atherosclerosis (I25.1-, I25.7-)

  I25.6 **Silent myocardial ischemia**

● **I25.7** **Atherosclerosis of coronary artery bypass graft(s) and
             coronary artery of transplanted heart with angina
             pectoris**

    Use additional code, if applicable, to identify:
     coronary atherosclerosis due to calcified coronary
                         lesion (I25.84)
     coronary atherosclerosis due to lipid rich plaque
                         (I25.83)

   Excludes1 atherosclerosis of bypass graft(s) of
                         transplanted heart without angina
                         pectoris (I25.812)
                         atherosclerosis of coronary artery bypass
                         graft(s) without angina pectoris
                         (I25.810)
                         atherosclerosis of native coronary artery
                         of transplanted heart without angina
                         pectoris (I25.811)

● **I25.70** **Atherosclerosis of coronary artery bypass
               graft(s), unspecified, with angina pectoris**

   I25.700 **Atherosclerosis of coronary artery
                         bypass graft(s), unspecified, with
                         unstable angina pectoris** 🐾   A

      Excludes1 unstable angina
                                              pectoris without
                                              atherosclerosis of
                                              coronary artery
                                              bypass graft
                                              (I20.0)

   I25.701 **Atherosclerosis of coronary artery
                         bypass graft(s), unspecified, with
                         angina pectoris with documented
                         spasm** 🐾   A

      Excludes1 angina pectoris with
                                              documented
                                              spasm without
                                              atherosclerosis of
                                              coronary artery
                                              bypass graft
                                              (I20.1)

   I25.708 **Atherosclerosis of coronary artery
                         bypass graft(s), unspecified, with
                         other forms of angina pectoris** 🐾   A

      Excludes1 other forms of angina
                                              pectoris without
                                              atherosclerosis of
                                              coronary artery
                                              bypass graft
                                              (I20.8)

   I25.709 **Atherosclerosis of coronary artery
                         bypass graft(s), unspecified, with
                         unspecified angina pectoris** 🐾   A

      Excludes1 unspecified angina
                                              pectoris without
                                              atherosclerosis of
                                              coronary artery
                                              bypass graft
                                              (I20.9)

CHAPTER 9 (I00-I99)

▶ New ⇒ Revised ~~deleted~~ Deleted Excludes 1 Excludes 2 Includes Use additional Code first Code also Key words
OGCR Official Guidelines X Assign placeholder X ● Use Additional Character(s) ▷ Manifestation Code 🐾 Hierarchical Condition Category **Coding Clinic**

● **I25.71**   **Atherosclerosis of autologous vein coronary artery bypass graft(s) with angina pectoris**

     I25.710   **Atherosclerosis of autologous vein coronary artery bypass graft(s) with unstable angina pectoris** 🗗   A

         Excludes1   unstable angina without atherosclerosis of autologous vein coronary artery bypass graft(s) (I20.0)

         Excludes2   embolism or thrombus of coronary artery bypass graft(s) (T82.8-)

     I25.711   **Atherosclerosis of autologous vein coronary artery bypass graft(s) with angina pectoris with documented spasm** 🗗   A

         Excludes1   angina pectoris with documented spasm without atherosclerosis of autologous vein coronary artery bypass graft(s) (I20.1)

     I25.718   **Atherosclerosis of autologous vein coronary artery bypass graft(s) with other forms of angina pectoris** 🗗   A

         Excludes1   other forms of angina pectoris without atherosclerosis of autologous vein coronary artery bypass graft(s) (I20.8)

     I25.719   **Atherosclerosis of autologous vein coronary artery bypass graft(s) with unspecified angina pectoris** 🗗   A

         Excludes1   unspecified angina pectoris without atherosclerosis of autologous vein coronary artery bypass graft(s) (I20.9)

● **I25.72**   **Atherosclerosis of autologous artery coronary artery bypass graft(s) with angina pectoris**

     Atherosclerosis of internal mammary artery graft with angina pectoris

     I25.720   **Atherosclerosis of autologous artery coronary artery bypass graft(s) with unstable angina pectoris** 🗗   A

         Excludes1   unstable angina without atherosclerosis of autologous artery coronary artery bypass graft(s) (I20.0)

     I25.721   **Atherosclerosis of autologous artery coronary artery bypass graft(s) with angina pectoris with documented spasm** 🗗   A

         Excludes1   angina pectoris with documented spasm without atherosclerosis of autologous artery coronary artery bypass graft(s) (I20.1)

     I25.728   **Atherosclerosis of autologous artery coronary artery bypass graft(s) with other forms of angina pectoris** 🗗   A

         Excludes1   other forms of angina pectoris without atherosclerosis of autologous artery coronary artery bypass graft(s) (I20.8)

     I25.729   **Atherosclerosis of autologous artery coronary artery bypass graft(s) with unspecified angina pectoris** 🗗   A

         Excludes1   unspecified angina pectoris without atherosclerosis of autologous artery coronary artery bypass graft(s) (I20.9)

● **I25.73**   **Atherosclerosis of nonautologous biological coronary artery bypass graft(s) with angina pectoris**

     I25.730   **Atherosclerosis of nonautologous biological coronary artery bypass graft(s) with unstable angina pectoris** 🗗   A

         Excludes1   unstable angina without atherosclerosis of nonautologous biological coronary artery bypass graft(s) (I20.0)

     I25.731   **Atherosclerosis of nonautologous biological coronary artery bypass graft(s) with angina pectoris with documented spasm** 🗗   A

         Excludes1   angina pectoris with documented spasm without atherosclerosis of nonautologous biological coronary artery bypass graft(s) (I20.1)

     I25.738   **Atherosclerosis of nonautologous biological coronary artery bypass graft(s) with other forms of angina pectoris** 🗗   A

         Excludes1   other forms of angina pectoris without atherosclerosis of nonautologous biological coronary artery bypass graft(s) (I20.8)

     I25.739   **Atherosclerosis of nonautologous biological coronary artery bypass graft(s) with unspecified angina pectoris** 🗗   A

         Excludes1   unspecified angina pectoris without atherosclerosis of nonautologous biological coronary artery bypass graft(s) (I20.9)

CHAPTER 9 (I00-I99)

● **I25.75**   **Atherosclerosis of native coronary artery of transplanted heart with angina pectoris**

Excludes1   atherosclerosis of native coronary artery of transplanted heart without angina pectoris (I25.811)

I25.750   **Atherosclerosis of native coronary artery of transplanted heart with unstable angina** 🦠

I25.751   **Atherosclerosis of native coronary artery of transplanted heart with angina pectoris with documented spasm** 🦠

I25.758   **Atherosclerosis of native coronary artery of transplanted heart with other forms of angina pectoris** 🦠

I25.759   **Atherosclerosis of native coronary artery of transplanted heart with unspecified angina pectoris** 🦠

● **I25.76**   **Atherosclerosis of bypass graft of coronary artery of transplanted heart with angina pectoris**

Excludes1   atherosclerosis of bypass graft of coronary artery of transplanted heart without angina pectoris (I25.812)

I25.760   **Atherosclerosis of bypass graft of coronary artery of transplanted heart with unstable angina** 🦠   A

I25.761   **Atherosclerosis of bypass graft of coronary artery of transplanted heart with angina pectoris with documented spasm** 🦠   A

I25.768   **Atherosclerosis of bypass graft of coronary artery of transplanted heart with other forms of angina pectoris** 🦠   A

I25.769   **Atherosclerosis of bypass graft of coronary artery of transplanted heart with unspecified angina pectoris** 🦠   A

● **I25.79**   **Atherosclerosis of other coronary artery bypass graft(s) with angina pectoris**   A

I25.790   **Atherosclerosis of other coronary artery bypass graft(s) with unstable angina pectoris** 🦠

Excludes1   unstable angina without atherosclerosis of other coronary artery bypass graft(s) (I20.0)

I25.791   **Atherosclerosis of other coronary artery bypass graft(s) with angina pectoris with documented spasm** 🦠   A

Excludes1   angina pectoris with documented spasm without atherosclerosis of other coronary artery bypass graft(s) (I20.1)

I25.798   **Atherosclerosis of other coronary artery bypass graft(s) with other forms of angina pectoris** 🦠   A

Excludes1   other forms of angina pectoris without atherosclerosis of other coronary artery bypass graft(s) (I20.8)

I25.799   **Atherosclerosis of other coronary artery bypass graft(s) with unspecified angina pectoris** 🦠   A

Excludes1   unspecified angina pectoris without atherosclerosis of other coronary artery bypass graft(s) (I20.9)

● **I25.8**   **Other forms of chronic ischemic heart disease**

● **I25.81**   **Atherosclerosis of other coronary vessels without angina pectoris**

Use additional code, if applicable, to identify: coronary atherosclerosis due to calcified coronary lesion (I25.84) coronary atherosclerosis due to lipid rich plaque (I25.83)

Excludes2   atherosclerotic heart disease of native coronary artery without angina pectoris (I25.10)

I25.810   **Atherosclerosis of coronary artery bypass graft(s) without angina pectoris**   A

Atherosclerosis of coronary artery bypass graft NOS

Excludes1   atherosclerosis of coronary bypass graft(s) with angina pectoris (I25.70- -I25.73-, I25.79-)

Coding Clinic: 2016, Q4, P86

I25.811   **Atherosclerosis of native coronary artery of transplanted heart without angina pectoris**

Atherosclerosis of native coronary artery of transplanted heart NOS

Excludes1   atherosclerosis of native coronary artery of transplanted heart with angina pectoris (I25.75-)

I25.812   **Atherosclerosis of bypass graft of coronary artery of transplanted heart without angina pectoris**   A

Atherosclerosis of bypass graft of transplanted heart NOS

Excludes1   atherosclerosis of bypass graft of transplanted heart with angina pectoris (I25.76)

I25.82 **Chronic total occlusion** of coronary artery
　　　Complete occlusion of coronary artery
　　　Total occlusion of coronary artery

　　　*Code first coronary atherosclerosis (I25.1-, I25.7-,
　　　　I25.81-)*

　　　Excludes1　acute coronary occlusion with
　　　　　　myocardial infarction
　　　　　　(I21.0-I21.9, I22.-)
　　　　　　acute coronary occlusion without
　　　　　　myocardial infarction (I24.0)

I25.83 Coronary atherosclerosis due to **lipid rich
　　　plaque**   A

　　　*Code first coronary atherosclerosis (I25.1-, I25.7-,
　　　　I25.81-)*

I25.84 Coronary atherosclerosis due to **calcified
　　　coronary lesion**
　　　　Coronary atherosclerosis due to severely
　　　　　calcified coronary lesion

　　　*Code first coronary atherosclerosis (I25.1-, I25.7-,
　　　　I25.81-)*

I25.89 **Other forms of chronic ischemic heart disease**

I25.9 **Chronic ischemic heart disease, unspecified**
　　　Ischemic heart disease (chronic) NOS

PULMONARY HEART DISEASE AND DISEASES OF PULMONARY CIRCULATION (I26-I28)

● **I26** **Pulmonary embolism**

　　　Includes　pulmonary (acute)(artery)(vein) infarction
　　　　　　pulmonary (acute)(artery)(vein)
　　　　　　　thromboembolism
　　　　　　pulmonary (acute)(artery)(vein) thrombosis

　　　Excludes2　chronic pulmonary embolism (I27.82)
　　　　　　personal history of pulmonary embolism (Z86.711)
　　　　　　pulmonary embolism due to trauma (T79.0, T79.1)
　　　　　　pulmonary embolism due to complications of
　　　　　　　surgical and medical care (T80.0, T81.7-, T82.8-)
　　　　　　pulmonary embolism complicating abortion,
　　　　　　　ectopic or molar pregnancy (O00-O07, O08.2)
　　　　　　pulmonary embolism complicating pregnancy,
　　　　　　　childbirth and the puerperium (O88.-)
　　　　　　septic (non-pulmonary) arterial embolism (I76)

　　　Coding Clinic: 2021, Q2, P10

● **I26.0** **Pulmonary embolism with acute cor pulmonale**

　　　I26.01 **Septic pulmonary embolism with acute cor
　　　　　pulmonale** ⚕
　　　　　　Code first underlying infection

　　　I26.02 **Saddle embolus of pulmonary artery with acute
　　　　　cor pulmonale** ⚕

　　　I26.09 **Other pulmonary embolism with acute cor
　　　　　pulmonale** ⚕
　　　　　　Acute cor pulmonale NOS

● **I26.9** **Pulmonary embolism without acute cor pulmonale**

　　　I26.90 **Septic pulmonary embolism without acute cor
　　　　　pulmonale** ⚕
　　　　　　Code first underlying infection

　　　I26.92 **Saddle embolus of pulmonary artery without
　　　　　acute cor pulmonale** ⚕

　　　I26.93 **Single subsegmental pulmonary embolism
　　　　　without acute cor pulmonale** ⚕
　　　　　　Subsegmental pulmonary embolism NOS

　　　I26.94 **Multiple subsegmental pulmonary emboli
　　　　　without acute cor pulmonale** ⚕
　　　　　　Coding Clinic: 2021, Q2, P10

　　　I26.99 **Other pulmonary embolism without acute cor
　　　　　pulmonale** ⚕
　　　　　　Acute pulmonary embolism NOS
　　　　　　Pulmonary embolism NOS
　　　　　　Coding Clinic: 2019, Q2, P22-23

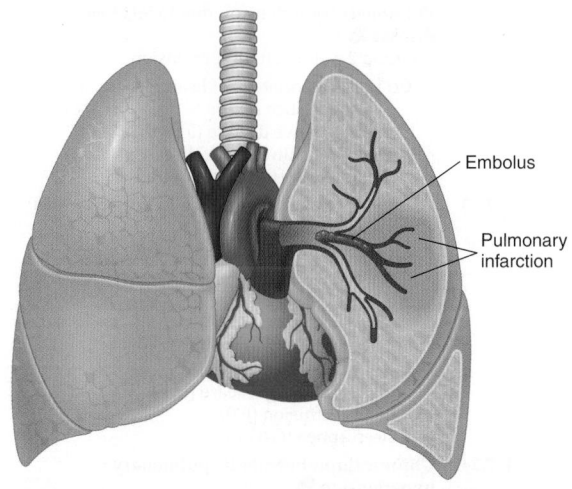

Figure 9-3　Pulmonary embolism. (From Chabner: The Language of
Medicine, ed 8, St. Louis, Saunders, 2007)

Item 9–7　Pulmonary heart disease or **cor pulmonale** is right ventricle
hypertrophy or RVH as a result of a respiratory disorder increasing back flow
pressure to the right ventricle. Left untreated, cor pulmonale leads to right-heart
failure and death.

● **I27** **Other pulmonary heart diseases**

　　　I27.0 **Primary pulmonary hypertension** ⚕
　　　　　Heritable pulmonary arterial hypertension
　　　　　Idiopathic pulmonary arterial hypertension
　　　　　Primary group 1 pulmonary hypertension
　　　　　Primary pulmonary arterial hypertension

　　　　　Excludes1　persistent pulmonary hypertension of
　　　　　　　newborn (P29.30)
　　　　　　　pulmonary hypertension NOS (I27.20)
　　　　　　　secondary pulmonary arterial
　　　　　　　　hypertension (I27.21)
　　　　　　　secondary pulmonary hypertension
　　　　　　　　(I27.29)

　　　I27.1 **Kyphoscoliotic heart disease** ⚕

● **I27.2** **Other secondary pulmonary hypertension**
　　　　　Code also associated underlying condition

　　　　　Excludes1　Eisenmenger's syndrome (I27.83)
　　　　　Coding Clinic: 2016, Q2, P8

　　　I27.20 **Pulmonary hypertension, unspecified** ⚕
　　　　　　Pulmonary hypertension NOS

　　　I27.21 **Secondary pulmonary arterial hypertension** ⚕
　　　　　　(Associated) (drug-induced) (toxin-induced)
　　　　　　　pulmonary arterial hypertension NOS
　　　　　　(Associated) (drug-induced) (toxin-induced)
　　　　　　　(secondary) group 1 pulmonary
　　　　　　　hypertension

　　　　　　Code also associated conditions if applicable, or
　　　　　　　adverse effects of drugs or toxins, such as:
　　　　　　adverse effect of appetite depressants
　　　　　　　(T50.5X5)
　　　　　　congenital heart disease (Q20-Q28)
　　　　　　human immunodeficiency virus [HIV]
　　　　　　　disease (B20)
　　　　　　polymyositis (M33.2-)
　　　　　　portal hypertension (K76.6)
　　　　　　rheumatoid arthritis (M05.-)
　　　　　　schistosomiasis (B65.-)
　　　　　　Sjögren syndrome (M35.0-)
　　　　　　systemic sclerosis (M34.-)

CHAPTER 9 (I00-I99)

I27.22 **Pulmonary hypertension due to left heart disease** 🐾
Group 2 pulmonary hypertension
Code also associated left heart disease, if known, such as:
multiple valve disease (I08.-)
rheumatic mitral valve diseases (I05.-)
rheumatic aortic valve diseases (I06.-)

I27.23 **Pulmonary hypertension due to lung diseases and hypoxia** 🐾
Group 3 pulmonary hypertension
Code also associated lung disease, if known, such as:
bronchiectasis (J47.-)
cystic fibrosis with pulmonary manifestations (E84.0)
interstitial lung disease (J84.-)
pleural effusion (J90)
sleep apnea (G47.3-)

I27.24 **Chronic thromboembolic pulmonary hypertension** 🐾
Group 4 pulmonary hypertension
Code also associated pulmonary embolism, if applicable (I26.-, I27.82)

I27.29 **Other secondary pulmonary hypertension** 🐾
Group 5 pulmonary hypertension
Pulmonary hypertension with unclear multifactorial mechanisms
Pulmonary hypertension due to hematologic disorders
Pulmonary hypertension due to metabolic disorders
Pulmonary hypertension due to other systemic disorders
Code also other associated disorders, if known, such as:
chronic myeloid leukemia (C92.10-C92.22)
essential thrombocythemia (D47.3)
Gaucher disease (E75.22)
hypertensive chronic kidney disease with end stage renal disease (I12.0, I13.11, I13.2)
hyperthyroidism (E05.-)
hypothyroidism (E00-E03)
polycythemia vera (D45)
sarcoidosis (D86.-)

● **I27.8** **Other specified pulmonary heart diseases**
I27.81 **Cor pulmonale (chronic)** 🐾
Cor pulmonale NOS
Excludes1 acute cor pulmonale (I26.0-)

I27.82 **Chronic pulmonary embolism** 🐾
Use additional code, if applicable, for associated long-term (current) use of anticoagulants (Z79.01)
Excludes1 personal history of pulmonary embolism (Z86.711)
Coding Clinic: 2021, Q2, P10

I27.83 **Eisenmenger's syndrome** 🐾
Eisenmenger's complex
(Irreversible) Eisenmenger's disease
Pulmonary hypertension with right to left shunt related to congenital heart disease
Code also underlying heart defect, if known, such as:
atrial septal defect (Q21.1)
Eisenmenger's defect (Q21.8)
patent ductus arteriosus (Q25.0)
ventricular septal defect (Q21.0)

I27.89 **Other specified pulmonary heart diseases** 🐾
I27.9 **Pulmonary heart disease, unspecified** 🐾
Chronic cardiopulmonary disease

● **I28** **Other diseases of pulmonary vessels**
I28.0 **Arteriovenous fistula of pulmonary vessels** 🐾
Excludes1 congenital arteriovenous fistula (Q25.72)

I28.1 **Aneurysm of pulmonary artery** 🐾
Excludes1 congenital aneurysm (Q25.79)
congenital arteriovenous aneurysm (Q25.72)

I28.8 **Other diseases of pulmonary vessels** 🐾
Pulmonary arteritis
Pulmonary endarteritis
Rupture of pulmonary vessels
Stenosis of pulmonary vessels
Stricture of pulmonary vessels

I28.9 **Disease of pulmonary vessels, unspecified** 🐾

~~OTHER FORMS OF HEART DISEASE (I30-I52)~~

▶ **OTHER FORMS OF HEART DISEASE (I30-I5A)**

● **I30** **Acute pericarditis**
Inflammation of pericardium (sac surrounding the heart) caused by an infection
Includes acute mediastinopericarditis
acute myopericarditis
acute pericardial effusion
acute pleuropericarditis
acute pneumopericarditis
Excludes1 Dressler's syndrome (I24.1)
rheumatic pericarditis (acute) (I01.0)
viral pericarditis due to Coxsakie virus (B33.23)

I30.0 **Acute nonspecific idiopathic pericarditis**
I30.1 **Infective pericarditis**
Pneumococcal pericarditis
Pneumopyopericardium
Purulent pericarditis
Pyopericarditis
Pyopericardium
Pyopneumopericardium
Staphylococcal pericarditis
Streptococcal pericarditis
Suppurative pericarditis
Viral pericarditis
Use additional code (B95-B97) to identify infectious agent

I30.8 **Other forms of acute pericarditis**
I30.9 **Acute pericarditis, unspecified**

● **I31** **Other diseases of pericardium**
Excludes1 diseases of pericardium specified as rheumatic (I09.2)
postcardiotomy syndrome (I97.0)
traumatic injury to pericardium (S26.-)

I31.0 **Chronic adhesive pericarditis**
Accretio cordis
Adherent pericardium
Adhesive mediastinopericarditis

I31.1 **Chronic constrictive pericarditis**
Concretio cordis
Pericardial calcification

I31.2 **Hemopericardium, not elsewhere classified**
Excludes1 hemopericardium as current complication following acute myocardial infarction (I23.0)

I31.3 **Pericardial effusion (noninflammatory)**
Chylopericardium
Excludes1 acute pericardial effusion (I30.9)
Coding Clinic: 2019, Q1, P16

I31.4 **Cardiac tamponade**
Code first underlying cause

I31.8 **Other specified diseases of pericardium**
Epicardial plaques
Focal pericardial adhesions

I31.9 **Disease of pericardium, unspecified**
Pericarditis (chronic) NOS

▶ New 🠒 Revised ~~deleted~~ Deleted Excludes 1 Excludes 2 Includes Use additional Code first Code also Key words
OGCR Official Guidelines X Assign placeholder X ● Use Additional Character(s) ▌ Manifestation Code 🐾 Hierarchical Condition Category Coding Clinic

▷ **I32**   *Pericarditis in diseases classified elsewhere*
  Code first underlying disease
  Excludes1   pericarditis (in):
  coxsackie (virus) (B33.23)
  gonococcal (A54.83)
  meningococcal (A39.53)
  rheumatoid (arthritis) (M05.31)
  syphilitic (A52.06)
  systemic lupus erythematosus (M32.12)
  tuberculosis (A18.84)

● **I33**   Acute and subacute endocarditis
  Inflammation/infection of lining of heart, affecting heart valves including replacement valves and is usually caused by a bacterial infection
  Excludes1   acute rheumatic endocarditis (I01.1)
  endocarditis NOS (I38)

   I33.0   **Acute and subacute infective endocarditis**
  Bacterial endocarditis (acute) (subacute)
  Infective endocarditis (acute) (subacute) NOS
  Endocarditis lenta (acute) (subacute)
  Malignant endocarditis (acute) (subacute)
  Purulent endocarditis (acute) (subacute)
  Septic endocarditis (acute) (subacute)
  Ulcerative endocarditis (acute) (subacute)
  Vegetative endocarditis (acute) (subacute)
  Use additional code (B95-B97) to identify infectious agent

   I33.9   **Acute and subacute endocarditis, unspecified**
  Acute endocarditis NOS
  Acute myoendocarditis NOS
  Acute periendocarditis NOS
  Subacute endocarditis NOS
  Subacute myoendocarditis NOS
  Subacute periendocarditis NOS

● **I34**   Nonrheumatic mitral valve disorders
  Excludes1   mitral valve disease (I05.9)
  mitral valve failure (I05.8)
  mitral valve stenosis (I05.0)
  mitral valve disorder of unspecified cause with diseases of aortic and/or tricuspid valve(s) (I08.-)
  mitral valve disorder of unspecified cause with mitral stenosis or obstruction (I05.0)
  mitral valve disorder specified as congenital (Q23.2, Q23.9)
  mitral valve disorder specified as rheumatic (I05.-)

   I34.0   **Nonrheumatic mitral (valve) insufficiency**
  Nonrheumatic mitral (valve) incompetence NOS
  Nonrheumatic mitral (valve) regurgitation NOS

   I34.1   **Nonrheumatic mitral (valve) prolapse**
  Floppy nonrheumatic mitral valve syndrome
  Excludes1   Marfan's syndrome (Q87.4-)

   I34.2   **Nonrheumatic mitral (valve) stenosis**
   I34.8   **Other nonrheumatic mitral valve disorders**
   I34.9   **Nonrheumatic mitral valve disorder, unspecified**

● **I35**   Nonrheumatic aortic valve disorders
  Excludes1   aortic valve disorder of unspecified cause but with diseases of mitral and/or tricuspid valve(s) (I08.-)
  aortic valve disorder specified as congenital (Q23.0, Q23.1)
  aortic valve disorder specified as rheumatic (I06.-)
  hypertrophic subaortic stenosis (I42.1)

   I35.0   **Nonrheumatic aortic (valve) stenosis**
   I35.1   **Nonrheumatic aortic (valve) insufficiency**
  Nonrheumatic aortic (valve) incompetence NOS
  Nonrheumatic aortic (valve) regurgitation NOS
   I35.2   **Nonrheumatic aortic (valve) stenosis with insufficiency**
   I35.8   **Other nonrheumatic aortic valve disorders**
   I35.9   **Nonrheumatic aortic valve disorder, unspecified**

● **I36**   Nonrheumatic tricuspid valve disorders
  Excludes1   tricuspid valve disorders of unspecified cause (I07.-)
  tricuspid valve disorders specified as congenital (Q22.4, Q22.8, Q22.9)
  tricuspid valve disorders specified as rheumatic (I07.-)
  tricuspid valve disorders with aortic and/or mitral valve involvement (I08.-)

   I36.0   **Nonrheumatic tricuspid (valve) stenosis**
   I36.1   **Nonrheumatic tricuspid (valve) insufficiency**
  Nonrheumatic tricuspid (valve) incompetence
  Nonrheumatic tricuspid (valve) regurgitation
   I36.2   **Nonrheumatic tricuspid (valve) stenosis with insufficiency**
   I36.8   **Other nonrheumatic tricuspid valve disorders**
   I36.9   **Nonrheumatic tricuspid valve disorder, unspecified**

● **I37**   Nonrheumatic pulmonary valve disorders
  Excludes1   pulmonary valve disorder specified as congenital (Q22.1, Q22.2, Q22.3)
  pulmonary valve disorder specified as rheumatic (I09.89)

   I37.0   **Nonrheumatic pulmonary valve stenosis**
   I37.1   **Nonrheumatic pulmonary valve insufficiency**
  Nonrheumatic pulmonary valve incompetence
  Nonrheumatic pulmonary valve regurgitation
   I37.2   **Nonrheumatic pulmonary valve stenosis with insufficiency**
   I37.8   **Other nonrheumatic pulmonary valve disorders**
   I37.9   **Nonrheumatic pulmonary valve disorder, unspecified**

   I38   Endocarditis, valve unspecified
  Includes   endocarditis (chronic) NOS
  valvular incompetence NOS
  valvular insufficiency NOS
  valvular regurgitation NOS
  valvular stenosis NOS
  valvulitis (chronic) NOS
  Excludes1   congenital insufficiency of cardiac valve NOS (Q24.8)
  congenital stenosis of cardiac valve NOS (Q24.8)
  endocardial fibroelastosis (I42.4)
  endocarditis specified as rheumatic (I09.1)

▷ **I39**   *Endocarditis and heart valve disorders in diseases classified elsewhere*
  Code first underlying disease, such as:
  Q fever (A78)
  Excludes1   endocardial involvement in:
  candidiasis (B37.6)
  gonococcal infection (A54.83)
  Libman-Sacks disease (M32.11)
  listerosis (A32.82)
  meningococcal infection (A39.51)
  rheumatoid arthritis (M05.31)
  syphilis (A52.03)
  tuberculosis (A18.84)
  typhoid fever (A01.02)

● **I40**   Acute myocarditis
  Inflammation of heart muscle due to infection (viral/bacterial)
  Includes   subacute myocarditis
  Excludes1   acute rheumatic myocarditis (I01.2)

   I40.0   **Infective myocarditis**
  Septic myocarditis
  Use additional code (B95-B97) to identify infectious agent

   I40.1   **Isolated myocarditis**
  Fiedler's myocarditis
  Giant cell myocarditis
  Idiopathic myocarditis

   I40.8   **Other acute myocarditis**
   I40.9   **Acute myocarditis, unspecified**

CHAPTER 9 (I00-I99)

CHAPTER 9 (I00-I99)

▶ **I41   Myocarditis in diseases classified elsewhere**

Code first underlying disease, such as:
    typhus (A75.0-A75.9)

    Excludes1   myocarditis (in):
                   Chagas' disease (chronic) (B57.2)
                   acute (B57.0)
                   coxsackie (virus) infection (B33.22)
                   diphtheritic (A36.81)
                   gonococcal (A54.83)
                   influenzal (J09.X9, J10.82, J11.82)
                   meningococcal (A39.52)
                   mumps (B26.82)
                   rheumatoid arthritis (M05.31)
                   sarcoid (D86.85)
                   syphilis (A52.06)
                   toxoplasmosis (B58.81)
                   tuberculous (A18.84)

● **I42 Cardiomyopathy**

Disease of the heart muscle resulting in an abnormally enlarged, weakened, thickened, and/or stiffened muscles

    Includes   myocardiopathy

Code first pre-existing cardiomyopathy complicating pregnancy and puerperium (O99.4)

    Excludes2   ischemic cardiomyopathy (I25.5)
                  peripartum cardiomyopathy (O90.3)
                  ventricular hypertrophy (I51.7)

    I42.0   **Dilated cardiomyopathy** 🅠
          Congestive cardiomyopathy

    I42.1   **Obstructive hypertrophic cardiomyopathy** 🅠
          Hypertrophic subaortic stenosis (idiopathic)

    I42.2   **Other hypertrophic cardiomyopathy** 🅠
          Nonobstructive hypertrophic cardiomyopathy

    I42.3   **Endomyocardial (eosinophilic) disease** 🅠
          Endomyocardial (tropical) fibrosis
          Löffler's endocarditis

    I42.4   **Endocardial fibroelastosis** 🅠
          Congenital cardiomyopathy
          Elastomyofibrosis

    I42.5   **Other restrictive cardiomyopathy** 🅠
          Constrictive cardiomyopathy NOS

    I42.6   **Alcoholic cardiomyopathy** 🅠
          Code also presence of alcoholism (F10.-)

    I42.7   **Cardiomyopathy due to drug and external agent** 🅠
          Code first poisoning due to drug or toxin, if applicable (T36-T65 with fifth or sixth character 1-4 or 6)
          Use additional code for adverse effect, if applicable, to identify drug (T36-T50 with fifth or sixth character 5)

    I42.8   **Other cardiomyopathies** 🅠

    I42.9   **Cardiomyopathy, unspecified** 🅠
          Cardiomyopathy (primary) (secondary) NOS

▶ **I43 Cardiomyopathy in diseases classified elsewhere** 🅠

Code first underlying disease, such as:
    amyloidosis (E85.-)
    glycogen storage disease (E74.0)
    gout (M10.0-)
    thyrotoxicosis (E05.0-E05.9-)

    Excludes1   cardiomyopathy (in):
                   coxsackie (virus) (B33.24)
                   diphtheria (A36.81)
                   sarcoidosis (D86.85)
                   tuberculosis (A18.84)

● **I44 Atrioventricular and left bundle-branch block**

Conduction problem resulting in arrhythmias/dysrhythmias due to a lack of electrical impulses being transmitted normally through the heart

    I44.0   **Atrioventricular block, first degree**

    I44.1   **Atrioventricular block, second degree**
          Atrioventricular block, type I and II
          Möbitz block, type I and II
          Second degree block, type I and II
          Wenckebach's block

    I44.2   **Atrioventricular block, complete** 🅠
          Complete heart block NOS
          Third degree block
          Coding Clinic: 2019, Q2, P4

●   **I44.3**   **Other and unspecified atrioventricular block**
          Atrioventricular block NOS

         I44.30   **Unspecified atrioventricular block**
         I44.39   **Other atrioventricular block**

    I44.4   **Left anterior fascicular block**

    I44.5   **Left posterior fascicular block**

●   **I44.6**   **Other and unspecified fascicular block**

         I44.60   **Unspecified fascicular block**
               Left bundle-branch hemiblock NOS

         I44.69   **Other fascicular block**

    I44.7   **Left bundle-branch block, unspecified**

● **I45 Other conduction disorders**

    I45.0   **Right fascicular block**

●   **I45.1**   **Other and unspecified right bundle-branch block**

         I45.10   **Unspecified right bundle-branch block**
               Right bundle-branch block NOS

         I45.19   **Other right bundle-branch block**

    I45.2   **Bifascicular block**

    I45.3   **Trifascicular block**

    I45.4   **Nonspecific intraventricular block**
          Bundle-branch block NOS

    I45.5   **Other specified heart block**
          Sinoatrial block
          Sinoauricular block

         Excludes1   heart block NOS (I45.9)

    I45.6   **Pre-excitation syndrome**
          Accelerated atrioventricular conduction
          Accessory atrioventricular conduction
          Anomalous atrioventricular excitation
          Lown-Ganong-Levine syndrome
          Pre-excitation atrioventricular conduction
          Wolff-Parkinson-White syndrome

●   **I45.8**   **Other specified conduction disorders**

         I45.81   **Long QT syndrome**

         I45.89   **Other specified conduction disorders**
               Atrioventricular [AV] dissociation
               Interference dissociation
               Isorhythmic dissociation
               Nonparoxysmal AV nodal tachycardia
               Coding Clinic: 2013, Q2, P32

    I45.9   **Conduction disorder, unspecified**
          Heart block NOS
          Stokes-Adams syndrome

● **I46 Cardiac arrest**

    Excludes2   cardiogenic shock (R57.0)

    I46.2   **Cardiac arrest due to underlying cardiac condition** 🅠
          Code first underlying cardiac condition

    I46.8   **Cardiac arrest due to other underlying condition** 🅠
          Code first underlying condition

    I46.9   **Cardiac arrest, cause unspecified** 🅠

● **I47 Paroxysmal tachycardia**

Code first tachycardia complicating:
    abortion or ectopic or molar pregnancy (O00-O07, O08.8)
    obstetric surgery and procedures (O75.4)

    Excludes1   tachycardia NOS (R00.0)
                   sinoauricular tachycardia NOS (R00.0)
                   sinus [sinusal] tachycardia NOS (R00.0)

    I47.0   **Re-entry ventricular arrhythmia** 🅠

    I47.1   **Supraventricular tachycardia** 🅠
          Atrial (paroxysmal) tachycardia
          Atrioventricular [AV] (paroxysmal) tachycardia
          Atrioventricular re-entrant (nodal) tachycardia [AVNRT] [AVRT]
          Junctional (paroxysmal) tachycardia
          Nodal (paroxysmal) tachycardia

▶ New   ⇒ Revised   ~~deleted~~ Deleted   Excludes 1   Excludes 2   Includes   Use additional   Code first   Code also   Key words

OGCR Official Guidelines   **X** Assign placeholder X   ● Use Additional Character(s)   ▶ Manifestation Code   🅠 Hierarchical Condition Category   **Coding Clinic**

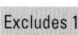

I47.2   Ventricular tachycardia 🦠
    Coding Clinic: 2013, Q3, P23

I47.9   Paroxysmal tachycardia, unspecified 🦠
    Bouveret (-Hoffman) syndrome

● **I48   Atrial fibrillation and flutter**
    *Most common abnormal heart rhythm (arrhythmia) presenting
    as irregular, rapid beating (tachycardia) of the heart's upper
    chamber.*

I48.0   Paroxysmal atrial fibrillation 🦠

● **I48.1   Persistent atrial fibrillation** 🦠
        Rapid contractions of the upper heart chamber

        Excludes1   Permanent atrial fibrillation (I48.21)
        Coding Clinic: 2019, Q2, P3-4

        I48.11   Longstanding persistent atrial fibrillation

        I48.19   Other persistent atrial fibrillation
                Chronic persistent atrial fibrillation
                Persistent atrial fibrillation, NOS

● **I48.2   Chronic atrial fibrillation** 🦠
        Coding Clinic: 2019, Q2, P3

        I48.20   Chronic atrial fibrillation, unspecified

                Excludes1   Chronic persistent atrial
                        fibrillation (I48.19)

        I48.21   Permanent atrial fibrillation

I48.3   Typical atrial flutter 🦠
        Type I atrial flutter

I48.4   Atypical atrial flutter 🦠
        Type II atrial flutter

● **I48.9   Unspecified atrial fibrillation and atrial flutter**

        I48.91   Unspecified atrial fibrillation 🦠

        I48.92   Unspecified atrial flutter 🦠

● **I49   Other cardiac arrhythmias**
    Code first cardiac arrhythmia complicating:
        abortion or ectopic or molar pregnancy (O00-O07, O08.8)
        obstetric surgery and procedures (O75.4)

        Excludes1   neonatal dysrhythmia (P29.1-)
                sinoatrial bradycardia (R00.1)
                sinus bradycardia (R00.1)
                vagal bradycardia (R00.1)

        Excludes2   bradycardia NOS (R00.1)

● **I49.0   Ventricular fibrillation and flutter**

        I49.01   Ventricular fibrillation 🦠

        I49.02   Ventricular flutter 🦠

I49.1   Atrial premature depolarization
        Atrial premature beats

I49.2   Junctional premature depolarization 🦠

I49.3   Ventricular premature depolarization

● **I49.4   Other and unspecified premature depolarization**

        I49.40   Unspecified premature depolarization
                Premature beats NOS

        I49.49   Other premature depolarization
                Ectopic beats
                Extrasystoles
                Extrasystolic arrhythmias
                Premature contractions

I49.5   Sick sinus syndrome 🦠
        Tachycardia-bradycardia syndrome
        Coding Clinic: 2019, Q1, P33

I49.8   Other specified cardiac arrhythmias
        Brugada syndrome
        Coronary sinus rhythm disorder
        Ectopic rhythm disorder
        Nodal rhythm disorder

I49.9   Cardiac arrhythmia, unspecified
        Arrhythmia (cardiac) NOS

● **I50   Heart failure**
    *Code first heart failure complicating abortion or ectopic or molar
        pregnancy (O00-O07, O08.8)*
        heart failure due to hypertension (I11.0)
        heart failure due to hypertension with chronic kidney disease
            (I13.-)
        heart failure following surgery (I97.13-)
        obstetric surgery and procedures (O75.4)
        rheumatic heart failure (I09.81)

        ~~Excludes1~~   ~~neonatal cardiac failure (P29.0)~~

        Excludes2   cardiac arrest (I46.-)

                ▶ neonatal cardiac failure (P20.0)
        Coding Clinic: 2017, Q1, P47; 2016, Q4, P122-123, Q1, P38; 2015, Q2, P15

I50.1   Left ventricular failure, unspecified 🦠
        Cardiac asthma
        Edema of lung with heart disease NOS
        Edema of lung with heart failure
        Left heart failure
        Pulmonary edema with heart disease NOS
        Pulmonary edema with heart failure

        Excludes1   edema of lung without heart disease or
                        heart failure (J81.-)
                pulmonary edema without heart disease
                        or failure (J81.-)

● **I50.2   Systolic (congestive) heart failure**
        Heart failure with reduced ejection fraction [HFrEF]
        Systolic left ventricular heart failure

        Code also end stage heart failure, if applicable (I50.84)

        Excludes1   combined systolic (congestive) and
                        diastolic (congestive) heart failure
                        (I50.4-)

        **I50.20   Unspecified systolic (congestive) heart
                failure** 🦠

        I50.21   Acute systolic (congestive) heart failure 🦠
                Presenting a short and relatively severe episode

        I50.22   Chronic systolic (congestive) heart failure 🦠
                Long-lasting, presenting over time

        **I50.23   Acute on chronic systolic (congestive) heart
                failure** 🦠
                *Combination code. What was a chronic condition
                        now has an acute exacerbation (to make more
                        severe).*
                Coding Clinic: 2013, Q2, P33

● **I50.3   Diastolic (congestive) heart failure**
        Diastolic left ventricular heart failure
        Heart failure with normal ejection fraction
        Heart failure with preserved ejection fraction [HFpEF]

        Code also end stage heart failure, if applicable (I50.84)

        Excludes1   combined systolic (congestive) and
                        diastolic (congestive) heart failure
                        (I50.4-)

        **I50.30   Unspecified diastolic (congestive) heart
                failure** 🦠

        I50.31   Acute diastolic (congestive) heart failure 🦠
                Coding Clinic: 2017, Q1, P46

        I50.32   Chronic diastolic (congestive) heart failure 🦠

        **I50.33   Acute on chronic diastolic (congestive) heart
                failure** 🦠

● **I50.4   Combined systolic (congestive) and diastolic
        (congestive) heart failure**
        Combined systolic and diastolic left ventricular heart
            failure
        Heart failure with reduced ejection fraction and
            diastolic dysfunction

        Code also end stage heart failure, if applicable (I50.84)

        **I50.40   Unspecified combined systolic (congestive) and
                diastolic (congestive) heart failure** 🦠

        **I50.41   Acute combined systolic (congestive) and
                diastolic (congestive) heart failure** 🦠

        **I50.42   Chronic combined systolic (congestive) and
                diastolic (congestive) heart failure** 🦠

        **I50.43   Acute on chronic combined systolic
                (congestive) and diastolic (congestive) heart
                failure** 🦠

CHAPTER 9 (I00-I99)

Item 9–8 Congestive heart failure (CHF) is a condition in which the left ventricle of the heart cannot pump enough blood to the body. The blood flow from the heart slows or returns to the heart from the venous system (back flow) resulting in congestion (fluid accumulation) particularly in the abdomen. Most commonly, fluid collects in the lungs and results in shortness of breath, especially when in a reclining position.

● I50.8   **Other heart failure**

   ● I50.81   **Right heart failure**
         Right ventricular failure

       I50.810   **Right heart failure, unspecified** 🐾
           Right heart failure without mention of left heart failure
           Right ventricular failure NOS

       I50.811   **Acute right heart failure** 🐾
           Acute isolated right heart failure
           Acute (isolated) right ventricular failure

       I50.812   **Chronic right heart failure** 🐾
           Chronic isolated right heart failure
           Chronic (isolated) right ventricular failure

       I50.813   **Acute on chronic right heart failure** 🐾
           Acute on chronic isolated right heart failure
           Acute on chronic (isolated) right ventricular failure
           Acute decompensation of chronic (isolated) right ventricular failure
           Acute exacerbation of chronic (isolated) right ventricular failure

       I50.814   **Right heart failure due to left heart failure** 🐾
           Right ventricular failure secondary to left ventricular failure
           Code also the type of left ventricular failure, if known (I50.2-I50.43)
           Excludes1   Right heart failure with but not due to left heart failure (I50.82)

    I50.82   **Biventricular heart failure** 🐾
       Code also the type of left ventricular failure as systolic, diastolic, or combined, if known **(I50.2-I50.43)**

    I50.83   **High output heart failure** 🐾

    I50.84   **End stage heart failure** 🐾
       Stage D heart failure
       Code also the type of heart failure as systolic, diastolic, or combined, if known (I50.2-I50.43)

    I50.89   **Other heart failure** 🐾

   I50.9   **Heart failure, unspecified** 🐾
      Cardiac, heart or myocardial failure NOS
      Congestive heart disease
      Congestive heart failure NOS
      Excludes2   fluid overload unrelated to congestive heart failure (E87.70)
      Coding Clinic: 2017, Q1, P45-46; 2015, Q2, P15; 2012, Q4, P92

● I51   **Complications and ill-defined descriptions of heart disease**
    Excludes1   any condition in I51.4-I51.9 due to hypertension (I11.-)
                any condition in I51.4-I51.9 due to hypertension and chronic kidney disease (I13.-)
                heart disease specified as rheumatic (I00-I09)

   I51.0   **Cardiac septal defect, acquired**   A
      Acquired septal atrial defect (old)
      Acquired septal auricular defect (old)
      Acquired septal ventricular defect (old)
      Excludes1   cardiac septal defect as current complication following acute myocardial infarction (I23.1, I23.2)

   I51.1   **Rupture of chordae tendineae, not elsewhere classified** 🐾
      Excludes1   rupture of chordae tendineae as current complication following acute myocardial infarction (I23.4)

   I51.2   **Rupture of papillary muscle, not elsewhere classified** 🐾
      Excludes1   rupture of papillary muscle as current complication following acute myocardial infarction (I23.5)

   I51.3   **Intracardiac thrombosis, not elsewhere classified**
      Apical thrombosis (old)
      Atrial thrombosis (old)
      Auricular thrombosis (old)
      Mural thrombosis (old)
      Ventricular thrombosis (old)
      Excludes1   intracardiac thrombosis as current complication following acute myocardial infarction (I23.6)
      Coding Clinic: 2013, Q1, P24

   I51.4   **Myocarditis, unspecified** 🐾
      Chronic (interstitial) myocarditis
      Myocardial fibrosis
      Myocarditis NOS
      Excludes1   acute or subacute myocarditis (I40.-)
      Coding Clinic: 2016, Q4, P122

   I51.5   **Myocardial degeneration** 🐾
      Fatty degeneration of heart or myocardium
      Myocardial disease
      Senile degeneration of heart or myocardium
      Coding Clinic: 2016, Q4, P122

   I51.7   **Cardiomegaly**
      Cardiac dilatation
      Cardiac hypertrophy
      Ventricular dilatation
      Coding Clinic: 2016, Q4, P122

● I51.8   **Other ill-defined heart diseases**
      Coding Clinic: 2016, Q4, P122

    I51.81   **Takotsubo syndrome**
       Reversible left ventricular dysfunction following sudden emotional stress
       Stress induced cardiomyopathy
       Takotsubo cardiomyopathy
       Transient left ventricular apical ballooning syndrome

    I51.89   **Other ill-defined heart diseases**
       Carditis (acute)(chronic)
       Pancarditis (acute)(chronic)
       Coding Clinic: 2019, Q2, P6

   I51.9   **Heart disease, unspecified**
      Coding Clinic: 2016, Q4, P122

▷ I52   *Other heart disorders in diseases classified elsewhere*
    Code first underlying disease, such as:
      congenital syphilis (A50.5)
      mucopolysaccharidosis (E76.3)
      schistosomiasis (B65.0-B65.9)
    Excludes1   heart disease (in):
              gonococcal infection (A54.83)
              meningococcal infection (A39.50)
              rheumatoid arthritis (M05.31)
              syphilis (A52.06)

▶ New   ⇒ Revised   ~~deleted~~ Deleted   Excludes 1   Excludes 2   Includes   Use additional   Code first   Code also   Key words
OGCR Official Guidelines   X Assign placeholder X   ● Use Additional Character(s)   ▷ Manifestation Code   🐾 Hierarchical Condition Category   **Coding Clinic**

CEREBROVASCULAR DISEASES (I60-I69)

Use additional code to identify presence of:
  alcohol abuse and dependence (F10.-)
  exposure to environmental tobacco smoke (Z77.22)
  history of tobacco dependence (Z87.891)
  hypertension (I10-I16)
  occupational exposure to environmental tobacco smoke
    (Z57.31)
  tobacco dependence (F17.-)
  tobacco use (Z72.0)

> **Excludes1**   traumatic intracranial hemorrhage (S06.-)

Coding Clinic: 2015, Q4, P40

▶**I5A   Non-ischemic myocardial injury (non-traumatic)**
  ▶Acute (non-ischemic) myocardial injury
  ▶Chronic (non-ischemic) myocardial injury
  ▶Unspecified (non-ischemic) myocardial injury
  ▶*Code first the underlying cause, if known and applicable, such as:*
    ▶acute kidney failure (N17.-)
    ▶acute myocarditis (I40.-)
    ▶cardiomyopathy (I42.-)
    ▶chronic kidney disease (CKD) (N18.-)
    ▶heart failure (I50.-)
    ▶hypertensive urgency (I16.0)
    ▶nonrheumatic aortic valve disorders (I35.-)
    ▶paroxysmal tachycardia (I47.-)
    ▶pulmonary embolism (I26.-)
    ▶pulmonary hypertension (I27.0, I27.2-)
    ▶sepsis (A41.-)
    ▶takotsubo syndrome (I51.81)

  ▶**Excludes1**   acute myocardial infarction (I21.-)
                  injury of heart (S26.-)

  ▶**Excludes2**   other acute ischemic heart diseases (I24.-)

● **I60   Nontraumatic subarachnoid hemorrhage**

> **Excludes1**   syphilitic ruptured cerebral aneurysm (A52.05)

> **Excludes2**   sequelae of subarachnoid hemorrhage (I69.0-)

● **I60.0   Nontraumatic subarachnoid hemorrhage from carotid siphon and bifurcation**

  I60.00   Nontraumatic subarachnoid hemorrhage from unspecified carotid siphon and bifurcation 🔖

  I60.01   Nontraumatic subarachnoid hemorrhage from right carotid siphon and bifurcation 🔖

  I60.02   Nontraumatic subarachnoid hemorrhage from left carotid siphon and bifurcation 🔖

● **I60.1   Nontraumatic subarachnoid hemorrhage from middle cerebral artery**

  I60.10   Nontraumatic subarachnoid hemorrhage from unspecified middle cerebral artery 🔖

  I60.11   Nontraumatic subarachnoid hemorrhage from right middle cerebral artery 🔖

  I60.12   Nontraumatic subarachnoid hemorrhage from left middle cerebral artery 🔖

I60.2   Nontraumatic subarachnoid hemorrhage from anterior communicating artery 🔖

● **I60.3   Nontraumatic subarachnoid hemorrhage from posterior communicating artery**

  I60.30   Nontraumatic subarachnoid hemorrhage from unspecified posterior communicating artery 🔖

  I60.31   Nontraumatic subarachnoid hemorrhage from right posterior communicating artery 🔖

  I60.32   Nontraumatic subarachnoid hemorrhage from left posterior communicating artery 🔖

I60.4   Nontraumatic subarachnoid hemorrhage from basilar artery 🔖

● **I60.5   Nontraumatic subarachnoid hemorrhage from vertebral artery**

  I60.50   Nontraumatic subarachnoid hemorrhage from unspecified vertebral artery 🔖

  I60.51   Nontraumatic subarachnoid hemorrhage from right vertebral artery 🔖

  I60.52   Nontraumatic subarachnoid hemorrhage from left vertebral artery 🔖

I60.6   Nontraumatic subarachnoid hemorrhage from other intracranial arteries 🔖

I60.7   Nontraumatic subarachnoid hemorrhage from unspecified intracranial artery 🔖
  Ruptured (congenital) berry aneurysm
  Ruptured (congenital) cerebral aneurysm
  Subarachnoid hemorrhage (nontraumatic) from cerebral artery NOS
  Subarachnoid hemorrhage (nontraumatic) from communicating artery NOS

> **Excludes1**   berry aneurysm, nonruptured (I67.1)

I60.8   Other nontraumatic subarachnoid hemorrhage 🔖
  Meningeal hemorrhage
  Rupture of cerebral arteriovenous malformation

I60.9   Nontraumatic subarachnoid hemorrhage, unspecified 🔖

● **I61   Nontraumatic intracerebral hemorrhage**

> **Excludes2**   sequelae of intracerebral hemorrhage (I69.1-)

Coding Clinic: 2017, Q2, P10

I61.0   Nontraumatic intracerebral hemorrhage in hemisphere, subcortical 🔖
  Deep intracerebral hemorrhage (nontraumatic)
  Coding Clinic: 2016, Q4, P27

I61.1   Nontraumatic intracerebral hemorrhage in hemisphere, cortical 🔖
  Cerebral lobe hemorrhage (nontraumatic)
  Superficial intracerebral hemorrhage (nontraumatic)
  Coding Clinic: 2016, Q4, P28

I61.2   Nontraumatic intracerebral hemorrhage in hemisphere, unspecified 🔖

I61.3   Nontraumatic intracerebral hemorrhage in brain stem 🔖

I61.4   Nontraumatic intracerebral hemorrhage in cerebellum 🔖

I61.5   Nontraumatic intracerebral hemorrhage, intraventricular 🔖

I61.6   Nontraumatic intracerebral hemorrhage, multiple localized 🔖

I61.8   Other nontraumatic intracerebral hemorrhage 🔖

I61.9   Nontraumatic intracerebral hemorrhage, unspecified 🔖

● **I62   Other and unspecified nontraumatic intracranial hemorrhage**

> **Excludes2**   sequelae of intracranial hemorrhage (I69.2)

● **I62.0   Nontraumatic subdural hemorrhage**

  I62.00   Nontraumatic subdural hemorrhage, unspecified 🔖

  I62.01   Nontraumatic acute subdural hemorrhage 🔖

  I62.02   Nontraumatic subacute subdural hemorrhage 🔖

  I62.03   Nontraumatic chronic subdural hemorrhage 🔖

I62.1   Nontraumatic extradural hemorrhage 🔖
  Nontraumatic epidural hemorrhage

I62.9   Nontraumatic intracranial hemorrhage, unspecified 🔖

★**(See Plate 31 of the Anatomy Illustrations.)**

● **I63   Cerebral infarction**

> **Excludes1**   neonatal cerebral infarction (P91.82-)

> **Includes**   occlusion and stenosis of cerebral and precerebral arteries, resulting in cerebral infarction

Use additional code, if applicable, to identify status post administration of tPA (rtPA) in a different facility within the last 24 hours prior to admission to current facility (Z92.82)

Use additional code, if known, to indicate National Institutes of Health Stroke Scale (NIHSS) score (R29.7-)

> **Excludes2**   sequelae of cerebral infarction (I69.3-)

Coding Clinic: 2016, Q4, P28, 61, 127

● **I63.0   Cerebral infarction due to thrombosis of precerebral arteries**

  I63.00   Cerebral infarction due to thrombosis of unspecified precerebral artery 🔖

Cerebral
embolus

Cerebral
hemorrhage

Cerebral
thrombosis

Figure 9-4 Events causing a stroke. (From Shiland: Mastering Healthcare Terminology, ed 1, St. Louis, Mosby, 2003)

● I63.01   Cerebral infarction due to thrombosis of vertebral artery
　　I63.011   Cerebral infarction due to thrombosis of right vertebral artery ⍟
　　I63.012   Cerebral infarction due to thrombosis of left vertebral artery ⍟
　　I63.013   Cerebral infarction due to thrombosis of bilateral vertebral arteries ⍟
　　I63.019   Cerebral infarction due to thrombosis of unspecified vertebral artery ⍟
　I63.02   Cerebral infarction due to thrombosis of basilar artery ⍟
● I63.03   Cerebral infarction due to thrombosis of carotid artery
　　I63.031   Cerebral infarction due to thrombosis of right carotid artery ⍟
　　I63.032   Cerebral infarction due to thrombosis of left carotid artery ⍟
　　I63.033   Cerebral infarction due to thrombosis of bilateral carotid arteries ⍟
　　I63.039   Cerebral infarction due to thrombosis of unspecified carotid artery ⍟
　I63.09   Cerebral infarction due to thrombosis of other precerebral artery ⍟
● I63.1   Cerebral infarction due to embolism of precerebral arteries
　I63.10   Cerebral infarction due to embolism of unspecified precerebral artery ⍟
● I63.11   Cerebral infarction due to embolism of vertebral artery
　　I63.111   Cerebral infarction due to embolism of right vertebral artery ⍟
　　I63.112   Cerebral infarction due to embolism of left vertebral artery ⍟
　　I63.113   Cerebral infarction due to embolism of bilateral vertebral arteries ⍟
　　I63.119   Cerebral infarction due to embolism of unspecified vertebral artery ⍟
　I63.12   Cerebral infarction due to embolism of basilar artery ⍟
● I63.13   Cerebral infarction due to embolism of carotid artery
　　I63.131   Cerebral infarction due to embolism of right carotid artery ⍟
　　I63.132   Cerebral infarction due to embolism of left carotid artery ⍟
　　I63.133   Cerebral infarction due to embolism of bilateral carotid arteries ⍟

　　I63.139   Cerebral infarction due to embolism of unspecified carotid artery ⍟
　I63.19   Cerebral infarction due to embolism of other precerebral artery ⍟
● I63.2   Cerebral infarction due to unspecified occlusion or stenosis of precerebral arteries
　I63.20   Cerebral infarction due to unspecified occlusion or stenosis of unspecified precerebral arteries ⍟
● I63.21   Cerebral infarction due to unspecified occlusion or stenosis of vertebral arteries
　　I63.211   Cerebral infarction due to unspecified occlusion or stenosis of right vertebral artery ⍟
　　I63.212   Cerebral infarction due to unspecified occlusion or stenosis of left vertebral artery ⍟
　　I63.213   Cerebral infarction due to unspecified occlusion or stenosis of bilateral vertebral arteries ⍟
　　I63.219   Cerebral infarction due to unspecified occlusion or stenosis of unspecified vertebral artery ⍟
　I63.22   Cerebral infarction due to unspecified occlusion or stenosis of basilar artery ⍟
● I63.23   Cerebral infarction due to unspecified occlusion or stenosis of carotid arteries
　　I63.231   Cerebral infarction due to unspecified occlusion or stenosis of right carotid arteries ⍟
　　I63.232   Cerebral infarction due to unspecified occlusion or stenosis of left carotid arteries ⍟
　　I63.233   Cerebral infarction due to unspecified occlusion or stenosis of bilateral carotid arteries ⍟
　　I63.239   Cerebral infarction due to unspecified occlusion or stenosis of unspecified carotid artery ⍟
　I63.29   Cerebral infarction due to unspecified occlusion or stenosis of other precerebral arteries ⍟
● I63.3   Cerebral infarction due to thrombosis of cerebral arteries
　I63.30   Cerebral infarction due to thrombosis of unspecified cerebral artery ⍟
● I63.31   Cerebral infarction due to thrombosis of middle cerebral artery
　　I63.311   Cerebral infarction due to thrombosis of right middle cerebral artery ⍟
　　I63.312   Cerebral infarction due to thrombosis of left middle cerebral artery ⍟
　　I63.313   Cerebral infarction due to thrombosis of bilateral middle cerebral arteries ⍟
　　I63.319   Cerebral infarction due to thrombosis of unspecified middle cerebral artery ⍟
● I63.32   Cerebral infarction due to thrombosis of anterior cerebral artery
　　I63.321   Cerebral infarction due to thrombosis of right anterior cerebral artery ⍟
　　I63.322   Cerebral infarction due to thrombosis of left anterior cerebral artery ⍟
　　I63.323   Cerebral infarction due to thrombosis of bilateral anterior cerebral arteries ⍟
　　I63.329   Cerebral infarction due to thrombosis of unspecified anterior cerebral artery ⍟
● I63.33   Cerebral infarction due to thrombosis of posterior cerebral artery
　　I63.331   Cerebral infarction due to thrombosis of right posterior cerebral artery ⍟

▶ New   ⇒ Revised   ~~deleted~~ Deleted   Excludes 1   Excludes 2   Includes   Use additional   Code first   Code also   Key words
OGCR Official Guidelines   X Assign placeholder X   ● Use Additional Character(s)   ▸ Manifestation Code   ⍟ Hierarchical Condition Category   **Coding Clinic**

I63.332 Cerebral infarction due to thrombosis of left posterior cerebral artery 🗫

I63.333 Cerebral infarction due to thrombosis of bilateral posterior cerebral arteries 🗫

I63.339 Cerebral infarction due to thrombosis of unspecified posterior cerebral artery 🗫

● I63.34 Cerebral infarction due to thrombosis of cerebellar artery

I63.341 Cerebral infarction due to thrombosis of right cerebellar artery 🗫

I63.342 Cerebral infarction due to thrombosis of left cerebellar artery 🗫

I63.343 Cerebral infarction due to thrombosis of bilateral cerebellar arteries 🗫

I63.349 Cerebral infarction due to thrombosis of unspecified cerebellar artery 🗫

I63.39 Cerebral infarction due to thrombosis of other cerebral artery 🗫

● I63.4 Cerebral infarction due to embolism of cerebral arteries

I63.40 Cerebral infarction due to embolism of unspecified cerebral artery 🗫

● I63.41 Cerebral infarction due to embolism of middle cerebral artery

I63.411 Cerebral infarction due to embolism of right middle cerebral artery 🗫

I63.412 Cerebral infarction due to embolism of left middle cerebral artery 🗫

I63.413 Cerebral infarction due to embolism of bilateral middle cerebral arteries 🗫

I63.419 Cerebral infarction due to embolism of unspecified middle cerebral artery 🗫

● I63.42 Cerebral infarction due to embolism of anterior cerebral artery

I63.421 Cerebral infarction due to embolism of right anterior cerebral artery 🗫

I63.422 Cerebral infarction due to embolism of left anterior cerebral artery 🗫

I63.423 Cerebral infarction due to embolism of bilateral anterior cerebral arteries 🗫

I63.429 Cerebral infarction due to embolism of unspecified anterior cerebral artery 🗫

● I63.43 Cerebral infarction due to embolism of posterior cerebral artery

I63.431 Cerebral infarction due to embolism of right posterior cerebral artery 🗫

I63.432 Cerebral infarction due to embolism of left posterior cerebral artery 🗫

I63.433 Cerebral infarction due to embolism of bilateral posterior cerebral arteries 🗫

I63.439 Cerebral infarction due to embolism of unspecified posterior cerebral artery 🗫

● I63.44 Cerebral infarction due to embolism of cerebellar artery

I63.441 Cerebral infarction due to embolism of right cerebellar artery 🗫

I63.442 Cerebral infarction due to embolism of left cerebellar artery 🗫

I63.443 Cerebral infarction due to embolism of bilateral cerebellar arteries 🗫

I63.449 Cerebral infarction due to embolism of unspecified cerebellar artery 🗫

I63.49 Cerebral infarction due to embolism of other cerebral artery 🗫

● I63.5 Cerebral infarction due to unspecified occlusion or stenosis of cerebral arteries

I63.50 Cerebral infarction due to unspecified occlusion or stenosis of unspecified cerebral artery 🗫

● I63.51 Cerebral infarction due to unspecified occlusion or stenosis of middle cerebral artery

I63.511 Cerebral infarction due to unspecified occlusion or stenosis of right middle cerebral artery 🗫

I63.512 Cerebral infarction due to unspecified occlusion or stenosis of left middle cerebral artery 🗫

I63.513 Cerebral infarction due to unspecified occlusion or stenosis of bilateral middle cerebral arteries 🗫

I63.519 Cerebral infarction due to unspecified occlusion or stenosis of unspecified middle cerebral artery 🗫

● I63.52 Cerebral infarction due to unspecified occlusion or stenosis of anterior cerebral artery

I63.521 Cerebral infarction due to unspecified occlusion or stenosis of right anterior cerebral artery 🗫

I63.522 Cerebral infarction due to unspecified occlusion or stenosis of left anterior cerebral artery 🗫

I63.523 Cerebral infarction due to unspecified occlusion or stenosis of bilateral anterior cerebral arteries 🗫

I63.529 Cerebral infarction due to unspecified occlusion or stenosis of unspecified anterior cerebral artery 🗫

● I63.53 Cerebral infarction due to unspecified occlusion or stenosis of posterior cerebral artery

I63.531 Cerebral infarction due to unspecified occlusion or stenosis of right posterior cerebral artery 🗫

I63.532 Cerebral infarction due to unspecified occlusion or stenosis of left posterior cerebral artery 🗫
Coding Clinic: 2017, Q2, P10

I63.533 Cerebral infarction due to unspecified occlusion or stenosis of bilateral posterior cerebral arteries 🗫

I63.539 Cerebral infarction due to unspecified occlusion or stenosis of unspecified posterior cerebral artery 🗫

● I63.54 Cerebral infarction due to unspecified occlusion or stenosis of cerebellar artery

I63.541 Cerebral infarction due to unspecified occlusion or stenosis of right cerebellar artery 🗫

I63.542 Cerebral infarction due to unspecified occlusion or stenosis of left cerebellar artery 🗫

I63.543 Cerebral infarction due to unspecified occlusion or stenosis of bilateral cerebellar arteries 🗫

I63.549 Cerebral infarction due to unspecified occlusion or stenosis of unspecified cerebellar artery 🗫

I63.59 Cerebral infarction due to unspecified occlusion or stenosis of other cerebral artery 🗫

I63.6 Cerebral infarction due to cerebral venous thrombosis, nonpyogenic 🗫

● I63.8 Other cerebral infarction 🗫

I63.81 Other cerebral infarction due to occlusion or stenosis of small artery 🗫
Lacunar infarction
Coding Clinic: 2018, Q4, P16

I63.89 Other cerebral infarction 🗫
Coding Clinic: 2017, Q2, P9

CHAPTER 9 (I00-I99)

I63.9   Cerebral infarction, unspecified 🅗
Stroke NOS
> **Excludes2**   transient cerebral ischemic attacks and related syndromes (G45.-)
> Coding Clinic: 2016, Q4, P62; 2015, Q1, P26

● **I65**   Occlusion and stenosis of precerebral arteries, not resulting in cerebral infarction
> **Includes**   embolism of precerebral artery
> narrowing of precerebral artery
> obstruction (complete) (partial) of precerebral artery
> thrombosis of precerebral artery
>
> **Excludes1**   insufficiency, NOS, of precerebral artery (G45.-)
> insufficiency of precerebral arteries causing cerebral infarction (I63.0-I63.2)

   ● **I65.0**   Occlusion and stenosis of vertebral artery
     I65.01   Occlusion and stenosis of right vertebral artery
     I65.02   Occlusion and stenosis of left vertebral artery
     I65.03   Occlusion and stenosis of bilateral vertebral arteries
     I65.09   Occlusion and stenosis of unspecified vertebral artery

   I65.1   Occlusion and stenosis of basilar artery
   ● **I65.2**   Occlusion and stenosis of carotid artery
     I65.21   Occlusion and stenosis of right carotid artery
     I65.22   Occlusion and stenosis of left carotid artery
     I65.23   Occlusion and stenosis of bilateral carotid arteries
       Coding Clinic: 2021, Q1, P4
     I65.29   Occlusion and stenosis of unspecified carotid artery

   I65.8   Occlusion and stenosis of other precerebral arteries
   I65.9   Occlusion and stenosis of unspecified precerebral artery
     Occlusion and stenosis of precerebral artery NOS

● **I66**   Occlusion and stenosis of cerebral arteries, not resulting in cerebral infarction
> **Includes**   embolism of cerebral artery
> narrowing of cerebral artery
> obstruction (complete) (partial) of cerebral artery
> thrombosis of cerebral artery
>
> **Excludes1**   occlusion and stenosis of cerebral artery causing cerebral infarction (I63.3-I63.5)

   ● **I66.0**   Occlusion and stenosis of middle cerebral artery
     I66.01   Occlusion and stenosis of right middle cerebral artery
     I66.02   Occlusion and stenosis of left middle cerebral artery
     I66.03   Occlusion and stenosis of bilateral middle cerebral arteries
     I66.09   Occlusion and stenosis of unspecified middle cerebral artery

   ● **I66.1**   Occlusion and stenosis of anterior cerebral artery
     I66.11   Occlusion and stenosis of right anterior cerebral artery
     I66.12   Occlusion and stenosis of left anterior cerebral artery
     I66.13   Occlusion and stenosis of bilateral anterior cerebral arteries
     I66.19   Occlusion and stenosis of unspecified anterior cerebral artery

   ● **I66.2**   Occlusion and stenosis of posterior cerebral artery
     I66.21   Occlusion and stenosis of right posterior cerebral artery
     I66.22   Occlusion and stenosis of left posterior cerebral artery
     I66.23   Occlusion and stenosis of bilateral posterior cerebral arteries

     I66.29   Occlusion and stenosis of unspecified posterior cerebral artery
   I66.3   Occlusion and stenosis of cerebellar arteries
   I66.8   Occlusion and stenosis of other cerebral arteries
     Occlusion and stenosis of perforating arteries
   I66.9   Occlusion and stenosis of unspecified cerebral artery

● **I67**   Other cerebrovascular diseases
> **Excludes2**   sequelae of the listed conditions (I69.8)

   I67.0   Dissection of cerebral arteries, nonruptured 🅗
> **Excludes1**   ruptured cerebral arteries (I60.7)

   I67.1   Cerebral aneurysm, nonruptured
     Cerebral aneurysm NOS
     Cerebral arteriovenous fistula, acquired
     Internal carotid artery aneurysm, intracranial portion
     Internal carotid artery aneurysm, NOS
> **Excludes1**   congenital cerebral aneurysm, nonruptured (Q28.-)
> ruptured cerebral aneurysm (I60.7)

   I67.2   Cerebral atherosclerosis   A
     Atheroma of cerebral and precerebral arteries

   I67.3   Progressive vascular leukoencephalopathy
     Binswanger's disease

   I67.4   Hypertensive encephalopathy
> **Excludes2**   insufficiency, NOS, of precerebral arteries (G45.2)

   I67.5   Moyamoya disease

   I67.6   Nonpyogenic thrombosis of intracranial venous system
     Nonpyogenic thrombosis of cerebral vein
     Nonpyogenic thrombosis of intracranial venous sinus
> **Excludes1**   nonpyogenic thrombosis of intracranial venous system causing infarction (I63.6)

   I67.7   Cerebral arteritis, not elsewhere classified
     Granulomatous angiitis of the nervous system
> **Excludes1**   allergic granulomatous angiitis (M30.1)

   ● **I67.8**   Other specified cerebrovascular diseases
     I67.81   Acute cerebrovascular insufficiency
       Acute cerebrovascular insufficiency unspecified as to location or reversibility
     I67.82   Cerebral ischemia
       Chronic cerebral ischemia
     I67.83   Posterior reversible encephalopathy syndrome
       PRES
     ● **I67.84**   Cerebral vasospasm and vasoconstriction
       I67.841   Reversible cerebrovascular vasoconstriction syndrome
         Call-Fleming syndrome
> *Code first underlying condition, if applicable, such as eclampsia (O15.00-O15.9)*

       I67.848   Other cerebrovascular vasospasm and vasoconstriction
     ● **I67.85**   Hereditary cerebrovascular diseases
       I67.850   Cerebral autosomal dominant arteriopathy with subcortical infarcts and leukoencephalopathy
         CADASIL
> Code also any associated diagnoses, such as:
> epilepsy (G40.-), stroke (I63.-)
> vascular dementia (F01.-)

       I67.858   Other hereditary cerebrovascular disease
     I67.89   Other cerebrovascular disease
   I67.9   Cerebrovascular disease, unspecified

I68   Cerebrovascular disorders in diseases classified elsewhere

▷ **I68.0   Cerebral amyloid angiopathy**
Code first underlying amyloidosis (E85.-)

▷ **I68.2   Cerebral arteritis in other diseases classified elsewhere**
Code first underlying disease
Excludes1 cerebral arteritis (in):
listerosis (A32.89)
systemic lupus erythematosus (M32.19)
syphilis (A52.04)
tuberculosis (A18.89)

▷ **I68.8   Other cerebrovascular disorders in diseases classified elsewhere**
Code first underlying disease
Excludes1 syphilitic cerebral aneurysm (A52.05)

OGCR Section I.c.9.d.

Sequelae of Cerebrovascular Disease

1) Category I69, Sequelae of Cerebrovascular disease

Category I69 is used to indicate conditions classifiable to categories I60-I67 as the causes of sequela (neurologic deficits), themselves classified elsewhere. These "late effects" include neurologic deficits that persist after initial onset of conditions classifiable to categories I60-I67. The neurologic deficits caused by cerebrovascular disease may be present from the onset of may arise at any time after the onset of the condition classifiable to categories I60-I67.

Codes from category I69, Sequelae of cerebrovascular disease, that specify hemiplegia, hemiparesis and monoplegia identify whether the dominant or nondominant side is affected. Should the affected side be documented, but not specified as dominant or nondominant, and the classification system does not indicate a default, code selection is as follows:

For ambidextrous patients, the default should be dominant.

If the left side is affected, the default is nondominant.

If the right side is affected, the default is dominant.

2) Codes from category I69 with codes from I60-I67

Codes from category I69 may be assigned on a health care record with codes from I60-I67, if the patient has a current cerebrovascular disease and deficits from an old cerebrovascular disease.

● **I69   Sequelae of cerebrovascular disease**
Note: Category I69 is to be used to indicate conditions in I60-I67 as the cause of sequelae. The 'sequelae' include conditions specified as such or as residuals which may occur at any time after the onset of the causal condition.

Excludes1 personal history of cerebral infarction without residual deficit (Z86.73)
personal history of prolonged reversible ischemic neurologic deficit (PRIND) (Z86.73)
personal history of reversible ischemic neurologcial deficit (RIND) (Z86.73)
sequelae of traumatic intracranial injury (S06.-)
Coding Clinic: 2016, Q4, P28; 2015, Q4, P40; 2012, Q4, P107

● **I69.0   Sequelae of nontraumatic subarachnoid hemorrhage**

I69.00   Unspecified sequelae of nontraumatic subarachnoid hemorrhage

● **I69.01   Cognitive deficits following nontraumatic subarachnoid hemorrhage**

I69.010   Attention and concentration deficit following nontraumatic subarachnoid hemorrhage

I69.011   Memory deficit following nontraumatic subarachnoid hemorrhage

I69.012   Visuospatial deficit and spatial neglect following nontraumatic subarachnoid hemorrhage

I69.013   Psychomotor deficit following nontraumatic subarachnoid hemorrhage

I69.014   Frontal lobe and executive function deficit following nontraumatic subarachnoid hemorrhage

I69.015   Cognitive social or emotional deficit following nontraumatic subarachnoid hemorrhage

I69.018   Other symptoms and signs involving cognitive functions following nontraumatic subarachnoid hemorrhage

I69.019   Unspecified symptoms and signs involving cognitive functions following nontraumatic subarachnoid hemorrhage

● **I69.02   Speech and language deficits following nontraumatic subarachnoid hemorrhage**

I69.020   Aphasia following nontraumatic subarachnoid hemorrhage

I69.021   Dysphasia following nontraumatic subarachnoid hemorrhage

I69.022   Dysarthria following nontraumatic subarachnoid hemorrhage

I69.023   Fluency disorder following nontraumatic subarachnoid hemorrhage
Stuttering following nontraumatic subarachnoid hemorrhage

I69.028   Other speech and language deficits following nontraumatic subarachnoid hemorrhage

● **I69.03   Monoplegia of upper limb following nontraumatic subarachnoid hemorrhage**

I69.031   Monoplegia of upper limb following nontraumatic subarachnoid hemorrhage affecting right dominant side 🦠

I69.032   Monoplegia of upper limb following nontraumatic subarachnoid hemorrhage affecting left dominant side 🦠

I69.033   Monoplegia of upper limb following nontraumatic subarachnoid hemorrhage affecting right non-dominant side 🦠

I69.034   Monoplegia of upper limb following nontraumatic subarachnoid hemorrhage affecting left non-dominant side 🦠

I69.039   Monoplegia of upper limb following nontraumatic subarachnoid hemorrhage affecting unspecified side 🦠

● **I69.04   Monoplegia of lower limb following nontraumatic subarachnoid hemorrhage**

I69.041   Monoplegia of lower limb following nontraumatic subarachnoid hemorrhage affecting right dominant side 🦠

I69.042   Monoplegia of lower limb following nontraumatic subarachnoid hemorrhage affecting left dominant side 🦠

I69.043   Monoplegia of lower limb following nontraumatic subarachnoid hemorrhage affecting right non-dominant side 🦠

I69.044   Monoplegia of lower limb following nontraumatic subarachnoid hemorrhage affecting left non-dominant side 🦠

I69.049   Monoplegia of lower limb following nontraumatic subarachnoid hemorrhage affecting unspecified side 🦠

CHAPTER 9 (I00-I99)

● I69.05   **Hemiplegia and hemiparesis** following nontraumatic subarachnoid hemorrhage

     I69.051   Hemiplegia and hemiparesis following nontraumatic subarachnoid hemorrhage affecting right dominant side 🐾

     I69.052   Hemiplegia and hemiparesis following nontraumatic subarachnoid hemorrhage affecting left dominant side 🐾

     I69.053   Hemiplegia and hemiparesis following nontraumatic subarachnoid hemorrhage affecting right non-dominant side 🐾

     I69.054   Hemiplegia and hemiparesis following nontraumatic subarachnoid hemorrhage affecting left non-dominant side 🐾

     I69.059   Hemiplegia and hemiparesis following nontraumatic subarachnoid hemorrhage affecting unspecified side 🐾

● I69.06   **Other paralytic syndrome** following nontraumatic subarachnoid hemorrhage

     Use additional code to identify type of paralytic syndrome, such as:
       locked-in state (G83.5)
       quadriplegia (G82.5-)

     Excludes1   hemiplegia/hemiparesis following nontraumatic subarachnoid hemorrhage (I69.05-)
                monoplegia of lower limb following nontraumatic subarachnoid hemorrhage (I69.04-)
                monoplegia of upper limb following nontraumatic subarachnoid hemorrhage (I69.03-)

     I69.061   Other paralytic syndrome following nontraumatic subarachnoid hemorrhage affecting right dominant side 🐾

     I69.062   Other paralytic syndrome following nontraumatic subarachnoid hemorrhage affecting left dominant side 🐾

     I69.063   Other paralytic syndrome following nontraumatic subarachnoid hemorrhage affecting right non-dominant side 🐾

     I69.064   Other paralytic syndrome following nontraumatic subarachnoid hemorrhage affecting left non-dominant side 🐾

     I69.065   Other paralytic syndrome following nontraumatic subarachnoid hemorrhage, bilateral 🐾

     I69.069   Other paralytic syndrome following nontraumatic subarachnoid hemorrhage affecting unspecified side 🐾

● I69.09   **Other sequelae of nontraumatic subarachnoid** hemorrhage

     I69.090   Apraxia following nontraumatic subarachnoid hemorrhage

     I69.091   Dysphagia following nontraumatic subarachnoid hemorrhage

         Use additional code to identify the type of dysphagia, if known (R13.1-)

     I69.092   Facial weakness following nontraumatic subarachnoid hemorrhage

         Facial droop following nontraumatic subarachnoid hemorrhage

     I69.093   Ataxia following nontraumatic subarachnoid hemorrhage

     I69.098   Other sequelae following nontraumatic subarachnoid hemorrhage

         Alterations of sensation following nontraumatic subarachnoid hemorrhage

         Disturbance of vision following nontraumatic subarachnoid hemorrhage

         Use additional code to identify the sequelae

● I69.1   **Sequelae of nontraumatic intracerebral hemorrhage**

     I69.10   Unspecified sequelae of nontraumatic intracerebral hemorrhage

● I69.11   **Cognitive deficits** following nontraumatic intracerebral hemorrhage

     I69.110   Attention and concentration deficit following nontraumatic intracerebral hemorrhage

     I69.111   Memory deficit following nontraumatic intracerebral hemorrhage

     I69.112   Visuospatial deficit and spatial neglect following nontraumatic intracerebral hemorrhage

     I69.113   Psychomotor deficit following nontraumatic intracerebral hemorrhage

     I69.114   Frontal lobe and executive function deficit following nontraumatic intracerebral hemorrhage

     I69.115   Cognitive social or emotional deficit following nontraumatic intracerebral hemorrhage

     I69.118   Other symptoms and signs involving cognitive functions following nontraumatic intracerebral hemorrhage

     I69.119   Unspecified symptoms and signs involving cognitive functions following nontraumatic intracerebral hemorrhage

● I69.12   **Speech and language deficits** following nontraumatic intracerebral hemorrhage

     I69.120   Aphasia following nontraumatic intracerebral hemorrhage

     I69.121   Dysphasia following nontraumatic intracerebral hemorrhage

     I69.122   Dysarthria following nontraumatic intracerebral hemorrhage

     I69.123   Fluency disorder following nontraumatic intracerebral hemorrhage

         Stuttering following nontraumatic intracerebral hemorrhage

     I69.128   Other speech and language deficits following nontraumatic intracerebral hemorrhage

● I69.13   **Monoplegia of upper limb** following nontraumatic intracerebral hemorrhage

     I69.131   Monoplegia of upper limb following nontraumatic intracerebral hemorrhage affecting right dominant side 🐾

     I69.132   Monoplegia of upper limb following nontraumatic intracerebral hemorrhage affecting left dominant side 🐾

I69.133   Monoplegia of upper limb following nontraumatic intracerebral hemorrhage affecting right non-dominant side 🦟

I69.134   Monoplegia of upper limb following nontraumatic intracerebral hemorrhage affecting left non-dominant side 🦟

I69.139   Monoplegia of upper limb following nontraumatic intracerebral hemorrhage affecting unspecified side 🦟

● I69.14   Monoplegia of lower limb following nontraumatic intracerebral hemorrhage

I69.141   Monoplegia of lower limb following nontraumatic intracerebral hemorrhage affecting right dominant side 🦟

I69.142   Monoplegia of lower limb following nontraumatic intracerebral hemorrhage affecting left dominant side 🦟

I69.143   Monoplegia of lower limb following nontraumatic intracerebral hemorrhage affecting right non-dominant side 🦟

I69.144   Monoplegia of lower limb following nontraumatic intracerebral hemorrhage affecting left non-dominant side 🦟

I69.149   Monoplegia of lower limb following nontraumatic intracerebral hemorrhage affecting unspecified side 🦟

● I69.15   Hemiplegia and hemiparesis following nontraumatic intracerebral hemorrhage

I69.151   Hemiplegia and hemiparesis following nontraumatic intracerebral hemorrhage affecting right dominant side 🦟

I69.152   Hemiplegia and hemiparesis following nontraumatic intracerebral hemorrhage affecting left dominant side 🦟

I69.153   Hemiplegia and hemiparesis following nontraumatic intracerebral hemorrhage affecting right non-dominant side 🦟

I69.154   Hemiplegia and hemiparesis following nontraumatic intracerebral hemorrhage affecting left non-dominant side 🦟

I69.159   Hemiplegia and hemiparesis following nontraumatic intracerebral hemorrhage affecting unspecified side 🦟

● I69.16   Other paralytic syndrome following nontraumatic intracerebral hemorrhage

Use additional code to identify type of paralytic syndrome, such as:
locked-in state (G83.5)
quadriplegia (G82.5-)

Excludes1   hemiplegia/hemiparesis following nontraumatic intracerebral hemorrhage (I69.15-)
monoplegia of lower limb following nontraumatic intracerebral hemorrhage (I69.14-)
monoplegia of upper limb following nontraumatic intracerebral hemorrhage (I69.13-)

I69.161   Other paralytic syndrome following nontraumatic intracerebral hemorrhage affecting right dominant side 🦟

I69.162   Other paralytic syndrome following nontraumatic intracerebral hemorrhage affecting left dominant side 🦟

I69.163   Other paralytic syndrome following nontraumatic intracerebral hemorrhage affecting right non-dominant side 🦟

I69.164   Other paralytic syndrome following nontraumatic intracerebral hemorrhage affecting left non-dominant side 🦟

I69.165   Other paralytic syndrome following nontraumatic intracerebral hemorrhage, bilateral 🦟

I69.169   Other paralytic syndrome following nontraumatic intracerebral hemorrhage affecting unspecified side 🦟

● I69.19   Other sequelae of nontraumatic intracerebral hemorrhage

I69.190   Apraxia following nontraumatic intracerebral hemorrhage

I69.191   Dysphagia following nontraumatic intracerebral hemorrhage

Use additional code to identify the type of dysphagia, if known (R13.1-)

I69.192   Facial weakness following nontraumatic intracerebral hemorrhage

Facial droop following nontraumatic intracerebral hemorrhage

I69.193   Ataxia following nontraumatic intracerebral hemorrhage

I69.198   Other sequelae of nontraumatic intracerebral hemorrhage

Alteration of sensations following nontraumatic intracerebral hemorrhage

Disturbance of vision following nontraumatic intracerebral hemorrhage

Use additional code to identify the sequelae

● I69.2   Sequelae of other nontraumatic intracranial hemorrhage

I69.20   Unspecified sequelae of other nontraumatic intracranial hemorrhage

● I69.21   Cognitive deficits following other nontraumatic intracranial hemorrhage

I69.210   Attention and concentration deficit following other nontraumatic intracranial hemorrhage

I69.211   Memory deficit following other nontraumatic intracranial hemorrhage

I69.212   Visuospatial deficit and spatial neglect following other nontraumatic intracranial hemorrhage

I69.213   Psychomotor deficit following other nontraumatic intracranial hemorrhage

I69.214   Frontal lobe and executive function deficit following other nontraumatic intracranial hemorrhage

I69.215   Cognitive social or emotional deficit following other nontraumatic intracranial hemorrhage

I69.218   Other symptoms and signs involving cognitive functions following other nontraumatic intracranial hemorrhage

I69.219   Unspecified symptoms and signs involving cognitive functions following other nontraumatic intracranial hemorrhage

CHAPTER 9 (I00-I99)

● **I69.22** **Speech and language deficits** following other nontraumatic intracranial hemorrhage

    I69.220 **Aphasia** following other nontraumatic intracranial hemorrhage

    I69.221 **Dysphasia** following other nontraumatic intracranial hemorrhage

    I69.222 **Dysarthria** following other nontraumatic intracranial hemorrhage

    I69.223 **Fluency disorder** following other nontraumatic intracranial hemorrhage
        Stuttering following other nontraumatic intracranial hemorrhage

    I69.228 **Other speech and language deficits** following other nontraumatic intracranial hemorrhage

● **I69.23** **Monoplegia of upper limb** following other nontraumatic intracranial hemorrhage

    I69.231 Monoplegia of upper limb following other nontraumatic intracranial hemorrhage affecting **right dominant side** 🏷

    I69.232 Monoplegia of upper limb following other nontraumatic intracranial hemorrhage affecting **left dominant side** 🏷

    I69.233 Monoplegia of upper limb following other nontraumatic intracranial hemorrhage affecting **right non-dominant side** 🏷

    I69.234 Monoplegia of upper limb following other nontraumatic intracranial hemorrhage affecting **left non-dominant side** 🏷

    I69.239 Monoplegia of upper limb following other nontraumatic intracranial hemorrhage affecting **unspecified side** 🏷

● **I69.24** **Monoplegia of lower limb** following other nontraumatic intracranial hemorrhage

    I69.241 Monoplegia of lower limb following other nontraumatic intracranial hemorrhage affecting **right dominant side** 🏷

    I69.242 Monoplegia of lower limb following other nontraumatic intracranial hemorrhage affecting **left dominant side** 🏷

    I69.243 Monoplegia of lower limb following other nontraumatic intracranial hemorrhage affecting **right non-dominant side** 🏷

    I69.244 Monoplegia of lower limb following other nontraumatic intracranial hemorrhage affecting **left non-dominant side** 🏷

    I69.249 Monoplegia of lower limb following other nontraumatic intracranial hemorrhage affecting **unspecified side** 🏷

● **I69.25** **Hemiplegia and hemiparesis** following other nontraumatic intracranial hemorrhage

    I69.251 Hemiplegia and hemiparesis following other nontraumatic intracranial hemorrhage affecting **right dominant side** 🏷

    I69.252 Hemiplegia and hemiparesis following other nontraumatic intracranial hemorrhage affecting **left dominant side** 🏷

    I69.253 Hemiplegia and hemiparesis following other nontraumatic intracranial hemorrhage affecting **right non-dominant side** 🏷

    I69.254 Hemiplegia and hemiparesis following other nontraumatic intracranial hemorrhage affecting **left non-dominant side** 🏷

    I69.259 Hemiplegia and hemiparesis following other nontraumatic intracranial hemorrhage affecting **unspecified side** 🏷

● **I69.26** **Other paralytic syndrome** following other nontraumatic intracranial hemorrhage
    Use additional code to identify type of paralytic syndrome, such as:
    locked-in state (G83.5)
    quadriplegia (G82.5-)

    Excludes1 hemiplegia/hemiparesis following other nontraumatic intracranial hemorrhage (I69.25-)
        monoplegia of lower limb following other nontraumatic intracranial hemorrhage (I69.24-)
        monoplegia of upper limb following other nontraumatic intracranial hemorrhage (I69.23-)

    I69.261 Other paralytic syndrome following other nontraumatic intracranial hemorrhage affecting **right dominant side** 🏷

    I69.262 Other paralytic syndrome following other nontraumatic intracranial hemorrhage affecting **left dominant side** 🏷

    I69.263 Other paralytic syndrome following other nontraumatic intracranial hemorrhage affecting **right non-dominant side** 🏷

    I69.264 Other paralytic syndrome following other nontraumatic intracranial hemorrhage affecting **left non-dominant side** 🏷

    I69.265 Other paralytic syndrome following other nontraumatic intracranial hemorrhage, **bilateral** 🏷

    I69.269 Other paralytic syndrome following other nontraumatic intracranial hemorrhage affecting **unspecified side** 🏷

● **I69.29** **Other sequelae** of other nontraumatic intracranial hemorrhage

    I69.290 **Apraxia** following other nontraumatic intracranial hemorrhage

    I69.291 **Dysphagia** following other nontraumatic intracranial hemorrhage
        Use additional code to identify the type of dysphagia, if known (R13.1-)

    I69.292 **Facial weakness** following other nontraumatic intracranial hemorrhage
        Facial droop following other nontraumatic intracranial hemorrhage

    I69.293 **Ataxia** following other nontraumatic intracranial hemorrhage

    I69.298 **Other sequelae** of other nontraumatic intracranial hemorrhage
        Alteration of sensation following other nontraumatic intracranial hemorrhage
        Disturbance of vision following other nontraumatic intracranial hemorrhage
        Use additional code to identify the sequelae

CHAPTER 9 (I00-I99)

▶ New   ⇒ Revised   ~~deleted~~ Deleted   Excludes 1   Excludes 2   Includes   Use additional   Code first   Code also   Key words

OGCR Official Guidelines   X Assign placeholder X   ● Use Additional Character(s)   ▷ Manifestation Code   🏷 Hierarchical Condition Category   **Coding Clinic**

● **I69.3**   **Sequelae of cerebral infarction**
Sequelae of stroke NOS
Coding Clinic: 2012, Q4, P92, 95

    I69.30   **Unspecified sequelae of cerebral infarction**

●   I69.31   **Cognitive deficits** following cerebral infarction

       I69.310   **Attention and concentration** deficit following cerebral infarction

       I69.311   **Memory** deficit following cerebral infarction

       I69.312   **Visuospatial** deficit and spatial neglect following cerebral infarction

       I69.313   **Psychomotor** deficit following cerebral infarction

       I69.314   **Frontal lobe and executive function** deficit following cerebral infarction

       I69.315   **Cognitive social or emotional** deficit following cerebral infarction

       I69.318   **Other symptoms and signs** involving cognitive functions following cerebral infarction

       I69.319   **Unspecified symptoms and signs** involving cognitive functions following cerebral infarction

●   I69.32   **Speech and language** deficits following cerebral infarction

       I69.320   **Aphasia** following cerebral infarction

       I69.321   **Dysphasia** following cerebral infarction
Coding Clinic: 2012, Q4, P91

       I69.322   **Dysarthria** following cerebral infarction

          Excludes2   transient ischemic attack (TIA) (G45.9)

       I69.323   **Fluency disorder** following cerebral infarction
Stuttering following cerebral infarction

       I69.328   **Other speech and language** deficits following cerebral infarction

●   I69.33   **Monoplegia of upper limb** following cerebral infarction
Coding Clinic: 2017, Q1, P47

       I69.331   Monoplegia of upper limb following cerebral infarction affecting **right dominant side** 🐾

       I69.332   Monoplegia of upper limb following cerebral infarction affecting **left dominant side** 🐾

       I69.333   Monoplegia of upper limb following cerebral infarction affecting **right non-dominant side** 🐾

       I69.334   Monoplegia of upper limb following cerebral infarction affecting **left non-dominant side** 🐾

       I69.339   Monoplegia of upper limb following cerebral infarction affecting unspecified side 🐾

●   I69.34   **Monoplegia of lower limb** following cerebral infarction
Coding Clinic: 2017, Q1, P47

       I69.341   Monoplegia of lower limb following cerebral infarction affecting **right dominant side** 🐾

       I69.342   Monoplegia of lower limb following cerebral infarction affecting **left dominant side** 🐾

       I69.343   Monoplegia of lower limb following cerebral infarction affecting **right non-dominant side** 🐾

       I69.344   Monoplegia of lower limb following cerebral infarction affecting **left non-dominant side** 🐾

       I69.349   Monoplegia of lower limb following cerebral infarction affecting unspecified side 🐾

●   I69.35   **Hemiplegia and hemiparesis** following cerebral infarction

       I69.351   Hemiplegia and hemiparesis following cerebral infarction affecting **right dominant side** 🐾

          Excludes2   transient ischemic attack (TIA) (G45.9)
Coding Clinic: 2015, Q1, P25

       I69.352   Hemiplegia and hemiparesis following cerebral infarction affecting **left dominant side** 🐾

       I69.353   Hemiplegia and hemiparesis following cerebral infarction affecting **right non-dominant side** 🐾

       I69.354   Hemiplegia and hemiparesis following cerebral infarction affecting **left non-dominant side** 🐾
Coding Clinic: 2012, Q4, P91

       I69.359   Hemiplegia and hemiparesis following cerebral infarction affecting unspecified side 🐾

●   I69.36   **Other paralytic syndrome** following cerebral infarction

       Use additional code to identify type of paralytic syndrome, such as:
locked-in state (G83.5)
quadriplegia (G82.5-)

       Excludes1   hemiplegia/hemiparesis following cerebral infarction (I69.35-)
monoplegia of lower limb following cerebral infarction (I69.34-)
monoplegia of upper limb following cerebral infarction (I69.33-)

       I69.361   Other paralytic syndrome following cerebral infarction affecting **right dominant side** 🐾

       I69.362   Other paralytic syndrome following cerebral infarction affecting **left dominant side** 🐾

       I69.363   Other paralytic syndrome following cerebral infarction affecting **right non-dominant side** 🐾

       I69.364   Other paralytic syndrome following cerebral infarction affecting **left non-dominant side** 🐾

       I69.365   Other paralytic syndrome following cerebral infarction, **bilateral** 🐾

       I69.369   Other paralytic syndrome following cerebral infarction affecting unspecified side 🐾

●   I69.39   **Other sequelae of cerebral infarction**

       I69.390   **Apraxia** following cerebral infarction

       I69.391   **Dysphagia** following cerebral infarction

          Use additional code to identify the type of dysphagia, if known (R13.1-)

       I69.392   **Facial weakness** following cerebral infarction
Facial droop following cerebral infarction

       I69.393   **Ataxia** following cerebral infarction

       I69.398   **Other sequelae** of cerebral infarction
Alteration of sensation following cerebral infarction
Disturbance of vision following cerebral infarction

          Use additional code to identify the sequelae

CHAPTER 9 (I00–I99)

● **I69.8 Sequelae of other cerebrovascular diseases**

   Excludes1 sequelae of traumatic intracranial injury (S06.-)

  I69.80 Unspecified sequelae of other cerebrovascular disease

● I69.81 Cognitive deficits following other cerebrovascular disease

    I69.810 Attention and concentration deficit following other cerebrovascular disease

    I69.811 Memory deficit following other cerebrovascular disease

    I69.812 Visuospatial deficit and spatial neglect following other cerebrovascular disease

    I69.813 Psychomotor deficit following other cerebrovascular disease

    I69.814 Frontal lobe and executive function deficit following other cerebrovascular disease

    I69.815 Cognitive social or emotional deficit following other cerebrovascular disease

    I69.818 Other symptoms and signs involving cognitive functions following other cerebrovascular disease

    I69.819 Unspecified symptoms and signs involving cognitive functions following other cerebrovascular disease

● I69.82 Speech and language deficits following other cerebrovascular disease

    I69.820 Aphasia following other cerebrovascular disease

    I69.821 Dysphasia following other cerebrovascular disease

    I69.822 Dysarthria following other cerebrovascular disease

    I69.823 Fluency disorder following other cerebrovascular disease
      Stuttering following other cerebrovascular disease
      Coding Clinic: 2019, Q3, P9

    I69.828 Other speech and language deficits following other cerebrovascular disease

● I69.83 Monoplegia of upper limb following other cerebrovascular disease

    I69.831 Monoplegia of upper limb following other cerebrovascular disease affecting right dominant side

    I69.832 Monoplegia of upper limb following other cerebrovascular disease affecting left dominant side

    I69.833 Monoplegia of upper limb following other cerebrovascular disease affecting right non-dominant side

    I69.834 Monoplegia of upper limb following other cerebrovascular disease affecting left non-dominant side

    I69.839 Monoplegia of upper limb following other cerebrovascular disease affecting unspecified side

● I69.84 Monoplegia of lower limb following other cerebrovascular disease

    I69.841 Monoplegia of lower limb following other cerebrovascular disease affecting right dominant side

    I69.842 Monoplegia of lower limb following other cerebrovascular disease affecting left dominant side

    I69.843 Monoplegia of lower limb following other cerebrovascular disease affecting right non-dominant side

    I69.844 Monoplegia of lower limb following other cerebrovascular disease affecting left non-dominant side

    I69.849 Monoplegia of lower limb following other cerebrovascular disease affecting unspecified side

● I69.85 Hemiplegia and hemiparesis following other cerebrovascular disease

    I69.851 Hemiplegia and hemiparesis following other cerebrovascular disease affecting right dominant side

    I69.852 Hemiplegia and hemiparesis following other cerebrovascular disease affecting left dominant side

    I69.853 Hemiplegia and hemiparesis following other cerebrovascular disease affecting right non-dominant side

    I69.854 Hemiplegia and hemiparesis following other cerebrovascular disease affecting left non-dominant side

    I69.859 Hemiplegia and hemiparesis following other cerebrovascular disease affecting unspecified side

● I69.86 Other paralytic syndrome following other cerebrovascular disease

   Use additional code to identify type of paralytic syndrome, such as:
   locked-in state (G83.5)
   quadriplegia (G82.5)

   Excludes1 hemiplegia/hemiparesis following other cerebrovascular disease (I69.85-)
     monoplegia of lower limb following other cerebrovascular disease (I69.84-)
     monoplegia of upper limb following other cerebrovascular disease (I69.83-)

    I69.861 Other paralytic syndrome following other cerebrovascular disease affecting right dominant side

    I69.862 Other paralytic syndrome following other cerebrovascular disease affecting left dominant side

    I69.863 Other paralytic syndrome following other cerebrovascular disease affecting right non-dominant side

    I69.864 Other paralytic syndrome following other cerebrovascular disease affecting left non-dominant side

    I69.865 Other paralytic syndrome following other cerebrovascular disease, bilateral

    I69.869 Other paralytic syndrome following other cerebrovascular disease affecting unspecified side

● I69.89 Other sequelae of other cerebrovascular disease

    I69.890 Apraxia following other cerebrovascular disease

    I69.891 Dysphagia following other cerebrovascular disease
      Use additional code to identify the type of dysphagia, if known (R13.1-)

CHAPTER 9 (I00-I99)

I69.892   **Facial weakness** following other cerebrovascular disease
          Facial droop following other cerebrovascular disease

I69.893   **Ataxia** following other cerebrovascular disease

I69.898   **Other sequelae** of other cerebrovascular disease
          Alteration of sensation following other cerebrovascular disease
          Disturbance of vision following other cerebrovascular disease
          Use additional code to identify the sequelae

● I69.9   Sequelae of unspecified cerebrovascular diseases
          Excludes1   sequelae of stroke (I69.3)
                          sequelae of traumatic intracranial injury (S06.-)

I69.90   **Unspecified** sequelae of unspecified cerebrovascular disease

● I69.91 **Cognitive deficits** following unspecified cerebrovascular disease

I69.910   **Attention and concentration** deficit following unspecified cerebrovascular disease

I69.911   **Memory** deficit following unspecified cerebrovascular disease

I69.912   **Visuospatial** deficit and spatial neglect following unspecified cerebrovascular disease

I69.913   **Psychomotor** deficit following unspecified cerebrovascular disease

I69.914   **Frontal lobe and executive function** deficit following unspecified cerebrovascular disease

I69.915   **Cognitive social or emotional** deficit following unspecified cerebrovascular disease

I69.918   **Other** symptoms and signs involving cognitive functions following unspecified cerebrovascular disease

I69.919   **Unspecified** symptoms and signs involving cognitive functions following unspecified cerebrovascular disease

● I69.92 **Speech and language** deficits following unspecified cerebrovascular disease

I69.920   **Aphasia** following unspecified cerebrovascular disease

I69.921   **Dysphasia** following unspecified cerebrovascular disease

I69.922   **Dysarthria** following unspecified cerebrovascular disease

I69.923   **Fluency disorder** following unspecified cerebrovascular disease
          Stuttering following unspecified cerebrovascular disease

I69.928   **Other speech and language deficits** following unspecified cerebrovascular disease

● I69.93 **Monoplegia of upper limb** following unspecified cerebrovascular disease

I69.931   Monoplegia of upper limb following unspecified cerebrovascular disease affecting right dominant side 🦠

I69.932   Monoplegia of upper limb following unspecified cerebrovascular disease affecting left dominant side 🦠

I69.933   Monoplegia of upper limb following unspecified cerebrovascular disease affecting right non-dominant side 🦠

I69.934   Monoplegia of upper limb following unspecified cerebrovascular disease affecting left non-dominant side 🦠

I69.939   Monoplegia of upper limb following unspecified cerebrovascular disease affecting unspecified side 🦠

● I69.94 **Monoplegia of lower limb** following unspecified cerebrovascular disease

I69.941   Monoplegia of lower limb following unspecified cerebrovascular disease affecting right dominant side 🦠

I69.942   Monoplegia of lower limb following unspecified cerebrovascular disease affecting left dominant side 🦠

I69.943   Monoplegia of lower limb following unspecified cerebrovascular disease affecting right non-dominant side 🦠

I69.944   Monoplegia of lower limb following unspecified cerebrovascular disease affecting left non-dominant side 🦠

I69.949   Monoplegia of lower limb following unspecified cerebrovascular disease affecting unspecified side 🦠

● I69.95 **Hemiplegia and hemiparesis** following unspecified cerebrovascular disease

I69.951   Hemiplegia and hemiparesis following unspecified cerebrovascular disease affecting right dominant side 🦠

I69.952   Hemiplegia and hemiparesis following unspecified cerebrovascular disease affecting left dominant side 🦠

I69.953   Hemiplegia and hemiparesis following unspecified cerebrovascular disease affecting right non-dominant side 🦠

I69.954   Hemiplegia and hemiparesis following unspecified cerebrovascular disease affecting left non-dominant side 🦠

I69.959   Hemiplegia and hemiparesis following unspecified cerebrovascular disease affecting unspecified side 🦠

● I69.96 **Other paralytic syndrome** following unspecified cerebrovascular disease
          Use additional code to identify type of paralytic syndrome, such as:
          locked-in state (G83.5)
          quadriplegia (G82.5-)
          Excludes1   hemiplegia/hemiparesis following unspecified cerebrovascular disease (I69.95-)
                          monoplegia of lower limb following unspecified cerebrovascular disease (I69.94-)
                          monoplegia of upper limb following unspecified cerebrovascular disease (I69.93-)

I69.961   Other paralytic syndrome following unspecified cerebrovascular disease affecting right dominant side 🦠

I69.962   Other paralytic syndrome following unspecified cerebrovascular disease affecting left dominant side 🦠

I69.963   Other paralytic syndrome following unspecified cerebrovascular disease affecting right non-dominant side 🦠

I69.964 Other paralytic syndrome following unspecified cerebrovascular disease affecting left non-dominant side 🦠

I69.965 Other paralytic syndrome following unspecified cerebrovascular disease, bilateral 🦠

I69.969 Other paralytic syndrome following unspecified cerebrovascular disease affecting unspecified side 🦠

● **I69.99** Other sequelae of unspecified cerebrovascular disease

I69.990 Apraxia following unspecified cerebrovascular disease

I69.991 Dysphagia following unspecified cerebrovascular disease

Use additional code to identify the type of dysphagia, if known (R13.1-)

I69.992 Facial weakness following unspecified cerebrovascular disease
Facial droop following unspecified cerebrovascular disease

I69.993 Ataxia following unspecified cerebrovascular disease

I69.998 Other sequelae following unspecified cerebrovascular disease
Alteration in sensation following unspecified cerebrovascular disease
Disturbance of vision following unspecified cerebrovascular disease
Use additional code to identify the sequelae

DISEASES OF ARTERIES, ARTERIOLES AND CAPILLARIES (I70-I79)

● **I70** Atherosclerosis

Includes arteriolosclerosis
arterial degeneration
arteriosclerosis
arteriosclerotic vascular disease
arteriovascular degeneration
atheroma
endarteritis deformans or obliterans
senile arteritis
senile endarteritis
vascular degeneration

Use additional code to identify:
exposure to environmental tobacco smoke (Z77.22)
history of tobacco dependence (Z87.891)
occupational exposure to environmental tobacco smoke (Z57.31)
tobacco dependence (F17.-)
tobacco use (Z72.0)

Excludes2 arteriosclerotic cardiovascular disease (I25.1-)
arteriosclerotic heart disease (I25.1-)
atheroembolism (I75.-)
cerebral atherosclerosis (I67.2)
coronary atherosclerosis (I25.1-)
mesenteric atherosclerosis (K55.1)
precerebral atherosclerosis (I67.2)
primary pulmonary atherosclerosis (I27.0)

I70.0 Atherosclerosis of aorta 🦠   A

I70.1 Atherosclerosis of renal artery 🦠   A
Goldblatt's kidney
Excludes2 atherosclerosis of renal arterioles (I12.-)

★ **(See Plates 500, 501, and 502 on pages 60 – 62.)**

● **I70.2** Atherosclerosis of native arteries of the extremities
Mönckeberg's (medial) sclerosis
Use additional code, if applicable, to identify chronic total occlusion of artery of extremity (I70.92)
Excludes2 atherosclerosis of bypass graft of extremities (I70.30-I70.79)

● **I70.20** Unspecified atherosclerosis of native arteries of extremities

I70.201 Unspecified atherosclerosis of native arteries of extremities, right leg 🦠   A

I70.202 Unspecified atherosclerosis of native arteries of extremities, left leg 🦠   A

I70.203 Unspecified atherosclerosis of native arteries of extremities, bilateral legs 🦠   A

I70.208 Unspecified atherosclerosis of native arteries of extremities, other extremity 🦠   A

I70.209 Unspecified atherosclerosis of native arteries of extremities, unspecified extremity 🦠   A

● **I70.21** Atherosclerosis of native arteries of extremities with intermittent claudication

I70.211 Atherosclerosis of native arteries of extremities with intermittent claudication, right leg 🦠   A

I70.212 Atherosclerosis of native arteries of extremities with intermittent claudication, left leg 🦠   A

I70.213 Atherosclerosis of native arteries of extremities with intermittent claudication, bilateral legs 🦠   A

I70.218 Atherosclerosis of native arteries of extremities with intermittent claudication, other extremity 🦠   A

I70.219 Atherosclerosis of native arteries of extremities with intermittent claudication, unspecified extremity 🦠   A

● **I70.22** Atherosclerosis of native arteries of extremities with rest pain
Includes any condition classifiable to I70.21-
chronic limb-threatening ischemia NOS of native arteries of extremities
chronic limb-threatening ischemia of native arteries of extremities with rest pain
critical limb ischemia NOS of native arteries of extremities
critical limb ischemia of native arteries of extremities with rest pain

I70.221 Atherosclerosis of native arteries of extremities with rest pain, right leg 🦠   A

I70.222 Atherosclerosis of native arteries of extremities with rest pain, left leg 🦠   A

I70.223 Atherosclerosis of native arteries of extremities with rest pain, bilateral legs 🦠   A

I70.228 Atherosclerosis of native arteries of extremities with rest pain, other extremity 🦠   A

I70.229 Atherosclerosis of native arteries of extremities with rest pain, unspecified extremity 🦠   A

● **I70.23**   Atherosclerosis of native arteries of right leg with ulceration

     Includes   any condition classifiable to I70.211 and I70.221
             chronic limb-threatening ischemia of native arteries of right leg with ulceration
             critical limb ischemia of native arteries of right leg with ulceration

     Use additional code to identify severity of ulcer (L97.-)

I70.231   Atherosclerosis of native arteries of right leg with ulceration of thigh 🔎 A

I70.232   Atherosclerosis of native arteries of right leg with ulceration of calf 🔎 A

I70.233   Atherosclerosis of native arteries of right leg with ulceration of ankle 🔎 A

I70.234   Atherosclerosis of native arteries of right leg with ulceration of heel and midfoot 🔎 A
     Atherosclerosis of native arteries of right leg with ulceration of plantar surface of midfoot

I70.235   Atherosclerosis of native arteries of right leg with ulceration of other part of foot 🔎 A
     Atherosclerosis of native arteries of right leg extremities with ulceration of toe

I70.238   Atherosclerosis of native arteries of right leg with ulceration of other part of lower leg 🔎 A

I70.239   Atherosclerosis of native arteries of right leg with ulceration of unspecified site 🔎 A

● **I70.24**   Atherosclerosis of native arteries of left leg with ulceration

     Includes   any condition classifiable to I70.212 and I70.222
             chronic limb-threatening ischemia of native arteries of left leg with ulceration
             critical limb ischemia of native arteries of left leg with ulceration

     Use additional code to identify severity of ulcer (L97.-)

I70.241   Atherosclerosis of native arteries of left leg with ulceration of thigh 🔎 A

I70.242   Atherosclerosis of native arteries of left leg with ulceration of calf 🔎 A

I70.243   Atherosclerosis of native arteries of left leg with ulceration of ankle 🔎 A

I70.244   Atherosclerosis of native arteries of left leg with ulceration of heel and midfoot 🔎 A
     Atherosclerosis of native arteries of left leg with ulceration of plantar surface of midfoot

I70.245   Atherosclerosis of native arteries of left leg with ulceration of other part of foot 🔎 A
     Atherosclerosis of native arteries of left leg extremities with ulceration of toe

I70.248   Atherosclerosis of native arteries of left leg with ulceration of other part of lower leg 🔎 A

I70.249   Atherosclerosis of native arteries of left leg with ulceration of unspecified site 🔎 A

I70.25   Atherosclerosis of native arteries of other extremities with ulceration 🔎 A

     Includes   any condition classifiable to I70.218 and I70.228

     Use additional code to identify the severity of the ulcer (L98.49-)

● **I70.26**   Atherosclerosis of native arteries of extremities with gangrene

     Includes   any condition classifiable to I70.21-, I70.22-, I70.23-, I70.24-, and I70.25-
             chronic limb-threatening ischemia of native arteries of extremities with gangrene
             critical limb ischemia of native arteries of extremities with gangrene

     Use additional code to identify the severity of any ulcer (L97.-, L98.49-), if applicable

I70.261   Atherosclerosis of native arteries of extremities with gangrene, right leg A

I70.262   Atherosclerosis of native arteries of extremities with gangrene, left leg 🔎 A

I70.263   Atherosclerosis of native arteries of extremities with gangrene, bilateral legs 🔎 A

I70.268   Atherosclerosis of native arteries of extremities with gangrene, other extremity 🔎 A

I70.269   Atherosclerosis of native arteries of extremities with gangrene, unspecified extremity 🔎 A

● **I70.29**   Other atherosclerosis of native arteries of extremities

I70.291   Other atherosclerosis of native arteries of extremities, right leg 🔎

I70.292   Other atherosclerosis of native arteries of extremities, left leg 🔎 A

I70.293   Other atherosclerosis of native arteries of extremities, bilateral legs 🔎 A

I70.298   Other atherosclerosis of native arteries of extremities, other extremity 🔎 A

I70.299   Other atherosclerosis of native arteries of extremities, unspecified extremity 🔎 A

● **I70.3**   Atherosclerosis of unspecified type of bypass graft(s) of the extremities

     Use additional code, if applicable, to identify chronic total occlusion of artery of extremity (I70.92)

     Excludes1   embolism or thrombus of bypass graft(s) of extremities (T82.8-)

● **I70.30**   Unspecified atherosclerosis of unspecified type of bypass graft(s) of the extremities

I70.301   Unspecified atherosclerosis of unspecified type of bypass graft(s) of the extremities, right leg 🔎 A

I70.302   Unspecified atherosclerosis of unspecified type of bypass graft(s) of the extremities, left leg 🔎 A

I70.303   Unspecified atherosclerosis of unspecified type of bypass graft(s) of the extremities, bilateral legs 🔎 A

I70.308   Unspecified atherosclerosis of unspecified type of bypass graft(s) of the extremities, other extremity 🔎 A

I70.309   Unspecified atherosclerosis of unspecified type of bypass graft(s) of the extremities, unspecified extremity 🔎 A

● **I70.31**   **Atherosclerosis of unspecified type of bypass graft(s) of the extremities with intermittent claudication**

    I70.311   Atherosclerosis of unspecified type of bypass graft(s) of the extremities with intermittent claudication, right leg 🦀   A

    I70.312   Atherosclerosis of unspecified type of bypass graft(s) of the extremities with intermittent claudication, left leg 🦀   A

    I70.313   Atherosclerosis of unspecified type of bypass graft(s) of the extremities with intermittent claudication, bilateral legs 🦀   A

    I70.318   Atherosclerosis of unspecified type of bypass graft(s) of the extremities with intermittent claudication, other extremity 🦀   A

    I70.319   Atherosclerosis of unspecified type of bypass graft(s) of the extremities with intermittent claudication, unspecified extremity 🦀   A

● **I70.32**   **Atherosclerosis of unspecified type of bypass graft(s) of the extremities with rest pain**

    Includes   any condition classifiable to I70.31-
chronic limb-threatening ischemia NOS of unspecified type of bypass graft(s) of the extremities
chronic limb-threatening ischemia of unspecified type of bypass graft(s) of the extremities with rest pain, right leg
critical limb ischemia NOS of unspecified type of bypass graft(s) of the extremities
critical limb ischemia of unspecified type of bypass graft(s) of the extremities with rest pain

    I70.321   Atherosclerosis of unspecified type of bypass graft(s) of the extremities with rest pain, right leg 🦀   A

    I70.322   Atherosclerosis of unspecified type of bypass graft(s) of the extremities with rest pain, left leg 🦀   A

    I70.323   Atherosclerosis of unspecified type of bypass graft(s) of the extremities with rest pain, bilateral legs 🦀   A

    I70.328   Atherosclerosis of unspecified type of bypass graft(s) of the extremities with rest pain, other extremity 🦀   A

    I70.329   Atherosclerosis of unspecified type of bypass graft(s) of the extremities with rest pain, unspecified extremity 🦀   A

● **I70.33**   **Atherosclerosis of unspecified type of bypass graft(s) of the right leg with ulceration**

    Includes   any condition classifiable to I70.311 and I70.321
chronic limb-threatening ischemia of unspecified type of bypass graft(s) of the right leg with ulceration
critical limb ischemia of unspecified type of bypass graft(s) of the right leg with ulceration

    Use additional code to identify severity of ulcer (L97.-)

    I70.331   Atherosclerosis of unspecified type of bypass graft(s) of the right leg with ulceration of thigh 🦀   A

I70.332   Atherosclerosis of unspecified type of bypass graft(s) of the right leg with ulceration of calf 🦀   A

I70.333   Atherosclerosis of unspecified type of bypass graft(s) of the right leg with ulceration of ankle 🦀   A

I70.334   Atherosclerosis of unspecified type of bypass graft(s) of the right leg with ulceration of heel and midfoot 🦀   A
Atherosclerosis of unspecified type of bypass graft(s) of right leg with ulceration of plantar surface of midfoot

I70.335   Atherosclerosis of unspecified type of bypass graft(s) of the right leg with ulceration of other part of foot 🦀   A
Atherosclerosis of unspecified type of bypass graft(s) of the right leg with ulceration of toe

I70.338   Atherosclerosis of unspecified type of bypass graft(s) of the right leg with ulceration of other part of lower leg 🦀   A

I70.339   Atherosclerosis of unspecified type of bypass graft(s) of the right leg with ulceration of unspecified site 🦀   A

● **I70.34**   **Atherosclerosis of unspecified type of bypass graft(s) of the left leg with ulceration**

    Includes   any condition classifiable to I70.312 and I70.322
chronic limb-threatening ischemia of unspecified type of bypass graft(s) of the left leg with ulceration
critical limb ischemia of unspecified type of bypass graft(s) of the left leg with ulceration

    Use additional code to identify severity of ulcer (L97.-)

    I70.341   Atherosclerosis of unspecified type of bypass graft(s) of the left leg with ulceration of thigh 🦀   A

    I70.342   Atherosclerosis of unspecified type of bypass graft(s) of the left leg with ulceration of calf 🦀   A

    I70.343   Atherosclerosis of unspecified type of bypass graft(s) of the left leg with ulceration of ankle 🦀   A

    I70.344   Atherosclerosis of unspecified type of bypass graft(s) of the left leg with ulceration of heel and midfoot 🦀   A
Atherosclerosis of unspecified type of bypass graft(s) of left leg with ulceration of plantar surface of midfoot

    I70.345   Atherosclerosis of unspecified type of bypass graft(s) of the left leg with ulceration of other part of foot 🦀   A
Atherosclerosis of unspecified type of bypass graft(s) of the left leg with ulceration of toe

    I70.348   Atherosclerosis of unspecified type of bypass graft(s) of the left leg with ulceration of other part of lower leg 🦀   A

    I70.349   Atherosclerosis of unspecified type of bypass graft(s) of the left leg with ulceration of unspecified site 🦀   A

▶ New   ⇒ Revised   ~~deleted~~ Deleted   Excludes 1   Excludes 2   Includes   Use additional   Code first   Code also   Key words
OGCR Official Guidelines   X Assign placeholder X   ● Use Additional Character(s)   ▷ Manifestation Code   🦀 Hierarchical Condition Category   **Coding Clinic**

I70.35   Atherosclerosis of unspecified type of bypass graft(s) of other extremity with ulceration 🔎 A

     Includes   any condition classifiable to I70.318 and I70.328

     Use additional code to identify severity of ulcer (L98.49-)

● I70.36   Atherosclerosis of unspecified type of bypass graft(s) of the extremities with gangrene

     Includes   any condition classifiable to I70.31-, I70.32-, I70.33-, I70.34-, I70.35
         chronic limb-threatening ischemia of unspecified type of bypass graft(s) of the extremities with gangrene
         critical limb ischemia of unspecified type of bypass graft(s) of the extremities with gangrene

     Use additional code to identify the severity of any ulcer (L97.-, L98.49-), if applicable

     I70.361   Atherosclerosis of unspecified type of bypass graft(s) of the extremities with gangrene, right leg 🔎   A

     I70.362   Atherosclerosis of unspecified type of bypass graft(s) of the extremities with gangrene, left leg 🔎   A

     I70.363   Atherosclerosis of unspecified type of bypass graft(s) of the extremities with gangrene, bilateral legs 🔎   A

     I70.368   Atherosclerosis of unspecified type of bypass graft(s) of the extremities with gangrene, other extremity 🔎   A

     I70.369   Atherosclerosis of unspecified type of bypass graft(s) of the extremities with gangrene, unspecified extremity 🔎   A

● I70.39   Other atherosclerosis of unspecified type of bypass graft(s) of the extremities

     I70.391   Other atherosclerosis of unspecified type of bypass graft(s) of the extremities, right leg 🔎   A

     I70.392   Other atherosclerosis of unspecified type of bypass graft(s) of the extremities, left leg 🔎   A

     I70.393   Other atherosclerosis of unspecified type of bypass graft(s) of the extremities, bilateral legs 🔎   A

     I70.398   Other atherosclerosis of unspecified type of bypass graft(s) of the extremities, other extremity 🔎   A

     I70.399   Other atherosclerosis of unspecified type of bypass graft(s) of the extremities, unspecified extremity 🔎 A

● I70.4   Atherosclerosis of autologous vein bypass graft(s) of the extremities

     Use additional code, if applicable, to identify chronic total occlusion of artery of extremity (I70.92)

● I70.40   Unspecified atherosclerosis of autologous vein bypass graft(s) of the extremities

     I70.401   Unspecified atherosclerosis of autologous vein bypass graft(s) of the extremities, right leg 🔎   A

     I70.402   Unspecified atherosclerosis of autologous vein bypass graft(s) of the extremities, left leg 🔎   A

     I70.403   Unspecified atherosclerosis of autologous vein bypass graft(s) of the extremities, bilateral legs 🔎   A

     I70.408   Unspecified atherosclerosis of autologous vein bypass graft(s) of the extremities, other extremity 🔎   A

     I70.409   Unspecified atherosclerosis of autologous vein bypass graft(s) of the extremities, unspecified extremity 🔎 A

● I70.41   Atherosclerosis of autologous vein bypass graft(s) of the extremities with intermittent claudication

     I70.411   Atherosclerosis of autologous vein bypass graft(s) of the extremities with intermittent claudication, right leg 🔎   A

     I70.412   Atherosclerosis of autologous vein bypass graft(s) of the extremities with intermittent claudication, left leg 🔎   A

     I70.413   Atherosclerosis of autologous vein bypass graft(s) of the extremities with intermittent claudication, bilateral legs 🔎   A

     I70.418   Atherosclerosis of autologous vein bypass graft(s) of the extremities with intermittent claudication, other extremity 🔎   A

     I70.419   Atherosclerosis of autologous vein bypass graft(s) of the extremities with intermittent claudication, unspecified extremity 🔎   A

● I70.42   Atherosclerosis of autologous vein bypass graft(s) of the extremities with rest pain

     Includes   any condition classifiable to I70.41-
         chronic limb-threatening ischemia NOS of autologous vein bypass graft(s) of the extremities
         chronic limb-threatening ischemia of autologous vein bypass graft(s) of the extremities with rest pain
         critical limb ischemia NOS of autologous vein bypass graft(s) of the extremities
         critical limb ischemia of autologous vein bypass graft(s) of the extremities with rest pain

     I70.421   Atherosclerosis of autologous vein bypass graft(s) of the extremities with rest pain, right leg 🔎   A

     I70.422   Atherosclerosis of autologous vein bypass graft(s) of the extremities with rest pain, left leg 🔎   A

     I70.423   Atherosclerosis of autologous vein bypass graft(s) of the extremities with rest pain, bilateral legs 🔎   A

     I70.428   Atherosclerosis of autologous vein bypass graft(s) of the extremities with rest pain, other extremity 🔎   A

     I70.429   Atherosclerosis of autologous vein bypass graft(s) of the extremities with rest pain, unspecified extremity 🔎   A

● I70.43   Atherosclerosis of autologous vein bypass graft(s) of the right leg with ulceration

     Includes   any condition classifiable to I70.411 and I70.421
         chronic limb-threatening ischemia of autologous vein bypass graft(s) of the right leg with ulceration
         critical limb ischemia of autologous vein bypass graft(s) of the right leg with ulceration

     Use additional code to identify severity of ulcer (L97.-)

     I70.431   Atherosclerosis of autologous vein bypass graft(s) of the right leg with ulceration of thigh 🔎   A

     I70.432   Atherosclerosis of autologous vein bypass graft(s) of the right leg with ulceration of calf 🔎   A

CHAPTER 9 (I00-I99)

I70.433   Atherosclerosis of autologous vein bypass graft(s) of the right leg with ulceration of ankle 🝙   A

I70.434   Atherosclerosis of autologous vein bypass graft(s) of the right leg with ulceration of heel and midfoot 🝙   A

    Atherosclerosis of autologous vein bypass graft(s) of right leg with ulceration of plantar surface of midfoot

I70.435   Atherosclerosis of autologous vein bypass graft(s) of the right leg with ulceration of other part of foot 🝙   A

    Atherosclerosis of autologous vein bypass graft(s) of right leg with ulceration of toe

I70.438   Atherosclerosis of autologous vein bypass graft(s) of the right leg with ulceration of other part of lower leg 🝙   A

I70.439   Atherosclerosis of autologous vein bypass graft(s) of the right leg with ulceration of unspecified site 🝙   A

● **I70.44**   Atherosclerosis of autologous vein bypass graft(s) of the left leg with ulceration

    Includes   any condition classifiable to I70.412 and I70.422

       chronic limb-threatening ischemia of autologous vein bypass graft(s) of the left leg with ulceration

       critical limb ischemia of autologous vein bypass graft(s) of the left leg with ulceration

    Use additional code to identify severity of ulcer (L97.-)

I70.441   Atherosclerosis of autologous vein bypass graft(s) of the left leg with ulceration of thigh 🝙   A

I70.442   Atherosclerosis of autologous vein bypass graft(s) of the left leg with ulceration of calf 🝙   A

I70.443   Atherosclerosis of autologous vein bypass graft(s) of the left leg with ulceration of ankle 🝙   A

I70.444   Atherosclerosis of autologous vein bypass graft(s) of the left leg with ulceration of heel and midfoot 🝙   A

    Atherosclerosis of autologous vein bypass graft(s) of left leg with ulceration of plantar surface of midfoot

I70.445   Atherosclerosis of autologous vein bypass graft(s) of the left leg with ulceration of other part of foot 🝙   A

    Atherosclerosis of autologous vein bypass graft(s) of left leg with ulceration of toe

I70.448   Atherosclerosis of autologous vein bypass graft(s) of the left leg with ulceration of other part of lower leg 🝙   A

I70.449   Atherosclerosis of autologous vein bypass graft(s) of the left leg with ulceration of unspecified site 🝙   A

I70.45   Atherosclerosis of autologous vein bypass graft(s) of other extremity with ulceration 🝙   A

    Includes   any condition classifiable to I70.418, I70.428, and I70.438

    Use additional code to identify severity of ulcer (L98.49-)

● **I70.46**   Atherosclerosis of autologous vein bypass graft(s) of the extremities with gangrene

    Includes   any condition classifiable to I70.41-, I70.42-, and I70.43-, I70.44-, I70.45

       chronic limb-threatening ischemia of autologous vein bypass graft(s) of the extremities with gangrene

       critical limb ischemia of autologous vein bypass graft(s) of the extremities with gangrene

    Use additional code to identify the severity of any ulcer (L97.-, L98.49-), if applicable

I70.461   Atherosclerosis of autologous vein bypass graft(s) of the extremities with gangrene, right leg   A

I70.462   Atherosclerosis of autologous vein bypass graft(s) of the extremities with gangrene, left leg 🝙   A

I70.463   Atherosclerosis of autologous vein bypass graft(s) of the extremities with gangrene, bilateral legs 🝙   A

I70.468   Atherosclerosis of autologous vein bypass graft(s) of the extremities with gangrene, other extremity 🝙   A

I70.469   Atherosclerosis of autologous vein bypass graft(s) of the extremities with gangrene, unspecified extremity 🝙   A

● **I70.49**   Other atherosclerosis of autologous vein bypass graft(s) of the extremities

I70.491   Other atherosclerosis of autologous vein bypass graft(s) of the extremities, right leg 🝙   A

I70.492   Other atherosclerosis of autologous vein bypass graft(s) of the extremities, left leg 🝙   A

I70.493   Other atherosclerosis of autologous vein bypass graft(s) of the extremities, bilateral legs 🝙   A

I70.498   Other atherosclerosis of autologous vein bypass graft(s) of the extremities, other extremity 🝙   A

I70.499   Other atherosclerosis of autologous vein bypass graft(s) of the extremities, unspecified extremity 🝙   A

● **I70.5**   Atherosclerosis of nonautologous biological bypass graft(s) of the extremities

    Use additional code, if applicable, to identify chronic total occlusion of artery of extremity (I70.92)

● **I70.50**   Unspecified atherosclerosis of nonautologous biological bypass graft(s) of the extremities

I70.501   Unspecified atherosclerosis of nonautologous biological bypass graft(s) of the extremities, right leg 🝙   A

I70.502   Unspecified atherosclerosis of nonautologous biological bypass graft(s) of the extremities, left leg 🝙 A

I70.503   Unspecified atherosclerosis of nonautologous biological bypass graft(s) of the extremities, bilateral legs 🝙   A

I70.508   Unspecified atherosclerosis of nonautologous biological bypass graft(s) of the extremities, other extremity 🝙   A

I70.509   Unspecified atherosclerosis of nonautologous biological bypass graft(s) of the extremities, unspecified extremity 🝙   A

▶ New   ⇒ Revised   ~~deleted~~ Deleted   Excludes 1   Excludes 2   Includes   Use additional   Code first   Code also   Key words

OGCR Official Guidelines   X Assign placeholder X   ● Use Additional Character(s)   ▶ Manifestation Code   🝙 Hierarchical Condition Category   **Coding Clinic**

● I70.51   Atherosclerosis of nonautologous biological bypass graft(s) of the extremities intermittent claudication

     I70.511   Atherosclerosis of nonautologous biological bypass graft(s) of the extremities with intermittent claudication, right leg 🔖   A

     I70.512   Atherosclerosis of nonautologous biological bypass graft(s) of the extremities with intermittent claudication, left leg 🔖   A

     I70.513   Atherosclerosis of nonautologous biological bypass graft(s) of the extremities with intermittent claudication, bilateral legs 🔖   A

     I70.518   Atherosclerosis of nonautologous biological bypass graft(s) of the extremities with intermittent claudication, other extremity 🔖   A

     I70.519   Atherosclerosis of nonautologous biological bypass graft(s) of the extremities with intermittent claudication, unspecified extremity 🔖   A

● I70.52   Atherosclerosis of nonautologous biological bypass graft(s) of the extremities with rest pain

    Includes   any condition classifiable to I70.51-
      chronic limb-threatening ischemia NOS of nonautologous biological bypass graft(s) of the extremities
      chronic limb-threatening ischemia of nonautologous biological bypass graft(s) of the extremities with rest pain
      critical limb ischemia NOS of nonautologous biological bypass graft(s) of the extremities
      critical limb ischemia of nonautologous biological bypass graft(s) of the extremities with rest pain

     I70.521   Atherosclerosis of nonautologous biological bypass graft(s) of the extremities with rest pain, right leg 🔖   A

     I70.522   Atherosclerosis of nonautologous biological bypass graft(s) of the extremities with rest pain, left leg 🔖   A

     I70.523   Atherosclerosis of nonautologous biological bypass graft(s) of the extremities with rest pain, bilateral legs 🔖   A

     I70.528   Atherosclerosis of nonautologous biological bypass graft(s) of the extremities with rest pain, other extremity 🔖   A

     I70.529   Atherosclerosis of nonautologous biological bypass graft(s) of the extremities with rest pain, unspecified extremity 🔖   A

● I70.53   Atherosclerosis of nonautologous biological bypass graft(s) of the right leg with ulceration

    Includes   any condition classifiable to I70.511 and I70.521
      chronic limb-threatening ischemia of nonautologous biological bypass graft(s) of the right leg with ulceration
      critical limb ischemia of nonautologous biological bypass graft(s) of the right leg with ulceration

    Use additional code to identify severity of ulcer (L97.-)

     I70.531   Atherosclerosis of nonautologous biological bypass graft(s) of the right leg with ulceration of thigh 🔖   A

     I70.532   Atherosclerosis of nonautologous biological bypass graft(s) of the right leg with ulceration of calf 🔖   A

     I70.533   Atherosclerosis of nonautologous biological bypass graft(s) of the right leg with ulceration of ankle 🔖   A

     I70.534   Atherosclerosis of nonautologous biological bypass graft(s) of the right leg with ulceration of heel and midfoot 🔖   A
       Atherosclerosis of nonautologous biological bypass graft(s) of right leg with ulceration of plantar surface of midfoot

     I70.535   Atherosclerosis of nonautologous biological bypass graft(s) of the right leg with ulceration of other part of foot 🔖   A
       Atherosclerosis of nonautologous biological bypass graft(s) of the right leg with ulceration of toe

     I70.538   Atherosclerosis of nonautologous biological bypass graft(s) of the right leg with ulceration of other part of lower leg 🔖   A

     I70.539   Atherosclerosis of nonautologous biological bypass graft(s) of the right leg with ulceration of unspecified site 🔖   A

● I70.54   Atherosclerosis of nonautologous biological bypass graft(s) of the left leg with ulceration

    Includes   any condition classifiable to I70.512 and I70.522
      chronic limb-threatening ischemia of nonautologous biological bypass graft(s) of the left leg with ulceration
      critical limb ischemia of nonautologous biological bypass graft(s) of the left leg with ulceration

    Use additional code to identify severity of ulcer (L97.-)

     I70.541   Atherosclerosis of nonautologous biological bypass graft(s) of the left leg with ulceration of thigh 🔖   A

     I70.542   Atherosclerosis of nonautologous biological bypass graft(s) of the left leg with ulceration of calf 🔖   A

     I70.543   Atherosclerosis of nonautologous biological bypass graft(s) of the left leg with ulceration of ankle 🔖   A

CHAPTER 9 (I00-I99)

I70.544   Atherosclerosis of nonautologous
           biological bypass graft(s) of the left
           leg with ulceration of heel and
           midfoot 🐾   A
               Atherosclerosis of nonautologous
                   biological bypass graft(s) of left
                   leg with ulceration of plantar
                   surface of midfoot
I70.545   Atherosclerosis of nonautologous
           biological bypass graft(s) of the left
           leg with ulceration of other part of
           foot 🐾   A
               Atherosclerosis of nonautologous
                   biological bypass graft(s) of the
                   left leg with ulceration of toe
I70.548   Atherosclerosis of nonautologous
           biological bypass graft(s) of the left
           leg with ulceration of other part of
           lower leg 🐾   A
I70.549   Atherosclerosis of nonautologous
           biological bypass graft(s) of the left
           leg with ulceration of unspecified
           site 🐾   A

I70.55   Atherosclerosis of nonautologous biological
          bypass graft(s) of other extremity with
          ulceration 🐾   A
          Includes   any condition classifiable to
                          I70.518, I70.528, and I70.538
          Use additional code to identify severity of
              ulcer (L98.49)

● I70.56   Atherosclerosis of nonautologous biological
           bypass graft(s) of the extremities with gangrene
           Includes   any condition classifiable to
                           I70.51-, I70.52-, and I70.53-,
                           I70.54-, I70.55
                           chronic limb-threatening
                               ischemia of nonautologous
                               biological bypass graft(s)
                               of the extremities with
                               gangrene
                           critical limb ischemia of
                               nonautologous biological
                               bypass graft(s) of the
                               extremities with gangrene
           Use additional code to identify the severity of
               any ulcer (L97.-, L98.49-), if applicable
           I70.561   Atherosclerosis of nonautologous
                      biological bypass graft(s) of the
                      extremities with gangrene, right
                      leg 🐾   A
           I70.562   Atherosclerosis of nonautologous
                      biological bypass graft(s) of the
                      extremities with gangrene, left leg 🐾 A
           I70.563   Atherosclerosis of nonautologous
                      biological bypass graft(s) of the
                      extremities with gangrene, bilateral
                      legs 🐾   A
           I70.568   Atherosclerosis of nonautologous
                      biological bypass graft(s) of the
                      extremities with gangrene, other
                      extremity 🐾   A
           I70.569   Atherosclerosis of nonautologous
                      biological bypass graft(s) of the
                      extremities with gangrene,
                      unspecified extremity 🐾   A

● I70.59   Other atherosclerosis of nonautologous
           biological bypass graft(s) of the extremities
           I70.591   Other atherosclerosis of nonautologous
                      biological bypass graft(s) of the
                      extremities, right leg 🐾   A
           I70.592   Other atherosclerosis of nonautologous
                      biological bypass graft(s) of the
                      extremities, left leg 🐾   A

I70.593   Other atherosclerosis of nonautologous
           biological bypass graft(s) of the
           extremities, bilateral legs 🐾   A
I70.598   Other atherosclerosis of nonautologous
           biological bypass graft(s) of the
           extremities, other extremity 🐾   A
I70.599   Other atherosclerosis of nonautologous
           biological bypass graft(s) of the
           extremities, unspecified extremity 🐾   A

● I70.6   Atherosclerosis of nonbiological bypass graft(s) of the
           extremities
           Use additional code, if applicable, to identify chronic
               total occlusion of artery of extremity (I70.92)
    ● I70.60   Unspecified atherosclerosis of nonbiological
                bypass graft(s) of the extremities
                I70.601   Unspecified atherosclerosis of
                           nonbiological bypass graft(s) of the
                           extremities, right leg 🐾   A
                I70.602   Unspecified atherosclerosis of
                           nonbiological bypass graft(s) of the
                           extremities, left leg 🐾   A
                I70.603   Unspecified atherosclerosis of
                           nonbiological bypass graft(s) of the
                           extremities, bilateral legs 🐾   A
                I70.608   Unspecified atherosclerosis of
                           nonbiological bypass graft(s) of the
                           extremities, other extremity 🐾   A
                I70.609   Unspecified atherosclerosis of
                           nonbiological bypass graft(s) of the
                           extremities, unspecified extremity 🐾 A

    ● I70.61   Atherosclerosis of nonbiological bypass graft(s)
                of the extremities with intermittent claudication
                I70.611   Atherosclerosis of nonbiological
                           bypass graft(s) of the extremities
                           with intermittent claudication,
                           right leg 🐾   A
                I70.612   Atherosclerosis of nonbiological
                           bypass graft(s) of the extremities with
                           intermittent claudication, left leg 🐾 A
                I70.613   Atherosclerosis of nonbiological
                           bypass graft(s) of the extremities with
                           intermittent claudication, bilateral
                           legs 🐾   A
                I70.618   Atherosclerosis of nonbiological
                           bypass graft(s) of the extremities with
                           intermittent claudication, other
                           extremity 🐾   A
                I70.619   Atherosclerosis of nonbiological
                           bypass graft(s) of the extremities with
                           intermittent claudication, unspecified
                           extremity 🐾   A

    ● I70.62   Atherosclerosis of nonbiological bypass graft(s)
                of the extremities with rest pain
                Includes   any condition classifiable to I70.61-
                                chronic limb-threatening
                                    ischemia NOS of
                                    nonbiological bypass
                                    graft(s) of the extremities
                                chronic limb-threatening
                                    ischemia of nonbiological
                                    bypass graft(s) of the
                                    extremities with rest pain
                                critical limb ischemia NOS
                                    of nonbiological bypass
                                    graft(s) of the extremities
                                critical limb ischemia of
                                    nonbiological bypass
                                    graft(s) of the extremities
                                    with rest pain
                I70.621   Atherosclerosis of nonbiological
                           bypass graft(s) of the extremities with
                           rest pain, right leg 🐾   A

I70.622   Atherosclerosis of nonbiological bypass graft(s) of the extremities with rest pain, left leg 🔗   A

I70.623   Atherosclerosis of nonbiological bypass graft(s) of the extremities with rest pain, bilateral legs 🔗   A

I70.628   Atherosclerosis of nonbiological bypass graft(s) of the extremities with rest pain, other extremity 🔗   A

I70.629   Atherosclerosis of nonbiological bypass graft(s) of the extremities with rest pain, unspecified extremity 🔗   A

● **I70.63**   Atherosclerosis of nonbiological bypass graft(s) of the right leg with ulceration

    Includes   any condition classifiable to I70.611 and I70.621
         chronic limb-threatening ischemia of nonbiological bypass graft(s) of the right leg with ulceration
         critical limb ischemia of nonbiological bypass graft(s) of the right leg with ulceration

    Use additional code to identify severity of ulcer (L97.-)

I70.631   Atherosclerosis of nonbiological bypass graft(s) of the right leg with ulceration of thigh 🔗   A

I70.632   Atherosclerosis of nonbiological bypass graft(s) of the right leg with ulceration of calf 🔗   A

I70.633   Atherosclerosis of nonbiological bypass graft(s) of the right leg with ulceration of ankle 🔗   A

I70.634   Atherosclerosis of nonbiological bypass graft(s) of the right leg with ulceration of heel and midfoot 🔗   A
    Atherosclerosis of nonbiological bypass graft(s) of right leg with ulceration of plantar surface of midfoot

I70.635   Atherosclerosis of nonbiological bypass graft(s) of the right leg with ulceration of other part of foot 🔗   A
    Atherosclerosis of nonbiological bypass graft(s) of the right leg with ulceration of toe

I70.638   Atherosclerosis of nonbiological bypass graft(s) of the right leg with ulceration of other part of lower leg 🔗   A

I70.639   Atherosclerosis of nonbiological bypass graft(s) of the right leg with ulceration of unspecified site 🔗   A

● **I70.64**   Atherosclerosis of nonbiological bypass graft(s) of the left leg with ulceration

    Includes   any condition classifiable to I70.612 and I70.622
         chronic limb-threatening ischemia of nonbiological bypass graft(s) of the left leg with ulceration
         critical limb ischemia of nonbiological bypass graft(s) of the left leg with ulceration

    Use additional code to identify severity of ulcer (L97.-)

I70.641   Atherosclerosis of nonbiological bypass graft(s) of the left leg with ulceration of thigh 🔗   A

I70.642   Atherosclerosis of nonbiological bypass graft(s) of the left leg with ulceration of calf 🔗   A

I70.643   Atherosclerosis of nonbiological bypass graft(s) of the left leg with ulceration of ankle 🔗   A

I70.644   Atherosclerosis of nonbiological bypass graft(s) of the left leg with ulceration of heel and midfoot 🔗   A
    Atherosclerosis of nonbiological bypass graft(s) of left leg with ulceration of plantar surface of midfoot

I70.645   Atherosclerosis of nonbiological bypass graft(s) of the left leg with ulceration of other part of foot 🔗   A
    Atherosclerosis of nonbiological bypass graft(s) of the left leg with ulceration of toe

I70.648   Atherosclerosis of nonbiological bypass graft(s) of the left leg with ulceration of other part of lower leg 🔗   A

I70.649   Atherosclerosis of nonbiological bypass graft(s) of the left leg with ulceration of unspecified site 🔗   A

I70.65   Atherosclerosis of nonbiological bypass graft(s) of other extremity with ulceration 🔗   A

    Includes   any condition classifiable to I70.618 and I70.628

    Use additional code to identify severity of ulcer (L98.49-)

● **I70.66**   Atherosclerosis of nonbiological bypass graft(s) of the extremities with gangrene

    Includes   any condition classifiable to I70.61-, I70.62-, I70.63-, I70.64-, I70.65
         chronic limb-threatening ischemia of nonbiological bypass graft(s) of the extremities with gangrene
         critical limb ischemia of nonbiological bypass graft(s) of the extremities with gangrene

    Use additional code to identify the severity of any ulcer (L97.-, L98.49-), if applicable

I70.661   Atherosclerosis of nonbiological bypass graft(s) of the extremities with gangrene, right leg 🔗   A

I70.662   Atherosclerosis of nonbiological bypass graft(s) of the extremities with gangrene, left leg 🔗   A

I70.663   Atherosclerosis of nonbiological bypass graft(s) of the extremities with gangrene, bilateral legs 🔗   A

I70.668   Atherosclerosis of nonbiological bypass graft(s) of the extremities with gangrene, other extremity 🔗   A

I70.669   Atherosclerosis of nonbiological bypass graft(s) of the extremities with gangrene, unspecified extremity 🔗   A

● **I70.69**   Other atherosclerosis of nonbiological bypass graft(s) of the extremities

I70.691   Other atherosclerosis of nonbiological bypass graft(s) of the extremities, right leg 🔗   A

I70.692   Other atherosclerosis of nonbiological bypass graft(s) of the extremities, left leg 🔗   A

I70.693   Other atherosclerosis of nonbiological bypass graft(s) of the extremities, bilateral legs 🔗   A

CHAPTER 9 (I00–I99)

I70.698   Other atherosclerosis of nonbiological bypass graft(s) of the extremities, other extremity 🐾   A

I70.699   Other atherosclerosis of nonbiological bypass graft(s) of the extremities, unspecified extremity 🐾   A

● I70.7   Atherosclerosis of other type of bypass graft(s) of the extremities

> Use additional code, if applicable, to identify chronic total occlusion of artery of extremity (I70.92)

● I70.70   Unspecified atherosclerosis of other type of bypass graft(s) of the extremities

I70.701   Unspecified atherosclerosis of other type of bypass graft(s) of the extremities, right leg 🐾   A

I70.702   Unspecified atherosclerosis of other type of bypass graft(s) of the extremities, left leg 🐾   A

I70.703   Unspecified atherosclerosis of other type of bypass graft(s) of the extremities, bilateral legs 🐾   A

I70.708   Unspecified atherosclerosis of other type of bypass graft(s) of the extremities, other extremity 🐾   A

I70.709   Unspecified atherosclerosis of other type of bypass graft(s) of the extremities, unspecified extremity 🐾 A

● I70.71   Atherosclerosis of other type of bypass graft(s) of the extremities with intermittent claudication

I70.711   Atherosclerosis of other type of bypass graft(s) of the extremities with intermittent claudication, right leg 🐾   A

I70.712   Atherosclerosis of other type of bypass graft(s) of the extremities with intermittent claudication, left leg 🐾 A

I70.713   Atherosclerosis of other type of bypass graft(s) of the extremities with intermittent claudication, bilateral legs 🐾   A

I70.718   Atherosclerosis of other type of bypass graft(s) of the extremities with intermittent claudication, other extremity 🐾   A

I70.719   Atherosclerosis of other type of bypass graft(s) of the extremities with intermittent claudication, unspecified extremity 🐾   A

● I70.72   Atherosclerosis of other type of bypass graft(s) of the extremities with rest pain

> **Includes**   any condition classifiable to I70.71-
> chronic limb-threatening ischemia NOS of other type of bypass graft(s) of the extremities
> chronic limb-threatening ischemia of other type of bypass graft(s) of the extremities with rest pain
> critical limb ischemia NOS of other type of bypass graft(s) of the extremities
> critical limb ischemia of other type of bypass graft(s) of the extremities with rest pain

I70.721   Atherosclerosis of other type of bypass graft(s) of the extremities with rest pain, right leg 🐾   A

I70.722   Atherosclerosis of other type of bypass graft(s) of the extremities with rest pain, left leg 🐾   A

I70.723   Atherosclerosis of other type of bypass graft(s) of the extremities with rest pain, bilateral legs 🐾   A

I70.728   Atherosclerosis of other type of bypass graft(s) of the extremities with rest pain, other extremity 🐾   A

I70.729   Atherosclerosis of other type of bypass graft(s) of the extremities with rest pain, unspecified extremity 🐾   A

● I70.73   Atherosclerosis of other type of bypass graft(s) of the right leg with ulceration

> **Includes**   any condition classifiable to I70.711 and I70.721
> chronic limb-threatening ischemia of other type of bypass graft(s) of the right leg with ulceration
> critical limb ischemia of other type of bypass graft(s) of the right leg with ulceration

> Use additional code to identify severity of ulcer (L97.-)

I70.731   Atherosclerosis of other type of bypass graft(s) of the right leg with ulceration of thigh 🐾   A

I70.732   Atherosclerosis of other type of bypass graft(s) of the right leg with ulceration of calf 🐾   A

I70.733   Atherosclerosis of other type of bypass graft(s) of the right leg with ulceration of ankle 🐾   A

I70.734   Atherosclerosis of other type of bypass graft(s) of the right leg with ulceration of heel and midfoot 🐾
> Atherosclerosis of other type of bypass graft(s) of right leg with ulceration of plantar surface of midfoot

I70.735   Atherosclerosis of other type of bypass graft(s) of the right leg with ulceration of other part of foot 🐾   A
> Atherosclerosis of other type of bypass graft(s) of right leg with ulceration of toe

I70.738   Atherosclerosis of other type of bypass graft(s) of the right leg with ulceration of other part of lower leg 🐾   A

I70.739   Atherosclerosis of other type of bypass graft(s) of the right leg with ulceration of unspecified site 🐾   A

● I70.74   Atherosclerosis of other type of bypass graft(s) of the left leg with ulceration

> **Includes**   any condition classifiable to I70.712 and I70.722
> chronic limb-threatening ischemia of other type of bypass graft(s) of the left leg with ulceration
> critical limb ischemia of other type of bypass graft(s) of the left leg with ulceration

> Use additional code to identify severity of ulcer (L97.-)

I70.741   Atherosclerosis of other type of bypass graft(s) of the left leg with ulceration of thigh 🐾   A

I70.742   Atherosclerosis of other type of bypass graft(s) of the left leg with ulceration of calf 🐾

I70.743   Atherosclerosis of other type of bypass graft(s) of the left leg with ulceration of ankle 🗗   A

I70.744   Atherosclerosis of other type of bypass graft(s) of the left leg with ulceration of heel and midfoot 🗗   A
           Atherosclerosis of other type of bypass graft(s) of left leg with ulceration of plantar surface of midfoot

I70.745   Atherosclerosis of other type of bypass graft(s) of the left leg with ulceration of other part of foot 🗗   A
           Atherosclerosis of other type of bypass graft(s) of left leg with ulceration of toe

I70.748   Atherosclerosis of other type of bypass graft(s) of the left leg with ulceration of other part of lower leg 🗗   A

I70.749   Atherosclerosis of other type of bypass graft(s) of the left leg with ulceration of unspecified site 🗗   A

I70.75   Atherosclerosis of other type of bypass graft(s) of other extremity with ulceration 🗗   A

    Includes   any condition classifiable to I70.718 and I70.728

    Use additional code to identify severity of ulcer (L98.49)

● I70.76   Atherosclerosis of other type of bypass graft(s) of the extremities with gangrene

    Includes   any condition classifiable to I70.71-, I70.72-, I70.73-, I70.74-, I70.75
                    chronic limb-threatening ischemia of other type of bypass graft(s) of the extremities with gangrene
                    critical limb ischemia of other type of bypass graft(s) of the extremities with gangrene

    Use additional code to identify the severity of any ulcer (L97.-, L98.49-), if applicable

I70.761   Atherosclerosis of other type of bypass graft(s) of the extremities with gangrene, right leg 🗗   A

I70.762   Atherosclerosis of other type of bypass graft(s) of the extremities with gangrene, left leg 🗗   A

I70.763   Atherosclerosis of other type of bypass graft(s) of the extremities with gangrene, bilateral legs 🗗   A

I70.768   Atherosclerosis of other type of bypass graft(s) of the extremities with gangrene, other extremity 🗗   A

I70.769   Atherosclerosis of other type of bypass graft(s) of the extremities with gangrene, unspecified extremity 🗗   A

● I70.79   Other atherosclerosis of other type of bypass graft(s) of the extremities

I70.791   Other atherosclerosis of other type of bypass graft(s) of the extremities, right leg 🗗   A

I70.792   Other atherosclerosis of other type of bypass graft(s) of the extremities, left leg 🗗   A

I70.793   Other atherosclerosis of other type of bypass graft(s) of the extremities, bilateral legs 🗗   A

I70.798   Other atherosclerosis of other type of bypass graft(s) of the extremities, other extremity 🗗   A

I70.799   Other atherosclerosis of other type of bypass graft(s) of the extremities, unspecified extremity 🗗   A

I70.8   Atherosclerosis of other arteries   A

● I70.9   Other and unspecified atherosclerosis

I70.90   Unspecified atherosclerosis   A

I70.91   Generalized atherosclerosis   A

I70.92   Chronic total occlusion of artery of the extremities 🗗   A
           Complete occlusion of artery of the extremities
           Total occlusion of artery of the extremities
           Code first atherosclerosis of arteries of the extremities (I70.2-, I70.3-, I70.4-, I70.5-, I70.6-, I70.7-)

● I71   **Aortic aneurysm and dissection**

    Excludes1   aortic ectasia (I77.81-)
                     syphilitic aortic aneurysm (A52.01)
                     traumatic aortic aneurysm (S25.09, S35.09)

● I71.0   **Dissection of aorta**

I71.00   Dissection of unspecified site of aorta 🗗

I71.01   Dissection of thoracic aorta 🗗

I71.02   Dissection of abdominal aorta 🗗

I71.03   Dissection of thoracoabdominal aorta 🗗

I71.1   Thoracic aortic aneurysm, ruptured 🗗

I71.2   Thoracic aortic aneurysm, without rupture 🗗

I71.3   Abdominal aortic aneurysm, ruptured 🗗

I71.4   Abdominal aortic aneurysm, without rupture 🗗

I71.5   Thoracoabdominal aortic aneurysm, ruptured 🗗

I71.6   Thoracoabdominal aortic aneurysm, without rupture 🗗

I71.8   Aortic aneurysm of unspecified site, ruptured 🗗
           Rupture of aorta NOS

I71.9   Aortic aneurysm of unspecified site, without rupture 🗗
           Aneurysm of aorta
           Dilatation of aorta
           Hyaline necrosis of aorta

● I72   **Other aneurysm**

    Includes   aneurysm (cirsoid) (false) (ruptured)

    Excludes2   acquired aneurysm (I77.0)
                     aneurysm (of) aorta (I71.-)
                     aneurysm (of) arteriovenous NOS (Q27.3-)
                     carotid artery dissection (I77.71)
                     cerebral (nonruptured) aneurysm (I67.1)
                     coronary aneurysm (I25.4)
                     coronary artery dissection (I25.42)
                     dissection of artery NEC (I77.79)
                     dissection of precerebral artery, congenital (nonruptured) (Q28.1)
                     heart aneurysm (I25.3)
                     iliac artery dissection (I77.72)
                     precerebral artery, congenital (nonruptured) (Q28.1)
                     pulmonary artery aneurysm (I28.1)
                     renal artery dissection (I77.73)
                     retinal aneurysm (H35.0)
                     ruptured cerebral aneurysm (I60.7)
                     varicose aneurysm (I77.0)
                     vertebral artery dissection (I77.74)

I72.0   Aneurysm of carotid artery 🗗
           Aneurysm of common carotid artery
           Aneurysm of external carotid artery
           Aneurysm of internal carotid artery, extracranial portion

    Excludes1   aneurysm of internal carotid artery, intracranial portion (I67.1)
                     aneurysm of internal carotid artery NOS (I67.1)

I72.1   Aneurysm of artery of upper extremity 🗗

I72.2   Aneurysm of renal artery 🗗

CHAPTER 9 (I00-I99)

I72.3   **Aneurysm of iliac artery**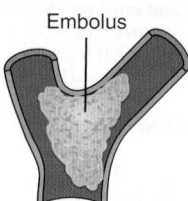

I72.4   **Aneurysm of artery of lower extremity**
      Coding Clinic: 2019, Q2, P22

I72.5   **Aneurysm of other precerebral arteries**
      Aneurysm of basilar artery (trunk)

      Excludes2   aneurysm of carotid artery (I72.0)
                   aneurysm of vertebral artery (I72.6)
                   dissection of carotid artery (I77.71)
                   dissection of other precerebral arteries
                     (I77.75)
                   dissection of vertebral artery (I77.74)
      Coding Clinic 2016, Q4, P28

I72.6   **Aneurysm of vertebral artery**

      Excludes2   dissection of vertebral artery (I77.74)
      Coding Clinic 2016, Q4, P28

I72.8   **Aneurysm of other specified arteries**

I72.9   **Aneurysm of unspecified site**

● I73   **Other peripheral vascular diseases**
      Excludes2   chilblains (T69.1)
                   frostbite (T33-T34)
                   immersion hand or foot (T69.0-)
                   spasm of cerebral artery (G45.9)
      Coding Clinic: 2018, Q4, P87-88

● I73.0   **Raynaud's syndrome**
      Diminishing oxygen supply to fingers, toes, nose, and ears
           when exposed to temperature changes or stress
      Raynaud's disease
      Raynaud's phenomenon (secondary)

      I73.00   **Raynaud's syndrome without gangrene**

      I73.01   **Raynaud's syndrome with gangrene**

I73.1   **Thromboangiitis obliterans [Buerger's disease]**
      Inflammatory occlusive disease resulting in poor circulation
           to the legs, feet, and sometimes the hands due to
           progressive inflammatory narrowing and eventually
           obliteration of the small arteries

● I73.8   **Other specified peripheral vascular diseases**
      Excludes1   diabetic (peripheral) angiopathy
                   (E08-E13 with .51-.52)

      I73.81   **Erythromelalgia**

      I73.89   **Other specified peripheral vascular diseases**
                   Acrocyanosis
                   Erythrocyanosis
                   Simple acroparesthesia [Schultze's type]
                   Vasomotor acroparesthesia [Nothnagel's type]

Figure 9-5   Raynaud's syndrome. (From Hallett: Comprehensive Vascular and Endovascular Surgery, ed 2, Philadelphia, Mosby Ltd., 2010)

Item 9–9   An **embolus** is a mass of undissolved matter present in the blood that is transported by the blood current. A **thrombus** is a blood clot that occludes or shuts off a vessel. When a thrombus is dislodged, it becomes an embolus.

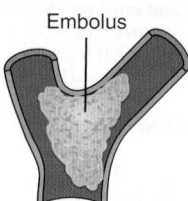

Figure 9-6   An arterial embolus.

I73.9   **Peripheral vascular disease, unspecified**
      Intermittent claudication
      Peripheral angiopathy NOS
      Spasm of artery

      Excludes1   atherosclerosis of the extremities
                   (I70.2—I70.7-)
      Coding Clinic: 2018, Q4, P87

● I74   **Arterial embolism and thrombosis**
      Includes   embolic infarction
                embolic occlusion
                thrombotic infarction
                thrombotic occlusion

      Code first embolism and thrombosis complicating abortion or
           ectopic or molar pregnancy (O00-O07, O08.2)
           embolism and thrombosis complicating pregnancy, childbirth
           and the puerperium (O88.-)

      Excludes2   atheroembolism (I75.-)
                   basilar embolism and thrombosis (I63.0-I63.2, I65.1)
                   carotid embolism and thrombosis (I63.0-I63.2, I65.2)
                   cerebral embolism and thrombosis (I63.3-I63.5,
                     I66.-)
                   coronary embolism and thrombosis (I21-I25)
                   mesenteric embolism and thrombosis (K55.0-)
                   ophthalmic embolism and thrombosis (H34.-)
                   precerebral embolism and thrombosis NOS
                     (I63.0-I63.2, I65.9)
                   pulmonary embolism and thrombosis (I26.-)
                   renal embolism and thrombosis (N28.0)
                   retinal embolism and thrombosis (H34.-)
                   septic embolism and thrombosis (I76)
                   vertebral embolism and thrombosis (I63.0-I63.2,
                     I65.0)

● I74.0   **Embolism and thrombosis of abdominal aorta**
      I74.01   **Saddle embolus of abdominal aorta**

      I74.09   **Other arterial embolism and thrombosis of abdominal aorta**
                   Aortic bifurcation syndrome
                   Aortoiliac obstruction
                   Leriche's syndrome

● I74.1   **Embolism and thrombosis of other and unspecified parts of aorta**
      I74.10   **Embolism and thrombosis of unspecified parts of aorta**

      I74.11   **Embolism and thrombosis of thoracic aorta**

      I74.19   **Embolism and thrombosis of other parts of aorta**

I74.2   **Embolism and thrombosis of arteries of the upper extremities**

I74.3   **Embolism and thrombosis of arteries of the lower extremities**

I74.4   **Embolism and thrombosis of arteries of extremities, unspecified**
      Peripheral arterial embolism NOS

I74.5   **Embolism and thrombosis of iliac artery**

I74.8   **Embolism and thrombosis of other arteries**

I74.9   **Embolism and thrombosis of unspecified artery**

▶ New   ⇒ Revised   ~~deleted~~ Deleted   Excludes 1   Excludes 2   Includes   Use additional   Code first   Code also   Key words

OGCR Official Guidelines   X Assign placeholder X   ● Use Additional Character(s)   ▶ Manifestation Code   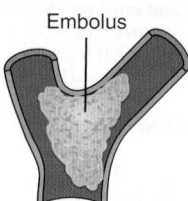 Hierarchical Condition Category   **Coding Clinic**

● **I75**   **Atheroembolism**
     Includes   atherothrombotic microembolism
                 cholesterol embolism

   ● **I75.0**   **Atheroembolism of extremities**
     ● **I75.01**   **Atheroembolism of upper extremity**
       I75.011   **Atheroembolism of right upper** extremity 🐾
       I75.012   **Atheroembolism of left upper** extremity 🐾
       I75.013   **Atheroembolism of bilateral upper** extremities 🐾
       I75.019   **Atheroembolism of unspecified upper** extremity 🐾

     ● **I75.02**   **Atheroembolism of lower extremity**
       I75.021   **Atheroembolism of right lower** extremity 🐾
       I75.022   **Atheroembolism of left lower** extremity 🐾
       I75.023   **Atheroembolism of bilateral lower** extremities 🐾
       I75.029   **Atheroembolism of unspecified lower** extremity 🐾

   ● **I75.8**   **Atheroembolism of other sites**
       I75.81   **Atheroembolism of kidney** 🐾
           Use additional code for any associated acute kidney failure and chronic kidney disease (N17.-, N18.-)
       I75.89   **Atheroembolism of other site** 🐾

I76   **Septic arterial embolism** 🐾
   Code first underlying infection, such as:
     infective endocarditis (I33.0)
     lung abscess (J85.-)
   Use additional code to identify the site of the embolism (I74.-)
   Excludes2   septic pulmonary embolism (I26.01, I26.90)

● **I77**   **Other disorders of arteries and arterioles**
   Excludes2   collagen (vascular) diseases (M30-M36)
                hypersensitivity angiitis (M31.0)
                pulmonary artery (I28.-)

   I77.0   **Arteriovenous fistula, acquired** 🐾
     Aneurysmal varix
     Arteriovenous aneurysm, acquired
     Excludes1   arteriovenous aneurysm NOS (Q27.3-)
                presence of arteriovenous shunt (fistula) for dialysis (Z99.2)
                traumatic - see injury of blood vessel by body region
     Excludes2   cerebral (I67.1)
                coronary (I25.4)

   I77.1   **Stricture of artery** 🐾
     Narrowing of artery

   I77.2   **Rupture of artery** 🐾
     Erosion of artery
     Fistula of artery
     Ulcer of artery
     Excludes1   traumatic rupture of artery - see injury of blood vessel by body region

   I77.3   **Arterial fibromuscular dysplasia** 🐾
     Fibromuscular hyperplasia (of) carotid artery
     Fibromuscular hyperplasia (of) renal artery

   I77.4   **Celiac artery compression syndrome** 🐾

   I77.5   **Necrosis of artery** 🐾

   I77.6   **Arteritis, unspecified** 🐾
     Aortitis NOS
     Endarteritis NOS
     Excludes1   arteritis or endarteritis:
                aortic arch (M31.4)
                cerebral NEC (I67.7)
                coronary (I25.89)
                deformans (I70.-)
                giant cell (M31.5, M31.6)
                obliterans (I70.-)
                senile (I70.-)

   ● **I77.7**   **Other arterial dissection**
     Excludes2   dissection of aorta (I71.0-)
                dissection of coronary artery (I25.42)
     I77.70   **Dissection of unspecified artery** 🐾
          Coding Clinic 2016, Q4, P28
     I77.71   **Dissection of carotid artery** 🐾
     I77.72   **Dissection of iliac artery** 🐾
     I77.73   **Dissection of renal artery** 🐾
     I77.74   **Dissection of vertebral artery** 🐾
       Excludes2   aneurysm of vertebral artery (I72.6)
     I77.75   **Dissection of other precerebral arteries** 🐾
       Dissection of basilar artery (trunk)
       Excludes2   aneurysm of carotid artery (I72.0)
                aneurysm of other precerebral arteries (I72.5)
                aneurysm of vertebral artery (I72.6)
                dissection of carotid artery (I77.71)
                dissection of vertebral artery (I77.74)
       Coding Clinic 2016, Q4, P28
     I77.76   **Dissection of artery of upper extremity** 🐾
       Coding Clinic 2016, Q4, P28
     I77.77   **Dissection of artery of lower extremity** 🐾
       Coding Clinic 2016, Q4, P28
     I77.79   **Dissection of other specified artery** 🐾
       Coding Clinic 2016, Q4, P28

   ● **I77.8**   **Other specified disorders of arteries and arterioles**
     I77.81   **Aortic ectasia**
       Ectasis aorta
       Excludes1   aortic aneurysm and dissection (I71.0-)
       I77.810   **Thoracic aortic ectasia** 🐾
       I77.811   **Abdominal aortic ectasia** 🐾
       I77.812   **Thoracoabdominal aortic ectasia** 🐾
       I77.819   **Aortic ectasia, unspecified site** 🐾
     I77.89   **Other specified disorders of arteries and arterioles** 🐾
       Coding Clinic 2021, Q1, P23

   I77.9   **Disorder of arteries and arterioles, unspecified** 🐾
     Coding Clinic 2021, Q1, P4

CHAPTER 9 (I00-I99)

CHAPTER 9 (I00-I99)

- I78 **Diseases of capillaries**
  - I78.0 **Hereditary hemorrhagic telangiectasia** 🦟
    - Rendu-Osler-Weber disease
  - I78.1 **Nevus, non-neoplastic**
    - Araneus nevus   Spider nevus
    - Senile nevus   Stellar nevus
      - **Excludes1** nevus NOS (D22.-)
        - vascular NOS (Q82.5)
      - **Excludes2** blue nevus (D22.-)
        - flammeus nevus (Q82.5)
        - hairy nevus (D22.-)
        - melanocytic nevus (D22.-)
        - pigmented nevus (D22.-)
        - portwine nevus (Q82.5)
        - sanguineous nevus (Q82.5)
        - strawberry nevus (Q82.5)
        - verrucous nevus (Q82.5)
    - Coding Clinic: 2019, Q1, P21
  - I78.8 **Other diseases of capillaries**
  - I78.9 **Disease of capillaries, unspecified**
- I79 **Disorders of arteries, arterioles and capillaries in diseases classified elsewhere**
  - ▷ I79.0 *Aneurysm of aorta in diseases classified elsewhere* 🦟
    - *Code first* underlying disease
      - **Excludes1** syphilitic aneurysm (A52.01)
  - ▷ I79.1 *Aortitis in diseases classified elsewhere* 🦟
    - *Code first* underlying disease
      - **Excludes1** syphilitic aortitis (A52.02)
  - ▷ I79.8 *Other disorders of arteries, arterioles and capillaries in diseases classified elsewhere*
    - *Code first* underlying disease, such as:
      - amyloidosis (E85.-)
      - **Excludes1** diabetic (peripheral) angiopathy
        - (E08-E13 with .51-.52)
        - syphilitic endarteritis (A52.09)
        - tuberculous endarteritis (A18.89)

DISEASES OF VEINS, LYMPHATIC VESSELS AND LYMPH NODES, NOT ELSEWHERE CLASSIFIED (I80-I89)

- I80 **Phlebitis and thrombophlebitis**
  - *Inflammation of a vein with infiltration of walls (phlebitis)*
    - **Includes** endophlebitis
      - inflammation, vein
      - periphlebitis
      - suppurative phlebitis
    - *Code first* phlebitis and thrombophlebitis complicating
      - abortion, ectopic or molar pregnancy (O00-O07, O08.7)
      - phlebitis and thrombophlebitis complicating pregnancy, childbirth and the puerperium (O22.-, O87.-)
    - **Excludes1** venous embolism and thrombosis of lower
      - extremities (I82.4-, I82.5-, I82.81-)
  - I80.0 **Phlebitis and thrombophlebitis of superficial vessels of lower extremities**
    - Phlebitis and thrombophlebitis of femoropopliteal vein
    - I80.00 **Phlebitis and thrombophlebitis of superficial vessels of unspecified lower extremity**
    - I80.01 **Phlebitis and thrombophlebitis of superficial vessels of right lower extremity**
    - I80.02 **Phlebitis and thrombophlebitis of superficial vessels of left lower extremity**
    - I80.03 **Phlebitis and thrombophlebitis of superficial vessels of lower extremities, bilateral**
  - I80.1 **Phlebitis and thrombophlebitis of femoral vein**
    - Phlebitis and thrombophlebitis of common femoral vein
    - Phlebitis and thrombophlebitis of deep femoral vein
    - I80.10 **Phlebitis and thrombophlebitis of unspecified femoral vein** 🦟
    - I80.11 **Phlebitis and thrombophlebitis of right femoral vein** 🦟

- I80.12 **Phlebitis and thrombophlebitis of left femoral vein** 🦟
- I80.13 **Phlebitis and thrombophlebitis of femoral vein, bilateral** 🦟
- I80.2 **Phlebitis and thrombophlebitis of other and unspecified deep vessels of lower extremities**
  - I80.20 **Phlebitis and thrombophlebitis of unspecified deep vessels of lower extremities**
    - I80.201 **Phlebitis and thrombophlebitis of unspecified deep vessels of right lower extremity** 🦟
    - I80.202 **Phlebitis and thrombophlebitis of unspecified deep vessels of left lower extremity** 🦟
    - I80.203 **Phlebitis and thrombophlebitis of unspecified deep vessels of lower extremities, bilateral** 🦟
    - I80.209 **Phlebitis and thrombophlebitis of unspecified deep vessels of unspecified lower extremity** 🦟
  - I80.21 **Phlebitis and thrombophlebitis of iliac vein**
    - Phlebitis and thrombophlebitis of common iliac vein
    - Phlebitis and thrombophlebitis of external iliac vein
    - Phlebitis and thrombophlebitis of internal iliac vein
    - I80.211 **Phlebitis and thrombophlebitis of right iliac vein** 🦟
    - I80.212 **Phlebitis and thrombophlebitis of left iliac vein** 🦟
    - I80.213 **Phlebitis and thrombophlebitis of iliac vein, bilateral** 🦟
    - I80.219 **Phlebitis and thrombophlebitis of unspecified iliac vein** 🦟
  - I80.22 **Phlebitis and thrombophlebitis of popliteal vein**
    - I80.221 **Phlebitis and thrombophlebitis of right popliteal vein** 🦟
    - I80.222 **Phlebitis and thrombophlebitis of left popliteal vein** 🦟
    - I80.223 **Phlebitis and thrombophlebitis of popliteal vein, bilateral** 🦟
    - I80.229 **Phlebitis and thrombophlebitis of unspecified popliteal vein** 🦟
  - I80.23 **Phlebitis and thrombophlebitis of tibial vein**
    - Phlebitis and thrombophlebitis of anterior tibial vein
    - Phlebitis and thrombophlebitis of posterior tibial vein
    - I80.231 **Phlebitis and thrombophlebitis of right tibial vein** 🦟
    - I80.232 **Phlebitis and thrombophlebitis of left tibial vein** 🦟
    - I80.233 **Phlebitis and thrombophlebitis of tibial vein, bilateral** 🦟
    - I80.239 **Phlebitis and thrombophlebitis of unspecified tibial vein** 🦟
  - I80.24 **Phlebitis and thrombophlebitis of peroneal vein**
    - I80.241 **Phlebitis and thrombophlebitis of right peroneal vein**
    - I80.242 **Phlebitis and thrombophlebitis of left peroneal vein**
    - I80.243 **Phlebitis and thrombophlebitis of peroneal vein, bilateral**
    - I80.249 **Phlebitis and thrombophlebitis of unspecified peroneal vein**

● I80.25   **Phlebitis and thrombophlebitis of calf muscular vein**
     Phlebitis and thrombophlebitis of calf muscular vein, NOS
     Phlebitis and thrombophlebitis of gastrocnemial vein
     Phlebitis and thrombophlebitis of soleal vein

     I80.251   **Phlebitis and thrombophlebitis of right calf muscular vein**

     I80.252   **Phlebitis and thrombophlebitis of left calf muscular vein**

     I80.253   **Phlebitis and thrombophlebitis of calf muscular vein, bilateral**

     I80.259   **Phlebitis and thrombophlebitis of unspecified calf muscular vein**

● I80.29   **Phlebitis and thrombophlebitis of other deep vessels of lower extremities**

     I80.291   **Phlebitis and thrombophlebitis of other deep vessels of right lower extremity** 🦟

     I80.292   **Phlebitis and thrombophlebitis of other deep vessels of left lower extremity** 🦟

     I80.293   **Phlebitis and thrombophlebitis of other deep vessels of lower extremity, bilateral** 🦟

     I80.299   **Phlebitis and thrombophlebitis of other deep vessels of unspecified lower extremity** 🦟

I80.3   **Phlebitis and thrombophlebitis of lower extremities, unspecified**

I80.8   **Phlebitis and thrombophlebitis of other sites**

I80.9   **Phlebitis and thrombophlebitis of unspecified site**

I81   **Portal vein thrombosis**
     Portal (vein) obstruction

     Excludes2   hepatic vein thrombosis (I82.0)
                 phlebitis of portal vein (K75.1)
     Coding Clinic: 2019, Q4, P68

● I82   **Other venous embolism and thrombosis**
     Code first venous embolism and thrombosis complicating:
         abortion, ectopic or molar pregnancy (O00-O07, O08.7)
         pregnancy, childbirth and the puerperium (O22.-, O87.-)

     Excludes2   venous embolism and thrombosis (of):
                 cerebral (I63.6, I67.6)
                 coronary (I21-I25)
                 intracranial and intraspinal, septic or NOS (G08)
                 intracranial, nonpyogenic (I67.6)
                 intraspinal, nonpyogenic (G95.1)
                 mesenteric (K55.0-)
                 portal (I81)
                 pulmonary (I26.-)

I82.0   **Budd-Chiari syndrome** 🦟
     Hepatic vein thrombosis

I82.1   **Thrombophlebitis migrans**
     "White leg" is the other term to describe a migrating thrombus.

● I82.2   **Embolism and thrombosis of vena cava and other thoracic veins**

   ● I82.21   **Embolism and thrombosis of superior vena cava**

     I82.210   **Acute embolism and thrombosis of superior vena cava** 🦟
         Embolism and thrombosis of superior vena cava NOS

     I82.211   **Chronic embolism and thrombosis of superior vena cava** 🦟

   ● I82.22   **Embolism and thrombosis of inferior vena cava**

     I82.220   **Acute embolism and thrombosis of inferior vena cava** 🦟
         Embolism and thrombosis of inferior vena cava NOS

     I82.221   **Chronic embolism and thrombosis of inferior vena cava** 🦟

   ● I82.29   **Embolism and thrombosis of other thoracic veins**
     Embolism and thrombosis of brachiocephalic (innominate) vein

     I82.290   **Acute embolism and thrombosis of other thoracic veins** 🦟

     I82.291   **Chronic embolism and thrombosis of other thoracic veins** 🦟

I82.3   **Embolism and thrombosis of renal vein** 🦟

● I82.4   **Acute embolism and thrombosis of deep veins of lower extremity**

     I82.40   **Acute embolism and thrombosis of unspecified deep veins of lower extremity**
     Deep vein thrombosis NOS
     DVT NOS

     Excludes1   acute embolism and thrombosis of unspecified deep veins of distal lower extremity (I82.4Z-)
                acute embolism and thrombosis of unspecified deep veins of proximal lower extremity (I82.4Y-)

     I82.401   **Acute embolism and thrombosis of unspecified deep veins of right lower extremity** 🦟

     I82.402   **Acute embolism and thrombosis of unspecified deep veins of left lower extremity** 🦟

     I82.403   **Acute embolism and thrombosis of unspecified deep veins of lower extremity, bilateral** 🦟

     I82.409   **Acute embolism and thrombosis of unspecified deep veins of unspecified lower extremity** 🦟

   ● I82.41   **Acute embolism and thrombosis of femoral vein**
     Acute embolism and thrombosis of common femoral vein
     Acute embolism and thrombosis of deep femoral vein

     I82.411   **Acute embolism and thrombosis of right femoral vein** 🦟

     I82.412   **Acute embolism and thrombosis of left femoral vein** 🦟

     I82.413   **Acute embolism and thrombosis of femoral vein, bilateral** 🦟

     I82.419   **Acute embolism and thrombosis of unspecified femoral vein** 🦟

   ● I82.42   **Acute embolism and thrombosis of iliac vein**
     Acute embolism and thrombosis of common iliac vein
     Acute embolism and thrombosis of external iliac vein
     Acute embolism and thrombosis of internal iliac vein

     I82.421   **Acute embolism and thrombosis of right iliac vein** 🦟

     I82.422   **Acute embolism and thrombosis of left iliac vein** 🦟

     I82.423   **Acute embolism and thrombosis of iliac vein, bilateral** 🦟

     I82.429   **Acute embolism and thrombosis of unspecified iliac vein** 🦟

CHAPTER 9 (I00-I99)

● **I82.43** Acute embolism and thrombosis of popliteal vein

    I82.431 Acute embolism and thrombosis of right popliteal vein 🔎

    I82.432 Acute embolism and thrombosis of left popliteal vein 🔎

    I82.433 Acute embolism and thrombosis of popliteal vein, bilateral 🔎

    I82.439 Acute embolism and thrombosis of unspecified popliteal vein 🔎

● **I82.44** Acute embolism and thrombosis of tibial vein

    Acute embolism and thrombosis of anterior tibial vein

    Acute embolism and thrombosis of posterior tibial vein

    I82.441 Acute embolism and thrombosis of right tibial vein 🔎

    I82.442 Acute embolism and thrombosis of left tibial vein 🔎

    I82.443 Acute embolism and thrombosis of tibial vein, bilateral 🔎

    I82.449 Acute embolism and thrombosis of unspecified tibial vein 🔎

● **I82.45** Acute embolism and thrombosis of peroneal vein

    I82.451 Acute embolism and thrombosis of right peroneal vein

    I82.452 Acute embolism and thrombosis of left peroneal vein

    I82.453 Acute embolism and thrombosis of peroneal vein, bilateral

    I82.459 Acute embolism and thrombosis of unspecified peroneal vein

● **I82.46** Acute embolism and thrombosis of calf muscular vein

    Acute embolism and thrombosis of calf muscular vein, NOS

    Acute embolism and thrombosis of gastrocnemial vein

    Acute embolism and thrombosis of soleal vein

    I82.461 Acute embolism and thrombosis of right calf muscular vein

    I82.462 Acute embolism and thrombosis of left calf muscular vein

    I82.463 Acute embolism and thrombosis of calf muscular vein, bilateral

    I82.469 Acute embolism and thrombosis of unspecified calf muscular vein

● **I82.49** Acute embolism and thrombosis of other specified deep vein of lower extremity

    I82.491 Acute embolism and thrombosis of other specified deep vein of right lower extremity 🔎

    I82.492 Acute embolism and thrombosis of other specified deep vein of left lower extremity 🔎

    I82.493 Acute embolism and thrombosis of other specified deep vein of lower extremity, bilateral 🔎

    I82.499 Acute embolism and thrombosis of other specified deep vein of unspecified lower extremity 🔎

● **I82.4Y** Acute embolism and thrombosis of unspecified deep veins of proximal lower extremity

    Acute embolism and thrombosis of deep vein of thigh NOS

    Acute embolism and thrombosis of deep vein of upper leg NOS

    I82.4Y1 Acute embolism and thrombosis of unspecified deep veins of right proximal lower extremity 🔎

    I82.4Y2 Acute embolism and thrombosis of unspecified deep veins of left proximal lower extremity 🔎

    I82.4Y3 Acute embolism and thrombosis of unspecified deep veins of proximal lower extremity, bilateral 🔎

    I82.4Y9 Acute embolism and thrombosis of unspecified deep veins of unspecified proximal lower extremity 🔎

● **I82.4Z** Acute embolism and thrombosis of unspecified deep veins of distal lower extremity

    Acute embolism and thrombosis of deep vein of calf NOS

    Acute embolism and thrombosis of deep vein of lower leg NOS

    I82.4Z1 Acute embolism and thrombosis of unspecified deep veins of right distal lower extremity 🔎

    I82.4Z2 Acute embolism and thrombosis of unspecified deep veins of left distal lower extremity 🔎

    I82.4Z3 Acute embolism and thrombosis of unspecified deep veins of distal lower extremity, bilateral 🔎

    I82.4Z9 Acute embolism and thrombosis of unspecified deep veins of unspecified distal lower extremity 🔎

● **I82.5** Chronic embolism and thrombosis of deep veins of lower extremity

    Use additional code, if applicable, for associated long-term (current) use of anticoagulants (Z79.01)

    Excludes1 personal history of venous embolism and thrombosis (Z86.718)

● **I82.50** Chronic embolism and thrombosis of unspecified deep veins of lower extremity

    Excludes1 chronic embolism and thrombosis of unspecified deep veins of distal lower extremity (I82.5Z-)

                 chronic embolism and thrombosis of unspecified deep veins of proximal lower extremity (I82.5Y-)

    I82.501 Chronic embolism and thrombosis of unspecified deep veins of right lower extremity 🔎

    I82.502 Chronic embolism and thrombosis of unspecified deep veins of left lower extremity 🔎

    I82.503 Chronic embolism and thrombosis of unspecified deep veins of lower extremity, bilateral 🔎

    I82.509 Chronic embolism and thrombosis of unspecified deep veins of unspecified lower extremity 🔎

●I82.51   **Chronic embolism and thrombosis of femoral vein**
> Chronic embolism and thrombosis of common femoral vein
> Chronic embolism and thrombosis of deep femoral vein

     I82.511   Chronic embolism and thrombosis of right femoral vein

     I82.512   Chronic embolism and thrombosis of left femoral vein

     I82.513   Chronic embolism and thrombosis of femoral vein, bilateral

     I82.519   Chronic embolism and thrombosis of unspecified femoral vein

●I82.52   **Chronic embolism and thrombosis of iliac vein**
> Chronic embolism and thrombosis of common iliac vein
> Chronic embolism and thrombosis of external iliac vein
> Chronic embolism and thrombosis of internal iliac vein

     I82.521   Chronic embolism and thrombosis of right iliac vein

     I82.522   Chronic embolism and thrombosis of left iliac vein

     I82.523   Chronic embolism and thrombosis of iliac vein, bilateral

     I82.529   Chronic embolism and thrombosis of unspecified iliac vein

●I82.53   **Chronic embolism and thrombosis of popliteal vein**

     I82.531   Chronic embolism and thrombosis of right popliteal vein

     I82.532   Chronic embolism and thrombosis of left popliteal vein

     I82.533   Chronic embolism and thrombosis of popliteal vein, bilateral

     I82.539   Chronic embolism and thrombosis of unspecified popliteal vein

●I82.54   **Chronic embolism and thrombosis of tibial vein**
> Chronic embolism and thrombosis of anterior tibial vein
> Chronic embolism and thrombosis of posterior tibial vein

     I82.541   Chronic embolism and thrombosis of right tibial vein

     I82.542   Chronic embolism and thrombosis of left tibial vein

     I82.543   Chronic embolism and thrombosis of tibial vein, bilateral

     I82.549   Chronic embolism and thrombosis of unspecified tibial vein

●I82.55   **Chronic embolism and thrombosis of peroneal vein**

     I82.551   Chronic embolism and thrombosis of right peroneal vein

     I82.552   Chronic embolism and thrombosis of left peroneal vein

     I82.553   Chronic embolism and thrombosis of peroneal vein, bilateral

     I82.559   Chronic embolism and thrombosis of unspecified peroneal vein

Item 9–10 Varicose/Varicosities (varix = singular, varices = plural): Enlarged, engorged, tortuous, twisted vascular vessels (veins, arteries, lymphatics). As such, the condition can present in various parts of the body, although the most familiar locations are the lower extremities. A common complication of varices is thrombophlebitis. Varicosities of the anus and rectum are called hemorrhoids.

Figure 9-7 Varicose veins of the legs. (Getty Image)

●I82.56   **Chronic embolism and thrombosis of calf muscular vein**
> Chronic embolism and thrombosis of calf muscular vein NOS
> Chronic embolism and thrombosis of gastrocnemial vein
> Chronic embolism and thrombosis of soleal vein

     I82.561   Chronic embolism and thrombosis of right calf muscular vein

     I82.562   Chronic embolism and thrombosis of left calf muscular vein

     I82.563   Chronic embolism and thrombosis of calf muscular vein, bilateral

     I82.569   Chronic embolism and thrombosis of unspecified calf muscular vein

●I82.59   **Chronic embolism and thrombosis of other specified deep vein of lower extremity**

     I82.591   Chronic embolism and thrombosis of other specified deep vein of right lower extremity

     I82.592   Chronic embolism and thrombosis of other specified deep vein of left lower extremity

     I82.593   Chronic embolism and thrombosis of other specified deep vein of lower extremity, bilateral

     I82.599   Chronic embolism and thrombosis of other specified deep vein of unspecified lower extremity

●I82.5Y   **Chronic embolism and thrombosis of unspecified deep veins of proximal lower extremity**
> Chronic embolism and thrombosis of deep veins of thigh NOS
> Chronic embolism and thrombosis of deep veins of upper leg NOS

     I82.5Y1   Chronic embolism and thrombosis of unspecified deep veins of right proximal lower extremity

     I82.5Y2   Chronic embolism and thrombosis of unspecified deep veins of left proximal lower extremity

     I82.5Y3   Chronic embolism and thrombosis of unspecified deep veins of proximal lower extremity, bilateral

     I82.5Y9   Chronic embolism and thrombosis of unspecified deep veins of unspecified proximal lower extremity

● **I82.5Z   Chronic embolism and thrombosis of unspecified deep veins of distal lower extremity**
　　　Chronic embolism and thrombosis of deep veins of calf NOS
　　　Chronic embolism and thrombosis of deep veins of lower leg NOS

　　I82.5Z1　Chronic embolism and thrombosis of unspecified deep veins of right distal lower extremity 🐾

　　I82.5Z2　Chronic embolism and thrombosis of unspecified deep veins of left distal lower extremity 🐾

　　I82.5Z3　Chronic embolism and thrombosis of unspecified deep veins of distal lower extremity, bilateral 🐾

　　I82.5Z9　Chronic embolism and thrombosis of unspecified deep veins of unspecified distal lower extremity 🐾

● **I82.6   Acute embolism and thrombosis of veins of upper extremity**

● **I82.60   Acute embolism and thrombosis of unspecified veins of upper extremity**

　　I82.601　Acute embolism and thrombosis of unspecified veins of right upper extremity

　　I82.602　Acute embolism and thrombosis of unspecified veins of left upper extremity

　　I82.603　Acute embolism and thrombosis of unspecified veins of upper extremity, bilateral

　　I82.609　Acute embolism and thrombosis of unspecified veins of unspecified upper extremity

● **I82.61   Acute embolism and thrombosis of superficial veins of upper extremity**
　　　Acute embolism and thrombosis of antecubital vein
　　　Acute embolism and thrombosis of basilic vein
　　　Acute embolism and thrombosis of cephalic vein

　　I82.611　Acute embolism and thrombosis of superficial veins of right upper extremity

　　I82.612　Acute embolism and thrombosis of superficial veins of left upper extremity

　　I82.613　Acute embolism and thrombosis of superficial veins of upper extremity, bilateral

　　I82.619　Acute embolism and thrombosis of superficial veins of unspecified upper extremity

● **I82.62   Acute embolism and thrombosis of deep veins of upper extremity**
　　　Acute embolism and thrombosis of brachial vein
　　　Acute embolism and thrombosis of radial vein
　　　Acute embolism and thrombosis of ulnar vein

　　I82.621　Acute embolism and thrombosis of deep veins of right upper extremity 🐾

　　I82.622　Acute embolism and thrombosis of deep veins of left upper extremity 🐾

　　I82.623　Acute embolism and thrombosis of deep veins of upper extremity, bilateral 🐾

　　I82.629　Acute embolism and thrombosis of deep veins of unspecified upper extremity 🐾

● **I82.7   Chronic embolism and thrombosis of veins of upper extremity**

　　Use additional code, if applicable, for associated long-term (current) use of anticoagulants (Z79.01)

　　Excludes1　personal history of venous embolism and thrombosis (Z86.718)

● **I82.70   Chronic embolism and thrombosis of unspecified veins of upper extremity**

　　I82.701　Chronic embolism and thrombosis of unspecified veins of right upper extremity

　　I82.702　Chronic embolism and thrombosis of unspecified veins of left upper extremity

　　I82.703　Chronic embolism and thrombosis of unspecified veins of upper extremity, bilateral

　　I82.709　Chronic embolism and thrombosis of unspecified veins of unspecified upper extremity

● **I82.71   Chronic embolism and thrombosis of superficial veins of upper extremity**
　　　Chronic embolism and thrombosis of antecubital vein
　　　Chronic embolism and thrombosis of basilic vein
　　　Chronic embolism and thrombosis of cephalic vein

　　I82.711　Chronic embolism and thrombosis of superficial veins of right upper extremity

　　I82.712　Chronic embolism and thrombosis of superficial veins of left upper extremity

　　I82.713　Chronic embolism and thrombosis of superficial veins of upper extremity, bilateral

　　I82.719　Chronic embolism and thrombosis of superficial veins of unspecified upper extremity

● **I82.72   Chronic embolism and thrombosis of deep veins of upper extremity**
　　　Chronic embolism and thrombosis of brachial vein
　　　Chronic embolism and thrombosis of radial vein
　　　Chronic embolism and thrombosis of ulnar vein

　　I82.721　Chronic embolism and thrombosis of deep veins of right upper extremity 🐾

　　I82.722　Chronic embolism and thrombosis of deep veins of left upper extremity 🐾

　　I82.723　Chronic embolism and thrombosis of deep veins of upper extremity, bilateral 🐾

　　I82.729　Chronic embolism and thrombosis of deep veins of unspecified upper extremity 🐾

● **I82.A   Embolism and thrombosis of axillary vein**

● **I82.A1   Acute embolism and thrombosis of axillary vein**

　　I82.A11　Acute embolism and thrombosis of right axillary vein 🐾

　　I82.A12　Acute embolism and thrombosis of left axillary vein 🐾

　　I82.A13　Acute embolism and thrombosis of axillary vein, bilateral 🐾

　　I82.A19　Acute embolism and thrombosis of unspecified axillary vein 🐾

▶ New　⇒ Revised　deleted Deleted　Excludes 1　Excludes 2　Includes　Use additional　Code first　Code also　Key words
OGCR Official Guidelines　X Assign placeholder X　● Use Additional Character(s)　▌ Manifestation Code　🐾 Hierarchical Condition Category　**Coding Clinic**

I82.A2   Chronic embolism and thrombosis of axillary vein

    I82.A21   Chronic embolism and thrombosis of right axillary vein 🔎

    I82.A22   Chronic embolism and thrombosis of left axillary vein 🔎

    I82.A23   Chronic embolism and thrombosis of axillary vein, bilateral 🔎

    I82.A29   Chronic embolism and thrombosis of unspecified axillary vein 🔎

I82.B   Embolism and thrombosis of subclavian vein

   I82.B1   Acute embolism and thrombosis of subclavian vein

    I82.B11   Acute embolism and thrombosis of right subclavian vein 🔎

    I82.B12   Acute embolism and thrombosis of left subclavian vein 🔎

    I82.B13   Acute embolism and thrombosis of subclavian vein, bilateral 🔎

    I82.B19   Acute embolism and thrombosis of unspecified subclavian vein 🔎

   I82.B2   Chronic embolism and thrombosis of subclavian vein

    I82.B21   Chronic embolism and thrombosis of right subclavian vein 🔎

    I82.B22   Chronic embolism and thrombosis of left subclavian vein 🔎

    I82.B23   Chronic embolism and thrombosis of subclavian vein, bilateral 🔎

    I82.B29   Chronic embolism and thrombosis of unspecified subclavian vein 🔎

I82.C   Embolism and thrombosis of internal jugular vein

   I82.C1   Acute embolism and thrombosis of internal jugular vein

    I82.C11   Acute embolism and thrombosis of right internal jugular vein 🔎

    I82.C12   Acute embolism and thrombosis of left internal jugular vein 🔎

    I82.C13   Acute embolism and thrombosis of internal jugular vein, bilateral 🔎

    I82.C19   Acute embolism and thrombosis of unspecified internal jugular vein 🔎

   I82.C2   Chronic embolism and thrombosis of internal jugular vein

    I82.C21   Chronic embolism and thrombosis of right internal jugular vein 🔎

    I82.C22   Chronic embolism and thrombosis of left internal jugular vein 🔎

    I82.C23   Chronic embolism and thrombosis of internal jugular vein, bilateral 🔎

    I82.C29   Chronic embolism and thrombosis of unspecified internal jugular vein 🔎

I82.8   Embolism and thrombosis of other specified veins

> Use additional code, if applicable, for associated long-term (current) use of anticoagulants (Z79.01)

   I82.81   Embolism and thrombosis of superficial veins of lower extremities

> Embolism and thrombosis of saphenous vein (greater) (lesser)

    I82.811   Embolism and thrombosis of superficial veins of right lower extremity

    I82.812   Embolism and thrombosis of superficial veins of left lower extremity

    I82.813   Embolism and thrombosis of superficial veins of lower extremities, bilateral

    I82.819   Embolism and thrombosis of superficial veins of unspecified lower extremity

   I82.89   Embolism and thrombosis of other specified veins

    I82.890   Acute embolism and thrombosis of other specified veins

    I82.891   Chronic embolism and thrombosis of other specified veins

I82.9   Embolism and thrombosis of unspecified vein

   I82.90   Acute embolism and thrombosis of unspecified vein

> Embolism of vein NOS
> Thrombosis (vein) NOS

   I82.91   Chronic embolism and thrombosis of unspecified vein

I83   Varicose veins of lower extremities

> ~~Excludes1   varicose veins complicating pregnancy (O22.0)~~
> ~~varicose veins complicating the puerperium (O87.4)~~

> ▶ **Excludes2**   varicose veins complicating pregnancy (O22.0-)
> ▶ varicose veins complicating the puerperium (O87.4)

I83.0   Varicose veins of lower extremities with ulcer

> Use additional code to identify severity of ulcer (L97.-)

   I83.00   Varicose veins of unspecified lower extremity with ulcer

    I83.001   Varicose veins of unspecified lower extremity with ulcer of thigh 🔎   A

    I83.002   Varicose veins of unspecified lower extremity with ulcer of calf 🔎   A

    I83.003   Varicose veins of unspecified lower extremity with ulcer of ankle 🔎   A

    I83.004   Varicose veins of unspecified lower extremity with ulcer of heel and midfoot 🔎   A

> Varicose veins of unspecified lower extremity with ulcer of plantar surface of midfoot

    I83.005   Varicose veins of unspecified lower extremity with ulcer other part of foot 🔎   A

> Varicose veins of unspecified lower extremity with ulcer of toe

    I83.008   Varicose veins of unspecified lower extremity with ulcer other part of lower leg 🔎   A

    I83.009   Varicose veins of unspecified lower extremity with ulcer of unspecified site 🔎   A

   I83.01   Varicose veins of right lower extremity with ulcer

    I83.011   Varicose veins of right lower extremity with ulcer of thigh 🔎   A

    I83.012   Varicose veins of right lower extremity with ulcer of calf 🔎   A

    I83.013   Varicose veins of right lower extremity with ulcer of ankle 🔎   A

    I83.014   Varicose veins of right lower extremity with ulcer of heel and midfoot 🔎   A

> Varicose veins of right lower extremity with ulcer of plantar surface of midfoot

Code	Description	
I83.015	Varicose veins of right lower extremity with ulcer other part of foot 🔸	A
	Varicose veins of right lower extremity with ulcer of toe	
I83.018	Varicose veins of right lower extremity with ulcer other part of lower leg 🔸	A
I83.019	Varicose veins of right lower extremity with ulcer of unspecified site 🔸	A
● I83.02	Varicose veins of left lower extremity with ulcer	
I83.021	Varicose veins of left lower extremity with ulcer of thigh 🔸	A
I83.022	Varicose veins of left lower extremity with ulcer of calf 🔸	A
I83.023	Varicose veins of left lower extremity with ulcer of ankle 🔸	A
I83.024	Varicose veins of left lower extremity with ulcer of heel and midfoot 🔸	A
	Varicose veins of left lower extremity with ulcer of plantar surface of midfoot	
I83.025	Varicose veins of left lower extremity with ulcer other part of foot 🔸	A
	Varicose veins of left lower extremity with ulcer of toe	
I83.028	Varicose veins of left lower extremity with ulcer other part of lower leg 🔸	A
I83.029	Varicose veins of left lower extremity with ulcer of unspecified site 🔸	A

● I83.1   Varicose veins of lower extremities with inflammation

Code	Description	
I83.10	Varicose veins of unspecified lower extremity with inflammation	A
I83.11	Varicose veins of right lower extremity with inflammation	A
I83.12	Varicose veins of left lower extremity with inflammation	A

● I83.2   Varicose veins of lower extremities with both ulcer and inflammation

Use additional code to identify severity of ulcer (L97.-)

Code	Description	
● I83.20	Varicose veins of unspecified lower extremity with both ulcer and inflammation	
I83.201	Varicose veins of unspecified lower extremity with both ulcer of thigh and inflammation 🔸	A
I83.202	Varicose veins of unspecified lower extremity with both ulcer of calf and inflammation 🔸	A
I83.203	Varicose veins of unspecified lower extremity with both ulcer of ankle and inflammation 🔸	A
I83.204	Varicose veins of unspecified lower extremity with both ulcer of heel and midfoot and inflammation 🔸	A
	Varicose veins of unspecified lower extremity with both ulcer of plantar surface of midfoot and inflammation	
I83.205	Varicose veins of unspecified lower extremity with both ulcer other part of foot and inflammation 🔸	A
	Varicose veins of unspecified lower extremity with both ulcer of toe and inflammation	
I83.208	Varicose veins of unspecified lower extremity with both ulcer of other part of lower extremity and inflammation 🔸	A
I83.209	Varicose veins of unspecified lower extremity with both ulcer of unspecified site and inflammation 🔸	A

Code	Description	
● I83.21	Varicose veins of right lower extremity with both ulcer and inflammation	
I83.211	Varicose veins of right lower extremity with both ulcer of thigh and inflammation 🔸	A
I83.212	Varicose veins of right lower extremity with both ulcer of calf and inflammation 🔸	A
I83.213	Varicose veins of right lower extremity with both ulcer of ankle and inflammation 🔸	A
I83.214	Varicose veins of right lower extremity with both ulcer of heel and midfoot and inflammation 🔸	A
	Varicose veins of right lower extremity with both ulcer of plantar surface of midfoot and inflammation	
I83.215	Varicose veins of right lower extremity with both ulcer other part of foot and inflammation 🔸	A
	Varicose veins of right lower extremity with both ulcer of toe and inflammation	
I83.218	Varicose veins of right lower extremity with both ulcer of other part of lower extremity and inflammation 🔸	A
I83.219	Varicose veins of right lower extremity with both ulcer of unspecified site and inflammation 🔸	A
● I83.22	Varicose veins of left lower extremity with both ulcer and inflammation	
I83.221	Varicose veins of left lower extremity with both ulcer of thigh and inflammation 🔸	A
I83.222	Varicose veins of left lower extremity with both ulcer of calf and inflammation 🔸	A
I83.223	Varicose veins of left lower extremity with both ulcer of ankle and inflammation 🔸	A
I83.224	Varicose veins of left lower extremity with both ulcer of heel and midfoot and inflammation 🔸	A
	Varicose veins of left lower extremity with both ulcer of plantar surface of midfoot and inflammation	
I83.225	Varicose veins of left lower extremity with both ulcer other part of foot and inflammation 🔸	A
	Varicose veins of left lower extremity with both ulcer of toe and inflammation	
I83.228	Varicose veins of left lower extremity with both ulcer of other part of lower extremity and inflammation 🔸	A
I83.229	Varicose veins of left lower extremity with both ulcer of unspecified site and inflammation 🔸	A

● I83.8   Varicose veins of lower extremities with other complications

Code	Description	
● I83.81	Varicose veins of lower extremities with pain	
I83.811	Varicose veins of right lower extremity with pain	A
I83.812	Varicose veins of left lower extremity with pain	A
I83.813	Varicose veins of bilateral lower extremities with pain	A
I83.819	Varicose veins of unspecified lower extremity with pain	A

▶ New   ➔ Revised   ~~deleted~~ Deleted   Excludes 1   Excludes 2   Includes   Use additional   Code first   Code also   Key words
OGCR Official Guidelines   X Assign placeholder X   ● Use Additional Character(s)   ▶ Manifestation Code   🔸 Hierarchical Condition Category   **Coding Clinic**

● I83.89   **Varicose veins of lower extremities with other complications**
     Varicose veins of lower extremities with edema
     Varicose veins of lower extremities with swelling

     I83.891   **Varicose veins of right lower extremity with other complications**   A

     I83.892   **Varicose veins of left lower extremity with other complications**   A

     I83.893   **Varicose veins of bilateral lower extremities with other complications** A

     I83.899   **Varicose veins of unspecified lower extremity with other complications**   A

● I83.9   **Asymptomatic varicose veins of lower extremities**
     Phlebectasia of lower extremities
     Varicose veins of lower extremities
     Varix of lower extremities

     I83.90   **Asymptomatic varicose veins of unspecified lower extremity**   A
        Varicose veins NOS

     I83.91   **Asymptomatic varicose veins of right lower extremity**   A

     I83.92   **Asymptomatic varicose veins of left lower extremity**   A

     I83.93   **Asymptomatic varicose veins of bilateral lower extremities**   A

● **I85**   **Esophageal varices**
     Use additional code to identify:
     alcohol abuse and dependence (F10.-)

● I85.0   **Esophageal varices**
     Idiopathic esophageal varices
     Primary esophageal varices

     I85.00   **Esophageal varices without bleeding** 🐾
        Esophageal varices NOS

     I85.01   **Esophageal varices with bleeding** 🐾

● I85.1   **Secondary esophageal varices**
     Esophageal varices secondary to alcoholic liver disease
     Esophageal varices secondary to cirrhosis of liver
     Esophageal varices secondary to schistosomiasis
     Esophageal varices secondary to toxic liver disease
     Code first underlying disease

     I85.10   **Secondary esophageal varices without bleeding** 🐾

     I85.11   **Secondary esophageal varices with bleeding** 🐾

● **I86**   **Varicose veins of other sites**
     Excludes1   varicose veins of unspecified site (I83.9-)
     Excludes2   retinal varices (H35.0-)

     I86.0   **Sublingual varices**
     I86.1   **Scrotal varices** ♂
        Varicocele
     I86.2   **Pelvic varices**
     I86.3   **Vulval varices** ♀
        Excludes1   vulval varices complicating childbirth and the puerperium (O87.8)
                 vulval varices complicating pregnancy (O22.1-)
     I86.4   **Gastric varices**
     I86.8   **Varicose veins of other specified sites**   A
        Varicose ulcer of nasal septum

● **I87**   **Other disorders of veins**
● I87.0   **Postthrombotic syndrome**
     Chronic venous hypertension due to deep vein thrombosis
     Postphlebitic syndrome
     Excludes1   chronic venous hypertension without deep vein thrombosis (I87.3-)

     ● I87.00   **Postthrombotic syndrome without complications**
        Asymptomatic Postthrombotic syndrome

     I87.001   Postthrombotic syndrome without complications of right lower extremity

     I87.002   Postthrombotic syndrome without complications of left lower extremity

     I87.003   Postthrombotic syndrome without complications of bilateral lower extremity

     I87.009   Postthrombotic syndrome without complications of unspecified extremity
        Postthrombotic syndrome NOS

● I87.01   **Postthrombotic syndrome with ulcer**
     Use additional code to specify site and severity of ulcer (L97.-)

     I87.011   Postthrombotic syndrome with ulcer of right lower extremity 🐾

     I87.012   Postthrombotic syndrome with ulcer of left lower extremity 🐾

     I87.013   Postthrombotic syndrome with ulcer of bilateral lower extremity 🐾

     I87.019   Postthrombotic syndrome with ulcer of unspecified lower extremity 🐾

● I87.02   **Postthrombotic syndrome with inflammation**

     I87.021   Postthrombotic syndrome with inflammation of right lower extremity

     I87.022   Postthrombotic syndrome with inflammation of left lower extremity

     I87.023   Postthrombotic syndrome with inflammation of bilateral lower extremity

     I87.029   Postthrombotic syndrome with inflammation of unspecified lower extremity

● I87.03   **Postthrombotic syndrome with ulcer and inflammation**
     Use additional code to specify site and severity of ulcer (L97.-)

     I87.031   Postthrombotic syndrome with ulcer and inflammation of right lower extremity 🐾

     I87.032   Postthrombotic syndrome with ulcer and inflammation of left lower extremity 🐾

     I87.033   Postthrombotic syndrome with ulcer and inflammation of bilateral lower extremity 🐾

     I87.039   Postthrombotic syndrome with ulcer and inflammation of unspecified lower extremity 🐾

● I87.09   **Postthrombotic syndrome with other complications**

     I87.091   Postthrombotic syndrome with other complications of right lower extremity

     I87.092   Postthrombotic syndrome with other complications of left lower extremity

     I87.093   Postthrombotic syndrome with other complications of bilateral lower extremity

     I87.099   Postthrombotic syndrome with other complications of unspecified lower extremity

I87.1   **Compression of vein**
     Stricture of vein
     Vena cava syndrome (inferior) (superior)
     Excludes2   compression of pulmonary vein (I28.8)

I87.2   **Venous insufficiency (chronic) (peripheral)**
     Stasis dermatitis
     Excludes1   stasis dermatitis with varicose veins of lower extremities (I83.1-, I83.2-)

● **I87.3** **Chronic venous hypertension (idiopathic)**
Stasis edema
> **Excludes1** chronic venous hypertension due to deep vein thrombosis (I87.0-)
> varicose veins of lower extremities (I83.-)

● **I87.30** **Chronic venous hypertension (idiopathic) without complications**
Asymptomatic chronic venous hypertension (idiopathic)

I87.301 **Chronic venous hypertension (idiopathic) without complications of right lower extremity**

I87.302 **Chronic venous hypertension (idiopathic) without complications of left lower extremity**

I87.303 **Chronic venous hypertension (idiopathic) without complications of bilateral lower extremity**

I87.309 **Chronic venous hypertension (idiopathic) without complications of unspecified lower extremity**
Chronic venous hypertension NOS

● **I87.31** **Chronic venous hypertension (idiopathic) with ulcer**
> Use additional code to specify site and severity of ulcer (L97.-)

I87.311 **Chronic venous hypertension (idiopathic) with ulcer of right lower extremity** 🐷

I87.312 **Chronic venous hypertension (idiopathic) with ulcer of left lower extremity** 🐷

I87.313 **Chronic venous hypertension (idiopathic) with ulcer of bilateral lower extremity** 🐷

I87.319 **Chronic venous hypertension (idiopathic) with ulcer of unspecified lower extremity** 🐷

● **I87.32** **Chronic venous hypertension (idiopathic) with inflammation**

I87.321 **Chronic venous hypertension (idiopathic) with inflammation of right lower extremity**

I87.322 **Chronic venous hypertension (idiopathic) with inflammation of left lower extremity**

I87.323 **Chronic venous hypertension (idiopathic) with inflammation of bilateral lower extremity**

I87.329 **Chronic venous hypertension (idiopathic) with inflammation of unspecified lower extremity**

● **I87.33** **Chronic venous hypertension (idiopathic) with ulcer and inflammation**
> Use additional code to specify site and severity of ulcer (L97.-)

I87.331 **Chronic venous hypertension (idiopathic) with ulcer and inflammation of right lower extremity** 🐷

I87.332 **Chronic venous hypertension (idiopathic) with ulcer and inflammation of left lower extremity** 🐷

I87.333 **Chronic venous hypertension (idiopathic) with ulcer and inflammation of bilateral lower extremity** 🐷

I87.339 **Chronic venous hypertension (idiopathic) with ulcer and inflammation of unspecified lower extremity** 🐷

● **I87.39** **Chronic venous hypertension (idiopathic) with other complications**

I87.391 **Chronic venous hypertension (idiopathic) with other complications of right lower extremity**

I87.392 **Chronic venous hypertension (idiopathic) with other complications of left lower extremity**

I87.393 **Chronic venous hypertension (idiopathic) with other complications of bilateral lower extremity**

I87.399 **Chronic venous hypertension (idiopathic) with other complications of unspecified lower extremity**

I87.8 **Other specified disorders of veins**
Phlebosclerosis
Venofibrosis

I87.9 **Disorder of vein, unspecified**

● **I88** **Nonspecific lymphadenitis**
> **Excludes1** acute lymphadenitis, except mesenteric (L04.-)
> enlarged lymph nodes NOS (R59.-)
> human immunodeficiency virus [HIV] disease resulting in generalized lymphadenopathy (B20)

I88.0 **Nonspecific mesenteric lymphadenitis**
Mesenteric lymphadenitis (acute)(chronic)

I88.1 **Chronic lymphadenitis, except mesenteric**
Adenitis
Lymphadenitis

I88.8 **Other nonspecific lymphadenitis**

I88.9 **Nonspecific lymphadenitis, unspecified**
Lymphadenitis NOS

● **I89** **Other noninfective disorders of lymphatic vessels and lymph nodes**
> **Excludes1** chylocele, tunica vaginalis (nonfilarial) NOS (N50.89)
> enlarged lymph nodes NOS (R59.-)
> filarial chylocele (B74.-)
> hereditary lymphedema (Q82.0)

I89.0 **Lymphedema, not elsewhere classified**
Elephantiasis (nonfilarial) NOS
Lymphangiectasis
Obliteration, lymphatic vessel
Praecox lymphedema
Secondary lymphedema
> **Excludes1** postmastectomy lymphedema (I97.2)

I89.1 **Lymphangitis**
Chronic lymphangitis
Lymphangitis NOS
Subacute lymphangitis
> **Excludes1** acute lymphangitis (L03.-)

I89.8 **Other specified noninfective disorders of lymphatic vessels and lymph nodes**
Chylocele (nonfilarial)
Chylous ascites
Chylous cyst
Lipomelanotic reticulosis
Lymph node or vessel fistula
Lymph node or vessel infarction
Lymph node or vessel rupture

I89.9 **Noninfective disorder of lymphatic vessels and lymph nodes, unspecified**
Disease of lymphatic vessels NOS

▶ New ⇒ Revised ~~deleted~~ Deleted Excludes 1 Excludes 2 Includes Use additional Code first Code also Key words
OGCR Official Guidelines X Assign placeholder X ● Use Additional Character(s) ❱ Manifestation Code 🐷 Hierarchical Condition Category **Coding Clinic**

OTHER AND UNSPECIFIED DISORDERS OF THE CIRCULATORY SYSTEM (I95-I99)

● **I95**   **Hypotension**
Subnormal arterial blood pressure

Excludes1   cardiovascular collapse (R57.9)
maternal hypotension syndrome (O26.5-)
nonspecific low blood pressure reading NOS
(R03.1)

I95.0   **Idiopathic hypotension**

I95.1   **Orthostatic hypotension**
Hypotension, postural
Moving from a sitting or reclining position to a standing
position precipitates a sudden drop in blood pressure
(hypotension).

Excludes1   neurogenic orthostatic hypotension [Shy-
Drager] (G90.3)
orthostatic hypotension due to drugs (I95.2)

I95.2   **Hypotension due to drugs**
Orthostatic hypotension due to drugs
Use additional code for adverse effect, if applicable,
to identify drug (T36-T50 with fifth or sixth
character 5)

I95.3   **Hypotension of hemodialysis**
Intra-dialytic hypotension

● I95.8   **Other hypotension**

I95.81   **Postprocedural hypotension**

I95.89   **Other hypotension**
Chronic hypotension

I95.9   **Hypotension, unspecified**

I96   **Gangrene, not elsewhere classified** ⚫
Gangrenous cellulitis

Excludes1   gangrene in atherosclerosis of native arteries of
the extremities (I70.26)
gangrene of certain specified sites - *see*
Alphabetical Index
gangrene in hernia (K40.1, K40.4, K41.1, K41.4,
K42.1, K43.1-, K44.1, K45.1, K46.1)
gangrene in other peripheral vascular diseases
(I73.-)
gas gangrene (A48.0)
pyoderma gangrenosum (L88)

Excludes2   gangrene in diabetes mellitus (E08-E13 with .52)
Coding Clinic: 2018, Q4, P87; 2017, Q3, P6; 2013, Q2, P35

● **I97**   **Intraoperative and postprocedural complications and disorders**
of circulatory system, not elsewhere classified

Excludes2   postprocedural shock (T81.1-)
Coding Clinic: 2019, Q2, P22

I97.0   **Postcardiotomy syndrome**

● I97.1   **Other postprocedural cardiac functional disturbances**

Excludes2   acute pulmonary insufficiency following
thoracic surgery (J95.1)
intraoperative cardiac functional
disturbances (I97.7-)

● I97.11   **Postprocedural cardiac insufficiency**

I97.110   **Postprocedural cardiac insufficiency**
following cardiac surgery

I97.111   **Postprocedural cardiac insufficiency**
following other surgery

● I97.12   **Postprocedural cardiac arrest**

I97.120   **Postprocedural cardiac arrest**
following cardiac surgery

I97.121   **Postprocedural cardiac arrest**
following other surgery

● I97.13   **Postprocedural heart failure**
Use additional code to identify the heart
failure (I50.-)

I97.130   **Postprocedural heart failure**
following cardiac surgery

I97.131   **Postprocedural heart failure**
following other surgery

● I97.19   **Other postprocedural cardiac functional**
disturbances
Use additional code, if applicable, to further
specify disorder

I97.190   **Other postprocedural cardiac**
functional disturbances following
cardiac surgery
Use Additional code, if applicable,
for type 4 or type 5 myocardial
infarction, to further specify
disorder
Coding Clinic: 2019, Q2, P32-33

I97.191   **Other postprocedural cardiac**
functional disturbances following
other surgery

I97.2   **Postmastectomy lymphedema syndrome**   A
Elephantiasis due to mastectomy
Obliteration of lymphatic vessels

I97.3   **Postprocedural hypertension**

● I97.4   **Intraoperative hemorrhage and hematoma of a**
circulatory system organ or structure complicating a
procedure

Excludes1   intraoperative hemorrhage and
hematoma of a circulatory system
organ or structure due to accidental
puncture and laceration during a
procedure (I97.5-)

Excludes2   intraoperative cerebrovascular
hemorrhage complicating a
procedure (G97.3-)

● I97.41   **Intraoperative hemorrhage and hematoma**
of a circulatory system organ or structure
complicating a circulatory system procedure

I97.410   **Intraoperative hemorrhage and**
hematoma of a circulatory system
organ or structure complicating a
cardiac catheterization

I97.411   **Intraoperative hemorrhage and**
hematoma of a circulatory system
organ or structure complicating a
cardiac bypass

I97.418   **Intraoperative hemorrhage and**
hematoma of a circulatory system
organ or structure complicating other
circulatory system procedure

I97.42   **Intraoperative hemorrhage and hematoma**
of a circulatory system organ or structure
complicating other procedure
Coding Clinic: 2020, Q1, P20; 2016, Q4, P100

● I97.5   **Accidental puncture and laceration of a circulatory**
system organ or structure during a procedure

Excludes2   accidental puncture and laceration of
brain during a procedure (G97.4-)

I97.51   **Accidental puncture and laceration of a**
circulatory system organ or structure during a
circulatory system procedure
Coding Clinic: 2019, Q2, P24

I97.52   **Accidental puncture and laceration of a**
circulatory system organ or structure during
other procedure

● I97.6   Postprocedural hemorrhage, hematoma and seroma
           of a circulatory system organ or structure following a
           procedure
           Excludes2   postprocedural cerebrovascular
                        hemorrhage complicating a
                        procedure (G97.5-)
           Coding Clinic: 2016, Q4, P10

● I97.61   Postprocedural hemorrhage of a circulatory
           system organ or structure following a
           circulatory system procedure
           I97.610   Postprocedural hemorrhage of a
                      circulatory system organ or structure
                      following a cardiac catheterization
           I97.611   Postprocedural hemorrhage of a
                      circulatory system organ or structure
                      following cardiac bypass
           I97.618   Postprocedural hemorrhage of a
                      circulatory system organ or structure
                      following other circulatory system
                      procedure

● I97.62   Postprocedural hemorrhage, hematoma
           and seroma of a circulatory system organ or
           structure following other procedure
           I97.620   Postprocedural hemorrhage of a
                      circulatory system organ or structure
                      following other procedure
           I97.621   Postprocedural hematoma of a
                      circulatory system organ or structure
                      following other procedure
           I97.622   Postprocedural seroma of a
                      circulatory system organ or structure
                      following other procedure

● I97.63   Postprocedural hematoma of a circulatory
           system organ or structure following a
           circulatory system procedure
           I97.630   Postprocedural hematoma of a
                      circulatory system organ or structure
                      following a cardiac catheterization
           I97.631   Postprocedural hematoma of a
                      circulatory system organ or structure
                      following cardiac bypass
           I97.638   Postprocedural hematoma of a
                      circulatory system organ or structure
                      following other circulatory system
                      procedure

● I97.64   Postprocedural seroma of a circulatory system
           organ or structure following a circulatory
           system procedure
           I97.640   Postprocedural seroma of a
                      circulatory system organ or structure
                      following a cardiac catheterization
           I97.641   Postprocedural seroma of a
                      circulatory system organ or structure
                      following cardiac bypass
           I97.648   Postprocedural seroma of a
                      circulatory system organ or structure
                      following other circulatory system
                      procedure

● I97.7   Intraoperative cardiac functional disturbances
           Excludes2   acute pulmonary insufficiency following
                        thoracic surgery (J95.1)
                        postprocedural cardiac functional
                        disturbances (I97.1-)
● I97.71   Intraoperative cardiac arrest
           I97.710   Intraoperative cardiac arrest during
                      cardiac surgery
           I97.711   Intraoperative cardiac arrest during
                      other surgery
● I97.79   Other intraoperative cardiac functional
           disturbances
           Use additional code, if applicable, to further
                specify disorder
           I97.790   Other intraoperative cardiac
                      functional disturbances during
                      cardiac surgery
           I97.791   Other intraoperative cardiac
                      functional disturbances during other
                      surgery

● I97.8   Other intraoperative and postprocedural complications
           and disorders of the circulatory system, not elsewhere
           classified
           Use additional code, if applicable, to further specify
                disorder
● I97.81   Intraoperative cerebrovascular infarction
           I97.810   Intraoperative cerebrovascular
                      infarction during cardiac surgery 🐾
           I97.811   Intraoperative cerebrovascular
                      infarction during other surgery 🐾
● I97.82   Postprocedural cerebrovascular infarction
           I97.820   Postprocedural cerebrovascular
                      infarction following cardiac
                      surgery 🐾
           I97.821   Postprocedural cerebrovascular
                      infarction following other surgery 🐾
           I97.88   Other intraoperative complications of the
                      circulatory system, not elsewhere classified
           I97.89   Other postprocedural complications and
                      disorders of the circulatory system, not
                      elsewhere classified
                      Coding Clinic: 2019, Q2, P32-33

● I99   Other and unspecified disorders of circulatory system
          I99.8   Other disorder of circulatory system
          I99.9   Unspecified disorder of circulatory system

▶ New   ⇨ Revised   ~~deleted~~ Deleted   Excludes 1   Excludes 2   Includes   Use additional   Code first   Code also   Key words
OGCR Official Guidelines   X Assign placeholder X   ● Use Additional Character(s)   ▷ Manifestation Code   🐾 Hierarchical Condition Category   Coding Clinic

CHAPTER 9 (I00-I99)

CHAPTER 10

DISEASES OF THE RESPIRATORY SYSTEM (J00-J99)

OGCR Chapter-Specific Coding Guidelines

10. **Chapter 10: Diseases of the Respiratory System (J00-J99)**

a. **Chronic Obstructive Pulmonary Disease [COPD] and Asthma**

1) **Acute exacerbation of chronic obstructive bronchitis and asthma**

The codes in categories J44 and J45 distinguish between uncomplicated cases and those in acute exacerbation. An acute exacerbation is a worsening or a decompensation of a chronic condition. An acute exacerbation is not equivalent to an infection superimposed on a chronic condition, though an exacerbation may be triggered by an infection.

b. **Acute Respiratory Failure**

1) **Acute respiratory failure as principal diagnosis**

A code from subcategory J96.0, Acute respiratory failure, or subcategory J96.2, Acute and chronic respiratory failure, may be assigned as a principal diagnosis when it is the condition established after study to be chiefly responsible for occasioning the admission to the hospital, and the selection is supported by the Alphabetic Index and Tabular List. However, chapter-specific coding guidelines (such as obstetrics, poisoning, HIV, newborn) that provide sequencing direction take precedence.

2) **Acute respiratory failure as secondary diagnosis**

Respiratory failure may be listed as a secondary diagnosis if it occurs after admission, or if it is present on admission, but does not meet the definition of principal diagnosis.

3) **Sequencing of acute respiratory failure and another acute condition**

When a patient is admitted with respiratory failure and another acute condition (e.g., myocardial infarction, cerebrovascular accident, aspiration pneumonia), the principal diagnosis will not be the same in every situation. This applies whether the other acute condition is a respiratory or nonrespiratory condition. Selection of the principal diagnosis will be dependent on the circumstances of admission. If both the respiratory failure and the other acute condition are equally responsible for occasioning the admission to the hospital, and there are no chapter-specific sequencing rules, the guideline regarding two or more diagnoses that equally meet the definition for principal diagnosis (*Section II, C.*) may be applied in these situations.

If the documentation is not clear as to whether acute respiratory failure and another condition are equally responsible for occasioning the admission, query the provider for clarification.

c. **Influenza due to certain identified influenza viruses**

Code only confirmed cases of influenza due to certain identified influenza viruses (category J09), and due to other identified influenza virus (category J10). This is an exception to the hospital inpatient guideline Section II, H. (Uncertain Diagnosis).

In this context, "confirmation" does not require documentation of positive laboratory testing specific for avian or other novel influenza A or other identified influenza virus. However, coding should be based on the provider's diagnostic statement that the patient has avian influenza, or other novel influenza A, for category J09, or has another particular identified strain of influenza, such as H1N1 or H3N2, but not identified as novel or variant, for category J10.

If the provider records "suspected" or "possible" or "probable" avian influenza, or novel influenza, or other identified influenza, then the appropriate influenza code from category J11, Influenza due to unidentified influenza virus, should be assigned. A code from category J09, Influenza due to certain identified influenza viruses, should not be assigned nor should a code from category J10, Influenza due to other identified influenza virus.

d. **Ventilator associated Pneumonia**

1) **Documentation of Ventilator associated Pneumonia**

As with all procedural or postprocedural complications, code assignment is based on the provider's documentation of the relationship between the condition and the procedure.

Code J95.851, Ventilator associated pneumonia, should be assigned only when the provider has documented ventilator associated pneumonia (VAP). An additional code to identify the organism (e.g., Pseudomonas aeruginosa, code B96.5) should also be assigned. Do not assign an additional code from categories J12-J18 to identify the type of pneumonia.

Code J95.851 should not be assigned for cases where the patient has pneumonia and is on a mechanical ventilator and the provider has not specifically stated that the pneumonia is ventilator associated pneumonia. If the documentation is unclear as to whether the patient has a pneumonia that is a complication attributable to the mechanical ventilator, query the provider.

2) **Ventilator associated Pneumonia Develops after Admission**

A patient may be admitted with one type of pneumonia (e.g., code J13, Pneumonia due to Streptococcus pneumonia) and subsequently develop VAP. In this instance, the principal diagnosis would be the appropriate code from categories J12-J18 for the pneumonia diagnosed at the time of admission. Code J95.851, Ventilator associated pneumonia, would be assigned as an additional diagnosis when the provider has also documented the presence of ventilator associated pneumonia.

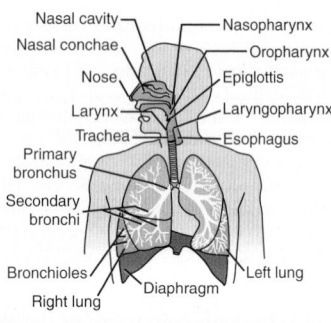

Figure 10-1 Respiratory system. (From Buck CJ: Step-by-Step Medical Coding, ed 2016, St. Louis, Elsevier, 2016)

Figure 10-2 Paranasal sinuses. (From Buck CJ: Step-by-Step Medical Coding, ed 2016, St. Louis, Elsevier, 2016)

Item 10-1 Pharyngitis is painful inflammation of the pharynx (sore throat). Ninety percent of the infections are caused by a virus with the remaining being bacterial and rarely a fungus (candidiasis). Other irritants such as pollutants, chemicals, or smoke may cause similar symptoms.

CHAPTER 10

DISEASES OF THE RESPIRATORY SYSTEM
(J00-J99)

> **Note:** When a respiratory condition is described as occurring in more than one site and is not specifically indexed, it should be classified to the lower anatomic site (e.g., tracheobronchitis to bronchitis in J40).

Use additional code, where applicable, to identify:
exposure to environmental tobacco smoke (Z77.22)
exposure to tobacco smoke in the perinatal period (P96.81)
history of tobacco dependence (Z87.891)
occupational exposure to environmental tobacco smoke (Z57.31)
tobacco dependence (F17.-)
tobacco use (Z72.0)

Excludes2 certain conditions originating in the perinatal period (P04-P96)
certain infectious and parasitic diseases (A00-B99)
complications of pregnancy, childbirth and the puerperium (O00-O99A)
congenital malformations, deformations and chromosomal abnormalities (Q00-Q99)
endocrine, nutritional and metabolic diseases (E00-E88)
injury, poisoning and certain other consequences of external causes (S00-T88)
neoplasms (C00-D49)
smoke inhalation (T59.81-)
symptoms, signs and abnormal clinical and laboratory findings, not elsewhere classified (R00-R94)

This chapter contains the following blocks:

J00-J06	Acute upper respiratory infections
J09-J18	Influenza and pneumonia
J20-J22	Other acute lower respiratory infections
J30-J39	Other diseases of upper respiratory tract
J40-J47	Chronic lower respiratory diseases
J60-J70	Lung diseases due to external agents
J80-J84	Other respiratory diseases principally affecting the interstitium
J85-J86	Suppurative and necrotic conditions of the lower respiratory tract
J90-J94	Other diseases of the pleura
J95	Intraoperative and postprocedural complications and disorders of respiratory system, not elsewhere classified
J96-J99	Other diseases of the respiratory system

ACUTE UPPER RESPIRATORY INFECTIONS (J00-J06)

Excludes1 chronic obstructive pulmonary disease with acute lower respiratory infection (J44.0)

J00 Acute nasopharyngitis [common cold]
Acute rhinitis
Coryza (acute)
Infective nasopharyngitis NOS
Infective rhinitis
Nasal catarrh, acute
Nasopharyngitis NOS

Excludes1 acute pharyngitis (J02.-)
acute sore throat NOS (J02.9)
influenza virus with other respiratory manifestations (J09.X2, J10.1, J11.1)
pharyngitis NOS (J02.9)
rhinitis NOS (J31.0)
sore throat NOS (J02.9)

Excludes2 allergic rhinitis (J30.1-J30.9)
chronic pharyngitis (J31.2)
chronic rhinitis (J31.0)
chronic sore throat (J31.2)
nasopharyngitis, chronic (J31.1)
vasomotor rhinitis (J30.0)

★ **(See Plate 27 of the Anatomy Illustrations.)**

● **J01 Acute sinusitis**
Includes acute abscess of sinus
acute empyema of sinus
acute infection of sinus
acute inflammation of sinus
acute suppuration of sinus

Use additional code (B95-B97) to identify infectious agent.
Excludes1 sinusitis NOS (J32.9)
Excludes2 chronic sinusitis (J32.0-J32.8)

● **J01.0 Acute maxillary sinusitis**
Acute antritis
J01.00 Acute maxillary sinusitis, unspecified
J01.01 Acute recurrent maxillary sinusitis

● **J01.1 Acute frontal sinusitis**
J01.10 Acute frontal sinusitis, unspecified
J01.11 Acute recurrent frontal sinusitis

● **J01.2 Acute ethmoidal sinusitis**
J01.20 Acute ethmoidal sinusitis, unspecified
J01.21 Acute recurrent ethmoidal sinusitis

● **J01.3 Acute sphenoidal sinusitis**
J01.30 Acute sphenoidal sinusitis, unspecified
J01.31 Acute recurrent sphenoidal sinusitis

● **J01.4 Acute pansinusitis**
J01.40 Acute pansinusitis, unspecified
J01.41 Acute recurrent pansinusitis

▶ New ⇒ Revised ~~deleted~~ Deleted Excludes 1 Excludes 2 Includes Use additional Code first Code also Key words
OGCR Official Guidelines X Assign placeholder X ● Use Additional Character(s) ▸ Manifestation Code 🔖 Hierarchical Condition Category Coding Clinic

● **J01.8** **Other acute sinusitis**

J01.80 Other acute sinusitis
Acute sinusitis involving more than one sinus but not pansinusitis

J01.81 Other acute recurrent sinusitis
Acute recurrent sinusitis involving more than one sinus but not pansinusitis

● **J01.9** **Acute sinusitis, unspecified**

J01.90 Acute sinusitis, unspecified

J01.91 Acute recurrent sinusitis, unspecified

● **J02** **Acute pharyngitis**

Includes acute sore throat

Excludes1 acute laryngopharyngitis (J06.0)
peritonsillar abscess (J36)
pharyngeal abscess (J39.1)
retropharyngeal abscess (J39.0)

Excludes2 chronic pharyngitis (J31.2)

J02.0 **Streptococcal pharyngitis**
Septic pharyngitis
Streptococcal sore throat

Excludes2 scarlet fever (A38.-)

J02.8 **Acute pharyngitis due to other specified organisms**
Use additional code (B95-B97) to identify infectious agent

Excludes1 pharyngitis due to coxsackie virus (B08.5)
pharyngitis due to gonococcus (A54.5)
acute pharyngitis due to herpes [simplex] virus (B00.2)
acute pharyngitis due to infectious mononucleosis (B27.-)
enteroviral vesicular pharyngitis (B08.5)

J02.9 **Acute pharyngitis, unspecified**
Gangrenous pharyngitis (acute)
Infective pharyngitis (acute) NOS
Pharyngitis (acute) NOS
Sore throat (acute) NOS
Suppurative pharyngitis (acute)
Ulcerative pharyngitis (acute)

Excludes1 influenza virus with other respiratory manifestations (J09.X2, J10.1, J11.1)

● **J03** **Acute tonsillitis**
Inflammation of pharyngeal tonsils caused by virus or bacteria

Excludes1 acute sore throat (J02.-)
hypertrophy of tonsils (J35.1)
peritonsillar abscess (J36)
sore throat NOS (J02.9)
streptococcal sore throat (J02.0)

Excludes2 chronic tonsillitis (J35.0)

● **J03.0** **Streptococcal tonsillitis**

J03.00 Acute streptococcal tonsillitis, unspecified

J03.01 Acute recurrent streptococcal tonsillitis

● **J03.8** **Acute tonsillitis due to other specified organisms**
Use additional code (B95-B97) to identify infectious agent.

Excludes1 diphtheritic tonsillitis (A36.0)
herpesviral pharyngotonsillitis (B00.2)
streptococcal tonsillitis (J03.0)
tuberculous tonsillitis (A15.8)
Vincent's tonsillitis (A69.1)

J03.80 Acute tonsillitis due to other specified organisms

J03.81 Acute recurrent tonsillitis due to other specified organisms

---

Item 10–2 **Laryngitis** is an inflammation of the larynx (voice box) resulting in hoarse voice or the complete loss of the voice. **Tracheitis** is an inflammation of the trachea (often following a URI) commonly caused by *staphylococcus aureus* resulting in inspiratory stridor (crowing sound on inspiration) and a crouplike cough.

● **J03.9** **Acute tonsillitis, unspecified**
Follicular tonsillitis (acute)
Gangrenous tonsillitis (acute)
Infective tonsillitis (acute)
Tonsillitis (acute) NOS
Ulcerative tonsillitis (acute)

Excludes1 influenza virus with other respiratory manifestations (J09.X2, J10.1, J11.1)

J03.90 Acute tonsillitis, unspecified

J03.91 Acute recurrent tonsillitis, unspecified

● **J04** **Acute laryngitis and tracheitis**
Use additional code (B95-B97) to identify infectious agent.
Code also influenza, if present, such as:
influenza due to identified novel influenza A virus with other respiratory manifestations (J09.X2)
influenza due to other identified influenza virus with other respiratory manifestations (J10.1)
influenza due to unidentified influenza virus with other respiratory manifestations (J11.1)

Excludes1 acute obstructive laryngitis [croup] and epiglottitis (J05.-)

Excludes2 laryngismus (stridulus) (J38.5)

J04.0 **Acute laryngitis**
Edematous laryngitis (acute)
Laryngitis (acute) NOS
Subglottic laryngitis (acute)
Suppurative laryngitis (acute)
Ulcerative laryngitis (acute)

Excludes1 acute obstructive laryngitis (J05.0)

Excludes2 chronic laryngitis (J37.0)

● **J04.1** **Acute tracheitis**
Acute viral tracheitis
Catarrhal tracheitis (acute)
Tracheitis (acute) NOS

Excludes2 chronic tracheitis (J42)

J04.10 Acute tracheitis without obstruction

J04.11 Acute tracheitis with obstruction

J04.2 **Acute laryngotracheitis**
Laryngotracheitis NOS
Tracheitis (acute) with laryngitis (acute)

Excludes1 acute obstructive laryngotracheitis (J05.0)

Excludes2 chronic laryngotracheitis (J37.1)

● **J04.3** **Supraglottitis, unspecified**

J04.30 Supraglottitis, unspecified, without obstruction

J04.31 Supraglottitis, unspecified, with obstruction

● **J05** **Acute obstructive laryngitis [croup] and epiglottitis**
Use additional code (B95-B97) to identify infectious agent.
⮕ Code also influenza, if present, such as:
influenza due to identified novel influenza A virus with other respiratory manifestations (J09.X2)
influenza due to other identified influenza virus with other respiratory manifestations (J10.1)
influenza due to unidentified influenza virus with other respiratory manifestations (J11.1)

J05.0 **Acute obstructive laryngitis [croup]**
Obstructive laryngitis (acute) NOS
Obstructive laryngotracheitis NOS

● **J05.1 Acute epiglottitis**
    Excludes2 epiglottitis, chronic (J37.0)
    J05.10 Acute epiglottitis without obstruction
        Epiglottitis NOS
    J05.11 Acute epiglottitis with obstruction

● **J06 Acute upper respiratory infections of multiple and unspecified sites**
    Excludes1 acute respiratory infection NOS (J22)
        influenza virus with other respiratory manifestations (J09.X2, J10.1, J11.1)
        streptococcal pharyngitis (J02.0)
    Coding Clinic: 2020, Q1, P22
  J06.0 Acute laryngopharyngitis
  J06.9 Acute upper respiratory infection, unspecified
    Upper respiratory disease, acute
    Upper respiratory infection NOS
    Use additional code (B95-B97) to identify infectious agent, if known, such as:
      respiratory syncytial virus (RSV) (B97.4)

INFLUENZA AND PNEUMONIA (J09-J18)

Excludes2 allergic or eosinophilic pneumonia (J82)
  aspiration pneumonia NOS (J69.0)
  meconium pneumonia (P24.01)
  neonatal aspiration pneumonia (P24.-)
  pneumonia due to solids and liquids (J69.-)
  congenital pneumonia (P23.9)
  lipid pneumonia (J69.1)
  rheumatic pneumonia (I00)
  ventilator associated pneumonia (J95.851)
Coding Clinic: 2020, Q1, P22

● **J09 Influenza due to certain identified influenza viruses**
  Excludes1 influenza A/H1N1 (J10.-)
    influenza due to other influenza viruses (J10.-)
    influenza due to unidentified influenza virus (J11.-)
    seasonal influenza due to other identified influenza virus (J10.-)
    seasonal influenza due to unidentified influenza virus (J11.-)

  ● **J09.X Influenza due to identified novel influenza A virus**
    Avian influenza
    Bird influenza
    Influenza A/H5N1
    Influenza of other animal origin, not bird or swine
    Swine influenza virus (viruses that normally cause infections in pigs)
    Coding Clinic: 2016, Q3, P11
    J09.X1 Influenza due to identified novel influenza A virus with pneumonia
      Code also, if applicable, associated:
        lung abscess (J85.1)
        other specified type of pneumonia
    J09.X2 Influenza due to identified novel influenza A virus with other respiratory manifestations
      Influenza due to identified novel influenza A virus NOS
      Influenza due to identified novel influenza A virus with laryngitis
      Influenza due to identified novel influenza A virus with pharyngitis
      Influenza due to identified novel influenza A virus with upper respiratory symptoms
      Use additional code, if applicable, for associated:
        pleural effusion (J91.8)
        sinusitis (J01.-)

    J09.X3 Influenza due to identified novel influenza A virus with gastrointestinal manifestations
      Influenza due to identified novel influenza A virus gastroenteritis
      Excludes1 'intestinal flu' [viral gastroenteritis] (A08.-)
    J09.X9 Influenza due to identified novel influenza A virus with other manifestations
      Influenza due to identified novel influenza A virus with encephalopathy
      Influenza due to identified novel influenza A virus with myocarditis
      Influenza due to identified novel influenza A virus with otitis media
      Use additional code to identify manifestation

● **J10 Influenza due to other identified influenza virus**
  Includes influenza A (non-novel)
    influenza B
    influenza C
  Excludes1 influenza due to avian influenza virus (J09.X-)
    influenza due to swine flu (J09.X-)
    influenza due to unidentified influenza virus (J11.-)

  ● **J10.0 Influenza due to other identified influenza virus with pneumonia**
    Code also associated lung abscess, if applicable (J85.1)
    J10.00 Influenza due to other identified influenza virus with unspecified type of pneumonia
    J10.01 Influenza due to other identified influenza virus with the same other identified influenza virus pneumonia
    J10.08 Influenza due to other identified influenza virus with other specified pneumonia
      Code also other specified type of pneumonia
      Coding Clinic: 2017, Q4, P96
  J10.1 Influenza due to other identified influenza virus with other respiratory manifestations
    Influenza due to other identified influenza virus NOS
    Influenza due to other identified influenza virus with laryngitis
    Influenza due to other identified influenza virus with pharyngitis
    Influenza due to other identified influenza virus with upper respiratory symptoms
    Use additional code for associated pleural effusion, if applicable (J91.8)
    Use additional code for associated sinusitis, if applicable (J01.-)
    Coding Clinic: 2016, Q3, P11
  J10.2 Influenza due to other identified influenza virus with gastrointestinal manifestations
    Influenza due to other identified influenza virus gastroenteritis
    Excludes1 'intestinal flu' [viral gastroenteritis] (A08.-)
  ● **J10.8 Influenza due to other identified influenza virus with other manifestations**
    J10.81 Influenza due to other identified influenza virus with encephalopathy
    J10.82 Influenza due to other identified influenza virus with myocarditis
    J10.83 Influenza due to other identified influenza virus with otitis media
      Use additional code for any associated perforated tympanic membrane (H72.-)
    J10.89 Influenza due to other identified influenza virus with other manifestations
      Use additional codes to identify the manifestations

● **J11   Influenza due to unidentified influenza virus**
  ● **J11.0   Influenza due to unidentified influenza virus with pneumonia**
      Code also associated lung abscess, if applicable (J85.1)

    J11.00   Influenza due to unidentified influenza virus with unspecified type of pneumonia
      Influenza with pneumonia NOS
      Coding Clinic: 2016, Q3, P12

    J11.08   Influenza due to unidentified influenza virus with specified pneumonia
      Code also other specified type of pneumonia

  J11.1   Influenza due to unidentified influenza virus with other respiratory manifestations
    Influenza NOS
    Influenzal laryngitis NOS
    Influenzal pharyngitis NOS
    Influenza with upper respiratory symptoms NOS
    Use additional code for associated pleural effusion, if applicable (J91.8)
    Use additional code for associated sinusitis, if applicable (J01.-)

  J11.2   Influenza due to unidentified influenza virus with gastrointestinal manifestations
    Influenza gastroenteritis NOS
    Excludes1 'intestinal flu' [viral gastroenteritis] (A08.-)

  ● **J11.8   Influenza due to unidentified influenza virus with other manifestations**

    J11.81   Influenza due to unidentified influenza virus with encephalopathy
      Influenzal encephalopathy NOS

    J11.82   Influenza due to unidentified influenza virus with myocarditis
      Influenzal myocarditis NOS

    J11.83   Influenza due to unidentified influenza virus with otitis media
      Influenzal otitis media NOS
      Use additional code for any associated perforated tympanic membrane (H72.-)

    J11.89   Influenza due to unidentified influenza virus with other manifestations
      Use additional codes to identify the manifestations

● **J12   Viral pneumonia, not elsewhere classified**
  Includes   bronchopneumonia due to viruses other than influenza viruses
  Code first associated influenza, if applicable (J09.X1, J10.0-, J11.0-)
  Code also associated abscess, if applicable (J85.1)
  Excludes1   aspiration pneumonia due to anesthesia during labor and delivery (O74.0)
    aspiration pneumonia due to anesthesia during pregnancy (O29)
    aspiration pneumonia due to anesthesia during puerperium (O89.0)
    aspiration pneumonia due to solids and liquids (J69.-)
    aspiration pneumonia NOS (J69.0)
    congenital pneumonia (P23.0)
    congenital rubella pneumonitis (P35.0)
    interstitial pneumonia NOS (J84.9)
    lipid pneumonia (J69.1)
    neonatal aspiration pneumonia (P24.-)
  Coding Clinic: 2021, Q1, P34

  J12.0   Adenoviral pneumonia
  J12.1   Respiratory syncytial virus pneumonia
    RSV pneumonia
  J12.2   Parainfluenza virus pneumonia
  J12.3   Human metapneumovirus pneumonia

Item 10–3 Pneumonia is an infection of the lungs, caused by a variety of microorganisms, including viruses, most commonly the Streptococcus pneumoniae (pneumococcus) bacteria, fungi, and parasites. Pneumonia occurs when the immune system is weakened, often by a URI or influenza.

  ● **J12.8   Other viral pneumonia**
    J12.81   Pneumonia due to SARS-associated coronavirus
      Severe acute respiratory syndrome NOS

    J12.82   Pneumonia due to coronavirus disease 2019
      Pneumonia due to 2019 novel coronavirus (SARS-CoV-2)
      Pneumonia due to COVID-19
      Code first COVID-19 (U07.1)
      Coding Clinic: 2021, Q1, P33-34, 42, 47, 49

    J12.89   Other viral pneumonia
      Coding Clinic: 2021, Q1, P33-34

  J12.9   Viral pneumonia, unspecified

J13   Pneumonia due to Streptococcus pneumoniae 🦠
  Bronchopneumonia due to S. pneumoniae
  Code first associated influenza, if applicable (J09.X1, J10.0-, J11.0-)
  Code also associated abscess, if applicable (J85.1)
  Excludes1   congenital pneumonia due to S. pneumoniae (P23.6)
    lobar pneumonia, unspecified organism (J18.1)
    pneumonia due to other streptococci (J15.3-J15.4)

J14   Pneumonia due to Hemophilus influenzae 🦠
  Bronchopneumonia due to H. influenzae
  Code first associated influenza, if applicable (J09.X1, J10.0-, J11.0-)
  Code also associated abscess, if applicable (J85.1)
  Excludes1   congenital pneumonia due to H. influenzae (P23.6)

● **J15   Bacterial pneumonia, not elsewhere classified**
  Includes   bronchopneumonia due to bacteria other than S. pneumoniae and H. influenzae
  Code first associated influenza, if applicable (J09.X1, J10.0-, J11.0-)
  Code also associated abscess, if applicable (J85.1)
  Excludes1   chlamydial pneumonia (J16.0)
    congenital pneumonia (P23.-)
    Legionnaires' disease (A48.1)
    spirochetal pneumonia (A69.8)

  J15.0   Pneumonia due to Klebsiella pneumoniae 🦠
  J15.1   Pneumonia due to Pseudomonas 🦠
  ● **J15.2   Pneumonia due to staphylococcus**
    J15.20   Pneumonia due to staphylococcus, unspecified 🦠
    ● **J15.21   Pneumonia due to staphylococcus aureus**
      J15.211   Pneumonia due to Methicillin susceptible Staphylococcus aureus 🦠
        MSSA pneumonia
        Pneumonia due to Staphylococcus aureus NOS
      J15.212   Pneumonia due to Methicillin resistant Staphylococcus aureus 🦠
    J15.29   Pneumonia due to other staphylococcus 🦠
  J15.3   Pneumonia due to streptococcus, group B 🦠
  J15.4   Pneumonia due to other streptococci 🦠
    Excludes1   pneumonia due to streptococcus, group B (J15.3)
      pneumonia due to Streptococcus pneumoniae (J13)

  J15.5   Pneumonia due to Escherichia coli 🦠
  J15.6   Pneumonia due to other Gram-negative bacteria 🦠
    Pneumonia due to other aerobic Gram-negative bacteria
    Pneumonia due to Serratia marcescens
  J15.7   Pneumonia due to Mycoplasma pneumoniae
  J15.8   Pneumonia due to other specified bacteria 🦠
  J15.9   Unspecified bacterial pneumonia
    Pneumonia due to gram-positive bacteria
    Coding Clinic: 2017, Q4, P96

CHAPTER 10 (J00-J99)

CHAPTER 10 (J00-J99)

● **J16**   **Pneumonia due to other infectious organisms, not elsewhere classified**

Code first associated influenza, if applicable (J09.X1, J10.0-, J11.0-)

Code also associated abscess, if applicable (J85.1)

Excludes1   congenital pneumonia (P23.-)
ornithosis (A70)
pneumocystosis (B59)
pneumonia NOS (J18.9)

J16.0   **Chlamydial pneumonia**

J16.8   **Pneumonia due to other specified infectious organisms**

▷ **J17**   *Pneumonia in diseases classified elsewhere*

Code first underlying disease, such as:
Q fever (A78)
rheumatic fever (I00)
schistosomiasis (B65.0-B65.9)

Excludes1   candidial pneumonia (B37.1)
chlamydial pneumonia (J16.0)
gonorrheal pneumonia (A54.84)
histoplasmosis pneumonia (B39.0-B39.2)
measles pneumonia (B05.2)
nocardiosis pneumonia (A43.0)
pneumocystosis (B59)
pneumonia due to Pneumocystis carinii (B59)
pneumonia due to Pneumocystis jiroveci (B59)
pneumonia in actinomycosis (A42.0)
pneumonia in anthrax (A22.1)
pneumonia in ascariasis (B77.81)
pneumonia in aspergillosis (B44.0-B44.1)
pneumonia in coccidioidomycosis (B38.0-B38.2)
pneumonia in cytomegalovirus disease (B25.0)
pneumonia in toxoplasmosis (B58.3)
rubella pneumonia (B06.81)
salmonella pneumonia (A02.22)
spirochetal infection NEC with pneumonia (A69.8)
tularemia pneumonia (A21.2)
typhoid fever with pneumonia (A01.03)
varicella pneumonia (B01.2)
whooping cough with pneumonia (A37 with fifth-character 1)

● **J18**   **Pneumonia, unspecified organism**

Code first associated influenza, if applicable (J09.X1, J10.0-, J11.0-)

Excludes1   abscess of lung with pneumonia (J85.1)
aspiration pneumonia due to anesthesia during labor and delivery (O74.0)
aspiration pneumonia due to anesthesia during pregnancy (O29)
aspiration pneumonia due to anesthesia during puerperium (O89.0)
aspiration pneumonia due to solids and liquids (J69.-)
aspiration pneumonia NOS (J69.0)
congenital pneumonia (P23.0)
drug-induced interstitial lung disorder (J70.2-J70.4)
interstitial pneumonia NOS (J84.9)
lipid pneumonia (J69.1)
neonatal aspiration pneumonia (P24.-)
pneumonitis due to external agents (J67-J70)
pneumonitis due to fumes and vapors (J68.0)
usual interstitial pneumonia (J84.178)

J18.0   **Bronchopneumonia, unspecified organism**

Excludes1   hypostatic bronchopneumonia (J18.2)
lipid pneumonia (J69.1)

Excludes2   acute bronchiolitis (J21.-)
chronic bronchiolitis (J44.9)

J18.1   **Lobar pneumonia, unspecified organism**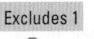
Coding Clinic: 2016, Q3, P15

J18.2   **Hypostatic pneumonia, unspecified organism**
Hypostatic bronchopneumonia
Passive pneumonia

J18.8   **Other pneumonia, unspecified organism**

J18.9   **Pneumonia, unspecified organism**
Coding Clinic: Q3, P15; 2019, Q2, P28; Q1, P36; 2016, Q3, P15; 2012, Q4, P94

OTHER ACUTE LOWER RESPIRATORY INFECTIONS (J20-J22)

Excludes2   chronic obstructive pulmonary disease with acute lower respiratory infection (J44.0)

● **J20**   **Acute bronchitis**
Inflammation/irritation of the bronchial tubes lasting 2-3 weeks, most commonly caused by a virus

Includes   acute and subacute bronchitis (with) bronchospasm
acute and subacute bronchitis (with) tracheitis
acute and subacute bronchitis (with) tracheobronchitis, acute
acute and subacute fibrinous bronchitis
acute and subacute membranous bronchitis
acute and subacute purulent bronchitis
acute and subacute septic bronchitis

Excludes1   bronchitis NOS (J40)
tracheobronchitis NOS (J40)

Excludes2   acute bronchitis with bronchiectasis (J47.0)
acute bronchitis with chronic obstructive asthma (J44.0)
acute bronchitis with chronic obstructive pulmonary disease (J44.0)
allergic bronchitis NOS (J45.909-)
bronchitis due to chemicals, fumes and vapors (J68.0)
chronic bronchitis NOS (J42)
chronic mucopurulent bronchitis (J41.1)
chronic obstructive bronchitis (J44.-)
chronic obstructive tracheobronchitis (J44.-)
chronic simple bronchitis (J41.0)
chronic tracheobronchitis (J42)

J20.0   **Acute bronchitis due to Mycoplasma pneumoniae**

J20.1   **Acute bronchitis due to Hemophilus influenzae**

J20.2   **Acute bronchitis due to streptococcus**

J20.3   **Acute bronchitis due to coxsackievirus**

J20.4   **Acute bronchitis due to parainfluenza virus**

J20.5   **Acute bronchitis due to respiratory syncytial virus**
Acute bronchitis due to RSV

J20.6   **Acute bronchitis due to rhinovirus**
Coding Clinic: 2016, Q3, P10

J20.7   **Acute bronchitis due to echovirus**

J20.8   **Acute bronchitis due to other specified organisms**
Coding Clinic: 2016, Q3, P11

J20.9   **Acute bronchitis, unspecified**
Coding Clinic: 2019, Q1, P35; 2016, Q3, P16

● **J21**   **Acute bronchiolitis**
Bronchiolitis obliterans with organizing pneumonia (BOOP) inflammation of bronchioles and surrounding tissue in lung

Includes   acute bronchiolitis with bronchospasm

Excludes2   respiratory bronchiolitis interstitial lung disease (J84.115)

J21.0   **Acute bronchiolitis due to respiratory syncytial virus**
Acute bronchitis due to RSV

J21.1   **Acute bronchiolitis due to human metapneumovirus**

J21.8   **Acute bronchiolitis due to other specified organisms**

J21.9   **Acute bronchiolitis, unspecified**
Bronchiolitis (acute)

Excludes1   chronic bronchiolitis (J44.-)

J22   **Unspecified acute lower respiratory infection**
Acute (lower) respiratory (tract) infection NOS

Excludes1   upper respiratory infection (acute) (J06.9)
Coding Clinic: 2020, Q1, P22-23

▶ New   ⇛ Revised   ~~deleted~~ Deleted   Excludes 1   Excludes 2   Includes   Use additional   Code first   Code also   Key words
OGCR Official Guidelines   X Assign placeholder X   ● Use Additional Character(s)   ▷ Manifestation Code   🕮 Hierarchical Condition Category   Coding Clinic

OTHER DISEASES OF UPPER RESPIRATORY TRACT (J30-J39)

● **J30**   **Vasomotor and allergic rhinitis**

> **Includes**   spasmodic rhinorrhea
>
> **Excludes1**   allergic rhinitis with asthma (bronchial) (J45.909)
> rhinitis NOS (J31.0)

    J30.0   **Vasomotor rhinitis**

    J30.1   **Allergic rhinitis due to pollen**
Allergy NOS due to pollen
Hay fever
Pollinosis

    J30.2   **Other seasonal allergic rhinitis**

    J30.5   **Allergic rhinitis due to food**

● **J30.8**   **Other allergic rhinitis**

       J30.81   **Allergic rhinitis due to animal (cat) (dog) hair and dander**

       J30.89   **Other allergic rhinitis**
Perennial allergic rhinitis

    J30.9   **Allergic rhinitis, unspecified**

● **J31**   **Chronic rhinitis, nasopharyngitis and pharyngitis**
Use additional code to identify:
exposure to environmental tobacco smoke (Z77.22)
exposure to tobacco smoke in the perinatal period (P96.81)
history of tobacco dependence (Z87.891)
occupational exposure to environmental tobacco smoke (Z57.31)
tobacco dependence (F17.-)
tobacco use (Z72.0)

    J31.0   **Chronic rhinitis**
Atrophic rhinitis (chronic)
Granulomatous rhinitis (chronic)
Hypertrophic rhinitis (chronic)
Obstructive rhinitis (chronic)
Ozena
Purulent rhinitis (chronic)
Rhinitis (chronic) NOS
Ulcerative rhinitis (chronic)

> **Excludes1**   allergic rhinitis (J30.1-J30.9)
> vasomotor rhinitis (J30.0)

    J31.1   **Chronic nasopharyngitis**

> **Excludes2**   acute nasopharyngitis (J00)

    J31.2   **Chronic pharyngitis**
Chronic sore throat
Atrophic pharyngitis (chronic)
Granular pharyngitis (chronic)
Hypertrophic pharyngitis (chronic)

> **Excludes2**   acute pharyngitis (J02.9)

● **J32**   **Chronic sinusitis**

> **Includes**   sinus abscess
> sinus empyema
> sinus infection
> sinus suppuration

Use additional code to identify:
exposure to environmental tobacco smoke (Z77.22)
exposure to tobacco smoke in the perinatal period (P96.81)
history of tobacco dependence (Z87.891)
infectious agent (B95-B97)
occupational exposure to environmental tobacco smoke (Z57.31)
tobacco dependence (F17.-)
tobacco use (Z72.0)

> **Excludes2**   acute sinusitis (J01.-)

    J32.0   **Chronic maxillary sinusitis**
Antritis (chronic)
Maxillary sinusitis NOS

    J32.1   **Chronic frontal sinusitis**
Frontal sinusitis NOS

Item 10-4 Nasal polyps are an abnormal growth of tissue (tumor) projecting from a mucous membrane and attached to the surface by a narrow elongated stalk (pedunculated). Nasal polyps usually originate in the ethmoid sinus but also may occur in the maxillary sinus. Symptoms are nasal block, sinusitis, anosmia, and secondary infections.

    J32.2   **Chronic ethmoidal sinusitis**
Ethmoidal sinusitis NOS

> **Excludes1**   Woakes' ethmoiditis (J33.1)

    J32.3   **Chronic sphenoidal sinusitis**
Sphenoidal sinusitis NOS

    J32.4   **Chronic pansinusitis**
Pansinusitis NOS

    J32.8   **Other chronic sinusitis**
Sinusitis (chronic) involving more than one sinus but not pansinusitis

    J32.9   **Chronic sinusitis, unspecified**
Sinusitis (chronic) NOS

● **J33**   **Nasal polyp**
Use additional code to identify:
exposure to environmental tobacco smoke (Z77.22)
exposure to tobacco smoke in the perinatal period (P96.81)
history of tobacco dependence (Z87.891)
occupational exposure to environmental tobacco smoke (Z57.31)
tobacco dependence (F17.-)
tobacco use (Z72.0)

> **Excludes1**   adenomatous polyps (D14.0)

    J33.0   **Polyp of nasal cavity**
Choanal polyp
Nasopharyngeal polyp

    J33.1   **Polypoid sinus degeneration**
Woakes' syndrome or ethmoiditis

    J33.8   **Other polyp of sinus**
Accessory polyp of sinus
Ethmoidal polyp of sinus
Maxillary polyp of sinus
Sphenoidal polyp of sinus

    J33.9   **Nasal polyp, unspecified**

● **J34**   **Other and unspecified disorders of nose and nasal sinuses**

> **Excludes2**   varicose ulcer of nasal septum (I86.8)

    J34.0   **Abscess, furuncle and carbuncle of nose**
Cellulitis of nose
Necrosis of nose
Ulceration of nose

    J34.1   **Cyst and mucocele of nose and nasal sinus**

    J34.2   **Deviated nasal septum**
Deflection or deviation of septum (nasal) (acquired)

> **Excludes1**   congenital deviated nasal septum (Q67.4)

    J34.3   **Hypertrophy of nasal turbinates**

Deviated septal cartilage

Figure 10-3 Deviated nasal septum.

Item 10-5 A **deviated nasal septum** is the displacement of the septal cartilage that separates the nares. This displacement causes obstructed air flow through the nasal passages. A child can be born with this displacement (congenital), or the condition may be acquired through trauma, such as a sports injury. Symptoms include nasal block, sinusitis, and related secondary infections. Septoplasty is surgical repair of this condition.

CHAPTER 10 (J00-J99)

● **J34.8** **Other specified disorders of nose and nasal sinuses**

J34.81 **Nasal mucositis (ulcerative)**

Code also type of associated therapy, such as:
antineoplastic and immunosuppressive
drugs (T45.1X-)
radiological procedure and radiotherapy
(Y84.2)

Excludes2 gastrointestinal mucositis
(ulcerative) (K92.81)
mucositis (ulcerative) of vagina
and vulva (N76.81)
oral mucositis (ulcerative)
(K12.3-)

J34.89 **Other specified disorders of nose and nasal
sinuses**

Perforation of nasal septum NOS
Rhinolith

J34.9 **Unspecified disorder of nose and nasal sinuses**

● **J35** **Chronic diseases of tonsils and adenoids**

Use additional code to identify:
exposure to environmental tobacco smoke (Z77.22)
exposure to tobacco smoke in the perinatal period (P96.81)
history of tobacco dependence (Z87.891)
occupational exposure to environmental tobacco smoke
(Z57.31)
tobacco dependence (F17.-)
tobacco use (Z72.0)

● **J35.0** **Chronic tonsillitis and adenoiditis**

Excludes2 acute tonsillitis (J03.-)

J35.01 **Chronic tonsillitis**

J35.02 **Chronic adenoiditis**

J35.03 **Chronic tonsillitis and adenoiditis**

J35.1 **Hypertrophy of tonsils**

Enlargement of tonsils

Excludes1 hypertrophy of tonsils with tonsillitis
(J35.0-)

J35.2 **Hypertrophy of adenoids**

Enlargement of adenoids

Excludes1 hypertrophy of adenoids with adenoiditis
(J35.0-)

J35.3 **Hypertrophy of tonsils with hypertrophy of adenoids**

Excludes1 hypertrophy of tonsils and adenoids with
tonsillitis and adenoiditis (J35.03)

J35.8 **Other chronic diseases of tonsils and adenoids**

Adenoid vegetations
Amygdalolith
Calculus, tonsil
Cicatrix of tonsil (and adenoid)
Tonsillar tag
Ulcer of tonsil

J35.9 **Chronic disease of tonsils and adenoids, unspecified**

Disease (chronic) of tonsils and adenoids NOS

J36 **Peritonsillar abscess**

Includes abscess of tonsil
peritonsillar cellulitis
quinsy

Use additional code (B95-B97) to identify infectious agent.

Excludes1 acute tonsillitis (J03.-)
chronic tonsillitis (J35.0)
retropharyngeal abscess (J39.0)
tonsillitis NOS (J03.9-)

● **J37** **Chronic laryngitis and laryngotracheitis**

Use additional code to identify:
exposure to environmental tobacco smoke (Z77.22)
exposure to tobacco smoke in the perinatal period (P96.81)
history of tobacco dependence (Z87.891)
infectious agent (B95-B97)
occupational exposure to environmental tobacco smoke
(Z57.31)
tobacco dependence (F17.-)
tobacco use (Z72.0)

J37.0 **Chronic laryngitis**

Catarrhal laryngitis
Hypertrophic laryngitis
Sicca laryngitis

Excludes2 acute laryngitis (J04.0)
obstructive (acute) laryngitis (J05.0)

J37.1 **Chronic laryngotracheitis**

Laryngitis, chronic, with tracheitis (chronic)
Tracheitis, chronic, with laryngitis

Excludes1 chronic tracheitis (J42)

Excludes2 acute laryngotracheitis (J04.2)
acute tracheitis (J04.1)

● **J38** **Diseases of vocal cords and larynx, not elsewhere classified**

Use additional code to identify:
exposure to environmental tobacco smoke (Z77.22)
exposure to tobacco smoke in the perinatal period (P96.81)
history of tobacco dependence (Z87.891)
occupational exposure to environmental tobacco smoke
(Z57.31)
tobacco dependence (F17.-)
tobacco use (Z72.0)

Excludes1 congenital laryngeal stridor (P28.89)
obstructive laryngitis (acute) (J05.0)
postprocedural subglottic stenosis (J95.5)
stridor (R06.1)
ulcerative laryngitis (J04.0)

● **J38.0** **Paralysis of vocal cords and larynx**

Laryngoplegia
Paralysis of glottis

J38.00 **Paralysis of vocal cords and larynx, unspecified**

J38.01 **Paralysis of vocal cords and larynx, unilateral**

J38.02 **Paralysis of vocal cords and larynx, bilateral**

J38.1 **Polyp of vocal cord and larynx**

Excludes1 adenomatous polyps (D14.1)

J38.2 **Nodules of vocal cords**

Chorditis (fibrinous)(nodosa)(tuberosa)
Singer's nodes
Teacher's nodes

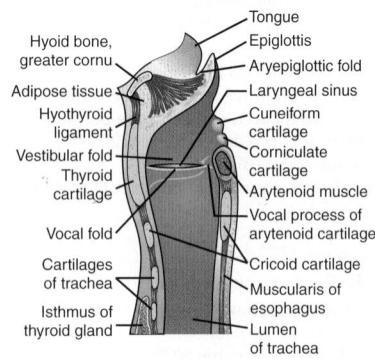

Figure 10-4 Coronal section of the larynx.

Item 10–6 The **larynx** extends from the tongue to the trachea and is
divided into an upper and lower portion separated by folds. The framework
of the larynx is cartilage composed of the single cricoid, thyroid, and epiglottic
cartilages, and the paired arytenoid, cuneiform, and corniculate cartilages.

▶ New　　⇒ Revised　　deleted Deleted　　Excludes 1　　Excludes 2　　Includes　　Use additional　　Code first　　Code also　　Key words

OGCR Official Guidelines　　X Assign placeholder X　　● Use Additional Character(s)　　▶ Manifestation Code　　🔖 Hierarchical Condition Category　　**Coding Clinic**

J38.3 Other diseases of vocal cords
Abscess of vocal cords
Cellulitis of vocal cords
Granuloma of vocal cords
Leukokeratosis of vocal cords
Leukoplakia of vocal cords

J38.4 Edema of larynx
Edema (of) glottis
Subglottic edema
Supraglottic edema
> **Excludes1** acute obstructive laryngitis [croup] (J05.0)
> edematous laryngitis (J04.0)

J38.5 Laryngeal spasm
Laryngismus (stridulus)

J38.6 Stenosis of larynx

J38.7 Other diseases of larynx
Abscess of larynx
Cellulitis of larynx
Disease of larynx NOS
Necrosis of larynx
Pachyderma of larynx
Perichondritis of larynx
Ulcer of larynx

● **J39 Other diseases of upper respiratory tract**
> **Excludes1** acute respiratory infection NOS (J22)
> acute upper respiratory infection (J06.9)
> upper respiratory inflammation due to chemicals, gases, fumes or vapors (J68.2)

J39.0 Retropharyngeal and parapharyngeal abscess
Peripharyngeal abscess
> **Excludes1** peritonsillar abscess (J36)

J39.1 Other abscess of pharynx
Cellulitis of pharynx
Nasopharyngeal abscess

J39.2 Other diseases of pharynx
Cyst of pharynx
Edema of pharynx
> **Excludes2** chronic pharyngitis (J31.2)
> ulcerative pharyngitis (J02.9)

J39.3 Upper respiratory tract hypersensitivity reaction, site unspecified
> **Excludes1** hypersensitivity reaction of upper respiratory tract, such as:
> extrinsic allergic alveolitis (J67.9)
> pneumoconiosis (J60-J67.9)

J39.8 Other specified diseases of upper respiratory tract

J39.9 Disease of upper respiratory tract, unspecified

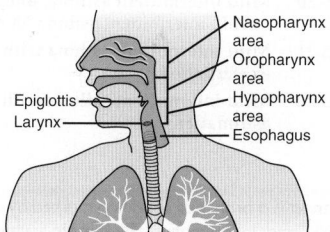

Figure 10-5 The pharynx.

Item 10–7 The **pharynx** is the passage for both food and air between the mouth and the esophagus and is divided into three areas: nasopharynx, oropharynx, and hypopharynx. The hypopharynx branches into the esophagus and the voice box.

Item 10–8 Chronic bronchitis is usually defined as being present in any patient who has persistent cough with sputum production for at least three months in at least two consecutive years. **Simple chronic bronchitis** is marked by a productive cough but no pathological airflow obstruction. **Chronic obstructive pulmonary disease (COPD)** is a group of conditions— bronchitis, emphysema, asthma, bronchiectasis, allergic alveolitis—marked by dyspnea. **Catarrhal** bronchitis is an acute form of bronchitis marked by profuse mucus and pus production (**mucopurulent** discharge). **Croupous** bronchitis, also known as pseudomembranous, fibrinous, plastic, exudative, or membranous, is marked by a violent cough and dyspnea.

CHRONIC LOWER RESPIRATORY DISEASES (J40-J47)
> **Excludes1** bronchitis due to chemicals, gases, fumes and vapors (J68.0)
> **Excludes2** cystic fibrosis (E84.-)

J40 Bronchitis, not specified as acute or chronic
Bronchitis NOS
Catarrhal bronchitis
Bronchitis with tracheitis NOS
Tracheobronchitis NOS
Use additional code to identify:
    exposure to environmental tobacco smoke (Z77.22)
    exposure to tobacco smoke in the perinatal period (P96.81)
    history of tobacco dependence (Z87.891)
    occupational exposure to environmental tobacco smoke (Z57.31)
    tobacco dependence (F17.-)
    tobacco use (Z72.0)
> **Excludes1** acute bronchitis (J20.-)
> allergic bronchitis NOS (J45.909-)
> asthmatic bronchitis NOS (J45.9-)
> bronchitis due to chemicals, gases, fumes and vapors (J68.0)

● **J41 Simple and mucopurulent chronic bronchitis**
Use additional code to identify:
    exposure to environmental tobacco smoke (Z77.22)
    exposure to tobacco smoke in the perinatal period (P96.81)
    history of tobacco dependence (Z87.891)
    occupational exposure to environmental tobacco smoke (Z57.31)
    tobacco dependence (F17.-)
    tobacco use (Z72.0)
> **Excludes1** chronic bronchitis NOS (J42)
> chronic obstructive bronchitis (J44.-)

J41.0 Simple chronic bronchitis 🐾

J41.1 Mucopurulent chronic bronchitis 🐾

J41.8 Mixed simple and mucopurulent chronic bronchitis 🐾

J42 Unspecified chronic bronchitis 🐾
Chronic bronchitis NOS
Chronic tracheitis
Chronic tracheobronchitis
Use additional code to identify:
    exposure to environmental tobacco smoke (Z77.22)
    exposure to tobacco smoke in the perinatal period (P96.81)
    history of tobacco dependence (Z87.891)
    occupational exposure to environmental tobacco smoke (Z57.31)
    tobacco dependence (F17.-)
    tobacco use (Z72.0)
> **Excludes1** chronic asthmatic bronchitis (J44.-)
> chronic bronchitis with airways obstruction (J44.-)
> chronic emphysematous bronchitis (J44.-)
> chronic obstructive pulmonary disease NOS (J44.9)
> simple and mucopurulent chronic bronchitis (J41.-)

● J43   Emphysema

Use additional code to identify:
     exposure to environmental tobacco smoke (Z77.22)
     history of tobacco dependence (Z87.891)
     occupational exposure to environmental tobacco smoke
        (Z57.31)
     tobacco dependence (F17.-)
     tobacco use (Z72.0)

> **Excludes1**   compensatory emphysema (J98.3)
>   emphysema due to inhalation of chemicals, gases,
>   fumes or vapors (J68.4)
>   emphysema with chronic (obstructive) bronchitis
>   (J44.-)
>   emphysematous (obstructive) bronchitis (J44.-)
>   interstitial emphysema (J98.2)
>   mediastinal emphysema (J98.2)
>   neonatal interstitial emphysema (P25.0)
>   surgical (subcutaneous) emphysema (T81.82)

> **Excludes2**   traumatic subcutaneous emphysema (T79.7)

J43.0   Unilateral pulmonary emphysema [MacLeod's syndrome]
     Swyer-James syndrome
     Unilateral emphysema
     Unilateral hyperlucent lung
     Unilateral pulmonary artery functional hypoplasia
     Unilateral transparency of lung

J43.1   Panlobular emphysema
     Panacinar emphysema

J43.2   Centrilobular emphysema

J43.8   Other emphysema

J43.9   Emphysema, unspecified
     Bullous emphysema (lung)(pulmonary)
     Emphysema (lung)(pulmonary) NOS
     Emphysematous bleb
     Vesicular emphysema (lung)(pulmonary)
     Coding Clinic: 2019, Q1, P35-37; 2017, Q4, P97-98

● J44   Other chronic obstructive pulmonary disease

> **Includes**   asthma with chronic obstructive pulmonary
>   disease
>   chronic asthmatic (obstructive) bronchitis
> ⇒ chronic bronchitis with airway obstruction
>   chronic bronchitis with emphysema
>   chronic emphysematous bronchitis
>   chronic obstructive asthma
>   chronic obstructive bronchitis
>   chronic obstructive tracheobronchitis

Code also type of asthma, if applicable (J45.-)

Use additional code to identify:
     exposure to environmental tobacco smoke (Z77.22)
     history of tobacco dependence (Z87.891)
     occupational exposure to environmental tobacco smoke
        (Z57.31)
     tobacco dependence (F17.-)
     tobacco use (Z72.0)

> **Excludes1**   bronchiectasis (J47.-)
>   chronic bronchitis NOS (J42)
>   chronic simple and mucopurulent bronchitis
>   (J41.-)
>   chronic tracheitis (J42)
>   chronic tracheobronchitis (J42)
>   emphysema without chronic bronchitis (J43.-)

Coding Clinic: 2019, Q1, P34-36; 2017, Q4, P97; 2017, Q1, P25; 2016, Q3, P16

J44.0   Chronic obstructive pulmonary disease with (acute) lower respiratory infection
     Code also to identify the infection
     Coding Clinic: 2019, Q1, P35-36; 2017, Q4, P96; 2017, Q2, P30, Q1, P24-25; 2016, Q3, P15-16

Figure 10-6   Emphysema. (From Shiland, BJ: Medical Terminology & Anatomy for ICD-10 Coding, ed 2, Mosby, 2015)

J44.1   Chronic obstructive pulmonary disease with (acute) exacerbation
     Decompensated COPD
     Decompensated COPD with (acute) exacerbation

> **Excludes2**   chronic obstructive pulmonary disease
>   [COPD] with acute bronchitis (J44.0)
>   lung diseases due to external agents
>   (J60-J70)

     Coding Clinic: 2019, Q1, P34-35; 2017, Q4, P96; 2017, Q1, P26; 2016, Q3, P15-16, Q1, P36

J44.9   Chronic obstructive pulmonary disease, unspecified
     Chronic obstructive airway disease NOS
     Chronic obstructive lung disease NOS

> **Excludes2**   lung diseases due to external agents
>   (J60-J70)

     Coding Clinic: 2019, Q1, P36; 2017, Q4, P96-97; 2017, Q1, P24-25; 2016, Q1, P37

● J45   Asthma
     Allergic (predominantly) asthma
     Allergic bronchitis NOS
     Allergic rhinitis with asthma
     Atopic asthma
     Extrinsic allergic asthma
     Hay fever with asthma
     Idiosyncratic asthma
     Intrinsic nonallergic asthma
     Nonallergic asthma

Use additional code to identify:
     eosinophilic asthma (J82.83)
     exposure to environmental tobacco smoke (Z77.22)
     exposure to tobacco smoke in the perinatal period (P96.81)
     history of tobacco dependence (Z87.891)
     occupational exposure to environmental tobacco smoke (Z57.31)
     tobacco dependence (F17.-)
     tobacco use (Z72.0)

> **Excludes1**   detergent asthma (J69.8)
>   eosinophilic asthma (J82)
>   miner's asthma (J60)
>   wheezing NOS (R06.2)
>   wood asthma (J67.8)

> **Excludes2**   asthma with chronic obstructive pulmonary
>   disease (J44.9)
>   chronic asthmatic (obstructive) bronchitis (J44.9)
>   chronic obstructive asthma (J44.9)

     Coding Clinic: 2019, Q1, P37; 2017, Q1, P25

● J45.2   Mild intermittent asthma

     J45.20   Mild intermittent asthma, uncomplicated
         Mild intermittent asthma NOS

     J45.21   Mild intermittent asthma with (acute) exacerbation

     J45.22   Mild intermittent asthma with status asthmaticus

Item 10-9   Asthma is a bronchial condition marked by airway obstruction, hyper-responsiveness, and inflammation. **Extrinsic** asthma, also known as allergic asthma, is characterized by the same symptoms that occur with exposure to allergens and is divided into the following types: **atopic, occupational,** and **allergic bronchopulmonary aspergillosis. Intrinsic** asthma occurs in patients who have no history of allergy or sensitivities to allergens and is divided into the following types: **nonreaginic** and **pharmacologic. Status asthmaticus** is the most severe form of asthma attack and can last for days or weeks.

▶ New   ⇒ Revised   ~~deleted~~ Deleted   Excludes 1   Excludes 2   Includes   Use additional   Code first   Code also   Key words

934   **OGCR** Official Guidelines   X Assign placeholder X   ● Use Additional Character(s)   ▶ Manifestation Code   Hierarchical Condition Category   **Coding Clinic**

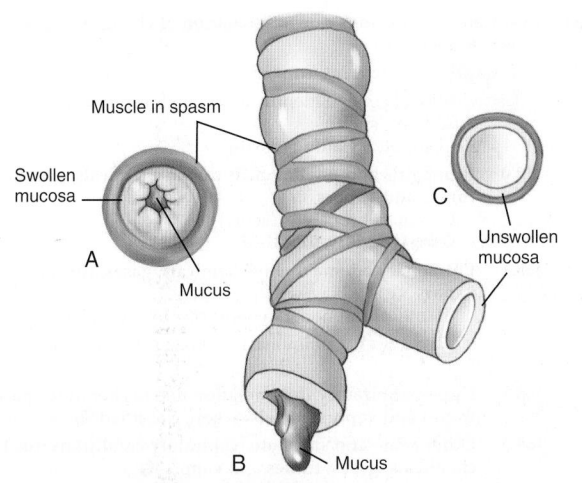

Figure 10-7   Factors causing expiratory obstruction in asthma. **A.** Cross section of a bronchiole occluded by muscle spasm, swollen mucosa, and mucus. **B.** Longitudinal section of an obstructed bronchiole. **C.** Cross section of a clear bronchiole. (From Shiland: Mastering Healthcare Terminology, ed 1, St. Louis, Mosby, 2003)

● **J45.3**   **Mild persistent asthma**
    J45.30   **Mild persistent asthma, uncomplicated**
        Mild persistent asthma NOS
    J45.31   **Mild persistent asthma with (acute) exacerbation**
        Coding Clinic: 2016, Q1, P35
    J45.32   **Mild persistent asthma with status asthmaticus**
● **J45.4**   **Moderate persistent asthma**
    J45.40   **Moderate persistent asthma, uncomplicated**
        Moderate persistent asthma NOS
    J45.41   **Moderate persistent asthma with (acute) exacerbation**
        Coding Clinic: 2017, Q1, P26
    J45.42   **Moderate persistent asthma with status asthmaticus**
● **J45.5**   **Severe persistent asthma**
    J45.50   **Severe persistent asthma, uncomplicated**
        Severe persistent asthma NOS
    J45.51   **Severe persistent asthma with (acute) exacerbation**
    J45.52   **Severe persistent asthma with status asthmaticus**
● **J45.9**   **Other and unspecified asthma**
  ● **J45.90**   **Unspecified asthma**
        Asthmatic bronchitis NOS
        Childhood asthma NOS
        Late onset asthma
      J45.901   **Unspecified asthma with (acute) exacerbation**
          Coding Clinic: 2017, Q4, P96
      J45.902   **Unspecified asthma with status asthmaticus**
      J45.909   **Unspecified asthma, uncomplicated**
        Asthma NOS
        Excludes2   lung diseases due to external agents (J60-J70)
        Coding Clinic: 2017, Q4, P96; 2017, Q1, P25
  ● **J45.99**   **Other asthma**
      J45.990   **Exercise induced bronchospasm**
      J45.991   **Cough variant asthma**
      J45.998   **Other asthma**

● **J47**   **Bronchiectasis**
    Includes   bronchiolectasis
    Use additional code to identify:
      exposure to environmental tobacco smoke (Z77.22)
      exposure to tobacco smoke in the perinatal period (P96.81)
      history of tobacco dependence (Z87.891)
      occupational exposure to environmental tobacco smoke (Z57.31)
      tobacco dependence (F17.-)
      tobacco use (Z72.0)
    Excludes1   congenital bronchiectasis (Q33.4)
        tuberculous bronchiectasis (current disease) (A15.0)
    J47.0   **Bronchiectasis with acute lower respiratory infection**
      Bronchiectasis with acute bronchitis
      ~~Use additional code to identify the infection~~
      ▶ Code also to identify infection, if applicable
    J47.1   **Bronchiectasis with (acute) exacerbation**
      Coding Clinic: 2021, Q1, P24
    J47.9   **Bronchiectasis, uncomplicated**
      Bronchiectasis NOS

LUNG DISEASES DUE TO EXTERNAL AGENTS (J60-J70)

    Excludes2   asthma (J45.-)
        malignant neoplasm of bronchus and lung (C34.-)
J60   **Coalworker's pneumoconiosis**   A
    Anthracosilicosis
    Anthracosis
    Black lung disease
    Coalworker's lung
    Excludes1   coalworker pneumoconiosis with tuberculosis, any type in A15 (J65)
J61   **Pneumoconiosis due to asbestos and other mineral fibers**   A
    Asbestosis
    Excludes1   pleural plaque with asbestosis (J92.0)
        pneumoconiosis with tuberculosis, any type in A15 (J65)
● **J62**   **Pneumoconiosis due to dust containing silica**
    Includes   silicotic fibrosis (massive) of lung
    Excludes1   pneumoconiosis with tuberculosis, any type in A15 (J65)
    J62.0   **Pneumoconiosis due to talc dust**
    J62.8   **Pneumoconiosis due to other dust containing silica**
      Silicosis NOS
● **J63**   **Pneumoconiosis due to other inorganic dusts**
    Excludes1   pneumoconiosis with tuberculosis, any type in A15 (J65)
    Coding Clinic: 2019, Q3, P8
    J63.0   **Aluminosis (of lung)**
    J63.1   **Bauxite fibrosis (of lung)**
    J63.2   **Berylliosis**
    J63.3   **Graphite fibrosis (of lung)**
    J63.4   **Siderosis**
      Coding Clinic: 2019, Q3, P8
    J63.5   **Stannosis**
    J63.6   **Pneumoconiosis due to other specified inorganic dusts**

Figure 10-8   Progressive massive fibrosis superimposed on coal workers' pneumoconiosis. The large, blackened scars are located principally in the upper lobe. (From Frazier MS, Drzymkowski JW: Essentials of Human Diseases and Conditions, St. Louis, MO, Saunders, 2004)

Item 10–10   Pneumoconiosis refers to a lung condition resulting from exposure to inorganic or organic airborne particles, such as coal dust or moldy hay, as well as chemical fumes and vapors, such as insecticides. In this condition, the lungs retain the airborne particles.

CHAPTER 10 (J00-J99)

J64   **Unspecified pneumoconiosis** 🔖

     Excludes1   pneumonoconiosis with tuberculosis, any type in A15 (J65)

J65   **Pneumoconiosis associated with tuberculosis** 🔖
     Any condition in J60-J64 with tuberculosis, any type in A15
     Silicotuberculosis

● **J66**   **Airway disease due to specific organic dust**

     Excludes2   allergic alveolitis (J67.-)
                     asbestosis (J61)
                     bagassosis (J67.1)
                     farmer's lung (J67.0)
                     hypersensitivity pneumonitis due to organic dust (J67.-)
                     reactive airways dysfunction syndrome (J68.3)

   J66.0   **Byssinosis** 🔖
        Airway disease due to cotton dust

   J66.1   **Flax-dressers' disease** 🔖

   J66.2   **Cannabinosis** 🔖

   J66.8   **Airway disease due to other specific organic dusts** 🔖

● **J67**   **Hypersensitivity pneumonitis due to organic dust**

     Includes   allergic alveolitis and pneumonitis due to inhaled organic dust and particles of fungal, actinomycetic or other origin

     Excludes1   pneumonitis due to inhalation of chemicals, gases, fumes or vapors (J68.0)

   J67.0   **Farmer's lung** 🔖
        Harvester's lung
        Haymaker's lung
        Moldy hay disease

   J67.1   **Bagassosis** 🔖
        Bagasse disease
        Bagasse pneumonitis

   J67.2   **Bird fancier's lung** 🔖
        Budgerigar fancier's disease or lung
        Pigeon fancier's disease or lung

   J67.3   **Suberosis** 🔖
        Corkhandler's disease or lung
        Corkworker's disease or lung

   J67.4   **Maltworker's lung** 🔖
        Alveolitis due to Aspergillus clavatus

   J67.5   **Mushroom-worker's lung** 🔖

   J67.6   **Maple-bark-stripper's lung** 🔖
        Alveolitis due to Cryptostroma corticale
        Cryptostromosis

   J67.7   **Air conditioner and humidifier lung** 🔖
        Allergic alveolitis due to fungal, thermophilic actinomycetes and other organisms growing in ventilation [air conditioning] systems

   J67.8   **Hypersensitivity pneumonitis due to other organic dusts** 🔖
        Cheese-washer's lung
        Coffee-worker's lung
        Fish-meal worker's lung
        Furrier's lung
        Sequoiosis

   J67.9   **Hypersensitivity pneumonitis due to unspecified organic dust** 🔖
        Allergic alveolitis (extrinsic) NOS
        Hypersensitivity pneumonitis NOS

● **J68**   **Respiratory conditions due to inhalation of chemicals, gases, fumes and vapors**

     Code first (T51-T65) to identify cause
     Use additional code to identify associated respiratory conditions, such as:
     acute respiratory failure (J96.0-)

   J68.0   **Bronchitis and pneumonitis due to chemicals, gases, fumes and vapors** 🔖
        Chemical bronchitis (acute)
        Coding Clinic: 2019, Q2, P31-32

   J68.1   **Pulmonary edema due to chemicals, gases, fumes and vapors** 🔖
        Chemical pulmonary edema (acute) (chronic)

        Excludes1   pulmonary edema (acute) (chronic) NOS (J81.-)

   J68.2   **Upper respiratory inflammation due to chemicals, gases, fumes and vapors, not elsewhere classified** 🔖

   J68.3   **Other acute and subacute respiratory conditions due to chemicals, gases, fumes and vapors** 🔖
        Reactive airways dysfunction syndrome

   J68.4   **Chronic respiratory conditions due to chemicals, gases, fumes and vapors** 🔖
        Emphysema (diffuse) (chronic) due to inhalation of chemicals, gases, fumes and vapors
        Obliterative bronchiolitis (chronic) (subacute) due to inhalation of chemicals, gases, fumes and vapors
        Pulmonary fibrosis (chronic) due to inhalation of chemicals, gases, fumes and vapors

        Excludes1   chronic pulmonary edema due to chemicals, gases, fumes and vapors (J68.1)

   J68.8   **Other respiratory conditions due to chemicals, gases, fumes and vapors** 🔖

   J68.9   **Unspecified respiratory condition due to chemicals, gases, fumes and vapors** 🔖

● **J69**   **Pneumonitis due to solids and liquids**

     Excludes1   neonatal aspiration syndromes (P24.-)
                     postprocedural pneumonitis (J95.4)

   J69.0   **Pneumonitis due to inhalation of food and vomit** 🔖
        Aspiration pneumonia NOS
        Aspiration pneumonia (due to) food (regurgitated)
        Aspiration pneumonia (due to) gastric secretions
        Aspiration pneumonia (due to) milk
        Aspiration pneumonia (due to) vomit

        Code also any associated foreign body in respiratory tract (T17.-)

        Excludes1   chemical pneumonitis due to anesthesia (J95.4)
                     obstetric aspiration pneumonia (O74.0)
        Coding Clinic: 2021, Q1, P34; 2019, Q2, P7, 31-32; 2017, Q1, P24

   J69.1   **Pneumonitis due to inhalation of oils and essences** 🔖
        Exogenous lipoid pneumonia
        Lipid pneumonia NOS

        Code first (T51-T65) to identify substance
        Excludes1   endogenous lipoid pneumonia (J84.89)

   J69.8   **Pneumonitis due to inhalation of other solids and liquids** 🔖
        Pneumonitis due to aspiration of blood
        Pneumonitis due to aspiration of detergent
        Code first (T51-T65) to identify substance

● **J70**   **Respiratory conditions due to other external agents**

   J70.0   **Acute pulmonary manifestations due to radiation** 🔊
      Radiation pneumonitis
      Use additional code (W88-W90, X39.0-) to identify the external cause

   J70.1   **Chronic and other pulmonary manifestations due to radiation** 🔊
      Fibrosis of lung following radiation
      Use additional code (W88-W90, X39.0-) to identify the external cause

   J70.2   **Acute drug-induced interstitial lung disorders** 🔊
      Use additional code for adverse effect, if applicable, to identify drug (T36-T50 with fifth or sixth character 5)
      Excludes1   interstitial pneumonia NOS (J84.9)
                lymphoid interstitial pneumonia (J84.2)
      Coding Clinic: 2019, Q2, P28

   J70.3   **Chronic drug-induced interstitial lung disorders** 🔊
      Use additional code for adverse effect, if applicable, to identify drug (T36-T50 with fifth or sixth character 5)
      Excludes1   interstitial pneumonia NOS (J84.9)
                lymphoid interstitial pneumonia (J84.2)

   J70.4   **Drug-induced interstitial lung disorders, unspecified** 🔊
      Use additional code for adverse effect, if applicable, to identify drug (T36-T50 with fifth or sixth character 5)
      Excludes1   interstitial pneumonia NOS (J84.9)
                lymphoid interstitial pneumonia (J84.2)
      Coding Clinic: 2019, Q2, P28

   J70.5   **Respiratory conditions due to smoke inhalation** 🔊
      Code first smoke inhalation (T59.81-)
      Excludes2   smoke inhalation due to chemicals, gases, fumes and vapors (J68.9)

   J70.8   **Respiratory conditions due to other specified external agents** 🔊
      Code first (T51-T65) to identify the external agent

   J70.9   **Respiratory conditions due to unspecified external agent** 🔊
      Code first (T51-T65) to identify the external agent

OTHER RESPIRATORY DISEASES PRINCIPALLY AFFECTING THE INTERSTITIUM (J80-J84)

● **J80**   **Acute respiratory distress syndrome** 🔊
     Acute respiratory distress syndrome in adult or child
     Adult hyaline membrane disease
     Excludes1   respiratory distress syndrome in newborn (perinatal) (P22.0)
     Coding Clinic: 2017, Q1, P26-27

● **J81**   **Pulmonary edema**
     Use additional code to identify:
      exposure to environmental tobacco smoke (Z77.22)
      history of tobacco dependence (Z87.891)
      occupational exposure to environmental tobacco smoke (Z57.31)
      tobacco dependence (F17.-)
      tobacco use (Z72.0)
     Excludes1   chemical (acute) pulmonary edema (J68.1)
               hypostatic pneumonia (J18.2)
               passive pneumonia (J18.2)
               pulmonary edema due to external agents (J60-J70)
               pulmonary edema with heart disease NOS (I50.1)
               pulmonary edema with heart failure (I50.1)

   J81.0   **Acute pulmonary edema** 🔊
      Acute edema of lung
      Coding Clinic: 2017, Q1, P26

   J81.1   **Chronic pulmonary edema**
      Pulmonary congestion (chronic) (passive)
      Pulmonary edema NOS

Figure 10-9   Bullous emphysema with large subpleural bullae *(upper left)*. (From Kumar: Robbins and Cotran: Pathologic Basis of Disease, ed 8, Saunders, An Imprint of Elsevier, 2009)

J82   **Pulmonary eosinophilia, not elsewhere classified** 🔊
     Excludes2   pulmonary eosinophilia due to aspergillosis (B44.-)
               pulmonary eosinophilia due to drugs (J70.2-J70.4)
               pulmonary eosinophilia due to specified parasitic infection (B50-B83)
               pulmonary eosinophilia due to systemic connective tissue disorders (M30-M36)
               pulmonary infiltrate NOS (R91.8)

● **J82.8**   **Pulmonary eosinophilia, not elsewhere classified**

   J82.81   **Chronic eosinophilic pneumonia**
      Eosinophilic pneumonia, NOS

   J82.82   **Acute eosinophilic pneumonia**

   J82.83   **Eosinophilic asthma**
      Code first asthma, by type, such as:
      mild intermittent asthma (J45.2-)
      mild persistent asthma (J45.3-)
      moderate persistent asthma (J45.4-)
      severe persistent asthma (J45.5-)

   J82.89   **Other pulmonary eosinophilia, not elsewhere classified**
      Allergic pneumonia
      Löffler's pneumonia
      Tropical (pulmonary) eosinophilia NOS

● **J84**   **Other interstitial pulmonary diseases**
     Excludes1   drug-induced interstitial lung disorders (J70.2-J70.4)
               interstitial emphysema (J98.2)
     Excludes2   lung diseases due to external agents (J60-J70)
     Coding Clinic: 2019, Q2, P28

● **J84.0**   **Alveolar and parieto-alveolar conditions**

   J84.01   **Alveolar proteinosis** 🔊

   J84.02   **Pulmonary alveolar microlithiasis** 🔊

▹ **J84.03**   *Idiopathic pulmonary hemosiderosis* 🔊
      Essential brown induration of lung
      Code first underlying disease, such as:
      disorders of iron metabolism (E83.1-)
      Excludes1   acute idiopathic pulmonary hemorrhage in infants [AIPHI] (R04.81)

   J84.09   **Other alveolar and parieto-alveolar conditions** 🔊

● **J84.1**   **Other interstitial pulmonary diseases with fibrosis**
     Excludes1   pulmonary fibrosis (chronic) due to inhalation of chemicals, gases, fumes or vapors (J68.4)
               pulmonary fibrosis (chronic) following radiation (J70.1)

J84.10   Pulmonary fibrosis, **unspecified** 🅦
    Capillary fibrosis of lung
    Cirrhosis of lung (chronic) NOS
    Fibrosis of lung (atrophic) (chronic) (confluent)
        (massive) (perialveolar) (peribronchial)
        NOS
    Induration of lung (chronic) NOS
    Postinflammatory pulmonary fibrosis

● **J84.11**   Idiopathic interstitial pneumonia
    Excludes1 lymphoid interstitial pneumonia
                  (J84.2)
               pneumocystis pneumonia (B59)

   J84.111   Idiopathic interstitial pneumonia, not
           otherwise specified 🅦

   J84.112   Idiopathic pulmonary fibrosis 🅦
           Cryptogenic fibrosing alveolitis
           Idiopathic fibrosing alveolitis

   J84.113   Idiopathic non-specific interstitial
           pneumonitis 🅦
           Excludes1 non-specific interstitial
                     pneumonia NOS,
                     or due to known
                     underlying cause
                     (J84.89)

   J84.114   Acute interstitial pneumonitis 🅦
           Hamman-Rich syndrome
           Excludes1 pneumocystis
                     pneumonia (B59)

   J84.115   Respiratory bronchiolitis interstitial
           lung disease 🅦

   J84.116   Cryptogenic organizing
           pneumonia 🅦
           Excludes1 organizing pneumonia
                     NOS, or due
                     to known
                     underlying cause
                     (J84.89)

   J84.117   Desquamative interstitial
           pneumonia 🅦

● ▸ *J84.17   Other interstitial pulmonary diseases with
    fibrosis in diseases classified elsewhere* 🅦

   ▸*J84.170   Interstitial lung disease with
           progressive fibrotic phenotype in
           diseases classified elsewhere*
             *Progressive fibrotic interstitial lung
               disease*

            Code first underlying disease, such as:
              lung diseases due to external agents
                (J60-J70)
              rheumatoid arthritis (M05.00-M06.9)
              sarcoidosis (D86)
              *systemic connective tissue disorders
                (M30-M36)*

   ▸**J84.178**   *Other interstitial pulmonary diseases
           with fibrosis in diseases classified
           elsewhere*
             *Interstitial pneumonia (nonspecific)
               (usual) due to collagen vascular
               disease*
             *Interstitial pneumonia (nonspecific)
               (usual) in diseases classified
               elsewhere*
             *Organizing pneumonia due to collagen
                vascular disease*
             *Organizing pneumonia in diseases
               classified elsewhere*

            Code first underlying disease, such as:
             progressive systemic sclerosis (M34.0)
             rheumatoid arthritis (M05.00-M06.9)
             *systemic lupus erythematosis
               (M32.0-M32.9)*

J84.2   Lymphoid interstitial pneumonia 🅦
    Lymphoid interstitial pneumonitis

● **J84.8**   Other specified interstitial pulmonary diseases
    Excludes1 exogenous lipoid pneumonia (J69.1)
               unspecified lipoid pneumonia (J69.1)

   J84.81   Lymphangioleiomyomatosis 🅦
           Lymphangiomyomatosis

   J84.82   Adult pulmonary Langerhans cell
           histiocytosis 🅦   A
           Adult PLCH

   J84.83   Surfactant mutations of the lung 🅦

● **J84.84**   Other interstitial lung diseases of childhood

   J84.841   Neuroendocrine cell hyperplasia of
           infancy 🅦

   J84.842   Pulmonary interstitial
           glycogenosis 🅦

   J84.843   Alveolar capillary dysplasia with vein
           misalignment 🅦

   J84.848   Other interstitial lung diseases of
           childhood 🅦

   J84.89   Other specified interstitial pulmonary diseases 🅦
           Endogenous lipoid pneumonia
           Interstitial pneumonitis
           Non-specific interstitial pneumonitis NOS
           Organizing pneumonia NOS
           Code first, if applicable:
             poisoning due to drug or toxin (T51-T65
               with fifth or sixth character to indicate
               intent), for toxic pneumonopathy
             underlying cause of pneumonopathy, if
             known

           Use additional code, for adverse effect, to
             identify drug (T36-T50 with fifth or sixth
             character 5), if drug-induced

           Excludes1 cryptogenic organizing
                     pneumonia (J84.116)
                   idiopathic non-specific interstitial
                     pneumonitis (J84.113)
                   lipoid pneumonia, exogenous or
                     unspecified (J69.1)
                   lymphoid interstitial pneumonia
                     (J84.2)

          Coding Clinic: 2021, Q1, P48; 2019, Q2, P28

J84.9   Interstitial pulmonary disease, **unspecified** 🅦
    Interstitial pneumonia NOS

▶ New   ⇒ Revised   ~~deleted~~ Deleted   Excludes 1   Excludes 2   Includes   Use additional   Code first   Code also   Key words

OGCR Official Guidelines   X Assign placeholder X   ● Use Additional Character(s)   ▸ Manifestation Code   🅦 Hierarchical Condition Category   **Coding Clinic**

SUPPURATIVE AND NECROTIC CONDITIONS OF THE LOWER RESPIRATORY TRACT (J85-J86)

● **J85   Abscess of lung and mediastinum**
Use additional code (B95-B97) to identify infectious agent.

J85.0   Gangrene and necrosis of lung 🔖

J85.1   Abscess of lung with pneumonia 🔖
Code also the type of pneumonia

J85.2   Abscess of lung without pneumonia 🔖
Abscess of lung NOS

J85.3   Abscess of mediastinum 🔖

● **J86   Pyothorax**
Use additional code (B95-B97) to identify infectious agent.
> **Excludes1**   abscess of lung (J85.-)
>   pyothorax due to tuberculosis (A15.6)

J86.0   Pyothorax with fistula 🔖
Bronchocutaneous fistula
Bronchopleural fistula
Hepatopleural fistula
Mediastinal fistula
Pleural fistula
Thoracic fistula
Any condition classifiable to J86.9 with fistula

J86.9   Pyothorax without fistula 🔖
Abscess of pleura
Abscess of thorax
Empyema (chest) (lung) (pleura)
Fibrinopurulent pleurisy
Purulent pleurisy
Pyopneumothorax
Septic pleurisy
Seropurulent pleurisy
Suppurative pleurisy

OTHER DISEASES OF THE PLEURA (J90-J94)

J90   Pleural effusion, not elsewhere classified
Encysted pleurisy
Pleural effusion NOS
Pleurisy with effusion (exudative) (serous)
> **Excludes1**   chylous (pleural) effusion (J94.0)
>   malignant pleural effusion (J91.0))
>   pleurisy NOS (R09.1)
>   tuberculous pleural effusion (A15.6)
Coding Clinic: 2015, Q2, P16

● **J91   Pleural effusion in conditions classified elsewhere**
> **Excludes2**   pleural effusion in heart failure (I50.-)
>   pleural effusion in systemic lupus erythematosus (M32.13)

▷ *J91.0   Malignant pleural effusion*
Code first underlying neoplasm

▷ *J91.8   Pleural effusion in other conditions classified elsewhere*
Code first underlying disease, such as:
filariasis (B74.0-B74.9)
influenza (J09.X2, J10.1, J11.1)
Coding Clinic: 2015, Q2, P16

● **J92   Pleural plaque**
> **Includes**   pleural thickening

J92.0   Pleural plaque with presence of asbestos

J92.9   Pleural plaque without asbestos
Pleural plaque NOS

● **J93   Pneumothorax and air leak**
Collapsed lung
> **Excludes1**   congenital or perinatal pneumothorax (P25.1)
>   postprocedural air leak (J95.812)
>   postprocedural pneumothorax (J95.811)
>   traumatic pneumothorax (S27.0)
>   tuberculous (current disease) pneumothorax (A15.-)
>   pyopneumothorax (J86.-)

J93.0   Spontaneous tension pneumothorax
Tension pneumothorax (most serious type) occurs when air (positive pressure) collects in the pleural space

Item 10–11   Empyema is a condition in which pus accumulates in a body cavity. Empyema **with fistula** occurs when the pus passes from one cavity to another organ or structure.

● **J93.1   Other spontaneous pneumothorax**

J93.11   Primary spontaneous pneumothorax

J93.12   Secondary spontaneous pneumothorax
Code first underlying condition, such as:
catamenial pneumothorax due to endometriosis (N80.8)
cystic fibrosis (E84.-)
eosinophilic pneumonia (J82)
lymphangioleiomyomatosis (J84.81)
malignant neoplasm of bronchus and lung (C34.-)
Marfan's syndrome (Q87.4)
pneumonia due to Pneumocystis carinii (B59)
secondary malignant neoplasm of lung (C78.0-)
spontaneous rupture of the esophagus (K22.3)

● **J93.8   Other pneumothorax and air leak**

J93.81   Chronic pneumothorax

J93.82   Other air leak
Persistent air leak

J93.83   Other pneumothorax
Acute pneumothorax
Spontaneous pneumothorax NOS

J93.9   Pneumothorax, unspecified
Pneumothorax NOS

● **J94   Other pleural conditions**
> **Excludes1**   pleurisy NOS (R09.1)
>   traumatic hemopneumothorax (S27.2)
>   traumatic hemothorax (S27.1)
>   tuberculous pleural conditions (current disease) (A15.-)

J94.0   Chylous effusion
Chyliform effusion

J94.1   Fibrothorax

J94.2   Hemothorax
Hemopneumothorax

J94.8   Other specified pleural conditions
Hydropneumothorax
Hydrothorax
Coding Clinic: 2021, Q1, P49

J94.9   Pleural condition, unspecified

INTRAOPERATIVE AND POSTPROCEDURAL COMPLICATIONS AND DISORDERS OF RESPIRATORY SYSTEM, NOT ELSEWHERE CLASSIFIED (J95)

● **J95**   **Intraoperative and postprocedural complications and disorders of respiratory system, not elsewhere classified**

     Excludes2   aspiration pneumonia (J69.-)
           emphysema (subcutaneous) resulting from a procedure (T81.82)
           hypostatic pneumonia (J18.2)
           pulmonary manifestations due to radiation (J70.0- J70.1)

● **J95.0**   **Tracheostomy complications**

     J95.00   **Unspecified tracheostomy complication** 🐾

     J95.01   **Hemorrhage from tracheostomy stoma** 🐾

     J95.02   **Infection of tracheostomy stoma** 🐾
         Use additional code to identify type of infection, such as:
           cellulitis of neck (L03.221)
           sepsis (A40, A41.-)

     J95.03   **Malfunction of tracheostomy stoma** 🐾
         Mechanical complication of tracheostomy stoma
         Obstruction of tracheostomy airway
         Tracheal stenosis due to tracheostomy

     J95.04   **Tracheo-esophageal fistula following tracheostomy** 🐾

     J95.09   **Other tracheostomy complication** 🐾

J95.1   **Acute pulmonary insufficiency following thoracic surgery** 🐾
     Excludes2   functional disturbances following cardiac surgery (I97.0, I97.1-)

J95.2   **Acute pulmonary insufficiency following nonthoracic surgery** 🐾
     Excludes2   functional disturbances following cardiac surgery (I97.0, I97.1-)

J95.3   **Chronic pulmonary insufficiency following surgery** 🐾
     Excludes2   functional disturbances following cardiac surgery (I97.0, I97.1-)

J95.4   **Chemical pneumonitis due to anesthesia**
     Mendelson's syndrome
     Postprocedural aspiration pneumonia
     Use additional code for adverse effect, if applicable, to identify drug (T41.- with fifth or sixth character 5)
     Excludes1   aspiration pneumonitis due to anesthesia complicating labor and delivery (O74.0)
           aspiration pneumonitis due to anesthesia complicating pregnancy (O29)
           aspiration pneumonitis due to anesthesia complicating the puerperium (O89.01)

J95.5   **Postprocedural subglottic stenosis**

● **J95.6**   **Intraoperative hemorrhage and hematoma of a respiratory system organ or structure complicating a procedure**
     Excludes1   intraoperative hemorrhage and hematoma of a respiratory system organ or structure due to accidental puncture and laceration during procedure (J95.7-)

     J95.61   **Intraoperative hemorrhage and hematoma of a respiratory system organ or structure complicating a respiratory system procedure**

     J95.62   **Intraoperative hemorrhage and hematoma of a respiratory system organ or structure complicating other procedure**

● **J95.7**   **Accidental puncture and laceration of a respiratory system organ or structure during a procedure**
     Excludes2   postprocedural pneumothorax (J95.811)

     J95.71   **Accidental puncture and laceration of a respiratory system organ or structure during a respiratory system procedure**

     J95.72   **Accidental puncture and laceration of a respiratory system organ or structure during other procedure**

● **J95.8**   **Other intraoperative and postprocedural complications and disorders of respiratory system, not elsewhere classified**
     Coding Clinic: 2016, Q4, P10

   ● **J95.81**   **Postprocedural pneumothorax and air leak**

     J95.811   **Postprocedural pneumothorax**
       Coding Clinic: 2021, Q1, P49

     J95.812   **Postprocedural air leak**

   ● **J95.82**   **Postprocedural respiratory failure**
     Excludes1   Respiratory failure in other conditions (J96.-)

     J95.821   **Acute postprocedural respiratory failure** 🐾
       Postprocedural respiratory failure NOS

     J95.822   **Acute and chronic postprocedural respiratory failure** 🐾

   ● **J95.83**   **Postprocedural hemorrhage of a respiratory system organ or structure following a procedure**

     J95.830   **Postprocedural hemorrhage of a respiratory system organ or structure following a respiratory system procedure**

     J95.831   **Postprocedural hemorrhage of a respiratory system organ or structure following other procedure**

     J95.84   **Transfusion-related acute lung injury (TRALI)**

   ● **J95.85**   **Complication of respirator [ventilator]**

     J95.850   **Mechanical complication of respirator** 🐾
       Excludes1   encounter for respirator [ventilator] dependence during power failure (Z99.12)

     J95.851   **Ventilator associated pneumonia** 🐾
       Ventilator associated pneumonitis
       Use additional code to identify the organism, if known (B95.-, B96.-, B97.-)
       Excludes1   ventilator lung in newborn (P27.8)
       Coding Clinic: 2017, Q1, P25

     J95.859   **Other complication of respirator [ventilator]** 🐾
       Coding Clinic: 2021, Q1, P49

● **J95.86** **Postprocedural hematoma and seroma of a respiratory system organ or structure following a procedure**

     J95.860 Postprocedural hematoma of a respiratory system organ or structure following a respiratory system procedure

     J95.861 Postprocedural hematoma of a respiratory system organ or structure following other procedure

     J95.862 Postprocedural seroma of a respiratory system organ or structure following a respiratory system procedure

     J95.863 Postprocedural seroma of a respiratory system organ or structure following other procedure

   J95.88 Other intraoperative complications of respiratory system, not elsewhere classified

   J95.89 Other postprocedural complications and disorders of respiratory system, not elsewhere classified

     Use additional code to identify disorder, such as:
       aspiration pneumonia (J69.-)
       bacterial or viral pneumonia (J12-J18)

     Excludes2   acute pulmonary insufficiency following thoracic surgery (J95.1)
                 postprocedural subglottic stenosis (J95.5)

OTHER DISEASES OF THE RESPIRATORY SYSTEM (J96-J99)

● **J96** **Respiratory failure, not elsewhere classified**

   Excludes1   acute respiratory distress syndrome (J80)
                cardiorespiratory failure (R09.2)
                newborn respiratory distress syndrome (P22.0)
                postprocedural respiratory failure (J95.82-)
                respiratory arrest (R09.2)
                respiratory arrest of newborn (P28.81)
                respiratory failure of newborn (P28.5)

● **J96.0** **Acute respiratory failure**

   J96.00 Acute respiratory failure, unspecified whether with hypoxia or hypercapnia 🔍
       Coding Clinic: 2016, Q3, P14

   J96.01 Acute respiratory failure with hypoxia 🔍

   J96.02 Acute respiratory failure with hypercapnia 🔍

● **J96.1** **Chronic respiratory failure**

   J96.10 Chronic respiratory failure, unspecified whether with hypoxia or hypercapnia 🔍
       Coding Clinic: 2021, Q1, P46; 2016, Q1, P38; 2015, Q1, P21

   J96.11 Chronic respiratory failure with hypoxia 🔍

   J96.12 Chronic respiratory failure with hypercapnia 🔍

● **J96.2** **Acute and chronic respiratory failure**
     Acute on chronic respiratory failure

   J96.20 Acute and chronic respiratory failure, unspecified whether with hypoxia or hypercapnia 🔍

   J96.21 Acute and chronic respiratory failure with hypoxia 🔍

   J96.22 Acute and chronic respiratory failure with hypercapnia 🔍

● **J96.9** **Respiratory failure, unspecified**

   J96.90 Respiratory failure, unspecified, unspecified whether with hypoxia or hypercapnia 🔍
       Coding Clinic: 2021, Q1, P44

   J96.91 Respiratory failure, unspecified with hypoxia 🔍

   J96.92 Respiratory failure, unspecified with hypercapnia 🔍

● **J98** **Other respiratory disorders**

   Use additional code to identify:
     exposure to environmental tobacco smoke (Z77.22)
     exposure to tobacco smoke in the perinatal period (P96.81)
     history of tobacco dependence (Z87.891)
     occupational exposure to environmental tobacco smoke (Z57.31)
     tobacco dependence (F17.-)
     tobacco use (Z72.0)

   Excludes1   newborn apnea (P28.4)
                newborn sleep apnea (P28.3)

   Excludes2   apnea NOS (R06.81)
                sleep apnea (G47.3-)

● **J98.0** **Diseases of bronchus, not elsewhere classified**

   J98.01 **Acute bronchospasm**

     Excludes1   acute bronchiolitis with bronchospasm (J21.-)
                acute bronchitis with bronchospasm (J20.-)
                asthma (J45.-)
                exercise induced bronchospasm (J45.990)

   J98.09 **Other diseases of bronchus, not elsewhere classified**
     Broncholithiasis
     Calcification of bronchus
     Stenosis of bronchus
     Tracheobronchial collapse
     Tracheobronchial dyskinesia
     Ulcer of bronchus

● **J98.1** **Pulmonary collapse**

   Excludes1   therapeutic collapse of lung status (Z98.3)

   J98.11 **Atelectasis**

     Excludes1   newborn atelectasis
                tuberculous atelectasis (current disease) (A15)

   J98.19 **Other pulmonary collapse**

● **J98.2** **Interstitial emphysema** 🔍
     Mediastinal emphysema

   Excludes1   emphysema NOS (J43.9)
                emphysema in newborn (P25.0)
                surgical emphysema (subcutaneous) (T81.82)
                traumatic subcutaneous emphysema (T79.7)

● **J98.3** **Compensatory emphysema** 🔍

● **J98.4** **Other disorders of lung**
     Calcification of lung
     Cystic lung disease (acquired)
     Lung disease NOS
     Pulmolithiasis

   Excludes1   acute interstitial pneumonitis (J84.114)
                pulmonary insufficiency following surgery (J95.1-J95.2)

CHAPTER 10 (J00-J99)

● **J98.5** **Diseases of mediastinum, not elsewhere classified**

     Excludes2   abscess of mediastinum (J85.3)

     Coding Clinic: 2016, Q4, P29

     J98.51   **Mediastinitis**

          Code first underlying condition, if applicable, such as postoperative mediastinitis (T81.-)

     J98.59   **Other diseases of mediastinum, not elsewhere classified**

          Fibrosis of mediastinum

          Hernia of mediastinum

          Retraction of mediastinum

J98.6 **Disorders of diaphragm**

     Diaphragmatitis

     Paralysis of diaphragm

     Relaxation of diaphragm

     Excludes1   congenital malformation of diaphragm NEC (Q79.1)

                   congenital diaphragmatic hernia (Q79.0)

     Excludes2   diaphragmatic hernia (K44.-)

J98.8 **Other specified respiratory disorders**

J98.9 **Respiratory disorder, unspecified**

     Respiratory disease (chronic) NOS

▶ *J99* ▷ *Respiratory disorders in diseases classified elsewhere* 🏷

     Code first underlying disease, such as:

         amyloidosis (E85.-)

         ankylosing spondylitis (M45)

         congenital syphilis (A50.5)

         cryoglobulinemia (D89.1)

         early congenital syphilis (A50.0)

         plasminogen deficiency (E88.02)

         schistosomiasis (B65.0-B65.9)

     Excludes1   respiratory disorders in:

         amebiasis (A06.5)

         blastomycosis (B40.0-B40.2)

         candidiasis (B37.1)

         coccidioidomycosis (B38.0-B38.2)

         cystic fibrosis with pulmonary manifestations (E84.0)

         dermatomyositis (M33.01, M33.11)

         histoplasmosis (B39.0-B39.2)

         late syphilis (A52.72, A52.73)

         polymyositis (M33.21)

    ▶ Sjögren syndrome (M35.02)

         systemic lupus erythematosus (M32.13)

         systemic sclerosis (M34.81)

         Wegener's granulomatosis (M31.30-M31.31)

▶ New   ⇒ Revised   ~~deleted~~ Deleted   Excludes 1   Excludes 2   Includes   Use additional   Code first   Code also   Key words

OGCR Official Guidelines   X Assign placeholder X   ● Use Additional Character(s)   ▷ Manifestation Code   🏷 Hierarchical Condition Category   **Coding Clinic**

CHAPTER 11

DISEASES OF THE DIGESTIVE SYSTEM
(K00-K95)

OGCR Chapter-Specific Coding Guidelines

11. Chapter 11: Diseases of the Digestive System (K00-K95)
    Reserved for future guideline expansion

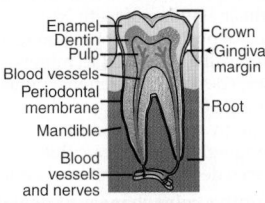

Figure 11-1 Anatomy of a tooth.

Item 11-1 Anodontia is the congenital absence of teeth. **Hypodontia** is partial anodontia. **Oligodontia** is the congenital absence of some teeth, whereas **supernumerary** is having more teeth than the normal number. **Mesiodens** are small extra teeth that often appear in pairs, although single small teeth are not uncommon.

CHAPTER 11

DISEASES OF THE DIGESTIVE SYSTEM
(K00-K95)

Excludes2   certain conditions originating in the perinatal period (P04-P96)
certain infectious and parasitic diseases (A00-B99)
complications of pregnancy, childbirth and the puerperium (O00-O9A)
congenital malformations, deformations and chromosomal abnormalities (Q00-Q99)
endocrine, nutritional and metabolic diseases (E00-E88)
injury, poisoning and certain other consequences of external causes (S00-T88)
neoplasms (C00-D49)
symptoms, signs and abnormal clinical and laboratory findings, not elsewhere classified (R00-R94)

This chapter contains the following blocks:

K00-K14	Diseases of oral cavity and salivary glands
K20-K31	Diseases of esophagus, stomach and duodenum
K35-K38	Diseases of appendix
K40-K46	Hernia
K50-K52	Noninfective enteritis and colitis
K55-K64	Other diseases of intestines
K65-K68	Diseases of peritoneum and retroperitoneum
K70-K77	Diseases of liver
K80-K87	Disorders of gallbladder, biliary tract and pancreas
K90-K95	Other diseases of the digestive system

DISEASES OF ORAL CAVITY AND SALIVARY GLANDS (K00-K14)

● **K00** **Disorders of tooth development and eruption**
   Excludes2   embedded and impacted teeth (K01.-)

   K00.0 Anodontia
      Hypodontia
      Oligodontia
      Excludes1   acquired absence of teeth (K08.1-)

   K00.1 Supernumerary teeth
      Distomolar
      Fourth molar
      Mesiodens
      Paramolar
      Supplementary teeth
      Excludes2   supernumerary roots (K00.2)

   K00.2 Abnormalities of size and form of teeth
      Concrescence of teeth
      Fusion of teeth
      Gemination of teeth
      Dens evaginatus
      Dens in dente
      Dens invaginatus
      Enamel pearls
      Macrodontia
      Microdontia
      Peg-shaped [conical] teeth
      Supernumerary roots
      Taurodontism
      Tuberculum paramolare
      Excludes1   abnormalities of teeth due to congenital syphilis (A50.5)
                 tuberculum Carabelli, which is regarded as a normal variation and should not be coded

   K00.3 Mottled teeth
      Dental fluorosis
      Mottling of enamel
      Nonfluoride enamel opacities
      Excludes2   deposits [accretions] on teeth (K03.6)

   K00.4 Disturbances in tooth formation
      Aplasia and hypoplasia of cementum
      Dilaceration of tooth
      Enamel hypoplasia (neonatal) (postnatal) (prenatal)
      Regional odontodysplasia
      Turner's tooth
      Excludes1   Hutchinson's teeth and mulberry molars in congenital syphilis (A50.5)
      Excludes2   mottled teeth (K00.3)

   K00.5 Hereditary disturbances in tooth structure, not elsewhere classified
      Amelogenesis imperfecta
      Dentinogenesis imperfecta
      Odontogenesis imperfecta
      Dentinal dysplasia
      Shell teeth

   K00.6 Disturbances in tooth eruption
      Dentia praecox
      Natal tooth
      Neonatal tooth
      Premature eruption of tooth
      Premature shedding of primary [deciduous] tooth
      Prenatal teeth
      Retained [persistent] primary tooth
      Excludes2   embedded and impacted teeth (K01.-)

   K00.7 Teething syndrome

   K00.8 Other disorders of tooth development
      Color changes during tooth formation
      Intrinsic staining of teeth NOS
      Excludes2   posteruptive color changes (K03.7)

   K00.9 Disorder of tooth development, unspecified
      Disorder of odontogenesis NOS

● **K01** **Embedded and impacted teeth**
   Excludes1   abnormal position of fully erupted teeth (M26.3-)
   K01.0 Embedded teeth
   K01.1 Impacted teeth

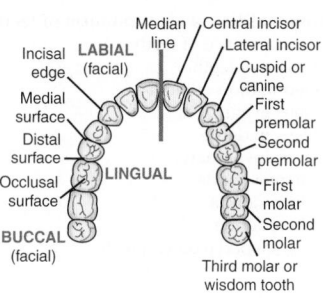

Figure 11-2 The permanent teeth within the dental arch.

Item 11-2 Each dental arch (jaw) normally contains 16 teeth. Tooth decay or **dental caries** is a disease of the enamel, dentin, and cementum of the tooth and can result in a cavity.

● **K02   Dental caries**

   Includes   caries of dentine
                   dental cavities
                   early childhood caries
                   pre-eruptive caries
                   recurrent caries (dentino enamel junction)
                      (enamel) (to the pulp)
                   tooth decay

   K02.3   Arrested dental caries
             Arrested coronal and root caries

   ● **K02.5   Dental caries on pit and fissure surface**
             Dental caries on chewing surface of tooth

       K02.51   Dental caries on pit and fissure surface limited to enamel
                   White spot lesions [initial caries] on pit and fissure surface of tooth

       K02.52   Dental caries on pit and fissure surface penetrating into dentin
                   Primary dental caries, cervical origin

       K02.53   Dental caries on pit and fissure surface penetrating into pulp

   ● **K02.6   Dental caries on smooth surface**

       K02.61   Dental caries on smooth surface limited to enamel
                   White spot lesions [initial caries] on smooth surface of tooth

       K02.62   Dental caries on smooth surface penetrating into dentin

       K02.63   Dental caries on smooth surface penetrating into pulp

   K02.7   Dental root caries

   K02.9   Dental caries, unspecified

● **K03   Other diseases of hard tissues of teeth**

   Excludes2   bruxism (F45.8)
                    dental caries (K02.-)
                    teeth-grinding NOS (F45.8)

   K03.0   Excessive attrition of teeth
             Approximal wear of teeth
             Occlusal wear of teeth

   K03.1   Abrasion of teeth
             Dentifrice abrasion of teeth
             Habitual abrasion of teeth
             Occupational abrasion of teeth
             Ritual abrasion of teeth
             Traditional abrasion of teeth
             Wedge defect NOS

   K03.2   Erosion of teeth
             Erosion of teeth due to diet
             Erosion of teeth due to drugs and medicaments
             Erosion of teeth due to persistent vomiting
             Erosion of teeth NOS
             Idiopathic erosion of teeth
             Occupational erosion of teeth

   K03.3   Pathological resorption of teeth
             Internal granuloma of pulp
             Resorption of teeth (external)

   K03.4   Hypercementosis
             Cementation hyperplasia

   K03.5   Ankylosis of teeth

   K03.6   Deposits [accretions] on teeth
             Betel deposits [accretions] on teeth
             Black deposits [accretions] on teeth
             Extrinsic staining of teeth NOS
             Green deposits [accretions] on teeth
             Materia alba deposits [accretions] on teeth
             Orange deposits [accretions] on teeth
             Staining of teeth NOS
             Subgingival dental calculus
             Supragingival dental calculus
             Tobacco deposits [accretions] on teeth

   K03.7   Posteruptive color changes of dental hard tissues
             Excludes2   deposits [accretions] on teeth (K03.6)

   ● **K03.8   Other specified diseases of hard tissues of teeth**
       K03.81   Cracked tooth
                   Excludes1   asymptomatic craze lines in enamel - omit code
                                    broken or fractured tooth due to trauma (S02.5)

       K03.89   Other specified diseases of hard tissues of teeth

   K03.9   Disease of hard tissues of teeth, unspecified

K04   Diseases of pulp and periapical tissues
        Coding Clinic: 2016, Q4, P29

   ● **K04.0   Pulpitis**
             Acute pulpitis
             Chronic (hyperplastic) (ulcerative) pulpitis

       K04.01   Reversible pulpitis

       K04.02   Irreversible pulpitis

   K04.1   Necrosis of pulp
             Pulpal gangrene

   K04.2   Pulp degeneration
             Denticles
             Pulpal calcifications
             Pulpal stones

   K04.3   Abnormal hard tissue formation in pulp
             Secondary or irregular dentine

   K04.4   Acute apical periodontitis of pulpal origin
             Acute apical periodontitis NOS
             Excludes1   acute periodontitis (K05.2-)

   K04.5   Chronic apical periodontitis
             Apical or periapical granuloma
             Apical periodontitis NOS
             Excludes1   chronic periodontitis (K05.3-)

   K04.6   Periapical abscess with sinus
             Dental abscess with sinus
             Dentoalveolar abscess with sinus

   K04.7   Periapical abscess without sinus
             Dental abscess without sinus
             Dentoalveolar abscess without sinus

   K04.8   Radicular cyst
             Apical (periodontal) cyst
             Periapical cyst
             Residual radicular cyst
             Excludes2   lateral periodontal cyst (K09.0)

   ● **K04.9   Other and unspecified diseases of pulp and periapical tissues**

       K04.90   Unspecified diseases of pulp and periapical tissues

       K04.99   Other diseases of pulp and periapical tissues

Item 11-3   Acute gingivitis, also known as orilitis or ulitis, is the short-term, severe inflammation of the gums (gingiva) caused by bacteria. **Chronic gingivitis** is persistent inflammation of the gums. When the gingivitis moves into the periodontium it is called periodontitis, also known as paradentitis.

▶ New   ⇒ Revised   ~~deleted~~ Deleted   Excludes 1   Excludes 2   Includes   Use additional   Code first   Code also   Key words

944   OGCR Official Guidelines   X Assign placeholder X   ● Use Additional Character(s)   ▌ Manifestation Code   🔖 Hierarchical Condition Category   **Coding Clinic**

● **K05**   **Gingivitis and periodontal diseases**
     Use additional code to identify:
        alcohol abuse and dependence (F10.-)
        exposure to environmental tobacco smoke (Z77.22)
        exposure to tobacco smoke in the perinatal period (P96.81)
        history of tobacco dependence (Z87.891)
        occupational exposure to environmental tobacco smoke
           (Z57.31)
        tobacco dependence (F17.-)
        tobacco use (Z72.0)
     Coding Clinic: 2016, Q4, P29

● **K05.0**   **Acute gingivitis**
       Excludes1   acute necrotizing ulcerative gingivitis
                (A69.1)
                herpesviral [herpes simplex]
                  gingivostomatitis (B00.2)

     K05.00   **Acute gingivitis, plaque induced**
         Acute gingivitis NOS
         Plaque induced gingival disease

     K05.01   **Acute gingivitis, non-plaque induced**

● **K05.1**   **Chronic gingivitis**
       Desquamative gingivitis (chronic)
       Gingivitis (chronic) NOS
       Hyperplastic gingivitis (chronic)
       Pregnancy associated gingivitis
       Simple marginal gingivitis (chronic)
       Ulcerative gingivitis (chronic)
       Code first, if applicable, diseases of the digestive system
         complicating pregnancy (O99.61-)

     K05.10   **Chronic gingivitis, plaque induced**
         Chronic gingivitis NOS
         Gingivitis NOS

     K05.11   **Chronic gingivitis, non-plaque induced**

● **K05.2**   **Aggressive periodontitis**
       Acute pericoronitis
       Excludes1   acute apical periodontitis (K04.4)
                periapical abscess (K04.7)
                periapical abscess with sinus (K04.6)

     K05.20   **Aggressive periodontitis, unspecified**

●   **K05.21**   **Aggressive periodontitis, localized**
         Periodontal abscess

         K05.211   **Aggressive periodontitis, localized,**
               slight

         K05.212   **Aggressive periodontitis, localized,**
               moderate

         K05.213   **Aggressive periodontitis, localized,**
               severe

         K05.219   **Aggressive periodontitis, localized,**
               unspecified severity

●   **K05.22**   **Aggressive periodontitis, generalized**

         K05.221   **Aggressive periodontitis, generalized,**
               slight

         K05.222   **Aggressive periodontitis, generalized,**
               moderate

         K05.223   **Aggressive periodontitis, generalized,**
               severe

         K05.229   **Aggressive periodontitis, generalized,**
               unspecified severity

● **K05.3**   **Chronic periodontitis**
       Chronic pericoronitis
       Complex periodontitis
       Periodontitis NOS
       Simplex periodontitis
       Excludes1   chronic apical periodontitis (K04.5)

     K05.30   **Chronic periodontitis, unspecified**

●   **K05.31**   **Chronic periodontitis, localized**

         K05.311   **Chronic periodontitis, localized,**
               slight

         K05.312   **Chronic periodontitis, localized,**
               moderate

         K05.313   **Chronic periodontitis, localized,**
               severe

         K05.319   **Chronic periodontitis, localized,**
               unspecified severity

●   **K05.32**   **Chronic periodontitis, generalized**

         K05.321   **Chronic periodontitis, generalized,**
               slight

         K05.322   **Chronic periodontitis, generalized,**
               moderate

         K05.323   **Chronic periodontitis, generalized,**
               severe

         K05.329   **Chronic periodontitis, generalized,**
               unspecified severity

  K05.4   **Periodontosis**
       Juvenile periodontosis

  K05.5   **Other periodontal diseases**
       Combined periodontic-endodontic lesion
       Narrow gingival width (of periodontal soft tissue)
       Excludes2   leukoplakia of gingiva (K13.21)

  K05.6   **Periodontal disease, unspecified**

● **K06**   **Other disorders of gingiva and edentulous alveolar ridge**
       Excludes2   acute gingivitis (K05.0)
                atrophy of edentulous alveolar ridge (K08.2)
                chronic gingivitis (K05.1)
                gingivitis NOS (K05.1)
     Coding Clinic: 2016, Q4, P29

● **K06.0**   **Gingival recession**
       Gingival recession (postinfective) (postprocedural)

●   **K06.01**   **Gingival recession, localized**

         K06.010   **Localized gingival recession,**
               unspecified
                 Localized gingival recession, NOS

         K06.011   **Localized gingival recession, minimal**

         K06.012   **Localized gingival recession,**
               moderate

         K06.013   **Localized gingival recession, severe**

●   **K06.02**   **Gingival recession, generalized**

         K06.020   **Generalized gingival recession,**
               unspecified
                 Generalized gingival recession, NOS

         K06.021   **Generalized gingival recession,**
               minimal

         K06.022   **Generalized gingival recession,**
               moderate

         K06.023   **Generalized gingival recession,**
               severe

  K06.1   **Gingival enlargement**
       Gingival fibromatosis

  K06.2   **Gingival and edentulous alveolar ridge lesions**
       associated with trauma
       Irritative hyperplasia of edentulous ridge [denture
         hyperplasia]
       Use additional code (Chapter 20) to identify external
         cause or denture status (Z97.2)

  K06.3   **Horizontal alveolar bone loss**

  K06.8   **Other specified disorders of gingiva and edentulous**
       alveolar ridge
       Fibrous epulis
       Flabby alveolar ridge
       Giant cell epulis
       Peripheral giant cell granuloma of gingiva
       Pyogenic granuloma of gingiva
       Vertical ridge deficiency
       Excludes2   gingival cyst (K09.0)

  K06.9   **Disorder of gingiva and edentulous alveolar ridge,**
       unspecified

● **K08**   **Other disorders of teeth and supporting structures**
       Excludes2   dentofacial anomalies [including malocclusion]
                (M26.-)
                disorders of jaw (M27.-)
     Coding Clinic: 2016, Q4, P29

  K08.0   **Exfoliation of teeth due to systemic causes**
       Code also underlying systemic condition

● **K08.1**   **Complete loss of teeth**
    Acquired loss of teeth, complete
    Excludes1   congenital absence of teeth (K00.0)
                exfoliation of teeth due to systemic causes
                   (K08.0)
                partial loss of teeth (K08.4-)

   ● **K08.10**   Complete loss of teeth, unspecified cause
      K08.101   Complete loss of teeth, unspecified cause, class I
      K08.102   Complete loss of teeth, unspecified cause, class II
      K08.103   Complete loss of teeth, unspecified cause, class III
      K08.104   Complete loss of teeth, unspecified cause, class IV
      K08.109   Complete loss of teeth, unspecified cause, unspecified class
            Edentulism NOS

   ● **K08.11**   Complete loss of teeth due to trauma
      K08.111   Complete loss of teeth due to trauma, class I
      K08.112   Complete loss of teeth due to trauma, class II
      K08.113   Complete loss of teeth due to trauma, class III
      K08.114   Complete loss of teeth due to trauma, class IV
      K08.119   Complete loss of teeth due to trauma, unspecified class

   ● **K08.12**   Complete loss of teeth due to periodontal diseases
      K08.121   Complete loss of teeth due to periodontal diseases, class I
      K08.122   Complete loss of teeth due to periodontal diseases, class II
      K08.123   Complete loss of teeth due to periodontal diseases, class III
      K08.124   Complete loss of teeth due to periodontal diseases, class IV
      K08.129   Complete loss of teeth due to periodontal diseases, unspecified class

   ● **K08.13**   Complete loss of teeth due to caries
      K08.131   Complete loss of teeth due to caries, class I
      K08.132   Complete loss of teeth due to caries, class II
      K08.133   Complete loss of teeth due to caries, class III
      K08.134   Complete loss of teeth due to caries, class IV
      K08.139   Complete loss of teeth due to caries, unspecified class

   ● **K08.19**   Complete loss of teeth due to other specified cause
      K08.191   Complete loss of teeth due to other specified cause, class I
      K08.192   Complete loss of teeth due to other specified cause, class II
      K08.193   Complete loss of teeth due to other specified cause, class III
      K08.194   Complete loss of teeth due to other specified cause, class IV
      K08.199   Complete loss of teeth due to other specified cause, unspecified class

● **K08.2**   **Atrophy of edentulous alveolar ridge**
    K08.20   Unspecified atrophy of edentulous alveolar ridge
            Atrophy of the mandible NOS
            Atrophy of the maxilla NOS
    K08.21   Minimal atrophy of the mandible
            Minimal atrophy of the edentulous mandible

    K08.22   Moderate atrophy of the mandible
            Moderate atrophy of the edentulous mandible
    K08.23   Severe atrophy of the mandible
            Severe atrophy of the edentulous mandible
    K08.24   Minimal atrophy of maxilla
            Minimal atrophy of the edentulous maxilla
    K08.25   Moderate atrophy of the maxilla
            Moderate atrophy of the edentulous maxilla
    K08.26   Severe atrophy of the maxilla
            Severe atrophy of the edentulous maxilla

  K08.3   **Retained dental root**

● **K08.4**   **Partial loss of teeth**
    Acquired loss of teeth, partial
    Excludes1   complete loss of teeth (K08.1-)
                congenital absence of teeth (K00.0)
    Excludes2   exfoliation of teeth due to systemic causes
                (K08.0)

   ● **K08.40**   Partial loss of teeth, unspecified cause
      K08.401   Partial loss of teeth, unspecified cause, class I
      K08.402   Partial loss of teeth, unspecified cause, class II
      K08.403   Partial loss of teeth, unspecified cause, class III
      K08.404   Partial loss of teeth, unspecified cause, class IV
      K08.409   Partial loss of teeth, unspecified cause, unspecified class
            Tooth extraction status NOS

   ● **K08.41**   Partial loss of teeth due to trauma
      K08.411   Partial loss of teeth due to trauma, class I
      K08.412   Partial loss of teeth due to trauma, class II
      K08.413   Partial loss of teeth due to trauma, class III
      K08.414   Partial loss of teeth due to trauma, class IV
      K08.419   Partial loss of teeth due to trauma, unspecified class

   ● **K08.42**   Partial loss of teeth due to periodontal diseases
      K08.421   Partial loss of teeth due to periodontal diseases, class I
      K08.422   Partial loss of teeth due to periodontal diseases, class II
      K08.423   Partial loss of teeth due to periodontal diseases, class III
      K08.424   Partial loss of teeth due to periodontal diseases, class IV
      K08.429   Partial loss of teeth due to periodontal diseases, unspecified class

   ● **K08.43**   Partial loss of teeth due to caries
      K08.431   Partial loss of teeth due to caries, class I
      K08.432   Partial loss of teeth due to caries, class II
      K08.433   Partial loss of teeth due to caries, class III
      K08.434   Partial loss of teeth due to caries, class IV
      K08.439   Partial loss of teeth due to caries, unspecified class

   ● **K08.49**   Partial loss of teeth due to other specified cause
      K08.491   Partial loss of teeth due to other specified cause, class I
      K08.492   Partial loss of teeth due to other specified cause, class II
      K08.493   Partial loss of teeth due to other specified cause, class III

▶ New   ➡ Revised   ~~deleted~~ Deleted   Excludes 1   Excludes 2   Includes   Use additional   Code first   Code also   Key words
OGCR Official Guidelines   X Assign placeholder X   ● Use Additional Character(s)   ▷ Manifestation Code   🔖 Hierarchical Condition Category   **Coding Clinic**

K08.494   Partial loss of teeth due to other specified cause, class IV

K08.499   Partial loss of teeth due to other specified cause, unspecified class

● **K08.5**   **Unsatisfactory restoration of tooth**
Defective bridge, crown, filling
Defective dental restoration

> **Excludes1**   dental restoration status (Z98.811)
>
> **Excludes2**   endosseous dental implant failure (M27.6-)
> unsatisfactory endodontic treatment (M27.5-)

K08.50   **Unsatisfactory restoration of tooth, unspecified**
Defective dental restoration NOS

K08.51   **Open restoration margins of tooth**
Dental restoration failure of marginal integrity
Open margin on tooth restoration
Poor gingival margin to tooth restoration

K08.52   **Unrepairable overhanging of dental restorative materials**
Overhanging of tooth restoration

● **K08.53**   **Fractured dental restorative material**

> **Excludes1**   cracked tooth (K03.81)
> traumatic fracture of tooth (S02.5)

K08.530   **Fractured dental restorative material without loss of material**

K08.531   **Fractured dental restorative material with loss of material**

K08.539   **Fractured dental restorative material, unspecified**

K08.54   **Contour of existing restoration of tooth biologically incompatible with oral health**
Dental restoration failure of periodontal anatomical integrity
Unacceptable contours of existing restoration of tooth
Unacceptable morphology of existing restoration of tooth

K08.55   **Allergy to existing dental restorative material**
Use additional code to identify the specific type of allergy

K08.56   **Poor aesthetic of existing restoration of tooth**
Dental restoration aesthetically inadequate or displeasing

K08.59   **Other unsatisfactory restoration of tooth**
Other defective dental restoration

● **K08.8**   **Other specified disorders of teeth and supporting structures**

K08.81   **Primary occlusal trauma**

K08.82   **Secondary occlusal trauma**

K08.89   **Other specified disorders of teeth and supporting structures**
Enlargement of alveolar ridge NOS
Insufficient anatomic crown height
Insufficient clinical crown length
Irregular alveolar process
Toothache NOS

K08.9   **Disorder of teeth and supporting structures, unspecified**

● **K09**   **Cysts of oral region, not elsewhere classified**

> **Includes**   lesions showing histological features both of aneurysmal cyst and of another fibro-osseous lesion
>
> **Excludes2**   cysts of jaw (M27.0-, M27.4-)
> radicular cyst (K04.8)

K09.0   **Developmental odontogenic cysts**
Dentigerous cyst
Eruption cyst
Follicular cyst
Gingival cyst
Lateral periodontal cyst
Primordial cyst

> **Excludes2**   keratocysts (D16.4, D16.5)
> odontogenic keratocystic tumors (D16.4, D16.5)

K09.1   **Developmental (nonodontogenic) cysts of oral region**
Cyst (of) incisive canal
Cyst (of) palatine of papilla
Globulomaxillary cyst
Median palatal cyst
Nasoalveolar cyst
Nasolabial cyst
Nasopalatine duct cyst

K09.8   **Other cysts of oral region, not elsewhere classified**
Dermoid cyst
Epidermoid cyst
Lymphoepithelial cyst
Epstein's pearl

K09.9   **Cyst of oral region, unspecified**

★ **(See Plate 28 of the Anatomy Illustrations.)**

● **K11**   **Diseases of salivary glands**
Use additional code to identify:
alcohol abuse and dependence (F10.-)
exposure to environmental tobacco smoke (Z77.22)
exposure to tobacco smoke in the perinatal period (P96.81)
history of tobacco dependence (Z87.891)
occupational exposure to environmental tobacco smoke (Z57.31)
tobacco dependence (F17.-)
tobacco use (Z72.0)

K11.0   **Atrophy of salivary gland**

K11.1   **Hypertrophy of salivary gland**

● **K11.2**   **Sialoadenitis**
Parotitis

> **Excludes1**   epidemic parotitis (B26.-)
> mumps (B26.-)
> uveoparotid fever [Heerfordt] (D86.89)

K11.20   **Sialoadenitis, unspecified**

K11.21   **Acute sialoadenitis**

> **Excludes1**   acute recurrent sialoadenitis (K11.22)

K11.22   **Acute recurrent sialoadenitis**

K11.23   **Chronic sialoadenitis**

K11.3   **Abscess of salivary gland**

K11.4   **Fistula of salivary gland**

> **Excludes1**   congenital fistula of salivary gland (Q38.4)

K11.5   **Sialolithiasis**
Calculus of salivary gland or duct
Stone of salivary gland or duct

K11.6   **Mucocele of salivary gland**
Mucous extravasation cyst of salivary gland
Mucous retention cyst of salivary gland
Ranula

K11.7   **Disturbances of salivary secretion**
Hypoptyalism
Ptyalism
Xerostomia

> **Excludes2**   dry mouth NOS (R68.2)

Figure 11-3   Major salivary glands.

Parotid gland
Sublingual gland
Submandibular gland

Item 11–4   **Atrophy** is wasting away of a tissue or organ, whereas **hypertrophy** is overdevelopment or enlargement of a tissue or organ. **Sialoadenitis** is salivary gland inflammation. **Parotitis** is the inflammation of the parotid gland. In the epidemic form, parotitis is also known as mumps. **Sialolithiasis** is the formation of calculus within a salivary gland. **Mucocele** is a polyp composed of mucus.

CHAPTER 11 (K00-K95)

K11.8   Other diseases of salivary glands
Benign lymphoepithelial lesion of salivary gland
Mikulicz' disease
Necrotizing sialometaplasia
Sialectasia
Stenosis of salivary duct
Stricture of salivary duct
> **Excludes1**   Sjögren syndrome (M35.0-)

K11.9   Disease of salivary gland, unspecified
Sialoadenopathy NOS

● **K12   Stomatitis and related lesions**
Use additional code to identify:
alcohol abuse and dependence (F10.-)
exposure to environmental tobacco smoke (Z77.22)
exposure to tobacco smoke in the perinatal period (P96.81)
history of tobacco dependence (Z87.891)
occupational exposure to environmental tobacco smoke (Z57.31)
tobacco dependence (F17.-)
tobacco use (Z72.0)
> **Excludes1**   cancrum oris (A69.0)
> cheilitis (K13.0)
> gangrenous stomatitis (A69.0)
> herpesviral [herpes simplex] gingivostomatitis (B00.2)
> noma (A69.0)

K12.0   Recurrent oral aphthae
Aphthous stomatitis (major) (minor)
Bednar's aphthae
Periadenitis mucosa necrotica recurrens
Recurrent aphthous ulcer
Stomatitis herpetiformis

K12.1   Other forms of stomatitis
Stomatitis NOS
Denture stomatitis
Ulcerative stomatitis
Vesicular stomatitis
> **Excludes1**   acute necrotizing ulcerative stomatitis (A69.1)
> Vincent's stomatitis (A69.1)

Item 11–5   Stomatitis is the inflammation of the oral mucosa. **Mucositis** is the inflammation of the mucous membranes lining the digestive tract from the mouth to the anus. It is a common side effect of chemotherapy and of radiotherapy that involves any part of the digestive tract.

K12.2   Cellulitis and abscess of mouth
Cellulitis of mouth (floor)
Submandibular abscess
> **Excludes2**   abscess of salivary gland (K11.3)
> abscess of tongue (K14.0)
> periapical abscess (K04.6-K04.7)
> periodontal abscess (K05.21)
> peritonsillar abscess (J36)

● **K12.3   Oral mucositis (ulcerative)**
Mucositis (oral) (oropharyneal)
> **Excludes2**   gastrointestinal mucositis (ulcerative) (K92.81)
> mucositis (ulcerative) of vagina and vulva (N76.81)
> nasal mucositis (ulcerative) (J34.81)

K12.30   Oral mucositis (ulcerative), unspecified

K12.31   Oral mucositis (ulcerative) due to antineoplastic therapy
Use additional code for adverse effect, if applicable, to identify antineoplastic and immunosuppressive drugs (T45.1X5)
Use additional code for other antineoplastic therapy, such as:
radiological procedure and radiotherapy (Y84.2)

K12.32   Oral mucositis (ulcerative) due to other drugs
Use additional code for adverse effect, if applicable, to identify drug (T36-T50 with fifth or sixth character 5)

K12.33   Oral mucositis (ulcerative) due to radiation
Use additional external cause code (W88-W90, X39.0-) to identify cause

K12.39   Other oral mucositis (ulcerative)
Viral oral mucositis (ulcerative)

● **K13   Other diseases of lip and oral mucosa**
Includes   epithelial disturbances of tongue
Use additional code to identify:
alcohol abuse and dependence (F10.-)
exposure to environmental tobacco smoke (Z77.22)
exposure to tobacco smoke in the perinatal period (P96.81)
history of tobacco dependence (Z87.891)
occupational exposure to environmental tobacco smoke (Z57.31)
tobacco dependence (F17.-)
tobacco use (Z72.0)
> **Excludes2**   certain disorders of gingiva and edentulous alveolar ridge (K05-K06)
> cysts of oral region (K09.-)
> diseases of tongue (K14.-)
> stomatitis and related lesions (K12.-)

K13.0   Diseases of lips

Abscess of lips	Exfoliative cheilitis
Angular cheilitis	Fistula of lips
Cellulitis of lips	Glandular cheilitis
Cheilitis NOS	Hypertrophy of lips
Cheilodynia	Perlèche NEC
Cheilosis	

> **Excludes1**   ariboflavinosis (E53.0)
> cheilitis due to radiation-related disorders (L55-L59)
> congenital fistula of lips (Q38.0)
> congenital hypertrophy of lips (Q18.6)
> Perlèche due to candidiasis (B37.83)
> Perlèche due to riboflavin deficiency (E53.0)

K13.1   Cheek and lip biting

● **K13.2   Leukoplakia and other disturbances of oral epithelium, including tongue**
> **Excludes1**   carcinoma in situ of oral epithelium (D00.0-)
> hairy leukoplakia (K13.3)

K13.21   Leukoplakia of oral mucosa, including tongue
Considered precancerous and evidenced by thickened white patches of epithelium on mucous membranes
Leukokeratosis of oral mucosa
Leukoplakia of gingiva, lips, tongue
> **Excludes1**   hairy leukoplakia (K13.3)
> leukokeratosis nicotina palati (K13.24)

K13.22   Minimal keratinized residual ridge mucosa
Minimal keratinization of alveolar ridge mucosa

K13.23   Excessive keratinized residual ridge mucosa
Excessive keratinization of alveolar ridge mucosa

K13.24   Leukokeratosis nicotina palati
Smoker's palate

K13.29   Other disturbances of oral epithelium, including tongue
Erythroplakia of mouth or tongue
Focal epithelial hyperplasia of mouth or tongue
Leukoedema of mouth or tongue
Other oral epithelium disturbances

Figure 11-4   Oral leukoplakia and associated. (From Swartz MH: Textbook of Physical Diagnosis: History and Examination, Philadelphia, PA, Saunders/Elsevier, 2010)

▶ New   ⇒ Revised   ~~deleted~~ Deleted   Excludes 1   Excludes 2   Includes   Use additional   Code first   Code also   Key words

OGCR Official Guidelines   X Assign placeholder X   ● Use Additional Character(s)   ▶ Manifestation Code   🦔 Hierarchical Condition Category   **Coding Clinic**

K13.3   Hairy leukoplakia

K13.4   Granuloma and granuloma-like lesions of oral mucosa
Eosinophilic granuloma
Granuloma pyogenicum
Verrucous xanthoma

K13.5   Oral submucous fibrosis
Submucous fibrosis of tongue

K13.6   Irritative hyperplasia of oral mucosa
Excludes2   irritative hyperplasia of edentulous ridge [denture hyperplasia] (K06.2)

● **K13.7   Other and unspecified lesions of oral mucosa**

K13.70   Unspecified lesions of oral mucosa

K13.79   Other lesions of oral mucosa
Focal oral mucinosis

★ **(See Plate 26 of the Anatomy Illustrations.)**

● **K14   Diseases of tongue**
Use additional code to identify:
alcohol abuse and dependence (F10.-)
exposure to environmental tobacco smoke (Z77.22)
history of tobacco dependence (Z87.891)
occupational exposure to environmental tobacco smoke (Z57.31)
tobacco dependence (F17.-)
tobacco use (Z72.0)

Excludes2   erythroplakia (K13.29)
focal epithelial hyperplasia (K13.29)
leukedema of tongue (K13.29)
leukoplakia of tongue (K13.21)
hairy leukoplakia (K13.3)
macroglossia (congenital) (Q38.2)
submucous fibrosis of tongue (K13.5)

K14.0   Glossitis
Abscess of tongue
Ulceration (traumatic) of tongue
Excludes1   atrophic glossitis (K14.4)

K14.1   Geographic tongue
Benign migratory glossitis
Glossitis areata exfoliativa

K14.2   Median rhomboid glossitis

K14.3   Hypertrophy of tongue papillae
Black hairy tongue
Coated tongue
Hypertrophy of foliate papillae
Lingua villosa nigra

K14.4   Atrophy of tongue papillae
Atrophic glossitis

K14.5   Plicated tongue
Fissured tongue   Scrotal tongue
Furrowed tongue
Excludes1   fissured tongue, congenital (Q38.3)

K14.6   Glossodynia
Glossopyrosis   Painful tongue
Glossopathy NOS

K14.8   Other diseases of tongue
Atrophy of tongue   Glossocele
Crenated tongue   Glossoptosis
Enlargement of tongue   Hypertrophy of tongue

K14.9   Disease of tongue, unspecified

DISEASES OF ESOPHAGUS, STOMACH AND DUODENUM (K20–K31)

Excludes2   hiatus hernia (K44.-)

● **K20   Esophagitis**
Use additional code to identify:
alcohol abuse and dependence (F10.-)
Excludes1   erosion of esophagus (K22.1-)
esophagitis with gastro-esophageal reflux disease (K21.0-)
reflux esophagitis (K21.0-)
ulcerative esophagitis (K22.1-)
Excludes2   eosinophilic gastritis or gastroenteritis (K52.81)

K20.0   Eosinophilic esophagitis

● **K20.8   Other esophagitis**

K20.80   Other esophagitis without bleeding
Abscess of esophagus
Other esophagitis NOS

K20.81   Other esophagitis with bleeding

● **K20.9   Esophagitis, unspecified**

K20.90   Esophagitis, unspecified without bleeding
Esophagitis NOS

K20.91   Esophagitis, unspecified with bleeding

● **K21   Gastro-esophageal reflux disease**
Excludes1   newborn esophageal reflux (P78.83)

● **K21.0   Gastro-esophageal reflux disease with esophagitis**

K21.00   Gastro-esophageal reflux disease with esophagitis, without bleeding
Reflux esophagitis

K21.01   Gastro-esophageal reflux disease with esophagitis, with bleeding

K21.9   Gastro-esophageal reflux disease without esophagitis
Esophageal reflux NOS
Coding Clinic: 2016, Q1, P18

● **K22   Other diseases of esophagus**
Excludes2   esophageal varices (I85.-)

K22.0   Achalasia of cardia
Achalasia NOS
Cardiospasm
Excludes1   congenital cardiospasm (Q39.5)

● **K22.1   Ulcer of esophagus**
Barrett's ulcer
Erosion of esophagus
Fungal ulcer of esophagus
Peptic ulcer of esophagus
Ulcer of esophagus due to ingestion of chemicals
Ulcer of esophagus due to ingestion of drugs and medicaments
Ulcerative esophagitis
Code first poisoning due to drug or toxin, if applicable (T36-T65 with fifth or sixth character 1-4 or 6)
Use additional code for adverse effect, if applicable, to identify drug (T36-T50 with fifth or sixth character 5)
Excludes1   Barrett's esophagus (K22.87-)

K22.10   Ulcer of esophagus without bleeding
Ulcer of esophagus NOS

K22.11   Ulcer of esophagus with bleeding
Excludes2   bleeding esophageal varices (I85.01, I85.11)

Item 11–6   Esophageal reflux is the return flow of the contents of the stomach to the esophagus and is referred to as GERD and/or "heartburn." **Gastroesophageal reflux** is the return flow of the contents of the stomach and duodenum to the esophagus. **Esophageal leukoplakia** are white areas on the mucous membrane of the esophagus for which no specific cause can be identified.

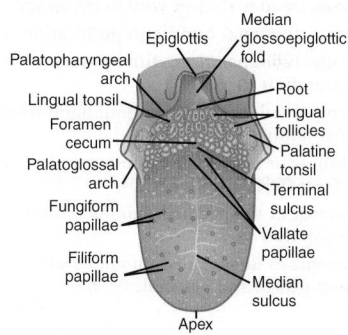

Figure 11-5   Structure of the tongue.

CHAPTER 11 (K00-K95)

K22.2   **Esophageal obstruction**
Compression of esophagus
Constriction of esophagus
Stenosis of esophagus
Stricture of esophagus
> **Excludes1**   congenital stenosis or stricture of esophagus (Q39.3)

K22.3   **Perforation of esophagus**
Rupture of esophagus
> **Excludes1**   traumatic perforation of (thoracic) esophagus (S27.8-)

K22.4   **Dyskinesia of esophagus**
Difficulty in moving
Corkscrew esophagus
Diffuse esophageal spasm
Spasm of esophagus
> **Excludes1**   cardiospasm (K22.0)

K22.5   **Diverticulum of esophagus, acquired**
Esophageal pouch, acquired
> **Excludes1**   diverticulum of esophagus (congenital) (Q39.6)

K22.6   **Gastro-esophageal laceration-hemorrhage syndrome**
Mallory-Weiss syndrome

● **K22.7**   **Barrett's esophagus**
Barrett's disease
Barrett's syndrome
> **Excludes1**   Barrett's ulcer (K22.1)
>   malignant neoplasm of esophagus (C15.-)

    K22.70   **Barrett's esophagus without dysplasia**
        Barrett's esophagus NOS

  ● **K22.71**   **Barrett's esophagus with dysplasia**
        K22.710   **Barrett's esophagus with low grade dysplasia**
        K22.711   **Barrett's esophagus with high grade dysplasia**
        K22.719   **Barrett's esophagus with dysplasia, unspecified**

● **K22.8**   **Other specified diseases of esophagus**
~~Hemorrhage of esophagus NOS~~

  ▶**K22.81**   **Esophageal polyp**
  ▶ **Excludes1**   benign neoplasm of esophagus (D13.0)

  ▶**K22.82** **Esophagogastric junction polyp**
  ▶ **Excludes1**   benign neoplasm of stomach (D13.1)

  ▶**K22.89**   **Other specified disease of esophagus**
        ▶Hemorrhage of esophagus NOS
> **Excludes2**   esophageal varices (I85.-)
>   Paterson-Kelly syndrome (D50.1)
> **Coding Clinic: 2020, Q1, P16**

K22.9   **Disease of esophagus, unspecified**

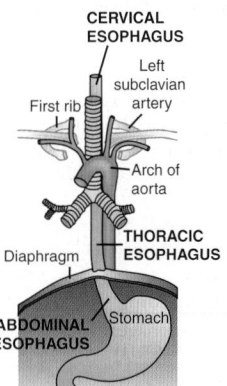

CERVICAL
ESOPHAGUS
Left subclavian artery
First rib
Arch of aorta
THORACIC ESOPHAGUS
Diaphragm
ABDOMINAL ESOPHAGUS
Stomach

Figure 11-6   The esophagus is the muscular tube that connects the pharynx and the stomach. The 10-inch (25 cm) long esophagus is divided into three parts: **cervical, thoracic,** and **abdominal.**

Item 11–7 **Achalasia** is a condition in which the smooth muscle fibers of the esophagus do not relax. Most frequently, this condition occurs at the esophagogastric sphincter. **Cardiospasm,** also known as **megaesophagus,** is achalasia of the thoracic esophagus.

Item 11–8 **Gastric ulcers** are lesions of the stomach that result in the death of the tissue and a defect of the surface. **Perforated ulcers** are those in which the lesion penetrates the gastric wall, leaving a hole. **Peptic ulcers** are lesions of the stomach or the duodenum. **Peptic** refers to the gastric juice, pepsin.

A   B   C

Figure 11-7 **A.** Ulcer. **B.** Perforated ulcer. **C.** Laparoscopic view of a perforated duodenal ulcer *(arrow)* with fibrinous exudate on the adjacent peritoneum. (**C** from Feldman: Sleisenger & Fordtran's Gastrointestinal and Liver Disease, ed 8, Saunders, An Imprint of Elsevier, 2006)

▶ **K23**   ***Disorders of esophagus in diseases classified elsewhere***
> *Code first* underlying disease, such as:
> congenital syphilis (A50.5)
> **Excludes1**   late syphilis (A52.79)
>   megaesophagus due to Chagas' disease (B57.31)
>
>   tuberculosis (A18.83)

● **K25**   **Gastric ulcer**
> **Includes**   erosion (acute) of stomach
>   pylorus ulcer (peptic)
>   stomach ulcer (peptic)
>
> Use additional code to identify:
> alcohol abuse and dependence (F10.-)
> **Excludes1**   acute gastritis (K29.0-)
>   peptic ulcer NOS (K27.-)

  K25.0   **Acute gastric ulcer with hemorrhage**
  K25.1   **Acute gastric ulcer with perforation** 🏷
  K25.2   **Acute gastric ulcer with both hemorrhage and perforation** 🏷
  K25.3   **Acute gastric ulcer without hemorrhage or perforation**
  K25.4   **Chronic or unspecified gastric ulcer with hemorrhage**
        Coding Clinic: 2017, Q3, P27
  K25.5   **Chronic or unspecified gastric ulcer with perforation** 🏷
  K25.6   **Chronic or unspecified gastric ulcer with both hemorrhage and perforation** 🏷
  K25.7   **Chronic gastric ulcer without hemorrhage or perforation**
  K25.9   **Gastric ulcer, unspecified as acute or chronic, without hemorrhage or perforation**
        Coding Clinic: 2021, Q1, P12

● **K26**   **Duodenal ulcer**
> **Includes**   erosion (acute) of duodenum
>   duodenum ulcer (peptic)
>   postpyloric ulcer (peptic)
>
> Use additional code to identify:
> alcohol abuse and dependence (F10.-)
> **Excludes1**   peptic ulcer NOS (K27.-)

  K26.0   **Acute duodenal ulcer with hemorrhage**
  K26.1   **Acute duodenal ulcer with perforation** 🏷
  K26.2   **Acute duodenal ulcer with both hemorrhage and perforation** 🏷
  K26.3   **Acute duodenal ulcer without hemorrhage or perforation**
  K26.4   **Chronic or unspecified duodenal ulcer with hemorrhage**
        Coding Clinic: 2016, Q1, P14
  K26.5   **Chronic or unspecified duodenal ulcer with perforation** 🏷
  K26.6   **Chronic or unspecified duodenal ulcer with both hemorrhage and perforation** 🏷

▶ New   ⇒ Revised   ~~deleted~~ Deleted   Excludes 1   Excludes 2   Includes   Use additional   Code first   Code also   Key words
OGCR Official Guidelines   X Assign placeholder X   ● Use Additional Character(s)   ▶ Manifestation Code   🏷 Hierarchical Condition Category   **Coding Clinic**

K26.7   Chronic duodenal ulcer without hemorrhage or perforation

K26.9   Duodenal ulcer, unspecified as acute or chronic, without hemorrhage or perforation

● **K27**   **Peptic ulcer, site unspecified**

> **Includes**   gastroduodenal ulcer NOS
> peptic ulcer NOS

> Use additional code to identify:
> alcohol abuse and dependence (F10.-)

> **Excludes1**   peptic ulcer of newborn (P78.82)

K27.0   Acute peptic ulcer, site unspecified, with hemorrhage

K27.1   Acute peptic ulcer, site unspecified, with perforation 🔗

K27.2   Acute peptic ulcer, site unspecified, with both hemorrhage and perforation 🔗

K27.3   Acute peptic ulcer, site unspecified, without hemorrhage or perforation

K27.4   Chronic or unspecified peptic ulcer, site unspecified, with hemorrhage

K27.5   Chronic or unspecified peptic ulcer, site unspecified, with perforation 🔗

K27.6   Chronic or unspecified peptic ulcer, site unspecified, with both hemorrhage and perforation 🔗

K27.7   Chronic peptic ulcer, site unspecified, without hemorrhage or perforation

K27.9   Peptic ulcer, site unspecified, unspecified as acute or chronic, without hemorrhage or perforation

● **K28**   **Gastrojejunal ulcer**

> **Includes**   anastomotic ulcer (peptic) or erosion
> gastrocolic ulcer (peptic) or erosion
> gastrointestinal ulcer (peptic) or erosion
> gastrojejunal ulcer (peptic) or erosion
> jejunal ulcer (peptic) or erosion
> marginal ulcer (peptic) or erosion
> stomal ulcer (peptic) or erosion

> Use additional code to identify:
> alcohol abuse and dependence (F10.-)

> **Excludes1**   primary ulcer of small intestine (K63.3)

K28.0   Acute gastrojejunal ulcer with hemorrhage

K28.1   Acute gastrojejunal ulcer with perforation 🔗

K28.2   Acute gastrojejunal ulcer with both hemorrhage and perforation 🔗

K28.3   Acute gastrojejunal ulcer without hemorrhage or perforation

K28.4   Chronic or unspecified gastrojejunal ulcer with hemorrhage

K28.5   Chronic or unspecified gastrojejunal ulcer with perforation 🔗

K28.6   Chronic or unspecified gastrojejunal ulcer with both hemorrhage and perforation 🔗

K28.7   Chronic gastrojejunal ulcer without hemorrhage or perforation

K28.9   Gastrojejunal ulcer, unspecified as acute or chronic, without hemorrhage or perforation

● **K29**   **Gastritis and duodenitis**

> **Excludes1**   eosinophilic gastritis or gastroenteritis (K52.81)
> Zollinger-Ellison syndrome (E16.4)

● **K29.0**   Acute gastritis

> Use additional code to identify:
> alcohol abuse and dependence (F10.-)

> **Excludes1**   erosion (acute) of stomach (K25.-)

K29.00   Acute gastritis without bleeding

K29.01   Acute gastritis with bleeding

Item 11–9   **Gastritis** is a severe inflammation of the stomach. **Atrophic gastritis** is a chronic inflammation of the stomach that results in destruction of the cells of the mucosa of the stomach. Duodenitis is an inflammation of the duodenum, the first section of the small intestine.

● **K29.2**   Alcoholic gastritis

> Use additional code to identify:
> alcohol abuse and dependence (F10.-)

K29.20   Alcoholic gastritis without bleeding

K29.21   Alcoholic gastritis with bleeding

● **K29.3**   Chronic superficial gastritis

K29.30   Chronic superficial gastritis without bleeding

K29.31   Chronic superficial gastritis with bleeding

● **K29.4**   Chronic atrophic gastritis

> Gastric atrophy

K29.40   Chronic atrophic gastritis without bleeding

K29.41   Chronic atrophic gastritis with bleeding

● **K29.5**   Unspecified chronic gastritis

> Chronic antral gastritis
> Chronic fundal gastritis

K29.50   Unspecified chronic gastritis without bleeding

K29.51   Unspecified chronic gastritis with bleeding

● **K29.6**   Other gastritis

> Giant hypertrophic gastritis
> Granulomatous gastritis
> Ménétrier's disease

K29.60   Other gastritis without bleeding

K29.61   Other gastritis with bleeding

● **K29.7**   Gastritis, unspecified

K29.70   Gastritis, unspecified, without bleeding

K29.71   Gastritis, unspecified, with bleeding

● **K29.8**   Duodenitis

K29.80   Duodenitis without bleeding

K29.81   Duodenitis with bleeding

● **K29.9**   Gastroduodenitis, unspecified

K29.90   Gastroduodenitis, unspecified, without bleeding

K29.91   Gastroduodenitis, unspecified, with bleeding

K30   **Functional dyspepsia**

> Indigestion

> **Excludes1**   dyspepsia NOS (R10.13)
> heartburn (R12)
> nervous dyspepsia (F45.8)
> neurotic dyspepsia (F45.8)
> psychogenic dyspepsia (F45.8)

● **K31**   **Other diseases of stomach and duodenum**

> Includes   functional disorders of stomach

> **Excludes2**   diabetic gastroparesis (E08.43, E09.43, E10.43, E11.43, E13.43)
> diverticulum of duodenum (K57.00-K57.13)

K31.0   Acute dilatation of stomach

> Acute distention of stomach

K31.1   Adult hypertrophic pyloric stenosis   A

> Pyloric stenosis NOS

> **Excludes1**   congenital or infantile pyloric stenosis (Q40.0)

K31.2   Hourglass stricture and stenosis of stomach

> **Excludes1**   congenital hourglass stomach (Q40.2)
> hourglass contraction of stomach (K31.89)

K31.3   Pylorospasm, not elsewhere classified

> **Excludes1**   congenital or infantile pylorospasm (Q40.0)
> neurotic pylorospasm (F45.8)
> psychogenic pylorospasm (F45.8)

K31.4   Gastric diverticulum

> **Excludes1**   congenital diverticulum of stomach (Q40.2)

K31.5   **Obstruction of duodenum**
            Constriction of duodenum
            Duodenal ileus (chronic)
            Stenosis of duodenum
                Narrowing
            Stricture of duodenum
                Narrowing
            Volvulus of duodenum
                Twisting/knotting
            Excludes1   congenital stenosis of duodenum (Q41.0)

K31.6   **Fistula of stomach and duodenum**
            Gastrocolic fistula
            Gastrojejunocolic fistula

Item 11–10 Achlorhydria, also known as gastric anacidity, is the absence of gastric acid.

K31.7   **Polyp of stomach and duodenum**
            Excludes1   adenomatous polyp of stomach (D13.1)
            Coding Clinic: 2020, Q1, P16

K31.8   **Other specified diseases of stomach and duodenum**
    K31.81   **Angiodysplasia of stomach and duodenum**
            K31.811   **Angiodysplasia of stomach and duodenum with bleeding**
            K31.819   **Angiodysplasia of stomach and duodenum without bleeding**
                    Angiodysplasia of stomach and duodenum NOS

    K31.82   **Dieulafoy lesion (hemorrhagic) of stomach and duodenum**
            Excludes2   Dieulafoy lesion of intestine (K63.81)

    K31.83   **Achlorhydria**

    K31.84   **Gastroparesis**
            Gastroparalysis
            Code first underlying disease, if known, such as:
                anorexia nervosa (F50.0-)
                diabetes mellitus (E08.43, E09.43, E10.43, E11.43, E13.43)
                scleroderma (M34.-)

    K31.89   **Other diseases of stomach and duodenum**
            Coding Clinic: 2020, Q1, P16; 2017, Q1, P28

K31.9   **Disease of stomach and duodenum, unspecified**

▶● K31.A   **Gastric intestinal metaplasia**
    ▶ K31.A0   **Gastric intestinal metaplasia, unspecified**
            ▶ Gastric intestinal metaplasia indefinite for dysplasia
            ▶ Gastric intestinal metaplasia NOS

    ▶● K31.A1   **Gastric intestinal metaplasia without dysplasia**
            ▶ K31.A11   **Gastric intestinal metaplasia without dysplasia, involving the antrum**
            ▶ K31.A12   **Gastric intestinal metaplasia without dysplasia, involving the body(corpus)**
            ▶ K31.A13   **Gastric intestinal metaplasia without dysplasia, involving the fundus involving the cardia**
            ▶ K31.A14   **Gastric intestinal metaplasia without dysplasia, involving the cardia**
            ▶ K31.A15   **Gastric intestinal metaplasia without dysplasia, involving multiple sites**
            ▶ K31.A19   **Gastric intestinal metaplasia without dysplasia, unspecified site**

    ▶● K31.A2   **Gastric intestinal metaplasia with dysplasia**
            ▶ K31.A21   **Gastric intestinal metaplasia with low grade dysplasia**
            ▶ K31.A22   **Gastric intestinal metaplasia with high grade dysplasia**
            ▶ K31.A29   **Gastric intestinal metaplasia with dysplasia, unspecified**

DISEASES OF APPENDIX (K35-K38)

● K35   **Acute appendicitis**
    ● K35.2   **Acute appendicitis with generalized peritonitis**
            Appendicitis (acute) with generalized (diffuse) peritonitis following rupture or perforation of appendix
            K35.20   **Acute appendicitis with generalized peritonitis, without abscess (Acute) appendicitis with generalized peritonitis NOS**
                    Coding Clinic: 2018, Q4, P18
            K35.21   **Acute appendicitis with generalized peritonitis, with abscess**

    ● K35.3   **Acute appendicitis with localized peritonitis**
            K35.30   **Acute appendicitis with localized peritonitis, without perforation or gangrene**
                    Acute appendicitis with localized peritonitis NOS
            K35.31   **Acute appendicitis with localized peritonitis and gangrene, without perforation**
            K35.32   **Acute appendicitis with perforation and localized peritonitis, without abscess**
                    (Acute) appendicitis with perforation NOS
                    Perforated appendix NOS
                    Ruptured appendix (with localized peritonitis) NOS
                    Coding Clinic: 2020, Q1, P16; 2018, Q4, P18
            K35.33   **Acute appendicitis with perforation and localized peritonitis, with abscess**
                    (Acute) appendicitis with (peritoneal) abscess NOS
                    Ruptured appendix with localized peritonitis and abscess

    ● K35.8   **Other and unspecified acute appendicitis**

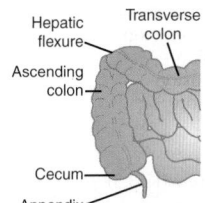

Figure 11-8 Acute appendicitis is the inflammation of the appendix, usually associated with obstruction. Most often this is a disease of adolescents and young adults.

            K35.80   **Unspecified acute appendicitis**
                    Acute appendicitis NOS
                    Acute appendicitis without (localized) (generalized) peritonitis
            ● K35.89   **Other acute appendicitis**
                    K35.890   **Other acute appendicitis without perforation or gangrene**
                    K35.891   **Other acute appendicitis without perforation, with gangrene**
                            (Acute) appendicitis with gangrene NOS

K36   **Other appendicitis**
        Chronic appendicitis
        Recurrent appendicitis

K37   **Unspecified appendicitis**
        Excludes1   unspecified appendicitis with peritonitis (K35.2-, K35.3)

● K38   **Other diseases of appendix**
    K38.0   **Hyperplasia of appendix**
    K38.1   **Appendicular concretions**
            Fecalith of appendix
            Stercolith of appendix
    K38.2   **Diverticulum of appendix**
    K38.3   **Fistula of appendix**
    K38.8   **Other specified diseases of appendix**
            Intussusception of appendix
    K38.9   **Disease of appendix, unspecified**

HERNIA (K40-K46)

Note: Hernia with both gangrene and obstruction is classified to hernia with gangrene.

Includes   acquired hernia
                congenital [except diaphragmatic or hiatus] hernia
                recurrent hernia

● **K40   Inguinal hernia**

Includes   bubonocele
                direct inguinal hernia
                double inguinal hernia
                indirect inguinal hernia
                inguinal hernia NOS
                oblique inguinal hernia
                scrotal hernia

● **K40.0   Bilateral inguinal hernia, with obstruction, without gangrene**

Inguinal hernia (bilateral) causing obstruction without gangrene
Incarcerated inguinal hernia (bilateral) without gangrene
Irreducible inguinal hernia (bilateral) without gangrene
Strangulated inguinal hernia (bilateral) without gangrene

K40.00   Bilateral inguinal hernia, with obstruction, without gangrene, not specified as recurrent
Bilateral inguinal hernia, with obstruction, without gangrene NOS

K40.01   Bilateral inguinal hernia, with obstruction, without gangrene, recurrent

● **K40.1   Bilateral inguinal hernia, with gangrene**

K40.10   Bilateral inguinal hernia, with gangrene, not specified as recurrent
Bilateral inguinal hernia, with gangrene NOS

K40.11   Bilateral inguinal hernia, with gangrene, recurrent

● **K40.2   Bilateral inguinal hernia, without obstruction or gangrene**

K40.20   Bilateral inguinal hernia, without obstruction or gangrene, not specified as recurrent
Bilateral inguinal hernia NOS

K40.21   Bilateral inguinal hernia, without obstruction or gangrene, recurrent

● **K40.3   Unilateral inguinal hernia, with obstruction, without gangrene**

Inguinal hernia (unilateral) causing obstruction without gangrene
Incarcerated inguinal hernia (unilateral) without gangrene
Irreducible inguinal hernia (unilateral) without gangrene
Strangulated inguinal hernia (unilateral) without gangrene

K40.30   Unilateral inguinal hernia, with obstruction, without gangrene, not specified as recurrent
Inguinal hernia, with obstruction NOS
Unilateral inguinal hernia, with obstruction, without gangrene NOS

K40.31   Unilateral inguinal hernia, with obstruction, without gangrene, recurrent

● **K40.4   Unilateral inguinal hernia, with gangrene**

K40.40   Unilateral inguinal hernia, with gangrene, not specified as recurrent
Inguinal hernia with gangrene NOS
Unilateral inguinal hernia with gangrene NOS

K40.41   Unilateral inguinal hernia, with gangrene, recurrent

● **K40.9   Unilateral inguinal hernia, without obstruction or gangrene**

K40.90   Unilateral inguinal hernia, without obstruction or gangrene, not specified as recurrent
Inguinal hernia NOS
Unilateral inguinal hernia NOS

K40.91   Unilateral inguinal hernia, without obstruction or gangrene, recurrent

● **K41   Femoral hernia**

● **K41.0   Bilateral femoral hernia, with obstruction, without gangrene**

Femoral hernia (bilateral) causing obstruction, without gangrene
Incarcerated femoral hernia (bilateral), without gangrene
Irreducible femoral hernia (bilateral), without gangrene
Strangulated femoral hernia (bilateral), without gangrene

K41.00   Bilateral femoral hernia, with obstruction, without gangrene, not specified as recurrent
Bilateral femoral hernia, with obstruction, without gangrene NOS

K41.01   Bilateral femoral hernia, with obstruction, without gangrene, recurrent

● **K41.1   Bilateral femoral hernia, with gangrene**

K41.10   Bilateral femoral hernia, with gangrene, not specified as recurrent
Bilateral femoral hernia, with gangrene NOS

K41.11   Bilateral femoral hernia, with gangrene, recurrent

● **K41.2   Bilateral femoral hernia, without obstruction or gangrene**

K41.20   Bilateral femoral hernia, without obstruction or gangrene, not specified as recurrent
Bilateral femoral hernia NOS

K41.21   Bilateral femoral hernia, without obstruction or gangrene, recurrent

Item 11-11   Hernias of the groin are the most common type, accounting for 80 percent of all hernias. There are two major types of inguinal hernias: indirect (oblique) affecting men only and direct. **Indirect inguinal hernias** result when the intestines emerge through the abdominal wall in an indirect fashion through the inguinal canal. **Direct inguinal hernias** penetrate through the abdominal wall in a direct fashion. **Femoral hernias** occur at the femoral ring where the femoral vessels enter the thigh and is most common in women. An abdominal wall hernia is also called a ventral or epigastric hernia and occurs in both sexes. Classification is based on location of the hernia and whether there is obstruction or gangrene.

Ventral, epigastric, or incisional hernia occurs on the abdominal surface caused by musculature weakness or a tear at a previous surgical site and is evidenced by a bulge that changes in size, becoming larger with exertion. An **incarcerated** hernia is one in which the intestines become trapped in the hernia. A **strangulated** hernia is one in which the blood supply to the intestines is lost. **Hiatal hernia** occurs when a loop of the stomach protrudes upward through the small opening in the diaphragm through which the esophagus passes, leaving the abdominal cavity and entering the chest. It occurs in both sexes.

Figure 11-9   Inguinal hernias are those that are located in the inguinal or iliac areas of the abdomen.

CHAPTER 11 (K00-K95)

● K41.3 **Unilateral femoral hernia, with obstruction, without gangrene**
Femoral hernia (unilateral) causing obstruction, without gangrene
Incarcerated femoral hernia (unilateral), without gangrene
Irreducible femoral hernia (unilateral), without gangrene
Strangulated femoral hernia (unilateral), without gangrene

  K41.30 **Unilateral femoral hernia, with obstruction, without gangrene, not specified as recurrent**
Femoral hernia, with obstruction NOS
Unilateral femoral hernia, with obstruction NOS

  K41.31 **Unilateral femoral hernia, with obstruction, without gangrene, recurrent**

● K41.4 **Unilateral femoral hernia, with gangrene**
  K41.40 **Unilateral femoral hernia, with gangrene, not specified as recurrent**
Femoral hernia, with gangrene NOS
Unilateral femoral hernia, with gangrene NOS

  K41.41 **Unilateral femoral hernia, with gangrene, recurrent**

● K41.9 **Unilateral femoral hernia, without obstruction or gangrene**
  K41.90 **Unilateral femoral hernia, without obstruction or gangrene, not specified as recurrent**
Femoral hernia NOS
Unilateral femoral hernia NOS

  K41.91 **Unilateral femoral hernia, without obstruction or gangrene, recurrent**

● K42 **Umbilical hernia**
  Includes paraumbilical hernia
  Excludes1 omphalocele (Q79.2)

  K42.0 **Umbilical hernia with obstruction, without gangrene**
Umbilical hernia causing obstruction, without gangrene
Incarcerated umbilical hernia, without gangrene
Irreducible umbilical hernia, without gangrene
Strangulated umbilical hernia, without gangrene

  K42.1 **Umbilical hernia with gangrene**
Gangrenous umbilical hernia

  K42.9 **Umbilical hernia without obstruction or gangrene**
Umbilical hernia NOS

● K43 **Ventral hernia**
  K43.0 **Incisional hernia with obstruction, without gangrene**
Incisional hernia causing obstruction, without gangrene
Incarcerated incisional hernia, without gangrene
Irreducible incisional hernia, without gangrene
Strangulated incisional hernia, without gangrene

  K43.1 **Incisional hernia with gangrene**
Gangrenous incisional hernia

  K43.2 **Incisional hernia without obstruction or gangrene**
Incisional hernia NOS

  K43.3 **Parastomal hernia with obstruction, without gangrene**
Incarcerated parastomal hernia, without gangrene
Irreducible parastomal hernia, without gangrene
Parastomal hernia causing obstruction, without gangrene
Strangulated parastomal hernia, without gangrene

  K43.4 **Parastomal hernia with gangrene**
Gangrenous parastomal hernia

  K43.5 **Parastomal hernia without obstruction or gangrene**
Parastomal hernia NOS

● K43.6 **Other and unspecified ventral hernia with obstruction, without gangrene**
Epigastric hernia causing obstruction, without gangrene
Hypogastric hernia causing obstruction, without gangrene
Incarcerated epigastric hernia without gangrene
Incarcerated hypogastric hernia without gangrene
Incarcerated midline hernia without gangrene
Incarcerated spigelian hernia without gangrene
Incarcerated subxiphoid hernia without gangrene
Irreducible epigastric hernia without gangrene
Irreducible hypogastric hernia without gangrene
Irreducible midline hernia without gangrene
Irreducible spigelian hernia without gangrene
Irreducible subxiphoid hernia without gangrene
Midline hernia causing obstruction, without gangrene
Spigelian hernia causing obstruction, without gangrene
Strangulated epigastric hernia without gangrene
Strangulated hypogastric hernia without gangrene
Strangulated midline hernia without gangrene
Strangulated spigelian hernia without gangrene
Strangulated subxiphoid hernia without gangrene
Subxiphoid hernia causing obstruction, without gangrene

● K43.7 **Other and unspecified ventral hernia with gangrene**
Any condition listed under K43.6 specified as gangrenous

● K43.9 **Ventral hernia without obstruction or gangrene**
Epigastric hernia
Ventral hernia NOS

● K44 **Diaphragmatic hernia**
  Includes hiatus hernia (esophageal) (sliding)
paraesophageal hernia
  Excludes1 congenital diaphragmatic hernia (Q79.0)
congenital hiatus hernia (Q40.1)

  K44.0 **Diaphragmatic hernia with obstruction, without gangrene**
Diaphragmatic hernia causing obstruction
Incarcerated diaphragmatic hernia
Irreducible diaphragmatic hernia
Strangulated diaphragmatic hernia

  K44.1 **Diaphragmatic hernia with gangrene**
Gangrenous diaphragmatic hernia

  K44.9 **Diaphragmatic hernia without obstruction or gangrene**
Diaphragmatic hernia NOS
Coding Clinic: 2017, Q1, P7

● K45 **Other abdominal hernia**
  Includes abdominal hernia, specified site NEC
lumbar hernia
obturator hernia
pudendal hernia
retroperitoneal hernia
sciatic hernia

  K45.0 **Other specified abdominal hernia with obstruction, without gangrene**
Other specified abdominal hernia causing obstruction
Other specified incarcerated abdominal hernia
Other specified irreducible abdominal hernia
Other specified strangulated abdominal hernia

  K45.1 **Other specified abdominal hernia with gangrene**
Any condition listed under K45 specified as gangrenous

  K45.8 **Other specified abdominal hernia without obstruction or gangrene**

● K46 **Unspecified abdominal hernia**
  Includes enterocele
epiplocele
hernia NOS
interstitial hernia
intestinal hernia
intra-abdominal hernia
  Excludes1 vaginal enterocele (N81.5)

K46.0 **Unspecified abdominal hernia** with obstruction, without gangrene
  Unspecified abdominal hernia causing obstruction
  Unspecified incarcerated abdominal hernia
  Unspecified irreducible abdominal hernia
  Unspecified strangulated abdominal hernia

K46.1 **Unspecified abdominal hernia** with gangrene
  Any condition listed under K46 specified as gangrenous

K46.9 **Unspecified abdominal hernia** without obstruction or gangrene
  Abdominal hernia NOS

★**(See Plate 32 of the Anatomy Illustrations.)**

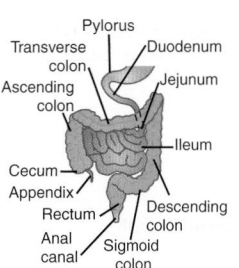

Pylorus
Transverse colon
Duodenum
Ascending colon
Jejunum
Ileum
Cecum
Appendix
Rectum
Descending colon
Anal canal
Sigmoid colon

Figure 11-10 Small and large intestines.

NONINFECTIVE ENTERITIS AND COLITIS (K50-K52)

Includes	noninfective inflammatory bowel disease
Excludes1	irritable bowel syndrome (K58.-)
	megacolon (K59.3-)

● **K50 Crohn's disease [regional enteritis]**
  Includes granulomatous enteritis
  Use additional code to identify manifestations, such as:
  pyoderma gangrenosum (L88)
  Excludes1 ulcerative colitis (K51.-)

● **K50.0 Crohn's disease of** small intestine
  Crohn's disease [regional enteritis] of duodenum
  Crohn's disease [regional enteritis] of ileum
  Crohn's disease [regional enteritis] of jejunum
  Regional ileitis
  Terminal ileitis
    Excludes1 Crohn's disease of both small and large intestine (K50.8-)

  K50.00 Crohn's disease of small intestine without complications

  ● **K50.01** Crohn's disease of small intestine with complications

    K50.011 Crohn's disease of small intestine with rectal bleeding

    K50.012 Crohn's disease of small intestine with intestinal obstruction

    K50.013 Crohn's disease of small intestine with fistula

    K50.014 Crohn's disease of small intestine with abscess
      Coding Clinic: 2012, Q4, P104

    K50.018 Crohn's disease of small intestine with other complication

    K50.019 Crohn's disease of small intestine with unspecified complications

● **K50.1 Crohn's disease of** large intestine
  Crohn's disease [regional enteritis] of colon
  Crohn's disease [regional enteritis] of large bowel
  Crohn's disease [regional enteritis] of rectum
  Granulomatous colitis
  Regional colitis
    Excludes1 Crohn's disease of both small and large intestine (K50.8)

  K50.10 Crohn's disease of large intestine without complications

  ● **K50.11** Crohn's disease of large intestine with complications

    K50.111 Crohn's disease of large intestine with rectal bleeding

    K50.112 Crohn's disease of large intestine with intestinal obstruction

    K50.113 Crohn's disease of large intestine with fistula

    K50.114 Crohn's disease of large intestine with abscess
      Coding Clinic: 2012, Q4, P104

    K50.118 Crohn's disease of large intestine with other complication

    K50.119 Crohn's disease of large intestine with unspecified complications

● **K50.8 Crohn's disease of** both small and large intestine

  K50.80 Crohn's disease of both small and large intestine without complications

  ● **K50.81** Crohn's disease of both small and large intestine with complications

    K50.811 Crohn's disease of both small and large intestine with rectal bleeding

    K50.812 Crohn's disease of both small and large intestine with intestinal obstruction

    K50.813 Crohn's disease of both small and large intestine with fistula

    K50.814 Crohn's disease of both small and large intestine with abscess
      Coding Clinic: 2012, Q4, P104

    K50.818 Crohn's disease of both small and large intestine with other complication

    K50.819 Crohn's disease of both small and large intestine with unspecified complications

● **K50.9 Crohn's disease,** unspecified

  K50.90 Crohn's disease, unspecified, without complications
    Crohn's disease NOS
    Regional enteritis NOS

  ● **K50.91** Crohn's disease, unspecified, with complications

    K50.911 Crohn's disease, unspecified, with rectal bleeding

    K50.912 Crohn's disease, unspecified, with intestinal obstruction

    K50.913 Crohn's disease, unspecified, with fistula

    K50.914 Crohn's disease, unspecified, with abscess
      Coding Clinic: 2012, Q4, P104

    K50.918 Crohn's disease, unspecified, with other complication

    K50.919 Crohn's disease, unspecified, with unspecified complications

● **K51 Ulcerative colitis**
  Use additional code to identify manifestations, such as:
  pyoderma gangrenosum (L88)
  Excludes1 Crohn's disease [regional enteritis] (K50.-)

● **K51.0 Ulcerative (chronic)** pancolitis
  Backwash ileitis

  K51.00 Ulcerative (chronic) pancolitis without complications
    Ulcerative (chronic) pancolitis NOS

Item 11-12 Crohn's disease, also known as **regional enteritis,** is a chronic inflammatory disease of the intestines. Classification is based on location in the small (duodenum, ileum, jejunum) or large (cecum, colon, rectum, anal canal) intestine.

CHAPTER 11 (K00-K95)

Item 11–13 Ulcerative colitis attacks the colonic mucosa and forms abscesses. The disease involves the intestines. Classification is based on the location:

- Enterocolitis: large and small intestine
- Ileocolitis: ileum and colon
- Proctitis: rectum
- Proctosigmoiditis: sigmoid colon and rectum

● K51.01   **Ulcerative (chronic) pancolitis with complications**
- K51.011   Ulcerative (chronic) pancolitis with **rectal bleeding** 🐾
- K51.012   Ulcerative (chronic) pancolitis with **intestinal obstruction** 🐾
- K51.013   Ulcerative (chronic) pancolitis with **fistula** 🐾
- K51.014   Ulcerative (chronic) pancolitis with **abscess** 🐾
- K51.018   Ulcerative (chronic) pancolitis with **other complication** 🐾
- K51.019   Ulcerative (chronic) pancolitis with **unspecified complications** 🐾

● K51.2   Ulcerative (chronic) **proctitis**
- K51.20   Ulcerative (chronic) proctitis **without complications** 🐾
  - Ulcerative (chronic) proctitis NOS
● K51.21   Ulcerative (chronic) proctitis **with complications**
- K51.211   Ulcerative (chronic) proctitis with **rectal bleeding** 🐾
- K51.212   Ulcerative (chronic) proctitis with **intestinal obstruction** 🐾
- K51.213   Ulcerative (chronic) proctitis with **fistula** 🐾
- K51.214   Ulcerative (chronic) proctitis with **abscess** 🐾
- K51.218   Ulcerative (chronic) proctitis with **other complication** 🐾
- K51.219   Ulcerative (chronic) proctitis with **unspecified complications** 🐾

● K51.3   Ulcerative (chronic) **rectosigmoiditis**
- K51.30   Ulcerative (chronic) rectosigmoiditis **without complications** 🐾
  - Ulcerative (chronic) rectosigmoiditis NOS
● K51.31   Ulcerative (chronic) rectosigmoiditis **with complications**
- K51.311   Ulcerative (chronic) rectosigmoiditis with **rectal bleeding** 🐾
- K51.312   Ulcerative (chronic) rectosigmoiditis with **intestinal obstruction** 🐾
- K51.313   Ulcerative (chronic) rectosigmoiditis with **fistula** 🐾
- K51.314   Ulcerative (chronic) rectosigmoiditis with **abscess** 🐾
- K51.318   Ulcerative (chronic) rectosigmoiditis with **other complication** 🐾
- K51.319   Ulcerative (chronic) rectosigmoiditis with **unspecified complications** 🐾

● K51.4   Inflammatory polyps of colon
> **Excludes1**   adenomatous polyp of colon (D12.6)
> polyposis of colon (D12.6)
> polyps of colon NOS (K63.5)

- K51.40   Inflammatory polyps of colon **without complications** 🐾
  - Inflammatory polyps of colon NOS
● K51.41   Inflammatory polyps of colon **with complications**
- K51.411   Inflammatory polyps of colon with **rectal bleeding** 🐾

- K51.412   Inflammatory polyps of colon with **intestinal obstruction** 🐾
- K51.413   Inflammatory polyps of colon with **fistula** 🐾
- K51.414   Inflammatory polyps of colon with **abscess** 🐾
- K51.418   Inflammatory polyps of colon with **other complication** 🐾
- K51.419   Inflammatory polyps of colon with **unspecified complications** 🐾

● K51.5   Left sided colitis
- Left hemicolitis
- K51.50   Left sided colitis **without complications** 🐾
  - Left sided colitis NOS
● K51.51   Left sided colitis **with complications**
- K51.511   Left sided colitis with **rectal bleeding** 🐾
- K51.512   Left sided colitis with **intestinal obstruction** 🐾
- K51.513   Left sided colitis with **fistula** 🐾
- K51.514   Left sided colitis with **abscess** 🐾
- K51.518   Left sided colitis with **other complication** 🐾
- K51.519   Left sided colitis with **unspecified complications** 🐾

● K51.8   Other ulcerative colitis
- K51.80   Other ulcerative colitis **without complications** 🐾
● K51.81   Other ulcerative colitis **with complications**
- K51.811   Other ulcerative colitis with **rectal bleeding** 🐾
- K51.812   Other ulcerative colitis with **intestinal obstruction** 🐾
- K51.813   Other ulcerative colitis with **fistula** 🐾
- K51.814   Other ulcerative colitis with **abscess** 🐾
- K51.818   Other ulcerative colitis with **other complication** 🐾
- K51.819   Other ulcerative colitis with **unspecified complications** 🐾

● K51.9   Ulcerative colitis, unspecified
- K51.90   Ulcerative colitis, unspecified, **without complications** 🐾
● K51.91   Ulcerative colitis, unspecified, **with complications**
- K51.911   Ulcerative colitis, unspecified with **rectal bleeding** 🐾
- K51.912   Ulcerative colitis, unspecified with **intestinal obstruction** 🐾
- K51.913   Ulcerative colitis, unspecified with **fistula** 🐾
- K51.914   Ulcerative colitis, unspecified with **abscess** 🐾
- K51.918   Ulcerative colitis, unspecified with **other complication** 🐾
- K51.919   Ulcerative colitis, unspecified with **unspecified complications** 🐾

● K52   **Other and unspecified noninfective gastroenteritis and colitis**
- K52.0   Gastroenteritis and colitis **due to radiation**
- K52.1   **Toxic gastroenteritis and colitis**
  - Drug-induced gastroenteritis and colitis
  - *Code first (T51-T65) to identify toxic agent*
  - Use additional code for adverse effect, if applicable, to identify drug (T36-T50 with fifth or sixth character 5)
  - **Coding Clinic: 2019, Q1, P17**

▶ New   ⏩ Revised   ~~deleted~~ Deleted   Excludes 1   Excludes 2   Includes   Use additional   Code first   Code also   Key words
OGCR Official Guidelines   X Assign placeholder X   ● Use Additional Character(s)   ▌ Manifestation Code   🐾 Hierarchical Condition Category   Coding Clinic

● **K52.2**   **Allergic and dietetic gastroenteritis and colitis**
Food hypersensitivity gastroenteritis or colitis

Use additional code to identify type of food allergy (Z91.01-, Z91.02-)

> **Excludes2**   allergic eosinophilic colitis (K52.82)
> allergic eosinophilic esophagitis (K20.0)
> allergic eosinophilic gastritis (K52.81)
> allergic eosinophilic gastroenteritis (K52.81)
> ~~food protein-induced proctocolitis (K52.82)~~

Coding Clinic: 2016, Q4, P30-31

K52.21   Food protein-induced **enterocolitis syndrome**
FPIES

Use additional code for hypovolemic shock, if present (R57.1)

K52.22   Food protein-induced **enteropathy**

K52.29   **Other** allergic and dietetic gastroenteritis and colitis
▶Allergic proctocolitis
Food hypersensitivity gastroenteritis or colitis
▶Food-induced eosinophilic proctocolitis
▶Food protein-induced proctocolitis
Immediate gastrointestinal hypersensitivity
▶Milk protein-induced proctocolitis

K52.3   **Indeterminate colitis**
Colonic inflammatory bowel disease unclassified (IBDU)

> **Excludes1**   unspecified colitis (K52.9)

● **K52.8**   Other specified noninfective gastroenteritis and colitis

K52.81   **Eosinophilic gastritis or gastroenteritis**
Eosinophilic enteritis

> **Excludes2**   eosinophilic esophagitis (K20.0)

K52.82   **Eosinophilic colitis**
~~Allergic proctocolitis~~
~~Food-induced eosinophilic proctocolitis~~
~~Food protein-induced proctocolitis~~
~~Milk protein-induced proctocolitis~~

> ▶ **Excludes2**   allergic proctocolitis (K52.29)
> ▶food-induced eosinophilic proctocolitis (K52.29)
> ▶food protein-induced enterocolitis syndrome (FPIES) (K52.21)
> ▶food protein-induced proctocolitis (K52.29)
> ▶milk protein-induced proctocolitis (K52.29)

● **K52.83**   Microscopic colitis
Coding Clinic: 2016, Q4, P30-31

K52.831   **Collagenous colitis**

K52.832   **Lymphocytic colitis**

K52.838   **Other** microscopic colitis

K52.839   **Microscopic colitis, unspecified**

K52.89   **Other specified** noninfective gastroenteritis and colitis
Coding Clinic: 2019, Q1, P21

K52.9   **Noninfective gastroenteritis and colitis, unspecified**

Colitis NOS	Ileitis NOS
Enteritis NOS	Jejunitis NOS
Gastroenteritis NOS	Sigmoiditis NOS

> **Excludes1**   diarrhea NOS (R19.7)
> functional diarrhea (K59.1)
> infectious gastroenteritis and colitis NOS (A09)
> neonatal diarrhea (noninfective) (P78.3)
> psychogenic diarrhea (F45.8)

OTHER DISEASES OF INTESTINES (K55-K64)

● **K55**   **Vascular disorders of intestine**

> **Excludes1**   necrotizing enterocolitis of newborn (P77.-)

● **K55.0**   **Acute vascular disorders of intestine**
Infarction of appendices epiploicae
Mesenteric (artery) (vein) embolism
Mesenteric (artery) (vein) infarction
Mesenteric (artery) (vein) thrombosis
Coding Clinic: 2019, Q4, P68

● **K55.01**   Acute (reversible) **ischemia of small intestine**
Coding Clinic: 2016, Q4, P32

K55.011   **Focal** (segmental) acute (reversible) ischemia of small intestine 🔖

K55.012   **Diffuse** acute (reversible) ischemia of small intestine 🔖

K55.019   Acute (reversible) ischemia of small intestine, extent **unspecified** 🔖

● **K55.02**   Acute **infarction of small intestine**
Gangrene of small intestine
Necrosis of small intestine
Coding Clinic: 2016, Q4, P32

K55.021   **Focal** (segmental) acute infarction of small intestine 🔖

K55.022   **Diffuse** acute infarction of small intestine 🔖

K55.029   Acute infarction of small intestine, extent **unspecified** 🔖

● **K55.03**   Acute (reversible) **ischemia of large intestine**
Acute fulminant ischemic colitis
Subacute ischemic colitis
Coding Clinic: 2016, Q4, P32

K55.031   **Focal** (segmental) acute (reversible) ischemia of large intestine 🔖

K55.032   **Diffuse** acute (reversible) ischemia of large intestine 🔖

K55.039   Acute (reversible) ischemia of large intestine, extent **unspecified** 🔖
Coding Clinic: 2019, Q4, P68

● **K55.04**   Acute **infarction of large intestine**
Gangrene of large intestine
Necrosis of large intestine
Coding Clinic: 2016, Q4, P32

K55.041   **Focal** (segmental) acute infarction of large intestine 🔖

K55.042   **Diffuse** acute infarction of large intestine 🔖

K55.049   Acute infarction of large intestine, extent **unspecified** 🔖

● **K55.05**   Acute (reversible) ischemia of intestine, part **unspecified**

K55.051   **Focal** (segmental) acute (reversible) ischemia of intestine, part unspecified 🔖

K55.052   **Diffuse** acute (reversible) ischemia of intestine, part unspecified 🔖

K55.059   Acute (reversible) ischemia of intestine, part and extent **unspecified** 🔖

● **K55.06**   Acute **infarction** of intestine, part **unspecified**
Acute intestinal infarction
Gangrene of intestine
Necrosis of intestine

K55.061   **Focal** (segmental) acute infarction of intestine, part unspecified 🔖

K55.062   **Diffuse** acute infarction of intestine, part unspecified 🔖

K55.069   Acute infarction of intestine, part and extent **unspecified** 🔖

K55.1   **Chronic** vascular disorders of intestine 🔖
Chronic ischemic colitis
Chronic ischemic enteritis
Chronic ischemic enterocolitis
Ischemic stricture of intestine
Mesenteric atherosclerosis
Mesenteric vascular insufficiency

● **K55.2**   **Angiodysplasia** of colon

K55.20   Angiodysplasia of colon **without hemorrhage**

K55.21   Angiodysplasia of colon **with hemorrhage**

CHAPTER 11 (KØØ-K95)

● **K55.3** **Necrotizing enterocolitis**
    Excludes1   necrotizing enterocolitis of newborn (P77.-)
    Excludes2   necrotizing enterocolitis due to
                 Clostridium difficile (A04.7-)

    K55.30   **Necrotizing enterocolitis, unspecified** 🐾
             Necrotizing enterocolitis, NOS

    K55.31   **Stage 1 necrotizing enterocolitis** 🐾
             Necrotizing enterocolitis without pneumatosis,
                without perforation
             Coding Clinic: 2016, Q4, P32

    K55.32   **Stage 2 necrotizing enterocolitis** 🐾
             Necrotizing enterocolitis with pneumatosis,
                without perforation
             Coding Clinic: 2016, Q4, P32

    K55.33   **Stage 3 necrotizing enterocolitis** 🐾
             Necrotizing enterocolitis with perforation
             Necrotizing enterocolitis with pneumatosis
                and perforation
             Coding Clinic: 2016, Q4, P32

  K55.8   **Other vascular disorders of intestine** 🐾

  K55.9   **Vascular disorder of intestine, unspecified** 🐾
         Ischemic colitis
         Ischemic enteritis
         Ischemic enterocolitis

● **K56** **Paralytic ileus and intestinal obstruction without hernia**
    Excludes1   congenital stricture or stenosis of intestine
                  (Q41-Q42)
                cystic fibrosis with meconium ileus (E84.11)
                ischemic stricture of intestine (K55.1)
                meconium ileus NOS (P76.0)
                neonatal intestinal obstructions classifiable to P76.-
                obstruction of duodenum (K31.5)
                postprocedural intestinal obstruction (K91.3-)
    Excludes2   stenosis of anus or rectum (K62.4)

  K56.0   **Paralytic ileus** 🐾
         Paralysis of bowel
         Paralysis of colon
         Paralysis of intestine
        Excludes1   gallstone ileus (K56.3)
                  ileus NOS (K56.7)
                  obstructive ileus NOS (K56.69-)

  K56.1   **Intussusception** 🐾
         Intussusception or invagination of bowel
         Intussusception or invagination of colon
         Intussusception or invagination of intestine
         Intussusception or invagination of rectum
        Excludes2   intussusception of appendix (K38.8)

SIMPLE TYPES   DOUBLE TYPES

Cecum and appendix

Ileum
Ileocecal valve   Ileum   Ileocecal valve

ILEOCOLIC

ILEOCECAL

Figure 11-11   Types of intussusception.

Item 11–14   **Intussusception** is the prolapse (telescoping) of a part of the intestine into another adjacent part of the intestine. Intussusception may be enteric (ileoileal, jejunoileal, jejunojejunal), colic (colocolic), or intracolic (ileocecal, ileocolic).

Item 11–15   **Volvulus** is the twisting of a segment of the intestine, resulting in obstruction. Paralytic ileus is paralysis of the intestine. It need not be a complete paralysis, but it must prohibit the passage of food through the intestine and lead to intestinal blockage. It is a common aftermath of some types of surgery.

  K56.2   **Volvulus** 🐾
         Strangulation of colon or intestine
         Torsion of colon or intestine
         Twist of colon or intestine
        Excludes2   volvulus of duodenum (K31.5)

  K56.3   **Gallstone ileus** 🐾
         Obstruction of intestine by gallstone

● **K56.4**   **Other impaction of intestine**
    K56.41   **Fecal impaction** 🐾
        Excludes1   constipation (K59.0-)
                  incomplete defecation (R15.0)

    K56.49   **Other impaction of intestine** 🐾

● **K56.5**   **Intestinal adhesions [bands] with obstruction (postinfection)**
         Abdominal hernia due to adhesions with obstruction
         Peritoneal adhesions [bands] with intestinal obstruction
           (postinfection)

    K56.50   **Intestinal adhesions [bands], unspecified as to partial versus complete obstruction** 🐾
             Intestinal adhesions with obstruction NOS

    K56.51   **Intestinal adhesions [bands], with partial obstruction** 🐾
             Intestinal adhesions with incomplete
                obstruction

    K56.52   **Intestinal adhesions [bands] with complete obstruction** 🐾

● **K56.6**   **Other and unspecified intestinal obstruction**
    ● **K56.60**   **Unspecified intestinal obstruction**
             Coding Clinic: 2017, Q2, P12

        K56.600   **Partial intestinal obstruction, unspecified as to cause** 🐾
                Incomplete intestinal obstruction, NOS

        K56.601   **Complete intestinal obstruction, unspecified as to cause** 🐾

        K56.609   **Unspecified intestinal obstruction, unspecified as to partial versus complete obstruction** 🐾
                Intestinal obstruction NOS

    ● **K56.69**   **Other intestinal obstruction**
             Enterostenosis NOS
             Obstructive ileus NOS
             Occlusion of colon or intestine NOS
             Stenosis of colon or intestine NOS
             Stricture of colon or intestine NOS
        Excludes1   intestinal obstruction due to specified condition-code to condition
             Coding Clinic: 2017, Q2, P12

        K56.690   **Other partial intestinal obstruction** 🐾
                Other incomplete intestinal obstruction

        K56.691   **Other complete intestinal obstruction** 🐾

        K56.699   **Other intestinal obstruction unspecified as to partial versus complete obstruction** 🐾
                Other intestinal obstruction, NEC

  K56.7   **Ileus, unspecified** 🐾
    Excludes1   obstructive ileus (K56.69-)
    Excludes2   intestinal obstruction with hernia (K40-K46)

  Coding Clinic: 2017, Q1, P41

● **K57   Diverticular disease of intestine**
    Code also if applicable peritonitis K65.-
    Excludes1   congenital diverticulum of intestine (Q43.8)
                 Meckel's diverticulum (Q43.0)
    Excludes2   diverticulum of appendix (K38.2)

● **K57.0   Diverticulitis of small intestine with perforation and abscess**
      Excludes1   diverticulitis of both small and large intestine with perforation and abscess (K57.4-)
    K57.00   Diverticulitis of small intestine with perforation and abscess without bleeding
    K57.01   Diverticulitis of small intestine with perforation and abscess with bleeding

● **K57.1   Diverticular disease of small intestine without perforation or abscess**
      Excludes1   diverticular disease of both small and large intestine without perforation or abscess (K57.5-)
    K57.10   Diverticulosis of small intestine without perforation or abscess without bleeding
           Diverticular disease of small intestine NOS
    K57.11   Diverticulosis of small intestine without perforation or abscess with bleeding
    K57.12   Diverticulitis of small intestine without perforation or abscess without bleeding
    K57.13   Diverticulitis of small intestine without perforation or abscess with bleeding

● **K57.2   Diverticulitis of large intestine with perforation and abscess**
      Excludes1   diverticulitis of both small and large intestine with perforation and abscess (K57.4-)
    K57.20   Diverticulitis of large intestine with perforation and abscess without bleeding
    K57.21   Diverticulitis of large intestine with perforation and abscess with bleeding

● **K57.3   Diverticular disease of large intestine without perforation or abscess**
      Excludes1   diverticular disease of both small and large intestine without perforation or abscess (K57.5-)
    K57.30   Diverticulosis of large intestine without perforation or abscess without bleeding
           Diverticular disease of colon NOS
    K57.31   Diverticulosis of large intestine without perforation or abscess with bleeding

Figure 11-12   Diverticulosis. (From Shiland: Mastering Healthcare Terminology, ed 4, St. Louis, Mosby, 2012)

Item 11–16   Diverticula of the intestines are acquired herniations of the mucosa. Diverticulum (singular): Pocket or pouch that bulges outward through a weak spot (herniation) in the colon. Diverticula (plural). **Diverticulosis** is the condition of having diverticula. **Diverticulitis** is inflammation of these pouches or herniations. Classification is based on location (small intestine or colon) and whether it occurs with or without hemorrhage.

    K57.32   Diverticulitis of large intestine without perforation or abscess without bleeding
    K57.33   Diverticulitis of large intestine without perforation or abscess with bleeding

● **K57.4   Diverticulitis of both small and large intestine with perforation and abscess**
    K57.40   Diverticulitis of both small and large intestine with perforation and abscess without bleeding
    K57.41   Diverticulitis of both small and large intestine with perforation and abscess with bleeding

● **K57.5   Diverticular disease of both small and large intestine without perforation or abscess**
    K57.50   Diverticulosis of both small and large intestine without perforation or abscess without bleeding
           Diverticular disease of both small and large intestine NOS
    K57.51   Diverticulosis of both small and large intestine without perforation or abscess with bleeding
    K57.52   Diverticulitis of both small and large intestine without perforation or abscess without bleeding
    K57.53   Diverticulitis of both small and large intestine without perforation or abscess with bleeding

● **K57.8   Diverticulitis of intestine, part unspecified, with perforation and abscess**
    K57.80   Diverticulitis of intestine, part unspecified, with perforation and abscess without bleeding
    K57.81   Diverticulitis of intestine, part unspecified, with perforation and abscess with bleeding

● **K57.9   Diverticular disease of intestine, part unspecified, without perforation or abscess**
    K57.90   Diverticulosis of intestine, part unspecified, without perforation or abscess without bleeding
           Diverticular disease of intestine NOS
           Coding Clinic: 2021, Q1, P12
    K57.91   Diverticulosis of intestine, part unspecified, without perforation or abscess with bleeding
    K57.92   Diverticulitis of intestine, part unspecified, without perforation or abscess without bleeding
    K57.93   Diverticulitis of intestine, part unspecified, without perforation or abscess with bleeding

● **K58   Irritable bowel syndrome**
    Includes   irritable colon
              spastic colon
    K58.0   Irritable bowel syndrome with diarrhea
    K58.1   Irritable bowel syndrome with constipation
           Coding Clinic: 2016, Q4, P32
    K58.2   Mixed irritable bowel syndrome
           Coding Clinic: 2016, Q4, P32
    K58.8   Other irritable bowel syndrome
           Coding Clinic: 2016, Q4, P32
    K58.9   Irritable bowel syndrome without diarrhea
           Irritable bowel syndrome NOS

● **K59   Other functional intestinal disorders**
    Excludes1   change in bowel habit NOS (R19.4)
               intestinal malabsorption (K90.-)
               psychogenic intestinal disorders (F45.8)
    Excludes2   functional disorders of stomach (K31.-)

● **K59.0   Constipation**
      Excludes1   fecal impaction (K56.41)
               incomplete defecation (R15.0)
    K59.00   Constipation, unspecified
    K59.01   Slow transit constipation
    K59.02   Outlet dysfunction constipation
    K59.03   Drug induced constipation
           Use additional code for adverse effect, if applicable, to identify drug (T36-T50 with fifth or sixth character 5)
           Coding Clinic: 2016, Q4, P33

K59.04   **Chronic idiopathic constipation**
Functional constipation
Coding Clinic: 2016, Q4, P33

K59.09   **Other constipation**
Chronic constipation

K59.1   **Functional diarrhea**
   Excludes1   diarrhea NOS (R19.7)
irritable bowel syndrome with diarrhea
(K58.0)

K59.2   **Neurogenic bowel, not elsewhere classified**

● **K59.3**   **Megacolon, not elsewhere classified**
Dilatation of colon
Code first, if applicable (T51-T65) to identify toxic agent
   Excludes1   congenital megacolon (aganglionic)
(Q43.1)
megacolon (due to) (in) Chagas' disease
(B57.32)
megacolon (due to) (in) Clostridium
difficile (A04.7-)
megacolon (due to) (in) Hirschsprung's
disease (Q43.1)
   Coding Clinic: 2016, Q4, P33

   K59.31   **Toxic megacolon** 🝆

   K59.39   **Other megacolon**
Megacolon NOS

K59.4   **Anal spasm**
Proctalgia fugax

● **K59.8**   **Other specified functional intestinal disorders**

   K59.81 Ogilvie syndrome
Acute colonic pseudo-obstruction (ACPO)

   K59.89 Other specified functional intestinal disorders
Atony of colon
Pseudo-obstruction (acute) (chronic) of
intestine

K59.9   **Functional intestinal disorder, unspecified**

● **K60**   **Fissure and fistula of anal and rectal regions**
   Excludes1   fissure and fistula of anal and rectal regions with
abscess or cellulitis (K61.-)
   Excludes2   anal sphincter tear (healed) (nontraumatic) (old)
(K62.81)

K60.0   **Acute anal fissure**

K60.1   **Chronic anal fissure**

K60.2   **Anal fissure, unspecified**

K60.3   **Anal fistula**

K60.4   **Rectal fistula**
Fistula of rectum to skin
   Excludes1   rectovaginal fistula (N82.3)
vesicorectal fistula (N32.1)

K60.5   **Anorectal fistula**

● **K61**   **Abscess of anal and rectal regions**
   Includes   abscess of anal and rectal regions
cellulitis of anal and rectal regions

K61.0   **Anal abscess**
Perianal abscess
   Excludes2   intrasphincteric abscess (K61.4)

K61.1   **Rectal abscess**
Perirectal abscess
   Excludes1   ischiorectal abscess (K61.39)
   Coding Clinic: 2012, Q4, P104

K61.2   **Anorectal abscess**

K61.3   **Ischiorectal abscess**

   K61.31   **Horseshoe abscess**

   K61.39   **Other ischiorectal abscess**
Abscess of ischiorectal fossa
Ischiorectal abscess, NOS

K61.4   **Intrasphincteric abscess**
Intersphincteric abscess

K61.5   **Supralevator abscess**

Item 11-17   A **fissure** is a groove in the surface, whereas a **fistula** is an abnormal passage. An **abscess** is an accumulation of pus in a tissue cavity resulting from a bacterial or parasitic infection.

● **K62**   **Other diseases of anus and rectum**
   Includes   anal canal
   Excludes2   colostomy and enterostomy malfunction (K94.0-,
K91.4-)
fecal incontinence (R15.-)
hemorrhoids (K64.-)

K62.0   **Anal polyp**
   Coding Clinic: 2018, Q1, P7

K62.1   **Rectal polyp**
   Excludes1   adenomatous polyp (D12.8)
   Coding Clinic: 2018, Q1, P7

K62.2   **Anal prolapse**
Prolapse of anal canal

K62.3   **Rectal prolapse**
Prolapse of rectal mucosa

K62.4   **Stenosis of anus and rectum**
Stricture of anus (sphincter)
   Coding Clinic: 2019, Q2, P13

K62.5   **Hemorrhage of anus and rectum**
   Excludes1   gastrointestinal bleeding NOS (K92.2)
melena (K92.1)
neonatal rectal hemorrhage (P54.2)

K62.6   **Ulcer of anus and rectum**
Solitary ulcer of anus and rectum
Stercoral ulcer of anus and rectum
   Excludes1   fissure and fistula of anus and rectum
(K60.-)
ulcerative colitis (K51.-)

K62.7   **Radiation proctitis**
Use additional code to identify the type of radiation
(W88.-) or radiation therapy (Y84.2)
   Coding Clinic: 2019, Q1, P21

● **K62.8**   **Other specified diseases of anus and rectum**
   Excludes2   ulcerative proctitis (K51.2)

   K62.81   **Anal sphincter tear (healed) (nontraumatic)
(old)**
Tear of anus, nontraumatic
Use additional code for any associated fecal
incontinence (R15.-)
    Excludes2   anal fissure (K60.-)
anal sphincter tear (healed)
(old) complicating delivery
(O34.7-)
traumatic tear of anal sphincter
(S31.831)

   K62.82   **Dysplasia of anus**
Anal intraepithelial neoplasia I and II (AIN I
and II) (histologically confirmed)
Dysplasia of anus NOS
Mild and moderate dysplasia of anus
(histologically confirmed)
    Excludes1   abnormal results from anal
cytologic examination
without histologic
confirmation (R85.61-)
anal intraepithelial neoplasia III
(D01.3)
carcinoma in situ of anus (D01.3)
HGSIL of anus (R85.613)
severe dysplasia of anus (D01.3)

   K62.89   **Other specified diseases of anus and rectum**
Proctitis NOS
Use additional code for any associated fecal
incontinence (R15.-)

K62.9   **Disease of anus and rectum, unspecified**

▶ New   ⇒ Revised   ~~deleted~~ Deleted   Excludes 1   Excludes 2   Includes   Use additional   Code first   Code also   Key words

OGCR Official Guidelines   X Assign placeholder X   ● Use Additional Character(s)   ▶ Manifestation Code   🝆 Hierarchical Condition Category   **Coding Clinic**

● **K63 Other diseases of intestine**

K63.0 Abscess of intestine

> **Excludes1** abscess of intestine with Crohn's disease (K50.014, K50.114, K50.814, K50.914)
> abscess of intestine with diverticular disease (K57.0, K57.2, K57.4, K57.8)
> abscess of intestine with ulcerative colitis (K51.014, K51.214, K51.314, K51.414, K51.514, K51.814, K51.914)

> **Excludes2** abscess of anal and rectal regions (K61.-)
> abscess of appendix (K35.3-)

K63.1 Perforation of intestine (nontraumatic)
Perforation (nontraumatic) of rectum

> **Excludes1** perforation (nontraumatic) of duodenum (K26.-)
> perforation (nontraumatic) of intestine with diverticular disease (K57.0, K57.2, K57.4, K57.8)

> **Excludes2** perforation (nontraumatic) of appendix (K35.2-, K35.3)

K63.2 Fistula of intestine

> **Excludes1** fistula of duodenum (K31.6)
> fistula of intestine with Crohn's disease (K50.013, K50.113, K50.813, K50.913)
> fistula of intestine with ulcerative colitis (K51.013, K51.213, K51.313, K51.413, K51.513, K51.813, K51.913)

> **Excludes2** fistula of anal and rectal regions (K60.-)
> fistula of appendix (K38.3)
> intestinal-genital fistula, female (N82.2-N82.4)
> vesicointestinal fistula (N32.1)

Coding Clinic: 2017, Q3, P4

K63.3 Ulcer of intestine
Primary ulcer of small intestine

> **Excludes1** duodenal ulcer (K26.-)
> gastrointestinal ulcer (K28.-)
> gastrojejunal ulcer (K28.-)
> jejunal ulcer (K28.-)
> peptic ulcer, site unspecified (K27.-)
> ulcer of intestine with perforation (K63.1)
> ulcer of anus or rectum (K62.6)
> ulcerative colitis (K51.-)

K63.4 Enteroptosis

K63.5 Polyp of colon

> **Excludes1** adenomatous polyp of colon (D12.-)
> inflammatory polyp of colon (K51.4-)
> polyposis of colon (D12.6)

Coding Clinic: 2019, Q1, P33; 2017, Q1, P15-16; 2015, Q2, P14

● **K63.8 Other specified diseases of intestine**

K63.81 Dieulafoy lesion of intestine

> **Excludes2** Dieulafoy lesion of stomach and duodenum (K31.82)

K63.89 Other specified diseases of intestine
Coding Clinic: 2013, Q2, P31

K63.9 Disease of intestine, unspecified

● **K64 Hemorrhoids and perianal venous thrombosis**

> **Includes** piles
> **Excludes1** hemorrhoids complicating childbirth and the puerperium (O87.2)
> hemorrhoids complicating pregnancy (O22.4)

K64.0 First degree hemorrhoids
Grade/stage I hemorrhoids
Hemorrhoids (bleeding) without prolapse outside of anal canal

K64.1 Second degree hemorrhoids
Grade/stage II hemorrhoids
Hemorrhoids (bleeding) that prolapse with straining, but retract spontaneously

K64.2 Third degree hemorrhoids
Grade/stage III hemorrhoids
Hemorrhoids (bleeding) that prolapse with straining and require manual replacement back inside anal canal

K64.3 Fourth degree hemorrhoids
Grade/stage IV hemorrhoids
Hemorrhoids (bleeding) with prolapsed tissue that cannot be manually replaced

K64.4 Residual hemorrhoidal skin tags
External hemorrhoids, NOS
Skin tags of anus

K64.5 Perianal venous thrombosis
External hemorrhoids with thrombosis
Perianal hematoma
Thrombosed hemorrhoids NOS

K64.8 Other hemorrhoids
Internal hemorrhoids, without mention of degree
Prolapsed hemorrhoids, degree not specified

K64.9 Unspecified hemorrhoids
Hemorrhoids (bleeding) NOS
Hemorrhoids (bleeding) without mention of degree

DISEASES OF PERITONEUM AND RETROPERITONEUM (K65-K68)

● **K65 Peritonitis**
Use additional code (B95-B97), to identify infectious agent, if known
Code also if applicable diverticular disease of intestine (K57.-)

> **Excludes1** acute appendicitis with generalized peritonitis (K35.2-)
> aseptic peritonitis (T81.6)
> benign paroxysmal peritonitis (E85.0)
> chemical peritonitis (T81.6)
> gonococcal peritonitis (A54.85)
> neonatal peritonitis (P78.0-P78.1)
> pelvic peritonitis, female (N73.3-N73.5)
> periodic familial peritonitis (E85.0)
> peritonitis due to talc or other foreign substance (T81.6)
> peritonitis in chlamydia (A74.81)
> peritonitis in diphtheria (A36.89)
> peritonitis in syphilis (late) (A52.74)
> peritonitis in tuberculosis (A18.31)
> peritonitis with or following abortion or ectopic or molar pregnancy (O00-O07, O08.0)
> peritonitis with or following appendicitis (K35.-)
> puerperal peritonitis (O85)
> retroperitoneal infections (K68.-)

K65.0 Generalized (acute) peritonitis
Pelvic peritonitis (acute), male
Subphrenic peritonitis (acute)
Suppurative peritonitis (acute)

K65.1 Peritoneal abscess
Abdominopelvic abscess
Abscess (of) omentum
Abscess (of) peritoneum
Mesenteric abscess
Retrocecal abscess
Subdiaphragmatic abscess
Subhepatic abscess
Subphrenic abscess
Coding Clinic: 2019, Q1, P15

K65.2 Spontaneous bacterial peritonitis

> **Excludes1** bacterial peritonitis NOS (K65.9)

K65.3 Choleperitonitis
Peritonitis due to bile

K65.4 Sclerosing mesenteritis
Fat necrosis of peritoneum
(Idiopathic) sclerosing mesenteric fibrosis
Mesenteric lipodystrophy
Mesenteric panniculitis
Retractile mesenteritis

Item 11-18 Peritonitis is an inflammation of the lining (peritoneum) of the abdominal cavity and surface of the intestines.

Item 11-19 **Retroperitoneal infections** occur between the posterior parietal peritoneum and posterior abdominal wall where the kidneys, adrenal glands, ureters, duodenum, ascending colon, descending colon, pancreas, and the large vessels and nerves are located.

K65.8   **Other peritonitis** 🔲
      Chronic proliferative peritonitis
      Peritonitis due to urine

K65.9   **Peritonitis, unspecified** 🔲
      Bacterial peritonitis NOS
      Coding Clinic: 2013, Q2, P31

● **K66**   **Other disorders of peritoneum**
      Excludes2   ascites (R18.-)
                    peritoneal effusion (chronic) (R18.8)

K66.0   **Peritoneal adhesions (postprocedural) (postinfection)**
      Adhesions (of) abdominal (wall)
      Adhesions (of) diaphragm
      Adhesions (of) intestine
      Adhesions (of) male pelvis
      Adhesions (of) omentum
      Adhesions (of) stomach
      Adhesive bands
      Mesenteric adhesions
      Excludes1   female pelvic adhesions [bands] (N73.6)
                    peritoneal adhesions with intestinal obstruction (K56.5-)

K66.1   **Hemoperitoneum**
      Excludes1   traumatic hemoperitoneum (S36.8-)

K66.8   **Other specified disorders of peritoneum**

K66.9   **Disorder of peritoneum, unspecified**

▷ **K67**   *Disorders of peritoneum in infectious diseases classified elsewhere* 🔲
      Code first underlying disease, such as:
      congenital syphilis (A50.0)
      helminthiasis (B65.0-B83.9)
      Excludes1   peritonitis in chlamydia (A74.81)
                    peritonitis in diphtheria (A36.89)
                    peritonitis in gonococcal (A54.85)
                    peritonitis in syphilis (late) (A52.74)
                    peritonitis in tuberculosis (A18.31)

● **K68**   **Disorders of retroperitoneum**
   ● K68.1   **Retroperitoneal abscess**
      K68.11   **Postprocedural retroperitoneal abscess**
          Excludes2   infection following procedure (T81.44)
      K68.12   **Psoas muscle abscess** 🔲
      K68.19   **Other retroperitoneal abscess** 🔲
          Coding Clinic: 2019, Q1, P15

   K68.9   **Other disorders of retroperitoneum**

DISEASES OF LIVER (K70-K77)

      Excludes1   jaundice NOS (R17)
      Excludes2   hemochromatosis (E83.11-)
                    Reye's syndrome (G93.7)
                    viral hepatitis (B15-B19)
                    Wilson's disease (E83.0)

● **K70**   **Alcoholic liver disease**
      Use additional code to identify:
      alcohol abuse and dependence (F10.-)
   K70.0   **Alcoholic fatty liver**   A
   ● K70.1   **Alcoholic hepatitis**
      K70.10   **Alcoholic hepatitis without ascites**   A
      K70.11   **Alcoholic hepatitis with ascites**   A
   K70.2   **Alcoholic fibrosis and sclerosis of liver**   A
   ● K70.3   **Alcoholic cirrhosis of liver**
      Alcoholic cirrhosis NOS
      K70.30   **Alcoholic cirrhosis of liver without ascites** 🔲   A
      K70.31   **Alcoholic cirrhosis of liver with ascites** 🔲   A
          Coding Clinic: 2018, Q1, P5

   ● K70.4   **Alcoholic hepatic failure**
      Acute alcoholic hepatic failure
      Alcoholic hepatic failure NOS
      Chronic alcoholic hepatic failure
      Subacute alcoholic hepatic failure
      K70.40   **Alcoholic hepatic failure without coma** 🔲   A
      K70.41   **Alcoholic hepatic failure with coma** 🔲   A
   K70.9   **Alcoholic liver disease, unspecified** 🔲   A

● **K71**   **Toxic liver disease**
      Includes   drug-induced idiosyncratic (unpredictable) liver disease
              drug-induced toxic (predictable) liver disease
      Code first poisoning due to drug or toxin, if applicable (T36-T65 with fifth or sixth character 1-4 or 6)
      Use additional code for adverse effect, if applicable, to identify drug (T36-T50 with fifth or sixth character 5)
      Excludes2   alcoholic liver disease (K70.-)
                    Budd-Chiari syndrome (I82.0)

   K71.0   **Toxic liver disease with cholestasis**
      Cholestasis with hepatocyte injury
      'Pure' cholestasis

   ● K71.1   **Toxic liver disease with hepatic necrosis**
      Hepatic failure (acute) (chronic) due to drugs
      K71.10   **Toxic liver disease with hepatic necrosis, without coma**
      K71.11   **Toxic liver disease with hepatic necrosis, with coma** 🔲

   K71.2   **Toxic liver disease with acute hepatitis**

   K71.3   **Toxic liver disease with chronic persistent hepatitis**

   K71.4   **Toxic liver disease with chronic lobular hepatitis**

   ● K71.5   **Toxic liver disease with chronic active hepatitis**
      Toxic liver disease with lupoid hepatitis
      K71.50   **Toxic liver disease with chronic active hepatitis without ascites**
      K71.51   **Toxic liver disease with chronic active hepatitis with ascites**
          Coding Clinic: 2018, Q1, P4

   K71.6   **Toxic liver disease with hepatitis, not elsewhere classified**

   K71.7   **Toxic liver disease with fibrosis and cirrhosis of liver**

   K71.8   **Toxic liver disease with other disorders of liver**
      Toxic liver disease with focal nodular hyperplasia
      Toxic liver disease with hepatic granulomas
      Toxic liver disease with peliosis hepatis
      Toxic liver disease with veno-occlusive disease of liver

   K71.9   **Toxic liver disease, unspecified**

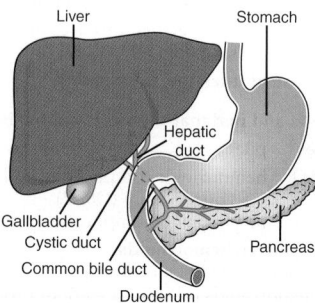

Figure 11-13   Liver and bile ducts.

Item 11–20   **Cirrhosis** is the progressive fibrosis of the liver resulting in loss of liver function. The main causes of cirrhosis of the liver are alcohol abuse, chronic hepatitis (inflammation of the liver), biliary disease, and excessive amounts of iron. **Alcoholic cirrhosis of the liver** is also called portal, Laënnec's, or fatty nutritional cirrhosis.

▶ New   ⇒ Revised   ~~deleted~~ Deleted   Excludes 1   Excludes 2   Includes   Use additional   Code first   Code also   Key words

OGCR Official Guidelines   X Assign placeholder X   ● Use Additional Character(s)   ▷ Manifestation Code   🔲 Hierarchical Condition Category   **Coding Clinic**

● **K72**   **Hepatic failure, not elsewhere classified**

      Includes   fulminant hepatitis NEC, with hepatic failure
                     hepatic encephalopathy NOS
                     liver (cell) necrosis with hepatic failure
                     malignant hepatitis NEC, with hepatic failure
                     yellow liver atrophy or dystrophy

      Excludes1   alcoholic hepatic failure (K70.4)
                     hepatic failure with toxic liver disease (K71.1-)
                     icterus of newborn (P55-P59)
                     postprocedural hepatic failure (K91.82)

      Excludes2   hepatic failure complicating abortion or ectopic
                        or molar pregnancy (O00-O07, O08.8)
                     hepatic failure complicating pregnancy, childbirth
                        and the puerperium (O26.6-)
                     viral hepatitis with hepatic coma (B15-B19)

● **K72.0**   **Acute and subacute hepatic failure**
         Acute non-viral hepatitis NOS
         Coding Clinic: 2015, Q2, P17

      K72.00   **Acute and subacute hepatic failure without
                    coma**
                    Coding Clinic: 2021, Q1, P13; 2015, Q2, P17

      K72.01   **Acute and subacute hepatic failure with
                    coma** 🦟

● **K72.1**   **Chronic hepatic failure**
      ▶End stage liver disease

      K72.10   **Chronic hepatic failure without coma** 🦟
                    Coding Clinic: 2021, Q1, P13; 2017, Q1, P41

      K72.11   **Chronic hepatic failure with coma** 🦟
                    Coding Clinic: 2020, Q1, P15

● **K72.9**   **Hepatic failure, unspecified**

      K72.90   **Hepatic failure, unspecified without coma** 🦟
                    Coding Clinic: 2018, Q4, P21

      K72.91   **Hepatic failure, unspecified with coma** 🦟
                  Hepatic coma NOS
                  Coding Clinic: 2016, Q2, P35

● **K73**   **Chronic hepatitis, not elsewhere classified**

      Excludes1   alcoholic hepatitis (chronic) (K70.1-)
                     drug-induced hepatitis (chronic) (K71.-)
                     granulomatous hepatitis (chronic) NEC (K75.3)
                     reactive, nonspecific hepatitis (chronic) (K75.2)
                     viral hepatitis (chronic) (B15-B19)

    K73.0   **Chronic persistent hepatitis, not elsewhere classified** 🦟
    K73.1   **Chronic lobular hepatitis, not elsewhere classified** 🦟
    K73.2   **Chronic active hepatitis, not elsewhere classified** 🦟
    K73.8   **Other chronic hepatitis, not elsewhere classified** 🦟
    K73.9   **Chronic hepatitis, unspecified** 🦟

● **K74**   **Fibrosis and cirrhosis of liver**
      Code also, if applicable, viral hepatitis (acute) (chronic)
         (B15-B19)

      Excludes1   alcoholic cirrhosis (of liver) (K70.3)
                     alcoholic fibrosis of liver (K70.2)
                     cardiac sclerosis of liver (K76.1)
                     cirrhosis (of liver) with toxic liver disease (K71.7)
                     congenital cirrhosis (of liver) (P78.81)
                     pigmentary cirrhosis (of liver) (E83.110)

● **K74.0**   **Hepatic fibrosis**
        Code first underlying liver disease, such as:
          nonalcoholic steatohepatitis (NASH) (K75.81)

      K74.00   **Hepatic fibrosis, unspecified**

      K74.01   **Hepatic fibrosis, early fibrosis**
             Hepatic fibrosis, stage F1 or stage F2

      K74.02   **Hepatic fibrosis, advanced fibrosis**
             Hepatic fibrosis, stage F3

            Excludes1   cirrhosis of liver (K74.6-)
                          hepatic fibrosis, stage F4 (K74.6-)

    K74.1   **Hepatic sclerosis**
    K74.2   **Hepatic fibrosis with hepatic sclerosis**

      K74.3   **Primary biliary cirrhosis** 🦟
         Chronic nonsuppurative destructive cholangitis
         Primary biliary cholangitis

         Excludes2   primary sclerosing cholangitis (K83.01)

      K74.4   **Secondary biliary cirrhosis** 🦟
      K74.5   **Biliary cirrhosis, unspecified** 🦟

● **K74.6**   **Other and unspecified cirrhosis of liver**

      K74.60   **Unspecified cirrhosis of liver** 🦟
            Cirrhosis (of liver) NOS
            Coding Clinic: 2018, Q1, P4

      K74.69   **Other cirrhosis of liver** 🦟
            Cryptogenic cirrhosis (of liver)
            Macronodular cirrhosis (of liver)
            Micronodular cirrhosis (of liver)
            Mixed type cirrhosis (of liver)
            Portal cirrhosis (of liver)
            Postnecrotic cirrhosis (of liver)

● **K75**   **Other inflammatory liver diseases**

      Excludes2   toxic liver disease (K71.-)

      K75.0   **Abscess of liver**
         Cholangitic hepatic abscess
         Hematogenic hepatic abscess
         Hepatic abscess NOS
         Lymphogenic hepatic abscess
         Pylephlebitic hepatic abscess

         Excludes1   amebic liver abscess (A06.4)
                        cholangitis without liver abscess (K83.09)
                        pylephlebitis without liver abscess (K75.1)

         Excludes2   acute or subacute hepatitis NOS (B17.9)
                        acute or subacute non-viral hepatitis
                           (K72.0)
                        chronic hepatitis NEC (K73.8)

      K75.1   **Phlebitis of portal vein**
         Pylephlebitis

         Excludes1   pylephlebitic liver abscess (K75.0)

      K75.2   **Nonspecific reactive hepatitis**

         Excludes1   acute or subacute hepatitis (K72.0-)
                        chronic hepatitis NEC (K73.-)
                        viral hepatitis (B15-B19)

      K75.3   **Granulomatous hepatitis, not elsewhere classified**

         Excludes1   acute or subacute hepatitis (K72.0-)
                        chronic hepatitis NEC (K73.-)
                        viral hepatitis (B15-B19)

      K75.4   **Autoimmune hepatitis** 🦟
         Lupoid hepatitis NEC

● **K75.8**   **Other specified inflammatory liver diseases**

      K75.81   **Nonalcoholic steatohepatitis (NASH)**
            Use additional code, if applicable, hepatic
               fibrosis (K74.0-)

      K75.89   **Other specified inflammatory liver diseases**

      K75.9   **Inflammatory liver disease, unspecified**
         Hepatitis NOS

         Excludes1   acute or subacute hepatitis (K72.0-)
                        chronic hepatitis NEC (K73.-)
                        viral hepatitis (B15-B19)
         Coding Clinic: 2015, Q2, P17

● **K76**   **Other diseases of liver**

      Excludes2   alcoholic liver disease (K70.-)
                     amyloid degeneration of liver (E85.-)
                     cystic disease of liver (congenital) (Q44.6)
                     hepatic vein thrombosis (I82.0)
                     hepatomegaly NOS (R16.0)
                     pigmentary cirrhosis (of liver) (E83.110)
                     portal vein thrombosis (I81)
                     toxic liver disease (K71.-)

      K76.0   **Fatty (change of) liver, not elsewhere classified**
         Nonalcoholic fatty liver disease (NAFLD)

         Excludes1   nonalcoholic steatohepatitis (NASH)
                        (K75.81)

K76.1   **Chronic passive congestion of liver**
Cardiac cirrhosis
Cardiac sclerosis

K76.2   **Central hemorrhagic necrosis of liver**
Excludes1   liver necrosis with hepatic failure (K72.-)

K76.3   **Infarction of liver**

K76.4   **Peliosis hepatis**
Hepatic angiomatosis

K76.5   **Hepatic veno-occlusive disease**
Excludes1   Budd-Chiari syndrome (I82.0)

K76.6   **Portal hypertension** 🅗
Use additional code for any associated complications,
such as:
portal hypertensive gastropathy (K31.89)
Coding Clinic: 2020, Q1, P15

K76.7   **Hepatorenal syndrome** 🅗
Excludes1   hepatorenal syndrome following labor
and delivery (O90.4)
postprocedural hepatorenal syndrome
(K91.83)

● **K76.8**   **Other specified diseases of liver**
K76.81   **Hepatopulmonary syndrome** 🅗
Code first underlying liver disease, such as:
alcoholic cirrhosis of liver (K70.3-)
cirrhosis of liver without mention of alcohol
(K74.6-)

K76.89   **Other specified diseases of liver**
Cyst (simple) of liver
Focal nodular hyperplasia of liver
Hepatoptosis

K76.9   **Liver disease, unspecified**

▶ *K77*   *Liver disorders in diseases classified elsewhere*
Code first underlying disease, such as:
amyloidosis (E85.-)
congenital syphilis (A50.0, A50.5)
congenital toxoplasmosis (P37.1)
▶infectious mononucleosis with liver disease (B27.0-B27.9
with .9)
schistosomiasis (B65.0-B65.9)
Excludes1   alcoholic hepatitis (K70.1-)
alcoholic liver disease (K70.-)
cytomegaloviral hepatitis (B25.1)
herpesviral [herpes simplex] hepatitis (B00.81)
~~infectious mononucleosis with liver disease~~
~~(B27.0-B27.9 with .9)~~
mumps hepatitis (B26.81)
sarcoidosis with liver disease (D86.89)
secondary syphilis with liver disease (A51.45)
syphilis (late) with liver disease (A52.74)
toxoplasmosis (acquired) hepatitis (B58.1)
tuberculosis with liver disease (A18.83)

DISORDERS OF GALLBLADDER, BILIARY TRACT AND PANCREAS (K80–K87)

● **K80**   **Cholelithiasis**
Presence or formation of gallstones
Excludes1   retained cholelithiasis following cholecystectomy
(K91.86)

● **K80.0**   **Calculus of gallbladder with acute cholecystitis**
Any condition listed in K80.2 with acute cholecystitis
Use additional code if applicable for associated
gangrene of gallbladder (K82.A1), or perforation of
gallbladder (K82.A2)
*Check documentation for acute/chronic gallbladder/common
bile duct either with or without obstruction.*
K80.00   **Calculus of gallbladder with acute cholecystitis
without obstruction**
Coding Clinic: 2018, Q4, P20

K80.01   **Calculus of gallbladder with acute cholecystitis
with obstruction**

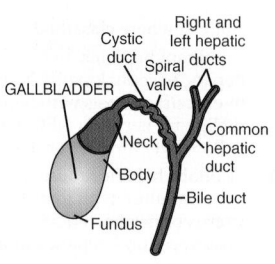

Figure 11-14   Gallbladder and bile ducts.

● **K80.1**   **Calculus of gallbladder with other cholecystitis**
Use additional code if applicable for associated
gangrene of gallbladder (K82.A1), or perforation of
gallbladder (K82.A2)

K80.10   **Calculus of gallbladder with chronic
cholecystitis without obstruction**
Cholelithiasis with cholecystitis NOS

K80.11   **Calculus of gallbladder with chronic
cholecystitis with obstruction**

K80.12   **Calculus of gallbladder with acute and chronic
cholecystitis without obstruction**

K80.13   **Calculus of gallbladder with acute and chronic
cholecystitis with obstruction**

K80.18   **Calculus of gallbladder with other cholecystitis
without obstruction**

K80.19   **Calculus of gallbladder with other cholecystitis
with obstruction**

● **K80.2**   **Calculus of gallbladder without cholecystitis**
Cholecystolithiasis without cholecystitis
Cholelithiasis (without cholecystitis)
Colic (recurrent) of gallbladder (without cholecystitis)
Gallstone (impacted) of cystic duct (without
cholecystitis)
Gallstone (impacted) of gallbladder (without
cholecystitis)

K80.20   **Calculus of gallbladder without cholecystitis
without obstruction**

K80.21   **Calculus of gallbladder without cholecystitis
with obstruction**

● **K80.3**   **Calculus of bile duct with cholangitis**
Any condition listed in K80.5 with cholangitis

K80.30   **Calculus of bile duct with cholangitis,
unspecified, without obstruction**

K80.31   **Calculus of bile duct with cholangitis,
unspecified, with obstruction**

K80.32   **Calculus of bile duct with acute cholangitis
without obstruction**

K80.33   **Calculus of bile duct with acute cholangitis
with obstruction**

K80.34   **Calculus of bile duct with chronic cholangitis
without obstruction**

K80.35   **Calculus of bile duct with chronic cholangitis
with obstruction**

K80.36   **Calculus of bile duct with acute and chronic
cholangitis without obstruction**

K80.37   **Calculus of bile duct with acute and chronic
cholangitis with obstruction**

● **K80.4**   **Calculus of bile duct with cholecystitis**
Any condition listed in K80.5 with cholecystitis (with
cholangitis)
Code also fistula of bile duct (K83.3)
Use additional code if applicable for associated
gangrene of gallbladder (K82.A1), or perforation of
gallbladder (K82.A2)

▶ New   ⇒ Revised   ~~deleted~~ Deleted   Excludes 1   Excludes 2   Includes   Use additional   Code first   Code also   Key words
OGCR Official Guidelines   X Assign placeholder X   ● Use Additional Character(s)   ▶ Manifestation Code   🅗 Hierarchical Condition Category   **Coding Clinic**

K80.40   Calculus of bile duct with cholecystitis, unspecified, without obstruction

K80.41   Calculus of bile duct with cholecystitis, unspecified, with obstruction
     Coding Clinic: 2019, Q1, P18

K80.42   Calculus of bile duct with acute cholecystitis without obstruction

K80.43   Calculus of bile duct with acute cholecystitis with obstruction

K80.44   Calculus of bile duct with chronic cholecystitis without obstruction

K80.45   Calculus of bile duct with chronic cholecystitis with obstruction

K80.46   Calculus of bile duct with acute and chronic cholecystitis without obstruction

K80.47   Calculus of bile duct with acute and chronic cholecystitis with obstruction

● K80.5   **Calculus of bile duct without cholangitis or cholecystitis**
Choledocholithiasis (without cholangitis or cholecystitis)
Gallstone (impacted) of bile duct NOS (without cholangitis or cholecystitis)
Gallstone (impacted) of common duct (without cholangitis or cholecystitis)
Gallstone (impacted) of hepatic duct (without cholangitis or cholecystitis)
Hepatic cholelithiasis (without cholangitis or cholecystitis)
Hepatic colic (recurrent) (without cholangitis or cholecystitis)

K80.50   Calculus of bile duct without cholangitis or cholecystitis without obstruction

K80.51   Calculus of bile duct without cholangitis or cholecystitis with obstruction

● K80.6   **Calculus of gallbladder and bile duct with cholecystitis**
Use additional code if applicable for associated gangrene of gallbladder (K82.A1), or perforation of gallbladder (K82.A2)

K80.60   Calculus of gallbladder and bile duct with cholecystitis, unspecified, without obstruction

K80.61   Calculus of gallbladder and bile duct with cholecystitis, unspecified, with obstruction

K80.62   Calculus of gallbladder and bile duct with acute cholecystitis without obstruction

K80.63   Calculus of gallbladder and bile duct with acute cholecystitis with obstruction

K80.64   Calculus of gallbladder and bile duct with chronic cholecystitis without obstruction

K80.65   Calculus of gallbladder and bile duct with chronic cholecystitis with obstruction

K80.66   Calculus of gallbladder and bile duct with acute and chronic cholecystitis without obstruction

K80.67   Calculus of gallbladder and bile duct with acute and chronic cholecystitis with obstruction

● K80.7   **Calculus of gallbladder and bile duct without cholecystitis**

K80.70   Calculus of gallbladder and bile duct without cholecystitis without obstruction

K80.71   Calculus of gallbladder and bile duct without cholecystitis with obstruction

● K80.8   **Other cholelithiasis**

K80.80   Other cholelithiasis without obstruction

K80.81   Other cholelithiasis with obstruction

● K81   **Cholecystitis**
Chronic or acute inflammation of the gallbladder
Use additional code if applicable for associated gangrene of gallbladder (K82.A1), or perforation of gallbladder (K82.A2)

   Excludes 1   cholecystitis with cholelithiasis (K80.-)

K81.0   **Acute cholecystitis**
Abscess of gallbladder
Angiocholecystitis
Emphysematous (acute) cholecystitis
Empyema of gallbladder
Gangrene of gallbladder
Gangrenous cholecystitis
Suppurative cholecystitis

K81.1   **Chronic cholecystitis**

K81.2   **Acute cholecystitis with chronic cholecystitis**

K81.9   **Cholecystitis, unspecified**

● K82   **Other diseases of gallbladder**

   Excludes 1   nonvisualization of gallbladder (R93.2)
postcholecystectomy syndrome (K91.5)

K82.0   **Obstruction of gallbladder**
Occlusion of cystic duct or gallbladder without cholelithiasis
Stenosis of cystic duct or gallbladder without cholelithiasis
Stricture of cystic duct or gallbladder without cholelithiasis

   Excludes 1   obstruction of gallbladder with cholelithiasis (K80.-)

K82.1   **Hydrops of gallbladder**
Mucocele of gallbladder

K82.2   **Perforation of gallbladder**
Rupture of cystic duct or gallbladder

   Excludes 1   Perforation of gallbladder in cholecystitis (K82.A2)

K82.3   **Fistula of gallbladder**
Cholecystocolic fistula
Cholecystoduodenal fistula
   Coding Clinic: 2019, Q1, P18

K82.4   **Cholesterolosis of gallbladder**
Strawberry gallbladder

   Excludes 1   cholesterolosis of gallbladder with cholecystitis (K81.-)
cholesterolosis of gallbladder with cholelithiasis (K80.-)

K82.8   **Other specified diseases of gallbladder**
Adhesions of cystic duct or gallbladder
Atrophy of cystic duct or gallbladder
Cyst of cystic duct or gallbladder
Dyskinesia of cystic duct or gallbladder
Hypertrophy of cystic duct or gallbladder
Nonfunctioning of cystic duct or gallbladder
Ulcer of cystic duct or gallbladder

K82.9   **Disease of gallbladder, unspecified**

● K82.A   **Disorders of gallbladder in diseases classified elsewhere**
Code first the type of cholecystitis (K81.-), or cholelithiasis with cholecystitis (K80.00-K80.19, K80.40-K80.47, K80.60-K80.67)

   ▶ *K82.A1*   *Gangrene of gallbladder in cholecystitis*
     Coding Clinic: 2018, Q4, P20

   ● **K82.A2**   **Perforation of gallbladder in cholecystitis**
     Coding Clinic: 2018, Q4, P20

CHAPTER 11 (K00-K95)

● **K83   Other diseases of biliary tract**
    Excludes1   postcholecystectomy syndrome (K91.5)
    Excludes2   conditions involving the gallbladder (K81-K82)
                 conditions involving the cystic duct (K81-K82)

  ● **K83.0   Cholangitis**
      Excludes1   cholangitic liver abscess (K75.0)
                 cholangitis with choledocholithiasis
                   (K80.3-, K80.4-)

      Excludes2   chronic nonsuppurative destructive
                 cholangitis (K74.3)
                 primary biliary cholangitis (K74.3)
                 primary biliary cirrhosis (K74.3)

    K83.01   Primary sclerosing cholangitis
        Coding Clinic: 2018, Q4, P21

    K83.09   Other cholangitis
        Ascending cholangitis
        Cholangitis NOS
        Primary cholangitis
        Recurrent cholangitis
        Sclerosing cholangitis
        Secondary cholangitis
        Stenosing cholangitis
        Suppurative cholangitis

  K83.1   Obstruction of bile duct
      Occlusion of bile duct without cholelithiasis
      Stenosis of bile duct without cholelithiasis
      Stricture of bile duct without cholelithiasis
      Excludes1   congenital obstruction of bile duct (Q44.3)
                 obstruction of bile duct with cholelithiasis
                   (K80.-)
      Coding Clinic: 2016, Q1, P18

  K83.2   Perforation of bile duct
      Rupture of bile duct

  K83.3   Fistula of bile duct
      Choledochoduodenal fistula

  K83.4   Spasm of sphincter of Oddi

  K83.5   Biliary cyst

  K83.8   Other specified diseases of biliary tract
      Adhesions of biliary tract
      Atrophy of biliary tract
      Hypertrophy of biliary tract
      Ulcer of biliary tract

  K83.9   Disease of biliary tract, unspecified

● **K85   Acute pancreatitis**
    Inflammatory process in which pancreatic enzymes autodigest the gland
    Includes   acute (recurrent) pancreatitis
             subacute pancreatitis
    Coding Clinic: 2016, Q4, P34

  ● **K85.0   Idiopathic acute pancreatitis**
    K85.00   Idiopathic acute pancreatitis without necrosis or infection
    K85.01   Idiopathic acute pancreatitis with uninfected necrosis
    K85.02   Idiopathic acute pancreatitis with infected necrosis

  ● **K85.1   Biliary acute pancreatitis**
      Gallstone pancreatitis
    K85.10   Biliary acute pancreatitis without necrosis or infection

    K85.11   Biliary acute pancreatitis with uninfected necrosis
    K85.12   Biliary acute pancreatitis with infected necrosis

  ● **K85.2   Alcohol induced acute pancreatitis**
      Excludes2   alcohol induced chronic pancreatitis
                 (K86.0)
    K85.20   Alcohol induced acute pancreatitis without necrosis or infection
        Coding Clinic: 2020, Q1, P9
    K85.21   Alcohol induced acute pancreatitis with uninfected necrosis
    K85.22   Alcohol induced acute pancreatitis with infected necrosis

  ● **K85.3   Drug induced acute pancreatitis**
      Use additional code for adverse effect, if applicable, to identify drug (T36-T50 with fifth or sixth character 5)
      Use additional code to identify drug abuse and dependence (F11.-F17.-)
    K85.30   Drug induced acute pancreatitis without necrosis or infection
    K85.31   Drug induced acute pancreatitis with uninfected necrosis
    K85.32   Drug induced acute pancreatitis with infected necrosis

  ● **K85.8   Other acute pancreatitis**
    K85.80   Other acute pancreatitis without necrosis or infection
    K85.81   Other acute pancreatitis with uninfected necrosis
    K85.82   Other acute pancreatitis with infected necrosis

  ● **K85.9   Acute pancreatitis, unspecified**
      Pancreatitis NOS
    K85.90   Acute pancreatitis without necrosis or infection, unspecified
    K85.91   Acute pancreatitis with uninfected necrosis, unspecified
    K85.92   Acute pancreatitis with infected necrosis, unspecified

● **K86   Other diseases of pancreas**
    Excludes2   fibrocystic disease of pancreas (E84.-)
               islet cell tumor (of pancreas) (D13.7)
               pancreatic steatorrhea (K90.3)

  K86.0   Alcohol-induced chronic pancreatitis 🐾
      Use additional code to identify:
        alcohol abuse and dependence (F10.-)
      Code also exocrine pancreatic insufficiency (K86.81)
      Excludes2   alcohol induced acute pancreatitis (K85.2-)

  K86.1   Other chronic pancreatitis 🐾
      Chronic pancreatitis NOS
      Infectious chronic pancreatitis
      Recurrent chronic pancreatitis
      Relapsing chronic pancreatitis
      Code also exocrine pancreatic insufficiency (K86.81)

  K86.2   Cyst of pancreas

  K86.3   Pseudocyst of pancreas

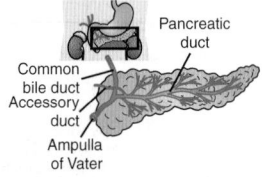

Figure 11-15   Pancreatic ductal system.

▶ New   ⇒ Revised   ~~deleted~~ Deleted   Excludes 1   Excludes 2   Includes   Use additional   Code first   Code also   Key words
OGCR Official Guidelines   X Assign placeholder X   ● Use Additional Character(s)   ▷ Manifestation Code   🐾 Hierarchical Condition Category   Coding Clinic

● **K86.8   Other specified diseases of pancreas**
Coding Clinic: 2016, Q4, P34

     K86.81   Exocrine pancreatic insufficiency

     K86.89   Other specified diseases of pancreas
         Aseptic pancreatic necrosis, unrelated to acute pancreatitis
         Atrophy of pancreas
         Calculus of pancreas
         Cirrhosis of pancreas
         Fibrosis of pancreas
         Pancreatic fat necrosis, unrelated to acute pancreatitis
         Pancreatic infantilism
         Pancreatic necrosis NOS, unrelated to acute pancreatitis

   K86.9   Disease of pancreas, unspecified

▸ *K87*   *Disorders of gallbladder, biliary tract and pancreas in diseases classified elsewhere*

     Code first underlying disease

     Excludes1   cytomegaloviral pancreatitis (B25.2)
                 mumps pancreatitis (B26.3)
                 syphilitic gallbladder (A52.74)
                 syphilitic pancreas (A52.74)
                 tuberculosis of gallbladder (A18.83)
                 tuberculosis of pancreas (A18.83)

OTHER DISEASES OF THE DIGESTIVE SYSTEM (K90-K95)

● **K90   Intestinal malabsorption**

     Excludes1   intestinal malabsorption following gastrointestinal surgery (K91.2)

   K90.0   Celiac disease
       Celiac disease with steatorrhea
       Celiac gluten-sensitive enteropathy
       Nontropical sprue

       Use additional code for associated disorders including:
         dermatitis herpetiformis (L13.0)
         gluten ataxia (G32.81)

       Code also exocrine pancreatic insufficiency (K86.81)

   K90.1   Tropical sprue
       Sprue NOS
       Tropical steatorrhea

   K90.2   Blind loop syndrome, not elsewhere classified
       Blind loop syndrome NOS

       Excludes1   congenital blind loop syndrome (Q43.8)
                 postsurgical blind loop syndrome (K91.2)

   K90.3   Pancreatic steatorrhea

● **K90.4   Other malabsorption due to intolerance**

       Excludes2   celiac gluten-sensitive enteropathy (K90.0)
                 lactose intolerance (E73.-)
       Coding Clinic: 2016, Q4, P35-36

     K90.41   Non-celiac gluten sensitivity
         Gluten sensitivity NOS
         Non-celiac gluten sensitive enteropathy

     K90.49   Malabsorption due to intolerance, not elsewhere classified
         Malabsorption due to intolerance to carbohydrate
         Malabsorption due to intolerance to fat
         Malabsorption due to intolerance to protein
         Malabsorption due to intolerance to starch

● **K90.8   Other intestinal malabsorption**

     K90.81   Whipple's disease

     K90.89   Other intestinal malabsorption

   K90.9   Intestinal malabsorption, unspecified
Coding Clinic: 2017, Q4, P108-109

● **K91   Intraoperative and postprocedural complications and disorders of digestive system, not elsewhere classified**

     Excludes2   complications of artificial opening of digestive system (K94.-)
                 complications of bariatric procedures (K95.-)
                 gastrojejunal ulcer (K28.-)
                 postprocedural (radiation) retroperitoneal abscess (K68.11)
                 radiation colitis (K52.0)
                 radiation gastroenteritis (K52.0)
                 radiation proctitis (K62.7)
     Coding Clinic: 2016, Q4, P10

   K91.0   Vomiting following gastrointestinal surgery

   K91.1   Postgastric surgery syndromes
       Dumping syndrome
       Postgastrectomy syndrome
       Postvagotomy syndrome

   K91.2   Postsurgical malabsorption, not elsewhere classified
       Postsurgical blind loop syndrome

       Excludes1   malabsorption osteomalacia in adults (M83.2)
                 malabsorption osteoporosis, postsurgical (M80.8-, M81.8)

● **K91.3   Postprocedural intestinal obstruction**
Coding Clinic: 2017, Q1, P40-41

     K91.30   Postprocedural intestinal obstruction, unspecified as to partial versus complete
         Postprocedural intestinal obstruction NOS

     K91.31   Postprocedural partial intestinal obstruction
         Postprocedural incomplete intestinal obstruction

     K91.32   Postprocedural complete intestinal obstruction

   K91.5   Postcholecystectomy syndrome

● **K91.6   Intraoperative hemorrhage and hematoma of a digestive system organ or structure complicating a procedure**

       Excludes1   intraoperative hemorrhage and hematoma of a digestive system organ or structure due to accidental puncture and laceration during a procedure (K91.7-)

     K91.61   Intraoperative hemorrhage and hematoma of a digestive system organ or structure complicating a digestive system procedure
Coding Clinic: 2020, Q1, P20

     K91.62   Intraoperative hemorrhage and hematoma of a digestive system organ or structure complicating other procedure

● **K91.7   Accidental puncture and laceration of a digestive system organ or structure during a procedure**

     K91.71   Accidental puncture and laceration of a digestive system organ or structure during a digestive system procedure
Coding Clinic: 2021, Q2, P12

     K91.72   Accidental puncture and laceration of a digestive system organ or structure during other procedure
Coding Clinic: 2019, Q2, P24

● **K91.8   Other intraoperative and postprocedural complications and disorders of digestive system**

     K91.81   Other intraoperative complications of digestive system

     K91.82   Postprocedural hepatic failure

     K91.83   Postprocedural hepatorenal syndrome

   ● **K91.84   Postprocedural hemorrhage of a digestive system organ or structure following a procedure**

       K91.840   Postprocedural hemorrhage of a digestive system organ or structure following a digestive system procedure
Coding Clinic: 2016, Q1, P15

       K91.841   Postprocedural hemorrhage of a digestive system organ or structure following other procedure

CHAPTER 11 (K00-K95)

● **K91.85** **Complications of intestinal pouch**
  K91.850 **Pouchitis** 🝔
    Inflammation of internal ileoanal pouch
  K91.858 **Other complications of intestinal pouch** 🝔
    Coding Clinic: 2019, Q2, P13
  K91.86 **Retained cholelithiasis** following cholecystectomy
● **K91.87** **Postprocedural hematoma and seroma** of a digestive system organ or structure following a procedure
  K91.870 **Postprocedural hematoma** of a digestive system organ or structure following a **digestive system procedure**
  K91.871 **Postprocedural hematoma** of a digestive system organ or structure following **other procedure**
  K91.872 **Postprocedural seroma** of a digestive system organ or structure following a digestive system procedure
  K91.873 **Postprocedural seroma** of a digestive system organ or structure following **other procedure**
  K91.89 **Other postprocedural complications** and disorders of digestive system
    Use additional code, if applicable, to further specify disorder
    Excludes2 postprocedural retroperitoneal abscess (K68.11)
    Coding Clinic: 2017, Q1, P41

● **K92** **Other diseases of digestive system**
  Excludes1 neonatal gastrointestinal hemorrhage (P54.0-P54.3)
  K92.0 **Hematemesis**
  K92.1 **Melena**
    Excludes1 occult blood in feces (R19.5)
  K92.2 **Gastrointestinal hemorrhage, unspecified**
    Gastric hemorrhage NOS
    Intestinal hemorrhage NOS
    Excludes1 acute hemorrhagic gastritis (K29.01)
    hemorrhage of anus and rectum (K62.5)
    angiodysplasia of stomach with hemorrhage (K31.811)
    diverticular disease with hemorrhage (K57.-)
    gastritis and duodenitis with hemorrhage (K29.-)
    peptic ulcer with hemorrhage (K25-K28)
    Coding Clinic: 2021, Q1, P12
  K92.8 **Other specified diseases of the digestive system**
    K92.81 **Gastrointestinal mucositis (ulcerative)**
      Code also type of associated therapy, such as:
      antineoplastic and immunosuppressive drugs (T45.1X-)
      radiological procedure and radiotherapy (Y84.2)
      Excludes2 mucositis (ulcerative) of vagina and vulva (N76.81)
      nasal mucositis (ulcerative) (J34.81)
      oral mucositis (ulcerative) (K12.3-)
    K92.89 **Other specified diseases of the digestive system**
  K92.9 **Disease of digestive system, unspecified**

● **K94** **Complications of artificial openings of the digestive system**
● **K94.0** **Colostomy complications**
  K94.00 **Colostomy complication, unspecified** 🝔
  K94.01 **Colostomy hemorrhage** 🝔
  K94.02 **Colostomy infection** 🝔
    Use additional code to specify type of infection, such as:
    cellulitis of abdominal wall (L03.311)
    sepsis (A40.-, A41.-)
  K94.03 **Colostomy malfunction** 🝔
    Mechanical complication of colostomy
  K94.09 **Other complications of colostomy** 🝔
● **K94.1** **Enterostomy complications**
  K94.10 **Enterostomy complication, unspecified** 🝔
  K94.11 **Enterostomy hemorrhage** 🝔
  K94.12 **Enterostomy infection** 🝔
    Use additional code to specify type of infection, such as:
    cellulitis of abdominal wall (L03.311)
    sepsis (A40.-, A41.-)
  K94.13 **Enterostomy malfunction** 🝔
    Mechanical complication of enterostomy
  K94.19 **Other complications of enterostomy** 🝔
● **K94.2** **Gastrostomy complications**
  K94.20 **Gastrostomy complication, unspecified** 🝔
  K94.21 **Gastrostomy hemorrhage** 🝔
  K94.22 **Gastrostomy infection** 🝔
    Use additional code to specify type of infection, such as:
    cellulitis of abdominal wall (L03.311)
    sepsis (A40.-, A41.-)
  K94.23 **Gastrostomy malfunction** 🝔
    Mechanical complication of gastrostomy
  K94.29 **Other complications of gastrostomy** 🝔
● **K94.3** **Esophagostomy complications**
  K94.30 **Esophagostomy complications, unspecified** 🝔
  K94.31 **Esophagostomy hemorrhage** 🝔
  K94.32 **Esophagostomy infection** 🝔
    Use additional code to identify the infection
  K94.33 **Esophagostomy malfunction** 🝔
    Mechanical complication of esophagostomy
  K94.39 **Other complications of esophagostomy** 🝔

● **K95** **Complications of bariatric procedures**
● **K95.0** **Complications of gastric band procedure**
  K95.01 **Infection due to gastric band procedure**
    Use additional code to specify type of infection or organism, such as:
    bacterial and viral infectious agents (B95.-, B96.-)
    cellulitis of abdominal wall (L03.311)
    sepsis (A40.-, A41.-)
  K95.09 **Other complications of gastric band procedure**
    Use additional code, if applicable, to further specify complication
● **K95.8** **Complications of other bariatric procedure**
  Excludes1 complications of gastric band surgery (K95.0-)
  K95.81 **Infection due to other bariatric procedure**
    Use additional code to specify type of infection or organism, such as:
    bacterial and viral infectious agents (B95.-, B96.-)
    cellulitis of abdominal wall (L03.311)
    sepsis (A40.-, A41.-)
  K95.89 **Other complications of other bariatric procedure**
    Use additional code, if applicable, to further specify complication

CHAPTER 12

DISEASES OF THE SKIN AND SUBCUTANEOUS TISSUE (L00-L99)

OGCR Chapter-Specific Coding Guidelines

12. Chapter 12: Diseases of the Skin and Subcutaneous Tissue (L00-L99)

a. Pressure ulcer stage codes

1) Pressure ulcer stages

Codes from category L89, Pressure ulcer, identify the site of the pressure ulcer as well as the stage of the ulcer.

The ICD-10-CM classifies pressure ulcer stages based on severity, which is designated by stages 1-4, unspecified stage and unstageable.

Assign as many codes from category L89 as needed to identify all the pressure ulcers the patient has, if applicable.

See Section I.B.14 for pressure ulcer stage documentation by clinicians other than patient's provider.

2) Unstageable pressure ulcers

Assignment of the code for unstageable pressure ulcer (L89.--0) should be based on the clinical documentation. These codes are used for pressure ulcers whose stage cannot be clinically determined (e.g., the ulcer is covered by eschar or has been treated with a skin or muscle graft) and pressure ulcers that are documented as deep tissue injury but not documented as due to trauma. This code should not be confused with the codes for unspecified stage (L89.--9). When there is no documentation regarding the stage of the pressure ulcer, assign the appropriate code for unspecified stage (L89.--9).

3) Documented pressure ulcer stage

Assignment of the pressure ulcer stage code should be guided by clinical documentation of the stage or documentation of the terms found in the Alphabetic Index. For clinical terms describing the stage that are not found in the Alphabetic Index, and there is no documentation of the stage, the provider should be queried.

4) Patients admitted with pressure ulcers documented as healed

No code is assigned if the documentation states that the pressure ulcer is completely healed.

5) Patients admitted with pressure ulcers documented as healing

Pressure ulcers described as healing should be assigned the appropriate pressure ulcer stage code based on the documentation in the medical record. If the documentation does not provide information about the stage of the healing pressure ulcer, assign the appropriate code for unspecified stage.

If the documentation is unclear as to whether the patient has a current (new) pressure ulcer or if the patient is being treated for a healing pressure ulcer, query the provider.

For ulcers that were present on admission but healed at the time of discharge, assign the code for the site and stage of the pressure ulcer at the time of admission.

6) Patient admitted with pressure ulcer evolving into another stage during the admission

If a patient is admitted to an inpatient hospital with a pressure ulcer at one stage and it progresses to a higher stage, two separate codes should be assigned: one code for the site and stage of the ulcer on admission and a second code for the same ulcer site and the highest stage reported during the stay.

b. Non-Pressure Chronic Ulcers

1) Patients admitted with non-pressure ulcers documented as healed

No code is assigned if the documentation states that the non-pressure ulcer is completely healed.

2) Patients admitted with non-pressure ulcers documented as healing

Non-pressure ulcers described as healing should be assigned the appropriate non-pressure ulcer code based on the documentation in the medical record. If the documentation does not provide information about the severity of the healing non-pressure ulcer, assign the appropriate code for unspecified severity.

If the documentation is unclear as to whether the patient has a current (new) non-pressure ulcer or if the patient is being treated for a healing non-pressure ulcer, query the provider.

For ulcers that were present on admission but healed at the time of discharge, assign the code for the site and severity of the non-pressure ulcer at the time of admission.

3) Patient admitted with non-pressure ulcer that progresses to another severity level during the admission

If a patient is admitted to an inpatient hospital with a non-pressure ulcer at one severity level and it progresses to a higher severity level, two separate codes should be assigned: one code for the site and severity level of the ulcer on admission and a second code for the same ulcer site and the highest severity level reported during the stay.

See Section I.B.14 for pressure ulcer stage documentation by clinicians other than patient's provider.

Figure 12-1 Furuncle, also known as a boil, is a staphylococcal infection. The organism enters the body through a hair follicle and so furuncles usually appear in hairy areas of the body. A cluster of furuncles is known as a carbuncle and involves infection into the deep subcutaneous fascia. These usually appear on the back and neck. (**B** from Habif TP, Binnick AN, Meyerson LB: Clinical Dermatology: A Color Guide to Diagnosis and Therapy, S.l., Mosby Elsevier, 2010)

CHAPTER 12

DISEASES OF THE SKIN AND SUBCUTANEOUS TISSUE (L00-L99)

Excludes2 certain conditions originating in the perinatal period (P04-P96)
certain infectious and parasitic diseases (A00-B99)
complications of pregnancy, childbirth and the puerperium (O00-O9A)
congenital malformations, deformations, and chromosomal abnormalities (Q00-Q99)
endocrine, nutritional and metabolic diseases (E00-E88)
lipomelanotic reticulosis (I89.8)
neoplasms (C00-D49)
symptoms, signs and abnormal clinical and laboratory findings, not elsewhere classified (R00-R94)
systemic connective tissue disorders (M30-M36)
viral warts (B07.-)

This chapter contains the following blocks:

L00-L08	Infections of the skin and subcutaneous tissue
L10-L14	Bullous disorders
L20-L30	Dermatitis and eczema
L40-L45	Papulosquamous disorders
L49-L54	Urticaria and erythema
L55-L59	Radiation-related disorders of the skin and subcutaneous tissue
L60-L75	Disorders of skin appendages
L76	Intraoperative and postprocedural complications of skin and subcutaneous tissue
L80-L99	Other disorders of the skin and subcutaneous tissue

INFECTIONS OF THE SKIN AND SUBCUTANEOUS TISSUE (L00-L08)

Use additional code (B95-B97) to identify infectious agent.

Excludes2   hordeolum (H00.0)
infective dermatitis (L30.3)
local infections of skin classified in Chapter 1
lupus panniculitis (L93.2)
panniculitis NOS (M79.3)
panniculitis of neck and back (M54.0-)
Perlèche NOS (K13.0)
Perlèche due to candidiasis (B37.0)
Perlèche due to riboflavin deficiency (E53.0)
pyogenic granuloma (L98.0)
relapsing panniculitis [Weber-Christian] (M35.6)
viral warts (B07.-)
zoster (B02.-)

L00   **Staphylococcal scalded skin syndrome**
Ritter's disease

Use additional code to identify percentage of skin exfoliation (L49.-)

Excludes1   bullous impetigo (L01.03)
pemphigus neonatorum (L01.03)
toxic epidermal necrolysis [Lyell] (L51.2)

● **L01**   **Impetigo**
Contagious skin infection caused by a streptococcus or staphylococcus aureus, common skin infections among children

Excludes1   impetigo herpetiformis (L40.1)

● **L01.0**   **Impetigo**
Impetigo contagiosa
Impetigo vulgaris

L01.00   **Impetigo, unspecified**
Impetigo NOS

L01.01   **Non-bullous impetigo**

L01.02   **Bockhart's impetigo**
Impetigo follicularis
Perifolliculitis NOS
Superficial pustular perifolliculitis

L01.03   **Bullous impetigo**
Impetigo neonatorum
Pemphigus neonatorum
Neonate = newborn

L01.09   **Other impetigo**
Ulcerative impetigo

L01.1   **Impetiginization of other dermatoses**

● **L02**   **Cutaneous abscess, furuncle and carbuncle**
Use additional code to identify organism (B95-B96)

Excludes2   abscess of anus and rectal regions (K61.-)
abscess of female genital organs (external) (N76.4)
abscess of male genital organs (external) (N48.2, N49.-)

● **L02.0**   **Cutaneous abscess, furuncle and carbuncle of face**

Excludes2   abscess of ear, external (H60.0)
abscess of eyelid (H00.0)
abscess of head [any part, except face] (L02.8)
abscess of lacrimal gland (H04.0)
abscess of lacrimal passages (H04.3)
abscess of mouth (K12.2)
abscess of nose (J34.0)
abscess of orbit (H05.0)
submandibular abscess (K12.2)

L02.01   **Cutaneous abscess of face**

Boil of face
Folliculitis of face

L02.03   **Carbuncle of face**

● **L02.1**   **Cutaneous abscess, furuncle and carbuncle of neck**

L02.11   **Cutaneous abscess of neck**

L02.12   **Furuncle of neck**
Boil of neck
Folliculitis of neck

L02.13   **Carbuncle of neck**

● **L02.2**   **Cutaneous abscess, furuncle and carbuncle of trunk**

Excludes1   non-newborn omphalitis (L08.82)
omphalitis of newborn (P38.-)

Excludes2   abscess of breast (N61.1)
abscess of buttocks (L02.3)
abscess of female external genital organs (N76.4)
abscess of male external genital organs (N48.2, N49.-)
abscess of hip (L02.4)

● **L02.21**   **Cutaneous abscess of trunk**

L02.211   **Cutaneous abscess of abdominal wall**

L02.212   **Cutaneous abscess of back [any part, except buttock]**

L02.213   **Cutaneous abscess of chest wall**

L02.214   **Cutaneous abscess of groin**

L02.215   **Cutaneous abscess of perineum**

L02.216   **Cutaneous abscess of umbilicus**

L02.219   **Cutaneous abscess of trunk, unspecified**

● **L02.22**   **Furuncle of trunk**
Boil of trunk
Folliculitis of trunk

L02.221   **Furuncle of abdominal wall**

L02.222   **Furuncle of back [any part, except buttock]**

L02.223   **Furuncle of chest wall**

L02.224   **Furuncle of groin**

L02.225   **Furuncle of perineum**

L02.226   **Furuncle of umbilicus**

L02.229   **Furuncle of trunk, unspecified**

● **L02.23**   **Carbuncle of trunk**

L02.231   **Carbuncle of abdominal wall**

L02.232   **Carbuncle of back [any part, except buttock]**

L02.233   **Carbuncle of chest wall**

L02.234   **Carbuncle of groin**

L02.235   **Carbuncle of perineum**

L02.236   **Carbuncle of umbilicus**

L02.239   **Carbuncle of trunk, unspecified**

● **L02.3**   **Cutaneous abscess, furuncle and carbuncle of buttock**

Excludes1   pilonidal cyst with abscess (L05.01)

L02.31   **Cutaneous abscess of buttock**
Cutaneous abscess of gluteal region

L02.32   **Furuncle of buttock**
Boil of buttock
Folliculitis of buttock
Furuncle of gluteal region

L02.33   **Carbuncle of buttock**
Carbuncle of gluteal region

Figure 12-2 Impetigo. A thick, honey-yellow adherent crust covers the entire eroded surface. (From James WD, Elston DM, Berger TG, Andrews GC: Andrews' Diseases of the Skin: Clinical Dermatology, London, Saunders/Elsevier, 2011)

L02.02   **Furuncle of face**

▶ New   ⇒ Revised   ~~deleted~~ Deleted   Excludes 1   Excludes 2   Includes   Use additional   Code first   Code also   Key words

OGCR Official Guidelines   X Assign placeholder X   ● Use Additional Character(s)   ❱ Manifestation Code   🔖 Hierarchical Condition Category   **Coding Clinic**

● **L02.4**   Cutaneous abscess, furuncle and carbuncle of limb
    Excludes2   Cutaneous abscess, furuncle and
        carbuncle of groin (L02.214, L02.224,
        L02.234)
        Cutaneous abscess, furuncle and
        carbuncle of hand (L02.5-)
        Cutaneous abscess, furuncle and
        carbuncle of foot (L02.6-)

  ● **L02.41**   Cutaneous abscess of limb
      L02.411   Cutaneous abscess of right axilla
      L02.412   Cutaneous abscess of left axilla
      L02.413   Cutaneous abscess of right upper limb
      L02.414   Cutaneous abscess of left upper limb
      L02.415   Cutaneous abscess of right lower limb
      L02.416   Cutaneous abscess of left lower limb
      L02.419   Cutaneous abscess of limb, unspecified

  ● **L02.42**   Furuncle of limb
      Boil of limb
      Folliculitis of limb
      L02.421   Furuncle of right axilla
      L02.422   Furuncle of left axilla
      L02.423   Furuncle of right upper limb
      L02.424   Furuncle of left upper limb
      L02.425   Furuncle of right lower limb
      L02.426   Furuncle of left lower limb
      L02.429   Furuncle of limb, unspecified

  ● **L02.43**   Carbuncle of limb
      L02.431   Carbuncle of right axilla
      L02.432   Carbuncle of left axilla
      L02.433   Carbuncle of right upper limb
      L02.434   Carbuncle of left upper limb
      L02.435   Carbuncle of right lower limb
      L02.436   Carbuncle of left lower limb
      L02.439   Carbuncle of limb, unspecified

● **L02.5**   Cutaneous abscess, furuncle and carbuncle of hand
  ● **L02.51**   Cutaneous abscess of hand
      L02.511   Cutaneous abscess of right hand
      L02.512   Cutaneous abscess of left hand
      L02.519   Cutaneous abscess of unspecified hand

  ● **L02.52**   Furuncle hand
      Boil of hand
      Folliculitis of hand
      L02.521   Furuncle right hand
      L02.522   Furuncle left hand
      L02.529   Furuncle unspecified hand

  ● **L02.53**   Carbuncle of hand
      L02.531   Carbuncle of right hand
      L02.532   Carbuncle of left hand
      L02.539   Carbuncle of unspecified hand

● **L02.6**   Cutaneous abscess, furuncle and carbuncle of foot
  ● **L02.61**   Cutaneous abscess of foot
      L02.611   Cutaneous abscess of right foot
      L02.612   Cutaneous abscess of left foot
      L02.619   Cutaneous abscess of unspecified foot

  ● **L02.62**   Furuncle of foot
      Boil of foot
      Folliculitis of foot
      L02.621   Furuncle of right foot
      L02.622   Furuncle of left foot
      L02.629   Furuncle of unspecified foot

  ● **L02.63**   Carbuncle of foot
      L02.631   Carbuncle of right foot
      L02.632   Carbuncle of left foot
      L02.639   Carbuncle of unspecified foot

● **L02.8**   Cutaneous abscess, furuncle and carbuncle of other sites
  ● **L02.81**   Cutaneous abscess of other sites
      L02.811   Cutaneous abscess of head [any part, except face]
      L02.818   Cutaneous abscess of other sites

  ● **L02.82**   Furuncle of other sites
      Boil of other sites
      Folliculitis of other sites
      L02.821   Furuncle of head [any part, except face]
      L02.828   Furuncle of other sites

  ● **L02.83**   Carbuncle of other sites
      L02.831   Carbuncle of head [any part, except face]
      L02.838   Carbuncle of other sites

● **L02.9**   Cutaneous abscess, furuncle and carbuncle, unspecified
    L02.91   Cutaneous abscess, unspecified
    L02.92   Furuncle, unspecified
      Boil NOS
      Furunculosis NOS
    L02.93   Carbuncle, unspecified

● **L03**   Cellulitis and acute lymphangitis
    Excludes2   cellulitis of anal and rectal region (K61.-)
        cellulitis of external auditory canal (H60.1)
        cellulitis of eyelid (H00.0)
        cellulitis of female external genital organs (N76.4)
        cellulitis of lacrimal apparatus (H04.3)
        cellulitis of male external genital organs (N48.2, N49.-)
        cellulitis of mouth (K12.2)
        cellulitis of nose (J34.0)
        eosinophilic cellulitis [Wells] (L98.3)
        febrile neutrophilic dermatosis [Sweet] (L98.2)
        lymphangitis (chronic) (subacute) (I89.1)

● **L03.0**   Cellulitis and acute lymphangitis of finger and toe
    Infection of nail
    Onychia
    Paronychia
    Perionychia

  ● **L03.01**   Cellulitis of finger
      Felon
      Whitlow
      Excludes1   herpetic whitlow (B00.89)
      L03.011   Cellulitis of right finger
      L03.012   Cellulitis of left finger
      L03.019   Cellulitis of unspecified finger

  ● **L03.02**   Acute lymphangitis of finger
      Hangnail with lymphangitis of finger
      L03.021   Acute lymphangitis of right finger
      L03.022   Acute lymphangitis of left finger
      L03.029   Acute lymphangitis of unspecified finger

  ● **L03.03**   Cellulitis of toe
      L03.031   Cellulitis of right toe
      L03.032   Cellulitis of left toe
      L03.039   Cellulitis of unspecified toe

  ● **L03.04**   Acute lymphangitis of toe
      Hangnail with lymphangitis of toe
      L03.041   Acute lymphangitis of right toe
      L03.042   Acute lymphangitis of left toe
      L03.049   Acute lymphangitis of unspecified toe

Item 12-1 Onychia is an inflammation of the tissue surrounding the nail with pus accumulation and loss of the nail, resulting from microscopic pathogens entering through small wounds. **Paronychia** is a nail disease also known as felon or whitlow and is a bacterial or fungal infection.

CHAPTER 12 (L00-L99)

Item 12-2 **Cellulitis** is an acute spreading bacterial infection below the surface of the skin characterized by redness (erythema), warmth, swelling, pain, fever, chills, and enlarged lymph nodes ("swollen glands").

- **L03.1**   Cellulitis and acute lymphangitis of other parts of limb
  - **L03.11**   Cellulitis of other parts of limb
    - **Excludes2**   cellulitis of fingers (L03.01-)
      cellulitis of toes (L03.03-)
      groin (L03.314)
    - L03.111   Cellulitis of right axilla
    - L03.112   Cellulitis of left axilla
    - L03.113   Cellulitis of right upper limb
    - L03.114   Cellulitis of left upper limb
      Coding Clinic: 2019, Q1, P13
    - L03.115   Cellulitis of right lower limb
    - L03.116   Cellulitis of left lower limb
    - L03.119   Cellulitis of unspecified part of limb
  - **L03.12**   Acute lymphangitis of other parts of limb
    - **Excludes2**   acute lymphangitis of fingers (L03.2-)
      acute lymphangitis of toes (L03.04-)
      acute lymphangitis of groin (L03.324)
    - L03.121   Acute lymphangitis of right axilla
    - L03.122   Acute lymphangitis of left axilla
    - L03.123   Acute lymphangitis of right upper limb
    - L03.124   Acute lymphangitis of left upper limb
    - L03.125   Acute lymphangitis of right lower limb
    - L03.126   Acute lymphangitis of left lower limb
    - L03.129   Acute lymphangitis of unspecified part of limb
- **L03.2**   Cellulitis and acute lymphangitis of face and neck
  - **L03.21**   Cellulitis and acute lymphangitis of face
    - L03.211   Cellulitis of face
      - **Excludes2**   abscess of orbit (H05.01-)
        cellulitis of ear (H60.1-)
        cellulitis of eyelid (H00.0-)
        cellulitis of head (L03.81)
        cellulitis of lacrimal apparatus (H04.3)
        cellulitis of lip (K13.0)
        cellulitis of mouth (K12.2)
        cellulitis of nose (internal) (J34.0)
        cellulitis of orbit (H05.01-)
        cellulitis of scalp (L03.81)
    - L03.212   Acute lymphangitis of face
    - L03.213   Periorbital cellulitis
      Preseptal cellulitis
      Coding Clinic: 2016, Q4, P36
  - **L03.22**   Cellulitis and acute lymphangitis of neck
    - L03.221   Cellulitis of neck
    - L03.222   Acute lymphangitis of neck
- **L03.3**   Cellulitis and acute lymphangitis of trunk
  - **L03.31**   Cellulitis of trunk
    - **Excludes2**   cellulitis of anal and rectal regions (K61.-)
      cellulitis of breast NOS (N61.0)
      cellulitis of female external genital organs (N76.4)
      cellulitis of male external genital organs (N48.2, N49.-)
      omphalitis of newborn (P38.-)
      puerperal cellulitis of breast (O91.2)
    - L03.311   Cellulitis of abdominal wall
      - **Excludes2**   cellulitis of umbilicus (L03.316)
        cellulitis of groin (L03.314)
    - L03.312   Cellulitis of back [any part except buttock]
    - L03.313   Cellulitis of chest wall
    - L03.314   Cellulitis of groin
    - L03.315   Cellulitis of perineum
    - L03.316   Cellulitis of umbilicus
    - L03.317   Cellulitis of buttock
    - L03.319   Cellulitis of trunk, unspecified
  - **L03.32**   Acute lymphangitis of trunk
    - L03.321   Acute lymphangitis of abdominal wall
    - L03.322   Acute lymphangitis of back [any part except buttock]
    - L03.323   Acute lymphangitis of chest wall
    - L03.324   Acute lymphangitis of groin
    - L03.325   Acute lymphangitis of perineum
    - L03.326   Acute lymphangitis of umbilicus
    - L03.327   Acute lymphangitis of buttock
    - L03.329   Acute lymphangitis of trunk, unspecified
- **L03.8**   Cellulitis and acute lymphangitis of other sites
  - **L03.81**   Cellulitis of other sites
    - L03.811   Cellulitis of head [any part, except face]
      Cellulitis of scalp
      - **Excludes2**   cellulitis of face (L03.211)
    - L03.818   Cellulitis of other sites
  - **L03.89**   Acute lymphangitis of other sites
    - L03.891   Acute lymphangitis of head [any part, except face]
    - L03.898   Acute lymphangitis of other sites
- **L03.9**   Cellulitis and acute lymphangitis, unspecified
  - L03.90   Cellulitis, unspecified
  - L03.91   Acute lymphangitis, unspecified
    - **Excludes1**   lymphangitis NOS (I89.1)

▶ New   ⟹ Revised   ~~deleted~~ Deleted   Excludes 1   Excludes 2   Includes   Use additional   Code first   Code also   Key words
OGCR Official Guidelines   X Assign placeholder X   ● Use Additional Character(s)   ▶ Manifestation Code   Hierarchical Condition Category   **Coding Clinic**

Item 12–3 **Abscess** is a localized collection of pus in tissues or organs and is a sign of infection, resulting in swelling and inflammation.

Item 12–4 **Pilonidal cyst,** also called a coccygeal cyst, is the result of a disorder called pilonidal disease. The cyst usually contains hair and pus.

● **L04** **Acute lymphadenitis**
   Short-term inflammation of lymph nodes which can be regionalized to involve a given area of the lymph system or systemic involving much of the body

   Includes abscess (acute) of lymph nodes, except mesenteric
   acute lymphadenitis, except mesenteric

   Excludes1 chronic or subacute lymphadenitis, except mesenteric (I88.1)
   enlarged lymph nodes (R59.-)
   human immunodeficiency virus [HIV] disease resulting in generalized lymphadenopathy (B20)
   lymphadenitis NOS (I88.9)
   nonspecific mesenteric lymphadenitis (I88.0)

   L04.0 **Acute lymphadenitis of face, head and neck**
   L04.1 **Acute lymphadenitis of trunk**
   L04.2 **Acute lymphadenitis of upper limb**
   Acute lymphadenitis of axilla
   Acute lymphadenitis of shoulder
   L04.3 **Acute lymphadenitis of lower limb**
   Acute lymphadenitis of hip
   Excludes2 acute lymphadenitis of groin (L04.1)
   L04.8 **Acute lymphadenitis of other sites**
   L04.9 **Acute lymphadenitis, unspecified**

● **L05** **Pilonidal cyst and sinus**
   ● L05.0 **Pilonidal cyst and sinus with abscess**
   L05.01 **Pilonidal cyst with abscess**
   Pilonidal abscess
   Pilonidal dimple with abscess
   Postanal dimple with abscess
   Excludes2 congenital sacral dimple (Q82.6)
   parasacral dimple (Q82.6)
   L05.02 **Pilonidal sinus with abscess**
   Coccygeal fistula with abscess
   Coccygeal sinus with abscess
   Pilonidal fistula with abscess
   ● L05.9 **Pilonidal cyst and sinus without abscess**
   L05.91 **Pilonidal cyst without abscess**
   Pilonidal dimple
   Postanal dimple
   Pilonidal cyst NOS
   Excludes2 congenital sacral dimple (Q82.6)
   parasacral dimple (Q82.6)
   L05.92 **Pilonidal sinus without abscess**
   Coccygeal fistula
   Coccygeal sinus without abscess
   Pilonidal fistula

● **L08** **Other local infections of skin and subcutaneous tissue**
   L08.0 **Pyoderma**
   Dermatitis gangrenosa
   Purulent dermatitis
   Septic dermatitis
   Suppurative dermatitis
   Excludes1 pyoderma gangrenosum (L88)
   pyoderma vegetans (L08.81)
   L08.1 **Erythrasma**

   L08.8 **Other specified local infections of the skin and subcutaneous tissue**
   L08.81 **Pyoderma vegetans**
   Excludes1 pyoderma gangrenosum (L88)
   pyoderma NOS (L08.0)
   L08.82 **Omphalitis not of newborn**
   Excludes1 omphalitis of newborn (P38.-)
   L08.89 **Other specified local infections of the skin and subcutaneous tissue**
   L08.9 **Local infection of the skin and subcutaneous tissue, unspecified**

BULLOUS DISORDERS (L10-L14)

   Excludes1 benign familial pemphigus [Hailey-Hailey] (Q82.8)
   staphylococcal scalded skin syndrome (L00)
   toxic epidermal necrolysis [Lyell] (L51.2)

● **L10** **Pemphigus**
   Excludes1 pemphigus neonatorum (L01.03)
   L10.0 **Pemphigus vulgaris**
   L10.1 **Pemphigus vegetans**
   L10.2 **Pemphigus foliaceous**
   L10.3 **Brazilian pemphigus [fogo selvagem]**
   L10.4 **Pemphigus erythematosus**
   Senear-Usher syndrome
   L10.5 **Drug-induced pemphigus**
   Use additional code for adverse effect, if applicable, to identify drug (T36-T50 with fifth or sixth character 5)
   L10.8 **Other pemphigus**
   L10.81 **Paraneoplastic pemphigus**
   L10.89 **Other pemphigus**
   L10.9 **Pemphigus, unspecified**

● **L11** **Other acantholytic disorders**
   L11.0 **Acquired keratosis follicularis**
   Excludes1 keratosis follicularis (congenital) [Darier-White] (Q82.8)
   L11.1 **Transient acantholytic dermatosis [Grover]**
   L11.8 **Other specified acantholytic disorders**
   L11.9 **Acantholytic disorder, unspecified**

● **L12** **Pemphigoid**
   Excludes1 herpes gestationis (O26.4-)
   impetigo herpetiformis (L40.1)
   L12.0 **Bullous pemphigoid**
   L12.1 **Cicatricial pemphigoid**
   Benign mucous membrane pemphigoid
   L12.2 **Chronic bullous disease of childhood**   P
   Juvenile dermatitis herpetiformis
   ● L12.3 **Acquired epidermolysis bullosa**
   Excludes1 epidermolysis bullosa (congenital) (Q81.-)
   L12.30 **Acquired epidermolysis bullosa, unspecified** 🔗
   L12.31 **Epidermolysis bullosa due to drug** 🔗
   Use additional code for adverse effect, if applicable, to identify drug (T36-T50 with fifth or sixth character 5)
   L12.35 **Other acquired epidermolysis bullosa** 🔗
   L12.8 **Other pemphigoid**
   L12.9 **Pemphigoid, unspecified**

CHAPTER 12 (L00-L99)

Item 12–5 Dermatitis herpetiformis, also known as Duhring's disease, is a systemic disease characterized by small blisters (3 to 5 mm) and occasionally large bullae (> 5 mm).

Figure 12-3 Dermatitis herpetiformis. (From Terhorst D: BASICS Dermatologie, München, Elsevier, Urban & Fischer, 2011)

● **L13 Other bullous disorders**

L13.0 Dermatitis herpetiformis
Duhring's disease
Hydroa herpetiformis
Excludes1 juvenile dermatitis herpetiformis (L12.2)
senile dermatitis herpetiformis (L12.0)

L13.1 Subcorneal pustular dermatitis
Sneddon-Wilkinson disease

L13.8 Other specified bullous disorders

L13.9 Bullous disorder, unspecified

▷ *L14 Bullous disorders in diseases classified elsewhere*
Code first underlying disease

DERMATITIS AND ECZEMA (L20-L30)

Note: In this block the terms dermatitis and eczema are used synonymously and interchangeably.
Excludes2 chronic (childhood) granulomatous disease (D71)
dermatitis gangrenosa (L08.0)
dermatitis herpetiformis (L13.0)
dry skin dermatitis (L85.3)
factitial dermatitis (L98.1)
perioral dermatitis (L71.0)
radiation-related disorders of the skin and
subcutaneous tissue (L55-L59)
stasis dermatitis (I87.2)

● **L20 Atopic dermatitis**

L20.0 Besnier's prurigo
● **L20.8 Other atopic dermatitis**
Excludes2 circumscribed neurodermatitis (L28.0)
L20.81 Atopic neurodermatitis
Diffuse neurodermatitis
L20.82 Flexural eczema
L20.83 Infantile (acute) (chronic) eczema   P
L20.84 Intrinsic (allergic) eczema
L20.89 Other atopic dermatitis
L20.9 Atopic dermatitis, unspecified

● **L21 Seborrheic dermatitis**
Excludes2 infective dermatitis (L30.3)
seborrheic keratosis (L82.-)

L21.0 Seborrhea capitis
Cradle cap
Coding Clinic: 2018, Q1, P6

L21.1 Seborrheic infantile dermatitis   P
L21.8 Other seborrheic dermatitis
L21.9 Seborrheic dermatitis, unspecified
Seborrhea NOS

L22 Diaper dermatitis
Diaper erythema
Diaper rash
Psoriasiform diaper rash

Item 12–6 Seborrheic dermatitis is characterized by greasy, scaly, red patches and is associated with oily skin and scalp.

Figure 12-4 Seborrheic dermatitis. (Getty Image)

Item 12–7 Atopic dermatitis, also known as atopic eczema, infantile eczema, disseminated neuro dermatitis, flexural eczema, and *prurigo diathesique* (Besnier), is characterized by intense itching and is often hereditary.

Figure 12-5 Atopic dermatitis. (From Chabner D-E: The Language of Medicine, St. Louis, MO, Saunders/Elsevier, 2007)

● **L23 Allergic contact dermatitis**
Excludes1 allergy NOS (T78.40)
contact dermatitis NOS (L25.9)
dermatitis NOS (L30.9)
Excludes2 dermatitis due to substances taken internally (L27.-)
dermatitis of eyelid (H01.1-)
diaper dermatitis (L22)
eczema of external ear (H60.5-)
irritant contact dermatitis (L24.-)
perioral dermatitis (L71.0)
radiation-related disorders of the skin and
subcutaneous tissue (L55-L59)

L23.0 Allergic contact dermatitis due to metals
Allergic contact dermatitis due to chromium
Allergic contact dermatitis due to nickel

L23.1 Allergic contact dermatitis due to adhesives
L23.2 Allergic contact dermatitis due to cosmetics
L23.3 Allergic contact dermatitis due to drugs in contact with skin

Use additional code for adverse effect, if applicable, to
identify drug (T36-T50 with fifth or sixth character 5)
Excludes2 dermatitis due to ingested drugs and
medicaments (L27.0-L27.1)

L23.4 Allergic contact dermatitis due to dyes
L23.5 Allergic contact dermatitis due to other chemical products
Allergic contact dermatitis due to cement
Allergic contact dermatitis due to insecticide
Allergic contact dermatitis due to plastic
Allergic contact dermatitis due to rubber

L23.6 Allergic contact dermatitis due to food in contact with the skin
Excludes2 dermatitis due to ingested food (L27.2)

L23.7 Allergic contact dermatitis due to plants, except food
Excludes2 allergy NOS due to pollen (J30.1)

● **L23.8 Allergic contact dermatitis due to other agents**
L23.81 Allergic contact dermatitis due to animal (cat) (dog) dander
Allergic contact dermatitis due to animal (cat) (dog) hair
L23.89 Allergic contact dermatitis due to other agents

L23.9 Allergic contact dermatitis, unspecified cause
Allergic contact eczema NOS

● **L24 Irritant contact dermatitis**
Excludes1 allergy NOS (T78.40)
contact dermatitis NOS (L25.9)
dermatitis NOS (L30.9)
Excludes2 allergic contact dermatitis (L23.-)
dermatitis due to substances taken internally (L27.-)
dermatitis of eyelid (H01.1-)
diaper dermatitis (L22)
eczema of external ear (H60.5-)
perioral dermatitis (L71.0)
radiation-related disorders of the skin and
subcutaneous tissue (L55-L59)

L24.0 Irritant contact dermatitis due to detergents
L24.1 Irritant contact dermatitis due to oils and greases

CHAPTER 12 (L00-L99)

▶ New   ⇒ Revised   ~~deleted~~ Deleted   Excludes 1   Excludes 2   Includes   Use additional   Code first   Code also   Key words
OGCR Official Guidelines   X Assign placeholder X   ● Use Additional Character(s)   ▷ Manifestation Code   🏷 Hierarchical Condition Category   **Coding Clinic**

L24.2 **Irritant contact dermatitis due to solvents**
Irritant contact dermatitis due to chlorocompound
Irritant contact dermatitis due to cyclohexane
Irritant contact dermatitis due to ester
Irritant contact dermatitis due to glycol
Irritant contact dermatitis due to hydrocarbon
Irritant contact dermatitis due to ketone

L24.3 **Irritant contact dermatitis due to cosmetics**

L24.4 **Irritant contact dermatitis due to drugs in contact with skin**
Use additional code for adverse effect, if applicable, to identify drug (T36-T50 with fifth or sixth character 5)

L24.5 **Irritant contact dermatitis due to other chemical products**
Irritant contact dermatitis due to cement
Irritant contact dermatitis due to insecticide
Irritant contact dermatitis due to plastic
Irritant contact dermatitis due to rubber

L24.6 **Irritant contact dermatitis due to food in contact with skin**
Excludes2 dermatitis due to ingested food (L27.2)

L24.7 **Irritant contact dermatitis due to plants, except food**
Excludes2 allergy NOS to pollen (J30.1)

● **L24.8** **Irritant contact dermatitis due to other agents**

L24.81 **Irritant contact dermatitis due to metals**
Irritant contact dermatitis due to chromium
Irritant contact dermatitis due to nickel

L24.89 **Irritant contact dermatitis due to other agents**
Irritant contact dermatitis due to dyes

L24.9 **Irritant contact dermatitis, unspecified cause**
Irritant contact eczema NOS

▶● **L24.A** **Irritant contact dermatitis due to friction or contact with body fluids**
▶**Excludes1** virritant contact dermatitis related to stoma or fistula (L24.B-)
▶**Excludes2** erythema intertrigo (L30.4)

▶ **L24.A0** **Irritant contact dermatitis due to friction or contact with body fluids, unspecified**

▶ **L24.A1** **Irritant contact dermatitis due to saliva**

▶ **L24.A2** **Irritant contact dermatitis due to fecal, urinary or dual incontinence**
▶**Excludes1** diaper dermatitis (L22)

▶ **L24.A9** **Irritant contact dermatitis due friction or contact with other specified body fluids**
▶Irritant contact dermatitis related to endotracheal tube
▶Wound fluids, exudate

▶● **L24.B** **Irritant contact dermatitis related to stoma or fistula**
▶Use additional code to identify any artificial opening status (Z93.-), if applicable, for contact dermatitis related to stoma secretions

▶ **L24.B0** **Irritant contact dermatitis related to unspecified stoma or fistula**
▶Irritant contact dermatitis related to fistula NOS
▶Irritant contact dermatitis related to stoma NOS

▶ **L24.B1** **Irritant contact dermatitis related to digestive stoma or fistula**
▶Irritant contact dermatitis related to gastrostomy
▶Irritant contact dermatitis related to jejunostomy
▶Irritant contact dermatitis related to saliva or spit fistula

▶ **L24.B2** **Irritant contact dermatitis related to respiratory stoma or fistula**
▶Irritant contact dermatitis related to tracheostomy

▶ **L24.B3** **Irritant contact dermatitis related to fecal or urinary stoma or fistula**
▶Irritant contact dermatitis related to colostomy
▶Irritant contact dermatitis related to enterocutaneous fistula
▶Irritant contact dermatitis related to ileostomy

● **L25** **Unspecified contact dermatitis**
Excludes1 allergic contact dermatitis (L23.-)
allergy NOS (T78.40)
dermatitis NOS (L30.9)
irritant contact dermatitis (L24.-)

Excludes2 dermatitis due to ingested substances (L27.-)
dermatitis of eyelid (H01.1-)
eczema of external ear (H60.5-)
perioral dermatitis (L71.0)
radiation-related disorders of the skin and subcutaneous tissue (L55-L59)

L25.0 **Unspecified contact dermatitis due to cosmetics**

L25.1 **Unspecified contact dermatitis due to drugs in contact with skin**
Use additional code for adverse effect, if applicable, to identify drug (T36-T50 with fifth or sixth character 5)
Excludes2 dermatitis due to ingested drugs and medicaments (L27.0-L27.1)

L25.2 **Unspecified contact dermatitis due to dyes**

L25.3 **Unspecified contact dermatitis due to other chemical products**
Unspecified contact dermatitis due to cement
Unspecified contact dermatitis due to insecticide

L25.4 **Unspecified contact dermatitis due to food in contact with skin**
Excludes2 dermatitis due to ingested food (L27.2)

L25.5 **Unspecified contact dermatitis due to plants, except food**
Excludes1 nettle rash (L50.9)
Excludes2 allergy NOS due to pollen (J30.1)

L25.8 **Unspecified contact dermatitis due to other agents**

L25.9 **Unspecified contact dermatitis, unspecified cause**
Contact dermatitis (occupational) NOS
Contact eczema (occupational) NOS

L26 **Exfoliative dermatitis**
Hebra's pityriasis
Excludes1 Ritter's disease (L00)

● **L27** **Dermatitis due to substances taken internally**
Excludes1 allergy NOS (T78.40)
Excludes2 adverse food reaction, except dermatitis (T78.0-T78.1)
contact dermatitis (L23-L25)
drug photoallergic response (L56.1)
drug phototoxic response (L56.0)
urticaria (L50.-)

L27.0 **Generalized skin eruption due to drugs and medicaments taken internally**
Use additional code for adverse effect, if applicable, to identify drug (T36-T50 with fifth or sixth character 5)

L27.1 **Localized skin eruption due to drugs and medicaments taken internally**
Use additional code for adverse effect, if applicable, to identify drug (T36-T50 with fifth or sixth character 5)

L27.2 **Dermatitis due to ingested food**
Excludes2 dermatitis due to food in contact with skin (L23.6, L24.6, L25.4)

L27.8 **Dermatitis due to other substances taken internally**

L27.9 **Dermatitis due to unspecified substance taken internally**

● **L28** **Lichen simplex chronicus and prurigo**

L28.0 **Lichen simplex chronicus**
Circumscribed neurodermatitis
Lichen NOS

L28.1 **Prurigo nodularis**

L28.2 **Other prurigo**
Prurigo NOS   Prurigo mitis
Prurigo Hebra   Urticaria papulosa

L29 Pruritus

Excludes1   neurotic excoriation (L98.1)
     psychogenic pruritus (F45.8)

L29.0   Pruritus ani
L29.1   Pruritus scroti ♂
L29.2   Pruritus vulvae ♀
L29.3   Anogenital pruritus, unspecified
L29.8   Other pruritus
L29.9   Pruritus, unspecified
     Itch NOS

L30 Other and unspecified dermatitis

Excludes2   contact dermatitis (L23-L25)
     dry skin dermatitis (L85.3)
     small plaque parapsoriasis (L41.3)
     stasis dermatitis (I87.2)

L30.0   Nummular dermatitis
L30.1   Dyshidrosis [pompholyx]
L30.2   Cutaneous autosensitization
     Candidid [levurid]   Eczematid
     Dermatophytid
L30.3   Infective dermatitis
     Infectious eczematoid dermatitis
L30.4   Erythema intertrigo
L30.5   Pityriasis alba
     Coding Clinic: 2018, Q1, P6
L30.8   Other specified dermatitis
L30.9   Dermatitis, unspecified
     Eczema NOS

PAPULOSQUAMOUS DISORDERS (L40-L45)

L40 Psoriasis

L40.0   Psoriasis vulgaris
     Nummular psoriasis   Plaque psoriasis
L40.1   Generalized pustular psoriasis
     Impetigo herpetiformis   Von Zumbusch's disease
L40.2   Acrodermatitis continua
L40.3   Pustulosis palmaris et plantaris
L40.4   Guttate psoriasis
L40.5   Arthropathic psoriasis
   L40.50   Arthropathic psoriasis, unspecified
   L40.51   Distal interphalangeal psoriatic arthropathy
   L40.52   Psoriatic arthritis mutilans
   L40.53   Psoriatic spondylitis
   L40.54   Psoriatic juvenile arthropathy
   L40.59   Other psoriatic arthropathy
L40.8   Other psoriasis
     Flexural psoriasis
L40.9   Psoriasis, unspecified

L41 Parapsoriasis

Excludes1   poikiloderma vasculare atrophicans (L94.5)

L41.0   Pityriasis lichenoides et varioliformis acuta
     Mucha-Habermann disease
L41.1   Pityriasis lichenoides chronica
L41.3   Small plaque parapsoriasis
L41.4   Large plaque parapsoriasis
L41.5   Retiform parapsoriasis
L41.8   Other parapsoriasis
L41.9   Parapsoriasis, unspecified

L42 Pityriasis rosea

L43 Lichen planus

Excludes1   lichen planopilaris (L66.1)

L43.0   Hypertrophic lichen planus
L43.1   Bullous lichen planus
L43.2   Lichenoid drug reaction
     Use additional code for adverse effect, if applicable, to identify drug (T36-T50 with fifth or sixth character 5)
L43.3   Subacute (active) lichen planus
     Lichen planus tropicus
L43.8   Other lichen planus
L43.9   Lichen planus, unspecified

L44 Other papulosquamous disorders

L44.0   Pityriasis rubra pilaris
L44.1   Lichen nitidus
L44.2   Lichen striatus
L44.3   Lichen ruber moniliformis
L44.4   Infantile papular acrodermatitis [Gianotti-Crosti]   P
L44.8   Other specified papulosquamous disorders
L44.9   Papulosquamous disorder, unspecified

L45 Papulosquamous disorders in diseases classified elsewhere
     Code first underlying disease

URTICARIA AND ERYTHEMA (L49-L54)

Excludes1   Lyme disease (A69.2-)
     rosacea (L71.-)

L49 Exfoliation due to erythematous conditions according to extent of body surface involved

Code first erythematous condition causing exfoliation, such as:
     Ritter's disease (L00)
     (Staphylococcal) scalded skin syndrome (L00)
     Stevens-Johnson syndrome (L51.1)
     Stevens-Johnson syndrome-toxic epidermal necrolysis overlap syndrome (L51.3)
     Toxic epidermal necrolysis (L51.2)

L49.0   Exfoliation due to erythematous condition involving less than 10 percent of body surface
     Exfoliation due to erythematous condition NOS
L49.1   Exfoliation due to erythematous condition involving 10-19 percent of body surface
L49.2   Exfoliation due to erythematous condition involving 20-29 percent of body surface
L49.3   Exfoliation due to erythematous condition involving 30-39 percent of body surface
L49.4   Exfoliation due to erythematous condition involving 40-49 percent of body surface
L49.5   Exfoliation due to erythematous condition involving 50-59 percent of body surface
L49.6   Exfoliation due to erythematous condition involving 60-69 percent of body surface
L49.7   Exfoliation due to erythematous condition involving 70-79 percent of body surface
L49.8   Exfoliation due to erythematous condition involving 80-89 percent of body surface
L49.9   Exfoliation due to erythematous condition involving 90 or more percent of body surface

Figure 12-6 Erythematous plaques with silvery scales in a patient with psoriasis. (Getty Image)

Item 12–8 Psoriasis is a chronic, recurrent inflammatory skin disease characterized by small patches covered with thick, silvery scales. **Parapsoriasis** is a treatment-resistant erythroderma. **Pityriasis rosea** is characterized by a herald patch that is a single large lesion and that usually appears on the trunk and is followed by scattered, smaller lesions.

New   Revised   ~~deleted~~ Deleted   Excludes 1   Excludes 2   Includes   Use additional   Code first   Code also   Key words
OGCR Official Guidelines   X Assign placeholder X   Use Additional Character(s)   Manifestation Code   Hierarchical Condition Category   Coding Clinic

Figure 12-7 Urticaria (hives). *(Courtesy of David Effron, MD.)* (Getty Image)

Item 12–9 Urticaria is a vascular reaction in which wheals surrounded by a red halo appear and cause severe itching. The causes of urticaria or hives are extensive and varied (e.g., food, heat, cold, drugs, stress, infections).

● **L50   Urticaria**
     Excludes1   allergic contact dermatitis (L23.-)
              angioneurotic edema (T78.3)
              giant urticaria (T78.3)
              hereditary angio-edema (D84.1)
              Quincke's edema (T78.3)
              serum urticaria (T80.6-)
              solar urticaria (L56.3)
              urticaria neonatorum (P83.8)
              urticaria papulosa (L28.2)
              urticaria pigmentosa (D47.01)

   L50.0   Allergic urticaria
   L50.1   Idiopathic urticaria
   L50.2   Urticaria due to cold and heat
       Excludes2   familial cold urticaria (M04.2)
   L50.3   Dermatographic urticaria
   L50.4   Vibratory urticaria
   L50.5   Cholinergic urticaria
   L50.6   Contact urticaria
   L50.8   Other urticaria
       Chronic urticaria
       Recurrent periodic urticaria
   L50.9   Urticaria, unspecified

● **L51   Erythema multiforme**
     Use additional code for adverse effect, if applicable, to identify drug (T36-T50 with fifth or sixth character 5)
     Use additional code to identify associated manifestations, such as:
       arthropathy associated with dermatological disorders (M14.8-)
       conjunctival edema (H11.42)
       conjunctivitis (H10.22-)
       corneal scars and opacities (H17.-)
       corneal ulcer (H16.0-)
       edema of eyelid (H02.84-)
       inflammation of eyelid (H01.8)
       keratoconjunctivitis sicca (H16.22-)
       mechanical lagophthalmos (H02.22-)
       stomatitis (K12.-)
       symblepharon (H11.23-)
     Use additional code to identify percentage of skin exfoliation (L49.-)
     Excludes1   staphylococcal scalded skin syndrome (L00)
              Ritter's disease (L00)
   L51.0   Nonbullous erythema multiforme
   L51.1   Stevens-Johnson syndrome 🔖
   L51.2   Toxic epidermal necrolysis [Lyell] 🔖
   L51.3   Stevens-Johnson syndrome-toxic epidermal necrolysis overlap syndrome 🔖
       SJS-TEN overlap syndrome
   L51.8   Other erythema multiforme
   L51.9   Erythema multiforme, unspecified
       Erythema iris
       Erythema multiforme major NOS
       Erythema multiforme minor NOS
       Herpes iris

L52   Erythema nodosum
     Excludes1   tuberculous erythema nodosum (A18.4)

● **L53   Other erythematous conditions**
     Excludes1   erythema ab igne (L59.0)
              erythema due to external agents in contact with skin (L23-L25)
              erythema intertrigo (L30.4)
   L53.0   Toxic erythema
       Code first poisoning due to drug or toxin, if applicable (T36-T65 with fifth or sixth character 1-4 or 6)
       Use additional code for adverse effect, if applicable, to identify drug (T36-T50 with fifth or sixth character 5)
       Excludes1   neonatal erythema toxicum (P83.1)
   L53.1   Erythema annulare centrifugum
   L53.2   Erythema marginatum
   L53.3   Other chronic figurate erythema
   L53.8   Other specified erythematous conditions
   L53.9   Erythematous condition, unspecified
       Erythema NOS
       Erythroderma NOS

▷ **L54   *Erythema in diseases classified elsewhere***
       Code first underlying disease

RADIATION-RELATED DISORDERS OF THE SKIN AND SUBCUTANEOUS TISSUE (L55-L59)

● **L55   Sunburn**
   L55.0   Sunburn of first degree
   L55.1   Sunburn of second degree
   L55.2   Sunburn of third degree
   L55.9   Sunburn, unspecified

● **L56   Other acute skin changes due to ultraviolet radiation**
     Use additional code to identify the source of the ultraviolet radiation (W89, X32)
   L56.0   Drug phototoxic response
       Use additional code for adverse effect, if applicable, to identify drug (T36-T50 with fifth or sixth character 5)
   L56.1   Drug photoallergic response
       Use additional code for adverse effect, if applicable, to identify drug (T36-T50 with fifth or sixth character 5)
   L56.2   Photocontact dermatitis [berloque dermatitis]
   L56.3   Solar urticaria
   L56.4   Polymorphous light eruption
   L56.5   Disseminated superficial actinic porokeratosis (DSAP)
   L56.8   Other specified acute skin changes due to ultraviolet radiation
   L56.9   Acute skin change due to ultraviolet radiation, unspecified

● **L57   Skin changes due to chronic exposure to nonionizing radiation**
     Use additional code to identify the source of the ultraviolet radiation (W89), or other nonionizing radiation (W90)
   L57.0   Actinic keratosis
       Keratosis NOS   Solar keratosis
       Senile keratosis
   L57.1   Actinic reticuloid
   L57.2   Cutis rhomboidalis nuchae
   L57.3   Poikiloderma of Civatte
   L57.4   Cutis laxa senilis
       Elastosis senilis
   L57.5   Actinic granuloma
   L57.8   Other skin changes due to chronic exposure to nonionizing radiation
       Farmer's skin   Solar dermatitis
       Sailor's skin
   L57.9   Skin changes due to chronic exposure to nonionizing radiation, unspecified

● **L58**   **Radiodermatitis**

> Use additional code to identify the source of the radiation (W88, W90)

    L58.0   **Acute** radiodermatitis

    L58.1   **Chronic** radiodermatitis

    L58.9   Radiodermatitis, **unspecified**

● **L59**   **Other disorders of skin and subcutaneous tissue related to radiation**

    L59.0   Erythema ab igne [dermatitis ab igne]

    L59.8   Other specified disorders of the skin and subcutaneous tissue related to radiation
> **Coding Clinic: 2017, Q1, P34**

    L59.9   Disorder of the skin and subcutaneous tissue related to radiation, **unspecified**

DISORDERS OF SKIN APPENDAGES (L60–L75)

Excludes1   congenital malformations of integument (Q84.-)

● **L60**   **Nail disorders**

Excludes2   clubbing of nails (R68.3)
> onychia and paronychia (L03.0-)

    L60.0   Ingrowing nail

    L60.1   Onycholysis

    L60.2   Onychogryphosis

    L60.3   Nail dystrophy

    L60.4   Beau's lines

    L60.5   Yellow nail syndrome

    L60.8   Other nail disorders

    L60.9   Nail disorder, **unspecified**

▷ *L62*   *Nail disorders in diseases classified elsewhere*

> *Code first* underlying disease, such as:
> pachydermoperiostosis (M89.4-)

● **L63**   **Alopecia areata**

    L63.0   Alopecia (capitis) **totalis**

    L63.1   Alopecia **universalis**

    L63.2   **Ophiasis**

    L63.8   **Other** alopecia areata

    L63.9   Alopecia areata, **unspecified**

● **L64**   **Androgenic alopecia**

Includes   male-pattern baldness

    L64.0   **Drug-induced** androgenic alopecia
> Use additional code for adverse effect, if applicable, to identify drug (T36-T50 with fifth or sixth character 5)

    L64.8   **Other** androgenic alopecia

    L64.9   Androgenic alopecia, **unspecified**

● **L65**   **Other nonscarring hair loss**

> Use additional code for adverse effect, if applicable, to identify drug (T36-T50 with fifth or sixth character 5)

Excludes1   trichotillomania (F63.3)

    L65.0   Telogen effluvium

    L65.1   Anagen effluvium

    L65.2   Alopecia mucinosa

    L65.8   Other specified nonscarring hair loss

    L65.9   Nonscarring hair loss, **unspecified**
> Alopecia NOS

● **L66**   **Cicatricial alopecia [scarring hair loss]**

    L66.0   Pseudopelade

    L66.1   Lichen planopilaris
> Follicular lichen planus

    L66.2   Folliculitis decalvans

    L66.3   Perifolliculitis capitis abscedens

    L66.4   Folliculitis ulerythematosa reticulata

    L66.8   Other cicatricial alopecia
> **Coding Clinic: 2015, Q1, P19**

    L66.9   Cicatricial alopecia, **unspecified**

● **L67**   **Hair color and hair shaft abnormalities**

Excludes1   monilethrix (Q84.1)
> pili annulati (Q84.1)
> telogen effluvium (L65.0)

    L67.0   **Trichorrhexis nodosa**

    L67.1   **Variations in hair color**
> Canities
> Greyness, hair (premature)
> Heterochromia of hair
> Poliosis circumscripta, acquired
> Poliosis NOS

    L67.8   **Other hair color and hair shaft abnormalities**
> Fragilitas crinium

    L67.9   **Hair color and hair shaft abnormality, unspecified**

● **L68**   **Hypertrichosis**

Includes   excess hair

Excludes1   congenital hypertrichosis (Q84.2)
> persistent lanugo (Q84.2)

    L68.0   **Hirsutism**
> *Excessive growth of hair*

    L68.1   **Acquired hypertrichosis lanuginosa**

    L68.2   **Localized hypertrichosis**

    L68.3   **Polytrichia**

    L68.8   **Other hypertrichosis**

    L68.9   **Hypertrichosis, unspecified**

Item 12–10   **Alopecia** is lack of hair and takes many forms. The most common is male pattern alopecia, also known as **androgenetic alopecia.** **Telogen effluvium** is early and excessive loss of hair resulting from a trauma to the hair follicle (fever, drugs, surgery, etc.).

Figure 12-8   Male pattern alopecia.

▶ New   ⇒ Revised   ~~deleted~~ Deleted   Excludes 1   Excludes 2   Includes   Use additional   Code first   Code also   Key words

OGCR Official Guidelines   X Assign placeholder X   ● Use Additional Character(s)   ▷ Manifestation Code   🍄 Hierarchical Condition Category   **Coding Clinic**

● **L70**   **Acne**
     Excludes2   acne keloid (L73.0)
     L70.0   Acne vulgaris
     L70.1   Acne conglobata
     L70.2   Acne varioliformis
              Acne necrotica miliaris
     L70.3   Acne tropica
     L70.4   Infantile acne   P
     L70.5   Acné excoriée
              Acné excoriée des jeunes filles
              Picker's acne
     L70.8   Other acne
     L70.9   Acne, unspecified

● **L71**   **Rosacea**
     Use additional code for adverse effect, if applicable, to identify drug (T36-T50 with fifth or sixth character 5)
     L71.0   Perioral dermatitis
     L71.1   Rhinophyma
     L71.8   Other rosacea
              Coding Clinic: 2018, Q4, P15
     L71.9   Rosacea, unspecified

● **L72**   **Follicular cysts of skin and subcutaneous tissue**
     L72.0   Epidermal cyst
●   L72.1   Pilar and trichodermal cyst
         L72.11   Pilar cyst
         L72.12   Trichodermal cyst
                 Trichilemmal (proliferating) cyst
     L72.3   Sebaceous cyst
         Excludes2   pilar cyst (L72.11)
                        trichilemmal (proliferating) cyst (L72.12)
     L72.2   Steatocystoma multiplex
     L72.8   Other follicular cysts of the skin and subcutaneous tissue
     L72.9   Follicular cyst of the skin and subcutaneous tissue, unspecified

● **L73**   **Other follicular disorders**
     L73.0   Acne keloid
     L73.1   Pseudofolliculitis barbae
     L73.2   Hidradenitis suppurativa
     L73.8   Other specified follicular disorders
              Sycosis barbae
     L73.9   Follicular disorder, unspecified

● **L74**   **Eccrine sweat disorders**
     Excludes2   generalized hyperhidrosis (R61)
     L74.0   Miliaria rubra
     L74.1   Miliaria crystallina
     L74.2   Miliaria profunda
              Miliaria tropicalis
     L74.3   Miliaria, unspecified
     L74.4   Anhidrosis
              Hypohidrosis
●   L74.5   Focal hyperhidrosis
●   L74.51   Primary focal hyperhidrosis
             L74.510   Primary focal hyperhidrosis, axilla
             L74.511   Primary focal hyperhidrosis, face
             L74.512   Primary focal hyperhidrosis, palms
             L74.513   Primary focal hyperhidrosis, soles
             L74.519   Primary focal hyperhidrosis, unspecified
         L74.52   Secondary focal hyperhidrosis
                 Frey's syndrome
     L74.8   Other eccrine sweat disorders
     L74.9   Eccrine sweat disorder, unspecified
             Sweat gland disorder NOS

● **L75**   **Apocrine sweat disorders**
     Excludes1   dyshidrosis (L30.1)
                        hidradenitis suppurativa (L73.2)
     L75.0   Bromhidrosis
     L75.1   Chromhidrosis
     L75.2   Apocrine miliaria
              Fox-Fordyce disease
     L75.8   Other apocrine sweat disorders
     L75.9   Apocrine sweat disorder, unspecified
              Intraoperative and postprocedural complications of skin and subcutaneous tissue (L76)

INTRAOPERATIVE AND POSTPROCEDURAL COMPLICATIONS OF SKIN AND SUBCUTANEOUS TISSUE (L76)

● **L76**   **Intraoperative and postprocedural complications of skin and subcutaneous tissue**
     Coding Clinic: 2016, Q4, P10
●   L76.0   Intraoperative hemorrhage and hematoma of skin and subcutaneous tissue complicating a procedure
         Excludes1   intraoperative hemorrhage and hematoma of skin and subcutaneous tissue due to accidental puncture and laceration during a procedure (L76.1-)
         L76.01   Intraoperative hemorrhage and hematoma of skin and subcutaneous tissue complicating a dermatologic procedure
         L76.02   Intraoperative hemorrhage and hematoma of skin and subcutaneous tissue complicating other procedure
●   L76.1   Accidental puncture and laceration of skin and subcutaneous tissue during a procedure
         L76.11   Accidental puncture and laceration of skin and subcutaneous tissue during a dermatologic procedure
         L76.12   Accidental puncture and laceration of skin and subcutaneous tissue during other procedure
●   L76.2   Postprocedural hemorrhage of skin and subcutaneous tissue following a procedure
         L76.21   Postprocedural hemorrhage of skin and subcutaneous tissue following a dermatologic procedure
         L76.22   Postprocedural hemorrhage of skin and subcutaneous tissue following other procedure
●   L76.3   Postprocedural hematoma and seroma of skin and subcutaneous tissue following a procedure
         L76.31   Postprocedural hematoma of skin and subcutaneous tissue following a dermatologic procedure
         L76.32   Postprocedural hematoma of skin and subcutaneous tissue following other procedure
         L76.33   Postprocedural seroma of skin and subcutaneous tissue following a dermatologic procedure
         L76.34   Postprocedural seroma of skin and subcutaneous tissue following other procedure
●   L76.8   Other intraoperative and postprocedural complications of skin and subcutaneous tissue
         Use additional code, if applicable, to further specify disorder
         L76.81   Other intraoperative complications of skin and subcutaneous tissue
         L76.82   Other postprocedural complications of skin and subcutaneous tissue
                 Coding Clinic: 2017, Q3, P6

OTHER DISORDERS OF THE SKIN AND SUBCUTANEOUS TISSUE (L80-L99)

L80   Vitiligo
   Excludes2 vitiligo of eyelids (H02.73-)
                vitiligo of vulva (N90.89)

L81   Other disorders of pigmentation
   Excludes1 birthmark NOS (Q82.5)
            Peutz-Jeghers syndrome (Q85.8)
   Excludes2 nevus - see Alphabetical Index
  L81.0 Postinflammatory hyperpigmentation
  L81.1 Chloasma
  L81.2 Freckles
  L81.3 Café au lait spots
  L81.4 Other melanin hyperpigmentation
       Lentigo
  L81.5 Leukoderma, not elsewhere classified
  L81.6 Other disorders of diminished melanin formation
  L81.7 Pigmented purpuric dermatosis
       Angioma serpiginosum
  L81.8 Other specified disorders of pigmentation
       Iron pigmentation
       Tattoo pigmentation
  L81.9 Disorder of pigmentation, **unspecified**

L82   Seborrheic keratosis
   Includes basal cell papilloma
          dermatosis papulosa nigra
          Leser-Trélat disease
   Excludes2 seborrheic dermatitis (L21.-)
  L82.0 Inflamed seborrheic keratosis
  L82.1 Other seborrheic keratosis
       Seborrheic keratosis NOS

L83   Acanthosis nigricans
    Confluent and reticulated papillomatosis

L84   Corns and callosities
    Callus
    Clavus

L85   Other epidermal thickening
   Excludes2 hypertrophic disorders of the skin (L91.-)
  L85.0 Acquired ichthyosis
    Excludes1 congenital ichthyosis (Q80.-)
  L85.1 Acquired keratosis [keratoderma] palmaris et plantaris
    Excludes1 inherited keratosis palmaris et plantaris (Q82.8)
  L85.2 Keratosis punctata (palmaris et plantaris)
  L85.3 Xerosis cutis
       Dry skin dermatitis
  L85.8 Other specified epidermal thickening
       Cutaneous horn
  L85.9 Epidermal thickening, **unspecified**

L86   Keratoderma in diseases classified elsewhere
   Firm horny papules that have a cobblestone appearance
   Code first underlying disease, such as:
    Reiter's disease (M02.3-)
   Excludes1 gonococcal keratoderma (A54.89)
           gonococcal keratosis (A54.89)
           keratoderma due to vitamin A deficiency (E50.8)
           keratosis due to vitamin A deficiency (E50.8)
           xeroderma due to vitamin A deficiency (E50.8)

L87   Transepidermal elimination disorders
   Excludes1 granuloma annulare (perforating) (L92.0)
  L87.0 Keratosis follicularis et parafollicularis in cutem penetrans
       Kyrle disease
       Hyperkeratosis follicularis penetrans
  L87.1 Reactive perforating collagenosis
  L87.2 Elastosis perforans serpiginosa
  L87.8 Other transepidermal elimination disorders
  L87.9 Transepidermal elimination disorder, **unspecified**

L88   Pyoderma gangrenosum
    Phagedenic pyoderma
   Excludes1 dermatitis gangrenosa (L08.0)

OGCR Section I.B.14.

General Coding Guidelines

Documentation for BMI, *Depth of* Non-pressure ulcers, Pressure Ulcer Stages, **Coma Scale, and** *NIH Stroke Scale*

For the Body Mass Index (BMI), depth of non-pressure chronic ulcers, pressure ulcer stage, **coma scale, and NIH stroke scale (NIHSS) codes,** code assignment may be based on medical record documentation from clinicians who are not the patient's provider (i.e., physician or other qualified healthcare practitioner legally accountable for establishing the patient's diagnosis), since this information is typically documented by other clinicians involved in the care of the patient (e.g., a dietitian often documents the BMI, a nurse often documents the pressure ulcer stages, **and an emergency medical technician often documents the coma scale**). However, the associated diagnosis (such as overweight, obesity, **acute stroke,** or pressure ulcer) must be documented by the patient's provider. If there is conflicting medical record documentation, either from the same clinician or different clinicians, the patient's attending provider should be queried for clarification. The BMI, **coma scale, and NHSS** codes should only be reported as secondary diagnoses.

L89   Pressure ulcer
   Includes bed sore   pressure area
           decubitus ulcer pressure sore
           plaster ulcer
   Code first any associated gangrene (I96)
   Excludes2 decubitus (trophic) ulcer of cervix (uteri) (N86)
           diabetic ulcers (E08.621, E08.622, E09.621, E09.622, E10.621, E10.622, E11.621, E11.622, E13.621, E13.622)
           non-pressure chronic ulcer of skin (L97.-)
           skin infections (L00-L08)
           varicose ulcer (I83.0, I83.2)
   Coding Clinic: 2019, Q4, P11; 2018, Q2, P22; 2016, Q4, P124

L89.0   Pressure ulcer of elbow
  L89.00 Pressure ulcer of **unspecified** elbow
    L89.000 Pressure ulcer of unspecified elbow, **unstageable**
    L89.001 Pressure ulcer of unspecified elbow, **stage 1**
       Healing pressure ulcer of unspecified elbow, stage 1
       Pressure pre-ulcer skin changes limited to persistent focal edema, unspecified elbow
    L89.002 Pressure ulcer of unspecified elbow, **stage 2**
       Healing pressure ulcer of unspecified elbow, stage 2
       Pressure ulcer with abrasion, blister, partial thickness skin loss involving epidermis and/or dermis, unspecified elbow

CHAPTER 12 (L00-L99)

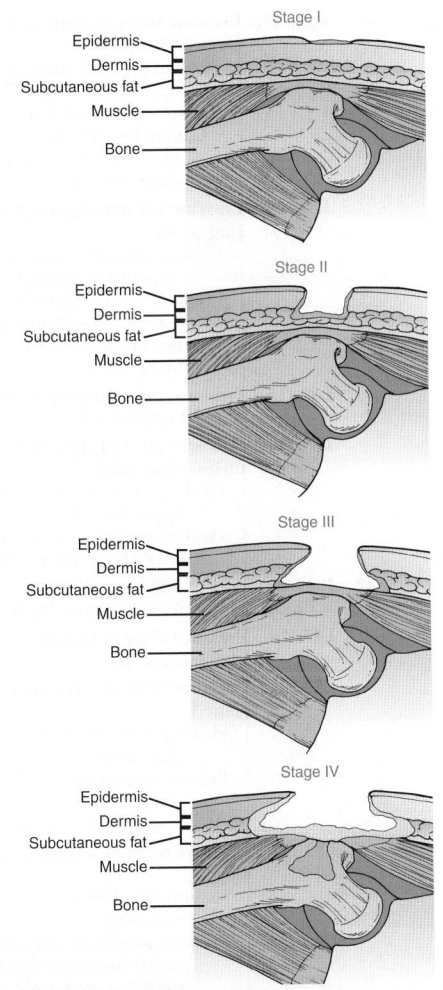

Stage I

Epidermis
Dermis
Subcutaneous fat
Muscle
Bone

Stage II

Epidermis
Dermis
Subcutaneous fat
Muscle
Bone

Stage III

Epidermis
Dermis
Subcutaneous fat
Muscle
Bone

Stage IV

Epidermis
Dermis
Subcutaneous fat
Muscle
Bone

Figure 12-9   Stage I, II, III, and IV of pressure ulcers.

L89.003   **Pressure ulcer of unspecified elbow, stage 3** 🔬
     Healing pressure ulcer of unspecified elbow, stage 3
     Pressure ulcer with full thickness skin loss involving damage or necrosis of subcutaneous tissue, unspecified elbow

L89.004   **Pressure ulcer of unspecified elbow, stage 4** 🔬
     Healing pressure ulcer of unspecified elbow, stage 4
     Pressure ulcer with necrosis of soft tissues through to underlying muscle, tendon, or bone, unspecified elbow

L89.006   **Pressure-induced deep tissue damage of unspecified elbow**

L89.009   **Pressure ulcer of unspecified elbow, unspecified stage**
     Healing pressure ulcer of elbow NOS
     Healing pressure ulcer of unspecified elbow, unspecified stage

⬤ **L89.01**   **Pressure ulcer of right elbow**

    L89.010   **Pressure ulcer of right elbow, unstageable** 🔬

    L89.011   **Pressure ulcer of right elbow, stage 1**
       Healing pressure ulcer of right elbow, stage 1
       Pressure pre-ulcer skin changes limited to persistent focal edema, right elbow

    L89.012   **Pressure ulcer of right elbow, stage 2**
       Healing pressure ulcer of right elbow, stage 2
       Pressure ulcer with abrasion, blister, partial thickness skin loss involving epidermis and/or dermis, right elbow

    L89.013   **Pressure ulcer of right elbow, stage 3** 🔬
       Healing pressure ulcer of right elbow, stage 3
       Pressure ulcer with full thickness skin loss involving damage or necrosis of subcutaneous tissue, right elbow

    L89.014   **Pressure ulcer of right elbow, stage 4** 🔬
       Healing pressure ulcer of right elbow, stage 4
       Pressure ulcer with necrosis of soft tissues through to underlying muscle, tendon, or bone, right elbow

    L89.016   **Pressure-induced deep tissue damage of right elbow**

    L89.019   **Pressure ulcer of right elbow, unspecified stage**
       ➠ Healing pressure ulcer of right elbow NOS
       Healing pressure ulcer of right elbow, unspecified stage

⬤ **L89.02**   **Pressure ulcer of left elbow**

    L89.020   **Pressure ulcer of left elbow, unstageable** 🔬

    L89.021   **Pressure ulcer of left elbow, stage 1**
       Healing pressure ulcer of left elbow, stage 1
       Pressure pre-ulcer skin changes limited to persistent focal edema, left elbow

    L89.022   **Pressure ulcer of left elbow, stage 2**
       Healing pressure ulcer of left elbow, stage 2
       Pressure ulcer with abrasion, blister, partial thickness skin loss involving epidermis and/or dermis, left elbow

    L89.023   **Pressure ulcer of left elbow, stage 3** 🔬
       Healing pressure ulcer of left elbow, stage 3
       Pressure ulcer with full thickness skin loss involving damage or necrosis of subcutaneous tissue, left elbow

    L89.024   **Pressure ulcer of left elbow, stage 4** 🔬
       Healing pressure ulcer of left elbow, stage 4
       Pressure ulcer with necrosis of soft tissues through to underlying muscle, tendon, or bone, left elbow

CHAPTER 12 (L00-L99)

      L89.026   **Pressure-induced deep tissue damage of left elbow**

      L89.029   **Pressure ulcer of left elbow, unspecified stage**

➡️ Healing pressure ulcer of left elbow NOS

~~Healing pressure ulcer of left elbow, unspecified stage~~

● **L89.1   Pressure ulcer of back**

  ● **L89.10   Pressure ulcer of unspecified part of back**

    L89.100   **Pressure ulcer of unspecified part of back, unstageable** 🐾

    L89.101   **Pressure ulcer of unspecified part of back, stage 1**

Healing pressure ulcer of unspecified part of back, stage 1

Pressure pre-ulcer skin changes limited to persistent focal edema, unspecified part of back

    L89.102   **Pressure ulcer of unspecified part of back, stage 2**

Healing pressure ulcer of unspecified part of back, stage 2

Pressure ulcer with abrasion, blister, partial thickness skin loss involving epidermis and/or dermis, unspecified part of back

    L89.103   **Pressure ulcer of unspecified part of back, stage 3** 🐾

Healing pressure ulcer of unspecified part of back, stage 3

Pressure ulcer with full thickness skin loss involving damage or necrosis of subcutaneous tissue, unspecified part of back

    L89.104   **Pressure ulcer of unspecified part of back, stage 4** 🐾

Healing pressure ulcer of unspecified part of back, stage 4

Pressure ulcer with necrosis of soft tissues through to underlying muscle, tendon, or bone, unspecified part of back

    L89.106   **Pressure-induced deep tissue damage of unspecified part of back**

    L89.109   **Pressure ulcer of unspecified part of back, unspecified stage**

Healing pressure ulcer of unspecified part of back NOS

Healing pressure ulcer of unspecified part of back, unspecified stage

  ● **L89.11   Pressure ulcer of right upper back**

Pressure ulcer of right shoulder blade

    L89.110   **Pressure ulcer of right upper back, unstageable** 🐾

    L89.111   **Pressure ulcer of right upper back, stage 1**

Healing pressure ulcer of right upper back, stage 1

Pressure pre-ulcer skin changes limited to persistent focal edema, right upper back

    L89.112   **Pressure ulcer of right upper back, stage 2**

Healing pressure ulcer of right upper back, stage 2

Pressure ulcer with abrasion, blister, partial thickness skin loss involving epidermis and/or dermis, right upper back

    L89.113   **Pressure ulcer of right upper back, stage 3** 🐾

Healing pressure ulcer of right upper back, stage 3

Pressure ulcer with full thickness skin loss involving damage or necrosis of subcutaneous tissue, right upper back

    L89.114   **Pressure ulcer of right upper back, stage 4** 🐾

Healing pressure ulcer of right upper back, stage 4

Pressure ulcer with necrosis of soft tissues through to underlying muscle, tendon, or bone, right upper back

    L89.116   **Pressure-induced deep tissue damage of right upper back**

    L89.119   **Pressure ulcer of right upper back, unspecified stage**

Healing pressure ulcer of right upper back NOS

Healing pressure ulcer of right upper back, unspecified stage

  ● **L89.12   Pressure ulcer of left upper back**

Pressure ulcer of left shoulder blade

    L89.120   **Pressure ulcer of left upper back, unstageable** 🐾

    L89.121   **Pressure ulcer of left upper back, stage 1**

Healing pressure ulcer of left upper back, stage 1

Pressure pre-ulcer skin changes limited to persistent focal edema, left upper back

    L89.122   **Pressure ulcer of left upper back, stage 2**

Healing pressure ulcer of left upper back, stage 2

Pressure ulcer with abrasion, blister, partial thickness skin loss involving epidermis and/or dermis, left upper back

    L89.123   **Pressure ulcer of left upper back, stage 3** 🐾

Healing pressure ulcer of left upper back, stage 3

Pressure ulcer with full thickness skin loss involving damage or necrosis of subcutaneous tissue, left upper back

    L89.124   **Pressure ulcer of left upper back, stage 4** 🐾

Healing pressure ulcer of left upper back, stage 4

Pressure ulcer with necrosis of soft tissues through to underlying muscle, tendon, or bone, left upper back

    L89.126   **Pressure-induced deep tissue damage of left upper back**

    L89.129   **Pressure ulcer of left upper back, unspecified stage**

Healing pressure ulcer of left upper back NOS

Healing pressure ulcer of left upper back, unspecified stage

▶ New   ➡️ Revised   ~~deleted~~ Deleted   Excludes 1   Excludes 2   Includes   Use additional   Code first   Code also   Key words

OGCR Official Guidelines   X Assign placeholder X   ● Use Additional Character(s)   ▶ Manifestation Code   🐾 Hierarchical Condition Category   **Coding Clinic**

● **L89.13**   Pressure ulcer of right lower back

    L89.130   **Pressure ulcer of right lower back, unstageable** 🔍

    L89.131   **Pressure ulcer of right lower back, stage 1**
        Healing pressure ulcer of right lower back, stage 1
        Pressure pre-ulcer skin changes limited to persistent focal edema, right lower back

    L89.132   **Pressure ulcer of right lower back, stage 2**
        Healing pressure ulcer of right lower back, stage 2
        Pressure ulcer with abrasion, blister, partial thickness skin loss involving epidermis and/or dermis, right lower back

    L89.133   **Pressure ulcer of right lower back, stage 3** 🔍
        Healing pressure ulcer of right lower back, stage 3
        Pressure ulcer with full thickness skin loss involving damage or necrosis of subcutaneous tissue, right lower back

    L89.134   **Pressure ulcer of right lower back, stage 4** 🔍
        Healing pressure ulcer of right lower back, stage 4
        Pressure ulcer with necrosis of soft tissues through to underlying muscle, tendon, or bone, right lower back

    L89.136   **Pressure-induced deep tissue damage of right lower back**

    L89.139   **Pressure ulcer of right lower back, unspecified stage**
        Healing pressure ulcer of right lower back NOS
        Healing pressure ulcer of right lower back, unspecified stage

● **L89.14**   Pressure ulcer of left lower back

    L89.140   **Pressure ulcer of left lower back, unstageable** 🔍

    L89.141   **Pressure ulcer of left lower back, stage 1**
        Healing pressure ulcer of left lower back, stage 1
        Pressure pre-ulcer skin changes limited to persistent focal edema, left lower back

    L89.142   **Pressure ulcer of left lower back, stage 2**
        Healing pressure ulcer of left lower back, stage 2
        Pressure ulcer with abrasion, blister, partial thickness skin loss involving epidermis and/or dermis, left lower back

    L89.143   **Pressure ulcer of left lower back, stage 3** 🔍
        Healing pressure ulcer of left lower back, stage 3
        Pressure ulcer with full thickness skin loss involving damage or necrosis of subcutaneous tissue, left lower back

    L89.144   **Pressure ulcer of left lower back, stage 4** 🔍
        Healing pressure ulcer of left lower back, stage 4
        Pressure ulcer with necrosis of soft tissues through to underlying muscle, tendon, or bone, left lower back

    L89.146   **Pressure-induced deep tissue damage of left lower back**

    L89.149   **Pressure ulcer of left lower back, unspecified stage**
        Healing pressure ulcer of left lower back NOS
        Healing pressure ulcer of left lower back, unspecified stage

● **L89.15**   Pressure ulcer of sacral region
     Pressure ulcer of coccyx
     Pressure ulcer of tailbone

    L89.150   **Pressure ulcer of sacral region, unstageable** 🔍

    L89.151   **Pressure ulcer of sacral region, stage 1**
        Healing pressure ulcer of sacral region, stage 1
        Pressure pre-ulcer skin changes limited to persistent focal edema, sacral region

    L89.152   **Pressure ulcer of sacral region, stage 2**
        Healing pressure ulcer of sacral region, stage 2
        Pressure ulcer with abrasion, blister, partial thickness skin loss involving epidermis and/or dermis, sacral region

    L89.153   **Pressure ulcer of sacral region, stage 3** 🔍
        Healing pressure ulcer of sacral region, stage 3
        Pressure ulcer with full thickness skin loss involving damage or necrosis of subcutaneous tissue, sacral region

    L89.154   **Pressure ulcer of sacral region, stage 4** 🔍
        Healing pressure ulcer of sacral region, stage 4
        Pressure ulcer with necrosis of soft tissues through to underlying muscle, tendon, or bone, sacral region
        Coding Clinic: 2021, Q1, P24

    L89.156   **Pressure-induced deep tissue damage of sacral region**

    L89.159   **Pressure ulcer of sacral region, unspecified stage**
        Healing pressure ulcer of sacral region NOS
        Healing pressure ulcer of sacral region, unspecified stage

● **L89.2**   Pressure ulcer of hip

   ● **L89.20**   Pressure ulcer of unspecified hip

    L89.200   **Pressure ulcer of unspecified hip, unstageable** 🔍

    L89.201   **Pressure ulcer of unspecified hip, stage 1**
        Healing pressure ulcer of unspecified hip back, stage 1
        Pressure pre-ulcer skin changes limited to persistent focal edema, unspecified hip

CHAPTER 12 (L00–L99)

CHAPTER 12 (L00-L99)

L89.202   **Pressure ulcer of unspecified hip, stage 2**
     Healing pressure ulcer of unspecified hip, stage 2
     Pressure ulcer with abrasion, blister, partial thickness skin loss involving epidermis and/or dermis, unspecified hip

L89.203   **Pressure ulcer of unspecified hip, stage 3** 🐾
     Healing pressure ulcer of unspecified hip, stage 3
     Pressure ulcer with full thickness skin loss involving damage or necrosis of subcutaneous tissue, unspecified hip

L89.204   **Pressure ulcer of unspecified hip, stage 4** 🐾
     Healing pressure ulcer of unspecified hip, stage 4
     Pressure ulcer with necrosis of soft tissues through to underlying muscle, tendon, or bone, unspecified hip

L89.206   **Pressure-induced deep tissue damage of unspecified hip**

L89.209   **Pressure ulcer of unspecified hip, unspecified stage**
     Healing pressure ulcer of unspecified hip NOS
     Healing pressure ulcer of unspecified hip, unspecified stage

● **L89.21**   **Pressure ulcer of right hip**

L89.210   **Pressure ulcer of right hip, unstageable** 🐾

L89.211   **Pressure ulcer of right hip, stage 1**
     Healing pressure ulcer of right hip back, stage 1
     Pressure pre-ulcer skin changes limited to persistent focal edema, right hip

L89.212   **Pressure ulcer of right hip, stage 2**
     Healing pressure ulcer of right hip, stage 2
     Pressure ulcer with abrasion, blister, partial thickness skin loss involving epidermis and/or dermis, right hip

L89.213   **Pressure ulcer of right hip, stage 3** 🐾
     Healing pressure ulcer of right hip, stage 3
     Pressure ulcer with full thickness skin loss involving damage or necrosis of subcutaneous tissue, right hip

L89.214   **Pressure ulcer of right hip, stage 4** 🐾
     Healing pressure ulcer of right hip, stage 4
     Pressure ulcer with necrosis of soft tissues through to underlying muscle, tendon, or bone, right hip

L89.216   **Pressure-induced deep tissue damage of right hip**

L89.219   **Pressure ulcer of right hip, unspecified stage**
     Healing pressure ulcer of right hip NOS
     Healing pressure ulcer of right hip, unspecified stage

● **L89.22**   **Pressure ulcer of left hip**

L89.220   **Pressure ulcer of left hip, unstageable** 🐾

L89.221   **Pressure ulcer of left hip, stage 1**
     Healing pressure ulcer of left hip back, stage 1
     Pressure pre-ulcer skin changes limited to persistent focal edema, left hip

L89.222   **Pressure ulcer of left hip, stage 2**
     Healing pressure ulcer of left hip, stage 2
     Pressure ulcer with abrasion, blister, partial thickness skin loss involving epidermis and/or dermis, left hip

L89.223   **Pressure ulcer of left hip, stage 3** 🐾
     Healing pressure ulcer of left hip, stage 3
     Pressure ulcer with full thickness skin loss involving damage or necrosis of subcutaneous tissue, left hip

L89.224   **Pressure ulcer of left hip, stage 4** 🐾
     Healing pressure ulcer of left hip, stage 4
     Pressure ulcer with necrosis of soft tissues through to underlying muscle, tendon, or bone, left hip

L89.226   **Pressure-induced deep tissue damage of left hip**

L89.229   **Pressure ulcer of left hip, unspecified stage**
     Healing pressure ulcer of left hip NOS
     Healing pressure ulcer of left hip, unspecified stage

● **L89.3**   **Pressure ulcer of buttock**

● **L89.30**   **Pressure ulcer of unspecified buttock**

L89.300   **Pressure ulcer of unspecified buttock, unstageable** 🐾

L89.301   **Pressure ulcer of unspecified buttock, stage 1**
     Healing pressure ulcer of unspecified buttock, stage 1
     Pressure pre-ulcer skin changes limited to persistent focal edema, unspecified buttock

L89.302   **Pressure ulcer of unspecified buttock, stage 2**
     Healing pressure ulcer of unspecified buttock, stage 2
     Pressure ulcer with abrasion, blister, partial thickness skin loss involving epidermis and/or dermis, unspecified buttock

L89.303   **Pressure ulcer of unspecified buttock, stage 3** 🐾
     Healing pressure ulcer of unspecified buttock, stage 3
     Pressure ulcer with full thickness skin loss involving damage or necrosis of subcutaneous tissue, unspecified buttock

L89.304   **Pressure ulcer of unspecified buttock, stage 4** 🐾
     Healing pressure ulcer of unspecified buttock, stage 4
     Pressure ulcer with necrosis of soft tissues through to underlying muscle, tendon, or bone, unspecified buttock

L89.306   **Pressure-induced deep tissue damage of unspecified buttock**

L89.309   **Pressure ulcer of unspecified buttock, unspecified stage**
Healing pressure ulcer of unspecified buttock NOS
Healing pressure ulcer of unspecified buttock, unspecified stage

● **L89.31**   **Pressure ulcer of right buttock**

L89.310   **Pressure ulcer of right buttock, unstageable** 🔖

L89.311   **Pressure ulcer of right buttock, stage 1**
Healing pressure ulcer of right buttock, stage 1
Pressure pre-ulcer skin changes limited to persistent focal edema, right buttock

L89.312   **Pressure ulcer of right buttock, stage 2**
Healing pressure ulcer of right buttock, stage 2
Pressure ulcer with abrasion, blister, partial thickness skin loss involving epidermis and/or dermis, right buttock

L89.313   **Pressure ulcer of right buttock, stage 3** 🔖
Healing pressure ulcer of right buttock, stage 3
Pressure ulcer with full thickness skin loss involving damage or necrosis of subcutaneous tissue, right buttock

L89.314   **Pressure ulcer of right buttock, stage 4** 🔖
Healing pressure ulcer of right buttock, stage 4
Pressure ulcer with necrosis of soft tissues through to underlying muscle, tendon, or bone, right buttock

L89.316   **Pressure-induced deep tissue damage of right buttock**

L89.319   **Pressure ulcer of right buttock, unspecified stage**
Healing pressure ulcer of right buttock NOS
Healing pressure ulcer of right buttock, unspecified stage

● **L89.32**   **Pressure ulcer of left buttock**

L89.320   **Pressure ulcer of left buttock, unstageable** 🔖

L89.321   **Pressure ulcer of left buttock, stage 1**
Healing pressure ulcer of left buttock, stage 1
Pressure pre-ulcer skin changes limited to persistent focal edema, left buttock

L89.322   **Pressure ulcer of left buttock, stage 2**
Healing pressure ulcer of left buttock, stage 2
Pressure ulcer with abrasion, blister, partial thickness skin loss involving epidermis and/or dermis, left buttock

L89.323   **Pressure ulcer of left buttock, stage 3** 🔖
Healing pressure ulcer of left buttock, stage 3
Pressure ulcer with full thickness skin loss involving damage or necrosis of subcutaneous tissue, left buttock

L89.324   **Pressure ulcer of left buttock, stage 4** 🔖
Healing pressure ulcer of left buttock, stage 4
Pressure ulcer with necrosis of soft tissues through to underlying muscle, tendon, or bone, left buttock

L89.326   **Pressure-induced deep tissue damage of left buttock**

L89.329   **Pressure ulcer of left buttock, unspecified stage**
Healing pressure ulcer of left buttock NOS
Healing pressure ulcer of left buttock, unspecified stage

● **L89.4**   **Pressure ulcer of contiguous site of back, buttock and hip**

L89.40   **Pressure ulcer of contiguous site of back, buttock and hip, unspecified stage**
Healing pressure ulcer of contiguous site of back, buttock and hip NOS
Healing pressure ulcer of contiguous site of back, buttock and hip, unspecified stage

L89.41   **Pressure ulcer of contiguous site of back, buttock and hip, stage 1**
Healing pressure ulcer of contiguous site of back, buttock and hip, stage 1
Pressure pre-ulcer skin changes limited to persistent focal edema, contiguous site of back, buttock and hip

L89.42   **Pressure ulcer of contiguous site of back, buttock and hip, stage 2**
Healing pressure ulcer of contiguous site of back, buttock and hip, stage 2
Pressure ulcer with abrasion, blister, partial thickness skin loss involving epidermis and/or dermis, contiguous site of back, buttock and hip

L89.43   **Pressure ulcer of contiguous site of back, buttock and hip, stage 3** 🔖
Healing pressure ulcer of contiguous site of back, buttock and hip, stage 3
Pressure ulcer with full thickness skin loss involving damage or necrosis of subcutaneous tissue, contiguous site of back, buttock and hip

L89.44   **Pressure ulcer of contiguous site of back, buttock and hip, stage 4** 🔖
Healing pressure ulcer of contiguous site of back, buttock and hip, stage 4
Pressure ulcer with necrosis of soft tissues through to underlying muscle, tendon, or bone, contiguous site of back, buttock and hip

L89.45   **Pressure ulcer of contiguous site of back, buttock and hip, unstageable** 🔖

L89.46   **Pressure-induced deep tissue damage of contiguous site of back, buttock and hip**

● **L89.5　Pressure ulcer of ankle**
　● **L89.50　Pressure ulcer of unspecified ankle**
　　　L89.500　Pressure ulcer of unspecified ankle, unstageable 🐾
　　　L89.501　Pressure ulcer of unspecified ankle, stage 1
　　　　　Healing pressure ulcer of unspecified ankle, stage 1
　　　　　Pressure pre-ulcer skin changes limited to persistent focal edema, unspecified ankle
　　　L89.502　Pressure ulcer of unspecified ankle, stage 2
　　　　　Healing pressure ulcer of unspecified ankle, stage 2
　　　　　Pressure ulcer with abrasion, blister, partial thickness skin loss involving epidermis and/or dermis, unspecified ankle
　　　L89.503　Pressure ulcer of unspecified ankle, stage 3 🐾
　　　　　Healing pressure ulcer of unspecified ankle, stage 3
　　　　　Pressure ulcer with full thickness skin loss involving damage or necrosis of subcutaneous tissue, unspecified ankle
　　　L89.504　Pressure ulcer of unspecified ankle, stage 4 🐾
　　　　　Healing pressure ulcer of unspecified ankle, stage 4
　　　　　Pressure ulcer with necrosis of soft tissues through to underlying muscle, tendon, or bone, unspecified ankle
　　　L89.506　Pressure-induced deep tissue damage of unspecified ankle
　　　L89.509　Pressure ulcer of unspecified ankle, unspecified stage
　　　　　Healing pressure ulcer of unspecified ankle NOS
　　　　　Healing pressure ulcer of unspecified ankle, unspecified stage
　● **L89.51　Pressure ulcer of right ankle**
　　　L89.510　Pressure ulcer of right ankle, unstageable 🐾
　　　L89.511　Pressure ulcer of right ankle, stage 1
　　　　　Healing pressure ulcer of right ankle, stage 1
　　　　　Pressure pre-ulcer skin changes limited to persistent focal edema, right ankle
　　　L89.512　Pressure ulcer of right ankle, stage 2
　　　　　Healing pressure ulcer of right ankle, stage 2
　　　　　Pressure ulcer with abrasion, blister, partial thickness skin loss involving epidermis and/or dermis, right ankle
　　　L89.513　Pressure ulcer of right ankle, stage 3 🐾
　　　　　Healing pressure ulcer of right ankle, stage 3
　　　　　Pressure ulcer with full thickness skin loss involving damage or necrosis of subcutaneous tissue, right ankle
　　　L89.514　Pressure ulcer of right ankle, stage 4 🐾
　　　　　Healing pressure ulcer of right ankle, stage 4
　　　　　Pressure ulcer with necrosis of soft tissues through to underlying muscle, tendon, or bone, right ankle

　　　L89.516　Pressure-induced deep tissue damage of right ankle
　　　L89.519　Pressure ulcer of right ankle, unspecified stage
　　　　　Healing pressure ulcer of right ankle NOS
　　　　　Healing pressure ulcer of right ankle, unspecified stage
　● **L89.52　Pressure ulcer of left ankle**
　　　L89.520　Pressure ulcer of left ankle, unstageable
　　　L89.521　Pressure ulcer of left ankle, stage 1
　　　　　Healing pressure ulcer of left ankle, stage 1
　　　　　Pressure pre-ulcer skin changes limited to persistent focal edema, left ankle
　　　L89.522　Pressure ulcer of left ankle, stage 2
　　　　　Healing pressure ulcer of left ankle, stage 2
　　　　　Pressure ulcer with abrasion, blister, partial thickness skin loss involving epidermis and/or dermis, left ankle
　　　L89.523　Pressure ulcer of left ankle, stage 3 🐾
　　　　　Healing pressure ulcer of left ankle, stage 3
　　　　　Pressure ulcer with full thickness skin loss involving damage or necrosis of subcutaneous tissue, left ankle
　　　L89.524　Pressure ulcer of left ankle, stage 4 🐾
　　　　　Healing pressure ulcer of left ankle, stage 4
　　　　　Pressure ulcer with necrosis of soft tissues through to underlying muscle, tendon, or bone, left ankle
　　　L89.526　Pressure-induced deep tissue damage of left ankle
　　　L89.529　Pressure ulcer of left ankle, unspecified stage
　　　　　Healing pressure ulcer of left ankle NOS
　　　　　Healing pressure ulcer of left ankle, unspecified stage
● **L89.6　Pressure ulcer of heel**
　● **L89.60　Pressure ulcer of unspecified heel**
　　　L89.600　Pressure ulcer of unspecified heel, unstageable 🐾
　　　L89.601　Pressure ulcer of unspecified heel, stage 1
　　　　　Healing pressure ulcer of unspecified heel, stage 1
　　　　　Pressure pre-ulcer skin changes limited to persistent focal edema, unspecified heel
　　　L89.602　Pressure ulcer of unspecified heel, stage 2
　　　　　Healing pressure ulcer of unspecified heel, stage 2
　　　　　Pressure ulcer with abrasion, blister, partial thickness skin loss involving epidermis and/or dermis, unspecified heel
　　　L89.603　Pressure ulcer of unspecified heel, stage 3 🐾
　　　　　Healing pressure ulcer of unspecified heel, stage 3
　　　　　Pressure ulcer with full thickness skin loss involving damage or necrosis of subcutaneous tissue, unspecified heel

▶ New　⇒ Revised　~~deleted~~ Deleted　Excludes 1　Excludes 2　Includes　Use additional　Code first　Code also　Key words
OGCR Official Guidelines　X Assign placeholder X　● Use Additional Character(s)　▶ Manifestation Code　🐾 Hierarchical Condition Category　**Coding Clinic**

CHAPTER 12 (L00-L99)

L89.604   Pressure ulcer of unspecified heel, stage 4 🔎
    Healing pressure ulcer of unspecified heel, stage 4
    Pressure ulcer with necrosis of soft tissues through to underlying muscle, tendon, or bone, unspecified heel

L89.606   Pressure-induced deep tissue damage of unspecified heel

L89.609   Pressure ulcer of unspecified heel, unspecified stage
    Healing pressure ulcer of unspecified heel NOS
    Healing pressure ulcer of unspecified heel, unspecified stage

● **L89.61   Pressure ulcer of right heel**

L89.610   Pressure ulcer of right heel, unstageable 🔎

L89.611   Pressure ulcer of right heel, stage 1
    Healing pressure ulcer of right heel, stage 1
    Pressure pre-ulcer skin changes limited to persistent focal edema, right heel

L89.612   Pressure ulcer of right heel, stage 2
    Healing pressure ulcer of right heel, stage 2
    Pressure ulcer with abrasion, blister, partial thickness skin loss involving epidermis and/or dermis, right heel

L89.613   Pressure ulcer of right heel, stage 3 🔎
    Healing pressure ulcer of right heel, stage 3
    Pressure ulcer with full thickness skin loss involving damage or necrosis of subcutaneous tissue, right heel

L89.614   Pressure ulcer of right heel, stage 4 🔎
    Healing pressure ulcer of right heel, stage 4
    Pressure ulcer with necrosis of soft tissues through to underlying muscle, tendon, or bone, right heel

L89.616   Pressure-induced deep tissue damage of right heel

L89.619   Pressure ulcer of right heel, unspecified stage
    Healing pressure ulcer of right heel NOS
    Healing pressure ulcer of right heel, unspecified stage

● **L89.62   Pressure ulcer of left heel**

L89.620   Pressure ulcer of left heel, unstageable 🔎

L89.621   Pressure ulcer of left heel, stage 1
    Healing pressure ulcer of left heel, stage 1
    Pressure pre-ulcer skin changes limited to persistent focal edema, left heel

L89.622   Pressure ulcer of left heel, stage 2
    Healing pressure ulcer of left heel, stage 2
    Pressure ulcer with abrasion, blister, partial thickness skin loss involving epidermis and/or dermis, left heel
    Coding Clinic: 2016, Q4, P142

L89.623   Pressure ulcer of left heel, stage 3 🔎
    Healing pressure ulcer of left heel, stage 3
    Pressure ulcer with full thickness skin loss involving damage or necrosis of subcutaneous tissue, left heel
    Coding Clinic: 2016, Q4, P142

L89.624   Pressure ulcer of left heel, stage 4 🔎
    Healing pressure ulcer of left heel, stage 4
    Pressure ulcer with necrosis of soft tissues through to underlying muscle, tendon, or bone, left heel

L89.626   Pressure-induced deep tissue damage of left heel

L89.629   Pressure ulcer of left heel, unspecified stage
    Healing pressure ulcer of left heel NOS
    Healing pressure ulcer of left heel, unspecified stage

● **L89.8   Pressure ulcer of other site**

● **L89.81   Pressure ulcer of head**
    Pressure ulcer of face

L89.810   Pressure ulcer of head, unstageable 🔎

L89.811   Pressure ulcer of head, stage 1
    Healing pressure ulcer of head, stage 1
    Pressure pre-ulcer skin changes limited to persistent focal edema, head

L89.812   Pressure ulcer of head, stage 2
    Healing pressure ulcer of head, stage 2
    Pressure ulcer with abrasion, blister, partial thickness skin loss involving epidermis and/or dermis, head

L89.813   Pressure ulcer of head, stage 3 🔎
    Healing pressure ulcer of head, stage 3
    Pressure ulcer with full thickness skin loss involving damage or necrosis of subcutaneous tissue, head

L89.814   Pressure ulcer of head, stage 4 🔎
    Healing pressure ulcer of head, stage 4
    Pressure ulcer with necrosis of soft tissues through to underlying muscle, tendon, or bone, head

L89.816   Pressure-induced deep tissue damage of head

L89.819   Pressure ulcer of head, unspecified stage
    Healing pressure ulcer of head NOS
    Healing pressure ulcer of head, unspecified stage

● **L89.89   Pressure ulcer of other site**

L89.890   Pressure ulcer of other site, unstageable 🔎

L89.891   Pressure ulcer of other site, stage 1
    Healing pressure ulcer of other site, stage 1
    Pressure pre-ulcer skin changes limited to persistent focal edema, other site

L89.892   Pressure ulcer of other site, stage 2
    Healing pressure ulcer of other site, stage 2
    Pressure ulcer with abrasion, blister, partial thickness skin loss involving epidermis and/or dermis, other site

CHAPTER 12 (L00-L99)

L89.893   **Pressure ulcer of other site, stage 3** 🐾
     Healing pressure ulcer of other site, stage 3
     Pressure ulcer with full thickness skin loss involving damage or necrosis of subcutaneous tissue, other site

L89.894   **Pressure ulcer of other site, stage 4** 🐾
     Healing pressure ulcer of other site, stage 4
     Pressure ulcer with necrosis of soft tissues through to underlying muscle, tendon, or bone, other site

L89.899   **Pressure ulcer of other site, unspecified stage**
     Healing pressure ulcer of other site NOS
     Healing pressure ulcer of other site, unspecified stage

● **L89.9   Pressure ulcer of unspecified site**

L89.90   **Pressure ulcer of unspecified site, unspecified stage**
     Healing pressure ulcer of unspecified site NOS
     Healing pressure ulcer of unspecified site, unspecified stage

L89.91   **Pressure ulcer of unspecified site, stage 1**
     Healing pressure ulcer of unspecified site, stage 1
     Pressure pre-ulcer skin changes limited to persistent focal edema, unspecified site

L89.92   **Pressure ulcer of unspecified site, stage 2**
     Healing pressure ulcer of unspecified site, stage 2
     Pressure ulcer with abrasion, blister, partial thickness skin loss involving epidermis and/or dermis, unspecified site

L89.93   **Pressure ulcer of unspecified site, stage 3** 🐾
     Healing pressure ulcer of unspecified site, stage 3
     Pressure ulcer with full thickness skin loss involving damage or necrosis of subcutaneous tissue, unspecified site

L89.94   **Pressure ulcer of unspecified site, stage 4** 🐾
     Healing pressure ulcer of unspecified site, stage 4
     Pressure ulcer with necrosis of soft tissues through to underlying muscle, tendon, or bone, unspecified site

L89.95   **Pressure ulcer of unspecified site, unstageable** 🐾

L89.96   **Pressure-induced deep tissue damage of unspecified site**

● **L90   Atrophic disorders of skin**

L90.0   **Lichen sclerosus et atrophicus**
     Excludes2   lichen sclerosus of external female genital organs (N90.4)
          lichen sclerosus of external male genital organs (N48.0)

L90.1   **Anetoderma of Schweninger-Buzzi**

L90.2   **Anetoderma of Jadassohn-Pellizzari**

L90.3   **Atrophoderma of Pasini and Pierini**

L90.4   **Acrodermatitis chronica atrophicans**

L90.5   **Scar conditions and fibrosis of skin**
     Adherent scar (skin)
     Cicatrix
     Disfigurement of skin due to scar
     Fibrosis of skin NOS
     Scar NOS
     Excludes2   hypertrophic scar (L91.0)
          keloid scar (L91.0)
     Coding Clinic: 2016, Q2, P5; 2015, Q1, P19

L90.6   **Striae atrophicae**

L90.8   **Other atrophic disorders of skin**

L90.9   **Atrophic disorder of skin, unspecified**

Item 12–11   Scleroderma means hard skin. It is a group of diseases that causes abnormal growth of connective tissues that support the skin and organs. There are two types: localized scleroderma affecting the skin and systemic scleroderma affecting blood vessels and internal organs and the skin.

● **L91   Hypertrophic disorders of skin**

L91.0   **Keloid scar**
     Hypertrophic scar
     Keloid
     Excludes2   acne keloid (L73.0)
          scar NOS (L90.5)

L91.8   **Other hypertrophic disorders of the skin**

L91.9   **Hypertrophic disorder of the skin, unspecified**

● **L92   Granulomatous disorders of skin and subcutaneous tissue**
     Excludes2   actinic granuloma (L57.5)

L92.0   **Granuloma annulare**
     Perforating granuloma annulare

L92.1   **Necrobiosis lipoidica, not elsewhere classified**
     Excludes1   necrobiosis lipoidica associated with diabetes mellitus (E08-E13 with .620)

L92.2   **Granuloma faciale [eosinophilic granuloma of skin]**

L92.3   **Foreign body granuloma of the skin and subcutaneous tissue**
     Use additional code to identify the type of retained foreign body (Z18.-)

L92.8   **Other granulomatous disorders of the skin and subcutaneous tissue**

L92.9   **Granulomatous disorder of the skin and subcutaneous tissue, unspecified**
     Excludes2   umbilical granuloma (P83.81)

● **L93   Lupus erythematosus**
     Use additional code for adverse effect, if applicable, to identify drug (T36-T50 with fifth or sixth character 5)
     Excludes1   lupus exedens (A18.4)
          lupus vulgaris (A18.4)
          scleroderma (M34.-)
          systemic lupus erythematosus (M32.-)

L93.0   **Discoid lupus erythematosus**
     Lupus erythematosus NOS

L93.1   **Subacute cutaneous lupus erythematosus**

L93.2   **Other local lupus erythematosus**
     Lupus erythematosus profundus
     Lupus panniculitis

● **L94   Other localized connective tissue disorders**
     Excludes1   systemic connective tissue disorders (M30-M36)

L94.0   **Localized scleroderma [morphea]**
     Circumscribed scleroderma

L94.1   **Linear scleroderma**
     En coup de sabre lesion

L94.2   **Calcinosis cutis**

L94.3   **Sclerodactyly**

L94.4   **Gottron's papules**

L94.5   **Poikiloderma vasculare atrophicans**

L94.6   **Ainhum**

L94.8   **Other specified localized connective tissue disorders**

L94.9   **Localized connective tissue disorder, unspecified**

● **L95   Vasculitis limited to skin, not elsewhere classified**
     Excludes1   angioma serpiginosum (L81.7)
          Henoch(-Schönlein) purpura (D69.0)
          hypersensitivity angiitis (M31.0)
          lupus panniculitis (L93.2)
          panniculitis NOS (M79.3)
          panniculitis of neck and back (M54.0-)
          polyarteritis nodosa (M30.0)
          relapsing panniculitis (M35.6)
          rheumatoid vasculitis (M05.2)
          serum sickness (T80.6-)
          urticaria (L50.-)
          Wegener's granulomatosis (M31.3-)

L95.0   Livedoid vasculitis
       Atrophie blanche (en plaque)

L95.1   Erythema elevatum diutinum

L95.8   Other vasculitis limited to the skin

L95.9   Vasculitis limited to the skin, unspecified

● **L97**   Non-pressure chronic ulcer of lower limb, not elsewhere classified

     Includes   chronic ulcer of skin of lower limb NOS
                   non-healing ulcer of skin
                   non-infected sinus of skin
                   trophic ulcer NOS
                   tropical ulcer NOS
                   ulcer of skin of lower limb NOS

     Code first any associated underlying condition, such as:
       any associated gangrene (I96)
       atherosclerosis of the lower extremities (I70.23-, I70.24-,
           I70.33-, I70.34-, I70.43-, I70.44-, I70.53-, I70.54-, I70.63-,
           I70.64-, I70.73-, I70.74-)
       chronic venous hypertension (I87.31-, I87.33-)
       diabetic ulcers (E08.621, E08.622, E09.621, E09.622, E10.621,
           E10.622, E11.621, E11.622, E13.621, E13.622)
       postphlebitic syndrome (I87.01-, I87.03-)
       postthrombotic syndrome (I87.01-, I87.03-)
       varicose ulcer (I83.0-, I83.2-)

     Excludes2   pressure ulcer (pressure area) (L89.-)
                   skin infections (L00-L08)
                   specific infections classified to A00-B99

● **L97.1**   Non-pressure chronic ulcer of thigh

   ● **L97.10**   Non-pressure chronic ulcer of unspecified thigh

       L97.101   Non-pressure chronic ulcer of unspecified thigh limited to breakdown of skin 🐾

       L97.102   Non-pressure chronic ulcer of unspecified thigh with fat layer exposed 🐾

       L97.103   Non-pressure chronic ulcer of unspecified thigh with necrosis of muscle 🐾

       L97.104   Non-pressure chronic ulcer of unspecified thigh with necrosis of bone 🐾

       L97.105   Non-pressure chronic ulcer of unspecified thigh with muscle involvement without evidence of necrosis 🐾

       L97.106   Non-pressure chronic ulcer of unspecified thigh with bone involvement without evidence of necrosis 🐾

       L97.108   Non-pressure chronic ulcer of unspecified thigh with other specified severity 🐾

       L97.109   Non-pressure chronic ulcer of unspecified thigh with unspecified severity 🐾

   ● **L97.11**   Non-pressure chronic ulcer of right thigh

       L97.111   Non-pressure chronic ulcer of right thigh limited to breakdown of skin 🐾

       L97.112   Non-pressure chronic ulcer of right thigh with fat layer exposed 🐾

       L97.113   Non-pressure chronic ulcer of right thigh with necrosis of muscle 🐾

       L97.114   Non-pressure chronic ulcer of right thigh with necrosis of bone 🐾

       L97.115   Non-pressure chronic ulcer of right thigh with muscle involvement without evidence of necrosis 🐾

       L97.116   Non-pressure chronic ulcer of right thigh with bone involvement without evidence of necrosis 🐾

       L97.118   Non-pressure chronic ulcer of right thigh with other specified severity 🐾

       L97.119   Non-pressure chronic ulcer of right thigh with unspecified severity 🐾

   ● **L97.12**   Non-pressure chronic ulcer of left thigh

       L97.121   Non-pressure chronic ulcer of left thigh limited to breakdown of skin 🐾

       L97.122   Non-pressure chronic ulcer of left thigh with fat layer exposed 🐾

       L97.123   Non-pressure chronic ulcer of left thigh with necrosis of muscle 🐾

       L97.124   Non-pressure chronic ulcer of left thigh with necrosis of bone 🐾

       L97.125   Non-pressure chronic ulcer of left thigh with muscle involvement without evidence of necrosis 🐾

       L97.126   Non-pressure chronic ulcer of left thigh with bone involvement without evidence of necrosis 🐾

       L97.128   Non-pressure chronic ulcer of left thigh with other specified severity 🐾

       L97.129   Non-pressure chronic ulcer of left thigh with unspecified severity 🐾

● **L97.2**   Non-pressure chronic ulcer of calf

   ● **L97.20**   Non-pressure chronic ulcer of unspecified calf

       L97.201   Non-pressure chronic ulcer of unspecified calf limited to breakdown of skin 🐾

       L97.202   Non-pressure chronic ulcer of unspecified calf with fat layer exposed 🐾

       L97.203   Non-pressure chronic ulcer of unspecified calf with necrosis of muscle 🐾

       L97.204   Non-pressure chronic ulcer of unspecified calf with necrosis of bone 🐾

       L97.205   Non-pressure chronic ulcer of unspecified calf with muscle involvement without evidence of necrosis 🐾

       L97.206   Non-pressure chronic ulcer of unspecified calf with bone involvement without evidence of necrosis 🐾

       L97.208   Non-pressure chronic ulcer of unspecified calf with other specified severity 🐾

       L97.209   Non-pressure chronic ulcer of unspecified calf with unspecified severity 🐾

   ● **L97.21**   Non-pressure chronic ulcer of right calf

       L97.211   Non-pressure chronic ulcer of right calf limited to breakdown of skin 🐾

       L97.212   Non-pressure chronic ulcer of right calf with fat layer exposed 🐾

       L97.213   Non-pressure chronic ulcer of right calf with necrosis of muscle 🐾

       L97.214   Non-pressure chronic ulcer of right calf with necrosis of bone 🐾

       L97.215   Non-pressure chronic ulcer of right calf with muscle involvement without evidence of necrosis 🐾

       L97.216   Non-pressure chronic ulcer of right calf with bone involvement without evidence of necrosis 🐾

       L97.218   Non-pressure chronic ulcer of right calf with other specified severity 🐾

       L97.219   Non-pressure chronic ulcer of right calf with unspecified severity 🐾

   ● **L97.22**   Non-pressure chronic ulcer of left calf

       L97.221   Non-pressure chronic ulcer of left calf limited to breakdown of skin 🐾

       L97.222   Non-pressure chronic ulcer of left calf with fat layer exposed 🐾

L97.223   Non-pressure chronic ulcer of left calf with necrosis of muscle 🐾

L97.224   Non-pressure chronic ulcer of left calf with necrosis of bone 🐾

L97.225   Non-pressure chronic ulcer of left calf with muscle involvement without evidence of necrosis 🐾

L97.226   Non-pressure chronic ulcer of left calf with bone involvement without evidence of necrosis 🐾

L97.228   Non-pressure chronic ulcer of left calf with other specified severity 🐾

L97.229   Non-pressure chronic ulcer of left calf with unspecified severity 🐾

● L97.3   Non-pressure chronic ulcer of ankle

  ● L97.30   Non-pressure chronic ulcer of unspecified ankle

L97.301   Non-pressure chronic ulcer of unspecified ankle limited to breakdown of skin 🐾

L97.302   Non-pressure chronic ulcer of unspecified ankle with fat layer exposed 🐾

L97.303   Non-pressure chronic ulcer of unspecified ankle with necrosis of muscle 🐾

L97.304   Non-pressure chronic ulcer of unspecified ankle with necrosis of bone 🐾

L97.305   Non-pressure chronic ulcer of unspecified ankle with muscle involvement without evidence of necrosis 🐾

L97.306   Non-pressure chronic ulcer of unspecified ankle with bone involvement without evidence of necrosis 🐾

L97.308   Non-pressure chronic ulcer of unspecified ankle with other specified severity 🐾

L97.309   Non-pressure chronic ulcer of unspecified ankle with unspecified severity 🐾

  ● L97.31   Non-pressure chronic ulcer of right ankle

L97.311   Non-pressure chronic ulcer of right ankle limited to breakdown of skin 🐾

L97.312   Non-pressure chronic ulcer of right ankle with fat layer exposed 🐾

L97.313   Non-pressure chronic ulcer of right ankle with necrosis of muscle 🐾

L97.314   Non-pressure chronic ulcer of right ankle with necrosis of bone 🐾

L97.315   Non-pressure chronic ulcer of right ankle with muscle involvement without evidence of necrosis 🐾
    Coding Clinic: 2017, Q4, P17

L97.316   Non-pressure chronic ulcer of right ankle with bone involvement without evidence of necrosis 🐾

L97.318   Non-pressure chronic ulcer of right ankle with other specified severity 🐾

L97.319   Non-pressure chronic ulcer of right ankle with unspecified severity 🐾

  ● L97.32   Non-pressure chronic ulcer of left ankle

L97.321   Non-pressure chronic ulcer of left ankle limited to breakdown of skin 🐾

L97.322   Non-pressure chronic ulcer of left ankle with fat layer exposed 🐾
    Coding Clinic: 2021, Q1, P8

L97.323   Non-pressure chronic ulcer of left ankle with necrosis of muscle 🐾

L97.324   Non-pressure chronic ulcer of left ankle with necrosis of bone 🐾

L97.325   Non-pressure chronic ulcer of left ankle with muscle involvement without evidence of necrosis 🐾

L97.326   Non-pressure chronic ulcer of left ankle with bone involvement without evidence of necrosis 🐾

L97.328   Non-pressure chronic ulcer of left ankle with other specified severity 🐾

L97.329   Non-pressure chronic ulcer of left ankle with unspecified severity 🐾

● L97.4   Non-pressure chronic ulcer of heel and midfoot
    Non-pressure chronic ulcer of plantar surface of midfoot

  ● L97.40   Non-pressure chronic ulcer of unspecified heel and midfoot

L97.401   Non-pressure chronic ulcer of unspecified heel and midfoot limited to breakdown of skin 🐾

L97.402   Non-pressure chronic ulcer of unspecified heel and midfoot with fat layer exposed 🐾

L97.403   Non-pressure chronic ulcer of unspecified heel and midfoot with necrosis of muscle 🐾

L97.404   Non-pressure chronic ulcer of unspecified heel and midfoot with necrosis of bone 🐾

L97.405   Non-pressure chronic ulcer of unspecified heel and midfoot with muscle involvement without evidence of necrosis 🐾

L97.406   Non-pressure chronic ulcer of unspecified heel and midfoot with bone involvement without evidence of necrosis 🐾

L97.408   Non-pressure chronic ulcer of unspecified heel and midfoot with other specified severity 🐾

L97.409   Non-pressure chronic ulcer of unspecified heel and midfoot with unspecified severity 🐾

  ● L97.41   Non-pressure chronic ulcer of right heel and midfoot

L97.411   Non-pressure chronic ulcer of right heel and midfoot limited to breakdown of skin 🐾

L97.412   Non-pressure chronic ulcer of right heel and midfoot with fat layer exposed 🐾

L97.413   Non-pressure chronic ulcer of right heel and midfoot with necrosis of muscle 🐾

L97.414   Non-pressure chronic ulcer of right heel and midfoot with necrosis of bone 🐾

L97.415   Non-pressure chronic ulcer of right heel and midfoot with muscle involvement without evidence of necrosis 🐾

L97.416   Non-pressure chronic ulcer of right heel and midfoot with bone involvement without evidence of necrosis 🐾

▶ New   ⇒ Revised   ~~deleted~~ Deleted   Excludes 1   Excludes 2   Includes   Use additional   Code first   Code also   Key words
OGCR Official Guidelines   X Assign placeholder X   ● Use Additional Character(s)   ▶ Manifestation Code   🐾 Hierarchical Condition Category   Coding Clinic

L97.418   Non-pressure chronic ulcer of right heel and midfoot with other specified severity 🔎

L97.419   Non-pressure chronic ulcer of right heel and midfoot with unspecified severity 🔎

● **L97.42**   Non-pressure chronic ulcer of left heel and midfoot

L97.421   Non-pressure chronic ulcer of left heel and midfoot limited to breakdown of skin 🔎
     Coding Clinic: 2016, Q1, P13

L97.422   Non-pressure chronic ulcer of left heel and midfoot with fat layer exposed 🔎

L97.423   Non-pressure chronic ulcer of left heel and midfoot with necrosis of muscle 🔎

L97.424   Non-pressure chronic ulcer of left heel and midfoot with necrosis of bone 🔎

L97.425   Non-pressure chronic ulcer of left heel and midfoot with muscle involvement without evidence of necrosis 🔎

L97.426   Non-pressure chronic ulcer of left heel and midfoot with bone involvement without evidence of necrosis 🔎

L97.428   Non-pressure chronic ulcer of left heel and midfoot with other specified severity 🔎

L97.429   Non-pressure chronic ulcer of left heel and midfoot with unspecified severity 🔎

● **L97.5**   Non-pressure chronic ulcer of other part of foot
     Non-pressure chronic ulcer of toe

● **L97.50**   Non-pressure chronic ulcer of other part of unspecified foot

L97.501   Non-pressure chronic ulcer of other part of unspecified foot limited to breakdown of skin 🔎

L97.502   Non-pressure chronic ulcer of other part of unspecified foot with fat layer exposed 🔎

L97.503   Non-pressure chronic ulcer of other part of unspecified foot with necrosis of muscle 🔎

L97.504   Non-pressure chronic ulcer of other part of unspecified foot with necrosis of bone 🔎

L97.505   Non-pressure chronic ulcer of other part of unspecified foot with muscle involvement without evidence of necrosis 🔎

L97.506   Non-pressure chronic ulcer of other part of unspecified foot with bone involvement without evidence of necrosis 🔎

L97.508   Non-pressure chronic ulcer of other part of unspecified foot with other specified severity 🔎

L97.509   Non-pressure chronic ulcer of other part of unspecified foot with unspecified severity 🔎

● **L97.51**   Non-pressure chronic ulcer of other part of right foot

L97.511   Non-pressure chronic ulcer of other part of right foot limited to breakdown of skin 🔎
     Coding Clinic: 2020, Q1, P12

L97.512   Non-pressure chronic ulcer of other part of right foot with fat layer exposed 🔎

L97.513   Non-pressure chronic ulcer of other part of right foot with necrosis of muscle 🔎

L97.514   Non-pressure chronic ulcer of other part of right foot with necrosis of bone 🔎

L97.515   Non-pressure chronic ulcer of other part of right foot with muscle involvement without evidence of necrosis 🔎

L97.516   Non-pressure chronic ulcer of other part of right foot with bone involvement without evidence of necrosis 🔎

L97.518   Non-pressure chronic ulcer of other part of right foot with other specified severity 🔎

L97.519   Non-pressure chronic ulcer of other part of right foot with unspecified severity 🔎

● **L97.52**   Non-pressure chronic ulcer of other part of left foot

L97.521   Non-pressure chronic ulcer of other part of left foot limited to breakdown of skin 🔎

L97.522   Non-pressure chronic ulcer of other part of left foot with fat layer exposed 🔎

L97.523   Non-pressure chronic ulcer of other part of left foot with necrosis of muscle 🔎

L97.524   Non-pressure chronic ulcer of other part of left foot with necrosis of bone 🔎

L97.525   Non-pressure chronic ulcer of other part of left foot with muscle involvement without evidence of necrosis 🔎

L97.526   Non-pressure chronic ulcer of other part of left foot with bone involvement without evidence of necrosis 🔎

L97.528   Non-pressure chronic ulcer of other part of left foot with other specified severity 🔎

L97.529   Non-pressure chronic ulcer of other part of left foot with unspecified severity 🔎

● **L97.8**   Non-pressure chronic ulcer of other part of lower leg

● **L97.80**   Non-pressure chronic ulcer of other part of unspecified lower leg

L97.801   Non-pressure chronic ulcer of other part of unspecified lower leg limited to breakdown of skin 🔎

L97.802   Non-pressure chronic ulcer of other part of unspecified lower leg with fat layer exposed 🔎

L97.803   Non-pressure chronic ulcer of other part of unspecified lower leg with necrosis of muscle 🔎

L97.804   Non-pressure chronic ulcer of other part of unspecified lower leg with necrosis of bone 🔎

L97.805   Non-pressure chronic ulcer of other part of unspecified lower leg with muscle involvement without evidence of necrosis 🔎

L97.806   Non-pressure chronic ulcer of other part of unspecified lower leg with bone involvement without evidence of necrosis 🔎

CHAPTER 12 (L00-L99)

L97.808   Non-pressure chronic ulcer of other part of unspecified lower leg with other specified severity 🐾

L97.809   Non-pressure chronic ulcer of other part of unspecified lower leg with unspecified severity 🐾

● L97.81   Non-pressure chronic ulcer of other part of right lower leg

L97.811   Non-pressure chronic ulcer of other part of right lower leg limited to breakdown of skin 🐾

L97.812   Non-pressure chronic ulcer of other part of right lower leg with fat layer exposed 🐾

L97.813   Non-pressure chronic ulcer of other part of right lower leg with necrosis of muscle 🐾

L97.814   Non-pressure chronic ulcer of other part of right lower leg with necrosis of bone 🐾

L97.815   Non-pressure chronic ulcer of other part of right lower leg with muscle involvement without evidence of necrosis 🐾

L97.816   Non-pressure chronic ulcer of other part of right lower leg with bone involvement without evidence of necrosis 🐾

L97.818   Non-pressure chronic ulcer of other part of right lower leg with other specified severity 🐾

L97.819   Non-pressure chronic ulcer of other part of right lower leg with unspecified severity 🐾

● L97.82   Non-pressure chronic ulcer of other part of left lower leg

L97.821   Non-pressure chronic ulcer of other part of left lower leg limited to breakdown of skin 🐾

L97.822   Non-pressure chronic ulcer of other part of left lower leg with fat layer exposed 🐾

L97.823   Non-pressure chronic ulcer of other part of left lower leg with necrosis of muscle 🐾

L97.824   Non-pressure chronic ulcer of other part of left lower leg with necrosis of bone 🐾

L97.825   Non-pressure chronic ulcer of other part of left lower leg with muscle involvement without evidence of necrosis 🐾

L97.826   Non-pressure chronic ulcer of other part of left lower leg with bone involvement without evidence of necrosis 🐾

L97.828   Non-pressure chronic ulcer of other part of left lower leg with other specified severity 🐾

L97.829   Non-pressure chronic ulcer of other part of left lower leg with unspecified severity 🐾

● L97.9   Non-pressure chronic ulcer of unspecified part of lower leg

● L97.90   Non-pressure chronic ulcer of unspecified part of unspecified lower leg

L97.901   Non-pressure chronic ulcer of unspecified part of unspecified lower leg limited to breakdown of skin 🐾

L97.902   Non-pressure chronic ulcer of unspecified part of unspecified lower leg with fat layer exposed 🐾

L97.903   Non-pressure chronic ulcer of unspecified part of unspecified lower leg with necrosis of muscle 🐾

L97.904   Non-pressure chronic ulcer of unspecified part of unspecified lower leg with necrosis of bone 🐾

L97.905   Non-pressure chronic ulcer of unspecified part of unspecified lower leg with muscle involvement without evidence of necrosis 🐾

L97.906   Non-pressure chronic ulcer of unspecified part of unspecified lower leg with bone involvement without evidence of necrosis 🐾

L97.908   Non-pressure chronic ulcer of unspecified part of unspecified lower leg with other specified severity 🐾

L97.909   Non-pressure chronic ulcer of unspecified part of unspecified lower leg with unspecified severity 🐾

● L97.91   Non-pressure chronic ulcer of unspecified part of right lower leg

L97.911   Non-pressure chronic ulcer of unspecified part of right lower leg limited to breakdown of skin 🐾

L97.912   Non-pressure chronic ulcer of unspecified part of right lower leg with fat layer exposed 🐾

L97.913   Non-pressure chronic ulcer of unspecified part of right lower leg with necrosis of muscle 🐾

L97.914   Non-pressure chronic ulcer of unspecified part of right lower leg with necrosis of bone 🐾

L97.915   Non-pressure chronic ulcer of unspecified part of right lower leg with muscle involvement without evidence of necrosis 🐾

L97.916   Non-pressure chronic ulcer of unspecified part of right lower leg with bone involvement without evidence of necrosis 🐾

L97.918   Non-pressure chronic ulcer of unspecified part of right lower leg with other specified severity 🐾

L97.919   Non-pressure chronic ulcer of unspecified part of right lower leg with unspecified severity 🐾

● L97.92   Non-pressure chronic ulcer of unspecified part of left lower leg

L97.921   Non-pressure chronic ulcer of unspecified part of left lower leg limited to breakdown of skin 🐾

L97.922   Non-pressure chronic ulcer of unspecified part of left lower leg with fat layer exposed 🐾

L97.923   Non-pressure chronic ulcer of unspecified part of left lower leg with necrosis of muscle 🐾

L97.924   Non-pressure chronic ulcer of unspecified part of left lower leg with necrosis of bone 🐾

L97.925   Non-pressure chronic ulcer of unspecified part of left lower leg with muscle involvement without evidence of necrosis 🐾

L97.926   Non-pressure chronic ulcer of unspecified part of left lower leg with bone involvement without evidence of necrosis 🐾

▶ New   ⇒ Revised   ~~deleted~~ Deleted   Excludes 1   Excludes 2   Includes   Use additional   Code first   Code also   Key words

OGCR Official Guidelines   X Assign placeholder X   ● Use Additional Character(s)   ▶ Manifestation Code   🐾 Hierarchical Condition Category   Coding Clinic

L97.928   **Non-pressure chronic ulcer of unspecified part of left lower leg with other specified severity** 🔖

L97.929   **Non-pressure chronic ulcer of unspecified part of left lower leg with unspecified severity** 🔖

● **L98   Other disorders of skin and subcutaneous tissue, not elsewhere classified**

L98.0   Pyogenic granuloma

> **Excludes2**   pyogenic granuloma of gingiva (K06.8)
> pyogenic granuloma of maxillary alveolar ridge (K04.5)
> pyogenic granuloma of oral mucosa (K13.4)

L98.1   Factitial dermatitis
Neurotic excoriation

> **Excludes1**   Excoriation (skin-picking) disorder (F42.4)

Coding Clinic: 2016, Q4, P15

L98.2   Febrile neutrophilic dermatosis [Sweet]

L98.3   Eosinophilic cellulitis [Wells]

● **L98.4   Non-pressure chronic ulcer of skin, not elsewhere classified**
Chronic ulcer of skin NOS
Tropical ulcer NOS
Ulcer of skin NOS

> **Excludes2**   pressure ulcer (pressure area) (L89.-)
> gangrene (I96) 🔖
> skin infections (L00-L08)
> specific infections classified to A00-B99
> ulcer of lower limb NEC (L97.-)
> varicose ulcer (I83.0-I83.93)

● **L98.41   Non-pressure chronic ulcer of buttock**

L98.411   **Non-pressure chronic ulcer of buttock limited to breakdown of skin** 🔖

L98.412   **Non-pressure chronic ulcer of buttock with fat layer exposed** 🔖

L98.413   **Non-pressure chronic ulcer of buttock with necrosis of muscle** 🔖

L98.414   **Non-pressure chronic ulcer of buttock with necrosis of bone** 🔖

L98.415   **Non-pressure chronic ulcer of buttock with muscle involvement without evidence of necrosis** 🔖

L98.416   **Non-pressure chronic ulcer of buttock with bone involvement without evidence of necrosis** 🔖

L98.418   **Non-pressure chronic ulcer of buttock with other specified severity** 🔖

L98.419   **Non-pressure chronic ulcer of buttock with unspecified severity** 🔖

● **L98.42   Non-pressure chronic ulcer of back**

L98.421   **Non-pressure chronic ulcer of back limited to breakdown of skin** 🔖

L98.422   **Non-pressure chronic ulcer of back with fat layer exposed** 🔖

L98.423   **Non-pressure chronic ulcer of back with necrosis of muscle** 🔖

L98.424   **Non-pressure chronic ulcer of back with necrosis of bone** 🔖

L98.425   **Non-pressure chronic ulcer of back with muscle involvement without evidence of necrosis** 🔖

L98.426   **Non-pressure chronic ulcer of back with bone involvement without evidence of necrosis** 🔖

L98.428   **Non-pressure chronic ulcer of back with other specified severity** 🔖

L98.429   **Non-pressure chronic ulcer of back with unspecified severity** 🔖

● **L98.49   Non-pressure chronic ulcer of skin of other sites**
Non-pressure chronic ulcer of skin NOS

L98.491   **Non-pressure chronic ulcer of skin of other sites limited to breakdown of skin** 🔖

L98.492   **Non-pressure chronic ulcer of skin of other sites with fat layer exposed** 🔖

L98.493   **Non-pressure chronic ulcer of skin of other sites with necrosis of muscle** 🔖

L98.494   **Non-pressure chronic ulcer of skin of other sites with necrosis of bone** 🔖

L98.495   **Non-pressure chronic ulcer of skin of other sites with muscle involvement without evidence of necrosis** 🔖

L98.496   **Non-pressure chronic ulcer of skin of other sites with bone involvement without evidence of necrosis** 🔖

L98.498   **Non-pressure chronic ulcer of skin of other sites with other specified severity** 🔖

L98.499   **Non-pressure chronic ulcer of skin of other sites with unspecified severity** 🔖

L98.5   Mucinosis of the skin
Focal mucinosis
Lichen myxedematosus
Reticular erythematous mucinosis

> **Excludes1**   focal oral mucinosis (K13.79)
> myxedema (E03.9)

L98.6   Other infiltrative disorders of the skin and subcutaneous tissue

> **Excludes1**   hyalinosis cutis et mucosae (E78.89)

L98.7   Excessive and redundant skin and subcutaneous tissue
Loose or sagging skin following bariatric surgery weight loss
Loose or sagging skin following dietary weight loss
Loose or sagging skin, NOS

> **Excludes2**   acquired excess or redundant skin of eyelid (H02.3-)
> congenital excess or redundant skin of eyelid (Q10.3)
> skin changes due to chronic exposure to nonionizing radiation (L57.-)

Coding Clinic: 2016, Q4, P36

L98.8   Other specified disorders of the skin and subcutaneous tissue
Coding Clinic: 2013, Q2, P32

L98.9   Disorder of the skin and subcutaneous tissue, unspecified

▶ *L99   Other disorders of skin and subcutaneous tissue in diseases classified elsewhere*
Code first underlying disease, such as:
amyloidosis (E85.-)

➡ **Excludes1**   skin disorders in diabetes (E08-E13 with .62-)
skin disorders in gonorrhea (A54.89)
skin disorders in syphilis (A51.31, A52.79)

CHAPTER 13

DISEASES OF THE MUSCULOSKELETAL SYSTEM AND CONNECTIVE TISSUE (M00-M99)

OGCR Chapter-Specific Coding Guidelines

13. **Chapter 13: Diseases of the Musculoskeletal System and Connective Tissue (M00-M99)**

   a. Site and laterality
   Most of the codes within Chapter 13 have site and laterality designations. The site represents the bone, joint or the muscle involved. For some conditions where more than one bone, joint or muscle is usually involved, such as osteoarthritis, there is a "multiple sites" code available. For categories where no multiple site code is provided and more than one bone, joint or muscle is involved, multiple codes should be used to indicate the different sites involved.

   1) Bone versus joint
   For certain conditions, the bone may be affected at the upper or lower end (e.g., avascular necrosis of bone, M87, Osteoporosis, M80, M81). Though the portion of the bone affected may be at the joint, the site designation will be the bone, not the joint.

   b. Acute traumatic versus chronic or recurrent musculoskeletal conditions
   Many musculoskeletal conditions are a result of previous injury or trauma to a site, or are recurrent conditions. Bone, joint or muscle conditions that are the result of a healed injury are usually found in Chapter 13. Recurrent bone, joint or muscle conditions are also usually found in Chapter 13. Any current, acute injury should be coded to the appropriate injury code from Chapter 19. Chronic or recurrent conditions should generally be coded with a code from Chapter 13. If it is difficult to determine from the documentation in the record which code is best to describe a condition, query the provider.

   c. Coding of Pathologic Fractures
   7th character A is for use as long as the patient is receiving active treatment for the fracture. While the patient may be seen by a new or different provider over the course of treatment for a pathological fracture, assignment of the 7th character is based on whether the patient is undergoing active treatment and not whether the provider is seeing the patient for the first time.

   7th character, D is to be used for encounters after the patient has completed active treatment for the fracture and is receiving routine care for the fracture during the healing or recovery phase. The other 7th characters, listed under each subcategory in the Tabular List, are to be used for subsequent encounters for treatment of problems associated with the healing, such as malunions, nonunions, and sequelae.

   Care for complications of surgical treatment for fracture repairs during the healing or recovery phase should be coded with the appropriate complication codes.

   See Section I.C.19. Coding of traumatic fractures.

   d. Osteoporosis
   Osteoporosis is a systemic condition, meaning that all bones of the musculoskeletal system are affected. Therefore, site is not a component of the codes under category M81, Osteoporosis without current pathological fracture. The site codes under category M80, Osteoporosis with current pathological fracture, identify the site of the fracture, not the osteoporosis.

   1) Osteoporosis without pathological fracture
   Category M81, Osteoporosis without current pathological fracture, is for use for patients with osteoporosis who do not currently have a pathologic fracture due to the osteoporosis, even if they have had a fracture in the past. For patients with a history of osteoporosis fractures, status code Z87.310, Personal history of (healed) osteoporosis fracture, should follow the code from M81.

   2) Osteoporosis with current pathological fracture
   Category M80, Osteoporosis with current pathological fracture, is for patients who have a current pathologic fracture at the time of an encounter. The codes under M80 identify the site of the fracture. A code from category M80, not a traumatic fracture code, should be used for any patient with known osteoporosis who suffers a fracture, even if the patient had a minor fall or trauma, if that fall or trauma would not usually break a normal, healthy bone.

CHAPTER 13

DISEASES OF THE MUSCULOSKELETAL SYSTEM AND CONNECTIVE TISSUE (M00-M99)

Note: Use an external cause code following the code for the musculoskeletal condition, if applicable, to identify the cause of the musculoskeletal condition

Excludes2   arthropathic psoriasis (L40.5-)
certain conditions originating in the perinatal period (P04-P96)
certain infectious and parasitic diseases (A00-B99)
compartment syndrome (traumatic) (T79.A-)
complications of pregnancy, childbirth and the puerperium (O00-O9A)
congenital malformations, deformations, and chromosomal abnormalities (Q00-Q99)
endocrine, nutritional and metabolic diseases (E00-E88)
injury, poisoning and certain other consequences of external causes (S00-T88)
neoplasms (C00-D49)
symptoms, signs and abnormal clinical and laboratory findings, not elsewhere classified (R00-R94)

This chapter contains the following blocks:

M00-M02	Infectious arthropathies
M04	Autoinflammatory syndromes
M05-M14	Inflammatory polyarthropathies
M15-M19	Osteoarthritis
M20-M25	Other joint disorders
M26-M27	Dentofacial anomalies [including malocclusion] and other disorders of jaw
M30-M36	Systemic connective tissue disorders
M40-M43	Deforming dorsopathies
M45-M49	Spondylopathies
M50-M54	Other dorsopathies
M60-M63	Disorders of muscles
M65-M67	Disorders of synovium and tendon
M70-M79	Other soft tissue disorders
M80-M85	Disorders of bone density and structure
M86-M90	Other osteopathies
M91-M94	Chondropathies
M95	Other disorders of the musculoskeletal system and connective tissue
M96	Intraoperative and postprocedural complications and disorders of musculoskeletal system, not elsewhere classified
M97	Periprosthetic fracture around internal prosthetic joint
M99	Biomechanical lesions, not elsewhere classified

Coding Clinic: 2016, Q4, P124

ARTHROPATHIES (M00-M25)

Includes   Disorders affecting predominantly peripheral (limb) joints

INFECTIOUS ARTHROPATHIES (M00-M02)

Note: This block comprises arthropathies due to microbiological agents.

Distinction is made between the following types of etiological relationship:

a) direct infection of joint, where organisms invade synovial tissue and microbial antigen is present in the joint;

b) indirect infection, which may be of two types: a reactive arthropathy, where microbial infection of the body is established but neither organisms nor antigens can be identified in the joint, and a postinfective arthropathy, where microbial antigen is present but recovery of an organism is inconstant and evidence of local multiplication is lacking.

▶ New   ⇒ Revised   ~~deleted~~ Deleted   Excludes 1   Excludes 2   Includes   Use additional   Code first   Code also   Key words
OGCR Official Guidelines   X Assign placeholder X   ● Use Additional Character(s)   ▶ Manifestation Code   🔖 Hierarchical Condition Category   Coding Clinic

● **M00   Pyogenic arthritis**

     Excludes2   infection and inflammatory reaction due to internal joint prosthesis (T84.5-)

● **M00.0   Staphylococcal arthritis and polyarthritis**

     Use additional code (B95.61-B95.8) to identify bacterial agent

     M00.00   Staphylococcal arthritis, unspecified joint 🦠

●   M00.01   Staphylococcal arthritis, shoulder

        M00.011   Staphylococcal arthritis, right shoulder 🦠

        M00.012   Staphylococcal arthritis, left shoulder 🦠

        M00.019   Staphylococcal arthritis, unspecified shoulder 🦠

●   M00.02   Staphylococcal arthritis, elbow

        M00.021   Staphylococcal arthritis, right elbow 🦠

        M00.022   Staphylococcal arthritis, left elbow 🦠

        M00.029   Staphylococcal arthritis, unspecified elbow 🦠

●   M00.03   Staphylococcal arthritis, wrist

        Staphylococcal arthritis of carpal bones

        M00.031   Staphylococcal arthritis, right wrist 🦠

        M00.032   Staphylococcal arthritis, left wrist 🦠

        M00.039   Staphylococcal arthritis, unspecified wrist 🦠

●   M00.04   Staphylococcal arthritis, hand

        Staphylococcal arthritis of metacarpus and phalanges

        M00.041   Staphylococcal arthritis, right hand 🦠

        M00.042   Staphylococcal arthritis, left hand 🦠

        M00.049   Staphylococcal arthritis, unspecified hand 🦠

●   M00.05   Staphylococcal arthritis, hip

        M00.051   Staphylococcal arthritis, right hip 🦠

        M00.052   Staphylococcal arthritis, left hip 🦠

        M00.059   Staphylococcal arthritis, unspecified hip 🦠

●   M00.06   Staphylococcal arthritis, knee

        M00.061   Staphylococcal arthritis, right knee 🦠

        M00.062   Staphylococcal arthritis, left knee 🦠

        M00.069   Staphylococcal arthritis, unspecified knee 🦠

●   M00.07   Staphylococcal arthritis, ankle and foot

        Staphylococcal arthritis, tarsus, metatarsus and phalanges

        M00.071   Staphylococcal arthritis, right ankle and foot 🦠

        M00.072   Staphylococcal arthritis, left ankle and foot 🦠

        M00.079   Staphylococcal arthritis, unspecified ankle and foot 🦠

     M00.08   Staphylococcal arthritis, vertebrae 🦠

     M00.09   Staphylococcal polyarthritis 🦠

● **M00.1   Pneumococcal arthritis and polyarthritis**

     M00.10   Pneumococcal arthritis, unspecified joint 🦠

●   M00.11   Pneumococcal arthritis, shoulder

        M00.111   Pneumococcal arthritis, right shoulder 🦠

        M00.112   Pneumococcal arthritis, left shoulder 🦠

        M00.119   Pneumococcal arthritis, unspecified shoulder 🦠

●   M00.12   Pneumococcal arthritis, elbow

        M00.121   Pneumococcal arthritis, right elbow 🦠

        M00.122   Pneumococcal arthritis, left elbow 🦠

        M00.129   Pneumococcal arthritis, unspecified elbow 🦠

●   M00.13   Pneumococcal arthritis, wrist

        Pneumococcal arthritis of carpal bones

        M00.131   Pneumococcal arthritis, right wrist 🦠

        M00.132   Pneumococcal arthritis, left wrist 🦠

        M00.139   Pneumococcal arthritis, unspecified wrist 🦠

●   M00.14   Pneumococcal arthritis, hand

        Pneumococcal arthritis of metacarpus and phalanges

        M00.141   Pneumococcal arthritis, right hand 🦠

        M00.142   Pneumococcal arthritis, left hand 🦠

        M00.149   Pneumococcal arthritis, unspecified hand 🦠

●   M00.15   Pneumococcal arthritis, hip

        M00.151   Pneumococcal arthritis, right hip 🦠

        M00.152   Pneumococcal arthritis, left hip 🦠

        M00.159   Pneumococcal arthritis, unspecified hip 🦠

●   M00.16   Pneumococcal arthritis, knee

        M00.161   Pneumococcal arthritis, right knee 🦠

        M00.162   Pneumococcal arthritis, left knee 🦠

        M00.169   Pneumococcal arthritis, unspecified knee 🦠

●   M00.17   Pneumococcal arthritis, ankle and foot

        Pneumococcal arthritis, tarsus, metatarsus and phalanges

        M00.171   Pneumococcal arthritis, right ankle and foot 🦠

        M00.172   Pneumococcal arthritis, left ankle and foot 🦠

        M00.179   Pneumococcal arthritis, unspecified ankle and foot 🦠

     M00.18   Pneumococcal arthritis, vertebrae 🦠

     M00.19   Pneumococcal polyarthritis 🦠

● **M00.2   Other streptococcal arthritis and polyarthritis**

     Use additional code (B95.0-B95.2, B95.4-B95.5) to identify bacterial agent

     M00.20   Other streptococcal arthritis, unspecified joint 🦠

●   M00.21   Other streptococcal arthritis, shoulder

        M00.211   Other streptococcal arthritis, right shoulder 🦠

        M00.212   Other streptococcal arthritis, left shoulder 🦠

        M00.219   Other streptococcal arthritis, unspecified shoulder 🦠

●   M00.22   Other streptococcal arthritis, elbow

        M00.221   Other streptococcal arthritis, right elbow 🦠

        M00.222   Other streptococcal arthritis, left elbow 🦠

        M00.229   Other streptococcal arthritis, unspecified elbow 🦠

●   M00.23   Other streptococcal arthritis, wrist

        Other streptococcal arthritis of carpal bones

        M00.231   Other streptococcal arthritis, right wrist 🦠

        M00.232   Other streptococcal arthritis, left wrist 🦠

        M00.239   Other streptococcal arthritis, unspecified wrist 🦠

● M00.24 Other streptococcal arthritis, hand
Other streptococcal arthritis metacarpus and phalanges
  - M00.241 Other streptococcal arthritis, right hand 🦠
  - M00.242 Other streptococcal arthritis, left hand 🦠
  - M00.249 Other streptococcal arthritis, unspecified hand 🦠

● M00.25 Other streptococcal arthritis, hip
  - M00.251 Other streptococcal arthritis, right hip 🦠
  - M00.252 Other streptococcal arthritis, left hip 🦠
  - M00.259 Other streptococcal arthritis, unspecified hip 🦠

● M00.26 Other streptococcal arthritis, knee
  - M00.261 Other streptococcal arthritis, right knee 🦠
  - M00.262 Other streptococcal arthritis, left knee 🦠
  - M00.269 Other streptococcal arthritis, unspecified knee 🦠

● M00.27 Other streptococcal arthritis, ankle and foot
Other streptococcal arthritis, tarsus, metatarsus and phalanges
  - M00.271 Other streptococcal arthritis, right ankle and foot 🦠
  - M00.272 Other streptococcal arthritis, left ankle and foot 🦠
  - M00.279 Other streptococcal arthritis, unspecified ankle and foot 🦠

M00.28 Other streptococcal arthritis, vertebrae 🦠

M00.29 Other streptococcal polyarthritis 🦠

● M00.8 Arthritis and polyarthritis due to other bacteria
Use additional code (B96) to identify bacteria

M00.80 Arthritis due to other bacteria, unspecified joint 🦠

● M00.81 Arthritis due to other bacteria, shoulder
  - M00.811 Arthritis due to other bacteria, right shoulder 🦠
  - M00.812 Arthritis due to other bacteria, left shoulder 🦠
  - M00.819 Arthritis due to other bacteria, unspecified shoulder 🦠

● M00.82 Arthritis due to other bacteria, elbow
  - M00.821 Arthritis due to other bacteria, right elbow 🦠
  - M00.822 Arthritis due to other bacteria, left elbow 🦠
  - M00.829 Arthritis due to other bacteria, unspecified elbow 🦠

● M00.83 Arthritis due to other bacteria, wrist
Arthritis due to other bacteria, carpal bones
  - M00.831 Arthritis due to other bacteria, right wrist 🦠
  - M00.832 Arthritis due to other bacteria, left wrist 🦠
  - M00.839 Arthritis due to other bacteria, unspecified wrist 🦠

● M00.84 Arthritis due to other bacteria, hand
Arthritis due to other bacteria, metacarpus and phalanges
  - M00.841 Arthritis due to other bacteria, right hand 🦠
  - M00.842 Arthritis due to other bacteria, left hand 🦠
  - M00.849 Arthritis due to other bacteria, unspecified hand 🦠

● M00.85 Arthritis due to other bacteria, hip
  - M00.851 Arthritis due to other bacteria, right hip 🦠
  - M00.852 Arthritis due to other bacteria, left hip 🦠
  - M00.859 Arthritis due to other bacteria, unspecified hip 🦠

● M00.86 Arthritis due to other bacteria, knee
  - M00.861 Arthritis due to other bacteria, right knee 🦠
  - M00.862 Arthritis due to other bacteria, left knee 🦠
    Coding Clinic: 2019, Q3, P16
  - M00.869 Arthritis due to other bacteria, unspecified knee 🦠

● M00.87 Arthritis due to other bacteria, ankle and foot
Arthritis due to other bacteria, tarsus, metatarsus, and phalanges
  - M00.871 Arthritis due to other bacteria, right ankle and foot 🦠
  - M00.872 Arthritis due to other bacteria, left ankle and foot 🦠
  - M00.879 Arthritis due to other bacteria, unspecified ankle and foot 🦠

M00.88 Arthritis due to other bacteria, vertebrae 🦠

M00.89 Polyarthritis due to other bacteria 🦠

M00.9 Pyogenic arthritis, unspecified 🦠
Infective arthritis NOS

● M01 Direct infections of joint in infectious and parasitic diseases classified elsewhere

Code first underlying disease, such as:
leprosy [Hansen's disease] (A30.-)
mycoses (B35-B49)
O'nyong-nyong fever (A92.1)
paratyphoid fever (A01.1-A01.4)

Excludes1 arthropathy in Lyme disease (A69.23)
gonococcal arthritis (A54.42)
meningococcal arthritis (A39.83)
mumps arthritis (B26.85)
postinfective arthropathy (M02.-)
postmeningococcal arthritis (A39.84)
reactive arthritis (M02.3)
rubella arthritis (B06.82)
sarcoidosis arthritis (D86.86)
typhoid fever arthritis (A01.04)
tuberculosis arthritis (A18.01-A18.02)

● M01.X Direct infection of joint in infectious and parasitic diseases classified elsewhere

▷ M01.X0 Direct infection of unspecified joint in infectious and parasitic diseases classified elsewhere 🦠

● M01.X1 Direct infection of shoulder joint in infectious and parasitic diseases classified elsewhere
  - ▷ M01.X11 Direct infection of right shoulder in infectious and parasitic diseases classified elsewhere 🦠
  - ▷ M01.X12 Direct infection of left shoulder in infectious and parasitic diseases classified elsewhere 🦠
  - ▷ M01.X19 Direct infection of unspecified shoulder in infectious and parasitic diseases classified elsewhere 🦠

● M01.X2 Direct infection of elbow in infectious and parasitic diseases classified elsewhere
  - ▷ M01.X21 Direct infection of right elbow in infectious and parasitic diseases classified elsewhere 🦠
  - ▷ M01.X22 Direct infection of left elbow in infectious and parasitic diseases classified elsewhere 🦠
  - ▷ M01.X29 Direct infection of unspecified elbow in infectious and parasitic diseases classified elsewhere 🦠

● **M01.X3** **Direct infection of wrist in infectious and parasitic diseases classified elsewhere**
> Direct infection of carpal bones in infectious and parasitic diseases classified elsewhere

  ▷ *M01.X31* *Direct infection of right wrist in infectious and parasitic diseases classified elsewhere* 🦠

  ▷ *M01.X32* *Direct infection of left wrist in infectious and parasitic diseases classified elsewhere* 🦠

  ▷ *M01.X39* *Direct infection of unspecified wrist in infectious and parasitic diseases classified elsewhere* 🦠

● **M01.X4** **Direct infection of hand in infectious and parasitic diseases classified elsewhere**
> Direct infection of metacarpus and phalanges in infectious and parasitic diseases classified elsewhere

  ▷ *M01.X41* *Direct infection of right hand in infectious and parasitic diseases classified elsewhere* 🦠

  ▷ *M01.X42* *Direct infection of left hand in infectious and parasitic diseases classified elsewhere* 🦠

  ▷ *M01.X49* *Direct infection of unspecified hand in infectious and parasitic diseases classified elsewhere* 🦠

● **M01.X5** **Direct infection of hip in infectious and parasitic diseases classified elsewhere**

  ▷ *M01.X51* *Direct infection of right hip in infectious and parasitic diseases classified elsewhere* 🦠

  ▷ *M01.X52* *Direct infection of left hip in infectious and parasitic diseases classified elsewhere* 🦠

  ▷ *M01.X59* *Direct infection of unspecified hip in infectious and parasitic diseases classified elsewhere* 🦠

● **M01.X6** **Direct infection of knee in infectious and parasitic diseases classified elsewhere**

  ▷ *M01.X61* *Direct infection of right knee in infectious and parasitic diseases classified elsewhere* 🦠

  ▷ *M01.X62* *Direct infection of left knee in infectious and parasitic diseases classified elsewhere* 🦠

  ▷ *M01.X69* *Direct infection of unspecified knee in infectious and parasitic diseases classified elsewhere* 🦠

● **M01.X7** **Direct infection of ankle and foot in infectious and parasitic diseases classified elsewhere**
> Direct infection of tarsus, metatarsus and phalanges in infectious and parasitic diseases classified elsewhere

  ▷ *M01.X71* *Direct infection of right ankle and foot in infectious and parasitic diseases classified elsewhere* 🦠

  ▷ *M01.X72* *Direct infection of left ankle and foot in infectious and parasitic diseases classified elsewhere* 🦠

  ▷ *M01.X79* *Direct infection of unspecified ankle and foot in infectious and parasitic diseases classified elsewhere* 🦠

  ▷ *M01.X8* *Direct infection of vertebrae in infectious and parasitic diseases classified elsewhere* 🦠

  ▷ *M01.X9* *Direct infection of multiple joints in infectious and parasitic diseases classified elsewhere* 🦠

● **M02** **Postinfective and reactive arthropathies**
> *Code first* underlying disease, such as:
> congenital syphilis [Clutton's joints] (A50.5)
> enteritis due to Yersinia enterocolitica (A04.6)
> infective endocarditis (I33.0)
> viral hepatitis (B15-B19)

  Excludes1   Behçet's disease (M35.2)
  > direct infections of joint in infectious and parasitic diseases classified elsewhere (M01.-)
  > postmeningococcal arthritis (A39.84)
  > mumps arthritis (B26.85)
  > rubella arthritis (B06.82)
  > syphilis arthritis (late) (A52.77)
  > rheumatic fever (I00)
  > tabetic arthropathy [Charcôt's] (A52.16)

● **M02.0** **Arthropathy following intestinal bypass**

  M02.00 **Arthropathy following intestinal bypass, unspecified site**

● **M02.01** **Arthropathy following intestinal bypass, shoulder**

  M02.011 **Arthropathy following intestinal bypass, right shoulder**

  M02.012 **Arthropathy following intestinal bypass, left shoulder**

  M02.019 **Arthropathy following intestinal bypass, unspecified shoulder**

● **M02.02** **Arthropathy following intestinal bypass, elbow**

  M02.021 **Arthropathy following intestinal bypass, right elbow**

  M02.022 **Arthropathy following intestinal bypass, left elbow**

  M02.029 **Arthropathy following intestinal bypass, unspecified elbow**

● **M02.03** **Arthropathy following intestinal bypass, wrist**
> Arthropathy following intestinal bypass, carpal bones

  M02.031 **Arthropathy following intestinal bypass, right wrist**

  M02.032 **Arthropathy following intestinal bypass, left wrist**

  M02.039 **Arthropathy following intestinal bypass, unspecified wrist**

● **M02.04** **Arthropathy following intestinal bypass, hand**
> Arthropathy following intestinal bypass, metacarpals and phalanges

  M02.041 **Arthropathy following intestinal bypass, right hand**

  M02.042 **Arthropathy following intestinal bypass, left hand**

  M02.049 **Arthropathy following intestinal bypass, unspecified hand**

● **M02.05** **Arthropathy following intestinal bypass, hip**

  M02.051 **Arthropathy following intestinal bypass, right hip**

  M02.052 **Arthropathy following intestinal bypass, left hip**

  M02.059 **Arthropathy following intestinal bypass, unspecified hip**

● **M02.06** **Arthropathy following intestinal bypass, knee**

  M02.061 **Arthropathy following intestinal bypass, right knee**

  M02.062 **Arthropathy following intestinal bypass, left knee**

  M02.069 **Arthropathy following intestinal bypass, unspecified knee**

CHAPTER 13 (M00-M99)

● **M02.07** Arthropathy following intestinal bypass, ankle and foot
> Arthropathy following intestinal bypass, tarsus, metatarsus and phalanges

     M02.071 Arthropathy following intestinal bypass, right ankle and foot

     M02.072 Arthropathy following intestinal bypass, left ankle and foot

     M02.079 Arthropathy following intestinal bypass, unspecified ankle and foot

   M02.08 Arthropathy following intestinal bypass, vertebrae

   M02.09 Arthropathy following intestinal bypass, multiple sites

● **M02.1** Postdysenteric arthropathy

   M02.10 Postdysenteric arthropathy, unspecified site 🐾

● **M02.11** Postdysenteric arthropathy, shoulder

     M02.111 Postdysenteric arthropathy, right shoulder 🐾

     M02.112 Postdysenteric arthropathy, left shoulder 🐾

     M02.119 Postdysenteric arthropathy, unspecified shoulder 🐾

● **M02.12** Postdysenteric arthropathy, elbow

     M02.121 Postdysenteric arthropathy, right elbow 🐾

     M02.122 Postdysenteric arthropathy, left elbow 🐾

     M02.129 Postdysenteric arthropathy, unspecified elbow 🐾

● **M02.13** Postdysenteric arthropathy, wrist
> Postdysenteric arthropathy, carpal bones

     M02.131 Postdysenteric arthropathy, right wrist 🐾

     M02.132 Postdysenteric arthropathy, left wrist 🐾

     M02.139 Postdysenteric arthropathy, unspecified wrist 🐾

● **M02.14** Postdysenteric arthropathy, hand
> Postdysenteric arthropathy, metacarpus and phalanges

     M02.141 Postdysenteric arthropathy, right hand 🐾

     M02.142 Postdysenteric arthropathy, left hand 🐾

     M02.149 Postdysenteric arthropathy, unspecified hand 🐾

● **M02.15** Postdysenteric arthropathy, hip

     M02.151 Postdysenteric arthropathy, right hip 🐾

     M02.152 Postdysenteric arthropathy, left hip 🐾

     M02.159 Postdysenteric arthropathy, unspecified hip 🐾

● **M02.16** Postdysenteric arthropathy, knee

     M02.161 Postdysenteric arthropathy, right knee 🐾

     M02.162 Postdysenteric arthropathy, left knee 🐾

     M02.169 Postdysenteric arthropathy, unspecified knee 🐾

● **M02.17** Postdysenteric arthropathy, ankle and foot
> Postdysenteric arthropathy, tarsus, metatarsus and phalanges

     M02.171 Postdysenteric arthropathy, right ankle and foot 🐾

     M02.172 Postdysenteric arthropathy, left ankle and foot 🐾

     M02.179 Postdysenteric arthropathy, unspecified ankle and foot 🐾

   M02.18 Postdysenteric arthropathy, vertebrae 🐾

   M02.19 Postdysenteric arthropathy, multiple sites 🐾

● **M02.2** Postimmunization arthropathy

   M02.20 Postimmunization arthropathy, unspecified site

● **M02.21** Postimmunization arthropathy, shoulder

     M02.211 Postimmunization arthropathy, right shoulder

     M02.212 Postimmunization arthropathy, left shoulder

     M02.219 Postimmunization arthropathy, unspecified shoulder

● **M02.22** Postimmunization arthropathy, elbow

     M02.221 Postimmunization arthropathy, right elbow

     M02.222 Postimmunization arthropathy, left elbow

     M02.229 Postimmunization arthropathy, unspecified elbow

● **M02.23** Postimmunization arthropathy, wrist
> Postimmunization arthropathy, carpal bones

     M02.231 Postimmunization arthropathy, right wrist

     M02.232 Postimmunization arthropathy, left wrist

     M02.239 Postimmunization arthropathy, unspecified wrist

● **M02.24** Postimmunization arthropathy, hand
> Postimmunization arthropathy, metacarpus and phalanges

     M02.241 Postimmunization arthropathy, right hand

     M02.242 Postimmunization arthropathy, left hand

     M02.249 Postimmunization arthropathy, unspecified hand

● **M02.25** Postimmunization arthropathy, hip

     M02.251 Postimmunization arthropathy, right hip

     M02.252 Postimmunization arthropathy, left hip

     M02.259 Postimmunization arthropathy, unspecified hip

● **M02.26** Postimmunization arthropathy, knee

     M02.261 Postimmunization arthropathy, right knee

     M02.262 Postimmunization arthropathy, left knee

     M02.269 Postimmunization arthropathy, unspecified knee

● **M02.27** Postimmunization arthropathy, ankle and foot
> Postimmunization arthropathy, tarsus, metatarsus and phalanges

     M02.271 Postimmunization arthropathy, right ankle and foot

     M02.272 Postimmunization arthropathy, left ankle and foot

     M02.279 Postimmunization arthropathy, unspecified ankle and foot

   M02.28 Postimmunization arthropathy, vertebrae

   M02.29 Postimmunization arthropathy, multiple sites

● **M02.3** Reiter's disease
> Reactive arthritis

   M02.30 Reiter's disease, unspecified site 🐾

● **M02.31** Reiter's disease, shoulder

     M02.311 Reiter's disease, right shoulder 🐾

     M02.312 Reiter's disease, left shoulder 🐾

     M02.319 Reiter's disease, unspecified shoulder 🐾

▶ New   ⇒ Revised   ~~deleted~~ Deleted   Excludes 1   Excludes 2   Includes   Use additional   Code first   Code also   Key words

OGCR Official Guidelines   X Assign placeholder X   ● Use Additional Character(s)   ▶ Manifestation Code   🐾 Hierarchical Condition Category   Coding Clinic

● M02.32   Reiter's disease, elbow
    M02.321   Reiter's disease, right elbow ℞
    M02.322   Reiter's disease, left elbow ℞
    M02.329   Reiter's disease, unspecified elbow ℞

● M02.33   Reiter's disease, wrist
     Reiter's disease, carpal bones
    M02.331   Reiter's disease, right wrist ℞
    M02.332   Reiter's disease, left wrist ℞
    M02.339   Reiter's disease, unspecified wrist ℞

● M02.34   Reiter's disease, hand
     Reiter's disease, metacarpus and phalanges
    M02.341   Reiter's disease, right hand ℞
    M02.342   Reiter's disease, left hand ℞
    M02.349   Reiter's disease, unspecified hand ℞

● M02.35   Reiter's disease, hip
    M02.351   Reiter's disease, right hip ℞
    M02.352   Reiter's disease, left hip ℞
    M02.359   Reiter's disease, unspecified hip ℞

● M02.36   Reiter's disease, knee
    M02.361   Reiter's disease, right knee ℞
    M02.362   Reiter's disease, left knee ℞
    M02.369   Reiter's disease, unspecified knee ℞

● M02.37   Reiter's disease, ankle and foot
     Reiter's disease, tarsus, metatarsus and
     phalanges
    M02.371   Reiter's disease, right ankle and foot ℞
    M02.372   Reiter's disease, left ankle and foot ℞
    M02.379   Reiter's disease, unspecified ankle and foot ℞

   M02.38   Reiter's disease, vertebrae ℞
   M02.39   Reiter's disease, multiple sites ℞

● M02.8   Other reactive arthropathies
   ▸ *M02.80*   *Other reactive arthropathies, unspecified site* ℞
  ● *M02.81*   Other reactive arthropathies, shoulder
    ▸ *M02.811*   *Other reactive arthropathies, right shoulder* ℞
    ▸ *M02.812*   *Other reactive arthropathies, left shoulder* ℞
    ▸ *M02.819*   *Other reactive arthropathies, unspecified shoulder* ℞
  ● M02.82   Other reactive arthropathies, elbow
    ▸ *M02.821*   *Other reactive arthropathies, right elbow* ℞
    ▸ *M02.822*   *Other reactive arthropathies, left elbow* ℞
    ▸ *M02.829*   *Other reactive arthropathies, unspecified elbow* ℞
  ● M02.83   Other reactive arthropathies, wrist
     Other reactive arthropathies, carpal bones
    ▸ *M02.831*   *Other reactive arthropathies, right wrist* ℞
    ▸ *M02.832*   *Other reactive arthropathies, left wrist* ℞
    ▸ *M02.839*   *Other reactive arthropathies, unspecified wrist* ℞
  ● M02.84   Other reactive arthropathies, hand
     Other reactive arthropathies, metacarpus and phalanges
    ▸ *M02.841*   *Other reactive arthropathies, right hand* ℞
    ▸ *M02.842*   *Other reactive arthropathies, left hand* ℞
    ▸ *M02.849*   *Other reactive arthropathies, unspecified hand* ℞

● M02.85   Other reactive arthropathies, hip
    ▸ *M02.851*   *Other reactive arthropathies, right hip* ℞
    ▸ *M02.852*   *Other reactive arthropathies, left hip* ℞
    ▸ *M02.859*   *Other reactive arthropathies, unspecified hip* ℞

● M02.86   Other reactive arthropathies, knee
    ▸ *M02.861*   *Other reactive arthropathies, right knee* ℞
    ▸ *M02.862*   *Other reactive arthropathies, left knee* ℞
    ▸ *M02.869*   *Other reactive arthropathies, unspecified knee* ℞

● M02.87   Other reactive arthropathies, ankle and foot
     Other reactive arthropathies, tarsus, metatarsus and phalanges
    ▸ *M02.871*   *Other reactive arthropathies, right ankle and foot* ℞
    ▸ *M02.872*   *Other reactive arthropathies, left ankle and foot* ℞
    ▸ *M02.879*   *Other reactive arthropathies, unspecified ankle and foot* ℞
   ▸ *M02.88*   *Other reactive arthropathies, vertebrae* ℞
   ▸ *M02.89*   *Other reactive arthropathies, multiple sites* ℞
  ▸ *M02.9*   *Reactive arthropathy, unspecified* ℞

AUTOINFLAMMATORY SYNDROMES (M04)

● M04   Autoinflammatory syndromes
    Excludes2   Crohn's disease (K50.-)
    Coding Clinic: 2016, Q4, P37

   M04.1   Periodic fever syndromes ℞
     Familial Mediterranean fever
     Hyperimmunoglobin D syndrome
     Mevalonate kinase deficiency
     Tumor necrosis factor receptor associated periodic syndrome [TRAPS]

   M04.2   Cryopyrin-associated periodic syndromes ℞
     Chronic infantile neurological, cutaneous and articular syndrome [CINCA]
     Familial cold autoinflammatory syndrome
     Familial cold urticaria
     Muckle-Wells syndrome
     Neonatal onset multisystemic inflammatory disorder [NOMID]

   M04.8   Other autoinflammatory syndromes ℞
     Blau syndrome
     Deficiency of interleukin 1 receptor antagonist [DIRA]
     Majeed syndrome
     Periodic fever, aphthous stomatitis, pharyngitis, and adenopathy syndrome [PFAPA]
     Pyogenic arthritis, pyoderma gangrenosum, and acne syndrome [PAPA]

   M04.9   Autoinflammatory syndrome, unspecified ℞

INFLAMMATORY POLYARTHROPATHIES (M05-M14)

● M05   Rheumatoid arthritis with rheumatoid factor
    Excludes1   rheumatic fever (I00)
          juvenile rheumatoid arthritis (M08.-)
          rheumatoid arthritis of spine (M45.-)

  ● M05.0   Felty's syndrome
     Rheumatoid arthritis with splenoadenomegaly and leukopenia
    M05.00   Felty's syndrome, unspecified site ℞
   ● M05.01   Felty's syndrome, shoulder
     M05.011   Felty's syndrome, right shoulder ℞
     M05.012   Felty's syndrome, left shoulder ℞
     M05.019   Felty's syndrome, unspecified shoulder ℞

CHAPTER 13 (M00-M99)

CHAPTER 13 (M00-M99)

● M05.02   Felty's syndrome, elbow
     M05.021   Felty's syndrome, right elbow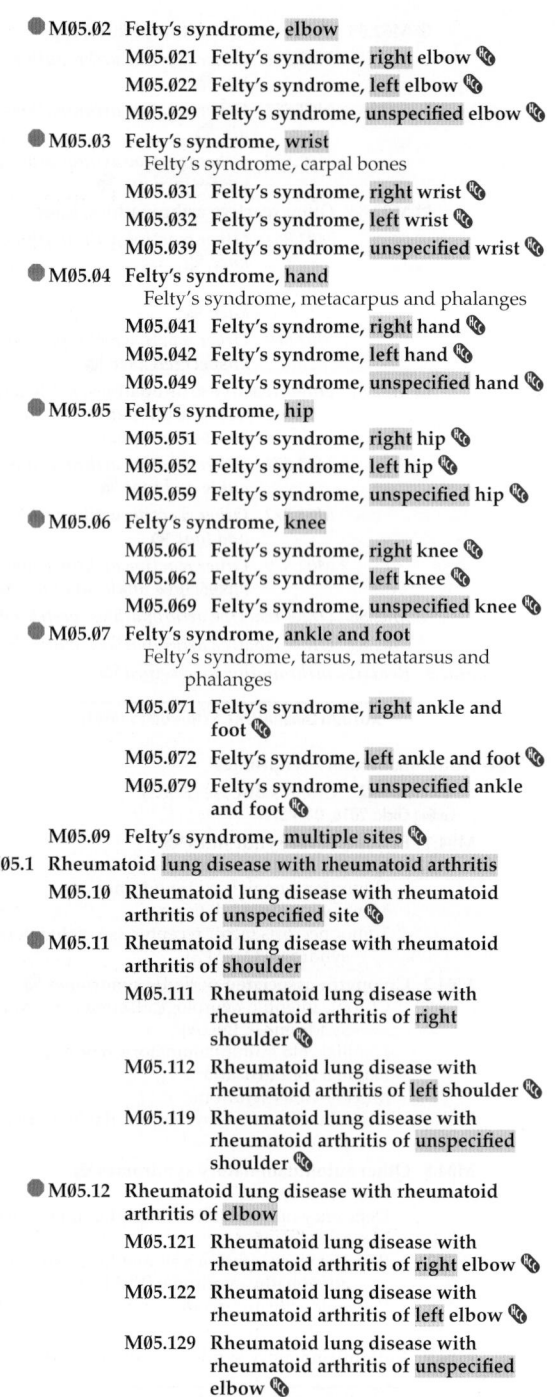
     M05.022   Felty's syndrome, left elbow
     M05.029   Felty's syndrome, unspecified elbow

● M05.03   Felty's syndrome, wrist
     Felty's syndrome, carpal bones
     M05.031   Felty's syndrome, right wrist
     M05.032   Felty's syndrome, left wrist
     M05.039   Felty's syndrome, unspecified wrist

● M05.04   Felty's syndrome, hand
     Felty's syndrome, metacarpus and phalanges
     M05.041   Felty's syndrome, right hand
     M05.042   Felty's syndrome, left hand
     M05.049   Felty's syndrome, unspecified hand

● M05.05   Felty's syndrome, hip
     M05.051   Felty's syndrome, right hip
     M05.052   Felty's syndrome, left hip
     M05.059   Felty's syndrome, unspecified hip

● M05.06   Felty's syndrome, knee
     M05.061   Felty's syndrome, right knee
     M05.062   Felty's syndrome, left knee
     M05.069   Felty's syndrome, unspecified knee

● M05.07   Felty's syndrome, ankle and foot
     Felty's syndrome, tarsus, metatarsus and phalanges
     M05.071   Felty's syndrome, right ankle and foot
     M05.072   Felty's syndrome, left ankle and foot
     M05.079   Felty's syndrome, unspecified ankle and foot

M05.09   Felty's syndrome, multiple sites

● M05.1   Rheumatoid lung disease with rheumatoid arthritis
     M05.10   Rheumatoid lung disease with rheumatoid arthritis of unspecified site

● M05.11   Rheumatoid lung disease with rheumatoid arthritis of shoulder
     M05.111   Rheumatoid lung disease with rheumatoid arthritis of right shoulder
     M05.112   Rheumatoid lung disease with rheumatoid arthritis of left shoulder
     M05.119   Rheumatoid lung disease with rheumatoid arthritis of unspecified shoulder

● M05.12   Rheumatoid lung disease with rheumatoid arthritis of elbow
     M05.121   Rheumatoid lung disease with rheumatoid arthritis of right elbow
     M05.122   Rheumatoid lung disease with rheumatoid arthritis of left elbow
     M05.129   Rheumatoid lung disease with rheumatoid arthritis of unspecified elbow

● M05.13   Rheumatoid lung disease with rheumatoid arthritis of wrist
     Rheumatoid lung disease with rheumatoid arthritis, carpal bones
     M05.131   Rheumatoid lung disease with rheumatoid arthritis of right wrist
     M05.132   Rheumatoid lung disease with rheumatoid arthritis of left wrist
     M05.139   Rheumatoid lung disease with rheumatoid arthritis of unspecified wrist

● M05.14   Rheumatoid lung disease with rheumatoid arthritis of hand
     Rheumatoid lung disease with rheumatoid arthritis, metacarpus and phalanges
     M05.141   Rheumatoid lung disease with rheumatoid arthritis of right hand
     M05.142   Rheumatoid lung disease with rheumatoid arthritis of left hand
     M05.149   Rheumatoid lung disease with rheumatoid arthritis of unspecified hand

● M05.15   Rheumatoid lung disease with rheumatoid arthritis of hip
     M05.151   Rheumatoid lung disease with rheumatoid arthritis of right hip
     M05.152   Rheumatoid lung disease with rheumatoid arthritis of left hip
     M05.159   Rheumatoid lung disease with rheumatoid arthritis of unspecified hip

● M05.16   Rheumatoid lung disease with rheumatoid arthritis of knee
     M05.161   Rheumatoid lung disease with rheumatoid arthritis of right knee
     M05.162   Rheumatoid lung disease with rheumatoid arthritis of left knee
     M05.169   Rheumatoid lung disease with rheumatoid arthritis of unspecified knee

● M05.17   Rheumatoid lung disease with rheumatoid arthritis of ankle and foot
     Rheumatoid lung disease with rheumatoid arthritis, tarsus, metatarsus and phalanges
     M05.171   Rheumatoid lung disease with rheumatoid arthritis of right ankle and foot
     M05.172   Rheumatoid lung disease with rheumatoid arthritis of left ankle and foot
     M05.179   Rheumatoid lung disease with rheumatoid arthritis of unspecified ankle and foot

M05.19   Rheumatoid lung disease with rheumatoid arthritis of multiple sites

● M05.2   Rheumatoid vasculitis with rheumatoid arthritis
     M05.20   Rheumatoid vasculitis with rheumatoid arthritis of unspecified site

● M05.21   Rheumatoid vasculitis with rheumatoid arthritis of shoulder
     M05.211   Rheumatoid vasculitis with rheumatoid arthritis of right shoulder
     M05.212   Rheumatoid vasculitis with rheumatoid arthritis of left shoulder
     M05.219   Rheumatoid vasculitis with rheumatoid arthritis of unspecified shoulder

Item 13-1   **Rheumatoid arthritis** (RA) is a chronic systemic inflammatory autoimmune disease of undetermined etiology involving primarily the synovial membranes and articular structures of multiple joints. It can also affect other organs, including the eyes, blood vessels, heart, and lungs. The disease is often progressive. In late stages, deformity, ankylosis, and other **inflammatory polyarthropathies** develop.

▶ New   ⇒ Revised   ~~deleted~~ Deleted   Excludes 1   Excludes 2   Includes   Use additional   Code first   Code also   Key words

OGCR Official Guidelines   X Assign placeholder X   ● Use Additional Character(s)   ▶ Manifestation Code   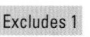 Hierarchical Condition Category   **Coding Clinic**

● **M05.22** **Rheumatoid vasculitis with rheumatoid arthritis of elbow**

    M05.221 Rheumatoid vasculitis with rheumatoid arthritis of right elbow 🐾

    M05.222 Rheumatoid vasculitis with rheumatoid arthritis of left elbow 🐾

    M05.229 Rheumatoid vasculitis with rheumatoid arthritis of unspecified elbow 🐾

● **M05.23** **Rheumatoid vasculitis with rheumatoid arthritis of wrist**

    Rheumatoid vasculitis with rheumatoid arthritis, carpal bones

    M05.231 Rheumatoid vasculitis with rheumatoid arthritis of right wrist 🐾

    M05.232 Rheumatoid vasculitis with rheumatoid arthritis of left wrist 🐾

    M05.239 Rheumatoid vasculitis with rheumatoid arthritis of unspecified wrist 🐾

● **M05.24** **Rheumatoid vasculitis with rheumatoid arthritis of hand**

    Rheumatoid vasculitis with rheumatoid arthritis, metacarpus and phalanges

    M05.241 Rheumatoid vasculitis with rheumatoid arthritis of right hand 🐾

    M05.242 Rheumatoid vasculitis with rheumatoid arthritis of left hand 🐾

    M05.249 Rheumatoid vasculitis with rheumatoid arthritis of unspecified hand 🐾

● **M05.25** **Rheumatoid vasculitis with rheumatoid arthritis of hip**

    M05.251 Rheumatoid vasculitis with rheumatoid arthritis of right hip 🐾

    M05.252 Rheumatoid vasculitis with rheumatoid arthritis of left hip 🐾

    M05.259 Rheumatoid vasculitis with rheumatoid arthritis of unspecified hip 🐾

● **M05.26** **Rheumatoid vasculitis with rheumatoid arthritis of knee**

    M05.261 Rheumatoid vasculitis with rheumatoid arthritis of right knee 🐾

    M05.262 Rheumatoid vasculitis with rheumatoid arthritis of left knee 🐾

    M05.269 Rheumatoid vasculitis with rheumatoid arthritis of unspecified knee 🐾

● **M05.27** **Rheumatoid vasculitis with rheumatoid arthritis of ankle and foot**

    Rheumatoid vasculitis with rheumatoid arthritis, tarsus, metatarsus and phalanges

    M05.271 Rheumatoid vasculitis with rheumatoid arthritis of right ankle and foot 🐾

    M05.272 Rheumatoid vasculitis with rheumatoid arthritis of left ankle and foot 🐾

    M05.279 Rheumatoid vasculitis with rheumatoid arthritis of unspecified ankle and foot 🐾

    M05.29 **Rheumatoid vasculitis with rheumatoid arthritis of multiple sites** 🐾

● **M05.3** **Rheumatoid heart disease with rheumatoid arthritis**

    Rheumatoid carditis

    Rheumatoid endocarditis

    Rheumatoid myocarditis

    Rheumatoid pericarditis

    M05.30 Rheumatoid heart disease with rheumatoid arthritis of unspecified site 🐾

● **M05.31** **Rheumatoid heart disease with rheumatoid arthritis of shoulder**

    M05.311 Rheumatoid heart disease with rheumatoid arthritis of right shoulder 🐾

    M05.312 Rheumatoid heart disease with rheumatoid arthritis of left shoulder 🐾

    M05.319 Rheumatoid heart disease with rheumatoid arthritis of unspecified shoulder 🐾

● **M05.32** **Rheumatoid heart disease with rheumatoid arthritis of elbow**

    M05.321 Rheumatoid heart disease with rheumatoid arthritis of right elbow 🐾

    M05.322 Rheumatoid heart disease with rheumatoid arthritis of left elbow 🐾

    M05.329 Rheumatoid heart disease with rheumatoid arthritis of unspecified elbow 🐾

● **M05.33** **Rheumatoid heart disease with rheumatoid arthritis of wrist**

    Rheumatoid heart disease with rheumatoid arthritis, carpal bones

    M05.331 Rheumatoid heart disease with rheumatoid arthritis of right wrist 🐾

    M05.332 Rheumatoid heart disease with rheumatoid arthritis of left wrist 🐾

    M05.339 Rheumatoid heart disease with rheumatoid arthritis of unspecified wrist 🐾

● **M05.34** **Rheumatoid heart disease with rheumatoid arthritis of hand**

    Rheumatoid heart disease with rheumatoid arthritis, metacarpus and phalanges

    M05.341 Rheumatoid heart disease with rheumatoid arthritis of right hand 🐾

    M05.342 Rheumatoid heart disease with rheumatoid arthritis of left hand 🐾

    M05.349 Rheumatoid heart disease with rheumatoid arthritis of unspecified hand 🐾

● **M05.35** **Rheumatoid heart disease with rheumatoid arthritis of hip**

    M05.351 Rheumatoid heart disease with rheumatoid arthritis of right hip 🐾

    M05.352 Rheumatoid heart disease with rheumatoid arthritis of left hip 🐾

    M05.359 Rheumatoid heart disease with rheumatoid arthritis of unspecified hip 🐾

● **M05.36** **Rheumatoid heart disease with rheumatoid arthritis of knee**

    M05.361 Rheumatoid heart disease with rheumatoid arthritis of right knee 🐾

    M05.362 Rheumatoid heart disease with rheumatoid arthritis of left knee 🐾

    M05.369 Rheumatoid heart disease with rheumatoid arthritis of unspecified knee 🐾

CHAPTER 13 (M00-M99)

● M05.37 **Rheumatoid heart disease with rheumatoid arthritis of** ==ankle and foot==
     Rheumatoid heart disease with rheumatoid arthritis, tarsus, metatarsus and phalanges

  M05.371 **Rheumatoid heart disease with rheumatoid arthritis of** ==right== **ankle and foot** 🐾

  M05.372 **Rheumatoid heart disease with rheumatoid arthritis of** ==left== **ankle and foot** 🐾

  M05.379 **Rheumatoid heart disease with rheumatoid arthritis of** ==unspecified== **ankle and foot** 🐾

  M05.39 **Rheumatoid heart disease with rheumatoid arthritis of** ==multiple sites== 🐾

● M05.4 **Rheumatoid** ==myopathy with rheumatoid arthritis==

  M05.40 **Rheumatoid myopathy with rheumatoid arthritis of** ==unspecified site== 🐾

● M05.41 **Rheumatoid myopathy with rheumatoid arthritis of** ==shoulder==

  M05.411 **Rheumatoid myopathy with rheumatoid arthritis of** ==right== **shoulder** 🐾

  M05.412 **Rheumatoid myopathy with rheumatoid arthritis of** ==left== **shoulder** 🐾

  M05.419 **Rheumatoid myopathy with rheumatoid arthritis of** ==unspecified== **shoulder** 🐾

● M05.42 **Rheumatoid myopathy with rheumatoid arthritis of** ==elbow==

  M05.421 **Rheumatoid myopathy with rheumatoid arthritis of** ==right== **elbow** 🐾

  M05.422 **Rheumatoid myopathy with rheumatoid arthritis of** ==left== **elbow** 🐾

  M05.429 **Rheumatoid myopathy with rheumatoid arthritis of** ==unspecified== **elbow** 🐾

● M05.43 **Rheumatoid myopathy with rheumatoid arthritis of** ==wrist==
     Rheumatoid myopathy with rheumatoid arthritis, carpal bones

  M05.431 **Rheumatoid myopathy with rheumatoid arthritis of** ==right== **wrist** 🐾

  M05.432 **Rheumatoid myopathy with rheumatoid arthritis of** ==left== **wrist** 🐾

  M05.439 **Rheumatoid myopathy with rheumatoid arthritis of** ==unspecified== **wrist** 🐾

● M05.44 **Rheumatoid myopathy with rheumatoid arthritis of** ==hand==
     Rheumatoid myopathy with rheumatoid arthritis, metacarpus and phalanges

  M05.441 **Rheumatoid myopathy with rheumatoid arthritis of** ==right== **hand** 🐾

  M05.442 **Rheumatoid myopathy with rheumatoid arthritis of** ==left== **hand** 🐾

  M05.449 **Rheumatoid myopathy with rheumatoid arthritis of** ==unspecified== **hand** 🐾

● M05.45 **Rheumatoid myopathy with rheumatoid arthritis of** ==hip==

  M05.451 **Rheumatoid myopathy with rheumatoid arthritis of** ==right== **hip** 🐾

  M05.452 **Rheumatoid myopathy with rheumatoid arthritis of** ==left== **hip** 🐾

  M05.459 **Rheumatoid myopathy with rheumatoid arthritis of** ==unspecified== **hip** 🐾

● M05.46 **Rheumatoid myopathy with rheumatoid arthritis of** ==knee==

  M05.461 **Rheumatoid myopathy with rheumatoid arthritis of** ==right== **knee** 🐾

  M05.462 **Rheumatoid myopathy with rheumatoid arthritis of** ==left== **knee** 🐾

  M05.469 **Rheumatoid myopathy with rheumatoid arthritis of** ==unspecified== **knee** 🐾

● M05.47 **Rheumatoid myopathy with rheumatoid arthritis of** ==ankle and foot==
     Rheumatoid myopathy with rheumatoid arthritis, tarsus, metatarsus and phalanges

  M05.471 **Rheumatoid myopathy with rheumatoid arthritis of** ==right== **ankle and foot** 🐾

  M05.472 **Rheumatoid myopathy with rheumatoid arthritis of** ==left== **ankle and foot** 🐾

  M05.479 **Rheumatoid myopathy with rheumatoid arthritis of** ==unspecified== **ankle and foot** 🐾

  M05.49 **Rheumatoid myopathy with rheumatoid arthritis of** ==multiple sites== 🐾

● M05.5 **Rheumatoid** ==polyneuropathy with rheumatoid arthritis==

  M05.50 **Rheumatoid polyneuropathy with rheumatoid arthritis of** ==unspecified site== 🐾

● M05.51 **Rheumatoid polyneuropathy with rheumatoid arthritis of** ==shoulder==

  M05.511 **Rheumatoid polyneuropathy with rheumatoid arthritis of** ==right== **shoulder** 🐾

  M05.512 **Rheumatoid polyneuropathy with rheumatoid arthritis of** ==left== **shoulder** 🐾

  M05.519 **Rheumatoid polyneuropathy with rheumatoid arthritis of** ==unspecified== **shoulder** 🐾

● M05.52 **Rheumatoid polyneuropathy with rheumatoid arthritis of** ==elbow==

  M05.521 **Rheumatoid polyneuropathy with rheumatoid arthritis of** ==right== **elbow** 🐾

  M05.522 **Rheumatoid polyneuropathy with rheumatoid arthritis of** ==left== **elbow** 🐾

  M05.529 **Rheumatoid polyneuropathy with rheumatoid arthritis of** ==unspecified== **elbow** 🐾

● M05.53 **Rheumatoid polyneuropathy with rheumatoid arthritis of** ==wrist==
     Rheumatoid polyneuropathy with rheumatoid arthritis, carpal bones

  M05.531 **Rheumatoid polyneuropathy with rheumatoid arthritis of** ==right== **wrist** 🐾

  M05.532 **Rheumatoid polyneuropathy with rheumatoid arthritis of** ==left== **wrist** 🐾

  M05.539 **Rheumatoid polyneuropathy with rheumatoid arthritis of** ==unspecified== **wrist** 🐾

● M05.54 **Rheumatoid polyneuropathy with rheumatoid arthritis of** ==hand==
     Rheumatoid polyneuropathy with rheumatoid arthritis, metacarpus and phalanges

  M05.541 **Rheumatoid polyneuropathy with rheumatoid arthritis of** ==right== **hand** 🐾

  M05.542 **Rheumatoid polyneuropathy with rheumatoid arthritis of** ==left== **hand** 🐾

  M05.549 **Rheumatoid polyneuropathy with rheumatoid arthritis of** ==unspecified== **hand** 🐾

▶ New   ⇒ Revised   ~~deleted~~ Deleted   Excludes 1   Excludes 2   Includes   Use additional   Code first   Code also   Key words
OGCR Official Guidelines   X Assign placeholder X   ● Use Additional Character(s)   ▶ Manifestation Code   🐾 Hierarchical Condition Category   **Coding Clinic**

● **M05.55** Rheumatoid polyneuropathy with rheumatoid arthritis of hip
  M05.551 Rheumatoid polyneuropathy with rheumatoid arthritis of right hip 🔗
  M05.552 Rheumatoid polyneuropathy with rheumatoid arthritis of left hip 🔗
  M05.559 Rheumatoid polyneuropathy with rheumatoid arthritis of unspecified hip 🔗

● **M05.56** Rheumatoid polyneuropathy with rheumatoid arthritis of knee
  M05.561 Rheumatoid polyneuropathy with rheumatoid arthritis of right knee 🔗
  M05.562 Rheumatoid polyneuropathy with rheumatoid arthritis of left knee 🔗
  M05.569 Rheumatoid polyneuropathy with rheumatoid arthritis of unspecified knee 🔗

● **M05.57** Rheumatoid polyneuropathy with rheumatoid arthritis of ankle and foot
      Rheumatoid polyneuropathy with rheumatoid arthritis, tarsus, metatarsus and phalanges
  M05.571 Rheumatoid polyneuropathy with rheumatoid arthritis of right ankle and foot 🔗
  M05.572 Rheumatoid polyneuropathy with rheumatoid arthritis of left ankle and foot 🔗
  M05.579 Rheumatoid polyneuropathy with rheumatoid arthritis of unspecified ankle and foot 🔗

  M05.59 Rheumatoid polyneuropathy with rheumatoid arthritis of multiple sites 🔗

● **M05.6** Rheumatoid arthritis with involvement of other organs and systems
  M05.60 Rheumatoid arthritis of unspecified site with involvement of other organs and systems 🔗

● **M05.61** Rheumatoid arthritis of shoulder with involvement of other organs and systems
  M05.611 Rheumatoid arthritis of right shoulder with involvement of other organs and systems 🔗
  M05.612 Rheumatoid arthritis of left shoulder with involvement of other organs and systems 🔗
  M05.619 Rheumatoid arthritis of unspecified shoulder with involvement of other organs and systems 🔗

● **M05.62** Rheumatoid arthritis of elbow with involvement of other organs and systems
  M05.621 Rheumatoid arthritis of right elbow with involvement of other organs and systems 🔗
  M05.622 Rheumatoid arthritis of left elbow with involvement of other organs and systems 🔗
  M05.629 Rheumatoid arthritis of unspecified elbow with involvement of other organs and systems 🔗

● **M05.63** Rheumatoid arthritis of wrist with involvement of other organs and systems
      Rheumatoid arthritis of carpal bones with involvement of other organs and systems
  M05.631 Rheumatoid arthritis of right wrist with involvement of other organs and systems 🔗
  M05.632 Rheumatoid arthritis of left wrist with involvement of other organs and systems 🔗
  M05.639 Rheumatoid arthritis of unspecified wrist with involvement of other organs and systems 🔗

● **M05.64** Rheumatoid arthritis of hand with involvement of other organs and systems
      Rheumatoid arthritis of metacarpus and phalanges with involvement of other organs and systems
  M05.641 Rheumatoid arthritis of right hand with involvement of other organs and systems 🔗
  M05.642 Rheumatoid arthritis of left hand with involvement of other organs and systems 🔗
  M05.649 Rheumatoid arthritis of unspecified hand with involvement of other organs and systems 🔗

● **M05.65** Rheumatoid arthritis of hip with involvement of other organs and systems
  M05.651 Rheumatoid arthritis of right hip with involvement of other organs and systems 🔗
  M05.652 Rheumatoid arthritis of left hip with involvement of other organs and systems 🔗
  M05.659 Rheumatoid arthritis of unspecified hip with involvement of other organs and systems 🔗

● **M05.66** Rheumatoid arthritis of knee with involvement of other organs and systems
  M05.661 Rheumatoid arthritis of right knee with involvement of other organs and systems 🔗
  M05.662 Rheumatoid arthritis of left knee with involvement of other organs and systems 🔗
  M05.669 Rheumatoid arthritis of unspecified knee with involvement of other organs and systems 🔗

● **M05.67** Rheumatoid arthritis of ankle and foot with involvement of other organs and systems
      Rheumatoid arthritis of tarsus, metatarsus and phalanges with involvement of other organs and systems
  M05.671 Rheumatoid arthritis of right ankle and foot with involvement of other organs and systems 🔗
  M05.672 Rheumatoid arthritis of left ankle and foot with involvement of other organs and systems 🔗
  M05.679 Rheumatoid arthritis of unspecified ankle and foot with involvement of other organs and systems 🔗

  M05.69 Rheumatoid arthritis of multiple sites with involvement of other organs and systems 🔗

● **M05.7** Rheumatoid arthritis with rheumatoid factor without organ or systems involvement
  M05.70 Rheumatoid arthritis with rheumatoid factor of unspecified site without organ or systems involvement 🔗

● **M05.71** Rheumatoid arthritis with rheumatoid factor of shoulder without organ or systems involvement
  M05.711 Rheumatoid arthritis with rheumatoid factor of right shoulder without organ or systems involvement 🔗
  M05.712 Rheumatoid arthritis with rheumatoid factor of left shoulder without organ or systems involvement 🔗
  M05.719 Rheumatoid arthritis with rheumatoid factor of unspecified shoulder without organ or systems involvement 🔗

CHAPTER 13 (M00-M99)

● **M05.72** Rheumatoid arthritis with rheumatoid factor of elbow without organ or systems involvement

     M05.721 Rheumatoid arthritis with rheumatoid factor of right elbow without organ or systems involvement 🦠

     M05.722 Rheumatoid arthritis with rheumatoid factor of left elbow without organ or systems involvement 🦠

     M05.729 Rheumatoid arthritis with rheumatoid factor of unspecified elbow without organ or systems involvement 🦠

● **M05.73** Rheumatoid arthritis with rheumatoid factor of wrist without organ or systems involvement

     M05.731 Rheumatoid arthritis with rheumatoid factor of right wrist without organ or systems involvement 🦠

     M05.732 Rheumatoid arthritis with rheumatoid factor of left wrist without organ or systems involvement 🦠

     M05.739 Rheumatoid arthritis with rheumatoid factor of unspecified wrist without organ or systems involvement 🦠

● **M05.74** Rheumatoid arthritis with rheumatoid factor of hand without organ or systems involvement

     M05.741 Rheumatoid arthritis with rheumatoid factor of right hand without organ or systems involvement 🦠

     M05.742 Rheumatoid arthritis with rheumatoid factor of left hand without organ or systems involvement 🦠

     M05.749 Rheumatoid arthritis with rheumatoid factor of unspecified hand without organ or systems involvement 🦠

● **M05.75** Rheumatoid arthritis with rheumatoid factor of hip without organ or systems involvement

     M05.751 Rheumatoid arthritis with rheumatoid factor of right hip without organ or systems involvement 🦠

     M05.752 Rheumatoid arthritis with rheumatoid factor of left hip without organ or systems involvement 🦠

     M05.759 Rheumatoid arthritis with rheumatoid factor of unspecified hip without organ or systems involvement 🦠

● **M05.76** Rheumatoid arthritis with rheumatoid factor of knee without organ or systems involvement

     M05.761 Rheumatoid arthritis with rheumatoid factor of right knee without organ or systems involvement 🦠

     M05.762 Rheumatoid arthritis with rheumatoid factor of left knee without organ or systems involvement 🦠

     M05.769 Rheumatoid arthritis with rheumatoid factor of unspecified knee without organ or systems involvement 🦠

● **M05.77** Rheumatoid arthritis with rheumatoid factor of ankle and foot without organ or systems involvement

     M05.771 Rheumatoid arthritis with rheumatoid factor of right ankle and foot without organ or systems involvement 🦠

     M05.772 Rheumatoid arthritis with rheumatoid factor of left ankle and foot without organ or systems involvement 🦠

     M05.779 Rheumatoid arthritis with rheumatoid factor of unspecified ankle and foot without organ or systems involvement 🦠

   M05.79 Rheumatoid arthritis with rheumatoid factor of multiple sites without organ or systems involvement 🦠

   M05.7A Rheumatoid arthritis with rheumatoid factor of other specified site without organ or systems involvement

● **M05.8** Other rheumatoid arthritis with rheumatoid factor

   M05.80 Other rheumatoid arthritis with rheumatoid factor of unspecified site 🦠

● **M05.81** Other rheumatoid arthritis with rheumatoid factor of shoulder

     M05.811 Other rheumatoid arthritis with rheumatoid factor of right shoulder 🦠

     M05.812 Other rheumatoid arthritis with rheumatoid factor of left shoulder 🦠

     M05.819 Other rheumatoid arthritis with rheumatoid factor of unspecified shoulder 🦠

● **M05.82** Other rheumatoid arthritis with rheumatoid factor of elbow

     M05.821 Other rheumatoid arthritis with rheumatoid factor of right elbow 🦠

     M05.822 Other rheumatoid arthritis with rheumatoid factor of left elbow 🦠

     M05.829 Other rheumatoid arthritis with rheumatoid factor of unspecified elbow 🦠

● **M05.83** Other rheumatoid arthritis with rheumatoid factor of wrist

     M05.831 Other rheumatoid arthritis with rheumatoid factor of right wrist 🦠

     M05.832 Other rheumatoid arthritis with rheumatoid factor of left wrist 🦠

     M05.839 Other rheumatoid arthritis with rheumatoid factor of unspecified wrist 🦠

● **M05.84** Other rheumatoid arthritis with rheumatoid factor of hand

     M05.841 Other rheumatoid arthritis with rheumatoid factor of right hand 🦠

     M05.842 Other rheumatoid arthritis with rheumatoid factor of left hand 🦠

     M05.849 Other rheumatoid arthritis with rheumatoid factor of unspecified hand 🦠

● **M05.85** Other rheumatoid arthritis with rheumatoid factor of hip

     M05.851 Other rheumatoid arthritis with rheumatoid factor of right hip 🦠

     M05.852 Other rheumatoid arthritis with rheumatoid factor of left hip 🦠

     M05.859 Other rheumatoid arthritis with rheumatoid factor of unspecified hip 🦠

▶ New   ⇒ Revised   ~~deleted~~ Deleted   Excludes 1   Excludes 2   Includes   Use additional   Code first   Code also   Key words

OGCR Official Guidelines   X Assign placeholder X   ● Use Additional Character(s)   ▶ Manifestation Code   🦠 Hierarchical Condition Category   **Coding Clinic**

● **M05.86** Other rheumatoid arthritis with rheumatoid factor of knee

    M05.861 Other rheumatoid arthritis with rheumatoid factor of right knee 🐾

    M05.862 Other rheumatoid arthritis with rheumatoid factor of left knee 🐾

    M05.869 Other rheumatoid arthritis with rheumatoid factor of unspecified knee 🐾

● **M05.87** Other rheumatoid arthritis with rheumatoid factor of ankle and foot

    M05.871 Other rheumatoid arthritis with rheumatoid factor of right ankle and foot 🐾

    M05.872 Other rheumatoid arthritis with rheumatoid factor of left ankle and foot 🐾

    M05.879 Other rheumatoid arthritis with rheumatoid factor of unspecified ankle and foot 🐾

  M05.89 Other rheumatoid arthritis with rheumatoid factor of multiple sites 🐾

  M05.8A Other rheumatoid arthritis with rheumatoid factor of other specified site

M05.9 Rheumatoid arthritis with rheumatoid factor, unspecified 🐾

● **M06** Other rheumatoid arthritis

  ● **M06.0** Rheumatoid arthritis without rheumatoid factor

    M06.00 Rheumatoid arthritis without rheumatoid factor, unspecified site 🐾

    ● M06.01 Rheumatoid arthritis without rheumatoid factor, shoulder

        M06.011 Rheumatoid arthritis without rheumatoid factor, right shoulder 🐾

        M06.012 Rheumatoid arthritis without rheumatoid factor, left shoulder 🐾

        M06.019 Rheumatoid arthritis without rheumatoid factor, unspecified shoulder 🐾

    ● M06.02 Rheumatoid arthritis without rheumatoid factor, elbow

        M06.021 Rheumatoid arthritis without rheumatoid factor, right elbow 🐾

        M06.022 Rheumatoid arthritis without rheumatoid factor, left elbow 🐾

        M06.029 Rheumatoid arthritis without rheumatoid factor, unspecified elbow 🐾

    ● M06.03 Rheumatoid arthritis without rheumatoid factor, wrist

        M06.031 Rheumatoid arthritis without rheumatoid factor, right wrist 🐾

        M06.032 Rheumatoid arthritis without rheumatoid factor, left wrist 🐾

        M06.039 Rheumatoid arthritis without rheumatoid factor, unspecified wrist 🐾

    ● M06.04 Rheumatoid arthritis without rheumatoid factor, hand

        M06.041 Rheumatoid arthritis without rheumatoid factor, right hand 🐾

        M06.042 Rheumatoid arthritis without rheumatoid factor, left hand 🐾

        M06.049 Rheumatoid arthritis without rheumatoid factor, unspecified hand 🐾

● M06.05 Rheumatoid arthritis without rheumatoid factor, hip

    M06.051 Rheumatoid arthritis without rheumatoid factor, right hip 🐾

    M06.052 Rheumatoid arthritis without rheumatoid factor, left hip 🐾

    M06.059 Rheumatoid arthritis without rheumatoid factor, unspecified hip 🐾

● M06.06 Rheumatoid arthritis without rheumatoid factor, knee

    M06.061 Rheumatoid arthritis without rheumatoid factor, right knee 🐾

    M06.062 Rheumatoid arthritis without rheumatoid factor, left knee 🐾

    M06.069 Rheumatoid arthritis without rheumatoid factor, unspecified knee 🐾

● M06.07 Rheumatoid arthritis without rheumatoid factor, ankle and foot

    M06.071 Rheumatoid arthritis without rheumatoid factor, right ankle and foot 🐾

    M06.072 Rheumatoid arthritis without rheumatoid factor, left ankle and foot 🐾

    M06.079 Rheumatoid arthritis without rheumatoid factor, unspecified ankle and foot 🐾

  M06.08 Rheumatoid arthritis without rheumatoid factor, vertebrae 🐾

  M06.09 Rheumatoid arthritis without rheumatoid factor, multiple sites 🐾

  M06.0A Rheumatoid arthritis without rheumatoid factor, other specified site

M06.1 **Adult-onset Still's disease** 🐾   A

    Excludes1   Still's disease NOS (M08.2-)

● **M06.2** Rheumatoid bursitis

  M06.20 Rheumatoid bursitis, unspecified site 🐾

  ● M06.21 Rheumatoid bursitis, shoulder

        M06.211 Rheumatoid bursitis, right shoulder 🐾

        M06.212 Rheumatoid bursitis, left shoulder 🐾

        M06.219 Rheumatoid bursitis, unspecified shoulder 🐾

  ● M06.22 Rheumatoid bursitis, elbow

        M06.221 Rheumatoid bursitis, right elbow 🐾

        M06.222 Rheumatoid bursitis, left elbow 🐾

        M06.229 Rheumatoid bursitis, unspecified elbow 🐾

  ● M06.23 Rheumatoid bursitis, wrist

        M06.231 Rheumatoid bursitis, right wrist 🐾

        M06.232 Rheumatoid bursitis, left wrist 🐾

        M06.239 Rheumatoid bursitis, unspecified wrist 🐾

  ● M06.24 Rheumatoid bursitis, hand

        M06.241 Rheumatoid bursitis, right hand 🐾

        M06.242 Rheumatoid bursitis, left hand 🐾

        M06.249 Rheumatoid bursitis, unspecified hand 🐾

  ● M06.25 Rheumatoid bursitis, hip

        M06.251 Rheumatoid bursitis, right hip 🐾

        M06.252 Rheumatoid bursitis, left hip 🐾

        M06.259 Rheumatoid bursitis, unspecified hip 🐾

  ● M06.26 Rheumatoid bursitis, knee

        M06.261 Rheumatoid bursitis, right knee 🐾

        M06.262 Rheumatoid bursitis, left knee 🐾

        M06.269 Rheumatoid bursitis, unspecified knee 🐾

● M06.27 Rheumatoid bursitis, ankle and foot
  M06.271 Rheumatoid bursitis, right ankle and foot 🅒
  M06.272 Rheumatoid bursitis, left ankle and foot 🅒
  M06.279 Rheumatoid bursitis, unspecified ankle and foot 🅒
 M06.28 Rheumatoid bursitis, vertebrae 🅒
 M06.29 Rheumatoid bursitis, multiple sites 🅒
● M06.3 Rheumatoid nodule
 M06.30 Rheumatoid nodule, unspecified site 🅒
● M06.31 Rheumatoid nodule, shoulder
  M06.311 Rheumatoid nodule, right shoulder 🅒
  M06.312 Rheumatoid nodule, left shoulder 🅒
  M06.319 Rheumatoid nodule, unspecified shoulder 🅒
● M06.32 Rheumatoid nodule, elbow
  M06.321 Rheumatoid nodule, right elbow 🅒
  M06.322 Rheumatoid nodule, left elbow 🅒
  M06.329 Rheumatoid nodule, unspecified elbow 🅒
● M06.33 Rheumatoid nodule, wrist
  M06.331 Rheumatoid nodule, right wrist 🅒
  M06.332 Rheumatoid nodule, left wrist 🅒
  M06.339 Rheumatoid nodule, unspecified wrist 🅒
● M06.34 Rheumatoid nodule, hand
  M06.341 Rheumatoid nodule, right hand 🅒
  M06.342 Rheumatoid nodule, left hand 🅒
  M06.349 Rheumatoid nodule, unspecified hand 🅒
● M06.35 Rheumatoid nodule, hip
  M06.351 Rheumatoid nodule, right hip 🅒
  M06.352 Rheumatoid nodule, left hip 🅒
  M06.359 Rheumatoid nodule, unspecified hip 🅒
● M06.36 Rheumatoid nodule, knee
  M06.361 Rheumatoid nodule, right knee 🅒
  M06.362 Rheumatoid nodule, left knee 🅒
  M06.369 Rheumatoid nodule, unspecified knee 🅒
● M06.37 Rheumatoid nodule, ankle and foot
  M06.371 Rheumatoid nodule, right ankle and foot 🅒
  M06.372 Rheumatoid nodule, left ankle and foot 🅒
  M06.379 Rheumatoid nodule, unspecified ankle and foot 🅒
 M06.38 Rheumatoid nodule, vertebrae 🅒
 M06.39 Rheumatoid nodule, multiple sites 🅒
 M06.4 Inflammatory polyarthropathy 🅒
   Excludes1   polyarthritis NOS (M13.0)
● M06.8 Other specified rheumatoid arthritis
 M06.80 Other specified rheumatoid arthritis, unspecified site 🅒
● M06.81 Other specified rheumatoid arthritis, shoulder
  M06.811 Other specified rheumatoid arthritis, right shoulder 🅒
  M06.812 Other specified rheumatoid arthritis, left shoulder 🅒
  M06.819 Other specified rheumatoid arthritis, unspecified shoulder 🅒

● M06.82 Other specified rheumatoid arthritis, elbow
  M06.821 Other specified rheumatoid arthritis, right elbow 🅒
  M06.822 Other specified rheumatoid arthritis, left elbow 🅒
  M06.829 Other specified rheumatoid arthritis, unspecified elbow 🅒
● M06.83 Other specified rheumatoid arthritis, wrist
  M06.831 Other specified rheumatoid arthritis, right wrist 🅒
  M06.832 Other specified rheumatoid arthritis, left wrist 🅒
  M06.839 Other specified rheumatoid arthritis, unspecified wrist 🅒
● M06.84 Other specified rheumatoid arthritis, hand
  M06.841 Other specified rheumatoid arthritis, right hand 🅒
  M06.842 Other specified rheumatoid arthritis, left hand 🅒
  M06.849 Other specified rheumatoid arthritis, unspecified hand 🅒
● M06.85 Other specified rheumatoid arthritis, hip
  M06.851 Other specified rheumatoid arthritis, right hip 🅒
  M06.852 Other specified rheumatoid arthritis, left hip 🅒
  M06.859 Other specified rheumatoid arthritis, unspecified hip 🅒
● M06.86 Other specified rheumatoid arthritis, knee
  M06.861 Other specified rheumatoid arthritis, right knee 🅒
  M06.862 Other specified rheumatoid arthritis, left knee 🅒
  M06.869 Other specified rheumatoid arthritis, unspecified knee 🅒
● M06.87 Other specified rheumatoid arthritis, ankle and foot
  M06.871 Other specified rheumatoid arthritis, right ankle and foot 🅒
  M06.872 Other specified rheumatoid arthritis, left ankle and foot 🅒
  M06.879 Other specified rheumatoid arthritis, unspecified ankle and foot 🅒
 M06.88 Other specified rheumatoid arthritis, vertebrae 🅒
 M06.89 Other specified rheumatoid arthritis, multiple sites 🅒
 M06.8A Other specified rheumatoid arthritis, other specified site
 M06.9 Rheumatoid arthritis, unspecified 🅒

● M07 Enteropathic arthropathies
   Code also associated enteropathy, such as:
     regional enteritis [Crohn's disease] (K50.-)
     ulcerative colitis (K51.-)
   Excludes1   psoriatic arthropathies (L40.5-)
● M07.6 Enteropathic arthropathies
 M07.60 Enteropathic arthropathies, unspecified site
● M07.61 Enteropathic arthropathies, shoulder
  M07.611 Enteropathic arthropathies, right shoulder
  M07.612 Enteropathic arthropathies, left shoulder
  M07.619 Enteropathic arthropathies, unspecified shoulder
● M07.62 Enteropathic arthropathies, elbow
  M07.621 Enteropathic arthropathies, right elbow
  M07.622 Enteropathic arthropathies, left elbow
  M07.629 Enteropathic arthropathies, unspecified elbow

● M07.63   Enteropathic arthropathies, wrist
    M07.631   Enteropathic arthropathies, right wrist
    M07.632   Enteropathic arthropathies, left wrist
    M07.639   Enteropathic arthropathies, unspecified wrist
● M07.64   Enteropathic arthropathies, hand
    M07.641   Enteropathic arthropathies, right hand
    M07.642   Enteropathic arthropathies, left hand
    M07.649   Enteropathic arthropathies, unspecified hand
● M07.65   Enteropathic arthropathies, hip
    M07.651   Enteropathic arthropathies, right hip
    M07.652   Enteropathic arthropathies, left hip
    M07.659   Enteropathic arthropathies, unspecified hip
● M07.66   Enteropathic arthropathies, knee
    M07.661   Enteropathic arthropathies, right knee
    M07.662   Enteropathic arthropathies, left knee
    M07.669   Enteropathic arthropathies, unspecified knee
● M07.67   Enteropathic arthropathies, ankle and foot
    M07.671   Enteropathic arthropathies, right ankle and foot
    M07.672   Enteropathic arthropathies, left ankle and foot
    M07.679   Enteropathic arthropathies, unspecified ankle and foot
  M07.68   Enteropathic arthropathies, vertebrae
  M07.69   Enteropathic arthropathies, multiple sites

● M08   **Juvenile arthritis**

    Code also any associated underlying condition, such as:
      regional enteritis [Crohn's disease] (K50.-)
      ulcerative colitis (K51.-)

    Excludes1   arthropathy in Whipple's disease (M14.8)
                 Felty's syndrome (M05.0)
                  juvenile dermatomyositis (M33.0-)
                  psoriatic juvenile arthropathy (L40.54)

● M08.0   **Unspecified juvenile rheumatoid arthritis**
    Juvenile rheumatoid arthritis with or without rheumatoid factor
    M08.00   **Unspecified juvenile rheumatoid arthritis of unspecified site** 🗊
● M08.01   **Unspecified juvenile rheumatoid arthritis, shoulder**
    M08.011   Unspecified juvenile rheumatoid arthritis, right shoulder 🗊
    M08.012   Unspecified juvenile rheumatoid arthritis, left shoulder 🗊
    M08.019   Unspecified juvenile rheumatoid arthritis, unspecified shoulder 🗊
● M08.02   **Unspecified juvenile rheumatoid arthritis of elbow**
    M08.021   Unspecified juvenile rheumatoid arthritis, right elbow 🗊
    M08.022   Unspecified juvenile rheumatoid arthritis, left elbow 🗊
    M08.029   Unspecified juvenile rheumatoid arthritis, unspecified elbow 🗊
● M08.03   **Unspecified juvenile rheumatoid arthritis, wrist**
    M08.031   Unspecified juvenile rheumatoid arthritis, right wrist 🗊
    M08.032   Unspecified juvenile rheumatoid arthritis, left wrist 🗊
    M08.039   Unspecified juvenile rheumatoid arthritis, unspecified wrist 🗊

● M08.04   **Unspecified juvenile rheumatoid arthritis, hand**
    M08.041   Unspecified juvenile rheumatoid arthritis, right hand 🗊
    M08.042   Unspecified juvenile rheumatoid arthritis, left hand 🗊
    M08.049   Unspecified juvenile rheumatoid arthritis, unspecified hand 🗊
● M08.05   **Unspecified juvenile rheumatoid arthritis, hip**
    M08.051   Unspecified juvenile rheumatoid arthritis, right hip 🗊
    M08.052   Unspecified juvenile rheumatoid arthritis, left hip 🗊
    M08.059   Unspecified juvenile rheumatoid arthritis, unspecified hip 🗊
● M08.06   **Unspecified juvenile rheumatoid arthritis, knee**
    M08.061   Unspecified juvenile rheumatoid arthritis, right knee 🗊
    M08.062   Unspecified juvenile rheumatoid arthritis, left knee 🗊
    M08.069   Unspecified juvenile rheumatoid arthritis, unspecified knee 🗊
● M08.07   **Unspecified juvenile rheumatoid arthritis, ankle and foot**
    M08.071   Unspecified juvenile rheumatoid arthritis, right ankle and foot 🗊
    M08.072   Unspecified juvenile rheumatoid arthritis, left ankle and foot 🗊
    M08.079   Unspecified juvenile rheumatoid arthritis, unspecified ankle and foot 🗊
  M08.08   **Unspecified juvenile rheumatoid arthritis, vertebrae** 🗊
  M08.09   **Unspecified juvenile rheumatoid arthritis, multiple sites** 🗊
  M08.0A   Unspecified juvenile rheumatoid arthritis, other specified site
  M08.1   **Juvenile ankylosing spondylitis** 🗊
    Excludes1   ankylosing spondylitis in adults (M45.0-)
● M08.2   **Juvenile rheumatoid arthritis with systemic onset**
    Still's disease NOS
    Excludes1   adult-onset Still's disease (M06.1-)
  M08.20   **Juvenile rheumatoid arthritis with systemic onset, unspecified site** 🗊
● M08.21   **Juvenile rheumatoid arthritis with systemic onset, shoulder**
    M08.211   Juvenile rheumatoid arthritis with systemic onset, right shoulder 🗊
    M08.212   Juvenile rheumatoid arthritis with systemic onset, left shoulder 🗊
    M08.219   Juvenile rheumatoid arthritis with systemic onset, unspecified shoulder 🗊
● M08.22   **Juvenile rheumatoid arthritis with systemic onset, elbow**
    M08.221   Juvenile rheumatoid arthritis with systemic onset, right elbow 🗊
    M08.222   Juvenile rheumatoid arthritis with systemic onset, left elbow 🗊
    M08.229   Juvenile rheumatoid arthritis with systemic onset, unspecified elbow 🗊
● M08.23   **Juvenile rheumatoid arthritis with systemic onset, wrist**
    M08.231   Juvenile rheumatoid arthritis with systemic onset, right wrist 🗊
    M08.232   Juvenile rheumatoid arthritis with systemic onset, left wrist 🗊
    M08.239   Juvenile rheumatoid arthritis with systemic onset, unspecified wrist 🗊

CHAPTER 13 (M00-M99)

● M08.24   Juvenile rheumatoid arthritis with systemic onset, hand

      M08.241   Juvenile rheumatoid arthritis with systemic onset, right hand 🦠

      M08.242   Juvenile rheumatoid arthritis with systemic onset, left hand 🦠

      M08.249   Juvenile rheumatoid arthritis with systemic onset, unspecified hand 🦠

● M08.25   Juvenile rheumatoid arthritis with systemic onset, hip

      M08.251   Juvenile rheumatoid arthritis with systemic onset, right hip 🦠

      M08.252   Juvenile rheumatoid arthritis with systemic onset, left hip 🦠

      M08.259   Juvenile rheumatoid arthritis with systemic onset, unspecified hip 🦠

● M08.26   Juvenile rheumatoid arthritis with systemic onset, knee

      M08.261   Juvenile rheumatoid arthritis with systemic onset, right knee 🦠

      M08.262   Juvenile rheumatoid arthritis with systemic onset, left knee 🦠

      M08.269   Juvenile rheumatoid arthritis with systemic onset, unspecified knee 🦠

● M08.27   Juvenile rheumatoid arthritis with systemic onset, ankle and foot

      M08.271   Juvenile rheumatoid arthritis with systemic onset, right ankle and foot 🦠

      M08.272   Juvenile rheumatoid arthritis with systemic onset, left ankle and foot 🦠

      M08.279   Juvenile rheumatoid arthritis with systemic onset, unspecified ankle and foot 🦠

   M08.28   Juvenile rheumatoid arthritis with systemic onset, vertebrae 🦠

   M08.29   Juvenile rheumatoid arthritis with systemic onset, multiple sites 🦠

   M08.2A   Juvenile rheumatoid arthritis with systemic onset, other specified site

   M08.3   Juvenile rheumatoid polyarthritis (seronegative)

● M08.4   Pauciarticular juvenile rheumatoid arthritis

   M08.40   Pauciarticular juvenile rheumatoid arthritis, unspecified site 🦠

● M08.41   Pauciarticular juvenile rheumatoid arthritis, shoulder

      M08.411   Pauciarticular juvenile rheumatoid arthritis, right shoulder 🦠

      M08.412   Pauciarticular juvenile rheumatoid arthritis, left shoulder 🦠

      M08.419   Pauciarticular juvenile rheumatoid arthritis, unspecified shoulder 🦠

● M08.42   Pauciarticular juvenile rheumatoid arthritis, elbow

      M08.421   Pauciarticular juvenile rheumatoid arthritis, right elbow 🦠

      M08.422   Pauciarticular juvenile rheumatoid arthritis, left elbow 🦠

      M08.429   Pauciarticular juvenile rheumatoid arthritis, unspecified elbow 🦠

● M08.43   Pauciarticular juvenile rheumatoid arthritis, wrist

      M08.431   Pauciarticular juvenile rheumatoid arthritis, right wrist 🦠

      M08.432   Pauciarticular juvenile rheumatoid arthritis, left wrist 🦠

      M08.439   Pauciarticular juvenile rheumatoid arthritis, unspecified wrist 🦠

● M08.44   Pauciarticular juvenile rheumatoid arthritis, hand

      M08.441   Pauciarticular juvenile rheumatoid arthritis, right hand 🦠

      M08.442   Pauciarticular juvenile rheumatoid arthritis, left hand 🦠

      M08.449   Pauciarticular juvenile rheumatoid arthritis, unspecified hand 🦠

● M08.45   Pauciarticular juvenile rheumatoid arthritis, hip

      M08.451   Pauciarticular juvenile rheumatoid arthritis, right hip 🦠

      M08.452   Pauciarticular juvenile rheumatoid arthritis, left hip 🦠

      M08.459   Pauciarticular juvenile rheumatoid arthritis, unspecified hip 🦠

● M08.46   Pauciarticular juvenile rheumatoid arthritis, knee

      M08.461   Pauciarticular juvenile rheumatoid arthritis, right knee 🦠

      M08.462   Pauciarticular juvenile rheumatoid arthritis, left knee 🦠

      M08.469   Pauciarticular juvenile rheumatoid arthritis, unspecified knee 🦠

● M08.47   Pauciarticular juvenile rheumatoid arthritis, ankle and foot

      M08.471   Pauciarticular juvenile rheumatoid arthritis, right ankle and foot 🦠

      M08.472   Pauciarticular juvenile rheumatoid arthritis, left ankle and foot 🦠

      M08.479   Pauciarticular juvenile rheumatoid arthritis, unspecified ankle and foot 🦠

   M08.48   Pauciarticular juvenile rheumatoid arthritis, vertebrae 🦠

   M08.4A   Pauciarticular juvenile rheumatoid arthritis, other specified site

● M08.8   Other juvenile arthritis

   M08.80   Other juvenile arthritis, unspecified site 🦠

● M08.81   Other juvenile arthritis, shoulder

      M08.811   Other juvenile arthritis, right shoulder 🦠

      M08.812   Other juvenile arthritis, left shoulder 🦠

      M08.819   Other juvenile arthritis, unspecified shoulder 🦠

● M08.82   Other juvenile arthritis, elbow

      M08.821   Other juvenile arthritis, right elbow 🦠

      M08.822   Other juvenile arthritis, left elbow 🦠

      M08.829   Other juvenile arthritis, unspecified elbow 🦠

● M08.83   Other juvenile arthritis, wrist

      M08.831   Other juvenile arthritis, right wrist 🦠

      M08.832   Other juvenile arthritis, left wrist 🦠

      M08.839   Other juvenile arthritis, unspecified wrist 🦠

● M08.84   Other juvenile arthritis, hand

      M08.841   Other juvenile arthritis, right hand 🦠

      M08.842   Other juvenile arthritis, left hand 🦠

      M08.849   Other juvenile arthritis, unspecified hand 🦠

● M08.85   Other juvenile arthritis, hip

      M08.851   Other juvenile arthritis, right hip 🦠

      M08.852   Other juvenile arthritis, left hip 🦠

      M08.859   Other juvenile arthritis, unspecified hip 🦠

▶ New   ⇒ Revised   ~~deleted~~ Deleted   Excludes 1   Excludes 2   Includes   Use additional   Code first   Code also   Key words

OGCR Official Guidelines   X Assign placeholder X   ● Use Additional Character(s)   ▶ Manifestation Code   🦠 Hierarchical Condition Category   Coding Clinic

● M08.86   Other juvenile arthritis, knee

    M08.861   Other juvenile arthritis, right knee 🐾

    M08.862   Other juvenile arthritis, left knee 🐾

    M08.869   Other juvenile arthritis, unspecified knee 🐾

● M08.87   Other juvenile arthritis, ankle and foot

    M08.871   Other juvenile arthritis, right ankle and foot 🐾

    M08.872   Other juvenile arthritis, left ankle and foot 🐾

    M08.879   Other juvenile arthritis, unspecified ankle and foot 🐾

   M08.88   Other juvenile arthritis, other specified site 🐾

           Other juvenile arthritis, vertebrae

   M08.89   Other juvenile arthritis, multiple sites 🐾

● M08.9   Juvenile arthritis, unspecified

> **Excludes1**   juvenile rheumatoid arthritis, unspecified (M08.0-)

   M08.90   Juvenile arthritis, unspecified, unspecified site 🐾

● M08.91   Juvenile arthritis, unspecified, shoulder

    M08.911   Juvenile arthritis, unspecified, right shoulder 🐾

    M08.912   Juvenile arthritis, unspecified, left shoulder 🐾

    M08.919   Juvenile arthritis, unspecified, unspecified shoulder 🐾

● M08.92   Juvenile arthritis, unspecified, elbow

    M08.921   Juvenile arthritis, unspecified, right elbow 🐾

    M08.922   Juvenile arthritis, unspecified, left elbow 🐾

    M08.929   Juvenile arthritis, unspecified, unspecified elbow 🐾

● M08.93   Juvenile arthritis, unspecified, wrist

    M08.931   Juvenile arthritis, unspecified, right wrist 🐾

    M08.932   Juvenile arthritis, unspecified, left wrist 🐾

    M08.939   Juvenile arthritis, unspecified, unspecified wrist 🐾

● M08.94   Juvenile arthritis, unspecified, hand

    M08.941   Juvenile arthritis, unspecified, right hand 🐾

    M08.942   Juvenile arthritis, unspecified, left hand 🐾

    M08.949   Juvenile arthritis, unspecified, unspecified hand 🐾

● M08.95   Juvenile arthritis, unspecified, hip

    M08.951   Juvenile arthritis, unspecified, right hip 🐾

    M08.952   Juvenile arthritis, unspecified, left hip 🐾

    M08.959   Juvenile arthritis, unspecified, unspecified hip 🐾

● M08.96   Juvenile arthritis, unspecified, knee

    M08.961   Juvenile arthritis, unspecified, right knee 🐾

    M08.962   Juvenile arthritis, unspecified, left knee 🐾

    M08.969   Juvenile arthritis, unspecified, unspecified knee 🐾

● M08.97   Juvenile arthritis, unspecified, ankle and foot

    M08.971   Juvenile arthritis, unspecified, right ankle and foot 🐾

    M08.972   Juvenile arthritis, unspecified, left ankle and foot 🐾

    M08.979   Juvenile arthritis, unspecified, unspecified ankle and foot 🐾

   M08.98   Juvenile arthritis, unspecified, vertebrae 🐾

   M08.99   Juvenile arthritis, unspecified, multiple sites 🐾

   M08.9A   Juvenile arthritis, unspecified, other specified site

● **M1A**   Chronic gout

> Use additional code to identify:
> Autonomic neuropathy in diseases classified elsewhere (G99.0)
> Calculus of urinary tract in diseases classified elsewhere (N22)
> Cardiomyopathy in diseases classified elsewhere (I43)
> Disorders of external ear in diseases classified elsewhere (H61.1-, H62.8-)
> Disorders of iris and ciliary body in diseases classified elsewhere (H22)
> Glomerular disorders in diseases classified elsewhere (N08)

> **Excludes1**   gout NOS (M10.-)

> **Excludes2**   acute gout (M10.-)

> The appropriate 7th character is to be added to each code from category M1A

0	without tophus (tophi)
1	with tophus (tophi)

● **M1A.0**   Idiopathic chronic gout

       Chronic gouty bursitis

       Primary chronic gout

   X ● M1A.00   Idiopathic chronic gout, unspecified site

   ● M1A.01   Idiopathic chronic gout, shoulder

     ● M1A.011   Idiopathic chronic gout, right shoulder

     ● M1A.012   Idiopathic chronic gout, left shoulder

     ● M1A.019   Idiopathic chronic gout, unspecified shoulder

   ● M1A.02   Idiopathic chronic gout, elbow

     ● M1A.021   Idiopathic chronic gout, right elbow

     ● M1A.022   Idiopathic chronic gout, left elbow

     ● M1A.029   Idiopathic chronic gout, unspecified elbow

   ● M1A.03   Idiopathic chronic gout, wrist

     ● M1A.031   Idiopathic chronic gout, right wrist

     ● M1A.032   Idiopathic chronic gout, left wrist

     ● M1A.039   Idiopathic chronic gout, unspecified wrist

   ● M1A.04   Idiopathic chronic gout, hand

     ● M1A.041   Idiopathic chronic gout, right hand

     ● M1A.042   Idiopathic chronic gout, left hand

     ● M1A.049   Idiopathic chronic gout, unspecified hand

   ● M1A.05   Idiopathic chronic gout, hip

     ● M1A.051   Idiopathic chronic gout, right hip

     ● M1A.052   Idiopathic chronic gout, left hip

     ● M1A.059   Idiopathic chronic gout, unspecified hip

   ● M1A.06   Idiopathic chronic gout, knee

     ● M1A.061   Idiopathic chronic gout, right knee

     ● M1A.062   Idiopathic chronic gout, left knee

     ● M1A.069   Idiopathic chronic gout, unspecified knee

   ● M1A.07   Idiopathic chronic gout, ankle and foot

     ● M1A.071   Idiopathic chronic gout, right ankle and foot

     ● M1A.072   Idiopathic chronic gout, left ankle and foot

     ● M1A.079   Idiopathic chronic gout, unspecified ankle and foot

   X ● M1A.08   Idiopathic chronic gout, vertebrae

   X ● M1A.09   Idiopathic chronic gout, multiple sites

CHAPTER 13 (M00-M99)

● **M1A.1** Lead-induced chronic gout
  Code first toxic effects of lead and its compounds (T56.0-)
X ● **M1A.10** Lead-induced chronic gout, unspecified site
● **M1A.11** Lead-induced chronic gout, shoulder
   ● **M1A.111** Lead-induced chronic gout, right shoulder
   ● **M1A.112** Lead-induced chronic gout, left shoulder
   ● **M1A.119** Lead-induced chronic gout, unspecified shoulder
● **M1A.12** Lead-induced chronic gout, elbow
   ● **M1A.121** Lead-induced chronic gout, right elbow
   ● **M1A.122** Lead-induced chronic gout, left elbow
   ● **M1A.129** Lead-induced chronic gout, unspecified elbow
● **M1A.13** Lead-induced chronic gout, wrist
   ● **M1A.131** Lead-induced chronic gout, right wrist
   ● **M1A.132** Lead-induced chronic gout, left wrist
   ● **M1A.139** Lead-induced chronic gout, unspecified wrist
● **M1A.14** Lead-induced chronic gout, hand
   ● **M1A.141** Lead-induced chronic gout, right hand
   ● **M1A.142** Lead-induced chronic gout, left hand
   ● **M1A.149** Lead-induced chronic gout, unspecified hand
● **M1A.15** Lead-induced chronic gout, hip
   ● **M1A.151** Lead-induced chronic gout, right hip
   ● **M1A.152** Lead-induced chronic gout, left hip
   ● **M1A.159** Lead-induced chronic gout, unspecified hip
● **M1A.16** Lead-induced chronic gout, knee
   ● **M1A.161** Lead-induced chronic gout, right knee
   ● **M1A.162** Lead-induced chronic gout, left knee
   ● **M1A.169** Lead-induced chronic gout, unspecified knee
● **M1A.17** Lead-induced chronic gout, ankle and foot
   ● **M1A.171** Lead-induced chronic gout, right ankle and foot
   ● **M1A.172** Lead-induced chronic gout, left ankle and foot
   ● **M1A.179** Lead-induced chronic gout, unspecified ankle and foot
X ● **M1A.18** Lead-induced chronic gout, vertebrae
X ● **M1A.19** Lead-induced chronic gout, multiple sites
● **M1A.2** Drug-induced chronic gout
  Use additional code for adverse effect, if applicable, to identify drug (T36-T50 with fifth or sixth character 5)
X ● **M1A.20** Drug-induced chronic gout, unspecified site
● **M1A.21** Drug-induced chronic gout, shoulder
   ● **M1A.211** Drug-induced chronic gout, right shoulder
   ● **M1A.212** Drug-induced chronic gout, left shoulder
   ● **M1A.219** Drug-induced chronic gout, unspecified shoulder
● **M1A.22** Drug-induced chronic gout, elbow
   ● **M1A.221** Drug-induced chronic gout, right elbow
   ● **M1A.222** Drug-induced chronic gout, left elbow
   ● **M1A.229** Drug-induced chronic gout, unspecified elbow

● **M1A.23** Drug-induced chronic gout, wrist
   ● **M1A.231** Drug-induced chronic gout, right wrist
   ● **M1A.232** Drug-induced chronic gout, left wrist
   ● **M1A.239** Drug-induced chronic gout, unspecified wrist
● **M1A.24** Drug-induced chronic gout, hand
   ● **M1A.241** Drug-induced chronic gout, right hand
   ● **M1A.242** Drug-induced chronic gout, left hand
   ● **M1A.249** Drug-induced chronic gout, unspecified hand
● **M1A.25** Drug-induced chronic gout, hip
   ● **M1A.251** Drug-induced chronic gout, right hip
   ● **M1A.252** Drug-induced chronic gout, left hip
   ● **M1A.259** Drug-induced chronic gout, unspecified hip
● **M1A.26** Drug-induced chronic gout, knee
   ● **M1A.261** Drug-induced chronic gout, right knee
   ● **M1A.262** Drug-induced chronic gout, left knee
   ● **M1A.269** Drug-induced chronic gout, unspecified knee
● **M1A.27** Drug-induced chronic gout, ankle and foot
   ● **M1A.271** Drug-induced chronic gout, right ankle and foot
   ● **M1A.272** Drug-induced chronic gout, left ankle and foot
   ● **M1A.279** Drug-induced chronic gout, unspecified ankle and foot
X ● **M1A.28** Drug-induced chronic gout, vertebrae
X ● **M1A.29** Drug-induced chronic gout, multiple sites
● **M1A.3** Chronic gout due to renal impairment
  Code first associated renal disease
X ● **M1A.30** Chronic gout due to renal impairment, unspecified site
● **M1A.31** Chronic gout due to renal impairment, shoulder
   ● **M1A.311** Chronic gout due to renal impairment, right shoulder
   ● **M1A.312** Chronic gout due to renal impairment, left shoulder
   ● **M1A.319** Chronic gout due to renal impairment, unspecified shoulder
● **M1A.32** Chronic gout due to renal impairment, elbow
   ● **M1A.321** Chronic gout due to renal impairment, right elbow
   ● **M1A.322** Chronic gout due to renal impairment, left elbow
   ● **M1A.329** Chronic gout due to renal impairment, unspecified elbow
● **M1A.33** Chronic gout due to renal impairment, wrist
   ● **M1A.331** Chronic gout due to renal impairment, right wrist
   ● **M1A.332** Chronic gout due to renal impairment, left wrist
   ● **M1A.339** Chronic gout due to renal impairment, unspecified wrist
● **M1A.34** Chronic gout due to renal impairment, hand
   ● **M1A.341** Chronic gout due to renal impairment, right hand
   ● **M1A.342** Chronic gout due to renal impairment, left hand
   ● **M1A.349** Chronic gout due to renal impairment, unspecified hand

▶ New   ⇒ Revised   ~~deleted~~ Deleted   Excludes 1   Excludes 2   Includes   Use additional   Code first   Code also   Key words
OGCR Official Guidelines   X Assign placeholder X   ● Use Additional Character(s)   ▶ Manifestation Code   🗴 Hierarchical Condition Category   **Coding Clinic**

● M1A.35 Chronic gout due to renal impairment, hip
  ● M1A.351 Chronic gout due to renal impairment, right hip
  ● M1A.352 Chronic gout due to renal impairment, left hip
  ● M1A.359 Chronic gout due to renal impairment, unspecified hip
● M1A.36 Chronic gout due to renal impairment, knee
  ● M1A.361 Chronic gout due to renal impairment, right knee
  ● M1A.362 Chronic gout due to renal impairment, left knee
  ● M1A.369 Chronic gout due to renal impairment, unspecified knee
● M1A.37 Chronic gout due to renal impairment, ankle and foot
  ● M1A.371 Chronic gout due to renal impairment, right ankle and foot
  ● M1A.372 Chronic gout due to renal impairment, left ankle and foot
  ● M1A.379 Chronic gout due to renal impairment, unspecified ankle and foot
X ● M1A.38 Chronic gout due to renal impairment, vertebrae
X ● M1A.39 Chronic gout due to renal impairment, multiple sites
● M1A.4 Other secondary chronic gout
  Code first associated condition
X ● M1A.40 Other secondary chronic gout, unspecified site
● M1A.41 Other secondary chronic gout, shoulder
  ● M1A.411 Other secondary chronic gout, right shoulder
  ● M1A.412 Other secondary chronic gout, left shoulder
  ● M1A.419 Other secondary chronic gout, unspecified shoulder
● M1A.42 Other secondary chronic gout, elbow
  ● M1A.421 Other secondary chronic gout, right elbow
  ● M1A.422 Other secondary chronic gout, left elbow
  ● M1A.429 Other secondary chronic gout, unspecified elbow
● M1A.43 Other secondary chronic gout, wrist
  ● M1A.431 Other secondary chronic gout, right wrist
  ● M1A.432 Other secondary chronic gout, left wrist
  ● M1A.439 Other secondary chronic gout, unspecified wrist
● M1A.44 Other secondary chronic gout, hand
  ● M1A.441 Other secondary chronic gout, right hand
  ● M1A.442 Other secondary chronic gout, left hand
  ● M1A.449 Other secondary chronic gout, unspecified hand
● M1A.45 Other secondary chronic gout, hip
  ● M1A.451 Other secondary chronic gout, right hip
  ● M1A.452 Other secondary chronic gout, left hip
  ● M1A.459 Other secondary chronic gout, unspecified hip

● M1A.46 Other secondary chronic gout, knee
  ● M1A.461 Other secondary chronic gout, right knee
  ● M1A.462 Other secondary chronic gout, left knee
  ● M1A.469 Other secondary chronic gout, unspecified knee
● M1A.47 Other secondary chronic gout, ankle and foot
  ● M1A.471 Other secondary chronic gout, right ankle and foot
  ● M1A.472 Other secondary chronic gout, left ankle and foot
  ● M1A.479 Other secondary chronic gout, unspecified ankle and foot
X ● M1A.48 Other secondary chronic gout, vertebrae
X ● M1A.49 Other secondary chronic gout, multiple sites
X ● M1A.9 Chronic gout, unspecified

● M10 Gout
  Accumulation of uric acid that results in swollen, red, hot, painful, stiff joints
  Acute gout
  Gout attack
  Gout flare
  Podagra
  Use additional code to identify:
    Autonomic neuropathy in diseases classified elsewhere (G99.0)
    Calculus of urinary tract in diseases classified elsewhere (N22)
    Cardiomyopathy in diseases classified elsewhere (I43)
    Disorders of external ear in diseases classified elsewhere (H61.1-, H62.8-)
    Disorders of iris and ciliary body in diseases classified elsewhere (H22)
    Glomerular disorders in diseases classified elsewhere (N08)
  Excludes2   chronic gout (M1A.-)
● M10.0 Idiopathic gout
  Gouty bursitis
  Primary gout
  M10.00 Idiopathic gout, unspecified site
  ● M10.01 Idiopathic gout, shoulder
    M10.011 Idiopathic gout, right shoulder
    M10.012 Idiopathic gout, left shoulder
    M10.019 Idiopathic gout, unspecified shoulder
  ● M10.02 Idiopathic gout, elbow
    M10.021 Idiopathic gout, right elbow
    M10.022 Idiopathic gout, left elbow
    M10.029 Idiopathic gout, unspecified elbow
  ● M10.03 Idiopathic gout, wrist
    M10.031 Idiopathic gout, right wrist
    M10.032 Idiopathic gout, left wrist
    M10.039 Idiopathic gout, unspecified wrist
  ● M10.04 Idiopathic gout, hand
    M10.041 Idiopathic gout, right hand
    M10.042 Idiopathic gout, left hand
    M10.049 Idiopathic gout, unspecified hand
  ● M10.05 Idiopathic gout, hip
    M10.051 Idiopathic gout, right hip
    M10.052 Idiopathic gout, left hip
    M10.059 Idiopathic gout, unspecified hip
  ● M10.06 Idiopathic gout, knee
    M10.061 Idiopathic gout, right knee
    M10.062 Idiopathic gout, left knee
    M10.069 Idiopathic gout, unspecified knee

CHAPTER 13 (M00-M99)

● M10.07 Idiopathic gout, ankle and foot
      M10.071 Idiopathic gout, right ankle and foot
      M10.072 Idiopathic gout, left ankle and foot
      M10.079 Idiopathic gout, unspecified ankle
               and foot
   M10.08 Idiopathic gout, vertebrae
   M10.09 Idiopathic gout, multiple sites
● M10.1 Lead-induced gout
      Code first toxic effects of lead and its compounds (T56.0-)
   M10.10 Lead-induced gout, unspecified site
● M10.11 Lead-induced gout, shoulder
      M10.111 Lead-induced gout, right shoulder
      M10.112 Lead-induced gout, left shoulder
      M10.119 Lead-induced gout, unspecified
               shoulder
● M10.12 Lead-induced gout, elbow
      M10.121 Lead-induced gout, right elbow
      M10.122 Lead-induced gout, left elbow
      M10.129 Lead-induced gout, unspecified elbow
● M10.13 Lead-induced gout, wrist
      M10.131 Lead-induced gout, right wrist
      M10.132 Lead-induced gout, left wrist
      M10.139 Lead-induced gout, unspecified wrist
● M10.14 Lead-induced gout, hand
      M10.141 Lead-induced gout, right hand
      M10.142 Lead-induced gout, left hand
      M10.149 Lead-induced gout, unspecified hand
● M10.15 Lead-induced gout, hip
      M10.151 Lead-induced gout, right hip
      M10.152 Lead-induced gout, left hip
      M10.159 Lead-induced gout, unspecified hip
● M10.16 Lead-induced gout, knee
      M10.161 Lead-induced gout, right knee
      M10.162 Lead-induced gout, left knee
      M10.169 Lead-induced gout, unspecified knee
● M10.17 Lead-induced gout, ankle and foot
      M10.171 Lead-induced gout, right ankle and
               foot
      M10.172 Lead-induced gout, left ankle and
               foot
      M10.179 Lead-induced gout, unspecified ankle
               and foot
   M10.18 Lead-induced gout, vertebrae
   M10.19 Lead-induced gout, multiple sites
● M10.2 Drug-induced gout
      Use additional code for adverse effect, if applicable,
         to identify drug (T36-T50 with fifth or sixth
         character 5)
   M10.20 Drug-induced gout, unspecified site
● M10.21 Drug-induced gout, shoulder
      M10.211 Drug-induced gout, right shoulder
      M10.212 Drug-induced gout, left shoulder
      M10.219 Drug-induced gout, unspecified
               shoulder
● M10.22 Drug-induced gout, elbow
      M10.221 Drug-induced gout, right elbow
      M10.222 Drug-induced gout, left elbow
      M10.229 Drug-induced gout, unspecified
               elbow
● M10.23 Drug-induced gout, wrist
      M10.231 Drug-induced gout, right wrist
      M10.232 Drug-induced gout, left wrist
      M10.239 Drug-induced gout, unspecified wrist

● M10.24 Drug-induced gout, hand
      M10.241 Drug-induced gout, right hand
      M10.242 Drug-induced gout, left hand
      M10.249 Drug-induced gout, unspecified hand
● M10.25 Drug-induced gout, hip
      M10.251 Drug-induced gout, right hip
      M10.252 Drug-induced gout, left hip
      M10.259 Drug-induced gout, unspecified hip
● M10.26 Drug-induced gout, knee
      M10.261 Drug-induced gout, right knee
      M10.262 Drug-induced gout, left knee
      M10.269 Drug-induced gout, unspecified knee
● M10.27 Drug-induced gout, ankle and foot
      M10.271 Drug-induced gout, right ankle and
               foot
      M10.272 Drug-induced gout, left ankle and
               foot
      M10.279 Drug-induced gout, unspecified ankle
               and foot
   M10.28 Drug-induced gout, vertebrae
   M10.29 Drug-induced gout, multiple sites
● M10.3 Gout due to renal impairment
      Code also associated renal disease
   M10.30 Gout due to renal impairment, unspecified site
● M10.31 Gout due to renal impairment, shoulder
      M10.311 Gout due to renal impairment, right
               shoulder
      M10.312 Gout due to renal impairment, left
               shoulder
      M10.319 Gout due to renal impairment,
               unspecified shoulder
● M10.32 Gout due to renal impairment, elbow
      M10.321 Gout due to renal impairment, right
               elbow
      M10.322 Gout due to renal impairment, left
               elbow
      M10.329 Gout due to renal impairment,
               unspecified elbow
● M10.33 Gout due to renal impairment, wrist
      M10.331 Gout due to renal impairment, right
               wrist
      M10.332 Gout due to renal impairment, left
               wrist
      M10.339 Gout due to renal impairment,
               unspecified wrist
● M10.34 Gout due to renal impairment, hand
      M10.341 Gout due to renal impairment, right
               hand
      M10.342 Gout due to renal impairment, left
               hand
      M10.349 Gout due to renal impairment,
               unspecified hand
● M10.35 Gout due to renal impairment, hip
      M10.351 Gout due to renal impairment, right
               hip
      M10.352 Gout due to renal impairment, left
               hip
      M10.359 Gout due to renal impairment,
               unspecified hip
● M10.36 Gout due to renal impairment, knee
      M10.361 Gout due to renal impairment, right
               knee
      M10.362 Gout due to renal impairment, left
               knee
      M10.369 Gout due to renal impairment,
               unspecified knee

▶ New   ⇒ Revised   ~~deleted~~ Deleted   Excludes 1   Excludes 2   Includes   Use additional   Code first   Code also   Key words
OGCR Official Guidelines   X Assign placeholder X   ● Use Additional Character(s)   ▷ Manifestation Code   🐾 Hierarchical Condition Category   Coding Clinic

● M10.37 Gout due to renal impairment, ankle and foot
    M10.371 Gout due to renal impairment, right ankle and foot
    M10.372 Gout due to renal impairment, left ankle and foot
    M10.379 Gout due to renal impairment, unspecified ankle and foot
  M10.38 Gout due to renal impairment, vertebrae
  M10.39 Gout due to renal impairment, multiple sites
● M10.4 Other secondary gout
    Code first associated condition
  M10.40 Other secondary gout, unspecified site
● M10.41 Other secondary gout, shoulder
    M10.411 Other secondary gout, right shoulder
    M10.412 Other secondary gout, left shoulder
    M10.419 Other secondary gout, unspecified shoulder
● M10.42 Other secondary gout, elbow
    M10.421 Other secondary gout, right elbow
    M10.422 Other secondary gout, left elbow
    M10.429 Other secondary gout, unspecified elbow
● M10.43 Other secondary gout, wrist
    M10.431 Other secondary gout, right wrist
    M10.432 Other secondary gout, left wrist
    M10.439 Other secondary gout, unspecified wrist
● M10.44 Other secondary gout, hand
    M10.441 Other secondary gout, right hand
    M10.442 Other secondary gout, left hand
    M10.449 Other secondary gout, unspecified hand
● M10.45 Other secondary gout, hip
    M10.451 Other secondary gout, right hip
    M10.452 Other secondary gout, left hip
    M10.459 Other secondary gout, unspecified hip
● M10.46 Other secondary gout, knee
    M10.461 Other secondary gout, right knee
    M10.462 Other secondary gout, left knee
    M10.469 Other secondary gout, unspecified knee
● M10.47 Other secondary gout, ankle and foot
    M10.471 Other secondary gout, right ankle and foot
    M10.472 Other secondary gout, left ankle and foot
    M10.479 Other secondary gout, unspecified ankle and foot
  M10.48 Other secondary gout, vertebrae
  M10.49 Other secondary gout, multiple sites
M10.9 Gout, unspecified
    Gout NOS

● M11 Other crystal arthropathies
● M11.0 Hydroxyapatite deposition disease
  M11.00 Hydroxyapatite deposition disease, unspecified site
● M11.01 Hydroxyapatite deposition disease, shoulder
    M11.011 Hydroxyapatite deposition disease, right shoulder
    M11.012 Hydroxyapatite deposition disease, left shoulder
    M11.019 Hydroxyapatite deposition disease, unspecified shoulder

● M11.02 Hydroxyapatite deposition disease, elbow
    M11.021 Hydroxyapatite deposition disease, right elbow
    M11.022 Hydroxyapatite deposition disease, left elbow
    M11.029 Hydroxyapatite deposition disease, unspecified elbow
● M11.03 Hydroxyapatite deposition disease, wrist
    M11.031 Hydroxyapatite deposition disease, right wrist
    M11.032 Hydroxyapatite deposition disease, left wrist
    M11.039 Hydroxyapatite deposition disease, unspecified wrist
● M11.04 Hydroxyapatite deposition disease, hand
    M11.041 Hydroxyapatite deposition disease, right hand
    M11.042 Hydroxyapatite deposition disease, left hand
    M11.049 Hydroxyapatite deposition disease, unspecified hand
● M11.05 Hydroxyapatite deposition disease, hip
    M11.051 Hydroxyapatite deposition disease, right hip
    M11.052 Hydroxyapatite deposition disease, left hip
    M11.059 Hydroxyapatite deposition disease, unspecified hip
● M11.06 Hydroxyapatite deposition disease, knee
    M11.061 Hydroxyapatite deposition disease, right knee
    M11.062 Hydroxyapatite deposition disease, left knee
    M11.069 Hydroxyapatite deposition disease, unspecified knee
● M11.07 Hydroxyapatite deposition disease, ankle and foot
    M11.071 Hydroxyapatite deposition disease, right ankle and foot
    M11.072 Hydroxyapatite deposition disease, left ankle and foot
    M11.079 Hydroxyapatite deposition disease, unspecified ankle and foot
  M11.08 Hydroxyapatite deposition disease, vertebrae
  M11.09 Hydroxyapatite deposition disease, multiple sites
● M11.1 Familial chondrocalcinosis
  M11.10 Familial chondrocalcinosis, unspecified site
● M11.11 Familial chondrocalcinosis, shoulder
    M11.111 Familial chondrocalcinosis, right shoulder
    M11.112 Familial chondrocalcinosis, left shoulder
    M11.119 Familial chondrocalcinosis, unspecified shoulder
● M11.12 Familial chondrocalcinosis, elbow
    M11.121 Familial chondrocalcinosis, right elbow
    M11.122 Familial chondrocalcinosis, left elbow
    M11.129 Familial chondrocalcinosis, unspecified elbow
● M11.13 Familial chondrocalcinosis, wrist
    M11.131 Familial chondrocalcinosis, right wrist
    M11.132 Familial chondrocalcinosis, left wrist
    M11.139 Familial chondrocalcinosis, unspecified wrist

CHAPTER 13 (M00-M99)

● M11.14   Familial chondrocalcinosis, hand
     M11.141   Familial chondrocalcinosis, right hand
     M11.142   Familial chondrocalcinosis, left hand
     M11.149   Familial chondrocalcinosis, unspecified hand

● M11.15   Familial chondrocalcinosis, hip
     M11.151   Familial chondrocalcinosis, right hip
     M11.152   Familial chondrocalcinosis, left hip
     M11.159   Familial chondrocalcinosis, unspecified hip

● M11.16   Familial chondrocalcinosis, knee
     M11.161   Familial chondrocalcinosis, right knee
     M11.162   Familial chondrocalcinosis, left knee
     M11.169   Familial chondrocalcinosis, unspecified knee

● M11.17   Familial chondrocalcinosis, ankle and foot
     M11.171   Familial chondrocalcinosis, right ankle and foot
     M11.172   Familial chondrocalcinosis, left ankle and foot
     M11.179   Familial chondrocalcinosis, unspecified ankle and foot

   M11.18   Familial chondrocalcinosis, vertebrae
   M11.19   Familial chondrocalcinosis, multiple sites

● M11.2   Other chondrocalcinosis
     Chondrocalcinosis NOS

   M11.20   Other chondrocalcinosis, unspecified site

● M11.21   Other chondrocalcinosis, shoulder
     M11.211   Other chondrocalcinosis, right shoulder
     M11.212   Other chondrocalcinosis, left shoulder
     M11.219   Other chondrocalcinosis, unspecified shoulder

● M11.22   Other chondrocalcinosis, elbow
     M11.221   Other chondrocalcinosis, right elbow
     M11.222   Other chondrocalcinosis, left elbow
     M11.229   Other chondrocalcinosis, unspecified elbow

● M11.23   Other chondrocalcinosis, wrist
     M11.231   Other chondrocalcinosis, right wrist
     M11.232   Other chondrocalcinosis, left wrist
     M11.239   Other chondrocalcinosis, unspecified wrist

● M11.24   Other chondrocalcinosis, hand
     M11.241   Other chondrocalcinosis, right hand
     M11.242   Other chondrocalcinosis, left hand
     M11.249   Other chondrocalcinosis, unspecified hand

● M11.25   Other chondrocalcinosis, hip
     M11.251   Other chondrocalcinosis, right hip
     M11.252   Other chondrocalcinosis, left hip
     M11.259   Other chondrocalcinosis, unspecified hip

● M11.26   Other chondrocalcinosis, knee
     M11.261   Other chondrocalcinosis, right knee
     M11.262   Other chondrocalcinosis, left knee
     M11.269   Other chondrocalcinosis, unspecified knee

● M11.27   Other chondrocalcinosis, ankle and foot
     M11.271   Other chondrocalcinosis, right ankle and foot
     M11.272   Other chondrocalcinosis, left ankle and foot
     M11.279   Other chondrocalcinosis, unspecified ankle and foot

   M11.28   Other chondrocalcinosis, vertebrae
   M11.29   Other chondrocalcinosis, multiple sites

● M11.8   Other specified crystal arthropathies

   M11.80   Other specified crystal arthropathies, unspecified site

● M11.81   Other specified crystal arthropathies, shoulder
     M11.811   Other specified crystal arthropathies, right shoulder
     M11.812   Other specified crystal arthropathies, left shoulder
     M11.819   Other specified crystal arthropathies, unspecified shoulder

● M11.82   Other specified crystal arthropathies, elbow
     M11.821   Other specified crystal arthropathies, right elbow
     M11.822   Other specified crystal arthropathies, left elbow
     M11.829   Other specified crystal arthropathies, unspecified elbow

● M11.83   Other specified crystal arthropathies, wrist
     M11.831   Other specified crystal arthropathies, right wrist
     M11.832   Other specified crystal arthropathies, left wrist
     M11.839   Other specified crystal arthropathies, unspecified wrist

● M11.84   Other specified crystal arthropathies, hand
     M11.841   Other specified crystal arthropathies, right hand
     M11.842   Other specified crystal arthropathies, left hand
     M11.849   Other specified crystal arthropathies, unspecified hand

● M11.85   Other specified crystal arthropathies, hip
     M11.851   Other specified crystal arthropathies, right hip
     M11.852   Other specified crystal arthropathies, left hip
     M11.859   Other specified crystal arthropathies, unspecified hip

● M11.86   Other specified crystal arthropathies, knee
     M11.861   Other specified crystal arthropathies, right knee
     M11.862   Other specified crystal arthropathies, left knee
     M11.869   Other specified crystal arthropathies, unspecified knee

● M11.87   Other specified crystal arthropathies, ankle and foot
     M11.871   Other specified crystal arthropathies, right ankle and foot
     M11.872   Other specified crystal arthropathies, left ankle and foot
     M11.879   Other specified crystal arthropathies, unspecified ankle and foot

   M11.88   Other specified crystal arthropathies, vertebrae
   M11.89   Other specified crystal arthropathies, multiple sites

  M11.9   Crystal arthropathy, unspecified

▶ New   ⇒ Revised   ~~deleted~~ Deleted   Excludes 1   Excludes 2   Includes   Use additional   Code first   Code also   Key words
OGCR Official Guidelines   X Assign placeholder X   ● Use Additional Character(s)   ▶ Manifestation Code   🏷 Hierarchical Condition Category   **Coding Clinic**

- **M12   Other and unspecified arthropathy**
  - **Excludes1**   arthrosis (M15-M19)
    - cricoarytenoid arthropathy (J38.7)
  - ● **M12.0   Chronic postrheumatic arthropathy [Jaccoud]**
    - **M12.00   Chronic postrheumatic arthropathy [Jaccoud], unspecified site** 🔗
    - ● **M12.01   Chronic postrheumatic arthropathy [Jaccoud], shoulder**
      - M12.011   Chronic postrheumatic arthropathy [Jaccoud], right shoulder 🔗
      - M12.012   Chronic postrheumatic arthropathy [Jaccoud], left shoulder 🔗
      - M12.019   Chronic postrheumatic arthropathy [Jaccoud], unspecified shoulder 🔗
    - ● **M12.02   Chronic postrheumatic arthropathy [Jaccoud], elbow**
      - M12.021   Chronic postrheumatic arthropathy [Jaccoud], right elbow 🔗
      - M12.022   Chronic postrheumatic arthropathy [Jaccoud], left elbow 🔗
      - M12.029   Chronic postrheumatic arthropathy [Jaccoud], unspecified elbow 🔗
    - ● **M12.03   Chronic postrheumatic arthropathy [Jaccoud], wrist**
      - M12.031   Chronic postrheumatic arthropathy [Jaccoud], right wrist 🔗
      - M12.032   Chronic postrheumatic arthropathy [Jaccoud], left wrist 🔗
      - M12.039   Chronic postrheumatic arthropathy [Jaccoud], unspecified wrist 🔗
    - ● **M12.04   Chronic postrheumatic arthropathy [Jaccoud], hand**
      - M12.041   Chronic postrheumatic arthropathy [Jaccoud], right hand 🔗
      - M12.042   Chronic postrheumatic arthropathy [Jaccoud], left hand 🔗
      - M12.049   Chronic postrheumatic arthropathy [Jaccoud], unspecified hand 🔗
    - ● **M12.05   Chronic postrheumatic arthropathy [Jaccoud], hip**
      - M12.051   Chronic postrheumatic arthropathy [Jaccoud], right hip 🔗
      - M12.052   Chronic postrheumatic arthropathy [Jaccoud], left hip 🔗
      - M12.059   Chronic postrheumatic arthropathy [Jaccoud], unspecified hip 🔗
    - ● **M12.06   Chronic postrheumatic arthropathy [Jaccoud], knee**
      - M12.061   Chronic postrheumatic arthropathy [Jaccoud], right knee 🔗
      - M12.062   Chronic postrheumatic arthropathy [Jaccoud], left knee 🔗
      - M12.069   Chronic postrheumatic arthropathy [Jaccoud], unspecified knee 🔗
    - ● **M12.07   Chronic postrheumatic arthropathy [Jaccoud], ankle and foot**
      - M12.071   Chronic postrheumatic arthropathy [Jaccoud], right ankle and foot 🔗
      - M12.072   Chronic postrheumatic arthropathy [Jaccoud], left ankle and foot 🔗
      - M12.079   Chronic postrheumatic arthropathy [Jaccoud], unspecified ankle and foot 🔗
    - **M12.08   Chronic postrheumatic arthropathy [Jaccoud], other specified site** 🔗
      - Chronic postrheumatic arthropathy [Jaccoud], vertebrae
    - **M12.09   Chronic postrheumatic arthropathy [Jaccoud], multiple sites** 🔗

- ● **M12.1   Kaschin-Beck disease**
  - Osteochondroarthrosis deformans endemica
  - **M12.10   Kaschin-Beck disease, unspecified site**
  - ● **M12.11   Kaschin-Beck disease, shoulder**
    - M12.111   Kaschin-Beck disease, right shoulder
    - M12.112   Kaschin-Beck disease, left shoulder
    - M12.119   Kaschin-Beck disease, unspecified shoulder
  - ● **M12.12   Kaschin-Beck disease, elbow**
    - M12.121   Kaschin-Beck disease, right elbow
    - M12.122   Kaschin-Beck disease, left elbow
    - M12.129   Kaschin-Beck disease, unspecified elbow
  - ● **M12.13   Kaschin-Beck disease, wrist**
    - M12.131   Kaschin-Beck disease, right wrist
    - M12.132   Kaschin-Beck disease, left wrist
    - M12.139   Kaschin-Beck disease, unspecified wrist
  - ● **M12.14   Kaschin-Beck disease, hand**
    - M12.141   Kaschin-Beck disease, right hand
    - M12.142   Kaschin-Beck disease, left hand
    - M12.149   Kaschin-Beck disease, unspecified hand
  - ● **M12.15   Kaschin-Beck disease, hip**
    - M12.151   Kaschin-Beck disease, right hip
    - M12.152   Kaschin-Beck disease, left hip
    - M12.159   Kaschin-Beck disease, unspecified hip
  - ● **M12.16   Kaschin-Beck disease, knee**
    - M12.161   Kaschin-Beck disease, right knee
    - M12.162   Kaschin-Beck disease, left knee
    - M12.169   Kaschin-Beck disease, unspecified knee
  - ● **M12.17   Kaschin-Beck disease, ankle and foot**
    - M12.171   Kaschin-Beck disease, right ankle and foot
    - M12.172   Kaschin-Beck disease, left ankle and foot
    - M12.179   Kaschin-Beck disease, unspecified ankle and foot
  - **M12.18   Kaschin-Beck disease, vertebrae**
  - **M12.19   Kaschin-Beck disease, multiple sites**
- ● **M12.2   Villonodular synovitis (pigmented)**
  - **M12.20   Villonodular synovitis (pigmented), unspecified site**
  - ● **M12.21   Villonodular synovitis (pigmented), shoulder**
    - M12.211   Villonodular synovitis (pigmented), right shoulder
    - M12.212   Villonodular synovitis (pigmented), left shoulder
    - M12.219   Villonodular synovitis (pigmented), unspecified shoulder
  - ● **M12.22   Villonodular synovitis (pigmented), elbow**
    - M12.221   Villonodular synovitis (pigmented), right elbow
    - M12.222   Villonodular synovitis (pigmented), left elbow
    - M12.229   Villonodular synovitis (pigmented), unspecified elbow
  - ● **M12.23   Villonodular synovitis (pigmented), wrist**
    - M12.231   Villonodular synovitis (pigmented), right wrist
    - M12.232   Villonodular synovitis (pigmented), left wrist
    - M12.239   Villonodular synovitis (pigmented), unspecified wrist

CHAPTER 13 (M00-M99)

CHAPTER 13 (M00-M99)

● M12.24 Villonodular synovitis (pigmented), hand
  M12.241 Villonodular synovitis (pigmented), right hand
  M12.242 Villonodular synovitis (pigmented), left hand
  M12.249 Villonodular synovitis (pigmented), unspecified hand
● M12.25 Villonodular synovitis (pigmented), hip
  M12.251 Villonodular synovitis (pigmented), right hip
  M12.252 Villonodular synovitis (pigmented), left hip
  M12.259 Villonodular synovitis (pigmented), unspecified hip
● M12.26 Villonodular synovitis (pigmented), knee
  M12.261 Villonodular synovitis (pigmented), right knee
  M12.262 Villonodular synovitis (pigmented), left knee
  M12.269 Villonodular synovitis (pigmented), unspecified knee
● M12.27 Villonodular synovitis (pigmented), ankle and foot
  M12.271 Villonodular synovitis (pigmented), right ankle and foot
  M12.272 Villonodular synovitis (pigmented), left ankle and foot
  M12.279 Villonodular synovitis (pigmented), unspecified ankle and foot
  M12.28 Villonodular synovitis (pigmented), other specified site
    Villonodular synovitis (pigmented), vertebrae
  M12.29 Villonodular synovitis (pigmented), multiple sites
● M12.3 Palindromic rheumatism
  M12.30 Palindromic rheumatism, unspecified site
● M12.31 Palindromic rheumatism, shoulder
  M12.311 Palindromic rheumatism, right shoulder
  M12.312 Palindromic rheumatism, left shoulder
  M12.319 Palindromic rheumatism, unspecified shoulder
● M12.32 Palindromic rheumatism, elbow
  M12.321 Palindromic rheumatism, right elbow
  M12.322 Palindromic rheumatism, left elbow
  M12.329 Palindromic rheumatism, unspecified elbow
● M12.33 Palindromic rheumatism, wrist
  M12.331 Palindromic rheumatism, right wrist
  M12.332 Palindromic rheumatism, left wrist
  M12.339 Palindromic rheumatism, unspecified wrist
● M12.34 Palindromic rheumatism, hand
  M12.341 Palindromic rheumatism, right hand
  M12.342 Palindromic rheumatism, left hand
  M12.349 Palindromic rheumatism, unspecified hand
● M12.35 Palindromic rheumatism, hip
  M12.351 Palindromic rheumatism, right hip
  M12.352 Palindromic rheumatism, left hip
  M12.359 Palindromic rheumatism, unspecified hip

● M12.36 Palindromic rheumatism, knee
  M12.361 Palindromic rheumatism, right knee
  M12.362 Palindromic rheumatism, left knee
  M12.369 Palindromic rheumatism, unspecified knee
● M12.37 Palindromic rheumatism, ankle and foot
  M12.371 Palindromic rheumatism, right ankle and foot
  M12.372 Palindromic rheumatism, left ankle and foot
  M12.379 Palindromic rheumatism, unspecified ankle and foot
  M12.38 Palindromic rheumatism, other specified site
    Palindromic rheumatism, vertebrae
  M12.39 Palindromic rheumatism, multiple sites
● M12.4 Intermittent hydrarthrosis
  M12.40 Intermittent hydrarthrosis, unspecified site
● M12.41 Intermittent hydrarthrosis, shoulder
  M12.411 Intermittent hydrarthrosis, right shoulder
  M12.412 Intermittent hydrarthrosis, left shoulder
  M12.419 Intermittent hydrarthrosis, unspecified shoulder
● M12.42 Intermittent hydrarthrosis, elbow
  M12.421 Intermittent hydrarthrosis, right elbow
  M12.422 Intermittent hydrarthrosis, left elbow
  M12.429 Intermittent hydrarthrosis, unspecified elbow
● M12.43 Intermittent hydrarthrosis, wrist
  M12.431 Intermittent hydrarthrosis, right wrist
  M12.432 Intermittent hydrarthrosis, left wrist
  M12.439 Intermittent hydrarthrosis, unspecified wrist
● M12.44 Intermittent hydrarthrosis, hand
  M12.441 Intermittent hydrarthrosis, right hand
  M12.442 Intermittent hydrarthrosis, left hand
  M12.449 Intermittent hydrarthrosis, unspecified hand
● M12.45 Intermittent hydrarthrosis, hip
  M12.451 Intermittent hydrarthrosis, right hip
  M12.452 Intermittent hydrarthrosis, left hip
  M12.459 Intermittent hydrarthrosis, unspecified hip
● M12.46 Intermittent hydrarthrosis, knee
  M12.461 Intermittent hydrarthrosis, right knee
  M12.462 Intermittent hydrarthrosis, left knee
  M12.469 Intermittent hydrarthrosis, unspecified knee
● M12.47 Intermittent hydrarthrosis, ankle and foot
  M12.471 Intermittent hydrarthrosis, right ankle and foot
  M12.472 Intermittent hydrarthrosis, left ankle and foot
  M12.479 Intermittent hydrarthrosis, unspecified ankle and foot
  M12.48 Intermittent hydrarthrosis, other site
  M12.49 Intermittent hydrarthrosis, multiple sites

▶ New   ⇒ Revised   ~~deleted~~ Deleted   Excludes 1   Excludes 2   Includes   Use additional   Code first   Code also   Key words
OGCR Official Guidelines   X Assign placeholder X   ● Use Additional Character(s)   ▶ Manifestation Code   🏷 Hierarchical Condition Category   Coding Clinic

● **M12.5**   Traumatic arthropathy
     Excludes1   current injury-see Alphabetic Index
                 post-traumatic osteoarthritis of first carpometacarpal joint (M18.2-M18.3)
                 post-traumatic osteoarthritis of hip (M16.4-M16.5)
                 post-traumatic osteoarthritis of knee (M17.2-M17.3)
                 post-traumatic osteoarthritis NOS (M19.1-)
                 post-traumatic osteoarthritis of other single joints (M19.1-)

   M12.50   Traumatic arthropathy, unspecified site
● M12.51   Traumatic arthropathy, shoulder
     M12.511   Traumatic arthropathy, right shoulder
     M12.512   Traumatic arthropathy, left shoulder
     M12.519   Traumatic arthropathy, unspecified shoulder
● M12.52   Traumatic arthropathy, elbow
     M12.521   Traumatic arthropathy, right elbow
     M12.522   Traumatic arthropathy, left elbow
     M12.529   Traumatic arthropathy, unspecified elbow
● M12.53   Traumatic arthropathy, wrist
     M12.531   Traumatic arthropathy, right wrist
     M12.532   Traumatic arthropathy, left wrist
     M12.539   Traumatic arthropathy, unspecified wrist
● M12.54   Traumatic arthropathy, hand
     M12.541   Traumatic arthropathy, right hand
     M12.542   Traumatic arthropathy, left hand
     M12.549   Traumatic arthropathy, unspecified hand
● M12.55   Traumatic arthropathy, hip
     M12.551   Traumatic arthropathy, right hip
     M12.552   Traumatic arthropathy, left hip
              Coding Clinic: 2015, Q1, P17
     M12.559   Traumatic arthropathy, unspecified hip
● M12.56   Traumatic arthropathy, knee
     M12.561   Traumatic arthropathy, right knee
     M12.562   Traumatic arthropathy, left knee
     M12.569   Traumatic arthropathy, unspecified knee
● M12.57   Traumatic arthropathy, ankle and foot
     M12.571   Traumatic arthropathy, right ankle and foot
     M12.572   Traumatic arthropathy, left ankle and foot
     M12.579   Traumatic arthropathy, unspecified ankle and foot
   M12.58   Traumatic arthropathy, other specified site
          Traumatic arthropathy, vertebrae
   M12.59   Traumatic arthropathy, multiple sites
● **M12.8**   Other specific arthropathies, not elsewhere classified
          Transient arthropathy
   M12.80   Other specific arthropathies, not elsewhere classified, unspecified site
● M12.81   Other specific arthropathies, not elsewhere classified, shoulder
     M12.811   Other specific arthropathies, not elsewhere classified, right shoulder
     M12.812   Other specific arthropathies, not elsewhere classified, left shoulder
     M12.819   Other specific arthropathies, not elsewhere classified, unspecified shoulder

● M12.82   Other specific arthropathies, not elsewhere classified, elbow
     M12.821   Other specific arthropathies, not elsewhere classified, right elbow
     M12.822   Other specific arthropathies, not elsewhere classified, left elbow
     M12.829   Other specific arthropathies, not elsewhere classified, unspecified elbow
● M12.83   Other specific arthropathies, not elsewhere classified, wrist
     M12.831   Other specific arthropathies, not elsewhere classified, right wrist
     M12.832   Other specific arthropathies, not elsewhere classified, left wrist
     M12.839   Other specific arthropathies, not elsewhere classified, unspecified wrist
● M12.84   Other specific arthropathies, not elsewhere classified, hand
     M12.841   Other specific arthropathies, not elsewhere classified, right hand
     M12.842   Other specific arthropathies, not elsewhere classified, left hand
     M12.849   Other specific arthropathies, not elsewhere classified, unspecified hand
● M12.85   Other specific arthropathies, not elsewhere classified, hip
     M12.851   Other specific arthropathies, not elsewhere classified, right hip
     M12.852   Other specific arthropathies, not elsewhere classified, left hip
     M12.859   Other specific arthropathies, not elsewhere classified, unspecified hip
● M12.86   Other specific arthropathies, not elsewhere classified, knee
     M12.861   Other specific arthropathies, not elsewhere classified, right knee
     M12.862   Other specific arthropathies, not elsewhere classified, left knee
     M12.869   Other specific arthropathies, not elsewhere classified, unspecified knee
● M12.87   Other specific arthropathies, not elsewhere classified, ankle and foot
     M12.871   Other specific arthropathies, not elsewhere classified, right ankle and foot
     M12.872   Other specific arthropathies, not elsewhere classified, left ankle and foot
     M12.879   Other specific arthropathies, not elsewhere classified, unspecified ankle and foot
   M12.88   Other specific arthropathies, not elsewhere classified, other specified site
          Other specific arthropathies, not elsewhere classified, vertebrae
   M12.89   Other specific arthropathies, not elsewhere classified, multiple sites

   M12.9   Arthropathy, unspecified

CHAPTER 13 (M00-M99)

CHAPTER 13 (M00-M99)

● M13   Other arthritis
     Excludes1   arthrosis (M15-M19)
                 osteoarthritis (M15-M19)

M13.0   Polyarthritis, unspecified

● M13.1   Monoarthritis, not elsewhere classified

     M13.10   Monoarthritis, not elsewhere classified, unspecified site

     ● M13.11   Monoarthritis, not elsewhere classified, shoulder

         M13.111   Monoarthritis, not elsewhere classified, right shoulder

         M13.112   Monoarthritis, not elsewhere classified, left shoulder

         M13.119   Monoarthritis, not elsewhere classified, unspecified shoulder

     ● M13.12   Monoarthritis, not elsewhere classified, elbow

         M13.121   Monoarthritis, not elsewhere classified, right elbow

         M13.122   Monoarthritis, not elsewhere classified, left elbow

         M13.129   Monoarthritis, not elsewhere classified, unspecified elbow

     ● M13.13   Monoarthritis, not elsewhere classified, wrist

         M13.131   Monoarthritis, not elsewhere classified, right wrist

         M13.132   Monoarthritis, not elsewhere classified, left wrist

         M13.139   Monoarthritis, not elsewhere classified, unspecified wrist

     ● M13.14   Monoarthritis, not elsewhere classified, hand

         M13.141   Monoarthritis, not elsewhere classified, right hand

         M13.142   Monoarthritis, not elsewhere classified, left hand

         M13.149   Monoarthritis, not elsewhere classified, unspecified hand

     ● M13.15   Monoarthritis, not elsewhere classified, hip

         M13.151   Monoarthritis, not elsewhere classified, right hip

         M13.152   Monoarthritis, not elsewhere classified, left hip

         M13.159   Monoarthritis, not elsewhere classified, unspecified hip

     ● M13.16   Monoarthritis, not elsewhere classified, knee

         M13.161   Monoarthritis, not elsewhere classified, right knee

         M13.162   Monoarthritis, not elsewhere classified, left knee

         M13.169   Monoarthritis, not elsewhere classified, unspecified knee

     ● M13.17   Monoarthritis, not elsewhere classified, ankle and foot

         M13.171   Monoarthritis, not elsewhere classified, right ankle and foot

         M13.172   Monoarthritis, not elsewhere classified, left ankle and foot

         M13.179   Monoarthritis, not elsewhere classified, unspecified ankle and foot

● M13.8   Other specified arthritis
     Allergic arthritis
     Excludes1   osteoarthritis (M15-M19)

     M13.80   Other specified arthritis, unspecified site

     ● M13.81   Other specified arthritis, shoulder

         M13.811   Other specified arthritis, right shoulder

         M13.812   Other specified arthritis, left shoulder

         M13.819   Other specified arthritis, unspecified shoulder

     ● M13.82   Other specified arthritis, elbow

         M13.821   Other specified arthritis, right elbow

         M13.822   Other specified arthritis, left elbow

         M13.829   Other specified arthritis, unspecified elbow

     ● M13.83   Other specified arthritis, wrist

         M13.831   Other specified arthritis, right wrist

         M13.832   Other specified arthritis, left wrist

         M13.839   Other specified arthritis, unspecified wrist

     ● M13.84   Other specified arthritis, hand

         M13.841   Other specified arthritis, right hand

         M13.842   Other specified arthritis, left hand

         M13.849   Other specified arthritis, unspecified hand

     ● M13.85   Other specified arthritis, hip

         M13.851   Other specified arthritis, right hip

         M13.852   Other specified arthritis, left hip

         M13.859   Other specified arthritis, unspecified hip

     ● M13.86   Other specified arthritis, knee

         M13.861   Other specified arthritis, right knee

         M13.862   Other specified arthritis, left knee

         M13.869   Other specified arthritis, unspecified knee

     ● M13.87   Other specified arthritis, ankle and foot

         M13.871   Other specified arthritis, right ankle and foot

         M13.872   Other specified arthritis, left ankle and foot

         M13.879   Other specified arthritis, unspecified ankle and foot

     M13.88   Other specified arthritis, other site

     M13.89   Other specified arthritis, multiple sites

● M14   Arthropathies in other diseases classified elsewhere
     Excludes1   arthropathy in:
                 diabetes mellitus (E08-E13 with .61-)
                 hematological disorders (M36.2-M36.3)
                 hypersensitivity reactions (M36.4)
                 neoplastic disease (M36.1)
                 neurosyphillis (A52.16)
                 sarcoidosis (D86.86)
         enteropathic arthropathies (M07.0-)
         juvenile psoriatic arthropathy (L40.54)
         lipoid dermatoarthritis (E78.81)

● M14.6   Charcôt's joint
     Neuropathic arthropathy
     Excludes1   Charcôt's joint in diabetes mellitus (E08-E13 with .610)
                 Charcôt's joint in tabes dorsalis (A52.16)

     M14.60   Charcôt's joint, unspecified site

     ● M14.61   Charcôt's joint, shoulder

         M14.611   Charcôt's joint, right shoulder

         M14.612   Charcôt's joint, left shoulder

         M14.619   Charcôt's joint, unspecified shoulder

     ● M14.62   Charcôt's joint, elbow

         M14.621   Charcôt's joint, right elbow

         M14.622   Charcôt's joint, left elbow

         M14.629   Charcôt's joint, unspecified elbow

     ● M14.63   Charcôt's joint, wrist

         M14.631   Charcôt's joint, right wrist

         M14.632   Charcôt's joint, left wrist

         M14.639   Charcôt's joint, unspecified wrist

▶ New   ▦ Revised   ~~deleted~~ Deleted   Excludes 1   Excludes 2   Includes   Use additional   Code first   Code also   Key words

OGCR Official Guidelines   X Assign placeholder X   ● Use Additional Character(s)   ▶ Manifestation Code   🍀 Hierarchical Condition Category   **Coding Clinic**

● M14.64   Charcôt's joint, hand
     M14.641   Charcôt's joint, right hand
     M14.642   Charcôt's joint, left hand
     M14.649   Charcôt's joint, unspecified hand

● M14.65   Charcôt's joint, hip
     M14.651   Charcôt's joint, right hip
     M14.652   Charcôt's joint, left hip
     M14.659   Charcôt's joint, unspecified hip

● M14.66   Charcôt's joint, knee
     M14.661   Charcôt's joint, right knee
     M14.662   Charcôt's joint, left knee
     M14.669   Charcôt's joint, unspecified knee

● M14.67   Charcôt's joint, ankle and foot
     M14.671   Charcôt's joint, right ankle and foot
     M14.672   Charcôt's joint, left ankle and foot
     M14.679   Charcôt's joint, unspecified ankle and foot

     M14.68   Charcôt's joint, vertebrae
     M14.69   Charcôt's joint, multiple sites

● M14.8   Arthropathies in other specified diseases classified elsewhere

     Code first underlying disease, such as:
       amyloidosis (E85.-)
       erythema multiforme (L51.-)
       erythema nodosum (L52)
       hemochromatosis (E83.11-)
       hyperparathyroidism (E21.-)
       hypothyroidism (E00-E03)
       sickle-cell disorders (D57.-)
       thyrotoxicosis [hyperthyroidism] (E05.-)
       Whipple's disease (K90.81)

    ▌ *M14.80*   *Arthropathies in other specified diseases classified elsewhere, unspecified site*

● M14.81   Arthropathies in other specified diseases classified elsewhere, shoulder
    ▌ *M14.811*   *Arthropathies in other specified diseases classified elsewhere, right shoulder*
    ▌ *M14.812*   *Arthropathies in other specified diseases classified elsewhere, left shoulder*
    ▌ *M14.819*   *Arthropathies in other specified diseases classified elsewhere, unspecified shoulder*

● M14.82   Arthropathies in other specified diseases classified elsewhere, elbow
    ▌ *M14.821*   *Arthropathies in other specified diseases classified elsewhere, right elbow*
    ▌ *M14.822*   *Arthropathies in other specified diseases classified elsewhere, left elbow*
    ▌ *M14.829*   *Arthropathies in other specified diseases classified elsewhere, unspecified elbow*

● M14.83   Arthropathies in other specified diseases classified elsewhere, wrist
    ▌ *M14.831*   *Arthropathies in other specified diseases classified elsewhere, right wrist*
    ▌ *M14.832*   *Arthropathies in other specified diseases classified elsewhere, left wrist*
    ▌ *M14.839*   *Arthropathies in other specified diseases classified elsewhere, unspecified wrist*

● M14.84   Arthropathies in other specified diseases classified elsewhere, hand
    ▌ *M14.841*   *Arthropathies in other specified diseases classified elsewhere, right hand*
    ▌ *M14.842*   *Arthropathies in other specified diseases classified elsewhere, left hand*
    ▌ *M14.849*   *Arthropathies in other specified diseases classified elsewhere, unspecified hand*

● M14.85   Arthropathies in other specified diseases classified elsewhere, hip
    ▌ *M14.851*   *Arthropathies in other specified diseases classified elsewhere, right hip*
    ▌ *M14.852*   *Arthropathies in other specified diseases classified elsewhere, left hip*
    ▌ *M14.859*   *Arthropathies in other specified diseases classified elsewhere, unspecified hip*

● M14.86   Arthropathies in other specified diseases classified elsewhere, knee
    ▌ *M14.861*   *Arthropathies in other specified diseases classified elsewhere, right knee*
    ▌ *M14.862*   *Arthropathies in other specified diseases classified elsewhere, left knee*
    ▌ *M14.869*   *Arthropathies in other specified diseases classified elsewhere, unspecified knee*

● M14.87   Arthropathies in other specified diseases classified elsewhere, ankle and foot
    ▌ *M14.871*   *Arthropathies in other specified diseases classified elsewhere, right ankle and foot*
    ▌ *M14.872*   *Arthropathies in other specified diseases classified elsewhere, left ankle and foot*
    ▌ *M14.879*   *Arthropathies in other specified diseases classified elsewhere, unspecified ankle and foot*

    ▌ *M14.88*   *Arthropathies in other specified diseases classified elsewhere, vertebrae*
    ▌ *M14.89*   *Arthropathies in other specified diseases classified elsewhere, multiple sites*

OSTEOARTHRITIS (M15-M19)

Osteoarthritis is the most common degenerative joint disease and form of arthritis that breaks down the cartilage causing pain, swelling, and reduced motion in the joints.

    Excludes2   osteoarthritis of spine (M47.-)

● M15   Polyosteoarthritis
    Includes   arthritis of multiple sites
    Excludes1   bilateral involvement of single joint (M16-M19)

    M15.0   Primary generalized (osteo)arthritis

    M15.1   Heberden's nodes (with arthropathy)
       Interphalangeal distal osteoarthritis

    M15.2   Bouchard's nodes (with arthropathy)
       Juxtaphalangeal distal osteoarthritis

    M15.3   Secondary multiple arthritis
       Post-traumatic polyosteoarthritis

    M15.4   Erosive (osteo)arthritis

    M15.8   Other polyosteoarthritis

    M15.9   Polyosteoarthritis, unspecified
       Generalized osteoarthritis NOS

CHAPTER 13 (M00-M99)

CHAPTER 13 (M00-M99)

● M16 **Osteoarthritis of hip**

    M16.0 **Bilateral primary** osteoarthritis of hip
            Coding Clinic: 2018, Q2, P15; 2016, Q4, P146

    ● M16.1 **Unilateral primary** osteoarthritis of hip
            Primary osteoarthritis of hip NOS

        M16.10 Unilateral primary osteoarthritis, **unspecified** hip

        M16.11 Unilateral primary osteoarthritis, **right** hip

        M16.12 Unilateral primary osteoarthritis, **left** hip

    M16.2 **Bilateral** osteoarthritis resulting from **hip dysplasia**

    ● M16.3 **Unilateral** osteoarthritis resulting from **hip dysplasia**
            Dysplastic osteoarthritis of hip NOS

        M16.30 Unilateral osteoarthritis resulting from hip dysplasia, **unspecified** hip

        M16.31 Unilateral osteoarthritis resulting from hip dysplasia, **right** hip

        M16.32 Unilateral osteoarthritis resulting from hip dysplasia, **left** hip

    M16.4 **Bilateral post-traumatic** osteoarthritis of hip

    ● M16.5 **Unilateral post-traumatic** osteoarthritis of hip
            Post-traumatic osteoarthritis of hip NOS

        M16.50 Unilateral post-traumatic osteoarthritis, **unspecified** hip

        M16.51 Unilateral post-traumatic osteoarthritis, **right** hip

        M16.52 Unilateral post-traumatic osteoarthritis, **left** hip

    M16.6 **Other bilateral secondary** osteoarthritis of hip

    M16.7 **Other unilateral secondary** osteoarthritis of hip
            Secondary osteoarthritis of hip NOS

    M16.9 **Osteoarthritis of hip, unspecified**

● M17 **Osteoarthritis of knee**

    M17.0 **Bilateral primary** osteoarthritis of knee

    ● M17.1 **Unilateral primary** osteoarthritis of knee
            Primary osteoarthritis of knee NOS

        M17.10 Unilateral primary osteoarthritis, **unspecified** knee
            Coding Clinic: 2016, Q4, P147

        M17.11 Unilateral primary osteoarthritis, **right** knee

        M17.12 Unilateral primary osteoarthritis, **left** knee
            Coding Clinic: 2016, Q4, P146

    M17.2 **Bilateral post-traumatic** osteoarthritis of knee

    ● M17.3 **Unilateral post-traumatic** osteoarthritis of knee
            Post-traumatic osteoarthritis of knee NOS

        M17.30 Unilateral post-traumatic osteoarthritis, **unspecified** knee

        M17.31 Unilateral post-traumatic osteoarthritis, **right** knee

        M17.32 Unilateral post-traumatic osteoarthritis, **left** knee

    M17.4 **Other bilateral secondary** osteoarthritis of knee

    M17.5 **Other unilateral secondary** osteoarthritis of knee
            Secondary osteoarthritis of knee NOS

    M17.9 **Osteoarthritis of knee, unspecified**
            Coding Clinic: 2016, Q4, P146

● M18 **Osteoarthritis of first carpometacarpal joint**

    M18.0 **Bilateral primary** osteoarthritis of first carpometacarpal joints

    ● M18.1 **Unilateral primary** osteoarthritis of first carpometacarpal joint
            Primary osteoarthritis of first carpometacarpal joint NOS

        M18.10 Unilateral primary osteoarthritis of first carpometacarpal joint, **unspecified** hand

        M18.11 Unilateral primary osteoarthritis of first carpometacarpal joint, **right** hand

        M18.12 Unilateral primary osteoarthritis of first carpometacarpal joint, **left** hand

    M18.2 **Bilateral post-traumatic** osteoarthritis of first carpometacarpal joints

    ● M18.3 **Unilateral post-traumatic** osteoarthritis of first carpometacarpal joint
            Post-traumatic osteoarthritis of first carpometacarpal joint NOS

        M18.30 Unilateral post-traumatic osteoarthritis of first carpometacarpal joint, **unspecified** hand

        M18.31 Unilateral post-traumatic osteoarthritis of first carpometacarpal joint, **right** hand

        M18.32 Unilateral post-traumatic osteoarthritis of first carpometacarpal joint, **left** hand

    M18.4 **Other bilateral secondary** osteoarthritis of first carpometacarpal joints

    ● M18.5 **Other unilateral secondary** osteoarthritis of first carpometacarpal joint
            Secondary osteoarthritis of first carpometacarpal joint NOS

        M18.50 Other unilateral secondary osteoarthritis of first carpometacarpal joint, **unspecified** hand

        M18.51 Other unilateral secondary osteoarthritis of first carpometacarpal joint, **right** hand

        M18.52 Other unilateral secondary osteoarthritis of first carpometacarpal joint, **left** hand

    M18.9 **Osteoarthritis of first carpometacarpal joint, unspecified**

● M19 **Other and unspecified osteoarthritis**

    Excludes1 polyarthritis (M15.-)
    Excludes2 arthrosis of spine (M47.-)
                hallux rigidus (M20.2)
                osteoarthritis of spine (M47.-)

    ● M19.0 **Primary osteoarthritis of other joints**

        ● M19.01 Primary osteoarthritis, **shoulder**

            M19.011 Primary osteoarthritis, **right shoulder**
                  Coding Clinic: 2016, Q4, P145

            M19.012 Primary osteoarthritis, **left shoulder**

            M19.019 Primary osteoarthritis, **unspecified** shoulder

        ● M19.02 Primary osteoarthritis, **elbow**

            M19.021 Primary osteoarthritis, **right elbow**

            M19.022 Primary osteoarthritis, **left elbow**

            M19.029 Primary osteoarthritis, **unspecified** elbow

        ● M19.03 Primary osteoarthritis, **wrist**

            M19.031 Primary osteoarthritis, **right wrist**

            M19.032 Primary osteoarthritis, **left wrist**

            M19.039 Primary osteoarthritis, **unspecified** wrist

        ● M19.04 Primary osteoarthritis, **hand**

            Excludes2 primary osteoarthritis of first carpometacarpal joint (M18.0-, M18.1-)

            M19.041 Primary osteoarthritis, **right hand**

            M19.042 Primary osteoarthritis, **left hand**

            M19.049 Primary osteoarthritis, **unspecified** hand

        ● M19.07 Primary osteoarthritis **ankle and foot**

            M19.071 Primary osteoarthritis, **right ankle and foot**

            M19.072 Primary osteoarthritis, **left ankle and foot**

            M19.079 Primary osteoarthritis, **unspecified** ankle and foot

        M19.09 Primary osteoarthritis, **other specified site**

▶ New   ⇒ Revised   deleted Deleted   Excludes 1   Excludes 2   Includes   Use additional   Code first   Code also   Key words

OGCR Official Guidelines   X Assign placeholder X   ● Use Additional Character(s)   ▶ Manifestation Code   🏷 Hierarchical Condition Category   **Coding Clinic**

● M19.1 Post-traumatic osteoarthritis of other joints
  ● M19.11 Post-traumatic osteoarthritis, shoulder
      M19.111 Post-traumatic osteoarthritis, right shoulder
      M19.112 Post-traumatic osteoarthritis, left shoulder
      M19.119 Post-traumatic osteoarthritis, unspecified shoulder
  ● M19.12 Post-traumatic osteoarthritis, elbow
      M19.121 Post-traumatic osteoarthritis, right elbow
      M19.122 Post-traumatic osteoarthritis, left elbow
      M19.129 Post-traumatic osteoarthritis, unspecified elbow
  ● M19.13 Post-traumatic osteoarthritis, wrist
      M19.131 Post-traumatic osteoarthritis, right wrist
      M19.132 Post-traumatic osteoarthritis, left wrist
      M19.139 Post-traumatic osteoarthritis, unspecified wrist
  ● M19.14 Post-traumatic osteoarthritis, hand
      Excludes2 post-traumatic osteoarthritis of first carpometacarpal joint (M18.2-, M18.3-)
      M19.141 Post-traumatic osteoarthritis, right hand
      M19.142 Post-traumatic osteoarthritis, left hand
      M19.149 Post-traumatic osteoarthritis, unspecified hand
  ● M19.17 Post-traumatic osteoarthritis, ankle and foot
      M19.171 Post-traumatic osteoarthritis, right ankle and foot
      M19.172 Post-traumatic osteoarthritis, left ankle and foot
      M19.179 Post-traumatic osteoarthritis, unspecified ankle and foot
    M19.19 Post-traumatic osteoarthritis, other specified site
● M19.2 Secondary osteoarthritis of other joints
  ● M19.21 Secondary osteoarthritis, shoulder
      M19.211 Secondary osteoarthritis, right shoulder
      M19.212 Secondary osteoarthritis, left shoulder
      M19.219 Secondary osteoarthritis, unspecified shoulder
  ● M19.22 Secondary osteoarthritis, elbow
      M19.221 Secondary osteoarthritis, right elbow
      M19.222 Secondary osteoarthritis, left elbow
      M19.229 Secondary osteoarthritis, unspecified elbow
  ● M19.23 Secondary osteoarthritis, wrist
      M19.231 Secondary osteoarthritis, right wrist
      M19.232 Secondary osteoarthritis, left wrist
      M19.239 Secondary osteoarthritis, unspecified wrist
  ● M19.24 Secondary osteoarthritis, hand
      M19.241 Secondary osteoarthritis, right hand
      M19.242 Secondary osteoarthritis, left hand
      M19.249 Secondary osteoarthritis, unspecified hand
  ● M19.27 Secondary osteoarthritis, ankle and foot
      M19.271 Secondary osteoarthritis, right ankle and foot
      M19.272 Secondary osteoarthritis, left ankle and foot
      M19.279 Secondary osteoarthritis, unspecified ankle and foot

    M19.29 Secondary osteoarthritis, other specified site
● M19.9 Osteoarthritis, unspecified site
    M19.90 Unspecified osteoarthritis, unspecified site
        Arthrosis NOS
        Arthritis NOS
        Osteoarthritis NOS
        Coding Clinic: 2016, Q4, P147
    M19.91 Primary osteoarthritis, unspecified site
        Primary osteoarthritis NOS
    M19.92 Post-traumatic osteoarthritis, unspecified site
        Post-traumatic osteoarthritis NOS
    M19.93 Secondary osteoarthritis, unspecified site
        Secondary osteoarthritis NOS

OTHER JOINT DISORDERS (M20-M25)

    Excludes2 joints of the spine (M40-M54)

● M20 Acquired deformities of fingers and toes
    Excludes1 acquired absence of fingers and toes (Z89.-)
        congenital absence of fingers and toes (Q71.3-, Q72.3-)
        congenital deformities and malformations of fingers and toes (Q66.-, Q68-Q70, Q74.-)
  ● M20.0 Deformity of finger(s)
      Excludes1 clubbing of fingers (R68.3)
          palmar fascial fibromatosis [Dupuytren] (M72.0)
          trigger finger (M65.3)
    ● M20.00 Unspecified deformity of finger(s)
        M20.001 Unspecified deformity of right finger(s)
        M20.002 Unspecified deformity of left finger(s)
        M20.009 Unspecified deformity of unspecified finger(s)
    ● M20.01 Mallet finger
        M20.011 Mallet finger of right finger(s)
        M20.012 Mallet finger of left finger(s)
        M20.019 Mallet finger of unspecified finger(s)
    ● M20.02 Boutonnière deformity
        M20.021 Boutonnière deformity of right finger(s)
        M20.022 Boutonnière deformity of left finger(s)
        M20.029 Boutonnière deformity of unspecified finger(s)
    ● M20.03 Swan-neck deformity
        M20.031 Swan-neck deformity of right finger(s)
        M20.032 Swan-neck deformity of left finger(s)
        M20.039 Swan-neck deformity of unspecified finger(s)
    ● M20.09 Other deformity of finger(s)
        M20.091 Other deformity of right finger(s)
        M20.092 Other deformity of left finger(s)
        M20.099 Other deformity of finger(s), unspecified finger(s)
  ● M20.1 Hallux valgus (acquired)
      Excludes2 bunion (M21.6-)
      Coding Clinic: 2016, Q4, P38
      M20.10 Hallux valgus (acquired), unspecified foot
      M20.11 Hallux valgus (acquired), right foot
      M20.12 Hallux valgus (acquired), left foot
  ● M20.2 Hallux rigidus
      M20.20 Hallux rigidus, unspecified foot
      M20.21 Hallux rigidus, right foot
      M20.22 Hallux rigidus, left foot

Figure 13-1   Hallux valgus.

Item 13-3 Cubitus valgus is a deformity of the elbow resulting in an increased carrying angle in which the arm extends at the side and the palm faces forward, which results in the forearm and hand extended at greater than 15 degrees.

Item 13-4 Cubitus varus is a deformity of the elbow resulting in the arm extended at the side and the palm facing forward so that the forearm and hand are held at less than 5 degrees, decreasing the carrying angle.

● M21.05 Valgus deformity, not elsewhere classified, hip
    M21.051 Valgus deformity, not elsewhere classified, right hip
    M21.052 Valgus deformity, not elsewhere classified, left hip
    M21.059 Valgus deformity, not elsewhere classified, unspecified hip
● M21.06 Valgus deformity, not elsewhere classified, knee
    Genu valgum
    Knock knee
    M21.061 Valgus deformity, not elsewhere classified, right knee
    M21.062 Valgus deformity, not elsewhere classified, left knee
    M21.069 Valgus deformity, not elsewhere classified, unspecified knee
● M21.07 Valgus deformity, not elsewhere classified, ankle
    M21.071 Valgus deformity, not elsewhere classified, right ankle
    M21.072 Valgus deformity, not elsewhere classified, left ankle
    M21.079 Valgus deformity, not elsewhere classified, unspecified ankle
● M21.1 Varus deformity, not elsewhere classified
    Excludes1 metatarsus varus (Q66.22-)
             tibia vara (M92.51-)
    M21.10 Varus deformity, not elsewhere classified, unspecified site
● M21.12 Varus deformity, not elsewhere classified, elbow
    Cubitus varus, elbow
    M21.121 Varus deformity, not elsewhere classified, right elbow
    M21.122 Varus deformity, not elsewhere classified, left elbow
    M21.129 Varus deformity, not elsewhere classified, unspecified elbow
● M21.15 Varus deformity, not elsewhere classified, hip
    M21.151 Varus deformity, not elsewhere classified, right hip
    M21.152 Varus deformity, not elsewhere classified, left hip
    M21.159 Varus deformity, not elsewhere classified, unspecified
● M21.16 Varus deformity, not elsewhere classified, knee
    Bow leg
    Genu varum
    M21.161 Varus deformity, not elsewhere classified, right knee
    M21.162 Varus deformity, not elsewhere classified, left knee
    M21.169 Varus deformity, not elsewhere classified, unspecified knee
● M21.17 Varus deformity, not elsewhere classified, ankle
    M21.171 Varus deformity, not elsewhere classified, right ankle
    M21.172 Varus deformity, not elsewhere classified, left ankle
    M21.179 Varus deformity, not elsewhere classified, unspecified ankle

Item 13-2 Hallux valgus is a sometimes painful structural deformity caused by an inflammation of the bursal sac at the base of the metatarsophalangeal joint (big toe). **Hallus varus** is a deviation of the great toe to the inner side of the foot or away from the next toe.

● M20.3 Hallux varus (acquired)
    M20.30 Hallux varus (acquired), unspecified foot
    M20.31 Hallux varus (acquired), right foot
    M20.32 Hallux varus (acquired), left foot
● M20.4 Other hammer toe(s) (acquired)
    M20.40 Other hammer toe(s) (acquired), unspecified foot
    M20.41 Other hammer toe(s) (acquired), right foot
    M20.42 Other hammer toe(s) (acquired), left foot
● M20.5 Other deformities of toe(s) (acquired)
  ● M20.5X Other deformities of toe(s) (acquired)
    M20.5X1 Other deformities of toe(s) (acquired), right foot
    M20.5X2 Other deformities of toe(s) (acquired), left foot
    M20.5X9 Other deformities of toe(s) (acquired), unspecified foot
● M20.6 Acquired deformities of toe(s), unspecified
    M20.60 Acquired deformities of toe(s), unspecified, unspecified foot
    M20.61 Acquired deformities of toe(s), unspecified, right foot
    M20.62 Acquired deformities of toe(s), unspecified, left foot
● M21 Other acquired deformities of limbs
    Excludes1 acquired absence of limb (Z89.-)
             congenital absence of limbs (Q71-Q73)
             congenital deformities and malformations of limbs (Q65-Q66, Q68-Q74)
    Excludes2 acquired deformities of fingers or toes (M20.-)
             coxa plana (M91.2)
● M21.0 Valgus deformity, not elsewhere classified
    Excludes1 metatarsus valgus (Q66.6)
             talipes calcaneovalgus (Q66.4-)
    M21.00 Valgus deformity, not elsewhere classified, unspecified site
  ● M21.02 Valgus deformity, not elsewhere classified, elbow
    Cubitus valgus
    M21.021 Valgus deformity, not elsewhere classified, right elbow
    M21.022 Valgus deformity, not elsewhere classified, left elbow
    M21.029 Valgus deformity, not elsewhere classified, unspecified elbow

▶ New ⇒ Revised ~~deleted~~ Deleted Excludes 1 Excludes 2 Includes Use additional Code first Code also Key words
OGCR Official Guidelines X Assign placeholder X ● Use Additional Character(s) ▶ Manifestation Code Hierarchical Condition Category **Coding Clinic**

● M21.2   Flexion deformity
    M21.20   Flexion deformity, unspecified site
   ● M21.21   Flexion deformity, shoulder
      M21.211   Flexion deformity, right shoulder
      M21.212   Flexion deformity, left shoulder
      M21.219   Flexion deformity, unspecified shoulder
   ● M21.22   Flexion deformity, elbow
      M21.221   Flexion deformity, right elbow
      M21.222   Flexion deformity, left elbow
      M21.229   Flexion deformity, unspecified elbow
   ● M21.23   Flexion deformity, wrist
      M21.231   Flexion deformity, right wrist
      M21.232   Flexion deformity, left wrist
      M21.239   Flexion deformity, unspecified wrist
   ● M21.24   Flexion deformity, finger joints
      M21.241   Flexion deformity, right finger joints
      M21.242   Flexion deformity, left finger joints
      M21.249   Flexion deformity, unspecified finger joints
   ● M21.25   Flexion deformity, hip
      M21.251   Flexion deformity, right hip
      M21.252   Flexion deformity, left hip
      M21.259   Flexion deformity, unspecified hip
   ● M21.26   Flexion deformity, knee
      M21.261   Flexion deformity, right knee
      M21.262   Flexion deformity, left knee
      M21.269   Flexion deformity, unspecified knee
   ● M21.27   Flexion deformity, ankle and toes
      M21.271   Flexion deformity, right ankle and toes
      M21.272   Flexion deformity, left ankle and toes
      M21.279   Flexion deformity, unspecified ankle and toes

● M21.3   Wrist or foot drop (acquired)
   ● M21.33   Wrist drop (acquired)
      M21.331   Wrist drop, right wrist
      M21.332   Wrist drop, left wrist
      M21.339   Wrist drop, unspecified wrist
   ● M21.37   Foot drop (acquired)
      M21.371   Foot drop, right foot
      M21.372   Foot drop, left foot
      M21.379   Foot drop, unspecified foot

● M21.4   Flat foot [pes planus] (acquired)
     Excludes1   congenital pes planus (Q66.5-)
    M21.40   Flat foot [pes planus] (acquired), unspecified foot
    M21.41   Flat foot [pes planus] (acquired), right foot
    M21.42   Flat foot [pes planus] (acquired), left foot

● M21.5   Acquired clawhand, clubhand, clawfoot and clubfoot
     Excludes1   clubfoot, not specified as acquired (Q66.89)
   ● M21.51   Acquired clawhand
      M21.511   Acquired clawhand, right hand
      M21.512   Acquired clawhand, left hand
      M21.519   Acquired clawhand, unspecified hand
   ● M21.52   Acquired clubhand
      M21.521   Acquired clubhand, right hand
      M21.522   Acquired clubhand, left hand
      M21.529   Acquired clubhand, unspecified hand
   ● M21.53   Acquired clawfoot
      M21.531   Acquired clawfoot, right foot
      M21.532   Acquired clawfoot, left foot
      M21.539   Acquired clawfoot, unspecified foot

   ● M21.54   Acquired clubfoot
      M21.541   Acquired clubfoot, right foot
      M21.542   Acquired clubfoot, left foot
      M21.549   Acquired clubfoot, unspecified foot

● M21.6   Other acquired deformities of foot
     Excludes2   deformities of toe (acquired) (M20.1-M20.6-)
   ● M21.61   Bunion
       Coding Clinic: 2016, Q4, P38
      M21.611   Bunion of right foot
      M21.612   Bunion of left foot
      M21.619   Bunion of unspecified foot
   ● M21.62   Bunionette
       Coding Clinic: 2016, Q4, P38
      M21.621   Bunionette of right foot
      M21.622   Bunionette of left foot
      M21.629   Bunionette of unspecified foot
   ● M21.6X   Other acquired deformities of foot
      M21.6X1   Other acquired deformities of right foot
      M21.6X2   Other acquired deformities of left foot
      M21.6X9   Other acquired deformities of unspecified foot

● M21.7   Unequal limb length (acquired)
     Note: The site used should correspond to the shorter limb.
    M21.70   Unequal limb length (acquired), unspecified site
   ● M21.72   Unequal limb length (acquired), humerus
      M21.721   Unequal limb length (acquired), right humerus
      M21.722   Unequal limb length (acquired), left humerus
      M21.729   Unequal limb length (acquired), unspecified humerus
   ● M21.73   Unequal limb length (acquired), ulna and radius
      M21.731   Unequal limb length (acquired), right ulna
      M21.732   Unequal limb length (acquired), left ulna
      M21.733   Unequal limb length (acquired), right radius
      M21.734   Unequal limb length (acquired), left radius
      M21.739   Unequal limb length (acquired), unspecified ulna and radius
   ● M21.75   Unequal limb length (acquired), femur
      M21.751   Unequal limb length (acquired), right femur
      M21.752   Unequal limb length (acquired), left femur
      M21.759   Unequal limb length (acquired), unspecified femur
   ● M21.76   Unequal limb length (acquired), tibia and fibula
      M21.761   Unequal limb length (acquired), right tibia
      M21.762   Unequal limb length (acquired), left tibia
      M21.763   Unequal limb length (acquired), right fibula
      M21.764   Unequal limb length (acquired), left fibula
      M21.769   Unequal limb length (acquired), unspecified tibia and fibula

- ● **M21.8** **Other specified acquired deformities of limbs**
  - **Excludes2**   coxa plana (M91.2)
  - **M21.80** Other specified acquired deformities of unspecified limb
  - ● **M21.82** Other specified acquired deformities of upper arm
    - **M21.821** Other specified acquired deformities of right upper arm
    - **M21.822** Other specified acquired deformities of left upper arm
    - **M21.829** Other specified acquired deformities of unspecified upper arm
  - ● **M21.83** Other specified acquired deformities of forearm
    - **M21.831** Other specified acquired deformities of right forearm
    - **M21.832** Other specified acquired deformities of left forearm
    - **M21.839** Other specified acquired deformities of unspecified forearm
  - ● **M21.85** Other specified acquired deformities of thigh
    - **M21.851** Other specified acquired deformities of right thigh
    - **M21.852** Other specified acquired deformities of left thigh
    - **M21.859** Other specified acquired deformities of unspecified thigh
  - ● **M21.86** Other specified acquired deformities of lower leg
    - **M21.861** Other specified acquired deformities of right lower leg
    - **M21.862** Other specified acquired deformities of left lower leg
    - **M21.869** Other specified acquired deformities of unspecified lower leg
- ● **M21.9** **Unspecified acquired deformity of limb and hand**
  - **M21.90** Unspecified acquired deformity of unspecified limb
  - ● **M21.92** Unspecified acquired deformity of upper arm
    - **M21.921** Unspecified acquired deformity of right upper arm
    - **M21.922** Unspecified acquired deformity of left upper arm
    - **M21.929** Unspecified acquired deformity of unspecified upper arm
  - ● **M21.93** Unspecified acquired deformity of forearm
    - **M21.931** Unspecified acquired deformity of right forearm
    - **M21.932** Unspecified acquired deformity of left forearm
    - **M21.939** Unspecified acquired deformity of unspecified forearm
  - ● **M21.94** Unspecified acquired deformity of hand
    - **M21.941** Unspecified acquired deformity of hand, right hand
    - **M21.942** Unspecified acquired deformity of hand, left hand
    - **M21.949** Unspecified acquired deformity of hand, unspecified hand
  - ● **M21.95** Unspecified acquired deformity of thigh
    - **M21.951** Unspecified acquired deformity of right thigh
    - **M21.952** Unspecified acquired deformity of left thigh
    - **M21.959** Unspecified acquired deformity of unspecified thigh
  - ● **M21.96** Unspecified acquired deformity of lower leg
    - **M21.961** Unspecified acquired deformity of right lower leg
    - **M21.962** Unspecified acquired deformity of left lower leg
    - **M21.969** Unspecified acquired deformity of unspecified lower leg

- ● **M22** **Disorder of patella**
  - **Excludes2**   traumatic dislocation of patella (S83.0-)
  - ● **M22.0** **Recurrent dislocation of patella**
    - **M22.00** Recurrent dislocation of patella, unspecified knee
    - **M22.01** Recurrent dislocation of patella, right knee
    - **M22.02** Recurrent dislocation of patella, left knee
  - ● **M22.1** **Recurrent subluxation of patella**
    - Incomplete dislocation of patella
    - **M22.10** Recurrent subluxation of patella, unspecified knee
    - **M22.11** Recurrent subluxation of patella, right knee
    - **M22.12** Recurrent subluxation of patella, left knee
  - ● **M22.2** **Patellofemoral disorders**
    - ● **M22.2X** Patellofemoral disorders
      - **M22.2X1** Patellofemoral disorders, right knee
      - **M22.2X2** Patellofemoral disorders, left knee
      - **M22.2X9** Patellofemoral disorders, unspecified knee
  - ● **M22.3** **Other derangements of patella**
    - ● **M22.3X** Other derangements of patella
      - **M22.3X1** Other derangements of patella, right knee
      - **M22.3X2** Other derangements of patella, left knee
      - **M22.3X9** Other derangements of patella, unspecified knee
  - ● **M22.4** **Chondromalacia patellae**
    - **M22.40** Chondromalacia patellae, unspecified knee
    - **M22.41** Chondromalacia patellae, right knee
    - **M22.42** Chondromalacia patellae, left knee
  - ● **M22.8** **Other disorders of patella**
    - ● **M22.8X** Other disorders of patella
      - **M22.8X1** Other disorders of patella, right knee
      - **M22.8X2** Other disorders of patella, left knee
      - **M22.8X9** Other disorders of patella, unspecified knee
  - ● **M22.9** **Unspecified disorder of patella**
    - **M22.90** Unspecified disorder of patella, unspecified knee
    - **M22.91** Unspecified disorder of patella, right knee
    - **M22.92** Unspecified disorder of patella, left knee

● **M23**   **Internal derangement of knee**

    Excludes1   ankylosis (M24.66)
                  deformity of knee (M21.-)
                  osteochondritis dissecans (M93.2)

    Excludes2   current injury - see injury of knee and lower leg
                    (S80-S89)
                  recurrent dislocation or subluxation of joints
                    (M24.4)
                  recurrent dislocation or subluxation of patella
                    (M22.0-M22.1)

     Coding Clinic: 2019, Q2, P26

● **M23.0**   **Cystic meniscus**

   ● **M23.00**   Cystic meniscus, unspecified meniscus
           Cystic meniscus, unspecified lateral meniscus
           Cystic meniscus, unspecified medial meniscus

      M23.000   Cystic meniscus, unspecified lateral meniscus, right knee

      M23.001   Cystic meniscus, unspecified lateral meniscus, left knee

      M23.002   Cystic meniscus, unspecified lateral meniscus, unspecified knee

      M23.003   Cystic meniscus, unspecified medial meniscus, right knee

      M23.004   Cystic meniscus, unspecified medial meniscus, left knee

      M23.005   Cystic meniscus, unspecified medial meniscus, unspecified knee

      M23.006   Cystic meniscus, unspecified meniscus, right knee

      M23.007   Cystic meniscus, unspecified meniscus, left knee

      M23.009   Cystic meniscus, unspecified meniscus, unspecified knee

   ● **M23.01**   Cystic meniscus, anterior horn of medial meniscus

      M23.011   Cystic meniscus, anterior horn of medial meniscus, right knee

      M23.012   Cystic meniscus, anterior horn of medial meniscus, left knee

      M23.019   Cystic meniscus, anterior horn of medial meniscus, unspecified knee

   ● **M23.02**   Cystic meniscus, posterior horn of medial meniscus

      M23.021   Cystic meniscus, posterior horn of medial meniscus, right knee

      M23.022   Cystic meniscus, posterior horn of medial meniscus, left knee

      M23.029   Cystic meniscus, posterior horn of medial meniscus, unspecified knee

   ● **M23.03**   Cystic meniscus, other medial meniscus

      M23.031   Cystic meniscus, other medial meniscus, right knee

      M23.032   Cystic meniscus, other medial meniscus, left knee

      M23.039   Cystic meniscus, other medial meniscus, unspecified knee

   ● **M23.04**   Cystic meniscus, anterior horn of lateral meniscus

      M23.041   Cystic meniscus, anterior horn of lateral meniscus, right knee

      M23.042   Cystic meniscus, anterior horn of lateral meniscus, left knee

      M23.049   Cystic meniscus, anterior horn of lateral meniscus, unspecified knee

   ● **M23.05**   Cystic meniscus, posterior horn of lateral meniscus

      M23.051   Cystic meniscus, posterior horn of lateral meniscus, right knee

      M23.052   Cystic meniscus, posterior horn of lateral meniscus, left knee

      M23.059   Cystic meniscus, posterior horn of lateral meniscus, unspecified knee

   ● **M23.06**   Cystic meniscus, other lateral meniscus

      M23.061   Cystic meniscus, other lateral meniscus, right knee

      M23.062   Cystic meniscus, other lateral meniscus, left knee

      M23.069   Cystic meniscus, other lateral meniscus, unspecified knee

★ **(See Plate 34 of the Anatomy Illustrations.)**

   ● **M23.2**   Derangement of meniscus due to old tear or injury
           Old bucket-handle tear

   ● **M23.20**   Derangement of unspecified meniscus due to old tear or injury
           Derangement of unspecified lateral meniscus due to old tear or injury
           Derangement of unspecified medial meniscus due to old tear or injury

      M23.200   Derangement of unspecified lateral meniscus due to old tear or injury, right knee

      M23.201   Derangement of unspecified lateral meniscus due to old tear or injury, left knee

      M23.202   Derangement of unspecified lateral meniscus due to old tear or injury, unspecified knee

      M23.203   Derangement of unspecified medial meniscus due to old tear or injury, right knee

      M23.204   Derangement of unspecified medial meniscus due to old tear or injury, left knee

      M23.205   Derangement of unspecified medial meniscus due to old tear or injury, unspecified knee

      M23.206   Derangement of unspecified meniscus due to old tear or injury, right knee

      M23.207   Derangement of unspecified meniscus due to old tear or injury, left knee

      M23.209   Derangement of unspecified meniscus due to old tear or injury, unspecified knee

   ● **M23.21**   Derangement of anterior horn of medial meniscus due to old tear or injury

      M23.211   Derangement of anterior horn of medial meniscus due to old tear or injury, right knee

      M23.212   Derangement of anterior horn of medial meniscus due to old tear or injury, left knee

      M23.219   Derangement of anterior horn of medial meniscus due to old tear or injury, unspecified knee

   ● **M23.22**   Derangement of posterior horn of medial meniscus due to old tear or injury

      M23.221   Derangement of posterior horn of medial meniscus due to old tear or injury, right knee

      M23.222   Derangement of posterior horn of medial meniscus due to old tear or injury, left knee

      M23.229   Derangement of posterior horn of medial meniscus due to old tear or injury, unspecified knee

● M23.23　Derangement of other medial meniscus due to old tear or injury
- M23.231　Derangement of other medial meniscus due to old tear or injury, right knee
- M23.232　Derangement of other medial meniscus due to old tear or injury, left knee
- M23.239　Derangement of other medial meniscus due to old tear or injury, unspecified knee

● M23.24　Derangement of anterior horn of lateral meniscus due to old tear or injury
- M23.241　Derangement of anterior horn of lateral meniscus due to old tear or injury, right knee
- M23.242　Derangement of anterior horn of lateral meniscus due to old tear or injury, left knee
- M23.249　Derangement of anterior horn of lateral meniscus due to old tear or injury, unspecified knee

● M23.25　Derangement of posterior horn of lateral meniscus due to old tear or injury
- M23.251　Derangement of posterior horn of lateral meniscus due to old tear or injury, right knee
- M23.252　Derangement of posterior horn of lateral meniscus due to old tear or injury, left knee
- M23.259　Derangement of posterior horn of lateral meniscus due to old tear or injury, unspecified knee

● M23.26　Derangement of other lateral meniscus due to old tear or injury
- M23.261　Derangement of other lateral meniscus due to old tear or injury, right knee
- M23.262　Derangement of other lateral meniscus due to old tear or injury, left knee
- M23.269　Derangement of other lateral meniscus due to old tear or injury, unspecified knee

● M23.3　Other meniscus derangements
Degenerate meniscus
Detached meniscus
Retained meniscus

● M23.30　Other meniscus derangements, unspecified meniscus
Other meniscus derangements, unspecified lateral meniscus
Other meniscus derangements, unspecified medial meniscus
- M23.300　Other meniscus derangements, unspecified lateral meniscus, right knee
- M23.301　Other meniscus derangements, unspecified lateral meniscus, left knee
- M23.302　Other meniscus derangements, unspecified lateral meniscus, unspecified knee
- M23.303　Other meniscus derangements, unspecified medial meniscus, right knee
- M23.304　Other meniscus derangements, unspecified medial meniscus, left knee
- M23.305　Other meniscus derangements, unspecified medial meniscus, unspecified knee
- M23.306　Other meniscus derangements, unspecified meniscus, right knee
- M23.307　Other meniscus derangements, unspecified meniscus, left knee
- M23.309　Other meniscus derangements, unspecified meniscus, unspecified knee

● M23.31　Other meniscus derangements, anterior horn of medial meniscus
- M23.311　Other meniscus derangements, anterior horn of medial meniscus, right knee
- M23.312　Other meniscus derangements, anterior horn of medial meniscus, left knee
- M23.319　Other meniscus derangements, anterior horn of medial meniscus, unspecified knee

● M23.32　Other meniscus derangements, posterior horn of medial meniscus
- M23.321　Other meniscus derangements, posterior horn of medial meniscus, right knee
- M23.322　Other meniscus derangements, posterior horn of medial meniscus, left knee
- M23.329　Other meniscus derangements, posterior horn of medial meniscus, unspecified knee

● M23.33　Other meniscus derangements, other medial meniscus
- M23.331　Other meniscus derangements, other medial meniscus, right knee
- M23.332　Other meniscus derangements, other medial meniscus, left knee
- M23.339　Other meniscus derangements, other medial meniscus, unspecified knee

● M23.34　Other meniscus derangements, anterior horn of lateral meniscus
- M23.341　Other meniscus derangements, anterior horn of lateral meniscus, right knee
- M23.342　Other meniscus derangements, anterior horn of lateral meniscus, left knee
- M23.349　Other meniscus derangements, anterior horn of lateral meniscus, unspecified knee

● M23.35　Other meniscus derangements, posterior horn of lateral meniscus
- M23.351　Other meniscus derangements, posterior horn of lateral meniscus, right knee
- M23.352　Other meniscus derangements, posterior horn of lateral meniscus, left knee
- M23.359　Other meniscus derangements, posterior horn of lateral meniscus, unspecified knee

● M23.36　Other meniscus derangements, other lateral meniscus
- M23.361　Other meniscus derangements, other lateral meniscus, right knee
- M23.362　Other meniscus derangements, other lateral meniscus, left knee
- M23.369　Other meniscus derangements, other lateral meniscus, unspecified knee

▶ New　　⇒ Revised　　deleted Deleted　　Excludes 1　　Excludes 2　　Includes　　Use additional　　Code first　　Code also　　Key words
OGCR Official Guidelines　　X Assign placeholder X　　● Use Additional Character(s)　　▶ Manifestation Code　　🦉 Hierarchical Condition Category　　Coding Clinic

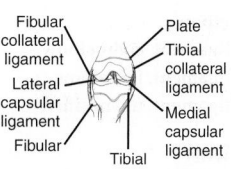

Fibular
collateral
ligament

Plate
Tibial
collateral
ligament

Lateral
capsular
ligament

Medial
capsular
ligament

Fibular

Tibial

Figure 13-2 Collateral and cruciate ligament of knee. (From DeLee: DeLee and Drez's Orthopaedic Sports Medicine, ed 3, Saunders, 2009)

● M23.4 **Loose body in knee**
    M23.40 Loose body in knee, unspecified knee
    M23.41 Loose body in knee, right knee
    M23.42 Loose body in knee, left knee
● M23.5 **Chronic instability of knee**
    M23.50 Chronic instability of knee, unspecified knee
    M23.51 Chronic instability of knee, right knee
    M23.52 Chronic instability of knee, left knee
● M23.6 Other spontaneous disruption of ligament(s) of knee
    ● M23.60 Other spontaneous disruption of unspecified ligament of knee
        M23.601 Other spontaneous disruption of unspecified ligament of right knee
        M23.602 Other spontaneous disruption of unspecified ligament of left knee
        M23.609 Other spontaneous disruption of unspecified ligament of unspecified knee
    ● M23.61 Other spontaneous disruption of anterior cruciate ligament of knee
        M23.611 Other spontaneous disruption of anterior cruciate ligament of right knee
        M23.612 Other spontaneous disruption of anterior cruciate ligament of left knee
        M23.619 Other spontaneous disruption of anterior cruciate ligament of unspecified knee
    ● M23.62 Other spontaneous disruption of posterior cruciate ligament of knee
        M23.621 Other spontaneous disruption of posterior cruciate ligament of right knee
        M23.622 Other spontaneous disruption of posterior cruciate ligament of left knee
        M23.629 Other spontaneous disruption of posterior cruciate ligament of unspecified knee
    ● M23.63 Other spontaneous disruption of medial collateral ligament of knee
        M23.631 Other spontaneous disruption of medial collateral ligament of right knee
        M23.632 Other spontaneous disruption of medial collateral ligament of left knee
        M23.639 Other spontaneous disruption of medial collateral ligament of unspecified knee
    ● M23.64 Other spontaneous disruption of lateral collateral ligament of knee
        M23.641 Other spontaneous disruption of lateral collateral ligament of right knee
        M23.642 Other spontaneous disruption of lateral collateral ligament of left knee
        M23.649 Other spontaneous disruption of lateral collateral ligament of unspecified knee

    ● M23.67 Other spontaneous disruption of capsular ligament of knee
        M23.671 Other spontaneous disruption of capsular ligament of right knee
        M23.672 Other spontaneous disruption of capsular ligament of left knee
        M23.679 Other spontaneous disruption of capsular ligament of unspecified knee
● M23.8 **Other internal derangements of knee**
    Laxity of ligament of knee
    Snapping knee
    ● M23.8X Other internal derangements of knee
        M23.8X1 Other internal derangements of right knee
        M23.8X2 Other internal derangements of left knee
        M23.8X9 Other internal derangements of unspecified knee
● M23.9 **Unspecified internal derangement of knee**
    M23.90 Unspecified internal derangement of unspecified knee
    M23.91 Unspecified internal derangement of right knee
    M23.92 Unspecified internal derangement of left knee
● M24 Other specific joint derangements
    Excludes1 current injury - see injury of joint by body region
    Excludes2 ganglion (M67.4)
        snapping knee (M23.8-)
        temporomandibular joint disorders (M26.6-)
● M24.0 **Loose body in joint**
    Excludes2 loose body in knee (M23.4)
    M24.00 Loose body in unspecified joint
    ● M24.01 Loose body in shoulder
        M24.011 Loose body in right shoulder
        M24.012 Loose body in left shoulder
        M24.019 Loose body in unspecified shoulder
    ● M24.02 Loose body in elbow
        M24.021 Loose body in right elbow
        M24.022 Loose body in left elbow
        M24.029 Loose body in unspecified elbow
    ● M24.03 Loose body in wrist
        M24.031 Loose body in right wrist
        M24.032 Loose body in left wrist
        M24.039 Loose body in unspecified wrist
    ● M24.04 Loose body in finger joints
        M24.041 Loose body in right finger joint(s)
        M24.042 Loose body in left finger joint(s)
        M24.049 Loose body in unspecified finger joint(s)
    ● M24.05 Loose body in hip
        M24.051 Loose body in right hip
        M24.052 Loose body in left hip
        M24.059 Loose body in unspecified hip
    ● M24.07 Loose body in ankle and toe joints
        M24.071 Loose body in right ankle
        M24.072 Loose body in left ankle
        M24.073 Loose body in unspecified ankle
        M24.074 Loose body in right toe joint(s)
        M24.075 Loose body in left toe joint(s)
        M24.076 Loose body in unspecified toe joints
    M24.08 Loose body, other site

● M24.1   Other articular cartilage disorders
> **Excludes2**   chondrocalcinosis (M11.1, M11.2-)
> internal derangement of knee (M23.-)
> metastatic calcification (E83.5)
> ochronosis (E70.2)

    M24.10   Other articular cartilage disorders, unspecified site

● M24.11   Other articular cartilage disorders, shoulder
      M24.111   Other articular cartilage disorders, right shoulder
      M24.112   Other articular cartilage disorders, left shoulder
      M24.119   Other articular cartilage disorders, unspecified shoulder

● M24.12   Other articular cartilage disorders, elbow
      M24.121   Other articular cartilage disorders, right elbow
      M24.122   Other articular cartilage disorders, left elbow
      M24.129   Other articular cartilage disorders, unspecified elbow

● M24.13   Other articular cartilage disorders, wrist
      M24.131   Other articular cartilage disorders, right wrist
      M24.132   Other articular cartilage disorders, left wrist
      M24.139   Other articular cartilage disorders, unspecified wrist

● M24.14   Other articular cartilage disorders, hand
      M24.141   Other articular cartilage disorders, right hand
      M24.142   Other articular cartilage disorders, left hand
      M24.149   Other articular cartilage disorders, unspecified hand

● M24.15   Other articular cartilage disorders, hip
      M24.151   Other articular cartilage disorders, right hip
      M24.152   Other articular cartilage disorders, left hip
      M24.159   Other articular cartilage disorders, unspecified hip

● M24.17   Other articular cartilage disorders, ankle and foot
      M24.171   Other articular cartilage disorders, right ankle
      M24.172   Other articular cartilage disorders, left ankle
      M24.173   Other articular cartilage disorders, unspecified ankle
      M24.174   Other articular cartilage disorders, right foot
      M24.175   Other articular cartilage disorders, left foot
      M24.176   Other articular cartilage disorders, unspecified foot

    M24.19   Other articular cartilage disorders, other specified site

● M24.2   Disorder of ligament
> Instability secondary to old ligament injury
> Ligamentous laxity NOS
> **Excludes1**   familial ligamentous laxity (M35.7)
> **Excludes2**   internal derangement of knee (M23.5-M23.8X9)

    M24.20   Disorder of ligament, unspecified site

● M24.21   Disorder of ligament, shoulder
      M24.211   Disorder of ligament, right shoulder
      M24.212   Disorder of ligament, left shoulder
      M24.219   Disorder of ligament, unspecified shoulder

● M24.22   Disorder of ligament, elbow
      M24.221   Disorder of ligament, right elbow
      M24.222   Disorder of ligament, left elbow
      M24.229   Disorder of ligament, unspecified elbow

● M24.23   Disorder of ligament, wrist
      M24.231   Disorder of ligament, right wrist
      M24.232   Disorder of ligament, left wrist
      M24.239   Disorder of ligament, unspecified wrist

● M24.24   Disorder of ligament, hand
      M24.241   Disorder of ligament, right hand
      M24.242   Disorder of ligament, left hand
      M24.249   Disorder of ligament, unspecified hand

● M24.25   Disorder of ligament, hip
      M24.251   Disorder of ligament, right hip
      M24.252   Disorder of ligament, left hip
      M24.259   Disorder of ligament, unspecified hip

● M24.27   Disorder of ligament, ankle and foot
      M24.271   Disorder of ligament, right ankle
      M24.272   Disorder of ligament, left ankle
      M24.273   Disorder of ligament, unspecified ankle
      M24.274   Disorder of ligament, right foot
      M24.275   Disorder of ligament, left foot
      M24.276   Disorder of ligament, unspecified foot

    M24.28   Disorder of ligament, vertebrae

    M24.29   Disorder of ligament, other specified site

● M24.3   Pathological dislocation of joint, not elsewhere classified
> **Excludes1**   congenital dislocation or displacement of joint - see congenital malformations and deformations of the musculoskeletal system (Q65-Q79)
> current injury - see injury of joints and ligaments by body region
> recurrent dislocation of joint (M24.4-)

    M24.30   Pathological dislocation of unspecified joint, not elsewhere classified

● M24.31   Pathological dislocation of shoulder, not elsewhere classified
      M24.311   Pathological dislocation of right shoulder, not elsewhere classified
      M24.312   Pathological dislocation of left shoulder, not elsewhere classified
      M24.319   Pathological dislocation of unspecified shoulder, not elsewhere classified

● M24.32   Pathological dislocation of elbow, not elsewhere classified
      M24.321   Pathological dislocation of right elbow, not elsewhere classified
      M24.322   Pathological dislocation of left elbow, not elsewhere classified
      M24.329   Pathological dislocation of unspecified elbow, not elsewhere classified

● M24.33   Pathological dislocation of wrist, not elsewhere classified
      M24.331   Pathological dislocation of right wrist, not elsewhere classified
      M24.332   Pathological dislocation of left wrist, not elsewhere classified
      M24.339   Pathological dislocation of unspecified wrist, not elsewhere classified

● M24.34 Pathological dislocation of hand, not elsewhere classified

    M24.341 Pathological dislocation of right hand, not elsewhere classified

    M24.342 Pathological dislocation of left hand, not elsewhere classified

    M24.349 Pathological dislocation of unspecified hand, not elsewhere classified

● M24.35 Pathological dislocation of hip, not elsewhere classified

    M24.351 Pathological dislocation of right hip, not elsewhere classified

    M24.352 Pathological dislocation of left hip, not elsewhere classified

    M24.359 Pathological dislocation of unspecified hip, not elsewhere classified

● M24.36 Pathological dislocation of knee, not elsewhere classified

    M24.361 Pathological dislocation of right knee, not elsewhere classified

    M24.362 Pathological dislocation of left knee, not elsewhere classified

    M24.369 Pathological dislocation of unspecified knee, not elsewhere classified

● M24.37 Pathological dislocation of ankle and foot, not elsewhere classified

    M24.371 Pathological dislocation of right ankle, not elsewhere classified

    M24.372 Pathological dislocation of left ankle, not elsewhere classified

    M24.373 Pathological dislocation of unspecified ankle, not elsewhere classified

    M24.374 Pathological dislocation of right foot, not elsewhere classified

    M24.375 Pathological dislocation of left foot, not elsewhere classified

    M24.376 Pathological dislocation of unspecified foot, not elsewhere classified

    M24.39 Pathological dislocation of other specified joint, not elsewhere classified

● M24.4 Recurrent dislocation of joint

    Recurrent subluxation of joint

    Excludes2 recurrent dislocation of patella (M22.0-M22.1)
          recurrent vertebral dislocation (M43.3-, M43.4, M43.5-)

    M24.40 Recurrent dislocation, unspecified joint

● M24.41 Recurrent dislocation, shoulder

    M24.411 Recurrent dislocation, right shoulder

    M24.412 Recurrent dislocation, left shoulder

    M24.419 Recurrent dislocation, unspecified shoulder

● M24.42 Recurrent dislocation, elbow

    M24.421 Recurrent dislocation, right elbow

    M24.422 Recurrent dislocation, left elbow

    M24.429 Recurrent dislocation, unspecified elbow

● M24.43 Recurrent dislocation, wrist

    M24.431 Recurrent dislocation, right wrist

    M24.432 Recurrent dislocation, left wrist

    M24.439 Recurrent dislocation, unspecified wrist

● M24.44 Recurrent dislocation, hand and finger(s)

    M24.441 Recurrent dislocation, right hand

    M24.442 Recurrent dislocation, left hand

    M24.443 Recurrent dislocation, unspecified hand

    M24.444 Recurrent dislocation, right finger

    M24.445 Recurrent dislocation, left finger

    M24.446 Recurrent dislocation, unspecified finger

● M24.45 Recurrent dislocation, hip

    M24.451 Recurrent dislocation, right hip

    M24.452 Recurrent dislocation, left hip

    M24.459 Recurrent dislocation, unspecified hip

● M24.46 Recurrent dislocation, knee

    M24.461 Recurrent dislocation, right knee

    M24.462 Recurrent dislocation, left knee

    M24.469 Recurrent dislocation, unspecified knee

● M24.47 Recurrent dislocation, ankle, foot and toes

    M24.471 Recurrent dislocation, right ankle

    M24.472 Recurrent dislocation, left ankle

    M24.473 Recurrent dislocation, unspecified ankle

    M24.474 Recurrent dislocation, right foot

    M24.475 Recurrent dislocation, left foot

    M24.476 Recurrent dislocation, unspecified foot

    M24.477 Recurrent dislocation, right toe(s)

    M24.478 Recurrent dislocation, left toe(s)

    M24.479 Recurrent dislocation, unspecified toe(s)

    M24.49 Recurrent dislocation, other specified joint

● M24.5 Contracture of joint

    Excludes1 contracture of muscle without contracture of joint (M62.4-)
          contracture of tendon (sheath) without contracture of joint (M62.4-)
          Dupuytren's contracture (M72.0)

    Excludes2 acquired deformities of limbs (M20-M21)

    M24.50 Contracture, unspecified joint

● M24.51 Contracture, shoulder

    M24.511 Contracture, right shoulder

    M24.512 Contracture, left shoulder

    M24.519 Contracture, unspecified shoulder

● M24.52 Contracture, elbow

    M24.521 Contracture, right elbow

    M24.522 Contracture, left elbow

    M24.529 Contracture, unspecified elbow

● M24.53 Contracture, wrist

    M24.531 Contracture, right wrist

    M24.532 Contracture, left wrist

    M24.539 Contracture, unspecified wrist

● M24.54 Contracture, hand

    M24.541 Contracture, right hand

    M24.542 Contracture, left hand

    M24.549 Contracture, unspecified hand

● M24.55 Contracture, hip

    M24.551 Contracture, right hip
        Coding Clinic: 2016, Q2, P6

    M24.552 Contracture, left hip
        Coding Clinic: 2016, Q2, P6

    M24.559 Contracture, unspecified hip

CHAPTER 13 (M00-M99)

Item 13-5 **Ankylosis** or arthrokleisis is a consolidation of a joint due to disease, injury, or surgical procedure. Spondylosis is the degeneration of the vertebral processes and formation of osteophytes and commonly occurs with age. **Spondylitis** or ankylosing spondylitis is a type of arthritis that affects the spine or backbone, causing back pain and stiffness.

⬤ M24.56   Contracture, knee
     M24.561   Contracture, right knee
          Coding Clinic: 2016, Q2, P6
     M24.562   Contracture, left knee
          Coding Clinic: 2016, Q2, P6
     M24.569   Contracture, unspecified knee

⬤ M24.57   Contracture, ankle and foot
     M24.571   Contracture, right ankle
     M24.572   Contracture, left ankle
     M24.573   Contracture, unspecified ankle
     M24.574   Contracture, right foot
     M24.575   Contracture, left foot
     M24.576   Contracture, unspecified foot

   M24.59   Contracture, other specified joint

⬤ M24.6   Ankylosis of joint
     Excludes1   stiffness of joint without ankylosis (M25.6-)
     Excludes2   spine (M43.2-)
   M24.60   Ankylosis, unspecified joint

⬤ M24.61   Ankylosis, shoulder
     M24.611   Ankylosis, right shoulder
     M24.612   Ankylosis, left shoulder
     M24.619   Ankylosis, unspecified shoulder

⬤ M24.62   Ankylosis, elbow
     M24.621   Ankylosis, right elbow
     M24.622   Ankylosis, left elbow
     M24.629   Ankylosis, unspecified elbow

⬤ M24.63   Ankylosis, wrist
     M24.631   Ankylosis, right wrist
     M24.632   Ankylosis, left wrist
     M24.639   Ankylosis, unspecified wrist

⬤ M24.64   Ankylosis, hand
     M24.641   Ankylosis, right hand
     M24.642   Ankylosis, left hand
     M24.649   Ankylosis, unspecified hand

⬤ M24.65   Ankylosis, hip
     M24.651   Ankylosis, right hip
     M24.652   Ankylosis, left hip
     M24.659   Ankylosis, unspecified hip

⬤ M24.66   Ankylosis, knee
     M24.661   Ankylosis, right knee
     M24.662   Ankylosis, left knee
     M24.669   Ankylosis, unspecified knee

⬤ M24.67   Ankylosis, ankle and foot
     M24.671   Ankylosis, right ankle
     M24.672   Ankylosis, left ankle
     M24.673   Ankylosis, unspecified ankle
     M24.674   Ankylosis, right foot
     M24.675   Ankylosis, left foot
     M24.676   Ankylosis, unspecified foot

   M24.69   Ankylosis, other specified joint

   M24.7   Protrusio acetabuli

⬤ M24.8   Other specific joint derangements, not elsewhere classified
     Excludes2   iliotibial band syndrome (M76.3)
   M24.80   Other specific joint derangements of unspecified joint, not elsewhere classified

⬤ M24.81   Other specific joint derangements of shoulder, not elsewhere classified
     M24.811   Other specific joint derangements of right shoulder, not elsewhere classified
     M24.812   Other specific joint derangements of left shoulder, not elsewhere classified
     M24.819   Other specific joint derangements of unspecified shoulder, not elsewhere classified

⬤ M24.82   Other specific joint derangements of elbow, not elsewhere classified
     M24.821   Other specific joint derangements of right elbow, not elsewhere classified
     M24.822   Other specific joint derangements of left elbow, not elsewhere classified
     M24.829   Other specific joint derangements of unspecified elbow, not elsewhere classified

⬤ M24.83   Other specific joint derangements of wrist, not elsewhere classified
     M24.831   Other specific joint derangements of right wrist, not elsewhere classified
     M24.832   Other specific joint derangements of left wrist, not elsewhere classified
     M24.839   Other specific joint derangements of unspecified wrist, not elsewhere classified

⬤ M24.84   Other specific joint derangements of hand, not elsewhere classified
     M24.841   Other specific joint derangements of right hand, not elsewhere classified
     M24.842   Other specific joint derangements of left hand, not elsewhere classified
     M24.849   Other specific joint derangements of unspecified hand, not elsewhere classified

⬤ M24.85   Other specific joint derangements of hip, not elsewhere classified
     Irritable hip
     M24.851   Other specific joint derangements of right hip, not elsewhere classified
     M24.852   Other specific joint derangements of left hip, not elsewhere classified
     M24.859   Other specific joint derangements of unspecified hip, not elsewhere classified

⬤ M24.87   Other specific joint derangements of ankle and foot, not elsewhere classified
     M24.871   Other specific joint derangements of right ankle, not elsewhere classified
     M24.872   Other specific joint derangements of left ankle, not elsewhere classified
     M24.873   Other specific joint derangements of unspecified ankle, not elsewhere classified
     M24.874   Other specific joint derangements of right foot, not elsewhere classified
     M24.875   Other specific joint derangements left foot, not elsewhere classified
     M24.876   Other specific joint derangements of unspecified foot, not elsewhere classified

   M24.89   Other specific joint derangement of other specified joint, not elsewhere classified

   M24.9   Joint derangement, unspecified

▶ New   ⬛▶ Revised   ~~deleted~~ Deleted   Excludes 1   Excludes 2   Includes   Use additional   Code first   Code also   Key words

OGCR Official Guidelines   X Assign placeholder X   ⬤ Use Additional Character(s)   ▷ Manifestation Code   🦠 Hierarchical Condition Category   **Coding Clinic**

● **M25   Other joint disorder, not elsewhere classified**
    Excludes2   abnormality of gait and mobility (R26.-)
                 acquired deformities of limb (M20-M21)
                 calcification of bursa (M71.4-)
                 calcification of shoulder (joint) (M75.3)
                 calcification of tendon (M65.2-)
                 difficulty in walking (R26.2)
                 temporomandibular joint disorder (M26.6-)

● **M25.0   Hemarthrosis**
    Excludes1   current injury - see injury of joint by body
                     region
                 hemophilic arthropathy (M36.2)
    M25.00   Hemarthrosis, unspecified joint
  ● M25.01   Hemarthrosis, shoulder
        M25.011   Hemarthrosis, right shoulder
        M25.012   Hemarthrosis, left shoulder
        M25.019   Hemarthrosis, unspecified shoulder
  ● M25.02   Hemarthrosis, elbow
        M25.021   Hemarthrosis, right elbow
        M25.022   Hemarthrosis, left elbow
        M25.029   Hemarthrosis, unspecified elbow
  ● M25.03   Hemarthrosis, wrist
        M25.031   Hemarthrosis, right wrist
        M25.032   Hemarthrosis, left wrist
        M25.039   Hemarthrosis, unspecified wrist
  ● M25.04   Hemarthrosis, hand
        M25.041   Hemarthrosis, right hand
        M25.042   Hemarthrosis, left hand
        M25.049   Hemarthrosis, unspecified hand
  ● M25.05   Hemarthrosis, hip
        M25.051   Hemarthrosis, right hip
        M25.052   Hemarthrosis, left hip
        M25.059   Hemarthrosis, unspecified hip
  ● M25.06   Hemarthrosis, knee
        M25.061   Hemarthrosis, right knee
        M25.062   Hemarthrosis, left knee
        M25.069   Hemarthrosis, unspecified knee
  ● M25.07   Hemarthrosis, ankle and foot
        M25.071   Hemarthrosis, right ankle
        M25.072   Hemarthrosis, left ankle
        M25.073   Hemarthrosis, unspecified ankle
        M25.074   Hemarthrosis, right foot
        M25.075   Hemarthrosis, left foot
        M25.076   Hemarthrosis, unspecified foot
    M25.08   Hemarthrosis, other specified site
            Hemarthrosis, vertebrae

● **M25.1   Fistula of joint**
    M25.10   Fistula, unspecified joint
  ● M25.11   Fistula, shoulder
        M25.111   Fistula, right shoulder
        M25.112   Fistula, left shoulder
        M25.119   Fistula, unspecified shoulder
  ● M25.12   Fistula, elbow
        M25.121   Fistula, right elbow
        M25.122   Fistula, left elbow
        M25.129   Fistula, unspecified elbow
  ● M25.13   Fistula, wrist
        M25.131   Fistula, right wrist
        M25.132   Fistula, left wrist
        M25.139   Fistula, unspecified wrist
  ● M25.14   Fistula, hand
        M25.141   Fistula, right hand
        M25.142   Fistula, left hand
        M25.149   Fistula, unspecified hand

● M25.15   Fistula, hip
        M25.151   Fistula, right hip
        M25.152   Fistula, left hip
        M25.159   Fistula, unspecified hip
● M25.16   Fistula, knee
        M25.161   Fistula, right knee
        M25.162   Fistula, left knee
        M25.169   Fistula, unspecified knee
● M25.17   Fistula, ankle and foot
        M25.171   Fistula, right ankle
        M25.172   Fistula, left ankle
        M25.173   Fistula, unspecified ankle
        M25.174   Fistula, right foot
        M25.175   Fistula, left foot
        M25.176   Fistula, unspecified foot
    M25.18   Fistula, other specified site
            Fistula, vertebrae

● **M25.2   Flail joint**
    M25.20   Flail joint, unspecified joint
  ● M25.21   Flail joint, shoulder
        M25.211   Flail joint, right shoulder
        M25.212   Flail joint, left shoulder
        M25.219   Flail joint, unspecified shoulder
  ● M25.22   Flail joint, elbow
        M25.221   Flail joint, right elbow
        M25.222   Flail joint, left elbow
        M25.229   Flail joint, unspecified elbow
  ● M25.23   Flail joint, wrist
        M25.231   Flail joint, right wrist
        M25.232   Flail joint, left wrist
        M25.239   Flail joint, unspecified wrist
  ● M25.24   Flail joint, hand
        M25.241   Flail joint, right hand
        M25.242   Flail joint, left hand
        M25.249   Flail joint, unspecified hand
  ● M25.25   Flail joint, hip
        M25.251   Flail joint, right hip
        M25.252   Flail joint, left hip
        M25.259   Flail joint, unspecified hip
  ● M25.26   Flail joint, knee
        M25.261   Flail joint, right knee
        M25.262   Flail joint, left knee
        M25.269   Flail joint, unspecified knee
  ● M25.27   Flail joint, ankle and foot
        M25.271   Flail joint, right ankle and foot
        M25.272   Flail joint, left ankle and foot
        M25.279   Flail joint, unspecified ankle and foot
    M25.28   Flail joint, other site

● **M25.3   Other instability of joint**
    Excludes1   instability of joint secondary to old
                     ligament injury (M24.2-)
                 instability of joint secondary to removal
                     of joint prosthesis (M96.8-)
    Excludes2   spinal instabilities (M53.2-)
    M25.30   Other instability, unspecified joint
  ● M25.31   Other instability, shoulder
        M25.311   Other instability, right shoulder
        M25.312   Other instability, left shoulder
        M25.319   Other instability, unspecified
                     shoulder
  ● M25.32   Other instability, elbow
        M25.321   Other instability, right elbow
        M25.322   Other instability, left elbow
        M25.329   Other instability, unspecified elbow

M25.33   Other instability, wrist
    M25.331   Other instability, right wrist
    M25.332   Other instability, left wrist
    M25.339   Other instability, unspecified wrist
M25.34   Other instability, hand
    M25.341   Other instability, right hand
    M25.342   Other instability, left hand
    M25.349   Other instability, unspecified hand
M25.35   Other instability, hip
    M25.351   Other instability, right hip
    M25.352   Other instability, left hip
    M25.359   Other instability, unspecified hip
M25.36   Other instability, knee
    M25.361   Other instability, right knee
    M25.362   Other instability, left knee
    M25.369   Other instability, unspecified knee
M25.37   Other instability, ankle and foot
    M25.371   Other instability, right ankle
    M25.372   Other instability, left ankle
    M25.373   Other instability, unspecified ankle
    M25.374   Other instability, right foot
    M25.375   Other instability, left foot
    M25.376   Other instability, unspecified foot
M25.39 Other instability of joint
M25.4   Effusion of joint
    Excludes1   hydrarthrosis in yaws (A66.6)
                 intermittent hydrarthrosis (M12.4-)
                 other infective (teno)synovitis (M65.1-)
M25.40   Effusion, unspecified joint
M25.41   Effusion, shoulder
    M25.411   Effusion, right shoulder
    M25.412   Effusion, left shoulder
    M25.419   Effusion, unspecified shoulder
M25.42   Effusion, elbow
    M25.421   Effusion, right elbow
    M25.422   Effusion, left elbow
    M25.429   Effusion, unspecified elbow
M25.43   Effusion, wrist
    M25.431   Effusion, right wrist
    M25.432   Effusion, left wrist
    M25.439   Effusion, unspecified wrist
M25.44   Effusion, hand
    M25.441   Effusion, right hand
    M25.442   Effusion, left hand
    M25.449   Effusion, unspecified hand
M25.45   Effusion, hip
    M25.451   Effusion, right hip
    M25.452   Effusion, left hip
    M25.459   Effusion, unspecified hip
M25.46   Effusion, knee
    M25.461   Effusion, right knee
    M25.462   Effusion, left knee
    M25.469   Effusion, unspecified knee
M25.47   Effusion, ankle and foot
    M25.471   Effusion, right ankle
    M25.472   Effusion, left ankle
    M25.473   Effusion, unspecified ankle
    M25.474   Effusion, right foot
    M25.475   Effusion, left foot
    M25.476   Effusion, unspecified foot
M25.48   Effusion, other site

M25.5   Pain in joint
    Excludes2   pain in hand (M79.64-)
                pain in fingers (M79.64-)
                pain in foot (M79.67-)
                pain in limb (M79.6-)
                pain in toes (M79.67-)
M25.50   Pain in unspecified joint
M25.51   Pain in shoulder
    M25.511   Pain in right shoulder
    M25.512   Pain in left shoulder
    M25.519   Pain in unspecified shoulder
M25.52   Pain in elbow
    M25.521   Pain in right elbow
    M25.522   Pain in left elbow
    M25.529   Pain in unspecified elbow
M25.53   Pain in wrist
    M25.531   Pain in right wrist
    M25.532   Pain in left wrist
    M25.539   Pain in unspecified wrist
M25.54   Pain in joints of hand
    Coding Clinic: 2016, Q4, P38
    M25.541   Pain in joints of right hand
    M25.542   Pain in joints of left hand
    M25.549   Pain in joints of unspecified hand
              Pain in joints of hand NOS
M25.55   Pain in hip
    M25.551   Pain in right hip
    M25.552   Pain in left hip
    M25.559   Pain in unspecified hip
M25.56   Pain in knee
    M25.561   Pain in right knee
    M25.562   Pain in left knee
    M25.569   Pain in unspecified knee
M25.57   Pain in ankle and joints of foot
    M25.571   Pain in right ankle and joints of right foot
    M25.572   Pain in left ankle and joints of left foot
    M25.579   Pain in unspecified ankle and joints of unspecified foot
M25.59   Pain in other specified joint
M25.6   Stiffness of joint, not elsewhere classified
    Excludes1   ankylosis of joint (M24.6-)
                 contracture of joint (M24.5-)
M25.60   Stiffness of unspecified joint, not elsewhere classified
M25.61   Stiffness of shoulder, not elsewhere classified
    M25.611   Stiffness of right shoulder, not elsewhere classified
    M25.612   Stiffness of left shoulder, not elsewhere classified
    M25.619   Stiffness of unspecified shoulder, not elsewhere classified
M25.62   Stiffness of elbow, not elsewhere classified
    M25.621   Stiffness of right elbow, not elsewhere classified
    M25.622   Stiffness of left elbow, not elsewhere classified
    M25.629   Stiffness of unspecified elbow, not elsewhere classified
M25.63   Stiffness of wrist, not elsewhere classified
    M25.631   Stiffness of right wrist, not elsewhere classified
    M25.632   Stiffness of left wrist, not elsewhere classified
    M25.639   Stiffness of unspecified wrist, not elsewhere classified

▶ New   ⇒ Revised   ~~deleted~~ Deleted   Excludes 1   Excludes 2   Includes   Use additional   Code first   Code also   Key words
OGCR Official Guidelines   X Assign placeholder X   ● Use Additional Character(s)   ▶ Manifestation Code   🏷 Hierarchical Condition Category   Coding Clinic

● M25.64   Stiffness of hand, not elsewhere classified
    M25.641   Stiffness of right hand, not elsewhere classified
    M25.642   Stiffness of left hand, not elsewhere classified
    M25.649   Stiffness of unspecified hand, not elsewhere classified
● M25.65   Stiffness of hip, not elsewhere classified
    M25.651   Stiffness of right hip, not elsewhere classified
    M25.652   Stiffness of left hip, not elsewhere classified
    M25.659   Stiffness of unspecified hip, not elsewhere classified
● M25.66   Stiffness of knee, not elsewhere classified
    M25.661   Stiffness of right knee, not elsewhere classified
    M25.662   Stiffness of left knee, not elsewhere classified
    M25.669   Stiffness of unspecified knee, not elsewhere classified
● M25.67   Stiffness of ankle and foot, not elsewhere classified
    M25.671   Stiffness of right ankle, not elsewhere classified
    M25.672   Stiffness of left ankle, not elsewhere classified
    M25.673   Stiffness of unspecified ankle, not elsewhere classified
    M25.674   Stiffness of right foot, not elsewhere classified
    M25.675   Stiffness of left foot, not elsewhere classified
    M25.676   Stiffness of unspecified foot, not elsewhere classified
    M25.69   Stiffness of other specified joint, not elsewhere classified
● M25.7   Osteophyte
    M25.70   Osteophyte, unspecified joint
● M25.71   Osteophyte, shoulder
    M25.711   Osteophyte, right shoulder
    M25.712   Osteophyte, left shoulder
    M25.719   Osteophyte, unspecified shoulder
● M25.72   Osteophyte, elbow
    M25.721   Osteophyte, right elbow
    M25.722   Osteophyte, left elbow
    M25.729   Osteophyte, unspecified elbow
● M25.73   Osteophyte, wrist
    M25.731   Osteophyte, right wrist
    M25.732   Osteophyte, left wrist
    M25.739   Osteophyte, unspecified wrist
● M25.74   Osteophyte, hand
    M25.741   Osteophyte, right hand
    M25.742   Osteophyte, left hand
    M25.749   Osteophyte, unspecified hand
● M25.75   Osteophyte, hip
    M25.751   Osteophyte, right hip
    M25.752   Osteophyte, left hip
    M25.759   Osteophyte, unspecified hip
● M25.76   Osteophyte, knee
    M25.761   Osteophyte, right knee
    M25.762   Osteophyte, left knee
    M25.769   Osteophyte, unspecified knee

● M25.77   Osteophyte, ankle and foot
    M25.771   Osteophyte, right ankle
    M25.772   Osteophyte, left ankle
    M25.773   Osteophyte, unspecified ankle
    M25.774   Osteophyte, right foot
    M25.775   Osteophyte, left foot
    M25.776   Osteophyte, unspecified foot
    M25.78   Osteophyte, vertebrae
● M25.8   Other specified joint disorders
    M25.80   Other specified joint disorders, unspecified joint
● M25.81   Other specified joint disorders, shoulder
    M25.811   Other specified joint disorders, right shoulder
    M25.812   Other specified joint disorders, left shoulder
    M25.819   Other specified joint disorders, unspecified shoulder
● M25.82   Other specified joint disorders, elbow
    M25.821   Other specified joint disorders, right elbow
    M25.822   Other specified joint disorders, left elbow
    M25.829   Other specified joint disorders, unspecified elbow
● M25.83   Other specified joint disorders, wrist
    M25.831   Other specified joint disorders, right wrist
    M25.832   Other specified joint disorders, left wrist
    M25.839   Other specified joint disorders, unspecified wrist
● M25.84   Other specified joint disorders, hand
    M25.841   Other specified joint disorders, right hand
    M25.842   Other specified joint disorders, left hand
    M25.849   Other specified joint disorders, unspecified hand
● M25.85   Other specified joint disorders, hip
    M25.851   Other specified joint disorders, right hip
    M25.852   Other specified joint disorders, left hip
    M25.859   Other specified joint disorders, unspecified hip
● M25.86   Other specified joint disorders, knee
    M25.861   Other specified joint disorders, right knee
    M25.862   Other specified joint disorders, left knee
    M25.869   Other specified joint disorders, unspecified knee
● M25.87   Other specified joint disorders, ankle and foot
    M25.871   Other specified joint disorders, right ankle and foot
    M25.872   Other specified joint disorders, left ankle and foot
    M25.879   Other specified joint disorders, unspecified ankle and foot
   M25.9   Joint disorder, unspecified

Figure 13-3   Dentofacial malocclusion.

Item 13–6 Hyperplasia is a condition of overdevelopment, whereas **hypoplasia** is a condition of underdevelopment. **Macrogenia** is overdevelopment of the chin, whereas **microgenia** is underdevelopment of the chin.

DENTOFACIAL ANOMALIES [INCLUDING MALOCCLUSION] AND OTHER DISORDERS OF JAW (M26-M27)

Excludes1   hemifacial atrophy or hypertrophy (Q67.4)
unilateral condylar hyperplasia or hypoplasia (M27.8)

● M26   Dentofacial anomalies [including malocclusion]
   ● M26.0   Major anomalies of jaw size
      Excludes1   acromegaly (E22.0)
         Robin's syndrome (Q87.0)
      M26.00   Unspecified anomaly of jaw size
      M26.01   Maxillary hyperplasia
      M26.02   Maxillary hypoplasia
      M26.03   Mandibular hyperplasia
      M26.04   Mandibular hypoplasia
      M26.05   Macrogenia
      M26.06   Microgenia
      M26.07   Excessive tuberosity of jaw
         Entire maxillary tuberosity
      M26.09   Other specified anomalies of jaw size
   ● M26.1   Anomalies of jaw-cranial base relationship
      M26.10   Unspecified anomaly of jaw-cranial base relationship
      M26.11   Maxillary asymmetry
      M26.12   Other jaw asymmetry
      M26.19   Other specified anomalies of jaw-cranial base relationship
         Coding Clinic: 2020, Q1, P21
   ● M26.2   Anomalies of dental arch relationship
      M26.20   Unspecified anomaly of dental arch relationship
      ● M26.21   Malocclusion, Angle's class
         M26.211   Malocclusion, Angle's class I
            Neutro-occlusion
         M26.212   Malocclusion, Angle's class II
            Disto-occlusion Division I
            Disto-occlusion Division II
         M26.213   Malocclusion, Angle's class III
            Mesio-occlusion
         M26.219   Malocclusion, Angle's class, unspecified
      ● M26.22   Open occlusal relationship
         M26.220   Open anterior occlusal relationship
            Anterior open bite
         M26.221   Open posterior occlusal relationship
            Posterior open bite
      M26.23   Excessive horizontal overlap
         Excessive horizontal overjet
      M26.24   Reverse articulation
         Crossbite (anterior) (posterior)

      M26.25   Anomalies of interarch distance
      M26.29   Other anomalies of dental arch relationship
         Midline deviation of dental arch
         Overbite (excessive) deep
         Overbite (excessive) horizontal
         Overbite (excessive) vertical
         Posterior lingual occlusion of mandibular teeth
   ● M26.3   Anomalies of tooth position of fully erupted tooth or teeth
      Excludes2   embedded and impacted teeth (K01.-)
      M26.30   Unspecified anomaly of tooth position of fully erupted tooth or teeth
         Abnormal spacing of fully erupted tooth or teeth NOS
         Displacement of fully erupted tooth or teeth NOS
         Transposition of fully erupted tooth or teeth NOS
      M26.31   Crowding of fully erupted teeth
      M26.32   Excessive spacing of fully erupted teeth
         Diastema of fully erupted tooth or teeth NOS
      M26.33   Horizontal displacement of fully erupted tooth or teeth
         Tipped tooth or teeth
         Tipping of fully erupted tooth
      M26.34   Vertical displacement of fully erupted tooth or teeth
         Extruded tooth
         Infraeruption of tooth or teeth
         Supraeruption of tooth or teeth
      M26.35   Rotation of fully erupted tooth or teeth
      M26.36   Insufficient interocclusal distance of fully erupted teeth (ridge)
         Lack of adequate intermaxillary vertical dimension of fully erupted teeth
      M26.37   Excessive interocclusal distance of fully erupted teeth
         Excessive intermaxillary vertical dimension of fully erupted teeth
         Loss of occlusal vertical dimension of fully erupted teeth
      M26.39   Other anomalies of tooth position of fully erupted tooth or teeth
   M26.4   Malocclusion, unspecified
   ● M26.5   Dentofacial functional abnormalities
      Excludes1   bruxism (F45.8)
         teeth-grinding NOS (F45.8)
      M26.50   Dentofacial functional abnormalities, unspecified
      M26.51   Abnormal jaw closure
      M26.52   Limited mandibular range of motion
      M26.53   Deviation in opening and closing of the mandible
      M26.54   Insufficient anterior guidance
         Insufficient anterior occlusal guidance
      M26.55   Centric occlusion maximum intercuspation discrepancy
         Excludes1   centric occlusion NOS (M26.59)
      M26.56   Non-working side interference
         Balancing side interference
      M26.57   Lack of posterior occlusal support
      M26.59   Other dentofacial functional abnormalities
         Centric occlusion (of teeth) NOS
         Malocclusion due to abnormal swallowing
         Malocclusion due to mouth breathing
         Malocclusion due to tongue, lip or finger habits

▶ New   ⇒ Revised   ~~deleted~~ Deleted   Excludes 1   Excludes 2   Includes   Use additional   Code first   Code also   Key words
OGCR Official Guidelines   X Assign placeholder X   ● Use Additional Character(s)   ▷ Manifestation Code   🔖 Hierarchical Condition Category   **Coding Clinic**

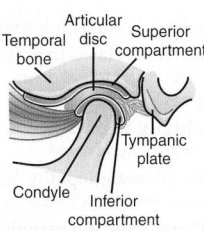

Figure 13-4 Temporomandibular joint.

Item 13-7 Dysfunction of the temporomandibular joint is termed **temporomandibular joint (TMJ) syndrome** and is characterized by pain and tenderness/spasm of the muscles of mastication, joint noise, and in the later stages, limited mandibular movement.

● M26.6 Temporomandibular joint disorders

     Excludes2   current temporomandibular joint dislocation (S03.0)
                        current temporomandibular joint sprain (S03.4)

     Coding Clinic: 2016, Q4, P38-39

   ● M26.60 Temporomandibular joint disorder, unspecified

       M26.601   Right temporomandibular joint disorder, unspecified

       M26.602   Left temporomandibular joint disorder, unspecified

       M26.603   Bilateral temporomandibular joint disorder, unspecified

       M26.609   Unspecified temporomandibular joint disorder, unspecified side
                   Temporomandibular joint disorder NOS

   ● M26.61 Adhesions and ankylosis of temporomandibular joint

       M26.611   Adhesions and ankylosis of right temporomandibular joint

       M26.612   Adhesions and ankylosis of left temporomandibular joint

       M26.613   Adhesions and ankylosis of bilateral temporomandibular joint

       M26.619   Adhesions and ankylosis of temporomandibular joint, unspecified side

   ● M26.62 Arthralgia of temporomandibular joint

       M26.621   Arthralgia of right temporomandibular joint

       M26.622   Arthralgia of left temporomandibular joint

       M26.623   Arthralgia of bilateral temporomandibular joint

       M26.629   Arthralgia of temporomandibular joint, unspecified side

   ● M26.63 Articular disc disorder of temporomandibular joint

       M26.631   Articular disc disorder of right temporomandibular joint

       M26.632   Articular disc disorder of left temporomandibular joint

       M26.633   Articular disc disorder of bilateral temporomandibular joint

       M26.639   Articular disc disorder of temporomandibular joint, unspecified side

   ● M26.64 Arthritis of temporomandibular joint

       M26.641   Arthritis of right temporomandibular joint

       M26.642   Arthritis of left temporomandibular joint

       M26.643   Arthritis of bilateral temporomandibular joint

       M26.649   Arthritis of unspecified temporomandibular joint

   ● M26.65 Arthropathy of temporomandibular joint

       M26.651   Arthropathy of right temporomandibular joint

       M26.652   Arthropathy of left temporomandibular joint

       M26.653   Arthropathy of bilateral temporomandibular joint

       M26.659   Arthropathy of unspecified temporomandibular joint

     M26.69   Other specified disorders of temporomandibular joint

  ● M26.7 Dental alveolar anomalies

     M26.70   Unspecified alveolar anomaly

     M26.71   Alveolar maxillary hyperplasia

     M26.72   Alveolar mandibular hyperplasia

     M26.73   Alveolar maxillary hypoplasia

     M26.74   Alveolar mandibular hypoplasia

     M26.79   Other specified alveolar anomalies

  ● M26.8 Other dentofacial anomalies

     M26.81   Anterior soft tissue impingement
                Anterior soft tissue impingement on teeth

     M26.82   Posterior soft tissue impingement
                Posterior soft tissue impingement on teeth

     M26.89   Other dentofacial anomalies

     M26.9   Dentofacial anomaly, unspecified

● M27   Other diseases of jaws

   M27.0   Developmental disorders of jaws
       Latent bone cyst of jaw
       Stafne's cyst
       Torus mandibularis
       Torus palatinus

   M27.1   Giant cell granuloma, central
       Giant cell granuloma NOS

     Excludes1   peripheral giant cell granuloma (K06.8)

   M27.2   Inflammatory conditions of jaws
       Osteitis of jaw(s)
       Osteomyelitis (neonatal) jaw(s)
       Osteoradionecrosis jaw(s)
       Periostitis jaw(s)
       Sequestrum of jaw bone
       Use additional code (W88-W90, X39.0) to identify radiation, if radiation-induced

     Excludes2   osteonecrosis of jaw due to drug (M87.180)

   M27.3   Alveolitis of jaws
       Alveolar osteitis
       Dry socket

  ● M27.4   Other and unspecified cysts of jaw

     Excludes1   cysts of oral region (K09.-)
                      latent bone cyst of jaw (M27.0)
                      Stafne's cyst (M27.0)

     M27.40   Unspecified cyst of jaw
            Cyst of jaw NOS

     M27.49   Other cysts of jaw
            Aneurysmal cyst of jaw
            Hemorrhagic cyst of jaw
            Traumatic cyst of jaw

  ● M27.5   Periradicular pathology associated with previous endodontic treatment

     M27.51   Perforation of root canal space due to endodontic treatment

CHAPTER 13 (M00-M99)

CHAPTER 13 (M00-M99)

M27.52   Endodontic overfill

M27.53   Endodontic underfill

M27.59   Other periradicular pathology associated with previous endodontic treatment

● M27.6   **Endosseous dental implant failure**

     M27.61   Osseointegration failure of dental implant
         Hemorrhagic complications of dental implant placement
         Iatrogenic osseointegration failure of dental implant
         Osseointegration failure of dental implant due to complications of systemic disease
         Osseointegration failure of dental implant due to poor bone quality
         Pre-integration failure of dental implant NOS
         Pre-osseointegration failure of dental implant

     M27.62   Post-osseointegration biological failure of dental implant
         Failure of dental implant due to lack of attached gingiva
         Failure of dental implant due to occlusal trauma (caused by poor prosthetic design)
         Failure of dental implant due to parafunctional habits
         Failure of dental implant due to periodontal infection (peri mplantitis)
         Failure of dental implant due to poor oral hygiene
         Iatrogenic post-osseointegration failure of dental implant
         Post-osseointegration failure of dental implant due to complications of systemic disease

     M27.63   Post-osseointegration mechanical failure of dental implant
         Failure of dental prosthesis causing loss of dental implant
         Fracture of dental implant

         Excludes2   cracked tooth (K03.81)
                  fractured dental restorative material with loss of material (K08.531)
                  fractured dental restorative material without loss of material (K08.530)
                  fractured tooth (S02.5)

     M27.69   Other endosseous dental implant failure
         Dental implant failure NOS

M27.8   **Other specified diseases of jaws**
     Cherubism
     Exostosis
     Fibrous dysplasia
     Unilateral condylar hyperplasia
     Unilateral condylar hypoplasia

     Excludes1   jaw pain (R68.84)

M27.9   **Disease of jaws, unspecified**

SYSTEMIC CONNECTIVE TISSUE DISORDERS (M30-M36)

     Includes   autoimmune disease NOS
                collagen (vascular) disease NOS
                systemic autoimmune disease
                systemic collagen (vascular) disease

     Excludes1   autoimmune disease, single organ or single cell-type - code to relevant condition category

● M30   **Polyarteritis nodosa and related conditions**

     Excludes1   microscopic polyarteritis (M31.7)

M30.0   **Polyarteritis nodosa** 🅱

M30.1   **Polyarteritis with lung involvement [Churg-Strauss]** 🅱
     Allergic granulomatous angiitis
     Eosinophilic granulomatosis with polyangiitis [EGPA]
     Coding Clinic: 2021, Q1, P23

M30.2   **Juvenile polyarteritis** 🅱

M30.3   Mucocutaneous lymph node syndrome [Kawasaki] 🅱

M30.8   Other conditions related to polyarteritis nodosa 🅱
     Polyangiitis overlap syndrome

● M31   **Other necrotizing vasculopathies**

M31.0   **Hypersensitivity angiitis** 🅱
     Goodpasture's syndrome

● M31.1   **Thrombotic microangiopathy** 🅱
     ~~Thrombotic thrombocytopenic purpura~~

     ▶ M31.10   Thrombotic microangiopathy, unspecified

     ▶ M31.11   Hematopoietic stem cell transplantation-associated thrombotic microangiopathy [HSCT-TMA]
         ▶ Transplant-associated thrombotic microangiopathy [TA-TMA]

         ▶ *Code first if applicable:*
         ▶ complications of bone marrow transplant (T86.0-)
         ▶ complications of stem cell transplant (T86.5)

         ▶ Use Additional code to identify specific organ dysfunction, such as:
                ▶ acute kidney failure (N17.-)
                ▶ acute respiratory distress syndrome (J80)
                ▶ capillary leak syndrome (I78.8)
                ▶ diffuse alveolar hemorrhage (R04.89)
                ▶ encephalopathy (metabolic) (septic) (G93.41)
                ▶ fluid overload, unspecified (E87.70)
                ▶ graft versus host disease (D89.81-)
                ▶ hemolytic uremic syndrome (D59.3)
                ▶ hepatic failure (K72.-)
                ▶ hepatic veno-occlusive disease (K76.5)
                ▶ idiopathic interstitial pneumonia (J84.11-)
                ▶ sinusoidal obstruction syndrome (K76.5)

     ▶ M31.19   Other thrombotic microangiopathy
         ▶ Thrombotic thrombocytopenic purpura

M31.2   **Lethal midline granuloma** 🅱

● M31.3   **Wegener's granulomatosis**
     Granulomatosis with polyangiitis
     Necrotizing respiratory granulomatosis
     Coding Clinic: 2021, Q1, P23

     M31.30   Wegener's granulomatosis without renal involvement 🅱
         Wegener's granulomatosis NOS
         Coding Clinic: 2021, Q2, P10

     M31.31   Wegener's granulomatosis with renal involvement 🅱

M31.4   **Aortic arch syndrome [Takayasu]** 🅱

M31.5   **Giant cell arteritis with polymyalgia rheumatica** 🅱

M31.6   **Other giant cell arteritis** 🅱

M31.7   **Microscopic polyangiitis** 🅱
     Microscopic polyarteritis

     Excludes1   polyarteritis nodosa (M30.0)
     Coding Clinic: 2021, Q1, P23

M31.8   **Other specified necrotizing vasculopathies** 🅱
     Hypocomplementemic vasculitis
     Septic vasculitis

M31.9   **Necrotizing vasculopathy, unspecified** 🅱

● M32   **Systemic lupus erythematosus (SLE)**
     Autoimmune inflammatory connective tissue disease of unknown cause that occurs most often in women

     Excludes1   lupus erythematosus (discoid) (NOS) (L93.0)

M32.0   **Drug-induced systemic lupus erythematosus** 🅱
     Use additional code for adverse effect, if applicable, to identify drug (T36-T50 with fifth or sixth character 5)

▶ New   ▦ Revised   ~~deleted~~ Deleted   Excludes 1   Excludes 2   Includes   Use additional   Code first   Code also   Key words

OGCR Official Guidelines   X Assign placeholder X   ● Use Additional Character(s)   ▶ Manifestation Code   🅱 Hierarchical Condition Category   **Coding Clinic**

- **M32.1 Systemic lupus erythematosus with organ or system involvement**
  - **M32.10 Systemic lupus erythematosus, organ or system involvement unspecified** 🔗
  - **M32.11 Endocarditis in systemic lupus erythematosus** 🔗
    - Libman-Sacks disease
  - **M32.12 Pericarditis in systemic lupus erythematosus** 🔗
    - Lupus pericarditis
  - **M32.13 Lung involvement in systemic lupus erythematosus** 🔗
    - Pleural effusion due to systemic lupus erythematosus
  - **M32.14 Glomerular disease in systemic lupus erythematosus** 🔗
    - Lupus renal disease NOS
  - **M32.15 Tubulo-interstitial nephropathy in systemic lupus erythematosus** 🔗
  - **M32.19 Other organ or system involvement in systemic lupus erythematosus** 🔗
- **M32.8 Other forms of systemic lupus erythematosus** 🔗
- **M32.9 Systemic lupus erythematosus, unspecified** 🔗
  - SLE NOS
  - Systemic lupus erythematosus NOS
  - Systemic lupus erythematosus without organ involvement

- **M33 Dermatopolymyositis**
  - **M33.0 Juvenile dermatomyositis**
    - **M33.00 Juvenile dermatomyositis, organ involvement unspecified** 🔗
    - **M33.01 Juvenile dermatomyositis with respiratory involvement** 🔗
    - **M33.02 Juvenile dermatomyositis with myopathy** 🔗
    - **M33.03 Juvenile dermatomyositis without myopathy** 🔗
    - **M33.09 Juvenile dermatomyositis with other organ involvement** 🔗
  - **M33.1 Other dermatomyositis**
    - Adult dermatomyositis
    - **M33.10 Other dermatomyositis, organ involvement unspecified** 🔗
    - **M33.11 Other dermatomyositis with respiratory involvement** 🔗
    - **M33.12 Other dermatomyositis with myopathy** 🔗
    - **M33.13 Other dermatomyositis without myopathy** 🔗
      - Dermatomyositis NOS
    - **M33.19 Other dermatomyositis with other organ involvement** 🔗
  - **M33.2 Polymyositis**
    - **M33.20 Polymyositis, organ involvement unspecified** 🔗
    - **M33.21 Polymyositis with respiratory involvement** 🔗
    - **M33.22 Polymyositis with myopathy** 🔗
    - **M33.29 Polymyositis with other organ involvement** 🔗
  - **M33.9 Dermatopolymyositis, unspecified**
    - **M33.90 Dermatopolymyositis, unspecified, organ involvement unspecified** 🔗
    - **M33.91 Dermatopolymyositis, unspecified with respiratory involvement** 🔗
    - **M33.92 Dermatopolymyositis, unspecified with myopathy** 🔗
    - **M33.93 Dermatopolymyositis, unspecified without myopathy** 🔗
    - **M33.99 Dermatopolymyositis, unspecified with other organ involvement** 🔗

- **M34 Systemic sclerosis [scleroderma]**
  - **Excludes1**   circumscribed scleroderma (L94.0)
    - neonatal scleroderma (P83.88)
  - **M34.0 Progressive systemic sclerosis** 🔗

- **M34.1 CR(E)ST syndrome** 🔗
  - Combination of calcinosis, Raynaud's phenomenon, esophageal dysfunction, sclerodactyly, telangiectasia
- **M34.2 Systemic sclerosis induced by drug and chemical** 🔗
  - *Code first poisoning due to drug or toxin, if applicable (T36-T65 with fifth or sixth character 1-4 or 6)*
  - Use additional code for adverse effect, if applicable, to identify drug (T36-T50 with fifth or sixth character 5)
- **M34.8 Other forms of systemic sclerosis**
  - **M34.81 Systemic sclerosis with lung involvement** 🔗
    - ▶Code also if applicable:
      - ▶other interstitial pulmonary diseases (J84.89)
      - ▶secondary pulmonary arterial hypertension (I27.21)
  - **M34.82 Systemic sclerosis with myopathy** 🔗
  - **M34.83 Systemic sclerosis with polyneuropathy** 🔗
  - **M34.89 Other systemic sclerosis** 🔗
- **M34.9 Systemic sclerosis, unspecified** 🔗

- **M35 Other systemic involvement of connective tissue**
  - **Excludes1**   reactive perforating collagenosis (L87.1)
  - ➡➡**M35.0 Sjögren syndrome**
    - ▶Sicca syndrome
    - ▶Use Additional code to identify associated manifestations
    - ▶**Excludes1**   dry mouth, unspecified (R68.2)
    - **M35.00 Sjögren syndrome, unspecified** 🔗
    - **M35.01 Sjögren syndrome with keratoconjunctivitis** 🔗
    - **M35.02 Sjögren syndrome with lung involvement** 🔗
    - **M35.03 Sjögren syndrome with myopathy** 🔗
    - **M35.04 Sjögren syndrome with tubulo-interstitial nephropathy** 🔗
      - Renal tubular acidosis in sicca syndrome
    - ▶**M35.05 Sjögren syndrome with inflammatory arthritis**
    - ▶**M35.06 Sjögren syndrome with peripheral nervous system involvement**
    - ▶**M35.07 Sjögren syndrome with central nervous system involvement**
    - ▶**M35.08 Sjögren syndrome with gastrointestinal involvement**
    - **M35.09 Sjögren syndrome with other organ involvement** 🔗
    - ▶**M35.0A Sjögren syndrome with glomerular disease**
    - ▶**M35.0B Sjögren syndrome with vasculitis**
    - ▶**M35.0C Sjögren syndrome with dental involvement**
  - **M35.1 Other overlap syndromes** 🔗
    - Mixed connective tissue disease
    - **Excludes1**   polyangiitis overlap syndrome (M30.8)
  - **M35.2 Behçet's disease** 🔗
  - **M35.3 Polymyalgia rheumatica** 🔗
    - **Excludes1**   polymyalgia rheumatica with giant cell arteritis (M31.5)
  - **M35.4 Diffuse (eosinophilic) fasciitis**
  - **M35.5 Multifocal fibrosclerosis** 🔗
  - **M35.6 Relapsing panniculitis [Weber-Christian]**
    - **Excludes1**   lupus panniculitis (L93.2)
      - panniculitis NOS (M79.3-)
  - **M35.7 Hypermobility syndrome**
    - Familial ligamentous laxity
    - **Excludes1**   ~~Ehlers-Danlos syndromes (Q79.6-)~~
      - ligamentous laxity, NOS (M24.2-)
    - **Excludes2**   Ehlers-Danlos syndromes (Q79.6-)

Item 13-8 Polymyalgia rheumatica is a syndrome characterized by aching and morning stiffness and is related to aging and hereditary predisposition.

● **M35.8** **Other specified systemic involvement of connective tissue** 🏥
    Coding Clinic: 2021, Q1, P36

    M35.81 **Multisystem inflammatory syndrome**
        MIS-A
        MIS-C
        Multisystem inflammatory syndrome in adults
        Multisystem inflammatory syndrome in children
        Pediatric inflammatory multisystem syndrome
        PIMS

        Code first, if applicable, COVID-19 (U07.1)
        Code also any associated complications such as:
            acute hepatic failure (K72.0-)
            acute kidney failure (N17.-)
            acute myocarditis (I40.-)
            acute respiratory distress syndrome (J80)
            cardiac arrhythmia (I47-I49.-)
            pneumonia due to COVID-19 (J12.82)
            severe sepsis (R65.2-)
            viral cardiomyopathy (B33.24)
            viral pericarditis (B33.23)
        Use additional code, if applicable, for:
            exposure to COVID-19 or SARS-C
            personal history of COVID-19 (Z86.16)
            ~~sequelae of COVID-19 (B94.8)~~
            post COVID-19 condition (U09.9)
        Coding Clinic: 2021, Q1, P36, 42

    M35.89 **Other specified systemic involvement of connective tissue**

● **M35.9** **Systemic involvement of connective tissue, unspecified** 🏥
    Autoimmune disease (systemic) NOS
    Collagen (vascular) disease NOS

● **M36** **Systemic disorders of connective tissue in diseases classified elsewhere**
    Excludes2 arthropathies in diseases classified elsewhere (M14.-)

▷ *M36.0* *Dermato(poly)myositis in neoplastic disease* 🏥
    Code first underlying neoplasm (C00-D49)

▷ *M36.1* *Arthropathy in neoplastic disease*
    Code first underlying neoplasm, such as:
      leukemia (C91-C95)
      malignant histiocytosis (C96.A)
      multiple myeloma (C90.0)

▷ *M36.2* *Hemophilic arthropathy*
    Hemarthrosis in hemophilic arthropathy
    Code first underlying disease, such as:
      factor VIII deficiency (D66)
      with vascular defect (D68.0)
      factor IX deficiency (D67)
      hemophilia (classical) (D66)
      hemophilia B (D67)
      hemophilia C (D68.1)

▷ *M36.3* *Arthropathy in other blood disorders*

▷ *M36.4* *Arthropathy in hypersensitivity reactions classified elsewhere*
    Code first underlying disease, such as:
      Henoch (-Schönlein) purpura (D69.0)
      serum sickness (T80.6-)

▷ *M36.8* *Systemic disorders of connective tissue in other diseases classified elsewhere* 🏥
    Code first underlying disease, such as:
      alkaptonuria (E70.2)
      hypogammaglobulinemia (D80.-)
      ochronosis (E70.2)

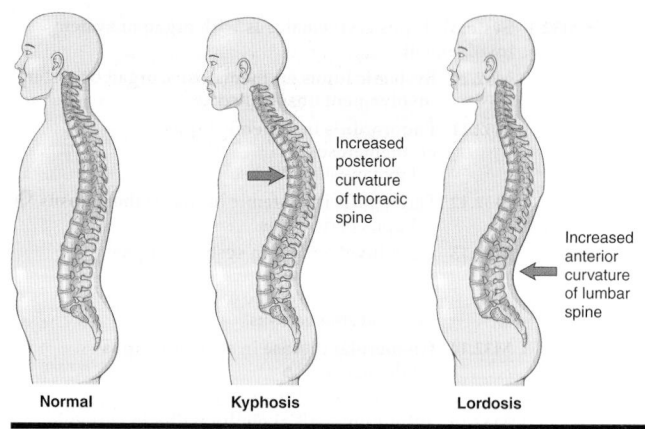

Figure 13-5   Kyphosis, Lordosis, Scoliosis. (From Chabner: The Language of Medicine, ed 8, St. Louis, Saunders, 2007)

Item 13–9 Kyphosis is an abnormal curvature of the spine. **Senile kyphosis** is a result of disc degeneration causing ossification (turning to bone). **Adolescent** or **juvenile** kyphosis is also known as **Scheuermann's disease,** a condition in which the discs of the lower thoracic spine herniate, causing the disc space to narrow and the spine to tilt forward. This condition is attributed to poor posture. **Lordosis or swayback** is an abnormal curvature of the spine resulting in an inward curve of the lumbar spine just above the buttocks. **Scoliosis** causes a sideways curve to the spine. The curves are S- or C-shaped, and it is most commonly acquired in late childhood and early teen years, when growth is fast.

DORSOPATHIES (M40-M54)

DEFORMING DORSOPATHIES (M40-M43)

● **M40** **Kyphosis and lordosis**
    Excludes1 congenital kyphosis and lordosis (Q76.4)
           kyphoscoliosis (M41.-)
           postprocedural kyphosis and lordosis (M96.-)
    ▷ *Code first* underlying disease

● **M40.0** **Postural kyphosis**
    Excludes1 osteochondrosis of spine (M42.-)
    M40.00 Postural kyphosis, site unspecified
    M40.03 Postural kyphosis, cervicothoracic region
    M40.04 Postural kyphosis, thoracic region
    M40.05 Postural kyphosis, thoracolumbar region

● **M40.1** **Other secondary kyphosis**
    M40.10 Other secondary kyphosis, site unspecified
    M40.12 Other secondary kyphosis, cervical region
    M40.13 Other secondary kyphosis, cervicothoracic region
    M40.14 Other secondary kyphosis, thoracic region
    M40.15 Other secondary kyphosis, thoracolumbar region

● **M40.2** **Other and unspecified kyphosis**
  ● **M40.20** **Unspecified kyphosis**
    M40.202 Unspecified kyphosis, cervical region
    M40.203 Unspecified kyphosis, cervicothoracic region
    M40.204 Unspecified kyphosis, thoracic region
    M40.205 Unspecified kyphosis, thoracolumbar region
    M40.209 Unspecified kyphosis, site unspecified
  ● **M40.29** **Other kyphosis**
    M40.292 Other kyphosis, cervical region
    M40.293 Other kyphosis, cervicothoracic region
    M40.294 Other kyphosis, thoracic region
    M40.295 Other kyphosis, thoracolumbar region
    M40.299 Other kyphosis, site unspecified

▶ New   ⇒ Revised   ~~deleted~~ Deleted   Excludes 1   Excludes 2   Includes   Use additional   Code first   Code also   Key words
OGCR Official Guidelines   X Assign placeholder X   ● Use Additional Character(s)   ▷ Manifestation Code   🏥 Hierarchical Condition Category   Coding Clinic

- M40.3 Flatback syndrome
  - M40.30 Flatback syndrome, site unspecified
  - M40.35 Flatback syndrome, thoracolumbar region
  - M40.36 Flatback syndrome, lumbar region
  - M40.37 Flatback syndrome, lumbosacral region
- M40.4 Postural lordosis
  - *Abnormal increase in the normal curvature of the lumbar spine (sway back)*
  - Acquired lordosis
  - M40.40 Postural lordosis, site unspecified
  - M40.45 Postural lordosis, thoracolumbar region
  - M40.46 Postural lordosis, lumbar region
  - M40.47 Postural lordosis, lumbosacral region
- M40.5 Lordosis, unspecified
  - M40.50 Lordosis, unspecified, site unspecified
  - M40.55 Lordosis, unspecified, thoracolumbar region
  - M40.56 Lordosis, unspecified, lumbar region
  - M40.57 Lordosis, unspecified, lumbosacral region
- M41 Scoliosis
  - **Includes** kyphoscoliosis
  - **Excludes1** congenital scoliosis NOS (Q67.5)
    - congenital scoliosis due to bony malformation (Q76.3)
    - postural congenital scoliosis (Q67.5)
    - kyphoscoliotic heart disease (I27.1)
    - ~~postprocedural scoliosis (M96.-)~~
  - ▶ **Excludes2** postprocedural scoliosis (M96.-)
- M41.0 Infantile idiopathic scoliosis
  - M41.00 Infantile idiopathic scoliosis, site unspecified
  - M41.02 Infantile idiopathic scoliosis, cervical region
  - M41.03 Infantile idiopathic scoliosis, cervicothoracic region
  - M41.04 Infantile idiopathic scoliosis, thoracic region
  - M41.05 Infantile idiopathic scoliosis, thoracolumbar region
  - M41.06 Infantile idiopathic scoliosis, lumbar region
  - M41.07 Infantile idiopathic scoliosis, lumbosacral region
  - M41.08 Infantile idiopathic scoliosis, sacral and sacrococcygeal region
- M41.1 Juvenile and adolescent idiopathic scoliosis
  - M41.11 Juvenile idiopathic scoliosis
    - M41.112 Juvenile idiopathic scoliosis, cervical region
    - M41.113 Juvenile idiopathic scoliosis, cervicothoracic region
    - M41.114 Juvenile idiopathic scoliosis, thoracic region
    - M41.115 Juvenile idiopathic scoliosis, thoracolumbar region
    - M41.116 Juvenile idiopathic scoliosis, lumbar region
    - M41.117 Juvenile idiopathic scoliosis, lumbosacral region
    - M41.119 Juvenile idiopathic scoliosis, site unspecified
  - M41.12 Adolescent scoliosis
    - M41.122 Adolescent idiopathic scoliosis, cervical region
    - M41.123 Adolescent idiopathic scoliosis, cervicothoracic region
    - M41.124 Adolescent idiopathic scoliosis, thoracic region
    - M41.125 Adolescent idiopathic scoliosis, thoracolumbar region
    - M41.126 Adolescent idiopathic scoliosis, lumbar region
    - M41.127 Adolescent idiopathic scoliosis, lumbosacral region
    - M41.129 Adolescent idiopathic scoliosis, site unspecified
- M41.2 Other idiopathic scoliosis
  - M41.20 Other idiopathic scoliosis, site unspecified
  - M41.22 Other idiopathic scoliosis, cervical region
  - M41.23 Other idiopathic scoliosis, cervicothoracic region
  - M41.24 Other idiopathic scoliosis, thoracic region
  - M41.25 Other idiopathic scoliosis, thoracolumbar region
  - M41.26 Other idiopathic scoliosis, lumbar region
  - M41.27 Other idiopathic scoliosis, lumbosacral region
- M41.3 Thoracogenic scoliosis
  - M41.30 Thoracogenic scoliosis, site unspecified
  - M41.34 Thoracogenic scoliosis, thoracic region
  - M41.35 Thoracogenic scoliosis, thoracolumbar region
- M41.4 Neuromuscular scoliosis
  - Scoliosis secondary to cerebral palsy, Friedreich's ataxia, poliomyelitis and other neuromuscular disorders
  - Code also underlying condition
  - M41.40 Neuromuscular scoliosis, site unspecified
  - M41.41 Neuromuscular scoliosis, occipito-atlanto-axial region
  - M41.42 Neuromuscular scoliosis, cervical region
  - M41.43 Neuromuscular scoliosis, cervicothoracic region
  - M41.44 Neuromuscular scoliosis, thoracic region
  - M41.45 Neuromuscular scoliosis, thoracolumbar region
  - M41.46 Neuromuscular scoliosis, lumbar region
  - M41.47 Neuromuscular scoliosis, lumbosacral region
- M41.5 Other secondary scoliosis
  - Coding Clinic: 2019, Q1, P19
  - ▶ Code first underlying disease
  - M41.50 Other secondary scoliosis, site unspecified
  - M41.52 Other secondary scoliosis, cervical region
  - M41.53 Other secondary scoliosis, cervicothoracic region
  - M41.54 Other secondary scoliosis, thoracic region
  - M41.55 Other secondary scoliosis, thoracolumbar region
  - M41.56 Other secondary scoliosis, lumbar region
  - M41.57 Other secondary scoliosis, lumbosacral region
- M41.8 Other forms of scoliosis
  - M41.80 Other forms of scoliosis, site unspecified
  - M41.82 Other forms of scoliosis, cervical region
  - M41.83 Other forms of scoliosis, cervicothoracic region
  - M41.84 Other forms of scoliosis, thoracic region
  - M41.85 Other forms of scoliosis, thoracolumbar region
  - M41.86 Other forms of scoliosis, lumbar region
  - M41.87 Other forms of scoliosis, lumbosacral region
- M41.9 Scoliosis, unspecified
- M42 Spinal osteochondrosis
  - M42.0 Juvenile osteochondrosis of spine
    - Calvé's disease
    - Scheuermann's disease
    - **Excludes1** postural kyphosis (M40.0)
    - M42.00 Juvenile osteochondrosis of spine, site unspecified
    - M42.01 Juvenile osteochondrosis of spine, occipito-atlanto-axial region
    - M42.02 Juvenile osteochondrosis of spine, cervical region
    - M42.03 Juvenile osteochondrosis of spine, cervicothoracic region
    - M42.04 Juvenile osteochondrosis of spine, thoracic region

CHAPTER 13 (M00-M99)

M42.05   Juvenile osteochondrosis of spine, thoracolumbar region

M42.06   Juvenile osteochondrosis of spine, lumbar region

M42.07   Juvenile osteochondrosis of spine, lumbosacral region

M42.08   Juvenile osteochondrosis of spine, sacral and sacrococcygeal region

M42.09   Juvenile osteochondrosis of spine, multiple sites in spine

● M42.1   Adult osteochondrosis of spine

M42.10   Adult osteochondrosis of spine, site unspecified   A

M42.11   Adult osteochondrosis of spine, occipitoatlanto-axial region   A

M42.12   Adult osteochondrosis of spine, cervical region   A

M42.13   Adult osteochondrosis of spine, cervicothoracic region   A

M42.14   Adult osteochondrosis of spine, thoracic region   A

M42.15   Adult osteochondrosis of spine, thoracolumbar region   A

M42.16   Adult osteochondrosis of spine, lumbar region   A

M42.17   Adult osteochondrosis of spine, lumbosacral region   A

M42.18   Adult osteochondrosis of spine, sacral and sacrococcygeal region   A

M42.19   Adult osteochondrosis of spine, multiple sites in spine   A

M42.9   Spinal osteochondrosis, unspecified

● M43   Other deforming dorsopathies

Excludes1   congenital spondylolysis and spondylolisthesis (Q76.2)
hemivertebra (Q76.3-Q76.4)
Klippel-Feil syndrome (Q76.1)
lumbarization and sacralization (Q76.4)
platyspondylisis (Q76.4)
spina bifida occulta (Q76.0)
spinal curvature in osteoporosis (M80.-)
spinal curvature in Paget's disease of bone [osteitis deformans] (M88.-)

● M43.0   Spondylolysis

Excludes1   congenital spondylolysis (Q76.2)
spondylolisthesis (M43.1)

M43.00   Spondylolysis, site unspecified

M43.01   Spondylolysis, occipito-atlanto-axial region

M43.02   Spondylolysis, cervical region

M43.03   Spondylolysis, cervicothoracic region

M43.04   Spondylolysis, thoracic region

M43.05   Spondylolysis, thoracolumbar region

M43.06   Spondylolysis, lumbar region

M43.07   Spondylolysis, lumbosacral region

M43.08   Spondylolysis, sacral and sacrococcygeal region

M43.09   Spondylolysis, multiple sites in spine

● M43.1   Spondylolisthesis

Excludes1   acute traumatic of lumbosacral region (S33.1)
acute traumatic of sites other than lumbosacral - code to Fracture, vertebra, by region
congenital spondylolisthesis (Q76.2)

M43.10   Spondylolisthesis, site unspecified

M43.11   Spondylolisthesis, occipito-atlanto-axial region

M43.12   Spondylolisthesis, cervical region

M43.13   Spondylolisthesis, cervicothoracic region

M43.14   Spondylolisthesis, thoracic region

M43.15   Spondylolisthesis, thoracolumbar region

M43.16   Spondylolisthesis, lumbar region

M43.17   Spondylolisthesis, lumbosacral region

M43.18   Spondylolisthesis, sacral and sacrococcygeal region

M43.19   Spondylolisthesis, multiple sites in spine

● M43.2   Fusion of spine
Ankylosis of spinal joint

Excludes1   ankylosing spondylitis (M45.0-)
congenital fusion of spine (Q76.4)

Excludes2   arthrodesis status (Z98.1)
pseudoarthrosis after fusion or arthrodesis (M96.0)

M43.20   Fusion of spine, site unspecified

M43.21   Fusion of spine, occipito-atlanto-axial region

M43.22   Fusion of spine, cervical region

M43.23   Fusion of spine, cervicothoracic region

M43.24   Fusion of spine, thoracic region

M43.25   Fusion of spine, thoracolumbar region

M43.26   Fusion of spine, lumbar region

M43.27   Fusion of spine, lumbosacral region

M43.28   Fusion of spine, sacral and sacrococcygeal region

M43.3   Recurrent atlantoaxial dislocation with myelopathy

M43.4   Other recurrent atlantoaxial dislocation

● M43.5   Other recurrent vertebral dislocation

Excludes1   biomechanical lesions NEC (M99.-)

● M43.5X   Other recurrent vertebral dislocation

M43.5X2   Other recurrent vertebral dislocation, cervical region

M43.5X3   Other recurrent vertebral dislocation, cervicothoracic region

M43.5X4   Other recurrent vertebral dislocation, thoracic region

M43.5X5   Other recurrent vertebral dislocation, thoracolumbar region

M43.5X6   Other recurrent vertebral dislocation, lumbar region

M43.5X7   Other recurrent vertebral dislocation, lumbosacral region

M43.5X8   Other recurrent vertebral dislocation, sacral and sacrococcygeal region

M43.5X9   Other recurrent vertebral dislocation, site unspecified

M43.6   Torticollis

Excludes1   congenital (sternomastoid) torticollis (Q68.0)
current injury - see Injury, of spine, by body region ocular torticollis (R29.891)
psychogenic torticollis (F45.8)
spasmodic torticollis (G24.3)
torticollis due to birth injury (P15.2)

● M43.8   Other specified deforming dorsopathies

Excludes2   kyphosis and lordosis (M40.-)
scoliosis (M41.-)

● M43.8X   Other specified deforming dorsopathies

M43.8X1   Other specified deforming dorsopathies, occipito-atlanto-axial region

M43.8X2   Other specified deforming dorsopathies, cervical region

M43.8X3   Other specified deforming dorsopathies, cervicothoracic region

M43.8X4   Other specified deforming dorsopathies, thoracic region

M43.8X5   Other specified deforming dorsopathies, thoracolumbar region

M43.8X6   Other specified deforming dorsopathies, lumbar region

M43.8X7   Other specified deforming dorsopathies, lumbosacral region

Item 13-10 Spondylolisthesis is a condition caused by the slipping forward of one disc over another.

▶ New   ⟱ Revised   ~~deleted~~ Deleted   Excludes 1   Excludes 2   Includes   Use additional   Code first   Code also   Key words

OGCR Official Guidelines   X Assign placeholder X   ● Use Additional Character(s)   ▌ Manifestation Code   🐧 Hierarchical Condition Category   **Coding Clinic**

M43.8X8   Other specified deforming dorsopathies, sacral and sacrococcygeal region

M43.8X9   Other specified deforming dorsopathies, site unspecified

M43.9   Deforming dorsopathy, unspecified
Curvature of spine NOS

SPONDYLOPATHIES (M45-M49)

● M45   Ankylosing spondylitis
Rheumatoid arthritis of spine

> **Excludes1**   arthropathy in Reiter's disease (M02.3-)
> juvenile (ankylosing) spondylitis (M08.1)

> **Excludes2**   Behçet's disease (M35.2)

M45.0   Ankylosing spondylitis of multiple sites in spine 🔒

M45.1   Ankylosing spondylitis of occipito-atlanto-axial region 🔒

M45.2   Ankylosing spondylitis of cervical region 🔒

M45.3   Ankylosing spondylitis of cervicothoracic region 🔒

M45.4   Ankylosing spondylitis of thoracic region 🔒

M45.5   Ankylosing spondylitis of thoracolumbar region 🔒

M45.6   Ankylosing spondylitis lumbar region 🔒

M45.7   Ankylosing spondylitis of lumbosacral region 🔒

M45.8   Ankylosing spondylitis sacral and sacrococcygeal region 🔒

M45.9   Ankylosing spondylitis of unspecified sites in spine 🔒

▶● M45.A   Non-radiographic axial spondyloarthritis

> ▶ M45.A0   Non-radiographic axial spondyloarthritis of unspecified sites in spine

> ▶ M45.A1   Non-radiographic axial spondyloarthritis of occipito-atlanto-axial region

> ▶ M45.A2   Non-radiographic axial spondyloarthritis of cervical region

> ▶ M45.A3   Non-radiographic axial spondyloarthritis of cervicothoracic region

> ▶ M45.A4   Non-radiographic axial spondyloarthritis of thoracic region

> ▶ M45.A5   Non-radiographic axial spondyloarthritis of thoracolumbar region

> ▶ M45.A6   Non-radiographic axial spondyloarthritis of lumbar region

> ▶ M45.A7   Non-radiographic axial spondyloarthritis of lumbosacral region

> ▶ M45.A8   Non-radiographic axial spondyloarthritis of sacral and sacrococcygeal region

> ▶ M45.AB   Non-radiographic axial spondyloarthritis of multiple sites in spine

● M46   Other inflammatory spondylopathies

● M46.0   Spinal enthesopathy
Disorder of ligamentous or muscular attachments of spine

M46.00   Spinal enthesopathy, site unspecified 🔒

M46.01   Spinal enthesopathy, occipito-atlanto-axial region 🔒

M46.02   Spinal enthesopathy, cervical region 🔒

M46.03   Spinal enthesopathy, cervicothoracic region 🔒

M46.04   Spinal enthesopathy, thoracic region 🔒

M46.05   Spinal enthesopathy, thoracolumbar region 🔒

M46.06   Spinal enthesopathy, lumbar region 🔒

M46.07   Spinal enthesopathy, lumbosacral region 🔒

M46.08   Spinal enthesopathy, sacral and sacrococcygeal region 🔒

M46.09   Spinal enthesopathy, multiple sites in spine 🔒

M46.1   Sacroiliitis, not elsewhere classified 🔒

● M46.2   Osteomyelitis of vertebra

M46.20   Osteomyelitis of vertebra, site unspecified 🔒

M46.21   Osteomyelitis of vertebra, occipito-atlanto-axial region 🔒

M46.22   Osteomyelitis of vertebra, cervical region 🔒

M46.23   Osteomyelitis of vertebra, cervicothoracic region 🔒

M46.24   Osteomyelitis of vertebra, thoracic region 🔒

M46.25   Osteomyelitis of vertebra, thoracolumbar region 🔒

M46.26   Osteomyelitis of vertebra, lumbar region 🔒

M46.27   Osteomyelitis of vertebra, lumbosacral region 🔒

M46.28   Osteomyelitis of vertebra, sacral and sacrococcygeal region 🔒

● M46.3   Infection of intervertebral disc (pyogenic)
Use additional code (B95-B97) to identify infectious agent

M46.30   Infection of intervertebral disc (pyogenic), site unspecified 🔒

M46.31   Infection of intervertebral disc (pyogenic), occipito-atlanto-axial region 🔒

M46.32   Infection of intervertebral disc (pyogenic), cervical region 🔒

M46.33   Infection of intervertebral disc (pyogenic), cervicothoracic region 🔒

M46.34   Infection of intervertebral disc (pyogenic), thoracic region 🔒

M46.35   Infection of intervertebral disc (pyogenic), thoracolumbar region 🔒

M46.36   Infection of intervertebral disc (pyogenic), lumbar region 🔒

M46.37   Infection of intervertebral disc (pyogenic), lumbosacral region 🔒

M46.38   Infection of intervertebral disc (pyogenic), sacral and sacrococcygeal region 🔒

M46.39   Infection of intervertebral disc (pyogenic), multiple sites in spine 🔒

● M46.4   Discitis, unspecified

M46.40   Discitis, unspecified, site unspecified

M46.41   Discitis, unspecified, occipito-atlanto-axial region

M46.42   Discitis, unspecified, cervical region

M46.43   Discitis, unspecified, cervicothoracic region

M46.44   Discitis, unspecified, thoracic region

M46.45   Discitis, unspecified, thoracolumbar region

M46.46   Discitis, unspecified, lumbar region

M46.47   Discitis, unspecified, lumbosacral region

M46.48   Discitis, unspecified, sacral and sacrococcygeal region

M46.49   Discitis, unspecified, multiple sites in spine

● M46.5   Other infective spondylopathies

M46.50   Other infective spondylopathies, site unspecified 🔒

M46.51   Other infective spondylopathies, occipitoatlanto-axial region 🔒

M46.52   Other infective spondylopathies, cervical region 🔒

M46.53   Other infective spondylopathies, cervicothoracic region 🔒

M46.54   Other infective spondylopathies, thoracic region 🔒

M46.55   Other infective spondylopathies, thoracolumbar region 🔒

M46.56   Other infective spondylopathies, lumbar region 🔒

M46.57   Other infective spondylopathies, lumbosacral region 🔒

M46.58   Other infective spondylopathies, sacral and sacrococcygeal region 🔒

M46.59   Other infective spondylopathies, multiple sites in spine 🔒

● M46.8   Other specified inflammatory spondylopathies

M46.80   Other specified inflammatory spondylopathies, site unspecified 🔒

M46.81   Other specified inflammatory spondylopathies, occipito-atlanto-axial region 🔒

M46.82　Other specified inflammatory spondylopathies, cervical region 🦠

M46.83　Other specified inflammatory spondylopathies, cervicothoracic region 🦠

M46.84　Other specified inflammatory spondylopathies, thoracic region 🦠

M46.85　Other specified inflammatory spondylopathies, thoracolumbar region 🦠

M46.86　Other specified inflammatory spondylopathies, lumbar region 🦠

M46.87　Other specified inflammatory spondylopathies, lumbosacral region 🦠

M46.88　Other specified inflammatory spondylopathies, sacral and sacrococcygeal region 🦠

M46.89　Other specified inflammatory spondylopathies, multiple sites in spine 🦠

● M46.9　Unspecified inflammatory spondylopathy

M46.90　Unspecified inflammatory spondylopathy, site unspecified 🦠

M46.91　Unspecified inflammatory spondylopathy, occipito-atlanto-axial region 🦠

M46.92　Unspecified inflammatory spondylopathy, cervical region 🦠
　　　　Coding Clinic: 2019, Q3, P10

M46.93　Unspecified inflammatory spondylopathy, cervicothoracic region 🦠

M46.94　Unspecified inflammatory spondylopathy, thoracic region 🦠

M46.95　Unspecified inflammatory spondylopathy, thoracolumbar region 🦠

M46.96　Unspecified inflammatory spondylopathy, lumbar region 🦠

M46.97　Unspecified inflammatory spondylopathy, lumbosacral region 🦠

M46.98　Unspecified inflammatory spondylopathy, sacral and sacrococcygeal region 🦠

M46.99　Unspecified inflammatory spondylopathy, multiple sites in spine 🦠

● M47　Spondylosis

Includes　arthrosis or osteoarthritis of spine
　　　　　　degeneration of facet joints

● M47.0　Anterior spinal and vertebral artery compression syndromes
　　　　Coding Clinic: 2019, Q3, P10

● M47.01　Anterior spinal artery compression syndromes

M47.011　Anterior spinal artery compression syndromes, occipito-atlanto-axial region

M47.012　Anterior spinal artery compression syndromes, cervical region

M47.013　Anterior spinal artery compression syndromes, cervicothoracic region

M47.014　Anterior spinal artery compression syndromes, thoracic region

M47.015　Anterior spinal artery compression syndromes, thoracolumbar region

M47.016　Anterior spinal artery compression syndromes, lumbar region

M47.019　Anterior spinal artery compression syndromes, site unspecified

● M47.02　Vertebral artery compression syndromes

M47.021　Vertebral artery compression syndromes, occipito-atlanto-axial region

M47.022　Vertebral artery compression syndromes, cervical region

M47.029　Vertebral artery compression syndromes, site unspecified

● M47.1　Other spondylosis with myelopathy
　　　　Spondylogenic compression of spinal cord
　　　　Excludes1　vertebral subluxation (M43.3-M43.5X9)

M47.10　Other spondylosis with myelopathy, site unspecified

M47.11　Other spondylosis with myelopathy, occipito-atlanto-axial region

M47.12　Other spondylosis with myelopathy, cervical region
　　　　Coding Clinic: 2020, Q1, P17

M47.13　Other spondylosis with myelopathy, cervicothoracic region

M47.14　Other spondylosis with myelopathy, thoracic region

M47.15　Other spondylosis with myelopathy, thoracolumbar region

M47.16　Other spondylosis with myelopathy, lumbar region

● M47.2　Other spondylosis with radiculopathy

M47.20　Other spondylosis with radiculopathy, site unspecified

M47.21　Other spondylosis with radiculopathy, occipito-atlanto-axial region

M47.22　Other spondylosis with radiculopathy, cervical region
　　　　Coding Clinic: 2020, Q1, P17

M47.23　Other spondylosis with radiculopathy, cervicothoracic region

M47.24　Other spondylosis with radiculopathy, thoracic region

M47.25　Other spondylosis with radiculopathy, thoracolumbar region

M47.26　Other spondylosis with radiculopathy, lumbar region

M47.27　Other spondylosis with radiculopathy, lumbosacral region

M47.28　Other spondylosis with radiculopathy, sacral and sacrococcygeal region

● M47.8　Other spondylosis

● M47.81　Spondylosis without myelopathy or radiculopathy

M47.811　Spondylosis without myelopathy or radiculopathy, occipito-atlanto-axial region

M47.812　Spondylosis without myelopathy or radiculopathy, cervical region
　　　　　Coding Clinic: 2019, Q3, P10-11; 2018, Q2, P15

M47.813　Spondylosis without myelopathy or radiculopathy, cervicothoracic region

M47.814　Spondylosis without myelopathy or radiculopathy, thoracic region

M47.815　Spondylosis without myelopathy or radiculopathy, thoracolumbar region

M47.816　Spondylosis without myelopathy or radiculopathy, lumbar region

M47.817　Spondylosis without myelopathy or radiculopathy, lumbosacral region

M47.818　Spondylosis without myelopathy or radiculopathy, sacral and sacrococcygeal region

M47.819　Spondylosis without myelopathy or radiculopathy, site unspecified

● M47.89　Other spondylosis

M47.891　Other spondylosis, occipito-atlanto-axial region

M47.892　Other spondylosis, cervical region

M47.893　Other spondylosis, cervicothoracic region

M47.894　Other spondylosis, thoracic region

M47.895　Other spondylosis, thoracolumbar region

▶ New　⇒ Revised　deleted Deleted　Excludes 1　Excludes 2　Includes　Use additional　Code first　Code also　Key words
OGCR Official Guidelines　X Assign placeholder X　● Use Additional Character(s)　▷ Manifestation Code　🦠 Hierarchical Condition Category　Coding Clinic

M47.896 Other spondylosis, lumbar region

M47.897 Other spondylosis, lumbosacral region

M47.898 Other spondylosis, sacral and sacrococcygeal region

M47.899 Other spondylosis, site unspecified

M47.9 Spondylosis, unspecified

● M48 Other spondylopathies

  ● M48.0 Spinal stenosis
    Caudal stenosis

M48.00 Spinal stenosis, site unspecified

M48.01 Spinal stenosis, occipito-atlanto-axial region

M48.02 Spinal stenosis, cervical region
    Coding Clinic: 2020, Q1, P17

M48.03 Spinal stenosis, cervicothoracic region

M48.04 Spinal stenosis, thoracic region

M48.05 Spinal stenosis, thoracolumbar region

  ● M48.06 Spinal stenosis, lumbar region
    Coding Clinic: 2017, Q3, P24

M48.061 Spinal stenosis, lumbar region without neurogenic claudication
    Spinal stenosis, lumbar region NOS

M48.062 Spinal stenosis, lumbar region with neurogenic claudication
    Coding Clinic: 2017, Q4, P19

M48.07 Spinal stenosis, lumbosacral region

M48.08 Spinal stenosis, sacral and sacrococcygeal region

  ● M48.1 Ankylosing hyperostosis [Forestier]
    Diffuse idiopathic skeletal hyperostosis [DISH]

M48.10 Ankylosing hyperostosis [Forestier], site unspecified

M48.11 Ankylosing hyperostosis [Forestier], occipito-atlanto-axial region

M48.12 Ankylosing hyperostosis [Forestier], cervical region

M48.13 Ankylosing hyperostosis [Forestier], cervicothoracic region

M48.14 Ankylosing hyperostosis [Forestier], thoracic region

M48.15 Ankylosing hyperostosis [Forestier], thoracolumbar region

M48.16 Ankylosing hyperostosis [Forestier], lumbar region

M48.17 Ankylosing hyperostosis [Forestier], lumbosacral region

M48.18 Ankylosing hyperostosis [Forestier], sacral and sacrococcygeal region

M48.19 Ankylosing hyperostosis [Forestier], multiple sites in spine

  ● M48.2 Kissing spine

M48.20 Kissing spine, site unspecified

M48.21 Kissing spine, occipito-atlanto-axial region

M48.22 Kissing spine, cervical region

M48.23 Kissing spine, cervicothoracic region

M48.24 Kissing spine, thoracic region

M48.25 Kissing spine, thoracolumbar region

M48.26 Kissing spine, lumbar region

M48.27 Kissing spine, lumbosacral region

  ● M48.3 Traumatic spondylopathy

M48.30 Traumatic spondylopathy, site unspecified

M48.31 Traumatic spondylopathy, occipito-atlanto-axial region

M48.32 Traumatic spondylopathy, cervical region

M48.33 Traumatic spondylopathy, cervicothoracic region

M48.34 Traumatic spondylopathy, thoracic region

M48.35 Traumatic spondylopathy, thoracolumbar region

M48.36 Traumatic spondylopathy, lumbar region

M48.37 Traumatic spondylopathy, lumbosacral region

M48.38 Traumatic spondylopathy, sacral and sacrococcygeal region

● M48.4 Fatigue fracture of vertebra
  Stress fracture of vertebra

> **Excludes1** pathological fracture NOS (M84.4-)
> pathological fracture of vertebra due to neoplasm (M84.58)
> pathological fracture of vertebra due to other diagnosis (M84.68)
> pathological fracture of vertebra due to osteoporosis (M80.-)
> traumatic fracture of vertebrae (S12.0-S12.3-, S22.0-, S32.0-)

The appropriate 7th character is to be added to each code from subcategory M48.4:

> A   initial encounter for fracture
> D   subsequent encounter for fracture with routine healing
> G   subsequent encounter for fracture with delayed healing
> S   sequela of fracture

X ● M48.40 Fatigue fracture of vertebra, site unspecified

X ● M48.41 Fatigue fracture of vertebra, occipitoatlanto-axial region

X ● M48.42 Fatigue fracture of vertebra, cervical region

X ● M48.43 Fatigue fracture of vertebra, cervicothoracic region

X ● M48.44 Fatigue fracture of vertebra, thoracic region

X ● M48.45 Fatigue fracture of vertebra, thoracolumbar region

X ● M48.46 Fatigue fracture of vertebra, lumbar region

X ● M48.47 Fatigue fracture of vertebra, lumbosacral region

X ● M48.48 Fatigue fracture of vertebra, sacral and sacrococcygeal region

● M48.5 Collapsed vertebra, not elsewhere classified
  Collapsed vertebra NOS
  Compression fracture of vertebra NOS
  Wedging of vertebra NOS

> **Excludes1** current injury - see Injury of spine, by body region
> fatigue fracture of vertebra (M48.4)
> pathological fracture of vertebra due to neoplasm (M84.58)
> pathological fracture of vertebra due to other diagnosis (M84.68)
> pathological fracture of vertebra due to osteoporosis (M80.-)
> pathological fracture NOS (M84.4-)
> stress fracture of vertebra (M48.4-)
> traumatic fracture of vertebra (S12.-, S22.-, S32.-)

The appropriate 7th character is to be added to each code from subcategory M48.5:

> A   initial encounter for fracture
> D   subsequent encounter for fracture with routine healing
> G   subsequent encounter for fracture with delayed healing
> S   sequela of fracture

X ● M48.50 Collapsed vertebra, not elsewhere classified, site unspecified A 🔒

X ● M48.51 Collapsed vertebra, not elsewhere classified, occipito-atlanto-axial region A 🔒

X ● M48.52 Collapsed vertebra, not elsewhere classified, cervical region A 🔒

X ● M48.53 Collapsed vertebra, not elsewhere classified, cervicothoracic region A 🔒

CHAPTER 13 (M00-M99)

X ● M48.54 Collapsed vertebra, not elsewhere classified, thoracic region A 🐾

X ● M48.55 Collapsed vertebra, not elsewhere classified, thoracolumbar region A 🐾

X ● M48.56 Collapsed vertebra, not elsewhere classified, lumbar region A 🐾

X ● M48.57 Collapsed vertebra, not elsewhere classified, lumbosacral region A 🐾

X ● M48.58 Collapsed vertebra, not elsewhere classified, sacral and sacrococcygeal region A 🐾

● M48.8 Other specified spondylopathies
　　　Ossification of posterior longitudinal ligament

　● M48.8X Other specified spondylopathies

　　　M48.8X1 Other specified spondylopathies, occipito-atlanto-axial region 🐾

　　　M48.8X2 Other specified spondylopathies, cervical region 🐾

　　　M48.8X3 Other specified spondylopathies, cervicothoracic region 🐾

　　　M48.8X4 Other specified spondylopathies, thoracic region 🐾

　　　M48.8X5 Other specified spondylopathies, thoracolumbar region 🐾

　　　M48.8X6 Other specified spondylopathies, lumbar region 🐾

　　　M48.8X7 Other specified spondylopathies, lumbosacral region 🐾

　　　M48.8X8 Other specified spondylopathies, sacral and sacrococcygeal region 🐾

　　　M48.8X9 Other specified spondylopathies, site unspecified 🐾

M48.9 Spondylopathy, unspecified

● M49 Spondylopathies in diseases classified elsewhere

　Includes   curvature of spine in diseases classified elsewhere
　　　　　　deformity of spine in diseases classified elsewhere
　　　　　　kyphosis in diseases classified elsewhere
　　　　　　scoliosis in diseases classified elsewhere
　　　　　　spondylopathy in diseases classified elsewhere

　Code first underlying disease, such as:
　　　brucellosis (A23.-)
　　　Charcot-Marie-Tooth disease (G60.0)
　　　enterobacterial infections (A01-A04)
　　　osteitis fibrosa cystica (E21.0)

　Excludes1   curvature of spine in tuberculosis [Pott's] (A18.01)
　　　　　　enteropathic arthropathies (M07.-)
　　　　　　gonococcal spondylitis (A54.41)
　　　　　　neuropathic [tabes dorsalis] spondylitis (A52.11)
　　　　　　neuropathic spondylopathy in syringomyelia (G95.0)
　　　　　　neuropathic spondylopathy in tabes dorsalis (A52.11)
　　　　　　nonsyphilitic neuropathic spondylopathy NEC (G98.0)
　　　　　　spondylitis in syphilis (acquired) (A52.77)
　　　　　　tuberculous spondylitis (A18.01)
　　　　　　typhoid fever spondylitis (A01.05)

● M49.8 Spondylopathy in diseases classified elsewhere

　▌ M49.80 Spondylopathy in diseases classified elsewhere, site unspecified 🐾

　▌ M49.81 Spondylopathy in diseases classified elsewhere, occipito-atlanto-axial region 🐾

　▌ M49.82 Spondylopathy in diseases classified elsewhere, cervical region 🐾

　▌ M49.83 Spondylopathy in diseases classified elsewhere, cervicothoracic region 🐾

　▌ M49.84 Spondylopathy in diseases classified elsewhere, thoracic region 🐾

　▌ M49.85 Spondylopathy in diseases classified elsewhere, thoracolumbar region 🐾

　▌ M49.86 Spondylopathy in diseases classified elsewhere, lumbar region 🐾

　▌ M49.87 Spondylopathy in diseases classified elsewhere, lumbosacral region 🐾

　▌ M49.88 Spondylopathy in diseases classified elsewhere, sacral and sacrococcygeal region 🐾

　▌ M49.89 Spondylopathy in diseases classified elsewhere, multiple sites in spine 🐾

OTHER DORSOPATHIES (M50-M54)

Excludes1   current injury - see injury of spine by body region
　　　　　　discitis NOS (M46.4-)

● M50 Cervical disc disorders
　Note: Code to the most superior level of disorder.
　Includes   cervicothoracic disc disorders with cervicalgia
　　　　　　cervicothoracic disc disorders
　Coding Clinic: 2016, Q1, P17

● M50.0 Cervical disc disorder with myelopathy

　　M50.00 Cervical disc disorder with myelopathy, unspecified cervical region

　　M50.01 Cervical disc disorder with myelopathy, high cervical region
　　　　　C2-C3 disc disorder with myelopathy
　　　　　C3-C4 disc disorder with myelopathy
　　　　　Coding Clinic: 2016, Q1, P17

　● M50.02 Cervical disc disorder with myelopathy, mid-cervical region
　　　　　Coding Clinic: 2016, Q4, P39-40

　　　M50.020 Cervical disc disorder with myelopathy, mid-cervical region, unspecified level

　　　M50.021 Cervical disc disorder at C4-C5 level with myelopathy
　　　　　　C4-C5 disc disorder with myelopathy

　　　M50.022 Cervical disc disorder at C5-C6 level with myelopathy
　　　　　　C5-C6 disc disorder with myelopathy

　　　M50.023 Cervical disc disorder at C6-C7 level with myelopathy
　　　　　　C6-C7 disc disorder with myelopathy

　　M50.03 Cervical disc disorder with myelopathy, cervicothoracic region
　　　　　C7-T1 disc disorder with myelopathy

● M50.1 Cervical disc disorder with radiculopathy

　Excludes2   brachial radiculitis NOS (M54.13)

　　M50.10 Cervical disc disorder with radiculopathy, unspecified cervical region

　　M50.11 Cervical disc disorder with radiculopathy, high cervical region
　　　　　C2-C3 disc disorder with radiculopathy
　　　　　C3 radiculopathy due to disc disorder
　　　　　C3-C4 disc disorder with radiculopathy
　　　　　C4 radiculopathy due to disc disorder

　● M50.12 Cervical disc disorder with radiculopathy, mid-cervical region
　　　　　Coding Clinic: 2016, Q4, P39-40

　　　M50.120 Mid-cervical disc disorder, unspecified level

　　　M50.121 Cervical disc disorder at C4-C5 level with radiculopathy
　　　　　　C4-C5 disc disorder with radiculopathy
　　　　　　C5 radiculopathy due to disc disorder

　　　M50.122 Cervical disc disorder at C5-C6 level with radiculopathy
　　　　　　C5-C6 disc disorder with radiculopathy
　　　　　　C6 radiculopathy due to disc disorder

▶ New   ⇒ Revised   ~~deleted~~ Deleted   Excludes 1   Excludes 2   Includes   Use additional   Code first   Code also   Key words

OGCR Official Guidelines   X Assign placeholder X   ● Use Additional Character(s)   ▌ Manifestation Code   🐾 Hierarchical Condition Category   Coding Clinic

M50.123 **Cervical disc disorder at C6-C7 level with radiculopathy**
C6-C7 disc disorder with radiculopathy
C7 radiculopathy due to disc disorder

M50.13 **Cervical disc disorder with radiculopathy, cervicothoracic region**
C7-T1 disc disorder with radiculopathy
C8 radiculopathy due to disc disorder

● M50.2 **Other cervical disc displacement**
Coding Clinic: 2016, Q4, P40

M50.20 **Other cervical disc displacement, unspecified cervical region**

M50.21 **Other cervical disc displacement, high cervical region**
Other C2-C3 cervical disc displacement
Other C3-C4 cervical disc displacement

● M50.22 **Other cervical disc displacement, mid-cervical region**

M50.220 **Other cervical disc displacement, mid-cervical region, unspecified level**

M50.221 **Other cervical disc displacement at C4-C5 level**
Other C4-C5 cervical disc displacement

M50.222 **Other cervical disc displacement at C5-C6 level**
Other C5-C6 cervical disc displacement

M50.223 **Other cervical disc displacement at C6-C7 level**
Other C6-C7 cervical disc displacement

M50.23 **Other cervical disc displacement, cervicothoracic region**
Other C7-T1 cervical disc displacement

● M50.3 **Other cervical disc degeneration**
Coding Clinic: 2016, Q4, P40

M50.30 **Other cervical disc degeneration, unspecified cervical region**

M50.31 **Other cervical disc degeneration, high cervical region**
Other C2-C3 cervical disc degeneration
Other C3-C4 cervical disc degeneration

● M50.32 **Other cervical disc degeneration, mid-cervical region**

M50.320 **Other cervical disc degeneration, mid-cervical region, unspecified level**

M50.321 **Other cervical disc degeneration at C4-C5 level**
Other C4-C5 cervical disc degeneration

M50.322 **Other cervical disc degeneration at C5-C6 level**
Other C5-C6 cervical disc degeneration

M50.323 **Other cervical disc degeneration at C6-C7 level**
Other C6-C7 cervical disc degeneration

M50.33 **Other cervical disc degeneration, cervicothoracic region**
Other C7-T1 cervical disc degeneration

● M50.8 **Other cervical disc disorders**
Coding Clinic: 2016, Q4, P40

M50.80 **Other cervical disc disorders, unspecified cervical region**

M50.81 **Other cervical disc disorders, high cervical region**
Other C2-C3 cervical disc disorders
Other C3-C4 cervical disc disorders

● M50.82 **Other cervical disc disorders, mid-cervical region**

M50.820 **Other cervical disc disorders, mid-cervical region, unspecified level**

M50.821 **Other cervical disc disorders at C4-C5 level**
Other C4-C5 cervical disc disorders

M50.822 **Other cervical disc disorders at C5-C6 level**
Other C5-C6 cervical disc disorders

M50.823 **Other cervical disc disorders at C6-C7 level**
Other C6-C7 cervical disc disorders

M50.83 **Other cervical disc disorders, cervicothoracic region**
Other C7-T1 cervical disc disorders

● M50.9 **Cervical disc disorder, unspecified**
Coding Clinic: 2016, Q4, P40

M50.90 **Cervical disc disorder, unspecified, unspecified cervical region**

M50.91 **Cervical disc disorder, unspecified, high cervical region**
C2-C3 cervical disc disorder, unspecified
C3-C4 cervical disc disorder, unspecified

● M50.92 **Cervical disc disorder, unspecified, mid-cervical region**

M50.920 **Unspecified cervical disc disorder, mid-cervical region, unspecified level**

M50.921 **Unspecified cervical disc disorder at C4-C5 level**
Unspecified C4-C5 cervical disc disorder

M50.922 **Unspecified cervical disc disorder at C5-C6 level**
Unspecified C5-C6 cervical disc disorder

M50.923 **Unspecified cervical disc disorder at C6-C7 level**
Unspecified C6-C7 cervical disc disorder

M50.93 **Cervical disc disorder, unspecified, cervicothoracic region**
C7-T1 cervical disc disorder, unspecified

● M51 **Thoracic, thoracolumbar, and lumbosacral intervertebral disc disorders**

Excludes2 cervical and cervicothoracic disc disorders (M50.-)
sacral and sacrococcygeal disorders (M53.3)

● M51.0 **Thoracic, thoracolumbar and lumbosacral intervertebral disc disorders with myelopathy**

M51.04 **Intervertebral disc disorders with myelopathy, thoracic region**

M51.05 **Intervertebral disc disorders with myelopathy, thoracolumbar region**

M51.06 **Intervertebral disc disorders with myelopathy, lumbar region**

● M51.1 **Thoracic, thoracolumbar and lumbosacral intervertebral disc disorders with radiculopathy**
Sciatica due to intervertebral disc disorder

Excludes1 lumbar radiculitis NOS (M54.16)
sciatica NOS (M54.3)

M51.14 **Intervertebral disc disorders with radiculopathy, thoracic region**

M51.15 **Intervertebral disc disorders with radiculopathy, thoracolumbar region**

M51.16 **Intervertebral disc disorders with radiculopathy, lumbar region**

M51.17 **Intervertebral disc disorders with radiculopathy, lumbosacral region**

CHAPTER 13 (M00-M99)

● **M51.2 Other thoracic, thoracolumbar and lumbosacral intervertebral disc displacement**
   Lumbago due to displacement of intervertebral disc

   M51.24 Other intervertebral disc displacement, thoracic region

   M51.25 Other intervertebral disc displacement, thoracolumbar region

   M51.26 Other intervertebral disc displacement, lumbar region

   M51.27 Other intervertebral disc displacement, lumbosacral region

● **M51.3 Other thoracic, thoracolumbar and lumbosacral intervertebral disc degeneration**
   Coding Clinic: 2013, Q3, P22

   M51.34 Other intervertebral disc degeneration, thoracic region

   M51.35 Other intervertebral disc degeneration, thoracolumbar region

   M51.36 Other intervertebral disc degeneration, lumbar region
   Coding Clinic: 2018, Q2, P15

   M51.37 Other intervertebral disc degeneration, lumbosacral region

● **M51.4 Schmorl's nodes**

   M51.44 Schmorl's nodes, thoracic region

   M51.45 Schmorl's nodes, thoracolumbar region

   M51.46 Schmorl's nodes, lumbar region

   M51.47 Schmorl's nodes, lumbosacral region

● **M51.8 Other thoracic, thoracolumbar and lumbosacral intervertebral disc disorders**

   M51.84 Other intervertebral disc disorders, thoracic region

   M51.85 Other intervertebral disc disorders, thoracolumbar region

   M51.86 Other intervertebral disc disorders, lumbar region

   M51.87 Other intervertebral disc disorders, lumbosacral region

   M51.9 Unspecified thoracic, thoracolumbar and lumbosacral intervertebral disc disorder

● **M53 Other and unspecified dorsopathies, not elsewhere classified**

   M53.0 Cervicocranial syndrome
      Posterior cervical sympathetic syndrome

   M53.1 Cervicobrachial syndrome

      Excludes2 cervical disc disorder (M50.-)
                     thoracic outlet syndrome (G54.0)

● **M53.2 Spinal instabilities**

   ● **M53.2X Spinal instabilities**

      M53.2X1 Spinal instabilities, occipito-atlanto-axial region

      M53.2X2 Spinal instabilities, cervical region

      M53.2X3 Spinal instabilities, cervicothoracic region

      M53.2X4 Spinal instabilities, thoracic region

      M53.2X5 Spinal instabilities, thoracolumbar region

      M53.2X6 Spinal instabilities, lumbar region

      M53.2X7 Spinal instabilities, lumbosacral region

      M53.2X8 Spinal instabilities, sacral and sacrococcygeal region

      M53.2X9 Spinal instabilities, site unspecified

   M53.3 Sacrococcygeal disorders, not elsewhere classified
      Coccygodynia

● **M53.8 Other specified dorsopathies**

   M53.80 Other specified dorsopathies, site unspecified

   M53.81 Other specified dorsopathies, occipito-atlanto-axial region

   M53.82 Other specified dorsopathies, cervical region

   M53.83 Other specified dorsopathies, cervicothoracic region

   M53.84 Other specified dorsopathies, thoracic region

   M53.85 Other specified dorsopathies, thoracolumbar region

   M53.86 Other specified dorsopathies, lumbar region

   M53.87 Other specified dorsopathies, lumbosacral region

   M53.88 Other specified dorsopathies, sacral and sacrococcygeal region

   M53.9 Dorsopathy, unspecified

● **M54 Dorsalgia**

   Excludes1 psychogenic dorsalgia (F45.41)

● **M54.0 Panniculitis affecting regions of neck and back**

   Excludes1 lupus panniculitis (L93.2)
                  panniculitis NOS (M79.3)
                  relapsing [Weber-Christian] panniculitis (M35.6)

   M54.00 Panniculitis affecting regions of neck and back, site unspecified

   M54.01 Panniculitis affecting regions of neck and back, occipito-atlanto-axial region

   M54.02 Panniculitis affecting regions of neck and back, cervical region

   M54.03 Panniculitis affecting regions of neck and back, cervicothoracic region

   M54.04 Panniculitis affecting regions of neck and back, thoracic region

   M54.05 Panniculitis affecting regions of neck and back, thoracolumbar region

   M54.06 Panniculitis affecting regions of neck and back, lumbar region

   M54.07 Panniculitis affecting regions of neck and back, lumbosacral region

   M54.08 Panniculitis affecting regions of neck and back, sacral and sacrococcygeal region

   M54.09 Panniculitis affecting regions, neck and back, multiple sites in spine

● **M54.1 Radiculopathy**
   Brachial neuritis or radiculitis NOS
   Lumbar neuritis or radiculitis NOS
   Lumbosacral neuritis or radiculitis NOS
   Thoracic neuritis or radiculitis NOS
   Radiculitis NOS

   Excludes1 neuralgia and neuritis NOS (M79.2)
                  radiculopathy with cervical disc disorder (M50.1)
                  radiculopathy with lumbar and other intervertebral disc disorder (M51.1-)
                  radiculopathy with spondylosis (M47.2-)

   M54.10 Radiculopathy, site unspecified

   M54.11 Radiculopathy, occipito-atlanto-axial region

   M54.12 Radiculopathy, cervical region

   M54.13 Radiculopathy, cervicothoracic region

   M54.14 Radiculopathy, thoracic region

   M54.15 Radiculopathy, thoracolumbar region

   M54.16 Radiculopathy, lumbar region

   M54.17 Radiculopathy, lumbosacral region

   M54.18 Radiculopathy, sacral and sacrococcygeal region

   M54.2 Cervicalgia

      Excludes1 cervicalgia due to intervertebral cervical disc disorder (M50.-)

● **M54.3 Sciatica**

      Excludes1 lesion of sciatic nerve (G57.0)
                     sciatica due to intervertebral disc disorder (M51.1-)
                     sciatica with lumbago (M54.4-)

   M54.30 Sciatica, unspecified side

   M54.31 Sciatica, right side

   M54.32 Sciatica, left side

▶ New   ⇒ Revised   ~~deleted~~ Deleted   Excludes 1   Excludes 2   Includes   Use additional   Code first   Code also   Key words

OGCR Official Guidelines   X Assign placeholder X   ● Use Additional Character(s)   ▌ Manifestation Code   🔍 Hierarchical Condition Category   Coding Clinic

● M54.4 Lumbago with sciatica
  Excludes1 lumbago with sciatica due to intervertebral disc disorder (M51.1-)
  M54.40 Lumbago with sciatica, unspecified side
  M54.41 Lumbago with sciatica, right side
  M54.42 Lumbago with sciatica, left side
    Coding Clinic: 2016, Q2, P7
● M54.5 Low back pain
  ~~Loin pain~~
  ~~Lumbago NOS~~
  Excludes1 low back strain (S39.012)
    lumbago due to intervertebral disc displacement (M51.2-)
    lumbago with sciatica (M54.4-)
  ▶ M54.50 Low back pain, unspecified
    ▶ Loin pain
    ▶ Lumbago NOS
  ▶ M54.51 Vertebrogenic low back pain
    ▶ Low back vertebral endplate pain
  ▶ M54.59 Other low back pain
  M54.6 Pain in thoracic spine
    Excludes1 pain in thoracic spine due to intervertebral disc disorder (M51.)
● M54.8 Other dorsalgia
    Excludes1 dorsalgia in thoracic region (M54.6)
      ▶ low back pain (M54.5-)
  M54.81 Occipital neuralgia
  M54.89 Other dorsalgia
  M54.9 Dorsalgia, unspecified
    Backache NOS
    Back pain NOS

SOFT TISSUE DISORDERS (M60-M79)

DISORDERS OF MUSCLES (M60-M63)

  Excludes1 dermatopolymyositis (M33.-)
    muscular dystrophies and myopathies (G71-G72)
    myopathy in amyloidosis (E85.-)
    myopathy in polyarteritis nodosa (M30.0)
    myopathy in rheumatoid arthritis (M05.32)
    myopathy in scleroderma (M34.-)
    myopathy in Sjögren's syndrome (M35.03)
    myopathy in systemic lupus erythematosus (M32.-)

● M60 Myositis
  Excludes2 inclusion body myositis [IBM] (G72.41)
● M60.0 Infective myositis
    Tropical pyomyositis
    Use additional code (B95-B97) to identify infectious agent
  ● M60.00 Infective myositis, unspecified site
    M60.000 Infective myositis, unspecified right arm
      Infective myositis, right upper limb NOS
    M60.001 Infective myositis, unspecified left arm
      Infective myositis, left upper limb NOS
    M60.002 Infective myositis, unspecified arm
      Infective myositis, upper limb NOS
    M60.003 Infective myositis, unspecified right leg
      Infective myositis, right lower limb NOS
    M60.004 Infective myositis, unspecified left leg
      Infective myositis, left lower limb NOS

    M60.005 Infective myositis, unspecified leg
      Infective myositis, lower limb NOS
    M60.009 Infective myositis, unspecified site
  ● M60.01 Infective myositis, shoulder
    M60.011 Infective myositis, right shoulder
    M60.012 Infective myositis, left shoulder
    M60.019 Infective myositis, unspecified shoulder
  ● M60.02 Infective myositis, upper arm
    M60.021 Infective myositis, right upper arm
    M60.022 Infective myositis, left upper arm
    M60.029 Infective myositis, unspecified upper arm
  ● M60.03 Infective myositis, forearm
    M60.031 Infective myositis, right forearm
    M60.032 Infective myositis, left forearm
    M60.039 Infective myositis, unspecified forearm
  ● M60.04 Infective myositis, hand and fingers
    M60.041 Infective myositis, right hand
    M60.042 Infective myositis, left hand
    M60.043 Infective myositis, unspecified hand
    M60.044 Infective myositis, right finger(s)
    M60.045 Infective myositis, left finger(s)
    M60.046 Infective myositis, unspecified finger(s)
  ● M60.05 Infective myositis, thigh
    M60.051 Infective myositis, right thigh
    M60.052 Infective myositis, left thigh
    M60.059 Infective myositis, unspecified thigh
  ● M60.06 Infective myositis, lower leg
    M60.061 Infective myositis, right lower leg
    M60.062 Infective myositis, left lower leg
    M60.069 Infective myositis, unspecified lower leg
  ● M60.07 Infective myositis, ankle, foot and toes
    M60.070 Infective myositis, right ankle
    M60.071 Infective myositis, left ankle
    M60.072 Infective myositis, unspecified ankle
    M60.073 Infective myositis, right foot
    M60.074 Infective myositis, left foot
    M60.075 Infective myositis, unspecified foot
    M60.076 Infective myositis, right toe(s)
    M60.077 Infective myositis, left toe(s)
    M60.078 Infective myositis, unspecified toe(s)
  M60.08 Infective myositis, other site
  M60.09 Infective myositis, multiple sites
● M60.1 Interstitial myositis
  M60.10 Interstitial myositis of unspecified site
  ● M60.11 Interstitial myositis, shoulder
    M60.111 Interstitial myositis, right shoulder
    M60.112 Interstitial myositis, left shoulder
    M60.119 Interstitial myositis, unspecified shoulder
  ● M60.12 Interstitial myositis, upper arm
    M60.121 Interstitial myositis, right upper arm
    M60.122 Interstitial myositis, left upper arm
    M60.129 Interstitial myositis, unspecified upper arm
  ● M60.13 Interstitial myositis, forearm
    M60.131 Interstitial myositis, right forearm
    M60.132 Interstitial myositis, left forearm
    M60.139 Interstitial myositis, unspecified forearm
  ● M60.14 Interstitial myositis, hand
    M60.141 Interstitial myositis, right hand

M60.142   Interstitial myositis, left hand
M60.149   Interstitial myositis, unspecified hand
● M60.15   Interstitial myositis, thigh
M60.151   Interstitial myositis, right thigh
M60.152   Interstitial myositis, left thigh
M60.159   Interstitial myositis, unspecified thigh
● M60.16   Interstitial myositis, lower leg
M60.161   Interstitial myositis, right lower leg
M60.162   Interstitial myositis, left lower leg
M60.169   Interstitial myositis, unspecified lower leg
● M60.17   Interstitial myositis, ankle and foot
M60.171   Interstitial myositis, right ankle and foot
M60.172   Interstitial myositis, left ankle and foot
M60.179   Interstitial myositis, unspecified ankle and foot
M60.18   Interstitial myositis, other site
M60.19   Interstitial myositis, multiple sites
● M60.2   Foreign body granuloma of soft tissue, not elsewhere classified

Use additional code to identify the type of retained foreign body (Z18.-)

Excludes1   foreign body granuloma of skin and subcutaneous tissue (L92.3)

M60.20   Foreign body granuloma of soft tissue, not elsewhere classified, unspecified site
● M60.21   Foreign body granuloma of soft tissue, not elsewhere classified, shoulder
M60.211   Foreign body granuloma of soft tissue, not elsewhere classified, right shoulder
M60.212   Foreign body granuloma of soft tissue, not elsewhere classified, left shoulder
M60.219   Foreign body granuloma of soft tissue, not elsewhere classified, unspecified shoulder
● M60.22   Foreign body granuloma of soft tissue, not elsewhere classified, upper arm
M60.221   Foreign body granuloma of soft tissue, not elsewhere classified, right upper arm
M60.222   Foreign body granuloma of soft tissue, not elsewhere classified, left upper arm
M60.229   Foreign body granuloma of soft tissue, not elsewhere classified, unspecified upper arm
● M60.23   Foreign body granuloma of soft tissue, not elsewhere classified, forearm
M60.231   Foreign body granuloma of soft tissue, not elsewhere classified, right forearm
M60.232   Foreign body granuloma of soft tissue, not elsewhere classified, left forearm
M60.239   Foreign body granuloma of soft tissue, not elsewhere classified, unspecified forearm
● M60.24   Foreign body granuloma of soft tissue, not elsewhere classified, hand
M60.241   Foreign body granuloma of soft tissue, not elsewhere classified, right hand
M60.242   Foreign body granuloma of soft tissue, not elsewhere classified, left hand
M60.249   Foreign body granuloma of soft tissue, not elsewhere classified, unspecified hand

● M60.25   Foreign body granuloma of soft tissue, not elsewhere classified, thigh
M60.251   Foreign body granuloma of soft tissue, not elsewhere classified, right thigh
M60.252   Foreign body granuloma of soft tissue, not elsewhere classified, left thigh
M60.259   Foreign body granuloma of soft tissue, not elsewhere classified, unspecified thigh
● M60.26   Foreign body granuloma of soft tissue, not elsewhere classified, lower leg
M60.261   Foreign body granuloma of soft tissue, not elsewhere classified, right lower leg
M60.262   Foreign body granuloma of soft tissue, not elsewhere classified, left lower leg
M60.269   Foreign body granuloma of soft tissue, not elsewhere classified, unspecified lower leg
● M60.27   Foreign body granuloma of soft tissue, not elsewhere classified, ankle and foot
M60.271   Foreign body granuloma of soft tissue, not elsewhere classified, right ankle and foot
M60.272   Foreign body granuloma of soft tissue, not elsewhere classified, left ankle and foot
M60.279   Foreign body granuloma of soft tissue, not elsewhere classified, unspecified ankle and foot
M60.28   Foreign body granuloma of soft tissue, not elsewhere classified, other site
● M60.8   Other myositis
M60.80   Other myositis, unspecified site
● M60.81   Other myositis shoulder
M60.811   Other myositis, right shoulder
M60.812   Other myositis, left shoulder
M60.819   Other myositis, unspecified shoulder
● M60.82   Other myositis, upper arm
M60.821   Other myositis, right upper arm
M60.822   Other myositis, left upper arm
M60.829   Other myositis, unspecified upper arm
● M60.83   Other myositis, forearm
M60.831   Other myositis, right forearm
M60.832   Other myositis, left forearm
M60.839   Other myositis, unspecified forearm
● M60.84   Other myositis, hand
M60.841   Other myositis, right hand
M60.842   Other myositis, left hand
M60.849   Other myositis, unspecified hand
● M60.85   Other myositis, thigh
M60.851   Other myositis, right thigh
M60.852   Other myositis, left thigh
M60.859   Other myositis, unspecified thigh
● M60.86   Other myositis, lower leg
M60.861   Other myositis, right lower leg
M60.862   Other myositis, left lower leg
M60.869   Other myositis, unspecified lower leg
● M60.87   Other myositis, ankle and foot
M60.871   Other myositis, right ankle and foot
M60.872   Other myositis, left ankle and foot
M60.879   Other myositis, unspecified ankle and foot
M60.88   Other myositis, other site
M60.89   Other myositis, multiple sites
M60.9   Myositis, unspecified

- M61 Calcification and ossification of muscle
  - M61.0 Myositis ossificans traumatica
    - M61.00 Myositis ossificans traumatica, unspecified site
    - M61.01 Myositis ossificans traumatica, shoulder
      - M61.011 Myositis ossificans traumatica, right shoulder
      - M61.012 Myositis ossificans traumatica, left shoulder
      - M61.019 Myositis ossificans traumatica, unspecified shoulder
    - M61.02 Myositis ossificans traumatica, upper arm
      - M61.021 Myositis ossificans traumatica, right upper arm
      - M61.022 Myositis ossificans traumatica, left upper arm
      - M61.029 Myositis ossificans traumatica, unspecified upper arm
    - M61.03 Myositis ossificans traumatica, forearm
      - M61.031 Myositis ossificans traumatica, right forearm
      - M61.032 Myositis ossificans traumatica, left forearm
      - M61.039 Myositis ossificans traumatica, unspecified forearm
    - M61.04 Myositis ossificans traumatica, hand
      - M61.041 Myositis ossificans traumatica, right hand
      - M61.042 Myositis ossificans traumatica, left hand
      - M61.049 Myositis ossificans traumatica, unspecified hand
    - M61.05 Myositis ossificans traumatica, thigh
      - M61.051 Myositis ossificans traumatica, right thigh
      - M61.052 Myositis ossificans traumatica, left thigh
      - M61.059 Myositis ossificans traumatica, unspecified thigh
    - M61.06 Myositis ossificans traumatica, lower leg
      - M61.061 Myositis ossificans traumatica, right lower leg
      - M61.062 Myositis ossificans traumatica, left lower leg
      - M61.069 Myositis ossificans traumatica, unspecified lower leg
    - M61.07 Myositis ossificans traumatica, ankle and foot
      - M61.071 Myositis ossificans traumatica, right ankle and foot
      - M61.072 Myositis ossificans traumatica, left ankle and foot
      - M61.079 Myositis ossificans traumatica, unspecified ankle and foot
    - M61.08 Myositis ossificans traumatica, other site
    - M61.09 Myositis ossificans traumatica, multiple sites
  - M61.1 Myositis ossificans progressiva
    Fibrodysplasia ossificans progressiva
    - M61.10 Myositis ossificans progressiva, unspecified site
    - M61.11 Myositis ossificans progressiva, shoulder
      - M61.111 Myositis ossificans progressiva, right shoulder
      - M61.112 Myositis ossificans progressiva, left shoulder
      - M61.119 Myositis ossificans progressiva, unspecified shoulder
  - M61.12 Myositis ossificans progressiva, upper arm
    - M61.121 Myositis ossificans progressiva, right upper arm
    - M61.122 Myositis ossificans progressiva, left upper arm
    - M61.129 Myositis ossificans progressiva, unspecified arm
  - M61.13 Myositis ossificans progressiva, forearm
    - M61.131 Myositis ossificans progressiva, right forearm
    - M61.132 Myositis ossificans progressiva, left forearm
    - M61.139 Myositis ossificans progressiva, unspecified forearm
  - M61.14 Myositis ossificans progressiva, hand and finger(s)
    - M61.141 Myositis ossificans progressiva, right hand
    - M61.142 Myositis ossificans progressiva, left hand
    - M61.143 Myositis ossificans progressiva, unspecified hand
    - M61.144 Myositis ossificans progressiva, right finger(s)
    - M61.145 Myositis ossificans progressiva, left finger(s)
    - M61.146 Myositis ossificans progressiva, unspecified finger(s)
  - M61.15 Myositis ossificans progressiva, thigh
    - M61.151 Myositis ossificans progressiva, right thigh
    - M61.152 Myositis ossificans progressiva, left thigh
    - M61.159 Myositis ossificans progressiva, unspecified thigh
  - M61.16 Myositis ossificans progressiva, lower leg
    - M61.161 Myositis ossificans progressiva, right lower leg
    - M61.162 Myositis ossificans progressiva, left lower leg
    - M61.169 Myositis ossificans progressiva, unspecified lower leg
  - M61.17 Myositis ossificans progressiva, ankle, foot and toe(s)
    - M61.171 Myositis ossificans progressiva, right ankle
    - M61.172 Myositis ossificans progressiva, left ankle
    - M61.173 Myositis ossificans progressiva, unspecified ankle
    - M61.174 Myositis ossificans progressiva, right foot
    - M61.175 Myositis ossificans progressiva, left foot
    - M61.176 Myositis ossificans progressiva, unspecified foot
    - M61.177 Myositis ossificans progressiva, right toe(s)
    - M61.178 Myositis ossificans progressiva, left toe(s)
    - M61.179 Myositis ossificans progressiva, unspecified toe(s)
  - M61.18 Myositis ossificans progressiva, other site
  - M61.19 Myositis ossificans progressiva, multiple sites
- M61.2 Paralytic calcification and ossification of muscle
  Myositis ossificans associated with quadriplegia or paraplegia
  - M61.20 Paralytic calcification and ossification of muscle, unspecified site

M61.21 Paralytic calcification and ossification of muscle, shoulder
    M61.211 Paralytic calcification and ossification of muscle, right shoulder
    M61.212 Paralytic calcification and ossification of muscle, left shoulder
    M61.219 Paralytic calcification and ossification of muscle, unspecified shoulder

M61.22 Paralytic calcification and ossification of muscle, upper arm
    M61.221 Paralytic calcification and ossification of muscle, right upper arm
    M61.222 Paralytic calcification and ossification of muscle, left upper arm
    M61.229 Paralytic calcification and ossification of muscle, unspecified upper arm

M61.23 Paralytic calcification and ossification of muscle, forearm
    M61.231 Paralytic calcification and ossification of muscle, right forearm
    M61.232 Paralytic calcification and ossification of muscle, left forearm
    M61.239 Paralytic calcification and ossification of muscle, unspecified forearm

M61.24 Paralytic calcification and ossification of muscle, hand
    M61.241 Paralytic calcification and ossification of muscle, right hand
    M61.242 Paralytic calcification and ossification of muscle, left hand
    M61.249 Paralytic calcification and ossification of muscle, unspecified hand

M61.25 Paralytic calcification and ossification of muscle, thigh
    M61.251 Paralytic calcification and ossification of muscle, right thigh
    M61.252 Paralytic calcification and ossification of muscle, left thigh
    M61.259 Paralytic calcification and ossification of muscle, unspecified thigh

M61.26 Paralytic calcification and ossification of muscle, lower leg
    M61.261 Paralytic calcification and ossification of muscle, right lower leg
    M61.262 Paralytic calcification and ossification of muscle, left lower leg
    M61.269 Paralytic calcification and ossification of muscle, unspecified lower leg

M61.27 Paralytic calcification and ossification of muscle, ankle and foot
    M61.271 Paralytic calcification and ossification of muscle, right ankle and foot
    M61.272 Paralytic calcification and ossification of muscle, left ankle and foot
    M61.279 Paralytic calcification and ossification of muscle, unspecified ankle and foot

M61.28 Paralytic calcification and ossification of muscle, other site

M61.29 Paralytic calcification and ossification of muscle, multiple sites

M61.3 Calcification and ossification of muscles associated with burns
    Myositis ossificans associated with burns

M61.30 Calcification and ossification of muscles associated with burns, unspecified site

M61.31 Calcification and ossification of muscles associated with burns, shoulder
    M61.311 Calcification and ossification of muscles associated with burns, right shoulder

M61.312 Calcification and ossification of muscles associated with burns, left shoulder
M61.319 Calcification and ossification of muscles associated with burns, unspecified shoulder

M61.32 Calcification and ossification of muscles associated with burns, upper arm
    M61.321 Calcification and ossification of muscles associated with burns, right upper arm
    M61.322 Calcification and ossification of muscles associated with burns, left upper arm
    M61.329 Calcification and ossification of muscles associated with burns, unspecified upper arm

M61.33 Calcification and ossification of muscles associated with burns, forearm
    M61.331 Calcification and ossification of muscles associated with burns, right forearm
    M61.332 Calcification and ossification of muscles associated with burns, left forearm
    M61.339 Calcification and ossification of muscles associated with burns, unspecified forearm

M61.34 Calcification and ossification of muscles associated with burns, hand
    M61.341 Calcification and ossification of muscles associated with burns, right hand
    M61.342 Calcification and ossification of muscles associated with burns, left hand
    M61.349 Calcification and ossification of muscles associated with burns, unspecified hand

M61.35 Calcification and ossification of muscles associated with burns, thigh
    M61.351 Calcification and ossification of muscles associated with burns, right thigh
    M61.352 Calcification and ossification of muscles associated with burns, left thigh
    M61.359 Calcification and ossification of muscles associated with burns, unspecified thigh

M61.36 Calcification and ossification of muscles associated with burns, lower leg
    M61.361 Calcification and ossification of muscles associated with burns, right lower leg
    M61.362 Calcification and ossification of muscles associated with burns, left lower leg
    M61.369 Calcification and ossification of muscles associated with burns, unspecified lower leg

M61.37 Calcification and ossification of muscles associated with burns, ankle and foot
    M61.371 Calcification and ossification of muscles associated with burns, right ankle and foot
    M61.372 Calcification and ossification of muscles associated with burns, left ankle and foot
    M61.379 Calcification and ossification of muscles associated with burns, unspecified ankle and foot

M61.38 Calcification and ossification of muscles associated with burns, other site

M61.39 Calcification and ossification of muscles associated with burns, multiple sites

● M61.4 Other calcification of muscle
  Excludes1 calcific tendinitis NOS (M65.2-)
       calcific tendinitis of shoulder (M75.3)

M61.40 Other calcification of muscle, unspecified site

● M61.41 Other calcification of muscle, shoulder
  M61.411 Other calcification of muscle, right shoulder
  M61.412 Other calcification of muscle, left shoulder
  M61.419 Other calcification of muscle, unspecified shoulder

● M61.42 Other calcification of muscle, upper arm
  M61.421 Other calcification of muscle, right upper arm
  M61.422 Other calcification of muscle, left upper arm
  M61.429 Other calcification of muscle, unspecified upper arm

● M61.43 Other calcification of muscle, forearm
  M61.431 Other calcification of muscle, right forearm
  M61.432 Other calcification of muscle, left forearm
  M61.439 Other calcification of muscle, unspecified forearm

● M61.44 Other calcification of muscle, hand
  M61.441 Other calcification of muscle, right hand
  M61.442 Other calcification of muscle, left hand
  M61.449 Other calcification of muscle, unspecified hand

● M61.45 Other calcification of muscle, thigh
  M61.451 Other calcification of muscle, right thigh
  M61.452 Other calcification of muscle, left thigh
  M61.459 Other calcification of muscle, unspecified thigh

● M61.46 Other calcification of muscle, lower leg
  M61.461 Other calcification of muscle, right lower leg
  M61.462 Other calcification of muscle, left lower leg
  M61.469 Other calcification of muscle, unspecified lower leg

● M61.47 Other calcification of muscle, ankle and foot
  M61.471 Other calcification of muscle, right ankle and foot
  M61.472 Other calcification of muscle, left ankle and foot
  M61.479 Other calcification of muscle, unspecified ankle and foot

M61.48 Other calcification of muscle, other site

M61.49 Other calcification of muscle, multiple sites

● M61.5 Other ossification of muscle

M61.50 Other ossification of muscle, unspecified site

● M61.51 Other ossification of muscle, shoulder
  M61.511 Other ossification of muscle, right shoulder
  M61.512 Other ossification of muscle, left shoulder
  M61.519 Other ossification of muscle, unspecified shoulder

● M61.52 Other ossification of muscle, upper arm
  M61.521 Other ossification of muscle, right upper arm
  M61.522 Other ossification of muscle, left upper arm
  M61.529 Other ossification of muscle, unspecified upper arm

● M61.53 Other ossification of muscle, forearm
  M61.531 Other ossification of muscle, right forearm
  M61.532 Other ossification of muscle, left forearm
  M61.539 Other ossification of muscle, unspecified forearm

● M61.54 Other ossification of muscle, hand
  M61.541 Other ossification of muscle, right hand
  M61.542 Other ossification of muscle, left hand
  M61.549 Other ossification of muscle, unspecified hand

● M61.55 Other ossification of muscle, thigh
  M61.551 Other ossification of muscle, right thigh
  M61.552 Other ossification of muscle, left thigh
  M61.559 Other ossification of muscle, unspecified thigh

● M61.56 Other ossification of muscle, lower leg
  M61.561 Other ossification of muscle, right lower leg
  M61.562 Other ossification of muscle, left lower leg
  M61.569 Other ossification of muscle, unspecified lower leg

● M61.57 Other ossification of muscle, ankle and foot
  M61.571 Other ossification of muscle, right ankle and foot
  M61.572 Other ossification of muscle, left ankle and foot
  M61.579 Other ossification of muscle, unspecified ankle and foot

M61.58 Other ossification of muscle, other site

M61.59 Other ossification of muscle, multiple sites

M61.9 Calcification and ossification of muscle, unspecified

● M62 Other disorders of muscle
  Excludes1 alcoholic myopathy (G72.1)
       cramp and spasm (R25.2)
       drug-induced myopathy (G72.0)
       myalgia (M79.1-)
       stiff-man syndrome (G25.82)
  Excludes2 nontraumatic hematoma of muscle (M79.81)

● M62.0 Separation of muscle (nontraumatic)
  Diastasis of muscle
  Excludes1 diastasis recti complicating pregnancy, labor and delivery (O71.8)
       traumatic separation of muscle - see strain of muscle by body region

M62.00 Separation of muscle (nontraumatic), unspecified site

● M62.01 Separation of muscle (nontraumatic), shoulder
  M62.011 Separation of muscle (nontraumatic), right shoulder
  M62.012 Separation of muscle (nontraumatic), left shoulder
  M62.019 Separation of muscle (nontraumatic), unspecified shoulder

CHAPTER 13 (M00-M99)

CHAPTER 13 (M00-M99)

● M62.02 Separation of muscle (nontraumatic), upper arm

   M62.021 Separation of muscle (nontraumatic), right upper arm

   M62.022 Separation of muscle (nontraumatic), left upper arm

   M62.029 Separation of muscle (nontraumatic), unspecified upper arm

● M62.03 Separation of muscle (nontraumatic), forearm

   M62.031 Separation of muscle (nontraumatic), right forearm

   M62.032 Separation of muscle (nontraumatic), left forearm

   M62.039 Separation of muscle (nontraumatic), unspecified forearm

● M62.04 Separation of muscle (nontraumatic), hand

   M62.041 Separation of muscle (nontraumatic), right hand

   M62.042 Separation of muscle (nontraumatic), left hand

   M62.049 Separation of muscle (nontraumatic), unspecified hand

● M62.05 Separation of muscle (nontraumatic), thigh

   M62.051 Separation of muscle (nontraumatic), right thigh

   M62.052 Separation of muscle (nontraumatic), left thigh

   M62.059 Separation of muscle (nontraumatic), unspecified thigh

● M62.06 Separation of muscle (nontraumatic), lower leg

   M62.061 Separation of muscle (nontraumatic), right lower leg

   M62.062 Separation of muscle (nontraumatic), left lower leg

   M62.069 Separation of muscle (nontraumatic), unspecified lower leg

● M62.07 Separation of muscle (nontraumatic), ankle and foot

   M62.071 Separation of muscle (nontraumatic), right ankle and foot

   M62.072 Separation of muscle (nontraumatic), left ankle and foot

   M62.079 Separation of muscle (nontraumatic), unspecified ankle and foot

   M62.08 Separation of muscle (nontraumatic), other site

● M62.1 Other rupture of muscle (nontraumatic)

   Excludes1   traumatic rupture of muscle - see strain of muscle by body region

   Excludes2   rupture of tendon (M66.-)

   M62.10 Other rupture of muscle (nontraumatic), unspecified site

● M62.11 Other rupture of muscle (nontraumatic), shoulder

   M62.111 Other rupture of muscle (nontraumatic), right shoulder

   M62.112 Other rupture of muscle (nontraumatic), left shoulder

   M62.119 Other rupture of muscle (nontraumatic), unspecified shoulder

● M62.12 Other rupture of muscle (nontraumatic), upper arm

   M62.121 Other rupture of muscle (nontraumatic), right upper arm

   M62.122 Other rupture of muscle (nontraumatic), left upper arm

   M62.129 Other rupture of muscle (nontraumatic), unspecified upper arm

● M62.13 Other rupture of muscle (nontraumatic), forearm

   M62.131 Other rupture of muscle (nontraumatic), right forearm

   M62.132 Other rupture of muscle (nontraumatic), left forearm

   M62.139 Other rupture of muscle (nontraumatic), unspecified forearm

● M62.14 Other rupture of muscle (nontraumatic), hand

   M62.141 Other rupture of muscle (nontraumatic), right hand

   M62.142 Other rupture of muscle (nontraumatic), left hand

   M62.149 Other rupture of muscle (nontraumatic), unspecified hand

● M62.15 Other rupture of muscle (nontraumatic), thigh

   M62.151 Other rupture of muscle (nontraumatic), right thigh

   M62.152 Other rupture of muscle (nontraumatic), left thigh

   M62.159 Other rupture of muscle (nontraumatic), unspecified thigh

● M62.16 Other rupture of muscle (nontraumatic), lower leg

   M62.161 Other rupture of muscle (nontraumatic), right lower leg

   M62.162 Other rupture of muscle (nontraumatic), left lower leg

   M62.169 Other rupture of muscle (nontraumatic), unspecified lower leg

● M62.17 Other rupture of muscle (nontraumatic), ankle and foot

   M62.171 Other rupture of muscle (nontraumatic), right ankle and foot

   M62.172 Other rupture of muscle (nontraumatic), left ankle and foot

   M62.179 Other rupture of muscle (nontraumatic), unspecified ankle and foot

   M62.18 Other rupture of muscle (nontraumatic), other site

● M62.2 Nontraumatic ischemic infarction of muscle

   Excludes1   compartment syndrome (traumatic) (T79.A-)
              nontraumatic compartment syndrome (M79.A-)
              traumatic ischemia of muscle (T79.6)
              rhabdomyolysis (M62.82)
              Volkmann's ischemic contracture (T79.6)

   M62.20 Nontraumatic ischemic infarction of muscle, unspecified site

● M62.21 Nontraumatic ischemic infarction of muscle, shoulder

   M62.211 Nontraumatic ischemic infarction of muscle, right shoulder

   M62.212 Nontraumatic ischemic infarction of muscle, left shoulder

   M62.219 Nontraumatic ischemic infarction of muscle, unspecified shoulder

● M62.22 Nontraumatic ischemic infarction of muscle, upper arm

   M62.221 Nontraumatic ischemic infarction of muscle, right upper arm

   M62.222 Nontraumatic ischemic infarction of muscle, left upper arm

   M62.229 Nontraumatic ischemic infarction of muscle, unspecified upper arm

● M62.23   Nontraumatic ischemic infarction of muscle, forearm
    M62.231   Nontraumatic ischemic infarction of muscle, right forearm
    M62.232   Nontraumatic ischemic infarction of muscle, left forearm
    M62.239   Nontraumatic ischemic infarction of muscle, unspecified forearm

● M62.24   Nontraumatic ischemic infarction of muscle, hand
    M62.241   Nontraumatic ischemic infarction of muscle, right hand
    M62.242   Nontraumatic ischemic infarction of muscle, left hand
    M62.249   Nontraumatic ischemic infarction of muscle, unspecified hand

● M62.25   Nontraumatic ischemic infarction of muscle, thigh
    M62.251   Nontraumatic ischemic infarction of muscle, right thigh
    M62.252   Nontraumatic ischemic infarction of muscle, left thigh
    M62.259   Nontraumatic ischemic infarction of muscle, unspecified thigh

● M62.26   Nontraumatic ischemic infarction of muscle, lower leg
    M62.261   Nontraumatic ischemic infarction of muscle, right lower leg
    M62.262   Nontraumatic ischemic infarction of muscle, left lower leg
    M62.269   Nontraumatic ischemic infarction of muscle, unspecified lower leg

● M62.27   Nontraumatic ischemic infarction of muscle, ankle and foot
    M62.271   Nontraumatic ischemic infarction of muscle, right ankle and foot
    M62.272   Nontraumatic ischemic infarction of muscle, left ankle and foot
    M62.279   Nontraumatic ischemic infarction of muscle, unspecified ankle and foot

    M62.28   Nontraumatic ischemic infarction of muscle, other site

M62.3   Immobility syndrome (paraplegic)

M62.4   Contracture of muscle
    Contracture of tendon (sheath)
    Excludes1   contracture of joint (M24.5-)

    M62.40   Contracture of muscle, unspecified site

● M62.41   Contracture of muscle, shoulder
    M62.411   Contracture of muscle, right shoulder
    M62.412   Contracture of muscle, left shoulder
    M62.419   Contracture of muscle, unspecified shoulder

● M62.42   Contracture of muscle, upper arm
    M62.421   Contracture of muscle, right upper arm
    M62.422   Contracture of muscle, left upper arm
    M62.429   Contracture of muscle, unspecified upper arm

● M62.43   Contracture of muscle, forearm
    M62.431   Contracture of muscle, right forearm
    M62.432   Contracture of muscle, left forearm
    M62.439   Contracture of muscle, unspecified forearm

● M62.44   Contracture of muscle, hand
    M62.441   Contracture of muscle, right hand
    M62.442   Contracture of muscle, left hand
    M62.449   Contracture of muscle, unspecified hand

● M62.45   Contracture of muscle, thigh
    M62.451   Contracture of muscle, right thigh
    M62.452   Contracture of muscle, left thigh
    M62.459   Contracture of muscle, unspecified thigh

● M62.46   Contracture of muscle, lower leg
    M62.461   Contracture of muscle, right lower leg
    M62.462   Contracture of muscle, left lower leg
    M62.469   Contracture of muscle, unspecified lower leg

● M62.47   Contracture of muscle, ankle and foot
    M62.471   Contracture of muscle, right ankle and foot
    M62.472   Contracture of muscle, left ankle and foot
    M62.479   Contracture of muscle, unspecified ankle and foot

    M62.48   Contracture of muscle, other site

    M62.49   Contracture of muscle, multiple sites

● M62.5   Muscle wasting and atrophy, not elsewhere classified
    Disuse atrophy NEC
    Excludes1   neuralgic amyotrophy (G54.5)
                progressive muscular atrophy (G12.21)
                sarcopenia (M62.84)
    Excludes2   pelvic muscle wasting (N81.84)

    M62.50   Muscle wasting and atrophy, not elsewhere classified, unspecified site

● M62.51   Muscle wasting and atrophy, not elsewhere classified, shoulder
    M62.511   Muscle wasting and atrophy, not elsewhere classified, right shoulder
    M62.512   Muscle wasting and atrophy, not elsewhere classified, left shoulder
    M62.519   Muscle wasting and atrophy, not elsewhere classified, unspecified shoulder

● M62.52   Muscle wasting and atrophy, not elsewhere classified, upper arm
    M62.521   Muscle wasting and atrophy, not elsewhere classified, right upper arm
    M62.522   Muscle wasting and atrophy, not elsewhere classified, left upper arm
    M62.529   Muscle wasting and atrophy, not elsewhere classified, unspecified upper arm

● M62.53   Muscle wasting and atrophy, not elsewhere classified, forearm
    M62.531   Muscle wasting and atrophy, not elsewhere classified, right forearm
    M62.532   Muscle wasting and atrophy, not elsewhere classified, left forearm
    M62.539   Muscle wasting and atrophy, not elsewhere classified, unspecified forearm

● M62.54   Muscle wasting and atrophy, not elsewhere classified, hand
    M62.541   Muscle wasting and atrophy, not elsewhere classified, right hand
    M62.542   Muscle wasting and atrophy, not elsewhere classified, left hand
    M62.549   Muscle wasting and atrophy, not elsewhere classified, unspecified hand

● M62.55   Muscle wasting and atrophy, not elsewhere classified, thigh
    M62.551   Muscle wasting and atrophy, not elsewhere classified, right thigh
    M62.552   Muscle wasting and atrophy, not elsewhere classified, left thigh
    M62.559   Muscle wasting and atrophy, not elsewhere classified, unspecified thigh

● M62.56 Muscle wasting and atrophy, not elsewhere classified, lower leg

    M62.561 Muscle wasting and atrophy, not elsewhere classified, right lower leg

    M62.562 Muscle wasting and atrophy, not elsewhere classified, left lower leg

    M62.569 Muscle wasting and atrophy, not elsewhere classified, unspecified lower leg

● M62.57 Muscle wasting and atrophy, not elsewhere classified, ankle and foot

    M62.571 Muscle wasting and atrophy, not elsewhere classified, right ankle and foot

    M62.572 Muscle wasting and atrophy, not elsewhere classified, left ankle and foot

    M62.579 Muscle wasting and atrophy, not elsewhere classified, unspecified ankle and foot

M62.58 Muscle wasting and atrophy, not elsewhere classified, other site

M62.59 Muscle wasting and atrophy, not elsewhere classified, multiple sites

● M62.8 Other specified disorders of muscle

    Excludes2   nontraumatic hematoma of muscle (M79.81)

  M62.81 Muscle weakness (generalized)

    Excludes1   muscle weakness in sarcopenia (M62.84)

  M62.82 Rhabdomyolysis

    Excludes1   traumatic rhabdomyolysis (T79.6)

    Coding Clinic: 2019, Q2, P12

● M62.83 Muscle spasm

    M62.830 Muscle spasm of back

    M62.831 Muscle spasm of calf

        Charley-horse

    M62.838 Other muscle spasm

  M62.84 Sarcopenia

    Age-related sarcopenia

    Code first underlying disease, if applicable, such as:
        disorders of myoneural junction and muscle disease in diseases classified elsewhere (G73.-)
        other and unspecified myopathies (G72.-)
        primary disorders of muscles (G71.-)

    Coding Clinic: 2016, Q4, P41

  M62.89 Other specified disorders of muscle

    Muscle (sheath) hernia

M62.9 Disorder of muscle, unspecified

● M63 Disorders of muscle in diseases classified elsewhere

  Code first underlying disease, such as:
    leprosy (A30.-)
    neoplasm (C49.-, C79.89, D21.-, D48.1)
    schistosomiasis (B65.-)
    trichinellosis (B75)

  Excludes1   myopathy in cysticercosis (B69.81)
        myopathy in endocrine diseases (G73.7)
        myopathy in metabolic diseases (G73.7)
        myopathy in sarcoidosis (D86.87)
        myopathy in secondary syphilis (A51.49)
        myopathy in syphilis (late) (A52.78)
        myopathy in toxoplasmosis (B58.82)
        myopathy in tuberculosis (A18.09)

● M63.8 Disorders of muscle in diseases classified elsewhere

  ▌ M63.80 Disorders of muscle in diseases classified elsewhere, unspecified site

● M63.81 Disorders of muscle in diseases classified elsewhere, shoulder

  ▌ M63.811 Disorders of muscle in diseases classified elsewhere, right shoulder

  ▌ M63.812 Disorders of muscle in diseases classified elsewhere, left shoulder

  ▌ M63.819 Disorders of muscle in diseases classified elsewhere, unspecified shoulder

● M63.82 Disorders of muscle in diseases classified elsewhere, upper arm

  ▌ M63.821 Disorders of muscle in diseases classified elsewhere, right upper arm

  ▌ M63.822 Disorders of muscle in diseases classified elsewhere, left upper arm

  ▌ M63.829 Disorders of muscle in diseases classified elsewhere, unspecified upper arm

● M63.83 Disorders of muscle in diseases classified elsewhere, forearm

  ▌ M63.831 Disorders of muscle in diseases classified elsewhere, right forearm

  ▌ M63.832 Disorders of muscle in diseases classified elsewhere, left forearm

  ▌ M63.839 Disorders of muscle in diseases classified elsewhere, unspecified forearm

● M63.84 Disorders of muscle in diseases classified elsewhere, hand

  ▌ M63.841 Disorders of muscle in diseases classified elsewhere, right hand

  ▌ M63.842 Disorders of muscle in diseases classified elsewhere, left hand

  ▌ M63.849 Disorders of muscle in diseases classified elsewhere, unspecified hand

● M63.85 Disorders of muscle in diseases classified elsewhere, thigh

  ▌ M63.851 Disorders of muscle in diseases classified elsewhere, right thigh

  ▌ M63.852 Disorders of muscle in diseases classified elsewhere, left thigh

  ▌ M63.859 Disorders of muscle in diseases classified elsewhere, unspecified thigh

● M63.86 Disorders of muscle in diseases classified elsewhere, lower leg

  ▌ M63.861 Disorders of muscle in diseases classified elsewhere, right lower leg

  ▌ M63.862 Disorders of muscle in diseases classified elsewhere, left lower leg

  ▌ M63.869 Disorders of muscle in diseases classified elsewhere, unspecified lower leg

● M63.87 Disorders of muscle in diseases classified elsewhere, ankle and foot

  ▌ M63.871 Disorders of muscle in diseases classified elsewhere, right ankle and foot

  ▌ M63.872 Disorders of muscle in diseases classified elsewhere, left ankle and foot

  ▌ M63.879 Disorders of muscle in diseases classified elsewhere, unspecified ankle and foot

  ▌ M63.88 Disorders of muscle in diseases classified elsewhere, other site

  ▌ M63.89 Disorders of muscle in diseases classified elsewhere, multiple sites

DISORDERS OF SYNOVIUM AND TENDON (M65-M67)

● M65   Synovitis and tenosynovitis

     Excludes1   chronic crepitant synovitis of hand and wrist (M70.0-)

                    current injury - see injury of ligament or tendon by body region

                    soft tissue disorders related to use, overuse and pressure (M70.-)

● M65.0   Abscess of tendon sheath

     Use additional code (B95-B96) to identify bacterial agent

     M65.00   Abscess of tendon sheath, unspecified site

●   M65.01   Abscess of tendon sheath, shoulder

         M65.011   Abscess of tendon sheath, right shoulder

         M65.012   Abscess of tendon sheath, left shoulder

         M65.019   Abscess of tendon sheath, unspecified shoulder

●   M65.02   Abscess of tendon sheath, upper arm

         M65.021   Abscess of tendon sheath, right upper arm

         M65.022   Abscess of tendon sheath, left upper arm

         M65.029   Abscess of tendon sheath, unspecified upper arm

●   M65.03   Abscess of tendon sheath, forearm

         M65.031   Abscess of tendon sheath, right forearm

         M65.032   Abscess of tendon sheath, left forearm

         M65.039   Abscess of tendon sheath, unspecified forearm

●   M65.04   Abscess of tendon sheath, hand

         M65.041   Abscess of tendon sheath, right hand

         M65.042   Abscess of tendon sheath, left hand

         M65.049   Abscess of tendon sheath, unspecified hand

●   M65.05   Abscess of tendon sheath, thigh

         M65.051   Abscess of tendon sheath, right thigh

         M65.052   Abscess of tendon sheath, left thigh

         M65.059   Abscess of tendon sheath, unspecified thigh

●   M65.06   Abscess of tendon sheath, lower leg

         M65.061   Abscess of tendon sheath, right lower leg

         M65.062   Abscess of tendon sheath, left lower leg

         M65.069   Abscess of tendon sheath, unspecified lower leg

●   M65.07   Abscess of tendon sheath, ankle and foot

         M65.071   Abscess of tendon sheath, right ankle and foot

         M65.072   Abscess of tendon sheath, left ankle and foot

         M65.079   Abscess of tendon sheath, unspecified ankle and foot

     M65.08   Abscess of tendon sheath, other site

● M65.1   Other infective (teno)synovitis

     M65.10   Other infective (teno)synovitis, unspecified site

●   M65.11   Other infective (teno)synovitis, shoulder

         M65.111   Other infective (teno)synovitis, right shoulder

         M65.112   Other infective (teno)synovitis, left shoulder

         M65.119   Other infective (teno)synovitis, unspecified shoulder

●   M65.12   Other infective (teno)synovitis, elbow

         M65.121   Other infective (teno)synovitis, right elbow

         M65.122   Other infective (teno)synovitis, left elbow

         M65.129   Other infective (teno)synovitis, unspecified elbow

●   M65.13   Other infective (teno)synovitis, wrist

         M65.131   Other infective (teno)synovitis, right wrist

         M65.132   Other infective (teno)synovitis, left wrist

         M65.139   Other infective (teno)synovitis, unspecified wrist

●   M65.14   Other infective (teno)synovitis, hand

         M65.141   Other infective (teno)synovitis, right hand

         M65.142   Other infective (teno)synovitis, left hand

         M65.149   Other infective (teno)synovitis, unspecified hand

●   M65.15   Other infective (teno)synovitis, hip

         M65.151   Other infective (teno)synovitis, right hip

         M65.152   Other infective (teno)synovitis, left hip

         M65.159   Other infective (teno)synovitis, unspecified hip

●   M65.16   Other infective (teno)synovitis, knee

         M65.161   Other infective (teno)synovitis, right knee

         M65.162   Other infective (teno)synovitis, left knee

         M65.169   Other infective (teno)synovitis, unspecified knee

●   M65.17   Other infective (teno)synovitis, ankle and foot

         M65.171   Other infective (teno)synovitis, right ankle and foot

         M65.172   Other infective (teno)synovitis, left ankle and foot

         M65.179   Other infective (teno)synovitis, unspecified ankle and foot

     M65.18   Other infective (teno)synovitis, other site

     M65.19   Other infective (teno)synovitis, multiple sites

● M65.2   Calcific tendinitis

     Excludes1   tendinitis as classified in M75-M77

                    calcified tendinitis of shoulder (M75.3)

     M65.20   Calcific tendinitis, unspecified site

●   M65.22   Calcific tendinitis, upper arm

         M65.221   Calcific tendinitis, right upper arm

         M65.222   Calcific tendinitis, left upper arm

         M65.229   Calcific tendinitis, unspecified upper arm

●   M65.23   Calcific tendinitis, forearm

         M65.231   Calcific tendinitis, right forearm

         M65.232   Calcific tendinitis, left forearm

         M65.239   Calcific tendinitis, unspecified forearm

Item 13-11   **Synovitis** is an inflammation of a synovial membrane resulting in pain on motion and is characterized by fluctuating swelling due to effusion in a synovial sac. **Tenosynovitis** is an inflammation of a tendon sheath and occurs most commonly in the wrists, hands, and feet. Bursitis is inflammation of a bursa (fluid-filled sac) caused by repetitive use, trauma, infection, or systemic inflammatory disease. Bursae act as protectors and facilitate movement between bones and overlapping muscles (deep bursae) or between bones and tendons/skin (superficial bursae).

CHAPTER 13 (M00-M99)

● M65.24　Calcific tendinitis, hand
　　　　　M65.241　Calcific tendinitis, right hand
　　　　　M65.242　Calcific tendinitis, left hand
　　　　　M65.249　Calcific tendinitis, unspecified hand
● M65.25　Calcific tendinitis, thigh
　　　　　M65.251　Calcific tendinitis, right thigh
　　　　　M65.252　Calcific tendinitis, left thigh
　　　　　M65.259　Calcific tendinitis, unspecified thigh
● M65.26　Calcific tendinitis, lower leg
　　　　　M65.261　Calcific tendinitis, right lower leg
　　　　　M65.262　Calcific tendinitis, left lower leg
　　　　　M65.269　Calcific tendinitis, unspecified lower leg
● M65.27　Calcific tendinitis, ankle and foot
　　　　　M65.271　Calcific tendinitis, right ankle and foot
　　　　　M65.272　Calcific tendinitis, left ankle and foot
　　　　　M65.279　Calcific tendinitis, unspecified ankle and foot
　　　　M65.28　Calcific tendinitis, other site
　　　　M65.29　Calcific tendinitis, multiple sites
● M65.3　Trigger finger
　　　　　Nodular tendinous disease
　　　　M65.30　Trigger finger, unspecified finger
● M65.31　Trigger thumb
　　　　　M65.311　Trigger thumb, right thumb
　　　　　M65.312　Trigger thumb, left thumb
　　　　　M65.319　Trigger thumb, unspecified thumb
● M65.32　Trigger finger, index finger
　　　　　M65.321　Trigger finger, right index finger
　　　　　M65.322　Trigger finger, left index finger
　　　　　M65.329　Trigger finger, unspecified index finger
● M65.33　Trigger finger, middle finger
　　　　　M65.331　Trigger finger, right middle finger
　　　　　M65.332　Trigger finger, left middle finger
　　　　　M65.339　Trigger finger, unspecified middle finger
● M65.34　Trigger finger, ring finger
　　　　　M65.341　Trigger finger, right ring finger
　　　　　M65.342　Trigger finger, left ring finger
　　　　　M65.349　Trigger finger, unspecified ring finger
● M65.35　Trigger finger, little finger
　　　　　M65.351　Trigger finger, right little finger
　　　　　M65.352　Trigger finger, left little finger
　　　　　M65.359　Trigger finger, unspecified little finger
　　　M65.4　Radial styloid tenosynovitis [de Quervain]
● M65.8　Other synovitis and tenosynovitis
　　　　M65.80　Other synovitis and tenosynovitis, unspecified site
● M65.81　Other synovitis and tenosynovitis, shoulder
　　　　　M65.811　Other synovitis and tenosynovitis, right shoulder
　　　　　M65.812　Other synovitis and tenosynovitis, left shoulder
　　　　　M65.819　Other synovitis and tenosynovitis, unspecified shoulder
● M65.82　Other synovitis and tenosynovitis, upper arm
　　　　　M65.821　Other synovitis and tenosynovitis, right upper arm
　　　　　M65.822　Other synovitis and tenosynovitis, left upper arm
　　　　　M65.829　Other synovitis and tenosynovitis, unspecified upper arm

● M65.83　Other synovitis and tenosynovitis, forearm
　　　　　M65.831　Other synovitis and tenosynovitis, right forearm
　　　　　M65.832　Other synovitis and tenosynovitis, left forearm
　　　　　M65.839　Other synovitis and tenosynovitis, unspecified forearm
● M65.84　Other synovitis and tenosynovitis, hand
　　　　　M65.841　Other synovitis and tenosynovitis, right hand
　　　　　M65.842　Other synovitis and tenosynovitis, left hand
　　　　　M65.849　Other synovitis and tenosynovitis, unspecified hand
● M65.85　Other synovitis and tenosynovitis, thigh
　　　　　M65.851　Other synovitis and tenosynovitis, right thigh
　　　　　M65.852　Other synovitis and tenosynovitis, left thigh
　　　　　M65.859　Other synovitis and tenosynovitis, unspecified thigh
● M65.86　Other synovitis and tenosynovitis, lower leg
　　　　　M65.861　Other synovitis and tenosynovitis, right lower leg
　　　　　M65.862　Other synovitis and tenosynovitis, left lower leg
　　　　　M65.869　Other synovitis and tenosynovitis, unspecified lower leg
● M65.87　Other synovitis and tenosynovitis, ankle and foot
　　　　　M65.871　Other synovitis and tenosynovitis, right ankle and foot
　　　　　M65.872　Other synovitis and tenosynovitis, left ankle and foot
　　　　　M65.879　Other synovitis and tenosynovitis, unspecified ankle and foot
　　　　M65.88　Other synovitis and tenosynovitis, other site
　　　　M65.89　Other synovitis and tenosynovitis, multiple sites
　　　M65.9　Synovitis and tenosynovitis, unspecified

● M66　Spontaneous rupture of synovium and tendon
　　　Includes　rupture that occurs when a normal force is applied to tissues that are inferred to have less than normal strength
　　　Excludes2　rotator cuff syndrome (M75.1-)
　　　　　　　　　rupture where an abnormal force is applied to normal tissue - see injury of tendon by body region
　　　M66.0　Rupture of popliteal cyst
● M66.1　Rupture of synovium
　　　　　Rupture of synovial cyst
　　　　Excludes2　rupture of popliteal cyst (M66.0)
　　　　M66.10　Rupture of synovium, unspecified joint
● M66.11　Rupture of synovium, shoulder
　　　　　M66.111　Rupture of synovium, right shoulder
　　　　　M66.112　Rupture of synovium, left shoulder
　　　　　M66.119　Rupture of synovium, unspecified shoulder
● M66.12　Rupture of synovium, elbow
　　　　　M66.121　Rupture of synovium, right elbow
　　　　　M66.122　Rupture of synovium, left elbow
　　　　　M66.129　Rupture of synovium, unspecified elbow
● M66.13　Rupture of synovium, wrist
　　　　　M66.131　Rupture of synovium, right wrist
　　　　　M66.132　Rupture of synovium, left wrist
　　　　　M66.139　Rupture of synovium, unspecified wrist

● M66.14   Rupture of synovium, hand and fingers
    M66.141   Rupture of synovium, right hand
    M66.142   Rupture of synovium, left hand
    M66.143   Rupture of synovium, unspecified hand
    M66.144   Rupture of synovium, right finger(s)
    M66.145   Rupture of synovium, left finger(s)
    M66.146   Rupture of synovium, unspecified finger(s)

● M66.15   Rupture of synovium, hip
    M66.151   Rupture of synovium, right hip
    M66.152   Rupture of synovium, left hip
    M66.159   Rupture of synovium, unspecified hip

● M66.17   Rupture of synovium, ankle, foot and toes
    M66.171   Rupture of synovium, right ankle
    M66.172   Rupture of synovium, left ankle
    M66.173   Rupture of synovium, unspecified ankle
    M66.174   Rupture of synovium, right foot
    M66.175   Rupture of synovium, left foot
    M66.176   Rupture of synovium, unspecified foot
    M66.177   Rupture of synovium, right toe(s)
    M66.178   Rupture of synovium, left toe(s)
    M66.179   Rupture of synovium, unspecified toe(s)

  M66.18   Rupture of synovium, other site

● M66.2   Spontaneous rupture of extensor tendons
  M66.20   Spontaneous rupture of extensor tendons, unspecified site

● M66.21   Spontaneous rupture of extensor tendons, shoulder
    M66.211   Spontaneous rupture of extensor tendons, right shoulder
    M66.212   Spontaneous rupture of extensor tendons, left shoulder
    M66.219   Spontaneous rupture of extensor tendons, unspecified shoulder

● M66.22   Spontaneous rupture of extensor tendons, upper arm
    M66.221   Spontaneous rupture of extensor tendons, right upper arm
    M66.222   Spontaneous rupture of extensor tendons, left upper arm
    M66.229   Spontaneous rupture of extensor tendons, unspecified upper arm

● M66.23   Spontaneous rupture of extensor tendons, forearm
    M66.231   Spontaneous rupture of extensor tendons, right forearm
    M66.232   Spontaneous rupture of extensor tendons, left forearm
    M66.239   Spontaneous rupture of extensor tendons, unspecified forearm

● M66.24   Spontaneous rupture of extensor tendons, hand
    M66.241   Spontaneous rupture of extensor tendons, right hand
    M66.242   Spontaneous rupture of extensor tendons, left hand
    M66.249   Spontaneous rupture of extensor tendons, unspecified hand

● M66.25   Spontaneous rupture of extensor tendons, thigh
    M66.251   Spontaneous rupture of extensor tendons, right thigh
    M66.252   Spontaneous rupture of extensor tendons, left thigh
    M66.259   Spontaneous rupture of extensor tendons, unspecified thigh

● M66.26   Spontaneous rupture of extensor tendons, lower leg
    M66.261   Spontaneous rupture of extensor tendons, right lower leg
    M66.262   Spontaneous rupture of extensor tendons, left lower leg
    M66.269   Spontaneous rupture of extensor tendons, unspecified lower leg

● M66.27   Spontaneous rupture of extensor tendons, ankle and foot
    M66.271   Spontaneous rupture of extensor tendons, right ankle and foot
    M66.272   Spontaneous rupture of extensor tendons, left ankle and foot
    M66.279   Spontaneous rupture of extensor tendons, unspecified ankle and foot

  M66.28   Spontaneous rupture of extensor tendons, other site

  M66.29   Spontaneous rupture of extensor tendons, multiple sites

● M66.3   Spontaneous rupture of flexor tendons
  M66.30   Spontaneous rupture of flexor tendons, unspecified site

● M66.31   Spontaneous rupture of flexor tendons, shoulder
    M66.311   Spontaneous rupture of flexor tendons, right shoulder
    M66.312   Spontaneous rupture of flexor tendons, left shoulder
    M66.319   Spontaneous rupture of flexor tendons, unspecified shoulder

● M66.32   Spontaneous rupture of flexor tendons, upper arm
    M66.321   Spontaneous rupture of flexor tendons, right upper arm
    M66.322   Spontaneous rupture of flexor tendons, left upper arm
    M66.329   Spontaneous rupture of flexor tendons, unspecified upper arm

● M66.33   Spontaneous rupture of flexor tendons, forearm
    M66.331   Spontaneous rupture of flexor tendons, right forearm
    M66.332   Spontaneous rupture of flexor tendons, left forearm
    M66.339   Spontaneous rupture of flexor tendons, unspecified forearm

● M66.34   Spontaneous rupture of flexor tendons, hand
    M66.341   Spontaneous rupture of flexor tendons, right hand
    M66.342   Spontaneous rupture of flexor tendons, left hand
    M66.349   Spontaneous rupture of flexor tendons, unspecified hand

● M66.35   Spontaneous rupture of flexor tendons, thigh
    M66.351   Spontaneous rupture of flexor tendons, right thigh
    M66.352   Spontaneous rupture of flexor tendons, left thigh
    M66.359   Spontaneous rupture of flexor tendons, unspecified thigh

● M66.36   Spontaneous rupture of flexor tendons, lower leg
    M66.361   Spontaneous rupture of flexor tendons, right lower leg
    M66.362   Spontaneous rupture of flexor tendons, left lower leg
    M66.369   Spontaneous rupture of flexor tendons, unspecified lower leg

CHAPTER 13 (M00–M99)

CHAPTER 13 (M00-M99)

- M66.37 **Spontaneous rupture of flexor tendons, ankle and foot**
  - M66.371 Spontaneous rupture of flexor tendons, right ankle and foot
  - M66.372 Spontaneous rupture of flexor tendons, left ankle and foot
  - M66.379 Spontaneous rupture of flexor tendons, unspecified ankle and foot
  - M66.38 Spontaneous rupture of flexor tendons, other site
  - M66.39 Spontaneous rupture of flexor tendons, multiple sites
- M66.8 **Spontaneous rupture of other tendons**
  - M66.80 Spontaneous rupture of other tendons, unspecified site
  - M66.81 Spontaneous rupture of other tendons, shoulder
    - M66.811 Spontaneous rupture of other tendons, right shoulder
    - M66.812 Spontaneous rupture of other tendons, left shoulder
    - M66.819 Spontaneous rupture of other tendons, unspecified shoulder
  - M66.82 Spontaneous rupture of other tendons, upper arm
    - M66.821 Spontaneous rupture of other tendons, right upper arm
    - M66.822 Spontaneous rupture of other tendons, left upper arm
    - M66.829 Spontaneous rupture of other tendons, unspecified upper arm
  - M66.83 Spontaneous rupture of other tendons, forearm
    - M66.831 Spontaneous rupture of other tendons, right forearm
    - M66.832 Spontaneous rupture of other tendons, left forearm
    - M66.839 Spontaneous rupture of other tendons, unspecified forearm
  - M66.84 Spontaneous rupture of other tendons, hand
    - M66.841 Spontaneous rupture of other tendons, right hand
    - M66.842 Spontaneous rupture of other tendons, left hand
    - M66.849 Spontaneous rupture of other tendons, unspecified hand
  - M66.85 Spontaneous rupture of other tendons, thigh
    - M66.851 Spontaneous rupture of other tendons, right thigh
    - M66.852 Spontaneous rupture of other tendons, left thigh
    - M66.859 Spontaneous rupture of other tendons, unspecified thigh
  - M66.86 Spontaneous rupture of other tendons, lower leg
    - M66.861 Spontaneous rupture of other tendons, right lower leg
    - M66.862 Spontaneous rupture of other tendons, left lower leg
    - M66.869 Spontaneous rupture of other tendons, unspecified lower leg
  - M66.87 Spontaneous rupture of other tendons, ankle and foot
    - M66.871 Spontaneous rupture of other tendons, right ankle and foot
    - M66.872 Spontaneous rupture of other tendons, left ankle and foot
    - M66.879 Spontaneous rupture of other tendons, unspecified ankle and foot

  - M66.88 Spontaneous rupture of other tendons, other sites
  - M66.89 Spontaneous rupture of other tendons, multiple sites
- M66.9 **Spontaneous rupture of unspecified tendon**
  Rupture at musculotendinous junction, nontraumatic

- M67 **Other disorders of synovium and tendon**
  - **Excludes1** palmar fascial fibromatosis [Dupuytren] (M72.0)
    tendinitis NOS (M77.9-)
    xanthomatosis localized to tendons (E78.2)
  - M67.0 **Short Achilles tendon (acquired)**
    - M67.00 Short Achilles tendon (acquired), unspecified ankle
    - M67.01 Short Achilles tendon (acquired), right ankle
    - M67.02 Short Achilles tendon (acquired), left ankle
  - M67.2 **Synovial hypertrophy, not elsewhere classified**
    - **Excludes1** villonodular synovitis (pigmented) (M12.2-)
    - M67.20 Synovial hypertrophy, not elsewhere classified, unspecified site
    - M67.21 Synovial hypertrophy, not elsewhere classified, shoulder
      - M67.211 Synovial hypertrophy, not elsewhere classified, right shoulder
      - M67.212 Synovial hypertrophy, not elsewhere classified, left shoulder
      - M67.219 Synovial hypertrophy, not elsewhere classified, unspecified shoulder
    - M67.22 Synovial hypertrophy, not elsewhere classified, upper arm
      - M67.221 Synovial hypertrophy, not elsewhere classified, right upper arm
      - M67.222 Synovial hypertrophy, not elsewhere classified, left upper arm
      - M67.229 Synovial hypertrophy, not elsewhere classified, unspecified upper arm
    - M67.23 Synovial hypertrophy, not elsewhere classified, forearm
      - M67.231 Synovial hypertrophy, not elsewhere classified, right forearm
      - M67.232 Synovial hypertrophy, not elsewhere classified, left forearm
      - M67.239 Synovial hypertrophy, not elsewhere classified, unspecified forearm
    - M67.24 Synovial hypertrophy, not elsewhere classified, hand
      - M67.241 Synovial hypertrophy, not elsewhere classified, right hand
      - M67.242 Synovial hypertrophy, not elsewhere classified, left hand
      - M67.249 Synovial hypertrophy, not elsewhere classified, unspecified hand
    - M67.25 Synovial hypertrophy, not elsewhere classified, thigh
      - M67.251 Synovial hypertrophy, not elsewhere classified, right thigh
      - M67.252 Synovial hypertrophy, not elsewhere classified, left thigh
      - M67.259 Synovial hypertrophy, not elsewhere classified, unspecified thigh
    - M67.26 Synovial hypertrophy, not elsewhere classified, lower leg
      - M67.261 Synovial hypertrophy, not elsewhere classified, right lower leg
      - M67.262 Synovial hypertrophy, not elsewhere classified, left lower leg
      - M67.269 Synovial hypertrophy, not elsewhere classified, unspecified lower leg

▶ New   ⮕ Revised   ~~deleted~~ Deleted   Excludes 1   Excludes 2   Includes   Use additional   Code first   Code also   Key words

OGCR Official Guidelines   X Assign placeholder X   ● Use Additional Character(s)   ▶ Manifestation Code   🐱 Hierarchical Condition Category   **Coding Clinic**

● M67.27 Synovial hypertrophy, not elsewhere classified, ankle and foot
   M67.271 Synovial hypertrophy, not elsewhere classified, right ankle and foot
   M67.272 Synovial hypertrophy, not elsewhere classified, left ankle and foot
   M67.279 Synovial hypertrophy, not elsewhere classified, unspecified ankle and foot
  M67.28 Synovial hypertrophy, not elsewhere classified, other site
  M67.29 Synovial hypertrophy, not elsewhere classified, multiple sites

● M67.3 Transient synovitis
   Toxic synovitis
   Excludes1 palindromic rheumatism (M12.3-)
  M67.30 Transient synovitis, unspecified site
● M67.31 Transient synovitis, shoulder
   M67.311 Transient synovitis, right shoulder
   M67.312 Transient synovitis, left shoulder
   M67.319 Transient synovitis, unspecified shoulder
● M67.32 Transient synovitis, elbow
   M67.321 Transient synovitis, right elbow
   M67.322 Transient synovitis, left elbow
   M67.329 Transient synovitis, unspecified elbow
● M67.33 Transient synovitis, wrist
   M67.331 Transient synovitis, right wrist
   M67.332 Transient synovitis, left wrist
   M67.339 Transient synovitis, unspecified wrist
● M67.34 Transient synovitis, hand
   M67.341 Transient synovitis, right hand
   M67.342 Transient synovitis, left hand
   M67.349 Transient synovitis, unspecified hand
● M67.35 Transient synovitis, hip
   M67.351 Transient synovitis, right hip
   M67.352 Transient synovitis, left hip
   M67.359 Transient synovitis, unspecified hip
● M67.36 Transient synovitis, knee
   M67.361 Transient synovitis, right knee
   M67.362 Transient synovitis, left knee
   M67.369 Transient synovitis, unspecified knee
● M67.37 Transient synovitis, ankle and foot
   M67.371 Transient synovitis, right ankle and foot
   M67.372 Transient synovitis, left ankle and foot
   M67.379 Transient synovitis, unspecified ankle and foot
  M67.38 Transient synovitis, other site
  M67.39 Transient synovitis, multiple sites

● M67.4 Ganglion
   Ganglion of joint or tendon (sheath)
   Excludes1 ganglion in yaws (A66.6)
   Excludes2 cyst of bursa (M71.2-M71.3)
        cyst of synovium (M71.2-M71.3)
  M67.40 Ganglion, unspecified site
● M67.41 Ganglion, shoulder
   M67.411 Ganglion, right shoulder
   M67.412 Ganglion, left shoulder
   M67.419 Ganglion, unspecified shoulder
● M67.42 Ganglion, elbow
   M67.421 Ganglion, right elbow
   M67.422 Ganglion, left elbow
   M67.429 Ganglion, unspecified elbow

● M67.43 Ganglion, wrist
   M67.431 Ganglion, right wrist
   M67.432 Ganglion, left wrist
   M67.439 Ganglion, unspecified wrist
● M67.44 Ganglion, hand
   M67.441 Ganglion, right hand
   M67.442 Ganglion, left hand
   M67.449 Ganglion, unspecified hand
● M67.45 Ganglion, hip
   M67.451 Ganglion, right hip
   M67.452 Ganglion, left hip
   M67.459 Ganglion, unspecified hip
● M67.46 Ganglion, knee
   M67.461 Ganglion, right knee
   M67.462 Ganglion, left knee
   M67.469 Ganglion, unspecified knee
● M67.47 Ganglion, ankle and foot
   M67.471 Ganglion, right ankle and foot
   M67.472 Ganglion, left ankle and foot
   M67.479 Ganglion, unspecified ankle and foot
  M67.48 Ganglion, other site
  M67.49 Ganglion, multiple sites

● M67.5 Plica syndrome
   Plica knee
  M67.50 Plica syndrome, unspecified knee
  M67.51 Plica syndrome, right knee
  M67.52 Plica syndrome, left knee

● M67.8 Other specified disorders of synovium and tendon
  M67.80 Other specified disorders of synovium and tendon, unspecified site
● M67.81 Other specified disorders of synovium and tendon, shoulder
   M67.811 Other specified disorders of synovium, right shoulder
   M67.812 Other specified disorders of synovium, left shoulder
   M67.813 Other specified disorders of tendon, right shoulder
   M67.814 Other specified disorders of tendon, left shoulder
   M67.819 Other specified disorders of synovium and tendon, unspecified shoulder
● M67.82 Other specified disorders of synovium and tendon, elbow
   M67.821 Other specified disorders of synovium, right elbow
   M67.822 Other specified disorders of synovium, left elbow
   M67.823 Other specified disorders of tendon, right elbow
   M67.824 Other specified disorders of tendon, left elbow
   M67.829 Other specified disorders of synovium and tendon, unspecified elbow
● M67.83 Other specified disorders of synovium and tendon, wrist
   M67.831 Other specified disorders of synovium, right wrist
   M67.832 Other specified disorders of synovium, left wrist
   M67.833 Other specified disorders of tendon, right wrist
   M67.834 Other specified disorders of tendon, left wrist
   M67.839 Other specified disorders of synovium and tendon, unspecified wrist

CHAPTER 13 (M00-M99)

● M67.84 Other specified disorders of synovium and tendon, hand
    M67.841 Other specified disorders of synovium, right hand
    M67.842 Other specified disorders of synovium, left hand
    M67.843 Other specified disorders of tendon, right hand
    M67.844 Other specified disorders of tendon, left hand
    M67.849 Other specified disorders of synovium and tendon, unspecified hand

● M67.85 Other specified disorders of synovium and tendon, hip
    M67.851 Other specified disorders of synovium, right hip
    M67.852 Other specified disorders of synovium, left hip
    M67.853 Other specified disorders of tendon, right hip
    M67.854 Other specified disorders of tendon, left hip
    M67.859 Other specified disorders of synovium and tendon, unspecified hip

● M67.86 Other specified disorders of synovium and tendon, knee
    M67.861 Other specified disorders of synovium, right knee
    M67.862 Other specified disorders of synovium, left knee
    M67.863 Other specified disorders of tendon, right knee
    M67.864 Other specified disorders of tendon, left knee
    M67.869 Other specified disorders of synovium and tendon, unspecified knee

● M67.87 Other specified disorders of synovium and tendon, ankle and foot
    M67.871 Other specified disorders of synovium, right ankle and foot
    M67.872 Other specified disorders of synovium, left ankle and foot
    M67.873 Other specified disorders of tendon, right ankle and foot
    M67.874 Other specified disorders of tendon, left ankle and foot
    M67.879 Other specified disorders of synovium and tendon, unspecified ankle and foot

    M67.88 Other specified disorders of synovium and tendon, other site
    M67.89 Other specified disorders of synovium and tendon, multiple sites

● M67.9 Unspecified disorder of synovium and tendon
    M67.90 Unspecified disorder of synovium and tendon, unspecified site
● M67.91 Unspecified disorder of synovium and tendon, shoulder
    M67.911 Unspecified disorder of synovium and tendon, right shoulder
    M67.912 Unspecified disorder of synovium and tendon, left shoulder
    M67.919 Unspecified disorder of synovium and tendon, unspecified shoulder

● M67.92 Unspecified disorder of synovium and tendon, upper arm
    M67.921 Unspecified disorder of synovium and tendon, right upper arm
    M67.922 Unspecified disorder of synovium and tendon, left upper arm
    M67.929 Unspecified disorder of synovium and tendon, unspecified upper arm

● M67.93 Unspecified disorder of synovium and tendon, forearm
    M67.931 Unspecified disorder of synovium and tendon, right forearm
    M67.932 Unspecified disorder of synovium and tendon, left forearm
    M67.939 Unspecified disorder of synovium and tendon, unspecified forearm

● M67.94 Unspecified disorder of synovium and tendon, hand
    M67.941 Unspecified disorder of synovium and tendon, right hand
    M67.942 Unspecified disorder of synovium and tendon, left hand
    M67.949 Unspecified disorder of synovium and tendon, unspecified hand

● M67.95 Unspecified disorder of synovium and tendon, thigh
    M67.951 Unspecified disorder of synovium and tendon, right thigh
    M67.952 Unspecified disorder of synovium and tendon, left thigh
    M67.959 Unspecified disorder of synovium and tendon, unspecified thigh

● M67.96 Unspecified disorder of synovium and tendon, lower leg
    M67.961 Unspecified disorder of synovium and tendon, right lower leg
    M67.962 Unspecified disorder of synovium and tendon, left lower leg
    M67.969 Unspecified disorder of synovium and tendon, unspecified lower leg

● M67.97 Unspecified disorder of synovium and tendon, ankle and foot
    M67.971 Unspecified disorder of synovium and tendon, right ankle and foot
    M67.972 Unspecified disorder of synovium and tendon, left ankle and foot
    M67.979 Unspecified disorder of synovium and tendon, unspecified ankle and foot

    M67.98 Unspecified disorder of synovium and tendon, other site
    M67.99 Unspecified disorder of synovium and tendon, multiple sites

OTHER SOFT TISSUE DISORDERS (M70-M79)

● M70 Soft tissue disorders related to use, overuse and pressure
    Includes soft tissue disorders of occupational origin
    Use additional external cause code to identify activity causing disorder (Y93.-)
    Excludes1 bursitis NOS (M71.9-)
    Excludes2 bursitis of shoulder (M75.5)
        enthesopathies (M76-M77)
        pressure ulcer (pressure area) (L89.-)

▶ New ⇒ Revised ~~deleted~~ Deleted Excludes 1 Excludes 2 Includes Use additional Code first Code also Key words
OGCR Official Guidelines X Assign placeholder X ● Use Additional Character(s) ▷ Manifestation Code 🔖 Hierarchical Condition Category Coding Clinic

● M70.0   Crepitant synovitis (acute) (chronic) of hand and wrist
     ● M70.03   Crepitant synovitis (acute) (chronic), wrist
         M70.031   Crepitant synovitis (acute) (chronic), right wrist
         M70.032   Crepitant synovitis (acute) (chronic), left wrist
         M70.039   Crepitant synovitis (acute) (chronic), unspecified wrist
     ● M70.04   Crepitant synovitis (acute) (chronic), hand
         M70.041   Crepitant synovitis (acute) (chronic), right hand
         M70.042   Crepitant synovitis (acute) (chronic), left hand
         M70.049   Crepitant synovitis (acute) (chronic), unspecified hand

● M70.1   Bursitis of hand
     M70.10   Bursitis, unspecified hand
     M70.11   Bursitis, right hand
     M70.12   Bursitis, left hand

● M70.2   Olecranon bursitis
     M70.20   Olecranon bursitis, unspecified elbow
     M70.21   Olecranon bursitis, right elbow
     M70.22   Olecranon bursitis, left elbow

● M70.3   Other bursitis of elbow
     M70.30   Other bursitis of elbow, unspecified elbow
     M70.31   Other bursitis of elbow, right elbow
     M70.32   Other bursitis of elbow, left elbow

● M70.4   Prepatellar bursitis
     M70.40   Prepatellar bursitis, unspecified knee
     M70.41   Prepatellar bursitis, right knee
     M70.42   Prepatellar bursitis, left knee

● M70.5   Other bursitis of knee
     M70.50   Other bursitis of knee, unspecified knee
     M70.51   Other bursitis of knee, right knee
     M70.52   Other bursitis of knee, left knee

● M70.6   Trochanteric bursitis
     Trochanteric tendinitis
     M70.60   Trochanteric bursitis, unspecified hip
     M70.61   Trochanteric bursitis, right hip
     M70.62   Trochanteric bursitis, left hip

● M70.7   Other bursitis of hip
     Ischial bursitis
     M70.70   Other bursitis of hip, unspecified hip
     M70.71   Other bursitis of hip, right hip
     M70.72   Other bursitis of hip, left hip

● M70.8   Other soft tissue disorders related to use, overuse and pressure
     M70.80   Other soft tissue disorders related to use, overuse and pressure of unspecified site
     ● M70.81   Other soft tissue disorders related to use, overuse and pressure of shoulder
         M70.811   Other soft tissue disorders related to use, overuse and pressure, right shoulder
         M70.812   Other soft tissue disorders related to use, overuse and pressure, left shoulder
         M70.819   Other soft tissue disorders related to use, overuse and pressure, unspecified shoulder

● M70.82   Other soft tissue disorders related to use, overuse and pressure of upper arm
     M70.821   Other soft tissue disorders related to use, overuse and pressure, right upper arm
     M70.822   Other soft tissue disorders related to use, overuse and pressure, left upper arm
     M70.829   Other soft tissue disorders related to use, overuse and pressure, unspecified upper arms

● M70.83   Other soft tissue disorders related to use, overuse and pressure of forearm
     M70.831   Other soft tissue disorders related to use, overuse and pressure, right forearm
     M70.832   Other soft tissue disorders related to use, overuse and pressure, left forearm
     M70.839   Other soft tissue disorders related to use, overuse and pressure, unspecified forearm

● M70.84   Other soft tissue disorders related to use, overuse and pressure of hand
     M70.841   Other soft tissue disorders related to use, overuse and pressure, right hand
     M70.842   Other soft tissue disorders related to use, overuse and pressure, left hand
     M70.849   Other soft tissue disorders related to use, overuse and pressure, unspecified hand

● M70.85   Other soft tissue disorders related to use, overuse and pressure of thigh
     M70.851   Other soft tissue disorders related to use, overuse and pressure, right thigh
     M70.852   Other soft tissue disorders related to use, overuse and pressure, left thigh
     M70.859   Other soft tissue disorders related to use, overuse and pressure, unspecified thigh

● M70.86   Other soft tissue disorders related to use, overuse and pressure lower leg
     M70.861   Other soft tissue disorders related to use, overuse and pressure, right lower leg
     M70.862   Other soft tissue disorders related to use, overuse and pressure, left lower leg
     M70.869   Other soft tissue disorders related to use, overuse and pressure, unspecified leg

● M70.87   Other soft tissue disorders related to use, overuse and pressure of ankle and foot
     M70.871   Other soft tissue disorders related to use, overuse and pressure, right ankle and foot
     M70.872   Other soft tissue disorders related to use, overuse and pressure, left ankle and foot
     M70.879   Other soft tissue disorders related to use, overuse and pressure, unspecified ankle and foot
     M70.88   Other soft tissue disorders related to use, overuse and pressure other site
     M70.89   Other soft tissue disorders related to use, overuse and pressure multiple sites

CHAPTER 13 (M00-M99)

● M70.9 Unspecified soft tissue disorder related to use, overuse and pressure

  M70.90 Unspecified soft tissue disorder related to use, overuse and pressure of unspecified site

● M70.91 Unspecified soft tissue disorder related to use, overuse and pressure of shoulder

  M70.911 Unspecified soft tissue disorder related to use, overuse and pressure, right shoulder

  M70.912 Unspecified soft tissue disorder related to use, overuse and pressure, left shoulder

  M70.919 Unspecified soft tissue disorder related to use, overuse and pressure, unspecified shoulder

● M70.92 Unspecified soft tissue disorder related to use, overuse and pressure of upper arm

  M70.921 Unspecified soft tissue disorder related to use, overuse and pressure, right upper arm

  M70.922 Unspecified soft tissue disorder related to use, overuse and pressure, left upper arm

  M70.929 Unspecified soft tissue disorder related to use, overuse and pressure, unspecified upper arm

● M70.93 Unspecified soft tissue disorder related to use, overuse and pressure of forearm

  M70.931 Unspecified soft tissue disorder related to use, overuse and pressure, right forearm

  M70.932 Unspecified soft tissue disorder related to use, overuse and pressure, left forearm

  M70.939 Unspecified soft tissue disorder related to use, overuse and pressure, unspecified forearm

● M70.94 Unspecified soft tissue disorder related to use, overuse and pressure of hand

  M70.941 Unspecified soft tissue disorder related to use, overuse and pressure, right hand

  M70.942 Unspecified soft tissue disorder related to use, overuse and pressure, left hand

  M70.949 Unspecified soft tissue disorder related to use, overuse and pressure, unspecified hand

● M70.95 Unspecified soft tissue disorder related to use, overuse and pressure of thigh

  M70.951 Unspecified soft tissue disorder related to use, overuse and pressure, right thigh

  M70.952 Unspecified soft tissue disorder related to use, overuse and pressure, left thigh

  M70.959 Unspecified soft tissue disorder related to use, overuse and pressure, unspecified thigh

● M70.96 Unspecified soft tissue disorder related to use, overuse and pressure lower leg

  M70.961 Unspecified soft tissue disorder related to use, overuse and pressure, right lower leg

  M70.962 Unspecified soft tissue disorder related to use, overuse and pressure, left lower leg

  M70.969 Unspecified soft tissue disorder related to use, overuse and pressure, unspecified lower leg

● M70.97 Unspecified soft tissue disorder related to use, overuse and pressure of ankle and foot

  M70.971 Unspecified soft tissue disorder related to use, overuse and pressure, right ankle and foot

  M70.972 Unspecified soft tissue disorder related to use, overuse and pressure, left ankle and foot

  M70.979 Unspecified soft tissue disorder related to use, overuse and pressure, unspecified ankle and foot

  M70.98 Unspecified soft tissue disorder related to use, overuse and pressure other

  M70.99 Unspecified soft tissue disorder related to use, overuse and pressure multiple sites

● M71 Other bursopathies

  Excludes1 bunion (M20.1)
            bursitis related to use, overuse or pressure (M70.-)
            enthesopathies (M76-M77)

● M71.0 Abscess of bursa

  Use additional code (B95.-, B96.-) to identify causative organism

  M71.00 Abscess of bursa, unspecified site

● M71.01 Abscess of bursa, shoulder

  M71.011 Abscess of bursa, right shoulder
  M71.012 Abscess of bursa, left shoulder
  M71.019 Abscess of bursa, unspecified shoulder

● M71.02 Abscess of bursa, elbow

  M71.021 Abscess of bursa, right elbow
  M71.022 Abscess of bursa, left elbow
  M71.029 Abscess of bursa, unspecified elbow

● M71.03 Abscess of bursa, wrist

  M71.031 Abscess of bursa, right wrist
  M71.032 Abscess of bursa, left wrist
  M71.039 Abscess of bursa, unspecified wrist

● M71.04 Abscess of bursa, hand

  M71.041 Abscess of bursa, right hand
  M71.042 Abscess of bursa, left hand
  M71.049 Abscess of bursa, unspecified hand

● M71.05 Abscess of bursa, hip

  M71.051 Abscess of bursa, right hip
  M71.052 Abscess of bursa, left hip
  M71.059 Abscess of bursa, unspecified hip

● M71.06 Abscess of bursa, knee

  M71.061 Abscess of bursa, right knee
  M71.062 Abscess of bursa, left knee
  M71.069 Abscess of bursa, unspecified knee

● M71.07 Abscess of bursa, ankle and foot

  M71.071 Abscess of bursa, right ankle and foot
  M71.072 Abscess of bursa, left ankle and foot
  M71.079 Abscess of bursa, unspecified ankle and foot

  M71.08 Abscess of bursa, other site

  M71.09 Abscess of bursa, multiple sites

● M71.1 Other infective bursitis

  Use additional code (B95.-, B96.-) to identify causative organism

  M71.10 Other infective bursitis, unspecified site

● M71.11 Other infective bursitis, shoulder

  M71.111 Other infective bursitis, right shoulder
  M71.112 Other infective bursitis, left shoulder
  M71.119 Other infective bursitis, unspecified shoulder

▶ New   ⇒ Revised   ~~deleted~~ Deleted   Excludes 1   Excludes 2   Includes   Use additional   Code first   Code also   Key words

OGCR Official Guidelines   X Assign placeholder X   ● Use Additional Character(s)   ⟩ Manifestation Code   ⟨⟩ Hierarchical Condition Category   Coding Clinic

● M71.12   Other infective bursitis, elbow
　　　　M71.121   Other infective bursitis, right elbow
　　　　M71.122   Other infective bursitis, left elbow
　　　　M71.129   Other infective bursitis, unspecified elbow
● M71.13   Other infective bursitis, wrist
　　　　M71.131   Other infective bursitis, right wrist
　　　　M71.132   Other infective bursitis, left wrist
　　　　M71.139   Other infective bursitis, unspecified wrist
● M71.14   Other infective bursitis, hand
　　　　M71.141   Other infective bursitis, right hand
　　　　M71.142   Other infective bursitis, left hand
　　　　M71.149   Other infective bursitis, unspecified hand
● M71.15   Other infective bursitis, hip
　　　　M71.151   Other infective bursitis, right hip
　　　　M71.152   Other infective bursitis, left hip
　　　　M71.159   Other infective bursitis, unspecified hip
● M71.16   Other infective bursitis, knee
　　　　M71.161   Other infective bursitis, right knee
　　　　M71.162   Other infective bursitis, left knee
　　　　M71.169   Other infective bursitis, unspecified knee
● M71.17   Other infective bursitis, ankle and foot
　　　　M71.171   Other infective bursitis, right ankle and foot
　　　　M71.172   Other infective bursitis, left ankle and foot
　　　　M71.179   Other infective bursitis, unspecified ankle and foot
　　　M71.18   Other infective bursitis, other site
　　　M71.19   Other infective bursitis, multiple sites
● M71.2   Synovial cyst of popliteal space [Baker]
　　　Popliteal space = popliteal cavity, popliteal fossa. Depression in the posterior aspect of the knee (behind the knee).
　　　Excludes1   synovial cyst of popliteal space with rupture (M66.0)
　　　M71.20   Synovial cyst of popliteal space [Baker], unspecified knee
　　　M71.21   Synovial cyst of popliteal space [Baker], right knee
　　　M71.22   Synovial cyst of popliteal space [Baker], left knee
● M71.3   Other bursal cyst
　　　Synovial cyst NOS
　　　Excludes1   synovial cyst with rupture (M66.1-)
　　　M71.30   Other bursal cyst, unspecified site
● M71.31   Other bursal cyst, shoulder
　　　　M71.311   Other bursal cyst, right shoulder
　　　　M71.312   Other bursal cyst, left shoulder
　　　　M71.319   Other bursal cyst, unspecified shoulder
● M71.32   Other bursal cyst, elbow
　　　　M71.321   Other bursal cyst, right elbow
　　　　M71.322   Other bursal cyst, left elbow
　　　　M71.329   Other bursal cyst, unspecified elbow
● M71.33   Other bursal cyst, wrist
　　　　M71.331   Other bursal cyst, right wrist
　　　　M71.332   Other bursal cyst, left wrist
　　　　M71.339   Other bursal cyst, unspecified wrist
● M71.34   Other bursal cyst, hand
　　　　M71.341   Other bursal cyst, right hand
　　　　M71.342   Other bursal cyst, left hand
　　　　M71.349   Other bursal cyst, unspecified hand

● M71.35   Other bursal cyst, hip
　　　　M71.351   Other bursal cyst, right hip
　　　　M71.352   Other bursal cyst, left hip
　　　　M71.359   Other bursal cyst, unspecified hip
● M71.37   Other bursal cyst, ankle and foot
　　　　M71.371   Other bursal cyst, right ankle and foot
　　　　M71.372   Other bursal cyst, left ankle and foot
　　　　M71.379   Other bursal cyst, unspecified ankle and foot
　　　M71.38   Other bursal cyst, other site
　　　M71.39   Other bursal cyst, multiple sites
● M71.4   Calcium deposit in bursa
　　　Excludes2   calcium deposit in bursa of shoulder (M75.3)
　　　M71.40   Calcium deposit in bursa, unspecified site
● M71.42   Calcium deposit in bursa, elbow
　　　　M71.421   Calcium deposit in bursa, right elbow
　　　　M71.422   Calcium deposit in bursa, left elbow
　　　　M71.429   Calcium deposit in bursa, unspecified elbow
● M71.43   Calcium deposit in bursa, wrist
　　　　M71.431   Calcium deposit in bursa, right wrist
　　　　M71.432   Calcium deposit in bursa, left wrist
　　　　M71.439   Calcium deposit in bursa, unspecified wrist
● M71.44   Calcium deposit in bursa, hand
　　　　M71.441   Calcium deposit in bursa, right hand
　　　　M71.442   Calcium deposit in bursa, left hand
　　　　M71.449   Calcium deposit in bursa, unspecified hand
● M71.45   Calcium deposit in bursa, hip
　　　　M71.451   Calcium deposit in bursa, right hip
　　　　M71.452   Calcium deposit in bursa, left hip
　　　　M71.459   Calcium deposit in bursa, unspecified hip
● M71.46   Calcium deposit in bursa, knee
　　　　M71.461   Calcium deposit in bursa, right knee
　　　　M71.462   Calcium deposit in bursa, left knee
　　　　M71.469   Calcium deposit in bursa, unspecified knee
● M71.47   Calcium deposit in bursa, ankle and foot
　　　　M71.471   Calcium deposit in bursa, right ankle and foot
　　　　M71.472   Calcium deposit in bursa, left ankle and foot
　　　　M71.479   Calcium deposit in bursa, unspecified ankle and foot
　　　M71.48   Calcium deposit in bursa, other site
　　　M71.49   Calcium deposit in bursa, multiple sites
● M71.5   Other bursitis, not elsewhere classified
　　　Excludes1   bursitis NOS (M71.9-)
　　　Excludes2   bursitis of shoulder (M75.5)
　　　　　　　　bursitis of tibial collateral [Pellegrini-Stieda] (M76.4-)
　　　M71.50   Other bursitis, not elsewhere classified, unspecified site
● M71.52   Other bursitis, not elsewhere classified, elbow
　　　　M71.521   Other bursitis, not elsewhere classified, right elbow
　　　　M71.522   Other bursitis, not elsewhere classified, left elbow
　　　　M71.529   Other bursitis, not elsewhere classified, unspecified elbow

● M71.53   Other bursitis, not elsewhere classified, wrist
    M71.531   Other bursitis, not elsewhere classified, right wrist
    M71.532   Other bursitis, not elsewhere classified, left wrist
    M71.539   Other bursitis, not elsewhere classified, unspecified wrist

● M71.54   Other bursitis, not elsewhere classified, hand
    M71.541   Other bursitis, not elsewhere classified, right hand
    M71.542   Other bursitis, not elsewhere classified, left hand
    M71.549   Other bursitis, not elsewhere classified, unspecified hand

● M71.55   Other bursitis, not elsewhere classified, hip
    M71.551   Other bursitis, not elsewhere classified, right hip
    M71.552   Other bursitis, not elsewhere classified, left hip
    M71.559   Other bursitis, not elsewhere classified, unspecified hip

● M71.56   Other bursitis, not elsewhere classified, knee
    M71.561   Other bursitis, not elsewhere classified, right knee
    M71.562   Other bursitis, not elsewhere classified, left knee
    M71.569   Other bursitis, not elsewhere classified, unspecified knee

● M71.57   Other bursitis, not elsewhere classified, ankle and foot
    M71.571   Other bursitis, not elsewhere classified, right ankle and foot
    M71.572   Other bursitis, not elsewhere classified, left ankle and foot
    M71.579   Other bursitis, not elsewhere classified, unspecified ankle and foot

   M71.58   Other bursitis, not elsewhere classified, other site

● M71.8   Other specified bursopathies
   M71.80   Other specified bursopathies, unspecified site
● M71.81   Other specified bursopathies, shoulder
    M71.811   Other specified bursopathies, right shoulder
    M71.812   Other specified bursopathies, left shoulder
    M71.819   Other specified bursopathies, unspecified shoulder

● M71.82   Other specified bursopathies, elbow
    M71.821   Other specified bursopathies, right elbow
    M71.822   Other specified bursopathies, left elbow
    M71.829   Other specified bursopathies, unspecified elbow

● M71.83   Other specified bursopathies, wrist
    M71.831   Other specified bursopathies, right wrist
    M71.832   Other specified bursopathies, left wrist
    M71.839   Other specified bursopathies, unspecified wrist

● M71.84   Other specified bursopathies, hand
    M71.841   Other specified bursopathies, right hand
    M71.842   Other specified bursopathies, left hand
    M71.849   Other specified bursopathies, unspecified hand

● M71.85   Other specified bursopathies, hip
    M71.851   Other specified bursopathies, right hip
    M71.852   Other specified bursopathies, left hip
    M71.859   Other specified bursopathies, unspecified hip

● M71.86   Other specified bursopathies, knee
    M71.861   Other specified bursopathies, right knee
    M71.862   Other specified bursopathies, left knee
    M71.869   Other specified bursopathies, unspecified knee

● M71.87   Other specified bursopathies, ankle and foot
    M71.871   Other specified bursopathies, right ankle and foot
    M71.872   Other specified bursopathies, left ankle and foot
    M71.879   Other specified bursopathies, unspecified ankle and foot

   M71.88   Other specified bursopathies, other site
   M71.89   Other specified bursopathies, multiple sites

M71.9   Bursopathy, unspecified
    Bursitis NOS

● M72   Fibroblastic disorders
   Excludes2   retroperitoneal fibromatosis (D48.3)

M72.0   Palmar fascial fibromatosis [Dupuytren]   A

M72.1   Knuckle pads

M72.2   Plantar fascial fibromatosis
    Plantar fasciitis

M72.4   Pseudosarcomatous fibromatosis
    Nodular fasciitis

M72.6   Necrotizing fasciitis 🅗
    Use additional code (B95.-, B96.-) to identify causative organism

M72.8   Other fibroblastic disorders
    Abscess of fascia
    Fasciitis NEC
    Other infective fasciitis
    Use additional code to (B95.-, B96.-) identify causative organism
    Excludes1   diffuse (eosinophilic) fasciitis (M35.4)
           necrotizing fasciitis (M72.6)
           nodular fasciitis (M72.4)
           perirenal fasciitis NOS (N13.5)
           perirenal fasciitis with infection (N13.6)
           plantar fasciitis (M72.2)

M72.9   Fibroblastic disorder, unspecified
    Fasciitis NOS
    Fibromatosis NOS

● M75   Shoulder lesions
   Excludes2   shoulder-hand syndrome (M89.0-)

● M75.0   Adhesive capsulitis of shoulder
    Frozen shoulder
    Periarthritis of shoulder
    M75.00   Adhesive capsulitis of unspecified shoulder
    M75.01   Adhesive capsulitis of right shoulder
    M75.02   Adhesive capsulitis of left shoulder
       Coding Clinic: 2015, Q2, P23

● M75.1   Rotator cuff tear or rupture, not specified as traumatic
    Rotator cuff syndrome
    Supraspinatus syndrome
    Supraspinatus tear or rupture, not specified as traumatic
    Excludes1   tear of rotator cuff, traumatic (S46.01-)
    Gradual onset due to repetitive stress to rotator cuff

● M75.10   Unspecified rotator cuff tear or rupture, not specified as traumatic
  - M75.100   Unspecified rotator cuff tear or rupture of unspecified shoulder, not specified as traumatic
  - M75.101   Unspecified rotator cuff tear or rupture of right shoulder, not specified as traumatic
  - M75.102   Unspecified rotator cuff tear or rupture of left shoulder, not specified as traumatic

● M75.11   Incomplete rotator cuff tear or rupture not specified as traumatic
  - M75.110   Incomplete rotator cuff tear or rupture of unspecified shoulder, not specified as traumatic
  - M75.111   Incomplete rotator cuff tear or rupture of right shoulder, not specified as traumatic
  - M75.112   Incomplete rotator cuff tear or rupture of left shoulder, not specified as traumatic

● M75.12   Complete rotator cuff tear or rupture not specified as traumatic
  - M75.120   Complete rotator cuff tear or rupture of unspecified shoulder, not specified as traumatic
  - M75.121   Complete rotator cuff tear or rupture of right shoulder, not specified as traumatic
  - M75.122   Complete rotator cuff tear or rupture of left shoulder, not specified as traumatic

● M75.2   Bicipital tendinitis
  - M75.20   Bicipital tendinitis, unspecified shoulder
  - M75.21   Bicipital tendinitis, right shoulder
  - M75.22   Bicipital tendinitis, left shoulder

● M75.3   Calcific tendinitis of shoulder
  Calcified bursa of shoulder
  - M75.30   Calcific tendinitis of unspecified shoulder
  - M75.31   Calcific tendinitis of right shoulder
  - M75.32   Calcific tendinitis of left shoulder

● M75.4   Impingement syndrome of shoulder
  - M75.40   Impingement syndrome of unspecified shoulder
  - M75.41   Impingement syndrome of right shoulder
  - M75.42   Impingement syndrome of left shoulder

● M75.5   Bursitis of shoulder
  - M75.50   Bursitis of unspecified shoulder
  - M75.51   Bursitis of right shoulder
  - M75.52   Bursitis of left shoulder

● M75.8   Other shoulder lesions
  - M75.80   Other shoulder lesions, unspecified shoulder
  - M75.81   Other shoulder lesions, right shoulder
  - M75.82   Other shoulder lesions, left shoulder

● M75.9   Shoulder lesion, unspecified
  - M75.90   Shoulder lesion, unspecified, unspecified shoulder
  - M75.91   Shoulder lesion, unspecified, right shoulder
  - M75.92   Shoulder lesion, unspecified, left shoulder

● M76   Enthesopathies, lower limb, excluding foot
  Excludes2   bursitis due to use, overuse and pressure (M70.-)
  enthesopathies of ankle and foot (M77.5-)

● M76.0   Gluteal tendinitis
  - M76.00   Gluteal tendinitis, unspecified hip
  - M76.01   Gluteal tendinitis, right hip
  - M76.02   Gluteal tendinitis, left hip

● M76.1   Psoas tendinitis
  - M76.10   Psoas tendinitis, unspecified hip
  - M76.11   Psoas tendinitis, right hip
  - M76.12   Psoas tendinitis, left hip

● M76.2   Iliac crest spur
  - M76.20   Iliac crest spur, unspecified hip
  - M76.21   Iliac crest spur, right hip
  - M76.22   Iliac crest spur, left hip

● M76.3   Iliotibial band syndrome
  - M76.30   Iliotibial band syndrome, unspecified leg
  - M76.31   Iliotibial band syndrome, right leg
  - M76.32   Iliotibial band syndrome, left leg

● M76.4   Tibial collateral bursitis [Pellegrini-Stieda]
  - M76.40   Tibial collateral bursitis [Pellegrini-Stieda], unspecified leg
  - M76.41   Tibial collateral bursitis [Pellegrini-Stieda], right leg
  - M76.42   Tibial collateral bursitis [Pellegrini-Stieda], left leg

● M76.5   Patellar tendinitis
  - M76.50   Patellar tendinitis, unspecified knee
  - M76.51   Patellar tendinitis, right knee
  - M76.52   Patellar tendinitis, left knee

● M76.6   Achilles tendinitis
  Achilles bursitis
  - M76.60   Achilles tendinitis, unspecified leg
  - M76.61   Achilles tendinitis, right leg
  - M76.62   Achilles tendinitis, left leg

● M76.7   Peroneal tendinitis
  - M76.70   Peroneal tendinitis, unspecified leg
  - M76.71   Peroneal tendinitis, right leg
  - M76.72   Peroneal tendinitis, left leg

● M76.8   Other specified enthesopathies of lower limb, excluding foot
  - ● M76.81   Anterior tibial syndrome
    - M76.811   Anterior tibial syndrome, right leg
    - M76.812   Anterior tibial syndrome, left leg
    - M76.819   Anterior tibial syndrome, unspecified leg
  - ● M76.82   Posterior tibial tendinitis
    - M76.821   Posterior tibial tendinitis, right leg
    - M76.822   Posterior tibial tendinitis, left leg
    - M76.829   Posterior tibial tendinitis, unspecified leg
  - ● M76.89   Other specified enthesopathies of lower limb, excluding foot
    - M76.891   Other specified enthesopathies of right lower limb, excluding foot
    - M76.892   Other specified enthesopathies of left lower limb, excluding foot
    - M76.899   Other specified enthesopathies of unspecified lower limb, excluding foot

● M76.9   Unspecified enthesopathy, lower limb, excluding foot

● M77   Other enthesopathies
  Excludes1   bursitis NOS (M71.9-)
  Excludes2   bursitis due to use, overuse and pressure (M70.-)
  osteophyte (M25.7)
  spinal enthesopathy (M46.0-)

● M77.0   Medial epicondylitis
  - M77.00   Medial epicondylitis, unspecified elbow
  - M77.01   Medial epicondylitis, right elbow
  - M77.02   Medial epicondylitis, left elbow

CHAPTER 13 (M00-M99)

● M77.1 Lateral epicondylitis
   Tennis elbow
   M77.10 Lateral epicondylitis, unspecified elbow
   M77.11 Lateral epicondylitis, right elbow
   M77.12 Lateral epicondylitis, left elbow
● M77.2 Periarthritis of wrist
   M77.20 Periarthritis, unspecified wrist
   M77.21 Periarthritis, right wrist
   M77.22 Periarthritis, left wrist
● M77.3 Calcaneal spur
   M77.30 Calcaneal spur, unspecified foot
   M77.31 Calcaneal spur, right foot
   M77.32 Calcaneal spur, left foot
● M77.4 Metatarsalgia
   Excludes1 Morton's metatarsalgia (G57.6)
   M77.40 Metatarsalgia, unspecified foot
   M77.41 Metatarsalgia, right foot
   M77.42 Metatarsalgia, left foot
● M77.5 Other enthesopathy of foot and ankle
   M77.50 Other enthesopathy of unspecified foot and ankle
   M77.51 Other enthesopathy of right foot and ankle
   M77.52 Other enthesopathy of left foot and ankle
  M77.8 Other enthesopathies, not elsewhere classified
  M77.9 Enthesopathy, unspecified
   Bone spur NOS
   Capsulitis NOS
   Periarthritis NOS
   Tendinitis NOS

● M79 Other and unspecified soft tissue disorders, not elsewhere classified
   Excludes1 psychogenic rheumatism (F45.8)
      soft tissue pain, psychogenic (F45.41)
  M79.0 Rheumatism, unspecified
   Excludes1 fibromyalgia (M79.7)
      palindromic rheumatism (M12.3-)
● M79.1 Myalgia
   Myofascial pain syndrome
   M79.10 Myalgia, unspecified site
   M79.11 Myalgia of mastication muscle
   M79.12 Myalgia of auxiliary muscles, head and neck
   M79.18 Myalgia, other site
     Excludes1 fibromyalgia (M79.7)
       myositis (M60.-)
  M79.2 Neuralgia and neuritis, unspecified
   Excludes1 brachial radiculitis NOS (M54.1)
      lumbosacral radiculitis NOS (M54.1)
      mononeuropathies (G56-G58)
      radiculitis NOS (M54.1)
      sciatica (M54.3-M54.4)
  M79.3 Panniculitis, unspecified
   Excludes1 lupus panniculitis (L93.2)
      neck and back panniculitis (M54.0-)
      relapsing [Weber-Christian] panniculitis (M35.6)
  M79.4 Hypertrophy of (infrapatellar) fat pad
  M79.5 Residual foreign body in soft tissue
   Excludes1 foreign body granuloma of skin and subcutaneous tissue (L92.3)
      foreign body granuloma of soft tissue (M60.2-)
● M79.6 Pain in limb, hand, foot, fingers and toes
   Excludes2 pain in joint (M25.5-)
  ● M79.60 Pain in limb, unspecified
   M79.601 Pain in right arm
     Pain in right upper limb NOS
   M79.602 Pain in left arm
     Pain in left upper limb NOS

   M79.603 Pain in arm, unspecified
     Pain in upper limb NOS
   M79.604 Pain in right leg
     Pain in right lower limb NOS
   M79.605 Pain in left leg
     Pain in left lower limb NOS
   M79.606 Pain in leg, unspecified
     Pain in lower limb NOS
   M79.609 Pain in unspecified limb
     Pain in limb NOS
● M79.62 Pain in upper arm
   Pain in axillary region
   M79.621 Pain in right upper arm
   M79.622 Pain in left upper arm
   M79.629 Pain in unspecified upper arm
● M79.63 Pain in forearm
   M79.631 Pain in right forearm
   M79.632 Pain in left forearm
   M79.639 Pain in unspecified forearm
● M79.64 Pain in hand and fingers
   M79.641 Pain in right hand
   M79.642 Pain in left hand
   M79.643 Pain in unspecified hand
   M79.644 Pain in right finger(s)
   M79.645 Pain in left finger(s)
   M79.646 Pain in unspecified finger(s)
● M79.65 Pain in thigh
   M79.651 Pain in right thigh
   M79.652 Pain in left thigh
   M79.659 Pain in unspecified thigh
● M79.66 Pain in lower leg
   M79.661 Pain in right lower leg
   M79.662 Pain in left lower leg
   M79.669 Pain in unspecified lower leg
● M79.67 Pain in foot and toes
   M79.671 Pain in right foot
   M79.672 Pain in left foot
   M79.673 Pain in unspecified foot
   M79.674 Pain in right toe(s)
   M79.675 Pain in left toe(s)
   M79.676 Pain in unspecified toe(s)
  M79.7 Fibromyalgia
   Fibromyositis
   Fibrositis
   Myofibrositis
● M79.A Nontraumatic compartment syndrome
   Code first, if applicable, associated postprocedural complication
   Excludes1 compartment syndrome NOS (T79.A-)
      fibromyalgia (M79.7) nontraumatic ischemic infarction of muscle (M62.2-)
      traumatic compartment syndrome (T79.A-)
● M79.A1 Nontraumatic compartment syndrome of upper extremity
   Nontraumatic compartment syndrome of shoulder, arm, forearm, wrist, hand, and fingers
   M79.A11 Nontraumatic compartment syndrome of right upper extremity
   M79.A12 Nontraumatic compartment syndrome of left upper extremity
   M79.A19 Nontraumatic compartment syndrome of unspecified upper extremity
● M79.A2 Nontraumatic compartment syndrome of lower extremity
   Nontraumatic compartment syndrome of hip, buttock, thigh, leg, foot, and toes
   M79.A21 Nontraumatic compartment syndrome of right lower extremity

▶ New ⇒ Revised ~~deleted~~ Deleted Excludes 1 Excludes 2 Includes Use additional Code first Code also Key words
OGCR Official Guidelines X Assign placeholder X ● Use Additional Character(s) ▷ Manifestation Code ⚙ Hierarchical Condition Category **Coding Clinic**

M79.A22 **Nontraumatic compartment syndrome of left lower extremity**

M79.A29 **Nontraumatic compartment syndrome of unspecified lower extremity**

M79.A3 **Nontraumatic compartment syndrome of abdomen**

M79.A9 **Nontraumatic compartment syndrome of other sites**

● M79.8 **Other specified soft tissue disorders**

M79.81 **Nontraumatic hematoma of soft tissue**
Nontraumatic hematoma of muscle
Nontraumatic seroma of muscle and soft tissue

M79.89 **Other specified soft tissue disorders**
Polyalgia

M79.9 **Soft tissue disorder, unspecified**

OGCR See Section I.C., Chapter 13.d.

Osteoporosis

Osteoporosis is a systemic condition, meaning that all bones of the musculoskeletal system are affected. Therefore, site is not a component of the codes under category M81, Osteoporosis without current pathological fracture. The site codes under category M80, Osteoporosis with current pathological fracture, identify the site of the fracture, not the osteoporosis.

1) Osteoporosis without pathological fracture

Category M81, Osteoporosis without current pathological fracture, is for use for patients with osteoporosis who do not currently have a pathologic fracture due to the osteoporosis, even if they have had a fracture in the past. For patients with a history of osteoporosis fractures, status code Z87.310, Personal history of (healed) osteoporosis fracture, should follow the code from M81.

2) Osteoporosis with current pathological fracture

Category M80, Osteoporosis with current pathological fracture, is for patients who have a current pathologic fracture at the time of an encounter. The codes under M80 identify the site of the fracture. A code from category M80, not a traumatic fracture code, should be used for any patient with known osteoporosis who suffers a fracture, even if the patient had a minor fall or trauma, if that fall or trauma would not usually break a normal, healthy bone.

OSTEOPATHIES AND CHONDROPATHIES (M80-M94)

DISORDERS OF BONE DENSITY AND STRUCTURE (M80-M85)

M80 **Osteoporosis with current pathological fracture**
Excessive skeletal fragility (porous bone) resulting in bone fractures

Includes   osteoporosis with current fragility fracture

Use additional code to identify major osseous defect, if applicable (M89.7-)

Excludes1   collapsed vertebra NOS (M48.5)
pathological fracture NOS (M84.4)
wedging of vertebra NOS (M48.5)

Excludes2   personal history of (healed) osteoporosis fracture (Z87.310)

Coding Clinic: 2018, Q2, P12

The appropriate 7th character is to be added to each code from category M80:

A	initial encounter for fracture *All encounters involving diagnosis and treatment*
D	subsequent encounter for fracture with routine healing
G	subsequent encounter for fracture with delayed healing *Encounters for attention to casting or fixation devices, medication, and follow-up visits during the healing phase*
K	subsequent encounter for fracture with nonunion *Total failure of fracture healing*
P	subsequent encounter for fracture with malunion *Fracture ends do not heal together correctly.*
S	sequela

● M80.0 **Age-related osteoporosis with current pathological fracture**
Involutional osteoporosis with current pathological fracture
Osteoporosis NOS with current pathological fracture
Postmenopausal osteoporosis with current pathological fracture
Senile osteoporosis with current pathological fracture

X ● M80.00 **Age-related osteoporosis with current pathological fracture, unspecified site**   A

● M80.01 **Age-related osteoporosis with current pathological fracture, shoulder**

● M80.011 **Age-related osteoporosis with current pathological fracture, right shoulder** A

● M80.012 **Age-related osteoporosis with current pathological fracture, left shoulder** A

● M80.019 **Age-related osteoporosis with current pathological fracture, unspecified shoulder** A

● M80.02 **Age-related osteoporosis with current pathological fracture, humerus**

● M80.021 **Age-related osteoporosis with current pathological fracture, right humerus** A

● M80.022 **Age-related osteoporosis with current pathological fracture, left humerus** A

● M80.029 **Age-related osteoporosis with current pathological fracture, unspecified humerus** A

● M80.03 **Age-related osteoporosis with current pathological fracture, forearm**
Age-related osteoporosis with current pathological fracture of wrist

● M80.031 **Age-related osteoporosis with current pathological fracture, right forearm** A

● M80.032 **Age-related osteoporosis with current pathological fracture, left forearm** A

● M80.039 **Age-related osteoporosis with current pathological fracture, unspecified forearm** A

● M80.04 **Age-related osteoporosis with current pathological fracture, hand**

● M80.041 **Age-related osteoporosis with current pathological fracture, right hand** A

● M80.042 **Age-related osteoporosis with current pathological fracture, left hand** A

● M80.049 **Age-related osteoporosis with current pathological fracture, unspecified hand** A

● M80.05 **Age-related osteoporosis with current pathological fracture, femur**
Age-related osteoporosis with current pathological fracture of hip

● M80.051 **Age-related osteoporosis with current pathological fracture, right femur** A 🖼   A

● M80.052 **Age-related osteoporosis with current pathological fracture, left femur** A 🖼 A
Coding Clinic: 2018, Q2, P12

● M80.059 **Age-related osteoporosis with current pathological fracture, unspecified femur** A 🖼   A

● M80.06 **Age-related osteoporosis with current pathological fracture, lower leg**

● M80.061 **Age-related osteoporosis with current pathological fracture, right lower leg** A

● M80.062 **Age-related osteoporosis with current pathological fracture, left lower leg** A

● M80.069 **Age-related osteoporosis with current pathological fracture, unspecified lower leg** A

M80.07   Age-related osteoporosis with current pathological fracture, ankle and foot

    M80.071   Age-related osteoporosis with current pathological fracture, right ankle and foot   A

    M80.072   Age-related osteoporosis with current pathological fracture, left ankle and foot   A

    M80.079   Age-related osteoporosis with current pathological fracture, unspecified ankle and foot   A

X **M80.08**   Age-related osteoporosis with current pathological fracture, vertebra(e)
    A 🦠   A

M80.0A   Age-related osteoporosis with current pathological fracture, other site
                     A

M80.8   Other osteoporosis with current pathological fracture

    Drug-induced osteoporosis with current pathological fracture

    Idiopathic osteoporosis with current pathological fracture

    Osteoporosis of disuse with current pathological fracture

    Postoophorectomy osteoporosis with current pathological fracture

    Postsurgical malabsorption osteoporosis with current pathological fracture

    Post-traumatic osteoporosis with current pathological fracture

    Use additional code for adverse effect, if applicable, to identify drug (T36-T50 with fifth or sixth character 5)

X **M80.80**   Other osteoporosis with current pathological fracture, unspecified site   A

M80.81   Other osteoporosis with pathological fracture, shoulder

    M80.811   Other osteoporosis with current pathological fracture, right shoulder

    M80.812   Other osteoporosis with current pathological fracture, left shoulder

    M80.819   Other osteoporosis with current pathological fracture, unspecified shoulder

M80.82   Other osteoporosis with current pathological fracture, humerus

    M80.821   Other osteoporosis with current pathological fracture, right humerus

    M80.822   Other osteoporosis with current pathological fracture, left humerus

    M80.829   Other osteoporosis with current pathological fracture, unspecified humerus

M80.83   Other osteoporosis with current pathological fracture, forearm

    Other osteoporosis with current pathological fracture of wrist

    M80.831   Other osteoporosis with current pathological fracture, right forearm

    M80.832   Other osteoporosis with current pathological fracture, left forearm

    M80.839   Other osteoporosis with current pathological fracture, unspecified forearm

M80.8A   Other osteoporosis with current pathological fracture, other site

M80.84   Other osteoporosis with current pathological fracture, hand

    M80.841   Other osteoporosis with current pathological fracture, right hand

    M80.842   Other osteoporosis with current pathological fracture, left hand

    M80.849   Other osteoporosis with current pathological fracture, unspecified hand

M80.85   Other osteoporosis with current pathological fracture, femur

    Other osteoporosis with current pathological fracture of hip

    M80.851   Other osteoporosis with current pathological fracture, right femur
    A 🦠

    M80.852   Other osteoporosis with current pathological fracture, left femur A 🦠

    M80.859   Other osteoporosis with current pathological fracture, unspecified femur A 🦠

M80.86   Other osteoporosis with current pathological fracture, lower leg

    M80.861   Other osteoporosis with current pathological fracture, right lower leg

    M80.862   Other osteoporosis with current pathological fracture, left lower leg

    M80.869   Other osteoporosis with current pathological fracture, unspecified lower leg

M80.87   Other osteoporosis with current pathological fracture, ankle and foot

    M80.871   Other osteoporosis with current pathological fracture, right ankle and foot

    M80.872   Other osteoporosis with current pathological fracture, left ankle and foot

    M80.879   Other osteoporosis with current pathological fracture, unspecified ankle and foot

X **M80.88**   Other osteoporosis with current pathological fracture, vertebra(e) A 🦠

M81   Osteoporosis without current pathological fracture

    Use additional code to identify:
    major osseous defect, if applicable (M89.7-)
    personal history of (healed) osteoporosis fracture, if applicable (Z87.310)

    Excludes1   osteoporosis with current pathological fracture (M80.-)
               Sudeck's atrophy (M89.0)

M81.0   Age-related osteoporosis without current pathological fracture   A

    Involutional osteoporosis without current pathological fracture

    Osteoporosis NOS

    Postmenopausal osteoporosis without current pathological fracture

    Senile osteoporosis without current pathological fracture

M81.6   Localized osteoporosis [Lequesne]

    Excludes1   Sudeck's atrophy (M89.0)

M81.8 Other osteoporosis without current pathological fracture
Drug-induced osteoporosis without current pathological fracture
Idiopathic osteoporosis without current pathological fracture
Osteoporosis of disuse without current pathological fracture
Postoophorectomy osteoporosis without current pathological fracture
Postsurgical malabsorption osteoporosis without current pathological fracture
Post-traumatic osteoporosis without current pathological fracture
Use additional code for adverse effect, if applicable, to identify drug (T36-T50 with fifth or sixth character 5)

● **M83 Adult osteomalacia**
     Excludes1   infantile and juvenile osteomalacia (E55.0)
                     renal osteodystrophy (N25.0)
                     rickets (active) (E55.0)
                     rickets (active) sequelae (E64.3)
                     vitamin D-resistant osteomalacia (E83.3)
                     vitamin D-resistant rickets (active) (E83.3)

   M83.0 **Puerperal osteomalacia** ♀   M

   M83.1 **Senile osteomalacia**   A

   M83.2 **Adult osteomalacia due to malabsorption**   A
          Postsurgical malabsorption osteomalacia in adults

   M83.3 **Adult osteomalacia due to malnutrition**   A

   M83.4 **Aluminum bone disease**

   M83.5 **Other drug-induced osteomalacia in adults**   A
          Use additional code for adverse effect, if applicable, to identify drug (T36-T50 with fifth or sixth character 5)

   M83.8 **Other adult osteomalacia**   A

   M83.9 **Adult osteomalacia, unspecified**   A

● **M84 Disorder of continuity of bone**
     Excludes2   traumatic fracture of bone-see fracture, by site

● **M84.3 Stress fracture**
     Fatigue fracture
     March fracture
     Stress fracture NOS
     Stress reaction
     Use additional external cause code(s) to identify the cause of the stress fracture
     Excludes1   pathological fracture NOS (M84.4.-)
                     pathological fracture due to osteoporosis (M80.-)
                     traumatic fracture (S12.-, S22.-, S32.-, S42.-, S52.-, S62.-, S72.-, S82.-, S92.-)
     Excludes2   personal history of (healed) stress (fatigue) fracture (Z87.312)
                     stress fracture of vertebra (M48.4-)

     The appropriate 7th character is to be added to each code from subcategory M84.3:

A	initial encounter for fracture
D	subsequent encounter for fracture with routine healing
G	subsequent encounter for fracture with delayed healing
K	subsequent encounter for fracture with nonunion
P	subsequent encounter for fracture with malunion
S	sequela

X ● **M84.30 Stress fracture, unspecified site**
   ● M84.31 **Stress fracture, shoulder**
     ● M84.311   Stress fracture, right shoulder
     ● M84.312   Stress fracture, left shoulder
     ● M84.319   Stress fracture, unspecified shoulder
   ● M84.32 **Stress fracture, humerus**
     ● M84.321   Stress fracture, right humerus
     ● M84.322   Stress fracture, left humerus
     ● M84.329   Stress fracture, unspecified humerus

● M84.33 **Stress fracture, ulna and radius**
   ● M84.331   Stress fracture, right ulna
   ● M84.332   Stress fracture, left ulna
   ● M84.333   Stress fracture, right radius
   ● M84.334   Stress fracture, left radius
   ● M84.339   Stress fracture, unspecified ulna and radius
● M84.34 **Stress fracture, hand and fingers**
   ● M84.341   Stress fracture, right hand
   ● M84.342   Stress fracture, left hand
   ● M84.343   Stress fracture, unspecified hand
   ● M84.344   Stress fracture, right finger(s)
   ● M84.345   Stress fracture, left finger(s)
   ● M84.346   Stress fracture, unspecified finger(s)
● M84.35 **Stress fracture, pelvis and femur**
     Stress fracture, hip
   ● M84.350   Stress fracture, pelvis
   ● M84.351   Stress fracture, right femur
   ● M84.352   Stress fracture, left femur
   ● M84.353   Stress fracture, unspecified femur
   ● M84.359   Stress fracture, hip, unspecified
● M84.36 **Stress fracture, tibia and fibula**
   ● M84.361   Stress fracture, right tibia
   ● M84.362   Stress fracture, left tibia
   ● M84.363   Stress fracture, right fibula
   ● M84.364   Stress fracture, left fibula
   ● M84.369   Stress fracture, unspecified tibia and fibula
● M84.37 **Stress fracture, ankle, foot and toes**
   ● M84.371   Stress fracture, right ankle
   ● M84.372   Stress fracture, left ankle
   ● M84.373   Stress fracture, unspecified ankle
   ● M84.374   Stress fracture, right foot
   ● M84.375   Stress fracture, left foot
   ● M84.376   Stress fracture, unspecified foot
   ● M84.377   Stress fracture, right toe(s)
   ● M84.378   Stress fracture, left toe(s)
   ● M84.379   Stress fracture, unspecified toe(s)
X ● M84.38 **Stress fracture, other site**
        Excludes2   stress fracture of vertebra (M48.4-)

● **M84.4 Pathological fracture, not elsewhere classified**
     Chronic fracture
     Pathological fracture NOS
     Excludes1   collapsed vertebra NEC (M48.5)
                     pathological fracture in neoplastic disease (M84.5-)
                     pathological fracture in osteoporosis (M80.-)
                     pathological fracture in other disease (M84.6-)
                     stress fracture (M84.3-)
                     traumatic fracture (S12.-, S22.-, S32.-, S42.-, S52.-, S62.-, S72.-, S82.-, S92.-)
     Excludes2   personal history of (healed) pathological fracture (Z87.311)

     The appropriate 7th character is to be added to each code from subcategory M84.4:

A	initial encounter for fracture
D	subsequent encounter for fracture with routine healing
G	subsequent encounter for fracture with delayed healing
K	subsequent encounter for fracture with nonunion
P	subsequent encounter for fracture with malunion
S	sequela

CHAPTER 13 (M00-M99)

X● M84.40   Pathological fracture, unspecified site

● M84.41   Pathological fracture, shoulder

     ● M84.411   Pathological fracture, right shoulder

     ● M84.412   Pathological fracture, left shoulder

     ● M84.419   Pathological fracture, unspecified shoulder

● M84.42   Pathological fracture, humerus

     ● M84.421   Pathological fracture, right humerus

     ● M84.422   Pathological fracture, left humerus

     ● M84.429   Pathological fracture, unspecified humerus

● M84.43   Pathological fracture, ulna and radius

     ● M84.431   Pathological fracture, right ulna

     ● M84.432   Pathological fracture, left ulna

     ● M84.433   Pathological fracture, right radius

     ● M84.434   Pathological fracture, left radius

     ● M84.439   Pathological fracture, unspecified ulna and radius

● M84.44   Pathological fracture, hand and fingers

     ● M84.441   Pathological fracture, right hand

     ● M84.442   Pathological fracture, left hand

     ● M84.443   Pathological fracture, unspecified hand

     ● M84.444   Pathological fracture, right finger(s)

     ● M84.445   Pathological fracture, left finger(s)

     ● M84.446   Pathological fracture, unspecified finger(s)

● M84.45   Pathological fracture, femur and pelvis

     ● M84.451   Pathological fracture, right femur A ⓗ

     ● M84.452   Pathological fracture, left femur A ⓗ

     ● M84.453   Pathological fracture, unspecified femur A ⓗ

     ● M84.454   Pathological fracture, pelvis A ⓗ
            Coding Clinic: 2016, Q4, P43

     ● M84.459   Pathological fracture, hip, unspecified A ⓗ

● M84.46   Pathological fracture, tibia and fibula

     ● M84.461   Pathological fracture, right tibia

     ● M84.462   Pathological fracture, left tibia

     ● M84.463   Pathological fracture, right fibula

     ● M84.464   Pathological fracture, left fibula

     ● M84.469   Pathological fracture, unspecified tibia and fibula

● M84.47   Pathological fracture, ankle, foot and toes

     ● M84.471   Pathological fracture, right ankle

     ● M84.472   Pathological fracture, left ankle

     ● M84.473   Pathological fracture, unspecified ankle

     ● M84.474   Pathological fracture, right foot

     ● M84.475   Pathological fracture, left foot

     ● M84.476   Pathological fracture, unspecified foot

     ● M84.477   Pathological fracture, right toe(s)

     ● M84.478   Pathological fracture, left toe(s)

     ● M84.479   Pathological fracture, unspecified toe(s)

X● M84.48   Pathological fracture, other site

OGCR Section I.C. 13.C.

Coding of Pathologic Fractures

7th character A is for use as long as the patient is receiving active treatment for the fracture. While the patient may be seen by a new or different provider over the course of treatment for a pathological fracture, assignment of the 7th character is based on whether the patient is undergoing active treatment and not whether the provider is seeing the patient for the first time.

7th character, D is to be used for encounters after the patient has completed active treatment for the fracture and is receiving routine care for the fracture during the healing or recovery phase. The other 7th characters, listed under each subcategory in the Tabular List, are to be used for subsequent encounters for treatment of problems associated with the healing, such as malunions, nonunions, and sequelae.

Care for complications of surgical treatment for fracture repairs during the healing or recovery phase should be coded with the appropriate complication codes.

See Section I.C.19. Coding of traumatic fractures.

● M84.5   Pathological fracture in neoplastic disease

     Code also underlying neoplasm

     The appropriate 7th character is to be added to each code from subcategory M84.5:

A	initial encounter for fracture
D	subsequent encounter for fracture with routine healing
G	subsequent encounter for fracture with delayed healing
K	subsequent encounter for fracture with nonunion
P	subsequent encounter for fracture with malunion
S	sequela

X● M84.50   Pathological fracture in neoplastic disease, unspecified site

● M84.51   Pathological fracture in neoplastic disease, shoulder

     ● M84.511   Pathological fracture in neoplastic disease, right shoulder

     ● M84.512   Pathological fracture in neoplastic disease, left shoulder

     ● M84.519   Pathological fracture in neoplastic disease, unspecified shoulder

● M84.52   Pathological fracture in neoplastic disease, humerus

     ● M84.521   Pathological fracture in neoplastic disease, right humerus

     ● M84.522   Pathological fracture in neoplastic disease, left humerus

     ● M84.529   Pathological fracture in neoplastic disease, unspecified humerus

● M84.53   Pathological fracture in neoplastic disease, ulna and radius

     ● M84.531   Pathological fracture in neoplastic disease, right ulna

     ● M84.532   Pathological fracture in neoplastic disease, left ulna

     ● M84.533   Pathological fracture in neoplastic disease, right radius

     ● M84.534   Pathological fracture in neoplastic disease, left radius

     ● M84.539   Pathological fracture in neoplastic disease, unspecified ulna and radius

● M84.54   Pathological fracture in neoplastic disease, hand

     ● M84.541   Pathological fracture in neoplastic disease, right hand

     ● M84.542   Pathological fracture in neoplastic disease, left hand

     ● M84.549   Pathological fracture in neoplastic disease, unspecified hand

---

▶ New   ⇒ Revised   ~~deleted~~ Deleted   Excludes 1   Excludes 2   Includes   Use additional   Code first   Code also   Key words

OGCR Official Guidelines   X Assign placeholder X   ● Use Additional Character(s)   ▶ Manifestation Code   ⓗ Hierarchical Condition Category   **Coding Clinic**

● M84.55   Pathological fracture in neoplastic disease, pelvis and femur
    ● M84.550   Pathological fracture in neoplastic disease, pelvis
    ● M84.551   Pathological fracture in neoplastic disease, right femur A 🐾
    ● M84.552   Pathological fracture in neoplastic disease, left femur A 🐾
    ● M84.553   Pathological fracture in neoplastic disease, unspecified femur A 🐾
    ● M84.559   Pathological fracture in neoplastic disease, hip, unspecified A 🐾

● M84.56   Pathological fracture in neoplastic disease, tibia and fibula
    ● M84.561   Pathological fracture in neoplastic disease, right tibia
    ● M84.562   Pathological fracture in neoplastic disease, left tibia
    ● M84.563   Pathological fracture in neoplastic disease, right fibula
    ● M84.564   Pathological fracture in neoplastic disease, left fibula
    ● M84.569   Pathological fracture in neoplastic disease, unspecified tibia and fibula

● M84.57   Pathological fracture in neoplastic disease, ankle and foot
    ● M84.571   Pathological fracture in neoplastic disease, right ankle
    ● M84.572   Pathological fracture in neoplastic disease, left ankle
    ● M84.573   Pathological fracture in neoplastic disease, unspecified ankle
    ● M84.574   Pathological fracture in neoplastic disease, right foot
    ● M84.575   Pathological fracture in neoplastic disease, left foot
    ● M84.576   Pathological fracture in neoplastic disease, unspecified foot

X ● M84.58   Pathological fracture in neoplastic disease, other specified site
      Pathological fracture in neoplastic disease, vertebrae

● M84.6   **Pathological fracture in other disease**
    Code also underlying condition
    Excludes1   pathological fracture in osteoporosis (M80.-)

    The appropriate 7th character is to be added to each code from subcategory M84.6:

> A   initial encounter for fracture
> D   subsequent encounter for fracture with routine healing
> G   subsequent encounter for fracture with delayed healing
> K   subsequent encounter for fracture with nonunion
> P   subsequent encounter for fracture with malunion
> S   sequela

X ● M84.60   Pathological fracture in other disease, unspecified site

● M84.61   Pathological fracture in other disease, shoulder
    ● M84.611   Pathological fracture in other disease, right shoulder
    ● M84.612   Pathological fracture in other disease, left shoulder
    ● M84.619   Pathological fracture in other disease, unspecified shoulder

● M84.62   Pathological fracture in other disease, humerus
    ● M84.621   Pathological fracture in other disease, right humerus
    ● M84.622   Pathological fracture in other disease, left humerus
    ● M84.629   Pathological fracture in other disease, unspecified humerus

● M84.63   Pathological fracture in other disease, ulna and radius
    ● M84.631   Pathological fracture in other disease, right ulna
    ● M84.632   Pathological fracture in other disease, left ulna
    ● M84.633   Pathological fracture in other disease, right radius
    ● M84.634   Pathological fracture in other disease, left radius
    ● M84.639   Pathological fracture in other disease, unspecified ulna and radius

● M84.64   Pathological fracture in other disease, hand
    ● M84.641   Pathological fracture in other disease, right hand
    ● M84.642   Pathological fracture in other disease, left hand
    ● M84.649   Pathological fracture in other disease, unspecified hand

● M84.65   Pathological fracture in other disease, pelvis and femur
    ● M84.650   Pathological fracture in other disease, pelvis
    ● M84.651   Pathological fracture in other disease, right femur A 🐾
    ● M84.652   Pathological fracture in other disease, left femur A 🐾
    ● M84.653   Pathological fracture in other disease, unspecified femur A 🐾
    ● M84.659   Pathological fracture in other disease, hip, unspecified A 🐾

● M84.66   Pathological fracture in other disease, tibia and fibula
    ● M84.661   Pathological fracture in other disease, right tibia
    ● M84.662   Pathological fracture in other disease, left tibia
    ● M84.663   Pathological fracture in other disease, right fibula
    ● M84.664   Pathological fracture in other disease, left fibula
    ● M84.669   Pathological fracture in other disease, unspecified tibia and fibula

● M84.67   Pathological fracture in other disease, ankle and foot
    ● M84.671   Pathological fracture in other disease, right ankle
    ● M84.672   Pathological fracture in other disease, left ankle
    ● M84.673   Pathological fracture in other disease, unspecified ankle
    ● M84.674   Pathological fracture in other disease, right foot
    ● M84.675   Pathological fracture in other disease, left foot
    ● M84.676   Pathological fracture in other disease, unspecified foot

X ● M84.68   Pathological fracture in other disease, other site

● **M84.7   Nontraumatic fracture, not elsewhere classified**
    ● **M84.75   Atypical femoral fracture**

The appropriate 7th character is to be added to each code from M84.75:

A	initial encounter for fracture
D	subsequent encounter for fracture with routine healing
G	subsequent encounter for fracture with delayed healing
K	subsequent encounter for fracture with nonunion
P	subsequent encounter for fracture with malunion
S	sequela

Coding Clinic: 2016, Q4, P41

      ● **M84.750   Atypical femoral fracture, unspecified**

      ● **M84.751   Incomplete atypical femoral fracture, right leg**

      ● **M84.752   Incomplete atypical femoral fracture, left leg**

      ● **M84.753   Incomplete atypical femoral fracture, unspecified leg**

      ● **M84.754   Complete transverse atypical femoral fracture, right leg A** 🝒

      ● **M84.755   Complete transverse atypical femoral fracture, left leg A** 🝒

      ● **M84.756   Complete transverse atypical femoral fracture, unspecified leg A** 🝒

      ● **M84.757   Complete oblique atypical femoral fracture, right leg A** 🝒

      ● **M84.758   Complete oblique atypical femoral fracture, left leg A** 🝒

      ● **M84.759   Complete oblique atypical femoral fracture, unspecified leg , A** 🝒

● **M84.8   Other disorders of continuity of bone**
    M84.80   Other disorders of continuity of bone, unspecified site

    ● **M84.81   Other disorders of continuity of bone, shoulder**

      M84.811   Other disorders of continuity of bone, right shoulder

      M84.812   Other disorders of continuity of bone, left shoulder

      M84.819   Other disorders of continuity of bone, unspecified shoulder

    ● **M84.82   Other disorders of continuity of bone, humerus**

      M84.821   Other disorders of continuity of bone, right humerus

      M84.822   Other disorders of continuity of bone, left humerus

      M84.829   Other disorders of continuity of bone, unspecified humerus

    ● **M84.83   Other disorders of continuity of bone, ulna and radius**

      M84.831   Other disorders of continuity of bone, right ulna

      M84.832   Other disorders of continuity of bone, left ulna

      M84.833   Other disorders of continuity of bone, right radius

      M84.834   Other disorders of continuity of bone, left radius

      M84.839   Other disorders of continuity of bone, unspecified ulna and radius

● **M84.84   Other disorders of continuity of bone, hand**

      M84.841   Other disorders of continuity of bone, right hand

      M84.842   Other disorders of continuity of bone, left hand

      M84.849   Other disorders of continuity of bone, unspecified hand

● **M84.85   Other disorders of continuity of bone, pelvic region and thigh**

      M84.851   Other disorders of continuity of bone, right pelvic region and thigh

      M84.852   Other disorders of continuity of bone, left pelvic region and thigh

      M84.859   Other disorders of continuity of bone, unspecified pelvic region and thigh

● **M84.86   Other disorders of continuity of bone, tibia and fibula**

      M84.861   Other disorders of continuity of bone, right tibia

      M84.862   Other disorders of continuity of bone, left tibia

      M84.863   Other disorders of continuity of bone, right fibula

      M84.864   Other disorders of continuity of bone, left fibula

      M84.869   Other disorders of continuity of bone, unspecified tibia and fibula

● **M84.87   Other disorders of continuity of bone, ankle and foot**

      M84.871   Other disorders of continuity of bone, right ankle and foot

      M84.872   Other disorders of continuity of bone, left ankle and foot

      M84.879   Other disorders of continuity of bone, unspecified ankle and foot

    M84.88   Other disorders of continuity of bone, other site

    M84.9   Disorder of continuity of bone, unspecified

● **M85   Other disorders of bone density and structure**

    Excludes1   osteogenesis imperfecta (Q78.0)
                osteopetrosis (Q78.2)
                osteopoikilosis (Q78.8)
                polyostotic fibrous dysplasia (Q78.1)

    ● **M85.0   Fibrous dysplasia (monostotic)**

      Excludes2   fibrous dysplasia of jaw (M27.8)

      M85.00   Fibrous dysplasia (monostotic), unspecified site

      ● **M85.01   Fibrous dysplasia (monostotic), shoulder**

        M85.011   Fibrous dysplasia (monostotic), right shoulder

        M85.012   Fibrous dysplasia (monostotic), left shoulder

        M85.019   Fibrous dysplasia (monostotic), unspecified shoulder

      ● **M85.02   Fibrous dysplasia (monostotic), upper arm**

        M85.021   Fibrous dysplasia (monostotic), right upper arm

        M85.022   Fibrous dysplasia (monostotic), left upper arm

        M85.029   Fibrous dysplasia (monostotic), unspecified upper arm

      ● **M85.03   Fibrous dysplasia (monostotic), forearm**

        M85.031   Fibrous dysplasia (monostotic), right forearm

        M85.032   Fibrous dysplasia (monostotic), left forearm

        M85.039   Fibrous dysplasia (monostotic), unspecified forearm

● M85.04   Fibrous dysplasia (monostotic), hand
     M85.041   Fibrous dysplasia (monostotic), right hand
     M85.042   Fibrous dysplasia (monostotic), left hand
     M85.049   Fibrous dysplasia (monostotic), unspecified hand
● M85.05   Fibrous dysplasia (monostotic), thigh
     M85.051   Fibrous dysplasia (monostotic), right thigh
     M85.052   Fibrous dysplasia (monostotic), left thigh
     M85.059   Fibrous dysplasia (monostotic), unspecified thigh
● M85.06   Fibrous dysplasia (monostotic), lower leg
     M85.061   Fibrous dysplasia (monostotic), right lower leg
     M85.062   Fibrous dysplasia (monostotic), left lower leg
     M85.069   Fibrous dysplasia (monostotic), unspecified lower leg
● M85.07   Fibrous dysplasia (monostotic), ankle and foot
     M85.071   Fibrous dysplasia (monostotic), right ankle and foot
     M85.072   Fibrous dysplasia (monostotic), left ankle and foot
     M85.079   Fibrous dysplasia (monostotic), unspecified ankle and foot
   M85.08   Fibrous dysplasia (monostotic), other site
   M85.09   Fibrous dysplasia (monostotic), multiple sites
● M85.1   Skeletal fluorosis
   M85.10   Skeletal fluorosis, unspecified site
● M85.11   Skeletal fluorosis, shoulder
     M85.111   Skeletal fluorosis, right shoulder
     M85.112   Skeletal fluorosis, left shoulder
     M85.119   Skeletal fluorosis, unspecified shoulder
● M85.12   Skeletal fluorosis, upper arm
     M85.121   Skeletal fluorosis, right upper arm
     M85.122   Skeletal fluorosis, left upper arm
     M85.129   Skeletal fluorosis, unspecified upper arm
● M85.13   Skeletal fluorosis, forearm
     M85.131   Skeletal fluorosis, right forearm
     M85.132   Skeletal fluorosis, left forearm
     M85.139   Skeletal fluorosis, unspecified forearm
● M85.14   Skeletal fluorosis, hand
     M85.141   Skeletal fluorosis, right hand
     M85.142   Skeletal fluorosis, left hand
     M85.149   Skeletal fluorosis, unspecified hand
● M85.15   Skeletal fluorosis, thigh
     M85.151   Skeletal fluorosis, right thigh
     M85.152   Skeletal fluorosis, left thigh
     M85.159   Skeletal fluorosis, unspecified thigh
● M85.16   Skeletal fluorosis, lower leg
     M85.161   Skeletal fluorosis, right lower leg
     M85.162   Skeletal fluorosis, left lower leg
     M85.169   Skeletal fluorosis, unspecified lower leg
● M85.17   Skeletal fluorosis, ankle and foot
     M85.171   Skeletal fluorosis, right ankle and foot
     M85.172   Skeletal fluorosis, left ankle and foot
     M85.179   Skeletal fluorosis, unspecified ankle and foot

   M85.18   Skeletal fluorosis, other site
   M85.19   Skeletal fluorosis, multiple sites
   M85.2   Hyperostosis of skull
● M85.3   Osteitis condensans
   M85.30   Osteitis condensans, unspecified site
● M85.31   Osteitis condensans, shoulder
     M85.311   Osteitis condensans, right shoulder
     M85.312   Osteitis condensans, left shoulder
     M85.319   Osteitis condensans, unspecified shoulder
● M85.32   Osteitis condensans, upper arm
     M85.321   Osteitis condensans, right upper arm
     M85.322   Osteitis condensans, left upper arm
     M85.329   Osteitis condensans, unspecified upper arm
● M85.33   Osteitis condensans, forearm
     M85.331   Osteitis condensans, right forearm
     M85.332   Osteitis condensans, left forearm
     M85.339   Osteitis condensans, unspecified forearm
● M85.34   Osteitis condensans, hand
     M85.341   Osteitis condensans, right hand
     M85.342   Osteitis condensans, left hand
     M85.349   Osteitis condensans, unspecified hand
● M85.35   Osteitis condensans, thigh
     M85.351   Osteitis condensans, right thigh
     M85.352   Osteitis condensans, left thigh
     M85.359   Osteitis condensans, unspecified thigh
● M85.36   Osteitis condensans, lower leg
     M85.361   Osteitis condensans, right lower leg
     M85.362   Osteitis condensans, left lower leg
     M85.369   Osteitis condensans, unspecified lower leg
● M85.37   Osteitis condensans, ankle and foot
     M85.371   Osteitis condensans, right ankle and foot
     M85.372   Osteitis condensans, left ankle and foot
     M85.379   Osteitis condensans, unspecified ankle and foot
   M85.38   Osteitis condensans, other site
   M85.39   Osteitis condensans, multiple sites
● M85.4   Solitary bone cyst
     Excludes2   solitary cyst of jaw (M27.4)
   M85.40   Solitary bone cyst, unspecified site
● M85.41   Solitary bone cyst, shoulder
     M85.411   Solitary bone cyst, right shoulder
     M85.412   Solitary bone cyst, left shoulder
     M85.419   Solitary bone cyst, unspecified shoulder
● M85.42   Solitary bone cyst, humerus
     M85.421   Solitary bone cyst, right humerus
     M85.422   Solitary bone cyst, left humerus
     M85.429   Solitary bone cyst, unspecified humerus
● M85.43   Solitary bone cyst, ulna and radius
     M85.431   Solitary bone cyst, right ulna and radius
     M85.432   Solitary bone cyst, left ulna and radius
     M85.439   Solitary bone cyst, unspecified ulna and radius

CHAPTER 13 (M00–M99)

CHAPTER 13 (M00-M99)

● M85.44   Solitary bone cyst, hand
     M85.441   Solitary bone cyst, right hand
     M85.442   Solitary bone cyst, left hand
     M85.449   Solitary bone cyst, unspecified hand
● M85.45   Solitary bone cyst, pelvis
     M85.451   Solitary bone cyst, right pelvis
     M85.452   Solitary bone cyst, left pelvis
     M85.459   Solitary bone cyst, unspecified pelvis
● M85.46   Solitary bone cyst, tibia and fibula
     M85.461   Solitary bone cyst, right tibia and fibula
     M85.462   Solitary bone cyst, left tibia and fibula
     M85.469   Solitary bone cyst, unspecified tibia and fibula
● M85.47   Solitary bone cyst, ankle and foot
     M85.471   Solitary bone cyst, right ankle and foot
     M85.472   Solitary bone cyst, left ankle and foot
     M85.479   Solitary bone cyst, unspecified ankle and foot
   M85.48   Solitary bone cyst, other site
● M85.5   Aneurysmal bone cyst
     Excludes2   aneurysmal cyst of jaw (M27.4)
   M85.50   Aneurysmal bone cyst, unspecified site
● M85.51   Aneurysmal bone cyst, shoulder
     M85.511   Aneurysmal bone cyst, right shoulder
     M85.512   Aneurysmal bone cyst, left shoulder
     M85.519   Aneurysmal bone cyst, unspecified shoulder
● M85.52   Aneurysmal bone cyst, upper arm
     M85.521   Aneurysmal bone cyst, right upper arm
     M85.522   Aneurysmal bone cyst, left upper arm
     M85.529   Aneurysmal bone cyst, unspecified upper arm
● M85.53   Aneurysmal bone cyst, forearm
     M85.531   Aneurysmal bone cyst, right forearm
     M85.532   Aneurysmal bone cyst, left forearm
     M85.539   Aneurysmal bone cyst, unspecified forearm
● M85.54   Aneurysmal bone cyst, hand
     M85.541   Aneurysmal bone cyst, right hand
     M85.542   Aneurysmal bone cyst, left hand
     M85.549   Aneurysmal bone cyst, unspecified hand
● M85.55   Aneurysmal bone cyst, thigh
     M85.551   Aneurysmal bone cyst, right thigh
     M85.552   Aneurysmal bone cyst, left thigh
     M85.559   Aneurysmal bone cyst, unspecified thigh
● M85.56   Aneurysmal bone cyst, lower leg
     M85.561   Aneurysmal bone cyst, right lower leg
     M85.562   Aneurysmal bone cyst, left lower leg
     M85.569   Aneurysmal bone cyst, unspecified lower leg
● M85.57   Aneurysmal bone cyst, ankle and foot
     M85.571   Aneurysmal bone cyst, right ankle and foot
     M85.572   Aneurysmal bone cyst, left ankle and foot
     M85.579   Aneurysmal bone cyst, unspecified ankle and foot
   M85.58   Aneurysmal bone cyst, other site
   M85.59   Aneurysmal bone cyst, multiple sites

● M85.6   Other cyst of bone
     Excludes1   cyst of jaw NEC (M27.4)
                 osteitis fibrosa cystica generalisata [von Recklinghausen's disease of bone] (E21.0)
   M85.60   Other cyst of bone, unspecified site
● M85.61   Other cyst of bone, shoulder
     M85.611   Other cyst of bone, right shoulder
     M85.612   Other cyst of bone, left shoulder
     M85.619   Other cyst of bone, unspecified shoulder
● M85.62   Other cyst of bone, upper arm
     M85.621   Other cyst of bone, right upper arm
     M85.622   Other cyst of bone, left upper arm
     M85.629   Other cyst of bone, unspecified upper arm
● M85.63   Other cyst of bone, forearm
     M85.631   Other cyst of bone, right forearm
     M85.632   Other cyst of bone, left forearm
     M85.639   Other cyst of bone, unspecified forearm
● M85.64   Other cyst of bone, hand
     M85.641   Other cyst of bone, right hand
     M85.642   Other cyst of bone, left hand
     M85.649   Other cyst of bone, unspecified hand
● M85.65   Other cyst of bone, thigh
     M85.651   Other cyst of bone, right thigh
     M85.652   Other cyst of bone, left thigh
     M85.659   Other cyst of bone, unspecified thigh
● M85.66   Other cyst of bone, lower leg
     M85.661   Other cyst of bone, right lower leg
     M85.662   Other cyst of bone, left lower leg
     M85.669   Other cyst of bone, unspecified lower leg
● M85.67   Other cyst of bone, ankle and foot
     M85.671   Other cyst of bone, right ankle and foot
     M85.672   Other cyst of bone, left ankle and foot
     M85.679   Other cyst of bone, unspecified ankle and foot
   M85.68   Other cyst of bone, other site
   M85.69   Other cyst of bone, multiple sites
● M85.8   Other specified disorders of bone density and structure
     Hyperostosis of bones, except skull
     Osteosclerosis, acquired
     Excludes1   diffuse idiopathic skeletal hyperostosis [DISH] (M48.1)
                 osteosclerosis congenita (Q77.4)
                 osteosclerosis fragilitas (generalista) (Q78.2)
                 osteosclerosis myelofibrosis (D75.81)
   M85.80   Other specified disorders of bone density and structure, unspecified site
● M85.81   Other specified disorders of bone density and structure, shoulder
     M85.811   Other specified disorders of bone density and structure, right shoulder
     M85.812   Other specified disorders of bone density and structure, left shoulder
     M85.819   Other specified disorders of bone density and structure, unspecified shoulder

▶ New   ⇒ Revised   ~~deleted~~ Deleted   Excludes 1   Excludes 2   Includes   Use additional   Code first   Code also   Key words
OGCR Official Guidelines   X Assign placeholder X   ● Use Additional Character(s)   ▷ Manifestation Code   ✿ Hierarchical Condition Category   **Coding Clinic**

● M85.82   Other specified disorders of bone density and structure, upper arm

    M85.821   Other specified disorders of bone density and structure, right upper arm

    M85.822   Other specified disorders of bone density and structure, left upper arm

    M85.829   Other specified disorders of bone density and structure, unspecified upper arm

● M85.83   Other specified disorders of bone density and structure, forearm

    M85.831   Other specified disorders of bone density and structure, right forearm

    M85.832   Other specified disorders of bone density and structure, left forearm

    M85.839   Other specified disorders of bone density and structure, unspecified forearm

● M85.84   Other specified disorders of bone density and structure, hand

    M85.841   Other specified disorders of bone density and structure, right hand

    M85.842   Other specified disorders of bone density and structure, left hand

    M85.849   Other specified disorders of bone density and structure, unspecified hand

● M85.85   Other specified disorders of bone density and structure, thigh

    M85.851   Other specified disorders of bone density and structure, right thigh

    M85.852   Other specified disorders of bone density and structure, left thigh

    M85.859   Other specified disorders of bone density and structure, unspecified thigh

● M85.86   Other specified disorders of bone density and structure, lower leg

    M85.861   Other specified disorders of bone density and structure, right lower leg

    M85.862   Other specified disorders of bone density and structure, left lower leg

    M85.869   Other specified disorders of bone density and structure, unspecified lower leg

● M85.87   Other specified disorders of bone density and structure, ankle and foot

    M85.871   Other specified disorders of bone density and structure, right ankle and foot

    M85.872   Other specified disorders of bone density and structure, left ankle and foot

    M85.879   Other specified disorders of bone density and structure, unspecified ankle and foot

   M85.88   Other specified disorders of bone density and structure, other site

   M85.89   Other specified disorders of bone density and structure, multiple sites

M85.9   Disorder of bone density and structure, unspecified

OTHER OSTEOPATHIES (M86-M90)

Excludes1	postprocedural osteopathies (M96.-)

● M86   **Osteomyelitis**

Use additional code (B95-B97) to identify infectious agent

Use additional code to identify major osseous defect, if applicable (M89.7-)

Excludes1	osteomyelitis due to:
	echinococcus (B67.2)
	gonococcus (A54.43)
	salmonella (A02.24)

Excludes2	ostemyelitis of:
	orbit (H05.0-)
	petrous bone (H70.2-)
	vertebra (M46.2-)

● M86.0   Acute hematogenous osteomyelitis

    M86.00   Acute hematogenous osteomyelitis, unspecified site 🦴

   ● M86.01   Acute hematogenous osteomyelitis, shoulder

     M86.011   Acute hematogenous osteomyelitis, right shoulder 🦴

     M86.012   Acute hematogenous osteomyelitis, left shoulder 🦴

     M86.019   Acute hematogenous osteomyelitis, unspecified shoulder 🦴

   ● M86.02   Acute hematogenous osteomyelitis, humerus

     M86.021   Acute hematogenous osteomyelitis, right humerus 🦴

     M86.022   Acute hematogenous osteomyelitis, left humerus 🦴

     M86.029   Acute hematogenous osteomyelitis, unspecified humerus 🦴

   ● M86.03   Acute hematogenous osteomyelitis, radius and ulna

     M86.031   Acute hematogenous osteomyelitis, right radius and ulna 🦴

     M86.032   Acute hematogenous osteomyelitis, left radius and ulna 🦴

     M86.039   Acute hematogenous osteomyelitis, unspecified radius and ulna 🦴

   ● M86.04   Acute hematogenous osteomyelitis, hand

     M86.041   Acute hematogenous osteomyelitis, right hand 🦴

     M86.042   Acute hematogenous osteomyelitis, left hand 🦴

     M86.049   Acute hematogenous osteomyelitis, unspecified hand 🦴

Figure 13-6   Osteomyelitis of the spine. A lateral view of the lower thoracic spine demonstrates destruction of the disk space *(arrow)* as well as destruction of the adjoining vertebral bodies. (From Mettler: Essentials of Radiology, ed 2, Saunders, An Imprint of Elsevier, 2005)

Item 13-12 Osteomyelitis is an inflammation of the bone. **Acute osteomyelitis** is a rapidly destructive, pus-producing infection capable of causing severe bone destruction. **Chronic osteomyelitis** can remain long after the initial acute episode has passed and may lead to a recurrence of the acute phase. **Brodie's abscess** is an encapsulated focal abscess that must be surgically drained. **Periostitis** is an inflammation of the periosteum, a dense membrane composed of fibrous connective tissue that closely wraps all bone, except those with articulating surfaces in joints, which are covered by synovial membranes.

CHAPTER 13 (M00-M99)

● M86.05   Acute hematogenous osteomyelitis, femur

     M86.051   Acute hematogenous osteomyelitis, right femur 🐾

     M86.052   Acute hematogenous osteomyelitis, left femur 🐾

     M86.059   Acute hematogenous osteomyelitis, unspecified femur 🐾

● M86.06   Acute hematogenous osteomyelitis, tibia and fibula

     M86.061   Acute hematogenous osteomyelitis, right tibia and fibula 🐾

     M86.062   Acute hematogenous osteomyelitis, left tibia and fibula 🐾

     M86.069   Acute hematogenous osteomyelitis, unspecified tibia and fibula 🐾

● M86.07   Acute hematogenous osteomyelitis, ankle and foot

     M86.071   Acute hematogenous osteomyelitis, right ankle and foot 🐾

     M86.072   Acute hematogenous osteomyelitis, left ankle and foot 🐾

     M86.079   Acute hematogenous osteomyelitis, unspecified ankle and foot 🐾

   M86.08   Acute hematogenous osteomyelitis, other sites 🐾

   M86.09   Acute hematogenous osteomyelitis, multiple sites 🐾

● M86.1   Other acute osteomyelitis

   M86.10   Other acute osteomyelitis, unspecified site 🐾

● M86.11   Other acute osteomyelitis, shoulder

     M86.111   Other acute osteomyelitis, right shoulder 🐾

     M86.112   Other acute osteomyelitis, left shoulder 🐾

     M86.119   Other acute osteomyelitis, unspecified shoulder 🐾

● M86.12   Other acute osteomyelitis, humerus

     M86.121   Other acute osteomyelitis, right humerus 🐾

     M86.122   Other acute osteomyelitis, left humerus 🐾

     M86.129   Other acute osteomyelitis, unspecified humerus 🐾

● M86.13   Other acute osteomyelitis, radius and ulna

     M86.131   Other acute osteomyelitis, right radius and ulna 🐾

     M86.132   Other acute osteomyelitis, left radius and ulna 🐾

     M86.139   Other acute osteomyelitis, unspecified radius and ulna 🐾

● M86.14   Other acute osteomyelitis, hand

     M86.141   Other acute osteomyelitis, right hand 🐾

     M86.142   Other acute osteomyelitis, left hand 🐾

     M86.149   Other acute osteomyelitis, unspecified hand 🐾

● M86.15   Other acute osteomyelitis, femur

     M86.151   Other acute osteomyelitis, right femur 🐾

     M86.152   Other acute osteomyelitis, left femur 🐾

     M86.159   Other acute osteomyelitis, unspecified femur 🐾

● M86.16   Other acute osteomyelitis, tibia and fibula

     M86.161   Other acute osteomyelitis, right tibia and fibula 🐾

     M86.162   Other acute osteomyelitis, left tibia and fibula 🐾

     M86.169   Other acute osteomyelitis, unspecified tibia and fibula 🐾

● M86.17   Other acute osteomyelitis, ankle and foot

     M86.171   Other acute osteomyelitis, right ankle and foot 🐾
        Coding Clinic: 2020, Q1, P12

     M86.172   Other acute osteomyelitis, left ankle and foot 🐾

     M86.179   Other acute osteomyelitis, unspecified ankle and foot 🐾

   M86.18   Other acute osteomyelitis, other site 🐾

   M86.19   Other acute osteomyelitis, multiple sites 🐾

● M86.2   Subacute osteomyelitis

   M86.20   Subacute osteomyelitis, unspecified site 🐾

● M86.21   Subacute osteomyelitis, shoulder

     M86.211   Subacute osteomyelitis, right shoulder 🐾

     M86.212   Subacute osteomyelitis, left shoulder 🐾

     M86.219   Subacute osteomyelitis, unspecified shoulder 🐾

● M86.22   Subacute osteomyelitis, humerus

     M86.221   Subacute osteomyelitis, right humerus 🐾

     M86.222   Subacute osteomyelitis, left humerus 🐾

     M86.229   Subacute osteomyelitis, unspecified humerus 🐾

● M86.23   Subacute osteomyelitis, radius and ulna

     M86.231   Subacute osteomyelitis, right radius and ulna 🐾

     M86.232   Subacute osteomyelitis, left radius and ulna 🐾

     M86.239   Subacute osteomyelitis, unspecified radius and ulna 🐾

● M86.24   Subacute osteomyelitis, hand

     M86.241   Subacute osteomyelitis, right hand 🐾

     M86.242   Subacute osteomyelitis, left hand 🐾

     M86.249   Subacute osteomyelitis, unspecified hand 🐾

● M86.25   Subacute osteomyelitis, femur

     M86.251   Subacute osteomyelitis, right femur 🐾

     M86.252   Subacute osteomyelitis, left femur 🐾

     M86.259   Subacute osteomyelitis, unspecified femur 🐾

● M86.26   Subacute osteomyelitis, tibia and fibula

     M86.261   Subacute osteomyelitis, right tibia and fibula 🐾

     M86.262   Subacute osteomyelitis, left tibia and fibula 🐾

     M86.269   Subacute osteomyelitis, unspecified tibia and fibula 🐾

● M86.27   Subacute osteomyelitis, ankle and foot

     M86.271   Subacute osteomyelitis, right ankle and foot 🐾

     M86.272   Subacute osteomyelitis, left ankle and foot 🐾

     M86.279   Subacute osteomyelitis, unspecified ankle and foot 🐾

   M86.28   Subacute osteomyelitis, other site 🐾

   M86.29   Subacute osteomyelitis, multiple sites 🐾

▶ New   ⟾ Revised   ~~deleted~~ Deleted   Excludes 1   Excludes 2   Includes   Use additional   Code first   Code also   Key words

OGCR Official Guidelines   X Assign placeholder X   ● Use Additional Character(s)   ▷ Manifestation Code   🐾 Hierarchical Condition Category   Coding Clinic

● **M86.3** Chronic multifocal osteomyelitis
    M86.30 Chronic multifocal osteomyelitis, unspecified site 🦴
    ● **M86.31** Chronic multifocal osteomyelitis, shoulder
        M86.311 Chronic multifocal osteomyelitis, right shoulder 🦴
        M86.312 Chronic multifocal osteomyelitis, left shoulder 🦴
        M86.319 Chronic multifocal osteomyelitis, unspecified shoulder 🦴
    ● **M86.32** Chronic multifocal osteomyelitis, humerus
        M86.321 Chronic multifocal osteomyelitis, right humerus 🦴
        M86.322 Chronic multifocal osteomyelitis, left humerus 🦴
        M86.329 Chronic multifocal osteomyelitis, unspecified humerus 🦴
    ● **M86.33** Chronic multifocal osteomyelitis, radius and ulna
        M86.331 Chronic multifocal osteomyelitis, right radius and ulna 🦴
        M86.332 Chronic multifocal osteomyelitis, left radius and ulna 🦴
        M86.339 Chronic multifocal osteomyelitis, unspecified radius and ulna 🦴
    ● **M86.34** Chronic multifocal osteomyelitis, hand
        M86.341 Chronic multifocal osteomyelitis, right hand 🦴
        M86.342 Chronic multifocal osteomyelitis, left hand 🦴
        M86.349 Chronic multifocal osteomyelitis, unspecified hand 🦴
    ● **M86.35** Chronic multifocal osteomyelitis, femur
        M86.351 Chronic multifocal osteomyelitis, right femur 🦴
        M86.352 Chronic multifocal osteomyelitis, left femur 🦴
        M86.359 Chronic multifocal osteomyelitis, unspecified femur 🦴
    ● **M86.36** Chronic multifocal osteomyelitis, tibia and fibula
        M86.361 Chronic multifocal osteomyelitis, right tibia and fibula 🦴
        M86.362 Chronic multifocal osteomyelitis, left tibia and fibula 🦴
        M86.369 Chronic multifocal osteomyelitis, unspecified tibia and fibula 🦴
    ● **M86.37** Chronic multifocal osteomyelitis, ankle and foot
        M86.371 Chronic multifocal osteomyelitis, right ankle and foot 🦴
        M86.372 Chronic multifocal osteomyelitis, left ankle and foot 🦴
        M86.379 Chronic multifocal osteomyelitis, unspecified ankle and foot 🦴
    M86.38 Chronic multifocal osteomyelitis, other site 🦴
    M86.39 Chronic multifocal osteomyelitis, multiple sites 🦴
● **M86.4** Chronic osteomyelitis with draining sinus
    M86.40 Chronic osteomyelitis with draining sinus, unspecified site 🦴
    ● **M86.41** Chronic osteomyelitis with draining sinus, shoulder
        M86.411 Chronic osteomyelitis with draining sinus, right shoulder 🦴
        M86.412 Chronic osteomyelitis with draining sinus, left shoulder 🦴
        M86.419 Chronic osteomyelitis with draining sinus, unspecified shoulder 🦴

● **M86.42** Chronic osteomyelitis with draining sinus, humerus
        M86.421 Chronic osteomyelitis with draining sinus, right humerus 🦴
        M86.422 Chronic osteomyelitis with draining sinus, left humerus 🦴
        M86.429 Chronic osteomyelitis with draining sinus, unspecified humerus 🦴
● **M86.43** Chronic osteomyelitis with draining sinus, radius and ulna
        M86.431 Chronic osteomyelitis with draining sinus, right radius and ulna 🦴
        M86.432 Chronic osteomyelitis with draining sinus, left radius and ulna 🦴
        M86.439 Chronic osteomyelitis with draining sinus, unspecified radius and ulna 🦴
● **M86.44** Chronic osteomyelitis with draining sinus, hand
        M86.441 Chronic osteomyelitis with draining sinus, right hand 🦴
        M86.442 Chronic osteomyelitis with draining sinus, left hand 🦴
        M86.449 Chronic osteomyelitis with draining sinus, unspecified hand 🦴
● **M86.45** Chronic osteomyelitis with draining sinus, femur
        M86.451 Chronic osteomyelitis with draining sinus, right femur 🦴
        M86.452 Chronic osteomyelitis with draining sinus, left femur 🦴
        M86.459 Chronic osteomyelitis with draining sinus, unspecified femur 🦴
● **M86.46** Chronic osteomyelitis with draining sinus, tibia and fibula
        M86.461 Chronic osteomyelitis with draining sinus, right tibia and fibula 🦴
        M86.462 Chronic osteomyelitis with draining sinus, left tibia and fibula 🦴
        M86.469 Chronic osteomyelitis with draining sinus, unspecified tibia and fibula 🦴
● **M86.47** Chronic osteomyelitis with draining sinus, ankle and foot
        M86.471 Chronic osteomyelitis with draining sinus, right ankle and foot 🦴
        M86.472 Chronic osteomyelitis with draining sinus, left ankle and foot 🦴
        M86.479 Chronic osteomyelitis with draining sinus, unspecified ankle and foot 🦴
    M86.48 Chronic osteomyelitis with draining sinus, other site 🦴
    M86.49 Chronic osteomyelitis with draining sinus, multiple sites 🦴
● **M86.5** Other chronic hematogenous osteomyelitis
    M86.50 Other chronic hematogenous osteomyelitis, unspecified site 🦴
    ● **M86.51** Other chronic hematogenous osteomyelitis, shoulder
        M86.511 Other chronic hematogenous osteomyelitis, right shoulder 🦴
        M86.512 Other chronic hematogenous osteomyelitis, left shoulder 🦴
        M86.519 Other chronic hematogenous osteomyelitis, unspecified shoulder 🦴

CHAPTER 13 (M00-M99)

CHAPTER 13 (M00-M99)

● M86.52   Other chronic hematogenous osteomyelitis, humerus
  - M86.521   Other chronic hematogenous osteomyelitis, right humerus 🐾
  - M86.522   Other chronic hematogenous osteomyelitis, left humerus 🐾
  - M86.529   Other chronic hematogenous osteomyelitis, unspecified humerus 🐾

● M86.53   Other chronic hematogenous osteomyelitis, radius and ulna
  - M86.531   Other chronic hematogenous osteomyelitis, right radius and ulna 🐾
  - M86.532   Other chronic hematogenous osteomyelitis, left radius and ulna 🐾
  - M86.539   Other chronic hematogenous osteomyelitis, unspecified radius and ulna 🐾

● M86.54   Other chronic hematogenous osteomyelitis, hand
  - M86.541   Other chronic hematogenous osteomyelitis, right hand 🐾
  - M86.542   Other chronic hematogenous osteomyelitis, left hand 🐾
  - M86.549   Other chronic hematogenous osteomyelitis, unspecified hand 🐾

● M86.55   Other chronic hematogenous osteomyelitis, femur
  - M86.551   Other chronic hematogenous osteomyelitis, right femur 🐾
  - M86.552   Other chronic hematogenous osteomyelitis, left femur 🐾
  - M86.559   Other chronic hematogenous osteomyelitis, unspecified femur 🐾

● M86.56   Other chronic hematogenous osteomyelitis, tibia and fibula
  - M86.561   Other chronic hematogenous osteomyelitis, right tibia and fibula 🐾
  - M86.562   Other chronic hematogenous osteomyelitis, left tibia and fibula 🐾
  - M86.569   Other chronic hematogenous osteomyelitis, unspecified tibia and fibula 🐾

● M86.57   Other chronic hematogenous osteomyelitis, ankle and foot
  - M86.571   Other chronic hematogenous osteomyelitis, right ankle and foot 🐾
  - M86.572   Other chronic hematogenous osteomyelitis, left ankle and foot 🐾
  - M86.579   Other chronic hematogenous osteomyelitis, unspecified ankle and foot 🐾

M86.58   Other chronic hematogenous osteomyelitis, other site 🐾

M86.59   Other chronic hematogenous osteomyelitis, multiple sites 🐾

● M86.6   **Other chronic osteomyelitis**
  - M86.60   Other chronic osteomyelitis, unspecified site 🐾
  - ● M86.61   Other chronic osteomyelitis, shoulder
    - M86.611   Other chronic osteomyelitis, right shoulder 🐾
    - M86.612   Other chronic osteomyelitis, left shoulder 🐾
    - M86.619   Other chronic osteomyelitis, unspecified shoulder 🐾

● M86.62   Other chronic osteomyelitis, humerus
  - M86.621   Other chronic osteomyelitis, right humerus 🐾
  - M86.622   Other chronic osteomyelitis, left humerus 🐾
  - M86.629   Other chronic osteomyelitis, unspecified humerus 🐾

● M86.63   Other chronic osteomyelitis, radius and ulna
  - M86.631   Other chronic osteomyelitis, right radius and ulna 🐾
  - M86.632   Other chronic osteomyelitis, left radius and ulna 🐾
  - M86.639   Other chronic osteomyelitis, unspecified radius and ulna 🐾

● M86.64   Other chronic osteomyelitis, hand
  - M86.641   Other chronic osteomyelitis, right hand 🐾
  - M86.642   Other chronic osteomyelitis, left hand 🐾
  - M86.649   Other chronic osteomyelitis, unspecified hand 🐾

● M86.65   Other chronic osteomyelitis, thigh
  - M86.651   Other chronic osteomyelitis, right thigh 🐾
  - M86.652   Other chronic osteomyelitis, left thigh 🐾
  - M86.659   Other chronic osteomyelitis, unspecified thigh 🐾

● M86.66   Other chronic osteomyelitis, tibia and fibula
  - M86.661   Other chronic osteomyelitis, right tibia and fibula 🐾
  - M86.662   Other chronic osteomyelitis, left tibia and fibula 🐾
  - M86.669   Other chronic osteomyelitis, unspecified tibia and fibula 🐾

● M86.67   Other chronic osteomyelitis, ankle and foot
  - M86.671   Other chronic osteomyelitis, right ankle and foot 🐾
    - Coding Clinic: 2016, Q1, P13
  - M86.672   Other chronic osteomyelitis, left ankle and foot 🐾
  - M86.679   Other chronic osteomyelitis, unspecified ankle and foot 🐾

M86.68   Other chronic osteomyelitis, other site 🐾

M86.69   Other chronic osteomyelitis, multiple sites 🐾

● M86.8   **Other osteomyelitis**
  Brodie's abscess
  - ● M86.8X   Other osteomyelitis
    - M86.8X0   Other osteomyelitis, multiple sites 🐾
    - M86.8X1   Other osteomyelitis, shoulder 🐾
    - M86.8X2   Other osteomyelitis, upper arm 🐾
    - M86.8X3   Other osteomyelitis, forearm 🐾
    - M86.8X4   Other osteomyelitis, hand 🐾
    - M86.8X5   Other osteomyelitis, thigh 🐾
    - M86.8X6   Other osteomyelitis, lower leg 🐾
    - M86.8X7   Other osteomyelitis, ankle and foot 🐾
    - M86.8X8   Other osteomyelitis, other site 🐾
    - M86.8X9   Other osteomyelitis, unspecified sites 🐾

M86.9   Osteomyelitis, unspecified 🐾
  Infection of bone NOS
  Periostitis without osteomyelitis

▶ New   ⇒ Revised   ~~deleted~~ Deleted   Excludes 1   Excludes 2   Includes   Use additional   Code first   Code also   Key words

OGCR Official Guidelines   X Assign placeholder X   ● Use Additional Character(s)   ▶ Manifestation Code   🐾 Hierarchical Condition Category   **Coding Clinic**

● **M87**   **Osteonecrosis**

> | **Includes** | avascular necrosis of bone |
> | --- | --- |

> Use additional code to identify major osseous defect, if applicable (M89.7-)

> | **Excludes1** | juvenile osteonecrosis (M91-M92) |
> | --- | --- |
> | | osteochondropathies (M90-M93) |

● **M87.0**   **Idiopathic aseptic necrosis of bone**

     M87.00   Idiopathic aseptic necrosis of unspecified bone 🔎

   ● **M87.01**   Idiopathic aseptic necrosis of shoulder
         Idiopathic aseptic necrosis of clavicle and scapula

         M87.011   Idiopathic aseptic necrosis of right shoulder 🔎

         M87.012   Idiopathic aseptic necrosis of left shoulder 🔎

         M87.019   Idiopathic aseptic necrosis of unspecified shoulder 🔎

   ● **M87.02**   Idiopathic aseptic necrosis of humerus

         M87.021   Idiopathic aseptic necrosis of right humerus 🔎

         M87.022   Idiopathic aseptic necrosis of left humerus 🔎

         M87.029   Idiopathic aseptic necrosis of unspecified humerus 🔎

   ● **M87.03**   Idiopathic aseptic necrosis of radius, ulna and carpus

         M87.031   Idiopathic aseptic necrosis of right radius 🔎

         M87.032   Idiopathic aseptic necrosis of left radius 🔎

         M87.033   Idiopathic aseptic necrosis of unspecified radius 🔎

         M87.034   Idiopathic aseptic necrosis of right ulna 🔎

         M87.035   Idiopathic aseptic necrosis of left ulna 🔎

         M87.036   Idiopathic aseptic necrosis of unspecified ulna 🔎

         M87.037   Idiopathic aseptic necrosis of right carpus 🔎

         M87.038   Idiopathic aseptic necrosis of left carpus 🔎

         M87.039   Idiopathic aseptic necrosis of unspecified carpus 🔎

   ● **M87.04**   Idiopathic aseptic necrosis of hand and fingers
         Idiopathic aseptic necrosis of metacarpals and phalanges of hands

         M87.041   Idiopathic aseptic necrosis of right hand 🔎

         M87.042   Idiopathic aseptic necrosis of left hand 🔎

         M87.043   Idiopathic aseptic necrosis of unspecified hand 🔎

         M87.044   Idiopathic aseptic necrosis of right finger(s) 🔎

         M87.045   Idiopathic aseptic necrosis of left finger(s) 🔎

         M87.046   Idiopathic aseptic necrosis of unspecified finger(s) 🔎

   ● **M87.05**   Idiopathic aseptic necrosis of pelvis and femur

         M87.050   Idiopathic aseptic necrosis of pelvis 🔎

         M87.051   Idiopathic aseptic necrosis of right femur 🔎

         M87.052   Idiopathic aseptic necrosis of left femur 🔎

         M87.059   Idiopathic aseptic necrosis of unspecified femur 🔎
           Idiopathic aseptic necrosis of hip NOS

● **M87.06**   Idiopathic aseptic necrosis of tibia and fibula

     M87.061   Idiopathic aseptic necrosis of right tibia 🔎

     M87.062   Idiopathic aseptic necrosis of left tibia 🔎

     M87.063   Idiopathic aseptic necrosis of unspecified tibia 🔎

     M87.064   Idiopathic aseptic necrosis of right fibula 🔎

     M87.065   Idiopathic aseptic necrosis of left fibula 🔎

     M87.066   Idiopathic aseptic necrosis of unspecified fibula 🔎

● **M87.07**   Idiopathic aseptic necrosis of ankle, foot and toes
      Idiopathic aseptic necrosis of metatarsus, tarsus, and phalanges of toes

     M87.071   Idiopathic aseptic necrosis of right ankle 🔎

     M87.072   Idiopathic aseptic necrosis of left ankle 🔎

     M87.073   Idiopathic aseptic necrosis of unspecified ankle 🔎

     M87.074   Idiopathic aseptic necrosis of right foot 🔎

     M87.075   Idiopathic aseptic necrosis of left foot 🔎

     M87.076   Idiopathic aseptic necrosis of unspecified foot 🔎

     M87.077   Idiopathic aseptic necrosis of right toe(s) 🔎

     M87.078   Idiopathic aseptic necrosis of left toe(s) 🔎

     M87.079   Idiopathic aseptic necrosis of unspecified toe(s) 🔎

     M87.08   Idiopathic aseptic necrosis of bone, other site 🔎

     M87.09   Idiopathic aseptic necrosis of bone, multiple sites 🔎

● **M87.1**   **Osteonecrosis due to drugs**

> Use additional code for adverse effect, if applicable, to identify drug (T36-T50 with fifth or sixth character 5)

     M87.10   Osteonecrosis due to drugs, unspecified bone 🔎

● **M87.11**   Osteonecrosis due to drugs, shoulder

     M87.111   Osteonecrosis due to drugs, right shoulder 🔎

     M87.112   Osteonecrosis due to drugs, left shoulder 🔎

     M87.119   Osteonecrosis due to drugs, unspecified shoulder 🔎

● **M87.12**   Osteonecrosis due to drugs, humerus

     M87.121   Osteonecrosis due to drugs, right humerus 🔎

     M87.122   Osteonecrosis due to drugs, left humerus 🔎

     M87.129   Osteonecrosis due to drugs, unspecified humerus 🔎

● **M87.13**   Osteonecrosis due to drugs of radius, ulna and carpus

     M87.131   Osteonecrosis due to drugs of right radius 🔎

     M87.132   Osteonecrosis due to drugs of left radius 🔎

     M87.133   Osteonecrosis due to drugs of unspecified radius 🔎

     M87.134   Osteonecrosis due to drugs of right ulna 🔎

     M87.135   Osteonecrosis due to drugs of left ulna 🔎

CHAPTER 13 (M00-M99)

CHAPTER 13 (M00-M99)

    M87.136   Osteonecrosis due to drugs of unspecified ulna 🦠

    M87.137   Osteonecrosis due to drugs of right carpus 🦠

    M87.138   Osteonecrosis due to drugs of left carpus 🦠

    M87.139   Osteonecrosis due to drugs of unspecified carpus 🦠

● M87.14   Osteonecrosis due to drugs, hand and fingers

    M87.141   Osteonecrosis due to drugs, right hand 🦠

    M87.142   Osteonecrosis due to drugs, left hand 🦠

    M87.143   Osteonecrosis due to drugs, unspecified hand 🦠

    M87.144   Osteonecrosis due to drugs, right finger(s) 🦠

    M87.145   Osteonecrosis due to drugs, left finger(s) 🦠

    M87.146   Osteonecrosis due to drugs, unspecified finger(s) 🦠

● M87.15   Osteonecrosis due to drugs, pelvis and femur

    M87.150   Osteonecrosis due to drugs, pelvis 🦠

    M87.151   Osteonecrosis due to drugs, right femur 🦠

    M87.152   Osteonecrosis due to drugs, left femur 🦠

    M87.159   Osteonecrosis due to drugs, unspecified femur 🦠

● M87.16   Osteonecrosis due to drugs, tibia and fibula

    M87.161   Osteonecrosis due to drugs, right tibia 🦠

    M87.162   Osteonecrosis due to drugs, left tibia 🦠

    M87.163   Osteonecrosis due to drugs, unspecified tibia 🦠

    M87.164   Osteonecrosis due to drugs, right fibula 🦠

    M87.165   Osteonecrosis due to drugs, left fibula 🦠

    M87.166   Osteonecrosis due to drugs, unspecified fibula 🦠

● M87.17   Osteonecrosis due to drugs, ankle, foot and toes

    M87.171   Osteonecrosis due to drugs, right ankle 🦠

    M87.172   Osteonecrosis due to drugs, left ankle 🦠

    M87.173   Osteonecrosis due to drugs, unspecified ankle 🦠

    M87.174   Osteonecrosis due to drugs, right foot 🦠

    M87.175   Osteonecrosis due to drugs, left foot 🦠

    M87.176   Osteonecrosis due to drugs, unspecified foot 🦠

    M87.177   Osteonecrosis due to drugs, right toe(s) 🦠

    M87.178   Osteonecrosis due to drugs, left toe(s) 🦠

    M87.179   Osteonecrosis due to drugs, unspecified toe(s) 🦠

● M87.18   Osteonecrosis due to drugs, other site

    M87.180   Osteonecrosis due to drugs, jaw 🦠

    M87.188   Osteonecrosis due to drugs, other site 🦠

  M87.19   Osteonecrosis due to drugs, multiple sites 🦠

● M87.2   Osteonecrosis due to previous trauma

  M87.20   Osteonecrosis due to previous trauma, unspecified bone 🦠

● M87.21   Osteonecrosis due to previous trauma, shoulder

    M87.211   Osteonecrosis due to previous trauma, right shoulder 🦠

    M87.212   Osteonecrosis due to previous trauma, left shoulder 🦠

    M87.219   Osteonecrosis due to previous trauma, unspecified shoulder 🦠

● M87.22   Osteonecrosis due to previous trauma, humerus

    M87.221   Osteonecrosis due to previous trauma, right humerus 🦠

    M87.222   Osteonecrosis due to previous trauma, left humerus 🦠

    M87.229   Osteonecrosis due to previous trauma, unspecified humerus 🦠

● M87.23   Osteonecrosis due to previous trauma of radius, ulna and carpus

    M87.231   Osteonecrosis due to previous trauma of right radius 🦠

    M87.232   Osteonecrosis due to previous trauma of left radius 🦠

    M87.233   Osteonecrosis due to previous trauma of unspecified radius 🦠

    M87.234   Osteonecrosis due to previous trauma of right ulna 🦠

    M87.235   Osteonecrosis due to previous trauma of left ulna 🦠

    M87.236   Osteonecrosis due to previous trauma of unspecified ulna 🦠

    M87.237   Osteonecrosis due to previous trauma of right carpus 🦠

    M87.238   Osteonecrosis due to previous trauma of left carpus 🦠

    M87.239   Osteonecrosis due to previous trauma of unspecified carpus 🦠

● M87.24   Osteonecrosis due to previous trauma, hand and fingers

    M87.241   Osteonecrosis due to previous trauma, right hand 🦠

    M87.242   Osteonecrosis due to previous trauma, left hand 🦠

    M87.243   Osteonecrosis due to previous trauma, unspecified hand 🦠

    M87.244   Osteonecrosis due to previous trauma, right finger(s) 🦠

    M87.245   Osteonecrosis due to previous trauma, left finger(s) 🦠

    M87.246   Osteonecrosis due to previous trauma, unspecified finger(s) 🦠

● M87.25   Osteonecrosis due to previous trauma, pelvis and femur

    M87.250   Osteonecrosis due to previous trauma, pelvis 🦠

    M87.251   Osteonecrosis due to previous trauma, right femur 🦠

    M87.252   Osteonecrosis due to previous trauma, left femur 🦠

    M87.256   Osteonecrosis due to previous trauma, unspecified femur 🦠

● M87.26   Osteonecrosis due to previous trauma, tibia and fibula

    M87.261   Osteonecrosis due to previous trauma, right tibia 🦠

    M87.262   Osteonecrosis due to previous trauma, left tibia 🦠

    M87.263   Osteonecrosis due to previous trauma, unspecified tibia 🦠

▶ New   ➡ Revised   ~~deleted~~ Deleted   Excludes 1   Excludes 2   Includes   Use additional   Code first   Code also   Key words

OGCR Official Guidelines   X Assign placeholder X   ● Use Additional Character(s)   ▶ Manifestation Code   🦠 Hierarchical Condition Category   **Coding Clinic**

M87.264   Osteonecrosis due to previous trauma, right fibula 🦴

M87.265   Osteonecrosis due to previous trauma, left fibula 🦴

M87.266   Osteonecrosis due to previous trauma, unspecified fibula 🦴

● M87.27   Osteonecrosis due to previous trauma, ankle, foot and toes

M87.271   Osteonecrosis due to previous trauma, right ankle 🦴

M87.272   Osteonecrosis due to previous trauma, left ankle 🦴

M87.273   Osteonecrosis due to previous trauma, unspecified ankle 🦴

M87.274   Osteonecrosis due to previous trauma, right foot 🦴

M87.275   Osteonecrosis due to previous trauma, left foot 🦴

M87.276   Osteonecrosis due to previous trauma, unspecified foot 🦴

M87.277   Osteonecrosis due to previous trauma, right toe(s) 🦴

M87.278   Osteonecrosis due to previous trauma, left toe(s) 🦴

M87.279   Osteonecrosis due to previous trauma, unspecified toe(s) 🦴

M87.28   Osteonecrosis due to previous trauma, other site 🦴

M87.29   Osteonecrosis due to previous trauma, multiple sites 🦴

● M87.3   Other secondary osteonecrosis

M87.30   Other secondary osteonecrosis, unspecified bone 🦴

● M87.31   Other secondary osteonecrosis, shoulder

M87.311   Other secondary osteonecrosis, right shoulder 🦴

M87.312   Other secondary osteonecrosis, left shoulder 🦴

M87.319   Other secondary osteonecrosis, unspecified shoulder 🦴

● M87.32   Other secondary osteonecrosis, humerus

M87.321   Other secondary osteonecrosis, right humerus 🦴

M87.322   Other secondary osteonecrosis, left humerus 🦴

M87.329   Other secondary osteonecrosis, unspecified humerus 🦴

● M87.33   Other secondary osteonecrosis of radius, ulna and carpus

M87.331   Other secondary osteonecrosis of right radius 🦴

M87.332   Other secondary osteonecrosis of left radius 🦴

M87.333   Other secondary osteonecrosis of unspecified radius 🦴

M87.334   Other secondary osteonecrosis of right ulna 🦴

M87.335   Other secondary osteonecrosis of left ulna 🦴

M87.336   Other secondary osteonecrosis of unspecified ulna 🦴

M87.337   Other secondary osteonecrosis of right carpus 🦴

M87.338   Other secondary osteonecrosis of left carpus 🦴

M87.339   Other secondary osteonecrosis of unspecified carpus 🦴

● M87.34   Other secondary osteonecrosis, hand and fingers

M87.341   Other secondary osteonecrosis, right hand 🦴

M87.342   Other secondary osteonecrosis, left hand 🦴

M87.343   Other secondary osteonecrosis, unspecified hand 🦴

M87.344   Other secondary osteonecrosis, right finger(s) 🦴

M87.345   Other secondary osteonecrosis, left finger(s) 🦴

M87.346   Other secondary osteonecrosis, unspecified finger(s) 🦴

● M87.35   Other secondary osteonecrosis, pelvis and femur

M87.350   Other secondary osteonecrosis, pelvis 🦴

M87.351   Other secondary osteonecrosis, right femur 🦴

M87.352   Other secondary osteonecrosis, left femur 🦴

M87.353   Other secondary osteonecrosis, unspecified femur 🦴

● M87.36   Other secondary osteonecrosis, tibia and fibula

M87.361   Other secondary osteonecrosis, right tibia 🦴

M87.362   Other secondary osteonecrosis, left tibia 🦴

M87.363   Other secondary osteonecrosis, unspecified tibia 🦴

M87.364   Other secondary osteonecrosis, right fibula 🦴

M87.365   Other secondary osteonecrosis, left fibula 🦴

M87.366   Other secondary osteonecrosis, unspecified fibula 🦴

● M87.37   Other secondary osteonecrosis, ankle and foot

M87.371   Other secondary osteonecrosis, right ankle 🦴

M87.372   Other secondary osteonecrosis, left ankle 🦴

M87.373   Other secondary osteonecrosis, unspecified ankle 🦴

M87.374   Other secondary osteonecrosis, right foot 🦴

M87.375   Other secondary osteonecrosis, left foot 🦴

M87.376   Other secondary osteonecrosis, unspecified foot 🦴

M87.377   Other secondary osteonecrosis, right toe(s) 🦴

M87.378   Other secondary osteonecrosis, left toe(s) 🦴

M87.379   Other secondary osteonecrosis, unspecified toe(s) 🦴

M87.38   Other secondary osteonecrosis, other site 🦴

M87.39   Other secondary osteonecrosis, multiple sites 🦴

● M87.8   Other osteonecrosis

M87.80   Other osteonecrosis, unspecified bone 🦴

● M87.81   Other osteonecrosis, shoulder

M87.811   Other osteonecrosis, right shoulder 🦴

M87.812   Other osteonecrosis, left shoulder 🦴

M87.819   Other osteonecrosis, unspecified shoulder 🦴

CHAPTER 13 (M00-M99)

CHAPTER 13 (M00–M99)

● M87.82   Other osteonecrosis, humerus
    M87.821   Other osteonecrosis, right humerus 🐾
    M87.822   Other osteonecrosis, left humerus 🐾
    M87.829   Other osteonecrosis, unspecified humerus 🐾

● M87.83   Other osteonecrosis of radius, ulna and carpus
    M87.831   Other osteonecrosis of right radius 🐾
    M87.832   Other osteonecrosis of left radius 🐾
    M87.833   Other osteonecrosis of unspecified radius 🐾
    M87.834   Other osteonecrosis of right ulna 🐾
    M87.835   Other osteonecrosis of left ulna 🐾
    M87.836   Other osteonecrosis of unspecified ulna 🐾
    M87.837   Other osteonecrosis of right carpus 🐾
    M87.838   Other osteonecrosis of left carpus 🐾
    M87.839   Other osteonecrosis of unspecified carpus 🐾

● M87.84   Other osteonecrosis, hand and fingers
    M87.841   Other osteonecrosis, right hand 🐾
    M87.842   Other osteonecrosis, left hand 🐾
    M87.843   Other osteonecrosis, unspecified hand 🐾
    M87.844   Other osteonecrosis, right finger(s) 🐾
    M87.845   Other osteonecrosis, left finger(s) 🐾
    M87.849   Other osteonecrosis, unspecified finger(s) 🐾

● M87.85   Other osteonecrosis, pelvis and femur
    M87.850   Other osteonecrosis, pelvis 🐾
    M87.851   Other osteonecrosis, right femur 🐾
    M87.852   Other osteonecrosis, left femur 🐾
    M87.859   Other osteonecrosis, unspecified femur 🐾

● M87.86   Other osteonecrosis, tibia and fibula
    M87.861   Other osteonecrosis, right tibia 🐾
    M87.862   Other osteonecrosis, left tibia 🐾
    M87.863   Other osteonecrosis, unspecified tibia 🐾
    M87.864   Other osteonecrosis, right fibula 🐾
    M87.865   Other osteonecrosis, left fibula 🐾
    M87.869   Other osteonecrosis, unspecified fibula 🐾

● M87.87   Other osteonecrosis, ankle, foot and toes
    M87.871   Other osteonecrosis, right ankle 🐾
    M87.872   Other osteonecrosis, left ankle 🐾
    M87.873   Other osteonecrosis, unspecified ankle 🐾
    M87.874   Other osteonecrosis, right foot 🐾
    M87.875   Other osteonecrosis, left foot 🐾
    M87.876   Other osteonecrosis, unspecified foot 🐾
    M87.877   Other osteonecrosis, right toe(s) 🐾
    M87.878   Other osteonecrosis, left toe(s) 🐾
    M87.879   Other osteonecrosis, unspecified toe(s) 🐾

   M87.88   Other osteonecrosis, other site 🐾
   M87.89   Other osteonecrosis, multiple sites 🐾

M87.9   Osteonecrosis, unspecified 🐾
    Necrosis of bone NOS

● M88   **Osteitis deformans [Paget's disease of bone]**
Chronic disorder that results in enlarged and deformed bones. The excessive breakdown and formation of bone tissue causes bones to weaken and results in bone pain, arthritis, deformities, and fractures.
    Excludes1   osteitis deformans in neoplastic disease (M90.6)

M88.0   Osteitis deformans of skull

M88.1   Osteitis deformans of vertebrae

● M88.8   Osteitis deformans of other bones
   ● M88.81   Osteitis deformans of shoulder
     M88.811   Osteitis deformans of right shoulder
     M88.812   Osteitis deformans of left shoulder
     M88.819   Osteitis deformans of unspecified shoulder

   ● M88.82   Osteitis deformans of upper arm
     M88.821   Osteitis deformans of right upper arm
     M88.822   Osteitis deformans of left upper arm
     M88.829   Osteitis deformans of unspecified upper arm

   ● M88.83   Osteitis deformans of forearm
     M88.831   Osteitis deformans of right forearm
     M88.832   Osteitis deformans of left forearm
     M88.839   Osteitis deformans of unspecified forearm

   ● M88.84   Osteitis deformans of hand
     M88.841   Osteitis deformans of right hand
     M88.842   Osteitis deformans of left hand
     M88.849   Osteitis deformans of unspecified hand

   ● M88.85   Osteitis deformans of thigh
     M88.851   Osteitis deformans of right thigh
     M88.852   Osteitis deformans of left thigh
     M88.859   Osteitis deformans of unspecified thigh

   ● M88.86   Osteitis deformans of lower leg
     M88.861   Osteitis deformans of right lower leg
     M88.862   Osteitis deformans of left lower leg
     M88.869   Osteitis deformans of unspecified lower leg

   ● M88.87   Osteitis deformans of ankle and foot
     M88.871   Osteitis deformans of right ankle and foot
     M88.872   Osteitis deformans of left ankle and foot
     M88.879   Osteitis deformans of unspecified ankle and foot

    M88.88   Osteitis deformans of other bones
      Excludes2   osteitis deformans of skull (M88.0)
           osteitis deformans of vertebrae (M88.1)

    M88.89   Osteitis deformans of multiple sites

M88.9   Osteitis deformans of unspecified bone

● M89   **Other disorders of bone**
   ● M89.0   Algoneurodystrophy
     Shoulder-hand syndrome
     Sudeck's atrophy
     Excludes1   causalgia, lower limb (G57.7-)
           causalgia, upper limb (G56.4-)
           complex regional pain syndrome II, lower limb (G57.7-)
           complex regional pain syndrome II, upper limb (G56.4-)
           reflex sympathetic dystrophy (G90.5-)

▶ New   ⟫ Revised   ~~deleted~~ Deleted   Excludes 1   Excludes 2   Includes   Use additional   Code first   Code also   Key words
OGCR Official Guidelines   X Assign placeholder X   ● Use Additional Character(s)   ▷ Manifestation Code   🐾 Hierarchical Condition Category   **Coding Clinic**

M89.00   Algoneurodystrophy, unspecified site

● M89.01   Algoneurodystrophy, shoulder

     M89.011   Algoneurodystrophy, right shoulder

     M89.012   Algoneurodystrophy, left shoulder

     M89.019   Algoneurodystrophy, unspecified shoulder

● M89.02   Algoneurodystrophy, upper arm

     M89.021   Algoneurodystrophy, right upper arm

     M89.022   Algoneurodystrophy, left upper arm

     M89.029   Algoneurodystrophy, unspecified upper arm

● M89.03   Algoneurodystrophy, forearm

     M89.031   Algoneurodystrophy, right forearm

     M89.032   Algoneurodystrophy, left forearm

     M89.039   Algoneurodystrophy, unspecified forearm

● M89.04   Algoneurodystrophy, hand

     M89.041   Algoneurodystrophy, right hand

     M89.042   Algoneurodystrophy, left hand

     M89.049   Algoneurodystrophy, unspecified hand

● M89.05   Algoneurodystrophy, thigh

     M89.051   Algoneurodystrophy, right thigh

     M89.052   Algoneurodystrophy, left thigh

     M89.059   Algoneurodystrophy, unspecified thigh

● M89.06   Algoneurodystrophy, lower leg

     M89.061   Algoneurodystrophy, right lower leg

     M89.062   Algoneurodystrophy, left lower leg

     M89.069   Algoneurodystrophy, unspecified lower leg

● M89.07   Algoneurodystrophy, ankle and foot

     M89.071   Algoneurodystrophy, right ankle and foot

     M89.072   Algoneurodystrophy, left ankle and foot

     M89.079   Algoneurodystrophy, unspecified ankle and foot

M89.08   Algoneurodystrophy, other site

M89.09   Algoneurodystrophy, multiple sites

● M89.1   Physeal arrest

     Arrest of growth plate

     Epiphyseal arrest

     Growth plate arrest

● M89.12   Physeal arrest, humerus

     M89.121   Complete physeal arrest, right proximal humerus

     M89.122   Complete physeal arrest, left proximal humerus

     M89.123   Partial physeal arrest, right proximal humerus

     M89.124   Partial physeal arrest, left proximal humerus

     M89.125   Complete physeal arrest, right distal humerus

     M89.126   Complete physeal arrest, left distal humerus

     M89.127   Partial physeal arrest, right distal humerus

     M89.128   Partial physeal arrest, left distal humerus

     M89.129   Physeal arrest, humerus, unspecified

● M89.13   Physeal arrest, forearm

     M89.131   Complete physeal arrest, right distal radius

     M89.132   Complete physeal arrest, left distal radius

     M89.133   Partial physeal arrest, right distal radius

     M89.134   Partial physeal arrest, left distal radius

     M89.138   Other physeal arrest of forearm

     M89.139   Physeal arrest, forearm, unspecified

● M89.15   Physeal arrest, femur

     M89.151   Complete physeal arrest, right proximal femur

     M89.152   Complete physeal arrest, left proximal femur

     M89.153   Partial physeal arrest, right proximal femur

     M89.154   Partial physeal arrest, left proximal femur

     M89.155   Complete physeal arrest, right distal femur

     M89.156   Complete physeal arrest, left distal femur

     M89.157   Partial physeal arrest, right distal femur

     M89.158   Partial physeal arrest, left distal femur

     M89.159   Physeal arrest, femur, unspecified

● M89.16   Physeal arrest, lower leg

     M89.160   Complete physeal arrest, right proximal tibia

     M89.161   Complete physeal arrest, left proximal tibia

     M89.162   Partial physeal arrest, right proximal tibia

     M89.163   Partial physeal arrest, left proximal tibia

     M89.164   Complete physeal arrest, right distal tibia

     M89.165   Complete physeal arrest, left distal tibia

     M89.166   Partial physeal arrest, right distal tibia

     M89.167   Partial physeal arrest, left distal tibia

     M89.168   Other physeal arrest of lower leg

     M89.169   Physeal arrest, lower leg, unspecified

M89.18   Physeal arrest, other site

● M89.2   Other disorders of bone development and growth

     M89.20   Other disorders of bone development and growth, unspecified site

● M89.21   Other disorders of bone development and growth, shoulder

     M89.211   Other disorders of bone development and growth, right shoulder

     M89.212   Other disorders of bone development and growth, left shoulder

     M89.219   Other disorders of bone development and growth, unspecified shoulder

● M89.22   Other disorders of bone development and growth, humerus

     M89.221   Other disorders of bone development and growth, right humerus

     M89.222   Other disorders of bone development and growth, left humerus

     M89.229   Other disorders of bone development and growth, unspecified humerus

● M89.23   Other disorders of bone development and growth, ulna and radius

     M89.231   Other disorders of bone development and growth, right ulna

     M89.232   Other disorders of bone development and growth, left ulna

     M89.233   Other disorders of bone development and growth, right radius

M89.234 Other disorders of bone development and growth, left radius

M89.239 Other disorders of bone development and growth, unspecified ulna and radius

● M89.24 Other disorders of bone development and growth, hand

M89.241 Other disorders of bone development and growth, right hand

M89.242 Other disorders of bone development and growth, left hand

M89.249 Other disorders of bone development and growth, unspecified hand

● M89.25 Other disorders of bone development and growth, femur

M89.251 Other disorders of bone development and growth, right femur

M89.252 Other disorders of bone development and growth, left femur

M89.259 Other disorders of bone development and growth, unspecified femur

● M89.26 Other disorders of bone development and growth, tibia and fibula

M89.261 Other disorders of bone development and growth, right tibia

M89.262 Other disorders of bone development and growth, left tibia

M89.263 Other disorders of bone development and growth, right fibula

M89.264 Other disorders of bone development and growth, left fibula

M89.269 Other disorders of bone development and growth, unspecified lower leg

● M89.27 Other disorders of bone development and growth, ankle and foot

M89.271 Other disorders of bone development and growth, right ankle and foot

M89.272 Other disorders of bone development and growth, left ankle and foot

M89.279 Other disorders of bone development and growth, unspecified ankle and foot

M89.28 Other disorders of bone development and growth, other site

M89.29 Other disorders of bone development and growth, multiple sites

● M89.3 Hypertrophy of bone

M89.30 Hypertrophy of bone, unspecified site

● M89.31 Hypertrophy of bone, shoulder

M89.311 Hypertrophy of bone, right shoulder

M89.312 Hypertrophy of bone, left shoulder

M89.319 Hypertrophy of bone, unspecified shoulder

● M89.32 Hypertrophy of bone, humerus

M89.321 Hypertrophy of bone, right humerus

M89.322 Hypertrophy of bone, left humerus

M89.329 Hypertrophy of bone, unspecified humerus

● M89.33 Hypertrophy of bone, ulna and radius

M89.331 Hypertrophy of bone, right ulna

M89.332 Hypertrophy of bone, left ulna

M89.333 Hypertrophy of bone, right radius

M89.334 Hypertrophy of bone, left radius

M89.339 Hypertrophy of bone, unspecified ulna and radius

● M89.34 Hypertrophy of bone, hand

M89.341 Hypertrophy of bone, right hand

M89.342 Hypertrophy of bone, left hand

M89.349 Hypertrophy of bone, unspecified hand

● M89.35 Hypertrophy of bone, femur

M89.351 Hypertrophy of bone, right femur

M89.352 Hypertrophy of bone, left femur

M89.359 Hypertrophy of bone, unspecified femur

● M89.36 Hypertrophy of bone, tibia and fibula

M89.361 Hypertrophy of bone, right tibia

M89.362 Hypertrophy of bone, left tibia

M89.363 Hypertrophy of bone, right fibula

M89.364 Hypertrophy of bone, left fibula

M89.369 Hypertrophy of bone, unspecified tibia and fibula

● M89.37 Hypertrophy of bone, ankle and foot

M89.371 Hypertrophy of bone, right ankle and foot

M89.372 Hypertrophy of bone, left ankle and foot

M89.379 Hypertrophy of bone, unspecified ankle and foot

M89.38 Hypertrophy of bone, other site

M89.39 Hypertrophy of bone, multiple sites

● M89.4 Other hypertrophic osteoarthropathy
Marie-Bamberger disease
Pachydermoperiostosis

M89.40 Other hypertrophic osteoarthropathy, unspecified site

● M89.41 Other hypertrophic osteoarthropathy, shoulder

M89.411 Other hypertrophic osteoarthropathy, right shoulder

M89.412 Other hypertrophic osteoarthropathy, left shoulder

M89.419 Other hypertrophic osteoarthropathy, unspecified shoulder

● M89.42 Other hypertrophic osteoarthropathy, upper arm

M89.421 Other hypertrophic osteoarthropathy, right upper arm

M89.422 Other hypertrophic osteoarthropathy, left upper arm

M89.429 Other hypertrophic osteoarthropathy, unspecified upper arm

● M89.43 Other hypertrophic osteoarthropathy, forearm

M89.431 Other hypertrophic osteoarthropathy, right forearm

M89.432 Other hypertrophic osteoarthropathy, left forearm

M89.439 Other hypertrophic osteoarthropathy, unspecified forearm

● M89.44 Other hypertrophic osteoarthropathy, hand

M89.441 Other hypertrophic osteoarthropathy, right hand

M89.442 Other hypertrophic osteoarthropathy, left hand

M89.449 Other hypertrophic osteoarthropathy, unspecified hand

● M89.45 Other hypertrophic osteoarthropathy, thigh

M89.451 Other hypertrophic osteoarthropathy, right thigh

M89.452 Other hypertrophic osteoarthropathy, left thigh

M89.459 Other hypertrophic osteoarthropathy, unspecified thigh

● M89.46 Other hypertrophic osteoarthropathy, lower leg
   M89.461   Other hypertrophic osteoarthropathy, right lower leg
   M89.462   Other hypertrophic osteoarthropathy, left lower leg
   M89.469   Other hypertrophic osteoarthropathy, unspecified lower leg

● M89.47 Other hypertrophic osteoarthropathy, ankle and foot
   M89.471   Other hypertrophic osteoarthropathy, right ankle and foot
   M89.472   Other hypertrophic osteoarthropathy, left ankle and foot
   M89.479   Other hypertrophic osteoarthropathy, unspecified ankle and foot

   M89.48   Other hypertrophic osteoarthropathy, other site
   M89.49   Other hypertrophic osteoarthropathy, multiple sites

● M89.5   Osteolysis
   Use additional code to identify major osseous defect, if applicable (M89.7-)
   Excludes2   periprosthetic osteolysis of internal prosthetic joint (T84.05-)

   M89.50   Osteolysis, unspecified site
● M89.51 Osteolysis, shoulder
   M89.511   Osteolysis, right shoulder
   M89.512   Osteolysis, left shoulder
   M89.519   Osteolysis, unspecified shoulder
● M89.52 Osteolysis, upper arm
   M89.521   Osteolysis, right upper arm
   M89.522   Osteolysis, left upper arm
   M89.529   Osteolysis, unspecified upper arm
● M89.53 Osteolysis, forearm
   M89.531   Osteolysis, right forearm
   M89.532   Osteolysis, left forearm
   M89.539   Osteolysis, unspecified forearm
● M89.54 Osteolysis, hand
   M89.541   Osteolysis, right hand
   M89.542   Osteolysis, left hand
   M89.549   Osteolysis, unspecified hand
● M89.55 Osteolysis, thigh
   M89.551   Osteolysis, right thigh
   M89.552   Osteolysis, left thigh
   M89.559   Osteolysis, unspecified thigh
● M89.56 Osteolysis, lower leg
   M89.561   Osteolysis, right lower leg
   M89.562   Osteolysis, left lower leg
   M89.569   Osteolysis, unspecified lower leg
● M89.57 Osteolysis, ankle and foot
   M89.571   Osteolysis, right ankle and foot
   M89.572   Osteolysis, left ankle and foot
   M89.579   Osteolysis, unspecified ankle and foot

   M89.58   Osteolysis, other site
   M89.59   Osteolysis, multiple sites
● M89.6   Osteopathy after poliomyelitis
   Use additional code (B91) to identify previous poliomyelitis
   Excludes1   postpolio syndrome (G14)
   M89.60   Osteopathy after poliomyelitis, unspecified site ✖
● M89.61 Osteopathy after poliomyelitis, shoulder
   M89.611   Osteopathy after poliomyelitis, right shoulder ✖
   M89.612   Osteopathy after poliomyelitis, left shoulder ✖
   M89.619   Osteopathy after poliomyelitis, unspecified shoulder ✖

● M89.62 Osteopathy after poliomyelitis, upper arm
   M89.621   Osteopathy after poliomyelitis, right upper arm ✖
   M89.622   Osteopathy after poliomyelitis, left upper arm ✖
   M89.629   Osteopathy after poliomyelitis, unspecified upper arm ✖
● M89.63 Osteopathy after poliomyelitis, forearm
   M89.631   Osteopathy after poliomyelitis, right forearm ✖
   M89.632   Osteopathy after poliomyelitis, left forearm ✖
   M89.639   Osteopathy after poliomyelitis, unspecified forearm ✖
● M89.64 Osteopathy after poliomyelitis, hand
   M89.641   Osteopathy after poliomyelitis, right hand ✖
   M89.642   Osteopathy after poliomyelitis, left hand ✖
   M89.649   Osteopathy after poliomyelitis, unspecified hand ✖
● M89.65 Osteopathy after poliomyelitis, thigh
   M89.651   Osteopathy after poliomyelitis, right thigh ✖
   M89.652   Osteopathy after poliomyelitis, left thigh ✖
   M89.659   Osteopathy after poliomyelitis, unspecified thigh ✖
● M89.66 Osteopathy after poliomyelitis, lower leg
   M89.661   Osteopathy after poliomyelitis, right lower leg ✖
   M89.662   Osteopathy after poliomyelitis, left lower leg ✖
   M89.669   Osteopathy after poliomyelitis, unspecified lower leg ✖
● M89.67 Osteopathy after poliomyelitis, ankle and foot
   M89.671   Osteopathy after poliomyelitis, right ankle and foot ✖
   M89.672   Osteopathy after poliomyelitis, left ankle and foot ✖
   M89.679   Osteopathy after poliomyelitis, unspecified ankle and foot ✖

   M89.68   Osteopathy after poliomyelitis, other site ✖
   M89.69   Osteopathy after poliomyelitis, multiple sites ✖

● M89.7   Major osseous defect
   Code first underlying disease, if known, such as:
      aseptic necrosis of bone (M87.-)
      malignant neoplasm of bone (C40.-)
      osteolysis (M89.5)
      osteomyelitis (M86.-)
      osteonecrosis (M87.-)
      osteoporosis (M80.-, M81.-)
      periprosthetic osteolysis (T84.05-)
   M89.70   Major osseous defect, unspecified site
● M89.71 Major osseous defect, shoulder region
      Major osseous defect clavicle or scapula
   M89.711   Major osseous defect, right shoulder region
   M89.712   Major osseous defect, left shoulder region
   M89.719   Major osseous defect, unspecified shoulder region
● M89.72 Major osseous defect, humerus
   M89.721   Major osseous defect, right humerus
   M89.722   Major osseous defect, left humerus
   M89.729   Major osseous defect, unspecified humerus

CHAPTER 13 (M00-M99)

M89.73 **Major osseous defect, forearm**
    Major osseous defect of radius and ulna
    M89.731 Major osseous defect, right forearm
    M89.732 Major osseous defect, left forearm
    M89.739 Major osseous defect, unspecified forearm

M89.74 **Major osseous defect, hand**
    Major osseous defect of carpus, fingers, metacarpus
    M89.741 Major osseous defect, right hand
    M89.742 Major osseous defect, left hand
    M89.749 Major osseous defect, unspecified hand

M89.75 **Major osseous defect, pelvic region and thigh**
    Major osseous defect of femur and pelvis
    M89.751 Major osseous defect, right pelvic region and thigh
    M89.752 Major osseous defect, left pelvic region and thigh
    M89.759 Major osseous defect, unspecified pelvic region and thigh

M89.76 **Major osseous defect, lower leg**
    Major osseous defect of fibula and tibia
    M89.761 Major osseous defect, right lower leg
    M89.762 Major osseous defect, left lower leg
    M89.769 Major osseous defect, unspecified lower leg

M89.77 **Major osseous defect, ankle and foot**
    Major osseous defect of metatarsus, tarsus, toes
    M89.771 Major osseous defect, right ankle and foot
    M89.772 Major osseous defect, left ankle and foot
    M89.779 Major osseous defect, unspecified ankle and foot

M89.78 Major osseous defect, other site
M89.79 Major osseous defect, multiple sites

M89.8 **Other specified disorders of bone**
    Infantile cortical hyperostoses
    Post-traumatic subperiosteal ossification

M89.8X **Other specified disorders of bone**
    M89.8X0 Other specified disorders of bone, multiple sites
    M89.8X1 Other specified disorders of bone, shoulder
    M89.8X2 Other specified disorders of bone, upper arm
    M89.8X3 Other specified disorders of bone, forearm
        Coding Clinic: 2019, Q3, P10
    M89.8X4 Other specified disorders of bone, hand
    M89.8X5 Other specified disorders of bone, thigh
    M89.8X6 Other specified disorders of bone, lower leg
    M89.8X7 Other specified disorders of bone, ankle and foot
    M89.8X8 Other specified disorders of bone, other site
    M89.8X9 Other specified disorders of bone, unspecified site

M89.9 Disorder of bone, unspecified

M90 **Osteopathies in diseases classified elsewhere**
    Excludes1 osteochondritis, osteomyelitis, and osteopathy (in):
        cryptococcosis (B45.3)
        diabetes mellitus (E08-E13 with .69-)
        gonococcal (A54.43)
        neurogenic syphilis (A52.11)
        renal osteodystrophy (N25.0)
        salmonellosis (A02.24)
        secondary syphilis (A51.46)
        syphilis (late) (A52.77)

M90.5 **Osteonecrosis in diseases classified elsewhere**
    Code first underlying disease, such as:
        caisson disease (T70.3)
        hemoglobinopathy (D50-D64)
    M90.50 *Osteonecrosis in diseases classified elsewhere, unspecified site* 🐾
    M90.51 **Osteonecrosis in diseases classified elsewhere, shoulder**
        M90.511 *Osteonecrosis in diseases classified elsewhere, right shoulder* 🐾
        M90.512 *Osteonecrosis in diseases classified elsewhere, left shoulder* 🐾
        M90.519 *Osteonecrosis in diseases classified elsewhere, unspecified shoulder* 🐾
    M90.52 **Osteonecrosis in diseases classified elsewhere, upper arm**
        M90.521 *Osteonecrosis in diseases classified elsewhere, right upper arm* 🐾
        M90.522 *Osteonecrosis in diseases classified elsewhere, left upper arm* 🐾
        M90.529 *Osteonecrosis in diseases classified elsewhere, unspecified upper arm* 🐾
    M90.53 **Osteonecrosis in diseases classified elsewhere, forearm**
        M90.531 *Osteonecrosis in diseases classified elsewhere, right forearm* 🐾
        M90.532 *Osteonecrosis in diseases classified elsewhere, left forearm* 🐾
        M90.539 *Osteonecrosis in diseases classified elsewhere, unspecified forearm* 🐾
    M90.54 **Osteonecrosis in diseases classified elsewhere, hand**
        M90.541 *Osteonecrosis in diseases classified elsewhere, right hand* 🐾
        M90.542 *Osteonecrosis in diseases classified elsewhere, left hand* 🐾
        M90.549 *Osteonecrosis in diseases classified elsewhere, unspecified hand* 🐾
    M90.55 **Osteonecrosis in diseases classified elsewhere, thigh**
        M90.551 *Osteonecrosis in diseases classified elsewhere, right thigh* 🐾
        M90.552 *Osteonecrosis in diseases classified elsewhere, left thigh* 🐾
        M90.559 *Osteonecrosis in diseases classified elsewhere, unspecified thigh* 🐾
    M90.56 **Osteonecrosis in diseases classified elsewhere, lower leg**
        M90.561 *Osteonecrosis in diseases classified elsewhere, right lower leg* 🐾
        M90.562 *Osteonecrosis in diseases classified elsewhere, left lower leg* 🐾
        M90.569 *Osteonecrosis in diseases classified elsewhere, unspecified lower leg* 🐾

▶ New   ▬▶ Revised   ~~deleted~~ Deleted   Excludes 1   Excludes 2   Includes   Use additional   Code first   Code also   Key words
OGCR Official Guidelines   X Assign placeholder X   ● Use Additional Character(s)   ▷ Manifestation Code   🐾 Hierarchical Condition Category   **Coding Clinic**

● **M90.57** **Osteonecrosis in diseases classified elsewhere, ankle and foot**

⟩ *M90.571 Osteonecrosis in diseases classified elsewhere, right ankle and foot* 🦴

⟩ *M90.572 Osteonecrosis in diseases classified elsewhere, left ankle and foot* 🦴

⟩ *M90.579 Osteonecrosis in diseases classified elsewhere, unspecified ankle and foot* 🦴

⟩ *M90.58 Osteonecrosis in diseases classified elsewhere, other site* 🦴

⟩ *M90.59 Osteonecrosis in diseases classified elsewhere, multiple sites* 🦴

● **M90.6** **Osteitis deformans in neoplastic diseases**
Osteitis deformans in malignant neoplasm of bone
Code first the neoplasm (C40.-, C41.-)

   Excludes1   osteitis deformans [Paget's disease of bone] (M88.-)

⟩ *M90.60 Osteitis deformans in neoplastic diseases, unspecified site*

● **M90.61** **Osteitis deformans in neoplastic diseases, shoulder**

⟩ *M90.611 Osteitis deformans in neoplastic diseases, right shoulder*

⟩ *M90.612 Osteitis deformans in neoplastic diseases, left shoulder*

⟩ *M90.619 Osteitis deformans in neoplastic diseases, unspecified shoulder*

● **M90.62** **Osteitis deformans in neoplastic diseases, upper arm**

⟩ *M90.621 Osteitis deformans in neoplastic diseases, right upper arm*

⟩ *M90.622 Osteitis deformans in neoplastic diseases, left upper arm*

⟩ *M90.629 Osteitis deformans in neoplastic diseases, unspecified upper arm*

● **M90.63** **Osteitis deformans in neoplastic diseases, forearm**

⟩ *M90.631 Osteitis deformans in neoplastic diseases, right forearm*

⟩ *M90.632 Osteitis deformans in neoplastic diseases, left forearm*

⟩ *M90.639 Osteitis deformans in neoplastic diseases, unspecified forearm*

● **M90.64** **Osteitis deformans in neoplastic diseases, hand**

⟩ *M90.641 Osteitis deformans in neoplastic diseases, right hand*

⟩ *M90.642 Osteitis deformans in neoplastic diseases, left hand*

⟩ *M90.649 Osteitis deformans in neoplastic diseases, unspecified hand*

● **M90.65** **Osteitis deformans in neoplastic diseases, thigh**

⟩ *M90.651 Osteitis deformans in neoplastic diseases, right thigh*

⟩ *M90.652 Osteitis deformans in neoplastic diseases, left thigh*

⟩ *M90.659 Osteitis deformans in neoplastic diseases, unspecified thigh*

● **M90.66** **Osteitis deformans in neoplastic diseases, lower leg**

⟩ *M90.661 Osteitis deformans in neoplastic diseases, right lower leg*

⟩ *M90.662 Osteitis deformans in neoplastic diseases, left lower leg*

⟩ *M90.669 Osteitis deformans in neoplastic diseases, unspecified lower leg*

● **M90.67** **Osteitis deformans in neoplastic diseases, ankle and foot**

⟩ *M90.671 Osteitis deformans in neoplastic diseases, right ankle and foot*

⟩ *M90.672 Osteitis deformans in neoplastic diseases, left ankle and foot*

⟩ *M90.679 Osteitis deformans in neoplastic diseases, unspecified ankle and foot*

⟩ *M90.68 Osteitis deformans in neoplastic diseases, other site*

⟩ *M90.69 Osteitis deformans in neoplastic diseases, multiple sites*

● **M90.8** **Osteopathy in diseases classified elsewhere**
Code first underlying disease, such as:
rickets (E55.0)
vitamin-D-resistant rickets (E83.3)

⟩ *M90.80 Osteopathy in diseases classified elsewhere, unspecified site*

● **M90.81** **Osteopathy in diseases classified elsewhere, shoulder**

⟩ *M90.811 Osteopathy in diseases classified elsewhere, right shoulder*

⟩ *M90.812 Osteopathy in diseases classified elsewhere, left shoulder*

⟩ *M90.819 Osteopathy in diseases classified elsewhere, unspecified shoulder*

● **M90.82** **Osteopathy in diseases classified elsewhere, upper arm**

⟩ *M90.821 Osteopathy in diseases classified elsewhere, right upper arm*

⟩ *M90.822 Osteopathy in diseases classified elsewhere, left upper arm*

⟩ *M90.829 Osteopathy in diseases classified elsewhere, unspecified upper arm*

● **M90.83** **Osteopathy in diseases classified elsewhere, forearm**

⟩ *M90.831 Osteopathy in diseases classified elsewhere, right forearm*

⟩ *M90.832 Osteopathy in diseases classified elsewhere, left forearm*

⟩ *M90.839 Osteopathy in diseases classified elsewhere, unspecified forearm*

● **M90.84** **Osteopathy in diseases classified elsewhere, hand**

⟩ *M90.841 Osteopathy in diseases classified elsewhere, right hand*

⟩ *M90.842 Osteopathy in diseases classified elsewhere, left hand*

⟩ *M90.849 Osteopathy in diseases classified elsewhere, unspecified hand*

● **M90.85** **Osteopathy in diseases classified elsewhere, thigh**

⟩ *M90.851 Osteopathy in diseases classified elsewhere, right thigh*

⟩ *M90.852 Osteopathy in diseases classified elsewhere, left thigh*

⟩ *M90.859 Osteopathy in diseases classified elsewhere, unspecified thigh*

● **M90.86** **Osteopathy in diseases classified elsewhere, lower leg**

⟩ *M90.861 Osteopathy in diseases classified elsewhere, right lower leg*

⟩ *M90.862 Osteopathy in diseases classified elsewhere, left lower leg*

⟩ *M90.869 Osteopathy in diseases classified elsewhere, unspecified lower leg*

CHAPTER 13 (M00-M99)

● M90.87 Osteopathy in diseases classified elsewhere, ankle and foot
  ▶ M90.871 Osteopathy in diseases classified elsewhere, right ankle and foot
  ▶ M90.872 Osteopathy in diseases classified elsewhere, left ankle and foot
  ▶ M90.879 Osteopathy in diseases classified elsewhere, unspecified ankle and foot
▶ M90.88 Osteopathy in diseases classified elsewhere, other site
▶ M90.89 Osteopathy in diseases classified elsewhere, multiple sites

CHONDROPATHIES (M91-M94)

Excludes1 postprocedural chondropathies (M96.-)

● M91 Juvenile osteochondrosis of hip and pelvis
  Excludes1 slipped upper femoral epiphysis (nontraumatic) (M93.0)

M91.0 Juvenile osteochondrosis of pelvis
  Osteochondrosis (juvenile) of acetabulum
  Osteochondrosis (juvenile) of iliac crest [Buchanan]
  Osteochondrosis (juvenile) of ischiopubic synchondrosis [van Neck]
  Osteochondrosis (juvenile) of symphysis pubis [Pierson]

● M91.1 Juvenile osteochondrosis of head of femur [Legg-Calvé-Perthes]
  M91.10 Juvenile osteochondrosis of head of femur [Legg-Calvé-Perthes], unspecified leg
  M91.11 Juvenile osteochondrosis of head of femur [Legg-Calvé-Perthes], right leg
  M91.12 Juvenile osteochondrosis of head of femur [Legg-Calvé-Perthes], left leg

● M91.2 Coxa plana
  Hip deformity due to previous juvenile osteochondrosis
  M91.20 Coxa plana, unspecified hip
  M91.21 Coxa plana, right hip
  M91.22 Coxa plana, left hip

● M91.3 Pseudocoxalgia
  M91.30 Pseudocoxalgia, unspecified hip
  M91.31 Pseudocoxalgia, right hip
  M91.32 Pseudocoxalgia, left hip

● M91.4 Coxa magna
  M91.40 Coxa magna, unspecified hip
  M91.41 Coxa magna, right hip
  M91.42 Coxa magna, left hip

● M91.8 Other juvenile osteochondrosis of hip and pelvis
  Juvenile osteochondrosis after reduction of congenital dislocation of hip
  M91.80 Other juvenile osteochondrosis of hip and pelvis, unspecified leg
  M91.81 Other juvenile osteochondrosis of hip and pelvis, right leg
  M91.82 Other juvenile osteochondrosis of hip and pelvis, left leg

● M91.9 Juvenile osteochondrosis of hip and pelvis, unspecified
  M91.90 Juvenile osteochondrosis of hip and pelvis, unspecified, unspecified leg
  M91.91 Juvenile osteochondrosis of hip and pelvis, unspecified, right leg
  M91.92 Juvenile osteochondrosis of hip and pelvis, unspecified, left leg

● M92 Other juvenile osteochondrosis
  ● M92.0 Juvenile osteochondrosis of humerus
    Osteochondrosis (juvenile) of capitulum of humerus [Panner]
    Osteochondrosis (juvenile) of head of humerus [Haas]
    M92.00 Juvenile osteochondrosis of humerus, unspecified arm
    M92.01 Juvenile osteochondrosis of humerus, right arm
    M92.02 Juvenile osteochondrosis of humerus, left arm

● M92.1 Juvenile osteochondrosis of radius and ulna
  Osteochondrosis (juvenile) of lower ulna [Burns]
  Osteochondrosis (juvenile) of radial head [Brailsford]
  M92.10 Juvenile osteochondrosis of radius and ulna, unspecified arm
  M92.11 Juvenile osteochondrosis of radius and ulna, right arm
  M92.12 Juvenile osteochondrosis of radius and ulna, left arm

● M92.2 Juvenile osteochondrosis, hand
  ● M92.20 Unspecified juvenile osteochondrosis, hand
    M92.201 Unspecified juvenile osteochondrosis, right hand
    M92.202 Unspecified juvenile osteochondrosis, left hand
    M92.209 Unspecified juvenile osteochondrosis, unspecified hand
  ● M92.21 Osteochondrosis (juvenile) of carpal lunate [Kienböck]
    M92.211 Osteochondrosis (juvenile) of carpal lunate [Kienböck], right hand
    M92.212 Osteochondrosis (juvenile) of carpal lunate [Kienböck], left hand
    M92.219 Osteochondrosis (juvenile) of carpal lunate [Kienböck], unspecified hand
  ● M92.22 Osteochondrosis (juvenile) of metacarpal heads [Mauclaire]
    M92.221 Osteochondrosis (juvenile) of metacarpal heads [Mauclaire], right hand
    M92.222 Osteochondrosis (juvenile) of metacarpal heads [Mauclaire], left hand
    M92.229 Osteochondrosis (juvenile) of metacarpal heads [Mauclaire], unspecified hand
  ● M92.29 Other juvenile osteochondrosis, hand
    M92.291 Other juvenile osteochondrosis, right hand
    M92.292 Other juvenile osteochondrosis, left hand
    M92.299 Other juvenile osteochondrosis, unspecified hand

● M92.3 Other juvenile osteochondrosis, upper limb
  M92.30 Other juvenile osteochondrosis, unspecified upper limb
  M92.31 Other juvenile osteochondrosis, right upper limb
  M92.32 Other juvenile osteochondrosis, left upper limb

● M92.4 Juvenile osteochondrosis of patella
  Osteochondrosis (juvenile) of primary patellar center [Köhler]
  Osteochondrosis (juvenile) of secondary patellar center [Sinding Larsen]
  M92.40 Juvenile osteochondrosis of patella, unspecified knee
  M92.41 Juvenile osteochondrosis of patella, right knee
  M92.42 Juvenile osteochondrosis of patella, left knee

● M92.5 Juvenile osteochondrosis of tibia and fibula
  ● M92.50 Unspecified juvenile osteochondrosis of tibia and fibula
    M92.501 Unspecified juvenile osteochondrosis, right leg
    M92.502 Unspecified juvenile osteochondrosis, left leg
    M92.503 Unspecified juvenile osteochondrosis, bilateral leg
    M92.509 Unspecified juvenile osteochondrosis, unspecified leg

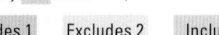

▶ New   ⇒ Revised   ~~deleted~~ Deleted   Excludes 1   Excludes 2   Includes   Use additional   Code first   Code also   Key words

OGCR Official Guidelines   X Assign placeholder X   ● Use Additional Character(s)   ▶ Manifestation Code   🏷 Hierarchical Condition Category   Coding Clinic

● M92.51 Juvenile osteochondrosis of proximal tibia
　　　　Blount disease
　　　　Tibia vara
　　　M92.511 Juvenile osteochondrosis of proximal tibia, right leg
　　　M92.512 Juvenile osteochondrosis of proximal tibia, left leg
　　　M92.513 Juvenile osteochondrosis of proximal tibia, bilateral
　　　M92.519 Juvenile osteochondrosis of proximal tibia, unspecified leg

● M92.52 Juvenile osteochondrosis of tibia tubercle
　　　　Osgood-Schlatter disease
　　　M92.521 Juvenile osteochondrosis of tibia tubercle, right leg
　　　M92.522 Juvenile osteochondrosis of tibia tubercle, left leg
　　　M92.523 Juvenile osteochondrosis of tibia tubercle, bilateral
　　　M92.529 Juvenile osteochondrosis of tibia tubercle, unspecified leg

　M92.59 Other juvenile osteochondrosis of tibia and fibula
　　　M92.591 Other juvenile osteochondrosis of tibia and fibula, right leg
　　　M92.592 Other juvenile osteochondrosis of tibia and fibula, left leg
　　　M92.593 Other juvenile osteochondrosis of tibia and fibula, bilateral
　　　M92.599 Other juvenile osteochondrosis of tibia and fibula, unspecified leg

● M92.6 Juvenile osteochondrosis of tarsus
　　　Osteochondrosis (juvenile) of calcaneum [Sever]
　　　Osteochondrosis (juvenile) of os tibiale externum [Haglund]
　　　Osteochondrosis (juvenile) of talus [Diaz]
　　　Osteochondrosis (juvenile) of tarsal navicular [Köhler]
　　M92.60 Juvenile osteochondrosis of tarsus, unspecified ankle
　　M92.61 Juvenile osteochondrosis of tarsus, right ankle
　　M92.62 Juvenile osteochondrosis of tarsus, left ankle

● M92.7 Juvenile osteochondrosis of metatarsus
　　　Osteochondrosis (juvenile) of fifth metatarsus [Iselin]
　　　Osteochondrosis (juvenile) of second metatarsus [Freiberg]
　　M92.70 Juvenile osteochondrosis of metatarsus, unspecified foot
　　M92.71 Juvenile osteochondrosis of metatarsus, right foot
　　M92.72 Juvenile osteochondrosis of metatarsus, left foot

　M92.8 Other specified juvenile osteochondrosis
　　　Calcaneal apophysitis

　M92.9 Juvenile osteochondrosis, unspecified
　　　Juvenile apophysitis NOS
　　　Juvenile epiphysitis NOS
　　　Juvenile osteochondritis NOS
　　　Juvenile osteochondrosis NOS

● M93 Other osteochondropathies
　　Excludes2　osteochondrosis of spine (M42.-)
● M93.0 Slipped upper femoral epiphysis (nontraumatic)
　　　Use additional code for associated chondrolysis (M94.3)
　● M93.00 Unspecified slipped upper femoral epiphysis (nontraumatic)
　　　M93.001 Unspecified slipped upper femoral epiphysis (nontraumatic), right hip
　　　M93.002 Unspecified slipped upper femoral epiphysis (nontraumatic), left hip
　　　M93.003 Unspecified slipped upper femoral epiphysis (nontraumatic), unspecified hip

● M93.01 Acute slipped upper femoral epiphysis (nontraumatic)
　　　M93.011 Acute slipped upper femoral epiphysis (nontraumatic), right hip
　　　M93.012 Acute slipped upper femoral epiphysis (nontraumatic), left hip
　　　M93.013 Acute slipped upper femoral epiphysis (nontraumatic), unspecified hip

● M93.02 Chronic slipped upper femoral epiphysis (nontraumatic)
　　　M93.021 Chronic slipped upper femoral epiphysis (nontraumatic), right hip
　　　M93.022 Chronic slipped upper femoral epiphysis (nontraumatic), left hip
　　　M93.023 Chronic slipped upper femoral epiphysis (nontraumatic), unspecified hip

● M93.03 Acute on chronic slipped upper femoral epiphysis (nontraumatic)
　　　M93.031 Acute on chronic slipped upper femoral epiphysis (nontraumatic), right hip
　　　M93.032 Acute on chronic slipped upper femoral epiphysis (nontraumatic), left hip
　　　M93.033 Acute on chronic slipped upper femoral epiphysis (nontraumatic), unspecified hip

　M93.1 Kienböck's disease of adults　　　　　　　　　A
　　　Adult osteochondrosis of carpal lunates

● M93.2 Osteochondritis dissecans
　　M93.20 Osteochondritis dissecans of unspecified site
　● M93.21 Osteochondritis dissecans of shoulder
　　　M93.211 Osteochondritis dissecans, right shoulder
　　　M93.212 Osteochondritis dissecans, left shoulder
　　　M93.219 Osteochondritis dissecans, unspecified shoulder
　● M93.22 Osteochondritis dissecans of elbow
　　　M93.221 Osteochondritis dissecans, right elbow
　　　M93.222 Osteochondritis dissecans, left elbow
　　　M93.229 Osteochondritis dissecans, unspecified elbow
　● M93.23 Osteochondritis dissecans of wrist
　　　M93.231 Osteochondritis dissecans, right wrist
　　　M93.232 Osteochondritis dissecans, left wrist
　　　M93.239 Osteochondritis dissecans, unspecified wrist
　● M93.24 Osteochondritis dissecans of joints of hand
　　　M93.241 Osteochondritis dissecans, joints of right hand
　　　M93.242 Osteochondritis dissecans, joints of left hand
　　　M93.249 Osteochondritis dissecans, joints of unspecified hand
　● M93.25 Osteochondritis dissecans of hip
　　　M93.251 Osteochondritis dissecans, right hip
　　　M93.252 Osteochondritis dissecans, left hip
　　　M93.259 Osteochondritis dissecans, unspecified hip
　● M93.26 Osteochondritis dissecans knee
　　　M93.261 Osteochondritis dissecans, right knee
　　　M93.262 Osteochondritis dissecans, left knee
　　　M93.269 Osteochondritis dissecans, unspecified knee

CHAPTER 13 (M00-M99)

● M93.27   **Osteochondritis dissecans of ankle and joints of foot**
     M93.271   Osteochondritis dissecans, right ankle and joints of right foot
     M93.272   Osteochondritis dissecans, left ankle and joints of left foot
     M93.279   Osteochondritis dissecans, unspecified ankle and joints of foot
   M93.28   Osteochondritis dissecans other site
   M93.29   Osteochondritis dissecans multiple sites
● M93.8   Other specified osteochondropathies
   M93.80   Other specified osteochondropathies of unspecified site
● M93.81   Other specified osteochondropathies of shoulder
     M93.811   Other specified osteochondropathies, right shoulder
     M93.812   Other specified osteochondropathies, left shoulder
     M93.819   Other specified osteochondropathies, unspecified shoulder
● M93.82   Other specified osteochondropathies of upper arm
     M93.821   Other specified osteochondropathies, right upper arm
     M93.822   Other specified osteochondropathies, left upper arm
     M93.829   Other specified osteochondropathies, unspecified upper arm
● M93.83   Other specified osteochondropathies of forearm
     M93.831   Other specified osteochondropathies, right forearm
     M93.832   Other specified osteochondropathies, left forearm
     M93.839   Other specified osteochondropathies, unspecified forearm
● M93.84   Other specified osteochondropathies of hand
     M93.841   Other specified osteochondropathies, right hand
     M93.842   Other specified osteochondropathies, left hand
     M93.849   Other specified osteochondropathies, unspecified hand
● M93.85   Other specified osteochondropathies of thigh
     M93.851   Other specified osteochondropathies, right thigh
     M93.852   Other specified osteochondropathies, left thigh
     M93.859   Other specified osteochondropathies, unspecified thigh
● M93.86   Other specified osteochondropathies lower leg
     M93.861   Other specified osteochondropathies, right lower leg
     M93.862   Other specified osteochondropathies, left lower leg
     M93.869   Other specified osteochondropathies, unspecified lower leg
● M93.87   Other specified osteochondropathies of ankle and foot
     M93.871   Other specified osteochondropathies, right ankle and foot
     M93.872   Other specified osteochondropathies, left ankle and foot
     M93.879   Other specified osteochondropathies, unspecified ankle and foot
   M93.88   Other specified osteochondropathies other
   M93.89   Other specified osteochondropathies multiple sites

M93.9   **Osteochondropathy, unspecified**
     Apophysitis NOS
     Epiphysitis NOS
     Osteochondritis NOS
     Osteochondrosis NOS
   M93.90   Osteochondropathy, unspecified of unspecified site
● M93.91   Osteochondropathy, unspecified of shoulder
     M93.911   Osteochondropathy, unspecified, right shoulder
     M93.912   Osteochondropathy, unspecified, left shoulder
     M93.919   Osteochondropathy, unspecified, unspecified shoulder
● M93.92   Osteochondropathy, unspecified of upper arm
     M93.921   Osteochondropathy, unspecified, right upper arm
     M93.922   Osteochondropathy, unspecified, left upper arm
     M93.929   Osteochondropathy, unspecified, unspecified upper arm
● M93.93   Osteochondropathy, unspecified of forearm
     M93.931   Osteochondropathy, unspecified, right forearm
     M93.932   Osteochondropathy, unspecified, left forearm
     M93.939   Osteochondropathy, unspecified, unspecified forearm
● M93.94   Osteochondropathy, unspecified of hand
     M93.941   Osteochondropathy, unspecified, right hand
     M93.942   Osteochondropathy, unspecified, left hand
     M93.949   Osteochondropathy, unspecified, unspecified hand
● M93.95   Osteochondropathy, unspecified of thigh
     M93.951   Osteochondropathy, unspecified, right thigh
     M93.952   Osteochondropathy, unspecified, left thigh
     M93.959   Osteochondropathy, unspecified, unspecified thigh
● M93.96   Osteochondropathy, unspecified lower leg
     M93.961   Osteochondropathy, unspecified, right lower leg
     M93.962   Osteochondropathy, unspecified, left lower leg
     M93.969   Osteochondropathy, unspecified, unspecified lower leg
● M93.97   Osteochondropathy, unspecified of ankle and foot
     M93.971   Osteochondropathy, unspecified, right ankle and foot
     M93.972   Osteochondropathy, unspecified, left ankle and foot
     M93.979   Osteochondropathy, unspecified, unspecified ankle and foot
   M93.98   Osteochondropathy, unspecified other
   M93.99   Osteochondropathy, unspecified multiple sites

● M94   **Other disorders of cartilage**
   M94.0   **Chondrocostal junction syndrome [Tietze]**
     Costochondritis
   M94.1   **Relapsing polychondritis**
● M94.2   **Chondromalacia**
     Excludes1   chondromalacia patellae (M22.4)
   M94.20   Chondromalacia, unspecified site
● M94.21   Chondromalacia, shoulder
     M94.211   Chondromalacia, right shoulder
     M94.212   Chondromalacia, left shoulder

　　　　　　M94.219　Chondromalacia, unspecified shoulder
　　　● M94.22　Chondromalacia, elbow
　　　　　　M94.221　Chondromalacia, right elbow
　　　　　　M94.222　Chondromalacia, left elbow
　　　　　　M94.229　Chondromalacia, unspecified elbow
　　　● M94.23　Chondromalacia, wrist
　　　　　　M94.231　Chondromalacia, right wrist
　　　　　　M94.232　Chondromalacia, left wrist
　　　　　　M94.239　Chondromalacia, unspecified wrist
　　　● M94.24　Chondromalacia, joints of hand
　　　　　　M94.241　Chondromalacia, joints of right hand
　　　　　　M94.242　Chondromalacia, joints of left hand
　　　　　　M94.249　Chondromalacia, joints of unspecified hand
　　　● M94.25　Chondromalacia, hip
　　　　　　M94.251　Chondromalacia, right hip
　　　　　　M94.252　Chondromalacia, left hip
　　　　　　M94.259　Chondromalacia, unspecified hip
　　　● M94.26　Chondromalacia, knee
　　　　　　M94.261　Chondromalacia, right knee
　　　　　　M94.262　Chondromalacia, left knee
　　　　　　M94.269　Chondromalacia, unspecified knee
　　　● M94.27　Chondromalacia, ankle and joints of foot
　　　　　　M94.271　Chondromalacia, right ankle and joints of right foot
　　　　　　M94.272　Chondromalacia, left ankle and joints of left foot
　　　　　　M94.279　Chondromalacia, unspecified ankle and joints of foot
　　　　　M94.28　Chondromalacia, other site
　　　　　M94.29　Chondromalacia, multiple sites
● M94.3　Chondrolysis
　　　　Code first any associated slipped upper femoral epiphysis (nontraumatic) (M93.0-)
　　　● M94.35　Chondrolysis, hip
　　　　　　M94.351　Chondrolysis, right hip
　　　　　　M94.352　Chondrolysis, left hip
　　　　　　M94.359　Chondrolysis, unspecified hip
● M94.8　Other specified disorders of cartilage
　　　● M94.8X　Other specified disorders of cartilage
　　　　　　M94.8X0　Other specified disorders of cartilage, multiple sites
　　　　　　M94.8X1　Other specified disorders of cartilage, shoulder
　　　　　　M94.8X2　Other specified disorders of cartilage, upper arm
　　　　　　M94.8X3　Other specified disorders of cartilage, forearm
　　　　　　M94.8X4　Other specified disorders of cartilage, hand
　　　　　　M94.8X5　Other specified disorders of cartilage, thigh
　　　　　　M94.8X6　Other specified disorders of cartilage, lower leg
　　　　　　M94.8X7　Other specified disorders of cartilage, ankle and foot
　　　　　　M94.8X8　Other specified disorders of cartilage, other site
　　　　　　M94.8X9　Other specified disorders of cartilage, unspecified sites
　　M94.9　Disorder of cartilage, unspecified

OTHER DISORDERS OF THE MUSCULOSKELETAL SYSTEM AND CONNECTIVE TISSUE (M95)

● M95　Other acquired deformities of musculoskeletal system and connective tissue
　　Excludes2　acquired absence of limbs and organs (Z89-Z90)
　　　　　　acquired deformities of limbs (M20-M21)
　　　　　　congenital malformations and deformations of the musculoskeletal system (Q65-Q79)
　　　　　　deforming dorsopathies (M40-M43)
　　　　　　dentofacial anomalies [including malocclusion] (M26.-)
　　　　　　postprocedural musculoskeletal disorders (M96.-)
　　M95.0　Acquired deformity of nose
　　　　Excludes2　deviated nasal septum (J34.2)
　● M95.1　Cauliflower ear
　　　　Excludes2　other acquired deformities of ear (H61.1)
　　　　　M95.10　Cauliflower ear, unspecified ear
　　　　　M95.11　Cauliflower ear, right ear
　　　　　M95.12　Cauliflower ear, left ear
　　M95.2　Other acquired deformity of head
　　M95.3　Acquired deformity of neck
　　M95.4　Acquired deformity of chest and rib
　　M95.5　Acquired deformity of pelvis
　　　　Excludes1　maternal care for known or suspected disproportion (O33.-)
　　M95.8　Other specified acquired deformities of musculoskeletal system
　　M95.9　Acquired deformity of musculoskeletal system, unspecified

INTRAOPERATIVE AND POSTPROCEDURAL COMPLICATIONS AND DISORDERS OF MUSCULOSKELETAL SYSTEM, NOT ELSEWHERE CLASSIFIED (M96)

● M96　Intraoperative and postprocedural complications and disorders of musculoskeletal system, not elsewhere classified
　　Excludes2　arthropathy following intestinal bypass (M02.0-)
　　　　　　complications of internal orthopedic prosthetic devices, implants and grafts (T84.-)
　　　　　　disorders associated with osteoporosis (M80)
　　　　　　periprosthetic fracture around internal prosthetic joint (M97.-)
　　　　　　presence of functional implants and other devices (Z96-Z97)
　　M96.0　Pseudarthrosis after fusion or arthrodesis
　　M96.1　Postlaminectomy syndrome, not elsewhere classified
　　M96.2　Postradiation kyphosis
　　M96.3　Postlaminectomy kyphosis
　　M96.4　Postsurgical lordosis
　　M96.5　Postradiation scoliosis
　● M96.6　Fracture of bone following insertion of orthopedic implant, joint prosthesis, or bone plate
　　　　Intraoperative fracture of bone during insertion of orthopedic implant, joint prosthesis, or bone plate
　　　　Excludes2　complication of internal orthopedic devices, implants or grafts (T84.-)
　　　● M96.62　Fracture of humerus following insertion of orthopedic implant, joint prosthesis, or bone plate
　　　　　　M96.621　Fracture of humerus following insertion of orthopedic implant, joint prosthesis, or bone plate, right arm 🦴
　　　　　　M96.622　Fracture of humerus following insertion of orthopedic implant, joint prosthesis, or bone plate, left arm 🦴
　　　　　　M96.629　Fracture of humerus following insertion of orthopedic implant, joint prosthesis, or bone plate, unspecified arm 🦴

CHAPTER 13 (M00-M99)

M96.63 Fracture of radius or ulna following insertion of orthopedic implant, joint prosthesis, or bone plate

    M96.631 Fracture of radius or ulna following insertion of orthopedic implant, joint prosthesis, or bone plate, right arm 🗝

    M96.632 Fracture of radius or ulna following insertion of orthopedic implant, joint prosthesis, or bone plate, left arm 🗝

    M96.639 Fracture of radius or ulna following insertion of orthopedic implant, joint prosthesis, or bone plate, unspecified arm 🗝

M96.65 Fracture of pelvis following insertion of orthopedic implant, joint prosthesis, or bone plate 🗝

M96.66 Fracture of femur following insertion of orthopedic implant, joint prosthesis, or bone plate

    M96.661 Fracture of femur following insertion of orthopedic implant, joint prosthesis, or bone plate, right leg 🗝

    M96.662 Fracture of femur following insertion of orthopedic implant, joint prosthesis, or bone plate, left leg 🗝

    M96.669 Fracture of femur following insertion of orthopedic implant, joint prosthesis, or bone plate, unspecified leg 🗝

M96.67 Fracture of tibia or fibula following insertion of orthopedic implant, joint prosthesis, or bone plate

    M96.671 Fracture of tibia or fibula following insertion of orthopedic implant, joint prosthesis, or bone plate, right leg 🗝

    M96.672 Fracture of tibia or fibula following insertion of orthopedic implant, joint prosthesis, or bone plate, left leg 🗝

    M96.679 Fracture of tibia or fibula following insertion of orthopedic implant, joint prosthesis, or bone plate, unspecified leg 🗝

M96.69 Fracture of other bone following insertion of orthopedic implant, joint prosthesis, or bone plate 🗝

M96.8 Other intraoperative and postprocedural complications and disorders of musculoskeletal system, not elsewhere classified
Coding Clinic: 2016, Q4, P10

M96.81 Intraoperative hemorrhage and hematoma of a musculoskeletal structure complicating a procedure

    Excludes1 intraoperative hemorrhage and hematoma of a musculoskeletal structure due to accidental puncture and laceration during a procedure (M96.82-)

    M96.810 Intraoperative hemorrhage and hematoma of a musculoskeletal structure complicating a musculoskeletal system procedure

    M96.811 Intraoperative hemorrhage and hematoma of a musculoskeletal structure complicating other procedure

M96.82 Accidental puncture and laceration of a musculoskeletal structure during a procedure

    M96.820 Accidental puncture and laceration of a musculoskeletal structure during a musculoskeletal system procedure

    M96.821 Accidental puncture and laceration of a musculoskeletal structure during other procedure

M96.83 Postprocedural hemorrhage of a musculoskeletal structure following a procedure

    M96.830 Postprocedural hemorrhage of a musculoskeletal structure following a musculoskeletal system procedure

    M96.831 Postprocedural hemorrhage of a musculoskeletal structure following other procedure

M96.84 Postprocedural hematoma and seroma of a musculoskeletal structure following a procedure

    M96.840 Postprocedural hematoma of a musculoskeletal structure following a musculoskeletal system procedure

    M96.841 Postprocedural hematoma of a musculoskeletal structure following other procedure
        Coding Clinic: 2016, Q4, P10

    M96.842 Postprocedural seroma of a musculoskeletal structure following a musculoskeletal system procedure

    M96.843 Postprocedural seroma of a musculoskeletal structure following other procedure

M96.89 Other intraoperative and postprocedural complications and disorders of the musculoskeletal system
    Instability of joint secondary to removal of joint prosthesis
    Use additional code, if applicable, to further specify disorder
    Coding Clinic: 2021, Q1, P5

PERIPROSTHETIC FRACTURE AROUND INTERNAL PROSTHETIC JOINT (M97)

M97 Periprosthetic fracture around internal prosthetic joint

    Excludes2 fracture of bone following insertion of orthopedic implant, joint prosthesis or bone plate (M96.6-)
        breakage (fracture) of prosthetic joint (T84.01-)
    Coding Clinic: 2016, Q4, P42

The appropriate 7th character is to be added to each code from category M97:

    A   initial encounter
    D   subsequent encounter
    S   sequela

M97.0 Periprosthetic fracture around internal prosthetic hip joint

    M97.01 Periprosthetic fracture around internal prosthetic right hip joint 🗝
        Coding Clinic: 2016, Q4, P43

    M97.02 Periprosthetic fracture around internal prosthetic left hip joint 🗝

M97.1 Periprosthetic fracture around internal prosthetic knee joint

    M97.11 Periprosthetic fracture around internal prosthetic right knee joint

    M97.12 Periprosthetic fracture around internal prosthetic left knee joint

M97.2 Periprosthetic fracture around internal prosthetic ankle joint

    M97.21 Periprosthetic fracture around internal prosthetic right ankle joint

    M97.22 Periprosthetic fracture around internal prosthetic left ankle joint

X ● **M97.3** **Periprosthetic fracture around internal prosthetic shoulder joint**

X ● **M97.31** **Periprosthetic fracture around internal prosthetic right shoulder joint**

X ● **M97.32** **Periprosthetic fracture around internal prosthetic left shoulder joint**

● **M97.4** **Periprosthetic fracture around internal prosthetic elbow joint**

X ● **M97.41** **Periprosthetic fracture around internal prosthetic right elbow joint**

X ● **M97.42** **Periprosthetic fracture around internal prosthetic left elbow joint**

X ● **M97.8** **Periprosthetic fracture around other internal prosthetic joint**

Periprosthetic fracture around internal prosthetic finger joint

Periprosthetic fracture around internal prosthetic spinal joint

Periprosthetic fracture around internal prosthetic toe joint

Periprosthetic fracture around internal prosthetic wrist joint

Use additional code to identify the joint (Z96.6-)

X ● **M97.9** **Periprosthetic fracture around unspecified internal prosthetic joint**

BIOMECHANICAL LESIONS, NOT ELSEWHERE CLASSIFIED (M99)

● **M99** **Biomechanical lesions, not elsewhere classified**

Note: This category should not be used if the condition can be classified elsewhere.

● **M99.0** **Segmental and somatic dysfunction**

M99.00 **Segmental and somatic dysfunction of head region**

M99.01 **Segmental and somatic dysfunction of cervical region**

M99.02 **Segmental and somatic dysfunction of thoracic region**

M99.03 **Segmental and somatic dysfunction of lumbar region**

M99.04 **Segmental and somatic dysfunction of sacral region**

M99.05 **Segmental and somatic dysfunction of pelvic region**

M99.06 **Segmental and somatic dysfunction of lower extremity**

M99.07 **Segmental and somatic dysfunction of upper extremity**

M99.08 **Segmental and somatic dysfunction of rib cage**

M99.09 **Segmental and somatic dysfunction of abdomen and other regions**

● **M99.1** **Subluxation complex (vertebral)**

M99.10 **Subluxation complex (vertebral) of head region**

M99.11 **Subluxation complex (vertebral) of cervical region**

M99.12 **Subluxation complex (vertebral) of thoracic region**

M99.13 **Subluxation complex (vertebral) of lumbar region**

M99.14 **Subluxation complex (vertebral) of sacral region**

M99.15 **Subluxation complex (vertebral) of pelvic region**

M99.16 **Subluxation complex (vertebral) of lower extremity**

M99.17 **Subluxation complex (vertebral) of upper extremity**

M99.18 **Subluxation complex (vertebral) of rib cage**

M99.19 **Subluxation complex (vertebral) of abdomen and other regions**

● **M99.2** **Subluxation stenosis of neural canal**

M99.20 **Subluxation stenosis of neural canal of head region**

M99.21 **Subluxation stenosis of neural canal of cervical region**

M99.22 **Subluxation stenosis of neural canal of thoracic region**

M99.23 **Subluxation stenosis of neural canal of lumbar region**

M99.24 **Subluxation stenosis of neural canal of sacral region**

M99.25 **Subluxation stenosis of neural canal of pelvic region**

M99.26 **Subluxation stenosis of neural canal of lower extremity**

M99.27 **Subluxation stenosis of neural canal of upper extremity**

M99.28 **Subluxation stenosis of neural canal of rib cage**

M99.29 **Subluxation stenosis of neural canal of abdomen and other regions**

● **M99.3** **Osseous stenosis of neural canal**

M99.30 **Osseous stenosis of neural canal of head region**

M99.31 **Osseous stenosis of neural canal of cervical region**

M99.32 **Osseous stenosis of neural canal of thoracic region**

M99.33 **Osseous stenosis of neural canal of lumbar region**

M99.34 **Osseous stenosis of neural canal of sacral region**

M99.35 **Osseous stenosis of neural canal of pelvic region**

M99.36 **Osseous stenosis of neural canal of lower extremity**

M99.37 **Osseous stenosis of neural canal of upper extremity**

M99.38 **Osseous stenosis of neural canal of rib cage**

M99.39 **Osseous stenosis of neural canal of abdomen and other regions**

● **M99.4** **Connective tissue stenosis of neural canal**

M99.40 **Connective tissue stenosis of neural canal of head region**

M99.41 **Connective tissue stenosis of neural canal of cervical region**

M99.42 **Connective tissue stenosis of neural canal of thoracic region**

M99.43 **Connective tissue stenosis of neural canal of lumbar region**

M99.44 **Connective tissue stenosis of neural canal of sacral region**

M99.45 **Connective tissue stenosis of neural canal of pelvic region**

M99.46 **Connective tissue stenosis of neural canal of lower extremity**

M99.47 **Connective tissue stenosis of neural canal of upper extremity**

M99.48 **Connective tissue stenosis of neural canal of rib cage**

M99.49 **Connective tissue stenosis of neural canal of abdomen and other regions**

● **M99.5** **Intervertebral disc stenosis of neural canal**

M99.50 **Intervertebral disc stenosis of neural canal of head region**

M99.51 **Intervertebral disc stenosis of neural canal of cervical region**

M99.52 **Intervertebral disc stenosis of neural canal of thoracic region**

M99.53 **Intervertebral disc stenosis of neural canal of lumbar region**

M99.54 **Intervertebral disc stenosis of neural canal of sacral region**

CHAPTER 13 (M00-M99)

    M99.55   Intervertebral disc stenosis of neural canal of pelvic region

    M99.56   Intervertebral disc stenosis of neural canal of lower extremity

    M99.57   Intervertebral disc stenosis of neural canal of upper extremity

    M99.58   Intervertebral disc stenosis of neural canal of rib cage

    M99.59   Intervertebral disc stenosis of neural canal of abdomen and other regions

● M99.6   Osseous and subluxation stenosis of intervertebral foramina

    M99.60   Osseous and subluxation stenosis of intervertebral foramina of head region

    M99.61   Osseous and subluxation stenosis of intervertebral foramina of cervical region

    M99.62   Osseous and subluxation stenosis of intervertebral foramina of thoracic region

    M99.63   Osseous and subluxation stenosis of intervertebral foramina of lumbar region

    M99.64   Osseous and subluxation stenosis of intervertebral foramina of sacral region

    M99.65   Osseous and subluxation stenosis of intervertebral foramina of pelvic region

    M99.66   Osseous and subluxation stenosis of intervertebral foramina of lower extremity

    M99.67   Osseous and subluxation stenosis of intervertebral foramina of upper extremity

    M99.68   Osseous and subluxation stenosis of intervertebral foramina of rib cage

    M99.69   Osseous and subluxation stenosis of intervertebral foramina of abdomen and other regions

● M99.7   Connective tissue and disc stenosis of intervertebral foramina

    M99.70   Connective tissue and disc stenosis of intervertebral foramina of head region

    M99.71   Connective tissue and disc stenosis of intervertebral foramina of cervical region

    M99.72   Connective tissue and disc stenosis of intervertebral foramina of thoracic region

    M99.73   Connective tissue and disc stenosis of intervertebral foramina of lumbar region

    M99.74   Connective tissue and disc stenosis of intervertebral foramina of sacral region

    M99.75   Connective tissue and disc stenosis of intervertebral foramina of pelvic region

    M99.76   Connective tissue and disc stenosis of intervertebral foramina of lower extremity

    M99.77   Connective tissue and disc stenosis of intervertebral foramina of upper extremity

    M99.78   Connective tissue and disc stenosis of intervertebral foramina of rib cage

    M99.79   Connective tissue and disc stenosis of intervertebral foramina of abdomen and other regions

● M99.8   Other biomechanical lesions

    M99.80   Other biomechanical lesions of head region

    M99.81   Other biomechanical lesions of cervical region

    M99.82   Other biomechanical lesions of thoracic region

    M99.83   Other biomechanical lesions of lumbar region

    M99.84   Other biomechanical lesions of sacral region

    M99.85   Other biomechanical lesions of pelvic region

    M99.86   Other biomechanical lesions of lower extremity

    M99.87   Other biomechanical lesions of upper extremity

    M99.88   Other biomechanical lesions of rib cage

    M99.89   Other biomechanical lesions of abdomen and other regions

  M99.9   Biomechanical lesion, unspecified

CHAPTER 14

DISEASES OF THE GENITOURINARY SYSTEM (N00-N99)

OGCR Chapter-Specific Coding Guidelines

> 14. **Chapter 14: Diseases of Genitourinary System (N00-N99)**
>
>   a. **Chronic kidney disease**
>
>   1) **Stages of chronic kidney disease (CKD)**
> The ICD-10-CM classifies CKD based on severity. The severity of CKD is designated by stages 1-5. Stage 2, code N18.2, equates to mild CKD; stage 3, code N18.3, equates to moderate CKD; and stage 4, code N18.4, equates to severe CKD. Code N18.6, End stage renal disease (ESRD), is assigned when the provider has documented end-stage-renal disease (ESRD).
>   If both a stage of CKD and ESRD are documented, assign code N18.6 only.
>
>   2) **Chronic kidney disease and kidney transplant status**
> Patients who have undergone kidney transplant may still have some form of chronic kidney disease CKD because the kidney transplant may not fully restore kidney function. Therefore, the presence of CKD alone does not constitute a transplant complication. Assign the appropriate N18 code for the patient's stage of CKD and code Z94.0, Kidney transplant status. If a transplant complication such as failure or rejection or other transplant complication is documented, see Section I.C.19.g for information on coding complications of a kidney transplant. If the documentation is unclear as to whether the patient has a complication of the transplant, query the provider.
>
>   3) **Chronic kidney disease with other conditions**
> Patients with CKD may also suffer from other serious conditions, most commonly diabetes mellitus and hypertension. The sequencing of the CKD code in relationship to codes for other contributing conditions is based on the conventions in the Tabular List.
>   *See I.C.9. Hypertensive chronic kidney disease.*
>   *See I.C.19. Chronic kidney disease and kidney transplant complications.*

Item 14–1 Nephritis (inflammation) or **nephropathy** (disease) **with lesion of proliferative glomerulonephritis** results from a streptococcal infection.

Nephritis (inflammation) or **nephropathy** (disease) **with lesion of membranous glomerulonephritis** is characterized by deposits along the epithelial side of the basement membrane.

Nephritis (inflammation) or **nephropathy** (disease) **with lesion of membranoproliferative glomerulonephritis** is characterized by alterations in the basement membranes of the kidney and the glomerular cells.

Nephritis (inflammation) or **nephropathy** (disease) **with lesion of rapidly progressive glomerulonephritis** is characterized by rapid and progressive decline in renal function.

Nephritis (inflammation) or **nephropathy** (disease) **with lesion of renal cortical necrosis** is characterized by death of the cortical tissues.

Nephritis (inflammation) or **nephropathy** (disease) **with lesion of renal medullary necrosis** is characterized by death of the tissues that collect urine.

Figure 14-1   Kidneys within the urinary system.

Item 14–2 Glomerulonephritis is nephritis accompanied by inflammation of the glomeruli of the kidney, resulting in the degeneration of the glomeruli and the nephrons.

Acute glomerulonephritis primarily affects children and young adults and is usually a result of a streptococcal infection.

Proliferative glomerulonephritis is the acute form of the disease resulting from a streptococcal infection.

Rapidly progressive glomerulonephritis, also known as **crescentic** or **malignant glomerulonephritis**, is the acute form of the disease, which leads quickly to rapid and progressive decline in renal function.

CHAPTER 14

DISEASES OF THE GENITOURINARY SYSTEM (N00-N99)

Excludes2 certain conditions originating in the perinatal period (P04-P96)
certain infectious and parasitic diseases (A00-B99)
complications of pregnancy, childbirth and the puerperium (O00-O9A)
congenital malformations, deformations and chromosomal abnormalities (Q00-Q99)
endocrine, nutritional and metabolic diseases (E00-E88)
injury, poisoning and certain other consequences of external causes (S00-T88)
neoplasms (C00-D49)
symptoms, signs and abnormal clinical and laboratory findings, not elsewhere classified (R00-R94)

This chapter contains the following blocks:

N00-N08	Glomerular diseases
N10-N16	Renal tubulo-interstitial diseases
N17-N19	Acute kidney failure and chronic kidney disease
N20-N23	Urolithiasis
N25-N29	Other disorders of kidney and ureter
N30-N39	Other diseases of the urinary system
N40-N53	Diseases of male genital organs
N60-N65	Disorders of breast
N70-N77	Inflammatory diseases of female pelvic organs
N80-N98	Noninflammatory disorders of female genital tract
N99	Intraoperative and postprocedural complications and disorders of genitourinary system, not elsewhere classified

GLOMERULAR DISEASES (N00-N08)

Code also any associated kidney failure (N17-N19)
Excludes1 hypertensive chronic kidney disease (I12.-)

● **N00 Acute nephritic syndrome**
  Includes   acute glomerular disease
                   acute glomerulonephritis
                   acute nephritis
  Excludes1   acute tubulo-interstitial nephritis (N10)
                     nephritic syndrome NOS (N05.-)

  N00.0 Acute nephritic syndrome with minor glomerular abnormality
    Acute nephritic syndrome with minimal change lesion

  N00.1 Acute nephritic syndrome with focal and segmental glomerular lesions
    Acute nephritic syndrome with focal and segmental hyalinosis
    Acute nephritic syndrome with focal and segmental sclerosis
    Acute nephritic syndrome with focal glomerulonephritis

  N00.2 Acute nephritic syndrome with diffuse membranous glomerulonephritis

  N00.3 Acute nephritic syndrome with diffuse mesangial proliferative glomerulonephritis

  N00.4 Acute nephritic syndrome with diffuse endocapillary proliferative glomerulonephritis

CHAPTER 14 (N00–N99)

N00.5 **Acute nephritic syndrome with diffuse mesangiocapillary glomerulonephritis**
Acute nephritic syndrome with membranoproliferative glomerulonephritis, types 1 and 3, or NOS

> **Excludes1**   Acute nephritic syndrome with C3 glomerulonephritis (N00.A)
> Acute nephritic syndrome with C3 glomerulopathy (N00.A)

N00.6 **Acute nephritic syndrome with dense deposit disease**
Acute nephritic syndrome with C3 glomerulopathy with dense deposit disease
Acute nephritic syndrome with membranoproliferative glomerulonephritis, type 2

N00.7 **Acute nephritic syndrome with diffuse crescentic glomerulonephritis**
Acute nephritic syndrome with extracapillary glomerulonephritis

N00.8 **Acute nephritic syndrome with other morphologic changes**
Acute nephritic syndrome with proliferative glomerulonephritis NOS

N00.9 **Acute nephritic syndrome with unspecified morphologic changes**

N00.A **Acute nephritic syndrome with C3 glomerulonephritis**
Acute nephritic syndrome with C3 glomerulopathy, NOS

> **Excludes1**   Acute nephritic syndrome (with C3 glomerulopathy) with dense deposit disease(N00.6)

● **N01** **Rapidly progressive nephritic syndrome**

> **Includes**   rapidly progressive glomerular disease
> rapidly progressive glomerulonephritis
> rapidly progressive nephritis

> **Excludes1**   nephritic syndrome NOS (N05.-)

N01.0 **Rapidly progressive nephritic syndrome with minor glomerular abnormality**
Rapidly progressive nephritic syndrome with minimal change lesion

N01.1 **Rapidly progressive nephritic syndrome with focal and segmental glomerular lesions**
Rapidly progressive nephritic syndrome with focal and segmental hyalinosis
Rapidly progressive nephritic syndrome with focal and segmental sclerosis
Rapidly progressive nephritic syndrome with focal glomerulonephritis

N01.2 **Rapidly progressive nephritic syndrome with diffuse membranous glomerulonephritis**

N01.3 **Rapidly progressive nephritic syndrome with diffuse mesangial proliferative glomerulonephritis**

N01.4 **Rapidly progressive nephritic syndrome with diffuse endocapillary proliferative glomerulonephritis**

N01.5 **Rapidly progressive nephritic syndrome with diffuse mesangiocapillary glomerulonephritis**
Rapidly progressive nephritic syndrome with membranoproliferative glomerulonephritis, types 1 and 3, or NOS

> **Excludes1**   Rapidly progressive nephritic syndrome with C3 glomerulonephritis (N01.A)
> Rapidly progressive nephritic syndrome with C3 glomerulopathy (N01.A)

N01.6 **Rapidly progressive nephritic syndrome with dense deposit disease**
Rapidly progressive nephritic syndrome with C3 glomerulopathy with dense deposit disease
Rapidly progressive nephritic syndrome with membranoproliferative glomerulonephritis, type 2

N01.7 **Rapidly progressive nephritic syndrome with diffuse crescentic glomerulonephritis**
Rapidly progressive nephritic syndrome with extracapillary glomerulonephritis

N01.8 **Rapidly progressive nephritic syndrome with other morphologic changes**
Rapidly progressive nephritic syndrome with proliferative glomerulonephritis NOS

N01.9 **Rapidly progressive nephritic syndrome with unspecified morphologic changes**

N01.A **Rapidly progressive nephritic syndrome with C3 glomerulonephritis**
Rapidly progressive nephritic syndrome with C3 glomerulopathy, NOS

> **Excludes1**   Rapidly progressive nephritic syndrome (with C3 glomerulopathy) with dense deposit disease (N01.6)

● **N02** **Recurrent and persistent hematuria**

> **Excludes1**   acute cystitis with hematuria (N30.01)
> hematuria NOS (R31.9)
> hematuria not associated with specified morphologic lesions (R31.-)

N02.0 **Recurrent and persistent hematuria with minor glomerular abnormality**
Recurrent and persistent hematuria with minimal change lesion

N02.1 **Recurrent and persistent hematuria with focal and segmental glomerular lesions**
Recurrent and persistent hematuria with focal and segmental hyalinosis
Recurrent and persistent hematuria with focal and segmental sclerosis
Recurrent and persistent hematuria with focal glomerulonephritis

N02.2 **Recurrent and persistent hematuria with diffuse membranous glomerulonephritis**

N02.3 **Recurrent and persistent hematuria with diffuse mesangial proliferative glomerulonephritis**

N02.4 **Recurrent and persistent hematuria with diffuse endocapillary proliferative glomerulonephritis**

N02.5 **Recurrent and persistent hematuria with diffuse mesangiocapillary glomerulonephritis**
Recurrent and persistent hematuria with membranoproliferative glomerulonephritis, types 1 and 3, or NOS

> **Excludes1**   Recurrent and persistent hematuria with C3 glomerulonephritis (N02.A)
> Recurrent and persistent hematuria with C3 glomerulopathy (N02.A)

N02.6 **Recurrent and persistent hematuria with dense deposit disease**
Recurrent and persistent hematuria with C3 glomerulopathy with dense deposit disease
Recurrent and persistent hematuria with membranoproliferative glomerulonephritis, type 2

N02.7 **Recurrent and persistent hematuria with diffuse crescentic glomerulonephritis**
Recurrent and persistent hematuria with extracapillary glomerulonephritis

N02.8 **Recurrent and persistent hematuria with other morphologic changes**
Recurrent and persistent hematuria with proliferative glomerulonephritis NOS

N02.9 **Recurrent and persistent hematuria with unspecified morphologic changes**
Coding Clinic: 2017, Q2, P5

N02.A **Recurrent and persistent hematuria with C3 glomerulonephritis**
Recurrent and persistent hematuria with C3 glomerulopathy

> **Excludes1**   Recurrent and persistent hematuria (with C3 glomerulopathy) with dense deposit disease (N02.6)

▶ New   ⇒ Revised   ~~deleted~~ Deleted   Excludes 1   Excludes 2   Includes   Use additional   Code first   Code also   Key words
OGCR Official Guidelines   X Assign placeholder X   ● Use Additional Character(s)   ▶ Manifestation Code   🗣 Hierarchical Condition Category   **Coding Clinic**

Item 14–3 Chronic glomerulonephritis (GN) persists over a period of years, with remissions and exacerbation.

Chronic GN with lesion of proliferative glomerulonephritis results from a streptococcal infection.

Chronic GN with lesion of membranous glomerulonephritis, also known as membranous nephropathy, is characterized by deposits along the epithelial side of the basement membrane.

Chronic GN with lesion of membrano-proliferative glomerulonephritis (MPGN) is a group of disorders characterized by alterations in the basement membranes of the kidney and the glomerular cells.

Chronic GN with lesion of rapidly progressive glomerulonephritis is characterized by necrosis, endothelial proliferation, and mesangial proliferation. The condition is marked by rapid and progressive decline in renal function.

● **N03**   **Chronic nephritic syndrome**

     Includes   chronic glomerular disease
                          chronic glomerulonephritis
                          chronic nephritis

     Excludes1   chronic tubulo-interstitial nephritis (N11.-)
                          diffuse sclerosing glomerulonephritis (N05.8-)
                          nephritic syndrome NOS (N05.-)

N03.0   **Chronic nephritic syndrome with minor glomerular abnormality**
        Chronic nephritic syndrome with minimal change lesion

N03.1   **Chronic nephritic syndrome with focal and segmental glomerular lesions**
        Chronic nephritic syndrome with focal and segmental hyalinosis
        Chronic nephritic syndrome with focal and segmental sclerosis
        Chronic nephritic syndrome with focal glomerulonephritis

N03.2   **Chronic nephritic syndrome with diffuse membranous glomerulonephritis**

N03.3   **Chronic nephritic syndrome with diffuse mesangial proliferative glomerulonephritis**

N03.4   **Chronic nephritic syndrome with diffuse endocapillary proliferative glomerulonephritis**

N03.5   **Chronic nephritic syndrome with diffuse mesangiocapillary glomerulonephritis**
        Chronic nephritic syndrome with membranoproliferative glomerulonephritis, types 1 and 3, or NOS

        Excludes1   Chronic nephritic syndrome with C3 glomerulonephritis (N03.A)
                      Chronic nephritic syndrome with C3 glomerulopathy (N03.A)

N03.6   **Chronic nephritic syndrome with dense deposit disease**
        Chronic nephritic syndrome with C3 glomerulopathy with dense deposit disease
        Chronic nephritic syndrome with membranoproliferative glomerulonephritis, type 2

N03.7   **Chronic nephritic syndrome with diffuse crescentic glomerulonephritis**
        Chronic nephritic syndrome with extracapillary glomerulonephritis

N03.8   **Chronic nephritic syndrome with other morphologic changes**
        Chronic nephritic syndrome with proliferative glomerulonephritis NOS

N03.9   **Chronic nephritic syndrome with unspecified morphologic changes**

N03.A   **Chronic nephritic syndrome with C3 glomerulonephritis**
        Chronic nephritic syndrome with C3 glomerulopathy

        Excludes1   Chronic nephritic syndrome (with C3 glomerulopathy) with dense deposit disease(N03.6)

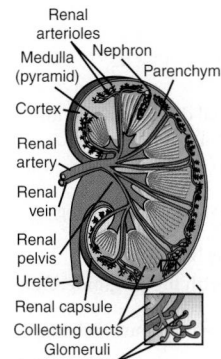

Figure 14-2   Kidney cross section.

Renal arterioles
Medulla (pyramid)
Nephron
Parenchyma
Cortex
Renal artery
Renal vein
Renal pelvis
Ureter
Renal capsule
Collecting ducts
Glomeruli (microscopic)

Item 14–4 Nephrotic syndrome (NS) is marked by massive proteinuria (protein in the urine) and water retention. Patients with NS are particularly vulnerable to staphylococcal and pneumococcal infections. NS with lesion of proliferative glomerulonephritis results from a streptococcal infection. NS with lesion of membranous glomerulonephritis results in thickening of the capillary walls. NS with lesion of minimal change glomerulonephritis is usually a benign disorder that occurs mostly in children and requires electron microscopy (biopsy) to verify changes in the glomeruli.

● **N04**   **Nephrotic syndrome**

     Includes   congenital nephrotic syndrome
                          lipoid nephrosis

N04.0   **Nephrotic syndrome with minor glomerular abnormality**
        Nephrotic syndrome with minimal change lesion

N04.1   **Nephrotic syndrome with focal and segmental glomerular lesions**
        Nephrotic syndrome with focal and segmental hyalinosis
        Nephrotic syndrome with focal and segmental sclerosis
        Nephrotic syndrome with focal glomerulonephritis

N04.2   **Nephrotic syndrome with diffuse membranous glomerulonephritis**

N04.3   **Nephrotic syndrome with diffuse mesangial proliferative glomerulonephritis**

N04.4   **Nephrotic syndrome with diffuse endocapillary proliferative glomerulonephritis**

N04.5   **Nephrotic syndrome with diffuse mesangiocapillary glomerulonephritis**
        Nephrotic syndrome with membranoproliferative glomerulonephritis, types 1 and 3, or NOS

        Excludes1   Nephrotic syndrome with C3 glomerulonephritis (N04.A)
                      Nephrotic syndrome with C3 glomerulopathy (N04.A)

N04.6   **Nephrotic syndrome with dense deposit disease**
        Nephrotic syndrome with C3 glomerulopathy with dense deposit disease
        Nephrotic syndrome with membranoproliferative glomerulonephritis, type 2

N04.7   **Nephrotic syndrome with diffuse crescentic glomerulonephritis**
        Nephrotic syndrome with extracapillary glomerulonephritis

N04.8   **Nephrotic syndrome with other morphologic changes**
        Nephrotic syndrome with proliferative glomerulonephritis NOS

N04.9   **Nephrotic syndrome with unspecified morphologic changes**

N04.A   **Nephrotic syndrome with C3 glomerulonephritis**
        Nephrotic syndrome with C3 glomerulopathy

        Excludes1   Nephrotic syndrome (with C3 glomerulopathy) with dense deposit disease (N04.6)

CHAPTER 14 (N00-N99)

● **N05   Unspecified nephritic syndrome**

     Includes   glomerular disease NOS
                 glomerulonephritis NOS
                 nephritis NOS
                 nephropathy NOS and renal disease NOS with
                     morphological lesion specified in .0-.8

     Excludes1   nephropathy NOS with no stated morphological
                    lesion (N28.9)
                    renal disease NOS with no stated morphological
                    lesion (N28.9)
                    tubulo-interstitial nephritis NOS (N12)

N05.0   Unspecified nephritic syndrome with minor glomerular abnormality
     Unspecified nephritic syndrome with minimal change lesion

N05.1   Unspecified nephritic syndrome with focal and segmental glomerular lesions
     Unspecified nephritic syndrome with focal and segmental hyalinosis
     Unspecified nephritic syndrome with focal and segmental sclerosis
     Unspecified nephritic syndrome with focal glomerulonephritis

N05.2   Unspecified nephritic syndrome with diffuse membranous glomerulonephritis

N05.3   Unspecified nephritic syndrome with diffuse mesangial proliferative glomerulonephritis

N05.4   Unspecified nephritic syndrome with diffuse endocapillary proliferative glomerulonephritis

N05.5   Unspecified nephritic syndrome with diffuse mesangiocapillary glomerulonephritis
     Unspecified nephritic syndrome with membranoproliferative glomerulonephritis, types 1 and 3, or NOS

     Excludes1   Unspecified nephritic syndrome with C3 glomerulonephritis (N05.A)
                    Unspecified nephritic syndrome with C3 glomerulopathy (N05.A)

N05.6   Unspecified nephritic syndrome with dense deposit disease
     Unspecified nephritic syndrome with C3 glomerulopathy with dense deposit disease
     Unspecified nephritic syndrome with membranoproliferative glomerulonephritis, type 2

N05.7   Unspecified nephritic syndrome with diffuse crescentic glomerulonephritis
     Unspecified nephritic syndrome with extracapillary glomerulonephritis

N05.8   Unspecified nephritic syndrome with other morphologic changes
     Unspecified nephritic syndrome with proliferative glomerulonephritis NOS

N05.9   Unspecified nephritic syndrome with unspecified morphologic changes

N05.A Unspecified nephritic syndrome with C3 glomerulonephritis
     Unspecified nephritic syndrome with C3 glomerulopathy

     Excludes1   Unspecified nephritic syndrome (with C3 glomerulopathy) with dense deposit disease(N05.6)

● **N06   Isolated proteinuria with specified morphological lesion**

     Excludes1   proteinuria not associated with specific morphologic lesions (R80.0)

N06.0   Isolated proteinuria with minor glomerular abnormality
     Isolated proteinuria with minimal change lesion

N06.1   Isolated proteinuria with focal and segmental glomerular lesions
     Isolated proteinuria with focal and segmental hyalinosis
     Isolated proteinuria with focal and segmental sclerosis
     Isolated proteinuria with focal glomerulonephritis

N06.2   Isolated proteinuria with diffuse membranous glomerulonephritis

N06.3   Isolated proteinuria with diffuse mesangial proliferative glomerulonephritis

N06.4   Isolated proteinuria with diffuse endocapillary proliferative glomerulonephritis

N06.5   Isolated proteinuria with diffuse mesangiocapillary glomerulonephritis
     Isolated proteinuria with membranoproliferative glomerulonephritis, types 1 and 3, or NOS

     Excludes1   Isolated proteinuria with C3 glomerulonephritis (N06.A)
                    Isolated proteinuria with C3 glomerulopathy (N06.A)

N06.6   Isolated proteinuria with dense deposit disease
     Isolated proteinuria with C3 glomerulopathy with dense deposit disease
     Isolated proteinuria with membranoproliferative glomerulonephritis, type 2

N06.7   Isolated proteinuria with diffuse crescentic glomerulonephritis
     Isolated proteinuria with extracapillary glomerulonephritis

N06.8   Isolated proteinuria with other morphologic lesion
     Isolated proteinuria with proliferative glomerulonephritis NOS

N06.9   Isolated proteinuria with unspecified morphologic lesion

N06.A Isolated proteinuria with C3 glomerulonephritis
     Isolated proteinuria with C3 glomerulopathy

     Excludes1   Isolated proteinuria (with C3 glomerulopathy) with dense deposit disease (N06.6)

● **N07   Hereditary nephropathy, not elsewhere classified**

     Excludes2   Alport's syndrome (Q87.81-)
                    hereditary amyloid nephropathy (E85.-)
                    nail patella syndrome (Q87.2)
                    non-neuropathic heredofamilial amyloidosis (E85.-)

N07.0   Hereditary nephropathy, not elsewhere classified with minor glomerular abnormality
     Hereditary nephropathy, not elsewhere classified with minimal change lesion

N07.1   Hereditary nephropathy, not elsewhere classified with focal and segmental glomerular lesions
     Hereditary nephropathy, not elsewhere classified with focal and segmental hyalinosis
     Hereditary nephropathy, not elsewhere classified with focal and segmental sclerosis
     Hereditary nephropathy, not elsewhere classified with focal glomerulonephritis

▶ New   ⇒ Revised   ~~deleted~~ Deleted   Excludes 1   Excludes 2   Includes   Use additional   Code first   Code also   Key words

OGCR Official Guidelines   X Assign placeholder X   ● Use Additional Character(s)   ▶ Manifestation Code   🏷 Hierarchical Condition Category   **Coding Clinic**

N07.2 **Hereditary nephropathy, not elsewhere classified with diffuse membranous glomerulonephritis**

N07.3 **Hereditary nephropathy, not elsewhere classified with diffuse mesangial proliferative glomerulonephritis**

N07.4 **Hereditary nephropathy, not elsewhere classified with diffuse endocapillary proliferative glomerulonephritis**

N07.5 **Hereditary nephropathy, not elsewhere classified with diffuse mesangiocapillary glomerulonephritis**
Hereditary nephropathy, not elsewhere classified with membranoproliferative glomerulonephritis, types 1 and 3, or NOS

> **Excludes1** Hereditary nephropathy, not elsewhere classified with C3 glomerulonephritis (N07.A)
> Hereditary nephropathy, not elsewhere classified with C3 glomerulopathy (N07.A)

N07.6 **Hereditary nephropathy, not elsewhere classified with dense deposit disease**
Hereditary nephropathy, not elsewhere classified with C3 glomerulopathy with dense deposit disease
Hereditary nephropathy, not elsewhere classified with membranoproliferative glomerulonephritis, type 2

N07.7 **Hereditary nephropathy, not elsewhere classified with diffuse crescentic glomerulonephritis**
Hereditary nephropathy, not elsewhere classified with extracapillary glomerulonephritis

N07.8 **Hereditary nephropathy, not elsewhere classified with other morphologic lesions**
Hereditary nephropathy, not elsewhere classified with proliferative glomerulonephritis NOS

N07.9 **Hereditary nephropathy, not elsewhere classified with unspecified morphologic lesions**

N07.A **Hereditary nephropathy, not elsewhere classified with C3 glomerulonephritis**
Hereditary nephropathy, not elsewhere classified with C3 glomerulopathy

> **Excludes1** Hereditary nephropathy, not elsewhere classified (with C3 glomerulopathy) with dense deposit disease (N07.6)

▷ **N08** *Glomerular disorders in diseases classified elsewhere*
Glomerulonephritis
Nephritis
Nephropathy
Code first underlying disease, such as:
amyloidosis (E85.-)
congenital syphilis (A50.5)
cryoglobulinemia (D89.1)
disseminated intravascular coagulation (D65)
gout (M1A.-, M10.-)
microscopic polyangiitis (M31.7)
multiple myeloma (C90.0-)
sepsis (A40.0-A41.9)
sickle-cell disease (D57.0-D57.8)

> **Excludes1** glomerulonephritis, nephritis and nephropathy (in):
> antiglomerular basement membrane disease (M31.0)
> diabetes (E08-E13 with .21)
> gonococcal (A54.21)
> Goodpasture's syndrome (M31.0)
> hemolytic-uremic syndrome (D59.3)
> lupus (M32.14)
> mumps (B26.83)
> syphilis (A52.75)
> systemic lupus erythematosus (M32.14)
> Wegener's granulomatosis (M31.31)
> pyelonephritis in diseases classified elsewhere (N16)
> renal tubulo-interstitial disorders classified elsewhere (N16)

Figure 14-3 Acute pyelonephritis. Cortical surface exhibits grayish white areas of inflammation and abscess formation. (From Frazier MS, Drzymkowski JW: Essentials of Human Diseases and Conditions, St. Louis, Saunders/Elsevier, 2009)

Item 14–5 Pyelonephritis is an infection of the kidneys and ureters and may be chronic or acute in one or both kidneys.

RENAL TUBULO-INTERSTITIAL DISEASES (N10-N16)

> **Includes** pyelonephritis
> **Excludes1** pyeloureteritis cystica (N28.85)

N10 **Acute pyelonephritis**
Acute infectious interstitial nephritis
Acute pyelitis
Acute tubulo-interstitial nephritis
Hemoglobin nephrosis
Myoglobin nephrosis
Use additional code (B95-B97), to identify infectious agent
Coding Clinic: 2019, Q3, P13-14

● **N11** **Chronic tubulo-interstitial nephritis**
> **Includes** chronic infectious interstitial nephritis
> chronic pyelitis
> chronic pyelonephritis

Use additional code (B95-B97), to identify infectious agent

N11.0 **Nonobstructive reflux-associated chronic pyelonephritis**
Pyelonephritis (chronic) associated with (vesicoureteral) reflux

> **Excludes1** vesicoureteral reflux NOS (N13.70)

N11.1 **Chronic obstructive pyelonephritis**
Pyelonephritis (chronic) associated with anomaly of pelviureteric junction
Pyelonephritis (chronic) associated with anomaly of pyeloureteric junction
Pyelonephritis (chronic) associated with crossing of vessel
Pyelonephritis (chronic) associated with kinking of ureter
Pyelonephritis (chronic) associated with obstruction of ureter
Pyelonephritis (chronic) associated with stricture of pelviureteric junction
Pyelonephritis (chronic) associated with stricture of ureter

> **Excludes1** calculous pyelonephritis (N20.9)
> obstructive uropathy (N13.-)

N11.8 **Other chronic tubulo-interstitial nephritis**
Nonobstructive chronic pyelonephritis NOS

N11.9 **Chronic tubulo-interstitial nephritis, unspecified**
Chronic interstitial nephritis NOS
Chronic pyelitis NOS
Chronic pyelonephritis NOS

N12 **Tubulo-interstitial nephritis, not specified as acute or chronic**
Interstitial nephritis NOS
Pyelitis NOS
Pyelonephritis NOS

> **Excludes1** calculous pyelonephritis (N20.9)

Figure 14-4 Hydronephrosis of the kidney, with marked dilatation of pelvis and calyces and thinning of renal parenchyma. (From Kumar: Robbins and Cotran: Pathologic Basis of Disease, ed 8, Saunders, An Imprint of Elsevier, 2009)

● N13 **Obstructive and reflux uropathy**

Excludes2   calculus of kidney and ureter without hydronephrosis (N20.-)
congenital obstructive defects of renal pelvis and ureter (Q62.0-Q62.3)
hydronephrosis with ureteropelvic junction obstruction (Q62.11)
obstructive pyelonephritis (N11.1)

N13.0 **Hydronephrosis with ureteropelvic junction obstruction**
Hydronephrosis due to acquired occlusion of ureteropelvic junction

Excludes2   Hydronephrosis with ureteropelvic junction obstruction due to calculus (N13.2)

Coding Clinic: 2016, Q4, P43

N13.1 **Hydronephrosis with ureteral stricture, not elsewhere classified**

Excludes1   hydronephrosis with ureteral stricture with infection (N13.6)

N13.2 **Hydronephrosis with renal and ureteral calculous obstruction**

Excludes1   hydronephrosis with renal and ureteral calculous obstruction with infection (N13.6)

● N13.3 **Other and unspecified hydronephrosis**

Excludes1   hydronephrosis with infection (N13.6)

N13.30 **Unspecified hydronephrosis**
N13.39 **Other hydronephrosis**

N13.4 **Hydroureter**

Excludes1   congenital hydroureter (Q62.3-)
hydroureter with infection (N13.6)
vesicoureteral-reflux with hydroureter (N13.73-)

N13.5 **Crossing vessel and stricture of ureter without hydronephrosis**
Kinking and stricture of ureter without hydronephrosis

Excludes1   crossing vessel and stricture of ureter without hydronephrosis with infection (N13.6)

Coding Clinic: 2016, Q4, P43

N13.6 **Pyonephrosis**
Conditions in N13.0-N13.5 with infection
Obstructive uropathy with infection

Use additional code (B95-B97), to identify infectious agent
Coding Clinic: 2018, Q2, P21

● N13.7 **Vesicoureteral-reflux**

Excludes1   reflux-associated pyelonephritis (N11.0)

N13.70 **Vesicoureteral-reflux, unspecified**
Occurs when urine flows from bladder back into ureters
Vesicoureteral-reflux NOS

N13.71 **Vesicoureteral-reflux without reflux nephropathy**

● N13.72 **Vesicoureteral-reflux with reflux nephropathy without hydroureter**

N13.721 **Vesicoureteral-reflux with reflux nephropathy without hydroureter, unilateral**

N13.722 **Vesicoureteral-reflux with reflux nephropathy without hydroureter, bilateral**

N13.729 **Vesicoureteral-reflux with reflux nephropathy without hydroureter, unspecified**

● N13.73 **Vesicoureteral-reflux with reflux nephropathy with hydroureter**

N13.731 **Vesicoureteral-reflux with reflux nephropathy with hydroureter, unilateral**

N13.732 **Vesicoureteral-reflux with reflux nephropathy with hydroureter, bilateral**

N13.739 **Vesicoureteral-reflux with reflux nephropathy with hydroureter, unspecified**

N13.8 **Other obstructive and reflux uropathy**
Urinary tract obstruction due to specified cause

Code first, if applicable, any causal condition first, such as:
enlarged prostate (N40.1)

N13.9 **Obstructive and reflux uropathy, unspecified**
Urinary tract obstruction NOS

● N14 **Drug- and heavy-metal-induced tubulo-interstitial and tubular conditions**

Code first poisoning due to drug or toxin, if applicable (T36-T65 with fifth or sixth character 1-4 or 6)

Use additional code for adverse effect, if applicable, to identify drug (T36-T50 with fifth or sixth character 5)

N14.0 **Analgesic nephropathy**
N14.1 **Nephropathy induced by other drugs, medicaments and biological substances**
N14.2 **Nephropathy induced by unspecified drug, medicament or biological substance**
N14.3 **Nephropathy induced by heavy metals**
N14.4 **Toxic nephropathy, not elsewhere classified**

● N15 **Other renal tubulo-interstitial diseases**
N15.0 **Balkan nephropathy**
Balkan endemic nephropathy
N15.1 **Renal and perinephric abscess**
N15.8 **Other specified renal tubulo-interstitial diseases**
N15.9 **Renal tubulo-interstitial disease, unspecified**
Infection of kidney NOS

Excludes1   urinary tract infection NOS (N39.0)

▶ New   ⇒ Revised   ~~deleted~~ Deleted   Excludes 1   Excludes 2   Includes   Use additional   Code first   Code also   Key words
OGCR Official Guidelines   X Assign placeholder X   ● Use Additional Character(s)   ▶ Manifestation Code   ✎ Hierarchical Condition Category   Coding Clinic

▶ N16   *Renal tubulo-interstitial disorders in diseases classified elsewhere*
        Pyelonephritis
        Tubulo-interstitial nephritis
        Code first underlying disease, such as:
            brucellosis (A23.0-A23.9)
            cryoglobulinemia (D89.1)
            glycogen storage disease (E74.0)
            leukemia (C91-C95)
            lymphoma (C81.0-C85.9, C96.0-C96.9)
            multiple myeloma (C90.0-)
            sepsis (A40.0-A41.9)
            Wilson's disease (E83.0)

Excludes1   diphtheritic pyelonephritis and tubulo-interstitial
                nephritis (A36.84)
                pyelonephritis and tubulo-interstitial nephritis in
                candidiasis (B37.49)
                pyelonephritis and tubulo-interstitial nephritis in
                cystinosis (E72.04)
                pyelonephritis and tubulo-interstitial nephritis in
                salmonella infection (A02.25)
                pyelonephritis and tubulo-interstitial nephritis in
                sarcoidosis (D86.84)
            ⇒ pyelonephritis and tubulo-interstitial nephritis in
                Sjögren syndrome (M35.04)
                pyelonephritis and tubulo-interstitial nephritis in
                systemic lupus erythematosus (M32.15)
                pyelonephritis and tubulo-interstitial nephritis in
                toxoplasmosis (B58.83)
                renal tubular degeneration in diabetes (E08-E13
                with .29)
                syphilitic pyelonephritis and tubulo-interstitial
                nephritis (A52.75)

ACUTE KIDNEY FAILURE AND CHRONIC KIDNEY DISEASE (N17-N19)

Excludes2   congenital renal failure (P96.0)
                drug- and heavy-metal-induced tubulo-
                interstitial and tubular conditions (N14.-)
                extrarenal uremia (R39.2)
                hemolytic-uremic syndrome (D59.3)
                hepatorenal syndrome (K76.7)
                postpartum hepatorenal syndrome (O90.4)
                posttraumatic renal failure (T79.5)
                prerenal uremia (R39.2)
                renal failure complicating abortion or ectopic or
                molar pregnancy (O00-O07, O08.4)
                renal failure following labor and delivery (O90.4)
                renal failure postprocedural (N99.0)

● N17   **Acute kidney failure**
        Code also associated underlying condition
        Excludes1   posttraumatic renal failure (T79.5)

N17.0   **Acute kidney failure with tubular necrosis** 🔗
            Acute tubular necrosis
            Renal tubular necrosis
            Tubular necrosis NOS

N17.1   **Acute kidney failure with acute cortical necrosis** 🔗
            Acute cortical necrosis
            Cortical necrosis NOS
            Renal cortical necrosis

N17.2   **Acute kidney failure with medullary necrosis** 🔗
            Medullary [papillary] necrosis NOS
            Acute medullary [papillary] necrosis
            Renal medullary [papillary] necrosis

N17.8   **Other acute kidney failure** 🔗

N17.9   **Acute kidney failure, unspecified** 🔗
            Acute kidney injury (nontraumatic)
            Excludes2   traumatic kidney injury (S37.0-)
            Coding Clinic: 2019, Q2, P7,25

● N18   **Chronic kidney disease (CKD)**
        Code first any associated:
            diabetic chronic kidney disease (E08.22, E09.22, E10.22,
            E11.22, E13.22)
            hypertensive chronic kidney disease (I12.-, I13.-)
        Use additional code to identify kidney transplant status, if
        applicable, (Z94.0)
        Coding Clinic: 2018, Q4, P89; 2016, Q4, P123

N18.1   **Chronic kidney disease, stage 1**
N18.2   **Chronic kidney disease, stage 2 (mild)**
● **N18.3**   **Chronic kidney disease, stage 3 (moderate)**
            N18.30   **Chronic kidney disease, stage 3 unspecified**
            N18.31   **Chronic kidney disease, stage 3a**
            N18.32   **Chronic kidney disease, stage 3b**
N18.4   **Chronic kidney disease, stage 4 (severe)** 🔗
            Coding Clinic: 2013, Q1, P24
N18.5   **Chronic kidney disease, stage 5** 🔗
            Excludes1   chronic kidney disease, stage 5 requiring
                            chronic dialysis (N18.6)
N18.6   **End stage renal disease** 🔗
            Chronic kidney disease requiring chronic dialysis
            Use additional code to identify dialysis status (Z99.2)
            Coding Clinic: 2016, Q3, P23, Q1, P13
N18.9   **Chronic kidney disease, unspecified**
            Chronic renal disease
            Chronic renal failure NOS
            Chronic renal insufficiency
            Chronic uremia NOS
            Diffuse sclerosing glomerulonephritis NOS
            Coding Clinic: 2018, Q4, P88

N19   **Unspecified kidney failure**
      Uremia NOS
      Excludes1   acute kidney failure (N17.-)
                      chronic kidney disease (N18.-)
                      chronic uremia (N18.9)
                      extrarenal uremia (R39.2)
                      prerenal uremia (R39.2)
                      renal insufficiency (acute) (N28.9)
                      uremia of newborn (P96.0)

UROLITHIASIS (N20-N23)

● N20   **Calculus of kidney and ureter**
        Calculous pyelonephritis
        Excludes1   nephrocalcinosis (E83.5)
                        that with hydronephrosis (N13.2)
        Coding Clinic: 2019, Q3, P14

N20.0   **Calculus of kidney**
            Nephrolithiasis NOS   Staghorn calculus
            Renal calculus   Stone in kidney
            Renal stone
            Coding Clinic: 2019, Q3, P13; 2017, Q1, P5

N20.1   **Calculus of ureter**
            Calculus of the ureteropelvic junction
            Ureteric stone
            Coding Clinic: 2016, Q3, P24

N20.2   **Calculus of kidney with calculus of ureter**
N20.9   **Urinary calculus, unspecified**

Multiple calculi

Figure 14-5   Multiple urinary calculi.

Item 14-6 Decreased blood flow is the usual cause of **acute renal failure**
that offers a good prognosis for recovery.
    Chronic renal failure is usually the result of long-standing kidney disease
and is a very serious condition that generally results in death.

CHAPTER 14 (N00-N99)

● N21 Calculus of lower urinary tract
   Includes   calculus of lower urinary tract with cystitis and urethritis
   N21.0 Calculus in bladder
      Calculus in diverticulum of bladder
      Urinary bladder stone
      Excludes2   staghorn calculus (N20.0)
      Coding Clinic: 2015, Q2, P9
   N21.1 Calculus in urethra
      Excludes2   calculus of prostate (N42.0)
   N21.8 Other lower urinary tract calculus
   N21.9 Calculus of lower urinary tract, unspecified
      Excludes1   calculus of urinary tract NOS (N20.9)

▷ N22 *Calculus of urinary tract in diseases classified elsewhere*
   Code first underlying disease, such as:
      gout (M1A.-, M10.-)
      schistosomiasis (B65.0-B65.9)

N23 Unspecified renal colic

OTHER DISORDERS OF KIDNEY AND URETER (N25-N29)
   Excludes2   disorders of kidney and ureter with urolithiasis (N20-N23)

● N25 Disorders resulting from impaired renal tubular function
   N25.0 Renal osteodystrophy
      Azotemic osteodystrophy
      Phosphate-losing tubular disorders
      Renal rickets
      Renal short stature
      Excludes2   metabolic disorders classifiable to E70-E88
   N25.1 Nephrogenic diabetes insipidus 🅗
      Excludes1   diabetes insipidus NOS (E23.2)
   ● N25.8 Other disorders resulting from impaired renal tubular function
      N25.81 Secondary hyperparathyroidism of renal origin 🅗
         Excludes1   secondary hyperparathyroidism, non-renal (E21.1)
         Excludes2   metabolic disorders classifiable to E70-E88
      N25.89 Other disorders resulting from impaired renal tubular function
         Hypokalemic nephropathy
         Lightwood-Albright syndrome
         Renal tubular acidosis NOS
   N25.9 Disorder resulting from impaired renal tubular function, unspecified

● N26 Unspecified contracted kidney
   Excludes1   contracted kidney due to hypertension (I12.-)
      diffuse sclerosing glomerulonephritis (N05.8.-)
      hypertensive nephrosclerosis (arteriolar) (arteriosclerotic) (I12.-)
      small kidney of unknown cause (N27.-)
   N26.1 Atrophy of kidney (terminal)
   N26.2 Page kidney
   N26.9 Renal sclerosis, unspecified

● N27 Small kidney of unknown cause
   Includes   oligonephronia
   N27.0 Small kidney, unilateral
   N27.1 Small kidney, bilateral
   N27.9 Small kidney, unspecified

● N28 Other disorders of kidney and ureter, not elsewhere classified
   N28.0 Ischemia and infarction of kidney 🅗
      Renal artery embolism
      Renal artery obstruction
      Renal artery occlusion
      Renal artery thrombosis
      Renal infarct
      Excludes1   atherosclerosis of renal artery (extrarenal part) (I70.1)
         congenital stenosis of renal artery (Q27.1)
         Goldblatt's kidney (I70.1)
   N28.1 Cyst of kidney, acquired
      Cyst (multiple) (solitary) of kidney, (acquired)
      Excludes1   cystic kidney disease (congenital) (Q61.-)
   ● N28.8 Other specified disorders of kidney and ureter
      Excludes1   hydroureter (N13.4)
         ureteric stricture with hydronephrosis (N13.1)
         ureteric stricture without hydronephrosis (N13.5)
      N28.81 Hypertrophy of kidney
      N28.82 Megaloureter
      N28.83 Nephroptosis
      N28.84 Pyelitis cystica
      N28.85 Pyeloureteritis cystica
      N28.86 Ureteritis cystica
      N28.89 Other specified disorders of kidney and ureter
   N28.9 Disorder of kidney and ureter, unspecified
      Nephropathy NOS
      Renal disease (acute) NOS
      Renal insufficiency (acute)
      Excludes1   chronic renal insufficiency (N18.9)
         unspecified nephritic syndrome (N05.-)
      Coding Clinic: 2016, Q1, P13

▷ N29 *Other disorders of kidney and ureter in diseases classified elsewhere*
   Code first underlying disease, such as:
      amyloidosis (E85.-)
      nephrocalcinosis (E83.5)
      schistosomiasis (B65.0-B65.9)
   Excludes1   disorders of kidney and ureter in:
      cystinosis (E72.0)
      gonorrhea (A54.21)
      syphilis (A52.75)
      tuberculosis (A18.11)

OTHER DISEASES OF THE URINARY SYSTEM (N30-N39)
   ~~**Excludes1**   urinary infection (complicating):~~
   ~~abortion or ectopic or molar pregnancy~~
   ~~(O00-O07, O08.8)~~
   ~~pregnancy, childbirth and the puerperium~~
   ~~(O23.-, O75.3, O86.2-)~~

   ▷ **Excludes2**   urinary infection (complicating):
      ▷abortion or ectopic or molar pregnancy (O00-O07, O08.8)
      ▷pregnancy, childbirth and the puerperium (O23.-, O75.3, O86.2-)

● N30 Cystitis
   Infection of bladder and irritation in lower urinary tract
   Use additional code to identify infectious agent (B95-B97)
   Excludes1   prostatocystitis (N41.3)
   ● N30.0 Acute cystitis
      Excludes1   irradiation cystitis (N30.4-)
         trigonitis (N30.3-)
      N30.00 Acute cystitis without hematuria
      N30.01 Acute cystitis with hematuria
   ● N30.1 Interstitial cystitis (chronic)
      Ongoing infection of kidney glomeruli and tubules
      N30.10 Interstitial cystitis (chronic) without hematuria
      N30.11 Interstitial cystitis (chronic) with hematuria

▶ New ⇒ Revised ~~deleted~~ Deleted Excludes 1 Excludes 2 Includes Use additional Code first Code also Key words

OGCR Official Guidelines X Assign placeholder X ● Use Additional Character(s) ▷ Manifestation Code 🅗 Hierarchical Condition Category **Coding Clinic**

● N30.2 Other chronic cystitis
    N30.20 Other chronic cystitis without hematuria
    N30.21 Other chronic cystitis with hematuria
● N30.3 Trigonitis
    Inflammation of triangular area of bladder (where the ureters and urethra come together)
    Urethrotrigonitis
    N30.30 Trigonitis without hematuria
    N30.31 Trigonitis with hematuria
● N30.4 Irradiation cystitis
    N30.40 Irradiation cystitis without hematuria
    N30.41 Irradiation cystitis with hematuria
● N30.8 Other cystitis
    Abscess of bladder
    N30.80 Other cystitis without hematuria
    N30.81 Other cystitis with hematuria
● N30.9 Cystitis, unspecified
    N30.90 Cystitis, unspecified without hematuria
    N30.91 Cystitis, unspecified with hematuria

● N31 **Neuromuscular dysfunction of bladder, not elsewhere classified**
    Use additional code to identify any associated urinary incontinence (N39.3-N39.4-)
    Excludes1 cord bladder NOS (G95.89)
            neurogenic bladder due to cauda equina syndrome (G83.4)
            neuromuscular dysfunction due to spinal cord lesion (G95.89)
  N31.0 **Uninhibited neuropathic bladder, not elsewhere classified**
  N31.1 **Reflex neuropathic bladder, not elsewhere classified**
  N31.2 **Flaccid neuropathic bladder, not elsewhere classified**
    Atonic (motor) (sensory) neuropathic bladder
    Diminished tone of bladder muscle
    Autonomous neuropathic bladder
    Nonreflex neuropathic bladder
  N31.8 **Other neuromuscular dysfunction of bladder**
  N31.9 **Neuromuscular dysfunction of bladder, unspecified**
    Neurogenic bladder dysfunction NOS

● N32 **Other disorders of bladder**
    Excludes2 calculus of bladder (N21.0)
            cystocele (N81.1-)
            hernia or prolapse of bladder, female (N81.1-)
  N32.0 **Bladder-neck obstruction**
    Bladder-neck stenosis (acquired)
    Excludes1 congenital bladder-neck obstruction (Q64.3-)
  N32.1 **Vesicointestinal fistula**
    Vesicorectal fistula
  N32.2 **Vesical fistula, not elsewhere classified**
    Excludes1 fistula between bladder and female genital tract (N82.0-N82.1)
  N32.3 **Diverticulum of bladder**
    Formation of sac from a herniation of wall of bladder
    Excludes1 congenital diverticulum of bladder (Q64.6)
            diverticulitis of bladder (N30.8-)
● N32.8 **Other specified disorders of bladder**
    N32.81 **Overactive bladder**
        Detrusor muscle hyperactivity
        Excludes1 frequent urination due to specified bladder condition-code to condition
    N32.89 **Other specified disorders of bladder**
        Bladder hemorrhage
        Bladder hypertrophy
        Calcified bladder
        Contracted bladder
  N32.9 **Bladder disorder, unspecified**

▷ N33 *Bladder disorders in diseases classified elsewhere*
    Code first underlying disease, such as:
    schistosomiasis (B65.0-B65.9)
    Excludes1 bladder disorder in syphilis (A52.76)
            bladder disorder in tuberculosis (A18.12)
            candidal cystitis (B37.41)
            chlamydial cystitis(A56.01)
            cystitis in gonorrhea (A54.01)
            cystitis in neurogenic bladder (N31.-)
            diphtheritic cystitis (A36.85)
            syphilitic cystitis (A52.76)
            trichomonal cystitis (A59.03)

● N34 **Urethritis and urethral syndrome**
    Use additional code (B95-B97), to identify infectious agent
    Excludes2 Reiter's disease (M02.3-)
            urethritis in diseases with a predominantly sexual mode of transmission (A50-A64)
            urethrotrigonitis (N30.3-)
  N34.0 **Urethral abscess**
    Abscess (of) Cowper's gland
    Abscess (of) Littré's gland
    Abscess (of) urethral (gland)
    Periurethral abscess
    Excludes1 urethral caruncle (N36.2)
  N34.1 **Nonspecific urethritis**
    Nongonococcal urethritis
    Nonvenereal urethritis
  N34.2 **Other urethritis**
    Inflammation of urethra
    Meatitis, urethral
    Postmenopausal urethritis
    Ulcer of urethra (meatus)
    Urethritis NOS
  N34.3 **Urethral syndrome, unspecified**

● N35 **Urethral stricture**
    Narrowing of lumen of urethra caused by scarring due to infection or injury
    Excludes1 congenital urethral stricture (Q64.3-)
            postprocedural urethral stricture (N99.1-)
● N35.0 **Post-traumatic urethral stricture**
    Urethral stricture due to injury
    Excludes1 postprocedural urethral stricture (N99.1-)
    ● N35.01 **Post-traumatic urethral stricture, male**
        N35.010 **Post-traumatic urethral stricture, male, meatal** ♂
        N35.011 **Post-traumatic bulbous urethral stricture** ♂
        N35.012 **Post-traumatic membranous urethral stricture** ♂
        N35.013 **Post-traumatic anterior urethral stricture** ♂
        N35.014 **Post-traumatic urethral stricture, male, unspecified** ♂
        N35.016 **Post-traumatic urethral stricture, male, overlapping sites** ♂
    ● N35.02 **Post-traumatic urethral stricture, female**
        N35.021 **Urethral stricture due to childbirth** ♀
        N35.028 **Other post-traumatic urethral stricture, female** ♀
● N35.1 **Postinfective urethral stricture, not elsewhere classified**
    Excludes1 urethral stricture associated with schistosomiasis (B65.-, N29)
            gonococcal urethral stricture (A54.01)
            syphilitic urethral stricture (A52.76)
    ● N35.11 **Postinfective urethral stricture, not elsewhere classified, male**
        N35.111 **Postinfective urethral stricture, not elsewhere classified, male, meatal** ♂
        N35.112 **Postinfective bulbous urethral stricture, not elsewhere classified, male** ♂

CHAPTER 14 (N00-N99)

N35.113   Postinfective membranous urethral stricture, not elsewhere classified, male ♂

N35.114   Postinfective anterior urethral stricture, not elsewhere classified, male ♂

N35.116   Postinfective urethral stricture, not elsewhere classified, male, overlapping sites ♂

N35.119   Postinfective urethral stricture, not elsewhere classified, male, unspecified ♂

N35.12   Postinfective urethral stricture, not elsewhere classified, female ♀

● **N35.8**   Other urethral stricture

     Excludes1   postprocedural urethral stricture (N99.1-)

   ● **N35.81**   Other urethral stricture, male

N35.811   Other urethral stricture, male, meatal ♂

N35.812   Other urethral bulbous stricture, male ♂

N35.813   Other membranous urethral stricture, male ♂

N35.814   Other anterior urethral stricture, male ♂

N35.816   Other urethral stricture, male, overlapping sites ♂

N35.819   Other urethral stricture, male, unspecified site ♂

N35.82   Other urethral stricture, female ♀

● **N35.9**   Urethral stricture, unspecified

   ● **N35.91**   Urethral stricture, unspecified, male

N35.911   Unspecified urethral stricture, male, meatal ♂

N35.912   Unspecified bulbous urethral stricture, male ♂

N35.913   Unspecified membranous urethral stricture, male ♂

N35.914   Unspecified anterior urethral stricture, male ♂

N35.916   Unspecified urethral stricture, male, overlapping sites ♂

N35.919   Unspecified urethral stricture, male, unspecified site ♂
       Pinhole meatus NOS
       Urethral stricture NOS

N35.92   Unspecified urethral stricture, female ♀

● **N36**   Other disorders of urethra

   N36.0   Urethral fistula
       Urethroperineal fistula
       Urethrorectal fistula
       Urinary fistula NOS

     Excludes1   urethroscrotal fistula (N50.89)
                   urethrovaginal fistula (N82.1)
                   urethrovesicovaginal fistula (N82.1)

   N36.1   Urethral diverticulum

   N36.2   Urethral caruncle

   ● **N36.4**   Urethral functional and muscular disorders
       Use additional code to identify associated urinary stress incontinence (N39.3)

N36.41   Hypermobility of urethra

N36.42   Intrinsic sphincter deficiency (ISD)

N36.43   Combined hypermobility of urethra and intrinsic sphincter deficiency

N36.44   Muscular disorders of urethra
       Bladder sphincter dyssynergy

N36.5   Urethral false passage

N36.8   Other specified disorders of urethra

     Excludes1   congenital urethrocele (Q64.7)
                   female urethrocele (N81.0)

N36.9   Urethral disorder, unspecified

▶ **N37**   *Urethral disorders in diseases classified elsewhere*
     Code first underlying disease

     Excludes1   urethritis (in):
                   candidal infection (B37.41)
                   chlamydial (A56.01)
                   gonorrhea (A54.01)
                   syphilis (A52.76)
                   trichomonal infection (A59.03)
                   tuberculosis (A18.13)

● **N39**   Other disorders of urinary system

     Excludes2   hematuria NOS (R31.-)
                   recurrent or persistent hematuria (N02.-)
                   recurrent or persistent hematuria with specified morphological lesion (N02.-)
                   proteinuria NOS (R80.-)

   N39.0   Urinary tract infection, site not specified
       Use additional code (B95-B97), to identify infectious agent

     Excludes1   candidiasis of urinary tract (B37.4-)
                   neonatal urinary tract infection (P39.3)
                   pyuria (R82.81)
                   urinary tract infection of specified site, such as:
                       cystitis (N30.-)
                       urethritis (N34.-)
     Coding Clinic: 2018, Q2, P22; Q1, P16; 2012, Q4, P94

   N39.3   Stress incontinence (female) (male)
       Code also any associated overactive bladder (N32.81)

     Excludes1   mixed incontinence (N39.46)

   ● **N39.4**   Other specified urinary incontinence
       Code also any associated overactive bladder (N32.81)

     Excludes1   enuresis NOS (R32)
                   functional urinary incontinence (R39.81)
                   urinary incontinence associated with cognitive impairment (R39.81)
                   urinary incontinence NOS (R32)
                   urinary incontinence of nonorganic origin (F98.0)

N39.41   Urge incontinence

     Excludes1   mixed incontinence (N39.46)

N39.42   Incontinence without sensory awareness
       Insensible (urinary) incontinence

N39.43   Post-void dribbling

N39.44   Nocturnal enuresis

  ▶ **Excludes2**   nocturnal polyuria (R35.81)

N39.45   Continuous leakage

N39.46   Mixed incontinence
       Urge and stress incontinence

   ● **N39.49**   Other specified urinary incontinence

N39.490   Overflow incontinence

N39.491   Coital incontinence
       Coding Clinic: 2016, Q4, P44

N39.492   Postural (urinary) incontinence
       Coding Clinic: 2016, Q4, P44

N39.498   Other specified urinary incontinence
       Reflex incontinence
       Total incontinence

   N39.8   Other specified disorders of urinary system

   N39.9   Disorder of urinary system, unspecified

1104

▶ New   ⇒ Revised   ~~deleted~~ Deleted   Excludes 1   Excludes 2   Includes   Use additional   Code first   Code also   Key words

OGCR Official Guidelines   X Assign placeholder X   ● Use Additional Character(s)   ▶ Manifestation Code   🔖 Hierarchical Condition Category   **Coding Clinic**

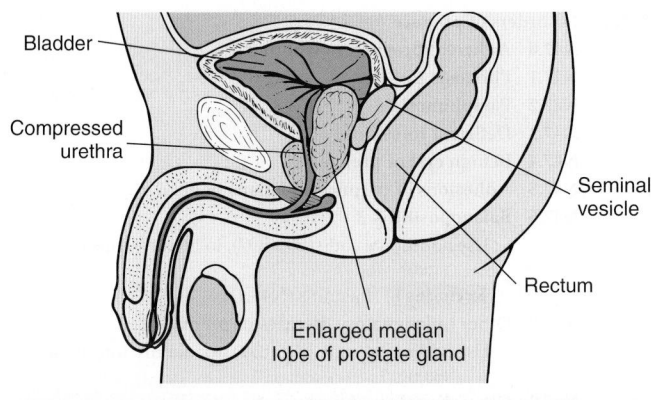

Bladder

Compressed
urethra

Seminal
vesicle

Rectum

Enlarged median
lobe of prostate gland

Figure 14-6 Benign prostatic hyperplasia. (From Shiland: Mastering Healthcare Terminology, ed 3, St. Louis, Mosby, 2010)

DISEASES OF MALE GENITAL ORGANS (N40-N53)

★**(See Plate 5 of the Anatomy Illustrations.)**

● **N40   Benign prostatic hyperplasia**

| **Includes** | adenofibromatous hypertrophy of prostate |
| | benign hypertrophy of the prostate |

Enlargement of prostate gland usually occurring with age and causing obstructed urine flow

benign prostatic hypertrophy
BPH
enlarged prostate
nodular prostate
polyp of prostate

| **Excludes1** | benign neoplasms of prostate (adenoma, benign) (fibroadenoma) (fibroma) (myoma) (D29.1) |
| | malignant neoplasm of prostate (C61) |

N40.0   Benign prostatic hyperplasia without lower urinary tract symptoms ♂   A
Enlarged prostate without LUTS
Enlarged prostate NOS

N40.1   Benign prostatic hyperplasia with lower urinary tract symptoms ♂   A
Enlarged prostate with LUTS
Use additional code for associated symptoms, when specified:
incomplete bladder emptying (R39.14)
nocturia (R35.1)
straining on urination (R39.16)
urinary frequency (R35.0)
urinary hesitancy (R39.11)
urinary incontinence (N39.4-)
urinary obstruction (N13.8)
urinary retention (R33.8)
urinary urgency (R39.15)
weak urinary stream (R39.12)
Coding Clinic: 2018, Q4, P55

N40.2   Nodular prostate without lower urinary tract symptoms ♂   A
Nodular prostate without LUTS

N40.3   Nodular prostate with lower urinary tract symptoms ♂   A
Use additional code for associated symptoms, when specified:
incomplete bladder emptying (R39.14)
nocturia (R35.1)
straining on urination (R39.16)
urinary frequency (R35.0)
urinary hesitancy (R39.11)
urinary incontinence (N39.4-)
urinary obstruction (N13.8)
urinary retention (R33.8)
urinary urgency (R39.15)
weak urinary stream (R39.12)

● **N41   Inflammatory diseases of prostate**
Use additional code (B95-B97), to identify infectious agent
N41.0   Acute prostatitis ♂   A
N41.1   Chronic prostatitis ♂   A
N41.2   Abscess of prostate ♂   A
N41.3   Prostatocystitis ♂   A
N41.4   Granulomatous prostatitis ♂   A
N41.8   Other inflammatory diseases of prostate ♂   A
N41.9   Inflammatory disease of prostate, unspecified ♂   A
Prostatitis NOS

● **N42   Other and unspecified disorders of prostate**
N42.0   Calculus of prostate ♂   A
Prostatic stone
N42.1   Congestion and hemorrhage of prostate ♂   A

Excludes1	enlarged prostate (N40.-)
	hematuria (R31.-)
	hyperplasia of prostate (N40.-)
	inflammatory diseases of prostate (N41.-)

● **N42.3   Dysplasia of prostate**
Coding Clinic: 2016, Q4, P44
N42.30   Unspecified dysplasia of prostate ♂
N42.31   Prostatic intraepithelial neoplasia ♂
PIN
Prostatic intraepithelial neoplasia I (PIN I)
Prostatic intraepithelial neoplasia II (PIN II)

| **Excludes1** | prostatic intraepithelial neoplasia III (PIN III) (D07.5) |

N42.32   Atypical small acinar proliferation of prostate ♂
N42.39   Other dysplasia of prostate ♂
● **N42.8   Other specified disorders of prostate**
N42.81   Prostatodynia syndrome ♂   A
Painful prostate syndrome
N42.82   Prostatosis syndrome ♂   A
N42.83   Cyst of prostate ♂   A
N42.89   Other specified disorders of prostate ♂   A
N42.9   Disorder of prostate, unspecified ♂   A

● **N43   Hydrocele and spermatocele**

| **Includes** | hydrocele of spermatic cord, testis or tunica vaginalis |

| **Excludes1** | congenital hydrocele (P83.5) |

N43.0   Encysted hydrocele ♂
N43.1   Infected hydrocele ♂
Use additional code (B95-B97), to identify infectious agent
N43.2   Other hydrocele ♂
N43.3   Hydrocele, unspecified ♂
● **N43.4   Spermatocele of epididymis** ♂
Spermatic cyst
N43.40   Spermatocele of epididymis, unspecified ♂
N43.41   Spermatocele of epididymis, single ♂
N43.42   Spermatocele of epididymis, multiple ♂

Item 14-7   Hydrocele is a sac of fluid accumulating in the testes membrane.

Blood vessels
Vas deferens
Epididymis
Testis
A
Hydrocele

Figure 14-7   A. Hydrocele. **B.** Newborn with large right hydrocele. (**B** from Nelson WE, Kliegman R: Nelson Textbook of Pediatrics, Philadelphia, Saunders Elsevier, 2011)

CHAPTER 14 (N00-N99)

● **N44 Noninflammatory disorders of testis**
  ● **N44.0 Torsion of testis**
      N44.00 Torsion of testis, unspecified ♂
      N44.01 Extravaginal torsion of spermatic cord ♂
      N44.02 Intravaginal torsion of spermatic cord ♂
              Torsion of spermatic cord NOS
      N44.03 Torsion of appendix testis ♂
      N44.04 Torsion of appendix epididymis ♂
    N44.1 Cyst of tunica albuginea testis ♂
    N44.2 Benign cyst of testis ♂
    N44.8 Other noninflammatory disorders of the testis ♂

● **N45 Orchitis and epididymitis**
      *Orchitis is inflammation of one or both of the testes as a result of
      mumps or other infection, trauma, or metastasis. **Epididymitis**
      is inflammation of the tubular structure that connects the testicle
      with the vas deferens.*
      Use additional code (B95-B97), to identify infectious agent
    N45.1 Epididymitis ♂
    N45.2 Orchitis ♂
    N45.3 Epididymo-orchitis ♂
    N45.4 Abscess of epididymis or testis ♂

● **N46 Male infertility**
      Excludes1   vasectomy status (Z98.52)
  ● **N46.0 Azoospermia**
          Absolute male infertility
          Male infertility due to germinal (cell) aplasia
          Male infertility due to spermatogenic arrest (complete)
      N46.01 Organic azoospermia ♂   A
              Azoospermia NOS
    ● **N46.02 Azoospermia due to extratesticular causes**
              Code also associated cause
          N46.021 Azoospermia due to drug therapy ♂ A
          N46.022 Azoospermia due to infection ♂   A
          **N46.023 Azoospermia due to obstruction of
                   efferent ducts** ♂   A
          N46.024 Azoospermia due to radiation ♂   A
          **N46.025 Azoospermia due to systemic
                   disease** ♂   A
          **N46.029 Azoospermia due to other
                   extratesticular causes** ♂   A
  ● **N46.1 Oligospermia**
          Male infertility due to germinal cell desquamation
          Male infertility due to hypospermatogenesis
          Male infertility due to incomplete spermatogenic arrest
      N46.11 Organic oligospermia ♂   A
              Oligospermia NOS
    ● **N46.12 Oligospermia due to extratesticular causes**
              Code also associated cause
          N46.121 Oligospermia due to drug therapy ♂ A
          N46.122 Oligospermia due to infection ♂   A
          **N46.123 Oligospermia due to obstruction of
                   efferent ducts** ♂   A
          N46.124 Oligospermia due to radiation ♂   A
          **N46.125 Oligospermia due to systemic
                   disease** ♂   A
          **N46.129 Oligospermia due to other
                   extratesticular causes** ♂   A
    N46.8 Other male infertility ♂   A
    N46.9 Male infertility, unspecified ♂   A

● **N47 Disorders of prepuce**
    N47.0 Adherent prepuce, newborn ♂   N
    N47.1 Phimosis ♂
    N47.2 Paraphimosis ♂
    N47.3 Deficient foreskin ♂
    N47.4 Benign cyst of prepuce ♂
    N47.5 Adhesions of prepuce and glans penis ♂
    N47.6 Balanoposthitis ♂
              Use additional code (B95-B97), to identify infectious
                agent
          Excludes1   balanitis (N48.1)
    N47.7 Other inflammatory diseases of prepuce ♂
              Use additional code (B95-B97), to identify infectious
                agent
    N47.8 Other disorders of prepuce ♂

● **N48 Other disorders of penis**
    N48.0 Leukoplakia of penis ♂
              Balanitis xerotica obliterans
              Kraurosis of penis
              Lichen sclerosus of external male genital organs
          Excludes1   carcinoma in situ of penis (D07.4)
    N48.1 Balanitis ♂
              Use additional code (B95-B97), to identify infectious
                agent
          Excludes1   amebic balanitis (A06.8)
                          balanitis xerotica obliterans (N48.0)
                          candidal balanitis (B37.42)
                          gonococcal balanitis (A54.23)
                          herpesviral [herpes simplex] balanitis
                            (A60.01)
  ● **N48.2 Other inflammatory disorders of penis**
              Use additional code (B95-B97), to identify infectious
                agent
          Excludes1   balanitis (N48.1)
                          balanitis xerotica obliterans (N48.0)
                          balanoposthitis (N47.6)
      N48.21 Abscess of corpus cavernosum and penis ♂
      N48.22 Cellulitis of corpus cavernosum and penis ♂
      N48.29 Other inflammatory disorders of penis ♂
  ● **N48.3 Priapism**
              Painful erection
              Code first underlying cause
      N48.30 Priapism, unspecified ♂
      N48.31 Priapism due to trauma ♂
    ▷ **N48.32 *Priapism due to disease classified elsewhere* ♂**
      N48.33 Priapism, drug-induced ♂
      N48.39 Other priapism ♂
    N48.5 Ulcer of penis ♂
    N48.6 Induration penis plastica ♂
              Peyronie's disease
              Plastic induration of penis
  ● **N48.8 Other specified disorders of penis**
      N48.81 Thrombosis of superficial vein of penis ♂
      N48.82 Acquired torsion of penis ♂
              Acquired torsion of penis NOS
          Excludes1   congenital torsion of penis
                            (Q55.63)
      N48.83 Acquired buried penis ♂
          Excludes1   congenital hidden penis (Q55.64)
      N48.89 Other specified disorders of penis ♂
    N48.9 Disorder of penis, unspecified ♂

Item 14-8 Male infertility is the inability of the female sex partner to conceive
after one year of unprotected intercourse.
   Azoospermia is no sperm ejaculated and **oligospermia** is few sperm
ejaculated—both resulting in infertility. Extratesticular causes such as injury,
infections, radiation, and chemotherapy may also cause male infertility.

▶ New   ⇒ Revised   ~~deleted~~ Deleted   Excludes 1   Excludes 2   Includes   Use additional   Code first   Code also   Key words
OGCR Official Guidelines   X Assign placeholder X   ● Use Additional Character(s)   ▷ Manifestation Code   🄷 Hierarchical Condition Category   **Coding Clinic**

● **N49 Inflammatory disorders of male genital organs, not elsewhere classified**
   Use additional code (B95-B97), to identify infectious agent
   Excludes1 inflammation of penis (N48.1, N48.2-)
   orchitis and epididymitis (N45.-)

N49.0 Inflammatory disorders of seminal vesicle ♂
   Vesiculitis NOS

N49.1 Inflammatory disorders of spermatic cord, tunica vaginalis and vas deferens ♂
   Vasitis

N49.2 Inflammatory disorders of scrotum ♂

N49.3 Fournier gangrene ♂

N49.8 Inflammatory disorders of other specified male genital organs ♂
   Inflammation of multiple sites in male genital organs

N49.9 Inflammatory disorder of unspecified male genital organ ♂
   Abscess of unspecified male genital organ
   Boil of unspecified male genital organ
   Carbuncle of unspecified male genital organ
   Cellulitis of unspecified male genital organ

● **N50 Other and unspecified disorders of male genital organs**
   Excludes2 torsion of testis (N44.0-)

N50.0 Atrophy of testis ♂

N50.1 Vascular disorders of male genital organs ♂
   Hematocele, NOS, of male genital organs
   Hemorrhage of male genital organs
   Thrombosis of male genital organs

N50.3 Cyst of epididymis ♂

● **N50.8 Other specified disorders of male genital organs**
   Coding Clinic: 2016, Q4, P45

   ● **N50.81 Testicular pain**
      N50.811 Right testicular pain ♂
      N50.812 Left testicular pain ♂
      N50.819 Testicular pain, unspecified ♂
   N50.82 Scrotal pain ♂
   N50.89 Other specified disorders of the male genital organs ♂
      Atrophy of scrotum, seminal vesicle, spermatic cord, tunica vaginalis and vas deferens
      Chylocele, tunica vaginalis (nonfilarial) NOS
      Edema of scrotum, seminal vesicle, spermatic cord, tunica vaginalis and vas deferens
      Hypertrophy of scrotum, seminal vesicle, spermatic cord, tunica vaginalis and vas deferens
      Stricture of spermatic cord, tunica vaginalis, and vas deferens
      Ulcer of scrotum, seminal vesicle, spermatic cord, testis, tunica vaginalis and vas deferens
      Urethroscrotal fistula

N50.9 Disorder of male genital organs, unspecified ♂

▶ **N51 Disorders of male genital organs in diseases classified elsewhere ♂**
   Code first underlying disease, such as:
   filariasis (B74.0-B74.9)
   Excludes1 amebic balanitis (A06.8)
   candidal balanitis (B37.42)
   gonococcal balanitis (A54.23)
   gonococcal prostatitis (A54.22)
   herpesviral [herpes simplex] balanitis (A60.01)
   trichomonal prostatitis (A59.02)
   tuberculous prostatitis (A18.14)

Item 14–9 Seminal vesiculitis is an inflammation of the seminal vesicle. **Spermatocele** is a benign cystic accumulation of sperm arising from the head of the epididymis. **Torsion of the testis** is a medical emergency occurring most commonly in boys 7 to 12 years of age and results from a congenital abnormality of the covering of the testis allowing the testis to twist within its sac and cutting off the blood supply to the testis.

Figure 14-8 A. Torsion of testis. **B.** Torsion of the testis. (**B** from Kliegman R, Nelson WE: Nelson Textbook of Pediatrics, Philadelphia, Saunders, 2007)

● **N52 Male erectile dysfunction**
   Excludes1 psychogenic impotence (F52.21)

● **N52.0 Vasculogenic erectile dysfunction**
   N52.01 Erectile dysfunction due to arterial insufficiency ♂   A
   N52.02 Corporo-venous occlusive erectile dysfunction ♂   A
   N52.03 Combined arterial insufficiency and corporo-venous occlusive erectile dysfunction ♂   A

▶ **N52.1 Erectile dysfunction due to diseases classified elsewhere ♂**   A
   Code first underlying disease

N52.2 Drug-induced erectile dysfunction ♂   A

● **N52.3 Postprocedural erectile dysfunction**
   N52.31 Erectile dysfunction following radical prostatectomy ♂   A
   N52.32 Erectile dysfunction following radical cystectomy ♂   A
   N52.33 Erectile dysfunction following urethral surgery ♂   A
   N52.34 Erectile dysfunction following simple prostatectomy ♂   A
   N52.35 Erectile dysfunction following radiation therapy ♂   A
      Coding Clinic: 2016, Q4, P45
   N52.36 Erectile dysfunction following interstitial seed therapy ♂   A
      Coding Clinic: 2016, Q4, P45
   N52.37 Erectile dysfunction following prostate ablative therapy ♂   A
      Erectile dysfunction following cryotherapy
      Erectile dysfunction following other prostate ablative therapies
      Erectile dysfunction following ultrasound ablative therapies
      Coding Clinic: 2016, Q4, P45
   N52.39 Other and unspecified postprocedural erectile dysfunction ♂   A

N52.8 Other male erectile dysfunction ♂   A

N52.9 Male erectile dysfunction, unspecified ♂   A
   Impotence NOS

CHAPTER 14 (N00-N99)

CHAPTER 14 (N00-N99)

● **N53** **Other male sexual dysfunction**

    Excludes1 psychogenic sexual dysfunction (F52.-)

  ● **N53.1** **Ejaculatory dysfunction**

    Excludes1 premature ejaculation (F52.4)

    N53.11 **Retarded ejaculation** ♂

    N53.12 **Painful ejaculation** ♂

    N53.13 **Anejaculatory orgasm** ♂

    N53.14 **Retrograde ejaculation** ♂

    N53.19 **Other ejaculatory dysfunction** ♂
        Ejaculatory dysfunction NOS

  N53.8 **Other male sexual dysfunction** ♂

  N53.9 **Unspecified male sexual dysfunction** ♂

DISORDERS OF BREAST (N60-N65)

    Excludes1 disorders of breast associated with childbirth
        (O91-O92)

● **N60** **Benign mammary dysplasia**
    Benign lumpiness of breast

    Includes fibrocystic mastopathy

  ● **N60.0** **Solitary cyst of breast**
    Cyst of breast

    N60.01 **Solitary cyst of right breast**

    N60.02 **Solitary cyst of left breast**

    N60.09 **Solitary cyst of unspecified breast**

  ● **N60.1** **Diffuse cystic mastopathy**
    Cystic breast
    Fibrocystic disease of breast

    Excludes1 diffuse cystic mastopathy with epithelial
        proliferation (N60.3-)

    N60.11 **Diffuse cystic mastopathy of right breast**   A

    N60.12 **Diffuse cystic mastopathy of left breast**   A

    N60.19 **Diffuse cystic mastopathy of unspecified
        breast**   A

  ● **N60.2** **Fibroadenosis of breast**
    Adenofibrosis of breast

    Excludes2 fibroadenoma of breast (D24.-)

    N60.21 **Fibroadenosis of right breast**

    N60.22 **Fibroadenosis of left breast**

    N60.29 **Fibroadenosis of unspecified breast**

  ● **N60.3** **Fibrosclerosis of breast**
    Cystic mastopathy with epithelial proliferation

    N60.31 **Fibrosclerosis of right breast**

    N60.32 **Fibrosclerosis of left breast**

    N60.39 **Fibrosclerosis of unspecified breast**

  ● **N60.4** **Mammary duct ectasia**

    N60.41 **Mammary duct ectasia of right breast**

    N60.42 **Mammary duct ectasia of left breast**

    N60.49 **Mammary duct ectasia of unspecified breast**

  ● **N60.8** **Other benign mammary dysplasias**

    N60.81 **Other benign mammary dysplasias of right
        breast**

    N60.82 **Other benign mammary dysplasias of left breast**

    N60.89 **Other benign mammary dysplasias of
        unspecified breast**

  ● **N60.9** **Unspecified benign mammary dysplasia**

    N60.91 **Unspecified benign mammary dysplasia of
        right breast**

    N60.92 **Unspecified benign mammary dysplasia of left
        breast**

    N60.99 **Unspecified benign mammary dysplasia of
        unspecified breast**

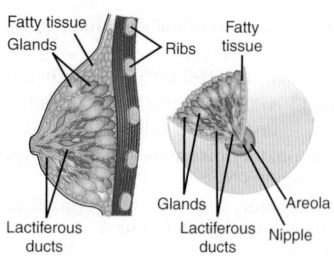

Figure 14-9 Breast.

● **N61** **Inflammatory disorders of breast**

    Excludes1 inflammatory carcinoma of breast (C50.9)
        inflammatory disorder of breast associated with
        childbirth (O91.-)
        neonatal infective mastitis (P39.0)
        thrombophlebitis of breast [Mondor's disease]
        (I80.8)

  N61.0 **Mastitis without abscess**
    Infective mastitis (acute) (nonpuerperal) (subacute)
    Mastitis (acute) (nonpuerperal) (subacute) NOS
    Cellulitis (acute) (nonpuerperal) (subacute) of breast NOS
    Cellulitis (acute) (nonpuerperal) (subacute) of nipple NOS

  N61.1 **Abscess of the breast and nipple**
    Abscess (acute) (chronic) (nonpuerperal) of areola
    Abscess (acute) (chronic) (nonpuerperal) of breast
    Carbuncle of breast
    Mastitis with abscess

  ● **N61.2** **Granulomatous mastitis**

    N61.20 **Granulomatous mastitis, unspecified breast**

    N61.21 **Granulomatous mastitis, right breast**

    N61.22 **Granulomatous mastitis, left breast**

    N61.23 **Granulomatous mastitis, bilateral breast**

● **N62** **Hypertrophy of breast**
    Gynecomastia
    Hypertrophy of breast NOS
    Massive pubertal hypertrophy of breast

    Excludes1 breast engorgement of newborn (P83.4)
        disproportion of reconstructed breast (N65.1)

● **N63** **Unspecified lump in breast**
    Nodule(s) NOS in breast

  N63.0 **Unspecified lump in unspecified breast**

  ● **N63.1** **Unspecified lump in the right breast**

    N63.10 **Unspecified lump in the right breast,
        unspecified quadrant**

    N63.11 **Unspecified lump in the right breast, upper
        outer quadrant**
        Coding Clinic: 2017, Q4, P19

    N63.12 **Unspecified lump in the right breast, upper
        inner quadrant**

    N63.13 **Unspecified lump in the right breast, lower
        outer quadrant**

    N63.14 **Unspecified lump in the right breast, lower
        inner quadrant**

    N63.15 **Unspecified lump in the right breast,
        overlapping quadrants**

  ● **N63.2** **Unspecified lump in the left breast**

    N63.20 **Unspecified lump in the left breast, unspecified
        quadrant**

    N63.21 **Unspecified lump in the left breast, upper outer
        quadrant**

    N63.22 **Unspecified lump in the left breast, upper inner
        quadrant**

    N63.23 **Unspecified lump in the left breast, lower outer
        quadrant**

    N63.24 **Unspecified lump in the left breast, lower inner
        quadrant**

    N63.25 **Unspecified lump in the left breast, overlapping
        quadrants**

● N63.3   Unspecified lump in axillary tail
     N63.31   Unspecified lump in axillary tail of the **right** breast
     N63.32   Unspecified lump in axillary tail of the **left** breast
● N63.4   Unspecified lump in breast, subareolar
     N63.41   Unspecified lump in **right** breast, subareolar
     N63.42   Unspecified lump in **left** breast, subareolar

● N64   Other disorders of breast
     Excludes2   mechanical complication of breast prosthesis and implant (T85.4-)
   N64.0   Fissure and fistula of nipple
   N64.1   Fat necrosis of breast
       Fat necrosis (segmental) of breast
       Code first breast necrosis due to breast graft (T85.898)
   N64.2   Atrophy of breast
   N64.3   Galactorrhea not associated with childbirth
       Excessive or spontaneous flow of milk
   N64.4   Mastodynia
● N64.5   Other signs and symptoms in breast
     Excludes2   abnormal findings on diagnostic imaging of breast (R92.-)
     N64.51   Induration of breast
     N64.52   Nipple discharge
       Excludes1   abnormal findings in nipple discharge (R89.-)
     N64.53   Retraction of nipple
     N64.59   Other signs and symptoms in breast
● N64.8   Other specified disorders of breast
     N64.81   Ptosis of breast   A
       Excludes1   ptosis of native breast in relation to reconstructed breast (N65.1)
     N64.82   Hypoplasia of breast   A
       Micromastia
       Excludes1   congenital absence of breast (Q83.0)
                 hypoplasia of native breast in relation to reconstructed breast (N65.1)
     N64.89   Other specified disorders of breast
       Galactocele
       Subinvolution of breast (postlactational)
       Coding Clinic: 2019, Q1, P32; 2018, Q1, P4
   N64.9   Disorder of breast, unspecified
       Coding Clinic: 2018, Q1, P4

● N65   Deformity and disproportion of reconstructed breast
   N65.0   Deformity of reconstructed breast   A
       Contour irregularity in reconstructed breast
       Excess tissue in reconstructed breast
       Misshapen reconstructed breast
   N65.1   Disproportion of reconstructed breast   A
       Breast asymmetry between native breast and reconstructed breast
       Disproportion between native breast and reconstructed breast

Figure 14-10 A. Female genital system. **B.** External female genital system. (From Buck CJ: Step-by-Step Medical Coding, ed 2016, St. Louis, Elsevier, 2016)

Item 14–10 Salpingitis is an infection of one or both fallopian tubes. **Oophoritis** is an infection of one or both ovaries.

INFLAMMATORY DISEASES OF FEMALE PELVIC ORGANS (N70-N77)

   Excludes1   inflammatory diseases of female pelvic organs complicating:
       abortion or ectopic or molar pregnancy (O00-O07, O08.0)
       pregnancy, childbirth and the puerperium (O23.-, O75.3, O85, O86.-)

★ **(See Plate 35 of the Anatomy Illustrations.)**

● N70   Salpingitis and oophoritis
       Oophoritis = inflammation of ovary
       Salpingitis = inflammation of falloplan tube
     Includes   abscess (of) fallopian tube
               abscess (of) ovary
               pyosalpinx
               salpingo-oophoritis
               tubo-ovarian abscess
               tubo-ovarian inflammatory disease
     Use additional code (B95-B97), to identify infectious agent
     Excludes1   gonococcal infection (A54.24)
                 tuberculous infection (A18.17)
   ● N70.0   Acute salpingitis and oophoritis
     N70.01   Acute salpingitis ♀
     N70.02   Acute oophoritis ♀
     N70.03   Acute salpingitis and oophoritis ♀
   ● N70.1   Chronic salpingitis and oophoritis
       Hydrosalpinx
     N70.11   Chronic salpingitis ♀
     N70.12   Chronic oophoritis ♀
     N70.13   Chronic salpingitis and oophoritis ♀
   ● N70.9   Salpingitis and oophoritis, unspecified
     N70.91   Salpingitis, unspecified ♀
     N70.92   Oophoritis, unspecified ♀
     N70.93   Salpingitis and oophoritis, unspecified ♀

CHAPTER 14 (N00-N99)

● **N71   Inflammatory disease of uterus, except cervix**

     Includes   endo (myo) metritis
                   metritis
                   myometritis
                   pyometra
                   uterine abscess

     Use additional code (B95-B97), to identify infectious agent

     Excludes1   hyperplastic endometritis (N85.0-)
                  infection of uterus following delivery (O85, O86.-)

   N71.0   Acute inflammatory disease of uterus ♀

   N71.1   Chronic inflammatory disease of uterus ♀

   N71.9   Inflammatory disease of uterus, unspecified ♀

  N72   Inflammatory disease of cervix uteri ♀

     Includes   cervicitis (with or without erosion or ectropion)
                   endocervicitis (with or without erosion or
                      ectropion)
                   exocervicitis (with or without erosion or ectropion)

     Use additional code (B95-B97), to identify infectious agent

     Excludes1   erosion and ectropion of cervix without cervicitis
                  (N86)

● **N73   Other female pelvic inflammatory diseases**

     Use additional code (B95-B97), to identify infectious agent

   N73.0   Acute parametritis and pelvic cellulitis ♀
          Abscess of broad ligament
          Abscess of parametrium
          Pelvic cellulitis, female

   N73.1   Chronic parametritis and pelvic cellulitis ♀
          Any condition in N73.0 specified as chronic

       Excludes1   tuberculous parametritis and pelvic
                    cellultis (A18.17)

   N73.2   Unspecified parametritis and pelvic cellulitis ♀
          Any condition in N73.0 unspecified whether acute or
          chronic

   N73.3   Female acute pelvic peritonitis ♀

   N73.4   Female chronic pelvic peritonitis ♀

       Excludes1   tuberculous pelvic (female) peritonitis
                    (A18.17)

   N73.5   Female pelvic peritonitis, unspecified ♀

   N73.6   Female pelvic peritoneal adhesions (postinfective) ♀

       Excludes2   postprocedural pelvic peritoneal
                    adhesions (N99.4)

   N73.8   Other specified female pelvic inflammatory diseases ♀

   N73.9   Female pelvic inflammatory disease, unspecified ♀
          Female pelvic infection or inflammation NOS

▷ *N74   Female pelvic inflammatory disorders in diseases classified*
     elsewhere ♀

     Code first underlying disease

     Excludes1   chlamydial cervicitis (A56.02)
                  chlamydial pelvic inflammatory disease (A56.11)
                  gonococcal cervicitis (A54.03)
                  gonococcal pelvic inflammatory disease (A54.24)
                  herpesviral [herpes simplex] cervicitis (A60.03)
                  herpesviral [herpes simplex] pelvic inflammatory
                    disease (A60.09)
                  syphilitic cervicitis (A52.76)
                  syphilitic pelvic inflammatory disease (A52.76)
                  trichomonal cervicitis (A59.09)
                  tuberculous cervicitis (A18.16)
                  tuberculous pelvic inflammatory disease (A18.17)

● **N75   Diseases of Bartholin's gland**

   N75.0   Cyst of Bartholin's gland ♀
          Cysts filled with liquid or semisolid material

   N75.1   Abscess of Bartholin's gland ♀
          Localized collection of pus

   N75.8   Other diseases of Bartholin's gland ♀
          Bartholinitis

   N75.9   Disease of Bartholin's gland, unspecified ♀

● **N76   Other inflammation of vagina and vulva**

     Use additional code (B95-B97), to identify infectious agent

     Excludes2   senile (atrophic) vaginitis (N95.2)
                  vulvar vestibulitis (N94.810)

   N76.0   Acute vaginitis ♀
          Acute vulvovaginitis
          Vaginitis NOS
          Vulvovaginitis NOS

   N76.1   Subacute and chronic vaginitis ♀
          Chronic vulvovaginitis
          Subacute vulvovaginitis

   N76.2   Acute vulvitis ♀
          Vulvitis NOS

   N76.3   Subacute and chronic vulvitis ♀

   N76.4   Abscess of vulva ♀
          Furuncle of vulva

   N76.5   Ulceration of vagina ♀

   N76.6   Ulceration of vulva ♀

● **N76.8**   Other specified inflammation of vagina and vulva

   N76.81   Mucositis (ulcerative) of vagina and vulva ♀

       Code also type of associated therapy, such as:
          antineoplastic and immunosuppressive
            drugs (T45.1X-)
          radiological procedure and radiotherapy
            (Y84.2)

         Excludes2   gastrointestinal mucositis
                    (ulcerative) (K92.81)
                    nasal mucositis (ulcerative)
                    (J34.81)
                    oral mucositis (ulcerative) (K12.3-)

   N76.89   Other specified inflammation of vagina and
          vulva ♀

● **N77   Vulvovaginal ulceration and inflammation in diseases classified**
     elsewhere

▷ *N77.0   Ulceration of vulva in diseases classified elsewhere ♀*

     Code first underlying disease, such as:
     Behçet's disease (M35.2)

     Excludes1   ulceration of vulva in gonococcal
                  infection (A54.02)
                  ulceration of vulva in herpesviral [herpes
                  simplex] infection (A60.04)
                  ulceration of vulva in syphilis (A51.0)
                  ulceration of vulva in tuberculosis (A18.18)

▷ *N77.1   Vaginitis, vulvitis and vulvovaginitis in diseases*
     classified elsewhere ♀

     Code first underlying disease, such as:
     pinworm (B80)

     Excludes1   candidial vulvovaginitis (B37.3)
                  chlamydial vulvovaginitis (A56.02)
                  gonococcal vulvovaginitis (A54.02)
                  herpesviral [herpes simplex]
                    vulvovaginitis (A60.04)
                  trichomonal vulvovaginitis (A59.01)
                  tuberculous vulvovaginitis (A18.18)
                  vulvovaginitis in early syphilis (A51.0)
                  vulvovaginitis in late syphilis (A52.76)

▶ New   ⇒ Revised   ~~deleted~~ Deleted   Excludes 1   Excludes 2   Includes   Use additional   Code first   Code also   Key words

OGCR Official Guidelines   **X** Assign placeholder X   ● Use Additional Character(s)   ▷ Manifestation Code   🐱 Hierarchical Condition Category   **Coding Clinic**

Item 14–11 Endometriosis is a condition for which no clear cause has been identified. Endometrial tissue is expelled from the uterus into the abdominal cavity and can implant onto a variety of organs. Classification is based on the site of implant of the endometrial tissue.

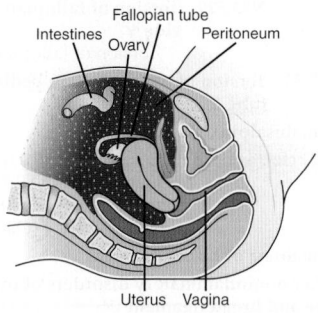

Figure 14-11 Sites of potential endometrial implants.

NONINFLAMMATORY DISORDERS OF FEMALE GENITAL TRACT (N80-N98)

● **N80 Endometriosis**

   N80.0 Endometriosis of uterus ♀
      Adenomyosis
      Excludes1 stromal endometriosis (D39.0)

   N80.1 Endometriosis of ovary ♀
   N80.2 Endometriosis of fallopian tube ♀
   N80.3 Endometriosis of pelvic peritoneum ♀
   N80.4 Endometriosis of rectovaginal septum and vagina ♀
   N80.5 Endometriosis of intestine ♀
   N80.6 Endometriosis in cutaneous scar ♀
   N80.8 Other endometriosis ♀
      Endometriosis of thorax

   N80.9 Endometriosis, unspecified ♀

● **N81 Female genital prolapse**

   Excludes1 genital prolapse complicating pregnancy, labor or delivery (O34.5-)
         prolapse and hernia of ovary and fallopian tube (N83.4-)
         prolapse of vaginal vault after hysterectomy (N99.3)

   N81.0 Urethrocele ♀
      Excludes1 urethrocele with cystocele (N81.1-)
         urethrocele with prolapse of uterus (N81.2-N81.4)

  ● **N81.1 Cystocele**
      Cystocele with urethrocele
      Cystourethrocele
      Excludes1 cystocele with prolapse of uterus (N81.2-N81.4)

     N81.10 Cystocele, unspecified ♀
        Prolapse of (anterior) vaginal wall NOS

     N81.11 Cystocele, midline ♀
     N81.12 Cystocele, lateral ♀
        Paravaginal cystocele

Figure 14-12 Three stages of uterine prolapse. **A.** Uterus is prolapsed. **B.** Vagina and uterus are prolapsed (incomplete uterovaginal prolapse). **C.** Vagina and uterus are completely prolapsed and are exposed through the external genitalia (complete uterovaginal prolapse).

   N81.2 Incomplete uterovaginal prolapse ♀
      First degree uterine prolapse
      Prolapse of cervix NOS
      Second degree uterine prolapse
      Excludes1 cervical stump prolapse (N81.85)

   N81.3 Complete uterovaginal prolapse ♀
      Procidentia (uteri) NOS
      Third degree uterine prolapse

   N81.4 Uterovaginal prolapse, unspecified ♀
      Prolapse of uterus NOS

   N81.5 Vaginal enterocele ♀
      Excludes1 enterocele with prolapse of uterus (N81.2-N81.4)

   N81.6 Rectocele ♀
      Prolapse of posterior vaginal wall
      Use additional code for any associated fecal incontinence, if applicable (R15.-)
      Excludes2 perineocele (N81.81)
         rectal prolapse (K62.3)
         rectocele with prolapse of uterus (N81.2-N81.4)

  ● **N81.8 Other female genital prolapse**
     N81.81 Perineocele ♀
     N81.82 Incompetence or weakening of pubocervical tissue ♀
     N81.83 Incompetence or weakening of rectovaginal tissue ♀
     N81.84 Pelvic muscle wasting ♀
        Disuse atrophy of pelvic muscles and anal sphincter
     N81.85 Cervical stump prolapse ♀
     N81.89 Other female genital prolapse ♀
        Deficient perineum
        Old laceration of muscles of pelvic floor

   N81.9 Female genital prolapse, unspecified ♀

● **N82 Fistulae involving female genital tract**
      Excludes1 vesicointestinal fistulae (N32.1)

   N82.0 Vesicovaginal fistula ♀
   N82.1 Other female urinary-genital tract fistulae ♀
      Cervicovesical fistula
      Ureterovaginal fistula
      Urethrovaginal fistula
      Uteroureteric fistula
      Uterovesical fistula
      Coding Clinic: 2017, Q3, P4

   N82.2 Fistula of vagina to small intestine ♀
   N82.3 Fistula of vagina to large intestine ♀
      Rectovaginal fistula

   N82.4 Other female intestinal-genital tract fistulae ♀
      Intestinouterine fistula

   N82.5 Female genital tract-skin fistulae ♀
      Uterus to abdominal wall fistula
      Vaginoperineal fistula

   N82.8 Other female genital tract fistulae ♀
   N82.9 Female genital tract fistula, unspecified ♀

● **N83 Noninflammatory disorders of ovary, fallopian tube and broad ligament**
      Excludes2 hydrosalpinx (N70.1-)

  ● **N83.0 Follicular cyst of ovary**
      Cyst of graafian follicle
      Hemorrhagic follicular cyst (of ovary)
      Coding Clinic: 2016, Q4, P46

     N83.00 Follicular cyst of ovary, unspecified side ♀
     N83.01 Follicular cyst of right ovary ♀
     N83.02 Follicular cyst of left ovary ♀

● **N83.1 Corpus luteum cyst**
Hemorrhagic corpus luteum cyst
Coding Clinic: 2016, Q4, P46

   N83.10 Corpus luteum cyst of ovary, unspecified side ♀
   N83.11 Corpus luteum cyst of right ovary ♀
   N83.12 Corpus luteum cyst of left ovary ♀

● **N83.2 Other and unspecified ovarian cysts**
   Excludes1   developmental ovarian cyst (Q50.1)
                  neoplastic ovarian cyst (D27.-)
                  polycystic ovarian syndrome (E28.2)
                  Stein-Leventhal syndrome (E28.2)
   Coding Clinic: 2016, Q4, P46

   ● **N83.20** Unspecified ovarian cysts
     N83.201 Unspecified ovarian cyst, right side ♀
     N83.202 Unspecified ovarian cyst, left side ♀
     N83.209 Unspecified ovarian cyst, unspecified side ♀
          Ovarian cyst, NOS

   ● **N83.29** Other ovarian cysts
      Retention cyst of ovary
      Simple cyst of ovary
     N83.291 Other ovarian cyst, right side ♀
     N83.292 Other ovarian cyst, left side ♀
     N83.299 Other ovarian cyst, unspecified side ♀

● **N83.3 Acquired atrophy of ovary and fallopian tube**
   Coding Clinic: 2016, Q4, P46

   ● **N83.31** Acquired atrophy of ovary
     N83.311 Acquired atrophy of right ovary ♀
     N83.312 Acquired atrophy of left ovary ♀
     N83.319 Acquired atrophy of ovary, unspecified side ♀
          Acquired atrophy of ovary, NOS

   ● **N83.32** Acquired atrophy of fallopian tube
     N83.321 Acquired atrophy of right fallopian tube ♀
     N83.322 Acquired atrophy of left fallopian tube ♀
     N83.329 Acquired atrophy of fallopian tube, unspecified side ♀
          Acquired atrophy of fallopian tube, NOS

   ● **N83.33** Acquired atrophy of ovary and fallopian tube
     N83.331 Acquired atrophy of right ovary and fallopian tube ♀
     N83.332 Acquired atrophy of left ovary and fallopian tube ♀
     N83.339 Acquired atrophy of ovary and fallopian tube, unspecified side ♀
          Acquired atrophy of ovary and fallopian tube, NOS

● **N83.4 Prolapse and hernia of ovary and fallopian tube**
   Coding Clinic: 2016, Q4, P46

   N83.40 Prolapse and hernia of ovary and fallopian tube, unspecified side ♀
          Prolapse and hernia of ovary and fallopian tube, NOS

   N83.41 Prolapse and hernia of right ovary and fallopian tube ♀
   N83.42 Prolapse and hernia of left ovary and fallopian tube ♀

● **N83.5 Torsion of ovary, ovarian pedicle and fallopian tube**
   Torsion of accessory tube
   Coding Clinic: 2016, Q4, P46

   ● **N83.51** Torsion of ovary and ovarian pedicle
     N83.511 Torsion of right ovary and ovarian pedicle ♀
     N83.512 Torsion of left ovary and ovarian pedicle ♀
     N83.519 Torsion of ovary and ovarian pedicle, unspecified side ♀
          Torsion of ovary and ovarian pedicle, NOS

   ● **N83.52** Torsion of fallopian tube
      Torsion of hydatid of Morgagni
     N83.521 Torsion of right fallopian tube ♀
     N83.522 Torsion of left fallopian tube ♀
     N83.529 Torsion of fallopian tube, unspecified side ♀
          Torsion of fallopian tube, NOS

   N83.53 Torsion of ovary, ovarian pedicle and fallopian tube ♀

● **N83.6 Hematosalpinx ♀**
   Excludes1   hematosalpinx (with) (in):
                  hematocolpos (N89.7)
                  hematometra (N85.7)
                  tubal pregnancy (O00.1-)

N83.7 Hematoma of broad ligament ♀

N83.8 Other noninflammatory disorders of ovary, fallopian tube and broad ligament ♀
   Broad ligament laceration syndrome [Allen-Masters]

N83.9 Noninflammatory disorder of ovary, fallopian tube and broad ligament, unspecified ♀

● **N84 Polyp of female genital tract**
   Excludes1   adenomatous polyp (D28.-)
                  placental polyp (O90.89)

N84.0 Polyp of corpus uteri ♀
   Polyp of endometrium
   Polyp of uterus NOS
   Excludes1   polypoid endometrial hyperplasia (N85.0-)

N84.1 Polyp of cervix uteri ♀
   Mucous polyp of cervix

N84.2 Polyp of vagina ♀

N84.3 Polyp of vulva ♀
   Polyp of labia

N84.8 Polyp of other parts of female genital tract ♀

N84.9 Polyp of female genital tract, unspecified ♀

● **N85 Other noninflammatory disorders of uterus, except cervix**
   Excludes1   endometriosis (N80.-)
                  inflammatory diseases of uterus (N71.-)
                  noninflammatory disorders of cervix, except malposition (N86-N88)
                  polyp of corpus uteri (N84.0)
                  uterine prolapse (N81.-)

   ● **N85.0 Endometrial hyperplasia**
     N85.00 Endometrial hyperplasia, unspecified ♀
        Hyperplasia (adenomatous) (cystic) (glandular) of endometrium
        Hyperplastic endometritis

     N85.01 Benign endometrial hyperplasia ♀
        Endometrial hyperplasia (complex) (simple) without atypia

     N85.02 Endometrial intraepithelial neoplasia [EIN] ♀
        Endometrial hyperplasia with atypia
        Excludes1   malignant neoplasm of endometrium (with endometrial intraepithelial neoplasia [EIN]) (C54.1)

N85.2 Hypertrophy of uterus ♀
   Bulky or enlarged uterus
   Excludes1   puerperal hypertrophy of uterus (O90.89)

N85.3 Subinvolution of uterus ♀
   Excludes1   puerperal subinvolution of uterus (O90.89)

N85.4 Malposition of uterus ♀
   Anteversion of uterus
   Retroflexion of uterus
   Retroversion of uterus
   Excludes1   malposition of uterus complicating pregnancy, labor or delivery (O34.5-, O65.5)

▶ New   ⇒ Revised   ~~deleted~~ Deleted   Excludes 1   Excludes 2   Includes   Use additional   Code first   Code also   Key words

OGCR Official Guidelines   **X** Assign placeholder X   ● Use Additional Character(s)   ▸ Manifestation Code   🏷 Hierarchical Condition Category   **Coding Clinic**

N85.5   **Inversion of uterus** ♀
> **Excludes1**   current obstetric trauma (O71.2)
>   postpartum inversion of uterus (O71.2)

N85.6   **Intrauterine synechiae** ♀

N85.7   **Hematometra** ♀
> Hematosalpinx with hematometra
> **Excludes1**   hematometra with hematocolpos (N89.7)

N85.8   **Other specified noninflammatory disorders of uterus** ♀
> Atrophy of uterus, acquired
> Fibrosis of uterus NOS

N85.9   **Noninflammatory disorder of uterus, unspecified** ♀
> Disorder of uterus NOS

N86   **Erosion and ectropion of cervix uteri** ♀
> Decubitus (trophic) ulcer of cervix
> Eversion of cervix
> **Excludes1**   erosion and ectropion of cervix with cervicitis
>   (N72)

● **N87**   **Dysplasia of cervix uteri**
> **Excludes1**   abnormal results from cervical cytologic
>   examination without histologic confirmation
>   (R87.61-)
>   carcinoma in situ of cervix uteri (D06.-)
>   cervical intraepithelial neoplasia III [CIN III]
>   (D06.-)
>   HGSIL of cervix (R87.613)
>   severe dysplasia of cervix uteri (D06.-)

N87.0   **Mild cervical dysplasia** ♀
> Cervical intraepithelial neoplasia I [CIN I]

N87.1   **Moderate cervical dysplasia** ♀
> Cervical intraepithelial neoplasia II [CIN II]

N87.9   **Dysplasia of cervix uteri, unspecified** ♀
> Anaplasia of cervix
> Cervical atypism
> Cervical dysplasia NOS

● **N88**   **Other noninflammatory disorders of cervix uteri**
> **Excludes2**   inflammatory disease of cervix (N72)
>   polyp of cervix (N84.1)

N88.0   **Leukoplakia of cervix uteri** ♀

N88.1   **Old laceration of cervix uteri** ♀
> Adhesions of cervix
> **Excludes1**   current obstetric trauma (O71.3)

N88.2   **Stricture and stenosis of cervix uteri** ♀
> **Excludes1**   stricture and stenosis of cervix uteri
>   complicating labor (O65.5)

N88.3   **Incompetence of cervix uteri** ♀
> Investigation and management of (suspected) cervical
> incompetence in a nonpregnant woman
> **Excludes1**   cervical incompetence complicating
>   pregnancy (O34.3-)

N88.4   **Hypertrophic elongation of cervix uteri** ♀

N88.8   **Other specified noninflammatory disorders of cervix uteri** ♀
> **Excludes1**   current obstetric trauma (O71.3)

N88.9   **Noninflammatory disorder of cervix uteri, unspecified** ♀

● **N89**   **Other noninflammatory disorders of vagina**
> **Excludes1**   abnormal results from vaginal cytologic
>   examination without histologic confirmation
>   (R87.62-)
>   carcinoma in situ of vagina (D07.2)
>   HGSIL of vagina (R87.623)
>   inflammation of vagina (N76.-)
>   senile (atrophic) vaginitis (N95.2)
>   severe dysplasia of vagina (D07.2)
>   trichomonal leukorrhea (A59.00)
>   vaginal intraepithelial neoplasia [VAIN], grade
>   III (D07.2)

N89.0   **Mild vaginal dysplasia** ♀
> Vaginal intraepithelial neoplasia [VAIN], grade I

N89.1   **Moderate vaginal dysplasia** ♀
> Vaginal intraepithelial neoplasia [VAIN], grade II

N89.3   **Dysplasia of vagina, unspecified** ♀

N89.4   **Leukoplakia of vagina** ♀

N89.5   **Stricture and atresia of vagina** ♀
> Vaginal adhesions   Vaginal stenosis
> **Excludes1**   congenital atresia or stricture (Q52.4)
>   postprocedural adhesions of vagina
>   (N99.2)

N89.6   **Tight hymenal ring** ♀
> Rigid hymen   Tight introitus
> **Excludes1**   imperforate hymen (Q52.3)

N89.7   **Hematocolpos** ♀
> Hematocolpos with hematometra or hematosalpinx
> **Coding Clinic: 2016, Q4, P59**

N89.8   **Other specified noninflammatory disorders of vagina** ♀
> Leukorrhea NOS
> Old vaginal laceration
> Pessary ulcer of vagina
> **Excludes1**   current obstetric trauma (O70.-, O71.4,
>   O71.7-O71.8)
>   old laceration involving muscles of pelvic
>   floor (N81.8)

N89.9   **Noninflammatory disorder of vagina, unspecified** ♀

● **N90**   **Other noninflammatory disorders of vulva and perineum**
> **Excludes1**   anogenital (venereal) warts (A63.0)
>   carcinoma in situ of vulva (D07.1)
>   condyloma acuminatum (A63.0)
>   current obstetric trauma (O70.-, O71.7-O71.8)
>   inflammation of vulva (N76.-)
>   severe dysplasia of vulva (D07.1)
>   vulvar intraepithelial neoplasm III [VIN III]
>   (D07.1)

N90.0   **Mild vulvar dysplasia** ♀
> Vulvar intraepithelial neoplasia [VIN], grade I

N90.1   **Moderate vulvar dysplasia** ♀
> Vulvar intraepithelial neoplasia [VIN], grade II

N90.3   **Dysplasia of vulva, unspecified** ♀

N90.4   **Leukoplakia of vulva** ♀
> Dystrophy of vulva
> Kraurosis of vulva
> Lichen sclerosus of external female genital organs

N90.5   **Atrophy of vulva** ♀
> Stenosis of vulva

● **N90.6**   **Hypertrophy of vulva**
> **Coding Clinic: 2016, Q4, P46**

     N90.60   **Unspecified hypertrophy of vulva** ♀
> Unspecified hypertrophy of labia

     N90.61   **Childhood asymmetric labium majus enlargement** ♀
> CALME

     N90.69   **Other specified hypertrophy of vulva** ♀
> Other specified hypertrophy of labia

N90.7   **Vulvar cyst** ♀

● **N90.8**   **Other specified noninflammatory disorders of vulva and perineum**

     ● **N90.81**   **Female genital mutilation status**
> Female genital cutting status

         N90.810   **Female genital mutilation status, unspecified** ♀
> Female genital cutting status, unspecified
> Female genital mutilation status NOS

         N90.811   **Female genital mutilation Type I status** ♀
> Clitorectomy status
> Female genital cutting Type I status

         N90.812   **Female genital mutilation Type II status** ♀
> Clitorectomy with excision of labia minora status
> Female genital cutting Type II status

CHAPTER 14 (N00–N99)

CHAPTER 14 (N00–N99)

N90.813   **Female genital mutilation** Type III **status** ♀
      Female genital cutting Type III status
      Infibulation status

N90.818   **Other female genital mutilation status** ♀
      Female genital cutting Type IV status
      Female genital mutilation Type IV status
      Other female genital cutting status

N90.89   **Other specified noninflammatory disorders of vulva and perineum** ♀
      Adhesions of vulva
      Hypertrophy of clitoris

N90.9   **Noninflammatory disorder of vulva and perineum, unspecified** ♀

● N91   **Absent, scanty and rare menstruation**
    Excludes1   ovarian dysfunction (E28.-)

N91.0   **Primary amenorrhea** ♀

N91.1   **Secondary amenorrhea** ♀

N91.2   **Amenorrhea, unspecified** ♀

N91.3   **Primary oligomenorrhea** ♀

N91.4   **Secondary oligomenorrhea** ♀

N91.5   **Oligomenorrhea, unspecified** ♀
      Hypomenorrhea NOS

● N92   **Excessive, frequent and irregular menstruation**
    Excludes1   postmenopausal bleeding (N95.0)
                   precocious puberty (menstruation) (E30.1)

N92.0   **Excessive and frequent menstruation with** regular cycle ♀
      Heavy periods NOS   Polymenorrhea
      Menorrhagia NOS

N92.1   **Excessive and frequent menstruation with** irregular **cycle** ♀
      Irregular intermenstrual bleeding
      Irregular, shortened intervals between menstrual bleeding
      Menometrorrhagia
      Metrorrhagia

N92.2   **Excessive menstruation at puberty** ♀   P
      Excessive bleeding associated with onset of menstrual periods
      Pubertal menorrhagia
      Puberty bleeding

N92.3   **Ovulation bleeding** ♀
      Regular intermenstrual bleeding

N92.4   **Excessive bleeding in the premenopausal period** ♀
      Climacteric menorrhagia or metrorrhagia
      Menopausal menorrhagia or metrorrhagia
      Perimenopausal bleeding
      Perimenopausal menorrhagia or metrorrhagia
      Preclimacteric menorrhagia or metrorrhagia
      Premenopausal menorrhagia or metrorrhagia

N92.5   **Other specified irregular menstruation** ♀

N92.6   **Irregular menstruation, unspecified** ♀
      Irregular bleeding NOS
      Irregular periods NOS
    Excludes1   irregular menstruation with:
           lengthened intervals or scanty bleeding (N91.3-N91.5)
           shortened intervals or excessive bleeding (N92.1)

● N93   **Other abnormal uterine and vaginal bleeding**
    Excludes1   neonatal vaginal hemorrhage (P54.6)
                   precocious puberty (menstruation) (E30.1)
                   pseudomenses (P54.6)

N93.0   **Postcoital and contact bleeding** ♀

N93.1   **Pre-pubertal vaginal bleeding** ♀
      Coding Clinic: 2016, Q4, P47

N93.8   **Other specified abnormal uterine and vaginal bleeding** ♀
      Dysfunctional or functional uterine or vaginal bleeding NOS

N93.9   **Abnormal uterine and vaginal bleeding, unspecified** ♀

● N94   **Pain and other conditions associated with female genital organs and menstrual cycle**

N94.0   **Mittelschmerz** ♀
      Ovulation pain

● N94.1   **Dyspareunia**
      Painful intercourse/coitus
    Excludes1   psychogenic dyspareunia (F52.6)
      Coding Clinic: 2016, Q4, P47

N94.10   **Unspecified dyspareunia** ♀

N94.11   **Superficial (introital) dyspareunia** ♀

N94.12   **Deep dyspareunia** ♀

N94.19   **Other specified dyspareunia** ♀

N94.2   **Vaginismus** ♀
      Vagina tightness
    Excludes1   psychogenic vaginismus (F52.5)

N94.3   **Premenstrual tension syndrome** ♀
      AKA: PMS
      Code also associated menstrual migraine (G43.82-, G43.83-)
    Excludes1   Premenstrual dysphoric disorder (F32.81)
      Coding Clinic: 2016, Q4, P14

N94.4   **Primary dysmenorrhea** ♀
      Lifelong painful menstruation

N94.5   **Secondary dysmenorrhea** ♀
      Later onset of painful menstruation

N94.6   **Dysmenorrhea, unspecified** ♀
    Excludes1   psychogenic dysmenorrhea (F45.8)

● N94.8   **Other specified conditions associated with female genital organs and menstrual cycle**

● N94.81   **Vulvodynia**

N94.810   **Vulvar vestibulitis** ♀

N94.818   **Other vulvodynia** ♀

N94.819   **Vulvodynia, unspecified** ♀
      Vulvodynia NOS

N94.89   **Other specified conditions associated with female genital organs and menstrual cycle** ♀

N94.9   **Unspecified condition associated with female genital organs and menstrual cycle** ♀

● N95   **Menopausal and other perimenopausal disorders**
      Menopausal and other perimenopausal disorders due to naturally occurring (age-related) menopause and perimenopause
    Excludes1   excessive bleeding in the premenopausal period (N92.4)
           menopausal and perimenopausal disorders due to artificial or premature menopause (E89.4-, E28.31-)
           premature menopause (E28.31-)
    Excludes2   postmenopausal osteoporosis (M81.0-)
           postmenopausal osteoporosis with current pathological fracture (M80.0-)
           postmenopausal urethritis (N34.2)

N95.0   **Postmenopausal bleeding** ♀

N95.1   **Menopausal and female climacteric states** ♀
      Symptoms such as flushing, sleeplessness, headache, lack of concentration, associated with natural (age-related) menopause
      Use additional code for associated symptoms
    Excludes1   asymptomatic menopausal state (Z78.0)
           symptoms associated with artificial menopause (E89.41)
           symptoms associated with premature menopause (E28.310)

N95.2   **Postmenopausal atrophic vaginitis** ♀
      Senile (atrophic) vaginitis

N95.8   **Other specified menopausal and perimenopausal disorders** ♀

N95.9   **Unspecified menopausal and perimenopausal disorder** ♀

▶ New   ⇒ Revised   ~~deleted~~ Deleted   Excludes 1   Excludes 2   Includes   Use additional   Code first   Code also   Key words

OGCR Official Guidelines   X Assign placeholder X   ● Use Additional Character(s)   ▶ Manifestation Code   🏷 Hierarchical Condition Category   **Coding Clinic**

N96   Recurrent pregnancy loss ♀
> Investigation or care in a nonpregnant woman with history of recurrent pregnancy loss
>
> **Excludes1**   recurrent pregnancy loss with current pregnancy (O26.2-)

● **N97   Female infertility**
> **Includes**   inability to achieve a pregnancy
> sterility, female NOS
>
> ~~**Excludes**   female infertility associated with:~~
> ~~hypopituitarism (E23.0)~~
> ~~Stein-Leventhal syndrome (E28.2)~~
>
> ▶ **Excludes2**   female infertility associated with:
> hypopituitarism (E23.0)
> Stein-Leventhal syndrome (E28.2)
> incompetence of cervix uteri (N88.3)

N97.0   Female infertility associated with anovulation ♀

N97.1   Female infertility of tubal origin ♀
> Female infertility associated with congenital anomaly of tube
> Female infertility due to tubal block
> Female infertility due to tubal occlusion
> Female infertility due to tubal stenosis

N97.2   Female infertility of uterine origin ♀
> Female infertility associated with congenital anomaly of uterus
> Female infertility due to nonimplantation of ovum

N97.8   Female infertility of other origin ♀

N97.9   Female infertility, unspecified ♀

● **N98   Complications associated with artificial fertilization**

N98.0   Infection associated with artificial insemination ♀

N98.1   Hyperstimulation of ovaries ♀
> Hyperstimulation of ovaries NOS
> Hyperstimulation of ovaries associated with induced ovulation

N98.2   Complications of attempted introduction of fertilized ovum following in vitro fertilization ♀

N98.3   Complications of attempted introduction of embryo in embryo transfer ♀

N98.8   Other complications associated with artificial fertilization ♀

N98.9   Complication associated with artificial fertilization, unspecified ♀

INTRAOPERATIVE AND POSTPROCEDURAL COMPLICATIONS AND DISORDERS OF GENITOURINARY SYSTEM, NOT ELSEWHERE CLASSIFIED (N99)

● **N99   Intraoperative and postprocedural complications and disorders of genitourinary system, not elsewhere classified**
> **Excludes2**   irradiation cystitis (N30.4-)
> postoophorectomy osteoporosis with current pathological fracture (M80.8-)
> postoophorectomy osteoporosis without current pathological fracture (M81.8)

N99.0   Postprocedural (acute) (chronic) kidney failure
> Use additional code to type of kidney disease

● **N99.1   Postprocedural urethral stricture**
> Postcatheterization urethral stricture

    ● **N99.11   Postprocedural urethral stricture, male ♂**

       N99.110   Postprocedural urethral stricture, male, meatal ♂

       N99.111   Postprocedural bulbous urethral stricture, male ♂

       N99.112   Postprocedural membranous urethral stricture, male ♂

       N99.113   Postprocedural anterior bulbous urethral stricture, male ♂
> Coding Clinic: 2016, Q4, P48

       N99.114   Postprocedural urethral stricture, male, unspecified ♂

       N99.115   Postprocedural fossa navicularis urethral stricture ♂
> Coding Clinic: 2016, Q4, P47

       N99.116   Postprocedural urethral stricture, male, overlapping sites ♂

    N99.12   Postprocedural urethral stricture, female ♀

N99.2   Postprocedural adhesions of vagina ♀

N99.3   Prolapse of vaginal vault after hysterectomy ♀

N99.4   Postprocedural pelvic peritoneal adhesions
> **Excludes2**   pelvic peritoneal adhesions NOS (N73.6)
> postinfective pelvic peritoneal adhesions (N73.6)

● **N99.5   Complications of stoma of urinary tract**
> **Excludes2**   mechanical complication of urinary catheter (T83.0-)

    ● **N99.51   Complication of cystostomy**

       N99.510   Cystostomy hemorrhage 🐾

       N99.511   Cystostomy infection 🐾

       N99.512   Cystostomy malfunction 🐾

       N99.518   Other cystostomy complication 🐾

    ● **N99.52   Complication of incontinent external stoma of urinary tract**

       N99.520   Hemorrhage of incontinent external stoma of urinary tract 🐾

       N99.521   Infection of incontinent external stoma of urinary tract 🐾
> Coding Clinic: 2016, Q4, P48

       N99.522   Malfunction of incontinent external stoma of urinary tract 🐾

       N99.523   Herniation of incontinent stoma of urinary tract 🐾
> Coding Clinic: 2016, Q4, P48

       N99.524   Stenosis of incontinent stoma of urinary tract 🐾
> Coding Clinic: 2016, Q4, P48

       N99.528   Other complication of incontinent external stoma of urinary tract 🐾

    ● **N99.53   Complication of continent stoma of urinary tract**

       N99.530   Hemorrhage of continent stoma of urinary tract 🐾

       N99.531   Infection of continent stoma of urinary tract 🐾

       N99.532   Malfunction of continent stoma of urinary tract 🐾

       N99.533   Herniation of continent stoma of urinary tract 🐾
> Coding Clinic: 2016, Q4, P48

       N99.534   Stenosis of continent stoma of urinary tract 🐾
> Coding Clinic: 2016, Q4, P48

       N99.538   Other complication of continent stoma of urinary tract 🐾

● **N99.6   Intraoperative hemorrhage and hematoma of a genitourinary system organ or structure complicating a procedure**
> **Excludes1**   intraoperative hemorrhage and hematoma of a genitourinary system organ or structure due to accidental puncture or laceration during a procedure (N99.7-)

    N99.61   Intraoperative hemorrhage and hematoma of a genitourinary system organ or structure complicating a genitourinary system procedure

    N99.62   Intraoperative hemorrhage and hematoma of a genitourinary system organ or structure complicating other procedure

● N99.7   Accidental puncture and laceration of a genitourinary system organ or structure during a procedure

    N99.71   Accidental puncture and laceration of a genitourinary system organ or structure during a genitourinary system procedure

    N99.72   Accidental puncture and laceration of a genitourinary system organ or structure during other procedure

● N99.8   Other intraoperative and postprocedural complications and disorders of genitourinary system
        Coding Clinic: 2016, Q4, P10

    N99.81   Other intraoperative complications of genitourinary system

  ● N99.82   Postprocedural hemorrhage of a genitourinary system organ or structure following a procedure

        N99.820   Postprocedural hemorrhage of a genitourinary system organ or structure following a genitourinary system procedure

        N99.821   Postprocedural hemorrhage of a genitourinary system organ or structure following other procedure

    N99.83   Residual ovary syndrome ♀

● N99.84   Postprocedural hematoma and seroma of a genitourinary system organ or structure following a procedure

        N99.840   Postprocedural hematoma of a genitourinary system organ or structure following a genitourinary system procedure

        N99.841   Postprocedural hematoma of a genitourinary system organ or structure following other procedure

        N99.842   Postprocedural seroma of a genitourinary system organ or structure following a genitourinary system procedure

        N99.843   Postprocedural seroma of a genitourinary system organ or structure following other procedure

    N99.85   Post endometrial ablation syndrome
         Coding Clinic: 2019, Q4, P12

    N99.89   Other postprocedural complications and disorders of genitourinary system

CHAPTER 15

PREGNANCY, CHILDBIRTH, AND THE PUERPERIUM (O00-O9A)

OGCR Chapter-Specific Coding Guidelines

15. Chapter 15: Pregnancy, Childbirth, and the Puerperium (O00-O9A)

a. General Rules for Obstetric Cases

1) Codes from Chapter 15 and sequencing priority
Obstetric cases require codes from Chapter 15, codes in the range O00-O9A, Pregnancy, Childbirth, and the Puerperium. Chapter 15 codes have sequencing priority over codes from other chapters. Additional codes from other chapters may be used in conjunction with Chapter 15 codes to further specify conditions. Should the provider document that the pregnancy is incidental to the encounter, then code Z33.1, Pregnant state, incidental, should be used in place of any Chapter 15 codes. It is the provider's responsibility to state that the condition being treated is not affecting the pregnancy.

2) Chapter 15 codes used only on the maternal record
Chapter 15 codes are to be used only on the maternal record, never on the record of the newborn.

3) Final character for trimester
The majority of codes in Chapter 15 have a final character indicating the trimester of pregnancy. The timeframes for the trimesters are indicated at the beginning of the chapter. If trimester is not a component of a code it is because the condition always occurs in a specific trimester, or the concept of trimester of pregnancy is not applicable. Certain codes have characters for only certain trimesters because the condition does not occur in all trimesters, but it may occur in more than just one.

Assignment of the final character for trimester should be based on the provider's documentation of the trimester (or number of weeks) for the current admission/encounter. This applies to the assignment of trimester for pre-existing conditions as well as those that develop during or are due to the pregnancy. The provider's documentation of the number of weeks may be used to assign the appropriate code identifying the trimester.

Whenever delivery occurs during the current admission, and there is an "in childbirth" option for the obstetric complication being coded, the "in childbirth" code should be assigned.

4) Selection of trimester for inpatient admissions that encompass more than one trimester
In instances when a patient is admitted to a hospital for complications of pregnancy during one trimester and remains in the hospital into a subsequent trimester, the trimester character for the antepartum complication code should be assigned on the basis of the trimester when the complication developed, not the trimester of the discharge. If the condition developed prior to the current admission/encounter or represents a pre-existing condition, the trimester character for the trimester at the time of the admission/encounter should be assigned.

5) Unspecified trimester
Each category that includes codes for trimester has a code for "unspecified trimester." The "unspecified trimester" code should rarely be used, such as when the documentation in the record is insufficient to determine the trimester and it is not possible to obtain clarification.

6) 7th character for Fetus Identification
Where applicable, a 7th character is to be assigned for certain categories (O31, O32, O33.3 - O33.6, O35, O36, O40, O41, O60.1, O60.2, O64, and O69) to identify the fetus for which the complication code applies.

Assign 7th character "0":
- For single gestations
- When the documentation in the record is insufficient to determine the fetus affected and it is not possible to obtain clarification.
- When it is not possible to clinically determine which fetus is affected.

b. Selection of OB Principal or First-listed Diagnosis

1) Routine outpatient prenatal visits
For routine outpatient prenatal visits when no complications are present, a code from category Z34, Encounter for supervision of normal pregnancy, should be used as the first-listed diagnosis. These codes should not be used in conjunction with Chapter 15 codes.

2) Supervision of High-Risk Pregnancy
Codes from category O09, Supervision of high-risk pregnancy, are intended for use only during the prenatal period. For complications during the labor or delivery episode as a result of a high-risk pregnancy, assign the applicable complication codes from Chapter 15. If there are no complications during the labor or delivery episode, assign code O80, Encounter for full-term uncomplicated delivery.

For routine prenatal outpatient visits for patients with high-risk pregnancies, a code from category O09, Supervision of high-risk pregnancy, should be used as the first-listed diagnosis. Secondary Chapter 15 codes may be used in conjunction with these codes if appropriate.

3) Episodes when no delivery occurs
In episodes when no delivery occurs, the principal diagnosis should correspond to the principal complication of the pregnancy which necessitated the encounter. Should more than one complication exist, all of which are treated or monitored, any of the complications codes may be sequenced first.

4) When a delivery occurs
When an obstetric patient is admitted and delivers during that admission, the condition that prompted the admission should be sequenced as the principal diagnosis. If multiple conditions prompted the admission, sequence the one most related to the delivery as the principal diagnosis. A code for any complication of the delivery should be assigned as an additional diagnosis. In cases of cesarean delivery, if the patient was admitted with a condition that resulted in the performance of a cesarean procedure, that condition should be selected as the principal diagnosis. If the reason for the admission was unrelated to the condition resulting in the cesarean delivery, the condition related to the reason for the admission should be selected as the principal diagnosis.

5) Outcome of delivery
A code from category Z37, Outcome of delivery, should be included on every maternal record when a delivery has occurred. These codes are not to be used on subsequent records or on the newborn record.

c. Pre-existing conditions versus conditions due to the pregnancy
Certain categories in Chapter 15 distinguish between conditions of the mother that existed prior to pregnancy (pre-existing) and those that are a direct result of pregnancy. When assigning codes from Chapter 15, it is important to assess if a condition was pre-existing prior to pregnancy or developed during or due to the pregnancy in order to assign the correct code.

Categories that do not distinguish between pre-existing and pregnancy-related conditions may be used for either. It is acceptable to use codes specifically for the puerperium with codes complicating pregnancy and childbirth if a condition arises postpartum during the delivery encounter.

d. Pre-existing hypertension in pregnancy
Category O10, Pre-existing hypertension complicating pregnancy, childbirth and the puerperium, includes codes for hypertensive heart and hypertensive chronic kidney disease. When assigning one of the O10 codes that includes hypertensive heart disease or hypertensive chronic kidney disease, it is necessary to add a secondary code from the appropriate hypertension category to specify the type of heart failure or chronic kidney disease.
See Section I.C.9. Hypertension.

e. Fetal Conditions Affecting the Management of the Mother

1) Codes from categories O35 and O36
Codes from categories O35, Maternal care for known or suspected fetal abnormality and damage, and O36, Maternal care for other fetal problems, are assigned only when the fetal condition is actually responsible for modifying the management of the mother, i.e., by requiring diagnostic studies, additional observation, special care, or termination of pregnancy. The fact that the fetal condition exists does not justify assigning a code from this series to the mother's record.

2) In utero surgery
In cases when surgery is performed on the fetus, a diagnosis code from category O35, Maternal care for known or suspected fetal abnormality and damage, should be assigned identifying the fetal condition. Assign the appropriate procedure code for the procedure performed.

No code from Chapter 16, the perinatal codes, should be used on the mother's record to identify fetal conditions. Surgery performed in utero on a fetus is still to be coded as an obstetric encounter.

f. HIV Infection in Pregnancy, Childbirth, and the Puerperium
During pregnancy, childbirth or the puerperium, a patient admitted because of an HIV-related illness should receive a principal diagnosis from subcategory O98.7-, Human immunodeficiency [HIV] disease complicating pregnancy, childbirth and the puerperium, followed by the code(s) for the HIV-related illness(es).

Patients with asymptomatic HIV infection status admitted during pregnancy, childbirth, or the puerperium should receive codes of O98.7- and Z21, Asymptomatic human immunodeficiency virus [HIV] infection status.

g. Diabetes mellitus in pregnancy
Diabetes mellitus is a significant complicating factor in pregnancy. Pregnant women who are diabetic should be assigned a code from category O24, Diabetes mellitus in pregnancy, childbirth, and the puerperium, first, followed by the appropriate diabetes code(s) (E08-E13) from Chapter 4.

h. Long-term use of insulin and oral hypoglycemics
See Section I.C.4.a.3 for information on the long-term use of insulin and oral hypoglycemic.

i. Gestational (pregnancy induced) diabetes
Gestational (pregnancy induced) diabetes can occur during the second and third trimester of pregnancy in women who were not diabetic prior to pregnancy. Gestational diabetes can cause complications in the pregnancy similar to those of pre-existing diabetes mellitus. It also puts the woman at greater risk of developing diabetes after the pregnancy. Codes for gestational diabetes are in subcategory O24.4, Gestational diabetes mellitus. No other code from category O24, Diabetes mellitus in pregnancy, childbirth, and the puerperium, should be used with a code from O24.4.

The codes under subcategory O24.4 include diet controlled, insulin controlled, and controlled by oral hypoglycemic drugs. If a patient with gestational diabetes is treated with both diet and insulin, only the code for insulin-controlled is required. If a patient with gestational diabetes is treated with both diet and oral hypoglycemic medications, only the code for "controlled by oral hypoglycemic drugs" is required. Code Z79.4, Long-term (current) use of insulin or code Z79.84, Long-term (current) use of oral hypoglycemic drugs, should not be assigned with codes from subcategory O24.4.

An abnormal glucose tolerance in pregnancy is assigned a code from subcategory O99.81, Abnormal glucose complicating pregnancy, childbirth, and the puerperium.

j. Sepsis and septic shock complicating abortion, pregnancy, childbirth and the puerperium
When assigning a Chapter 15 code for sepsis complicating abortion, pregnancy, childbirth, and the puerperium, a code for the specific type of infection should be assigned as an additional diagnosis. If severe sepsis is present, a code from subcategory R65.2, Severe sepsis, and code(s) for associated organ dysfunction(s) should also be assigned as additional diagnoses.

k. Puerperal sepsis
Code O85, Puerperal sepsis, should be assigned with a secondary code to identify the causal organism (e.g., for a bacterial infection, assign a code from category B95-B96, Bacterial infections in conditions classified elsewhere). A code from category A40, Streptococcal sepsis, or A41, Other sepsis, should not be used for puerperal sepsis. If applicable, use additional codes to identify severe sepsis (R65.2-) and any associated acute organ dysfunction.

l. Alcohol, tobacco and drug use during pregnancy, childbirth and the puerperium

1) Alcohol use during pregnancy, childbirth and the puerperium
Codes under subcategory O99.31, Alcohol use complicating pregnancy, childbirth, and the puerperium, should be assigned for any pregnancy case when a mother uses alcohol during the pregnancy or postpartum. A secondary code from category F10, Alcohol-related disorders, should also be assigned to identify manifestations of the alcohol use.

2) Tobacco use during pregnancy, childbirth, and the puerperium
Codes under subcategory O99.33, Smoking (tobacco) complicating pregnancy, childbirth, and the puerperium, should be assigned for any pregnancy case when a mother uses any type of tobacco product during the pregnancy or postpartum. A secondary code from category F17, Nicotine dependence, should also be assigned to identify the type of nicotine dependence.

3) Drug use during pregnancy, childbirth and the puerperium
Codes under subcategory O99.32, Drug use complicating pregnancy, childbirth, and the puerperium, should be assigned for any pregnancy case when a mother uses drugs during the pregnancy or postpartum. This can involve illegal drugs, or inappropriate use or abuse of prescription drugs. Secondary code(s) from categories F11-F16 and F18F19 should also be assigned to identify manifestations of the drug use.

m. Poisoning, toxic effects, adverse effects and underdosing in a pregnant patient
A code from subcategory O9A.2, Injury, poisoning and certain other consequences of external causes complicating pregnancy, childbirth, and the puerperium, should be sequenced first, followed by the appropriate injury, poisoning, toxic effect, adverse effect or underdosing code, and then the additional code(s) that specifies the condition caused by the poisoning, toxic effect, adverse effect or underdosing.
See Section I.C.19. Adverse effects, poisoning, underdosing and toxic effects.

n. Normal Delivery, Code O80

1) Encounter for full-term uncomplicated delivery
Code O80 should be assigned when a woman is admitted for a full-term normal delivery and delivers a single, healthy infant without any complications antepartum, during the delivery, or postpartum during the delivery episode. Code O80 is always a principal

diagnosis. It is not to be used if any other code from Chapter 15 is needed to describe a current complication of the antenatal, delivery, or perinatal period. Additional codes from other chapters may be used with code O80 if they are not related to or are in any way complicating the pregnancy.

2) Uncomplicated delivery with resolved antepartum complication
Code O80 may be used if the patient had a complication at some point during the pregnancy, but the complication is not present at the time of the admission for delivery.

3) Outcome of delivery for O80
Z37.0, Single live birth, is the only outcome of delivery code appropriate for use with O80.

o. The Peripartum and Postpartum Periods

1) Peripartum and Postpartum periods
The postpartum period begins immediately after delivery and continues for six weeks following delivery. The peripartum period is defined as the last month of pregnancy to five months postpartum.

2) Peripartum and postpartum complication
A postpartum complication is any complication occurring within the six-week period.

3) Pregnancy-related complications after 6 week period
Chapter 15 codes may also be used to describe pregnancy-related complications after the peripartum or postpartum period if the provider documents that a condition is pregnancy related.

4) Admission for routine postpartum care following delivery outside hospital
When the mother delivers outside the hospital prior to admission and is admitted for routine postpartum care and no complications are noted, code Z39.0, Encounter for care and examination of mother immediately after delivery, should be assigned as the principal diagnosis.

5) Pregnancy associated cardiomyopathy
Pregnancy associated cardiomyopathy, code O90.3, is unique in that it may be diagnosed in the third trimester of pregnancy but may continue to progress months after delivery. For this reason, it is referred to as peripartum cardiomyopathy. Code O90.3 is only for use when the cardiomyopathy develops as a result of pregnancy in a woman who did not have pre-existing heart disease.

p. Code O94, Sequelae of complication of pregnancy, childbirth, and the puerperium

1) Code O94
Code O94, Sequelae of complication of pregnancy, childbirth, and the puerperium, is for use in those cases when an initial complication of a pregnancy develops a sequelae requiring care or treatment at a future date.

2) After the initial postpartum period
This code may be used at any time after the initial postpartum period.

3) Sequencing of Code O94
This code, like all sequela codes, is to be sequenced following the code describing the sequelae of the complication.

q. Termination of Pregnancy and Spontaneous abortions

1) Abortion with Liveborn Fetus
When an attempted termination of pregnancy results in a liveborn fetus assign code Z33.2, Encounter for elective termination of pregnancy and a code from category Z37, Outcome of Delivery.

2) Retained Products of Conception following an abortion
Subsequent encounters for retained products of conception following a spontaneous abortion or elective termination of pregnancy, without complications are assigned O03.4, Incomplete spontaneous, abortion without complication, or codes O07.4, Failed attempted termination of pregnancy without complication. This advice is appropriate even when the patient was discharged previously with a discharge diagnosis of complete abortion. If the patient has a specific complication associated with the spontaneous abortion or elective termination of pregnancy in addition to retained products of conception, assign the appropriate complication in category O03 or O07 instead of code O03.4 or O07.4

3) Complications leading to abortion
Codes from Chapter 15 may be used as additional codes to identify any documented complications of the pregnancy in conjunction with codes in categories in O04, O07 and O08.

r. Abuse in a pregnant patient
For suspected or confirmed cases of abuse of a pregnant patient, a code(s) from subcategories O9A.3, Physical abuse complicating pregnancy, childbirth, and the puerperium, O9A.4, Sexual abuse complicating pregnancy, childbirth, and the puerperium, and O9A.5, Psychological abuse complicating pregnancy, childbirth, and the puerperium, should be sequenced first, followed by the appropriate codes (if applicable) to identify any associated current injury due to physical abuse, sexual abuse, and the perpetrator of abuse.
See Section I.C.19. Adult and child abuse, neglect and other maltreatment.

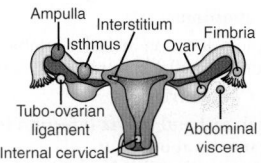

Figure 15-1 Implantation sites of ectopic pregnancy.

Item 15-1 Ectopic pregnancy most often occurs in the fallopian tube. Pregnancy outside the uterus may end in a lifethreatening rupture.

★ **(See Plate 4 of the Anatomy Illustrations.)**

CHAPTER 15

PREGNANCY, CHILDBIRTH, AND THE PUERPERIUM (O00-O9A)

Note: CODES FROM THIS CHAPTER ARE FOR USE ONLY ON MATERNAL RECORDS, NEVER ON NEWBORN RECORDS

Codes from this chapter are for use for conditions related to or aggravated by the pregnancy, childbirth, or by the puerperium (maternal causes or obstetric causes)

Trimesters are counted from the first day of the last menstrual period. They are defined as follows:

1st trimester - less than 14 weeks 0 days

2nd trimester - 14 weeks 0 days to less than 28 weeks 0 days

3rd trimester - 28 weeks 0 days until delivery

Use additional code from category Z3A, Weeks of gestation, to identify the specific week of the pregnancy, if known.

Excludes1 supervision of normal pregnancy (Z34.-)
Excludes2 mental and behavioral disorders associated with the puerperium (F53.-)
     obstetrical tetanus (A34)
     postpartum necrosis of pituitary gland (E23.0)
     puerperal osteomalacia (M83.0)

This chapter contains the following blocks:

O00-O08	Pregnancy with abortive outcome
O09	Supervision of high risk pregnancy
O10-O16	Edema, proteinuria and hypertensive disorders in pregnancy, childbirth and the puerperium
O20-O29	Other maternal disorders predominantly related to pregnancy
O30-O48	Maternal care related to the fetus and amniotic cavity and possible delivery problems
O60-O77	Complications of labor and delivery
O80, O82	Encounter for delivery
O85-O92	Complications predominantly related to the puerperium
O94-O9A	Other obstetric conditions, not elsewhere classified

PREGNANCY WITH ABORTIVE OUTCOME (O00-O08)

Excludes1 continuing pregnancy in multiple gestation after abortion of one fetus or more (O31.1-, O31.3-)
Coding Clinic: 2016, Q4, P130

● **O00 Ectopic pregnancy**
     Includes ruptured ectopic pregnancy
     Use additional code from category O08 to identify any associated complication

● **O00.0 Abdominal pregnancy**
     Excludes1 maternal care for viable fetus in abdominal pregnancy (O36.7-)
     Coding Clinic: 2016, Q4, P49

     O00.00 Abdominal pregnancy **without intrauterine pregnancy** ♀   M
        Abdominal pregnancy NOS

     O00.01 Abdominal pregnancy **with intrauterine pregnancy** ♀   M

● **O00.1 Tubal pregnancy**
     Fallopian pregnancy
     Rupture of (fallopian) tube due to pregnancy
     Tubal abortion
     Coding Clinic: 2016, Q4, P49

   ● O00.10 Tubal pregnancy **without intrauterine pregnancy**
        Tubal pregnancy NOS

     O00.101 **Right** tubal pregnancy without intrauterine pregnancy ♀   M

     O00.102 **Left** tubal pregnancy without intrauterine pregnancy ♀   M

     O00.109 **Unspecified** tubal pregnancy without intrauterine pregnancy ♀   M

   ● O00.11 Tubal pregnancy **with intrauterine pregnancy**

     O00.111 **Right** tubal pregnancy with intrauterine pregnancy ♀   M

     O00.112 **Left** tubal pregnancy with intrauterine pregnancy ♀   M

     O00.119 **Unspecified** tubal pregnancy with intrauterine pregnancy ♀   M

● **O00.2 Ovarian pregnancy**
     Coding Clinic: 2016, Q4, P49

   ● O00.20 Ovarian pregnancy **without intrauterine pregnancy**
        Ovarian pregnancy NOS

     O00.201 **Right** ovarian pregnancy without intrauterine pregnancy ♀   M

     O00.202 **Left** ovarian pregnancy without intrauterine pregnancy ♀   M

     O00.209 **Unspecified** ovarian pregnancy without intrauterine pregnancy ♀   M

   ● O00.21 Ovarian pregnancy **with intrauterine pregnancy**

     O00.211 **Right** ovarian pregnancy with intrauterine pregnancy ♀   M

     O00.212 **Left** ovarian pregnancy with intrauterine pregnancy ♀   M

     O00.219 **Unspecified** ovarian pregnancy with intrauterine pregnancy ♀   M

● **O00.8 Other ectopic pregnancy**
     Cervical pregnancy
     Cornual pregnancy
     Intraligamentous pregnancy
     Mural pregnancy
     Coding Clinic: 2016, Q4, P49

     O00.80 Other ectopic pregnancy **without intrauterine pregnancy** ♀   M
        Other ectopic pregnancy NOS

     O00.81 Other ectopic pregnancy **with intrauterine pregnancy** ♀   M

CHAPTER 15 (O00-O9A)

● O00.9   **Ectopic pregnancy, unspecified**
Coding Clinic: 2016, Q4, P49

     O00.90   **Unspecified ectopic pregnancy without intrauterine pregnancy** ♀   M
Ectopic pregnancy NOS

     O00.91   **Unspecified ectopic pregnancy with intrauterine pregnancy** ♀   M

● O01   **Hydatidiform mole**
Use additional code from category O08 to identify any associated complication

     Excludes1   chorioadenoma (destruens) (D39.2)
                  malignant hydatidiform mole (D39.2)

     O01.0   **Classical hydatidiform mole**   M
Complete hydatidiform mole

     O01.1   **Incomplete and partial hydatidiform mole** ♀   M

     O01.9   **Hydatidiform mole, unspecified** ♀   M
Trophoblastic disease NOS
Vesicular mole NOS

● O02   **Other abnormal products of conception**
Use additional code from category O08 to identify any associated complication

     Excludes1   papyraceous fetus (O31.0-)

     O02.0   **Blighted ovum and nonhydatidiform mole** ♀   M
Carneous mole   Molar pregnancy NEC
Fleshy mole   Pathological ovum
Intrauterine mole NOS

     O02.1   **Missed abortion** ♀   M
Early fetal death, before completion of 20 weeks of gestation, with retention of dead fetus

         Excludes1   failed induced abortion (O07.-)
                  fetal death (intrauterine) (late) (O36.4)
                  missed abortion with blighted ovum (O02.0)
                  missed abortion with hydatidiform mole (O01.-)
                  missed abortion with nonhydatidiform (O02.0)
                  missed abortion with other abnormal products of conception (O02.8-)
                  missed delivery (O36.4)
                  stillbirth (P95)

         Coding Clinic: 2019, Q3, P12

● O02.8   **Other specified abnormal products of conception**

         Excludes1   abnormal products of conception with blighted ovum (O02.0)
                  abnormal products of conception with hydatidiform mole (O01.-)
                  abnormal products of conception with nonhydatidiform mole (O02.0)

     O02.81   **Inappropriate change in quantitative human chorionic gonadotropin (hCG) in early pregnancy** ♀   M
Biochemical pregnancy
Chemical pregnancy
Inappropriate level of quantitative human chorionic gonadotropin (hCG) for gestational age in early pregnancy

     O02.89   **Other abnormal products of conception** ♀   M

     O02.9   **Abnormal product of conception, unspecified** ♀   M

● O03   **Spontaneous abortion**
Note: Incomplete abortion includes retained products of conception following spontaneous abortion.

     Includes   miscarriage

     O03.0   **Genital tract and pelvic infection following incomplete spontaneous abortion** ♀   M
Endometritis following incomplete spontaneous abortion
Oophoritis following incomplete spontaneous abortion
Parametritis following incomplete spontaneous abortion
Pelvic peritonitis following incomplete spontaneous abortion
Salpingitis following incomplete spontaneous abortion
Salpingo-oophoritis following incomplete spontaneous abortion

         Excludes1   sepsis following incomplete spontaneous abortion (O03.37)
                  urinary tract infection following incomplete spontaneous abortion (O03.38)

     O03.1   **Delayed or excessive hemorrhage following incomplete spontaneous abortion** ♀   M
Afibrinogenemia following incomplete spontaneous abortion
Defibrination syndrome following incomplete spontaneous abortion
Hemolysis following incomplete spontaneous abortion
Intravascular coagulation following incomplete spontaneous abortion

     O03.2   **Embolism following incomplete spontaneous abortion** ♀   M
Air embolism following incomplete spontaneous abortion
Amniotic fluid embolism following incomplete spontaneous abortion
Blood-clot embolism following incomplete spontaneous abortion
Embolism NOS following incomplete spontaneous abortion
Fat embolism following incomplete spontaneous abortion
Pulmonary embolism following incomplete spontaneous abortion
Pyemic embolism following incomplete spontaneous abortion
Septic or septicopyemic embolism following incomplete spontaneous abortion
Soap embolism following incomplete spontaneous abortion

● O03.3   **Other and unspecified complications following incomplete spontaneous abortion**

     O03.30   **Unspecified complication following incomplete spontaneous abortion** ♀   M

     O03.31   **Shock following incomplete spontaneous abortion** ♀   M
Circulatory collapse following incomplete spontaneous abortion
Shock (postprocedural) following incomplete spontaneous abortion

         Excludes1   shock due to infection following incomplete spontaneous abortion (O03.37)

     O03.32   **Renal failure following incomplete spontaneous abortion** ♀   M
Kidney failure (acute) following incomplete spontaneous abortion
Oliguria following incomplete spontaneous abortion
Renal shutdown following incomplete spontaneous abortion
Renal tubular necrosis following incomplete spontaneous abortion
Uremia following incomplete spontaneous abortion

Item 15–2 A **hydatidiform** mole is an overproduction of placental tissue. The tumor secretes a hormone, chorionic gonadotropic hormone (CGH), that indicates a positive pregnancy test. There is no viable fetus. More than 80% of hydatidiform moles are noncancerous.

▶ New   ⇒ Revised   ~~deleted~~ Deleted   Excludes 1   Excludes 2   Includes   Use additional   Code first   Code also   Key words
OGCR Official Guidelines   X Assign placeholder X   ● Use Additional Character(s)   ▶ Manifestation Code   🅗 Hierarchical Condition Category   **Coding Clinic**

O03.33   **Metabolic disorder** following incomplete spontaneous abortion ♀   **M**

O03.34   **Damage to pelvic organs** following incomplete spontaneous abortion ♀   **M**
> Laceration, perforation, tear or chemical damage of bladder following incomplete spontaneous abortion
> Laceration, perforation, tear or chemical damage of bowel following incomplete spontaneous abortion
> Laceration, perforation, tear or chemical damage of broad ligament following incomplete spontaneous abortion
> Laceration, perforation, tear or chemical damage of cervix following incomplete spontaneous abortion
> Laceration, perforation, tear or chemical damage of periurethral tissue following incomplete spontaneous abortion
> Laceration, perforation, tear or chemical damage of uterus following incomplete spontaneous abortion
> Laceration, perforation, tear or chemical damage of vagina following incomplete spontaneous abortion

O03.35   **Other venous complications** following incomplete spontaneous abortion ♀   **M**

O03.36   **Cardiac arrest** following incomplete spontaneous abortion ♀   **M**

O03.37   **Sepsis** following incomplete spontaneous abortion ♀   **M**
> Use additional code to identify infectious agent (B95-B97)
> Use additional code to identify severe sepsis, if applicable (R65.2-)
> **Excludes1**   septic or septicopyemic embolism following incomplete spontaneous abortion (O03.2)

O03.38   **Urinary tract infection** following incomplete spontaneous abortion ♀   **M**
> Cystitis following incomplete spontaneous abortion

O03.39   **Incomplete spontaneous abortion with other complications** ♀   **M**

O03.4   **Incomplete spontaneous abortion without complication** ♀   **M**

O03.5   **Genital tract and pelvic infection** following complete or unspecified spontaneous abortion ♀   **M**
> Endometritis following complete or unspecified spontaneous abortion
> Oophoritis following complete or unspecified spontaneous abortion
> Parametritis following complete or unspecified spontaneous abortion
> Pelvic peritonitis following complete or unspecified spontaneous abortion
> Salpingitis following complete or unspecified spontaneous abortion
> Salpingo-oophoritis following complete or unspecified spontaneous abortion
> **Excludes1**   sepsis following complete or unspecified spontaneous abortion (O03.87)
> urinary tract infection following complete or unspecified spontaneous abortion (O03.88)

O03.6   **Delayed or excessive hemorrhage** following complete or unspecified spontaneous abortion ♀   **M**
> Afibrinogenemia following complete or unspecified spontaneous abortion
> Defibrination syndrome following complete or unspecified spontaneous abortion
> Hemolysis following complete or unspecified spontaneous abortion
> Intravascular coagulation following complete or unspecified spontaneous abortion

O03.7   **Embolism** following complete or unspecified spontaneous abortion ♀   **M**
> Air embolism following complete or unspecified spontaneous abortion
> Amniotic fluid embolism following complete or unspecified spontaneous abortion
> Blood-clot embolism following complete or unspecified spontaneous abortion
> Embolism NOS following complete or unspecified spontaneous abortion
> Fat embolism following complete or unspecified spontaneous abortion
> Pulmonary embolism following complete or unspecified spontaneous abortion
> Pyemic embolism following complete or unspecified spontaneous abortion
> Septic or septicopyemic embolism following complete or unspecified spontaneous abortion
> Soap embolism following complete or unspecified spontaneous abortion

● O03.8   **Other and unspecified complications following complete or unspecified spontaneous abortion**

O03.80   **Unspecified complication** following complete or unspecified spontaneous abortion ♀   **M**

O03.81   **Shock** following complete or unspecified spontaneous abortion ♀   **M**
> Circulatory collapse following complete or unspecified spontaneous abortion
> Shock (postprocedural) following complete or unspecified spontaneous abortion
> **Excludes1**   shock due to infection following complete or unspecified spontaneous abortion (O03.87)

O03.82   **Renal failure** following complete or unspecified spontaneous abortion ♀   **M**
> Kidney failure (acute) following complete or unspecified spontaneous abortion
> Oliguria following complete or unspecified spontaneous abortion
> Renal shutdown following complete or unspecified spontaneous abortion
> Renal tubular necrosis following complete or unspecified spontaneous abortion
> Uremia following complete or unspecified spontaneous abortion

O03.83   **Metabolic disorder** following complete or unspecified spontaneous abortion ♀   **M**

O03.84   **Damage to pelvic organs** following complete or unspecified spontaneous abortion ♀   **M**
> Laceration, perforation, tear or chemical damage of bladder following complete or unspecified spontaneous abortion
> Laceration, perforation, tear or chemical damage of bowel following complete or unspecified spontaneous abortion
> Laceration, perforation, tear or chemical damage of broad ligament following complete or unspecified spontaneous abortion
> Laceration, perforation, tear or chemical damage of cervix following complete or unspecified spontaneous abortion
> Laceration, perforation, tear or chemical damage of periurethral tissue following complete or unspecified spontaneous abortion
> Laceration, perforation, tear or chemical damage of uterus following complete or unspecified spontaneous abortion
> Laceration, perforation, tear or chemical damage of vagina following complete or unspecified spontaneous abortion

O03.85 **Other venous complications following complete or unspecified spontaneous abortion** ♀ M

O03.86 **Cardiac arrest following complete or unspecified spontaneous abortion** ♀ M

O03.87 **Sepsis following complete or unspecified spontaneous abortion** ♀ M

Use additional code to identify infectious agent (B95-B97)

Use additional code to identify severe sepsis, if applicable (R65.2-)

Excludes1 septic or septicopyemic embolism following complete or unspecified spontaneous abortion (O03.7)

O03.88 **Urinary tract infection following complete or unspecified spontaneous abortion** ♀ M

Cystitis following complete or unspecified spontaneous abortion

O03.89 **Complete or unspecified spontaneous abortion with other complications** ♀ M

O03.9 **Complete or unspecified spontaneous abortion without complication** ♀ M

Miscarriage NOS
Spontaneous abortion NOS

● O04 **Complications following (induced) termination of pregnancy**

Includes complications following (induced) termination of pregnancy

Excludes1 encounter for elective termination of pregnancy, uncomplicated (Z33.2)

failed attempted termination of pregnancy (O07.-)

O04.5 **Genital tract and pelvic infection following (induced) termination of pregnancy** ♀ M

Endometritis following (induced) termination of pregnancy
Oophoritis following (induced) termination of pregnancy
Parametritis following (induced) termination of pregnancy
Pelvic peritonitis following (induced) termination of pregnancy
Salpingitis following (induced) termination of pregnancy
Salpingo-oophoritis following (induced) termination of pregnancy

Excludes1 sepsis following (induced) termination of pregnancy (O04.87)

urinary tract infection following (induced) termination of pregnancy (O04.88)

O04.6 **Delayed or excessive hemorrhage following (induced) termination of pregnancy** ♀ M

Afibrinogenemia following (induced) termination of pregnancy
Defibrination syndrome following (induced) termination of pregnancy
Hemolysis following (induced) termination of pregnancy
Intravascular coagulation following (induced) termination of pregnancy

Coding Clinic: 2019, Q3, P12

O04.7 **Embolism following (induced) termination of pregnancy** ♀ M

Air embolism following (induced) termination of pregnancy
Amniotic fluid embolism following (induced) termination of pregnancy
Blood-clot embolism following (induced) termination of pregnancy
Embolism NOS following (induced) termination of pregnancy
Fat embolism following (induced) termination of pregnancy
Pulmonary embolism following (induced) termination of pregnancy
Pyemic embolism following (induced) termination of pregnancy
Septic or septicopyemic embolism following (induced) termination of pregnancy
Soap embolism following (induced) termination of pregnancy

● O04.8 **(Induced) termination of pregnancy with other and unspecified complications**

O04.80 **(Induced) termination of pregnancy with unspecified complications** ♀ M

O04.81 **Shock following (induced) termination of pregnancy** ♀ M

Circulatory collapse following (induced) termination of pregnancy
Shock (postprocedural) following (induced) termination of pregnancy

Excludes1 shock due to infection following (induced) termination of pregnancy (O04.87)

O04.82 **Renal failure following (induced) termination of pregnancy** ♀ M

Kidney failure (acute) following (induced) termination of pregnancy
Oliguria following (induced) termination of pregnancy
Renal shutdown following (induced) termination of pregnancy
Renal tubular necrosis following (induced) termination of pregnancy
Uremia following (induced) termination of pregnancy

O04.83 **Metabolic disorder following (induced) termination of pregnancy** ♀ M

O04.84 **Damage to pelvic organs following (induced) termination of pregnancy** ♀ M

Laceration, perforation, tear or chemical damage of bladder following (induced) termination of pregnancy
Laceration, perforation, tear or chemical damage of bowel following (induced) termination of pregnancy
Laceration, perforation, tear or chemical damage of broad ligament following (induced) termination of pregnancy
Laceration, perforation, tear or chemical damage of cervix following (induced) termination of pregnancy
Laceration, perforation, tear or chemical damage of periurethral tissue following (induced) termination of pregnancy
Laceration, perforation, tear or chemical damage of uterus following (induced) termination of pregnancy
Laceration, perforation, tear or chemical damage of vagina following (induced) termination of pregnancy

O04.85　**Other venous complications** following (induced) termination of pregnancy ♀　　M

O04.86　**Cardiac arrest** following (induced) termination of pregnancy ♀　　M

O04.87　**Sepsis** following (induced) termination of pregnancy ♀　　M

　　Use additional code to identify infectious agent (B95-B97)

　　Use additional code to identify severe sepsis, if applicable (R65.2-)

　　Excludes1　septic or septicopyemic embolism following (induced) termination of pregnancy (O04.7)

O04.88　**Urinary tract infection** following (induced) termination of pregnancy ♀　　M

　　Cystitis following (induced) termination of pregnancy

O04.89　(Induced) termination of pregnancy with **other** complications ♀　　M

● **O07**　**Failed attempted termination** of pregnancy

　　Includes　failure of attempted induction of termination of pregnancy

　　　　incomplete elective abortion

　　Excludes1　incomplete spontaneous abortion (O03.0-)

O07.0　**Genital tract and pelvic infection** following failed attempted termination of pregnancy ♀　　M

　　Endometritis following failed attempted termination of pregnancy

　　Oophoritis following failed attempted termination of pregnancy

　　Parametritis following failed attempted termination of pregnancy

　　Pelvic peritonitis following failed attempted termination of pregnancy

　　Salpingitis following failed attempted termination of pregnancy

　　Salpingo-oophoritis following failed attempted termination of pregnancy

　　Excludes1　sepsis following failed attempted termination of pregnancy (O07.37)

　　　　urinary tract infection following failed attempted termination of pregnancy (O07.38)

O07.1　**Delayed or excessive hemorrhage** following failed attempted termination of pregnancy ♀　　M

　　Afibrinogenemia following failed attempted termination of pregnancy

　　Defibrination syndrome following failed attempted termination of pregnancy

　　Hemolysis following failed attempted termination of pregnancy

　　Intravascular coagulation following failed attempted termination of pregnancy

O07.2　**Embolism** following failed attempted termination of pregnancy ♀　　M

　　Air embolism following failed attempted termination of pregnancy

　　Amniotic fluid embolism following failed attempted termination of pregnancy

　　Blood-clot embolism following failed attempted termination of pregnancy

　　Embolism NOS following failed attempted termination of pregnancy

　　Fat embolism following failed attempted termination of pregnancy

　　Pulmonary embolism following failed attempted termination of pregnancy

　　Pyemic embolism following failed attempted termination of pregnancy

　　Septic or septicopyemic embolism following failed attempted termination of pregnancy

　　Soap embolism following failed attempted termination of pregnancy

● O07.3　**Failed attempted termination of pregnancy with other and unspecified complications**

O07.30　**Failed attempted termination of pregnancy with unspecified complications** ♀　　M

O07.31　**Shock** following failed attempted termination of pregnancy ♀　　M

　　Circulatory collapse following failed attempted termination of pregnancy

　　Shock (postprocedural) following failed attempted termination of pregnancy

　　Excludes1　shock due to infection following failed attempted termination of pregnancy (O07.37)

O07.32　**Renal failure** following failed attempted termination of pregnancy ♀　　M

　　Kidney failure (acute) following failed attempted termination of pregnancy

　　Oliguria following failed attempted termination of pregnancy

　　Renal shutdown following failed attempted termination of pregnancy

　　Renal tubular necrosis following failed attempted termination of pregnancy

　　Uremia following failed attempted termination of pregnancy

O07.33　**Metabolic disorder** following failed attempted termination of pregnancy ♀　　M

O07.34　**Damage to pelvic organs** following failed attempted termination of pregnancy ♀　　M

　　Laceration, perforation, tear or chemical damage of bladder following failed attempted termination of pregnancy

　　Laceration, perforation, tear or chemical damage of bowel following failed attempted termination of pregnancy

　　Laceration, perforation, tear or chemical damage of broad ligament following failed attempted termination of pregnancy

　　Laceration, perforation, tear or chemical damage of cervix following failed attempted termination of pregnancy

　　Laceration, perforation, tear or chemical damage of periurethral tissue following failed attempted termination of pregnancy

　　Laceration, perforation, tear or chemical damage of uterus following failed attempted termination of pregnancy

　　Laceration, perforation, tear or chemical damage of vagina following failed attempted termination of pregnancy

O07.35　**Other venous complications** following failed attempted termination of pregnancy ♀　　M

O07.36　**Cardiac arrest** following failed attempted termination of pregnancy ♀　　M

O07.37　**Sepsis** following failed attempted termination of pregnancy ♀　　M

　　Use additional code (B95-B97), to identify infectious agent

　　Use additional code (R65.2-) to identify severe sepsis, if applicable

　　Excludes1　septic or septicopyemic embolism following failed attempted termination of pregnancy (O07.2)

O07.38　**Urinary tract infection** following failed attempted termination of pregnancy ♀　　M

　　Cystitis following failed attempted termination of pregnancy

O07.39　**Failed attempted termination of pregnancy with other complications** ♀　　M

O07.4　**Failed attempted termination of pregnancy without complication** ♀　　M

CHAPTER 15 (O00-O9A)

● **O08 Complications following ectopic and molar pregnancy**
This category is for use with categories O00-O02 to identify any associated complications.

O08.0 Genital tract and pelvic infection following ectopic and molar pregnancy ♀   M
Endometritis following ectopic and molar pregnancy
Oophoritis following ectopic and molar pregnancy
Parametritis following ectopic and molar pregnancy
Pelvic peritonitis following ectopic and molar pregnancy
Salpingitis following ectopic and molar pregnancy
Salpingo-oophoritis following ectopic and molar pregnancy
> **Excludes1**   sepsis following ectopic and molar pregnancy (O08.82)
> urinary tract infection (O08.83)

O08.1 Delayed or excessive hemorrhage following ectopic and molar pregnancy ♀   M
Afibrinogenemia following ectopic and molar pregnancy
Defibrination syndrome following ectopic and molar pregnancy
Hemolysis following ectopic and molar pregnancy
Intravascular coagulation following ectopic and molar pregnancy
> **Excludes1**   delayed or excessive hemorrhage due to incomplete abortion (O03.1)

O08.2 Embolism following ectopic and molar pregnancy ♀   M
Air embolism following ectopic and molar pregnancy
Amniotic fluid embolism following ectopic and molar pregnancy
Blood-clot embolism following ectopic and molar pregnancy
Embolism NOS following ectopic and molar pregnancy
Fat embolism following ectopic and molar pregnancy
Pulmonary embolism following ectopic and molar pregnancy
Pyemic embolism following ectopic and molar pregnancy
Septic or septicopyemic embolism following ectopic and molar pregnancy
Soap embolism following ectopic and molar pregnancy

O08.3 Shock following ectopic and molar pregnancy ♀   M
Circulatory collapse following ectopic and molar pregnancy
Shock (postprocedural) following ectopic and molar pregnancy
> **Excludes1**   shock due to infection following ectopic and molar pregnancy (O08.82)

O08.4 Renal failure following ectopic and molar pregnancy ♀   M
Kidney failure (acute) following ectopic and molar pregnancy
Oliguria following ectopic and molar pregnancy
Renal shutdown following ectopic and molar pregnancy
Renal tubular necrosis following ectopic and molar pregnancy
Uremia following ectopic and molar pregnancy

O08.5 Metabolic disorders following an ectopic and molar pregnancy ♀   M

O08.6 Damage to pelvic organs and tissues following an ectopic and molar pregnancy ♀   M
Laceration, perforation, tear or chemical damage of bladder following an ectopic and molar pregnancy
Laceration, perforation, tear or chemical damage of bowel following an ectopic and molar pregnancy
Laceration, perforation, tear or chemical damage of broad ligament following an ectopic and molar pregnancy
Laceration, perforation, tear or chemical damage of cervix following an ectopic and molar pregnancy
Laceration, perforation, tear or chemical damage of periurethral tissue following an ectopic and molar pregnancy
Laceration, perforation, tear or chemical damage of uterus following an ectopic and molar pregnancy
Laceration, perforation, tear or chemical damage of vagina following an ectopic and molar pregnancy

O08.7 Other venous complications following an ectopic and molar pregnancy ♀   M

● **O08.8 Other complications following an ectopic and molar pregnancy**

O08.81 Cardiac arrest following an ectopic and molar pregnancy ♀   M

O08.82 Sepsis following ectopic and molar pregnancy ♀   M
> Use additional code (B95-B97), to identify infectious agent
> Use additional code (R65.2-) to identify severe sepsis, if applicable
> **Excludes1**   septic or septicopyemic embolism following ectopic and molar pregnancy (O08.2)

O08.83 Urinary tract infection following an ectopic and molar pregnancy ♀   M
Cystitis following an ectopic and molar pregnancy

O08.89 Other complications following an ectopic and molar pregnancy ♀   M

O08.9 Unspecified complication following an ectopic and molar pregnancy ♀   M

SUPERVISION OF HIGH RISK PREGNANCY (O09)

● **O09 Supervision of high risk pregnancy**
Coding Clinic: 2016, Q4, P125, 150

● **O09.0 Supervision of pregnancy with history of infertility**

O09.00 Supervision of pregnancy with history of infertility, unspecified trimester ♀   M

O09.01 Supervision of pregnancy with history of infertility, first trimester ♀   M

O09.02 Supervision of pregnancy with history of infertility, second trimester ♀   M

O09.03 Supervision of pregnancy with history of infertility, third trimester ♀   M

● **O09.1 Supervision of pregnancy with history of ectopic pregnancy**
Coding Clinic: 2016, Q4, P49-50

O09.10 Supervision of pregnancy with history of ectopic pregnancy, unspecified trimester ♀   M

O09.11 Supervision of pregnancy with history of ectopic pregnancy, first trimester ♀   M

O09.12 Supervision of pregnancy with history of ectopic pregnancy, second trimester ♀   M

O09.13 Supervision of pregnancy with history of ectopic pregnancy, third trimester ♀   M

● **O09.A Supervision of pregnancy with history of molar pregnancy**
Coding Clinic: 2016, Q4, P50

O09.A0 Supervision of pregnancy with history of molar pregnancy, unspecified trimester ♀   M

O09.A1 Supervision of pregnancy with history of molar pregnancy, first trimester ♀   M

O09.A2 Supervision of pregnancy with history of molar pregnancy, second trimester ♀   M

O09.A3 Supervision of pregnancy with history of molar pregnancy, third trimester ♀   M

▶ New   ⇒ Revised   ~~deleted~~ Deleted   Excludes 1   Excludes 2   Includes   Use additional   Code first   Code also   Key words
OGCR Official Guidelines   X Assign placeholder X   ● Use Additional Character(s)   ▶ Manifestation Code   🐧 Hierarchical Condition Category   **Coding Clinic**

● **O09.2   Supervision of pregnancy with other poor reproductive or obstetric history**

    Excludes2   pregnancy care for patient with history of recurrent pregnancy loss (O26.2-)

  ● **O09.21   Supervision of pregnancy with history of pre-term labor**

     O09.211   Supervision of pregnancy with history of pre-term labor, first trimester ♀   M

     O09.212   Supervision of pregnancy with history of pre-term labor, second trimester ♀ M

     O09.213   Supervision of pregnancy with history of pre-term labor, third trimester ♀   M

     O09.219   Supervision of pregnancy with history of pre-term labor, unspecified trimester ♀   M

  ● **O09.29   Supervision of pregnancy with other poor reproductive or obstetric history**

     Supervision of pregnancy with history of neonatal death

     Supervision of pregnancy with history of stillbirth

     O09.291   Supervision of pregnancy with other poor reproductive or obstetric history, first trimester ♀   M

     O09.292   Supervision of pregnancy with other poor reproductive or obstetric history, second trimester ♀   M

     O09.293   Supervision of pregnancy with other poor reproductive or obstetric history, third trimester ♀   M

     O09.299   Supervision of pregnancy with other poor reproductive or obstetric history, unspecified trimester ♀   M

● **O09.3   Supervision of pregnancy with insufficient antenatal care**

     Supervision of concealed pregnancy

     Supervision of hidden pregnancy

   O09.30   Supervision of pregnancy with insufficient antenatal care, unspecified trimester ♀   M

   O09.31   Supervision of pregnancy with insufficient antenatal care, first trimester ♀   M

   O09.32   Supervision of pregnancy with insufficient antenatal care, second trimester ♀   M

   O09.33   Supervision of pregnancy with insufficient antenatal care, third trimester ♀   M

● **O09.4   Supervision of pregnancy with grand multiparity**

   O09.40   Supervision of pregnancy with grand multiparity, unspecified trimester ♀   M

   O09.41   Supervision of pregnancy with grand multiparity, first trimester ♀   M

   O09.42   Supervision of pregnancy with grand multiparity, second trimester ♀   M

   O09.43   Supervision of pregnancy with grand multiparity, third trimester ♀   M

● **O09.5   Supervision of elderly primigravida and multigravida**

     Pregnancy for a female 35 years and older at expected date of delivery

  ● **O09.51   Supervision of elderly primigravida**

     O09.511   Supervision of elderly primigravida, first trimester ♀   M

     O09.512   Supervision of elderly primigravida, second trimester ♀   M

     O09.513   Supervision of elderly primigravida, third trimester ♀   M

     O09.519   Supervision of elderly primigravida, unspecified trimester ♀   M

● **O09.52   Supervision of elderly multigravida**

     O09.521   Supervision of elderly multigravida, first trimester ♀   M

     O09.522   Supervision of elderly multigravida, second trimester ♀   M

     O09.523   Supervision of elderly multigravida, third trimester ♀   M

       Coding Clinic: 2016, Q4, P150

     O09.529   Supervision of elderly multigravida, unspecified trimester ♀   M

● **O09.6   Supervision of young primigravida and multigravida**

     Supervision of pregnancy for a female less than 16 years old at expected date of delivery

  ● **O09.61   Supervision of young primigravida**

     O09.611   Supervision of young primigravida, first trimester ♀   M

     O09.612   Supervision of young primigravida, second trimester ♀   M

     O09.613   Supervision of young primigravida, third trimester ♀   M

     O09.619   Supervision of young primigravida, unspecified trimester ♀   M

  ● **O09.62   Supervision of young multigravida**

     O09.621   Supervision of young multigravida, first trimester ♀   M

     O09.622   Supervision of young multigravida, second trimester ♀   M

     O09.623   Supervision of young multigravida, third trimester ♀   M

     O09.629   Supervision of young multigravida, unspecified trimester ♀   M

● **O09.7   Supervision of high risk pregnancy due to social problems**

   O09.70   Supervision of high risk pregnancy due to social problems, unspecified trimester ♀   M

   O09.71   Supervision of high risk pregnancy due to social problems, first trimester ♀   M

   O09.72   Supervision of high risk pregnancy due to social problems, second trimester ♀   M

   O09.73   Supervision of high risk pregnancy due to social problems, third trimester ♀   M

● **O09.8   Supervision of other high risk pregnancies**

  ● **O09.81   Supervision of pregnancy resulting from assisted reproductive technology**

     Supervision of pregnancy resulting from in-vitro fertilization

    Excludes2   gestational carrier status (Z33.3)

     O09.811   Supervision of pregnancy resulting from assisted reproductive technology, first trimester ♀   M

     O09.812   Supervision of pregnancy resulting from assisted reproductive technology, second trimester ♀   M

     O09.813   Supervision of pregnancy resulting from assisted reproductive technology, third trimester ♀   M

     O09.819   Supervision of pregnancy resulting from assisted reproductive technology, unspecified trimester ♀   M

● **O09.82   Supervision of pregnancy with history of in utero procedure during previous pregnancy**

 O09.821   Supervision of pregnancy with history of in utero procedure during previous pregnancy, **first trimester** ♀ M

 O09.822   Supervision of pregnancy with history of in utero procedure during previous pregnancy, **second trimester** ♀ M

 O09.823   Supervision of pregnancy with history of in utero procedure during previous pregnancy, **third trimester** ♀ M

 O09.829   Supervision of pregnancy with history of in utero procedure during previous pregnancy, **unspecified trimester** ♀ M

  Excludes1 supervision of pregnancy affected by in utero procedure during current pregnancy (O35.7)

● **O09.89   Supervision of other high risk pregnancies**

 O09.891   Supervision of other high risk pregnancies, **first trimester** ♀ M

 O09.892   Supervision of other high risk pregnancies, **second trimester** ♀ M

 O09.893   Supervision of other high risk pregnancies, **third trimester** ♀ M

 O09.899   Supervision of other high risk pregnancies, **unspecified trimester** ♀ M

● **O09.9   Supervision of high risk pregnancy, unspecified**

 O09.90   Supervision of high risk pregnancy, unspecified, **unspecified trimester** ♀ M

 O09.91   Supervision of high risk pregnancy, unspecified, **first trimester** ♀ M

 O09.92   Supervision of high risk pregnancy, unspecified, **second trimester** ♀ M

 O09.93   Supervision of high risk pregnancy, unspecified, **third trimester** ♀ M

EDEMA, PROTEINURIA AND HYPERTENSIVE DISORDERS IN PREGNANCY, CHILDBIRTH AND THE PUERPERIUM (O10-O16)

● **O10   Pre-existing hypertension complicating pregnancy, childbirth and the puerperium**

 Includes pre-existing hypertension with pre-existing proteinuria complicating pregnancy, childbirth and the puerperium

 Excludes2 pre-existing hypertension with superimposed pre-eclampsia complicating pregnancy, childbirth and the puerperium (O11.-)

 Coding Clinic: 2016, Q4, P50

● **O10.0   Pre-existing essential hypertension complicating pregnancy, childbirth and the puerperium**

 Any condition in I10 specified as a reason for obstetric care during pregnancy, childbirth or the puerperium

 ● **O10.01   Pre-existing essential hypertension complicating pregnancy**

  O10.011   Pre-existing essential hypertension complicating pregnancy, **first trimester** ♀ M

  O10.012   Pre-existing essential hypertension complicating pregnancy, **second trimester** ♀ M

  O10.013   Pre-existing essential hypertension complicating pregnancy, **third trimester** ♀ M

  O10.019   Pre-existing essential hypertension complicating pregnancy, **unspecified trimester** ♀ M

 O10.02   Pre-existing essential hypertension complicating **childbirth** ♀ M

 O10.03   Pre-existing essential hypertension complicating the **puerperium** ♀ M

● **O10.1   Pre-existing hypertensive heart disease complicating pregnancy, childbirth and the puerperium**

 Any condition in I11 specified as a reason for obstetric care during pregnancy, childbirth or the puerperium

 Use additional code from I11 to identify the type of hypertensive heart disease

 ● **O10.11   Pre-existing hypertensive heart disease complicating pregnancy**

  O10.111   Pre-existing hypertensive heart disease complicating pregnancy, **first trimester** ♀ M

  O10.112   Pre-existing hypertensive heart disease complicating pregnancy, **second trimester** ♀ M

  O10.113   Pre-existing hypertensive heart disease complicating pregnancy, **third trimester** ♀ M

  O10.119   Pre-existing hypertensive heart disease complicating pregnancy, **unspecified trimester** ♀ M

 O10.12   Pre-existing hypertensive heart disease complicating **childbirth** ♀ M

 O10.13   Pre-existing hypertensive heart disease complicating the **puerperium** ♀ M

● **O10.2   Pre-existing hypertensive chronic kidney disease complicating pregnancy, childbirth and the puerperium**

 Any condition in I12 specified as a reason for obstetric care during pregnancy, childbirth or the puerperium

 Use additional code from I12 to identify the type of hypertensive chronic kidney disease

 ● **O10.21   Pre-existing hypertensive chronic kidney disease complicating pregnancy**

  O10.211   Pre-existing hypertensive chronic kidney disease complicating pregnancy, **first trimester** ♀ M

  O10.212   Pre-existing hypertensive chronic kidney disease complicating pregnancy, **second trimester** ♀ M

  O10.213   Pre-existing hypertensive chronic kidney disease complicating pregnancy, **third trimester** ♀ M

  O10.219   Pre-existing hypertensive chronic kidney disease complicating pregnancy, **unspecified trimester** ♀ M

 O10.22   Pre-existing hypertensive chronic kidney disease complicating **childbirth** ♀ M

 O10.23   Pre-existing hypertensive chronic kidney disease complicating the **puerperium** ♀ M

● **O10.3**   Pre-existing hypertensive heart and chronic kidney disease complicating pregnancy, childbirth and the puerperium

     Any condition in I13 specified as a reason for obstetric care during pregnancy, childbirth or the puerperium

     Use additional code from I13 to identify the type of hypertensive heart and chronic kidney disease

    ● **O10.31**   Pre-existing hypertensive heart and chronic kidney disease complicating pregnancy

       O10.311   Pre-existing hypertensive heart and chronic kidney disease complicating pregnancy, first trimester ♀   M

       O10.312   Pre-existing hypertensive heart and chronic kidney disease complicating pregnancy, second trimester ♀   M

       O10.313   Pre-existing hypertensive heart and chronic kidney disease complicating pregnancy, third trimester ♀   M

       O10.319   Pre-existing hypertensive heart and chronic kidney disease complicating pregnancy, unspecified trimester ♀   M

    O10.32   Pre-existing hypertensive heart and chronic kidney disease complicating childbirth ♀   M

    O10.33   Pre-existing hypertensive heart and chronic kidney disease complicating the puerperium ♀   M

● **O10.4**   Pre-existing secondary hypertension complicating pregnancy, childbirth and the puerperium

     Any condition in I15 specified as a reason for obstetric care during pregnancy, childbirth or the puerperium

     Use additional code from I15 to identify the type of secondary hypertension

    ● **O10.41**   Pre-existing secondary hypertension complicating pregnancy

       O10.411   Pre-existing secondary hypertension complicating pregnancy, first trimester ♀   M

       O10.412   Pre-existing secondary hypertension complicating pregnancy, second trimester ♀   M

       O10.413   Pre-existing secondary hypertension complicating pregnancy, third trimester ♀   M

       O10.419   Pre-existing secondary hypertension complicating pregnancy, unspecified trimester ♀   M

    O10.42   Pre-existing secondary hypertension complicating childbirth ♀   M

    O10.43   Pre-existing secondary hypertension complicating the puerperium ♀   M

● **O10.9**   Unspecified pre-existing hypertension complicating pregnancy, childbirth and the puerperium

    ● **O10.91**   Unspecified pre-existing hypertension complicating pregnancy

       O10.911   Unspecified pre-existing hypertension complicating pregnancy, first trimester ♀   M

       O10.912   Unspecified pre-existing hypertension complicating pregnancy, second trimester ♀   M

       O10.913   Unspecified pre-existing hypertension complicating pregnancy, third trimester ♀   M

       O10.919   Unspecified pre-existing hypertension complicating pregnancy, unspecified trimester ♀   M

    O10.92   Unspecified pre-existing hypertension complicating childbirth ♀   M

    O10.93   Unspecified pre-existing hypertension complicating the puerperium ♀   M

● **O11**   Pre-existing hypertension with pre-eclampsia

    Includes   conditions in O10 complicated by pre-eclampsia pre-eclampsia superimposed pre-existing hypertension

     Use additional code from O10 to identify the type of hypertension

     Coding Clinic: 2016, Q4, P50

    O11.1   Pre-existing hypertension with pre-eclampsia, first trimester ♀   M

    O11.2   Pre-existing hypertension with pre-eclampsia, second trimester ♀   M

    O11.3   Pre-existing hypertension with pre-eclampsia, third trimester ♀   M

    O11.4   Pre-existing hypertension with pre-eclampsia, complicating childbirth ♀   M

    O11.5   Pre-existing hypertension with pre-eclampsia, complicating the puerperium ♀   M

    O11.9   Pre-existing hypertension with pre-eclampsia, unspecified trimester ♀   M

● **O12**   Gestational [pregnancy-induced] edema and proteinuria without hypertension

     Coding Clinic: 2016, Q4, P50

    ● **O12.0**   Gestational edema

       O12.00   Gestational edema, unspecified trimester ♀   M

       O12.01   Gestational edema, first trimester ♀   M

       O12.02   Gestational edema, second trimester ♀   M

       O12.03   Gestational edema, third trimester ♀   M

       O12.04   Gestational edema, complicating childbirth ♀   M

       O12.05   Gestational edema, complicating the puerperium ♀   M

    ● **O12.1**   Gestational proteinuria

       O12.10   Gestational proteinuria, unspecified trimester ♀   M

       O12.11   Gestational proteinuria, first trimester ♀   M

       O12.12   Gestational proteinuria, second trimester ♀   M

       O12.13   Gestational proteinuria, third trimester ♀   M

       O12.14   Gestational proteinuria, complicating childbirth ♀   M

       O12.15   Gestational proteinuria, complicating the puerperium ♀   M

    ● **O12.2**   Gestational edema with proteinuria

       O12.20   Gestational edema with proteinuria, unspecified trimester ♀   M

       O12.21   Gestational edema with proteinuria, first trimester ♀   M

       O12.22   Gestational edema with proteinuria, second trimester ♀   M

       O12.23   Gestational edema with proteinuria, third trimester ♀   M

       O12.24   Gestational edema with proteinuria, complicating childbirth ♀   M

       O12.25   Gestational edema with proteinuria, complicating the puerperium ♀   M

CHAPTER 15 (O00-O9A)

● O13 Gestational [pregnancy-induced] hypertension without significant proteinuria
    Includes   gestational hypertension NOS
                transient hypertension of pregnancy ♀
    Coding Clinic: 2016, Q4, P50

O13.1 Gestational [pregnancy-induced] hypertension without significant proteinuria, first trimester ♀   M

O13.2 Gestational [pregnancy-induced] hypertension without significant proteinuria, second trimester ♀   M

O13.3 Gestational [pregnancy-induced] hypertension without significant proteinuria, third trimester ♀   M

O13.4 Gestational [pregnancy-induced] hypertension without significant proteinuria, complicating childbirth ♀   M

O13.5 Gestational [pregnancy-induced] hypertension without significant proteinuria, complicating the puerperium ♀   M

O13.9 Gestational [pregnancy-induced] hypertension without significant proteinuria, unspecified trimester ♀   M

● O14 Pre-eclampsia
    Excludes1   pre-existing hypertension with pre-eclampsia (O11)
    Coding Clinic: 2016, Q4, P50

● O14.0 Mild to moderate pre-eclampsia

    O14.00 Mild to moderate pre-eclampsia, unspecified trimester ♀   M

    O14.02 Mild to moderate pre-eclampsia, second trimester ♀   M

    O14.03 Mild to moderate pre-eclampsia, third trimester ♀   M

    O14.04 Mild to moderate pre-eclampsia, complicating childbirth ♀
            Coding Clinic: 2019, Q2, P8   M

    O14.05 Mild to moderate pre-eclampsia, complicating the puerperium ♀   M

● O14.1 Severe pre-eclampsia
    Excludes1   HELLP syndrome (O14.2-)
    H=hemolysis, EL=elevated liver enzymes, LP=low platelet count
    Coding Clinic: 2019, Q3, P12

    O14.10 Severe pre-eclampsia, unspecified trimester ♀ M

    O14.12 Severe pre-eclampsia, second trimester ♀ M

    O14.13 Severe pre-eclampsia, third trimester ♀ M

    O14.14 Severe pre-eclampsia complicating childbirth ♀   M

    O14.15 Severe pre-eclampsia, complicating the puerperium ♀   M

● O14.2 HELLP syndrome
    Severe pre-eclampsia with hemolysis, elevated liver enzymes and low platelet count (HELLP)

    O14.20 HELLP syndrome (HELLP), unspecified trimester ♀   M

    O14.22 HELLP syndrome (HELLP), second trimester ♀   M

    O14.23 HELLP syndrome (HELLP), third trimester ♀ M

    O14.24 HELLP syndrome, complicating childbirth ♀ M

    O14.25 HELLP syndrome, complicating the puerperium ♀   M

● O14.9 Unspecified pre-eclampsia

    O14.90 Unspecified pre-eclampsia, unspecified trimester ♀   M

    O14.92 Unspecified pre-eclampsia, second trimester ♀   M

    O14.93 Unspecified pre-eclampsia, third trimester ♀   M

    O14.94 Unspecified pre-eclampsia, complicating childbirth ♀   M

    O14.95 Unspecified pre-eclampsia, complicating the puerperium ♀   M

● O15 Eclampsia
    Includes   convulsions following conditions in O10-O14 and O16

● O15.0 Eclampsia complicating pregnancy
    Coding Clinic: 2016, Q4, P50

    O15.00 Eclampsia complicating pregnancy, unspecified trimester ♀   M

    O15.02 Eclampsia complicating pregnancy, second trimester ♀   M

    O15.03 Eclampsia complicating pregnancy, third trimester ♀   M

O15.1 Eclampsia complicating labor ♀   M

O15.2 Eclampsia complicating the puerperium ♀   M

O15.9 Eclampsia, unspecified as to time period ♀   M
    Eclampsia NOS

● O16 Unspecified maternal hypertension
    Coding Clinic: 2016, Q4, P50

O16.1 Unspecified maternal hypertension, first trimester ♀   M

O16.2 Unspecified maternal hypertension, second trimester ♀   M

O16.3 Unspecified maternal hypertension, third trimester ♀ M

O16.4 Unspecified maternal hypertension, complicating childbirth ♀   M

O16.5 Unspecified maternal hypertension, complicating the puerperium ♀   M

O16.9 Unspecified maternal hypertension, unspecified trimester ♀   M

OTHER MATERNAL DISORDERS PREDOMINANTLY RELATED TO PREGNANCY (O20-O29)

    Excludes2   maternal care related to the fetus and amniotic cavity and possible delivery problems (O30-O48)
                maternal diseases classifiable elsewhere but complicating pregnancy, labor and delivery, and the puerperium (O98-O99)

● O20 Hemorrhage in early pregnancy
    Includes   hemorrhage before completion of 20 weeks gestation
    Excludes1   pregnancy with abortive outcome (O00-O08)

O20.0 Threatened abortion ♀   M
    Hemorrhage specified as due to threatened abortion

O20.8 Other hemorrhage in early pregnancy ♀   M

O20.9 Hemorrhage in early pregnancy, unspecified ♀   M

● O21 Excessive vomiting in pregnancy

O21.0 Mild hyperemesis gravidarum ♀   M
    Hyperemesis gravidarum, mild or unspecified, starting before the end of the 20th week of gestation

O21.1 Hyperemesis gravidarum with metabolic disturbance ♀   M
    Hyperemesis gravidarum, starting before the end of the 20th week of gestation, with metabolic disturbance such as carbohydrate depletion
    Hyperemesis gravidarum, starting before the end of the 20th week of gestation, with metabolic disturbance such as dehydration
    Hyperemesis gravidarum, starting before the end of the 20th week of gestation, with metabolic disturbance such as electrolyte imbalance

O21.2 Late vomiting of pregnancy ♀   M
    Excessive vomiting starting after 20 completed weeks of gestation

O21.8 Other vomiting complicating pregnancy ♀   M
    Vomiting due to diseases classified elsewhere, complicating pregnancy
    Use additional code, to identify cause

O21.9 Vomiting of pregnancy, unspecified ♀   M

▶ New   ⇒ Revised   ~~deleted~~ Deleted   Excludes 1   Excludes 2   Includes   Use additional   Code first   Code also   Key words
OGCR Official Guidelines   X Assign placeholder X   ● Use Additional Character(s)   ▶ Manifestation Code   🐾 Hierarchical Condition Category   **Coding Clinic**

● **O22 Venous complications and hemorrhoids in pregnancy**

    Excludes1 venous complications of:
            abortion NOS (O03.9)
            ectopic or molar pregnancy (O08.7)
            failed attempted abortion (O07.35)
            induced abortion (O04.85)
            spontaneous abortion (O03.89)

    Excludes2 obstetric pulmonary embolism (O88.-)
            venous complications and hemorrhoids of
              childbirth and the puerperium (O87.-)

● **O22.0 Varicose veins of lower extremity in pregnancy**
      Varicose veins NOS in pregnancy

    O22.00 **Varicose veins of lower extremity in pregnancy, unspecified trimester** ♀   M

    O22.01 **Varicose veins of lower extremity in pregnancy, first trimester** ♀   M

    O22.02 **Varicose veins of lower extremity in pregnancy, second trimester** ♀   M

    O22.03 **Varicose veins of lower extremity in pregnancy, third trimester** ♀   M

● **O22.1 Genital varices in pregnancy**
      Perineal varices in pregnancy
      Vaginal varices in pregnancy
      Vulval varices in pregnancy

    O22.10 **Genital varices in pregnancy, unspecified trimester** ♀   M

    O22.11 **Genital varices in pregnancy, first trimester** ♀ M

    O22.12 **Genital varices in pregnancy, second trimester** ♀   M

    O22.13 **Genital varices in pregnancy, third trimester** ♀ M

● **O22.2 Superficial thrombophlebitis in pregnancy**
      Phlebitis in pregnancy NOS
      Thrombophlebitis of legs in pregnancy
      Thrombosis in pregnancy NOS

      Use additional code to identify the superficial
         thrombophlebitis (I80.0-)

    O22.20 **Superficial thrombophlebitis in pregnancy, unspecified trimester** ♀   M

    O22.21 **Superficial thrombophlebitis in pregnancy, first trimester** ♀   M

    O22.22 **Superficial thrombophlebitis in pregnancy, second trimester** ♀   M

    O22.23 **Superficial thrombophlebitis in pregnancy, third trimester** ♀   M

● **O22.3 Deep phlebothrombosis in pregnancy**
      Deep vein thrombosis, antepartum

  ⇒ Use additional code to identify the deep vein
        thrombosis (I82.4-, I82.5-, I82.62-, I82.72-)

      Use additional code, if applicable, for associated long-
        term (current) use of anticoagulants (Z79.01)

    O22.30 **Deep phlebothrombosis in pregnancy, unspecified trimester** ♀   M

    O22.31 **Deep phlebothrombosis in pregnancy, first trimester** ♀   M

    O22.32 **Deep phlebothrombosis in pregnancy, second trimester** ♀   M

    O22.33 **Deep phlebothrombosis in pregnancy, third trimester** ♀   M

● **O22.4 Hemorrhoids in pregnancy**

    O22.40 **Hemorrhoids in pregnancy, unspecified trimester** ♀   M

    O22.41 **Hemorrhoids in pregnancy, first trimester** ♀ M

    O22.42 **Hemorrhoids in pregnancy, second trimester** ♀   M

    O22.43 **Hemorrhoids in pregnancy, third trimester** ♀ M

● **O22.5 Cerebral venous thrombosis in pregnancy**
      Cerebrovenous sinus thrombosis in pregnancy

    O22.50 **Cerebral venous thrombosis in pregnancy, unspecified trimester** ♀   M

    O22.51 **Cerebral venous thrombosis in pregnancy, first trimester** ♀   M

    O22.52 **Cerebral venous thrombosis in pregnancy, second trimester** ♀   M

    O22.53 **Cerebral venous thrombosis in pregnancy, third trimester** ♀   M

● **O22.8 Other venous complications in pregnancy**

  ● **O22.8X Other venous complications in pregnancy**

        O22.8X1 **Other venous complications in pregnancy, first trimester** ♀   M

        O22.8X2 **Other venous complications in pregnancy, second trimester** ♀   M

        O22.8X3 **Other venous complications in pregnancy, third trimester** ♀   M

        O22.8X9 **Other venous complications in pregnancy, unspecified trimester** ♀   M

● **O22.9 Venous complication in pregnancy, unspecified**
      Gestational phlebitis NOS
      Gestational phlebopathy NOS
      Gestational thrombosis NOS

    O22.90 **Venous complication in pregnancy, unspecified, unspecified trimester** ♀   M

    O22.91 **Venous complication in pregnancy, unspecified, first trimester** ♀   M

    O22.92 **Venous complication in pregnancy, unspecified, second trimester** ♀   M

    O22.93 **Venous complication in pregnancy, unspecified, third trimester** ♀   M

● **O23 Infections of genitourinary tract in pregnancy**

      Use additional code to identify organism (B95.-, B96.-)

    Excludes2 gonococcal infections complicating pregnancy,
              childbirth and the puerperium (O98.2)
            infections with a predominantly sexual mode of
              transmission NOS complicating pregnancy,
              childbirth and the puerperium (O98.3)
            syphilis complicating pregnancy, childbirth and
              the puerperium (O98.1)
            tuberculosis of genitourinary system
              complicating pregnancy, childbirth and the
              puerperium (O98.0)
            venereal disease NOS complicating pregnancy,
              childbirth and the puerperium (O98.3)

● **O23.0 Infections of kidney in pregnancy**
      Pyelonephritis in pregnancy

    O23.00 **Infections of kidney in pregnancy, unspecified trimester** ♀   M

    O23.01 **Infections of kidney in pregnancy, first trimester** ♀   M

    O23.02 **Infections of kidney in pregnancy, second trimester** ♀   M

    O23.03 **Infections of kidney in pregnancy, third trimester** ♀   M

● **O23.1 Infections of bladder in pregnancy**

    O23.10 **Infections of bladder in pregnancy, unspecified trimester** ♀   M

    O23.11 **Infections of bladder in pregnancy, first trimester** ♀   M

    O23.12 **Infections of bladder in pregnancy, second trimester** ♀   M

    O23.13 **Infections of bladder in pregnancy, third trimester** ♀   M

● **O23.2**   Infections of urethra in pregnancy

    O23.20   Infections of urethra in pregnancy, unspecified trimester ♀   M

    O23.21   Infections of urethra in pregnancy, first trimester ♀   M

    O23.22   Infections of urethra in pregnancy, second trimester ♀   M

    O23.23   Infections of urethra in pregnancy, third trimester ♀   M

● **O23.3**   Infections of other parts of urinary tract in pregnancy

    O23.30   Infections of other parts of urinary tract in pregnancy, unspecified trimester ♀   M

    O23.31   Infections of other parts of urinary tract in pregnancy, first trimester ♀   M

    O23.32   Infections of other parts of urinary tract in pregnancy, second trimester ♀   M

    O23.33   Infections of other parts of urinary tract in pregnancy, third trimester ♀   M

● **O23.4**   Unspecified infection of urinary tract in pregnancy

    O23.40   Unspecified infection of urinary tract in pregnancy, unspecified trimester ♀   M

    O23.41   Unspecified infection of urinary tract in pregnancy, first trimester ♀   M

    O23.42   Unspecified infection of urinary tract in pregnancy, second trimester ♀   M

    O23.43   Unspecified infection of urinary tract in pregnancy, third trimester ♀   M

● **O23.5**   Infections of the genital tract in pregnancy

   ● **O23.51**   Infection of cervix in pregnancy

      O23.511   Infections of cervix in pregnancy, first trimester ♀   M

      O23.512   Infections of cervix in pregnancy, second trimester ♀   M

      O23.513   Infections of cervix in pregnancy, third trimester ♀   M

      O23.519   Infections of cervix in pregnancy, unspecified trimester ♀   M

   ● **O23.52**   Salpingo-oophoritis in pregnancy

       Oophoritis = inflammation of ovary
       Salpingitis = inflammation of fallopian tube
       Oophoritis in pregnancy
       Salpingitis in pregnancy

      O23.521   Salpingo-oophoritis in pregnancy, first trimester ♀   M

      O23.522   Salpingo-oophoritis in pregnancy, second trimester ♀   M

      O23.523   Salpingo-oophoritis in pregnancy, third trimester ♀   M

      O23.529   Salpingo-oophoritis in pregnancy, unspecified trimester ♀   M

   ● **O23.59**   Infection of other part of genital tract in pregnancy

      O23.591   Infection of other part of genital tract in pregnancy, first trimester ♀   M

      O23.592   Infection of other part of genital tract in pregnancy, second trimester ♀   M

      O23.593   Infection of other part of genital tract in pregnancy, third trimester ♀   M

      O23.599   Infection of other part of genital tract in pregnancy, unspecified trimester ♀   M

● **O23.9**   Unspecified genitourinary tract infection in pregnancy

       Genitourinary tract infection in pregnancy NOS

    O23.90   Unspecified genitourinary tract infection in pregnancy, unspecified trimester ♀   M

    O23.91   Unspecified genitourinary tract infection in pregnancy, first trimester ♀   M

    O23.92   Unspecified genitourinary tract infection in pregnancy, second trimester ♀   M

    O23.93   Unspecified genitourinary tract infection in pregnancy, third trimester ♀   M

OGCR   Section I.C.15.g.

> Diabetes mellitus in pregnancy
>
> Diabetes mellitus is a significant complicating factor in pregnancy. Pregnant women who are diabetic should be assigned a code from category O24, Diabetes mellitus in pregnancy, childbirth, and the puerperium, first, followed by the appropriate diabetes code(s) (E08-E13) from Chapter 4.

● **O24**   Diabetes mellitus in pregnancy, childbirth, and the puerperium

   ● **O24.0**   Pre-existing type 1 diabetes mellitus, in pregnancy, childbirth and the puerperium

       Juvenile onset diabetes mellitus, in pregnancy, childbirth and the puerperium
       Ketosis-prone diabetes mellitus in pregnancy, childbirth and the puerperium

       Use additional code from category E10 to further identify any manifestations

    ● **O24.01**   Pre-existing type 1 diabetes mellitus, in pregnancy

      O24.011   Pre-existing type 1 diabetes mellitus, in pregnancy, first trimester ♀   M

      O24.012   Pre-existing type 1 diabetes mellitus, in pregnancy, second trimester ♀   M

      O24.013   Pre-existing type 1 diabetes mellitus, in pregnancy, third trimester ♀   M

      O24.019   Pre-existing type 1 diabetes mellitus, in pregnancy, unspecified trimester ♀   M

    O24.02   Pre-existing type 1 diabetes mellitus, in childbirth ♀   M

    O24.03   Pre-existing type 1 diabetes mellitus, in the puerperium ♀   M

   ● **O24.1**   Pre-existing type 2 diabetes mellitus, in pregnancy, childbirth and the puerperium

       Insulin-resistant diabetes mellitus in pregnancy, childbirth and the puerperium

       Use additional code (for):
          from category E11 to further identify any manifestations
          long-term (current) use of insulin (Z79.4)

    ● **O24.11**   Pre-existing type 2 diabetes mellitus, in pregnancy

      O24.111   Pre-existing type 2 diabetes mellitus, in pregnancy, first trimester ♀   M

      O24.112   Pre-existing type 2 diabetes mellitus, in pregnancy, second trimester ♀   M

      O24.113   Pre-existing type 2 diabetes mellitus, in pregnancy, third trimester ♀   M

      O24.119   Pre-existing type 2 diabetes mellitus, in pregnancy, unspecified trimester ♀   M

    O24.12   Pre-existing type 2 diabetes mellitus, in childbirth ♀   M

    O24.13   Pre-existing type 2 diabetes mellitus, in the puerperium ♀   M

▶ New   ⇒ Revised   ~~deleted~~ Deleted   Excludes 1   Excludes 2   Includes   Use additional   Code first   Code also   Key words

OGCR Official Guidelines   X Assign placeholder X   ● Use Additional Character(s)   ▶ Manifestation Code   🐄 Hierarchical Condition Category   **Coding Clinic**

● **O24.3**   Unspecified pre-existing diabetes mellitus in pregnancy, childbirth and the puerperium

> Use additional code (for):
> from category E11 to further identify any manifestation
> long-term (current) use of insulin (Z79.4)

  ● **O24.31**   Unspecified pre-existing diabetes mellitus in pregnancy

     O24.311   Unspecified pre-existing diabetes mellitus in pregnancy, first trimester ♀   M

     O24.312   Unspecified pre-existing diabetes mellitus in pregnancy, second trimester ♀   M

     O24.313   Unspecified pre-existing diabetes mellitus in pregnancy, third trimester ♀   M

     O24.319   Unspecified pre-existing diabetes mellitus in pregnancy, unspecified trimester ♀   M

   O24.32   Unspecified pre-existing diabetes mellitus in childbirth ♀   M

   O24.33   Unspecified pre-existing diabetes mellitus in the puerperium ♀   M

● **O24.4**   **Gestational diabetes mellitus**

> Diabetes mellitus arising in pregnancy
> Gestational diabetes mellitus NOS
> **Coding Clinic: 2016, Q4, P50, 126**

  ● **O24.41**   Gestational diabetes mellitus in pregnancy

     O24.410   Gestational diabetes mellitus in pregnancy, diet controlled ♀   M

     O24.414   Gestational diabetes mellitus in pregnancy, insulin controlled ♀   M

     O24.415   Gestational diabetes mellitus in pregnancy, controlled by oral hypoglycemic drugs ♀   M

> Gestational diabetes mellitus in pregnancy, controlled by oral antidiabetic drugs
> **Coding Clinic: 2016, Q4, P50**

     O24.419   Gestational diabetes mellitus in pregnancy, unspecified control ♀   M

> **Coding Clinic: 2015, Q4, P34**

  ● **O24.42**   Gestational diabetes mellitus in childbirth

     O24.420   Gestational diabetes mellitus in childbirth, diet controlled ♀   M

     O24.424   Gestational diabetes mellitus in childbirth, insulin controlled ♀   M

     O24.425   Gestational diabetes mellitus in childbirth, controlled by oral hypoglycemic drugs ♀   M

> Gestational diabetes mellitus in childbirth, controlled by oral antidiabetic drugs
> **Coding Clinic: 2016, Q4, P50**

     O24.429   Gestational diabetes mellitus in childbirth, unspecified control ♀   M

OGCR Section I.C.15.i.

Gestational (pregnancy induced) diabetes

Gestational (pregnancy induced) diabetes can occur during the second and third trimester of pregnancy in women who were not diabetic prior to pregnancy. Gestational diabetes can cause complications in the pregnancy similar to those of pre-existing diabetes mellitus. It also puts the woman at greater risk of developing diabetes after the pregnancy. Codes for gestational diabetes are in subcategory O24.4, Gestational diabetes mellitus. No other code from category O24, Diabetes mellitus in pregnancy, childbirth, and the puerperium, should be used with a code from O24.4

The codes under subcategory O24.4 include diet controlled, insulin controlled, **and controlled by oral hypoglycemic drugs.** If a patient with gestational diabetes is treated with both diet and insulin, only the code for insulin-controlled is required. **If a patient with gestational diabetes is treated with both diet and oral hypoglycemic medications, only the code for "controlled by oral hypoglycemic drugs" is required.** Code Z79.4, Long-term (current) use of insulin **or code Z79.84, Long-term (current) use of oral hypoglycemic drugs,** should not be assigned with codes from subcategory O24.4.

An abnormal glucose tolerance in pregnancy is assigned a code from subcategory O99.81, Abnormal glucose complicating pregnancy, childbirth, and the puerperium.

  ● **O24.43**   Gestational diabetes mellitus in the puerperium

     O24.430   Gestational diabetes mellitus in the puerperium, diet controlled ♀   M

     O24.434   Gestational diabetes mellitus in the puerperium, insulin controlled ♀   M

     O24.435   Gestational diabetes mellitus in puerperium, controlled by oral hypoglycemic drugs ♀   M

> Gestational diabetes mellitus in puerperium, controlled by oral antidiabetic drugs
> **Coding Clinic: 2016, Q4, P50**

     O24.439   Gestational diabetes mellitus in the puerperium, unspecified control ♀   M

● **O24.8**   **Other pre-existing diabetes mellitus in pregnancy, childbirth, and the puerperium**

> Use additional code (for):
> from categories E08, E09 and E13 to further identify any manifestation
> long-term (current) use of insulin (Z79.4)

  ● **O24.81**   Other pre-existing diabetes mellitus in pregnancy

     O24.811   Other pre-existing diabetes mellitus in pregnancy, first trimester ♀   M

     O24.812   Other pre-existing diabetes mellitus in pregnancy, second trimester ♀   M

     O24.813   Other pre-existing diabetes mellitus in pregnancy, third trimester ♀   M

     O24.819   Other pre-existing diabetes mellitus in pregnancy, unspecified trimester ♀   M

   O24.82   Other pre-existing diabetes mellitus in childbirth ♀   M

   O24.83   Other pre-existing diabetes mellitus in the puerperium ♀   M

● **O24.9**   **Unspecified diabetes mellitus in pregnancy, childbirth and the puerperium**

> Use additional code for long-term (current) use of insulin (Z79.4)
> *Unknown whether patient was diabetic before pregnancy occurred*

  ● **O24.91**   Unspecified diabetes mellitus in pregnancy

     O24.911   Unspecified diabetes mellitus in pregnancy, first trimester ♀   M

     O24.912   Unspecified diabetes mellitus in pregnancy, second trimester ♀   M

CHAPTER 15 (O00-O9A)

O24.913	Unspecified diabetes mellitus in pregnancy, third trimester ♀	M
O24.919	Unspecified diabetes mellitus in pregnancy, unspecified trimester ♀	M
O24.92	Unspecified diabetes mellitus in childbirth ♀	M
O24.93	Unspecified diabetes mellitus in the puerperium ♀	M

● **O25   Malnutrition in pregnancy, childbirth and the puerperium**
  ● **O25.1   Malnutrition in pregnancy**

O25.10	Malnutrition in pregnancy, unspecified trimester ♀	M
O25.11	Malnutrition in pregnancy, first trimester ♀	M
O25.12	Malnutrition in pregnancy, second trimester ♀	M
O25.13	Malnutrition in pregnancy, third trimester ♀	M

     O25.2   Malnutrition in childbirth ♀   M
     O25.3   Malnutrition in the puerperium ♀   M

● **O26   Maternal care for other conditions predominantly related to pregnancy**
  ● **O26.0   Excessive weight gain in pregnancy**

         Excludes2   gestational edema (O12.0, O12.2)

O26.00	Excessive weight gain in pregnancy, unspecified trimester ♀	M
O26.01	Excessive weight gain in pregnancy, first trimester ♀	M
O26.02	Excessive weight gain in pregnancy, second trimester ♀	M
O26.03	Excessive weight gain in pregnancy, third trimester ♀	M

  ● **O26.1   Low weight gain in pregnancy**

O26.10	Low weight gain in pregnancy, unspecified trimester ♀	M
O26.11	Low weight gain in pregnancy, first trimester ♀	M
O26.12	Low weight gain in pregnancy, second trimester ♀	M
O26.13	Low weight gain in pregnancy, third trimester ♀	M

  ● **O26.2   Pregnancy care for patient with recurrent pregnancy loss**

O26.20	Pregnancy care for patient with recurrent pregnancy loss, unspecified trimester ♀	M
O26.21	Pregnancy care for patient with recurrent pregnancy loss, first trimester ♀	M
O26.22	Pregnancy care for patient with recurrent pregnancy loss, second trimester ♀	M
O26.23	Pregnancy care for patient with recurrent pregnancy loss, third trimester ♀	M

  ● **O26.3   Retained intrauterine contraceptive device in pregnancy**

O26.30	Retained intrauterine contraceptive device in pregnancy, unspecified trimester ♀	M
O26.31	Retained intrauterine contraceptive device in pregnancy, first trimester ♀	M
O26.32	Retained intrauterine contraceptive device in pregnancy, second trimester ♀	M
O26.33	Retained intrauterine contraceptive device in pregnancy, third trimester ♀	M

  ● **O26.4   Herpes gestationis**

O26.40	Herpes gestationis, unspecified trimester ♀	M
O26.41	Herpes gestationis, first trimester ♀	M
O26.42	Herpes gestationis, second trimester ♀	M
O26.43	Herpes gestationis, third trimester ♀	M

● **O26.5   Maternal hypotension syndrome**
         Supine hypotensive syndrome

O26.50	Maternal hypotension syndrome, unspecified trimester ♀	M
O26.51	Maternal hypotension syndrome, first trimester ♀	M
O26.52	Maternal hypotension syndrome, second trimester ♀	M
O26.53	Maternal hypotension syndrome, third trimester ♀	M

● **O26.6   Liver and biliary tract disorders in pregnancy, childbirth and the puerperium**

         Use additional code to identify the specific disorder

         Excludes2   hepatorenal syndrome following labor and delivery (O90.4)

  ● **O26.61   Liver and biliary tract disorders in pregnancy**

O26.611	Liver and biliary tract disorders in pregnancy, first trimester ♀	M
O26.612	Liver and biliary tract disorders in pregnancy, second trimester ♀	M
O26.613	Liver and biliary tract disorders in pregnancy, third trimester ♀	M
O26.619	Liver and biliary tract disorders in pregnancy, unspecified trimester ♀	M

     O26.62   Liver and biliary tract disorders in childbirth ♀   M
     O26.63   Liver and biliary tract disorders in the puerperium ♀   M

● **O26.7   Subluxation of symphysis (pubis) in pregnancy, childbirth and the puerperium**

         Excludes1   traumatic separation of symphysis (pubis) during childbirth (O71.6)

  ● **O26.71   Subluxation of symphysis (pubis) in pregnancy**

O26.711	Subluxation of symphysis (pubis) in pregnancy, first trimester ♀	M
O26.712	Subluxation of symphysis (pubis) in pregnancy, second trimester ♀	M
O26.713	Subluxation of symphysis (pubis) in pregnancy, third trimester ♀	M
O26.719	Subluxation of symphysis (pubis) in pregnancy, unspecified trimester ♀	M

     O26.72   Subluxation of symphysis (pubis) in childbirth ♀   M
     O26.73   Subluxation of symphysis (pubis) in the puerperium ♀   M

● **O26.8   Other specified pregnancy related conditions**
  ● **O26.81   Pregnancy related exhaustion and fatigue**

O26.811	Pregnancy related exhaustion and fatigue, first trimester ♀	M
O26.812	Pregnancy related exhaustion and fatigue, second trimester ♀	M
O26.813	Pregnancy related exhaustion and fatigue, third trimester ♀	M
O26.819	Pregnancy related exhaustion and fatigue, unspecified trimester ♀	M

  ● **O26.82   Pregnancy related peripheral neuritis**

O26.821	Pregnancy related peripheral neuritis, first trimester ♀	M
O26.822	Pregnancy related peripheral neuritis, second trimester ♀	M
O26.823	Pregnancy related peripheral neuritis, third trimester ♀	M
O26.829	Pregnancy related peripheral neuritis, unspecified trimester ♀	M

▶ New   ⇒ Revised   ~~deleted~~ Deleted   Excludes 1   Excludes 2   Includes   Use additional   Code first   Code also   Key words

1132   OGCR Official Guidelines   X Assign placeholder X   ● Use Additional Character(s)   ▷ Manifestation Code   🔖 Hierarchical Condition Category   Coding Clinic

● O26.83 Pregnancy related renal disease
  Use additional code to identify the specific
  disorder
  O26.831 Pregnancy related renal disease, first
  trimester ♀   M
  O26.832 Pregnancy related renal disease,
  second trimester ♀   M
  O26.833 Pregnancy related renal disease, third
  trimester ♀   M
  O26.839 Pregnancy related renal disease,
  unspecified trimester ♀   M
● O26.84 Uterine size-date discrepancy complicating
  pregnancy
  Excludes1 encounter for suspected problem
  with fetal growth ruled out
  (Z03.74)
  O26.841 Uterine size-date discrepancy, first
  trimester ♀   M
  O26.842 Uterine size-date discrepancy, second
  trimester ♀   M
  O26.843 Uterine size-date discrepancy, third
  trimester ♀   M
  O26.849 Uterine size-date discrepancy,
  unspecified trimester ♀   M
● O26.85 Spotting complicating pregnancy
  O26.851 Spotting complicating pregnancy, first
  trimester ♀   M
  O26.852 Spotting complicating pregnancy,
  second trimester ♀   M
  O26.853 Spotting complicating pregnancy,
  third trimester ♀   M
  O26.859 Spotting complicating pregnancy,
  unspecified trimester ♀   M
  O26.86 Pruritic urticarial papules and plaques of
  pregnancy (PUPPP) ♀   M
  Polymorphic eruption of pregnancy
● O26.87 Cervical shortening
  Excludes1 encounter for suspected cervical
  shortening ruled out
  (Z03.75)
  O26.872 Cervical shortening, second
  trimester ♀   M
  O26.873 Cervical shortening, third
  trimester ♀   M
  O26.879 Cervical shortening, unspecified
  trimester ♀   M
● O26.89 Other specified pregnancy related conditions
  O26.891 Other specified pregnancy related
  conditions, first trimester ♀   M
  O26.892 Other specified pregnancy related
  conditions, second trimester ♀   M
  O26.893 Other specified pregnancy related
  conditions, third trimester ♀   M
  Coding Clinic: 2015, Q3, P40
  O26.899 Other specified pregnancy related
  conditions, unspecified trimester ♀   M
● O26.9 Pregnancy related conditions, unspecified
  O26.90 Pregnancy related conditions, unspecified,
  unspecified trimester ♀   M
  O26.91 Pregnancy related conditions, unspecified, first
  trimester ♀   M
  O26.92 Pregnancy related conditions, unspecified,
  second trimester ♀   M
  O26.93 Pregnancy related conditions, unspecified, third
  trimester ♀   M

● O28 Abnormal findings on antenatal screening of mother
  Excludes1 diagnostic findings classified elsewhere - see
  Alphabetical Index
  O28.0 Abnormal hematological finding on antenatal screening
  of mother ♀   M
  O28.1 Abnormal biochemical finding on antenatal screening of
  mother ♀   M
  O28.2 Abnormal cytological finding on antenatal screening of
  mother ♀   M
  O28.3 Abnormal ultrasonic finding on antenatal screening of
  mother ♀   M
  Coding Clinic: 2016, Q4, P5
  O28.4 Abnormal radiological finding on antenatal screening of
  mother ♀   M
  O28.5 Abnormal chromosomal and genetic finding on
  antenatal screening of mother ♀   M
  O28.8 Other abnormal findings on antenatal screening of
  mother ♀   M
  O28.9 Unspecified abnormal findings on antenatal screening of
  mother ♀   M
● O29 Complications of anesthesia during pregnancy
  Includes maternal complications arising from the
  administration of a general, regional or
  local anesthetic, analgesic or other sedation
  during pregnancy
  Use additional code, if necessary, to identify the complication
  Excludes2 complications of anesthesia during labor and
  delivery (O74.-)
  complications of anesthesia during the
  puerperium (O89.-)
● O29.0 Pulmonary complications of anesthesia during
  pregnancy
  ● O29.01 Aspiration pneumonitis due to anesthesia
  during pregnancy
  Inhalation of stomach contents or secretions
  NOS due to anesthesia during pregnancy
  Mendelson's syndrome due to anesthesia
  during pregnancy
    O29.011 Aspiration pneumonitis due to
  anesthesia during pregnancy, first
  trimester ♀   M
    O29.012 Aspiration pneumonitis due to
  anesthesia during pregnancy, second
  trimester ♀   M
    O29.013 Aspiration pneumonitis due to
  anesthesia during pregnancy, third
  trimester ♀   M
    O29.019 Aspiration pneumonitis due to
  anesthesia during pregnancy,
  unspecified trimester ♀   M
  ● O29.02 Pressure collapse of lung due to anesthesia
  during pregnancy
    O29.021 Pressure collapse of lung due to
  anesthesia during pregnancy, first
  trimester ♀   M
    O29.022 Pressure collapse of lung due to
  anesthesia during pregnancy, second
  trimester ♀   M
    O29.023 Pressure collapse of lung due to
  anesthesia during pregnancy, third
  trimester ♀   M
    O29.029 Pressure collapse of lung due
  to anesthesia during pregnancy,
  unspecified trimester ♀   M
  ● O29.09 Other pulmonary complications of anesthesia
  during pregnancy
    O29.091 Other pulmonary complications of
  anesthesia during pregnancy, first
  trimester ♀   M
    O29.092 Other pulmonary complications of
  anesthesia during pregnancy, second
  trimester ♀   M

      O29.093   Other pulmonary complications of anesthesia during pregnancy, third trimester ♀   M

      O29.099   Other pulmonary complications of anesthesia during pregnancy, unspecified trimester ♀   M

● O29.1   Cardiac complications of anesthesia during pregnancy

  ● O29.11   Cardiac arrest due to anesthesia during pregnancy

      O29.111   Cardiac arrest due to anesthesia during pregnancy, first trimester ♀   M

      O29.112   Cardiac arrest due to anesthesia during pregnancy, second trimester ♀   M

      O29.113   Cardiac arrest due to anesthesia during pregnancy, third trimester ♀   M

      O29.119   Cardiac arrest due to anesthesia during pregnancy, unspecified trimester ♀   M

  ● O29.12   Cardiac failure due to anesthesia during pregnancy

      O29.121   Cardiac failure due to anesthesia during pregnancy, first trimester ♀   M

      O29.122   Cardiac failure due to anesthesia during pregnancy, second trimester ♀   M

      O29.123   Cardiac failure due to anesthesia during pregnancy, third trimester ♀   M

      O29.129   Cardiac failure due to anesthesia during pregnancy, unspecified trimester ♀   M

  ● O29.19   Other cardiac complications of anesthesia during pregnancy

      O29.191   Other cardiac complications of anesthesia during pregnancy, first trimester ♀   M

      O29.192   Other cardiac complications of anesthesia during pregnancy, second trimester ♀   M

      O29.193   Other cardiac complications of anesthesia during pregnancy, third trimester ♀   M

      O29.199   Other cardiac complications of anesthesia during pregnancy, unspecified trimester ♀   M

● O29.2   Central nervous system complications of anesthesia during pregnancy

  ● O29.21   Cerebral anoxia due to anesthesia during pregnancy

      O29.211   Cerebral anoxia due to anesthesia during pregnancy, first trimester ♀   M

      O29.212   Cerebral anoxia due to anesthesia during pregnancy, second trimester ♀   M

      O29.213   Cerebral anoxia due to anesthesia during pregnancy, third trimester ♀   M

      O29.219   Cerebral anoxia due to anesthesia during pregnancy, unspecified trimester ♀   M

  ● O29.29   Other central nervous system complications of anesthesia during pregnancy

      O29.291   Other central nervous system complications of anesthesia during pregnancy, first trimester ♀   M

      O29.292   Other central nervous system complications of anesthesia during pregnancy, second trimester ♀   M

      O29.293   Other central nervous system complications of anesthesia during pregnancy, third trimester ♀   M

      O29.299   Other central nervous system complications of anesthesia during pregnancy, unspecified trimester ♀   M

● O29.3   Toxic reaction to local anesthesia during pregnancy

  ● O29.3X   Toxic reaction to local anesthesia during pregnancy

      O29.3X1   Toxic reaction to local anesthesia during pregnancy, first trimester ♀   M

      O29.3X2   Toxic reaction to local anesthesia during pregnancy, second trimester ♀   M

      O29.3X3   Toxic reaction to local anesthesia during pregnancy, third trimester ♀   M

      O29.3X9   Toxic reaction to local anesthesia during pregnancy, unspecified trimester ♀   M

● O29.4   Spinal and epidural anesthesia induced headache during pregnancy

      O29.40   Spinal and epidural anesthesia induced headache during pregnancy, unspecified trimester ♀   M

      O29.41   Spinal and epidural anesthesia induced headache during pregnancy, first trimester ♀   M

      O29.42   Spinal and epidural anesthesia induced headache during pregnancy, second trimester ♀   M

      O29.43   Spinal and epidural anesthesia induced headache during pregnancy, third trimester ♀   M

● O29.5   Other complications of spinal and epidural anesthesia during pregnancy

  ● O29.5X   Other complications of spinal and epidural anesthesia during pregnancy

      O29.5X1   Other complications of spinal and epidural anesthesia during pregnancy, first trimester ♀   M

      O29.5X2   Other complications of spinal and epidural anesthesia during pregnancy, second trimester ♀   M

      O29.5X3   Other complications of spinal and epidural anesthesia during pregnancy, third trimester ♀   M

      O29.5X9   Other complications of spinal and epidural anesthesia during pregnancy, unspecified trimester ♀   M

● O29.6   Failed or difficult intubation for anesthesia during pregnancy

      O29.60   Failed or difficult intubation for anesthesia during pregnancy, unspecified trimester ♀   M

      O29.61   Failed or difficult intubation for anesthesia during pregnancy, first trimester ♀   M

      O29.62   Failed or difficult intubation for anesthesia during pregnancy, second trimester ♀   M

      O29.63   Failed or difficult intubation for anesthesia during pregnancy, third trimester ♀   M

● O29.8   Other complications of anesthesia during pregnancy

  ● O29.8X   Other complications of anesthesia during pregnancy

      O29.8X1   Other complications of anesthesia during pregnancy, first trimester ♀   M

      O29.8X2   Other complications of anesthesia during pregnancy, second trimester ♀   M

      O29.8X3   Other complications of anesthesia during pregnancy, third trimester ♀   M

      O29.8X9   Other complications of anesthesia during pregnancy, unspecified trimester ♀   M

▶ New   ⇒ Revised   ~~deleted~~ Deleted   Excludes 1   Excludes 2   Includes   Use additional   Code first   Code also   Key words

OGCR Official Guidelines   X Assign placeholder X   ● Use Additional Character(s)   ▶ Manifestation Code   🦠 Hierarchical Condition Category   **Coding Clinic**

● O29.9   Unspecified complication of anesthesia during pregnancy
    O29.90   Unspecified complication of anesthesia during pregnancy, unspecified trimester ♀   M
    O29.91   Unspecified complication of anesthesia during pregnancy, first trimester ♀   M
    O29.92   Unspecified complication of anesthesia during pregnancy, second trimester ♀   M
    O29.93   Unspecified complication of anesthesia during pregnancy, third trimester ♀   M

MATERNAL CARE RELATED TO THE FETUS AND AMNIOTIC CAVITY AND POSSIBLE DELIVERY PROBLEMS (O30-O48)

● O30   Multiple gestation
    Code also any complications specific to multiple gestation
    Coding Clinic: 2016, Q4, P51
  ● O30.0   Twin pregnancy
    ● O30.00   Twin pregnancy, unspecified number of placenta and unspecified number of amniotic sacs
        O30.001   Twin pregnancy, unspecified number of placenta and unspecified number of amniotic sacs, first trimester ♀   M
        O30.002   Twin pregnancy, unspecified number of placenta and unspecified number of amniotic sacs, second trimester ♀ M
        O30.003   Twin pregnancy, unspecified number of placenta and unspecified number of amniotic sacs, third trimester ♀   M
        O30.009   Twin pregnancy, unspecified number of placenta and unspecified number of amniotic sacs, unspecified trimester ♀
    ● O30.01   Twin pregnancy, monochorionic/monoamniotic
        Twin pregnancy, one placenta, one amniotic sac
        Excludes1   conjoined twins (O30.02-)
        O30.011   Twin pregnancy, monochorionic/monoamniotic, first trimester ♀   M
        O30.012   Twin pregnancy, monochorionic/monoamniotic, second trimester ♀   M
        O30.013   Twin pregnancy, monochorionic/monoamniotic, third trimester ♀   M
        O30.019   Twin pregnancy, monochorionic/monoamniotic, unspecified trimester ♀   M
    ● O30.02   Conjoined twin pregnancy
        O30.021   Conjoined twin pregnancy, first trimester ♀   M
        O30.022   Conjoined twin pregnancy, second trimester ♀   M
        O30.023   Conjoined twin pregnancy, third trimester ♀   M
        O30.029   Conjoined twin pregnancy, unspecified trimester ♀   M
    ● O30.03   Twin pregnancy, monochorionic/diamniotic
        Twin pregnancy, one placenta, two amniotic sacs
        O30.031   Twin pregnancy, monochorionic/diamniotic, first trimester ♀   M
        O30.032   Twin pregnancy, monochorionic/diamniotic, second trimester ♀   M
        O30.033   Twin pregnancy, monochorionic/diamniotic, third trimester ♀   M
        O30.039   Twin pregnancy, monochorionic/diamniotic, unspecified trimester ♀   M

● O30.04   Twin pregnancy, dichorionic/diamniotic
    Twin pregnancy, two placentae, two amniotic sacs
    O30.041   Twin pregnancy, dichorionic/diamniotic, first trimester ♀   M
    O30.042   Twin pregnancy, dichorionic/diamniotic, second trimester ♀   M
    O30.043   Twin pregnancy, dichorionic/diamniotic, third trimester ♀   M
    O30.049   Twin pregnancy, dichorionic/diamniotic, unspecified trimester ♀ M
● O30.09   Twin pregnancy, unable to determine number of placenta and number of amniotic sacs
    O30.091   Twin pregnancy, unable to determine number of placenta and number of amniotic sacs, first trimester ♀   M
    O30.092   Twin pregnancy, unable to determine number of placenta and number of amniotic sacs, second trimester ♀   M
    O30.093   Twin pregnancy, unable to determine number of placenta and number of amniotic sacs, third trimester ♀   M
    O30.099   Twin pregnancy, unable to determine number of placenta and number of amniotic sacs, unspecified trimester ♀
  ● O30.1   Triplet pregnancy
    ● O30.10   Triplet pregnancy, unspecified number of placenta and unspecified number of amniotic sacs
        O30.101   Triplet pregnancy, unspecified number of placenta and unspecified number of amniotic sacs, first trimester ♀   M
        O30.102   Triplet pregnancy, unspecified number of placenta and unspecified number of amniotic sacs, second trimester ♀   M
        O30.103   Triplet pregnancy, unspecified number of placenta and unspecified number of amniotic sacs, third trimester ♀   M
        Coding Clinic: 2016, Q2, P8
        O30.109   Triplet pregnancy, unspecified number of placenta and unspecified number of amniotic sacs, unspecified trimester ♀   M
    ● O30.11   Triplet pregnancy with two or more monochorionic fetuses
        O30.111   Triplet pregnancy with two or more monochorionic fetuses, first trimester ♀   M
        O30.112   Triplet pregnancy with two or more monochorionic fetuses, second trimester ♀   M
        O30.113   Triplet pregnancy with two or more monochorionic fetuses, third trimester ♀   M
        O30.119   Triplet pregnancy with two or more monochorionic fetuses, unspecified trimester ♀   M
    ● O30.12   Triplet pregnancy with two or more monoamniotic fetuses
        O30.121   Triplet pregnancy with two or more monoamniotic fetuses, first trimester ♀   M
        O30.122   Triplet pregnancy with two or more monoamniotic fetuses, second trimester ♀   M

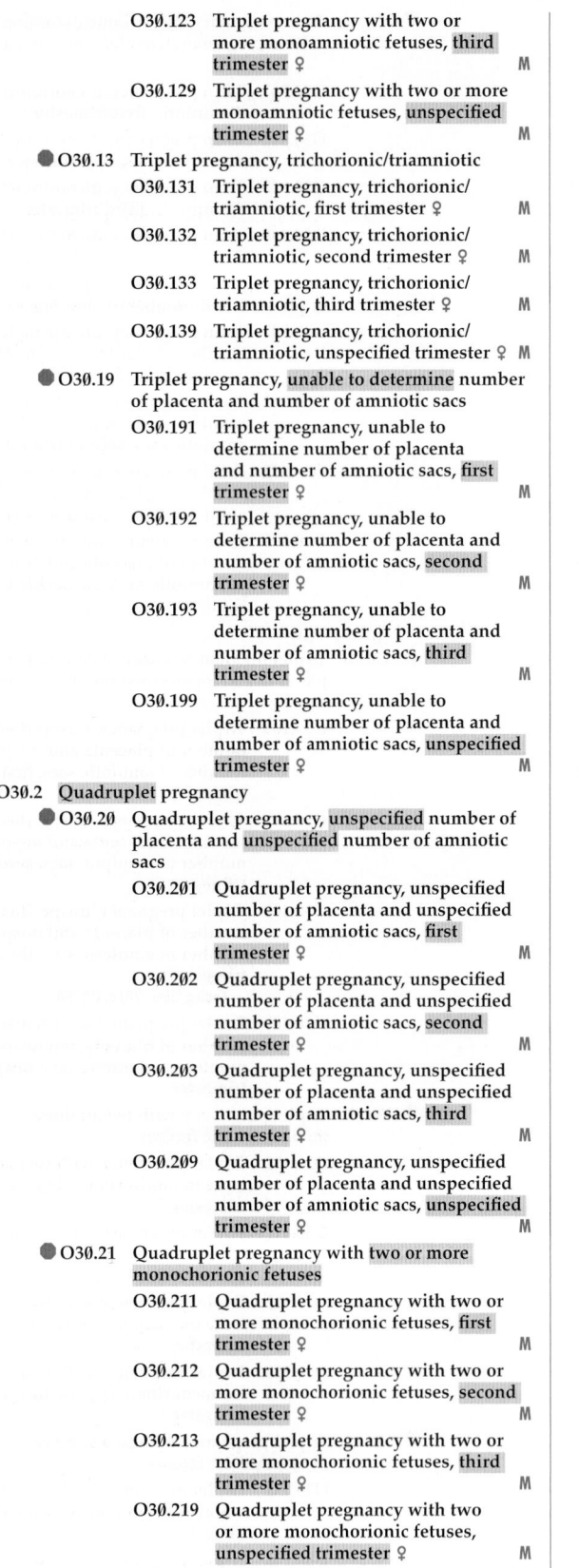

O30.123   Triplet pregnancy with two or
          more monoamniotic fetuses, third
          trimester ♀   M
O30.129   Triplet pregnancy with two or more
          monoamniotic fetuses, unspecified
          trimester ♀   M
● O30.13 Triplet pregnancy, trichorionic/triamniotic
O30.131   Triplet pregnancy, trichorionic/
          triamniotic, first trimester ♀   M
O30.132   Triplet pregnancy, trichorionic/
          triamniotic, second trimester ♀   M
O30.133   Triplet pregnancy, trichorionic/
          triamniotic, third trimester ♀   M
O30.139   Triplet pregnancy, trichorionic/
          triamniotic, unspecified trimester ♀ M
● O30.19 Triplet pregnancy, unable to determine number
          of placenta and number of amniotic sacs
O30.191   Triplet pregnancy, unable to
          determine number of placenta
          and number of amniotic sacs, first
          trimester ♀   M
O30.192   Triplet pregnancy, unable to
          determine number of placenta and
          number of amniotic sacs, second
          trimester ♀   M
O30.193   Triplet pregnancy, unable to
          determine number of placenta and
          number of amniotic sacs, third
          trimester ♀   M
O30.199   Triplet pregnancy, unable to
          determine number of placenta and
          number of amniotic sacs, unspecified
          trimester ♀   M
● O30.2   Quadruplet pregnancy
  ● O30.20 Quadruplet pregnancy, unspecified number of
            placenta and unspecified number of amniotic
            sacs
O30.201   Quadruplet pregnancy, unspecified
          number of placenta and unspecified
          number of amniotic sacs, first
          trimester ♀   M
O30.202   Quadruplet pregnancy, unspecified
          number of placenta and unspecified
          number of amniotic sacs, second
          trimester ♀   M
O30.203   Quadruplet pregnancy, unspecified
          number of placenta and unspecified
          number of amniotic sacs, third
          trimester ♀   M
O30.209   Quadruplet pregnancy, unspecified
          number of placenta and unspecified
          number of amniotic sacs, unspecified
          trimester ♀   M
  ● O30.21 Quadruplet pregnancy with two or more
            monochorionic fetuses
O30.211   Quadruplet pregnancy with two or
          more monochorionic fetuses, first
          trimester ♀   M
O30.212   Quadruplet pregnancy with two or
          more monochorionic fetuses, second
          trimester ♀   M
O30.213   Quadruplet pregnancy with two or
          more monochorionic fetuses, third
          trimester ♀   M
O30.219   Quadruplet pregnancy with two
          or more monochorionic fetuses,
          unspecified trimester ♀   M

● O30.22 Quadruplet pregnancy with two or more
          monoamniotic fetuses
O30.221   Quadruplet pregnancy with two or
          more monoamniotic fetuses, first
          trimester ♀   M
O30.222   Quadruplet pregnancy with two or
          more monoamniotic fetuses, second
          trimester ♀   M
O30.223   Quadruplet pregnancy with two or
          more monoamniotic fetuses, third
          trimester ♀   M
O30.229   Quadruplet pregnancy with two
          or more monoamniotic fetuses,
          unspecified trimester ♀   M
● O30.23 Quadruplet pregnancy, quadrachorionic/
          quadra-amniotic
O30.231   Quadruplet pregnancy,
          quadrachorionic/quadra-amniotic,
          first trimester ♀   M
O30.232   Quadruplet pregnancy,
          quadrachorionic/quadra-amniotic,
          second trimester ♀   M
O30.233   Quadruplet pregnancy,
          quadrachorionic/quadra-amniotic,
          third trimester ♀   M
O30.239   Quadruplet pregnancy,
          quadrachorionic/quadra-amniotic,
          unspecifiedtrimester ♀   M
● O30.29 Quadruplet pregnancy, unable to determine
          number of placenta and number of amniotic sacs
O30.291   Quadruplet pregnancy, unable
          to determine number of placenta
          and number of amniotic sacs, first
          trimester ♀   M
O30.292   Quadruplet pregnancy, unable to
          determine number of placenta and
          number of amniotic sacs, second
          trimester ♀   M
O30.293   Quadruplet pregnancy, unable to
          determine number of placenta and
          number of amniotic sacs, third
          trimester ♀   M
O30.299   Quadruplet pregnancy, unable to
          determine number of placenta and
          number of amniotic sacs, unspecified
          trimester ♀   M
● O30.8   Other specified multiple gestation
          Multiple gestation pregnancy greater then quadruplets
  ● O30.80 Other specified multiple gestation, unspecified
            number of placenta and unspecified number of
            amniotic sacs
O30.801   Other specified multiple gestation,
          unspecified number of placenta and
          unspecified number of amniotic sacs,
          first trimester ♀   M
O30.802   Other specified multiple gestation,
          unspecified number of placenta and
          unspecified number of amniotic sacs,
          second trimester ♀   M
O30.803   Other specified multiple gestation,
          unspecified number of placenta and
          unspecified number of amniotic sacs,
          third trimester ♀   M
O30.809   Other specified multiple gestation,
          unspecified number of placenta and
          unspecified number of amniotic sacs,
          unspecified trimester ♀   M

▶ New ▦ Revised ~~deleted~~ Deleted   Excludes 1   Excludes 2   Includes   Use additional   Code first   Code also   Key words

1136   OGCR Official Guidelines   X Assign placeholder X   ● Use Additional Character(s)   ▶ Manifestation Code   🐾 Hierarchical Condition Category   Coding Clinic

● **O30.81**   **Other specified multiple gestation with two or more monochorionic fetuses**

    O30.811   Other specified multiple gestation with two or more monochorionic fetuses, first trimester ♀   M

    O30.812   Other specified multiple gestation with two or more monochorionic fetuses, second trimester ♀   M

    O30.813   Other specified multiple gestation with two or more monochorionic fetuses, third trimester ♀   M

    O30.819   Other specified multiple gestation with two or more monochorionic fetuses, unspecified trimester ♀   M

● **O30.82**   **Other specified multiple gestation with two or more monoamniotic fetuses**

    O30.821   Other specified multiple gestation with two or more monoamniotic fetuses, first trimester ♀   M

    O30.822   Other specified multiple gestation with two or more monoamniotic fetuses, second trimester ♀   M

    O30.823   Other specified multiple gestation with two or more monoamniotic fetuses, third trimester ♀   M

    O30.829   Other specified multiple gestation with two or more monoamniotic fetuses, unspecified trimester ♀   M

● **O30.83**   **Other specified multiple gestation, number of chorions and amnions are both equal to the number of fetuses**

    Pentachorionic, penta-amniotic pregnancy (quintuplets)

    Hexachorionic, hexa-amniotic pregnancy (sextuplets)

    Heptachorionic, hepta-amniotic pregnancy (septuplets)

    O30.831   Other specified multiple gestation, number of chorions and amnions are both equal to the number of fetuses, first trimester ♀   M

    O30.832   Other specified multiple gestation, number of chorions and amnions are both equal to the number of fetuses, second trimester ♀   M

    O30.833   Other specified multiple gestation, number of chorions and amnions are both equal to the number of fetuses, third trimester ♀   M

    O30.839   Other specified multiple gestation, number of chorions and amnions are both equal to the number of fetuses, unspecified trimester ♀   M

● **O30.89**   **Other specified multiple gestation, unable to determine number of placenta and number of amniotic sacs**

    O30.891   Other specified multiple gestation, unable to determine number of placenta and number of amniotic sacs, first trimester ♀   M

    O30.892   Other specified multiple gestation, unable to determine number of placenta and number of amniotic sacs, second trimester ♀   M

    O30.893   Other specified multiple gestation, unable to determine number of placenta and number of amniotic sacs, third trimester ♀   M

    O30.899   Other specified multiple gestation, unable to determine number of placenta and number of amniotic sacs, unspecified trimester ♀   M

● **O30.9**   **Multiple gestation, unspecified**

    Multiple pregnancy NOS

    O30.90   Multiple gestation, unspecified, unspecified trimester ♀   M

    O30.91   Multiple gestation, unspecified, first trimester ♀   M

    O30.92   Multiple gestation, unspecified, second trimester ♀   M

    O30.93   Multiple gestation, unspecified, third trimester ♀   M

● **O31**   **Complications specific to multiple gestation**

    Excludes2   delayed delivery of second twin, triplet, etc. (O63.2)

                malpresentation of one fetus or more (O32.9)

                placental transfusion syndromes (O43.0-)

    Coding Clinic: 2012, Q4, P107

    One of the following 7th characters is to be assigned to each code under category O31. 7th character Ø is for single gestations and multiple gestations where the fetus is unspecified. 7th characters 1 through 9 are for cases of multiple gestations to identify the fetus for which the code applies. The appropriate code from category O30, Multiple gestation, must also be assigned when assigning a code from category O31 that has a 7th character of 1 through 9.

Ø	not applicable or unspecified
1	fetus 1
2	fetus 2
3	fetus 3
4	fetus 4
5	fetus 5
9	other fetus

● **O31.0**   **Papyraceous fetus**

    Fetus compressus

X ● O31.00   Papyraceous fetus, unspecified trimester ♀   M

X ● O31.01   Papyraceous fetus, first trimester ♀   M

X ● O31.02   Papyraceous fetus, second trimester ♀   M

X ● O31.03   Papyraceous fetus, third trimester ♀   M

● **O31.1**   **Continuing pregnancy after spontaneous abortion of one fetus or more**

X ● O31.10   Continuing pregnancy after spontaneous abortion of one fetus or more, unspecified trimester ♀   M

X ● O31.11   Continuing pregnancy after spontaneous abortion of one fetus or more, first trimester ♀ M

X ● O31.12   Continuing pregnancy after spontaneous abortion of one fetus or more, second trimester ♀   M

X ● O31.13   Continuing pregnancy after spontaneous abortion of one fetus or more, third trimester ♀   M

● **O31.2**   **Continuing pregnancy after intrauterine death of one fetus or more**

X ● O31.20   Continuing pregnancy after intrauterine death of one fetus or more, unspecified trimester ♀   M

X ● O31.21   Continuing pregnancy after intrauterine death of one fetus or more, first trimester ♀   M

X ● O31.22   Continuing pregnancy after intrauterine death of one fetus or more, second trimester ♀   M

X ● O31.23   Continuing pregnancy after intrauterine death of one fetus or more, third trimester ♀   M

● **O31.3**   **Continuing pregnancy after elective fetal reduction of one fetus or more**

    Continuing pregnancy after selective termination of one fetus or more

X ● O31.30   Continuing pregnancy after elective fetal reduction of one fetus or more, unspecified trimester ♀   M

X ● O31.31   Continuing pregnancy after elective fetal reduction of one fetus or more, first trimester ♀   M

X ● **O31.32** **Continuing pregnancy after elective fetal reduction of one fetus or more, second trimester** ♀   M

X ● **O31.33** **Continuing pregnancy after elective fetal reduction of one fetus or more, third trimester** ♀

● **O31.8** **Other complications specific to multiple gestation**

  ● **O31.8X** **Other complications specific to multiple gestation**

    ● **O31.8X1** **Other complications specific to multiple gestation, first trimester** ♀ M

    ● **O31.8X2** **Other complications specific to multiple gestation, second trimester** ♀   M

    ● **O31.8X3** **Other complications specific to multiple gestation, third trimester** ♀ M

    ● **O31.8X9** **Other complications specific to multiple gestation, unspecified trimester** ♀   M

● **O32** **Maternal care for malpresentation of fetus**

  Includes   the listed conditions as a reason for observation, hospitalization or other obstetric care of the mother, or for cesarean delivery before onset of labor

  Excludes1   malpresentation of fetus with obstructed labor (O64.-)

Coding Clinic: 2012, Q4, P107

One of the following 7th characters is to be assigned to each code under category O32. 7th character Ø is for single gestations and multiple gestations where the fetus is unspecified. 7th characters 1 through 9 are for cases of multiple gestations to identify the fetus for which the code applies. The appropriate code from category O30, Multiple gestation, must also be assigned when assigning a code from category O32 that has a 7th character of 1 through 9.

Ø	not applicable or unspecified
1	fetus 1
2	fetus 2
3	fetus 3
4	fetus 4
5	fetus 5
9	other fetus

X ● **O32.0** **Maternal care for unstable lie** ♀   M

X ● **O32.1** **Maternal care for breech presentation** ♀   M
     Maternal care for buttocks presentation
     Maternal care for complete breech
     Maternal care for frank breech

    Excludes1   footling presentation (O32.8)
                   incomplete breech (O32.8)

X ● **O32.2** **Maternal care for transverse and oblique lie** ♀   M
     Maternal care for oblique presentation
     Maternal care for transverse presentation

X ● **O32.3** **Maternal care for face, brow and chin presentation** ♀   M

X ● **O32.4** **Maternal care for high head at term** ♀   M
     Maternal care for failure of head to enter pelvic brim

X ● **O32.6** **Maternal care for compound presentation** ♀   M

X ● **O32.8** **Maternal care for other malpresentation of fetus** ♀   M
     Maternal care for footling presentation
     Maternal care for incomplete breech

X ● **O32.9** **Maternal care for malpresentation of fetus, unspecified** ♀   M

● **O33** **Maternal care for disproportion**

  Includes   the listed conditions as a reason for observation, hospitalization or other obstetric care of the mother, or for cesarean delivery before onset of labor

  Excludes1   disproportion with obstructed labor (O65-O66)

● **O33.0** **Maternal care for disproportion due to deformity of maternal pelvic bones** ♀   M
     Maternal care for disproportion due to pelvic deformity causing disproportion NOS

● **O33.1** **Maternal care for disproportion due to generally contracted pelvis** ♀   M
     Maternal care for disproportion due to contracted pelvis NOS causing disproportion

● **O33.2** **Maternal care for disproportion due to inlet contraction of pelvis** ♀   M
     Maternal care for disproportion due to inlet contraction (pelvis) causing disproportion

X ● **O33.3** **Maternal care for disproportion due to outlet contraction of pelvis** ♀   M
     Maternal care for disproportion due to mid-cavity contraction (pelvis)
     Maternal care for disproportion due to outlet contraction (pelvis)

One of the following 7th characters is to be assigned to code O33.3. 7th character Ø is for single gestations and multiple gestations where the fetus is unspecified. 7th characters 1 through 9 are for cases of multiple gestations to identify the fetus for which the code applies. The appropriate code from category O30, Multiple gestation, must also be assigned when assigning code O33.3 with a 7th character of 1 through 9.

Ø	not applicable or unspecified
1	fetus 1
2	fetus 2
3	fetus 3
4	fetus 4
5	fetus 5
9	other fetus

X ● **O33.4** **Maternal care for disproportion of mixed maternal and fetal origin** ♀   M

One of the following 7th characters is to be assigned to code O33.4. 7th character Ø is for single gestations and multiple gestations where the fetus is unspecified. 7th characters 1 through 9 are for cases of multiple gestations to identify the fetus for which the code applies. The appropriate code from category O30, Multiple gestation, must also be assigned when assigning code O33.4 with a 7th character of 1 through 9.

Ø	not applicable or unspecified
1	fetus 1
2	fetus 2
3	fetus 3
4	fetus 4
5	fetus 5
9	other fetus

X ● **O33.5** **Maternal care for disproportion due to unusually large fetus** ♀   M
     Maternal care for disproportion due to disproportion of fetal origin with normally formed fetus
     Maternal care for disproportion due to fetal disproportion NOS

One of the following 7th characters is to be assigned to code O33.5. 7th character Ø is for single gestations and multiple gestations where the fetus is unspecified. 7th characters 1 through 9 are for cases of multiple gestations to identify the fetus for which the code applies. The appropriate code from category O30, Multiple gestation, must also be assigned when assigning code O33.5 with a 7th character of 1 through 9.

Ø	not applicable or unspecified
1	fetus 1
2	fetus 2
3	fetus 3
4	fetus 4
5	fetus 5
9	other fetus

▶ New   ⇒ Revised   ~~deleted~~ Deleted   Excludes 1   Excludes 2   Includes   Use additional   Code first   Code also   Key words

OGCR Official Guidelines   X Assign placeholder X   ● Use Additional Character(s)   ▶ Manifestation Code   🐾 Hierarchical Condition Category   Coding Clinic

X ● **O33.6** **Maternal care for disproportion due to hydrocephalic fetus** ♀   M

One of the following 7th characters is to be assigned to code O33.6. 7th character Ø is for single gestations and multiple gestations where the fetus is unspecified. 7th characters 1 through 9 are for cases of multiple gestations to identify the fetus for which the code applies. The appropriate code from category O30, Multiple gestation, must also be assigned when assigning code O33.6 with a 7th character of 1 through 9.

Ø	not applicable or unspecified
1	fetus 1
2	fetus 2
3	fetus 3
4	fetus 4
5	fetus 5
9	other fetus

X ● **O33.7** **Maternal care for disproportion due to other fetal deformities** ♀   M

Maternal care for disproportion due to fetal ascites
Maternal care for disproportion due to fetal hydrops
Maternal care for disproportion due to fetal meningomyelocele
Maternal care for disproportion due to fetal sacral teratoma
Maternal care for disproportion due to fetal tumor

Excludes1   obstructed labor due to other fetal deformities (O66.3)

Coding Clinic: 2016, Q4, P51

One of the following 7th characters is to be assigned to code O33.7. 7th character Ø is for single gestations and multiple gestations where the fetus is unspecified. 7th characters 1 through 9 are for cases of multiple gestations to identify the fetus for which the code applies. The appropriate code from category O30, Multiple gestation, must also be assigned when assigning code O33.7 with a 7th character of 1 through 9.

Ø	not applicable or unspecified
1	fetus 1
2	fetus 2
3	fetus 3
4	fetus 4
5	fetus 5
9	other fetus

O33.8 **Maternal care for disproportion of other origin** ♀   M

O33.9 **Maternal care for disproportion, unspecified** ♀   M
Maternal care for disproportion due to cephalopelvic disproportion NOS
Maternal care for disproportion due to fetopelvic disproportion NOS

● **O34** **Maternal care for abnormality of pelvic organs**

Includes   the listed conditions as a reason for hospitalization or other obstetric care of the mother, or for cesarean delivery before onset of labor

Code first any associated obstructed labor (O65.5)
Use additional code for specific condition

● **O34.0** **Maternal care for congenital malformation of uterus**
Maternal care for double uterus
Maternal care for uterus bicornis

O34.00 **Maternal care for unspecified congenital malformation of uterus, unspecified trimester** ♀   M

O34.01 **Maternal care for unspecified congenital malformation of uterus, first trimester** ♀   M

O34.02 **Maternal care for unspecified congenital malformation of uterus, second trimester** ♀   M

O34.03 **Maternal care for unspecified congenital malformation of uterus, third trimester** ♀   M

● **O34.1** **Maternal care for benign tumor of corpus uteri**

Excludes2   maternal care for benign tumor of cervix (O34.4-)
maternal care for malignant neoplasm of uterus (O9A.1-)

O34.10 **Maternal care for benign tumor of corpus uteri, unspecified trimester** ♀   M

O34.11 **Maternal care for benign tumor of corpus uteri, first trimester** ♀   M

O34.12 **Maternal care for benign tumor of corpus uteri, second trimester** ♀   M

O34.13 **Maternal care for benign tumor of corpus uteri, third trimester** ♀   M

● **O34.2** **Maternal care due to uterine scar from previous surgery**
Coding Clinic: 2016, Q4, P76

● **O34.21** **Maternal care for scar from previous cesarean delivery**
Coding Clinic: 2016, Q4, P51

O34.211 **Maternal care for low transverse scar from previous cesarean delivery** ♀   M

O34.212 **Maternal care for vertical scar from previous cesarean delivery** ♀   M
Maternal care for classical scar from previous cesarean delivery

O34.218 **Maternal care for other type scar from previous cesarean delivery** ♀   M
Mid-transverse T incision

O34.219 **Maternal care for unspecified type scar from previous cesarean delivery** ♀   M

O34.22 **Maternal care for cesarean scar defect (isthmocele)** ♀   M

O34.29 **Maternal care due to uterine scar from other previous surgery** ♀   M
Maternal care due to uterine scar from other transmural uterine incision

● **O34.3** **Maternal care for cervical incompetence**
Maternal care for cerclage with or without cervical incompetence
Maternal care for Shirodkar suture with or without cervical incompetence

O34.30 **Maternal care for cervical incompetence, unspecified trimester** ♀   M

O34.31 **Maternal care for cervical incompetence, first trimester** ♀   M

O34.32 **Maternal care for cervical incompetence, second trimester** ♀   M

O34.33 **Maternal care for cervical incompetence, third trimester** ♀   M

● **O34.4** **Maternal care for other abnormalities of cervix**

O34.40 **Maternal care for other abnormalities of cervix, unspecified trimester** ♀   M

O34.41 **Maternal care for other abnormalities of cervix, first trimester** ♀   M

O34.42 **Maternal care for other abnormalities of cervix, second trimester** ♀   M

O34.43 **Maternal care for other abnormalities of cervix, third trimester** ♀   M

● **O34.5** **Maternal care for other abnormalities of gravid uterus**

● **O34.51** **Maternal care for incarceration of gravid uterus**

O34.511 **Maternal care for incarceration of gravid uterus, first trimester** ♀   M

O34.512 **Maternal care for incarceration of gravid uterus, second trimester** ♀   M

O34.513 **Maternal care for incarceration of gravid uterus, third trimester** ♀   M

O34.519 **Maternal care for incarceration of gravid uterus, unspecified trimester** ♀   M

CHAPTER 15 (O00-O9A)

● O34.52   Maternal care for prolapse of gravid uterus

    O34.521   Maternal care for prolapse of gravid uterus, first trimester ♀   M

    O34.522   Maternal care for prolapse of gravid uterus, second trimester ♀   M

    O34.523   Maternal care for prolapse of gravid uterus, third trimester ♀   M

    O34.529   Maternal care for prolapse of gravid uterus, unspecified trimester ♀   M

● O34.53   Maternal care for retroversion of gravid uterus

    O34.531   Maternal care for retroversion of gravid uterus, first trimester ♀   M

    O34.532   Maternal care for retroversion of gravid uterus, second trimester ♀   M

    O34.533   Maternal care for retroversion of gravid uterus, third trimester ♀   M

    O34.539   Maternal care for retroversion of gravid uterus, unspecified trimester ♀   M

● O34.59   Maternal care for other abnormalities of gravid uterus

    O34.591   Maternal care for other abnormalities of gravid uterus, first trimester ♀   M

    O34.592   Maternal care for other abnormalities of gravid uterus, second trimester ♀ M

    O34.593   Maternal care for other abnormalities of gravid uterus, third trimester ♀   M

    O34.599   Maternal care for other abnormalities of gravid uterus, unspecified trimester ♀   M

● O34.6   Maternal care for abnormality of vagina

    Excludes2   maternal care for vaginal varices in pregnancy (O22.1-)

    O34.60   Maternal care for abnormality of vagina, unspecified trimester ♀   M

    O34.61   Maternal care for abnormality of vagina, first trimester ♀   M

    O34.62   Maternal care for abnormality of vagina, second trimester ♀   M

    O34.63   Maternal care for abnormality of vagina, third trimester ♀   M

● O34.7   Maternal care for abnormality of vulva and perineum

    Excludes2   maternal care for perineal and vulval varices in pregnancy (O22.1-)

    O34.70   Maternal care for abnormality of vulva and perineum, unspecified trimester ♀   M

    O34.71   Maternal care for abnormality of vulva and perineum, first trimester ♀   M

    O34.72   Maternal care for abnormality of vulva and perineum, second trimester ♀   M

    O34.73   Maternal care for abnormality of vulva and perineum, third trimester ♀   M

● O34.8   Maternal care for other abnormalities of pelvic organs

    O34.80   Maternal care for other abnormalities of pelvic organs, unspecified trimester ♀   M

    O34.81   Maternal care for other abnormalities of pelvic organs, first trimester ♀   M

    O34.82   Maternal care for other abnormalities of pelvic organs, second trimester ♀   M

    O34.83   Maternal care for other abnormalities of pelvic organs, third trimester ♀   M

● O34.9   Maternal care for abnormality of pelvic organ, unspecified

    O34.90   Maternal care for abnormality of pelvic organ, unspecified, unspecified trimester ♀   M

    O34.91   Maternal care for abnormality of pelvic organ, unspecified, first trimester ♀   M

    O34.92   Maternal care for abnormality of pelvic organ, unspecified, second trimester ♀   M

    O34.93   Maternal care for abnormality of pelvic organ, unspecified, third trimester ♀   M

● O35   Maternal care for known or suspected fetal abnormality and damage

    Includes   the listed conditions in the fetus as a reason for hospitalization or other obstetric care to the mother, or for termination of pregnancy

    Code also any associated maternal condition

    Excludes1   encounter for suspected maternal and fetal conditions ruled out (Z03.7-)

    One of the following 7th characters is to be assigned to each code under category O35. 7th character Ø is for single gestations and multiple gestations where the fetus is unspecified. 7th characters 1 through 9 are for cases of multiple gestations to identify the fetus for which the code applies. The appropriate code from category O30, Multiple gestation, must also be assigned when assigning a code from category O35 that has a 7th character of 1 through 9.

Ø	not applicable or unspecified
1	fetus 1
2	fetus 2
3	fetus 3
4	fetus 4
5	fetus 5
9	other fetus

X ● O35.0   Maternal care for (suspected) central nervous system malformation in fetus ♀   M

    Maternal care for fetal anencephaly
    Maternal care for fetal hydrocephalus
    Maternal care for fetal spina bifida

    Excludes2   chromosomal abnormality in fetus (O35.1)

X ● O35.1   Maternal care for (suspected) chromosomal abnormality in fetus ♀   M

X ● O35.2   Maternal care for (suspected) hereditary disease in fetus ♀   M

    Excludes2   chromosomal abnormality in fetus (O35.1)

X ● O35.3   Maternal care for (suspected) damage to fetus from viral disease in mother ♀   M

    Maternal care for damage to fetus from maternal cytomegalovirus infection
    Maternal care for damage to fetus from maternal rubella
    Coding Clinic: 2016, Q4, P6

X ● O35.4   Maternal care for (suspected) damage to fetus from alcohol ♀   M

X ● O35.5   Maternal care for (suspected) damage to fetus by drugs ♀   M

    Maternal care for damage to fetus from drug addiction

X ● O35.6   Maternal care for (suspected) damage to fetus by radiation ♀   M

X ● O35.7   Maternal care for (suspected) damage to fetus by other medical procedures ♀   M

    Maternal care for damage to fetus by amniocentesis
    Maternal care for damage to fetus by biopsy procedures
    Maternal care for damage to fetus by hematological investigation
    Maternal care for damage to fetus by intrauterine contraceptive device
    Maternal care for damage to fetus by intrauterine surgery

X ● O35.8   Maternal care for other (suspected) fetal abnormality and damage ♀   M

    Maternal care for damage to fetus from maternal listeriosis
    Maternal care for damage to fetus from maternal toxoplasmosis

X ● O35.9   Maternal care for (suspected) fetal abnormality and damage, unspecified ♀   M

▶ New   ⇒ Revised   ~~deleted~~ Deleted   Excludes 1   Excludes 2   Includes   Use additional   Code first   Code also   Key words

OGCR Official Guidelines   X Assign placeholder X   ● Use Additional Character(s)   ▶ Manifestation Code   🔑 Hierarchical Condition Category   **Coding Clinic**

OGCR Section I.C.15.e.l.

Fetal Conditions Affecting the Management of the Mother
1) Code from categories O35 and O36
Codes from categories O35, Maternal care for known or suspected fetal abnormality and damage, and O36, Maternal care for other fetal problems, are assigned only when the fetal condition is actually responsible for modifying the management of the mother, i.e., by requiring diagnostic studies, additional observation, special care, or termination of pregnancy. The fact that the fetal condition exists does not justify assigning a code from this series to the mother's record.
2) In utero surgery
In cases when surgery is performed on the fetus, a diagnosis code from category O35, Maternal care for known or suspected fetal abnormality and damage, should be assigned identifying the fetal condition. Assign the appropriate procedure code for the procedure performed.
No code from Chapter 16, the perinatal codes, should be used on the mother's record to identify fetal conditions. Surgery performed in utero on a fetus is still to be coded as an obstetric encounter.

● O36 Maternal care for other fetal problems

Includes	the listed conditions in the fetus as a reason for hospitalization or other obstetric care of the mother, or for termination of pregnancy
Excludes1	encounter for suspected maternal and fetal conditions ruled out (Z03.7-) placental transfusion syndromes (O43.0-)
Excludes2	labor and delivery complicated by fetal stress (O77.-)

One of the following 7th characters is to be assigned to each code under category O36. 7th character Ø is for single gestations and multiple gestations where the fetus is unspecified. 7th characters 1 through 9 are for cases of multiple gestations to identify the fetus for which the code applies. The appropriate code from category O30, Multiple gestation, must also be assigned when assigning a code from category O36 that has a 7th character of 1 through 9.

Ø	not applicable or unspecified
1	fetus 1
2	fetus 2
3	fetus 3
4	fetus 4
5	fetus 5
9	other fetus

Coding Clinic: 2015, Q3, P40

● O36.0 Maternal care for rhesus isoimmunization
       Maternal care for Rh incompatibility (with hydrops fetalis)

  ● O36.01   Maternal care for anti-D [Rh] antibodies

    ● O36.011   Maternal care for anti-D [Rh] antibodies, first trimester ♀   M

    ● O36.012   Maternal care for anti-D [Rh] antibodies, second trimester ♀ M

    ● O36.013   Maternal care for anti-D [Rh] antibodies, third trimester ♀   M

    ● O36.019   Maternal care for anti-D [Rh] antibodies, unspecified trimester ♀ M

  ● O36.09   Maternal care for other rhesus isoimmunization

    ● O36.091   Maternal care for other rhesus isoimmunization, first trimester ♀   M

    ● O36.092   Maternal care for other rhesus isoimmunization, second trimester ♀ M

    ● O36.093   Maternal care for other rhesus isoimmunization, third trimester ♀ M
             Coding Clinic: 2015, Q3, P40

    ● O36.099   Maternal care for other rhesus isoimmunization, unspecified trimester ♀ M

● O36.1 Maternal care for other isoimmunization
      Maternal care for ABO isoimmunization

  ● O36.11   Maternal care for Anti-A sensitization
          Maternal care for isoimmunization NOS (with hydrops fetalis)

    ● O36.111   Maternal care for Anti-A sensitization, first trimester ♀   M

    ● O36.112   Maternal care for Anti-A sensitization, second trimester ♀ M

    ● O36.113   Maternal care for Anti-A sensitization, third trimester ♀   M

    ● O36.119   Maternal care for Anti-A sensitization, unspecified trimester ♀   M

  ● O36.19   Maternal care for other isoimmunization
         Maternal care for Anti-B sensitization

    ● O36.191   Maternal care for other isoimmunization, first trimester ♀   M

    ● O36.192   Maternal care for other isoimmunization, second trimester ♀ M

    ● O36.193   Maternal care for other isoimmunization, third trimester ♀ M

    ● O36.199   Maternal care for other isoimmunization, unspecified trimester ♀ M

● O36.2 Maternal care for hydrops fetalis
      Maternal care for hydrops fetalis NOS
      Maternal care for hydrops fetalis not associated with isoimmunization

Excludes1	hydrops fetalis associated with ABO isoimmunization (O36.1-) hydrops fetalis associated with rhesus isoimmunization (O36.0-)

  ● O36.20   Maternal care for hydrops fetalis, unspecified trimester ♀ M

  ● O36.21   Maternal care for hydrops fetalis, first trimester ♀ M

  ● O36.22   Maternal care for hydrops fetalis, second trimester ♀ M

  ● O36.23   Maternal care for hydrops fetalis, third trimester ♀ M

● O36.4 Maternal care for intrauterine death ♀ M
      Maternal care for intrauterine fetal death NOS
      Maternal care for intrauterine fetal death after completion of 20 weeks of gestation
      Maternal care for late fetal death
      Maternal care for missed delivery

Excludes1	missed abortion (O02.1) stillbirth (P95)

● O36.5 Maternal care for known or suspected poor fetal growth

  ● O36.51   Maternal care for known or suspected placental insufficiency

    ● O36.511   Maternal care for known or suspected placental insufficiency, first trimester ♀ M

    ● O36.512   Maternal care for known or suspected placental insufficiency, second trimester ♀

    ● O36.513   Maternal care for known or suspected placental insufficiency, third trimester ♀ M

    ● O36.519   Maternal care for known or suspected placental insufficiency, unspecified trimester ♀ M

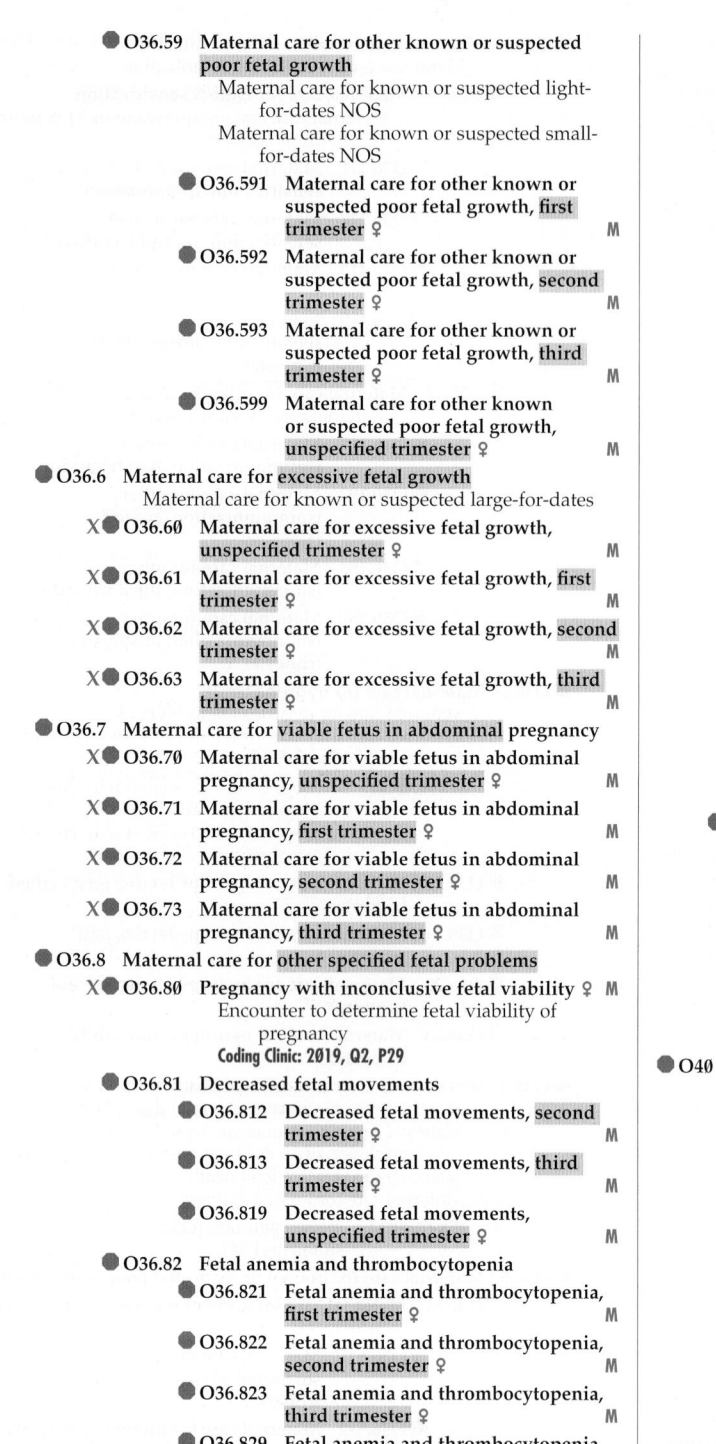

● O36.59   **Maternal care for other known or suspected poor fetal growth**
           Maternal care for known or suspected light-for-dates NOS
           Maternal care for known or suspected small-for-dates NOS
　　● O36.591   **Maternal care for other known or suspected poor fetal growth, first trimester** ♀   M
　　● O36.592   **Maternal care for other known or suspected poor fetal growth, second trimester** ♀   M
　　● O36.593   **Maternal care for other known or suspected poor fetal growth, third trimester** ♀   M
　　● O36.599   **Maternal care for other known or suspected poor fetal growth, unspecified trimester** ♀   M

● O36.6   **Maternal care for excessive fetal growth**
           Maternal care for known or suspected large-for-dates
X ● O36.60   **Maternal care for excessive fetal growth, unspecified trimester** ♀   M
X ● O36.61   **Maternal care for excessive fetal growth, first trimester** ♀   M
X ● O36.62   **Maternal care for excessive fetal growth, second trimester** ♀   M
X ● O36.63   **Maternal care for excessive fetal growth, third trimester** ♀   M

● O36.7   **Maternal care for viable fetus in abdominal pregnancy**
X ● O36.70   **Maternal care for viable fetus in abdominal pregnancy, unspecified trimester** ♀   M
X ● O36.71   **Maternal care for viable fetus in abdominal pregnancy, first trimester** ♀   M
X ● O36.72   **Maternal care for viable fetus in abdominal pregnancy, second trimester** ♀   M
X ● O36.73   **Maternal care for viable fetus in abdominal pregnancy, third trimester** ♀   M

● O36.8   **Maternal care for other specified fetal problems**
X ● O36.80   **Pregnancy with inconclusive fetal viability** ♀ M
           Encounter to determine fetal viability of pregnancy
           Coding Clinic: 2019, Q2, P29
● O36.81   **Decreased fetal movements**
　　● O36.812   **Decreased fetal movements, second trimester** ♀   M
　　● O36.813   **Decreased fetal movements, third trimester** ♀   M
　　● O36.819   **Decreased fetal movements, unspecified trimester** ♀   M
● O36.82   **Fetal anemia and thrombocytopenia**
　　● O36.821   **Fetal anemia and thrombocytopenia, first trimester** ♀   M
　　● O36.822   **Fetal anemia and thrombocytopenia, second trimester** ♀   M
　　● O36.823   **Fetal anemia and thrombocytopenia, third trimester** ♀   M
　　● O36.829   **Fetal anemia and thrombocytopenia, unspecified trimester** ♀   M

● O36.83   **Maternal care for abnormalities of the fetal heart rate or rhythm**
           Maternal care for depressed fetal heart rate tones
           Maternal care for fetal bradycardia
           Maternal care for fetal heart rate abnormal variability
           Maternal care for fetal heart rate decelerations
           Maternal care for fetal heart rate irregularity
           Maternal care for fetal tachycardia
           Maternal care for non-reassuring fetal heart rate or rhythm
　　● O36.831   **Maternal care for abnormalities of the fetal heart rate or rhythm, first trimester** ♀   M
　　● O36.832   **Maternal care for abnormalities of the fetal heart rate or rhythm, second trimester** ♀   M
　　● O36.833   **Maternal care for abnormalities of the fetal heart rate or rhythm, third trimester** ♀   M
　　● O36.839   **Maternal care for abnormalities of the fetal heart rate or rhythm, unspecified trimester** ♀   M

● O36.89   **Maternal care for other specified fetal problems**
　　● O36.891   **Maternal care for other specified fetal problems, first trimester** ♀   M
　　● O36.892   **Maternal care for other specified fetal problems, second trimester** ♀   M
　　● O36.893   **Maternal care for other specified fetal problems, third trimester** ♀   M
　　● O36.899   **Maternal care for other specified fetal problems, unspecified trimester** ♀ M

● O36.9   **Maternal care for fetal problem, unspecified**
X ● O36.90   **Maternal care for fetal problem, unspecified, unspecified trimester** ♀   M
X ● O36.91   **Maternal care for fetal problem, unspecified, first trimester** ♀   M
X ● O36.92   **Maternal care for fetal problem, unspecified, second trimester** ♀   M
X ● O36.93   **Maternal care for fetal problem, unspecified, third trimester** ♀   M

● O40   **Polyhydramnios**
       Overabundance of amniotic fluid

Includes	hydramnios
Excludes1	encounter for suspected maternal and fetal conditions ruled out (Z03.7-)

One of the following 7th characters is to be assigned to each code under category O40. 7th character 0 is for single gestations and multiple gestations where the fetus is unspecified. 7th characters 1 through 9 are for cases of multiple gestations to identify the fetus for which the code applies. The appropriate code from category O30, Multiple gestation, must also be assigned when assigning a code from category O40 that has a 7th character of 1 through 9.

0	not applicable or unspecified
1	fetus 1
2	fetus 2
3	fetus 3
4	fetus 4
5	fetus 5
9	other fetus

X ● O40.1   **Polyhydramnios, first trimester** ♀   M
X ● O40.2   **Polyhydramnios, second trimester** ♀   M
X ● O40.3   **Polyhydramnios, third trimester** ♀   M
X ● O40.9   **Polyhydramnios, unspecified trimester** ♀   M

● **O41**   **Other disorders of amniotic fluid and membranes**

    Excludes1   encounter for suspected maternal and fetal conditions ruled out (Z03.7-)

    One of the following 7th characters is to be assigned to each code under category O41. 7th character Ø is for single gestations and multiple gestations where the fetus is unspecified. 7th characters 1 through 9 are for cases of multiple gestations to identify the fetus for which the code applies. The appropriate code from category O30, Multiple gestation, must also be assigned when assigning a code from category O41 that has a 7th character of 1 through 9.

Ø	not applicable or unspecified
1	fetus 1
2	fetus 2
3	fetus 3
4	fetus 4
5	fetus 5
9	other fetus

● **O41.0**   **Oligohydramnios**
     Scant volume of amniotic fluid
     ● Oligohydramnios without rupture of membranes
    X ● **O41.00**   Oligohydramnios, unspecified trimester ♀   M
    X ● **O41.01**   Oligohydramnios, first trimester ♀   M
    X ● **O41.02**   Oligohydramnios, second trimester ♀   M
    X ● **O41.03**   Oligohydramnios, third trimester ♀   M

● **O41.1**   **Infection of amniotic sac and membranes**
   ● **O41.10**   Infection of amniotic sac and membranes, unspecified
     ● **O41.101**   Infection of amniotic sac and membranes, unspecified, first trimester ♀   M
     ● **O41.102**   Infection of amniotic sac and membranes, unspecified, second trimester ♀   M
     ● **O41.103**   Infection of amniotic sac and membranes, unspecified, third trimester ♀   M
     ● **O41.109**   Infection of amniotic sac and membranes, unspecified, unspecified trimester ♀   M
   ● **O41.12**   Chorioamnionitis
     Coding Clinic: 2019, Q2, P34-35
     ● **O41.121**   Chorioamnionitis, first trimester ♀   M
     ● **O41.122**   Chorioamnionitis, second trimester ♀   M
     ● **O41.123**   Chorioamnionitis, third trimester ♀   M
     ● **O41.129**   Chorioamnionitis, unspecified trimester ♀   M
   ● **O41.14**   Placentitis
     ● **O41.141**   Placentitis, first trimester ♀   M
     ● **O41.142**   Placentitis, second trimester ♀   M
     ● **O41.143**   Placentitis, third trimester ♀   M
     ● **O41.149**   Placentitis, unspecified trimester ♀   M

● **O41.8**   **Other specified disorders of amniotic fluid and membranes**
   ● **O41.8X**   Other specified disorders of amniotic fluid and membranes
     ● **O41.8X1**   Other specified disorders of amniotic fluid and membranes, first trimester ♀   M
     ● **O41.8X2**   Other specified disorders of amniotic fluid and membranes, second trimester ♀   M
     ● **O41.8X3**   Other specified disorders of amniotic fluid and membranes, third trimester ♀   M
     ● **O41.8X9**   Other specified disorders of amniotic fluid and membranes, unspecified trimester ♀   M

● **O41.9**   **Disorder of amniotic fluid and membranes, unspecified**
   X ● **O41.90**   Disorder of amniotic fluid and membranes, unspecified, unspecified trimester ♀   M
   X ● **O41.91**   Disorder of amniotic fluid and membranes, unspecified, first trimester ♀   M
   X ● **O41.92**   Disorder of amniotic fluid and membranes, unspecified, second trimester ♀   M
   X ● **O41.93**   Disorder of amniotic fluid and membranes, unspecified, third trimester ♀   M

● **O42**   **Premature rupture of membranes**
   ● **O42.0**   **Premature rupture of membranes, onset of labor within 24 hours of rupture**
     O42.00   Premature rupture of membranes, onset of labor within 24 hours of rupture, unspecified weeks of gestation ♀   M
     ● **O42.01**   Preterm premature rupture of membranes, onset of labor within 24 hours of rupture
       Premature rupture of membranes before 37 completed weeks of gestation
       O42.011   Preterm premature rupture of membranes, onset of labor within 24 hours of rupture, first trimester ♀   M
       O42.012   Preterm premature rupture of membranes, onset of labor within 24 hours of rupture, second trimester ♀ M
       O42.013   Preterm premature rupture of membranes, onset of labor within 24 hours of rupture, third trimester ♀ M
       O42.019   Preterm premature rupture of membranes, onset of labor within 24 hours of rupture, unspecified trimester ♀   M
     O42.02   Full-term premature rupture of membranes, onset of labor within 24 hours of rupture ♀   M
       Premature rupture of membranes at or after 37 completed weeks of gestation, onset of labor within 24 hours of rupture
   ● **O42.1**   **Premature rupture of membranes, onset of labor more than 24 hours following rupture**
     O42.10   Premature rupture of membranes, onset of labor more than 24 hours following rupture, unspecified weeks of gestation ♀   M
     ● **O42.11**   Preterm premature rupture of membranes, onset of labor more than 24 hours following rupture
       Premature rupture of membranes before 37 completed weeks of gestation
       O42.111   Preterm premature rupture of membranes, onset of labor more than 24 hours following rupture, first trimester ♀   M
       O42.112   Preterm premature rupture of membranes, onset of labor more than 24 hours following rupture, second trimester ♀   M
       O42.113   Preterm premature rupture of membranes, onset of labor more than 24 hours following rupture, third trimester ♀   M
       O42.119   Preterm premature rupture of membranes, onset of labor more than 24 hours following rupture, unspecified trimester ♀   M
     O42.12   Full-term premature rupture of membranes, onset of labor more than 24 hours following rupture ♀   M
       Premature rupture of membranes at or after 37 completed weeks of gestation, onset of labor more than 24 hours following rupture

● **O42.9** **Premature rupture of membranes, unspecified as to length of time between rupture and onset of labor**

    O42.90 Premature rupture of membranes, unspecified as to length of time between rupture and onset of labor, unspecified weeks of gestation ♀   M

    ● **O42.91** Preterm premature rupture of membranes, unspecified as to length of time between rupture and onset of labor
        Premature rupture of membranes before 37 completed weeks of gestation

        O42.911 Preterm premature rupture of membranes, unspecified as to length of time between rupture and onset of labor, first trimester ♀   M

        O42.912 Preterm premature rupture of membranes, unspecified as to length of time between rupture and onset of labor, second trimester ♀   M

        O42.913 Preterm premature rupture of membranes, unspecified as to length of time between rupture and onset of labor, third trimester ♀   M

        O42.919 Preterm premature rupture of membranes, unspecified as to length of time between rupture and onset of labor, unspecified trimester ♀   M

    O42.92 Full-term premature rupture of membranes, unspecified as to length of time between rupture and onset of labor ♀   M
        Premature rupture of membranes at or after 37 completed weeks of gestation, unspecified as to length of time between rupture and onset of labor

● **O43** **Placental disorders**

    Excludes2 maternal care for poor fetal growth due to placental insufficiency (O36.5-)
        placenta previa (O44.-)
        placental polyp (O90.89)
        placentitis (O41.14-)
        premature separation of placenta [abruptio placentae] (O45.-)

    ● **O43.0** **Placental transfusion syndromes**

        ● **O43.01** Fetomaternal placental transfusion syndrome
            Maternofetal placental transfusion syndrome

            O43.011 Fetomaternal placental transfusion syndrome, first trimester ♀   M

            O43.012 Fetomaternal placental transfusion syndrome, second trimester ♀   M

            O43.013 Fetomaternal placental transfusion syndrome, third trimester ♀   M

            O43.019 Fetomaternal placental transfusion syndrome, unspecified trimester ♀   M

        ● **O43.02** Fetus-to-fetus placental transfusion syndrome

            O43.021 Fetus-to-fetus placental transfusion syndrome, first trimester ♀   M

            O43.022 Fetus-to-fetus placental transfusion syndrome, second trimester ♀   M

            O43.023 Fetus-to-fetus placental transfusion syndrome, third trimester ♀   M

            O43.029 Fetus-to-fetus placental transfusion syndrome, unspecified trimester ♀   M

    ● **O43.1** **Malformation of placenta**

        ● **O43.10** Malformation of placenta, unspecified
            Abnormal placenta NOS

            O43.101 Malformation of placenta, unspecified, first trimester ♀   M

            O43.102 Malformation of placenta, unspecified, second trimester ♀   M

            O43.103 Malformation of placenta, unspecified, third trimester ♀   M

            O43.109 Malformation of placenta, unspecified, unspecified trimester ♀ M

    ● **O43.11** Circumvallate placenta

        O43.111 Circumvallate placenta, first trimester ♀   M

        O43.112 Circumvallate placenta, second trimester ♀   M

        O43.113 Circumvallate placenta, third trimester ♀   M

        O43.119 Circumvallate placenta, unspecified trimester ♀   M

    ● **O43.12** Velamentous insertion of umbilical cord

        O43.121 Velamentous insertion of umbilical cord, first trimester ♀   M

        O43.122 Velamentous insertion of umbilical cord, second trimester ♀   M

        O43.123 Velamentous insertion of umbilical cord, third trimester ♀   M

        O43.129 Velamentous insertion of umbilical cord, unspecified trimester ♀   M

    ● **O43.19** Other malformation of placenta

        O43.191 Other malformation of placenta, first trimester ♀   M

        O43.192 Other malformation of placenta, second trimester ♀   M

        O43.193 Other malformation of placenta, third trimester ♀   M

        O43.199 Other malformation of placenta, unspecified trimester ♀   M

● **O43.2** **Morbidly adherent placenta**

    Code also associated third stage postpartum hemorrhage, if applicable (O72.0)

    Excludes1 retained placenta (O73.-)

    ● **O43.21** Placenta accreta

        O43.211 Placenta accreta, first trimester ♀   M

        O43.212 Placenta accreta, second trimester ♀ M

        O43.213 Placenta accreta, third trimester ♀   M

        O43.219 Placenta accreta, unspecified trimester ♀   M

    ● **O43.22** Placenta increta

        O43.221 Placenta increta, first trimester ♀   M

        O43.222 Placenta increta, second trimester ♀ M

        O43.223 Placenta increta, third trimester ♀   M

        O43.229 Placenta increta, unspecified trimester ♀   M

    ● **O43.23** Placenta percreta

        O43.231 Placenta percreta, first trimester ♀   M

        O43.232 Placenta percreta, second trimester ♀M

        O43.233 Placenta percreta, third trimester ♀   M

        O43.239 Placenta percreta, unspecified trimester ♀   M

● **O43.8** **Other placental disorders**

    ● **O43.81** Placental infarction

        O43.811 Placental infarction, first trimester ♀ M

        O43.812 Placental infarction, second trimester ♀   M

        O43.813 Placental infarction, third trimester ♀   M

        O43.819 Placental infarction, unspecified trimester ♀   M

    ● **O43.89** Other placental disorders
        Placental dysfunction

        O43.891 Other placental disorders, first trimester ♀   M

        O43.892 Other placental disorders, second trimester ♀   M

        O43.893 Other placental disorders, third trimester ♀   M

        O43.899 Other placental disorders, unspecified trimester ♀   M

▶ New   ⇒ Revised   ~~deleted~~ Deleted   Excludes 1   Excludes 2   Includes   Use additional   Code first   Code also   Key words

OGCR Official Guidelines   X Assign placeholder X   ● Use Additional Character(s)   ▶ Manifestation Code   🦚 Hierarchical Condition Category   **Coding Clinic**

● O43.9 Unspecified placental disorder
    O43.90 Unspecified placental disorder, unspecified trimester ♀ M
    O43.91 Unspecified placental disorder, first trimester ♀ M
    O43.92 Unspecified placental disorder, second trimester ♀ M
    O43.93 Unspecified placental disorder, third trimester ♀ M

● O44 Placenta previa
    Coding Clinic: 2016, Q4, P52

● O44.0 Complete placenta previa NOS or without hemorrhage
    Placenta previa NOS
    O44.00 Complete placenta previa NOS or without hemorrhage, unspecified trimester ♀ M
    O44.01 Complete placenta previa NOS or without hemorrhage, first trimester ♀ M
    O44.02 Complete placenta previa NOS or without hemorrhage, second trimester ♀ M
    O44.03 Complete placenta previa NOS or without hemorrhage, third trimester ♀ M

● O44.1 Complete placenta previa with hemorrhage
    Excludes1 labor and delivery complicated by hemorrhage from vasa previa (O69.4)
    O44.10 Complete placenta previa with hemorrhage, unspecified trimester ♀ M
    O44.11 Complete placenta previa with hemorrhage, first trimester ♀ M
    O44.12 Complete placenta previa with hemorrhage, second trimester ♀ M
    O44.13 Complete placenta previa with hemorrhage, third trimester ♀ M

● O44.2 Partial placenta previa without hemorrhage
    Marginal placenta previa, NOS or without hemorrhage
    O44.20 Partial placenta previa NOS or without hemorrhage, unspecified trimester ♀ M
    O44.21 Partial placenta previa NOS or without hemorrhage, first trimester ♀ M
    O44.22 Partial placenta previa NOS or without hemorrhage, second trimester ♀ M
    O44.23 Partial placenta previa NOS or without hemorrhage, third trimester ♀ M

● O44.3 Partial placenta previa with hemorrhage
    Marginal placenta previa with hemorrhage
    O44.30 Partial placenta previa with hemorrhage, unspecified trimester ♀ M
    O44.31 Partial placenta previa with hemorrhage, first trimester ♀ M
    O44.32 Partial placenta previa with hemorrhage, second trimester ♀ M
    O44.33 Partial placenta previa with hemorrhage, third trimester ♀ M

● O44.4 Low lying placenta NOS or without hemorrhage
    Low implantation of placenta NOS or without hemorrhage
    O44.40 Low lying placenta NOS or without hemorrhage, unspecified trimester ♀ M
    O44.41 Low lying placenta NOS or without hemorrhage, first trimester ♀ M
    O44.42 Low lying placenta NOS or without hemorrhage, second trimester ♀ M
    O44.43 Low lying placenta NOS or without hemorrhage, third trimester ♀ M

● O44.5 Low lying placenta with hemorrhage
    Low implantation of placenta with hemorrhage
    O44.50 Low lying placenta with hemorrhage, unspecified trimester ♀ M
    O44.51 Low lying placenta with hemorrhage, first trimester ♀ M
    O44.52 Low lying placenta with hemorrhage, second trimester ♀ M
    O44.53 Low lying placenta with hemorrhage, third trimester ♀ M

● O45 Premature separation of placenta [abruptio placentae]
  ● O45.0 Premature separation of placenta with coagulation defect
    ● O45.00 Premature separation of placenta with coagulation defect, unspecified
      O45.001 Premature separation of placenta with coagulation defect, unspecified, first trimester ♀ M
      O45.002 Premature separation of placenta with coagulation defect, unspecified, second trimester ♀ M
      O45.003 Premature separation of placenta with coagulation defect, unspecified, third trimester ♀ M
      O45.009 Premature separation of placenta with coagulation defect, unspecified, unspecified trimester ♀ M
    ● O45.01 Premature separation of placenta with afibrinogenemia
      Premature separation of placenta with hypofibrinogenemia
      O45.011 Premature separation of placenta with afibrinogenemia, first trimester ♀ M
      O45.012 Premature separation of placenta with afibrinogenemia, second trimester ♀ M
      O45.013 Premature separation of placenta with afibrinogenemia, third trimester ♀ M
      O45.019 Premature separation of placenta with afibrinogenemia, unspecified trimester ♀ M

Figure 15-2 **A.** Marginal placento previa. **B.** Partial placenta previa. **C.** Total placento previa.

Item 15–3 **Placenta previa** is a condition in which the opening of the cervix is obstructed by the displaced placenta. The three types, marginal, partial, and total, are varying degrees of placenta displacement. Placenta abruption is the premature breaking away of the placenta from the site of the uterine implant before the delivery of the fetus.

Figure 15-3 Abruptio placentae is classified according to the grade of separation of the placenta from the uterine wall. **A.** Mild separation in which hemorrhage is internal. **B.** Moderate separation in which there is external hemorrhage. **C.** Severe separation in which there is external hemorrhage and extreme separation.

CHAPTER 15 (O00-O9A)

● O45.02 Premature separation of placenta with disseminated intravascular coagulation

   O45.021 Premature separation of placenta with disseminated intravascular coagulation, first trimester ♀   M

   O45.022 Premature separation of placenta with disseminated intravascular coagulation, second trimester ♀   M

   O45.023 Premature separation of placenta with disseminated intravascular coagulation, third trimester ♀   M

   O45.029 Premature separation of placenta with disseminated intravascular coagulation, unspecified trimester ♀ M

● O45.09 Premature separation of placenta with other coagulation defect

   O45.091 Premature separation of placenta with other coagulation defect, first trimester ♀   M

   O45.092 Premature separation of placenta with other coagulation defect, second trimester ♀   M

   O45.093 Premature separation of placenta with other coagulation defect, third trimester ♀   M

   O45.099 Premature separation of placenta with other coagulation defect, unspecified trimester ♀   M

● O45.8 Other premature separation of placenta

  ● O45.8X Other premature separation of placenta

   O45.8X1 Other premature separation of placenta, first trimester ♀   M

   O45.8X2 Other premature separation of placenta, second trimester ♀   M

   O45.8X3 Other premature separation of placenta, third trimester ♀   M

   O45.8X9 Other premature separation of placenta, unspecified trimester ♀   M

● O45.9 Premature separation of placenta, unspecified
   Abruptio placentae NOS

   O45.90 Premature separation of placenta, unspecified, unspecified trimester ♀   M

   O45.91 Premature separation of placenta, unspecified, first trimester ♀   M

   O45.92 Premature separation of placenta, unspecified, second trimester ♀   M

   O45.93 Premature separation of placenta, unspecified, third trimester ♀   M

● O46 Antepartum hemorrhage, not elsewhere classified

  Excludes1 hemorrhage in early pregnancy (O20.-)
            intrapartum hemorrhage NEC (O67.-)
            placenta previa (O44.-)
            premature separation of placenta [abruptio placentae] (O45.-)

● O46.0 Antepartum hemorrhage with coagulation defect

  ● O46.00 Antepartum hemorrhage with coagulation defect, unspecified

   O46.001 Antepartum hemorrhage with coagulation defect, unspecified, first trimester ♀   M

   O46.002 Antepartum hemorrhage with coagulation defect, unspecified, second trimester ♀   M

   O46.003 Antepartum hemorrhage with coagulation defect, unspecified, third trimester ♀   M

   O46.009 Antepartum hemorrhage with coagulation defect, unspecified, unspecified trimester ♀   M

● O46.01 Antepartum hemorrhage with afibrinogenemia
   Antepartum hemorrhage with hypofibrinogenemia

   O46.011 Antepartum hemorrhage with afibrinogenemia, first trimester ♀   M

   O46.012 Antepartum hemorrhage with afibrinogenemia, second trimester ♀ M

   O46.013 Antepartum hemorrhage with afibrinogenemia, third trimester ♀   M

   O46.019 Antepartum hemorrhage with afibrinogenemia, unspecified trimester ♀   M

● O46.02 Antepartum hemorrhage with disseminated intravascular coagulation

   O46.021 Antepartum hemorrhage with disseminated intravascular coagulation, first trimester ♀   M

   O46.022 Antepartum hemorrhage with disseminated intravascular coagulation, second trimester ♀   M

   O46.023 Antepartum hemorrhage with disseminated intravascular coagulation, third trimester ♀   M

   O46.029 Antepartum hemorrhage with disseminated intravascular coagulation, unspecified trimester ♀ M

● O46.09 Antepartum hemorrhage with other coagulation defect

   O46.091 Antepartum hemorrhage with other coagulation defect, first trimester ♀   M

   O46.092 Antepartum hemorrhage with other coagulation defect, second trimester ♀   M

   O46.093 Antepartum hemorrhage with other coagulation defect, third trimester ♀ M

   O46.099 Antepartum hemorrhage with other coagulation defect, unspecified trimester ♀   M

● O46.8 Other antepartum hemorrhage

  ● O46.8x Other antepartum hemorrhage

   O46.8x1 Other antepartum hemorrhage, first trimester ♀   M

   O46.8x2 Other antepartum hemorrhage, second trimester ♀   M

   O46.8x3 Other antepartum hemorrhage, third trimester ♀   M

   O46.8x9 Other antepartum hemorrhage, unspecified trimester ♀   M

● O46.9 Antepartum hemorrhage, unspecified

   O46.90 Antepartum hemorrhage, unspecified, unspecified trimester ♀   M

   O46.91 Antepartum hemorrhage, unspecified, first trimester ♀   M

   O46.92 Antepartum hemorrhage, unspecified, second trimester ♀   M

   O46.93 Antepartum hemorrhage, unspecified, third trimester ♀   M

▶ New   ⇒ Revised   ~~deleted~~ Deleted   Excludes 1   Excludes 2   Includes   Use additional   Code first   Code also   Key words

OGCR Official Guidelines   X Assign placeholder X   ● Use Additional Character(s)   ▌ Manifestation Code   🦊 Hierarchical Condition Category   **Coding Clinic**

● O47   **False labor**
        Includes   Braxton Hicks contractions
                        threatened labor
        Excludes1   preterm labor (O60.-)

   ● O47.0   **False labor before 37 completed weeks of gestation**
         O47.00   **False labor before 37 completed weeks of gestation, unspecified trimester** ♀   M
         O47.02   **False labor before 37 completed weeks of gestation, second trimester** ♀   M
         O47.03   **False labor before 37 completed weeks of gestation, third trimester** ♀   M
      O47.1   **False labor at or after 37 completed weeks of gestation** ♀   M
               Coding Clinic: 2021, Q1, P10
      O47.9   **False labor, unspecified** ♀   M

● O48   **Late pregnancy**
      O48.0   **Post-term pregnancy** ♀   M
               Pregnancy over 40 completed weeks to 42 completed weeks gestation
      O48.1   **Prolonged pregnancy** ♀   M
               Pregnancy which has advanced beyond 42 completed weeks gestation

---

COMPLICATIONS OF LABOR AND DELIVERY (O60-O77)

● O60   **Preterm labor**
        Includes   onset (spontaneous) of labor before 37 completed
                        weeks of gestation
        Excludes1   false labor (O47.0-)
                        threatened labor NOS (O47.0-)

   ● O60.0   **Preterm labor without delivery**
         O60.00   **Preterm labor without delivery, unspecified trimester** ♀   M
         O60.02   **Preterm labor without delivery, second trimester** ♀   M
         O60.03   **Preterm labor without delivery, third trimester** ♀   M

   ● O60.1   **Preterm labor with preterm delivery**
         One of the following 7th characters is to be assigned to
         each code under subcategory O60.1. 7th character 0
         is for single gestations and multiple gestations
         where the fetus is unspecified. 7th characters 1
         through 9 are for cases of multiple gestations to
         identify the fetus for which the code applies. The
         appropriate code from category O30, Multiple
         gestation, must also be assigned when assigning
         a code from subcategory O60.1 that has a 7th
         character of 1 through 9.

0	not applicable or unspecified
1	fetus 1
2	fetus 2
3	fetus 3
4	fetus 4
5	fetus 5
9	other fetus

         Coding Clinic: 2016, Q2, P11

      X● O60.10   **Preterm labor with preterm delivery, unspecified trimester** ♀   M
                  Preterm labor with delivery NOS
      X● O60.12   **Preterm labor second trimester with preterm delivery second trimester** ♀   M
      X● O60.13   **Preterm labor second trimester with preterm delivery third trimester** ♀   M
      X● O60.14   **Preterm labor third trimester with preterm delivery third trimester** ♀   M
                  Coding Clinic: 2016, Q2, P10

● O60.2   **Term delivery with preterm labor**
         One of the following 7th characters is to be assigned to
         each code under subcategory O60.2. 7th character 0
         is for single gestations and multiple gestations
         where the fetus is unspecified. 7th characters 1
         through 9 are for cases of multiple gestations to
         identify the fetus for which the code applies. The
         appropriate code from category O30, Multiple
         gestation, must also be assigned when assigning
         a code from subcategory O60.2 that has a 7th
         character of 1 through 9.

0	not applicable or unspecified
1	fetus 1
2	fetus 2
3	fetus 3
4	fetus 4
5	fetus 5
9	other fetus

      X● O60.20   **Term delivery with preterm labor, unspecified trimester** ♀   M
      X● O60.22   **Term delivery with preterm labor, second trimester** ♀   M
      X● O60.23   **Term delivery with preterm labor, third trimester** ♀   M

● O61   **Failed induction of labor**
      O61.0   **Failed medical induction of labor** ♀   M
               Failed induction (of labor) by oxytocin
               Failed induction (of labor) by prostaglandins
      O61.1   **Failed instrumental induction of labor** ♀   M
               Failed mechanical induction (of labor)
               Failed surgical induction (of labor)
      O61.8   **Other failed induction of labor** ♀   M
      O61.9   **Failed induction of labor, unspecified** ♀   M

● O62   **Abnormalities of forces of labor**
      O62.0   **Primary inadequate contractions** ♀   M
               Failure of cervical dilatation
               Primary hypotonic uterine dysfunction
               Uterine inertia during latent phase of labor
      O62.1   **Secondary uterine inertia** ♀   M
               Arrested active phase of labor
               Secondary hypotonic uterine dysfunction
      O62.2   **Other uterine inertia** ♀   M
               Atony of uterus without hemorrhage
               Atony of uterus NOS
               Desultory labor
               Hypotonic uterine dysfunction NOS
               Irregular labor
               Poor contractions
               Slow slope active phase of labor
               Uterine inertia NOS
               Excludes1   atony of uterus with hemorrhage
                               (postpartum) (O72.1)
                               postpartum atony of uterus without
                               hemorrhage (O75.89)
      O62.3   **Precipitate labor** ♀   M
      O62.4   **Hypertonic, incoordinate, and prolonged uterine contractions** ♀   M
               Cervical spasm
               Contraction ring dystocia
               Dyscoordinate labor
               Hour-glass contraction of uterus
               Hypertonic uterine dysfunction
               Incoordinate uterine action
               Tetanic contractions
               Uterine dystocia NOS
               Uterine spasm
               Excludes1   dystocia (fetal) (maternal) NOS (O66.9)
      O62.8   **Other abnormalities of forces of labor** ♀   M
      O62.9   **Abnormality of forces of labor, unspecified** ♀   M

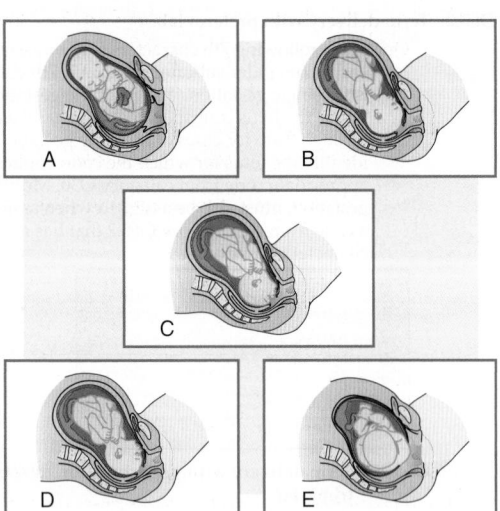

Figure 15-4 Five types of malposition and malpresentation of the fetus:
A. Breech. **B.** Vertex. **C.** Face. **D.** Brow. **E.** Shoulder.

● **O63**   **Long labor**

     O63.0   Prolonged first stage (of labor) ♀   M

     O63.1   Prolonged second stage (of labor) ♀   M

     O63.2   Delayed delivery of second twin, triplet, etc. ♀   M

     O63.9   Long labor, unspecified ♀   M
            Prolonged labor NOS

● **O64**   **Obstructed labor due to malposition and malpresentation of fetus**

     One of the following 7th characters is to be assigned to each code under category O64. 7th character Ø is for single gestations and multiple gestations where the fetus is unspecified. 7th characters 1 through 9 are for cases of multiple gestations to identify the fetus for which the code applies. The appropriate code from category O3Ø, Multiple gestation, must also be assigned when assigning a code from category O64 that has a 7th character of 1 through 9.

Ø	not applicable or unspecified
1	fetus 1
2	fetus 2
3	fetus 3
4	fetus 4
5	fetus 5
9	other fetus

  X ● **O64.0**   Obstructed labor due to incomplete rotation of fetal head ♀   M
            Deep transverse arrest
            Obstructed labor due to persistent occipitoiliac (position)
            Obstructed labor due to persistent occipitoposterior (position)
            Obstructed labor due to persistent occipitosacral (position)
            Obstructed labor due to persistent occipitotransverse (position)

  X ● **O64.1**   Obstructed labor due to breech presentation ♀   M
            Obstructed labor due to buttocks presentation
            Obstructed labor due to complete breech presentation
            Obstructed labor due to frank breech presentation

  X ● **O64.2**   Obstructed labor due to face presentation ♀   M
            Obstructed labor due to chin presentation

  X ● **O64.3**   Obstructed labor due to brow presentation ♀   M

  X ● **O64.4**   Obstructed labor due to shoulder presentation ♀   M
            Prolapsed arm
            Excludes1   impacted shoulders (O66.0)
                        shoulder dystocia (O66.0)

  X ● **O64.5**   Obstructed labor due to compound presentation ♀   M

  X ● **O64.8**   Obstructed labor due to other malposition and malpresentation ♀   M
            Obstructed labor due to footling presentation
            Obstructed labor due to incomplete breech presentation

  X ● **O64.9**   Obstructed labor due to malposition and malpresentation, unspecified ♀   M

● **O65**   **Obstructed labor due to maternal pelvic abnormality**

     O65.0   Obstructed labor due to deformed pelvis ♀   M

     O65.1   Obstructed labor due to generally contracted pelvis ♀   M

     O65.2   Obstructed labor due to pelvic inlet contraction ♀   M

     O65.3   Obstructed labor due to pelvic outlet and mid-cavity contraction ♀   M

     O65.4   Obstructed labor due to fetopelvic disproportion, unspecified ♀   M
            Excludes1   dystocia due to abnormality of fetus (O66.2-O66.3)

     O65.5   Obstructed labor due to abnormality of maternal pelvic organs ♀   M
            Obstructed labor due to conditions listed in O34.-
            Use additional code to identify abnormality of pelvic organs O34.-

     O65.8   Obstructed labor due to other maternal pelvic abnormalities ♀   M

     O65.9   Obstructed labor due to maternal pelvic abnormality, unspecified ♀   M

● **O66**   **Other obstructed labor**

     O66.0   Obstructed labor due to shoulder dystocia ♀   M
            Impacted shoulders

     O66.1   Obstructed labor due to locked twins ♀   M

     O66.2   Obstructed labor due to unusually large fetus ♀   M

     O66.3   Obstructed labor due to other abnormalities of fetus ♀ M
            Dystocia due to fetal ascites
            Dystocia due to fetal hydrops
            Dystocia due to fetal meningomyelocele
            Dystocia due to fetal sacral teratoma
            Dystocia due to fetal tumor
            Dystocia due to hydrocephalic fetus
            Use additional code to identify cause of obstruction

    ● **O66.4**   **Failed trial of labor**

        O66.40   Failed trial of labor, unspecified ♀   M

        O66.41   Failed attempted vaginal birth after previous cesarean delivery ♀   M
                Code first rupture of uterus, if applicable (O71.0-, O71.1)

     O66.5   Attempted application of vacuum extractor and forceps ♀   M
            Attempted application of vacuum or forceps, with subsequent delivery by forceps or cesarean delivery

     O66.6   Obstructed labor due to other multiple fetuses ♀   M

     O66.8   Other specified obstructed labor ♀   M
            Use additional code to identify cause of obstruction

     O66.9   Obstructed labor, unspecified ♀   M
            Dystocia NOS
            Fetal dystocia NOS
            Maternal dystocia NOS

Figure 15-5 Hydrocephalic fetus causing disproportion.

▶ New   ⇒ Revised   ~~deleted~~ Deleted   Excludes 1   Excludes 2   Includes   Use additional   Code first   Code also   Key words
OGCR Official Guidelines   X Assign placeholder X   ● Use Additional Character(s)   ▶ Manifestation Code   🝔 Hierarchical Condition Category   **Coding Clinic**

● **O67 Labor and delivery complicated by intrapartum hemorrhage, not elsewhere classified**

    Excludes1   antepartum hemorrhage NEC (O46.-)
                    placenta previa (O44.-)
                    premature separation of placenta [abruptio placentae] (O45.-)

    Excludes2   postpartum hemorrhage (O72.-)

    O67.0 Intrapartum hemorrhage with coagulation defect ♀   M
         Intrapartum hemorrhage (excessive) associated with afibrinogenemia
         Intrapartum hemorrhage (excessive) associated with disseminated intravascular coagulation
         Intrapartum hemorrhage (excessive) associated with hyperfibrinolysis
         Intrapartum hemorrhage (excessive) associated with hypofibrinogenemia

    O67.8 Other intrapartum hemorrhage ♀   M
         Excessive intrapartum hemorrhage

    O67.9 Intrapartum hemorrhage, unspecified ♀   M

● **O68 Labor and delivery complicated by abnormality of fetal acid-base balance ♀**   M
         Fetal acidemia complicating labor and delivery
         Fetal acidosis complicating labor and delivery
         Fetal alkalosis complicating labor and delivery
         Fetal metabolic acidemia complicating labor and delivery

    Excludes1   fetal stress NOS (O77.9)
                    labor and delivery complicated by electrocardiographic evidence of fetal stress (O77.8)
                    labor and delivery complicated by ultrasonic evidence of fetal stress (O77.8)

    Excludes2   abnormality in fetal heart rate or rhythm (O76)
                    labor and delivery complicated by meconium in amniotic fluid (O77.0)

● **O69 Labor and delivery complicated by umbilical cord complications**

     One of the following 7th characters is to be assigned to each code under category O69. 7th character Ø is for single gestations and multiple gestations where the fetus is unspecified. 7th characters 1 through 9 are for cases of multiple gestations to identify the fetus for which the code applies. The appropriate code from category O30, Multiple gestation, must also be assigned when assigning a code from category O69 that has a 7th character of 1 through 9.

Ø	not applicable or unspecified
1	fetus 1
2	fetus 2
3	fetus 3
4	fetus 4
5	fetus 5
9	other fetus

X● **O69.0 Labor and delivery complicated by prolapse of cord ♀**   M

X● **O69.1 Labor and delivery complicated by cord around neck, with compression ♀**   M
    Excludes1   labor and delivery complicated by cord around neck, without compression (O69.81)

X● **O69.2 Labor and delivery complicated by other cord entanglement, with compression ♀**   M
         Labor and delivery complicated by compression of cord NOS
         Labor and delivery complicated by entanglement of cords of twins in monoamniotic sac
         Labor and delivery complicated by knot in cord
    Excludes1   labor and delivery complicated by other cord entanglement, without compression (O69.82)

X● **O69.3 Labor and delivery complicated by short cord ♀**   M

X● **O69.4 Labor and delivery complicated by vasa previa ♀**   M
         Labor and delivery complicated by hemorrhage from vasa previa

X● **O69.5 Labor and delivery complicated by vascular lesion of cord ♀**   M
         Labor and delivery complicated by cord bruising
         Labor and delivery complicated by cord hematoma
         Labor and delivery complicated by thrombosis of umbilical vessels

● **O69.8 Labor and delivery complicated by other cord complications**

X● **O69.81 Labor and delivery complicated by cord around neck, without compression ♀**   M

X● **O69.82 Labor and delivery complicated by other cord entanglement, without compression ♀**   M

X● **O69.89 Labor and delivery complicated by other cord complications ♀**   M

X● **O69.9 Labor and delivery complicated by cord complication, unspecified ♀**   M

● **O70 Perineal laceration during delivery**

    Includes   episiotomy extended by laceration
    Excludes1   obstetric high vaginal laceration alone (O71.4)

    O70.0 First degree perineal laceration during delivery ♀   M
         Perineal laceration, rupture or tear involving fourchette during delivery
         Perineal laceration, rupture or tear involving labia during delivery
         Perineal laceration, rupture or tear involving skin during delivery
         Perineal laceration, rupture or tear involving vagina during delivery
         Perineal laceration, rupture or tear involving vulva during delivery
         Slight perineal laceration, rupture or tear during delivery

    O70.1 Second degree perineal laceration during delivery ♀   M
         Perineal laceration, rupture or tear during delivery as in O70.0, also involving pelvic floor
         Perineal laceration, rupture or tear during delivery as in O70.0, also involving perineal muscles
         Perineal laceration, rupture or tear during delivery as in O70.0, also involving vaginal muscles
    Excludes1   perineal laceration involving anal sphincter (O70.2)
    Coding Clinic: 2016, CODING CIQ4, P53, Q2, P34

● **O70.2 Third degree perineal laceration during delivery**
         Perineal laceration, rupture or tear during delivery as in O70.1, also involving anal sphincter
         Perineal laceration, rupture or tear during delivery as in O70.1, also involving rectovaginal septum
         Perineal laceration, rupture or tear during delivery as in O70.1, also involving sphincter NOS
    Excludes1   anal sphincter tear during delivery without third degree perineal laceration (O70.4)
                  perineal laceration involving anal or rectal mucosa (O70.3)

    O70.20 Third degree perineal laceration during delivery, unspecified ♀   M

    O70.21 Third degree perineal laceration during delivery, IIIa ♀   M
         Third degree perineal laceration during delivery with less than 50% of external anal sphincter (EAS) thickness torn

    O70.22 Third degree perineal laceration during delivery, IIIb ♀   M
         Third degree perineal laceration during delivery with more than 50% external anal sphincter (EAS) thickness torn

    O70.23 Third degree perineal laceration during delivery, IIIc ♀   M
         Third degree perineal laceration during delivery with both external anal sphincter (EAS) and internal anal sphincter (IAS) torn

Vaginal   Urethral
opening   opening

A
B
C
D

Anus

Figure 15-6 Perineal lacerations: **A.** First-degree is laceration of superficial tissues. **B.** Second-degree is limited to the pelvic floor and may involve the perineal or vaginal muscles. **C.** Third-degree involves the anal sphincter. **D.** Fourth-degree involves anal or rectal mucosa.

O70.3   **Fourth degree perineal laceration during delivery** ♀   M
Perineal laceration, rupture or tear during delivery as in O70.2, also involving anal mucosa
Perineal laceration, rupture or tear during delivery as in O70.2, also involving rectal mucosa

O70.4   **Anal sphincter tear complicating delivery, not associated with third degree laceration** ♀   M
Excludes1   anal sphincter tear with third degree perineal laceration (O70.2)

O70.9   **Perineal laceration during delivery, unspecified** ♀   M

● O71   **Other obstetric trauma**
Includes   obstetric damage from instruments

● O71.0   **Rupture of uterus (spontaneous) before onset of labor**
Excludes1   disruption of (current) cesarean delivery wound (O90.0)
laceration of uterus, NEC (O71.81)

O71.00   **Rupture of uterus before onset of labor, unspecified trimester** ♀   M

O71.02   **Rupture of uterus before onset of labor, second trimester** ♀   M

O71.03   **Rupture of uterus before onset of labor, third trimester** ♀   M

O71.1   **Rupture of uterus during labor** ♀   M
Rupture of uterus not stated as occurring before onset of labor
Excludes1   disruption of cesarean delivery wound (O90.0)
laceration of uterus, NEC (O71.81)

O71.2   **Postpartum inversion of uterus** ♀   M

O71.3   **Obstetric laceration of cervix** ♀   M
Annular detachment of cervix

O71.4   **Obstetric high vaginal laceration alone** ♀   M
Laceration of vaginal wall without perineal laceration
Excludes1   obstetric high vaginal laceration with perineal laceration (O70.-)

O71.5   **Other obstetric injury to pelvic organs** ♀   M
Obstetric injury to bladder
Obstetric injury to urethra
Excludes2   obstetric periurethral trauma (O71.82)

O71.6   **Obstetric damage to pelvic joints and ligaments** ♀   M
Obstetric avulsion of inner symphyseal cartilage
Obstetric damage to coccyx
Obstetric traumatic separation of symphysis (pubis)

O71.7   **Obstetric hematoma of pelvis** ♀   M
Obstetric hematoma of perineum
Obstetric hematoma of vagina
Obstetric hematoma of vulva

● O71.8   **Other specified obstetric trauma**

O71.81   **Laceration of uterus, not elsewhere classified** ♀   M

O71.82   **Other specified trauma to perineum and vulva** ♀   M
Obstetric periurethral trauma

O71.89   **Other specified obstetric trauma** ♀   M

O71.9   **Obstetric trauma, unspecified** ♀   M

● O72   **Postpartum hemorrhage**
Includes   hemorrhage after delivery of fetus or infant

O72.0   **Third-stage hemorrhage** ♀   M
Hemorrhage associated with retained, trapped or adherent placenta
Retained placenta NOS
Code also type of adherent placenta (O43.2-)

O72.1   **Other immediate postpartum hemorrhage** ♀   M
Hemorrhage following delivery of placenta
Postpartum hemorrhage (atonic) NOS
Uterine atony with hemorrhage
Excludes1   uterine atony NOS (O62.2)
uterine atony without hemorrhage (O62.2)
postpartum atony of uterus without hemorrhage (O75.89)

O72.2   **Delayed and secondary postpartum hemorrhage** ♀   M
Hemorrhage associated with retained portions of placenta or membranes after the first 24 hours following delivery of placenta
Retained products of conception NOS, following delivery

O72.3   **Postpartum coagulation defects** ♀   M
Postpartum afibrinogenemia
Postpartum fibrinolysis

● O73   **Retained placenta and membranes, without hemorrhage**
Excludes1   placenta accreta (O43.21-)
placenta increta (O43.22-)
placenta percreta (O43.23-)

O73.0   **Retained placenta without hemorrhage** ♀   M
Adherent placenta, without hemorrhage
Trapped placenta without hemorrhage

O73.1   **Retained portions of placenta and membranes, without hemorrhage** ♀   M
Retained products of conception following delivery, without hemorrhage

● O74   **Complications of anesthesia during labor and delivery**
Includes   maternal complications arising from the administration of a general, regional or local anesthetic, analgesic or other sedation during labor and delivery
Use additional code, if applicable, to identify specific complication

O74.0   **Aspiration pneumonitis due to anesthesia during labor and delivery** ♀   M
Inhalation of stomach contents or secretions NOS due to anesthesia during labor and delivery
Mendelson's syndrome due to anesthesia during labor and delivery

O74.1   **Other pulmonary complications of anesthesia during labor and delivery** ♀   M

O74.2   **Cardiac complications of anesthesia during labor and delivery** ♀   M

O74.3   **Central nervous system complications of anesthesia during labor and delivery** ♀   M

O74.4   **Toxic reaction to local anesthesia during labor and delivery** ♀   M

O74.5   **Spinal and epidural anesthesia-induced headache during labor and delivery** ♀   M

O74.6   **Other complications of spinal and epidural anesthesia during labor and delivery** ♀   M

O74.7   **Failed or difficult intubation for anesthesia during labor and delivery** ♀   M

O74.8   **Other complications of anesthesia during labor and delivery** ♀   M

O74.9   **Complication of anesthesia during labor and delivery, unspecified** ♀   M

CHAPTER 15 (O00-O9A)

● **O75   Other complications of labor and delivery, not elsewhere classified**

    Excludes2   puerperal (postpartum) infection (O86.-)
                  puerperal (postpartum) sepsis (O85)

   O75.0   Maternal distress during labor and delivery ♀   M

   O75.1   Shock during or following labor and delivery ♀   M
       Obstetric shock following labor and delivery

   O75.2   Pyrexia during labor, not elsewhere classified ♀   M

   O75.3   Other infection during labor ♀   M
       Sepsis during labor
       Use additional code (B95-B97), to identify infectious agent

   O75.4   Other complications of obstetric surgery and procedures ♀   M
       Cardiac arrest following obstetric surgery or procedures
       Cardiac failure following obstetric surgery or procedures
       Cerebral anoxia following obstetric surgery or procedures
       Pulmonary edema following obstetric surgery or procedures
       Use additional code to identify specific complication

      Excludes2   complications of anesthesia during labor and delivery (O74.-)
                  disruption of obstetrical (surgical) wound (O90.0-O90.1)
                  hematoma of obstetrical (surgical) wound (O90.2)
                  infection of obstetrical (surgical) wound (O86.0-)

   O75.5   Delayed delivery after artificial rupture of membranes ♀   M

●   **O75.8   Other specified complications of labor and delivery**

      O75.81   Maternal exhaustion complicating labor and delivery ♀   M

      O75.82   Onset (spontaneous) of labor after 37 completed weeks of gestation but before 39 completed weeks gestation, with delivery by (planned) cesarean section ♀   M
         Delivery by (planned) cesarean section occurring after 37 completed weeks of gestation but before 39 completed weeks gestation due to (spontaneous) onset of labor
         Code first to specify reason for planned cesarean section such as:
            cephalopelvic disproportion (normally formed fetus) (O33.9)
            previous cesarean delivery (O34.21)

      O75.89   Other specified complications of labor and delivery ♀   M

   O75.9   Complication of labor and delivery, unspecified ♀   M

O76   Abnormality in fetal heart rate and rhythm complicating labor and delivery ♀   M
   Depressed fetal heart rate tones complicating labor and delivery
   Fetal bradycardia complicating labor and delivery
   Fetal heart rate decelerations complicating labor and delivery
   Fetal heart rate irregularity complicating labor and delivery
   Fetal heart rate abnormal variability complicating labor and delivery
   Fetal tachycardia complicating labor and delivery
   Non-reassuring fetal heart rate or rhythm complicating labor and delivery

   Excludes1   fetal stress NOS (O77.9)
               labor and delivery complicated by electrocardiographic evidence of fetal stress (O77.8)
               labor and delivery complicated by ultrasonic evidence of fetal stress (O77.8)

   Excludes2   fetal metabolic acidemia (O68)
               other fetal stress (O77.0-O77.1)

● **O77   Other fetal stress complicating labor and delivery**

   O77.0   Labor and delivery complicated by meconium in amniotic fluid ♀   M

   O77.1   Fetal stress in labor or delivery due to drug administration ♀   M

   O77.8   Labor and delivery complicated by other evidence of fetal stress ♀   M
       Labor and delivery complicated by electrocardiographic evidence of fetal stress
       Labor and delivery complicated by ultrasonic evidence of fetal stress

      Excludes1   abnormality of fetal acid-base balance (O68)
                  abnormality in fetal heart rate or rhythm (O76)
                  fetal metabolic acidemia (O68)

   O77.9   Labor and delivery complicated by fetal stress, unspecified ♀   M
      Excludes1   abnormality of fetal acid-base balance (O68)
                  abnormality in fetal heart rate or rhythm (O76)
                  fetal metabolic acidemia (O68)

OGCR Section I.C., Chapter 15.n.

Normal Delivery, Code O80

1) Encounter for full-term uncomplicated delivery

Code O80 should be assigned when a woman is admitted for a full-term normal delivery and delivers a single, healthy infant without any complications antepartum, during the delivery, or postpartum during the delivery episode. Code O80 is always a principal diagnosis. It is not to be used if any other code from Chapter 15 is needed to describe a current complication of the antenatal, delivery, or perinatal period. Additional codes from other chapters may be used with code O80 if they are not related to or are in any way complicating the pregnancy.

2) Uncomplicated delivery with resolved antepartum complication

Code O80 may be used if the patient had a complication at some point during the pregnancy, but the complication is not present at the time of the admission for delivery.

3) Outcome of delivery for O80

Z37.0, Single live brith, is the only outcome of delivery code appropriate for use with O80.

ENCOUNTER FOR DELIVERY (O80-O82)

O80   Encounter for full-term uncomplicated delivery ♀   M
   Delivery requiring minimal or no assistance, with or without episiotomy, without fetal manipulation [e.g., rotation version] or instrumentation [forceps] of a spontaneous, cephalic, vaginal, full-term, single, live-born infant. This code is for use as a single diagnosis code and is not to be used with any other code from Chapter 15.

   Use additional code to indicate outcome of delivery (Z37.0)
   Coding Clinic: 2016, Q4, P124, 150

O82   Encounter for cesarean delivery without indication ♀   M
   Use additional code to indicate outcome of delivery (Z37.0)

Figure 15-7 The four stages of normal delivery: **I.** Lightening, which occurs 2 to 4 weeks before birth, at which time the fetus turns with head toward the vagina. **II.** Regular contractions begin, the amniotic sac ruptures, and dilation is complete. **III.** Delivery of the head and rotation. **IV.** Expulsion of placenta.

CHAPTER 15 (O00-O9A)

COMPLICATIONS PREDOMINANTLY RELATED TO THE PUERPERIUM (O85-O92)

Excludes2   mental and behavioral disorders associated with the puerperium (F53.-)
obstetrical tetanus (A34)
puerperal osteomalacia (M83.0)

O85   **Puerperal sepsis** ♀   M
Postpartum sepsis
Puerperal peritonitis
Puerperal pyemia
Use additional code (B95-B97), to identify infectious agent
Use additional code (R65.2-) to identify severe sepsis, if applicable

Excludes1   fever of unknown origin following delivery (O86.4)
genital tract infection following delivery (O86.1-)
obstetric pyemic and septic embolism (O88.3-)
puerperal septic thrombophlebitis (O86.81)
urinary tract infection following delivery (O86.2-)

Excludes2   sepsis during labor (O75.3)
Coding Clinic: 2018, Q4, P23

● **O86**   **Other puerperal infections**
Use additional code (B95-B97), to identify infectious agent
Excludes2   infection during labor (O75.3)
obstetrical tetanus (A34)

   ● **O86.0**   **Infection of obstetric surgical wound**
Infected cesarean delivery wound following delivery
Infected perineal repair following delivery
Excludes1   complications of procedures, not elsewhere classified (T81.44)
postprocedural fever NOS (R50.82)
postprocedural retroperitoneal abscess (K68.11)

     O86.00   **Infection of obstetric surgical wound, unspecified** ♀   M

     O86.01   **Infection of obstetric surgical wound, superficial incisional site** ♀   M
Subcutaneous abscess following an obstetrical procedure
Stitch abscess following an obstetrical procedure

     O86.02   **Infection of obstetric surgical wound, deep incisional site** ♀   M
Intramuscular abscess following an obstetrical procedure
Sub-fascial abscess following an obstetrical procedure
Coding Clinic: 2018, Q4, P23

     O86.03   **Infection of obstetric surgical wound, organ and space site** ♀   M
Intraabdominal abscess following an obstetrical procedure
Subphrenic abscess following an obstetrical procedure

     O86.04   **Sepsis following an obstetrical procedure** ♀   M
Use additional code to identify the sepsis

     O86.09   **Infection of obstetric surgical wound, other surgical site** ♀   M

   ● **O86.1**   **Other infection of genital tract following delivery**
     O86.11   **Cervicitis following delivery** ♀   M
     O86.12   **Endometritis following delivery** ♀   M
     O86.13   **Vaginitis following delivery** ♀   M
     O86.19   **Other infection of genital tract following delivery** ♀   M

   ● **O86.2**   **Urinary tract infection following delivery**
     O86.20   **Urinary tract infection following delivery, unspecified** ♀   M
Puerperal urinary tract infection NOS
     O86.21   **Infection of kidney following delivery** ♀   M

     O86.22   **Infection of bladder following delivery** ♀   M
Infection of urethra following delivery
     O86.29   **Other urinary tract infection following delivery** ♀   M

   O86.4   **Pyrexia of unknown origin following delivery** ♀   M
Puerperal infection NOS following delivery
Puerperal pyrexia NOS following delivery
Excludes2   pyrexia during labor (O75.2)

   ● **O86.8**   **Other specified puerperal infections**
     O86.81   **Puerperal septic thrombophlebitis** ♀   M
     O86.89   **Other specified puerperal infections** ♀   M

● **O87**   **Venous complications and hemorrhoids in the puerperium**
Includes   venous complications in labor, delivery and the puerperium
Excludes2   obstetric embolism (O88.-)
puerperal septic thrombophlebitis (O86.81)
venous complications in pregnancy (O22.-)

   O87.0   **Superficial thrombophlebitis in the puerperium** ♀   M
Puerperal phlebitis NOS
Puerperal thrombosis NOS

   O87.1   **Deep phlebothrombosis in the puerperium** ♀   M
Deep vein thrombosis, postpartum
Pelvic thrombophlebitis, postpartum
⟹ Use additional code to identify the deep vein thrombosis (I82.4-, I82.5-, I82.62-, I82.72-)
Use additional code, if applicable, for associated long-term (current) use of anticoagulants (Z79.01)

   O87.2   **Hemorrhoids in the puerperium** ♀   M
   O87.3   **Cerebral venous thrombosis in the puerperium** ♀   M
Cerebrovenous sinus thrombosis in the puerperium

   O87.4   **Varicose veins of lower extremity in the puerperium** ♀   M
   O87.8   **Other venous complications in the puerperium** ♀   M
Genital varices in the puerperium

   O87.9   **Venous complication in the puerperium, unspecified** ♀   M
Puerperal phlebopathy NOS

O88   **Obstetric embolism**
Excludes1   embolism complicating abortion NOS (O03.2)
embolism complicating ectopic or molar pregnancy (O08.2)
embolism complicating failed attempted abortion (O07.2)
embolism complicating induced abortion (O04.7)
embolism complicating spontaneous abortion (O03.2, O03.7)

   ● **O88.0**   **Obstetric air embolism**
     ● **O88.01**   **Obstetric air embolism in pregnancy**
        O88.011   **Air embolism in pregnancy, first trimester** ♀   M
        O88.012   **Air embolism in pregnancy, second trimester** ♀   M
        O88.013   **Air embolism in pregnancy, third trimester** ♀   M
        O88.019   **Air embolism in pregnancy, unspecified trimester** ♀   M
     O88.02   **Air embolism in childbirth** ♀   M
     O88.03   **Air embolism in the puerperium** ♀   M

   ● **O88.1**   **Amniotic fluid embolism**
Anaphylactoid syndrome in pregnancy
     ● **O88.11**   **Amniotic fluid embolism in pregnancy**
        O88.111   **Amniotic fluid embolism in pregnancy, first trimester** ♀   M
        O88.112   **Amniotic fluid embolism in pregnancy, second trimester** ♀   M
        O88.113   **Amniotic fluid embolism in pregnancy, third trimester** ♀   M
        O88.119   **Amniotic fluid embolism in pregnancy, unspecified trimester** ♀   M
     O88.12   **Amniotic fluid embolism in childbirth** ♀   M
     O88.13   **Amniotic fluid embolism in the puerperium** ♀   M

▶ New   ⟹ Revised   ~~deleted~~ Deleted   Excludes 1   Excludes 2   Includes   Use additional   Code first   Code also   Key words
OGCR Official Guidelines   X Assign placeholder X   ● Use Additional Character(s)   ▌ Manifestation Code   🅒🅒 Hierarchical Condition Category   **Coding Clinic**

● **O88.2 Obstetric thromboembolism**
  ● **O88.21 Thromboembolism in pregnancy**
    Obstetric (pulmonary) embolism NOS
    O88.211 Thromboembolism in pregnancy, first trimester ♀   M
    O88.212 Thromboembolism in pregnancy, second trimester ♀   M
    O88.213 Thromboembolism in pregnancy, third trimester ♀   M
    O88.219 Thromboembolism in pregnancy, unspecified trimester ♀   M
  O88.22 Thromboembolism in childbirth ♀   M
  O88.23 Thromboembolism in the puerperium ♀   M
    Puerperal (pulmonary) embolism NOS

● **O88.3 Obstetric pyemic and septic embolism**
  ● **O88.31 Pyemic and septic embolism in pregnancy**
    O88.311 Pyemic and septic embolism in pregnancy, first trimester ♀   M
    O88.312 Pyemic and septic embolism in pregnancy, second trimester ♀   M
    O88.313 Pyemic and septic embolism in pregnancy, third trimester ♀   M
    O88.319 Pyemic and septic embolism in pregnancy, unspecified trimester ♀   M
  O88.32 Pyemic and septic embolism in childbirth ♀   M
  O88.33 Pyemic and septic embolism in the puerperium ♀   M

● **O88.8 Other obstetric embolism**
    Obstetric fat embolism
  ● **O88.81 Other embolism in pregnancy**
    O88.811 Other embolism in pregnancy, first trimester ♀   M
    O88.812 Other embolism in pregnancy, second trimester ♀   M
    O88.813 Other embolism in pregnancy, third trimester ♀   M
    O88.819 Other embolism in pregnancy, unspecified trimester ♀   M
  O88.82 Other embolism in childbirth ♀   M
  O88.83 Other embolism in the puerperium ♀   M

● **O89 Complications of anesthesia during the puerperium**
  Includes   maternal complications arising from the administration of a general, regional or local anesthetic, analgesic or other sedation during the puerperium
  Use additional code, if applicable, to identify specific complication

  ● **O89.0 Pulmonary complications of anesthesia during the puerperium**
    O89.01 Aspiration pneumonitis due to anesthesia during the puerperium ♀   M
    Inhalation of stomach contents or secretions NOS due to anesthesia during the puerperium
    Mendelson's syndrome due to anesthesia during the puerperium
    O89.09 Other pulmonary complications of anesthesia during the puerperium ♀   M
  O89.1 Cardiac complications of anesthesia during the puerperium ♀   M
  O89.2 Central nervous system complications of anesthesia during the puerperium ♀   M
  O89.3 Toxic reaction to local anesthesia during the puerperium ♀   M
  O89.4 Spinal and epidural anesthesia-induced headache during the puerperium ♀   M
  O89.5 Other complications of spinal and epidural anesthesia during the puerperium ♀   M
  O89.6 Failed or difficult intubation for anesthesia during the puerperium ♀   M
  O89.8 Other complications of anesthesia during the puerperium ♀   M
  O89.9 Complication of anesthesia during the puerperium, unspecified ♀   M

● **O90 Complications of the puerperium, not elsewhere classified**
  O90.0 Disruption of cesarean delivery wound ♀   M
    Dehiscence of cesarean delivery wound
    Excludes1   rupture of uterus (spontaneous) before onset of labor (O71.0-)
        rupture of uterus during labor (O71.1)
  O90.1 Disruption of perineal obstetric wound ♀   M
    Disruption of wound of episiotomy
    Disruption of wound of perineal laceration
    Secondary perineal tear
  O90.2 Hematoma of obstetric wound ♀   M
  O90.3 Peripartum cardiomyopathy ♀   M
    Conditions in I42.- arising during pregnancy and the puerperium
    Excludes1   pre-existing heart disease complicating pregnancy and the puerperium (O99.4-)
  O90.4 Postpartum acute kidney failure ♀   M
    Hepatorenal syndrome following labor and delivery
  O90.5 Postpartum thyroiditis ♀   M
  O90.6 Postpartum mood disturbance ♀   M
    Postpartum blues   Postpartum sadness
    Postpartum dysphoria
    Excludes1   postpartum depression (F53.0)
        puerperal psychosis (F53.1)
  ● **O90.8 Other complications of the puerperium, not elsewhere classified**
    O90.81 Anemia of the puerperium ♀   M
    Postpartum anemia NOS
      Excludes1   pre-existing anemia complicating the puerperium (O99.03)
    O90.89 Other complications of the puerperium, not elsewhere classified ♀   M
    Placental polyp
  O90.9 Complication of the puerperium, unspecified ♀   M

● **O91 Infections of breast associated with pregnancy, the puerperium and lactation**
  Use additional code to identify infection
  ● **O91.0 Infection of nipple associated with pregnancy, the puerperium and lactation**
  ● **O91.01 Infection of nipple associated with pregnancy**
    Gestational abscess of nipple
    O91.011 Infection of nipple associated with pregnancy, first trimester ♀   M
    O91.012 Infection of nipple associated with pregnancy, second trimester ♀   M
    O91.013 Infection of nipple associated with pregnancy, third trimester ♀   M
    O91.019 Infection of nipple associated with pregnancy, unspecified trimester ♀   M
    O91.02 Infection of nipple associated with the puerperium ♀   M
    Puerperal abscess of nipple
    O91.03 Infection of nipple associated with lactation ♀ M
    Abscess of nipple associated with lactation
  ● **O91.1 Abscess of breast associated with pregnancy, the puerperium and lactation**
  ● **O91.11 Abscess of breast associated with pregnancy**
    Gestational mammary abscess
    Gestational purulent mastitis
    Gestational subareolar abscess
    O91.111 Abscess of breast associated with pregnancy, first trimester ♀   M
    O91.112 Abscess of breast associated with pregnancy, second trimester ♀   M
    O91.113 Abscess of breast associated with pregnancy, third trimester ♀   M
    O91.119 Abscess of breast associated with pregnancy, unspecified trimester ♀   M

CHAPTER 15 (O00–O9A)

O91.12   Abscess of breast associated with the puerperium ♀   M
     Puerperal mammary abscess
     Puerperal purulent mastitis
     Puerperal subareolar abscess

O91.13   Abscess of breast associated with lactation ♀   M
     Mammary abscess associated with lactation
     Purulent mastitis associated with lactation
     Subareolar abscess associated with lactation

● O91.2   Nonpurulent mastitis associated with pregnancy, the puerperium and lactation

  ● O91.21   Nonpurulent mastitis associated with pregnancy
       Gestational interstitial mastitis
       Gestational lymphangitis of breast
       Gestational mastitis NOS
       Gestational parenchymatous mastitis

      O91.211   Nonpurulent mastitis associated with pregnancy, first trimester ♀   M

      O91.212   Nonpurulent mastitis associated with pregnancy, second trimester ♀   M

      O91.213   Nonpurulent mastitis associated with pregnancy, third trimester ♀   M

      O91.219   Nonpurulent mastitis associated with pregnancy, unspecified trimester ♀   M

     O91.22   Nonpurulent mastitis associated with the puerperium ♀   M
       Puerperal interstitial mastitis
       Puerperal lymphangitis of breast
       Puerperal mastitis NOS
       Puerperal parenchymatous mastitis

     O91.23   Nonpurulent mastitis associated with lactation ♀   M
       Interstitial mastitis associated with lactation
       Lymphangitis of breast associated with lactation
       Mastitis NOS associated with lactation
       Parenchymatous mastitis associated with lactation

● O92   Other disorders of breast and disorders of lactation associated with pregnancy and the puerperium

  ● O92.0   Retracted nipple associated with pregnancy, the puerperium, and lactation

    ● O92.01   Retracted nipple associated with pregnancy

       O92.011   Retracted nipple associated with pregnancy, first trimester ♀   M

       O92.012   Retracted nipple associated with pregnancy, second trimester ♀   M

       O92.013   Retracted nipple associated with pregnancy, third trimester ♀   M

       O92.019   Retracted nipple associated with pregnancy, unspecified trimester ♀   M

     O92.02   Retracted nipple associated with the puerperium ♀   M

     O92.03   Retracted nipple associated with lactation ♀   M

  ● O92.1   Cracked nipple associated with pregnancy, the puerperium, and lactation
      Fissure of nipple, gestational or puerperal

    ● O92.11   Cracked nipple associated with pregnancy

       O92.111   Cracked nipple associated with pregnancy, first trimester ♀   M

       O92.112   Cracked nipple associated with pregnancy, second trimester ♀   M

       O92.113   Cracked nipple associated with pregnancy, third trimester ♀   M

       O92.119   Cracked nipple associated with pregnancy, unspecified trimester ♀   M

     O92.12   Cracked nipple associated with the puerperium ♀   M

     O92.13   Cracked nipple associated with lactation ♀   M

  ● O92.2   Other and unspecified disorders of breast associated with pregnancy and the puerperium

     O92.20   Unspecified disorder of breast associated with pregnancy and the puerperium ♀   M

     O92.29   Other disorders of breast associated with pregnancy and the puerperium ♀   M

   O92.3   Agalactia ♀   M
      Primary agalactia

     Excludes1   elective agalactia (O92.5)
              secondary agalactia (O92.5)
              therapeutic agalactia (O92.5)

   O92.4   Hypogalactia ♀   M

   O92.5   Suppressed lactation ♀   M
      Elective agalactia   Therapeutic agalactia
      Secondary agalactia

     Excludes1   primary agalactia (O92.3)

   O92.6   Galactorrhea ♀   M

  ● O92.7   Other and unspecified disorders of lactation

     O92.70   Unspecified disorders of lactation ♀   M

     O92.79   Other disorders of lactation ♀   M
       Puerperal galactocele

OTHER OBSTETRIC CONDITIONS, NOT ELSEWHERE CLASSIFIED (O94-O9A)

O94   Sequelae of complication of pregnancy, childbirth, and the puerperium ♀   M

   Note: This category is to be used to indicate conditions in O00-O77.-, O85-O94 and O98-O9A.- as the cause of late effects. The "sequelae" include conditions specified as such, or as late effects, which may occur at any time after the puerperium.

   Code first condition resulting from (sequela) of complication of pregnancy, childbirth, and the puerperium

O98   Maternal infectious and parasitic diseases classifiable elsewhere but complicating pregnancy, childbirth and the puerperium

   Includes   the listed conditions when complicating the pregnant state, when aggravated by the pregnancy, or as a reason for obstetric care

   Use additional code (Chapter 1), to identify specific infectious or parasitic disease

   Excludes2   herpes gestationis (O26.4-)
            infectious carrier state (O99.82-, O99.83-)
            obstetrical tetanus (A34)
            puerperal infection (O86.-)
            puerperal sepsis (O85)
            when the reason for maternal care is that the disease is known or suspected to have affected the fetus (O35-O36)

  ● O98.0   Tuberculosis complicating pregnancy, childbirth and the puerperium
      Conditions in A15-A19

    ● O98.01   Tuberculosis complicating pregnancy

       O98.011   Tuberculosis complicating pregnancy, first trimester ♀   M

       O98.012   Tuberculosis complicating pregnancy, second trimester ♀   M

       O98.013   Tuberculosis complicating pregnancy, third trimester ♀   M

       O98.019   Tuberculosis complicating pregnancy, unspecified trimester ♀   M

     O98.02   Tuberculosis complicating childbirth ♀   M

     O98.03   Tuberculosis complicating the puerperium ♀   M

  ● O98.1   Syphilis complicating pregnancy, childbirth and the puerperium
      Conditions in A50-A53

    ● O98.11   Syphilis complicating pregnancy

       O98.111   Syphilis complicating pregnancy, first trimester ♀   M

       O98.112   Syphilis complicating pregnancy, second trimester ♀   M

O98.113 Syphilis complicating pregnancy, third trimester ♀ M

O98.119 Syphilis complicating pregnancy, unspecified trimester ♀ M

O98.12 Syphilis complicating childbirth ♀ M

O98.13 Syphilis complicating the puerperium ♀ M

● O98.2 Gonorrhea complicating pregnancy, childbirth and the puerperium
    Conditions in A54.-

  ● O98.21 Gonorrhea complicating pregnancy

O98.211 Gonorrhea complicating pregnancy, first trimester ♀ M

O98.212 Gonorrhea complicating pregnancy, second trimester ♀ M

O98.213 Gonorrhea complicating pregnancy, third trimester ♀ M

O98.219 Gonorrhea complicating pregnancy, unspecified trimester ♀ M

O98.22 Gonorrhea complicating childbirth ♀ M

O98.23 Gonorrhea complicating the puerperium ♀ M

● O98.3 Other infections with a predominantly sexual mode of transmission complicating pregnancy, childbirth and the puerperium
    Conditions in A55-A64

  ● O98.31 Other infections with a predominantly sexual mode of transmission complicating pregnancy

O98.311 Other infections with a predominantly sexual mode of transmission complicating pregnancy, first trimester ♀ M

O98.312 Other infections with a predominantly sexual mode of transmission complicating pregnancy, second trimester ♀ M

O98.313 Other infections with a predominantly sexual mode of transmission complicating pregnancy, third trimester ♀ M

O98.319 Other infections with a predominantly sexual mode of transmission complicating pregnancy, unspecified trimester ♀ M

O98.32 Other infections with a predominantly sexual mode of transmission complicating childbirth ♀ M
    Coding Clinic: 2020, Q1, P20

O98.33 Other infections with a predominantly sexual mode of transmission complicating the puerperium ♀ M

● O98.4 Viral hepatitis complicating pregnancy, childbirth and the puerperium
    Conditions in B15-B19

  ● O98.41 Viral hepatitis complicating pregnancy

O98.411 Viral hepatitis complicating pregnancy, first trimester ♀ M

O98.412 Viral hepatitis complicating pregnancy, second trimester ♀ M

O98.413 Viral hepatitis complicating pregnancy, third trimester ♀ M

O98.419 Viral hepatitis complicating pregnancy, unspecified trimester ♀ M

O98.42 Viral hepatitis complicating childbirth ♀ M

O98.43 Viral hepatitis complicating the puerperium ♀ M

● O98.5 Other viral diseases complicating pregnancy, childbirth and the puerperium
    Conditions in A80-B09, B25-B34, R87.81-, R87.82-

    Excludes:1 human immunodeficiency virus [HIV] disease complicating pregnancy, childbirth and the puerperium (O98.7-)

● O98.51 Other viral diseases complicating pregnancy

O98.511 Other viral diseases complicating pregnancy, first trimester ♀ M

O98.512 Other viral diseases complicating pregnancy, second trimester ♀ M
    Coding Clinic: 2016, Q4, P5-6

O98.513 Other viral diseases complicating pregnancy, third trimester ♀ M
    Coding Clinic: 2016, Q4, P6

O98.519 Other viral diseases complicating pregnancy, unspecified trimester ♀ M

O98.52 Other viral diseases complicating childbirth ♀ M

O98.53 Other viral diseases complicating the puerperium ♀ M

● O98.6 Protozoal diseases complicating pregnancy, childbirth and the puerperium
    Conditions in B50-B64

  ● O98.61 Protozoal diseases complicating pregnancy

O98.611 Protozoal diseases complicating pregnancy, first trimester ♀ M

O98.612 Protozoal diseases complicating pregnancy, second trimester ♀ M

O98.613 Protozoal diseases complicating pregnancy, third trimester ♀ M

O98.619 Protozoal diseases complicating pregnancy, unspecified trimester ♀ M

O98.62 Protozoal diseases complicating childbirth ♀ M

O98.63 Protozoal diseases complicating the puerperium ♀ M

● O98.7 Human immunodeficiency virus [HIV] disease complicating pregnancy, childbirth and the puerperium
    Use additional code to identify the type of HIV disease:
    Acquired immune deficiency syndrome (AIDS) (B20)
    Asymptomatic HIV status (Z21)
    HIV positive NOS (Z21)
    Symptomatic HIV disease (B20)

    OGCR Section I.C.15.f.

    HIV Infection in Pregnancy, Childbirth and the Puerperium

    During pregnancy, childbirth or the puerperium, a patient admitted because of an HIV-related illness should receive a principal diagnosis from subcategory O98.7-. Human immunodeficiency [HIV] disease complicating pregnancy, childbirth and the puerperium, followed by the code(s) for the HIV-related illness(es).

    Patients with asymptomatic HIV infection status admitted during pregnancy, childbirth, or the puerperium should receive codes of O98.7- and Z21, Asymptomatic human immunodeficiency virus [HIV] infection status.

  ● O98.71 Human immunodeficiency virus [HIV] disease complicating pregnancy

O98.711 Human immunodeficiency virus [HIV] disease complicating pregnancy, first trimester ♀ M

O98.712 Human immunodeficiency virus [HIV] disease complicating pregnancy, second trimester ♀ M

O98.713 Human immunodeficiency virus [HIV] disease complicating pregnancy, third trimester ♀ M

O98.719 Human immunodeficiency virus [HIV] disease complicating pregnancy, unspecified trimester ♀ M

O98.72 Human immunodeficiency virus [HIV] disease complicating childbirth ♀ M

O98.73 Human immunodeficiency virus [HIV] disease complicating the puerperium ♀ M

● O98.8 Other maternal infectious and parasitic diseases complicating pregnancy, childbirth and the puerperium

● **O98.81**   **Other maternal infectious and parasitic diseases complicating pregnancy**

     O98.811   Other maternal infectious and parasitic diseases complicating pregnancy, **first trimester** ♀   M

     O98.812   Other maternal infectious and parasitic diseases complicating pregnancy, **second trimester** ♀   M

     O98.813   Other maternal infectious and parasitic diseases complicating pregnancy, **third trimester** ♀   M

     O98.819   Other maternal infectious and parasitic diseases complicating pregnancy, **unspecified trimester** ♀   M

    O98.82   Other maternal infectious and parasitic diseases complicating **childbirth** ♀   M
        Coding Clinic: 2020, Q1, P10

    O98.83   Other maternal infectious and parasitic diseases complicating the **puerperium** ♀   M

● **O98.9**   **Unspecified maternal infectious and parasitic disease complicating pregnancy, childbirth and the puerperium**

   ● **O98.91**   **Unspecified** maternal infectious and parasitic disease complicating **pregnancy**

     O98.911   Unspecified maternal infectious and parasitic disease complicating pregnancy, **first trimester** ♀   M

     O98.912   Unspecified maternal infectious and parasitic disease complicating pregnancy, **second trimester** ♀   M

     O98.913   Unspecified maternal infectious and parasitic disease complicating pregnancy, **third trimester** ♀   M

     O98.919   Unspecified maternal infectious and parasitic disease complicating pregnancy, **unspecified trimester** ♀   M

    O98.92   **Unspecified** maternal infectious and parasitic disease complicating **childbirth** ♀   M

    O98.93   **Unspecified** maternal infectious and parasitic disease complicating the **puerperium** ♀   M

● **O99**   **Other maternal diseases** classifiable elsewhere but complicating pregnancy, childbirth and the puerperium

    Includes: conditions which complicate the pregnant state, are aggravated by the pregnancy or are a main reason for obstetric care

    Use additional code to identify specific condition

    Excludes2   when the reason for maternal care is that the condition is known or suspected to have affected the fetus (O35-O36)

    Coding Clinic: 2018, Q4, P8-9

   ● **O99.0**   **Anemia complicating pregnancy, childbirth and the puerperium**
        Conditions in D50-D64

     Excludes1   anemia arising in the puerperium (O90.81)
                postpartum anemia NOS (O90.81)

    ● **O99.01**   Anemia complicating **pregnancy**

     O99.011   Anemia complicating pregnancy, **first trimester** ♀   M

     O99.012   Anemia complicating pregnancy, **second trimester** ♀   M

     O99.013   Anemia complicating pregnancy, **third trimester** ♀   M

     O99.019   Anemia complicating pregnancy, **unspecified trimester** ♀   M

    O99.02   Anemia complicating **childbirth** ♀   M

    O99.03   Anemia complicating the **puerperium** ♀   M

     Excludes1   postpartum anemia not pre-existing prior to delivery (O90.81)

● **O99.1**   **Other diseases of the blood and blood-forming organs and certain disorders involving the immune mechanism complicating pregnancy, childbirth and the puerperium**
        Conditions in D65-D89

    Excludes1   hemorrhage with coagulation defects (O45.-, O46.0-, O67.0, O72.3)

   ● **O99.11**   Other diseases of the blood and blood-forming organs and certain disorders involving the immune mechanism complicating **pregnancy**

     O99.111   Other diseases of the blood and blood-forming organs and certain disorders involving the immune mechanism complicating pregnancy, **first trimester** ♀   M

     O99.112   Other diseases of the blood and blood-forming organs and certain disorders involving the immune mechanism complicating pregnancy, **second trimester** ♀   M

     O99.113   Other diseases of the blood and blood-forming organs and certain disorders involving the immune mechanism complicating pregnancy, **third trimester** ♀   M

     O99.119   Other diseases of the blood and blood-forming organs and certain disorders involving the immune mechanism complicating pregnancy, **unspecified trimester** ♀   M

    O99.12   Other diseases of the blood and blood-forming organs and certain disorders involving the immune mechanism complicating **childbirth** ♀   M

    O99.13   Other diseases of the blood and blood-forming organs and certain disorders involving the immune mechanism complicating the **puerperium** ♀   M

● **O99.2**   **Endocrine, nutritional and metabolic diseases complicating pregnancy, childbirth and the puerperium**
        Conditions in E00-E89

    Excludes2   diabetes mellitus (O24.-)
                malnutrition (O25.-)
                postpartum thyroiditis (O90.5)

   ● **O99.21**   **Obesity complicating pregnancy, childbirth and the puerperium**

     Use additional code to identify the type of obesity (E66.-)

     O99.210   Obesity complicating pregnancy, **unspecified trimester** ♀   M

     O99.211   Obesity complicating pregnancy, **first trimester** ♀   M

     O99.212   Obesity complicating pregnancy, **second trimester** ♀   M

     O99.213   Obesity complicating pregnancy, **third trimester** ♀   M

     O99.214   Obesity complicating **childbirth** ♀   M
        Coding Clinic: 2021, Q2, P10-11; 2018, Q4, P80

     O99.215   Obesity complicating the **puerperium** ♀   M

   ● **O99.28**   Other endocrine, nutritional and metabolic diseases complicating pregnancy, childbirth and the puerperium

     O99.280   Endocrine, nutritional and metabolic diseases complicating pregnancy, **unspecified trimester** ♀   M

     O99.281   Endocrine, nutritional and metabolic diseases complicating pregnancy, **first trimester** ♀   M

     O99.282   Endocrine, nutritional and metabolic diseases complicating pregnancy, **second trimester** ♀   M

▶ New   ⇒ Revised   ~~deleted~~ Deleted   Excludes 1   Excludes 2   Includes   Use additional   Code first   Code also   Key words
OGCR Official Guidelines   X Assign placeholder X   ● Use Additional Character(s)   ▶ Manifestation Code   🔾 Hierarchical Condition Category   **Coding Clinic**

O99.283 Endocrine, nutritional and metabolic diseases complicating pregnancy, third trimester ♀ M

O99.284 Endocrine, nutritional and metabolic diseases complicating childbirth ♀ M

O99.285 Endocrine, nutritional and metabolic diseases complicating the puerperium ♀ M
  Coding Clinic: 2021, Q1, P9

● O99.3 Mental disorders and diseases of the nervous system complicating pregnancy, childbirth and the puerperium

  ● O99.31 Alcohol use complicating pregnancy, childbirth, and the puerperium
    Use additional code(s) from F10 to identify manifestations of the alcohol use

    O99.310 Alcohol use complicating pregnancy, unspecified trimester ♀ M

    O99.311 Alcohol use complicating pregnancy, first trimester ♀ M

    O99.312 Alcohol use complicating pregnancy, second trimester ♀ M

    O99.313 Alcohol use complicating pregnancy, third trimester ♀ M

    O99.314 Alcohol use complicating childbirth ♀ M

    O99.315 Alcohol use complicating the puerperium ♀ M

  ● O99.32 Drug use complicating pregnancy, childbirth, and the puerperium
    Use additional code(s) from F11-F16 and F18-F19 to identify manifestations of the drug use

    O99.320 Drug use complicating pregnancy, unspecified trimester ♀ M

    O99.321 Drug use complicating pregnancy, first trimester ♀ M

    O99.322 Drug use complicating pregnancy, second trimester ♀ M

    O99.323 Drug use complicating pregnancy, third trimester ♀ M

    O99.324 Drug use complicating childbirth ♀ M

    O99.325 Drug use complicating the puerperium ♀ M

  ● O99.33 Tobacco use disorder complicating pregnancy, childbirth, and the puerperium
    Smoking complicating pregnancy, childbirth, and the puerperium
    Use additional code from category F17 to identify type of tobacco nicotine dependence

    O99.330 Smoking (tobacco) complicating pregnancy, unspecified trimester ♀ M

    O99.331 Smoking (tobacco) complicating pregnancy, first trimester ♀ M

    O99.332 Smoking (tobacco) complicating pregnancy, second trimester ♀ M

    O99.333 Smoking (tobacco) complicating pregnancy, third trimester ♀ M

    O99.334 Smoking (tobacco) complicating childbirth ♀ M

    O99.335 Smoking (tobacco) complicating the puerperium ♀ M

  ● O99.34 Other mental disorders complicating pregnancy, childbirth, and the puerperium
    Conditions in F01-F09, F20-F52 and F54-F99

    Excludes2 postpartum mood disturbance (O90.6)
    postnatal psychosis (F53.1)
    puerperal psychosis (F53.1)
    Coding Clinic: 2018, Q4, P9

    O99.340 Other mental disorders complicating pregnancy, unspecified trimester ♀ M

    O99.341 Other mental disorders complicating pregnancy, first trimester ♀ M

    O99.342 Other mental disorders complicating pregnancy, second trimester ♀ M

    O99.343 Other mental disorders complicating pregnancy, third trimester ♀ M

    O99.344 Other mental disorders complicating childbirth ♀ M

    O99.345 Other mental disorders complicating the puerperium ♀ M
    Coding Clinic: 2018, Q4, P8-9

  ● O99.35 Diseases of the nervous system complicating pregnancy, childbirth, and the puerperium
    Conditions in G00-G99

    Excludes2 pregnancy related peripheral neuritis (O26.8-)

    O99.350 Diseases of the nervous system complicating pregnancy, unspecified trimester ♀ M

    O99.351 Diseases of the nervous system complicating pregnancy, first trimester ♀ M

    O99.352 Diseases of the nervous system complicating pregnancy, second trimester ♀ M

    O99.353 Diseases of the nervous system complicating pregnancy, third trimester ♀ M

    O99.354 Diseases of the nervous system complicating childbirth ♀ M

    O99.355 Diseases of the nervous system complicating the puerperium ♀ M

● O99.4 Diseases of the circulatory system complicating pregnancy, childbirth and the puerperium
  Conditions in I00-I99

  Excludes1 peripartum cardiomyopathy (O90.3)
  Excludes2 hypertensive disorders (O10-O16)
  obstetric embolism (O88.-)
  venous complications and cerebrovenous sinus thrombosis in labor, childbirth and the puerperium (O87.-)
  venous complications and cerebrovenous sinus thrombosis in pregnancy (O22.-)

  ● O99.41 Diseases of the circulatory system complicating pregnancy
    Coding Clinic: 2016, Q2, P8

    O99.411 Diseases of the circulatory system complicating pregnancy, first trimester ♀ M

    O99.412 Diseases of the circulatory system complicating pregnancy, second trimester ♀ M

    O99.413 Diseases of the circulatory system complicating pregnancy, third trimester ♀ M

    O99.419 Diseases of the circulatory system complicating pregnancy, unspecified trimester ♀ M

    O99.42 Diseases of the circulatory system complicating childbirth ♀ M

    O99.43 Diseases of the circulatory system complicating the puerperium ♀ M

● O99.5 Diseases of the respiratory system complicating pregnancy, childbirth and the puerperium
  Conditions in J00-J99

  ● O99.51 Diseases of the respiratory system complicating pregnancy

    O99.511 Diseases of the respiratory system complicating pregnancy, first trimester ♀ M

    O99.512 Diseases of the respiratory system complicating pregnancy, second trimester ♀ M

O99.513   Diseases of the respiratory system complicating pregnancy, **third trimester** ♀   M

O99.519   Diseases of the respiratory system complicating pregnancy, **unspecified trimester** ♀   M

O99.52   Diseases of the respiratory system complicating **childbirth** ♀   M

O99.53   Diseases of the respiratory system complicating the **puerperium** ♀   M

● O99.6   **Diseases of the digestive system** complicating pregnancy, childbirth and the puerperium
     Conditions in K00-K93

     Excludes2   hemorrhoids in pregnancy (O22.4-)
           liver and biliary tract disorders in pregnancy, childbirth and the puerperium (O26.6-)

   ● O99.61   Diseases of the digestive system complicating **pregnancy**

     O99.611   Diseases of the digestive system complicating pregnancy, **first trimester** ♀   M

     O99.612   Diseases of the digestive system complicating pregnancy, **second trimester** ♀   M

     O99.613   Diseases of the digestive system complicating pregnancy, **third trimester** ♀   M

     O99.619   Diseases of the digestive system complicating pregnancy, **unspecified trimester** ♀   M

   O99.62   Diseases of the digestive system complicating **childbirth** ♀   M

   O99.63   Diseases of the digestive system complicating the **puerperium** ♀   M

● O99.7   **Diseases of the skin and subcutaneous tissue** complicating pregnancy, childbirth and the puerperium
     Conditions in L00-L99

     Excludes2   herpes gestationis (O26.4)
           pruritic urticarial papules and plaques of pregnancy (PUPPP) (O26.86)

   ● O99.71   Diseases of the skin and subcutaneous tissue complicating **pregnancy**

     O99.711   Diseases of the skin and subcutaneous tissue complicating pregnancy, **first trimester** ♀   M

     O99.712   Diseases of the skin and subcutaneous tissue complicating pregnancy, **second trimester** ♀   M

     O99.713   Diseases of the skin and subcutaneous tissue complicating pregnancy, **third trimester** ♀   M

     O99.719   Diseases of the skin and subcutaneous tissue complicating pregnancy, **unspecified trimester** ♀   M

   O99.72   Diseases of the skin and subcutaneous tissue complicating **childbirth** ♀   M

   O99.73   Diseases of the skin and subcutaneous tissue complicating the **puerperium** ♀   M

● O99.8   **Other specified diseases and conditions** complicating pregnancy, childbirth and the puerperium
     Conditions in D00-D48, H00-H95, M00-N99, and Q00-Q99

     Use additional code to identify condition

     Excludes2   genitourinary infections in pregnancy (O23.-)
           infection of genitourinary tract following delivery (O86.1-O86.4)
           malignant neoplasm complicating pregnancy, childbirth and the puerperium (O9A.1-)
           maternal care for known or suspected abnormality of maternal pelvic organs (O34.-)
           postpartum acute kidney failure (O90.4)
           traumatic injuries in pregnancy (O9A.2-)

● O99.81   **Abnormal glucose** complicating pregnancy, childbirth and the puerperium

     Excludes1   gestational diabetes (O24.4-)

   O99.810   Abnormal glucose complicating **pregnancy** ♀   M

   O99.814   Abnormal glucose complicating **childbirth** ♀   M

   O99.815   Abnormal glucose complicating the **puerperium** ♀   M

● O99.82   **Streptococcus B carrier state** complicating pregnancy, childbirth and the puerperium

     Excludes1   Carrier of streptococcus group B (GBS) in a nonpregnant woman (Z22.330)

   O99.820   Streptococcus B carrier state complicating **pregnancy** ♀   M

   O99.824   Streptococcus B carrier state complicating **childbirth** ♀   M
       Coding Clinic: 2019, Q2, P9

   O99.825   Streptococcus B carrier state complicating the **puerperium** ♀   M

● O99.83   **Other infection carrier state** complicating pregnancy, childbirth and the puerperium

     Use additional code to identify the carrier state (Z22.-)

   O99.830   Other infection carrier state complicating **pregnancy** ♀   M

   O99.834   Other infection carrier state complicating **childbirth** ♀   M

   O99.835   Other infection carrier state complicating the **puerperium** ♀   M

● O99.84   **Bariatric surgery status** complicating pregnancy, childbirth and the puerperium
     Gastric banding status complicating pregnancy, childbirth and the puerperium
     Gastric bypass status for obesity complicating pregnancy, childbirth and the puerperium
     Obesity surgery status complicating pregnancy, childbirth and the puerperium

   O99.840   Bariatric surgery status complicating pregnancy, **unspecified trimester** ♀   M

   O99.841   Bariatric surgery status complicating pregnancy, **first trimester** ♀   M

   O99.842   Bariatric surgery status complicating pregnancy, **second trimester** ♀   M

   O99.843   Bariatric surgery status complicating pregnancy, **third trimester** ♀   M

   O99.844   Bariatric surgery status complicating **childbirth** ♀   M

   O99.845   Bariatric surgery status complicating the **puerperium** ♀   M

● O99.89   **Other specified diseases and conditions** complicating pregnancy, childbirth and the puerperium ♀   M

   O99.891   Other specified diseases and conditions complicating **pregnancy** ♀   M

   O99.892   Other specified diseases and conditions complicating **childbirth** ♀   M

   O99.893   Other specified diseases and conditions complicating **puerperium** ♀   M

OGCR Section I.C.2.I.3.

Malignant neoplasm in a pregnant patient

When a pregnant woman has a malignant neoplasm, a code from subcategory O9A.1-, Malignant neoplasm complicating pregnancy, childbirth, and the puerperium, should be sequenced first, followed by the appropriate code from Chapter 2 to indicate the type of neoplasm.

▶ New   ⇛ Revised   ~~deleted~~ Deleted   Excludes 1   Excludes 2   Includes   Use additional   Code first   Code also   Key words

OGCR Official Guidelines   X Assign placeholder X   ● Use Additional Character(s)   ⟩ Manifestation Code   ⚕ Hierarchical Condition Category   **Coding Clinic**

● O9A   Maternal malignant neoplasms, traumatic injuries and abuse classifiable elsewhere but complicating pregnancy, childbirth and the puerperium

  ● O9A.1   Malignant neoplasm complicating pregnancy, childbirth and the puerperium
         Conditions in C00-C96

         Use additional code to identify neoplasm

         Excludes2   maternal care for benign tumor of corpus uteri (O34.1-)
                         maternal care for benign tumor of cervix (O34.4-)

    ● O9A.11   Malignant neoplasm complicating pregnancy

         O9A.111   Malignant neoplasm complicating pregnancy, first trimester ♀   M

         O9A.112   Malignant neoplasm complicating pregnancy, second trimester ♀   M

         O9A.113   Malignant neoplasm complicating pregnancy, third trimester ♀   M

         O9A.119   Malignant neoplasm complicating pregnancy, unspecified trimester ♀   M

     O9A.12   Malignant neoplasm complicating childbirth ♀   M

     O9A.13   Malignant neoplasm complicating the puerperium ♀   M
         Coding Clinic: 2015, Q3, P19

  ● O9A.2   Injury, poisoning and certain other consequences of external causes complicating pregnancy, childbirth and the puerperium
         Conditions in S00-T88, except T74 and T76

         Use additional code(s) to identify the injury or poisoning

         Excludes2   physical, sexual and psychological abuse complicating pregnancy, childbirth and the puerperium (O9A.3-, O9A.4-, O9A.5-)

    ● O9A.21   Injury, poisoning and certain other consequences of external causes complicating pregnancy

         O9A.211   Injury, poisoning and certain other consequences of external causes complicating pregnancy, first trimester ♀   M

         O9A.212   Injury, poisoning and certain other consequences of external causes complicating pregnancy, second trimester ♀   M

         O9A.213   Injury, poisoning and certain other consequences of external causes complicating pregnancy, third trimester ♀   M

         O9A.219   Injury, poisoning and certain other consequences of external causes complicating pregnancy, unspecified trimester ♀   M

     O9A.22   Injury, poisoning and certain other consequences of external causes complicating childbirth ♀   M

     O9A.23   Injury, poisoning and certain other consequences of external causes complicating the puerperium ♀   M

  ● O9A.3   Physical abuse complicating pregnancy, childbirth and the puerperium
         Conditions in T74.11 or T76.11

         Use additional code (if applicable):
         to identify any associated current injury due to physical abuse
         to identify the perpetrator of abuse (Y07.-)

         Excludes2   sexual abuse complicating pregnancy, childbirth and the puerperium (O9A.4)

    ● O9A.31   Physical abuse complicating pregnancy

         O9A.311   Physical abuse complicating pregnancy, first trimester ♀   M

         O9A.312   Physical abuse complicating pregnancy, second trimester ♀   M

         O9A.313   Physical abuse complicating pregnancy, third trimester ♀   M

         O9A.319   Physical abuse complicating pregnancy, unspecified trimester ♀   M

     O9A.32   Physical abuse complicating childbirth ♀   M

     O9A.33   Physical abuse complicating the puerperium ♀   M

  ● O9A.4   Sexual abuse complicating pregnancy, childbirth and the puerperium
         Conditions in T74.21 or T76.21

         Use additional code (if applicable):
         to identify any associated current injury due to sexual abuse
         to identify the perpetrator of abuse (Y07.-)

    ● O9A.41   Sexual abuse complicating pregnancy

         O9A.411   Sexual abuse complicating pregnancy, first trimester ♀   M

         O9A.412   Sexual abuse complicating pregnancy, second trimester ♀   M

         O9A.413   Sexual abuse complicating pregnancy, third trimester ♀   M

         O9A.419   Sexual abuse complicating pregnancy, unspecified trimester ♀   M

     O9A.42   Sexual abuse complicating childbirth ♀   M

     O9A.43   Sexual abuse complicating the puerperium ♀   M

  ● O9A.5   Psychological abuse complicating pregnancy, childbirth and the puerperium
         Conditions in T74.31 or T76.31

         Use additional code to identify the perpetrator of abuse (Y07.-)

    ● O9A.51   Psychological abuse complicating pregnancy

         O9A.511   Psychological abuse complicating pregnancy, first trimester ♀   M

         O9A.512   Psychological abuse complicating pregnancy, second trimester ♀   M

         O9A.513   Psychological abuse complicating pregnancy, third trimester ♀   M

         O9A.519   Psychological abuse complicating pregnancy, unspecified trimester ♀   M

     O9A.52   Psychological abuse complicating childbirth ♀ M

     O9A.53   Psychological abuse complicating the puerperium ♀   M

CHAPTER 16

CERTAIN CONDITIONS ORIGINATING IN THE PERINATAL PERIOD (P00-P96)

OGCR Chapter-Specific Coding Guidelines

16. Chapter 16: Certain Conditions Originating in the Perinatal Period (P00-P96)
For coding and reporting purposes the perinatal period is defined as before birth through the 28th day following birth. The following guidelines are provided for reporting purposes

a. General Perinatal Rules

1) Use of Chapter 16 Codes
Codes in this chapter are <u>never</u> for use on the maternal record. Codes from Chapter 15, the obstetric chapter, are never permitted on the newborn record. Chapter 16 codes may be used throughout the life of the patient if the condition is still present.

2) Principal Diagnosis for Birth Record
When coding the birth episode in a newborn record, assign a code from category Z38, Liveborn infants according to place of birth and type of delivery, as the principal diagnosis. A code from category Z38 is assigned only once, to a newborn at the time of birth. If a newborn is transferred to another institution, a code from category Z38 should not be used at the receiving hospital.

A code from category Z38 is used only on the newborn record, not on the mother's record.

3) Use of Codes from other Chapters with Codes from Chapter 16
Codes from other chapters may be used with codes from chapter 16 if the codes from the other chapters provide more specific detail. Codes for signs and symptoms may be assigned when a definitive diagnosis has not been established. If the reason for the encounter is a perinatal condition, the code from Chapter 16 should be sequenced first.

4) Use of Chapter 16 Codes after the Perinatal Period
Should a condition originate in the perinatal period, and continue throughout the life of the patient, the perinatal code should continue to be used regardless of the patient's age.

5) Birth process or community acquired conditions
If a newborn has a condition that may be either due to the birth process or community acquired and the documentation does not indicate which it is, the default is due to the birth process and the code from Chapter 16 should be used. If the condition is community-acquired, a code from Chapter 16 should not be assigned.

6) Code all clinically significant conditions
All clinically significant conditions noted on routine newborn examination should be coded. A condition is clinically significant if it requires:
- clinical evaluation; or
- therapeutic treatment; or
- diagnostic procedures; or
- extended length of hospital stay; or
- increased nursing care and/or monitoring; or
- has implications for future health care needs

Note: The perinatal guidelines listed above are the same as the general coding guidelines for "additional diagnoses", except for the final point regarding implications for future health care needs. Codes should be assigned for conditions that have been specified by the provider as having implications for future health care needs.

b. Observation and Evaluation of Newborns for Suspected Conditions Not Found

1) Use of Z05 codes
Assign a code from category Z05, Observation and evaluation of newborns and infants for suspected conditions ruled out, to identify those instances when a healthy newborn is evaluated for a suspected condition that is determined after study not to be present. Do not use a code from category Z05 when the patient has identified signs or symptoms of a suspected problem; in such cases code the sign or symptom.

2) Z05 on Other than the Birth Record
A code from category Z05 may also be assigned as a principal or first-listed code for readmissions or encounters when the code from category Z38 code no longer applies. Codes from category Z05 are for use only for healthy newborns and infants for which no condition after study is found to be present.

3) Z05 on a birth record
A code from category Z05 is to be used as a secondary code after the code from category Z38, Liveborn infants according to place of birth and type of delivery.

c. Coding Additional Perinatal Diagnoses

1) Assigning codes for conditions that require treatment
Assign codes for conditions that require treatment or further investigation, prolong the length of stay, or require resource utilization.

2) Codes for conditions specified as having implications for future health care needs
Assign codes for conditions that have been specified by the provider as having implications for future health care needs.
Note: This guideline should not be used for adult patients.

d. Prematurity and Fetal Growth Retardation
Providers utilize different criteria in determining prematurity. A code for prematurity should not be assigned unless it is documented. Assignment of codes in categories P05, Disorders of newborn related to slow fetal growth and fetal malnutrition, and P07, Disorders of newborn related to short gestation and low birth weight, not elsewhere classified, should be based on the recorded birth weight and estimated gestational age.

When both birth weight and gestational age are available, two codes from category P07 should be assigned, with the code for birth weight sequenced before the code for gestational age.

e. Low birth weight and immaturity status
Codes from category P07, Disorders of newborn related to short gestation and low birth weight, not elsewhere classified, are for use for a child or adult who was premature or had a low birth weight as a newborn and this is affecting the patient's current health status.
See Section I.C.21. Factors influencing health status and contact with health services, Status.

f. Bacterial Sepsis of Newborn
Category P36, Bacterial sepsis of newborn, includes congenital sepsis. If a perinate is documented as having sepsis without documentation of congenital or community acquired, the default is congenital and a code from category P36 should be assigned. If the P36 code includes the causal organism, an additional code from category B95, Streptococcus, Staphylococcus, and Enterococcus as the cause of diseases classified elsewhere, or B96, Other bacterial agents as the cause of diseases classified elsewhere, should not be assigned. If the P36 code does not include the causal organism, assign an additional code from category B96. If applicable, use additional codes to identify severe sepsis (R65.2-) and any associated acute organ dysfunction.

g. Stillbirth
Code P95, Stillbirth, is only for use in institutions that maintain separate records for stillbirths. No other code should be used with P95. Code P95 should not be used on the mother's record.

CHAPTER 16

CERTAIN CONDITIONS ORIGINATING IN THE PERINATAL PERIOD (P00-P96)

Note: Codes from this chapter are for use on newborn records only, never on maternal records.

Includes   conditions that have their origin in the fetal or perinatal period (before birth through the first 28 days after birth) even if morbidity occurs later

Excludes2   congenital malformations, deformations and chromosomal abnormalities (Q00-Q99)
endocrine, nutritional and metabolic diseases (E00-E88)
injury, poisoning and certain other consequences of external causes (S00-T88)
neoplasms (C00-D49)
tetanus neonatorum (A33)

This chapter contains the following blocks:

P00-P04	Newborn affected by maternal factors and by complications of pregnancy, labor, and delivery
P05-P08	Disorders of newborns related to length of gestation and fetal growth
P09	Abnormal findings on neonatal screening
P10-P15	Birth trauma
P19-P29	Respiratory and cardiovascular disorders specific to the perinatal period
P35-P39	Infections specific to the perinatal period
P50-P61	Hemorrhagic and hematological disorders of newborn
P70-P74	Transitory endocrine and metabolic disorders specific to newborn
P76-P78	Digestive system disorders of newborn
P80-P83	Conditions involving the integument and temperature regulation of newborn
P84	Other problems with newborn
P90-P96	Other disorders originating in the perinatal period

NEWBORN AFFECTED BY MATERNAL FACTORS AND BY COMPLICATIONS OF PREGNANCY, LABOR, AND DELIVERY (P00–P04)

Note: These codes are for use when the listed maternal conditions are specified as the cause of confirmed morbidity or potential morbidity which have their origin in the perinatal period (before birth through the first 28 days after birth).

● **P00**   **Newborn affected by maternal conditions that may be unrelated to present pregnancy**

Code first any current condition in newborn

Excludes2   encounter for observation of newborn for suspected diseases and conditions ruled out (Z05.-)
newborn affected by maternal complications of pregnancy (P01.-)
newborn affected by maternal endocrine and metabolic disorders (P70–P74)
newborn affected by noxious substances transmitted via placenta or breast milk (P04.-)

Coding Clinic: 2016, Q4, P54

P00.0   **Newborn affected by maternal hypertensive disorders**
Newborn affected by maternal conditions classifiable to O10-O11, O13-O16

P00.1   **Newborn affected by maternal renal and urinary tract diseases**
Newborn affected by maternal conditions classifiable to N00-N39

P00.2   **Newborn affected by maternal infectious and parasitic diseases**
Newborn affected by maternal infectious disease classifiable to A00-B99, J09 and J10

     Excludes1   maternal genital tract or other localized infections (P00.8)

     Excludes2   infections specific to the perinatal period (P35-P39)

      ▶newborn affected by (positive) maternal group B streptococcus (GBS) colonization (P00.82)

Coding Clinic: 2019, Q2, P10; 2015, Q3, P21

P00.3   **Newborn affected by other maternal circulatory and respiratory diseases**
Newborn affected by maternal conditions classifiable to I00-I99, J00-J99, Q20-Q34 and not included in P00.0, P00.2

P00.4   **Newborn affected by maternal nutritional disorders**
Newborn affected by maternal disorders classifiable to E40-E64
Maternal malnutrition NOS

P00.5   **Newborn affected by maternal injury**
Newborn affected by maternal conditions classifiable to O9A.2-

P00.6   **Newborn affected by surgical procedure on mother**
Newborn affected by amniocentesis

     Excludes1   Cesarean delivery for present delivery (P03.4)
damage to placenta from amniocentesis, cesarean delivery or surgical induction (P02.1)
previous surgery to uterus or pelvic organs (P03.89)

     Excludes2   newborn affected by complication of (fetal) intrauterine procedure (P96.5)

P00.7   **Newborn affected by other medical procedures on mother, not elsewhere classified**
Newborn affected by radiation to mother

     Excludes1   damage to placenta from amniocentesis, cesarean delivery or surgical induction (P02.1)
newborn affected by other complications of labor and delivery (P03.-)

● **P00.8**   **Newborn affected by other maternal conditions**

     P00.81   **Newborn affected by periodontal disease in mother**

  ▶**P00.82**   **Newborn affected by (positive) maternal group B streptococcus (GBS) colonization**
    ▶Contact with positive maternal group B streptococcus

     P00.89   **Newborn affected by other maternal conditions**
Newborn affected by conditions classifiable to T80-T88
Newborn affected by maternal genital tract or other localized infections
Newborn affected by maternal systemic lupus erythematosus
Use additional code to identify infectious agent, if known

       ▶**Excludes2**   newborn affected by positive maternal group B streptococcus (GBS) colonization (P00.82)

Coding Clinic: 2019, Q2, P9

P00.9   **Newborn affected by unspecified maternal condition**

● **P01**   **Newborn affected by maternal complications of pregnancy**

Code first any current condition in newborn

     Excludes2   encounter for observation of newborn for suspected diseases and conditions ruled out (Z05.-)

Coding Clinic: 2016, Q4, P54

P01.0   **Newborn affected by incompetent cervix**

P01.1   **Newborn affected by premature rupture of membranes**

P01.2   Newborn affected by oligohydramnios
>   **Excludes1**   oligohydramnios due to premature
>   rupture of membranes (P01.1)

P01.3   Newborn affected by polyhydramnios
>   *Excess of amniotic fluid, usually > 2000 mL*
>   Newborn affected by hydramnios

P01.4   Newborn affected by ectopic pregnancy
>   Newborn affected by abdominal pregnancy

P01.5   Newborn affected by multiple pregnancy
>   Newborn affected by triplet (pregnancy)
>   Newborn affected by twin (pregnancy)

P01.6   Newborn affected by maternal death

P01.7   Newborn affected by malpresentation before labor
>   Newborn affected by breech presentation before labor
>   Newborn affected by external version before labor
>   Newborn affected by face presentation before labor
>   Newborn affected by transverse lie before labor
>   Newborn affected by unstable lie before labor

P01.8   Newborn affected by other maternal complications of pregnancy

P01.9   Newborn affected by maternal complication of pregnancy, unspecified

● **P02**   Newborn affected by complications of placenta, cord and membranes
>   *Code first any current condition in newborn*
>   **Excludes2**   encounter for observation of newborn for
>   suspected diseases and conditions ruled out
>   (Z05.-)
>   Coding Clinic: 2016, Q4, P54

P02.0   Newborn affected by placenta previa

P02.1   Newborn affected by other forms of placental separation and hemorrhage
>   Newborn affected by abruptio placenta
>   Newborn affected by accidental hemorrhage
>   Newborn affected by antepartum hemorrhage
>   Newborn affected by damage to placenta from
>   amniocentesis, cesarean delivery or surgical
>   induction
>   Newborn affected by maternal blood loss
>   Newborn affected by premature separation of placenta

● **P02.2**   Newborn affected by other and unspecified morphological and functional abnormalities of placenta
>   **P02.20**   Newborn affected by unspecified
>   morphological and functional abnormalities of
>   placenta
>   **P02.29**   Newborn affected by other morphological and
>   functional abnormalities of placenta
>   Newborn affected by placental dysfunction
>   Newborn affected by placental infarction
>   Newborn affected by placental insufficiency

P02.3   Newborn affected by placental transfusion syndromes
>   Newborn affected by placental and cord abnormalities
>   resulting in twin-to-twin or other transplacental
>   transfusion

P02.4   Newborn affected by prolapsed cord

P02.5   Newborn affected by other compression of umbilical cord
>   Newborn affected by umbilical cord (tightly) around
>   neck
>   Newborn affected by entanglement of umbilical cord
>   Newborn affected by knot in umbilical cord

● **P02.6**   Newborn affected by other and unspecified conditions of umbilical cord
>   **P02.60**   Newborn affected by unspecified conditions of
>   umbilical cord
>   **P02.69**   Newborn affected by other conditions of
>   umbilical cord
>   Newborn affected by short umbilical cord
>   Newborn affected by vasa previa
>   **Excludes1**   newborn affected by single
>   umbilical artery (Q27.0)

● **P02.7**   Newborn affected by chorioamnionitis
>   *Inflammation of chorion and amnion*
>   **P02.70**   Newborn affected by fetal inflammatory
>   response syndrome 🝝
>   Newborn affected by FIRS
>   **P02.78**   Newborn affected by other conditions from
>   chorioamnionitis
>   Newborn affected by amnionitis
>   Newborn affected by membranitis
>   Newborn affected by placentitis

P02.8   Newborn affected by other abnormalities of membranes

P02.9   Newborn affected by abnormality of membranes, unspecified

● **P03**   Newborn affected by other complications of labor and delivery
>   *Code first any current condition in newborn*
>   **Excludes2**   encounter for observation of newborn for
>   suspected diseases and conditions ruled out
>   (Z05.-)
>   Coding Clinic: 2016, Q4, P54

P03.0   Newborn affected by breech delivery and extraction

P03.1   Newborn affected by other malpresentation, malposition and disproportion during labor and delivery
>   Newborn affected by contracted pelvis
>   Newborn affected by conditions classifiable to O64-O66
>   Newborn affected by persistent occipitoposterior
>   Newborn affected by transverse lie

P03.2   Newborn affected by forceps delivery

P03.3   Newborn affected by delivery by vacuum extractor [ventouse]

P03.4   Newborn affected by Cesarean delivery

P03.5   Newborn affected by precipitate delivery
>   Newborn affected by rapid second stage

P03.6   Newborn affected by abnormal uterine contractions
>   Newborn affected by conditions classifiable to O62.-,
>   except O62.3
>   Newborn affected by hypertonic labor
>   Newborn affected by uterine inertia

● **P03.8**   Newborn affected by other specified complications of labor and delivery
>   ● **P03.81**   Newborn affected by abnormality in fetal
>   (intrauterine) heart rate or rhythm
>   **Excludes1**   neonatal cardiac dysrhythmia
>   (P29.1-)
>   **P03.810**   Newborn affected by abnormality
>   in fetal (intrauterine) heart rate or
>   rhythm before the onset of labor
>   **P03.811**   Newborn affected by abnormality
>   in fetal (intrauterine) heart rate or
>   rhythm during labor
>   **P03.819**   Newborn affected by abnormality
>   in fetal (intrauterine) heart rate or
>   rhythm, unspecified as to time of
>   onset
>   **P03.82**   Meconium passage during delivery
>   **Excludes1**   meconium aspiration (P24.00,
>   P24.01)
>   meconium staining (P96.83)
>   **P03.89**   Newborn affected by other specified
>   complications of labor and delivery
>   Newborn affected by abnormality of maternal
>   soft tissues
>   Newborn affected by conditions classifiable to
>   O60-O75 and by procedures used in labor
>   and delivery not included in P02.- and
>   P03.0-P03.6
>   Newborn affected by induction of labor

P03.9   Newborn affected by complication of labor and delivery, unspecified

---

▶ New   ⮞ Revised   ~~deleted~~ Deleted   Excludes 1   Excludes 2   Includes   Use additional   Code first   Code also   Key words
OGCR Official Guidelines   X Assign placeholder X   ● Use Additional Character(s)   ▷ Manifestation Code   🝝 Hierarchical Condition Category   **Coding Clinic**

● **P04**   **Newborn affected by noxious substances transmitted via placenta or breast milk**

> *Code first any current condition in newborn, if applicable*

Includes   nonteratogenic effects of substances transmitted via placenta

Excludes2   congenital malformations (Q00-Q99)
encounter for observation of newborn for suspected diseases and conditions ruled out (Z05.-)
neonatal jaundice from excessive hemolysis due to drugs or toxins transmitted from mother (P58.4)
newborn in contact with and (suspected) exposures hazardous to health not transmitted via placenta or breast milk (Z77.-)

     Coding Clinic: 2016, Q4, P54

P04.0   **Newborn affected by maternal anesthesia and analgesia in pregnancy, labor and delivery**

Newborn affected by reactions and intoxications from maternal opiates and tranquilizers administered for procedures during pregnancy or labor and delivery

Excludes2   newborn affected by other maternal medication (P04.1-)

● **P04.1**   **Newborn affected by other maternal medication**

> *Code first withdrawal symptoms from maternal use of drugs of addiction, if applicable (P96.1)*

Excludes1   dysmorphism due to warfarin (Q86.2)
fetal hydantoin syndrome (Q86.1)

Excludes2   maternal anesthesia and analgesia in pregnancy, labor and delivery (P04.0)
maternal use of drugs of addiction (P04.4-)

P04.11   Newborn affected by maternal antineoplastic chemotherapy

P04.12   Newborn affected by maternal cytotoxic drugs

P04.13   Newborn affected by maternal use of anticonvulsants

P04.14   Newborn affected by maternal use of opiates

P04.15   Newborn affected by maternal use of antidepressants

P04.16   Newborn affected by maternal use of amphetamines

P04.17   Newborn affected by maternal use of sedative-hypnotics

P04.1A   Newborn affected by maternal use of anxiolytics

P04.18   Newborn affected by other maternal medication

P04.19   Newborn affected by maternal use of unspecified medication

     Coding Clinic: 2016, Q4, P55

P04.2   **Newborn affected by maternal use of tobacco**

Newborn affected by exposure in utero to tobacco smoke

Excludes2   newborn exposure to environmental tobacco smoke (P96.81)

P04.3   **Newborn affected by maternal use of alcohol**

Excludes1   fetal alcohol syndrome (Q86.0)

● **P04.4**   **Newborn affected by maternal use of drugs of addiction**

P04.40   Newborn affected by maternal use of unspecified drugs of addiction

P04.41   Newborn affected by maternal use of cocaine

P04.42   Newborn affected by maternal use of hallucinogens

Excludes2   newborn affected by other maternal medication (P04.1-)

P04.49   Newborn affected by maternal use of other drugs of addiction

Excludes2   newborn affected by maternal anesthesia and analgesia (P04.0)
withdrawal symptoms from maternal use of drugs of addiction (P96.1)

P04.5   **Newborn affected by maternal use of nutritional chemical substances**

P04.6   **Newborn affected by maternal exposure to environmental chemical substances**

● **P04.8**   **Newborn affected by other maternal noxious substances**

P04.81   Newborn affected by maternal use of cannabis

P04.89   Newborn affected by other maternal noxious substances

P04.9   **Newborn affected by maternal noxious substance, unspecified**

OGCR Section I.C.16.d.

> Prematurity and Fetal Growth Retardation
>
> Providers utilize different criteria in determining prematurity. A code for prematurity should not be assigned unless it is documented. Assignment of codes in categories P05, Disorders of newborn related to slow fetal growth and fetal malnutrition, and P07, Disorders of newborn related to short gestation and low birth weight, not elsewhere classified, should be based on the recorded birth weight and estimated gestational age.
>
> When both birth weight and gestational age are available, two codes from category P07 should be assigned, with the code for birth weight sequenced before the code for gestational age.

DISORDERS OF NEWBORN RELATED TO LENGTH OF GESTATION AND FETAL GROWTH (P05-P08)

● **P05**   **Disorders of newborn related to slow fetal growth and fetal malnutrition**

     Coding Clinic: 2016, Q4, P56

● **P05.0**   **Newborn light for gestational age**

Newborn light-for-dates
Weight below but length above 10th percentile for gestational age

P05.00   Newborn light for gestational age, unspecified weight

P05.01   Newborn light for gestational age, less than 500 grams

P05.02   Newborn light for gestational age, 500-749 grams

P05.03   Newborn light for gestational age, 750-999 grams

P05.04   Newborn light for gestational age, 1000-1249 grams

P05.05   Newborn light for gestational age, 1250-1499 grams

P05.06   Newborn light for gestational age, 1500-1749 grams

P05.07   Newborn light for gestational age, 1750-1999 grams

P05.08   Newborn light for gestational age, 2000-2499 grams

P05.09   Newborn light for gestational age, 2500 grams and over

Newborn light for gestational age, other
     Coding Clinic: 2016, Q4, P55

● **P05.1 Newborn small for gestational age**
Newborn small-and-light-for-dates
Newborn small-for-dates
Weight and length below 10th percentile for gestational age

P05.10 Newborn small for gestational age, unspecified weight

P05.11 Newborn small for gestational age, less than 500 grams

P05.12 Newborn small for gestational age, 500-749 grams

P05.13 Newborn small for gestational age, 750-999 grams

P05.14 Newborn small for gestational age, 1000-1249 grams

P05.15 Newborn small for gestational age, 1250-1499 grams

P05.16 Newborn small for gestational age, 1500-1749 grams

P05.17 Newborn small for gestational age, 1750-1999 grams

P05.18 Newborn small for gestational age, 2000-2499 grams

P05.19 Newborn small for gestational age, other
Newborn small for gestational age, 2500 grams and over
Coding Clinic: 2016, Q4, P55

P05.2 Newborn affected by fetal (intrauterine) malnutrition not light or small for gestational age
Infant, not light or small for gestational age, showing signs of fetal malnutrition, such as dry, peeling skin and loss of subcutaneous tissue

> **Excludes1** newborn affected by fetal malnutrition with light for gestational age (P05.0-)
> newborn affected by fetal malnutrition with small for gestational age (P05.1-)

P05.9 Newborn affected by slow intrauterine growth, unspecified
Newborn affected by fetal growth retardation NOS

● **P07 Disorders of newborn related to short gestation and low birth weight, not elsewhere classified**
Note: When both birth weight and gestational age of the newborn are available, both should be coded with birth weight sequenced before gestational age.

> **Includes** the listed conditions, without further specification, as the cause of morbidity or additional care, in newborn

● **P07.0 Extremely low birth weight newborn**
Newborn birth weight 999 g. or less

> **Excludes1** low birth weight due to slow fetal growth and fetal malnutrition (P05.-)

P07.00 Extremely low birth weight newborn, unspecified weight

P07.01 Extremely low birth weight newborn, less than 500 grams

P07.02 Extremely low birth weight newborn, 500-749 grams

P07.03 Extremely low birth weight newborn, 750-999 grams

● **P07.1 Other low birth weight newborn**
Newborn birth weight 1000-2499 g.

> **Excludes1** low birth weight due to slow fetal growth and fetal malnutrition (P05.-)

P07.10 Other low birth weight newborn, unspecified weight

P07.14 Other low birth weight newborn, 1000-1249 grams

P07.15 Other low birth weight newborn, 1250-1499 grams

P07.16 Other low birth weight newborn, 1500-1749 grams

P07.17 Other low birth weight newborn, 1750-1999 grams

P07.18 Other low birth weight newborn, 2000-2499 grams

● **P07.2 Extreme immaturity of newborn**
Less than 28 completed weeks (less than 196 completed days) of gestation

P07.20 Extreme immaturity of newborn, unspecified weeks of gestation
Gestational age less than 28 completed weeks NOS

P07.21 Extreme immaturity of newborn, gestational age less than 23 completed weeks
Extreme immaturity of newborn, gestational age less than 23 weeks, 0 days

P07.22 Extreme immaturity of newborn, gestational age 23 completed weeks
Extreme immaturity of newborn, gestational age 23 weeks, 0 days through 23 weeks, 6 days

P07.23 Extreme immaturity of newborn, gestational age 24 completed weeks
Extreme immaturity of newborn, gestational age 24 weeks, 0 days through 24 weeks, 6 days

P07.24 Extreme immaturity of newborn, gestational age 25 completed weeks
Extreme immaturity of newborn, gestational age 25 weeks, 0 days through 25 weeks, 6 days

P07.25 Extreme immaturity of newborn, gestational age 26 completed weeks
Extreme immaturity of newborn, gestational age 26 weeks, 0 days through 26 weeks, 6 days

P07.26 Extreme immaturity of newborn, gestational age 27 completed weeks
Extreme immaturity of newborn, gestational age 27 weeks, 0 days through 27 weeks, 6 days

● **P07.3 Preterm [premature] newborn [other]**
28 completed weeks or more but less than 37 completed weeks (196 completed days but less than 259 completed days) of gestation
Prematurity NOS

P07.30 Preterm newborn, unspecified weeks of gestation

P07.31 Preterm newborn, gestational age 28 completed weeks
Preterm newborn, gestational age 28 weeks, 0 days through 28 weeks, 6 days

P07.32 Preterm newborn, gestational age 29 completed weeks
Preterm newborn, gestational age 29 weeks, 0 days through 29 weeks, 6 days

P07.33 Preterm newborn, gestational age 30 completed weeks
Preterm newborn, gestational age 30 weeks, 0 days through 30 weeks, 6 days

P07.34 Preterm newborn, gestational age 31 completed weeks
Preterm newborn, gestational age 31 weeks, 0 days through 31 weeks, 6 days

P07.35 Preterm newborn, gestational age 32 completed weeks
Preterm newborn, gestational age 32 weeks, 0 days through 32 weeks, 6 days

P07.36 Preterm newborn, gestational age 33 completed weeks
Preterm newborn, gestational age 33 weeks, 0 days through 33 weeks, 6 days

▶ New   ⇒ Revised   ~~deleted~~ Deleted   Excludes 1   Excludes 2   Includes   Use additional   Code first   Code also   Key words

OGCR Official Guidelines   X Assign placeholder X   ● Use Additional Character(s)   ▶ Manifestation Code   ❧ Hierarchical Condition Category   **Coding Clinic**

P07.37 **Preterm newborn, gestational age 34 completed weeks**
Preterm newborn, gestational age 34 weeks, 0 days through 34 weeks, 6 days
Coding Clinic: 2017, Q2, P7

P07.38 **Preterm newborn, gestational age 35 completed weeks**
Preterm newborn, gestational age 35 weeks, 0 days through 35 weeks, 6 days

P07.39 **Preterm newborn, gestational age 36 completed weeks**
Preterm newborn, gestational age 36 weeks, 0 days through 36 weeks, 6 days
Coding Clinic: 2017, Q3, P26

● P08 **Disorders of newborn related to long gestation and high birth weight**
Note: When both birth weight and gestational age of the newborn are available, priority of assignment should be given to birth weight.
Includes the listed conditions, without further specification, as causes of morbidity or additional care, in newborn

P08.0 **Exceptionally large newborn baby**
Usually implies a birth weight of 4500 g. or more
Excludes1 syndrome of infant of diabetic mother (P70.1)
syndrome of infant of mother with gestational diabetes (P70.0)

P08.1 **Other heavy for gestational age newborn**
Other newborn heavy- or large-for-dates regardless of period of gestation
Usually implies a birth weight of 4000 g. to 4499 g.
Excludes1 newborn with a birth weight of 4500 or more (P08.0)
syndrome of infant of diabetic mother (P70.1)
syndrome of infant of mother with gestational diabetes (P70.0)

● P08.2 **Late newborn, not heavy for gestational age**
P08.21 **Post-term newborn**
Newborn with gestation period over 40 completed weeks to 42 completed weeks
P08.22 **Prolonged gestation of newborn**
Newborn with gestation period over 42 completed weeks (294 days or more), not heavy- or large-for-dates
Postmaturity NOS

ABNORMAL FINDINGS ON NEONATAL SCREENING (P09)

● P09 **Abnormal findings on neonatal screening**
Use additional code to identify signs, symptoms and conditions associated with the screening
▶Includes: Abnormal findings on state mandated newborn screens
▶Failed newborn screening
Excludes2 nonspecific serologic evidence of human immunodeficiency virus [HIV] (R75)

▶P09.1 **Abnormal findings on neonatal screening for inborn errors of metabolism**

▶P09.2 **Abnormal findings on neonatal screening for congenital endocrine disease**
▶Abnormal findings on neonatal screening for congenital adrenal hyperplasia
▶Abnormal findings on neonatal screening for hypothyroidism screen

▶P09.3 **Abnormal findings on neonatal screening for congenital hematologic disorders**
▶Abnormal findings for hemoglobinothies screen
▶Abnormal findings on red cell membrane defects screen
▶Abnormal findings on sickle cell screen

▶P09.4 **Abnormal findings on neonatal screening for cystic fibrosis**

▶P09.5 **Abnormal findings on neonatal screening for critical congenital heart disease**
▶Neonatal congenital heart disease screening failure

▶P09.6 **Abnormal findings on neonatal screening for neonatal hearing loss**
▶**Excludes2** encounter for hearing examination following failed hearing screening (Z01.110)

▶P09.8 **Other abnormal findings on neonatal screening**

▶P09.9 **Abnormal findings on neonatal screening, unspecified**

BIRTH TRAUMA (P10-P15)

● P10 **Intracranial laceration and hemorrhage due to birth injury**
Excludes1 intracranial hemorrhage of newborn NOS (P52.9)
intracranial hemorrhage of newborn due to anoxia or hypoxia (P52.-)
nontraumatic intracranial hemorrhage of newborn (P52.-)

P10.0 **Subdural hemorrhage due to birth injury**
Subdural hematoma (localized) due to birth injury
Excludes1 subdural hemorrhage accompanying tentorial tear (P10.4)

P10.1 **Cerebral hemorrhage due to birth injury**

P10.2 **Intraventricular hemorrhage due to birth injury**

P10.3 **Subarachnoid hemorrhage due to birth injury**

P10.4 **Tentorial tear due to birth injury**
Pertaining to tentorium of cerebellum (extension of dura mater that separates cerebellum from inferior portion of occipital lobes)

P10.8 **Other intracranial lacerations and hemorrhages due to birth injury**

P10.9 **Unspecified intracranial laceration and hemorrhage due to birth injury**

● P11 **Other birth injuries to central nervous system**
P11.0 **Cerebral edema due to birth injury**
P11.1 **Other specified brain damage due to birth injury**
P11.2 **Unspecified brain damage due to birth injury**
P11.3 **Birth injury to facial nerve**
Facial palsy due to birth injury
P11.4 **Birth injury to other cranial nerves**
P11.5 **Birth injury to spine and spinal cord**
Fracture of spine due to birth injury
P11.9 **Birth injury to central nervous system, unspecified**

● P12 **Birth injury to scalp**
P12.0 **Cephalhematoma due to birth injury**
P12.1 **Chignon (from vacuum extraction) due to birth injury**
P12.2 **Epicranial subaponeurotic hemorrhage due to birth injury**
Subgaleal hemorrhage
P12.3 **Bruising of scalp due to birth injury**
P12.4 **Injury of scalp of newborn due to monitoring equipment**
Sampling incision of scalp of newborn
Scalp clip (electrode) injury of newborn
● P12.8 **Other birth injuries to scalp**
P12.81 **Caput succedaneum**
P12.89 **Other birth injuries to scalp**
P12.9 **Birth injury to scalp, unspecified**

● P13 **Birth injury to skeleton**
Excludes2 birth injury to spine (P11.5)
P13.0 **Fracture of skull due to birth injury**
P13.1 **Other birth injuries to skull**
Excludes1 cephalhematoma (P12.0)

CHAPTER 16 (P00-P96)

Item 16–1 The **peripheral nervous system** consists of 31 pairs of spinal nerves, 12 pairs of cranial nerves, and the autonomic nerves, which are divided into the parasympathetic and sympathetic nerves. The cranial nerves are: olfactory (I), optic (II), oculomotor (III), trochlear (IV), trigeminal (V), abducens (VI), facial (VII), vestibulocochlear (VIII), glossopharyngeal (IX), vagus (X), accessory (XI), and hypoglossal (XII).

Central Nervous System

• Brain
• Spinal cord

Peripheral Nervous System

• Cranial nerves (12)
• Spinal nerves
   cervical (8)
   thoracic (12)
   lumbar (5)
   sacral (5)
   coccyx (1)

Figure 16-1 The central nervous system consists of the brain and spinal cord. The peripheral nervous system consists of nerves that lie outside the skull and spinal cord. (From Stoy: Mosby's EMT-Basic Textbook, ed 2, St. Louis, Mosby, 2007)

P13.2 Birth injury to femur
P13.3 Birth injury to other long bones
P13.4 Fracture of clavicle due to birth injury
P13.8 Birth injuries to other parts of skeleton
P13.9 Birth injury to skeleton, unspecified

● P14 Birth injury to peripheral nervous system
P14.0 Erb's paralysis due to birth injury
P14.1 Klumpke's paralysis due to birth injury
P14.2 Phrenic nerve paralysis due to birth injury
P14.3 Other brachial plexus birth injuries
P14.8 Birth injuries to other parts of peripheral nervous system
P14.9 Birth injury to peripheral nervous system, unspecified

● P15 Other birth injuries
P15.0 Birth injury to liver
       Rupture of liver due to birth injury
P15.1 Birth injury to spleen
       Rupture of spleen due to birth injury
P15.2 Sternomastoid injury due to birth injury

P15.3 Birth injury to eye
       Subconjunctival hemorrhage due to birth injury
       Traumatic glaucoma due to birth injury
P15.4 Birth injury to face
       Facial congestion due to birth injury
P15.5 Birth injury to external genitalia
P15.6 Subcutaneous fat necrosis due to birth injury
P15.8 Other specified birth injuries
P15.9 Birth injury, unspecified

RESPIRATORY AND CARDIOVASCULAR DISORDERS SPECIFIC TO THE PERINATAL PERIOD (P19-P29)

● P19 Metabolic acidemia in newborn
   Includes metabolic acidemia in newborn
P19.0 Metabolic acidemia in newborn first noted before onset of labor
P19.1 Metabolic acidemia in newborn first noted during labor
P19.2 Metabolic acidemia noted at birth
P19.9 Metabolic acidemia, unspecified

● P22 Respiratory distress of newborn
   Coding Clinic: 2019, Q2, P29
P22.0 Respiratory distress syndrome of newborn
       Cardiorespiratory distress syndrome of newborn
       Hyaline membrane disease
       Idiopathic respiratory distress syndrome [IRDS or RDS] of newborn
       Pulmonary hypoperfusion syndrome
       Respiratory distress syndrome, type I
       Excludes2 respiratory arrest of newborn (P28.81)
                     respiratory failure of newborn NOS (P28.5)
       Coding Clinic: 2019, Q2, P29
P22.1 Transient tachypnea of newborn
       Idiopathic tachypnea of newborn
       Respiratory distress syndrome, type II
       Wet lung syndrome
P22.8 Other respiratory distress of newborn
       Excludes1 respiratory arrest of newborn (P28.81)
                     respiratory failure of newborn NOS (P28.5)
P22.9 Respiratory distress of newborn, unspecified
       Excludes1 respiratory arrest of newborn (P28.81)
                     respiratory failure of newborn NOS (P28.5)

● P23 Congenital pneumonia
   Includes infective pneumonia acquired in utero or during birth
   Excludes1 neonatal pneumonia resulting from aspiration (P24.-)
P23.0 Congenital pneumonia due to viral agent
       Use additional code (B97) to identify organism
       Excludes1 congenital rubella pneumonitis (P35.0)
P23.1 Congenital pneumonia due to Chlamydia
P23.2 Congenital pneumonia due to staphylococcus
P23.3 Congenital pneumonia due to streptococcus, group B
P23.4 Congenital pneumonia due to Escherichia coli
P23.5 Congenital pneumonia due to Pseudomonas
P23.6 Congenital pneumonia due to other bacterial agents
       Congenital pneumonia due to Hemophilus influenzae
       Congenital pneumonia due to Klebsiella pneumoniae
       Congenital pneumonia due to Mycoplasma
       Congenital pneumonia due to Streptococcus, except group B
       Use additional code (B95-B96) to identify organism
P23.8 Congenital pneumonia due to other organisms
P23.9 Congenital pneumonia, unspecified

▶ New   ⇒ Revised   ~~deleted~~ Deleted   Excludes 1   Excludes 2   Includes   Use additional   Code first   Code also   Key words
OGCR Official Guidelines   X Assign placeholder X   ● Use Additional Character(s)   ▌ Manifestation Code   ☜ Hierarchical Condition Category   Coding Clinic

● **P24**   **Neonatal aspiration**
> **Includes**   aspiration in utero and during delivery

● **P24.0**   **Meconium aspiration**
> **Excludes1**   meconium passage (without aspiration) during delivery (P03.82)
> meconium staining (P96.83)

     P24.00   **Meconium aspiration without respiratory symptoms**
         Meconium aspiration NOS

     P24.01   **Meconium aspiration with respiratory symptoms**
         Meconium aspiration pneumonia
         Meconium aspiration pneumonitis
         Meconium aspiration syndrome NOS

         Use additional code to identify any secondary pulmonary hypertension, if applicable (I27.2-)

● **P24.1**   **Neonatal aspiration of (clear) amniotic fluid and mucus**
     Neonatal aspiration of liquor (amnii)

     P24.10   **Neonatal aspiration of (clear) amniotic fluid and mucus without respiratory symptoms**
         Neonatal aspiration of amniotic fluid and mucus NOS

     P24.11   **Neonatal aspiration of (clear) amniotic fluid and mucus with respiratory symptoms**
         Neonatal aspiration of amniotic fluid and mucus with pneumonia
         Neonatal aspiration of amniotic fluid and mucus with pneumonitis

         Use additional code to identify any secondary pulmonary hypertension, if applicable (I27.2-)

● **P24.2**   **Neonatal aspiration of blood**

     P24.20   **Neonatal aspiration of blood without respiratory symptoms**
         Neonatal aspiration of blood NOS

     P24.21   **Neonatal aspiration of blood with respiratory symptoms**
         Neonatal aspiration of blood with pneumonia
         Neonatal aspiration of blood with pneumonitis
         Use additional code to identify any secondary pulmonary hypertension, if applicable (I27.2-)

● **P24.3**   **Neonatal aspiration of milk and regurgitated food**
     Neonatal aspiration of stomach contents

     P24.30   **Neonatal aspiration of milk and regurgitated food without respiratory symptoms**
         Neonatal aspiration of milk and regurgitated food NOS

     P24.31   **Neonatal aspiration of milk and regurgitated food with respiratory symptoms**
         Neonatal aspiration of milk and regurgitated food with pneumonia
         Neonatal aspiration of milk and regurgitated food with pneumonitis

         Use additional code to identify any secondary pulmonary hypertension, if applicable (I27.2-)

● **P24.8**   **Other neonatal aspiration**

     P24.80   **Other neonatal aspiration without respiratory symptoms**
         Neonatal aspiration NEC

     P24.81   **Other neonatal aspiration with respiratory symptoms**
         Neonatal aspiration pneumonia NEC
         Neonatal aspiration with pneumonitis NEC
         Neonatal aspiration with pneumonia NOS
         Neonatal aspiration with pneumonitis NOS

         Use additional code to identify any secondary pulmonary hypertension, if applicable (I27.2-)

P24.9   **Neonatal aspiration, unspecified**

● **P25**   **Interstitial emphysema and related conditions originating in the perinatal period**

     P25.0   **Interstitial emphysema originating in the perinatal period**

     P25.1   **Pneumothorax originating in the perinatal period**

     P25.2   **Pneumomediastinum originating in the perinatal period**

     P25.3   **Pneumopericardium originating in the perinatal period**

     P25.8   **Other conditions related to interstitial emphysema originating in the perinatal period**

● **P26**   **Pulmonary hemorrhage originating in the perinatal period**
> **Excludes1**   acute idiopathic hemorrhage in infants over 28 days old (R04.81)

     P26.0   **Tracheobronchial hemorrhage originating in the perinatal period**

     P26.1   **Massive pulmonary hemorrhage originating in the perinatal period**

     P26.8   **Other pulmonary hemorrhages originating in the perinatal period**

     P26.9   **Unspecified pulmonary hemorrhage originating in the perinatal period**

● **P27**   **Chronic respiratory disease originating in the perinatal period**
> **Excludes2**   respiratory distress of newborn (P22.0-P22.9)

     P27.0   **Wilson-Mikity syndrome**
         Pulmonary dysmaturity

     P27.1   **Bronchopulmonary dysplasia originating in the perinatal period**

     P27.8   **Other chronic respiratory diseases originating in the perinatal period**
         Congenital pulmonary fibrosis
         Ventilator lung in newborn

     P27.9   **Unspecified chronic respiratory disease originating in the perinatal period**

● **P28**   **Other respiratory conditions originating in the perinatal period**
> **Excludes1**   congenital malformations of the respiratory system (Q30-Q34)

     P28.0   **Primary atelectasis of newborn**
         Failure of lungs to expand properly at birth
         Primary failure to expand terminal respiratory units
         Pulmonary hypoplasia associated with short gestation
         Pulmonary immaturity NOS

●   **P28.1**   **Other and unspecified atelectasis of newborn**

     P28.10   **Unspecified atelectasis of newborn**
         Atelectasis of newborn NOS

     P28.11   **Resorption atelectasis without respiratory distress syndrome**
> **Excludes1**   resorption atelectasis with respiratory distress syndrome (P22.0)

     P28.19   **Other atelectasis of newborn**
         Partial atelectasis of newborn
         Secondary atelectasis of newborn

     P28.2   **Cyanotic attacks of newborn**
> **Excludes1**   apnea of newborn (P28.3-P28.4)

     P28.3   **Primary sleep apnea of newborn**
         Central sleep apnea of newborn
         Obstructive sleep apnea of newborn
         Sleep apnea of newborn NOS

     P28.4   **Other apnea of newborn**
         Apnea of prematurity
         Obstructive apnea of newborn
> **Excludes1**   obstructive sleep apnea of newborn (P28.3)

     P28.5   **Respiratory failure of newborn**
> **Excludes1**   respiratory arrest of newborn (P28.81)
> respiratory distress of newborn (P22.0-)

     Coding Clinic: 2019, Q2, P29

- **P28.8**   Other specified respiratory conditions of newborn
  - **P28.81**   **Respiratory arrest of newborn**
    Coding Clinic: 2017, Q2, P6
  - **P28.89**   **Other specified respiratory conditions of newborn**
    Congenital laryngeal stridor
    Sniffles in newborn
    Snuffles in newborn
    - **Excludes1**   early congenital syphilitic rhinitis (A50.05)
- **P28.9**   Respiratory condition of newborn, **unspecified**
  Respiratory depression in newborn
- **P29**   Cardiovascular disorders originating in the perinatal period
  - ~~**Excludes1** congenital malformations of the circulatory system (Q20-Q28)~~
  - ▶ **Excludes2**   congenital malformations of the circulatory system (Q20-Q28)
  - **P29.0**   Neonatal cardiac failure
  - **P29.1**   Neonatal cardiac dysrhythmia
    - **P29.11**   Neonatal **tachycardia**
    - **P29.12**   Neonatal **bradycardia**
  - **P29.2**   Neonatal hypertension
  - **P29.3**   Persistent fetal circulation
    - **P29.30**   **Pulmonary hypertension of newborn**
      Persistent pulmonary hypertension of newborn
    - **P29.38**   **Other persistent fetal circulation**
      Delayed closure of ductus arteriosus
  - **P29.4**   Transient myocardial ischemia in newborn
  - **P29.8**   Other cardiovascular disorders originating in the perinatal period
    - **P29.81**   **Cardiac arrest of newborn**
    - **P29.89**   **Other cardiovascular disorders originating in the perinatal period**
  - **P29.9**   Cardiovascular disorder originating in the perinatal period, **unspecified**

INFECTIONS SPECIFIC TO THE PERINATAL PERIOD (P35-P39)

Infections acquired in utero, during birth via the umbilicus, or during the first 28 days after birth

Excludes2   asymptomatic human immunodeficiency virus [HIV] infection status (Z21)
congenital gonococcal infection (A54.-)
congenital pneumonia (P23.-)
congenital syphilis (A50.-)
human immunodeficiency virus [HIV] disease (B20)
infant botulism (A48.51)
infectious diseases not specific to the perinatal period (A00-B99, J09, J10.-)
intestinal infectious disease (A00-A09)
laboratory evidence of human immunodeficiency virus [HIV] (R75)
tetanus neonatorum (A33)

- **P35**   Congenital viral diseases
  - **Includes**   infections acquired in utero or during birth
  - **P35.0**   Congenital **rubella syndrome**
    Congenital rubella pneumonitis
  - **P35.1**   Congenital **cytomegalovirus infection**
    Viruses transmitted by multiple routes that cause mild/subclinical infection
  - **P35.2**   Congenital **herpesviral [herpes simplex] infection**
  - **P35.3**   Congenital **viral hepatitis**
  - **P35.4**   Congenital **Zika virus disease**
    Use additional code to identify manifestations of congenital Zika virus disease
    Coding Clinic: 2018, Q4, P26
  - **P35.8**   **Other congenital viral diseases**
    Congenital varicella [chickenpox]
    Coding Clinic: 2016, Q4, P7
  - **P35.9**   Congenital viral disease, **unspecified**

- **P36**   Bacterial sepsis of newborn
  - **Includes**   congenital sepsis
  - Use additional code(s), if applicable, to identify severe sepsis (R65.2-) and associated acute organ dysfunction(s)
  - **P36.0**   Sepsis of newborn due to **streptococcus, group B** 🏷
  - **P36.1**   Sepsis of newborn due to other and unspecified **streptococci**
    - **P36.10**   **Sepsis of newborn due to unspecified streptococci** 🏷
    - **P36.19**   **Sepsis of newborn due to other streptococci** 🏷
  - **P36.2**   Sepsis of newborn due to **Staphylococcus aureus** 🏷
  - **P36.3**   Sepsis of newborn due to other and unspecified **staphylococci**
    - **P36.30**   **Sepsis of newborn due to unspecified staphylococci** 🏷
    - **P36.39**   **Sepsis of newborn due to other staphylococci** 🏷
  - **P36.4**   Sepsis of newborn due to **Escherichia coli** 🏷
  - **P36.5**   Sepsis of newborn due to **anaerobes** 🏷
  - **P36.8**   **Other bacterial sepsis of newborn** 🏷
    Use additional code from category B96 to identify organism
  - **P36.9**   Bacterial sepsis of newborn, **unspecified** 🏷

- **P37**   Other congenital infectious and parasitic diseases
  - **Excludes2**   congenital syphilis (A50.-)
    infectious neonatal diarrhea (A00-A09)
    necrotizing enterocolitis in newborn (P77.-)
    noninfectious neonatal diarrhea (P78.3)
    ophthalmia neonatorum due to gonococcus (A54.31)
    tetanus neonatorum (A33)
  - **P37.0**   Congenital **tuberculosis**
  - **P37.1**   Congenital **toxoplasmosis**
    Parasitic infection, often causing mild flu-like illness
    Hydrocephalus due to congenital toxoplasmosis
  - **P37.2**   Neonatal (disseminated) **listeriosis**
    Acquired transplacentally or during/after parturition in which symptoms are those of sepsis
  - **P37.3**   Congenital **falciparum malaria**
  - **P37.4**   **Other congenital malaria**
  - **P37.5**   Neonatal **candidiasis**
  - **P37.8**   **Other specified congenital infectious and parasitic diseases**
  - **P37.9**   Congenital infectious or parasitic disease, **unspecified**

- **P38**   Omphalitis of newborn
  Inflammation of umbilicus
  - **Excludes1**   omphalitis not of newborn (L08.82)
    tetanus omphalitis (A33)
    umbilical hemorrhage of newborn (P51.-)
  - **P38.1**   Omphalitis **with mild hemorrhage**
  - **P38.9**   Omphalitis **without hemorrhage**
    Omphalitis of newborn NOS

- **P39**   Other infections specific to the perinatal period
  Use additional code to identify organism or specific infection
  - **P39.0**   Neonatal infective **mastitis**
    - **Excludes1**   breast engorgement of newborn (P83.4)
      noninfective mastitis of newborn (P83.4)
  - **P39.1**   Neonatal **conjunctivitis and dacryocystitis**
    Neonatal chlamydial conjunctivitis
    Ophthalmia neonatorum NOS
    Neonate = newborn
    - **Excludes1**   gonococcal conjunctivitis (A54.31)
  - **P39.2**   **Intra-amniotic infection affecting newborn, not elsewhere classified**
  - **P39.3**   Neonatal **urinary tract infection**

▶ New   ⇒ Revised   ~~deleted~~ Deleted   Excludes 1   Excludes 2   Includes   Use additional   Code first   Code also   Key words

OGCR Official Guidelines   X Assign placeholder X   ● Use Additional Character(s)   ▌ Manifestation Code   🏷 Hierarchical Condition Category   **Coding Clinic**

P39.4   Neonatal skin infection
Neonatal pyoderma

> **Excludes1**   pemphigus neonatorum (L00)
> staphylococcal scalded skin syndrome
> (L00)

P39.8   Other specified infections specific to the perinatal period

P39.9   Infection specific to the perinatal period, unspecified

HEMORRHAGIC AND HEMATOLOGICAL DISORDERS OF NEWBORN (P50-P61)

> **Excludes1**   congenital stenosis and stricture of bile ducts (Q44.3)
> Crigler-Najjar syndrome (E80.5)
> Dubin-Johnson syndrome (E80.6)
> Gilbert syndrome (E80.4)
> hereditary hemolytic anemias (D55-D58)

● **P50**   Newborn affected by intrauterine (fetal) blood loss

> **Excludes1**   congenital anemia from intrauterine (fetal) blood
> loss (P61.3)

P50.0   Newborn affected by intrauterine (fetal) blood loss from vasa previa

P50.1   Newborn affected by intrauterine (fetal) blood loss from ruptured cord

P50.2   Newborn affected by intrauterine (fetal) blood loss from placenta

P50.3   Newborn affected by hemorrhage into co-twin

P50.4   Newborn affected by hemorrhage into maternal circulation

P50.5   Newborn affected by intrauterine (fetal) blood loss from cut end of co-twin's cord

P50.8   Newborn affected by other intrauterine (fetal) blood loss

P50.9   Newborn affected by intrauterine (fetal) blood loss, unspecified
Newborn affected by fetal hemorrhage NOS

● **P51**   Umbilical hemorrhage of newborn

> **Excludes1**   omphalitis with mild hemorrhage (P38.1)
> umbilical hemorrhage from cut end of co-twins
> cord (P50.5)

P51.0   Massive umbilical hemorrhage of newborn

P51.8   Other umbilical hemorrhages of newborn
Slipped umbilical ligature NOS

P51.9   Umbilical hemorrhage of newborn, unspecified

● **P52**   Intracranial nontraumatic hemorrhage of newborn

> **Includes**   intracranial hemorrhage due to anoxia or hypoxia
> **Excludes1**   intracranial hemorrhage due to birth injury
> (P10.-)
> intracranial hemorrhage due to other injury
> (S06.-)

P52.0   Intraventricular (nontraumatic) hemorrhage, grade 1, of newborn
Subependymal hemorrhage (without intraventricular extension)
Bleeding into germinal matrix

P52.1   Intraventricular (nontraumatic) hemorrhage, grade 2, of newborn
Subependymal hemorrhage with intraventricular extension
Bleeding into ventricle

● **P52.2**   Intraventricular (nontraumatic) hemorrhage, grade 3 and grade 4, of newborn

P52.21   Intraventricular (nontraumatic) hemorrhage, grade 3, of newborn
Subependymal hemorrhage with intraventricular extension with enlargement of ventricle

P52.22   Intraventricular (nontraumatic) hemorrhage, grade 4, of newborn
Bleeding into cerebral cortex
Subependymal hemorrhage with intracerebral extension

P52.3   Unspecified intraventricular (nontraumatic) hemorrhage of newborn

P52.4   Intracerebral (nontraumatic) hemorrhage of newborn

P52.5   Subarachnoid (nontraumatic) hemorrhage of newborn

P52.6   Cerebellar (nontraumatic) and posterior fossa hemorrhage of newborn

P52.8   Other intracranial (nontraumatic) hemorrhages of newborn

P52.9   Intracranial (nontraumatic) hemorrhage of newborn, unspecified

● **P53**   Hemorrhagic disease of newborn
Vitamin K deficiency of newborn

● **P54**   Other neonatal hemorrhages

> **Excludes1**   newborn affected by (intrauterine) blood loss
> (P50.-)
> pulmonary hemorrhage originating in the
> perinatal period (P26.-)

P54.0   Neonatal hematemesis
Vomiting of blood

> **Excludes1**   neonatal hematemesis due to swallowed
> maternal blood (P78.2)

P54.1   Neonatal melena
Dark-colored feces stained with blood pigments

> **Excludes1**   neonatal melena due to swallowed
> maternal blood (P78.2)

P54.2   Neonatal rectal hemorrhage

P54.3   Other neonatal gastrointestinal hemorrhage

P54.4   Neonatal adrenal hemorrhage

P54.5   Neonatal cutaneous hemorrhage
Neonatal bruising
Neonatal ecchymoses
Neonatal petechiae
Neonatal superficial hematomata

> **Excludes2**   bruising of scalp due to birth injury
> (P12.3)
> cephalhematoma due to birth injury
> (P12.0)

P54.6   Neonatal vaginal hemorrhage ♀
Neonatal pseudomenses

P54.8   Other specified neonatal hemorrhages

P54.9   Neonatal hemorrhage, unspecified

● **P55**   Hemolytic disease of newborn
AKA erythroblastosis fetalis and is due to Rh isoimmunization, result of Rh blood factor incompatibilities between mother (Rh negative) and fetus (Rh positive)

P55.0   Rh isoimmunization of newborn

P55.1   ABO isoimmunization of newborn
Coding Clinic: 2015, Q3, P20

P55.8   Other hemolytic diseases of newborn

P55.9   Hemolytic disease of newborn, unspecified

● **P56**   Hydrops fetalis due to hemolytic disease
Caused by maternal sensitization to fetal blood group antigen

> **Excludes1**   hydrops fetalis NOS (P83.2)

P56.0   Hydrops fetalis due to isoimmunization

● **P56.9**   Hydrops fetalis due to other and unspecified hemolytic disease

P56.90   Hydrops fetalis due to unspecified hemolytic disease

P56.99   Hydrops fetalis due to other hemolytic disease

● **P57**   Kernicterus
High levels of bilirubin in blood, with severe neural symptoms

P57.0   Kernicterus due to isoimmunization

P57.8   Other specified kernicterus

> **Excludes1**   Crigler-Najjar syndrome (E80.5)

P57.9   Kernicterus, unspecified

CHAPTER 16 (P00-P96)

● **P58** **Neonatal jaundice due to other excessive hemolysis**

> **Excludes1** jaundice due to isoimmunization (P55-P57)

P58.0 Neonatal jaundice due to bruising

P58.1 Neonatal jaundice due to bleeding

P58.2 Neonatal jaundice due to infection

P58.3 Neonatal jaundice due to polycythemia

● P58.4 Neonatal jaundice due to drugs or toxins transmitted from mother or given to newborn

> *Code first poisoning due to drug or toxin, if applicable (T36-T65 with fifth or sixth character 1-4 or 6)*
>
> *Use additional code for adverse effect, if applicable, to identify drug (T36-T50 with fifth or sixth character 5)*

P58.41 Neonatal jaundice due to drugs or toxins transmitted from mother

P58.42 Neonatal jaundice due to drugs or toxins given to newborn

P58.5 Neonatal jaundice due to swallowed maternal blood

P58.8 Neonatal jaundice due to other specified excessive hemolysis

P58.9 Neonatal jaundice due to excessive hemolysis, unspecified

● **P59** **Neonatal jaundice from other and unspecified causes**

> **Excludes1** jaundice due to inborn errors of metabolism (E70-E88)
> kernicterus (P57.-)

P59.0 Neonatal jaundice associated with preterm delivery
Hyperbilirubinemia of prematurity
Jaundice due to delayed conjugation associated with preterm delivery

P59.1 Inspissated bile syndrome

● P59.2 Neonatal jaundice from other and unspecified hepatocellular damage

> **Excludes1** congenital viral hepatitis (P35.3)

P59.20 Neonatal jaundice from unspecified hepatocellular damage

P59.29 Neonatal jaundice from other hepatocellular damage
Neonatal giant cell hepatitis
Neonatal (idiopathic) hepatitis

P59.3 Neonatal jaundice from breast milk inhibitor

P59.8 Neonatal jaundice from other specified causes

P59.9 Neonatal jaundice, unspecified
Neonatal physiological jaundice (intense)(prolonged) NOS
Coding Clinic: 2015, Q3, P20

P60 **Disseminated intravascular coagulation of newborn**
Defibrination syndrome of newborn

● **P61** **Other perinatal hematological disorders**

> **Excludes1** transient hypogammaglobulinemia of infancy (D80.7)

P61.0 Transient neonatal thrombocytopenia
Lack of sufficient numbers of circulating thrombocytes (platelets)
Neonatal thrombocytopenia due to exchange transfusion
Neonatal thrombocytopenia due to idiopathic maternal thrombocytopenia
Neonatal thrombocytopenia due to isoimmunization

P61.1 Polycythemia neonatorum
Neonate = newborn

P61.2 Anemia of prematurity

P61.3 Congenital anemia from fetal blood loss

P61.4 Other congenital anemias, not elsewhere classified
Congenital anemia NOS

P61.5 Transient neonatal neutropenia
Low levels of granulocytic neutrophilic white blood cells

> **Excludes1** congenital neutropenia (nontransient) (D70.0)

P61.6 Other transient neonatal disorders of coagulation

P61.8 Other specified perinatal hematological disorders

P61.9 Perinatal hematological disorder, unspecified

TRANSITORY ENDOCRINE AND METABOLIC DISORDERS SPECIFIC TO NEWBORN (P70-P74)

> **Includes** transitory endocrine and metabolic disturbances caused by the infant's response to maternal endocrine and metabolic factors, or its adjustment to extrauterine environment

● **P70** **Transitory disorders of carbohydrate metabolism specific to newborn**

P70.0 Syndrome of infant of mother with gestational diabetes
Newborn (with hypoglycemia) affected by maternal gestational diabetes

> **Excludes1** newborn (with hypoglycemia) affected by maternal (pre-existing) diabetes mellitus (P70.1)
> syndrome of infant of a diabetic mother (P70.1)

P70.1 Syndrome of infant of a diabetic mother
Newborn (with hypoglycemia) affected by maternal (pre-existing) diabetes mellitus

> **Excludes1** newborn (with hypoglycemia) affected by maternal gestational diabetes (P70.0)
> syndrome of infant of mother with gestational diabetes (P70.0)

P70.2 Neonatal diabetes mellitus

P70.3 Iatrogenic neonatal hypoglycemia

P70.4 Other neonatal hypoglycemia
Transitory neonatal hypoglycemia

P70.8 Other transitory disorders of carbohydrate metabolism of newborn

P70.9 Transitory disorder of carbohydrate metabolism of newborn, unspecified

● **P71** **Transitory neonatal disorders of calcium and magnesium metabolism**

P71.0 Cow's milk hypocalcemia in newborn

P71.1 Other neonatal hypocalcemia

> **Excludes1** neonatal hypoparathyroidism (P71.4)

P71.2 Neonatal hypomagnesemia

P71.3 Neonatal tetany without calcium or magnesium deficiency
Neonatal tetany NOS

P71.4 Transitory neonatal hypoparathyroidism

P71.8 Other transitory neonatal disorders of calcium and magnesium metabolism
Coding Clinic: 2016, Q4, P55

P71.9 Transitory neonatal disorder of calcium and magnesium metabolism, unspecified

● **P72** **Other transitory neonatal endocrine disorders**

> **Excludes1** congenital hypothyroidism with or without goiter (E03.0-E03.1)
> dyshormogenetic goiter (E07.1)
> Pendred's syndrome (E07.1)

P72.0 Neonatal goiter, not elsewhere classified
Transitory congenital goiter with normal functioning

P72.1 Transitory neonatal hyperthyroidism
Neonatal thyrotoxicosis

P72.2 Other transitory neonatal disorders of thyroid function, not elsewhere classified
Transitory neonatal hypothyroidism

P72.8 Other specified transitory neonatal endocrine disorders

P72.9 Transitory neonatal endocrine disorder, unspecified

● **P74** **Other transitory neonatal electrolyte and metabolic disturbances**

P74.0 Late metabolic acidosis of newborn

> **Excludes1** (fetal) metabolic acidosis of newborn (P19)

P74.1 Dehydration of newborn

▶ New   ⇒ Revised   ~~deleted~~ Deleted   Excludes 1   Excludes 2   Includes   Use additional   Code first   Code also   Key words

OGCR Official Guidelines   **X** Assign placeholder X   ● Use Additional Character(s)   ▌ Manifestation Code   🔖 Hierarchical Condition Category   **Coding Clinic**

● **P74.2   Disturbances of sodium balance of newborn**
            Coding Clinic: 2018, Q2, P6
      P74.21   Hypernatremia of newborn
      P74.22   Hyponatremia of newborn
● **P74.3   Disturbances of potassium balance of newborn**
      P74.31   Hyperkalemia of newborn
      P74.32   Hypokalemia of newborn
● **P74.4   Other transitory electrolyte disturbances of newborn**
      P74.41   **Alkalosis of newborn**
            Hyperbicarbonatemia
    ● P74.42   **Disturbances of chlorine balance of newborn**
          P74.421   Hyperchloremia of newborn
                 Hyperchloremic metabolic acidosis

> **Excludes2** late metabolic acidosis of the newborn (P74.0)

          P74.422   Hypochloremia of newborn
      P74.49   **Other transitory electrolyte disturbance of newborn**
    P74.5   Transitory **tyrosinemia** of newborn
    P74.6   Transitory **hyperammonemia** of newborn
    P74.8   **Other transitory metabolic disturbances of newborn**
         Amino-acid metabolic disorders described as transitory
    P74.9   **Transitory metabolic disturbance of newborn, unspecified**

DIGESTIVE SYSTEM DISORDERS OF NEWBORN (P76-P78)

● **P76   Other intestinal obstruction of newborn**
    P76.0   **Meconium plug syndrome**
        Fetal stool obstruction in large intestine, present at birth; may be symptom of organic disease.
        Meconium ileus NOS

> **Excludes1** meconium ileus in cystic fibrosis (E84.11)

    P76.1   **Transitory ileus of newborn**
        Temporary obstruction of ileus (small intestine)

> **Excludes1** Hirschsprung's disease (Q43.1)

    P76.2   **Intestinal obstruction due to inspissated milk**
        Being thickened, dried, or made less fluid
    P76.8   **Other specified intestinal obstruction of newborn**

> **Excludes1** intestinal obstruction classifiable to K56.-

    P76.9   **Intestinal obstruction of newborn, unspecified**

● **P77   Necrotizing enterocolitis of newborn**
    P77.1   **Stage 1 necrotizing enterocolitis in newborn**
        Necrotizing enterocolitis without pneumatosis, without perforation
    P77.2   **Stage 2 necrotizing enterocolitis in newborn**
        Necrotizing enterocolitis with pneumatosis, without perforation
    P77.3   **Stage 3 necrotizing enterocolitis in newborn**
        Necrotizing enterocolitis with perforation
        Necrotizing enterocolitis with pneumatosis and perforation
    P77.9   **Necrotizing enterocolitis in newborn, unspecified**
        Necrotizing enterocolitis in newborn, NOS

● **P78   Other perinatal digestive system disorders**

> **Excludes1** cystic fibrosis (E84.0-E84.9)
> neonatal gastrointestinal hemorrhages (P54.0-P54.3)

    P78.0   **Perinatal intestinal perforation**
        Meconium peritonitis
    P78.1   **Other neonatal peritonitis**
        Neonatal peritonitis NOS
    P78.2   **Neonatal hematemesis and melena due to swallowed maternal blood**
    P78.3   **Noninfective neonatal diarrhea**
        Neonatal diarrhea NOS

● **P78.8   Other specified perinatal digestive system disorders**
      P78.81   **Congenital cirrhosis (of liver)**
      P78.82   **Peptic ulcer of newborn**
      P78.83   **Newborn esophageal reflux**
            Neonatal esophageal reflux
      P78.84   **Gestational alloimmune liver disease**
            GALD
            Neonatal hemochromatosis

> **Excludes1** hemochromatosis (E83.11-)

      P78.89   **Other specified perinatal digestive system disorders**
    P78.9   **Perinatal digestive system disorder, unspecified**

CONDITIONS INVOLVING THE INTEGUMENT AND TEMPERATURE REGULATION OF NEWBORN (P80-P83)

● **P80   Hypothermia of newborn**
    P80.0   **Cold injury syndrome**
        Severe and usually chronic hypothermia associated with a pink flushed appearance, edema and neurological and biochemical abnormalities.

> **Excludes1** mild hypothermia of newborn (P80.8)

    P80.8   **Other hypothermia of newborn**
        Mild hypothermia of newborn
    P80.9   **Hypothermia of newborn, unspecified**

● **P81   Other disturbances of temperature regulation of newborn**
    P81.0   **Environmental hyperthermia of newborn**
    P81.8   **Other specified disturbances of temperature regulation of newborn**
    P81.9   **Disturbance of temperature regulation of newborn, unspecified**
        Fever of newborn NOS

● **P83   Other conditions of integument specific to newborn**

> **Excludes1** congenital malformations of skin and integument (Q80-Q84)
> hydrops fetalis due to hemolytic disease (P56.-)
> neonatal skin infection (P39.4)
> staphylococcal scalded skin syndrome (L00)

> **Excludes2** cradle cap (L21.0)
> diaper [napkin] dermatitis (L22)

    P83.0   **Sclerema neonatorum**
        Neonate = newborn
    P83.1   **Neonatal erythema toxicum**
        Benign, generalized, transient pustules that become firm vesicles
    P83.2   **Hydrops fetalis not due to hemolytic disease**
        Severe, life-threatening problem of severe edema (swelling) as a result of too much fluid leaving blood and entering tissue
        Hydrops fetalis NOS
● **P83.3   Other and unspecified edema specific to newborn**
      P83.30   **Unspecified edema specific to newborn**
      P83.39   **Other edema specific to newborn**
    P83.4   **Breast engorgement of newborn**
        Noninfective mastitis of newborn
    P83.5   **Congenital hydrocele** ♂
    P83.6   **Umbilical polyp of newborn**
● **P83.8   Other specified conditions of integument specific to newborn**
      P83.81   **Umbilical granuloma**

> **Excludes2** Granulomatous disorder of the skin and subcutaneous tissue, unspecified (L92.9)

      P83.88   **Other specified conditions of integument specific to newborn**
          Bronze baby syndrome
          Neonatal scleroderma
          Urticaria neonatorum
    P83.9   **Condition of the integument specific to newborn, unspecified**

CHAPTER 16 (P00-P96)

OTHER PROBLEMS WITH NEWBORN (P84)

P84   Other problems with newborn
   Acidemia of newborn
   Acidosis of newborn
   Anoxia of newborn NOS
   Asphyxia of newborn NOS
   Hypercapnia of newborn
   Hypoxemia of newborn
   Hypoxia of newborn NOS
   Mixed metabolic and respiratory acidosis of newborn

   Excludes1   intracranial hemorrhage due to anoxia or hypoxia
                        (P52.-)
                    hypoxic ischemic encephalopathy [HIE] (P91.6-)
                    late metabolic acidosis of newborn (P74.0)

OTHER DISORDERS ORIGINATING IN THE PERINATAL PERIOD (P90-P96)

P90   Convulsions of newborn

   Excludes1   benign myoclonic epilepsy in infancy (G40.3-)
                    benign neonatal convulsions (familial) (G40.3-)

● **P91   Other disturbances of cerebral status of newborn**

   P91.0   Neonatal cerebral ischemia

      Excludes1   Neonatal cerebral infarction (P91.82-)

   P91.1   Acquired periventricular cysts of newborn

   P91.2   Neonatal cerebral leukomalacia
      *Degeneration of white matter adjacent to cerebral ventricles
         following cerebral hypoxia or brain ischemia in neonates*
      Periventricular leukomalacia

   P91.3   Neonatal cerebral irritability

   P91.4   Neonatal cerebral depression

   P91.5   Neonatal coma

● **P91.6   Hypoxic ischemic encephalopathy [HIE]**

      Excludes1   Neonatal cerebral depression (P91.4)
                       Neonatal cerebral irritability (P91.3)
                       Neonatal coma (P91.5)

      **P91.60   Hypoxic ischemic encephalopathy [HIE],
                  unspecified**

      **P91.61   Mild hypoxic ischemic encephalopathy
                  [HIE]**

      **P91.62   Moderate hypoxic ischemic encephalopathy
                  [HIE]**

      P91.63   Severe hypoxic ischemic encephalopathy [HIE]

● **P91.8   Other specified disturbances of cerebral status of
            newborn**

   ● **P91.81   Neonatal encephalopathy**

      ▸ *P91.811   Neonatal encephalopathy in diseases
                    classified elsewhere*

         Code first underlying condition, if known,
               such as:
            congenital cirrhosis (of liver) (P78.81)
            intracranial nontraumatic
                  hemorrhage of newborn (P52.-)
            kernicterus (P57.-)

      P91.819   Neonatal encephalopathy, unspecified

● **P91.82   Neonatal cerebral infarction**
   Neonatal stroke
   Perinatal arterial ischemic stroke
   Perinatal cerebral infarction

   Excludes1   cerebral infarction (I63.-)

   Excludes2   intracranial hemorrhage of
                    newborn (P52.-)

   **P91.821   Neonatal cerebral infarction, right
               side of brain**

   **P91.822   Neonatal cerebral infarction, left side
               of brain**

   P91.823   Neonatal cerebral infarction, bilateral

   **P91.829   Neonatal cerebral infarction,
               unspecified side**

   **P91.88   Other specified disturbances of cerebral status
              of newborn**

   P91.9   Disturbance of cerebral status of newborn, unspecified

● **P92   Feeding problems of newborn**

   ~~**Excludes1**   eating disorders (F50.-)~~
   ~~feeding problems in child over 28 days old~~
   ~~(R63.3)~~

   ▸ **Excludes2**   feeding problems in child over 28 days old
                    (R63.3)

   Coding Clinic: 2017, Q1, P28; 2016, Q3, P19

● **P92.0   Vomiting of newborn**

   Excludes1   vomiting of child over 28 days old (R11.-)

   P92.01   Bilious vomiting of newborn

      Excludes1   bilious vomiting in child over
                       28 days old (R11.14)

   P92.09   Other vomiting of newborn

      Excludes1   regurgitation of food in newborn
                       (P92.1)

   P92.1   Regurgitation and rumination of newborn

   P92.2   Slow feeding of newborn

   P92.3   Underfeeding of newborn

   P92.4   Overfeeding of newborn

   P92.5   Neonatal difficulty in feeding at breast
      Coding Clinic: 2017, Q1, P28; 2016, Q3, P19

   P92.6   Failure to thrive in newborn

      Excludes1   failure to thrive in child over 28 days old
                       (R62.51)

   P92.8   Other feeding problems of newborn

   P92.9   Feeding problem of newborn, unspecified

● **P93   Reactions and intoxications due to drugs administered to
          newborn**

   Includes   reactions and intoxications due to drugs
                  administered to fetus affecting newborn

   Excludes1   jaundice due to drugs or toxins transmitted from
                    mother or given to newborn (P58.4-)
                    reactions and intoxications from maternal
                       opiates, tranquilizers and other medication
                       (P04.0-P04.1, P04.4-)
                    withdrawal symptoms from maternal use of
                       drugs of addiction (P96.1)
                    withdrawal symptoms from therapeutic use of
                       drugs in newborn (P96.2)

   P93.0   Grey baby syndrome
      Grey syndrome from chloramphenicol administration
         in newborn

   **P93.8   Other reactions and intoxications due to drugs
              administered to newborn**

         Use additional code for adverse effect, if applicable,
            to identify drug (T36-T50 with fifth or sixth
            character 5)

▸ New   ⇒ Revised   ~~deleted~~ Deleted   Excludes 1   Excludes 2   Includes   Use additional   Code first   Code also   Key words

OGCR Official Guidelines   X Assign placeholder X   ● Use Additional Character(s)   ▸ Manifestation Code   🔖 Hierarchical Condition Category   **Coding Clinic**

● P94   **Disorders of muscle tone of newborn**

P94.0   Transient neonatal myasthenia gravis

    Excludes1   myasthenia gravis (G70.0)

P94.1   **Congenital hypertonia**

P94.2   **Congenital hypotonia**

    Floppy baby syndrome, unspecified

P94.8   **Other disorders of muscle tone of newborn**

P94.9   **Disorder of muscle tone of newborn, unspecified**

OGCR Section I.C.16.g.

Stillbirth

Code P95, Stillbirth, is only for use for institutions that maintain separate records for stillbirths. No other code should be used with P95. Code P95 should not be used on the mother's record.

P95   **Stillbirth**

    Deadborn fetus NOS
    Fetal death of unspecified cause
    Stillbirth NOS

    Excludes1   maternal care for intrauterine death (O36.4)
                    missed abortion (O02.1)
                    outcome of delivery, stillbirth (Z37.1, Z37.3,
                        Z37.4, Z37.7)

● P96   **Other conditions originating in the perinatal period**

P96.0   **Congenital renal failure**

    Uremia of newborn

P96.1   **Neonatal withdrawal symptoms from maternal use of drugs of addiction**

    Drug withdrawal syndrome in infant of dependent
        mother
    Neonatal abstinence syndrome

    Excludes1   reactions and intoxications from
                    maternal opiates and tranquilizers
                    administered during labor and
                    delivery (P04.0)

P96.2   **Withdrawal symptoms from therapeutic use of drugs in newborn**

P96.3   **Wide cranial sutures of newborn**

    Neonatal craniotabes

P96.5   **Complication to newborn due to (fetal) intrauterine procedure**

    Excludes2   newborn affected by amniocentesis
                    (P00.6)

● P96.8   **Other specified conditions originating in the perinatal period**

P96.81   **Exposure to (parental) (environmental) tobacco smoke in the perinatal period**

    Excludes2   newborn affected by in utero
                    exposure to tobacco (P04.2)
                    exposure to environmental
                    tobacco smoke after the
                    perinatal period (Z77.22)

P96.82   **Delayed separation of umbilical cord**

P96.83   **Meconium staining**

    Excludes1   meconium aspiration (P24.00,
                    P24.01)
                    meconium passage during
                    delivery (P03.82)

P96.89   **Other specified conditions originating in the perinatal period**

    Use additional code to specify condition

P96.9   **Condition originating in the perinatal period, unspecified**

    Congenital debility NOS

CHAPTER 17

CONGENITAL MALFORMATIONS, DEFORMATIONS, AND CHROMOSOMAL ABNORMALITIES (Q00-Q99)

OGCR Chapter-Specific Coding Guidelines

17. **Chapter 17: Congenital malformations, deformations, and chromosomal abnormalities (Q00-Q99)**

Assign an appropriate code(s) from categories Q00-Q99, Congenital malformations, deformations, and chromosomal abnormalities when a malformation/deformation or chromosomal abnormality is documented. A malformation/deformation/or chromosomal abnormality may be the principal/first-listed diagnosis on a record or a secondary diagnosis.

When a malformation/deformation/or chromosomal abnormality does not have a unique code assignment, assign additional code(s) for any manifestations that may be present.

When the code assignment specifically identifies the malformation/deformation/or chromosomal abnormality, manifestations that are an inherent component of the anomaly should not be coded separately. Additional codes should be assigned for manifestations that are not an inherent component.

Codes from Chapter 17 may be used throughout the life of the patient. If a congenital malformation or deformity has been corrected, a personal history code should be used to identify the history of the malformation or deformity. Although present at birth, malformation/deformation/or chromosomal abnormality may not be identified until later in life. Whenever the condition is diagnosed by the physician, it is appropriate to assign a code from codes Q00-Q99.

For the birth admission, the appropriate code from category Z38, Liveborn infants, according to place of birth and type of delivery, should be sequenced as the principal diagnosis, followed by any congenital anomaly codes, Q00-Q99.

CHAPTER 17

CONGENITAL MALFORMATIONS, DEFORMATIONS, AND CHROMOSOMAL ABNORMALITIES (Q00-Q99)

Note: Codes from this chapter are not for use on maternal records

Excludes2 inborn errors of metabolism (E70-E88)

This chapter contains the following blocks:

Q00-Q07	Congenital malformations of the nervous system
Q10-Q18	Congenital malformations of eye, ear, face and neck
Q20-Q28	Congenital malformations of the circulatory system
Q30-Q34	Congenital malformations of the respiratory system
Q35-Q37	Cleft lip and cleft palate
Q38-Q45	Other congenital malformations of the digestive system
Q50-Q56	Congenital malformations of genital organs
Q60-Q64	Congenital malformations of the urinary system
Q65-Q79	Congenital malformations and deformations of the musculoskeletal system
Q80-Q89	Other congenital malformations
Q90-Q99	Chromosomal abnormalities, not elsewhere classified

Figure 17-1 An infant with a large occipital encephalocele. The large skin-covered encephalocele is visible. (From Swaiman KF, Ashwal S, Ferriero DM: Pediatric Neurology: Principles and Practice, Philadelphia, Saunders, 2012)

CONGENITAL MALFORMATIONS OF THE NERVOUS SYSTEM (Q00–Q07)

● **Q00 Anencephaly and similar malformations**

Q00.0 Anencephaly 🐾
Absence of skull with cerebral hemispheres missing or reduced to small masses attached to base of cranium
Acephaly
Acrania
Amyelencephaly
Hemianencephaly
Hemicephaly

Q00.1 Craniorachischisis 🐾
Developmental anomaly consisting of fissure of cranium and vertebral column

Q00.2 Iniencephaly 🐾
Developmental anomaly characterized by enlargement of foramen magnum and absence of laminae and spinous processes of cervical, dorsal

● **Q01 Encephalocele**
Sac-like protrusions of brain and membranes visible through an opening in skull

Includes	Arnold-Chiari syndrome, type III encephalocystocele encephalomyelocele hydroencephalocele hydromeningocele, cranial meningocele, cerebral meningoencephalocele
Excludes1	Meckel-Gruber syndrome (Q61.9)

Q01.0 Frontal encephalocele 🐾
Q01.1 Nasofrontal encephalocele 🐾
Q01.2 Occipital encephalocele 🐾
Q01.8 Encephalocele of other sites 🐾
Q01.9 Encephalocele, unspecified 🐾

Q02 Microcephaly 🐾
Head size measures significantly below normal based on standardized charts

Includes	hydromicrocephaly micrencephalon

Code first, if applicable, congenital Zika virus disease

Excludes1	Meckel-Gruber syndrome (Q61.9)

Coding Clinic: 2018, Q4, P26; 2016, Q4, P7

● **Q03 Congenital hydrocephalus**
Accumulation of cerebrospinal fluid in ventricles resulting in swelling and enlargement

Includes	hydrocephalus in newborn
Excludes1	Arnold-Chiari syndrome, type II (Q07.0-) acquired hydrocephalus (G91.-) hydrocephalus due to congenital toxoplasmosis (P37.1) hydrocephalus with spina bifida (Q05.0-Q05.4)

Q03.0 Malformations of aqueduct of Sylvius 🐾
Anomaly of aqueduct of Sylvius
Obstruction of aqueduct of Sylvius, congenital
Stenosis of aqueduct of Sylvius

Q03.1 Atresia of foramina of Magendie and Luschka 🐾
Dandy-Walker syndrome

Q03.8 Other congenital hydrocephalus 🐾

Q03.9 Congenital hydrocephalus, unspecified 🐾

▶ New   ⟹ Revised   ~~deleted~~ Deleted   Excludes 1   Excludes 2   Includes   Use additional   Code first   Code also   Key words
OGCR Official Guidelines   X Assign placeholder X   ● Use Additional Character(s)   ▶ Manifestation Code   🐾 Hierarchical Condition Category   **Coding Clinic**

● **Q04   Other congenital malformations of brain**

> **Excludes1**   cyclopia (Q87.0)
> macrocephaly (Q75.3)

Q04.0   Congenital malformations of corpus callosum 🔍
Agenesis of corpus callosum

Q04.1   Arhinencephaly 🔍
Congenital absence of olfactory bulbs, tract, or nerves

Q04.2   Holoprosencephaly 🔍
Failure of cleavage of forebrain (prosencephalon) resulting in incomplete or absent cortical separation and deficits in midline facial development

Q04.3   Other reduction deformities of brain 🔍
Absence of part of brain
Agenesis of part of brain
> *Cerebral cortex are not fully formed, brain surface is smooth*

Agyria
Aplasia of part of brain
Hydranencephaly
Hypoplasia of part of brain
Lissencephaly
> *Congenital malformation or absence of convolutions of cerebral cortex*

Microgyria
> *Malformation of brain characterized by excessive number of small convolutions (gyri) on surface*

Pachygyria
> *Reduction in number of sulci of cerebrum*

> **Excludes1**   congenital malformations of corpus callosum (Q04.0)

Q04.4   Septo-optic dysplasia of brain 🔍
Q04.5   Megalencephaly 🔍
Abnormally large brain

Q04.6   Congenital cerebral cysts 🔍
Porencephaly   Schizencephaly
> **Excludes1**   acquired porencephalic cyst (G93.0)

Q04.8   Other specified congenital malformations of brain 🔍
Arnold-Chiari syndrome, type IV
Macrogyria

Q04.9   Congenital malformation of brain, unspecified 🔍
Congenital anomaly NOS of brain
Congenital deformity NOS of brain
Congenital disease or lesion NOS of brain
Multiple anomalies NOS of brain, congenital

● **Q05   Spina bifida**
Developmental anomaly characterized by defective closure of vertebral arch, through which spinal cord and meninges may protrude

> **Includes**   hydromeningocele (spinal)
> meningocele (spinal)
> meningomyelocele
> myelocele
> myelomeningocele
> rachischisis
> spina bifida (aperta)(cystica)
> syringomyelocele

Use additional code for any associated paraplegia (paraparesis) (G82.2-)

> **Excludes1**   Arnold-Chiari syndrome, type II (Q07.0-)
> spina bifida occulta (Q76.0)

Q05.0   Cervical spina bifida with hydrocephalus 🔍
Q05.1   Thoracic spina bifida with hydrocephalus 🔍
Dorsal spina bifida with hydrocephalus
Thoracolumbar spina bifida with hydrocephalus

Q05.2   Lumbar spina bifida with hydrocephalus 🔍
Lumbosacral spina bifida with hydrocephalus

Q05.3   Sacral spina bifida with hydrocephalus 🔍
Q05.4   Unspecified spina bifida with hydrocephalus 🔍
Q05.5   Cervical spina bifida without hydrocephalus 🔍
Q05.6   Thoracic spina bifida without hydrocephalus 🔍
Dorsal spina bifida NOS
Thoracolumbar spina bifida NOS

Q05.7   Lumbar spina bifida without hydrocephalus 🔍
Lumbosacral spina bifida NOS

Q05.8   Sacral spina bifida without hydrocephalus 🔍
Q05.9   Spina bifida, unspecified 🔍

● **Q06   Other congenital malformations of spinal cord**

Q06.0   Amyelia 🔍
Congenital absence of spinal cord

Q06.1   Hypoplasia and dysplasia of spinal cord 🔍
Underdevelopment of spinal cord
Atelomyelia
> *Congenitally incomplete development of spinal cord*
Myelatelia
Myelodysplasia of spinal cord
> *Defective development of spinal cord, especially lower segments*

Q06.2   Diastematomyelia 🔍
Congenital anomaly, associated with spina bifida, in which spinal cord is split into halves and surrounded by dural sac

Q06.3   Other congenital cauda equina malformations 🔍
Q06.4   Hydromyelia 🔍
Dilation of central canal of spinal cord with increased fluid accumulation
Hydrorachis

Q06.8   Other specified congenital malformations of spinal cord 🔍

Q06.9   Congenital malformation of spinal cord, unspecified 🔍
Congenital anomaly NOS of spinal cord
Congenital deformity NOS of spinal cord
Congenital disease or lesion NOS of spinal cord

● **Q07   Other congenital malformations of nervous system**

> **Excludes2**   congenital central alveolar hypoventilation syndrome (G47.35)
> familial dysautonomia [Riley-Day] (G90.1)
> neurofibromatosis (nonmalignant) (Q85.0-)

● **Q07.0   Arnold-Chiari syndrome**
Herniation of cerebellar tonsils and vermis through foramen magnum into spinal canal
Arnold-Chiari syndrome, type II
> **Excludes1**   Arnold-Chiari syndrome, type III (Q01.-)
> Arnold-Chiari syndrome, type IV (Q04.8)

Q07.00   Arnold-Chiari syndrome without spina bifida or hydrocephalus 🔍

Q07.01   Arnold-Chiari syndrome with spina bifida 🔍

Q07.02   Arnold-Chiari syndrome with hydrocephalus 🔍

Q07.03   Arnold-Chiari syndrome with spina bifida and hydrocephalus 🔍

Q07.8   Other specified congenital malformations of nervous system 🔍
Agenesis of nerve
Displacement of brachial plexus
Jaw-winking syndrome
Marcus Gunn's syndrome

Q07.9   Congenital malformation of nervous system, unspecified 🔍
Congenital anomaly NOS of nervous system
Congenital deformity NOS of nervous system
Congenital disease or lesion NOS of nervous system

CONGENITAL MALFORMATIONS OF EYE, EAR, FACE AND NECK (Q10-Q18)

> **Excludes2**   cleft lip and cleft palate (Q35-Q37)
> congenital malformation of cervical spine (Q05.0, Q05.5, Q67.5, Q76.0-Q76.4)
> congenital malformation of larynx (Q31.-)
> congenital malformation of lip NEC (Q38.0)
> congenital malformation of nose (Q30.-)
> congenital malformation of parathyroid gland (Q89.2)
> congenital malformation of thyroid gland (Q89.2)

● **Q10**   Congenital malformations of eyelid, lacrimal apparatus and orbit
> **Excludes1**   cryptophthalmos NOS (Q11.2)
> cryptophthalmos syndrome (Q87.0)

Q10.0   Congenital ptosis
> *Prolapse or drooping of upper eyelid from paralysis of third nerve or from sympathetic innervations*

Q10.1   Congenital ectropion
> *Outward turning of eyelid*

Q10.2   Congenital entropion
> *Inward turning of eyelid*

Q10.3   Other congenital malformations of eyelid
> Ablepharon
> Blepharophimosis, congenital
> Coloboma of eyelid
> Congenital absence or agenesis of cilia
> Congenital absence or agenesis of eyelid
> Congenital accessory eyelid
> Congenital accessory eye muscle
> Congenital malformation of eyelid NOS

Q10.4   Absence and agenesis of lacrimal apparatus
> Congenital absence of punctum lacrimale

Q10.5   Congenital stenosis and stricture of lacrimal duct

Q10.6   Other congenital malformations of lacrimal apparatus
> Congenital malformation of lacrimal apparatus NOS

Q10.7   Congenital malformation of orbit

● **Q11**   Anophthalmos, microphthalmos and macrophthalmos
> *Absence of eye and optic pit*

Q11.0   Cystic eyeball

Q11.1   Other anophthalmos
> Anophthalmos NOS
> Agenesis of eye
> > *Absence of eye*
> Aplasia of eye

Q11.2   Microphthalmos
> *Partial absence of eye and optic pit*
> Cryptophthalmos NOS
> Dysplasia of eye
> Hypoplasia of eye
> Rudimentary eye
> > **Excludes1**   cryptophthalmos syndrome (Q87.0)

Q11.3   Macrophthalmos
> *Congenital enlargement of eyes*
> > **Excludes1**   macrophthalmos in congenital glaucoma (Q15.0)

● **Q12**   Congenital lens malformations

Q12.0   Congenital cataract

Q12.1   Congenital displaced lens

Q12.2   Coloboma of lens

Q12.3   Congenital aphakia

Q12.4   Spherophakia
> *Smaller, more spherical optic lens than normal*

Q12.8   Other congenital lens malformations
> Microphakia

Q12.9   Congenital lens malformation, unspecified

● **Q13**   Congenital malformations of anterior segment of eye

Q13.0   Coloboma of iris
> Coloboma NOS

Q13.1   Absence of iris
> Aniridia
> Use additional code for associated glaucoma (H42)

Q13.2   Other congenital malformations of iris
> Anisocoria, congenital
> Atresia of pupil
> Congenital malformation of iris NOS
> Corectopia

Q13.3   Congenital corneal opacity

Q13.4   Other congenital corneal malformations
> Congenital malformation of cornea NOS
> Microcornea
> Peter's anomaly

Q13.5   Blue sclera
> *Condition of unusual blueness of sclera; not harmful*

● **Q13.8**   Other congenital malformations of anterior segment of eye

Q13.81   Rieger's anomaly
> Use additional code for associated glaucoma (H42)

Q13.89   Other congenital malformations of anterior segment of eye

Q13.9   Congenital malformation of anterior segment of eye, unspecified

● **Q14**   Congenital malformations of posterior segment of eye
> **Excludes2**   optic nerve hypoplasia (H47.03-)

Q14.0   Congenital malformation of vitreous humor
> Congenital vitreous opacity

Q14.1   Congenital malformation of retina
> Congenital retinal aneurysm

Q14.2   Congenital malformation of optic disc
> Coloboma of optic disc

Q14.3   Congenital malformation of choroid

Q14.8   Other congenital malformations of posterior segment of eye
> Coloboma of the fundus

Q14.9   Congenital malformation of posterior segment of eye, unspecified

● **Q15**   Other congenital malformations of eye
> **Excludes1**   congenital nystagmus (H55.01)
> ocular albinism (E70.31-)
> optic nerve hypoplasia (H47.03-)
> retinitis pigmentosa (H35.52)

Q15.0   Congenital glaucoma
> Axenfeld's anomaly
> Buphthalmos
> > *Congenital syndrome characterized by enlargement of the eye with symptoms of glaucoma.*
> Glaucoma of childhood
> Glaucoma of newborn
> Hydrophthalmos
> Keratoglobus, congenital, with glaucoma
> Macrocornea with glaucoma
> Macrophthalmos in congenital glaucoma
> Megalocornea with glaucoma

Q15.8   Other specified congenital malformations of eye

Q15.9   Congenital malformation of eye, unspecified
> Congenital anomaly of eye
> Congenital deformity of eye

● **Q16**   Congenital malformations of ear causing impairment of hearing
> **Excludes1**   congenital deafness (H90.-)

Q16.0   Congenital absence of (ear) auricle

Q16.1   Congenital absence, atresia and stricture of auditory canal (external)
> Congenital atresia or stricture of osseous meatus

Q16.2   Absence of eustachian tube

Q16.3   Congenital malformation of ear ossicles
> Congenital fusion of ear ossicles

Q16.4   Other congenital malformations of middle ear
> Congenital malformation of middle ear NOS

Figure 17-2 Bilateral congenital **hydrophthalmia,** in which the eyes are very large in comparison to the other facial features due to glaucoma.

Q16.5   **Congenital malformation of inner ear**
Congenital anomaly of membranous labyrinth
Congenital anomaly of organ of Corti

Q16.9   **Congenital malformation of ear causing impairment of hearing, unspecified**
Congenital absence of ear NOS

● **Q17   Other congenital malformations of ear**

     Excludes1   congenital malformations of ear with impairment of hearing (Q16.0-Q16.9)
preauricular sinus (Q18.1)

Q17.0   **Accessory auricle**
Accessory tragus
Polyotia
Preauricular appendage or tag
Supernumerary ear
Supernumerary lobule

Q17.1   **Macrotia**
Enlarged ears

Q17.2   **Microtia**
An abnormally small or underdeveloped external ear

Q17.3   **Other misshapen ear**
Pointed ear

Q17.4   **Misplaced ear**
Low-set ears
     Excludes1   cervical auricle (Q18.2)

Q17.5   **Prominent ear**
Bat ear

Q17.8   **Other specified congenital malformations of ear**
Congenital absence of lobe of ear

Q17.9   **Congenital malformation of ear, unspecified**
Congenital anomaly of ear NOS

● **Q18   Other congenital malformations of face and neck**

     Excludes1   cleft lip and cleft palate (Q35-Q37)
conditions classified to Q67.0-Q67.4
congenital malformations of skull and face bones (Q75.-)
cyclopia (Q87.0)
dentofacial anomalies [including malocclusion] (M26.-)
malformation syndromes affecting facial appearance (Q87.0)
persistent thyroglossal duct (Q89.2)

Q18.0   **Sinus, fistula and cyst of branchial cleft**
Branchial vestige
Branchial remnants (cysts, fistula, skin tags) that are developmental anomalies

Q18.1   **Preauricular sinus and cyst**
Fistula of auricle, congenital
Cervicoaural fistula
Abnormal passage in neck originating from first branchial cleft

Q18.2   **Other branchial cleft malformations**
Branchial cleft malformation NOS
Cervical auricle
Otocephaly

Q18.3   **Webbing of neck**
Pterygium colli
Thick fold of skin on side of neck

Q18.4   **Macrostomia**
Results from failure of union of maxillary and mandibular processes, results in abnormally large mouth

Q18.5   **Microstomia**

Q18.6   **Macrocheilia**
Excessive size of lips
Hypertrophy of lip, congenital

Q18.7   **Microcheilia**
Abnormal smallness of lips

Q18.8   **Other specified congenital malformations of face and neck**
Medial cyst of face and neck
Medial fistula of face and neck
Medial sinus of face and neck

Q18.9   **Congenital malformation of face and neck, unspecified**
Congenital anomaly NOS of face and neck

CONGENITAL MALFORMATIONS OF THE CIRCULATORY SYSTEM (Q20-Q28)

● **Q20   Congenital malformations of cardiac chambers and connections**

     Excludes1   dextrocardia with situs inversus (Q89.3)
mirror-image atrial arrangement with situs inversus (Q89.3)

Q20.0   **Common arterial trunk**
Persistent truncus arteriosus
     Excludes1   aortic septal defect (Q21.4)

Q20.1   **Double outlet right ventricle**
Taussig-Bing syndrome

Q20.2   **Double outlet left ventricle**

Q20.3   **Discordant ventriculoarterial connection**
Dextrotransposition of aorta
Transposition of great vessels (complete)

Q20.4   **Double inlet ventricle**
Common ventricle
Cor triloculare biatriatum
Single ventricle

Q20.5   **Discordant atrioventricular connection**
Corrected transposition
Levotransposition
Ventricular inversion

Q20.6   **Isomerism of atrial appendages**
Isomerism of atrial appendages with asplenia or polysplenia

Q20.8   **Other congenital malformations of cardiac chambers and connections**
Cor binoculare

Q20.9   **Congenital malformation of cardiac chambers and connections, unspecified**

● **Q21   Congenital malformations of cardiac septa**

     Excludes1   acquired cardiac septal defect (I51.0)

Q21.0   **Ventricular septal defect**
Roger's disease

Q21.1   **Atrial septal defect**
Coronary sinus defect
Patent or persistent foramen ovale
Patent or persistent ostium secundum defect (type II)
Patent or persistent sinus venosus defect

Q21.2   **Atrioventricular septal defect**
Common atrioventricular canal
Endocardial cushion defect
Ostium primum atrial septal defect (type I)

Q21.3   **Tetralogy of Fallot**
Ventricular septal defect with pulmonary stenosis or atresia, dextroposition of aorta and hypertrophy of right ventricle.

Q21.4   **Aortopulmonary septal defect**
Aortic septal defect
Aortopulmonary window

Q21.8   **Other congenital malformations of cardiac septa**
Eisenmenger's defect
Pentalogy of Fallot
⇒ Code also, if applicable:
Eisenmenger's complex (I27.83)
Eisenmenger's syndrome (I27.83)

Q21.9   **Congenital malformation of cardiac septum, unspecified**
Septal (heart) defect NOS

● **Q22   Congenital malformations of pulmonary and tricuspid valves**

Q22.0   **Pulmonary valve atresia**

Q22.1   **Congenital pulmonary valve stenosis**

Q22.2   **Congenital pulmonary valve insufficiency**
Congenital pulmonary valve regurgitation

Q22.3   **Other congenital malformations of pulmonary valve**
Congenital malformation of pulmonary valve NOS
Supernumerary cusps of pulmonary valve

Q22.4   **Congenital tricuspid stenosis**
Congenital tricuspid atresia

Q22.5   **Ebstein's anomaly**
Malformation of tricuspid valve

CHAPTER 17 (Q00-Q99)

Q22.6 **Hypoplastic right heart syndrome**
Q22.8 **Other congenital malformations of tricuspid valve**
Q22.9 **Congenital malformation of tricuspid valve, unspecified**

● Q23 **Congenital malformations of aortic and mitral valves**
Q23.0 **Congenital stenosis of aortic valve**
Congenital aortic atresia
Congenital aortic stenosis NOS
Excludes1 congenital stenosis of aortic valve in hypoplastic left heart syndrome (Q23.4)
congenital subaortic stenosis (Q24.4)
supravalvular aortic stenosis (congenital) (Q25.3)

Q23.1 **Congenital insufficiency of aortic valve**
Bicuspid aortic valve
Congenital aortic insufficiency

Q23.2 **Congenital mitral stenosis**
Congenital mitral atresia

Q23.3 **Congenital mitral insufficiency**

Q23.4 **Hypoplastic left heart syndrome**

Q23.8 **Other congenital malformations of aortic and mitral valves**

Q23.9 **Congenital malformation of aortic and mitral valves, unspecified**

● Q24 **Other congenital malformations of heart**
Excludes1 endocardial fibroelastosis (I42.4)

Q24.0 **Dextrocardia**
Heart is located in right hemithorax
Excludes1 dextrocardia with situs inversus (Q89.3)
isomerism of atrial appendages (with asplenia or polysplenia) (Q20.6)
mirror-image atrial arrangement with situs inversus (Q89.3)

Q24.1 **Levocardia**
Normal position of heart but related structures on wrong side

Q24.2 **Cor triatriatum**
Congenital heart defect; left atrium is subdivided

Q24.3 **Pulmonary infundibular stenosis**
Subvalvular pulmonic stenosis

Q24.4 **Congenital subaortic stenosis**

Q24.5 **Malformation of coronary vessels**
Congenital coronary (artery) aneurysm

Q24.6 **Congenital heart block**

Q24.8 **Other specified congenital malformations of heart**
Congenital diverticulum of left ventricle
Congenital malformation of myocardium
Congenital malformation of pericardium
Malposition of heart
Uhl's disease

Q24.9 **Congenital malformation of heart, unspecified**
Congenital anomaly of heart
Congenital disease of heart

● Q25 **Congenital malformations of great arteries**
Q25.0 **Patent ductus arteriosus**
Fetal blood vessel connecting left pulmonary artery directly to descending aorta
Patent ductus Botallo
Persistent ductus arteriosus

Q25.1 **Coarctation of aorta**
Coarctation of aorta (preductal) (postductal)
Stenosis of aorta
Coding Clinic: 2016, Q4, P56-57

● Q25.2 **Atresia of aorta**
Coding Clinic: 2016, Q4, P56
Q25.21 **Interruption of aortic arch**
Atresia of aortic arch
Q25.29 **Other atresia of aorta**
Atresia of aorta

Q25.3 **Supravalvular aortic stenosis**
Excludes1 congenital aortic stenosis NOS (Q23.0)
congenital stenosis of aortic valve (Q23.0)

● Q25.4 **Other congenital malformations of aorta**
Excludes1 hypoplasia of aorta in hypoplastic left heart syndrome (Q23.4)
Coding Clinic: 2016, Q4, P57
Q25.40 **Congenital malformation of aorta unspecified**
Q25.41 **Absence and aplasia of aorta**
Q25.42 **Hypoplasia of aorta**
Q25.43 **Congenital aneurysm of aorta**
Congenital aneurysm of aortic root
Congenital aneurysm of aortic sinus
Q25.44 **Congenital dilation of aorta**
Q25.45 **Double aortic arch**
Vascular ring of aorta
Q25.46 **Tortuous aortic arch**
Persistent convolutions of aortic arch
Q25.47 **Right aortic arch**
Persistent right aortic arch
Q25.48 **Anomalous origin of subclavian artery**
Q25.49 **Other congenital malformations of aorta**
Aortic arch
Bovine arch

Q25.5 **Atresia of pulmonary artery**

Q25.6 **Stenosis of pulmonary artery**
Supravalvular pulmonary stenosis

● Q25.7 **Other congenital malformations of pulmonary artery**
Q25.71 **Coarctation of pulmonary artery**
Q25.72 **Congenital pulmonary arteriovenous malformation**
Congenital pulmonary arteriovenous aneurysm
Q25.79 **Other congenital malformations of pulmonary artery**
Aberrant pulmonary artery
Agenesis of pulmonary artery
Congenital aneurysm of pulmonary artery
Congenital anomaly of pulmonary artery
Hypoplasia of pulmonary artery

Q25.8 **Other congenital malformations of other great arteries**

Q25.9 **Congenital malformation of great arteries, unspecified**

● Q26 **Congenital malformations of great veins**
Q26.0 **Congenital stenosis of vena cava**
Congenital stenosis of vena cava (inferior)(superior)

Q26.1 **Persistent left superior vena cava**

Q26.2 **Total anomalous pulmonary venous connection**
Total anomalous pulmonary venous return [TAPVR], subdiaphragmatic
Total anomalous pulmonary venous return [TAPVR], supradiaphragmatic

Q26.3 **Partial anomalous pulmonary venous connection**
Partial anomalous pulmonary venous return

Q26.4 **Anomalous pulmonary venous connection, unspecified**

Q26.5 **Anomalous portal venous connection**

Q26.6 **Portal vein-hepatic artery fistula**

Q26.8 **Other congenital malformations of great veins**
Absence of vena cava (inferior) (superior)
Azygos continuation of inferior vena cava
Persistent left posterior cardinal vein
Scimitar syndrome

Q26.9 **Congenital malformation of great vein, unspecified**
Congenital anomaly of vena cava (inferior) (superior) NOS

● Q27 **Other congenital malformations of peripheral vascular system**
Excludes2 anomalies of cerebral and precerebral vessels (Q28.0-Q28.3)
anomalies of coronary vessels (Q24.5)
anomalies of pulmonary artery (Q25.5-Q25.7)
congenital retinal aneurysm (Q14.1)
hemangioma and lymphangioma (D18.-)

▶ New   ⇒ Revised   ~~deleted~~ Deleted | Excludes 1 | | Excludes 2 | | Includes | | Use additional | | Code first | | Code also | | Key words |
OGCR Official Guidelines   X Assign placeholder X   ● Use Additional Character(s)   ▶ Manifestation Code   Hierarchical Condition Category   **Coding Clinic**

Q27.0   Congenital absence and hypoplasia of umbilical artery
       Single umbilical artery

Q27.1   Congenital renal artery stenosis

Q27.2   Other congenital malformations of renal artery
       Congenital malformation of renal artery NOS
       Multiple renal arteries

● Q27.3   Arteriovenous malformation (peripheral)
       Arteriovenous aneurysm

       Excludes1   acquired arteriovenous aneurysm (I77.0)

       Excludes2   arteriovenous malformation of cerebral
                 vessels (Q28.2)
                 arteriovenous malformation of
                 precerebral vessels (Q28.0)

      Q27.30   Arteriovenous malformation, site unspecified

      Q27.31   Arteriovenous malformation of vessel of upper limb

      Q27.32   Arteriovenous malformation of vessel of lower limb

      Q27.33   Arteriovenous malformation of digestive system vessel

      Q27.34   Arteriovenous malformation of renal vessel

      Q27.39   Arteriovenous malformation, other site

Q27.4   Congenital phlebectasia

Q27.8   Other specified congenital malformations of peripheral vascular system
       Absence of peripheral vascular system
       Atresia of peripheral vascular system
       Congenital aneurysm (peripheral)
       Congenital stricture, artery
       Congenital varix

       Excludes1   arteriovenous malformation (Q27.3-)

Q27.9   Congenital malformation of peripheral vascular system, unspecified
       Anomaly of artery or vein NOS

● Q28   Other congenital malformations of circulatory system

       Excludes1   congenital aneurysm NOS (Q27.8)
                 congenital coronary aneurysm (Q24.5)
                 ruptured cerebral arteriovenous malformation
                 (I60.8)
                 ruptured malformation of precerebral vessels
                 (I72.0)

       Excludes2   congenital peripheral aneurysm (Q27.8)
                 congenital pulmonary aneurysm (Q25.79)
                 congenital retinal aneurysm (Q14.1)

Q28.0   Arteriovenous malformation of precerebral vessels
       Congenital arteriovenous precerebral aneurysm
       (nonruptured)

Q28.1   Other malformations of precerebral vessels
       Congenital malformation of precerebral vessels NOS
       Congenital precerebral aneurysm (nonruptured)

Q28.2   Arteriovenous malformation of cerebral vessels
       Arteriovenous malformation of brain NOS
       Congenital arteriovenous cerebral aneurysm
       (nonruptured)

Q28.3   Other malformations of cerebral vessels
       Congenital cerebral aneurysm (nonruptured)
       Congenital malformation of cerebral vessels NOS
       Developmental venous anomaly

Q28.8   Other specified congenital malformations of circulatory system
       Congenital aneurysm, specified site NEC
       Spinal vessel anomaly

Q28.9   Congenital malformation of circulatory system, unspecified

---

CONGENITAL MALFORMATIONS OF THE RESPIRATORY SYSTEM (Q30-Q34)

● Q30   Congenital malformations of nose

       Excludes1   congenital deviation of nasal septum (Q67.4)

Q30.0   Choanal atresia
       Atresia of nares (anterior) (posterior)
       Congenital stenosis of nares (anterior) (posterior)

Q30.1   Agenesis and underdevelopment of nose
       Congenital absent of nose

Q30.2   Fissured, notched and cleft nose

Q30.3   Congenital perforated nasal septum

Q30.8   Other congenital malformations of nose
       Accessory nose
       Congenital anomaly of nasal sinus wall

Q30.9   Congenital malformation of nose, unspecified

● Q31   Congenital malformations of larynx

       Excludes1   congenital laryngeal stridor NOS (P28.89)

Q31.0   Web of larynx
       Glottic web of larynx
       Subglottic web of larynx
       Web of larynx NOS

Q31.1   Congenital subglottic stenosis

Q31.2   Laryngeal hypoplasia

Q31.3   Laryngocele

Q31.5   Congenital laryngomalacia

Q31.8   Other congenital malformations of larynx
       Absence of larynx
       Agenesis of larynx
       Atresia of larynx
       Congenital cleft thyroid cartilage
       Congenital fissure of epiglottis
       Congenital stenosis of larynx NEC
       Posterior cleft of cricoid cartilage

Q31.9   Congenital malformation of larynx, unspecified

● Q32   Congenital malformations of trachea and bronchus

       Excludes1   congenital bronchiectasis (Q33.4)

Q32.0   Congenital tracheomalacia

Q32.1   Other congenital malformations of trachea
       Atresia of trachea
       Congenital anomaly of tracheal cartilage
       Congenital dilatation of trachea
       Congenital malformation of trachea
       Congenital stenosis of trachea
       Congenital tracheocele

Q32.2   Congenital bronchomalacia

Q32.3   Congenital stenosis of bronchus

Q32.4   Other congenital malformations of bronchus
       Absence of bronchus
       Agenesis of bronchus
       Atresia of bronchus
       Congenital diverticulum of bronchus
       Congenital malformation of bronchus NOS

● Q33   Congenital malformations of lung

Q33.0   Congenital cystic lung
       Congenital cystic lung disease
       Congenital honeycomb lung
       Congenital polycystic lung disease

       Excludes1   cystic fibrosis (E84.0)
                 cystic lung disease, acquired or
                 unspecified (J98.4)

Q33.1   Accessory lobe of lung
       Azygos lobe (fissured), lung

Q33.2   Sequestration of lung

Q33.3   Agenesis of lung
       Congenital absence of lung (lobe)

Q33.4   Congenital bronchiectasis

Q33.5   Ectopic tissue in lung

Q33.6   Congenital hypoplasia and dysplasia of lung

       Excludes1   pulmonary hypoplasia associated with
                 short gestation (P28.0)

Q33.8   Other congenital malformations of lung

Q33.9   Congenital malformation of lung, unspecified

● Q34   Other congenital malformations of respiratory system

       Excludes2   congenital central alveolar hypoventilation
                 syndrome (G47.35)

Q34.0   Anomaly of pleura

Q34.1   Congenital cyst of mediastinum

CHAPTER 17 (Q00-Q99)

Figure 17-3 Cleft palate.

Q34.8   Other specified congenital malformations of respiratory system
     Atresia of nasopharynx

Q34.9   Congenital malformation of respiratory system, unspecified
     Congenital absence of respiratory system
     Congenital anomaly of respiratory system NOS

CLEFT LIP AND CLEFT PALATE (Q35-Q37)

Use additional code to identify associated malformation of the nose (Q30.2)

~~Excludes1   Robin's syndrome (Q87.0)~~

Excludes2   Robin's syndrome (Q87.0)

● **Q35   Cleft palate**
     Includes   fissure of palate
                   palatoschisis
     Excludes1   cleft palate with cleft lip (Q37.-)

Q35.1   Cleft hard palate

Q35.3   Cleft soft palate

Q35.5   Cleft hard palate with cleft soft palate

Q35.7   Cleft uvula

Q35.9   Cleft palate, unspecified
     Cleft palate NOS

● **Q36   Cleft lip**
     Includes   cheiloschisis
                   congenital fissure of lip
                   harelip
                   labium leporinum
     Excludes1   cleft lip with cleft palate (Q37.-)

Q36.0   Cleft lip, bilateral

Q36.1   Cleft lip, median

Q36.9   Cleft lip, unilateral
     Cleft lip NOS

● **Q37   Cleft palate with cleft lip**
     Includes   cheilopalatoschisis

Q37.0   Cleft hard palate with bilateral cleft lip

Q37.1   Cleft hard palate with unilateral cleft lip
     Cleft hard palate with cleft lip NOS

Q37.2   Cleft soft palate with bilateral cleft lip

Q37.3   Cleft soft palate with unilateral cleft lip
     Cleft soft palate with cleft lip NOS

Q37.4   Cleft hard and soft palate with bilateral cleft lip

Q37.5   Cleft hard and soft palate with unilateral cleft lip
     Cleft hard and soft palate with cleft lip NOS

Q37.8   Unspecified cleft palate with bilateral cleft lip

Q37.9   Unspecified cleft palate with unilateral cleft lip
     Cleft palate with cleft lip NOS

OTHER CONGENITAL MALFORMATIONS OF THE DIGESTIVE SYSTEM (Q38-Q45)

● **Q38   Other congenital malformations of tongue, mouth and pharynx**
     Excludes1   dentofacial anomalies (M26.-)
                        macrostomia (Q18.4)
                        microstomia (Q18.5)

Q38.0   Congenital malformations of lips, not elsewhere classified
     Congenital fistula of lip
     Congenital malformation of lip NOS
     Van der Woude's syndrome
     Excludes1   cleft lip (Q36.-)
                        cleft lip with cleft palate (Q37.-)
                        macrocheilia (Q18.6)
                        microcheilia (Q18.7)

Q38.1   Ankyloglossia
     Restricted movement of tongue resulting in speech difficulty
     Tongue tie

Q38.2   Macroglossia
     Excessive size of tongue
     Congenital hypertrophy of tongue

Q38.3   Other congenital malformations of tongue
     Aglossia
     Bifid tongue
     Congenital adhesion of tongue
     Congenital fissure of tongue
     Congenital malformation of tongue NOS
     Double tongue
     Hypoglossia
     Hypoplasia of tongue
     Microglossia

Q38.4   Congenital malformations of salivary glands and ducts
     Atresia of salivary glands and ducts
     Congenital absence of salivary glands and ducts
     Congenital accessory salivary glands and ducts
     Congenital fistula of salivary gland

Q38.5   Congenital malformations of palate, not elsewhere classified
     Congenital absence of uvula
     Congenital malformation of palate NOS
     Congenital high arched palate
     Excludes1   cleft palate (Q35.-)
                        cleft palate with cleft lip (Q37.-)

Q38.6   Other congenital malformations of mouth
     Congenital malformation of mouth NOS

Q38.7   Congenital pharyngeal pouch
     Congenital diverticulum of pharynx
     Excludes1   pharyngeal pouch syndrome (D82.1)

Q38.8   Other congenital malformations of pharynx
     Congenital malformation of pharynx NOS
     Imperforate pharynx

● **Q39   Congenital malformations of esophagus**

Q39.0   Atresia of esophagus without fistula
     Atresia of esophagus NOS

Q39.1   Atresia of esophagus with tracheo-esophageal fistula
     Atresia of esophagus with broncho-esophageal fistula

Q39.2   Congenital tracheo-esophageal fistula without atresia
     Congenital tracheo-esophageal fistula NOS

Q39.3   Congenital stenosis and stricture of esophagus

Q39.4   Esophageal web

Q39.5   Congenital dilatation of esophagus
     Congenital cardiospasm

Q39.6   Congenital diverticulum of esophagus
     Congenital esophageal pouch

Q39.8   Other congenital malformations of esophagus
     Congenital absence of esophagus
     Congenital displacement of esophagus
     Congenital duplication of esophagus

Q39.9   Congenital malformation of esophagus, unspecified

● **Q40   Other congenital malformations of upper alimentary tract**

Q40.0   Congenital hypertrophic pyloric stenosis
     Congenital or infantile constriction
     Congenital or infantile hypertrophy
     Congenital or infantile spasm
     Congenital or infantile stenosis
     Congenital or infantile stricture

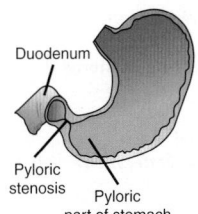

Duodenum

Pyloric
stenosis

Pyloric
part of stomach

Figure 17-4 Pyloric stenosis.

Q40.1 Congenital hiatus hernia
Congenital displacement of cardia through esophageal hiatus

> **Excludes1** congenital diaphragmatic hernia (Q79.0)

Q40.2 Other specified congenital malformations of stomach
Congenital displacement of stomach
Congenital diverticulum of stomach
Congenital hourglass stomach
Congenital duplication of stomach
Megalogastria
Microgastria

Q40.3 Congenital malformation of stomach, unspecified

Q40.8 Other specified congenital malformations of upper alimentary tract

Q40.9 Congenital malformation of upper alimentary tract, unspecified
Congenital anomaly of upper alimentary tract
Congenital deformity of upper alimentary tract

● **Q41 Congenital absence, atresia and stenosis of small intestine**

> **Includes** congenital obstruction, occlusion or stricture of small intestine or intestine NOS

> **Excludes1** cystic fibrosis with intestinal manifestation (E84.11)
> meconium ileus NOS (without cystic fibrosis) (P76.0)

Q41.0 Congenital absence, atresia and stenosis of duodenum

Q41.1 Congenital absence, atresia and stenosis of jejunum
Apple peel syndrome
Imperforate jejunum

Q41.2 Congenital absence, atresia and stenosis of ileum

Q41.8 Congenital absence, atresia and stenosis of other specified parts of small intestine

Q41.9 Congenital absence, atresia and stenosis of small intestine, part unspecified
Congenital absence, atresia and stenosis of intestine NOS

● **Q42 Congenital absence, atresia and stenosis of large intestine**

> **Includes** congenital obstruction, occlusion and stricture of large intestine

Q42.0 Congenital absence, atresia and stenosis of rectum with fistula

Q42.1 Congenital absence, atresia and stenosis of rectum without fistula
Imperforate rectum

Q42.2 Congenital absence, atresia and stenosis of anus with fistula

Q42.3 Congenital absence, atresia and stenosis of anus without fistula
Imperforate anus

Q42.8 Congenital absence, atresia and stenosis of other parts of large intestine

Q42.9 Congenital absence, atresia and stenosis of large intestine, part unspecified

● **Q43 Other congenital malformations of intestine**

Q43.0 Meckel's diverticulum (displaced) (hypertrophic)
Congenital abnormality in which a pouch remains on the lower end of the small intestine
Persistent omphalomesenteric duct
Persistent vitelline duct

Q43.1 Hirschsprung's disease
Developmental disorder of enteric nervous system characterized by absence of ganglion cells in distal colon resulting in functional obstruction
Aganglionosis
Congenital (aganglionic) megacolon

Q43.2 Other congenital functional disorders of colon
Congenital dilatation of colon

Q43.3 Congenital malformations of intestinal fixation
Congenital omental, anomalous adhesions [bands]
Congenital peritoneal adhesions [bands]
Incomplete rotation of cecum and colon
Insufficient rotation of cecum and colon
Jackson's membrane
Malrotation of colon
Rotation failure of cecum and colon
Universal mesentery

Q43.4 Duplication of intestine

Q43.5 Ectopic anus
Anal opening in abnormal location

Q43.6 Congenital fistula of rectum and anus

> **Excludes1** congenital fistula of anus with absence, atresia and stenosis (Q42.2)
> congenital fistula of rectum with absence, atresia and stenosis (Q42.0)
> congenital rectovaginal fistula (Q52.2)
> congenital urethrorectal fistula (Q64.73)
> pilonidal fistula or sinus (L05.-)

Q43.7 Persistent cloaca
Malformation in which rectum, vagina, and urinary tract form one channel; AKA congenital cloaca
Cloaca NOS

Q43.8 Other specified congenital malformations of intestine
Congenital blind loop syndrome
Congenital diverticulitis, colon
Congenital diverticulum, intestine
Dolichocolon
Megaloappendix
Megaloduodenum
Microcolon
Transposition of appendix
Transposition of colon
Transposition of intestine

Q43.9 Congenital malformation of intestine, unspecified

● **Q44 Congenital malformations of gallbladder, bile ducts and liver**

Q44.0 Agenesis, aplasia and hypoplasia of gallbladder
Congenital absence of gallbladder

Q44.1 Other congenital malformations of gallbladder
Congenital malformation of gallbladder NOS
Intrahepatic gallbladder

Q44.2 Atresia of bile ducts

Q44.3 Congenital stenosis and stricture of bile ducts

Q44.4 Choledochal cyst

Q44.5 Other congenital malformations of bile ducts
Accessory hepatic duct
Biliary duct duplication
Congenital malformation of bile duct NOS
Cystic duct duplication

Q44.6 Cystic disease of liver
Fibrocystic disease of liver

Q44.7 Other congenital malformations of liver
Accessory liver
Alagille's syndrome
Congenital absence of liver
Congenital hepatomegaly
Congenital malformation of liver NOS

● **Q45 Other congenital malformations of digestive system**

> **Excludes2** congenital diaphragmatic hernia (Q79.0)
> congenital hiatus hernia (Q40.1)

Q45.0 Agenesis, aplasia and hypoplasia of pancreas
Congenital absence of pancreas

Q45.1 Annular pancreas

Q45.2 Congenital pancreatic cyst

CHAPTER 17 (Q00-Q99)

Q45.3   **Other congenital malformations of pancreas and pancreatic duct**
     Accessory pancreas
     Congenital malformation of pancreas or pancreatic duct NOS

     Excludes1   congenital diabetes mellitus (E10.-)
                     cystic fibrosis (E84.0-E84.9)
                     fibrocystic disease of pancreas (E84.-)
                     neonatal diabetes mellitus (P70.2)

Q45.8   **Other specified congenital malformations of digestive system**
     Absence (complete) (partial) of alimentary tract NOS
     Duplication of digestive system
     Malposition, congenital of digestive system

Q45.9   **Congenital malformation of digestive system, unspecified**
     Congenital anomaly of digestive system
     Congenital deformity of digestive system

CONGENITAL MALFORMATIONS OF GENITAL ORGANS (Q50-Q56)

     Excludes1   androgen insensitivity syndrome (E34.5-)
                     syndromes associated with anomalies in the number and form of chromosomes (Q90-Q99)

● Q50   **Congenital malformations of ovaries, fallopian tubes and broad ligaments**

  ● Q50.0   **Congenital absence of ovary**

       Excludes1   Turner's syndrome (Q96.-)

       Q50.01   Congenital absence of ovary, unilateral ♀

       Q50.02   Congenital absence of ovary, bilateral ♀

   Q50.1   Developmental ovarian cyst ♀

   Q50.2   Congenital torsion of ovary ♀

  ● Q50.3   Other congenital malformations of ovary

       Q50.31   Accessory ovary ♀

       Q50.32   Ovarian streak ♀
           Inadequate ovaries with absent follicular and hormonal function
           46, XX with streak gonads

       Q50.39   Other congenital malformation of ovary ♀
           Congenital malformation of ovary NOS

   Q50.4   Embryonic cyst of fallopian tube ♀
       Fimbrial cyst

   Q50.5   Embryonic cyst of broad ligament ♀
       Epoophoron cyst
       Parovarian cyst

   Q50.6   Other congenital malformations of fallopian tube and broad ligament ♀
       Absence of fallopian tube and broad ligament
       Accessory fallopian tube and broad ligament
       Atresia of fallopian tube and broad ligament
       Congenital malformation of fallopian tube or broad ligament NOS

● Q51   **Congenital malformations of uterus and cervix**

   Q51.0   **Agenesis and aplasia of uterus** ♀
       Congenital absence of uterus

  ● Q51.1   **Doubling of uterus with doubling of cervix and vagina**

       Q51.10   Doubling of uterus with doubling of cervix and vagina without obstruction ♀
           Doubling of uterus with doubling of cervix and vagina NOS

       Q51.11   Doubling of uterus with doubling of cervix and vagina with obstruction ♀

  ● Q51.2   **Other doubling of uterus**
       Doubling of uterus NOS
       Septate uterus

       ~~Q51.20   Other doubling of uterus, unspecified~~
           ~~Septate uterus, unspecified~~

       Q51.21   Complete doubling of uterus ♀
           Complete septate uterus

       Q51.22   Partial doubling of uterus ♀
           Partial septate uterus

       Q51.28   Other and unspecified doubling of uterus ♀
           Septate uterus NOS

   Q51.3   **Bicornate uterus** ♀
       Bicornate uterus, complete or partial
       Birth defect in which uterus has two separate "horns" that form top of uterus

   Q51.4   **Unicornate uterus** ♀
       Unicornate uterus with or without a separate uterine horn
       Uterus with only one functioning horn
       Uterus with half being undeveloped

   Q51.5   **Agenesis and aplasia of cervix** ♀
       Congenital absence of cervix

   Q51.6   **Embryonic cyst of cervix** ♀

   Q51.7   **Congenital fistulae between uterus and digestive and urinary tracts** ♀

  ● Q51.8   **Other congenital malformations of uterus and cervix**

    ● Q51.81   **Other congenital malformations of uterus**

       Q51.810   Arcuate uterus ♀
           Arcuatus uterus

       Q51.811   Hypoplasia of uterus ♀

       Q51.818   Other congenital malformations of uterus ♀
           Müllerian anomaly of uterus NEC

    ● Q51.82   **Other congenital malformations of cervix**

       Q51.820   Cervical duplication ♀

       Q51.821   Hypoplasia of cervix ♀

       Q51.828   Other congenital malformations of cervix ♀

   Q51.9   **Congenital malformation of uterus and cervix, unspecified** ♀

● Q52   **Other congenital malformations of female genitalia**

   Q52.0   **Congenital absence of vagina** ♀
       Vaginal agenesis, total or partial

  ● Q52.1   **Doubling of vagina**

       Excludes1   doubling of vagina with doubling of uterus and cervix (Q51.1-)

       Q52.10   Doubling of vagina, unspecified ♀
           Septate vagina NOS

       Q52.11   Transverse vaginal septum ♀

    ● Q52.12   Longitudinal vaginal septum
           Coding Clinic: 2016, Q4, P58

       Q52.120   Longitudinal vaginal septum, nonobstructing ♀

       Q52.121   Longitudinal vaginal septum, obstructing, right side ♀

       Q52.122   Longitudinal vaginal septum, obstructing, left side ♀

       Q52.123   Longitudinal vaginal septum, microperforate, right side ♀

       Q52.124   Longitudinal vaginal septum, microperforate, left side ♀
           Coding Clinic: 2016, Q4, P59

       Q52.129   Other and unspecified longitudinal vaginal septum ♀

   Q52.2   Congenital rectovaginal fistula ♀

       Excludes1   cloaca (Q43.7)

   Q52.3   Imperforate hymen ♀
       Membrane (hymen) completely closes vaginal orifice

   Q52.4   Other congenital malformations of vagina ♀
       Canal of Nuck cyst, congenital
       Congenital malformation of vagina NOS
       Embryonic vaginal cyst
       Gartner's duct cyst

   Q52.5   Fusion of labia ♀

   Q52.6   Congenital malformation of clitoris ♀

▶ New   ⇒ Revised   ~~deleted~~ Deleted   Excludes 1   Excludes 2   Includes   Use additional   Code first   Code also   Key words

OGCR Official Guidelines   X Assign placeholder X   ● Use Additional Character(s)   ▶ Manifestation Code   🐾 Hierarchical Condition Category   **Coding Clinic**

- **Q52.7** **Other and unspecified congenital malformations of vulva**
  - **Q52.70** **Unspecified** congenital malformations of vulva ♀
    - Congenital malformation of vulva NOS
  - **Q52.71** Congenital **absence of vulva** ♀
  - **Q52.79** **Other** congenital malformations of **vulva** ♀
    - Congenital cyst of vulva
  - **Q52.8** **Other specified congenital malformations of female genitalia** ♀
  - **Q52.9** **Congenital malformation of female genitalia, unspecified** ♀

- **Q53** **Undescended and ectopic testicle**
  - **Q53.0** **Ectopic testis**
    - **Q53.00** Ectopic testis, **unspecified** ♂
    - **Q53.01** Ectopic testis, **unilateral** ♂
    - **Q53.02** Ectopic **testes, bilateral** ♂
  - **Q53.1** **Undescended testicle, unilateral**
    - **Q53.10** **Unspecified** undescended testicle, unilateral ♂
    - **Q53.11** **Abdominal** testis, unilateral
      - **Q53.111** Unilateral **intraabdominal testis** ♂
      - **Q53.112** Unilateral **inguinal testis** ♂
    - **Q53.12** Ectopic **perineal testis, unilateral** ♂
    - **Q53.13** Unilateral **high scrotal testis** ♂
  - **Q53.2** **Undescended testicle, bilateral**
    - **Q53.20** Undescended testicle, **unspecified, bilateral** ♂
    - **Q53.21** **Abdominal** testis, bilateral
      - **Q53.211** Bilateral **intraabdominal testes** ♂
      - **Q53.212** Bilateral **inguinal testes** ♂
    - **Q53.22** Ectopic **perineal testis, bilateral** ♂
    - **Q53.23** Bilateral **high scrotal testes** ♂
  - **Q53.9** **Undescended testicle, unspecified** ♂
    - Cryptorchism NOS

- **Q54** **Hypospadias**
  - *Birth defect of male; urethra opens in abnormal location on shaft*
  - **Excludes1**   epispadias (Q64.0)
  - **Q54.0** **Hypospadias, balanic** ♂
    - Hypospadias, coronal
    - Hypospadias, glandular
  - **Q54.1** **Hypospadias, penile** ♂
  - **Q54.2** **Hypospadias, penoscrotal** ♂
  - **Q54.3** **Hypospadias, perineal** ♂
  - **Q54.4** **Congenital chordee** ♂
    - Chordee without hypospadias
  - **Q54.8** **Other hypospadias** ♂
    - Hypospadias with intersex state
  - **Q54.9** **Hypospadias, unspecified** ♂

Item 17-1   Testes form in the abdomen of the male and only descend into the scrotum during normal embryonic development. "Ectopic" testes are out of their normal place or "retained" (left behind) in the abdomen. Crypto (hidden) orchism (testicle) is a major risk factor for testicular cancer.

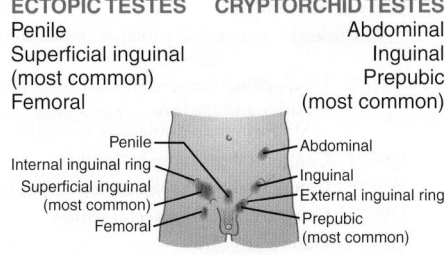

ECTOPIC TESTES	CRYPTORCHID TESTES
Penile	Abdominal
Superficial inguinal	Inguinal
(most common)	Prepubic
Femoral	(most common)

Penile
Internal inguinal ring
Superficial inguinal
(most common)
Femoral

Abdominal
Inguinal
External inguinal ring
Prepubic
(most common)

Figure 17-5   Undescended testes and the positions of the testes in various types of cryptorchidism or abnormal paths of descent.

- **Q55** **Other congenital malformations of male genital organs**
  - **Excludes1**   congenital hydrocele (P83.5)
    - hypospadias (Q54.-)
  - **Q55.0** **Absence and aplasia of testis** ♂
    - Monorchism
  - **Q55.1** **Hypoplasia of testis and scrotum** ♂
    - Fusion of testes
  - **Q55.2** **Other and unspecified congenital malformations of testis and scrotum**
    - **Q55.20** **Unspecified congenital malformation of testis and scrotum** ♂
      - Congenital malformation of testis or scrotum NOS
    - **Q55.21** **Polyorchism** ♂
      - *Developmental anomaly characterized by presence of more than two testes*
    - **Q55.22** **Retractile testis** ♂
    - **Q55.23** Scrotal **transposition** ♂
    - **Q55.29** **Other** congenital malformations of testis and scrotum ♂
  - **Q55.3** **Atresia of vas deferens** ♂
    - *Code first any associated cystic fibrosis (E84.-)*
  - **Q55.4** **Other congenital malformations of vas deferens, epididymis, seminal vesicles and prostate** ♂
    - Absence or aplasia of prostate
    - Absence or aplasia of spermatic cord
    - Congenital malformation of vas deferens, epididymis, seminal vesicles or prostate NOS
  - **Q55.5** Congenital **absence and aplasia of penis** ♂
  - **Q55.6** **Other congenital malformations of penis**
    - **Q55.61** **Curvature of penis (lateral)** ♂
    - **Q55.62** **Hypoplasia of penis** ♂
      - *Underdevelopment penis*
      - Micropenis
    - **Q55.63** **Congenital torsion of penis** ♂
      - **Excludes1**   acquired torsion of penis (N48.82)
    - **Q55.64** **Hidden penis** ♂
      - Buried penis
      - Concealed penis
      - **Excludes1**   acquired buried penis (N48.83)
    - **Q55.69** **Other** congenital malformation of penis ♂
      - Congenital malformation of penis NOS
  - **Q55.7** Congenital **vasocutaneous fistula** ♂
    - *Abnormal opening between vas deferens and skin*
  - **Q55.8** **Other specified congenital malformations of male genital organs** ♂
  - **Q55.9** **Congenital malformation of male genital organ, unspecified** ♂
    - Congenital anomaly of male genital organ
    - Congenital deformity of male genital organ

- **Q56** **Indeterminate sex and pseudohermaphroditism**
  - *Internal reproductive organs are opposite external physical characteristics.*
  - **Excludes1**   46,XX true hermaphrodite (Q99.1)
    - androgen insensitivity syndrome (E34.5-)
    - chimera 46,XX/46,XY true hermaphrodite (Q99.0)
    - female pseudohermaphroditism with adrenocortical disorder (E25.-)
    - pseudohermaphroditism with specified chromosomal anomaly (Q96-Q99)
    - pure gonadal dysgenesis (Q99.1)
  - **Q56.0** **Hermaphroditism, not elsewhere classified**
    - Ovotestis
  - **Q56.1** **Male pseudohermaphroditism, not elsewhere classified** ♂
    - 46, XY with streak gonads
    - Male pseudohermaphroditism NOS
  - **Q56.2** **Female pseudohermaphroditism, not elsewhere classified** ♀
    - Female pseudohermaphroditism NOS

CHAPTER 17 (Q00-Q99)

Q56.3   Pseudohermaphroditism, unspecified

Q56.4   Indeterminate sex, unspecified
      Ambiguous genitalia

CONGENITAL MALFORMATIONS OF THE URINARY SYSTEM (Q60–Q64)

● Q60   Renal agenesis and other reduction defects of kidney

    Includes   congenital absence of kidney
                congenital atrophy of kidney
                infantile atrophy of kidney

Q60.0   Renal agenesis, unilateral

Q60.1   Renal agenesis, bilateral

Q60.2   Renal agenesis, unspecified

Q60.3   Renal hypoplasia, unilateral

Q60.4   Renal hypoplasia, bilateral

Q60.5   Renal hypoplasia, unspecified

Q60.6   Potter's syndrome

● Q61   Cystic kidney disease
    Cysts that develop in failing kidney due to end-stage renal disease

    Excludes1   acquired cyst of kidney (N28.1)
                 Potter's syndrome (Q60.6)

● Q61.0   Congenital renal cyst

    Q61.00   Congenital renal cyst, unspecified
          Cyst of kidney NOS (congenital)

    Q61.01   Congenital single renal cyst

    Q61.02   Congenital multiple renal cysts

● Q61.1   Polycystic kidney, infantile type
    Polycystic kidney, autosomal recessive

    Q61.11   Cystic dilatation of collecting ducts

    Q61.19   Other polycystic kidney, infantile type

Q61.2   Polycystic kidney, adult type
    Polycystic kidney, autosomal dominant

Q61.3   Polycystic kidney, unspecified
    Coding Clinic: 2016, Q3, P23

Q61.4   Renal dysplasia
    Multicystic dysplastic kidney
    Multicystic kidney (development)
    Multicystic kidney disease
    Multicystic renal dysplasia

    Excludes1   polycystic kidney disease (Q61.11–Q61.3)

Q61.5   Medullary cystic kidney
    ➡ Nephronophthisis
    Sponge kidney NOS

Q61.8   Other cystic kidney diseases
    Fibrocystic kidney
    Fibrocystic renal degeneration or disease

Q61.9   Cystic kidney disease, unspecified
    Meckel-Gruber syndrome

● Q62   Congenital obstructive defects of renal pelvis and congenital malformations of ureter

Q62.0   Congenital hydronephrosis

● Q62.1   Congenital occlusion of ureter
    Atresia and stenosis of ureter

    Q62.10   Congenital occlusion of ureter, unspecified

    Q62.11   Congenital occlusion of ureteropelvic junction

    Q62.12   Congenital occlusion of ureterovesical orifice

Q62.2   Congenital megaureter
    Congenital dilatation of ureter

● Q62.3   Other obstructive defects of renal pelvis and ureter

    Q62.31   Congenital ureterocele, orthotopic

    Q62.32   Cecoureterocele
          Ectopic ureterocele

    Q62.39   Other obstructive defects of renal pelvis and ureter
          Ureteropelvic junction obstruction NOS

Q62.4   Agenesis of ureter
    Congenital absence ureter

Q62.5   Duplication of ureter
    Accessory ureter
    Double ureter

● Q62.6   Malposition of ureter

    Q62.60   Malposition of ureter, unspecified

    Q62.61   Deviation of ureter

    Q62.62   Displacement of ureter

    Q62.63   Anomalous implantation of ureter
          Ectopia of ureter
          Ectopic ureter

    Q62.69   Other malposition of ureter

Q62.7   Congenital vesico-uretero-renal reflux

Q62.8   Other congenital malformations of ureter
    Anomaly of ureter NOS

● Q63   Other congenital malformations of kidney

    Excludes1   congenital nephrotic syndrome (N04.-)

Q63.0   Accessory kidney

Q63.1   Lobulated, fused and horseshoe kidney

Q63.2   Ectopic kidney
    Congenital displaced kidney
    Malrotation of kidney

Q63.3   Hyperplastic and giant kidney
    Compensatory hypertrophy of kidney

Q63.8   Other specified congenital malformations of kidney
    Congenital renal calculi

Q63.9   Congenital malformation of kidney, unspecified

● Q64   Other congenital malformations of urinary system

Q64.0   Epispadias
    Urethral opening somewhere on dorsum of penis

    Excludes1   hypospadias (Q54.-)

● Q64.1   Exstrophy of urinary bladder
    Bladder is exposed, inside out, and protrudes through abdominal wall

    Q64.10   Exstrophy of urinary bladder, unspecified
          Ectopia vesicae

    Q64.11   Supravesical fissure of urinary bladder

    Q64.12   Cloacal exstrophy of urinary bladder

    Q64.19   Other exstrophy of urinary bladder
          Extroversion of bladder

Q64.2   Congenital posterior urethral valves

● Q64.3   Other atresia and stenosis of urethra and bladder neck

    Q64.31   Congenital bladder neck obstruction
          Congenital obstruction of vesicourethral orifice

    Q64.32   Congenital stricture of urethra

    Q64.33   Congenital stricture of urinary meatus

    Q64.39   Other atresia and stenosis of urethra and bladder neck
          Atresia and stenosis of urethra and bladder neck NOS

Q64.4   Malformation of urachus
    Cyst of urachus
    Patent urachus
    Prolapse of urachus

Q64.5   Congenital absence of bladder and urethra

Q64.6   Congenital diverticulum of bladder

● Q64.7   Other and unspecified congenital malformations of bladder and urethra

    Excludes1   congenital prolapse of bladder (mucosa) (Q79.4)

    Q64.70   Unspecified congenital malformation of bladder and urethra
          Malformation of bladder or urethra NOS

    Q64.71   Congenital prolapse of urethra

    Q64.72   Congenital prolapse of urinary meatus

    Q64.73   Congenital urethrorectal fistula

    Q64.74   Double urethra

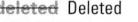

▶ New   ⇒ Revised   ~~deleted~~ Deleted   Excludes 1   Excludes 2   Includes   Use additional   Code first   Code also   Key words

OGCR Official Guidelines   X Assign placeholder X   ● Use Additional Character(s)   ▷ Manifestation Code   🅗🅒 Hierarchical Condition Category   **Coding Clinic**

Q64.75   Double urinary meatus

Q64.79   Other congenital malformations of bladder and
         urethra

Q64.8   Other specified congenital malformations of urinary
        system

Q64.9   Congenital malformation of urinary system, unspecified
        Congenital anomaly NOS of urinary system
        Congenital deformity NOS of urinary system

CONGENITAL MALFORMATIONS AND DEFORMATIONS OF THE MUSCULOSKELETAL SYSTEM (Q65-Q79)

● Q65   Congenital deformities of hip
        Excludes1   clicking hip (R29.4)

● Q65.0   Congenital dislocation of hip, unilateral
          Q65.00   Congenital dislocation of unspecified hip,
                   unilateral
          Q65.01   Congenital dislocation of right hip, unilateral
          Q65.02   Congenital dislocation of left hip, unilateral

Q65.1   Congenital dislocation of hip, bilateral
Q65.2   Congenital dislocation of hip, unspecified

● Q65.3   Congenital partial dislocation of hip, unilateral
          Q65.30   Congenital partial dislocation of unspecified
                   hip, unilateral
          Q65.31   Congenital partial dislocation of right
                   hip, unilateral
          Q65.32   Congenital partial dislocation of left
                   hip, unilateral

Q65.4   Congenital partial dislocation of hip, bilateral
Q65.5   Congenital partial dislocation of hip, unspecified
Q65.6   Congenital unstable hip
        Congenital dislocatable hip

● Q65.8   Other congenital deformities of hip
          Q65.81   Congenital coxa valga
          Q65.82   Congenital coxa vara
          Q65.89   Other specified congenital deformities of hip
                   Anteversion of femoral neck
                   Congenital acetabular dysplasia

Q65.9   Congenital deformity of hip, unspecified

● Q66   Congenital deformities of feet
        Excludes1   reduction defects of feet (Q72.-)
                        valgus deformities (acquired) (M21.0-)
                        varus deformities (acquired) (M21.1-)

● Q66.0   Congenital talipes equinovarus
          Heel is turned inward from midline and foot is plantar flexed;
          AKA clubfoot
          Q66.00   Congenital talipes equinovarus, unspecified
                   foot
          Q66.01   Congenital talipes equinovarus, right foot
          Q66.02   Congenital talipes equinovarus, left foot

Item 17-2   Equinus foot is a term referring to the hoof of a horse. The deformity is usually congenital or spastic. **Talipes equinovarus** is referred to as clubfoot. The foot tends to be smaller than normal, with the heel pointing downward and the forefoot turning inward. The heel cord (Achilles tendon) is tight, causing the heel to be drawn up toward the leg.

Figure 17-6   Supination and cavus deformity of forefoot. (From Kliegman R, Nelson WE: Nelson Textbook of Pediatrics, Philadelphia, Saunders, 2007)

● Q66.1   Congenital talipes calcaneovarus
          Deformity of foot in which heel is turned toward midline of
          body and anterior of foot is elevated
          Q66.10   Congenital talipes calcaneovarus, unspecified
                   foot
          Q66.11   Congenital talipes calcaneovarus, right foot
          Q66.12   Congenital talipes calcaneovarus, left foot

● Q66.2   Congenital metatarsus (primus) varus
          Angulation of first metatarsal bone toward midline of body
          Coding Clinic: 2016, Q4, P59
          ● Q66.21   Congenital metatarsus primus varus
                     Q66.211   Congenital metatarsus primus varus,
                               right foot
                     Q66.212   Congenital metatarsus primus varus,
                               left foot
                     Q66.219   Congenital metatarsus primus varus,
                               unspecified foot
          ● Q66.22   Congenital metatarsus adductus
                     Congenital metatarsus varus
                     Q66.221   Congenital metatarsus adductus, right
                               foot
                     Q66.222   Congenital metatarsus adductus, left
                               foot
                     Q66.229   Congenital metatarsus adductus,
                               unspecified foot

● Q66.3   Other congenital varus deformities of feet
          Hallux varus, congenital
          Q66.30   Other congenital varus deformities of feet,
                   unspecified foot
          Q66.31   Other congenital varus deformities of feet, right
                   foot
          Q66.32   Other congenital varus deformities of feet, left
                   foot

● Q66.4   Congenital talipes calcaneovalgus
          Q66.40   Congenital talipes calcaneovalgus, unspecified
                   foot
          Q66.41   Congenital talipes calcaneovalgus, right foot
          Q66.42   Congenital talipes calcaneovalgus, left foot

● Q66.5   Congenital pes planus
          Congenital flat foot
          Congenital rigid flat foot
          Congenital spastic (everted) flat foot
          Excludes1   pes planus, acquired (M21.4)
          Q66.50   Congenital pes planus, unspecified foot
          Q66.51   Congenital pes planus, right foot
          Q66.52   Congenital pes planus, left foot

Q66.6   Other congenital valgus deformities of feet
        Inward angulation
        Congenital metatarsus valgus

Talipes   Talipes   Talipes
cavus   equinus   calcaneus

Talipes   Talipes   Talipes
valgus   equinovalgus   calcaneovalgus

Talipes
varus

Talipes   Talipes   Talipes
cavovarus   equinovarus   calcaneocavus

Figure 17-7   Talipes. (From Dorland: Dorland's Illustrated Medical Dictionary, ed 31, Saunders, 2007, p 1893)

CHAPTER 17 (Q00-Q99)

● Q66.7   Congenital pes cavus
     Q66.70   Congenital pes cavus, unspecified foot
     Q66.71   Congenital pes cavus, right foot
     Q66.72   Congenital pes cavus, left foot
● Q66.8   Other congenital deformities of feet
     Q66.80   Congenital vertical talus deformity, unspecified foot
     Q66.81   Congenital vertical talus deformity, right foot
     Q66.82   Congenital vertical talus deformity, left foot
     Q66.89   Other specified congenital deformities of feet
         Congenital asymmetric talipes
         Congenital clubfoot NOS
         Congenital talipes NOS
         Congenital tarsal coalition
         Hammer toe, congenital
● Q66.9   Congenital deformity of feet, unspecified
     Q66.90   Congenital deformity of feet, unspecified, unspecified foot
     Q66.91   Congenital deformity of feet, unspecified, right foot
     Q66.92   Congenital deformity of feet, unspecified, left foot

● Q67   Congenital musculoskeletal deformities of head, face, spine and chest

> **Excludes1**   congenital malformation syndromes classified to Q87.-
>   Potter's syndrome (Q60.6)

   Q67.0   Congenital facial asymmetry
   Q67.1   Congenital compression facies
   Q67.2   Dolichocephaly
        Long head dimension
   Q67.3   Plagiocephaly
        Asymmetric shape of head resulting from irregular closure of cranial sutures
   Q67.4   Other congenital deformities of skull, face and jaw
        Congenital depressions in skull
        Congenital hemifacial atrophy or hypertrophy
        Deviation of nasal septum, congenital
        Squashed or bent nose, congenital

> **Excludes1**   dentofacial anomalies [including malocclusion] (M26.-)
>   syphilitic saddle nose (A50.5)

   Q67.5   Congenital deformity of spine
        Congenital postural scoliosis
        Congenital scoliosis NOS

> **Excludes1**   infantile idiopathic scoliosis (M41.0)
>   scoliosis due to congenital bony malformation (Q76.3)

   Q67.6   Pectus excavatum
        Congenital funnel chest
        Funnel-shaped chest depression
   Q67.7   Pectus carinatum
        Congenital pigeon chest
   Q67.8   Other congenital deformities of chest
        Congenital deformity of chest wall NOS

Figure 17-8   Mild to moderate inbowing of the lower leg. (From Lissauer T, Clayden G: Illustrated Textbook of Paediatrics, Edinburgh, Mosby, 2011)

● Q68   Other congenital musculoskeletal deformities

> **Excludes1**   reduction defects of limb(s) (Q71-Q73)
> **Excludes2**   congenital myotonic chondrodystrophy (G71.13)

   Q68.0   Congenital deformity of sternocleidomastoid muscle
        Congenital contracture of sternocleidomastoid (muscle)
        Congenital (sternomastoid) torticollis
        Sternomastoid tumor (congenital)
   Q68.1   Congenital deformity of finger(s) and hand
        Congenital clubfinger
        Spade-like hand (congenital)
   Q68.2   Congenital deformity of knee
        Congenital dislocation of knee
        Congenital genu recurvatum
        Hyperextension of knee resulting from hypermobility
   Q68.3   Congenital bowing of femur

> **Excludes1**   anteversion of femur (neck) (Q65.89)

   Q68.4   Congenital bowing of tibia and fibula
   Q68.5   Congenital bowing of long bones of leg, unspecified
   Q68.6   Discoid meniscus
   Q68.8   Other specified congenital musculoskeletal deformities
        Congenital deformity of clavicle
        Congenital deformity of elbow
        Congenital deformity of forearm
        Congenital deformity of scapula
        Congenital deformity of wrist
        Congenital dislocation of elbow
        Congenital dislocation of shoulder
        Congenital dislocation of wrist

● Q69   Polydactyly
        AKA hyperdactyly, consists of supernumerary fingers or toes
   Q69.0   Accessory finger(s)
   Q69.1   Accessory thumb(s)
   Q69.2   Accessory toe(s)
        Accessory hallux
   Q69.9   Polydactyly, unspecified
        Supernumerary digit(s) NOS

● Q70   Syndactyly
        Webbing between distal phalanges of adjacent digits
● Q70.0   Fused fingers
        Complex syndactyly of fingers with synostosis
     Q70.00   Fused fingers, unspecified hand
     Q70.01   Fused fingers, right hand
     Q70.02   Fused fingers, left hand
     Q70.03   Fused fingers, bilateral
● Q70.1   Webbed fingers
        Simple syndactyly of fingers without synostosis
     Q70.10   Webbed fingers, unspecified hand
     Q70.11   Webbed fingers, right hand
     Q70.12   Webbed fingers, left hand
     Q70.13   Webbed fingers, bilateral
● Q70.2   Fused toes
        Complex syndactyly of toes with synostosis
     Q70.20   Fused toes, unspecified foot
     Q70.21   Fused toes, right foot
     Q70.22   Fused toes, left foot
     Q70.23   Fused toes, bilateral
● Q70.3   Webbed toes
        Simple syndactyly of toes without synostosis
     Q70.30   Webbed toes, unspecified foot
     Q70.31   Webbed toes, right foot
     Q70.32   Webbed toes, left foot
     Q70.33   Webbed toes, bilateral
   Q70.4   Polysyndactyly, unspecified

> **Excludes1**   specified syndactyly of hand and feet - code to specified conditions (Q70.0- -Q70.3-)

        Extra and webbed digits
   Q70.9   Syndactyly, unspecified
        Symphalangy NOS

Figure 17-9 Thumb and index finger. (From Chung K: Hand and Upper Extremity Reconstruction, 1e, Saunders, 2008)

● Q71   Reduction defects of upper limb
  ● Q71.0   Congenital complete absence of upper limb
    Q71.00   Congenital complete absence of unspecified upper limb
    Q71.01   Congenital complete absence of right upper limb
    Q71.02   Congenital complete absence of left upper limb
    Q71.03   Congenital complete absence of upper limb, bilateral
  ● Q71.1   Congenital absence of upper arm and forearm with hand present
    Q71.10   Congenital absence of unspecified upper arm and forearm with hand present
    Q71.11   Congenital absence of right upper arm and forearm with hand present
    Q71.12   Congenital absence of left upper arm and forearm with hand present
    Q71.13   Congenital absence of upper arm and forearm with hand present, bilateral
  ● Q71.2   Congenital absence of both forearm and hand
    Q71.20   Congenital absence of both forearm and hand, unspecified upper limb
    Q71.21   Congenital absence of both forearm and hand, right upper limb
    Q71.22   Congenital absence of both forearm and hand, left upper limb
    Q71.23   Congenital absence of both forearm and hand, bilateral
  ● Q71.3   Congenital absence of hand and finger
    Q71.30   Congenital absence of unspecified hand and finger
    Q71.31   Congenital absence of right hand and finger
    Q71.32   Congenital absence of left hand and finger
    Q71.33   Congenital absence of hand and finger, bilateral
  ● Q71.4   Longitudinal reduction defect of radius
    Clubhand (congenital)
    Radial clubhand
    Q71.40   Longitudinal reduction defect of unspecified radius
    Q71.41   Longitudinal reduction defect of right radius
    Q71.42   Longitudinal reduction defect of left radius
    Q71.43   Longitudinal reduction defect of radius, bilateral
  ● Q71.5   Longitudinal reduction defect of ulna
    Q71.50   Longitudinal reduction defect of unspecified ulna
    Q71.51   Longitudinal reduction defect of right ulna
    Q71.52   Longitudinal reduction defect of left ulna
    Q71.53   Longitudinal reduction defect of ulna, bilateral
  ● Q71.6   Lobster-claw hand
    Q71.60   Lobster-claw hand, unspecified hand
    Q71.61   Lobster-claw right hand

    Q71.62   Lobster-claw left hand
    Q71.63   Lobster-claw hand, bilateral
  ● Q71.8   Other reduction defects of upper limb
    ● Q71.81   Congenital shortening of upper limb
      Q71.811   Congenital shortening of right upper limb
      Q71.812   Congenital shortening of left upper limb
      Q71.813   Congenital shortening of upper limb, bilateral
      Q71.819   Congenital shortening of unspecified upper limb
    ● Q71.89   Other reduction defects of upper limb
      Q71.891   Other reduction defects of right upper limb
      Q71.892   Other reduction defects of left upper limb
      Q71.893   Other reduction defects of upper limb, bilateral
      Q71.899   Other reduction defects of unspecified upper limb
  ● Q71.9   Unspecified reduction defect of upper limb
    Q71.90   Unspecified reduction defect of unspecified upper limb
    Q71.91   Unspecified reduction defect of right upper limb
    Q71.92   Unspecified reduction defect of left upper limb
    Q71.93   Unspecified reduction defect of upper limb, bilateral

● Q72   Reduction defects of lower limb
  ● Q72.0   Congenital complete absence of lower limb
    Q72.00   Congenital complete absence of unspecified lower limb
    Q72.01   Congenital complete absence of right lower limb
    Q72.02   Congenital complete absence of left lower limb
    Q72.03   Congenital complete absence of lower limb, bilateral
  ● Q72.1   Congenital absence of thigh and lower leg with foot present
    Q72.10   Congenital absence of unspecified thigh and lower leg with foot present
    Q72.11   Congenital absence of right thigh and lower leg with foot present
    Q72.12   Congenital absence of left thigh and lower leg with foot present
    Q72.13   Congenital absence of thigh and lower leg with foot present, bilateral
  ● Q72.2   Congenital absence of both lower leg and foot
    Q72.20   Congenital absence of both lower leg and foot, unspecified lower limb
    Q72.21   Congenital absence of both lower leg and foot, right lower limb
    Q72.22   Congenital absence of both left lower leg and foot, left lower limb
    Q72.23   Congenital absence of both lower leg and foot, bilateral
  ● Q72.3   Congenital absence of foot and toe(s)
    Q72.30   Congenital absence of unspecified foot and toe(s)
    Q72.31   Congenital absence of right foot and toe(s)
    Q72.32   Congenital absence of left foot and toe(s)
    Q72.33   Congenital absence of foot and toe(s), bilateral

● **Q72.4 Longitudinal reduction defect of femur**
Proximal femoral focal deficiency
- Q72.40 Longitudinal reduction defect of unspecified femur
- Q72.41 Longitudinal reduction defect of right femur
- Q72.42 Longitudinal reduction defect of left femur
- Q72.43 Longitudinal reduction defect of femur, bilateral

● **Q72.5 Longitudinal reduction defect of tibia**
- Q72.50 Longitudinal reduction defect of unspecified tibia
- Q72.51 Longitudinal reduction defect of right tibia
- Q72.52 Longitudinal reduction defect of left tibia
- Q72.53 Longitudinal reduction defect of tibia, bilateral

● **Q72.6 Longitudinal reduction defect of fibula**
- Q72.60 Longitudinal reduction defect of unspecified fibula
- Q72.61 Longitudinal reduction defect of right fibula
- Q72.62 Longitudinal reduction defect of left fibula
- Q72.63 Longitudinal reduction defect of fibula, bilateral

● **Q72.7 Split foot**
- Q72.70 Split foot, unspecified lower limb
- Q72.71 Split foot, right lower limb
- Q72.72 Split foot, left lower limb
- Q72.73 Split foot, bilateral

● **Q72.8 Other reduction defects of lower limb**
- ● Q72.81 Congenital shortening of lower limb
  - Q72.811 Congenital shortening of right lower limb
  - Q72.812 Congenital shortening of left lower limb
  - Q72.813 Congenital shortening of lower limb, bilateral
  - Q72.819 Congenital shortening of unspecified lower limb
- ● Q72.89 Other reduction defects of lower limb
  - Q72.891 Other reduction defects of right lower limb
  - Q72.892 Other reduction defects of left lower limb
  - Q72.893 Other reduction defects of lower limb, bilateral
  - Q72.899 Other reduction defects of unspecified lower limb

● **Q72.9 Unspecified reduction defect of lower limb**
- Q72.90 Unspecified reduction defect of unspecified lower limb
- Q72.91 Unspecified reduction defect of right lower limb
- Q72.92 Unspecified reduction defect of left lower limb
- Q72.93 Unspecified reduction defect of lower limb, bilateral

● **Q73 Reduction defects of unspecified limb**
- **Q73.0 Congenital absence of unspecified limb(s)**
  Amelia NOS
- **Q73.1 Phocomelia, unspecified limb(s)**
  Phocomelia NOS
  Absence/shortening of long bones primarily as a result of thalidomide
- **Q73.8 Other reduction defects of unspecified limb(s)**
  Longitudinal reduction deformity of unspecified limb(s)
  Ectromelia of limb NOS
  Gross hypoplasia or aplasia of one or more long bones of limb(s)
  Hemimelia of limb NOS
  Absence of one-half of long bone
  Reduction defect of limb NOS

● **Q74 Other congenital malformations of limb(s)**
- **Excludes1** polydactyly (Q69.-)
  reduction defect of limb (Q71-Q73)
  syndactyly (Q70.-)
- **Q74.0 Other congenital malformations of upper limb(s), including shoulder girdle**
  Accessory carpal bones
  Cleidocranial dysostosis
  Congenital pseudarthrosis of clavicle
  Macrodactylia (fingers)
  Madelung's deformity
  Radioulnar synostosis
  Sprengel's deformity
  Triphalangeal thumb
- **Q74.1 Congenital malformation of knee**
  Congenital absence of patella
  Congenital dislocation of patella
  Congenital genu valgum
  Congenital genu varum
  Rudimentary patella
  - **Excludes1** congenital dislocation of knee (Q68.2)
    congenital genu recurvatum (Q68.2)
    nail patella syndrome (Q87.2)
- **Q74.2 Other congenital malformations of lower limb(s), including pelvic girdle**
  Congenital fusion of sacroiliac joint
  Congenital malformation of ankle joint
  Congenital malformation of sacroiliac joint
  - **Excludes1** anteversion of femur (neck) (Q65.89)
- **Q74.3 Arthrogryposis multiplex congenita**
- **Q74.8 Other specified congenital malformations of limb(s)**
- **Q74.9 Unspecified congenital malformation of limb(s)**
  Congenital anomaly of limb(s) NOS

● **Q75 Other congenital malformations of skull and face bones**
- **Excludes1** congenital malformation of face NOS (Q18.-)
  congenital malformation syndromes classified to Q87.-
  dentofacial anomalies [including malocclusion] (M26.-)
  musculoskeletal deformities of head and face (Q67.0-Q67.4)
  skull defects associated with congenital anomalies of brain such as:
  anencephaly (Q00.0)
  encephalocele (Q01.-)
  hydrocephalus (Q03.-)
  microcephaly (Q02)
- **Q75.0 Craniosynostosis**
  Premature closure of sutures of skull
  Acrocephaly
  Imperfect fusion of skull
  Oxycephaly
  Trigonocephaly
- **Q75.1 Craniofacial dysostosis**
  Congenital deformity of head
  Crouzon's disease
- **Q75.2 Hypertelorism**

Item 17-3 Anencephalus is a congenital deformity of the cranial vault. **Craniosynostosis,** also known as craniostenosis and stenocephaly, signifies any form of congenital deformity of the skull that results from the premature closing of the sutures of the skull. **Iniencephaly** is a deformity in which the head and neck are flexed backward to a great extent and the head is very large in comparison to the shortened body.

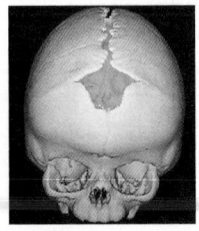

Figure 17-10 Generalized craniosynostosis without symptoms or signs of increased intracranial pressure. (From Goetz C: Textbook of Clinical Neurology, St. Louis, MO, Elsevier, 2007)

▶ New   ⇒ Revised   ~~deleted~~ Deleted   Excludes 1   Excludes 2   Includes   Use additional   Code first   Code also   Key words
OGCR Official Guidelines   X Assign placeholder X   ● Use Additional Character(s)   ▷ Manifestation Code   🐾 Hierarchical Condition Category   **Coding Clinic**

Q75.3 Macrocephaly
Unusually large size of head; AKA megalocephaly

Q75.4 Mandibulofacial dysostosis
Franceschetti syndrome
Treacher Collins syndrome

Q75.5 Oculomandibular dysostosis
Ossification of occular and mandibular bones

Q75.8 Other specified congenital malformations of skull and face bones
Absence of skull bone, congenital
Congenital deformity of forehead
Platybasia

Q75.9 Congenital malformation of skull and face bones, unspecified
Congenital anomaly of face bones NOS
Congenital anomaly of skull NOS

● **Q76 Congenital malformations of spine and bony thorax**
Excludes1   congenital musculoskeletal deformities of spine and chest (Q67.5-Q67.8)

Q76.0 Spina bifida occulta
Excludes1   meningocele (spinal) (Q05.-)
spina bifida (aperta) (cystica) (Q05.-)

Q76.1 Klippel-Feil syndrome
Cervical fusion syndrome

Q76.2 Congenital spondylolisthesis
Congenital spondylolysis
Excludes1   spondylolisthesis (acquired) (M43.1-)
spondylolysis (acquired) (M43.0-)

Q76.3 Congenital scoliosis due to congenital bony malformation
Hemivertebra fusion or failure of segmentation with scoliosis

● **Q76.4 Other congenital malformations of spine, not associated with scoliosis**

   ● **Q76.41 Congenital kyphosis**
Abnormal increase in convexity curvature of thoracic spinal column; AKA humpback

     Q76.411 Congenital kyphosis, occipito-atlanto-axial region

     Q76.412 Congenital kyphosis, cervical region

     Q76.413 Congenital kyphosis, cervicothoracic region

     Q76.414 Congenital kyphosis, thoracic region

     Q76.415 Congenital kyphosis, thoracolumbar region

     Q76.419 Congenital kyphosis, unspecified region

   ● **Q76.42 Congenital lordosis**
An abnormal increase in curvature of lumbar spine (sway back)

     Q76.425 Congenital lordosis, thoracolumbar region

     Q76.426 Congenital lordosis, lumbar region

     Q76.427 Congenital lordosis, lumbosacral region

     Q76.428 Congenital lordosis, sacral and sacrococcygeal region

     Q76.429 Congenital lordosis, unspecified region

   Q76.49 Other congenital malformations of spine, not associated with scoliosis
Congenital absence of vertebra NOS
Congenital fusion of spine NOS
Congenital malformation of lumbosacral (joint) (region) NOS
Congenital malformation of spine NOS
Hemivertebra NOS
Malformation of spine NOS
Platyspondylisis NOS
Supernumerary vertebra NOS

Q76.5 Cervical rib
Supernumerary rib in cervical region

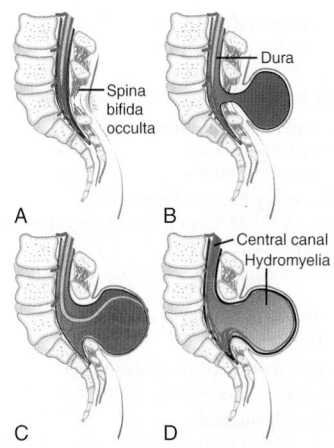

Figure 17-11   **A.** Spina bifida occulta. **B.** Meningocele. **C.** Myelomeningocele. **D.** Myelocystocele (syringomyelocele) or hydromyelia.

Item 17–4   **Spina bifida** is a midline spinal defect in which one or more vertebrae fail to fuse, leaving an opening in the vertebral canal. When the defect is not visible, it is called spina bifida occulta, and when it is visible, it is called spina bifida cystica.

Q76.6 Other congenital malformations of ribs
Accessory rib
Congenital absence of rib
Congenital fusion of ribs
Congenital malformation of ribs NOS
Excludes1   short rib syndrome (Q77.2)

Q76.7 Congenital malformation of sternum
Congenital absence of sternum
Sternum bifidum

Q76.8 Other congenital malformations of bony thorax

Q76.9 Congenital malformation of bony thorax, unspecified

● **Q77 Osteochondrodysplasia with defects of growth of tubular bones and spine**
Excludes1   mucopolysaccharidosis (E76.0-E76.3)
Excludes2   congenital myotonic chondrodystrophy (G71.13)

Q77.0 Achondrogenesis
Hypochondrogenesis

Q77.1 Thanatophoric short stature

Q77.2 Short rib syndrome
Asphyxiating thoracic dysplasia [Jeune]

Q77.3 Chondrodysplasia punctata
Benign cartilaginous neoplasms
Excludes1   rhizomelic chondrodysplasia punctata (E71.43)

Q77.4 Achondroplasia
Disturbance of epiphyseal chondroblastic growth and maturation, results in dwarfism
Hypochondroplasia
Osteosclerosis congenita

Q77.5 Diastrophic dysplasia

Q77.6 Chondroectodermal dysplasia
Defective development of skin, hair, teeth, with polydactyly and defect of cardiac septum
Ellis-van Creveld syndrome

Q77.7 Spondyloepiphyseal dysplasia

Q77.8 Other osteochondrodysplasia with defects of growth of tubular bones and spine

Q77.9 Osteochondrodysplasia with defects of growth of tubular bones and spine, unspecified

CHAPTER 17 (Q00-Q99)

● **Q78**   **Other osteochondrodysplasias**
Disorder of development of bone and cartilage; common cause of dwarfism

> **Excludes2**   congenital myotonic chondrodystrophy (G71.13)

Q78.0   **Osteogenesis imperfecta**
Fragilitas ossium
Osteopsathyrosis

Q78.1   **Polyostotic fibrous dysplasia**
Albright(-McCune)(-Sternberg) syndrome

Q78.2   **Osteopetrosis**
Abnormally dense bone; AKA marble bones disease, ivory bones
Albers-Schönberg syndrome
Osteosclerosis NOS

Q78.3   **Progressive diaphyseal dysplasia**
Camurati-Engelmann syndrome

Q78.4   **Enchondromatosis**
Thinning of overlying cortex of bone and distorted length
Maffucci's syndrome
Ollier's disease

Q78.5   **Metaphyseal dysplasia**
Disturbance in enchondral bone growth, causing ends of shafts to remain larger than normal in circumference
Pyle's syndrome

Q78.6   **Multiple congenital exostoses**
Diaphyseal aclasis

Q78.8   **Other specified osteochondrodysplasias**
Osteopoikilosis

Q78.9   **Osteochondrodysplasia, unspecified**
Chondrodystrophy NOS
AKA skeletal dysplasia (dwarfism) caused by genetic mutations affecting hyaline cartilage capping long bones and vertebrae
Osteodystrophy NOS

● **Q79**   **Congenital malformations of musculoskeletal system, not elsewhere classified**

> **Excludes2**   congenital (sternomastoid) torticollis (Q68.0)

Q79.0   **Congenital diaphragmatic hernia**

> **Excludes1**   congenital hiatus hernia (Q40.1)

Q79.1   **Other congenital malformations of diaphragm**
Absence of diaphragm
Congenital malformation of diaphragm NOS
Eventration of diaphragm

Q79.2   **Exomphalos**
Abdominal hernia in which part of intestine protrudes at umbilicus; AKA exomphalos and exumbilication
Omphalocele

> **Excludes1**   umbilical hernia (K42.-)

Q79.3   **Gastroschisis**
Congenital fissure of anterior abdominal wall often with protrusion of small/large intestine

Q79.4   **Prune belly syndrome**
Congenital prolapse of bladder mucosa
Eagle-Barrett syndrome

● **Q79.5**   **Other congenital malformations of abdominal wall**

> **Excludes1**   umbilical hernia (K42.-)

Q79.51   **Congenital hernia of bladder**

Q79.59   **Other congenital malformations of abdominal wall**

● **Q79.6**   **Ehlers-Danlos syndromes**
Group of inherited disorders of connective tissue; AKA cutis hyperelastica

Q79.60   **Ehlers-Danlos syndrome, unspecified**

Q79.61   **Classical Ehlers-Danlos syndrome**
Classical EDS (cEDS)

Q79.62   **Hypermobile Ehlers-Danlos syndrome**
Hypermobile EDS (hEDS)

Q79.63   **Vascular Ehlers-Danlos syndrome**
Vascular EDS (vEDS)

Q79.69   **Other Ehlers-Danlos syndromes**

Q79.8   **Other congenital malformations of musculoskeletal system**
Absence of muscle
Absence of tendon
Accessory muscle
Amyotrophia congenita
Congenital constricting bands
Congenital shortening of tendon
Poland syndrome

Q79.9   **Congenital malformation of musculoskeletal system, unspecified**
Congenital anomaly of musculoskeletal system NOS
Congenital deformity of musculoskeletal system NOS

OTHER CONGENITAL MALFORMATIONS (Q80-Q89)

● **Q80**   **Congenital ichthyosis**
Characterized by increased keratinization, resulting in noninflammatory scaling of skin

> **Excludes1**   Refsum's disease (G60.1)

Q80.0   **Ichthyosis vulgaris**

Q80.1   **X-linked ichthyosis**

Q80.2   **Lamellar ichthyosis**
Collodion baby

Q80.3   **Congenital bullous ichthyosiform erythroderma**

Q80.4   **Harlequin fetus**

Q80.8   **Other congenital ichthyosis**

Q80.9   **Congenital ichthyosis, unspecified**

● **Q81**   **Epidermolysis bullosa**
Loosening of epidermis

Q81.0   **Epidermolysis bullosa simplex**

> **Excludes1**   Cockayne's syndrome (Q87.19)

Q81.1   **Epidermolysis bullosa letalis**
Herlitz' syndrome

Q81.2   **Epidermolysis bullosa dystrophica**

Q81.8   **Other epidermolysis bullosa**

Q81.9   **Epidermolysis bullosa, unspecified**

● **Q82**   **Other congenital malformations of skin**

> **Excludes1**   acrodermatitis enteropathica (E83.2)
> congenital erythropoietic porphyria (E80.0)
> pilonidal cyst or sinus (L05.-)
> Sturge-Weber (-Dimitri) syndrome (Q85.8)

Q82.0   **Hereditary lymphedema**
Characterized by swelling of subcutaneous tissue caused by obstruction of lymphatic vessels and resulting edema of lymph fluid

Q82.1   **Xeroderma pigmentosum**
Extreme sensitivity to ultraviolet rays that most commonly affects the eyes and skin, but may also involve the nervous system

Q82.2   **Congenital cutaneous mastocytosis**
Characterized by infiltrates of mast cells in tissues/organs
Congenital diffuse cutaneous mastocytosis
Congenital maculopapular cutaneous mastocytosis
Congenital urticaria pigmentosa

> **Excludes1**   cutaneous mastocytosis NOS (D47.01)
> diffuse cutaneous mastocytosis (with onset after newborn period) (D47.01)
> malignant mastocytosis (C96.2-)
> systemic mastocytosis (D47.02)
> urticaria pigmentosa (non-congenital) (with onset after newborn period) (D47.01)

Q82.3   **Incontinentia pigmenti**
Characterized by hypopigmented cutaneous in adults and early childhood

Q82.4   **Ectodermal dysplasia (anhidrotic)**
Absence/deficiency of tissues/structures, including teeth, hair, nails, and certain glands

> **Excludes1**   Ellis-van Creveld syndrome (Q77.6)

▶ New   ⇒ Revised   ~~deleted~~ Deleted   Excludes 1   Excludes 2   Includes   Use additional   Code first   Code also   Key words
OGCR Official Guidelines   X Assign placeholder X   ● Use Additional Character(s)   ▶ Manifestation Code   🅒 Hierarchical Condition Category   **Coding Clinic**

Q82.5   **Congenital non-neoplastic nevus**
Birthmark NOS
Flammeus Nevus
Portwine Nevus
Sanguineous Nevus
Strawberry Nevus
Vascular Nevus NOS
Verrucous Nevus
> **Excludes2**   Café au lait spots (L81.3)
> lentigo (L81.4)
> nevus NOS (D22.-)
> araneus nevus (I78.1)
> melanocytic nevus (D22.-)
> pigmented nevus (D22.-)
> spider nevus (I78.1)
> stellar nevus (I78.1)

Q82.6   **Congenital sacral dimple**
Parasacral dimple
> **Excludes2**   pilonidal cyst with abscess (L05.01)
> pilonidal cyst without abscess (L05.91)

Coding Clinic: 2016, Q4, P60

Q82.8   **Other specified congenital malformations of skin**
Abnormal palmar creases
Accessory skin tags
Benign familial pemphigus [Hailey-Hailey]
Congenital poikiloderma
Cutis laxa (hyperelastica)
Dermatoglyphic anomalies
Inherited keratosis palmaris et plantaris
Keratosis follicularis [Darier-White]
> **Excludes1**   Ehlers-Danlos syndromes (Q79.6-)

Coding Clinic: 2016, Q1, P17

Q82.9   **Congenital malformation of skin, unspecified**

● **Q83**   **Congenital malformations of breast**
> **Excludes2**   absence of pectoral muscle (Q79.8)
> hypoplasia of breast (N64.82)
> micromastia (N64.82)

Q83.0   **Congenital absence of breast with absent nipple**

Q83.1   **Accessory breast**
Supernumerary breast

Q83.2   **Absent nipple**

Q83.3   **Accessory nipple**
Supernumerary nipple

Q83.8   **Other congenital malformations of breast**

Q83.9   **Congenital malformation of breast, unspecified**

● **Q84**   **Other congenital malformations of integument**
Q84.0   **Congenital alopecia**
Congenital atrichosis

Q84.1   **Congenital morphological disturbances of hair, not elsewhere classified**
Beaded hair
Monilethrix
Pili annulati
> **Excludes1**   Menkes' kinky hair syndrome (E83.0)

Q84.2   **Other congenital malformations of hair**
Congenital hypertrichosis
Congenital malformation of hair NOS
Persistent lanugo

Q84.3   **Anonychia**
Absence of nail
> **Excludes1**   nail patella syndrome (Q87.2)

Q84.4   **Congenital leukonychia**
Opaque, whitish discoloration of nails; AKA leukopathia unguium

Q84.5   **Enlarged and hypertrophic nails**
Congenital onychauxis
Pachyonychia

Q84.6   **Other congenital malformations of nails**
Congenital clubnail
Congenital koilonychia
Congenital malformation of nail NOS

Q84.8   **Other specified congenital malformations of integument**
Aplasia cutis congenita

Q84.9   **Congenital malformation of integument, unspecified**
Congenital anomaly of integument NOS
Congenital deformity of integument NOS

● **Q85**   **Phakomatoses, not elsewhere classified**
> **Excludes1**   ataxia telangiectasia [Louis-Bar] (G11.3)
> familial dysautonomia [Riley-Day] (G90.1)

● **Q85.0**   **Neurofibromatosis (nonmalignant)**
Developmental changes in nervous system and other structures, with formation of neurofibromas

   Q85.00   **Neurofibromatosis, unspecified** 🔗

   Q85.01   **Neurofibromatosis, type 1** 🔗
Von Recklinghausen disease

   Q85.02   **Neurofibromatosis, type 2** 🔗
Acoustic neurofibromatosis

   Q85.03   **Schwannomatosis**

   Q85.09   **Other neurofibromatosis** 🔗

Q85.1   **Tuberous sclerosis** 🔗
Bourneville's disease
Epiloia

Q85.8   **Other phakomatoses, not elsewhere classified** 🔗
Peutz-Jeghers Syndrome
Sturge-Weber(-Dimitri) syndrome
von Hippel-Lindau syndrome
> **Excludes1**   Meckel-Gruber syndrome (Q61.9)

Q85.9   **Phakomatosis, unspecified** 🔗
Hamartosis NOS

● **Q86**   **Congenital malformation syndromes due to known exogenous causes, not elsewhere classified**
> **Excludes2**   iodine-deficiency-related hypothyroidism (E00-E02)
> nonteratogenic effects of substances transmitted via placenta or breast milk (P04.-)

Q86.0   **Fetal alcohol syndrome (dysmorphic)**

Q86.1   **Fetal hydantoin syndrome**
Meadow's syndrome

Q86.2   **Dysmorphism due to warfarin**

Q86.8   **Other congenital malformation syndromes due to known exogenous causes**

● **Q87**   **Other specified congenital malformation syndromes affecting multiple systems**
Use additional code(s) to identify all associated manifestations

Q87.0   **Congenital malformation syndromes predominantly affecting facial appearance**
Acrocephalopolysyndactyly
Acrocephalosyndactyly [Apert]
Cryptophthalmos syndrome
Cyclopia
Goldenhar syndrome
Moebius syndrome
Oro-facial-digital syndrome
Robin syndrome
Whistling face

● **Q87.1**   **Congenital malformation syndromes predominantly associated with short stature**

   Q87.11   **Prader-Willi syndrome**

   Q87.19   **Other congenital malformation syndromes predominantly associated with short stature**
Aarskog syndrome
Cockayne syndrome
De Lange syndrome
Dubowitz syndrome
Noonan syndrome
Robinow-Silverman-Smith syndrome
Russell-Silver syndrome
Seckel syndrome
> **Excludes1**   Ellis-van Creveld syndrome (Q77.6)
> Smith-Lemli-Opitz syndrome (E78.72)

CHAPTER 17 (Q00-Q99)

Q87.2   Congenital malformation syndromes predominantly involving limbs
  Holt-Oram syndrome
  Klippel-Trenaunay-Weber syndrome
  Nail patella syndrome
  Rubinstein-Taybi syndrome
  Sirenomelia syndrome
  Thrombocytopenia with absent radius [TAR] syndrome
  VATER syndrome

Q87.3   Congenital malformation syndromes involving early overgrowth
  Beckwith-Wiedemann syndrome
  Sotos' syndrome
  Weaver syndrome

● **Q87.4   Marfan's syndrome**

  Q87.40   Marfan's syndrome, unspecified

  ● **Q87.41   Marfan's syndrome with cardiovascular manifestations**

      Q87.410   Marfan's syndrome with aortic dilation

      Q87.418   Marfan's syndrome with other cardiovascular manifestations

  Q87.42   Marfan's syndrome with ocular manifestations

  Q87.43   Marfan's syndrome with skeletal manifestation

Q87.5   Other congenital malformation syndromes with other skeletal changes

● **Q87.8   Other specified congenital malformation syndromes, not elsewhere classified**

  Excludes1   Zellweger syndrome (E71.510)

  Q87.81   Alport syndrome
      Progressive sensorineural hearing loss, progressive pyelonephritis or glomerulonephritis, and ocular defects

      Use additional code to identify stage of chronic kidney disease (N18.1-N18.6)

  Q87.82   Arterial tortuosity syndrome
      Coding Clinic: 2016, Q4, P60-61

  Q87.89   Other specified congenital malformation syndromes, not elsewhere classified
      Laurence-Moon (-Bardet)-Biedl syndrome

● **Q89   Other congenital malformations, not elsewhere classified**

  ● **Q89.0   Congenital absence and malformations of spleen**

      Excludes1   isomerism of atrial appendages (with asplenia or polysplenia) (Q20.6)

      Q89.01   Asplenia (congenital)

      Q89.09   Congenital malformations of spleen
          Congenital splenomegaly

  Q89.1   Congenital malformations of adrenal gland

      Excludes1   adrenogenital disorders (E25.-)
                  congenital adrenal hyperplasia (E25.0)

  Q89.2   Congenital malformations of other endocrine glands
      Congenital malformation of parathyroid or thyroid gland
      Persistent thyroglossal duct
      Thyroglossal cyst

      Excludes1   congenital goiter (E03.0)
                  congenital hypothyroidism (E03.1)

  Q89.3   Situs inversus
      Lateral transposition of viscera of thorax and abdomen
      Dextrocardia with situs inversus
      Mirror-image atrial arrangement with situs inversus
      Situs inversus or transversus abdominalis
      Situs inversus or transversus thoracis
      Transposition of abdominal viscera
      Transposition of thoracic viscera

      Excludes1   dextrocardia NOS (Q24.0)

  Q89.4   Conjoined twins
      Craniopagus
      Dicephaly
      Pygopagus
      Thoracopagus

Q89.7   Multiple congenital malformations, not elsewhere classified
  Multiple congenital anomalies NOS
  Multiple congenital deformities NOS

  Excludes1   congenital malformation syndromes affecting multiple systems (Q87.-)

Q89.8   Other specified congenital malformations
  Use additional code(s) to identify all associated manifestations

Q89.9   Congenital malformation, unspecified
  Congenital anomaly NOS
  Congenital deformity NOS

CHROMOSOMAL ABNORMALITIES, NOT ELSEWHERE CLASSIFIED (Q90-Q99)

  Excludes2   mitochondrial metabolic disorders (E88.4-)

● **Q90   Down syndrome**
  Use additional code(s) to identify any associated physical conditions and degree of intellectual disabilities (F70-F79)

  Q90.0   Trisomy 21, nonmosaicism (meiotic nondisjunction)
      Trisomy 21, nondisjunction, accounts for 95% of Downs syndrome cases

  Q90.1   Trisomy 21, mosaicism (mitotic nondisjunction)

  Q90.2   Trisomy 21, translocation

  Q90.9   Down syndrome, unspecified
      Trisomy 21 NOS

● **Q91   Trisomy 18 and Trisomy 13**

  Q91.0   Trisomy 18, nonmosaicism (meiotic nondisjunction)

  Q91.1   Trisomy 18, mosaicism (mitotic nondisjunction)

  Q91.2   Trisomy 18, translocation

  Q91.3   Trisomy 18, unspecified

  Q91.4   Trisomy 13, nonmosaicism (meiotic nondisjunction)

  Q91.5   Trisomy 13, mosaicism (mitotic nondisjunction)

  Q91.6   Trisomy 13, translocation

  Q91.7   Trisomy 13, unspecified

● **Q92   Other trisomies and partial trisomies of the autosomes, not elsewhere classified**

  Includes   unbalanced translocations and insertions
  Excludes1   trisomies of chromosomes 13, 18, 21 (Q90-Q91)

  Q92.0   Whole chromosome trisomy, nonmosaicism (meiotic nondisjunction)

  Q92.1   Whole chromosome trisomy, mosaicism (mitotic nondisjunction)

  Q92.2   Partial trisomy
      Less than whole arm duplicated
      Whole arm or more duplicated

      Excludes1   partial trisomy due to unbalanced translocation (Q92.5)

  Q92.5   Duplications with other complex rearrangements
      Partial trisomy due to unbalanced translocations

      Code also any associated deletions due to unbalanced translocations, inversions and insertions (Q93.7)

  ● **Q92.6   Marker chromosomes**
      Trisomies due to dicentrics
      Trisomies due to extra rings
      Trisomies due to isochromosomes
      Individual with marker heterochromatin

      Q92.61   Marker chromosomes in normal individual

      Q92.62   Marker chromosomes in abnormal individual

  Q92.7   Triploidy and polyploidy

  Q92.8   Other specified trisomies and partial trisomies of autosomes
      Duplications identified by fluorescence in situ hybridization (FISH)
      Duplications identified by in situ hybridization (ISH)
      Duplications seen only at prometaphase

  Q92.9   Trisomy and partial trisomy of autosomes, unspecified

▶ New   ⇒ Revised   ~~deleted~~ Deleted   Excludes 1   Excludes 2   Includes   Use additional   Code first   Code also   Key words
OGCR Official Guidelines   X Assign placeholder X   ● Use Additional Character(s)   ▶ Manifestation Code   🔖 Hierarchical Condition Category   **Coding Clinic**

- Q93 Monosomies and deletions from the autosomes, not elsewhere classified

  Q93.0 Whole chromosome monosomy, nonmosaicism (meiotic nondisjunction)

  Q93.1 Whole chromosome monosomy, mosaicism (mitotic nondisjunction)

  Q93.2 Chromosome replaced with ring, dicentric or isochromosome

  Q93.3 Deletion of short arm of chromosome 4
  Wolff-Hirschorn syndrome

  Q93.4 Deletion of short arm of chromosome 5
  Cri-du-chat syndrome

  - Q93.5 Other deletions of part of a chromosome

    Q93.51 Angelman syndrome

    Q93.59 Other deletions of part of a chromosome

  Q93.7 Deletions with other complex rearrangements
  Deletions due to unbalanced translocations, inversions and insertions
  Code also any associated duplications due to unbalanced translocations, inversions and insertions (Q92.5)

  - Q93.8 Other deletions from the autosomes

    Q93.81 Velo-cardio-facial syndrome
    Deletion 22q11.2
    Coding Clinic: 2019, Q3, P14

    Q93.82 Williams syndrome

    Q93.88 Other microdeletions Miller-Dieker syndrome
    Smith-Magenis syndrome

    Q93.89 Other deletions from the autosomes
    Deletions identified by fluorescence in situ hybridization (FISH)
    Deletions identified by in situ hybridization (ISH)
    Deletions seen only at prometaphase

  Q93.9 Deletion from autosomes, unspecified

- Q95 Balanced rearrangements and structural markers, not elsewhere classified

  Includes Robertsonian and balanced reciprocal translocations and insertions

  Q95.0 Balanced translocation and insertion in normal individual

  Q95.1 Chromosome inversion in normal individual

  Q95.2 Balanced autosomal rearrangement in abnormal individual

  Q95.3 Balanced sex/autosomal rearrangement in abnormal individual

  Q95.5 Individual with autosomal fragile site

  Q95.8 Other balanced rearrangements and structural markers

  Q95.9 Balanced rearrangement and structural marker, unspecified

- Q96 Turner's syndrome
  Caused by missing or incomplete X chromosome affecting growth and sexual development

  Excludes1 Noonan syndrome (Q87.19)

  Q96.0 Karyotype 45, X ♀

  Q96.1 Karyotype 46, X iso (Xq) ♀
  Karyotype 46, isochromosome Xq

  Q96.2 Karyotype 46, X with abnormal sex chromosome, except iso (Xq) ♀
  Karyotype 46, X with abnormal sex chromosome, except isochromosome Xq

  Q96.3 Mosaicism, 45, X/46, XX or XY ♀

  Q96.4 Mosaicism, 45, X/other cell line(s) with abnormal sex chromosome ♀

  Q96.8 Other variants of Turner's syndrome ♀

  Q96.9 Turner's syndrome, unspecified ♀

- Q97 Other sex chromosome abnormalities, female phenotype, not elsewhere classified

  Excludes1 Turner's syndrome (Q96.-)

  Q97.0 Karyotype 47, XXX ♀

  Q97.1 Female with more than three X chromosomes ♀

  Q97.2 Mosaicism, lines with various numbers of X chromosomes ♀

  Q97.3 Female with 46, XY karyotype ♀

  Q97.8 Other specified sex chromosome abnormalities, female phenotype ♀

  Q97.9 Sex chromosome abnormality, female phenotype, unspecified ♀

- Q98 Other sex chromosome abnormalities, male phenotype, not elsewhere classified

  Q98.0 Klinefelter syndrome karyotype 47, XXY ♂

  Q98.1 Klinefelter syndrome, male with more than two X chromosomes ♂

  Q98.3 Other male with 46, XX karyotype ♂

  Q98.4 Klinefelter syndrome, unspecified ♂

  Q98.5 Karyotype 47, XYY

  Q98.6 Male with structurally abnormal sex chromosome ♂

  Q98.7 Male with sex chromosome mosaicism ♂

  Q98.8 Other specified sex chromosome abnormalities, male phenotype ♂

  Q98.9 Sex chromosome abnormality, male phenotype, unspecified ♂

- Q99 Other chromosome abnormalities, not elsewhere classified

  Q99.0 Chimera 46, XX/46, XY
  Chimera 46, XX/46, XY true hermaphrodite

  Q99.1 46, XX true hermaphrodite
  46, XX with streak gonads
  46, XY with streak gonads
  Pure gonadal dysgenesis

  Q99.2 Fragile X chromosome
  Fragile X syndrome

  Q99.8 Other specified chromosome abnormalities

  Q99.9 Chromosomal abnormality, unspecified

CHAPTER 17 (Q00-Q99)

CHAPTER 18

SYMPTOMS, SIGNS, AND ABNORMAL CLINICAL AND LABORATORY FINDINGS, NOT ELSEWHERE CLASSIFIED (R00-R99)

OGCR Chapter-Specific Coding Guidelines

18. **Chapter 18: Symptoms, signs, and abnormal clinical and laboratory findings, not elsewhere classified (R00-R99)**
Chapter 18 includes symptoms, signs, abnormal results of clinical or other investigative procedures, and ill-defined conditions regarding which no diagnosis classifiable elsewhere is recorded. Signs and symptoms that point to a specific diagnosis have been assigned to a category in other chapters of the classification.

   a. **Use of symptom codes**
   Codes that describe symptoms and signs are acceptable for reporting purposes when a related definitive diagnosis has not been established (confirmed) by the provider.

   b. **Use of a symptom code with a definitive diagnosis code**
   Codes for signs and symptoms may be reported in addition to a related definitive diagnosis when the sign or symptom is not routinely associated with that diagnosis, such as the various signs and symptoms associated with complex syndromes. The definitive diagnosis code should be sequenced before the symptom code.
   Signs or symptoms that are associated routinely with a disease process should not be assigned as additional codes, unless otherwise instructed by the classification.

   c. **Combination codes that include symptoms**
   ICD-10-CM contains a number of combination codes that identify both the definitive diagnosis and common symptoms of that diagnosis. When using one of these combination codes, an additional code should not be assigned for the symptom.

   d. **Repeated falls**
   Code R29.6, Repeated falls, is for use for encounters when a patient has recently fallen and the reason for the fall is being investigated.
   Code Z91.81, History of falling, is for use when a patient has fallen in the past and is at risk for future falls. When appropriate, both codes R29.6 and Z91.81 may be assigned together.

   e. **Coma scale**
   The coma scale codes (R40.2-) can be used in conjunction with traumatic brain injury codes, acute cerebrovascular disease or sequelae of cerebrovascular disease codes. These codes are primarily for use by trauma registries, but they may be used in any setting where this information is collected. The coma scale may also be used to assess the status of the central nervous system for other non-trauma conditions, such as monitoring patients in the intensive care unit regardless of medical condition. The coma scale codes should be sequenced after the diagnosis code(s).
   These codes, one from each subcategory, are needed to complete the scale. The 7th character indicates when the scale was recorded. The 7th character should match for all three codes.

At a minimum, report the initial score documented on presentation at your facility. This may be a score from the emergency medicine technician (EMT) or in the emergency department. If desired, a facility may choose to capture multiple coma scale scores.
   Assign code R40.24, Glasgow coma scale, total score, when only the total score is documented in the medical record and not the individual score(s).
   Do not report codes for individual or total Glasgow coma scale scores for a patient with a medically induced coma or a sedated patient.
   See Section I.B.14 for coma scale documentation by clinicians other than patient's provider.

   f. **Functional quadriplegia**
   GUIDELINE HAS BEEN DELETED EFFECTIVE OCTOBER 1, 2017

   g. **SIRS due to Non-Infectious Process**
   The systemic inflammatory response syndrome (SIRS) can develop as a result of certain non-infectious disease processes, such as trauma, malignant neoplasm, or pancreatitis. When SIRS is documented with a noninfectious condition, and no subsequent infection is documented, the code for the underlying condition, such as an injury, should be assigned, followed by code R65.10, Systemic inflammatory response syndrome (SIRS) of non-infectious origin without acute organ dysfunction, or code R65.11, Systemic inflammatory response syndrome (SIRS) of non-infectious origin with acute organ dysfunction. If an associated acute organ dysfunction is documented, the appropriate code(s) for the specific type of organ dysfunction(s) should be assigned in addition to code R65.11. If acute organ dysfunction is documented, but it cannot be determined if the acute organ dysfunction is associated with SIRS or due to another condition (e.g., directly due to the trauma), the provider should be queried.

   h. **Death NOS**
   Code R99, Ill-defined and unknown cause of mortality, is only for use in the very limited circumstance when a patient who has already died is brought into an emergency department or other healthcare facility and is pronounced dead upon arrival. It does not represent the discharge disposition of death.

   i. **NIHSS Stroke Scale**
   The NIH stroke scale (NIHSS) codes (R29.7- -) can be used in conjunction with acute stroke codes (I63) to identify the patient's neurological status and the severity of the stroke. The stroke scale codes should be sequenced after the acute stroke diagnosis code(s).
   At a minimum, report the initial score documented. If desired, a facility may choose to capture multiple stroke scale scores.
   See Section I.B.14 for NIHSS stroke scale documentation by clinicians other than patient's provider.

CHAPTER 18

SYMPTOMS, SIGNS, AND ABNORMAL CLINICAL AND LABORATORY FINDINGS, NOT ELSEWHERE CLASSIFIED (R00-R99)

Note: This chapter includes symptoms, signs, abnormal results of clinical or other investigative procedures, and ill-defined conditions regarding which no diagnosis classifiable elsewhere is recorded.

Signs and symptoms that point rather definitely to a given diagnosis have been assigned to a category in other chapters of the classification. In general, categories in this chapter include the less well-defined conditions and symptoms that, without the necessary study of the case to establish a final diagnosis, point perhaps equally to two or more diseases or to two or more systems of the body. Practically all categories in the chapter could be designated "not otherwise specified", "unknown etiology" or "transient". The Alphabetical Index should be consulted to determine which symptoms and signs are to be allocated here and which to other chapters. The residual subcategories, numbered .8, are generally provided for other relevant symptoms that cannot be allocated elsewhere in the classification.

The conditions and signs or symptoms included in categories R00-R94 consist of:
(a) cases for which no more specific diagnosis can be made even after all the facts bearing on the case have been investigated;
(b) signs or symptoms existing at the time of initial encounter that proved to be transient and whose causes could not be determined;
(c) provisional diagnosis in a patient who failed to return for further investigation or care;
(d) cases referred elsewhere for investigation or treatment before the diagnosis was made;
(e) cases in which a more precise diagnosis was not available for any other reason;
(f) certain symptoms, for which supplementary information is provided, that represent important problems in medical care in their own right.

Excludes2   abnormal findings on antenatal screening of mother (O28.-)
       certain conditions originating in the perinatal period (P04-P96)
       signs and symptoms classified in the body system chapters
       signs and symptoms of breast (N63, N64.5)

This chapter contains the following blocks:

R00-R09	Symptoms and signs involving the circulatory and respiratory systems
R10-R19	Symptoms and signs involving the digestive system and abdomen
R20-R23	Symptoms and signs involving the skin and subcutaneous tissue
R25-R29	Symptoms and signs involving the nervous and musculoskeletal systems
R30-R39	Symptoms and signs involving the genitourinary system
R40-R46	Symptoms and signs involving cognition, perception, emotional state and behavior
R47-R49	Symptoms and signs involving speech and voice
R50-R69	General symptoms and signs
R70-R79	Abnormal findings on examination of blood, without diagnosis
R80-R82	Abnormal findings on examination of urine, without diagnosis
R83-R89	Abnormal findings on examination of other body fluids, substances and tissues, without diagnosis
R90-R94	Abnormal findings on diagnostic imaging and in function studies, without diagnosis
R97	Abnormal tumor markers
R99	Ill-defined and unknown cause of mortality

SYMPTOMS AND SIGNS INVOLVING THE CIRCULATORY AND RESPIRATORY SYSTEMS (R00-R09)

● **R00**   **Abnormalities of heart beat**
     Excludes1   abnormalities originating in the perinatal period (P29.1-)
     Excludes2   specified arrhythmias (I47-I49)

     R00.0   **Tachycardia, unspecified**
         Rapid heart rate >100 beats
         Rapid heart beat
         Sinoauricular tachycardia NOS
         Sinus [sinusal] tachycardia NOS
         Excludes1   neonatal tachycardia (P29.11)
                         paroxysmal tachycardia (I47.-)

     R00.1   **Bradycardia, unspecified**
         Slow heart rate, <60
         Sinoatrial bradycardia
         Sinus bradycardia
         Slow heart beat
         Vagal bradycardia
         Use additional code for adverse effect, if applicable, to identify drug (T36-T50 with fifth or sixth character 5)
         Excludes1   neonatal bradycardia (P29.12)

     R00.2   **Palpitations**
         Awareness of heart beat

     R00.8   **Other abnormalities of heart beat**

     R00.9   **Unspecified abnormalities of heart beat**

● **R01   Cardiac murmurs and other cardiac sounds**

> **Excludes1**   cardiac murmurs and sounds originating in the
> perinatal period (P29.8)

R01.0   Benign and innocent cardiac murmurs
Functional cardiac murmur

R01.1   Cardiac murmur, unspecified
Cardiac bruit NOS
Heart murmur NOS
Systolic murmur NOS

R01.2   Other cardiac sounds
Cardiac dullness, increased or decreased
Precordial friction

OGCR Section I.C.9.a.7.

> Hypertension, Transient
> Assign code R03.0, Elevated blood pressure reading without
> diagnosis of hypertension, unless patient has an established
> diagnosis of hypertension. Assign code O13.-, Gestational
> [pregnancy-induced] hypertension with significant
> proteinuria, or O14.-, Pre-eclampsia, for transient hypertension
> of pregnancy.

● **R03   Abnormal blood-pressure reading, without diagnosis**

**R03.0   Elevated blood-pressure reading, without diagnosis of
hypertension**

> **Note:** This category is to be used to record an episode
> of elevated blood pressure in a patient in whom no
> formal diagnosis of hypertension has been made,
> or as an isolated incidental finding.

R03.1   Nonspecific low blood-pressure reading

> **Excludes1**   hypotension (I95.-)
> maternal hypotension syndrome (O26.5-)
> neurogenic orthostatic hypotension
> (G90.3)

● **R04   Hemorrhage from respiratory passages**

R04.0   Epistaxis
Hemorrhage from nose
Nosebleed
Coding Clinic: 2018, Q4, P38

R04.1   Hemorrhage from throat

> **Excludes2**   hemoptysis (R04.2)

R04.2   Hemoptysis
Blood-stained sputum
Cough with hemorrhage

● **R04.8   Hemorrhage from other sites in respiratory passages**

**R04.81   Acute idiopathic pulmonary hemorrhage in
infants**   P
AIPHI
Acute idiopathic hemorrhage in infants over
28 days old

> **Excludes1**   perinatal pulmonary
> hemorrhage (P26.-)
> von Willebrand's disease (D68.0)

**R04.89   Hemorrhage from other sites in respiratory
passages**
Pulmonary hemorrhage NOS

R04.9   Hemorrhage from respiratory passages, unspecified

● **R05   Cough**

> **Excludes1**   ~~cough with hemorrhage (R04.2)~~
> ▶paroxysmal cough due to Bordetella pertussis
> (A37.0-)
> smoker's cough (J41.0)
>
> ▶**Excludes2**   cough with hemorrhage (R04.2))

▶ **R05.1   Acute cough**

▶ **R05.2   Subacute cough**

▶ **R05.3   Chronic cough**
▶Persistent cough
▶Refractory cough
▶Unexplained cough

▶ **R05.4   Cough syncope**
> ▶*Code first syncope and collapse (R55)*

▶ **R05.8   Other specified cough**

▶ **R05.9   Cough, unspecified**

● **R06   Abnormalities of breathing**

> **Excludes1**   acute respiratory distress syndrome (J80)
> respiratory arrest (R09.2)
> respiratory arrest of newborn (P28.81)
> respiratory distress syndrome of newborn (P22.-)
> respiratory failure (J96.-)
> respiratory failure of newborn (P28.5)

● **R06.0   Dyspnea**

> **Excludes1**   tachypnea NOS (R06.82)
> transient tachypnea of newborn (P22.1)

R06.00   Dyspnea, unspecified
Coding Clinic: 2017, Q1, P26-27

R06.01   Orthopnea

R06.02   Shortness of breath

R06.03   Acute respiratory distress

R06.09   Other forms of dyspnea

R06.1   Stridor
Harsh, high-pitched breath sound

> **Excludes1**   congenital laryngeal stridor (P28.89)
> laryngismus (stridulus) (J38.5)

R06.2   Wheezing

> **Excludes1**   Asthma (J45.-)

Coding Clinic: 2016, Q2, P34

R06.3   Periodic breathing
Cheyne-Stokes breathing
*An abnormal pattern of breathing with gradually
increasing and decreasing tidal volume with some
periods of apnea*

R06.4   Hyperventilation

> **Excludes1**   psychogenic hyperventilation (F45.8)

R06.5   Mouth breathing

> **Excludes2**   dry mouth NOS (R68.2)

R06.6   Hiccough

> **Excludes1**   psychogenic hiccough (F45.8)

R06.7   Sneezing

● **R06.8   Other abnormalities of breathing**

R06.81   Apnea, not elsewhere classified
Apnea NOS

> **Excludes1**   apnea (of) newborn (P28.4)
> sleep apnea (G47.3-)
> sleep apnea of newborn
> (primary) (P28.3)

R06.82   Tachypnea, not elsewhere classified
Tachypnea NOS

> **Excludes1**   transitory tachypnea of newborn
> (P22.1)

R06.83   Snoring

R06.89   Other abnormalities of breathing
Breath-holding (spells)
Sighing

R06.9   Unspecified abnormalities of breathing

● **R07   Pain in throat and chest**

> **Excludes1**   epidemic myalgia (B33.0)
>
> **Excludes2**   jaw pain R68.84
> pain in breast (N64.4)

R07.0   Pain in throat

> **Excludes1**   chronic sore throat (J31.2)
> sore throat (acute) NOS (J02.9)
>
> **Excludes2**   dysphagia (R13.1-)
> pain in neck (M54.2)

R07.1   Chest pain on breathing
Painful respiration

R07.2   Precordial pain

▶ New   ⫸ Revised   ~~deleted~~ Deleted   Excludes 1   Excludes 2   Includes   Use additional   Code first   Code also   Key words

1196   **OGCR** Official Guidelines   X Assign placeholder X   ● Use Additional Character(s)   ▶ Manifestation Code   🅲 Hierarchical Condition Category   **Coding Clinic**

● R07.8   **Other chest pain**

     R07.81   **Pleurodynia**

         Pleurodynia NOS

         Excludes1   epidemic pleurodynia (B33.0)

     R07.82   **Intercostal pain**

     R07.89   **Other chest pain**

         Anterior chest-wall pain NOS

         Coding Clinic: 2021, Q1, P42

     R07.9   **Chest pain, unspecified**

● R09   **Other symptoms and signs involving the circulatory and respiratory system**

     Excludes1   acute respiratory distress syndrome (J80)

         respiratory arrest of newborn (P28.81)

         respiratory distress syndrome of newborn (P22.0)

         respiratory failure (J96.-)

         respiratory failure of newborn (P28.5)

● R09.0   **Asphyxia and hypoxemia**

     Excludes1   asphyxia due to carbon monoxide (T58.-)

         asphyxia due to foreign body in respiratory tract (T17.-)

         birth (intrauterine) asphyxia (P84)

         hyperventilation (R06.4)

         traumatic asphyxia (T71.-)

     Excludes2   hypercapnia (R06.89)

     R09.01   **Asphyxia**

     R09.02   **Hypoxemia**

         Coding Clinic: 2019, Q3, P15

     R09.1   **Pleurisy**

         Occurs when double membrane (pleura) lining chest cavity and lung surface becomes inflamed, causing sharp pain on inspiration/expiration

         Excludes1   pleurisy with effusion (J90)

     R09.2   **Respiratory arrest** 🔊

         Cardiorespiratory failure

         Excludes1   cardiac arrest (I46.-)

         respiratory arrest of newborn (P28.81)

         respiratory distress of newborn (P22.0)

         respiratory failure (J96.-)

         respiratory failure of newborn (P28.5)

         respiratory insufficiency (R06.89)

         respiratory insufficiency of newborn (P28.5)

     R09.3   **Abnormal sputum**

         Abnormal amount of sputum

         Abnormal color of sputum

         Abnormal odor of sputum

         Excessive sputum

     Excludes1   blood-stained sputum (R04.2)

● R09.8   **Other specified symptoms and signs involving the circulatory and respiratory systems**

     R09.81   **Nasal congestion**

     R09.82   **Postnasal drip**

     R09.89   **Other specified symptoms and signs involving the circulatory and respiratory systems**

         Bruit (arterial)

         Abnormal chest percussion

         Feeling of foreign body in throat

         Friction sounds in chest

         Chest tympany

         Choking sensation

         Rales

         Wet rattling, clicking, crackling sounds on auscultation

         Weak pulse

     Excludes2   foreign body in throat (T17.2-)

         wheezing (R06.2)

     Coding Clinic: 2021, Q1, P42

SYMPTOMS AND SIGNS INVOLVING THE DIGESTIVE SYSTEM AND ABDOMEN (R10-R19)

     Excludes2   congenital or infantile pylorospasm (Q40.0)

         gastrointestinal hemorrhage (K92.0-K92.2)

         intestinal obstruction (K56.-)

         newborn gastrointestinal hemorrhage (P54.0-P54.3)

         newborn intestinal obstruction (P76.-)

         pylorospasm (K31.3)

         signs and symptoms involving the urinary system (R30-R39)

         symptoms referable to female genital organs (N94.-)

         symptoms referable to male genital organs (N48-N50)

● R10   **Abdominal and pelvic pain**

     Excludes1   renal colic (N23)

     Excludes2   dorsalgia (M54.-)

         flatulence and related conditions (R14.-)

     R10.0   **Acute abdomen**

         Severe abdominal pain (generalized) (with abdominal rigidity)

     Excludes1   abdominal rigidity NOS (R19.3)

         generalized abdominal pain NOS (R10.84)

         localized abdominal pain (R10.1-R10.3-)

● R10.1   **Pain localized to upper abdomen**

     R10.10   **Upper abdominal pain, unspecified**

     R10.11   **Right upper quadrant pain**

     R10.12   **Left upper quadrant pain**

     R10.13   **Epigastric pain**

         Dyspepsia

         Excludes1   functional dyspepsia (K30)

     R10.2   **Pelvic and perineal pain**

         Excludes1   vulvodynia (N94.81)

● R10.3   **Pain localized to other parts of lower abdomen**

     R10.30   **Lower abdominal pain, unspecified**

     R10.31   **Right lower quadrant pain**

     R10.32   **Left lower quadrant pain**

     R10.33   **Periumbilical pain**

● R10.8   **Other abdominal pain**

     ● R10.81   **Abdominal tenderness**

         Abdominal tenderness NOS

         R10.811   **Right upper quadrant abdominal tenderness**

         R10.812   **Left upper quadrant abdominal tenderness**

         R10.813   **Right lower quadrant abdominal tenderness**

         R10.814   **Left lower quadrant abdominal tenderness**

         R10.815   **Periumbilic abdominal tenderness**

         R10.816   **Epigastric abdominal tenderness**

         R10.817   **Generalized abdominal tenderness**

         R10.819   **Abdominal tenderness, unspecified site**

     ● R10.82   **Rebound abdominal tenderness**

         R10.821   **Right upper quadrant rebound abdominal tenderness**

         R10.822   **Left upper quadrant rebound abdominal tenderness**

         R10.823   **Right lower quadrant rebound abdominal tenderness**

         R10.824   **Left lower quadrant rebound abdominal tenderness**

         R10.825   **Periumbilic rebound abdominal tenderness**

         R10.826   **Epigastric rebound abdominal tenderness**

CHAPTER 18 (R00-R99)

CHAPTER 18 (R00-R99)

R10.827   **Generalized** rebound abdominal tenderness

R10.829   Rebound abdominal tenderness, **unspecified site**

R10.83   **Colic**   P
     Colic NOS
     Infantile colic
     Excludes1   colic in adult and child over 12 months old (R10.84)

R10.84   **Generalized abdominal pain**
     Excludes1   generalized abdominal pain associated with acute abdomen (R10.0)

R10.9   **Unspecified abdominal pain**

● R11   **Nausea and vomiting**
     Excludes1   cyclical vomiting associated with migraine (G43.A-)
                   excessive vomiting in pregnancy (O21.-)
                   hematemesis (K92.0)
                   neonatal hematemesis (P54.0)
                   newborn vomiting (P92.0-)
                   psychogenic vomiting (F50.89)
                   vomiting associated with bulimia nervosa (F50.2)
                   vomiting following gastrointestinal surgery (K91.0)
     Coding Clinic: 2017, Q1, P27

R11.0   **Nausea**
     Nausea NOS
     Nausea without vomiting

● R11.1   **Vomiting**

R11.10   **Vomiting, unspecified**
     Vomiting NOS

R11.11   **Vomiting without nausea**

R11.12   **Projectile vomiting**

R11.13   **Vomiting of fecal matter**

R11.14   **Bilious vomiting**
     Bilious emesis

R11.15   **Cyclical vomiting syndrome unrelated to migraine**
     Cyclic vomiting syndrome NOS
     Persistent vomiting
     Excludes1   cyclical vomiting in migraine (G43.A-)
     Excludes2   bulimia nervosa (F50.2)
                diabetes mellitus due to underlying condition (E08.-)

R11.2   **Nausea with vomiting, unspecified**
     Persistent nausea with vomiting NOS
     Coding Clinic: 2020, Q1, P8

R12   **Heartburn**
     Excludes1   dyspepsia NOS (R10.13)
                functional dyspepsia (K30)

● R13   **Aphagia and dysphagia**

R13.0   **Aphagia**
     Inability to swallow
     Excludes1   psychogenic aphagia (F50.9)

● R13.1   **Dysphagia**
     Difficulty swallowing
     Code first, if applicable, dysphagia following cerebrovascular disease (I69. with final characters -91)
     Excludes1   psychogenic dysphagia (F45.8)

R13.10   **Dysphagia, unspecified**
     Difficulty in swallowing NOS

R13.11   **Dysphagia, oral phase**

R13.12   **Dysphagia, oropharyngeal phase**

R13.13   **Dysphagia, pharyngeal phase**

R13.14   **Dysphagia, pharyngoesophageal phase**

R13.19   **Other dysphagia**
     Cervical dysphagia
     Neurogenic dysphagia

● R14   **Flatulence and related conditions**
     Excludes1   psychogenic aerophagy (F45.8)

R14.0   **Abdominal distension (gaseous)**
     Bloating
     Tympanites (abdominal) (intestinal)

R14.1   **Gas pain**

R14.2   **Eructation**
     Belching air from stomach through mouth

R14.3   **Flatulence**

● R15   **Fecal incontinence**
     Includes   encopresis NOS
     Excludes1   fecal incontinence of nonorganic origin (F98.1)

R15.0   **Incomplete defecation**
     Excludes1   constipation (K59.0-)
                fecal impaction (K56.41)

R15.1   **Fecal smearing**
     Fecal soiling

R15.2   **Fecal urgency**

R15.9   **Full incontinence of feces**
     Fecal incontinence NOS

● R16   **Hepatomegaly and splenomegaly, not elsewhere classified**
     Enlargement of liver or spleen

R16.0   **Hepatomegaly, not elsewhere classified**
     Hepatomegaly NOS

R16.1   **Splenomegaly, not elsewhere classified**
     Splenomegaly NOS

R16.2   **Hepatomegaly with splenomegaly, not elsewhere classified**
     Hepatosplenomegaly NOS

R17   **Unspecified jaundice**
     Excludes1   neonatal jaundice (P55, P57-P59)

● R18   **Ascites**
     Includes   fluid in peritoneal cavity
     Excludes1   ascites in alcoholic cirrhosis (K70.31)
                ascites in alcoholic hepatitis (K70.11)
                ascites in toxic liver disease with chronic active hepatitis (K71.51)

R18.0   **Malignant ascites**
     Code first malignancy, such as:
     malignant neoplasm of ovary (C56.-)
     secondary malignant neoplasm of retroperitoneum and peritoneum (C78.6)

R18.8   **Other ascites**
     Ascites NOS
     Peritoneal effusion (chronic)
     Coding Clinic: 2018, Q1, P4

● R19   **Other symptoms and signs involving the digestive system and abdomen**
     Excludes1   acute abdomen (R10.0)

● R19.0   **Intra-abdominal and pelvic swelling, mass and lump**
     Excludes1   abdominal distension (gaseous) (R14.-)
                ascites (R18.-)

R19.00   **Intra-abdominal and pelvic swelling, mass and lump, unspecified site**

R19.01   **Right upper quadrant abdominal swelling, mass and lump**

R19.02   **Left upper quadrant abdominal swelling, mass and lump**

R19.03   **Right lower quadrant abdominal swelling, mass and lump**

R19.04   **Left lower quadrant abdominal swelling, mass and lump**

R19.05   **Periumbilic swelling, mass or lump**
     Diffuse or generalized umbilical swelling or mass

▶ New   ⇛ Revised   ~~deleted~~ Deleted   Excludes 1   Excludes 2   Includes   Use additional   Code first   Code also   Key words

OGCR Official Guidelines   X Assign placeholder X   ● Use Additional Character(s)   ▶ Manifestation Code   🅱 Hierarchical Condition Category   **Coding Clinic**

R19.06   Epigastric swelling, mass or lump
R19.07   Generalized intra-abdominal and pelvic swelling, mass and lump
     Diffuse or generalized intra-abdominal swelling or mass NOS
     Diffuse or generalized pelvic swelling or mass NOS
R19.09   Other intra-abdominal and pelvic swelling, mass and lump

● R19.1   Abnormal bowel sounds
R19.11   **Absent** bowel sounds
R19.12   **Hyperactive** bowel sounds
R19.15   **Other** abnormal bowel sounds
     Abnormal bowel sounds NOS

R19.2   Visible peristalsis
     Hyperperistalsis

● R19.3   Abdominal rigidity
     Excludes1   abdominal rigidity with severe abdominal pain (R10.0)
R19.30   Abdominal rigidity, **unspecified** site
R19.31   **Right upper** quadrant abdominal rigidity
R19.32   **Left upper** quadrant abdominal rigidity
R19.33   **Right lower** quadrant abdominal rigidity
R19.34   **Left lower** quadrant abdominal rigidity
R19.35   **Periumbilic** abdominal rigidity
R19.36   **Epigastric** abdominal rigidity
R19.37   **Generalized** abdominal rigidity

R19.4   Change in bowel habit
     Excludes1   constipation (K59.0-)
     functional diarrhea (K59.1)

R19.5   Other fecal abnormalities
     Abnormal stool color
     Bulky stools
     Mucus in stools
     Occult blood in feces
     Occult blood in stools
     Excludes1   melena (K92.1)
     neonatal melena (P54.1)
     Coding Clinic: 2021, Q1, P10; 2019, Q1, P32

R19.6   Halitosis

R19.7   Diarrhea, **unspecified**
     Diarrhea NOS
     Excludes1   functional diarrhea (K59.1)
     neonatal diarrhea (P78.3)
     psychogenic diarrhea (F45.8)

R19.8   Other specified symptoms and signs involving the digestive system and abdomen

SYMPTOMS AND SIGNS INVOLVING THE SKIN AND SUBCUTANEOUS TISSUE (R20-R23)

     Excludes2   symptoms relating to breast (N64.4-N64.5)

● R20   Disturbances of skin sensation
     Excludes1   dissociative anesthesia and sensory loss (F44.6)
     psychogenic disturbances (F45.8)
R20.0   **Anesthesia** of skin
     Loss of sensation
R20.1   **Hypoesthesia** of skin
     Unpleasant abnormal sensation
R20.2   **Paresthesia** of skin
     Abnormal touch sensation, including burning, prickling, often in absence of external stimulus
     Formication   Tingling skin
     Pins and needles
     Excludes1   acroparesthesia (I73.8)
R20.3   **Hyperesthesia**
R20.8   **Other** disturbances of skin sensation
R20.9   **Unspecified** disturbances of skin sensation

R21   Rash and other nonspecific skin eruption
     Includes   rash NOS
     Excludes1   specified type of rash- code to condition
     vesicular eruption (R23.8)

● R22   Localized swelling, mass and lump of skin and subcutaneous tissue
     Includes   subcutaneous nodules (localized) (superficial)
     Excludes1   abnormal findings on diagnostic imaging (R90-R93)
     edema (R60.-)
     enlarged lymph nodes (R59.-)
     localized adiposity (E65)
     swelling of joint (M25.4-)
R22.0   Localized swelling, mass and lump, **head**
R22.1   Localized swelling, mass and lump, **neck**
R22.2   Localized swelling, mass and lump, **trunk**
     Excludes1   intra-abdominal or pelvic mass and lump (R19.0-)
     intra-abdominal or pelvic swelling (R19.0-)
     Excludes2   breast mass and lump (N63)

● R22.3   Localized swelling, mass and lump, **upper limb**
R22.30   Localized swelling, mass and lump, **unspecified** upper limb
R22.31   Localized swelling, mass and lump, **right** upper limb
R22.32   Localized swelling, mass and lump, **left** upper limb
R22.33   Localized swelling, mass and lump, upper limb, **bilateral**

● R22.4   Localized swelling, mass and lump, **lower limb**
R22.40   Localized swelling, mass and lump, **unspecified** lower limb
R22.41   Localized swelling, mass and lump, **right** lower limb
R22.42   Localized swelling, mass and lump, **left** lower limb
R22.43   Localized swelling, mass and lump, lower limb, **bilateral**

R22.9   Localized swelling, mass and lump, **unspecified**

● R23   Other skin changes
R23.0   Cyanosis
     Excludes1   acrocyanosis (I73.8)
     cyanotic attacks of newborn (P28.2)
R23.1   Pallor
     Clammy skin
R23.2   Flushing
     Excessive blushing
     Code first, if applicable, menopausal and female climacteric states (N95.1)
R23.3   Spontaneous ecchymoses
     Small hemorrhagic spot of skin; AKA black and blue spot
     Petechiae
     Excludes1   ecchymoses of newborn (P54.5)
     purpura (D69.-)
R23.4   Changes in skin texture
     Desquamation of skin   Scaling of skin
     Induration of skin
     Excludes1   epidermal thickening NOS (L85.9)
R23.8   **Other** skin changes
R23.9   **Unspecified** skin changes

CHAPTER 18 (R00-R99)

SYMPTOMS AND SIGNS INVOLVING THE NERVOUS AND MUSCULOSKELETAL SYSTEMS (R25-R29)

● **R25**   **Abnormal involuntary movements**
> **Excludes1**   specific movement disorders (G20-G26)
> stereotyped movement disorders (F98.4)
> tic disorders (F95.-)

R25.0   **Abnormal head movements**

R25.1   **Tremor, unspecified**
> **Excludes1**   chorea NOS (G25.5)
> essential tremor (G25.0)
> hysterical tremor (F44.4)
> intention tremor (G25.2)

R25.2   **Cramp and spasm**
> **Excludes2**   carpopedal spasm (R29.0)
> charley-horse (M62.831)
> infantile spasms (G40.4-)
> muscle spasm of back (M62.830)
> muscle spasm of calf (M62.831)

R25.3   **Fasciculation**
> Twitching NOS

R25.8   **Other abnormal involuntary movements**

R25.9   **Unspecified abnormal involuntary movements**

● **R26**   **Abnormalities of gait and mobility**
> **Excludes1**   ataxia NOS (R27.0)
> hereditary ataxia (G11.-)
> locomotor (syphilitic) ataxia (A52.11)
> immobility syndrome (paraplegic) (M62.3)

R26.0   **Ataxic gait**
> Staggering gait

R26.1   **Paralytic gait**
> Spastic gait

R26.2   **Difficulty in walking, not elsewhere classified**
> **Excludes1**   falling (R29.6)
> unsteadiness on feet (R26.81)
>
> Coding Clinic: 2016, Q2, P7

● **R26.8**   **Other abnormalities of gait and mobility**

R26.81   **Unsteadiness on feet**

R26.89   **Other abnormalities of gait and mobility**

R26.9   **Unspecified abnormalities of gait and mobility**

● **R27**   **Other lack of coordination**
> **Excludes1**   ataxic gait (R26.0)
> hereditary ataxia (G11.-)
> vertigo NOS (R42)

R27.0   **Ataxia, unspecified**
> **Excludes1**   ataxia following cerebrovascular disease (I69. with final characters -93)

R27.8   **Other lack of coordination**

R27.9   **Unspecified lack of coordination**

● **R29**   **Other symptoms and signs involving the nervous and musculoskeletal systems**

R29.0   **Tetany**
> *Hyperexcitability of nerves and muscles characterized by spasm, twitching, and cramps*
> Carpopedal spasm
> **Excludes1**   hysterical tetany (F44.5)
> neonatal tetany (P71.3)
> parathyroid tetany (E20.9)
> post-thyroidectomy tetany (E89.2)

R29.1   **Meningismus**

R29.2   **Abnormal reflex**
> **Excludes2**   abnormal pupillary reflex (H57.0)
> hyperactive gag reflex (J39.2)
> vasovagal reaction or syncope (R55)

R29.3   **Abnormal posture**

R29.4   **Clicking hip**
> **Excludes1**   congenital deformities of hip (Q65.-)

R29.5   **Transient paralysis**
> *Code first any associated spinal cord injury (S14.0, S14.1-, S24.0, S24.1-, S34.0-, S34.1-)*
> **Excludes1**   transient ischemic attack (G45.9)

R29.6   **Repeated falls**
> Falling
> Tendency to fall
> **Excludes2**   at risk for falling (Z91.81)
> history of falling (Z91.81)

OGCR   Section I.C.18.d.

> Repeated falls
>
> Code R29.6, Repeated falls, is for use for encounters when a patient has recently fallen and the reason for the fall is being investigated.
>
> Code Z91.81, History of falling, is for use when a patient has fallen in the past and is at risk for future falls. When appropriate, both codes R29.6 and Z91.81 may be assigned together.

Coding Clinic: 2016, Q2, P7

● **R29.7**   **National Institutes of Health Stroke Scale (NIHSS) score**
> *Code first the type of cerebral infarction (I63.-)*
> Coding Clinic: 2016, Q4, P61, 127

● **R29.70**   **NIHSS score 0-9**

    R29.700   NIHSS score 0
    R29.701   NIHSS score 1
    R29.702   NIHSS score 2
    R29.703   NIHSS score 3
    R29.704   NIHSS score 4
    R29.705   NIHSS score 5
    R29.706   NIHSS score 6
    R29.707   NIHSS score 7
    R29.708   NIHSS score 8
    R29.709   NIHSS score 9

● **R29.71**   **NIHSS score 10-19**

    R29.710   NIHSS score 10
    R29.711   NIHSS score 11
    R29.712   NIHSS score 12
    R29.713   NIHSS score 13
    R29.714   NIHSS score 14
    R29.715   NIHSS score 15
    R29.716   NIHSS score 16
    R29.717   NIHSS score 17
    R29.718   NIHSS score 18
    R29.719   NIHSS score 19

● **R29.72**   **NIHSS score 20-29**

    R29.720   NIHSS score 20
    R29.721   NIHSS score 21
    R29.722   NIHSS score 22
    R29.723   NIHSS score 23
    R29.724   NIHSS score 24
    R29.725   NIHSS score 25
    R29.726   NIHSS score 26
    R29.727   NIHSS score 27
    R29.728   NIHSS score 28
    R29.729   NIHSS score 29

OGCR   Section I.C.18.i.

> NIHSS Stroke Scale
>
> The NIH stroke scale (NIHSS) codes (R29.7- -) can be used in conjunction with acute stroke codes (I63) to identify the patient's neurological status and the severity of the stroke. The stroke scale codes should be sequenced after the acute stroke diagnosis code(s).
>
> At a minimum, report the initial score documented. If desired, a facility may choose to capture multiple stroke scale scores.

▶ New   ⇒ Revised   ~~deleted~~ Deleted   Excludes 1   Excludes 2   Includes   Use additional   Code first   Code also   Key words

OGCR Official Guidelines   X Assign placeholder X   ● Use Additional Character(s)   ▮ Manifestation Code   🅗🅒 Hierarchical Condition Category   **Coding Clinic**

● R29.73   NIHSS score 30-39
    R29.730   NIHSS score 30
            Coding Clinic: 2016, Q4, P62
    R29.731   NIHSS score 31
    R29.732   NIHSS score 32
    R29.733   NIHSS score 33
    R29.734   NIHSS score 34
    R29.735   NIHSS score 35
    R29.736   NIHSS score 36
    R29.737   NIHSS score 37
    R29.738   NIHSS score 38
    R29.739   NIHSS score 39
● R29.74   NIHSS score 40-42
    R29.740   NIHSS score 40
    R29.741   NIHSS score 41
    R29.742   NIHSS score 42
● R29.8   **Other symptoms and signs involving the nervous and musculoskeletal systems**
   ● R29.81   **Other symptoms and signs involving the nervous system**
     R29.810   **Facial weakness**
           Facial droop
           Excludes1   Bell's palsy (G51.0)
                         facial weakness following cerebrovascular disease (I69. with final characters -92)
     R29.818   **Other symptoms and signs involving the nervous system**
   ● R29.89   **Other symptoms and signs involving the musculoskeletal system**
        Excludes2   pain in limb (M79.6-)
     R29.890   **Loss of height**
           Excludes1   osteoporosis (M80-M81)
     R29.891   **Ocular torticollis**
           Excludes1   congenital (sterno-mastoid) torticollis Q68.0
                         psychogenic torticollis (F45.8)
                         spasmodic torticollis (G24.3)
                         torticollis due to birth injury (P15.8)
                         torticollis NOS M43.6
     R29.898   **Other symptoms and signs involving the musculoskeletal system**
● R29.9   **Unspecified symptoms and signs involving the nervous and musculoskeletal systems**
    R29.90   Unspecified symptoms and signs involving the nervous system
    R29.91   Unspecified symptoms and signs involving the musculoskeletal system

SYMPTOMS AND SIGNS INVOLVING THE GENITOURINARY SYSTEM (R30-R39)

● R30   **Pain associated with micturition**
    Excludes1   psychogenic pain associated with micturition (F45.8)
    R30.0   **Dysuria**
        Painful urination
        Strangury
    R30.1   **Vesical tenesmus**
        Straining to urinate, with sensation of a full bladder even when empty
    R30.9   **Painful micturition, unspecified**
        Painful urination NOS

● R31   **Hematuria**
    Excludes1   hematuria included with underlying conditions, such as:
                  acute cystitis with hematuria (N30.01)
                  recurrent and persistent hematuria in glomerular diseases (N02.-)
    R31.0   **Gross hematuria**
        Coding Clinic: 2017, Q1, P17
    R31.1   **Benign essential microscopic hematuria**
   ● R31.2   **Other microscopic hematuria**
        Coding Clinic: 2016, Q4, P62
     R31.21   **Asymptomatic microscopic hematuria**
           AMH
     R31.29   **Other microscopic hematuria**
    R31.9   **Hematuria, unspecified**
        Coding Clinic: 2017, Q1, P6

R32   **Unspecified urinary incontinence**
    Enuresis NOS
    Excludes1   functional urinary incontinence (R39.81)
                  nonorganic enuresis (F98.0)
                  stress incontinence and other specified urinary incontinence (N39.3-N39.4-)
                  urinary incontinence associated with cognitive impairment (R39.81)

● R33   **Retention of urine**
    Excludes1   psychogenic retention of urine (F45.8)
    R33.0   **Drug induced retention of urine**
        Use additional code for adverse effect, if applicable, to identify drug (T36-T50 with fifth or sixth character 5)
    R33.8   **Other retention of urine**
        Code first, if applicable, any causal condition, such as:
        enlarged prostate (N40.1)
        Coding Clinic: 2018, Q4, P55
    R33.9   **Retention of urine, unspecified**

R34   **Anuria and oliguria**
    Excludes1   anuria and oliguria complicating abortion or ectopic or molar pregnancy (O00-O07, O08.4)
                  anuria and oliguria complicating pregnancy (O26.83-)
                  anuria and oliguria complicating the puerperium (O90.4)

● R35   **Polyuria**
    Passage of excessive volume of urine
    Code first, if applicable, any causal condition, such as:
    enlarged prostate (N40.1)
    Excludes1   psychogenic polyuria (F45.8)
    R35.0   **Frequency of micturition**
        Discharge or passage of urine; AKA uresis
    R35.1   **Nocturia**
        Urinary frequency at night
   ● R35.8   **Other polyuria**
        ~~Polyuria NOS~~
     ▶R35.81   **Nocturnal polyuria**
        ▶**Excludes2**   nocturnal enuresis (N39.44)
     ▶R35.89   **Other polyuria**
        ▶Polyuria NOS

● R36   **Urethral discharge**
    R36.0   **Urethral discharge without blood**
    R36.1   **Hematospermia** ♂
        Presence of blood in semen
    R36.9   **Urethral discharge, unspecified**
        Penile discharge NOS
        Urethrorrhea

R37   **Sexual dysfunction, unspecified**

CHAPTER 18 (R00-R99)

CHAPTER 18 (R00-R99)

● **R39   Other and unspecified symptoms and signs involving the genitourinary system**

     R39.0   Extravasation of urine
         Leakage, discharge

   ● **R39.1   Other difficulties with micturition**
         Code first, if applicable, any causal condition, such as:
         enlarged prostate (N40.1)

         R39.11   Hesitancy of micturition

         R39.12   Poor urinary stream
                Weak urinary steam

         R39.13   Splitting of urinary stream

         R39.14   Feeling of incomplete bladder emptying

         R39.15   Urgency of urination
                Excludes1   urge incontinence (N39.41, N39.46)

         R39.16   Straining to void

     ● **R39.19   Other difficulties with micturition**
                Coding Clinic: 2016, Q4, P63

            R39.191   Need to immediately re-void

            R39.192   Position dependent micturition

            R39.198   Other difficulties with micturition

     R39.2   Extrarenal uremia
         Prerenal uremia
         Excludes1   uremia NOS (N19)

   ● **R39.8   Other symptoms and signs involving the genitourinary system**

         R39.81   Functional urinary incontinence
                Urinary incontinence due to cognitive impairment, or severe physical disability or immobility
                Excludes1   stress incontinence and other specified urinary incontinence (N39.3-N39.4-)
                         urinary incontinence NOS (R32)

         R39.82   Chronic bladder pain
                Coding Clinic: 2016, Q4, P64

         R39.83   Unilateral non-palpable testicle ♂

         R39.84   Bilateral non-palpable testicles ♂

         R39.89   Other symptoms and signs involving the genitourinary system
                Coding Clinic: 2016, Q4, P64

     R39.9   Unspecified symptoms and signs involving the genitourinary system

---

SYMPTOMS AND SIGNS INVOLVING COGNITION, PERCEPTION, EMOTIONAL STATE AND BEHAVIOR (R40-R46)

     Excludes2   symptoms and signs constituting part of a pattern of mental disorder (F01-F99)
     Coding Clinic: 2015, Q4, P40

● **R40   Somnolence, stupor and coma**
     Excludes1   neonatal coma (P91.5)
                   somnolence, stupor and coma in diabetes (E08-E13)
                   somnolence, stupor and coma in hepatic failure (K72.-)
                   somnolence, stupor and coma in hypoglycemia (nondiabetic) (E15)

     R40.0   Somnolence
         Drowsiness
         Excludes1   coma (R40.2-)

     R40.1   Stupor
         Lowered level of consciousness
         Catatonic stupor
         Semicoma
         Excludes1   catatonic schizophrenia (F20.2)
                   coma (R40.2-)
                   depressive stupor (F31-F33)
                   dissociative stupor (F44.2)
                   manic stupor (F30.2)

OGCR   Section I.C.18.e.

> **Coma scale**
>
> The coma scale codes (R40.2-) can be used in conjunction with traumatic brain injury codes, acute cerebrovascular disease or sequelae of cerebrovascular disease codes. These codes are primarily for use by trauma registries, but they may be used in any setting where this information is collected. The coma scale may also be used to assess the status of the central nervous system for other non-trauma conditions, such as monitoring patients in the intensive care unit regardless of medical condition. The coma scale codes should be sequenced after the diagnosis code(s).
>
> These codes, one from each subcategory, are needed to complete the scale. The 7th character indicates when the scale was recorded. The 7th character should match for all three codes.
>
> At a minimum, report the initial score documented on presentation at your facility. This may be a score from the emergency medicine technician (EMT) or in the emergency department. If desired, a facility may choose to capture multiple coma scale scores.
>
> Assign code R40.24, Glasgow coma scale, total score, when only the total score is documented in the medical record and not the individual score(s).

● **R40.2   Coma**
     Code first any associated:
         fracture of skull (S02.-)
         intracranial injury (S06.-)
     Note: One code from each subcategory R40.21-R40-23 is required to complete the coma scale
     Coding Clinic: 2016, Q4, P127

     R40.20   Unspecified coma 🗝
         Coma NOS
         Unconsciousness NOS

   ● **R40.21   Coma scale, eyes open**

         The following appropriate 7th character is to be added to subcategory R40.21-:

0	unspecified time
1	in the field [EMT or ambulance]
2	at arrival to emergency department
3	at hospital admission
4	24 hours or more after hospital admission

         Coding Clinic: 2017, Q4, P25; 2015, Q2, P18

     ● **R40.211   Coma scale, eyes open, never** 🗝
                Coma scale eye opening score of 1

     ● **R40.212   Coma scale, eyes open, to pain** 🗝
                Coma scale eye opening score of 2

     ● **R40.213   Coma scale, eyes open, to sound**
                Coma scale eye opening score of 3

     ● **R40.214   Coma scale, eyes open, spontaneous**
                Coma scale eye opening score of 4

   ● **R40.22   Coma scale, best verbal response**

         The following appropriate 7th character is to be added to subcategory R40.22-:

0	unspecified time
1	in the field [EMT or ambulance]
2	at arrival to emergency department
3	at hospital admission
4	24 hours or more after hospital admission

         Coding Clinic: 2017, Q4, P25; 2015, Q2, P18

     ● **R40.221   Coma scale, best verbal response, none** 🗝
                Coma scale verbal score of 1

     ● **R40.222   Coma scale, best verbal response, incomprehensible words** 🗝
                Coma scale verbal score of 2
                Incomprehensible sounds (2-5 years of age)
                Moans/grunts to pain; restless (<2 years old)

▶ New   ⇒ Revised   ~~deleted~~ Deleted   Excludes 1   Excludes 2   Includes   Use additional   Code first   Code also   Key words

OGCR Official Guidelines   X Assign placeholder X   ● Use Additional Character(s)   ▶ Manifestation Code   🗝 Hierarchical Condition Category   Coding Clinic

Glasgow Coma Scale

Eye Opening Response	
• Spontaneous--open with blinking at baseline	4 points
• To verbal stimuli, command, speech	3 points
• To pain only (not applied to face)	2 points
• No response	1 point
Verbal Response	
• Oriented	5 points
• Confused conversation, but able to answer questions	4 points
• Inappropriate words	3 points
• Incomprehensible speech	2 points
• No response	1 point
Motor Response	
• Obeys commands for movement	6 points
• Purposeful movement to painful stimulus	5 points
• Withdraws in response to pain	4 points
• Flexion in response to pain (decorticate posturing)	3 points
• Extension response in response to pain (decerebrate posturing)	2 points
• No response	1 point
Categorization: Coma: No eye opening, no ability to follow commands, no word verbalizations (3-8)	
Head Injury Classification: Severe Head Injury--GCS score of 8 or less Moderate Head Injury--GCS score of 9 to 12 Mild head injury--GCS score of 13 to 15	
(Adapted from: Advanced Trauma Life Support: Course for Physicians, American College of Surgeons, 1993). http://www.bt.cdc.gov/masscasulatires/gscale.asp	

Figure 18-1

● R40.223 **Coma scale, best verbal response, inappropriate words**
  Coma scale verbal score of 3
  Inappropriate crying or screaming (< 2 years of age)
  Screaming (2-5 years of age)

● R40.224 **Coma scale, best verbal response, confused conversation**
  Coma scale verbal score of 4
  Inappropriate words (2-5 years of age)
  Irritable cries (< 2 years of age)

● R40.225 **Coma scale, best verbal response, oriented**
  Coma scale verbal score of 5
  Cooing or babbling or crying appropriately (< 2 years of age)
  Uses appropriate words (2- 5 years of age)

● R40.23 **Coma scale, best motor response**
  The following appropriate 7th character is to be added to subcategory R40.23-:

0	unspecified time
1	in the field [EMT or ambulance]
2	at arrival to emergency department
3	at hospital admission
4	24 hours or more after hospital admission

  Coding Clinic: 2017, Q4, P25; 2015, Q2, P18

● R40.231 **Coma scale, best motor response, none** 🔘
  Coma scale motor score of 1

● R40.232 **Coma scale, best motor response, extension** 🔘
  Abnormal extensor posturing to pain or noxious stimuli (< 2 years of age)
  Coma scale motor score of 2
  Extensor posturing to pain or noxious stimuli (2-5 years of age)

● R40.233 **Coma scale, best motor response, abnormal flexion**
  Coma scale motor score of 3
  Abnormal flexure posturing to pain or noxious stimuli (2-5 years of age)
  Flexion/decorticate posturing (< 2 years of age)

● R40.234 **Coma scale, best motor response, flexion withdrawal** 🔘
  Coma scale motor score of 4
  Withdraws from pain or noxious stimuli (2-5 years of age)

● R40.235 **Coma scale, best motor response, localizes pain**
  Coma scale motor score of 5
  Localizes pain (2-5 years of age)
  Withdraws to touch (< 2 years of age)

● R40.236 **Coma scale, best motor response, obeys commands**
  Coma scale motor score of 6
  Normal or spontaneous movement (< 2 years of age)
  Obeys commands (2-5 years of age)

● R40.24 **Glasgow coma scale, total score**
  Note: Assign a code from subcategory R40.24, when only the total coma score is documented
  The following appropriate 7th character is to be added to subcategory R40.24-:

0	unspecified time
1	in the field [EMT or ambulance]
2	at arrival to emergency department
3	at hospital admission
4	24 hours or more after hospital admission

  Coding Clinic: 2016, Q4, P64; 2015, Q2, P18

● R40.241 **Glasgow coma scale score 13-15**
● R40.242 **Glasgow coma scale score 9-12**
● R40.243 **Glasgow coma scale score 3-8** 🔘
● R40.244 **Other coma, without documented Glasgow coma scale score, or with partial score reported** 🔘

R40.3 **Persistent vegetative state** 🔘

R40.4 **Transient alteration of awareness**

● R41 **Other symptoms and signs involving cognitive functions and awareness**
  Excludes1 dissociative [conversion] disorders (F44.-)
  mild cognitive impairment, so stated (G31.84)

R41.0 **Disorientation, unspecified**
  Confusion NOS   Delirium NOS
  Coding Clinic: 2019, Q2, P34; 2016, Q4, P71

R41.1 **Anterograde amnesia**

R41.2 **Retrograde amnesia**

R41.3   Other amnesia
Amnesia NOS
Memory loss NOS

> **Excludes1**   amnestic disorder due to known physiologic condition (F04)
> amnestic syndrome due to psychoactive substance use (F10-F19 with 5th character .6)
> mild memory disturbance due to known physiological condition (F06.8)
> transient global amnesia (G45.4)

R41.4   Neurologic neglect syndrome
Asomatognosia   Left-sided neglect
Hemi-akinesia   Sensory neglect
Hemi-inattention   Visuospatial neglect
Hemispatial neglect

> **Excludes1**   visuospatial deficit (R41.842)

● **R41.8   Other symptoms and signs involving cognitive functions and awareness**

   R41.81   Age-related cognitive decline   A
   Senility NOS

   R41.82   Altered mental status, unspecified
   Change in mental status NOS

   > **Excludes1**   altered level of consciousness (R40.-)
   > altered mental status due to known condition - code to condition
   > delirium NOS (R41.0)

   Coding Clinic: 2012, Q4, P98

   R41.83   Borderline intellectual functioning
   IQ level 71 to 84

   > **Excludes1**   intellectual disabilities (F70-F79)

● **R41.84   Other specified cognitive deficit**

   > **Excludes1**   cognitive deficits as sequelae of cerebrovascular disease (I69.01-, I69.11-, I69.21-, I69.31-, I69.81-, I69.91-)

      R41.840   Attention and concentration deficit

      > **Excludes1**   attention-deficit hyperactivity disorders (F90.-)

      R41.841   Cognitive communication deficit
      R41.842   Visuospatial deficit
      R41.843   Psychomotor deficit
      R41.844   Frontal lobe and executive function deficit

   R41.89   Other symptoms and signs involving cognitive functions and awareness
   Anosognosia

R41.9   Unspecified symptoms and signs involving cognitive functions and awareness
Unspecified neurocognitive disorder

R42   Dizziness and giddiness
Light-headedness
Vertigo NOS

> **Excludes1**   vertiginous syndromes (H81.-)
> vertigo from infrasound (T75.23)

Coding Clinic: 2015, Q4, P40

● **R43   Disturbances of smell and taste**

   R43.0   Anosmia
   Absence of sense of smell; AKA anosphresia and olfactory anesthesia

   R43.1   Parosmia

   R43.2   Parageusia
   Perversion of sense of taste or bad taste in mouth; AKA dysgeusia

   R43.8   Other disturbances of smell and taste
   Mixed disturbance of smell and taste

   R43.9   Unspecified disturbances of smell and taste

● **R44   Other symptoms and signs involving general sensations and perceptions**

   > **Excludes1**   alcoholic hallucinations (F10.151, F10.251, F10.951)
   > hallucinations in drug psychosis (F11-F19 with fifth to sixth characters 51)
   > hallucinations in mood disorders with psychotic symptoms (F30.2, F31.5, F32.3, F33.3)
   > hallucinations in schizophrenia, schizotypal and delusional disorders (F20-F29)

   > **Excludes2**   disturbances of skin sensation (R20.-)

   R44.0   Auditory hallucinations
   R44.1   Visual hallucinations
   R44.2   Other hallucinations
   R44.3   Hallucinations, unspecified
   R44.8   Other symptoms and signs involving general sensations and perceptions
   R44.9   Unspecified symptoms and signs involving general sensations and perceptions

● **R45   Symptoms and signs involving emotional state**

   R45.0   Nervousness
   Nervous tension

   R45.1   Restlessness and agitation
   R45.2   Unhappiness
   R45.3   Demoralization and apathy

   > **Excludes1**   anhedonia (R45.84)

   R45.4   Irritability and anger
   R45.5   Hostility
   R45.6   Violent behavior
   R45.7   State of emotional shock and stress, unspecified

● **R45.8   Other symptoms and signs involving emotional state**

   R45.81   Low self-esteem
   R45.82   Worries
   R45.83   Excessive crying of child, adolescent or adult

   > **Excludes1**   excessive crying of infant (baby) R68.11

   R45.84   Anhedonia
   Total loss of feeling of pleasure in pleasurable acts

● **R45.85   Homicidal and suicidal ideations**

   > **Excludes1**   suicide attempt (T14.91)

   R45.850   Homicidal ideations
   R45.851   Suicidal ideations

   R45.86   Emotional lability
   R45.87   Impulsiveness
▶ **R45.88   Nonsuicidal self-harm**
   ▶ Nonsuicidal self-injury
   ▶ Nonsuicidal self-mutilation
   ▶ Self-inflicted injury without suicidal intent
   ▶ Code also injury, if known

   R45.89   Other symptoms and signs involving emotional state

● **R46   Symptoms and signs involving appearance and behavior**

   > **Excludes1**   appearance and behavior in schizophrenia, schizotypal and delusional disorders (F20-F29)
   > mental and behavioral disorders (F01-F99)

   R46.0   Very low level of personal hygiene
   R46.1   Bizarre personal appearance
   R46.2   Strange and inexplicable behavior
   R46.3   Overactivity
   R46.4   Slowness and poor responsiveness

   > **Excludes1**   stupor (R40.1)

   R46.5   Suspiciousness and marked evasiveness
   R46.6   Undue concern and preoccupation with stressful events

▶ New   ⇛ Revised   ~~deleted~~ Deleted   Excludes 1   Excludes 2   Includes   Use additional   Code first   Code also   Key words

OGCR Official Guidelines   X Assign placeholder X   ● Use Additional Character(s)   ▷ Manifestation Code   🝆 Hierarchical Condition Category   Coding Clinic

R46.7   Verbosity and circumstantial detail obscuring reason for contact

● R46.8   Other symptoms and signs involving appearance and behavior

   R46.81   Obsessive-compulsive behavior
            Excludes1   obsessive-compulsive disorder (F42.-)

   R46.89   Other symptoms and signs involving appearance and behavior

SYMPTOMS AND SIGNS INVOLVING SPEECH AND VOICE (R47-R49)

● R47   Speech disturbances, not elsewhere classified
         Excludes1   autism (F84.0)
                         cluttering (F80.81)
                         specific developmental disorders of speech and language (F80.-)
                         stuttering (F80.81)

● R47.0   Dysphasia and aphasia
   R47.01   Aphasia
            Excludes1   aphasia following cerebrovascular disease (I69. with final characters -20)
                            progressive isolated aphasia (G31.01)

   R47.02   Dysphasia
            Impairment in comprehension of speech, caused by left-sided brain damage
            Excludes1   dysphasia following cerebrovascular disease (I69. with final characters -21)

   R47.1   Dysarthria and anarthria
            Motor speech disorder
            Excludes1   dysarthria following cerebrovascular disease (I69. with final characters -22)

● R47.8   Other speech disturbances
            Excludes1   dysarthria following cerebrovascular disease (I69. with final characters -28)

   R47.81   Slurred speech
   ▌R47.82   *Fluency disorder in conditions classified elsewhere*
            Stuttering in conditions classified elsewhere
            Code first underlying disease or condition, such as:
            Parkinson's disease (G20)
            Excludes1   adult onset fluency disorder (F98.5)
                            childhood onset fluency disorder (F80.81)
                            fluency disorder (stuttering) following cerebrovascular disease (I69. with final characters -23)

   R47.89   Other speech disturbances
   R47.9   Unspecified speech disturbances

● R48   Dyslexia and other symbolic dysfunctions, not elsewhere classified
         Excludes1   specific developmental disorders of scholastic skills (F81.-)

   R48.0   Dyslexia and alexia
   R48.1   Agnosia
            Loss of ability to recognize objects, persons, sounds, shapes, or smells
            Astereognosis (astereognosis)
            Autotopagnosia
            Excludes1   visual object agnosia (R48.3)

   R48.2   Apraxia
            Loss of ability to execute or carry out learned purposeful movements
            Excludes1   apraxia following cerebrovascular disease (I69. with final characters -90)

R48.3   Visual agnosia
         Prosopagnosia
         Simultagnosia (asimultagnosia)

R48.8   Other symbolic dysfunctions
         Acalculia
         Difficulty performing simple mathematical tasks resulting from neurological injury
         Agraphia
         Coding Clinic: 2017, Q1, P27

R48.9   Unspecified symbolic dysfunctions

● R49   Voice and resonance disorders
         Excludes1   psychogenic voice and resonance disorders (F44.4)

R49.0   Dysphonia
         Hoarseness

R49.1   Aphonia
         Loss of voice

● R49.2   Hypernasality and hyponasality
   R49.21   Hypernasality
   R49.22   Hyponasality

R49.8   Other voice and resonance disorders
R49.9   Unspecified voice and resonance disorder
         Change in voice NOS
         Resonance disorder NOS

GENERAL SYMPTOMS AND SIGNS (R50-R69)

● R50   Fever of other and unknown origin
         Excludes1   chills without fever (R68.83)
                         febrile convulsions (R56.0-)
                         fever of unknown origin during labor (O75.2)
                         fever of unknown origin in newborn (P81.9)
                         hypothermia due to illness (R68.0)
                         malignant hyperthermia due to anesthesia (T88.3)
                         puerperal pyrexia NOS (O86.4)

R50.2   Drug induced fever
         Use additional code for adverse effect, if applicable, to identify drug (T36-T50 with fifth or sixth character 5)
         Excludes1   postvaccination (postimmunization) fever (R50.83)

● R50.8   Other specified fever
   ▌R50.81   *Fever presenting with conditions classified elsewhere*
            Code first underlying condition when associated fever is present, such as with:
            leukemia (C91-C95)
            neutropenia (D70.-)
            sickle-cell disease (D57.-)
            Coding Clinic: 2019, Q2, P25

   R50.82   Postprocedural fever
            Excludes1   postprocedural infection (T81.44)
                            posttransfusion fever (R50.84)
                            postvaccination (postimmunization) fever (R50.83)

   R50.83   Postvaccination fever
            Postimmunization fever

   R50.84   Febrile nonhemolytic transfusion reaction
            FNHTR
            Posttransfusion fever

R50.9   Fever, unspecified
         Fever NOS
         Fever of unknown origin [FUO]
         Fever with chills
         Fever with rigors
         Hyperpyrexia NOS
         Persistent fever
         Pyrexia NOS

● **R51   Headache**

> **Excludes2**   atypical face pain (G50.1)
>   migraine and other headache syndromes
>   (G43-G44)
>   trigeminal neuralgia (G50.0)

R51.0   Headache with orthostatic component, not elsewhere classified
> Headache with positional component, not elsewhere classified

R51.9 Headache, unspecified
> Facial pain NOS

R52   Pain, unspecified
> Acute pain NOS
> Generalized pain NOS

> **Excludes1**   acute and chronic pain, not elsewhere classified
>   (G89.-)
>   localized pain, unspecified type - code to pain by
>   site, such as:
>   abdomen pain (R10.-)
>   back pain (M54.9)
>   breast pain (N64.4)
>   chest pain (R07.1-R07.9)
>   ear pain (H92.0-)
>   eye pain (H57.1)
>   headache (R51.9)
>   joint pain (M25.5-)
>   limb pain (M79.6-)
> ➠   lumbar region pain (M54.5-)
>   pelvic and perineal pain (R10.2)
>   shoulder pain (M25.51-)
>   spine pain (M54.-)
>   throat pain (R07.0)
>   tongue pain (K14.6)
>   tooth pain (K08.8)
>   renal colic (N23)
>   pain disorders exclusively related to
>   psychological factors (F45.41)

● **R53   Malaise and fatigue**

R53.0   Neoplastic (malignant) related fatigue
> *Code first associated neoplasm*

R53.1   Weakness
> Asthenia NOS

> **Excludes1**   age-related weakness (R54)
>   muscle weakness (generalized) (M62.81)
>   sarcopenia (M62.84)
>   senile asthenia (R54)
> **Coding Clinic: 2017, Q1, P7**

R53.2   Functional quadriplegia 🅦
> Complete immobility due to severe physical disability
>   or frailty

> **Excludes1**   frailty NOS (R54)
>   hysterical paralysis (F44.4)
>   immobility syndrome (M62.3)
>   neurologic quadriplegia (G82.5-)
>   quadriplegia (G82.50)
> **Coding Clinic: 2016, Q2, P6**

● **R53.8   Other malaise and fatigue**

> **Excludes1**   combat exhaustion and fatigue (F43.0)
>   congenital debility (P96.9)
>   exhaustion and fatigue due to excessive
>   exertion (T73.3)
>   exhaustion and fatigue due to exposure
>   (T73.2)
>   exhaustion and fatigue due to heat (T67.-)
>   exhaustion and fatigue due to pregnancy
>   (O26.8-)
>   exhaustion and fatigue due to recurrent
>   depressive episode (F33)
>   exhaustion and fatigue due to senile
>   debility (R54)

R53.81   Other malaise
> Chronic debility
> Debility NOS
> General physical deterioration
> Malaise NOS
> Nervous debility

> **Excludes1**   age-related physical debility
>   (R54)
> **Coding Clinic: 2021, Q1, P43**

R53.82   Chronic fatigue, unspecified
> Chronic fatigue syndrome NOS

> **Excludes1**   postviral fatigue syndrome
>   (G93.3)

R53.83   Other fatigue
> Fatigue NOS   Lethargy
> Lack of energy   Tiredness

> **Excludes2**   exhaustion and fatigue due to
>   depressive episode (F32.-)
> **Coding Clinic: 2017, Q1, P7**

R54   Age-related physical debility   A
> Frailty   Senile asthenia
> Old age   Senile debility
> Senescence

> **Excludes1**   age-related cognitive decline (R41.81)
>   sarcopenia (M62.84)
>   senile psychosis (F03)
>   senility NOS (R41.81)

R55   Syncope and collapse
> Blackout
> Fainting
> Vasovagal attack

> **Excludes1**   cardiogenic shock (R57.0)
>   carotid sinus syncope (G90.01)
>   heat syncope (T67.1)
>   neurocirculatory asthenia (F45.8)
>   neurogenic orthostatic hypotension (G90.3)
>   orthostatic hypotension (I95.1)
>   postprocedural shock (T81.1-)
>   psychogenic syncope (F48.8)
>   shock NOS (R57.9)
>   shock complicating or following abortion or
>   ectopic or molar pregnancy (O00-O07, O08.3)
>   shock complicating or following labor and
>   delivery (O75.1)
>   Stokes-Adams attack (I45.9)
>   unconsciousness NOS (R40.2-)

● **R56   Convulsions, not elsewhere classified**

> **Excludes1**   dissociative convulsions and seizures (F44.5)
>   epileptic convulsions and seizures (G40.-)
>   newborn convulsions and seizures (P90)

● **R56.0   Febrile convulsions**

R56.00   Simple febrile convulsions 🅦
> Febrile convulsion NOS
> Febrile seizure NOS

R56.01   Complex febrile convulsions 🅦
> Atypical febrile seizure
> Complex febrile seizure
> Complicated febrile seizure

> **Excludes1**   status epilepticus (G40.901)

R56.1 **Post traumatic seizures** 🔖
> **Excludes1**   post traumatic epilepsy (G40.-)

R56.9 **Unspecified convulsions** 🔖
Convulsion disorder   Recurrent convulsions
Fit NOS   Seizure(s) (convulsive) NOS
Coding Clinic: 2021, Q1, P3; 2019, Q4, P18

● R57 **Shock, not elsewhere classified**
> **Excludes1**   anaphylactic shock NOS (T78.2)
> anaphylactic reaction or shock due to adverse
>   food reaction (T78.0-)
> anaphylactic shock due to adverse effect of
>   correct drug or medicament properly
>   administered (T88.6)
> anaphylactic shock due to serum (T80.5-)
> ~~anesthetic shock (T88.3)~~
> electric shock (T75.4)
> obstetric shock (O75.1)
> postprocedural shock (T81.1-)
> psychic shock (F43.0)
> shock complicating or following ectopic or molar
>   pregnancy (O00-O07, O08.3)
> ▶shock due to anesthesia (T88.2)
> shock due to lightning (T75.01)
> traumatic shock (T79.4)
> toxic shock syndrome (A48.3)

R57.0 **Cardiogenic shock** 🔖
> **Excludes2**   septic shock (R65.21)

R57.1 **Hypovolemic shock** 🔖
Decreased blood volume (loss)
Coding Clinic: 2019, Q2, P7-8

R57.8 **Other shock** 🔖

R57.9 **Shock, unspecified** 🔖
Failure of peripheral circulation NOS
Resulting in significant blood pressure drop

R58 **Hemorrhage, not elsewhere classified**
Hemorrhage NOS
> **Excludes1**   hemorrhage included with underlying
>   conditions, such as:
>   acute duodenal ulcer with hemorrhage (K26.0)
>   acute gastritis with bleeding (K29.01)
>   ulcerative enterocolitis with rectal bleeding
>   (K51.01)

● R59 **Enlarged lymph nodes**
> **Includes**   swollen glands
> **Excludes1**   lymphadenitis NOS (I88.9)
> acute lymphadenitis (L04.-)
> chronic lymphadenitis (I88.1)
> mesenteric (acute) (chronic) lymphadenitis (I88.0)

R59.0 **Localized enlarged lymph nodes**

R59.1 **Generalized enlarged lymph nodes**
Lymphadenopathy NOS

R59.9 **Enlarged lymph nodes, unspecified**

● R60 **Edema, not elsewhere classified**
> **Excludes1**   angioneurotic edema (T78.3)
> ascites (R18.-)
> cerebral edema (G93.6)
> cerebral edema due to birth injury (P11.0)
> edema of larynx (J38.4)
> edema of nasopharynx (J39.2)
> edema of pharynx (J39.2)
> gestational edema (O12.0-)
> hereditary edema (Q82.0)
> hydrops fetalis NOS (P83.2)
> hydrothorax (J94.8)
> hydrops fetalis NOS (P83.2)
> newborn edema (P83.3)
> pulmonary edema (J81.-)

R60.0 **Localized edema**

R60.1 **Generalized edema**
> **Excludes2**   nutritional edema (E40-E46)

R60.9 **Edema, unspecified**
Fluid retention NOS

R61 **Generalized hyperhidrosis**
Excessive sweating
Night sweats
Secondary hyperhidrosis
Code first, if applicable, menopausal and female climacteric states
(N95.1)
> **Excludes1**   focal (primary) (secondary) hyperhidrosis
>   (L74.5-)
> Frey's syndrome (L74.52)
> localized (primary) (secondary) hyperhidrosis
>   (L74.5-)

● R62 **Lack of expected normal physiological development in childhood and adults**
> **Excludes1**   delayed puberty (E30.0)
> gonadal dysgenesis (Q99.1)
> hypopituitarism (E23.0)

R62.0 **Delayed milestone in childhood**   P
Delayed attainment of expected physiological
    developmental stage
Late talker
Late walker

● R62.5 **Other and unspecified lack of expected normal physiological development in childhood**
> **Excludes1**   HIV disease resulting in failure to thrive
>   (B20)
> physical retardation due to malnutrition
>   (E45)

R62.50 **Unspecified lack of expected normal physiological development in childhood**
Infantilism NOS

R62.51 **Failure to thrive (child)**   P
Failure to gain weight
> **Excludes1**   failure to thrive in child under 28
>   days old (P92.6)

Coding Clinic: 2018, Q4, P82

R62.52 **Short stature (child)**
Lack of growth   Short stature NOS
Physical retardation
> **Excludes1**   short stature due to endocrine
>   disorder (E34.3)

R62.59 **Other lack of expected normal physiological development in childhood**

R62.7 **Adult failure to thrive**   A

CHAPTER 18 (R00-R99)

CHAPTER 18 (R00-R99)

● **R63**   **Symptoms and signs concerning food and fluid intake**
> **Excludes1**   bulimia NOS (F50.2)

R63.0   **Anorexia**
> Loss of appetite
> > **Excludes1**   anorexia nervosa (F50.0-)
> > loss of appetite of nonorganic origin (F50.89)

R63.1   **Polydipsia**
> Excessive thirst

R63.2   **Polyphagia**
> Excessive eating   Hyperalimentation NOS

● **R63.3**   **Feeding difficulties**
> ~~Feeding problem (elderly) (infant) NOS~~
> ~~Picky eater~~
> > ~~**Excludes1** eating disorders (F50.-)~~
> > ~~feeding problems of newborn (P92.-)~~
> > ~~infant feeding disorder of nonorganic origin (F98.2-)~~
> > ▶ **Excludes2**   eating disorders (F50.-)
> > ▶ feeding problems of newborn (P92.-)
> > ▶ infant feeding disorder of nonorganic origin (F98.2-)

▶ **R63.30**   **Feeding difficulties, unspecified**

▶ **R63.31**   **Pediatric feeding disorder, acute**
> ▶ Pediatric feeding dysfunction, acute
> ▶ Code also, if applicable, associated conditions such as:
> ▶ aspiration pneumonia (J69.0)
> ▶ dysphagia (R13.1-)
> ▶ gastro-esophageal reflux disease (K21.-)
> ▶ malnutrition (E40-E46)

▶ **R63.32**   **Pediatric feeding disorder, chronic**
> ▶ Pediatric feeding dysfunction, chronic
> ▶ Code also, if applicable, associated conditions such as:
> ▶ aspiration pneumonia (J69.0)
> ▶ dysphagia (R13.1-)
> ▶ gastro-esophageal reflux disease (K21.-)
> ▶ malnutrition (E40-E46)

▶ **R63.39**   **Other feeding difficulties**
> ▶ Feeding problem (elderly) (infant) NOS
> ▶ Picky eater

Coding Clinic: 2017, Q1, P27; 2016, Q3, P19

R63.4   **Abnormal weight loss**

R63.5   **Abnormal weight gain**
> > **Excludes1**   excessive weight gain in pregnancy (O26.0-)
> > obesity (E66.-)

R63.6   **Underweight**
> Use additional code to identify body mass index (BMI), if known (Z68.-)
> > **Excludes1**   abnormal weight loss (R63.4)
> > anorexia nervosa (F50.0-)
> > malnutrition (E40-E46)

R63.8   **Other symptoms and signs concerning food and fluid intake**

R64   **Cachexia** 🅗
> Wasting syndrome
> *Code first* underlying condition, if known
> > **Excludes1**   abnormal weight loss (R63.4)
> > nutritional marasmus (E41)

Coding Clinic: 2017, Q3, P25

● **R65**   **Symptoms and signs specifically associated with systemic inflammation and infection**

● **R65.1**   **Systemic inflammatory response syndrome (SIRS) of non-infectious origin**
> *Code first* underlying condition, such as:
> heatstroke (T67.0-)
> injury and trauma (S00-T88)
> > **Excludes1**   sepsis - code to infection
> > severe sepsis (R65.2)

Coding Clinic: 2019, Q2, P38

R65.10   **Systemic inflammatory response syndrome (SIRS) of non-infectious origin without acute organ dysfunction** 🅗
> Systemic inflammatory response syndrome (SIRS) NOS

Coding Clinic: 2019, Q2, P25, 38

R65.11   **Systemic inflammatory response syndrome (SIRS) of non-infectious origin with acute organ dysfunction** 🅗
> Use additional code to identify specific acute organ dysfunction, such as:
> acute kidney failure (N17.-)
> acute respiratory failure (J96.0-)
> critical illness myopathy (G72.81)
> critical illness polyneuropathy (G62.81)
> disseminated intravascular coagulopathy [DIC] (D65)
> encephalopathy (metabolic) (septic) (G93.41)
> hepatic failure (K72.0-)

OGCR Section I.C.18.g.

> SIRS due to Non-Infectious Process
>
> The systemic inflammatory response syndrome (SIRS) can develop as a result of certain non-infectious disease processes, such as trauma, malignant neoplasm, or pancreatitis. When SIRS is documented with a noninfectious condition, and no subsequent infection is documented, the code for the underlying condition, such as an injury, should be assigned, followed by code R65.10, Systemic inflammatory response syndrome (SIRS) of non-infectious origin without acute organ dysfunction, or code R65.11, Systemic inflammatory response syndrome (SIRS) of non-infectious origin with acute organ dysfunction. If an associated acute organ dysfunction is documented, the appropriate code(s) for the specific type of organ dysfunction(s) should be assigned in addition to code R65.11. If acute organ dysfunction is documented, but it cannot be determined if the acute organ dysfunction is associated with SIRS or due to another condition (e.g., directly due to the trauma), the provider should be queried.

● **R65.2**   **Severe sepsis**
> Infection with associated acute organ dysfunction
> Sepsis with acute organ dysfunction
> Sepsis with multiple organ dysfunction
> Systemic inflammatory response syndrome due to infectious process with acute organ dysfunction
>
> *Code first* underlying infection, such as:
> infection following a procedure (T81.44)
> infections following infusion, transfusion and therapeutic injection (T80.2-)
> puerperal sepsis (O85)
> sepsis following complete or unspecified spontaneous abortion (O03.87)
> sepsis following ectopic and molar pregnancy (O08.82)
> sepsis following incomplete spontaneous abortion (O03.37)
> sepsis following (induced) termination of pregnancy (O04.87)
> sepsis NOS (A41.9)
>
> Use additional code to identify specific acute organ dysfunction, such as:
> acute kidney failure (N17.-)
> acute respiratory failure (J96.0-)
> critical illness myopathy (G72.81)
> critical illness polyneuropathy (G62.81)
> disseminated intravascular coagulopathy [DIC] (D65)
> encephalopathy (metabolic) (septic) (G93.41)
> hepatic failure (K72.0-)

Coding Clinic: 2017, Q4, P99; 2016, Q3, P8

R65.20   **Severe sepsis without septic shock** 🅗
> Severe sepsis NOS

Coding Clinic: 2019, Q1, P14; 2018, Q4, P90; 2016, Q3, P14

R65.21   **Severe sepsis with septic shock** 🅗

▶ New   ⟹ Revised   ~~deleted~~ Deleted   Excludes 1   Excludes 2   Includes   Use additional   Code first   Code also   Key words

OGCR Official Guidelines   X Assign placeholder X   ● Use Additional Character(s)   ▶ Manifestation Code   🅗 Hierarchical Condition Category   **Coding Clinic**

● R68   Other general symptoms and signs

     R68.0   **Hypothermia, not associated with low environmental temperature**

         Excludes1   hypothermia NOS (accidental) (T68)
                        hypothermia due to anesthesia (T88.51)
                        hypothermia due to low environmental temperature (T68)
                        newborn hypothermia (P80.-)

   ● R68.1   **Nonspecific symptoms peculiar to infancy**

         Excludes1   colic, infantile (R10.83)
                        neonatal cerebral irritability (P91.3)
                        teething syndrome (K00.7)

       R68.11   **Excessive crying of infant (baby)**   P

           Excludes1   excessive crying of child, adolescent, or adult (R45.83)

       R68.12   **Fussy infant (baby)**   P
             Irritable infant

       R68.13   **Apparent life threatening event in infant (ALTE)**   P
             Apparent life threatening event in newborn
             Brief resolved unexplained event (BRUE)
             Code first confirmed diagnosis, if known
             Use additional code(s) for associated signs and symptoms if no confirmed diagnosis established, or if signs and symptoms are not associated routinely with confirmed diagnosis, or provide additional information for cause of ALTE

       R68.19   **Other nonspecific symptoms peculiar to infancy**   P

     R68.2   **Dry mouth, unspecified**

         Excludes1   dry mouth due to dehydration (E86.0)
                  �》dry mouth due to Sjögren syndrome (M35.0-)
                  salivary gland hyposecretion (K11.7)

     R68.3   **Clubbing of fingers**
         Clubbing of nails

         Excludes1   congenital clubfinger (Q68.1)

   ● R68.8   **Other general symptoms and signs**

       R68.81   **Early satiety**

       R68.82   **Decreased libido**   A
           Decreased sexual desire

       R68.83   **Chills (without fever)**
           Chills NOS

           Excludes1   chills with fever (R50.9)

       R68.84   **Jaw pain**
           Mandibular pain
           Maxilla pain

           Excludes1   temporomandibular joint arthralgia (M26.62-)

       R68.89   **Other general symptoms and signs**

R69   **Illness, unspecified**
     Unknown and unspecified cases of morbidity

ABNORMAL FINDINGS ON EXAMINATION OF BLOOD, WITHOUT DIAGNOSIS (R70-R79)

     Excludes2   abnormal findings on antenatal screening of mother (O28.-)
                   abnormalities of lipids (E78.-)
                   abnormalities of platelets and thrombocytes (D69.-)
                   abnormalities of white blood cells classified elsewhere (D70-D72)
                   coagulation hemorrhagic disorders (D65-D68)
                   diagnostic abnormal findings classified elsewhere —*see* Alphabetical Index
                   hemorrhagic and hematological disorders of newborn (P50-P61)

● R70   **Elevated erythrocyte sedimentation rate and abnormality of plasma viscosity**

     R70.0   **Elevated erythrocyte sedimentation rate**

     R70.1   **Abnormal plasma viscosity**

● R71   **Abnormality of red blood cells**

     Excludes1   anemias (D50-D64)
                anemia of premature infant (P61.2)
                benign (familial) polycythemia (D75.0)
                congenital anemias (P61.2-P61.4)
                newborn anemia due to isoimmunization (P55.-)
                polycythemia neonatorum (P61.1)
                polycythemia NOS (D75.1)
                polycythemia vera (D45)
                secondary polycythemia (D75.1)

     R71.0   **Precipitous drop in hematocrit**
         Drop (precipitous) in hemoglobin
         Drop in hematocrit
         Blood volume that has decreased red blood cells

     R71.8   **Other abnormality of red blood cells**
         Abnormal red-cell morphology NOS
         Abnormal red-cell volume NOS
         Anisocytosis
         Red blood cells of unequal size
         Poikilocytosis
         Red blood cells of abnormal shape

● R73   **Elevated blood glucose level**

     Excludes1   diabetes mellitus (E08-E13)
                diabetes mellitus in pregnancy, childbirth and the puerperium (O24.-)
                neonatal disorders (P70.0-P70.2)
                postsurgical hypoinsulinemia (E89.1)

   ● R73.0   **Abnormal glucose**

         Excludes1   abnormal glucose in pregnancy (O99.81-)
                  diabetes mellitus (E08-E13)
                  dysmetabolic syndrome X (E88.81)
                  gestational diabetes (O24.4-)
                  glycosuria (R81)
                  hypoglycemia (E16.2)

       R73.01   **Impaired fasting glucose**
           Elevated fasting glucose

       R73.02   **Impaired glucose tolerance (oral)**
           Elevated glucose tolerance

       R73.03   **Prediabetes**
           Latent diabetes
           Coding Clinic: 2016, Q4, P65

       R73.09   **Other abnormal glucose**
           Abnormal glucose NOS
           Abnormal non-fasting glucose tolerance
           Coding Clinic: 2016, Q4, P65

     R73.9   **Hyperglycemia, unspecified**

● R74   **Abnormal serum enzyme levels**

   ● R74.0   **Nonspecific elevation of levels of transaminase and lactic acid dehydrogenase [LDH]**

       R74.01   **Elevation of levels of liver transaminase levels**
           Elevation of levels of alanine transaminase (ALT)
           Elevation of levels of aspartate transaminase (AST)

       R74.02   **Elevation of levels of lactic acid dehydrogenase [LDH]**

     R74.8   **Abnormal levels of other serum enzymes**
         Abnormal level of acid phosphatase
         Abnormal level of alkaline phosphatase
         Abnormal level of amylase
         Abnormal level of lipase [triacylglycerol lipase]
         Coding Clinic: 2019, Q2, P6

     R74.9   **Abnormal serum enzyme level, unspecified**

R75   **Inconclusive laboratory evidence of human immunodeficiency virus [HIV]**
     Nonconclusive HIV-test finding in infants

     Excludes1   asymptomatic human immunodeficiency virus [HIV] infection status (Z21)
                human immunodeficiency virus [HIV] disease (B20)

OGCR Section I.C.1.e and f.

Patients with inconclusive HIV serology

e. Patients with inconclusive HIV serology, but no definitive diagnosis or manifestations of the illness, may be assigned code R75, Inconclusive laboratory evidence of human immunodeficiency virus [HIV].

f. Previously diagnosed HIV-related illness

Patients with any known prior diagnosis of an HIV-related illness should be coded to B20. Once a patient has developed an HIV-related illness, the patient should always be assigned code B20 on every subsequent admission/encounter. Patients previously diagnosed with any HIV illness (B20) should never be assigned to R75 or Z21, Asymptomatic human immunodeficiency virus [HIV] infection status.

● R76   Other abnormal immunological findings in serum

    R76.0   Raised antibody titer

       Excludes1   isoimmunization in pregnancy (O36.0-O36.1)

                isoimmunization affecting newborn (P55.-)

       Coding Clinic: 2021, Q1, P7

● R76.1   Nonspecific reaction to test for tuberculosis

       R76.11   Nonspecific reaction to tuberculin skin test without active tuberculosis

             Abnormal result of Mantoux test

             PPD positive

             Tuberculin (skin test) positive

             Tuberculin (skin test) reactor

             Excludes1   nonspecific reaction to cell mediated immunity measurement of gamma interferon antigen response without active tuberculosis (R76.12)

       R76.12   Nonspecific reaction to cell mediated immunity measurement of gamma interferon antigen response without active tuberculosis

             Nonspecific reaction to QuantiFERON-TB test (QFT) without active tuberculosis

             Excludes1   nonspecific reaction to tuberculin skin test without active tuberculosis (R76.11)

                        positive tuberculin skin test (R76.11)

    R76.8   Other specified abnormal immunological findings in serum

       Raised level of immunoglobulins NOS

       Coding Clinic: 2021, Q1, P7

    R76.9   Abnormal immunological finding in serum, unspecified

● R77   Other abnormalities of plasma proteins

       Excludes1   disorders of plasma-protein metabolism (E88.0-)

    R77.0   Abnormality of albumin

    R77.1   Abnormality of globulin

       Hyperglobulinemia NOS

    R77.2   Abnormality of alphafetoprotein

    R77.8   Other specified abnormalities of plasma proteins

       Coding Clinic: 2019, Q2, P6

    R77.9   Abnormality of plasma protein, unspecified

       Coding Clinic: 2019, Q2, P6

● R78   Findings of drugs and other substances, not normally found in blood

       Use additional code to identify any retained foreign body, if applicable (Z18.-)

       Excludes1   mental or behavioral disorders due to psychoactive substance use (F10-F19)

    R78.0   Finding of alcohol in blood

       Use additional external cause code (Y90.-), for detail regarding alcohol level.

    R78.1   Finding of opiate drug in blood

    R78.2   Finding of cocaine in blood

    R78.3   Finding of hallucinogen in blood

    R78.4   Finding of other drugs of addictive potential in blood

    R78.5   Finding of other psychotropic drug in blood

    R78.6   Finding of steroid agent in blood

● R78.7   Finding of abnormal level of heavy metals in blood

       R78.71   Abnormal lead level in blood

             Excludes1   lead poisoning (T56.0-)

       R78.79   Finding of abnormal level of heavy metals in blood

● R78.8   Finding of other specified substances, not normally found in blood

       R78.81   Bacteremia

             Blood poisoning/bacteremia

             Excludes1   sepsis-code to specified infection

       R78.89   Finding of other specified substances, not normally found in blood

             Finding of abnormal level of lithium in blood

    R78.9   Finding of unspecified substance, not normally found in blood

● R79   Other abnormal findings of blood chemistry

       Use additional code to identify any retained foreign body, if applicable (Z18.-)

       Excludes1   asymptomatic hyperuricemia (E79.0)

               hyperglycemia NOS (R73.9)

               hypoglycemia NOS (E16.2)

               neonatal hypoglycemia (P70.3-P70.4)

               specific findings indicating disorder of amino-acid metabolism (E70-E72)

               specific findings indicating disorder of carbohydrate metabolism (E73-E74)

               specific findings indicating disorder of lipid metabolism (E75.-)

    R79.0   Abnormal level of blood mineral

       Abnormal blood level of cobalt

       Abnormal blood level of copper

       Abnormal blood level of iron

       Abnormal blood level of magnesium

       Abnormal blood level of mineral NEC

       Abnormal blood level of zinc

       Excludes1   abnormal level of lithium (R78.89)

               disorders of mineral metabolism (E83.-)

               neonatal hypomagnesemia (P71.2)

               nutritional mineral deficiency (E58-E61)

    R79.1   Abnormal coagulation profile

       Abnormal or prolonged bleeding time

       Abnormal or prolonged coagulation time

       Abnormal or prolonged partial thromboplastin time [PTT]

       Abnormal or prolonged prothrombin time [PT]

       Excludes1   coagulation defects (D68.-)

       Excludes2   abnormality of fluid, electrolyte or acid-base balance (E86-E87)

● R79.8   Other specified abnormal findings of blood chemistry

       R79.81   Abnormal blood-gas level

       R79.82   Elevated C-reactive protein (CRP)

▶   R79.83   Abnormal findings of blood amino-acid level

▶   Homocysteinemia

       ▶ **Excludes1**   disorders of amino-acid metabolism (E70-E72)

       R79.89   Other specified abnormal findings of blood chemistry

             Coding Clinic: 2019, Q2, P6

    R79.9   Abnormal finding of blood chemistry, unspecified

ABNORMAL FINDINGS ON EXAMINATION OF URINE, WITHOUT DIAGNOSIS (R80-R82)

       Excludes1   abnormal findings on antenatal screening of mother (O28.-)

               diagnostic abnormal findings classified elsewhere - see Alphabetical Index

               specific findings indicating disorder of amino-acid metabolism (E70-E72)

               specific findings indicating disorder of carbohydrate metabolism (E73-E74)

▶ New   ▥ Revised   ~~deleted~~ Deleted   Excludes 1   Excludes 2   Includes   Use additional   Code first   Code also   Key words

OGCR Official Guidelines   X Assign placeholder X   ● Use Additional Character(s)   ▶ Manifestation Code   ◕ Hierarchical Condition Category   Coding Clinic

● **R80   Proteinuria**
    Excludes1   gestational proteinuria (O12.1-)
  R80.0   Isolated proteinuria
      Idiopathic proteinuria
      Excludes1   isolated proteinuria with specific
                 morphological lesion (N06.-)
  R80.1   Persistent proteinuria, unspecified
  R80.2   Orthostatic proteinuria, unspecified
      Postural proteinuria
  R80.3   Bence Jones proteinuria
  R80.8   Other proteinuria
  R80.9   Proteinuria, unspecified
      Albuminuria NOS

  R81   Glycosuria
    Excludes1   renal glycosuria (E74.818)

● **R82   Other and unspecified abnormal findings in urine**
    Includes   chromoabnormalities in urine
    Use additional code to identify any retained foreign body, if
    applicable (Z18.-)
    Excludes2   hematuria (R31.-)
  R82.0   Chyluria
      White milky urine
      Excludes1   filarial chyluria (B74.-)
  R82.1   Myoglobinuria
      Presence of myoglobin (iron containing protein) in urine
  R82.2   Biliuria
      Presence of bile pigments/salts in urine
  R82.3   Hemoglobinuria
      Presence of hemoglobin in urine
      Excludes1   hemoglobinuria due to hemolysis from
                 external causes NEC (D59.6)
                 hemoglobinuria due to paroxysmal
                    nocturnal [Marchiafava-Micheli]
                    (D59.5)
  R82.4   Acetonuria
      Ketonuria
  **R82.5   Elevated urine levels of drugs, medicaments and
      biological substances**
      Elevated urine levels of catecholamines
      Elevated urine levels of indoleacetic acid
      Elevated urine levels of 17-ketosteroids
      Elevated urine levels of steroids
  **R82.6   Abnormal urine levels of substances chiefly
      nonmedicinal as to source**
      Abnormal urine level of heavy metals
● **R82.7   Abnormal findings on microbiological examination of
      urine**
      Excludes1   colonization status (Z22.-)
      Coding Clinic: 2016, Q4, P65
    R82.71   Bacteriuria
    **R82.79   Other abnormal findings on microbiological
         examination of urine**
         Positive culture findings of urine
● **R82.8   Abnormal findings on cytological and histological
      examination of urine**
    R82.81   Pyuria
         Sterile pyuria
         Coding Clinic: 2019, Q4, P16
    **R82.89   Other abnormal findings on cytological and
         histological examination of urine**
● **R82.9   Other and unspecified abnormal findings in urine**
    R82.90   Unspecified abnormal findings in urine
    R82.91   Other chromoabnormalities of urine
         Chromoconversion (dipstick)
         Idiopathic dipstick converts positive for blood
           with no cellular forms in sediment
         Excludes1   hemoglobinuria (R82.3)
                    myoglobinuria (R82.1)

● **R82.99   Other abnormal findings in urine**
    R82.991   Hypocitraturia
    R82.992   Hyperoxaluria
         Excludes1   Primary hyperoxaluria
                   (E72.53)
    R82.993   Hyperuricosuria
    R82.994   Hypercalciuria
         Idiopathic hypercalciuria
    R82.998   Other abnormal findings in urine
         Cells and casts in urine
         Crystalluria
         Melanuria

**ABNORMAL FINDINGS ON EXAMINATION OF OTHER BODY FLUIDS,
SUBSTANCES AND TISSUES, WITHOUT DIAGNOSIS (R83-R89)**

    Excludes1   abnormal findings on antenatal screening of
               mother (O28.-)
         diagnostic abnormal findings classified elsewhere
         - see Alphabetical Index
    Excludes2   abnormal findings on examination of blood,
               without diagnosis (R70-R79)
         abnormal findings on examination of urine,
               without diagnosis (R80-R82)
         abnormal tumor markers (R97.-)

● **R83   Abnormal findings in cerebrospinal fluid**
  R83.0   Abnormal level of enzymes in cerebrospinal fluid
  R83.1   Abnormal level of hormones in cerebrospinal fluid
  **R83.2   Abnormal level of other drugs, medicaments and
      biological substances in cerebrospinal fluid**
  **R83.3   Abnormal level of substances chiefly nonmedicinal as to
      source in cerebrospinal fluid**
  **R83.4   Abnormal immunological findings in cerebrospinal
      fluid**
  **R83.5   Abnormal microbiological findings in cerebrospinal
      fluid**
      Positive culture findings in cerebrospinal fluid
      Excludes1   colonization status (Z22.-)
  R83.6   Abnormal cytological findings in cerebrospinal fluid
  R83.8   Other abnormal findings in cerebrospinal fluid
      Abnormal chromosomal findings in cerebrospinal fluid
  R83.9   Unspecified abnormal finding in cerebrospinal fluid

● **R84   Abnormal findings in specimens from respiratory organs and
    thorax**
    Includes   abnormal findings in bronchial washings
         abnormal findings in nasal secretions
         abnormal findings in pleural fluid
         abnormal findings in sputum
         abnormal findings in throat scrapings
    Excludes1   blood-stained sputum (R04.2)
  **R84.0   Abnormal level of enzymes in specimens from
      respiratory organs and thorax**
  **R84.1   Abnormal level of hormones in specimens from
      respiratory organs and thorax**
  **R84.2   Abnormal level of other drugs, medicaments and
      biological substances in specimens from respiratory
      organs and thorax**
  **R84.3   Abnormal level of substances chiefly nonmedicinal as to
      source in specimens from respiratory organs and thorax**
  **R84.4   Abnormal immunological findings in specimens from
      respiratory organs and thorax**
  **R84.5   Abnormal microbiological findings in specimens from
      respiratory organs and thorax**
      Positive culture findings in specimens from respiratory
      organs and thorax
    Excludes1   colonization status (Z22.-)

R84.6 Abnormal cytological findings in specimens from respiratory organs and thorax

R84.7 Abnormal histological findings in specimens from respiratory organs and thorax

R84.8 Other abnormal findings in specimens from respiratory organs and thorax
    Abnormal chromosomal findings in specimens from respiratory organs and thorax

R84.9 Unspecified abnormal finding in specimens from respiratory organs and thorax

● **R85** Abnormal findings in specimens from digestive organs and abdominal cavity

   Includes abnormal findings in peritoneal fluid
              abnormal findings in saliva

   Excludes1 cloudy peritoneal dialysis effluent (R88.0)
              fecal abnormalities (R19.5)

R85.0 Abnormal level of enzymes in specimens from digestive organs and abdominal cavity

R85.1 Abnormal level of hormones in specimens from digestive organs and abdominal cavity

R85.2 Abnormal level of other drugs, medicaments and biological substances in specimens from digestive organs and abdominal cavity

R85.3 Abnormal level of substances chiefly nonmedicinal as to source in specimens from digestive organs and abdominal cavity

R85.4 Abnormal immunological findings in specimens from digestive organs and abdominal cavity

R85.5 Abnormal microbiological findings in specimens from digestive organs and abdominal cavity
    Positive culture findings in specimens from digestive organs and abdominal cavity

   Excludes1 colonization status (Z22.-)

● **R85.6** Abnormal cytological findings in specimens from digestive organs and abdominal cavity

   ● **R85.61** Abnormal cytologic smear of anus

      Excludes1 abnormal cytological findings in specimens from other digestive organs and abdominal cavity (R85.69)
                  carcinoma in situ of anus (histologically confirmed) (D01.3)
                  anal intraepithelial neoplasia I [AIN I] (K62.82)
                  anal intraepithelial neoplasia II [AIN II] (K62.82)
                  anal intraepithelial neoplasia III [AIN III] (D01.3)
                  dysplasia (mild) (moderate) of anus (histologically confirmed) (K62.82)
                  severe dysplasia of anus (histologically confirmed) (D01.3)

      Excludes2 anal high risk human papillomavirus (HPV) DNA test positive (R85.81)
                  anal low risk human papillomavirus (HPV) DNA test positive (R85.82)

   R85.610 Atypical squamous cells of undetermined significance on cytologic smear of anus (ASC-US)

   R85.611 Atypical squamous cells cannot exclude high grade squamous intraepithelial lesion on cytologic smear of anus (ASC-H)

   R85.612 Low grade squamous intraepithelial lesion on cytologic smear of anus (LGSIL)

   R85.613 High grade squamous intraepithelial lesion on cytologic smear of anus (HGSIL)

   R85.614 Cytologic evidence of malignancy on smear of anus

   R85.615 Unsatisfactory cytologic smear of anus
       Inadequate sample of cytologic smear of anus

   R85.616 Satisfactory anal smear but lacking transformation zone

   R85.618 Other abnormal cytological findings on specimens from anus

   R85.619 Unspecified abnormal cytological findings in specimens from anus
       Abnormal anal cytology NOS
       Atypical glandular cells of anus NOS

   R85.69 Abnormal cytological findings in specimens from other digestive organs and abdominal cavity

R85.7 Abnormal histological findings in specimens from digestive organs and abdominal cavity

● **R85.8** Other abnormal findings in specimens from digestive organs and abdominal cavity

   R85.81 Anal high risk human papillomavirus (HPV) DNA test positive

      Excludes1 anogenital warts due to human papillomavirus (HPV) (A63.0)
                  condyloma acuminatum (A63.0)

   R85.82 Anal low risk human papillomavirus (HPV) DNA test positive
       Use additional code for associated human papillomavirus (B97.7)

   R85.89 Other abnormal findings in specimens from digestive organs and abdominal cavity
       Abnormal chromosomal findings in specimens from digestive organs and abdominal cavity

R85.9 Unspecified abnormal finding in specimens from digestive organs and abdominal cavity

● **R86** Abnormal findings in specimens from male genital organs

   Includes abnormal findings in prostatic secretions
              abnormal findings in semen, seminal fluid
              abnormal spermatozoa

   Excludes1 azoospermia (N46.0-)
              oligospermia (N46.1-)

R86.0 Abnormal level of enzymes in specimens from male genital organs ♂

R86.1 Abnormal level of hormones in specimens from male genital organs ♂

R86.2 Abnormal level of other drugs, medicaments and biological substances in specimens from male genital organs ♂

R86.3 Abnormal level of substances chiefly nonmedicinal as to source in specimens from male genital organs ♂

R86.4 Abnormal immunological findings in specimens from male genital organs ♂

R86.5 Abnormal microbiological findings in specimens from male genital organs ♂
    Positive culture findings in specimens from male genital organs

   Excludes1 colonization status (Z22.-)

R86.6 Abnormal cytological findings in specimens from male genital organs ♂

R86.7 Abnormal histological findings in specimens from male genital organs ♂

R86.8 Other abnormal findings in specimens from male genital organs ♂
    Abnormal chromosomal findings in specimens from male genital organs

R86.9 Unspecified abnormal finding in specimens from male genital organs ♂

▶ New   ⇒ Revised   ~~deleted~~ Deleted   Excludes 1   Excludes 2   Includes   Use additional   Code first   Code also   Key words

OGCR Official Guidelines   **X** Assign placeholder X   ● Use Additional Character(s)   ▶ Manifestation Code   🏥 Hierarchical Condition Category   **Coding Clinic**

● **R87**   **Abnormal findings in specimens from female genital organs**

     Includes   abnormal findings in secretion and smears from cervix uteri

                   abnormal findings in secretion and smears from vagina

                   abnormal findings in secretion and smears from vulva

R87.0   **Abnormal level of enzymes in specimens from female genital organs** ♀

R87.1   **Abnormal level of hormones in specimens from female genital organs** ♀

R87.2   **Abnormal level of other drugs, medicaments and biological substances in specimens from female genital organs** ♀

R87.3   **Abnormal level of substances chiefly nonmedicinal as to source in specimens from female genital organs** ♀

R87.4   **Abnormal immunological findings in specimens from female genital organs** ♀

R87.5   **Abnormal microbiological findings in specimens from female genital organs** ♀

     Positive culture findings in specimens from female genital organs

     Excludes1   colonization status (Z22.-)

● **R87.6**   **Abnormal cytological findings in specimens from female genital organs**

   ● **R87.61**   **Abnormal cytological findings in specimens from cervix uteri**

       Excludes1   abnormal cytological findings in specimens from other female genital organs (R87.69)

                abnormal cytological findings in specimens from vagina (R87.62-)

                carcinoma in situ of cervix uteri (histologically confirmed) (D06.-)

                cervical intraepithelial neoplasia I [CIN I] (N87.0)

                cervical intraepithelial neoplasia II [CIN II] (N87.1)

                cervical intraepithelial neoplasia III [CIN III] (D06.-)

                dysplasia (mild) (moderate) of cervix uteri (histologically confirmed) (N87.-)

                severe dysplasia of cervix uteri (histologically confirmed) (D06.-)

       Excludes2   cervical high risk human papillomavirus (HPV) DNA test positive (R87.810)

                cervical low risk human papillomavirus (HPV) DNA test positive (R87.820)

     R87.610   **Atypical squamous cells of undetermined significance on cytologic smear of cervix (ASC-US)** ♀

     R87.611   **Atypical squamous cells cannot exclude high grade squamous intraepithelial lesion on cytologic smear of cervix (ASC-H)** ♀

     R87.612   **Low grade squamous intraepithelial lesion on cytologic smear of cervix (LGSIL)** ♀

     R87.613   **High grade squamous intraepithelial lesion on cytologic smear of cervix (HGSIL)** ♀

     R87.614   **Cytologic evidence of malignancy on smear of cervix** ♀

     R87.615   **Unsatisfactory cytologic smear of cervix** ♀

       Inadequate sample of cytologic smear of cervix

     R87.616   **Satisfactory cervical smear but lacking transformation zone** ♀

     R87.618   **Other abnormal cytological findings on specimens from cervix uteri** ♀

     R87.619   **Unspecified abnormal cytological findings in specimens from cervix uteri** ♀

       Abnormal cervical cytology NOS

       Abnormal Papanicolaou smear of cervix NOS

       Abnormal thin preparation smear of cervix NOS

       Atypical endocervial cells of cervix NOS

       Atypical endometrial cells of cervix NOS

       Atypical glandular cells of cervix NOS

● **R87.62**   **Abnormal cytological findings in specimens from vagina**

     Use additional code to identify acquired absence of uterus and cervix, if applicable (Z90.71-)

     Excludes1   abnormal cytological findings in specimens from cervix uteri (R87.61-)

                abnormal cytological findings in specimens from other female genital organs (R87.69)

                carcinoma in situ of vagina (histologically confirmed) (D07.2)

                vaginal intraepithelial neoplasia I [VAIN I] (N89.0)

                vaginal intraepithelial neoplasia II [VAIN II] (N89.1)

                vaginal intraepithelial neoplasia III [VAIN III] (D07.2)

                dysplasia (mild) (moderate) of vagina (histologically confirmed) (N89.-)

                severe dysplasia of vagina (histologically confirmed) (D07.2)

     Excludes2   vaginal high risk human papillomavirus (HPV) DNA test positive (R87.811)

                vaginal low risk human papillomavirus (HPV) DNA test positive (R87.821)

     R87.620   **Atypical squamous cells of undetermined significance on cytologic smear of vagina (ASC-US)** ♀

     R87.621   **Atypical squamous cells cannot exclude high grade squamous intraepithelial lesion on cytologic smear of vagina (ASC-H)** ♀

     R87.622   **Low grade squamous intraepithelial lesion on cytologic smear of vagina (LGSIL)** ♀

     R87.623   **High grade squamous intraepithelial lesion on cytologic smear of vagina (HGSIL)** ♀

     R87.624   **Cytologic evidence of malignancy on smear of vagina** ♀

     R87.625   **Unsatisfactory cytologic smear of vagina** ♀

       Inadequate sample of cytologic smear of vagina

     R87.628   **Other abnormal cytological findings on specimens from vagina** ♀

R87.629   **Unspecified** abnormal cytological
findings in specimens from vagina ♀
    Abnormal Papanicolaou smear of
vagina NOS
    Abnormal thin preparation smear of
vagina NOS
    Abnormal vaginal cytology NOS
    Atypical endocervical cells of vagina
NOS
    Atypical endometrial cells of vagina
NOS
    Atypical glandular cells of vagina
NOS

R87.69   **Abnormal** cytological findings in specimens
from **other female genital organs** ♀
    Abnormal cytological findings in specimens
from female genital organs NOS
    Excludes1   dysplasia of vulva (histologically
confirmed) (N90.0-N90.3)

R87.7   Abnormal **histological** findings in specimens from
female genital organs ♀
    Excludes1   carcinoma in situ (histologically
confirmed) of female genital organs
(D06-D07.3)
    cervical intraepithelial neoplasia I [CIN
I] (N87.0)
    cervical intraepithelial neoplasia II [CIN
II] (N87.1)
    cervical intraepithelial neoplasia III [CIN
III] (D06.-)
    dysplasia (mild) (moderate) of cervix
uteri (histologically confirmed)
(N87.-)
    dysplasia (mild) (moderate) of vagina
(histologically confirmed) (N89.-)
    vaginal intraepithelial neoplasia I [VAIN
I] (N89.0)
    vaginal intraepithelial neoplasia II [VAIN
II] (N89.1)
    vaginal intraepithelial neoplasia III [VAIN
III] (D07.2)
    severe dysplasia of cervix uteri
(histologically confirmed) (D06.-)
    severe dysplasia of vagina (histologically
confirmed) (D07.2)

● R87.8   **Other** abnormal findings in specimens from female
genital organs
  ● R87.81   **High risk human papillomavirus (HPV) DNA
test positive from female genital organs**
    Excludes1   anogenital warts due to human
papillomavirus (HPV)
(A63.0)
    condyloma acuminatum (A63.0)

    R87.810   **Cervical high risk human
papillomavirus (HPV) DNA test
positive** ♀

    R87.811   **Vaginal high risk human
papillomavirus (HPV) DNA test
positive** ♀

  ● R87.82   **Low risk human papillomavirus (HPV) DNA
test positive from female genital organs**
    Use additional code for associated human
papillomavirus (B97.7)

    R87.820   **Cervical low risk human
papillomavirus (HPV) DNA test
positive** ♀

    R87.821   **Vaginal low risk human
papillomavirus (HPV) DNA test
positive** ♀

  R87.89   **Other** abnormal findings in specimens from
female genital organs ♀
    Abnormal chromosomal findings in specimens
from female genital organs

R87.9   **Unspecified** abnormal finding in specimens from female
genital organs ♀

● R88   Abnormal findings in other body fluids and substances
  R88.0   Cloudy (hemodialysis) (peritoneal) dialysis effluent
  R88.8   Abnormal findings in other body fluids and substances

● R89   Abnormal findings in specimens from **other organs, systems
and tissues**
    Includes   abnormal findings in nipple discharge
abnormal findings in synovial fluid
abnormal findings in wound secretions

  R89.0   Abnormal level of **enzymes** in specimens from other
organs, systems and tissues

  R89.1   Abnormal level of **hormones** in specimens from other
organs, systems and tissues

  R89.2   Abnormal level of **other drugs, medicaments and
biological substances** in specimens from other organs,
systems and tissues

  R89.3   Abnormal level of **substances chiefly nonmedicinal** as
to source in specimens from other organs, systems and
tissues

  R89.4   Abnormal **immunological** findings in specimens from
other organs, systems and tissues

  R89.5   Abnormal **microbiological** findings in specimens from
other organs, systems and tissues
    Positive culture findings in specimens from other
organs, systems and tissues
    Excludes1   colonization status (Z22.-)

  R89.6   Abnormal **cytological** findings in specimens from other
organs, systems and tissues

  R89.7   Abnormal **histological** findings in specimens from other
organs, systems and tissues

  R89.8   **Other** abnormal findings in specimens from other
organs, systems and tissues
    Abnormal chromosomal findings in specimens from
other organs, systems and tissues

  R89.9   **Unspecified** abnormal finding in specimens from other
organs, systems and tissues

ABNORMAL FINDINGS ON DIAGNOSTIC IMAGING AND IN
FUNCTION STUDIES, WITHOUT DIAGNOSIS (R90-R94)

    Includes   nonspecific abnormal findings on diagnostic
imaging by computerized axial tomography
[CAT scan]
nonspecific abnormal findings on diagnostic
imaging by magnetic resonance imaging
[MRI][NMR]
nonspecific abnormal findings on diagnostic
imaging by positron emission tomography
[PET scan]
nonspecific abnormal findings on diagnostic
imaging by thermography
nonspecific abnormal findings on diagnostic
imaging by ultrasound [echogram]
nonspecific abnormal findings on diagnostic
imaging by X-ray examination

    Excludes1   abnormal findings on antenatal screening of
mother (O28.-)
diagnostic abnormal findings classified elsewhere
- see Alphabetical Index

● R90   Abnormal findings on **diagnostic imaging of central nervous
system**
  R90.0   **Intracranial** space-occupying lesion found on diagnostic
imaging of central nervous system
  ● R90.8   Other abnormal findings on diagnostic imaging of
central nervous system
    R90.81   Abnormal echoencephalogram
    R90.82   White matter disease, **unspecified**
    R90.89   **Other** abnormal findings on diagnostic imaging
of central nervous system
    Other cerebrovascular abnormality found on
diagnostic imaging of central nervous
system

▶ New   ⇒ Revised   ~~deleted~~ Deleted   Excludes 1   Excludes 2   Includes   Use additional   Code first   Code also   Key words
OGCR Official Guidelines   X Assign placeholder X   ● Use Additional Character(s)   ▌ Manifestation Code   🅒🅒 Hierarchical Condition Category   **Coding Clinic**

● **R91**   **Abnormal findings on diagnostic imaging of lung**

     R91.1   **Solitary pulmonary nodule**
          Coin lesion lung
          Solitary pulmonary nodule, subsegmental branch of the bronchial tree

     R91.8   **Other nonspecific abnormal finding of lung field**
          Lung mass NOS found on diagnostic imaging of lung
          Pulmonary infiltrate NOS
          Shadow, lung

● **R92**   **Abnormal and inconclusive findings on diagnostic imaging of breast**

     R92.0   **Mammographic microcalcification found on diagnostic imaging of breast**
          Excludes2   mammographic calcification (calculus) found on diagnostic imaging of breast (R92.1)

     R92.1   **Mammographic calcification found on diagnostic imaging of breast**
          Mammographic calculus found on diagnostic imaging of breast

     R92.2   **Inconclusive mammogram**
          Dense breasts NOS
          Inconclusive mammogram NEC
          Inconclusive mammography due to dense breasts
          Inconclusive mammography NEC
          Coding Clinic: 2015, Q1, P24

     R92.8   **Other abnormal and inconclusive findings on diagnostic imaging of breast**

● **R93**   **Abnormal findings on diagnostic imaging of other body structures**

     R93.0   **Abnormal findings on diagnostic imaging of skull and head, not elsewhere classified**
          Excludes1   intracranial space-occupying lesion found on diagnostic imaging (R90.0)

     R93.1   **Abnormal findings on diagnostic imaging of heart and coronary circulation**
          Abnormal echocardiogram NOS
          Abnormal heart shadow

     R93.2   **Abnormal findings on diagnostic imaging of liver and biliary tract**
          Nonvisualization of gallbladder

     R93.3   **Abnormal findings on diagnostic imaging of other parts of digestive tract**

    ● **R93.4**   **Abnormal findings on diagnostic imaging of urinary organs**
          Excludes2   hypertrophy of kidney (N28.81)
          Coding Clinic: 2016, Q4, P66

         R93.41   **Abnormal radiologic findings on diagnostic imaging of renal pelvis, ureter, or bladder**
             Filling defect of bladder found on diagnostic imaging
             Filling defect of renal pelvis found on diagnostic imaging
             Filling defect of ureter found on diagnostic imaging

      ● **R93.42**   **Abnormal radiologic findings on diagnostic imaging of kidney**
            R93.421   **Abnormal radiologic findings on diagnostic imaging of right kidney**
            R93.422   **Abnormal radiologic findings on diagnostic imaging of left kidney**
            R93.429   **Abnormal radiologic findings on diagnostic imaging of unspecified kidney**

         R93.49   **Abnormal radiologic findings on diagnostic imaging of other urinary organs**

     R93.5   **Abnormal findings on diagnostic imaging of other abdominal regions, including retroperitoneum**

     R93.6   **Abnormal findings on diagnostic imaging of limbs**
          Excludes2   abnormal finding in skin and subcutaneous tissue (R93.8-)
          Coding Clinic: 2020, Q1, P14

     R93.7   **Abnormal findings on diagnostic imaging of other parts of musculoskeletal system**
          Excludes2   abnormal findings on diagnostic imaging of skull (R93.0)

    ● **R93.8**   **Abnormal findings on diagnostic imaging of other specified body structures**

      ● **R93.81**   **Abnormal radiologic findings on diagnostic imaging of testis**
            R93.811   **Abnormal radiologic findings on diagnostic imaging of right testicle** ♂
            R93.812   **Abnormal radiologic findings on diagnostic imaging of left testicle** ♂
            R93.813   **Abnormal radiologic findings on diagnostic imaging of testicles, bilateral** ♂
            R93.819   **Abnormal radiologic findings on diagnostic imaging of unspecified testicle** ♂

         R93.89   **Abnormal findings on diagnostic imaging of other specified body structures**
             Abnormal finding by radioisotope localization of placenta
             Abnormal radiological finding in skin and subcutaneous tissue
             Mediastinal shift

     R93.9   **Diagnostic imaging inconclusive due to excess body fat of patient**

● **R94**   **Abnormal results of function studies**
        Includes   abnormal results of radionuclide [radioisotope] uptake studies
             abnormal results of scintigraphy

    ● **R94.0**   **Abnormal results of function studies of central nervous system**
         R94.01   **Abnormal electroencephalogram [EEG]**
         R94.02   **Abnormal brain scan**
         R94.09   **Abnormal results of other function studies of central nervous system**

    ● **R94.1**   **Abnormal results of function studies of peripheral nervous system and special senses**

      ● **R94.11**   **Abnormal results of function studies of eye**
            R94.110   **Abnormal electro-oculogram [EOG]**
            R94.111   **Abnormal electroretinogram [ERG]**
               Abnormal retinal function study
            R94.112   **Abnormal visually evoked potential [VEP]**
            R94.113   **Abnormal oculomotor study**
            R94.118   **Abnormal results of other function studies of eye**

      ● **R94.12**   **Abnormal results of function studies of ear and other special senses**
            R94.120   **Abnormal auditory function study**
               Coding Clinic: 2016, Q3, P17
            R94.121   **Abnormal vestibular function study**
            R94.128   **Abnormal results of other function studies of ear and other special senses**

Figure 18-2 Cranial nerves. (From Patton and Thibodeau: Anatomy and physiology, ed 7, St. Louis, Mosby, 2009)

Trochlear nerve (IV)
Optic nerve (II)
Olfactory nerve (I)
Abducens nerve (VI)
Oculomotor nerve (III)
Facial nerve (VII)
Trigeminal nerve (V)
Vestibulocochlear nerve (VIII)
Glossopharyngeal nerve (IX)
Vagus nerve (X)
Accessory nerve (XI)
Hypoglossal nerve (XII)

CHAPTER 18 (R00-R99)

Item 18-1 The **peripheral nervous system** consists of 31 pairs of spinal nerves, 12 pairs of cranial nerves, and the autonomic nerves, which are divided into the parasympathetic and sympathetic nerves. The cranial nerves are: olfactory (I), optic (II), oculomotor (III), trochlear (IV), trigeminal (V), abducens (VI), facial (VII), vestibulocochlear (VIII), glossopharyngeal (IX), vagus (X), accessory (XI), and hypoglossal (XII).

● R94.13　Abnormal results of function studies of peripheral nervous system

　　R94.130　Abnormal response to nerve stimulation, unspecified

　　R94.131　Abnormal electromyogram [EMG]
　　　　　　Excludes1　electromyogram of eye (R94.113)

　　R94.138　Abnormal results of other function studies of peripheral nervous system

　R94.2　Abnormal results of pulmonary function studies
　　　　Reduced ventilatory capacity
　　　　Reduced vital capacity

● R94.3　Abnormal results of cardiovascular function studies

　　R94.30　Abnormal result of cardiovascular function study, unspecified

　　R94.31　Abnormal electrocardiogram [ECG] [EKG]
　　　　　　Excludes1　long QT syndrome (I45.81)

　　R94.39　Abnormal result of other cardiovascular function study
　　　　　　Abnormal electrophysiological intracardiac studies
　　　　　　Abnormal phonocardiogram
　　　　　　Abnormal vectorcardiogram

　R94.4　Abnormal results of kidney function studies
　　　　Abnormal renal function test

　R94.5　Abnormal results of liver function studies

　R94.6　Abnormal results of thyroid function studies

　R94.7　Abnormal results of other endocrine function studies
　　　　　　Excludes2　abnormal glucose (R73.0-)

　R94.8　Abnormal results of function studies of other organs and systems
　　　　Abnormal basal metabolic rate [BMR]
　　　　Abnormal bladder function test
　　　　Abnormal splenic function test

ABNORMAL TUMOR MARKERS (R97)

● R97　Abnormal tumor markers
　　　Elevated tumor associated antigens [TAA]
　　　Elevated tumor specific antigens [TSA]

　R97.0　Elevated carcinoembryonic antigen [CEA]

　R97.1　Elevated cancer antigen 125 [CA 125]

● R97.2　Elevated prostate specific antigen [PSA]
　　　　Coding Clinic: 2016, Q4, P66

　　　R97.20　Elevated prostate specific antigen [PSA] ♂　　A

　　　R97.21　Rising PSA following treatment for malignant neoplasm of prostate ♂　　A

　R97.8　Other abnormal tumor markers

ILL-DEFINED AND UNKNOWN CAUSE OF MORTALITY (R99)

R99　Ill-defined and unknown cause of mortality
　　　Death (unexplained) NOS
　　　Unspecified cause of mortality

OGCR Section I.C.18.h.

Death NOS

Code R99, Ill-defined and unknown cause of mortality, is only for use in the very limited circumstance when a patient who has already died is brought into the emergency department or other healthcare facility and is pronounced dead upon arrival. It does not represent the discharge disposition of death.

▶ New　⇒ Revised　~~deleted~~ Deleted　Excludes 1　Excludes 2　Includes　Use additional　Code first　Code also　Key words
OGCR Official Guidelines　X Assign placeholder X　● Use Additional Character(s)　▷ Manifestation Code　🐾 Hierarchical Condition Category　**Coding Clinic**

CHAPTER 19

INJURY, POISONING AND CERTAIN OTHER CONSEQUENCES OF EXTERNAL CAUSES (S00-T88)

OGCR Chapter-Specific Coding Guidelines

19. Chapter 19: Injury, poisoning, and certain other consequences of external causes (S00-T88)

a. Application of 7th Characters in Chapter 19

Most categories in Chapter 19 have a 7th character requirement for each applicable code. Most categories in this chapter have three 7th character values (with the exception of fractures): A, initial encounter, D, subsequent encounter and S, sequela. Categories for traumatic fractures have additional 7th character values. While the patient may be seen by a new or different provider over the course of treatment for an injury, assignment of the 7th character is based on whether the patient is undergoing active treatment and not whether the provider is seeing the patient for the first time.

For complication codes, active treatment refers to treatment for the condition described by the code, even though it may be related to an earlier precipitating problem. For example, code T84.50XA, Infection and inflammatory reaction due to unspecified internal joint prosthesis, initial encounter, is used when active treatment is provided for the infection, even though the condition relates to the prosthetic device, implant or graft that was placed at a previous encounter.

7th character "A", initial encounter is used for each encounter where the patient is receiving active treatment for the condition.

7th character "D" subsequent encounter is used for encounters after the patient has completed active treatment of the condition and is receiving routine care for the condition during the healing or recovery phase.

The aftercare Z codes should not be used for aftercare for conditions such as injuries or poisonings, where 7th characters are provided to identify subsequent care. For example, for aftercare of an injury, assign the acute injury code with the 7th character "D" (subsequent encounter).

7th character "S", sequela, is for use for complications or conditions that arise as a direct result of a condition, such as scar formation after a burn. The scars are sequelae of the burn. When using 7th character "S", it is necessary to use both the injury code that precipitated the sequela and the code for the sequela itself. The "S" is added only to the injury code, not the sequela code. The 7th character "S" identifies the injury responsible for the sequela. The specific type of sequela (e.g. scar) is sequenced first, followed by the injury code.

See Section I.B.10. Sequelae, (Late Effects).

b. Coding of Injuries

When coding injuries, assign separate codes for each injury unless a combination code is provided, in which case the combination code is assigned. Codes from category T07, Unspecified multiple injuries should not be assigned in the inpatient setting unless information for a more specific code is not available. Traumatic injury codes (S00-T14.9) are not to be used for normal, healing surgical wounds or to identify complications of surgical wounds.

The code for the most serious injury, as determined by the provider and the focus of treatment, is sequenced first.

1) Superficial injuries

Superficial injuries such as abrasions or contusions are not coded when associated with more severe injuries of the same site.

2) Primary injury with damage to nerves/blood vessels

When a primary injury results in minor damage to peripheral nerves or blood vessels, the primary injury is sequenced first with additional code(s) for injuries to nerves and spinal cord (such as category S04), and/or injury to blood vessels (such as category S15). When the primary injury is to the blood vessels or nerves, that injury should be sequenced first.

c. Coding of Traumatic Fractures

The principles of multiple coding of injuries should be followed in coding fractures. Fractures of specified sites are coded individually by site in accordance with both the provisions within categories S02, S12, S22, S32, S42, S49, S52, S59, S62, S72, S79, S82, S89, S92 and the level of detail furnished by medical record content.

A fracture not indicated as open or closed should be coded to closed. A fracture not indicated whether displaced or not displaced should be coded to displaced.

More specific guidelines are as follows:

1) Initial vs. Subsequent Encounter for Fractures

Traumatic fractures are coded using the appropriate 7th character for initial encounter (A, B, C) for each encounter where the patient is receiving active treatment for the fracture. The appropriate 7th character for initial encounter should also be assigned for a patient who delayed seeking treatment for the fracture or nonunion.

Fractures are coded using the appropriate 7th character for subsequent care for encounters after the patient has completed active treatment of the fracture and is receiving routine care for the fracture during the healing or recovery phase.

Care for complications of surgical treatment for fracture repairs during the healing or recovery phase should be coded with the appropriate complication codes.

Care of complications of fractures, such as malunion and nonunion, should be reported with the appropriate 7th character for subsequent care with nonunion (K, M, N,) or subsequent care with malunion (P, Q, R).

Malunion/nonunion: The appropriate 7th character for initial encounter should also be assigned for a patient who delayed seeking treatment for the fracture or nonunion.

The open fracture designations in the assignment of the 7th character for fractures of the forearm, femur and lower leg, including ankle are based on the Gustilo open fracture classification. When the Gustilo classification type is not specified for an open fracture, the 7th character for open fracture type I or II should be assigned (B, E, H, M, Q).

A code from category M80, not a traumatic fracture code, should be used for any patient with known osteoporosis who suffers a fracture, even if the patient had a minor fall or trauma, if that fall or trauma would not usually break a normal, healthy bone.

See Section I.C.13. Osteoporosis.

The aftercare Z codes should not be used for aftercare for traumatic fractures. For aftercare of a traumatic fracture, assign the acute fracture code with the appropriate 7th character.

2) Multiple fractures sequencing

Multiple fractures are sequenced in accordance with the severity of the fracture.

d. Coding of Burns and Corrosions

The ICD-10-CM makes a distinction between burns and corrosions. The burn codes are for thermal burns, except sunburns, that come from a heat source, such as a fire or hot appliance. The burn codes are also for burns resulting from electricity and radiation. Corrosions are burns due to chemicals. The guidelines are the same for burns and corrosions.

Current burns (T20-T25) are classified by depth, extent and by agent (X code). Burns are classified by depth as first degree (erythema), second degree (blistering), and third degree (full-thickness involvement). Burns of the eye and internal organs (T26-T28) are classified by site, but not by degree.

1) Sequencing of burn and related condition codes

Sequence first the code that reflects the highest degree of burn when more than one burn is present.

    a. When the reason for the admission or encounter is for treatment of external multiple burns, sequence first the code that reflects the burn of the highest degree.

    b. When a patient has both internal and external burns, the circumstances of admission govern the selection of the principal diagnosis or first-listed diagnosis.

    c. When a patient is admitted for burn injuries and other related conditions such as smoke inhalation and/or respiratory failure, the circumstances of admission govern the selection of the principal or first-listed diagnosis.

2) Burns of the same *anatomic* site

Classify burns of the same anatomic site and on the same side but of different degrees to the subcategory identifying the highest degree recorded in the diagnosis (e.g., for second- and third-degree burns of right thigh, assign only code T24.311-).

3) Non-healing burns

Non-healing burns are coded as acute burns.

Necrosis of burned skin should be coded as a non-healed burn.

4) Infected Burn

For any documented infected burn site, use an additional code for the infection.

5) Assign separate codes for each burn site

When coding burns, assign separate codes for each burn site. Category T30, Burn and corrosion, body region unspecified is extremely vague and should rarely be used.

Codes for burns of "multiple sites" should only be assigned when the medical record documentation does not specify the individual sites.

6) Burns and Corrosions Classified According to Extent of Body Surface Involved

Assign codes from category T31, Burns classified according to extent of body surface involved, or T32, Corrosions classified according to extent of body surface involved, when the site of the burn is not specified or when there is a need for additional data. It is advisable to use category T31 as additional coding when needed to provide data for evaluating burn mortality, such as that needed by burn units. It is also advisable to use category T31 as an additional code for reporting purposes when there is mention of a third-degree burn involving 20 percent or more of the body surface.

Categories T31 and T32 are based on the classic "rule of nines" in estimating body surface involved: head and neck are assigned nine percent, each arm nine percent, each leg 18 percent, the anterior trunk 18 percent, posterior trunk 18 percent, and genitalia one percent. Providers may change these percentage assignments where necessary to accommodate infants and children who have proportionally larger heads than adults, and patients who have large buttocks, thighs, or abdomen that involve burns.

7) Encounters for treatment of sequela of burns

Encounters for the treatment of the late effects of burns or corrosions (i.e., scars or joint contractures) should be coded with a burn or corrosion code with the 7th character "S" for sequela.

8) Sequelae with a late effect code and current burn

When appropriate, both a code for a current burn or corrosion with 7th character "A" or "D" and a burn or corrosion code with 7th character "S" may be assigned on the same record (when both a current burn and sequelae of an old burn exist). Burns and corrosions do not heal at the same rate and a current healing wound may still exist with sequela of a healed burn or corrosion.
See Section I.B.10. Sequela, (Late Effects).

9) Use of an external cause code with burns and corrosions

An external cause code should be used with burns and corrosions to identify the source and intent of the burn, as well as the place where it occurred.

e. Adverse Effects, Poisoning , Underdosing and Toxic Effects

Codes in categories T36-T65 are combination codes that include the substance that was taken as well as the intent. No additional external cause code is required for poisonings, toxic effects, adverse effects and underdosing codes.

1) Do not code directly from the Table of Drugs

Do not code directly from the Table of Drugs and Chemicals. Always refer back to the Tabular List.

2) Use as many codes as necessary to describe

Use as many codes as necessary to describe completely all drugs, medicinal or biological substances.

3) If the same code would describe the causative agent

If the same code would describe the causative agent for more than one adverse reaction, poisoning, toxic effect or underdosing, assign the code only once.

4) If two or more drugs, medicinal or biological substances

If two or more drugs, medicinal or biological substances are reported, code each individually unless a combination code is listed in the Table of Drugs and Chemicals.

5) The occurrence of drug toxicity is classified in ICD-10-CM as follows:

(a) Adverse Effect

When coding an adverse effect of a drug that has been correctly prescribed and properly administered, assign the appropriate code for the nature of the adverse effect followed by the appropriate code for the adverse effect of the drug (T36-T50). The code for the drug should have a 5th or 6th character "5" (for example T36.0X5-) Examples of the nature of an adverse effect are tachycardia, delirium, gastrointestinal hemorrhaging, vomiting, hypokalemia, hepatitis, renal failure, or respiratory failure.

(b) Poisoning

When coding a poisoning or reaction to the improper use of a medication (e.g., overdose, wrong substance given or taken in error, wrong route of administration), first assign the appropriate code from categories T36-T50. The poisoning codes have an associated intent as their 5th or 6th character (accidental, intentional self-harm, assault and undetermined). If the intent of the poisoning is unknown or unspecified, code the intent as accidental intent. The undetermined intent is only for use if the documentation in the record specifies that the intent cannot be determined. Use additional code(s) for all manifestations of poisonings.

If there is also a diagnosis of abuse or dependence of the substance, the abuse or dependence is assigned as an additional code.

Examples of poisoning include:

(i) Error was made in drug prescription
Errors made in drug prescription or in the administration of the drug by provider, nurse, patient, or other person.

(ii) Overdose of a drug intentionally taken If an overdose of a drug was intentionally taken or administered and resulted in drug toxicity, it would be coded as a poisoning.

(iii) Nonprescribed drug taken with correctly prescribed and properly administered drug. If a nonprescribed drug or medicinal agent was taken in combination with a correctly prescribed and properly administered drug, any drug toxicity or other reaction resulting from the interaction of the two drugs would be classified as a poisoning.

(iv) Interaction of drug(s) and alcohol.
When a reaction results from the interaction of a drug(s) and alcohol, this would be classified as poisoning.

See Section I.C.4. if poisoning is the result of insulin pump malfunctions.

(c) Underdosing

Underdosing refers to taking less of a medication than is prescribed by a provider or a manufacturer's instruction. Discontinuing the use of a prescribed medication on the patient's own initiative (not directed by the patient's provider) is also classified as an underdosing. For underdosing, assign the code from categories T36-T50 (fifth or sixth character "6").

Codes for underdosing should never be assigned as principal or first-listed codes. If a patient has a relapse or exacerbation of the medical condition for which the drug is prescribed because of the reduction in dose, then the medical condition itself should be coded.

Noncompliance (Z91.12-, Z91.13- and Z91.14-) or complication of care (Y63.6-Y63.9) codes are to be used with an underdosing code to indicate intent, if known.

(d) Toxic Effects
When a harmful substance is ingested or comes in contact with a person, this is classified as a toxic effect. The toxic effect codes are in categories T51-T65.

Toxic effect codes have an associated intent: accidental, intentional self-harm, assault and undetermined.

f. Adult and child abuse, neglect and other maltreatment
Sequence first the appropriate code from categories T74 (Adult and child abuse, neglect and other maltreatment, confirmed) or T76 (Adult and child abuse, neglect and other maltreatment, suspected) for abuse, neglect and other maltreatment, followed by any accompanying mental health or injury code(s).

If the documentation in the medical record states abuse or neglect it is coded as confirmed (T74.-). It is coded as suspected if it is documented as suspected (T76.-).

For cases of confirmed abuse or neglect an external cause code from the assault section (X92-Y09) should be added to identify the cause of any physical injuries. A perpetrator code (Y07) should be added when the perpetrator of the abuse is known. For suspected cases of abuse or neglect, do not report external cause or perpetrator code.

If a suspected case of abuse, neglect or mistreatment is ruled out during an encounter code Z04.71, Encounter for examination and observation following alleged physical adult abuse, ruled out, or code Z04.72, Encounter for examination and observation following alleged child physical abuse, ruled out, should be used, not a code from T76.

If a suspected case of alleged rape or sexual abuse is ruled out during an encounter code Z04.41, Encounter for examination and observation following alleged adult rape or code Z04.42, Encounter for examination and observation following alleged child rape, should be used, not a code from T76.

If a suspected case of forced sexual exploitation or forced labor exploitation is ruled out during an encounter, code Z04.81, Encounter for examination and observation of victim following forced sexual exploitation, or code Z04.82, Encounter for examination and observation of victim following forced labor exploitation, should be used, not a code from T76.

See Section I.C.15. Abuse in a pregnant patient.

g. Complications of care
1) General guidelines for complications of care
(a) Documentation of complications of care
See Section I.B.16. for information on documentation of complications of care.

2) Pain due to medical devices
Pain associated with devices, implants or grafts left in a surgical site (for example painful hip prosthesis) is assigned to the appropriate code(s) found in Chapter 19, Injury, poisoning, and certain other consequences of external causes. Specific codes for pain due to medical devices are found in the T code section of the ICD-10-CM. Use additional code(s) from category G89 to identify acute or chronic pain due to presence of the device, implant or graft (G89.18 or G89.28).

3) Transplant complications
(a) Transplant complications other than kidney
Codes under category T86, Complications of transplanted organs and tissues, are for use for both complications and rejection of transplanted organs. A transplant complication code is only assigned if the complication affects the function of the transplanted organ. Two codes are required to fully describe a transplant complication: the appropriate code from category T86 and a secondary code that identifies the complication.

Pre-existing conditions or conditions that develop after the transplant are not coded as complications unless they affect the function of the transplanted organs.

See I.C.21. for transplant organ removal status.
See I.C.2. for malignant neoplasm associated with transplanted organ.

(b) Kidney transplant complications
Patients who have undergone kidney transplant may still have some form of chronic kidney disease (CKD) because the kidney transplant may not fully restore kidney function. Code T86.1- should be assigned for documented complications of a kidney transplant, such as transplant failure or rejection or other transplant complication. Code T86.1- should not be assigned for post kidney transplant patients who have chronic kidney (CKD) unless a transplant complication such as transplant failure or rejection is documented. If the documentation is unclear as to whether the patient has a complication of the transplant, query the provider.

Conditions that affect the function of the transplanted kidney, other than CKD, should be assigned a code from subcategory T86.1, Complications of transplanted organ, Kidney, and a secondary code that identifies the complication.

For patients with CKD following a kidney transplant, but who do not have a complication such as failure or rejection, *see Section I.C.14. Chronic kidney disease and kidney transplant status.*

4) Complication codes that include the external cause
As with certain other T codes, some of the complications of care codes have the external cause included in the code. The code includes the nature of the complication as well as the type of procedure that caused the complication. No external cause code indicating the type of procedure is necessary for these codes.

5) Complications of care codes within the body system chapters
Intraoperative and postprocedural complication codes are found within the body system chapters with codes specific to the organs and structures of that body system. These codes should be sequenced first, followed by a code(s) for the specific complication, if applicable.

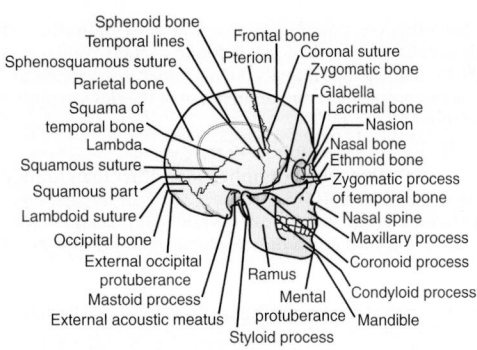

Figure 19-1 Lateral view of skull.

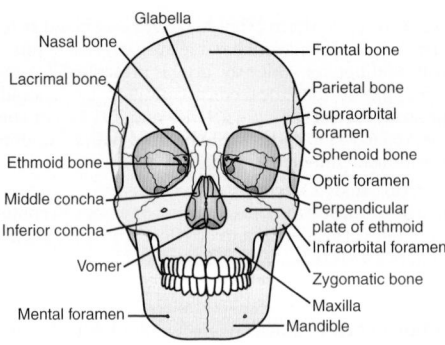

Figure 19-2 Frontal view of skull.

Figure 19-3 Anterior view of vertebral column.

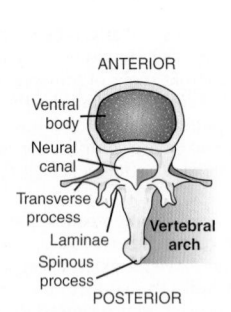

Figure 19-4 Vertebra viewed from above.

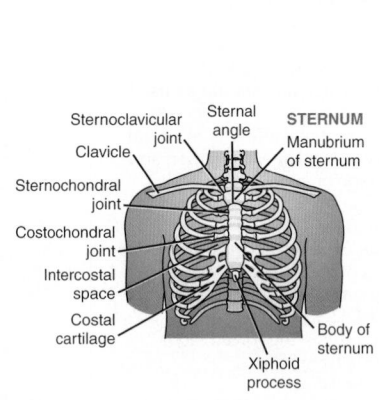

Figure 19-5 Anterior view of rib cage.

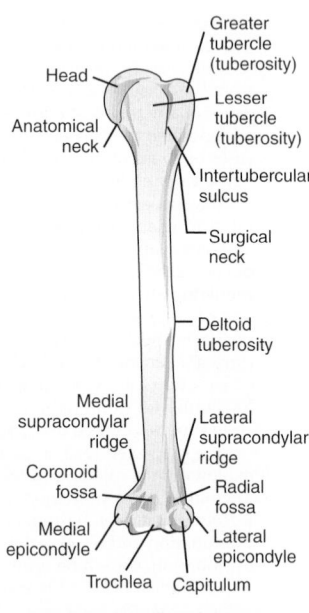

Figure 19-6 Anterior aspect of left humerus.

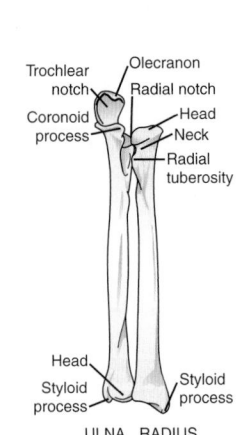

Figure 19-7 Anterior aspect of left radius and ulna.

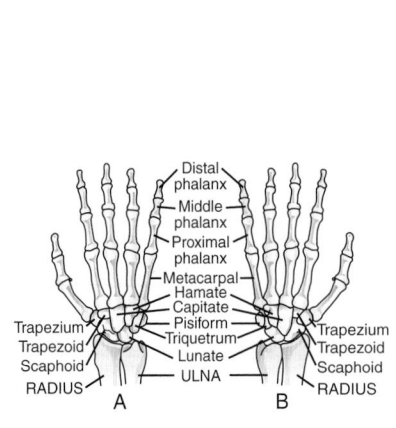

Figure 19-8 Right hand and wrist: **A.** Dorsal surface. **B.** Palmar surface.

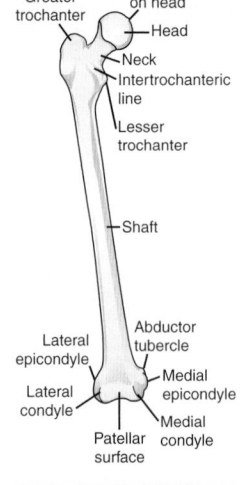

Figure 19-9 Anterior aspect of right femur.

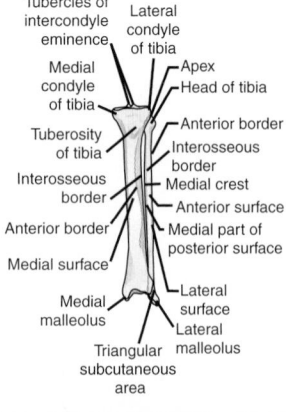

Figure 19-10 Anterior aspect of left tibia and fibula.

▶ New   ⇒ Revised   deleted Deleted   Excludes 1   Excludes 2   Includes   Use additional   Code first   Code also   Key words

OGCR Official Guidelines   X Assign placeholder X   ● Use Additional Character(s)   ▶ Manifestation Code   Hierarchical Condition Category   **Coding Clinic**

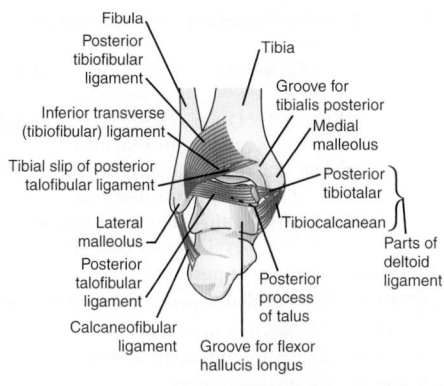

Figure 19-11 Posterior aspect of the left ankle joint.

Figure 19-12 Right foot viewed from above.

CHAPTER 19

INJURY, POISONING AND CERTAIN OTHER CONSEQUENCES OF EXTERNAL CAUSES (S00-T88)

Note: Use secondary code(s) from Chapter 20, External causes of morbidity, to indicate cause of injury. Codes within the T section that include the external cause do not require an additional external cause code.

Use additional code to identify any retained foreign body, if applicable (Z18.-)

Excludes1   birth trauma (P10-P15)
               obstetric trauma (O70-O71)

Note: The chapter uses the S-section for coding different types of injuries related to single body regions and the T-section to cover injuries to unspecified body regions as well as poisoning and certain other consequences of external causes.

This chapter contains the following blocks:

S00-S09	Injuries to the head
S10-S19	Injuries to the neck
S20-S29	Injuries to the thorax
S30-S39	Injuries to the abdomen, lower back, lumbar spine, pelvis and external genitals
S40-S49	Injuries to the shoulder and upper arm
S50-S59	Injuries to the elbow and forearm
S60-S69	Injuries to the wrist, hand, and fingers
S70-S79	Injuries to the hip and thigh
S80-S89	Injuries to the knee and lower leg
S90-S99	Injuries to the ankle and foot

T07	Injuries involving multiple body regions
T14	Injury of unspecified body region
T15-T19	Effects of foreign body entering through natural orifice
T20-T25	Burns and corrosions of external body surface, specified by site
T26-T28	Burns and corrosions confined to eye and internal organs
T30-T32	Burns and corrosions of multiple and unspecified body regions
T33-T34	Frostbite
T36-T50	Poisoning by, adverse effect of and underdosing of drugs, medicaments and biological substances
T51-T65	Toxic effects of substances chiefly nonmedicinal as to source
T66-T78	Other and unspecified effects of external causes
T79	Certain early complications of trauma
T80-T88	Complications of surgical and medical care, not elsewhere classified

INJURIES TO THE HEAD (S00-S09)

Includes   injuries of ear
               injuries of eye
               injuries of face [any part]
               injuries of gum
               injuries of jaw
               injuries of oral cavity
               injuries of palate
               injuries of periocular area
               injuries of scalp
               injuries of temporomandibular joint area
               injuries of tongue
               injuries of tooth

Code also for any associated infection

Excludes2   burns and corrosions (T20-T32)
             effects of foreign body in ear (T16)
             effects of foreign body in larynx (T17.3)
             effects of foreign body in mouth NOS (T18.0)
             effects of foreign body in nose (T17.0-T17.1)
             effects of foreign body in pharynx (T17.2)
             effects of foreign body on external eye (T15.-)
             frostbite (T33-T34)
             insect bite or sting, venomous (T63.4)

● **S00**   **Superficial injury of head**

    Excludes1   diffuse cerebral contusion (S06.2-)
             focal cerebral contusion (S06.3-)
             injury of eye and orbit (S05.-)
             open wound of head (S01.-)

The appropriate 7th character is to be added to each code from category S00

A	initial encounter *All encounters involving diagnosis and treatment*
D	subsequent encounter *Encounters during the healing phase*
S	sequela

● **S00.0**   **Superficial injury of scalp**

  X ● **S00.00**   **Unspecified superficial injury of scalp**

  X ● **S00.01**   **Abrasion of scalp**

  X ● **S00.02**   **Blister (nonthermal) of scalp**

  X ● **S00.03**   **Contusion of scalp**
                  Bruise of scalp
                  Hematoma of scalp

  X ● **S00.04**   **External constriction of part of scalp**

  X ● **S00.05**   **Superficial foreign body of scalp**
                  Splinter in the scalp

  X ● **S00.06**   **Insect bite (nonvenomous) of scalp**

  X ● **S00.07**   **Other superficial bite of scalp**

        Excludes1   open bite of scalp (S01.05)

● **S00.1** ▸ Contusion of eyelid and periocular area
       Black eye
     ⇨ **Excludes2**   contusion of eyeball and orbital tissues
                         (S05.1-)

X ● **S00.10**   Contusion of unspecified eyelid and periocular area

X ● **S00.11**   Contusion of right eyelid and periocular area

X ● **S00.12**   Contusion of left eyelid and periocular area

● **S00.2**   Other and unspecified superficial injuries of eyelid and periocular area
     Excludes2   superficial injury of conjunctiva and
                       cornea (S05.0-)

   ● **S00.20**   Unspecified superficial injury of eyelid and periocular area

     ● **S00.201**   Unspecified superficial injury of right eyelid and periocular area

     ● **S00.202**   Unspecified superficial injury of left eyelid and periocular area

     ● **S00.209**   Unspecified superficial injury of unspecified eyelid and periocular area

   ● **S00.21**   Abrasion of eyelid and periocular area

     ● **S00.211**   Abrasion of right eyelid and periocular area

     ● **S00.212**   Abrasion of left eyelid and periocular area

     ● **S00.219**   Abrasion of unspecified eyelid and periocular area

   ● **S00.22**   Blister (nonthermal) of eyelid and periocular area

     ● **S00.221**   Blister (nonthermal) of right eyelid and periocular area

     ● **S00.222**   Blister (nonthermal) of left eyelid and periocular area

     ● **S00.229**   Blister (nonthermal) of unspecified eyelid and periocular area

   ● **S00.24**   External constriction of eyelid and periocular area

     ● **S00.241**   External constriction of right eyelid and periocular area

     ● **S00.242**   External constriction of left eyelid and periocular area

     ● **S00.249**   External constriction of unspecified eyelid and periocular area

   ● **S00.25**   Superficial foreign body of eyelid and periocular area
          Splinter of eyelid and periocular area
       Excludes2   retained foreign body in eyelid
                       (H02.81-)

     ● **S00.251**   Superficial foreign body of right eyelid and periocular area

     ● **S00.252**   Superficial foreign body of left eyelid and periocular area

     ● **S00.259**   Superficial foreign body of unspecified eyelid and periocular area

   ● **S00.26**   Insect bite (nonvenomous) of eyelid and periocular area

     ● **S00.261**   Insect bite (nonvenomous) of right eyelid and periocular area

     ● **S00.262**   Insect bite (nonvenomous) of left eyelid and periocular area

     ● **S00.269**   Insect bite (nonvenomous) of unspecified eyelid and periocular area

● **S00.27**   Other superficial bite of eyelid and periocular area
     Excludes1   open bite of eyelid and
                       periocular area (S01.15)

   ● **S00.271**   Other superficial bite of right eyelid and periocular area

   ● **S00.272**   Other superficial bite of left eyelid and periocular area

   ● **S00.279**   Other superficial bite of unspecified eyelid and periocular area

● **S00.3**   Superficial injury of nose

X ● **S00.30**   Unspecified superficial injury of nose

X ● **S00.31**   Abrasion of nose

X ● **S00.32**   Blister (nonthermal) of nose

X ● **S00.33**   Contusion of nose
          Bruise of nose
          Hematoma of nose

X ● **S00.34**   External constriction of nose

X ● **S00.35**   Superficial foreign body of nose
          Splinter in the nose

X ● **S00.36**   Insect bite (nonvenomous) of nose

X ● **S00.37**   Other superficial bite of nose
     Excludes1   open bite of nose (S01.25)

● **S00.4**   Superficial injury of ear

   ● **S00.40**   Unspecified superficial injury of ear

     ● **S00.401**   Unspecified superficial injury of right ear

     ● **S00.402**   Unspecified superficial injury of left ear

     ● **S00.409**   Unspecified superficial injury of unspecified ear

   ● **S00.41**   Abrasion of ear

     ● **S00.411**   Abrasion of right ear

     ● **S00.412**   Abrasion of left ear

     ● **S00.419**   Abrasion of unspecified ear

   ● **S00.42**   Blister (nonthermal) of ear

     ● **S00.421**   Blister (nonthermal) of right ear

     ● **S00.422**   Blister (nonthermal) of left ear

     ● **S00.429**   Blister (nonthermal) of unspecified ear

   ● **S00.43**   Contusion of ear
          Bruise of ear
          Hematoma of ear

     ● **S00.431**   Contusion of right ear

     ● **S00.432**   Contusion of left ear

     ● **S00.439**   Contusion of unspecified ear

   ● **S00.44**   External constriction of ear

     ● **S00.441**   External constriction of right ear

     ● **S00.442**   External constriction of left ear

     ● **S00.449**   External constriction of unspecified ear

   ● **S00.45**   Superficial foreign body of ear
          Splinter in the ear

     ● **S00.451**   Superficial foreign body of right ear

     ● **S00.452**   Superficial foreign body of left ear

     ● **S00.459**   Superficial foreign body of unspecified ear

   ● **S00.46**   Insect bite (nonvenomous) of ear

     ● **S00.461**   Insect bite (nonvenomous) of right ear

     ● **S00.462**   Insect bite (nonvenomous) of left ear

     ● **S00.469**   Insect bite (nonvenomous) of unspecified ear

● S00.47 **Other superficial bite** of ear
        Excludes1   open bite of ear (S01.35)
   ● S00.471 Other superficial bite of **right** ear
   ● S00.472 Other superficial bite of **left** ear
   ● S00.479 Other superficial bite of **unspecified** ear

● S00.5 **Superficial injury of lip and oral cavity**
  ● S00.50 **Unspecified** superficial injury of lip and oral cavity
   ● S00.501 Unspecified superficial injury of **lip**
   ● S00.502 Unspecified superficial injury of **oral cavity**
  ● S00.51 **Abrasion** of lip and oral cavity
   ● S00.511 Abrasion of **lip**
   ● S00.512 Abrasion of **oral cavity**
  ● S00.52 **Blister (nonthermal)** of lip and oral cavity
   ● S00.521 Blister (nonthermal) of **lip**
   ● S00.522 Blister (nonthermal) of **oral cavity**
  ● S00.53 **Contusion** of lip and oral cavity
   ● S00.531 Contusion of **lip**
      Bruise of lip
      Hematoma of lip
   ● S00.532 Contusion of **oral cavity**
      Bruise of oral cavity
      Hematoma of oral cavity
  ● S00.54 **External constriction** of lip and oral cavity
   ● S00.541 External constriction of **lip**
   ● S00.542 External constriction of **oral cavity**
  ● S00.55 **Superficial foreign body** of lip and oral cavity
   ● S00.551 Superficial foreign body of **lip**
      Splinter of lip and oral cavity
   ● S00.552 Superficial foreign body of **oral cavity**
      Splinter of lip and oral cavity
  ● S00.56 **Insect bite (nonvenomous)** of lip and oral cavity
   ● S00.561 Insect bite (nonvenomous) of **lip**
   ● S00.562 Insect bite (nonvenomous) of **oral cavity**
  ● S00.57 **Other superficial bite** of lip and oral cavity
   ● S00.571 Other superficial bite of **lip**
      Excludes1   open bite of lip (S01.551)
   ● S00.572 Other superficial bite of **oral cavity**
      Excludes1   open bite of oral cavity (S01.552)

● S00.8 **Superficial injury of other parts of head**
  Superficial injuries of face [any part]
  X ● S00.80 **Unspecified** superficial injury of other part of head
  X ● S00.81 **Abrasion** of other part of head
  X ● S00.82 **Blister (nonthermal)** of other part of head
  X ● S00.83 **Contusion** of other part of head
      Bruise of other part of head
      Hematoma of other part of head
  X ● S00.84 **External constriction** of other part of head
  X ● S00.85 **Superficial foreign body** of other part of head
      Splinter in other part of head
  X ● S00.86 **Insect bite (nonvenomous)** of other part of head
  X ● S00.87 **Other superficial bite** of other part of head
      Excludes1   open bite of other part of head (S01.85)

● S00.9 **Superficial injury of unspecified part of head**
  X ● S00.90 **Unspecified** superficial injury of unspecified part of head
  X ● S00.91 **Abrasion** of unspecified part of head
  X ● S00.92 **Blister (nonthermal)** of unspecified part of head

X ● S00.93 **Contusion** of unspecified part of head
     Bruise of head
     Hematoma of head
X ● S00.94 **External constriction** of unspecified part of head
X ● S00.95 **Superficial foreign body** of unspecified part of head
     Splinter of head
X ● S00.96 **Insect bite (nonvenomous)** of unspecified part of head
X ● S00.97 **Other superficial bite** of unspecified part of head
      Excludes1   open bite of head (S01.95)

● S01 **Open wound of head**
  Code also any associated:
    injury of cranial nerve (S04.-)
    injury of muscle and tendon of head (S09.1-)
    intracranial injury (S06.-)
    wound infection
    Excludes1   open skull fracture (S02.- with 7th character B)
    Excludes2   injury of eye and orbit (S05.-)
                traumatic amputation of part of head (S08.-)
  The appropriate 7th character is to be added to each code from category S01

    A   initial encounter
    D   subsequent encounter
    S   sequela

  ● S01.0 **Open wound of scalp**
    ➠ **Excludes1**   avulsion of scalp (S08.0-)
  X ● S01.00 **Unspecified** open wound of scalp
  X ● S01.01 **Laceration without foreign body** of scalp
  X ● S01.02 **Laceration with foreign body** of scalp
      Coding Clinic: 2015, Q1, P5-7
  X ● S01.03 **Puncture wound without foreign body** of scalp
  X ● S01.04 **Puncture wound with foreign body** of scalp
  X ● S01.05 **Open bite** of scalp
      Bite of scalp NOS
      Excludes1   superficial bite of scalp (S00.06, S00.07-)

  ● S01.1 **Open wound of eyelid and periocular area**
    Open wound of eyelid and periocular area with or without involvement of lacrimal passages
   ● S01.10 **Unspecified** open wound of eyelid and periocular area
    ● S01.101 Unspecified open wound of **right** eyelid and periocular area
    ● S01.102 Unspecified open wound of **left** eyelid and periocular area
    ● S01.109 Unspecified open wound of **unspecified** eyelid and periocular area
   ● S01.11 **Laceration without foreign body** of eyelid and periocular area
    ● S01.111 Laceration without foreign body of **right** eyelid and periocular area
    ● S01.112 Laceration without foreign body of **left** eyelid and periocular area
    ● S01.119 Laceration without foreign body of **unspecified** eyelid and periocular area
   ● S01.12 **Laceration with foreign body** of eyelid and periocular area
    ● S01.121 Laceration with foreign body of **right** eyelid and periocular area
    ● S01.122 Laceration with foreign body of **left** eyelid and periocular area
    ● S01.129 Laceration with foreign body of **unspecified** eyelid and periocular area

CHAPTER 19 (S00-T88)

- S01.13 **Puncture wound without foreign body** of eyelid and periocular area
  - S01.131 Puncture wound without foreign body of **right** eyelid and periocular area
  - S01.132 Puncture wound without foreign body of **left** eyelid and periocular area
  - S01.139 Puncture wound without foreign body of **unspecified** eyelid and periocular area
- S01.14 **Puncture wound with foreign body** of eyelid and periocular area
  - S01.141 Puncture wound with foreign body of **right** eyelid and periocular area
  - S01.142 Puncture wound with foreign body of **left** eyelid and periocular area
  - S01.149 Puncture wound with foreign body of **unspecified** eyelid and periocular area
- S01.15 **Open bite** of eyelid and periocular area
  Bite of eyelid and periocular area NOS
  Excludes1 superficial bite of eyelid and periocular area (S00.26, S00.27)
  - S01.151 Open bite of **right** eyelid and periocular area
  - S01.152 Open bite of **left** eyelid and periocular area
  - S01.159 Open bite of **unspecified** eyelid and periocular area
- S01.2 **Open wound of nose**
  - X● S01.20 **Unspecified** open wound of nose
  - X● S01.21 **Laceration without foreign body** of nose
    Coding Clinic: 2015, Q1, P5-6
  - X● S01.22 **Laceration with foreign body** of nose
  - X● S01.23 **Puncture wound without foreign body** of nose
  - X● S01.24 **Puncture wound with foreign body** of nose
  - X● S01.25 **Open bite** of nose
    Bite of nose NOS
    Excludes1 superficial bite of nose (S00.36, S00.37)
- S01.3 **Open wound of ear**
  - S01.30 **Unspecified** open wound of ear
    - S01.301 Unspecified open wound of **right** ear
    - S01.302 Unspecified open wound of **left** ear
    - S01.309 Unspecified open wound of **unspecified** ear
  - S01.31 **Laceration without foreign body** of ear
    - S01.311 Laceration without foreign body of **right** ear
    - S01.312 Laceration without foreign body of **left** ear
    - S01.319 Laceration without foreign body of **unspecified** ear
  - S01.32 **Laceration with foreign body** of ear
    - S01.321 Laceration with foreign body of **right** ear
    - S01.322 Laceration with foreign body of **left** ear
    - S01.329 Laceration with foreign body of **unspecified** ear

- S01.33 **Puncture wound without foreign body** of ear
  - S01.331 Puncture wound without foreign body of **right** ear
  - S01.332 Puncture wound without foreign body of **left** ear
  - S01.339 Puncture wound without foreign body of **unspecified** ear
- S01.34 **Puncture wound with foreign body** of ear
  - S01.341 Puncture wound with foreign body of **right** ear
  - S01.342 Puncture wound with foreign body of **left** ear
  - S01.349 Puncture wound with foreign body of **unspecified** ear
- S01.35 **Open bite** of ear
  Bite of ear NOS
  Excludes1 superficial bite of ear (S00.46, S00.47)
  - S01.351 Open bite of **right** ear
  - S01.352 Open bite of **left** ear
  - S01.359 Open bite of **unspecified** ear
- S01.4 **Open wound of cheek and temporomandibular area**
  - S01.40 **Unspecified** open wound of cheek and temporomandibular area
    - S01.401 Unspecified open wound of **right** cheek and temporomandibular area
    - S01.402 Unspecified open wound of **left** cheek and temporomandibular area
    - S01.409 Unspecified open wound of **unspecified** cheek and temporomandibular area
  - S01.41 **Laceration without foreign body** of cheek and temporomandibular area
    - S01.411 Laceration without foreign body of **right** cheek and temporomandibular area
      Coding Clinic: 2015, Q1, P5-7
    - S01.412 Laceration without foreign body of **left** cheek and temporomandibular area
    - S01.419 Laceration without foreign body of **unspecified** cheek and temporomandibular area
  - S01.42 **Laceration with foreign body** of cheek and temporomandibular area
    - S01.421 Laceration with foreign body of **right** cheek and temporomandibular area
    - S01.422 Laceration with foreign body of **left** cheek and temporomandibular area
    - S01.429 Laceration with foreign body of **unspecified** cheek and temporomandibular area
  - S01.43 **Puncture wound without foreign body** of cheek and temporomandibular area
    - S01.431 Puncture wound without foreign body of **right** cheek and temporomandibular area
    - S01.432 Puncture wound without foreign body of **left** cheek and temporomandibular area
    - S01.439 Puncture wound without foreign body of **unspecified** cheek and temporomandibular area

● S01.44   **Puncture wound with foreign body of cheek and temporomandibular area**
    ● S01.441   Puncture wound with foreign body of right cheek and temporomandibular area
    ● S01.442   Puncture wound with foreign body of left cheek and temporomandibular area
    ● S01.449   Puncture wound with foreign body of unspecified cheek and temporomandibular area

● S01.45   **Open bite of cheek and temporomandibular area**
    Bite of cheek and temporomandibular area NOS
      Excludes2   superficial bite of cheek and temporomandibular area (S00.86, S00.87)
    ● S01.451   Open bite of right cheek and temporomandibular area
    ● S01.452   Open bite of left cheek and temporomandibular area
    ● S01.459   Open bite of unspecified cheek and temporomandibular area

● S01.5   **Open wound of lip and oral cavity**
     Excludes2   tooth dislocation (S03.2)
                 tooth fracture (S02.5)
    ● S01.50   **Unspecified open wound of lip and oral cavity**
      ● S01.501   Unspecified open wound of lip
      ● S01.502   Unspecified open wound of oral cavity
    ● S01.51   **Laceration of lip and oral cavity without foreign body**
      ● S01.511   Laceration without foreign body of lip
      ● S01.512   Laceration without foreign body of oral cavity
    ● S01.52   **Laceration of lip and oral cavity with foreign body**
      ● S01.521   Laceration with foreign body of lip
      ● S01.522   Laceration with foreign body of oral cavity
    ● S01.53   **Puncture wound of lip and oral cavity without foreign body**
      ● S01.531   Puncture wound without foreign body of lip
      ● S01.532   Puncture wound without foreign body of oral cavity
    ● S01.54   **Puncture wound of lip and oral cavity with foreign body**
      ● S01.541   Puncture wound with foreign body of lip
      ● S01.542   Puncture wound with foreign body of oral cavity
    ● S01.55   **Open bite of lip and oral cavity**
      ● S01.551   Open bite of lip
          Bite of lip NOS
            Excludes1   superficial bite of lip (S00.571)
      ● S01.552   Open bite of oral cavity
          Bite of oral cavity NOS
            Excludes1   superficial bite of oral cavity (S00.572)

● S01.8   **Open wound of other parts of head**
    X ● S01.80   Unspecified open wound of other part of head
    X ● S01.81   Laceration without foreign body of other part of head
    X ● S01.82   Laceration with foreign body of other part of head

X ● S01.83   Puncture wound without foreign body of other part of head
X ● S01.84   Puncture wound with foreign body of other part of head
X ● S01.85   Open bite of other part of head
    Bite of other part of head NOS
      Excludes1   superficial bite of other part of head (S00.87)

● S01.9   **Open wound of unspecified part of head**
    X ● S01.90   Unspecified open wound of unspecified part of head
    X ● S01.91   Laceration without foreign body of unspecified part of head
    X ● S01.92   Laceration with foreign body of unspecified part of head
    X ● S01.93   Puncture wound without foreign body of unspecified part of head
    X ● S01.94   Puncture wound with foreign body of unspecified part of head
    X ● S01.95   Open bite of unspecified part of head
      Bite of head NOS
        Excludes1   superficial bite of head NOS (S00.97)

● S02   **Fracture of skull and facial bones**
    Note: A fracture not indicated as open or closed should be coded to closed
    The appropriate 7th character is to be added to each code from category S02

A	initial encounter for closed fracture
B	initial encounter for open fracture
D	subsequent encounter for fracture with routine healing
G	subsequent encounter for fracture with delayed healing
K	subsequent encounter for fracture with nonunion
S	sequela

    Code also any associated intracranial injury (S06.-)

X ● S02.0   **Fracture of vault of skull A, B, S 🔁**
    Fracture of frontal bone
    Fracture of parietal bone

● S02.1   **Fracture of base of skull**
     Excludes2   lateral orbital wall (S02.84-)
                 medial orbital wall (S02.83-)
                 orbital floor (S02.3-)
    Coding Clinic: 2016, Q4, P66
    ● S02.10   **Unspecified fracture of base of skull**
      ● S02.101   Fracture of base of skull, right side A, B, S 🔁
      ● S02.102   Fracture of base of skull, left side A, B, S 🔁
      ● S02.109   Fracture of base of skull, unspecified side A, B, S 🔁
    ● S02.11   **Fracture of occiput**
      ● S02.110   Type I occipital condyle fracture, unspecified side A, B, S 🔁
      ● S02.111   Type II occipital condyle fracture, unspecified side A, B, S 🔁
      ● S02.112   Type III occipital condyle fracture, unspecified side A, B, S 🔁
      ● S02.113   Unspecified occipital condyle fracture A, B, S 🔁
      ● S02.118   Other fracture of occiput, unspecified side A, B, S 🔁
      ● S02.119   Unspecified fracture of occiput A, B, S 🔁

● S02.11A   Type I occipital condyle fracture, right side A, B, S 🐾

● S02.11B   Type I occipital condyle fracture, left side A, B, S 🐾

● S02.11C   Type II occipital condyle fracture, right side A, B, S 🐾

● S02.11D   Type II occipital condyle fracture, left side A, B, S 🐾

● S02.11E   Type III occipital condyle fracture, right side A, B, S 🐾

● S02.11F   Type III occipital condyle fracture, left side A, B, S 🐾

● S02.11G   Other fracture of occiput, right side A, B, S 🐾

● S02.11H   Other fracture of occiput, left side A, B, S 🐾

S02.12   Fracture of orbital roof

    S02.121   Fracture of orbital roof, right side

    S02.122   Fracture of orbital roof, left side

    S02.129   Fracture of orbital roof, unspecified side

X ● S02.19   Other fracture of base of skull A, B, S 🐾
     Fracture of anterior fossa of base of skull
     Fracture of ethmoid sinus
     Fracture of frontal sinus
     Fracture of middle fossa of base of skull
     Fracture of posterior fossa of base of skull
     Fracture of sphenoid
     Fracture of temporal bone

X ● S02.2   Fracture of nasal bones

● S02.3   Fracture of orbital floor
     Fracture of inferior orbital wall

     Excludes1   orbit NOS (S02.85)

     Excludes2   lateral orbital wall (S02.84-)
                medial orbital wall (S02.83-)
                orbital roof (S02.1-)

     Coding Clinic: 2016, Q4, P66

X ● S02.30   Fracture of orbital floor, unspecified side A, B, S 🐾

X ● S02.31   Fracture of orbital floor, right side A, B, S 🐾

X ● S02.32   Fracture of orbital floor, left side A, B, S 🐾

● S02.4   Fracture of malar, maxillary and zygoma bones
     Fracture of superior maxilla
     Fracture of upper jaw (bone)
     Fracture of zygomatic process of temporal bone
     Coding Clinic: 2016, Q4, P66

● S02.40   Fracture of malar, maxillary and zygoma bones, unspecified

    ● S02.400   Malar fracture unspecified side A, B, S 🐾

    ● S02.401   Maxillary fracture, unspecified side A, B, S 🐾

    ● S02.402   Zygomatic fracture, unspecified side A, B, S 🐾

    ● S02.40A   Malar fracture, right side A, B, S 🐾

    ● S02.40B   Malar fracture, left side A, B, S 🐾

    ● S02.40C   Maxillary fracture, right side A, B, S 🐾

    ● S02.40D   Maxillary fracture, left side A, B, S 🐾

    ● S02.40E   Zygomatic fracture, right side A, B, S 🐾

    ● S02.40F   Zygomatic fracture, left side A, B, S 🐾

● S02.41   LeFort fracture

    ● S02.411   LeFort I fracture A, B, S 🐾

    ● S02.412   LeFort II fracture A, B, S 🐾

    ● S02.413   LeFort III fracture A, B, S 🐾

X ● S02.42   Fracture of alveolus of maxilla A, B, S 🐾

X ● S02.5   Fracture of tooth (traumatic) Broken tooth

     Excludes1   cracked tooth (nontraumatic) (K03.81)

● S02.6   Fracture of mandible
     Fracture of lower jaw (bone)
     Coding Clinic: 2016, Q4, P66

● S02.60   Fracture of mandible of unspecified site

    ● S02.600   Fracture of unspecified part of body of mandible, unspecified side A, B, S 🐾

    ● S02.601   Fracture of unspecified part of body of right mandible A, B, S 🐾

    ● S02.602   Fracture of unspecified part of body of left mandible A, B, S 🐾

    ● S02.609   Fracture of mandible, unspecified A, B, S 🐾

● S02.61   Fracture of condylar process of mandible

    ● S02.610   Fracture of condylar process of mandible, unspecified side A, B, S 🐾

    ● S02.611   Fracture of condylar process of right mandible A, B, S 🐾
         Coding Clinic: 2021, Q1, P6

    ● S02.612   Fracture of condylar process of left mandible A, B, S 🐾

● S02.62   Fracture of subcondylar process of mandible

    ● S02.620   Fracture of subcondylar process of mandible, unspecified side A, B, S 🐾

    ● S02.621   Fracture of subcondylar process of right mandible A, B, S 🐾

    ● S02.622   Fracture of subcondylar process of left mandible A, B, S 🐾

● S02.63   Fracture of coronoid process of mandible

    ● S02.630   Fracture of coronoid process of mandible, unspecified side A, B, S 🐾

    ● S02.631   Fracture of coronoid process of right mandible A, B, S 🐾

    ● S02.632   Fracture of coronoid process of left mandible A, B, S 🐾

● S02.64   Fracture of ramus of mandible

    ● S02.640   Fracture of ramus of mandible, unspecified side A, B, S 🐾

    ● S02.641   Fracture of ramus of right mandible A, B, S 🐾

    ● S02.642   Fracture of ramus of left mandible A, B, S 🐾

● S02.65   Fracture of angle of mandible

    ● S02.650   Fracture of angle of mandible, unspecified side A, B, S 🐾

    ● S02.651   Fracture of angle of right mandible A, B, S 🐾

    ● S02.652   Fracture of angle of left mandible A, B, S 🐾

X ● S02.66   Fracture of symphysis of mandible A, B, S 🐾
     Coding Clinic: 2021, Q1, P6

● S02.67   Fracture of alveolus of mandible

    ● S02.670   Fracture of alveolus of mandible, unspecified side A, B, S 🐾

    ● S02.671   Fracture of alveolus of right mandible A, B, S 🐾

    ● S02.672   Fracture of alveolus of left mandible A, B, S 🐾

X ● S02.69   Fracture of mandible of other specified site A, B, S 🐾

▶ New   ➡ Revised   ~~deleted~~ Deleted   Excludes 1   Excludes 2   Includes   Use additional   Code first   Code also   Key words

OGCR Official Guidelines   X Assign placeholder X   ● Use Additional Character(s)   ▶ Manifestation Code   🐾 Hierarchical Condition Category   **Coding Clinic**

● **S02.8**   **Fractures of other specified skull and facial bones**
Fracture of palate
    Excludes2   lateral orbital wall (S02.84-)
                medial orbital wall (S02.83-)
    Coding Clinic: 2016, Q4, P66

X ● **S02.80**   Fracture of other specified skull and facial bones, unspecified side A, B, S 🔗

X ● **S02.81**   Fracture of other specified skull and facial bones, right side A, B, S 🔗

X ● **S02.82**   Fracture of other specified skull and facial bones, left side A, B, S 🔗

   ● **S02.83 Fracture of medial orbital wall**
      Excludes2   orbital floor (S02.3-)
                  orbital roof (S02.12-)

     S02.831   Fracture of medial orbital wall, right side

     S02.832   Fracture of medial orbital wall, left side

     S02.839   Fracture of medial orbital wall, unspecified side

   ● **S02.84 Fracture of lateral orbital wall**
      Excludes2   orbital floor (S02.3-)
                  orbital roof (S02.12-)

     S02.841   Fracture of lateral orbital wall, right side

     S02.842   Fracture of lateral orbital wall, left side

     S02.849   Fracture of lateral orbital wall, unspecified side

   S02.85 Fracture of orbit, unspecified
     Fracture of orbit NOS
     Fracture of orbit wall NOS
      Excludes1   lateral orbital wall (S02.84-)
                  medial orbital wall (S02.83-)
                  orbital floor (S02.3-)
                  orbital roof (S02.12-)

● **S02.9**   **Fracture of unspecified skull and facial bones**

X ● **S02.91**   Unspecified fracture of skull A, B, S 🔗

X ● **S02.92**   Unspecified fracture of facial bones A, B, S 🔗

● **S03**   **Dislocation and sprain of joints and ligaments of head**
    Includes   avulsion of joint (capsule) or ligament of head
            laceration of cartilage, joint (capsule) or ligament of head
            sprain of cartilage, joint (capsule) or ligament of head
            traumatic hemarthrosis of joint or ligament of head
            traumatic rupture of joint or ligament of head
            traumatic subluxation of joint or ligament of head
            traumatic tear of joint or ligament of head
  Code also any associated open wound
    Excludes2   Strain of muscle or tendon of head (S09.1)
  The appropriate 7th character is to be added to each code from category S03

    | | |
    A   initial encounter
    D   subsequent encounter
    S   sequela

● **S03.0**   **Dislocation of jaw**
    Dislocation of jaw (cartilage) (meniscus)
    Dislocation of mandible
    Dislocation of temporomandibular (joint)
    Coding Clinic: 2016, Q4, P67

X ● **S03.00**   Dislocation of jaw, unspecified side

X ● **S03.01**   Dislocation of jaw, right side

X ● **S03.02**   Dislocation of jaw, left side

X ● **S03.03**   Dislocation of jaw, bilateral side

X ● **S03.1**   Dislocation of septal cartilage of nose

X ● **S03.2**   Dislocation of tooth

● **S03.4**   **Sprain of jaw**
    Sprain of temporomandibular (joint) (ligament)
    Coding Clinic: 2016, Q4, P67

X ● **S03.40**   Sprain of jaw, unspecified side

X ● **S03.41**   Sprain of jaw, right side

X ● **S03.42**   Sprain of jaw, left side

X ● **S03.43**   Sprain of jaw, bilateral side

X ● **S03.8**   Sprain of joints and ligaments of other parts of head

X ● **S03.9**   Sprain of joints and ligaments of unspecified parts of head

● **S04**   **Injury of cranial nerve**
    The selection of side should be based on the side of the body being affected
    Code first any associated intracranial injury (S06.-)
    Code also any associated:
      open wound of head (S01.-)
      skull fracture (S02.-)
    The appropriate 7th character is to be added to each code from category S04

    A   initial encounter
    D   subsequent encounter
    S   sequela

● **S04.0**   **Injury of optic nerve and pathways**
    Use additional code to identify any visual field defect or blindness (H53.4-, H54.-)

   ● **S04.01**   **Injury of optic nerve**
      Injury of 2nd cranial nerve

     ● **S04.011**   Injury of optic nerve, right eye

     ● **S04.012**   Injury of optic nerve, left eye

     ● **S04.019**   Injury of optic nerve, unspecified eye
        Injury of optic nerve NOS

X ● **S04.02**   Injury of optic chiasm

   ● **S04.03**   **Injury of optic tract and pathways**
      Injury of optic radiation

     ● **S04.031**   Injury of optic tract and pathways, right side

     ● **S04.032**   Injury of optic tract and pathways, left side

     ● **S04.039**   Injury of optic tract and pathways, unspecified side
        Injury of optic tract and pathways NOS

   ● **S04.04**   **Injury of visual cortex**

     ● **S04.041**   Injury of visual cortex, right side

     ● **S04.042**   Injury of visual cortex, left side

     ● **S04.049**   Injury of visual cortex, unspecified side
        Injury of visual cortex NOS

● **S04.1**   **Injury of oculomotor nerve**
    Injury of 3rd cranial nerve

X ● **S04.10**   Injury of oculomotor nerve, unspecified side

X ● **S04.11**   Injury of oculomotor nerve, right side

X ● **S04.12**   Injury of oculomotor nerve, left side

● **S04.2**   **Injury of trochlear nerve**
    Injury of 4th cranial nerve

X ● **S04.20**   Injury of trochlear nerve, unspecified side

X ● **S04.21**   Injury of trochlear nerve, right side

X ● **S04.22**   Injury of trochlear nerve, left side

● **S04.3**   **Injury of trigeminal nerve**
    Injury of 5th cranial nerve

X ● **S04.30**   Injury of trigeminal nerve, unspecified side

X ● **S04.31**   Injury of trigeminal nerve, right side

X ● **S04.32**   Injury of trigeminal nerve, left side

● **S04.4**   **Injury of abducent nerve**
    Injury of 6th cranial nerve

X ● **S04.40**   Injury of abducent nerve, unspecified side

X ● **S04.41**   Injury of abducent nerve, right side

X ● **S04.42**   Injury of abducent nerve, left side

CHAPTER 19 (S00-T88)

Figure 19-13 Cranial nerves. (From Patton and Thibodeau: Anatomy and physiology, ed 7, St. Louis, Mosby, 2009)

● **S04.5**   **Injury of facial nerve**
      Injury of 7th cranial nerve
   X ● **S04.50**   **Injury of facial nerve, unspecified side**
   X ● **S04.51**   **Injury of facial nerve, right side**
   X ● **S04.52**   **Injury of facial nerve, left side**

● **S04.6**   **Injury of acoustic nerve**
      Injury of auditory nerve
      Injury of 8th cranial nerve
   X ● **S04.60**   **Injury of acoustic nerve, unspecified side**
   X ● **S04.61**   **Injury of acoustic nerve, right side**
   X ● **S04.62**   **Injury of acoustic nerve, left side**

● **S04.7**   **Injury of accessory nerve**
      Injury of 11th cranial nerve
   X ● **S04.70**   **Injury of accessory nerve, unspecified side**
   X ● **S04.71**   **Injury of accessory nerve, right side**
   X ● **S04.72**   **Injury of accessory nerve, left side**

● **S04.8**   **Injury of other cranial nerves**
   ● **S04.81**   **Injury of olfactory [1st] nerve**
     ● **S04.811**   **Injury of olfactory [1st] nerve, right side**
     ● **S04.812**   **Injury of olfactory [1st] nerve, left side**
     ● **S04.819**   **Injury of olfactory [1st] nerve, unspecified side**
   ● **S04.89**   **Injury of other cranial nerves**
      Injury of vagus [10th] nerve
     ● **S04.891**   **Injury of other cranial nerves, right side**
     ● **S04.892**   **Injury of other cranial nerves, left side**
     ● **S04.899**   **Injury of other cranial nerves, unspecified side**

   X ● **S04.9**   **Injury of unspecified cranial nerve**

● **S05**   **Injury of eye and orbit**
   Includes   open wound of eye and orbit
   Excludes2   2nd cranial [optic] nerve injury (S04.0-)
           3rd cranial [oculomotor] nerve injury (S04.1-)
           open wound of eyelid and periocular area (S01.1-)
           orbital bone fracture (S02.1-, S02.3-, S02.8-)
           superficial injury of eyelid (S00.1-S00.2)

The appropriate 7th character is to be added to each code from category S05

A	initial encounter
D	subsequent encounter
S	sequela

● **S05.0**   **Injury of conjunctiva and corneal abrasion without foreign body**
     Excludes1   foreign body in conjunctival sac (T15.1)
             foreign body in cornea (T15.0)
   X ● **S05.00**   **Injury of conjunctiva and corneal abrasion without foreign body, unspecified eye**
   X ● **S05.01**   **Injury of conjunctiva and corneal abrasion without foreign body, right eye**
   X ● **S05.02**   **Injury of conjunctiva and corneal abrasion without foreign body, left eye**

● **S05.1**   **Contusion of eyeball and orbital tissues**
      Traumatic hyphema
     Excludes2   black eye NOS (S00.1)
             contusion of eyelid and periocular area (S00.1)
   X ● **S05.10**   **Contusion of eyeball and orbital tissues, unspecified eye**
   X ● **S05.11**   **Contusion of eyeball and orbital tissues, right eye**
   X ● **S05.12**   **Contusion of eyeball and orbital tissues, left eye**

● **S05.2**   **Ocular laceration and rupture with prolapse or loss of intraocular tissue**
- X● **S05.20**   Ocular laceration and rupture with prolapse or loss of intraocular tissue, unspecified eye
- X● **S05.21**   Ocular laceration and rupture with prolapse or loss of intraocular tissue, right eye
- X● **S05.22**   Ocular laceration and rupture with prolapse or loss of intraocular tissue, left eye

● **S05.3**   **Ocular laceration without prolapse or loss of intraocular tissue**
    Laceration of eye NOS
- X● **S05.30**   Ocular laceration without prolapse or loss of intraocular tissue, unspecified eye
- X● **S05.31**   Ocular laceration without prolapse or loss of intraocular tissue, right eye
- X● **S05.32**   Ocular laceration without prolapse or loss of intraocular tissue, left eye

● **S05.4**   **Penetrating wound of orbit with or without foreign body**
    Excludes2   retained (old) foreign body following penetrating wound in orbit (H05.5-)
- X● **S05.40**   Penetrating wound of orbit with or without foreign body, unspecified eye
- X● **S05.41**   Penetrating wound of orbit with or without foreign body, right eye
- X● **S05.42**   Penetrating wound of orbit with or without foreign body, left eye

● **S05.5**   **Penetrating wound with foreign body of eyeball**
    Excludes2   retained (old) intraocular foreign body (H44.6-, H44.7)
- X● **S05.50**   Penetrating wound with foreign body of unspecified eyeball
- X● **S05.51**   Penetrating wound with foreign body of right eyeball
- X● **S05.52**   Penetrating wound with foreign body of left eyeball

● **S05.6**   **Penetrating wound without foreign body of eyeball**
    Ocular penetration NOS
- X● **S05.60**   Penetrating wound without foreign body of unspecified eyeball
- X● **S05.61**   Penetrating wound without foreign body of right eyeball
- X● **S05.62**   Penetrating wound without foreign body of left eyeball

● **S05.7**   **Avulsion of eye**
    Traumatic enucleation
- X● **S05.70**   Avulsion of unspecified eye
- X● **S05.71**   Avulsion of right eye
- X● **S05.72**   Avulsion of left eye

● **S05.8**   **Other injuries of eye and orbit**
    Lacrimal duct injury
- ● **S05.8X**   Other injuries of eye and orbit
  - ● **S05.8X1**   Other injuries of right eye and orbit
  - ● **S05.8X2**   Other injuries of left eye and orbit
  - ● **S05.8X9**   Other injuries of unspecified eye and orbit

● **S05.9**   **Unspecified injury of eye and orbit**
    Injury of eye NOS
- X● **S05.90**   Unspecified injury of unspecified eye and orbit
- X● **S05.91**   Unspecified injury of right eye and orbit
- X● **S05.92**   Unspecified injury of left eye and orbit

● **S06**   **Intracranial injury**
    Includes   traumatic brain injury
    Code also any associated:
      open wound of head (S01.-)
      skull fracture (S02.-)
    Excludes1   head injury NOS (S09.90)
    The appropriate 7th character is to be added to each code from category S06

A	initial encounter
D	subsequent encounter
S	sequela

    Note: 7th characters D and S do not apply to codes in category S06 with 6th character 7 - death due to brain injury prior to regaining consciousness, or 8 - death due to other cause prior to regaining consciousness.
    Coding Clinic: 2015, Q4, P40

● **S06.0**   **Concussion**
    Commotio cerebri
    Excludes1   concussion with other intracranial injuries classified in subcategories S06.1- to S06.6- , S06.81- and S06.82- code to specified intracranial injury
    Coding Clinic: 2016, Q4, P67
- ● **S06.0X**   Concussion
  - ● **S06.0X0**   Concussion without loss of consciousness S 🔗
  - ● **S06.0X1**   Concussion with loss of consciousness of 30 minutes or less S 🔗
  - ● **S06.0X9**   Concussion with loss of consciousness of unspecified duration S 🔗
        Concussion NOS
        Coding Clinic: 2016, Q4, P68

● **S06.1**   **Traumatic cerebral edema**
    Diffuse traumatic cerebral edema
    Focal traumatic cerebral edema
    Coding Clinic: 2016, Q4, P67
- ● **S06.1X**   Traumatic cerebral edema
  - ● **S06.1X0**   Traumatic cerebral edema without loss of consciousness A, S 🔗
        Coding Clinic: 2015, Q1, P12
  - ● **S06.1X1**   Traumatic cerebral edema with loss of consciousness of 30 minutes or less A, S 🔗
  - ● **S06.1X2**   Traumatic cerebral edema with loss of consciousness of 31 minutes to 59 minutes A, S 🔗
  - ● **S06.1X3**   Traumatic cerebral edema with loss of consciousness of 1 hour to 5 hours 59 minutes A, S 🔗
  - ● **S06.1X4**   Traumatic cerebral edema with loss of consciousness of 6 hours to 24 hours A, S 🔗
  - ● **S06.1X5**   Traumatic cerebral edema with loss of consciousness greater than 24 hours with return to pre-existing conscious level A, S 🔗
  - ● **S06.1X6**   Traumatic cerebral edema with loss of consciousness greater than 24 hours without return to pre-existing conscious level with patient surviving A, S 🔗

CHAPTER 19 (S00-T88)

● S06.1X7   Traumatic cerebral edema with loss of consciousness of any duration with death due to brain injury prior to regaining consciousness

● S06.1X8   Traumatic cerebral edema with loss of consciousness of any duration with death due to other cause prior to regaining consciousness

● S06.1X9   Traumatic cerebral edema with loss of consciousness of unspecified duration A, S 🐾
       Traumatic cerebral edema NOS

● S06.2   **Diffuse traumatic brain injury**
     Diffuse axonal brain injury

     Excludes1   traumatic diffuse cerebral edema (S06.1X-)

▶ Use Additional code, if applicable, for traumatic brain compression or herniation (S06.A-)

● S06.2X   Diffuse traumatic brain injury

    ● S06.2X0   Diffuse traumatic brain injury without loss of consciousness A, S 🐾

    ● S06.2X1   Diffuse traumatic brain injury with loss of consciousness of 30 minutes or less A, S 🐾

    ● S06.2X2   Diffuse traumatic brain injury with loss of consciousness of 31 minutes to 59 minutes A, S 🐾

    ● S06.2X3   Diffuse traumatic brain injury with loss of consciousness of 1 hour to 5 hours 59 minutes A, S 🐾

    ● S06.2X4   Diffuse traumatic brain injury with loss of consciousness of 6 hours to 24 hours A, S 🐾

    ● S06.2X5   Diffuse traumatic brain injury with loss of consciousness greater than 24 hours with return to pre-existing conscious levels A, S 🐾

    ● S06.2X6   Diffuse traumatic brain injury with loss of consciousness greater than 24 hours without return to pre-existing conscious level with patient surviving A, S 🐾

    ● S06.2X7   Diffuse traumatic brain injury with loss of consciousness of any duration with death due to brain injury prior to regaining consciousness

    ● S06.2X8   Diffuse traumatic brain injury with loss of consciousness of any duration with death due to other cause prior to regaining consciousness

    ● S06.2X9   Diffuse traumatic brain injury with loss of consciousness of unspecified duration A, S 🐾
       Diffuse traumatic brain injury NOS

● S06.3   **Focal traumatic brain injury**

     Excludes1   any condition classifiable to S06.4-S06.6

     Excludes2   focal cerebral edema (S06.1)

▶ Use Additional code, if applicable, for traumatic brain compression or herniation (S06.A-)

● S06.30   Unspecified focal traumatic brain injury

    ● S06.300   Unspecified focal traumatic brain injury without loss of consciousness A, S 🐾

    ● S06.301   Unspecified focal traumatic brain injury with loss of consciousness of 30 minutes or less A, S 🐾

    ● S06.302   Unspecified focal traumatic brain injury with loss of consciousness of 31 minutes to 59 minutes A, S 🐾

    ● S06.303   Unspecified focal traumatic brain injury with loss of consciousness of 1 hour to 5 hours 59 minutes A, S 🐾

● S06.304   Unspecified focal traumatic brain injury with loss of consciousness of 6 hours to 24 hours A, S 🐾

● S06.305   Unspecified focal traumatic brain injury with loss of consciousness greater than 24 hours with return to pre-existing conscious level A, S 🐾

● S06.306   Unspecified focal traumatic brain injury with loss of consciousness greater than 24 hours without return to pre-existing conscious level with patient surviving A, S 🐾

● S06.307   Unspecified focal traumatic brain injury with loss of consciousness of any duration with death due to brain injury prior to regaining consciousness

● S06.308   Unspecified focal traumatic brain injury with loss of consciousness of any duration with death due to other cause prior to regaining consciousness

● S06.309   Unspecified focal traumatic brain injury with loss of consciousness of unspecified duration A, S 🐾
       Unspecified focal traumatic brain injury NOS

● S06.31   Contusion and laceration of right cerebrum

    ● S06.310   Contusion and laceration of right cerebrum without loss of consciousness A, S 🐾

    ● S06.311   Contusion and laceration of right cerebrum with loss of consciousness of 30 minutes or less A, S 🐾

    ● S06.312   Contusion and laceration of right cerebrum with loss of consciousness of 31 minutes to 59 minutes A, S 🐾

    ● S06.313   Contusion and laceration of right cerebrum with loss of consciousness of 1 hour to 5 hours 59 minutes A, S 🐾

    ● S06.314   Contusion and laceration of right cerebrum with loss of consciousness of 6 hours to 24 hours A, S 🐾

    ● S06.315   Contusion and laceration of right cerebrum with loss of consciousness greater than 24 hours with return to pre-existing conscious level A, S 🐾

    ● S06.316   Contusion and laceration of right cerebrum with loss of consciousness greater than 24 hours without return to pre-existing conscious level with patient surviving A, S 🐾

    ● S06.317   Contusion and laceration of right cerebrum with loss of consciousness of any duration with death due to brain injury prior to regaining consciousness

    ● S06.318   Contusion and laceration of right cerebrum with loss of consciousness of any duration with death due to other cause prior to regaining consciousness

    ● S06.319   Contusion and laceration of right cerebrum with loss of consciousness of unspecified duration A, S 🐾
       Contusion and laceration of right cerebrum NOS

▶ New   ⇒ Revised   ~~deleted~~ Deleted   Excludes 1   Excludes 2   Includes   Use additional   Code first   Code also   Key words

OGCR Official Guidelines   X Assign placeholder X   ● Use Additional Character(s)   ▶ Manifestation Code   🐾 Hierarchical Condition Category   **Coding Clinic**

1230

● S06.32   Contusion and laceration of left cerebrum
   ● S06.320   Contusion and laceration of left cerebrum without loss of consciousness A, S 🐾
   ● S06.321   Contusion and laceration of left cerebrum with loss of consciousness of 30 minutes or less A, S 🐾
   ● S06.322   Contusion and laceration of left cerebrum with loss of consciousness of 31 minutes to 59 minutes A, S 🐾
   ● S06.323   Contusion and laceration of left cerebrum with loss of consciousness of 1 hour to 5 hours 59 minutes A, S 🐾
   ● S06.324   Contusion and laceration of left cerebrum with loss of consciousness of 6 hours to 24 hours A, S 🐾
   ● S06.325   Contusion and laceration of left cerebrum with loss of consciousness greater than 24 hours with return to pre-existing conscious level A, S 🐾
   ● S06.326   Contusion and laceration of left cerebrum with loss of consciousness greater than 24 hours without return to pre-existing conscious level with patient surviving A, S 🐾
   ● S06.327   Contusion and laceration of left cerebrum with loss of consciousness of any duration with death due to brain injury prior to regaining consciousness
   ● S06.328   Contusion and laceration of left cerebrum with loss of consciousness of any duration with death due to other cause prior to regaining consciousness
   ● S06.329   Contusion and laceration of left cerebrum with loss of consciousness of unspecified duration A, S 🐾
        Contusion and laceration of left cerebrum NOS

● S06.33   Contusion and laceration of cerebrum, unspecified
   ● S06.330   Contusion and laceration of cerebrum, unspecified, without loss of consciousness A, S 🐾
   ● S06.331   Contusion and laceration of cerebrum, unspecified, with loss of consciousness of 30 minutes or less A, S 🐾
   ● S06.332   Contusion and laceration of cerebrum, unspecified, with loss of consciousness of 31 minutes to 59 minutes A, S 🐾
   ● S06.333   Contusion and laceration of cerebrum, unspecified, with loss of consciousness of 1 hour to 5 hours 59 minutes A, S 🐾
   ● S06.334   Contusion and laceration of cerebrum, unspecified, with loss of consciousness of 6 hours to 24 hours A, S 🐾
   ● S06.335   Contusion and laceration of cerebrum, unspecified, with loss of consciousness greater than 24 hours with return to pre-existing conscious level A, S 🐾

● S06.336   Contusion and laceration of cerebrum, unspecified, with loss of consciousness greater than 24 hours without return to pre-existing conscious level with patient surviving A, S 🐾
● S06.337   Contusion and laceration of cerebrum, unspecified, with loss of consciousness of any duration with death due to brain injury prior to regaining consciousness
● S06.338   Contusion and laceration of cerebrum, unspecified, with loss of consciousness of any duration with death due to other cause prior to regaining consciousness
● S06.339   Contusion and laceration of cerebrum, unspecified, with loss of consciousness of unspecified duration A, S 🐾
        Contusion and laceration of cerebrum NOS

● S06.34   Traumatic hemorrhage of right cerebrum
       Traumatic intracerebral hemorrhage and hematoma of right cerebrum
   ● S06.340   Traumatic hemorrhage of right cerebrum without loss of consciousness A, S 🐾
        Coding Clinic: 2015, Q1, P12
   ● S06.341   Traumatic hemorrhage of right cerebrum with loss of consciousness of 30 minutes or less A, S 🐾
   ● S06.342   Traumatic hemorrhage of right cerebrum with loss of consciousness of 31 minutes to 59 minutes A, S 🐾
   ● S06.343   Traumatic hemorrhage of right cerebrum with loss of consciousness of 1 hours to 5 hours 59 minutes A, S 🐾
   ● S06.344   Traumatic hemorrhage of right cerebrum with loss of consciousness of 6 hours to 24 hours A, S 🐾
   ● S06.345   Traumatic hemorrhage of right cerebrum with loss of consciousness greater than 24 hours with return to pre-existing conscious level A, S 🐾
   ● S06.346   Traumatic hemorrhage of right cerebrum with loss of consciousness greater than 24 hours without return to pre-existing conscious level with patient surviving A, S 🐾
   ● S06.347   Traumatic hemorrhage of right cerebrum with loss of consciousness of any duration with death due to brain injury prior to regaining consciousness
   ● S06.348   Traumatic hemorrhage of right cerebrum with loss of consciousness of any duration with death due to other cause prior to regaining consciousness
   ● S06.349   Traumatic hemorrhage of right cerebrum with loss of consciousness of unspecified duration A, S 🐾
        Traumatic hemorrhage of right cerebrum NOS

CHAPTER 19 (S00–T88)

● S06.35   **Traumatic hemorrhage of left cerebrum**
Traumatic intracerebral hemorrhage and hematoma of left cerebrum

● S06.350   Traumatic hemorrhage of left cerebrum without loss of consciousness A, S 🐾

● S06.351   Traumatic hemorrhage of left cerebrum with loss of consciousness of 30 minutes or less A, S 🐾

● S06.352   Traumatic hemorrhage of left cerebrum with loss of consciousness of 31 minutes to 59 minutes A, S 🐾

● S06.353   Traumatic hemorrhage of left cerebrum with loss of consciousness of 1 hours to 5 hours 59 minutes A, S 🐾

● S06.354   Traumatic hemorrhage of left cerebrum with loss of consciousness of 6 hours to 24 hours A, S 🐾

● S06.355   Traumatic hemorrhage of left cerebrum with loss of consciousness greater than 24 hours with return to pre-existing conscious level A, S 🐾

● S06.356   Traumatic hemorrhage of left cerebrum with loss of consciousness greater than 24 hours without return to pre-existing conscious level with patient surviving A, S 🐾

● S06.357   Traumatic hemorrhage of left cerebrum with loss of consciousness of any duration with death due to brain injury prior to regaining consciousness

● S06.358   Traumatic hemorrhage of left cerebrum with loss of consciousness of any duration with death due to other cause prior to regaining consciousness

● S06.359   Traumatic hemorrhage of left cerebrum with loss of consciousness of unspecified duration A, S 🐾
Traumatic hemorrhage of left cerebrum NOS

● S06.36   **Traumatic hemorrhage of cerebrum, unspecified**
Traumatic intracerebral hemorrhage and hematoma, unspecified

● S06.360   Traumatic hemorrhage of cerebrum, unspecified, without loss of consciousness A, S 🐾

● S06.361   Traumatic hemorrhage of cerebrum, unspecified, with loss of consciousness of 30 minutes or less A, S 🐾

● S06.362   Traumatic hemorrhage of cerebrum, unspecified, with loss of consciousness of 31 minutes to 59 minutes A, S 🐾

● S06.363   Traumatic hemorrhage of cerebrum, unspecified, with loss of consciousness of 1 hours to 5 hours 59 minutes A, S 🐾

● S06.364   Traumatic hemorrhage of cerebrum, unspecified, with loss of consciousness of 6 hours to 24 hours A, S 🐾

● S06.365   Traumatic hemorrhage of cerebrum, unspecified, with loss of consciousness greater than 24 hours with return to pre-existing conscious level A, S 🐾

● S06.366   Traumatic hemorrhage of cerebrum, unspecified, with loss of consciousness greater than 24 hours without return to pre-existing conscious level with patient surviving A, S 🐾

● S06.367   Traumatic hemorrhage of cerebrum, unspecified, with loss of consciousness of any duration with death due to brain injury prior to regaining consciousness

● S06.368   Traumatic hemorrhage of cerebrum, unspecified, with loss of consciousness of any duration with death due to other cause prior to regaining consciousness

● S06.369   Traumatic hemorrhage of cerebrum, unspecified, with loss of consciousness of unspecified duration A, S 🐾
Traumatic hemorrhage of cerebrum NOS

● S06.37   **Contusion, laceration, and hemorrhage of cerebellum**

● S06.370   Contusion, laceration, and hemorrhage of cerebellum without loss of consciousness A, S 🐾

● S06.371   Contusion, laceration, and hemorrhage of cerebellum with loss of consciousness of 30 minutes or less A, S 🐾

● S06.372   Contusion, laceration, and hemorrhage of cerebellum with loss of consciousness of 31 minutes to 59 minutes A, S 🐾

● S06.373   Contusion, laceration, and hemorrhage of cerebellum with loss of consciousness of 1 hour to 5 hours 59 minutes A, S 🐾

● S06.374   Contusion, laceration, and hemorrhage of cerebellum with loss of consciousness of 6 hours to 24 hours A, S 🐾

● S06.375   Contusion, laceration, and hemorrhage of cerebellum with loss of consciousness greater than 24 hours with return to pre-existing conscious level A, S 🐾

● S06.376   Contusion, laceration, and hemorrhage of cerebellum with loss of consciousness greater than 24 hours without return to pre-existing conscious level with patient surviving A, S 🐾

● S06.377   Contusion, laceration, and hemorrhage of cerebellum with loss of consciousness of any duration with death due to brain injury prior to regaining consciousness

● S06.378   Contusion, laceration, and hemorrhage of cerebellum with loss of consciousness of any duration with death due to other cause prior to regaining consciousness

● S06.379   Contusion, laceration, and hemorrhage of cerebellum with loss of consciousness of unspecified duration A, S 🐾
Contusion, laceration, and hemorrhage of cerebellum NOS

● S06.38   **Contusion, laceration, and hemorrhage of brainstem**

● S06.380   Contusion, laceration, and hemorrhage of brainstem without loss of consciousness A, S 🐾

● S06.381   Contusion, laceration, and hemorrhage of brainstem with loss of consciousness of 30 minutes or less A, S 🐾

▶ New   ⇛ Revised   ~~deleted~~ Deleted   Excludes 1   Excludes 2   Includes   Use additional   Code first   Code also   Key words

OGCR Official Guidelines   X Assign placeholder X   ● Use Additional Character(s)   ▶ Manifestation Code   🐾 Hierarchical Condition Category   **Coding Clinic**

● S06.382 Contusion, laceration, and hemorrhage of brainstem with loss of consciousness of 31 minutes to 59 minutes A, S 🐾

● S06.383 Contusion, laceration, and hemorrhage of brainstem with loss of consciousness of 1 hour to 5 hours 59 minutes A, S 🐾

● S06.384 Contusion, laceration, and hemorrhage of brainstem with loss of consciousness of 6 hours to 24 hours A, S 🐾

● S06.385 Contusion, laceration, and hemorrhage of brainstem with loss of consciousness greater than 24 hours with return to pre-existing conscious level A, S 🐾

● S06.386 Contusion, laceration, and hemorrhage of brainstem with loss of consciousness greater than 24 hours without return to pre-existing conscious level with patient surviving A, S 🐾

● S06.387 Contusion, laceration, and hemorrhage of brainstem with loss of consciousness of any duration with death due to brain injury prior to regaining consciousness

● S06.388 Contusion, laceration, and hemorrhage of brainstem with loss of consciousness of any duration with death due to other cause prior to regaining consciousness

● S06.389 Contusion, laceration, and hemorrhage of brainstem with loss of consciousness of unspecified duration A, S 🐾

Contusion, laceration, and hemorrhage of brainstem NOS

● S06.4 Epidural hemorrhage
Situated outside dura mater
Extradural hemorrhage NOS
Intracranial hemorrhage due to trauma
Extradural hemorrhage (traumatic)

● S06.4X Epidural hemorrhage

● S06.4X0 Epidural hemorrhage without loss of consciousness A, S 🐾

● S06.4X1 Epidural hemorrhage with loss of consciousness of 30 minutes or less A, S 🐾

● S06.4X2 Epidural hemorrhage with loss of consciousness of 31 minutes to 59 minutes A, S 🐾

● S06.4X3 Epidural hemorrhage with loss of consciousness of 1 hour to 5 hours 59 minutes A, S 🐾

● S06.4X4 Epidural hemorrhage with loss of consciousness of 6 hours to 24 hours A, S 🐾

● S06.4X5 Epidural hemorrhage with loss of consciousness greater than 24 hours with return to pre-existing conscious level A, S 🐾

● S06.4X6 Epidural hemorrhage with loss of consciousness greater than 24 hours without return to pre-existing conscious level with patient surviving A, S 🐾

● S06.4X7 Epidural hemorrhage with loss of consciousness of any duration with death due to brain injury prior to regaining consciousness

● S06.4X8 Epidural hemorrhage with loss of consciousness of any duration with death due to other causes prior to regaining consciousness

● S06.4X9 Epidural hemorrhage with loss of consciousness of unspecified duration A, S 🐾
Epidural hemorrhage NOS

● S06.5 Traumatic subdural hemorrhage
▶ Use Additional code, if applicable, for traumatic brain compression or herniation (S06.A-)

● S06.5X Traumatic subdural hemorrhage

● S06.5X0 Traumatic subdural hemorrhage without loss of consciousness A, S 🐾
Coding Clinic: 2021, Q1, P4; 2018, Q2, P13; 2015, Q3, P37

● S06.5X1 Traumatic subdural hemorrhage with loss of consciousness of 30 minutes or less A, S 🐾

● S06.5X2 Traumatic subdural hemorrhage with loss of consciousness of 31 minutes to 59 minutes A, S 🐾

● S06.5X3 Traumatic subdural hemorrhage with loss of consciousness of 1 hour to 5 hours 59 minutes A, S 🐾

● S06.5X4 Traumatic subdural hemorrhage with loss of consciousness of 6 hours to 24 hours A, S 🐾

● S06.5X5 Traumatic subdural hemorrhage with loss of consciousness greater than 24 hours with return to pre-existing conscious level A, S 🐾

● S06.5X6 Traumatic subdural hemorrhage with loss of consciousness greater than 24 hours without return to pre-existing conscious level with patient surviving A, S 🐾
Coding Clinic: 2021, Q2, P5

● S06.5X7 Traumatic subdural hemorrhage with loss of consciousness of any duration with death due to brain injury before regaining consciousness

● S06.5X8 Traumatic subdural hemorrhage with loss of consciousness of any duration with death due to other cause before regaining consciousness

● S06.5X9 Traumatic subdural hemorrhage with loss of consciousness of unspecified duration A, S 🐾
Traumatic subdural hemorrhage NOS

● S06.6 Traumatic subarachnoid hemorrhage
Between arachnoid and pia mater
▶ Use Additional code, if applicable, for traumatic brain compression or herniation (S06.A-)
Coding Clinic: 2016, Q4, P67

● S06.6X Traumatic subarachnoid hemorrhage

● S06.6X0 Traumatic subarachnoid hemorrhage without loss of consciousness A, S 🐾
Coding Clinic: 2015, Q3, P37

● S06.6X1 Traumatic subarachnoid hemorrhage with loss of consciousness of 30 minutes or less A, S 🐾

● S06.6X2 Traumatic subarachnoid hemorrhage with loss of consciousness of 31 minutes to 59 minutes A, S 🐾

● S06.6X3 Traumatic subarachnoid hemorrhage with loss of consciousness of 1 hour to 5 hours 59 minutes A, S 🐾

CHAPTER 19 (S00-T88)

● S06.6X4   Traumatic subarachnoid hemorrhage with loss of consciousness of 6 hours to 24 hours A, S 🍪

● S06.6X5   Traumatic subarachnoid hemorrhage with loss of consciousness greater than 24 hours with return to pre-existing conscious level A, S 🍪

● S06.6X6   Traumatic subarachnoid hemorrhage with loss of consciousness greater than 24 hours without return to pre-existing conscious level with patient surviving A, S 🍪
         Coding Clinic: 2021, Q2, P5

● S06.6X7   Traumatic subarachnoid hemorrhage with loss of consciousness of any duration with death due to brain injury prior to regaining consciousness

● S06.6X8   Traumatic subarachnoid hemorrhage with loss of consciousness of any duration with death due to other cause prior to regaining consciousness

● S06.6X9   Traumatic subarachnoid hemorrhage with loss of consciousness of unspecified duration A, S 🍪
         Traumatic subarachnoid hemorrhage NOS

● S06.8   Other specified intracranial injuries

  ● S06.81   Injury of right internal carotid artery, intracranial portion, not elsewhere classified
         Coding Clinic: 2016, Q4, P67

    ● S06.810   Injury of right internal carotid artery, intracranial portion, not elsewhere classified without loss of consciousness A, S 🍪

    ● S06.811   Injury of right internal carotid artery, intracranial portion, not elsewhere classified with loss of consciousness of 30 minutes or less A, S 🍪

    ● S06.812   Injury of right internal carotid artery, intracranial portion, not elsewhere classified with loss of consciousness of 31 minutes to 59 minutes A, S 🍪

    ● S06.813   Injury of right internal carotid artery, intracranial portion, not elsewhere classified with loss of consciousness of 1 hour to 5 hours 59 minutes A, S 🍪

    ● S06.814   Injury of right internal carotid artery, intracranial portion, not elsewhere classified with loss of consciousness of 6 hours to 24 hours A, S 🍪

    ● S06.815   Injury of right internal carotid artery, intracranial portion, not elsewhere classified with loss of consciousness greater than 24 hours with return to pre-existing conscious level A, S 🍪

    ● S06.816   Injury of right internal carotid artery, intracranial portion, not elsewhere classified with loss of consciousness greater than 24 hours without return to pre-existing conscious level with patient surviving A, S 🍪

    ● S06.817   Injury of right internal carotid artery, intracranial portion, not elsewhere classified with loss of consciousness of any duration with death due to brain injury prior to regaining consciousness

● S06.818   Injury of right internal carotid artery, intracranial portion, not elsewhere classified with loss of consciousness of any duration with death due to other cause prior to regaining consciousness

● S06.819   Injury of right internal carotid artery, intracranial portion, not elsewhere classified with loss of consciousness of unspecified duration A, S 🍪
         Injury of right internal carotid artery, intracranial portion, not elsewhere classified NOS

  ● S06.82   Injury of left internal carotid artery, intracranial portion, not elsewhere classified
         Coding Clinic: 2016, Q4, P67

    ● S06.820   Injury of left internal carotid artery, intracranial portion, not elsewhere classified without loss of consciousness A, S 🍪

    ● S06.821   Injury of left internal carotid artery, intracranial portion, not elsewhere classified with loss of consciousness of 30 minutes or less A, S 🍪

    ● S06.822   Injury of left internal carotid artery, intracranial portion, not elsewhere classified with loss of consciousness of 31 minutes to 59 minutes A, S 🍪

    ● S06.823   Injury of left internal carotid artery, intracranial portion, not elsewhere classified with loss of consciousness of 1 hour to 5 hours 59 minutes A, S 🍪

    ● S06.824   Injury of left internal carotid artery, intracranial portion, not elsewhere classified with loss of consciousness of 6 hours to 24 hours A, S 🍪

    ● S06.825   Injury of left internal carotid artery, intracranial portion, not elsewhere classified with loss of consciousness greater than 24 hours with return to pre-existing conscious level

    ● S06.826   Injury of left internal carotid artery, intracranial portion, not elsewhere classified with loss of consciousness greater than 24 hours without return to pre-existing conscious level with patient surviving A, S 🍪

    ● S06.827   Injury of left internal carotid artery, intracranial portion, not elsewhere classified with loss of consciousness of any duration with death due to brain injury prior to regaining consciousness

    ● S06.828   Injury of left internal carotid artery, intracranial portion, not elsewhere classified with loss of consciousness of any duration with death due to other cause prior to regaining consciousness

    ● S06.829   Injury of left internal carotid artery, intracranial portion, not elsewhere classified with loss of consciousness of unspecified duration A, S 🍪
         Injury of left internal carotid artery, intracranial portion, not elsewhere classified NOS

▶ New   ⇒ Revised   ~~deleted~~ Deleted   Excludes 1   Excludes 2   Includes   Use additional   Code first   Code also   Key words
OGCR Official Guidelines   X Assign placeholder X   ● Use Additional Character(s)   ▶ Manifestation Code   🍪 Hierarchical Condition Category   Coding Clinic

● **S06.89**   **Other specified intracranial injury**
     Excludes1   concussion (S06.0X-)

   ● **S06.890**   Other specified intracranial injury without loss of consciousness A, S 🔄

   ● **S06.891**   Other specified intracranial injury with loss of consciousness of 30 minutes or less A, S 🔄

   ● **S06.892**   Other specified intracranial injury with loss of consciousness of 31 minutes to 59 minutes A, S 🔄

   ● **S06.893**   Other specified intracranial injury with loss of consciousness of 1 hour to 5 hours 59 minutes A, S 🔄

   ● **S06.894**   Other specified intracranial injury with loss of consciousness of 6 hours to 24 hours A, S 🔄

   ● **S06.895**   Other specified intracranial injury with loss of consciousness greater than 24 hours with return to pre-existing conscious level A, S 🔄

   ● **S06.896**   Other specified intracranial injury with loss of consciousness greater than 24 hours without return to pre-existing conscious level with patient surviving A, S 🔄

   ● **S06.897**   Other specified intracranial injury with loss of consciousness of any duration with death due to brain injury prior to regaining consciousness

   ● **S06.898**   Other specified intracranial injury with loss of consciousness of any duration with death due to other cause prior to regaining consciousness

   ● **S06.899**   Other specified intracranial injury with loss of consciousness of unspecified duration A, S 🔄

● **S06.9**   **Unspecified intracranial injury**
     Brain injury NOS
     Head injury NOS with loss of consciousness
     Traumatic brain injury NOS

     Excludes1   conditions classifiable to S06.0- to S06.8- code to specified intracranial injury head injury NOS (S09.90)

   ● **S06.9X**   **Unspecified intracranial injury**

     ● **S06.9X0**   Unspecified intracranial injury without loss of consciousness A, S 🔄

     ● **S06.9X1**   Unspecified intracranial injury with loss of consciousness of 30 minutes or less A, S 🔄

     ● **S06.9X2**   Unspecified intracranial injury with loss of consciousness of 31 minutes to 59 minutes A, S 🔄

     ● **S06.9X3**   Unspecified intracranial injury with loss of consciousness of 1 hour to 5 hours 59 minutes A, S 🔄

     ● **S06.9X4**   Unspecified intracranial injury with loss of consciousness of 6 hours to 24 hours A, S 🔄

     ● **S06.9X5**   Unspecified intracranial injury with loss of consciousness greater than 24 hours with return to pre-existing conscious level A, S 🔄

     ● **S06.9X6**   Unspecified intracranial injury with loss of consciousness greater than 24 hours without return to pre-existing conscious level with patient surviving A, S 🔄

     ● **S06.9X7**   Unspecified intracranial injury with loss of consciousness of any duration with death due to brain injury prior to regaining consciousness

     ● **S06.9X8**   Unspecified intracranial injury with loss of consciousness of any duration with death due to other cause prior to regaining consciousness

     ● **S06.9X9**   Unspecified intracranial injury with loss of consciousness of unspecified duration A, S 🔄

▶ ● **S06.A**   **Traumatic brain compression and herniation**
   ▶ Traumatic cerebral compression
   ▶ *Code first the underlying traumatic brain injury, such as:*
     ▶ diffuse traumatic brain injury (S06.2-)
     ▶ focal traumatic brain injury (S06.3-)
     ▶ traumatic subdural hemorrhage (S06.5-)
     ▶ traumatic subarachnoid hemorrhage (S06.6-)

▶   **S06.A0**   **Traumatic brain compression without herniation**
   ▶ Traumatic brain compression NOS
   ▶ Traumatic cerebral compression NOS

▶   **S06.A1**   **Traumatic brain compression with herniation**
   ▶ Traumatic brain herniation
   ▶ Traumatic brainstem compression with herniation
   ▶ Traumatic cerebellar compression with herniation
   ▶ Traumatic cerebral compression with herniation

● **S07**   **Crushing injury of head**
     Use additional code for all associated injuries, such as:
       intracranial injuries (S06.-)
       skull fractures (S02.-)
     The appropriate 7th character is to be added to each code from category S07

A	initial encounter
D	subsequent encounter
S	sequela

X ● **S07.0**   **Crushing injury of face**

X ● **S07.1**   **Crushing injury of skull**

X ● **S07.8**   **Crushing injury of other parts of head**

X ● **S07.9**   **Crushing injury of head, part unspecified**

● **S08**   **Avulsion and traumatic amputation of part of head**
     An amputation not identified as partial or complete should be coded to complete
     The appropriate 7th character is to be added to each code from category S08

A	initial encounter
D	subsequent encounter
S	sequela

X ● **S08.0**   **Avulsion of scalp**

● **S08.1**   **Traumatic amputation of ear**

   ● **S08.11**   **Complete traumatic amputation of ear**

     ● **S08.111**   Complete traumatic amputation of right ear

     ● **S08.112**   Complete traumatic amputation of left ear

     ● **S08.119**   Complete traumatic amputation of unspecified ear

   ● **S08.12**   **Partial traumatic amputation of ear**

     ● **S08.121**   Partial traumatic amputation of right ear

     ● **S08.122**   Partial traumatic amputation of left ear

     ● **S08.129**   Partial traumatic amputation of unspecified ear

● **S08.8**   **Traumatic amputation of other parts of head**

   ● **S08.81**   **Traumatic amputation of nose**

     ● **S08.811**   Complete traumatic amputation of nose

     ● **S08.812**   Partial traumatic amputation of nose

X ● **S08.89**   **Traumatic amputation of other parts of head**

CHAPTER 19 (S00-T88)

CHAPTER 19 (S00-T88)

● **S09**   **Other and unspecified injuries of head**

The appropriate 7th character is to be added to each code from category S09

A	initial encounter
D	subsequent encounter
S	sequela

X● **S09.0**   **Injury of blood vessels of head, not elsewhere classified**

    Excludes1   injury of cerebral blood vessels (S06.-)
                      injury of precerebral blood vessels (S15.-)

● **S09.1**   **Injury of muscle and tendon of head**

    Code also any associated open wound (S01.-)

    Excludes2   sprain to joints and ligament of head (S03.9)

   X● **S09.10**   **Unspecified injury of muscle and tendon of head**
           Injury of muscle and tendon of head NOS

   X● **S09.11**   **Strain of muscle and tendon of head**

   X● **S09.12**   **Laceration of muscle and tendon of head**

   X● **S09.19**   **Other specified injury of muscle and tendon of head**

● **S09.2**   **Traumatic rupture of ear drum**

    Excludes1   traumatic rupture of ear drum due to blast injury (S09.31-)

   X● **S09.20**   **Traumatic rupture of unspecified ear drum**

   X● **S09.21**   **Traumatic rupture of right ear drum**

   X● **S09.22**   **Traumatic rupture of left ear drum**

● **S09.3**   **Other specified and unspecified injury of middle and inner ear**

    Excludes1   injury to ear NOS (S09.91-)

    Excludes2   injury to external ear (S00.4-, S01.3-, S08.1-)

   ● **S09.30**   **Unspecified injury of middle and inner ear**

     ● **S09.301**   **Unspecified injury of right middle and inner ear**

     ● **S09.302**   **Unspecified injury of left middle and inner ear**

     ● **S09.309**   **Unspecified injury of unspecified middle and inner ear**

   ● **S09.31**   **Primary blast injury of ear**
           Blast injury of ear NOS

     ● **S09.311**   **Primary blast injury of right ear**

     ● **S09.312**   **Primary blast injury of left ear**

     ● **S09.313**   **Primary blast injury of ear, bilateral**

     ● **S09.319**   **Primary blast injury of unspecified ear**

   ● **S09.39**   **Other specified injury of middle and inner ear**
           Secondary blast injury to ear

     ● **S09.391**   **Other specified injury of right middle and inner ear**

     ● **S09.392**   **Other specified injury of left middle and inner ear**

     ● **S09.399**   **Other specified injury of unspecified middle and inner ear**

X● **S09.8**   **Other specified injuries of head**

● **S09.9**   **Unspecified injury of face and head**

   X● **S09.90**   **Unspecified injury of head**
           Head injury NOS

     Excludes1   brain injury NOS (S06.9-)
                  head injury NOS with loss of consciousness (S06.9-)
                  intracranial injury NOS (S06.9-)

   X● **S09.91**   **Unspecified injury of ear**
           Injury of ear NOS

   X● **S09.92**   **Unspecified injury of nose**
           Injury of nose NOS

   X● **S09.93**   **Unspecified injury of face**
           Injury of face NOS

INJURIES TO THE NECK (S10-S19)

Includes   injuries of nape
            injuries of supraclavicular region
            injuries of throat

Excludes2   burns and corrosions (T20-T32)
             effects of foreign body in esophagus (T18.1)
             effects of foreign body in larynx (T17.3)
             effects of foreign body in pharynx (T17.2)
             effects of foreign body in trachea (T17.4)
             frostbite (T33-T34)
             insect bite or sting, venomous (T63.4)

● **S10**   **Superficial injury of neck**

The appropriate 7th character is to be added to each code from category S10

A	initial encounter
D	subsequent encounter
S	sequela

X● **S10.0**   **Contusion of throat**
         Contusion of cervical esophagus
         Contusion of larynx
         Contusion of pharynx
         Contusion of trachea

● **S10.1**   **Other and unspecified superficial injuries of throat**

   X● **S10.10**   **Unspecified superficial injuries of throat**

   X● **S10.11**   **Abrasion of throat**

   X● **S10.12**   **Blister (nonthermal) of throat**

   X● **S10.14**   **External constriction of part of throat**

   X● **S10.15**   **Superficial foreign body of throat**
           Splinter in the throat

   X● **S10.16**   **Insect bite (nonvenomous) of throat**

   X● **S10.17**   **Other superficial bite of throat**

     Excludes1   open bite of throat (S11.85)

● **S10.8**   **Superficial injury of other specified parts of neck**

   X● **S10.80**   **Unspecified superficial injury of other specified part of neck**

   X● **S10.81**   **Abrasion of other specified part of neck**

   X● **S10.82**   **Blister (nonthermal) of other specified part of neck**

   X● **S10.83**   **Contusion of other specified part of neck**

   X● **S10.84**   **External constriction of other specified part of neck**

   X● **S10.85**   **Superficial foreign body of other specified part of neck**
           Splinter in other part of neck

   X● **S10.86**   **Insect bite of other specified part of neck**

   X● **S10.87**   **Other superficial bite of other specified part of neck**

     Excludes1   open bite of other specified parts of neck (S11.85)

● **S10.9**   **Superficial injury of unspecified part of neck**

   X● **S10.90**   **Unspecified superficial injury of unspecified part of neck**

   X● **S10.91**   **Abrasion of unspecified part of neck**

   X● **S10.92**   **Blister (nonthermal) of unspecified part of neck**

   X● **S10.93**   **Contusion of unspecified part of neck**

   X● **S10.94**   **External constriction of unspecified part of neck**

   X● **S10.95**   **Superficial foreign body of unspecified part of neck**

   X● **S10.96**   **Insect bite of unspecified part of neck**

   X● **S10.97**   **Other superficial bite of unspecified part of neck**

▶ New   ⫸ Revised   ~~deleted~~ Deleted   Excludes 1   Excludes 2   Includes   Use additional   Code first   Code also   Key words

OGCR Official Guidelines   X Assign placeholder X   ● Use Additional Character(s)   ▶ Manifestation Code   Hierarchical Condition Category   **Coding Clinic**

● **S11   Open wound of neck**

Code also any associated:
     spinal cord injury (S14.0, S14.1-)
     wound infection

Excludes2   open fracture of vertebra (S12.- with 7th character B)

The appropriate 7th character is to be added to each code from category S11

> A   initial encounter
> D   subsequent encounter
> S   sequela

● **S11.0   Open wound of larynx and trachea**

   ● **S11.01   Open wound of larynx**

       Excludes2   open wound of vocal cord (S11.03)

     ● **S11.011   Laceration without foreign body of larynx**

     ● **S11.012   Laceration with foreign body of larynx**

     ● **S11.013   Puncture wound without foreign body of larynx**

     ● **S11.014   Puncture wound with foreign body of larynx**

     ● **S11.015   Open bite of larynx**
         Bite of larynx NOS

     ● **S11.019   Unspecified open wound of larynx**

   ● **S11.02   Open wound of trachea**
      Open wound of cervical trachea
      Open wound of trachea NOS

       Excludes2   open wound of thoracic trachea (S27.5-)

     ● **S11.021   Laceration without foreign body of trachea**

     ● **S11.022   Laceration with foreign body of trachea**

     ● **S11.023   Puncture wound without foreign body of trachea**

     ● **S11.024   Puncture wound with foreign body of trachea**

     ● **S11.025   Open bite of trachea**
         Bite of trachea NOS

     ● **S11.029   Unspecified open wound of trachea**

   ● **S11.03   Open wound of vocal cord**

     ● **S11.031   Laceration without foreign body of vocal cord**

     ● **S11.032   Laceration with foreign body of vocal cord**

     ● **S11.033   Puncture wound without foreign body of vocal cord**

     ● **S11.034   Puncture wound with foreign body of vocal cord**

     ● **S11.035   Open bite of vocal cord**
         Bite of vocal cord NOS

     ● **S11.039   Unspecified open wound of vocal cord**

● **S11.1   Open wound of thyroid gland**

   X ● **S11.10   Unspecified open wound of thyroid gland**

   X ● **S11.11   Laceration without foreign body of thyroid gland**

   X ● **S11.12   Laceration with foreign body of thyroid gland**

   X ● **S11.13   Puncture wound without foreign body of thyroid gland**

   X ● **S11.14   Puncture wound with foreign body of thyroid gland**

   X ● **S11.15   Open bite of thyroid gland**
         Bite of thyroid gland NOS

● **S11.2   Open wound of pharynx and cervical esophagus**

       Excludes1   open wound of esophagus NOS (S27.8-)

   X ● **S11.20   Unspecified open wound of pharynx and cervical esophagus**

   X ● **S11.21   Laceration without foreign body of pharynx and cervical esophagus**

   X ● **S11.22   Laceration with foreign body of pharynx and cervical esophagus**

   X ● **S11.23   Puncture wound without foreign body of pharynx and cervical esophagus**

   X ● **S11.24   Puncture wound with foreign body of pharynx and cervical esophagus**

   X ● **S11.25   Open bite of pharynx and cervical esophagus**
         Bite of pharynx and cervical esophagus NOS

● **S11.8   Open wound of other specified parts of neck**

   X ● **S11.80   Unspecified open specified wound of other part of neck**

   X ● **S11.81   Laceration without foreign body of other specified part of neck**

   X ● **S11.82   Laceration with foreign body of other specified part of neck**

   X ● **S11.83   Puncture wound without foreign body of other specified part of neck**

   X ● **S11.84   Puncture wound with foreign body of other specified part of neck**

   X ● **S11.85   Open bite of other specified part of neck**
         Bite of other part of neck NOS

         Excludes1   superficial bite of other specified part of neck (S10.87)

   X ● **S11.89   Other open wound of other part of neck**

● **S11.9   Open wound of unspecified part of neck**

   X ● **S11.90   Unspecified open wound of unspecified part of neck**

   X ● **S11.91   Laceration without foreign body of unspecified part of neck**

   X ● **S11.92   Laceration with foreign body of unspecified part of neck**

   X ● **S11.93   Puncture wound without foreign body of unspecified part of neck**

   X ● **S11.94   Puncture wound with foreign body of unspecified part of neck**

   X ● **S11.95   Open bite of unspecified part of neck**
         Bite of neck NOS

         Excludes1   superficial bite of neck (S10.97)

CHAPTER 19 (S00-T88)

● S12   **Fracture of cervical vertebra and other parts of neck**

     Note: A fracture not indicated as displaced or nondisplaced should be coded to displaced

         A fracture not indicated as open or closed should be coded to closed

     Includes   fracture of cervical neural arch
                  fracture of cervical spine
                  fracture of cervical spinous process
                  fracture of cervical transverse process
                  fracture of cervical vertebral arch
                  fracture of neck

     Code first any associated cervical spinal cord injury (S14.0, S14.1-)

     The appropriate 7th character is to be added to all codes from subcategories S12.0-S12.6

A	initial encounter for closed fracture
B	initial encounter for open fracture
D	subsequent encounter for fracture with routine healing
G	subsequent encounter for fracture with delayed healing
K	subsequent encounter for fracture with nonunion
S	sequela

● S12.0   **Fracture of first cervical vertebra**
     Atlas

   ● S12.00   Unspecified fracture of first cervical vertebra

     ● S12.000   Unspecified displaced fracture of first cervical vertebra A, B 🐷

     ● S12.001   Unspecified nondisplaced fracture of first cervical vertebra A, B 🐷

   X ● S12.01   Stable burst fracture of first cervical vertebra A, B 🐷

   X ● S12.02   Unstable burst fracture of first cervical vertebra A, B 🐷

   ● S12.03   Posterior arch fracture of first cervical vertebra

     ● S12.030   Displaced posterior arch fracture of first cervical vertebra A, B 🐷

     ● S12.031   Nondisplaced posterior arch fracture of first cervical vertebra A, B 🐷

   ● S12.04   Lateral mass fracture of first cervical vertebra

     ● S12.040   Displaced lateral mass fracture of first cervical vertebra A, B 🐷

     ● S12.041   Nondisplaced lateral mass fracture of first cervical vertebra A, B 🐷

   ● S12.09   Other fracture of first cervical vertebra

     ● S12.090   Other displaced fracture of first cervical vertebra A, B 🐷

     ● S12.091   Other nondisplaced fracture of first cervical vertebra A, B 🐷

● S12.1   **Fracture of second cervical vertebra**
     Axis

   ● S12.10   Unspecified fracture of second cervical vertebra

     ● S12.100   Unspecified displaced fracture of second cervical vertebra A, B 🐷

     ● S12.101   Unspecified nondisplaced fracture of second cervical vertebra A, B 🐷

   ● S12.11   Type II dens fracture

     ● S12.110   Anterior displaced Type II dens fracture A, B 🐷

     ● S12.111   Posterior displaced Type II dens fracture A, B 🐷

     ● S12.112   Nondisplaced Type II dens fracture A, B 🐷

   ● S12.12   Other dens fracture

     ● S12.120   Other displaced dens fracture A, B 🐷

     ● S12.121   Other nondisplaced dens fracture A, B 🐷

   ● S12.13   Unspecified traumatic spondylolisthesis of second cervical vertebra

     ● S12.130   Unspecified traumatic displaced spondylolisthesis of second cervical vertebra A, B 🐷

     ● S12.131   Unspecified traumatic nondisplaced spondylolisthesis of second cervical vertebra A, B 🐷

   X ● S12.14   Type III traumatic spondylolisthesis of second cervical vertebra A, B 🐷

   ● S12.15   Other traumatic spondylolisthesis of second cervical vertebra

     ● S12.150   Other traumatic displaced spondylolisthesis of second cervical vertebra A, B 🐷

     ● S12.151   Other traumatic nondisplaced spondylolisthesis of second cervical vertebra A, B 🐷

   ● S12.19   Other fracture of second cervical vertebra

     ● S12.190   Other displaced fracture of second cervical vertebra A, B 🐷

     ● S12.191   Other nondisplaced fracture of second cervical vertebra A, B 🐷

● S12.2   **Fracture of third cervical vertebra**

   ● S12.20   Unspecified fracture of third cervical vertebra

     ● S12.200   Unspecified displaced fracture of third cervical vertebra A, B 🐷

     ● S12.201   Unspecified nondisplaced fracture of third cervical vertebra A, B 🐷

   ● S12.23   Unspecified traumatic spondylolisthesis of third cervical vertebra

     ● S12.230   Unspecified traumatic displaced spondylolisthesis of third cervical vertebra A, B 🐷

     ● S12.231   Unspecified traumatic nondisplaced spondylolisthesis of third cervical vertebra A, B 🐷

   X ● S12.24   Type III traumatic spondylolisthesis of third cervical vertebra A, B 🐷

   ● S12.25   Other traumatic spondylolisthesis of third cervical vertebra

     ● S12.250   Other traumatic displaced spondylolisthesis of third cervical vertebra A, B 🐷

     ● S12.251   Other traumatic nondisplaced spondylolisthesis of third cervical vertebra A, B 🐷

   ● S12.29   Other fracture of third cervical vertebra

     ● S12.290   Other displaced fracture of third cervical vertebra A, B 🐷

     ● S12.291   Other nondisplaced fracture of third cervical vertebra A, B 🐷

● S12.3   **Fracture of fourth cervical vertebra**

   ● S12.30   Unspecified fracture of fourth cervical vertebra

     ● S12.300   Unspecified displaced fracture of fourth cervical vertebra A, B 🐷

     ● S12.301   Unspecified nondisplaced fracture of fourth cervical vertebra A, B 🐷

▶ New   ⇒ Revised   ~~deleted~~ Deleted   Excludes 1   Excludes 2   Includes   Use additional   Code first   Code also   Key words

OGCR Official Guidelines   X Assign placeholder X   ● Use Additional Character(s)   ▸ Manifestation Code   🐷 Hierarchical Condition Category   **Coding Clinic**

● S12.33 Unspecified traumatic spondylolisthesis of fourth cervical vertebra

  ● S12.330 Unspecified traumatic displaced spondylolisthesis of fourth cervical vertebra A, B 🏷

  ● S12.331 Unspecified traumatic nondisplaced spondylolisthesis of fourth cervical vertebra A, B 🏷

X ● S12.34 Type III traumatic spondylolisthesis of fourth cervical vertebra A, B 🏷

● S12.35 Other traumatic spondylolisthesis of fourth cervical vertebra

  ● S12.350 Other traumatic displaced spondylolisthesis of fourth cervical vertebra A, B 🏷

  ● S12.351 Other traumatic nondisplaced spondylolisthesis of fourth cervical vertebra A, B 🏷

● S12.39 Other fracture of fourth cervical vertebra

  ● S12.390 Other displaced fracture of fourth cervical vertebra A, B 🏷

  ● S12.391 Other nondisplaced fracture of fourth cervical vertebra A, B 🏷

● S12.4 Fracture of fifth cervical vertebra

  ● S12.40 Unspecified fracture of fifth cervical vertebra

    ● S12.400 Unspecified displaced fracture of fifth cervical vertebra A, B 🏷

    ● S12.401 Unspecified nondisplaced fracture of fifth cervical vertebra A, B 🏷

  ● S12.43 Unspecified traumatic spondylolisthesis of fifth cervical vertebra

    ● S12.430 Unspecified traumatic displaced spondylolisthesis of fifth cervical vertebra A, B 🏷

    ● S12.431 Unspecified traumatic nondisplaced spondylolisthesis of fifth cervical vertebra A, B 🏷

X ● S12.44 Type III traumatic spondylolisthesis of fifth cervical vertebra A, B 🏷

  ● S12.45 Other traumatic spondylolisthesis of fifth cervical vertebra

    ● S12.450 Other traumatic displaced spondylolisthesis of fifth cervical vertebra A, B 🏷

    ● S12.451 Other traumatic nondisplaced spondylolisthesis of fifth cervical vertebra A, B 🏷

  ● S12.49 Other fracture of fifth cervical vertebra

    ● S12.490 Other displaced fracture of fifth cervical vertebra A, B 🏷

    ● S12.491 Other nondisplaced fracture of fifth cervical vertebra A, B 🏷

● S12.5 Fracture of sixth cervical vertebra

  ● S12.50 Unspecified fracture of sixth cervical vertebra

    ● S12.500 Unspecified displaced fracture of sixth cervical vertebra A, B 🏷

    ● S12.501 Unspecified nondisplaced fracture of sixth cervical vertebra A, B 🏷

  ● S12.53 Unspecified traumatic spondylolisthesis of sixth cervical vertebra

    ● S12.530 Unspecified traumatic displaced spondylolisthesis of sixth cervical vertebra A, B 🏷

    ● S12.531 Unspecified traumatic nondisplaced spondylolisthesis of sixth cervical vertebra A, B 🏷

X ● S12.54 Type III traumatic spondylolisthesis of sixth cervical vertebra A, B 🏷

● S12.55 Other traumatic spondylolisthesis of sixth cervical vertebra

  ● S12.550 Other traumatic displaced spondylolisthesis of sixth cervical vertebra A, B 🏷

  ● S12.551 Other traumatic nondisplaced spondylolisthesis of sixth cervical vertebra A, B 🏷

● S12.59 Other fracture of sixth cervical vertebra

  ● S12.590 Other displaced fracture of sixth cervical vertebra A, B 🏷

  ● S12.591 Other nondisplaced fracture of sixth cervical vertebra A, B 🏷

● S12.6 Fracture of seventh cervical vertebra

  ● S12.60 Unspecified fracture of seventh cervical vertebra

    ● S12.600 Unspecified displaced fracture of seventh cervical vertebra A, B 🏷

    ● S12.601 Unspecified nondisplaced fracture of seventh cervical vertebra A, B 🏷

  ● S12.63 Unspecified traumatic spondylolisthesis of seventh cervical vertebra

    ● S12.630 Unspecified traumatic displaced spondylolisthesis of seventh cervical vertebra A, B 🏷

    ● S12.631 Unspecified traumatic nondisplaced spondylolisthesis of seventh cervical vertebra A, B 🏷

X ● S12.64 Type III traumatic spondylolisthesis of seventh cervical vertebra A, B 🏷

● S12.65 Other traumatic spondylolisthesis of seventh cervical vertebra

  ● S12.650 Other traumatic displaced spondylolisthesis of seventh cervical vertebra A, B 🏷

  ● S12.651 Other traumatic nondisplaced spondylolisthesis of seventh cervical vertebra A, B 🏷

● S12.69 Other fracture of seventh cervical vertebra

  ● S12.690 Other displaced fracture of seventh cervical vertebra A, B 🏷

  ● S12.691 Other nondisplaced fracture of seventh cervical vertebra A, B 🏷

X ● S12.8 Fracture of other parts of neck A 🏷

  Hyoid bone   Thyroid cartilage
  Larynx   Trachea

The appropriate 7th character is to be added to code S12.8

A	initial encounter
D	subsequent encounter
S	sequela

X ● S12.9 Fracture of neck, unspecified A 🏷

  Fracture of neck NOS
  Fracture of cervical spine NOS
  Fracture of cervical vertebra NOS

The appropriate 7th character is to be added to code S12.9

A	initial encounter
D	subsequent encounter
S	sequela

● S13   **Dislocation and sprain of joints and ligaments at neck level**

    Includes   avulsion of joint or ligament at neck level

               laceration of cartilage, joint or ligament at neck level

               sprain of cartilage, joint or ligament at neck level

               traumatic hemarthrosis of joint or ligament at neck level

               traumatic rupture of joint or ligament at neck level

               traumatic subluxation of joint or ligament at neck level

               traumatic tear of joint or ligament at neck level

    Code also any associated open wound

    Excludes2   strain of muscle or tendon at neck level (S16.1)

    The appropriate 7th character is to be added to each code from category S13

> A   initial encounter
> D   subsequent encounter
> S   sequela

X ● **S13.0**   **Traumatic rupture of cervical intervertebral disc**

    Excludes1   rupture or displacement (nontraumatic) of cervical intervertebral disc NOS (M50.-)

● **S13.1**   **Subluxation and dislocation of cervical vertebrae**

    Code also any associated:

       open wound of neck (S11.-)

       spinal cord injury (S14.1-)

    Excludes2   fracture of cervical vertebrae (S12.0-S12.3-)

   ● **S13.10**   **Subluxation and dislocation of unspecified cervical vertebrae**

      ● **S13.100**   **Subluxation of unspecified cervical vertebrae**

      ● **S13.101**   **Dislocation of unspecified cervical vertebrae**

   ● **S13.11**   **Subluxation and dislocation of C0/C1 cervical vertebrae**

        Subluxation and dislocation of atlantooccipital joint

        Subluxation and dislocation of atloidooccipital joint

        Subluxation and dislocation of occipitoatloid joint

      ● **S13.110**   **Subluxation of C0/C1 cervical vertebrae**

      ● **S13.111**   **Dislocation of C0/C1 cervical vertebrae**

   ● **S13.12**   **Subluxation and dislocation of C1/C2 cervical vertebrae**

        Subluxation and dislocation of atlantoaxial joint

      ● **S13.120**   **Subluxation of C1/C2 cervical vertebrae**

      ● **S13.121**   **Dislocation of C1/C2 cervical vertebrae**

   ● **S13.13**   **Subluxation and dislocation of C2/C3 cervical vertebrae**

      ● **S13.130**   **Subluxation of C2/C3 cervical vertebrae**

      ● **S13.131**   **Dislocation of C2/C3 cervical vertebrae**

   ● **S13.14**   **Subluxation and dislocation of C3/C4 cervical vertebrae**

      ● **S13.140**   **Subluxation of C3/C4 cervical vertebrae**

      ● **S13.141**   **Dislocation of C3/C4 cervical vertebrae**

● **S13.15**   **Subluxation and dislocation of C4/C5 cervical vertebrae**

    ● **S13.150**   **Subluxation of C4/C5 cervical vertebrae**

    ● **S13.151**   **Dislocation of C4/C5 cervical vertebrae**

● **S13.16**   **Subluxation and dislocation of C5/C6 cervical vertebrae**

    ● **S13.160**   **Subluxation of C5/C6 cervical vertebrae**

    ● **S13.161**   **Dislocation of C5/C6 cervical vertebrae**

● **S13.17**   **Subluxation and dislocation of C6/C7 cervical vertebrae**

    ● **S13.170**   **Subluxation of C6/C7 cervical vertebrae**

    ● **S13.171**   **Dislocation of C6/C7 cervical vertebrae**

● **S13.18**   **Subluxation and dislocation of C7/T1 cervical vertebrae**

    ● **S13.180**   **Subluxation of C7/T1 cervical vertebrae**

    ● **S13.181**   **Dislocation of C7/T1 cervical vertebrae**

  ● **S13.2**   **Dislocation of other and unspecified parts of neck**

   X ● **S13.20**   **Dislocation of unspecified parts of neck**

   X ● **S13.29**   **Dislocation of other parts of neck**

X ● **S13.4**   **Sprain of ligaments of cervical spine**

    Sprain of anterior longitudinal (ligament), cervical

    Sprain of atlanto-axial (joints)

    Sprain of atlanto-occipital (joints)

    Whiplash injury of cervical spine

X ● **S13.5**   **Sprain of thyroid region**

    Sprain of cricoarytenoid (joint) (ligament)

    Sprain of cricothyroid (joint) (ligament)

    Sprain of thyroid cartilage

X ● **S13.8**   **Sprain of joints and ligaments of other parts of neck**

X ● **S13.9**   **Sprain of joints and ligaments of unspecified parts of neck**

● S14   **Injury of nerves and spinal cord at neck level**

    Note: Code to highest level of cervical cord injury

    Code also any associated:

       fracture of cervical vertebra (S12.0--S12.6.-)

       open wound of neck (S11.-)

       transient paralysis (R29.5)

    The appropriate 7th character is to be added to each code from category S14

> A   initial encounter
> D   subsequent encounter
> S   sequela

X ● **S14.0**   **Concussion and edema of cervical spinal cord** A, D, S 🦠

  ● **S14.1**   **Other and unspecified injuries of cervical spinal cord**

   ● **S14.10**   **Unspecified injury of cervical spinal cord**

      ● **S14.101**   **Unspecified injury at C1 level of cervical spinal cord** A, D, S 🦠

      ● **S14.102**   **Unspecified injury at C2 level of cervical spinal cord** A, D, S 🦠

      ● **S14.103**   **Unspecified injury at C3 level of cervical spinal cord** A, D, S 🦠

      ● **S14.104**   **Unspecified injury at C4 level of cervical spinal cord** A, D, S 🦠

      ● **S14.105**   **Unspecified injury at C5 level of cervical spinal cord** A, D, S 🦠

      ● **S14.106**   **Unspecified injury at C6 level of cervical spinal cord** A, D, S 🦠

▶ New   ⇒ Revised   ~~deleted~~ Deleted   Excludes 1   Excludes 2   Includes   Use additional   Code first   Code also   Key words

OGCR Official Guidelines   X Assign placeholder X   ● Use Additional Character(s)   ▶ Manifestation Code   🦠 Hierarchical Condition Category   **Coding Clinic**

● S14.107   Unspecified injury at C7 level of cervical spinal cord A, D, S 🔗

● S14.108   Unspecified injury at C8 level of cervical spinal cord A, D, S 🔗

● S14.109   Unspecified injury at unspecified level of cervical spinal cord A, D, S 🔗
Injury of cervical spinal cord NOS

● S14.11   Complete lesion of cervical spinal cord

  ● S14.111   Complete lesion at C1 level of cervical spinal cord A, D, S 🔗

  ● S14.112   Complete lesion at C2 level of cervical spinal cord A, D, S 🔗

  ● S14.113   Complete lesion at C3 level of cervical spinal cord A, D, S 🔗

  ● S14.114   Complete lesion at C4 level of cervical spinal cord A, D, S 🔗

  ● S14.115   Complete lesion at C5 level of cervical spinal cord A, D, S 🔗

  ● S14.116   Complete lesion at C6 level of cervical spinal cord A, D, S 🔗

  ● S14.117   Complete lesion at C7 level of cervical spinal cord A, D, S 🔗

  ● S14.118   Complete lesion at C8 level of cervical spinal cord A, D, S 🔗

  ● S14.119   Complete lesion at unspecified level of cervical spinal cord A, D, S 🔗

● S14.12   Central cord syndrome of cervical spinal cord

  ● S14.121   Central cord syndrome at C1 level of cervical spinal cord A, D, S 🔗

  ● S14.122   Central cord syndrome at C2 level of cervical spinal cord A, D, S 🔗

  ● S14.123   Central cord syndrome at C3 level of cervical spinal cord A, D, S 🔗

  ● S14.124   Central cord syndrome at C4 level of cervical spinal cord A, D, S 🔗

  ● S14.125   Central cord syndrome at C5 level of cervical spinal cord A, D, S 🔗

  ● S14.126   Central cord syndrome at C6 level of cervical spinal cord A, D, S 🔗

  ● S14.127   Central cord syndrome at C7 level of cervical spinal cord A, D, S 🔗

  ● S14.128   Central cord syndrome at C8 level of cervical spinal cord A, D, S 🔗

  ● S14.129   Central cord syndrome at unspecified level of cervical spinal cord A, D, S 🔗

● S14.13   Anterior cord syndrome of cervical spinal cord

  ● S14.131   Anterior cord syndrome at C1 level of cervical spinal cord A, D, S 🔗

  ● S14.132   Anterior cord syndrome at C2 level of cervical spinal cord A, D, S 🔗

  ● S14.133   Anterior cord syndrome at C3 level of cervical spinal cord A, D, S 🔗

  ● S14.134   Anterior cord syndrome at C4 level of cervical spinal cord A, D, S 🔗

  ● S14.135   Anterior cord syndrome at C5 level of cervical spinal cord A, D, S 🔗

  ● S14.136   Anterior cord syndrome at C6 level of cervical spinal cord A, D, S 🔗

  ● S14.137   Anterior cord syndrome at C7 level of cervical spinal cord A, D, S 🔗

  ● S14.138   Anterior cord syndrome at C8 level of cervical spinal cord A, D, S 🔗

  ● S14.139   Anterior cord syndrome at unspecified level of cervical spinal cord A, D, S 🔗

● S14.14   Brown-Séquard syndrome of cervical spinal cord

  ● S14.141   Brown-Séquard syndrome at C1 level of cervical spinal cord A, D, S 🔗

  ● S14.142   Brown-Séquard syndrome at C2 level of cervical spinal cord A, D, S 🔗

  ● S14.143   Brown-Séquard syndrome at C3 level of cervical spinal cord A, D, S 🔗

  ● S14.144   Brown-Séquard syndrome at C4 level of cervical spinal cord A, D, S 🔗

  ● S14.145   Brown-Séquard syndrome at C5 level of cervical spinal cord A, D, S 🔗

  ● S14.146   Brown-Séquard syndrome at C6 level of cervical spinal cord A, D, S 🔗

  ● S14.147   Brown-Séquard syndrome at C7 level of cervical spinal cord A, D, S 🔗

  ● S14.148   Brown-Séquard syndrome at C8 level of cervical spinal cord A, D, S 🔗

  ● S14.149   Brown-Séquard syndrome at unspecified level of cervical spinal cord A, D, S 🔗

● S14.15   Other incomplete lesions of cervical spinal cord
Incomplete lesion of cervical spinal cord NOS
Posterior cord syndrome of cervical spinal cord

  ● S14.151   Other incomplete lesion at C1 level of cervical spinal cord A, D, S 🔗

  ● S14.152   Other incomplete lesion at C2 level of cervical spinal cord A, D, S 🔗

  ● S14.153   Other incomplete lesion at C3 level of cervical spinal cord A, D, S 🔗

  ● S14.154   Other incomplete lesion at C4 level of cervical spinal cord A, D, S 🔗

  ● S14.155   Other incomplete lesion at C5 level of cervical spinal cord A, D, S 🔗

  ● S14.156   Other incomplete lesion at C6 level of cervical spinal cord A, D, S 🔗

  ● S14.157   Other incomplete lesion at C7 level of cervical spinal cord A, D, S 🔗

  ● S14.158   Other incomplete lesion at C8 level of cervical spinal cord A, D, S 🔗

  ● S14.159   Other incomplete lesion at unspecified level of cervical spinal cord A, D, S 🔗

X ● S14.2   Injury of nerve root of cervical spine

X ● S14.3   Injury of brachial plexus

X ● S14.4   Injury of peripheral nerves of neck

X ● S14.5   Injury of cervical sympathetic nerves

X ● S14.8   Injury of other specified nerves of neck

X ● S14.9   Injury of unspecified nerves of neck

● S15   **Injury of blood vessels at neck level**

Code also any associated open wound (S11.-)

The appropriate 7th character is to be added to each code from category S15

A	initial encounter
D	subsequent encounter
S	sequela

● S15.0   **Injury of carotid artery of neck**
Injury of carotid artery (common) (external) (internal, extracranial portion)
Injury of carotid artery NOS

Excludes1   injury of internal carotid artery, intracranial portion (S06.8)

● S15.00   Unspecified injury of carotid artery
  ● S15.001   Unspecified injury of right carotid artery
  ● S15.002   Unspecified injury of left carotid artery
  ● S15.009   Unspecified injury of unspecified carotid artery
● S15.01   Minor laceration of carotid artery
            Incomplete transection of carotid artery
            Laceration of carotid artery NOS
            Superficial laceration of carotid artery
  ● S15.011   Minor laceration of right carotid artery
  ● S15.012   Minor laceration of left carotid artery
  ● S15.019   Minor laceration of unspecified carotid artery
● S15.02   Major laceration of carotid artery
            Complete transection of carotid artery
            Traumatic rupture of carotid artery
  ● S15.021   Major laceration of right carotid artery
  ● S15.022   Major laceration of left carotid artery
  ● S15.029   Major laceration of unspecified carotid artery
● S15.09   Other specified injury of carotid artery
  ● S15.091   Other specified injury of right carotid artery
  ● S15.092   Other specified injury of left carotid artery
  ● S15.099   Other specified injury of unspecified carotid artery
● S15.1   Injury of vertebral artery
  ● S15.10   Unspecified injury of vertebral artery
    ● S15.101   Unspecified injury of right vertebral artery
    ● S15.102   Unspecified injury of left vertebral artery
    ● S15.109   Unspecified injury of unspecified vertebral artery
  ● S15.11   Minor laceration of vertebral artery
              Incomplete transection of vertebral artery
              Laceration of vertebral artery NOS
              Superficial laceration of vertebral artery
    ● S15.111   Minor laceration of right vertebral artery
    ● S15.112   Minor laceration of left vertebral artery
    ● S15.119   Minor laceration of unspecified vertebral artery
  ● S15.12   Major laceration of vertebral artery
              Complete transection of vertebral artery
              Traumatic rupture of vertebral artery
    ● S15.121   Major laceration of right vertebral artery
    ● S15.122   Major laceration of left vertebral artery
    ● S15.129   Major laceration of unspecified vertebral artery

● S15.19   Other specified injury of vertebral artery
  ● S15.191   Other specified injury of right vertebral artery
  ● S15.192   Other specified injury of left vertebral artery
  ● S15.199   Other specified injury of unspecified vertebral artery
● S15.2   Injury of external jugular vein
  ● S15.20   Unspecified injury of external jugular vein
    ● S15.201   Unspecified injury of right external jugular vein
    ● S15.202   Unspecified injury of left external jugular vein
    ● S15.209   Unspecified injury of unspecified external jugular vein
  ● S15.21   Minor laceration of external jugular vein
              Incomplete transection of external jugular vein
              Laceration of external jugular vein NOS
              Superficial laceration of external jugular vein
    ● S15.211   Minor laceration of right external jugular vein
    ● S15.212   Minor laceration of left external jugular vein
    ● S15.219   Minor laceration of unspecified external jugular vein
  ● S15.22   Major laceration of external jugular vein
              Complete transection of external jugular vein
              Traumatic rupture of external jugular vein
    ● S15.221   Major laceration of right external jugular vein
    ● S15.222   Major laceration of left external jugular vein
    ● S15.229   Major laceration of unspecified external jugular vein
  ● S15.29   Other specified injury of external jugular vein
    ● S15.291   Other specified injury of right external jugular vein
    ● S15.292   Other specified injury of left external jugular vein
    ● S15.299   Other specified injury of unspecified external jugular vein
● S15.3   Injury of internal jugular vein
  ● S15.30   Unspecified injury of internal jugular vein
    ● S15.301   Unspecified injury of right internal jugular vein
    ● S15.302   Unspecified injury of left internal jugular vein
    ● S15.309   Unspecified injury of unspecified internal jugular vein
  ● S15.31   Minor laceration of internal jugular vein
              Incomplete transection of internal jugular vein
              Laceration of internal jugular vein NOS
              Superficial laceration of internal jugular vein
    ● S15.311   Minor laceration of right internal jugular vein
    ● S15.312   Minor laceration of left internal jugular vein
    ● S15.319   Minor laceration of unspecified internal jugular vein

▶ New   ⟳ Revised   ~~deleted~~ Deleted   Excludes 1   Excludes 2   Includes   Use additional   Code first   Code also   Key words
OGCR Official Guidelines   X Assign placeholder X   ● Use Additional Character(s)   ▶ Manifestation Code   ℞ Hierarchical Condition Category   Coding Clinic

● **S15.32** Major laceration of internal jugular vein
　　　　Complete transection of internal jugular vein
　　　　Traumatic rupture of internal jugular vein

　● **S15.321** Major laceration of right internal jugular vein
　● **S15.322** Major laceration of left internal jugular vein
　● **S15.329** Major laceration of unspecified internal jugular vein

● **S15.39** Other specified injury of internal jugular vein

　● **S15.391** Other specified injury of right internal jugular vein
　● **S15.392** Other specified injury of left internal jugular vein
　● **S15.399** Other specified injury of unspecified internal jugular vein

X● **S15.8** Injury of other specified blood vessels at neck level
X● **S15.9** Injury of unspecified blood vessel at neck level

● **S16** Injury of muscle, fascia and tendon at neck level
　Code also any associated open wound (S11.-)
　Excludes2 sprain of joint or ligament at neck level (S13.9)

　The appropriate 7th character is to be added to each code from category S16

A	initial encounter
D	subsequent encounter
S	sequela

X● **S16.1** Strain of muscle, fascia and tendon at neck level
X● **S16.2** Laceration of muscle, fascia and tendon at neck level
X● **S16.8** Other specified injury of muscle, fascia and tendon at neck level
X● **S16.9** Unspecified injury of muscle, fascia and tendon at neck level

● **S17** Crushing injury of neck
　Use additional code for all associated injuries, such as:
　　injury of blood vessels (S15.-)
　　open wound of neck (S11.-)
　　spinal cord injury (S14.0, S14.1-)
　　vertebral fracture (S12.0--S12.3-)

　The appropriate 7th character is to be added to each code from category S17

A	initial encounter
D	subsequent encounter
S	sequela

X● **S17.0** Crushing injury of larynx and trachea
X● **S17.8** Crushing injury of other specified parts of neck
X● **S17.9** Crushing injury of neck, part unspecified

● **S19** Other and unspecified injuries of neck

　The appropriate 7th character is to be added to each code from category S19

A	initial encounter
D	subsequent encounter
S	sequela

● **S19.8** Other specified injuries of neck
　X● **S19.80** Other specified injuries of unspecified part of neck
　X● **S19.81** Other specified injuries of larynx
　X● **S19.82** Other specified injuries of cervical trachea
　　　Excludes2 other specified injury of thoracic trachea (S27.5-)
　X● **S19.83** Other specified injuries of vocal cord

X● **S19.84** Other specified injuries of thyroid gland
X● **S19.85** Other specified injuries of pharynx and cervical esophagus
X● **S19.89** Other specified injuries of other specified part of neck

X● **S19.9** Unspecified injury of neck

INJURIES TO THE THORAX (S20-S29)

Includes injuries of breast
　　　　injuries of chest (wall)
　　　　injuries of interscapular area

Excludes2 burns and corrosions (T20-T32)
　　　　effects of foreign body in bronchus (T17.5)
　　　　effects of foreign body in esophagus (T18.1)
　　　　effects of foreign body in lung (T17.8)
　　　　effects of foreign body in trachea (T17.4)
　　　　frostbite (T33-T34)
　　　　injuries of axilla
　　　　injuries of clavicle
　　　　injuries of scapular region
　　　　injuries of shoulder
　　　　insect bite or sting, venomous (T63.4)

● **S20** Superficial injury of thorax
　The appropriate 7th character is to be added to each code from category S20

A	initial encounter
D	subsequent encounter
S	sequela

● **S20.0** Contusion of breast
　X● **S20.00** Contusion of breast, unspecified breast
　X● **S20.01** Contusion of right breast
　X● **S20.02** Contusion of left breast

● **S20.1** Other and unspecified superficial injuries of breast
　● **S20.10** Unspecified superficial injuries of breast
　　● **S20.101** Unspecified superficial injuries of breast, right breast
　　● **S20.102** Unspecified superficial injuries of breast, left breast
　　● **S20.109** Unspecified superficial injuries of breast, unspecified breast

　● **S20.11** Abrasion of breast
　　● **S20.111** Abrasion of breast, right breast
　　● **S20.112** Abrasion of breast, left breast
　　● **S20.119** Abrasion of breast, unspecified breast

　● **S20.12** Blister (nonthermal) of breast
　　● **S20.121** Blister (nonthermal) of breast, right breast
　　● **S20.122** Blister (nonthermal) of breast, left breast
　　● **S20.129** Blister (nonthermal) of breast, unspecified breast

　● **S20.14** External constriction of part of breast
　　● **S20.141** External constriction of part of breast, right breast
　　● **S20.142** External constriction of part of breast, left breast
　　● **S20.149** External constriction of part of breast, unspecified breast

　● **S20.15** Superficial foreign body of breast
　　　Splinter in the breast
　　● **S20.151** Superficial foreign body of breast, right breast
　　● **S20.152** Superficial foreign body of breast, left breast
　　● **S20.159** Superficial foreign body of breast, unspecified breast

CHAPTER 19 (S00-T88)

● S20.16   Insect bite (nonvenomous) of breast
   ● S20.161   Insect bite (nonvenomous) of breast, right breast
   ● S20.162   Insect bite (nonvenomous) of breast, left breast
   ● S20.169   Insect bite (nonvenomous) of breast, unspecified breast
● S20.17   Other superficial bite of breast
     Excludes1   open bite of breast (S21.05-)
   ● S20.171   Other superficial bite of breast, right breast
   ● S20.172   Other superficial bite of breast, left breast
   ● S20.179   Other superficial bite of breast, unspecified breast
● S20.2   Contusion of thorax
 X ● S20.20   Contusion of thorax, unspecified
  ● S20.21   Contusion of front wall of thorax
   ● S20.211   Contusion of right front wall of thorax
   ● S20.212   Contusion of left front wall of thorax
    S20.213   Contusion of bilateral front wall of thorax
    S20.214   Contusion of middle front wall of thorax
   ● S20.219   Contusion of unspecified front wall of thorax
  ● S20.22   Contusion of back wall of thorax
   ● S20.221   Contusion of right back wall of thorax
   ● S20.222   Contusion of left back wall of thorax
    S20.223   Contusion of bilateral back wall of thorax
    S20.224   Contusion of middle back wall of thorax
   ● S20.229   Contusion of unspecified back wall of thorax
● S20.3   Other and unspecified superficial injuries of front wall of thorax
  ● S20.30   Unspecified superficial injuries of front wall of thorax
   ● S20.301   Unspecified superficial injuries of right front wall of thorax
   ● S20.302   Unspecified superficial injuries of left front wall of thorax
    S20.303   Unspecified superficial injuries of bilateral front wall of thorax
    S20.304   Unspecified superficial injuries of middle front wall of thorax
   ● S20.309   Unspecified superficial injuries of unspecified front wall of thorax
  ● S20.31   Abrasion of front wall of thorax
   ● S20.311   Abrasion of right front wall of thorax
   ● S20.312   Abrasion of left front wall of thorax
    S20.313   Abrasion of bilateral front wall of thorax
    S20.314   Abrasion of middle front wall of thorax
   ● S20.319   Abrasion of unspecified front wall of thorax
  ● S20.32   Blister (nonthermal) of front wall of thorax
   ● S20.321   Blister (nonthermal) of right front wall of thorax
   ● S20.322   Blister (nonthermal) of left front wall of thorax

    S20.323   Blister (nonthermal) of bilateral front wall of thorax
    S20.324   Blister (nonthermal) of middle front wall of thorax
   ● S20.329   Blister (nonthermal) of unspecified front wall of thorax
  ● S20.34   External constriction of front wall of thorax
   ● S20.341   External constriction of right front wall of thorax
   ● S20.342   External constriction of left front wall of thorax
    S20.343   External constriction of bilateral front wall of thorax
    S20.344   External constriction of middle front wall of thorax
   ● S20.349   External constriction of unspecified front wall of thorax
  ● S20.35   Superficial foreign body of front wall of thorax
    Splinter in front wall of thorax
   ● S20.351   Superficial foreign body of right front wall of thorax
   ● S20.352   Superficial foreign body of left front wall of thorax
    S20.353   Superficial foreign body of bilateral front wall of thorax
    S20.354   Superficial foreign body of middle front wall of thorax
   ● S20.359   Superficial foreign body of unspecified front wall of thorax
  ● S20.36   Insect bite (nonvenomous) of front wall of thorax
   ● S20.361   Insect bite (nonvenomous) of right front wall of thorax
   ● S20.362   Insect bite (nonvenomous) of left front wall of thorax
    S20.363   Insect bite (nonvenomous) of bilateral front wall of thorax
    S20.364   Insect bite (nonvenomous) of middle front wall of thorax
   ● S20.369   Insect bite (nonvenomous) of unspecified front wall of thorax
  ● S20.37   Other superficial bite of front wall of thorax
     Excludes1   open bite of front wall of thorax (S21.14)
   ● S20.371   Other superficial bite of right front wall of thorax
   ● S20.372   Other superficial bite of left front wall of thorax
    S20.373   Other superficial bite of bilateral front wall of thorax
    S20.374   Other superficial bite of middle front wall of thorax
   ● S20.379   Other superficial bite of unspecified front wall of thorax
● S20.4   Other and unspecified superficial injuries of back wall of thorax
  ● S20.40   Unspecified superficial injuries of back wall of thorax
   ● S20.401   Unspecified superficial injuries of right back wall of thorax
   ● S20.402   Unspecified superficial injuries of left back wall of thorax
   ● S20.409   Unspecified superficial injuries of unspecified back wall of thorax

● **S20.41**   **Abrasion** of back wall of thorax
    ● **S20.411**   Abrasion of **right** back wall of thorax
    ● **S20.412**   Abrasion of **left** back wall of thorax
    ● **S20.419**   Abrasion of **unspecified** back wall of thorax

● **S20.42**   **Blister** (nonthermal) of back wall of thorax
    ● **S20.421**   Blister (nonthermal) of **right** back wall of thorax
    ● **S20.422**   Blister (nonthermal) of **left** back wall of thorax
    ● **S20.429**   Blister (nonthermal) of **unspecified** back wall of thorax

● **S20.44**   **External constriction** of back wall of thorax
    ● **S20.441**   External constriction of **right** back wall of thorax
    ● **S20.442**   External constriction of **left** back wall of thorax
    ● **S20.449**   External constriction of **unspecified** back wall of thorax

● **S20.45**   **Superficial foreign body** of back wall of thorax
    Splinter of back wall of thorax
    ● **S20.451**   Superficial foreign body of **right** back wall of thorax
    ● **S20.452**   Superficial foreign body of **left** back wall of thorax
    ● **S20.459**   Superficial foreign body of **unspecified** back wall of thorax

● **S20.46**   **Insect bite** (nonvenomous) of back wall of thorax
    ● **S20.461**   Insect bite (nonvenomous) of **right** back wall of thorax
    ● **S20.462**   Insect bite (nonvenomous) of **left** back wall of thorax
    ● **S20.469**   Insect bite (nonvenomous) of **unspecified** back wall of thorax

● **S20.47**   **Other superficial bite** of back wall of thorax
    Excludes1   open bite of back wall of thorax (S21.24)
    ● **S20.471**   Other superficial bite of **right** back wall of thorax
    ● **S20.472**   Other superficial bite of **left** back wall of thorax
    ● **S20.479**   Other superficial bite of **unspecified** back wall of thorax

● **S20.9**   **Superficial injury** of unspecified parts of thorax
    Excludes1   contusion of thorax NOS (S20.20)
X ● **S20.90**   Unspecified superficial injury of unspecified parts of thorax
    Superficial injury of thoracic wall NOS
X ● **S20.91**   **Abrasion** of unspecified parts of thorax
X ● **S20.92**   **Blister** (nonthermal) of unspecified parts of thorax
X ● **S20.94**   **External constriction** of unspecified parts of thorax
X ● **S20.95**   **Superficial foreign body** of unspecified parts of thorax
    Splinter in thorax NOS
X ● **S20.96**   **Insect bite** (nonvenomous) of unspecified parts of thorax
X ● **S20.97**   **Other** superficial bite of unspecified parts of thorax
    Excludes1   open bite of thorax NOS (S21.95)

● **S21**   **Open wound of thorax**
    Code also any associated injury such as:
      injury of heart (S26.-)
      injury of intrathoracic organs (S27.-)
      rib fracture (S22.3-, S22.4-)
      spinal cord injury (S24.0-, S24.1-)
      traumatic hemothorax (S27.1)
      traumatic hemopneumothorax (S27.3)
      traumatic pneumothorax (S27.0)
      wound infection
    Excludes1   traumatic amputation (partial) of thorax (S28.1)
    The appropriate 7th character is to be added to each code from category S21

A	initial encounter
D	subsequent encounter
S	sequela

● **S21.0**   **Open wound of breast**
    ● **S21.00**   **Unspecified** open wound of breast
        ● **S21.001**   Unspecified open wound of **right** breast
        ● **S21.002**   Unspecified open wound of **left** breast
        ● **S21.009**   Unspecified open wound of **unspecified** breast
    ● **S21.01**   **Laceration without foreign body** of breast
        ● **S21.011**   Laceration without foreign body of **right** breast
        ● **S21.012**   Laceration without foreign body of **left** breast
        ● **S21.019**   Laceration without foreign body of **unspecified** breast
    ● **S21.02**   **Laceration with foreign body** of breast
        ● **S21.021**   Laceration with foreign body of **right** breast
        ● **S21.022**   Laceration with foreign body of **left** breast
        ● **S21.029**   Laceration with foreign body of **unspecified** breast
    ● **S21.03**   **Puncture wound without foreign body** of breast
        ● **S21.031**   Puncture wound without foreign body of **right** breast
        ● **S21.032**   Puncture wound without foreign body of **left** breast
        ● **S21.039**   Puncture wound without foreign body of **unspecified** breast
    ● **S21.04**   **Puncture wound with foreign body** of breast
        ● **S21.041**   Puncture wound with foreign body of **right** breast
        ● **S21.042**   Puncture wound with foreign body of **left** breast
        ● **S21.049**   Puncture wound with foreign body of **unspecified** breast

Item 19–1 Pneumothorax is a collection of gas (positive air pressure) in the pleural space, resulting in the lung collapsing. A **tension pneumothorax** is life-threatening and is a result of air in the pleural space causing a displacement in the mediastinal structures and cardiopulmonary function compromise. A **traumatic pneumothorax** results from blunt or penetrating injury that disrupts the parietal/visceral pleura. **Hemothorax** is blood or bloody fluid in the pleural cavity as a result of traumatic blood vessel rupture or inflammation of the lungs from pneumonia.

CHAPTER 19 (S00-T88)

CHAPTER 19 (S00-T88)

● **S21.05**   **Open bite of breast**
Bite of breast NOS

> **Excludes1**   superficial bite of breast (S20.17)

  ● **S21.051**   Open bite of right breast
  ● **S21.052**   Open bite of left breast
  ● **S21.059**   Open bite of unspecified breast

● **S21.1**   **Open wound of front wall of thorax without penetration into thoracic cavity**
Open wound of chest without penetration into thoracic cavity

  ● **S21.10**   **Unspecified open wound of front wall of thorax without penetration into thoracic cavity**

    ● **S21.101**   Unspecified open wound of right front wall of thorax without penetration into thoracic cavity

    ● **S21.102**   Unspecified open wound of left front wall of thorax without penetration into thoracic cavity

    ● **S21.109**   Unspecified open wound of unspecified front wall of thorax without penetration into thoracic cavity

  ● **S21.11**   **Laceration without foreign body of front wall of thorax without penetration into thoracic cavity**

    ● **S21.111**   Laceration without foreign body of right front wall of thorax without penetration into thoracic cavity

    ● **S21.112**   Laceration without foreign body of left front wall of thorax without penetration into thoracic cavity

    ● **S21.119**   Laceration without foreign body of unspecified front wall of thorax without penetration into thoracic cavity

  ● **S21.12**   **Laceration with foreign body of front wall of thorax without penetration into thoracic cavity**

    ● **S21.121**   Laceration with foreign body of right front wall of thorax without penetration into thoracic cavity

    ● **S21.122**   Laceration with foreign body of left front wall of thorax without penetration into thoracic cavity

    ● **S21.129**   Laceration with foreign body of unspecified front wall of thorax without penetration into thoracic cavity

  ● **S21.13**   **Puncture wound without foreign body of front wall of thorax without penetration into thoracic cavity**

    ● **S21.131**   Puncture wound without foreign body of right front wall of thorax without penetration into thoracic cavity

    ● **S21.132**   Puncture wound without foreign body of left front wall of thorax without penetration into thoracic cavity

    ● **S21.139**   Puncture wound without foreign body of unspecified front wall of thorax without penetration into thoracic cavity

● **S21.14**   **Puncture wound with foreign body of front wall of thorax without penetration into thoracic cavity**

  ● **S21.141**   Puncture wound with foreign body of right front wall of thorax without penetration into thoracic cavity

  ● **S21.142**   Puncture wound with foreign body of left front wall of thorax without penetration into thoracic cavity

  ● **S21.149**   Puncture wound with foreign body of unspecified front wall of thorax without penetration into thoracic cavity

● **S21.15**   **Open bite of front wall of thorax without penetration into thoracic cavity**
Bite of front wall of thorax NOS

> **Excludes1**   superficial bite of front wall of thorax (S20.37)

  ● **S21.151**   Open bite of right front wall of thorax without penetration into thoracic cavity

  ● **S21.152**   Open bite of left front wall of thorax without penetration into thoracic cavity

  ● **S21.159**   Open bite of unspecified front wall of thorax without penetration into thoracic cavity

● **S21.2**   **Open wound of back wall of thorax without penetration into thoracic cavity**

  ● **S21.20**   **Unspecified open wound of back wall of thorax without penetration into thoracic cavity**

    ● **S21.201**   Unspecified open wound of right back wall of thorax without penetration into thoracic cavity

    ● **S21.202**   Unspecified open wound of left back wall of thorax without penetration into thoracic cavity

    ● **S21.209**   Unspecified open wound of unspecified back wall of thorax without penetration into thoracic cavity

  ● **S21.21**   **Laceration without foreign body of back wall of thorax without penetration into thoracic cavity**

    ● **S21.211**   Laceration without foreign body of right back wall of thorax without penetration into thoracic cavity

    ● **S21.212**   Laceration without foreign body of left back wall of thorax without penetration into thoracic cavity

    ● **S21.219**   Laceration without foreign body of unspecified back wall of thorax without penetration into thoracic cavity

  ● **S21.22**   **Laceration with foreign body of back wall of thorax without penetration into thoracic cavity**

    ● **S21.221**   Laceration with foreign body of right back wall of thorax without penetration into thoracic cavity

    ● **S21.222**   Laceration with foreign body of left back wall of thorax without penetration into thoracic cavity

    ● **S21.229**   Laceration with foreign body of unspecified back wall of thorax without penetration into thoracic cavity

● S21.23 Puncture wound without foreign body of back wall of thorax without penetration into thoracic cavity

   ● S21.231 Puncture wound without foreign body of right back wall of thorax without penetration into thoracic cavity

   ● S21.232 Puncture wound without foreign body of left back wall of thorax without penetration into thoracic cavity

   ● S21.239 Puncture wound without foreign body of unspecified back wall of thorax without penetration into thoracic cavity

● S21.24 Puncture wound with foreign body of back wall of thorax without penetration into thoracic cavity

   ● S21.241 Puncture wound with foreign body of right back wall of thorax without penetration into thoracic cavity

   ● S21.242 Puncture wound with foreign body of left back wall of thorax without penetration into thoracic cavity

   ● S21.249 Puncture wound with foreign body of unspecified back wall of thorax without penetration into thoracic cavity

● S21.25 Open bite of back wall of thorax without penetration into thoracic cavity

   Bite of back wall of thorax NOS

   Excludes1   superficial bite of back wall of thorax (S20.47)

   ● S21.251 Open bite of right back wall of thorax without penetration into thoracic cavity

   ● S21.252 Open bite of left back wall of thorax without penetration into thoracic cavity

   ● S21.259 Open bite of unspecified back wall of thorax without penetration into thoracic cavity

● S21.3 Open wound of front wall of thorax with penetration into thoracic cavity

   Open wound of chest with penetration into thoracic cavity

   ● S21.30 Unspecified open wound of front wall of thorax with penetration into thoracic cavity

     ● S21.301 Unspecified open wound of right front wall of thorax with penetration into thoracic cavity

     ● S21.302 Unspecified open wound of left front wall of thorax with penetration into thoracic cavity

     ● S21.309 Unspecified open wound of unspecified front wall of thorax with penetration into thoracic cavity

   ● S21.31 Laceration without foreign body of front wall of thorax with penetration into thoracic cavity

     ● S21.311 Laceration without foreign body of right front wall of thorax with penetration into thoracic cavity

     ● S21.312 Laceration without foreign body of left front wall of thorax with penetration into thoracic cavity

     ● S21.319 Laceration without foreign body of unspecified front wall of thorax with penetration into thoracic cavity

● S21.32 Laceration with foreign body of front wall of thorax with penetration into thoracic cavity

   ● S21.321 Laceration with foreign body of right front wall of thorax with penetration into thoracic cavity

   ● S21.322 Laceration with foreign body of left front wall of thorax with penetration into thoracic cavity

   ● S21.329 Laceration with foreign body of unspecified front wall of thorax with penetration into thoracic cavity

● S21.33 Puncture wound without foreign body of front wall of thorax with penetration into thoracic cavity

   ● S21.331 Puncture wound without foreign body of right front wall of thorax with penetration into thoracic cavity

   ● S21.332 Puncture wound without foreign body of left front wall of thorax with penetration into thoracic cavity

   ● S21.339 Puncture wound without foreign body of unspecified front wall of thorax with penetration into thoracic cavity

● S21.34 Puncture wound with foreign body of front wall of thorax with penetration into thoracic cavity

   ● S21.341 Puncture wound with foreign body of right front wall of thorax with penetration into thoracic cavity

   ● S21.342 Puncture wound with foreign body of left front wall of thorax with penetration into thoracic cavity

   ● S21.349 Puncture wound with foreign body of unspecified front wall of thorax with penetration into thoracic cavity

● S21.35 Open bite of front wall of thorax with penetration into thoracic cavity

   Excludes1   superficial bite of front wall of thorax (S20.37)

   ● S21.351 Open bite of right front wall of thorax with penetration into thoracic cavity

   ● S21.352 Open bite of left front wall of thorax with penetration into thoracic cavity

   ● S21.359 Open bite of unspecified front wall of thorax with penetration into thoracic cavity

● S21.4 Open wound of back wall of thorax with penetration into thoracic cavity

   ● S21.40 Unspecified open wound of back wall of thorax with penetration into thoracic cavity

     ● S21.401 Unspecified open wound of right back wall of thorax with penetration into thoracic cavity

     ● S21.402 Unspecified open wound of left back wall of thorax with penetration into thoracic cavity

     ● S21.409 Unspecified open wound of unspecified back wall of thorax with penetration into thoracic cavity

   ● S21.41 Laceration without foreign body of back wall of thorax with penetration into thoracic cavity

     ● S21.411 Laceration without foreign body of right back wall of thorax with penetration into thoracic cavity

     ● S21.412 Laceration without foreign body of left back wall of thorax with penetration into thoracic cavity

     ● S21.419 Laceration without foreign body of unspecified back wall of thorax with penetration into thoracic cavity

● S21.42   **Laceration with foreign body** of back wall of thorax with penetration into thoracic cavity
     ● S21.421   Laceration with foreign body of **right** back wall of thorax with penetration into thoracic cavity
     ● S21.422   Laceration with foreign body of **left** back wall of thorax with penetration into thoracic cavity
     ● S21.429   Laceration with foreign body of **unspecified** back wall of thorax with penetration into thoracic cavity

● S21.43   **Puncture wound without foreign body** of back wall of thorax with penetration into thoracic cavity
     ● S21.431   Puncture wound without foreign body of **right** back wall of thorax with penetration into thoracic cavity
     ● S21.432   Puncture wound without foreign body of **left** back wall of thorax with penetration into thoracic cavity
     ● S21.439   Puncture wound without foreign body of **unspecified** back wall of thorax with penetration into thoracic cavity

● S21.44   **Puncture wound with foreign body** of back wall of thorax with penetration into thoracic cavity
     ● S21.441   Puncture wound with foreign body of **right** back wall of thorax with penetration into thoracic cavity
     ● S21.442   Puncture wound with foreign body of **left** back wall of thorax with penetration into thoracic cavity
     ● S21.449   Puncture wound with foreign body of **unspecified** back wall of thorax with penetration into thoracic cavity

● S21.45   **Open bite** of back wall of thorax with penetration into thoracic cavity
     Bite of back wall of thorax NOS
     Excludes1   superficial bite of back wall of thorax (S20.47)
     ● S21.451   Open bite of **right** back wall of thorax with penetration into thoracic cavity
     ● S21.452   Open bite of **left** back wall of thorax with penetration into thoracic cavity
     ● S21.459   Open bite of **unspecified** back wall of thorax with penetration into thoracic cavity

● S21.9   Open wound of **unspecified part** of thorax
     Open wound of thoracic wall NOS
   X ● S21.90   **Unspecified** open wound of unspecified part of thorax
   X ● S21.91   **Laceration without foreign body** of unspecified part of thorax
   X ● S21.92   **Laceration with foreign body** of unspecified part of thorax
   X ● S21.93   **Puncture wound without foreign body** of unspecified part of thorax
   X ● S21.94   **Puncture wound with foreign body** of unspecified part of thorax
   X ● S21.95   **Open bite** of unspecified part of thorax
       Excludes1   superficial bite of thorax (S20.97)

● S22   **Fracture of rib(s), sternum and thoracic spine**
   Note: A fracture not indicated as displaced or nondisplaced should be coded to displaced
      A fracture not indicated as open or closed should be coded to closed
   Includes   fracture of thoracic neural arch
                fracture of thoracic spinous process
                fracture of thoracic transverse process
                fracture of thoracic vertebra
                fracture of thoracic vertebral arch
   Code first any associated:
     injury of intrathoracic organ (S27.-)
     spinal cord injury (S24.0-, S24.1-)
   Excludes1   transection of thorax (S28.1)
   Excludes2   fracture of clavicle (S42.0-)
                 fracture of scapula (S42.1-)
   The appropriate 7th character is to be added to each code from category S22

> A   initial encounter for closed fracture
> B   initial encounter for open fracture
> D   subsequent encounter for fracture with routine healing
> G   subsequent encounter for fracture with delayed healing
> K   subsequent encounter for fracture with nonunion
> S   sequela

● S22.0   **Fracture of thoracic vertebra**
   ● S22.00   Fracture of **unspecified** thoracic vertebra
     ● S22.000   **Wedge compression** fracture of unspecified thoracic vertebra A, B 🐾
     ● S22.001   **Stable burst** fracture of unspecified thoracic vertebra A, B 🐾
     ● S22.002   **Unstable burst** fracture of unspecified thoracic vertebra A, B 🐾
     ● S22.008   **Other** fracture of unspecified thoracic vertebra A, B 🐾
     ● S22.009   **Unspecified** fracture of unspecified thoracic vertebra A, B 🐾
   ● S22.01   Fracture of **first** thoracic vertebra
     ● S22.010   **Wedge compression** fracture of first thoracic vertebra A, B 🐾
     ● S22.011   **Stable burst** fracture of first thoracic vertebra A, B 🐾
     ● S22.012   **Unstable burst** fracture of first thoracic vertebra A, B 🐾
     ● S22.018   **Other** fracture of first thoracic vertebra A, B 🐾
     ● S22.019   **Unspecified** fracture of first thoracic vertebra A, B 🐾
   ● S22.02   Fracture of **second** thoracic vertebra
     ● S22.020   **Wedge compression** fracture of second thoracic vertebra A, B 🐾
     ● S22.021   **Stable burst** fracture of second thoracic vertebra A, B 🐾
     ● S22.022   **Unstable burst** fracture of second thoracic vertebra A, B 🐾
     ● S22.028   **Other** fracture of second thoracic vertebra A, B 🐾
     ● S22.029   **Unspecified** fracture of second thoracic vertebra A, B 🐾
   ● S22.03   Fracture of **third** thoracic vertebra
     ● S22.030   **Wedge compression** fracture of third thoracic vertebra A, B 🐾
     ● S22.031   **Stable burst** fracture of third thoracic vertebra A, B 🐾

- S22.Ø32   Unstable burst fracture of third thoracic vertebra A, B 🔖
- S22.Ø38   Other fracture of third thoracic vertebra A, B 🔖
- S22.Ø39   Unspecified fracture of third thoracic vertebra A, B 🔖
- S22.Ø4   Fracture of fourth thoracic vertebra
  - S22.Ø4Ø   Wedge compression fracture of fourth thoracic vertebra A, B 🔖
  - S22.Ø41   Stable burst fracture of fourth thoracic vertebra A, B 🔖
  - S22.Ø42   Unstable burst fracture of fourth thoracic vertebra A, B 🔖
  - S22.Ø48   Other fracture of fourth thoracic vertebra A, B 🔖
  - S22.Ø49   Unspecified fracture of fourth thoracic vertebra A, B 🔖
- S22.Ø5   Fracture of T5-T6 vertebra
  - S22.Ø5Ø   Wedge compression fracture of T5-T6 vertebra A, B 🔖
  - S22.Ø51   Stable burst fracture of T5-T6 vertebra A, B 🔖
  - S22.Ø52   Unstable burst fracture of T5-T6 vertebra A, B 🔖
  - S22.Ø58   Other fracture of T5-T6 vertebra A, B 🔖
  - S22.Ø59   Unspecified fracture of T5-T6 vertebra A, B 🔖
- S22.Ø6   Fracture of T7-T8 vertebra
  - S22.Ø6Ø   Wedge compression fracture of T7-T8 vertebra A, B 🔖
  - S22.Ø61   Stable burst fracture of T7-T8 vertebra A, B 🔖
  - S22.Ø62   Unstable burst fracture of T7-T8 vertebra A, B 🔖
  - S22.Ø68   Other fracture of T7-T8 thoracic vertebra A, B 🔖
  - S22.Ø69   Unspecified fracture of T7-T8 vertebra A, B 🔖
- S22.Ø7   Fracture of T9-T1Ø vertebra
  - S22.Ø7Ø   Wedge compression fracture of T9-T1Ø vertebra A, B 🔖
  - S22.Ø71   Stable burst fracture of T9-T1Ø vertebra A, B 🔖
  - S22.Ø72   Unstable burst fracture of T9-T1Ø vertebra A, B 🔖
  - S22.Ø78   Other fracture of T9-T1Ø vertebra A, B 🔖
  - S22.Ø79   Unspecified fracture of T9-T1Ø vertebra A, B 🔖
- S22.Ø8   Fracture of T11-T12 vertebra
  - S22.Ø8Ø   Wedge compression fracture of T11-T12 vertebra A, B 🔖
  - S22.Ø81   Stable burst fracture of T11-T12 vertebra A, B 🔖
  - S22.Ø82   Unstable burst fracture of T11-T12 vertebra A, B 🔖
  - S22.Ø88   Other fracture of T11-T12 vertebra A, B 🔖
  - S22.Ø89   Unspecified fracture of T11-T12 vertebra A, B 🔖

- S22.2   Fracture of sternum
  - X● S22.2Ø   Unspecified fracture of sternum
  - X● S22.21   Fracture of manubrium
  - X● S22.22   Fracture of body of sternum
  - X● S22.23   Sternal manubrial dissociation
  - X● S22.24   Fracture of xiphoid process
- S22.3   Fracture of one rib
  - X● S22.31   Fracture of one rib, right side
  - X● S22.32   Fracture of one rib, left side
  - X● S22.39   Fracture of one rib, unspecified side
- S22.4   Multiple fractures of ribs

  Fractures of two or more ribs

  > **Excludes1**   flail chest (S22.5-)

  - X● S22.41   Multiple fractures of ribs, right side
  - X● S22.42   Multiple fractures of ribs, left side
  - X● S22.43   Multiple fractures of ribs, bilateral
  - X● S22.49   Multiple fractures of ribs, unspecified side
- X● S22.5   Flail chest

  Unstable chest due to sternum and/or rib fracture
- X● S22.9   Fracture of bony thorax, part unspecified

- S23   **Dislocation and sprain of joints and ligaments of thorax**

  > **Includes**   avulsion of joint or ligament of thorax
  > laceration of cartilage, joint or ligament of thorax
  > sprain of cartilage, joint or ligament of thorax
  > traumatic hemarthrosis of joint or ligament of thorax
  > traumatic rupture of joint or ligament of thorax
  > traumatic subluxation of joint or ligament of thorax
  > traumatic tear of joint or ligament of thorax

  ▰▻ Code also any associated: open wound

  > **Excludes2**   dislocation, sprain of sternoclavicular joint (S43.2, S43.6)
  > strain of muscle or tendon of thorax (S29.Ø1-)

  The appropriate 7th character is to be added to each code from category S23

A	initial encounter
D	subsequent encounter
S	sequela

  - X● S23.Ø   **Traumatic rupture of thoracic intervertebral disc**

    > **Excludes1**   rupture or displacement (nontraumatic) of thoracic intervertebral disc NOS (M51.- with fifth character 4)

  - S23.1   **Subluxation and dislocation of thoracic vertebra**

    Code also any associated
        open wound of thorax (S21.-)
        spinal cord injury (S24.Ø-, S24.1-)

    > **Excludes2**   fracture of thoracic vertebrae (S22.Ø-)

    - S23.1Ø   Subluxation and dislocation of unspecified thoracic vertebra
      - S23.1ØØ   Subluxation of unspecified thoracic vertebra
      - S23.1Ø1   Dislocation of unspecified thoracic vertebra
    - S23.11   Subluxation and dislocation of T1/T2 thoracic vertebra
      - S23.11Ø   Subluxation of T1/T2 thoracic vertebra
      - S23.111   Dislocation of T1/T2 thoracic vertebra

CHAPTER 19 (SØØ-T88)

● S23.12   Subluxation and dislocation of T2/T3-T3/T4 thoracic vertebra
   ● S23.120   Subluxation of T2/T3 thoracic vertebra
   ● S23.121   Dislocation of T2/T3 thoracic vertebra
   ● S23.122   Subluxation of T3/T4 thoracic vertebra
   ● S23.123   Dislocation of T3/T4 thoracic vertebra

● S23.13   Subluxation and dislocation of T4/T5-T5/T6 thoracic vertebra
   ● S23.130   Subluxation of T4/T5 thoracic vertebra
   ● S23.131   Dislocation of T4/T5 thoracic vertebra
   ● S23.132   Subluxation of T5/T6 thoracic vertebra
   ● S23.133   Dislocation of T5/T6 thoracic vertebra

● S23.14   Subluxation and dislocation of T6/T7-T7/T8 thoracic vertebra
   ● S23.140   Subluxation of T6/T7 thoracic vertebra
   ● S23.141   Dislocation of T6/T7 thoracic vertebra
   ● S23.142   Subluxation of T7/T8 thoracic vertebra
   ● S23.143   Dislocation of T7/T8 thoracic vertebra

● S23.15   Subluxation and dislocation of T8/T9-T9/T10 thoracic vertebra
   ● S23.150   Subluxation of T8/T9 thoracic vertebra
   ● S23.151   Dislocation of T8/T9 thoracic vertebra
   ● S23.152   Subluxation of T9/T10 thoracic vertebra
   ● S23.153   Dislocation of T9/T10 thoracic vertebra

● S23.16   Subluxation and dislocation of T10/T11-T11/T12 thoracic vertebra
   ● S23.160   Subluxation of T10/T11 thoracic vertebra
   ● S23.161   Dislocation of T10/T11 thoracic vertebra
   ● S23.162   Subluxation of T11/T12 thoracic vertebra
   ● S23.163   Dislocation of T11/T12 thoracic vertebra

● S23.17   Subluxation and dislocation of T12/L1 thoracic vertebra
   ● S23.170   Subluxation of T12/L1 thoracic vertebra
   ● S23.171   Dislocation of T12/L1 thoracic vertebra

● S23.2   Dislocation of other and unspecified parts of thorax
  X ● S23.20   Dislocation of unspecified part of thorax
  X ● S23.29   Dislocation of other parts of thorax

X ● S23.3   Sprain of ligaments of thoracic spine

● S23.4   Sprain of ribs and sternum
  X ● S23.41   Sprain of ribs
  ● S23.42   Sprain of sternum
   ● S23.420   Sprain of sternoclavicular (joint) (ligament)
   ● S23.421   Sprain of chondrosternal joint
   ● S23.428   Other sprain of sternum
   ● S23.429   Unspecified sprain of sternum

X ● S23.8   Sprain of other specified parts of thorax

X ● S23.9   Sprain of unspecified parts of thorax

● S24   Injury of nerves and spinal cord at thorax level

Note: Code to highest level of thoracic spinal cord injury.

Injuries to the spinal cord (S24.0 and S24.1) refer to the cord level and not bone level injury, and can affect nerve roots at and below the level given.

Code also any associated:
fracture of thoracic vertebra (S22.0-)
open wound of thorax (S21.-)
transient paralysis (R29.5)

Excludes2   injury of brachial plexus (S14.3)

The appropriate 7th character is to be added to each code from category S24

A	initial encounter
D	subsequent encounter
S	sequela

X ● S24.0   Concussion and edema of thoracic spinal cord A, D, S 🐾

● S24.1   Other and unspecified injuries of thoracic spinal cord
  ● S24.10   Unspecified injury of thoracic spinal cord
   ● S24.101   Unspecified injury at T1 level of thoracic spinal cord A, D, S 🐾
   ● S24.102   Unspecified injury at T2-T6 level of thoracic spinal cord A, D, S 🐾
   ● S24.103   Unspecified injury at T7-T10 level of thoracic spinal cord A, D, S 🐾
   ● S24.104   Unspecified injury at T11-T12 level of thoracic spinal cord A, D, S 🐾
   ● S24.109   Unspecified injury at unspecified level of thoracic spinal cord A, D, S 🐾
      Injury of thoracic spinal cord NOS

  ● S24.11   Complete lesion of thoracic spinal cord
   ● S24.111   Complete lesion at T1 level of thoracic spinal cord A, D, S 🐾
   ● S24.112   Complete lesion at T2-T6 level of thoracic spinal cord A, D, S 🐾
   ● S24.113   Complete lesion at T7-T10 level of thoracic spinal cord A, D, S 🐾
   ● S24.114   Complete lesion at T11-T12 level of thoracic spinal cord A, D, S 🐾
   ● S24.119   Complete lesion at unspecified level of thoracic spinal cord A, D, S 🐾

  ● S24.13   Anterior cord syndrome of thoracic spinal cord
   ● S24.131   Anterior cord syndrome at T1 level of thoracic spinal cord A, D, S 🐾
   ● S24.132   Anterior cord syndrome at T2-T6 level of thoracic spinal cord A, D, S 🐾
   ● S24.133   Anterior cord syndrome at T7-T10 level of thoracic spinal cord A, D, S 🐾
   ● S24.134   Anterior cord syndrome at T11-T12 level of thoracic spinal cord A, D, S 🐾
   ● S24.139   Anterior cord syndrome at unspecified level of thoracic spinal cord A, D, S 🐾

  ● S24.14   Brown-Séquard syndrome of thoracic spinal cord
   ● S24.141   Brown-Séquard syndrome at T1 level of thoracic spinal cord A, D, S 🐾
   ● S24.142   Brown-Séquard syndrome at T2-T6 level of thoracic spinal cord A, D, S 🐾
   ● S24.143   Brown-Séquard syndrome at T7-T10 level of thoracic spinal cord A, D, S 🐾
   ● S24.144   Brown-Séquard syndrome at T11-T12 level of thoracic spinal cord A, D, S 🐾
   ● S24.149   Brown-Séquard syndrome at unspecified level of thoracic spinal cord A, D, S 🐾

● **S24.15**   **Other incomplete lesions of thoracic spinal cord**
Incomplete lesion of thoracic spinal cord NOS
Posterior cord syndrome of thoracic spinal cord

   ● **S24.151**   **Other incomplete lesion at T1 level of thoracic spinal cord** A, D, S 🔗

   ● **S24.152**   **Other incomplete lesion at T2-T6 level of thoracic spinal cord** A, D, S 🔗

   ● **S24.153**   **Other incomplete lesion at T7-T10 level of thoracic spinal cord** A, D, S 🔗

   ● **S24.154**   **Other incomplete lesion at T11-T12 level of thoracic spinal cord** A, D, S 🔗

   ● **S24.159**   **Other incomplete lesion at unspecified level of thoracic spinal cord** A, D, S 🔗

X ● **S24.2**   **Injury of nerve root of thoracic spine**

X ● **S24.3**   **Injury of peripheral nerves of thorax**

X ● **S24.4**   **Injury of thoracic sympathetic nervous system**
Injury of cardiac plexus
Injury of esophageal plexus
Injury of pulmonary plexus
Injury of stellate ganglion
Injury of thoracic sympathetic ganglion

X ● **S24.8**   **Injury of other specified nerves of thorax**

X ● **S24.9**   **Injury of unspecified nerve of thorax**

● **S25**   **Injury of blood vessels of thorax**
The appropriate 7th character is to be added to each code from category S25

> | | |
> |---|---|
> | A | initial encounter |
> | D | subsequent encounter |
> | S | sequela |

Code also any associated open wound (S21.-)

● **S25.0**   **Injury of thoracic aorta**
Injury of aorta NOS

  X ● **S25.00**   **Unspecified injury of thoracic aorta**

  X ● **S25.01**   **Minor laceration of thoracic aorta**
Incomplete transection of thoracic aorta
Laceration of thoracic aorta NOS
Superficial laceration of thoracic aorta

  X ● **S25.02**   **Major laceration of thoracic aorta**
Complete transection of thoracic aorta
Traumatic rupture of thoracic aorta

  X ● **S25.09**   **Other specified injury of thoracic aorta**

● **S25.1**   **Injury of innominate or subclavian artery**

  ● **S25.10**   **Unspecified injury of innominate or subclavian artery**

   ● **S25.101**   **Unspecified injury of right innominate or subclavian artery**

   ● **S25.102**   **Unspecified injury of left innominate or subclavian artery**

   ● **S25.109**   **Unspecified injury of unspecified innominate or subclavian artery**

  ● **S25.11**   **Minor laceration of innominate or subclavian artery**
Incomplete transection of innominate or subclavian artery
Laceration of innominate or subclavian artery NOS
Superficial laceration of innominate or subclavian artery

   ● **S25.111**   **Minor laceration of right innominate or subclavian artery**

   ● **S25.112**   **Minor laceration of left innominate or subclavian artery**

   ● **S25.119**   **Minor laceration of unspecified innominate or subclavian artery**

  ● **S25.12**   **Major laceration of innominate or subclavian artery**
Complete transection of innominate or subclavian artery
Traumatic rupture of innominate or subclavian artery

   ● **S25.121**   **Major laceration of right innominate or subclavian artery**

   ● **S25.122**   **Major laceration of left innominate or subclavian artery**

   ● **S25.129**   **Major laceration of unspecified innominate or subclavian artery**

  ● **S25.19**   **Other specified injury of innominate or subclavian artery**

   ● **S25.191**   **Other specified injury of right innominate or subclavian artery**

   ● **S25.192**   **Other specified injury of left innominate or subclavian artery**

   ● **S25.199**   **Other specified injury of unspecified innominate or subclavian artery**

● **S25.2**   **Injury of superior vena cava**
Injury of vena cava NOS

  X ● **S25.20**   **Unspecified injury of superior vena cava**

  X ● **S25.21**   **Minor laceration of superior vena cava**
Incomplete transection of superior vena cava
Laceration of superior vena cava NOS
Superficial laceration of superior vena cava

  X ● **S25.22**   **Major laceration of superior vena cava**
Complete transection of superior vena cava
Traumatic rupture of superior vena cava

  X ● **S25.29**   **Other specified injury of superior vena cava**

● **S25.3**   **Injury of innominate or subclavian vein**

  ● **S25.30**   **Unspecified injury of innominate or subclavian vein**

   ● **S25.301**   **Unspecified injury of right innominate or subclavian vein**

   ● **S25.302**   **Unspecified injury of left innominate or subclavian vein**

   ● **S25.309**   **Unspecified injury of unspecified innominate or subclavian vein**

  ● **S25.31**   **Minor laceration of innominate or subclavian vein**
Incomplete transection of innominate or subclavian vein
Laceration of innominate or subclavian vein NOS
Superficial laceration of innominate or subclavian vein

   ● **S25.311**   **Minor laceration of right innominate or subclavian vein**

   ● **S25.312**   **Minor laceration of left innominate or subclavian vein**

   ● **S25.319**   **Minor laceration of unspecified innominate or subclavian vein**

  ● **S25.32**   **Major laceration of innominate or subclavian vein**
Complete transection of innominate or subclavian vein
Traumatic rupture of innominate or subclavian vein

   ● **S25.321**   **Major laceration of right innominate or subclavian vein**

   ● **S25.322**   **Major laceration of left innominate or subclavian vein**

   ● **S25.329**   **Major laceration of unspecified innominate or subclavian vein**

CHAPTER 19 (S00-T88)

● S25.39   Other specified injury of innominate or subclavian vein
    ● S25.391   Other specified injury of right innominate or subclavian vein
    ● S25.392   Other specified injury of left innominate or subclavian vein
    ● S25.399   Other specified injury of unspecified innominate or subclavian vein

● S25.4   Injury of pulmonary blood vessels
   ● S25.40   Unspecified injury of pulmonary blood vessels
    ● S25.401   Unspecified injury of right pulmonary blood vessels
    ● S25.402   Unspecified injury of left pulmonary blood vessels
    ● S25.409   Unspecified injury of unspecified pulmonary blood vessels
   ● S25.41   Minor laceration of pulmonary blood vessels
      Incomplete transection of pulmonary blood vessels
      Laceration of pulmonary blood vessels NOS
      Superficial laceration of pulmonary blood vessels
    ● S25.411   Minor laceration of right pulmonary blood vessels
    ● S25.412   Minor laceration of left pulmonary blood vessels
    ● S25.419   Minor laceration of unspecified pulmonary blood vessels
   ● S25.42   Major laceration of pulmonary blood vessels
      Complete transection of pulmonary blood vessels
      Traumatic rupture of pulmonary blood vessels
    ● S25.421   Major laceration of right pulmonary blood vessels
    ● S25.422   Major laceration of left pulmonary blood vessels
    ● S25.429   Major laceration of unspecified pulmonary blood vessels
   ● S25.49   Other specified injury of pulmonary blood vessels
    ● S25.491   Other specified injury of right pulmonary blood vessels
    ● S25.492   Other specified injury of left pulmonary blood vessels
    ● S25.499   Other specified injury of unspecified pulmonary blood vessels

● S25.5   Injury of intercostal blood vessels
   ● S25.50   Unspecified injury of intercostal blood vessels
    ● S25.501   Unspecified injury of intercostal blood vessels, right side
    ● S25.502   Unspecified injury of intercostal blood vessels, left side
    ● S25.509   Unspecified injury of intercostal blood vessels, unspecified side
   ● S25.51   Laceration of intercostal blood vessels
    ● S25.511   Laceration of intercostal blood vessels, right side
    ● S25.512   Laceration of intercostal blood vessels, left side
    ● S25.519   Laceration of intercostal blood vessels, unspecified side

● S25.59   Other specified injury of intercostal blood vessels
    ● S25.591   Other specified injury of intercostal blood vessels, right side
    ● S25.592   Other specified injury of intercostal blood vessels, left side
    ● S25.599   Other specified injury of intercostal blood vessels, unspecified side

● S25.8   Injury of other blood vessels of thorax
      Injury of azygos vein
      Injury of mammary artery or vein
   ● S25.80   Unspecified injury of other blood vessels of thorax
    ● S25.801   Unspecified injury of other blood vessels of thorax, right side
    ● S25.802   Unspecified injury of other blood vessels of thorax, left side
    ● S25.809   Unspecified injury of other blood vessels of thorax, unspecified side
   ● S25.81   Laceration of other blood vessels of thorax
    ● S25.811   Laceration of other blood vessels of thorax, right side
    ● S25.812   Laceration of other blood vessels of thorax, left side
    ● S25.819   Laceration of other blood vessels of thorax, unspecified side
   ● S25.89   Other specified injury of other blood vessels of thorax
    ● S25.891   Other specified injury of other blood vessels of thorax, right side
    ● S25.892   Other specified injury of other blood vessels of thorax, left side
    ● S25.899   Other specified injury of other blood vessels of thorax, unspecified side

● S25.9   Injury of unspecified blood vessel of thorax
  X ● S25.90   Unspecified injury of unspecified blood vessel of thorax
  X ● S25.91   Laceration of unspecified blood vessel of thorax
  X ● S25.99   Other specified injury of unspecified blood vessel of thorax

● S26   Injury of heart
      The appropriate 7th character is to be added to each code from category S26

A	initial encounter
D	subsequent encounter
S	sequela

      Code also any associated:
        open wound of thorax (S21.-)
        traumatic hemopneumothorax (S27.2)
        traumatic hemothorax (S27.1)
        traumatic pneumothorax (S27.Ø)

● S26.Ø   Injury of heart with hemopericardium
      Hemopericardium: effusion of blood within pericardium
  X ● S26.00   Unspecified injury of heart with hemopericardium
  X ● S26.01   Contusion of heart with hemopericardium

● **S26.02**   **Laceration of heart with hemopericardium**
    ● **S26.020**   **Mild laceration of heart with hemopericardium**
       Laceration of heart without penetration of heart chamber
    ● **S26.021**   **Moderate laceration of heart with hemopericardium**
       Laceration of heart with penetration of heart chamber
    ● **S26.022**   **Major laceration of heart with hemopericardium**
       Laceration of heart with penetration of multiple heart chambers
X ● **S26.09**   **Other injury of heart with hemopericardium**
● **S26.1**   **Injury of heart without hemopericardium**
    Hemopericardium: effusion of blood within pericardium
X ● **S26.10**   **Unspecified injury of heart without hemopericardium**
X ● **S26.11**   **Contusion of heart without hemopericardium**
X ● **S26.12**   **Laceration of heart without hemopericardium**
X ● **S26.19**   **Other injury of heart without hemopericardium**
● **S26.9**   **Injury of heart, unspecified with or without hemopericardium**
    Hemopericardium: effusion of blood within pericardium
X ● **S26.90**   **Unspecified injury of heart, unspecified with or without hemopericardium**
X ● **S26.91**   **Contusion of heart, unspecified with or without hemopericardium**
X ● **S26.92**   **Laceration of heart, unspecified with or without hemopericardium**
       Laceration of heart NOS
X ● **S26.99**   **Other injury of heart, unspecified with or without hemopericardium**

● **S27**   **Injury of other and unspecified intrathoracic organs**
    Code also any associated open wound of thorax (S21.-)
    Excludes2   injury of cervical esophagus (S10-S19)
            injury of trachea (cervical) (S10-S19)
    The appropriate 7th character is to be added to each code from category S27

A	initial encounter
D	subsequent encounter
S	sequela

X ● **S27.0**   **Traumatic pneumothorax**
    Excludes1   spontaneous pneumothorax (J93.-)
X ● **S27.1**   **Traumatic hemothorax**
X ● **S27.2**   **Traumatic hemopneumothorax**
● **S27.3**   **Other and unspecified injuries of lung**
    ● **S27.30**   **Unspecified injury of lung**
       ● **S27.301**   **Unspecified injury of lung, unilateral**
       ● **S27.302**   **Unspecified injury of lung, bilateral**
       ● **S27.309**   **Unspecified injury of lung, unspecified**
    ● **S27.31**   **Primary blast injury of lung**
       Blast injury of lung NOS
       ● **S27.311**   **Primary blast injury of lung, unilateral**
       ● **S27.312**   **Primary blast injury of lung, bilateral**
       ● **S27.319**   **Primary blast injury of lung, unspecified**

Item 19-2 Pneumothorax is a collection of gas (positive air pressure) in the pleural space resulting in the lung collapsing. A **tension pneumothorax** is life-threatening and is a result of air in the pleural space causing a displacement in the mediastinal structures and cardiopulmonary function compromise. A **traumatic pneumothorax** results from blunt or penetrating injury that disrupts the parietal/visceral pleura. **Hemothorax** is blood or bloody fluid in the pleural cavity as a result of traumatic blood vessel rupture or inflammation of the lungs from pneumonia.

    ● **S27.32**   **Contusion of lung**
       ● **S27.321**   **Contusion of lung, unilateral**
       ● **S27.322**   **Contusion of lung, bilateral**
       ● **S27.329**   **Contusion of lung, unspecified**
    ● **S27.33**   **Laceration of lung**
       ● **S27.331**   **Laceration of lung, unilateral**
       ● **S27.332**   **Laceration of lung, bilateral**
       ● **S27.339**   **Laceration of lung, unspecified**
    ● **S27.39**   **Other injuries of lung**
       Secondary blast injury of lung
       ● **S27.391**   **Other injuries of lung, unilateral**
       ● **S27.392**   **Other injuries of lung, bilateral**
       ● **S27.399**   **Other injuries of lung, unspecified**
● **S27.4**   **Injury of bronchus**
    ● **S27.40**   **Unspecified injury of bronchus**
       ● **S27.401**   **Unspecified injury of bronchus, unilateral**
       ● **S27.402**   **Unspecified injury of bronchus, bilateral**
       ● **S27.409**   **Unspecified injury of bronchus, unspecified**
    ● **S27.41**   **Primary blast injury of bronchus**
       Blast injury of bronchus NOS
       ● **S27.411**   **Primary blast injury of bronchus, unilateral**
       ● **S27.412**   **Primary blast injury of bronchus, bilateral**
       ● **S27.419**   **Primary blast injury of bronchus, unspecified**
    ● **S27.42**   **Contusion of bronchus**
       ● **S27.421**   **Contusion of bronchus, unilateral**
       ● **S27.422**   **Contusion of bronchus, bilateral**
       ● **S27.429**   **Contusion of bronchus, unspecified**
    ● **S27.43**   **Laceration of bronchus**
       ● **S27.431**   **Laceration of bronchus, unilateral**
       ● **S27.432**   **Laceration of bronchus, bilateral**
       ● **S27.439**   **Laceration of bronchus, unspecified**
    ● **S27.49**   **Other injury of bronchus**
       Secondary blast injury of bronchus
       ● **S27.491**   **Other injury of bronchus, unilateral**
       ● **S27.492**   **Other injury of bronchus, bilateral**
       ● **S27.499**   **Other injury of bronchus, unspecified**
● **S27.5**   **Injury of thoracic trachea**
    X ● **S27.50**   **Unspecified injury of thoracic trachea**
    X ● **S27.51**   **Primary blast injury of thoracic trachea**
       Blast injury of thoracic trachea NOS
    X ● **S27.52**   **Contusion of thoracic trachea**
    X ● **S27.53**   **Laceration of thoracic trachea**
    X ● **S27.59**   **Other injury of thoracic trachea**
       Secondary blast injury of thoracic trachea

CHAPTER 19 (S00-T88)

X● S27.6　Injury of pleura
　　X● S27.60　Unspecified injury of pleura
　　X● S27.63　Laceration of pleura
　　X● S27.69　Other injury of pleura
● S27.8　Injury of other specified intrathoracic organs
　　● S27.80　Injury of diaphragm
　　　　● S27.802　Contusion of diaphragm
　　　　● S27.803　Laceration of diaphragm
　　　　● S27.808　Other injury of diaphragm
　　　　● S27.809　Unspecified injury of diaphragm
　　● S27.81　Injury of esophagus (thoracic part)
　　　　● S27.812　Contusion of esophagus (thoracic part)
　　　　● S27.813　Laceration of esophagus (thoracic part)
　　　　● S27.818　Other injury of esophagus (thoracic part)
　　　　● S27.819　Unspecified injury of esophagus (thoracic part)
　　● S27.89　Injury of other specified intrathoracic organs
　　　　　　　Injury of lymphatic thoracic duct
　　　　　　　Injury of thymus gland
　　　　● S27.892　Contusion of other specified intrathoracic organs
　　　　● S27.893　Laceration of other specified intrathoracic organs
　　　　● S27.898　Other injury of other specified intrathoracic organs
　　　　● S27.899　Unspecified injury of other specified intrathoracic organs
X● S27.9　Injury of unspecified intrathoracic organ

● S28　Crushing injury of thorax, and traumatic amputation of part of thorax
　　　　The appropriate 7th character is to be added to each code from category S28

A	initial encounter
D	subsequent encounter
S	sequela

X● S28.0　Crushed chest
　　　　　Use additional code for all associated injuries
　　　　　Excludes1　flail chest (S22.5)
X● S28.1　Traumatic amputation (partial) of part of thorax, except breast
● S28.2　Traumatic amputation of breast
　　● S28.21　Complete traumatic amputation of breast
　　　　　　　Traumatic amputation of breast NOS
　　　　● S28.211　Complete traumatic amputation of right breast
　　　　● S28.212　Complete traumatic amputation of left breast
　　　　● S28.219　Complete traumatic amputation of unspecified breast
　　● S28.22　Partial traumatic amputation of breast
　　　　● S28.221　Partial traumatic amputation of right breast
　　　　● S28.222　Partial traumatic amputation of left breast
　　　　● S28.229　Partial traumatic amputation of unspecified breast

● S29　Other and unspecified injuries of thorax
　　　　Code also any associated open wound (S21.-)
　　　　The appropriate 7th character is to be added to each code from category S29

A	initial encounter
D	subsequent encounter
S	sequela

● S29.0　Injury of muscle and tendon at thorax level
　　● S29.00　Unspecified injury of muscle and tendon of thorax
　　　　● S29.001　Unspecified injury of muscle and tendon of front wall of thorax
　　　　● S29.002　Unspecified injury of muscle and tendon of back wall of thorax
　　　　● S29.009　Unspecified injury of muscle and tendon of unspecified wall of thorax
　　● S29.01　Strain of muscle and tendon of thorax
　　　　● S29.011　Strain of muscle and tendon of front wall of thorax
　　　　● S29.012　Strain of muscle and tendon of back wall of thorax
　　　　● S29.019　Strain of muscle and tendon of unspecified wall of thorax
　　● S29.02　Laceration of muscle and tendon of thorax
　　　　● S29.021　Laceration of muscle and tendon of front wall of thorax
　　　　● S29.022　Laceration of muscle and tendon of back wall of thorax
　　　　● S29.029　Laceration of muscle and tendon of unspecified wall of thorax
　　● S29.09　Other injury of muscle and tendon of thorax
　　　　● S29.091　Other injury of muscle and tendon of front wall of thorax
　　　　● S29.092　Other injury of muscle and tendon of back wall of thorax
　　　　● S29.099　Other injury of muscle and tendon of unspecified wall of thorax
X● S29.8　Other specified injuries of thorax
X● S29.9　Unspecified injury of thorax

INJURIES TO THE ABDOMEN, LOWER BACK, LUMBAR SPINE PELVIS AND EXTERNAL GENITALS (S30-S39)

Includes　injuries to the abdominal wall
　　　　　　injuries to the anus
　　　　　　injuries to the buttock
　　　　　　injuries to the external genitalia
　　　　　　injuries to the flank
　　　　　　injuries to the groin

Excludes2　burns and corrosions (T20-T32)
　　　　　　effects of foreign body in anus and rectum (T18.5)
　　　　　　effects of foreign body in genitourinary tract (T19.-)
　　　　　　effects of foreign body in stomach, small intestine and colon (T18.2-T18.4)
　　　　　　frostbite (T33-T34)
　　　　　　insect bite or sting, venomous (T63.4)

● S30　Superficial injury of abdomen, lower back, pelvis and external genitals
　　　　Excludes2　superficial injury of hip (S70.-)
　　　　The appropriate 7th character is to be added to each code from category S30

A	initial encounter
D	subsequent encounter
S	sequela

X● S30.0　Contusion of lower back and pelvis
　　　　　Contusion of buttock

CHAPTER 19 (S00-T88)

X● **S30.1**   Contusion of abdominal wall
     Contusion of flank
     Contusion of groin

● **S30.2**   Contusion of external genital organs

   ● **S30.20**   Contusion of unspecified external genital organ

     ● **S30.201**   Contusion of unspecified external genital organ, male ♂

     ● **S30.202**   Contusion of unspecified external genital organ, female ♀

   X● **S30.21**   Contusion of penis ♂

   X● **S30.22**   Contusion of scrotum and testes ♂

   X● **S30.23**   Contusion of vagina and vulva ♀

X● **S30.3**   Contusion of anus

● **S30.8**   Other superficial injuries of abdomen, lower back, pelvis and external genitals

   ● **S30.81**   Abrasion of abdomen, lower back, pelvis and external genitals

     ● **S30.810**   Abrasion of lower back and pelvis

     ● **S30.811**   Abrasion of abdominal wall

     ● **S30.812**   Abrasion of penis ♂

     ● **S30.813**   Abrasion of scrotum and testes ♂

     ● **S30.814**   Abrasion of vagina and vulva ♀

     ● **S30.815**   Abrasion of unspecified external genital organs, male ♂

     ● **S30.816**   Abrasion of unspecified external genital organs, female ♀

     ● **S30.817**   Abrasion of anus

   ● **S30.82**   Blister (nonthermal) of abdomen, lower back, pelvis and external genitals

     ● **S30.820**   Blister (nonthermal) of lower back and pelvis

     ● **S30.821**   Blister (nonthermal) of abdominal wall

     ● **S30.822**   Blister (nonthermal) of penis ♂

     ● **S30.823**   Blister (nonthermal) of scrotum and testes ♂

     ● **S30.824**   Blister (nonthermal) of vagina and vulva ♀

     ● **S30.825**   Blister (nonthermal) of unspecified external genital organs, male ♂

     ● **S30.826**   Blister (nonthermal) of unspecified external genital organs, female ♀

     ● **S30.827**   Blister (nonthermal) of anus

   ● **S30.84**   External constriction of abdomen, lower back, pelvis and external genitals

     ● **S30.840**   External constriction of lower back and pelvis

     ● **S30.841**   External constriction of abdominal wall

     ● **S30.842**   External constriction of penis ♂
         Hair tourniquet syndrome of penis
         Use additional cause code to identify the constricting item (W49.0-)

     ● **S30.843**   External constriction of scrotum and testes ♂

     ● **S30.844**   External constriction of vagina and vulva ♀

     ● **S30.845**   External constriction of unspecified external genital organs, male ♂

     ● **S30.846**   External constriction of unspecified external genital organs, female ♀

   ● **S30.85**   Superficial foreign body of abdomen, lower back, pelvis and external genitals
     Splinter in the abdomen, lower back, pelvis and external genitals

     ● **S30.850**   Superficial foreign body of lower back and pelvis

     ● **S30.851**   Superficial foreign body of abdominal wall

     ● **S30.852**   Superficial foreign body of penis ♂

     ● **S30.853**   Superficial foreign body of scrotum and testes ♂

     ● **S30.854**   Superficial foreign body of vagina and vulva ♀

     ● **S30.855**   Superficial foreign body of unspecified external genital organs, male ♂

     ● **S30.856**   Superficial foreign body of unspecified external genital organs, female ♀

     ● **S30.857**   Superficial foreign body of anus

   ● **S30.86**   Insect bite (nonvenomous) of abdomen, lower back, pelvis and external genitals

     ● **S30.860**   Insect bite (nonvenomous) of lower back and pelvis

     ● **S30.861**   Insect bite (nonvenomous) of abdominal wall

     ● **S30.862**   Insect bite (nonvenomous) of penis ♂

     ● **S30.863**   Insect bite (nonvenomous) of scrotum and testes ♂

     ● **S30.864**   Insect bite (nonvenomous) of vagina and vulva ♀

     ● **S30.865**   Insect bite (nonvenomous) of unspecified external genital organs, male ♂

     ● **S30.866**   Insect bite (nonvenomous) of unspecified external genital organs, female ♀

     ● **S30.867**   Insect bite (nonvenomous) of anus

   ● **S30.87**   Other superficial bite of abdomen, lower back, pelvis and external genitals

     Excludes1   open bite of abdomen, lower back, pelvis and external genitals (S31.05, S31.15, S31.25, S31.35, S31.45, S31.55)

     ● **S30.870**   Other superficial bite of lower back and pelvis

     ● **S30.871**   Other superficial bite of abdominal wall

     ● **S30.872**   Other superficial bite of penis ♂

     ● **S30.873**   Other superficial bite of scrotum and testes ♂

     ● **S30.874**   Other superficial bite of vagina and vulva ♀

     ● **S30.875**   Other superficial bite of unspecified external genital organs, male ♂

     ● **S30.876**   Other superficial bite of unspecified external genital organs, female ♀

     ● **S30.877**   Other superficial bite of anus

● **S30.9**   Unspecified superficial injury of abdomen, lower back, pelvis and external genitals

   X● **S30.91**   Unspecified superficial injury of lower back and pelvis

   X● **S30.92**   Unspecified superficial injury of abdominal wall

   X● **S30.93**   Unspecified superficial injury of penis ♂

   X● **S30.94**   Unspecified superficial injury of scrotum and testes ♂

   X● **S30.95**   Unspecified superficial injury of vagina and vulva ♀

   X● **S30.96**   Unspecified superficial injury of unspecified external genital organs, male ♂

   X● **S30.97**   Unspecified superficial injury of unspecified external genital organs, female ♀

   X● **S30.98**   Unspecified superficial injury of anus

N Newborn Age: 0   **P** Pediatric Age: 0–17   **M** Maternity DX: 9–64   **A** Adult Age: 15–124   ♀ Females Only   ♂ Males Only

● S31   Open wound of abdomen, lower back, pelvis and external genitals

Code also any associated:
   spinal cord injury (S24.0, S24.1-, S34.0-, S34.1-)
   wound infection

Excludes1   traumatic amputation of part of abdomen, lower back and pelvis (S38.2-, S38.3)

Excludes2   open wound of hip (S71.00-S71.02)
   open fracture of pelvis (S32.1--S32.9 with 7th character B)

The appropriate 7th character is to be added to each code from category S31

> A   initial encounter
> D   subsequent encounter
> S   sequela

● S31.0   Open wound of lower back and pelvis

  ● S31.00   Unspecified open wound of lower back and pelvis

    ● S31.000   Unspecified open wound of lower back and pelvis without penetration into retroperitoneum
         Unspecified open wound of lower back and pelvis NOS

    ● S31.001   Unspecified open wound of lower back and pelvis with penetration into retroperitoneum

  ● S31.01   Laceration without foreign body of lower back and pelvis

    ● S31.010   Laceration without foreign body of lower back and pelvis without penetration into retroperitoneum
         Laceration without foreign body of lower back and pelvis NOS

    ● S31.011   Laceration without foreign body of lower back and pelvis with penetration into retroperitoneum

  ● S31.02   Laceration with foreign body of lower back and pelvis

    ● S31.020   Laceration with foreign body of lower back and pelvis without penetration into retroperitoneum
         Laceration with foreign body of lower back and pelvis NOS

    ● S31.021   Laceration with foreign body of lower back and pelvis with penetration into retroperitoneum

● S31.03   Puncture wound without foreign body of lower back and pelvis

  ● S31.030   Puncture wound without foreign body of lower back and pelvis without penetration into retroperitoneum
       Puncture wound without foreign body of lower back and pelvis NOS

  ● S31.031   Puncture wound without foreign body of lower back and pelvis with penetration into retroperitoneum

● S31.04   Puncture wound with foreign body of lower back and pelvis

  ● S31.040   Puncture wound with foreign body of lower back and pelvis without penetration into retroperitoneum
       Puncture wound with foreign body of lower back and pelvis NOS

  ● S31.041   Puncture wound with foreign body of lower back and pelvis with penetration into retroperitoneum

● S31.05   Open bite of lower back and pelvis
    Bite of lower back and pelvis NOS

    Excludes1   superficial bite of lower back and pelvis (S30.860, S30.870)

  ● S31.050   Open bite of lower back and pelvis without penetration into retroperitoneum
       Open bite of lower back and pelvis NOS

  ● S31.051   Open bite of lower back and pelvis with penetration into retroperitoneum

● S31.1   Open wound of abdominal wall without penetration into peritoneal cavity
    Open wound of abdominal wall NOS

    Excludes2   open wound of abdominal wall with penetration into peritoneal cavity (S31.6-)

  ● S31.10   Unspecified open wound of abdominal wall without penetration into peritoneal cavity

    ● S31.100   Unspecified open wound of abdominal wall, right upper quadrant without penetration into peritoneal cavity

    ● S31.101   Unspecified open wound of abdominal wall, left upper quadrant without penetration into peritoneal cavity

● S31.102   Unspecified open wound of abdominal wall, epigastric region without penetration into peritoneal cavity

● S31.103   Unspecified open wound of abdominal wall, right lower quadrant without penetration into peritoneal cavity

● S31.104   Unspecified open wound of abdominal wall, left lower quadrant without penetration into peritoneal cavity

● S31.105   Unspecified open wound of abdominal wall, periumbilic region without penetration into peritoneal cavity

● S31.109   Unspecified open wound of abdominal wall, unspecified quadrant without penetration into peritoneal cavity

     Unspecified open wound of abdominal wall NOS

● S31.11   Laceration without foreign body of abdominal wall without penetration into peritoneal cavity

● S31.110   Laceration without foreign body of abdominal wall, right upper quadrant without penetration into peritoneal cavity

● S31.111   Laceration without foreign body of abdominal wall, left upper quadrant without penetration into peritoneal cavity

● S31.112   Laceration without foreign body of abdominal wall, epigastric region without penetration into peritoneal cavity

● S31.113   Laceration without foreign body of abdominal wall, right lower quadrant without penetration into peritoneal cavity

● S31.114   Laceration without foreign body of abdominal wall, left lower quadrant without penetration into peritoneal cavity

● S31.115   Laceration without foreign body of abdominal wall, periumbilic region without penetration into peritoneal cavity

● S31.119   Laceration without foreign body of abdominal wall, unspecified quadrant without penetration into peritoneal cavity

● S31.12   Laceration with foreign body of abdominal wall without penetration into peritoneal cavity

● S31.120   Laceration of abdominal wall with foreign body, right upper quadrant without penetration into peritoneal cavity

● S31.121   Laceration of abdominal wall with foreign body, left upper quadrant without penetration into peritoneal cavity

● S31.122   Laceration of abdominal wall with foreign body, epigastric region without penetration into peritoneal cavity

● S31.123   Laceration of abdominal wall with foreign body, right lower quadrant without penetration into peritoneal cavity

● S31.124   Laceration of abdominal wall with foreign body, left lower quadrant without penetration into peritoneal cavity

● S31.125   Laceration of abdominal wall with foreign body, periumbilic region without penetration into peritoneal cavity

● S31.129   Laceration of abdominal wall with foreign body, unspecified quadrant without penetration into peritoneal cavity

● S31.13   Puncture wound of abdominal wall without foreign body without penetration into peritoneal cavity

● S31.130   Puncture wound of abdominal wall without foreign body, right upper quadrant without penetration into peritoneal cavity

● S31.131   Puncture wound of abdominal wall without foreign body, left upper quadrant without penetration into peritoneal cavity

● S31.132   Puncture wound of abdominal wall without foreign body, epigastric region without penetration into peritoneal cavity

● S31.133   Puncture wound of abdominal wall without foreign body, right lower quadrant without penetration into peritoneal cavity

● S31.134   Puncture wound of abdominal wall without foreign body, left lower quadrant without penetration into peritoneal cavity

● S31.135   Puncture wound of abdominal wall without foreign body, periumbilic region without penetration into peritoneal cavity

● S31.139   Puncture wound of abdominal wall without foreign body, unspecified quadrant without penetration into peritoneal cavity

● S31.14   Puncture wound of abdominal wall with foreign body without penetration into peritoneal cavity

● S31.140   Puncture wound of abdominal wall with foreign body, right upper quadrant without penetration into peritoneal cavity

● S31.141   Puncture wound of abdominal wall with foreign body, left upper quadrant without penetration into peritoneal cavity

● S31.142   Puncture wound of abdominal wall with foreign body, epigastric region without penetration into peritoneal cavity

● S31.143   Puncture wound of abdominal wall with foreign body, right lower quadrant without penetration into peritoneal cavity

● S31.144   Puncture wound of abdominal wall with foreign body, left lower quadrant without penetration into peritoneal cavity

● S31.145   Puncture wound of abdominal wall with foreign body, periumbilic region without penetration into peritoneal cavity

● S31.149   Puncture wound of abdominal wall with foreign body, unspecified quadrant without penetration into peritoneal cavity

CHAPTER 19 (S00-T88)

● S31.15   Open bite of abdominal wall without penetration into peritoneal cavity
Bite of abdominal wall NOS

> **Excludes1**   superficial bite of abdominal wall (S30.871)

● S31.150   Open bite of abdominal wall, right upper quadrant without penetration into peritoneal cavity

● S31.151   Open bite of abdominal wall, left upper quadrant without penetration into peritoneal cavity

● S31.152   Open bite of abdominal wall, epigastric region without penetration into peritoneal cavity

● S31.153   Open bite of abdominal wall, right lower quadrant without penetration into peritoneal cavity

● S31.154   Open bite of abdominal wall, left lower quadrant without penetration into peritoneal cavity

● S31.155   Open bite of abdominal wall, periumbilic region without penetration into peritoneal cavity

● S31.159   Open bite of abdominal wall, unspecified quadrant without penetration into peritoneal cavity

● S31.2   Open wound of penis

X ● S31.20   Unspecified open wound of penis ♂

X ● S31.21   Laceration without foreign body of penis ♂

X ● S31.22   Laceration with foreign body of penis ♂

X ● S31.23   Puncture wound without foreign body of penis ♂

X ● S31.24   Puncture wound with foreign body of penis ♂

X ● S31.25   Open bite of penis ♂
Bite of penis NOS

> **Excludes1**   superficial bite of penis (S30.862, S30.872)

● S31.3   Open wound of scrotum and testes

X ● S31.30   Unspecified open wound of scrotum and testes ♂

X ● S31.31   Laceration without foreign body of scrotum and testes ♂

X ● S31.32   Laceration with foreign body of scrotum and testes ♂

X ● S31.33   Puncture wound without foreign body of scrotum and testes ♂

X ● S31.34   Puncture wound with foreign body of scrotum and testes ♂

X ● S31.35   Open bite of scrotum and testes ♂
Bite of scrotum and testes NOS

> **Excludes1**   superficial bite of scrotum and testes (S30.863, S30.873)

● S31.4   Open wound of vagina and vulva

> **Excludes1**   injury to vagina and vulva during delivery (O70.-, O71.4)

X ● S31.40   Unspecified open wound of vagina and vulva ♀

X ● S31.41   Laceration without foreign body of vagina and vulva ♀

X ● S31.42   Laceration with foreign body of vagina and vulva ♀

X ● S31.43   Puncture wound without foreign body of vagina and vulva ♀

X ● S31.44   Puncture wound with foreign body of vagina and vulva ♀

X ● S31.45   Open bite of vagina and vulva ♀
Bite of vagina and vulva NOS

> **Excludes1**   superficial bite of vagina and vulva (S30.864, S30.874)

● S31.5   Open wound of unspecified external genital organs

> **Excludes1**   traumatic amputation of external genital organs (S38.21, S38.22)

● S31.50   Unspecified open wound of unspecified external genital organs

● S31.501   Unspecified open wound of unspecified external genital organs, male ♂

● S31.502   Unspecified open wound of unspecified external genital organs, female ♀

● S31.51   Laceration without foreign body of unspecified external genital organs

● S31.511   Laceration without foreign body of unspecified external genital organs, male ♂

● S31.512   Laceration without foreign body of unspecified external genital organs, female ♀

● S31.52   Laceration with foreign body of unspecified external genital organs

● S31.521   Laceration with foreign body of unspecified external genital organs, male ♂

● S31.522   Laceration with foreign body of unspecified external genital organs, female ♀

● S31.53   Puncture wound without foreign body of unspecified external genital organs

● S31.531   Puncture wound without foreign body of unspecified external genital organs, male ♂

● S31.532   Puncture wound without foreign body of unspecified external genital organs, female ♀

● S31.54   Puncture wound with foreign body of unspecified external genital organs

● S31.541   Puncture wound with foreign body of unspecified external genital organs, male ♂

● S31.542   Puncture wound with foreign body of unspecified external genital organs, female ♀

● S31.55   Open bite of unspecified external genital organs
Bite of unspecified external genital organs NOS

> **Excludes1**   superficial bite of unspecified external genital organs (S30.865, S30.866, S30.875, S30.876)

● S31.551   Open bite of unspecified external genital organs, male ♂

● S31.552   Open bite of unspecified external genital organs, female ♀

● S31.6   Open wound of abdominal wall with penetration into peritoneal cavity

● S31.60   Unspecified open wound of abdominal wall with penetration into peritoneal cavity

● S31.600   Unspecified open wound of abdominal wall, right upper quadrant with penetration into peritoneal cavity

● S31.601   Unspecified open wound of abdominal wall, left upper quadrant with penetration into peritoneal cavity

● S31.602   Unspecified open wound of abdominal wall, epigastric region with penetration into peritoneal cavity

▶ New   ⇒ Revised   ~~deleted~~ Deleted   Excludes 1   Excludes 2   Includes   Use additional   Code first   Code also   Key words

OGCR Official Guidelines   X Assign placeholder X   ● Use Additional Character(s)   ▷ Manifestation Code   🐾 Hierarchical Condition Category   **Coding Clinic**

● S31.603   Unspecified open wound of abdominal wall, right lower quadrant with penetration into peritoneal cavity

● S31.604   Unspecified open wound of abdominal wall, left lower quadrant with penetration into peritoneal cavity

● S31.605   Unspecified open wound of abdominal wall, periumbilic region with penetration into peritoneal cavity

● S31.609   Unspecified open wound of abdominal wall, unspecified quadrant with penetration into peritoneal cavity

● S31.61   Laceration without foreign body of abdominal wall with penetration into peritoneal cavity

● S31.610   Laceration without foreign body of abdominal wall, right upper quadrant with penetration into peritoneal cavity

● S31.611   Laceration without foreign body of abdominal wall, left upper quadrant with penetration into peritoneal cavity

● S31.612   Laceration without foreign body of abdominal wall, epigastric region with penetration into peritoneal cavity

● S31.613   Laceration without foreign body of abdominal wall, right lower quadrant with penetration into peritoneal cavity

     Coding Clinic: 2015, Q4, P37

● S31.614   Laceration without foreign body of abdominal wall, left lower quadrant with penetration into peritoneal cavity

● S31.615   Laceration without foreign body of abdominal wall, periumbilic region with penetration into peritoneal cavity

● S31.619   Laceration without foreign body of abdominal wall, unspecified quadrant with penetration into peritoneal cavity

● S31.62   Laceration with foreign body of abdominal wall with penetration into peritoneal cavity

● S31.620   Laceration with foreign body of abdominal wall, right upper quadrant with penetration into peritoneal cavity

● S31.621   Laceration with foreign body of abdominal wall, left upper quadrant with penetration into peritoneal cavity

● S31.622   Laceration with foreign body of abdominal wall, epigastric region with penetration into peritoneal cavity

● S31.623   Laceration with foreign body of abdominal wall, right lower quadrant with penetration into peritoneal cavity

● S31.624   Laceration with foreign body of abdominal wall, left lower quadrant with penetration into peritoneal cavity

● S31.625   Laceration with foreign body of abdominal wall, periumbilic region with penetration into peritoneal cavity

● S31.629   Laceration with foreign body of abdominal wall, unspecified quadrant with penetration into peritoneal cavity

● S31.63   Puncture wound without foreign body of abdominal wall with penetration into peritoneal cavity

● S31.630   Puncture wound without foreign body of abdominal wall, right upper quadrant with penetration into peritoneal cavity

● S31.631   Puncture wound without foreign body of abdominal wall, left upper quadrant with penetration into peritoneal cavity

● S31.632   Puncture wound without foreign body of abdominal wall, epigastric region with penetration into peritoneal cavity

● S31.633   Puncture wound without foreign body of abdominal wall, right lower quadrant with penetration into peritoneal cavity

● S31.634   Puncture wound without foreign body of abdominal wall, left lower quadrant with penetration into peritoneal cavity

● S31.635   Puncture wound without foreign body of abdominal wall, periumbilic region with penetration into peritoneal cavity

● S31.639   Puncture wound without foreign body of abdominal wall, unspecified quadrant with penetration into peritoneal cavity

● S31.64   Puncture wound with foreign body of abdominal wall with penetration into peritoneal cavity

● S31.640   Puncture wound with foreign body of abdominal wall, right upper quadrant with penetration into peritoneal cavity

● S31.641   Puncture wound with foreign body of abdominal wall, left upper quadrant with penetration into peritoneal cavity

● S31.642   Puncture wound with foreign body of abdominal wall, epigastric region with penetration into peritoneal cavity

● S31.643   Puncture wound with foreign body of abdominal wall, right lower quadrant with penetration into peritoneal cavity

● S31.644   Puncture wound with foreign body of abdominal wall, left lower quadrant with penetration into peritoneal cavity

● S31.645   Puncture wound with foreign body of abdominal wall, periumbilic region with penetration into peritoneal cavity

● S31.649   Puncture wound with foreign body of abdominal wall, unspecified quadrant with penetration into peritoneal cavity

CHAPTER 19 (S00-T88)

● S31.65   **Open bite of abdominal wall with penetration into peritoneal cavity**

> **Excludes1**   superficial bite of abdominal wall (S30.861, S30.871)

● S31.650   Open bite of abdominal wall, **right upper** quadrant with penetration into peritoneal cavity

● S31.651   Open bite of abdominal wall, **left upper** quadrant with penetration into peritoneal cavity

● S31.652   Open bite of abdominal wall, **epigastric region** with penetration into peritoneal cavity

● S31.653   Open bite of abdominal wall, **right lower** quadrant with penetration into peritoneal cavity

● S31.654   Open bite of abdominal wall, **left lower** quadrant with penetration into peritoneal cavity

● S31.655   Open bite of abdominal wall, **periumbilic region** with penetration into peritoneal cavity

● S31.659   Open bite of abdominal wall, **unspecified** quadrant with penetration into peritoneal cavity

● S31.8   **Open wound of other parts of abdomen, lower back and pelvis**

● S31.80   Open wound of **unspecified buttock**

● S31.801   Laceration **without foreign** body of unspecified buttock

● S31.802   Laceration **with foreign** body of unspecified buttock

● S31.803   **Puncture wound without foreign** body of unspecified buttock

● S31.804   **Puncture wound with foreign** body of unspecified buttock

● S31.805   **Open bite of** unspecified buttock
> Bite of buttock NOS
> > **Excludes1**   superficial bite of buttock (S30.870)

● S31.809   **Unspecified** open wound of unspecified buttock

● S31.81   Open wound of **right buttock**

● S31.811   Laceration **without foreign** body of right buttock

● S31.812   Laceration **with foreign** body of right buttock

● S31.813   **Puncture wound without foreign** body of right buttock

● S31.814   **Puncture wound with foreign** body of right buttock

● S31.815   **Open bite of** right buttock
> Bite of right buttock NOS
> > **Excludes1**   superficial bite of buttock (S30.870)

● S31.819   **Unspecified** open wound of right buttock

● S31.82   Open wound of **left buttock**

● S31.821   Laceration **without foreign** body of left buttock

● S31.822   Laceration **with foreign** body of left buttock

● S31.823   **Puncture wound without foreign** body of left buttock

● S31.824   **Puncture wound with foreign** body of left buttock

● S31.825   **Open bite of** left buttock
> Bite of left buttock NOS
> > **Excludes1**   superficial bite of buttock (S30.870)

● S31.829   **Unspecified** open wound of left buttock

● S31.83   **Open wound of anus**

● S31.831   Laceration **without foreign** body of anus

● S31.832   Laceration **with foreign** body of anus

● S31.833   **Puncture wound without foreign** body of anus

● S31.834   **Puncture wound with foreign** body of anus

● S31.835   **Open bite of anus**
> Bite of anus NOS
> > **Excludes1**   superficial bite of anus (S30.877)

● S31.839   **Unspecified** open wound of anus

● S32   **Fracture of lumbar spine and pelvis**

Note: A fracture not indicated as displaced or nondisplaced should be coded to displaced

A fracture not indicated as opened or closed should be coded to closed

> **Includes**   fracture of lumbosacral neural arch
> fracture of lumbosacral spinous process
> fracture of lumbosacral transverse process
> fracture of lumbosacral vertebra
> fracture of lumbosacral vertebral arch

Code first any associated spinal cord and spinal nerve injury (S34.-)

> **Excludes1**   transection of abdomen (S38.3)
> **Excludes2**   fracture of hip NOS (S72.0-)

The appropriate 7th character is to be added to each code from category S32

> A   initial encounter for closed fracture
> B   initial encounter for open fracture
> D   subsequent encounter for fracture with routine healing
> G   subsequent encounter for fracture with delayed healing
> K   subsequent encounter for fracture with nonunion
> S   sequela

● S32.0   **Fracture of lumbar vertebra**
> Fracture of lumbar spine NOS

● S32.00   Fracture of **unspecified** lumbar vertebra

● S32.000   **Wedge compression** fracture of unspecified lumbar vertebra A, B 🐾

● S32.001   **Stable burst** fracture of unspecified lumbar vertebra A, B 🐾

● S32.002   **Unstable burst** fracture of unspecified lumbar vertebra A, B 🐾

● S32.008   **Other** fracture of unspecified lumbar vertebra A, B 🐾

● S32.009   **Unspecified** fracture of unspecified lumbar vertebra A, B 🐾

● S32.01   Fracture of **first** lumbar vertebra

● S32.010   **Wedge compression** fracture of first lumbar vertebra A, B 🐾

● S32.011   **Stable burst** fracture of first lumbar vertebra A, B 🐾

● S32.012   **Unstable burst** fracture of first lumbar vertebra A, B 🐾

● S32.018   **Other** fracture of first lumbar vertebra A, B 🐾

● S32.019   **Unspecified** fracture of first lumbar vertebra A, B 🐾

● S32.02   Fracture of **second** lumbar vertebra

● S32.020   **Wedge compression** fracture of second lumbar vertebra A, B 🐾

● S32.021   **Stable burst** fracture of second lumbar vertebra A, B 🐾

● S32.022   **Unstable burst** fracture of second lumbar vertebra A, B 🐾

● S32.028   **Other** fracture of second lumbar vertebra A, B 🐾

● S32.029   **Unspecified** fracture of second lumbar vertebra A, B 🐾

▶ New   ⇒ Revised   ~~deleted~~ Deleted   Excludes 1   Excludes 2   Includes   Use additional   Code first   Code also   Key words

OGCR Official Guidelines   X Assign placeholder X   ● Use Additional Character(s)   ▶ Manifestation Code   🐾 Hierarchical Condition Category   **Coding Clinic**

● S32.03   Fracture of third lumbar vertebra
   ● S32.030   Wedge compression fracture of third lumbar vertebra A, B 🦴
   ● S32.031   Stable burst fracture of third lumbar vertebra A, B 🦴
   ● S32.032   Unstable burst fracture of third lumbar vertebra A, B 🦴
   ● S32.038   Other fracture of third lumbar vertebra A, B 🦴
   ● S32.039   Unspecified fracture of third lumbar vertebra A, B 🦴

● S32.04   Fracture of fourth lumbar vertebra
   ● S32.040   Wedge compression fracture of fourth lumbar vertebra A, B 🦴
   ● S32.041   Stable burst fracture of fourth lumbar vertebra A, B 🦴
   ● S32.042   Unstable burst fracture of fourth lumbar vertebra A, B 🦴
   ● S32.048   Other fracture of fourth lumbar vertebra A, B 🦴
   ● S32.049   Unspecified fracture of fourth lumbar vertebra A, B 🦴

● S32.05   Fracture of fifth lumbar vertebra
   ● S32.050   Wedge compression fracture of fifth lumbar vertebra A, B 🦴
   ● S32.051   Stable burst fracture of fifth lumbar vertebra A, B 🦴
   ● S32.052   Unstable burst fracture of fifth lumbar vertebra A, B 🦴
   ● S32.058   Other fracture of fifth lumbar vertebra A, B 🦴
   ● S32.059   Unspecified fracture of fifth lumbar vertebra A, B 🦴

● S32.1   Fracture of sacrum
   For vertical fractures, code to most medial fracture extension
   Use two codes if both a vertical and transverse fracture are present
   Code also any associated fracture of pelvic ring (S32.8-)

X ● S32.10   Unspecified fracture of sacrum A, B 🦴

● S32.11   Zone I fracture of sacrum
   Vertical sacral ala fracture of sacrum
   ● S32.110   Nondisplaced Zone I fracture of sacrum A, B 🦴
   ● S32.111   Minimally displaced Zone I fracture of sacrum A, B 🦴
   ● S32.112   Severely displaced Zone I fracture of sacrum A, B 🦴
   ● S32.119   Unspecified Zone I fracture of sacrum A, B 🦴

● S32.12   Zone II fracture of sacrum
   Vertical foraminal region fracture of sacrum
   ● S32.120   Nondisplaced Zone II fracture of sacrum A, B 🦴
   ● S32.121   Minimally displaced Zone II fracture of sacrum A, B 🦴
   ● S32.122   Severely displaced Zone II fracture of sacrum A, B 🦴
   ● S32.129   Unspecified Zone II fracture of sacrum A, B 🦴

● S32.13   Zone III fracture of sacrum
   Vertical fracture into spinal canal region of sacrum
   ● S32.130   Nondisplaced Zone III fracture of sacrum A, B 🦴
   ● S32.131   Minimally displaced Zone III fracture of sacrum A, B 🦴
   ● S32.132   Severely displaced Zone III fracture of sacrum A, B 🦴
   ● S32.139   Unspecified Zone III fracture of sacrum A, B 🦴

X ● S32.14   Type 1 fracture of sacrum A, B 🦴
   Transverse flexion fracture of sacrum without displacement
X ● S32.15   Type 2 fracture of sacrum A, B 🦴
   Transverse flexion fracture of sacrum with posterior displacement
X ● S32.16   Type 3 fracture of sacrum A, B 🦴
   Transverse extension fracture of sacrum with anterior displacement
X ● S32.17   Type 4 fracture of sacrum A, B 🦴
   Transverse segmental comminution of upper sacrum
X ● S32.19   Other fracture of sacrum A, B 🦴

X ● S32.2   Fracture of coccyx A, B 🦴

● S32.3   Fracture of ilium
   Excludes1   fracture of ilium with associated disruption of pelvic ring (S32.8-)
   ● S32.30   Unspecified fracture of ilium
      ● S32.301   Unspecified fracture of right ilium A, B 🦴
      ● S32.302   Unspecified fracture of left ilium A, B 🦴
      ● S32.309   Unspecified fracture of unspecified ilium A, B 🦴

   ● S32.31   Avulsion fracture of ilium
      ● S32.311   Displaced avulsion fracture of right ilium A, B 🦴
      ● S32.312   Displaced avulsion fracture of left ilium A, B 🦴
      ● S32.313   Displaced avulsion fracture of unspecified ilium A, B 🦴
      ● S32.314   Nondisplaced avulsion fracture of right ilium A, B 🦴
      ● S32.315   Nondisplaced avulsion fracture of left ilium A, B 🦴
      ● S32.316   Nondisplaced avulsion fracture of unspecified ilium A, B 🦴

   ● S32.39   Other fracture of ilium
      ● S32.391   Other fracture of right ilium A, B 🦴
      ● S32.392   Other fracture of left ilium A, B 🦴
      ● S32.399   Other fracture of unspecified ilium A, B 🦴

● S32.4   Fracture of acetabulum
   Code also any associated fracture of pelvic ring (S32.8-)
   ● S32.40   Unspecified fracture of acetabulum
      ● S32.401   Unspecified fracture of right acetabulum A, B 🦴
      ● S32.402   Unspecified fracture of left acetabulum A, B 🦴
      ● S32.409   Unspecified fracture of unspecified acetabulum A, B 🦴

   ● S32.41   Fracture of anterior wall of acetabulum
      ● S32.411   Displaced fracture of anterior wall of right acetabulum A, B 🦴
      ● S32.412   Displaced fracture of anterior wall of left acetabulum A, B 🦴
      ● S32.413   Displaced fracture of anterior wall of unspecified acetabulum A, B 🦴
      ● S32.414   Nondisplaced fracture of anterior wall of right acetabulum A, B 🦴
      ● S32.415   Nondisplaced fracture of anterior wall of left acetabulum A, B 🦴
      ● S32.416   Nondisplaced fracture of anterior wall of unspecified acetabulum A, B 🦴

- S32.42   Fracture of posterior wall of acetabulum
  - S32.421   Displaced fracture of posterior wall of right acetabulum A, B 🦁
  - S32.422   Displaced fracture of posterior wall of left acetabulum A, B 🦁
  - S32.423   Displaced fracture of posterior wall of unspecified acetabulum A, B 🦁
  - S32.424   Nondisplaced fracture of posterior wall of right acetabulum A, B 🦁
  - S32.425   Nondisplaced fracture of posterior wall of left acetabulum A, B 🦁
  - S32.426   Nondisplaced fracture of posterior wall of unspecified acetabulum A, B 🦁
- S32.43   Fracture of anterior column [iliopubic] of acetabulum
  - S32.431   Displaced fracture of anterior column [iliopubic] of right acetabulum A, B 🦁
  - S32.432   Displaced fracture of anterior column [iliopubic] of left acetabulum A, B 🦁
  - S32.433   Displaced fracture of anterior column [iliopubic] of unspecified acetabulum A, B 🦁
  - S32.434   Nondisplaced fracture of anterior column [iliopubic] of right acetabulum A, B 🦁
  - S32.435   Nondisplaced fracture of anterior column [iliopubic] of left acetabulum A, B 🦁
  - S32.436   Nondisplaced fracture of anterior column [iliopubic] of unspecified acetabulum A, B 🦁
- S32.44   Fracture of posterior column [ilioischial] of acetabulum
  - S32.441   Displaced fracture of posterior column [ilioischial] of right acetabulum A, B 🦁
  - S32.442   Displaced fracture of posterior column [ilioischial] of left acetabulum A, B 🦁
  - S32.443   Displaced fracture of posterior column [ilioischial] of unspecified acetabulum A, B 🦁
  - S32.444   Nondisplaced fracture of posterior column [ilioischial] of right acetabulum A, B 🦁
  - S32.445   Nondisplaced fracture of posterior column [ilioischial] of left acetabulum A, B 🦁
  - S32.446   Nondisplaced fracture of posterior column [ilioischial] of unspecified acetabulum A, B 🦁
- S32.45   Transverse fracture of acetabulum
  - S32.451   Displaced transverse fracture of right acetabulum A, B 🦁
  - S32.452   Displaced transverse fracture of left acetabulum A, B 🦁
  - S32.453   Displaced transverse fracture of unspecified acetabulum A, B 🦁
  - S32.454   Nondisplaced transverse fracture of right acetabulum A, B 🦁
  - S32.455   Nondisplaced transverse fracture of left acetabulum A, B 🦁
  - S32.456   Nondisplaced transverse fracture of unspecified acetabulum A, B 🦁

- S32.46   Associated transverse-posterior fracture of acetabulum
  - S32.461   Displaced associated transverse-posterior fracture of right acetabulum A, B 🦁
  - S32.462   Displaced associated transverse-posterior fracture of left acetabulum A, B 🦁
  - S32.463   Displaced associated transverse-posterior fracture of unspecified acetabulum A, B 🦁
  - S32.464   Nondisplaced associated transverse-posterior fracture of right acetabulum A, B 🦁
  - S32.465   Nondisplaced associated transverse-posterior fracture of left acetabulum A, B 🦁
  - S32.466   Nondisplaced associated transverse-posterior fracture of unspecified acetabulum A, B 🦁
- S32.47   Fracture of medial wall of acetabulum
  - S32.471   Displaced fracture of medial wall of right acetabulum A, B 🦁
  - S32.472   Displaced fracture of medial wall of left acetabulum A, B 🦁
  - S32.473   Displaced fracture of medial wall of unspecified acetabulum A, B 🦁
  - S32.474   Nondisplaced fracture of medial wall of right acetabulum A, B 🦁
  - S32.475   Nondisplaced fracture of medial wall of left acetabulum A, B 🦁
  - S32.476   Nondisplaced fracture of medial wall of unspecified acetabulum A, B 🦁
- S32.48   Dome fracture of acetabulum
  - S32.481   Displaced dome fracture of right acetabulum A, B 🦁
  - S32.482   Displaced dome fracture of left acetabulum A, B 🦁
  - S32.483   Displaced dome fracture of unspecified acetabulum A, B 🦁
  - S32.484   Nondisplaced dome fracture of right acetabulum A, B 🦁
  - S32.485   Nondisplaced dome fracture of left acetabulum A, B 🦁
  - S32.486   Nondisplaced dome fracture of unspecified acetabulum A, B 🦁
- S32.49   Other fracture of acetabulum
  - S32.491   Other fracture of right acetabulum A, B 🦁
  - S32.492   Other fracture of left acetabulum A, B 🦁
  - S32.499   Other fracture of unspecified acetabulum A, B 🦁
- S32.5   Fracture of pubis
  - **Excludes 1**   fracture of pubis with associated disruption of pelvic ring (S32.8-)
  - S32.50   Unspecified fracture of pubis
    - S32.501   Unspecified fracture of right pubis A, B 🦁
    - S32.502   Unspecified fracture of left pubis A, B 🦁
    - S32.509   Unspecified fracture of unspecified pubis A, B 🦁
  - S32.51   Fracture of superior rim of pubis
    - S32.511   Fracture of superior rim of right pubis A, B 🦁
    - S32.512   Fracture of superior rim of left pubis A, B 🦁
    - S32.519   Fracture of superior rim of unspecified pubis A, B 🦁

▶ New   ⇒ Revised   ~~deleted~~ Deleted   Excludes 1   Excludes 2   Includes   Use additional   Code first   Code also   Key words
OGCR Official Guidelines   X Assign placeholder X   ● Use Additional Character(s)   ▷ Manifestation Code   🦁 Hierarchical Condition Category   **Coding Clinic**

● S32.59   Other specified fracture of pubis
   ● S32.591   Other specified fracture of right pubis A, B 🔍
   ● S32.592   Other specified fracture of left pubis A, B 🔍
   ● S32.599   Other specified fracture of unspecified pubis A, B 🔍

● S32.6   Fracture of ischium
   Excludes1   fracture of ischium with associated disruption of pelvic ring (S32.8-)
  ● S32.60   Unspecified fracture of ischium
   ● S32.601   Unspecified fracture of right ischium A, B 🔍
   ● S32.602   Unspecified fracture of left ischium A, B 🔍
   ● S32.609   Unspecified fracture of unspecified ischium A, B 🔍
  ● S32.61   Avulsion fracture of ischium
   ● S32.611   Displaced avulsion fracture of right ischium A, B 🔍
   ● S32.612   Displaced avulsion fracture of left ischium A, B 🔍
   ● S32.613   Displaced avulsion fracture of unspecified ischium A, B 🔍
   ● S32.614   Nondisplaced avulsion fracture of right ischium A, B 🔍
   ● S32.615   Nondisplaced avulsion fracture of left ischium A, B 🔍
   ● S32.616   Nondisplaced avulsion fracture of unspecified ischium A, B 🔍
  ● S32.69   Other specified fracture of ischium
   ● S32.691   Other specified fracture of right ischium A, B 🔍
   ● S32.692   Other specified fracture of left ischium A, B 🔍
   ● S32.699   Other specified fracture of unspecified ischium A, B 🔍

● S32.8   Fracture of other parts of pelvis
   Code also any associated:
     fracture of acetabulum (S32.4-)
     sacral fracture (S32.1-)
  ● S32.81   Multiple fractures of pelvis with disruption of pelvic ring
     Multiple pelvic fractures with disruption of pelvic circle
   ● S32.810   Multiple fractures of pelvis with stable disruption of pelvic ring A, B 🔍
   ● S32.811   Multiple fractures of pelvis with unstable disruption of pelvic ring A, B 🔍
  X ● S32.82   Multiple fractures of pelvis without disruption of pelvic ring A, B 🔍
     Multiple pelvic fractures without disruption of pelvic circle
  X ● S32.89   Fracture of other parts of pelvis A, B 🔍
X ● S32.9   Fracture of unspecified parts of lumbosacral spine and pelvis A, B 🔍
   Fracture of lumbosacral spine NOS
   Fracture of pelvis NOS
   Coding Clinic: 2012, Q4, P93

● S33   Dislocation and sprain of joints and ligaments of lumbar spine and pelvis
   Includes   avulsion of joint or ligament of lumbar spine and pelvis
     laceration of cartilage, joint or ligament of lumbar spine and pelvis
     sprain of cartilage, joint or ligament of lumbar spine and pelvis
     traumatic hemarthrosis of joint or ligament of lumbar spine and pelvis
     traumatic rupture of joint or ligament of lumbar spine and pelvis
     traumatic subluxation of joint or ligament of lumbar spine and pelvis
     traumatic tear of joint or ligament of lumbar spine and pelvis
   Code also any associated open wound
   Excludes1   nontraumatic rupture or displacement of lumbar intervertebral disc NOS (M51.-)
     obstetric damage to pelvic joints and ligaments (O71.6)
   Excludes2   dislocation and sprain of joints and ligaments of hip (S73.-)
     strain of muscle of lower back and pelvis (S39.01-)
   The appropriate 7th character is to be added to each code from category S33

A	initial encounter
D	subsequent encounter
S	sequela

X ● S33.0   Traumatic rupture of lumbar intervertebral disc
   Excludes1   rupture or displacement (nontraumatic) of lumbar intervertebral disc NOS (M51.- with fifth character 6)
● S33.1   Subluxation and dislocation of lumbar vertebra
   Code also any associated:
     open wound of abdomen, lower back and pelvis (S31)
     spinal cord injury (S24.0, S24.1-, S34.0-, S34.1-)
   Excludes2   fracture of lumbar vertebrae (S32.0-)
  ● S33.10   Subluxation and dislocation of unspecified lumbar vertebra
   ● S33.100   Subluxation of unspecified lumbar vertebra
   ● S33.101   Dislocation of unspecified lumbar vertebra
  ● S33.11   Subluxation and dislocation of L1/L2 lumbar vertebra
   ● S33.110   Subluxation of L1/L2 lumbar vertebra
   ● S33.111   Dislocation of L1/L2 lumbar vertebra
  ● S33.12   Subluxation and dislocation of L2/L3 lumbar vertebra
   ● S33.120   Subluxation of L2/L3 lumbar vertebra
   ● S33.121   Dislocation of L2/L3 lumbar vertebra
  ● S33.13   Subluxation and dislocation of L3/L4 lumbar vertebra
   ● S33.130   Subluxation of L3/L4 lumbar vertebra
   ● S33.131   Dislocation of L3/L4 lumbar vertebra
  ● S33.14   Subluxation and dislocation of L4/L5 lumbar vertebra
   ● S33.140   Subluxation of L4/L5 lumbar vertebra
   ● S33.141   Dislocation of L4/L5 lumbar vertebra
X ● S33.2   Dislocation of sacroiliac and sacrococcygeal joint

- ● S33.3   **Dislocation of other and unspecified parts of lumbar spine and pelvis**
  - X ● S33.30   Dislocation of unspecified parts of lumbar spine and pelvis
  - X ● S33.39   Dislocation of other parts of lumbar spine and pelvis
- X ● S33.4   Traumatic rupture of symphysis pubis
- X ● S33.5   Sprain of ligaments of lumbar spine
- X ● S33.6   Sprain of sacroiliac joint
- X ● S33.8   Sprain of other parts of lumbar spine and pelvis
- X ● S33.9   Sprain of unspecified parts of lumbar spine and pelvis

- ● S34   **Injury of lumbar and sacral spinal cord and nerves at abdomen, lower back and pelvis level**

  Note: Code to highest level of lumbar cord injury

  Injuries to the spinal cord (S34.0 and S34.1) refer to the cord level and not bone level injury, and can affect nerve roots at and below the level given.

  The appropriate 7th character is to be added to each code from category S34

A	initial encounter
D	subsequent encounter
S	sequela

  Code also any associated:
  fracture of vertebra (S22.0-, S32.0-)
  open wound of abdomen, lower back and pelvis (S31.-)
  transient paralysis (R29.5)

  - ● S34.0   **Concussion and edema of lumbar and sacral spinal cord**
    - X ● S34.01   Concussion and edema of lumbar spinal cord A, D, S 🐾
    - X ● S34.02   Concussion and edema of sacral spinal cord A, D, S 🐾
      Concussion and edema of conus medullaris
  - ● S34.1   **Other and unspecified injury of lumbar and sacral spinal cord**
    - ● S34.10   Unspecified injury to lumbar spinal cord
      - ● S34.101   Unspecified injury to L_1 level of lumbar spinal cord A, D, S 🐾
        Unspecified injury to lumbar spinal cord level 1
      - ● S34.102   Unspecified injury to L_2 level of lumbar spinal cord A, D, S 🐾
        Unspecified injury to lumbar spinal cord level 2
      - ● S34.103   Unspecified injury to L_3 level of lumbar spinal cord A, D, S 🐾
        Unspecified injury to lumbar spinal cord level 3
      - ● S34.104   Unspecified injury to L_4 level of lumbar spinal cord A, D, S 🐾
        Unspecified injury to lumbar spinal cord level 4
      - ● S34.105   Unspecified injury to L_5 level of lumbar spinal cord A, D, S 🐾
        Unspecified injury to lumbar spinal cord level 5
      - ● S34.109   Unspecified injury to unspecified level of lumbar spinal cord A, D, S 🐾
    - ● S34.11   Complete lesion of lumbar spinal cord
      - ● S34.111   Complete lesion of L_1 level of lumbar spinal cord A, D, S 🐾
        Complete lesion of lumbar spinal cord level 1
      - ● S34.112   Complete lesion of L_2 level of lumbar spinal cord A, D, S 🐾

Complete lesion of lumbar spinal cord level 2
- ● S34.113   Complete lesion of L_3 level of lumbar spinal cord A, D, S 🐾
  Complete lesion of lumbar spinal cord level 3
- ● S34.114   Complete lesion of L_4 level of lumbar spinal cord A, D, S 🐾
  Complete lesion of lumbar spinal cord level 4
- ● S34.115   Complete lesion of L_5 level of lumbar spinal cord A, D, S 🐾
  Complete lesion of lumbar spinal cord level 5
- ● S34.119   Complete lesion of unspecified level of lumbar spinal cord A, D, S 🐾
- ● S34.12   Incomplete lesion of lumbar spinal cord
  - ● S34.121   Incomplete lesion of L_1 level of lumbar spinal cord A, D, S 🐾
    Incomplete lesion of lumbar spinal cord level 1
  - ● S34.122   Incomplete lesion of L_2 level of lumbar spinal cord A, D, S 🐾
    Incomplete lesion of lumbar spinal cord level 2
  - ● S34.123   Incomplete lesion of L_3 level of lumbar spinal cord A, D, S 🐾
    Incomplete lesion of lumbar spinal cord level 3
  - ● S34.124   Incomplete lesion of L_4 level of lumbar spinal cord A, D, S 🐾
    Incomplete lesion of lumbar spinal cord level 4
  - ● S34.125   Incomplete lesion of L_5 level of lumbar spinal cord A, D, S 🐾
    Incomplete lesion of lumbar spinal cord level 5
  - ● S34.129   Incomplete lesion of unspecified level of lumbar spinal cord A, D, S 🐾
- ● S34.13   Other and unspecified injury to sacral spinal cord
  Other injury to conus medullaris
  - ● S34.131   Complete lesion of sacral spinal cord A, D, S 🐾
    Complete lesion of conus medullaris
  - ● S34.132   Incomplete lesion of sacral spinal cord A, D, S 🐾
    Incomplete lesion of conus medullaris
  - ● S34.139   Unspecified injury to sacral spinal cord A, D, S 🐾
    Unspecified injury of conus medullaris
- ● S34.2   Injury of nerve root of lumbar and sacral spine
  - X ● S34.21   Injury of nerve root of lumbar spine
  - X ● S34.22   Injury of nerve root of sacral spine
- X ● S34.3   Injury of cauda equina A, D, S 🐾
- X ● S34.4   Injury of lumbosacral plexus
- X ● S34.5   Injury of lumbar, sacral and pelvic sympathetic nerves
  Injury of celiac ganglion or plexus
  Injury of hypogastric plexus
  Injury of mesenteric plexus (inferior) (superior)
  Injury of splanchnic nerve
- X ● S34.6   Injury of peripheral nerve(s) at abdomen, lower back and pelvis level
- X ● S34.8   Injury of other nerves at abdomen, lower back and pelvis level
- X ● S34.9   Injury of unspecified nerves at abdomen, lower back and pelvis level

▶ New   ⇒ Revised   ~~deleted~~ Deleted   Excludes 1   Excludes 2   Includes   Use additional   Code first   Code also   Key words

OGCR Official Guidelines   X Assign placeholder X   ● Use Additional Character(s)   ▶ Manifestation Code   🐾 Hierarchical Condition Category   **Coding Clinic**

CHAPTER 19 (S00-T88)

● S35   **Injury of blood vessels at abdomen, lower back and pelvis level**
The appropriate 7th character is to be added to each code from category S35

A	initial encounter
D	subsequent encounter
S	sequela

Code also any associated open wound (S31.-)

● **S35.0   Injury of abdominal aorta**
    Excludes1   injury of aorta NOS (S25.0)

X● **S35.00   Unspecified injury of abdominal aorta**

X● **S35.01   Minor laceration of abdominal aorta**
    Incomplete transection of abdominal aorta
    Laceration of abdominal aorta NOS
    Superficial laceration of abdominal aorta

X● **S35.02   Major laceration of abdominal aorta**
    Complete transection of abdominal aorta
    Traumatic rupture of abdominal aorta

X● **S35.09   Other injury of abdominal aorta**

● **S35.1   Injury of inferior vena cava**
    Injury of hepatic vein
    Excludes1   injury of vena cava NOS (S25.2)

X● **S35.10   Unspecified injury of inferior vena cava**

X● **S35.11   Minor laceration of inferior vena cava**
    Incomplete transection of inferior vena cava
    Laceration of inferior vena cava NOS
    Superficial laceration of inferior vena cava

X● **S35.12   Major laceration of inferior vena cava**
    Complete transection of inferior vena cava
    Traumatic rupture of inferior vena cava

X● **S35.19   Other injury of inferior vena cava**

● **S35.2   Injury of celiac or mesenteric artery and branches**

  ● **S35.21   Injury of celiac artery**

    ● **S35.211   Minor laceration of celiac artery**
      Incomplete transection of celiac artery
      Laceration of celiac artery NOS
      Superficial laceration of celiac artery

    ● **S35.212   Major laceration of celiac artery**
      Complete transection of celiac artery
      Traumatic rupture of celiac artery

    ● **S35.218   Other injury of celiac artery**

    ● **S35.219   Unspecified injury of celiac artery**

  ● **S35.22   Injury of superior mesenteric artery**

    ● **S35.221   Minor laceration of superior mesenteric artery**
      Incomplete transection of superior mesenteric artery
      Laceration of superior mesenteric artery NOS
      Superficial laceration of superior mesenteric artery

    ● **S35.222   Major laceration of superior mesenteric artery**
      Complete transection of superior mesenteric artery
      Traumatic rupture of superior mesenteric artery

    ● **S35.228   Other injury of superior mesenteric artery**

    ● **S35.229   Unspecified injury of superior mesenteric artery**

● **S35.23   Injury of inferior mesenteric artery**

  ● **S35.231   Minor laceration of inferior mesenteric artery**
    Incomplete transection of inferior mesenteric artery
    Laceration of inferior mesenteric artery NOS
    Superficial laceration of inferior mesenteric artery

  ● **S35.232   Major laceration of inferior mesenteric artery**
    Complete transection of inferior mesenteric artery
    Traumatic rupture of inferior mesenteric artery

  ● **S35.238   Other injury of inferior mesenteric artery**

  ● **S35.239   Unspecified injury of inferior mesenteric artery**

● **S35.29   Injury of branches of celiac and mesenteric artery**
    Injury of gastric artery
    Injury of gastroduodenal artery
    Injury of hepatic artery
    Injury of splenic artery

  ● **S35.291   Minor laceration of branches of celiac and mesenteric artery**
    Incomplete transection of branches of celiac and mesenteric artery
    Laceration of branches of celiac and mesenteric artery NOS
    Superficial laceration of branches of celiac and mesenteric artery

  ● **S35.292   Major laceration of branches of celiac and mesenteric artery**
    Complete transection of branches of celiac and mesenteric artery
    Traumatic rupture of branches of celiac and mesenteric artery

  ● **S35.298   Other injury of branches of celiac and mesenteric artery**

  ● **S35.299   Unspecified injury of branches of celiac and mesenteric artery**

● **S35.3   Injury of portal or splenic vein and branches**

  ● **S35.31   Injury of portal vein**

    ● **S35.311   Laceration of portal vein**

    ● **S35.318   Other specified injury of portal vein**

    ● **S35.319   Unspecified injury of portal vein**

  ● **S35.32   Injury of splenic vein**

    ● **S35.321   Laceration of splenic vein**

    ● **S35.328   Other specified injury of splenic vein**

    ● **S35.329   Unspecified injury of splenic vein**

  ● **S35.33   Injury of superior mesenteric vein**

    ● **S35.331   Laceration of superior mesenteric vein**

    ● **S35.338   Other specified injury of superior mesenteric vein**

    ● **S35.339   Unspecified injury of superior mesenteric vein**

  ● **S35.34   Injury of inferior mesenteric vein**

    ● **S35.341   Laceration of inferior mesenteric vein**

    ● **S35.348   Other specified injury of inferior mesenteric vein**

    ● **S35.349   Unspecified injury of inferior mesenteric vein**

CHAPTER 19 (S00-T88)

● S35.4   Injury of renal blood vessels
  ● S35.40   Unspecified injury of renal blood vessel
    ● S35.401   Unspecified injury of right renal artery
    ● S35.402   Unspecified injury of left renal artery
    ● S35.403   Unspecified injury of unspecified renal artery
    ● S35.404   Unspecified injury of right renal vein
    ● S35.405   Unspecified injury of left renal vein
    ● S35.406   Unspecified injury of unspecified renal vein
  ● S35.41   Laceration of renal blood vessel
    ● S35.411   Laceration of right renal artery
    ● S35.412   Laceration of left renal artery
    ● S35.413   Laceration of unspecified renal artery
    ● S35.414   Laceration of right renal vein
    ● S35.415   Laceration of left renal vein
    ● S35.416   Laceration of unspecified renal vein
  ● S35.49   Other specified injury of renal blood vessel
    ● S35.491   Other specified injury of right renal artery
    ● S35.492   Other specified injury of left renal artery
    ● S35.493   Other specified injury of unspecified renal artery
    ● S35.494   Other specified injury of right renal vein
    ● S35.495   Other specified injury of left renal vein
    ● S35.496   Other specified injury of unspecified renal vein
● S35.5   Injury of iliac blood vessels
  X ● S35.50   Injury of unspecified iliac blood vessel(s)
  ● S35.51   Injury of iliac artery or vein
    Injury of hypogastric artery or vein
    ● S35.511   Injury of right iliac artery
    ● S35.512   Injury of left iliac artery
    ● S35.513   Injury of unspecified iliac artery
    ● S35.514   Injury of right iliac vein
    ● S35.515   Injury of left iliac vein
    ● S35.516   Injury of unspecified iliac vein
  ● S35.53   Injury of uterine artery or vein
    ● S35.531   Injury of right uterine artery ♀
    ● S35.532   Injury of left uterine artery ♀
    ● S35.533   Injury of unspecified uterine artery ♀
    ● S35.534   Injury of right uterine vein ♀
    ● S35.535   Injury of left uterine vein ♀
    ● S35.536   Injury of unspecified uterine vein ♀
  X ● S35.59   Injury of other iliac blood vessels
● S35.8   Injury of other blood vessels at abdomen, lower back and pelvis level
    Injury of ovarian artery or vein
  ● S35.8X   Injury of other blood vessels at abdomen, lower back and pelvis level
    ● S35.8X1   Laceration of other blood vessels at abdomen, lower back and pelvis level
    ● S35.8X8   Other specified injury of other blood vessels at abdomen, lower back and pelvis level
    ● S35.8X9   Unspecified injury of other blood vessels at abdomen, lower back and pelvis level

● S35.9   Injury of unspecified blood vessel at abdomen, lower back and pelvis level
  X ● S35.90   Unspecified injury of unspecified blood vessel at abdomen, lower back and pelvis level
  X ● S35.91   Laceration of unspecified blood vessel at abdomen, lower back and pelvis level
  X ● S35.99   Other specified injury of unspecified blood vessel at abdomen, lower back and pelvis level
● S36   Injury of intra-abdominal organs
  The appropriate 7th character is to be added to each code from category S36

A	initial encounter
D	subsequent encounter
S	sequela

  Code also any associated open wound (S31.-)
● S36.0   Injury of spleen
  X ● S36.00   Unspecified injury of spleen
  ● S36.02   Contusion of spleen
    ● S36.020   Minor contusion of spleen
      Contusion of spleen less than 2 cm
    ● S36.021   Major contusion of spleen
      Contusion of spleen greater than 2 cm
    ● S36.029   Unspecified contusion of spleen
      Coding Clinic: 2015, Q2, P36, Q1, P11
  ● S36.03   Laceration of spleen
    ● S36.030   Superficial (capsular) laceration of spleen
      Laceration of spleen less than 1 cm
      Minor laceration of spleen
    ● S36.031   Moderate laceration of spleen
      Laceration of spleen 1 to 3 cm
      Coding Clinic: 2015, Q2, P36, Q1, P11
    ● S36.032   Major laceration of spleen
      Avulsion of spleen
      Laceration of spleen greater than 3 cm
      Massive laceration of spleen
      Multiple moderate lacerations of spleen
      Stellate laceration of spleen
    ● S36.039   Unspecified laceration of spleen
  X ● S36.09   Other injury of spleen
● S36.1   Injury of liver and gallbladder and bile duct
  ● S36.11   Injury of liver
    ● S36.112   Contusion of liver
    ● S36.113   Laceration of liver, unspecified degree
    ● S36.114   Minor laceration of liver
      Laceration involving capsule only, or, without significant involvement of hepatic parenchyma [i.e., less than 1 cm deep]
    ● S36.115   Moderate laceration of liver
      Laceration involving parenchyma but without major disruption of parenchyma [i.e., less than 10 cm long and less than 3 cm deep]
    ● S36.116   Major laceration of liver
      Laceration with significant disruption of hepatic parenchyma [i.e., greater than 10 cm long and 3 cm deep]
      Multiple moderate lacerations, with or without hematoma
      Stellate laceration of liver
    ● S36.118   Other injury of liver
    ● S36.119   Unspecified injury of liver
      Coding Clinic: 2015, Q2, P17

▶ New   ⇨ Revised   ~~deleted~~ Deleted   Excludes 1   Excludes 2   Includes   Use additional   Code first   Code also   Key words
OGCR Official Guidelines   X Assign placeholder X   ● Use Additional Character(s)   ▷ Manifestation Code   🐾 Hierarchical Condition Category   Coding Clinic

- ● S36.12   Injury of gallbladder
  - ● S36.122   Contusion of gallbladder
  - ● S36.123   Laceration of gallbladder
  - ● S36.128   Other injury of gallbladder
  - ● S36.129   Unspecified injury of gallbladder
- X ● S36.13   Injury of bile duct
- ● S36.2   Injury of pancreas
  - ● S36.20   Unspecified injury of pancreas
    - ● S36.200   Unspecified injury of head of pancreas
    - ● S36.201   Unspecified injury of body of pancreas
    - ● S36.202   Unspecified injury of tail of pancreas
    - ● S36.209   Unspecified injury of unspecified part of pancreas
  - ● S36.22   Contusion of pancreas
    - ● S36.220   Contusion of head of pancreas
    - ● S36.221   Contusion of body of pancreas
    - ● S36.222   Contusion of tail of pancreas
    - ● S36.229   Contusion of unspecified part of pancreas
  - ● S36.23   Laceration of pancreas, unspecified degree
    - ● S36.230   Laceration of head of pancreas, unspecified degree
    - ● S36.231   Laceration of body of pancreas, unspecified degree
    - ● S36.232   Laceration of tail of pancreas, unspecified degree
    - ● S36.239   Laceration of unspecified part of pancreas, unspecified degree
  - ● S36.24   Minor laceration of pancreas
    - ● S36.240   Minor laceration of head of pancreas
    - ● S36.241   Minor laceration of body of pancreas
    - ● S36.242   Minor laceration of tail of pancreas
    - ● S36.249   Minor laceration of unspecified part of pancreas
  - ● S36.25   Moderate laceration of pancreas
    - ● S36.250   Moderate laceration of head of pancreas
    - ● S36.251   Moderate laceration of body of pancreas
    - ● S36.252   Moderate laceration of tail of pancreas
    - ● S36.259   Moderate laceration of unspecified part of pancreas
  - ● S36.26   Major laceration of pancreas
    - ● S36.260   Major laceration of head of pancreas
    - ● S36.261   Major laceration of body of pancreas
    - ● S36.262   Major laceration of tail of pancreas
    - ● S36.269   Major laceration of unspecified part of pancreas
  - ● S36.29   Other injury of pancreas
    - ● S36.290   Other injury of head of pancreas
    - ● S36.291   Other injury of body of pancreas
    - ● S36.292   Other injury of tail of pancreas
    - ● S36.299   Other injury of unspecified part of pancreas
- ● S36.3   Injury of stomach
  - X ● S36.30   Unspecified injury of stomach
  - X ● S36.32   Contusion of stomach
  - X ● S36.33   Laceration of stomach
  - X ● S36.39   Other injury of stomach

- ● S36.4   Injury of small intestine
  - ● S36.40   Unspecified injury of small intestine
    - ● S36.400   Unspecified injury of duodenum
    - ● S36.408   Unspecified injury of other part of small intestine
    - ● S36.409   Unspecified injury of unspecified part of small intestine
  - ● S36.41   Primary blast injury of small intestine
    Blast injury of small intestine NOS
    - ● S36.410   Primary blast injury of duodenum
    - ● S36.418   Primary blast injury of other part of small intestine
    - ● S36.419   Primary blast injury of unspecified part of small intestine
  - ● S36.42   Contusion of small intestine
    - ● S36.420   Contusion of duodenum
    - ● S36.428   Contusion of other part of small intestine
    - ● S36.429   Contusion of unspecified part of small intestine
  - ● S36.43   Laceration of small intestine
    - ● S36.430   Laceration of duodenum
    - ● S36.438   Laceration of other part of small intestine
    - ● S36.439   Laceration of unspecified part of small intestine
  - ● S36.49   Other injury of small intestine
    - ● S36.490   Other injury of duodenum
    - ● S36.498   Other injury of other part of small intestine
    - ● S36.499   Other injury of unspecified part of small intestine
- ● S36.5   Injury of colon
  - **Excludes2**   injury of rectum (S36.6-)
  - ● S36.50   Unspecified injury of colon
    - ● S36.500   Unspecified injury of ascending [right] colon
    - ● S36.501   Unspecified injury of transverse colon
    - ● S36.502   Unspecified injury of descending [left] colon
    - ● S36.503   Unspecified injury of sigmoid colon
    - ● S36.508   Unspecified injury of other part of colon
    - ● S36.509   Unspecified injury of unspecified part of colon
  - ● S36.51   Primary blast injury of colon
    Blast injury of colon NOS
    - ● S36.510   Primary blast injury of ascending [right] colon
    - ● S36.511   Primary blast injury of transverse colon
    - ● S36.512   Primary blast injury of descending [left] colon
    - ● S36.513   Primary blast injury of sigmoid colon
    - ● S36.518   Primary blast injury of other part of colon
    - ● S36.519   Primary blast injury of unspecified part of colon
  - ● S36.52   Contusion of colon
    - ● S36.520   Contusion of ascending [right] colon
    - ● S36.521   Contusion of transverse colon
    - ● S36.522   Contusion of descending [left] colon
    - ● S36.523   Contusion of sigmoid colon
    - ● S36.528   Contusion of other part of colon
    - ● S36.529   Contusion of unspecified part of colon

CHAPTER 19 (S00-T88)

CHAPTER 19 (S00-T88)

● S36.53   Laceration of colon
  ● S36.530   Laceration of ascending [right] colon
  ● S36.531   Laceration of transverse colon
  ● S36.532   Laceration of descending [left] colon
  ● S36.533   Laceration of sigmoid colon
  ● S36.538   Laceration of other part of colon
    S36.539   Laceration of unspecified part of colon
● S36.59   Other injury of colon
              Secondary blast injury of colon
  ● S36.590   Other injury of ascending [right] colon
  ● S36.591   Other injury of transverse colon
  ● S36.592   Other injury of descending [left] colon
  ● S36.593   Other injury of sigmoid colon
  ● S36.598   Other injury of other part of colon
  ● S36.599   Other injury of unspecified part of colon

● S36.6   Injury of rectum
  X ● S36.60   Unspecified injury of rectum
  X ● S36.61   Primary blast injury of rectum
                  Blast injury of rectum NOS
  X ● S36.62   Contusion of rectum
  X ● S36.63   Laceration of rectum
  X ● S36.69   Other injury of rectum
                  Secondary blast injury of rectum
● S36.8   Injury of other intra-abdominal organs
  X ● S36.81   Injury of peritoneum
    ● S36.89   Injury of other intra-abdominal organs
                  Injury of retroperitoneum
      ● S36.892   Contusion of other intra-abdominal organs
      ● S36.893   Laceration of other intra-abdominal organs
      ● S36.898   Other injury of other intra-abdominal organs
        S36.899   Unspecified injury of other intra-abdominal organs
● S36.9   Injury of unspecified intra-abdominal organ
  X ● S36.90   Unspecified injury of unspecified intra-abdominal organ
  X ● S36.92   Contusion of unspecified intra-abdominal organ
  X ● S36.93   Laceration of unspecified intra-abdominal organ
  X ● S36.99   Other injury of unspecified intra-abdominal organ

● S37   Injury of urinary and pelvic organs
         Code also any associated open wound (S31.-)
         Excludes1   obstetric trauma to pelvic organs (O71.-)
         Excludes2   injury of peritoneum (S36.81)
                      injury of retroperitoneum (S36.89-)
         The appropriate 7th character is to be added to each code from
             category S37

         ┌─────────────────────────────────────┐
         │ A   initial encounter   │
         │ D   subsequent encounter   │
         │ S   sequela   │
         └─────────────────────────────────────┘

● S37.0   Injury of kidney
           Excludes2   acute kidney injury (nontraumatic) (N17.9)
  ● S37.00   Unspecified injury of kidney
    ● S37.001   Unspecified injury of right kidney
    ● S37.002   Unspecified injury of left kidney
    ● S37.009   Unspecified injury of unspecified kidney

● S37.01   Minor contusion of kidney
              Contusion of kidney less than 2 cm
              Contusion of kidney NOS
  ● S37.011   Minor contusion of right kidney
  ● S37.012   Minor contusion of left kidney
  ● S37.019   Minor contusion of unspecified kidney
● S37.02   Major contusion of kidney
              Contusion of kidney greater than 2 cm
  ● S37.021   Major contusion of right kidney
  ● S37.022   Major contusion of left kidney
  ● S37.029   Major contusion of unspecified kidney
● S37.03   Laceration of kidney, unspecified degree
  ● S37.031   Laceration of right kidney, unspecified degree
  ● S37.032   Laceration of left kidney, unspecified degree
  ● S37.039   Laceration of unspecified kidney, unspecified degree
● S37.04   Minor laceration of kidney
              Laceration of kidney less than 1 cm
  ● S37.041   Minor laceration of right kidney
  ● S37.042   Minor laceration of left kidney
  ● S37.049   Minor laceration of unspecified kidney
● S37.05   Moderate laceration of kidney
              Laceration of kidney 1 to 3 cm
  ● S37.051   Moderate laceration of right kidney
  ● S37.052   Moderate laceration of left kidney
  ● S37.059   Moderate laceration of unspecified kidney
● S37.06   Major laceration of kidney
              Avulsion of kidney
              Laceration of kidney greater than 3 cm
              Massive laceration of kidney
              Multiple moderate lacerations of kidney
              Stellate laceration of kidney
  ● S37.061   Major laceration of right kidney
  ● S37.062   Major laceration of left kidney
  ● S37.069   Major laceration of unspecified kidney
● S37.09   Other injury of kidney
  ● S37.091   Other injury of right kidney
  ● S37.092   Other injury of left kidney
  ● S37.099   Other injury of unspecified kidney

● S37.1   Injury of ureter
  X ● S37.10   Unspecified injury of ureter
  X ● S37.12   Contusion of ureter
  X ● S37.13   Laceration of ureter
  X ● S37.19   Other injury of ureter
● S37.2   Injury of bladder
  X ● S37.20   Unspecified injury of bladder
  X ● S37.22   Contusion of bladder
  X ● S37.23   Laceration of bladder
  X ● S37.29   Other injury of bladder
● S37.3   Injury of urethra
  X ● S37.30   Unspecified injury of urethra
  X ● S37.32   Contusion of urethra
  X ● S37.33   Laceration of urethra
  X ● S37.39   Other injury of urethra
● S37.4   Injury of ovary
  ● S37.40   Unspecified injury of ovary
    ● S37.401   Unspecified injury of ovary, unilateral ♀
    ● S37.402   Unspecified injury of ovary, bilateral ♀
    ● S37.409   Unspecified injury of ovary, unspecified ♀

▶ New   ⇒ Revised   deleted Deleted   Excludes 1   Excludes 2   Includes   Use additional   Code first   Code also   Key words
OGCR Official Guidelines   X Assign placeholder X   ● Use Additional Character(s)   ▷ Manifestation Code   🔖 Hierarchical Condition Category   Coding Clinic

- ● S37.42   Contusion of ovary
  - ● S37.421   Contusion of ovary, unilateral ♀
  - ● S37.422   Contusion of ovary, bilateral ♀
  - ● S37.429   Contusion of ovary, unspecified ♀
- ● S37.43   Laceration of ovary
  - ● S37.431   Laceration of ovary, unilateral ♀
  - ● S37.432   Laceration of ovary, bilateral ♀
  - ● S37.439   Laceration of ovary, unspecified ♀
- ● S37.49   Other injury of ovary
  - ● S37.491   Other injury of ovary, unilateral ♀
  - ● S37.492   Other injury of ovary, bilateral ♀
  - ● S37.499   Other injury of ovary, unspecified ♀
- ● S37.5   Injury of fallopian tube
  - ● S37.50   Unspecified injury of fallopian tube
    - ● S37.501   Unspecified injury of fallopian tube, unilateral ♀
    - ● S37.502   Unspecified injury of fallopian tube, bilateral ♀
    - ● S37.509   Unspecified injury of fallopian tube, unspecified ♀
  - ● S37.51   Primary blast injury of fallopian tube
    - Blast injury of fallopian tube NOS
    - ● S37.511   Primary blast injury of fallopian tube, unilateral ♀
    - ● S37.512   Primary blast injury of fallopian tube, bilateral ♀
    - ● S37.519   Primary blast injury of fallopian tube, unspecified ♀
  - ● S37.52   Contusion of fallopian tube
    - ● S37.521   Contusion of fallopian tube, unilateral ♀
    - ● S37.522   Contusion of fallopian tube, bilateral ♀
    - ● S37.529   Contusion of fallopian tube, unspecified ♀
  - ● S37.53   Laceration of fallopian tube
    - ● S37.531   Laceration of fallopian tube, unilateral ♀
    - ● S37.532   Laceration of fallopian tube, bilateral ♀
    - ● S37.539   Laceration of fallopian tube, unspecified ♀
  - ● S37.59   Other injury of fallopian tube
    - Secondary blast injury of fallopian tube
    - ● S37.591   Other injury of fallopian tube, unilateral ♀
    - ● S37.592   Other injury of fallopian tube, bilateral ♀
    - ● S37.599   Other injury of fallopian tube, unspecified ♀
- ● S37.6   Injury of uterus

  Excludes1   injury to gravid uterus (O9A.2-)
               injury to uterus during delivery (O71.-)

  - X ● S37.60   Unspecified injury of uterus ♀
  - X ● S37.62   Contusion of uterus ♀
  - X ● S37.63   Laceration of uterus ♀
  - X ● S37.69   Other injury of uterus ♀
- ● S37.8   Injury of other urinary and pelvic organs
  - ● S37.81   Injury of adrenal gland
    - ● S37.812   Contusion of adrenal gland
    - ● S37.813   Laceration of adrenal gland
    - ● S37.818   Other injury of adrenal gland
    - ● S37.819   Unspecified injury of adrenal gland
  - ● S37.82   Injury of prostate
    - ● S37.822   Contusion of prostate ♂
    - ● S37.823   Laceration of prostate ♂
    - ● S37.828   Other injury of prostate ♂
    - ● S37.829   Unspecified injury of prostate ♂

- ● S37.89   Injury of other urinary and pelvic organ
  - ● S37.892   Contusion of other urinary and pelvic organ
  - ● S37.893   Laceration of other urinary and pelvic organ
  - ● S37.898   Other injury of other urinary and pelvic organ
  - ● S37.899   Unspecified injury of other urinary and pelvic organ
- ● S37.9   Injury of unspecified urinary and pelvic organ
  - X ● S37.90   Unspecified injury of unspecified urinary and pelvic organ
  - X ● S37.92   Contusion of unspecified urinary and pelvic organ
  - X ● S37.93   Laceration of unspecified urinary and pelvic organ
  - X ● S37.99   Other injury of unspecified urinary and pelvic organ
- ● S38   Crushing injury and traumatic amputation of abdomen, lower back, pelvis and external genitals

  An amputation not identified as partial or complete should be coded to complete

  The appropriate 7th character is to be added to each code from category S38

A	initial encounter
D	subsequent encounter
S	sequela

  - ● S38.0   Crushing injury of external genital organs

    Use additional code for any associated injuries

    - ● S38.00   Crushing injury of unspecified external genital organs
      - ● S38.001   Crushing injury of unspecified external genital organs, male ♂
      - ● S38.002   Crushing injury of unspecified external genital organs, female ♀
    - X ● S38.01   Crushing injury of penis ♂
    - X ● S38.02   Crushing injury of scrotum and testis ♂
    - X ● S38.03   Crushing injury of vulva ♀
  - X ● S38.1   Crushing injury of abdomen, lower back, and pelvis

    Use additional code for all associated injuries, such as:
    fracture of thoracic or lumbar spine and pelvis (S22.0-, S32.-)
    injury to intra-abdominal organs (S36.-)
    injury to urinary and pelvic organs (S37.-)
    open wound of abdominal wall (S31.-)
    spinal cord injury (S34.0, S34.1-)

    Excludes2   crushing injury of external genital organs (S38.0-)

  - ● S38.2   Traumatic amputation of external genital organs
    - ● S38.21   Traumatic amputation of female external genital organs

      Traumatic amputation of clitoris
      Traumatic amputation of labium (majus) (minus)
      Traumatic amputation of vulva

      - ● S38.211   Complete traumatic amputation of female external genital organs ♀
      - ● S38.212   Partial traumatic amputation of female external genital organs ♀
    - ● S38.22   Traumatic amputation of penis
      - ● S38.221   Complete traumatic amputation of penis ♂
      - ● S38.222   Partial traumatic amputation of penis ♂
    - ● S38.23   Traumatic amputation of scrotum and testis
      - ● S38.231   Complete traumatic amputation of scrotum and testis ♂
      - ● S38.232   Partial traumatic amputation of scrotum and testis ♂
  - X ● S38.3   Transection (partial) of abdomen

CHAPTER 19 (S00–T88)

● **S39**   **Other and unspecified injuries of abdomen, lower back, pelvis and external genitals**

Code also any associated open wound (S31.-)

Excludes2   sprain of joints and ligaments of lumbar spine and pelvis (S33.-)

The appropriate 7th character is to be added to each code from category S39

A	initial encounter
D	subsequent encounter
S	sequela

● **S39.0**   Injury of muscle, fascia and tendon of abdomen, lower back and pelvis

   ● **S39.00**   Unspecified injury of muscle, fascia and tendon of abdomen, lower back and pelvis

     ● **S39.001**   Unspecified injury of muscle, fascia and tendon of abdomen

     ● **S39.002**   Unspecified injury of muscle, fascia and tendon of lower back

     ● **S39.003**   Unspecified injury of muscle, fascia and tendon of pelvis

   ● **S39.01**   Strain of muscle, fascia and tendon of abdomen, lower back and pelvis

     ● **S39.011**   Strain of muscle, fascia and tendon of abdomen

     ● **S39.012**   Strain of muscle, fascia and tendon of lower back
          Coding Clinic: 2016, Q4, P74

     ● **S39.013**   Strain of muscle, fascia and tendon of pelvis

   ● **S39.02**   Laceration of muscle, fascia and tendon of abdomen, lower back and pelvis

     ● **S39.021**   Laceration of muscle, fascia and tendon of abdomen

     ● **S39.022**   Laceration of muscle, fascia and tendon of lower back

     ● **S39.023**   Laceration of muscle, fascia and tendon of pelvis

   ● **S39.09**   Other injury of muscle, fascia and tendon of abdomen, lower back and pelvis

     ● **S39.091**   Other injury of muscle, fascia and tendon of abdomen

     ● **S39.092**   Other injury of muscle, fascia and tendon of lower back

     ● **S39.093**   Other injury of muscle, fascia and tendon of pelvis

● **S39.8**   Other specified injuries of abdomen, lower back, pelvis and external genitals

   X ● **S39.81**   Other specified injuries of abdomen

   X ● **S39.82**   Other specified injuries of lower back

   X ● **S39.83**   Other specified injuries of pelvis

   ● **S39.84**   Other specified injuries of external genitals

     ● **S39.840**   Fracture of corpus cavernosum penis ♂

     ● **S39.848**   Other specified injuries of external genitals

● **S39.9**   Unspecified injury of abdomen, lower back, pelvis and external genitals

   X ● **S39.91**   Unspecified injury of abdomen

   X ● **S39.92**   Unspecified injury of lower back

   X ● **S39.93**   Unspecified injury of pelvis

   X ● **S39.94**   Unspecified injury of external genitals

INJURIES TO THE SHOULDER AND UPPER ARM (S40-S49)

Includes	injuries of axilla injuries of scapular region
Excludes2	burns and corrosions (T20-T32)
	frostbite (T33-T34)
	injuries of elbow (S50-S59)
	insect bite or sting, venomous (T63.4)

● **S40**   Superficial injury of shoulder and upper arm

The appropriate 7th character is to be added to each code from category S40

A	initial encounter
D	subsequent encounter
S	sequela

● **S40.0**   Contusion of shoulder and upper arm

   ● **S40.01**   Contusion of shoulder

     ● **S40.011**   Contusion of right shoulder

     ● **S40.012**   Contusion of left shoulder

     ● **S40.019**   Contusion of unspecified shoulder

   ● **S40.02**   Contusion of upper arm

     ● **S40.021**   Contusion of right upper arm

     ● **S40.022**   Contusion of left upper arm

     ● **S40.029**   Contusion of unspecified upper arm

● **S40.2**   Other superficial injuries of shoulder

   ● **S40.21**   Abrasion of shoulder

     ● **S40.211**   Abrasion of right shoulder

     ● **S40.212**   Abrasion of left shoulder

     ● **S40.219**   Abrasion of unspecified shoulder

   ● **S40.22**   Blister (nonthermal) of shoulder

     ● **S40.221**   Blister (nonthermal) of right shoulder

     ● **S40.222**   Blister (nonthermal) of left shoulder

     ● **S40.229**   Blister (nonthermal) of unspecified shoulder

   ● **S40.24**   External constriction of shoulder

     ● **S40.241**   External constriction of right shoulder

     ● **S40.242**   External constriction of left shoulder

     ● **S40.249**   External constriction of unspecified shoulder

   ● **S40.25**   Superficial foreign body of shoulder
       Splinter in the shoulder

     ● **S40.251**   Superficial foreign body of right shoulder

     ● **S40.252**   Superficial foreign body of left shoulder

     ● **S40.259**   Superficial foreign body of unspecified shoulder

   ● **S40.26**   Insect bite (nonvenomous) of shoulder

     ● **S40.261**   Insect bite (nonvenomous) of right shoulder

     ● **S40.262**   Insect bite (nonvenomous) of left shoulder

     ● **S40.269**   Insect bite (nonvenomous) of unspecified shoulder

   ● **S40.27**   Other superficial bite of shoulder
       Excludes1   open bite of shoulder (S41.05)

     ● **S40.271**   Other superficial bite of right shoulder

     ● **S40.272**   Other superficial bite of left shoulder

     ● **S40.279**   Other superficial bite of unspecified shoulder

● S40.8 Other superficial injuries of upper arm
  ● S40.81   Abrasion of upper arm
    ● S40.811   Abrasion of right upper arm
    ● S40.812   Abrasion of left upper arm
    ● S40.819   Abrasion of unspecified upper arm
  ● S40.82   Blister (nonthermal) of upper arm
    ● S40.821   Blister (nonthermal) of right upper arm
    ● S40.822   Blister (nonthermal) of left upper arm
    ● S40.829   Blister (nonthermal) of unspecified upper arm
  ● S40.84   External constriction of upper arm
    ● S40.841   External constriction of right upper arm
    ● S40.842   External constriction of left upper arm
    ● S40.849   External constriction of unspecified upper arm
  ● S40.85   Superficial foreign body of upper arm
            Splinter in the upper arm
    ● S40.851   Superficial foreign body of right upper arm
    ● S40.852   Superficial foreign body of left upper arm
    ● S40.859   Superficial foreign body of unspecified upper arm
  ● S40.86   Insect bite (nonvenomous) of upper arm
    ● S40.861   Insect bite (nonvenomous) of right upper arm
    ● S40.862   Insect bite (nonvenomous) of left upper arm
    ● S40.869   Insect bite (nonvenomous) of unspecified upper arm
  ● S40.87   Other superficial bite of upper arm
            Excludes1   open bite of upper arm (S41.14)
            Excludes2   other superficial bite of shoulder (S40.27-)
    ● S40.871   Other superficial bite of right upper arm
    ● S40.872   Other superficial bite of left upper arm
    ● S40.879   Other superficial bite of unspecified upper arm
● S40.9 Unspecified superficial injury of shoulder and upper arm
  ● S40.91   Unspecified superficial injury of shoulder
    ● S40.911   Unspecified superficial injury of right shoulder
    ● S40.912   Unspecified superficial injury of left shoulder
    ● S40.919   Unspecified superficial injury of unspecified shoulder
  ● S40.92   Unspecified superficial injury of upper arm
    ● S40.921   Unspecified superficial injury of right upper arm
    ● S40.922   Unspecified superficial injury of left upper arm
    ● S40.929   Unspecified superficial injury of unspecified upper arm

● S41 Open wound of shoulder and upper arm
       Code also any associated wound infection
       Excludes1   traumatic amputation of shoulder and upper arm (S48.-)
       Excludes2   open fracture of shoulder and upper arm (S42.- with 7th character B or C)
       The appropriate 7th character is to be added to each code from category S41

       | A | initial encounter |
       | D | subsequent encounter |
       | S | sequela |

  ● S41.0 Open wound of shoulder
    ● S41.00   Unspecified open wound of shoulder
      ● S41.001   Unspecified open wound of right shoulder
      ● S41.002   Unspecified open wound of left shoulder
      ● S41.009   Unspecified open wound of unspecified shoulder
    ● S41.01   Laceration without foreign body of shoulder
      ● S41.011   Laceration without foreign body of right shoulder
      ● S41.012   Laceration without foreign body of left shoulder
      ● S41.019   Laceration without foreign body of unspecified shoulder
    ● S41.02   Laceration with foreign body of shoulder
      ● S41.021   Laceration with foreign body of right shoulder
      ● S41.022   Laceration with foreign body of left shoulder
      ● S41.029   Laceration with foreign body of unspecified shoulder
    ● S41.03   Puncture wound without foreign body of shoulder
      ● S41.031   Puncture wound without foreign body of right shoulder
      ● S41.032   Puncture wound without foreign body of left shoulder
      ● S41.039   Puncture wound without foreign body of unspecified shoulder
    ● S41.04   Puncture wound with foreign body of shoulder
      ● S41.041   Puncture wound with foreign body of right shoulder
      ● S41.042   Puncture wound with foreign body of left shoulder
      ● S41.049   Puncture wound with foreign body of unspecified shoulder
    ● S41.05   Open bite of shoulder
              Bite of shoulder NOS
              Excludes1   superficial bite of shoulder (S40.27)
      ● S41.051   Open bite of right shoulder
      ● S41.052   Open bite of left shoulder
      ● S41.059   Open bite of unspecified shoulder
  ● S41.1 Open wound of upper arm
    ● S41.10   Unspecified open wound of upper arm
      ● S41.101   Unspecified open wound of right upper arm
      ● S41.102   Unspecified open wound of left upper arm
      ● S41.109   Unspecified open wound of unspecified upper arm

CHAPTER 19 (S00-T88)

- **S41.11** Laceration without foreign body of upper arm
  - **S41.111** Laceration without foreign body of right upper arm
  - **S41.112** Laceration without foreign body of left upper arm
  - **S41.119** Laceration without foreign body of unspecified upper arm
- **S41.12** Laceration with foreign body of upper arm
  - **S41.121** Laceration with foreign body of right upper arm
  - **S41.122** Laceration with foreign body of left upper arm
  - **S41.129** Laceration with foreign body of unspecified upper arm
- **S41.13** Puncture wound without foreign body of upper arm
  - **S41.131** Puncture wound without foreign body of right upper arm
  - **S41.132** Puncture wound without foreign body of left upper arm
  - **S41.139** Puncture wound without foreign body of unspecified upper arm
- **S41.14** Puncture wound with foreign body of upper arm
  - **S41.141** Puncture wound with foreign body of right upper arm
  - **S41.142** Puncture wound with foreign body of left upper arm
  - **S41.149** Puncture wound with foreign body of unspecified upper arm
- **S41.15** Open bite of upper arm
  Bite of upper arm NOS
  - **Excludes1** superficial bite of upper arm (S40.87)
  - **S41.151** Open bite of right upper arm
  - **S41.152** Open bite of left upper arm
  - **S41.159** Open bite of unspecified upper arm

- **S42 Fracture of shoulder and upper arm**
  Note: A fracture not indicated as displaced or nondisplaced should be coded to displaced
  A fracture not indicated as open or closed should be coded to closed
  - **Excludes1** traumatic amputation of shoulder and upper arm (S48.-)

  The appropriate 7th character is to be added to all codes from category S42

A	initial encounter for closed fracture
B	initial encounter for open fracture
D	subsequent encounter for fracture with routine healing
G	subsequent encounter for fracture with delayed healing
K	subsequent encounter for fracture with nonunion
P	subsequent encounter for fracture with malunion
S	sequela

- **S42.0** Fracture of clavicle
  - **S42.00** Fracture of unspecified part of clavicle
    - **S42.001** Fracture of unspecified part of right clavicle
    - **S42.002** Fracture of unspecified part of left clavicle
    - **S42.009** Fracture of unspecified part of unspecified clavicle
      Coding Clinic: 2012, Q4, P3

- **S42.01** Fracture of sternal end of clavicle
  - **S42.011** Anterior displaced fracture of sternal end of right clavicle
  - **S42.012** Anterior displaced fracture of sternal end of left clavicle
  - **S42.013** Anterior displaced fracture of sternal end of unspecified clavicle
    Displaced fracture of sternal end of clavicle NOS
  - **S42.014** Posterior displaced fracture of sternal end of right clavicle
  - **S42.015** Posterior displaced fracture of sternal end of left clavicle
  - **S42.016** Posterior displaced fracture of sternal end of unspecified clavicle
  - **S42.017** Nondisplaced fracture of sternal end of right clavicle
  - **S42.018** Nondisplaced fracture of sternal end of left clavicle
  - **S42.019** Nondisplaced fracture of sternal end of unspecified clavicle
- **S42.02** Fracture of shaft of clavicle
  - **S42.021** Displaced fracture of shaft of right clavicle
  - **S42.022** Displaced fracture of shaft of left clavicle
  - **S42.023** Displaced fracture of shaft of unspecified clavicle
  - **S42.024** Nondisplaced fracture of shaft of right clavicle
  - **S42.025** Nondisplaced fracture of shaft of left clavicle
  - **S42.026** Nondisplaced fracture of shaft of unspecified clavicle
- **S42.03** Fracture of lateral end of clavicle
  Fracture of acromial end of clavicle
  - **S42.031** Displaced fracture of lateral end of right clavicle
  - **S42.032** Displaced fracture of lateral end of left clavicle
  - **S42.033** Displaced fracture of lateral end of unspecified clavicle
  - **S42.034** Nondisplaced fracture of lateral end of right clavicle
  - **S42.035** Nondisplaced fracture of lateral end of left clavicle
  - **S42.036** Nondisplaced fracture of lateral end of unspecified clavicle
- **S42.1** Fracture of scapula
  - **S42.10** Fracture of unspecified part of scapula
    - **S42.101** Fracture of unspecified part of scapula, right shoulder
    - **S42.102** Fracture of unspecified part of scapula, left shoulder
    - **S42.109** Fracture of unspecified part of scapula, unspecified shoulder
  - **S42.11** Fracture of body of scapula
    - **S42.111** Displaced fracture of body of scapula, right shoulder
    - **S42.112** Displaced fracture of body of scapula, left shoulder
    - **S42.113** Displaced fracture of body of scapula, unspecified shoulder
    - **S42.114** Nondisplaced fracture of body of scapula, right shoulder
    - **S42.115** Nondisplaced fracture of body of scapula, left shoulder
    - **S42.116** Nondisplaced fracture of body of scapula, unspecified shoulder

- S42.12   Fracture of acromial process
  - S42.121   Displaced fracture of acromial process, right shoulder
  - S42.122   Displaced fracture of acromial process, left shoulder
  - S42.123   Displaced fracture of acromial process, unspecified shoulder
  - S42.124   Nondisplaced fracture of acromial process, right shoulder
  - S42.125   Nondisplaced fracture of acromial process, left shoulder
  - S42.126   Nondisplaced fracture, of acromial process, unspecified shoulder
- S42.13   Fracture of coracoid process
  - S42.131   Displaced fracture of coracoid process, right shoulder
  - S42.132   Displaced fracture of coracoid process, left shoulder
  - S42.133   Displaced fracture of coracoid process, unspecified shoulder
  - S42.134   Nondisplaced fracture of coracoid process, right shoulder
  - S42.135   Nondisplaced fracture of coracoid process, left shoulder
  - S42.136   Nondisplaced fracture of coracoid process, unspecified shoulder
- S42.14   Fracture of glenoid cavity of scapula
  - S42.141   Displaced fracture of glenoid cavity of scapula, right shoulder
  - S42.142   Displaced fracture of glenoid cavity of scapula, left shoulder
  - S42.143   Displaced fracture of glenoid cavity of scapula, unspecified shoulder
  - S42.144   Nondisplaced fracture of glenoid cavity of scapula, right shoulder
  - S42.145   Nondisplaced fracture of glenoid cavity of scapula, left shoulder
  - S42.146   Nondisplaced fracture of glenoid cavity of scapula, unspecified shoulder
- S42.15   Fracture of neck of scapula
  - S42.151   Displaced fracture of neck of scapula, right shoulder
  - S42.152   Displaced fracture of neck of scapula, left shoulder
  - S42.153   Displaced fracture of neck of scapula, unspecified shoulder
  - S42.154   Nondisplaced fracture of neck of scapula, right shoulder
  - S42.155   Nondisplaced fracture of neck of scapula, left shoulder
  - S42.156   Nondisplaced fracture of neck of scapula, unspecified shoulder
- S42.19   Fracture of other part of scapula
  - S42.191   Fracture of other part of scapula, right shoulder
  - S42.192   Fracture of other part of scapula, left shoulder
  - S42.199   Fracture of other part of scapula, unspecified shoulder
- S42.2   Fracture of upper end of humerus
  Fracture of proximal end of humerus
  - **Excludes2**   fracture of shaft of humerus (S42.3-)
    physeal fracture of upper end of humerus (S49.0-)
- S42.20   Unspecified fracture of upper end of humerus
  - S42.201   Unspecified fracture of upper end of right humerus
  - S42.202   Unspecified fracture of upper end of left humerus
  - S42.209   Unspecified fracture of upper end of unspecified humerus

- S42.21   Unspecified fracture of surgical neck of humerus
  Fracture of neck of humerus NOS
  - S42.211   Unspecified displaced fracture of surgical neck of right humerus
  - S42.212   Unspecified displaced fracture of surgical neck of left humerus
  - S42.213   Unspecified displaced fracture of surgical neck of unspecified humerus
  - S42.214   Unspecified nondisplaced fracture of surgical neck of right humerus
  - S42.215   Unspecified nondisplaced fracture of surgical neck of left humerus
  - S42.216   Unspecified nondisplaced fracture of surgical neck of unspecified humerus
- S42.22   2-part fracture of surgical neck of humerus
  - S42.221   2-part displaced fracture of surgical neck of right humerus
  - S42.222   2-part displaced fracture of surgical neck of left humerus
  - S42.223   2-part displaced fracture of surgical neck of unspecified humerus
  - S42.224   2-part nondisplaced fracture of surgical neck of right humerus
  - S42.225   2-part nondisplaced fracture of surgical neck of left humerus
  - S42.226   2-part nondisplaced fracture of surgical neck of unspecified humerus
- S42.23   3-part fracture of surgical neck of humerus
  - S42.231   3-part fracture of surgical neck of right humerus
  - S42.232   3-part fracture of surgical neck of left humerus
  - S42.239   3-part fracture of surgical neck of unspecified humerus
- S42.24   4-part fracture of surgical neck of humerus
  - S42.241   4-part fracture of surgical neck of right humerus
  - S42.242   4-part fracture of surgical neck of left humerus
  - S42.249   4-part fracture of surgical neck of unspecified humerus
- S42.25   Fracture of greater tuberosity of humerus
  - S42.251   Displaced fracture of greater tuberosity of right humerus
  - S42.252   Displaced fracture of greater tuberosity of left humerus
  - S42.253   Displaced fracture of greater tuberosity of unspecified humerus
  - S42.254   Nondisplaced fracture of greater tuberosity of right humerus
  - S42.255   Nondisplaced fracture of greater tuberosity of left humerus
  - S42.256   Nondisplaced fracture of greater tuberosity of unspecified humerus
- S42.26   Fracture of lesser tuberosity of humerus
  - S42.261   Displaced fracture of lesser tuberosity of right humerus
  - S42.262   Displaced fracture of lesser tuberosity of left humerus
  - S42.263   Displaced fracture of lesser tuberosity of unspecified humerus
  - S42.264   Nondisplaced fracture of lesser tuberosity of right humerus
  - S42.265   Nondisplaced fracture of lesser tuberosity of left humerus
  - S42.266   Nondisplaced fracture of lesser tuberosity of unspecified humerus

● **S42.27**   **Torus** fracture of upper end of humerus

The appropriate 7th character is to be added to all codes in subcategory S42.27

A	initial encounter for closed fracture
D	subsequent encounter for fracture with routine healing
G	subsequent encounter for fracture with delayed healing
K	subsequent encounter for fracture with nonunion
P	subsequent encounter for fracture with malunion
S	sequela

  ● **S42.271**   Torus fracture of upper end of **right** humerus

  ● **S42.272**   Torus fracture of upper end of **left** humerus

  ● **S42.279**   Torus fracture of upper end of **unspecified** humerus

● **S42.29**   Other fracture of upper end of humerus

    Fracture of anatomical neck of humerus
    Fracture of articular head of humerus

  ● **S42.291**   Other **displaced** fracture of upper end of **right** humerus

  ● **S42.292**   Other **displaced** fracture of upper end of **left** humerus

  ● **S42.293**   Other **displaced** fracture of upper end of **unspecified** humerus

  ● **S42.294**   Other **nondisplaced** fracture of upper end of right humerus

  ● **S42.295**   Other **nondisplaced** fracture of upper end of left humerus
         Coding Clinic: 2019, Q1, P19

  ● **S42.296**   Other **nondisplaced** fracture of upper end of **unspecified** humerus

● **S42.3**   Fracture of **shaft** of humerus

    Fracture of humerus NOS
    Fracture of upper arm NOS

    Excludes2   physeal fractures of upper end of humerus (S49.0-)
                physeal fractures of lower end of humerus (S49.1-)

  ● **S42.30**   Unspecified fracture of shaft of humerus

    ● **S42.301**   Unspecified fracture of shaft of humerus, **right** arm

    ● **S42.302**   Unspecified fracture of shaft of humerus, **left** arm

    ● **S42.309**   Unspecified fracture of shaft of humerus, **unspecified** arm

  ● **S42.31**   **Greenstick** fracture of shaft of humerus

The appropriate 7th character is to be added to all codes in subcategory S42.31

A	initial encounter for closed fracture
D	subsequent encounter for fracture with routine healing
G	subsequent encounter for fracture with delayed healing
K	subsequent encounter for fracture with nonunion
P	subsequent encounter for fracture with malunion
S	sequela

    ● **S42.311**   Greenstick fracture of shaft of humerus, **right** arm

    ● **S42.312**   Greenstick fracture of shaft of humerus, **left** arm

    ● **S42.319**   Greenstick fracture of shaft of humerus, **unspecified** arm

  ● **S42.32**   **Transverse** fracture of shaft of humerus

    ● **S42.321**   **Displaced** transverse fracture of shaft of humerus, **right** arm

    ● **S42.322**   **Displaced** transverse fracture of shaft of humerus, **left** arm

    ● **S42.323**   **Displaced** transverse fracture of shaft of humerus, **unspecified** arm

    ● **S42.324**   **Nondisplaced** transverse fracture of shaft of humerus, **right** arm

    ● **S42.325**   **Nondisplaced** transverse fracture of shaft of humerus, **left** arm

    ● **S42.326**   **Nondisplaced** transverse fracture of shaft of humerus, **unspecified** arm

  ● **S42.33**   **Oblique** fracture of shaft of humerus

    ● **S42.331**   **Displaced** oblique fracture of shaft of humerus, **right** arm

    ● **S42.332**   **Displaced** oblique fracture of shaft of humerus, **left** arm

    ● **S42.333**   **Displaced** oblique fracture of shaft of humerus, **unspecified** arm

    ● **S42.334**   **Nondisplaced** oblique fracture of shaft of humerus, **right** arm

    ● **S42.335**   **Nondisplaced** oblique fracture of shaft of humerus, **left** arm

    ● **S42.336**   **Nondisplaced** oblique fracture of shaft of humerus, **unspecified** arm

  ● **S42.34**   **Spiral** fracture of shaft of humerus

    ● **S42.341**   **Displaced** spiral fracture of shaft of humerus, **right** arm

    ● **S42.342**   **Displaced** spiral fracture of shaft of humerus, **left** arm

    ● **S42.343**   **Displaced** spiral fracture of shaft of humerus, **unspecified** arm

    ● **S42.344**   **Nondisplaced** spiral fracture of shaft of humerus, **right** arm

    ● **S42.345**   **Nondisplaced** spiral fracture of shaft of humerus, **left** arm

    ● **S42.346**   **Nondisplaced** spiral fracture of shaft of humerus, **unspecified** arm

  ● **S42.35**   **Comminuted** fracture of shaft of humerus

    ● **S42.351**   **Displaced** comminuted fracture of shaft of humerus, **right** arm

    ● **S42.352**   **Displaced** comminuted fracture of shaft of humerus, **left** arm

    ● **S42.353**   **Displaced** comminuted fracture of shaft of humerus, **unspecified** arm

    ● **S42.354**   **Nondisplaced** comminuted fracture of shaft of humerus, **right** arm

    ● **S42.355**   **Nondisplaced** comminuted fracture of shaft of humerus, **left** arm

    ● **S42.356**   **Nondisplaced** comminuted fracture of shaft of humerus, **unspecified** arm

  ● **S42.36**   **Segmental** fracture of shaft of humerus

    ● **S42.361**   **Displaced** segmental fracture of shaft of humerus, **right** arm

    ● **S42.362**   **Displaced** segmental fracture of shaft of humerus, **left** arm

    ● **S42.363**   **Displaced** segmental fracture of shaft of humerus, **unspecified** arm

    ● **S42.364**   **Nondisplaced** segmental fracture of shaft of humerus, **right** arm

    ● **S42.365**   **Nondisplaced** segmental fracture of shaft of humerus, **left** arm

    ● **S42.366**   **Nondisplaced** segmental fracture of shaft of humerus, **unspecified** arm

- S42.39   Other fracture of shaft of humerus
  - S42.391   Other fracture of shaft of right humerus
  - S42.392   Other fracture of shaft of left humerus
  - S42.399   Other fracture of shaft of unspecified humerus
- S42.4   Fracture of lower end of humerus
  Fracture of distal end of humerus
  - **Excludes2**   fracture of shaft of humerus (S42.3-)
  physeal fracture of lower end of humerus (S49.1-)
- S42.40   Unspecified fracture of lower end of humerus
  Fracture of elbow NOS
  - S42.401   Unspecified fracture of lower end of right humerus
  - S42.402   Unspecified fracture of lower end of left humerus
  - S42.409   Unspecified fracture of lower end of unspecified humerus
- S42.41   Simple supracondylar fracture without intercondylar fracture of humerus
  - S42.411   Displaced simple supracondylar fracture without intercondylar fracture of right humerus
  - S42.412   Displaced simple supracondylar fracture without intercondylar fracture of left humerus
  - S42.413   Displaced simple supracondylar fracture without intercondylar fracture of unspecified humerus
  - S42.414   Nondisplaced simple supracondylar fracture without intercondylar fracture of right humerus
  - S42.415   Nondisplaced simple supracondylar fracture without intercondylar fracture of left humerus
  - S42.416   Nondisplaced simple supracondylar fracture without intercondylar fracture of unspecified humerus
- S42.42   Comminuted supracondylar fracture without intercondylar fracture of humerus
  - S42.421   Displaced comminuted supracondylar fracture without intercondylar fracture of right humerus
  - S42.422   Displaced comminuted supracondylar fracture without intercondylar fracture of left humerus
  - S42.423   Displaced comminuted supracondylar fracture without intercondylar fracture of unspecified humerus
  - S42.424   Nondisplaced comminuted supracondylar fracture without intercondylar fracture of right humerus
  - S42.425   Nondisplaced comminuted supracondylar fracture without intercondylar fracture of left humerus
  - S42.426   Nondisplaced comminuted supracondylar fracture without intercondylar fracture of unspecified humerus

- S42.43   Fracture (avulsion) of lateral epicondyle of humerus
  - S42.431   Displaced fracture (avulsion) of lateral epicondyle of right humerus
  - S42.432   Displaced fracture (avulsion) of lateral epicondyle of left humerus
  - S42.433   Displaced fracture (avulsion) of lateral epicondyle of unspecified humerus
  - S42.434   Nondisplaced fracture (avulsion) of lateral epicondyle of right humerus
  - S42.435   Nondisplaced fracture (avulsion) of lateral epicondyle of left humerus
  - S42.436   Nondisplaced fracture (avulsion) of lateral epicondyle of unspecified humerus
- S42.44   Fracture (avulsion) of medial epicondyle of humerus
  - S42.441   Displaced fracture (avulsion) of medial epicondyle of right humerus
  - S42.442   Displaced fracture (avulsion) of medial epicondyle of left humerus
  - S42.443   Displaced fracture (avulsion) of medial epicondyle of unspecified humerus
  - S42.444   Nondisplaced fracture (avulsion) of medial epicondyle of right humerus
  - S42.445   Nondisplaced fracture (avulsion) of medial epicondyle of left humerus
  - S42.446   Nondisplaced fracture (avulsion) of medial epicondyle of unspecified humerus
  - S42.447   Incarcerated fracture (avulsion) of medial epicondyle of right humerus
  - S42.448   Incarcerated fracture (avulsion) of medial epicondyle of left humerus
  - S42.449   Incarcerated fracture (avulsion) of medial epicondyle of unspecified humerus
- S42.45   Fracture of lateral condyle of humerus
  Fracture of capitellum of humerus
  - S42.451   Displaced fracture of lateral condyle of right humerus
  - S42.452   Displaced fracture of lateral condyle of left humerus
  - S42.453   Displaced fracture of lateral condyle of unspecified humerus
  - S42.454   Nondisplaced fracture of lateral condyle of right humerus
  - S42.455   Nondisplaced fracture of lateral condyle of left humerus
  - S42.456   Nondisplaced fracture of lateral condyle of unspecified humerus
- S42.46   Fracture of medial condyle of humerus
  Trochlea fracture of humerus
  - S42.461   Displaced fracture of medial condyle of right humerus
  - S42.462   Displaced fracture of medial condyle of left humerus
  - S42.463   Displaced fracture of medial condyle of unspecified humerus
  - S42.464   Nondisplaced fracture of medial condyle of right humerus
  - S42.465   Nondisplaced fracture of medial condyle of left humerus
  - S42.466   Nondisplaced fracture of medial condyle of unspecified humerus

- S42.47 Transcondylar fracture of humerus
  - S42.471 Displaced transcondylar fracture of right humerus
  - S42.472 Displaced transcondylar fracture of left humerus
  - S42.473 Displaced transcondylar fracture of unspecified humerus
  - S42.474 Nondisplaced transcondylar fracture of right humerus
  - S42.475 Nondisplaced transcondylar fracture of left humerus
  - S42.476 Nondisplaced transcondylar fracture of unspecified humerus
- S42.48 Torus fracture of lower end of humerus

  The appropriate 7th character is to be added to all codes in subcategory S42.48

A	initial encounter for closed fracture
D	subsequent encounter for fracture with routine healing
G	subsequent encounter for fracture with delayed healing
K	subsequent encounter for fracture with nonunion
P	subsequent encounter for fracture with malunion
S	sequela

  - S42.481 Torus fracture of lower end of right humerus
  - S42.482 Torus fracture of lower end of left humerus
  - S42.489 Torus fracture of lower end of unspecified humerus
- S42.49 Other fracture of lower end of humerus
  - S42.491 Other displaced fracture of lower end of right humerus
  - S42.492 Other displaced fracture of lower end of left humerus
  - S42.493 Other displaced fracture of lower end of unspecified humerus
  - S42.494 Other nondisplaced fracture of lower end of right humerus
  - S42.495 Other nondisplaced fracture of lower end of left humerus
  - S42.496 Other nondisplaced fracture of lower end of unspecified humerus
- S42.9 Fracture of shoulder girdle, part unspecified
  Fracture of shoulder NOS
  - X S42.90 Fracture of unspecified shoulder girdle, part unspecified
  - X S42.91 Fracture of right shoulder girdle, part unspecified
  - X S42.92 Fracture of left shoulder girdle, part unspecified

- S43 Dislocation and sprain of joints and ligaments of shoulder girdle

  Includes avulsion of joint or ligament of shoulder girdle
  laceration of cartilage, joint or ligament of shoulder girdle
  sprain of cartilage, joint or ligament of shoulder girdle
  traumatic hemarthrosis of joint or ligament of shoulder girdle
  traumatic rupture of joint or ligament of shoulder girdle
  traumatic subluxation of joint or ligament of shoulder girdle
  traumatic tear of joint or ligament of shoulder girdle

  Code also any associated open wound

  Excludes2 strain of muscle, fascia and tendon of shoulder and upper arm (S46.-)

  The appropriate 7th character is to be added to each code from category S43

A	initial encounter
D	subsequent encounter
S	sequela

  - S43.0 Subluxation and dislocation of shoulder joint
    Dislocation of glenohumeral joint
    Subluxation of glenohumeral joint
    - S43.00 Unspecified subluxation and dislocation of shoulder joint
      Dislocation of humerus NOS
      Subluxation of humerus NOS
      - S43.001 Unspecified subluxation of right shoulder joint
      - S43.002 Unspecified subluxation of left shoulder joint
      - S43.003 Unspecified subluxation of unspecified shoulder joint
      - S43.004 Unspecified dislocation of right shoulder joint
      - S43.005 Unspecified dislocation of left shoulder joint
      - S43.006 Unspecified dislocation of unspecified shoulder joint
    - S43.01 Anterior subluxation and dislocation of humerus
      - S43.011 Anterior subluxation of right humerus
      - S43.012 Anterior subluxation of left humerus
      - S43.013 Anterior subluxation of unspecified humerus
      - S43.014 Anterior dislocation of right humerus
      - S43.015 Anterior dislocation of left humerus
      - S43.016 Anterior dislocation of unspecified humerus
    - S43.02 Posterior subluxation and dislocation of humerus
      - S43.021 Posterior subluxation of right humerus
      - S43.022 Posterior subluxation of left humerus
      - S43.023 Posterior subluxation of unspecified humerus
      - S43.024 Posterior dislocation of right humerus
      - S43.025 Posterior dislocation of left humerus
      - S43.026 Posterior dislocation of unspecified humerus

● **S43.03**   Inferior subluxation and dislocation of humerus
- ● S43.031   Inferior subluxation of right humerus
- ● S43.032   Inferior subluxation of left humerus
- ● S43.033   Inferior subluxation of unspecified humerus
- ● S43.034   Inferior dislocation of right humerus
- ● S43.035   Inferior dislocation of left humerus
- ● S43.036   Inferior dislocation of unspecified humerus

● **S43.08**   Other subluxation and dislocation of shoulder joint
- ● S43.081   Other subluxation of right shoulder joint
- ● S43.082   Other subluxation of left shoulder joint
- ● S43.083   Other subluxation of unspecified shoulder joint
- ● S43.084   Other dislocation of right shoulder joint
- ● S43.085   Other dislocation of left shoulder joint
- ● S43.086   Other dislocation of unspecified shoulder joint

● **S43.1**   Subluxation and dislocation of acromioclavicular joint
  ● **S43.10**   Unspecified dislocation of acromioclavicular joint
- ● S43.101   Unspecified dislocation of right acromioclavicular joint
- ● S43.102   Unspecified dislocation of left acromioclavicular joint
- ● S43.109   Unspecified dislocation of unspecified acromioclavicular joint

  ● **S43.11**   Subluxation of acromioclavicular joint
- ● S43.111   Subluxation of right acromioclavicular joint
- ● S43.112   Subluxation of left acromioclavicular joint
- ● S43.119   Subluxation of unspecified acromioclavicular joint

  ● **S43.12**   Dislocation of acromioclavicular joint, 100%-200% displacement
- ● S43.121   Dislocation of right acromioclavicular joint, 100%-200% displacement
- ● S43.122   Dislocation of left acromioclavicular joint, 100%-200% displacement
- ● S43.129   Dislocation of unspecified acromioclavicular joint, 100%-200% displacement

  ● **S43.13**   Dislocation of acromioclavicular joint, greater than 200% displacement
- ● S43.131   Dislocation of right acromioclavicular joint, greater than 200% displacement
- ● S43.132   Dislocation of left acromioclavicular joint, greater than 200% displacement
- ● S43.139   Dislocation of unspecified acromioclavicular joint, greater than 200% displacement

  ● **S43.14**   Inferior dislocation of acromioclavicular joint
- ● S43.141   Inferior dislocation of right acromioclavicular joint
- ● S43.142   Inferior dislocation of left acromioclavicular joint
- ● S43.149   Inferior dislocation of unspecified acromioclavicular joint

  ● **S43.15**   Posterior dislocation of acromioclavicular joint
- ● S43.151   Posterior dislocation of right acromioclavicular joint
- ● S43.152   Posterior dislocation of left acromioclavicular joint
- ● S43.159   Posterior dislocation of unspecified acromioclavicular joint

● **S43.2**   Subluxation and dislocation of sternoclavicular joint
  ● **S43.20**   Unspecified subluxation and dislocation of sternoclavicular joint
- ● S43.201   Unspecified subluxation of right sternoclavicular joint
- ● S43.202   Unspecified subluxation of left sternoclavicular joint
- ● S43.203   Unspecified subluxation of unspecified sternoclavicular joint
- ● S43.204   Unspecified dislocation of right sternoclavicular joint
- ● S43.205   Unspecified dislocation of left sternoclavicular joint
- ● S43.206   Unspecified dislocation of unspecified sternoclavicular joint

  ● **S43.21**   Anterior subluxation and dislocation of sternoclavicular joint
- ● S43.211   Anterior subluxation of right sternoclavicular joint
- ● S43.212   Anterior subluxation of left sternoclavicular joint
- ● S43.213   Anterior subluxation of unspecified sternoclavicular joint
- ● S43.214   Anterior dislocation of right sternoclavicular joint
- ● S43.215   Anterior dislocation of left sternoclavicular joint
- ● S43.216   Anterior dislocation of unspecified sternoclavicular joint

  ● **S43.22**   Posterior subluxation and dislocation of sternoclavicular joint
- ● S43.221   Posterior subluxation of right sternoclavicular joint
- ● S43.222   Posterior subluxation of left sternoclavicular joint
- ● S43.223   Posterior subluxation of unspecified sternoclavicular joint
- ● S43.224   Posterior dislocation of right sternoclavicular joint
- ● S43.225   Posterior dislocation of left sternoclavicular joint
- ● S43.226   Posterior dislocation of unspecified sternoclavicular joint

● **S43.3**   Subluxation and dislocation of other and unspecified parts of shoulder girdle
  ● **S43.30**   Subluxation and dislocation of unspecified parts of shoulder girdle
        Dislocation of shoulder girdle NOS
        Subluxation of shoulder girdle NOS
- ● S43.301   Subluxation of unspecified parts of right shoulder girdle
- ● S43.302   Subluxation of unspecified parts of left shoulder girdle
- ● S43.303   Subluxation of unspecified parts of unspecified shoulder girdle
- ● S43.304   Dislocation of unspecified parts of right shoulder girdle
- ● S43.305   Dislocation of unspecified parts of left shoulder girdle
- ● S43.306   Dislocation of unspecified parts of unspecified shoulder girdle

CHAPTER 19 (S00-T88)

- ● S43.31   Subluxation and dislocation of scapula
  - ● S43.311   Subluxation of right scapula
  - ● S43.312   Subluxation of left scapula
  - ● S43.313   Subluxation of unspecified scapula
  - ● S43.314   Dislocation of right scapula
  - ● S43.315   Dislocation of left scapula
  - ● S43.316   Dislocation of unspecified scapula
- ● S43.39   Subluxation and dislocation of other parts of shoulder girdle
  - ● S43.391   Subluxation of other parts of right shoulder girdle
  - ● S43.392   Subluxation of other parts of left shoulder girdle
  - ● S43.393   Subluxation of other parts of unspecified shoulder girdle
  - ● S43.394   Dislocation of other parts of right shoulder girdle
  - ● S43.395   Dislocation of other parts of left shoulder girdle
  - ● S43.396   Dislocation of other parts of unspecified shoulder girdle
- ● S43.4   Sprain of shoulder joint
  - ● S43.40   Unspecified sprain of shoulder joint
    - ● S43.401   Unspecified sprain of right shoulder joint
    - ● S43.402   Unspecified sprain of left shoulder joint
    - ● S43.409   Unspecified sprain of unspecified shoulder joint
  - ● S43.41   Sprain of coracohumeral (ligament)
    - ● S43.411   Sprain of right coracohumeral (ligament)
    - ● S43.412   Sprain of left coracohumeral (ligament)
    - ● S43.419   Sprain of unspecified coracohumeral (ligament)
  - ● S43.42   Sprain of rotator cuff capsule
    Encounters during the healing phase
    > **Excludes1**   rotator cuff syndrome (complete) (incomplete), not specified as traumatic (M75.1-)
    > **Excludes2**   injury of tendon of rotator cuff (S46.0-)
    - ● S43.421   Sprain of right rotator cuff capsule
    - ● S43.422   Sprain of left rotator cuff capsule
    - ● S43.429   Sprain of unspecified rotator cuff capsule
  - ● S43.43   Superior glenoid labrum lesion
    SLAP lesion
    Coding Clinic: 2019, Q2, P27
    - ● S43.431   Superior glenoid labrum lesion of right shoulder
    - ● S43.432   Superior glenoid labrum lesion of left shoulder
    - ● S43.439   Superior glenoid labrum lesion of unspecified shoulder
  - ● S43.49   Other sprain of shoulder joint
    - ● S43.491   Other sprain of right shoulder joint
    - ● S43.492   Other sprain of left shoulder joint
    - ● S43.499   Other sprain of unspecified shoulder joint
- ● S43.5   Sprain of acromioclavicular joint
  Sprain of acromioclavicular ligament
  - X ● S43.50   Sprain of unspecified acromioclavicular joint
  - X ● S43.51   Sprain of right acromioclavicular joint
  - X ● S43.52   Sprain of left acromioclavicular joint

- ● S43.6   Sprain of sternoclavicular joint
  - X ● S43.60   Sprain of unspecified sternoclavicular joint
  - X ● S43.61   Sprain of right sternoclavicular joint
  - X ● S43.62   Sprain of left sternoclavicular joint
- ● S43.8   Sprain of other specified parts of shoulder girdle
  - X ● S43.80   Sprain of other specified parts of unspecified shoulder girdle
  - X ● S43.81   Sprain of other specified parts of right shoulder girdle
  - X ● S43.82   Sprain of other specified parts of left shoulder girdle
- ● S43.9   Sprain of unspecified parts of shoulder girdle
  - X ● S43.90   Sprain of unspecified parts of unspecified shoulder girdle
    Sprain of shoulder girdle NOS
  - X ● S43.91   Sprain of unspecified parts of right shoulder girdle
  - X ● S43.92   Sprain of unspecified parts of left shoulder girdle

- ● S44   Injury of nerves at shoulder and upper arm level
  Code also any associated open wound (S41.-)
  > **Excludes2**   injury of brachial plexus (S14.3-)
  The appropriate 7th character is to be added to each code from category S44

A	initial encounter
D	subsequent encounter
S	sequela

  - ● S44.0   Injury of ulnar nerve at upper arm level
    > **Excludes1**   ulnar nerve NOS (S54.0)
    - X ● S44.00   Injury of ulnar nerve at upper arm level, unspecified arm
    - X ● S44.01   Injury of ulnar nerve at upper arm level, right arm
    - X ● S44.02   Injury of ulnar nerve at upper arm level, left arm
  - ● S44.1   Injury of median nerve at upper arm level
    > **Excludes1**   median nerve NOS (S54.1)
    - X ● S44.10   Injury of median nerve at upper arm level, unspecified arm
    - X ● S44.11   Injury of median nerve at upper arm level, right arm
    - X ● S44.12   Injury of median nerve at upper arm level, left arm
  - ● S44.2   Injury of radial nerve at upper arm level
    > **Excludes1**   radial nerve NOS (S54.2)
    - X ● S44.20   Injury of radial nerve at upper arm level, unspecified arm
    - X ● S44.21   Injury of radial nerve at upper arm level, right arm
    - X ● S44.22   Injury of radial nerve at upper arm level, left arm
  - ● S44.3   Injury of axillary nerve
    - X ● S44.30   Injury of axillary nerve, unspecified arm
    - X ● S44.31   Injury of axillary nerve, right arm
    - X ● S44.32   Injury of axillary nerve, left arm
  - ● S44.4   Injury of musculocutaneous nerve
    - X ● S44.40   Injury of musculocutaneous nerve, unspecified arm
    - X ● S44.41   Injury of musculocutaneous nerve, right arm
    - X ● S44.42   Injury of musculocutaneous nerve, left arm

▶ New   ⇛ Revised   ~~deleted~~ Deleted   Excludes 1   Excludes 2   Includes   Use additional   Code first   Code also   Key words

OGCR Official Guidelines   X Assign placeholder X   ● Use Additional Character(s)   ⟩ Manifestation Code   🝖 Hierarchical Condition Category   **Coding Clinic**

● **S44.5**   Injury of cutaneous sensory nerve at shoulder and upper arm level

   X● **S44.50**   Injury of cutaneous sensory nerve at shoulder and upper arm level, unspecified arm

   X● **S44.51**   Injury of cutaneous sensory nerve at shoulder and upper arm level, right arm

   X● **S44.52**   Injury of cutaneous sensory nerve at shoulder and upper arm level, left arm

● **S44.8**   Injury of other nerves at shoulder and upper arm level

   ● **S44.8X**   Injury of other nerves at shoulder and upper arm level

     ● **S44.8X1**   Injury of other nerves at shoulder and upper arm level, right arm

     ● **S44.8X2**   Injury of other nerves at shoulder and upper arm level, left arm

     ● **S44.8X9**   Injury of other nerves at shoulder and upper arm level, unspecified arm

● **S44.9**   Injury of unspecified nerve at shoulder and upper arm level

   X● **S44.90**   Injury of unspecified nerve at shoulder and upper arm level, unspecified arm

   X● **S44.91**   Injury of unspecified nerve at shoulder and upper arm level, right arm

   X● **S44.92**   Injury of unspecified nerve at shoulder and upper arm level, left arm

● **S45**   **Injury of blood vessels at shoulder and upper arm level**

   Code also any associated open wound (S41.-)

   Excludes2   injury of subclavian artery (S25.1)
                 injury of subclavian vein (S25.3)

   The appropriate 7th character is to be added to each code from category S45

A	initial encounter
D	subsequent encounter
S	sequela

● **S45.0**   Injury of axillary artery

   ● **S45.00**   Unspecified injury of axillary artery

     ● **S45.001**   Unspecified injury of axillary artery, right side

     ● **S45.002**   Unspecified injury of axillary artery, left side

     ● **S45.009**   Unspecified injury of axillary artery, unspecified side

   ● **S45.01**   Laceration of axillary artery

     ● **S45.011**   Laceration of axillary artery, right side

     ● **S45.012**   Laceration of axillary artery, left side

     ● **S45.019**   Laceration of axillary artery, unspecified side

   ● **S45.09**   Other specified injury of axillary artery

     ● **S45.091**   Other specified injury of axillary artery, right side

     ● **S45.092**   Other specified injury of axillary artery, left side

     ● **S45.099**   Other specified injury of axillary artery, unspecified side

● **S45.1**   Injury of brachial artery

   ● **S45.10**   Unspecified injury of brachial artery

     ● **S45.101**   Unspecified injury of brachial artery, right side

     ● **S45.102**   Unspecified injury of brachial artery, left side

     ● **S45.109**   Unspecified injury of brachial artery, unspecified side

● **S45.11**   Laceration of brachial artery

     ● **S45.111**   Laceration of brachial artery, right side

     ● **S45.112**   Laceration of brachial artery, left side

     ● **S45.119**   Laceration of brachial artery, unspecified side

   ● **S45.19**   Other specified injury of brachial artery

     ● **S45.191**   Other specified injury of brachial artery, right side

     ● **S45.192**   Other specified injury of brachial artery, left side

     ● **S45.199**   Other specified injury of brachial artery, unspecified side

● **S45.2**   Injury of axillary or brachial vein

   ● **S45.20**   Unspecified injury of axillary or brachial vein

     ● **S45.201**   Unspecified injury of axillary or brachial vein, right side

     ● **S45.202**   Unspecified injury of axillary or brachial vein, left side

     ● **S45.209**   Unspecified injury of axillary or brachial vein, unspecified side

   ● **S45.21**   Laceration of axillary or brachial vein

     ● **S45.211**   Laceration of axillary or brachial vein, right side

     ● **S45.212**   Laceration of axillary or brachial vein, left side

     ● **S45.219**   Laceration of axillary or brachial vein, unspecified side

   ● **S45.29**   Other specified injury of axillary or brachial vein

     ● **S45.291**   Other specified injury of axillary or brachial vein, right side

     ● **S45.292**   Other specified injury of axillary or brachial vein, left side

     ● **S45.299**   Other specified injury of axillary or brachial vein, unspecified side

● **S45.3**   Injury of superficial vein at shoulder and upper arm level

   ● **S45.30**   Unspecified injury of superficial vein at shoulder and upper arm level

     ● **S45.301**   Unspecified injury of superficial vein at shoulder and upper arm level, right arm

     ● **S45.302**   Unspecified injury of superficial vein at shoulder and upper arm level, left arm

     ● **S45.309**   Unspecified injury of superficial vein at shoulder and upper arm level, unspecified arm

   ● **S45.31**   Laceration of superficial vein at shoulder and upper arm level

     ● **S45.311**   Laceration of superficial vein at shoulder and upper arm level, right arm

     ● **S45.312**   Laceration of superficial vein at shoulder and upper arm level, left arm

     ● **S45.319**   Laceration of superficial vein at shoulder and upper arm level, unspecified arm

   ● **S45.39**   Other specified injury of superficial vein at shoulder and upper arm level

     ● **S45.391**   Other specified injury of superficial vein at shoulder and upper arm level, right arm

     ● **S45.392**   Other specified injury of superficial vein at shoulder and upper arm level, left arm

     ● **S45.399**   Other specified injury of superficial vein at shoulder and upper arm level, unspecified arm

● **S45.8** Injury of other specified blood vessels at shoulder and upper arm level

  ● **S45.80** Unspecified injury of other specified blood vessels at shoulder and upper arm level

   ● **S45.801** Unspecified injury of other specified blood vessels at shoulder and upper arm level, right arm

   ● **S45.802** Unspecified injury of other specified blood vessels at shoulder and upper arm level, left arm

   ● **S45.809** Unspecified injury of other specified blood vessels at shoulder and upper arm level, unspecified arm

  ● **S45.81** Laceration of other specified blood vessels at shoulder and upper arm level

   ● **S45.811** Laceration of other specified blood vessels at shoulder and upper arm level, right arm

   ● **S45.812** Laceration of other specified blood vessels at shoulder and upper arm level, left arm

   ● **S45.819** Laceration of other specified blood vessels at shoulder and upper arm level, unspecified arm

  ● **S45.89** Other specified injury of other specified blood vessels at shoulder and upper arm level

   ● **S45.891** Other specified injury of other specified blood vessels at shoulder and upper arm level, right arm

   ● **S45.892** Other specified injury of other specified blood vessels at shoulder and upper arm level, left arm

   ● **S45.899** Other specified injury of other specified blood vessels at shoulder and upper arm level, unspecified arm

● **S45.9** Injury of unspecified blood vessel at shoulder and upper arm level

  ● **S45.90** Unspecified injury of unspecified blood vessel at shoulder and upper arm level

   ● **S45.901** Unspecified injury of unspecified blood vessel at shoulder and upper arm level, right arm

   ● **S45.902** Unspecified injury of unspecified blood vessel at shoulder and upper arm level, left arm

   ● **S45.909** Unspecified injury of unspecified blood vessel at shoulder and upper arm level, unspecified arm

  ● **S45.91** Laceration of unspecified blood vessel at shoulder and upper arm level

   ● **S45.911** Laceration of unspecified blood vessel at shoulder and upper arm level, right arm

   ● **S45.912** Laceration of unspecified blood vessel at shoulder and upper arm level, left arm

   ● **S45.919** Laceration of unspecified blood vessel at shoulder and upper arm level, unspecified arm

  ● **S45.99** Other specified injury of unspecified blood vessel at shoulder and upper arm level

   ● **S45.991** Other specified injury of unspecified blood vessel at shoulder and upper arm level, right arm

   ● **S45.992** Other specified injury of unspecified blood vessel at shoulder and upper arm level, left arm

   ● **S45.999** Other specified injury of unspecified blood vessel at shoulder and upper arm level, unspecified arm

● **S46** Injury of muscle, fascia and tendon at shoulder and upper arm level

  Code also any associated open wound (S41.-)

  Excludes2 injury of muscle, fascia and tendon at elbow (S56.-)
  sprain of joints and ligaments of shoulder girdle (S43.9)

  The appropriate 7th character is to be added to each code from category S46

A	initial encounter
D	subsequent encounter
S	sequela

  ● **S46.0** Injury of muscle(s) and tendon(s) of the rotator cuff of shoulder

   ● **S46.00** Unspecified injury of muscle(s) and tendon(s) of the rotator cuff of shoulder

    ● **S46.001** Unspecified injury of muscle(s) and tendon(s) of the rotator cuff of right shoulder

    ● **S46.002** Unspecified injury of muscle(s) and tendon(s) of the rotator cuff of left shoulder

    ● **S46.009** Unspecified injury of muscle(s) and tendon(s) of the rotator cuff of unspecified shoulder

   ● **S46.01** Strain of muscle(s) and tendon(s) of the rotator cuff of shoulder
    Acute onset due to trauma to rotator cuff muscle/tendon

    ● **S46.011** Strain of muscle(s) and tendon(s) of the rotator cuff of right shoulder

    ● **S46.012** Strain of muscle(s) and tendon(s) of the rotator cuff of left shoulder

    ● **S46.019** Strain of muscle(s) and tendon(s) of the rotator cuff of unspecified shoulder

   ● **S46.02** Laceration of muscle(s) and tendon(s) of the rotator cuff of shoulder

    ● **S46.021** Laceration of muscle(s) and tendon(s) of the rotator cuff of right shoulder

    ● **S46.022** Laceration of muscle(s) and tendon(s) of the rotator cuff of left shoulder

    ● **S46.029** Laceration of muscle(s) and tendon(s) of the rotator cuff of unspecified shoulder

   ● **S46.09** Other injury of muscle(s) and tendon(s) of the rotator cuff of shoulder

    ● **S46.091** Other injury of muscle(s) and tendon(s) of the rotator cuff of right shoulder

    ● **S46.092** Other injury of muscle(s) and tendon(s) of the rotator cuff of left shoulder

    ● **S46.099** Other injury of muscle(s) and tendon(s) of the rotator cuff of unspecified shoulder

  ● **S46.1** Injury of muscle, fascia and tendon of long head of biceps

   ● **S46.10** Unspecified injury of muscle, fascia and tendon of long head of biceps

    ● **S46.101** Unspecified injury of muscle, fascia and tendon of long head of biceps, right arm

    ● **S46.102** Unspecified injury of muscle, fascia and tendon of long head of biceps, left arm

    ● **S46.109** Unspecified injury of muscle, fascia and tendon of long head of biceps, unspecified arm

▶ New   ⇒ Revised   ~~deleted~~ Deleted   Excludes 1   Excludes 2   Includes   Use additional   Code first   Code also   Key words

OGCR Official Guidelines   X Assign placeholder X   ● Use Additional Character(s)   ▶ Manifestation Code   🐄 Hierarchical Condition Category   **Coding Clinic**

● S46.11   Strain of muscle, fascia and tendon of long head of biceps
      Coding Clinic: 2019, Q2, P27
   ● S46.111   Strain of muscle, fascia and tendon of long head of biceps, right arm
   ● S46.112   Strain of muscle, fascia and tendon of long head of biceps, left arm
   ● S46.119   Strain of muscle, fascia and tendon of long head of biceps, unspecified arm

● S46.12   Laceration of muscle, fascia and tendon of long head of biceps
   ● S46.121   Laceration of muscle, fascia and tendon of long head of biceps, right arm
   ● S46.122   Laceration of muscle, fascia and tendon of long head of biceps, left arm
   ● S46.129   Laceration of muscle, fascia and tendon of long head of biceps, unspecified arm

● S46.19   Other injury of muscle, fascia and tendon of long head of biceps
   ● S46.191   Other injury of muscle, fascia and tendon of long head of biceps, right arm
   ● S46.192   Other injury of muscle, fascia and tendon of long head of biceps, left arm
   ● S46.199   Other injury of muscle, fascia and tendon of long head of biceps, unspecified arm

● S46.2   Injury of muscle, fascia and tendon of other parts of biceps
  ● S46.20   Unspecified injury of muscle, fascia and tendon of other parts of biceps
   ● S46.201   Unspecified injury of muscle, fascia and tendon of other parts of biceps, right arm
   ● S46.202   Unspecified injury of muscle, fascia and tendon of other parts of biceps, left arm
   ● S46.209   Unspecified injury of muscle, fascia and tendon of other parts of biceps, unspecified arm

  ● S46.21   Strain of muscle, fascia and tendon of other parts of biceps
   ● S46.211   Strain of muscle, fascia and tendon of other parts of biceps, right arm
   ● S46.212   Strain of muscle, fascia and tendon of other parts of biceps, left arm
   ● S46.219   Strain of muscle, fascia and tendon of other parts of biceps, unspecified arm

  ● S46.22   Laceration of muscle, fascia and tendon of other parts of biceps
   ● S46.221   Laceration of muscle, fascia and tendon of other parts of biceps, right arm
   ● S46.222   Laceration of muscle, fascia and tendon of other parts of biceps, left arm
   ● S46.229   Laceration of muscle, fascia and tendon of other parts of biceps, unspecified arm

  ● S46.29   Other injury of muscle, fascia and tendon of other parts of biceps
   ● S46.291   Other injury of muscle, fascia and tendon of other parts of biceps, right arm
   ● S46.292   Other injury of muscle, fascia and tendon of other parts of biceps, left arm
   ● S46.299   Other injury of muscle, fascia and tendon of other parts of biceps, unspecified arm

● S46.3   Injury of muscle, fascia and tendon of triceps
  ● S46.30   Unspecified injury of muscle, fascia and tendon of triceps
   ● S46.301   Unspecified injury of muscle, fascia and tendon of triceps, right arm
   ● S46.302   Unspecified injury of muscle, fascia and tendon of triceps, left arm
   ● S46.309   Unspecified injury of muscle, fascia and tendon of triceps, unspecified arm

  ● S46.31   Strain of muscle, fascia and tendon of triceps
   ● S46.311   Strain of muscle, fascia and tendon of triceps, right arm
   ● S46.312   Strain of muscle, fascia and tendon of triceps, left arm
   ● S46.319   Strain of muscle, fascia and tendon of triceps, unspecified arm

  ● S46.32   Laceration of muscle, fascia and tendon of triceps
   ● S46.321   Laceration of muscle, fascia and tendon of triceps, right arm
   ● S46.322   Laceration of muscle, fascia and tendon of triceps, left arm
   ● S46.329   Laceration of muscle, fascia and tendon of triceps, unspecified arm

  ● S46.39   Other injury of muscle, fascia and tendon of triceps
   ● S46.391   Other injury of muscle, fascia and tendon of triceps, right arm
   ● S46.392   Other injury of muscle, fascia and tendon of triceps, left arm
   ● S46.399   Other injury of muscle, fascia and tendon of triceps, unspecified arm

● S46.8   Injury of other muscles, fascia and tendons at shoulder and upper arm level
  ● S46.80   Unspecified injury of other muscles, fascia and tendons at shoulder and upper arm level
   ● S46.801   Unspecified injury of other muscles, fascia and tendons at shoulder and upper arm level, right arm
   ● S46.802   Unspecified injury of other muscles, fascia and tendons at shoulder and upper arm level, left arm
   ● S46.809   Unspecified injury of other muscles, fascia and tendons at shoulder and upper arm level, unspecified arm

  ● S46.81   Strain of other muscles, fascia and tendons at shoulder and upper arm level
   ● S46.811   Strain of other muscles, fascia and tendons at shoulder and upper arm level, right arm
   ● S46.812   Strain of other muscles, fascia and tendons at shoulder and upper arm level, left arm
   ● S46.819   Strain of other muscles, fascia and tendons at shoulder and upper arm level, unspecified arm

  ● S46.82   Laceration of other muscles, fascia and tendons at shoulder and upper arm level
   ● S46.821   Laceration of other muscles, fascia and tendons at shoulder and upper arm level, right arm
   ● S46.822   Laceration of other muscles, fascia and tendons at shoulder and upper arm level, left arm
   ● S46.829   Laceration of other muscles, fascia and tendons at shoulder and upper arm level, unspecified arm

CHAPTER 19 (S00-T88)

● S46.89   Other injury of other muscles, fascia and tendons at shoulder and upper arm level
- ● S46.891   Other injury of other muscles, fascia and tendons at shoulder and upper arm level, right arm
- ● S46.892   Other injury of other muscles, fascia and tendons at shoulder and upper arm level, left arm
- ● S46.899   Other injury of other muscles, fascia and tendons at shoulder and upper arm level, unspecified arm

● S46.9   Injury of unspecified muscle, fascia and tendon at shoulder and upper arm level
- ● S46.90   Unspecified injury of unspecified muscle, fascia and tendon at shoulder and upper arm level
  - ● S46.901   Unspecified injury of unspecified muscle, fascia and tendon at shoulder and upper arm level, right arm
  - ● S46.902   Unspecified injury of unspecified muscle, fascia and tendon at shoulder and upper arm level, left arm
  - ● S46.909   Unspecified injury of unspecified muscle, fascia and tendon at shoulder and upper arm level, unspecified arm
- ● S46.91   Strain of unspecified muscle, fascia and tendon at shoulder and upper arm level
  - ● S46.911   Strain of unspecified muscle, fascia and tendon at shoulder and upper arm level, right arm
  - ● S46.912   Strain of unspecified muscle, fascia and tendon at shoulder and upper arm level, left arm
  - ● S46.919   Strain of unspecified muscle, fascia and tendon at shoulder and upper arm level, unspecified arm
- ● S46.92   Laceration of unspecified muscle, fascia and tendon at shoulder and upper arm level
  - ● S46.921   Laceration of unspecified muscle, fascia and tendon at shoulder and upper arm level, right arm
  - ● S46.922   Laceration of unspecified muscle, fascia and tendon at shoulder and upper arm level, left arm
  - ● S46.929   Laceration of unspecified muscle, fascia and tendon at shoulder and upper arm level, unspecified arm
- ● S46.99   Other injury of unspecified muscle, fascia and tendon at shoulder and upper arm level
  - ● S46.991   Other injury of unspecified muscle, fascia and tendon at shoulder and upper arm level, right arm
  - ● S46.992   Other injury of unspecified muscle, fascia and tendon at shoulder and upper arm level, left arm
  - ● S46.999   Other injury of unspecified muscle, fascia and tendon at shoulder and upper arm level, unspecified arm

● S47   Crushing injury of shoulder and upper arm

    Use additional code for all associated injuries

    Excludes2   crushing injury of elbow (S57.0-)

    The appropriate 7th character is to be added to each code from category S47

A	initial encounter
D	subsequent encounter
S	sequela

X ● S47.1   Crushing injury of right shoulder and upper arm

X ● S47.2   Crushing injury of left shoulder and upper arm

X ● S47.9   Crushing injury of shoulder and upper arm, unspecified arm

● S48   Traumatic amputation of shoulder and upper arm

    An amputation not identified as partial or complete should be coded to complete

    Excludes1   traumatic amputation at elbow level (S58.0)

    The appropriate 7th character is to be added to each code from category S48

A	initial encounter
D	subsequent encounter
S	sequela

● S48.0   Traumatic amputation at shoulder joint
- ● S48.01   Complete traumatic amputation at shoulder joint
  - ● S48.011   Complete traumatic amputation at right shoulder joint A, S 🅗🅒
  - ● S48.012   Complete traumatic amputation at left shoulder joint A, S 🅗🅒
  - ● S48.019   Complete traumatic amputation at unspecified shoulder joint A, S 🅗🅒
- ● S48.02   Partial traumatic amputation at shoulder joint
  - ● S48.021   Partial traumatic amputation at right shoulder joint A, S 🅗🅒
  - ● S48.022   Partial traumatic amputation at left shoulder joint A, S 🅗🅒
  - ● S48.029   Partial traumatic amputation at unspecified shoulder joint A, S 🅗🅒

● S48.1   Traumatic amputation at level between shoulder and elbow
- ● S48.11   Complete traumatic amputation at level between shoulder and elbow
  - ● S48.111   Complete traumatic amputation at level between right shoulder and elbow A, S 🅗🅒
  - ● S48.112   Complete traumatic amputation at level between left shoulder and elbow A, S 🅗🅒
  - ● S48.119   Complete traumatic amputation at level between unspecified shoulder and elbow A, S 🅗🅒
- ● S48.12   Partial traumatic amputation at level between shoulder and elbow
  - ● S48.121   Partial traumatic amputation at level between right shoulder and elbow A, S 🅗🅒
  - ● S48.122   Partial traumatic amputation at level between left shoulder and elbow A, S 🅗🅒
  - ● S48.129   Partial traumatic amputation at level between unspecified shoulder and elbow A, S 🅗🅒

● S48.9   Traumatic amputation of shoulder and upper arm, level unspecified
- ● S48.91   Complete traumatic amputation of shoulder and upper arm, level unspecified
  - ● S48.911   Complete traumatic amputation of right shoulder and upper arm, level unspecified A, S 🅗🅒
  - ● S48.912   Complete traumatic amputation of left shoulder and upper arm, level unspecified A, S 🅗🅒
  - ● S48.919   Complete traumatic amputation of unspecified shoulder and upper arm, level unspecified A, S 🅗🅒
- ● S48.92   Partial traumatic amputation of shoulder and upper arm, level unspecified
  - ● S48.921   Partial traumatic amputation of right shoulder and upper arm, level unspecified A, S 🅗🅒
  - ● S48.922   Partial traumatic amputation of left shoulder and upper arm, level unspecified A, S 🅗🅒
  - ● S48.929   Partial traumatic amputation of unspecified shoulder and upper arm, level unspecified A, S 🅗🅒

▶ New   ⇒ Revised   ~~deleted~~ Deleted   Excludes 1   Excludes 2   Includes   Use additional   Code first   Code also   Key words

OGCR Official Guidelines   X Assign placeholder X   ● Use Additional Character(s)   ▶ Manifestation Code   🅗🅒 Hierarchical Condition Category   **Coding Clinic**

Item 19–3 SALTER-HARRIS TYPE 1: epiphysis is completely separated from end of bone, or metaphysic growth plate remains attached to epiphysis

SALTER-HARRIS TYPE 2: epiphysis and growth plate are partially separated from metaphysis, which is cracked—most common type

SALTER-HARRIS TYPE 3: fracture occurring through epiphysis and separates part of epiphysis and growth plate from metaphysis fracture, usually at distal end of tibia

SALTER-HARRIS TYPE 4: fracture runs through epiphysis, across growth plate, into metaphysic, surgery is required to restore joint surface to normal and align growth plate

● **S49**   **Other and unspecified injuries of shoulder and upper arm**

The appropriate 7th character is to be added to each code from subcategories S49.0 and S49.1

A	initial encounter for closed fracture
D	subsequent encounter for fracture with routine healing
G	subsequent encounter for fracture with delayed healing
K	subsequent encounter for fracture with nonunion
P	subsequent encounter for fracture with malunion
S	sequela

● **S49.0**   **Physeal fracture of upper end of humerus**

  ● **S49.00**   **Unspecified** physeal fracture of upper end of humerus

    ● S49.001   Unspecified physeal fracture of upper end of humerus, right arm

    ● S49.002   Unspecified physeal fracture of upper end of humerus, left arm

    ● S49.009   Unspecified physeal fracture of upper end of humerus, unspecified arm

  ● **S49.01**   **Salter-Harris Type I** physeal fracture of upper end of humerus

    ● S49.011   Salter-Harris Type I physeal fracture of upper end of humerus, right arm

    ● S49.012   Salter-Harris Type I physeal fracture of upper end of humerus, left arm

    ● S49.019   Salter-Harris Type I physeal fracture of upper end of humerus, unspecified arm

  ● **S49.02**   **Salter-Harris Type II** physeal fracture of upper end of humerus

    ● S49.021   Salter-Harris Type II physeal fracture of upper end of humerus, right arm

    ● S49.022   Salter-Harris Type II physeal fracture of upper end of humerus, left arm

    ● S49.029   Salter-Harris Type II physeal fracture of upper end of humerus, unspecified arm

  ● **S49.03**   **Salter-Harris Type III** physeal fracture of upper end of humerus

    ● S49.031   Salter-Harris Type III physeal fracture of upper end of humerus, right arm

    ● S49.032   Salter-Harris Type III physeal fracture of upper end of humerus, left arm

    ● S49.039   Salter-Harris Type III physeal fracture of upper end of humerus, unspecified arm

  ● **S49.04**   **Salter-Harris Type IV** physeal fracture of upper end of humerus

    ● S49.041   Salter-Harris Type IV physeal fracture of upper end of humerus, right arm

    ● S49.042   Salter-Harris Type IV physeal fracture of upper end of humerus, left arm

    ● S49.049   Salter-Harris Type IV physeal fracture of upper end of humerus, unspecified arm

  ● **S49.09**   **Other** physeal fracture of upper end of humerus

    ● S49.091   Other physeal fracture of upper end of humerus, right arm

    ● S49.092   Other physeal fracture of upper end of humerus, left arm

    ● S49.099   Other physeal fracture of upper end of humerus, unspecified arm

● **S49.1**   **Physeal fracture of lower end of humerus**

  ● **S49.10**   **Unspecified** physeal fracture of lower end of humerus

    ● S49.101   Unspecified physeal fracture of lower end of humerus, right arm

    ● S49.102   Unspecified physeal fracture of lower end of humerus, left arm

    ● S49.109   Unspecified physeal fracture of lower end of humerus, unspecified arm

  ● **S49.11**   **Salter-Harris Type I** physeal fracture of lower end of humerus

    ● S49.111   Salter-Harris Type I physeal fracture of lower end of humerus, right arm

    ● S49.112   Salter-Harris Type I physeal fracture of lower end of humerus, left arm

    ● S49.119   Salter-Harris Type I physeal fracture of lower end of humerus, unspecified arm

  ● **S49.12**   **Salter-Harris Type II** physeal fracture of lower end of humerus

    ● S49.121   Salter-Harris Type II physeal fracture of lower end of humerus, right arm

    ● S49.122   Salter-Harris Type II physeal fracture of lower end of humerus, left arm

    ● S49.129   Salter-Harris Type II physeal fracture of lower end of humerus, unspecified arm

  ● **S49.13**   **Salter-Harris Type III** physeal fracture of lower end of humerus

    ● S49.131   Salter-Harris Type III physeal fracture of lower end of humerus, right arm

    ● S49.132   Salter-Harris Type III physeal fracture of lower end of humerus, left arm

    ● S49.139   Salter-Harris Type III physeal fracture of lower end of humerus, unspecified arm

  ● **S49.14**   **Salter-Harris Type IV** physeal fracture of lower end of humerus

    ● S49.141   Salter-Harris Type IV physeal fracture of lower end of humerus, right arm

    ● S49.142   Salter-Harris Type IV physeal fracture of lower end of humerus, left arm

    ● S49.149   Salter-Harris Type IV physeal fracture of lower end of humerus, unspecified arm

  ● **S49.19**   **Other** physeal fracture of lower end of humerus

    ● S49.191   Other physeal fracture of lower end of humerus, right arm

    ● S49.192   Other physeal fracture of lower end of humerus, left arm

    ● S49.199   Other physeal fracture of lower end of humerus, unspecified arm

CHAPTER 19 (S00-T88)

CHAPTER 19 (S00-T88)

● **S49.8 Other specified injuries of shoulder and upper arm**

The appropriate 7th character is to be added to each code in subcategory S49.8

A	initial encounter
D	subsequent encounter
S	sequela

X ● **S49.80 Other specified injuries of shoulder and upper arm, unspecified arm**

X ● **S49.81 Other specified injuries of right shoulder and upper arm**

X ● **S49.82 Other specified injuries of left shoulder and upper arm**

● **S49.9 Unspecified injury of shoulder and upper arm**

The appropriate 7th character is to be added to each code in subcategory S49.9

A	initial encounter
D	subsequent encounter
S	sequela

X ● **S49.90 Unspecified injury of shoulder and upper arm, unspecified arm**

X ● **S49.91 Unspecified injury of right shoulder and upper arm**

X ● **S49.92 Unspecified injury of left shoulder and upper arm**

INJURIES TO THE ELBOW AND FOREARM (S50-S59)

Excludes2   burns and corrosions (T20-T32)
frostbite (T33-T34)
injuries of wrist and hand (S60-S69)
insect bite or sting, venomous (T63.4)

● **S50 Superficial injury of elbow and forearm**

Excludes2   superficial injury of wrist and hand (S60.-)

The appropriate 7th character is to be added to each code from category S50

A	initial encounter
D	subsequent encounter
S	sequela

● **S50.0 Contusion of elbow**

X ● **S50.00 Contusion of unspecified elbow**

X ● **S50.01 Contusion of right elbow**

X ● **S50.02 Contusion of left elbow**

● **S50.1 Contusion of forearm**

X ● **S50.10 Contusion of unspecified forearm**

X ● **S50.11 Contusion of right forearm**

X ● **S50.12 Contusion of left forearm**

● **S50.3 Other superficial injuries of elbow**

● **S50.31 Abrasion of elbow**

● **S50.311 Abrasion of right elbow**

● **S50.312 Abrasion of left elbow**

● **S50.319 Abrasion of unspecified elbow**

● **S50.32 Blister (nonthermal) of elbow**

● **S50.321 Blister (nonthermal) of right elbow**

● **S50.322 Blister (nonthermal) of left elbow**

● **S50.329 Blister (nonthermal) of unspecified elbow**

● **S50.34 External constriction of elbow**

● **S50.341 External constriction of right elbow**

● **S50.342 External constriction of left elbow**

● **S50.349 External constriction of unspecified elbow**

● **S50.35 Superficial foreign body of elbow**
Splinter in the elbow

● **S50.351 Superficial foreign body of right elbow**

● **S50.352 Superficial foreign body of left elbow**

● **S50.359 Superficial foreign body of unspecified elbow**

● **S50.36 Insect bite (nonvenomous) of elbow**

● **S50.361 Insect bite (nonvenomous) of right elbow**

● **S50.362 Insect bite (nonvenomous) of left elbow**

● **S50.369 Insect bite (nonvenomous) of unspecified elbow**

● **S50.37 Other superficial bite of elbow**

Excludes1   open bite of elbow (S51.04)

● **S50.371 Other superficial bite of right elbow**

● **S50.372 Other superficial bite of left elbow**

● **S50.379 Other superficial bite of unspecified elbow**

● **S50.8 Other superficial injuries of forearm**

● **S50.81 Abrasion of forearm**

● **S50.811 Abrasion of right forearm**

● **S50.812 Abrasion of left forearm**

● **S50.819 Abrasion of unspecified forearm**

● **S50.82 Blister (nonthermal) of forearm**

● **S50.821 Blister (nonthermal) of right forearm**

● **S50.822 Blister (nonthermal) of left forearm**

● **S50.829 Blister (nonthermal) of unspecified forearm**

● **S50.84 External constriction of forearm**

● **S50.841 External constriction of right forearm**

● **S50.842 External constriction of left forearm**

● **S50.849 External constriction of unspecified forearm**

● **S50.85 Superficial foreign body of forearm**
Splinter in the forearm

● **S50.851 Superficial foreign body of right forearm**

● **S50.852 Superficial foreign body of left forearm**

● **S50.859 Superficial foreign body of unspecified forearm**

● **S50.86 Insect bite (nonvenomous) of forearm**

● **S50.861 Insect bite (nonvenomous) of right forearm**

● **S50.862 Insect bite (nonvenomous) of left forearm**

● **S50.869 Insect bite (nonvenomous) of unspecified forearm**

● **S50.87 Other superficial bite of forearm**

Excludes1   open bite of forearm (S51.84)

● **S50.871 Other superficial bite of right forearm**

● **S50.872 Other superficial bite of left forearm**

● **S50.879 Other superficial bite of unspecified forearm**

● **S50.9 Unspecified superficial injury of elbow and forearm**

● **S50.90 Unspecified superficial injury of elbow**

● **S50.901 Unspecified superficial injury of right elbow**

● **S50.902 Unspecified superficial injury of left elbow**

● **S50.909 Unspecified superficial injury of unspecified elbow**

▶ New   ⇒ Revised   ~~deleted~~ Deleted   Excludes 1   Excludes 2   Includes   Use additional   Code first   Code also   Key words

OGCR Official Guidelines   X Assign placeholder X   ● Use Additional Character(s)   ▷ Manifestation Code   🔖 Hierarchical Condition Category   **Coding Clinic**

- S50.91   Unspecified superficial injury of forearm
  - S50.911   Unspecified superficial injury of right forearm
  - S50.912   Unspecified superficial injury of left forearm
  - S50.919   Unspecified superficial injury of unspecified forearm

- S51   Open wound of elbow and forearm

  Code also any associated wound infection

  Excludes1   open fracture of elbow and forearm (S52.- with open fracture 7th character)
  traumatic amputation of elbow and forearm (S58.-)

  Excludes2   open wound of wrist and hand (S61.-)

  The appropriate 7th character is to be added to each code from category S51

A	initial encounter
D	subsequent encounter
S	sequela

  - S51.0   Open wound of elbow
    - S51.00   Unspecified open wound of elbow
      - S51.001   Unspecified open wound of right elbow

        Coding Clinic: 2012, Q4, P108
      - S51.002   Unspecified open wound of left elbow
      - S51.009   Unspecified open wound of unspecified elbow

        Open wound of elbow NOS
    - S51.01   Laceration without foreign body of elbow
      - S51.011   Laceration without foreign body of right elbow
      - S51.012   Laceration without foreign body of left elbow
      - S51.019   Laceration without foreign body of unspecified elbow
    - S51.02   Laceration with foreign body of elbow
      - S51.021   Laceration with foreign body of right elbow
      - S51.022   Laceration with foreign body of left elbow
      - S51.029   Laceration with foreign body of unspecified elbow
    - S51.03   Puncture wound without foreign body of elbow
      - S51.031   Puncture wound without foreign body of right elbow
      - S51.032   Puncture wound without foreign body of left elbow
      - S51.039   Puncture wound without foreign body of unspecified elbow
    - S51.04   Puncture wound with foreign body of elbow
      - S51.041   Puncture wound with foreign body of right elbow
      - S51.042   Puncture wound with foreign body of left elbow
      - S51.049   Puncture wound with foreign body of unspecified elbow

- S51.05   Open bite of elbow

  Bite of elbow NOS

  Excludes1   superficial bite of elbow (S50.36, S50.37)
  - S51.051   Open bite, right elbow
  - S51.052   Open bite, left elbow
  - S51.059   Open bite, unspecified elbow

- S51.8   Open wound of forearm

  Excludes2   open wound of elbow (S51.0-)
  - S51.80   Unspecified open wound of forearm
    - S51.801   Unspecified open wound of right forearm
    - S51.802   Unspecified open wound of left forearm
    - S51.809   Unspecified open wound of unspecified forearm

      Open wound of forearm NOS
  - S51.81   Laceration without foreign body of forearm
    - S51.811   Laceration without foreign body of right forearm
    - S51.812   Laceration without foreign body of left forearm
    - S51.819   Laceration without foreign body of unspecified forearm
  - S51.82   Laceration with foreign body of forearm
    - S51.821   Laceration with foreign body of right forearm
    - S51.822   Laceration with foreign body of left forearm
    - S51.829   Laceration with foreign body of unspecified forearm
  - S51.83   Puncture wound without foreign body of forearm
    - S51.831   Puncture wound without foreign body of right forearm
    - S51.832   Puncture wound without foreign body of left forearm
    - S51.839   Puncture wound without foreign body of unspecified forearm
  - S51.84   Puncture wound with foreign body of forearm
    - S51.841   Puncture wound with foreign body of right forearm
    - S51.842   Puncture wound with foreign body of left forearm
    - S51.849   Puncture wound with foreign body of unspecified forearm
  - S51.85   Open bite of forearm

    Bite of forearm NOS

    Excludes1   superficial bite of forearm (S50.86, S50.87)
    - S51.851   Open bite of right forearm
    - S51.852   Open bite of left forearm
    - S51.859   Open bite of unspecified forearm

● **S52   Fracture of forearm**

> **Note:** A fracture not identified as displaced or nondisplaced should be coded to displaced
>
> A fracture not designated as open or closed should be coded to closed
>
> The open fracture designations are based on the Gustilo open fracture classification

Excludes1   traumatic amputation of forearm (S58.-)

Excludes2   fracture at wrist and hand level (S62.-)

The appropriate 7th character is to be added to all codes from category S52

A	initial encounter for closed fracture
B	initial encounter for open fracture type I or II
	initial encounter for open fracture NOS
C	initial encounter for open fracture type IIIA, IIIB, or IIIC
D	subsequent encounter for closed fracture with routine healing
E	subsequent encounter for open fracture type I or II with routine healing
F	subsequent encounter for open fracture type IIIA, IIIB, or IIIC with routine healing
G	subsequent encounter for closed fracture with delayed healing
H	subsequent encounter for open fracture type I or II with delayed healing
J	subsequent encounter for open fracture type IIIA, IIIB, or IIIC with delayed healing
K	subsequent encounter for closed fracture with nonunion
M	subsequent encounter for open fracture type I or II with nonunion
N	subsequent encounter for open fracture type IIIA, IIIB, or IIIC with nonunion
P	subsequent encounter for closed fracture with malunion
Q	subsequent encounter for open fracture type I or II with malunion
R	subsequent encounter for open fracture type IIIA, IIIB, or IIIC with malunion
S	sequela

Coding Clinic: 2016, Q1, P33

● **S52.0   Fracture of upper end of ulna**

> Fracture of proximal end of ulna

Excludes2   fracture of elbow NOS (S42.40-)
fractures of shaft of ulna (S52.2-)

● **S52.00   Unspecified fracture of upper end of ulna**

● S52.001   Unspecified fracture of upper end of right ulna

● S52.002   Unspecified fracture of upper end of left ulna

● S52.009   Unspecified fracture of upper end of unspecified ulna

● **S52.01   Torus fracture of upper end of ulna**

> The appropriate 7th character is to be added to all codes in subcategory S52.01

A	initial encounter for closed fracture
D	subsequent encounter for fracture with routine healing
G	subsequent encounter for fracture with delayed healing
K	subsequent encounter for fracture with nonunion
P	subsequent encounter for fracture with malunion
S	sequela

● S52.011   Torus fracture of upper end of right ulna

● S52.012   Torus fracture of upper end of left ulna

● S52.019   Torus fracture of upper end of unspecified ulna

● **S52.02   Fracture of olecranon process without intraarticular extension of ulna**

● S52.021   Displaced fracture of olecranon process without intraarticular extension of right ulna

● S52.022   Displaced fracture of olecranon process without intraarticular extension of left ulna

● S52.023   Displaced fracture of olecranon process without intraarticular extension of unspecified ulna

● S52.024   Nondisplaced fracture of olecranon process without intraarticular extension of right ulna

● S52.025   Nondisplaced fracture of olecranon process without intraarticular extension of left ulna

● S52.026   Nondisplaced fracture of olecranon process without intraarticular extension of unspecified ulna

● **S52.03   Fracture of olecranon process with intraarticular extension of ulna**

● S52.031   Displaced fracture of olecranon process with intraarticular extension of right ulna

● S52.032   Displaced fracture of olecranon process with intraarticular extension of left ulna

● S52.033   Displaced fracture of olecranon process with intraarticular extension of unspecified ulna

● S52.034   Nondisplaced fracture of olecranon process with intraarticular extension of right ulna

● S52.035   Nondisplaced fracture of olecranon process with intraarticular extension of left ulna

● S52.036   Nondisplaced fracture of olecranon process with intraarticular extension of unspecified ulna

● **S52.04   Fracture of coronoid process of ulna**

● S52.041   Displaced fracture of coronoid process of right ulna

● S52.042   Displaced fracture of coronoid process of left ulna

● S52.043   Displaced fracture of coronoid process of unspecified ulna

● S52.044   Nondisplaced fracture of coronoid process of right ulna

● S52.045   Nondisplaced fracture of coronoid process of left ulna

● S52.046   Nondisplaced fracture of coronoid process of unspecified ulna

● **S52.09   Other fracture of upper end of ulna**

● S52.091   Other fracture of upper end of right ulna

● S52.092   Other fracture of upper end of left ulna

● S52.099   Other fracture of upper end of unspecified ulna

● **S52.1   Fracture of upper end of radius**

> Fracture of proximal end of radius

Excludes2   physeal fractures of upper end of radius (S59.2-)
fracture of shaft of radius (S52.3-)

● **S52.10   Unspecified fracture of upper end of radius**

● S52.101   Unspecified fracture of upper end of right radius

● S52.102   Unspecified fracture of upper end of left radius

● S52.109   Unspecified fracture of upper end of unspecified radius

▶ New   ⇒ Revised   ~~deleted~~ Deleted   Excludes 1   Excludes 2   Includes   Use additional   Code first   Code also   Key words

OGCR Official Guidelines   X Assign placeholder X   ● Use Additional Character(s)   ▷ Manifestation Code   ℞ Hierarchical Condition Category   Coding Clinic

● **S52.11**   Torus fracture of upper end of radius

The appropriate 7th character is to be added to all codes in subcategory S52.11

A	initial encounter for closed fracture
D	subsequent encounter for fracture with routine healing
G	subsequent encounter for fracture with delayed healing
K	subsequent encounter for fracture with nonunion
P	subsequent encounter for fracture with malunion
S	sequela

   ● **S52.111**   Torus fracture of upper end of right radius

   ● **S52.112**   Torus fracture of upper end of left radius

   ● **S52.119**   Torus fracture of upper end of unspecified radius

● **S52.12**   Fracture of head of radius

   ● **S52.121**   Displaced fracture of head of right radius

   ● **S52.122**   Displaced fracture of head of left radius

   ● **S52.123**   Displaced fracture of head of unspecified radius

   ● **S52.124**   Nondisplaced fracture of head of right radius

   ● **S52.125**   Nondisplaced fracture of head of left radius

   ● **S52.126**   Nondisplaced fracture of head of unspecified radius

● **S52.13**   Fracture of neck of radius

   ● **S52.131**   Displaced fracture of neck of right radius

   ● **S52.132**   Displaced fracture of neck of left radius

   ● **S52.133**   Displaced fracture of neck of unspecified radius

   ● **S52.134**   Nondisplaced fracture of neck of right radius

   ● **S52.135**   Nondisplaced fracture of neck of left radius

   ● **S52.136**   Nondisplaced fracture of neck of unspecified radius

● **S52.18**   Other fracture of upper end of radius

   ● **S52.181**   Other fracture of upper end of right radius

   ● **S52.182**   Other fracture of upper end of left radius

   ● **S52.189**   Other fracture of upper end of unspecified radius

● **S52.2**   Fracture of shaft of ulna

   ● **S52.20**   Unspecified fracture of shaft of ulna
             Fracture of ulna NOS

   ● **S52.201**   Unspecified fracture of shaft of right ulna

   ● **S52.202**   Unspecified fracture of shaft of left ulna

   ● **S52.209**   Unspecified fracture of shaft of unspecified ulna

● **S52.21**   Greenstick fracture of shaft of ulna

The appropriate 7th character is to be added to all codes in subcategory S52.21

A	initial encounter for closed fracture
D	subsequent encounter for fracture with routine healing
G	subsequent encounter for fracture with delayed healing
K	subsequent encounter for fracture with nonunion
P	subsequent encounter for fracture with malunion
S	sequela

   ● **S52.211**   Greenstick fracture of shaft of right ulna

   ● **S52.212**   Greenstick fracture of shaft of left ulna

   ● **S52.219**   Greenstick fracture of shaft of unspecified ulna

● **S52.22**   Transverse fracture of shaft of ulna

   ● **S52.221**   Displaced transverse fracture of shaft of right ulna

   ● **S52.222**   Displaced transverse fracture of shaft of left ulna

   ● **S52.223**   Displaced transverse fracture of shaft of unspecified ulna

   ● **S52.224**   Nondisplaced transverse fracture of shaft of right ulna

   ● **S52.225**   Nondisplaced transverse fracture of shaft of left ulna

   ● **S52.226**   Nondisplaced transverse fracture of shaft of unspecified ulna

● **S52.23**   Oblique fracture of shaft of ulna

   ● **S52.231**   Displaced oblique fracture of shaft of right ulna

   ● **S52.232**   Displaced oblique fracture of shaft of left ulna

   ● **S52.233**   Displaced oblique fracture of shaft of unspecified ulna

   ● **S52.234**   Nondisplaced oblique fracture of shaft of right ulna

   ● **S52.235**   Nondisplaced oblique fracture of shaft of left ulna

   ● **S52.236**   Nondisplaced oblique fracture of shaft of unspecified ulna

● **S52.24**   Spiral fracture of shaft of ulna

   ● **S52.241**   Displaced spiral fracture of shaft of ulna, right arm

   ● **S52.242**   Displaced spiral fracture of shaft of ulna, left arm

   ● **S52.243**   Displaced spiral fracture of shaft of ulna, unspecified arm

   ● **S52.244**   Nondisplaced spiral fracture of shaft of ulna, right arm

   ● **S52.245**   Nondisplaced spiral fracture of shaft of ulna, left arm

   ● **S52.246**   Nondisplaced spiral fracture of shaft of ulna, unspecified arm

● **S52.25**   Comminuted fracture of shaft of ulna

   ● **S52.251**   Displaced comminuted fracture of shaft of ulna, right arm

   ● **S52.252**   Displaced comminuted fracture of shaft of ulna, left arm

   ● **S52.253**   Displaced comminuted fracture of shaft of ulna, unspecified arm

   ● **S52.254**   Nondisplaced comminuted fracture of shaft of ulna, right arm

   ● **S52.255**   Nondisplaced comminuted fracture of shaft of ulna, left arm

   ● **S52.256**   Nondisplaced comminuted fracture of shaft of ulna, unspecified arm

CHAPTER 19 (S00-T88)

- ● S52.26   Segmental fracture of shaft of ulna
  - ● S52.261   Displaced segmental fracture of shaft of ulna, right arm
  - ● S52.262   Displaced segmental fracture of shaft of ulna, left arm
  - ● S52.263   Displaced segmental fracture of shaft of ulna, unspecified arm
  - ● S52.264   Nondisplaced segmental fracture of shaft of ulna, right arm
  - ● S52.265   Nondisplaced segmental fracture of shaft of ulna, left arm
  - ● S52.266   Nondisplaced segmental fracture of shaft of ulna, unspecified arm
- ● S52.27   Monteggia's fracture of ulna
  Fracture of upper shaft of ulna with dislocation of radial head
  - ● S52.271   Monteggia's fracture of right ulna
  - ● S52.272   Monteggia's fracture of left ulna
  - ● S52.279   Monteggia's fracture of unspecified ulna
- ● S52.28   Bent bone of ulna
  - ● S52.281   Bent bone of right ulna
  - ● S52.282   Bent bone of left ulna
  - ● S52.283   Bent bone of unspecified ulna
- ● S52.29   Other fracture of shaft of ulna
  - ● S52.291   Other fracture of shaft of right ulna
  - ● S52.292   Other fracture of shaft of left ulna
  - ● S52.299   Other fracture of shaft of unspecified ulna
- ● S52.3   Fracture of shaft of radius
  - ● S52.30   Unspecified fracture of shaft of radius
    - ● S52.301   Unspecified fracture of shaft of right radius
    - ● S52.302   Unspecified fracture of shaft of left radius
    - ● S52.309   Unspecified fracture of shaft of unspecified radius
  - ● S52.31   Greenstick fracture of shaft of radius

    The appropriate 7th character is to be added to all codes in subcategory S52.31

A	initial encounter for closed fracture
D	subsequent encounter for fracture with routine healing
G	subsequent encounter for fracture with delayed healing
K	subsequent encounter for fracture with nonunion
P	subsequent encounter for fracture with malunion
S	sequela

    - ● S52.311   Greenstick fracture of shaft of radius, right arm
    - ● S52.312   Greenstick fracture of shaft of radius, left arm
    - ● S52.319   Greenstick fracture of shaft of radius, unspecified arm
  - ● S52.32   Transverse fracture of shaft of radius
    - ● S52.321   Displaced transverse fracture of shaft of right radius
    - ● S52.322   Displaced transverse fracture of shaft of left radius
    - ● S52.323   Displaced transverse fracture of shaft of unspecified radius
    - ● S52.324   Nondisplaced transverse fracture of shaft of right radius
    - ● S52.325   Nondisplaced transverse fracture of shaft of left radius
    - ● S52.326   Nondisplaced transverse fracture of shaft of unspecified radius

- ● S52.33   Oblique fracture of shaft of radius
  - ● S52.331   Displaced oblique fracture of shaft of right radius
  - ● S52.332   Displaced oblique fracture of shaft of left radius
  - ● S52.333   Displaced oblique fracture of shaft of unspecified radius
  - ● S52.334   Nondisplaced oblique fracture of shaft of right radius
  - ● S52.335   Nondisplaced oblique fracture of shaft of left radius
  - ● S52.336   Nondisplaced oblique fracture of shaft of unspecified radius
- ● S52.34   Spiral fracture of shaft of radius
  - ● S52.341   Displaced spiral fracture of shaft of radius, right arm
  - ● S52.342   Displaced spiral fracture of shaft of radius, left arm
  - ● S52.343   Displaced spiral fracture of shaft of radius, unspecified arm
  - ● S52.344   Nondisplaced spiral fracture of shaft of radius, right arm
  - ● S52.345   Nondisplaced spiral fracture of shaft of radius, left arm
  - ● S52.346   Nondisplaced spiral fracture of shaft of radius, unspecified arm
- ● S52.35   Comminuted fracture of shaft of radius
  - ● S52.351   Displaced comminuted fracture of shaft of radius, right arm
  - ● S52.352   Displaced comminuted fracture of shaft of radius, left arm
  - ● S52.353   Displaced comminuted fracture of shaft of radius, unspecified arm
  - ● S52.354   Nondisplaced comminuted fracture of shaft of radius, right arm
  - ● S52.355   Nondisplaced comminuted fracture of shaft of radius, left arm
  - ● S52.356   Nondisplaced comminuted fracture of shaft of radius, unspecified arm
- ● S52.36   Segmental fracture of shaft of radius
  - ● S52.361   Displaced segmental fracture of shaft of radius, right arm
  - ● S52.362   Displaced segmental fracture of shaft of radius, left arm
  - ● S52.363   Displaced segmental fracture of shaft of radius, unspecified arm
  - ● S52.364   Nondisplaced segmental fracture of shaft of radius, right arm
  - ● S52.365   Nondisplaced segmental fracture of shaft of radius, left arm
  - ● S52.366   Nondisplaced segmental fracture of shaft of radius, unspecified arm
- ● S52.37   Galeazzi's fracture
  Fracture of lower shaft of radius with radioulnar joint dislocation
  - ● S52.371   Galeazzi's fracture of right radius
  - ● S52.372   Galeazzi's fracture of left radius
  - ● S52.379   Galeazzi's fracture of unspecified radius
- ● S52.38   Bent bone of radius
  - ● S52.381   Bent bone of right radius
  - ● S52.382   Bent bone of left radius
  - ● S52.389   Bent bone of unspecified radius
- ● S52.39   Other fracture of shaft of radius
  - ● S52.391   Other fracture of shaft of radius, right arm
  - ● S52.392   Other fracture of shaft of radius, left arm
  - ● S52.399   Other fracture of shaft of radius, unspecified arm

▶ New   ⇒ Revised   ~~deleted~~ Deleted   Excludes 1   Excludes 2   Includes   Use additional   Code first   Code also   Key words

OGCR Official Guidelines   X Assign placeholder X   ● Use Additional Character(s)   ▷ Manifestation Code   🗝 Hierarchical Condition Category   **Coding Clinic**

● **S52.5**   Fracture of lower end of radius
Fracture of distal end of radius

> **Excludes2**   physeal fractures of lower end of radius
> (S59.2-)

● **S52.50**   Unspecified fracture of the lower end of radius
- ● **S52.501**   Unspecified fracture of the lower end of right radius
- ● **S52.502**   Unspecified fracture of the lower end of left radius
- ● **S52.509**   Unspecified fracture of the lower end of unspecified radius

● **S52.51**   Fracture of radial styloid process
- ● **S52.511**   Displaced fracture of right radial styloid process
- ● **S52.512**   Displaced fracture of left radial styloid process
- ● **S52.513**   Displaced fracture of unspecified radial styloid process
- ● **S52.514**   Nondisplaced fracture of right radial styloid process
- ● **S52.515**   Nondisplaced fracture of left radial styloid process
- ● **S52.516**   Nondisplaced fracture of unspecified radial styloid process

● **S52.52**   Torus fracture of lower end of radius

The appropriate 7th character is to be added to all codes in subcategory S52.52

A	initial encounter for closed fracture
D	subsequent encounter for fracture with routine healing
G	subsequent encounter for fracture with delayed healing
K	subsequent encounter for fracture with nonunion
P	subsequent encounter for fracture with malunion
S	sequela

- ● **S52.521**   Torus fracture of lower end of right radius
- ● **S52.522**   Torus fracture of lower end of left radius
- ● **S52.529**   Torus fracture of lower end of unspecified radius

● **S52.53**   Colles' fracture
- ● **S52.531**   Colles' fracture of right radius
- ● **S52.532**   Colles' fracture of left radius
  > **Coding Clinic: 2016, Q2, P5**
- ● **S52.539**   Colles' fracture of unspecified radius

● **S52.54**   Smith's fracture
- ● **S52.541**   Smith's fracture of right radius
- ● **S52.542**   Smith's fracture of left radius
- ● **S52.549**   Smith's fracture of unspecified radius

● **S52.55**   Other extraarticular fracture of lower end of radius
- ● **S52.551**   Other extraarticular fracture of lower end of right radius
- ● **S52.552**   Other extraarticular fracture of lower end of left radius
- ● **S52.559**   Other extraarticular fracture of lower end of unspecified radius

● **S52.56**   Barton's fracture
- ● **S52.561**   Barton's fracture of right radius
- ● **S52.562**   Barton's fracture of left radius
- ● **S52.569**   Barton's fracture of unspecified radius

● **S52.57**   Other intraarticular fracture of lower end of radius
- ● **S52.571**   Other intraarticular fracture of lower end of right radius
- ● **S52.572**   Other intraarticular fracture of lower end of left radius
- ● **S52.579**   Other intraarticular fracture of lower end of unspecified radius

● **S52.59**   Other fractures of lower end of radius
- ● **S52.591**   Other fractures of lower end of right radius
  > **Coding Clinic: 2019, Q3, P10**
- ● **S52.592**   Other fractures of lower end of left radius
- ● **S52.599**   Other fractures of lower end of unspecified radius

● **S52.6**   Fracture of lower end of ulna
● **S52.60**   Unspecified fracture of lower end of ulna
- ● **S52.601**   Unspecified fracture of lower end of right ulna
- ● **S52.602**   Unspecified fracture of lower end of left ulna
- ● **S52.609**   Unspecified fracture of lower end of unspecified ulna

● **S52.61**   Fracture of ulna styloid process
- ● **S52.611**   Displaced fracture of right ulna styloid process
- ● **S52.612**   Displaced fracture of left ulna styloid process
- ● **S52.613**   Displaced fracture of unspecified ulna styloid process
- ● **S52.614**   Nondisplaced fracture of right ulna styloid process
- ● **S52.615**   Nondisplaced fracture of left ulna styloid process
- ● **S52.616**   Nondisplaced fracture of unspecified ulna styloid process

● **S52.62**   Torus fracture of lower end of ulna

The appropriate 7th character is to be added to all codes in subcategory S52.62

A	initial encounter for closed fracture
D	subsequent encounter for fracture with routine healing
G	subsequent encounter for fracture with delayed healing
K	subsequent encounter for fracture with nonunion
P	subsequent encounter for fracture with malunion
S	sequela

- ● **S52.621**   Torus fracture of lower end of right ulna
- ● **S52.622**   Torus fracture of lower end of left ulna
- ● **S52.629**   Torus fracture of lower end of unspecified ulna

● **S52.69**   Other fracture of lower end of ulna
- ● **S52.691**   Other fracture of lower end of right ulna
  > **Coding Clinic: 2019, Q3, P10**
- ● **S52.692**   Other fracture of lower end of left ulna
- ● **S52.699**   Other fracture of lower end of unspecified ulna

● **S52.9**   Unspecified fracture of forearm
- X ● **S52.90**   Unspecified fracture of unspecified forearm
- X ● **S52.91**   Unspecified fracture of right forearm
- X ● **S52.92**   Unspecified fracture of left forearm

CHAPTER 19 (S00-T88)

CHAPTER 19 (S00-T88)

● **S53**   **Dislocation and sprain of joints and ligaments of elbow**

     Includes   avulsion of joint or ligament of elbow
                    laceration of cartilage, joint or ligament of elbow
                    sprain of cartilage, joint or ligament of elbow
                    traumatic hemarthrosis of joint or ligament of elbow
                    traumatic rupture of joint or ligament of elbow
                    traumatic subluxation of joint or ligament of elbow
                    traumatic tear of joint or ligament of elbow

     Code also any associated open wound

     Excludes2   strain of muscle, fascia and tendon at forearm level (S56.-)

     The appropriate 7th character is to be added to each code from category S53

       A   initial encounter
       D   subsequent encounter
       S   sequela

● **S53.0**   **Subluxation and dislocation of radial head**
       Dislocation of radiohumeral joint
       Subluxation of radiohumeral joint

       Excludes1   Monteggia's fracture-dislocation (S52.27-)

   ● **S53.00**   **Unspecified subluxation and dislocation of radial head**

     ● **S53.001**   Unspecified subluxation of right radial head
     ● **S53.002**   Unspecified subluxation of left radial head
     ● **S53.003**   Unspecified subluxation of unspecified radial head
     ● **S53.004**   Unspecified dislocation of right radial head
     ● **S53.005**   Unspecified dislocation of left radial head
     ● **S53.006**   Unspecified dislocation of unspecified radial head

   ● **S53.01**   **Anterior subluxation and dislocation of radial head**
       Anteriomedial subluxation and dislocation of radial head

     ● **S53.011**   Anterior subluxation of right radial head
     ● **S53.012**   Anterior subluxation of left radial head
     ● **S53.013**   Anterior subluxation of unspecified radial head
     ● **S53.014**   Anterior dislocation of right radial head
     ● **S53.015**   Anterior dislocation of left radial head
     ● **S53.016**   Anterior dislocation of unspecified radial head

   ● **S53.02**   **Posterior subluxation and dislocation of radial head**
       Posteriolateral subluxation and dislocation of radial head

     ● **S53.021**   Posterior subluxation of right radial head
     ● **S53.022**   Posterior subluxation of left radial head
     ● **S53.023**   Posterior subluxation of unspecified radial head
     ● **S53.024**   Posterior dislocation of right radial head
     ● **S53.025**   Posterior dislocation of left radial head
     ● **S53.026**   Posterior dislocation of unspecified radial head

   ● **S53.03**   **Nursemaid's elbow**

     ● **S53.031**   Nursemaid's elbow, right elbow
                Coding Clinic: 2015, Q1, P7-8
     ● **S53.032**   Nursemaid's elbow, left elbow
     ● **S53.033**   Nursemaid's elbow, unspecified elbow

   ● **S53.09**   **Other subluxation and dislocation of radial head**

     ● **S53.091**   Other subluxation of right radial head
     ● **S53.092**   Other subluxation of left radial head
     ● **S53.093**   Other subluxation of unspecified radial head
     ● **S53.094**   Other dislocation of right radial head
     ● **S53.095**   Other dislocation of left radial head
     ● **S53.096**   Other dislocation of unspecified radial head

● **S53.1**   **Subluxation and dislocation of ulnohumeral joint**
       Subluxation and dislocation of elbow NOS

       Excludes1   dislocation of radial head alone (S53.0-)

   ● **S53.10**   **Unspecified subluxation and dislocation of ulnohumeral joint**

     ● **S53.101**   Unspecified subluxation of right ulnohumeral joint
     ● **S53.102**   Unspecified subluxation of left ulnohumeral joint
     ● **S53.103**   Unspecified subluxation of unspecified ulnohumeral joint
     ● **S53.104**   Unspecified dislocation of right ulnohumeral joint
     ● **S53.105**   Unspecified dislocation of left ulnohumeral joint
     ● **S53.106**   Unspecified dislocation of unspecified ulnohumeral joint

   ● **S53.11**   **Anterior subluxation and dislocation of ulnohumeral joint**

     ● **S53.111**   Anterior subluxation of right ulnohumeral joint
     ● **S53.112**   Anterior subluxation of left ulnohumeral joint
     ● **S53.113**   Anterior subluxation of unspecified ulnohumeral joint
     ● **S53.114**   Anterior dislocation of right ulnohumeral joint
                Coding Clinic: 2012, Q4, P108
     ● **S53.115**   Anterior dislocation of left ulnohumeral joint
     ● **S53.116**   Anterior dislocation of unspecified ulnohumeral joint

   ● **S53.12**   **Posterior subluxation and dislocation of ulnohumeral joint**

     ● **S53.121**   Posterior subluxation of right ulnohumeral joint
     ● **S53.122**   Posterior subluxation of left ulnohumeral joint
     ● **S53.123**   Posterior subluxation of unspecified ulnohumeral joint
     ● **S53.124**   Posterior dislocation of right ulnohumeral joint
     ● **S53.125**   Posterior dislocation of left ulnohumeral joint
     ● **S53.126**   Posterior dislocation of unspecified ulnohumeral joint

▶ New   ⇒ Revised   ~~deleted~~ Deleted   Excludes 1   Excludes 2   Includes   Use additional   Code first   Code also   Key words

OGCR Official Guidelines   X Assign placeholder X   ● Use Additional Character(s)   ▶ Manifestation Code   Hierarchical Condition Category   **Coding Clinic**

● **S53.13**   Medial subluxation and dislocation of ulnohumeral joint
    ● **S53.131**   Medial subluxation of right ulnohumeral joint
    ● **S53.132**   Medial subluxation of left ulnohumeral joint
    ● **S53.133**   Medial subluxation of unspecified ulnohumeral joint
    ● **S53.134**   Medial dislocation of right ulnohumeral joint
    ● **S53.135**   Medial dislocation of left ulnohumeral joint
    ● **S53.136**   Medial dislocation of unspecified ulnohumeral joint
● **S53.14**   Lateral subluxation and dislocation of ulnohumeral joint
    ● **S53.141**   Lateral subluxation of right ulnohumeral joint
    ● **S53.142**   Lateral subluxation of left ulnohumeral joint
    ● **S53.143**   Lateral subluxation of unspecified ulnohumeral joint
    ● **S53.144**   Lateral dislocation of right ulnohumeral joint
    ● **S53.145**   Lateral dislocation of left ulnohumeral joint
    ● **S53.146**   Lateral dislocation of unspecified ulnohumeral joint
● **S53.19**   Other subluxation and dislocation of ulnohumeral joint
    ● **S53.191**   Other subluxation of right ulnohumeral joint
    ● **S53.192**   Other subluxation of left ulnohumeral joint
    ● **S53.193**   Other subluxation of unspecified ulnohumeral joint
    ● **S53.194**   Other dislocation of right ulnohumeral joint
    ● **S53.195**   Other dislocation of left ulnohumeral joint
    ● **S53.196**   Other dislocation of unspecified ulnohumeral joint
● **S53.2**   Traumatic rupture of radial collateral ligament
    Excludes1   sprain of radial collateral ligament NOS (S53.43-)
X● **S53.20**   Traumatic rupture of unspecified radial collateral ligament
X● **S53.21**   Traumatic rupture of right radial collateral ligament
X● **S53.22**   Traumatic rupture of left radial collateral ligament
● **S53.3**   Traumatic rupture of ulnar collateral ligament
    Excludes1   sprain of ulnar collateral ligament (S53.44-)
X● **S53.30**   Traumatic rupture of unspecified ulnar collateral ligament
X● **S53.31**   Traumatic rupture of right ulnar collateral ligament
X● **S53.32**   Traumatic rupture of left ulnar collateral ligament
● **S53.4**   Sprain of elbow
    Excludes2   traumatic rupture of radial collateral ligament (S53.2-)
              traumatic rupture of ulnar collateral ligament (S53.3-)
    ● **S53.40**   Unspecified sprain of elbow
       ● **S53.401**   Unspecified sprain of right elbow
       ● **S53.402**   Unspecified sprain of left elbow
       ● **S53.409**   Unspecified sprain of unspecified elbow
             Sprain of elbow NOS

● **S53.41**   Radiohumeral (joint) sprain
    ● **S53.411**   Radiohumeral (joint) sprain of right elbow
    ● **S53.412**   Radiohumeral (joint) sprain of left elbow
    ● **S53.419**   Radiohumeral (joint) sprain of unspecified elbow
● **S53.42**   Ulnohumeral (joint) sprain
    ● **S53.421**   Ulnohumeral (joint) sprain of right elbow
    ● **S53.422**   Ulnohumeral (joint) sprain of left elbow
    ● **S53.429**   Ulnohumeral (joint) sprain of unspecified elbow
● **S53.43**   Radial collateral ligament sprain
    ● **S53.431**   Radial collateral ligament sprain of right elbow
    ● **S53.432**   Radial collateral ligament sprain of left elbow
    ● **S53.439**   Radial collateral ligament sprain of unspecified elbow
● **S53.44**   Ulnar collateral ligament sprain
    ● **S53.441**   Ulnar collateral ligament sprain of right elbow
    ● **S53.442**   Ulnar collateral ligament sprain of left elbow
    ● **S53.449**   Ulnar collateral ligament sprain of unspecified elbow
● **S53.49**   Other sprain of elbow
    ● **S53.491**   Other sprain of right elbow
    ● **S53.492**   Other sprain of left elbow
    ● **S53.499**   Other sprain of unspecified elbow

● **S54**   **Injury of nerves at forearm level**
    Code also any associated open wound (S51.-)
    Excludes2   injury of nerves at wrist and hand level (S64.-)
    The appropriate 7th character is to be added to each code from category S54

A	initial encounter
D	subsequent encounter
S	sequela

● **S54.0**   Injury of ulnar nerve at forearm level
            Injury of ulnar nerve NOS
    X● **S54.00**   Injury of ulnar nerve at forearm level, unspecified arm
    X● **S54.01**   Injury of ulnar nerve at forearm level, right arm
    X● **S54.02**   Injury of ulnar nerve at forearm level, left arm
● **S54.1**   Injury of median nerve at forearm level
            Injury of median nerve NOS
    X● **S54.10**   Injury of median nerve at forearm level, unspecified arm
    X● **S54.11**   Injury of median nerve at forearm level, right arm
    X● **S54.12**   Injury of median nerve at forearm level, left arm
● **S54.2**   Injury of radial nerve at forearm level
            Injury of radial nerve NOS
    X● **S54.20**   Injury of radial nerve at forearm level, unspecified arm
    X● **S54.21**   Injury of radial nerve at forearm level, right arm
    X● **S54.22**   Injury of radial nerve at forearm level, left arm
● **S54.3**   Injury of cutaneous sensory nerve at forearm level
    X● **S54.30**   Injury of cutaneous sensory nerve at forearm level, unspecified arm
    X● **S54.31**   Injury of cutaneous sensory nerve at forearm level, right arm
    X● **S54.32**   Injury of cutaneous sensory nerve at forearm level, left arm

CHAPTER 19 (S00-T88)

- ● S54.8   Injury of other nerves at forearm level
  - ● S54.8X   Injury of other nerves at forearm level
    - ● S54.8X1   Injury of other nerves at forearm level, right arm
    - ● S54.8X2   Injury of other nerves at forearm level, left arm
    - ● S54.8X9   Injury of other nerves at forearm level, unspecified arm
- ● S54.9   Injury of unspecified nerve at forearm level
  - X ● S54.90   Injury of unspecified nerve at forearm level, unspecified arm
  - X ● S54.91   Injury of unspecified nerve at forearm level, right arm
  - X ● S54.92   Injury of unspecified nerve at forearm level, left arm

- ● S55   Injury of blood vessels at forearm level

  Code also any associated open wound (S51.-)

  Excludes2   injury of blood vessels at wrist and hand level (S65.-)
                 injury of brachial vessels (S45.1-S45.2)

  The appropriate 7th character is to be added to each code from category S55

A	initial encounter
D	subsequent encounter
S	sequela

  - ● S55.0   Injury of ulnar artery at forearm level
    - ● S55.00   Unspecified injury of ulnar artery at forearm level
      - ● S55.001   Unspecified injury of ulnar artery at forearm level, right arm
      - ● S55.002   Unspecified injury of ulnar artery at forearm level, left arm
      - ● S55.009   Unspecified injury of ulnar artery at forearm level, unspecified arm
    - ● S55.01   Laceration of ulnar artery at forearm level
      - ● S55.011   Laceration of ulnar artery at forearm level, right arm
      - ● S55.012   Laceration of ulnar artery at forearm level, left arm
      - ● S55.019   Laceration of ulnar artery at forearm level, unspecified arm
    - ● S55.09   Other specified injury of ulnar artery at forearm level
      - ● S55.091   Other specified injury of ulnar artery at forearm level, right arm
      - ● S55.092   Other specified injury of ulnar artery at forearm level, left arm
      - ● S55.099   Other specified injury of ulnar artery at forearm level, unspecified arm
  - ● S55.1   Injury of radial artery at forearm level
    - ● S55.10   Unspecified injury of radial artery at forearm level
      - ● S55.101   Unspecified injury of radial artery at forearm level, right arm
      - ● S55.102   Unspecified injury of radial artery at forearm level, left arm
      - ● S55.109   Unspecified injury of radial artery at forearm level, unspecified arm
    - ● S55.11   Laceration of radial artery at forearm level
      - ● S55.111   Laceration of radial artery at forearm level, right arm
      - ● S55.112   Laceration of radial artery at forearm level, left arm
      - ● S55.119   Laceration of radial artery at forearm level, unspecified arm

  - ● S55.19   Other specified injury of radial artery at forearm level
    - ● S55.191   Other specified injury of radial artery at forearm level, right arm
    - ● S55.192   Other specified injury of radial artery at forearm level, left arm
    - ● S55.199   Other specified injury of radial artery at forearm level, unspecified arm
  - ● S55.2   Injury of vein at forearm level
    - ● S55.20   Unspecified injury of vein at forearm level
      - ● S55.201   Unspecified injury of vein at forearm level, right arm
      - ● S55.202   Unspecified injury of vein at forearm level, left arm
      - ● S55.209   Unspecified injury of vein at forearm level, unspecified arm
    - ● S55.21   Laceration of vein at forearm level
      - ● S55.211   Laceration of vein at forearm level, right arm
      - ● S55.212   Laceration of vein at forearm level, left arm
      - ● S55.219   Laceration of vein at forearm level, unspecified arm
    - ● S55.29   Other specified injury of vein at forearm level
      - ● S55.291   Other specified injury of vein at forearm level, right arm
      - ● S55.292   Other specified injury of vein at forearm level, left arm
      - ● S55.299   Other specified injury of vein at forearm level, unspecified arm
  - ● S55.8   Injury of other blood vessels at forearm level
    - ● S55.80   Unspecified injury of other blood vessels at forearm level
      - ● S55.801   Unspecified injury of other blood vessels at forearm level, right arm
      - ● S55.802   Unspecified injury of other blood vessels at forearm level, left arm
      - ● S55.809   Unspecified injury of other blood vessels at forearm level, unspecified arm
    - ● S55.81   Laceration of other blood vessels at forearm level
      - ● S55.811   Laceration of other blood vessels at forearm level, right arm
      - ● S55.812   Laceration of other blood vessels at forearm level, left arm
      - ● S55.819   Laceration of other blood vessels at forearm level, unspecified arm
    - ● S55.89   Other specified injury of other blood vessels at forearm level
      - ● S55.891   Other specified injury of other blood vessels at forearm level, right arm
      - ● S55.892   Other specified injury of other blood vessels at forearm level, left arm
      - ● S55.899   Other specified injury of other blood vessels at forearm level, unspecified arm
  - ● S55.9   Injury of unspecified blood vessel at forearm level
    - ● S55.90   Unspecified injury of unspecified blood vessel at forearm level
      - ● S55.901   Unspecified injury of unspecified blood vessel at forearm level, right arm
      - ● S55.902   Unspecified injury of unspecified blood vessel at forearm level, left arm
      - ● S55.909   Unspecified injury of unspecified blood vessel at forearm level, unspecified arm

● S55.91   Laceration of unspecified blood vessel at forearm level
     ● S55.911   Laceration of unspecified blood vessel at forearm level, right arm
     ● S55.912   Laceration of unspecified blood vessel at forearm level, left arm
     ● S55.919   Laceration of unspecified blood vessel at forearm level, unspecified arm
● S55.99   Other specified injury of unspecified blood vessel at forearm level
     ● S55.991   Other specified injury of unspecified blood vessel at forearm level, right arm
     ● S55.992   Other specified injury of unspecified blood vessel at forearm level, left arm
     ● S55.999   Other specified injury of unspecified blood vessel at forearm level, unspecified arm

● S56   Injury of muscle, fascia and tendon at forearm level
     Code also any associated open wound (S51.-)
     Excludes2   injury of muscle, fascia and tendon at or below wrist (S66.-)
              sprain of joints and ligaments of elbow (S53.4-)
     The appropriate 7th character is to be added to each code from category S56

     | | |
     A   initial encounter
     D   subsequent encounter
     S   sequela

● S56.0   Injury of flexor muscle, fascia and tendon of thumb at forearm level
     ● S56.00   Unspecified injury of flexor muscle, fascia and tendon of thumb at forearm level
         ● S56.001   Unspecified injury of flexor muscle, fascia and tendon of right thumb at forearm level
         ● S56.002   Unspecified injury of flexor muscle, fascia and tendon of left thumb at forearm level
         ● S56.009   Unspecified injury of flexor muscle, fascia and tendon of unspecified thumb at forearm level
     ● S56.01   Strain of flexor muscle, fascia and tendon of thumb at forearm level
         ● S56.011   Strain of flexor muscle, fascia and tendon of right thumb at forearm level
         ● S56.012   Strain of flexor muscle, fascia and tendon of left thumb at forearm level
         ● S56.019   Strain of flexor muscle, fascia and tendon of unspecified thumb at forearm level
     ● S56.02   Laceration of flexor muscle, fascia and tendon of thumb at forearm level
         ● S56.021   Laceration of flexor muscle, fascia and tendon of right thumb at forearm level
         ● S56.022   Laceration of flexor muscle, fascia and tendon of left thumb at forearm level
         ● S56.029   Laceration of flexor muscle, fascia and tendon of unspecified thumb at forearm level

● S56.09   Other injury of flexor muscle, fascia and tendon of thumb at forearm level
     ● S56.091   Other injury of flexor muscle, fascia and tendon of right thumb at forearm level
     ● S56.092   Other injury of flexor muscle, fascia and tendon of left thumb at forearm level
     ● S56.099   Other injury of flexor muscle, fascia and tendon of unspecified thumb at forearm level

● S56.1   Injury of flexor muscle, fascia and tendon of other and unspecified finger at forearm level
     ● S56.10   Unspecified injury of flexor muscle, fascia and tendon of other and unspecified finger at forearm level
         ● S56.101   Unspecified injury of flexor muscle, fascia and tendon of right index finger at forearm level
         ● S56.102   Unspecified injury of flexor muscle, fascia and tendon of left index finger at forearm level
         ● S56.103   Unspecified injury of flexor muscle, fascia and tendon of right middle finger at forearm level
         ● S56.104   Unspecified injury of flexor muscle, fascia and tendon of left middle finger at forearm level
         ● S56.105   Unspecified injury of flexor muscle, fascia and tendon of right ring finger at forearm level
         ● S56.106   Unspecified injury of flexor muscle, fascia and tendon of left ring finger at forearm level
         ● S56.107   Unspecified injury of flexor muscle, fascia and tendon of right little finger at forearm level
         ● S56.108   Unspecified injury of flexor muscle, fascia and tendon of left little finger at forearm level
         ● S56.109   Unspecified injury of flexor muscle, fascia and tendon of unspecified finger at forearm level
     ● S56.11   Strain of flexor muscle, fascia and tendon of other and unspecified finger at forearm level
         ● S56.111   Strain of flexor muscle, fascia and tendon of right index finger at forearm level
         ● S56.112   Strain of flexor muscle, fascia and tendon of left index finger at forearm level
         ● S56.113   Strain of flexor muscle, fascia and tendon of right middle finger at forearm level
         ● S56.114   Strain of flexor muscle, fascia and tendon of left middle finger at forearm level
         ● S56.115   Strain of flexor muscle, fascia and tendon of right ring finger at forearm level
         ● S56.116   Strain of flexor muscle, fascia and tendon of left ring finger at forearm level
         ● S56.117   Strain of flexor muscle, fascia and tendon of right little finger at forearm level

CHAPTER 19 (S00-T88)

- S56.118   Strain of flexor muscle, fascia and tendon of left little finger at forearm level
- S56.119   Strain of flexor muscle, fascia and tendon of finger of unspecified finger at forearm level
- S56.12   Laceration of flexor muscle, fascia and tendon of other and unspecified finger at forearm level
  - S56.121   Laceration of flexor muscle, fascia and tendon of right index finger at forearm level
  - S56.122   Laceration of flexor muscle, fascia and tendon of left index finger at forearm level
  - S56.123   Laceration of flexor muscle, fascia and tendon of right middle finger at forearm level
  - S56.124   Laceration of flexor muscle, fascia and tendon of left middle finger at forearm level
  - S56.125   Laceration of flexor muscle, fascia and tendon of right ring finger at forearm level
  - S56.126   Laceration of flexor muscle, fascia and tendon of left ring finger at forearm level
  - S56.127   Laceration of flexor muscle, fascia and tendon of right little finger at forearm level
  - S56.128   Laceration of flexor muscle, fascia and tendon of left little finger at forearm level
  - S56.129   Laceration of flexor muscle, fascia and tendon of unspecified finger at forearm level
- S56.19   Other injury of flexor muscle, fascia and tendon of other and unspecified finger at forearm level
  - S56.191   Other injury of flexor muscle, fascia and tendon of right index finger at forearm level
  - S56.192   Other injury of flexor muscle, fascia and tendon of left index finger at forearm level
  - S56.193   Other injury of flexor muscle, fascia and tendon of right middle finger at forearm level
  - S56.194   Other injury of flexor muscle, fascia and tendon of left middle finger at forearm level
  - S56.195   Other injury of flexor muscle, fascia and tendon of right ring finger at forearm level
  - S56.196   Other injury of flexor muscle, fascia and tendon of left ring finger at forearm level
  - S56.197   Other injury of flexor muscle, fascia and tendon of right little finger at forearm level
  - S56.198   Other injury of flexor muscle, fascia and tendon of left little finger at forearm level
  - S56.199   Other injury of flexor muscle, fascia and tendon of unspecified finger at forearm level

- S56.2   Injury of other flexor muscle, fascia and tendon at forearm level
  - S56.20   Unspecified injury of other flexor muscle, fascia and tendon at forearm level
    - S56.201   Unspecified injury of other flexor muscle, fascia and tendon at forearm level, right arm
    - S56.202   Unspecified injury of other flexor muscle, fascia and tendon at forearm level, left arm
    - S56.209   Unspecified injury of other flexor muscle, fascia and tendon at forearm level, unspecified arm
  - S56.21   Strain of other flexor muscle, fascia and tendon at forearm level
    - S56.211   Strain of other flexor muscle, fascia and tendon at forearm level, right arm
    - S56.212   Strain of other flexor muscle, fascia and tendon at forearm level, left arm
    - S56.219   Strain of other flexor muscle, fascia and tendon at forearm level, unspecified arm
  - S56.22   Laceration of other flexor muscle, fascia and tendon at forearm level
    - S56.221   Laceration of other flexor muscle, fascia and tendon at forearm level, right arm
    - S56.222   Laceration of other flexor muscle, fascia and tendon at forearm level, left arm
    - S56.229   Laceration of other flexor muscle, fascia and tendon at forearm level, unspecified arm
  - S56.29   Other injury of other flexor muscle, fascia and tendon at forearm level
    - S56.291   Other injury of other flexor muscle, fascia and tendon at forearm level, right arm
    - S56.292   Other injury of other flexor muscle, fascia and tendon at forearm level, left arm
    - S56.299   Other injury of other flexor muscle, fascia and tendon at forearm level, unspecified arm
- S56.3   Injury of extensor or abductor muscles, fascia and tendons of thumb at forearm level
  - S56.30   Unspecified injury of extensor or abductor muscles, fascia and tendons of thumb at forearm level
    - S56.301   Unspecified injury of extensor or abductor muscles, fascia and tendons of right thumb at forearm level
    - S56.302   Unspecified injury of extensor or abductor muscles, fascia and tendons of left thumb at forearm level
    - S56.309   Unspecified injury of extensor or abductor muscles, fascia and tendons of unspecified thumb at forearm level
  - S56.31   Strain of extensor or abductor muscles, fascia and tendons of thumb at forearm level
    - S56.311   Strain of extensor or abductor muscles, fascia and tendons of right thumb at forearm level
    - S56.312   Strain of extensor or abductor muscles, fascia and tendons of left thumb at forearm level
    - S56.319   Strain of extensor or abductor muscles, fascia and tendons of unspecified thumb at forearm level

▶ New   ⇒ Revised   deleted Deleted   Excludes 1   Excludes 2   Includes   Use additional   Code first   Code also   Key words

OGCR Official Guidelines   X Assign placeholder X   ● Use Additional Character(s)   ▷ Manifestation Code   🏷 Hierarchical Condition Category   Coding Clinic

● S56.32 Laceration of extensor or abductor muscles, fascia and tendons of thumb at forearm level
  ● S56.321 Laceration of extensor or abductor muscles, fascia and tendons of right thumb at forearm level
  ● S56.322 Laceration of extensor or abductor muscles, fascia and tendons of left thumb at forearm level
  ● S56.329 Laceration of extensor or abductor muscles, fascia and tendons of unspecified thumb at forearm level

● S56.39 Other injury of extensor or abductor muscles, fascia and tendons of thumb at forearm level
  ● S56.391 Other injury of extensor or abductor muscles, fascia and tendons of right thumb at forearm level
  ● S56.392 Other injury of extensor or abductor muscles, fascia and tendons of left thumb at forearm level
  ● S56.399 Other injury of extensor or abductor muscles, fascia and tendons of unspecified thumb at forearm level

● S56.4 Injury of extensor muscle, fascia and tendon of other and unspecified finger at forearm level
  ● S56.40 Unspecified injury of extensor muscle, fascia and tendon of other and unspecified finger at forearm level
    ● S56.401 Unspecified injury of extensor muscle, fascia and tendon of right index finger at forearm level
    ● S56.402 Unspecified injury of extensor muscle, fascia and tendon of left index finger at forearm level
    ● S56.403 Unspecified injury of extensor muscle, fascia and tendon of right middle finger at forearm level
    ● S56.404 Unspecified injury of extensor muscle, fascia and tendon of left middle finger at forearm level
    ● S56.405 Unspecified injury of extensor muscle, fascia and tendon of right ring finger at forearm level
    ● S56.406 Unspecified injury of extensor muscle, fascia and tendon of left ring finger at forearm level
    ● S56.407 Unspecified injury of extensor muscle, fascia and tendon of right little finger at forearm level
    ● S56.408 Unspecified injury of extensor muscle, fascia and tendon of left little finger at forearm level
    ● S56.409 Unspecified injury of extensor muscle, fascia and tendon of unspecified finger at forearm level

  ● S56.41 Strain of extensor muscle, fascia and tendon of other and unspecified finger at forearm level
    ● S56.411 Strain of extensor muscle, fascia and tendon of right index finger at forearm level
    ● S56.412 Strain of extensor muscle, fascia and tendon of left index finger at forearm level
    ● S56.413 Strain of extensor muscle, fascia and tendon of right middle finger at forearm level

    ● S56.414 Strain of extensor muscle, fascia and tendon of left middle finger at forearm level
    ● S56.415 Strain of extensor muscle, fascia and tendon of right ring finger at forearm level
    ● S56.416 Strain of extensor muscle, fascia and tendon of left ring finger at forearm level
    ● S56.417 Strain of extensor muscle, fascia and tendon of right little finger at forearm level
    ● S56.418 Strain of extensor muscle, fascia and tendon of left little finger at forearm level
    ● S56.419 Strain of extensor muscle, fascia and tendon of finger, unspecified finger at forearm level

● S56.42 Laceration of extensor muscle, fascia and tendon of other and unspecified finger at forearm level
  ● S56.421 Laceration of extensor muscle, fascia and tendon of right index finger at forearm level
  ● S56.422 Laceration of extensor muscle, fascia and tendon of left index finger at forearm level
  ● S56.423 Laceration of extensor muscle, fascia and tendon of right middle finger at forearm level
  ● S56.424 Laceration of extensor muscle, fascia and tendon of left middle finger at forearm level
  ● S56.425 Laceration of extensor muscle, fascia and tendon of right ring finger at forearm level
  ● S56.426 Laceration of extensor muscle, fascia and tendon of left ring finger at forearm level
  ● S56.427 Laceration of extensor muscle, fascia and tendon of right little finger at forearm level
  ● S56.428 Laceration of extensor muscle, fascia and tendon of left little finger at forearm level
  ● S56.429 Laceration of extensor muscle, fascia and tendon of unspecified finger at forearm level

● S56.49 Other injury of extensor muscle, fascia and tendon of other and unspecified finger at forearm level
  ● S56.491 Other injury of extensor muscle, fascia and tendon of right index finger at forearm level
  ● S56.492 Other injury of extensor muscle, fascia and tendon of left index finger at forearm level
  ● S56.493 Other injury of extensor muscle, fascia and tendon of right middle finger at forearm level
  ● S56.494 Other injury of extensor muscle, fascia and tendon of left middle finger at forearm level
  ● S56.495 Other injury of extensor muscle, fascia and tendon of right ring finger at forearm level

● S56.496   Other injury of extensor muscle, fascia and tendon of left ring finger at forearm level

● S56.497   Other injury of extensor muscle, fascia and tendon of right little finger at forearm level

● S56.498   Other injury of extensor muscle, fascia and tendon of left little finger at forearm level

● S56.499   Other injury of extensor muscle, fascia and tendon of unspecified finger at forearm level

● S56.5   Injury of other extensor muscle, fascia and tendon at forearm level

  ● S56.50   Unspecified injury of other extensor muscle, fascia and tendon at forearm level

    ● S56.501   Unspecified injury of other extensor muscle, fascia and tendon at forearm level, right arm

    ● S56.502   Unspecified injury of other extensor muscle, fascia and tendon at forearm level, left arm

    ● S56.509   Unspecified injury of other extensor muscle, fascia and tendon at forearm level, unspecified arm

  ● S56.51   Strain of other extensor muscle, fascia and tendon at forearm level

    ● S56.511   Strain of other extensor muscle, fascia and tendon at forearm level, right arm

    ● S56.512   Strain of other extensor muscle, fascia and tendon at forearm level, left arm

    ● S56.519   Strain of other extensor muscle, fascia and tendon at forearm level, unspecified arm

  ● S56.52   Laceration of other extensor muscle, fascia and tendon at forearm level

    ● S56.521   Laceration of other extensor muscle, fascia and tendon at forearm level, right arm

    ● S56.522   Laceration of other extensor muscle, fascia and tendon at forearm level, left arm

    ● S56.529   Laceration of other extensor muscle, fascia and tendon at forearm level, unspecified arm

  ● S56.59   Other injury of other extensor muscle, fascia and tendon at forearm level

    ● S56.591   Other injury of other extensor muscle, fascia and tendon at forearm level, right arm

    ● S56.592   Other injury of other extensor muscle, fascia and tendon at forearm level, left arm

    ● S56.599   Other injury of other extensor muscle, fascia and tendon at forearm level, unspecified arm

● S56.8   Injury of other muscles, fascia and tendons at forearm level

  ● S56.80   Unspecified injury of other muscles, fascia and tendons at forearm level

    ● S56.801   Unspecified injury of other muscles, fascia and tendons at forearm level, right arm

    ● S56.802   Unspecified injury of other muscles, fascia and tendons at forearm level, left arm

    ● S56.809   Unspecified injury of other muscles, fascia and tendons at forearm level, unspecified arm

● S56.81   Strain of other muscles, fascia and tendons at forearm level

  ● S56.811   Strain of other muscles, fascia and tendons at forearm level, right arm

  ● S56.812   Strain of other muscles, fascia and tendons at forearm level, left arm

  ● S56.819   Strain of other muscles, fascia and tendons at forearm level, unspecified arm

● S56.82   Laceration of other muscles, fascia and tendons at forearm level

  ● S56.821   Laceration of other muscles, fascia and tendons at forearm level, right arm

  ● S56.822   Laceration of other muscles, fascia and tendons at forearm level, left arm

  ● S56.829   Laceration of other muscles, fascia and tendons at forearm level, unspecified arm

● S56.89   Other injury of other muscles, fascia and tendons at forearm level

  ● S56.891   Other injury of other muscles, fascia and tendons at forearm level, right arm

  ● S56.892   Other injury of other muscles, fascia and tendons at forearm level, left arm

  ● S56.899   Other injury of other muscles, fascia and tendons at forearm level, unspecified arm

● S56.9   Injury of unspecified muscles, fascia and tendons at forearm level

  ● S56.90   Unspecified injury of unspecified muscles, fascia and tendons at forearm level

    ● S56.901   Unspecified injury of unspecified muscles, fascia and tendons at forearm level, right arm

    ● S56.902   Unspecified injury of unspecified muscles, fascia and tendons at forearm level, left arm

    ● S56.909   Unspecified injury of unspecified muscles, fascia and tendons at forearm level, unspecified arm

  ● S56.91   Strain of unspecified muscles, fascia and tendons at forearm level

    ● S56.911   Strain of unspecified muscles, fascia and tendons at forearm level, right arm

    ● S56.912   Strain of unspecified muscles, fascia and tendons at forearm level, left arm

    ● S56.919   Strain of unspecified muscles, fascia and tendons at forearm level, unspecified arm

  ● S56.92   Laceration of unspecified muscles, fascia and tendons at forearm level

    ● S56.921   Laceration of unspecified muscles, fascia and tendons at forearm level, right arm

    ● S56.922   Laceration of unspecified muscles, fascia and tendons at forearm level, left arm

    ● S56.929   Laceration of unspecified muscles, fascia and tendons at forearm level, unspecified arm

S56.99   Other injury of unspecified muscles, fascia and tendons at forearm level

● S56.991   Other injury of unspecified muscles, fascia and tendons at forearm level, right arm

● S56.992   Other injury of unspecified muscles, fascia and tendons at forearm level, left arm

● S56.999   Other injury of unspecified muscles, fascia and tendons at forearm level, unspecified arm

● **S57   Crushing injury of elbow and forearm**

Use additional code(s) for all associated injuries

Excludes2   crushing injury of wrist and hand (S67.-)

The appropriate 7th character is to be added to each code from category S57

A	initial encounter
D	subsequent encounter
S	sequela

● S57.0   Crushing injury of elbow

X ● S57.00   Crushing injury of unspecified elbow

X ● S57.01   Crushing injury of right elbow

X ● S57.02   Crushing injury of left elbow

● S57.8   Crushing injury of forearm

X ● S57.80   Crushing injury of unspecified forearm

X ● S57.81   Crushing injury of right forearm

X ● S57.82   Crushing injury of left forearm

● **S58   Traumatic amputation of elbow and forearm**

An amputation not identified as partial or complete should be coded to complete

Excludes1   traumatic amputation of wrist and hand (S68.-)

The appropriate 7th character is to be added to each code from category S58

A	initial encounter
D	subsequent encounter
S	sequela

● S58.0   Traumatic amputation at elbow level

● S58.01   Complete traumatic amputation at elbow level

● S58.011   Complete traumatic amputation at elbow level, right arm A, S 🔾

● S58.012   Complete traumatic amputation at elbow level, left arm A, S 🔾

● S58.019   Complete traumatic amputation at elbow level, unspecified arm A, S 🔾

● S58.02   Partial traumatic amputation at elbow level

● S58.021   Partial traumatic amputation at elbow level, right arm A, S 🔾

● S58.022   Partial traumatic amputation at elbow level, left arm A, S 🔾

● S58.029   Partial traumatic amputation at elbow level, unspecified arm A, S 🔾

● S58.1   Traumatic amputation at level between elbow and wrist

● S58.11   Complete traumatic amputation at level between elbow and wrist

● S58.111   Complete traumatic amputation at level between elbow and wrist, right arm A, S 🔾

● S58.112   Complete traumatic amputation at level between elbow and wrist, left arm A, S 🔾

● S58.119   Complete traumatic amputation at level between elbow and wrist, unspecified arm A, S 🔾

Item 19–4   SALTER-HARRIS TYPE 1: epiphysis is completely separated from end of bone, or metaphysic growth plate remains attached to epiphysis

SALTER-HARRIS TYPE 2: epiphysis and growth plate are partially separated from metaphysis, which is cracked—most common type

SALTER-HARRIS TYPE 3: fracture occurring through epiphysis and separates part of epiphysis and growth plate from metaphysis fracture, usually at distal end of tibia

SALTER-HARRIS TYPE 4: fracture runs through epiphysis, across growth plate, into metaphysic, surgery is required to restore joint surface to normal and align growth plate

● S58.12   Partial traumatic amputation at level between elbow and wrist

● S58.121   Partial traumatic amputation at level between elbow and wrist, right arm A, S 🔾

● S58.122   Partial traumatic amputation at level between elbow and wrist, left arm A, S 🔾

● S58.129   Partial traumatic amputation at level between elbow and wrist, unspecified arm A, S 🔾

● S58.9   Traumatic amputation of forearm, level unspecified

Excludes1   traumatic amputation of wrist (S68.-)

● S58.91   Complete traumatic amputation of forearm, level unspecified

● S58.911   Complete traumatic amputation of right forearm, level unspecified A, S 🔾

● S58.912   Complete traumatic amputation of left forearm, level unspecified A, S 🔾

● S58.919   Complete traumatic amputation of unspecified forearm, level unspecified A, S 🔾

● S58.92   Partial traumatic amputation of forearm, level unspecified

● S58.921   Partial traumatic amputation of right forearm, level unspecified A, S 🔾

● S58.922   Partial traumatic amputation of left forearm, level unspecified A, S 🔾

● S58.929   Partial traumatic amputation of unspecified forearm, level unspecified A, S 🔾

● **S59   Other and unspecified injuries of elbow and forearm**

Excludes2   other and unspecified injuries of wrist and hand (S69.-)

The appropriate 7th character is to be added to each code from subcategories S59.0, S59.1, and S59.2

A	initial encounter for closed fracture
D	subsequent encounter for fracture with routine healing
G	subsequent encounter for fracture with delayed healing
K	subsequent encounter for fracture with nonunion
P	subsequent encounter for fracture with malunion
S	sequela

● S59.0   Physeal fracture of lower end of ulna

● S59.00   Unspecified physeal fracture of lower end of ulna

● S59.001   Unspecified physeal fracture of lower end of ulna, right arm

● S59.002   Unspecified physeal fracture of lower end of ulna, left arm

● S59.009   Unspecified physeal fracture of lower end of ulna, unspecified arm

CHAPTER 19 (S00-T88)

- S59.01   Salter-Harris Type I physeal fracture of lower end of ulna
  - S59.011   Salter-Harris Type I physeal fracture of lower end of ulna, right arm
  - S59.012   Salter-Harris Type I physeal fracture of lower end of ulna, left arm
  - S59.019   Salter-Harris Type I physeal fracture of lower end of ulna, unspecified arm
- S59.02   Salter-Harris Type II physeal fracture of lower end of ulna
  - S59.021   Salter-Harris Type II physeal fracture of lower end of ulna, right arm
  - S59.022   Salter-Harris Type II physeal fracture of lower end of ulna, left arm
  - S59.029   Salter-Harris Type II physeal fracture of lower end of ulna, unspecified arm
- S59.03   Salter-Harris Type III physeal fracture of lower end of ulna
  - S59.031   Salter-Harris Type III physeal fracture of lower end of ulna, right arm
  - S59.032   Salter-Harris Type III physeal fracture of lower end of ulna, left arm
  - S59.039   Salter-Harris Type III physeal fracture of lower end of ulna, unspecified arm
- S59.04   Salter-Harris Type IV physeal fracture of lower end of ulna
  - S59.041   Salter-Harris Type IV physeal fracture of lower end of ulna, right arm
  - S59.042   Salter-Harris Type IV physeal fracture of lower end of ulna, left arm
  - S59.049   Salter-Harris Type IV physeal fracture of lower end of ulna, unspecified arm
- S59.09   Other physeal fracture of lower end of ulna
  - S59.091   Other physeal fracture of lower end of ulna, right arm
  - S59.092   Other physeal fracture of lower end of ulna, left arm
  - S59.099   Other physeal fracture of lower end of ulna, unspecified arm
- S59.1   Physeal fracture of upper end of radius
  - S59.10   Unspecified physeal fracture of upper end of radius
    - S59.101   Unspecified physeal fracture of upper end of radius, right arm
    - S59.102   Unspecified physeal fracture of upper end of radius, left arm
    - S59.109   Unspecified physeal fracture of upper end of radius, unspecified arm
  - S59.11   Salter-Harris Type I physeal fracture of upper end of radius
    - S59.111   Salter-Harris Type I physeal fracture of upper end of radius, right arm
    - S59.112   Salter-Harris Type I physeal fracture of upper end of radius, left arm
    - S59.119   Salter-Harris Type I physeal fracture of upper end of radius, unspecified arm
  - S59.12   Salter-Harris Type II physeal fracture of upper end of radius
    - S59.121   Salter-Harris Type II physeal fracture of upper end of radius, right arm
    - S59.122   Salter-Harris Type II physeal fracture of upper end of radius, left arm
    - S59.129   Salter-Harris Type II physeal fracture of upper end of radius, unspecified arm

- S59.13   Salter-Harris Type III physeal fracture of upper end of radius
  - S59.131   Salter-Harris Type III physeal fracture of upper end of radius, right arm
  - S59.132   Salter-Harris Type III physeal fracture of upper end of radius, left arm
  - S59.139   Salter-Harris Type III physeal fracture of upper end of radius, unspecified arm
- S59.14   Salter-Harris Type IV physeal fracture of upper end of radius
  - S59.141   Salter-Harris Type IV physeal fracture of upper end of radius, right arm
  - S59.142   Salter-Harris Type IV physeal fracture of upper end of radius, left arm
  - S59.149   Salter-Harris Type IV physeal fracture of upper end of radius, unspecified arm
- S59.19   Other physeal fracture of upper end of radius
  - S59.191   Other physeal fracture of upper end of radius, right arm
  - S59.192   Other physeal fracture of upper end of radius, left arm
  - S59.199   Other physeal fracture of upper end of radius, unspecified arm
- S59.2   Physeal fracture of lower end of radius
  - S59.20   Unspecified physeal fracture of lower end of radius
    - S59.201   Unspecified physeal fracture of lower end of radius, right arm
    - S59.202   Unspecified physeal fracture of lower end of radius, left arm
    - S59.209   Unspecified physeal fracture of lower end of radius, unspecified arm
  - S59.21   Salter-Harris Type I physeal fracture of lower end of radius
    - S59.211   Salter-Harris Type I physeal fracture of lower end of radius, right arm
    - S59.212   Salter-Harris Type I physeal fracture of lower end of radius, left arm
    - S59.219   Salter-Harris Type I physeal fracture of lower end of radius, unspecified arm
  - S59.22   Salter-Harris Type II physeal fracture of lower end of radius
    - S59.221   Salter-Harris Type II physeal fracture of lower end of radius, right arm
    - S59.222   Salter-Harris Type II physeal fracture of lower end of radius, left arm
    - S59.229   Salter-Harris Type II physeal fracture of lower end of radius, unspecified arm
  - S59.23   Salter-Harris Type III physeal fracture of lower end of radius
    - S59.231   Salter-Harris Type III physeal fracture of lower end of radius, right arm
    - S59.232   Salter-Harris Type III physeal fracture of lower end of radius, left arm
    - S59.239   Salter-Harris Type III physeal fracture of lower end of radius, unspecified arm

▶ New   ⇒ Revised   ~~deleted~~ Deleted   Excludes 1   Excludes 2   Includes   Use additional   Code first   Code also   Key words

OGCR Official Guidelines   X Assign placeholder X   ● Use Additional Character(s)   ▶ Manifestation Code   Hierarchical Condition Category   Coding Clinic

● S59.24   Salter-Harris Type IV physeal fracture of lower end of radius
  ● S59.241   Salter-Harris Type IV physeal fracture of lower end of radius, right arm
  ● S59.242   Salter-Harris Type IV physeal fracture of lower end of radius, left arm
  ● S59.249   Salter-Harris Type IV physeal fracture of lower end of radius, unspecified arm
● S59.29   Other physeal fracture of lower end of radius
  ● S59.291   Other physeal fracture of lower end of radius, right arm
  ● S59.292   Other physeal fracture of lower end of radius, left arm
  ● S59.299   Other physeal fracture of lower end of radius, unspecified arm

● S59.8   Other specified injuries of elbow and forearm

The appropriate 7th character is to be added to each code in subcategory S59.8

> A   initial encounter
> D   subsequent encounter
> S   sequela

  ● S59.80   Other specified injuries of elbow
    ● S59.801   Other specified injuries of right elbow
    ● S59.802   Other specified injuries of left elbow
    ● S59.809   Other specified injuries of unspecified elbow

  ● S59.81   Other specified injuries of forearm
    ● S59.811   Other specified injuries right forearm
    ● S59.812   Other specified injuries left forearm
    ● S59.819   Other specified injuries unspecified forearm

● S59.9   Unspecified injury of elbow and forearm

The appropriate 7th character is to be added to each code in subcategory S59.9

> A   initial encounter
> D   subsequent encounter
> S   sequela

  ● S59.90   Unspecified injury of elbow
    ● S59.901   Unspecified injury of right elbow
    ● S59.902   Unspecified injury of left elbow
    ● S59.909   Unspecified injury of unspecified elbow

  ● S59.91   Unspecified injury of forearm
    ● S59.911   Unspecified injury of right forearm
    ● S59.912   Unspecified injury of left forearm
    ● S59.919   Unspecified injury of unspecified forearm

INJURIES TO THE WRIST, HAND AND FINGERS (S60-S69)

Excludes2   burns and corrosions (T20-T32)
frostbite (T33-T34)
insect bite or sting, venomous (T63.4)

● **S60**   Superficial injury of wrist, hand and fingers

The appropriate 7th character is to be added to each code from category S60

A   initial encounter
D   subsequent encounter
S   sequela

● **S60.0**   Contusion of finger without damage to nail
Excludes1   contusion involving nail (matrix) (S60.1)

X● **S60.00**   Contusion of unspecified finger without damage to nail
Contusion of finger(s) NOS

● **S60.01**   Contusion of thumb without damage to nail
● S60.011   Contusion of right thumb without damage to nail
● S60.012   Contusion of left thumb without damage to nail
● S60.019   Contusion of unspecified thumb without damage to nail

● **S60.02**   Contusion of index finger without damage to nail
● S60.021   Contusion of right index finger without damage to nail
● S60.022   Contusion of left index finger without damage to nail
● S60.029   Contusion of unspecified index finger without damage to nail

● **S60.03**   Contusion of middle finger without damage to nail
● S60.031   Contusion of right middle finger without damage to nail
● S60.032   Contusion of left middle finger without damage to nail
● S60.039   Contusion of unspecified middle finger without damage to nail

● **S60.04**   Contusion of ring finger without damage to nail
● S60.041   Contusion of right ring finger without damage to nail
● S60.042   Contusion of left ring finger without damage to nail
● S60.049   Contusion of unspecified ring finger without damage to nail

● **S60.05**   Contusion of little finger without damage to nail
● S60.051   Contusion of right little finger without damage to nail
● S60.052   Contusion of left little finger without damage to nail
● S60.059   Contusion of unspecified little finger without damage to nail

● **S60.1**   Contusion of finger with damage to nail
X● **S60.10**   Contusion of unspecified finger with damage to nail
● **S60.11**   Contusion of thumb with damage to nail
● S60.111   Contusion of right thumb with damage to nail
● S60.112   Contusion of left thumb with damage to nail
● S60.119   Contusion of unspecified thumb with damage to nail

● **S60.12**   Contusion of index finger with damage to nail
● S60.121   Contusion of right index finger with damage to nail
● S60.122   Contusion of left index finger with damage to nail
● S60.129   Contusion of unspecified index finger with damage to nail

● **S60.13**   Contusion of middle finger with damage to nail
● S60.131   Contusion of right middle finger with damage to nail
● S60.132   Contusion of left middle finger with damage to nail
● S60.139   Contusion of unspecified middle finger with damage to nail

● **S60.14**   Contusion of ring finger with damage to nail
● S60.141   Contusion of right ring finger with damage to nail
● S60.142   Contusion of left ring finger with damage to nail
● S60.149   Contusion of unspecified ring finger with damage to nail

● **S60.15**   Contusion of little finger with damage to nail
● S60.151   Contusion of right little finger with damage to nail
● S60.152   Contusion of left little finger with damage to nail
● S60.159   Contusion of unspecified little finger with damage to nail

● **S60.2**   Contusion of wrist and hand
Excludes2   contusion of fingers (S60.0-, S60.1-)
● **S60.21**   Contusion of wrist
● S60.211   Contusion of right wrist
● S60.212   Contusion of left wrist
● S60.219   Contusion of unspecified wrist
● **S60.22**   Contusion of hand
● S60.221   Contusion of right hand
● S60.222   Contusion of left hand
● S60.229   Contusion of unspecified hand

● **S60.3**   Other superficial injuries of thumb
● **S60.31**   Abrasion of thumb
● S60.311   Abrasion of right thumb
● S60.312   Abrasion of left thumb
● S60.319   Abrasion of unspecified thumb
● **S60.32**   Blister (nonthermal) of thumb
● S60.321   Blister (nonthermal) of right thumb
● S60.322   Blister (nonthermal) of left thumb
● S60.329   Blister (nonthermal) of unspecified thumb
● **S60.34**   External constriction of thumb
Hair tourniquet syndrome of thumb
Use additional cause code to identify the constricting item (W49.0-)
● S60.341   External constriction of right thumb
● S60.342   External constriction of left thumb
● S60.349   External constriction of unspecified thumb
● **S60.35**   Superficial foreign body of thumb
Splinter in the thumb
● S60.351   Superficial foreign body of right thumb
● S60.352   Superficial foreign body of left thumb
● S60.359   Superficial foreign body of unspecified thumb

CHAPTER 19 (S00-T88)

● S60.36 Insect bite (nonvenomous) of thumb
  ● S60.361 Insect bite (nonvenomous) of right thumb
  ● S60.362 Insect bite (nonvenomous) of left thumb
  ● S60.369 Insect bite (nonvenomous) of unspecified thumb
● S60.37 Other superficial bite of thumb
  Excludes1 open bite of thumb (S61.05-, S61.15-)
  ● S60.371 Other superficial bite of right thumb
  ● S60.372 Other superficial bite of left thumb
  ● S60.379 Other superficial bite of unspecified thumb
● S60.39 Other superficial injuries of thumb
  ● S60.391 Other superficial injuries of right thumb
  ● S60.392 Other superficial injuries of left thumb
  ● S60.399 Other superficial injuries of unspecified thumb
● S60.4 Other superficial injuries of other fingers
  ● S60.41 Abrasion of fingers
    ● S60.410 Abrasion of right index finger
    ● S60.411 Abrasion of left index finger
    ● S60.412 Abrasion of right middle finger
    ● S60.413 Abrasion of left middle finger
    ● S60.414 Abrasion of right ring finger
    ● S60.415 Abrasion of left ring finger
    ● S60.416 Abrasion of right little finger
    ● S60.417 Abrasion of left little finger
    ● S60.418 Abrasion of other finger
             Abrasion of specified finger with unspecified laterality
    ● S60.419 Abrasion of unspecified finger
  ● S60.42 Blister (nonthermal) of fingers
    ● S60.420 Blister (nonthermal) of right index finger
    ● S60.421 Blister (nonthermal) of left index finger
    ● S60.422 Blister (nonthermal) of right middle finger
    ● S60.423 Blister (nonthermal) of left middle finger
    ● S60.424 Blister (nonthermal) of right ring finger
    ● S60.425 Blister (nonthermal) of left ring finger
    ● S60.426 Blister (nonthermal) of right little finger
    ● S60.427 Blister (nonthermal) of left little finger
    ● S60.428 Blister (nonthermal) of other finger
             Blister (nonthermal) of specified finger with unspecified laterality
    ● S60.429 Blister (nonthermal) of unspecified finger
  ● S60.44 External constriction of fingers
           Hair tourniquet syndrome of finger
           Use additional cause code to identify the constricting item (W49.0-)
    ● S60.440 External constriction of right index finger
    ● S60.441 External constriction of left index finger

● S60.442 External constriction of right middle finger
● S60.443 External constriction of left middle finger
● S60.444 External constriction of right ring finger
● S60.445 External constriction of left ring finger
● S60.446 External constriction of right little finger
● S60.447 External constriction of left little finger
● S60.448 External constriction of other finger
           External constriction of specified finger with unspecified laterality
● S60.449 External constriction of unspecified finger
● S60.45 Superficial foreign body of fingers
         Splinter in the finger(s)
  ● S60.450 Superficial foreign body of right index finger
  ● S60.451 Superficial foreign body of left index finger
  ● S60.452 Superficial foreign body of right middle finger
  ● S60.453 Superficial foreign body of left middle finger
  ● S60.454 Superficial foreign body of right ring finger
  ● S60.455 Superficial foreign body of left ring finger
  ● S60.456 Superficial foreign body of right little finger
  ● S60.457 Superficial foreign body of left little finger
  ● S60.458 Superficial foreign body of other finger
           Superficial foreign body of specified finger with unspecified laterality
  ● S60.459 Superficial foreign body of unspecified finger
● S60.46 Insect bite (nonvenomous) of fingers
  ● S60.460 Insect bite (nonvenomous) of right index finger
  ● S60.461 Insect bite (nonvenomous) of left index finger
  ● S60.462 Insect bite (nonvenomous) of right middle finger
  ● S60.463 Insect bite (nonvenomous) of left middle finger
  ● S60.464 Insect bite (nonvenomous) of right ring finger
  ● S60.465 Insect bite (nonvenomous) of left ring finger
  ● S60.466 Insect bite (nonvenomous) of right little finger
  ● S60.467 Insect bite (nonvenomous) of left little finger
  ● S60.468 Insect bite (nonvenomous) of other finger
           Insect bite (nonvenomous) of specified finger with unspecified laterality
  ● S60.469 Insect bite (nonvenomous) of unspecified finger

CHAPTER 19 (S00-T88)

● **S60.47** Other superficial bite of fingers

    Excludes1   open bite of fingers (S61.25-, S61.35-)

  ● **S60.470** Other superficial bite of right index finger

  ● **S60.471** Other superficial bite of left index finger

  ● **S60.472** Other superficial bite of right middle finger

  ● **S60.473** Other superficial bite of left middle finger

  ● **S60.474** Other superficial bite of right ring finger

  ● **S60.475** Other superficial bite of left ring finger

  ● **S60.476** Other superficial bite of right little finger

  ● **S60.477** Other superficial bite of left little finger

  ● **S60.478** Other superficial bite of other finger

       Other superficial bite of specified finger with unspecified laterality

  ● **S60.479** Other superficial bite of unspecified finger

● **S60.5** Other superficial injuries of hand

    Excludes2   superficial injuries of fingers (S60.3-, S60.4-)

  ● **S60.51** Abrasion of hand

    ● **S60.511** Abrasion of right hand

    ● **S60.512** Abrasion of left hand

    ● **S60.519** Abrasion of unspecified hand

  ● **S60.52** Blister (nonthermal) of hand

    ● **S60.521** Blister (nonthermal) of right hand

    ● **S60.522** Blister (nonthermal) of left hand

    ● **S60.529** Blister (nonthermal) of unspecified hand

  ● **S60.54** External constriction of hand

    ● **S60.541** External constriction of right hand

    ● **S60.542** External constriction of left hand

    ● **S60.549** External constriction of unspecified hand

  ● **S60.55** Superficial foreign body of hand

     Splinter in the hand

    ● **S60.551** Superficial foreign body of right hand

    ● **S60.552** Superficial foreign body of left hand

    ● **S60.559** Superficial foreign body of unspecified hand

  ● **S60.56** Insect bite (nonvenomous) of hand

    ● **S60.561** Insect bite (nonvenomous) of right hand

    ● **S60.562** Insect bite (nonvenomous) of left hand

    ● **S60.569** Insect bite (nonvenomous) of unspecified hand

  ● **S60.57** Other superficial bite of hand

    Excludes1   open bite of hand (S61.45-)

    ● **S60.571** Other superficial bite of hand of right hand

    ● **S60.572** Other superficial bite of hand of left hand

    ● **S60.579** Other superficial bite of hand of unspecified hand

● **S60.8** Other superficial injuries of wrist

  ● **S60.81** Abrasion of wrist

    ● **S60.811** Abrasion of right wrist

    ● **S60.812** Abrasion of left wrist

    ● **S60.819** Abrasion of unspecified wrist

  ● **S60.82** Blister (nonthermal) of wrist

    ● **S60.821** Blister (nonthermal) of right wrist

    ● **S60.822** Blister (nonthermal) of left wrist

    ● **S60.829** Blister (nonthermal) of unspecified wrist

  ● **S60.84** External constriction of wrist

    ● **S60.841** External constriction of right wrist

    ● **S60.842** External constriction of left wrist

    ● **S60.849** External constriction of unspecified wrist

  ● **S60.85** Superficial foreign body of wrist

     Splinter in the wrist

    ● **S60.851** Superficial foreign body of right wrist

    ● **S60.852** Superficial foreign body of left wrist

    ● **S60.859** Superficial foreign body of unspecified wrist

  ● **S60.86** Insect bite (nonvenomous) of wrist

    ● **S60.861** Insect bite (nonvenomous) of right wrist

    ● **S60.862** Insect bite (nonvenomous) of left wrist

    ● **S60.869** Insect bite (nonvenomous) of unspecified wrist

  ● **S60.87** Other superficial bite of wrist

    Excludes1   open bite of wrist (S61.55)

    ● **S60.871** Other superficial bite of right wrist

    ● **S60.872** Other superficial bite of left wrist

    ● **S60.879** Other superficial bite of unspecified wrist

● **S60.9** Unspecified superficial injury of wrist, hand and fingers

  ● **S60.91** Unspecified superficial injury of wrist

    ● **S60.911** Unspecified superficial injury of right wrist

    ● **S60.912** Unspecified superficial injury of left wrist

    ● **S60.919** Unspecified superficial injury of unspecified wrist

  ● **S60.92** Unspecified superficial injury of hand

    ● **S60.921** Unspecified superficial injury of right hand

    ● **S60.922** Unspecified superficial injury of left hand

    ● **S60.929** Unspecified superficial injury of unspecified hand

  ● **S60.93** Unspecified superficial injury of thumb

    ● **S60.931** Unspecified superficial injury of right thumb

    ● **S60.932** Unspecified superficial injury of left thumb

    ● **S60.939** Unspecified superficial injury of unspecified thumb

▶ New   ⇒ Revised   ~~deleted~~ Deleted   Excludes 1   Excludes 2   Includes   Use additional   Code first   Code also   Key words

OGCR Official Guidelines   X Assign placeholder X   ● Use Additional Character(s)   ▷ Manifestation Code   🅿️ Hierarchical Condition Category   **Coding Clinic**

● **S60.94**   Unspecified superficial injury of other fingers
     ● S60.940   Unspecified superficial injury of right index finger
     ● S60.941   Unspecified superficial injury of left index finger
     ● S60.942   Unspecified superficial injury of right middle finger
     ● S60.943   Unspecified superficial injury of left middle finger
     ● S60.944   Unspecified superficial injury of right ring finger
     ● S60.945   Unspecified superficial injury of left ring finger
     ● S60.946   Unspecified superficial injury of right little finger
     ● S60.947   Unspecified superficial injury of left little finger
     ● S60.948   Unspecified superficial injury of other finger
         Unspecified superficial injury of specified finger with unspecified laterality
     ● S60.949   Unspecified superficial injury of unspecified finger

● **S61**   Open wound of wrist, hand and fingers
     Code also any associated wound infection
     Excludes1   open fracture of wrist, hand and finger (S62.- with 7th character B)
         traumatic amputation of wrist and hand (S68.-)
     The appropriate 7th character is to be added to each code from category S61

A	initial encounter
D	subsequent encounter
S	sequela

● **S61.0**   Open wound of thumb without damage to nail
     Excludes1   open wound of thumb with damage to nail (S61.1-)
     ● S61.00   Unspecified open wound of thumb without damage to nail
         ● S61.001   Unspecified open wound of right thumb without damage to nail
         ● S61.002   Unspecified open wound of left thumb without damage to nail
         ● S61.009   Unspecified open wound of unspecified thumb without damage to nail
     ● S61.01   Laceration without foreign body of thumb without damage to nail
         ● S61.011   Laceration without foreign body of right thumb without damage to nail
         ● S61.012   Laceration without foreign body of left thumb without damage to nail
         ● S61.019   Laceration without foreign body of unspecified thumb without damage to nail
     ● S61.02   Laceration with foreign body of thumb without damage to nail
         ● S61.021   Laceration with foreign body of right thumb without damage to nail
         ● S61.022   Laceration with foreign body of left thumb without damage to nail
         ● S61.029   Laceration with foreign body of unspecified thumb without damage to nail

● **S61.03**   Puncture wound without foreign body of thumb without damage to nail
     ● S61.031   Puncture wound without foreign body of right thumb without damage to nail
     ● S61.032   Puncture wound without foreign body of left thumb without damage to nail
     ● S61.039   Puncture wound without foreign body of unspecified thumb without damage to nail
● **S61.04**   Puncture wound with foreign body of thumb without damage to nail
     ● S61.041   Puncture wound with foreign body of right thumb without damage to nail
     ● S61.042   Puncture wound with foreign body of left thumb without damage to nail
     ● S61.049   Puncture wound with foreign body of unspecified thumb without damage to nail
● **S61.05**   Open bite of thumb without damage to nail
     Bite of thumb NOS
     Excludes1   superficial bite of thumb (S60.36-, S60.37-)
     ● S61.051   Open bite of right thumb without damage to nail
     ● S61.052   Open bite of left thumb without damage to nail
     ● S61.059   Open bite of unspecified thumb without damage to nail

● **S61.1**   Open wound of thumb with damage to nail
     ● S61.10   Unspecified open wound of thumb with damage to nail
         ● S61.101   Unspecified open wound of right thumb with damage to nail
         ● S61.102   Unspecified open wound of left thumb with damage to nail
         ● S61.109   Unspecified open wound of unspecified thumb with damage to nail
     ● S61.11   Laceration without foreign body of thumb with damage to nail
         ● S61.111   Laceration without foreign body of right thumb with damage to nail
         ● S61.112   Laceration without foreign body of left thumb with damage to nail
         ● S61.119   Laceration without foreign body of unspecified thumb with damage to nail
     ● S61.12   Laceration with foreign body of thumb with damage to nail
         ● S61.121   Laceration with foreign body of right thumb with damage to nail
         ● S61.122   Laceration with foreign body of left thumb with damage to nail
         ● S61.129   Laceration with foreign body of unspecified thumb with damage to nail

CHAPTER 19 (S00-T88)

- S61.13   Puncture wound without foreign body of thumb with damage to nail
  - S61.131   Puncture wound without foreign body of right thumb with damage to nail
  - S61.132   Puncture wound without foreign body of left thumb with damage to nail
  - S61.139   Puncture wound without foreign body of unspecified thumb with damage to nail
- S61.14   Puncture wound with foreign body of thumb with damage to nail
  - S61.141   Puncture wound with foreign body of right thumb with damage to nail
  - S61.142   Puncture wound with foreign body of left thumb with damage to nail
  - S61.149   Puncture wound with foreign body of unspecified thumb with damage to nail
- S61.15   Open bite of thumb with damage to nail
  Bite of thumb with damage to nail NOS

  Excludes1   superficial bite of thumb (S60.36-, S60.37-)
  - S61.151   Open bite of right thumb with damage to nail
  - S61.152   Open bite of left thumb with damage to nail
  - S61.159   Open bite of unspecified thumb with damage to nail
- S61.2   Open wound of other finger without damage to nail

  Excludes1   open wound of finger involving nail (matrix) (S61.3-)

  Excludes2   open wound of thumb without damage to nail (S61.0-)
  - S61.20   Unspecified open wound of other finger without damage to nail
    - S61.200   Unspecified open wound of right index finger without damage to nail
    - S61.201   Unspecified open wound of left index finger without damage to nail
    - S61.202   Unspecified open wound of right middle finger without damage to nail
    - S61.203   Unspecified open wound of left middle finger without damage to nail
    - S61.204   Unspecified open wound of right ring finger without damage to nail
    - S61.205   Unspecified open wound of left ring finger without damage to nail
    - S61.206   Unspecified open wound of right little finger without damage to nail
    - S61.207   Unspecified open wound of left little finger without damage to nail
    - S61.208   Unspecified open wound of other finger without damage to nail
      Unspecified open wound of specified finger with unspecified laterality without damage to nail
    - S61.209   Unspecified open wound of unspecified finger without damage to nail
  - S61.21   Laceration without foreign body of finger without damage to nail
    - S61.210   Laceration without foreign body of right index finger without damage to nail
    - S61.211   Laceration without foreign body of left index finger without damage to nail
    - S61.212   Laceration without foreign body of right middle finger without damage to nail
    - S61.213   Laceration without foreign body of left middle finger without damage to nail
    - S61.214   Laceration without foreign body of right ring finger without damage to nail
    - S61.215   Laceration without foreign body of left ring finger without damage to nail
    - S61.216   Laceration without foreign body of right little finger without damage to nail
    - S61.217   Laceration without foreign body of left little finger without damage to nail
    - S61.218   Laceration without foreign body of other finger without damage to nail
      Laceration without foreign body of specified finger with unspecified laterality without damage to nail
    - S61.219   Laceration without foreign body of unspecified finger without damage to nail
  - S61.22   Laceration with foreign body of finger without damage to nail
    - S61.220   Laceration with foreign body of right index finger without damage to nail
    - S61.221   Laceration with foreign body of left index finger without damage to nail
    - S61.222   Laceration with foreign body of right middle finger without damage to nail
    - S61.223   Laceration with foreign body of left middle finger without damage to nail
    - S61.224   Laceration with foreign body of right ring finger without damage to nail
    - S61.225   Laceration with foreign body of left ring finger without damage to nail
    - S61.226   Laceration with foreign body of right little finger without damage to nail
    - S61.227   Laceration with foreign body of left little finger without damage to nail
    - S61.228   Laceration with foreign body of other finger without damage to nail
      Laceration with foreign body of specified finger with unspecified laterality without damage to nail
    - S61.229   Laceration with foreign body of unspecified finger without damage to nail
  - S61.23   Puncture wound without foreign body of finger without damage to nail
    - S61.230   Puncture wound without foreign body of right index finger without damage to nail
    - S61.231   Puncture wound without foreign body of left index finger without damage to nail
    - S61.232   Puncture wound without foreign body of right middle finger without damage to nail
    - S61.233   Puncture wound without foreign body of left middle finger without damage to nail
    - S61.234   Puncture wound without foreign body of right ring finger without damage to nail

▶ New   ⇒ Revised   ~~deleted~~ Deleted   Excludes 1   Excludes 2   Includes   Use additional   Code first   Code also   Key words

OGCR Official Guidelines   X Assign placeholder X   ● Use Additional Character(s)   ▶ Manifestation Code   🔖 Hierarchical Condition Category   **Coding Clinic**

● S61.235 Puncture wound without foreign body of left ring finger without damage to nail

● S61.236 Puncture wound without foreign body of right little finger without damage to nail

● S61.237 Puncture wound without foreign body of left little finger without damage to nail

● S61.238 Puncture wound without foreign body of other finger without damage to nail

      Puncture wound without foreign body of specified finger with unspecified laterality without damage to nail

● S61.239 Puncture wound without foreign body of unspecified finger without damage to nail

● S61.24 Puncture wound with foreign body of finger without damage to nail

● S61.240 Puncture wound with foreign body of right index finger without damage to nail

● S61.241 Puncture wound with foreign body of left index finger without damage to nail

● S61.242 Puncture wound with foreign body of right middle finger without damage to nail

● S61.243 Puncture wound with foreign body of left middle finger without damage to nail

● S61.244 Puncture wound with foreign body of right ring finger without damage to nail

● S61.245 Puncture wound with foreign body of left ring finger without damage to nail

● S61.246 Puncture wound with foreign body of right little finger without damage to nail

● S61.247 Puncture wound with foreign body of left little finger without damage to nail

● S61.248 Puncture wound with foreign body of other finger without damage to nail

      Puncture wound with foreign body of specified finger with unspecified laterality without damage to nail

● S61.249 Puncture wound with foreign body of unspecified finger without damage to nail

● S61.25 Open bite of finger without damage to nail

      Bite of finger without damage to nail NOS

      Excludes1 superficial bite of finger (S60.46-, S60.47-)

● S61.250 Open bite of right index finger without damage to nail

● S61.251 Open bite of left index finger without damage to nail

● S61.252 Open bite of right middle finger without damage to nail

● S61.253 Open bite of left middle finger without damage to nail

● S61.254 Open bite of right ring finger without damage to nail

● S61.255 Open bite of left ring finger without damage to nail

● S61.256 Open bite of right little finger without damage to nail

● S61.257 Open bite of left little finger without damage to nail

● S61.258 Open bite of other finger without damage to nail

      Open bite of specified finger with unspecified laterality without damage to nail

● S61.259 Open bite of unspecified finger without damage to nail

● S61.3 Open wound of other finger with damage to nail

● S61.30 Unspecified open wound of finger with damage to nail

● S61.300 Unspecified open wound of right index finger with damage to nail

● S61.301 Unspecified open wound of left index finger with damage to nail

● S61.302 Unspecified open wound of right middle finger with damage to nail

● S61.303 Unspecified open wound of left middle finger with damage to nail

● S61.304 Unspecified open wound of right ring finger with damage to nail

● S61.305 Unspecified open wound of left ring finger with damage to nail

● S61.306 Unspecified open wound of right little finger with damage to nail

● S61.307 Unspecified open wound of left little finger with damage to nail

● S61.308 Unspecified open wound of other finger with damage to nail

      Unspecified open wound of specified finger with unspecified laterality with damage to nail

● S61.309 Unspecified open wound of unspecified finger with damage to nail

● S61.31 Laceration without foreign body of finger with damage to nail

● S61.310 Laceration without foreign body of right index finger with damage to nail

● S61.311 Laceration without foreign body of left index finger with damage to nail

● S61.312 Laceration without foreign body of right middle finger with damage to nail

● S61.313 Laceration without foreign body of left middle finger with damage to nail

● S61.314 Laceration without foreign body of right ring finger with damage to nail

● S61.315 Laceration without foreign body of left ring finger with damage to nail

● S61.316 Laceration without foreign body of right little finger with damage to nail

● S61.317 Laceration without foreign body of left little finger with damage to nail

● S61.318 Laceration without foreign body of other finger with damage to nail

      Laceration without foreign body of specified finger with unspecified laterality with damage to nail

● S61.319 Laceration without foreign body of unspecified finger with damage to nail

CHAPTER 19 (S00-T88)

● **S61.32**   Laceration with foreign body of finger with damage to nail
    ● **S61.320**   Laceration with foreign body of right index finger with damage to nail
    ● **S61.321**   Laceration with foreign body of left index finger with damage to nail
    ● **S61.322**   Laceration with foreign body of right middle finger with damage to nail
    ● **S61.323**   Laceration with foreign body of left middle finger with damage to nail
    ● **S61.324**   Laceration with foreign body of right ring finger with damage to nail
    ● **S61.325**   Laceration with foreign body of left ring finger with damage to nail
    ● **S61.326**   Laceration with foreign body of right little finger with damage to nail
    ● **S61.327**   Laceration with foreign body of left little finger with damage to nail
    ● **S61.328**   Laceration with foreign body of other finger with damage to nail
        Laceration with foreign body of specified finger with unspecified laterality with damage to nail
    ● **S61.329**   Laceration with foreign body of unspecified finger with damage to nail
● **S61.33**   Puncture wound without foreign body of finger with damage to nail
    ● **S61.330**   Puncture wound without foreign body of right index finger with damage to nail
    ● **S61.331**   Puncture wound without foreign body of left index finger with damage to nail
    ● **S61.332**   Puncture wound without foreign body of right middle finger with damage to nail
    ● **S61.333**   Puncture wound without foreign body of left middle finger with damage to nail
    ● **S61.334**   Puncture wound without foreign body of right ring finger with damage to nail
    ● **S61.335**   Puncture wound without foreign body of left ring finger with damage to nail
    ● **S61.336**   Puncture wound without foreign body of right little finger with damage to nail
    ● **S61.337**   Puncture wound without foreign body of left little finger with damage to nail
    ● **S61.338**   Puncture wound without foreign body of other finger with damage to nail
        Puncture wound without foreign body of specified finger with unspecified laterality with damage to nail
    ● **S61.339**   Puncture wound without foreign body of unspecified finger with damage to nail

● **S61.34**   Puncture wound with foreign body of finger with damage to nail
    ● **S61.340**   Puncture wound with foreign body of right index finger with damage to nail
    ● **S61.341**   Puncture wound with foreign body of left index finger with damage to nail
    ● **S61.342**   Puncture wound with foreign body of right middle finger with damage to nail
    ● **S61.343**   Puncture wound with foreign body of left middle finger with damage to nail
    ● **S61.344**   Puncture wound with foreign body of right ring finger with damage to nail
    ● **S61.345**   Puncture wound with foreign body of left ring finger with damage to nail
    ● **S61.346**   Puncture wound with foreign body of right little finger with damage to nail
    ● **S61.347**   Puncture wound with foreign body of left little finger with damage to nail
    ● **S61.348**   Puncture wound with foreign body of other finger with damage to nail
        Puncture wound with foreign body of specified finger with unspecified laterality with damage to nail
    ● **S61.349**   Puncture wound with foreign body of unspecified finger with damage to nail
● **S61.35**   Open bite of finger with damage to nail
        Bite of finger with damage to nail NOS
        Excludes1   superficial bite of finger (S60.46-, S60.47-)
    ● **S61.350**   Open bite of right index finger with damage to nail
    ● **S61.351**   Open bite of left index finger with damage to nail
    ● **S61.352**   Open bite of right middle finger with damage to nail
    ● **S61.353**   Open bite of left middle finger with damage to nail
    ● **S61.354**   Open bite of right ring finger with damage to nail
    ● **S61.355**   Open bite of left ring finger with damage to nail
    ● **S61.356**   Open bite of right little finger with damage to nail
    ● **S61.357**   Open bite of left little finger with damage to nail
    ● **S61.358**   Open bite of other finger with damage to nail
        Open bite of specified finger with unspecified laterality with damage to nail
    ● **S61.359**   Open bite of unspecified finger with damage to nail
● **S61.4**   Open wound of hand
    ● **S61.40**   Unspecified open wound of hand
       ● **S61.401**   Unspecified open wound of right hand
       ● **S61.402**   Unspecified open wound of left hand
       ● **S61.409**   Unspecified open wound of unspecified hand
    ● **S61.41**   Laceration without foreign body of hand
       ● **S61.411**   Laceration without foreign body of right hand
       ● **S61.412**   Laceration without foreign body of left hand
       ● **S61.419**   Laceration without foreign body of unspecified hand

S61.42 Laceration with foreign body of hand
- S61.421 Laceration with foreign body of right hand
- S61.422 Laceration with foreign body of left hand
- S61.429 Laceration with foreign body of unspecified hand

S61.43 Puncture wound without foreign body of hand
- S61.431 Puncture wound without foreign body of right hand
- S61.432 Puncture wound without foreign body of left hand
- S61.439 Puncture wound without foreign body of unspecified hand

S61.44 Puncture wound with foreign body of hand
- S61.441 Puncture wound with foreign body of right hand
- S61.442 Puncture wound with foreign body of left hand
- S61.449 Puncture wound with foreign body of unspecified hand

S61.45 Open bite of hand
Bite of hand NOS
> **Excludes1** superficial bite of hand (S60.56-, S60.57-)
- S61.451 Open bite of right hand
- S61.452 Open bite of left hand
- S61.459 Open bite of unspecified hand

S61.5 Open wound of wrist
- S61.50 Unspecified open wound of wrist
  - S61.501 Unspecified open wound of right wrist
  - S61.502 Unspecified open wound of left wrist
  - S61.509 Unspecified open wound of unspecified wrist
- S61.51 Laceration without foreign body of wrist
  - S61.511 Laceration without foreign body of right wrist
  - S61.512 Laceration without foreign body of left wrist
  - S61.519 Laceration without foreign body of unspecified wrist
- S61.52 Laceration with foreign body of wrist
  - S61.521 Laceration with foreign body of right wrist
  - S61.522 Laceration with foreign body of left wrist
  - S61.529 Laceration with foreign body of unspecified wrist
- S61.53 Puncture wound without foreign body of wrist
  - S61.531 Puncture wound without foreign body of right wrist
  - S61.532 Puncture wound without foreign body of left wrist
  - S61.539 Puncture wound without foreign body of unspecified wrist
- S61.54 Puncture wound with foreign body of wrist
  - S61.541 Puncture wound with foreign body of right wrist
  - S61.542 Puncture wound with foreign body of left wrist
  - S61.549 Puncture wound with foreign body of unspecified wrist

S61.55 Open bite of wrist
Bite of wrist NOS
> **Excludes1** superficial bite of wrist (S60.86-, S60.87-)
- S61.551 Open bite of right wrist
- S61.552 Open bite of left wrist
- S61.559 Open bite of unspecified wrist

S62 Fracture at wrist and hand level
Note: A fracture not indicated as displaced or nondisplaced should be coded to displaced

A fracture not indicated as open or closed should be coded to closed

Excludes1 traumatic amputation of wrist and hand (S68.-)
Excludes2 fracture of distal parts of ulna and radius (S52.-)

The appropriate 7th character is to be added to each code from category S62

A	initial encounter for closed fracture
B	initial encounter for open fracture
D	subsequent encounter for fracture with routine healing
G	subsequent encounter for fracture with delayed healing
K	subsequent encounter for fracture with nonunion
P	subsequent encounter for fracture with malunion
S	sequela

S62.0 Fracture of navicular [scaphoid] bone of wrist
- S62.00 Unspecified fracture of navicular [scaphoid] bone of wrist
  - S62.001 Unspecified fracture of navicular [scaphoid] bone of right wrist
  - S62.002 Unspecified fracture of navicular [scaphoid] bone of left wrist
    Coding Clinic: 2012, Q4, P106
  - S62.009 Unspecified fracture of navicular [scaphoid] bone of unspecified wrist
- S62.01 Fracture of distal pole of navicular [scaphoid] bone of wrist
  Fracture of volar tuberosity of navicular [scaphoid] bone of wrist
  - S62.011 Displaced fracture of distal pole of navicular [scaphoid] bone of right wrist
  - S62.012 Displaced fracture of distal pole of navicular [scaphoid] bone of left wrist
  - S62.013 Displaced fracture of distal pole of navicular [scaphoid] bone of unspecified wrist
  - S62.014 Nondisplaced fracture of distal pole of navicular [scaphoid] bone of right wrist
  - S62.015 Nondisplaced fracture of distal pole of navicular [scaphoid] bone of left wrist
  - S62.016 Nondisplaced fracture of distal pole of navicular [scaphoid] bone of unspecified wrist
- S62.02 Fracture of middle third of navicular [scaphoid] bone of wrist
  - S62.021 Displaced fracture of middle third of navicular [scaphoid] bone of right wrist
  - S62.022 Displaced fracture of middle third of navicular [scaphoid] bone of left wrist
  - S62.023 Displaced fracture of middle third of navicular [scaphoid] bone of unspecified wrist
  - S62.024 Nondisplaced fracture of middle third of navicular [scaphoid] bone of right wrist

● S62.025   Nondisplaced fracture of middle third of navicular [scaphoid] bone of left wrist

● S62.026   Nondisplaced fracture of middle third of navicular [scaphoid] bone of unspecified wrist

● S62.03   Fracture of proximal third of navicular [scaphoid] bone of wrist

● S62.031   Displaced fracture of proximal third of navicular [scaphoid] bone of right wrist

● S62.032   Displaced fracture of proximal third of navicular [scaphoid] bone of left wrist

● S62.033   Displaced fracture of proximal third of navicular [scaphoid] bone of unspecified wrist

● S62.034   Nondisplaced fracture of proximal third of navicular [scaphoid] bone of right wrist

● S62.035   Nondisplaced fracture of proximal third of navicular [scaphoid] bone of left wrist

● S62.036   Nondisplaced fracture of proximal third of navicular [scaphoid] bone of unspecified wrist

● S62.1   Fracture of other and unspecified carpal bone(s)

  Excludes2   fracture of scaphoid of wrist (S62.0-)

● S62.10   Fracture of unspecified carpal bone
  Fracture of wrist NOS

● S62.101   Fracture of unspecified carpal bone, right wrist

● S62.102   Fracture of unspecified carpal bone, left wrist
  Coding Clinic: 2012, Q4, P95

● S62.109   Fracture of unspecified carpal bone, unspecified wrist

● S62.11   Fracture of triquetrum [cuneiform] bone of wrist

● S62.111   Displaced fracture of triquetrum [cuneiform] bone, right wrist

● S62.112   Displaced fracture of triquetrum [cuneiform] bone, left wrist

● S62.113   Displaced fracture of triquetrum [cuneiform] bone, unspecified wrist

● S62.114   Nondisplaced fracture of triquetrum [cuneiform] bone, right wrist

● S62.115   Nondisplaced fracture of triquetrum [cuneiform] bone, left wrist

● S62.116   Nondisplaced fracture of triquetrum [cuneiform] bone, unspecified wrist

● S62.12   Fracture of lunate [semilunar]

● S62.121   Displaced fracture of lunate [semilunar], right wrist

● S62.122   Displaced fracture of lunate [semilunar], left wrist

● S62.123   Displaced fracture of lunate [semilunar], unspecified wrist

● S62.124   Nondisplaced fracture of lunate [semilunar], right wrist

● S62.125   Nondisplaced fracture of lunate [semilunar], left wrist

● S62.126   Nondisplaced fracture of lunate [semilunar], unspecified wrist

● S62.13   Fracture of capitate [os magnum] bone

● S62.131   Displaced fracture of capitate [os magnum] bone, right wrist

● S62.132   Displaced fracture of capitate [os magnum] bone, left wrist

● S62.133   Displaced fracture of capitate [os magnum] bone, unspecified wrist

● S62.134   Nondisplaced fracture of capitate [os magnum] bone, right wrist

● S62.135   Nondisplaced fracture of capitate [os magnum] bone, left wrist

● S62.136   Nondisplaced fracture of capitate [os magnum] bone, unspecified wrist

● S62.14   Fracture of body of hamate [unciform] bone
  Fracture of hamate [unciform] bone NOS

● S62.141   Displaced fracture of body of hamate [unciform] bone, right wrist

● S62.142   Displaced fracture of body of hamate [unciform] bone, left wrist

● S62.143   Displaced fracture of body of hamate [unciform] bone, unspecified wrist

● S62.144   Nondisplaced fracture of body of hamate [unciform] bone, right wrist

● S62.145   Nondisplaced fracture of body of hamate [unciform] bone, left wrist

● S62.146   Nondisplaced fracture of body of hamate [unciform] bone, unspecified wrist

● S62.15   Fracture of hook process of hamate [unciform] bone
  Fracture of unciform process of hamate [unciform] bone

● S62.151   Displaced fracture of hook process of hamate [unciform] bone, right wrist

● S62.152   Displaced fracture of hook process of hamate [unciform] bone, left wrist

● S62.153   Displaced fracture of hook process of hamate [unciform] bone, unspecified wrist

● S62.154   Nondisplaced fracture of hook process of hamate [unciform] bone, right wrist

● S62.155   Nondisplaced fracture of hook process of hamate [unciform] bone, left wrist

● S62.156   Nondisplaced fracture of hook process of hamate [unciform] bone, unspecified wrist

● S62.16   Fracture of pisiform

● S62.161   Displaced fracture of pisiform, right wrist

● S62.162   Displaced fracture of pisiform, left wrist

● S62.163   Displaced fracture of pisiform, unspecified wrist

● S62.164   Nondisplaced fracture of pisiform, right wrist

● S62.165   Nondisplaced fracture of pisiform, left wrist

● S62.166   Nondisplaced fracture of pisiform, unspecified wrist

● S62.17   Fracture of trapezium [larger multangular]

● S62.171   Displaced fracture of trapezium [larger multangular], right wrist

● S62.172   Displaced fracture of trapezium [larger multangular], left wrist

● S62.173   Displaced fracture of trapezium [larger multangular], unspecified wrist

● S62.174   Nondisplaced fracture of trapezium [larger multangular], right wrist

● S62.175   Nondisplaced fracture of trapezium [larger multangular], left wrist

● S62.176   Nondisplaced fracture of trapezium [larger multangular], unspecified wrist

▶ New   ⇒ Revised   ~~deleted~~ Deleted   Excludes 1   Excludes 2   Includes   Use additional   Code first   Code also   Key words

OGCR Official Guidelines   X Assign placeholder X   ● Use Additional Character(s)   ▷ Manifestation Code   🐾 Hierarchical Condition Category   **Coding Clinic**

● S62.18 Fracture of trapezoid [smaller multangular]
  ● S62.181 Displaced fracture of trapezoid [smaller multangular], right wrist
  ● S62.182 Displaced fracture of trapezoid [smaller multangular], left wrist
  ● S62.183 Displaced fracture of trapezoid [smaller multangular], unspecified wrist
  ● S62.184 Nondisplaced fracture of trapezoid [smaller multangular], right wrist
  ● S62.185 Nondisplaced fracture of trapezoid [smaller multangular], left wrist
  ● S62.186 Nondisplaced fracture of trapezoid [smaller multangular], unspecified wrist

● S62.2 Fracture of first metacarpal bone
  ● S62.20 Unspecified fracture of first metacarpal bone
    ● S62.201 Unspecified fracture of first metacarpal bone, right hand
    ● S62.202 Unspecified fracture of first metacarpal bone, left hand
    ● S62.209 Unspecified fracture of first metacarpal bone, unspecified hand
  ● S62.21 Bennett's fracture
    ● S62.211 Bennett's fracture, right hand
    ● S62.212 Bennett's fracture, left hand
    ● S62.213 Bennett's fracture, unspecified hand
  ● S62.22 Rolando's fracture
    ● S62.221 Displaced Rolando's fracture, right hand
    ● S62.222 Displaced Rolando's fracture, left hand
    ● S62.223 Displaced Rolando's fracture, unspecified hand
    ● S62.224 Nondisplaced Rolando's fracture, right hand
    ● S62.225 Nondisplaced Rolando's fracture, left hand
    ● S62.226 Nondisplaced Rolando's fracture, unspecified hand
  ● S62.23 Other fracture of base of first metacarpal bone
    ● S62.231 Other displaced fracture of base of first metacarpal bone, right hand
    ● S62.232 Other displaced fracture of base of first metacarpal bone, left hand
    ● S62.233 Other displaced fracture of base of first metacarpal bone, unspecified hand
    ● S62.234 Other nondisplaced fracture of base of first metacarpal bone, right hand
    ● S62.235 Other nondisplaced fracture of base of first metacarpal bone, left hand
    ● S62.236 Other nondisplaced fracture of base of first metacarpal bone, unspecified hand
  ● S62.24 Fracture of shaft of first metacarpal bone
    ● S62.241 Displaced fracture of shaft of first metacarpal bone, right hand
    ● S62.242 Displaced fracture of shaft of first metacarpal bone, left hand
    ● S62.243 Displaced fracture of shaft of first metacarpal bone, unspecified hand
    ● S62.244 Nondisplaced fracture of shaft of first metacarpal bone, right hand

    ● S62.245 Nondisplaced fracture of shaft of first metacarpal bone, left hand
    ● S62.246 Nondisplaced fracture of shaft of first metacarpal bone, unspecified hand
  ● S62.25 Fracture of neck of first metacarpal bone
    ● S62.251 Displaced fracture of neck of first metacarpal bone, right hand
    ● S62.252 Displaced fracture of neck of first metacarpal bone, left hand
    ● S62.253 Displaced fracture of neck of first metacarpal bone, unspecified hand
    ● S62.254 Nondisplaced fracture of neck of first metacarpal bone, right hand
    ● S62.255 Nondisplaced fracture of neck of first metacarpal bone, left hand
    ● S62.256 Nondisplaced fracture of neck of first metacarpal bone, unspecified hand
  ● S62.29 Other fracture of first metacarpal bone
    ● S62.291 Other fracture of first metacarpal bone, right hand
    ● S62.292 Other fracture of first metacarpal bone, left hand
    ● S62.299 Other fracture of first metacarpal bone, unspecified hand

● S62.3 Fracture of other and unspecified metacarpal bone
    Excludes2   fracture of first metacarpal bone (S62.2-)
  ● S62.30 Unspecified fracture of other metacarpal bone
    ● S62.300 Unspecified fracture of second metacarpal bone, right hand
    ● S62.301 Unspecified fracture of second metacarpal bone, left hand
    ● S62.302 Unspecified fracture of third metacarpal bone, right hand
    ● S62.303 Unspecified fracture of third metacarpal bone, left hand
    ● S62.304 Unspecified fracture of fourth metacarpal bone, right hand
    ● S62.305 Unspecified fracture of fourth metacarpal bone, left hand
    ● S62.306 Unspecified fracture of fifth metacarpal bone, right hand
    ● S62.307 Unspecified fracture of fifth metacarpal bone, left hand
    ● S62.308 Unspecified fracture of other metacarpal bone
              Unspecified fracture of specified metacarpal bone with unspecified laterality
    ● S62.309 Unspecified fracture of unspecified metacarpal bone
  ● S62.31 Displaced fracture of base of other metacarpal bone
    ● S62.310 Displaced fracture of base of second metacarpal bone, right hand
    ● S62.311 Displaced fracture of base of second metacarpal bone, left hand
    ● S62.312 Displaced fracture of base of third metacarpal bone, right hand
    ● S62.313 Displaced fracture of base of third metacarpal bone, left hand
    ● S62.314 Displaced fracture of base of fourth metacarpal bone, right hand

● S62.315   Displaced fracture of base of fourth metacarpal bone, left hand

● S62.316   Displaced fracture of base of fifth metacarpal bone, right hand

● S62.317   Displaced fracture of base of fifth metacarpal bone, left hand

● S62.318   Displaced fracture of base of other metacarpal bone
     Displaced fracture of base of specified metacarpal bone with unspecified laterality

● S62.319   Displaced fracture of base of unspecified metacarpal bone

● S62.32   Displaced fracture of shaft of other metacarpal bone

● S62.320   Displaced fracture of shaft of second metacarpal bone, right hand

● S62.321   Displaced fracture of shaft of second metacarpal bone, left hand

● S62.322   Displaced fracture of shaft of third metacarpal bone, right hand

● S62.323   Displaced fracture of shaft of third metacarpal bone, left hand

● S62.324   Displaced fracture of shaft of fourth metacarpal bone, right hand

● S62.325   Displaced fracture of shaft of fourth metacarpal bone, left hand

● S62.326   Displaced fracture of shaft of fifth metacarpal bone, right hand

● S62.327   Displaced fracture of shaft of fifth metacarpal bone, left hand

● S62.328   Displaced fracture of shaft of other metacarpal bone
     Displaced fracture of shaft of specified metacarpal bone with unspecified laterality

● S62.329   Displaced fracture of shaft of unspecified metacarpal bone

● S62.33   Displaced fracture of neck of other metacarpal bone

● S62.330   Displaced fracture of neck of second metacarpal bone, right hand

● S62.331   Displaced fracture of neck of second metacarpal bone, left hand

● S62.332   Displaced fracture of neck of third metacarpal bone, right hand

● S62.333   Displaced fracture of neck of third metacarpal bone, left hand

● S62.334   Displaced fracture of neck of fourth metacarpal bone, right hand

● S62.335   Displaced fracture of neck of fourth metacarpal bone, left hand

● S62.336   Displaced fracture of neck of fifth metacarpal bone, right hand

● S62.337   Displaced fracture of neck of fifth metacarpal bone, left hand

● S62.338   Displaced fracture of neck of other metacarpal bone
     Displaced fracture of neck of specified metacarpal bone with unspecified laterality

● S62.339   Displaced fracture of neck of unspecified metacarpal bone

● S62.34   Nondisplaced fracture of base of other metacarpal bone

● S62.340   Nondisplaced fracture of base of second metacarpal bone, right hand

● S62.341   Nondisplaced fracture of base of second metacarpal bone, left hand

● S62.342   Nondisplaced fracture of base of third metacarpal bone, right hand

● S62.343   Nondisplaced fracture of base of third metacarpal bone, left hand

● S62.344   Nondisplaced fracture of base of fourth metacarpal bone, right hand

● S62.345   Nondisplaced fracture of base of fourth metacarpal bone, left hand

● S62.346   Nondisplaced fracture of base of fifth metacarpal bone, right hand

● S62.347   Nondisplaced fracture of base of fifth metacarpal bone, left hand

● S62.348   Nondisplaced fracture of base of other metacarpal bone
     Nondisplaced fracture of base of specified metacarpal bone with unspecified laterality

● S62.349   Nondisplaced fracture of base of unspecified metacarpal bone

● S62.35   Nondisplaced fracture of shaft of other metacarpal bone

● S62.350   Nondisplaced fracture of shaft of second metacarpal bone, right hand

● S62.351   Nondisplaced fracture of shaft of second metacarpal bone, left hand

● S62.352   Nondisplaced fracture of shaft of third metacarpal bone, right hand

● S62.353   Nondisplaced fracture of shaft of third metacarpal bone, left hand

● S62.354   Nondisplaced fracture of shaft of fourth metacarpal bone, right hand

● S62.355   Nondisplaced fracture of shaft of fourth metacarpal bone, left hand

● S62.356   Nondisplaced fracture of shaft of fifth metacarpal bone, right hand

● S62.357   Nondisplaced fracture of shaft of fifth metacarpal bone, left hand

● S62.358   Nondisplaced fracture of shaft of other metacarpal bone
     Nondisplaced fracture of shaft of specified metacarpal bone with unspecified laterality

● S62.359   Nondisplaced fracture of shaft of unspecified metacarpal bone

● S62.36   Nondisplaced fracture of neck of other metacarpal bone

● S62.360   Nondisplaced fracture of neck of second metacarpal bone, right hand

● S62.361   Nondisplaced fracture of neck of second metacarpal bone, left hand

● S62.362   Nondisplaced fracture of neck of third metacarpal bone, right hand

● S62.363   Nondisplaced fracture of neck of third metacarpal bone, left hand

● S62.364   Nondisplaced fracture of neck of fourth metacarpal bone, right hand

● S62.365   Nondisplaced fracture of neck of fourth metacarpal bone, left hand

▶ New   ⮕ Revised   ~~deleted~~ Deleted   Excludes 1   Excludes 2   Includes   Use additional   Code first   Code also   Key words

OGCR Official Guidelines   X Assign placeholder X   ● Use Additional Character(s)   ⫶ Manifestation Code   🔖 Hierarchical Condition Category   Coding Clinic

● S62.366   Nondisplaced fracture of neck of fifth metacarpal bone, right hand
● S62.367   Nondisplaced fracture of neck of fifth metacarpal bone, left hand
● S62.368   Nondisplaced fracture of neck of other metacarpal bone
        Nondisplaced fracture of neck of specified metacarpal bone with unspecified laterality
● S62.369   Nondisplaced fracture of neck of unspecified metacarpal bone

● S62.39   Other fracture of other metacarpal bone
   ● S62.390   Other fracture of second metacarpal bone, right hand
   ● S62.391   Other fracture of second metacarpal bone, left hand
   ● S62.392   Other fracture of third metacarpal bone, right hand
   ● S62.393   Other fracture of third metacarpal bone, left hand
   ● S62.394   Other fracture of fourth metacarpal bone, right hand
   ● S62.395   Other fracture of fourth metacarpal bone, left hand
   ● S62.396   Other fracture of fifth metacarpal bone, right hand
   ● S62.397   Other fracture of fifth metacarpal bone, left hand
   ● S62.398   Other fracture of other metacarpal bone
           Other fracture of specified metacarpal bone with unspecified laterality
   ● S62.399   Other fracture of unspecified metacarpal bone

● S62.5   Fracture of thumb
  ● S62.50   Fracture of unspecified phalanx of thumb
   ● S62.501   Fracture of unspecified phalanx of right thumb
   ● S62.502   Fracture of unspecified phalanx of left thumb
   ● S62.509   Fracture of unspecified phalanx of unspecified thumb
  ● S62.51   Fracture of proximal phalanx of thumb
   ● S62.511   Displaced fracture of proximal phalanx of right thumb
   ● S62.512   Displaced fracture of proximal phalanx of left thumb
   ● S62.513   Displaced fracture of proximal phalanx of unspecified thumb
   ● S62.514   Nondisplaced fracture of proximal phalanx of right thumb
   ● S62.515   Nondisplaced fracture of proximal phalanx of left thumb
   ● S62.516   Nondisplaced fracture of proximal phalanx of unspecified thumb
  ● S62.52   Fracture of distal phalanx of thumb
   ● S62.521   Displaced fracture of distal phalanx of right thumb
   ● S62.522   Displaced fracture of distal phalanx of left thumb
   ● S62.523   Displaced fracture of distal phalanx of unspecified thumb

● S62.524   Nondisplaced fracture of distal phalanx of right thumb
● S62.525   Nondisplaced fracture of distal phalanx of left thumb
● S62.526   Nondisplaced fracture of distal phalanx of unspecified thumb

● S62.6   Fracture of other and unspecified finger(s)
    Excludes2   fracture of thumb (S62.5-)
  ● S62.60   Fracture of unspecified phalanx of finger
   ● S62.600   Fracture of unspecified phalanx of right index finger
   ● S62.601   Fracture of unspecified phalanx of left index finger
   ● S62.602   Fracture of unspecified phalanx of right middle finger
   ● S62.603   Fracture of unspecified phalanx of left middle finger
   ● S62.604   Fracture of unspecified phalanx of right ring finger
   ● S62.605   Fracture of unspecified phalanx of left ring finger
   ● S62.606   Fracture of unspecified phalanx of right little finger
   ● S62.607   Fracture of unspecified phalanx of left little finger
   ● S62.608   Fracture of unspecified phalanx of other finger
           Fracture of unspecified phalanx of specified finger with unspecified laterality
   ● S62.609   Fracture of unspecified phalanx of unspecified finger
  ● S62.61   Displaced fracture of proximal phalanx of finger
   ● S62.610   Displaced fracture of proximal phalanx of right index finger
   ● S62.611   Displaced fracture of proximal phalanx of left index finger
   ● S62.612   Displaced fracture of proximal phalanx of right middle finger
   ● S62.613   Displaced fracture of proximal phalanx of left middle finger

Figure 19-14 Dorsal dislocation of the distal phalanx of the index finger. (From Hardy M, Snaith B: Musculoskeletal Trauma: A Guide to Assessment and Diagnosis, 1e, Elsevier, 2011)

CHAPTER 19 (S00-T88)

● S62.614   Displaced fracture of proximal
            phalanx of right ring finger

● S62.615   Displaced fracture of proximal
            phalanx of left ring finger

● S62.616   Displaced fracture of proximal
            phalanx of right little finger

● S62.617   Displaced fracture of proximal
            phalanx of left little finger

● S62.618   Displaced fracture of proximal
            phalanx of other finger
              Displaced fracture of proximal
                phalanx of specified finger with
                unspecified laterality

● S62.619   Displaced fracture of proximal
            phalanx of unspecified finger

● S62.62   Displaced fracture of middle phalanx of finger

   ● S62.620   Displaced fracture of middle phalanx
               of right index finger

   ● S62.621   Displaced fracture of middle phalanx
               of left index finger

   ● S62.622   Displaced fracture of middle phalanx
               of right middle finger

   ● S62.623   Displaced fracture of middle phalanx
               of left middle finger

   ● S62.624   Displaced fracture of middle phalanx
               of right ring finger

   ● S62.625   Displaced fracture of middle phalanx
               of left ring finger

   ● S62.626   Displaced fracture of middle phalanx
               of right little finger

   ● S62.627   Displaced fracture of middle phalanx
               of left little finger

   ● S62.628   Displaced fracture of middle phalanx
               of other finger
                 Displaced fracture of middle
                   phalanx of specified finger with
                   unspecified laterality

   ● S62.629   Displaced fracture of middle phalanx
               of unspecified finger

● S62.63   Displaced fracture of distal phalanx of finger

   ● S62.630   Displaced fracture of distal phalanx
               of right index finger

   ● S62.631   Displaced fracture of distal phalanx
               of left index finger

   ● S62.632   Displaced fracture of distal phalanx
               of right middle finger

   ● S62.633   Displaced fracture of distal phalanx
               of left middle finger

   ● S62.634   Displaced fracture of distal phalanx
               of right ring finger

   ● S62.635   Displaced fracture of distal phalanx
               of left ring finger

   ● S62.636   Displaced fracture of distal phalanx
               of right little finger

   ● S62.637   Displaced fracture of distal phalanx
               of left little finger

   ● S62.638   Displaced fracture of distal phalanx
               of other finger
                 Displaced fracture of distal phalanx
                   of specified finger with
                   unspecified laterality

   ● S62.639   Displaced fracture of distal phalanx
               of unspecified finger

● S62.64   Nondisplaced fracture of proximal phalanx of
           finger

   ● S62.640   Nondisplaced fracture of proximal
               phalanx of right index finger

   ● S62.641   Nondisplaced fracture of proximal
               phalanx of left index finger

● S62.642   Nondisplaced fracture of proximal
            phalanx of right middle finger

● S62.643   Nondisplaced fracture of proximal
            phalanx of left middle finger

● S62.644   Nondisplaced fracture of proximal
            phalanx of right ring finger

● S62.645   Nondisplaced fracture of proximal
            phalanx of left ring finger

● S62.646   Nondisplaced fracture of proximal
            phalanx of right little finger

● S62.647   Nondisplaced fracture of proximal
            phalanx of left little finger

● S62.648   Nondisplaced fracture of proximal
            phalanx of other finger
              Nondisplaced fracture of proximal
                phalanx of specified finger with
                unspecified laterality

● S62.649   Nondisplaced fracture of proximal
            phalanx of unspecified finger

● S62.65   Nondisplaced fracture of middle phalanx of
           finger

   ● S62.650   Nondisplaced fracture of middle
               phalanx of right index finger

   ● S62.651   Nondisplaced fracture of middle
               phalanx of left index finger

   ● S62.652   Nondisplaced fracture of middle
               phalanx of right middle finger

   ● S62.653   Nondisplaced fracture of middle
               phalanx of left middle finger

   ● S62.654   Nondisplaced fracture of middle
               phalanx of right ring finger

   ● S62.655   Nondisplaced fracture of middle
               phalanx of left ring finger

   ● S62.656   Nondisplaced fracture of middle
               phalanx of right little finger

   ● S62.657   Nondisplaced fracture of middle
               phalanx of left little finger

   ● S62.658   Nondisplaced fracture of middle
               phalanx of other finger
                 Nondisplaced fracture of middle
                   phalanx of specified finger with
                   unspecified laterality

   ● S62.659   Nondisplaced fracture of middle
               phalanx of unspecified finger

● S62.66   Nondisplaced fracture of distal phalanx of finger

   ● S62.660   Nondisplaced fracture of distal
               phalanx of right index finger

   ● S62.661   Nondisplaced fracture of distal
               phalanx of left index finger

   ● S62.662   Nondisplaced fracture of distal
               phalanx of right middle finger

   ● S62.663   Nondisplaced fracture of distal
               phalanx of left middle finger

   ● S62.664   Nondisplaced fracture of distal
               phalanx of right ring finger

   ● S62.665   Nondisplaced fracture of distal
               phalanx of left ring finger

   ● S62.666   Nondisplaced fracture of distal
               phalanx of right little finger

   ● S62.667   Nondisplaced fracture of distal
               phalanx of left little finger

   ● S62.668   Nondisplaced fracture of distal
               phalanx of other finger
                 Nondisplaced fracture of distal
                   phalanx of specified finger with
                   unspecified laterality

   ● S62.669   Nondisplaced fracture of distal
               phalanx of unspecified finger

▶ New   ⇒ Revised   ~~deleted~~ Deleted   Excludes 1   Excludes 2   Includes   Use additional   Code first   Code also   Key words

OGCR Official Guidelines   X Assign placeholder X   ● Use Additional Character(s)   ▌ Manifestation Code   🏷 Hierarchical Condition Category   Coding Clinic

● S62.9   Unspecified fracture of wrist and hand
   X ● S62.90   Unspecified fracture of unspecified wrist and hand
   X ● S62.91   Unspecified fracture of right wrist and hand
   X ● S62.92   Unspecified fracture of left wrist and hand

● S63   Dislocation and sprain of joints and ligaments at wrist and hand level

Includes	avulsion of joint or ligament at wrist and hand level
	laceration of cartilage, joint or ligament at wrist and hand level
	sprain of cartilage, joint or ligament at wrist and hand level
	traumatic hemarthrosis of joint or ligament at wrist and hand level
	traumatic rupture of joint or ligament at wrist and hand level
	traumatic subluxation of joint or ligament at wrist and hand level
	traumatic tear of joint or ligament at wrist and hand level

Code also any associated open wound

Excludes2	strain of muscle, fascia and tendon of wrist and hand (S66.-)

The appropriate 7th character is to be added to each code from category S63

A	initial encounter
D	subsequent encounter
S	sequela

● S63.0   Subluxation and dislocation of wrist and hand joints
   ● S63.00   Unspecified subluxation and dislocation of wrist and hand
     Dislocation of carpal bone NOS
     Dislocation of distal end of radius NOS
     Subluxation of carpal bone NOS
     Subluxation of distal end of radius NOS
     ● S63.001   Unspecified subluxation of right wrist and hand
     ● S63.002   Unspecified subluxation of left wrist and hand
     ● S63.003   Unspecified subluxation of unspecified wrist and hand
     ● S63.004   Unspecified dislocation of right wrist and hand
     ● S63.005   Unspecified dislocation of left wrist and hand
     ● S63.006   Unspecified dislocation of unspecified wrist and hand
   ● S63.01   Subluxation and dislocation of distal radioulnar joint
     ● S63.011   Subluxation of distal radioulnar joint of right wrist
     ● S63.012   Subluxation of distal radioulnar joint of left wrist
     ● S63.013   Subluxation of distal radioulnar joint of unspecified wrist
     ● S63.014   Dislocation of distal radioulnar joint of right wrist
     ● S63.015   Dislocation of distal radioulnar joint of left wrist
     ● S63.016   Dislocation of distal radioulnar joint of unspecified wrist
   ● S63.02   Subluxation and dislocation of radiocarpal joint
     ● S63.021   Subluxation of radiocarpal joint of right wrist
     ● S63.022   Subluxation of radiocarpal joint of left wrist
     ● S63.023   Subluxation of radiocarpal joint of unspecified wrist

     ● S63.024   Dislocation of radiocarpal joint of right wrist
     ● S63.025   Dislocation of radiocarpal joint of left wrist
     ● S63.026   Dislocation of radiocarpal joint of unspecified wrist
   ● S63.03   Subluxation and dislocation of midcarpal joint
     ● S63.031   Subluxation of midcarpal joint of right wrist
     ● S63.032   Subluxation of midcarpal joint of left wrist
     ● S63.033   Subluxation of midcarpal joint of unspecified wrist
     ● S63.034   Dislocation of midcarpal joint of right wrist
     ● S63.035   Dislocation of midcarpal joint of left wrist
     ● S63.036   Dislocation of midcarpal joint of unspecified wrist
   ● S63.04   Subluxation and dislocation of carpometacarpal joint of thumb

Excludes2	interphalangeal subluxation and dislocation of thumb (S63.1-)

     ● S63.041   Subluxation of carpometacarpal joint of right thumb
     ● S63.042   Subluxation of carpometacarpal joint of left thumb
     ● S63.043   Subluxation of carpometacarpal joint of unspecified thumb
     ● S63.044   Dislocation of carpometacarpal joint of right thumb
     ● S63.045   Dislocation of carpometacarpal joint of left thumb
     ● S63.046   Dislocation of carpometacarpal joint of unspecified thumb
   ● S63.05   Subluxation and dislocation of other carpometacarpal joint

Excludes2	subluxation and dislocation of carpometacarpal joint of thumb (S63.04-)

     ● S63.051   Subluxation of other carpometacarpal joint of right hand
     ● S63.052   Subluxation of other carpometacarpal joint of left hand
     ● S63.053   Subluxation of other carpometacarpal joint of unspecified hand
     ● S63.054   Dislocation of other carpometacarpal joint of right hand
     ● S63.055   Dislocation of other carpometacarpal joint of left hand
     ● S63.056   Dislocation of other carpometacarpal joint of unspecified hand
   ● S63.06   Subluxation and dislocation of metacarpal (bone), proximal end
     ● S63.061   Subluxation of metacarpal (bone), proximal end of right hand
     ● S63.062   Subluxation of metacarpal (bone), proximal end of left hand
     ● S63.063   Subluxation of metacarpal (bone), proximal end of unspecified hand
     ● S63.064   Dislocation of metacarpal (bone), proximal end of right hand
     ● S63.065   Dislocation of metacarpal (bone), proximal end of left hand
     ● S63.066   Dislocation of metacarpal (bone), proximal end of unspecified hand

CHAPTER 19 (S00-T88)

- ● S63.07 Subluxation and dislocation of distal end of ulna
  - ● S63.071 Subluxation of distal end of right ulna
  - ● S63.072 Subluxation of distal end of left ulna
  - ● S63.073 Subluxation of distal end of unspecified ulna
  - ● S63.074 Dislocation of distal end of right ulna
  - ● S63.075 Dislocation of distal end of left ulna
  - ● S63.076 Dislocation of distal end of unspecified ulna
- ● S63.09 Other subluxation and dislocation of wrist and hand
  - ● S63.091 Other subluxation of right wrist and hand
  - ● S63.092 Other subluxation of left wrist and hand
  - ● S63.093 Other subluxation of unspecified wrist and hand
  - ● S63.094 Other dislocation of right wrist and hand
  - ● S63.095 Other dislocation of left wrist and hand
  - ● S63.096 Other dislocation of unspecified wrist and hand
- ● S63.1 Subluxation and dislocation of thumb
  - ● S63.10 Unspecified subluxation and dislocation of thumb
    - ● S63.101 Unspecified subluxation of right thumb
    - ● S63.102 Unspecified subluxation of left thumb
    - ● S63.103 Unspecified subluxation of unspecified thumb
    - ● S63.104 Unspecified dislocation of right thumb
    - ● S63.105 Unspecified dislocation of left thumb
    - ● S63.106 Unspecified dislocation of unspecified thumb
  - ● S63.11 Subluxation and dislocation of metacarpophalangeal joint of thumb
    - ● S63.111 Subluxation of metacarpophalangeal joint of right thumb
    - ● S63.112 Subluxation of metacarpophalangeal joint of left thumb
    - ● S63.113 Subluxation of metacarpophalangeal joint of unspecified thumb
    - ● S63.114 Dislocation of metacarpophalangeal joint of right thumb
    - ● S63.115 Dislocation of metacarpophalangeal joint of left thumb
    - ● S63.116 Dislocation of metacarpophalangeal joint of unspecified thumb
  - ● S63.12 Subluxation and dislocation of interphalangeal joint of thumb
    - ● S63.121 Subluxation of interphalangeal joint of right thumb
    - ● S63.122 Subluxation of interphalangeal joint of left thumb
    - ● S63.123 Subluxation of interphalangeal joint of unspecified thumb
    - ● S63.124 Dislocation of interphalangeal joint of right thumb
    - ● S63.125 Dislocation of interphalangeal joint of left thumb
    - ● S63.126 Dislocation of interphalangeal joint of unspecified thumb

- ● S63.2 Subluxation and dislocation of other finger(s)
  - **Excludes2** subluxation and dislocation of thumb (S63.1-)
  - ● S63.20 Unspecified subluxation of other finger
    - ● S63.200 Unspecified subluxation of right index finger
    - ● S63.201 Unspecified subluxation of left index finger
    - ● S63.202 Unspecified subluxation of right middle finger
    - ● S63.203 Unspecified subluxation of left middle finger
    - ● S63.204 Unspecified subluxation of right ring finger
    - ● S63.205 Unspecified subluxation of left ring finger
    - ● S63.206 Unspecified subluxation of right little finger
    - ● S63.207 Unspecified subluxation of left little finger
    - ● S63.208 Unspecified subluxation of other finger
      Unspecified subluxation of specified finger with unspecified laterality
    - ● S63.209 Unspecified subluxation of unspecified finger
  - ● S63.21 Subluxation of metacarpophalangeal joint of finger
    - ● S63.210 Subluxation of metacarpophalangeal joint of right index finger
    - ● S63.211 Subluxation of metacarpophalangeal joint of left index finger
    - ● S63.212 Subluxation of metacarpophalangeal joint of right middle finger
    - ● S63.213 Subluxation of metacarpophalangeal joint of left middle finger
    - ● S63.214 Subluxation of metacarpophalangeal joint of right ring finger
    - ● S63.215 Subluxation of metacarpophalangeal joint of left ring finger
    - ● S63.216 Subluxation of metacarpophalangeal joint of right little finger
    - ● S63.217 Subluxation of metacarpophalangeal joint of left little finger
    - ● S63.218 Subluxation of metacarpophalangeal joint of other finger
      Subluxation of metacarpophalangeal joint of specified finger with unspecified laterality
    - ● S63.219 Subluxation of metacarpophalangeal joint of unspecified finger
  - ● S63.22 Subluxation of unspecified interphalangeal joint of finger
    - ● S63.220 Subluxation of unspecified interphalangeal joint of right index finger
    - ● S63.221 Subluxation of unspecified interphalangeal joint of left index finger
    - ● S63.222 Subluxation of unspecified interphalangeal joint of right middle finger
    - ● S63.223 Subluxation of unspecified interphalangeal joint of left middle finger
    - ● S63.224 Subluxation of unspecified interphalangeal joint of right ring finger

▶ New ⇒ Revised ~~deleted~~ Deleted Excludes 1 Excludes 2 Includes Use additional Code first Code also Key words
OGCR Official Guidelines X Assign placeholder X ● Use Additional Character(s) ▷ Manifestation Code 🅚 Hierarchical Condition Category **Coding Clinic**

● S63.225   Subluxation of unspecified interphalangeal joint of left ring finger

● S63.226   Subluxation of unspecified interphalangeal joint of right little finger

● S63.227   Subluxation of unspecified interphalangeal joint of left little finger

● S63.228   Subluxation of unspecified interphalangeal joint of other finger
       Subluxation of unspecified interphalangeal joint of specified finger with unspecified laterality

● S63.229   Subluxation of unspecified interphalangeal joint of unspecified finger

● S63.23   Subluxation of proximal interphalangeal joint of finger

  ● S63.230   Subluxation of proximal interphalangeal joint of right index finger

  ● S63.231   Subluxation of proximal interphalangeal joint of left index finger

  ● S63.232   Subluxation of proximal interphalangeal joint of right middle finger

  ● S63.233   Subluxation of proximal interphalangeal joint of left middle finger

  ● S63.234   Subluxation of proximal interphalangeal joint of right ring finger

  ● S63.235   Subluxation of proximal interphalangeal joint of left ring finger

  ● S63.236   Subluxation of proximal interphalangeal joint of right little finger

  ● S63.237   Subluxation of proximal interphalangeal joint of left little finger

  ● S63.238   Subluxation of proximal interphalangeal joint of other finger
       Subluxation of proximal interphalangeal joint of specified finger with unspecified laterality

  ● S63.239   Subluxation of proximal interphalangeal joint of unspecified finger

● S63.24   Subluxation of distal interphalangeal joint of finger

  ● S63.240   Subluxation of distal interphalangeal joint of right index finger

  ● S63.241   Subluxation of distal interphalangeal joint of left index finger

  ● S63.242   Subluxation of distal interphalangeal joint of right middle finger

  ● S63.243   Subluxation of distal interphalangeal joint of left middle finger

  ● S63.244   Subluxation of distal interphalangeal joint of right ring finger

  ● S63.245   Subluxation of distal interphalangeal joint of left ring finger

  ● S63.246   Subluxation of distal interphalangeal joint of right little finger

  ● S63.247   Subluxation of distal interphalangeal joint of left little finger

  ● S63.248   Subluxation of distal interphalangeal joint of other finger
       Subluxation of distal interphalangeal joint of specified finger with unspecified laterality

  ● S63.249   Subluxation of distal interphalangeal joint of unspecified finger

● S63.25   Unspecified dislocation of other finger

  ● S63.250   Unspecified dislocation of right index finger

  ● S63.251   Unspecified dislocation of left index finger

  ● S63.252   Unspecified dislocation of right middle finger

  ● S63.253   Unspecified dislocation of left middle finger

  ● S63.254   Unspecified dislocation of right ring finger

  ● S63.255   Unspecified dislocation of left ring finger

  ● S63.256   Unspecified dislocation of right little finger

  ● S63.257   Unspecified dislocation of left little finger

  ● S63.258   Unspecified dislocation of other finger
       Unspecified dislocation of specified finger with unspecified laterality

  ● S63.259   Unspecified dislocation of unspecified finger
       Unspecified dislocation of unspecified finger with unspecified laterality

● S63.26   Dislocation of metacarpophalangeal joint of finger

  ● S63.260   Dislocation of metacarpophalangeal joint of right index finger

  ● S63.261   Dislocation of metacarpophalangeal joint of left index finger

  ● S63.262   Dislocation of metacarpophalangeal joint of right middle finger

  ● S63.263   Dislocation of metacarpophalangeal joint of left middle finger

  ● S63.264   Dislocation of metacarpophalangeal joint of right ring finger

  ● S63.265   Dislocation of metacarpophalangeal joint of left ring finger

  ● S63.266   Dislocation of metacarpophalangeal joint of right little finger

  ● S63.267   Dislocation of metacarpophalangeal joint of left little finger

  ● S63.268   Dislocation of metacarpophalangeal joint of other finger
       Dislocation of metacarpophalangeal joint of specified finger with unspecified laterality

  ● S63.269   Dislocation of metacarpophalangeal joint of unspecified finger

● S63.27   Dislocation of unspecified interphalangeal joint of finger

  ● S63.270   Dislocation of unspecified interphalangeal joint of right index finger

  ● S63.271   Dislocation of unspecified interphalangeal joint of left index finger

● S63.272 Dislocation of unspecified interphalangeal joint of right middle finger

● S63.273 Dislocation of unspecified interphalangeal joint of left middle finger

● S63.274 Dislocation of unspecified interphalangeal joint of right ring finger

● S63.275 Dislocation of unspecified interphalangeal joint of left ring finger

● S63.276 Dislocation of unspecified interphalangeal joint of right little finger

● S63.277 Dislocation of unspecified interphalangeal joint of left little finger

● S63.278 Dislocation of unspecified interphalangeal joint of other finger
　　　　　　Dislocation of unspecified interphalangeal joint of specified finger with unspecified laterality

● S63.279 Dislocation of unspecified interphalangeal joint of unspecified finger
　　　　　　Dislocation of unspecified interphalangeal joint of unspecified finger without specified laterality

● S63.28 Dislocation of proximal interphalangeal joint of finger

● S63.280 Dislocation of proximal interphalangeal joint of right index finger

● S63.281 Dislocation of proximal interphalangeal joint of left index finger

● S63.282 Dislocation of proximal interphalangeal joint of right middle finger

● S63.283 Dislocation of proximal interphalangeal joint of left middle finger

● S63.284 Dislocation of proximal interphalangeal joint of right ring finger

● S63.285 Dislocation of proximal interphalangeal joint of left ring finger

● S63.286 Dislocation of proximal interphalangeal joint of right little finger

● S63.287 Dislocation of proximal interphalangeal joint of left little finger

● S63.288 Dislocation of proximal interphalangeal joint of other finger
　　　　　　Dislocation of proximal interphalangeal joint of specified finger with unspecified laterality

● S63.289 Dislocation of proximal interphalangeal joint of unspecified finger

● S63.29 Dislocation of distal interphalangeal joint of finger

● S63.290 Dislocation of distal interphalangeal joint of right index finger

● S63.291 Dislocation of distal interphalangeal joint of left index finger

● S63.292 Dislocation of distal interphalangeal joint of right middle finger

● S63.293 Dislocation of distal interphalangeal joint of left middle finger

● S63.294 Dislocation of distal interphalangeal joint of right ring finger

● S63.295 Dislocation of distal interphalangeal joint of left ring finger

● S63.296 Dislocation of distal interphalangeal joint of right little finger

● S63.297 Dislocation of distal interphalangeal joint of left little finger

● S63.298 Dislocation of distal interphalangeal joint of other finger
　　　　　　Dislocation of distal interphalangeal joint of specified finger with unspecified laterality

● S63.299 Dislocation of distal interphalangeal joint of unspecified finger

● S63.3 Traumatic rupture of ligament of wrist

● S63.30 Traumatic rupture of unspecified ligament of wrist

● S63.301 Traumatic rupture of unspecified ligament of right wrist

● S63.302 Traumatic rupture of unspecified ligament of left wrist

● S63.309 Traumatic rupture of unspecified ligament of unspecified wrist

● S63.31 Traumatic rupture of collateral ligament of wrist

● S63.311 Traumatic rupture of collateral ligament of right wrist

● S63.312 Traumatic rupture of collateral ligament of left wrist

● S63.319 Traumatic rupture of collateral ligament of unspecified wrist

● S63.32 Traumatic rupture of radiocarpal ligament

● S63.321 Traumatic rupture of right radiocarpal ligament

● S63.322 Traumatic rupture of left radiocarpal ligament

● S63.329 Traumatic rupture of unspecified radiocarpal ligament

● S63.33 Traumatic rupture of ulnocarpal (palmar) ligament

● S63.331 Traumatic rupture of right ulnocarpal (palmar) ligament

● S63.332 Traumatic rupture of left ulnocarpal (palmar) ligament

● S63.339 Traumatic rupture of unspecified ulnocarpal (palmar) ligament

● S63.39 Traumatic rupture of other ligament of wrist

● S63.391 Traumatic rupture of other ligament of right wrist

● S63.392 Traumatic rupture of other ligament of left wrist

● S63.399 Traumatic rupture of other ligament of unspecified wrist

● S63.4 Traumatic rupture of ligament of finger at metacarpophalangeal and interphalangeal joint(s)

● S63.40 Traumatic rupture of unspecified ligament of finger at metacarpophalangeal and interphalangeal joint

● S63.400 Traumatic rupture of unspecified ligament of right index finger at metacarpophalangeal and interphalangeal joint

● S63.401 Traumatic rupture of unspecified ligament of left index finger at metacarpophalangeal and interphalangeal joint

● S63.402 Traumatic rupture of unspecified ligament of right middle finger at metacarpophalangeal and interphalangeal joint

● S63.403 Traumatic rupture of unspecified ligament of left middle finger at metacarpophalangeal and interphalangeal joint

● S63.404 Traumatic rupture of unspecified ligament of right ring finger at metacarpophalangeal and interphalangeal joint

● S63.405 Traumatic rupture of unspecified ligament of left ring finger at metacarpophalangeal and interphalangeal joint

● S63.406 Traumatic rupture of unspecified ligament of right little finger at metacarpophalangeal and interphalangeal joint

● S63.407 Traumatic rupture of unspecified ligament of left little finger at metacarpophalangeal and interphalangeal joint

● S63.408 Traumatic rupture of unspecified ligament of other finger at metacarpophalangeal and interphalangeal joint
    Traumatic rupture of unspecified ligament of specified finger with unspecified laterality at metacarpophalangeal and interphalangeal joint

● S63.409 Traumatic rupture of unspecified ligament of unspecified finger at metacarpophalangeal and interphalangeal joint

● S63.41 Traumatic rupture of collateral ligament of finger at metacarpophalangeal and interphalangeal joint

● S63.410 Traumatic rupture of collateral ligament of right index finger at metacarpophalangeal and interphalangeal joint

● S63.411 Traumatic rupture of collateral ligament of left index finger at metacarpophalangeal and interphalangeal joint

● S63.412 Traumatic rupture of collateral ligament of right middle finger at metacarpophalangeal and interphalangeal joint

● S63.413 Traumatic rupture of collateral ligament of left middle finger at metacarpophalangeal and interphalangeal joint

● S63.414 Traumatic rupture of collateral ligament of right ring finger at metacarpophalangeal and interphalangeal joint

● S63.415 Traumatic rupture of collateral ligament of left ring finger at metacarpophalangeal and interphalangeal joint

● S63.416 Traumatic rupture of collateral ligament of right little finger at metacarpophalangeal and interphalangeal joint

● S63.417 Traumatic rupture of collateral ligament of left little finger at metacarpophalangeal and interphalangeal joint

● S63.418 Traumatic rupture of collateral ligament of other finger at metacarpophalangeal and interphalangeal joint
    Traumatic rupture of collateral ligament of specified finger with unspecified laterality at metacarpophalangeal and interphalangeal joint

● S63.419 Traumatic rupture of collateral ligament of unspecified finger at metacarpophalangeal and interphalangeal joint

● S63.42 Traumatic rupture of palmar ligament of finger at metacarpophalangeal and interphalangeal joint

● S63.420 Traumatic rupture of palmar ligament of right index finger at metacarpophalangeal and interphalangeal joint

● S63.421 Traumatic rupture of palmar ligament of left index finger at metacarpophalangeal and interphalangeal joint

● S63.422 Traumatic rupture of palmar ligament of right middle finger at metacarpophalangeal and interphalangeal joint

● S63.423 Traumatic rupture of palmar ligament of left middle finger at metacarpophalangeal and interphalangeal joint

● S63.424 Traumatic rupture of palmar ligament of right ring finger at metacarpophalangeal and interphalangeal joint

● S63.425 Traumatic rupture of palmar ligament of left ring finger at metacarpophalangeal and interphalangeal joint

● S63.426 Traumatic rupture of palmar ligament of right little finger at metacarpophalangeal and interphalangeal joint

● S63.427 Traumatic rupture of palmar ligament of left little finger at metacarpophalangeal and interphalangeal joint

● S63.428 Traumatic rupture of palmar ligament of other finger at metacarpophalangeal and interphalangeal joint
    Traumatic rupture of palmar ligament of specified finger with unspecified laterality at metacarpophalangeal and interphalangeal joint

● S63.429 Traumatic rupture of palmar ligament of unspecified finger at metacarpophalangeal and interphalangeal joint

CHAPTER 19 (S00-T88)

● S63.43 Traumatic rupture of volar plate of finger at metacarpophalangeal and interphalangeal joint
- ● S63.430 Traumatic rupture of volar plate of right index finger at metacarpophalangeal and interphalangeal joint
- ● S63.431 Traumatic rupture of volar plate of left index finger at metacarpophalangeal and interphalangeal joint
- ● S63.432 Traumatic rupture of volar plate of right middle finger at metacarpophalangeal and interphalangeal joint
- ● S63.433 Traumatic rupture of volar plate of left middle finger at metacarpophalangeal and interphalangeal joint
- ● S63.434 Traumatic rupture of volar plate of right ring finger at metacarpophalangeal and interphalangeal joint
- ● S63.435 Traumatic rupture of volar plate of left ring finger at metacarpophalangeal and interphalangeal joint
- ● S63.436 Traumatic rupture of volar plate of right little finger at metacarpophalangeal and interphalangeal joint
- ● S63.437 Traumatic rupture of volar plate of left little finger at metacarpophalangeal and interphalangeal joint
- ● S63.438 Traumatic rupture of volar plate of other finger at metacarpophalangeal and interphalangeal joint
  Traumatic rupture of volar plate of specified finger with unspecified laterality at metacarpophalangeal and interphalangeal joint
- ● S63.439 Traumatic rupture of volar plate of unspecified finger at metacarpophalangeal and interphalangeal joint

● S63.49 Traumatic rupture of other ligament of finger at metacarpophalangeal and interphalangeal joint
- ● S63.490 Traumatic rupture of other ligament of right index finger at metacarpophalangeal and interphalangeal joint
- ● S63.491 Traumatic rupture of other ligament of left index finger at metacarpophalangeal and interphalangeal joint
- ● S63.492 Traumatic rupture of other ligament of right middle finger at metacarpophalangeal and interphalangeal joint
- ● S63.493 Traumatic rupture of other ligament of left middle finger at metacarpophalangeal and interphalangeal joint
- ● S63.494 Traumatic rupture of other ligament of right ring finger at metacarpophalangeal and interphalangeal joint
- ● S63.495 Traumatic rupture of other ligament of left ring finger at metacarpophalangeal and interphalangeal joint
- ● S63.496 Traumatic rupture of other ligament of right little finger at metacarpophalangeal and interphalangeal joint
- ● S63.497 Traumatic rupture of other ligament of left little finger at metacarpophalangeal and interphalangeal joint
- ● S63.498 Traumatic rupture of other ligament of other finger at metacarpophalangeal and interphalangeal joint
  Traumatic rupture of ligament of specified finger with unspecified laterality at metacarpophalangeal and interphalangeal joint
- ● S63.499 Traumatic rupture of other ligament of unspecified finger at metacarpophalangeal and interphalangeal joint

● S63.5 Other and unspecified sprain of wrist
- ● S63.50 Unspecified sprain of wrist
  - ● S63.501 Unspecified sprain of right wrist
  - ● S63.502 Unspecified sprain of left wrist
  - ● S63.509 Unspecified sprain of unspecified wrist
- ● S63.51 Sprain of carpal (joint)
  - ● S63.511 Sprain of carpal joint of right wrist
  - ● S63.512 Sprain of carpal joint of left wrist
  - ● S63.519 Sprain of carpal joint of unspecified wrist
- ● S63.52 Sprain of radiocarpal joint
  Excludes1 traumatic rupture of radiocarpal ligament (S63.32-)
  - ● S63.521 Sprain of radiocarpal joint of right wrist
  - ● S63.522 Sprain of radiocarpal joint of left wrist
  - ● S63.529 Sprain of radiocarpal joint of unspecified wrist
- ● S63.59 Other specified sprain of wrist
  - ● S63.591 Other specified sprain of right wrist
  - ● S63.592 Other specified sprain of left wrist
  - ● S63.599 Other specified sprain of unspecified wrist

● S63.6 Other and unspecified sprain of finger(s)
  Excludes1 traumatic rupture of ligament of finger at metacarpophalangeal and interphalangeal joint(s) (S63.4-)
- ● S63.60 Unspecified sprain of thumb
  - ● S63.601 Unspecified sprain of right thumb
  - ● S63.602 Unspecified sprain of left thumb
  - ● S63.609 Unspecified sprain of unspecified thumb
- ● S63.61 Unspecified sprain of other and unspecified finger(s)
  - ● S63.610 Unspecified sprain of right index finger
  - ● S63.611 Unspecified sprain of left index finger

● S63.612   Unspecified sprain of right middle finger

● S63.613   Unspecified sprain of left middle finger

● S63.614   Unspecified sprain of right ring finger

● S63.615   Unspecified sprain of left ring finger

● S63.616   Unspecified sprain of right little finger

● S63.617   Unspecified sprain of left little finger

● S63.618   Unspecified sprain of other finger
    Unspecified sprain of specified finger with unspecified laterality

● S63.619   Unspecified sprain of unspecified finger

● S63.62   Sprain of interphalangeal joint of thumb

● S63.621   Sprain of interphalangeal joint of right thumb

● S63.622   Sprain of interphalangeal joint of left thumb

● S63.629   Sprain of interphalangeal joint of unspecified thumb

● S63.63   Sprain of interphalangeal joint of other and unspecified finger(s)

● S63.630   Sprain of interphalangeal joint of right index finger

● S63.631   Sprain of interphalangeal joint of left index finger

● S63.632   Sprain of interphalangeal joint of right middle finger

● S63.633   Sprain of interphalangeal joint of left middle finger

● S63.634   Sprain of interphalangeal joint of right ring finger

● S63.635   Sprain of interphalangeal joint of left ring finger

● S63.636   Sprain of interphalangeal joint of right little finger

● S63.637   Sprain of interphalangeal joint of left little finger

● S63.638   Sprain of interphalangeal joint of other finger

● S63.639   Sprain of interphalangeal joint of unspecified finger

● S63.64   Sprain of metacarpophalangeal joint of thumb

● S63.641   Sprain of metacarpophalangeal joint of right thumb

● S63.642   Sprain of metacarpophalangeal joint of left thumb

● S63.649   Sprain of metacarpophalangeal joint of unspecified thumb

● S63.65   Sprain of metacarpophalangeal joint of other and unspecified finger(s)

● S63.650   Sprain of metacarpophalangeal joint of right index finger

● S63.651   Sprain of metacarpophalangeal joint of left index finger

● S63.652   Sprain of metacarpophalangeal joint of right middle finger

● S63.653   Sprain of metacarpophalangeal joint of left middle finger

● S63.654   Sprain of metacarpophalangeal joint of right ring finger

● S63.655   Sprain of metacarpophalangeal joint of left ring finger

● S63.656   Sprain of metacarpophalangeal joint of right little finger

● S63.657   Sprain of metacarpophalangeal joint of left little finger

● S63.658   Sprain of metacarpophalangeal joint of other finger
    Sprain of metacarpophalangeal joint of specified finger with unspecified laterality

● S63.659   Sprain of metacarpophalangeal joint of unspecified finger

● S63.68   Other sprain of thumb

● S63.681   Other sprain of right thumb

● S63.682   Other sprain of left thumb

● S63.689   Other sprain of unspecified thumb

● S63.69   Other sprain of other and unspecified finger(s)

● S63.690   Other sprain of right index finger

● S63.691   Other sprain of left index finger

● S63.692   Other sprain of right middle finger

● S63.693   Other sprain of left middle finger

● S63.694   Other sprain of right ring finger

● S63.695   Other sprain of left ring finger

● S63.696   Other sprain of right little finger

● S63.697   Other sprain of left little finger

● S63.698   Other sprain of other finger
    Other sprain of specified finger with unspecified laterality

● S63.699   Other sprain of unspecified finger

● S63.8   Sprain of other part of wrist and hand

● S63.8X   Sprain of other part of wrist and hand

● S63.8X1   Sprain of other part of right wrist and hand

● S63.8X2   Sprain of other part of left wrist and hand

● S63.8X9   Sprain of other part of unspecified wrist and hand

● S63.9   Sprain of unspecified part of wrist and hand

X ● S63.90   Sprain of unspecified part of unspecified wrist and hand

X ● S63.91   Sprain of unspecified part of right wrist and hand

X ● S63.92   Sprain of unspecified part of left wrist and hand

● S64   Injury of nerves at wrist and hand level

The appropriate 7th character is to be added to each code from category S64

A	initial encounter
D	subsequent encounter
S	sequela

Code also any associated open wound (S61.-)

● S64.0   Injury of ulnar nerve at wrist and hand level

X ● S64.00   Injury of ulnar nerve at wrist and hand level of unspecified arm

X ● S64.01   Injury of ulnar nerve at wrist and hand level of right arm

X ● S64.02   Injury of ulnar nerve at wrist and hand level of left arm

● S64.1   Injury of median nerve at wrist and hand level

X ● S64.10   Injury of median nerve at wrist and hand level of unspecified arm

X ● S64.11   Injury of median nerve at wrist and hand level of right arm

X ● S64.12   Injury of median nerve at wrist and hand level of left arm

CHAPTER 19 (S00-T88)

● S64.2   Injury of radial nerve at wrist and hand level
- X ● S64.20   Injury of radial nerve at wrist and hand level of unspecified arm
- X ● S64.21   Injury of radial nerve at wrist and hand level of right arm
- X ● S64.22   Injury of radial nerve at wrist and hand level of left arm

● S64.3   Injury of digital nerve of thumb
- X ● S64.30   Injury of digital nerve of unspecified thumb
- X ● S64.31   Injury of digital nerve of right thumb
- X ● S64.32   Injury of digital nerve of left thumb

● S64.4   Injury of digital nerve of other and unspecified finger
- X ● S64.40   Injury of digital nerve of unspecified finger
- ● S64.49   Injury of digital nerve of other finger
  - ● S64.490   Injury of digital nerve of right index finger
  - ● S64.491   Injury of digital nerve of left index finger
  - ● S64.492   Injury of digital nerve of right middle finger
  - ● S64.493   Injury of digital nerve of left middle finger
  - ● S64.494   Injury of digital nerve of right ring finger
  - ● S64.495   Injury of digital nerve of left ring finger
  - ● S64.496   Injury of digital nerve of right little finger
  - ● S64.497   Injury of digital nerve of left little finger
  - ● S64.498   Injury of digital nerve of other finger
    Injury of digital nerve of specified finger with unspecified laterality

● S64.8   Injury of other nerves at wrist and hand level
- ● S64.8X   Injury of other nerves at wrist and hand level
  - ● S64.8X1   Injury of other nerves at wrist and hand level of right arm
  - ● S64.8X2   Injury of other nerves at wrist and hand level of left arm
  - ● S64.8X9   Injury of other nerves at wrist and hand level of unspecified arm

● S64.9   Injury of unspecified nerve at wrist and hand level
- X ● S64.90   Injury of unspecified nerve at wrist and hand level of unspecified arm
- X ● S64.91   Injury of unspecified nerve at wrist and hand level of right arm
- X ● S64.92   Injury of unspecified nerve at wrist and hand level of left arm

● S65   Injury of blood vessels at wrist and hand level

The appropriate 7th character is to be added to each code from category S65

> A   initial encounter
> D   subsequent encounter
> S   sequela

Code also any associated open wound (S61.-)

● S65.0   Injury of ulnar artery at wrist and hand level
- ● S65.00   Unspecified injury of ulnar artery at wrist and hand level
  - ● S65.001   Unspecified injury of ulnar artery at wrist and hand level of right arm
  - ● S65.002   Unspecified injury of ulnar artery at wrist and hand level of left arm
  - ● S65.009   Unspecified injury of ulnar artery at wrist and hand level of unspecified arm

- ● S65.01   Laceration of ulnar artery at wrist and hand level
  - ● S65.011   Laceration of ulnar artery at wrist and hand level of right arm
  - ● S65.012   Laceration of ulnar artery at wrist and hand level of left arm
  - ● S65.019   Laceration of ulnar artery at wrist and hand level of unspecified arm

- ● S65.09   Other specified injury of ulnar artery at wrist and hand level
  - ● S65.091   Other specified injury of ulnar artery at wrist and hand level of right arm
  - ● S65.092   Other specified injury of ulnar artery at wrist and hand level of left arm
  - ● S65.099   Other specified injury of ulnar artery at wrist and hand level of unspecified arm

● S65.1   Injury of radial artery at wrist and hand level
- ● S65.10   Unspecified injury of radial artery at wrist and hand level
  - ● S65.101   Unspecified injury of radial artery at wrist and hand level of right arm
  - ● S65.102   Unspecified injury of radial artery at wrist and hand level of left arm
  - ● S65.109   Unspecified injury of radial artery at wrist and hand level of unspecified arm

- ● S65.11   Laceration of radial artery at wrist and hand level
  - ● S65.111   Laceration of radial artery at wrist and hand level of right arm
  - ● S65.112   Laceration of radial artery at wrist and hand level of left arm
  - ● S65.119   Laceration of radial artery at wrist and hand level of unspecified arm

- ● S65.19   Other specified injury of radial artery at wrist and hand level
  - ● S65.191   Other specified injury of radial artery at wrist and hand level of right arm
  - ● S65.192   Other specified injury of radial artery at wrist and hand level of left arm
  - ● S65.199   Other specified injury of radial artery at wrist and hand level of unspecified arm

● S65.2   Injury of superficial palmar arch
- ● S65.20   Unspecified injury of superficial palmar arch
  - ● S65.201   Unspecified injury of superficial palmar arch of right hand
  - ● S65.202   Unspecified injury of superficial palmar arch of left hand
  - ● S65.209   Unspecified injury of superficial palmar arch of unspecified hand

- ● S65.21   Laceration of superficial palmar arch
  - ● S65.211   Laceration of superficial palmar arch of right hand
  - ● S65.212   Laceration of superficial palmar arch of left hand
  - ● S65.219   Laceration of superficial palmar arch of unspecified hand

- ● S65.29   Other specified injury of superficial palmar arch
  - ● S65.291   Other specified injury of superficial palmar arch of right hand
  - ● S65.292   Other specified injury of superficial palmar arch of left hand
  - ● S65.299   Other specified injury of superficial palmar arch of unspecified hand

▶ New   ⇒ Revised   ~~deleted~~ Deleted   Excludes 1   Excludes 2   Includes   Use additional   Code first   Code also   Key words

OGCR Official Guidelines   X Assign placeholder X   ● Use Additional Character(s)   ▶ Manifestation Code   🅗 Hierarchical Condition Category   **Coding Clinic**

● S65.3   Injury of deep palmar arch
  ● S65.30   Unspecified injury of deep palmar arch
    ● S65.301   Unspecified injury of deep palmar arch of right hand
    ● S65.302   Unspecified injury of deep palmar arch of left hand
    ● S65.309   Unspecified injury of deep palmar arch of unspecified hand
  ● S65.31   Laceration of deep palmar arch
    ● S65.311   Laceration of deep palmar arch of right hand
    ● S65.312   Laceration of deep palmar arch of left hand
    ● S65.319   Laceration of deep palmar arch of unspecified hand
  ● S65.39   Other specified injury of deep palmar arch
    ● S65.391   Other specified injury of deep palmar arch of right hand
    ● S65.392   Other specified injury of deep palmar arch of left hand
    ● S65.399   Other specified injury of deep palmar arch of unspecified hand

● S65.4   Injury of blood vessel of thumb
  ● S65.40   Unspecified injury of blood vessel of thumb
    ● S65.401   Unspecified injury of blood vessel of right thumb
    ● S65.402   Unspecified injury of blood vessel of left thumb
    ● S65.409   Unspecified injury of blood vessel of unspecified thumb
  ● S65.41   Laceration of blood vessel of thumb
    ● S65.411   Laceration of blood vessel of right thumb
    ● S65.412   Laceration of blood vessel of left thumb
    ● S65.419   Laceration of blood vessel of unspecified thumb
  ● S65.49   Other specified injury of blood vessel of thumb
    ● S65.491   Other specified injury of blood vessel of right thumb
    ● S65.492   Other specified injury of blood vessel of left thumb
    ● S65.499   Other specified injury of blood vessel of unspecified thumb

● S65.5   Injury of blood vessel of other and unspecified finger
  ● S65.50   Unspecified injury of blood vessel of other and unspecified finger
    ● S65.500   Unspecified injury of blood vessel of right index finger
    ● S65.501   Unspecified injury of blood vessel of left index finger
    ● S65.502   Unspecified injury of blood vessel of right middle finger
    ● S65.503   Unspecified injury of blood vessel of left middle finger
    ● S65.504   Unspecified injury of blood vessel of right ring finger
    ● S65.505   Unspecified injury of blood vessel of left ring finger
    ● S65.506   Unspecified injury of blood vessel of right little finger
    ● S65.507   Unspecified injury of blood vessel of left little finger

    ● S65.508   Unspecified injury of blood vessel of other finger
       Unspecified injury of blood vessel of specified finger with unspecified laterality
    ● S65.509   Unspecified injury of blood vessel of unspecified finger
  ● S65.51   Laceration of blood vessel of other and unspecified finger
    ● S65.510   Laceration of blood vessel of right index finger
    ● S65.511   Laceration of blood vessel of left index finger
    ● S65.512   Laceration of blood vessel of right middle finger
    ● S65.513   Laceration of blood vessel of left middle finger
    ● S65.514   Laceration of blood vessel of right ring finger
    ● S65.515   Laceration of blood vessel of left ring finger
    ● S65.516   Laceration of blood vessel of right little finger
    ● S65.517   Laceration of blood vessel of left little finger
    ● S65.518   Laceration of blood vessel of other finger
       Laceration of blood vessel of specified finger with unspecified laterality
    ● S65.519   Laceration of blood vessel of unspecified finger
  ● S65.59   Other specified injury of blood vessel of other and unspecified finger
    ● S65.590   Other specified injury of blood vessel of right index finger
    ● S65.591   Other specified injury of blood vessel of left index finger
    ● S65.592   Other specified injury of blood vessel of right middle finger
    ● S65.593   Other specified injury of blood vessel of left middle finger
    ● S65.594   Other specified injury of blood vessel of right ring finger
    ● S65.595   Other specified injury of blood vessel of left ring finger
    ● S65.596   Other specified injury of blood vessel of right little finger
    ● S65.597   Other specified injury of blood vessel of left little finger
    ● S65.598   Other specified injury of blood vessel of other finger
       Other specified injury of blood vessel of specified finger with unspecified laterality
    ● S65.599   Other specified injury of blood vessel of unspecified finger

● S65.8   Injury of other blood vessels at wrist and hand level
  ● S65.80   Unspecified injury of other blood vessels at wrist and hand level
    ● S65.801   Unspecified injury of other blood vessels at wrist and hand level of right arm
    ● S65.802   Unspecified injury of other blood vessels at wrist and hand level of left arm
    ● S65.809   Unspecified injury of other blood vessels at wrist and hand level of unspecified arm

- S65.81   Laceration of other blood vessels at wrist and hand level
    - S65.811   Laceration of other blood vessels at wrist and hand level of right arm
    - S65.812   Laceration of other blood vessels at wrist and hand level of left arm
    - S65.819   Laceration of other blood vessels at wrist and hand level of unspecified arm
- S65.89   Other specified injury of other blood vessels at wrist and hand level
    - S65.891   Other specified injury of other blood vessels at wrist and hand level of right arm
    - S65.892   Other specified injury of other blood vessels at wrist and hand level of left arm
    - S65.899   Other specified injury of other blood vessels at wrist and hand level of unspecified arm
- S65.9   Injury of unspecified blood vessel at wrist and hand level
    - S65.90   Unspecified injury of unspecified blood vessel at wrist and hand level
        - S65.901   Unspecified injury of unspecified blood vessel at wrist and hand level of right arm
        - S65.902   Unspecified injury of unspecified blood vessel at wrist and hand level of left arm
        - S65.909   Unspecified injury of unspecified blood vessel at wrist and hand level of unspecified arm
    - S65.91   Laceration of unspecified blood vessel at wrist and hand level
        - S65.911   Laceration of unspecified blood vessel at wrist and hand level of right arm
        - S65.912   Laceration of unspecified blood vessel at wrist and hand level of left arm
        - S65.919   Laceration of unspecified blood vessel at wrist and hand level of unspecified arm
    - S65.99   Other specified injury of unspecified blood vessel at wrist and hand level
        - S65.991   Other specified injury of unspecified blood vessel at wrist and hand of right arm
        - S65.992   Other specified injury of unspecified blood vessel at wrist and hand of left arm
        - S65.999   Other specified injury of unspecified blood vessel at wrist and hand of unspecified arm

- S66   **Injury of muscle, fascia and tendon at wrist and hand level**

    Code also any associated open wound (S61.-)

    Excludes2   sprain of joints and ligaments of wrist and hand (S63.-)

    The appropriate 7th character is to be added to each code from category S66

A	initial encounter
D	subsequent encounter
S	sequela

    - S66.0   Injury of long flexor muscle, fascia and tendon of thumb at wrist and hand level
        - S66.00   Unspecified injury of long flexor muscle, fascia and tendon of thumb at wrist and hand level
            - S66.001   Unspecified injury of long flexor muscle, fascia and tendon of right thumb at wrist and hand level

---

- S66.002   Unspecified injury of long flexor muscle, fascia and tendon of left thumb at wrist and hand level
- S66.009   Unspecified injury of long flexor muscle, fascia and tendon of unspecified thumb at wrist and hand level
- S66.01   Strain of long flexor muscle, fascia and tendon of thumb at wrist and hand level
    - S66.011   Strain of long flexor muscle, fascia and tendon of right thumb at wrist and hand level
    - S66.012   Strain of long flexor muscle, fascia and tendon of left thumb at wrist and hand level
    - S66.019   Strain of long flexor muscle, fascia and tendon of unspecified thumb at wrist and hand level
- S66.02   Laceration of long flexor muscle, fascia and tendon of thumb at wrist and hand level
    - S66.021   Laceration of long flexor muscle, fascia and tendon of right thumb at wrist and hand level
    - S66.022   Laceration of long flexor muscle, fascia and tendon of left thumb at wrist and hand level
    - S66.029   Laceration of long flexor muscle, fascia and tendon of unspecified thumb at wrist and hand level
- S66.09   Other specified injury of long flexor muscle, fascia and tendon of thumb at wrist and hand level
    - S66.091   Other specified injury of long flexor muscle, fascia and tendon of right thumb at wrist and hand level
    - S66.092   Other specified injury of long flexor muscle, fascia and tendon of left thumb at wrist and hand level
    - S66.099   Other specified injury of long flexor muscle, fascia and tendon of unspecified thumb at wrist and hand level
- S66.1   Injury of flexor muscle, fascia and tendon of other and unspecified finger at wrist and hand level

    Excludes2   injury of long flexor muscle, fascia and tendon of thumb at wrist and hand level (S66.0-)

    - S66.10   Unspecified injury of flexor muscle, fascia and tendon of other and unspecified finger at wrist and hand level
        - S66.100   Unspecified injury of flexor muscle, fascia and tendon of right index finger at wrist and hand level
        - S66.101   Unspecified injury of flexor muscle, fascia and tendon of left index finger at wrist and hand level
        - S66.102   Unspecified injury of flexor muscle, fascia and tendon of right middle finger at wrist and hand level
        - S66.103   Unspecified injury of flexor muscle, fascia and tendon of left middle finger at wrist and hand level
        - S66.104   Unspecified injury of flexor muscle, fascia and tendon of right ring finger at wrist and hand level

▶ New   ⇒ Revised   ~~deleted~~ Deleted   Excludes 1   Excludes 2   Includes   Use additional   Code first   Code also   Key words

OGCR Official Guidelines   X Assign placeholder X   ● Use Additional Character(s)   ▷ Manifestation Code   🝒 Hierarchical Condition Category   **Coding Clinic**

● S66.105   Unspecified injury of flexor muscle, fascia and tendon of left ring finger at wrist and hand level

● S66.106   Unspecified injury of flexor muscle, fascia and tendon of right little finger at wrist and hand level

● S66.107   Unspecified injury of flexor muscle, fascia and tendon of left little finger at wrist and hand level

● S66.108   Unspecified injury of flexor muscle, fascia and tendon of other finger at wrist and hand level

> Unspecified injury of flexor muscle, fascia and tendon of specified finger with unspecified laterality at wrist and hand level

● S66.109   Unspecified injury of flexor muscle, fascia and tendon of unspecified finger at wrist and hand level

● S66.11   Strain of flexor muscle, fascia and tendon of other and unspecified finger at wrist and hand level

● S66.110   Strain of flexor muscle, fascia and tendon of right index finger at wrist and hand level

● S66.111   Strain of flexor muscle, fascia and tendon of left index finger at wrist and hand level

● S66.112   Strain of flexor muscle, fascia and tendon of right middle finger at wrist and hand level

● S66.113   Strain of flexor muscle, fascia and tendon of left middle finger at wrist and hand level

● S66.114   Strain of flexor muscle, fascia and tendon of right ring finger at wrist and hand level

● S66.115   Strain of flexor muscle, fascia and tendon of left ring finger at wrist and hand level

● S66.116   Strain of flexor muscle, fascia and tendon of right little finger at wrist and hand level

● S66.117   Strain of flexor muscle, fascia and tendon of left little finger at wrist and hand level

● S66.118   Strain of flexor muscle, fascia and tendon of other finger at wrist and hand level

> Strain of flexor muscle, fascia and tendon of specified finger with unspecified laterality at wrist and hand level

● S66.119   Strain of flexor muscle, fascia and tendon of unspecified finger at wrist and hand level

● S66.12   Laceration of flexor muscle, fascia and tendon of other and unspecified finger at wrist and hand level

● S66.120   Laceration of flexor muscle, fascia and tendon of right index finger at wrist and hand level

● S66.121   Laceration of flexor muscle, fascia and tendon of left index finger at wrist and hand level

● S66.122   Laceration of flexor muscle, fascia and tendon of right middle finger at wrist and hand level

● S66.123   Laceration of flexor muscle, fascia and tendon of left middle finger at wrist and hand level

● S66.124   Laceration of flexor muscle, fascia and tendon of right ring finger at wrist and hand level

● S66.125   Laceration of flexor muscle, fascia and tendon of left ring finger at wrist and hand level

● S66.126   Laceration of flexor muscle, fascia and tendon of right little finger at wrist and hand level

● S66.127   Laceration of flexor muscle, fascia and tendon of left little finger at wrist and hand level

● S66.128   Laceration of flexor muscle, fascia and tendon of other finger at wrist and hand level

> Laceration of flexor muscle, fascia and tendon of specified finger with unspecified laterality at wrist and hand level

● S66.129   Laceration of flexor muscle, fascia and tendon of unspecified finger at wrist and hand level

● S66.19   Other injury of flexor muscle, fascia and tendon of other and unspecified finger at wrist and hand level

● S66.190   Other injury of flexor muscle, fascia and tendon of right index finger at wrist and hand level

● S66.191   Other injury of flexor muscle, fascia and tendon of left index finger at wrist and hand level

● S66.192   Other injury of flexor muscle, fascia and tendon of right middle finger at wrist and hand level

● S66.193   Other injury of flexor muscle, fascia and tendon of left middle finger at wrist and hand level

● S66.194   Other injury of flexor muscle, fascia and tendon of right ring finger at wrist and hand level

● S66.195   Other injury of flexor muscle, fascia and tendon of left ring finger at wrist and hand level

● S66.196   Other injury of flexor muscle, fascia and tendon of right little finger at wrist and hand level

● S66.197   Other injury of flexor muscle, fascia and tendon of left little finger at wrist and hand level

● S66.198   Other injury of flexor muscle, fascia and tendon of other finger at wrist and hand level

> Other injury of flexor muscle, fascia and tendon of specified finger with unspecified laterality at wrist and hand level

● S66.199   Other injury of flexor muscle, fascia and tendon of unspecified finger at wrist and hand level

CHAPTER 19 (S00-T88)

● **S66.2** Injury of extensor muscle, fascia and tendon of thumb at wrist and hand level

- ● **S66.20** Unspecified injury of extensor muscle, fascia and tendon of thumb at wrist and hand level
  - ● **S66.201** Unspecified injury of extensor muscle, fascia and tendon of right thumb at wrist and hand level
  - ● **S66.202** Unspecified injury of extensor muscle, fascia and tendon of left thumb at wrist and hand level
  - ● **S66.209** Unspecified injury of extensor muscle, fascia and tendon of unspecified thumb at wrist and hand level

- ● **S66.21** Strain of extensor muscle, fascia and tendon of thumb at wrist and hand level
  - ● **S66.211** Strain of extensor muscle, fascia and tendon of right thumb at wrist and hand level
  - ● **S66.212** Strain of extensor muscle, fascia and tendon of left thumb at wrist and hand level
  - ● **S66.219** Strain of extensor muscle, fascia and tendon of unspecified thumb at wrist and hand level

- ● **S66.22** Laceration of extensor muscle, fascia and tendon of thumb at wrist and hand level
  - ● **S66.221** Laceration of extensor muscle, fascia and tendon of right thumb at wrist and hand level
  - ● **S66.222** Laceration of extensor muscle, fascia and tendon of left thumb at wrist and hand level
  - ● **S66.229** Laceration of extensor muscle, fascia and tendon of unspecified thumb at wrist and hand level

- ● **S66.29** Other specified injury of extensor muscle, fascia and tendon of thumb at wrist and hand level
  - ● **S66.291** Other specified injury of extensor muscle, fascia and tendon of right thumb at wrist and hand level
  - ● **S66.292** Other specified injury of extensor muscle, fascia and tendon of left thumb at wrist and hand level
  - ● **S66.299** Other specified injury of extensor muscle, fascia and tendon of unspecified thumb at wrist and hand level

● **S66.3** Injury of extensor muscle, fascia and tendon of other and unspecified finger at wrist and hand level

   Excludes2   injury of extensor muscle, fascia and tendon of thumb at wrist and hand level (S66.2-)

- ● **S66.30** Unspecified injury of extensor muscle, fascia and tendon of other and unspecified finger at wrist and hand level
  - ● **S66.300** Unspecified injury of extensor muscle, fascia and tendon of right index finger at wrist and hand level
  - ● **S66.301** Unspecified injury of extensor muscle, fascia and tendon of left index finger at wrist and hand level
  - ● **S66.302** Unspecified injury of extensor muscle, fascia and tendon of right middle finger at wrist and hand level
  - ● **S66.303** Unspecified injury of extensor muscle, fascia and tendon of left middle finger at wrist and hand level
  - ● **S66.304** Unspecified injury of extensor muscle, fascia and tendon of right ring finger at wrist and hand level
  - ● **S66.305** Unspecified injury of extensor muscle, fascia and tendon of left ring finger at wrist and hand level
  - ● **S66.306** Unspecified injury of extensor muscle, fascia and tendon of right little finger at wrist and hand level
  - ● **S66.307** Unspecified injury of extensor muscle, fascia and tendon of left little finger at wrist and hand level
  - ● **S66.308** Unspecified injury of extensor muscle, fascia and tendon of other finger at wrist and hand level

    Unspecified injury of extensor muscle, fascia and tendon of specified finger with unspecified laterality at wrist and hand level
  - ● **S66.309** Unspecified injury of extensor muscle, fascia and tendon of unspecified finger at wrist and hand level

- ● **S66.31** Strain of extensor muscle, fascia and tendon of other and unspecified finger at wrist and hand level
  - ● **S66.310** Strain of extensor muscle, fascia and tendon of right index finger at wrist and hand level
  - ● **S66.311** Strain of extensor muscle, fascia and tendon of left index finger at wrist and hand level
  - ● **S66.312** Strain of extensor muscle, fascia and tendon of right middle finger at wrist and hand level
  - ● **S66.313** Strain of extensor muscle, fascia and tendon of left middle finger at wrist and hand level
  - ● **S66.314** Strain of extensor muscle, fascia and tendon of right ring finger at wrist and hand level
  - ● **S66.315** Strain of extensor muscle, fascia and tendon of left ring finger at wrist and hand level
  - ● **S66.316** Strain of extensor muscle, fascia and tendon of right little finger at wrist and hand level
  - ● **S66.317** Strain of extensor muscle, fascia and tendon of left little finger at wrist and hand level
  - ● **S66.318** Strain of extensor muscle, fascia and tendon of other finger at wrist and hand level

    Strain of extensor muscle, fascia and tendon of specified finger with unspecified laterality at wrist and hand level
  - ● **S66.319** Strain of extensor muscle, fascia and tendon of unspecified finger at wrist and hand level

▶ New   ⇒ Revised   ~~deleted~~ Deleted   Excludes 1   Excludes 2   Includes   Use additional   Code first   Code also   Key words

OGCR Official Guidelines   X Assign placeholder X   ● Use Additional Character(s)   ▷ Manifestation Code   ℞ Hierarchical Condition Category   Coding Clinic

● **S66.32** Laceration of extensor muscle, fascia and tendon of other and unspecified finger at wrist and hand level

   ● **S66.320** Laceration of extensor muscle, fascia and tendon of right index finger at wrist and hand level

   ● **S66.321** Laceration of extensor muscle, fascia and tendon of left index finger at wrist and hand level

   ● **S66.322** Laceration of extensor muscle, fascia and tendon of right middle finger at wrist and hand level

   ● **S66.323** Laceration of extensor muscle, fascia and tendon of left middle finger at wrist and hand level

   ● **S66.324** Laceration of extensor muscle, fascia and tendon of right ring finger at wrist and hand level

   ● **S66.325** Laceration of extensor muscle, fascia and tendon of left ring finger at wrist and hand level

   ● **S66.326** Laceration of extensor muscle, fascia and tendon of right little finger at wrist and hand level

   ● **S66.327** Laceration of extensor muscle, fascia and tendon of left little finger at wrist and hand level

   ● **S66.328** Laceration of extensor muscle, fascia and tendon of other finger at wrist and hand level

       Laceration of extensor muscle, fascia and tendon of specified finger with unspecified laterality at wrist and hand level

   ● **S66.329** Laceration of extensor muscle, fascia and tendon of unspecified finger at wrist and hand level

● **S66.39** Other injury of extensor muscle, fascia and tendon of other and unspecified finger at wrist and hand level

   ● **S66.390** Other injury of extensor muscle, fascia and tendon of right index finger at wrist and hand level

   ● **S66.391** Other injury of extensor muscle, fascia and tendon of left index finger at wrist and hand level

   ● **S66.392** Other injury of extensor muscle, fascia and tendon of right middle finger at wrist and hand level

   ● **S66.393** Other injury of extensor muscle, fascia and tendon of left middle finger at wrist and hand level

   ● **S66.394** Other injury of extensor muscle, fascia and tendon of right ring finger at wrist and hand level

   ● **S66.395** Other injury of extensor muscle, fascia and tendon of left ring finger at wrist and hand level

   ● **S66.396** Other injury of extensor muscle, fascia and tendon of right little finger at wrist and hand level

   ● **S66.397** Other injury of extensor muscle, fascia and tendon of left little finger at wrist and hand level

   ● **S66.398** Other injury of extensor muscle, fascia and tendon of other finger at wrist and hand level

       Other injury of extensor muscle, fascia and tendon of specified finger with unspecified laterality at wrist and hand level

   ● **S66.399** Other injury of extensor muscle, fascia and tendon of unspecified finger at wrist and hand level

● **S66.4** Injury of intrinsic muscle, fascia and tendon of thumb at wrist and hand level

   ● **S66.40** Unspecified injury of intrinsic muscle, fascia and tendon of thumb at wrist and hand level

      ● **S66.401** Unspecified injury of intrinsic muscle, fascia and tendon of right thumb at wrist and hand level

      ● **S66.402** Unspecified injury of intrinsic muscle, fascia and tendon of left thumb at wrist and hand level

      ● **S66.409** Unspecified injury of intrinsic muscle, fascia and tendon of unspecified thumb at wrist and hand level

   ● **S66.41** Strain of intrinsic muscle, fascia and tendon of thumb at wrist and hand level

      ● **S66.411** Strain of intrinsic muscle, fascia and tendon of right thumb at wrist and hand level

      ● **S66.412** Strain of intrinsic muscle, fascia and tendon of left thumb at wrist and hand level

      ● **S66.419** Strain of intrinsic muscle, fascia and tendon of unspecified thumb at wrist and hand level

   ● **S66.42** Laceration of intrinsic muscle, fascia and tendon of thumb at wrist and hand level

      ● **S66.421** Laceration of intrinsic muscle, fascia and tendon of right thumb at wrist and hand level

      ● **S66.422** Laceration of intrinsic muscle, fascia and tendon of left thumb at wrist and hand level

      ● **S66.429** Laceration of intrinsic muscle, fascia and tendon of unspecified thumb at wrist and hand level

   ● **S66.49** Other specified injury of intrinsic muscle, fascia and tendon of thumb at wrist and hand level

      ● **S66.491** Other specified injury of intrinsic muscle, fascia and tendon of right thumb at wrist and hand level

      ● **S66.492** Other specified injury of intrinsic muscle, fascia and tendon of left thumb at wrist and hand level

      ● **S66.499** Other specified injury of intrinsic muscle, fascia and tendon of unspecified thumb at wrist and hand level

● S66.5   Injury of intrinsic muscle, fascia and tendon of other and unspecified finger at wrist and hand level

     Excludes2   injury of intrinsic muscle, fascia and tendon of thumb at wrist and hand level (S66.4-)

● S66.50   Unspecified injury of intrinsic muscle, fascia and tendon of other and unspecified finger at wrist and hand level

    ● S66.500   Unspecified injury of intrinsic muscle, fascia and tendon of right index finger at wrist and hand level

    ● S66.501   Unspecified injury of intrinsic muscle, fascia and tendon of left index finger at wrist and hand level

    ● S66.502   Unspecified injury of intrinsic muscle, fascia and tendon of right middle finger at wrist and hand level

    ● S66.503   Unspecified injury of intrinsic muscle, fascia and tendon of left middle finger at wrist and hand level

    ● S66.504   Unspecified injury of intrinsic muscle, fascia and tendon of right ring finger at wrist and hand level

    ● S66.505   Unspecified injury of intrinsic muscle, fascia and tendon of left ring finger at wrist and hand level

    ● S66.506   Unspecified injury of intrinsic muscle, fascia and tendon of right little finger at wrist and hand level

    ● S66.507   Unspecified injury of intrinsic muscle, fascia and tendon of left little finger at wrist and hand level

    ● S66.508   Unspecified injury of intrinsic muscle, fascia and tendon of other finger at wrist and hand level

        Unspecified injury of intrinsic muscle, fascia and tendon of specified finger with unspecified laterality at wrist and hand level

    ● S66.509   Unspecified injury of intrinsic muscle, fascia and tendon of unspecified finger at wrist and hand level

● S66.51   Strain of intrinsic muscle, fascia and tendon of other and unspecified finger at wrist and hand level

    ● S66.510   Strain of intrinsic muscle, fascia and tendon of right index finger at wrist and hand level

    ● S66.511   Strain of intrinsic muscle, fascia and tendon of left index finger at wrist and hand level

    ● S66.512   Strain of intrinsic muscle, fascia and tendon of right middle finger at wrist and hand level

    ● S66.513   Strain of intrinsic muscle, fascia and tendon of left middle finger at wrist and hand level

    ● S66.514   Strain of intrinsic muscle, fascia and tendon of right ring finger at wrist and hand level

    ● S66.515   Strain of intrinsic muscle, fascia and tendon of left ring finger at wrist and hand level

    ● S66.516   Strain of intrinsic muscle, fascia and tendon of right little finger at wrist and hand level

    ● S66.517   Strain of intrinsic muscle, fascia and tendon of left little finger at wrist and hand level

    ● S66.518   Strain of intrinsic muscle, fascia and tendon of other finger at wrist and hand level

        Strain of intrinsic muscle, fascia and tendon of specified finger with unspecified laterality at wrist and hand level

    ● S66.519   Strain of intrinsic muscle, fascia and tendon of unspecified finger at wrist and hand level

● S66.52   Laceration of intrinsic muscle, fascia and tendon of other and unspecified finger at wrist and hand level

    ● S66.520   Laceration of intrinsic muscle, fascia and tendon of right index finger at wrist and hand level

    ● S66.521   Laceration of intrinsic muscle, fascia and tendon of left index finger at wrist and hand level

    ● S66.522   Laceration of intrinsic muscle, fascia and tendon of right middle finger at wrist and hand level

    ● S66.523   Laceration of intrinsic muscle, fascia and tendon of left middle finger at wrist and hand level

    ● S66.524   Laceration of intrinsic muscle, fascia and tendon of right ring finger at wrist and hand level

    ● S66.525   Laceration of intrinsic muscle, fascia and tendon of left ring finger at wrist and hand level

    ● S66.526   Laceration of intrinsic muscle, fascia and tendon of right little finger at wrist and hand level

    ● S66.527   Laceration of intrinsic muscle, fascia and tendon of left little finger at wrist and hand level

    ● S66.528   Laceration of intrinsic muscle, fascia and tendon of other finger at wrist and hand level

        Laceration of intrinsic muscle, fascia and tendon of specified finger with unspecified laterality at wrist and hand level

    ● S66.529   Laceration of intrinsic muscle, fascia and tendon of unspecified finger at wrist and hand level

● S66.59   Other injury of intrinsic muscle, fascia and tendon of other and unspecified finger at wrist and hand level

    ● S66.590   Other injury of intrinsic muscle, fascia and tendon of right index finger at wrist and hand level

    ● S66.591   Other injury of intrinsic muscle, fascia and tendon of left index finger at wrist and hand level

    ● S66.592   Other injury of intrinsic muscle, fascia and tendon of right middle finger at wrist and hand level

    ● S66.593   Other injury of intrinsic muscle, fascia and tendon of left middle finger at wrist and hand level

▶ New   ⟹ Revised   ~~deleted~~ Deleted   Excludes 1   Excludes 2   Includes   Use additional   Code first   Code also   Key words

OGCR Official Guidelines   X Assign placeholder X   ● Use Additional Character(s)   ▶ Manifestation Code   ℞ Hierarchical Condition Category   **Coding Clinic**

● S66.594   Other injury of intrinsic muscle, fascia and tendon of right ring finger at wrist and hand level

● S66.595   Other injury of intrinsic muscle, fascia and tendon of left ring finger at wrist and hand level

● S66.596   Other injury of intrinsic muscle, fascia and tendon of right little finger at wrist and hand level

● S66.597   Other injury of intrinsic muscle, fascia and tendon of left little finger at wrist and hand level

● S66.598   Other injury of intrinsic muscle, fascia and tendon of other finger at wrist and hand level

> Other injury of intrinsic muscle, fascia and tendon of specified finger with unspecified laterality at wrist and hand level

● S66.599   Other injury of intrinsic muscle, fascia and tendon of unspecified finger at wrist and hand level

● S66.8   Injury of other specified muscles, fascia and tendons at wrist and hand level

   ● S66.80   Unspecified injury of other specified muscles, fascia and tendons at wrist and hand level

     ● S66.801   Unspecified injury of other specified muscles, fascia and tendons at wrist and hand level, right hand

     ● S66.802   Unspecified injury of other specified muscles, fascia and tendons at wrist and hand level, left hand

     ● S66.809   Unspecified injury of other specified muscles, fascia and tendons at wrist and hand level, unspecified hand

   ● S66.81   Strain of other specified muscles, fascia and tendons at wrist and hand level

     ● S66.811   Strain of other specified muscles, fascia and tendons at wrist and hand level, right hand

     ● S66.812   Strain of other specified muscles, fascia and tendons at wrist and hand level, left hand

     ● S66.819   Strain of other specified muscles, fascia and tendons at wrist and hand level, unspecified hand

   ● S66.82   Laceration of other specified muscles, fascia and tendons at wrist and hand level

     ● S66.821   Laceration of other specified muscles, fascia and tendons at wrist and hand level, right hand

     ● S66.822   Laceration of other specified muscles, fascia and tendons at wrist and hand level, left hand

     ● S66.829   Laceration of other specified muscles, fascia and tendons at wrist and hand level, unspecified hand

   ● S66.89   Other injury of other specified muscles, fascia and tendons at wrist and hand level

     ● S66.891   Other injury of other specified muscles, fascia and tendons at wrist and hand level, right hand

     ● S66.892   Other injury of other specified muscles, fascia and tendons at wrist and hand level, left hand

     ● S66.899   Other injury of other specified muscles, fascia and tendons at wrist and hand level, unspecified hand

● S66.9   Injury of unspecified muscle, fascia and tendon at wrist and hand level

   ● S66.90   Unspecified injury of unspecified muscle, fascia and tendon at wrist and hand level

     ● S66.901   Unspecified injury of unspecified muscle, fascia and tendon at wrist and hand level, right hand

     ● S66.902   Unspecified injury of unspecified muscle, fascia and tendon at wrist and hand level, left hand

     ● S66.909   Unspecified injury of unspecified muscle, fascia and tendon at wrist and hand level, unspecified hand

   ● S66.91   Strain of unspecified muscle, fascia and tendon at wrist and hand level

     ● S66.911   Strain of unspecified muscle, fascia and tendon at wrist and hand level, right hand

     ● S66.912   Strain of unspecified muscle, fascia and tendon at wrist and hand level, left hand

     ● S66.919   Strain of unspecified muscle, fascia and tendon at wrist and hand level, unspecified hand

   ● S66.92   Laceration of unspecified muscle, fascia and tendon at wrist and hand level

     ● S66.921   Laceration of unspecified muscle, fascia and tendon at wrist and hand level, right hand

     ● S66.922   Laceration of unspecified muscle, fascia and tendon at wrist and hand level, left hand

     ● S66.929   Laceration of unspecified muscle, fascia and tendon at wrist and hand level, unspecified hand

   ● S66.99   Other injury of unspecified muscle, fascia and tendon at wrist and hand level

     ● S66.991   Other injury of unspecified muscle, fascia and tendon at wrist and hand level, right hand

     ● S66.992   Other injury of unspecified muscle, fascia and tendon at wrist and hand level, left hand

     ● S66.999   Other injury of unspecified muscle, fascia and tendon at wrist and hand level, unspecified hand

● S67   **Crushing injury of wrist, hand and fingers**

> Use additional code for all associated injuries, such as:
> fracture of wrist and hand (S62.-)
> open wound of wrist and hand (S61.-)

> The appropriate 7th character is to be added to each code from category S67

A	initial encounter
D	subsequent encounter
S	sequela

● S67.0   Crushing injury of thumb

   X ● S67.00   Crushing injury of unspecified thumb

   X ● S67.01   Crushing injury of right thumb

   X ● S67.02   Crushing injury of left thumb

● S67.1   Crushing injury of other and unspecified finger(s)

> **Excludes2**   crushing injury of thumb (S67.0-)

   X ● S67.10   Crushing injury of unspecified finger(s)

   ● S67.19   Crushing injury of other finger(s)

     ● S67.190   Crushing injury of right index finger

     ● S67.191   Crushing injury of left index finger

● S67.192　Crushing injury of right middle finger

● S67.193　Crushing injury of left middle finger

● S67.194　Crushing injury of right ring finger

● S67.195　Crushing injury of left ring finger

● S67.196　Crushing injury of right little finger

● S67.197　Crushing injury of left little finger

● S67.198　Crushing injury of other finger
　　　　　Crushing injury of specified finger with unspecified laterality

● S67.2　Crushing injury of hand

　　Excludes2　crushing injury of fingers (S67.1-)
　　　　　　　crushing injury of thumb (S67.0-)

X ● S67.20　Crushing injury of unspecified hand

X ● S67.21　Crushing injury of right hand

X ● S67.22　Crushing injury of left hand

● S67.3　Crushing injury of wrist

X ● S67.30　Crushing injury of unspecified wrist

X ● S67.31　Crushing injury of right wrist

X ● S67.32　Crushing injury of left wrist

● S67.4　Crushing injury of wrist and hand

　　Excludes1　crushing injury of hand alone (S67.2-)
　　　　　　　crushing injury of wrist alone (S67.3-)

　　Excludes2　crushing injury of fingers (S67.1-)
　　　　　　　crushing injury of thumb (S67.0-)

X ● S67.40　Crushing injury of unspecified wrist and hand

X ● S67.41　Crushing injury of right wrist and hand

X ● S67.42　Crushing injury of left wrist and hand

● S67.9　Crushing injury of unspecified part(s) of wrist, hand and fingers

X ● S67.90　Crushing injury of unspecified part(s) of unspecified wrist, hand and fingers

X ● S67.91　Crushing injury of unspecified part(s) of right wrist, hand and fingers

X ● S67.92　Crushing injury of unspecified part(s) of left wrist, hand and fingers

● S68　Traumatic amputation of wrist, hand and fingers
　　An amputation not identified as partial or complete should be coded to complete
　　The appropriate 7th character is to be added to each code from category S68

A	initial encounter
D	subsequent encounter
S	sequela

● S68.0　Traumatic metacarpophalangeal amputation of thumb
　　Traumatic amputation of thumb NOS

● S68.01　Complete traumatic metacarpophalangeal amputation of thumb

● S68.011　Complete traumatic metacarpophalangeal amputation of right thumb S 🐾

● S68.012　Complete traumatic metacarpophalangeal amputation of left thumb S 🐾

● S68.019　Complete traumatic metacarpophalangeal amputation of unspecified thumb S 🐾

● S68.02　Partial traumatic metacarpophalangeal amputation of thumb

● S68.021　Partial traumatic metacarpophalangeal amputation of right thumb S 🐾

● S68.022　Partial traumatic metacarpophalangeal amputation of left thumb S 🐾

● S68.029　Partial traumatic metacarpophalangeal amputation of unspecified thumb S 🐾

● S68.1　Traumatic metacarpophalangeal amputation of other and unspecified finger
　　Traumatic amputation of finger NOS

　　Excludes2　traumatic metacarpophalangeal amputation of thumb (S68.0-)

● S68.11　Complete traumatic metacarpophalangeal amputation of other and unspecified finger

● S68.110　Complete traumatic metacarpophalangeal amputation of right index finger S 🐾

● S68.111　Complete traumatic metacarpophalangeal amputation of left index finger S 🐾

● S68.112　Complete traumatic metacarpophalangeal amputation of right middle finger S 🐾

● S68.113　Complete traumatic metacarpophalangeal amputation of left middle finger S 🐾

● S68.114　Complete traumatic metacarpophalangeal amputation of right ring finger S 🐾

● S68.115　Complete traumatic metacarpophalangeal amputation of left ring finger S 🐾

● S68.116　Complete traumatic metacarpophalangeal amputation of right little finger S 🐾

● S68.117　Complete traumatic metacarpophalangeal amputation of left little finger S 🐾

● S68.118　Complete traumatic metacarpophalangeal amputation of other finger S 🐾
　　　　　Complete traumatic metacarpophalangeal amputation of specified finger with unspecified laterality

● S68.119　Complete traumatic metacarpophalangeal amputation of unspecified finger S 🐾

● S68.12　Partial traumatic metacarpophalangeal amputation of other and unspecified finger

● S68.120　Partial traumatic metacarpophalangeal amputation of right index finger S 🐾

● S68.121　Partial traumatic metacarpophalangeal amputation of left index finger S 🐾

● S68.122　Partial traumatic metacarpophalangeal amputation of right middle finger S 🐾

● S68.123　Partial traumatic metacarpophalangeal amputation of left middle finger S 🐾

● S68.124　Partial traumatic metacarpophalangeal amputation of right ring finger S 🐾

● S68.125　Partial traumatic metacarpophalangeal amputation of left ring finger S 🐾

● S68.126　Partial traumatic metacarpophalangeal amputation of right little finger S 🐾

● S68.127　Partial traumatic metacarpophalangeal amputation of left little finger S 🐾

● S68.128   Partial traumatic
            metacarpophalangeal amputation of
            other finger S ⟐
                Partial traumatic
                metacarpophalangeal
                amputation of specified finger
                with unspecified laterality
● S68.129   Partial traumatic
            metacarpophalangeal amputation of
            unspecified finger S ⟐

● S68.4 **Traumatic amputation of hand at wrist level**
         Traumatic amputation of hand NOS
         Traumatic amputation of wrist

   ● S68.41 **Complete traumatic amputation of hand at
             wrist level**
      ● S68.411   Complete traumatic amputation of
                  right hand at wrist level A, S ⟐
      ● S68.412   Complete traumatic amputation of
                  left hand at wrist level A, S ⟐
      ● S68.419   Complete traumatic amputation of
                  unspecified hand at wrist level A, S ⟐

   ● S68.42 **Partial traumatic amputation of hand at wrist
             level**
      ● S68.421   Partial traumatic amputation of right
                  hand at wrist level A, S ⟐
      ● S68.422   Partial traumatic amputation of left
                  hand at wrist level A, S ⟐
      ● S68.429   Partial traumatic amputation of
                  unspecified hand at wrist level A, S ⟐

● S68.5 **Traumatic transphalangeal amputation of thumb**
         Traumatic interphalangeal joint amputation of thumb

   ● S68.51 **Complete traumatic transphalangeal
             amputation of thumb**
      ● S68.511   Complete traumatic transphalangeal
                  amputation of right thumb S ⟐
      ● S68.512   Complete traumatic transphalangeal
                  amputation of left thumb S ⟐
      ● S68.519   Complete traumatic transphalangeal
                  amputation of unspecified thumb S ⟐

   ● S68.52 **Partial traumatic transphalangeal amputation of
             thumb**
      ● S68.521   Partial traumatic transphalangeal
                  amputation of right thumb S ⟐
      ● S68.522   Partial traumatic transphalangeal
                  amputation of left thumb S ⟐
      ● S68.529   Partial traumatic transphalangeal
                  amputation of unspecified thumb S ⟐

● S68.6 **Traumatic transphalangeal amputation of other and
         unspecified finger**

   ● S68.61 **Complete traumatic transphalangeal
             amputation of other and unspecified finger(s)**
      ● S68.610   Complete traumatic transphalangeal
                  amputation of right index finger S ⟐
      ● S68.611   Complete traumatic transphalangeal
                  amputation of left index finger S ⟐
      ● S68.612   Complete traumatic transphalangeal
                  amputation of right middle
                  finger S ⟐
      ● S68.613   Complete traumatic transphalangeal
                  amputation of left middle finger S ⟐

      ● S68.614   Complete traumatic transphalangeal
                  amputation of right ring finger S ⟐
      ● S68.615   Complete traumatic transphalangeal
                  amputation of left ring finger S ⟐
      ● S68.616   Complete traumatic transphalangeal
                  amputation of right little finger S ⟐
      ● S68.617   Complete traumatic transphalangeal
                  amputation of left little finger S ⟐
      ● S68.618   Complete traumatic transphalangeal
                  amputation of other finger S ⟐
                      Complete traumatic transphalangeal
                      amputation of specified finger
                      with unspecified laterality
      ● S68.619   Complete traumatic transphalangeal
                  amputation of unspecified finger S ⟐

   ● S68.62 **Partial traumatic transphalangeal amputation of
             other and unspecified finger**
      ● S68.620   Partial traumatic transphalangeal
                  amputation of right index finger S ⟐
      ● S68.621   Partial traumatic transphalangeal
                  amputation of left index finger S ⟐
      ● S68.622   Partial traumatic transphalangeal
                  amputation of right middle
                  finger S ⟐
      ● S68.623   Partial traumatic transphalangeal
                  amputation of left middle finger S ⟐
      ● S68.624   Partial traumatic transphalangeal
                  amputation of right ring finger S ⟐
      ● S68.625   Partial traumatic transphalangeal
                  amputation of left ring finger S ⟐
      ● S68.626   Partial traumatic transphalangeal
                  amputation of right little finger S ⟐
      ● S68.627   Partial traumatic transphalangeal
                  amputation of left little finger S ⟐
      ● S68.628   Partial traumatic transphalangeal
                  amputation of other finger S ⟐
                      Partial traumatic transphalangeal
                      amputation of specified finger
                      with unspecified laterality
      ● S68.629   Partial traumatic transphalangeal
                  amputation of unspecified finger S ⟐

● S68.7 **Traumatic transmetacarpal amputation of hand**

   ● S68.71 **Complete traumatic transmetacarpal
             amputation of hand**
      ● S68.711   Complete traumatic transmetacarpal
                  amputation of right hand A, S ⟐
      ● S68.712   Complete traumatic transmetacarpal
                  amputation of left hand A, S ⟐
      ● S68.719   Complete traumatic transmetacarpal
                  amputation of unspecified hand
                  A, S ⟐

   ● S68.72 **Partial traumatic transmetacarpal amputation of
             hand**
      ● S68.721   Partial traumatic transmetacarpal
                  amputation of right hand A, S ⟐
      ● S68.722   Partial traumatic transmetacarpal
                  amputation of left hand A, S ⟐
      ● S68.729   Partial traumatic transmetacarpal
                  amputation of unspecified hand
                  A, S ⟐

CHAPTER 19 (S00–T88)

● **S69**   **Other and unspecified injuries of wrist, hand and finger(s)**

The appropriate 7th character is to be added to each code from category S69

A	initial encounter
D	subsequent encounter
S	sequela

● **S69.8**   Other specified injuries of wrist, hand and finger(s)
   X ● **S69.80**   Other specified injuries of unspecified wrist, hand and finger(s)
   X ● **S69.81**   Other specified injuries of right wrist, hand and finger(s)
   X ● **S69.82**   Other specified injuries of left wrist, hand and finger(s)

● **S69.9**   Unspecified injury of wrist, hand and finger(s)
   X ● **S69.90**   Unspecified injury of unspecified wrist, hand and finger(s)
   X ● **S69.91**   Unspecified injury of right wrist, hand and finger(s)
   X ● **S69.92**   Unspecified injury of left wrist, hand and finger(s)

INJURIES TO THE HIP AND THIGH (S70-S79)

Excludes2   burns and corrosions (T20-T32)
                   frostbite (T33-T34)
                   snake bite (T63.0-)
                   venomous insect bite or sting (T63.4-)

● **S70**   **Superficial injury of hip and thigh**

The appropriate 7th character is to be added to each code from category S70

A	initial encounter
D	subsequent encounter
S	sequela

● **S70.0**   Contusion of hip
   X ● **S70.00**   Contusion of unspecified hip
   X ● **S70.01**   Contusion of right hip
   X ● **S70.02**   Contusion of left hip

● **S70.1**   Contusion of thigh
   X ● **S70.10**   Contusion of unspecified thigh
   X ● **S70.11**   Contusion of right thigh
   X ● **S70.12**   Contusion of left thigh

● **S70.2**   Other superficial injuries of hip
   ● **S70.21**   Abrasion of hip
     ● **S70.211**   Abrasion, right hip
     ● **S70.212**   Abrasion, left hip
     ● **S70.219**   Abrasion, unspecified hip
   ● **S70.22**   Blister (nonthermal) of hip
     ● **S70.221**   Blister (nonthermal), right hip
     ● **S70.222**   Blister (nonthermal), left hip
     ● **S70.229**   Blister (nonthermal), unspecified hip
   ● **S70.24**   External constriction of hip
     ● **S70.241**   External constriction, right hip
     ● **S70.242**   External constriction, left hip
     ● **S70.249**   External constriction, unspecified hip
   ● **S70.25**   Superficial foreign body of hip
       Splinter in the hip
     ● **S70.251**   Superficial foreign body, right hip
     ● **S70.252**   Superficial foreign body, left hip
     ● **S70.259**   Superficial foreign body, unspecified hip
   ● **S70.26**   Insect bite (nonvenomous) of hip
     ● **S70.261**   Insect bite (nonvenomous), right hip
     ● **S70.262**   Insect bite (nonvenomous), left hip
     ● **S70.269**   Insect bite (nonvenomous), unspecified hip

   ● **S70.27**   Other superficial bite of hip
       Excludes1   open bite of hip (S71.05-)
     ● **S70.271**   Other superficial bite of hip, right hip
     ● **S70.272**   Other superficial bite of hip, left hip
     ● **S70.279**   Other superficial bite of hip, unspecified hip

● **S70.3**   Other superficial injuries of thigh
   ● **S70.31**   Abrasion of thigh
     ● **S70.311**   Abrasion, right thigh
     ● **S70.312**   Abrasion, left thigh
     ● **S70.319**   Abrasion, unspecified thigh
   ● **S70.32**   Blister (nonthermal) of thigh
     ● **S70.321**   Blister (nonthermal), right thigh
     ● **S70.322**   Blister (nonthermal), left thigh
     ● **S70.329**   Blister (nonthermal), unspecified thigh
   ● **S70.34**   External constriction of thigh
     ● **S70.341**   External constriction, right thigh
     ● **S70.342**   External constriction, left thigh
     ● **S70.349**   External constriction, unspecified thigh
   ● **S70.35**   Superficial foreign body of thigh
       Splinter in the thigh
     ● **S70.351**   Superficial foreign body, right thigh
     ● **S70.352**   Superficial foreign body, left thigh
     ● **S70.359**   Superficial foreign body, unspecified thigh
   ● **S70.36**   Insect bite (nonvenomous) of thigh
     ● **S70.361**   Insect bite (nonvenomous), right thigh
     ● **S70.362**   Insect bite (nonvenomous), left thigh
     ● **S70.369**   Insect bite (nonvenomous), unspecified thigh
   ● **S70.37**   Other superficial bite of thigh
       Excludes1   open bite of thigh (S71.15)
     ● **S70.371**   Other superficial bite of right thigh
     ● **S70.372**   Other superficial bite of left thigh
     ● **S70.379**   Other superficial bite of unspecified thigh

● **S70.9**   Unspecified superficial injury of hip and thigh
   ● **S70.91**   Unspecified superficial injury of hip
     ● **S70.911**   Unspecified superficial injury of right hip
     ● **S70.912**   Unspecified superficial injury of left hip
     ● **S70.919**   Unspecified superficial injury of unspecified hip
   ● **S70.92**   Unspecified superficial injury of thigh
     ● **S70.921**   Unspecified superficial injury of right thigh
     ● **S70.922**   Unspecified superficial injury of left thigh
     ● **S70.929**   Unspecified superficial injury of unspecified thigh

● **S71**   **Open wound of hip and thigh**

Code also any associated wound infection

Excludes1   open fracture of hip and thigh (S72.-)
             traumatic amputation of hip and thigh (S78.-)

Excludes2   bite of venomous animal (T63.-)
             open wound of ankle, foot and toes (S91.-)
             open wound of knee and lower leg (S81.-)

The appropriate 7th character is to be added to each code from category S71

A	initial encounter
D	subsequent encounter
S	sequela

▶ New   ⇒ Revised   ~~deleted~~ Deleted   Excludes 1   Excludes 2   Includes   Use additional   Code first   Code also   Key words

OGCR Official Guidelines   X Assign placeholder X   ● Use Additional Character(s)   ▶ Manifestation Code   🐾 Hierarchical Condition Category   **Coding Clinic**

● **S71.0**   **Open wound of hip**
    ● **S71.00**   Unspecified open wound of hip
       ● S71.001   Unspecified open wound, right hip
       ● S71.002   Unspecified open wound, left hip
       ● S71.009   Unspecified open wound, unspecified hip
    ● **S71.01**   Laceration without foreign body of hip
       ● S71.011   Laceration without foreign body, right hip
       ● S71.012   Laceration without foreign body, left hip
       ● S71.019   Laceration without foreign body, unspecified hip
    ● **S71.02**   Laceration with foreign body of hip
       ● S71.021   Laceration with foreign body, right hip
       ● S71.022   Laceration with foreign body, left hip
       ● S71.029   Laceration with foreign body, unspecified hip
    ● **S71.03**   Puncture wound without foreign body of hip
       ● S71.031   Puncture wound without foreign body, right hip
       ● S71.032   Puncture wound without foreign body, left hip
       ● S71.039   Puncture wound without foreign body, unspecified hip
    ● **S71.04**   Puncture wound with foreign body of hip
       ● S71.041   Puncture wound with foreign body, right hip
       ● S71.042   Puncture wound with foreign body, left hip
       ● S71.049   Puncture wound with foreign body, unspecified hip
    ● **S71.05**   Open bite of hip
       Bite of hip NOS
       Excludes1   superficial bite of hip (S70.26, S70.27)
       ● S71.051   Open bite, right hip
       ● S71.052   Open bite, left hip
       ● S71.059   Open bite, unspecified hip
● **S71.1**   **Open wound of thigh**
    ● **S71.10**   Unspecified open wound of thigh
       ● S71.101   Unspecified open wound, right thigh
       ● S71.102   Unspecified open wound, left thigh
       ● S71.109   Unspecified open wound, unspecified thigh
    ● **S71.11**   Laceration without foreign body of thigh
       ● S71.111   Laceration without foreign body, right thigh
       ● S71.112   Laceration without foreign body, left thigh
       ● S71.119   Laceration without foreign body, unspecified thigh
    ● **S71.12**   Laceration with foreign body of thigh
       ● S71.121   Laceration with foreign body, right thigh
       ● S71.122   Laceration with foreign body, left thigh
       ● S71.129   Laceration with foreign body, unspecified thigh

● **S71.13**   Puncture wound without foreign body of thigh
       ● S71.131   Puncture wound without foreign body, right thigh
       ● S71.132   Puncture wound without foreign body, left thigh
       ● S71.139   Puncture wound without foreign body, unspecified thigh
● **S71.14**   Puncture wound with foreign body of thigh
       ● S71.141   Puncture wound with foreign body, right thigh
       ● S71.142   Puncture wound with foreign body, left thigh
       ● S71.149   Puncture wound with foreign body, unspecified thigh
● **S71.15**   Open bite of thigh
       Bite of thigh NOS
       Excludes1   superficial bite of thigh (S70.37-)
       ● S71.151   Open bite, right thigh
       ● S71.152   Open bite, left thigh
       ● S71.159   Open bite, unspecified thigh

● S72   **Fracture of femur**
    Note: A fracture not indicated as displaced or nondisplaced should be coded to displaced
       A fracture not indicated as open or closed should be coded to closed
       The open fracture designations are based on the Gustilo open fracture classification
    Excludes1   traumatic amputation of hip and thigh (S78.-)
    Excludes2   fracture of lower leg and ankle (S82.-)
       fracture of foot (S92.-)
       periprosthetic fracture of prosthetic implant of hip (M97.0-)
    The appropriate 7th character is to be added to all codes from category S72

A	initial encounter for closed fracture
B	initial encounter for open fracture type I or II
	initial encounter for open fracture NOS
C	initial encounter for open fracture type IIIA, IIIB, or IIIC
D	subsequent encounter for closed fracture with routine healing
E	subsequent encounter for open fracture type I or II with routine healing
F	subsequent encounter for open fracture type IIIA, IIIB, or IIIC with routine healing
G	subsequent encounter for closed fracture with delayed healing
H	subsequent encounter for open fracture type I or II with delayed healing
J	subsequent encounter for open fracture type IIIA, IIIB, or IIIC with delayed healing
K	subsequent encounter for closed fracture with nonunion
M	subsequent encounter for open fracture type I or II with nonunion
N	subsequent encounter for open fracture type IIIA, IIIB, or IIIC with nonunion
P	subsequent encounter for closed fracture with malunion
Q	subsequent encounter for open fracture type I or II with malunion
R	subsequent encounter for open fracture type IIIA, IIIB, or IIIC with malunion
S	sequela

● **S72.0** Fracture of head and neck of femur

> **Excludes2** physeal fracture of upper end of femur (S79.0-)

● **S72.00** Fracture of unspecified part of neck of femur

> Fracture of hip NOS
> Fracture of neck of femur NOS

● **S72.001** Fracture of unspecified part of neck of right femur A, B, C 🐾

● **S72.002** Fracture of unspecified part of neck of left femur A, B, C 🐾
> **Coding Clinic: 2015, Q4, P37, Q1, P17**

● **S72.009** Fracture of unspecified part of neck of unspecified femur A, B, C 🐾

● **S72.01** Unspecified intracapsular fracture of femur

> Subcapital fracture of femur

● **S72.011** Unspecified intracapsular fracture of right femur A, B, C 🐾

● **S72.012** Unspecified intracapsular fracture of left femur A, B, C 🐾

● **S72.019** Unspecified intracapsular fracture of unspecified femur A, B, C 🐾

● **S72.02** Fracture of epiphysis (separation) (upper) of femur

> Transepiphyseal fracture of femur
> *Fracture and separation across growth plate*

> **Excludes1** capital femoral epiphyseal fracture (pediatric) of femur (S79.01-)
> Salter-Harris Type I physeal fracture of upper end of femur (S79.01-)

● **S72.021** Displaced fracture of epiphysis (separation) (upper) of right femur A, B, C 🐾

● **S72.022** Displaced fracture of epiphysis (separation) (upper) of left femur A, B, C 🐾

● **S72.023** Displaced fracture of epiphysis (separation) (upper) of unspecified femur A, B, C 🐾

● **S72.024** Nondisplaced fracture of epiphysis (separation) (upper) of right femur A, B, C 🐾

● **S72.025** Nondisplaced fracture of epiphysis (separation) (upper) of left femur A, B, C 🐾

● **S72.026** Nondisplaced fracture of epiphysis (separation) (upper) of unspecified femur A, B, C 🐾

● **S72.03 Midcervical** fracture of femur
Transcervical fracture of femur NOS
  ● **S72.031 Displaced** midcervical fracture of **right** femur A, B, C 🔧
  ● **S72.032 Displaced** midcervical fracture of **left** femur A, B, C 🔧
  ● **S72.033 Displaced** midcervical fracture of **unspecified** femur A, B, C 🔧
  ● **S72.034 Nondisplaced** midcervical fracture of **right** femur A, B, C 🔧
  ● **S72.035 Nondisplaced** midcervical fracture of **left** femur A, B, C 🔧
  ● **S72.036 Nondisplaced** midcervical fracture of **unspecified** femur A, B, C 🔧
● **S72.04 Fracture** of base of neck of femur
Cervicotrochanteric fracture of femur
  ● **S72.041 Displaced** fracture of base of neck of **right** femur A, B, C 🔧
  ● **S72.042 Displaced** fracture of base of neck of **left** femur A, B, C 🔧
  ● **S72.043 Displaced** fracture of base of neck of **unspecified** femur A, B, C 🔧
  ● **S72.044 Nondisplaced** fracture of base of neck of **right** femur A, B, C 🔧
  ● **S72.045 Nondisplaced** fracture of base of neck of **left** femur A, B, C 🔧
  ● **S72.046 Nondisplaced** fracture of base of neck of **unspecified** femur A, B, C 🔧
● **S72.05 Unspecified** fracture of head of femur
Fracture of head of femur NOS
  ● **S72.051 Unspecified** fracture of head of **right** femur A, B, C 🔧
  ● **S72.052 Unspecified** fracture of head of **left** femur A, B, C 🔧
  ● **S72.059 Unspecified** fracture of head of **unspecified** femur A, B, C 🔧
● **S72.06 Articular** fracture of head of femur
  ● **S72.061 Displaced** articular fracture of head of **right** femur A, B, C 🔧
  ● **S72.062 Displaced** articular fracture of head of **left** femur A, B, C 🔧
  ● **S72.063 Displaced** articular fracture of head of **unspecified** femur A, B, C 🔧
  ● **S72.064 Nondisplaced** articular fracture of head of **right** femur A, B, C 🔧
  ● **S72.065 Nondisplaced** articular fracture of head of **left** femur A, B, C 🔧
  ● **S72.066 Nondisplaced** articular fracture of head of **unspecified** femur A, B, C 🔧
● **S72.09 Other** fracture of head and neck of femur
  ● **S72.091 Other** fracture of head and neck of **right** femur A, B, C 🔧
  ● **S72.092 Other** fracture of head and neck of **left** femur A, B, C 🔧
  ● **S72.099 Other** fracture of head and neck of **unspecified** femur A, B, C 🔧
● **S72.1 Pertrochanteric** fracture
Fracture extending close to, but not into, joint
  ● **S72.10 Unspecified** trochanteric fracture of femur
Fracture of trochanter NOS
    ● **S72.101 Unspecified** trochanteric fracture of **right** femur A, B, C 🔧
    ● **S72.102 Unspecified** trochanteric fracture of **left** femur A, B, C 🔧
    ● **S72.109 Unspecified** trochanteric fracture of **unspecified** femur A, B, C 🔧

● **S72.11 Fracture** of greater trochanter of femur
  ● **S72.111 Displaced** fracture of greater trochanter of **right** femur A, B, C 🔧
  ● **S72.112 Displaced** fracture of greater trochanter of **left** femur A, B, C 🔧
  ● **S72.113 Displaced** fracture of greater trochanter of **unspecified** femur A, B, C 🔧
  ● **S72.114 Nondisplaced** fracture of greater trochanter of **right** femur A, B, C 🔧
  ● **S72.115 Nondisplaced** fracture of greater trochanter of **left** femur A, B, C 🔧
  ● **S72.116 Nondisplaced** fracture of greater trochanter of **unspecified** femur A, B, C 🔧
● **S72.12 Fracture** of lesser trochanter of femur
  ● **S72.121 Displaced** fracture of lesser trochanter of **right** femur A, B, C 🔧
  ● **S72.122 Displaced** fracture of lesser trochanter of **left** femur A, B, C 🔧
  ● **S72.123 Displaced** fracture of lesser trochanter of **unspecified** femur A, B, C 🔧
  ● **S72.124 Nondisplaced** fracture of lesser trochanter of **right** femur A, B, C 🔧
  ● **S72.125 Nondisplaced** fracture of lesser trochanter of **left** femur A, B, C 🔧
  ● **S72.126 Nondisplaced** fracture of lesser trochanter of **unspecified** femur A, B, C 🔧
● **S72.13 Apophyseal** fracture of femur
Pertaining to articulations between articular facets of adjacent vertebrae
  Excludes1 chronic (nontraumatic) slipped upper femoral epiphysis (M93.0-)
  ● **S72.131 Displaced** apophyseal fracture of **right** femur A, B, C 🔧
  ● **S72.132 Displaced** apophyseal fracture of **left** femur A, B, C 🔧
  ● **S72.133 Displaced** apophyseal fracture of **unspecified** femur A, B, C 🔧
  ● **S72.134 Nondisplaced** apophyseal fracture of **right** femur A, B, C 🔧
  ● **S72.135 Nondisplaced** apophyseal fracture of **left** femur A, B, C 🔧
  ● **S72.136 Nondisplaced** apophyseal fracture of **unspecified** femur A, B, C 🔧
● **S72.14 Intertrochanteric** fracture of femur
  ● **S72.141 Displaced** intertrochanteric fracture of **right** femur A, B, C 🔧
    Coding Clinic: 2016, Q3, P17
  ● **S72.142 Displaced** intertrochanteric fracture of **left** femur A, B, C 🔧
  ● **S72.143 Displaced** intertrochanteric fracture of **unspecified** femur A, B, C 🔧
  ● **S72.144 Nondisplaced** intertrochanteric fracture of **right** femur A, B, C 🔧
  ● **S72.145 Nondisplaced** intertrochanteric fracture of **left** femur A, B, C 🔧
  ● **S72.146 Nondisplaced** intertrochanteric fracture of **unspecified** femur A, B, C 🔧
● **S72.2 Subtrochanteric** fracture of femur
Subtrochanteric: inferior to trochanter
  X ● **S72.21 Displaced** subtrochanteric fracture of **right** femur A, B, C 🔧
  X ● **S72.22 Displaced** subtrochanteric fracture of **left** femur A, B, C 🔧

CHAPTER 19 (S00-T88)

CHAPTER 19 (S00-T88)

X ● S72.23   Displaced subtrochanteric fracture of unspecified femur A, B, C 🦴

X ● S72.24   Nondisplaced subtrochanteric fracture of right femur A, B, C 🦴

X ● S72.25   Nondisplaced subtrochanteric fracture of left femur A, B, C 🦴

X ● S72.26   Nondisplaced subtrochanteric fracture of unspecified femur A, B, C 🦴

● S72.3   Fracture of shaft of femur

  ● S72.30   Unspecified fracture of shaft of femur

    ● S72.301   Unspecified fracture of shaft of right femur A, B, C 🦴
           Coding Clinic: 2018, Q2, P12

    ● S72.302   Unspecified fracture of shaft of left femur A, B, C 🦴

    ● S72.309   Unspecified fracture of shaft of unspecified femur A, B, C 🦴

  ● S72.32   Transverse fracture of shaft of femur

    ● S72.321   Displaced transverse fracture of shaft of right femur A, B, C 🦴

    ● S72.322   Displaced transverse fracture of shaft of left femur A, B, C 🦴

    ● S72.323   Displaced transverse fracture of shaft of unspecified femur A, B, C 🦴

    ● S72.324   Nondisplaced transverse fracture of shaft of right femur A, B, C 🦴

    ● S72.325   Nondisplaced transverse fracture of shaft of left femur A, B, C 🦴

    ● S72.326   Nondisplaced transverse fracture of shaft of unspecified femur A, B, C 🦴

  ● S72.33   Oblique fracture of shaft of femur

    ● S72.331   Displaced oblique fracture of shaft of right femur A, B, C 🦴

    ● S72.332   Displaced oblique fracture of shaft of left femur A, B, C 🦴

    ● S72.333   Displaced oblique fracture of shaft of unspecified femur A, B, C 🦴

    ● S72.334   Nondisplaced oblique fracture of shaft of right femur A, B, C 🦴

    ● S72.335   Nondisplaced oblique fracture of shaft of left femur A, B, C 🦴

    ● S72.336   Nondisplaced oblique fracture of shaft of unspecified femur A, B, C 🦴

  ● S72.34   Spiral fracture of shaft of femur

    ● S72.341   Displaced spiral fracture of shaft of right femur A, B, C 🦴

    ● S72.342   Displaced spiral fracture of shaft of left femur A, B, C 🦴

    ● S72.343   Displaced spiral fracture of shaft of unspecified femur A, B, C 🦴

    ● S72.344   Nondisplaced spiral fracture of shaft of right femur A, B, C 🦴

    ● S72.345   Nondisplaced spiral fracture of shaft of left femur A, B, C 🦴

    ● S72.346   Nondisplaced spiral fracture of shaft of unspecified femur A, B, C 🦴

  ● S72.35   Comminuted fracture of shaft of femur

    ● S72.351   Displaced comminuted fracture of shaft of right femur A, B, C 🦴

    ● S72.352   Displaced comminuted fracture of shaft of left femur A, B, C 🦴

    ● S72.353   Displaced comminuted fracture of shaft of unspecified femur A, B, C 🦴

    ● S72.354   Nondisplaced comminuted fracture of shaft of right femur A, B, C 🦴

    ● S72.355   Nondisplaced comminuted fracture of shaft of left femur A, B, C 🦴

    ● S72.356   Nondisplaced comminuted fracture of shaft of unspecified femur A, B, C 🦴

  ● S72.36   Segmental fracture of shaft of femur

    ● S72.361   Displaced segmental fracture of shaft of right femur A, B, C 🦴

    ● S72.362   Displaced segmental fracture of shaft of left femur A, B, C 🦴

    ● S72.363   Displaced segmental fracture of shaft of unspecified femur A, B, C 🦴

    ● S72.364   Nondisplaced segmental fracture of shaft of right femur A, B, C 🦴

    ● S72.365   Nondisplaced segmental fracture of shaft of left femur A, B, C 🦴

    ● S72.366   Nondisplaced segmental fracture of shaft of unspecified femur A, B, C 🦴

  ● S72.39   Other fracture of shaft of femur

    ● S72.391   Other fracture of shaft of right femur A, B, C 🦴

    ● S72.392   Other fracture of shaft of left femur A, B, C 🦴

    ● S72.399   Other fracture of shaft of unspecified femur A, B, C 🦴

● S72.4   Fracture of lower end of femur
     Fracture of distal end of femur

     Excludes2   fracture of shaft of femur (S72.3-)
                physeal fracture of lower end of femur (S79.1-)

  ● S72.40   Unspecified fracture of lower end of femur

    ● S72.401   Unspecified fracture of lower end of right femur A, B, C 🦴
           Coding Clinic: 2016, Q4, P43

    ● S72.402   Unspecified fracture of lower end of left femur A, B, C 🦴

    ● S72.409   Unspecified fracture of lower end of unspecified femur A, B, C 🦴

  ● S72.41   Unspecified condyle fracture of lower end of femur
       Condyle fracture of femur NOS

    ● S72.411   Displaced unspecified condyle fracture of lower end of right femur A, B, C 🦴

    ● S72.412   Displaced unspecified condyle fracture of lower end of left femur A, B, C 🦴

    ● S72.413   Displaced unspecified condyle fracture of lower end of unspecified femur A, B, C 🦴

    ● S72.414   Nondisplaced unspecified condyle fracture of lower end of right femur A, B, C 🦴

    ● S72.415   Nondisplaced unspecified condyle fracture of lower end of left femur A, B, C 🦴

    ● S72.416   Nondisplaced unspecified condyle fracture of lower end of unspecified femur A, B, C 🦴

  ● S72.42   Fracture of lateral condyle of femur

    ● S72.421   Displaced fracture of lateral condyle of right femur A, B, C 🦴

    ● S72.422   Displaced fracture of lateral condyle of left femur A, B, C 🦴

    ● S72.423   Displaced fracture of lateral condyle of unspecified femur A, B, C 🦴

    ● S72.424   Nondisplaced fracture of lateral condyle of right femur A, B, C 🦴

    ● S72.425   Nondisplaced fracture of lateral condyle of left femur A, B, C 🦴

    ● S72.426   Nondisplaced fracture of lateral condyle of unspecified femur A, B, C 🦴

▶ New   ⇒ Revised   ~~deleted~~ Deleted   Excludes 1   Excludes 2   Includes   Use additional   Code first   Code also   Key words

OGCR Official Guidelines   X Assign placeholder X   ● Use Additional Character(s)   ▸ Manifestation Code   🦴 Hierarchical Condition Category   **Coding Clinic**

● S72.43   Fracture of medial condyle of femur

    ● S72.431   Displaced fracture of medial condyle of right femur A, B, C 🔗

    ● S72.432   Displaced fracture of medial condyle of left femur A, B, C 🔗

    ● S72.433   Displaced fracture of medial condyle of unspecified femur A, B, C 🔗

    ● S72.434   Nondisplaced fracture of medial condyle of right femur A, B, C 🔗

    ● S72.435   Nondisplaced fracture of medial condyle of left femur A, B, C 🔗

    ● S72.436   Nondisplaced fracture of medial condyle of unspecified femur A, B, C 🔗

● S72.44   Fracture of lower epiphysis (separation) of femur

    Excludes1   Salter-Harris Type I physeal fracture of lower end of femur (S79.11-)

    ● S72.441   Displaced fracture of lower epiphysis (separation) of right femur A, B, C 🔗

    ● S72.442   Displaced fracture of lower epiphysis (separation) of left femur A, B, C 🔗

    ● S72.443   Displaced fracture of lower epiphysis (separation) of unspecified femur A, B, C 🔗

    ● S72.444   Nondisplaced fracture of lower epiphysis (separation) of right femur A, B, C 🔗

    ● S72.445   Nondisplaced fracture of lower epiphysis (separation) of left femur A, B, C 🔗

    ● S72.446   Nondisplaced fracture of lower epiphysis (separation) of unspecified femur A, B, C 🔗

● S72.45   Supracondylar fracture without intracondylar extension of lower end of femur

    Supracondylar fracture of lower end of femur NOS

    Excludes1   supracondylar fracture with intracondylar extension of lower end of femur (S72.46-)

    ● S72.451   Displaced supracondylar fracture without intracondylar extension of lower end of right femur A, B, C 🔗

    ● S72.452   Displaced supracondylar fracture without intracondylar extension of lower end of left femur A, B, C 🔗

    ● S72.453   Displaced supracondylar fracture without intracondylar extension of lower end of unspecified femur A, B, C 🔗

    ● S72.454   Nondisplaced supracondylar fracture without intracondylar extension of lower end of right femur A, B, C 🔗

    ● S72.455   Nondisplaced supracondylar fracture without intracondylar extension of lower end of left femur A, B, C 🔗

    ● S72.456   Nondisplaced supracondylar fracture without intracondylar extension of lower end of unspecified femur A, B, C 🔗

● S72.46   Supracondylar fracture with intracondylar extension of lower end of femur

    Excludes1   supracondylar fracture without intracondylar extension of lower end of femur (S72.45-)

    ● S72.461   Displaced supracondylar fracture with intracondylar extension of lower end of right femur A, B, C 🔗

    ● S72.462   Displaced supracondylar fracture with intracondylar extension of lower end of left femur A, B, C 🔗

    ● S72.463   Displaced supracondylar fracture with intracondylar extension of lower end of unspecified femur A, B, C 🔗

    ● S72.464   Nondisplaced supracondylar fracture with intracondylar extension of lower end of right femur A, B, C 🔗

    ● S72.465   Nondisplaced supracondylar fracture with intracondylar extension of lower end of left femur A, B, C 🔗

    ● S72.466   Nondisplaced supracondylar fracture with intracondylar extension of lower end of unspecified femur A, B, C 🔗

● S72.47   Torus fracture of lower end of femur

    The appropriate 7th character is to be added to all codes in subcategory S72.47

A	initial encounter for closed fracture
D	subsequent encounter for fracture with routine healing
G	subsequent encounter for fracture with delayed healing
K	subsequent encounter for fracture with nonunion
P	subsequent encounter for fracture with malunion
S	sequela

    ● S72.471   Torus fracture of lower end of right femur A 🔗

    ● S72.472   Torus fracture of lower end of left femur A 🔗

    ● S72.479   Torus fracture of lower end of unspecified femur A 🔗

● S72.49   Other fracture of lower end of femur

    ● S72.491   Other fracture of lower end of right femur A, B, C 🔗

    ● S72.492   Other fracture of lower end of left femur A, B, C 🔗

    ● S72.499   Other fracture of lower end of unspecified femur A, B, C 🔗

● S72.8   Other fracture of femur

    ● S72.8X   Other fracture of femur

      ● S72.8X1   Other fracture of right femur A, B, C 🔗

      ● S72.8X2   Other fracture of left femur A, B, C 🔗

      ● S72.8X9   Other fracture of unspecified femur A, B, C 🔗

● S72.9   Unspecified fracture of femur

    Fracture of thigh NOS

    Fracture of upper leg NOS

    Excludes1   fracture of hip NOS (S72.00-, S72.01-)

    X ● S72.90   Unspecified fracture of unspecified femur A, B, C 🔗

       Coding Clinic: 2012, Q4, P94

    X ● S72.91   Unspecified fracture of right femur A, B, C 🔗

    X ● S72.92   Unspecified fracture of left femur A, B, C 🔗

● S73   Dislocation and sprain of joint and ligaments of hip

    Includes   avulsion of joint or ligament of hip

       laceration of cartilage, joint or ligament of hip

       sprain of cartilage, joint or ligament of hip

       traumatic hemarthrosis of joint or ligament of hip

       traumatic rupture of joint or ligament of hip

       traumatic subluxation of joint or ligament of hip

       traumatic tear of joint or ligament of hip

    Code also any associated open wound

    Excludes2   strain of muscle, fascia and tendon of hip and thigh (S76.-)

    The appropriate 7th character is to be added to each code from category S73

A	initial encounter
D	subsequent encounter
S	sequela

● S73.0   Subluxation and dislocation of hip
     Out of position
     Excludes2   dislocation and subluxation of hip
                 prosthesis (T84.020, T84.021)

  ● S73.00   Unspecified subluxation and dislocation of hip
       Dislocation of hip NOS
       Subluxation of hip NOS

    ● S73.001   Unspecified subluxation of right hip A 🐾

    ● S73.002   Unspecified subluxation of left hip A 🐾

    ● S73.003   Unspecified subluxation of unspecified hip A 🐾

    ● S73.004   Unspecified dislocation of right hip A 🐾

    ● S73.005   Unspecified dislocation of left hip A 🐾

    ● S73.006   Unspecified dislocation of unspecified hip A 🐾

  ● S73.01   Posterior subluxation and dislocation of hip

    ● S73.011   Posterior subluxation of right hip A 🐾

    ● S73.012   Posterior subluxation of left hip A 🐾

    ● S73.013   Posterior subluxation of unspecified hip A 🐾

    ● S73.014   Posterior dislocation of right hip A 🐾

    ● S73.015   Posterior dislocation of left hip A 🐾

    ● S73.016   Posterior dislocation of unspecified hip A 🐾

  ● S73.02   Obturator subluxation and dislocation of hip

    ● S73.021   Obturator subluxation of right hip A 🐾

    ● S73.022   Obturator subluxation of left hip A 🐾

    ● S73.023   Obturator subluxation of unspecified hip A 🐾

    ● S73.024   Obturator dislocation of right hip A 🐾

    ● S73.025   Obturator dislocation of left hip A 🐾

    ● S73.026   Obturator dislocation of unspecified hip A 🐾

  ● S73.03   Other anterior subluxation and dislocation of hip

    ● S73.031   Other anterior subluxation of right hip A 🐾

    ● S73.032   Other anterior subluxation of left hip A 🐾

    ● S73.033   Other anterior subluxation of unspecified hip A 🐾

    ● S73.034   Other anterior dislocation of right hip A 🐾

    ● S73.035   Other anterior dislocation of left hip A 🐾

    ● S73.036   Other anterior dislocation of unspecified hip A 🐾

  ● S73.04   Central subluxation and dislocation of hip

    ● S73.041   Central subluxation of right hip A 🐾

    ● S73.042   Central subluxation of left hip A 🐾

    ● S73.043   Central subluxation of unspecified hip A 🐾

    ● S73.044   Central dislocation of right hip A 🐾

    ● S73.045   Central dislocation of left hip A 🐾

    ● S73.046   Central dislocation of unspecified hip A 🐾

● S73.1   Sprain of hip

  ● S73.10   Unspecified sprain of hip

    ● S73.101   Unspecified sprain of right hip

    ● S73.102   Unspecified sprain of left hip

    ● S73.109   Unspecified sprain of unspecified hip

  ● S73.11   Iliofemoral ligament sprain of hip

    ● S73.111   Iliofemoral ligament sprain of right hip

    ● S73.112   Iliofemoral ligament sprain of left hip

    ● S73.119   Iliofemoral ligament sprain of unspecified hip

  ● S73.12   Ischiocapsular (ligament) sprain of hip

    ● S73.121   Ischiocapsular ligament sprain of right hip

    ● S73.122   Ischiocapsular ligament sprain of left hip

    ● S73.129   Ischiocapsular ligament sprain of unspecified hip

  ● S73.19   Other sprain of hip

    ● S73.191   Other sprain of right hip

    ● S73.192   Other sprain of left hip

    ● S73.199   Other sprain of unspecified hip

● S74   Injury of nerves at hip and thigh level
     Code also any associated open wound (S71.-)
     Excludes2   injury of nerves at ankle and foot level (S94.-)
                 injury of nerves at lower leg level (S84.-)

     The appropriate 7th character is to be added to each code from category S74

A	initial encounter
D	subsequent encounter
S	sequela

  ● S74.0   Injury of sciatic nerve at hip and thigh level

     X ● **S74.00   Injury of sciatic nerve at hip and thigh level, unspecified leg**

     X ● **S74.01   Injury of sciatic nerve at hip and thigh level, right leg**

     X ● **S74.02   Injury of sciatic nerve at hip and thigh level, left leg**

  ● S74.1   Injury of femoral nerve at hip and thigh level

     X ● **S74.10   Injury of femoral nerve at hip and thigh level, unspecified leg**

     X ● **S74.11   Injury of femoral nerve at hip and thigh level, right leg**

     X ● **S74.12   Injury of femoral nerve at hip and thigh level, left leg**

  ● S74.2   Injury of cutaneous sensory nerve at hip and thigh level

     X ● **S74.20   Injury of cutaneous sensory nerve at hip and thigh level, unspecified leg**

     X ● **S74.21   Injury of cutaneous sensory nerve at hip and high level, right leg**

     X ● **S74.22   Injury of cutaneous sensory nerve at hip and thigh level, left leg**

  ● S74.8   Injury of other nerves at hip and thigh level

     ● **S74.8X   Injury of other nerves at hip and thigh level**

       ● **S74.8X1   Injury of other nerves at hip and thigh level, right leg**

       ● **S74.8X2   Injury of other nerves at hip and thigh level, left leg**

       ● **S74.8X9   Injury of other nerves at hip and thigh level, unspecified leg**

  ● S74.9   Injury of unspecified nerve at hip and thigh level

     X ● **S74.90   Injury of unspecified nerve at hip and thigh level, unspecified leg**

     X ● **S74.91   Injury of unspecified nerve at hip and thigh level, right leg**

     X ● **S74.92   Injury of unspecified nerve at hip and thigh level, left leg**

▶ New   ⇒ Revised   ~~deleted~~ Deleted   Excludes 1   Excludes 2   Includes   Use additional   Code first   Code also   Key words

OGCR Official Guidelines   X Assign placeholder X   ● Use Additional Character(s)   ▷ Manifestation Code   🐾 Hierarchical Condition Category   **Coding Clinic**

● **S75** **Injury of blood vessels at hip and thigh level**

Code also any associated open wound (S71.-)

> **Excludes2** injury of blood vessels at lower leg level (S85.-)
> injury of popliteal artery (S85.0)

The appropriate 7th character is to be added to each code from category S75

> | A | initial encounter |
> |---|---|
> | D | subsequent encounter |
> | S | sequela |

● **S75.0** **Injury of femoral artery**

　● **S75.00** **Unspecified injury of femoral artery**

　　● S75.001 **Unspecified injury of femoral artery, right leg**

　　● S75.002 **Unspecified injury of femoral artery, left leg**

　　● S75.009 **Unspecified injury of femoral artery, unspecified leg**

　● **S75.01** **Minor laceration of femoral artery**

　　Incomplete transection of femoral artery
　　Laceration of femoral artery NOS
　　Superficial laceration of femoral artery

　　● S75.011 **Minor laceration of femoral artery, right leg**

　　● S75.012 **Minor laceration of femoral artery, left leg**

　　● S75.019 **Minor laceration of femoral artery, unspecified leg**

　● **S75.02** **Major laceration of femoral artery**

　　Complete transection of femoral artery
　　Traumatic rupture of femoral artery

　　● S75.021 **Major laceration of femoral artery, right leg**

　　● S75.022 **Major laceration of femoral artery, left leg**

　　● S75.029 **Major laceration of femoral artery, unspecified leg**

　● **S75.09** **Other specified injury of femoral artery**

　　● S75.091 **Other specified injury of femoral artery, right leg**

　　● S75.092 **Other specified injury of femoral artery, left leg**

　　● S75.099 **Other specified injury of femoral artery, unspecified leg**

● **S75.1** **Injury of femoral vein at hip and thigh level**

　● **S75.10** **Unspecified injury of femoral vein at hip and thigh level**

　　● S75.101 **Unspecified injury of femoral vein at hip and thigh level, right leg**

　　● S75.102 **Unspecified injury of femoral vein at hip and thigh level, left leg**

　　● S75.109 **Unspecified injury of femoral vein at hip and thigh level, unspecified leg**

　● **S75.11** **Minor laceration of femoral vein at hip and thigh level**

　　Incomplete transection of femoral vein at hip and thigh level
　　Laceration of femoral vein at hip and thigh level NOS
　　Superficial laceration of femoral vein at hip and thigh level

　　● S75.111 **Minor laceration of femoral vein at hip and thigh level, right leg**

　　● S75.112 **Minor laceration of femoral vein at hip and thigh level, left leg**

　　● S75.119 **Minor laceration of femoral vein at hip and thigh level, unspecified leg**

● **S75.12** **Major laceration of femoral vein at hip and thigh level**

Complete transection of femoral vein at hip and thigh level
Traumatic rupture of femoral vein at hip and thigh level

　● S75.121 **Major laceration of femoral vein at hip and thigh level, right leg**

　● S75.122 **Major laceration of femoral vein at hip and thigh level, left leg**

　● S75.129 **Major laceration of femoral vein at hip and thigh level, unspecified leg**

● **S75.19** **Other specified injury of femoral vein at hip and thigh level**

　● S75.191 **Other specified injury of femoral vein at hip and thigh level, right leg**

　● S75.192 **Other specified injury of femoral vein at hip and thigh level, left leg**

　● S75.199 **Other specified injury of femoral vein at hip and thigh level, unspecified leg**

● **S75.2** **Injury of greater saphenous vein at hip and thigh level**

> **Excludes1** greater saphenous vein NOS (S85.3)

　● **S75.20** **Unspecified injury of greater saphenous vein at hip and thigh level**

　　● S75.201 **Unspecified injury of greater saphenous vein at hip and thigh level, right leg**

　　● S75.202 **Unspecified injury of greater saphenous vein at hip and thigh level, left leg**

　　● S75.209 **Unspecified injury of greater saphenous vein at hip and thigh level, unspecified leg**

　● **S75.21** **Minor laceration of greater saphenous vein at hip and thigh level**

　　Incomplete transection of greater saphenous vein at hip and thigh level
　　Laceration of greater saphenous vein at hip and thigh level NOS
　　Superficial laceration of greater saphenous vein at hip and thigh level

　　● S75.211 **Minor laceration of greater saphenous vein at hip and thigh level, right leg**

　　● S75.212 **Minor laceration of greater saphenous vein at hip and thigh level, left leg**

　　● S75.219 **Minor laceration of greater saphenous vein at hip and thigh level, unspecified leg**

　● **S75.22** **Major laceration of greater saphenous vein at hip and thigh level**

　　Complete transection of greater saphenous vein at hip and thigh level
　　Traumatic rupture of greater saphenous vein at hip and thigh level

　　● S75.221 **Major laceration of greater saphenous vein at hip and thigh level, right leg**

　　● S75.222 **Major laceration of greater saphenous vein at hip and thigh level, left leg**

　　● S75.229 **Major laceration of greater saphenous vein at hip and thigh level, unspecified leg**

　● **S75.29** **Other specified injury of greater saphenous vein at hip and thigh level**

　　● S75.291 **Other specified injury of greater saphenous vein at hip and thigh level, right leg**

　　● S75.292 **Other specified injury of greater saphenous vein at hip and thigh level, left leg**

　　● S75.299 **Other specified injury of greater saphenous vein at hip and thigh level, unspecified leg**

- S75.8   Injury of other blood vessels at hip and thigh level
  - S75.80   Unspecified injury of other blood vessels at hip and thigh level
    - S75.801   Unspecified injury of other blood vessels at hip and thigh level, right leg
    - S75.802   Unspecified injury of other blood vessels at hip and thigh level, left leg
    - S75.809   Unspecified injury of other blood vessels at hip and thigh level, unspecified leg
  - S75.81   Laceration of other blood vessels at hip and thigh level
    - S75.811   Laceration of other blood vessels at hip and thigh level, right leg
    - S75.812   Laceration of other blood vessels at hip and thigh level, left leg
    - S75.819   Laceration of other blood vessels at hip and thigh level, unspecified leg
  - S75.89   Other specified injury of other blood vessels at hip and thigh level
    - S75.891   Other specified injury of other blood vessels at hip and thigh level, right leg
    - S75.892   Other specified injury of other blood vessels at hip and thigh level, left leg
    - S75.899   Other specified injury of other blood vessels at hip and thigh level, unspecified leg
- S75.9   Injury of unspecified blood vessel at hip and thigh level
  - S75.90   Unspecified injury of unspecified blood vessel at hip and thigh level
    - S75.901   Unspecified injury of unspecified blood vessel at hip and thigh level, right leg
    - S75.902   Unspecified injury of unspecified blood vessel at hip and thigh level, left leg
    - S75.909   Unspecified injury of unspecified blood vessel at hip and thigh level, unspecified leg
  - S75.91   Laceration of unspecified blood vessel at hip and thigh level
    - S75.911   Laceration of unspecified blood vessel at hip and thigh level, right leg
    - S75.912   Laceration of unspecified blood vessel at hip and thigh level, left leg
    - S75.919   Laceration of unspecified blood vessel at hip and thigh level, unspecified leg
  - S75.99   Other specified injury of unspecified blood vessel at hip and thigh level
    - S75.991   Other specified injury of unspecified blood vessel at hip and thigh level, right leg
    - S75.992   Other specified injury of unspecified blood vessel at hip and thigh level, left leg
    - S75.999   Other specified injury of unspecified blood vessel at hip and thigh level, unspecified leg

- S76   Injury of muscle, fascia and tendon at hip and thigh level

  Code also any associated open wound (S71.-)

  Excludes2   injury of muscle, fascia and tendon at lower leg level (S86)

  sprain of joint and ligament of hip (S73.1)

  The appropriate 7th character is to be added to each code from category S76

A	initial encounter
D	subsequent encounter
S	sequela

- S76.0   Injury of muscle, fascia and tendon of hip
  - S76.00   Unspecified injury of muscle, fascia and tendon of hip
    - S76.001   Unspecified injury of muscle, fascia and tendon of right hip
    - S76.002   Unspecified injury of muscle, fascia and tendon of left hip
    - S76.009   Unspecified injury of muscle, fascia and tendon of unspecified hip
  - S76.01   Strain of muscle, fascia and tendon of hip
    - S76.011   Strain of muscle, fascia and tendon of right hip
    - S76.012   Strain of muscle, fascia and tendon of left hip
    - S76.019   Strain of muscle, fascia and tendon of unspecified hip
  - S76.02   Laceration of muscle, fascia and tendon of hip
    - S76.021   Laceration of muscle, fascia and tendon of right hip
    - S76.022   Laceration of muscle, fascia and tendon of left hip
    - S76.029   Laceration of muscle, fascia and tendon of unspecified hip
  - S76.09   Other specified injury of muscle, fascia and tendon of hip
    - S76.091   Other specified injury of muscle, fascia and tendon of right hip
    - S76.092   Other specified injury of muscle, fascia and tendon of left hip
    - S76.099   Other specified injury of muscle, fascia and tendon of unspecified hip
- S76.1   Injury of quadriceps muscle, fascia and tendon

  Injury of patellar ligament (tendon)
  - S76.10   Unspecified injury of quadriceps muscle, fascia and tendon
    - S76.101   Unspecified injury of right quadriceps muscle, fascia and tendon
    - S76.102   Unspecified injury of left quadriceps muscle, fascia and tendon
    - S76.109   Unspecified injury of unspecified quadriceps muscle, fascia and tendon
  - S76.11   Strain of quadriceps muscle, fascia and tendon
    - S76.111   Strain of right quadriceps muscle, fascia and tendon
    - S76.112   Strain of left quadriceps muscle, fascia and tendon
    - S76.119   Strain of unspecified quadriceps muscle, fascia and tendon
  - S76.12   Laceration of quadriceps muscle, fascia and tendon
    - S76.121   Laceration of right quadriceps muscle, fascia and tendon
    - S76.122   Laceration of left quadriceps muscle, fascia and tendon
    - S76.129   Laceration of unspecified quadriceps muscle, fascia and tendon
  - S76.19   Other specified injury of quadriceps muscle, fascia and tendon
    - S76.191   Other specified injury of right quadriceps muscle, fascia and tendon
    - S76.192   Other specified injury of left quadriceps muscle, fascia and tendon
    - S76.199   Other specified injury of unspecified quadriceps muscle, fascia and tendon

▶ New   ⏩ Revised   ~~deleted~~ Deleted   Excludes 1   Excludes 2   Includes   Use additional   Code first   Code also   Key words

OGCR Official Guidelines   X Assign placeholder X   ● Use Additional Character(s)   ▶ Manifestation Code   🐾 Hierarchical Condition Category   Coding Clinic

- S76.2   Injury of adductor muscle, fascia and tendon of thigh
  - S76.20   Unspecified injury of adductor muscle, fascia and tendon of thigh
    - S76.201   Unspecified injury of adductor muscle, fascia and tendon of right thigh
    - S76.202   Unspecified injury of adductor muscle, fascia and tendon of left thigh
    - S76.209   Unspecified injury of adductor muscle, fascia and tendon of unspecified thigh
  - S76.21   Strain of adductor muscle, fascia and tendon of thigh
    - S76.211   Strain of adductor muscle, fascia and tendon of right thigh
    - S76.212   Strain of adductor muscle, fascia and tendon of left thigh
    - S76.219   Strain of adductor muscle, fascia and tendon of unspecified thigh
  - S76.22   Laceration of adductor muscle, fascia and tendon of thigh
    - S76.221   Laceration of adductor muscle, fascia and tendon of right thigh
    - S76.222   Laceration of adductor muscle, fascia and tendon of left thigh
    - S76.229   Laceration of adductor muscle, fascia and tendon of unspecified thigh
  - S76.29   Other injury of adductor muscle, fascia and tendon of thigh
    - S76.291   Other injury of adductor muscle, fascia and tendon of right thigh
    - S76.292   Other injury of adductor muscle, fascia and tendon of left thigh
    - S76.299   Other injury of adductor muscle, fascia and tendon of unspecified thigh
- S76.3   Injury of muscle, fascia and tendon of the posterior muscle group at thigh level
  - S76.30   Unspecified injury of muscle, fascia and tendon of the posterior muscle group at thigh level
    - S76.301   Unspecified injury of muscle, fascia and tendon of the posterior muscle group at thigh level, right thigh
    - S76.302   Unspecified injury of muscle, fascia and tendon of the posterior muscle group at thigh level, left thigh
    - S76.309   Unspecified injury of muscle, fascia and tendon of the posterior muscle group at thigh level, unspecified thigh
  - S76.31   Strain of muscle, fascia and tendon of the posterior muscle group at thigh level
    - S76.311   Strain of muscle, fascia and tendon of the posterior muscle group at thigh level, right thigh
    - S76.312   Strain of muscle, fascia and tendon of the posterior muscle group at thigh level, left thigh
    - S76.319   Strain of muscle, fascia and tendon of the posterior muscle group at thigh level, unspecified thigh

- S76.32   Laceration of muscle, fascia and tendon of the posterior muscle group at thigh level
    - S76.321   Laceration of muscle, fascia and tendon of the posterior muscle group at thigh level, right thigh
    - S76.322   Laceration of muscle, fascia and tendon of the posterior muscle group at thigh level, left thigh
    - S76.329   Laceration of muscle, fascia and tendon of the posterior muscle group at thigh level, unspecified thigh
  - S76.39   Other specified injury of muscle, fascia and tendon of the posterior muscle group at thigh level
    - S76.391   Other specified injury of muscle, fascia and tendon of the posterior muscle group at thigh level, right thigh
    - S76.392   Other specified injury of muscle, fascia and tendon of the posterior muscle group at thigh level, left thigh
    - S76.399   Other specified injury of muscle, fascia and tendon of the posterior muscle group at thigh level, unspecified thigh
- S76.8   Injury of other specified muscles, fascia and tendons at thigh level
  - S76.80   Unspecified injury of other specified muscles, fascia and tendons at thigh level
    - S76.801   Unspecified injury of other specified muscles, fascia and tendons at thigh level, right thigh
    - S76.802   Unspecified injury of other specified muscles, fascia and tendons at thigh level, left thigh
    - S76.809   Unspecified injury of other specified muscles, fascia and tendons at thigh level, unspecified thigh
  - S76.81   Strain of other specified specified muscles, fascia and tendons at thigh level
    - S76.811   Strain of other specified muscles, fascia and tendons at thigh level, right thigh
    - S76.812   Strain of other specified muscles, fascia and tendons at thigh level, left thigh
    - S76.819   Strain of other specified muscles, fascia and tendons at thigh level, unspecified thigh
  - S76.82   Laceration of other specified muscles, fascia and tendons at thigh level
    - S76.821   Laceration of other specified muscles, fascia and tendons at thigh level, right thigh
    - S76.822   Laceration of other specified muscles, fascia and tendons at thigh level, left thigh
    - S76.829   Laceration of other specified muscles, fascia and tendons at thigh level, unspecified thigh

CHAPTER 19 (S00-T88)

- S76.89   Other injury of other specified muscles, fascia and tendons at thigh level
  - S76.891   Other injury of other specified muscles, fascia and tendons at thigh level, right thigh
  - S76.892   Other injury of other specified muscles, fascia and tendons at thigh level, left thigh
  - S76.899   Other injury of other specified muscles, fascia and tendons at thigh level, unspecified thigh
- S76.9   Injury of unspecified muscles, fascia and tendons at thigh level
  - S76.90   Unspecified injury of unspecified muscles, fascia and tendons at thigh level
    - S76.901   Unspecified injury of unspecified muscles, fascia and tendons at thigh level, right thigh
    - S76.902   Unspecified injury of unspecified muscles, fascia and tendons at thigh level, left thigh
    - S76.909   Unspecified injury of unspecified muscles, fascia and tendons at thigh level, unspecified thigh
  - S76.91   Strain of unspecified muscles, fascia and tendons at thigh level
    - S76.911   Strain of unspecified muscles, fascia and tendons at thigh level, right thigh
    - S76.912   Strain of unspecified muscles, fascia and tendons at thigh level, left thigh
    - S76.919   Strain of unspecified muscles fascia and tendons at thigh level, unspecified thigh
  - S76.92   Laceration of unspecified muscles, fascia and tendons at thigh level
    - S76.921   Laceration of unspecified muscles, fascia and tendons at thigh level, right thigh
    - S76.922   Laceration of unspecified muscles, fascia and tendons at thigh level, left thigh
    - S76.929   Laceration of unspecified muscles, fascia and tendons at thigh level, unspecified thigh
  - S76.99   Other specified injury of unspecified muscles, fascia and tendons at thigh level
    - S76.991   Other specified injury of unspecified muscles, fascia and tendons at thigh level, right thigh
    - S76.992   Other specified injury of unspecified muscles, fascia and tendons at thigh level, left thigh
    - S76.999   Other specified injury of unspecified muscles, fascia and tendons at thigh level, unspecified thigh

- S77   **Crushing injury of hip and thigh**

  Use additional code(s) for all associated injuries

  Excludes2   crushing injury of ankle and foot (S97.-)
  crushing injury of lower leg (S87.-)

  The appropriate 7th character is to be added to each code from category S77

A	initial encounter
D	subsequent encounter
S	sequela

  - S77.0   Crushing injury of hip
    - X S77.00   Crushing injury of unspecified hip
    - X S77.01   Crushing injury of right hip
    - X S77.02   Crushing injury of left hip

- S77.1   Crushing injury of thigh
  - X S77.10   Crushing injury of unspecified thigh
  - X S77.11   Crushing injury of right thigh
  - X S77.12   Crushing injury of left thigh
- S77.2   Crushing injury of hip with thigh
  - X S77.20   Crushing injury of unspecified hip with thigh
  - X S77.21   Crushing injury of right hip with thigh
  - X S77.22   Crushing injury of left hip with thigh

- S78   **Traumatic amputation of hip and thigh**

  An amputation not identified as partial or complete should be coded to complete

  Excludes1   traumatic amputation of knee (S88.0-)

  The appropriate 7th character is to be added to each code from category S78

A	initial encounter
D	subsequent encounter
S	sequela

  - S78.0   Traumatic amputation at hip joint
    - S78.01   Complete traumatic amputation at hip joint
      - S78.011   Complete traumatic amputation at right hip joint A, D, S 🦠
      - S78.012   Complete traumatic amputation at left hip joint A, D, S 🦠
      - S78.019   Complete traumatic amputation at unspecified hip joint A, D, S 🦠
    - S78.02   Partial traumatic amputation at hip joint
      - S78.021   Partial traumatic amputation at right hip joint A, D, S 🦠
      - S78.022   Partial traumatic amputation at left hip joint A, D, S 🦠
      - S78.029   Partial traumatic amputation at unspecified hip joint A, D, S 🦠
  - S78.1   Traumatic amputation at level between hip and knee

    Excludes1   traumatic amputation of knee (S88.0-)

    - S78.11   Complete traumatic amputation at level between hip and knee
      - S78.111   Complete traumatic amputation at level between right hip and knee A, D, S 🦠
      - S78.112   Complete traumatic amputation at level between left hip and knee A, D, S 🦠
      - S78.119   Complete traumatic amputation at level between unspecified hip and knee A, D, S 🦠
    - S78.12   Partial traumatic amputation at level between hip and knee
      - S78.121   Partial traumatic amputation at level between right hip and knee A, D, S 🦠
      - S78.122   Partial traumatic amputation at level between left hip and knee A, D, S 🦠
      - S78.129   Partial traumatic amputation at level between unspecified hip and knee A, D, S 🦠
  - S78.9   Traumatic amputation of hip and thigh, level unspecified
    - S78.91   Complete traumatic amputation of hip and thigh, level unspecified
      - S78.911   Complete traumatic amputation of right hip and thigh, level unspecified A, D, S 🦠
      - S78.912   Complete traumatic amputation of left hip and thigh, level unspecified A, D, S 🦠
      - S78.919   Complete traumatic amputation of unspecified hip and thigh, level unspecified A, D, S 🦠

▶ New   ⇒ Revised   ~~deleted~~ Deleted   Excludes 1   Excludes 2   Includes   Use additional   Code first   Code also   Key words

OGCR Official Guidelines   X Assign placeholder X   ● Use Additional Character(s)   ▌ Manifestation Code   🦠 Hierarchical Condition Category   **Coding Clinic**

● S78.92   Partial traumatic amputation of hip and thigh, level unspecified

     ● S78.921   Partial traumatic amputation of right hip and thigh, level unspecified A, D, S 🕮

     ● S78.922   Partial traumatic amputation of left hip and thigh, level unspecified A, D, S 🕮

     ● S78.929   Partial traumatic amputation of unspecified hip and thigh, level unspecified A, D, S 🕮

● S79   Other and unspecified injuries of hip and thigh

     Note: A fracture not indicated as open or closed should be coded to closed

     The appropriate 7th character is to be added to each code from subcategories S79.0 and S79.1

A	initial encounter for closed fracture
D	subsequent encounter for fracture with routine healing
G	subsequent encounter for fracture with delayed healing
K	subsequent encounter for fracture with nonunion
P	subsequent encounter for fracture with malunion
S	sequela

● S79.0   Physeal fracture of upper end of femur

     Excludes1   apophyseal fracture of upper end of femur (S72.13-)

                   nontraumatic slipped upper femoral epiphysis (M93.0-)

     ● S79.00   Unspecified physeal fracture of upper end of femur

         ● S79.001   Unspecified physeal fracture of upper end of right femur A 🕮

         ● S79.002   Unspecified physeal fracture of upper end of left femur A 🕮

         ● S79.009   Unspecified physeal fracture of upper end of unspecified femur A 🕮

     ● S79.01   Salter-Harris Type I physeal fracture of upper end of femur

            Acute on chronic slipped capital femoral epiphysis (traumatic)

            Acute slipped capital femoral epiphysis (traumatic)

            Capital femoral epiphyseal fracture

            Excludes1   chronic slipped upper femoral epiphysis (nontraumatic) (M93.02-)

         ● S79.011   Salter-Harris Type I physeal fracture of upper end of right femur A 🕮

         ● S79.012   Salter-Harris Type I physeal fracture of upper end of left femur A 🕮

         ● S79.019   Salter-Harris Type I physeal fracture of upper end of unspecified femur A 🕮

● S79.09   Other physeal fracture of upper end of femur

     ● S79.091   Other physeal fracture of upper end of right femur A 🕮

     ● S79.092   Other physeal fracture of upper end of left femur A 🕮

     ● S79.099   Other physeal fracture of upper end of unspecified femur A 🕮

● S79.1   Physeal fracture of lower end of femur

     ● S79.10   Unspecified physeal fracture of lower end of femur

         ● S79.101   Unspecified physeal fracture of lower end of right femur A 🕮

         ● S79.102   Unspecified physeal fracture of lower end of left femur A 🕮

         ● S79.109   Unspecified physeal fracture of lower end of unspecified femur A 🕮

     ● S79.11   Salter-Harris Type I physeal fracture of lower end of femur

         ● S79.111   Salter-Harris Type I physeal fracture of lower end of right femur A 🕮

         ● S79.112   Salter-Harris Type I physeal fracture of lower end of left femur A 🕮

         ● S79.119   Salter-Harris Type I physeal fracture of lower end of unspecified femur A 🕮

     ● S79.12   Salter-Harris Type II physeal fracture of lower end of femur

         ● S79.121   Salter-Harris Type II physeal fracture of lower end of right femur A 🕮

         ● S79.122   Salter-Harris Type II physeal fracture of lower end of left femur A 🕮

         ● S79.129   Salter-Harris Type II physeal fracture of lower end of unspecified femur A 🕮

     ● S79.13   Salter-Harris Type III physeal fracture of lower end of femur

         ● S79.131   Salter-Harris Type III physeal fracture of lower end of right femur A 🕮

         ● S79.132   Salter-Harris Type III physeal fracture of lower end of left femur A 🕮

         ● S79.139   Salter-Harris Type III physeal fracture of lower end of unspecified femur A 🕮

     ● S79.14   Salter-Harris Type IV physeal fracture of lower end of femur

         ● S79.141   Salter-Harris Type IV physeal fracture of lower end of right femur A 🕮

         ● S79.142   Salter-Harris Type IV physeal fracture of lower end of left femur A 🕮

         ● S79.149   Salter-Harris Type IV physeal fracture of lower end of unspecified femur A 🕮

     ● S79.19   Other physeal fracture of lower end of femur

         ● S79.191   Other physeal fracture of lower end of right femur A 🕮

         ● S79.192   Other physeal fracture of lower end of left femur A 🕮

         ● S79.199   Other physeal fracture of lower end of unspecified femur A 🕮

CHAPTER 19 (S00-T88)

Item 19–5   SALTER-HARRIS TYPE 1: epiphysis is completely separated from end of bone, or metaphysic growth plate remains attached to epiphysis

    SALTER-HARRIS TYPE 2: epiphysis and growth plate are partially separated from metaphysis, which is cracked—most common type

    SALTER-HARRIS TYPE 3: fracture occurring through epiphysis and separates part of epiphysis and growth plate from metaphysis fracture, usually at distal end of tibia

    SALTER-HARRIS TYPE 4: fracture runs through epiphysis, across growth plate, into metaphysic; surgery is required to restore joint surface to normal and align growth plate

CHAPTER 19 (S00-T88)

● **S79.8 Other specified injuries of hip and thigh**

The appropriate 7th character is to be added to each code in subcategory S79.8

A	initial encounter
D	subsequent encounter
S	sequela

● **S79.81   Other specified injuries of hip**
- ● S79.811   Other specified injuries of right hip
- ● S79.812   Other specified injuries of left hip
- ● S79.819   Other specified injuries of unspecified hip

● **S79.82   Other specified injuries of thigh**
- ● S79.821   Other specified injuries of right thigh
- ● S79.822   Other specified injuries of left thigh
- ● S79.829   Other specified injuries of unspecified thigh

● **S79.9   Unspecified injury of hip and thigh**

The appropriate 7th character is to be added to each code in subcategory S79.9

A	initial encounter
D	subsequent encounter
S	sequela

● **S79.91   Unspecified injury of hip**
- ● S79.911   Unspecified injury of right hip
- ● S79.912   Unspecified injury of left hip
- ● S79.919   Unspecified injury of unspecified hip

● **S79.92   Unspecified injury of thigh**
- ● S79.921   Unspecified injury of right thigh
- ● S79.922   Unspecified injury of left thigh
- ● S79.929   Unspecified injury of unspecified thigh

INJURIES TO THE KNEE AND LOWER LEG (S80-S89)

Excludes2   burns and corrosions (T20-T32)
       frostbite (T33-T34)
       injuries of ankle and foot, except fracture of ankle and malleolus (S90-S99)
       insect bite or sting, venomous (T63.4)

● **S80   Superficial injury of knee and lower leg**

Excludes2   superficial injury of ankle and foot (S90.-)

The appropriate 7th character is to be added to each code from category S80

A	initial encounter
D	subsequent encounter
S	sequela

● **S80.0   Contusion of knee**
- X ● S80.00   Contusion of unspecified knee
- X ● S80.01   Contusion of right knee
- X ● S80.02   Contusion of left knee

● **S80.1   Contusion of lower leg**
- X ● S80.10   Contusion of unspecified lower leg
- X ● S80.11   Contusion of right lower leg
- X ● S80.12   Contusion of left lower leg

● **S80.2   Other superficial injuries of knee**

● **S80.21   Abrasion of knee**
- ● S80.211   Abrasion, right knee
- ● S80.212   Abrasion, left knee
- ● S80.219   Abrasion, unspecified knee

● **S80.22   Blister (nonthermal) of knee**
- ● S80.221   Blister (nonthermal), right knee
- ● S80.222   Blister (nonthermal), left knee
- ● S80.229   Blister (nonthermal), unspecified knee

● **S80.24   External constriction of knee**
- ● S80.241   External constriction, right knee
- ● S80.242   External constriction, left knee
- ● S80.249   External constriction, unspecified knee

● **S80.25   Superficial foreign body of knee**
      Splinter in the knee
- ● S80.251   Superficial foreign body, right knee
- ● S80.252   Superficial foreign body, left knee
- ● S80.259   Superficial foreign body, unspecified knee

● **S80.26   Insect bite (nonvenomous) of knee**
- ● S80.261   Insect bite (nonvenomous), right knee
- ● S80.262   Insect bite (nonvenomous), left knee
- ● S80.269   Insect bite (nonvenomous), unspecified knee

● **S80.27   Other superficial bite of knee**
      Excludes1   open bite of knee (S81.05-)
- ● S80.271   Other superficial bite of right knee
- ● S80.272   Other superficial bite of left knee
- ● S80.279   Other superficial bite of unspecified knee

● **S80.8   Other superficial injuries of lower leg**

● **S80.81   Abrasion of lower leg**
- ● S80.811   Abrasion, right lower leg
- ● S80.812   Abrasion, left lower leg
- ● S80.819   Abrasion, unspecified lower leg

● **S80.82   Blister (nonthermal) of lower leg**
- ● S80.821   Blister (nonthermal), right lower leg
- ● S80.822   Blister (nonthermal), left lower leg
- ● S80.829   Blister (nonthermal), unspecified lower leg

● **S80.84   External constriction of lower leg**
- ● S80.841   External constriction, right lower leg
- ● S80.842   External constriction, left lower leg
- ● S80.849   External constriction, unspecified lower leg

● **S80.85   Superficial foreign body of lower leg**
      Splinter in the lower leg
- ● S80.851   Superficial foreign body, right lower leg
- ● S80.852   Superficial foreign body, left lower leg
- ● S80.859   Superficial foreign body, unspecified lower leg

▶ New   ⮞ Revised   ~~deleted~~ Deleted   Excludes 1   Excludes 2   Includes   Use additional   Code first   Code also   Key words
OGCR Official Guidelines   X Assign placeholder X   ● Use Additional Character(s)   ▶ Manifestation Code   🗝 Hierarchical Condition Category   **Coding Clinic**

● S80.86   Insect bite (nonvenomous) of lower leg
    ● S80.861   Insect bite (nonvenomous), right lower leg
    ● S80.862   Insect bite (nonvenomous), left lower leg
    ● S80.869   Insect bite (nonvenomous), unspecified lower leg
● S80.87   Other superficial bite of lower leg
    Excludes1   open bite of lower leg (S81.85-)
    ● S80.871   Other superficial bite, right lower leg
    ● S80.872   Other superficial bite, left lower leg
    ● S80.879   Other superficial bite, unspecified lower leg
● S80.9   Unspecified superficial injury of knee and lower leg
    ● S80.91   Unspecified superficial injury of knee
        ● S80.911   Unspecified superficial injury of right knee
        ● S80.912   Unspecified superficial injury of left knee
        ● S80.919   Unspecified superficial injury of unspecified knee
    ● S80.92   Unspecified superficial injury of lower leg
        ● S80.921   Unspecified superficial injury of right lower leg
        ● S80.922   Unspecified superficial injury of left lower leg
        ● S80.929   Unspecified superficial injury of unspecified lower leg

● S81   Open wound of knee and lower leg
    Code also any associated wound infection
    Excludes1   open fracture of knee and lower leg (S82.-)
                traumatic amputation of lower leg (S88.-)
    Excludes2   open wound of ankle and foot (S91.-)
    The appropriate 7th character is to be added to each code from category S81

A	initial encounter
D	subsequent encounter
S	sequela

    ● S81.0   Open wound of knee
        ● S81.00   Unspecified open wound of knee
            ● S81.001   Unspecified open wound, right knee
            ● S81.002   Unspecified open wound, left knee
            ● S81.009   Unspecified open wound, unspecified knee
        ● S81.01   Laceration without foreign body of knee
            ● S81.011   Laceration without foreign body, right knee
            ● S81.012   Laceration without foreign body, left knee
            ● S81.019   Laceration without foreign body, unspecified knee
        ● S81.02   Laceration with foreign body of knee
            ● S81.021   Laceration with foreign body, right knee
            ● S81.022   Laceration with foreign body, left knee
            ● S81.029   Laceration with foreign body, unspecified knee

● S81.03   Puncture wound without foreign body of knee
    ● S81.031   Puncture wound without foreign body, right knee
    ● S81.032   Puncture wound without foreign body, left knee
    ● S81.039   Puncture wound without foreign body, unspecified knee
● S81.04   Puncture wound with foreign body of knee
    ● S81.041   Puncture wound with foreign body, right knee
    ● S81.042   Puncture wound with foreign body, left knee
    ● S81.049   Puncture wound with foreign body, unspecified knee
● S81.05   Open bite of knee
    Bite of knee NOS
    Excludes1   superficial bite of knee (S80.27-)
    ● S81.051   Open bite, right knee
    ● S81.052   Open bite, left knee
    ● S81.059   Open bite, unspecified knee
● S81.8   Open wound of lower leg
    ● S81.80   Unspecified open wound of lower leg
        ● S81.801   Unspecified open wound, right lower leg
        ● S81.802   Unspecified open wound, left lower leg
        ● S81.809   Unspecified open wound, unspecified lower leg
    ● S81.81   Laceration without foreign body of lower leg
        ● S81.811   Laceration without foreign body, right lower leg
        ● S81.812   Laceration without foreign body, left lower leg
        ● S81.819   Laceration without foreign body, unspecified lower leg
    ● S81.82   Laceration with foreign body of lower leg
        ● S81.821   Laceration with foreign body, right lower leg
        ● S81.822   Laceration with foreign body, left lower leg
        ● S81.829   Laceration with foreign body, unspecified lower leg
    ● S81.83   Puncture wound without foreign body of lower leg
        ● S81.831   Puncture wound without foreign body, right lower leg
        ● S81.832   Puncture wound without foreign body, left lower leg
        ● S81.839   Puncture wound without foreign body, unspecified lower leg
    ● S81.84   Puncture wound with foreign body of lower leg
        ● S81.841   Puncture wound with foreign body, right lower leg
            Coding Clinic: 2016, Q3, P46
        ● S81.842   Puncture wound with foreign body, left lower leg
        ● S81.849   Puncture wound with foreign body, unspecified lower leg
    ● S81.85   Open bite of lower leg
        Bite of lower leg NOS
        Excludes1   superficial bite of lower leg (S80.86-, S80.87-)
        ● S81.851   Open bite, right lower leg
        ● S81.852   Open bite, left lower leg
        ● S81.859   Open bite, unspecified lower leg

CHAPTER 19 (S00-T88)

● **S82   Fracture of lower leg, including ankle**

    Note: A fracture not indicated as displaced or nondisplaced should be coded to displaced

    A fracture not indicated as open or closed should be coded to closed

    The open fracture designations are based on the Gustilo open fracture classification

    Includes   fracture of malleolus

    Excludes1 traumatic amputation of lower leg (S88.-)

    Excludes2 fracture of foot, except ankle (S92.-)

       ⇒ periprosthetic fracture around internal of prosthetic implant of knee joint (M97.1-)

    The appropriate 7th character is to be added to all codes from category S82

A	initial encounter for closed fracture
B	initial encounter for open fracture type I or II initial encounter for open fracture NOS
C	initial encounter for open fracture type IIIA, IIIB, or IIIC
D	subsequent encounter for closed fracture with routine healing
E	subsequent encounter for open fracture type I or II with routine healing
F	subsequent encounter for open fracture type IIIA, IIIB, or IIIC with routine healing
G	subsequent encounter for closed fracture with delayed healing
H	subsequent encounter for open fracture type I or II with delayed healing
J	subsequent encounter for open fracture type IIIA, IIIB, or IIIC with delayed healing
K	subsequent encounter for closed fracture with nonunion
M	subsequent encounter for open fracture type I or II with nonunion
N	subsequent encounter for open fracture type IIIA, IIIB, or IIIC with nonunion
P	subsequent encounter for closed fracture with malunion
Q	subsequent encounter for open fracture type I or II with malunion
R	subsequent encounter for open fracture type IIIA, IIIB, or IIIC with malunion
S	sequela

● **S82.0   Fracture of patella**
    Knee cap

  ● **S82.00   Unspecified fracture of patella**

    ● S82.001   Unspecified fracture of right patella

    ● S82.002   Unspecified fracture of left patella

    ● S82.009   Unspecified fracture of unspecified patella

  ● **S82.01   Osteochondral fracture of patella**

    ● S82.011   Displaced osteochondral fracture of right patella

    ● S82.012   Displaced osteochondral fracture of left patella

    ● S82.013   Displaced osteochondral fracture of unspecified patella

    ● S82.014   Nondisplaced osteochondral fracture of right patella

    ● S82.015   Nondisplaced osteochondral fracture of left patella

    ● S82.016   Nondisplaced osteochondral fracture of unspecified patella

● **S82.02   Longitudinal fracture of patella**

    ● S82.021   Displaced longitudinal fracture of right patella

    ● S82.022   Displaced longitudinal fracture of left patella

    ● S82.023   Displaced longitudinal fracture of unspecified patella

    ● S82.024   Nondisplaced longitudinal fracture of right patella

    ● S82.025   Nondisplaced longitudinal fracture of left patella

    ● S82.026   Nondisplaced longitudinal fracture of unspecified patella

● **S82.03   Transverse fracture of patella**

    ● S82.031   Displaced transverse fracture of right patella

    ● S82.032   Displaced transverse fracture of left patella

    ● S82.033   Displaced transverse fracture of unspecified patella

    ● S82.034   Nondisplaced transverse fracture of right patella

    ● S82.035   Nondisplaced transverse fracture of left patella

    ● S82.036   Nondisplaced transverse fracture of unspecified patella

● **S82.04   Comminuted fracture of patella**

    ● S82.041   Displaced comminuted fracture of right patella

    ● S82.042   Displaced comminuted fracture of left patella

    ● S82.043   Displaced comminuted fracture of unspecified patella

    ● S82.044   Nondisplaced comminuted fracture of right patella

    ● S82.045   Nondisplaced comminuted fracture of left patella

    ● S82.046   Nondisplaced comminuted fracture of unspecified patella

● **S82.09   Other fracture of patella**

    ● S82.091   Other fracture of right patella

    ● S82.092   Other fracture of left patella

    ● S82.099   Other fracture of unspecified patella

● **S82.1   Fracture of upper end of tibia**
    Fracture of proximal end of tibia

    Excludes2 fracture of shaft of tibia (S82.2-)
              physeal fracture of upper end of tibia (S89.0-)

  ● **S82.10   Unspecified fracture of upper end of tibia**

    ● S82.101   Unspecified fracture of upper end of right tibia

    ● S82.102   Unspecified fracture of upper end of left tibia

    ● S82.109   Unspecified fracture of upper end of unspecified tibia

  ● **S82.11   Fracture of tibial spine**

    ● S82.111   Displaced fracture of right tibial spine

    ● S82.112   Displaced fracture of left tibial spine

    ● S82.113   Displaced fracture of unspecified tibial spine

▶ New   ⇒ Revised   ~~deleted~~ Deleted   Excludes 1   Excludes 2   Includes   Use additional   Code first   Code also   Key words

OGCR Official Guidelines   X Assign placeholder X   ● Use Additional Character(s)   ▷ Manifestation Code   🅗 Hierarchical Condition Category   Coding Clinic

● S82.114   Nondisplaced fracture of **right** tibial spine

● S82.115   Nondisplaced fracture of **left** tibial spine

● S82.116   Nondisplaced fracture of **unspecified** tibial spine

● S82.12   Fracture of lateral condyle of tibia

  ● S82.121   Displaced fracture of lateral condyle of **right** tibia

  ● S82.122   Displaced fracture of lateral condyle of **left** tibia

  ● S82.123   Displaced fracture of lateral condyle of **unspecified** tibia

  ● S82.124   Nondisplaced fracture of lateral condyle of **right** tibia

  ● S82.125   Nondisplaced fracture of lateral condyle of **left** tibia

  ● S82.126   Nondisplaced fracture of lateral condyle of **unspecified** tibia

● S82.13   Fracture of medial condyle of tibia

  ● S82.131   Displaced fracture of medial condyle of **right** tibia

  ● S82.132   Displaced fracture of medial condyle of **left** tibia

  ● S82.133   Displaced fracture of medial condyle of **unspecified** tibia

  ● S82.134   Nondisplaced fracture of medial condyle of **right** tibia

  ● S82.135   Nondisplaced fracture of medial condyle of **left** tibia

  ● S82.136   Nondisplaced fracture of medial condyle of **unspecified** tibia

● S82.14   Bicondylar fracture of tibia
      Fracture of tibial plateau NOS

  ● S82.141   Displaced bicondylar fracture of **right** tibia

  ● S82.142   Displaced bicondylar fracture of **left** tibia

  ● S82.143   Displaced bicondylar fracture of **unspecified** tibia

  ● S82.144   Nondisplaced bicondylar fracture of **right** tibia

  ● S82.145   Nondisplaced bicondylar fracture of **left** tibia

  ● S82.146   Nondisplaced bicondylar fracture of **unspecified** tibia

● S82.15   Fracture of tibial tuberosity

  ● S82.151   Displaced fracture of **right** tibial tuberosity

  ● S82.152   Displaced fracture of **left** tibial tuberosity

  ● S82.153   Displaced fracture of **unspecified** tibial tuberosity

  ● S82.154   Nondisplaced fracture of **right** tibial tuberosity

  ● S82.155   Nondisplaced fracture of **left** tibial tuberosity

  ● S82.156   Nondisplaced fracture of **unspecified** tibial tuberosity

● S82.16   Torus fracture of **upper end** of tibia

     The appropriate 7th character is to be added to all codes in subcategory S82.16

A	initial encounter for closed fracture
D	subsequent encounter for fracture with routine healing
G	subsequent encounter for fracture with delayed healing
K	subsequent encounter for fracture with nonunion
P	subsequent encounter for fracture with malunion
S	sequela

  ● S82.161   Torus fracture of upper end of **right** tibia

  ● S82.162   Torus fracture of upper end of **left** tibia

  ● S82.169   Torus fracture of upper end of **unspecified** tibia

● S82.19   Other fracture of upper end of tibia

  ● S82.191   Other fracture of upper end of **right** tibia

  ● S82.192   Other fracture of upper end of **left** tibia

  ● S82.199   Other fracture of upper end of **unspecified** tibia

● S82.2   Fracture of **shaft** of tibia

  ● S82.20   **Unspecified** fracture of shaft of tibia
      Fracture of tibia NOS

    ● S82.201   Unspecified fracture of shaft of **right** tibia

    ● S82.202   Unspecified fracture of shaft of **left** tibia

    ● S82.209   Unspecified fracture of shaft of **unspecified** tibia

  ● S82.22   **Transverse** fracture of shaft of tibia

    ● S82.221   Displaced transverse fracture of shaft of **right** tibia

    ● S82.222   Displaced transverse fracture of shaft of **left** tibia

    ● S82.223   Displaced transverse fracture of shaft of **unspecified** tibia

    ● S82.224   Nondisplaced transverse fracture of shaft of **right** tibia

    ● S82.225   Nondisplaced transverse fracture of shaft of **left** tibia

    ● S82.226   Nondisplaced transverse fracture of shaft of **unspecified** tibia

  ● S82.23   **Oblique** fracture of shaft of tibia

    ● S82.231   Displaced oblique fracture of shaft of **right** tibia

    ● S82.232   Displaced oblique fracture of shaft of **left** tibia

    ● S82.233   Displaced oblique fracture of shaft of **unspecified** tibia

    ● S82.234   Nondisplaced oblique fracture of shaft of **right** tibia
       Coding Clinic: 2015, Q1, P9-10

    ● S82.235   Nondisplaced oblique fracture of shaft of **left** tibia

    ● S82.236   Nondisplaced oblique fracture of shaft of **unspecified** tibia

  ● S82.24   **Spiral** fracture of shaft of tibia
      Toddler fracture

    ● S82.241   Displaced spiral fracture of shaft of **right** tibia

    ● S82.242   Displaced spiral fracture of shaft of **left** tibia

CHAPTER 19 (S00-T88)

CHAPTER 19 (S00-T88)

- S82.243   Displaced spiral fracture of shaft of unspecified tibia
- S82.244   Nondisplaced spiral fracture of shaft of right tibia
- S82.245   Nondisplaced spiral fracture of shaft of left tibia
- S82.246   Nondisplaced spiral fracture of shaft of unspecified tibia
- S82.25   Comminuted fracture of shaft of tibia
  - S82.251   Displaced comminuted fracture of shaft of right tibia
    Coding Clinic: 2015, Q2, P6
  - S82.252   Displaced comminuted fracture of shaft of left tibia
  - S82.253   Displaced comminuted fracture of shaft of unspecified tibia
  - S82.254   Nondisplaced comminuted fracture of shaft of right tibia
  - S82.255   Nondisplaced comminuted fracture of shaft of left tibia
  - S82.256   Nondisplaced comminuted fracture of shaft of unspecified tibia
- S82.26   Segmental fracture of shaft of tibia
  - S82.261   Displaced segmental fracture of shaft of right tibia
  - S82.262   Displaced segmental fracture of shaft of left tibia
  - S82.263   Displaced segmental fracture of shaft of unspecified tibia
  - S82.264   Nondisplaced segmental fracture of shaft of right tibia
  - S82.265   Nondisplaced segmental fracture of shaft of left tibia
  - S82.266   Nondisplaced segmental fracture of shaft of unspecified tibia
- S82.29   Other fracture of shaft of tibia
  - S82.291   Other fracture of shaft of right tibia
  - S82.292   Other fracture of shaft of left tibia
  - S82.299   Other fracture of shaft of unspecified tibia
- S82.3   Fracture of lower end of tibia

  Excludes1   bimalleolar fracture of lower leg (S82.84-)
  fracture of medial malleolus alone (S82.5-)
  Maisonneuve's fracture (S82.86-)
  pilon fracture of distal tibia (S82.87-)
  trimalleolar fractures of lower leg (S82.85-)

- S82.30   Unspecified fracture of lower end of tibia
  - S82.301   Unspecified fracture of lower end of right tibia
  - S82.302   Unspecified fracture of lower end of left tibia
  - S82.309   Unspecified fracture of lower end of unspecified tibia
- S82.31   Torus fracture of lower end of tibia

  The appropriate 7th character is to be added to all codes in subcategory S82.31

A	initial encounter for closed fracture
D	subsequent encounter for fracture with routine healing
G	subsequent encounter for fracture with delayed healing
K	subsequent encounter for fracture with nonunion
P	subsequent encounter for fracture with malunion
S	sequela

- S82.311   Torus fracture of lower end of right tibia
- S82.312   Torus fracture of lower end of left tibia
- S82.319   Torus fracture of lower end of unspecified tibia
- S82.39   Other fracture of lower end of tibia
  - S82.391   Other fracture of lower end of right tibia
  - S82.392   Other fracture of lower end of left tibia
    Coding Clinic: 2015, Q1, P25
  - S82.399   Other fracture of lower end of unspecified tibia
- S82.4   Fracture of shaft of fibula

  Excludes2   fracture of lateral malleolus alone (S82.6-)

- S82.40   Unspecified fracture of shaft of fibula
  - S82.401   Unspecified fracture of shaft of right fibula
  - S82.402   Unspecified fracture of shaft of left fibula
  - S82.409   Unspecified fracture of shaft of unspecified fibula
- S82.42   Transverse fracture of shaft of fibula
  - S82.421   Displaced transverse fracture of shaft of right fibula
  - S82.422   Displaced transverse fracture of shaft of left fibula
  - S82.423   Displaced transverse fracture of shaft of unspecified fibula
  - S82.424   Nondisplaced transverse fracture of shaft of right fibula
  - S82.425   Nondisplaced transverse fracture of shaft of left fibula
  - S82.426   Nondisplaced transverse fracture of shaft of unspecified fibula
- S82.43   Oblique fracture of shaft of fibula
  - S82.431   Displaced oblique fracture of shaft of right fibula
  - S82.432   Displaced oblique fracture of shaft of left fibula
  - S82.433   Displaced oblique fracture of shaft of unspecified fibula
  - S82.434   Nondisplaced oblique fracture of shaft of right fibula
  - S82.435   Nondisplaced oblique fracture of shaft of left fibula
  - S82.436   Nondisplaced oblique fracture of shaft of unspecified fibula
- S82.44   Spiral fracture of shaft of fibula
  - S82.441   Displaced spiral fracture of shaft of right fibula
  - S82.442   Displaced spiral fracture of shaft of left fibula
  - S82.443   Displaced spiral fracture of shaft of unspecified fibula
  - S82.444   Nondisplaced spiral fracture of shaft of right fibula

● S82.445   Nondisplaced spiral fracture of shaft of left fibula

● S82.446   Nondisplaced spiral fracture of shaft of unspecified fibula

● S82.45   Comminuted fracture of shaft of fibula

● S82.451   Displaced comminuted fracture of shaft of right fibula

● S82.452   Displaced comminuted fracture of shaft of left fibula

● S82.453   Displaced comminuted fracture of shaft of unspecified fibula

● S82.454   Nondisplaced comminuted fracture of shaft of right fibula

● S82.455   Nondisplaced comminuted fracture of shaft of left fibula

● S82.456   Nondisplaced comminuted fracture of shaft of unspecified fibula

● S82.46   Segmental fracture of shaft of fibula

● S82.461   Displaced segmental fracture of shaft of right fibula

● S82.462   Displaced segmental fracture of shaft of left fibula

● S82.463   Displaced segmental fracture of shaft of unspecified fibula

● S82.464   Nondisplaced segmental fracture of shaft of right fibula

● S82.465   Nondisplaced segmental fracture of shaft of left fibula

● S82.466   Nondisplaced segmental fracture of shaft of unspecified fibula

● S82.49   Other fracture of shaft of fibula

● S82.491   Other fracture of shaft of right fibula

● S82.492   Other fracture of shaft of left fibula

● S82.499   Other fracture of shaft of unspecified fibula

● S82.5   Fracture of medial malleolus

Excludes1   pilon fracture of distal tibia (S82.87-)
Salter-Harris type III of lower end of tibia (S89.13-)
Salter-Harris type IV of lower end of tibia (S89.14-)

X● S82.51   Displaced fracture of medial malleolus of right tibia

X● S82.52   Displaced fracture of medial malleolus of left tibia

X● S82.53   Displaced fracture of medial malleolus of unspecified tibia

X● S82.54   Nondisplaced fracture of medial malleolus of right tibia

X● S82.55   Nondisplaced fracture of medial malleolus of left tibia

X● S82.56   Nondisplaced fracture of medial malleolus of unspecified tibia

● S82.6   Fracture of lateral malleolus

Excludes1   pilon fracture of distal tibia (S82.87-)

X● S82.61   Displaced fracture of lateral malleolus of right fibula

X● S82.62   Displaced fracture of lateral malleolus of left fibula

X● S82.63   Displaced fracture of lateral malleolus of unspecified fibula

X● S82.64   Nondisplaced fracture of lateral malleolus of right fibula

X● S82.65   Nondisplaced fracture of lateral malleolus of left fibula

X● S82.66   Nondisplaced fracture of lateral malleolus of unspecified fibula

● S82.8   Other fractures of lower leg

● S82.81   Torus fracture of upper end of fibula

The appropriate 7th character is to be added to all codes in subcategory S82.81

A	initial encounter for closed fracture
D	subsequent encounter for fracture with routine healing
G	subsequent encounter for fracture with delayed healing
K	subsequent encounter for fracture with nonunion
P	subsequent encounter for fracture with malunion
S	sequela

● S82.811   Torus fracture of upper end of right fibula

● S82.812   Torus fracture of upper end of left fibula

● S82.819   Torus fracture of upper end of unspecified fibula

● S82.82   Torus fracture of lower end of fibula

The appropriate 7th character is to be added to all codes in subcategory S82.82

A	initial encounter for closed fracture
D	subsequent encounter for fracture with routine healing
G	subsequent encounter for fracture with delayed healing
K	subsequent encounter for fracture with nonunion
P	subsequent encounter for fracture with malunion
S	sequela

● S82.821   Torus fracture of lower end of right fibula

● S82.822   Torus fracture of lower end of left fibula

● S82.829   Torus fracture of lower end of unspecified fibula

● S82.83   Other fracture of upper and lower end of fibula

● S82.831   Other fracture of upper and lower end of right fibula

● S82.832   Other fracture of upper and lower end of left fibula
Coding Clinic: 2015, Q1, P9-10

● S82.839   Other fracture of upper and lower end of unspecified fibula

● S82.84   Bimalleolar fracture of lower leg

● S82.841   Displaced bimalleolar fracture of right lower leg

● S82.842   Displaced bimalleolar fracture of left lower leg

● S82.843   Displaced bimalleolar fracture of unspecified lower leg

● S82.844   Nondisplaced bimalleolar fracture of right lower leg

● S82.845   Nondisplaced bimalleolar fracture of left lower leg

● S82.846   Nondisplaced bimalleolar fracture of unspecified lower leg

● S82.85   Trimalleolar fracture of lower leg

● S82.851   Displaced trimalleolar fracture of right lower leg

● S82.852   Displaced trimalleolar fracture of left lower leg

● S82.853   Displaced trimalleolar fracture of unspecified lower leg

● S82.854   Nondisplaced trimalleolar fracture of right lower leg

● S82.855   Nondisplaced trimalleolar fracture of left lower leg

● S82.856   Nondisplaced trimalleolar fracture of unspecified lower leg

● S82.86   Maisonneuve's fracture

● S82.861   Displaced Maisonneuve's fracture of right leg

● S82.862   Displaced Maisonneuve's fracture of left leg

● S82.863   Displaced Maisonneuve's fracture of unspecified leg

● S82.864   Nondisplaced Maisonneuve's fracture of right leg

● S82.865   Nondisplaced Maisonneuve's fracture of left leg

● S82.866   Nondisplaced Maisonneuve's fracture of unspecified leg

● S82.87   Pilon fracture of tibia

● S82.871   Displaced pilon fracture of right tibia

● S82.872   Displaced pilon fracture of left tibia

● S82.873   Displaced pilon fracture of unspecified tibia

● S82.874   Nondisplaced pilon fracture of right tibia

● S82.875   Nondisplaced pilon fracture of left tibia

● S82.876   Nondisplaced pilon fracture of unspecified tibia

● S82.89   Other fractures of lower leg
            Fracture of ankle NOS

● S82.891   Other fracture of right lower leg

● S82.892   Other fracture of left lower leg

● S82.899   Other fracture of unspecified lower leg

● S82.9   Unspecified fracture of lower leg

X ● S82.90   Unspecified fracture of unspecified lower leg

X ● S82.91   Unspecified fracture of right lower leg

X ● S82.92   Unspecified fracture of left lower leg

● S83   Dislocation and sprain of joints and ligaments of knee

    Includes   avulsion of joint or ligament of knee
                    laceration of cartilage, joint or ligament of knee
                    sprain of cartilage, joint or ligament of knee
                    traumatic hemarthrosis of joint or ligament of knee
                    traumatic rupture of joint or ligament of knee
                    traumatic subluxation of joint or ligament of knee
                    traumatic tear of joint or ligament of knee

    Code also any associated open wound

    Excludes2   derangement of patella (M22.0-M22.3)
                    injury of patellar ligament (tendon) (S76.1-)
                    internal derangement of knee (M23.-)
                    old dislocation of knee (M24.36)
                    pathological dislocation of knee (M24.36)
                    recurrent dislocation of knee (M22.0)
                    strain of muscle, fascia and tendon of lower leg (S86.-)

    Coding Clinic: 2019, Q2, P26

    The appropriate 7th character is to be added to each code from category S83

A	initial encounter
D	subsequent encounter
S	sequela

● S83.0   Subluxation and dislocation of patella

● S83.00   Unspecified subluxation and dislocation of patella

● S83.001   Unspecified subluxation of right patella

● S83.002   Unspecified subluxation of left patella

● S83.003   Unspecified subluxation of unspecified patella

● S83.004   Unspecified dislocation of right patella

● S83.005   Unspecified dislocation of left patella

● S83.006   Unspecified dislocation of unspecified patella

● S83.01   Lateral subluxation and dislocation of patella

● S83.011   Lateral subluxation of right patella

● S83.012   Lateral subluxation of left patella

● S83.013   Lateral subluxation of unspecified patella

● S83.014   Lateral dislocation of right patella

● S83.015   Lateral dislocation of left patella

● S83.016   Lateral dislocation of unspecified patella

● S83.09   Other subluxation and dislocation of patella

● S83.091   Other subluxation of right patella

● S83.092   Other subluxation of left patella

● S83.093   Other subluxation of unspecified patella

● S83.094   Other dislocation of right patella

● S83.095   Other dislocation of left patella

● S83.096   Other dislocation of unspecified patella

● S83.1   Subluxation and dislocation of knee

    Excludes2   instability of knee prosthesis (T84.022, T84.023)

● S83.10   Unspecified subluxation and dislocation of knee

● S83.101   Unspecified subluxation of right knee

● S83.102   Unspecified subluxation of left knee

● S83.103   Unspecified subluxation of unspecified knee

● S83.104   Unspecified dislocation of right knee

● S83.105   Unspecified dislocation of left knee

● S83.106   Unspecified dislocation of unspecified knee

● S83.11   Anterior subluxation and dislocation of proximal end of tibia
            Posterior subluxation and dislocation of distal end of femur

● S83.111   Anterior subluxation of proximal end of tibia, right knee

● S83.112   Anterior subluxation of proximal end of tibia, left knee

● S83.113   Anterior subluxation of proximal end of tibia, unspecified knee

● S83.114   Anterior dislocation of proximal end of tibia, right knee

● S83.115   Anterior dislocation of proximal end of tibia, left knee

● S83.116   Anterior dislocation of proximal end of tibia, unspecified knee

● S83.12   Posterior subluxation and dislocation of proximal end of tibia
     Anterior dislocation of distal end of femur

    ● S83.121   Posterior subluxation of proximal end of tibia, right knee

    ● S83.122   Posterior subluxation of proximal end of tibia, left knee

    ● S83.123   Posterior subluxation of proximal end of tibia, unspecified knee

    ● S83.124   Posterior dislocation of proximal end of tibia, right knee

    ● S83.125   Posterior dislocation of proximal end of tibia, left knee

    ● S83.126   Posterior dislocation of proximal end of tibia, unspecified knee

● S83.13   Medial subluxation and dislocation of proximal end of tibia

    ● S83.131   Medial subluxation of proximal end of tibia, right knee

    ● S83.132   Medial subluxation of proximal end of tibia, left knee

    ● S83.133   Medial subluxation of proximal end of tibia, unspecified knee

    ● S83.134   Medial dislocation of proximal end of tibia, right knee

    ● S83.135   Medial dislocation of proximal end of tibia, left knee

    ● S83.136   Medial dislocation of proximal end of tibia, unspecified knee

● S83.14   Lateral subluxation and dislocation of proximal end of tibia

    ● S83.141   Lateral subluxation of proximal end of tibia, right knee

    ● S83.142   Lateral subluxation of proximal end of tibia, left knee

    ● S83.143   Lateral subluxation of proximal end of tibia, unspecified knee

    ● S83.144   Lateral dislocation of proximal end of tibia, right knee

    ● S83.145   Lateral dislocation of proximal end of tibia, left knee

    ● S83.146   Lateral dislocation of proximal end of tibia, unspecified knee

● S83.19   Other subluxation and dislocation of knee

    ● S83.191   Other subluxation of right knee

    ● S83.192   Other subluxation of left knee

    ● S83.193   Other subluxation of unspecified knee

    ● S83.194   Other dislocation of right knee

    ● S83.195   Other dislocation of left knee

    ● S83.196   Other dislocation of unspecified knee

● S83.2   Tear of meniscus, current injury

    Excludes1   old bucket-handle tear (M23.2)

● S83.20   Tear of unspecified meniscus, current injury
    Tear of meniscus of knee NOS

    ● S83.200   Bucket-handle tear of unspecified meniscus, current injury, right knee

    ● S83.201   Bucket-handle tear of unspecified meniscus, current injury, left knee

    ● S83.202   Bucket-handle tear of unspecified meniscus, current injury, unspecified knee

    ● S83.203   Other tear of unspecified meniscus, current injury, right knee

    ● S83.204   Other tear of unspecified meniscus, current injury, left knee

    ● S83.205   Other tear of unspecified meniscus, current injury, unspecified knee

    ● S83.206   Unspecified tear of unspecified meniscus, current injury, right knee

    ● S83.207   Unspecified tear of unspecified meniscus, current injury, left knee

    ● S83.209   Unspecified tear of unspecified meniscus, current injury, unspecified knee

● S83.21   Bucket-handle tear of medial meniscus, current injury

    ● S83.211   Bucket-handle tear of medial meniscus, current injury, right knee

    ● S83.212   Bucket-handle tear of medial meniscus, current injury, left knee

    ● S83.219   Bucket-handle tear of medial meniscus, current injury, unspecified knee

● S83.22   Peripheral tear of medial meniscus, current injury

    ● S83.221   Peripheral tear of medial meniscus, current injury, right knee

    ● S83.222   Peripheral tear of medial meniscus, current injury, left knee

    ● S83.229   Peripheral tear of medial meniscus, current injury, unspecified knee

● S83.23   Complex tear of medial meniscus, current injury

    ● S83.231   Complex tear of medial meniscus, current injury, right knee

    ● S83.232   Complex tear of medial meniscus, current injury, left knee
       Coding Clinic: 2019, Q2, P26

    ● S83.239   Complex tear of medial meniscus, current injury, unspecified knee

● S83.24   Other tear of medial meniscus, current injury

    ● S83.241   Other tear of medial meniscus, current injury, right knee

    ● S83.242   Other tear of medial meniscus, current injury, left knee

    ● S83.249   Other tear of medial meniscus, current injury, unspecified knee

● S83.25   Bucket-handle tear of lateral meniscus, current injury

    ● S83.251   Bucket-handle tear of lateral meniscus, current injury, right knee

    ● S83.252   Bucket-handle tear of lateral meniscus, current injury, left knee

    ● S83.259   Bucket-handle tear of lateral meniscus, current injury, unspecified knee

● S83.26   Peripheral tear of lateral meniscus, current injury

    ● S83.261   Peripheral tear of lateral meniscus, current injury, right knee

    ● S83.262   Peripheral tear of lateral meniscus, current injury, left knee

    ● S83.269   Peripheral tear of lateral meniscus, current injury, unspecified knee

- ● S83.27 Complex tear of lateral meniscus, current injury
  - ● S83.271 Complex tear of lateral meniscus, current injury, right knee
  - ● S83.272 Complex tear of lateral meniscus, current injury, left knee
  - ● S83.279 Complex tear of lateral meniscus, current injury, unspecified knee
- ● S83.28 Other tear of lateral meniscus, current injury
  - ● S83.281 Other tear of lateral meniscus, current injury, right knee
  - ● S83.282 Other tear of lateral meniscus, current injury, left knee
  - ● S83.289 Other tear of lateral meniscus, current injury, unspecified knee
- ● S83.3 Tear of articular cartilage of knee, current
  - X ● S83.30 Tear of articular cartilage of unspecified knee, current
  - X ● S83.31 Tear of articular cartilage of right knee, current
  - X ● S83.32 Tear of articular cartilage of left knee, current
- ● S83.4 Sprain of collateral ligament of knee
  - ● S83.40 Sprain of unspecified collateral ligament of knee
    - ● S83.401 Sprain of unspecified collateral ligament of right knee
    - ● S83.402 Sprain of unspecified collateral ligament of left knee
    - ● S83.409 Sprain of unspecified collateral ligament of unspecified knee
  - ● S83.41 Sprain of medial collateral ligament of knee
    Sprain of tibial collateral ligament
    - ● S83.411 Sprain of medial collateral ligament of right knee
    - ● S83.412 Sprain of medial collateral ligament of left knee
    - ● S83.419 Sprain of medial collateral ligament of unspecified knee
  - ● S83.42 Sprain of lateral collateral ligament of knee
    Sprain of fibular collateral ligament
    - ● S83.421 Sprain of lateral collateral ligament of right knee
    - ● S83.422 Sprain of lateral collateral ligament of left knee
    - ● S83.429 Sprain of lateral collateral ligament of unspecified knee
- ● S83.5 Sprain of cruciate ligament of knee
  - ● S83.50 Sprain of unspecified cruciate ligament of knee
    - ● S83.501 Sprain of unspecified cruciate ligament of right knee
    - ● S83.502 Sprain of unspecified cruciate ligament of left knee
    - ● S83.509 Sprain of unspecified cruciate ligament of unspecified knee
  - ● S83.51 Sprain of anterior cruciate ligament of knee
    - ● S83.511 Sprain of anterior cruciate ligament of right knee
      Coding Clinic: 2016, Q2, P4
    - ● S83.512 Sprain of anterior cruciate ligament of left knee
    - ● S83.519 Sprain of anterior cruciate ligament of unspecified knee

- ● S83.52 Sprain of posterior cruciate ligament of knee
  - ● S83.521 Sprain of posterior cruciate ligament of right knee
  - ● S83.522 Sprain of posterior cruciate ligament of left knee
  - ● S83.529 Sprain of posterior cruciate ligament of unspecified knee
- ● S83.6 Sprain of the superior tibiofibular joint and ligament
  - X ● S83.60 Sprain of the superior tibiofibular joint and ligament, unspecified knee
  - X ● S83.61 Sprain of the superior tibiofibular joint and ligament, right knee
  - X ● S83.62 Sprain of the superior tibiofibular joint and ligament, left knee
- ● S83.8 Sprain of other specified parts of knee
  - ● S83.8X Sprain of other specified parts of knee
    - ● S83.8X1 Sprain of other specified parts of right knee
    - ● S83.8X2 Sprain of other specified parts of left knee
    - ● S83.8X9 Sprain of other specified parts of unspecified knee
- ● S83.9 Sprain of unspecified site of knee
  - X ● S83.90 Sprain of unspecified site of unspecified knee
  - X ● S83.91 Sprain of unspecified site of right knee
  - X ● S83.92 Sprain of unspecified site of left knee

- ● S84 Injury of nerves at lower leg level
  Code also any associated open wound (S81.-)
  Excludes2 injury of nerves at ankle and foot level (S94.-)
  The appropriate 7th character is to be added to each code from category S84

A	initial encounter
D	subsequent encounter
S	sequela

- ● S84.0 Injury of tibial nerve at lower leg level
  - X ● S84.00 Injury of tibial nerve at lower leg level, unspecified leg
  - X ● S84.01 Injury of tibial nerve at lower leg level, right leg
  - X ● S84.02 Injury of tibial nerve at lower leg level, left leg
- ● S84.1 Injury of peroneal nerve at lower leg level
  - X ● S84.10 Injury of peroneal nerve at lower leg level, unspecified leg
  - X ● S84.11 Injury of peroneal nerve at lower leg level, right leg
  - X ● S84.12 Injury of peroneal nerve at lower leg level, left leg
- ● S84.2 Injury of cutaneous sensory nerve at lower leg level
  - X ● S84.20 Injury of cutaneous sensory nerve at lower leg level, unspecified leg
  - X ● S84.21 Injury of cutaneous sensory nerve at lower leg level, right leg
  - X ● S84.22 Injury of cutaneous sensory nerve at lower leg level, left leg
- ● S84.8 Injury of other nerves at lower leg level
  - ● S84.80 Injury of other nerves at lower leg level
    - ● S84.801 Injury of other nerves at lower leg level, right leg
    - ● S84.802 Injury of other nerves at lower leg level, left leg
    - ● S84.809 Injury of other nerves at lower leg level, unspecified leg

● **S84.9**   Injury of unspecified nerve at lower leg level
   X● **S84.90**   Injury of unspecified nerve at lower leg level, unspecified leg
   X● **S84.91**   Injury of unspecified nerve at lower leg level, right leg
   X● **S84.92**   Injury of unspecified nerve at lower leg level, left leg

● **S85**   Injury of blood vessels at lower leg level
   Code also any associated open wound (S81.-)
   Excludes2   injury of blood vessels at ankle and foot level (S95.-)
   The appropriate 7th character is to be added to each code from category S85

A	initial encounter
D	subsequent encounter
S	sequela

 ● **S85.0**   Injury of popliteal artery
  ● **S85.00**   Unspecified injury of popliteal artery
   ● **S85.001**   Unspecified injury of popliteal artery, right leg
   ● **S85.002**   Unspecified injury of popliteal artery, left leg
   ● **S85.009**   Unspecified injury of popliteal artery, unspecified leg
  ● **S85.01**   Laceration of popliteal artery
   ● **S85.011**   Laceration of popliteal artery, right leg
   ● **S85.012**   Laceration of popliteal artery, left leg
   ● **S85.019**   Laceration of popliteal artery, unspecified leg
  ● **S85.09**   Other specified injury of popliteal artery
   ● **S85.091**   Other specified injury of popliteal artery, right leg
   ● **S85.092**   Other specified injury of popliteal artery, left leg
   ● **S85.099**   Other specified injury of popliteal artery, unspecified leg

 ● **S85.1**   Injury of tibial artery
  ● **S85.10**   Unspecified injury of unspecified tibial artery
    Injury of tibial artery NOS
   ● **S85.101**   Unspecified injury of unspecified tibial artery, right leg
   ● **S85.102**   Unspecified injury of unspecified tibial artery, left leg
   ● **S85.109**   Unspecified injury of unspecified tibial artery, unspecified leg
  ● **S85.11**   Laceration of unspecified tibial artery
   ● **S85.111**   Laceration of unspecified tibial artery, right leg
   ● **S85.112**   Laceration of unspecified tibial artery, left leg
   ● **S85.119**   Laceration of unspecified tibial artery, unspecified leg
  ● **S85.12**   Other specified injury of unspecified tibial artery
   ● **S85.121**   Other specified injury of unspecified tibial artery, right leg
   ● **S85.122**   Other specified injury of unspecified tibial artery, left leg
   ● **S85.129**   Other specified injury of unspecified tibial artery, unspecified leg

 ● **S85.13**   Unspecified injury of anterior tibial artery
  ● **S85.131**   Unspecified injury of anterior tibial artery, right leg
  ● **S85.132**   Unspecified injury of anterior tibial artery, left leg
  ● **S85.139**   Unspecified injury of anterior tibial artery, unspecified leg
 ● **S85.14**   Laceration of anterior tibial artery
  ● **S85.141**   Laceration of anterior tibial artery, right leg
  ● **S85.142**   Laceration of anterior tibial artery, left leg
  ● **S85.149**   Laceration of anterior tibial artery, unspecified leg
 ● **S85.15**   Other specified injury of anterior tibial artery
  ● **S85.151**   Other specified injury of anterior tibial artery, right leg
  ● **S85.152**   Other specified injury of anterior tibial artery, left leg
  ● **S85.159**   Other specified injury of anterior tibial artery, unspecified leg
 ● **S85.16**   Unspecified injury of posterior tibial artery
  ● **S85.161**   Unspecified injury of posterior tibial artery, right leg
  ● **S85.162**   Unspecified injury of posterior tibial artery, left leg
  ● **S85.169**   Unspecified injury of posterior tibial artery, unspecified leg
 ● **S85.17**   Laceration of posterior tibial artery
  ● **S85.171**   Laceration of posterior tibial artery, right leg
  ● **S85.172**   Laceration of posterior tibial artery, left leg
  ● **S85.179**   Laceration of posterior tibial artery, unspecified leg
 ● **S85.18**   Other specified injury of posterior tibial artery
  ● **S85.181**   Other specified injury of posterior tibial artery, right leg
  ● **S85.182**   Other specified injury of posterior tibial artery, left leg
  ● **S85.189**   Other specified injury of posterior tibial artery, unspecified leg
● **S85.2**   Injury of peroneal artery
 ● **S85.20**   Unspecified injury of peroneal artery
  ● **S85.201**   Unspecified injury of peroneal artery, right leg
  ● **S85.202**   Unspecified injury of peroneal artery, left leg
  ● **S85.209**   Unspecified injury of peroneal artery, unspecified leg
 ● **S85.21**   Laceration of peroneal artery
  ● **S85.211**   Laceration of peroneal artery, right leg
  ● **S85.212**   Laceration of peroneal artery, left leg
  ● **S85.219**   Laceration of peroneal artery, unspecified leg
 ● **S85.29**   Other specified injury of peroneal artery
  ● **S85.291**   Other specified injury of peroneal artery, right leg
  ● **S85.292**   Other specified injury of peroneal artery, left leg
  ● **S85.299**   Other specified injury of peroneal artery, unspecified leg

- S85.3   Injury of greater saphenous vein at lower leg level
  - Injury of greater saphenous vein NOS
  - Injury of saphenous vein NOS
  - S85.30   Unspecified injury of greater saphenous vein at lower leg level
    - S85.301   Unspecified injury of greater saphenous vein at lower leg level, right leg
    - S85.302   Unspecified injury of greater saphenous vein at lower leg level, left leg
    - S85.309   Unspecified injury of greater saphenous vein at lower leg level, unspecified leg
  - S85.31   Laceration of greater saphenous vein at lower leg level
    - S85.311   Laceration of greater saphenous vein at lower leg level, right leg
    - S85.312   Laceration of greater saphenous vein at lower leg level, left leg
    - S85.319   Laceration of greater saphenous vein at lower leg level, unspecified leg
  - S85.39   Other specified injury of greater saphenous vein at lower leg level
    - S85.391   Other specified injury of greater saphenous vein at lower leg level, right leg
    - S85.392   Other specified injury of greater saphenous vein at lower leg level, left leg
    - S85.399   Other specified injury of greater saphenous vein at lower leg level, unspecified leg
- S85.4   Injury of lesser saphenous vein at lower leg level
  - S85.40   Unspecified injury of lesser saphenous vein at lower leg level
    - S85.401   Unspecified injury of lesser saphenous vein at lower leg level, right leg
    - S85.402   Unspecified injury of lesser saphenous vein at lower leg level, left leg
    - S85.409   Unspecified injury of lesser saphenous vein at lower leg level, unspecified leg
  - S85.41   Laceration of lesser saphenous vein at lower leg level
    - S85.411   Laceration of lesser saphenous vein at lower leg level, right leg
    - S85.412   Laceration of lesser saphenous vein at lower leg level, left leg
    - S85.419   Laceration of lesser saphenous vein at lower leg level, unspecified leg
  - S85.49   Other specified injury of lesser saphenous vein at lower leg level
    - S85.491   Other specified injury of lesser saphenous vein at lower leg level, right leg
    - S85.492   Other specified injury of lesser saphenous vein at lower leg level, left leg
    - S85.499   Other specified injury of lesser saphenous vein at lower leg level, unspecified leg
- S85.5   Injury of popliteal vein
  - S85.50   Unspecified injury of popliteal vein
    - S85.501   Unspecified injury of popliteal vein, right leg
    - S85.502   Unspecified injury of popliteal vein, left leg
    - S85.509   Unspecified injury of popliteal vein, unspecified leg
  - S85.51   Laceration of popliteal vein
    - S85.511   Laceration of popliteal vein, right leg
    - S85.512   Laceration of popliteal vein, left leg
    - S85.519   Laceration of popliteal vein, unspecified leg
  - S85.59   Other specified injury of popliteal vein
    - S85.591   Other specified injury of popliteal vein, right leg
    - S85.592   Other specified injury of popliteal vein, left leg
    - S85.599   Other specified injury of popliteal vein, unspecified leg
- S85.8   Injury of other blood vessels at lower leg level
  - S85.80   Unspecified injury of other blood vessels at lower leg level
    - S85.801   Unspecified injury of other blood vessels at lower leg level, right leg
    - S85.802   Unspecified injury of other blood vessels at lower leg level, left leg
    - S85.809   Unspecified injury of other blood vessels at lower leg level, unspecified leg
  - S85.81   Laceration of other blood vessels at lower leg level
    - S85.811   Laceration of other blood vessels at lower leg level, right leg
    - S85.812   Laceration of other blood vessels at lower leg level, left leg
    - S85.819   Laceration of other blood vessels at lower leg level, unspecified leg
  - S85.89   Other specified injury of other blood vessels at lower leg level
    - S85.891   Other specified injury of other blood vessels at lower leg level, right leg
    - S85.892   Other specified injury of other blood vessels at lower leg level, left leg
    - S85.899   Other specified injury of other blood vessels at lower leg level, unspecified leg
- S85.9   Injury of unspecified blood vessel at lower leg level
  - S85.90   Unspecified injury of unspecified blood vessel at lower leg level
    - S85.901   Unspecified injury of unspecified blood vessel at lower leg level, right leg
    - S85.902   Unspecified injury of unspecified blood vessel at lower leg level, left leg
    - S85.909   Unspecified injury of unspecified blood vessel at lower leg level, unspecified leg

▶ New   ⇒ Revised   ~~deleted~~ Deleted   Excludes 1   Excludes 2   Includes   Use additional   Code first   Code also   Key words
OGCR Official Guidelines   X Assign placeholder X   ● Use Additional Character(s)   ▶ Manifestation Code   🐍 Hierarchical Condition Category   **Coding Clinic**

- **S85.91** Laceration of unspecified blood vessel at lower leg level
  - **S85.911** Laceration of unspecified blood vessel at lower leg level, right leg
  - **S85.912** Laceration of unspecified blood vessel at lower leg level, left leg
  - **S85.919** Laceration of unspecified blood vessel at lower leg level, unspecified leg
- **S85.99** Other specified injury of unspecified blood vessel at lower leg level
  - **S85.991** Other specified injury of unspecified blood vessel at lower leg level, right leg
  - **S85.992** Other specified injury of unspecified blood vessel at lower leg level, left leg
  - **S85.999** Other specified injury of unspecified blood vessel at lower leg level, unspecified leg

- **S86** Injury of muscle, fascia and tendon at lower leg level

  Code also any associated open wound (S81.-)

  Excludes2   injury of muscle, fascia and tendon at ankle (S96.-)
  injury of patellar ligament (tendon) (S76.1-)
  sprain of joints and ligaments of knee (S83.-)

  The appropriate 7th character is to be added to each code from category S86

A	initial encounter
D	subsequent encounter
S	sequela

  - **S86.0** Injury of Achilles tendon
    - **S86.00** Unspecified injury of Achilles tendon
      - **S86.001** Unspecified injury of right Achilles tendon
      - **S86.002** Unspecified injury of left Achilles tendon
      - **S86.009** Unspecified injury of unspecified Achilles tendon
    - **S86.01** Strain of Achilles tendon
      - **S86.011** Strain of right Achilles tendon
      - **S86.012** Strain of left Achilles tendon
      - **S86.019** Strain of unspecified Achilles tendon
    - **S86.02** Laceration of Achilles tendon
      - **S86.021** Laceration of right Achilles tendon
      - **S86.022** Laceration of left Achilles tendon
      - **S86.029** Laceration of unspecified Achilles tendon
    - **S86.09** Other specified injury of Achilles tendon
      - **S86.091** Other specified injury of right Achilles tendon
      - **S86.092** Other specified injury of left Achilles tendon
      - **S86.099** Other specified injury of unspecified Achilles tendon
  - **S86.1** Injury of other muscle(s) and tendon(s) of posterior muscle group at lower leg level
    - **S86.10** Unspecified injury of other muscle(s) and tendon(s) of posterior muscle group at lower leg level
      - **S86.101** Unspecified injury of other muscle(s) and tendon(s) of posterior muscle group at lower leg level, right leg
      - **S86.102** Unspecified injury of other muscle(s) and tendon(s) of posterior muscle group at lower leg level, left leg
      - **S86.109** Unspecified injury of other muscle(s) and tendon(s) of posterior muscle group at lower leg level, unspecified leg

- **S86.11** Strain of other muscle(s) and tendon(s) of posterior muscle group at lower leg level
  - **S86.111** Strain of other muscle(s) and tendon(s) of posterior muscle group at lower leg level, right leg
  - **S86.112** Strain of other muscle(s) and tendon(s) of posterior muscle group at lower leg level, left leg
  - **S86.119** Strain of other muscle(s) and tendon(s) of posterior muscle group at lower leg level, unspecified leg
- **S86.12** Laceration of other muscle(s) and tendon(s) of posterior muscle group at lower leg level
  - **S86.121** Laceration of other muscle(s) and tendon(s) of posterior muscle group at lower leg level, right leg
  - **S86.122** Laceration of other muscle(s) and tendon(s) of posterior muscle group at lower leg level, left leg
  - **S86.129** Laceration of other muscle(s) and tendon(s) of posterior muscle group at lower leg level, unspecified leg
- **S86.19** Other injury of other muscle(s) and tendon(s) of posterior muscle group at lower leg level
  - **S86.191** Other injury of other muscle(s) and tendon(s) of posterior muscle group at lower leg level, right leg
  - **S86.192** Other injury of other muscle(s) and tendon(s) of posterior muscle group at lower leg level, left leg
  - **S86.199** Other injury of other muscle(s) and tendon(s) of posterior muscle group at lower leg level, unspecified leg
- **S86.2** Injury of muscle(s) and tendon(s) of anterior muscle group at lower leg level
  - **S86.20** Unspecified injury of muscle(s) and tendon(s) of anterior muscle group at lower leg level
    - **S86.201** Unspecified injury of muscle(s) and tendon(s) of anterior muscle group at lower leg level, right leg
    - **S86.202** Unspecified injury of muscle(s) and tendon(s) of anterior muscle group at lower leg level, left leg
    - **S86.209** Unspecified injury of muscle(s) and tendon(s) of anterior muscle group at lower leg level, unspecified leg
  - **S86.21** Strain of muscle(s) and tendon(s) of anterior muscle group at lower leg level
    - **S86.211** Strain of muscle(s) and tendon(s) of anterior muscle group at lower leg level, right leg
    - **S86.212** Strain of muscle(s) and tendon(s) of anterior muscle group at lower leg level, left leg
    - **S86.219** Strain of muscle(s) and tendon(s) of anterior muscle group at lower leg level, unspecified leg
  - **S86.22** Laceration of muscle(s) and tendon(s) of anterior muscle group at lower leg level
    - **S86.221** Laceration of muscle(s) and tendon(s) of anterior muscle group at lower leg level, right leg
    - **S86.222** Laceration of muscle(s) and tendon(s) of anterior muscle group at lower leg level, left leg
    - **S86.229** Laceration of muscle(s) and tendon(s) of anterior muscle group at lower leg level, unspecified leg

● S86.29   Other injury of muscle(s) and tendon(s) of anterior muscle group at lower leg level

    ● S86.291   Other injury of muscle(s) and tendon(s) of anterior muscle group at lower leg level, right leg

    ● S86.292   Other injury of muscle(s) and tendon(s) of anterior muscle group at lower leg level, left leg

    ● S86.299   Other injury of muscle(s) and tendon(s) of anterior muscle group at lower leg level, unspecified leg

● S86.3   Injury of muscle(s) and tendon(s) of peroneal muscle group at lower leg level

    ● S86.30   Unspecified injury of muscle(s) and tendon(s) of peroneal muscle group at lower leg level

      ● S86.301   Unspecified injury of muscle(s) and tendon(s) of peroneal muscle group at lower leg level, right leg

      ● S86.302   Unspecified injury of muscle(s) and tendon(s) of peroneal muscle group at lower leg level, left leg

      ● S86.309   Unspecified injury of muscle(s) and tendon(s) of peroneal muscle group at lower leg level, unspecified leg

    ● S86.31   Strain of muscle(s) and tendon(s) of peroneal muscle group at lower leg level

      ● S86.311   Strain of muscle(s) and tendon(s) of peroneal muscle group at lower leg level, right leg

      ● S86.312   Strain of muscle(s) and tendon(s) of peroneal muscle group at lower leg level, left leg

      ● S86.319   Strain of muscle(s) and tendon(s) of peroneal muscle group at lower leg level, unspecified leg

    ● S86.32   Laceration of muscle(s) and tendon(s) of peroneal muscle group at lower leg level

      ● S86.321   Laceration of muscle(s) and tendon(s) of peroneal muscle group at lower leg level, right leg

      ● S86.322   Laceration of muscle(s) and tendon(s) of peroneal muscle group at lower leg level, left leg

      ● S86.329   Laceration of muscle(s) and tendon(s) of peroneal muscle group at lower leg level, unspecified leg

    ● S86.39   Other injury of muscle(s) and tendon(s) of peroneal muscle group at lower leg level

      ● S86.391   Other injury of muscle(s) and tendon(s) of peroneal muscle group at lower leg level, right leg

      ● S86.392   Other injury of muscle(s) and tendon(s) of peroneal muscle group at lower leg level, left leg

      ● S86.399   Other injury of muscle(s) and tendon(s) of peroneal muscle group at lower leg level, unspecified leg

● S86.8   Injury of other muscles and tendons at lower leg level

    ● S86.80   Unspecified injury of other muscles and tendons at lower leg level

      ● S86.801   Unspecified injury of other muscle(s) and tendon(s) at lower leg level, right leg

      ● S86.802   Unspecified injury of other muscle(s) and tendon(s) at lower leg level, left leg

      ● S86.809   Unspecified injury of other muscle(s) and tendon(s) at lower leg level, unspecified leg

● S86.81   Strain of other muscles and tendons at lower leg level

    ● S86.811   Strain of other muscle(s) and tendon(s) at lower leg level, right leg

    ● S86.812   Strain of other muscle(s) and tendon(s) at lower leg level, left leg

    ● S86.819   Strain of other muscle(s) and tendon(s) at lower leg level, unspecified leg

● S86.82   Laceration of other muscles and tendons at lower leg level

    ● S86.821   Laceration of other muscle(s) and tendon(s) at lower leg level, right leg

    ● S86.822   Laceration of other muscle(s) and tendon(s) at lower leg level, left leg

    ● S86.829   Laceration of other muscle(s) and tendon(s) at lower leg level, unspecified leg

● S86.89   Other injury of other muscles and tendons at lower leg level

    ● S86.891   Other injury of other muscle(s) and tendon(s) at lower leg level, right leg

    ● S86.892   Other injury of other muscle(s) and tendon(s) at lower leg level, left leg

    ● S86.899   Other injury of other muscle(s) and tendon(s) at lower leg level, unspecified leg

● S86.9   Injury of unspecified muscle and tendon at lower leg level

    ● S86.90   Unspecified injury of unspecified muscle and tendon at lower leg level

      ● S86.901   Unspecified injury of unspecified muscle(s) and tendon(s) at lower leg level, right leg

      ● S86.902   Unspecified injury of unspecified muscle(s) and tendon(s) at lower leg level, left leg

      ● S86.909   Unspecified injury of unspecified muscle(s) and tendon(s) at lower leg level, unspecified leg

    ● S86.91   Strain of unspecified muscle and tendon at lower leg level

      ● S86.911   Strain of unspecified muscle(s) and tendon(s) at lower leg level, right leg

      ● S86.912   Strain of unspecified muscle(s) and tendon(s) at lower leg level, left leg

      ● S86.919   Strain of unspecified muscle(s) and tendon(s) at lower leg level, unspecified leg

    ● S86.92   Laceration of unspecified muscle and tendon at lower leg level

      ● S86.921   Laceration of unspecified muscle(s) and tendon(s) at lower leg level, right leg

      ● S86.922   Laceration of unspecified muscle(s) and tendon(s) at lower leg level, left leg

      ● S86.929   Laceration of unspecified muscle(s) and tendon(s) at lower leg level, unspecified leg

▶ New   ⫸ Revised   ~~deleted~~ Deleted   Excludes 1   Excludes 2   Includes   Use additional   Code first   Code also   Key words

OGCR Official Guidelines   X Assign placeholder X   ● Use Additional Character(s)   ▮ Manifestation Code   🝖 Hierarchical Condition Category   Coding Clinic

● S86.99   Other injury of unspecified muscle and tendon at lower leg level
   ● S86.991   Other injury of unspecified muscle(s) and tendon(s) at lower leg level, right leg
   ● S86.992   Other injury of unspecified muscle(s) and tendon(s) at lower leg level, left leg
   ● S86.999   Other injury of unspecified muscle(s) and tendon(s) at lower leg level, unspecified leg

● S87   Crushing injury of lower leg
   Use additional code(s) for all associated injuries
   Excludes2   crushing injury of ankle and foot (S97.-)
   The appropriate 7th character is to be added to each code from category S87

A	initial encounter
D	subsequent encounter
S	sequela

  ● S87.0   Crushing injury of knee
   X ● S87.00   Crushing injury of unspecified knee
   X ● S87.01   Crushing injury of right knee
   X ● S87.02   Crushing injury of left knee
  ● S87.8   Crushing injury of lower leg
   X ● S87.80   Crushing injury of unspecified lower leg
   X ● S87.81   Crushing injury of right lower leg
   X ● S87.82   Crushing injury of left lower leg

● S88   Traumatic amputation of lower leg
   An amputation not identified as partial or complete should be coded to complete
   Excludes1   traumatic amputation of ankle and foot (S98.-)
   The appropriate 7th character is to be added to each code from category S88

A	initial encounter
D	subsequent encounter
S	sequela

  ● S88.0   Traumatic amputation at knee level
   ● S88.01   Complete traumatic amputation at knee level
     ● S88.011   Complete traumatic amputation at knee level, right lower leg A, D, S 🔾
     ● S88.012   Complete traumatic amputation at knee level, left lower leg A, D, S 🔾
     ● S88.019   Complete traumatic amputation at knee level, unspecified lower leg A, D, S 🔾
   ● S88.02   Partial traumatic amputation at knee level
     ● S88.021   Partial traumatic amputation at knee level, right lower leg A, D, S 🔾
     ● S88.022   Partial traumatic amputation at knee level, left lower leg A, D, S 🔾
     ● S88.029   Partial traumatic amputation at knee level, unspecified lower leg A, D, S 🔾
  ● S88.1   Traumatic amputation at level between knee and ankle
   ● S88.11   Complete traumatic amputation at level between knee and ankle
     ● S88.111   Complete traumatic amputation at level between knee and ankle, right lower leg A, D, S 🔾
     ● S88.112   Complete traumatic amputation at level between knee and ankle, left lower leg A, D, S 🔾
     ● S88.119   Complete traumatic amputation at level between knee and ankle, unspecified lower leg A, D, S 🔾

● S88.12   Partial traumatic amputation at level between knee and ankle
   ● S88.121   Partial traumatic amputation at level between knee and ankle, right lower leg A, D, S 🔾
   ● S88.122   Partial traumatic amputation at level between knee and ankle, left lower leg A, D, S 🔾
   ● S88.129   Partial traumatic amputation at level between knee and ankle, unspecified lower leg A, D, S 🔾
● S88.9   Traumatic amputation of lower leg, level unspecified
  ● S88.91   Complete traumatic amputation of lower leg, level unspecified
   ● S88.911   Complete traumatic amputation of right lower leg, level unspecified A, D, S 🔾
   ● S88.912   Complete traumatic amputation of left lower leg, level unspecified A, D, S 🔾
   ● S88.919   Complete traumatic amputation of unspecified lower leg, level unspecified A, D, S 🔾
  ● S88.92   Partial traumatic amputation of lower leg, level unspecified
   ● S88.921   Partial traumatic amputation of right lower leg, level unspecified A, D, S 🔾
   ● S88.922   Partial traumatic amputation of left lower leg, level unspecified A, D, S 🔾
   ● S88.929   Partial traumatic amputation of unspecified lower leg, level unspecified A, D, S 🔾

● S89   Other and unspecified injuries of lower leg
   Note: A fracture not indicated as open or closed should be coded to closed
   Excludes2   other and unspecified injuries of ankle and foot (S99.-)
   The appropriate 7th character is to be added to each code from subcategories S89.0, S89.1, S89.2, and S89.3

A	initial encounter for closed fracture
D	subsequent encounter for fracture with routine healing
G	subsequent encounter for fracture with delayed healing
K	subsequent encounter for fracture with nonunion
P	subsequent encounter for fracture with malunion
S	sequela

  ● S89.0   Physeal fracture of upper end of tibia
   ● S89.00   Unspecified physeal fracture of upper end of tibia
     ● S89.001   Unspecified physeal fracture of upper end of right tibia
     ● S89.002   Unspecified physeal fracture of upper end of left tibia
     ● S89.009   Unspecified physeal fracture of upper end of unspecified tibia
   ● S89.01   Salter-Harris Type I physeal fracture of upper end of tibia
     ● S89.011   Salter-Harris Type I physeal fracture of upper end of right tibia
     ● S89.012   Salter-Harris Type I physeal fracture of upper end of left tibia
     ● S89.019   Salter-Harris Type I physeal fracture of upper end of unspecified tibia

CHAPTER 19 (S00–T88)

● S89.02   Salter-Harris Type II physeal fracture of upper end of tibia
- ● S89.021   Salter-Harris Type II physeal fracture of upper end of right tibia
- ● S89.022   Salter-Harris Type II physeal fracture of upper end of left tibia
- ● S89.029   Salter-Harris Type II physeal fracture of upper end of unspecified tibia

● S89.03   Salter-Harris Type III physeal fracture of upper end of tibia
- ● S89.031   Salter-Harris Type III physeal fracture of upper end of right tibia
- ● S89.032   Salter-Harris Type III physeal fracture of upper end of left tibia
- ● S89.039   Salter-Harris Type III physeal fracture of upper end of unspecified tibia

● S89.04   Salter-Harris Type IV physeal fracture of upper end of tibia
- ● S89.041   Salter-Harris Type IV physeal fracture of upper end of right tibia
- ● S89.042   Salter-Harris Type IV physeal fracture of upper end of left tibia
- ● S89.049   Salter-Harris Type IV physeal fracture of upper end of unspecified tibia

● S89.09   Other physeal fracture of upper end of tibia
- ● S89.091   Other physeal fracture of upper end of right tibia
- ● S89.092   Other physeal fracture of upper end of left tibia
- ● S89.099   Other physeal fracture of upper end of unspecified tibia

● S89.1   Physeal fracture of lower end of tibia

● S89.10   Unspecified physeal fracture of lower end of tibia
- ● S89.101   Unspecified physeal fracture of lower end of right tibia
- ● S89.102   Unspecified physeal fracture of lower end of left tibia
- ● S89.109   Unspecified physeal fracture of lower end of unspecified tibia

● S89.11   Salter-Harris Type I physeal fracture of lower end of tibia
- ● S89.111   Salter-Harris Type I physeal fracture of lower end of right tibia
- ● S89.112   Salter-Harris Type I physeal fracture of lower end of left tibia
- ● S89.119   Salter-Harris Type I physeal fracture of lower end of unspecified tibia

● S89.12   Salter-Harris Type II physeal fracture of lower end of tibia
- ● S89.121   Salter-Harris Type II physeal fracture of lower end of right tibia
- ● S89.122   Salter-Harris Type II physeal fracture of lower end of left tibia
- ● S89.129   Salter-Harris Type II physeal fracture of lower end of unspecified tibia

● S89.13   Salter-Harris Type III physeal fracture of lower end of tibia

     Excludes1   fracture of medial malleolus (adult) (S82.5-)

- ● S89.131   Salter-Harris Type III physeal fracture of lower end of right tibia
- ● S89.132   Salter-Harris Type III physeal fracture of lower end of left tibia
- ● S89.139   Salter-Harris Type III physeal fracture of lower end of unspecified tibia

● S89.14   Salter-Harris Type IV physeal fracture of lower end of tibia

     Excludes1   fracture of medial malleolus (adult) (S82.5-)

- ● S89.141   Salter-Harris Type IV physeal fracture of lower end of right tibia
- ● S89.142   Salter-Harris Type IV physeal fracture of lower end of left tibia
- ● S89.149   Salter-Harris Type IV physeal fracture of lower end of unspecified tibia

● S89.19   Other physeal fracture of lower end of tibia
- ● S89.191   Other physeal fracture of lower end of right tibia
- ● S89.192   Other physeal fracture of lower end of left tibia
- ● S89.199   Other physeal fracture of lower end of unspecified tibia

● S89.2   Physeal fracture of upper end of fibula

● S89.20   Unspecified physeal fracture of upper end of fibula
- ● S89.201   Unspecified physeal fracture of upper end of right fibula
- ● S89.202   Unspecified physeal fracture of upper end of left fibula
- ● S89.209   Unspecified physeal fracture of upper end of unspecified fibula

● S89.21   Salter-Harris Type I physeal fracture of upper end of fibula
- ● S89.211   Salter-Harris Type I physeal fracture of upper end of right fibula
- ● S89.212   Salter-Harris Type I physeal fracture of upper end of left fibula
- ● S89.219   Salter-Harris Type I physeal fracture of upper end of unspecified fibula

● S89.22   Salter-Harris Type II physeal fracture of upper end of fibula
- ● S89.221   Salter-Harris Type II physeal fracture of upper end of right fibula
- ● S89.222   Salter-Harris Type II physeal fracture of upper end of left fibula
- ● S89.229   Salter-Harris Type II physeal fracture of upper end of unspecified fibula

● S89.29   Other physeal fracture of upper end of fibula
- ● S89.291   Other physeal fracture of upper end of right fibula
- ● S89.292   Other physeal fracture of upper end of left fibula
- ● S89.299   Other physeal fracture of upper end of unspecified fibula

● S89.3   Physeal fracture of lower end of fibula

● S89.30   Unspecified physeal fracture of lower end of fibula
- ● S89.301   Unspecified physeal fracture of lower end of right fibula
- ● S89.302   Unspecified physeal fracture of lower end of left fibula
- ● S89.309   Unspecified physeal fracture of lower end of unspecified fibula

● S89.31   Salter-Harris Type I physeal fracture of lower end of fibula
- ● S89.311   Salter-Harris Type I physeal fracture of lower end of right fibula
- ● S89.312   Salter-Harris Type I physeal fracture of lower end of left fibula
- ● S89.319   Salter-Harris Type I physeal fracture of lower end of unspecified fibula

● S89.32   Salter-Harris Type II physeal fracture of lower end of fibula

     ● S89.321   Salter-Harris Type II physeal fracture of lower end of right fibula

     ● S89.322   Salter-Harris Type II physeal fracture of lower end of left fibula

     ● S89.329   Salter-Harris Type II physeal fracture of lower end of unspecified fibula

● S89.39   Other physeal fracture of lower end of fibula

     ● S89.391   Other physeal fracture of lower end of right fibula

     ● S89.392   Other physeal fracture of lower end of left fibula

     ● S89.399   Other physeal fracture of lower end of unspecified fibula

● S89.8   Other specified injuries of lower leg

     The appropriate 7th character is to be added to each code in subcategory S89.8

A	initial encounter
D	subsequent encounter
S	sequela

X● S89.80   Other specified injuries of unspecified lower leg

X● S89.81   Other specified injuries of right lower leg

X● S89.82   Other specified injuries of left lower leg

● S89.9   Unspecified injury of lower leg

     The appropriate 7th character is to be added to each code in subcategory S89.9

A	initial encounter
D	subsequent encounter
S	sequela

X● S89.90   Unspecified injury of unspecified lower leg

X● S89.91   Unspecified injury of right lower leg

X● S89.92   Unspecified injury of left lower leg

INJURIES TO THE ANKLE AND FOOT (S90-S99)

Excludes2   burns and corrosions (T20-T32)
             fracture of ankle and malleolus (S82.-)
             frostbite (T33-T34)
             insect bite or sting, venomous (T63.4)

● S90   Superficial injury of ankle, foot and toes

     The appropriate 7th character is to be added to each code from category S90

A	initial encounter
D	subsequent encounter
S	sequela

● S90.0   Contusion of ankle

X● S90.00   Contusion of unspecified ankle

X● S90.01   Contusion of right ankle

X● S90.02   Contusion of left ankle

● S90.1   Contusion of toe without damage to nail

     ● S90.11   Contusion of great toe without damage to nail

         ● S90.111   Contusion of right great toe without damage to nail

         ● S90.112   Contusion of left great toe without damage to nail

         ● S90.119   Contusion of unspecified great toe without damage to nail

     ● S90.12   Contusion of lesser toe without damage to nail

         ● S90.121   Contusion of right lesser toe(s) without damage to nail

         ● S90.122   Contusion of left lesser toe(s) without damage to nail

         ● S90.129   Contusion of unspecified lesser toe(s) without damage to nail
             Contusion of toe NOS

● S90.2   Contusion of toe with damage to nail

     ● S90.21   Contusion of great toe with damage to nail

         ● S90.211   Contusion of right great toe with damage to nail

         ● S90.212   Contusion of left great toe with damage to nail

         ● S90.219   Contusion of unspecified great toe with damage to nail

     ● S90.22   Contusion of lesser toe with damage to nail

         ● S90.221   Contusion of right lesser toe(s) with damage to nail

         ● S90.222   Contusion of left lesser toe(s) with damage to nail

         ● S90.229   Contusion of unspecified lesser toe(s) with damage to nail

● S90.3   Contusion of foot

     Excludes2   contusion of toes (S90.1-, S90.2-)

X● S90.30   Contusion of unspecified foot
         Contusion of foot NOS

X● S90.31   Contusion of right foot

X● S90.32   Contusion of left foot

● S90.4   Other superficial injuries of toe

     ● S90.41   Abrasion of toe

         ● S90.411   Abrasion, right great toe

         ● S90.412   Abrasion, left great toe

         ● S90.413   Abrasion, unspecified great toe

         ● S90.414   Abrasion, right lesser toe(s)

         ● S90.415   Abrasion, left lesser toe(s)

         ● S90.416   Abrasion, unspecified lesser toe(s)

     ● S90.42   Blister (nonthermal) of toe

         ● S90.421   Blister (nonthermal), right great toe

         ● S90.422   Blister (nonthermal), left great toe

         ● S90.423   Blister (nonthermal), unspecified great toe

         ● S90.424   Blister (nonthermal), right lesser toe(s)

         ● S90.425   Blister (nonthermal), left lesser toe(s)

         ● S90.426   Blister (nonthermal), unspecified lesser toe(s)

     ● S90.44   External constriction of toe
         Hair tourniquet syndrome of toe

         ● S90.441   External constriction, right great toe

         ● S90.442   External constriction, left great toe

         ● S90.443   External constriction, unspecified great toe

         ● S90.444   External constriction, right lesser toe(s)

         ● S90.445   External constriction, left lesser toe(s)

         ● S90.446   External constriction, unspecified lesser toe(s)

     ● S90.45   Superficial foreign body of toe
         Splinter in the toe

         ● S90.451   Superficial foreign body, right great toe

         ● S90.452   Superficial foreign body, left great toe

● S90.453   Superficial foreign body, unspecified great toe

● S90.454   Superficial foreign body, right lesser toe(s)

● S90.455   Superficial foreign body, left lesser toe(s)

● S90.456   Superficial foreign body, unspecified lesser toe(s)

● S90.46   Insect bite (nonvenomous) of toe

  ● S90.461   Insect bite (nonvenomous), right great toe

  ● S90.462   Insect bite (nonvenomous), left great toe

  ● S90.463   Insect bite (nonvenomous), unspecified great toe

  ● S90.464   Insect bite (nonvenomous), right lesser toe(s)

  ● S90.465   Insect bite (nonvenomous), left lesser toe(s)

  ● S90.466   Insect bite (nonvenomous), unspecified lesser toe(s)

● S90.47   Other superficial bite of toe

    Excludes1   open bite of toe (S91.15-, S91.25-)

  ● S90.471   Other superficial bite of right great toe

  ● S90.472   Other superficial bite of left great toe

  ● S90.473   Other superficial bite of unspecified great toe

  ● S90.474   Other superficial bite of right lesser toe(s)

  ● S90.475   Other superficial bite of left lesser toe(s)

  ● S90.476   Other superficial bite of unspecified lesser toe(s)

● S90.5   Other superficial injuries of ankle

 ● S90.51   Abrasion of ankle

  ● S90.511   Abrasion, right ankle

  ● S90.512   Abrasion, left ankle

  ● S90.519   Abrasion, unspecified ankle

 ● S90.52   Blister (nonthermal) of ankle

  ● S90.521   Blister (nonthermal), right ankle

  ● S90.522   Blister (nonthermal), left ankle

  ● S90.529   Blister (nonthermal), unspecified ankle

 ● S90.54   External constriction of ankle

  ● S90.541   External constriction, right ankle

  ● S90.542   External constriction, left ankle

  ● S90.549   External constriction, unspecified ankle

 ● S90.55   Superficial foreign body of ankle

  Splinter in the ankle

  ● S90.551   Superficial foreign body, right ankle

  ● S90.552   Superficial foreign body, left ankle

  ● S90.559   Superficial foreign body, unspecified ankle

 ● S90.56   Insect bite (nonvenomous) of ankle

  ● S90.561   Insect bite (nonvenomous), right ankle

  ● S90.562   Insect bite (nonvenomous), left ankle

  ● S90.569   Insect bite (nonvenomous), unspecified ankle

● S90.57   Other superficial bite of ankle

    Excludes1   open bite of ankle (S91.05-)

  ● S90.571   Other superficial bite of ankle, right ankle

  ● S90.572   Other superficial bite of ankle, left ankle

  ● S90.579   Other superficial bite of ankle, unspecified ankle

● S90.8   Other superficial injuries of foot

 ● S90.81   Abrasion of foot

  ● S90.811   Abrasion, right foot

  ● S90.812   Abrasion, left foot

  ● S90.819   Abrasion, unspecified foot

 ● S90.82   Blister (nonthermal) of foot

  ● S90.821   Blister (nonthermal), right foot

  ● S90.822   Blister (nonthermal), left foot

  ● S90.829   Blister (nonthermal), unspecified foot

 ● S90.84   External constriction of foot

  ● S90.841   External constriction, right foot

  ● S90.842   External constriction, left foot

  ● S90.849   External constriction, unspecified foot

 ● S90.85   Superficial foreign body of foot

  Splinter in the foot

  ● S90.851   Superficial foreign body, right foot

  ● S90.852   Superficial foreign body, left foot

  ● S90.859   Superficial foreign body, unspecified foot

 ● S90.86   Insect bite (nonvenomous) of foot

  ● S90.861   Insect bite (nonvenomous), right foot

  ● S90.862   Insect bite (nonvenomous), left foot

  ● S90.869   Insect bite (nonvenomous), unspecified foot

 ● S90.87   Other superficial bite of foot

    Excludes1   open bite of foot (S91.35-)

  ● S90.871   Other superficial bite of right foot

  ● S90.872   Other superficial bite of left foot

  ● S90.879   Other superficial bite of unspecified foot

● S90.9   Unspecified superficial injury of ankle, foot and toe

 ● S90.91   Unspecified superficial injury of ankle

  ● S90.911   Unspecified superficial injury of right ankle

  ● S90.912   Unspecified superficial injury of left ankle

  ● S90.919   Unspecified superficial injury of unspecified ankle

 ● S90.92   Unspecified superficial injury of foot

  ● S90.921   Unspecified superficial injury of right foot

  ● S90.922   Unspecified superficial injury of left foot

  ● S90.929   Unspecified superficial injury of unspecified foot

 S90.93   Unspecified superficial injury of toes

  ● S90.931   Unspecified superficial injury of right great toe

  ● S90.932   Unspecified superficial injury of left great toe

  ● S90.933   Unspecified superficial injury of unspecified great toe

  ● S90.934   Unspecified superficial injury of right lesser toe(s)

  ● S90.935   Unspecified superficial injury of left lesser toe(s)

  ● S90.936   Unspecified superficial injury of unspecified lesser toe(s)

▶ New   ⇒ Revised   ~~deleted~~ Deleted   Excludes 1   Excludes 2   Includes   Use additional   Code first   Code also   Key words

OGCR Official Guidelines   X Assign placeholder X   ● Use Additional Character(s)   ▶ Manifestation Code   🝙 Hierarchical Condition Category   **Coding Clinic**

● S91   **Open wound of ankle, foot and toes**

Code also any associated wound infection

Excludes1   open fracture of ankle, foot and toes (S92.-with 7th character B)

traumatic amputation of ankle and foot (S98.-)

The appropriate 7th character is to be added to each code from category S91

A	initial encounter
D	subsequent encounter
S	sequela

● S91.0   **Open wound of ankle**

   ● S91.00   **Unspecified** open wound of ankle

     ● S91.001   Unspecified open wound, **right ankle**

     ● S91.002   Unspecified open wound, **left ankle**

     ● S91.009   Unspecified open wound, **unspecified ankle**

   ● S91.01   **Laceration without foreign body of ankle**

     ● S91.011   Laceration without foreign body, **right ankle**

     ● S91.012   Laceration without foreign body, **left ankle**

         Coding Clinic: 2021, Q1, P8

     ● S91.019   Laceration without foreign body, **unspecified ankle**

   ● S91.02   **Laceration with foreign body of ankle**

     ● S91.021   Laceration with foreign body, **right ankle**

     ● S91.022   Laceration with foreign body, **left ankle**

     ● S91.029   Laceration with foreign body, **unspecified ankle**

   ● S91.03   **Puncture wound without foreign body of ankle**

     ● S91.031   Puncture wound without foreign body, **right ankle**

     ● S91.032   Puncture wound without foreign body, **left ankle**

     ● S91.039   Puncture wound without foreign body, **unspecified ankle**

   ● S91.04   **Puncture wound with foreign body of ankle**

     ● S91.041   Puncture wound with foreign body, **right ankle**

     ● S91.042   Puncture wound with foreign body, **left ankle**

     ● S91.049   Puncture wound with foreign body, **unspecified ankle**

   ● S91.05   **Open bite of ankle**

       Excludes1   superficial bite of ankle (S90.56-, S90.57-)

     ● S91.051   Open bite, **right ankle**

     ● S91.052   Open bite, **left ankle**

     ● S91.059   Open bite, **unspecified ankle**

● S91.1   **Open wound of toe without damage to nail**

   ● S91.10   **Unspecified** open wound of toe without damage to nail

     ● S91.101   Unspecified open wound of **right great** toe without damage to nail

     ● S91.102   Unspecified open wound of **left great** toe without damage to nail

     ● S91.103   Unspecified open wound of **unspecified great** toe without damage to nail

     ● S91.104   Unspecified open wound of **right lesser** toe(s) without damage to nail

     ● S91.105   Unspecified open wound of **left lesser** toe(s) without damage to nail

     ● S91.106   Unspecified open wound of **unspecified lesser** toe(s) without damage to nail

     ● S91.109   Unspecified open wound of **unspecified toe**(s) without damage to nail

   ● S91.11   **Laceration without foreign body** of toe without damage to nail

     ● S91.111   Laceration without foreign body of **right great** toe without damage to nail

     ● S91.112   Laceration without foreign body of **left great** toe without damage to nail

     ● S91.113   Laceration without foreign body of **unspecified great** toe without damage to nail

     ● S91.114   Laceration without foreign body of **right lesser** toe(s) without damage to nail

     ● S91.115   Laceration without foreign body of **left lesser** toe(s) without damage to nail

     ● S91.116   Laceration without foreign body of **unspecified lesser** toe(s) without damage to nail

     ● S91.119   Laceration without foreign body of **unspecified toe** without damage to nail

   ● S91.12   **Laceration with foreign body** of toe without damage to nail

     ● S91.121   Laceration with foreign body of **right great** toe without damage to nail

     ● S91.122   Laceration with foreign body of **left great** toe without damage to nail

     ● S91.123   Laceration with foreign body of **unspecified great** toe without damage to nail

     ● S91.124   Laceration with foreign body of **right lesser** toe(s) without damage to nail

     ● S91.125   Laceration with foreign body of **left lesser** toe(s) without damage to nail

     ● S91.126   Laceration with foreign body of **unspecified lesser** toe(s) without damage to nail

     ● S91.129   Laceration with foreign body of **unspecified toe**(s) without damage to nail

   ● S91.13   **Puncture wound without foreign body** of toe without damage to nail

     ● S91.131   Puncture wound without foreign body of **right great** toe without damage to nail

     ● S91.132   Puncture wound without foreign body of **left great** toe without damage to nail

     ● S91.133   Puncture wound without foreign body of **unspecified great** toe without damage to nail

     ● S91.134   Puncture wound without foreign body of **right lesser** toe(s) without damage to nail

     ● S91.135   Puncture wound without foreign body of **left lesser** toe(s) without damage to nail

     ● S91.136   Puncture wound without foreign body of **unspecified lesser** toe(s) without damage to nail

     ● S91.139   Puncture wound without foreign body of **unspecified toe**(s) without damage to nail

● **S91.14**   **Puncture wound with foreign body** of toe without damage to nail

- ● S91.141   Puncture wound with foreign body of right great toe without damage to nail
- ● S91.142   Puncture wound with foreign body of left great toe without damage to nail
- ● S91.143   Puncture wound with foreign body of unspecified great toe without damage to nail
- ● S91.144   Puncture wound with foreign body of right lesser toe(s) without damage to nail
- ● S91.145   Puncture wound with foreign body of left lesser toe(s) without damage to nail
- ● S91.146   Puncture wound with foreign body of unspecified lesser toe(s) without damage to nail
- ● S91.149   Puncture wound with foreign body of unspecified toe(s) without damage to nail

● **S91.15**   **Open bite of toe** without damage to nail
    Bite of toe NOS

> **Excludes1**   superficial bite of toe (S90.46-, S90.47-)

- ● S91.151   Open bite of right great toe without damage to nail
- ● S91.152   Open bite of left great toe without damage to nail
- ● S91.153   Open bite of unspecified great toe without damage to nail
- ● S91.154   Open bite of right lesser toe(s) without damage to nail
- ● S91.155   Open bite of left lesser toe(s) without damage to nail
- ● S91.156   Open bite of unspecified lesser toe(s) without damage to nail
- ● S91.159   Open bite of unspecified toe(s) without damage to nail

● **S91.2**   **Open wound of toe with damage to nail**

- ● **S91.20**   Unspecified open wound of toe with damage to nail
  - ● S91.201   Unspecified open wound of right great toe with damage to nail
  - ● S91.202   Unspecified open wound of left great toe with damage to nail
  - ● S91.203   Unspecified open wound of unspecified great toe with damage to nail
  - ● S91.204   Unspecified open wound of right lesser toe(s) with damage to nail
  - ● S91.205   Unspecified open wound of left lesser toe(s) with damage to nail
  - ● S91.206   Unspecified open wound of unspecified lesser toe(s) with damage to nail
  - ● S91.209   Unspecified open wound of unspecified toe(s) with damage to nail
- ● **S91.21**   Laceration without foreign body of toe with damage to nail
  - ● S91.211   Laceration without foreign body of right great toe with damage to nail
  - ● S91.212   Laceration without foreign body of left great toe with damage to nail
  - ● S91.213   Laceration without foreign body of unspecified great toe with damage to nail
  - ● S91.214   Laceration without foreign body of right lesser toe(s) with damage to nail
  - ● S91.215   Laceration without foreign body of left lesser toe(s) with damage to nail

- ● S91.216   Laceration without foreign body of unspecified lesser toe(s) with damage to nail
- ● S91.219   Laceration without foreign body of unspecified toe(s) with damage to nail

● **S91.22**   **Laceration with foreign body** of toe with damage to nail

- ● S91.221   Laceration with foreign body of right great toe with damage to nail
- ● S91.222   Laceration with foreign body of left great toe with damage to nail
- ● S91.223   Laceration with foreign body of unspecified great toe with damage to nail
- ● S91.224   Laceration with foreign body of right lesser toe(s) with damage to nail
- ● S91.225   Laceration with foreign body of left lesser toe(s) with damage to nail
- ● S91.226   Laceration with foreign body of unspecified lesser toe(s) with damage to nail
- ● S91.229   Laceration with foreign body of unspecified toe(s) with damage to nail

● **S91.23**   **Puncture wound without foreign body** of toe with damage to nail

- ● S91.231   Puncture wound without foreign body of right great toe with damage to nail
- ● S91.232   Puncture wound without foreign body of left great toe with damage to nail
- ● S91.233   Puncture wound without foreign body of unspecified great toe with damage to nail
- ● S91.234   Puncture wound without foreign body of right lesser toe(s) with damage to nail
- ● S91.235   Puncture wound without foreign body of left lesser toe(s) with damage to nail
- ● S91.236   Puncture wound without foreign body of unspecified lesser toe(s) with damage to nail
- ● S91.239   Puncture wound without foreign body of unspecified toe(s) with damage to nail

● **S91.24**   **Puncture wound with foreign body** of toe with damage to nail

- ● S91.241   Puncture wound with foreign body of right great toe with damage to nail
- ● S91.242   Puncture wound with foreign body of left great toe with damage to nail
- ● S91.243   Puncture wound with foreign body of unspecified great toe with damage to nail
- ● S91.244   Puncture wound with foreign body of right lesser toe(s) with damage to nail
- ● S91.245   Puncture wound with foreign body of left lesser toe(s) with damage to nail
- ● S91.246   Puncture wound with foreign body of unspecified lesser toe(s) with damage to nail
- ● S91.249   Puncture wound with foreign body of unspecified toe(s) with damage to nail

● **S91.25**   **Open bite of toe** with damage to nail
    Bite of toe with damage to nail NOS

> **Excludes1**   superficial bite of toe (S90.46-, S90.47-)

- ● S91.251   Open bite of right great toe with damage to nail
- ● S91.252   Open bite of left great toe with damage to nail

- S91.253   Open bite of unspecified great toe with damage to nail
- S91.254   Open bite of right lesser toe(s) with damage to nail
- S91.255   Open bite of left lesser toe(s) with damage to nail
- S91.256   Open bite of unspecified lesser toe(s) with damage to nail
- S91.259   Open bite of unspecified toe(s) with damage to nail

- S91.3   **Open wound of foot**
  - S91.30   Unspecified open wound of foot
    - S91.301   Unspecified open wound, right foot
    - S91.302   Unspecified open wound, left foot
    - S91.309   Unspecified open wound, unspecified foot
  - S91.31   Laceration without foreign body of foot
    - S91.311   Laceration without foreign body, right foot
    - S91.312   Laceration without foreign body, left foot
    - S91.319   Laceration without foreign body, unspecified foot
  - S91.32   Laceration with foreign body of foot
    - S91.321   Laceration with foreign body, right foot
    - S91.322   Laceration with foreign body, left foot
    - S91.329   Laceration with foreign body, unspecified foot
  - S91.33   Puncture wound without foreign body of foot
    - S91.331   Puncture wound without foreign body, right foot
    - S91.332   Puncture wound without foreign body, left foot
    - S91.339   Puncture wound without foreign body, unspecified foot
  - S91.34   Puncture wound with foreign body of foot
    - S91.341   Puncture wound with foreign body, right foot
    - S91.342   Puncture wound with foreign body, left foot
    - S91.349   Puncture wound with foreign body, unspecified foot
  - S91.35   Open bite of foot
    - **Excludes1**   superficial bite of foot (S90.86-, S90.87-)
    - S91.351   Open bite, right foot
    - S91.352   Open bite, left foot
    - S91.359   Open bite, unspecified foot

- S92   **Fracture of foot and toe, except ankle**
  - **Note:** A fracture not indicated as displaced or nondisplaced should be coded to displaced

    A fracture not indicated as open or closed should be coded to closed

    ~~**Excludes1**   traumatic amputation of ankle and foot (S98.-)~~

    Excludes2   fracture of ankle (S82.-)

    fracture of malleolus (S82.-)

    ▶traumatic amputation of ankle and foot (S98.-)

    The appropriate 7th character is to be added to each code from category S92

A	initial encounter for closed fracture
B	initial encounter for open fracture
D	subsequent encounter for fracture with routine healing
G	subsequent encounter for fracture with delayed healing
K	subsequent encounter for fracture with nonunion
P	subsequent encounter for fracture with malunion
S	sequela

- S92.0   **Fracture of calcaneus**
  - Heel bone   Os calcis
  - **Excludes2**   Physeal fracture of calcaneus (S99.0-)
  - S92.00   Unspecified fracture of calcaneus
    - S92.001   Unspecified fracture of right calcaneus
    - S92.002   Unspecified fracture of left calcaneus
    - S92.009   Unspecified fracture of unspecified calcaneus
  - S92.01   Fracture of body of calcaneus
    - S92.011   Displaced fracture of body of right calcaneus
    - S92.012   Displaced fracture of body of left calcaneus
    - S92.013   Displaced fracture of body of unspecified calcaneus
    - S92.014   Nondisplaced fracture of body of right calcaneus
    - S92.015   Nondisplaced fracture of body of left calcaneus
    - S92.016   Nondisplaced fracture of body of unspecified calcaneus
  - S92.02   Fracture of anterior process of calcaneus
    - S92.021   Displaced fracture of anterior process of right calcaneus
    - S92.022   Displaced fracture of anterior process of left calcaneus
    - S92.023   Displaced fracture of anterior process of unspecified calcaneus
    - S92.024   Nondisplaced fracture of anterior process of right calcaneus
    - S92.025   Nondisplaced fracture of anterior process of left calcaneus
    - S92.026   Nondisplaced fracture of anterior process of unspecified calcaneus
  - S92.03   Avulsion fracture of tuberosity of calcaneus
    - S92.031   Displaced avulsion fracture of tuberosity of right calcaneus
    - S92.032   Displaced avulsion fracture of tuberosity of left calcaneus
    - S92.033   Displaced avulsion fracture of tuberosity of unspecified calcaneus
    - S92.034   Nondisplaced avulsion fracture of tuberosity of right calcaneus
    - S92.035   Nondisplaced avulsion fracture of tuberosity of left calcaneus
    - S92.036   Nondisplaced avulsion fracture of tuberosity of unspecified calcaneus
  - S92.04   Other fracture of tuberosity of calcaneus
    - S92.041   Displaced other fracture of tuberosity of right calcaneus
    - S92.042   Displaced other fracture of tuberosity of left calcaneus
    - S92.043   Displaced other fracture of tuberosity of unspecified calcaneus
    - S92.044   Nondisplaced other fracture of tuberosity of right calcaneus
    - S92.045   Nondisplaced other fracture of tuberosity of left calcaneus
    - S92.046   Nondisplaced other fracture of tuberosity of unspecified calcaneus
  - S92.05   Other extraarticular fracture of calcaneus
    - S92.051   Displaced other extraarticular fracture of right calcaneus
    - S92.052   Displaced other extraarticular fracture of left calcaneus
    - S92.053   Displaced other extraarticular fracture of unspecified calcaneus
    - S92.054   Nondisplaced other extraarticular fracture of right calcaneus

- ● S92.055   Nondisplaced other extraarticular fracture of left calcaneus
- ● S92.056   Nondisplaced other extraarticular fracture of unspecified calcaneus
- ● S92.06   Intraarticular fracture of calcaneus
  - ● S92.061   Displaced intraarticular fracture of right calcaneus
  - ● S92.062   Displaced intraarticular fracture of left calcaneus
  - ● S92.063   Displaced intraarticular fracture of unspecified calcaneus
  - ● S92.064   Nondisplaced intraarticular fracture of right calcaneus
  - ● S92.065   Nondisplaced intraarticular fracture of left calcaneus
  - ● S92.066   Nondisplaced intraarticular fracture of unspecified calcaneus
- ● S92.1   Fracture of talus
  Astragalus
  - ● S92.10   Unspecified fracture of talus
    - ● S92.101   Unspecified fracture of right talus
    - ● S92.102   Unspecified fracture of left talus
    - ● S92.109   Unspecified fracture of unspecified talus
  - ● S92.11   Fracture of neck of talus
    - ● S92.111   Displaced fracture of neck of right talus
    - ● S92.112   Displaced fracture of neck of left talus
    - ● S92.113   Displaced fracture of neck of unspecified talus
    - ● S92.114   Nondisplaced fracture of neck of right talus
    - ● S92.115   Nondisplaced fracture of neck of left talus
    - ● S92.116   Nondisplaced fracture of neck of unspecified talus
  - ● S92.12   Fracture of body of talus
    - ● S92.121   Displaced fracture of body of right talus
    - ● S92.122   Displaced fracture of body of left talus
    - ● S92.123   Displaced fracture of body of unspecified talus
    - ● S92.124   Nondisplaced fracture of body of right talus
    - ● S92.125   Nondisplaced fracture of body of left talus
    - ● S92.126   Nondisplaced fracture of body of unspecified talus
  - ● S92.13   Fracture of posterior process of talus
    - ● S92.131   Displaced fracture of posterior process of right talus
    - ● S92.132   Displaced fracture of posterior process of left talus
    - ● S92.133   Displaced fracture of posterior process of unspecified talus
    - ● S92.134   Nondisplaced fracture of posterior process of right talus
    - ● S92.135   Nondisplaced fracture of posterior process of left talus
    - ● S92.136   Nondisplaced fracture of posterior process of unspecified talus
  - ● S92.14   Dome fracture of talus
    - **Excludes1**   osteochondritis dissecans (M93.2)
    - ● S92.141   Displaced dome fracture of right talus
    - ● S92.142   Displaced dome fracture of left talus

- ● S92.143   Displaced dome fracture of unspecified talus
- ● S92.144   Nondisplaced dome fracture of right talus
- ● S92.145   Nondisplaced dome fracture of left talus
- ● S92.146   Nondisplaced dome fracture of unspecified talus
- ● S92.15   Avulsion fracture (chip fracture) of talus
  - ● S92.151   Displaced avulsion fracture (chip fracture) of right talus
  - ● S92.152   Displaced avulsion fracture (chip fracture) of left talus
  - ● S92.153   Displaced avulsion fracture (chip fracture) of unspecified talus
  - ● S92.154   Nondisplaced avulsion fracture (chip fracture) of right talus
  - ● S92.155   Nondisplaced avulsion fracture (chip fracture) of left talus
  - ● S92.156   Nondisplaced avulsion fracture (chip fracture) of unspecified talus
- ● S92.19   Other fracture of talus
  - ● S92.191   Other fracture of right talus
  - ● S92.192   Other fracture of left talus
  - ● S92.199   Other fracture of unspecified talus
- ● S92.2   Fracture of other and unspecified tarsal bone(s)
  - ● S92.20   Fracture of unspecified tarsal bone(s)
    - ● S92.201   Fracture of unspecified tarsal bone(s) of right foot
    - ● S92.202   Fracture of unspecified tarsal bone(s) of left foot
    - ● S92.209   Fracture of unspecified tarsal bone(s) of unspecified foot
  - ● S92.21   Fracture of cuboid bone
    - ● S92.211   Displaced fracture of cuboid bone of right foot
    - ● S92.212   Displaced fracture of cuboid bone of left foot
    - ● S92.213   Displaced fracture of cuboid bone of unspecified foot
    - ● S92.214   Nondisplaced fracture of cuboid bone of right foot
    - ● S92.215   Nondisplaced fracture of cuboid bone of left foot
    - ● S92.216   Nondisplaced fracture of cuboid bone of unspecified foot
  - ◖ S92.22   Fracture of lateral cuneiform
    - ● S92.221   Displaced fracture of lateral cuneiform of right foot
    - ● S92.222   Displaced fracture of lateral cuneiform of left foot
    - ● S92.223   Displaced fracture of lateral cuneiform of unspecified foot
    - ● S92.224   Nondisplaced fracture of lateral cuneiform of right foot
    - ● S92.225   Nondisplaced fracture of lateral cuneiform of left foot
    - ● S92.226   Nondisplaced fracture of lateral cuneiform of unspecified foot
  - ● S92.23   Fracture of intermediate cuneiform
    - ● S92.231   Displaced fracture of intermediate cuneiform of right foot
    - ● S92.232   Displaced fracture of intermediate cuneiform of left foot
    - ● S92.233   Displaced fracture of intermediate cuneiform of unspecified foot
    - ● S92.234   Nondisplaced fracture of intermediate cuneiform of right foot

▶ New   ⇒ Revised   ~~deleted~~ Deleted   Excludes 1   Excludes 2   Includes   Use additional   Code first   Code also   Key words

OGCR Official Guidelines   X Assign placeholder X   ● Use Additional Character(s)   ▶ Manifestation Code   🔒 Hierarchical Condition Category   **Coding Clinic**

● S92.235   Nondisplaced fracture of intermediate cuneiform of left foot

● S92.236   Nondisplaced fracture of intermediate cuneiform of unspecified foot

● S92.24   Fracture of medial cuneiform

　● S92.241   Displaced fracture of medial cuneiform of right foot

　● S92.242   Displaced fracture of medial cuneiform of left foot

　● S92.243   Displaced fracture of medial cuneiform of unspecified foot

　● S92.244   Nondisplaced fracture of medial cuneiform of right foot

　● S92.245   Nondisplaced fracture of medial cuneiform of left foot

　● S92.246   Nondisplaced fracture of medial cuneiform of unspecified foot

● S92.25   Fracture of navicular [scaphoid] of foot

　● S92.251   Displaced fracture of navicular [scaphoid] of right foot

　● S92.252   Displaced fracture of navicular [scaphoid] of left foot

　● S92.253   Displaced fracture of navicular [scaphoid] of unspecified foot

　● S92.254   Nondisplaced fracture of navicular [scaphoid] of right foot

　● S92.255   Nondisplaced fracture of navicular [scaphoid] of left foot

　● S92.256   Nondisplaced fracture of navicular [scaphoid] of unspecified foot

● S92.3   Fracture of metatarsal bone(s)

　Excludes2   Physeal fracture of metatarsal (S99.1-)

● S92.30   Fracture of unspecified metatarsal bone(s)

　● S92.301   Fracture of unspecified metatarsal bone(s), right foot

　● S92.302   Fracture of unspecified metatarsal bone(s), left foot

　● S92.309   Fracture of unspecified metatarsal bone(s), unspecified foot

● S92.31   Fracture of first metatarsal bone

　● S92.311   Displaced fracture of first metatarsal bone, right foot

　● S92.312   Displaced fracture of first metatarsal bone, left foot

　● S92.313   Displaced fracture of first metatarsal bone, unspecified foot

　● S92.314   Nondisplaced fracture of first metatarsal bone, right foot

　● S92.315   Nondisplaced fracture of first metatarsal bone, left foot

　● S92.316   Nondisplaced fracture of first metatarsal bone, unspecified foot

● S92.32   Fracture of second metatarsal bone

　● S92.321   Displaced fracture of second metatarsal bone, right foot

　● S92.322   Displaced fracture of second metatarsal bone, left foot

　● S92.323   Displaced fracture of second metatarsal bone, unspecified foot

　● S92.324   Nondisplaced fracture of second metatarsal bone, right foot

　● S92.325   Nondisplaced fracture of second metatarsal bone, left foot

　● S92.326   Nondisplaced fracture of second metatarsal bone, unspecified foot

● S92.33   Fracture of third metatarsal bone
　Coding Clinic: 2018, Q1, P3

　● S92.331   Displaced fracture of third metatarsal bone, right foot

　● S92.332   Displaced fracture of third metatarsal bone, left foot

　● S92.333   Displaced fracture of third metatarsal bone, unspecified foot

　● S92.334   Nondisplaced fracture of third metatarsal bone, right foot

　● S92.335   Nondisplaced fracture of third metatarsal bone, left foot

　● S92.336   Nondisplaced fracture of third metatarsal bone, unspecified foot

● S92.34   Fracture of fourth metatarsal bone

　● S92.341   Displaced fracture of fourth metatarsal bone, right foot

　● S92.342   Displaced fracture of fourth metatarsal bone, left foot

　● S92.343   Displaced fracture of fourth metatarsal bone, unspecified foot

　● S92.344   Nondisplaced fracture of fourth metatarsal bone, right foot

　● S92.345   Nondisplaced fracture of fourth metatarsal bone, left foot

　● S92.346   Nondisplaced fracture of fourth metatarsal bone, unspecified foot

● S92.35   Fracture of fifth metatarsal bone

　● S92.351   Displaced fracture of fifth metatarsal bone, right foot

　● S92.352   Displaced fracture of fifth metatarsal bone, left foot

　● S92.353   Displaced fracture of fifth metatarsal bone, unspecified foot

　● S92.354   Nondisplaced fracture of fifth metatarsal bone, right foot

　● S92.355   Nondisplaced fracture of fifth metatarsal bone, left foot

　● S92.356   Nondisplaced fracture of fifth metatarsal bone, unspecified foot

● S92.4   Fracture of great toe

　Excludes2   Physeal fracture of phalanx of toe (S99.2-)

● S92.40   Unspecified fracture of great toe

　● S92.401   Displaced unspecified fracture of right great toe

　● S92.402   Displaced unspecified fracture of left great toe

　● S92.403   Displaced unspecified fracture of unspecified great toe

　● S92.404   Nondisplaced unspecified fracture of right great toe

　● S92.405   Nondisplaced unspecified fracture of left great toe

　● S92.406   Nondisplaced unspecified fracture of unspecified great toe

● S92.41   Fracture of proximal phalanx of great toe

　● S92.411   Displaced fracture of proximal phalanx of right great toe

　● S92.412   Displaced fracture of proximal phalanx of left great toe

　● S92.413   Displaced fracture of proximal phalanx of unspecified great toe

　● S92.414   Nondisplaced fracture of proximal phalanx of right great toe

　● S92.415   Nondisplaced fracture of proximal phalanx of left great toe

　● S92.416   Nondisplaced fracture of proximal phalanx of unspecified great toe

CHAPTER 19 (S00-T88)

● S92.42   Fracture of distal phalanx of great toe
  ● S92.421   Displaced fracture of distal phalanx of right great toe
  ● S92.422   Displaced fracture of distal phalanx of left great toe
  ● S92.423   Displaced fracture of distal phalanx of unspecified great toe
  ● S92.424   Nondisplaced fracture of distal phalanx of right great toe
  ● S92.425   Nondisplaced fracture of distal phalanx of left great toe
  ● S92.426   Nondisplaced fracture of distal phalanx of unspecified great toe

● S92.49   Other fracture of great toe
  ● S92.491   Other fracture of right great toe
  ● S92.492   Other fracture of left great toe
  ● S92.499   Other fracture of unspecified great toe

● S92.5   Fracture of lesser toe(s)
  Excludes2   Physeal fracture of phalanx of toe (S99.2-)

  ● S92.50   Unspecified fracture of lesser toe(s)
    ● S92.501   Displaced unspecified fracture of right lesser toe(s)
    ● S92.502   Displaced unspecified fracture of left lesser toe(s)
    ● S92.503   Displaced unspecified fracture of unspecified lesser toe(s)
    ● S92.504   Nondisplaced unspecified fracture of right lesser toe(s)
    ● S92.505   Nondisplaced unspecified fracture of left lesser toe(s)
    ● S92.506   Nondisplaced unspecified fracture of unspecified lesser toe(s)

  ● S92.51   Fracture of proximal phalanx of lesser toe(s)
    ● S92.511   Displaced fracture of proximal phalanx of right lesser toe(s)
    ● S92.512   Displaced fracture of proximal phalanx of left lesser toe(s)
    ● S92.513   Displaced fracture of proximal phalanx of unspecified lesser toe(s)
    ● S92.514   Nondisplaced fracture of proximal phalanx of right lesser toe(s)
    ● S92.515   Nondisplaced fracture of proximal phalanx of left lesser toe(s)
    ● S92.516   Nondisplaced fracture of proximal phalanx of unspecified lesser toe(s)

  ● S92.52   Fracture of middle phalanx of lesser toe(s)
    ● S92.521   Displaced fracture of middle phalanx of right lesser toe(s)
    ● S92.522   Displaced fracture of middle phalanx of left lesser toe(s)
    ● S92.523   Displaced fracture of middle phalanx of unspecified lesser toe(s)
    ● S92.524   Nondisplaced fracture of middle phalanx of right lesser toe(s)
    ● S92.525   Nondisplaced fracture of middle phalanx of left lesser toe(s)
    ● S92.526   Nondisplaced fracture of middle phalanx of unspecified lesser toe(s)

  ● S92.53   Fracture of distal phalanx of lesser toe(s)
    ● S92.531   Displaced fracture of distal phalanx of right lesser toe(s)
    ● S92.532   Displaced fracture of distal phalanx of left lesser toe(s)
    ● S92.533   Displaced fracture of distal phalanx of unspecified lesser toe(s)
    ● S92.534   Nondisplaced fracture of distal phalanx of right lesser toe(s)

● S92.535   Nondisplaced fracture of distal phalanx of left lesser toe(s)
● S92.536   Nondisplaced fracture of distal phalanx of unspecified lesser toe(s)

● S92.59   Other fracture of lesser toe(s)
  ● S92.591   Other fracture of right lesser toe(s)
  ● S92.592   Other fracture of left lesser toe(s)
  ● S92.599   Other fracture of unspecified lesser toe(s)

● S92.8   Other fracture of foot, except ankle
  ● S92.81   Other fracture of foot
    Sesamoid fracture of foot
    Coding Clinic: 2016, Q4, P68
    ● S92.811   Other fracture of right foot
    ● S92.812   Other fracture of left foot
    ● S92.819   Other fracture of unspecified foot

● S92.9   Unspecified fracture of foot and toe
  ● S92.90   Unspecified fracture of foot
    ● S92.901   Unspecified fracture of right foot
    ● S92.902   Unspecified fracture of left foot
    ● S92.909   Unspecified fracture of unspecified foot
  ● S92.91   Unspecified fracture of toe
    ● S92.911   Unspecified fracture of right toe(s)
    ● S92.912   Unspecified fracture of left toe(s)
    ● S92.919   Unspecified fracture of unspecified toe(s)

● S93   Dislocation and sprain of joints and ligaments at ankle, foot and toe level
  Includes   avulsion of joint or ligament of ankle, foot and toe
    laceration of cartilage, joint or ligament of ankle, foot and toe
    sprain of cartilage, joint or ligament of ankle, foot and toe
    traumatic hemarthrosis of joint or ligament of ankle, foot and toe
    traumatic rupture of joint or ligament of ankle, foot and toe
    traumatic subluxation of joint or ligament of ankle, foot and toe
    traumatic tear of joint or ligament of ankle, foot and toe

  Code also any associated open wound
  Excludes2   strain of muscle and tendon of ankle and foot (S96.-)

  The appropriate 7th character is to be added to each code from category S93

A	initial encounter
D	subsequent encounter
S	sequela

● S93.0   Subluxation and dislocation of ankle joint
  Subluxation and dislocation of astragalus
  Subluxation and dislocation of fibula, lower end
  Subluxation and dislocation of talus
  Subluxation and dislocation of tibia, lower end
  X ● S93.01   Subluxation of right ankle joint
  X ● S93.02   Subluxation of left ankle joint
  X ● S93.03   Subluxation of unspecified ankle joint
  X ● S93.04   Dislocation of right ankle joint
  X ● S93.05   Dislocation of left ankle joint
  X ● S93.06   Dislocation of unspecified ankle joint

● S93.1   Subluxation and dislocation of toe
  ● S93.10   Unspecified subluxation and dislocation of toe
    Dislocation of toe NOS
    Subluxation of toe NOS
    ● S93.101   Unspecified subluxation of right toe(s)

● S93.102   Unspecified subluxation of left toe(s)
● S93.103   Unspecified subluxation of unspecified toe(s)
● S93.104   Unspecified dislocation of right toe(s)
● S93.105   Unspecified dislocation of left toe(s)
● S93.106   Unspecified dislocation of unspecified toe(s)

● S93.11   Dislocation of interphalangeal joint
  ● S93.111   Dislocation of interphalangeal joint of right great toe
  ● S93.112   Dislocation of interphalangeal joint of left great toe
  ● S93.113   Dislocation of interphalangeal joint of unspecified great toe
  ● S93.114   Dislocation of interphalangeal joint of right lesser toe(s)
  ● S93.115   Dislocation of interphalangeal joint of left lesser toe(s)
  ● S93.116   Dislocation of interphalangeal joint of unspecified lesser toe(s)
  ● S93.119   Dislocation of interphalangeal joint of unspecified toe(s)

● S93.12   Dislocation of metatarsophalangeal joint
  ● S93.121   Dislocation of metatarsophalangeal joint of right great toe
  ● S93.122   Dislocation of metatarsophalangeal joint of left great toe
  ● S93.123   Dislocation of metatarsophalangeal joint of unspecified great toe
  ● S93.124   Dislocation of metatarsophalangeal joint of right lesser toe(s)
  ● S93.125   Dislocation of metatarsophalangeal joint of left lesser toe(s)
  ● S93.126   Dislocation of metatarsophalangeal joint of unspecified lesser toe(s)
  ● S93.129   Dislocation of metatarsophalangeal joint of unspecified toe(s)

● S93.13   Subluxation of interphalangeal joint
  ● S93.131   Subluxation of interphalangeal joint of right great toe
  ● S93.132   Subluxation of interphalangeal joint of left great toe
  ● S93.133   Subluxation of interphalangeal joint of unspecified great toe
  ● S93.134   Subluxation of interphalangeal joint of right lesser toe(s)
  ● S93.135   Subluxation of interphalangeal joint of left lesser toe(s)
  ● S93.136   Subluxation of interphalangeal joint of unspecified lesser toe(s)
  ● S93.139   Subluxation of interphalangeal joint of unspecified toe(s)

● S93.14   Subluxation of metatarsophalangeal joint
  ● S93.141   Subluxation of metatarsophalangeal joint of right great toe
  ● S93.142   Subluxation of metatarsophalangeal joint of left great toe
  ● S93.143   Subluxation of metatarsophalangeal joint of unspecified great toe
  ● S93.144   Subluxation of metatarsophalangeal joint of right lesser toe(s)
  ● S93.145   Subluxation of metatarsophalangeal joint of left lesser toe(s)
  ● S93.146   Subluxation of metatarsophalangeal joint of unspecified lesser toe(s)
  ● S93.149   Subluxation of metatarsophalangeal joint of unspecified toe(s)

● S93.3   Subluxation and dislocation of foot
  Excludes2   dislocation of toe (S93.1-)
  ● S93.30   Unspecified subluxation and dislocation of foot
    Dislocation of foot NOS
    Subluxation of foot NOS
    ● S93.301   Unspecified subluxation of right foot
    ● S93.302   Unspecified subluxation of left foot
    ● S93.303   Unspecified subluxation of unspecified foot
    ● S93.304   Unspecified dislocation of right foot
    ● S93.305   Unspecified dislocation of left foot
    ● S93.306   Unspecified dislocation of unspecified foot

  ● S93.31   Subluxation and dislocation of tarsal joint
    ● S93.311   Subluxation of tarsal joint of right foot
    ● S93.312   Subluxation of tarsal joint of left foot
    ● S93.313   Subluxation of tarsal joint of unspecified foot
    ● S93.314   Dislocation of tarsal joint of right foot
    ● S93.315   Dislocation of tarsal joint of left foot
    ● S93.316   Dislocation of tarsal joint of unspecified foot

  ● S93.32   Subluxation and dislocation of tarsometatarsal joint
    ● S93.321   Subluxation of tarsometatarsal joint of right foot
    ● S93.322   Subluxation of tarsometatarsal joint of left foot
    ● S93.323   Subluxation of tarsometatarsal joint of unspecified foot
    ● S93.324   Dislocation of tarsometatarsal joint of right foot
    ● S93.325   Dislocation of tarsometatarsal joint of left foot
    ● S93.326   Dislocation of tarsometatarsal joint of unspecified foot

  ● S93.33   Other subluxation and dislocation of foot
    ● S93.331   Other subluxation of right foot
    ● S93.332   Other subluxation of left foot
    ● S93.333   Other subluxation of unspecified foot
    ● S93.334   Other dislocation of right foot
    ● S93.335   Other dislocation of left foot
    ● S93.336   Other dislocation of unspecified foot

● S93.4   Sprain of ankle
  Injury to ligaments when one or more is stretched/torn
  Excludes2   injury of Achilles tendon (S86.0-)
  ● S93.40   Sprain of unspecified ligament of ankle
    Sprain of ankle NOS
    Sprained ankle NOS
    ● S93.401   Sprain of unspecified ligament of right ankle
    ● S93.402   Sprain of unspecified ligament of left ankle
    ● S93.409   Sprain of unspecified ligament of unspecified ankle

  ● S93.41   Sprain of calcaneofibular ligament
    ● S93.411   Sprain of calcaneofibular ligament of right ankle
    ● S93.412   Sprain of calcaneofibular ligament of left ankle
    ● S93.419   Sprain of calcaneofibular ligament of unspecified ankle

CHAPTER 19 (S00-T88)

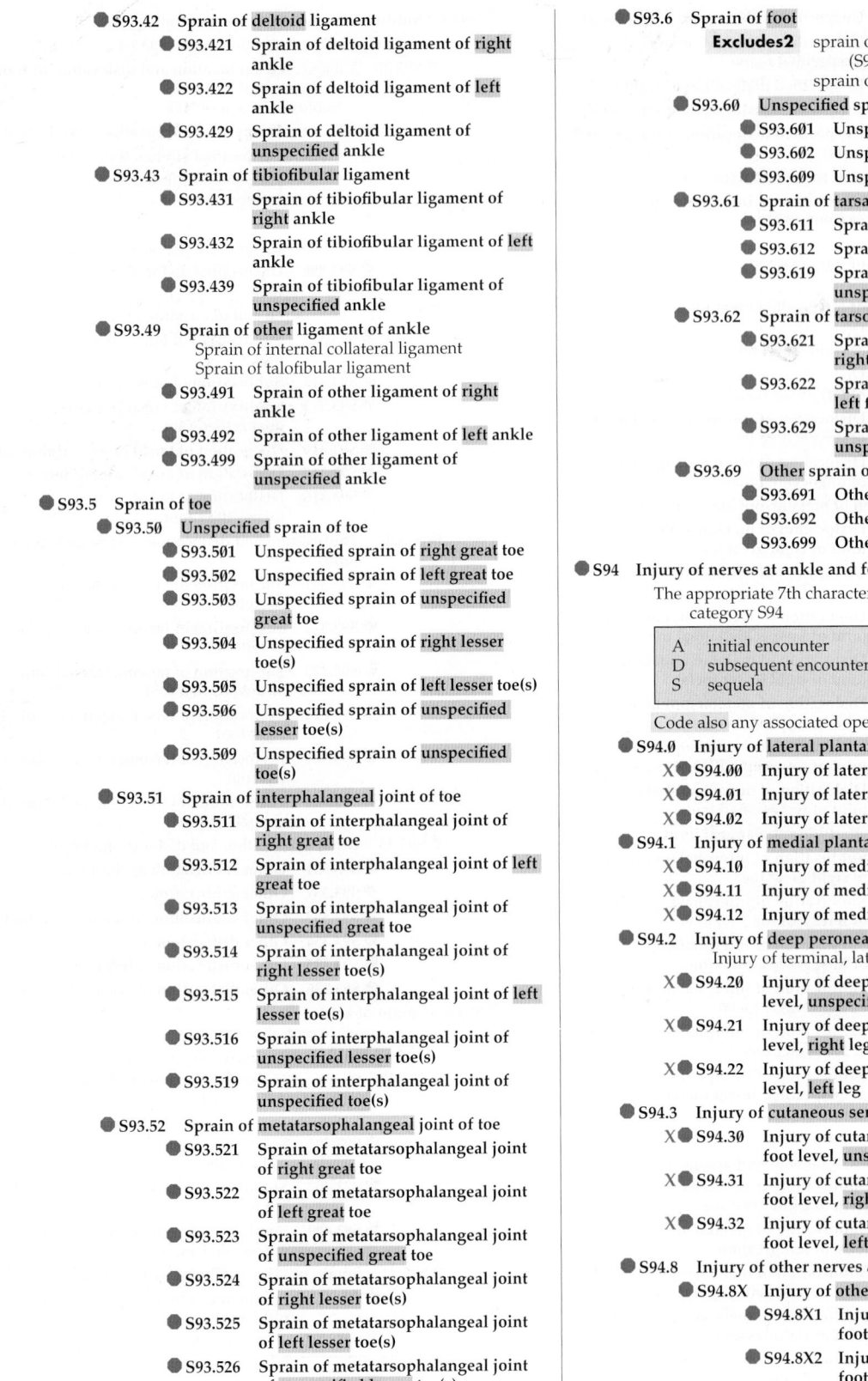

CHAPTER 19 (S00–T88)

● S93.42   Sprain of deltoid ligament
- ● S93.421   Sprain of deltoid ligament of right ankle
- ● S93.422   Sprain of deltoid ligament of left ankle
- ● S93.429   Sprain of deltoid ligament of unspecified ankle

● S93.43   Sprain of tibiofibular ligament
- ● S93.431   Sprain of tibiofibular ligament of right ankle
- ● S93.432   Sprain of tibiofibular ligament of left ankle
- ● S93.439   Sprain of tibiofibular ligament of unspecified ankle

● S93.49   Sprain of other ligament of ankle
     Sprain of internal collateral ligament
     Sprain of talofibular ligament
- ● S93.491   Sprain of other ligament of right ankle
- ● S93.492   Sprain of other ligament of left ankle
- ● S93.499   Sprain of other ligament of unspecified ankle

● S93.5   Sprain of toe
- ● S93.50   Unspecified sprain of toe
  - ● S93.501   Unspecified sprain of right great toe
  - ● S93.502   Unspecified sprain of left great toe
  - ● S93.503   Unspecified sprain of unspecified great toe
  - ● S93.504   Unspecified sprain of right lesser toe(s)
  - ● S93.505   Unspecified sprain of left lesser toe(s)
  - ● S93.506   Unspecified sprain of unspecified lesser toe(s)
  - ● S93.509   Unspecified sprain of unspecified toe(s)
- ● S93.51   Sprain of interphalangeal joint of toe
  - ● S93.511   Sprain of interphalangeal joint of right great toe
  - ● S93.512   Sprain of interphalangeal joint of left great toe
  - ● S93.513   Sprain of interphalangeal joint of unspecified great toe
  - ● S93.514   Sprain of interphalangeal joint of right lesser toe(s)
  - ● S93.515   Sprain of interphalangeal joint of left lesser toe(s)
  - ● S93.516   Sprain of interphalangeal joint of unspecified lesser toe(s)
  - ● S93.519   Sprain of interphalangeal joint of unspecified toe(s)
- ● S93.52   Sprain of metatarsophalangeal joint of toe
  - ● S93.521   Sprain of metatarsophalangeal joint of right great toe
  - ● S93.522   Sprain of metatarsophalangeal joint of left great toe
  - ● S93.523   Sprain of metatarsophalangeal joint of unspecified great toe
  - ● S93.524   Sprain of metatarsophalangeal joint of right lesser toe(s)
  - ● S93.525   Sprain of metatarsophalangeal joint of left lesser toe(s)
  - ● S93.526   Sprain of metatarsophalangeal joint of unspecified lesser toe(s)
  - ● S93.529   Sprain of metatarsophalangeal joint of unspecified toe(s)

● S93.6   Sprain of foot
    Excludes2   sprain of metatarsophalangeal joint of toe (S93.52-)
                 sprain of toe (S93.5-)
- ● S93.60   Unspecified sprain of foot
  - ● S93.601   Unspecified sprain of right foot
  - ● S93.602   Unspecified sprain of left foot
  - ● S93.609   Unspecified sprain of unspecified foot
- ● S93.61   Sprain of tarsal ligament of foot
  - ● S93.611   Sprain of tarsal ligament of right foot
  - ● S93.612   Sprain of tarsal ligament of left foot
  - ● S93.619   Sprain of tarsal ligament of unspecified foot
- ● S93.62   Sprain of tarsometatarsal ligament of foot
  - ● S93.621   Sprain of tarsometatarsal ligament of right foot
  - ● S93.622   Sprain of tarsometatarsal ligament of left foot
  - ● S93.629   Sprain of tarsometatarsal ligament of unspecified foot
- ● S93.69   Other sprain of foot
  - ● S93.691   Other sprain of right foot
  - ● S93.692   Other sprain of left foot
  - ● S93.699   Other sprain of unspecified foot

● S94   Injury of nerves at ankle and foot level
    The appropriate 7th character is to be added to each code from category S94

A	initial encounter
D	subsequent encounter
S	sequela

    Code also any associated open wound (S91.-)
- ● S94.0   Injury of lateral plantar nerve
  - X ● S94.00   Injury of lateral plantar nerve, unspecified leg
  - X ● S94.01   Injury of lateral plantar nerve, right leg
  - X ● S94.02   Injury of lateral plantar nerve, left leg
- ● S94.1   Injury of medial plantar nerve
  - X ● S94.10   Injury of medial plantar nerve, unspecified leg
  - X ● S94.11   Injury of medial plantar nerve, right leg
  - X ● S94.12   Injury of medial plantar nerve, left leg
- ● S94.2   Injury of deep peroneal nerve at ankle and foot level
      Injury of terminal, lateral branch of deep peroneal nerve
  - X ● S94.20   Injury of deep peroneal nerve at ankle and foot level, unspecified leg
  - X ● S94.21   Injury of deep peroneal nerve at ankle and foot level, right leg
  - X ● S94.22   Injury of deep peroneal nerve at ankle and foot level, left leg
- ● S94.3   Injury of cutaneous sensory nerve at ankle and foot level
  - X ● S94.30   Injury of cutaneous sensory nerve at ankle and foot level, unspecified leg
  - X ● S94.31   Injury of cutaneous sensory nerve at ankle and foot level, right leg
  - X ● S94.32   Injury of cutaneous sensory nerve at ankle and foot level, left leg
- ● S94.8   Injury of other nerves at ankle and foot level
  - ● S94.8X   Injury of other nerves at ankle and foot level
    - ● S94.8X1   Injury of other nerves at ankle and foot level, right leg
    - ● S94.8X2   Injury of other nerves at ankle and foot level, left leg
    - ● S94.8X9   Injury of other nerves at ankle and foot level, unspecified leg

▶ New   ⇒ Revised   ~~deleted~~ Deleted   Excludes 1   Excludes 2   Includes   Use additional   Code first   Code also   Key words

OGCR Official Guidelines   X Assign placeholder X   ● Use Additional Character(s)   ▶ Manifestation Code   🐄 Hierarchical Condition Category   **Coding Clinic**

S94.9   Injury of unspecified nerve at ankle and foot level

   X⬤ S94.90   Injury of unspecified nerve at ankle and foot level, unspecified leg

   X⬤ S94.91   Injury of unspecified nerve at ankle and foot level, right leg

   X⬤ S94.92   Injury of unspecified nerve at ankle and foot level, left leg

⬤ S95   Injury of blood vessels at ankle and foot level

   Code also any associated open wound (S91.-)

   Excludes2   injury of posterior tibial artery and vein (S85.1-, S85.8-)

   The appropriate 7th character is to be added to each code from category S95

A	initial encounter
D	subsequent encounter
S	sequela

⬤ S95.0   Injury of dorsal artery of foot

  ⬤ S95.00   Unspecified injury of dorsal artery of foot

    ⬤ S95.001   Unspecified injury of dorsal artery of right foot

    ⬤ S95.002   Unspecified injury of dorsal artery of left foot

    ⬤ S95.009   Unspecified injury of dorsal artery of unspecified foot

  ⬤ S95.01   Laceration of dorsal artery of foot

    ⬤ S95.011   Laceration of dorsal artery of right foot

    ⬤ S95.012   Laceration of dorsal artery of left foot

    ⬤ S95.019   Laceration of dorsal artery of unspecified foot

  ⬤ S95.09   Other specified injury of dorsal artery of foot

    ⬤ S95.091   Other specified injury of dorsal artery of right foot

    ⬤ S95.092   Other specified injury of dorsal artery of left foot

    ⬤ S95.099   Other specified injury of dorsal artery of unspecified foot

⬤ S95.1   Injury of plantar artery of foot

  ⬤ S95.10   Unspecified injury of plantar artery of foot

    ⬤ S95.101   Unspecified injury of plantar artery of right foot

    ⬤ S95.102   Unspecified injury of plantar artery of left foot

    ⬤ S95.109   Unspecified injury of plantar artery of unspecified foot

  ⬤ S95.11   Laceration of plantar artery of foot

    ⬤ S95.111   Laceration of plantar artery of right foot

    ⬤ S95.112   Laceration of plantar artery of left foot

    ⬤ S95.119   Laceration of plantar artery of unspecified foot

  ⬤ S95.19   Other specified injury of plantar artery of foot

    ⬤ S95.191   Other specified injury of plantar artery of right foot

    ⬤ S95.192   Other specified injury of plantar artery of left foot

    ⬤ S95.199   Other specified injury of plantar artery of unspecified foot

⬤ S95.2   Injury of dorsal vein of foot

  ⬤ S95.20   Unspecified injury of dorsal vein of foot

    ⬤ S95.201   Unspecified injury of dorsal vein of right foot

    ⬤ S95.202   Unspecified injury of dorsal vein of left foot

    ⬤ S95.209   Unspecified injury of dorsal vein of unspecified foot

  ⬤ S95.21   Laceration of dorsal vein of foot

    ⬤ S95.211   Laceration of dorsal vein of right foot

    ⬤ S95.212   Laceration of dorsal vein of left foot

    ⬤ S95.219   Laceration of dorsal vein of unspecified foot

  ⬤ S95.29   Other specified injury of dorsal vein of foot

    ⬤ S95.291   Other specified injury of dorsal vein of right foot

    ⬤ S95.292   Other specified injury of dorsal vein of left foot

    ⬤ S95.299   Other specified injury of dorsal vein of unspecified foot

⬤ S95.8   Injury of other blood vessels at ankle and foot level

  ⬤ S95.80   Unspecified injury of other blood vessels at ankle and foot level

    ⬤ S95.801   Unspecified injury of other blood vessels at ankle and foot level, right leg

    ⬤ S95.802   Unspecified injury of other blood vessels at ankle and foot level, left leg

    ⬤ S95.809   Unspecified injury of other blood vessels at ankle and foot level, unspecified leg

  ⬤ S95.81   Laceration of other blood vessels at ankle and foot level

    ⬤ S95.811   Laceration of other blood vessels at ankle and foot level, right leg

    ⬤ S95.812   Laceration of other blood vessels at ankle and foot level, left leg

    ⬤ S95.819   Laceration of other blood vessels at ankle and foot level, unspecified leg

  ⬤ S95.89   Other specified injury of other blood vessels at ankle and foot level

    ⬤ S95.891   Other specified injury of other blood vessels at ankle and foot level, right leg

    ⬤ S95.892   Other specified injury of other blood vessels at ankle and foot level, left leg

    ⬤ S95.899   Other specified injury of other blood vessels at ankle and foot level, unspecified leg

⬤ S95.9   Injury of unspecified blood vessel at ankle and foot level

  ⬤ S95.90   Unspecified injury of unspecified blood vessel at ankle and foot level

    ⬤ S95.901   Unspecified injury of unspecified blood vessel at ankle and foot level, right leg

    ⬤ S95.902   Unspecified injury of unspecified blood vessel at ankle and foot level, left leg

    ⬤ S95.909   Unspecified injury of unspecified blood vessel at ankle and foot level, unspecified leg

  ⬤ S95.91   Laceration of unspecified blood vessel at ankle and foot level

    ⬤ S95.911   Laceration of unspecified blood vessel at ankle and foot level, right leg

    ⬤ S95.912   Laceration of unspecified blood vessel at ankle and foot level, left leg

    ⬤ S95.919   Laceration of unspecified blood vessel at ankle and foot level, unspecified leg

CHAPTER 19 (S00-T88)

● S95.99   Other specified injury of unspecified blood vessel at ankle and foot level
   ● S95.991   Other specified injury of unspecified blood vessel at ankle and foot level, right leg
   ● S95.992   Other specified injury of unspecified blood vessel at ankle and foot level, left leg
   ● S95.999   Other specified injury of unspecified blood vessel at ankle and foot level, unspecified leg

● S96   Injury of muscle and tendon at ankle and foot level
   Code also any associated open wound (S91.-)
   Excludes2   injury of Achilles tendon (S86.0-)
                   sprain of joints and ligaments of ankle and foot (S93.-)

   The appropriate 7th character is to be added to each code from category S96

A	initial encounter
D	subsequent encounter
S	sequela

● S96.0   Injury of muscle and tendon of long flexor muscle of toe at ankle and foot level
   ● S96.00   Unspecified injury of muscle and tendon of long flexor muscle of toe at ankle and foot level
      ● S96.001   Unspecified injury of muscle and tendon of long flexor muscle of toe at ankle and foot level, right foot
      ● S96.002   Unspecified injury of muscle and tendon of long flexor muscle of toe at ankle and foot level, left foot
      ● S96.009   Unspecified injury of muscle and tendon of long flexor muscle of toe at ankle and foot level, unspecified foot
   ● S96.01   Strain of muscle and tendon of long flexor muscle of toe at ankle and foot level
      ● S96.011   Strain of muscle and tendon of long flexor muscle of toe at ankle and foot level, right foot
      ● S96.012   Strain of muscle and tendon of long flexor muscle of toe at ankle and foot level, left foot
      ● S96.019   Strain of muscle and tendon of long flexor muscle of toe at ankle and foot level, unspecified foot
   ● S96.02   Laceration of muscle and tendon of long flexor muscle of toe at ankle and foot level
      ● S96.021   Laceration of muscle and tendon of long flexor muscle of toe at ankle and foot level, right foot
      ● S96.022   Laceration of muscle and tendon of long flexor muscle of toe at ankle and foot level, left foot
      ● S96.029   Laceration of muscle and tendon of long flexor muscle of toe at ankle and foot level, unspecified foot
   ● S96.09   Other injury of muscle and tendon of long flexor muscle of toe at ankle and foot level
      ● S96.091   Other injury of muscle and tendon of long flexor muscle of toe at ankle and foot level, right foot
      ● S96.092   Other injury of muscle and tendon of long flexor muscle of toe at ankle and foot level, left foot
      ● S96.099   Other injury of muscle and tendon of long flexor muscle of toe at ankle and foot level, unspecified foot

● S96.1   Injury of muscle and tendon of long extensor muscle of toe at ankle and foot level
   ● S96.10   Unspecified injury of muscle and tendon of long extensor muscle of toe at ankle and foot level
      ● S96.101   Unspecified injury of muscle and tendon of long extensor muscle of toe at ankle and foot level, right foot
      ● S96.102   Unspecified injury of muscle and tendon of long extensor muscle of toe at ankle and foot level, left foot
      ● S96.109   Unspecified injury of muscle and tendon of long extensor muscle of toe at ankle and foot level, unspecified foot
   ● S96.11   Strain of muscle and tendon of long extensor muscle of toe at ankle and foot level
      ● S96.111   Strain of muscle and tendon of long extensor muscle of toe at ankle and foot level, right foot
      ● S96.112   Strain of muscle and tendon of long extensor muscle of toe at ankle and foot level, left foot
      ● S96.119   Strain of muscle and tendon of long extensor muscle of toe at ankle and foot level, unspecified foot
   ● S96.12   Laceration of muscle and tendon of long extensor muscle of toe at ankle and foot level
      ● S96.121   Laceration of muscle and tendon of long extensor muscle of toe at ankle and foot level, right foot
      ● S96.122   Laceration of muscle and tendon of long extensor muscle of toe at ankle and foot level, left foot
      ● S96.129   Laceration of muscle and tendon of long extensor muscle of toe at ankle and foot level, unspecified foot
   ● S96.19   Other specified injury of muscle and tendon of long extensor muscle of toe at ankle and foot level
      ● S96.191   Other specified injury of muscle and tendon of long extensor muscle of toe at ankle and foot level, right foot
      ● S96.192   Other specified injury of muscle and tendon of long extensor muscle of toe at ankle and foot level, left foot
      ● S96.199   Other specified injury of muscle and tendon of long extensor muscle of toe at ankle and foot level, unspecified foot

● S96.2   Injury of intrinsic muscle and tendon at ankle and foot level
   ● S96.20   Unspecified injury of intrinsic muscle and tendon at ankle and foot level
      ● S96.201   Unspecified injury of intrinsic muscle and tendon at ankle and foot level, right foot
      ● S96.202   Unspecified injury of intrinsic muscle and tendon at ankle and foot level, left foot
      ● S96.209   Unspecified injury of intrinsic muscle and tendon at ankle and foot level, unspecified foot
   ● S96.21   Strain of intrinsic muscle and tendon at ankle and foot level
      ● S96.211   Strain of intrinsic muscle and tendon at ankle and foot level, right foot
      ● S96.212   Strain of intrinsic muscle and tendon at ankle and foot level, left foot
      ● S96.219   Strain of intrinsic muscle and tendon at ankle and foot level, unspecified foot

▶ New   ⇒ Revised   ~~deleted~~ Deleted   Excludes 1   Excludes 2   Includes   Use additional   Code first   Code also   Key words

OGCR Official Guidelines   X Assign placeholder X   ● Use Additional Character(s)   ▶ Manifestation Code   🍄 Hierarchical Condition Category   **Coding Clinic**

● S96.22   Laceration of intrinsic muscle and tendon at ankle and foot level

    ● S96.221   Laceration of intrinsic muscle and tendon at ankle and foot level, right foot

    ● S96.222   Laceration of intrinsic muscle and tendon at left ankle and foot level, left foot

    ● S96.229   Laceration of intrinsic muscle and tendon at ankle and foot level, unspecified foot

● S96.29   Other specified injury of intrinsic muscle and tendon at ankle and foot level

    ● S96.291   Other specified injury of intrinsic muscle and tendon at ankle and foot level, right foot

    ● S96.292   Other specified injury of intrinsic muscle and tendon at ankle and foot level, left foot

    ● S96.299   Other specified injury of intrinsic muscle and tendon at ankle and foot level, unspecified foot

● S96.8   Injury of other specified muscles and tendons at ankle and foot level

    ● S96.80   Unspecified injury of other specified muscles and tendons at ankle and foot level

       ● S96.801   Unspecified injury of other specified muscles and tendons at ankle and foot level, right foot

       ● S96.802   Unspecified injury of other specified muscles and tendons at ankle and foot level, left foot

       ● S96.809   Unspecified injury of other specified muscles and tendons at ankle and foot level, unspecified foot

    ● S96.81   Strain of other specified muscles and tendons at ankle and foot level

       ● S96.811   Strain of other specified muscles and tendons at ankle and foot level, right foot

       ● S96.812   Strain of other specified muscles and tendons at ankle and foot level, left foot

       ● S96.819   Strain of other specified muscles and tendons at ankle and foot level, unspecified foot

    ● S96.82   Laceration of other specified muscles and tendons at ankle and foot level

       ● S96.821   Laceration of other specified muscles and tendons at ankle and foot level, right foot

       ● S96.822   Laceration of other specified muscles and tendons at ankle and foot level, left foot

       ● S96.829   Laceration of other specified muscles and tendons at ankle and foot level, unspecified foot

    ● S96.89   Other specified injury of other specified muscles and tendons at ankle and foot level

       ● S96.891   Other specified injury of other specified muscles and tendons at ankle and foot level, right foot

       ● S96.892   Other specified injury of other specified muscles and tendons at ankle and foot level, left foot

       ● S96.899   Other specified injury of other specified muscles and tendons at ankle and foot level, unspecified foot

● S96.9   Injury of unspecified muscle and tendon at ankle and foot level

    ● S96.90   Unspecified injury of unspecified muscle and tendon at ankle and foot level

       ● S96.901   Unspecified injury of unspecified muscle and tendon at ankle and foot level, right foot

       ● S96.902   Unspecified injury of unspecified muscle and tendon at ankle and foot level, left foot

       ● S96.909   Unspecified injury of unspecified muscle and tendon at ankle and foot level, unspecified foot

    ● S96.91   Strain of unspecified muscle and tendon at ankle and foot level

       ● S96.911   Strain of unspecified muscle and tendon at ankle and foot level, right foot

       ● S96.912   Strain of unspecified muscle and tendon at ankle and foot level, left foot

       ● S96.919   Strain of unspecified muscle and tendon at ankle and foot level, unspecified foot

    ● S96.92   Laceration of unspecified muscle and tendon at ankle and foot level

       ● S96.921   Laceration of unspecified muscle and tendon at ankle and foot level, right foot

       ● S96.922   Laceration of unspecified muscle and tendon at ankle and foot level, left foot

       ● S96.929   Laceration of unspecified muscle and tendon at ankle and foot level, unspecified foot

    ● S96.99   Other specified injury of unspecified muscle and tendon at ankle and foot level

       ● S96.991   Other specified injury of unspecified muscle and tendon at ankle and foot level, right foot

       ● S96.992   Other specified injury of unspecified muscle and tendon at ankle and foot level, left foot

       ● S96.999   Other specified injury of unspecified muscle and tendon at ankle and foot level, unspecified foot

● S97   Crushing injury of ankle and foot

    Use additional code(s) for all associated injuries

    The appropriate 7th character is to be added to each code from category S97

A	initial encounter
D	subsequent encounter
S	sequela

● S97.0   Crushing injury of ankle

    X ● S97.00   Crushing injury of unspecified ankle

    X ● S97.01   Crushing injury of right ankle

    X ● S97.02   Crushing injury of left ankle

● S97.1   Crushing injury of toe

    ● S97.10   Crushing injury of unspecified toe(s)

       ● S97.101   Crushing injury of unspecified right toe(s)

       ● S97.102   Crushing injury of unspecified left toe(s)

       ● S97.109   Crushing injury of unspecified toe(s)
                Crushing injury of toe NOS

    ● S97.11   Crushing injury of great toe

       ● S97.111   Crushing injury of right great toe

       ● S97.112   Crushing injury of left great toe

       ● S97.119   Crushing injury of unspecified great toe

CHAPTER 19 (S00–T88)

CHAPTER 19 (S00-T88)

- S97.12 Crushing injury of lesser toe(s)
  - S97.121 Crushing injury of right lesser toe(s)
  - S97.122 Crushing injury of left lesser toe(s)
  - S97.129 Crushing injury of lesser toe(s), unspecified toe(s)
- S97.8 Crushing injury of foot
  - X S97.80 Crushing injury of foot, unspecified side
    Crushing injury of foot NOS
  - X S97.81 Crushing injury of right foot
  - X S97.82 Crushing injury of left foot
- S98 Traumatic amputation of ankle and foot
  An amputation not identified as partial or complete should be coded to complete

  The appropriate 7th character is to be added to each code from category S98

  A initial encounter
  D subsequent encounter
  S sequela

- S98.0 Traumatic amputation of foot at ankle level
  - S98.01 Complete traumatic amputation of foot at ankle level
    - S98.011 Complete traumatic amputation of right foot at ankle level A, D, S
    - S98.012 Complete traumatic amputation of left foot at ankle level A, D, S
    - S98.019 Complete traumatic amputation of unspecified foot at ankle level A, D, S
  - S98.02 Partial traumatic amputation of foot at ankle level
    - S98.021 Partial traumatic amputation of right foot at ankle level A, D, S
    - S98.022 Partial traumatic amputation of left foot at ankle level A, D, S
    - S98.029 Partial traumatic amputation of unspecified foot at ankle level A, D, S
- S98.1 Traumatic amputation of one toe
  - S98.11 Complete traumatic amputation of great toe
    - S98.111 Complete traumatic amputation of right great toe A, D, S
    - S98.112 Complete traumatic amputation of left great toe A, D, S
    - S98.119 Complete traumatic amputation of unspecified great toe A, D, S
  - S98.12 Partial traumatic amputation of great toe
    - S98.121 Partial traumatic amputation of right great toe A, D, S
    - S98.122 Partial traumatic amputation of left great toe A, D, S
    - S98.129 Partial traumatic amputation of unspecified great toe A, D, S
  - S98.13 Complete traumatic amputation of one lesser toe
    Traumatic amputation of toe NOS
    - S98.131 Complete traumatic amputation of one right lesser toe A, D, S
    - S98.132 Complete traumatic amputation of one left lesser toe A, D, S
    - S98.139 Complete traumatic amputation of one unspecified lesser toe A, D, S

- S98.14 Partial traumatic amputation of one lesser toe
  - S98.141 Partial traumatic amputation of one right lesser toe A, D, S
  - S98.142 Partial traumatic amputation of one left lesser toe A, D, S
  - S98.149 Partial traumatic amputation of one unspecified lesser toe A, D, S
- S98.2 Traumatic amputation of two or more lesser toes
  - S98.21 Complete traumatic amputation of two or more lesser toes
    - S98.211 Complete traumatic amputation of two or more right lesser toes A, D, S
    - S98.212 Complete traumatic amputation of two or more left lesser toes A, D, S
    - S98.219 Complete traumatic amputation of two or more unspecified lesser toes A, D, S
  - S98.22 Partial traumatic amputation of two or more lesser toes
    - S98.221 Partial traumatic amputation of two or more right lesser toes A, D, S
    - S98.222 Partial traumatic amputation of two or more left lesser toes A, D, S
    - S98.229 Partial traumatic amputation of two or more unspecified lesser toes A, D, S
- S98.3 Traumatic amputation of midfoot
  - S98.31 Complete traumatic amputation of midfoot
    - S98.311 Complete traumatic amputation of right midfoot A, D, S
    - S98.312 Complete traumatic amputation of left midfoot A, D, S
    - S98.319 Complete traumatic amputation of unspecified midfoot A, D, S
  - S98.32 Partial traumatic amputation of midfoot
    - S98.321 Partial traumatic amputation of right midfoot A, D, S
    - S98.322 Partial traumatic amputation of left midfoot A, D, S
    - S98.329 Partial traumatic amputation of unspecified midfoot A, D, S
- S98.9 Traumatic amputation of foot, level unspecified
  - S98.91 Complete traumatic amputation of foot, level unspecified
    - S98.911 Complete traumatic amputation of right foot, level unspecified A, D, S
    - S98.912 Complete traumatic amputation of left foot, level unspecified A, D, S
    - S98.919 Complete traumatic amputation of unspecified foot, level unspecified A, D, S
  - S98.92 Partial traumatic amputation of foot, level unspecified
    - S98.921 Partial traumatic amputation of right foot, level unspecified A, D, S
    - S98.922 Partial traumatic amputation of left foot, level unspecified A, D, S
    - S98.929 Partial traumatic amputation of unspecified foot, level unspecified A, D, S

● **S99** **Other and unspecified injuries of ankle and foot**
    Coding Clinic: 2016, Q4, P68
  ● **S99.0** **Physeal fracture of calcaneus**

    The appropriate 7th character is to be added to each
    code from subcategories S99.0

A	initial encounter for closed fracture
B	initial encounter for open fracture
D	subsequent encounter for fracture with routine healing
G	subsequent encounter for fracture with delayed healing
K	subsequent encounter for fracture with nonunion
P	subsequent encounter for fracture with malunion
S	sequela

    ● **S99.00** Unspecified physeal fracture of calcaneus
      ● S99.001 Unspecified physeal fracture of right calcaneus
      ● S99.002 Unspecified physeal fracture of left calcaneus
      ● S99.009 Unspecified physeal fracture of unspecified calcaneus
    ● **S99.01** Salter-Harris Type I physeal fracture of calcaneus
        Coding Clinic: 2016, Q4, P69
      ● S99.011 Salter-Harris Type I physeal fracture of right calcaneus
      ● S99.012 Salter-Harris Type I physeal fracture of left calcaneus
      ● S99.019 Salter-Harris Type I physeal fracture of unspecified calcaneus
    ● **S99.02** Salter-Harris Type II physeal fracture of calcaneus
        Coding Clinic: 2016, Q4, P69
      ● S99.021 Salter-Harris Type II physeal fracture of right calcaneus
      ● S99.022 Salter-Harris Type II physeal fracture of left calcaneus
      ● S99.029 Salter-Harris Type II physeal fracture of unspecified calcaneus
    ● **S99.03** Salter-Harris Type III physeal fracture of calcaneus
        Coding Clinic: 2016, Q4, P69
      ● S99.031 Salter-Harris Type III physeal fracture of right calcaneus
      ● S99.032 Salter-Harris Type III physeal fracture of left calcaneus
      ● S99.039 Salter-Harris Type III physeal fracture of unspecified calcaneus
    ● **S99.04** Salter-Harris Type IV physeal fracture of calcaneus
        Coding Clinic: 2016, Q4, P69
      ● S99.041 Salter-Harris Type IV physeal fracture of right calcaneus
      ● S99.042 Salter-Harris Type IV physeal fracture of left calcaneus
      ● S99.049 Salter-Harris Type IV physeal fracture of unspecified calcaneus
    ● **S99.09** Other physeal fracture of calcaneus
        Coding Clinic: 2016, Q4, P69
      ● S99.091 Other physeal fracture of right calcaneus
      ● S99.092 Other physeal fracture of left calcaneus
      ● S99.099 Other physeal fracture of unspecified calcaneus

  ● **S99.1** **Physeal fracture of metatarsal**

    The appropriate 7th character is to be added to each
    code from subcategories S99.1

A	initial encounter for closed fracture
B	initial encounter for open fracture
D	subsequent encounter for fracture with routine healing
G	subsequent encounter for fracture with delayed healing
K	subsequent encounter for fracture with nonunion
P	subsequent encounter for fracture with malunion
S	sequela

    ● **S99.10** Unspecified physeal fracture of metatarsal
      ● S99.101 Unspecified physeal fracture of right metatarsal
      ● S99.102 Unspecified physeal fracture of left metatarsal
      ● S99.109 Unspecified physeal fracture of unspecified metatarsal
    ● **S99.11** Salter-Harris Type I physeal fracture of metatarsal
        Coding Clinic: 2016, Q4, P69
      ● S99.111 Salter-Harris Type I physeal fracture of right metatarsal
      ● S99.112 Salter-Harris Type I physeal fracture of left metatarsal
          Coding Clinic: 2018, Q1, P3
      ● S99.119 Salter-Harris Type I physeal fracture of unspecified metatarsal
    ● **S99.12** Salter-Harris Type II physeal fracture of metatarsal
        Coding Clinic: 2016, Q4, P69
      ● S99.121 Salter-Harris Type II physeal fracture of right metatarsal
      ● S99.122 Salter-Harris Type II physeal fracture of left metatarsal
      ● S99.129 Salter-Harris Type II physeal fracture of unspecified metatarsal
    ● **S99.13** Salter-Harris Type III physeal fracture of metatarsal
        Coding Clinic: 2016, Q4, P69
      ● S99.131 Salter-Harris Type III physeal fracture of right metatarsal
      ● S99.132 Salter-Harris Type III physeal fracture of left metatarsal
      ● S99.139 Salter-Harris Type III physeal fracture of unspecified metatarsal
    ● **S99.14** Salter-Harris Type IV physeal fracture of metatarsal
        Coding Clinic: 2016, Q4, P69
      ● S99.141 Salter-Harris Type IV physeal fracture of right metatarsal
      ● S99.142 Salter-Harris Type IV physeal fracture of left metatarsal
      ● S99.149 Salter-Harris Type IV physeal fracture of unspecified metatarsal
    ● **S99.19** Other physeal fracture of metatarsal
        Coding Clinic: 2016, Q4, P69
      ● S99.191 Other physeal fracture of right metatarsal
      ● S99.192 Other physeal fracture of left metatarsal
      ● S99.199 Other physeal fracture of unspecified metatarsal

CHAPTER 19 (S00-T88)

● **S99.2**   Physeal fracture of phalanx of toe

The appropriate 7th character is to be added to each code from subcategories S99.2

A	initial encounter for closed fracture
B	initial encounter for open fracture
D	subsequent encounter for fracture with routine healing
G	subsequent encounter for fracture with delayed healing
K	subsequent encounter for fracture with nonunion
P	subsequent encounter for fracture with malunion
S	sequela

● **S99.20**   Unspecified physeal fracture of phalanx of toe
- ● S99.201   Unspecified physeal fracture of phalanx of right toe
- ● S99.202   Unspecified physeal fracture of phalanx of right toe
- ● S99.209   Unspecified physeal fracture of phalanx of unspecified toe

● **S99.21**   Salter-Harris Type I physeal fracture of phalanx of toe
        Coding Clinic: 2016, Q4, P69
- ● S99.211   Salter-Harris Type I physeal fracture of phalanx of right toe
- ● S99.212   Salter-Harris Type I physeal fracture of phalanx of left toe
- ● S99.219   Salter-Harris Type I physeal fracture of phalanx of unspecified toe

● **S99.22**   Salter-Harris Type II physeal fracture of phalanx of toe
        Coding Clinic: 2016, Q4, P69
- ● S99.221   Salter-Harris Type II physeal fracture of phalanx of right toe
- ● S99.222   Salter-Harris Type II physeal fracture of phalanx of left toe
- ● S99.229   Salter-Harris Type II physeal fracture of phalanx of unspecified toe

● **S99.23**   Salter-Harris Type III physeal fracture of phalanx of toe
        Coding Clinic: 2016, Q4, P69
- ● S99.231   Salter-Harris Type III physeal fracture of phalanx of right toe
- ● S99.232   Salter-Harris Type III physeal fracture of phalanx of left toe
- ● S99.239   Salter-Harris Type III physeal fracture of phalanx of unspecified toe

● **S99.24**   Salter-Harris Type IV physeal fracture of phalanx of toe
        Coding Clinic: 2016, Q4, P69
- ● S99.241   Salter-Harris Type IV physeal fracture of phalanx of right toe
- ● S99.242   Salter-Harris Type IV physeal fracture of phalanx of left toe
- ● S99.249   Salter-Harris Type IV physeal fracture of phalanx of unspecified toe

● **S99.29**   Other physeal fracture of phalanx of toe
        Coding Clinic: 2016, Q4, P69
- ● S99.291   Other physeal fracture of phalanx of right toe
- ● S99.292   Other physeal fracture of phalanx of left toe
- ● S99.299   Other physeal fracture of phalanx of unspecified toe

● **S99.8**   Other specified injuries of ankle and foot

The appropriate 7th character is to be added to each code from subcategory S99.8

A	initial encounter
D	subsequent encounter
S	sequela

● **S99.81**   Other specified injuries of ankle
- ● S99.811   Other specified injuries of right ankle
- ● S99.812   Other specified injuries of left ankle
- ● S99.819   Other specified injuries of unspecified ankle

● **S99.82**   Other specified injuries of foot
- ● S99.821   Other specified injuries of right foot
- ● S99.822   Other specified injuries of left foot
- ● S99.829   Other specified injuries of unspecified foot

● **S99.9**   Unspecified injury of ankle and foot

The appropriate 7th character is to be added to each code from subcategory S99.9

A	initial encounter
D	subsequent encounter
S	sequela

● **S99.91**   Unspecified injury of ankle
- ● S99.911   Unspecified injury of right ankle
- ● S99.912   Unspecified injury of left ankle
- ● S99.919   Unspecified injury of unspecified ankle

● **S99.92**   Unspecified injury of foot
- ● S99.921   Unspecified injury of right foot
- ● S99.922   Unspecified injury of left foot
- ● S99.929   Unspecified injury of unspecified foot

INJURY, POISONING AND CERTAIN OTHER CONSEQUENCES OF EXTERNAL CAUSES (T07-T88)

INJURIES INVOLVING MULTIPLE BODY REGIONS (T07)

Excludes1   burns and corrosions (T20-T32)
               frostbite (T33-T34)
               insect bite or sting, venomous (T63.4)
               sunburn (L55.-)

X ● **T07**   Unspecified multiple injuries

The appropriate 7th character is to be added to code T07

A	initial encounter
D	subsequent encounter
S	sequela

Excludes1   injury NOS (T14.90)

INJURY OF UNSPECIFIED BODY REGION (T14)

● **T14**   Injury of unspecified body region

The appropriate 7th character is to be added to each code from category T14

A	initial encounter
D	subsequent encounter
S	sequela

Excludes1   multiple unspecified injuries (T07)

X ● **T14.8**   Other injury of unspecified body region
    Abrasion NOS   Skin injury NOS
    Contusion NOS   Vascular injury NOS
    Crush injury NOS   Wound NOS
    Fracture NOS

● **T14.9**   Unspecified injury

X ● **T14.90**   Injury, unspecified
         Injury NOS

X ● **T14.91**   Suicide attempt A, D, S 🔖
         Attempted suicide NOS

▶ New   ⇒ Revised   ~~deleted~~ Deleted   Excludes 1   Excludes 2   Includes   Use additional   Code first   Code also   Key words

OGCR Official Guidelines   X Assign placeholder X   ● Use Additional Character(s)   ▶ Manifestation Code   🔖 Hierarchical Condition Category   **Coding Clinic**

EFFECTS OF FOREIGN BODY ENTERING THROUGH NATURAL ORIFICE (T15-T19)

     Excludes2   foreign body accidentally left in operation wound (T81.5-)
                        foreign body in penetrating wound - see open wound by body region
                        residual foreign body in soft tissue (M79.5)
                        splinter, without open wound - see superficial injury by body region

● T15   **Foreign body on external eye**
     Excludes2   foreign body in penetrating wound of orbit and eye ball (S05.4-, S05.5-)
                        open wound of eyelid and periocular area (S01.1-)
                        retained foreign body in eyelid (H02.8-)
                        retained (old) foreign body in penetrating wound of orbit and eye ball (H05.5-, H44.6-, H44.7-)
                        superficial foreign body of eyelid and periocular area (S00.25-)

The appropriate 7th character is to be added to each code from category T15

A	initial encounter
D	subsequent encounter
S	sequela

● T15.0   Foreign body in cornea
   X ● T15.00   Foreign body in cornea, unspecified eye
   X ● T15.01   Foreign body in cornea, right eye
   X ● T15.02   Foreign body in cornea, left eye
● T15.1   Foreign body in conjunctival sac
   X ● T15.10   Foreign body in conjunctival sac, unspecified eye
   X ● T15.11   Foreign body in conjunctival sac, right eye
   X ● T15.12   Foreign body in conjunctival sac, left eye
● T15.8   Foreign body in other and multiple parts of external eye
        Foreign body in lacrimal punctum
   X ● T15.80   Foreign body in other and multiple parts of external eye, unspecified eye
   X ● T15.81   Foreign body in other and multiple parts of external eye, right eye
   X ● T15.82   Foreign body in other and multiple parts of external eye, left eye
● T15.9   Foreign body on external eye, part unspecified
   X ● T15.90   Foreign body on external eye, part unspecified, unspecified eye
   X ● T15.91   Foreign body on external eye, part unspecified, right eye
   X ● T15.92   Foreign body on external eye, part unspecified, left eye

● T16   **Foreign body in ear**
     Includes   foreign body in auditory canal
The appropriate 7th character is to be added to each code from category T16

A	initial encounter
D	subsequent encounter
S	sequela

   X ● T16.1   Foreign body in right ear
   X ● T16.2   Foreign body in left ear
   X ● T16.9   Foreign body in ear, unspecified ear

● T17   **Foreign body in respiratory tract**
The appropriate 7th character is to be added to each code from category T17

A	initial encounter
D	subsequent encounter
S	sequela

X ● T17.0   Foreign body in nasal sinus
X ● T17.1   Foreign body in nostril
         Foreign body in nose NOS
● T17.2   Foreign body in pharynx
         Foreign body in nasopharynx
         Foreign body in throat NOS
   ● T17.20   Unspecified foreign body in pharynx
     ● T17.200   Unspecified foreign body in pharynx causing asphyxiation
     ● T17.208   Unspecified foreign body in pharynx causing other injury
   ● T17.21   Gastric contents in pharynx
        Aspiration of gastric contents into pharynx
        Vomitus in pharynx
     ● T17.210   Gastric contents in pharynx causing asphyxiation
     ● T17.218   Gastric contents in pharynx causing other injury
   ● T17.22   Food in pharynx
        Bones in pharynx
        Seeds in pharynx
     ● T17.220   Food in pharynx causing asphyxiation
     ● T17.228   Food in pharynx causing other injury
   ● T17.29   Other foreign object in pharynx
     ● T17.290   Other foreign object in pharynx causing asphyxiation
     ● T17.298   Other foreign object in pharynx causing other injury
● T17.3   Foreign body in larynx
   ● T17.30   Unspecified foreign body in larynx
     ● T17.300   Unspecified foreign body in larynx causing asphyxiation
     ● T17.308   Unspecified foreign body in larynx causing other injury
   ● T17.31   Gastric contents in larynx
        Aspiration of gastric contents into larynx
        Vomitus in larynx
     ● T17.310   Gastric contents in larynx causing asphyxiation
     ● T17.318   Gastric contents in larynx causing other injury
   ● T17.32   Food in larynx
        Bones in larynx
        Seeds in larynx
     ● T17.320   Food in larynx causing asphyxiation
     ● T17.328   Food in larynx causing other injury
   ● T17.39   Other foreign object in larynx
     ● T17.390   Other foreign object in larynx causing asphyxiation
     ● T17.398   Other foreign object in larynx causing other injury
● T17.4   Foreign body in trachea
   ● T17.40   Unspecified foreign body in trachea
     ● T17.400   Unspecified foreign body in trachea causing asphyxiation
     ● T17.408   Unspecified foreign body in trachea causing other injury

CHAPTER 19 (S00-T88)

CHAPTER 19 (S00-T88)

● T17.41   Gastric contents in trachea
   Aspiration of gastric contents into trachea
   Vomitus in trachea
  ● T17.410   Gastric contents in trachea causing asphyxiation
  ● T17.418   Gastric contents in trachea causing other injury
● T17.42   Food in trachea
   Bones in trachea
   Seeds in trachea
  ● T17.420   Food in trachea causing asphyxiation
  ● T17.428   Food in trachea causing other injury
● T17.49   Other foreign object in trachea
  ● T17.490   Other foreign object in trachea causing asphyxiation
  ● T17.498   Other foreign object in trachea causing other injury

● T17.5   Foreign body in bronchus
 ● T17.50   Unspecified foreign body in bronchus
  ● T17.500   Unspecified foreign body in bronchus causing asphyxiation
  ● T17.508   Unspecified foreign body in bronchus causing other injury
 ● T17.51   Gastric contents in bronchus
   Aspiration of gastric contents into bronchus
   Vomitus in bronchus
  ● T17.510   Gastric contents in bronchus causing asphyxiation
  ● T17.518   Gastric contents in bronchus causing other injury
 ● T17.52   Food in bronchus
   Bones in bronchus
   Seeds in bronchus
  ● T17.520   Food in bronchus causing asphyxiation
  ● T17.528   Food in bronchus causing other injury
 ● T17.59   Other foreign object in bronchus
  ● T17.590   Other foreign object in bronchus causing asphyxiation
  ● T17.598   Other foreign object in bronchus causing other injury

● T17.8   Foreign body in other parts of respiratory tract
  Foreign body in bronchioles
  Foreign body in lung
 ● T17.80   Unspecified foreign body in other parts of respiratory tract
  ● T17.800   Unspecified foreign body in other parts of respiratory tract causing asphyxiation
  ● T17.808   Unspecified foreign body in other parts of respiratory tract causing other injury
 ● T17.81   Gastric contents in other parts of respiratory tract
   Aspiration of gastric contents into other parts of respiratory tract
   Vomitus in other parts of respiratory tract
  ● T17.810   Gastric contents in other parts of respiratory tract causing asphyxiation
  ● T17.818   Gastric contents in other parts of respiratory tract causing other injury
 ● T17.82   Food in other parts of respiratory tract
   Bones in other parts of respiratory tract
   Seeds in other parts of respiratory tract
  ● T17.820   Food in other parts of respiratory tract causing asphyxiation
  ● T17.828   Food in other parts of respiratory tract causing other injury

● T17.89   Other foreign object in other parts of respiratory tract
  ● T17.890   Other foreign object in other parts of respiratory tract causing asphyxiation
  ● T17.898   Other foreign object in other parts of respiratory tract causing other injury

● T17.9   Foreign body in respiratory tract, part unspecified
 ● T17.90   Unspecified foreign body in respiratory tract, part unspecified
  ● T17.900   Unspecified foreign body in respiratory tract, part unspecified causing asphyxiation
  ● T17.908   Unspecified foreign body in respiratory tract, part unspecified causing other injury
 ● T17.91   Gastric contents in respiratory tract, part unspecified
   Aspiration of gastric contents into respiratory tract, part unspecified
   Vomitus in trachea respiratory tract, part unspecified
  ● T17.910   Gastric contents in respiratory tract, part unspecified causing asphyxiation
  ● T17.918   Gastric contents in respiratory tract, part unspecified causing other injury
 ● T17.92   Food in respiratory tract, part unspecified
   Bones in respiratory tract, part unspecified
   Seeds in respiratory tract, part unspecified
  ● T17.920   Food in respiratory tract, part unspecified causing asphyxiation
  ● T17.928   Food in respiratory tract, part unspecified causing other injury
 ● T17.99   Other foreign object in respiratory tract, part unspecified
  ● T17.990   Other foreign object in respiratory tract, part unspecified in causing asphyxiation
    Coding Clinic: 2019, Q3, P15
  ● T17.998   Other foreign object in respiratory tract, part unspecified causing other injury

● T18   Foreign body in alimentary tract
 Excludes2   foreign body in pharynx (T17.2-)
 The appropriate 7th character is to be added to each code from category T18

A	initial encounter
D	subsequent encounter
S	sequela

X ● T18.0   Foreign body in mouth
X ● T18.1   Foreign body in esophagus
 Excludes2   foreign body in respiratory tract (T17.-)
 ● T18.10   Unspecified foreign body in esophagus
  ● T18.100   Unspecified foreign body in esophagus causing compression of trachea
   Unspecified foreign body in esophagus causing obstruction of respiration
  ● T18.108   Unspecified foreign body in esophagus causing other injury
 ● T18.11   Gastric contents in esophagus
   Vomitus in esophagus
  ● T18.110   Gastric contents in esophagus causing compression of trachea
   Gastric contents in esophagus causing obstruction of respiration
  ● T18.118   Gastric contents in esophagus causing other injury

▶ New   ⇒ Revised   ~~deleted~~ Deleted   Excludes 1   Excludes 2   Includes   Use additional   Code first   Code also   Key words
OGCR Official Guidelines   X Assign placeholder X   ● Use Additional Character(s)   ▶ Manifestation Code   🐾 Hierarchical Condition Category   **Coding Clinic**

● T18.12   **Food in esophagus**
       Bones in esophagus
       Seeds in esophagus

  ● T18.120   **Food in esophagus causing compression of trachea**
           Food in esophagus causing obstruction of respiration

  ● T18.128   **Food in esophagus causing other injury**

● T18.19   **Other foreign object in esophagus**

  ● T18.190   **Other foreign object in esophagus causing compression of trachea**
           Other foreign body in esophagus causing obstruction of respiration
           Coding Clinic: 2015, Q1, P24

  ● T18.198   **Other foreign object in esophagus causing other injury**
           Coding Clinic: 2015, Q1, P24

X● T18.2   **Foreign body in stomach**

X● T18.3   **Foreign body in small intestine**

X● T18.4   **Foreign body in colon**

X● T18.5   **Foreign body in anus and rectum**
       Foreign body in rectosigmoid (junction)

X● T18.8   **Foreign body in other parts of alimentary tract**

X● T18.9   **Foreign body of alimentary tract, part unspecified**
       Foreign body in digestive system NOS
       Swallowed foreign body NOS

● T19   **Foreign body in genitourinary tract**

  Excludes2   complications due to implanted mesh (T83.7-)
          mechanical complications of contraceptive device (intrauterine) (vaginal) (T83.3-)
          presence of contraceptive device (intrauterine) (vaginal) (Z97.5)

  The appropriate 7th character is to be added to each code from category T19

A	initial encounter
D	subsequent encounter
S	sequela

X● T19.0   **Foreign body in urethra**

X● T19.1   **Foreign body in bladder**

X● T19.2   **Foreign body in vulva and vagina ♀**

X● T19.3   **Foreign body in uterus ♀**

X● T19.4   **Foreign body in penis ♂**

X● T19.8   **Foreign body in other parts of genitourinary tract**

X● T19.9   **Foreign body in genitourinary tract, part unspecified**

BURNS AND CORROSIONS (T20-T32)

Includes   burns (thermal) from electrical heating appliances
         burns (thermal) from electricity
         burns (thermal) from flame
         burns (thermal) from friction
         burns (thermal) from hot air and hot gases
         burns (thermal) from hot objects
         burns (thermal) from lightning
         burns (thermal) from radiation chemical
         burn [corrosion] (external) (internal) scalds

Excludes2   erythema [dermatitis] ab igne (L59.0)
         radiation-related disorders of the skin and subcutaneous tissue (L55-L59)
         sunburn (L55.-)

BURNS AND CORROSIONS OF EXTERNAL BODY SURFACE, SPECIFIED BY SITE (T20-T25)

Includes   burns and corrosions of first degree [erythema]
         burns and corrosions of second degree [blisters] [epidermal loss]
         burns and corrosions of third degree [deep necrosis of underlying tissue] [full-thickness skin loss]

Use additional code from category T31 or T32 to identify extent of body surface involved

● T20   **Burn and corrosion of head, face, and neck**

  Excludes2   burn and corrosion of ear drum (T28.41, T28.91)
          burn and corrosion of eye and adnexa (T26.-)
          burn and corrosion of mouth and pharynx (T28.0)

  The appropriate 7th character is to be added to each code from category T20

A	initial encounter
D	subsequent encounter
S	sequela

● T20.0   **Burn of unspecified degree of head, face, and neck**
       Use additional external cause code to identify the source, place and intent of the burn (X00-X19, X75-X77, X96-X98, Y92)

  X● T20.00   **Burn of unspecified degree of head, face, and neck, unspecified site**

  ● T20.01   **Burn of unspecified degree of ear [any part, except ear drum]**
         Excludes2   burn of ear drum (T28.41-)

    ● T20.011   **Burn of unspecified degree of right ear [any part, except ear drum]**

    ● T20.012   **Burn of unspecified degree of left ear [any part, except ear drum]**

    ● T20.019   **Burn of unspecified degree of unspecified ear [any part, except ear drum]**

Figure 19-15 A. Second-degree burn. **B.** Third-degree burn. (A. From Black J, Hawks J: Medical-Surgical Nursing: Clinical Management for Positive Outcomes, 8e, Saunders, 2008. B. From Marx J, Hockberger R, Walls R: Rosen's Emergency Medicine - Concepts and Clinical Practice, 7e, Mosby, 2009)

X ● T20.02   Burn of unspecified degree of lip(s)

X ● T20.03   Burn of unspecified degree of chin

X ● T20.04   Burn of unspecified degree of nose (septum)

X ● T20.05   Burn of unspecified degree of scalp [any part]

X ● T20.06   Burn of unspecified degree of forehead and cheek

X ● T20.07   Burn of unspecified degree of neck

X ● T20.09   Burn of unspecified degree of multiple sites of head, face, and neck

● T20.1   Burn of first degree of head, face, and neck

Use additional external cause code to identify the source, place and intent of the burn (X00-X19, X75-X77, X96-X98, Y92)

X ● T20.10   Burn of first degree of head, face, and neck, unspecified site

● T20.11   Burn of first degree of ear [any part, except ear drum]

Excludes2   burn of ear drum (T28.41-)

● T20.111   Burn of first degree of right ear [any part, except ear drum]

● T20.112   Burn of first degree of left ear [any part, except ear drum]

● T20.119   Burn of first degree of unspecified ear [any part, except ear drum]

X ● T20.12   Burn of first degree of lip(s)

X ● T20.13   Burn of first degree of chin

X ● T20.14   Burn of first degree of nose (septum)

X ● T20.15   Burn of first degree of scalp [any part]

X ● T20.16   Burn of first degree of forehead and cheek

X ● T20.17   Burn of first degree of neck

X ● T20.19   Burn of first degree of multiple sites of head, face, and neck

● T20.2   Burn of second degree of head, face, and neck

Use additional external cause code to identify the source, place and intent of the burn (X00-X19, X75-X77, X96-X98, Y92)

X ● T20.20   Burn of second degree of head, face, and neck, unspecified site

● T20.21   Burn of second degree of ear [any part, except ear drum]

Excludes2   burn of ear drum (T28.41-)

● T20.211   Burn of second degree of right ear [any part, except ear drum]

● T20.212   Burn of second degree of left ear [any part, except ear drum]

● T20.219   Burn of second degree of unspecified ear [any part, except ear drum]

X ● T20.22   Burn of second degree of lip(s)

X ● T20.23   Burn of second degree of chin

X ● T20.24   Burn of second degree of nose (septum)

X ● T20.25   Burn of second degree of scalp [any part]
Coding Clinic: 2015, Q1, P19

X ● T20.26   Burn of second degree of forehead and cheek

X ● T20.27   Burn of second degree of neck

X ● T20.29   Burn of second degree of multiple sites of head, face, and neck

● T20.3   Burn of third degree of head, face, and neck

Use additional external cause code to identify the source, place and intent of the burn (X00-X19, X75-X77, X96-X98, Y92)

X ● T20.30   Burn of third degree of head, face, and neck, unspecified site

● T20.31   Burn of third degree of ear [any part, except ear drum]

Excludes2   burn of ear drum (T28.41-)

● T20.311   Burn of third degree of right ear [any part, except ear drum]

● T20.312   Burn of third degree of left ear [any part, except ear drum]
Coding Clinic: 2015, Q1, P18

● T20.319   Burn of third degree of unspecified ear [any part, except ear drum]

X ● T20.32   Burn of third degree of lip(s)

X ● T20.33   Burn of third degree of chin

X ● T20.34   Burn of third degree of nose (septum)

X ● T20.35   Burn of third degree of scalp [any part]

X ● T20.36   Burn of third degree of forehead and cheek

X ● T20.37   Burn of third degree of neck

X ● T20.39   Burn of third degree of multiple sites of head, face, and neck

● T20.4   Corrosion of unspecified degree of head, face, and neck

Code first (T51-T65) to identify chemical and intent

Use additional external cause code to identify place (Y92)

X ● T20.40   Corrosion of unspecified degree of head, face, and neck, unspecified site

● T20.41   Corrosion of unspecified degree of ear [any part, except ear drum]

Excludes2   corrosion of ear drum (T28.91-)

● T20.411   Corrosion of unspecified degree of right ear [any part, except ear drum]

● T20.412   Corrosion of unspecified degree of left ear [any part, except ear drum]

● T20.419   Corrosion of unspecified degree of unspecified ear [any part, except ear drum]

X ● T20.42   Corrosion of unspecified degree of lip(s)

X ● T20.43   Corrosion of unspecified degree of chin

X ● T20.44   Corrosion of unspecified degree of nose (septum)

X ● T20.45   Corrosion of unspecified degree of scalp [any part]

X ● T20.46   Corrosion of unspecified degree of forehead and cheek

X ● T20.47   Corrosion of unspecified degree of neck

X ● T20.49   Corrosion of unspecified degree of multiple sites of head, face, and neck

● T20.5   Corrosion of first degree of head, face, and neck

Code first (T51-T65) to identify chemical and intent

Use additional external cause code to identify place (Y92)

X ● T20.50   Corrosion of first degree of head, face, and neck, unspecified site

● T20.51   Corrosion of first degree of ear [any part, except ear drum]

Excludes2   corrosion of ear drum (T28.91-)

▶ New   ⇒ Revised   ~~deleted~~ Deleted   Excludes 1   Excludes 2   Includes   Use additional   Code first   Code also   Key words

OGCR Official Guidelines   X Assign placeholder X   ● Use Additional Character(s)   ▶ Manifestation Code   🔖 Hierarchical Condition Category   **Coding Clinic**

1376

● **T20.511** Corrosion of first degree of right ear [any part, except ear drum]

● **T20.512** Corrosion of first degree of left ear [any part, except ear drum]

● **T20.519** Corrosion of first degree of unspecified ear [any part, except ear drum]

X ● **T20.52** Corrosion of first degree of lip(s)

X ● **T20.53** Corrosion of first degree of chin

X ● **T20.54** Corrosion of first degree of nose (septum)

X ● **T20.55** Corrosion of first degree of scalp [any part]

X ● **T20.56** Corrosion of first degree of forehead and cheek

X ● **T20.57** Corrosion of first degree of neck

X ● **T20.59** Corrosion of first degree of multiple sites of head, face, and neck

● **T20.6** Corrosion of second degree of head, face, and neck

     Code first (T51-T65) to identify chemical and intent

     Use additional external cause code to identify place (Y92)

X ● **T20.60** Corrosion of second degree of head, face, and neck, unspecified site

● **T20.61** Corrosion of second degree of ear [any part, except ear drum]

     Excludes2 corrosion of ear drum (T28.91-)

● **T20.611** Corrosion of second degree of right ear [any part, except ear drum]

● **T20.612** Corrosion of second degree of left ear [any part, except ear drum]

● **T20.619** Corrosion of second degree of unspecified ear [any part, except ear drum]

X ● **T20.62** Corrosion of second degree of lip(s)

X ● **T20.63** Corrosion of second degree of chin

X ● **T20.64** Corrosion of second degree of nose (septum)

X ● **T20.65** Corrosion of second degree of scalp [any part]

X ● **T20.66** Corrosion of second degree of forehead and cheek

X ● **T20.67** Corrosion of second degree of neck

X ● **T20.69** Corrosion of second degree of multiple sites of head, face, and neck

● **T20.7** Corrosion of third degree of head, face, and neck

     Code first (T51-T65) to identify chemical and intent

     Use additional external cause code to identify place (Y92)

X ● **T20.70** Corrosion of third degree of head, face, and neck, unspecified site

● **T20.71** Corrosion of third degree of ear [any part, except ear drum]

     Excludes2 corrosion of ear drum (T28.91-)

● **T20.711** Corrosion of third degree of right ear [any part, except ear drum]

● **T20.712** Corrosion of third degree of left ear [any part, except ear drum]

● **T20.719** Corrosion of third degree of unspecified ear [any part, except ear drum]

X ● **T20.72** Corrosion of third degree of lip(s)

X ● **T20.73** Corrosion of third degree of chin

X ● **T20.74** Corrosion of third degree of nose (septum)

X ● **T20.75** Corrosion of third degree of scalp [any part]

X ● **T20.76** Corrosion of third degree of forehead and cheek

X ● **T20.77** Corrosion of third degree of neck

X ● **T20.79** Corrosion of third degree of multiple sites of head, face, and neck

● **T21** Burn and corrosion of trunk

     Includes burns and corrosion of hip region

     Excludes2 burns and corrosion of axilla (T22.- with fifth character 4)

         burns and corrosion of scapular region (T22.- with fifth character 6)

         burns and corrosion of shoulder (T22.- with fifth character 5)

The appropriate 7th character is to be added to each code from category T21

A	initial encounter
D	subsequent encounter
S	sequela

● **T21.0** Burn of unspecified degree of trunk

     Use additional external cause code to identify the source, place and intent of the burn (X00-X19, X75-X77, X96-X98, Y92)

X ● **T21.00** Burn of unspecified degree of trunk, unspecified site

X ● **T21.01** Burn of unspecified degree of chest wall

     Burn of unspecified degree of breast

X ● **T21.02** Burn of unspecified degree of abdominal wall

     Burn of unspecified degree of flank

     Burn of unspecified degree of groin

X ● **T21.03** Burn of unspecified degree of upper back

     Burn of unspecified degree of interscapular region

X ● **T21.04** Burn of unspecified degree of lower back

X ● **T21.05** Burn of unspecified degree of buttock

     Burn of unspecified degree of anus

X ● **T21.06** Burn of unspecified degree of male genital region ♂

     Burn of unspecified degree of penis

     Burn of unspecified degree of scrotum

     Burn of unspecified degree of testis

X ● **T21.07** Burn of unspecified degree of female genital region ♀

     Burn of unspecified degree of labium (majus) (minus)

     Burn of unspecified degree of perineum

     Burn of unspecified degree of vulva

     Excludes2 burn of vagina (T28.3)

X ● **T21.09** Burn of unspecified degree of other site of trunk

● **T21.1** Burn of first degree of trunk

     Use additional external cause code to identify the source, place and intent of the burn (X00-X19, X75-X77, X96-X98, Y92)

X ● **T21.10** Burn of first degree of trunk, unspecified site

X ● **T21.11** Burn of first degree of chest wall

     Burn of first degree of breast

X ● **T21.12** Burn of first degree of abdominal wall

     Burn of first degree of flank

     Burn of first degree of groin

X ● **T21.13** Burn of first degree of upper back

     Burn of first degree of interscapular region

X ● **T21.14** Burn of first degree of lower back

X ● **T21.15** Burn of first degree of buttock

     Burn of first degree of anus

X ● **T21.16** Burn of first degree of male genital region ♂

     Burn of first degree of penis

     Burn of first degree of scrotum

     Burn of first degree of testis

X ● **T21.17** Burn of first degree of female genital region ♀

     Burn of first degree of labium (majus) (minus)

     Burn of first degree of perineum

     Burn of first degree of vulva

     Excludes2 burn of vagina (T28.3)

CHAPTER 19 (S00-T88)

CHAPTER 19 (S00-T88)

X ● **T21.19**   Burn of first degree of other site of trunk
● **T21.2**   Burn of second degree of trunk
  Use additional external cause code to identify the
  source, place and intent of the burn (X00-X19,
  X75-X77, X96-X98, Y92)
X ● **T21.20**   Burn of second degree of trunk, unspecified site
X ● **T21.21**   Burn of second degree of chest wall
  Burn of second degree of breast
X ● **T21.22**   Burn of second degree of abdominal wall
  Burn of second degree of flank
  Burn of second degree of groin
X ● **T21.23**   Burn of second degree of upper back
  Burn of second degree of interscapular region
X ● **T21.24**   Burn of second degree of lower back
X ● **T21.25**   Burn of second degree of buttock
  Burn of second degree of anus
X ● **T21.26**   Burn of second degree of male genital region ♂
  Burn of second degree of penis
  Burn of second degree of scrotum
  Burn of second degree of testis
X ● **T21.27**   Burn of second degree of female genital
  region ♀
  Burn of second degree of labium (majus)
    (minus)
  Burn of second degree of perineum
  Burn of second degree of vulva
  Excludes2   burn of vagina (T28.3)
X ● **T21.29**   Burn of second degree of other site of trunk
● **T21.3**   Burn of third degree of trunk
  Use additional external cause code to identify the
  source, place and intent of the burn (X00-X19,
  X75-X77, X96-X98, Y92)
X ● **T21.30**   Burn of third degree of trunk, unspecified site
X ● **T21.31**   Burn of third degree of chest wall
  Burn of third degree of breast
  Coding Clinic: 2016, Q2, P6
X ● **T21.32**   Burn of third degree of abdominal wall
  Burn of third degree of flank
  Burn of third degree of groin
X ● **T21.33**   Burn of third degree of upper back
  Burn of third degree of interscapular region
X ● **T21.34**   Burn of third degree of lower back
X ● **T21.35**   Burn of third degree of buttock
  Burn of third degree of anus
X ● **T21.36**   Burn of third degree of male genital region ♂
  Burn of third degree of penis
  Burn of third degree of scrotum
  Burn of third degree of testis
X ● **T21.37**   Burn of third degree of female genital region ♀
  Burn of third degree of labium (majus) (minus)
  Burn of third degree of perineum
  Burn of third degree of vulva
  Excludes2   burn of vagina (T28.3)
X ● **T21.39**   Burn of third degree of other site of trunk
● **T21.4**   Corrosion of unspecified degree of trunk
  Code first (T51-T65) to identify chemical and intent
  Use additional external cause code to identify
  place (Y92)
X ● **T21.40**   Corrosion of unspecified degree of trunk,
  unspecified site
X ● **T21.41**   Corrosion of unspecified degree of chest wall
  Corrosion of unspecified degree of breast

X ● **T21.42**   Corrosion of unspecified degree of abdominal
  wall
  Corrosion of unspecified degree of flank
  Corrosion of unspecified degree of groin
X ● **T21.43**   Corrosion of unspecified degree of upper back
  Corrosion of unspecified degree of
    interscapular region
X ● **T21.44**   Corrosion of unspecified degree of lower back
X ● **T21.45**   Corrosion of unspecified degree of buttock
  Corrosion of unspecified degree of anus
X ● **T21.46**   Corrosion of unspecified degree of male genital
  region ♂
  Corrosion of unspecified degree of penis
  Corrosion of unspecified degree of scrotum
  Corrosion of unspecified degree of testis
X ● **T21.47**   Corrosion of unspecified degree of female
  genital region ♀
  Corrosion of unspecified degree of labium
    (majus) (minus)
  Corrosion of unspecified degree of perineum
  Corrosion of unspecified degree of vulva
  Excludes2   corrosion of vagina (T28.8)
X ● **T21.49**   Corrosion of unspecified degree of other site of
  trunk
● **T21.5**   Corrosion of first degree of trunk
  Code first (T51-T65) to identify chemical and intent
  Use additional external cause code to identify
  place (Y92)
X ● **T21.50**   Corrosion of first degree of trunk, unspecified
  site
X ● **T21.51**   Corrosion of first degree of chest wall
  Corrosion of first degree of breast
X ● **T21.52**   Corrosion of first degree of abdominal wall
  Corrosion of first degree of flank
  Corrosion of first degree of groin
X ● **T21.53**   Corrosion of first degree of upper back
  Corrosion of first degree of interscapular
    region
X ● **T21.54**   Corrosion of first degree of lower back
X ● **T21.55**   Corrosion of first degree of buttock
  Corrosion of first degree of anus
X ● **T21.56**   Corrosion of first degree of male genital
  region ♂
  Corrosion of first degree of penis
  Corrosion of first degree of scrotum
  Corrosion of first degree of testis
X ● **T21.57**   Corrosion of first degree of female genital
  region ♀
  Corrosion of first degree of labium (majus)
    (minus)
  Corrosion of first degree of perineum
  Corrosion of first degree of vulva
  Excludes2   corrosion of vagina (T28.8)
X ● **T21.59**   Corrosion of first degree of other site of trunk
● **T21.6**   Corrosion of second degree of trunk
  Code first (T51-T65) to identify chemical and intent
  Use additional external cause code to identify
  place (Y92)
X ● **T21.60**   Corrosion of second degree of trunk,
  unspecified site
X ● **T21.61**   Corrosion of second degree of chest wall
  Corrosion of second degree of breast
X ● **T21.62**   Corrosion of second degree of abdominal wall
  Corrosion of second degree of flank
  Corrosion of second degree of groin

X ● **T21.63** **Corrosion of second degree of** upper back
Corrosion of second degree of interscapular region

X ● **T21.64** **Corrosion of second degree of** lower back

X ● **T21.65** **Corrosion of second degree of** buttock
Corrosion of second degree of anus

X ● **T21.66** **Corrosion of second degree of** male genital region ♂
Corrosion of second degree of penis
Corrosion of second degree of scrotum
Corrosion of second degree of testis

X ● **T21.67** **Corrosion of second degree of** female genital region ♀
Corrosion of second degree of labium (majus) (minus)
Corrosion of second degree of perineum
Corrosion of second degree of vulva

Excludes2 corrosion of vagina (T28.8)

X ● **T21.69** **Corrosion of second degree of** other site of trunk

● **T21.7** **Corrosion of** third degree of trunk
Code first (T51-T65) to identify chemical and intent
Use additional external cause code to identify place (Y92)

X ● **T21.70** **Corrosion of third degree of trunk,** unspecified site

X ● **T21.71** **Corrosion of third degree of** chest wall
Corrosion of third degree of breast

X ● **T21.72** **Corrosion of third degree of** abdominal wall
Corrosion of third degree of flank
Corrosion of third degree of groin

X ● **T21.73** **Corrosion of third degree of** upper back
Corrosion of third degree of interscapular region

X ● **T21.74** **Corrosion of third degree of** lower back

X ● **T21.75** **Corrosion of third degree of** buttock
Corrosion of third degree of anus

X ● **T21.76** **Corrosion of third degree of** male genital region ♂
Corrosion of third degree of penis
Corrosion of third degree of scrotum
Corrosion of third degree of testis

X ● **T21.77** **Corrosion of third degree of** female genital region ♀
Corrosion of third degree of labium (majus) (minus)
Corrosion of third degree of perineum
Corrosion of third degree of vulva

Excludes2 corrosion of vagina (T28.8)

X ● **T21.79** **Corrosion of third degree of** other site of trunk

● **T22** **Burn and corrosion of shoulder and upper limb, except wrist and hand**

Excludes2 burn and corrosion of interscapular region (T21.-)
burn and corrosion of wrist and hand (T23.-)

The appropriate 7th character is to be added to each code from category T22

A	initial encounter
D	subsequent encounter
S	sequela

● **T22.0** **Burn of** unspecified degree of shoulder and upper limb, except wrist and hand
Use additional external cause code to identify the source, place and intent of the burn (X00-X19, X75-X77, X96-X98, Y92)

X ● **T22.00** **Burn of unspecified degree of shoulder and upper limb, except wrist and hand,** unspecified site

● **T22.01** **Burn of unspecified degree of** forearm

● **T22.011** Burn of unspecified degree of right forearm

● **T22.012** Burn of unspecified degree of left forearm

● **T22.019** Burn of unspecified degree of unspecified forearm

● **T22.02** **Burn of unspecified degree of** elbow

● **T22.021** Burn of unspecified degree of right elbow

● **T22.022** Burn of unspecified degree of left elbow

● **T22.029** Burn of unspecified degree of unspecified elbow

● **T22.03** **Burn of unspecified degree of** upper arm

● **T22.031** Burn of unspecified degree of right upper arm

● **T22.032** Burn of unspecified degree of left upper arm

● **T22.039** Burn of unspecified degree of unspecified upper arm

● **T22.04** **Burn of unspecified degree of** axilla

● **T22.041** Burn of unspecified degree of right axilla

● **T22.042** Burn of unspecified degree of left axilla

● **T22.049** Burn of unspecified degree of unspecified axilla

● **T22.05** **Burn of unspecified degree of** shoulder

● **T22.051** Burn of unspecified degree of right shoulder

● **T22.052** Burn of unspecified degree of left shoulder

● **T22.059** Burn of unspecified degree of unspecified shoulder

● **T22.06** **Burn of unspecified degree of** scapular region

● **T22.061** Burn of unspecified degree of right scapular region

● **T22.062** Burn of unspecified degree of left scapular region

● **T22.069** Burn of unspecified degree of unspecified scapular region

● **T22.09** **Burn of unspecified degree of** multiple sites of shoulder and upper limb, except wrist and hand

● **T22.091** Burn of unspecified degree of multiple sites of right shoulder and upper limb, except wrist and hand

● **T22.092** Burn of unspecified degree of multiple sites of left shoulder and upper limb, except wrist and hand

● **T22.099** Burn of unspecified degree of multiple sites of unspecified shoulder and upper limb, except wrist and hand

CHAPTER 19 (S00-T88)

CHAPTER 19 (S00-T88)

● T22.1   Burn of first degree of shoulder and upper limb, except wrist and hand

Use additional external cause code to identify the source, place and intent of the burn (X00-X19, X75-X77, X96-X98, Y92)

X ● T22.10   Burn of first degree of shoulder and upper limb, except wrist and hand, unspecified site

● T22.11   Burn of first degree of forearm
- ● T22.111   Burn of first degree of right forearm
- ● T22.112   Burn of first degree of left forearm
- ● T22.119   Burn of first degree of unspecified forearm

● T22.12   Burn of first degree of elbow
- ● T22.121   Burn of first degree of right elbow
- ● T22.122   Burn of first degree of left elbow
- ● T22.129   Burn of first degree of unspecified elbow

● T22.13   Burn of first degree of upper arm
- ● T22.131   Burn of first degree of right upper arm
- ● T22.132   Burn of first degree of left upper arm
- ● T22.139   Burn of first degree of unspecified upper arm

● T22.14   Burn of first degree of axilla
- ● T22.141   Burn of first degree of right axilla
- ● T22.142   Burn of first degree of left axilla
- ● T22.149   Burn of first degree of unspecified axilla

● T22.15   Burn of first degree of shoulder
- ● T22.151   Burn of first degree of right shoulder
- ● T22.152   Burn of first degree of left shoulder
- ● T22.159   Burn of first degree of unspecified shoulder

● T22.16   Burn of first degree of scapular region
- ● T22.161   Burn of first degree of right scapular region
- ● T22.162   Burn of first degree of left scapular region
- ● T22.169   Burn of first degree of unspecified scapular region

● T22.19   Burn of first degree of multiple sites of shoulder and upper limb, except wrist and hand
- ● T22.191   Burn of first degree of multiple sites of right shoulder and upper limb, except wrist and hand
- ● T22.192   Burn of first degree of multiple sites of left shoulder and upper limb, except wrist and hand
- ● T22.199   Burn of first degree of multiple sites of unspecified shoulder and upper limb, except wrist and hand

● T22.2   Burn of second degree of shoulder and upper limb, except wrist and hand

Use additional external cause code to identify the source, place and intent of the burn (X00-X19, X75-X77, X96-X98, Y92)

X ● T22.20   Burn of second degree of shoulder and upper limb, except wrist and hand, unspecified site

● T22.21   Burn of second degree of forearm
- ● T22.211   Burn of second degree of right forearm
- ● T22.212   Burn of second degree of left forearm
- ● T22.219   Burn of second degree of unspecified forearm

● T22.22   Burn of second degree of elbow

- ● T22.221   Burn of second degree of right elbow
- ● T22.222   Burn of second degree of left elbow
- ● T22.229   Burn of second degree of unspecified elbow

● T22.23   Burn of second degree of upper arm
- ● T22.231   Burn of second degree of right upper arm
- ● T22.232   Burn of second degree of left upper arm
- ● T22.239   Burn of second degree of unspecified upper arm

● T22.24   Burn of second degree of axilla
- ● T22.241   Burn of second degree of right axilla
- ● T22.242   Burn of second degree of left axilla
- ● T22.249   Burn of second degree of unspecified axilla

● T22.25   Burn of second degree of shoulder
- ● T22.251   Burn of second degree of right shoulder
- ● T22.252   Burn of second degree of left shoulder
- ● T22.259   Burn of second degree of unspecified shoulder

● T22.26   Burn of second degree of scapular region
- ● T22.261   Burn of second degree of right scapular region
- ● T22.262   Burn of second degree of left scapular region
- ● T22.269   Burn of second degree of unspecified scapular region

● T22.29   Burn of second degree of multiple sites of shoulder and upper limb, except wrist and hand
- ● T22.291   Burn of second degree of multiple sites of right shoulder and upper limb, except wrist and hand
- ● T22.292   Burn of second degree of multiple sites of left shoulder and upper limb, except wrist and hand
- ● T22.299   Burn of second degree of multiple sites of unspecified shoulder and upper limb, except wrist and hand

● T22.3   Burn of third degree of shoulder and upper limb, except wrist and hand

Use additional external cause code to identify the source, place and intent of the burn (X00-X19, X75-X77, X96-X98, Y92)

X ● T22.30   Burn of third degree of shoulder and upper limb, except wrist and hand, unspecified site

● T22.31   Burn of third degree of forearm
- ● T22.311   Burn of third degree of right forearm
- ● T22.312   Burn of third degree of left forearm
- ● T22.319   Burn of third degree of unspecified forearm

● T22.32   Burn of third degree of elbow
- ● T22.321   Burn of third degree of right elbow
- ● T22.322   Burn of third degree of left elbow
- ● T22.329   Burn of third degree of unspecified elbow

● T22.33   Burn of third degree of upper arm
- ● T22.331   Burn of third degree of right upper arm
- ● T22.332   Burn of third degree of left upper arm
- ● T22.339   Burn of third degree of unspecified upper arm

● T22.34   Burn of third degree of axilla
    ● T22.341   Burn of third degree of right axilla
    ● T22.342   Burn of third degree of left axilla
    ● T22.349   Burn of third degree of unspecified axilla

● T22.35   Burn of third degree of shoulder
    ● T22.351   Burn of third degree of right shoulder
    ● T22.352   Burn of third degree of left shoulder
    ● T22.359   Burn of third degree of unspecified shoulder

● T22.36   Burn of third degree of scapular region
    ● T22.361   Burn of third degree of right scapular region
    ● T22.362   Burn of third degree of left scapular region
    ● T22.369   Burn of third degree of unspecified scapular region

● T22.39   Burn of third degree of multiple sites of shoulder and upper limb, except wrist and hand
    ● T22.391   Burn of third degree of multiple sites of right shoulder and upper limb, except wrist and hand
    ● T22.392   Burn of third degree of multiple sites of left shoulder and upper limb, except wrist and hand
    ● T22.399   Burn of third degree of multiple sites of unspecified shoulder and upper limb, except wrist and hand

● T22.4   Corrosion of unspecified degree of shoulder and upper limb, except wrist and hand
    Code first (T51-T65) to identify chemical and intent
    Use additional external cause code to identify place (Y92)

X ● T22.40   Corrosion of unspecified degree of shoulder and upper limb, except wrist and hand, unspecified site

● T22.41   Corrosion of unspecified degree of forearm
    ● T22.411   Corrosion of unspecified degree of right forearm
    ● T22.412   Corrosion of unspecified degree of left forearm
    ● T22.419   Corrosion of unspecified degree of unspecified forearm

● T22.42   Corrosion of unspecified degree of elbow
    ● T22.421   Corrosion of unspecified degree of right elbow
    ● T22.422   Corrosion of unspecified degree of left elbow
    ● T22.429   Corrosion of unspecified degree of unspecified elbow

● T22.43   Corrosion of unspecified degree of upper arm
    ● T22.431   Corrosion of unspecified degree of right upper arm
    ● T22.432   Corrosion of unspecified degree of left upper arm
    ● T22.439   Corrosion of unspecified degree of unspecified upper arm

● T22.44   Corrosion of unspecified degree of axilla
    ● T22.441   Corrosion of unspecified degree of right axilla
    ● T22.442   Corrosion of unspecified degree of left axilla
    ● T22.449   Corrosion of unspecified degree of unspecified axilla

● T22.45   Corrosion of unspecified degree of shoulder
    ● T22.451   Corrosion of unspecified degree of right shoulder
    ● T22.452   Corrosion of unspecified degree of left shoulder
    ● T22.459   Corrosion of unspecified degree of unspecified shoulder

● T22.46   Corrosion of unspecified degree of scapular region
    ● T22.461   Corrosion of unspecified degree of right scapular region
    ● T22.462   Corrosion of unspecified degree of left scapular region
    ● T22.469   Corrosion of unspecified degree of unspecified scapular region

● T22.49   Corrosion of unspecified degree of multiple sites of shoulder and upper limb, except wrist and hand
    ● T22.491   Corrosion of unspecified degree of multiple sites of right shoulder and upper limb, except wrist and hand
    ● T22.492   Corrosion of unspecified degree of multiple sites of left shoulder and upper limb, except wrist and hand
    ● T22.499   Corrosion of unspecified degree of multiple sites of unspecified shoulder and upper limb, except wrist and hand

● T22.5   Corrosion of first degree of shoulder and upper limb, except wrist and hand
    Code first (T51-T65) to identify chemical and intent
    Use additional external cause code to identify place (Y92)

X ● T22.50   Corrosion of first degree of shoulder and upper limb, except wrist and hand unspecified site

● T22.51   Corrosion of first degree of forearm
    ● T22.511   Corrosion of first degree of right forearm
    ● T22.512   Corrosion of first degree of left forearm
    ● T22.519   Corrosion of first degree of unspecified forearm

● T22.52   Corrosion of first degree of elbow
    ● T22.521   Corrosion of first degree of right elbow
    ● T22.522   Corrosion of first degree of left elbow
    ● T22.529   Corrosion of first degree of unspecified elbow

● T22.53   Corrosion of first degree of upper arm
    ● T22.531   Corrosion of first degree of right upper arm
    ● T22.532   Corrosion of first degree of left upper arm
    ● T22.539   Corrosion of first degree of unspecified upper arm

● T22.54   Corrosion of first degree of axilla
    ● T22.541   Corrosion of first degree of right axilla
    ● T22.542   Corrosion of first degree of left axilla
    ● T22.549   Corrosion of first degree of unspecified axilla

● T22.55   Corrosion of first degree of shoulder
    ● T22.551   Corrosion of first degree of right shoulder
    ● T22.552   Corrosion of first degree of left shoulder
    ● T22.559   Corrosion of first degree of unspecified shoulder

CHAPTER 19 (S00-T88)

● **T22.56**   Corrosion of first degree of scapular region
- ● **T22.561**   Corrosion of first degree of right scapular region
- ● **T22.562**   Corrosion of first degree of left scapular region
- ● **T22.569**   Corrosion of first degree of unspecified scapular region

● **T22.59**   Corrosion of first degree of multiple sites of shoulder and upper limb, except wrist and hand
- ● **T22.591**   Corrosion of first degree of multiple sites of right shoulder and upper limb, except wrist and hand
- ● **T22.592**   Corrosion of first degree of multiple sites of left shoulder and upper limb, except wrist and hand
- ● **T22.599**   Corrosion of first degree of multiple sites of unspecified shoulder and upper limb, except wrist and hand

● **T22.6**   Corrosion of second degree of shoulder and upper limb, except wrist and hand

     Code first (T51-T65) *to identify chemical and intent*

     Use additional external cause code to identify place (Y92)

   X ● **T22.60**   Corrosion of second degree of shoulder and upper limb, except wrist and hand, unspecified site

● **T22.61**   Corrosion of second degree of forearm
- ● **T22.611**   Corrosion of second degree of right forearm
- ● **T22.612**   Corrosion of second degree of left forearm
- ● **T22.619**   Corrosion of second degree of unspecified forearm

● **T22.62**   Corrosion of second degree of elbow
- ● **T22.621**   Corrosion of second degree of right elbow
- ● **T22.622**   Corrosion of second degree of left elbow
- ● **T22.629**   Corrosion of second degree of unspecified elbow

● **T22.63**   Corrosion of second degree of upper arm
- ● **T22.631**   Corrosion of second degree of right upper arm
- ● **T22.632**   Corrosion of second degree of left upper arm
- ● **T22.639**   Corrosion of second degree of unspecified upper arm

● **T22.64**   Corrosion of second degree of axilla
- ● **T22.641**   Corrosion of second degree of right axilla
- ● **T22.642**   Corrosion of second degree of left axilla
- ● **T22.649**   Corrosion of second degree of unspecified axilla

● **T22.65**   Corrosion of second degree of shoulder
- ● **T22.651**   Corrosion of second degree of right shoulder
- ● **T22.652**   Corrosion of second degree of left shoulder
- ● **T22.659**   Corrosion of second degree of unspecified shoulder

● **T22.66**   Corrosion of second degree of scapular region
- ● **T22.661**   Corrosion of second degree of right scapular region
- ● **T22.662**   Corrosion of second degree of left scapular region
- ● **T22.669**   Corrosion of second degree of unspecified scapular region

● **T22.69**   Corrosion of second degree of multiple sites of shoulder and upper limb, except wrist and hand
- ● **T22.691**   Corrosion of second degree of multiple sites of right shoulder and upper limb, except wrist and hand
- ● **T22.692**   Corrosion of second degree of multiple sites of left shoulder and upper limb, except wrist and hand
- ● **T22.699**   Corrosion of second degree of multiple sites of unspecified shoulder and upper limb, except wrist and hand

● **T22.7**   Corrosion of third degree of shoulder and upper limb, except wrist and hand

     Code first (T51-T65) *to identify chemical and intent*

     Use additional external cause code to identify place (Y92)

   X ● **T22.70**   Corrosion of third degree of shoulder and upper limb, except wrist and hand, unspecified site

● **T22.71**   Corrosion of third degree of forearm
- ● **T22.711**   Corrosion of third degree of right forearm
- ● **T22.712**   Corrosion of third degree of left forearm
- ● **T22.719**   Corrosion of third degree of unspecified forearm

● **T22.72**   Corrosion of third degree of elbow
- ● **T22.721**   Corrosion of third degree of right elbow
- ● **T22.722**   Corrosion of third degree of left elbow
- ● **T22.729**   Corrosion of third degree of unspecified elbow

● **T22.73**   Corrosion of third degree of upper arm
- ● **T22.731**   Corrosion of third degree of right upper arm
- ● **T22.732**   Corrosion of third degree of left upper arm
- ● **T22.739**   Corrosion of third degree of unspecified upper arm

● **T22.74**   Corrosion of third degree of axilla
- ● **T22.741**   Corrosion of third degree of right axilla
- ● **T22.742**   Corrosion of third degree of left axilla
- ● **T22.749**   Corrosion of third degree of unspecified axilla

● **T22.75**   Corrosion of third degree of shoulder
- ● **T22.751**   Corrosion of third degree of right shoulder
- ● **T22.752**   Corrosion of third degree of left shoulder
- ● **T22.759**   Corrosion of third degree of unspecified shoulder

● T22.76   Corrosion of third degree of scapular region
    ● T22.761   Corrosion of third degree of right scapular region
    ● T22.762   Corrosion of third degree of left scapular region
    ● T22.769   Corrosion of third degree of unspecified scapular region
● T22.79   Corrosion of third degree of multiple sites of shoulder and upper limb, except wrist and hand
    ● T22.791   Corrosion of third degree of multiple sites of right shoulder and upper limb, except wrist and hand
    ● T22.792   Corrosion of third degree of multiple sites of left shoulder and upper limb, except wrist and hand
    ● T22.799   Corrosion of third degree of multiple sites of unspecified shoulder and upper limb, except wrist and hand

● T23   Burn and corrosion of wrist and hand

> The appropriate 7th character is to be added to each code from category T23

> | | |
> |---|---|
> | A | initial encounter |
> | D | subsequent encounter |
> | S | sequela |

● T23.0   Burn of unspecified degree of wrist and hand

> Use additional external cause code to identify the source, place and intent of the burn (X00-X19, X75-X77, X96-X98, Y92)

    ● T23.00   Burn of unspecified degree of hand, unspecified site
       ● T23.001   Burn of unspecified degree of right hand, unspecified site
       ● T23.002   Burn of unspecified degree of left hand, unspecified site
       ● T23.009   Burn of unspecified degree of unspecified hand, unspecified site
    ● T23.01   Burn of unspecified degree of thumb (nail)
       ● T23.011   Burn of unspecified degree of right thumb (nail)
       ● T23.012   Burn of unspecified degree of left thumb (nail)
       ● T23.019   Burn of unspecified degree of unspecified thumb (nail)
    ● T23.02   Burn of unspecified degree of single finger (nail) except thumb
       ● T23.021   Burn of unspecified degree of single right finger (nail) except thumb
       ● T23.022   Burn of unspecified degree of single left finger (nail) except thumb
       ● T23.029   Burn of unspecified degree of unspecified single finger (nail) except thumb
    ● T23.03   Burn of unspecified degree of multiple fingers (nail), not including thumb
       ● T23.031   Burn of unspecified degree of multiple right fingers (nail), not including thumb
       ● T23.032   Burn of unspecified degree of multiple left fingers (nail), not including thumb
       ● T23.039   Burn of unspecified degree of unspecified multiple fingers (nail), not including thumb

● T23.04   Burn of unspecified degree of multiple fingers (nail), including thumb
    ● T23.041   Burn of unspecified degree of multiple right fingers (nail), including thumb
    ● T23.042   Burn of unspecified degree of multiple left fingers (nail), including thumb
    ● T23.049   Burn of unspecified degree of unspecified multiple fingers (nail), including thumb
● T23.05   Burn of unspecified degree of palm
    ● T23.051   Burn of unspecified degree of right palm
    ● T23.052   Burn of unspecified degree of left palm
    ● T23.059   Burn of unspecified degree of unspecified palm
● T23.06   Burn of unspecified degree of back of hand
    ● T23.061   Burn of unspecified degree of back of right hand
    ● T23.062   Burn of unspecified degree of back of left hand
    ● T23.069   Burn of unspecified degree of back of unspecified hand
● T23.07   Burn of unspecified degree of wrist
    ● T23.071   Burn of unspecified degree of right wrist
    ● T23.072   Burn of unspecified degree of left wrist
    ● T23.079   Burn of unspecified degree of unspecified wrist
● T23.09   Burn of unspecified degree of multiple sites of wrist and hand
    ● T23.091   Burn of unspecified degree of multiple sites of right wrist and hand
    ● T23.092   Burn of unspecified degree of multiple sites of left wrist and hand
    ● T23.099   Burn of unspecified degree of multiple sites of unspecified wrist and hand
● T23.1   Burn of first degree of wrist and hand

> Use additional external cause code to identify the source, place and intent of the burn (X00-X19, X75-X77, X96-X98, Y92)

    ● T23.10   Burn of first degree of hand, unspecified site
       ● T23.101   Burn of first degree of right hand, unspecified site
       ● T23.102   Burn of first degree of left hand, unspecified site
       ● T23.109   Burn of first degree of unspecified hand, unspecified site
    ● T23.11   Burn of first degree of thumb (nail)
       ● T23.111   Burn of first degree of right thumb (nail)
       ● T23.112   Burn of first degree of left thumb (nail)
       ● T23.119   Burn of first degree of unspecified thumb (nail)
    ● T23.12   Burn of first degree of single finger (nail) except thumb
       ● T23.121   Burn of first degree of single right finger (nail) except thumb
       ● T23.122   Burn of first degree of single left finger (nail) except thumb
       ● T23.129   Burn of first degree of unspecified single finger (nail) except thumb

CHAPTER 19 (S00-T88)

CHAPTER 19 (S00-T88)

- T23.13   Burn of first degree of multiple fingers (nail), not including thumb
  - T23.131   Burn of first degree of multiple right fingers (nail), not including thumb
  - T23.132   Burn of first degree of multiple left fingers (nail), not including thumb
  - T23.139   Burn of first degree of unspecified multiple fingers (nail), not including thumb
- T23.14   Burn of first degree of multiple fingers (nail), including thumb
  - T23.141   Burn of first degree of multiple right fingers (nail), including thumb
  - T23.142   Burn of first degree of multiple left fingers (nail), including thumb
  - T23.149   Burn of first degree of unspecified multiple fingers (nail), including thumb
- T23.15   Burn of first degree of palm
  - T23.151   Burn of first degree of right palm
  - T23.152   Burn of first degree of left palm
  - T23.159   Burn of first degree of unspecified palm
- T23.16   Burn of first degree of back of hand
  - T23.161   Burn of first degree of back of right hand
  - T23.162   Burn of first degree of back of left hand
  - T23.169   Burn of first degree of back of unspecified hand
- T23.17   Burn of first degree of wrist
  - T23.171   Burn of first degree of right wrist
  - T23.172   Burn of first degree of left wrist
  - T23.179   Burn of first degree of unspecified wrist
- T23.19   Burn of first degree of multiple sites of wrist and hand
  - T23.191   Burn of first degree of multiple sites of right wrist and hand
  - T23.192   Burn of first degree of multiple sites of left wrist and hand
  - T23.199   Burn of first degree of multiple sites of unspecified wrist and hand
- T23.2   Burn of second degree of wrist and hand

  Use additional external cause code to identify the source, place and intent of the burn (X00-X19, X75-X77, X96-X98, Y92)
  - T23.20   Burn of second degree of hand, unspecified site
    - T23.201   Burn of second degree of right hand, unspecified site
    - T23.202   Burn of second degree of left hand, unspecified site
    - T23.209   Burn of second degree of unspecified hand, unspecified site
  - T23.21   Burn of second degree of thumb (nail)
    - T23.211   Burn of second degree of right thumb (nail)
    - T23.212   Burn of second degree of left thumb (nail)
    - T23.219   Burn of second degree of unspecified thumb (nail)

- T23.22   Burn of second degree of single finger (nail) except thumb
  - T23.221   Burn of second degree of single right finger (nail) except thumb
  - T23.222   Burn of second degree of single left finger (nail) except thumb
  - T23.229   Burn of second degree of unspecified single finger (nail) except thumb
- T23.23   Burn of second degree of multiple fingers (nail), not including thumb
  - T23.231   Burn of second degree of multiple right fingers (nail), not including thumb
  - T23.232   Burn of second degree of multiple left fingers (nail), not including thumb
  - T23.239   Burn of second degree of unspecified multiple fingers (nail), not including thumb
- T23.24   Burn of second degree of multiple fingers (nail), including thumb
  - T23.241   Burn of second degree of multiple right fingers (nail), including thumb
  - T23.242   Burn of second degree of multiple left fingers (nail), including thumb
  - T23.249   Burn of second degree of unspecified multiple fingers (nail), including thumb
- T23.25   Burn of second degree of palm
  - T23.251   Burn of second degree of right palm
  - T23.252   Burn of second degree of left palm
  - T23.259   Burn of second degree of unspecified palm
- T23.26   Burn of second degree of back of hand
  - T23.261   Burn of second degree of back of right hand
  - T23.262   Burn of second degree of back of left hand
  - T23.269   Burn of second degree of back of unspecified hand
- T23.27   Burn of second degree of wrist
  - T23.271   Burn of second degree of right wrist
  - T23.272   Burn of second degree of left wrist
  - T23.279   Burn of second degree of unspecified wrist
- T23.29   Burn of second degree of multiple sites of wrist and hand
  - T23.291   Burn of second degree of multiple sites of right wrist and hand
  - T23.292   Burn of second degree of multiple sites of left wrist and hand
  - T23.299   Burn of second degree of multiple sites of unspecified wrist and hand
- T23.3   Burn of third degree of wrist and hand

  Use additional external cause code to identify the source, place and intent of the burn (X00-X19, X75-X77, X96-X98, Y92)
  - T23.30   Burn of third degree of hand, unspecified site
    - T23.301   Burn of third degree of right hand, unspecified site
      Coding Clinic: 2015, Q1, P19
    - T23.302   Burn of third degree of left hand, unspecified site
      Coding Clinic: 2016, Q2, P5
    - T23.309   Burn of third degree of unspecified hand, unspecified site

▶ New   ⇛ Revised   ~~deleted~~ Deleted   Excludes 1   Excludes 2   Includes   Use additional   Code first   Code also   Key words

OGCR Official Guidelines   X Assign placeholder X   ● Use Additional Character(s)   ▷ Manifestation Code   ⬥ Hierarchical Condition Category   **Coding Clinic**

- ● T23.31   Burn of third degree of thumb (nail)
  - ● T23.311   Burn of third degree of right thumb (nail)
  - ● T23.312   Burn of third degree of left thumb (nail)
  - ● T23.319   Burn of third degree of unspecified thumb (nail)
- ● T23.32   Burn of third degree of single finger (nail) except thumb
  - ● T23.321   Burn of third degree of single right finger (nail) except thumb
  - ● T23.322   Burn of third degree of single left finger (nail) except thumb
  - ● T23.329   Burn of third degree of unspecified single finger (nail) except thumb
- ● T23.33   Burn of third degree of multiple fingers (nail), not including thumb
  - ● T23.331   Burn of third degree of multiple right fingers (nail), not including thumb
  - ● T23.332   Burn of third degree of multiple left fingers (nail), not including thumb
  - ● T23.339   Burn of third degree of unspecified multiple fingers (nail), not including thumb
- ● T23.34   Burn of third degree of multiple fingers (nail), including thumb
  - ● T23.341   Burn of third degree of multiple right fingers (nail), including thumb
  - ● T23.342   Burn of third degree of multiple left fingers (nail), including thumb
  - ● T23.349   Burn of third degree of unspecified multiple fingers (nail), including thumb
- ● T23.35   Burn of third degree of palm
  - ● T23.351   Burn of third degree of right palm
  - ● T23.352   Burn of third degree of left palm
  - ● T23.359   Burn of third degree of unspecified palm
- ● T23.36   Burn of third degree of back of hand
  - ● T23.361   Burn of third degree of back of right hand
  - ● T23.362   Burn of third degree of back of left hand
  - ● T23.369   Burn of third degree of back of unspecified hand
- ● T23.37   Burn of third degree of wrist
  - ● T23.371   Burn of third degree of right wrist
  - ● T23.372   Burn of third degree of left wrist
  - ● T23.379   Burn of third degree of unspecified wrist
- ● T23.39   Burn of third degree of multiple sites of wrist and hand
  - ● T23.391   Burn of third degree of multiple sites of right wrist and hand
  - ● T23.392   Burn of third degree of multiple sites of left wrist and hand
  - ● T23.399   Burn of third degree of multiple sites of unspecified wrist and hand

- ● T23.4   Corrosion of unspecified degree of wrist and hand
  Code first (T51-T65) to identify chemical and intent
  Use additional external cause code to identify place (Y92)
  - ● T23.40   Corrosion of unspecified degree of hand, unspecified site
    - ● T23.401   Corrosion of unspecified degree of right hand, unspecified site
    - ● T23.402   Corrosion of unspecified degree of left hand, unspecified site
    - ● T23.409   Corrosion of unspecified degree of unspecified hand, unspecified site
  - ● T23.41   Corrosion of unspecified degree of thumb (nail)
    - ● T23.411   Corrosion of unspecified degree of right thumb (nail)
    - ● T23.412   Corrosion of unspecified degree of left thumb (nail)
    - ● T23.419   Corrosion of unspecified degree of unspecified thumb (nail)
  - ● T23.42   Corrosion of unspecified degree of single finger (nail) except thumb
    - ● T23.421   Corrosion of unspecified degree of single right finger (nail) except thumb
    - ● T23.422   Corrosion of unspecified degree of single left finger (nail) except thumb
    - ● T23.429   Corrosion of unspecified degree of unspecified single finger (nail) except thumb
  - ● T23.43   Corrosion of unspecified degree of multiple fingers (nail), not including thumb
    - ● T23.431   Corrosion of unspecified degree of multiple right fingers (nail), not including thumb
    - ● T23.432   Corrosion of unspecified degree of multiple left fingers (nail), not including thumb
    - ● T23.439   Corrosion of unspecified degree of unspecified multiple fingers (nail), not including thumb
  - ● T23.44   Corrosion of unspecified degree of multiple fingers (nail), including thumb
    - ● T23.441   Corrosion of unspecified degree of multiple right fingers (nail), including thumb
    - ● T23.442   Corrosion of unspecified degree of multiple left fingers (nail), including thumb
    - ● T23.449   Corrosion of unspecified degree of unspecified multiple fingers (nail), including thumb
  - ● T23.45   Corrosion of unspecified degree of palm
    - ● T23.451   Corrosion of unspecified degree of right palm
    - ● T23.452   Corrosion of unspecified degree of left palm
    - ● T23.459   Corrosion of unspecified degree of unspecified palm
  - ● T23.46   Corrosion of unspecified degree of back of hand
    - ● T23.461   Corrosion of unspecified degree of back of right hand
    - ● T23.462   Corrosion of unspecified degree of back of left hand
    - ● T23.469   Corrosion of unspecified degree of back of unspecified hand

CHAPTER 19 (S00-T88)

● T23.47   Corrosion of unspecified degree of wrist
- ● T23.471   Corrosion of unspecified degree of right wrist
- ● T23.472   Corrosion of unspecified degree of left wrist
- ● T23.479   Corrosion of unspecified degree of unspecified wrist

● T23.49   Corrosion of unspecified degree of multiple sites of wrist and hand
- ● T23.491   Corrosion of unspecified degree of multiple sites of right wrist and hand
- ● T23.492   Corrosion of unspecified degree of multiple sites of left wrist and hand
- ● T23.499   Corrosion of unspecified degree of multiple sites of unspecified wrist and hand

● T23.5   Corrosion of first degree of wrist and hand

Code first (T51-T65) to identify chemical and intent

Use additional external cause code to identify place (Y92)

● T23.50   Corrosion of first degree of hand, unspecified site
- ● T23.501   Corrosion of first degree of right hand, unspecified site
- ● T23.502   Corrosion of first degree of left hand, unspecified site
- ● T23.509   Corrosion of first degree of unspecified hand, unspecified site

● T23.51   Corrosion of first degree of thumb (nail)
- ● T23.511   Corrosion of first degree of right thumb (nail)
- ● T23.512   Corrosion of first degree of left thumb (nail)
- ● T23.519   Corrosion of first degree of unspecified thumb (nail)

● T23.52   Corrosion of first degree of single finger (nail) except thumb
- ● T23.521   Corrosion of first degree of single right finger (nail) except thumb
- ● T23.522   Corrosion of first degree of single left finger (nail) except thumb
- ● T23.529   Corrosion of first degree of unspecified single finger (nail) except thumb

● T23.53   Corrosion of first degree of multiple fingers (nail), not including thumb
- ● T23.531   Corrosion of first degree of multiple right fingers (nail), not including thumb
- ● T23.532   Corrosion of first degree of multiple left fingers (nail), not including thumb
- ● T23.539   Corrosion of first degree of unspecified multiple fingers (nail), not including thumb

● T23.54   Corrosion of first degree of multiple fingers (nail), including thumb
- ● T23.541   Corrosion of first degree of multiple right fingers (nail), including thumb
- ● T23.542   Corrosion of first degree of multiple left fingers (nail), including thumb
- ● T23.549   Corrosion of first degree of unspecified multiple fingers (nail), including thumb

● T23.55   Corrosion of first degree of palm
- ● T23.551   Corrosion of first degree of right palm
- ● T23.552   Corrosion of first degree of left palm
- ● T23.559   Corrosion of first degree of unspecified palm

● T23.56   Corrosion of first degree of back of hand
- ● T23.561   Corrosion of first degree of back of right hand
- ● T23.562   Corrosion of first degree of back of left hand
- ● T23.569   Corrosion of first degree of back of unspecified hand

● T23.57   Corrosion of first degree of wrist
- ● T23.571   Corrosion of first degree of right wrist
- ● T23.572   Corrosion of first degree of left wrist
- ● T23.579   Corrosion of first degree of unspecified wrist

● T23.59   Corrosion of first degree of multiple sites of wrist and hand
- ● T23.591   Corrosion of first degree of multiple sites of right wrist and hand
- ● T23.592   Corrosion of first degree of multiple sites of left wrist and hand
- ● T23.599   Corrosion of first degree of multiple sites of unspecified wrist and hand

● T23.6   Corrosion of second degree of wrist and hand

Code first (T51-T65) to identify chemical and intent

Use additional external cause code to identify place (Y92)

● T23.60   Corrosion of second degree of hand, unspecified site
- ● T23.601   Corrosion of second degree of right hand, unspecified site
- ● T23.602   Corrosion of second degree of left hand, unspecified site
- ● T23.609   Corrosion of second degree of unspecified hand, unspecified site

● T23.61   Corrosion of second degree of thumb (nail)
- ● T23.611   Corrosion of second degree of right thumb (nail)
- ● T23.612   Corrosion of second degree of left thumb (nail)
- ● T23.619   Corrosion of second degree of unspecified thumb (nail)

● T23.62   Corrosion of second degree of single finger (nail) except thumb
- ● T23.621   Corrosion of second degree of single right finger (nail) except thumb
- ● T23.622   Corrosion of second degree of single left finger (nail) except thumb
- ● T23.629   Corrosion of second degree of unspecified single finger (nail) except thumb

● T23.63   Corrosion of second degree of multiple fingers (nail), not including thumb
- ● T23.631   Corrosion of second degree of multiple right fingers (nail), not including thumb
- ● T23.632   Corrosion of second degree of multiple left fingers (nail), not including thumb
- ● T23.639   Corrosion of second degree of unspecified multiple fingers (nail), not including thumb

● T23.64   Corrosion of second degree of multiple fingers (nail), including thumb
- ● T23.641   Corrosion of second degree of multiple right fingers (nail), including thumb
- ● T23.642   Corrosion of second degree of multiple left fingers (nail), including thumb
- ● T23.649   Corrosion of second degree of unspecified multiple fingers (nail), including thumb

- **T23.65** Corrosion of second degree of palm
  - **T23.651** Corrosion of second degree of right palm
  - **T23.652** Corrosion of second degree of left palm
  - **T23.659** Corrosion of second degree of unspecified palm
- **T23.66** Corrosion of second degree of back of hand
  - **T23.661** Corrosion of second degree back of right hand
  - **T23.662** Corrosion of second degree back of left hand
  - **T23.669** Corrosion of second degree back of unspecified hand
- **T23.67** Corrosion of second degree of wrist
  - **T23.671** Corrosion of second degree of right wrist
  - **T23.672** Corrosion of second degree of left wrist
  - **T23.679** Corrosion of second degree of unspecified wrist
- **T23.69** Corrosion of second degree of multiple sites of wrist and hand
  - **T23.691** Corrosion of second degree of multiple sites of right wrist and hand
  - **T23.692** Corrosion of second degree of multiple sites of left wrist and hand
  - **T23.699** Corrosion of second degree of multiple sites of unspecified wrist and hand
- **T23.7** Corrosion of third degree of wrist and hand

  Code first (T51-T65) to identify chemical and intent

  Use additional external cause code to identify place (Y92)

  - **T23.70** Corrosion of third degree of hand, unspecified site
    - **T23.701** Corrosion of third degree of right hand, unspecified site
    - **T23.702** Corrosion of third degree of left hand, unspecified site
    - **T23.709** Corrosion of third degree of unspecified hand, unspecified site
  - **T23.71** Corrosion of third degree of thumb (nail)
    - **T23.711** Corrosion of third degree of right thumb (nail)
    - **T23.712** Corrosion of third degree of left thumb (nail)
    - **T23.719** Corrosion of third degree of unspecified thumb (nail)
  - **T23.72** Corrosion of third degree of single finger (nail) except thumb
    - **T23.721** Corrosion of third degree of single right finger (nail) except thumb
    - **T23.722** Corrosion of third degree of single left finger (nail) except thumb
    - **T23.729** Corrosion of third degree of unspecified single finger (nail) except thumb
  - **T23.73** Corrosion of third degree of multiple fingers (nail), not including thumb
    - **T23.731** Corrosion of third degree of multiple right fingers (nail), not including thumb
    - **T23.732** Corrosion of third degree of multiple left fingers (nail), not including thumb
    - **T23.739** Corrosion of third degree of unspecified multiple fingers (nail), not including thumb

- **T23.74** Corrosion of third degree of multiple fingers (nail), including thumb
  - **T23.741** Corrosion of third degree of multiple right fingers (nail), including thumb
  - **T23.742** Corrosion of third degree of multiple left fingers (nail), including thumb
  - **T23.749** Corrosion of third degree of unspecified multiple fingers (nail), including thumb
- **T23.75** Corrosion of third degree of palm
  - **T23.751** Corrosion of third degree of right palm
  - **T23.752** Corrosion of third degree of left palm
  - **T23.759** Corrosion of third degree of unspecified palm
- **T23.76** Corrosion of third degree of back of hand
  - **T23.761** Corrosion of third degree of back of right hand
  - **T23.762** Corrosion of third degree of back of left hand
  - **T23.769** Corrosion of third degree of back of unspecified hand
- **T23.77** Corrosion of third degree of wrist
  - **T23.771** Corrosion of third degree of right wrist
  - **T23.772** Corrosion of third degree of left wrist
  - **T23.779** Corrosion of third degree of unspecified wrist
- **T23.79** Corrosion of third degree of multiple sites of wrist and hand
  - **T23.791** Corrosion of third degree of multiple sites of right wrist and hand
  - **T23.792** Corrosion of third degree of multiple sites of left wrist and hand
  - **T23.799** Corrosion of third degree of multiple sites of unspecified wrist and hand

- **T24** Burn and corrosion of lower limb, except ankle and foot

  Excludes2   burn and corrosion of ankle and foot (T25.-)
  burn and corrosion of hip region (T21.-)

  The appropriate 7th character is to be added to each code from category T24

A	initial encounter
D	subsequent encounter
S	sequela

  - **T24.0** Burn of unspecified degree of lower limb, except ankle and foot

    Use additional external cause code to identify the source, place and intent of the burn (X00-X19, X75-X77, X96-X98, Y92)

    - **T24.00** Burn of unspecified degree of unspecified site of lower limb, except ankle and foot
      - **T24.001** Burn of unspecified degree of unspecified site of right lower limb, except ankle and foot
      - **T24.002** Burn of unspecified degree of unspecified site of left lower limb, except ankle and foot
      - **T24.009** Burn of unspecified degree of unspecified site of unspecified lower limb, except ankle and foot
    - **T24.01** Burn of unspecified degree of thigh
      - **T24.011** Burn of unspecified degree of right thigh
      - **T24.012** Burn of unspecified degree of left thigh
      - **T24.019** Burn of unspecified degree of unspecified thigh

- ● T24.02   Burn of unspecified degree of knee
  - ● T24.021   Burn of unspecified degree of right knee
  - ● T24.022   Burn of unspecified degree of left knee
  - ● T24.029   Burn of unspecified degree of unspecified knee
- ● T24.03   Burn of unspecified degree of lower leg
  - ● T24.031   Burn of unspecified degree of right lower leg
  - ● T24.032   Burn of unspecified degree of left lower leg
  - ● T24.039   Burn of unspecified degree of unspecified lower leg
- ● T24.09   Burn of unspecified degree of multiple sites of lower limb, except ankle and foot
  - ● T24.091   Burn of unspecified degree of multiple sites of right lower limb, except ankle and foot
  - ● T24.092   Burn of unspecified degree of multiple sites of left lower limb, except ankle and foot
  - ● T24.099   Burn of unspecified degree of multiple sites of unspecified lower limb, except ankle and foot
- ● T24.1   Burn of first degree of lower limb, except ankle and foot

  Use additional external cause code to identify the source, place and intent of the burn (X00-X19, X75-X77, X96-X98, Y92)

  - ● T24.10   Burn of first degree of unspecified site of lower limb, except ankle and foot
    - ● T24.101   Burn of first degree of unspecified site of right lower limb, except ankle and foot
    - ● T24.102   Burn of first degree of unspecified site of left lower limb, except ankle and foot
    - ● T24.109   Burn of first degree of unspecified site of unspecified lower limb, except ankle and foot
  - ● T24.11   Burn of first degree of thigh
    - ● T24.111   Burn of first degree of right thigh
    - ● T24.112   Burn of first degree of left thigh
    - ● T24.119   Burn of first degree of unspecified thigh
  - ● T24.12   Burn of first degree of knee
    - ● T24.121   Burn of first degree of right knee
    - ● T24.122   Burn of first degree of left knee
    - ● T24.129   Burn of first degree of unspecified knee
  - ● T24.13   Burn of first degree of lower leg
    - ● T24.131   Burn of first degree of right lower leg
    - ● T24.132   Burn of first degree of left lower leg
    - ● T24.139   Burn of first degree of unspecified lower leg
  - ● T24.19   Burn of first degree of multiple sites of lower limb, except ankle and foot
    - ● T24.191   Burn of first degree of multiple sites of right lower limb, except ankle and foot
    - ● T24.192   Burn of first degree of multiple sites of left lower limb, except ankle and foot
    - ● T24.199   Burn of first degree of multiple sites of unspecified lower limb, except ankle and foot

- ● T24.2   Burn of second degree of lower limb, except ankle and foot

  Use additional external cause code to identify the source, place and intent of the burn (X00-X19, X75-X77, X96-X98, Y92)

  - ● T24.20   Burn of second degree of unspecified site of lower limb, except ankle and foot
    - ● T24.201   Burn of second degree of unspecified site of right lower limb, except ankle and foot
    - ● T24.202   Burn of second degree of unspecified site of left lower limb, except ankle and foot
    - ● T24.209   Burn of second degree of unspecified site of unspecified lower limb, except ankle and foot
  - ● T24.21   Burn of second degree of thigh
    - ● T24.211   Burn of second degree of right thigh
    - ● T24.212   Burn of second degree of left thigh
    - ● T24.219   Burn of second degree of unspecified thigh
  - ● T24.22   Burn of second degree of knee
    - ● T24.221   Burn of second degree of right knee
    - ● T24.222   Burn of second degree of left knee
    - ● T24.229   Burn of second degree of unspecified knee
  - ● T24.23   Burn of second degree of lower leg
    - ● T24.231   Burn of second degree of right lower leg
    - ● T24.232   Burn of second degree of left lower leg
    - ● T24.239   Burn of second degree of unspecified lower leg
  - ● T24.29   Burn of second degree of multiple sites of lower limb, except ankle and foot
    - ● T24.291   Burn of second degree of multiple sites of right lower limb, except ankle and foot
    - ● T24.292   Burn of second degree of multiple sites of left lower limb, except ankle and foot
    - ● T24.299   Burn of second degree of multiple sites of unspecified lower limb, except ankle and foot
- ● T24.3   Burn of third degree of lower limb, except ankle and foot

  Use additional external cause code to identify the source, place and intent of the burn (X00-X19, X75-X77, X96-X98, Y92)

  - ● T24.30   Burn of third degree of unspecified site of lower limb, except ankle and foot
    - ● T24.301   Burn of third degree of unspecified site of right lower limb, except ankle and foot
    - ● T24.302   Burn of third degree of unspecified site of left lower limb, except ankle and foot
    - ● T24.309   Burn of third degree of unspecified site of unspecified lower limb, except ankle and foot
  - ● T24.31   Burn of third degree of thigh
    - ● T24.311   Burn of third degree of right thigh
    - ● T24.312   Burn of third degree of left thigh
    - ● T24.319   Burn of third degree of unspecified thigh

● T24.32　Burn of third degree of knee
- ● T24.321　Burn of third degree of right knee
- ● T24.322　Burn of third degree of left knee
- ● T24.329　Burn of third degree of unspecified knee

● T24.33　Burn of third degree of lower leg
- ● T24.331　Burn of third degree of right lower leg
- ● T24.332　Burn of third degree of left lower leg
- ● T24.339　Burn of third degree of unspecified lower leg

● T24.39　Burn of third degree of multiple sites of lower limb, except ankle and foot
- ● T24.391　Burn of third degree of multiple sites of right lower limb, except ankle and foot
  - **Coding Clinic: 2016, Q2, P5**
- ● T24.392　Burn of third degree of multiple sites of left lower limb, except ankle and foot
- ● T24.399　Burn of third degree of multiple sites of unspecified lower limb, except ankle and foot

● T24.4　Corrosion of unspecified degree of lower limb, except ankle and foot

　Code first (T51-T65) to identify chemical and intent
　Use additional external cause code to identify place (Y92)

- ● T24.40　Corrosion of unspecified degree of unspecified site of lower limb, except ankle and foot
  - ● T24.401　Corrosion of unspecified degree of unspecified site of right lower limb, except ankle and foot
  - ● T24.402　Corrosion of unspecified degree of unspecified site of left lower limb, except ankle and foot
  - ● T24.409　Corrosion of unspecified degree of unspecified site of unspecified lower limb, except ankle and foot
- ● T24.41　Corrosion of unspecified degree of thigh
  - ● T24.411　Corrosion of unspecified degree of right thigh
  - ● T24.412　Corrosion of unspecified degree of left thigh
  - ● T24.419　Corrosion of unspecified degree of unspecified thigh
- ● T24.42　Corrosion of unspecified degree of knee
  - ● T24.421　Corrosion of unspecified degree of right knee
  - ● T24.422　Corrosion of unspecified degree of left knee
  - ● T24.429　Corrosion of unspecified degree of unspecified knee
- ● T24.43　Corrosion of unspecified degree of lower leg
  - ● T24.431　Corrosion of unspecified degree of right lower leg
  - ● T24.432　Corrosion of unspecified degree of left lower leg
  - ● T24.439　Corrosion of unspecified degree of unspecified lower leg
- ● T24.49　Corrosion of unspecified degree of multiple sites of lower limb, except ankle and foot
  - ● T24.491　Corrosion of unspecified degree of multiple sites of right lower limb, except ankle and foot
  - ● T24.492　Corrosion of unspecified degree of multiple sites of left lower limb, except ankle and foot
  - ● T24.499　Corrosion of unspecified degree of multiple sites of unspecified lower limb, except ankle and foot

● T24.5　Corrosion of first degree of lower limb, except ankle and foot

　Code first (T51-T65) to identify chemical and intent
　Use additional external cause code to identify place (Y92)

- ● T24.50　Corrosion of first degree of unspecified site of lower limb, except ankle and foot
  - ● T24.501　Corrosion of first degree of unspecified site of right lower limb, except ankle and foot
  - ● T24.502　Corrosion of first degree of unspecified site of left lower limb, except ankle and foot
  - ● T24.509　Corrosion of first degree of unspecified site of unspecified lower limb, except ankle and foot
- ● T24.51　Corrosion of first degree of thigh
  - ● T24.511　Corrosion of first degree of right thigh
  - ● T24.512　Corrosion of first degree of left thigh
  - ● T24.519　Corrosion of first degree of unspecified thigh
- ● T24.52　Corrosion of first degree of knee
  - ● T24.521　Corrosion of first degree of right knee
  - ● T24.522　Corrosion of first degree of left knee
  - ● T24.529　Corrosion of first degree of unspecified knee
- ● T24.53　Corrosion of first degree of lower leg
  - ● T24.531　Corrosion of first degree of right lower leg
  - ● T24.532　Corrosion of first degree of left lower leg
  - ● T24.539　Corrosion of first degree of unspecified lower leg
- ● T24.59　Corrosion of first degree of multiple sites of lower limb, except ankle and foot
  - ● T24.591　Corrosion of first degree of multiple sites of right lower limb, except ankle and foot
  - ● T24.592　Corrosion of first degree of multiple sites of left lower limb, except ankle and foot
  - ● T24.599　Corrosion of first degree of multiple sites of unspecified lower limb, except ankle and foot

● T24.6　Corrosion of second degree of lower limb, except ankle and foot

　Code first (T51-T65) to identify chemical and intent
　Use additional external cause code to identify place (Y92)

- ● T24.60　Corrosion of second degree of unspecified site of lower limb, except ankle and foot
  - ● T24.601　Corrosion of second degree of unspecified site of right lower limb, except ankle and foot
  - ● T24.602　Corrosion of second degree of unspecified site of left lower limb, except ankle and foot
  - ● T24.609　Corrosion of second degree of unspecified site of unspecified lower limb, except ankle and foot
- ● T24.61　Corrosion of second degree of thigh
  - ● T24.611　Corrosion of second degree of right thigh
  - ● T24.612　Corrosion of second degree of left thigh
  - ● T24.619　Corrosion of second degree of unspecified thigh

CHAPTER 19 (S00-T88)

- T24.62 Corrosion of second degree of knee
  - T24.621 Corrosion of second degree of right knee
  - T24.622 Corrosion of second degree of left knee
  - T24.629 Corrosion of second degree of unspecified knee
- T24.63 Corrosion of second degree of lower leg
  - T24.631 Corrosion of second degree of right lower leg
  - T24.632 Corrosion of second degree of left lower leg
  - T24.639 Corrosion of second degree of unspecified lower leg
- T24.69 Corrosion of second degree of multiple sites of lower limb, except ankle and foot
  - T24.691 Corrosion of second degree of multiple sites of right lower limb, except ankle and foot
  - T24.692 Corrosion of second degree of multiple sites of left lower limb, except ankle and foot
  - T24.699 Corrosion of second degree of multiple sites of unspecified lower limb, except ankle and foot
- T24.7 Corrosion of third degree of lower limb, except ankle and foot

  Code first (T51-T65) to identify chemical and intent

  Use additional external cause code to identify place (Y92)

  - T24.70 Corrosion of third degree of unspecified site of lower limb, except ankle and foot
    - T24.701 Corrosion of third degree of unspecified site of right lower limb, except ankle and foot
    - T24.702 Corrosion of third degree of unspecified site of left lower limb, except ankle and foot
    - T24.709 Corrosion of third degree of unspecified site of unspecified lower limb, except ankle and foot
  - T24.71 Corrosion of third degree of thigh
    - T24.711 Corrosion of third degree of right thigh
    - T24.712 Corrosion of third degree of left thigh
    - T24.719 Corrosion of third degree of unspecified thigh
  - T24.72 Corrosion of third degree of knee
    - T24.721 Corrosion of third degree of right knee
    - T24.722 Corrosion of third degree of left knee
    - T24.729 Corrosion of third degree of unspecified knee
  - T24.73 Corrosion of third degree of lower leg
    - T24.731 Corrosion of third degree of right lower leg
    - T24.732 Corrosion of third degree of left lower leg
    - T24.739 Corrosion of third degree of unspecified lower leg
  - T24.79 Corrosion of third degree of multiple sites of lower limb, except ankle and foot
    - T24.791 Corrosion of third degree of multiple sites of right lower limb, except ankle and foot
    - T24.792 Corrosion of third degree of multiple sites of left lower limb, except ankle and foot
    - T24.799 Corrosion of third degree of multiple sites of unspecified lower limb, except ankle and foot

- T25 Burn and corrosion of ankle and foot

  The appropriate 7th character is to be added to each code from category T25

A	initial encounter
D	subsequent encounter
S	sequela

- T25.0 Burn of unspecified degree of ankle and foot

  Use additional external cause code to identify the source, place and intent of the burn (X00-X19, X75-X77, X96-X98, Y92)

  - T25.01 Burn of unspecified degree of ankle
    - T25.011 Burn of unspecified degree of right ankle
    - T25.012 Burn of unspecified degree of left ankle
    - T25.019 Burn of unspecified degree of unspecified ankle
  - T25.02 Burn of unspecified degree of foot

    Excludes2 burn of unspecified degree of toe(s) (nail) (T25.03-)

    - T25.021 Burn of unspecified degree of right foot
    - T25.022 Burn of unspecified degree of left foot
    - T25.029 Burn of unspecified degree of unspecified foot
  - T25.03 Burn of unspecified degree of toe(s) (nail)
    - T25.031 Burn of unspecified degree of right toe(s) (nail)
    - T25.032 Burn of unspecified degree of left toe(s) (nail)
    - T25.039 Burn of unspecified degree of unspecified toe(s) (nail)
  - T25.09 Burn of unspecified degree of multiple sites of ankle and foot
    - T25.091 Burn of unspecified degree of multiple sites of right ankle and foot
    - T25.092 Burn of unspecified degree of multiple sites of left ankle and foot
    - T25.099 Burn of unspecified degree of multiple sites of unspecified ankle and foot
- T25.1 Burn of first degree of ankle and foot

  Use additional external cause code to identify the source, place and intent of the burn (X00-X19, X75-X77, X96-X98, Y92)

  - T25.11 Burn of first degree of ankle
    - T25.111 Burn of first degree of right ankle
    - T25.112 Burn of first degree of left ankle
    - T25.119 Burn of first degree of unspecified ankle
  - T25.12 Burn of first degree of foot

    Excludes2 burn of first degree of toe(s) (nail) (T25.13-)

    - T25.121 Burn of first degree of right foot
    - T25.122 Burn of first degree of left foot
    - T25.129 Burn of first degree of unspecified foot
  - T25.13 Burn of first degree of toe(s) (nail)
    - T25.131 Burn of first degree of right toe(s) (nail)
    - T25.132 Burn of first degree of left toe(s) (nail)
    - T25.139 Burn of first degree of unspecified toe(s) (nail)

▶ New   ⇒ Revised   deleted Deleted   Excludes 1   Excludes 2   Includes   Use additional   Code first   Code also   Key words

OGCR Official Guidelines   X Assign placeholder X   ● Use Additional Character(s)   ▶ Manifestation Code   🐾 Hierarchical Condition Category   Coding Clinic

● T25.19   Burn of first degree of multiple sites of ankle and foot

  ● T25.191   Burn of first degree of multiple sites of right ankle and foot

  ● T25.192   Burn of first degree of multiple sites of left ankle and foot

  ● T25.199   Burn of first degree of multiple sites of unspecified ankle and foot

● T25.2   Burn of second degree of ankle and foot

  Use additional external cause code to identify the source, place and intent of the burn (X00-X19, X75-X77, X96-X98, Y92)

  ● T25.21   Burn of second degree of ankle

    ● T25.211   Burn of second degree of right ankle

    ● T25.212   Burn of second degree of left ankle

    ● T25.219   Burn of second degree of unspecified ankle

  ● T25.22   Burn of second degree of foot

    Excludes2   burn of second degree of toe(s) (nail) (T25.23-)

    ● T25.221   Burn of second degree of right foot

    ● T25.222   Burn of second degree of left foot

    ● T25.229   Burn of second degree of unspecified foot

  ● T25.23   Burn of second degree of toe(s) (nail)

    ● T25.231   Burn of second degree of right toe(s) (nail)

    ● T25.232   Burn of second degree of left toe(s) (nail)

    ● T25.239   Burn of second degree of unspecified toe(s) (nail)

  ● T25.29   Burn of second degree of multiple sites of ankle and foot

    ● T25.291   Burn of second degree of multiple sites of right ankle and foot

    ● T25.292   Burn of second degree of multiple sites of left ankle and foot

    ● T25.299   Burn of second degree of multiple sites of unspecified ankle and foot

● T25.3   Burn of third degree of ankle and foot

  Use additional external cause code to identify the source, place and intent of the burn (X00-X19, X75-X77, X96-X98, Y92)

  ● T25.31   Burn of third degree of ankle

    ● T25.311   Burn of third degree of right ankle

    ● T25.312   Burn of third degree of left ankle

    ● T25.319   Burn of third degree of unspecified ankle

  ● T25.32   Burn of third degree of foot

    Excludes2   burn of third degree of toe(s) (nail) (T25.33-)

    ● T25.321   Burn of third degree of right foot

    ● T25.322   Burn of third degree of left foot

    ● T25.329   Burn of third degree of unspecified foot

  ● T25.33   Burn of third degree of toe(s) (nail)

    ● T25.331   Burn of third degree of right toe(s) (nail)

    ● T25.332   Burn of third degree of left toe(s) (nail)

    ● T25.339   Burn of third degree of unspecified toe(s) (nail)

● T25.39   Burn of third degree of multiple sites of ankle and foot

  ● T25.391   Burn of third degree of multiple sites of right ankle and foot

  ● T25.392   Burn of third degree of multiple sites of left ankle and foot

  ● T25.399   Burn of third degree of multiple sites of unspecified ankle and foot

● T25.4   Corrosion of unspecified degree of ankle and foot

  Code first (T51-T65) to identify chemical and intent

  Use additional external cause code to identify place (Y92)

  ● T25.41   Corrosion of unspecified degree of ankle

    ● T25.411   Corrosion of unspecified degree of right ankle

    ● T25.412   Corrosion of unspecified degree of left ankle

    ● T25.419   Corrosion of unspecified degree of unspecified ankle

  ● T25.42   Corrosion of unspecified degree of foot

    Excludes2   corrosion of unspecified degree of toe(s) (nail) (T25.43-)

    ● T25.421   Corrosion of unspecified degree of right foot

    ● T25.422   Corrosion of unspecified degree of left foot

    ● T25.429   Corrosion of unspecified degree of unspecified foot

  ● T25.43   Corrosion of unspecified degree of toe(s) (nail)

    ● T25.431   Corrosion of unspecified degree of right toe(s) (nail)

    ● T25.432   Corrosion of unspecified degree of left toe(s) (nail)

    ● T25.439   Corrosion of unspecified degree of unspecified toe(s) (nail)

  ● T25.49   Corrosion of unspecified degree of multiple sites of ankle and foot

    ● T25.491   Corrosion of unspecified degree of multiple sites of right ankle and foot

    ● T25.492   Corrosion of unspecified degree of multiple sites of left ankle and foot

    ● T25.499   Corrosion of unspecified degree of multiple sites of unspecified ankle and foot

● T25.5   Corrosion of first degree of ankle and foot

  Code first (T51-T65) to identify chemical and intent

  Use additional external cause code to identify place (Y92)

  ● T25.51   Corrosion of first degree of ankle

    ● T25.511   Corrosion of first degree of right ankle

    ● T25.512   Corrosion of first degree of left ankle

    ● T25.519   Corrosion of first degree of unspecified ankle

  ● T25.52   Corrosion of first degree of foot

    Excludes2   corrosion of first degree of toe(s) (nail) (T25.53-)

    ● T25.521   Corrosion of first degree of right foot

    ● T25.522   Corrosion of first degree of left foot

    ● T25.529   Corrosion of first degree of unspecified foot

CHAPTER 19 (S00-T88)

- ● T25.53 Corrosion of first degree of toe(s) (nail)
  - ● T25.531 Corrosion of first degree of right toe(s) (nail)
  - ● T25.532 Corrosion of first degree of left toe(s) (nail)
  - ● T25.539 Corrosion of first degree of unspecified toe(s) (nail)
- ● T25.59 Corrosion of first degree of multiple sites of ankle and foot
  - ● T25.591 Corrosion of first degree of multiple sites of right ankle and foot
  - ● T25.592 Corrosion of first degree of multiple sites of left ankle and foot
  - ● T25.599 Corrosion of first degree of multiple sites of unspecified ankle and foot
- ● T25.6 Corrosion of second degree of ankle and foot

  Code first (T51-T65) to identify chemical and intent

  Use additional external cause code to identify place (Y92)
  - ● T25.61 Corrosion of second degree of ankle
    - ● T25.611 Corrosion of second degree of right ankle
    - ● T25.612 Corrosion of second degree of left ankle
    - ● T25.619 Corrosion of second degree of unspecified ankle
  - ● T25.62 Corrosion of second degree of foot

    Excludes2 corrosion of second degree of toe(s) (nail) (T25.63-)
    - ● T25.621 Corrosion of second degree of right foot
    - ● T25.622 Corrosion of second degree of left foot
    - ● T25.629 Corrosion of second degree of unspecified foot
  - ● T25.63 Corrosion of second degree of toe(s) (nail)
    - ● T25.631 Corrosion of second degree of right toe(s) (nail)
    - ● T25.632 Corrosion of second degree of left toe(s) (nail)
    - ● T25.639 Corrosion of second degree of unspecified toe(s) (nail)
  - ● T25.69 Corrosion of second degree of multiple sites of ankle and foot
    - ● T25.691 Corrosion of second degree of right ankle and foot
    - ● T25.692 Corrosion of second degree of left ankle and foot
    - ● T25.699 Corrosion of second degree of unspecified ankle and foot
- ● T25.7 Corrosion of third degree of ankle and foot

  Code first (T51-T65) to identify chemical and intent

  Use additional external cause code to identify place (Y92)
  - ● T25.71 Corrosion of third degree of ankle
    - ● T25.711 Corrosion of third degree of right ankle
    - ● T25.712 Corrosion of third degree of left ankle
    - ● T25.719 Corrosion of third degree of unspecified ankle
  - ● T25.72 Corrosion of third degree of foot

    Excludes2 corrosion of third degree of toe(s) (nail) (T25.73-)
    - ● T25.721 Corrosion of third degree of right foot
    - ● T25.722 Corrosion of third degree of left foot
    - ● T25.729 Corrosion of third degree of unspecified foot

- ● T25.73 Corrosion of third degree of toe(s) (nail)
  - ● T25.731 Corrosion of third degree of right toe(s) (nail)
  - ● T25.732 Corrosion of third degree of left toe(s) (nail)
  - ● T25.739 Corrosion of third degree of unspecified toe(s) (nail)
- ● T25.79 Corrosion of third degree of multiple sites of ankle and foot
  - ● T25.791 Corrosion of third degree of multiple sites of right ankle and foot
  - ● T25.792 Corrosion of third degree of multiple sites of left ankle and foot
  - ● T25.799 Corrosion of third degree of multiple sites of unspecified ankle and foot

BURNS AND CORROSIONS CONFINED TO EYE AND INTERNAL ORGANS (T26-T28)

- ● T26 Burn and corrosion confined to eye and adnexa

  The appropriate 7th character is to be added to each code from category T26

A	initial encounter
D	subsequent encounter
S	sequela

- ● T26.0 Burn of eyelid and periocular area

  Use additional external cause code to identify the source, place and intent of the burn (X00-X19, X75-X77, X96-X98, Y92)
  - X● T26.00 Burn of unspecified eyelid and periocular area
  - X● T26.01 Burn of right eyelid and periocular area
  - X● T26.02 Burn of left eyelid and periocular area
- ● T26.1 Burn of cornea and conjunctival sac

  Use additional external cause code to identify the source, place and intent of the burn (X00-X19, X75-X77, X96-X98, Y92)
  - X● T26.10 Burn of cornea and conjunctival sac, unspecified eye
  - X● T26.11 Burn of cornea and conjunctival sac, right eye
  - X● T26.12 Burn of cornea and conjunctival sac, left eye
- ● T26.2 Burn with resulting rupture and destruction of eyeball

  Use additional external cause code to identify the source, place and intent of the burn (X00-X19, X75-X77, X96-X98, Y92)
  - X● T26.20 Burn with resulting rupture and destruction of unspecified eyeball
  - X● T26.21 Burn with resulting rupture and destruction of right eyeball
  - X● T26.22 Burn with resulting rupture and destruction of left eyeball
- ● T26.3 Burns of other specified parts of eye and adnexa

  Use additional external cause code to identify the source, place and intent of the burn (X00-X19, X75-X77, X96-X98, Y92)
  - X● T26.30 Burns of other specified parts of unspecified eye and adnexa
  - X● T26.31 Burns of other specified parts of right eye and adnexa
  - X● T26.32 Burns of other specified parts of left eye and adnexa
- ● T26.4 Burn of eye and adnexa, part unspecified

  Use additional external cause code to identify the source, place and intent of the burn (X00-X19, X75-X77, X96-X98, Y92)
  - X● T26.40 Burn of unspecified eye and adnexa, part unspecified
  - X● T26.41 Burn of right eye and adnexa, part unspecified
  - X● T26.42 Burn of left eye and adnexa, part unspecified

● **T26.5**   Corrosion of eyelid and periocular area
>   *Code first (T51-T65) to identify chemical and intent*
>   Use additional external cause code to identify place (Y92)

  X● **T26.50**   Corrosion of unspecified eyelid and periocular area

  X● **T26.51**   Corrosion of right eyelid and periocular area

  X● **T26.52**   Corrosion of left eyelid and periocular area

● **T26.6**   Corrosion of cornea and conjunctival sac
>   *Code first (T51-T65) to identify chemical and intent*
>   Use additional external cause code to identify place (Y92)

  X● **T26.60**   Corrosion of cornea and conjunctival sac, unspecified eye

  X● **T26.61**   Corrosion of cornea and conjunctival sac, right eye

  X● **T26.62**   Corrosion of cornea and conjunctival sac, left eye

● **T26.7**   Corrosion with resulting rupture and destruction of eyeball
>   *Code first (T51-T65) to identify chemical and intent*
>   Use additional external cause code to identify place (Y92)

  X● **T26.70**   Corrosion with resulting rupture and destruction of unspecified eyeball

  X● **T26.71**   Corrosion with resulting rupture and destruction of right eyeball

  X● **T26.72**   Corrosion with resulting rupture and destruction of left eyeball

● **T26.8**   Corrosions of other specified parts of eye and adnexa
>   *Code first (T51-T65) to identify chemical and intent*
>   Use additional external cause code to identify place (Y92)

  X● **T26.80**   Corrosions of other specified parts of unspecified eye and adnexa

  X● **T26.81**   Corrosions of other specified parts of right eye and adnexa

  X● **T26.82**   Corrosions of other specified parts of left eye and adnexa

● **T26.9**   Corrosion of eye and adnexa, part unspecified
>   *Code first (T51-T65) to identify chemical and intent*
>   Use additional external cause code to identify place (Y92)

  X● **T26.90**   Corrosion of unspecified eye and adnexa, part unspecified

  X● **T26.91**   Corrosion of right eye and adnexa, part unspecified

  X● **T26.92**   Corrosion of left eye and adnexa, part unspecified

● **T27**   Burn and corrosion of respiratory tract
>   Use additional external cause code to identify the source and intent of the burn (X00-X19, X75-X77, X96-X98)
>   Use additional external cause code to identify place (Y92)
>   The appropriate 7th character is to be added to each code from category T27

A	initial encounter
D	subsequent encounter
S	sequela

  X● **T27.0**   Burn of larynx and trachea

  X● **T27.1**   Burn involving larynx and trachea with lung

  X● **T27.2**   Burn of other parts of respiratory tract
>   Burn of thoracic cavity

  X● **T27.3**   Burn of respiratory tract, part unspecified

  X● **T27.4**   Corrosion of larynx and trachea
>   *Code first (T51-T65) to identify chemical and intent*

  X● **T27.5**   Corrosion involving larynx and trachea with lung
>   *Code first (T51-T65) to identify chemical and intent*

  X● **T27.6**   Corrosion of other parts of respiratory tract
>   *Code first (T51-T65) to identify chemical and intent*

  X● **T27.7**   Corrosion of respiratory tract, part unspecified
>   *Code first (T51-T65) to identify chemical and intent*

● **T28**   Burn and corrosion of other internal organs
>   Use additional external cause code to identify the source and intent of the burn (X00-X19, X75-X77, X96-X98)
>   Use additional external cause code to identify place (Y92)
>   The appropriate 7th character is to be added to each code from category T28

A	initial encounter
D	subsequent encounter
S	sequela

  X● **T28.0**   Burn of mouth and pharynx

  X● **T28.1**   Burn of esophagus

  X● **T28.2**   Burn of other parts of alimentary tract

  X● **T28.3**   Burn of internal genitourinary organs

  X● **T28.4**   Burns of other and unspecified internal organs

  X● **T28.40**   Burn of unspecified internal organ

  ● **T28.41**   Burn of ear drum

  ● **T28.411**   Burn of right ear drum

  ● **T28.412**   Burn of left ear drum

  ● **T28.419**   Burn of unspecified ear drum

  X● **T28.49**   Burn of other internal organ

  X● **T28.5**   Corrosion of mouth and pharynx
>   *Code first (T51-T65) to identify chemical and intent*

  X● **T28.6**   Corrosion of esophagus
>   *Code first (T51-T65) to identify chemical and intent*

  X● **T28.7**   Corrosion of other parts of alimentary tract
>   *Code first (T51-T65) to identify chemical and intent*

  X● **T28.8**   Corrosion of internal genitourinary organs
>   *Code first (T51-T65) to identify chemical and intent*

  ● **T28.9**   Corrosions of other and unspecified internal organs
>   *Code first (T51-T65) to identify chemical and intent*

  X● **T28.90**   Corrosions of unspecified internal organs

  ● **T28.91**   Corrosions of ear drum

  ● **T28.911**   Corrosions of right ear drum

  ● **T28.912**   Corrosions of left ear drum

  ● **T28.919**   Corrosions of unspecified ear drum

  X● **T28.99**   Corrosions of other internal organs

OGCR Section I.C.19.d.5.

Assign separate code for each burn site

When coding burns, assign separate codes for each burn site. Category T30, Burn and corrosion, body region unspecified is extremely vague and should rarely be used.

BURNS AND CORROSIONS OF MULTIPLE AND UNSPECIFIED BODY REGIONS (T30-T32)

● **T30**   Burn and corrosion, body region unspecified

  T30.0   Burn of unspecified body region, unspecified degree
>   This code is not for inpatient use. Code to specified site and degree of burns
>   Burn NOS
>   Multiple burns NOS

  T30.4   Corrosion of unspecified body region, unspecified degree
>   This code is not for inpatient use. Code to specified site and degree of corrosion
>   Corrosion NOS
>   Multiple corrosion NOS

CHAPTER 19 (S00-T88)

CHAPTER 19 (S00-T88)

● **T31**   Burns classified according to extent of body surface involved

     Note: This category is to be used as the primary code only when the site of the burn is unspecified. It should be used as a supplementary code with categories T20-T25 when the site is specified.

    T31.0   Burns involving less than 10% of body surface

● **T31.1**   Burns involving 10-19% of body surface

      T31.10   Burns involving 10-19% of body surface with 0% to 9% third degree burns
          Burns involving 10-19% of body surface NOS

      T31.11   Burns involving 10-19% of body surface with 10-19% third degree burns

● **T31.2**   Burns involving 20-29% of body surface

      T31.20   Burns involving 20-29% of body surface with 0% to 9% third degree burns
          Burns involving 20-29% of body surface NOS

      T31.21   Burns involving 20-29% of body surface with 10-19% third degree burns

      T31.22   Burns involving 20-29% of body surface with 20-29% third degree burns

● **T31.3**   Burns involving 30-39% of body surface

      T31.30   Burns involving 30-39% of body surface with 0% to 9% third degree burns
          Burns involving 30-39% of body surface NOS

      T31.31   Burns involving 30-39% of body surface with 10-19% third degree burns

      T31.32   Burns involving 30-39% of body surface with 20-29% third degree burns

      T31.33   Burns involving 30-39% of body surface with 30-39% third degree burns

● **T31.4**   Burns involving 40-49% of body surface

      T31.40   Burns involving 40-49% of body surface with 0% to 9% third degree burns
          Burns involving 40-49% of body surface NOS

      T31.41   Burns involving 40-49% of body surface with 10-19% third degree burns

      T31.42   Burns involving 40-49% of body surface with 20-29% third degree burns

      T31.43   Burns involving 40-49% of body surface with 30-39% third degree burns

      T31.44   Burns involving 40-49% of body surface with 40-49% third degree burns

● **T31.5**   Burns involving 50-59% of body surface

      T31.50   Burns involving 50-59% of body surface with 0% to 9% third degree burns
          Burns involving 50-59% of body surface NOS

      T31.51   Burns involving 50-59% of body surface with 10-19% third degree burns

      T31.52   Burns involving 50-59% of body surface with 20-29% third degree burns

      T31.53   Burns involving 50-59% of body surface with 30-39% third degree burns

      T31.54   Burns involving 50-59% of body surface with 40-49% third degree burns

      T31.55   Burns involving 50-59% of body surface with 50-59% third degree burns

● **T31.6**   Burns involving 60-69% of body surface

      T31.60   Burns involving 60-69% of body surface with 0% to 9% third degree burns
          Burns involving 60-69% of body surface NOS

      T31.61   Burns involving 60-69% of body surface with 10-19% third degree burns

      T31.62   Burns involving 60-69% of body surface with 20-29% third degree burns

      T31.63   Burns involving 60-69% of body surface with 30-39% third degree burns

      T31.64   Burns involving 60-69% of body surface with 40-49% third degree burns

      T31.65   Burns involving 60-69% of body surface with 50-59% third degree burns

      T31.66   Burns involving 60-69% of body surface with 60-69% third degree burns

● **T31.7**   Burns involving 70-79% of body surface

      T31.70   Burns involving 70-79% of body surface with 0% to 9% third degree burns
          Burns involving 70-79% of body surface NOS

      T31.71   Burns involving 70-79% of body surface with 10-19% third degree burns

      T31.72   Burns involving 70-79% of body surface with 20-29% third degree burns

      T31.73   Burns involving 70-79% of body surface with 30-39% third degree burns

      T31.74   Burns involving 70-79% of body surface with 40-49% third degree burns

      T31.75   Burns involving 70-79% of body surface with 50-59% third degree burns

      T31.76   Burns involving 70-79% of body surface with 60-69% third degree burns

      T31.77   Burns involving 70-79% of body surface with 70-79% third degree burns

● **T31.8**   Burns involving 80-89% of body surface

      T31.80   Burns involving 80-89% of body surface with 0% to 9% third degree burns
          Burns involving 80-89% of body surface NOS

      T31.81   Burns involving 80-89% of body surface with 10-19% third degree burns

      T31.82   Burns involving 80-89% of body surface with 20-29% third degree burns

      T31.83   Burns involving 80-89% of body surface with 30-39% third degree burns

      T31.84   Burns involving 80-89% of body surface with 40-49% third degree burns

      T31.85   Burns involving 80-89% of body surface with 50-59% third degree burns

      T31.86   Burns involving 80-89% of body surface with 60-69% third degree burns

      T31.87   Burns involving 80-89% of body surface with 70-79% third degree burns

      T31.88   Burns involving 80-89% of body surface with 80-89% third degree burns

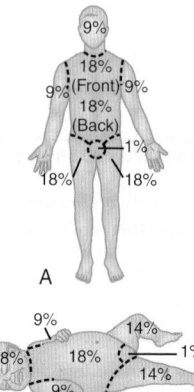

Figure 19-16   Rule of nines: percentages of total body area. (From Marx: Rosen's Emergency Medicine: Concepts and Clinical Practice, ed 6, Mosby, 2006)

▶ New   ⇒ Revised   ~~deleted~~ Deleted   Excludes 1   Excludes 2   Includes   Use additional   Code first   Code also   Key words

OGCR Official Guidelines   **X** Assign placeholder X   ● Use Additional Character(s)   ▷ Manifestation Code   🐾 Hierarchical Condition Category   **Coding Clinic**

● **T31.9**   Burns involving 90% or more of body surface

     T31.90   Burns involving 90% or more of body surface with 0% to 9% third degree burns
         Burns involving 90% or more of body surface NOS

     T31.91   Burns involving 90% or more of body surface with 10-19% third degree burns 🔾

     T31.92   Burns involving 90% or more of body surface with 20-29% third degree burns 🔾

     T31.93   Burns involving 90% or more of body surface with 30-39% third degree burns 🔾

     T31.94   Burns involving 90% or more of body surface with 40-49% third degree burns 🔾

     T31.95   Burns involving 90% or more of body surface with 50-59% third degree burns 🔾

     T31.96   Burns involving 90% or more of body surface with 60-69% third degree burns 🔾

     T31.97   Burns involving 90% or more of body surface with 70-79% third degree burns 🔾

     T31.98   Burns involving 90% or more of body surface with 80-89% third degree burns 🔾

     T31.99   Burns involving 90% or more of body surface with 90% or more third degree burns 🔾

● **T32**   Corrosions classified according to extent of body surface involved

     Note: This category is to be used as the primary code only when the site of the corrosion is unspecified. It may be used as a supplementary code with categories T20-T25 when the site is specified.

   T32.0   Corrosions involving less than 10% of body surface

● T32.1   Corrosions involving 10-19% of body surface

     T32.10   Corrosions involving 10-19% of body surface with 0% to 9% third degree corrosion
         Corrosions involving 10-19% of body surface NOS

     T32.11   Corrosions involving 10-19% of body surface with 10-19% third degree corrosion 🔾

● T32.2   Corrosions involving 20-29% of body surface

     T32.20   Corrosions involving 20-29% of body surface with 0% to 9% third degree corrosion

     T32.21   Corrosions involving 20-29% of body surface with 10-19% third degree corrosion 🔾

     T32.22   Corrosions involving 20-29% of body surface with 20-29% third degree corrosion 🔾

● T32.3   Corrosions involving 30-39% of body surface

     T32.30   Corrosions involving 30-39% of body surface with 0% to 9% third degree corrosion

     T32.31   Corrosions involving 30-39% of body surface with 10-19% third degree corrosion 🔾

     T32.32   Corrosions involving 30-39% of body surface with 20-29% third degree corrosion 🔾

     T32.33   Corrosions involving 30-39% of body surface with 30-39% third degree corrosion 🔾

● T32.4   Corrosions involving 40-49% of body surface

     T32.40   Corrosions involving 40-49% of body surface with 0% to 9% third degree corrosion

     T32.41   Corrosions involving 40-49% of body surface with 10-19% third degree corrosion 🔾

     T32.42   Corrosions involving 40-49% of body surface with 20-29% third degree corrosion 🔾

     T32.43   Corrosions involving 40-49% of body surface with 30-39% third degree corrosion 🔾

     T32.44   Corrosions involving 40-49% of body surface with 40-49% third degree corrosion 🔾

● T32.5   Corrosions involving 50-59% of body surface

     T32.50   Corrosions involving 50-59% of body surface with 0% to 9% third degree corrosion

     T32.51   Corrosions involving 50-59% of body surface with 10-19% third degree corrosion 🔾

     T32.52   Corrosions involving 50-59% of body surface with 20-29% third degree corrosion 🔾

     T32.53   Corrosions involving 50-59% of body surface with 30-39% third degree corrosion 🔾

     T32.54   Corrosions involving 50-59% of body surface with 40-49% third degree corrosion 🔾

     T32.55   Corrosions involving 50-59% of body surface with 50-59% third degree corrosion 🔾

● T32.6   Corrosions involving 60-69% of body surface

     T32.60   Corrosions involving 60-69% of body surface with 0% to 9% third degree corrosion

     T32.61   Corrosions involving 60-69% of body surface with 10-19% third degree corrosion 🔾

     T32.62   Corrosions involving 60-69% of body surface with 20-29% third degree corrosion 🔾

     T32.63   Corrosions involving 60-69% of body surface with 30-39% third degree corrosion 🔾

     T32.64   Corrosions involving 60-69% of body surface with 40-49% third degree corrosion 🔾

     T32.65   Corrosions involving 60-69% of body surface with 50-59% third degree corrosion 🔾

     T32.66   Corrosions involving 60-69% of body surface with 60-69% third degree corrosion 🔾

● T32.7   Corrosions involving 70-79% of body surface

     T32.70   Corrosions involving 70-79% of body surface with 0% to 9% third degree corrosion

     T32.71   Corrosions involving 70-79% of body surface with 10-19% third degree corrosion 🔾

     T32.72   Corrosions involving 70-79% of body surface with 20-29% third degree corrosion 🔾

     T32.73   Corrosions involving 70-79% of body surface with 30-39% third degree corrosion 🔾

     T32.74   Corrosions involving 70-79% of body surface with 40-49% third degree corrosion 🔾

     T32.75   Corrosions involving 70-79% of body surface with 50-59% third degree corrosion 🔾

     T32.76   Corrosions involving 70-79% of body surface with 60-69% third degree corrosion 🔾

     T32.77   Corrosions involving 70-79% of body surface with 70-79% third degree corrosion 🔾

● T32.8   Corrosions involving 80-89% of body surface

     T32.80   Corrosions involving 80-89% of body surface with 0% to 9% third degree corrosion

     T32.81   Corrosions involving 80-89% of body surface with 10-19% third degree corrosion 🔾

     T32.82   Corrosions involving 80-89% of body surface with 20-29% third degree corrosion 🔾

     T32.83   Corrosions involving 80-89% of body surface with 30-39% third degree corrosion 🔾

     T32.84   Corrosions involving 80-89% of body surface with 40-49% third degree corrosion 🔾

     T32.85   Corrosions involving 80-89% of body surface with 50-59% third degree corrosion 🔾

     T32.86   Corrosions involving 80-89% of body surface with 60-69% third degree corrosion 🔾

     T32.87   Corrosions involving 80-89% of body surface with 70-79% third degree corrosion 🔾

     T32.88   Corrosions involving 80-89% of body surface with 80-89% third degree corrosion 🔾

● T32.9   Corrosions involving 90% or more of body surface

     T32.90   Corrosions involving 90% or more of body surface with 0% to 9% third degree corrosion

     T32.91   Corrosions involving 90% or more of body surface with 10-19% third degree corrosion 🔾

     T32.92   Corrosions involving 90% or more of body surface with 20-29% third degree corrosion 🔾

     T32.93   Corrosions involving 90% or more of body surface with 30-39% third degree corrosion 🔾

T32.94   Corrosions involving 90% or more of body
          surface with 40-49% third degree corrosion ❦

T32.95   Corrosions involving 90% or more of body
          surface with 50-59% third degree corrosion ❦

T32.96   Corrosions involving 90% or more of body
          surface with 60-69% third degree corrosion ❦

T32.97   Corrosions involving 90% or more of body
          surface with 70-79% third degree corrosion ❦

T32.98   Corrosions involving 90% or more of body
          surface with 80-89% third degree corrosion ❦

T32.99   Corrosions involving 90% or more of body
          surface with 90% or more third degree
          corrosion ❦

FROSTBITE (T33-T34)

Excludes2   hypothermia and other effects of reduced
                 temperature (T68, T69.-)

● T33   **Superficial frostbite**

    Includes   frostbite with partial thickness skin loss

    The appropriate 7th character is to be added to each code from
    category T33

A	initial encounter
D	subsequent encounter
S	sequela

  ● T33.0   Superficial frostbite of head
    ● T33.01   Superficial frostbite of ear
      ● T33.011   Superficial frostbite of right ear
      ● T33.012   Superficial frostbite of left ear
      ● T33.019   Superficial frostbite of unspecified ear
  X ● T33.02   Superficial frostbite of nose
  X ● T33.09   Superficial frostbite of other part of head
X ● T33.1   Superficial frostbite of neck
X ● T33.2   Superficial frostbite of thorax
X ● T33.3   Superficial frostbite of abdominal wall, lower back and
    pelvis
  ● T33.4   Superficial frostbite of arm

    Excludes2   superficial frostbite of wrist and hand
               (T33.5-)

  X ● T33.40   Superficial frostbite of unspecified arm
  X ● T33.41   Superficial frostbite of right arm
  X ● T33.42   Superficial frostbite of left arm
  ● T33.5   Superficial frostbite of wrist, hand, and fingers
    ● T33.51   Superficial frostbite of wrist
      ● T33.511   Superficial frostbite of right wrist
      ● T33.512   Superficial frostbite of left wrist
      ● T33.519   Superficial frostbite of unspecified
              wrist
    ● T33.52   Superficial frostbite of hand

      Excludes2   superficial frostbite of fingers
               (T33.53-)

      ● T33.521   Superficial frostbite of right hand
      ● T33.522   Superficial frostbite of left hand
      ● T33.529   Superficial frostbite of unspecified
              hand
    ● T33.53   Superficial frostbite of finger(s)
      ● T33.531   Superficial frostbite of right finger(s)
      ● T33.532   Superficial frostbite of left finger(s)
      ● T33.539   Superficial frostbite of unspecified
              finger(s)

● T33.6   Superficial frostbite of hip and thigh
  X ● T33.60   Superficial frostbite of unspecified hip and
            thigh
  X ● T33.61   Superficial frostbite of right hip and thigh
  X ● T33.62   Superficial frostbite of left hip and thigh
● T33.7   Superficial frostbite of knee and lower leg

    Excludes2   superficial frostbite of ankle and foot
               (T33.8-)

  X ● T33.70   Superficial frostbite of unspecified knee and
            lower leg
  X ● T33.71   Superficial frostbite of right knee and lower leg
  X ● T33.72   Superficial frostbite of left knee and lower leg
● T33.8   Superficial frostbite of ankle, foot, and toe(s)
  ● T33.81   Superficial frostbite of ankle
    ● T33.811   Superficial frostbite of right ankle
    ● T33.812   Superficial frostbite of left ankle
    ● T33.819   Superficial frostbite of unspecified
            ankle
  ● T33.82   Superficial frostbite of foot
    ● T33.821   Superficial frostbite of right foot
    ● T33.822   Superficial frostbite of left foot
    ● T33.829   Superficial frostbite of unspecified
            foot
  ● T33.83   Superficial frostbite of toe(s)
    ● T33.831   Superficial frostbite of right toe(s)
    ● T33.832   Superficial frostbite of left toe(s)
    ● T33.839   Superficial frostbite of unspecified
            toe(s)
● T33.9   Superficial frostbite of other and unspecified sites
  X ● T33.90   Superficial frostbite of unspecified sites
          Superficial frostbite NOS

  X ● T33.99   Superficial frostbite of other sites
          Superficial frostbite of leg NOS
          Superficial frostbite of trunk NOS

● T34   **Frostbite with tissue necrosis**

    The appropriate 7th character is to be added to each code from
    category T34

A	initial encounter
D	subsequent encounter
S	sequela

  ● T34.0   Frostbite with tissue necrosis of head
    ● T34.01   Frostbite with tissue necrosis of ear
      ● T34.011   Frostbite with tissue necrosis of right
              ear
      ● T34.012   Frostbite with tissue necrosis of left
              ear
      ● T34.019   Frostbite with tissue necrosis of
              unspecified ear
  X ● T34.02   Frostbite with tissue necrosis of nose
  X ● T34.09   Frostbite with tissue necrosis of other part of
            head
X ● T34.1   Frostbite with tissue necrosis of neck
X ● T34.2   Frostbite with tissue necrosis of thorax
X ● T34.3   Frostbite with tissue necrosis of abdominal wall, lower
    back and pelvis
  ● T34.4   Frostbite with tissue necrosis of arm

      Excludes2   frostbite with tissue necrosis of wrist and
               hand (T34.5-)

  X ● T34.40   Frostbite with tissue necrosis of unspecified
            arm
  X ● T34.41   Frostbite with tissue necrosis of right arm
  X ● T34.42   Frostbite with tissue necrosis of left arm

▶ New   ⇒ Revised   ~~deleted~~ Deleted   Excludes 1   Excludes 2   Includes   Use additional   Code first   Code also   Key words

OGCR Official Guidelines   X Assign placeholder X   ● Use Additional Character(s)   ▷ Manifestation Code   ❦ Hierarchical Condition Category   **Coding Clinic**

● T34.5　Frostbite with tissue necrosis of wrist, hand, and finger(s)
　　● T34.51　Frostbite with tissue necrosis of wrist
　　　　● T34.511　Frostbite with tissue necrosis of right wrist
　　　　● T34.512　Frostbite with tissue necrosis of left wrist
　　　　● T34.519　Frostbite with tissue necrosis of unspecified wrist
　　● T34.52　Frostbite with tissue necrosis of hand
　　　　　　Excludes2　frostbite with tissue necrosis of finger(s) (T34.53-)
　　　　● T34.521　Frostbite with tissue necrosis of right hand
　　　　● T34.522　Frostbite with tissue necrosis of left hand
　　　　● T34.529　Frostbite with tissue necrosis of unspecified hand
　　● T34.53　Frostbite with tissue necrosis of finger(s)
　　　　● T34.531　Frostbite with tissue necrosis of right finger(s)
　　　　● T34.532　Frostbite with tissue necrosis of left finger(s)
　　　　● T34.539　Frostbite with tissue necrosis of unspecified finger(s)
● T34.6　Frostbite with tissue necrosis of hip and thigh
　X● T34.60　Frostbite with tissue necrosis of unspecified hip and thigh
　X● T34.61　Frostbite with tissue necrosis of right hip and thigh
　X● T34.62　Frostbite with tissue necrosis of left hip and thigh
● T34.7　Frostbite with tissue necrosis of knee and lower leg
　　　Excludes2　frostbite with tissue necrosis of ankle and foot (T34.8-)
　X● T34.70　Frostbite with tissue necrosis of unspecified knee and lower leg
　X● T34.71　Frostbite with tissue necrosis of right knee and lower leg
　X● T34.72　Frostbite with tissue necrosis of left knee and lower leg
● T34.8　Frostbite with tissue necrosis of ankle, foot, and toe(s)
　　● T34.81　Frostbite with tissue necrosis of ankle
　　　　● T34.811　Frostbite with tissue necrosis of right ankle
　　　　● T34.812　Frostbite with tissue necrosis of left ankle
　　　　● T34.819　Frostbite with tissue necrosis of unspecified ankle
　　● T34.82　Frostbite with tissue necrosis of foot
　　　　● T34.821　Frostbite with tissue necrosis of right foot
　　　　● T34.822　Frostbite with tissue necrosis of left foot
　　　　● T34.829　Frostbite with tissue necrosis of unspecified foot
　　● T34.83　Frostbite with tissue necrosis of toe(s)
　　　　● T34.831　Frostbite with tissue necrosis of right toe(s)
　　　　● T34.832　Frostbite with tissue necrosis of left toe(s)
　　　　● T34.839　Frostbite with tissue necrosis of unspecified toe(s)

● T34.9　Frostbite with tissue necrosis of other and unspecified sites
　X● T34.90　Frostbite with tissue necrosis of unspecified sites
　　　　　　Frostbite with tissue necrosis NOS
　X● T34.99　Frostbite with tissue necrosis of other sites
　　　　　　Frostbite with tissue necrosis of leg NOS
　　　　　　Frostbite with tissue necrosis of trunk NOS

OGCR　See Section I.C.19.e.

Adverse Effects, Poisoning, Underdosing and Toxic Effects
Codes in categories T36-T65 are combination codes that include the substance that was taken as well as the intent. No additional external cause code is required for poisonings, toxic effects, adverse effects and underdosing codes.

POISONING BY, ADVERSE EFFECTS OF AND UNDERDOSING OF DRUGS MEDICAMENTS AND BIOLOGICAL SUBSTANCES (T36-T50)

Includes　adverse effect of correct substance properly administered
　　　　　poisoning by overdose of substance
　　　　　poisoning by wrong substance given or taken in error
　　　　　underdosing by (inadvertently) (deliberately) taking less substance than prescribed or instructed

Code first, for adverse effects, the nature of the adverse effect, such as:
　　adverse effect NOS (T88.7)
　　aspirin gastritis (K29.-)
　　blood disorders (D56-D76)
　　contact dermatitis (L23-L25)
　　dermatitis due to substances taken internally (L27.-)
　　nephropathy (N14.0-N14.2)

Note:　The drug giving rise to the adverse effect should be identified by use of codes from categories T36-T50 with fifth or sixth character 5.

Use additional code(s) to specify:
　　manifestations of poisoning
　　underdosing or failure in dosage during medical and surgical care (Y63.6, Y63.8-Y63.9)
　　underdosing of medication regimen (Z91.12-, Z91.13-)

Excludes1　toxic reaction to local anesthesia in pregnancy (O29.3-)

Excludes2　abuse and dependence of psychoactive substances (F10-F19)
　　　　　abuse of non-dependence-producing substances (F55.-)
　　　　　drug reaction and poisoning affecting newborn (P00-P96)
　　　　　immunodeficiency due to drugs (D84.821)
　　　　　pathological drug intoxication (inebriation) (F10-F19)

● T36　Poisoning by, adverse effect of and underdosing of systemic antibiotics
　　Excludes1　antineoplastic antibiotics (T45.1-)
　　　　　locally applied antibiotic NEC (T49.0)
　　　　　topically used antibiotic for ear, nose and throat (T49.6)
　　　　　topically used antibiotic for eye (T49.5)

The appropriate 7th character is to be added to each code from category T36

A	initial encounter
D	subsequent encounter
S	sequela

● **T36.0**   Poisoning by, adverse effect of and underdosing of penicillins

   ● **T36.0X**   Poisoning by, adverse effect of and underdosing of penicillins

      ● **T36.0X1**   Poisoning by penicillins, accidental (unintentional)
           Poisoning by penicillins NOS

      ● **T36.0X2**   Poisoning by penicillins, intentional self-harm A, S 🐾

      ● **T36.0X3**   Poisoning by penicillins, assault

      ● **T36.0X4**   Poisoning by penicillins, undetermined

      ● **T36.0X5**   Adverse effect of penicillins

      ● **T36.0X6**   Underdosing of penicillins

● **T36.1**   Poisoning by, adverse effect of and underdosing of cephalosporins and other betalactam antibiotics

   ● **T36.1X**   Poisoning by, adverse effect of and underdosing of cephalosporins and other beta-lactam antibiotics

      ● **T36.1X1**   Poisoning by cephalosporins and other beta-lactam antibiotics, accidental (unintentional)
           Poisoning by cephalosporins and other beta-lactam antibiotics NOS

      ● **T36.1X2**   Poisoning by cephalosporins and other beta-lactam antibiotics, intentional self-harm A, S 🐾

      ● **T36.1X3**   Poisoning by cephalosporins and other beta-lactam antibiotics, assault

      ● **T36.1X4**   Poisoning by cephalosporins and other beta-lactam antibiotics, undetermined

      ● **T36.1X5**   Adverse effect of cephalosporins and other beta-lactam antibiotics

      ● **T36.1X6**   Underdosing of cephalosporins and other beta-lactam antibiotics

● **T36.2**   Poisoning by, adverse effect of and underdosing of chloramphenicol group

   ● **T36.2X**   Poisoning by, adverse effect of and underdosing of chloramphenicol group

      ● **T36.2X1**   Poisoning by chloramphenicol group, accidental (unintentional)
           Poisoning by chloramphenicol group NOS

      ● **T36.2X2**   Poisoning by chloramphenicol group, intentional self-harm A, S 🐾

      ● **T36.2X3**   Poisoning by chloramphenicol group, assault

      ● **T36.2X4**   Poisoning by chloramphenicol group, undetermined

      ● **T36.2X5**   Adverse effect of chloramphenicol group

      ● **T36.2X6**   Underdosing of chloramphenicol group

● **T36.3**   Poisoning by, adverse effect of and underdosing of macrolides

   ● **T36.3X**   Poisoning by, adverse effect of and underdosing of macrolides

      ● **T36.3X1**   Poisoning by macrolides, accidental (unintentional)
           Poisoning by macrolides NOS

      ● **T36.3X2**   Poisoning by macrolides, intentional self-harm A, S 🐾

      ● **T36.3X3**   Poisoning by macrolides, assault

      ● **T36.3X4**   Poisoning by macrolides, undetermined

      ● **T36.3X5**   Adverse effect of macrolides

      ● **T36.3X6**   Underdosing of macrolides

● **T36.4**   Poisoning by, adverse effect of and underdosing of tetracyclines

   ● **T36.4X**   Poisoning by, adverse effect of and underdosing of tetracyclines

      ● **T36.4X1**   Poisoning by tetracyclines, accidental (unintentional)
           Poisoning by tetracyclines NOS

      ● **T36.4X2**   Poisoning by tetracyclines, intentional self-harm A, S 🐾

      ● **T36.4X3**   Poisoning by tetracyclines, assault

      ● **T36.4X4**   Poisoning by tetracyclines, undetermined

      ● **T36.4X5**   Adverse effect of tetracyclines

      ● **T36.4X6**   Underdosing of tetracyclines

● **T36.5**   Poisoning by, adverse effect of and underdosing of aminoglycosides
     Poisoning by, adverse effect of and underdosing of streptomycin

   ● **T36.5X**   Poisoning by, adverse effect of and underdosing of aminoglycosides

      ● **T36.5X1**   Poisoning by aminoglycosides, accidental (unintentional)
           Poisoning by aminoglycosides NOS

      ● **T36.5X2**   Poisoning by aminoglycosides, intentional self-harm A, S 🐾

      ● **T36.5X3**   Poisoning by aminoglycosides, assault

      ● **T36.5X4**   Poisoning by aminoglycosides, undetermined

      ● **T36.5X5**   Adverse effect of aminoglycosides

      ● **T36.5X6**   Underdosing of aminoglycosides

● **T36.6**   Poisoning by, adverse effect of and underdosing of rifampicins

   ● **T36.6X**   Poisoning by, adverse effect of and underdosing of rifampicins

      ● **T36.6X1**   Poisoning by rifampicins, accidental (unintentional)
           Poisoning by rifampicins NOS

      ● **T36.6X2**   Poisoning by rifampicins, intentional self-harm A, S 🐾

      ● **T36.6X3**   Poisoning by rifampicins, assault

      ● **T36.6X4**   Poisoning by rifampicins, undetermined

      ● **T36.6X5**   Adverse effect of rifampicins

      ● **T36.6X6**   Underdosing of rifampicins

● **T36.7**   Poisoning by, adverse effect of and underdosing of antifungal antibiotics, systemically used

   ● **T36.7X**   Poisoning by, adverse effect of and underdosing of antifungal antibiotics, systemically used

      ● **T36.7X1**   Poisoning by antifungal antibiotics, systemically used, accidental (unintentional)
           Poisoning by antifungal antibiotics, systemically used NOS

      ● **T36.7X2**   Poisoning by antifungal antibiotics, systemically used, intentional self-harm A, S 🐾

      ● **T36.7X3**   Poisoning by antifungal antibiotics, systemically used, assault

      ● **T36.7X4**   Poisoning by antifungal antibiotics, systemically used, undetermined

      ● **T36.7X5**   Adverse effect of antifungal antibiotics, systemically used

      ● **T36.7X6**   Underdosing of antifungal antibiotics, systemically used

▶ New   ⇒ Revised   ~~deleted~~ Deleted   Excludes 1   Excludes 2   Includes   Use additional   Code first   Code also   Key words

OGCR Official Guidelines   X Assign placeholder X   ● Use Additional Character(s)   ▌ Manifestation Code   🐾 Hierarchical Condition Category   **Coding Clinic**

● **T36.8** Poisoning by, adverse effect of and underdosing of other systemic antibiotics

  ● **T36.8X** Poisoning by, adverse effect of and underdosing of other systemic antibiotics

    ● **T36.8X1** Poisoning by other systemic antibiotics, accidental (unintentional)
      Poisoning by other systemic antibiotics NOS

    ● **T36.8X2** Poisoning by other systemic antibiotics, intentional self-harm A, S 🐾

    ● **T36.8X3** Poisoning by other systemic antibiotics, assault

    ● **T36.8X4** Poisoning by other systemic antibiotics, undetermined

    ● **T36.8X5** Adverse effect of other systemic antibiotics
      Coding Clinic: 2017, Q1, P39

    ● **T36.8X6** Underdosing of other systemic antibiotics

● **T36.9** Poisoning by, adverse effect of and underdosing of unspecified systemic antibiotic

  X ● **T36.91** Poisoning by unspecified systemic antibiotic, accidental (unintentional)
      Poisoning by systemic antibiotic NOS

  X ● **T36.92** Poisoning by unspecified systemic antibiotic, intentional self-harm A, S 🐾

  X ● **T36.93** Poisoning by unspecified systemic antibiotic, assault

  X ● **T36.94** Poisoning by unspecified systemic antibiotic, undetermined

  X ● **T36.95** Adverse effect of unspecified systemic antibiotic

  X ● **T36.96** Underdosing of unspecified systemic antibiotic

● **T37** Poisoning by, adverse effect of and underdosing of other systemic anti-infectives and antiparasitics

  Excludes1 anti-infectives topically used for ear, nose and throat (T49.6-)
    anti-infectives topically used for eye (T49.5-)
    locally applied anti-infectives NEC (T49.0-)

  The appropriate 7th character is to be added to each code from category T37

A	initial encounter
D	subsequent encounter
S	sequela

● **T37.0** Poisoning by, adverse effect of and underdosing of sulfonamides

  ● **T37.0X** Poisoning by, adverse effect of and underdosing of sulfonamides

    ● **T37.0X1** Poisoning by sulfonamides, accidental (unintentional)
      Poisoning by sulfonamides NOS

    ● **T37.0X2** Poisoning by sulfonamides, intentional self-harm A, S 🐾

    ● **T37.0X3** Poisoning by sulfonamides, assault

    ● **T37.0X4** Poisoning by sulfonamides, undetermined

    ● **T37.0X5** Adverse effect of sulfonamides

    ● **T37.0X6** Underdosing of sulfonamides

● **T37.1** Poisoning by, adverse effect of and underdosing of antimycobacterial drugs

  Excludes1 rifampicins (T36.6-) streptomycin (T36.5-)

  ● **T37.1X** Poisoning by, adverse effect of and underdosing of antimycobacterial drugs

    ● **T37.1X1** Poisoning by antimycobacterial drugs, accidental (unintentional)
      Poisoning by antimycobacterial drugs NOS

    ● **T37.1X2** Poisoning by antimycobacterial drugs, intentional self-harm A, S 🐾

    ● **T37.1X3** Poisoning by antimycobacterial drugs, assault

    ● **T37.1X4** Poisoning by antimycobacterial drugs, undetermined

    ● **T37.1X5** Adverse effect of antimycobacterial drugs

    ● **T37.1X6** Underdosing of antimycobacterial drugs

● **T37.2** Poisoning by, adverse effect of and underdosing of antimalarials and drugs acting on other blood protozoa

  Excludes1 hydroxyquinoline derivatives (T37.8-)

  ● **T37.2X** Poisoning by, adverse effect of and underdosing of antimalarials and drugs acting on other blood protozoa

    ● **T37.2X1** Poisoning by antimalarials and drugs acting on other blood protozoa, accidental (unintentional)
      Poisoning by antimalarials and drugs acting on other blood protozoa NOS

    ● **T37.2X2** Poisoning by antimalarials and drugs acting on other blood protozoa, intentional self-harm A, S 🐾

    ● **T37.2X3** Poisoning by antimalarials and drugs acting on other blood protozoa, assault

    ● **T37.2X4** Poisoning by antimalarials and drugs acting on other blood protozoa, undetermined

    ● **T37.2X5** Adverse effect of antimalarials and drugs acting on other blood protozoa

    ● **T37.2X6** Underdosing of antimalarials and drugs acting on other blood protozoa

● **T37.3** Poisoning by, adverse effect of and underdosing of other antiprotozoal drugs

  ● **T37.3X** Poisoning by, adverse effect of and underdosing of other antiprotozoal drugs

    ● **T37.3X1** Poisoning by other antiprotozoal drugs, accidental (unintentional)
      Poisoning by other antiprotozoal drugs NOS

    ● **T37.3X2** Poisoning by other antiprotozoal drugs, intentional self-harm A, S 🐾

    ● **T37.3X3** Poisoning by other antiprotozoal drugs, assault

    ● **T37.3X4** Poisoning by other antiprotozoal drugs, undetermined

    ● **T37.3X5** Adverse effect of other antiprotozoal drugs

    ● **T37.3X6** Underdosing of other antiprotozoal drugs

● **T37.4** Poisoning by, adverse effect of and underdosing of anthelminthics

  ● **T37.4X** Poisoning by, adverse effect of and underdosing of anthelminthics

    ● **T37.4X1** Poisoning by anthelminthics, accidental (unintentional)
      Poisoning by anthelminthics NOS

    ● **T37.4X2** Poisoning by anthelminthics, intentional self-harm A, S 🐾

    ● **T37.4X3** Poisoning by anthelminthics, assault

    ● **T37.4X4** Poisoning by anthelminthics, undetermined

    ● **T37.4X5** Adverse effect of anthelminthics

    ● **T37.4X6** Underdosing of anthelminthics

CHAPTER 19 (S00–T88)

● **T37.5** **Poisoning by, adverse effect of and underdosing of antiviral drugs**
    Excludes1   amantadine (T42.8-)
               cytarabine (T45.1-)

  ● **T37.5X** **Poisoning by, adverse effect of and underdosing of antiviral drugs**

    ● **T37.5X1** **Poisoning by antiviral drugs, accidental (unintentional)**
            Poisoning by antiviral drugs NOS

    ● **T37.5X2** **Poisoning by antiviral drugs, intentional self-harm A, S**

    ● **T37.5X3** **Poisoning by antiviral drugs, assault**

    ● **T37.5X4** **Poisoning by antiviral drugs, undetermined**

    ● **T37.5X5** **Adverse effect of antiviral drugs**

    ● **T37.5X6** **Underdosing of antiviral drugs**

● **T37.8** **Poisoning by, adverse effect of and underdosing of other specified systemic anti-infectives and antiparasitics**
     Poisoning by, adverse effect of and underdosing of hydroxyquinoline derivatives
    Excludes1   antimalarial drugs (T37.2-)

  ● **T37.8X** **Poisoning by, adverse effect of and underdosing of other specified systemic anti-infectives and antiparasitics**

    ● **T37.8X1** **Poisoning by other specified systemic anti-infectives and antiparasitics, accidental (unintentional)**
            Poisoning by other specified systemic anti-infectives and antiparasitics NOS

    ● **T37.8X2** **Poisoning by other specified systemic anti-infectives and antiparasitics, intentional self-harm A, S**

    ● **T37.8X3** **Poisoning by other specified systemic anti-infectives and antiparasitics, assault**

    ● **T37.8X4** **Poisoning by other specified systemic anti-infectives and antiparasitics, undetermined**

    ● **T37.8X5** **Adverse effect of other specified systemic anti-infectives and antiparasitics**

    ● **T37.8X6** **Underdosing of other specified systemic anti-infectives and antiparasitics**

● **T37.9** **Poisoning by, adverse effect of and underdosing of unspecified systemic anti-infective and antiparasitics**

  X ● **T37.91** **Poisoning by unspecified systemic anti-infective and antiparasitics, accidental (unintentional)**
          Poisoning by, adverse effect of and underdosing of systemic anti-infective and antiparasitics NOS

  X ● **T37.92** **Poisoning by unspecified systemic anti-infective and antiparasitics, intentional self-harm A, S**

  X ● **T37.93** **Poisoning by unspecified systemic anti-infective and antiparasitics, assault**

  X ● **T37.94** **Poisoning by unspecified systemic anti-infective and antiparasitics, undetermined**

  X ● **T37.95** **Adverse effect of unspecified systemic anti-infective and antiparasitic**

  X ● **T37.96** **Underdosing of unspecified systemic anti-infectives and antiparasitics**

● **T38** **Poisoning by, adverse effect of and underdosing of hormones and their synthetic substitutes and antagonists, not elsewhere classified**
    Excludes1   mineralocorticoids and their antagonists (T50.0-)
               oxytocic hormones (T48.0-)
               parathyroid hormones and derivatives (T50.9-)
     The appropriate 7th character is to be added to each code from category T38

> A   initial encounter
> D   subsequent encounter
> S   sequela

● **T38.0** **Poisoning by, adverse effect of and underdosing of glucocorticoids and synthetic analogues**
    Excludes1   glucocorticoids, topically used (T49.-)

  ● **T38.0X** **Poisoning by, adverse effect of and underdosing of glucocorticoids and synthetic analogues**

    ● **T38.0X1** **Poisoning by glucocorticoids and synthetic analogues, accidental (unintentional)**
            Poisoning by glucocorticoids and synthetic analogues NOS

    ● **T38.0X2** **Poisoning by glucocorticoids and synthetic analogues, intentional self-harm A, S**

    ● **T38.0X3** **Poisoning by glucocorticoids and synthetic analogues, assault**

    ● **T38.0X4** **Poisoning by glucocorticoids and synthetic analogues, undetermined**

    ● **T38.0X5** **Adverse effect of glucocorticoids and synthetic analogues**

    ● **T38.0X6** **Underdosing of glucocorticoids and synthetic analogues**

● **T38.1** **Poisoning by, adverse effect of and underdosing of thyroid hormones and substitutes**

  ● **T38.1X** **Poisoning by, adverse effect of and underdosing of thyroid hormones and substitutes**

    ● **T38.1X1** **Poisoning by thyroid hormones and substitutes, accidental (unintentional)**
            Poisoning by thyroid hormones and substitutes NOS

    ● **T38.1X2** **Poisoning by thyroid hormones and substitutes, intentional self-harm A, S**

    ● **T38.1X3** **Poisoning by thyroid hormones and substitutes, assault**

    ● **T38.1X4** **Poisoning by thyroid hormones and substitutes, undetermined**

    ● **T38.1X5** **Adverse effect of thyroid hormones and substitutes**

    ● **T38.1X6** **Underdosing of thyroid hormones and substitutes**

● **T38.2** **Poisoning by, adverse effect of and underdosing of antithyroid drugs**

  ● **T38.2X** **Poisoning by, adverse effect of and underdosing of antithyroid drugs**

    ● **T38.2X1** **Poisoning by antithyroid drugs, accidental (unintentional)**
            Poisoning by antithyroid drugs NOS

    ● **T38.2X2** **Poisoning by antithyroid drugs, intentional self-harm A, S**

    ● **T38.2X3** **Poisoning by antithyroid drugs, assault**

CHAPTER 19 (S00-T88)

● T38.2X4 Poisoning by antithyroid drugs, undetermined
● T38.2X5 Adverse effect of antithyroid drugs
● T38.2X6 Underdosing of antithyroid drugs

● T38.3 Poisoning by, adverse effect of and underdosing of insulin and oral hypoglycemic [antidiabetic] drugs

 ● T38.3X Poisoning by, adverse effect of and underdosing of insulin and oral hypoglycemic [antidiabetic] drugs

  ● T38.3X1 Poisoning by insulin and oral hypoglycemic [antidiabetic] drugs, accidental (unintentional)
       Poisoning by insulin and oral hypoglycemic [antidiabetic] drugs NOS

  ● T38.3X2 Poisoning by insulin and oral hypoglycemic [antidiabetic] drugs, intentional self-harm

  ● T38.3X3 Poisoning by insulin and oral hypoglycemic [antidiabetic] drugs, assault A, S 🔊

  ● T38.3X4 Poisoning by insulin and oral hypoglycemic [antidiabetic] drugs, undetermined

  ● T38.3X5 Adverse effect of insulin and oral hypoglycemic [antidiabetic] drugs

  ● T38.3X6 Underdosing of insulin and oral hypoglycemic [antidiabetic] drugs

● T38.4 Poisoning by, adverse effect of and underdosing of oral contraceptives
     Poisoning by, adverse effect of and underdosing of multiple- and single-ingredient oral contraceptive preparations

 ● T38.4X Poisoning by, adverse effect of and underdosing of oral contraceptives

  ● T38.4X1 Poisoning by oral contraceptives, accidental (unintentional)
       Poisoning by oral contraceptives NOS

  ● T38.4X2 Poisoning by oral contraceptives, intentional self-harm A, S 🔊

  ● T38.4X3 Poisoning by oral contraceptives, assault

  ● T38.4X4 Poisoning by oral contraceptives, undetermined

  ● T38.4X5 Adverse effect of oral contraceptives

  ● T38.4X6 Underdosing of oral contraceptives

● T38.5 Poisoning by, adverse effect of and underdosing of other estrogens and progestogens
     Poisoning by, adverse effect of and underdosing of estrogens and progestogens mixtures and substitutes

 ● T38.5X Poisoning by, adverse effect of and underdosing of other estrogens and progestogens

  ● T38.5X1 Poisoning by other estrogens and progestogens, accidental (unintentional)
       Poisoning by other estrogens and progestogens NOS

  ● T38.5X2 Poisoning by other estrogens and progestogens, intentional self-harm A, S 🔊

  ● T38.5X3 Poisoning by other estrogens and progestogens, assault

  ● T38.5X4 Poisoning by other estrogens and progestogens, undetermined

● T38.5X5 Adverse effect of other estrogens and progestogens
● T38.5X6 Underdosing of other estrogens and progestogens

● T38.6 Poisoning by, adverse effect of and underdosing of antigonadotrophins, antiestrogens, antiandrogens, not elsewhere classified
     Poisoning by, adverse effect of and underdosing of tamoxifen

 ● T38.6X Poisoning by, adverse effect of and underdosing of antigonadotrophins, antiestrogens, antiandrogens, not elsewhere classified

  ● T38.6X1 Poisoning by antigonadotrophins, antiestrogens, antiandrogens, not elsewhere classified, accidental (unintentional)
       Poisoning by antigonadotrophins, antiestrogens, antiandrogens, not elsewhere classified NOS

  ● T38.6X2 Poisoning by antigonadotrophins, antiestrogens, antiandrogens, not elsewhere classified, intentional self-harm A, S 🔊

  ● T38.6X3 Poisoning by antigonadotrophins, antiestrogens, antiandrogens, not elsewhere classified, assault

  ● T38.6X4 Poisoning by antigonadotrophins, antiestrogens, antiandrogens, not elsewhere classified, undetermined

  ● T38.6X5 Adverse effect of antigonadotrophins, antiestrogens, antiandrogens, not elsewhere classified

  ● T38.6X6 Underdosing of antigonadotrophins, antiestrogens, antiandrogens, not elsewhere classified

● T38.7 Poisoning by, adverse effect of and underdosing of androgens and anabolic congeners

 ● T38.7X Poisoning by, adverse effect of and underdosing of androgens and anabolic congeners

  ● T38.7X1 Poisoning by androgens and anabolic congeners, accidental (unintentional)
       Poisoning by androgens and anabolic congeners NOS

  ● T38.7X2 Poisoning by androgens and anabolic congeners, intentional self-harm A, S 🔊

  ● T38.7X3 Poisoning by androgens and anabolic congeners, assault

  ● T38.7X4 Poisoning by androgens and anabolic congeners, undetermined

  ● T38.7X5 Adverse effect of androgens and anabolic congeners

  ● T38.7X6 Underdosing of androgens and anabolic congeners

● T38.8 Poisoning by, adverse effect of and underdosing of other and unspecified hormones and synthetic substitutes

 ● T38.80 Poisoning by, adverse effect of and underdosing of unspecified hormones and synthetic substitutes

  ● T38.801 Poisoning by unspecified hormones and synthetic substitutes, accidental (unintentional)
       Poisoning by unspecified hormones and synthetic substitutes NOS

  ● T38.802 Poisoning by unspecified hormones and synthetic substitutes, intentional self-harm A, S 🔊

CHAPTER 19 (S00-T88)

● T38.803 Poisoning by unspecified hormones and synthetic substitutes, assault

● T38.804 Poisoning by unspecified hormones and synthetic substitutes, undetermined

● T38.805 Adverse effect of unspecified hormones and synthetic substitutes

● T38.806 Underdosing of unspecified hormones and synthetic substitutes

● T38.81 Poisoning by, adverse effect of and underdosing of anterior pituitary [adenohypophyseal] hormones

● T38.811 Poisoning by anterior pituitary [adenohypophyseal] hormones, accidental (unintentional)
Poisoning by anterior pituitary [adenohypophyseal] hormones NOS

● T38.812 Poisoning by anterior pituitary [adenohypophyseal] hormones, intentional self-harm A, S 🐾

● T38.813 Poisoning by anterior pituitary [adenohypophyseal] hormones, assault

● T38.814 Poisoning by anterior pituitary [adenohypophyseal] hormones, undetermined

● T38.815 Adverse effect of anterior pituitary [adenohypophyseal] hormones

● T38.816 Underdosing of anterior pituitary [adenohypophyseal] hormones

● T38.89 Poisoning by, adverse effect of and underdosing of other hormones and synthetic substitutes

● T38.891 Poisoning by other hormones and synthetic substitutes, accidental (unintentional)
Poisoning by other hormones and synthetic substitutes NOS

● T38.892 Poisoning by other hormones and synthetic substitutes, intentional self-harm A, S 🐾

● T38.893 Poisoning by other hormones and synthetic substitutes, assault

● T38.894 Poisoning by other hormones and synthetic substitutes, undetermined

● T38.895 Adverse effect of other hormones and synthetic substitutes

● T38.896 Underdosing of other hormones and synthetic substitutes

● T38.9 Poisoning by, adverse effect of and underdosing of other and unspecified hormone antagonists

● T38.90 Poisoning by, adverse effect of and underdosing of unspecified hormone antagonists

● T38.901 Poisoning by unspecified hormone antagonists, accidental (unintentional)
Poisoning by unspecified hormone antagonists NOS

● T38.902 Poisoning by unspecified hormone antagonists, intentional self-harm A, S 🐾

● T38.903 Poisoning by unspecified hormone antagonists, assault

● T38.904 Poisoning by unspecified hormone antagonists, undetermined

● T38.905 Adverse effect of unspecified hormone antagonists

● T38.906 Underdosing of unspecified hormone antagonists

● T38.99 Poisoning by, adverse effect of and underdosing of other hormone antagonists

● T38.991 Poisoning by other hormone antagonists, accidental (unintentional)
Poisoning by other hormone antagonists NOS

● T38.992 Poisoning by other hormone antagonists, intentional self-harm A, S 🐾

● T38.993 Poisoning by other hormone antagonists, assault

● T38.994 Poisoning by other hormone antagonists, undetermined

● T38.995 Adverse effect of other hormone antagonists

● T38.996 Underdosing of other hormone antagonists

● T39 Poisoning by, adverse effect of and underdosing of nonopioid analgesics, antipyretics and antirheumatics
The appropriate 7th character is to be added to each code from category T39

A	initial encounter
D	subsequent encounter
S	sequela

● T39.0 Poisoning by, adverse effect of and underdosing of salicylates

● T39.01 Poisoning by, adverse effect of and underdosing of aspirin
Poisoning by, adverse effect of and underdosing of acetylsalicylic acid

● T39.011 Poisoning by aspirin, accidental (unintentional)

● T39.012 Poisoning by aspirin, intentional self-harm A, S 🐾

● T39.013 Poisoning by aspirin, assault

● T39.014 Poisoning by aspirin, undetermined

● T39.015 Adverse effect of aspirin
Coding Clinic: 2016, Q1, P15

● T39.016 Underdosing of aspirin

● T39.09 Poisoning by, adverse effect of and underdosing of other salicylates

● T39.091 Poisoning by salicylates, accidental (unintentional)
Poisoning by salicylates NOS

● T39.092 Poisoning by salicylates, intentional self-harm A, S 🐾

● T39.093 Poisoning by salicylates, assault

● T39.094 Poisoning by salicylates, undetermined

● T39.095 Adverse effect of salicylates

● T39.096 Underdosing of salicylates

● T39.1 Poisoning by, adverse effect of and underdosing of 4-Aminophenol derivatives

● T39.1X Poisoning by, adverse effect of and underdosing of 4-Aminophenol derivatives

● T39.1X1 Poisoning by 4-Aminophenol derivatives, accidental (unintentional)
Poisoning by 4-Aminophenol derivatives NOS

● T39.1X2 Poisoning by 4-Aminophenol derivatives, intentional self-harm A, S 🐾

▶ New   ⇒ Revised   ~~deleted~~ Deleted   Excludes 1   Excludes 2   Includes   Use additional   Code first   Code also   Key words
OGCR Official Guidelines   X Assign placeholder X   ● Use Additional Character(s)   ▶ Manifestation Code   🐾 Hierarchical Condition Category   Coding Clinic

● T39.1X3   Poisoning by 4-Aminophenol derivatives, assault

● T39.1X4   Poisoning by 4-Aminophenol derivatives, undetermined

● T39.1X5   Adverse effect of 4-Aminophenol derivatives

● T39.1X6   Underdosing of 4-Aminophenol derivatives

● T39.2   Poisoning by, adverse effect of and underdosing of pyrazolone derivatives

  ● T39.2X   Poisoning by, adverse effect of and underdosing of pyrazolone derivatives

    ● T39.2X1   Poisoning by pyrazolone derivatives, accidental (unintentional)
          Poisoning by pyrazolone derivatives NOS

    ● T39.2X2   Poisoning by pyrazolone derivatives, intentional self-harm A, S 🔗

    ● T39.2X3   Poisoning by pyrazolone derivatives, assault

    ● T39.2X4   Poisoning by pyrazolone derivatives, undetermined

    ● T39.2X5   Adverse effect of pyrazolone derivatives

    ● T39.2X6   Underdosing of pyrazolone derivatives

● T39.3   Poisoning by, adverse effect of and underdosing of other nonsteroidal anti-inflammatory drugs [NSAID]

  ● T39.31   Poisoning by, adverse effect of and underdosing of propionic acid derivatives
      Poisoning by, adverse effect of and underdosing of fenoprofen
      Poisoning by, adverse effect of and underdosing of flurbiprofen
      Poisoning by, adverse effect of and underdosing of ibuprofen
      Poisoning by, adverse effect of and underdosing of ketoprofen
      Poisoning by, adverse effect of and underdosing of naproxen
      Poisoning by, adverse effect of and underdosing of oxaprozin

    ● T39.311   Poisoning by propionic acid derivatives, accidental (unintentional)

    ● T39.312   Poisoning by propionic acid derivatives, intentional self-harm A, S 🔗

    ● T39.313   Poisoning by propionic acid derivatives, assault

    ● T39.314   Poisoning by propionic acid derivatives, undetermined

    ● T39.315   Adverse effect of propionic acid derivatives

    ● T39.316   Underdosing of propionic acid derivatives

  ● T39.39   Poisoning by, adverse effect of and underdosing of other nonsteroidal anti-inflammatory drugs [NSAID]

    ● T39.391   Poisoning by other nonsteroidal anti-inflammatory drugs [NSAID], accidental (unintentional)
          Poisoning by other nonsteroidal anti-inflammatory drugs NOS

    ● T39.392   Poisoning by other nonsteroidal anti-inflammatory drugs [NSAID], intentional self-harm A, S 🔗

● T39.393   Poisoning by other nonsteroidal anti-inflammatory drugs [NSAID], assault

● T39.394   Poisoning by other nonsteroidal anti-inflammatory drugs [NSAID], undetermined

● T39.395   Adverse effect of other nonsteroidal anti-inflammatory drugs [NSAID]

● T39.396   Underdosing of other nonsteroidal anti-inflammatory drugs [NSAID]

● T39.4   Poisoning by, adverse effect of and underdosing of antirheumatics, not elsewhere classified

    Excludes1   poisoning by, adverse effect of and underdosing of glucocorticoids (T38.Ø-)
            poisoning by, adverse effect of and underdosing of salicylates (T39.Ø-)

  ● T39.4X   Poisoning by, adverse effect of and underdosing of antirheumatics, not elsewhere classified

    ● T39.4X1   Poisoning by antirheumatics, not elsewhere classified, accidental (unintentional)
          Poisoning by antirheumatics, not elsewhere classified NOS

    ● T39.4X2   Poisoning by antirheumatics, not elsewhere classified, intentional self-harm A, S 🔗

    ● T39.4X3   Poisoning by antirheumatics, not elsewhere classified, assault

    ● T39.4X4   Poisoning by antirheumatics, not elsewhere classified, undetermined

    ● T39.4X5   Adverse effect of antirheumatics, not elsewhere classified

    ● T39.4X6   Underdosing of antirheumatics, not elsewhere classified

● T39.8   Poisoning by, adverse effect of and underdosing of other nonopioid analgesics and antipyretics, not elsewhere classified

  ● T39.8X   Poisoning by, adverse effect of and underdosing of other nonopioid analgesics and antipyretics, not elsewhere classified

    ● T39.8X1   Poisoning by other nonopioid analgesics and antipyretics, not elsewhere classified, accidental (unintentional)
          Poisoning by other nonopioid analgesics and antipyretics, not elsewhere classified NOS

    ● T39.8X2   Poisoning by other nonopioid analgesics and antipyretics, not elsewhere classified, intentional self-harm A, S 🔗

    ● T39.8X3   Poisoning by other nonopioid analgesics and antipyretics, not elsewhere classified, assault

    ● T39.8X4   Poisoning by other nonopioid analgesics and antipyretics, not elsewhere classified, undetermined

    ● T39.8X5   Adverse effect of other nonopioid analgesics and antipyretics, not elsewhere classified

    ● T39.8X6   Underdosing of other nonopioid analgesics and antipyretics, not elsewhere classified

CHAPTER 19 (SØØ-T88)

●T39.9 Poisoning by, adverse effect of and underdosing of unspecified nonopioid analgesic, antipyretic and antirheumatic

X●T39.91 Poisoning by unspecified nonopioid analgesic, antipyretic and antirheumatic, accidental (unintentional)
  Poisoning by nonopioid analgesic, antipyretic and antirheumatic NOS

X●T39.92 Poisoning by unspecified nonopioid analgesic, antipyretic and antirheumatic, intentional self-harm A, S 🐾

X●T39.93 Poisoning by unspecified nonopioid analgesic, antipyretic and antirheumatic, assault

X●T39.94 Poisoning by unspecified nonopioid analgesic, antipyretic and antirheumatic, undetermined

X●T39.95 Adverse effect of unspecified nonopioid analgesic, antipyretic and antirheumatic

X●T39.96 Underdosing of unspecified nonopioid analgesic, antipyretic and antirheumatic

●T40 Poisoning by, adverse effect of and underdosing of narcotics and psychodysleptics [hallucinogens]

  Excludes2 drug dependence and related mental and behavioral disorders due to psychoactive substance use (F10.-F19.-)

  The appropriate 7th character is to be added to each code from category T40

A	initial encounter
D	subsequent encounter
S	sequela

●T40.0 Poisoning by, adverse effect of and underdosing of opium

  ●T40.0X Poisoning by, adverse effect of and underdosing of opium

    ●T40.0X1 Poisoning by opium, accidental (unintentional)
      Poisoning by opium NOS

    ●T40.0X2 Poisoning by opium, intentional self-harm A, S 🐾

    ●T40.0X3 Poisoning by opium, assault

    ●T40.0X4 Poisoning by opium, undetermined

    ●T40.0X5 Adverse effect of opium

    ●T40.0X6 Underdosing of opium

●T40.1 Poisoning by and adverse effect of heroin

  ●T40.1X Poisoning by and adverse effect of heroin

    ●T40.1X1 Poisoning by heroin, accidental (unintentional)
      Poisoning by heroin NOS

    ●T40.1X2 Poisoning by heroin, intentional self-harm A, S 🐾

    ●T40.1X3 Poisoning by heroin, assault

    ●T40.1X4 Poisoning by heroin, undetermined

●T40.2 Poisoning by, adverse effect of and underdosing of other opioids

  ●T40.2X Poisoning by, adverse effect of and underdosing of other opioids

    ●T40.2X1 Poisoning by other opioids, accidental (unintentional)
      Poisoning by other opioids NOS

    ●T40.2X2 Poisoning by other opioids, intentional self-harm A, S 🐾

    ●T40.2X3 Poisoning by other opioids, assault

    ●T40.2X4 Poisoning by other opioids, undetermined

    ●T40.2X5 Adverse effect of other opioids

    ●T40.2X6 Underdosing of other opioids

●T40.3 Poisoning by, adverse effect of and underdosing of methadone

  ●T40.3X Poisoning by, adverse effect of and underdosing of methadone

    ●T40.3X1 Poisoning by methadone, accidental (unintentional)
      Poisoning by methadone NOS

    ●T40.3X2 Poisoning by methadone, intentional self-harm A, S 🐾

    ●T40.3X3 Poisoning by methadone, assault

    ●T40.3X4 Poisoning by methadone, undetermined

    ●T40.3X5 Adverse effect of methadone

    ●T40.3X6 Underdosing of methadone

●T40.4 Poisoning by, adverse effect of and underdosing of other synthetic narcotics

  ●T40.41 Poisoning by, adverse effect of and underdosing of fentanyl or fentanyl analogs

    T40.411 Poisoning by fentanyl or fentanyl analogs, accidental (unintentional)

    T40.412 Poisoning by fentanyl or fentanyl analogs, intentional self-harm

    T40.413 Poisoning by fentanyl or fentanyl analogs, assault

    T40.414 Poisoning by fentanyl or fentanyl analogs, undetermined

    T40.415 Adverse effect of fentanyl or fentanyl analogs

    T40.416 Underdosing of fentanyl or fentanyl analogs

  ●T40.42 Poisoning by, adverse effect of and underdosing of tramadol

    T40.421 Poisoning by tramadol, accidental (unintentional)

    T40.422 Poisoning by tramadol, intentional self-harm

    T40.423 Poisoning by tramadol, assault

    T40.424 Poisoning by tramadol, undetermined

    T40.425 Adverse effect of tramadol

    T40.426 Underdosing of tramadol

  ●T40.49 Poisoning by, adverse effect of and underdosing of other synthetic narcotics

    T40.491 Poisoning by other synthetic narcotics, accidental (unintentional)

    T40.492 Poisoning by other synthetic narcotics, intentional self-harm

    T40.493 Poisoning by other synthetic narcotics, assault

    T40.494 Poisoning by other synthetic narcotics, undetermined

    T40.495 Adverse effect of other synthetic narcotics

    T40.496 Underdosing of other synthetic narcotics

●T40.5 Poisoning by, adverse effect of and underdosing of cocaine

  ●T40.5X Poisoning by, adverse effect of and underdosing of cocaine

    ●T40.5X1 Poisoning by cocaine, accidental (unintentional)
      Poisoning by cocaine NOS
      Coding Clinic: 2016, Q2, P9

    ●T40.5X2 Poisoning by cocaine, intentional self-harm A, S 🐾

    ●T40.5X3 Poisoning by cocaine, assault

    ●T40.5X4 Poisoning by cocaine, undetermined

    ●T40.5X5 Adverse effect of cocaine

    ●T40.5X6 Underdosing of cocaine

▶ New ⇒ Revised ~~deleted~~ Deleted Excludes 1 Excludes 2 Includes Use additional Code first Code also Key words

OGCR Official Guidelines X Assign placeholder X ● Use Additional Character(s) ▌Manifestation Code 🐾 Hierarchical Condition Category **Coding Clinic**

● **T40.6 Poisoning by, adverse effect of and underdosing of other and unspecified narcotics**
  ● **T40.60 Poisoning by, adverse effect of and underdosing of unspecified narcotics**
    ● **T40.601 Poisoning by unspecified narcotics, accidental (unintentional)**
        Poisoning by narcotics NOS
    ● **T40.602 Poisoning by unspecified narcotics, intentional self-harm A, S** 🔖
    ● **T40.603 Poisoning by unspecified narcotics, assault**
    ● **T40.604 Poisoning by unspecified narcotics, undetermined**
    ● **T40.605 Adverse effect of unspecified narcotics**
    ● **T40.606 Underdosing of unspecified narcotics**
  ● **T40.69 Poisoning by, adverse effect of and underdosing of other narcotics**
    ● **T40.691 Poisoning by other narcotics, accidental (unintentional)**
        Poisoning by other narcotics NOS
    ● **T40.692 Poisoning by other narcotics, intentional self-harm A, S** 🔖
    ● **T40.693 Poisoning by other narcotics, assault**
    ● **T40.694 Poisoning by other narcotics, undetermined**
    ● **T40.695 Adverse effect of other narcotics**
    ● **T40.696 Underdosing of other narcotics**
● **T40.7 Poisoning by, adverse effect of and underdosing of cannabis (derivatives)**
  ▶● **T40.71 Poisoning by, adverse effect of and underdosing of cannabis (derivatives)**
    ▶ **T40.711 Poisoning by cannabis, accidental (unintentional)**
    ▶ **T40.712 Poisoning by cannabis, intentional self-harm**
    ▶ **T40.713 Poisoning by cannabis, assault**
    ▶ **T40.714 Poisoning by cannabis, undetermined**
    ▶ **T40.715 Adverse effect of cannabis**
    ▶ **T40.716 Underdosing of cannabis**
  ▶● **T40.72 Poisoning by, adverse effect of and underdosing of synthetic cannabinoids**
    ▶ **T40.721 Poisoning by synthetic cannabinoids, accidental (unintentional)**
    ▶ **T40.722 Poisoning by synthetic cannabinoids, intentional self-harm**
    ▶ **T40.723 Poisoning by synthetic cannabinoids, assault**
    ▶ **T40.724 Poisoning by synthetic cannabinoids, undetermined**
    ▶ **T40.725 Adverse effect of synthetic cannabinoids**
    ▶ **T40.726 Underdosing of synthetic cannabinoids**

~~T40.7X Poisoning by, adverse effect of and underdosing of cannabis (derivatives)~~
  ~~T40.7X1 Poisoning by cannabis (derivatives), accidental (unintentional)~~
      ~~Poisoning by cannabis NOS~~
      ~~Coding Clinic: 2020, Q1, P8~~
  ~~T40.7X2 Poisoning by cannabis (derivatives), intentional self-harm A, S~~
  ~~T40.7X3 Poisoning by cannabis (derivatives), assault~~
  ~~T40.7X4 Poisoning by cannabis (derivatives), undetermined~~
  ~~T40.7X5 Adverse effect of cannabis (derivatives)~~
  ~~T40.7X6 Underdosing of cannabis (derivatives)~~

● **T40.8 Poisoning by and adverse effect of lysergide [LSD]**
  ● **T40.8X Poisoning by and adverse effect of lysergide [LSD]**
    ● **T40.8X1 Poisoning by lysergide [LSD], accidental (unintentional)**
        Poisoning by lysergide [LSD] NOS
    ● **T40.8X2 Poisoning by lysergide [LSD], intentional self-harm A, S** 🔖
    ● **T40.8X3 Poisoning by lysergide [LSD], assault**
    ● **T40.8X4 Poisoning by lysergide [LSD], undetermined**
● **T40.9 Poisoning by, adverse effect of and underdosing of other and unspecified psychodysleptics [hallucinogens]**
  ● **T40.90 Poisoning by, adverse effect of and underdosing of unspecified psychodysleptics [hallucinogens]**
    ● **T40.901 Poisoning by unspecified psychodysleptics [hallucinogens], accidental (unintentional)**
    ● **T40.902 Poisoning by unspecified psychodysleptics [hallucinogens], intentional self-harm A, S** 🔖
    ● **T40.903 Poisoning by unspecified psychodysleptics [hallucinogens], assault**
    ● **T40.904 Poisoning by unspecified psychodysleptics [hallucinogens], undetermined**
    ● **T40.905 Adverse effect of unspecified psychodysleptics [hallucinogens]**
    ● **T40.906 Underdosing of unspecified psychodysleptics [hallucinogens]**
  ● **T40.99 Poisoning by, adverse effect of and underdosing of other psychodysleptics [hallucinogens]**
    ● **T40.991 Poisoning by other psychodysleptics [hallucinogens], accidental (unintentional)**
        Poisoning by other psychodysleptics [hallucinogens] NOS
    ● **T40.992 Poisoning by other psychodysleptics [hallucinogens], intentional self-harm A, S** 🔖
    ● **T40.993 Poisoning by other psychodysleptics [hallucinogens], assault**
    ● **T40.994 Poisoning by other psychodysleptics [hallucinogens], undetermined**
    ● **T40.995 Adverse effect of other psychodysleptics [hallucinogens]**
    ● **T40.996 Underdosing of other psychodysleptics [hallucinogens]**

● **T41 Poisoning by, adverse effect of and underdosing of anesthetics and therapeutic gases**

Excludes1   benzodiazepines (T42.4-)
              cocaine (T40.5-)
              complications of anesthesia during pregnancy (O29.-)
              complications of anesthesia during labor and delivery (O74.-)
              complications of anesthesia during the puerperium (O89.-) opioids (T40.0-T40.2-)

The appropriate 7th character is to be added to each code from category T41

A	initial encounter
D	subsequent encounter
S	sequela

● **T41.0 Poisoning by, adverse effect of and underdosing of inhaled anesthetics**

Excludes1   oxygen (T41.5-)

● **T41.0X** Poisoning by, adverse effect of and underdosing of inhaled anesthetics

   ● **T41.0X1** Poisoning by inhaled anesthetics, accidental (unintentional)
      Poisoning by inhaled anesthetics NOS

   ● **T41.0X2** Poisoning by inhaled anesthetics, intentional self-harm A, S 🐾

   ● **T41.0X3** Poisoning by inhaled anesthetics, assault

   ● **T41.0X4** Poisoning by inhaled anesthetics, undetermined

   ● **T41.0X5** Adverse effect of inhaled anesthetics

   ● **T41.0X6** Underdosing of inhaled anesthetics

● **T41.1** Poisoning by, adverse effect of and underdosing of intravenous anesthetics
   Poisoning by, adverse effect of and underdosing of thiobarbiturates

  ● **T41.1X** Poisoning by, adverse effect of and underdosing of intravenous anesthetics

   ● **T41.1X1** Poisoning by intravenous anesthetics, accidental (unintentional)
      Poisoning by intravenous anesthetics NOS

   ● **T41.1X2** Poisoning by intravenous anesthetics, intentional self-harm A, S 🐾

   ● **T41.1X3** Poisoning by intravenous anesthetics, assault

   ● **T41.1X4** Poisoning by intravenous anesthetics, undetermined

   ● **T41.1X5** Adverse effect of intravenous anesthetics

   ● **T41.1X6** Underdosing of intravenous anesthetics

● **T41.2** Poisoning by, adverse effect of and underdosing of other and unspecified general anesthetics

  ● **T41.20** Poisoning by, adverse effect of and underdosing of unspecified general anesthetics

   ● **T41.201** Poisoning by unspecified general anesthetics, accidental (unintentional)
      Poisoning by general anesthetics NOS

   ● **T41.202** Poisoning by unspecified general anesthetics, intentional self-harm A, S 🐾

   ● **T41.203** Poisoning by unspecified general anesthetics, assault

   ● **T41.204** Poisoning by unspecified general anesthetics, undetermined

   ● **T41.205** Adverse effect of unspecified general anesthetics
      Coding Clinic: 2016, Q4, P73

   ● **T41.206** Underdosing of unspecified general anesthetics

  ● **T41.29** Poisoning by, adverse effect of and underdosing of other general anesthetics

   ● **T41.291** Poisoning by other general anesthetics, accidental (unintentional)
      Poisoning by other general anesthetics NOS

   ● **T41.292** Poisoning by other general anesthetics, intentional self-harm A, S 🐾

   ● **T41.293** Poisoning by other general anesthetics, assault

   ● **T41.294** Poisoning by other general anesthetics, undetermined

   ● **T41.295** Adverse effect of other general anesthetics

   ● **T41.296** Underdosing of other general anesthetics

● **T41.3** Poisoning by, adverse effect of and underdosing of local anesthetics
   Cocaine (topical)

   Excludes2 poisoning by cocaine used as a central nervous system stimulant (T40.5X1-T40.5X4)

  ● **T41.3X** Poisoning by, adverse effect of and underdosing of local anesthetics

   ● **T41.3X1** Poisoning by local anesthetics, accidental (unintentional)
      Poisoning by local anesthetics NOS

   ● **T41.3X2** Poisoning by local anesthetics, intentional self-harm A, S 🐾

   ● **T41.3X3** Poisoning by local anesthetics, assault

   ● **T41.3X4** Poisoning by local anesthetics, undetermined

   ● **T41.3X5** Adverse effect of local anesthetics

   ● **T41.3X6** Underdosing of local anesthetics

● **T41.4** Poisoning by, adverse effect of and underdosing of unspecified anesthetic

  X● **T41.41** Poisoning by unspecified anesthetic, accidental (unintentional)
      Poisoning by anesthetic NOS

  X● **T41.42** Poisoning by unspecified anesthetic, intentional self-harm A, S 🐾

  X● **T41.43** Poisoning by unspecified anesthetic, assault

  X● **T41.44** Poisoning by unspecified anesthetic, undetermined

  X● **T41.45** Adverse effect of unspecified anesthetic

  X● **T41.46** Underdosing of unspecified anesthetics

● **T41.5** Poisoning by, adverse effect of and underdosing of therapeutic gases

  ● **T41.5X** Poisoning by, adverse effect of and underdosing of therapeutic gases

   ● **T41.5X1** Poisoning by therapeutic gases, accidental (unintentional)
      Poisoning by therapeutic gases NOS

   ● **T41.5X2** Poisoning by therapeutic gases, intentional self-harm A, S 🐾

   ● **T41.5X3** Poisoning by therapeutic gases, assault

   ● **T41.5X4** Poisoning by therapeutic gases, undetermined

   ● **T41.5X5** Adverse effect of therapeutic gases

   ● **T41.5X6** Underdosing of therapeutic gases

● **T42** Poisoning by, adverse effect of and underdosing of antiepileptic, sedative-hypnotic and antiparkinsonism drugs

   Excludes2 drug dependence and related mental and behavioral disorders due to psychoactive substance use (F10.--F19.-)

   The appropriate 7th character is to be added to each code from category T42

A	initial encounter
D	subsequent encounter
S	sequela

● **T42.0** Poisoning by, adverse effect of and underdosing of hydantoin derivatives

  ● **T42.0X** Poisoning by, adverse effect of and underdosing of hydantoin derivatives

   ● **T42.0X1** Poisoning by hydantoin derivatives, accidental (unintentional)
      Poisoning by hydantoin derivatives NOS

   ● **T42.0X2** Poisoning by hydantoin derivatives, intentional self-harm A, S 🐾

   ● **T42.0X3** Poisoning by hydantoin derivatives, assault

▶ New   ⇒ Revised   ~~deleted~~ Deleted   Excludes 1   Excludes 2   Includes   Use additional   Code first   Code also   Key words
OGCR Official Guidelines   X Assign placeholder X   ● Use Additional Character(s)   ▶ Manifestation Code   🐾 Hierarchical Condition Category   **Coding Clinic**

- ● T42.0X4   Poisoning by hydantoin derivatives, undetermined
- ● T42.0X5   Adverse effect of hydantoin derivatives
- ● T42.0X6   Underdosing of hydantoin derivatives
- ● T42.1   Poisoning by, adverse effect of and underdosing of iminostilbenes
  - Poisoning by, adverse effect of and underdosing of carbamazepine
  - ● T42.1X   Poisoning by, adverse effect of and underdosing of iminostilbenes
    - ● T42.1X1   Poisoning by iminostilbenes, accidental (unintentional)
      - Poisoning by iminostilbenes NOS
    - ● T42.1X2   Poisoning by iminostilbenes, intentional self-harm A, S 🔖
    - ● T42.1X3   Poisoning by iminostilbenes, assault
    - ● T42.1X4   Poisoning by iminostilbenes, undetermined
    - ● T42.1X5   Adverse effect of iminostilbenes
    - ● T42.1X6   Underdosing of iminostilbenes
- ● T42.2   Poisoning by, adverse effect of and underdosing of succinimides and oxazolidinediones
  - ● T42.2X   Poisoning by, adverse effect of and underdosing of succinimides and oxazolidinediones
    - ● T42.2X1   Poisoning by succinimides and oxazolidinediones, accidental (unintentional)
      - Poisoning by succinimides and oxazolidinediones NOS
    - ● T42.2X2   Poisoning by succinimides and oxazolidinediones, intentional self-harm A, S 🔖
    - ● T42.2X3   Poisoning by succinimides and oxazolidinediones, assault
    - ● T42.2X4   Poisoning by succinimides and oxazolidinediones, undetermined
    - ● T42.2X5   Adverse effect of succinimides and oxazolidinediones
    - ● T42.2X6   Underdosing of succinimides and oxazolidinediones
- ● T42.3   Poisoning by, adverse effect of and underdosing of barbiturates
  - **Excludes1**   poisoning by, adverse effect of and underdosing of thiobarbiturates (T41.1-)
  - ● T42.3X   Poisoning by, adverse effect of and underdosing of barbiturates
    - ● T42.3X1   Poisoning by barbiturates, accidental (unintentional)
      - Poisoning by barbiturates NOS
    - ● T42.3X2   Poisoning by barbiturates, intentional self-harm A, S 🔖
    - ● T42.3X3   Poisoning by barbiturates, assault
    - ● T42.3X4   Poisoning by barbiturates, undetermined
    - ● T42.3X5   Adverse effect of barbiturates
    - ● T42.3X6   Underdosing of barbiturates
- ● T42.4   Poisoning by, adverse effect of and underdosing of benzodiazepines
  - ● T42.4X   Poisoning by, adverse effect of and underdosing of benzodiazepines
    - ● T42.4X1   Poisoning by benzodiazepines, accidental (unintentional)
      - Poisoning by benzodiazepines NOS
    - ● T42.4X2   Poisoning by benzodiazepines, intentional self-harm A, S 🔖
    - ● T42.4X3   Poisoning by benzodiazepines, assault

- ● T42.4X4   Poisoning by benzodiazepines, undetermined
- ● T42.4X5   Adverse effect of benzodiazepines
- ● T42.4X6   Underdosing of benzodiazepines
- ● T42.5   Poisoning by, adverse effect of and underdosing of mixed antiepileptics
  - ● T42.5X   Poisoning by, adverse effect of and underdosing of antiepileptics
    - ● T42.5X1   Poisoning by mixed antiepileptics, accidental (unintentional)
      - Poisoning by mixed antiepileptics NOS
    - ● T42.5X2   Poisoning by mixed antiepileptics, intentional self-harm A, S 🔖
    - ● T42.5X3   Poisoning by mixed antiepileptics, assault
    - ● T42.5X4   Poisoning by mixed antiepileptics, undetermined
    - ● T42.5X5   Adverse effect of mixed antiepileptics
    - ● T42.5X6   Underdosing of mixed antiepileptics
- ● T42.6   Poisoning by, adverse effect of and underdosing of other antiepileptic and sedative-hypnotic drugs
  - Poisoning by, adverse effect of and underdosing of methaqualone
  - Poisoning by, adverse effect of and underdosing of valproic acid
  - **Excludes1**   poisoning by, adverse effect of and underdosing of carbamazepine (T42.1-)
  - ● T42.6X   Poisoning by, adverse effect of and underdosing of other antiepileptic and sedative-hypnotic drugs
    - ● T42.6X1   Poisoning by other antiepileptic and sedative-hypnotic drugs, accidental (unintentional)
      - Poisoning by other antiepileptic and sedative-hypnotic drugs NOS
    - ● T42.6X2   Poisoning by other antiepileptic and sedative-hypnotic drugs, intentional self-harm A, S 🔖
    - ● T42.6X3   Poisoning by other antiepileptic and sedative-hypnotic drugs, assault
    - ● T42.6X4   Poisoning by other antiepileptic and sedative-hypnotic drugs, undetermined
    - ● T42.6X5   Adverse effect of other antiepileptic and sedative-hypnotic drugs
    - ● T42.6X6   Underdosing of other antiepileptic and sedative-hypnotic drugs
- ● T42.7   Poisoning by, adverse effect of and underdosing of unspecified antiepileptic and sedative-hypnotic drugs
  - X ● T42.71   Poisoning by unspecified antiepileptic and sedative-hypnotic drugs, accidental (unintentional)
    - Poisoning by antiepileptic and sedative-hypnotic drugs NOS
  - X ● T42.72   Poisoning by unspecified antiepileptic and sedative-hypnotic drugs, intentional self-harm A, S 🔖
  - X ● T42.73   Poisoning by unspecified antiepileptic and sedative-hypnotic drugs, assault
  - X ● T42.74   Poisoning by unspecified antiepileptic and sedative-hypnotic drugs, undetermined
  - X ● T42.75   Adverse effect of unspecified antiepileptic and sedative-hypnotic drugs
  - X ● T42.76   Underdosing of unspecified antiepileptic and sedative-hypnotic drugs

CHAPTER 19 (S00-T88)

CHAPTER 19 (S00-T88)

● **T42.8** Poisoning by, adverse effect of and underdosing of antiparkinsonism drugs and other central muscle-tone depressants

Poisoning by, adverse effect of and underdosing of amantadine

  ● **T42.8X** Poisoning by, adverse effect of and underdosing of antiparkinsonism drugs and other central muscle-tone depressants

    ● **T42.8X1** Poisoning by antiparkinsonism drugs and other central muscle-tone depressants, accidental (unintentional)

Poisoning by antiparkinsonism drugs and other central muscle-tone depressants NOS

    ● **T42.8X2** Poisoning by antiparkinsonism drugs and other central muscle-tone depressants, intentional self-harm A, S 🐾

    ● **T42.8X3** Poisoning by antiparkinsonism drugs and other central muscle-tone depressants, assault

    ● **T42.8X4** Poisoning by antiparkinsonism drugs and other central muscle-tone depressants, undetermined

    ● **T42.8X5** Adverse effect of antiparkinsonism drugs and other central muscle-tone depressants

    ● **T42.8X6** Underdosing of antiparkinsonism drugs and other central muscle-tone depressants

● **T43** Poisoning by, adverse effect of and underdosing of psychotropic drugs, not elsewhere classified

  Excludes1   appetite depressants (T50.5-)
                   barbiturates (T42.3-)
                   benzodiazepines (T42.4-)
                   methaqualone (T42.6-)
                   psychodysleptics [hallucinogens] (T40.7-T40.9-)

  Excludes2   drug dependence and related mental and behavioral disorders due to psychoactive substance use (F10.--F19.-)

The appropriate 7th character is to be added to each code from category T43

        A   initial encounter
        D   subsequent encounter
        S   sequela

  ● **T43.0** Poisoning by, adverse effect of and underdosing of tricyclic and tetracyclic antidepressants

    ● **T43.01** Poisoning by, adverse effect of and underdosing of tricyclic antidepressants

      ● **T43.011** Poisoning by tricyclic antidepressants, accidental (unintentional)

Poisoning by tricyclic antidepressants NOS

      ● **T43.012** Poisoning by tricyclic antidepressants, intentional self-harm A, S 🐾

      ● **T43.013** Poisoning by tricyclic antidepressants, assault

      ● **T43.014** Poisoning by tricyclic antidepressants, undetermined

      ● **T43.015** Adverse effect of tricyclic antidepressants

      ● **T43.016** Underdosing of tricyclic antidepressants

● **T43.02** Poisoning by, adverse effect of and underdosing of tetracyclic antidepressants

  ● **T43.021** Poisoning by tetracyclic antidepressants, accidental (unintentional)

Poisoning by tetracyclic antidepressants NOS

  ● **T43.022** Poisoning by tetracyclic antidepressants, intentional self-harm A, S 🐾

  ● **T43.023** Poisoning by tetracyclic antidepressants, assault

  ● **T43.024** Poisoning by tetracyclic antidepressants, undetermined

  ● **T43.025** Adverse effect of tetracyclic antidepressants

  ● **T43.026** Underdosing of tetracyclic antidepressants

● **T43.1** Poisoning by, adverse effect of and underdosing of monoamine-oxidase-inhibitor antidepressants

  ● **T43.1X** Poisoning by, adverse effect of and underdosing of monoamine-oxidase-inhibitor antidepressants

    ● **T43.1X1** Poisoning by monoamine-oxidase-inhibitor antidepressants, accidental (unintentional)

Poisoning by monoamine-oxidase-inhibitor antidepressants NOS

    ● **T43.1X2** Poisoning by monoamine-oxidase-inhibitor antidepressants, intentional self-harm A, S 🐾

    ● **T43.1X3** Poisoning by monoamine-oxidase-inhibitor antidepressants, assault

    ● **T43.1X4** Poisoning by monoamine-oxidase-inhibitor antidepressants, undetermined

    ● **T43.1X5** Adverse effect of monoamine-oxidase-inhibitor antidepressants

    ● **T43.1X6** Underdosing of monoamine-oxidase-inhibitor antidepressants

● **T43.2** Poisoning by, adverse effect of and underdosing of other and unspecified antidepressants

  ● **T43.20** Poisoning by, adverse effect of and underdosing of unspecified antidepressants

    ● **T43.201** Poisoning by unspecified antidepressants, accidental (unintentional)

Poisoning by antidepressants NOS

    ● **T43.202** Poisoning by unspecified antidepressants, intentional self-harm A, S 🐾

    ● **T43.203** Poisoning by unspecified antidepressants, assault

    ● **T43.204** Poisoning by unspecified antidepressants, undetermined

    ● **T43.205** Adverse effect of unspecified antidepressants

Antidepressant discontinuation syndrome

    ● **T43.206** Underdosing of unspecified antidepressants

▶ New   ⫸ Revised   ~~deleted~~ Deleted   Excludes 1   Excludes 2   Includes   Use additional   Code first   Code also   Key words

OGCR Official Guidelines   **X** Assign placeholder X   ● Use Additional Character(s)   ▶ Manifestation Code   🐾 Hierarchical Condition Category   **Coding Clinic**

● T43.21   Poisoning by, adverse effect of and underdosing of selective serotonin and norepinephrine reuptake inhibitors

Poisoning by, adverse effect of and underdosing of SSNRI antidepressants

   ● T43.211   Poisoning by selective serotonin and norepinephrine reuptake inhibitors, accidental (unintentional)

   ● T43.212   Poisoning by selective serotonin and norepinephrine reuptake inhibitors, intentional self-harm A, S 🐾

   ● T43.213   Poisoning by selective serotonin and norepinephrine reuptake inhibitors, assault

   ● T43.214   Poisoning by selective serotonin and norepinephrine reuptake inhibitors, undetermined

   ● T43.215   Adverse effect of selective serotonin and norepinephrine reuptake inhibitors

   ● T43.216   Underdosing of selective serotonin and norepinephrine reuptake inhibitors

● T43.22   Poisoning by, adverse effect of and underdosing of selective serotonin reuptake inhibitors

Poisoning by, adverse effect of and underdosing of SSRI antidepressants

   ● T43.221   Poisoning by selective serotonin reuptake inhibitors, accidental (unintentional)

   ● T43.222   Poisoning by selective serotonin reuptake inhibitors, intentional self-harm A, S 🐾

   ● T43.223   Poisoning by selective serotonin reuptake inhibitors, assault

   ● T43.224   Poisoning by selective serotonin reuptake inhibitors, undetermined

   ● T43.225   Adverse effect of selective serotonin reuptake inhibitors

   ● T43.226   Underdosing of selective serotonin reuptake inhibitors

● T43.29   Poisoning by, adverse effect of and underdosing of other antidepressants

   ● T43.291   Poisoning by other antidepressants, accidental (unintentional)

Poisoning by other antidepressants NOS

   ● T43.292   Poisoning by other antidepressants, intentional self-harm A, S 🐾

   ● T43.293   Poisoning by other antidepressants, assault

   ● T43.294   Poisoning by other antidepressants, undetermined

   ● T43.295   Adverse effect of other antidepressants

   ● T43.296   Underdosing of other antidepressants

● T43.3   Poisoning by, adverse effect of and underdosing of phenothiazine antipsychotics and neuroleptics

   ● T43.3X   Poisoning by, adverse effect of and underdosing of phenothiazine antipsychotics and neuroleptics

   ● T43.3X1   Poisoning by phenothiazine antipsychotics and neuroleptics, accidental (unintentional)

Poisoning by phenothiazine antipsychotics and neuroleptics NOS

   ● T43.3X2   Poisoning by phenothiazine antipsychotics and neuroleptics, intentional self-harm A, S 🐾

   ● T43.3X3   Poisoning by phenothiazine antipsychotics and neuroleptics, assault

   ● T43.3X4   Poisoning by phenothiazine antipsychotics and neuroleptics, undetermined

   ● T43.3X5   Adverse effect of phenothiazine antipsychotics and neuroleptics

   ● T43.3X6   Underdosing of phenothiazine antipsychotics and neuroleptics

● T43.4   Poisoning by, adverse effect of and underdosing of butyrophenone and thiothixene neuroleptics

   ● T43.4X   Poisoning by, adverse effect of and underdosing of butyrophenone and thiothixene neuroleptics

   ● T43.4X1   Poisoning by butyrophenone and thiothixene neuroleptics, accidental (unintentional)

Poisoning by butyrophenone and thiothixene neuroleptics NOS

   ● T43.4X2   Poisoning by butyrophenone and thiothixene neuroleptics, intentional self-harm A, S 🐾

   ● T43.4X3   Poisoning by butyrophenone and thiothixene neuroleptics, assault

   ● T43.4X4   Poisoning by butyrophenone and thiothixene neuroleptics, undetermined

   ● T43.4X5   Adverse effect of butyrophenone and thiothixene neuroleptics

   ● T43.4X6   Underdosing of butyrophenone and thiothixene neuroleptics

● T43.5   Poisoning by, adverse effect of and underdosing of other and unspecified antipsychotics and neuroleptics

   Excludes1   poisoning by, adverse effect of and underdosing of rauwolfia (T46.5-)

   ● T43.50   Poisoning by, adverse effect of and underdosing of unspecified antipsychotics and neuroleptics

   ● T43.501   Poisoning by unspecified antipsychotics and neuroleptics, accidental (unintentional)

Poisoning by antipsychotics and neuroleptics NOS

   ● T43.502   Poisoning by unspecified antipsychotics and neuroleptics, intentional self-harm A, S 🐾

   ● T43.503   Poisoning by unspecified antipsychotics and neuroleptics, assault

   ● T43.504   Poisoning by unspecified antipsychotics and neuroleptics, undetermined

   ● T43.505   Adverse effect of unspecified antipsychotics and neuroleptics

   ● T43.506   Underdosing of unspecified antipsychotics and neuroleptics

   ● T43.59   Poisoning by, adverse effect of and underdosing of other antipsychotics and neuroleptics

   ● T43.591   Poisoning by other antipsychotics and neuroleptics, accidental (unintentional)

Poisoning by other antipsychotics and neuroleptics NOS

   ● T43.592   Poisoning by other antipsychotics and neuroleptics, intentional self-harm A, S 🐾

   Coding Clinic: 2017, Q1, P40

   ● T43.593   Poisoning by other antipsychotics and neuroleptics, assault

● T43.594 Poisoning by other antipsychotics and neuroleptics, undetermined

● T43.595 Adverse effect of other antipsychotics and neuroleptics

● T43.596 Underdosing of other antipsychotics and neuroleptics

● T43.6 Poisoning by, adverse effect of and underdosing of psychostimulants

  Excludes1 poisoning by, adverse effect of and underdosing of cocaine (T40.5-)

● T43.60 Poisoning by, adverse effect of and underdosing of unspecified psychostimulant

● T43.601 Poisoning by unspecified psychostimulants, accidental (unintentional)
  Poisoning by psychostimulants NOS

● T43.602 Poisoning by unspecified psychostimulants, intentional self-harm A, S 🦚

● T43.603 Poisoning by unspecified psychostimulants, assault

● T43.604 Poisoning by unspecified psychostimulants, undetermined

● T43.605 Adverse effect of unspecified psychostimulants

● T43.606 Underdosing of unspecified psychostimulants

● T43.61 Poisoning by, adverse effect of and underdosing of caffeine

● T43.611 Poisoning by caffeine, accidental (unintentional)
  Poisoning by caffeine NOS

● T43.612 Poisoning by caffeine, intentional self-harm A, S 🦚

● T43.613 Poisoning by caffeine, assault

● T43.614 Poisoning by caffeine, undetermined

● T43.615 Adverse effect of caffeine

● T43.616 Underdosing of caffeine

● T43.62 Poisoning by, adverse effect of and underdosing of amphetamines
  Poisoning by, adverse effect of and underdosing of methamphetamines

● T43.621 Poisoning by amphetamines, accidental (unintentional)
  Poisoning by amphetamines NOS

● T43.622 Poisoning by amphetamines, intentional self-harm A, S 🦚

● T43.623 Poisoning by amphetamines, assault

● T43.624 Poisoning by amphetamines, undetermined

● T43.625 Adverse effect of amphetamines

● T43.626 Underdosing of amphetamines

● T43.63 Poisoning by, adverse effect of and underdosing of methylphenidate

● T43.631 Poisoning by methylphenidate, accidental (unintentional)
  Poisoning by methylphenidate NOS

● T43.632 Poisoning by methylphenidate, intentional self-harm A, S 🦚

● T43.633 Poisoning by methylphenidate, assault

● T43.634 Poisoning by methylphenidate, undetermined

● T43.635 Adverse effect of methylphenidate

● T43.636 Underdosing of methylphenidate

● T43.64 Poisoning by ecstasy
  Poisoning by MDMA
  Poisoning by 3,4-methylenedioxymethamphetamine

● T43.641 Poisoning by ecstasy, accidental (unintentional)
  Poisoning by ecstasy NOS
  Coding Clinic: 2018, Q4, P31

● T43.642 Poisoning by ecstasy, intentional self-harm A, S 🦚

● T43.643 Poisoning by ecstasy, assault

● T43.644 Poisoning by ecstasy, undetermined

● T43.69 Poisoning by, adverse effect of and underdosing of other psychostimulants

● T43.691 Poisoning by other psychostimulants, accidental (unintentional)
  Poisoning by other psychostimulants NOS

● T43.692 Poisoning by other psychostimulants, intentional self-harm A, S 🦚

● T43.693 Poisoning by other psychostimulants, assault

● T43.694 Poisoning by other psychostimulants, undetermined

● T43.695 Adverse effect of other psychostimulants

● T43.696 Underdosing of other psychostimulants

● T43.8 Poisoning by, adverse effect of and underdosing of other psychotropic drugs

● T43.8X Poisoning by, adverse effect of and underdosing of other psychotropic drugs

● T43.8X1 Poisoning by other psychotropic drugs, accidental (unintentional)
  Poisoning by other psychotropic drugs NOS

● T43.8X2 Poisoning by other psychotropic drugs, intentional self-harm A, S 🦚

● T43.8X3 Poisoning by other psychotropic drugs, assault

● T43.8X4 Poisoning by other psychotropic drugs, undetermined

● T43.8X5 Adverse effect of other psychotropic drugs

● T43.8X6 Underdosing of other psychotropic drugs

● T43.9 Poisoning by, adverse effect of and underdosing of unspecified psychotropic drug

X ● T43.91 Poisoning by unspecified psychotropic drug, accidental (unintentional)
  Poisoning by psychotropic drug NOS

X ● T43.92 Poisoning by unspecified psychotropic drug, intentional self-harm A, S 🦚

X ● T43.93 Poisoning by unspecified psychotropic drug, assault

X ● T43.94 Poisoning by unspecified psychotropic drug, undetermined

X ● T43.95 Adverse effect of unspecified psychotropic drug

X ● T43.96 Underdosing of unspecified psychotropic drug

- **T44   Poisoning by, adverse effect of and underdosing of drugs primarily affecting the autonomic nervous system**

   The appropriate 7th character is to be added to each code from category T44

A	initial encounter
D	subsequent encounter
S	sequela

   - **T44.0   Poisoning by, adverse effect of and underdosing of anticholinesterase agents**
      - **T44.0X   Poisoning by, adverse effect of and underdosing of anticholinesterase agents**
         - **T44.0X1   Poisoning by anticholinesterase agents, accidental (unintentional)**
            Poisoning by anticholinesterase agents NOS
         - **T44.0X2   Poisoning by anticholinesterase agents, intentional self-harm A, S 🐾**
         - **T44.0X3   Poisoning by anticholinesterase agents, assault**
         - **T44.0X4   Poisoning by anticholinesterase agents, undetermined**
         - **T44.0X5   Adverse effect of anticholinesterase agents**
         - **T44.0X6   Underdosing of anticholinesterase agents**

   - **T44.1   Poisoning by, adverse effect of and underdosing of other parasympathomimetics [cholinergics]**
      - **T44.1X   Poisoning by, adverse effect of and underdosing of other parasympathomimetics [cholinergics]**
         - **T44.1X1   Poisoning by other parasympathomimetics [cholinergics], accidental (unintentional)**
            Poisoning by other parasympathomimetics [cholinergics] NOS
         - **T44.1X2   Poisoning by other parasympathomimetics [cholinergics], intentional self-harm A, S 🐾**
         - **T44.1X3   Poisoning by other parasympathomimetics [cholinergics], assault**
         - **T44.1X4   Poisoning by other parasympathomimetics [cholinergics], undetermined**
         - **T44.1X5   Adverse effect of other parasympathomimetics [cholinergics]**
         - **T44.1X6   Underdosing of other parasympathomimetics [cholinergics]**

   - **T44.2   Poisoning by, adverse effect of and underdosing of ganglionic blocking drugs**
      - **T44.2X   Poisoning by, adverse effect of and underdosing of ganglionic blocking drugs**
         - **T44.2X1   Poisoning by ganglionic blocking drugs, accidental (unintentional)**
            Poisoning by ganglionic blocking drugs NOS
         - **T44.2X2   Poisoning by ganglionic blocking drugs, intentional self-harm A, S 🐾**
         - **T44.2X3   Poisoning by ganglionic blocking drugs, assault**
         - **T44.2X4   Poisoning by ganglionic blocking drugs, undetermined**
         - **T44.2X5   Adverse effect of ganglionic blocking drugs**
         - **T44.2X6   Underdosing of ganglionic blocking drugs**

   - **T44.3   Poisoning by, adverse effect of and underdosing of other parasympatholytics [anticholinergics and antimuscarinics] and spasmolytics**
      Poisoning by, adverse effect of and underdosing of papaverine
      - **T44.3X   Poisoning by, adverse effect of and underdosing of other parasympatholytics [anticholinergics and antimuscarinics] and spasmolytics**
         - **T44.3X1   Poisoning by other parasympatholytics [anticholinergics and antimuscarinics] and spasmolytics, accidental (unintentional)**
            Poisoning by other parasympatholytics [anticholinergics and antimuscarinics] and spasmolytics NOS
         - **T44.3X2   Poisoning by other parasympatholytics [anticholinergics and antimuscarinics] and spasmolytics, intentional self-harm A, S 🐾**
         - **T44.3X3   Poisoning by other parasympatholytics [anticholinergics and antimuscarinics] and spasmolytics, assault**
         - **T44.3X4   Poisoning by other parasympatholytics [anticholinergics and antimuscarinics] and spasmolytics, undetermined**
         - **T44.3X5   Adverse effect of other parasympatholytics [anticholinergics and antimuscarinics] and spasmolytics**
         - **T44.3X6   Underdosing of other parasympatholytics [anticholinergics and antimuscarinics] and spasmolytics**

   - **T44.4   Poisoning by, adverse effect of and underdosing of predominantly alpha-adrenoreceptor agonists**
      Poisoning by, adverse effect of and underdosing of metaraminol
      - **T44.4X   Poisoning by, adverse effect of and underdosing of predominantly alpha-adrenoreceptor agonists**
         - **T44.4X1   Poisoning by predominantly alpha-adrenoreceptor agonists, accidental (unintentional)**
            Poisoning by predominantly alpha-adrenoreceptor agonists NOS
         - **T44.4X2   Poisoning by predominantly alpha-adrenoreceptor agonists, intentional self-harm A, S 🐾**
         - **T44.4X3   Poisoning by predominantly alpha-adrenoreceptor agonists, assault**
         - **T44.4X4   Poisoning by predominantly alpha-adrenoreceptor agonists, undetermined**
         - **T44.4X5   Adverse effect of predominantly alpha-adrenoreceptor agonists**
         - **T44.4X6   Underdosing of predominantly alpha-adrenoreceptor agonists**

● **T44.5 Poisoning by, adverse effect of and underdosing of predominantly beta-adrenoreceptor agonists**

> **Excludes1** poisoning by, adverse effect of and underdosing of beta-adrenoreceptor agonists used in asthma therapy (T48.6-)

● **T44.5X Poisoning by, adverse effect of and underdosing of predominantly beta-adrenoreceptor agonists**

● **T44.5X1 Poisoning by predominantly beta-adrenoreceptor agonists, accidental (unintentional)**
Poisoning by predominantly beta-adrenoreceptor agonists NOS

● **T44.5X2 Poisoning by predominantly beta-adrenoreceptor agonists, intentional self-harm A, S** 🐾

● **T44.5X3 Poisoning by predominantly beta-adrenoreceptor agonists, assault**

● **T44.5X4 Poisoning by predominantly beta-adrenoreceptor agonists, undetermined**

● **T44.5X5 Adverse effect of predominantly beta-adrenoreceptor agonists**

● **T44.5X6 Underdosing of predominantly beta-adrenoreceptor agonists**

● **T44.6 Poisoning by, adverse effect of and underdosing of alpha-adrenoreceptor antagonists**

> **Excludes1** poisoning by, adverse effect of and underdosing of ergot alkaloids (T48.0)

● **T44.6X Poisoning by, adverse effect of and underdosing of alpha-adrenoreceptor antagonists**

● **T44.6X1 Poisoning by alpha-adrenoreceptor antagonists, accidental (unintentional)**
Poisoning by alpha-adrenoreceptor antagonists NOS

● **T44.6X2 Poisoning by alpha-adrenoreceptor antagonists, intentional self-harm A, S** 🐾

● **T44.6X3 Poisoning by alpha-adrenoreceptor antagonists, assault**

● **T44.6X4 Poisoning by alpha-adrenoreceptor antagonists, undetermined**

● **T44.6X5 Adverse effect of alpha-adrenoreceptor antagonists**

● **T44.6X6 Underdosing of alpha-adrenoreceptor antagonists**

● **T44.7 Poisoning by, adverse effect of and underdosing of beta-adrenoreceptor antagonists**

● **T44.7X Poisoning by, adverse effect of and underdosing of beta-adrenoreceptor antagonists**

● **T44.7X1 Poisoning by beta-adrenoreceptor antagonists, accidental (unintentional)**
Poisoning by beta-adrenoreceptor antagonists NOS

● **T44.7X2 Poisoning by beta-adrenoreceptor antagonists, intentional self-harm A, S** 🐾

● **T44.7X3 Poisoning by beta-adrenoreceptor antagonists, assault**

● **T44.7X4 Poisoning by beta-adrenoreceptor antagonists, undetermined**

● **T44.7X5 Adverse effect of beta-adrenoreceptor antagonists**

● **T44.7X6 Underdosing of beta-adrenoreceptor antagonists**

● **T44.8 Poisoning by, adverse effect of and underdosing of centrally-acting and adrenergic-neuron-blocking agents**

> ~~**Excludes1** poisoning by, adverse effect of and underdosing of clonidine (T46.5) poisoning by, adverse effect of and underdosing of guanethidine (T46.5)~~

▶ **Excludes2** poisoning by, adverse effect of and underdosing of clonidine (T46.5)
▶ poisoning by, adverse effect of and underdosing of guanethidine (T46.5)

● **T44.8X Poisoning by, adverse effect of and underdosing of centrally-acting and adrenergic-neuron-blocking agents**

● **T44.8X1 Poisoning by centrally-acting and adrenergic-neuron-blocking agents, accidental (unintentional)**
Poisoning by centrally-acting and adrenergic-neuron-blocking agents NOS

● **T44.8X2 Poisoning by centrally-acting and adrenergic-neuron-blocking agents, intentional self-harm A, S** 🐾

● **T44.8X3 Poisoning by centrally-acting and adrenergic-neuron-blocking agents, assault**

● **T44.8X4 Poisoning by centrally-acting and adrenergic-neuron-blocking agents, undetermined**

● **T44.8X5 Adverse effect of centrally-acting and adrenergic-neuron-blocking agents**

● **T44.8X6 Underdosing of centrally-acting and adrenergic-neuron-blocking agents**

● **T44.9 Poisoning by, adverse effect of and underdosing of other and unspecified drugs primarily affecting the autonomic nervous system**
Poisoning by, adverse effect of and underdosing of drug stimulating both alpha and beta-adrenoreceptors

● **T44.90 Poisoning by, adverse effect of and underdosing of unspecified drugs primarily affecting the autonomic nervous system**

● **T44.901 Poisoning by unspecified drugs primarily affecting the autonomic nervous system, accidental (unintentional)**
Poisoning by unspecified drugs primarily affecting the autonomic nervous system NOS

● **T44.902 Poisoning by unspecified drugs primarily affecting the autonomic nervous system, intentional self-harm A, S** 🐾

● **T44.903 Poisoning by unspecified drugs primarily affecting the autonomic nervous system, assault**

● **T44.904 Poisoning by unspecified drugs primarily affecting the autonomic nervous system, undetermined**

● **T44.905 Adverse effect of unspecified drugs primarily affecting the autonomic nervous system**

● **T44.906 Underdosing of unspecified drugs primarily affecting the autonomic nervous system**

▶ New ⇒ Revised ~~deleted~~ Deleted | Excludes 1 | Excludes 2 | Includes | Use additional | Code first | Code also | Key words
OGCR Official Guidelines X Assign placeholder X ● Use Additional Character(s) ▶ Manifestation Code 🐾 Hierarchical Condition Category **Coding Clinic**

● T44.99 Poisoning by, adverse effect of and underdosing of other drugs primarily affecting the autonomic nervous system

  ● T44.991 Poisoning by other drug primarily affecting the autonomic nervous system, accidental (unintentional)
             Poisoning by other drugs primarily affecting the autonomic nervous system NOS

  ● T44.992 Poisoning by other drug primarily affecting the autonomic nervous system, intentional self-harm A, S 🐾

  ● T44.993 Poisoning by other drug primarily affecting the autonomic nervous system, assault

  ● T44.994 Poisoning by other drug primarily affecting the autonomic nervous system, undetermined

  ● T44.995 Adverse effect of other drug primarily affecting the autonomic nervous system

  ● T44.996 Underdosing of other drug primarily affecting the autonomic nervous system

● T45 Poisoning by, adverse effect of and underdosing of primarily systemic and hematological agents, not elsewhere classified

      The appropriate 7th character is to be added to each code from category T45

A	initial encounter
D	subsequent encounter
S	sequela

● T45.0 Poisoning by, adverse effect of and underdosing of antiallergic and antiemetic drugs
      Excludes1 poisoning by, adverse effect of and underdosing of phenothiazine-based neuroleptics (T43.3)

  ● T45.0X Poisoning by, adverse effect of and underdosing of antiallergic and antiemetic drugs

    ● T45.0X1 Poisoning by antiallergic and antiemetic drugs, accidental (unintentional)
               Poisoning by antiallergic and antiemetic drugs NOS

    ● T45.0X2 Poisoning by antiallergic and antiemetic drugs, intentional self-harm A, S 🐾

    ● T45.0X3 Poisoning by antiallergic and antiemetic drugs, assault

    ● T45.0X4 Poisoning by antiallergic and antiemetic drugs, undetermined

    ● T45.0X5 Adverse effect of antiallergic and antiemetic drugs

    ● T45.0X6 Underdosing of antiallergic and antiemetic drugs

● T45.1 Poisoning by, adverse effect of and underdosing of antineoplastic and immunosuppressive drugs
      Excludes1 poisoning by, adverse effect of and underdosing of tamoxifen (T38.6)

  ● T45.1X Poisoning by, adverse effect of and underdosing of antineoplastic and immunosuppressive drugs

    ● T45.1X1 Poisoning by antineoplastic and immunosuppressive drugs, accidental (unintentional)
               Poisoning by antineoplastic and immunosuppressive drugs NOS

    ● T45.1X2 Poisoning by antineoplastic and immunosuppressive drugs, intentional self-harm A, S 🐾

    ● T45.1X3 Poisoning by antineoplastic and immunosuppressive drugs, assault

    ● T45.1X4 Poisoning by antineoplastic and immunosuppressive drugs, undetermined

    ● T45.1X5 Adverse effect of antineoplastic and immunosuppressive drugs
               Coding Clinic: 2019, Q2, P25, 28; Q1, P17, 21

    ● T45.1X6 Underdosing of antineoplastic and immunosuppressive drugs

● T45.2 Poisoning by, adverse effect of and underdosing of vitamins
      Excludes2 poisoning by, adverse effect of and underdosing of nicotinic acid (derivatives) (T46.7)
                 poisoning by, adverse effect of and underdosing of iron (T45.4)
                 poisoning by, adverse effect of and underdosing of vitamin K (T45.7)

  ● T45.2X Poisoning by, adverse effect of and underdosing of vitamins

    ● T45.2X1 Poisoning by vitamins, accidental (unintentional)
               Poisoning by vitamins NOS

    ● T45.2X2 Poisoning by vitamins, intentional self-harm A, S 🐾

    ● T45.2X3 Poisoning by vitamins, assault

    ● T45.2X4 Poisoning by vitamins, undetermined

    ● T45.2X5 Adverse effect of vitamins

    ● T45.2X6 Underdosing of vitamins
               Excludes1 vitamin deficiencies (E50-E56)

● T45.3 Poisoning by, adverse effect of and underdosing of enzymes

  ● T45.3X Poisoning by, adverse effect of and underdosing of enzymes

    ● T45.3X1 Poisoning by enzymes, accidental (unintentional)
               Poisoning by enzymes NOS

    ● T45.3X2 Poisoning by enzymes, intentional self-harm A, S 🐾

    ● T45.3X3 Poisoning by enzymes, assault

    ● T45.3X4 Poisoning by enzymes, undetermined

    ● T45.3X5 Adverse effect of enzymes

    ● T45.3X6 Underdosing of enzymes

● T45.4 Poisoning by, adverse effect of and underdosing of iron and its compounds

  ● T45.4X Poisoning by, adverse effect of and underdosing of iron and its compounds

    ● T45.4X1 Poisoning by iron and its compounds, accidental (unintentional)
               Poisoning by iron and its compounds NOS

    ● T45.4X2 Poisoning by iron and its compounds, intentional self-harm A, S 🐾

    ● T45.4X3 Poisoning by iron and its compounds, assault

    ● T45.4X4 Poisoning by iron and its compounds, undetermined

    ● T45.4X5 Adverse effect of iron and its compounds

    ● T45.4X6 Underdosing of iron and its compounds
               Excludes1 iron deficiency (E61.1)

CHAPTER 19 (S00–T88)

- T45.5 Poisoning by, adverse effect of and underdosing of anticoagulants and antithrombotic drugs
  - T45.51 Poisoning by, adverse effect of and underdosing of anticoagulants
    - T45.511 Poisoning by anticoagulants, accidental (unintentional)
      Poisoning by anticoagulants NOS
    - T45.512 Poisoning by anticoagulants, intentional self-harm A, S 🐾
    - T45.513 Poisoning by anticoagulants, assault
    - T45.514 Poisoning by anticoagulants, undetermined
    - T45.515 Adverse effect of anticoagulants
      Coding Clinic: 2021, Q1, P5; 2016, Q1, P14; 2013, Q2, P35
    - T45.516 Underdosing of anticoagulants
  - T45.52 Poisoning by, adverse effect of and underdosing of antithrombotic drugs
    Poisoning by, adverse effect of and underdosing of antiplatelet drugs
    - Excludes2 poisoning by, adverse effect of and underdosing of aspirin (T39.01-)
      poisoning by, adverse effect of and underdosing of acetylsalicylic acid (T39.01-)
    - T45.521 Poisoning by antithrombotic drugs, accidental (unintentional)
      Poisoning by antithrombotic drug NOS
    - T45.522 Poisoning by antithrombotic drugs, intentional self-harm A, S 🐾
    - T45.523 Poisoning by antithrombotic drugs, assault
    - T45.524 Poisoning by antithrombotic drugs, undetermined
    - T45.525 Adverse effect of antithrombotic drugs
      Coding Clinic: 2016, Q1, P15
    - T45.526 Underdosing of antithrombotic drugs
- T45.6 Poisoning by, adverse effect of and underdosing of fibrinolysis-affecting drugs
  - T45.60 Poisoning by, adverse effect of and underdosing of unspecified fibrinolysis-affecting drugs
    - T45.601 Poisoning by unspecified fibrinolysis-affecting drugs, accidental (unintentional)
      Poisoning by fibrinolysis-affecting drug NOS
    - T45.602 Poisoning by unspecified fibrinolysis-affecting drugs, intentional self-harm A, S 🐾
    - T45.603 Poisoning by unspecified fibrinolysis-affecting drugs, assault
    - T45.604 Poisoning by unspecified fibrinolysis-affecting drugs, undetermined
    - T45.605 Adverse effect of unspecified fibrinolysis-affecting drugs
    - T45.606 Underdosing of unspecified fibrinolysis-affecting drugs
  - T45.61 Poisoning by, adverse effect of and underdosing of thrombolytic drugs
    - T45.611 Poisoning by thrombolytic drug, accidental (unintentional)
      Poisoning by thrombolytic drug NOS
    - T45.612 Poisoning by thrombolytic drug, intentional self-harm A, S 🐾

- T45.613 Poisoning by thrombolytic drug, assault
- T45.614 Poisoning by thrombolytic drug, undetermined
- T45.615 Adverse effect of thrombolytic drugs
  Coding Clinic: 2017, Q2, P10
- T45.616 Underdosing of thrombolytic drugs
- T45.62 Poisoning by, adverse effect of and underdosing of hemostatic drugs
  - T45.621 Poisoning by hemostatic drug, accidental (unintentional)
    Poisoning by hemostatic drug NOS
  - T45.622 Poisoning by hemostatic drug, intentional self-harm A, S 🐾
  - T45.623 Poisoning by hemostatic drug, assault
  - T45.624 Poisoning by hemostatic drug, undetermined
  - T45.625 Adverse effect of hemostatic drug
  - T45.626 Underdosing of hemostatic drugs
- T45.69 Poisoning by, adverse effect of and underdosing of other fibrinolysis-affecting drugs
  - T45.691 Poisoning by other fibrinolysis-affecting drugs, accidental (unintentional)
    Poisoning by other fibrinolysis-affecting drug NOS
  - T45.692 Poisoning by other fibrinolysis-affecting drugs, intentional self-harm A, S 🐾
  - T45.693 Poisoning by other fibrinolysis-affecting drugs, assault
  - T45.694 Poisoning by other fibrinolysis-affecting drugs, undetermined
  - T45.695 Adverse effect of other fibrinolysis-affecting drugs
  - T45.696 Underdosing of other fibrinolysis-affecting drugs
- T45.7 Poisoning by, adverse effect of and underdosing of anticoagulant antagonists, vitamin K and other coagulants
  - T45.7X Poisoning by, adverse effect of and underdosing of anticoagulant antagonists, vitamin K and other coagulants
    - T45.7X1 Poisoning by anticoagulant antagonists, vitamin K and other coagulants, accidental (unintentional)
      Poisoning by anticoagulant antagonists, vitamin K and other coagulants NOS
    - T45.7X2 Poisoning by anticoagulant antagonists, vitamin K and other coagulants, intentional self-harm A, S 🐾
    - T45.7X3 Poisoning by anticoagulant antagonists, vitamin K and other coagulants, assault
    - T45.7X4 Poisoning by anticoagulant antagonists, vitamin K and other coagulants, undetermined
    - T45.7X5 Adverse effect of anticoagulant antagonists, vitamin K and other coagulants
    - T45.7X6 Underdosing of anticoagulant antagonist, vitamin K and other coagulants
      - Excludes1 vitamin K deficiency (E56.1)

▶ New   ⇒ Revised   ~~deleted~~ Deleted   Excludes 1   Excludes 2   Includes   Use additional   Code first   Code also   Key words

OGCR Official Guidelines   X Assign placeholder X   ● Use Additional Character(s)   ▶ Manifestation Code   🐾 Hierarchical Condition Category   **Coding Clinic**

- **T45.8** **Poisoning by, adverse effect of and underdosing of other primarily systemic and hematological agents**
  Poisoning by, adverse effect of and underdosing of liver preparations and other antianemic agents
  Poisoning by, adverse effect of and underdosing of natural blood and blood products
  Poisoning by, adverse effect of and underdosing of plasma substitute
  Excludes2   poisoning by, adverse effect of and underdosing of immunoglobulin (T50.Z1)
  poisoning by, adverse effect of and underdosing of iron (T45.4)
  transfusion reactions (T80.-)
  - **T45.8X** **Poisoning by, adverse effect of and underdosing of other primarily systemic and hematological agents**
    - **T45.8X1** **Poisoning by other primarily systemic and hematological agents, accidental (unintentional)**
      Poisoning by other primarily systemic and hematological agents NOS
    - **T45.8X2** **Poisoning by other primarily systemic and hematological agents, intentional self-harm A, S** 🔒
    - **T45.8X3** **Poisoning by other primarily systemic and hematological agents, assault**
    - **T45.8X4** **Poisoning by other primarily systemic and hematological agents, undetermined**
    - **T45.8X5** **Adverse effect of other primarily systemic and hematological agents**
      Coding Clinic: 2016, Q4, P42
    - **T45.8X6** **Underdosing of other primarily systemic and hematological agents**
- **T45.9** **Poisoning by, adverse effect of and underdosing of unspecified primarily systemic and hematological agent**
  - X● **T45.91** **Poisoning by unspecified primarily systemic and hematological agent, accidental (unintentional)**
    Poisoning by primarily systemic and hematological agent NOS
  - X● **T45.92** **Poisoning by unspecified primarily systemic and hematological agent, intentional self-harm A, S** 🔒
  - X● **T45.93** **Poisoning by unspecified primarily systemic and hematological agent, assault**
  - X● **T45.94** **Poisoning by unspecified primarily systemic and hematological agent, undetermined**
  - X● **T45.95** **Adverse effect of unspecified primarily systemic and hematological agent**
  - X● **T45.96** **Underdosing of unspecified primarily systemic and hematological agent**

- **T46** **Poisoning by, adverse effect of and underdosing of agents primarily affecting the cardiovascular system**
  Excludes1   poisoning by, adverse effect of and underdosing of metaraminol (T44.4)
  The appropriate 7th character is to be added to each code from category T46

A	initial encounter
D	subsequent encounter
S	sequela

- **T46.0** **Poisoning by, adverse effect of and underdosing of cardiac-stimulant glycosides and drugs of similar action**
  - **T46.0X** **Poisoning by, adverse effect of and underdosing of cardiac-stimulant glycosides and drugs of similar action**
    - **T46.0X1** **Poisoning by cardiac-stimulant glycosides and drugs of similar action, accidental (unintentional)**
      Poisoning by cardiac-stimulant glycosides and drugs of similar action NOS
    - **T46.0X2** **Poisoning by cardiac-stimulant glycosides and drugs of similar action, intentional self-harm A, S** 🔒
    - **T46.0X3** **Poisoning by cardiac-stimulant glycosides and drugs of similar action, assault**
    - **T46.0X4** **Poisoning by cardiac-stimulant glycosides and drugs of similar action, undetermined**
    - **T46.0X5** **Adverse effect of cardiac-stimulant glycosides and drugs of similar action**
    - **T46.0X6** **Underdosing of cardiac-stimulant glycosides and drugs of similar action**
- **T46.1** **Poisoning by, adverse effect of and underdosing of calcium-channel blockers**
  - **T46.1X** **Poisoning by, adverse effect of and underdosing of calcium-channel blockers**
    - **T46.1X1** **Poisoning by calcium-channel blockers, accidental (unintentional)**
      Poisoning by calcium-channel blockers NOS
    - **T46.1X2** **Poisoning by calcium-channel blockers, intentional self-harm A, S** 🔒
    - **T46.1X3** **Poisoning by calcium-channel blockers, assault**
    - **T46.1X4** **Poisoning by calcium-channel blockers, undetermined**
    - **T46.1X5** **Adverse effect of calcium-channel blockers**
    - **T46.1X6** **Underdosing of calcium-channel blockers**
- **T46.2** **Poisoning by, adverse effect of and underdosing of other antidysrhythmic drugs, not elsewhere classified**
  Excludes1   poisoning by, adverse effect of and underdosing of beta-adrenoreceptor antagonists (T44.7-)
  - **T46.2X** **Poisoning by, adverse effect of and underdosing of other antidysrhythmic drugs**
    - **T46.2X1** **Poisoning by other antidysrhythmic drugs, accidental (unintentional)**
      Poisoning by other antidysrhythmic drugs NOS
    - **T46.2X2** **Poisoning by other antidysrhythmic drugs, intentional self-harm A, S** 🔒
    - **T46.2X3** **Poisoning by other antidysrhythmic drugs, assault**
    - **T46.2X4** **Poisoning by other antidysrhythmic drugs, undetermined**
    - **T46.2X5** **Adverse effect of other antidysrhythmic drugs**
    - **T46.2X6** **Underdosing of other antidysrhythmic drugs**
- **T46.3** **Poisoning by, adverse effect of and underdosing of coronary vasodilators**
  Poisoning by, adverse effect of and underdosing of dipyridamole
  Excludes1   poisoning by, adverse effect of and underdosing of calcium-channel blockers (T46.1)
  - **T46.3X** **Poisoning by, adverse effect of and underdosing of coronary vasodilators**

● T46.3X1   **Poisoning by coronary vasodilators, accidental** (unintentional)
> Poisoning by coronary vasodilators NOS

● T46.3X2   **Poisoning by coronary vasodilators, intentional self-harm** A, S 🐾

● T46.3X3   **Poisoning by coronary vasodilators, assault**

● T46.3X4   **Poisoning by coronary vasodilators, undetermined**

● T46.3X5   **Adverse effect of coronary vasodilators**

● T46.3X6   **Underdosing of coronary vasodilators**

● T46.4   **Poisoning by, adverse effect of and underdosing of angiotensin-converting-enzyme inhibitors**

  ● T46.4X   **Poisoning by, adverse effect of and underdosing of angiotensin-converting-enzyme inhibitors**

    ● T46.4X1   **Poisoning by angiotensin-converting-enzyme inhibitors, accidental** (unintentional)
> Poisoning by angiotensin-converting-enzyme inhibitors NOS

    ● T46.4X2   **Poisoning by angiotensin-converting-enzyme inhibitors, intentional self-harm** A, S 🐾

    ● T46.4X3   **Poisoning by angiotensin-converting-enzyme inhibitors, assault**

    ● T46.4X4   **Poisoning by angiotensin-converting-enzyme inhibitors, undetermined**

    ● T46.4X5   **Adverse effect of angiotensin-converting-enzyme inhibitors**

    ● T46.4X6   **Underdosing of angiotensin-converting-enzyme inhibitors**

● T46.5   **Poisoning by, adverse effect of and underdosing of other antihypertensive drugs**

> **Excludes2**   poisoning by, adverse effect of and underdosing of beta-adrenoreceptor antagonists (T44.7)
> poisoning by, adverse effect of and underdosing of calcium-channel blockers (T46.1)
> poisoning by, adverse effect of and underdosing of diuretics (T50.Ø-T50.2)

  ● T46.5X   **Poisoning by, adverse effect of and underdosing of other antihypertensive drugs**

    ● T46.5X1   **Poisoning by other antihypertensive drugs, accidental** (unintentional)
> Poisoning by other antihypertensive drugs NOS

    ● T46.5X2   **Poisoning by other antihypertensive drugs, intentional self-harm** A, S 🐾

    ● T46.5X3   **Poisoning by other antihypertensive drugs, assault**

    ● T46.5X4   **Poisoning by other antihypertensive drugs, undetermined**

    ● T46.5X5   **Adverse effect of other antihypertensive drugs**

    ● T46.5X6   **Underdosing of other antihypertensive drugs**

● T46.6   **Poisoning by, adverse effect of and underdosing of antihyperlipidemic and antiarteriosclerotic drugs**

  ● T46.6X   **Poisoning by, adverse effect of and underdosing of antihyperlipidemic and antiarteriosclerotic drugs**

    ● T46.6X1   **Poisoning by antihyperlipidemic and antiarteriosclerotic drugs, accidental (unintentional)**
> Poisoning by antihyperlipidemic and antiarteriosclerotic drugs NOS

    ● T46.6X2   **Poisoning by antihyperlipidemic and antiarteriosclerotic drugs, intentional self-harm** A, S 🐾

    ● T46.6X3   **Poisoning by antihyperlipidemic and antiarteriosclerotic drugs, assault**

    ● T46.6X4   **Poisoning by antihyperlipidemic and antiarteriosclerotic drugs, undetermined**

    ● T46.6X5   **Adverse effect of antihyperlipidemic and antiarteriosclerotic drugs**

    ● T46.6X6   **Underdosing of antihyperlipidemic and antiarteriosclerotic drugs**

● T46.7   **Poisoning by, adverse effect of and underdosing of peripheral vasodilators**
> Poisoning by, adverse effect of and underdosing of nicotinic acid (derivatives)

> **Excludes1**   poisoning by, adverse effect of and underdosing of papaverine (T44.3)

  ● T46.7X   **Poisoning by, adverse effect of and underdosing of peripheral vasodilators**

    ● T46.7X1   **Poisoning by peripheral vasodilators, accidental** (unintentional)
> Poisoning by peripheral vasodilators NOS

    ● T46.7X2   **Poisoning by peripheral vasodilators, intentional self-harm** A, S 🐾

    ● T46.7X3   **Poisoning by peripheral vasodilators, assault**

    ● T46.7X4   **Poisoning by peripheral vasodilators, undetermined**

    ● T46.7X5   **Adverse effect of peripheral vasodilators**

    ● T46.7X6   **Underdosing of peripheral vasodilators**

● T46.8   **Poisoning by, adverse effect of and underdosing of antivaricose drugs, including sclerosing agents**

  ● T46.8X   **Poisoning by, adverse effect of and underdosing of antivaricose drugs, including sclerosing agents**

    ● T46.8X1   **Poisoning by antivaricose drugs, including sclerosing agents, accidental (unintentional)**
> Poisoning by antivaricose drugs, including sclerosing agents NOS

    ● T46.8X2   **Poisoning by antivaricose drugs, including sclerosing agents, intentional self-harm** A, S 🐾

    ● T46.8X3   **Poisoning by antivaricose drugs, including sclerosing agents, assault**

    ● T46.8X4   **Poisoning by antivaricose drugs, including sclerosing agents, undetermined**

    ● T46.8X5   **Adverse effect of antivaricose drugs, including sclerosing agents**

    ● T46.8X6   **Underdosing of antivaricose drugs, including sclerosing agents**

- T46.9   Poisoning by, adverse effect of and underdosing of other and unspecified agents primarily affecting the cardiovascular system
  - T46.90   Poisoning by, adverse effect of and underdosing of unspecified agents primarily affecting the cardiovascular system
    - T46.901   Poisoning by unspecified agents primarily affecting the cardiovascular system, accidental (unintentional)
    - T46.902   Poisoning by unspecified agents primarily affecting the cardiovascular system, intentional self-harm A, S 🔖
    - T46.903   Poisoning by unspecified agents primarily affecting the cardiovascular system, assault
    - T46.904   Poisoning by unspecified agents primarily affecting the cardiovascular system, undetermined
    - T46.905   Adverse effect of unspecified agents primarily affecting the cardiovascular system
    - T46.906   Underdosing of unspecified agents primarily affecting the cardiovascular system
  - T46.99   Poisoning by, adverse effect of and underdosing of other agents primarily affecting the cardiovascular system
    - T46.991   Poisoning by other agents primarily affecting the cardiovascular system, accidental (unintentional)
    - T46.992   Poisoning by other agents primarily affecting the cardiovascular system, intentional self-harm A, S 🔖
    - T46.993   Poisoning by other agents primarily affecting the cardiovascular system, assault
    - T46.994   Poisoning by other agents primarily affecting the cardiovascular system, undetermined
    - T46.995   Adverse effect of other agents primarily affecting the cardiovascular system
    - T46.996   Underdosing of other agents primarily affecting the cardiovascular system

- T47   Poisoning by, adverse effect of and underdosing of agents primarily affecting the gastrointestinal system

  The appropriate 7th character is to be added to each code from category T47

A	initial encounter
D	subsequent encounter
S	sequela

  - T47.0   Poisoning by, adverse effect of and underdosing of histamine H2-receptor blockers
    - T47.0X   Poisoning by, adverse effect of and underdosing of histamine H2-receptor blockers
      - T47.0X1   Poisoning by histamine H2-receptor blockers, accidental (unintentional)
        Poisoning by histamine H2-receptor blockers NOS
      - T47.0X2   Poisoning by histamine H2-receptor blockers, intentional self-harm A, S 🔖

      - T47.0X3   Poisoning by histamine H2-receptor blockers, assault
      - T47.0X4   Poisoning by histamine H2-receptor blockers, undetermined
      - T47.0X5   Adverse effect of histamine H2-receptor blockers
      - T47.0X6   Underdosing of histamine H2-receptor blockers
  - T47.1   Poisoning by, adverse effect of and underdosing of other antacids and anti-gastric-secretion drugs
    - T47.1X   Poisoning by, adverse effect of and underdosing of other antacids and anti-gastric-secretion drugs
      - T47.1X1   Poisoning by other antacids and anti-gastric-secretion drugs, accidental (unintentional)
        Poisoning by other antacids and anti-gastric-secretion drugs NOS
      - T47.1X2   Poisoning by other antacids and anti-gastric-secretion drugs, intentional self-harm A, S 🔖
      - T47.1X3   Poisoning by other antacids and anti-gastric-secretion drugs, assault
      - T47.1X4   Poisoning by other antacids and anti-gastric-secretion drugs, undetermined
      - T47.1X5   Adverse effect of other antacids and anti-gastric-secretion drugs
      - T47.1X6   Underdosing of other antacids and anti-gastric-secretion drugs
  - T47.2   Poisoning by, adverse effect of and underdosing of stimulant laxatives
    - T47.2X   Poisoning by, adverse effect of and underdosing of stimulant laxatives
      - T47.2X1   Poisoning by stimulant laxatives, accidental (unintentional)
        Poisoning by stimulant laxatives NOS
      - T47.2X2   Poisoning by stimulant laxatives, intentional self-harm A, S 🔖
      - T47.2X3   Poisoning by stimulant laxatives, assault
      - T47.2X4   Poisoning by stimulant laxatives, undetermined
      - T47.2X5   Adverse effect of stimulant laxatives
      - T47.2X6   Underdosing of stimulant laxatives
  - T47.3   Poisoning by, adverse effect of and underdosing of saline and osmotic laxatives
    - T47.3X   Poisoning by and adverse effect of saline and osmotic laxatives
      - T47.3X1   Poisoning by saline and osmotic laxatives, accidental (unintentional)
        Poisoning by saline and osmotic laxatives NOS
      - T47.3X2   Poisoning by saline and osmotic laxatives, intentional self-harm
      - T47.3X3   Poisoning by saline and osmotic laxatives, assault A, S 🔖
      - T47.3X4   Poisoning by saline and osmotic laxatives, undetermined
      - T47.3X5   Adverse effect of saline and osmotic laxatives
      - T47.3X6   Underdosing of saline and osmotic laxatives

- **T47.4** **Poisoning by, adverse effect of and underdosing of other laxatives**
  - **T47.4X** **Poisoning by, adverse effect of and underdosing of other laxatives**
    - **T47.4X1** Poisoning by other laxatives, accidental (unintentional)
      Poisoning by other laxatives NOS
    - **T47.4X2** Poisoning by other laxatives, intentional self-harm A, S 🐾
    - **T47.4X3** Poisoning by other laxatives, assault
    - **T47.4X4** Poisoning by other laxatives, undetermined
    - **T47.4X5** Adverse effect of other laxatives
    - **T47.4X6** Underdosing of other laxatives
- **T47.5** **Poisoning by, adverse effect of and underdosing of digestants**
  - **T47.5X** **Poisoning by, adverse effect of and underdosing of digestants**
    - **T47.5X1** Poisoning by digestants, accidental (unintentional)
      Poisoning by digestants NOS
    - **T47.5X2** Poisoning by digestants, intentional self-harm A, S 🐾
    - **T47.5X3** Poisoning by digestants, assault
    - **T47.5X4** Poisoning by digestants, undetermined
    - **T47.5X5** Adverse effect of digestants
    - **T47.5X6** Underdosing of digestants
- **T47.6** **Poisoning by, adverse effect of and underdosing of antidiarrheal drugs**
  - **Excludes2** poisoning by, adverse effect of and underdosing of systemic antibiotics and other anti-infectives (T36-T37)
  - **T47.6X** **Poisoning by, adverse effect of and underdosing of antidiarrheal drugs**
    - **T47.6X1** Poisoning by antidiarrheal drugs, accidental (unintentional)
      Poisoning by antidiarrheal drugs NOS
    - **T47.6X2** Poisoning by antidiarrheal drugs, intentional self-harm A, S 🐾
    - **T47.6X3** Poisoning by antidiarrheal drugs, assault
    - **T47.6X4** Poisoning by antidiarrheal drugs, undetermined
    - **T47.6X5** Adverse effect of antidiarrheal drugs
    - **T47.6X6** Underdosing of antidiarrheal drugs
- **T47.7** **Poisoning by, adverse effect of and underdosing of emetics**
  - **T47.7X** **Poisoning by, adverse effect of and underdosing of emetics**
    - **T47.7X1** Poisoning by emetics, accidental (unintentional)
      Poisoning by emetics NOS
    - **T47.7X2** Poisoning by emetics, intentional self-harm A, S 🐾
    - **T47.7X3** Poisoning by emetics, assault
    - **T47.7X4** Poisoning by emetics, undetermined
    - **T47.7X5** Adverse effect of emetics
    - **T47.7X6** Underdosing of emetics

- **T47.8** **Poisoning by, adverse effect of and underdosing of other agents primarily affecting gastrointestinal system**
  - **T47.8X** **Poisoning by, adverse effect of and underdosing of other agents primarily affecting gastrointestinal system**
    - **T47.8X1** Poisoning by other agents primarily affecting gastrointestinal system, accidental (unintentional)
      Poisoning by other agents primarily affecting gastrointestinal system NOS
    - **T47.8X2** Poisoning by other agents primarily affecting gastrointestinal system, intentional self-harm A, S 🐾
    - **T47.8X3** Poisoning by other agents primarily affecting gastrointestinal system, assault
    - **T47.8X4** Poisoning by other agents primarily affecting gastrointestinal system, undetermined
    - **T47.8X5** Adverse effect of other agents primarily affecting gastrointestinal system
    - **T47.8X6** Underdosing of other agents primarily affecting gastrointestinal system
- **T47.9** **Poisoning by, adverse effect of and underdosing of unspecified agents primarily affecting the gastrointestinal system**
  - X **T47.91** Poisoning by unspecified agents primarily affecting the gastrointestinal system, accidental (unintentional)
    Poisoning by agents primarily affecting the gastrointestinal system NOS
  - X **T47.92** Poisoning by unspecified agents primarily affecting the gastrointestinal system, intentional self-harm A, S 🐾
  - X **T47.93** Poisoning by unspecified agents primarily affecting the gastrointestinal system, assault
  - X **T47.94** Poisoning by unspecified agents primarily affecting the gastrointestinal system, undetermined
  - X **T47.95** Adverse effect of unspecified agents primarily affecting the gastrointestinal system
  - X **T47.96** Underdosing of unspecified agents primarily affecting the gastrointestinal system
- **T48** **Poisoning by, adverse effect of and underdosing of agents primarily acting on smooth and skeletal muscles and the respiratory system**
  - The appropriate 7th character is to be added to each code from category T48

A	initial encounter
D	subsequent encounter
S	sequela

  - **T48.0** **Poisoning by, adverse effect of and underdosing of oxytocic drugs**
    - **Excludes1** poisoning by, adverse effect of and underdosing of estrogens, progestogens and antagonists (T38.4-T38.6)
    - **T48.0X** **Poisoning by, adverse effect of and underdosing of oxytocic drugs**
      - **T48.0X1** Poisoning by oxytocic drugs, accidental (unintentional)
        Poisoning by oxytocic drugs NOS
      - **T48.0X2** Poisoning by oxytocic drugs, intentional self-harm A, S 🐾
      - **T48.0X3** Poisoning by oxytocic drugs, assault

▶ New   ⟫ Revised   ~~deleted~~ Deleted   Excludes 1   Excludes 2   Includes   Use additional   Code first   Code also   Key words

OGCR Official Guidelines   X Assign placeholder X   ● Use Additional Character(s)   ▶ Manifestation Code   🐾 Hierarchical Condition Category   **Coding Clinic**

● T48.0X4   Poisoning by oxytocic drugs, undetermined
● T48.0X5   Adverse effect of oxytocic drugs
● T48.0X6   Underdosing of oxytocic drugs

● T48.1   Poisoning by, adverse effect of and underdosing of skeletal muscle relaxants [neuromuscular blocking agents]

   ● T48.1X   Poisoning by, adverse effect of and underdosing of skeletal muscle relaxants [neuromuscular blocking agents]

     ● T48.1X1   Poisoning by skeletal muscle relaxants [neuromuscular blocking agents], accidental (unintentional)
       Poisoning by skeletal muscle relaxants [neuromuscular blocking agents] NOS

     ● T48.1X2   Poisoning by skeletal muscle relaxants [neuromuscular blocking agents], intentional self-harm A, S 🔒

     ● T48.1X3   Poisoning by skeletal muscle relaxants [neuromuscular blocking agents], assault

     ● T48.1X4   Poisoning by skeletal muscle relaxants [neuromuscular blocking agents], undetermined

     ● T48.1X5   Adverse effect of skeletal muscle relaxants [neuromuscular blocking agents]

     ● T48.1X6   Underdosing of skeletal muscle relaxants [neuromuscular blocking agents]

● T48.2   Poisoning by, adverse effect of and underdosing of other and unspecified drugs acting on muscles

   ● T48.20   Poisoning by, adverse effect of and underdosing of unspecified drugs acting on muscles

     ● T48.201   Poisoning by unspecified drugs acting on muscles, accidental (unintentional)
       Poisoning by unspecified drugs acting on muscles NOS

     ● T48.202   Poisoning by unspecified drugs acting on muscles, intentional self-harm A, S 🔒

     ● T48.203   Poisoning by unspecified drugs acting on muscles, assault

     ● T48.204   Poisoning by unspecified drugs acting on muscles, undetermined

     ● T48.205   Adverse effect of unspecified drugs acting on muscles

     ● T48.206   Underdosing of unspecified drugs acting on muscles

   ● T48.29   Poisoning by, adverse effect of and underdosing of other drugs acting on muscles

     ● T48.291   Poisoning by other drugs acting on muscles, accidental (unintentional)
       Poisoning by other drugs acting on muscles NOS

     ● T48.292   Poisoning by other drugs acting on muscles, intentional self-harm A, S 🔒

     ● T48.293   Poisoning by other drugs acting on muscles, assault

     ● T48.294   Poisoning by other drugs acting on muscles, undetermined

     ● T48.295   Adverse effect of other drugs acting on muscles

     ● T48.296   Underdosing of other drugs acting on muscles

● T48.3   Poisoning by, adverse effect of and underdosing of antitussives

   ● T48.3X   Poisoning by, adverse effect of and underdosing of antitussives

     ● T48.3X1   Poisoning by antitussives, accidental (unintentional)
       Poisoning by antitussives NOS

     ● T48.3X2   Poisoning by antitussives, intentional self-harm A, S 🔒

     ● T48.3X3   Poisoning by antitussives, assault

     ● T48.3X4   Poisoning by antitussives, undetermined

     ● T48.3X5   Adverse effect of antitussives

     ● T48.3X6   Underdosing of antitussives

● T48.4   Poisoning by, adverse effect of and underdosing of expectorants

   ● T48.4X   Poisoning by, adverse effect of and underdosing of expectorants

     ● T48.4X1   Poisoning by expectorants, accidental (unintentional)
       Poisoning by expectorants NOS

     ● T48.4X2   Poisoning by expectorants, intentional self-harm A, S 🔒

     ● T48.4X3   Poisoning by expectorants, assault

     ● T48.4X4   Poisoning by expectorants, undetermined

     ● T48.4X5   Adverse effect of expectorants

     ● T48.4X6   Underdosing of expectorants

● T48.5   Poisoning by, adverse effect of and underdosing of other anti-common-cold drugs
   Poisoning by, adverse effect of and underdosing of decongestants

   Excludes2   poisoning by, adverse effect of and underdosing of antipyretics, NEC (T39.9-)
     poisoning by, adverse effect of and underdosing of non-steroidal antiinflammatory drugs (T39.3-)
     poisoning by, adverse effect of and underdosing of salicylates (T39.0-)

   ● T48.5X   Poisoning by, adverse effect of and underdosing of other anti-common-cold drugs

     ● T48.5X1   Poisoning by other anti-common-cold drugs, accidental (unintentional)
       Poisoning by other anti-common-cold drugs NOS

     ● T48.5X2   Poisoning by other anti-common-cold drugs, intentional self-harm A, S 🔒

     ● T48.5X3   Poisoning by other anti-common-cold drugs, assault

     ● T48.5X4   Poisoning by other anti-common-cold drugs, undetermined

     ● T48.5X5   Adverse effect of other anti-common-cold drugs

     ● T48.5X6   Underdosing of other anti-common-cold drugs

CHAPTER 19 (S00-T88)

● **T48.6   Poisoning by, adverse effect of and underdosing of antiasthmatics, not elsewhere classified**
Poisoning by, adverse effect of and underdosing of beta-adrenoreceptor agonists used in asthma therapy

> **Excludes1**   poisoning by, adverse effect of and underdosing of beta-adrenoreceptor agonists not used in asthma therapy (T44.5)
> poisoning by, adverse effect of and underdosing of anterior pituitary [adenohypophyseal] hormones (T38.8)

● T48.6X   **Poisoning by, adverse effect of and underdosing of antiasthmatics**
● T48.6X1   **Poisoning by antiasthmatics, accidental (unintentional)**
Poisoning by antiasthmatics NOS
● T48.6X2   **Poisoning by antiasthmatics, intentional self-harm** A, S 🕮
● T48.6X3   **Poisoning by antiasthmatics, assault**
● T48.6X4   **Poisoning by antiasthmatics, undetermined**
● T48.6X5   **Adverse effect of antiasthmatics**
● T48.6X6   **Underdosing of antiasthmatics**

● **T48.9   Poisoning by, adverse effect of and underdosing of other and unspecified agents primarily acting on the respiratory system**
● T48.90   **Poisoning by, adverse effect of and underdosing of unspecified agents primarily acting on the respiratory system**
● T48.901   **Poisoning by unspecified agents primarily acting on the respiratory system, accidental (unintentional)**
● T48.902   **Poisoning by unspecified agents primarily acting on the respiratory system, intentional self-harm** A, S 🕮
● T48.903   **Poisoning by unspecified agents primarily acting on the respiratory system, assault**
● T48.904   **Poisoning by unspecified agents primarily acting on the respiratory system, undetermined**
● T48.905   **Adverse effect of unspecified agents primarily acting on the respiratory system**
● T48.906   **Underdosing of unspecified agents primarily acting on the respiratory system**
● T48.99   **Poisoning by, adverse effect of and underdosing of other agents primarily acting on the respiratory system**
● T48.991   **Poisoning by other agents primarily acting on the respiratory system, accidental (unintentional)**
● T48.992   **Poisoning by other agents primarily acting on the respiratory system, intentional self-harm** A, S 🕮
● T48.993   **Poisoning by other agents primarily acting on the respiratory system, assault**
● T48.994   **Poisoning by other agents primarily acting on the respiratory system, undetermined**
● T48.995   **Adverse effect of other agents primarily acting on the respiratory system**
● T48.996   **Underdosing of other agents primarily acting on the respiratory system**

● **T49   Poisoning by, adverse effect of and underdosing of topical agents primarily affecting skin and mucous membrane and by ophthalmological, otorhinolaryngological and dental drugs**

> **Includes**   poisoning by, adverse effect of and underdosing of glucocorticoids, topically used

The appropriate 7th character is to be added to each code from category T49

A	initial encounter
D	subsequent encounter
S	sequela

● **T49.0   Poisoning by, adverse effect of and underdosing of local antifungal, anti-infective and anti-inflammatory drugs**
● T49.0X   **Poisoning by, adverse effect of and underdosing of local antifungal, anti-infective and anti-inflammatory drugs**
● T49.0X1   **Poisoning by local antifungal, anti-infective and anti-inflammatory drugs, accidental (unintentional)**
Poisoning by local antifungal, anti-infective and anti-inflammatory drugs NOS
● T49.0X2   **Poisoning by local antifungal, anti-infective and anti-inflammatory drugs, intentional self-harm** A, S 🕮
● T49.0X3   **Poisoning by local antifungal, anti-infective and anti-inflammatory drugs, assault**
● T49.0X4   **Poisoning by local antifungal, anti-infective and anti-inflammatory drugs, undetermined**
● T49.0X5   **Adverse effect of local antifungal, anti-infective and anti-inflammatory drugs**
● T49.0X6   **Underdosing of local antifungal, anti-infective and anti-inflammatory drugs**

● **T49.1   Poisoning by, adverse effect of and underdosing of antipruritics**
● T49.1X   **Poisoning by, adverse effect of and underdosing of antipruritics**
● T49.1X1   **Poisoning by antipruritics, accidental (unintentional)**
Poisoning by antipruritics NOS
● T49.1X2   **Poisoning by antipruritics, intentional self-harm** A, S 🕮
● T49.1X3   **Poisoning by antipruritics, assault**
● T49.1X4   **Poisoning by antipruritics, undetermined**
● T49.1X5   **Adverse effect of antipruritics**
● T49.1X6   **Underdosing of antipruritics**

● **T49.2   Poisoning by, adverse effect of and underdosing of local astringents and local detergents**
● T49.2X   **Poisoning by, adverse effect of and underdosing of local astringents and local detergents**
● T49.2X1   **Poisoning by local astringents and local detergents, accidental (unintentional)**
Poisoning by local astringents and local detergents NOS
● T49.2X2   **Poisoning by local astringents and local detergents, intentional self-harm** A, S 🕮
● T49.2X3   **Poisoning by local astringents and local detergents, assault**
● T49.2X4   **Poisoning by local astringents and local detergents, undetermined**

● T49.2X5   Adverse effect of local astringents and local detergents

● T49.2X6   Underdosing of local astringents and local detergents

● T49.3   Poisoning by, adverse effect of and underdosing of emollients, demulcents and protectants

  ● T49.3X   Poisoning by, adverse effect of and underdosing of emollients, demulcents and protectants

    ● T49.3X1   Poisoning by emollients, demulcents and protectants, accidental (unintentional)
         Poisoning by emollients, demulcents and protectants NOS

    ● T49.3X2   Poisoning by emollients, demulcents and protectants, intentional self-harm A, S 🔎

    ● T49.3X3   Poisoning by emollients, demulcents and protectants, assault

    ● T49.3X4   Poisoning by emollients, demulcents and protectants, undetermined

    ● T49.3X5   Adverse effect of emollients, demulcents and protectants

    ● T49.3X6   Underdosing of emollients, demulcents and protectants

● T49.4   Poisoning by, adverse effect of and underdosing of keratolytics, keratoplastics, and other hair treatment drugs and preparations

  ● T49.4X   Poisoning by, adverse effect of and underdosing of keratolytics, keratoplastics, and other hair treatment drugs and preparations

    ● T49.4X1   Poisoning by keratolytics, keratoplastics, and other hair treatment drugs and preparations, accidental (unintentional)
         Poisoning by keratolytics, keratoplastics, and other hair treatment drugs and preparations NOS

    ● T49.4X2   Poisoning by keratolytics, keratoplastics, and other hair treatment drugs and preparations, intentional self-harm A, S 🔎

    ● T49.4X3   Poisoning by keratolytics, keratoplastics, and other hair treatment drugs and preparations, assault

    ● T49.4X4   Poisoning by keratolytics, keratoplastics, and other hair treatment drugs and preparations, undetermined

    ● T49.4X5   Adverse effect of keratolytics, keratoplastics, and other hair treatment drugs and preparations

    ● T49.4X6   Underdosing of keratolytics, keratoplastics, and other hair treatment drugs and preparations

● T49.5   Poisoning by, adverse effect of and underdosing of ophthalmological drugs and preparations

  ● T49.5X   Poisoning by, adverse effect of and underdosing of ophthalmological drugs and preparations

    ● T49.5X1   Poisoning by ophthalmological drugs and preparations, accidental (unintentional)
         Poisoning by ophthalmological drugs and preparations NOS

    ● T49.5X2   Poisoning by ophthalmological drugs and preparations, intentional self-harm A, S 🔎

    ● T49.5X3   Poisoning by ophthalmological drugs and preparations, assault

    ● T49.5X4   Poisoning by ophthalmological drugs and preparations, undetermined

    ● T49.5X5   Adverse effect of ophthalmological drugs and preparations

    ● T49.5X6   Underdosing of ophthalmological drugs and preparations

● T49.6   Poisoning by, adverse effect of and underdosing of otorhinolaryngological drugs and preparations

  ● T49.6X   Poisoning by, adverse effect of and underdosing of otorhinolaryngological drugs and preparations

    ● T49.6X1   Poisoning by otorhinolaryngological drugs and preparations, accidental (unintentional)
         Poisoning by otorhinolaryngological drugs and preparations NOS

    ● T49.6X2   Poisoning by otorhinolaryngological drugs and preparations, intentional self-harm A, S 🔎

    ● T49.6X3   Poisoning by otorhinolaryngological drugs and preparations, assault

    ● T49.6X4   Poisoning by otorhinolaryngological drugs and preparations, undetermined

    ● T49.6X5   Adverse effect of otorhinolaryngological drugs and preparations

    ● T49.6X6   Underdosing of otorhinolaryngological drugs and preparations

● T49.7   Poisoning by, adverse effect of and underdosing of dental drugs, topically applied

  ● T49.7X   Poisoning by, adverse effect of and underdosing of dental drugs, topically applied

    ● T49.7X1   Poisoning by dental drugs, topically applied, accidental (unintentional)
         Poisoning by dental drugs, topically applied NOS

    ● T49.7X2   Poisoning by dental drugs, topically applied, intentional self-harm A, S 🔎

    ● T49.7X3   Poisoning by dental drugs, topically applied, assault

    ● T49.7X4   Poisoning by dental drugs, topically applied, undetermined

    ● T49.7X5   Adverse effect of dental drugs, topically applied

    ● T49.7X6   Underdosing of dental drugs, topically applied

● T49.8   Poisoning by, adverse effect of and underdosing of other topical agents
      Poisoning by, adverse effect of and underdosing of spermicides

  ● T49.8X   Poisoning by, adverse effect of and underdosing of other topical agents

    ● T49.8X1   Poisoning by other topical agents, accidental (unintentional)
         Poisoning by other topical agents NOS

    ● T49.8X2   Poisoning by other topical agents, intentional self-harm A, S 🔎

    ● T49.8X3   Poisoning by other topical agents, assault

    ● T49.8X4   Poisoning by other topical agents, undetermined

    ● T49.8X5   Adverse effect of other topical agents

    ● T49.8X6   Underdosing of other topical agents

CHAPTER 19 (S00-T88)

● T49.9   Poisoning by, adverse effect of and underdosing of unspecified topical agent

  X ● T49.91   Poisoning by unspecified topical agent, accidental (unintentional)

  X ● T49.92   Poisoning by unspecified topical agent, intentional self-harm A, S 🦠

  X ● T49.93   Poisoning by unspecified topical agent, assault

  X ● T49.94   Poisoning by unspecified topical agent, undetermined

  X ● T49.95   Adverse effect of unspecified topical agent

  X ● T49.96   Underdosing of unspecified topical agent

● T50   Poisoning by, adverse effect of and underdosing of diuretics and other and unspecified drugs, medicaments and biological substances

    The appropriate 7th character is to be added to each code from category T50

A	initial encounter
D	subsequent encounter
S	sequela

  ● T50.0   Poisoning by, adverse effect of and underdosing of mineralocorticoids and their antagonists

    ● T50.0X   Poisoning by, adverse effect of and underdosing of mineralocorticoids and their antagonists

      ● T50.0X1   Poisoning by mineralocorticoids and their antagonists, accidental (unintentional)
        Poisoning by mineralocorticoids and their antagonists NOS

      ● T50.0X2   Poisoning by mineralocorticoids and their antagonists, intentional self-harm A, S 🦠

      ● T50.0X3   Poisoning by mineralocorticoids and their antagonists, assault

      ● T50.0X4   Poisoning by mineralocorticoids and their antagonists, undetermined

      ● T50.0X5   Adverse effect of mineralocorticoids and their antagonists

      ● T50.0X6   Underdosing of mineralocorticoids and their antagonists

  ● T50.1   Poisoning by, adverse effect of and underdosing of loop [high-ceiling] diuretics

    ● T50.1X   Poisoning by, adverse effect of and underdosing of loop [high-ceiling] diuretics

      ● T50.1X1   Poisoning by loop [high-ceiling] diuretics, accidental (unintentional)
        Poisoning by loop [high-ceiling] diuretics NOS

      ● T50.1X2   Poisoning by loop [high-ceiling] diuretics, intentional self-harm A, S 🦠

      ● T50.1X3   Poisoning by loop [high-ceiling] diuretics, assault

      ● T50.1X4   Poisoning by loop [high-ceiling] diuretics, undetermined

      ● T50.1X5   Adverse effect of loop [high-ceiling] diuretics

      ● T50.1X6   Underdosing of loop [high-ceiling] diuretics

● T50.2   Poisoning by, adverse effect of and underdosing of carbonic-anhydrase inhibitors, benzothiadiazides and other diuretics
    Poisoning by, adverse effect of and underdosing of acetazolamide

  ● T50.2X   Poisoning by, adverse effect of and underdosing of carbonic-anhydrase inhibitors, benzothiadiazides and other diuretics

    ● T50.2X1   Poisoning by carbonic-anhydrase inhibitors, benzothiadiazides and other diuretics, accidental (unintentional)
      Poisoning by carbonic-anhydrase inhibitors, benzothiadiazides and other diuretics NOS

    ● T50.2X2   Poisoning by carbonic-anhydrase inhibitors, benzothiadiazides and other diuretics, intentional self-harm A, S 🦠

    ● T50.2X3   Poisoning by carbonic-anhydrase inhibitors, benzothiadiazides and other diuretics, assault

    ● T50.2X4   Poisoning by carbonic-anhydrase inhibitors, benzothiadiazides and other diuretics, undetermined

    ● T50.2X5   Adverse effect of carbonic-anhydrase inhibitors, benzothiadiazides and other diuretics

    ● T50.2X6   Underdosing of carbonic-anhydrase inhibitors, benzothiadiazides and other diuretics

● T50.3   Poisoning by, adverse effect of and underdosing of electrolytic, caloric and water-balance agents
    Poisoning by, adverse effect of and underdosing of oral rehydration salts

  ● T50.3X   Poisoning by, adverse effect of and underdosing of electrolytic, caloric and water-balance agents

    ● T50.3X1   Poisoning by electrolytic, caloric and water-balance agents, accidental (unintentional)
      Poisoning by electrolytic, caloric and water-balance agents NOS

    ● T50.3X2   Poisoning by electrolytic, caloric and water-balance agents, intentional self-harm A, S 🦠

    ● T50.3X3   Poisoning by electrolytic, caloric and water-balance agents, assault

    ● T50.3X4   Poisoning by electrolytic, caloric and water-balance agents, undetermined

    ● T50.3X5   Adverse effect of electrolytic, caloric and water-balance agents

    ● T50.3X6   Underdosing of electrolytic, caloric and water-balance agents

● T50.4   Poisoning by, adverse effect of and underdosing of drugs affecting uric acid metabolism

  ● T50.4X   Poisoning by, adverse effect of and underdosing of drugs affecting uric acid metabolism

    ● T50.4X1   Poisoning by drugs affecting uric acid metabolism, accidental (unintentional)
      Poisoning by drugs affecting uric acid metabolism NOS

    ● T50.4X2   Poisoning by drugs affecting uric acid metabolism, intentional self-harm A, S 🦠

▶ New   ⇒ Revised   deleted Deleted   Excludes 1   Excludes 2   Includes   Use additional   Code first   Code also   Key words
OGCR Official Guidelines   X Assign placeholder X   ● Use Additional Character(s)   ▶ Manifestation Code   🦠 Hierarchical Condition Category   Coding Clinic

● T50.4X3   Poisoning by drugs affecting uric acid metabolism, assault

● T50.4X4   Poisoning by drugs affecting uric acid metabolism, undetermined

● T50.4X5   Adverse effect of drugs affecting uric acid metabolism

● T50.4X6   Underdosing of drugs affecting uric acid metabolism

● T50.5   Poisoning by, adverse effect of and underdosing of appetite depressants

   ● T50.5X   Poisoning by, adverse effect of and underdosing of appetite depressants

     ● T50.5X1   Poisoning by appetite depressants, accidental (unintentional)
         Poisoning by appetite depressants NOS

     ● T50.5X2   Poisoning by appetite depressants, intentional self-harm A, S 🦠

     ● T50.5X3   Poisoning by appetite depressants, assault

     ● T50.5X4   Poisoning by appetite depressants, undetermined

     ● T50.5X5   Adverse effect of appetite depressants

     ● T50.5X6   Underdosing of appetite depressants

● T50.6   Poisoning by, adverse effect of and underdosing of antidotes and chelating agents
     Poisoning by, adverse effect of and underdosing of alcohol deterrents

   ● T50.6X   Poisoning by, adverse effect of and underdosing of antidotes and chelating agents

     ● T50.6X1   Poisoning by antidotes and chelating agents, accidental (unintentional)
         Poisoning by antidotes and chelating agents NOS

     ● T50.6X2   Poisoning by antidotes and chelating agents, intentional self-harm A, S 🦠

     ● T50.6X3   Poisoning by antidotes and chelating agents, assault

     ● T50.6X4   Poisoning by antidotes and chelating agents, undetermined

     ● T50.6X5   Adverse effect of antidotes and chelating agents

     ● T50.6X6   Underdosing of antidotes and chelating agents

● T50.7   Poisoning by, adverse effect of and underdosing of analeptics and opioid receptor antagonists

   ● T50.7X   Poisoning by, adverse effect of and underdosing of analeptics and opioid receptor antagonists

     ● T50.7X1   Poisoning by analeptics and opioid receptor antagonists, accidental (unintentional)
         Poisoning by analeptics and opioid receptor antagonists NOS

     ● T50.7X2   Poisoning by analeptics and opioid receptor antagonists, intentional self-harm A, S 🦠

     ● T50.7X3   Poisoning by analeptics and opioid receptor antagonists, assault

     ● T50.7X4   Poisoning by analeptics and opioid receptor antagonists, undetermined

     ● T50.7X5   Adverse effect of analeptics and opioid receptor antagonists

     ● T50.7X6   Underdosing of analeptics and opioid receptor antagonists

● T50.8   Poisoning by, adverse effect of and underdosing of diagnostic agents

   ● T50.8X   Poisoning by, adverse effect of and underdosing of diagnostic agents

     ● T50.8X1   Poisoning by diagnostic agents, accidental (unintentional)
         Poisoning by diagnostic agents NOS

     ● T50.8X2   Poisoning by diagnostic agents, intentional self-harm A, S 🦠

     ● T50.8X3   Poisoning by diagnostic agents, assault

     ● T50.8X4   Poisoning by diagnostic agents, undetermined

     ● T50.8X5   Adverse effect of diagnostic agents

     ● T50.8X6   Underdosing of diagnostic agents

● T50.A   Poisoning by, adverse effect of and underdosing of bacterial vaccines

   ● T50.A1   Poisoning by, adverse effect of and underdosing of pertussis vaccine, including combinations with a pertussis component

     ● T50.A11   Poisoning by pertussis vaccine, including combinations with a pertussis component, accidental (unintentional)

     ● T50.A12   Poisoning by pertussis vaccine, including combinations with a pertussis component, intentional self-harm A, S 🦠

     ● T50.A13   Poisoning by pertussis vaccine, including combinations with a pertussis component, assault

     ● T50.A14   Poisoning by pertussis vaccine, including combinations with a pertussis component, undetermined

     ● T50.A15   Adverse effect of pertussis vaccine, including combinations with a pertussis component

     ● T50.A16   Underdosing of pertussis vaccine, including combinations with a pertussis component

   ● T50.A2   Poisoning by, adverse effect of and underdosing of mixed bacterial vaccines without a pertussis component

     ● T50.A21   Poisoning by mixed bacterial vaccines without a pertussis component, accidental (unintentional)

     ● T50.A22   Poisoning by mixed bacterial vaccines without a pertussis component, intentional self-harm A, S 🦠

     ● T50.A23   Poisoning by mixed bacterial vaccines without a pertussis component, assault

     ● T50.A24   Poisoning by mixed bacterial vaccines without a pertussis component, undetermined

     ● T50.A25   Adverse effect of mixed bacterial vaccines without a pertussis component

     ● T50.A26   Underdosing of mixed bacterial vaccines without a pertussis component

   ● T50.A9   Poisoning by, adverse effect of and underdosing of other bacterial vaccines

     ● T50.A91   Poisoning by other bacterial vaccines, accidental (unintentional)

     ● T50.A92   Poisoning by other bacterial vaccines, intentional self-harm A, S 🦠

● T50.A93   Poisoning by other bacterial vaccines, assault

● T50.A94   Poisoning by other bacterial vaccines, undetermined

● T50.A95   Adverse effect of other bacterial vaccines

● T50.A96   Underdosing of other bacterial vaccines

● T50.B   Poisoning by, adverse effect of and underdosing of viral vaccines

    ● T50.B1   Poisoning by, adverse effect of and underdosing of smallpox vaccines

       ● T50.B11   Poisoning by smallpox vaccines, accidental (unintentional)

       ● T50.B12   Poisoning by smallpox vaccines, intentional self-harm A, S 🐾

       ● T50.B13   Poisoning by smallpox vaccines, assault

       ● T50.B14   Poisoning by smallpox vaccines, undetermined

       ● T50.B15   Adverse effect of smallpox vaccines

       ● T50.B16   Underdosing of smallpox vaccines

    ● T50.B9   Poisoning by, adverse effect of and underdosing of other viral vaccines

       ● T50.B91   Poisoning by other viral vaccines, accidental (unintentional)

       ● T50.B92   Poisoning by other viral vaccines, intentional self-harm A, S 🐾

       ● T50.B93   Poisoning by other viral vaccines, assault

       ● T50.B94   Poisoning by other viral vaccines, undetermined

       ● T50.B95   Adverse effect of other viral vaccines
          Coding Clinic: 2021, Q1, P43-44

       ● T50.B96   Underdosing of other viral vaccines

● T50.Z   Poisoning by, adverse effect of and underdosing of other vaccines and biological substances

    ● T50.Z1   Poisoning by, adverse effect of and underdosing of immunoglobulin

       ● T50.Z11   Poisoning by immunoglobulin, accidental (unintentional)

       ● T50.Z12   Poisoning by immunoglobulin, intentional self-harm A, S 🐾

       ● T50.Z13   Poisoning by immunoglobulin, assault

       ● T50.Z14   Poisoning by immunoglobulin, undetermined

       ● T50.Z15   Adverse effect of immunoglobulin

       ● T50.Z16   Underdosing of immunoglobulin

    ● T50.Z9   Poisoning by, adverse effect of and underdosing of other vaccines and biological substances

       ● T50.Z91   Poisoning by other vaccines and biological substances, accidental (unintentional)

       ● T50.Z92   Poisoning by other vaccines and biological substances, intentional self-harm A, S 🐾

       ● T50.Z93   Poisoning by other vaccines and biological substances, assault

       ● T50.Z94   Poisoning by other vaccines and biological substances, undetermined

       ● T50.Z95   Adverse effect of other vaccines and biological substances
          Coding Clinic: 2020, Q1, P19

       ● T50.Z96   Underdosing of other vaccines and biological substances

● T50.9   Poisoning by, adverse effect of and underdosing of other and unspecified drugs, medicaments and biological substances

    ● T50.90   Poisoning by, adverse effect of and underdosing of unspecified drugs, medicaments and biological substances

       ● T50.901   Poisoning by unspecified drugs, medicaments and biological substances, accidental (unintentional)
          Coding Clinic: 2015, Q1, P21

       ● T50.902   Poisoning by unspecified drugs, medicaments and biological substances, intentional self-harm A, S 🐾

       ● T50.903   Poisoning by unspecified drugs, medicaments and biological substances, assault

       ● T50.904   Poisoning by unspecified drugs, medicaments and biological substances, undetermined

       ● T50.905   Adverse effect of unspecified drugs, medicaments and biological substances

       ● T50.906   Underdosing of unspecified drugs, medicaments and biological substances

    ● T50.91   Poisoning by, adverse effect of and underdosing of multiple unspecified drugs, medicaments and biological substances
       Multiple drug ingestion NOS
       Code also any specific drugs, medicaments and biological substances

       ● T50.911   Poisoning by multiple unspecified drugs, medicaments and biological substances, accidental (unintentional)

       ● T50.912   Poisoning by multiple unspecified drugs, medicaments and biological substances, intentional self-harm

       ● T50.913   Poisoning by multiple unspecified drugs, medicaments and biological substances, assault

       ● T50.914   Poisoning by multiple unspecified drugs, medicaments and biological substances, undetermined

       ● T50.915   Adverse effect of multiple unspecified drugs, medicaments and biological substances

       ● T50.916   Underdosing of multiple unspecified drugs, medicaments and biological substances

    ● T50.99   Poisoning by, adverse effect of and underdosing of other drugs, medicaments and biological substances

       ● T50.991   Poisoning by other drugs, medicaments and biological substances, accidental (unintentional)

       ● T50.992   Poisoning by other drugs, medicaments and biological substances, intentional self-harm A, S 🐾

       ● T50.993   Poisoning by other drugs, medicaments and biological substances, assault

       ● T50.994   Poisoning by other drugs, medicaments and biological substances, undetermined

       ● T50.995   Adverse effect of other drugs, medicaments and biological substances

       ● T50.996   Underdosing of other drugs, medicaments and biological substances

▶ New   ⇒ Revised   ~~deleted~~ Deleted   Excludes 1   Excludes 2   Includes   Use additional   Code first   Code also   Key words
OGCR Official Guidelines   X Assign placeholder X   ● Use Additional Character(s)   ▷ Manifestation Code   🐾 Hierarchical Condition Category   **Coding Clinic**

TOXIC EFFECTS OF SUBSTANCES CHIEFLY NONMEDICINAL AS TO SOURCE (T51-T65)

Note: When no intent is indicated code to accidental.
Undetermined intent is only for use when there is specific
documentation in the record that the intent of the toxic
effect cannot be determined.

Use additional code(s): for all associated manifestations of toxic
effect, such as:
respiratory conditions due to external agents (J60-J70)
personal history of foreign body fully removed (Z87.821)
to identify any retained foreign body, if applicable (Z18.-)

Excludes1   contact with and (suspected) exposure to toxic
substances (Z77.-)

● **T51**   **Toxic effect of alcohol**

The appropriate 7th character is to be added to each code from
category T51

A	initial encounter
D	subsequent encounter
S	sequela

● **T51.0**   **Toxic effect of ethanol**
Toxic effect of ethyl alcohol

     Excludes2   acute alcohol intoxication or 'hangover'
effects (F10.129, F10.229, F10.929)
drunkenness (F10.129, F10.229, F10.929)
pathological alcohol intoxication (F10.129,
F10.229, F10.929)

   ● **T51.0X**   **Toxic effect of ethanol**

     ● **T51.0X1**   Toxic effect of ethanol, **accidental (unintentional)**
Toxic effect of ethanol NOS

     ● **T51.0X2**   Toxic effect of ethanol, **intentional self-harm** A, S 🐾

     ● **T51.0X3**   Toxic effect of ethanol, **assault**

     ● **T51.0X4**   Toxic effect of ethanol, **undetermined**

● **T51.1**   **Toxic effect of methanol**
Toxic effect of methyl alcohol

   ● **T51.1X**   **Toxic effect of methanol**

     ● **T51.1X1**   Toxic effect of methanol, **accidental (unintentional)**
Toxic effect of methanol NOS

     ● **T51.1X2**   Toxic effect of methanol, **intentional self-harm** A, S 🐾

     ● **T51.1X3**   Toxic effect of methanol, **assault**

     ● **T51.1X4**   Toxic effect of methanol, **undetermined**

● **T51.2**   **Toxic effect of 2-Propanol**
Toxic effect of isopropyl alcohol

   ● **T51.2X**   **Toxic effect of 2-Propanol**

     ● **T51.2X1**   Toxic effect of 2-Propanol, **accidental (unintentional)**
Toxic effect of 2-Propanol NOS

     ● **T51.2X2**   Toxic effect of 2-Propanol, **intentional self-harm** A, S 🐾

     ● **T51.2X3**   Toxic effect of 2-Propanol, **assault**

     ● **T51.2X4**   Toxic effect of 2-Propanol, **undetermined**

● **T51.3**   **Toxic effect of fusel oil**
Toxic effect of amyl alcohol
Toxic effect of butyl [1-butanol] alcohol
Toxic effect of propyl [1-propanol] alcohol

   ● **T51.3X**   **Toxic effect of fusel oil**

     ● **T51.3X1**   Toxic effect of fusel oil, **accidental (unintentional)**
Toxic effect of fusel oil NOS

     ● **T51.3X2**   Toxic effect of fusel oil, **intentional self-harm** A, S 🐾

     ● **T51.3X3**   Toxic effect of fusel oil, **assault**

     ● **T51.3X4**   Toxic effect of fusel oil, **undetermined**

● **T51.8**   **Toxic effect of other alcohols**

   ● **T51.8X**   **Toxic effect of other alcohols**

     ● **T51.8X1**   Toxic effect of other alcohols, **accidental (unintentional)**
Toxic effect of other alcohols NOS

     ● **T51.8X2**   Toxic effect of other alcohols, **intentional self-harm** A, S 🐾

     ● **T51.8X3**   Toxic effect of other alcohols, **assault**

     ● **T51.8X4**   Toxic effect of other alcohols, **undetermined**

● **T51.9**   **Toxic effect of unspecified alcohol**

   X ● **T51.91**   Toxic effect of unspecified alcohol, **accidental (unintentional)**

   X ● **T51.92**   Toxic effect of unspecified alcohol, **intentional self-harm** A, S 🐾

   X ● **T51.93**   Toxic effect of unspecified alcohol, **assault**

   X ● **T51.94**   Toxic effect of unspecified alcohol, **undetermined**

● **T52**   **Toxic effect of organic solvents**

     Excludes1   halogen derivatives of aliphatic and aromatic
hydrocarbons (T53.-)

The appropriate 7th character is to be added to each code from
category T52

A	initial encounter
D	subsequent encounter
S	sequela

● **T52.0**   **Toxic effects of petroleum products**
Toxic effects of gasoline [petrol]
Toxic effects of kerosene [paraffin oil]
Toxic effects of paraffin wax
Toxic effects of ether petroleum
Toxic effects of naphtha petroleum
Toxic effects of spirit petroleum

   ● **T52.0X**   **Toxic effects of petroleum products**

     ● **T52.0X1**   Toxic effect of petroleum products, **accidental (unintentional)**
Toxic effects of petroleum products NOS

     ● **T52.0X2**   Toxic effect of petroleum products, **intentional self-harm** A, S 🐾

     ● **T52.0X3**   Toxic effect of petroleum products, **assault**

     ● **T52.0X4**   Toxic effect of petroleum products, **undetermined**

● **T52.1**   **Toxic effects of benzene**

     Excludes1   homologues of benzene (T52.2)
nitroderivatives and aminoderivatives of
benzene and its homologues (T65.3)

   ● **T52.1X**   **Toxic effects of benzene**

     ● **T52.1X1**   Toxic effect of benzene, **accidental (unintentional)**
Toxic effects of benzene NOS

     ● **T52.1X2**   Toxic effect of benzene, **intentional self-harm** A, S 🐾

     ● **T52.1X3**   Toxic effect of benzene, **assault**

     ● **T52.1X4**   Toxic effect of benzene, **undetermined**

● **T52.2   Toxic effects of homologues of benzene**
Toxic effects of toluene [methylbenzene]
Toxic effects of xylene [dimethylbenzene]

● **T52.2X   Toxic effects of homologues of benzene**

● **T52.2X1   Toxic effect of homologues of benzene, accidental (unintentional)**
Toxic effects of homologues of benzene NOS

● **T52.2X2   Toxic effect of homologues of benzene, intentional self-harm A, S** 🐾

● **T52.2X3   Toxic effect of homologues of benzene, assault**

● **T52.2X4   Toxic effect of homologues of benzene, undetermined**

● **T52.3   Toxic effects of glycols**

● **T52.3X   Toxic effects of glycols**

● **T52.3X1   Toxic effect of glycols, accidental (unintentional)**
Toxic effects of glycols NOS

● **T52.3X2   Toxic effect of glycols, intentional self-harm A, S** 🐾

● **T52.3X3   Toxic effect of glycols, assault**

● **T52.3X4   Toxic effect of glycols, undetermined**

● **T52.4   Toxic effects of ketones**

● **T52.4X   Toxic effects of ketones**

● **T52.4X1   Toxic effect of ketones, accidental (unintentional)**
Toxic effects of ketones NOS

● **T52.4X2   Toxic effect of ketones, intentional self-harm A, S** 🐾

● **T52.4X3   Toxic effect of ketones, assault**

● **T52.4X4   Toxic effect of ketones, undetermined**

● **T52.8   Toxic effects of other organic solvents**

● **T52.8X   Toxic effects of other organic solvents**

● **T52.8X1   Toxic effect of other organic solvents, accidental (unintentional)**
Toxic effects of other organic solvents NOS

● **T52.8X2   Toxic effect of other organic solvents, intentional self-harm A, S** 🐾

● **T52.8X3   Toxic effect of other organic solvents, assault**

● **T52.8X4   Toxic effect of other organic solvents, undetermined**

● **T52.9   Toxic effects of unspecified organic solvent**

X ● **T52.91   Toxic effect of unspecified organic solvent, accidental (unintentional)**

X ● **T52.92   Toxic effect of unspecified organic solvent, intentional self-harm A, S** 🐾

X ● **T52.93   Toxic effect of unspecified organic solvent, assault**

X ● **T52.94   Toxic effect of unspecified organic solvent, undetermined**

● **T53   Toxic effect of halogen derivatives of aliphatic and aromatic hydrocarbons**
The appropriate 7th character is to be added to each code from category T53

> A   initial encounter
> D   subsequent encounter
> S   sequela

● **T53.0   Toxic effects of carbon tetrachloride**
Toxic effects of tetrachloromethane

● **T53.0X   Toxic effects of carbon tetrachloride**

● **T53.0X1   Toxic effect of carbon tetrachloride, accidental (unintentional)**
Toxic effects of carbon tetrachloride NOS

● **T53.0X2   Toxic effect of carbon tetrachloride, intentional self-harm A, S** 🐾

● **T53.0X3   Toxic effect of carbon tetrachloride, assault**

● **T53.0X4   Toxic effect of carbon tetrachloride, undetermined**

● **T53.1   Toxic effects of chloroform**
Toxic effects of trichloromethane

● **T53.1X   Toxic effects of chloroform**

● **T53.1X1   Toxic effect of chloroform, accidental (unintentional)**
Toxic effects of chloroform NOS

● **T53.1X2   Toxic effect of chloroform, intentional self-harm A, S** 🐾

● **T53.1X3   Toxic effect of chloroform, assault**

● **T53.1X4   Toxic effect of chloroform, undetermined**

● **T53.2   Toxic effects of trichloroethylene**
Toxic effects of trichloroethene

● **T53.2X   Toxic effects of trichloroethylene**

● **T53.2X1   Toxic effect of trichloroethylene, accidental (unintentional)**
Toxic effects of trichloroethylene NOS

● **T53.2X2   Toxic effect of trichloroethylene, intentional self-harm A, S** 🐾

● **T53.2X3   Toxic effect of trichloroethylene, assault**

● **T53.2X4   Toxic effect of trichloroethylene, undetermined**

● **T53.3   Toxic effects of tetrachloroethylene**
Toxic effects of perchloroethylene
Toxic effect of tetrachloroethene

● **T53.3X   Toxic effects of tetrachloroethylene**

● **T53.3X1   Toxic effect of tetrachloroethylene, accidental (unintentional)**
Toxic effects of tetrachloroethylene NOS

● **T53.3X2   Toxic effect of tetrachloroethylene, intentional self-harm A, S** 🐾

● **T53.3X3   Toxic effect of tetrachloroethylene, assault**

● **T53.3X4   Toxic effect of tetrachloroethylene, undetermined**

▶ New   ⇒ Revised   ~~deleted~~ Deleted   Excludes 1   Excludes 2   Includes   Use additional   Code first   Code also   Key words
OGCR Official Guidelines   X Assign placeholder X   ● Use Additional Character(s)   ▷ Manifestation Code   🐾 Hierarchical Condition Category   **Coding Clinic**

● **T53.4**   Toxic effects of dichloromethane
     Toxic effects of methylene chloride
   ● **T53.4X**   Toxic effects of dichloromethane
     ● **T53.4X1**   Toxic effect of dichloromethane, accidental (unintentional)
         Toxic effects of dichloromethane NOS
     ● **T53.4X2**   Toxic effect of dichloromethane, intentional self-harm A, S 🐾
     ● **T53.4X3**   Toxic effect of dichloromethane, assault
     ● **T53.4X4**   Toxic effect of dichloromethane, undetermined

● **T53.5**   Toxic effects of chlorofluorocarbons
   ● **T53.5X**   Toxic effects of chlorofluorocarbons
     ● **T53.5X1**   Toxic effect of chlorofluorocarbons, accidental (unintentional)
         Toxic effects of chlorofluorocarbons NOS
     ● **T53.5X2**   Toxic effect of chlorofluorocarbons, intentional self-harm A, S 🐾
     ● **T53.5X3**   Toxic effect of chlorofluorocarbons, assault
     ● **T53.5X4**   Toxic effect of chlorofluorocarbons, undetermined

● **T53.6**   Toxic effects of other halogen derivatives of aliphatic hydrocarbons
   ● **T53.6X**   Toxic effects of other halogen derivatives of aliphatic hydrocarbons
     ● **T53.6X1**   Toxic effect of other halogen derivatives of aliphatic hydrocarbons, accidental (unintentional)
         Toxic effects of other halogen derivatives of aliphatic hydrocarbons NOS
     ● **T53.6X2**   Toxic effect of other halogen derivatives of aliphatic hydrocarbons, intentional self-harm A, S 🐾
     ● **T53.6X3**   Toxic effect of other halogen derivatives of aliphatic hydrocarbons, assault
     ● **T53.6X4**   Toxic effect of other halogen derivatives of aliphatic hydrocarbons, undetermined

● **T53.7**   Toxic effects of other halogen derivatives of aromatic hydrocarbons
   ● **T53.7X**   Toxic effects of other halogen derivatives of aromatic hydrocarbons
     ● **T53.7X1**   Toxic effect of other halogen derivatives of aromatic hydrocarbons, accidental (unintentional)
         Toxic effects of other halogen derivatives of aromatic hydrocarbons NOS
     ● **T53.7X2**   Toxic effect of other halogen derivatives of aromatic hydrocarbons, intentional self-harm A, S 🐾
     ● **T53.7X3**   Toxic effect of other halogen derivatives of aromatic hydrocarbons, assault
     ● **T53.7X4**   Toxic effect of other halogen derivatives of aromatic hydrocarbons, undetermined

● **T53.9**   Toxic effects of unspecified halogen derivatives of aliphatic and aromatic hydrocarbons
   X ● **T53.91**   Toxic effect of unspecified halogen derivatives of aliphatic and aromatic hydrocarbons, accidental (unintentional)
   X ● **T53.92**   Toxic effect of unspecified halogen derivatives of aliphatic and aromatic hydrocarbons, intentional self-harm A, S 🐾
   X ● **T53.93**   Toxic effect of unspecified halogen derivatives of aliphatic and aromatic hydrocarbons, assault
   X ● **T53.94**   Toxic effect of unspecified halogen derivatives of aliphatic and aromatic hydrocarbons, undetermined

● **T54**   Toxic effect of corrosive substances
     The appropriate 7th character is to be added to each code from category T54

> A   initial encounter
> D   subsequent encounter
> S   sequela

   ● **T54.0**   Toxic effects of phenol and phenol homologues
     ● **T54.0X**   Toxic effects of phenol and phenol homologues
       ● **T54.0X1**   Toxic effect of phenol and phenol homologues, accidental (unintentional)
         Toxic effects of phenol and phenol homologues NOS
       ● **T54.0X2**   Toxic effect of phenol and phenol homologues, intentional self-harm A, S 🐾
       ● **T54.0X3**   Toxic effect of phenol and phenol homologues, assault
       ● **T54.0X4**   Toxic effect of phenol and phenol homologues, undetermined

   ● **T54.1**   Toxic effects of other corrosive organic compounds
     ● **T54.1X**   Toxic effects of other corrosive organic compounds
       ● **T54.1X1**   Toxic effect of other corrosive organic compounds, accidental (unintentional)
         Toxic effects of other corrosive organic compounds NOS
       ● **T54.1X2**   Toxic effect of other corrosive organic compounds, intentional self-harm A, S 🐾
       ● **T54.1X3**   Toxic effect of other corrosive organic compounds, assault
       ● **T54.1X4**   Toxic effect of other corrosive organic compounds, undetermined

   ● **T54.2**   Toxic effects of corrosive acids and acid-like substances
     Toxic effects of hydrochloric acid
     Toxic effects of sulfuric acid
     ● **T54.2X**   Toxic effects of corrosive acids and acid-like substances
       ● **T54.2X1**   Toxic effect of corrosive acids and acid-like substances, accidental (unintentional)
         Toxic effects of corrosive acids and acid-like substances NOS
       ● **T54.2X2**   Toxic effect of corrosive acids and acid-like substances, intentional self-harm A, S 🐾
       ● **T54.2X3**   Toxic effect of corrosive acids and acid-like substances, assault
       ● **T54.2X4**   Toxic effect of corrosive acids and acid-like substances, undetermined

CHAPTER 19 (S00-T88)

CHAPTER 19 (S00-T88)

● **T54.3**   **Toxic effects of corrosive alkalis and alkali-like substances**
     Toxic effects of potassium hydroxide
     Toxic effects of sodium hydroxide
   ● **T54.3X**   Toxic effects of corrosive alkalis and alkali-like substances
     ● **T54.3X1**   Toxic effect of corrosive alkalis and alkali-like substances, accidental (unintentional)
         Toxic effects of corrosive alkalis and alkali-like substances NOS
     ● **T54.3X2**   Toxic effect of corrosive alkalis and alkali-like substances, intentional self-harm A, S 🐱
     ● **T54.3X3**   Toxic effect of corrosive alkalis and alkali-like substances, assault
     ● **T54.3X4**   Toxic effect of corrosive alkalis and alkali-like substances, undetermined

● **T54.9**   Toxic effects of unspecified corrosive substance
   X ● **T54.91**   Toxic effect of unspecified corrosive substance, accidental (unintentional)
   X ● **T54.92**   Toxic effect of unspecified corrosive substance, intentional self-harm A, S 🐱
   X ● **T54.93**   Toxic effect of unspecified corrosive substance, assault
   X ● **T54.94**   Toxic effect of unspecified corrosive substance, undetermined

● **T55**   **Toxic effect of soaps and detergents**
     The appropriate 7th character is to be added to each code from category T55

A	initial encounter
D	subsequent encounter
S	sequela

   ● **T55.0**   Toxic effect of soaps
     ● **T55.0X**   Toxic effect of soaps
       ● **T55.0X1**   Toxic effect of soaps, accidental (unintentional)
         Toxic effect of soaps NOS
       ● **T55.0X2**   Toxic effect of soaps, intentional self-harm A, S 🐱
       ● **T55.0X3**   Toxic effect of soaps, assault
       ● **T55.0X4**   Toxic effect of soaps, undetermined
   ● **T55.1**   Toxic effect of detergents
     ● **T55.1X**   Toxic effect of detergents
       ● **T55.1X1**   Toxic effect of detergents, accidental (unintentional)
         Toxic effect of detergents NOS
       ● **T55.1X2**   Toxic effect of detergents, intentional self-harm A, S 🐱
       ● **T55.1X3**   Toxic effect of detergents, assault
       ● **T55.1X4**   Toxic effect of detergents, undetermined

● **T56**   **Toxic effect of metals**

Includes	toxic effects of fumes and vapors of metals
	toxic effects of metals from all sources, except medicinal substances

     Use additional code to identify any retained metal foreign body, if applicable (Z18.0-, T18.1-)

Excludes1	arsenic and its compounds (T57.0)
	manganese and its compounds (T57.2)

     The appropriate 7th character is to be added to each code from category T56

A	initial encounter
D	subsequent encounter
S	sequela

● **T56.0**   Toxic effects of lead and its compounds
   ● **T56.0X**   Toxic effects of lead and its compounds
     ● **T56.0X1**   Toxic effect of lead and its compounds, accidental (unintentional)
       Toxic effects of lead and its compounds NOS
     ● **T56.0X2**   Toxic effect of lead and its compounds, intentional self-harm A, S 🐱
     ● **T56.0X3**   Toxic effect of lead and its compounds, assault
     ● **T56.0X4**   Toxic effect of lead and its compounds, undetermined

● **T56.1**   Toxic effects of mercury and its compounds
   ● **T56.1X**   Toxic effects of mercury and its compounds
     ● **T56.1X1**   Toxic effect of mercury and its compounds, accidental (unintentional)
       Toxic effects of mercury and its compounds NOS
     ● **T56.1X2**   Toxic effect of mercury and its compounds, intentional self-harm A, S 🐱
     ● **T56.1X3**   Toxic effect of mercury and its compounds, assault
     ● **T56.1X4**   Toxic effect of mercury and its compounds, undetermined

● **T56.2**   Toxic effects of chromium and its compounds
   ● **T56.2X**   Toxic effects of chromium and its compounds
     ● **T56.2X1**   Toxic effect of chromium and its compounds, accidental (unintentional)
       Toxic effects of chromium and its compounds NOS
     ● **T56.2X2**   Toxic effect of chromium and its compounds, intentional self-harm A, S 🐱
     ● **T56.2X3**   Toxic effect of chromium and its compounds, assault
     ● **T56.2X4**   Toxic effect of chromium and its compounds, undetermined

● **T56.3**   Toxic effects of cadmium and its compounds
   ● **T56.3X**   Toxic effects of cadmium and its compounds
     ● **T56.3X1**   Toxic effect of cadmium and its compounds, accidental (unintentional)
       Toxic effects of cadmium and its compounds NOS
     ● **T56.3X2**   Toxic effect of cadmium and its compounds, intentional self-harm A, S 🐱
     ● **T56.3X3**   Toxic effect of cadmium and its compounds, assault
     ● **T56.3X4**   Toxic effect of cadmium and its compounds, undetermined

● **T56.4**   Toxic effects of copper and its compounds
   ● **T56.4X**   Toxic effects of copper and its compounds
     ● **T56.4X1**   Toxic effect of copper and its compounds, accidental (unintentional)
       Toxic effects of copper and its compounds NOS
     ● **T56.4X2**   Toxic effect of copper and its compounds, intentional self-harm A, S 🐱
     ● **T56.4X3**   Toxic effect of copper and its compounds, assault
     ● **T56.4X4**   Toxic effect of copper and its compounds, undetermined

▶ New   ⇒ Revised   ~~deleted~~ Deleted   Excludes 1   Excludes 2   Includes   Use additional   Code first   Code also   Key words
OGCR Official Guidelines   X Assign placeholder X   ● Use Additional Character(s)   ▶ Manifestation Code   🐱 Hierarchical Condition Category   **Coding Clinic**

● **T56.5**   Toxic effects of zinc and its compounds
   ● **T56.5X**   Toxic effects of zinc and its compounds
     ● **T56.5X1**   Toxic effect of zinc and its compounds, accidental (unintentional)
        Toxic effects of zinc and its compounds NOS
     ● **T56.5X2**   Toxic effect of zinc and its compounds, intentional self-harm A, S 🌊
     ● **T56.5X3**   Toxic effect of zinc and its compounds, assault
     ● **T56.5X4**   Toxic effect of zinc and its compounds, undetermined

● **T56.6**   Toxic effects of tin and its compounds
   ● **T56.6X**   Toxic effects of tin and its compounds
     ● **T56.6X1**   Toxic effect of tin and its compounds, accidental (unintentional)
        Toxic effects of tin and its compounds NOS
     ● **T56.6X2**   Toxic effect of tin and its compounds, intentional self-harm A, S 🌊
     ● **T56.6X3**   Toxic effect of tin and its compounds, assault
     ● **T56.6X4**   Toxic effect of tin and its compounds, undetermined

● **T56.7**   Toxic effects of beryllium and its compounds
   ● **T56.7X**   Toxic effects of beryllium and its compounds
     ● **T56.7X1**   Toxic effect of beryllium and its compounds, accidental (unintentional)
        Toxic effects of beryllium and its compounds NOS
     ● **T56.7X2**   Toxic effect of beryllium and its compounds, intentional self-harm A, S 🌊
     ● **T56.7X3**   Toxic effect of beryllium and its compounds, assault
     ● **T56.7X4**   Toxic effect of beryllium and its compounds, undetermined

● **T56.8**   Toxic effects of other metals
   ● **T56.81**   Toxic effect of thallium
     ● **T56.811**   Toxic effect of thallium, accidental (unintentional)
        Toxic effect of thallium NOS
     ● **T56.812**   Toxic effect of thallium, intentional self-harm A, S 🌊
     ● **T56.813**   Toxic effect of thallium, assault
     ● **T56.814**   Toxic effect of thallium, undetermined
   ● **T56.89**   Toxic effects of other metals
     ● **T56.891**   Toxic effect of other metals, accidental (unintentional)
        Toxic effects of other metals NOS
     ● **T56.892**   Toxic effect of other metals, intentional self-harm A, S 🌊
     ● **T56.893**   Toxic effect of other metals, assault
     ● **T56.894**   Toxic effect of other metals, undetermined

● **T56.9**   Toxic effects of unspecified metal
  X ● **T56.91**   Toxic effect of unspecified metal, accidental (unintentional)
  X ● **T56.92**   Toxic effect of unspecified metal, intentional self-harm A, S 🌊
  X ● **T56.93**   Toxic effect of unspecified metal, assault
  X ● **T56.94**   Toxic effect of unspecified metal, undetermined

● **T57**   Toxic effect of other inorganic substances
   The appropriate 7th character is to be added to each code from category T57

A	initial encounter
D	subsequent encounter
S	sequela

● **T57.0**   Toxic effect of arsenic and its compounds
   ● **T57.0X**   Toxic effect of arsenic and its compounds
     ● **T57.0X1**   Toxic effect of arsenic and its compounds, accidental (unintentional)
        Toxic effect of arsenic and its compounds NOS
     ● **T57.0X2**   Toxic effect of arsenic and its compounds, intentional self-harm A, S 🌊
     ● **T57.0X3**   Toxic effect of arsenic and its compounds, assault
     ● **T57.0X4**   Toxic effect of arsenic and its compounds, undetermined

● **T57.1**   Toxic effect of phosphorus and its compounds
   Excludes1   organophosphate insecticides (T60.0)
   ● **T57.1X**   Toxic effect of phosphorus and its compounds
     ● **T57.1X1**   Toxic effect of phosphorus and its compounds, accidental (unintentional)
        Toxic effect of phosphorus and its compounds NOS
     ● **T57.1X2**   Toxic effect of phosphorus and its compounds, intentional self-harm A, S 🌊
     ● **T57.1X3**   Toxic effect of phosphorus and its compounds, assault
     ● **T57.1X4**   Toxic effect of phosphorus and its compounds, undetermined

● **T57.2**   Toxic effect of manganese and its compounds
   ● **T57.2X**   Toxic effect of manganese and its compounds
     ● **T57.2X1**   Toxic effect of manganese and its compounds, accidental (unintentional)
        Toxic effect of manganese and its compounds NOS
     ● **T57.2X2**   Toxic effect of manganese and its compounds, intentional self-harm A, S 🌊
     ● **T57.2X3**   Toxic effect of manganese and its compounds, assault
     ● **T57.2X4**   Toxic effect of manganese and its compounds, undetermined

● **T57.3**   Toxic effect of hydrogen cyanide
   ● **T57.3X**   Toxic effect of hydrogen cyanide
     ● **T57.3X1**   Toxic effect of hydrogen cyanide, accidental (unintentional)
        Toxic effect of hydrogen cyanide NOS
     ● **T57.3X2**   Toxic effect of hydrogen cyanide, intentional self-harm A, S 🌊
     ● **T57.3X3**   Toxic effect of hydrogen cyanide, assault
     ● **T57.3X4**   Toxic effect of hydrogen cyanide, undetermined

CHAPTER 19 (S00-T88)

● T57.8   Toxic effect of other specified inorganic substances
   ● T57.8X   Toxic effect of other specified inorganic substances
     ● T57.8X1   Toxic effect of other specified inorganic substances, accidental (unintentional)
          Toxic effect of other specified inorganic substances NOS
     ● T57.8X2   Toxic effect of other specified inorganic substances, intentional self-harm A, S 🐷
     ● T57.8X3   Toxic effect of other specified inorganic substances, assault
     ● T57.8X4   Toxic effect of other specified inorganic substances, undetermined

● T57.9   Toxic effect of unspecified inorganic substance
  X ● T57.91   Toxic effect of unspecified inorganic substance, accidental (unintentional)
  X ● T57.92   Toxic effect of unspecified inorganic substance, intentional self-harm A, S 🐷
  X ● T57.93   Toxic effect of unspecified inorganic substance, assault
  X ● T57.94   Toxic effect of unspecified inorganic substance, undetermined

● T58   Toxic effect of carbon monoxide

Includes   asphyxiation from carbon monoxide
        toxic effect of carbon monoxide from all sources

The appropriate 7th character is to be added to each code from category T58

A	initial encounter
D	subsequent encounter
S	sequela

● T58.0   Toxic effect of carbon monoxide from motor vehicle exhaust
        Toxic effect of exhaust gas from gas engine
        Toxic effect of exhaust gas from motor pump
  X ● T58.01   Toxic effect of carbon monoxide from motor vehicle exhaust, accidental (unintentional)
  X ● T58.02   Toxic effect of carbon monoxide from motor vehicle exhaust, intentional self-harm A, S 🐷
  X ● T58.03   Toxic effect of carbon monoxide from motor vehicle exhaust, assault
  X ● T58.04   Toxic effect of carbon monoxide from motor vehicle exhaust, undetermined

● T58.1   Toxic effect of carbon monoxide from utility gas
        Toxic effect of acetylene
        Toxic effect of gas NOS used for lighting, heating, cooking
        Toxic effect of water gas
  X ● T58.11   Toxic effect of carbon monoxide from utility gas, accidental (unintentional)
  X ● T58.12   Toxic effect of carbon monoxide from utility gas, intentional self-harm A, S 🐷
  X ● T58.13   Toxic effect of carbon monoxide from utility gas, assault
  X ● T58.14   Toxic effect of carbon monoxide from utility gas, undetermined

● T58.2   Toxic effect of carbon monoxide from incomplete combustion of other domestic fuels
        Toxic effect of carbon monoxide from incomplete combustion of coal, coke, kerosene, wood
   ● T58.2X   Toxic effect of carbon monoxide from incomplete combustion of other domestic fuels
     ● T58.2X1   Toxic effect of carbon monoxide from incomplete combustion of other domestic fuels, accidental (unintentional)
     ● T58.2X2   Toxic effect of carbon monoxide from incomplete combustion of other domestic fuels, intentional self-harm A, S 🐷
     ● T58.2X3   Toxic effect of carbon monoxide from incomplete combustion of other domestic fuels, assault
     ● T58.2X4   Toxic effect of carbon monoxide from incomplete combustion of other domestic fuels, undetermined

● T58.8   Toxic effect of carbon monoxide from other source
        Toxic effect of carbon monoxide from blast furnace gas
        Toxic effect of carbon monoxide from fuels in industrial use
        Toxic effect of carbon monoxide from kiln vapor
   ● T58.8X   Toxic effect of carbon monoxide from other source
     ● T58.8X1   Toxic effect of carbon monoxide from other source, accidental (unintentional)
     ● T58.8X2   Toxic effect of carbon monoxide from other source, intentional self-harm A, S 🐷
     ● T58.8X3   Toxic effect of carbon monoxide from other source, assault
     ● T58.8X4   Toxic effect of carbon monoxide from other source, undetermined

● T58.9   Toxic effect of carbon monoxide from unspecified source
  X ● T58.91   Toxic effect of carbon monoxide from unspecified source, accidental (unintentional)
  X ● T58.92   Toxic effect of carbon monoxide from unspecified source, intentional self-harm A, S 🐷
  X ● T58.93   Toxic effect of carbon monoxide from unspecified source, assault
  X ● T58.94   Toxic effect of carbon monoxide from unspecified source, undetermined

● T59   Toxic effect of other gases, fumes and vapors

Includes   aerosol propellants
Excludes1   chlorofluorocarbons (T53.5)

The appropriate 7th character is to be added to each code from category T59

A	initial encounter
D	subsequent encounter
S	sequela

● T59.0   Toxic effect of nitrogen oxides
   ● T59.0X   Toxic effect of nitrogen oxides
     ● T59.0X1   Toxic effect of nitrogen oxides, accidental (unintentional)
          Toxic effect of nitrogen oxides NOS
     ● T59.0X2   Toxic effect of nitrogen oxides, intentional self-harm A, S 🐷

● T59.0X3   Toxic effect of nitrogen oxides, assault

● T59.0X4   Toxic effect of nitrogen oxides, undetermined

● T59.1   Toxic effect of sulfur dioxide

　● T59.1X   Toxic effect of sulfur dioxide

　　● T59.1X1   Toxic effect of sulfur dioxide, accidental (unintentional)
　　　　　　Toxic effect of sulfur dioxide NOS

　　● T59.1X2   Toxic effect of sulfur dioxide, intentional self-harm A, S 🎗

　　● T59.1X3   Toxic effect of sulfur dioxide, assault

　　● T59.1X4   Toxic effect of sulfur dioxide, undetermined

● T59.2   Toxic effect of formaldehyde

　● T59.2X   Toxic effect of formaldehyde

　　● T59.2X1   Toxic effect of formaldehyde, accidental (unintentional)
　　　　　　Toxic effect of formaldehyde NOS

　　● T59.2X2   Toxic effect of formaldehyde, intentional self-harm A, S 🎗

　　● T59.2X3   Toxic effect of formaldehyde, assault

　　● T59.2X4   Toxic effect of formaldehyde, undetermined

● T59.3   Toxic effect of lacrimogenic gas
　　Toxic effect of tear gas

　● T59.3X   Toxic effect of lacrimogenic gas

　　● T59.3X1   Toxic effect of lacrimogenic gas, accidental (unintentional)
　　　　　　Toxic effect of lacrimogenic gas NOS

　　● T59.3X2   Toxic effect of lacrimogenic gas, intentional self-harm A, S 🎗

　　● T59.3X3   Toxic effect of lacrimogenic gas, assault

　　● T59.3X4   Toxic effect of lacrimogenic gas, undetermined

● T59.4   Toxic effect of chlorine gas

　● T59.4X   Toxic effect of chlorine gas

　　● T59.4X1   Toxic effect of chlorine gas, accidental (unintentional)
　　　　　　Toxic effect of chlorine gas NOS

　　● T59.4X2   Toxic effect of chlorine gas, intentional self-harm A, S 🎗

　　● T59.4X3   Toxic effect of chlorine gas, assault

　　● T59.4X4   Toxic effect of chlorine gas, undetermined

● T59.5   Toxic effect of fluorine gas and hydrogen fluoride

　● T59.5X   Toxic effect of fluorine gas and hydrogen fluoride

　　● T59.5X1   Toxic effect of fluorine gas and hydrogen fluoride, accidental (unintentional)
　　　　　　Toxic effect of fluorine gas and hydrogen fluoride NOS

　　● T59.5X2   Toxic effect of fluorine gas and hydrogen fluoride, intentional self-harm A, S 🎗

　　● T59.5X3   Toxic effect of fluorine gas and hydrogen fluoride, assault

　　● T59.5X4   Toxic effect of fluorine gas and hydrogen fluoride, undetermined

● T59.6   Toxic effect of hydrogen sulfide

　● T59.6X   Toxic effect of hydrogen sulfide

　　● T59.6X1   Toxic effect of hydrogen sulfide, accidental (unintentional)
　　　　　　Toxic effect of hydrogen sulfide NOS

　　● T59.6X2   Toxic effect of hydrogen sulfide, intentional self-harm A, S 🎗

　　● T59.6X3   Toxic effect of hydrogen sulfide, assault

　　● T59.6X4   Toxic effect of hydrogen sulfide, undetermined

● T59.7   Toxic effect of carbon dioxide

　● T59.7X   Toxic effect of carbon dioxide

　　● T59.7X1   Toxic effect of carbon dioxide, accidental (unintentional)
　　　　　　Toxic effect of carbon dioxide NOS

　　● T59.7X2   Toxic effect of carbon dioxide, intentional self-harm A, S 🎗

　　● T59.7X3   Toxic effect of carbon dioxide, assault

　　● T59.7X4   Toxic effect of carbon dioxide, undetermined

● T59.8   Toxic effect of other specified gases, fumes and vapors

　● T59.81   Toxic effect of smoke
　　　Smoke inhalation

　　　Excludes2   toxic effect of cigarette (tobacco) smoke (T65.22-)

　　● T59.811   Toxic effect of smoke, accidental (unintentional)
　　　　　　Toxic effect of smoke NOS

　　● T59.812   Toxic effect of smoke, intentional self-harm A, S 🎗

　　● T59.813   Toxic effect of smoke, assault

　　● T59.814   Toxic effect of smoke, undetermined

　● T59.89   Toxic effect of other specified gases, fumes and vapors

　　● T59.891   Toxic effect of other specified gases, fumes and vapors, accidental (unintentional)

　　● T59.892   Toxic effect of other specified gases, fumes and vapors, intentional self-harm A, S 🎗

　　● T59.893   Toxic effect of other specified gases, fumes and vapors, assault

　　● T59.894   Toxic effect of other specified gases, fumes and vapors, undetermined

● T59.9   Toxic effect of unspecified gases, fumes and vapors

　X ● T59.91   Toxic effect of unspecified gases, fumes and vapors, accidental (unintentional)

　X ● T59.92   Toxic effect of unspecified gases, fumes and vapors, intentional self-harm A, S 🎗

　X ● T59.93   Toxic effect of unspecified gases, fumes and vapors, assault

　X ● T59.94   Toxic effect of unspecified gases, fumes and vapors, undetermined

CHAPTER 19 (S00-T88)

● **T60**   **Toxic effect of pesticides**

> **Includes**   toxic effect of wood preservatives

> The appropriate 7th character is to be added to each code from category T60

> | | |
> |---|---|
> | A | initial encounter |
> | D | subsequent encounter |
> | S | sequela |

● **T60.0**   **Toxic effect of organophosphate and carbamate insecticides**

   ● **T60.0X**   Toxic effect of organophosphate and carbamate insecticides

     ● **T60.0X1**   Toxic effect of organophosphate and carbamate insecticides, accidental (unintentional)
       Toxic effect of organophosphate and carbamate insecticides NOS

     ● **T60.0X2**   Toxic effect of organophosphate and carbamate insecticides, intentional self-harm A, S

     ● **T60.0X3**   Toxic effect of organophosphate and carbamate insecticides, assault

     ● **T60.0X4**   Toxic effect of organophosphate and carbamate insecticides, undetermined

● **T60.1**   **Toxic effect of halogenated insecticides**

> **Excludes1**   chlorinated hydrocarbon (T53.-)

   ● **T60.1X**   Toxic effect of halogenated insecticides

     ● **T60.1X1**   Toxic effect of halogenated insecticides, accidental (unintentional)
       Toxic effect of halogenated insecticides NOS

     ● **T60.1X2**   Toxic effect of halogenated insecticides, intentional self-harm A, S

     ● **T60.1X3**   Toxic effect of halogenated insecticides, assault

     ● **T60.1X4**   Toxic effect of halogenated insecticides, undetermined

● **T60.2**   **Toxic effect of other insecticides**

   ● **T60.2X**   Toxic effect of other insecticides

     ● **T60.2X1**   Toxic effect of other insecticides, accidental (unintentional)
       Toxic effect of other insecticides NOS

     ● **T60.2X2**   Toxic effect of other insecticides, intentional self-harm A, S

     ● **T60.2X3**   Toxic effect of other insecticides, assault

     ● **T60.2X4**   Toxic effect of other insecticides, undetermined

● **T60.3**   **Toxic effect of herbicides and fungicides**

   ● **T60.3X**   Toxic effect of herbicides and fungicides

     ● **T60.3X1**   Toxic effect of herbicides and fungicides, accidental (unintentional)
       Toxic effect of herbicides and fungicides NOS

     ● **T60.3X2**   Toxic effect of herbicides and fungicides, intentional self-harm A, S

     ● **T60.3X3**   Toxic effect of herbicides and fungicides, assault

     ● **T60.3X4**   Toxic effect of herbicides and fungicides, undetermined

● **T60.4**   **Toxic effect of rodenticides**

> **Excludes1**   strychnine and its salts (T65.1)
> thallium (T56.81-)

   ● **T60.4X**   Toxic effect of rodenticides

     ● **T60.4X1**   Toxic effect of rodenticides, accidental (unintentional)
       Toxic effect of rodenticides NOS

     ● **T60.4X2**   Toxic effect of rodenticides, intentional self-harm A, S

     ● **T60.4X3**   Toxic effect of rodenticides, assault

     ● **T60.4X4**   Toxic effect of rodenticides, undetermined

● **T60.8**   **Toxic effect of other pesticides**

   ● **T60.8X**   Toxic effect of other pesticides

     ● **T60.8X1**   Toxic effect of other pesticides, accidental (unintentional)
       Toxic effect of other pesticides NOS

     ● **T60.8X2**   Toxic effect of other pesticides, intentional self-harm A, S

     ● **T60.8X3**   Toxic effect of other pesticides, assault

     ● **T60.8X4**   Toxic effect of other pesticides, undetermined

● **T60.9**   **Toxic effect of unspecified pesticide**

   X ● **T60.91**   Toxic effect of unspecified pesticide, accidental (unintentional)

   X ● **T60.92**   Toxic effect of unspecified pesticide, intentional self-harm A, S

   X ● **T60.93**   Toxic effect of unspecified pesticide, assault

   X ● **T60.94**   Toxic effect of unspecified pesticide, undetermined

● **T61**   **Toxic effect of noxious substances eaten as seafood**

> **Excludes1**   allergic reaction to food, such as:
>   anaphylactic reaction or shock due to adverse food reaction (T78.0-)
>   bacterial foodborne intoxications (A05.-)
>   dermatitis (L23.6, L25.4, L27.2)
>   food protein-induced enterocolitis syndrome (K52.21)
>   food protein-induced enteropathy (K52.22)
>   gastroenteritis (noninfective) (K52.29)
>   toxic effect of aflatoxin and other mycotoxins (T64)
>   toxic effect of cyanides (T65.0-)
>   toxic effect of harmful algae bloom (T65.82-)
>   toxic effect of hydrogen cyanide (T57.3-)
>   toxic effect of mercury (T56.1-)
>   toxic effect of red tide (T65.82-)

> The appropriate 7th character is to be added to each code from category T61

> | | |
> |---|---|
> | A | initial encounter |
> | D | subsequent encounter |
> | S | sequela |

● **T61.0**   **Ciguatera fish poisoning**

   X ● **T61.01**   Ciguatera fish poisoning, accidental (unintentional)

   X ● **T61.02**   Ciguatera fish poisoning, intentional self-harm A, S

   X ● **T61.03**   Ciguatera fish poisoning, assault

   X ● **T61.04**   Ciguatera fish poisoning, undetermined

● **T61.1**   **Scombroid fish poisoning**
   Histamine-like syndrome

   X ● **T61.11**   Scombroid fish poisoning, accidental (unintentional)

   X ● **T61.12**   Scombroid fish poisoning, intentional self-harm A, S

   X ● **T61.13**   Scombroid fish poisoning, assault

   X ● **T61.14**   Scombroid fish poisoning, undetermined

● **T61.7**   **Other fish and shellfish poisoning**

   ● **T61.77**   Other fish poisoning

     ● **T61.771**   Other fish poisoning, accidental (unintentional)

     ● **T61.772**   Other fish poisoning, intentional self-harm A, S

     ● **T61.773**   Other fish poisoning, assault

     ● **T61.774**   Other fish poisoning, undetermined

▶ New   ⯈ Revised   ~~deleted~~ Deleted   Excludes 1   Excludes 2   Includes   Use additional   Code first   Code also   Key words

1432   OGCR Official Guidelines   X Assign placeholder X   ● Use Additional Character(s)   ▶ Manifestation Code   Hierarchical Condition Category   **Coding Clinic**

● T61.78   Other shellfish poisoning
  ● T61.781   Other shellfish poisoning, accidental (unintentional)
  ● T61.782   Other shellfish poisoning, intentional self-harm A, S 🏷
  ● T61.783   Other shellfish poisoning, assault
  ● T61.784   Other shellfish poisoning, undetermined
● T61.8   Toxic effect of other seafood
  ● T61.8X   Toxic effect of other seafood
    ● T61.8X1   Toxic effect of other seafood, accidental (unintentional)
    ● T61.8X2   Toxic effect of other seafood, intentional self-harm A, S 🏷
    ● T61.8X3   Toxic effect of other seafood, assault
    ● T61.8X4   Toxic effect of other seafood, undetermined
● T61.9   Toxic effect of unspecified seafood
  X ● T61.91   Toxic effect of unspecified seafood, accidental (unintentional)
  X ● T61.92   Toxic effect of unspecified seafood, intentional self-harm A, S 🏷
  X ● T61.93   Toxic effect of unspecified seafood, assault
  X ● T61.94   Toxic effect of unspecified seafood, undetermined

● T62   Toxic effect of other noxious substances eaten as food
    Excludes1   allergic reaction to food, such as:
                    anaphylactic shock (reaction) due to adverse food reaction (T78.0-)
                    dermatitis (L23.6, L25.4, L27.2)
                    food protein-induced enterocolitis syndrome (K52.21)
                    food protein-induced enteropathy (K52.22)
                    gastroenteritis (noninfective) (K52.29)
                    bacterial food borne intoxications (A05.-)
                    toxic effect of aflatoxin and other mycotoxins (T64)
                    toxic effect of cyanides (T65.0-)
                    toxic effect of hydrogen cyanide (T57.3-)
                    toxic effect of mercury (T56.1-)
    The appropriate 7th character is to be added to each code from category T62

A	initial encounter
D	subsequent encounter
S	sequela

● T62.0   Toxic effect of ingested mushrooms
  ● T62.0X   Toxic effect of ingested mushrooms
    ● T62.0X1   Toxic effect of ingested mushrooms, accidental (unintentional)
                    Toxic effect of ingested mushrooms NOS
    ● T62.0X2   Toxic effect of ingested mushrooms, intentional self-harm A, S 🏷
    ● T62.0X3   Toxic effect of ingested mushrooms, assault
    ● T62.0X4   Toxic effect of ingested mushrooms, undetermined
● T62.1   Toxic effect of ingested berries
  ● T62.1X   Toxic effect of ingested berries
    ● T62.1X1   Toxic effect of ingested berries, accidental (unintentional)
                    Toxic effect of ingested berries NOS
    ● T62.1X2   Toxic effect of ingested berries, intentional self-harm A, S 🏷
    ● T62.1X3   Toxic effect of ingested berries, assault
    ● T62.1X4   Toxic effect of ingested berries, undetermined

● T62.2   Toxic effect of other ingested (parts of) plant(s)
  ● T62.2X   Toxic effect of other ingested (parts of) plant(s)
    ● T62.2X1   Toxic effect of other ingested (parts of) plant(s), accidental (unintentional)
                    Toxic effect of other ingested (parts of) plant(s) NOS
    ● T62.2X2   Toxic effect of other ingested (parts of) plant(s), intentional self-harm A, S 🏷
    ● T62.2X3   Toxic effect of other ingested (parts of) plant(s), assault
    ● T62.2X4   Toxic effect of other ingested (parts of) plant(s), undetermined
● T62.8   Toxic effect of other specified noxious substances eaten as food
  ● T62.8X   Toxic effect of other specified noxious substances eaten as food
    ● T62.8X1   Toxic effect of other specified noxious substances eaten as food, accidental (unintentional)
                    Toxic effect of other specified noxious substances eaten as food NOS
    ● T62.8X2   Toxic effect of other specified noxious substances eaten as food, intentional self-harm A, S 🏷
    ● T62.8X3   Toxic effect of other specified noxious substances eaten as food, assault
    ● T62.8X4   Toxic effect of other specified noxious substances eaten as food, undetermined
● T62.9   Toxic effect of unspecified noxious substance eaten as food
  X ● T62.91   Toxic effect of unspecified noxious substance eaten as food, accidental (unintentional)
                    Toxic effect of unspecified noxious substance eaten as food NOS
  X ● T62.92   Toxic effect of unspecified noxious substance eaten as food, intentional self-harm A, S 🏷
  X ● T62.93   Toxic effect of unspecified noxious substance eaten as food, assault
  X ● T62.94   Toxic effect of unspecified noxious substance eaten as food, undetermined

● T63   Toxic effect of contact with venomous animals and plants
    Includes   bite or touch of venomous animal
                    pricked or stuck by thorn or leaf
    Excludes2   ingestion of toxic animal or plant (T61.-, T62.-)
    The appropriate 7th character is to be added to each code from category T63

A	initial encounter
D	subsequent encounter
S	sequela

● T63.0   Toxic effect of snake venom
  ● T63.00   Toxic effect of unspecified snake venom
    ● T63.001   Toxic effect of unspecified snake venom, accidental (unintentional)
                    Toxic effect of unspecified snake venom NOS
    ● T63.002   Toxic effect of unspecified snake venom, intentional self-harm A, S 🏷
    ● T63.003   Toxic effect of unspecified snake venom, assault
    ● T63.004   Toxic effect of unspecified snake venom, undetermined

- T63.01 Toxic effect of rattlesnake venom
  - T63.011 Toxic effect of rattlesnake venom, accidental (unintentional)
    Toxic effect of rattlesnake venom NOS
  - T63.012 Toxic effect of rattlesnake venom, intentional self-harm A, S 🐾
  - T63.013 Toxic effect of rattlesnake venom, assault
  - T63.014 Toxic effect of rattlesnake venom, undetermined
- T63.02 Toxic effect of coral snake venom
  - T63.021 Toxic effect of coral snake venom, accidental (unintentional)
    Toxic effect of coral snake venom NOS
  - T63.022 Toxic effect of coral snake venom, intentional self-harm A, S 🐾
  - T63.023 Toxic effect of coral snake venom, assault
  - T63.024 Toxic effect of coral snake venom, undetermined
- T63.03 Toxic effect of taipan venom
  - T63.031 Toxic effect of taipan venom, accidental (unintentional)
    Toxic effect of taipan venom NOS
  - T63.032 Toxic effect of taipan venom, intentional self-harm A, S 🐾
  - T63.033 Toxic effect of taipan venom, assault
  - T63.034 Toxic effect of taipan venom, undetermined
- T63.04 Toxic effect of cobra venom
  - T63.041 Toxic effect of cobra venom, accidental (unintentional)
    Toxic effect of cobra venom NOS
  - T63.042 Toxic effect of cobra venom, intentional self-harm A, S 🐾
  - T63.043 Toxic effect of cobra venom, assault
  - T63.044 Toxic effect of cobra venom, undetermined
- T63.06 Toxic effect of venom of other North and South American snake
  - T63.061 Toxic effect of venom of other North and South American snake, accidental (unintentional)
    Toxic effect of venom of other North and South American snake NOS
  - T63.062 Toxic effect of venom of other North and South American snake, intentional self-harm A, S 🐾
  - T63.063 Toxic effect of venom of other North and South American snake, assault
  - T63.064 Toxic effect of venom of other North and South American snake, undetermined
- T63.07 Toxic effect of venom of other Australian snake
  - T63.071 Toxic effect of venom of other Australian snake, accidental (unintentional)
    Toxic effect of venom of other Australian snake NOS
  - T63.072 Toxic effect of venom of other Australian snake, intentional self-harm A, S 🐾
  - T63.073 Toxic effect of venom of other Australian snake, assault
  - T63.074 Toxic effect of venom of other Australian snake, undetermined

- T63.08 Toxic effect of venom of other African and Asian snake
  - T63.081 Toxic effect of venom of other African and Asian snake, accidental (unintentional)
    Toxic effect of venom of other African and Asian snake NOS
  - T63.082 Toxic effect of venom of other African and Asian snake, intentional self-harm A, S 🐾
  - T63.083 Toxic effect of venom of other African and Asian snake, assault
  - T63.084 Toxic effect of venom of other African and Asian snake, undetermined
- T63.09 Toxic effect of venom of other snake
  - T63.091 Toxic effect of venom of other snake, accidental (unintentional)
    Toxic effect of venom of other snake NOS
  - T63.092 Toxic effect of venom of other snake, intentional self-harm A, S 🐾
  - T63.093 Toxic effect of venom of other snake, assault
  - T63.094 Toxic effect of venom of other snake, undetermined
- T63.1 Toxic effect of venom of other reptiles
  - T63.11 Toxic effect of venom of gila monster
    - T63.111 Toxic effect of venom of gila monster, accidental (unintentional)
      Toxic effect of venom of gila monster NOS
    - T63.112 Toxic effect of venom of gila monster, intentional self-harm A, S 🐾
    - T63.113 Toxic effect of venom of gila monster, assault
    - T63.114 Toxic effect of venom of gila monster, undetermined
  - T63.12 Toxic effect of venom of other venomous lizard
    - T63.121 Toxic effect of venom of other venomous lizard, accidental (unintentional)
      Toxic effect of venom of other venomous lizard NOS
    - T63.122 Toxic effect of venom of other venomous lizard, intentional self-harm A, S 🐾
    - T63.123 Toxic effect of venom of other venomous lizard, assault
    - T63.124 Toxic effect of venom of other venomous lizard, undetermined
  - T63.19 Toxic effect of venom of other reptiles
    - T63.191 Toxic effect of venom of other reptiles, accidental (unintentional)
      Toxic effect of venom of other reptiles NOS
    - T63.192 Toxic effect of venom of other reptiles, intentional self-harm A, S 🐾
    - T63.193 Toxic effect of venom of other reptiles, assault
    - T63.194 Toxic effect of venom of other reptiles, undetermined
- T63.2 Toxic effect of venom of scorpion
  - T63.2X Toxic effect of venom of scorpion
    - T63.2X1 Toxic effect of venom of scorpion, accidental (unintentional)
      Toxic effect of venom of scorpion NOS
    - T63.2X2 Toxic effect of venom of scorpion, intentional self-harm A, S 🐾

▶ New ⇒ Revised ~~deleted~~ Deleted | Excludes 1 | Excludes 2 | Includes | Use additional | Code first | Code also | Key words
OGCR Official Guidelines   X Assign placeholder X   ● Use Additional Character(s)   ▶ Manifestation Code   🐾 Hierarchical Condition Category   **Coding Clinic**

- T63.2X3 Toxic effect of venom of scorpion, assault
- T63.2X4 Toxic effect of venom of scorpion, undetermined
- T63.3 Toxic effect of venom of spider
  - T63.30 Toxic effect of unspecified spider venom
    - T63.301 Toxic effect of unspecified spider venom, accidental (unintentional)
    - T63.302 Toxic effect of unspecified spider venom, intentional self-harm A, S 🔖
    - T63.303 Toxic effect of unspecified spider venom, assault
    - T63.304 Toxic effect of unspecified spider venom, undetermined
  - T63.31 Toxic effect of venom of black widow spider
    - T63.311 Toxic effect of venom of black widow spider, accidental (unintentional)
    - T63.312 Toxic effect of venom of black widow spider, intentional self-harm A, S 🔖
    - T63.313 Toxic effect of venom of black widow spider, assault
    - T63.314 Toxic effect of venom of black widow spider, undetermined
  - T63.32 Toxic effect of venom of tarantula
    - T63.321 Toxic effect of venom of tarantula, accidental (unintentional)
    - T63.322 Toxic effect of venom of tarantula, intentional self-harm A, S 🔖
    - T63.323 Toxic effect of venom of tarantula, assault
    - T63.324 Toxic effect of venom of tarantula, undetermined
  - T63.33 Toxic effect of venom of brown recluse spider
    - T63.331 Toxic effect of venom of brown recluse spider, accidental (unintentional)
    - T63.332 Toxic effect of venom of brown recluse spider, intentional self-harm A, S 🔖
    - T63.333 Toxic effect of venom of brown recluse spider, assault
    - T63.334 Toxic effect of venom of brown recluse spider, undetermined
  - T63.39 Toxic effect of venom of other spider
    - T63.391 Toxic effect of venom of other spider, accidental (unintentional)
    - T63.392 Toxic effect of venom of other spider, intentional self-harm A, S 🔖
    - T63.393 Toxic effect of venom of other spider, assault
    - T63.394 Toxic effect of venom of other spider, undetermined
- T63.4 Toxic effect of venom of other arthropods
  - T63.41 Toxic effect of venom of centipedes and venomous millipedes
    - T63.411 Toxic effect of venom of centipedes and venomous millipedes, accidental (unintentional)
    - T63.412 Toxic effect of venom of centipedes and venomous millipedes, intentional self-harm A, S 🔖
    - T63.413 Toxic effect of venom of centipedes and venomous millipedes, assault
    - T63.414 Toxic effect of venom of centipedes and venomous millipedes, undetermined
- T63.42 Toxic effect of venom of ants
  - T63.421 Toxic effect of venom of ants, accidental (unintentional)
  - T63.422 Toxic effect of venom of ants, intentional self-harm A, S 🔖
  - T63.423 Toxic effect of venom of ants, assault
  - T63.424 Toxic effect of venom of ants, undetermined
- T63.43 Toxic effect of venom of caterpillars
  - T63.431 Toxic effect of venom of caterpillars, accidental (unintentional)
  - T63.432 Toxic effect of venom of caterpillars, intentional self-harm A, S 🔖
  - T63.433 Toxic effect of venom of caterpillars, assault
  - T63.434 Toxic effect of venom of caterpillars, undetermined
- T63.44 Toxic effect of venom of bees
  - T63.441 Toxic effect of venom of bees, accidental (unintentional)
  - T63.442 Toxic effect of venom of bees, intentional self-harm A, S 🔖
  - T63.443 Toxic effect of venom of bees, assault
  - T63.444 Toxic effect of venom of bees, undetermined
- T63.45 Toxic effect of venom of hornets
  - T63.451 Toxic effect of venom of hornets, accidental (unintentional)
  - T63.452 Toxic effect of venom of hornets, intentional self-harm A, S 🔖
  - T63.453 Toxic effect of venom of hornets, assault
  - T63.454 Toxic effect of venom of hornets, undetermined
- T63.46 Toxic effect of venom of wasps
  Toxic effect of yellow jacket
  - T63.461 Toxic effect of venom of wasps, accidental (unintentional)
  - T63.462 Toxic effect of venom of wasps, intentional self-harm A, S 🔖
  - T63.463 Toxic effect of venom of wasps, assault
  - T63.464 Toxic effect of venom of wasps, undetermined
- T63.48 Toxic effect of venom of other arthropod
  - T63.481 Toxic effect of venom of other arthropod, accidental (unintentional)
  - T63.482 Toxic effect of venom of other arthropod, intentional self-harm A, S 🔖
  - T63.483 Toxic effect of venom of other arthropod, assault
  - T63.484 Toxic effect of venom of other arthropod, undetermined
- T63.5 Toxic effect of contact with venomous fish
  Excludes2 poisoning by ingestion of fish (T61.-)
  - T63.51 Toxic effect of contact with stingray
    - T63.511 Toxic effect of contact with stingray, accidental (unintentional)
    - T63.512 Toxic effect of contact with stingray, intentional self-harm A, S 🔖
    - T63.513 Toxic effect of contact with stingray, assault
    - T63.514 Toxic effect of contact with stingray, undetermined

CHAPTER 19 (S00-T88)

● T63.59   Toxic effect of contact with other venomous fish
  ● T63.591   Toxic effect of contact with other venomous fish, accidental (unintentional)
  ● T63.592   Toxic effect of contact with other venomous fish, intentional self-harm A, S 🐷
  ● T63.593   Toxic effect of contact with other venomous fish, assault
  ● T63.594   Toxic effect of contact with other venomous fish, undetermined

● T63.6   Toxic effect of contact with other venomous marine animals
  Excludes1   sea-snake venom (T63.09)
  Excludes2   poisoning by ingestion of shellfish (T61.78-)

⇒● T63.61   Toxic effect of contact with Portuguese Man-o-war
          Toxic effect of contact with bluebottle
  ⇒● T63.611   Toxic effect of contact with Portuguese Man-o-war, accidental (unintentional)
  ⇒● T63.612   Toxic effect of contact with Portuguese Man-o-war, intentional self-harm A, S 🐷
  ⇒● T63.613   Toxic effect of contact with Portuguese Man-o-war, assault
  ⇒● T63.614   Toxic effect of contact with Portuguese Man-o-war, undetermined

  ● T63.62   Toxic effect of contact with other jellyfish
    ● T63.621   Toxic effect of contact with other jellyfish, accidental (unintentional)
    ● T63.622   Toxic effect of contact with other jellyfish, intentional self-harm A, S 🐷
    ● T63.623   Toxic effect of contact with other jellyfish, assault
    ● T63.624   Toxic effect of contact with other jellyfish, undetermined

  ● T63.63   Toxic effect of contact with sea anemone
    ● T63.631   Toxic effect of contact with sea anemone, accidental (unintentional)
    ● T63.632   Toxic effect of contact with sea anemone, intentional self-harm A, S 🐷
    ● T63.633   Toxic effect of contact with sea anemone, assault
    ● T63.634   Toxic effect of contact with sea anemone, undetermined

  ● T63.69   Toxic effect of contact with other venomous marine animals
    ● T63.691   Toxic effect of contact with other venomous marine animals, accidental (unintentional)
    ● T63.692   Toxic effect of contact with other venomous marine animals, intentional self-harm A, S 🐷
    ● T63.693   Toxic effect of contact with other venomous marine animals, assault
    ● T63.694   Toxic effect of contact with other venomous marine animals, undetermined

● T63.7   Toxic effect of contact with venomous plant
  ● T63.71   Toxic effect of contact with venomous marine plant
    ● T63.711   Toxic effect of contact with venomous marine plant, accidental (unintentional)
    ● T63.712   Toxic effect of contact with venomous marine plant, intentional self-harm A, S 🐷
    ● T63.713   Toxic effect of contact with venomous marine plant, assault
    ● T63.714   Toxic effect of contact with venomous marine plant, undetermined

● T63.79   Toxic effect of contact with other venomous plant
  ● T63.791   Toxic effect of contact with other venomous plant, accidental (unintentional)
  ● T63.792   Toxic effect of contact with other venomous plant, intentional self-harm A, S 🐷
  ● T63.793   Toxic effect of contact with other venomous plant, assault
  ● T63.794   Toxic effect of contact with other venomous plant, undetermined

● T63.8   Toxic effect of contact with other venomous animals
  ● T63.81   Toxic effect of contact with venomous frog
    Excludes1   contact with nonvenomous frog (W62.0)
    ● T63.811   Toxic effect of contact with venomous frog, accidental (unintentional)
    ● T63.812   Toxic effect of contact with venomous frog, intentional self-harm A, S 🐷
    ● T63.813   Toxic effect of contact with venomous frog, assault
    ● T63.814   Toxic effect of contact with venomous frog, undetermined

  ● T63.82   Toxic effect of contact with venomous toad
    Excludes1   contact with nonvenomous toad (W62.1)
    ● T63.821   Toxic effect of contact with venomous toad, accidental (unintentional)
    ● T63.822   Toxic effect of contact with venomous toad, intentional self-harm A, S 🐷
    ● T63.823   Toxic effect of contact with venomous toad, assault
    ● T63.824   Toxic effect of contact with venomous toad, undetermined

  ● T63.83   Toxic effect of contact with other venomous amphibian
    Excludes1   contact with nonvenomous amphibian (W62.9)
    ● T63.831   Toxic effect of contact with other venomous amphibian, accidental (unintentional)
    ● T63.832   Toxic effect of contact with other venomous amphibian, intentional self-harm A, S 🐷
    ● T63.833   Toxic effect of contact with other venomous amphibian, assault
    ● T63.834   Toxic effect of contact with other venomous amphibian, undetermined

  ● T63.89   Toxic effect of contact with other venomous animals
    ● T63.891   Toxic effect of contact with other venomous animals, accidental (unintentional)
    ● T63.892   Toxic effect of contact with other venomous animals, intentional self-harm A, S 🐷
    ● T63.893   Toxic effect of contact with other venomous animals, assault
    ● T63.894   Toxic effect of contact with other venomous animals, undetermined

● T63.9   Toxic effect of contact with unspecified venomous animal
  X ● T63.91   Toxic effect of contact with unspecified venomous animal, accidental (unintentional)
  X ● T63.92   Toxic effect of contact with unspecified venomous animal, intentional self-harm A, S 🐷
  X ● T63.93   Toxic effect of contact with unspecified venomous animal, assault
  X ● T63.94   Toxic effect of contact with unspecified venomous animal, undetermined

▶ New   ⇒ Revised   ~~deleted~~ Deleted   Excludes 1   Excludes 2   Includes   Use additional   Code first   Code also   Key words
OGCR Official Guidelines   X Assign placeholder X   ● Use Additional Character(s)   ▷ Manifestation Code   🐷 Hierarchical Condition Category   **Coding Clinic**

● T64 Toxic effect of aflatoxin and other mycotoxin food contaminants

The appropriate 7th character is to be added to each code from category T64

> A initial encounter
> D subsequent encounter
> S sequela

● T64.0 Toxic effect of aflatoxin

X ● T64.01 Toxic effect of aflatoxin, accidental (unintentional)

X ● T64.02 Toxic effect of aflatoxin, intentional self-harm A, S 🔒

X ● T64.03 Toxic effect of aflatoxin, assault

X ● T64.04 Toxic effect of aflatoxin, undetermined

● T64.8 Toxic effect of other mycotoxin food contaminants

X ● T64.81 Toxic effect of other mycotoxin food contaminants, accidental (unintentional)

X ● T64.82 Toxic effect of other mycotoxin food contaminants, intentional self-harm A, S 🔒

X ● T64.83 Toxic effect of other mycotoxin food contaminants, assault

X ● T64.84 Toxic effect of other mycotoxin food contaminants, undetermined

● T65 Toxic effect of other and unspecified substances

The appropriate 7th character is to be added to each code from category T65

> A initial encounter
> D subsequent encounter
> S sequela

● T65.0 Toxic effect of cyanides

Excludes1 hydrogen cyanide (T57.3-)

● T65.0X Toxic effect of cyanides

● T65.0X1 Toxic effect of cyanides, accidental (unintentional)
Toxic effect of cyanides NOS

● T65.0X2 Toxic effect of cyanides, intentional self-harm A, S 🔒

● T65.0X3 Toxic effect of cyanides, assault

● T65.0X4 Toxic effect of cyanides, undetermined

● T65.1 Toxic effect of strychnine and its salts

● T65.1X Toxic effect of strychnine and its salts

● T65.1X1 Toxic effect of strychnine and its salts, accidental (unintentional)
Toxic effect of strychnine and its salts NOS

● T65.1X2 Toxic effect of strychnine and its salts, intentional self-harm A, S 🔒

● T65.1X3 Toxic effect of strychnine and its salts, assault

● T65.1X4 Toxic effect of strychnine and its salts, undetermined

● T65.2 Toxic effect of tobacco and nicotine

Excludes2 nicotine dependence (F17.-)

● T65.21 Toxic effect of chewing tobacco

● T65.211 Toxic effect of chewing tobacco, accidental (unintentional)
Toxic effect of chewing tobacco NOS

● T65.212 Toxic effect of chewing tobacco, intentional self-harm A, S 🔒

● T65.213 Toxic effect of chewing tobacco, assault

● T65.214 Toxic effect of chewing tobacco, undetermined

● T65.22 Toxic effect of tobacco cigarettes
Toxic effect of tobacco smoke

Use additional code for exposure to second hand tobacco smoke (Z57.31, Z77.22)

● T65.221 Toxic effect of tobacco cigarettes, accidental (unintentional)
Toxic effect of tobacco cigarettes NOS

● T65.222 Toxic effect of tobacco cigarettes, intentional self-harm A, S 🔒

● T65.223 Toxic effect of tobacco cigarettes, assault

● T65.224 Toxic effect of tobacco cigarettes, undetermined

● T65.29 Toxic effect of other tobacco and nicotine

● T65.291 Toxic effect of other tobacco and nicotine, accidental (unintentional)
Toxic effect of other tobacco and nicotine NOS

● T65.292 Toxic effect of other tobacco and nicotine, intentional self-harm A, S 🔒

● T65.293 Toxic effect of other tobacco and nicotine, assault

● T65.294 Toxic effect of other tobacco and nicotine, undetermined

● T65.3 Toxic effect of nitroderivatives and aminoderivatives of benzene and its homologues
Toxic effect of anilin [benzenamine]
Toxic effect of nitrobenzene
Toxic effect of trinitrotoluene

● T65.3X Toxic effect of nitroderivatives and aminoderivatives of benzene and its homologues

● T65.3X1 Toxic effect of nitroderivatives and aminoderivatives of benzene and its homologues, accidental (unintentional)
Toxic effect of nitroderivatives and aminoderivatives of benzene and its homologues NOS

● T65.3X2 Toxic effect of nitroderivatives and aminoderivatives of benzene and its homologues, intentional self-harm A, S 🔒

● T65.3X3 Toxic effect of nitroderivatives and aminoderivatives of benzene and its homologues, assault

● T65.3X4 Toxic effect of nitroderivatives and aminoderivatives of benzene and its homologues, undetermined

● T65.4 Toxic effect of carbon disulfide

● T65.4X Toxic effect of carbon disulfide

● T65.4X1 Toxic effect of carbon disulfide, accidental (unintentional)
Toxic effect of carbon disulfide NOS

● T65.4X2 Toxic effect of carbon disulfide, intentional self-harm A, S 🔒

● T65.4X3 Toxic effect of carbon disulfide, assault

● T65.4X4 Toxic effect of carbon disulfide, undetermined

CHAPTER 19 (S00-T88)

- **T65.5** Toxic effect of nitroglycerin and other nitric acids and esters
  - Toxic effect of 1,2,3-Propanetriol trinitrate
  - **T65.5X** Toxic effect of nitroglycerin and other nitric acids and esters
    - **T65.5X1** Toxic effect of nitroglycerin and other nitric acids and esters, accidental (unintentional)
      - Toxic effect of nitroglycerin and other nitric acids and esters NOS
    - **T65.5X2** Toxic effect of nitroglycerin and other nitric acids and esters, intentional self-harm A, S 🔒
    - **T65.5X3** Toxic effect of nitroglycerin and other nitric acids and esters, assault
    - **T65.5X4** Toxic effect of nitroglycerin and other nitric acids and esters, undetermined
- **T65.6** Toxic effect of paints and dyes, not elsewhere classified
  - **T65.6X** Toxic effect of paints and dyes, not elsewhere classified
    - **T65.6X1** Toxic effect of paints and dyes, not elsewhere classified, accidental (unintentional)
      - Toxic effect of paints and dyes NOS
    - **T65.6X2** Toxic effect of paints and dyes, not elsewhere classified, intentional self-harm A, S 🔒
    - **T65.6X3** Toxic effect of paints and dyes, not elsewhere classified, assault
    - **T65.6X4** Toxic effect of paints and dyes, not elsewhere classified, undetermined
- **T65.8** Toxic effect of other specified substances
  - **T65.81** Toxic effect of latex
    - **T65.811** Toxic effect of latex, accidental (unintentional)
      - Toxic effect of latex NOS
    - **T65.812** Toxic effect of latex, intentional self-harm A, S 🔒
    - **T65.813** Toxic effect of latex, assault
    - **T65.814** Toxic effect of latex, undetermined
  - **T65.82** Toxic effect of harmful algae and algae toxins
    - Toxic effect of (harmful) algae bloom NOS
    - Toxic effect of blue-green algae bloom
    - Toxic effect of brown tide
    - Toxic effect of cyanobacteria bloom
    - Toxic effect of Florida red tide
    - Toxic effect of pfiesteria piscicida
    - Toxic effect of red tide

- **T65.821** Toxic effect of harmful algae and algae toxins, accidental (unintentional)
  - Toxic effect of harmful algae and algae toxins NOS
- **T65.822** Toxic effect of harmful algae and algae toxins, intentional self-harm A, S 🔒
- **T65.823** Toxic effect of harmful algae and algae toxins, assault
- **T65.824** Toxic effect of harmful algae and algae toxins, undetermined
- **T65.83** Toxic effect of fiberglass
  - **T65.831** Toxic effect of fiberglass, accidental (unintentional)
    - Toxic effect of fiberglass NOS
  - **T65.832** Toxic effect of fiberglass, intentional self-harm A, S 🔒
  - **T65.833** Toxic effect of fiberglass, assault
  - **T65.834** Toxic effect of fiberglass, undetermined
- **T65.89** Toxic effect of other specified substances
  - **T65.891** Toxic effect of other specified substances, accidental (unintentional)
    - Toxic effect of other specified substances NOS
    - **Coding Clinic: 2018, Q1, P5**
  - **T65.892** Toxic effect of other specified substances, intentional self-harm A, S 🔒
  - **T65.893** Toxic effect of other specified substances, assault
  - **T65.894** Toxic effect of other specified substances, undetermined
- **T65.9** Toxic effect of unspecified substance
  - X **T65.91** Toxic effect of unspecified substance, accidental (unintentional)
    - Poisoning NOS
  - X **T65.92** Toxic effect of unspecified substance, intentional self-harm A, S 🔒
  - X **T65.93** Toxic effect of unspecified substance, assault
  - X **T65.94** Toxic effect of unspecified substance, undetermined

▶ New   ⇒ Revised   ~~deleted~~ Deleted   Excludes 1   Excludes 2   Includes   Use additional   Code first   Code also   Key words

OGCR Official Guidelines   X Assign placeholder X   ● Use Additional Character(s)   ▶ Manifestation Code   🔒 Hierarchical Condition Category   **Coding Clinic**

OTHER AND UNSPECIFIED EFFECTS OF EXTERNAL CAUSES (T66-T78)

● T66   Radiation sickness, unspecified

       Excludes1   specified adverse effects of radiation, such as:
                burns (T20-T31)
                leukemia (C91-C95)
                radiation gastroenteritis and colitis (K52.0)
                radiation pneumonitis (J70.0)
                radiation related disorders of the skin and
                    subcutaneous tissue (L55-L59)
                sunburn (L55.-)

       The appropriate 7th character is to be added to code T66

A	initial encounter
D	subsequent encounter
S	sequela

● T67   Effects of heat and light

       Excludes1   erythema [dermatitis] ab igne (L59.0)
                malignant hyperpyrexia due to anesthesia (T88.3)
                radiation-related disorders of the skin and
                    subcutaneous tissue (L55-L59)

       Excludes2   burns (T20-T31)
                sunburn (L55.-)
                sweat disorder due to heat (L74-L75)

       The appropriate 7th character is to be added to each code from
          category T67

A	initial encounter
D	subsequent encounter
S	sequela

X ● T67.0   Heatstroke and sunstroke

           Use additional code(s) to identify any associated
               complications of heatstroke, such as:
               coma and stupor (R40.-)
               rhabdomyolysis (M62.82)
               systemic inflammatory response syndrome (R65.1-)
           Coding Clinic: 2019, Q4, P18

     X ● T67.01   Heatstroke and sunstroke
                 Heat apoplexy
                 Heat pyrexia
                 Siriasis
                 Thermoplegia

     X ● T67.02   Exertional heatstroke
                 Coding Clinic: 2019, Q4, P18

     X ● T67.09   Other heatstroke and sunstroke

X ● T67.1   Heat syncope
          Heat collapse

X ● T67.2   Heat cramp

X ● T67.3   Heat exhaustion, anhydrotic
          Heat prostration due to water depletion

          Excludes1   heat exhaustion due to salt depletion
                    (T67.4)

X ● T67.4   Heat exhaustion due to salt depletion
          Heat prostration due to salt (and water) depletion

X ● T67.5   Heat exhaustion, unspecified
          Heat prostration NOS

X ● T67.6   Heat fatigue, transient

X ● T67.7   Heat edema

X ● T67.8   Other effects of heat and light

X ● T67.9   Effect of heat and light, unspecified

X ● T68   Hypothermia
       Accidental hypothermia
       Hypothermia NOS

       Use additional code to identify source of exposure:
          Exposure to excessive cold of man-made origin (W93)
          Exposure to excessive cold of natural origin (X31)

       Excludes1   hypothermia following anesthesia (T88.51)
                hypothermia not associated with low
                    environmental temperature (R68.0)
                hypothermia of newborn (P80.-)

       Excludes2   frostbite (T33-T34)

       The appropriate 7th character is to be added to code T68

A	initial encounter
D	subsequent encounter
S	sequela

● T69   Other effects of reduced temperature

       Use additional code to identify source of exposure:
          Exposure to excessive cold of man-made origin (W93)
          Exposure to excessive cold of natural origin (X31)

       Excludes2   frostbite (T33-T34)

       The appropriate 7th character is to be added to each code from
          category T69

A	initial encounter
D	subsequent encounter
S	sequela

  ● T69.0   Immersion hand and foot

     ● T69.01   Immersion hand

        ● T69.011   Immersion hand, right hand
        ● T69.012   Immersion hand, left hand
        ● T69.019   Immersion hand, unspecified hand

     ● T69.02   Immersion foot
           Trench foot

        ● T69.021   Immersion foot, right foot
        ● T69.022   Immersion foot, left foot
        ● T69.029   Immersion foot, unspecified foot

X ● T69.1   Chilblains

X ● T69.8   Other specified effects of reduced temperature

X ● T69.9   Effect of reduced temperature, unspecified

● T70   Effects of air pressure and water pressure

       The appropriate 7th character is to be added to each code from
          category T70

A	initial encounter
D	subsequent encounter
S	sequela

X ● T70.0   Otitic barotrauma
          Aero-otitis media
          Effects of change in ambient atmospheric pressure or
            water pressure on ears

X ● T70.1   Sinus barotrauma
          Aerosinusitis
          Effects of change in ambient atmospheric pressure on
            sinuses

● T70.2   Other and unspecified effects of high altitude

       Excludes2   polycythemia due to high altitude (D75.1)

     X ● T70.20   Unspecified effects of high altitude

     X ● T70.29   Other effects of high altitude
             Alpine sickness
             Anoxia due to high altitude
             Barotrauma NOS
             Hypobaropathy
             Mountain sickness

CHAPTER 19 (S00-T88)

X● **T70.3**   **Caisson disease [decompression sickness]**
         Compressed-air disease
         Diver's palsy or paralysis

X● **T70.4**   **Effects of high-pressure fluids**
         Hydraulic jet injection (industrial)
         Pneumatic jet injection (industrial)
         Traumatic jet injection (industrial)

X● **T70.8**   **Other effects of air pressure and water pressure**

X● **T70.9**   **Effect of air pressure and water pressure, unspecified**

● **T71**   **Asphyxiation**
         Mechanical suffocation
         Traumatic suffocation

     Excludes1   acute respiratory distress (syndrome) (J80)
                 anoxia due to high altitude (T70.2)
                 asphyxia NOS (R09.01)
                 asphyxia from carbon monoxide (T58.-)
                 asphyxia from inhalation of food or foreign body
                     (T17.-)
                 asphyxia from other gases, fumes and vapors
                     (T59.-)
                 respiratory distress (syndrome) in newborn
                     (P22.-)

     The appropriate 7th character is to be added to each code from
        category T71

> A   initial encounter
> D   subsequent encounter
> S   sequela

● **T71.1**   **Asphyxiation due to mechanical threat to breathing**
         Suffocation due to mechanical threat to breathing

   ● **T71.11**   **Asphyxiation due to smothering under pillow**

     ● **T71.111**   **Asphyxiation due to smothering
                 under pillow, accidental**
                 Asphyxiation due to smothering
                     under pillow NOS

     ● **T71.112**   **Asphyxiation due to smothering
                 under pillow, intentional self-harm
                 A, S** 🐾

     ● **T71.113**   **Asphyxiation due to smothering
                 under pillow, assault**

     ● **T71.114**   **Asphyxiation due to smothering
                 under pillow, undetermined**

   ● **T71.12**   **Asphyxiation due to plastic bag**

     ● **T71.121**   **Asphyxiation due to plastic bag,
                 accidental**
                 Asphyxiation due to plastic bag
                     NOS

     ● **T71.122**   **Asphyxiation due to plastic bag,
                 intentional self-harm A, S** 🐾

     ● **T71.123**   **Asphyxiation due to plastic bag,
                 assault**

     ● **T71.124**   **Asphyxiation due to plastic bag,
                 undetermined**

   ● **T71.13**   **Asphyxiation due to being trapped in bed
               linens**

     ● **T71.131**   **Asphyxiation due to being trapped in
                 bed linens, accidental**
                 Asphyxiation due to being trapped
                     in bed linens NOS

     ● **T71.132**   **Asphyxiation due to being trapped in
                 bed linens, intentional self-harm
                 A, S** 🐾

     ● **T71.133**   **Asphyxiation due to being trapped in
                 bed linens, assault**

     ● **T71.134**   **Asphyxiation due to being trapped in
                 bed linens, undetermined**

   ● **T71.14**   **Asphyxiation due to smothering under another
              person's body (in bed)**

     ● **T71.141**   **Asphyxiation due to smothering
                 under another person's body (in bed),
                 accidental**
                 Asphyxiation due to smothering
                     under another person's body
                     (in bed) NOS

     ● **T71.143**   **Asphyxiation due to smothering
                 under another person's body (in bed),
                 assault**

     ● **T71.144**   **Asphyxiation due to smothering
                 under another person's body (in bed),
                 undetermined**

   ● **T71.15**   **Asphyxiation due to smothering in furniture**

     ● **T71.151**   **Asphyxiation due to smothering in
                 furniture, accidental**
                 Asphyxiation due to smothering in
                     furniture NOS

     ● **T71.152**   **Asphyxiation due to smothering in
                 furniture, intentional self-harm
                 A, S** 🐾

     ● **T71.153**   **Asphyxiation due to smothering in
                 furniture, assault**

     ● **T71.154**   **Asphyxiation due to smothering in
                 furniture, undetermined**

   ● **T71.16**   **Asphyxiation due to hanging**
              Hanging by window shade cord
              Use additional code for any associated injuries,
                 such as:
              crushing injury of neck (S17.-)
              fracture of cervical vertebrae (S12.0-S12.2-)
              open wound of neck (S11.-)

     ● **T71.161**   **Asphyxiation due to hanging,
                 accidental**
                 Asphyxiation due to hanging NOS
                 Hanging NOS

     ● **T71.162**   **Asphyxiation due to hanging,
                 intentional self-harm A, S** 🐾

     ● **T71.163**   **Asphyxiation due to hanging, assault**

     ● **T71.164**   **Asphyxiation due to hanging,
                 undetermined**

   ● **T71.19**   **Asphyxiation due to mechanical**
              Threat to breathing due to other causes

     ● **T71.191**   **Asphyxiation due to mechanical
                 threat to breathing due to other
                 causes, accidental**
                 Asphyxiation due to other causes
                     NOS
                 Coding Clinic: 2016, Q4, P76

     ● **T71.192**   **Asphyxiation due to mechanical
                 threat to breathing due to other
                 causes, intentional self-harm A, S** 🐾

     ● **T71.193**   **Asphyxiation due to mechanical
                 threat to breathing due to other
                 causes, assault**

     ● **T71.194**   **Asphyxiation due to mechanical
                 threat to breathing due to other
                 causes, undetermined**

● **T71.2**   **Asphyxiation due to systemic oxygen deficiency due to
         low oxygen content in ambient air**
         Suffocation due to systemic oxygen deficiency due to
             low oxygen content in ambient air

   X● **T71.20**   **Asphyxiation due to systemic oxygen deficiency
              due to low oxygen content in ambient air due to
              unspecified cause**

   X● **T71.21**   **Asphyxiation due to cave-in or falling earth**
              Use additional code for any associated
                 cataclysm (X34-X38)

▶ New   ⇒ Revised   ~~deleted~~ Deleted   Excludes 1   Excludes 2   Includes   Use additional   Code first   Code also   Key words

1440   **OGCR** Official Guidelines   X Assign placeholder X   ● Use Additional Character(s)   ▌ Manifestation Code   🐾 Hierarchical Condition Category   **Coding Clinic**

● **T71.22**   Asphyxiation due to being trapped in a car trunk
    ● **T71.221**   Asphyxiation due to being trapped in a car trunk, accidental
    ● **T71.222**   Asphyxiation due to being trapped in a car trunk, intentional self-harm A, S 🔖
    ● **T71.223**   Asphyxiation due to being trapped in a car trunk, assault
    ● **T71.224**   Asphyxiation due to being trapped in a car trunk, undetermined

● **T71.23**   Asphyxiation due to being trapped in a (discarded) refrigerator
    ● **T71.231**   Asphyxiation due to being trapped in a (discarded) refrigerator, accidental
    ● **T71.232**   Asphyxiation due to being trapped in a (discarded) refrigerator, intentional self-harm A, S 🔖
    ● **T71.233**   Asphyxiation due to being trapped in a (discarded) refrigerator, assault
    ● **T71.234**   Asphyxiation due to being trapped in a (discarded) refrigerator, undetermined

X ● **T71.29**   Asphyxiation due to being trapped in other low oxygen environment

X ● **T71.9**   Asphyxiation due to unspecified cause
    Suffocation (by strangulation) due to unspecified cause
    Suffocation NOS
    Systemic oxygen deficiency due to low oxygen content in ambient air due to unspecified cause
    Systemic oxygen deficiency due to mechanical threat to breathing due to unspecified cause
    Traumatic asphyxia NOS

● **T73**   **Effects of other deprivation**
    The appropriate 7th character is to be added to each code from category T73

A	initial encounter
D	subsequent encounter
S	sequela

X ● **T73.0**   **Starvation**
    Deprivation of food
X ● **T73.1**   **Deprivation of water**
X ● **T73.2**   **Exhaustion due to exposure**
X ● **T73.3**   **Exhaustion due to excessive exertion**
    Exhaustion due to overexertion
X ● **T73.8**   **Other effects of deprivation**
X ● **T73.9**   **Effect of deprivation, unspecified**

● **T74**   **Adult and child abuse, neglect and other maltreatment, confirmed**
    Use additional code, if applicable, to identify any associated current injury
    Use additional external cause code to identify perpetrator, if known (Y07.-)
    Excludes1   abuse and maltreatment in pregnancy (O9A.3-, O9A.4-, O9A.5-)
               adult and child maltreatment, suspected (T76.-)
    The appropriate 7th character is to be added to each code from category T74

A	initial encounter
D	subsequent encounter
S	sequela

● **T74.0**   **Neglect or abandonment, confirmed**
    X ● **T74.01**   Adult neglect or abandonment, confirmed   A
    X ● **T74.02**   Child neglect or abandonment, confirmed   P

● **T74.1**   **Physical abuse, confirmed**
    Excludes2   sexual abuse (T74.2-)
    X ● **T74.11**   Adult physical abuse, confirmed   A
    X ● **T74.12**   Child physical abuse, confirmed   P
         Excludes2   shaken infant syndrome (T74.4)

● **T74.2**   **Sexual abuse, confirmed**
    Rape, confirmed
    Sexual assault, confirmed
    X ● **T74.21**   Adult sexual abuse, confirmed   A
    X ● **T74.22**   Child sexual abuse, confirmed   P

● **T74.3**   **Psychological abuse, confirmed**
    Bullying and intimidation, confirmed
    Intimidation through social media, confirmed
    X ● **T74.31**   Adult psychological abuse, confirmed   A
    X ● **T74.32**   Child psychological abuse, confirmed   P

X ● **T74.4**   **Shaken infant syndrome**   P

● **T74.5**   **Forced sexual exploitation, confirmed**
    X ● **T74.51**   Adult forced sexual exploitation, confirmed   P
    X ● **T74.52**   Child sexual exploitation, confirmed   P

● **T74.6**   **Forced labor exploitation, confirmed**
    X ● **T74.61**   Adult forced labor exploitation, confirmed   P
    X ● **T74.62**   Child forced labor exploitation, confirmed   P

● **T74.9**   **Unspecified maltreatment, confirmed**
    X ● **T74.91**   Unspecified adult maltreatment, confirmed   A
    X ● **T74.92**   Unspecified child maltreatment, confirmed   P

● **T75**   **Other and unspecified effects of other external causes**
    Excludes1   adverse effects NEC (T78.-)
    Excludes2   burns (electric) (T20-T31)
    The appropriate 7th character is to be added to each code from category T75

A	initial encounter
D	subsequent encounter
S	sequela

● **T75.0**   **Effects of lightning**
    Struck by lightning
    X ● **T75.00**   Unspecified effects of lightning
         Struck by lightning NOS
    X ● **T75.01**   Shock due to being struck by lightning
    X ● **T75.09**   Other effects of lightning
         Use additional code for other effects of lightning

X ● **T75.1**   **Unspecified effects of drowning and nonfatal submersion**
    Immersion
    Excludes1   specified effects of drowning code to effects

● **T75.2**   **Effects of vibration**
    X ● **T75.20**   Unspecified effects of vibration
    X ● **T75.21**   Pneumatic hammer syndrome
    X ● **T75.22**   Traumatic vasospastic syndrome
    X ● **T75.23**   Vertigo from infrasound
         Excludes1   vertigo NOS (R42)
    X ● **T75.29**   Other effects of vibration

X ● **T75.3**   **Motion sickness**
     Airsickness   Travel sickness
     Seasickness
     Use additional external cause code to identify vehicle or
       type of motion (Y92.81-, Y93.5-)

X ● **T75.4**   **Electrocution**
     Shock from electric current
     Shock from electroshock gun (taser)

● **T75.8**   **Other specified effects of external causes**

    X ● **T75.81**   **Effects of abnormal gravitation [G] forces**

    X ● **T75.82**   **Effects of weightlessness**

    X ● **T75.89**   **Other specified effects of external causes**

● **T76**   **Adult and child abuse, neglect and other maltreatment, suspected**
     Use additional code, if applicable, to identify any associated
       current injury

     Excludes1   adult and child maltreatment, confirmed (T74.-)
                 suspected abuse and maltreatment in pregnancy
                   (O9A.3-, O9A.4-, O9A.5-)
                 suspected adult physical abuse, ruled out (Z04.71)
                 suspected adult sexual abuse, ruled out (Z04.41)
                 suspected child physical abuse, ruled out (Z04.72)
                 suspected child sexual abuse, ruled out (Z04.42)

     The appropriate 7th character is to be added to each code from
       category T76

     A   initial encounter
     D   subsequent encounter
     S   sequela

     Coding Clinic: 2016, Q4, P129

● **T76.0**   **Neglect or abandonment, suspected**

    X ● **T76.01**   **Adult neglect or abandonment, suspected**   A

    X ● **T76.02**   **Child neglect or abandonment, suspected**   P

● **T76.1**   **Physical abuse, suspected**

    X ● **T76.11**   **Adult physical abuse, suspected**   A

    X ● **T76.12**   **Child physical abuse, suspected**   P
               Coding Clinic: 2019, Q2, P12

● **T76.2**   **Sexual abuse, suspected**
     Rape, suspected

     Excludes1   alleged abuse, ruled out (Z04.7)

    X ● **T76.21**   **Adult sexual abuse, suspected**   A

    X ● **T76.22**   **Child sexual abuse, suspected**   P

● **T76.3**   **Psychological abuse, suspected**
     Bullying and intimidation, suspected
     Intimidation through social media, suspected

    X ● **T76.31**   **Adult psychological abuse, suspected**   A

    X ● **T76.32**   **Child psychological abuse, suspected**   P

● **T76.5**   **Forced sexual exploitation, suspected**

    X ● **T76.51**   **Adult forced sexual exploitation, suspected**   P

    X ● **T76.52**   **Child sexual exploitation, suspected**   P

● **T76.6**   **Forced labor exploitation, suspected**

    X ● **T76.61**   **Adult forced labor exploitation, suspected**   P

    X ● **T76.62**   **Child forced labor exploitation, suspected**   P

● **T76.9**   **Unspecified maltreatment, suspected**

    X ● **T76.91**   **Unspecified adult maltreatment, suspected**   A

    X ● **T76.92**   **Unspecified child maltreatment, suspected**   P

● **T78**   **Adverse effects, not elsewhere classified**

     Excludes2   complications of surgical and medical care NEC
                 (T80-T88)

     The appropriate 7th character is to be added to each code from
       category T78

     A   initial encounter
     D   subsequent encounter
     S   sequela

● **T78.0**   **Anaphylactic reaction due to food**
     Anaphylactic reaction due to adverse food reaction
     Anaphylactic shock or reaction due to nonpoisonous
       foods
     Anaphylactoid reaction due to food

    X ● **T78.00**   **Anaphylactic reaction due to unspecified food**

    X ● **T78.01**   **Anaphylactic reaction due to peanuts**

    X ● **T78.02**   **Anaphylactic reaction due to shellfish (crustaceans)**

    X ● **T78.03**   **Anaphylactic reaction due to other fish**

    X ● **T78.04**   **Anaphylactic reaction due to fruits and vegetables**

    X ● **T78.05**   **Anaphylactic reaction due to tree nuts and seeds**

       Excludes2   anaphylactic reaction due to peanuts (T78.01)

    X ● **T78.06**   **Anaphylactic reaction due to food additives**

    X ● **T78.07**   **Anaphylactic reaction due to milk and dairy products**

    X ● **T78.08**   **Anaphylactic reaction due to eggs**

    X ● **T78.09**   **Anaphylactic reaction due to other food products**

X ● **T78.1**   **Other adverse food reactions, not elsewhere classified**
     Use additional code to identify the type of reaction, if
       applicable

     Excludes1   anaphylactic reaction or shock due to
                 adverse food reaction (T78.0-)
                 anaphylactic reaction due to food (T78.0-)
                 bacterial food borne intoxications (A05.-)

     Excludes2   allergic and dietetic gastroenteritis and
                 colitis (K52.29)
                 allergic rhinitis due to food (J30.5)
                 dermatitis due to food in contact with
                   skin (L23.6, L24.6, L25.4)
                 dermatitis due to ingested food (L27.2)
                 food protein-induced enterocolitis
                   syndrome (K52.21)
                 food protein-induced enteropathy
                   (K52.22)

X ● **T78.2**   **Anaphylactic shock, unspecified**
     *Occurs when allergic response triggers large quantities of
       histamines, prostaglandins, leukotrienes resulting in
       systemic vasodilation*
     Allergic shock
     Anaphylactic reaction
     Anaphylaxis

     Excludes1   anaphylactic reaction or shock due to
                 adverse effect of correct medicinal
                   substance properly administered
                   (T88.6)
                 anaphylactic reaction or shock due to
                   adverse food reaction (T78.0-)
                 anaphylactic reaction or shock due to
                   serum (T80.5-)

▶ New   ⇒ Revised   ~~deleted~~ Deleted   Excludes 1   Excludes 2   Includes   Use additional   Code first   Code also   Key words

OGCR Official Guidelines   X Assign placeholder X   ● Use Additional Character(s)   ▶ Manifestation Code   🅗 Hierarchical Condition Category   **Coding Clinic**

X● **T78.3** **Angioneurotic edema**
     Allergic angioedema
     Giant urticaria
     Vascular disorder resulting from abnormalities of autonomic
     nervous system fibers supplying blood vessels
     Quincke's edema
     Excludes1   serum urticaria (T80.6-)
                    urticaria (L50.-)

● **T78.4** **Other and unspecified allergy**
     Excludes1   specified types of allergic reaction
                    such as:
                    allergic diarrhea (K52.29)
                    allergic gastroenteritis and colitis
                       (K52.29)
                    dermatitis (L23-L25, L27.-)
                    food protein-induced enterocolitis
                       syndrome (K52.21)
                    food protein-induced enteropathy
                       (K52.22)
                    hay fever (J30.1)

     X● **T78.40** **Allergy, unspecified**
           Allergic reaction NOS
           Hypersensitivity NOS

     X● **T78.41** **Arthus phenomenon**
           Arthus reaction

     X● **T78.49** **Other allergy**
           Coding Clinic: 2021, Q1, P42

X● **T78.8**   **Other adverse effects, not elsewhere classified**

CERTAIN EARLY COMPLICATIONS OF TRAUMA (T79)

● **T79**   **Certain early complications of trauma, not elsewhere classified**
     Excludes2   acute respiratory distress syndrome (J80)
                    complications occurring during or following
                       medical procedures (T80-T88)
                    complications of surgical and medical care NEC
                       (T80-T88)
                    newborn respiratory distress syndrome (P22.0)

     The appropriate 7th character is to be added to each code from
     category T79

A	initial encounter
D	subsequent encounter
S	sequela

X●● **T79.0** **Air embolism (traumatic)** A 🚫
     Excludes1   air embolism complicating abortion
                    or ectopic or molar pregnancy
                       (O00-O07, O08.2)
                    air embolism complicating pregnancy,
                       childbirth and the puerperium
                       (O88.0)
                    air embolism following infusion,
                       transfusion, and therapeutic injection
                       (T80.0)
                    air embolism following procedure NEC
                       (T81.7-)

X● **T79.1** **Fat embolism (traumatic)** A 🚫
     Excludes1   fat embolism complicating:
                    abortion or ectopic or molar pregnancy
                       (O00-O07, O08.2)
                    pregnancy, childbirth and the
                       puerperium (O88.8)

X● **T79.2** **Traumatic secondary and recurrent hemorrhage and**
     seroma A 🚫

X● **T79.4** **Traumatic shock** A 🚫
     Shock (immediate) (delayed) following injury
     Excludes1   anaphylactic shock due to adverse food
                    reaction (T78.0-)
                    anaphylactic shock due to correct
                       medicinal substance properly
                       administered (T88.6)
                    anaphylactic shock due to serum (T80.5-)
                    anaphylactic shock NOS (T78.2)
                    ~~anesthetic shock (T88.2)~~
                    electric shock (T75.4)
                    nontraumatic shock NEC (R57.-)
                    obstetric shock (O75.1)
                    postprocedural shock (T81.1-)
                    septic shock (R65.21)
                    shock complicating abortion or ectopic or
                       molar pregnancy (O00-O07, O08.3)
          ▶ shock due to anesthesia (T88.2)
                    shock due to lightning (T75.01)
                    shock NOS (R57.9)

X● **T79.5** **Traumatic anuria** A 🚫
     Crush syndrome
     Renal failure following crushing

X● **T79.6** **Traumatic ischemia of muscle** A 🚫
     Traumatic rhabdomyolysis
     Volkmann's ischemic contracture
     Excludes2   anterior tibial syndrome (M76.8)
                    compartment syndrome (traumatic)
                       (T79.A-)
                    nontraumatic ischemia of muscle (M62.2-)

X● **T79.7** **Traumatic subcutaneous emphysema** A 🚫
     Excludes2   emphysema NOS (J43)
                    emphysema (subcutaneous) resulting
                       from a procedure (T81.82)

● **T79.A** **Traumatic compartment syndrome**
     Excludes1   fibromyalgia (M79.7)
                    nontraumatic compartment syndrome
                       (M79.A-)
     Excludes2   traumatic ischemic infarction of muscle
                    (T79.6)

     X● **T79.A0** **Compartment syndrome, unspecified**
           Compartment syndrome NOS

     ● **T79.A1** **Traumatic compartment syndrome of upper**
           extremity
           Traumatic compartment syndrome of shoulder,
             arm, forearm, wrist, hand, and fingers

         ● **T79.A11** **Traumatic compartment syndrome of**
              right upper extremity A 🚫

         ● **T79.A12** **Traumatic compartment syndrome of**
              left upper extremity A 🚫

         ● **T79.A19** **Traumatic compartment syndrome of**
              unspecified upper extremity A 🚫

     ● **T79.A2** **Traumatic compartment syndrome of lower**
           extremity
           Traumatic compartment syndrome of hip,
             buttock, thigh, leg, foot, and toes

         ● **T79.A21** **Traumatic compartment syndrome of**
              right lower extremity A 🚫

         ● **T79.A22** **Traumatic compartment syndrome of**
              left lower extremity A 🚫

         ● **T79.A29** **Traumatic compartment syndrome of**
              unspecified lower extremity

     X● **T79.A3** **Traumatic compartment syndrome of abdomen**
           A 🚫

     X● **T79.A9** **Traumatic compartment syndrome of other sites**
           A 🚫

X● **T79.8**   **Other early complications of trauma** A 🚫

X● **T79.9**   **Unspecified early complication of trauma** A 🚫

CHAPTER 19 (S00-T88)

COMPLICATIONS OF SURGICAL AND MEDICAL CARE NOT ELSEWHERE CLASSIFIED (T80-T88)

Use additional code for adverse effect, if applicable, to identify drug (T36-T50 with fifth or sixth character 5)

Use additional code(s) to identify the specified condition resulting from the complication.

Use additional code to identify devices involved and details of circumstances (Y62-Y82)

Excludes2   any encounters with medical care for postprocedural conditions in which no complications are present, such as:
artificial opening status (Z93.-)
closure of external stoma (Z43.-)
fitting and adjustment of external prosthetic device (Z44.-)
burns and corrosions from local applications and irradiation (T20-T32)
complications of surgical procedures during pregnancy, childbirth and the puerperium (O00-O9A)
mechanical complication of respirator [ventilator] (J95.850)
poisoning and toxic effects of drugs and chemicals (T36-T65 with fifth or sixth character 1-4 or 6)
postprocedural fever (R50.82)
specified complications classified elsewhere, such as:
cerebrospinal fluid leak from spinal puncture (G97.0)
colostomy malfunction (K94.0-)
disorders of fluid and electrolyte imbalance (E86-E87)
functional disturbances following cardiac surgery (I97.0-I97.1)
intraoperative and postprocedural complications of specified body systems (D78.-, E36.-, E89.-, G97.3-, G97.4, H59.3-, H59.-, H95.2-, H95.3, I97.4-, I97.5, J95.6-, J95.7, K91.6-, L76.-, M96.-, N99.-)
ostomy complications (J95.0-, K94.-, N99.5-)
postgastric surgery syndromes (K91.1)
postlaminectomy syndrome NEC (M96.1)
postmastectomy lymphedema syndrome (I97.2)
postsurgical blind-loop syndrome (K91.2)
ventilator associated pneumonia (J95.851)

● **T80**   **Complications following infusion, transfusion and therapeutic injection**

Includes   complications following perfusion

Excludes2   bone marrow transplant rejection (T86.01)
febrile nonhemolytic transfusion reaction (R50.84)
fluid overload due to transfusion (E87.71)
posttransfusion purpura (D69.51)
transfusion associated circulatory overload (TACO) (E87.71)
transfusion (red blood cell) associated hemochromatosis (E83.111)
transfusion related acute lung injury (TRALI) (J95.84)

The appropriate 7th character is to be added to each code from category T80

A	initial encounter
D	subsequent encounter
S	sequela

X ● **T80.0**   **Air embolism following infusion, transfusion and therapeutic injection**

X ● **T80.1**   **Vascular complications following infusion, transfusion and therapeutic injection**

Use additional code to identify the vascular complication

Excludes2   extravasation of vesicant agent (T80.81-)
infiltration of vesicant agent (T80.81-)
vascular complications specified as due to prosthetic devices, implants and grafts (T82.8- T83.8-, T84.8-, T85.8-)
postprocedural vascular complications (T81.7-)

● **T80.2**   **Infections following infusion, transfusion and therapeutic injection**

Use additional code to identify the specific infection, such as:
sepsis (A41.9)

Use additional code (R65.2-) to identify severe sepsis, if applicable

Excludes2   infections specified as due to prosthetic devices, implants and grafts (T82.6-T82.7, T83.5-T83.6, T84.5-T84.7, T85.7)
postprocedural infections (T81.44)

Coding Clinic: 2018, Q4, P89

● **T80.21**   **Infection due to central venous catheter**

Infection due to pulmonary artery catheter (Swan-Ganz catheter)

Coding Clinic: 2019, Q1, P13-14; 2018, Q4, P89

● **T80.211**   **Bloodstream infection due to central venous catheter**

Catheter-related bloodstream infection (CRBSI) NOS
Central line-associated bloodstream infection (CLABSI)
Bloodstream infection due to Hickman catheter
Bloodstream infection due to peripherally inserted central catheter (PICC)
Bloodstream infection due to portacath (port-a-cath)
Bloodstream infection due to pulmonary artery catheter
Bloodstream infection due to triple lumen catheter
Bloodstream infection due to umbilical venous catheter

Coding Clinic: 2018, Q4, P89

● **T80.212**   **Local infection due to central venous catheter**

Exit or insertion site infection
Local infection due to Hickman catheter
Local infection due to peripherally inserted central catheter (PICC)
Local infection due to portacath (port-a-cath)
Local infection due to pulmonary artery catheter
Local infection due to triple lumen catheter
Local infection due to umbilical venous catheter
Port or reservoir infection
Tunnel infection

● **T80.218** **Other infection due to central venous catheter**
Other central line-associated infection
Other infection due to Hickman catheter
Other infection due to peripherally inserted central catheter (PICC)
Other infection due to portacath (port-a-cath)
Other infection due to pulmonary artery catheter
Other infection due to triple lumen catheter
Other infection due to umbilical venous catheter

● **T80.219** **Unspecified infection due to central venous catheter**
Central line-associated infection NOS
Unspecified infection due to Hickman catheter
Unspecified infection due to peripherally inserted central catheter (PICC)
Unspecified infection due to portacath (port-a-cath)
Unspecified infection due to pulmonary artery catheter
Unspecified infection due to triple lumen catheter
Unspecified infection due to umbilical venous catheter

X● **T80.22** **Acute infection following transfusion, infusion, or injection of blood and blood products**

X● **T80.29** **Infection following other infusion, transfusion and therapeutic injection**

● **T80.3** **ABO incompatibility reaction due to transfusion of blood or blood products**

Excludes1   minor blood group antigens reactions (Duffy) (E) (K) (Kell) (Kidd) (Lewis) (M) (N) (P) (S) (T80.A-)

X● **T80.30** **ABO incompatibility reaction due to transfusion of blood or blood products, unspecified**
ABO incompatibility blood transfusion NOS
Reaction to ABO incompatibility from transfusion NOS

● **T80.31** **ABO incompatibility with hemolytic transfusion reaction**

● **T80.310** **ABO incompatibility with acute hemolytic transfusion reaction**
ABO incompatibility with hemolytic transfusion reaction less than 24 hours after transfusion
Acute hemolytic transfusion reaction (AHTR) due to ABO incompatibility

● **T80.311** **ABO incompatibility with delayed hemolytic transfusion reaction**
ABO incompatibility with hemolytic transfusion reaction 24 hours or more after transfusion
Delayed hemolytic transfusion reaction (DHTR) due to ABO incompatibility

● **T80.319** **ABO incompatibility with hemolytic transfusion reaction, unspecified**
ABO incompatibility with hemolytic transfusion reaction at unspecified time after transfusion
Hemolytic transfusion reaction (HTR) due to ABO incompatibility NOS

X● **T80.39** **Other ABO incompatibility reaction due to transfusion of blood or blood products**
Delayed serologic transfusion reaction (DSTR) from ABO incompatibility
Other ABO incompatible blood transfusion
Other reaction to ABO incompatible blood transfusion

● **T80.4** **Rh incompatibility reaction due to transfusion of blood or blood products**
Reaction due to incompatibility of Rh antigens (C) (c) (D) (E) (e)

X● **T80.40** **Rh incompatibility reaction due to transfusion of blood or blood products, unspecified**
Reaction due to Rh factor in transfusion NOS
Rh incompatible blood transfusion NOS

● **T80.41** **Rh incompatibility with hemolytic transfusion reaction**

● **T80.410** **Rh incompatibility with acute hemolytic transfusion reaction**
Acute hemolytic transfusion reaction (AHTR) due to Rh incompatibility
Rh incompatibility with hemolytic transfusion reaction less than 24 hours after transfusion

● **T80.411** **Rh incompatibility with delayed hemolytic transfusion reaction**
Delayed hemolytic transfusion reaction (DHTR) due to Rh incompatibility
Rh incompatibility with hemolytic transfusion reaction 24 hours or more after transfusion

● **T80.419** **Rh incompatibility with hemolytic transfusion reaction, unspecified**
Rh incompatibility with hemolytic transfusion reaction at unspecified time after transfusion
Hemolytic transfusion reaction (HTR) due to Rh incompatibility NOS

X● **T80.49** **Other Rh incompatibility reaction due to transfusion of blood or blood products**
Delayed serologic transfusion reaction (DSTR) from Rh incompatibility
Other reaction to Rh incompatible blood transfusion

● **T80.A** **Non-ABO incompatibility reaction due to transfusion of blood or blood products**
Reaction due to incompatibility of minor antigens (Duffy) (Kell) (Kidd) (Lewis) (M) (N) (P) (S)

X● **T80.A0** **Non-ABO incompatibility reaction due to transfusion of blood or blood products, unspecified**
Non-ABO antigen incompatibility reaction from transfusion NOS

● **T80.A1** **Non-ABO incompatibility with hemolytic transfusion reaction**

● **T80.A10** **Non-ABO incompatibility with acute hemolytic transfusion reaction**
Acute hemolytic transfusion reaction (AHTR) due to non-ABO incompatibility
Non-ABO incompatibility with hemolytic transfusion reaction less than 24 hours after transfusion

● **T80.A11**   **Non-ABO incompatibility with delayed hemolytic transfusion reaction**
> Delayed hemolytic transfusion reaction (DHTR) due to non-ABO incompatibility
> Non-ABO incompatibility with hemolytic transfusion reaction 24 or more hours after transfusion

● **T80.A19**   **Non-ABO incompatibility with hemolytic transfusion reaction, unspecified**
> Hemolytic transfusion reaction (HTR) due to non-ABO incompatibility NOS
> Non-ABO incompatibility with hemolytic transfusion reaction at unspecified time after transfusion

X ● **T80.A9**   **Other non-ABO incompatibility reaction due to transfusion of blood or blood products**
> Delayed serologic transfusion reaction (DSTR) from non-ABO incompatibility
> Other reaction to non-ABO incompatible blood transfusion

● **T80.5**   **Anaphylactic reaction due to serum**
> Allergic reaction due to serum
> Anaphylactic shock due to serum
> Anaphylactoid reaction due to serum
> Anaphylaxis due to serum

> **Excludes1**   ABO incompatibility reaction due to transfusion of blood or blood products (T80.3-)
> allergic reaction or shock NOS (T78.2)
> anaphylactic reaction or shock NOS (T78.2)
> anaphylactic reaction or shock due to adverse effect of correct medicinal substance properly administered (T88.6)
> other serum reaction (T80.6-)

X ● **T80.51**   **Anaphylactic reaction due to administration of blood and blood products**

X ● **T80.52**   **Anaphylactic reaction due to vaccination**
> Coding Clinic: 2021, Q1, P43

X ● **T80.59**   **Anaphylactic reaction due to other serum**

● **T80.6**   **Other serum reactions**
> Intoxication by serum   Serum sickness
> Protein sickness   Serum urticaria
> Serum rash

> **Excludes2**   serum hepatitis (B16-B19)

X ● **T80.61**   **Other serum reaction due to administration of blood and blood products**

X ● **T80.62**   **Other serum reaction due to vaccination**
> Coding Clinic: 2021, Q1, P42

X ● **T80.69**   **Other serum reaction due to other serum**
> Code also, if applicable, arthropathy in hypersensitivity reactions classified elsewhere (M36.4)

● **T80.8**   **Other complications following infusion, transfusion and therapeutic injection**

● **T80.81**   **Extravasation of vesicant agent**
> Infiltration of vesicant agent

● **T80.810**   **Extravasation of vesicant antineoplastic chemotherapy**
> Infiltration of vesicant antineoplastic chemotherapy

● **T80.818**   **Extravasation of other vesicant agent**
> Infiltration of other vesicant agent

▶ **T80.82**   **Complication of immune effector cellular therapy**
> ▶Complication of chimeric antigen receptor (CAR-T) cell therapy
> ▶Complication of IEC therapy

> ▶ **Excludes2**   complication of bone marrow transplant (T86.0)
>   ▶complication of stem cell transplant (T86.5)

> ▶Use additional code to identify the specific complication, such as:
>   ▶cytokine release syndrome (D89.83-)
>   ▶immune effector cell-associated neurotoxicity syndrome (G92.0-)

X ● **T80.89**   **Other complications following infusion, transfusion and therapeutic injection**
> Delayed serologic transfusion reaction (DSTR), unspecified incompatibility

> Use additional code to identify graft-versus-host reaction, if applicable, (D89.81-)

● **T80.9**   **Unspecified complication following infusion, transfusion and therapeutic injection**

X ● **T80.90**   **Unspecified complication following infusion and therapeutic injection**

● **T80.91**   **Hemolytic transfusion reaction, unspecified incompatibility**

> **Excludes1**   ABO incompatibility with hemolytic transfusion reaction (T80.31-)
> Non-ABO incompatibility with hemolytic transfusion reaction (T80.A1-)
> Rh incompatibility with hemolytic transfusion reaction (T80.41-)

● **T80.910**   **Acute hemolytic transfusion reaction, unspecified incompatibility**

● **T80.911**   **Delayed hemolytic transfusion reaction, unspecified incompatibility**

● **T80.919**   **Hemolytic transfusion reaction, unspecified incompatibility, unspecified as acute or delayed**
> Hemolytic transfusion reaction NOS

X ● **T80.92**   **Unspecified transfusion reaction**
> Transfusion reaction NOS

● **T81**   **Complications of procedures, not elsewhere classified**

Use additional code for adverse effect, if applicable, to identify drug (T36-T50 with fifth or sixth character 5)

Excludes2   complications following immunization (T88.0-T88.1)

complications following infusion, transfusion and therapeutic injection (T80.-)

complications of transplanted organs and tissue (T86.-)

poisoning and toxic effects of drugs and chemicals (T36-T65 with fifth or sixth character 1-4 or 6)

specified complications classified elsewhere, such as:

complication of prosthetic devices, implants and grafts (T82-T85)

dermatitis due to drugs and medicaments (L23.3, L24.4, L25.1, L27.0-L27.1)

endosseous dental implant failure (M27.6-)

floppy iris syndrome (IFIS) (intraoperative) H21.81

intraoperative and postprocedural complications of specific body system (D78.-, E36.-, E89.-, G97.3-, G97.4, H59.3-, H59.-, H95.2-, H95.3, I97.4-, I97.5, J95, K91.-, L76.-, M96.-, N99.-)

ostomy complications (J95.0-, K94.-, N99.5-)

plateau iris syndrome (post-iridectomy) (postprocedural) H21.82

Coding Clinic: 2019, Q2, P21-22; 2016, Q4, P29

The appropriate 7th character is to be added to each code from category T81

A	initial encounter
D	subsequent encounter
S	sequela

● **T81.1**   **Postprocedural shock**

Shock during or resulting from a procedure, not elsewhere classified

Excludes1   anaphylactic shock NOS (T78.2)

anaphylactic shock due to correct substance properly administered (T88.6)

anaphylactic shock due to serum (T80.5-)

~~anesthetic shock (T88.2)~~

electric shock (T75.4)

obstetric shock (O75.1)

septic shock (R65.21)

▶shock due to anesthesia (T88.2)

shock following abortion or ectopic or molar pregnancy (O00-O07, O08.3)

traumatic shock (T79.4)

X● **T81.10**   **Postprocedural shock unspecified**

Collapse NOS during or resulting from a procedure, not elsewhere classified

Postprocedural failure of peripheral circulation

Postprocedural shock NOS

X● **T81.11**   **Postprocedural cardiogenic shock A** 🔊

X● **T81.12**   **Postprocedural septic shock A** 🔊

Postprocedural endotoxic shock resulting from a procedure, not elsewhere classified

Postprocedural gram-negative shock resulting from a procedure, not elsewhere classified

Code first underlying infection

Use additional code, to identify any associated acute organ dysfunction, if applicable

X● **T81.19**   **Other postprocedural shock**

Postprocedural hypovolemic shock

Coding Clinic: 2021, Q1, P14

● **T81.3**   **Disruption of wound, not elsewhere classified**

Disruption of any suture materials or other closure methods

Excludes1   breakdown (mechanical) of permanent sutures (T85.612)

displacement of permanent sutures (T85.622)

disruption of cesarean delivery wound (O90.0)

disruption of perineal obstetric wound (O90.1)

mechanical complication of permanent sutures NEC (T85.692)

X● **T81.30**   **Disruption of wound, unspecified**

Disruption of wound NOS

X● **T81.31**   **Disruption of external operation (surgical) wound, not elsewhere classified**

Excludes1   dehiscence of amputation stump (T87.81)

Dehiscence of operation wound NOS

Disruption of operation wound NOS

Disruption or dehiscence of closure of cornea

Disruption or dehiscence of closure of mucosa

Disruption or dehiscence of closure of skin and subcutaneous tissue

Full-thickness skin disruption or dehiscence

Superficial disruption or dehiscence of operation wound

Coding Clinic: 2015, Q1, P20

X● **T81.32**   **Disruption of internal operation (surgical) wound, not elsewhere classified**

Deep disruption or dehiscence of operation wound NOS

Disruption or dehiscence of closure of internal organ or other internal tissue

Disruption or dehiscence of closure of muscle or muscle flap

Disruption or dehiscence of closure of ribs or rib cage

Disruption or dehiscence of closure of skull or craniotomy

Disruption or dehiscence of closure of sternum or sternotomy

Disruption or dehiscence of closure of tendon or ligament

Disruption or dehiscence of closure of superficial or muscular fascia

Coding Clinic: 2017, Q3, P4

X● **T81.33**   **Disruption of traumatic injury wound repair**

Disruption or dehiscence of closure of traumatic laceration (external) (internal)

● **T81.4**   **Infection following a procedure**

Use additional code to identify infection

Use additional code (R65.2-) to identify severe sepsis, if applicable

Excludes2   bleb associated endophthalmitis (H59.4-)

infection due to infusion, transfusion and therapeutic injection (T80.2-)

infection due to prosthetic devices, implants and grafts (T82.6-T82.7, T83.5-T83.6, T84.5-T84.7, T85.7)

obstetric surgical wound infection (O86.0-)

postprocedural fever NOS (R50.82)

postprocedural retroperitoneal abscess (K68.11)

X ● **T81.40**   Infection following a procedure, unspecified

X ● **T81.41**   Infection following a procedure, superficial incisional surgical site
     Subcutaneous abscess following a procedure
     Stitch abscess following a procedure
     Coding Clinic: 2018, Q4, P34

X ● **T81.42**   Infection following a procedure, deep incisional surgical site
     Intra-muscular abscess following a procedure

X ● **T81.43**   Infection following a procedure, organ and space surgical site
     Intra-abdominal abscess following a procedure
     Subphrenic abscess following a procedure

X ● **T81.44**   Sepsis following a procedure A 🦠
     Use additional code to identify the sepsis

X ● **T81.49**   Infection following a procedure, other surgical site
     Coding Clinic: 2015, Q4, P37

● **T81.5**   Complications of foreign body accidentally left in body following procedure

   ● **T81.50**   Unspecified complication of foreign body accidentally left in body following procedure

     ● **T81.500**   Unspecified complication of foreign body accidentally left in body following surgical operation

     ● **T81.501**   Unspecified complication of foreign body accidentally left in body following infusion or transfusion

     ● **T81.502**   Unspecified complication of foreign body accidentally left in body following kidney dialysis A, D, S 🦠

     ● **T81.503**   Unspecified complication of foreign body accidentally left in body following injection or immunization

     ● **T81.504**   Unspecified complication of foreign body accidentally left in body following endoscopic examination

     ● **T81.505**   Unspecified complication of foreign body accidentally left in body following heart catheterization

     ● **T81.506**   Unspecified complication of foreign body accidentally left in body following aspiration, puncture or other catheterization

     ● **T81.507**   Unspecified complication of foreign body accidentally left in body following removal of catheter or packing

     ● **T81.508**   Unspecified complication of foreign body accidentally left in body following other procedure

     ● **T81.509**   Unspecified complication of foreign body accidentally left in body following unspecified procedure

   ● **T81.51**   Adhesions due to foreign body accidentally left in body following procedure

     ● **T81.510**   Adhesions due to foreign body accidentally left in body following surgical operation

     ● **T81.511**   Adhesions due to foreign body accidentally left in body following infusion or transfusion

     ● **T81.512**   Adhesions due to foreign body accidentally left in body following kidney dialysis A, D, S 🦠

● **T81.513**   Adhesions due to foreign body accidentally left in body following injection or immunization

● **T81.514**   Adhesions due to foreign body accidentally left in body following endoscopic examination

● **T81.515**   Adhesions due to foreign body accidentally left in body following heart catheterization

● **T81.516**   Adhesions due to foreign body accidentally left in body following aspiration, puncture or other catheterization

● **T81.517**   Adhesions due to foreign body accidentally left in body following removal of catheter or packing

● **T81.518**   Adhesions due to foreign body accidentally left in body following other procedure

● **T81.519**   Adhesions due to foreign body accidentally left in body following unspecified procedure

● **T81.52**   Obstruction due to foreign body accidentally left in body following procedure

   ● **T81.520**   Obstruction due to foreign body accidentally left in body following surgical operation

   ● **T81.521**   Obstruction due to foreign body accidentally left in body following infusion or transfusion

   ● **T81.522**   Obstruction due to foreign body accidentally left in body following kidney dialysis A, D, S 🦠

   ● **T81.523**   Obstruction due to foreign body accidentally left in body following injection or immunization

   ● **T81.524**   Obstruction due to foreign body accidentally left in body following endoscopic examination

   ● **T81.525**   Obstruction due to foreign body accidentally left in body following heart catheterization

   ● **T81.526**   Obstruction due to foreign body accidentally left in body following aspiration, puncture or other catheterization

   ● **T81.527**   Obstruction due to foreign body accidentally left in body following removal of catheter or packing

   ● **T81.528**   Obstruction due to foreign body accidentally left in body following other procedure

   ● **T81.529**   Obstruction due to foreign body accidentally left in body following unspecified procedure

● **T81.53**   Perforation due to foreign body accidentally left in body following procedure

   ● **T81.530**   Perforation due to foreign body accidentally left in body following surgical operation

   ● **T81.531**   Perforation due to foreign body accidentally left in body following infusion or transfusion

   ● **T81.532**   Perforation due to foreign body accidentally left in body following kidney dialysis A, D, S 🦠

● T81.533   Perforation due to foreign body accidentally left in body following injection or immunization

● T81.534   Perforation due to foreign body accidentally left in body following endoscopic examination

● T81.535   Perforation due to foreign body accidentally left in body following heart catheterization

● T81.536   Perforation due to foreign body accidentally left in body following aspiration, puncture or other catheterization

● T81.537   Perforation due to foreign body accidentally left in body following removal of catheter or packing

● T81.538   Perforation due to foreign body accidentally left in body following other procedure

● T81.539   Perforation due to foreign body accidentally left in body following unspecified procedure

● T81.59   Other complications of foreign body accidentally left in body following procedure

Excludes2   obstruction or perforation due to prosthetic devices and implants intentionally left in body (T82.0-T82.5, T83.0-T83.4, T83.7, T84.0-T84.4, T85.0-T85.6)

● T81.590   Other complications of foreign body accidentally left in body following surgical operation

● T81.591   Other complications of foreign body accidentally left in body following infusion or transfusion

● T81.592   Other complications of foreign body accidentally left in body following kidney dialysis A, D, S 🔄

● T81.593   Other complications of foreign body accidentally left in body following injection or immunization

● T81.594   Other complications of foreign body accidentally left in body following endoscopic examination

● T81.595   Other complications of foreign body accidentally left in body following heart catheterization

● T81.596   Other complications of foreign body accidentally left in body following aspiration, puncture or other catheterization

● T81.597   Other complications of foreign body accidentally left in body following removal of catheter or packing

● T81.598   Other complications of foreign body accidentally left in body following other procedure

● T81.599   Other complications of foreign body accidentally left in body following unspecified procedure

● T81.6   Acute reaction to foreign substance accidentally left during a procedure

Excludes2   complications of foreign body accidentally left in body cavity or operation wound following procedure (T81.5-)

X ● T81.60   Unspecified acute reaction to foreign substance accidentally left during a procedure

X ● T81.61   Aseptic peritonitis due to foreign substance accidentally left during a procedure
Chemical peritonitis

X ● T81.69   Other acute reaction to foreign substance accidentally left during a procedure

● T81.7   Vascular complications following a procedure, not elsewhere classified
Air embolism following procedure NEC
Phlebitis or thrombophlebitis resulting from a procedure

Excludes1   embolism complicating abortion or ectopic or molar pregnancy (O00-O07, O08.2)
embolism complicating pregnancy, childbirth and the puerperium (O88.-)
traumatic embolism (T79.0)

Excludes2   embolism due to prosthetic devices, implants and grafts (T82.8, T83.81, T84.8-, T85.1-)
embolism following infusion, transfusion and therapeutic injection (T80.0)

Coding Clinic: 2019, Q2, P23

● T81.71   Complication of artery following a procedure, not elsewhere classified
Coding Clinic: 2019, Q2, P22

● T81.710   Complication of mesenteric artery following a procedure, not elsewhere classified

● T81.711   Complication of renal artery following a procedure, not elsewhere classified

● T81.718   Complication of other artery following a procedure, not elsewhere classified
Coding Clinic: 2019, Q2, P22-23

● T81.719   Complication of unspecified artery following a procedure, not elsewhere classified

X ● T81.72   Complication of vein following a procedure, not elsewhere classified
Coding Clinic: 2019, Q2, P22

● T81.8   Other complications of procedures, not elsewhere classified

Excludes2   hypothermia following anesthesia (T88.51)
malignant hyperpyrexia due to anesthesia (T88.3)

X ● T81.81   Complication of inhalation therapy

X ● T81.82   Emphysema (subcutaneous) resulting from a procedure

X ● T81.83   Persistent postprocedural fistula
Coding Clinic: 2017, Q3, P3-5

X ● T81.89   Other complications of procedures, not elsewhere classified
Use additional code to specify complication, such as:
postprocedural delirium (F05)

X ● T81.9   Unspecified complication of procedure

● **T82   Complications of cardiac and vascular prosthetic devices, implants and grafts**

Excludes2   failure and rejection of transplanted organs and tissue (T86.-)

The appropriate 7th character is to be added to each code from category T82

> A   initial encounter
> D   subsequent encounter
> S   sequela

● **T82.0   Mechanical complication of heart valve prosthesis**
Mechanical complication of artificial heart valve

> **Excludes1**   mechanical complication of biological heart valve graft (T82.22-)

X ● **T82.01   Breakdown (mechanical) of heart valve prosthesis**

X ● **T82.02   Displacement of heart valve prosthesis**
Malposition of heart valve prosthesis

X ● **T82.03   Leakage of heart valve prosthesis**

X ● **T82.09   Other mechanical complication of heart valve prosthesis**
Obstruction (mechanical) of heart valve prosthesis
Perforation of heart valve prosthesis
Protrusion of heart valve prosthesis

● **T82.1   Mechanical complication of cardiac electronic device**
● **T82.11   Breakdown (mechanical) of cardiac electronic device**
● T82.110   Breakdown (mechanical) of cardiac electrode
● T82.111   Breakdown (mechanical) of cardiac pulse generator (battery)
● T82.118   Breakdown (mechanical) of other cardiac electronic device
● T82.119   Breakdown (mechanical) of unspecified cardiac electronic device

● **T82.12   Displacement of cardiac electronic device**
Malposition of cardiac electronic device
● T82.120   Displacement of cardiac electrode
● T82.121   Displacement of cardiac pulse generator (battery)
● T82.128   Displacement of other cardiac electronic device
● T82.129   Displacement of unspecified cardiac electronic device

● **T82.19   Other mechanical complication of cardiac electronic device**
Leakage of cardiac electronic device
Obstruction of cardiac electronic device
Perforation of cardiac electronic device
Protrusion of cardiac electronic device
● T82.190   Other mechanical complication of cardiac electrode
● T82.191   Other mechanical complication of cardiac pulse generator (battery)
● T82.198   Other mechanical complication of other cardiac electronic device
● T82.199   Other mechanical complication of unspecified cardiac device

● **T82.2   Mechanical complication of coronary artery bypass graft and biological heart valve graft**

> **Excludes1**   mechanical complication of artificial heart valve prosthesis (T82.0-)

● **T82.21   Mechanical complication of coronary artery bypass graft**
● T82.211   Breakdown (mechanical) of coronary artery bypass graft
● T82.212   Displacement of coronary artery bypass graft
Malposition of coronary artery bypass graft
● T82.213   Leakage of coronary artery bypass graft
● T82.218   Other mechanical complication of coronary artery bypass graft
Obstruction, mechanical of coronary artery bypass graft
Perforation of coronary artery bypass graft
Protrusion of coronary artery bypass graft

● **T82.22   Mechanical complication of biological heart valve graft**
● T82.221   Breakdown (mechanical) of biological heart valve graft
● T82.222   Displacement of biological heart valve graft
Malposition of biological heart valve graft
● T82.223   Leakage of biological heart valve graft
● T82.228   Other mechanical complication of biological heart valve graft
Obstruction of biological heart valve graft
Perforation of biological heart valve graft
Protrusion of biological heart valve graft

● **T82.3   Mechanical complication of other vascular grafts**
● **T82.31   Breakdown (mechanical) of other vascular grafts**
● T82.310   Breakdown (mechanical) of aortic (bifurcation) graft (replacement) A 🐾
● T82.311   Breakdown (mechanical) of carotid arterial graft (bypass) A 🐾
● T82.312   Breakdown (mechanical) of femoral arterial graft (bypass) A 🐾
● T82.318   Breakdown (mechanical) of other vascular grafts A 🐾
● T82.319   Breakdown (mechanical) of unspecified vascular grafts A 🐾

● **T82.32   Displacement of other vascular grafts**
Malposition of other vascular grafts
● T82.320   Displacement of aortic (bifurcation) graft (replacement) A 🐾
● T82.321   Displacement of carotid arterial graft (bypass) A 🐾
● T82.322   Displacement of femoral arterial graft (bypass) A 🐾
● T82.328   Displacement of other vascular grafts A 🐾
● T82.329   Displacement of unspecified vascular grafts A 🐾

● T82.33   Leakage of other vascular grafts
   ● T82.330   Leakage of aortic (bifurcation) graft (replacement) A 🐾
   ● T82.331   Leakage of carotid arterial graft (bypass) A 🐾
   ● T82.332   Leakage of femoral arterial graft (bypass) A 🐾
   ● T82.338   Leakage of other vascular grafts A 🐾
   ● T82.339   Leakage of unspecified vascular graft A 🐾

● T82.39   Other mechanical complication of other vascular grafts
      Obstruction (mechanical) of other vascular grafts
      Perforation of other vascular grafts
      Protrusion of other vascular grafts
   ● T82.390   Other mechanical complication of aortic (bifurcation) graft (replacement) A 🐾
   ● T82.391   Other mechanical complication of carotid arterial graft (bypass) A 🐾
   ● T82.392   Other mechanical complication of femoral arterial graft (bypass) A 🐾
   ● T82.398   Other mechanical complication of other vascular grafts A 🐾
   ● T82.399   Other mechanical complication of unspecified vascular grafts A 🐾

● T82.4   Mechanical complication of vascular dialysis catheter
      Mechanical complication of hemodialysis catheter
      Excludes1   mechanical complication of intraperitoneal dialysis catheter (T85.62)
   X ● T82.41   Breakdown (mechanical) of vascular dialysis catheter A, D, S 🐾
   X ● T82.42   Displacement of vascular dialysis catheter A, D, S 🐾
      Malposition of vascular dialysis catheter
   X ● T82.43   Leakage of vascular dialysis catheter A, D, S 🐾
   X ● T82.49   Other complication of vascular dialysis catheter A, D, S 🐾
      Obstruction (mechanical) of vascular dialysis catheter
      Perforation of vascular dialysis catheter
      Protrusion of vascular dialysis catheter

● T82.5   Mechanical complication of other cardiac and vascular devices and implants
      Excludes2   mechanical complication of epidural and subdural infusion catheter (T85.61)
   ● T82.51   Breakdown (mechanical) of other cardiac and vascular devices and implants
      ● T82.510   Breakdown (mechanical) of surgically created arteriovenous fistula A 🐾
      ● T82.511   Breakdown (mechanical) of surgically created arteriovenous shunt A 🐾
      ● T82.512   Breakdown (mechanical) of artificial heart
      ● T82.513   Breakdown (mechanical) of balloon (counterpulsation) device A 🐾
      ● T82.514   Breakdown (mechanical) of infusion catheter A 🐾
      ● T82.515   Breakdown (mechanical) of umbrella device A 🐾
      ● T82.518   Breakdown (mechanical) of other cardiac and vascular devices and implants A 🐾
      ● T82.519   Breakdown (mechanical) of unspecified cardiac and vascular devices and implants

● T82.52   Displacement of other cardiac and vascular devices and implants
      Malposition of other cardiac and vascular devices and implants
   ● T82.520   Displacement of surgically created arteriovenous fistula A 🐾
   ● T82.521   Displacement of surgically created arteriovenous shunt A 🐾
   ● T82.522   Displacement of artificial heart
   ● T82.523   Displacement of balloon (counterpulsation) device A 🐾
   ● T82.524   Displacement of infusion catheter A 🐾
      Coding Clinic: 2019, Q3, P15
   ● T82.525   Displacement of umbrella device A 🐾
   ● T82.528   Displacement of other cardiac and vascular devices and implants A 🐾
   ● T82.529   Displacement of unspecified cardiac and vascular devices and implants

● T82.53   Leakage of other cardiac and vascular devices and implants
   ● T82.530   Leakage of surgically created arteriovenous fistula A 🐾
   ● T82.531   Leakage of surgically created arteriovenous shunt A 🐾
   ● T82.532   Leakage of artificial heart
   ● T82.533   Leakage of balloon (counterpulsation) device A 🐾
   ● T82.534   Leakage of infusion catheter A 🐾
   ● T82.535   Leakage of umbrella device A 🐾
   ● T82.538   Leakage of other cardiac and vascular devices and implants A 🐾
   ● T82.539   Leakage of unspecified cardiac and vascular devices and implants

● T82.59   Other mechanical complication of other cardiac and vascular devices and implants
      Obstruction (mechanical) of other cardiac and vascular devices and implants
      Perforation of other cardiac and vascular devices and implants
      Protrusion of other cardiac and vascular devices and implants
   ● T82.590   Other mechanical complication of surgically created arteriovenous fistula A 🐾
   ● T82.591   Other mechanical complication of surgically created arteriovenous shunt A 🐾
   ● T82.592   Other mechanical complication of artificial heart
   ● T82.593   Other mechanical complication of balloon (counterpulsation) device A 🐾
   ● T82.594   Other mechanical complication of infusion catheter A 🐾
   ● T82.595   Other mechanical complication of umbrella device A 🐾
   ● T82.598   Other mechanical complication of other cardiac and vascular devices and implants A 🐾
   ● T82.599   Other mechanical complication of unspecified cardiac and vascular devices and implants

CHAPTER 19 (S00-T88)

X ● **T82.6**   Infection and inflammatory reaction due to cardiac valve prosthesis A 🐾
    Use additional code to identify infection

X ● **T82.7**   Infection and inflammatory reaction due to other cardiac and vascular devices, implants and grafts A 🐾
    Use additional code to identify infection
    Coding Clinic: 2019, Q1, P13-14; 2018, Q4, P89

● **T82.8**   Other specified complications of cardiac and vascular prosthetic devices, implants and grafts

   ● **T82.81**   Embolism due to cardiac and vascular prosthetic devices, implants and grafts
       Coding Clinic: 2016, Q4, P70

     ● **T82.817**   Embolism due to cardiac prosthetic devices, implants and grafts
         Coding Clinic: 2016, Q4, P70; 2015, Q1, P20

     ● **T82.818**   Embolism due to vascular prosthetic devices, implants and grafts A 🐾

   ● **T82.82**   Fibrosis due to cardiac and vascular prosthetic devices, implants and grafts
       Coding Clinic: 2016, Q4, P70

     ● **T82.827**   Fibrosis due to cardiac prosthetic devices, implants and grafts

     ● **T82.828**   Fibrosis due to vascular prosthetic devices, implants and grafts A 🐾

   ● **T82.83**   Hemorrhage due to cardiac and vascular prosthetic devices, implants and grafts
       Coding Clinic: 2016, Q4, P70

     ● **T82.837**   Hemorrhage due to cardiac prosthetic devices, implants and grafts

     ● **T82.838**   Hemorrhage due to vascular prosthetic devices, implants and grafts A 🐾

   ● **T82.84**   Pain due to cardiac and vascular prosthetic devices, implants and grafts
       Coding Clinic: 2016, Q4, P70

     ● **T82.847**   Pain due to cardiac prosthetic devices, implants and grafts

     ● **T82.848**   Pain due to vascular prosthetic devices, implants and grafts A 🐾

   ● **T82.85**   Stenosis due to cardiac and vascular prosthetic devices, implants and grafts

     ● **T82.855**   Stenosis of coronary artery stent
         In-stent stenosis (restenosis) of coronary artery stent
         Restenosis of coronary artery stent
         Coding Clinic: 2016, Q4, P70

     ● **T82.856**   Stenosis of peripheral vascular stent A 🐾
         In-stent stenosis (restenosis) of peripheral vascular stent
         Restenosis of peripheral vascular stent
         Coding Clinic: 2016, Q4, P70

     ● **T82.857**   Stenosis of other cardiac prosthetic devices, implants and grafts
         Coding Clinic: 2016, Q4, P70

     ● **T82.858**   Stenosis of other vascular prosthetic devices, implants and grafts A 🐾
         Coding Clinic: 2016, Q4, P70

   ● **T82.86**   Thrombosis of cardiac and vascular prosthetic devices, implants and grafts

     ● **T82.867**   Thrombosis due to cardiac prosthetic devices, implants and grafts

     ● **T82.868**   Thrombosis due to vascular prosthetic devices, implants and grafts A 🐾

   ● **T82.89**   Other specified complication of cardiac and vascular prosthetic devices, implants and grafts

     ● **T82.897**   Other specified complication of cardiac prosthetic devices, implants and grafts
         Coding Clinic: 2019, Q2, P32-33

     ● **T82.898**   Other specified complication of vascular prosthetic devices, implants and grafts A 🐾

X ● **T82.9**   Unspecified complication of cardiac and vascular prosthetic device, implant and graft

● **T83**   Complications of genitourinary prosthetic devices, implants and grafts

    Excludes2   failure and rejection of transplanted organs and tissue (T86.-)

    The appropriate 7th character is to be added to each code from category T83

A	initial encounter
D	subsequent encounter
S	sequela

    Coding Clinic: 2016, Q4, P70-71

   ● **T83.0**   Mechanical complication of urinary catheter
      Excludes2   complications of stoma of urinary tract (N99.5-)
      Coding Clinic: 2016, Q4, P70

     ● **T83.01**   Breakdown (mechanical) of urinary catheter

       ● **T83.010**   Breakdown (mechanical) of cystostomy catheter A 🐾

       ● **T83.011**   Breakdown (mechanical) of indwelling urethral catheter A 🐾

       ● **T83.012**   Breakdown (mechanical) of nephrostomy catheter A 🐾

       ● **T83.018**   Breakdown (mechanical) of other urinary catheter A 🐾
          Breakdown (mechanical) of Hopkins catheter
          Breakdown (mechanical) of ileostomy catheter
          Breakdown (mechanical) urostomy catheter

     ● **T83.02**   Displacement of urinary catheter
       Malposition of urinary catheter

       ● **T83.020**   Displacement of cystostomy catheter A 🐾

       ● **T83.021**   Displacement of indwelling urethral catheter A 🐾

       ● **T83.022**   Displacement of nephrostomy catheter A 🐾

       ● **T83.028**   Displacement of other urinary catheter A 🐾
          Displacement of Hopkins catheter
          Displacement of ileostomy catheter
          Displacement of urostomy catheter

     ● **T83.03**   Leakage of urinary catheter

       ● **T83.030**   Leakage of cystostomy catheter A 🐾

       ● **T83.031**   Leakage of indwelling urethral catheter A 🐾

       ● **T83.032**   Leakage of nephrostomy catheter A 🐾

       ● **T83.038**   Leakage of other urinary catheter A 🐾
          Leakage of Hopkins catheter
          Leakage of ileostomy catheter
          Leakage of urostomy catheter

▶ New   ⇒ Revised   ~~deleted~~ Deleted   Excludes 1   Excludes 2   Includes   Use additional   Code first   Code also   Key words

OGCR Official Guidelines   X Assign placeholder X   ● Use Additional Character(s)   ▶ Manifestation Code   🐾 Hierarchical Condition Category   Coding Clinic

● **T83.09**   Other mechanical complication of urinary catheter
     Obstruction (mechanical) of urinary catheter
     Perforation of urinary catheter
     Protrusion of urinary catheter

  ● **T83.090**   Other mechanical complication of cystostomy catheter A 🗫

  ● **T83.091**   Other mechanical complication of indwelling urethral catheter A 🗫

  ● **T83.092**   Other mechanical complication of nephrostomy catheter A 🗫

  ● **T83.098**   Other mechanical complication of other urinary catheter A 🗫
       Other mechanical complication of Hopkins catheter
       Other mechanical complication of ileostomy catheter
       Other mechanical complication of urostomy catheter

● **T83.1**   Mechanical complication of other urinary devices and implants
    Coding Clinic: 2016, Q4, P70

 ● **T83.11**   Breakdown (mechanical) of other urinary devices and implants

  ● **T83.110**   Breakdown (mechanical) of urinary electronic stimulator device A 🗫
       Excludes2   Breakdown (mechanical) of electrode (lead) for sacral nerve neurostimulator (T85.111)
             Breakdown (mechanical) of implanted electronic sacral neurostimulator, pulse generator or receiver (T85.113)

  ● **T83.111**   Breakdown (mechanical) of implanted urinary sphincter A 🗫

  ● **T83.112**   Breakdown (mechanical) of indwelling ureteral stent A 🗫

  ● **T83.113**   Breakdown (mechanical) of other urinary stents A 🗫
       Breakdown (mechanical) of ileal conduit stent
       Breakdown (mechanical) of nephroureteral stent

  ● **T83.118**   Breakdown (mechanical) of other urinary devices and implants A 🗫

 ● **T83.12**   Displacement of other urinary devices and implants
     Malposition of other urinary devices and implants

  ● **T83.120**   Displacement of urinary electronic stimulator device A 🗫
       Excludes2   Displacement of electrode (lead) for sacral nerve neurostimulator (T85.121)
             Displacement of implanted electronic sacral neurostimulator, pulse generator or receiver (T85.123)

  ● **T83.121**   Displacement of implanted urinary sphincter A 🗫

  ● **T83.122**   Displacement of indwelling ureteral stent A 🗫

  ● **T83.123**   Displacement of other urinary stents A 🗫
       Displacement of ileal conduit stent
       Displacement of nephroureteral stent

  ● **T83.128**   Displacement of other urinary devices and implants A 🗫

 ● **T83.19**   Other mechanical complication of other urinary devices and implants
     Leakage of other urinary devices and implants
     Obstruction (mechanical) of other urinary devices and implants
     Perforation of other urinary devices and implants
     Protrusion of other urinary devices and implants

  ● **T83.190**   Other mechanical complication of urinary electronic stimulator device A 🗫
       Excludes2   Other mechanical complication of electrode (lead) for sacral nerve neurostimulator (T85.191)
             Other mechanical complication of implanted electronic sacral neurostimulator, pulse generator or receiver (T85.193)

  ● **T83.191**   Other mechanical complication of implanted urinary sphincter A 🗫

  ● **T83.192**   Other mechanical complication of indwelling ureteral stent A 🗫

  ● **T83.193**   Other mechanical complication of other urinary stent A 🗫
       Other mechanical complication of ileal conduit stent
       Other mechanical complication of nephroureteral stent

  ● **T83.198**   Other mechanical complication of other urinary devices and implants A 🗫

● **T83.2**   Mechanical complication of graft of urinary organ
    Coding Clinic: 2016, Q4, P70

 X ● **T83.21**   Breakdown (mechanical) of graft of urinary organ A 🗫

 X ● **T83.22**   Displacement of graft of urinary organ A 🗫
     Malposition of graft of urinary organ

 X ● **T83.23**   Leakage of graft of urinary organ A 🗫

 X ● **T83.24**   Erosion of graft of urinary organ A 🗫
     Coding Clinic: 2016, Q4, P70

 X ● **T83.25**   Exposure of graft of urinary organ A 🗫
     Coding Clinic: 2016, Q4, P70

 X ● **T83.29**   Other mechanical complication of graft of urinary organ A 🗫
     Obstruction (mechanical) of graft of urinary organ
     Perforation of graft of urinary organ
     Protrusion of graft of urinary organ

● **T83.3**   **Mechanical complication of intrauterine contraceptive device**

X● **T83.31**   **Breakdown (mechanical) of intrauterine contraceptive device** ♀

X● **T83.32**   **Displacement of intrauterine contraceptive device** ♀
     Malposition of intrauterine contraceptive device
     Missing string of intrauterine contraceptive device

X● **T83.39**   **Other mechanical complication of intrauterine contraceptive device** ♀
     Leakage of intrauterine contraceptive device
     Obstruction (mechanical) of intrauterine contraceptive device
     Perforation of intrauterine contraceptive device
     Protrusion of intrauterine contraceptive device

● **T83.4**   **Mechanical complication of other prosthetic devices, implants and grafts of genital tract**
     Coding Clinic: 2016, Q4, P71

● **T83.41**   **Breakdown (mechanical) of other prosthetic devices, implants and grafts of genital tract**

     ● **T83.410**   **Breakdown (mechanical) of implanted penile prosthesis** ♂ A ⚕
         Breakdown (mechanical) of penile prosthesis cylinder
         Breakdown (mechanical) of penile prosthesis pump
         Breakdown (mechanical) of penile prosthesis reservoir

     ● **T83.411**   **Breakdown (mechanical) of implanted testicular prosthesis** A ⚕

     ● **T83.418**   **Breakdown (mechanical) of other prosthetic devices, implants and grafts of genital tract** A ⚕

● **T83.42**   **Displacement of other prosthetic devices, implants and grafts of genital tract**
     Malposition of other prosthetic devices, implants and grafts of genital tract

     ● **T83.420**   **Displacement of implanted penile prosthesis** ♂ A ⚕
         Displacement of penile prosthesis cylinder
         Displacement of penile prosthesis pump
         Displacement of penile prosthesis reservoir

     ● **T83.421**   **Displacement of implanted testicular prosthesis** A ⚕

     ● **T83.428**   **Displacement of other prosthetic devices, implants and grafts of genital tract** A ⚕
         Coding Clinic: 2018, Q1, P6

● **T83.49**   **Other mechanical complication of other prosthetic devices, implants and grafts of genital tract**
     Leakage of other prosthetic devices, implants and grafts of genital tract
     Obstruction, mechanical of other prosthetic devices, implants and grafts of genital tract
     Perforation of other prosthetic devices, implants and grafts of genital tract
     Protrusion of other prosthetic devices, implants and grafts of genital tract

     ● **T83.490**   **Other mechanical complication of implanted penile prosthesis** ♂ A ⚕
         Other mechanical complication of penile prosthesis cylinder
         Other mechanical complication of penile prosthesis pump
         Other mechanical complication of penile prosthesis reservoir

     ● **T83.491**   **Other mechanical complication of implanted testicular prosthesis** A ⚕

     ● **T83.498**   **Other mechanical complication of other prosthetic devices, implants and grafts of genital tract** A ⚕

● **T83.5**   **Infection and inflammatory reaction due to prosthetic device, implant and graft in urinary system**
     Use additional code to identify infection
     Coding Clinic: 2016, Q4, P71

● **T83.51**   **Infection and inflammatory reaction due to urinary catheter**
     Excludes2   complications of stoma of urinary tract (N99.5-)

     ● **T83.510**   **Infection and inflammatory reaction due to cystostomy catheter** A ⚕

     ● **T83.511**   **Infection and inflammatory reaction due to indwelling urethral catheter** A ⚕

     ● **T83.512**   **Infection and inflammatory reaction due to nephrostomy catheter** A ⚕

     ● **T83.518**   **Infection and inflammatory reaction due to other urinary catheter** A ⚕
         Infection and inflammatory reaction due to Hopkins catheter
         Infection and inflammatory reaction due to ileostomy catheter
         Infection and inflammatory reaction due to urostomy catheter

● **T83.59**   **Infection and inflammatory reaction due to prosthetic device, implant and graft in urinary system**

     ● **T83.590**   **Infection and inflammatory reaction due to implanted urinary neurostimulation device** A ⚕
         Excludes2   Infection and inflammatory reaction due to electrode lead of sacral nerve neurostimulator (T85.732)
             Infection and inflammatory reaction due to pulse generator or receiver of sacral nerve neurostimulator (T85.734)

     ● **T83.591**   **Infection and inflammatory reaction due to implanted urinary sphincter** A ⚕

▶ New   ⇒ Revised   ~~deleted~~ Deleted   Excludes 1   Excludes 2   Includes   Use additional   Code first   Code also   Key words
OGCR Official Guidelines   X Assign placeholder X   ● Use Additional Character(s)   ▶ Manifestation Code   ⚕ Hierarchical Condition Category   **Coding Clinic**

● **T83.592** Infection and inflammatory reaction due to indwelling ureteral stent A 🔎

● **T83.593** Infection and inflammatory reaction due to other urinary stents A 🔎
    Infection and inflammatory reaction due to ileal conduit stents
    Infection and inflammatory reaction due to nephroureteral stent

● **T83.598** Infection and inflammatory reaction due to other prosthetic device, implant and graft in urinary system A 🔎

● **T83.6** Infection and inflammatory reaction due to prosthetic device, implant and graft in genital tract
    Use additional code to identify infection
    Coding Clinic: 2016, Q4, P71

● **T83.61** Infection and inflammatory reaction due to implanted penile prosthesis A 🔎
    Infection and inflammatory reaction due to penile prosthesis cylinder
    Infection and inflammatory reaction due to penile prosthesis pump
    Infection and inflammatory reaction due to penile prosthesis reservoir

● **T83.62** Infection and inflammatory reaction due to implanted testicular prosthesis A 🔎

● **T83.69** Infection and inflammatory reaction due to other prosthetic device, implant and graft in genital tract A 🔎

● **T83.7** Complications due to implanted mesh and other prosthetic materials
    Coding Clinic: 2016, Q4, P71

● **T83.71** Erosion of implanted mesh and other prosthetic materials to surrounding organ or tissue
    Coding Clinic: 2016, Q4, P71

● **T83.711** Erosion of implanted vaginal mesh to surrounding organ or tissue ♀ A 🔎
    Erosion of implanted vaginal mesh into pelvic floor muscles
    Coding Clinic: 2016, Q4, P71

● **T83.712** Erosion of implanted urethral mesh to surrounding organ or tissue A 🔎
    Erosion of implanted female urethral sling
    Erosion of implanted male urethral sling
    Erosion of implanted urethral mesh into pelvic floor muscles

● **T83.713** Erosion of implanted urethral bulking agent to surrounding organ or tissue A 🔎

● **T83.714** Erosion of implanted ureteral bulking agent to surrounding organ or tissue A 🔎

● **T83.718** Erosion of other implanted mesh to organ or tissue A 🔎
    Coding Clinic: 2016, Q4, P71

● **T83.719** Erosion of other prosthetic materials to surrounding organ or tissue A 🔎
    Coding Clinic: 2016, Q4, P71

● **T83.72** Exposure of implanted mesh and other prosthetic materials into surrounding organ or tissue
    Extrusion of implanted mesh
    Coding Clinic: 2016, Q4, P71

● **T83.721** Exposure of implanted vaginal mesh into vagina ♀ A 🔎
    Exposure of implanted vaginal mesh through vaginal wall

● **T83.722** Exposure of implanted urethral mesh into urethra A 🔎
    Exposure of implanted female urethral sling
    Exposure of implanted male urethral sling
    Exposure of implanted urethral mesh through urethral wall

● **T83.723** Exposure of implanted urethral bulking agent into urethra A 🔎

● **T83.724** Exposure of implanted ureteral bulking agent into ureter A 🔎

● **T83.728** Exposure of other implanted mesh into organ or tissue A 🔎
    Coding Clinic: 2016, Q4, P71

● **T83.729** Exposure of other prosthetic materials into organ or tissue A 🔎
    Coding Clinic: 2016, Q4, P71

X ● **T83.79** Other specified complications due to other genitourinary prosthetic materials A 🔎

● **T83.8** Other specified complications of genitourinary prosthetic devices, implants and grafts

X ● **T83.81** Embolism due to genitourinary prosthetic devices, implants and grafts A 🔎

X ● **T83.82** Fibrosis due to genitourinary prosthetic devices, implants and grafts A 🔎

X ● **T83.83** Hemorrhage due to genitourinary prosthetic devices, implants and grafts A 🔎

X ● **T83.84** Pain due to genitourinary prosthetic devices, implants and grafts A 🔎

X ● **T83.85** Stenosis due to genitourinary prosthetic devices, implants and grafts A 🔎

X ● **T83.86** Thrombosis due to genitourinary prosthetic devices, implants and grafts A 🔎

X ● **T83.89** Other specified complication of genitourinary prosthetic devices, implants and grafts A 🔎

X ● **T83.9** Unspecified complication of genitourinary prosthetic device, implant and graft A 🔎

● **T84** Complications of internal orthopedic prosthetic devices, implants and grafts
    Excludes2   failure and rejection of transplanted organs and tissues (T86.-)
                fracture of bone following insertion of orthopedic implant, joint prosthesis or bone plate (M96.6)

The appropriate 7th character is to be added to each code from category T84

A	initial encounter
D	subsequent encounter
S	sequela

CHAPTER 19 (S00-T88)

● **T84.0   Mechanical complication of internal joint prosthesis**

  ● **T84.01   Broken internal joint prosthesis**

      Breakage (fracture) of prosthetic joint

      Broken prosthetic joint implant

      Excludes1   periprosthetic joint implant fracture (M97.-)

      Coding Clinic: 2016, Q4, P42

    ● **T84.010   Broken internal right hip prosthesis** A 🐾

    ● **T84.011   Broken internal left hip prosthesis** A 🐾

    ● **T84.012   Broken internal right knee prosthesis** A 🐾

    ● **T84.013   Broken internal left knee prosthesis** A 🐾

    ● **T84.018   Broken internal joint prosthesis, other site** A 🐾

       Use additional code to identify the joint (Z96.6-)

    ● **T84.019   Broken internal joint prosthesis, unspecified site** A 🐾

  ● **T84.02   Dislocation of internal joint prosthesis**

      Instability of internal joint prosthesis

      Subluxation of internal joint prosthesis

    ● **T84.020   Dislocation of internal right hip prosthesis** A 🐾

    ● **T84.021   Dislocation of internal left hip prosthesis** A 🐾

       Coding Clinic: 2019, Q2, P27

    ● **T84.022   Instability of internal right knee prosthesis** A 🐾

    ● **T84.023   Instability of internal left knee prosthesis** A 🐾

    ● **T84.028   Dislocation of other internal joint prosthesis** A 🐾

       Use additional code to identify the joint (Z96.6-)

    ● **T84.029   Dislocation of unspecified internal joint prosthesis** A 🐾

  ● **T84.03   Mechanical loosening of internal prosthetic joint**

      Aseptic loosening of prosthetic joint

    ● **T84.030   Mechanical loosening of internal right hip prosthetic joint** A 🐾

    ● **T84.031   Mechanical loosening of internal left hip prosthetic joint** A 🐾

    ● **T84.032   Mechanical loosening of internal right knee prosthetic joint** A 🐾

    ● **T84.033   Mechanical loosening of internal left knee prosthetic joint** A 🐾

    ● **T84.038   Mechanical loosening of other internal prosthetic joint** A 🐾

       Use additional code to identify the joint (Z96.6-)

    ● **T84.039   Mechanical loosening of unspecified internal prosthetic joint** A 🐾

  ● **T84.05   Periprosthetic osteolysis of internal prosthetic joint**

      Use additional code to identify major osseous defect, if applicable (M89.7-)

    ● **T84.050   Periprosthetic osteolysis of internal prosthetic right hip joint** A 🐾

    ● **T84.051   Periprosthetic osteolysis of internal prosthetic left hip joint** A 🐾

    ● **T84.052   Periprosthetic osteolysis of internal prosthetic right knee joint** A 🐾

    ● **T84.053   Periprosthetic osteolysis of internal prosthetic left knee joint** A 🐾

    ● **T84.058   Periprosthetic osteolysis of other internal prosthetic joint** A 🐾

       Use additional code to identify the joint (Z96.6-)

    ● **T84.059   Periprosthetic osteolysis of unspecified internal prosthetic joint** A 🐾

  ● **T84.06   Wear of articular bearing surface of internal prosthetic joint**

    ● **T84.060   Wear of articular bearing surface of internal prosthetic right hip joint** A 🐾

    ● **T84.061   Wear of articular bearing surface of internal prosthetic left hip joint** A 🐾

    ● **T84.062   Wear of articular bearing surface of internal prosthetic right knee joint** A 🐾

    ● **T84.063   Wear of articular bearing surface of internal prosthetic left knee joint** A 🐾

    ● **T84.068   Wear of articular bearing surface of other internal prosthetic joint** A 🐾

       Use additional code to identify the joint (Z96.6-)

    ● **T84.069   Wear of articular bearing surface of unspecified internal prosthetic joint** A 🐾

  ● **T84.09   Other mechanical complication of internal joint prosthesis**

      Prosthetic joint implant failure NOS

    ● **T84.090   Other mechanical complication of internal right hip prosthesis** A 🐾

       Coding Clinic: 2019, Q1, P20

    ● **T84.091   Other mechanical complication of internal left hip prosthesis** A 🐾

    ● **T84.092   Other mechanical complication of internal right knee prosthesis** A 🐾

    ● **T84.093   Other mechanical complication of internal left knee prosthesis** A 🐾

    ● **T84.098   Other mechanical complication of other internal joint prosthesis** A 🐾

       Use additional code to identify the joint (Z96.6-)

    ● **T84.099   Other mechanical complication of unspecified internal joint prosthesis** A 🐾

● **T84.1   Mechanical complication of internal fixation device of bones of limb**

      Excludes2   mechanical complication of internal fixation device of bones of feet (T84.2-)

               mechanical complication of internal fixation device of bones of fingers (T84.2-)

               mechanical complication of internal fixation device of bones of hands (T84.2-)

               mechanical complication of internal fixation device of bones of toes (T84.2-)

● **T84.11**   Breakdown (mechanical) of internal fixation device of bones of limb
- ● **T84.110**   Breakdown (mechanical) of internal fixation device of right humerus A 🦴
- ● **T84.111**   Breakdown (mechanical) of internal fixation device of left humerus A 🦴
- ● **T84.112**   Breakdown (mechanical) of internal fixation device of bone of right forearm A 🦴
- ● **T84.113**   Breakdown (mechanical) of internal fixation device of bone of left forearm A 🦴
- ● **T84.114**   Breakdown (mechanical) of internal fixation device of right femur A 🦴
- ● **T84.115**   Breakdown (mechanical) of internal fixation device of left femur A 🦴
- ● **T84.116**   Breakdown (mechanical) of internal fixation device of bone of right lower leg A 🦴
- ● **T84.117**   Breakdown (mechanical) of internal fixation device of bone of left lower leg A 🦴
- ● **T84.119**   Breakdown (mechanical) of internal fixation device of unspecified bone of limb A 🦴

● **T84.12**   Displacement of internal fixation device of bones of limb
> Malposition of internal fixation device of bones of limb
- ● **T84.120**   Displacement of internal fixation device of right humerus A 🦴
- ● **T84.121**   Displacement of internal fixation device of left humerus A 🦴
- ● **T84.122**   Displacement of internal fixation device of bone of right forearm A 🦴
- ● **T84.123**   Displacement of internal fixation device of bone of left forearm A 🦴
- ● **T84.124**   Displacement of internal fixation device of right femur A 🦴
- ● **T84.125**   Displacement of internal fixation device of left femur A 🦴
- ● **T84.126**   Displacement of internal fixation device of bone of right lower leg A 🦴
- ● **T84.127**   Displacement of internal fixation device of bone of left lower leg A 🦴
- ● **T84.129**   Displacement of internal fixation device of unspecified bone of limb A 🦴

● **T84.19**   Other mechanical complication of internal fixation device of bones of limb
> Obstruction (mechanical) of internal fixation device of bones of limb
> Perforation of internal fixation device of bones of limb
> Protrusion of internal fixation device of bones of limb
- ● **T84.190**   Other mechanical complication of internal fixation device of right humerus A 🦴
- ● **T84.191**   Other mechanical complication of internal fixation device of left humerus A 🦴
- ● **T84.192**   Other mechanical complication of internal fixation device of bone of right forearm A 🦴
- ● **T84.193**   Other mechanical complication of internal fixation device of bone of left forearm A 🦴
- ● **T84.194**   Other mechanical complication of internal fixation device of right femur A 🦴
- ● **T84.195**   Other mechanical complication of internal fixation device of left femur A 🦴
- ● **T84.196**   Other mechanical complication of internal fixation device of bone of right lower leg A 🦴
- ● **T84.197**   Other mechanical complication of internal fixation device of bone of left lower leg A 🦴
- ● **T84.199**   Other mechanical complication of internal fixation device of unspecified bone of limb A 🦴

● **T84.2**   Mechanical complication of internal fixation device of other bones

● **T84.21**   Breakdown (mechanical) of internal fixation device of other bones
- ● **T84.210**   Breakdown (mechanical) of internal fixation device of bones of hand and fingers A 🦴
- ● **T84.213**   Breakdown (mechanical) of internal fixation device of bones of foot and toes A 🦴
- ● **T84.216**   Breakdown (mechanical) of internal fixation device of vertebrae A 🦴
- ● **T84.218**   Breakdown (mechanical) of internal fixation device of other bones A 🦴

● **T84.22**   Displacement of internal fixation device of other bones
> Malposition of internal fixation device of other bones
- ● **T84.220**   Displacement of internal fixation device of bones of hand and fingers A 🦴
- ● **T84.223**   Displacement of internal fixation device of bones of foot and toes A 🦴
- ● **T84.226**   Displacement of internal fixation device of vertebrae A 🦴
- ● **T84.228**   Displacement of internal fixation device of other bones A 🦴

● **T84.29**   Other mechanical complication of internal fixation device of other bones
> Obstruction (mechanical) of internal fixation device of other bones
> Perforation of internal fixation device of other bones
> Protrusion of internal fixation device of other bones
- ● **T84.290**   Other mechanical complication of internal fixation device of bones of hand and fingers A 🦴
- ● **T84.293**   Other mechanical complication of internal fixation device of bones of foot and toes A 🦴

CHAPTER 19 (S00-T88)

● T84.296   Other mechanical complication of internal fixation device of vertebrae A 🐾

● T84.298   Other mechanical complication of internal fixation device of other bones A 🐾

● T84.3   Mechanical complication of other bone devices, implants and grafts

   Excludes2   other complications of bone graft (T86.83-)

● T84.31   Breakdown (mechanical) of other bone devices, implants and grafts

   ● T84.310   Breakdown (mechanical) of electronic bone stimulator A 🐾

   ● T84.318   Breakdown (mechanical) of other bone devices, implants and grafts A 🐾

● T84.32   Displacement of other bone devices, implants and grafts

   Malposition of other bone devices, implants and grafts

   ● T84.320   Displacement of electronic bone stimulator A 🐾

   ● T84.328   Displacement of other bone devices, implants and grafts A 🐾

● T84.39   Other mechanical complication of other bone devices, implants and grafts

   Obstruction (mechanical) of other bone devices, implants and grafts

   Perforation of other bone devices, implants and grafts

   Protrusion of other bone devices, implants and grafts

   ● T84.390   Other mechanical complication of electronic bone stimulator A 🐾

   ● T84.398   Other mechanical complication of other bone devices, implants and grafts A 🐾

● T84.4   Mechanical complication of other internal orthopedic devices, implants and grafts

● T84.41   Breakdown (mechanical) of other internal orthopedic devices, implants and grafts

   ● T84.410   Breakdown (mechanical) of muscle and tendon graft A 🐾

   ● T84.418   Breakdown (mechanical) of other internal orthopedic devices, implants and grafts A 🐾

● T84.42   Displacement of other internal orthopedic devices, implants and grafts

   Malposition of other internal orthopedic devices, implants and grafts

   ● T84.420   Displacement of muscle and tendon graft A 🐾

   ● T84.428   Displacement of other internal orthopedic devices, implants and grafts A 🐾

● T84.49   Other mechanical complication of other internal orthopedic devices, implants and grafts

   Mechanical complication of other internal orthopedic devices, implants and grafts NOS

   Obstruction (mechanical) of other internal orthopedic devices, implants and grafts

   Perforation of other internal orthopedic devices, implants and grafts

   Protrusion of other internal orthopedic devices, implants and grafts

   ● T84.490   Other mechanical complication of muscle and tendon graft A 🐾

   ● T84.498   Other mechanical complication of other internal orthopedic devices, implants and grafts A 🐾

● T84.5   Infection and inflammatory reaction due to internal joint prosthesis

   Use additional code to identify infection
   Coding Clinic: 2015, Q1, P16

   X ● T84.50   Infection and inflammatory reaction due to unspecified internal joint prosthesis A 🐾
   Coding Clinic: 2015, Q1, P3

   X ● T84.51   Infection and inflammatory reaction due to internal right hip prosthesis A 🐾
   Coding Clinic: 2015, Q4, P36

   X ● T84.52   Infection and inflammatory reaction due to internal left hip prosthesis A 🐾
   Coding Clinic: 2015, Q1, P16-17

   X ● T84.53   Infection and inflammatory reaction due to internal right knee prosthesis A 🐾

   X ● T84.54   Infection and inflammatory reaction due to internal left knee prosthesis A 🐾
   Coding Clinic: 2019, Q3, P16

   X ● T84.59   Infection and inflammatory reaction due to other internal joint prosthesis A 🐾

● T84.6   Infection and inflammatory reaction due to internal fixation device

   Use additional code to identify infection

   X ● T84.60   Infection and inflammatory reaction due to internal fixation device of unspecified site A 🐾

   ● T84.61   Infection and inflammatory reaction due to internal fixation device of arm

      ● T84.610   Infection and inflammatory reaction due to internal fixation device of right humerus A 🐾

      ● T84.611   Infection and inflammatory reaction due to internal fixation device of left humerus A 🐾

      ● T84.612   Infection and inflammatory reaction due to internal fixation device of right radius A 🐾

      ● T84.613   Infection and inflammatory reaction due to internal fixation device of left radius A 🐾

      ● T84.614   Infection and inflammatory reaction due to internal fixation device of right ulna A 🐾

      ● T84.615   Infection and inflammatory reaction due to internal fixation device of left ulna A 🐾

      ● T84.619   Infection and inflammatory reaction due to internal fixation device of unspecified bone of arm A 🐾

   ● T84.62   Infection and inflammatory reaction due to internal fixation device of leg

      ● T84.620   Infection and inflammatory reaction due to internal fixation device of right femur A 🐾

      ● T84.621   Infection and inflammatory reaction due to internal fixation device of left femur A 🐾

      ● T84.622   Infection and inflammatory reaction due to internal fixation device of right tibia A 🐾

▶ New   ⟾ Revised   ~~deleted~~ Deleted   Excludes 1   Excludes 2   Includes   Use additional   Code first   Code also   Key words
OGCR Official Guidelines   X Assign placeholder X   ● Use Additional Character(s)   ▶ Manifestation Code   🐾 Hierarchical Condition Category   **Coding Clinic**

● T84.623 Infection and inflammatory reaction due to internal fixation device of left tibia A 🦠

● T84.624 Infection and inflammatory reaction due to internal fixation device of right fibula A 🦠

● T84.625 Infection and inflammatory reaction due to internal fixation device of left fibula A 🦠

● T84.629 Infection and inflammatory reaction due to internal fixation device of unspecified bone of leg A 🦠

X● T84.63 Infection and inflammatory reaction due to internal fixation device of spine A 🦠

X● T84.69 Infection and inflammatory reaction due to internal fixation device of other site A 🦠

● T84.7 Infection and inflammatory reaction due to other internal orthopedic prosthetic devices, implants and grafts A 🦠

Use additional code to identify infection

● T84.8 Other specified complications of internal orthopedic prosthetic devices, implants and grafts

X● T84.81 Embolism due to internal orthopedic prosthetic devices, implants and grafts A 🦠

X● T84.82 Fibrosis due to internal orthopedic prosthetic devices, implants and grafts A 🦠

X● T84.83 Hemorrhage due to internal orthopedic prosthetic devices, implants and grafts A 🦠

X● T84.84 Pain due to internal orthopedic prosthetic devices, implants and grafts A 🦠

X● T84.85 Stenosis due to internal orthopedic prosthetic devices, implants and grafts A 🦠

X● T84.86 Thrombosis due to internal orthopedic prosthetic devices, implants and grafts A 🦠

X● T84.89 Other specified complication of internal orthopedic prosthetic devices, implants and grafts A 🦠

X● T84.9 Unspecified complication of internal orthopedic prosthetic device, implant and graft A 🦠

● T85 Complications of other internal prosthetic devices, implants and grafts

Excludes2 failure and rejection of transplanted organs and tissue (T86.-)

The appropriate 7th character is to be added to each code from category T85

A	initial encounter
D	subsequent encounter
S	sequela

Coding Clinic: 2016, Q4, P71

● T85.0 Mechanical complication of ventricular intracranial (communicating) shunt

X● T85.01 Breakdown (mechanical) of ventricular intracranial (communicating) shunt A 🦠

X● T85.02 Displacement of ventricular intracranial (communicating) shunt A 🦠

Malposition of ventricular intracranial (communicating) shunt

X● T85.03 Leakage of ventricular intracranial (communicating) shunt A 🦠

X● T85.09 Other mechanical complication of ventricular intracranial (communicating) shunt A 🦠

Obstruction (mechanical) of ventricular intracranial (communicating) shunt
Perforation of ventricular intracranial (communicating) shunt
Protrusion of ventricular intracranial (communicating) shunt

● T85.1 Mechanical complication of implanted electronic stimulator of nervous system
Coding Clinic: 2016, Q4, P71

● T85.11 Breakdown (mechanical) of implanted electronic stimulator of nervous system

● T85.110 Breakdown (mechanical) of implanted electronic neurostimulator of brain electrode (lead) A 🦠

● T85.111 Breakdown (mechanical) of implanted electronic neurostimulator of peripheral nerve electrode (lead) A 🦠

Breakdown of electrode (lead) for cranial nerve neurostimulators
Breakdown of electrode (lead) for gastric neurostimulator
Breakdown of electrode (lead) for sacral nerve neurostimulator
Breakdown of electrode (lead) for vagal nerve neurostimulators

● T85.112 Breakdown (mechanical) of implanted electronic neurostimulator of spinal cord electrode (lead) A 🦠

● T85.113 Breakdown (mechanical) of implanted electronic neurostimulator, generator A 🦠

Breakdown (mechanical) of implanted electronic neurostimulator generator, brain, peripheral, gastric, spinal
Breakdown (mechanical) of implanted electronic sacral neurostimulator, pulse generator or receiver

● T85.118 Breakdown (mechanical) of other implanted electronic stimulator of nervous system A 🦠

● T85.12 Displacement of implanted electronic stimulator of nervous system

Malposition of implanted electronic stimulator of nervous system

● T85.120 Displacement of implanted electronic neurostimulator of brain electrode (lead) A 🦠

● T85.121 Displacement of implanted electronic neurostimulator of peripheral nerve electrode (lead) A 🦠

Displacement of electrode (lead) for cranial nerve neurostimulators
Displacement of electrode (lead) for gastric neurostimulator
Displacement of electrode (lead) for sacral nerve neurostimulator
Displacement of electrode (lead) for vagal nerve neurostimulators

CHAPTER 19 (S00-T88)

● T85.122   Displacement of implanted electronic neurostimulator of spinal cord electrode (lead) A 🔖

● T85.123   Displacement of implanted electronic neurostimulator, generator A 🔖
     Displacement of implanted electronic neurostimulator generator, brain, peripheral, gastric, spinal
     Displacement of implanted electronic sacral neurostimulator, pulse generator or receiver

● T85.128   Displacement of other implanted electronic stimulator of nervous system A 🔖

● T85.19   Other mechanical complication of implanted electronic stimulator of nervous system
     Leakage of implanted electronic stimulator of nervous system
     Obstruction (mechanical) of implanted electronic stimulator of nervous system
     Perforation of implanted electronic stimulator of nervous system
     Protrusion of implanted electronic stimulator of nervous system

● T85.190   Other mechanical complication of implanted electronic neurostimulator of brain electrode (lead) A 🔖

● T85.191   Other mechanical complication of implanted electronic neurostimulator of peripheral nerve electrode (lead) A 🔖
     Other mechanical complication of electrode (lead) for cranial nerve neurostimulators
     Other mechanical complication of electrode (lead) for gastric neurostimulator
     Other mechanical complication of electrode (lead) for sacral nerve neurostimulator
     Other mechanical complication of electrode (lead) for vagal nerve neurostimulators

● T85.192   Other mechanical complication of implanted electronic neurostimulator of spinal cord electrode (lead) A 🔖

● T85.193   Other mechanical complication of implanted electronic neurostimulator, generator A 🔖
     Other mechanical complication of implanted electronic neurostimulator generator, brain, peripheral, gastric, spinal
     Other mechanical complication of implanted electronic sacral neurostimulator, pulse generator or receiver

● T85.199   Other mechanical complication of other implanted electronic stimulator of nervous system A 🔖

● T85.2   Mechanical complication of intraocular lens
   X ● T85.21   Breakdown (mechanical) of intraocular lens
   X ● T85.22   Displacement of intraocular lens
     Malposition of intraocular lens
   X ● T85.29   Other mechanical complication of intraocular lens
     Obstruction (mechanical) of intraocular lens
     Perforation of intraocular lens
     Protrusion of intraocular lens

● T85.3   Mechanical complication of other ocular prosthetic devices, implants and grafts
     Excludes2   other complications of corneal graft (T86.84-)

● T85.31   Breakdown (mechanical) of other ocular prosthetic devices, implants and grafts
   ● T85.310   Breakdown (mechanical) of prosthetic orbit of right eye
   ● T85.311   Breakdown (mechanical) of prosthetic orbit of left eye
   ● T85.318   Breakdown (mechanical) of other ocular prosthetic devices, implants and grafts

● T85.32   Displacement of other ocular prosthetic devices, implants and grafts
     Malposition of other ocular prosthetic devices, implants and grafts
   ● T85.320   Displacement of prosthetic orbit of right eye
   ● T85.321   Displacement of prosthetic orbit of left eye
   ● T85.328   Displacement of other ocular prosthetic devices, implants and grafts

● T85.39   Other mechanical complication of other ocular prosthetic devices, implants and grafts
     Obstruction (mechanical) of other ocular prosthetic devices, implants and grafts
     Perforation of other ocular prosthetic devices, implants and grafts
     Protrusion of other ocular prosthetic devices, implants and grafts
   ● T85.390   Other mechanical complication of prosthetic orbit of right eye
   ● T85.391   Other mechanical complication of prosthetic orbit of left eye
   ● T85.398   Other mechanical complication of other ocular prosthetic devices, implants and grafts

● T85.4   Mechanical complication of breast prosthesis and implant
   X ● T85.41   Breakdown (mechanical) of breast prosthesis and implant
   X ● T85.42   Displacement of breast prosthesis and implant
     Malposition of breast prosthesis and implant
   X ● T85.43   Leakage of breast prosthesis and implant
   X ● T85.44   Capsular contracture of breast implant
   X ● T85.49   Other mechanical complication of breast prosthesis and implant
     Obstruction (mechanical) of breast prosthesis and implant
     Perforation of breast prosthesis and implant
     Protrusion of breast prosthesis and implant

- T85.5   Mechanical complication of gastrointestinal prosthetic devices, implants and grafts
  - T85.51   Breakdown (mechanical) of gastrointestinal prosthetic devices, implants and grafts
    - T85.510   Breakdown (mechanical) of bile duct prosthesis
    - T85.511   Breakdown (mechanical) of esophageal anti-reflux device
    - T85.518   Breakdown (mechanical) of other gastrointestinal prosthetic devices, implants and grafts
  - T85.52   Displacement of gastrointestinal prosthetic devices, implants and grafts
    Malposition of gastrointestinal prosthetic devices, implants and grafts
    - T85.520   Displacement of bile duct prosthesis
    - T85.521   Displacement of esophageal anti-reflux device
    - T85.528   Displacement of other gastrointestinal prosthetic devices, implants and grafts
  - T85.59   Other mechanical complication of gastrointestinal prosthetic devices, implants and
    Obstruction, mechanical of gastrointestinal prosthetic devices, implants and grafts
    Perforation of gastrointestinal prosthetic devices, implants and grafts
    Protrusion of gastrointestinal prosthetic devices, implants and grafts
    - T85.590   Other mechanical complication of bile duct prosthesis
    - T85.591   Other mechanical complication of esophageal anti-reflux device
    - T85.598   Other mechanical complication of other gastrointestinal prosthetic devices, implants and grafts
- T85.6   Mechanical complication of other specified internal and external prosthetic devices, implants and grafts
  Coding Clinic: 2016, Q4, P71
  - T85.61   Breakdown (mechanical) of other specified internal prosthetic devices, implants and grafts
    - T85.610   Breakdown (mechanical) of cranial or spinal infusion catheter
      Breakdown (mechanical) of epidural infusion catheter
      Breakdown (mechanical) of intrathecal infusion catheter
      Breakdown (mechanical) of subarachnoid infusion catheter
      Breakdown (mechanical) of subdural infusion catheter
    - T85.611   Breakdown (mechanical) of intraperitoneal dialysis catheter A, D, S 🔁
      Excludes1   mechanical complication of vascular dialysis catheter (T82.4-)
    - T85.612   Breakdown (mechanical) of permanent sutures
      Excludes1   mechanical complication of permanent (wire) suture used in bone repair (T84.1-T84.2)

- T85.613   Breakdown (mechanical) of artificial skin graft and decellularized allodermis
  Failure of artificial skin graft and decellularized allodermis
  Non-adherence of artificial skin graft and decellularized allodermis
  Poor incorporation of artificial skin graft and decellularized allodermis
  Shearing of artificial skin graft and decellularized allodermis
- T85.614   Breakdown (mechanical) of insulin pump
- T85.615   Breakdown (mechanical) of other nervous system device, implant or graft A 🔁
  Breakdown (mechanical) of intrathecal infusion pump
- T85.618   Breakdown (mechanical) of other specified internal prosthetic devices, implants and grafts
- T85.62   Displacement of other specified internal prosthetic devices, implants and grafts
  Malposition of other specified internal prosthetic devices, implants and grafts
  - T85.620   Displacement of cranial or spinal infusion catheter
    Displacement of epidural infusion catheter
    Displacement of intrathecal infusion catheter
    Displacement of subarachnoid infusion catheter
    Displacement of subdural infusion catheter
  - T85.621   Displacement of intraperitoneal dialysis catheter A, D, S 🔁
    Excludes1   mechanical complication of vascular dialysis catheter (T82.4-)
  - T85.622   Displacement of permanent sutures
    Excludes1   mechanical complication of permanent (wire) suture used in bone repair (T84.1-T84.2)
  - T85.623   Displacement of artificial skin graft and decellularized allodermis
    Dislodgement of artificial skin graft and decellularized allodermis
  - T85.624   Displacement of insulin pump
  - T85.625   Displacement of other nervous system device, implant or graft A 🔁
    Displacement of intrathecal infusion pump
  - T85.628   Displacement of other specified internal prosthetic devices, implants and grafts
    Coding Clinic: 2015, Q1, P15

CHAPTER 19 (S00-T88)

● **T85.63** Leakage of other specified internal prosthetic devices, implants and grafts
- ● **T85.630** Leakage of cranial or spinal infusion catheter
  - Leakage of epidural infusion catheter
  - Leakage of intrathecal infusion catheter
  - Leakage of subdural infusion catheter
  - Leakage of subarachnoid infusion catheter
- ● **T85.631** Leakage of intraperitoneal dialysis catheter A, D, S 🐾
  - **Excludes1** mechanical complication of vascular dialysis catheter (T82.4)
- ● **T85.633** Leakage of insulin pump
- ● **T85.635** Leakage of other nervous system device, implant or graft A 🐾
  - Leakage of intrathecal infusion pump
- ● **T85.638** Leakage of other specified internal prosthetic devices, implants and grafts

● **T85.69** Other mechanical complication of other specified internal prosthetic devices, implants and grafts
- Obstruction, mechanical of other specified internal prosthetic devices, implants and grafts
- Perforation of other specified internal prosthetic devices, implants and grafts
- Protrusion of other specified internal prosthetic devices, implants and grafts
- ● **T85.690** Other mechanical complication of cranial or spinal infusion catheter
  - Other mechanical complication of epidural infusion catheter
  - Other mechanical complication of intrathecal infusion catheter
  - Other mechanical complication of subarachnoid infusion catheter
  - Other mechanical complication of subdural infusion catheter
- ● **T85.691** Other mechanical complication of intraperitoneal dialysis catheter A, D, S 🐾
  - **Excludes1** mechanical complication of vascular dialysis catheter (T82.4)
- ● **T85.692** Other mechanical complication of permanent sutures
  - **Excludes1** mechanical complication of permanent (wire) suture used in bone repair (T84.1-T84.2)
- ● **T85.693** Other mechanical complication of artificial skin graft and decellularized allodermis
- ● **T85.694** Other mechanical complication of insulin pump

● **T85.695** Other mechanical complication of other nervous system device, implant or graft A 🐾
  - Other mechanical complication of intrathecal infusion pump
● **T85.698** Other mechanical complication of other specified internal prosthetic devices, implants and grafts
  - Mechanical complication of nonabsorbable surgical material NOS

● **T85.7** Infection and inflammatory reaction due to other internal prosthetic devices, implants and grafts
  - Use additional code to identify infection
  - Coding Clinic: 2016, Q4, P72
- X● **T85.71** Infection and inflammatory reaction due to peritoneal dialysis catheter A, D, S 🐾
- X● **T85.72** Infection and inflammatory reaction due to insulin pump A 🐾
- ● **T85.73** Infection and inflammatory reaction due to nervous system devices, implants and graft
  - ● **T85.730** Infection and inflammatory reaction due to ventricular intracranial (communicating) shunt A 🐾
  - ● **T85.731** Infection and inflammatory reaction due to implanted electronic neurostimulator of brain, electrode (lead) A 🐾
  - ● **T85.732** Infection and inflammatory reaction due to implanted electronic neurostimulator of peripheral nerve, electrode (lead) A 🐾
    - Infection and inflammatory reaction due to electrode (lead) for cranial nerve neurostimulators
    - Infection and inflammatory reaction due to electrode (lead) for gastric neurostimulator
    - Infection and inflammatory reaction due to electrode (lead) for sacral nerve neurostimulator
    - Infection and inflammatory reaction due to electrode (lead) for vagal nerve neurostimulators
  - ● **T85.733** Infection and inflammatory reaction due to implanted electronic neurostimulator of spinal cord, electrode (lead) A 🐾
  - ● **T85.734** Infection and inflammatory reaction due to implanted electronic neurostimulator, generator A 🐾
    - Generator pocket infection
  - ● **T85.735** Infection and inflammatory reaction due to cranial or spinal infusion catheter A 🐾
    - Infection and inflammatory reaction due to epidural catheter
    - Infection and inflammatory reaction due to intrathecal infusion catheter
    - Infection and inflammatory reaction due to subarachnoid catheter
    - Infection and inflammatory reaction due to subdural catheter
  - ● **T85.738** Infection and inflammatory reaction due to other nervous system device, implant or graft A 🐾
    - Infection and inflammatory reaction due to intrathecal infusion pump

X● T85.79   Infection and inflammatory reaction due to other internal prosthetic devices, implants and grafts A 🐾
     Coding Clinic: 2016, Q4, P72

● T85.8   Other specified complications of internal prosthetic devices, implants and grafts, not elsewhere classified
     Coding Clinic: 2016, Q4, P72

   ● T85.81   Embolism due to internal prosthetic devices, implants and grafts, not elsewhere classified

     ● T85.810   Embolism due to nervous system prosthetic devices, implants and grafts A 🐾

     ● T85.818   Embolism due to other internal prosthetic devices, implants and grafts

   ● T85.82   Fibrosis due to internal prosthetic devices, implants and grafts, not elsewhere classified

     ● T85.820   Fibrosis due to nervous system prosthetic devices, implants and grafts A 🐾

     ● T85.828   Fibrosis due to other internal prosthetic devices, implants and grafts

   ● T85.83   Hemorrhage due to internal prosthetic devices, implants and grafts, not elsewhere classified

     ● T85.830   Hemorrhage due to nervous system prosthetic devices, implants and grafts A 🐾

     ● T85.838   Hemorrhage due to other internal prosthetic devices, implants and grafts

   ● T85.84   Pain due to internal prosthetic devices, implants and grafts, not elsewhere classified

     ● T85.840   Pain due to nervous system prosthetic devices, implants and grafts A 🐾

     ● T85.848   Pain due to other internal prosthetic devices, implants and grafts

   ● T85.85   Stenosis due to internal prosthetic devices, implants and grafts, not elsewhere classified

     ● T85.850   Stenosis due to nervous system prosthetic devices, implants and grafts A 🐾

     ● T85.858   Stenosis due to other internal prosthetic devices, implants and grafts

   ● T85.86   Thrombosis due to internal prosthetic devices, implants and grafts, not elsewhere classified

     ● T85.860   Thrombosis due to nervous system prosthetic devices, implants and grafts A 🐾

     ● T85.868   Thrombosis due to other internal prosthetic devices, implants and grafts

   ● T85.89   Other specified complication of internal prosthetic devices, implants and grafts, not elsewhere classified
     Coding Clinic: 2016, Q4, P72

     ● T85.890   Other specified complication of nervous system prosthetic devices, implants and grafts A 🐾

     ● T85.898   Other specified complication of other internal prosthetic devices, implants and grafts

X● T85.9   Unspecified complication of internal prosthetic device, implant and graft
     Complication of internal prosthetic device, implant and graft NOS

OGCR Section I.C.19.g.3.

Organ Transplant Complications
Transplant Complications

(a) Transplant complications other than kidney

Codes under category T86, Complications of transplanted organs and tissues, are for use for both complications and rejection of transplanted organs. A transplant complication code is only assigned if the complication affects the function of the transplanted organ. Two codes are required to fully describe a transplant complication: the appropriate code from category T86 and a secondary code that identifies the complication.

Pre-existing conditions or conditions that develop after the transplant are not coded as complications unless they affect the function of the transplanted organs.

See I.C.21 for transplant organ removal status.

See I.C.2 for malignant neoplasm associated with transplanted organ.

● T86   Complications of transplanted organs and tissue
     Use additional code to identify other transplant complications, such as:
       graft-versus-host disease (D89.81-)
       malignancy associated with organ transplant (C80.2)
       post-transplant lymphoproliferative disorders (PTLD) (D47.Z1)

   ● T86.0   Complications of bone marrow transplant

     T86.00   Unspecified complication of bone marrow transplant 🐾

     T86.01   Bone marrow transplant rejection 🐾

     T86.02   Bone marrow transplant failure 🐾

     T86.03   Bone marrow transplant infection 🐾

     T86.09   Other complications of bone marrow transplant 🐾

   ● T86.1   Complications of kidney transplant

     T86.10   Unspecified complication of kidney transplant

     T86.11   Kidney transplant rejection

     T86.12   Kidney transplant failure
       Coding Clinic: 2013, Q1, P24

     T86.13   Kidney transplant infection
       Use additional code to specify infection

     T86.19   Other complication of kidney transplant
       Coding Clinic: 2019, Q2, P7

   ● T86.2   Complications of heart transplant

     Excludes1   complication of:
       ▸artificial heart device (T82.5-)
       ▸heart-lung transplant (T86.3-)

     T86.20   Unspecified complication of heart transplant 🐾

     T86.21   Heart transplant rejection 🐾

     T86.22   Heart transplant failure 🐾

     T86.23   Heart transplant infection 🐾
       Use additional code to specify infection

     ● T86.29   Other complications of heart transplant

       T86.290   Cardiac allograft vasculopathy 🐾
         Excludes1   atherosclerosis of coronary arteries (I25.75-, I25.76-, I25.81-)

       T86.298   Other complications of heart transplant 🐾

   ● T86.3   Complications of heart-lung transplant

     T86.30   Unspecified complication of heart-lung transplant 🐾

     T86.31   Heart-lung transplant rejection 🐾

     T86.32   Heart-lung transplant failure 🐾

T86.33   Heart-lung transplant infection 🅗
       Use additional code to specify infection

T86.39   Other complications of heart-lung transplant 🅗

● **T86.4**   Complications of liver transplant

     T86.40   Unspecified complication of liver transplant 🅗

     T86.41   Liver transplant rejection 🅗

     T86.42   Liver transplant failure 🅗

     T86.43   Liver transplant infection 🅗
         Use additional code to identify infection, such as:
            Cytomegalovirus (CMV) infection (B25.-)

     T86.49   Other complications of liver transplant 🅗

● **T86.5**   Complications of stem cell transplant 🅗
       Complications from stem cells from peripheral blood
       Complications from stem cells from umbilical cord

● **T86.8**   Complications of other transplanted organs and tissues

   ● **T86.81**   Complications of lung transplant

       Excludes1   complication of heart-lung transplant (T86.3-)

     T86.810   Lung transplant rejection 🅗

     T86.811   Lung transplant failure 🅗

     T86.812   Lung transplant infection 🅗
         Use additional code to specify infection

     T86.818   Other complications of lung transplant 🅗
         Coding Clinic: 2019, Q2, P7

     T86.819   Unspecified complication of lung transplant 🅗

   ● **T86.82**   Complications of skin graft (allograft) (autograft)

       Excludes2   complication of artificial skin graft (T85.693)

     T86.820   Skin graft (allograft) rejection

     T86.821   Skin graft (allograft) (autograft) failure

     T86.822   Skin graft (allograft) (autograft) infection
         Use additional code to specify infection

     T86.828   Other complications of skin graft (allograft) (autograft)

     T86.829   Unspecified complication of skin graft (allograft) (autograft)

   ● **T86.83**   Complications of bone graft

       Excludes2   mechanical complications of bone graft (T84.3-)

     T86.830   Bone graft rejection

     T86.831   Bone graft failure

     T86.832   Bone graft infection
         Use additional code to specify infection

     T86.838   Other complications of bone graft

     T86.839   Unspecified complication of bone graft

   ● **T86.84**   Complications of corneal transplant

       Excludes2   mechanical complications of corneal graft (T85.3-)

   ● **T86.840**   Corneal transplant rejection

     T86.8401   Corneal transplant rejection, right eye

     T86.8402   Corneal transplant rejection, left eye

     T86.8403   Corneal transplant rejection, bilateral

     T86.8409   Corneal transplant rejection, unspecified eye

   ● **T86.841**   Corneal transplant failure

     T86.8411   Corneal transplant failure, right eye

     T86.8412   Corneal transplant failure, left eye

     T86.8413   Corneal transplant failure, bilateral

     T86.8419   Corneal transplant failure, unspecified eye

   ● **T86.842**   Corneal transplant infection 🅗
         Use additional code to specify infection

     T86.8421   Corneal transplant infection, right eye

     T86.8422   Corneal transplant infection, left eye

     T86.8423   Corneal transplant infection, bilateral

     T86.8429   Corneal transplant infection, unspecified eye

   ● **T86.848**   Other complications of corneal transplant

     T86.8481   Other complications of corneal transplant, right eye

     T86.8482   Other complications of corneal transplant, left eye

     T86.8483   Other complications of corneal transplant, bilateral

     T86.8489   Other complications of corneal transplant, unspecified eye

   ● **T86.849**   Unspecified complication of corneal transplant

     T86.8491   Unspecified complication of corneal transplant, right eye

     T86.8492   Unspecified complication of corneal transplant, left eye

     T86.8493   Unspecified complication of corneal transplant, bilateral

     T86.8499   Unspecified complication of corneal transplant, unspecified eye

   ● **T86.85**   Complication of intestine transplant

     T86.850   Intestine transplant rejection 🅗

     T86.851   Intestine transplant failure 🅗

     T86.852   Intestine transplant infection 🅗
         Use additional code to specify infection

     T86.858   Other complications of intestine transplant 🅗

     T86.859   Unspecified complication of intestine transplant 🅗

   ● **T86.89**   Complications of other transplanted tissue
       Transplant failure or rejection of pancreas

     T86.890   Other transplanted tissue rejection

     T86.891   Other transplanted tissue failure

     T86.892   Other transplanted tissue infection
         Use additional code to specify infection

     T86.898   Other complications of other transplanted tissue

     T86.899   Unspecified complication of other transplanted tissue

▶ New   ⇒ Revised   ~~deleted~~ Deleted   Excludes 1   Excludes 2   Includes   Use additional   Code first   Code also   Key words

OGCR Official Guidelines   X Assign placeholder X   ● Use Additional Character(s)   ▶ Manifestation Code   🅗 Hierarchical Condition Category   **Coding Clinic**

● **T86.9**   Complication of unspecified transplanted organ and tissue

    T86.90   Unspecified complication of unspecified transplanted organ and tissue

    T86.91   Unspecified transplanted organ and tissue rejection

    T86.92   Unspecified transplanted organ and tissue failure

    T86.93   Unspecified transplanted organ and tissue infection

       Use additional code to specify infection

    T86.99   Other complications of unspecified transplanted organ and tissue

● **T87**   Complications peculiar to reattachment and amputation

 ● **T87.0**   Complications of reattached (part of) upper extremity

  ● **T87.0X**   Complications of reattached (part of) upper extremity

     T87.0X1   Complications of reattached (part of) right upper extremity 🔊

     T87.0X2   Complications of reattached (part of) left upper extremity 🔊

     T87.0X9   Complications of reattached (part of) unspecified upper extremity 🔊

 ● **T87.1**   Complications of reattached (part of) lower extremity

  ● **T87.1X**   Complications of reattached (part of) lower extremity

     T87.1X1   Complications of reattached (part of) right lower extremity 🔊

     T87.1X2   Complications of reattached (part of) left lower extremity 🔊

     T87.1X9   Complications of reattached (part of) unspecified lower extremity 🔊

    T87.2   Complications of other reattached body part 🔊

 ● **T87.3**   Neuroma of amputation stump

    T87.30   Neuroma of amputation stump, unspecified extremity 🔊

    T87.31   Neuroma of amputation stump, right upper extremity 🔊

    T87.32   Neuroma of amputation stump, left upper extremity 🔊

    T87.33   Neuroma of amputation stump, right lower extremity 🔊

    T87.34   Neuroma of amputation stump, left lower extremity 🔊

 ● **T87.4**   Infection of amputation stump

    T87.40   Infection of amputation stump, unspecified extremity 🔊

    T87.41   Infection of amputation stump, right upper extremity 🔊

    T87.42   Infection of amputation stump, left upper extremity 🔊

    T87.43   Infection of amputation stump, right lower extremity 🔊

    T87.44   Infection of amputation stump, left lower extremity 🔊

 ● **T87.5**   Necrosis of amputation stump

    T87.50   Necrosis of amputation stump, unspecified extremity 🔊

    T87.51   Necrosis of amputation stump, right upper extremity 🔊

    T87.52   Necrosis of amputation stump, left upper extremity 🔊

    T87.53   Necrosis of amputation stump, right lower extremity 🔊

    T87.54   Necrosis of amputation stump, left lower extremity 🔊

● **T87.8**   Other complications of amputation stump

    T87.81   Dehiscence of amputation stump 🔊

    T87.89   Other complications of amputation stump 🔊

       Amputation stump contracture

       Amputation stump contracture of next proximal joint

       Amputation stump flexion

       Amputation stump edema

       Amputation stump hematoma

       Excludes2   phantom limb syndrome (G54.6-G54.7)

    T87.9   Unspecified complications of amputation stump 🔊

● **T88**   Other complications of surgical and medical care, not elsewhere classified

    Excludes2   complication following infusion, transfusion and therapeutic injection (T80.-)

            complication following procedure NEC (T81.-)

            complications of anesthesia in labor and delivery (O74.-)

            complications of anesthesia in pregnancy (O29.-)

            complications of anesthesia in puerperium (O89.-)

            complications of devices, implants and grafts (T82-T85)

            complications of obstetric surgery and procedure (O75.4)

            dermatitis due to drugs and medicaments (L23.3, L24.4, L25.1, L27.0-L27.1)

            poisoning and toxic effects of drugs and chemicals (T36-T65 with fifth or sixth character 1-4 or 6)

            specified complications classified elsewhere

    The appropriate 7th character is to be added to each code from category T88

A	initial encounter
D	subsequent encounter
S	sequela

X● **T88.0**   Infection following immunization

       Sepsis following immunization

       Coding Clinic: 2019, Q1, P14;2018, Q4, P90

X● **T88.1**   Other complications following immunization, not elsewhere classified

       Generalized vaccinia

       Rash following immunization

       Excludes1   vaccinia not from vaccine (B08.011)

       Excludes2   anaphylactic shock due to serum (T80.5-)

            other serum reactions (T80.6-)

            postimmunization arthropathy (M02.2)

            postimmunization encephalitis (G04.02)

            postimmunization fever (R50.83)

X● **T88.2**   Shock due to anesthesia

       Use additional code for adverse effect, if applicable, to identify drug (T41.- with fifth or sixth character 5)

       Excludes1   complications of anesthesia (in):

            labor and delivery (O74.-)

            pregnancy (O29.-)

            puerperium (O89.-)

            postprocedural shock NOS (T81.1-)

X● **T88.3**   Malignant hyperthermia due to anesthesia

       Use additional code for adverse effect, if applicable, to identify drug (T41.- with fifth or sixth character 5)

X● **T88.4**   Failed or difficult intubation

● **T88.5**   Other complications of anesthesia

       Use additional code for adverse effect, if applicable, to identify drug (T41.- with fifth or sixth character 5)

       Coding Clinic: 2016, Q4, P72

X● **T88.51**   Hypothermia following anesthesia

X● **T88.52**   Failed moderate sedation during procedure

       Failed conscious sedation during procedure

       Excludes2   personal history of failed moderate sedation (Z92.83)

X● **T88.53** **Unintended awareness under general anesthesia during procedure**
     Excludes2 personal history of unintended awareness under general anesthesia (Z92.84)
     Coding Clinic: 2016, Q4, P72-73

X● **T88.59** **Other complications of anesthesia**

X● **T88.6** **Anaphylactic reaction due to adverse effect of correct drug or medicament properly administered**
     Anaphylactic shock due to adverse effect of correct drug or medicament properly administered
     Anaphylactoid reaction NOS
     Use additional code for adverse effect, if applicable, to identify drug (T36-T50 with fifth or sixth character 5)
     Excludes1 anaphylactic reaction due to serum (T80.5-)
         anaphylactic shock or reaction due to adverse food reaction (T78.0-)
     Coding Clinic: 2020, Q1, P18

X● **T88.7** **Unspecified adverse effect of drug or medicament**
     Drug hypersensitivity NOS
     Drug reaction NOS
     Use additional code for adverse effect, if applicable, to identify drug (T36-T50 with fifth or sixth character 5)
     Excludes1 specified adverse effects of drugs and medicaments (A00-R94 and T80-T88.6, T88.8)

X● **T88.8** **Other specified complications of surgical and medical care, not elsewhere classified**
     Use additional code to identify the complication

X● **T88.9** **Complication of surgical and medical care, unspecified**

CHAPTER 19 (S00-T88)

CHAPTER 20

EXTERNAL CAUSES OF MORBIDITY (V00-Y99)

OGCR Chapter-Specific Coding Guidelines

20. Chapter 20: External Causes of Morbidity (V00-Y99)
The external causes of morbidity codes should never be sequenced as the first-listed or principal diagnosis.

External cause codes are intended to provide data for injury research and evaluation of injury prevention strategies. These codes capture how the injury or health condition happened (cause), the intent (unintentional or accidental; or intentional, such as suicide or assault), the place where the event occurred the activity of the patient at the time of the event, and the person's status (e.g., civilian, military).

There is no national requirement for mandatory ICD-10-CM external cause code reporting. Unless a provider is subject to a state-based external cause code reporting mandate or these codes are required by a particular payer, reporting of ICD-10-CM codes in Chapter 20, External Causes of Morbidity, is not required. In the absence of a mandatory reporting requirement, providers are encouraged to voluntarily report external cause codes, as they provide valuable data for injury research and evaluation of injury prevention strategies.

a. General External Cause Coding Guidelines

1) Used with any code in the range of A00.0-T88.9, Z00-Z99
An external cause code may be used with any code in the range of A00.0-T88.9, Z00-Z99, classification that represents a health condition due to an external cause. Though they are most applicable to injuries, they are also valid for use with such things as infections or diseases due to an external source, and other health conditions, such as a heart attack that occurs during strenuous physical activity.

2) External cause code used for length of treatment
Assign the external cause code, with the appropriate 7th character (initial encounter, subsequent encounter or sequela) for each encounter for which the injury or condition is being treated.

Most categories in Chapter 20 have a 7th character requirement for each applicable code. Most categories in this chapter have three 7th character values: A, initial encounter, D, subsequent encounter and S, sequela. While the patient may be seen by a new or different provider over the course of treatment for an injury or condition, assignment of the 7th character for external cause should match the 7th character of the code assigned for the associated injury or condition for the encounter.

3) Use the full range of external cause codes
Use the full range of external cause codes to completely describe the cause, the intent, the place of occurrence and if applicable, the activity of the patient at the time of the event, and the patient's status, for all injuries, and other health conditions due to an external cause.

4) Assign as many external cause codes as necessary
Assign as many external cause codes as necessary to fully explain each cause. If only one external code can be recorded, assign the code most related to the principal diagnosis.

5) The selection of the appropriate external cause code
The selection of the appropriate external cause code is guided by the Alphabetic Index of External Causes and by Inclusion and Exclusion notes in the Tabular List.

6) External cause code can never be a principal diagnosis
An external cause code can never be a principal (first-listed) diagnosis.

7) Combination external cause codes
Certain of the external cause codes are combination codes that identify sequential events that result in an injury, such as a fall which results in striking against an object. The injury may be due to either event or both. The combination external cause code used should correspond to the sequence of events regardless of which caused the most serious injury.

8) No external cause code needed in certain circumstances
No external cause code from Chapter 20 is needed if the external cause and intent are included in a code from another chapter (e.g., T36.0X1- Poisoning by penicillins, accidental (unintentional)).

b. Place of Occurrence Guideline
Codes from category Y92, Place of occurrence of the external cause, are secondary codes for use after other external cause codes to identify the location of the patient at the time of injury or other condition.

Generally, a place of occurrence code is assigned only once, at the initial encounter for treatment. However, in the rare instance that a new injury occurs during hospitalization, an additional place of occurrence code may be assigned. No 7th characters are used for Y92. Only one code from Y92 should be recorded on a medical record.

Do not use place of occurrence code Y92.9 if the place is not stated or is not applicable.

c. Activity Code
Assign a code from category Y93, Activity code, to describe the activity of the patient at the time the injury or other health condition occurred.

An activity code is used only once, at the initial encounter for treatment. Only one code from Y93 should be recorded on a medical record.

The activity codes are not applicable to poisonings, adverse effects, misadventures or sequela.

Do not assign Y93.9, Unspecified activity, if the activity is not stated.

A code from category Y93 is appropriate for use with external cause and intent codes if identifying the activity provides additional information about the event.

d. Place of Occurrence, Activity, and Status Codes Used with Other External Cause Code
When applicable, place of occurrence, activity, and external cause status codes are sequenced after the main external cause code(s). Regardless of the number of external cause codes assigned, there should be only one place of occurrence code, one activity code, and one external cause status code assigned to an encounter.

e. If the Reporting Format Limits the Number of External Cause Codes

If the reporting format limits the number of external cause codes that can be used in reporting clinical data, report the code for the cause/intent most related to the principal diagnosis. If the format permits capture of additional external cause codes, the cause/intent, including medical misadventures, of the additional events should be reported rather than the codes for place, activity, or external status.

f. Multiple External Cause Coding Guidelines

More than one external cause code is required to fully describe the external cause of an illness or injury. The assignment of external cause codes should be sequenced in the following priority:

If two or more events cause separate injuries, an external cause code should be assigned for each cause. The first-listed external cause code will be selected in the following order:

External codes for child and adult abuse take priority over all other external cause codes.

See Section I.C.19., Child and Adult abuse guidelines.

External codes for terrorism events take priority over all other external cause codes except child and adult abuse.

External cause codes for cataclysmic events take priority over all other external cause codes except child and adult abuse and terrorism.

External cause codes for transport accidents take priority over all other external cause codes except cataclysmic events, child and adult abuse and terrorism.

Activity and external cause status codes are assigned following all causal (intent) external cause codes.

The first-listed external cause code should correspond to the cause of the most serious diagnosis due to an assault, accident, or self-harm, following the order of hierarchy listed above.

g. Child and Adult Abuse Guideline

Adult and child abuse, neglect and maltreatment are classified as assault. Any of the assault codes may be used to indicate the external cause of any injury resulting from the confirmed abuse.

For confirmed cases of abuse, neglect and maltreatment, when the perpetrator is known, a code from Y07, Perpetrator of maltreatment and neglect, should accompany any other assault codes.

See Section I.C.19. Adult and child abuse, neglect and other maltreatment

h. Unknown or Undetermined Intent Guideline

If the intent (accident, self-harm, assault) of the cause of an injury or other condition is unknown or unspecified, code the intent as accidental intent. All transport accident categories assume accidental intent.

1) Use of undetermined intent

External cause codes for events of undetermined intent are only for use if the documentation in the record specifies that the intent cannot be determined.

i. Sequelae (Late Effects) of External Cause Guidelines

1) Sequelae external cause codes

Sequela are reported using the external cause code with the 7th character "S" for sequela. These codes should be used with any report of a late effect or sequela resulting from a previous injury.

See Section I.B.10. Sequela, (Late Effects).

2) Sequela external cause code with a related current injury

A sequela external cause code should never be used with a related current nature of injury code.

3) Use of sequela external cause codes for subsequent visits

Use a late effect external cause code for subsequent visits when a late effect of the initial injury is being treated. Do not use a late effect external cause code for subsequent visits for follow-up care (e.g., to assess healing, to receive rehabilitative therapy) of the injury when no late effect of the injury has been documented.

j. Terrorism Guidelines

1) Cause of injury identified by the Federal Government (FBI) as terrorism

When the cause of an injury is identified by the Federal Government (FBI) as terrorism, the first-listed external cause code should be a code from category Y38, Terrorism. The definition of terrorism employed by the FBI is found at the inclusion note at the beginning of category Y38. Use additional code for place of occurrence (Y92.-). More than one Y38 code may be assigned if the injury is the result of more than one mechanism of terrorism.

2) Cause of an injury is suspected to be the result of terrorism

When the cause of an injury is suspected to be the result of terrorism a code from category Y38 should not be assigned. Suspected cases should be classified as assault.

3) Code Y38.9, Terrorism, secondary effects

Assign code Y38.9, Terrorism, secondary effects, for conditions occurring subsequent to the terrorist event. This code should not be assigned for conditions that are due to the initial terrorist act.

It is acceptable to assign code Y38.9 with another code from Y38 if there is an injury due to the initial terrorist event and an injury that is a subsequent result of the terrorist event.

k. External cause status

A code from category Y99, External cause status, should be assigned whenever any other external cause code is assigned for an encounter, including an Activity code, except for the events noted below. Assign a code from category Y99, External cause status, to indicate the work status of the person at the time the event occurred. The status code indicates whether the event occurred during military activity, whether a non-military person was at work, whether an individual including a student or volunteer was involved in a non-work activity at the time of the causal event.

A code from Y99, External cause status, should be assigned, when applicable, with other external cause codes, such as transport accidents and falls. The external cause status codes are not applicable to poisonings, adverse effects, misadventures or late effects.

Do not assign a code from category Y99 if no other external cause codes (cause, activity) are applicable for the encounter.

An external cause status code is used only once, at the initial encounter for treatment. Only one code from Y99 should be recorded on a medical record.

Do not assign code Y99.9, Unspecified external cause status, if the status is not stated.

CHAPTER 2Ø

EXTERNAL CAUSES OF MORBIDITY (VØØ-Y99)

Note: This chapter permits the classification of environmental events and circumstances as the cause of injury, and other adverse effects. Where a code from this section is applicable, it is intended that it shall be used secondary to a code from another chapter of the Classification indicating the nature of the condition. Most often, the condition will be classifiable to Chapter 19, Injury, poisoning and certain other consequences of external causes (SØØ-T88). Other conditions that may be stated to be due to external causes are classified in Chapters 1 to 18. For these conditions, codes from Chapter 2Ø should be used to provide additional information as to the cause of the condition.

This chapter contains the following blocks:

VØØ-X58	Accidents
VØØ-V99	Transport accidents
VØØ-VØ9	Pedestrian injured in transport accident
V1Ø-V19	Pedal cycle rider injured in transport accident
V2Ø-V29	Motorcycle rider injured in transport accident
V3Ø-V39	Occupant of three-wheeled motor vehicle injured in transport accident
V4Ø-V49	Car occupant injured in transport accident
V5Ø-V59	Occupant of pick-up truck or van injured in transport accident
V6Ø-V69	Occupant of heavy transport vehicle injured in transport accident
V7Ø-V79	Bus occupant injured in transport accident
V8Ø-V89	Other land transport accidents
V9Ø-V94	Water transport accidents
V95-V97	Air and space transport accidents
V98-V99	Other and unspecified transport accidents
WØØ-X58	Other external causes of accidental injury
WØØ-W19	Slipping, tripping, stumbling and falls
W2Ø-W49	Exposure to inanimate mechanical forces
W5Ø-W64	Exposure to animate mechanical forces
W65-W74	Accidental non-transport drowning and submersion
W85-W99	Exposure to electric current, radiation and extreme ambient air temperature and pressure
XØØ-XØ8	Exposure to smoke, fire and flames
X1Ø-X19	Contact with heat and hot substances
X3Ø-X39	Exposure to forces of nature
X5Ø	Overexertion and strenuous or repetitive movements
X52, X58	Accidental exposure to other specified factors
X71-X83	Intentional self-harm
X92-YØ9	Assault
Y21-Y33	Event of undetermined intent
Y35-Y38	Legal intervention, operations of war, military operations, and terrorism
Y62-Y84	Complications of medical and surgical care
Y62-Y69	Misadventures to patients during surgical and medical care
Y7Ø-Y82	Medical devices associated with adverse incidents in diagnostic and therapeutic use
Y83-Y84	Surgical and other medical procedures as the cause of abnormal reaction of the patient, or of later complication, without mention of misadventure at the time of the procedure
Y9Ø-Y99	Supplementary factors related to causes of morbidity classified elsewhere

ACCIDENTS (VØØ-X58)

TRANSPORT ACCIDENTS (VØØ-V99)

Note: This section is structured in 12 groups. Those relating to land transport accidents (VØØ-V89) reflect the victim's mode of transport and are subdivided to identify the victim's 'counterpart' or the type of event. The vehicle of which the injured person is an occupant is identified in the first two characters since it is seen as the most important factor to identify for prevention purposes. A transport accident is one in which the vehicle involved must be moving or running or in use for transport purposes at the time of the accident.

Use additional code to identify:
Airbag injury (W22.1)
Type of street or road (Y92.4-)
Use of cellular telephone and other electronic equipment at the time of the transport accident (Y93.C-)

Excludes1 agricultural vehicles in stationary use or maintenance (W31.-)
assault by crashing of motor vehicle (YØ3.-)
automobile or motor cycle in stationary use or maintenance - code to type of accident
crashing of motor vehicle, undetermined intent (Y32)
intentional self-harm by crashing of motor vehicle (X82)

Excludes2 transport accidents due to cataclysm (X34-X38)

Note: Definitions related to transport accidents:

(a) A transport accident (VØØ-V99) is any accident involving a device designed primarily for, or used at the time primarily for, conveying persons or good from one place to another.

(b) A public highway [trafficway] or street is the entire width between property lines (or other boundary lines) of land open to the public as a matter of right or custom for purposes of moving persons or property from one place to another. A roadway is that part of the public highway designed, improved and customarily used for vehicular traffic.

(c) A traffic accident is any vehicle accident occurring on the public highway [i.e., originating on, terminating on, or involving a vehicle partially on the highway]. A vehicle accident is assumed to have occurred on the public highway unless another place is specified, except in the case of accidents involving only off-road motor vehicles, which are classified as nontraffic accidents unless the contrary is stated.

(d) A nontraffic accident is any vehicle accident that occurs entirely in any place other than a public highway.

(e) A pedestrian is any person involved in an accident who was not at the time of the accident riding in or on a motor vehicle, railway train, streetcar or animal-drawn or other vehicle, or on a pedal cycle or animal. This includes, a person changing a tire, working on a parked car, or a person on foot. It also includes the user of a pedestrian conveyance such as a baby stroller, ice-skates, skis, sled, roller skates, a skateboard, nonmotorized or motorized wheelchair, motorized mobility scooter, or nonmotorized scooter.

(f) A driver is an occupant of a transport vehicle who is operating or intending to operate it.

(g) A passenger is any occupant of a transport vehicle other than the driver, except a person traveling on the outside of the vehicle.

(h) A person on the outside of a vehicle is any person being transported by a vehicle but not occupying the space normally reserved for the driver or passengers, or the space intended for the transport of property. This includes a person travelling on the bodywork, bumper, fender, roof, running board or step of a vehicle, as well as, hanging on the outside of the vehicle.

(i) A pedal cycle is any land transport vehicle operated solely by nonmotorized pedals including a bicycle or tricycle.

(j) A pedal cyclist is any person riding a pedal cycle or in a sidecar or trailer attached to a pedal cycle.

(k) A motorcycle is a two-wheeled motor vehicle with one or two riding saddles and sometimes with a third wheel for the support of a sidecar. The sidecar is considered part of the motorcycle. This includes a moped, motor scooter, or motorized bicycle.

(l) A motorcycle rider is any person riding a motorcycle or in a sidecar or trailer attached to the motorcycle.

(m) A three-wheeled motor vehicle is a motorized tricycle designed primarily for on-road use. This includes a motor-driven tricycle, a motorized rickshaw, or a three-wheeled motor car.

(n) A car [automobile] is a four-wheeled motor vehicle designed primarily for carrying up to 7 persons. A trailer being towed by the car is considered part of the car. It does not include a van or minivan—see definition (o)

(o) A pick-up truck or van is a four or six-wheeled motor vehicle designed for carrying passengers as well as property or cargo weighing less than the local limit for classification as a heavy goods vehicle, and not requiring a special driver's license. This includes a minivan and a sport-utility vehicle (SUV).

(p) A heavy transport vehicle is a motor vehicle designed primarily for carrying property, meeting local criteria for classification as a heavy goods vehicle in terms of weight and requiring a special driver's license.

(q) A bus (coach) is a motor vehicle designed or adapted primarily for carrying more than 10 passengers, and requiring a special driver's license.

(r) A railway train or railway vehicle is any device, with or without freight or passenger cars coupled to it, designed for traffic on a railway track. This includes subterranean (subways) or elevated trains.

(s) A streetcar is a device designed and used primarily for transporting passengers within a municipality, running on rails, usually subject to normal traffic control signals, and operated principally on a right-of-way that forms part of the roadway. This includes a tram or trolley that runs on rails. A trailer being towed by a streetcar is considered part of the streetcar.

(t) A special vehicle mainly used on industrial premises is a motor vehicle designed primarily for use within the buildings and premises of industrial or commercial establishments. This includes battery-powered airport passenger vehicles or baggage/mail trucks, forklifts, coal-cars in a coal mine, logging cars and trucks used in mines or quarries.

(u) A special vehicle mainly used in agriculture is a motor vehicle designed specifically for use in farming and agriculture (horticulture), to work the land, tend and harvest crops and transport materials on the farm. This includes harvesters, farm machinery and tractor and trailers.

(v) A special construction vehicle is a motor vehicle designed specifically for use on construction and demolition sites. This includes bulldozers, diggers, earth levellers, dump trucks, backhoes, front-end loaders, pavers, and mechanical shovels.

(w) A special all-terrain vehicle is a motor vehicle of special design to enable it to negotiate over rough or soft terrain, snow or sand. Examples of special design are high construction, special wheels and tires, tracks, and support on a cushion of air. This includes snow mobiles, all-terrain vehicles (ATV), and dune buggies. It does not include passenger vehicle designated as sport utility vehicles (SUV).

(x) A watercraft is any device designed for transporting passengers or goods on water. This includes motor or sail boats, ships, and hovercraft.

(y) An aircraft is any device for transporting passengers or goods in the air. This includes hot-air balloons, gliders, helicopters and airplanes.

(z) A military vehicle is any motorized vehicle operating on a public roadway owned by the military and being operated by a member of the military.

PEDESTRIAN INJURED IN TRANSPORT ACCIDENT (V00-V09)

Includes   person changing tire on transport vehicle
person examining engine of vehicle broken down in (on side of) road

Excludes1   fall due to non-transport collision with other person (W03)
pedestrian on foot falling (slipping) on ice and snow (W00.-)
struck or bumped by another person (W51)

● **V00**   Pedestrian conveyance accident

Use additional place of occurrence and activity external cause codes, if known (Y92.-, Y93.-)

Excludes1   collision with another person without fall (W51)
fall due to person on foot colliding with another person on foot (W03)
fall from non-moving wheelchair, nonmotorized scooter and motorized mobility scooter without collision (W05.-)
pedestrian (conveyance) collision with other land transport vehicle (V01-V09)
pedestrian on foot falling (slipping) on ice and snow (W00.-)

The appropriate 7th character is to be added to each code from category V00

A	initial encounter
D	subsequent encounter
S	sequela

● **V00.0**   Pedestrian on foot injured in collision with pedestrian conveyance

X ● **V00.01**   Pedestrian on foot injured in collision with roller-skater

X ● **V00.02**   Pedestrian on foot injured in collision with skateboarder

● **V00.03**   Pedestrian on foot injured in collision with standing micro-mobility pedestrian conveyance

   V00.031   Pedestrian on foot injured in collision with rider of standing electric scooter

   V00.038   Pedestrian on foot injured in collision with rider of other standing micro-mobility pedestrian conveyance
Pedestrian on foot injured in collision with rider of hoverboard
Pedestrian on foot injured in collision with rider of segway

X ● **V00.09**   Pedestrian on foot injured in collision with other pedestrian conveyance

● **V00.1**   Rolling-type pedestrian conveyance accident

Excludes1   accident with baby stroller (V00.82-)
accident with wheelchair (powered) (V00.81-)
accident with motorized mobility scooter (V00.83-)

● **V00.11**   In-line roller-skate accident

● **V00.111**   Fall from in-line roller-skates

● **V00.112**   In-line roller-skater colliding with stationary object

● **V00.118**   Other in-line roller-skate accident

Excludes1   roller-skater collision with other land transport vehicle (V01-V09 with 5th character 1)

CHAPTER 20 (V00-Y99)

- ● V00.12   **Non-in-line roller-skate** accident
  - ● V00.121   **Fall from non-in-line roller-skates**
  - ● V00.122   **Non-in-line roller-skater colliding with stationary object**
  - ● V00.128   **Other non-in-line roller-skating** accident
    - **Excludes1**   roller-skater collision with other land transport vehicle (V01-V09 with 5th character 1)
- ● V00.13   **Skateboard** accident
  - ● V00.131   **Fall from skateboard**
  - ● V00.132   **Skateboarder colliding with stationary object**
  - ● V00.138   **Other skateboard** accident
    - **Excludes1**   skateboarder collision with other land transport vehicle (V01-V09 with 5th character 2)
- ● V00.14   **Scooter (nonmotorized)** accident
  - **Excludes1**   motor scooter accident (V20-V29)
  - ● V00.141   **Fall from scooter (nonmotorized)**
  - ● V00.142   **Scooter (nonmotorized) colliding with stationary object**
  - ● V00.148   **Other scooter (nonmotorized)** accident
    - **Excludes1**   scooter (non-motorized) collision with other land transport vehicle (V01-V09 with fifth character 9)
- ● V00.15   **Heelies** accident
  - Rolling shoe
  - Wheeled shoe
  - Wheelies accident
  - ● V00.151   **Fall from heelies**
  - ● V00.152   **Heelies colliding with stationary object**
  - ● V00.158   **Other heelies** accident
- ● V00.18   Accident on **other rolling-type pedestrian conveyance**
  - ● V00.181   **Fall from other rolling-type pedestrian conveyance**
  - ● V00.182   **Pedestrian on other rolling-type pedestrian conveyance colliding with stationary object**
  - ● V00.188   **Other accident on other rolling-type pedestrian conveyance**
- ● V00.2   Gliding-type pedestrian conveyance accident
  - ● V00.21   **Ice-skates** accident
    - ● V00.211   **Fall from ice-skates**
    - ● V00.212   **Ice-skater colliding with stationary object**
    - ● V00.218   **Other ice-skates** accident
      - **Excludes1**   ice-skater collision with other land transport vehicle (V01-V09 with 5th character 9)
  - ● V00.22   **Sled** accident
    - ● V00.221   **Fall from sled**
    - ● V00.222   **Sledder colliding with stationary object**
    - ● V00.228   **Other sled** accident
      - **Excludes1**   sled collision with other land transport vehicle (V01-V09 with 5th character 9)
- ● V00.28   Other **gliding-type pedestrian conveyance** accident
  - ● V00.281   **Fall from other gliding-type pedestrian conveyance**
  - ● V00.282   **Pedestrian on other gliding-type pedestrian conveyance colliding with stationary object**
  - ● V00.288   **Other accident on other gliding-type pedestrian conveyance**
    - **Excludes1**   gliding-type pedestrian conveyance collision with other land transport vehicle (V01-V09 with 5th character 9)
- ● V00.3   **Flat-bottomed pedestrian conveyance accident**
  - ● V00.31   **Snowboard** accident
    - ● V00.311   **Fall from snowboard**
    - ● V00.312   **Snowboarder colliding with stationary object**
    - ● V00.318   **Other snowboard** accident
      - **Excludes1**   snowboarder collision with other land transport vehicle (V01-V09 with 5th character 9)
  - ● V00.32   **Snow-ski** accident
    - ● V00.321   **Fall from snow-skis**
      - **Coding Clinic: 2015, Q1, P12**
    - ● V00.322   **Snow-skier colliding with stationary object**
    - ● V00.328   **Other snow-ski** accident
      - **Excludes1**   snow-skier collision with other land transport vehicle (V01-V09 with 5th character 9)
  - ● V00.38   **Other flat-bottomed pedestrian conveyance** accident
    - ● V00.381   **Fall from other flat-bottomed pedestrian conveyance**
    - ● V00.382   **Pedestrian on other flat-bottomed pedestrian conveyance colliding with stationary object**
    - ● V00.388   **Other accident on other flat-bottomed pedestrian conveyance**
- ● V00.8   Accident on other pedestrian conveyance
  - ● V00.81   Accident with **wheelchair (powered)**
    - ● V00.811   **Fall from moving wheelchair (powered)**
      - **Excludes1**   fall from non-moving wheelchair (W05.0)
    - ● V00.812   **Wheelchair (powered) colliding with stationary object**
    - ● V00.818   **Other accident with wheelchair (powered)**
  - ● V00.82   Accident with **baby stroller**
    - ● V00.821   **Fall from baby stroller**
    - ● V00.822   **Baby stroller colliding with stationary object**
    - ● V00.828   **Other accident with baby stroller**

CHAPTER 20 (V00-Y99)

CHAPTER 20 (V00-Y99)

● **V00.83　Accident with motorized mobility scooter**
　　● **V00.831　Fall from motorized mobility scooter**
　　　　Excludes1　fall from non-moving motorized mobility scooter (W05.2)
　　● **V00.832　Motorized mobility scooter colliding with stationary object**
　　● **V00.838　Other accident with motorized mobility scooter**
● **V00.84　Accident with standing micro-mobility pedestrian conveyance**
　　V00.841　Fall from standing electric scooter
　　V00.842　Pedestrian on standing electric scooter colliding with stationary object
　　V00.848　Other accident with standing micro-mobility pedestrian conveyance
　　　　Accident with hoverboard
　　　　Accident with segway
● **V00.89　Accident on other pedestrian conveyance**
　　● **V00.891　Fall from other pedestrian conveyance**
　　● **V00.892　Pedestrian on other pedestrian conveyance colliding with stationary object**
　　● **V00.898　Other accident on other pedestrian conveyance**
　　　　Excludes1　other pedestrian (conveyance) collision with other land transport vehicle (V01-V09 with 5th character 9)

● **V01　Pedestrian injured in collision with pedal cycle**
　　The appropriate 7th character is to be added to each code from category V01

A	initial encounter
D	subsequent encounter
S	sequela

　● **V01.0　Pedestrian injured in collision with pedal cycle in nontraffic accident**
　　X● **V01.00　Pedestrian on foot injured in collision with pedal cycle in nontraffic accident**
　　　　Pedestrian NOS injured in collision with pedal cycle in nontraffic accident
　　X● **V01.01　Pedestrian on roller-skates injured in collision with pedal cycle in nontraffic accident**
　　X● **V01.02　Pedestrian on skateboard injured in collision with pedal cycle in nontraffic accident**
　　● **V01.03　Pedestrian on standing micro-mobility pedestrian conveyance injured in collision with pedal cycle in nontraffic accident**
　　　　V01.031　Pedestrian on standing electric scooter injured in collision with pedal cycle in nontraffic accident
　　　　V01.038　Pedestrian on other standing micro-mobility pedestrian conveyance injured in collision with pedal cycle in nontraffic accident
　　　　　　Pedestrian on hoverboard injured in collision with pedal cycle in nontraffic accident
　　　　　　Pedestrian on segway injured in collision with pedal cycle in nontraffic accident

X● **V01.09　Pedestrian with other conveyance injured in collision with pedal cycle in nontraffic accident**
　　Pedestrian with baby stroller injured in collision with pedal cycle in nontraffic accident
　　Pedestrian in wheelchair (powered) injured in collision with pedal cycle in nontraffic accident
　　Pedestrian in motorized mobility scooter injured in collision with pedal cycle in nontraffic accident
　　Pedestrian on ice-skates injured in collision with pedal cycle in nontraffic accident
　　Pedestrian on nonmotorized scooter injured in collision with pedal cycle in nontraffic accident
　　Pedestrian on sled injured in collision with pedal cycle in nontraffic accident
　　Pedestrian on snowboard injured in collision with pedal cycle in nontraffic accident
　　Pedestrian on snow-skis injured in collision with pedal cycle in nontraffic accident
● **V01.1　Pedestrian injured in collision with pedal cycle in traffic accident**
　　X● **V01.10　Pedestrian on foot injured in collision with pedal cycle in traffic accident**
　　　　Pedestrian NOS injured in collision with pedal cycle in traffic accident
　　X● **V01.11　Pedestrian on roller-skates injured in collision with pedal cycle in traffic accident**
　　X● **V01.12　Pedestrian on skateboard injured in collision with pedal cycle in traffic accident**
　　● **V01.13　Pedestrian on standing micro-mobility pedestrian conveyance injured in collision with pedal cycle in traffic accident**
　　　　V01.131　Pedestrian on standing electric scooter injured in collision with pedal cycle in traffic accident
　　　　V01.138　Pedestrian on other standing micro-mobility pedestrian conveyance injured in collision with pedal cycle in traffic accident
　　　　　　Pedestrian on hoverboard injured in collision with pedal cycle in traffic accident
　　　　　　Pedestrian on segway injured in collision with pedal cycle in traffic accident
　　X● **V01.19　Pedestrian with other conveyance injured in collision with pedal cycle in traffic accident**
　　　　Pedestrian with baby stroller injured in collision with pedal cycle in traffic accident
　　　　Pedestrian in wheelchair (powered) injured in collision with pedal cycle in traffic accident
　　　　Pedestrian in motorized mobility scooter injured in collision with pedal cycle in traffic accident
　　　　Pedestrian on ice-skates injured in collision with pedal cycle in traffic accident
　　　　Pedestrian on nonmotorized scooter injured in collision with pedal cycle in traffic accident
　　　　Pedestrian on sled injured in collision with pedal cycle in traffic accident
　　　　Pedestrian on snowboard injured in collision with pedal cycle in traffic accident
　　　　Pedestrian on snow-skis injured in collision with pedal cycle in traffic accident

▶ New　⇒ Revised　deleted Deleted　Excludes 1　Excludes 2　Includes　Use additional　Code first　Code also　Key words
OGCR Official Guidelines　X Assign placeholder X　● Use Additional Character(s)　❱ Manifestation Code　🝜 Hierarchical Condition Category　**Coding Clinic**

● **V01.9** Pedestrian injured in collision with pedal cycle, unspecified whether traffic or nontraffic accident

X● **V01.90** Pedestrian on foot injured in collision with pedal cycle, unspecified whether traffic or nontraffic accident
      Pedestrian NOS injured in collision with pedal cycle, unspecified whether traffic or nontraffic accident

X● **V01.91** Pedestrian on roller-skates injured in collision with pedal cycle, unspecified whether traffic or nontraffic accident

X● **V01.92** Pedestrian on skateboard injured in collision with pedal cycle, unspecified whether traffic or nontraffic accident

● **V01.93** Pedestrian on standing micro-mobility pedestrian conveyance injured in collision with pedal cycle, unspecified whether traffic or nontraffic accident

  V01.931 Pedestrian on standing electric scooter injured in collision with pedal cycle, unspecified whether traffic or nontraffic accident

  V01.938 Pedestrian on other standing micro-mobility pedestrian conveyance injured in collision with pedal cycle, unspecified whether traffic or nontraffic accident
      Pedestrian on hoverboard injured in collision with pedal cycle, unspecified whether traffic or nontraffic accident
      Pedestrian on segway injured in collision with pedal cycle, unspecified whether traffic or nontraffic accident

X● **V01.99** Pedestrian with other conveyance injured in collision with pedal cycle, unspecified whether traffic or nontraffic accident
      Pedestrian with baby stroller injured in collision with pedal cycle, unspecified whether traffic or nontraffic accident
      Pedestrian in wheelchair (powered) injured in collision with pedal cycle, unspecified whether traffic or nontraffic accident
      Pedestrian in motorized mobility scooter injured in collision with pedal cycle, unspecified whether traffic or nontraffic accident
      Pedestrian on ice-skates injured in collision with pedal cycle unspecified, whether traffic or nontraffic accident
      Pedestrian on nonmotorized scooter injured in collision with pedal cycle, unspecified whether traffic or nontraffic accident
      Pedestrian on sled injured in collision with pedal cycle unspecified, whether traffic or nontraffic accident
      Pedestrian on snowboard injured in collision with pedal cycle, unspecified whether traffic or nontraffic accident
      Pedestrian on snow-skis injured in collision with pedal cycle, unspecified whether traffic or nontraffic accident

● **V02** Pedestrian injured in collision with two- or three-wheeled motor vehicle

The appropriate 7th character is to be added to each code from category V02

A	initial encounter
D	subsequent encounter
S	sequela

● **V02.0** Pedestrian injured in collision with two- or three-wheeled motor vehicle in nontraffic accident

X● **V02.00** Pedestrian on foot injured in collision with two- or three-wheeled motor vehicle in nontraffic accident
      Pedestrian NOS injured in collision with two- or three-wheeled motor vehicle in nontraffic accident

X● **V02.01** Pedestrian on roller-skates injured in collision with two- or three-wheeled motor vehicle in nontraffic accident

X● **V02.02** Pedestrian on skateboard injured in collision with two- or three-wheeled motor vehicle in nontraffic accident

● **V02.03** Pedestrian on standing micro-mobility pedestrian conveyance injured in collision with two- or three-wheeled motor vehicle in nontraffic accident

  V02.031 Pedestrian on standing electric scooter injured in collision with two- or three-wheeled motor vehicle in nontraffic accident

  V02.038 Pedestrian on other standing micro-mobility pedestrian conveyance injured in collision with two- or three-wheeled motor vehicle in nontraffic accident
      Pedestrian on hoverboard injured in collision with two-or three wheeled motor vehicle in nontraffic accident
      Pedestrian on segway injured in collision with two- or three-wheeled motor vehicle in nontraffic accident

X● **V02.09** Pedestrian with other conveyance injured in collision with two- or three-wheeled motor vehicle in nontraffic accident
      Pedestrian with baby stroller injured in collision with two- or three-wheeled motor vehicle in nontraffic accident
      Pedestrian on ice-skates injured in collision with two- or three-wheeled motor vehicle in nontraffic accident
      Pedestrian in wheelchair (powered) injured in collision with two- or three-wheeled motor vehicle in nontraffic accident
      Pedestrian in motorized mobility scooter injured in collision with two- or three-wheeled motor vehicle in nontraffic accident
      Pedestrian on nonmotorized scooter injured in collision with two- or three-wheeled motor vehicle in nontraffic accident
      Pedestrian on sled injured in collision with two- or three-wheeled motor vehicle in nontraffic accident
      Pedestrian on snowboard injured in collision with two- or three-wheeled motor vehicle in nontraffic accident
      Pedestrian on snow-skis injured in collision with two- or three-wheeled motor vehicle in nontraffic accident

● **V02.1** Pedestrian injured in collision with two- or three-wheeled motor vehicle in traffic accident

X● **V02.10** Pedestrian on foot injured in collision with two- or three-wheeled motor vehicle in traffic accident

Pedestrian NOS injured in collision with two- or three-wheeled motor vehicle in traffic accident

X● **V02.11** Pedestrian on roller-skates injured in collision with two- or three-wheeled motor vehicle in traffic accident

X● **V02.12** Pedestrian on skateboard injured in collision with two- or three-wheeled motor vehicle in traffic accident

● **V02.13** Pedestrian on standing micro-mobility pedestrian conveyance injured in collision with two- or three-wheeled motor vehicle in traffic accident

V02.131 Pedestrian on standing electric scooter injured in collision with two- or three-wheeled motor vehicle in traffic accident

V02.138 Pedestrian on other standing micro-mobility pedestrian conveyance injured in collision with two- or three-wheeled motor vehicle in traffic accident

Pedestrian on hoverboard injured in collision with two-or three wheeled motor vehicle in traffic accident

Pedestrian on segway injured in collision with two- or three-wheeled motor vehicle in traffic accident

X● **V02.19** Pedestrian with other conveyance injured in collision with two- or three-wheeled motor vehicle in traffic accident

Pedestrian with baby stroller injured in collision with two- or three-wheeled motor vehicle in traffic accident

Pedestrian in wheelchair (powered) injured in collision with two- or three-wheeled motor vehicle in traffic accident

Pedestrian in motorized mobility scooter injured in collision with two- or three-wheeled motor vehicle in traffic accident

Pedestrian on ice-skates injured in collision with two- or three-wheeled motor vehicle in traffic accident

Pedestrian on nonmotorized scooter injured in collision with two- or three-wheeled motor vehicle in traffic accident

Pedestrian on sled injured in collision with two- or three-wheeled motor vehicle in traffic accident

Pedestrian on snowboard injured in collision with two- or three-wheeled motor vehicle in traffic accident

Pedestrian on snow-skis injured in collision with two- or three-wheeled motor vehicle in traffic accident

● **V02.9** Pedestrian injured in collision with two- or three-wheeled motor vehicle, unspecified whether traffic or nontraffic accident

X● **V02.90** Pedestrian on foot injured in collision with two- or three-wheeled motor vehicle, unspecified whether traffic or nontraffic accident

Pedestrian NOS injured in collision with two- or three-wheeled motor vehicle, unspecified whether traffic or nontraffic accident

X● **V02.91** Pedestrian on roller-skates injured in collision with two- or three-wheeled motor vehicle, unspecified whether traffic or nontraffic accident

X● **V02.92** Pedestrian on skateboard injured in collision with two- or three-wheeled motor vehicle, unspecified whether traffic or nontraffic accident

● **V02.93** Pedestrian on standing micro-mobility pedestrian conveyance injured in collision with two-or three-wheeled motor vehicle, unspecified whether traffic or nontraffic accident

V02.931 Pedestrian on standing electric scooter injured in collision with two- or three wheeled motor vehicle, unspecified whether traffic or nontraffic accident

V02.938 Pedestrian on other standing micro-mobility pedestrian conveyance injured in collision with two- or three wheeled motor vehicle, unspecified whether traffic or nontraffic accident

Pedestrian on hoverboard injured in collision with two-three-wheeled motor vehicle, unspecified whether traffic or nontraffic accident

Pedestrian on segway injured in collision with two- or three wheeled motor vehicle, unspecified whether traffic or nontraffic accident

X● **V02.99** Pedestrian with other conveyance injured in collision with two- or three-wheeled motor vehicle, unspecified whether traffic or nontraffic accident

Pedestrian with baby stroller injured in collision with two- or three-wheeled motor vehicle, unspecified whether traffic or nontraffic accident

Pedestrian in wheelchair (powered) injured in collision with two- or three-wheeled motor vehicle, unspecified whether traffic or nontraffic accident

Pedestrian in motorized mobility scooter injured in collision with two- or three-wheeled motor vehicle, unspecified whether traffic or nontraffic accident

Pedestrian on ice-skates injured in collision with two- or three-wheeled motor vehicle, unspecified whether traffic or nontraffic accident

Pedestrian on nonmotorized scooter injured in collision with two- or three-wheeled motor vehicle, unspecified whether traffic or nontraffic accident

Pedestrian on sled injured in collision with two- or three-wheeled motor vehicle, unspecified whether traffic or nontraffic accident

Pedestrian on snowboard injured in collision with two- or three-wheeled motor vehicle, unspecified whether traffic or nontraffic accident

Pedestrian on snow-skis injured in collision with two- or three-wheeled motor vehicle, unspecified whether traffic or nontraffic accident

▶ New   ⇒ Revised   ~~deleted~~ Deleted   Excludes 1   Excludes 2   Includes   Use additional   Code first   Code also   Key words

OGCR Official Guidelines   X Assign placeholder X   ● Use Additional Character(s)   ▶ Manifestation Code   🦠 Hierarchical Condition Category   **Coding Clinic**

● **V03** **Pedestrian injured in collision with car, pick-up truck or van**

> The appropriate 7th character is to be added to each code from category V03

> | | |
> |---|---|
> | A | initial encounter |
> | D | subsequent encounter |
> | S | sequela |

● **V03.0** **Pedestrian injured in collision with car, pick-up truck or van in** nontraffic accident

X ● **V03.00** **Pedestrian on foot injured in collision with car, pick-up truck or van in nontraffic accident**

> Pedestrian NOS injured in collision with car, pick-up truck or van in nontraffic accident

X ● **V03.01** **Pedestrian on roller-skates injured in collision with car, pick-up truck or van in nontraffic accident**

X ● **V03.02** **Pedestrian on skateboard injured in collision with car, pick-up truck or van in nontraffic accident**

● **V03.03** **Pedestrian on standing micro-mobility pedestrian conveyance injured in collision with car, pick-up or van in nontraffic accident**

V03.031 **Pedestrian on standing electric scooter injured in collision with car, pick-up or van in nontraffic accident**

V03.038 **Pedestrian on other standing micro-mobility pedestrian conveyance injured in collision with car, pick-up or van in nontraffic accident**

> Pedestrian on hoverboard injured in collision with car, pick-up or van in nontraffic accident
> Pedestrian on segway injured in collision with car, pick-up or van in nontraffic accident

X ● **V03.09** **Pedestrian with other conveyance injured in collision with car, pick-up truck or van in nontraffic accident**

> Pedestrian with baby stroller injured in collision with car, pick-up truck or van in nontraffic accident
> Pedestrian in wheelchair (powered) injured in collision with car, pick-up truck or van in nontraffic accident
> Pedestrian in motorized mobility scooter injured in collision with car, pick-up truck or van in nontraffic accident
> Pedestrian on ice-skates injured in collision with car, pick-up truck or van in nontraffic accident
> Pedestrian on nonmotorized scooter injured in collision with car, pick-up truck or van in nontraffic accident
> Pedestrian on sled injured in collision with car, pick-up truck or van in nontraffic accident
> Pedestrian on snowboard injured in collision with car, pick-up truck or van in nontraffic accident
> Pedestrian on snow-skis injured in collision with car, pick-up truck or van in nontraffic accident

● **V03.1** **Pedestrian injured in collision with car, pick-up truck or van in** traffic accident

X ● **V03.10** **Pedestrian on foot injured in collision with car, pick-up truck or van in traffic accident**

> Pedestrian NOS injured in collision with car, pick-up truck or van in traffic accident

X ● **V03.11** **Pedestrian on roller-skates injured in collision with car, pick-up truck or van in traffic accident**

X ● **V03.12** **Pedestrian on skateboard injured in collision with car, pick-up truck or van in traffic accident**

● **V03.13** **Pedestrian on standing micro-mobility pedestrian conveyance injured in collision with car, pick-up or van in traffic accident**

V03.131 **Pedestrian on standing electric scooter injured in collision with car, pick-up or van in traffic accident**

V03.138 **Pedestrian on other standing micro-mobility pedestrian conveyance injured in collision with car, pick-up or van in traffic accident**

> Pedestrian on hoverboard injured in collision with car, pick-up or van in traffic accident
> Pedestrian on segway injured in collision with car, pick-up or van in traffic accident

X ● **V03.19** **Pedestrian with other conveyance injured in collision with car, pick-up truck or van in traffic accident**

> Pedestrian with baby stroller injured in collision with car, pick-up truck or van in traffic accident
> Pedestrian in wheelchair (powered) injured in collision with car, pick-up truck or van in traffic accident
> Pedestrian in motorized mobility scooter injured in collision with car, pick-up truck or van in traffic accident
> Pedestrian on ice-skates injured in collision with car, pick-up truck or van in traffic accident
> Pedestrian on nonmotorized scooter injured in collision with car, pick-up truck or van in traffic accident
> Pedestrian on sled injured in collision with car, pick-up truck or van in traffic accident
> Pedestrian on snowboard injured in collision with car, pick-up truck or van in traffic accident
> Pedestrian on snow-skis injured in collision with car, pick-up truck or van in traffic accident

● **V03.9** **Pedestrian injured in collision with car, pick-up truck or van, unspecified whether traffic or nontraffic accident**

X ● **V03.90** **Pedestrian on foot injured in collision with car, pick-up truck or van, unspecified whether traffic or nontraffic accident**

> Pedestrian NOS injured in collision with car, pick-up truck or van, unspecified whether traffic or nontraffic accident

X ● **V03.91** **Pedestrian on roller-skates injured in collision with car, pick-up truck or van, unspecified whether traffic or nontraffic accident**

X ● **V03.92** **Pedestrian on skateboard injured in collision with car, pick-up truck or van, unspecified whether traffic or nontraffic accident**

● **V03.93** **Pedestrian on standing micro-mobility pedestrian conveyance injured in collision with car, pick-up or van, unspecified whether traffic or nontraffic accident**

V03.931 **Pedestrian on standing electric scooter injured in collision with car, pick-up or van, unspecified whether traffic or nontraffic accident**

V03.938 **Pedestrian on other standing micro-mobility pedestrian conveyance injured in collision with car, pick-up or van, unspecified whether traffic or nontraffic accident**

> Pedestrian on hoverboard injured in collision with car, pick-up or van, unspecified whether traffic or nontraffic accident
> Pedestrian on segway injured in collision with car, pick-up or van, unspecified whether traffic or nontraffic accident

X● **V03.99** Pedestrian with other conveyance injured in collision with car, pick-up truck or van, unspecified whether traffic or nontraffic accident

Pedestrian with baby stroller injured in collision with car, pick-up truck or van, unspecified whether traffic or nontraffic accident

Pedestrian in wheelchair (powered) injured in collision with car, pick-up truck or van, unspecified whether traffic or nontraffic accident

Pedestrian in motorized mobility scooter injured in collision with car, pick-up truck or van, unspecified whether traffic or nontraffic accident

Pedestrian on ice-skates injured in collision with car, pick-up truck or van, unspecified whether traffic or nontraffic accident

Pedestrian on nonmotorized scooter injured in collision with car, pick-up truck or van, unspecified whether traffic or nontraffic accident

Pedestrian on sled injured in collision with car, pick-up truck or van in nontraffic accident

Pedestrian on snowboard injured in collision with car, pick-up truck or van, unspecified whether traffic or nontraffic accident

Pedestrian on snow-skis injured in collision with car, pick-up truck or van, unspecified whether traffic or nontraffic accident

● **V04** Pedestrian injured in collision with heavy transport vehicle or bus

> **Excludes1** pedestrian injured in collision with military vehicle (V09.01, V09.21)

The appropriate 7th character is to be added to each code from category V04

> A initial encounter
> D subsequent encounter
> S sequela

● **V04.0** Pedestrian injured in collision with heavy transport vehicle or bus in nontraffic accident

X● **V04.00** Pedestrian on foot injured in collision with heavy transport vehicle or bus in nontraffic accident

Pedestrian NOS injured in collision with heavy transport vehicle or bus in nontraffic accident

X● **V04.01** Pedestrian on roller-skates injured in collision with heavy transport vehicle or bus in nontraffic accident

X● **V04.02** Pedestrian on skateboard injured in collision with heavy transport vehicle or bus in nontraffic accident

● **V04.03** Pedestrian on standing micro-mobility pedestrian conveyance injured in collision with heavy transport vehicle or bus in nontraffic accident

V04.031 Pedestrian on standing electric scooter injured in collision with heavy transport vehicle or bus in nontraffic accident

V04.038 Pedestrian on other standing micro-mobility pedestrian conveyance injured in collision with heavy transport vehicle or bus in nontraffic accident

Pedestrian on hoverboard injured in collision with heavy transport vehicle or bus in nontraffic accident

Pedestrian on segway injured in collision with heavy transport vehicle or bus in nontraffic accident

X● **V04.09** Pedestrian with other conveyance injured in collision with heavy transport vehicle or bus in nontraffic accident

Pedestrian with baby stroller injured in collision with heavy transport vehicle or bus in nontraffic accident

Pedestrian in wheelchair (powered) injured in collision with heavy transport vehicle or bus in nontraffic accident

Pedestrian in motorized mobility scooter injured in collision with heavy transport vehicle or bus in nontraffic accident

Pedestrian on ice-skates injured in collision with heavy transport vehicle or bus in nontraffic accident

Pedestrian on nonmotorized scooter injured in collision with heavy transport vehicle or bus in nontraffic accident

Pedestrian on sled injured in collision with heavy transport vehicle or bus in nontraffic accident

Pedestrian on snowboard injured in collision with heavy transport vehicle or bus in nontraffic accident

Pedestrian on snow-skis injured in collision with heavy transport vehicle or bus in nontraffic accident

● **V04.1** Pedestrian injured in collision with heavy transport vehicle or bus in traffic accident

X● **V04.10** Pedestrian on foot injured in collision with heavy transport vehicle or bus in traffic accident

Pedestrian NOS injured in collision with heavy transport vehicle or bus in traffic accident

X● **V04.11** Pedestrian on roller-skates injured in collision with heavy transport vehicle or bus in traffic accident

X● **V04.12** Pedestrian on skateboard injured in collision with heavy transport vehicle or bus in traffic accident

● **V04.13** Pedestrian on standing micro-mobility pedestrian conveyance injured in collision with heavy transport vehicle or bus in traffic accident

V04.131 Pedestrian on standing electric scooter injured in collision with heavy transport vehicle or bus in traffic accident

V04.138 Pedestrian on other standing micro-mobility pedestrian conveyance injured in collision with heavy transport vehicle or bus in traffic accident

Pedestrian on hoverboard injured in collision with heavy transport vehicle or bus in traffic accident

Pedestrian on segway injured in collision with heavy transport vehicle or bus in traffic accident

▶ New　🡆 Revised　deleted Deleted　Excludes 1　Excludes 2　Includes　Use additional　Code first　Code also　Key words

OGCR Official Guidelines　X Assign placeholder X　● Use Additional Character(s)　▸ Manifestation Code　🝔 Hierarchical Condition Category　**Coding Clinic**

X ● **V04.19** **Pedestrian with other conveyance injured in collision with heavy transport vehicle or bus in traffic accident**

Pedestrian with baby stroller injured in collision with heavy transport vehicle or bus in traffic accident

Pedestrian in wheelchair (powered) injured in collision with heavy transport vehicle or bus in traffic accident

Pedestrian in motorized mobility scooter injured in collision with heavy transport vehicle or bus in traffic accident

Pedestrian on ice-skates injured in collision with heavy transport vehicle or bus in traffic accident

Pedestrian on nonmotorized scooter injured in collision with heavy transport vehicle or bus in traffic accident

Pedestrian on sled injured in collision with heavy transport vehicle or bus in traffic accident

Pedestrian on snowboard injured in collision with heavy transport vehicle or bus in traffic accident

Pedestrian on snow-skis injured in collision with heavy transport vehicle or bus in traffic accident

● **V04.9** **Pedestrian injured in collision with heavy transport vehicle or bus, unspecified whether traffic or nontraffic accident**

X ● **V04.90** **Pedestrian on foot injured in collision with heavy transport vehicle or bus, unspecified whether traffic or nontraffic accident**

Pedestrian NOS injured in collision with heavy transport vehicle or bus, unspecified whether traffic or nontraffic accident

X ● **V04.91** **Pedestrian on roller-skates injured in collision with heavy transport vehicle or bus, unspecified whether traffic or nontraffic accident**

X ● **V04.92** **Pedestrian on skateboard injured in collision with heavy transport vehicle or bus, unspecified whether traffic or nontraffic accident**

● **V04.93** **Pedestrian on standing micro-mobility pedestrian conveyance injured in collision with heavy transport vehicle or bus, unspecified whether traffic or nontraffic accident**

V04.931 **Pedestrian on standing electric scooter injured in collision with heavy transport vehicle or bus, unspecified whether traffic or nontraffic accident**

V04.938 **Pedestrian on other standing micro-mobility pedestrian conveyance injured in collision with heavy transport vehicle or bus, unspecified whether traffic or nontraffic accident**

Pedestrian on hoverboard injured in collision with heavy transport vehicle or bus, unspecified whether traffic or nontraffic accident

Pedestrian on segway injured in collision with heavy transport vehicle or bus, unspecified whether traffic or nontraffic accident

X ● **V04.99** **Pedestrian with other conveyance injured in collision with heavy transport vehicle or bus, unspecified whether traffic or nontraffic accident**

Pedestrian with baby stroller injured in collision with heavy transport vehicle or bus, unspecified whether traffic or nontraffic accident

Pedestrian in wheelchair (powered) injured in collision with heavy transport vehicle or bus, unspecified whether traffic or nontraffic accident

Pedestrian in motorized mobility scooter injured in collision with heavy transport vehicle or bus, unspecified whether traffic or nontraffic accident

Pedestrian on ice-skates injured in collision with heavy transport vehicle or bus, unspecified whether traffic or nontraffic accident

Pedestrian on nonmotorized scooter injured in collision with heavy transport vehicle or bus, unspecified whether traffic or nontraffic accident

Pedestrian on sled injured in collision with heavy transport vehicle or bus, unspecified whether traffic or nontraffic accident

Pedestrian on snowboard injured in collision with heavy transport vehicle or bus, unspecified whether traffic or nontraffic accident

Pedestrian on snow-skis injured in collision with heavy transport vehicle or bus, unspecified whether traffic or nontraffic accident

● **V05** **Pedestrian injured in collision with railway train or railway vehicle**

The appropriate 7th character is to be added to each code from category V05

A	initial encounter
D	subsequent encounter
S	sequela

● **V05.0** **Pedestrian injured in collision with railway train or railway vehicle in nontraffic accident**

X ● **V05.00** **Pedestrian on foot injured in collision with railway train or railway vehicle in nontraffic accident**

Pedestrian NOS injured in collision with railway train or railway vehicle in nontraffic accident

X ● **V05.01** **Pedestrian on roller-skates injured in collision with railway train or railway vehicle in nontraffic accident**

X ● **V05.02** **Pedestrian on skateboard injured in collision with railway train or railway vehicle in nontraffic accident**

● **V05.03** **Pedestrian on standing micro-mobility pedestrian conveyance injured in collision with railway train or railway vehicle in nontraffic accident**

V05.031 **Pedestrian on standing electric scooter injured in collision with railway train or railway vehicle in nontraffic accident**

V05.038 **Pedestrian on other standing micro-mobility pedestrian conveyance injured in collision with railway train or railway vehicle in nontraffic accident**

Pedestrian on hoverboard injured in collision with railway train or railway vehicle in nontraffic accident

Pedestrian on segway injured in collision with railway train or railway vehicle in nontraffic accident

X ● **V05.09** **Pedestrian with other conveyance injured in collision with railway train or railway vehicle in nontraffic accident**
　　Pedestrian with baby stroller injured in collision with railway train or railway vehicle in nontraffic accident
　　Pedestrian in wheelchair (powered) injured in collision with railway train or railway vehicle in nontraffic accident
　　Pedestrian in motorized mobility scooter injured in collision with railway train or railway vehicle in nontraffic accident
　　Pedestrian on ice-skates injured in collision with railway train or railway vehicle in nontraffic accident
　　Pedestrian on nonmotorized scooter injured in collision with railway train or railway vehicle in nontraffic accident
　　Pedestrian on sled injured in collision with railway train or railway vehicle in nontraffic accident
　　Pedestrian on snowboard injured in collision with railway train or railway vehicle in nontraffic accident
　　Pedestrian on snow-skis injured in collision with railway train or railway vehicle in nontraffic accident

● **V05.1** **Pedestrian injured in collision with railway train or railway vehicle in traffic accident**

X ● **V05.10** **Pedestrian on foot injured in collision with railway train or railway vehicle in traffic accident**
　　Pedestrian NOS injured in collision with railway train or railway vehicle in traffic accident

X ● **V05.11** **Pedestrian on roller-skates injured in collision with railway train or railway vehicle in traffic accident**

X ● **V05.12** **Pedestrian on skateboard injured in collision with railway train or railway vehicle in traffic accident**

● **V05.13** **Pedestrian on standing micro-mobility pedestrian conveyance injured in collision with railway train or railway vehicle in traffic accident**

　　V05.131 **Pedestrian on standing electric scooter injured in collision with railway train or railway vehicle in traffic accident**

　　V05.138 **Pedestrian on other standing micro-mobility pedestrian conveyance injured in collision with railway train or railway vehicle in traffic accident**
　　　　Pedestrian on hoverboard injured in collision with railway train or railway vehicle in traffic accident
　　　　Pedestrian on segway injured in collision with railway train or railway vehicle in traffic accident

X ● **V05.19** **Pedestrian with other conveyance injured in collision with railway train or railway vehicle in traffic accident**
　　Pedestrian with baby stroller injured in collision with railway train or railway vehicle in traffic accident
　　Pedestrian in wheelchair (powered) injured in collision with railway train or railway vehicle in traffic accident
　　Pedestrian in motorized mobility scooter injured in collision with railway train or railway vehicle in traffic accident
　　Pedestrian on ice-skates injured in collision with railway train or railway vehicle in traffic accident
　　Pedestrian on nonmotorized scooter injured in collision with railway train or railway vehicle in traffic accident
　　Pedestrian on sled injured in collision with railway train or railway vehicle in traffic accident
　　Pedestrian on snowboard injured in collision with railway train or railway vehicle in traffic accident
　　Pedestrian on snow-skis injured in collision with railway train or railway vehicle in traffic accident

● **V05.9** **Pedestrian injured in collision with railway train or railway vehicle, unspecified whether traffic or nontraffic accident**

X ● **V05.90** **Pedestrian on foot injured in collision with railway train or railway vehicle, unspecified whether traffic or nontraffic accident**
　　Pedestrian NOS injured in collision with railway train or railway vehicle, unspecified whether traffic or nontraffic accident

X ● **V05.91** **Pedestrian on roller-skates injured in collision with railway train or railway vehicle, unspecified whether traffic or nontraffic accident**

X ● **V05.92** **Pedestrian on skateboard injured in collision with railway train or railway vehicle, unspecified whether traffic or nontraffic accident**

● **V05.93** **Pedestrian on standing micro-mobility pedestrian conveyance injured in collision with railway train or railway vehicle, unspecified whether traffic or nontraffic accident**

　　V05.931 **Pedestrian on standing electric scooter injured in collision with railway train or railway vehicle, unspecified whether traffic or nontraffic accident**

　　V05.938 **Pedestrian on other standing micro-mobility pedestrian conveyance injured in collision with railway train or railway vehicle, unspecified whether traffic or nontraffic accident**
　　　　Pedestrian on hoverboard injured in collision with railway train or railway vehicle, unspecified whether traffic or nontraffic accident
　　　　Pedestrian on segway injured in collision with railway train or railway vehicle, unspecified whether traffic or nontraffic accident

X ● **V05.99 Pedestrian with other conveyance injured in collision with railway train or railway vehicle, unspecified whether traffic or nontraffic accident**

> Pedestrian with baby stroller injured in collision with railway train or railway vehicle, unspecified whether traffic or nontraffic
>
> Pedestrian in wheelchair (powered) injured in collision with railway train or railway vehicle, unspecified whether traffic or nontraffic
>
> Pedestrian in motorized mobility scooter injured in collision with railway train or railway vehicle, unspecified whether traffic or nontraffic
>
> Pedestrian on ice-skates injured in collision with railway train or railway vehicle, unspecified whether traffic or nontraffic
>
> Pedestrian on nonmotorized scooter injured in collision with railway train or railway vehicle, unspecified whether traffic or nontraffic
>
> Pedestrian on sled injured in collision with railway train or railway vehicle, unspecified whether traffic or nontraffic
>
> Pedestrian on snowboard injured in collision with railway train or railway vehicle, unspecified whether traffic or nontraffic
>
> Pedestrian on snow-skis injured in collision with railway train or railway vehicle, unspecified whether traffic or nontraffic

● **V06 Pedestrian injured in collision with other nonmotor vehicle**

| **Includes** | collision with animal-drawn vehicle, animal being ridden, nonpowered streetcar |
| **Excludes1** | pedestrian injured in collision with pedestrian conveyance (V00.0-) |

The appropriate 7th character is to be added to each code from category V06

> A   initial encounter
> D   subsequent encounter
> S   sequela

● **V06.0 Pedestrian injured in collision with other nonmotor vehicle in nontraffic accident**

X ● **V06.00 Pedestrian on foot injured in collision with other nonmotor vehicle in nontraffic accident**

> Pedestrian NOS injured in collision with other nonmotor vehicle in nontraffic accident

X ● **V06.01 Pedestrian on roller-skates injured in collision with other nonmotor vehicle in nontraffic accident**

X ● **V06.02 Pedestrian on skateboard injured in collision with other nonmotor vehicle in nontraffic accident**

● **V06.03 Pedestrian on standing micro-mobility pedestrian conveyance injured in collision with other nonmotor vehicle in nontraffic accident**

> **V06.031 Pedestrian on standing electric scooter injured in collision with other nonmotor vehicle in nontraffic accident**
>
> **V06.038 Pedestrian on other standing micro-mobility pedestrian conveyance injured in collision with other nonmotor vehicle in nontraffic accident**
>
>> Pedestrian on hoverboard injured in collision with other nonmotor vehicle in nontraffic accident
>>
>> Pedestrian on segway injured in collision with other nonmotor vehicle in nontraffic accident

X ● **V06.09 Pedestrian with other conveyance injured in collision with other nonmotor vehicle in nontraffic accident**

> Pedestrian with baby stroller injured in collision with other nonmotor vehicle in nontraffic accident
>
> Pedestrian in wheelchair (powered) injured in collision with other nonmotor vehicle in nontraffic accident
>
> Pedestrian in motorized mobility scooter injured in collision with other nonmotor vehicle in nontraffic accident
>
> Pedestrian on ice-skates injured in collision with other nonmotor vehicle in nontraffic accident
>
> Pedestrian on nonmotorized scooter injured in collision with other nonmotor vehicle in nontraffic accident
>
> Pedestrian on sled injured in collision with other nonmotor vehicle in nontraffic accident
>
> Pedestrian on snowboard injured in collision with other nonmotor vehicle in nontraffic accident
>
> Pedestrian on snow-skis injured in collision with other nonmotor vehicle in nontraffic accident

● **V06.1 Pedestrian injured in collision with other nonmotor vehicle in traffic accident**

X ● **V06.10 Pedestrian on foot injured in collision with other nonmotor vehicle in traffic accident**

> Pedestrian NOS injured in collision with other nonmotor vehicle in traffic accident

X ● **V06.11 Pedestrian on roller-skates injured in collision with other nonmotor vehicle in traffic accident**

X ● **V06.12 Pedestrian on skateboard injured in collision with other nonmotor vehicle in traffic accident**

● **V06.13 Pedestrian on standing micro-mobility pedestrian conveyance injured in collision with other nonmotor vehicle in traffic accident**

> **V06.131 Pedestrian on standing electric scooter injured in collision with other nonmotor vehicle in traffic accident**
>
> **V06.138 Pedestrian on other standing micro-mobility pedestrian conveyance injured in collision with other nonmotor vehicle in traffic accident**
>
>> Pedestrian on hoverboard injured in collision with other nonmotor vehicle in traffic accident
>>
>> Pedestrian on segway injured in collision with other nonmotor vehicle in traffic accident

X ● **V06.19 Pedestrian with other conveyance injured in collision with other nonmotor vehicle in traffic accident**

> Pedestrian with baby stroller injured in collision with other nonmotor vehicle in nontraffic accident
>
> Pedestrian in wheelchair (powered) injured in collision with other nonmotor vehicle in traffic accident
>
> Pedestrian in motorized mobility scooter injured in collision with other nonmotor vehicle in traffic accident
>
> Pedestrian on ice-skates injured in collision with other nonmotor vehicle in traffic accident
>
> Pedestrian on nonmotorized scooter injured in collision with other nonmotor vehicle in traffic accident
>
> Pedestrian on sled injured in collision with other nonmotor vehicle in traffic accident
>
> Pedestrian on snowboard injured in collision with other nonmotor vehicle in traffic accident
>
> Pedestrian on snow-skis injured in collision with other nonmotor vehicle in traffic accident

CHAPTER 20 (V00-Y99)

- ● V06.9 **Pedestrian injured in collision with other nonmotor vehicle, unspecified whether traffic or nontraffic accident**

X ● V06.90 **Pedestrian on foot injured in collision with other nonmotor vehicle, unspecified whether traffic or nontraffic accident**
   Pedestrian NOS injured in collision with other nonmotor vehicle, unspecified whether traffic or nontraffic accident

X ● V06.91 **Pedestrian on roller-skates injured in collision with other nonmotor vehicle, unspecified whether traffic or nontraffic accident**

X ● V06.92 **Pedestrian on skateboard injured in collision with other nonmotor vehicle, unspecified whether traffic or nontraffic accident**

● V06.93 **Pedestrian on standing micro-mobility pedestrian conveyance injured in collision with other nonmotor vehicle, unspecified whether traffic or nontraffic accident**

   V06.931 **Pedestrian on standing electric scooter injured in collision with other nonmotor vehicle, unspecified whether traffic or nontraffic accident**

   V06.938 **Pedestrian on other standing micro-mobility pedestrian conveyance injured in collision with other nonmotor vehicle, unspecified whether traffic or nontraffic accident**
      Pedestrian on hoverboard injured in collision with other nonmotor, unspecified whether traffic or nontraffic accident
      Pedestrian on segway injured in collision with other nonmotor vehicle, unspecified whether traffic or nontraffic accident

X ● V06.99 **Pedestrian with other conveyance injured in collision with other nonmotor vehicle, unspecified whether traffic or nontraffic accident**
      Pedestrian with baby stroller injured in collision with other nonmotor vehicle, unspecified whether traffic or nontraffic accident
      Pedestrian in wheelchair (powered) injured in collision with other nonmotor vehicle, unspecified whether traffic or nontraffic accident
      Pedestrian in motorized mobility scooter injured in collision with other nonmotor vehicle, unspecified whether traffic or nontraffic accident
      Pedestrian on ice-skates injured in collision with other nonmotor vehicle, unspecified whether traffic or nontraffic accident
      Pedestrian on nonmotorized scooter injured in collision with other nonmotor vehicle, unspecified whether traffic or nontraffic accident
      Pedestrian on sled injured in collision with other nonmotor vehicle, unspecified whether traffic or nontraffic accident
      Pedestrian on snowboard injured in collision with other nonmotor vehicle, unspecified whether traffic or nontraffic accident
      Pedestrian on snow-skis injured in collision with other nonmotor vehicle, unspecified whether traffic or nontraffic accident

- ● V09 **Pedestrian injured in other and unspecified transport accidents**
   The appropriate 7th character is to be added to each code from category V09

A	initial encounter
D	subsequent encounter
S	sequela

● V09.0 **Pedestrian injured in nontraffic accident involving other and unspecified motor vehicles**

X ● V09.00 **Pedestrian injured in nontraffic accident involving unspecified motor vehicles**

X ● V09.01 **Pedestrian injured in nontraffic accident involving military vehicle**

X ● V09.09 **Pedestrian injured in nontraffic accident involving other motor vehicles**
   Pedestrian injured in nontraffic accident by special vehicle

X ● V09.1 **Pedestrian injured in unspecified nontraffic accident**

● V09.2 **Pedestrian injured in traffic accident involving other and unspecified motor vehicles**

X ● V09.20 **Pedestrian injured in traffic accident involving unspecified motor vehicles**

X ● V09.21 **Pedestrian injured in traffic accident involving military vehicle**

X ● V09.29 **Pedestrian injured in traffic accident involving other motor vehicles**

X ● V09.3 **Pedestrian injured in unspecified traffic accident**

X ● V09.9 **Pedestrian injured in unspecified transport accident**

PEDAL CYCLE RIDER INJURED IN TRANSPORT ACCIDENT (V10-V19)

Includes any non-motorized vehicle, excluding an animal-drawn vehicle, or a sidecar or trailer attached to the pedal cycle

Excludes2 rupture of pedal cycle tire (W37.0)

● V10 **Pedal cycle rider injured in collision with pedestrian or animal**
   Excludes1 pedal cycle rider collision with animal-drawn vehicle or animal being ridden (V16.-)
   The appropriate 7th character is to be added to each code from category V10

A	initial encounter
D	subsequent encounter
S	sequela

X ● V10.0 **Pedal cycle driver injured in collision with pedestrian or animal in nontraffic accident**

X ● V10.1 **Pedal cycle passenger injured in collision with pedestrian or animal in nontraffic accident**

X ● V10.2 **Unspecified pedal cyclist injured in collision with pedestrian or animal in nontraffic accident**

X ● V10.3 **Person boarding or alighting a pedal cycle injured in collision with pedestrian or animal**

X ● V10.4 **Pedal cycle driver injured in collision with pedestrian or animal in traffic accident**

X ● V10.5 **Pedal cycle passenger injured in collision with pedestrian or animal in traffic accident**

X ● V10.9 **Unspecified pedal cyclist injured in collision with pedestrian or animal in traffic accident**

▶ New   ⇒ Revised   ~~deleted~~ Deleted   Excludes 1   Excludes 2   Includes   Use additional   Code first   Code also   Key words

OGCR Official Guidelines   X Assign placeholder X   ● Use Additional Character(s)   ▷ Manifestation Code   ⬤ Hierarchical Condition Category   **Coding Clinic**

● **V11**   **Pedal cycle rider injured in collision with other pedal cycle**

The appropriate 7th character is to be added to each code from category V11

> A   initial encounter
> D   subsequent encounter
> S   sequela

X● **V11.0**   Pedal cycle driver injured in collision with other pedal cycle in nontraffic accident

X● **V11.1**   Pedal cycle passenger injured in collision with other pedal cycle in nontraffic accident

X● **V11.2**   Unspecified pedal cyclist injured in collision with other pedal cycle in nontraffic accident

X● **V11.3**   Person boarding or alighting a pedal cycle injured in collision with other pedal cycle

X● **V11.4**   Pedal cycle driver injured in collision with other pedal cycle in traffic accident

X● **V11.5**   Pedal cycle passenger injured in collision with other pedal cycle in traffic accident

X● **V11.9**   Unspecified pedal cyclist injured in collision with other pedal cycle in traffic accident

● **V12**   **Pedal cycle rider injured in collision with two- or three-wheeled motor vehicle**

The appropriate 7th character is to be added to each code from category V12

> A   initial encounter
> D   subsequent encounter
> S   sequela

X● **V12.0**   Pedal cycle driver injured in collision with two- or three-wheeled motor vehicle in nontraffic accident

X● **V12.1**   Pedal cycle passenger injured in collision with two- or three-wheeled motor vehicle in nontraffic accident

X● **V12.2**   Unspecified pedal cyclist injured in collision with two- or three-wheeled motor vehicle in nontraffic accident

X● **V12.3**   Person boarding or alighting a pedal cycle injured in collision with two- or three-wheeled motor vehicle

X● **V12.4**   Pedal cycle driver injured in collision with two- or three-wheeled motor vehicle in traffic accident

X● **V12.5**   Pedal cycle passenger injured in collision with two- or three-wheeled motor vehicle in traffic accident

X● **V12.9**   Unspecified pedal cyclist injured in collision with two- or three-wheeled motor vehicle in traffic accident

● **V13**   **Pedal cycle rider injured in collision with car, pick-up truck or van**

The appropriate 7th character is to be added to each code from category V13

> A   initial encounter
> D   subsequent encounter
> S   sequela

X● **V13.0**   Pedal cycle driver injured in collision with car, pick-up truck or van in nontraffic accident

X● **V13.1**   Pedal cycle passenger injured in collision with car, pick-up truck or van in nontraffic accident

X● **V13.2**   Unspecified pedal cyclist injured in collision with car, pick-up truck or van in nontraffic accident

X● **V13.3**   Person boarding or alighting a pedal cycle injured in collision with car, pick-up truck or van

X● **V13.4**   Pedal cycle driver injured in collision with car, pick-up truck or van in traffic accident

X● **V13.5**   Pedal cycle passenger injured in collision with car, pick-up truck or van in traffic accident

X● **V13.9**   Unspecified pedal cyclist injured in collision with car, pick-up truck or van in traffic accident

● **V14**   **Pedal cycle rider injured in collision with heavy transport vehicle or bus**

> **Excludes1**   pedal cycle rider injured in collision with military vehicle (V19.81)

The appropriate 7th character is to be added to each code from category V14

> A   initial encounter
> D   subsequent encounter
> S   sequela

X● **V14.0**   Pedal cycle driver injured in collision with heavy transport vehicle or bus in nontraffic accident

X● **V14.1**   Pedal cycle passenger injured in collision with heavy transport vehicle or bus in nontraffic accident

X● **V14.2**   Unspecified pedal cyclist injured in collision with heavy transport vehicle or bus in nontraffic accident

X● **V14.3**   Person boarding or alighting a pedal cycle injured in collision with heavy transport vehicle or bus

X● **V14.4**   Pedal cycle driver injured in collision with heavy transport vehicle or bus in traffic accident

X● **V14.5**   Pedal cycle passenger injured in collision with heavy transport vehicle or bus in traffic accident

X● **V14.9**   Unspecified pedal cyclist injured in collision with heavy transport vehicle or bus in traffic accident

● **V15**   **Pedal cycle rider injured in collision with railway train or railway vehicle**

The appropriate 7th character is to be added to each code from category V15

> A   initial encounter
> D   subsequent encounter
> S   sequela

X● **V15.0**   Pedal cycle driver injured in collision with railway train or railway vehicle in nontraffic accident

X● **V15.1**   Pedal cycle passenger injured in collision with railway train or railway vehicle in nontraffic accident

X● **V15.2**   Unspecified pedal cyclist injured in collision with railway train or railway vehicle in nontraffic accident

X● **V15.3**   Person boarding or alighting a pedal cycle injured in collision with railway train or railway vehicle

X● **V15.4**   Pedal cycle driver injured in collision with railway train or railway vehicle in traffic accident

X● **V15.5**   Pedal cycle passenger injured in collision with railway train or railway vehicle in traffic accident

X● **V15.9**   Unspecified pedal cyclist injured in collision with railway train or railway vehicle in traffic accident

● **V16**   **Pedal cycle rider injured in collision with other nonmotor vehicle**

> **Includes**   collision with animal-drawn vehicle, animal being ridden, streetcar

The appropriate 7th character is to be added to each code from category V16

> A   initial encounter
> D   subsequent encounter
> S   sequela

X● **V16.0**   Pedal cycle driver injured in collision with other nonmotor vehicle in nontraffic accident

X● **V16.1**   Pedal cycle passenger injured in collision with other nonmotor vehicle in nontraffic accident

X● **V16.2**   Unspecified pedal cyclist injured in collision with other nonmotor vehicle in nontraffic accident

X● **V16.3**   Person boarding or alighting a pedal cycle injured in collision with other nonmotor vehicle in nontraffic accident

X● **V16.4**   Pedal cycle driver injured in collision with other nonmotor vehicle in traffic accident

CHAPTER 20 (V00-Y99)

X ● **V16.5** Pedal cycle passenger injured in collision with other nonmotor vehicle in traffic accident

X ● **V16.9** Unspecified pedal cyclist injured in collision with other nonmotor vehicle in traffic accident

● **V17** Pedal cycle rider injured in collision with fixed or stationary object

The appropriate 7th character is to be added to each code from category V17

A	initial encounter
D	subsequent encounter
S	sequela

X ● **V17.0** Pedal cycle driver injured in collision with fixed or stationary object in nontraffic accident

X ● **V17.1** Pedal cycle passenger injured in collision with fixed or stationary object in nontraffic accident

X ● **V17.2** Unspecified pedal cyclist injured in collision with fixed or stationary object in nontraffic accident

X ● **V17.3** Person boarding or alighting a pedal cycle injured in collision with fixed or stationary object

X ● **V17.4** Pedal cycle driver injured in collision with fixed or stationary object in traffic accident

X ● **V17.5** Pedal cycle passenger injured in collision with fixed or stationary object in traffic accident

X ● **V17.9** Unspecified pedal cyclist injured in collision with fixed or stationary object in traffic accident

● **V18** Pedal cycle rider injured in noncollision transport accident

Includes fall or thrown from pedal cycle (without antecedent collision)
overturning pedal cycle NOS
overturning pedal cycle without collision

The appropriate 7th character is to be added to each code from category V18

A	initial encounter
D	subsequent encounter
S	sequela

X ● **V18.0** Pedal cycle driver injured in noncollision transport accident in nontraffic accident

X ● **V18.1** Pedal cycle passenger injured in noncollision transport accident in nontraffic accident

X ● **V18.2** Unspecified pedal cyclist injured in noncollision transport accident in nontraffic accident

X ● **V18.3** Person boarding or alighting a pedal cycle injured in noncollision transport accident

X ● **V18.4** Pedal cycle driver injured in noncollision transport accident in traffic accident

X ● **V18.5** Pedal cycle passenger injured in noncollision transport accident in traffic accident

X ● **V18.9** Unspecified pedal cyclist injured in noncollision transport accident in traffic accident

● **V19** Pedal cycle rider injured in other and unspecified transport accidents

The appropriate 7th character is to be added to each code from category V19

A	initial encounter
D	subsequent encounter
S	sequela

● **V19.0** Pedal cycle driver injured in collision with other and unspecified motor vehicles in nontraffic accident

X ● **V19.00** Pedal cycle driver injured in collision with unspecified motor vehicles in nontraffic accident

X ● **V19.09** Pedal cycle driver injured in collision with other motor vehicles in nontraffic accident

● **V19.1** Pedal cycle passenger injured in collision with other and unspecified motor vehicles in nontraffic accident

X ● **V19.10** Pedal cycle passenger injured in collision with unspecified motor vehicles in nontraffic accident

X ● **V19.19** Pedal cycle passenger injured in collision with other motor vehicles in nontraffic accident

● **V19.2** Unspecified pedal cyclist injured in collision with other and unspecified motor vehicles in nontraffic accident

X ● **V19.20** Unspecified pedal cyclist injured in collision with unspecified motor vehicles in nontraffic accident
Pedal cycle collision NOS, nontraffic

X ● **V19.29** Unspecified pedal cyclist injured in collision with other motor vehicles in nontraffic accident

X ● **V19.3** Pedal cyclist (driver) (passenger) injured in unspecified nontraffic accident
Pedal cycle accident NOS, nontraffic
Pedal cyclist injured in nontraffic accident NOS

● **V19.4** Pedal cycle driver injured in collision with other and unspecified motor vehicles in traffic accident

X ● **V19.40** Pedal cycle driver injured in collision with unspecified motor vehicles in traffic accident

X ● **V19.49** Pedal cycle driver injured in collision with other motor vehicles in traffic accident

● **V19.5** Pedal cycle passenger injured in collision with other and unspecified motor vehicles in traffic accident

X ● **V19.50** Pedal cycle passenger injured in collision with unspecified motor vehicles in traffic accident

X ● **V19.59** Pedal cycle passenger injured in collision with other motor vehicles in traffic accident

● **V19.6** Unspecified pedal cyclist injured in collision with other and unspecified motor vehicles in traffic accident

X ● **V19.60** Unspecified pedal cyclist injured in collision with unspecified motor vehicles in traffic accident
Pedal cycle collision NOS (traffic)

X ● **V19.69** Unspecified pedal cyclist injured in collision with other motor vehicles in traffic accident

● **V19.8** Pedal cyclist (driver) (passenger) injured in other specified transport accidents

X ● **V19.81** Pedal cyclist (driver) (passenger) injured in transport accident with military vehicle

X ● **V19.88** Pedal cyclist (driver) (passenger) injured in other specified transport accidents

X ● **V19.9** Pedal cyclist (driver) (passenger) injured in unspecified traffic accident
Pedal cycle accident NOS

MOTORCYCLE RIDER INJURED IN TRANSPORT ACCIDENT (V20-V29)

Includes moped motorcycle with sidecar motorized bicycle motor scooter

Excludes1 three-wheeled motor vehicle (V30-V39)

● **V20** Motorcycle rider injured in collision with pedestrian or animal

Excludes1 motorcycle rider collision with animal-drawn vehicle or animal being ridden (V26.-)

The appropriate 7th character is to be added to each code from category V20

A	initial encounter
D	subsequent encounter
S	sequela

X ● **V20.0** Motorcycle driver injured in collision with pedestrian or animal in nontraffic accident

X ● **V20.1** Motorcycle passenger injured in collision with pedestrian or animal in nontraffic accident

X ● **V20.2** Unspecified motorcycle rider injured in collision with pedestrian or animal in nontraffic accident

X ● **V20.3** Person boarding or alighting a motorcycle injured in collision with pedestrian or animal

X ● **V20.4** Motorcycle driver injured in collision with pedestrian or animal in traffic accident

X ● **V20.5** Motorcycle passenger injured in collision with pedestrian or animal in traffic accident

X ● **V20.9** Unspecified motorcycle rider injured in collision with pedestrian or animal in traffic accident

● **V21** Motorcycle rider injured in collision with pedal cycle

> The appropriate 7th character is to be added to each code from category V21

> | A | initial encounter |
> |---|---|
> | D | subsequent encounter |
> | S | sequela |

X ● **V21.0** Motorcycle driver injured in collision with pedal cycle in nontraffic accident

X ● **V21.1** Motorcycle passenger injured in collision with pedal cycle in nontraffic accident

X ● **V21.2** Unspecified motorcycle rider injured in collision with pedal cycle in nontraffic accident

X ● **V21.3** Person boarding or alighting a motorcycle injured in collision with pedal cycle

X ● **V21.4** Motorcycle driver injured in collision with pedal cycle in traffic accident

X ● **V21.5** Motorcycle passenger injured in collision with pedal cycle in traffic accident

X ● **V21.9** Unspecified motorcycle rider injured in collision with pedal cycle in traffic accident

● **V22** Motorcycle rider injured in collision with two- or three-wheeled motor vehicle

> The appropriate 7th character is to be added to each code from category V22

> | A | initial encounter |
> |---|---|
> | D | subsequent encounter |
> | S | sequela |

X ● **V22.0** Motorcycle driver injured in collision with two- or three-wheeled motor vehicle in nontraffic accident

X ● **V22.1** Motorcycle passenger injured in collision with two- or three-wheeled motor vehicle in nontraffic accident

X ● **V22.2** Unspecified motorcycle rider injured in collision with two- or three-wheeled motor vehicle in nontraffic accident

X ● **V22.3** Person boarding or alighting a motorcycle injured in collision with two- or three-wheeled motor vehicle

X ● **V22.4** Motorcycle driver injured in collision with two- or three-wheeled motor vehicle in traffic accident

X ● **V22.5** Motorcycle passenger injured in collision with two- or three-wheeled motor vehicle in traffic accident

X ● **V22.9** Unspecified motorcycle rider injured in collision with two- or three-wheeled motor vehicle in traffic accident

● **V23** Motorcycle rider injured in collision with car, pick-up truck or van

> The appropriate 7th character is to be added to each code from category V23

> | A | initial encounter |
> |---|---|
> | D | subsequent encounter |
> | S | sequela |

X ● **V23.0** Motorcycle driver injured in collision with car, pick-up truck or van in nontraffic accident

X ● **V23.1** Motorcycle passenger injured in collision with car, pick-up truck or van in nontraffic accident

X ● **V23.2** Unspecified motorcycle rider injured in collision with car, pick-up truck or van in nontraffic accident

X ● **V23.3** Person boarding or alighting a motorcycle injured in collision with car, pick-up truck or van

X ● **V23.4** Motorcycle driver injured in collision with car, pick-up truck or van in traffic accident

X ● **V23.5** Motorcycle passenger injured in collision with car, pick-up truck or van in traffic accident

X ● **V23.9** Unspecified motorcycle rider injured in collision with car, pick-up truck or van in traffic accident

● **V24** Motorcycle rider injured in collision with heavy transport vehicle or bus

> **Excludes 1**   motorcycle rider injured in collision with military vehicle (V29.81)

> The appropriate 7th character is to be added to each code from category V24

> | A | initial encounter |
> |---|---|
> | D | subsequent encounter |
> | S | sequela |

X ● **V24.0** Motorcycle driver injured in collision with heavy transport vehicle or bus in nontraffic accident

X ● **V24.1** Motorcycle passenger injured in collision with heavy transport vehicle or bus in nontraffic accident

X ● **V24.2** Unspecified motorcycle rider injured in collision with heavy transport vehicle or bus in nontraffic accident

X ● **V24.3** Person boarding or alighting a motorcycle injured in collision with heavy transport vehicle or bus

X ● **V24.4** Motorcycle driver injured in collision with heavy transport vehicle or bus in traffic accident

X ● **V24.5** Motorcycle passenger injured in collision with heavy transport vehicle or bus in traffic accident

X ● **V24.9** Unspecified motorcycle rider injured in collision with heavy transport vehicle or bus in traffic accident

● **V25** Motorcycle rider injured in collision with railway train or railway vehicle

> The appropriate 7th character is to be added to each code from category V25

> | A | initial encounter |
> |---|---|
> | D | subsequent encounter |
> | S | sequela |

X ● **V25.0** Motorcycle driver injured in collision with railway train or railway vehicle in nontraffic accident

X ● **V25.1** Motorcycle passenger injured in collision with railway train or railway vehicle in nontraffic accident

X ● **V25.2** Unspecified motorcycle rider injured in collision with railway train or railway vehicle in nontraffic accident

X ● **V25.3** Person boarding or alighting a motorcycle injured in collision with railway train or railway vehicle

X ● **V25.4** Motorcycle driver injured in collision with railway train or railway vehicle in traffic accident

X ● **V25.5** Motorcycle passenger injured in collision with railway train or railway vehicle in traffic accident

X ● **V25.9** Unspecified motorcycle rider injured in collision with railway train or railway vehicle in traffic accident

CHAPTER 20 (V00-Y99)

CHAPTER 20 (V00-Y99)

● **V26 Motorcycle rider injured in collision with other nonmotor vehicle**

> **Includes**   collision with animal-drawn vehicle, animal being ridden, streetcar

> The appropriate 7th character is to be added to each code from category V26

> > A   initial encounter
> > D   subsequent encounter
> > S   sequela

X● **V26.0** Motorcycle driver injured in collision with other nonmotor vehicle in nontraffic accident

X● **V26.1** Motorcycle passenger injured in collision with other nonmotor vehicle in nontraffic accident

X● **V26.2** Unspecified motorcycle rider injured in collision with other nonmotor vehicle in nontraffic accident

X● **V26.3** Person boarding or alighting a motorcycle injured in collision with other nonmotor vehicle

X● **V26.4** Motorcycle driver injured in collision with other nonmotor vehicle in traffic accident

X● **V26.5** Motorcycle passenger injured in collision with other nonmotor vehicle in traffic accident

X● **V26.9** Unspecified motorcycle rider injured in collision with other nonmotor vehicle in traffic accident

● **V27 Motorcycle rider injured in collision with fixed or stationary object**

> The appropriate 7th character is to be added to each code from category V27

> > A   initial encounter
> > D   subsequent encounter
> > S   sequela

X● **V27.0** Motorcycle driver injured in collision with fixed or stationary object in nontraffic accident

X● **V27.1** Motorcycle passenger injured in collision with fixed or stationary object in nontraffic accident

X● **V27.2** Unspecified motorcycle rider injured in collision with fixed or stationary object in nontraffic accident

X● **V27.3** Person boarding or alighting a motorcycle injured in collision with fixed or stationary object

X● **V27.4** Motorcycle driver injured in collision with fixed or stationary object in traffic accident

X● **V27.5** Motorcycle passenger injured in collision with fixed or stationary object in traffic accident

X● **V27.9** Unspecified motorcycle rider injured in collision with fixed or stationary object in traffic accident

● **V28 Motorcycle rider injured in noncollision transport accident**

> **Includes**   fall or thrown from motorcycle (without antecedent collision)
> > overturning motorcycle NOS
> > overturning motorcycle without collision

> The appropriate 7th character is to be added to each code from category V28

> > A   initial encounter
> > D   subsequent encounter
> > S   sequela

X● **V28.0** Motorcycle driver injured in noncollision transport accident in nontraffic accident

X● **V28.1** Motorcycle passenger injured in noncollision transport accident in nontraffic accident

X● **V28.2** Unspecified motorcycle rider injured in noncollision transport accident in nontraffic accident

X● **V28.3** Person boarding or alighting a motorcycle injured in noncollision transport accident

X● **V28.4** Motorcycle driver injured in noncollision transport accident in traffic accident

X● **V28.5** Motorcycle passenger injured in noncollision transport accident in traffic accident

X● **V28.9** Unspecified motorcycle rider injured in noncollision transport accident in traffic accident

● **V29 Motorcycle rider injured in other and unspecified transport accidents**

> The appropriate 7th character is to be added to each code from category V29

> > A   initial encounter
> > D   subsequent encounter
> > S   sequela

> **Coding Clinic: 2015, Q3, P20**

● **V29.0** Motorcycle driver injured in collision with other and unspecified motor vehicles in nontraffic accident

X● **V29.00** Motorcycle driver injured in collision with unspecified motor vehicles in nontraffic accident

X● **V29.09** Motorcycle driver injured in collision with other motor vehicles in nontraffic accident

● **V29.1** Motorcycle passenger injured in collision with other and unspecified motor vehicles in nontraffic accident

X● **V29.10** Motorcycle passenger injured in collision with unspecified motor vehicles in nontraffic accident

X● **V29.19** Motorcycle passenger injured in collision with other motor vehicles in nontraffic accident

● **V29.2** Unspecified motorcycle rider injured in collision with other and unspecified motor vehicles in nontraffic accident

X● **V29.20** Unspecified motorcycle rider injured in collision with unspecified motor vehicles in nontraffic accident
> Motorcycle collision NOS, nontraffic

X● **V29.29** Unspecified motorcycle rider injured in collision with other motor vehicles in nontraffic accident

X● **V29.3** Motorcycle rider (driver) (passenger) injured in unspecified nontraffic accident
> Motorcycle accident NOS, nontraffic
> Motorcycle rider injured in nontraffic accident NOS

● **V29.4** Motorcycle driver injured in collision with other and unspecified motor vehicles in traffic accident

X● **V29.40** Motorcycle driver injured in collision with unspecified motor vehicles in traffic accident

X● **V29.49** Motorcycle driver injured in collision with other motor vehicles in traffic accident

● **V29.5** Motorcycle passenger injured in collision with other and unspecified motor vehicles in traffic accident

X● **V29.50** Motorcycle passenger injured in collision with unspecified motor vehicles in traffic accident

X● **V29.59** Motorcycle passenger injured in collision with other motor vehicles in traffic accident

● **V29.6** Unspecified motorcycle rider injured in collision with other and unspecified motor vehicles in traffic accident

X● **V29.60** Unspecified motorcycle rider injured in collision with unspecified motor vehicles in traffic accident
> Motorcycle collision NOS (traffic)

X● **V29.69** Unspecified motorcycle rider injured in collision with other motor vehicles in traffic accident

● **V29.8** Motorcycle rider (driver) (passenger) injured in other specified transport accidents

X● **V29.81** Motorcycle rider (driver) (passenger) injured in transport accident with military vehicle

X● **V29.88** Motorcycle rider (driver) (passenger) injured in other specified transport accidents

X● **V29.9** Motorcycle rider (driver) (passenger) injured in unspecified traffic accident
> Motorcycle accident NOS

OCCUPANT OF THREE-WHEELED MOTOR VEHICLE INJURED IN TRANSPORT ACCIDENT (V30-V39)

Includes	motorized tricycle
	motorized rickshaw
	three-wheeled motor car
Excludes1	all-terrain vehicles (V86.-)
	motorcycle with sidecar (V20-V29)
	vehicle designed primarily for off-road use (V86.-)

● **V30**   Occupant of three-wheeled motor vehicle injured in collision with pedestrian or animal

    Excludes1   three-wheeled motor vehicle collision with animal-drawn vehicle or animal being ridden (V36.-)

    The appropriate 7th character is to be added to each code from category V30

A	initial encounter
D	subsequent encounter
S	sequela

X● **V30.0**   Driver of three-wheeled motor vehicle injured in collision with pedestrian or animal in nontraffic accident

X● **V30.1**   Passenger in three-wheeled motor vehicle injured in collision with pedestrian or animal in nontraffic accident

X● **V30.2**   Person on outside of three-wheeled motor vehicle injured in collision with pedestrian or animal in nontraffic accident

X● **V30.3**   Unspecified occupant of three-wheeled motor vehicle injured in collision with pedestrian or animal in nontraffic accident

X● **V30.4**   Person boarding or alighting a three-wheeled motor vehicle injured in collision with pedestrian or animal

X● **V30.5**   Driver of three-wheeled motor vehicle injured in collision with pedestrian or animal in traffic accident

X● **V30.6**   Passenger in three-wheeled motor vehicle injured in collision with pedestrian or animal in traffic accident

X● **V30.7**   Person on outside of three-wheeled motor vehicle injured in collision with pedestrian or animal in traffic accident

X● **V30.9**   Unspecified occupant of three-wheeled motor vehicle injured in collision with pedestrian or animal in traffic accident

● **V31**   Occupant of three-wheeled motor vehicle injured in collision with pedal cycle

    The appropriate 7th character is to be added to each code from category V31

A	initial encounter
D	subsequent encounter
S	sequela

X● **V31.0**   Driver of three-wheeled motor vehicle injured in collision with pedal cycle in nontraffic accident

X● **V31.1**   Passenger in three-wheeled motor vehicle injured in collision with pedal cycle in nontraffic accident

X● **V31.2**   Person on outside of three-wheeled motor vehicle injured in collision with pedal cycle in nontraffic accident

X● **V31.3**   Unspecified occupant of three-wheeled motor vehicle injured in collision with pedal cycle in nontraffic accident

X● **V31.4**   Person boarding or alighting a three-wheeled motor vehicle injured in collision with pedal cycle

X● **V31.5**   Driver of three-wheeled motor vehicle injured in collision with pedal cycle in traffic accident

X● **V31.6**   Passenger in three-wheeled motor vehicle injured in collision with pedal cycle in traffic accident

X● **V31.7**   Person on outside of three-wheeled motor vehicle injured in collision with pedal cycle in traffic accident

X● **V31.9**   Unspecified occupant of three-wheeled motor vehicle injured in collision with pedal cycle in traffic accident

● **V32**   Occupant of three-wheeled motor vehicle injured in collision with two- or three-wheeled motor vehicle

    The appropriate 7th character is to be added to each code from category V32

A	initial encounter
D	subsequent encounter
S	sequela

X● **V32.0**   Driver of three-wheeled motor vehicle injured in collision with two- or three-wheeled motor vehicle in nontraffic accident

X● **V32.1**   Passenger in three-wheeled motor vehicle injured in collision with two- or three-wheeled motor vehicle in nontraffic accident

X● **V32.2**   Person on outside of three-wheeled motor vehicle injured in collision with two- or three-wheeled motor vehicle in nontraffic accident

X● **V32.3**   Unspecified occupant of three-wheeled motor vehicle injured in collision with two- or three-wheeled motor vehicle in nontraffic accident

X● **V32.4**   Person boarding or alighting a three-wheeled motor vehicle injured in collision with two- or three-wheeled motor vehicle

X● **V32.5**   Driver of three-wheeled motor vehicle injured in collision with two- or three-wheeled motor vehicle in traffic accident

X● **V32.6**   Passenger in three-wheeled motor vehicle injured in collision with two- or three-wheeled motor vehicle in traffic accident

X● **V32.7**   Person on outside of three-wheeled motor vehicle injured in collision with two- or three-wheeled motor vehicle in traffic accident

X● **V32.9**   Unspecified occupant of three-wheeled motor vehicle injured in collision with two- or three-wheeled motor vehicle in traffic accident

● **V33**   Occupant of three-wheeled motor vehicle injured in collision with car, pick-up truck or van

    The appropriate 7th character is to be added to each code from category V33

A	initial encounter
D	subsequent encounter
S	sequela

X● **V33.0**   Driver of three-wheeled motor vehicle injured in collision with car, pick-up truck or van in nontraffic accident

X● **V33.1**   Passenger in three-wheeled motor vehicle injured in collision with car, pick-up truck or van in nontraffic accident

X● **V33.2**   Person on outside of three-wheeled motor vehicle injured in collision with car, pick-up truck or van in nontraffic accident

X● **V33.3**   Unspecified occupant of three-wheeled motor vehicle injured in collision with car, pick-up truck or van in nontraffic accident

X● **V33.4**   Person boarding or alighting a three-wheeled motor vehicle injured in collision with car, pick-up truck or van

X● **V33.5**   Driver of three-wheeled motor vehicle injured in collision with car, pick-up truck or van in traffic accident

X● **V33.6**   Passenger in three-wheeled motor vehicle injured in collision with car, pick-up truck or van in traffic accident

X● **V33.7**   Person on outside of three-wheeled motor vehicle injured in collision with car, pick-up truck or van in traffic accident

X● **V33.9**   Unspecified occupant of three-wheeled motor vehicle injured in collision with car, pick-up truck or van in traffic accident

● V34 **Occupant of three-wheeled motor vehicle injured in collision with heavy transport vehicle or bus**

> Excludes1   occupant of three-wheeled motor vehicle injured in collision with military vehicle (V39.81)

> The appropriate 7th character is to be added to each code from category V34

> | A | initial encounter |
> |---|---|
> | D | subsequent encounter |
> | S | sequela |

X ● V34.0   Driver of three-wheeled motor vehicle injured in collision with heavy transport vehicle or bus in nontraffic accident

X ● V34.1   Passenger in three-wheeled motor vehicle injured in collision with heavy transport vehicle or bus in nontraffic accident

X ● V34.2   Person on outside of three-wheeled motor vehicle injured in collision with heavy transport vehicle or bus in nontraffic accident

X ● V34.3   Unspecified occupant of three-wheeled motor vehicle injured in collision with heavy transport vehicle or bus in nontraffic accident

X ● V34.4   Person boarding or alighting a three-wheeled motor vehicle injured in collision with heavy transport vehicle or bus

X ● V34.5   Driver of three-wheeled motor vehicle injured in collision with heavy transport vehicle or bus in traffic accident

X ● V34.6   Passenger in three-wheeled motor vehicle injured in collision with heavy transport vehicle or bus in traffic accident

X ● V34.7   Person on outside of three-wheeled motor vehicle injured in collision with heavy transport vehicle or bus in traffic accident

X ● V34.9   Unspecified occupant of three-wheeled motor vehicle injured in collision with heavy transport vehicle or bus in traffic accident

● V35 **Occupant of three-wheeled motor vehicle injured in collision with railway train or railway vehicle**

> The appropriate 7th character is to be added to each code from category V35

> | A | initial encounter |
> |---|---|
> | D | subsequent encounter |
> | S | sequela |

X ● V35.0   Driver of three-wheeled motor vehicle injured in collision with railway train or railway vehicle in nontraffic accident

X ● V35.1   Passenger in three-wheeled motor vehicle injured in collision with railway train or railway vehicle in nontraffic accident

X ● V35.2   Person on outside of three-wheeled motor vehicle injured in collision with railway train or railway vehicle in nontraffic accident

X ● V35.3   Unspecified occupant of three-wheeled motor vehicle injured in collision with railway train or railway vehicle in nontraffic accident

X ● V35.4   Person boarding or alighting a three-wheeled motor vehicle injured in collision with railway train or railway vehicle

X ● V35.5   Driver of three-wheeled motor vehicle injured in collision with railway train or railway vehicle in traffic accident

X ● V35.6   Passenger in three-wheeled motor vehicle injured in collision with railway train or railway vehicle in traffic accident

X ● V35.7   Person on outside of three-wheeled motor vehicle injured in collision with railway train or railway vehicle in traffic accident

X ● V35.9   Unspecified occupant of three-wheeled motor vehicle injured in collision with railway train or railway vehicle in traffic accident

● V36 **Occupant of three-wheeled motor vehicle injured in collision with other nonmotor vehicle**

> Includes   collision with animal-drawn vehicle, animal being ridden, streetcar

> The appropriate 7th character is to be added to each code from category V36

> | A | initial encounter |
> |---|---|
> | D | subsequent encounter |
> | S | sequela |

X ● V36.0   Driver of three-wheeled motor vehicle injured in collision with other nonmotor vehicle in nontraffic accident

X ● V36.1   Passenger in three-wheeled motor vehicle injured in collision with other nonmotor vehicle in nontraffic accident

X ● V36.2   Person on outside of three-wheeled motor vehicle injured in collision with other nonmotor vehicle in nontraffic accident

X ● V36.3   Unspecified occupant of three-wheeled motor vehicle injured in collision with other nonmotor vehicle in nontraffic accident

X ● V36.4   Person boarding or alighting a three-wheeled motor vehicle injured in collision with other nonmotor vehicle

X ● V36.5   Driver of three-wheeled motor vehicle injured in collision with other nonmotor vehicle in traffic accident

X ● V36.6   Passenger in three-wheeled motor vehicle injured in collision with other nonmotor vehicle in traffic accident

X ● V36.7   Person on outside of three-wheeled motor vehicle injured in collision with other nonmotor vehicle in traffic accident

X ● V36.9   Unspecified occupant of three-wheeled motor vehicle injured in collision with other nonmotor vehicle in traffic accident

● V37 **Occupant of three-wheeled motor vehicle injured in collision with fixed or stationary object**

> The appropriate 7th character is to be added to each code from category V37

> | A | initial encounter |
> |---|---|
> | D | subsequent encounter |
> | S | sequela |

X ● V37.0   Driver of three-wheeled motor vehicle injured in collision with fixed or stationary object in nontraffic accident

X ● V37.1   Passenger in three-wheeled motor vehicle injured in collision with fixed or stationary object in nontraffic accident

X ● V37.2   Person on outside of three-wheeled motor vehicle injured in collision with fixed or stationary object in nontraffic accident

X ● V37.3   Unspecified occupant of three-wheeled motor vehicle injured in collision with fixed or stationary object in nontraffic accident

X ● V37.4   Person boarding or alighting a three-wheeled motor vehicle injured in collision with fixed or stationary object

X ● V37.5   Driver of three-wheeled motor vehicle injured in collision with fixed or stationary object in traffic accident

X ● V37.6   Passenger in three-wheeled motor vehicle injured in collision with fixed or stationary object in traffic accident

X ● V37.7   Person on outside of three-wheeled motor vehicle injured in collision with fixed or stationary object in traffic accident

X ● V37.9   Unspecified occupant of three-wheeled motor vehicle injured in collision with fixed or stationary object in traffic accident

▶ New   ⇒ Revised   ~~deleted~~ Deleted   Excludes 1   Excludes 2   Includes   Use additional   Code first   Code also   Key words

OGCR Official Guidelines   X Assign placeholder X   ● Use Additional Character(s)   ▶ Manifestation Code   🐾 Hierarchical Condition Category   **Coding Clinic**

● V38   Occupant of three-wheeled motor vehicle injured in noncollision transport accident

     Includes   fall or thrown from three-wheeled motor vehicle
                      overturning of three-wheeled motor vehicle NOS
                      overturning of three-wheeled motor vehicle
                        without collision

    The appropriate 7th character is to be added to each code from category V38

A	initial encounter
D	subsequent encounter
S	sequela

X ● V38.0 Driver of three-wheeled motor vehicle injured in noncollision transport accident in nontraffic accident

X ● V38.1 Passenger in three-wheeled motor vehicle injured in noncollision transport accident in nontraffic accident

X ● V38.2 Person on outside of three-wheeled motor vehicle injured in noncollision transport accident in nontraffic accident

X ● V38.3 Unspecified occupant of three-wheeled motor vehicle injured in noncollision transport accident in nontraffic accident

X ● V38.4 Person boarding or alighting a three-wheeled motor vehicle injured in noncollision transport accident

X ● V38.5 Driver of three-wheeled motor vehicle injured in noncollision transport accident in traffic accident

X ● V38.6 Passenger in three-wheeled motor vehicle injured in noncollision transport accident in traffic accident

X ● V38.7 Person on outside of three-wheeled motor vehicle injured in noncollision transport accident in traffic accident

X ● V38.9 Unspecified occupant of three-wheeled motor vehicle injured in noncollision transport accident in traffic accident

● V39   Occupant of three-wheeled motor vehicle injured in other and unspecified transport accidents

    The appropriate 7th character is to be added to each code from category V39

A	initial encounter
D	subsequent encounter
S	sequela

● V39.0 Driver of three-wheeled motor vehicle injured in collision with other and unspecified motor vehicles in nontraffic accident

  X ● V39.00 Driver of three-wheeled motor vehicle injured in collision with unspecified motor vehicles in nontraffic accident

  X ● V39.09 Driver of three-wheeled motor vehicle injured in collision with other motor vehicles in nontraffic accident

● V39.1 Passenger in three-wheeled motor vehicle injured in collision with other and unspecified motor vehicles in nontraffic accident

  X ● V39.10 Passenger in three-wheeled motor vehicle injured in collision with unspecified motor vehicles in nontraffic accident

  X ● V39.19 Passenger in three-wheeled motor vehicle injured in collision with other motor vehicles in nontraffic accident

● V39.2 Unspecified occupant of three-wheeled motor vehicle injured in collision with other and unspecified motor vehicles in nontraffic accident

  X ● V39.20 Unspecified occupant of three-wheeled motor vehicle injured in collision with unspecified motor vehicles in nontraffic accident

      Collision NOS involving three-wheeled motor vehicle, nontraffic

  X ● V39.29 Unspecified occupant of three-wheeled motor vehicle injured in collision with other motor vehicles in nontraffic accident

X ● V39.3 Occupant (driver) (passenger) of three-wheeled motor vehicle injured in unspecified nontraffic accident

     Accident NOS involving three-wheeled motor vehicle, nontraffic

     Occupant of three-wheeled motor vehicle injured in nontraffic accident NOS

● V39.4 Driver of three-wheeled motor vehicle injured in collision with other and unspecified motor vehicles in traffic accident

  X ● V39.40 Driver of three-wheeled motor vehicle injured in collision with unspecified motor vehicles in traffic accident

  X ● V39.49 Driver of three-wheeled motor vehicle injured in collision with other motor vehicles in traffic accident

● V39.5 Passenger in three-wheeled motor vehicle injured in collision with other and unspecified motor vehicles in traffic accident

  X ● V39.50 Passenger in three-wheeled motor vehicle injured in collision with unspecified motor vehicles in traffic accident

  X ● V39.59 Passenger in three-wheeled motor vehicle injured in collision with other motor vehicles in traffic accident

● V39.6 Unspecified occupant of three-wheeled motor vehicle injured in collision with other and unspecified motor vehicles in traffic accident

  X ● V39.60 Unspecified occupant of three-wheeled motor vehicle injured in collision with unspecified motor vehicles in traffic accident

      Collision NOS involving three-wheeled motor vehicle (traffic)

  X ● V39.69 Unspecified occupant of three-wheeled motor vehicle injured in collision with other motor vehicles in traffic accident

● V39.8 Occupant (driver) (passenger) of three-wheeled motor vehicle injured in other specified transport accidents

  X ● V39.81 Occupant (driver) (passenger) of three-wheeled motor vehicle injured in transport accident with military vehicle

  X ● V39.89 Occupant (driver) (passenger) of three-wheeled motor vehicle injured in other specified transport accidents

X ● V39.9 Occupant (driver) (passenger) of three-wheeled motor vehicle injured in unspecified traffic accident

     Accident NOS involving three-wheeled motor vehicle

CAR OCCUPANT INJURED IN TRANSPORT ACCIDENT (V40-V49)

     Includes   a four-wheeled motor vehicle designed primarily for carrying passengers
                     automobile (pulling a trailer or camper)

     Excludes1   bus (V50-V59)
                   minibus (V50-V59)
                   minivan (V50-V59)
                   motorcoach (V70-V79)
                   pick-up truck (V50-V59)
                   sport utility vehicle (SUV) (V50-V59)

● V40   Car occupant injured in collision with pedestrian or animal

     Excludes1   car collision with animal-drawn vehicle or animal being ridden (V46.-)

    The appropriate 7th character is to be added to each code from category V40

A	initial encounter
D	subsequent encounter
S	sequela

X ● V40.0 Car driver injured in collision with pedestrian or animal in nontraffic accident

X ● V40.1 Car passenger injured in collision with pedestrian or animal in nontraffic accident

X● **V40.2** Person on outside of car injured in collision with pedestrian or animal in nontraffic accident

X● **V40.3** Unspecified car occupant injured in collision with pedestrian or animal in nontraffic accident

X● **V40.4** Person boarding or alighting a car injured in collision with pedestrian or animal

X● **V40.5** Car driver injured in collision with pedestrian or animal in traffic accident

X● **V40.6** Car passenger injured in collision with pedestrian or animal in traffic accident

X● **V40.7** Person on outside of car injured in collision with pedestrian or animal in traffic accident

X● **V40.9** Unspecified car occupant injured in collision with pedestrian or animal in traffic accident

● **V41** Car occupant injured in collision with pedal cycle

The appropriate 7th character is to be added to each code from category V41

> A   initial encounter
> D   subsequent encounter
> S   sequela

X● **V41.0** Car driver injured in collision with pedal cycle in nontraffic accident

X● **V41.1** Car passenger injured in collision with pedal cycle in nontraffic accident

X● **V41.2** Person on outside of car injured in collision with pedal cycle in nontraffic accident

X● **V41.3** Unspecified car occupant injured in collision with pedal cycle in nontraffic accident

X● **V41.4** Person boarding or alighting a car injured in collision with pedal cycle

X● **V41.5** Car driver injured in collision with pedal cycle in traffic accident

X● **V41.6** Car passenger injured in collision with pedal cycle in traffic accident

X● **V41.7** Person on outside of car injured in collision with pedal cycle in traffic accident

X● **V41.9** Unspecified car occupant injured in collision with pedal cycle in traffic accident

● **V42** Car occupant injured in collision with two- or three-wheeled motor vehicle

The appropriate 7th character is to be added to each code from category V42

> A   initial encounter
> D   subsequent encounter
> S   sequela

X● **V42.0** Car driver injured in collision with two- or three-wheeled motor vehicle in nontraffic accident

X● **V42.1** Car passenger injured in collision with two- or three-wheeled motor vehicle in nontraffic accident

X● **V42.2** Person on outside of car injured in collision with two- or three-wheeled motor vehicle in nontraffic accident

X● **V42.3** Unspecified car occupant injured in collision with two- or three-wheeled motor vehicle in nontraffic accident

X● **V42.4** Person boarding or alighting a car injured in collision with two- or three-wheeled motor vehicle

X● **V42.5** Car driver injured in collision with two- or three-wheeled motor vehicle in traffic accident

X● **V42.6** Car passenger injured in collision with two- or three-wheeled motor vehicle in traffic accident

X● **V42.7** Person on outside of car injured in collision with two- or three-wheeled motor vehicle in traffic accident

X● **V42.9** Unspecified car occupant injured in collision with two- or three-wheeled motor vehicle in traffic accident

● **V43** Car occupant injured in collision with car, pick-up truck or van

The appropriate 7th character is to be added to each code from category V43

> A   initial encounter
> D   subsequent encounter
> S   sequela

● **V43.0** Car driver injured in collision with car, pick-up truck or van in nontraffic accident

X● **V43.01** Car driver injured in collision with sport utility vehicle in nontraffic accident

X● **V43.02** Car driver injured in collision with other type car in nontraffic accident

X● **V43.03** Car driver injured in collision with pick-up truck in nontraffic accident

X● **V43.04** Car driver injured in collision with van in nontraffic accident

● **V43.1** Car passenger injured in collision with car, pick-up truck or van in nontraffic accident

X● **V43.11** Car passenger injured in collision with sport utility vehicle in nontraffic accident

X● **V43.12** Car passenger injured in collision with other type car in nontraffic accident

X● **V43.13** Car passenger injured in collision with pick-up truck in nontraffic accident

X● **V43.14** Car passenger injured in collision with van in nontraffic accident

● **V43.2** Person on outside of car injured in collision with car, pick-up truck or van in nontraffic accident

X● **V43.21** Person on outside of car injured in collision with sport utility vehicle in nontraffic accident

X● **V43.22** Person on outside of car injured in collision with other type car in nontraffic accident

X● **V43.23** Person on outside of car injured in collision with pick-up truck in nontraffic accident

X● **V43.24** Person on outside of car injured in collision with van in nontraffic accident

● **V43.3** Unspecified car occupant injured in collision with car, pick-up truck or van in nontraffic accident

X● **V43.31** Unspecified car occupant injured in collision with sport utility vehicle in nontraffic accident

X● **V43.32** Unspecified car occupant injured in collision with other type car in nontraffic accident

X● **V43.33** Unspecified car occupant injured in collision with pick-up truck in nontraffic accident

X● **V43.34** Unspecified car occupant injured in collision with van in nontraffic accident

● **V43.4** Person boarding or alighting a car injured in collision with car, pick-up truck or van

X● **V43.41** Person boarding or alighting a car injured in collision with sport utility vehicle

X● **V43.42** Person boarding or alighting a car injured in collision with other type car

X● **V43.43** Person boarding or alighting a car injured in collision with pick-up truck

X● **V43.44** Person boarding or alighting a car injured in collision with van

● **V43.5** Car driver injured in collision with car, pick-up truck or van in traffic accident

X● **V43.51** Car driver injured in collision with sport utility vehicle in traffic accident

X● **V43.52** Car driver injured in collision with other type car in traffic accident

X● **V43.53** Car driver injured in collision with pick-up truck in traffic accident

X● **V43.54** Car driver injured in collision with van in traffic accident

▶ New   ⇒ Revised   ~~deleted~~ Deleted   Excludes 1   Excludes 2   Includes   Use additional   Code first   Code also   Key words

OGCR Official Guidelines   X Assign placeholder X   ● Use Additional Character(s)   ▸ Manifestation Code   🦚 Hierarchical Condition Category   **Coding Clinic**

● V43.6   Car passenger injured in collision with car, pick-up truck or van in traffic accident

   X● V43.61   Car passenger injured in collision with sport utility vehicle in traffic accident
       Coding Clinic: 2015, Q1, P5-7

   X● V43.62   Car passenger injured in collision with other type car in traffic accident

   X● V43.63   Car passenger injured in collision with pick-up truck in traffic accident

   X● V43.64   Car passenger injured in collision with van in traffic accident

● V43.7   Person on outside of car injured in collision with car, pick-up truck or van in traffic accident

   X● V43.71   Person on outside of car injured in collision with sport utility vehicle in traffic accident

   X● V43.72   Person on outside of car injured in collision with other type car in traffic accident

   X● V43.73   Person on outside of car injured in collision with pick-up truck in traffic accident

   X● V43.74   Person on outside of car injured in collision with van in traffic accident

● V43.9   Unspecified car occupant injured in collision with car, pick-up truck or van in traffic accident

   X● V43.91   Unspecified car occupant injured in collision with sport utility vehicle in traffic accident

   X● V43.92   Unspecified car occupant injured in collision with other type car in traffic accident

   X● V43.93   Unspecified car occupant injured in collision with pick-up truck in traffic accident

   X● V43.94   Unspecified car occupant injured in collision with van in traffic accident

● V44   Car occupant injured in collision with heavy transport vehicle or bus

   Excludes1   car occupant injured in collision with military vehicle (V49.81)

   The appropriate 7th character is to be added to each code from category V44

> A   initial encounter
> D   subsequent encounter
> S   sequela

   X● V44.0   Car driver injured in collision with heavy transport vehicle or bus in nontraffic accident

   X● V44.1   Car passenger injured in collision with heavy transport vehicle or bus in nontraffic accident

   X● V44.2   Person on outside of car injured in collision with heavy transport vehicle or bus in nontraffic accident

   X● V44.3   Unspecified car occupant injured in collision with heavy transport vehicle or bus in nontraffic accident

   X● V44.4   Person boarding or alighting a car injured in collision with heavy transport vehicle or bus

   X● V44.5   Car driver injured in collision with heavy transport vehicle or bus in traffic accident

   X● V44.6   Car passenger injured in collision with heavy transport vehicle or bus in traffic accident

   X● V44.7   Person on outside of car injured in collision with heavy transport vehicle or bus in traffic accident

   X● V44.9   Unspecified car occupant injured in collision with heavy transport vehicle or bus in traffic accident

● V45   Car occupant injured in collision with railway train or railway vehicle

   The appropriate 7th character is to be added to each code from category V45

> A   initial encounter
> D   subsequent encounter
> S   sequela

   X● V45.0   Car driver injured in collision with railway train or railway vehicle in nontraffic accident

   X● V45.1   Car passenger injured in collision with railway train or railway vehicle in nontraffic accident

   X● V45.2   Person on outside of car injured in collision with railway train or railway vehicle in nontraffic accident

   X● V45.3   Unspecified car occupant injured in collision with railway train or railway vehicle in nontraffic accident

   X● V45.4   Person boarding or alighting a car injured in collision with railway train or railway vehicle

   X● V45.5   Car driver injured in collision with railway train or railway vehicle in traffic accident

   X● V45.6   Car passenger injured in collision with railway train or railway vehicle in traffic accident

   X● V45.7   Person on outside of car injured in collision with railway train or railway vehicle in traffic accident

   X● V45.9   Unspecified car occupant injured in collision with railway train or railway vehicle in traffic accident

● V46   Car occupant injured in collision with other nonmotor vehicle

   Includes   collision with animal-drawn vehicle, animal being ridden, streetcar

   The appropriate 7th character is to be added to each code from category V46

> A   initial encounter
> D   subsequent encounter
> S   sequela

   X● V46.0   Car driver injured in collision with other nonmotor vehicle in nontraffic accident

   X● V46.1   Car passenger injured in collision with other nonmotor vehicle in nontraffic accident

   X● V46.2   Person on outside of car injured in collision with other nonmotor vehicle in nontraffic accident

   X● V46.3   Unspecified car occupant injured in collision with other nonmotor vehicle in nontraffic accident

   X● V46.4   Person boarding or alighting a car injured in collision with other nonmotor vehicle

   X● V46.5   Car driver injured in collision with other nonmotor vehicle in traffic accident

   X● V46.6   Car passenger injured in collision with other nonmotor vehicle in traffic accident

   X● V46.7   Person on outside of car injured in collision with other nonmotor vehicle in traffic accident

   X● V46.9   Unspecified car occupant injured in collision with other nonmotor vehicle in traffic accident

● V47   Car occupant injured in collision with fixed or stationary object

   The appropriate 7th character is to be added to each code from category V47

> A   initial encounter
> D   subsequent encounter
> S   sequela

   Coding Clinic: 2016, Q4, P73

   X● V47.0   Car driver injured in collision with fixed or stationary object in nontraffic accident

   X● V47.1   Car passenger injured in collision with fixed or stationary object in nontraffic accident

   X● V47.2   Person on outside of car injured in collision with fixed or stationary object in nontraffic accident

   X● V47.3   Unspecified car occupant injured in collision with fixed or stationary object in nontraffic accident

   X● V47.4   Person boarding or alighting a car injured in collision with fixed or stationary object

   X● V47.5   Car driver injured in collision with fixed or stationary object in traffic accident

   X● V47.6   Car passenger injured in collision with fixed or stationary object in traffic accident

   X● V47.7   Person on outside of car injured in collision with fixed or stationary object in traffic accident

   X● V47.9   Unspecified car occupant injured in collision with fixed or stationary object in traffic accident

CHAPTER 20 (V00-Y99)

● **V48**   Car occupant injured in noncollision transport accident

    Includes   overturning car NOS
                      overturning car without collision

The appropriate 7th character is to be added to each code from category V48

A	initial encounter
D	subsequent encounter
S	sequela

X● **V48.0**   Car driver injured in noncollision transport accident in nontraffic accident

X● **V48.1**   Car passenger injured in noncollision transport accident in nontraffic accident

X● **V48.2**   Person on outside of car injured in noncollision transport accident in nontraffic accident

X● **V48.3**   Unspecified car occupant injured in noncollision transport accident in nontraffic accident

X● **V48.4**   Person boarding or alighting a car injured in noncollision transport accident

X● **V48.5**   Car driver injured in noncollision transport accident in traffic accident

X● **V48.6**   Car passenger injured in noncollision transport accident in traffic accident

X● **V48.7**   Person on outside of car injured in noncollision transport accident in traffic accident

X● **V48.9**   Unspecified car occupant injured in noncollision transport accident in traffic accident

● **V49**   Car occupant injured in other and unspecified transport accidents

The appropriate 7th character is to be added to each code from category V49

A	initial encounter
D	subsequent encounter
S	sequela

● **V49.0**   Driver injured in collision with other and unspecified motor vehicles in nontraffic accident

   X● **V49.00**   Driver injured in collision with unspecified motor vehicles in nontraffic accident

   X● **V49.09**   Driver injured in collision with other motor vehicles in nontraffic accident

● **V49.1**   Passenger injured in collision with other and unspecified motor vehicles in nontraffic accident

   X● **V49.10**   Passenger injured in collision with unspecified motor vehicles in nontraffic accident

   X● **V49.19**   Passenger injured in collision with other motor vehicles in nontraffic accident

● **V49.2**   Unspecified car occupant injured in collision with other and unspecified motor vehicles in nontraffic accident

   X● **V49.20**   Unspecified car occupant injured in collision with unspecified motor vehicles in nontraffic accident
                Car collision NOS, nontraffic

   X● **V49.29**   Unspecified car occupant injured in collision with other motor vehicles in nontraffic accident

X● **V49.3**   Car occupant (driver) (passenger) injured in unspecified nontraffic accident
        Car accident NOS, nontraffic
        Car occupant injured in nontraffic accident NOS

● **V49.4**   Driver injured in collision with other and unspecified motor vehicles in traffic accident

   X● **V49.40**   Driver injured in collision with unspecified motor vehicles in traffic accident

   X● **V49.49**   Driver injured in collision with other motor vehicles in traffic accident

● **V49.5**   Passenger injured in collision with other and unspecified motor vehicles in traffic accident

   X● **V49.50**   Passenger injured in collision with unspecified motor vehicles in traffic accident

   X● **V49.59**   Passenger injured in collision with other motor vehicles in traffic accident

● **V49.6**   Unspecified car occupant injured in collision with other and unspecified motor vehicles in traffic accident

   X● **V49.60**   Unspecified car occupant injured in collision with unspecified motor vehicles in traffic accident
                Car collision NOS (traffic)

   X● **V49.69**   Unspecified car occupant injured in collision with other motor vehicles in traffic accident

● **V49.8**   Car occupant (driver) (passenger) injured in other specified transport accidents

   X● **V49.81**   Car occupant (driver) (passenger) injured in transport accident with military vehicle

   X● **V49.88**   Car occupant (driver) (passenger) injured in other specified transport accidents

X● **V49.9**   Car occupant (driver) (passenger) injured in unspecified traffic accident
        Car accident NOS
        Coding Clinic: 2015, Q1, P11

OCCUPANT OF PICK-UP TRUCK OR VAN INJURED IN TRANSPORT ACCIDENT (V50-V59)

   Includes   a four- or six-wheel motor vehicle designed primarily for carrying passengers and property but weighing less than the local limit for classification as a heavy goods vehicle
                minibus
                minivan
                sport utility vehicle (SUV)
                truck
                van

   Excludes 1   heavy transport vehicle (V60-V69)

● **V50**   Occupant of pick-up truck or van injured in collision with pedestrian or animal

   Excludes 1   pick-up truck or van collision with animal-drawn vehicle or animal being ridden (V56.-)

The appropriate 7th character is to be added to each code from category V50

A	initial encounter
D	subsequent encounter
S	sequela

X● **V50.0**   Driver of pick-up truck or van injured in collision with pedestrian or animal in nontraffic accident

X● **V50.1**   Passenger in pick-up truck or van injured in collision with pedestrian or animal in nontraffic accident

X● **V50.2**   Person on outside of pick-up truck or van injured in collision with pedestrian or animal in nontraffic accident

X● **V50.3**   Unspecified occupant of pick-up truck or van injured in collision with pedestrian or animal in nontraffic accident

X● **V50.4**   Person boarding or alighting a pick-up truck or van injured in collision with pedestrian or animal

X● **V50.5**   Driver of pick-up truck or van injured in collision with pedestrian or animal in traffic accident

X● **V50.6**   Passenger in pick-up truck or van injured in collision with pedestrian or animal in traffic accident

X● **V50.7**   Person on outside of pick-up truck or van injured in collision with pedestrian or animal in traffic accident

X● **V50.9**   Unspecified occupant of pick-up truck or van injured in collision with pedestrian or animal in traffic accident

● **V51**   **Occupant of pick-up truck or van injured in collision with pedal cycle**

The appropriate 7th character is to be added to each code from category V51

> A   initial encounter
> D   subsequent encounter
> S   sequela

X● **V51.0**   Driver of pick-up truck or van injured in collision with pedal cycle in nontraffic accident

X● **V51.1**   Passenger in pick-up truck or van injured in collision with pedal cycle in nontraffic accident

X● **V51.2**   Person on outside of pick-up truck or van injured in collision with pedal cycle in nontraffic accident

X● **V51.3**   Unspecified occupant of pick-up truck or van injured in collision with pedal cycle in nontraffic accident

X● **V51.4**   Person boarding or alighting a pick-up truck or van injured in collision with pedal cycle

X● **V51.5**   Driver of pick-up truck or van injured in collision with pedal cycle in traffic accident

X● **V51.6**   Passenger in pick-up truck or van injured in collision with pedal cycle in traffic accident

X● **V51.7**   Person on outside of pick-up truck or van injured in collision with pedal cycle in traffic accident

X● **V51.9**   Unspecified occupant of pick-up truck or van injured in collision with pedal cycle in traffic accident

● **V52**   **Occupant of pick-up truck or van injured in collision with two- or three-wheeled motor vehicle**

The appropriate 7th character is to be added to each code from category V52

> A   initial encounter
> D   subsequent encounter
> S   sequela

X● **V52.0**   Driver of pick-up truck or van injured in collision with two- or three-wheeled motor vehicle in nontraffic accident

X● **V52.1**   Passenger in pick-up truck or van injured in collision with two- or three-wheeled motor vehicle in nontraffic accident

X● **V52.2**   Person on outside of pick-up truck or van injured in collision with two- or three-wheeled motor vehicle in nontraffic accident

X● **V52.3**   Unspecified occupant of pick-up truck or van injured in collision with two- or three-wheeled motor vehicle in nontraffic accident

X● **V52.4**   Person boarding or alighting a pick-up truck or van injured in collision with two- or three-wheeled motor vehicle

X● **V52.5**   Driver of pick-up truck or van injured in collision with two- or three-wheeled motor vehicle in traffic accident

X● **V52.6**   Passenger in pick-up truck or van injured in collision with two- or three-wheeled motor vehicle in traffic accident

X● **V52.7**   Person on outside of pick-up truck or van injured in collision with two- or three-wheeled motor vehicle in traffic accident

X● **V52.9**   Unspecified occupant of pick-up truck or van injured in collision with two- or three-wheeled motor vehicle in traffic accident

● **V53**   **Occupant of pick-up truck or van injured in collision with car, pick-up truck or van**

The appropriate 7th character is to be added to each code from category V53

> A   initial encounter
> D   subsequent encounter
> S   sequela

X● **V53.0**   Driver of pick-up truck or van injured in collision with car, pick-up truck or van in nontraffic accident

X● **V53.1**   Passenger in pick-up truck or van injured in collision with car, pick-up truck or van in nontraffic accident

X● **V53.2**   Person on outside of pick-up truck or van injured in collision with car, pick-up truck or van in nontraffic accident

X● **V53.3**   Unspecified occupant of pick-up truck or van injured in collision with car, pick-up truck or van in nontraffic accident

X● **V53.4**   Person boarding or alighting a pick-up truck or van injured in collision with car, pick-up truck or van

X● **V53.5**   Driver of pick-up truck or van injured in collision with car, pick-up truck or van in traffic accident

X● **V53.6**   Passenger in pick-up truck or van injured in collision with car, pick-up truck or van in traffic accident

X● **V53.7**   Person on outside of pick-up truck or van injured in collision with car, pick-up truck or van in traffic accident

X● **V53.9**   Unspecified occupant of pick-up truck or van injured in collision with car, pick-up truck or van in traffic accident

● **V54**   **Occupant of pick-up truck or van injured in collision with heavy transport vehicle or bus**

> **Excludes 1**   occupant of pick-up truck or van injured in collision with military vehicle (V59.81)

The appropriate 7th character is to be added to each code from category V54

> A   initial encounter
> D   subsequent encounter
> S   sequela

X● **V54.0**   Driver of pick-up truck or van injured in collision with heavy transport vehicle or bus in nontraffic accident

X● **V54.1**   Passenger in pick-up truck or van injured in collision with heavy transport vehicle or bus in nontraffic accident

X● **V54.2**   Person on outside of pick-up truck or van injured in collision with heavy transport vehicle or bus in nontraffic accident

X● **V54.3**   Unspecified occupant of pick-up truck or van injured in collision with heavy transport vehicle or bus in nontraffic accident

X● **V54.4**   Person boarding or alighting a pick-up truck or van injured in collision with heavy transport vehicle or bus

X● **V54.5**   Driver of pick-up truck or van injured in collision with heavy transport vehicle or bus in traffic accident

X● **V54.6**   Passenger in pick-up truck or van injured in collision with heavy transport vehicle or bus in traffic accident

X● **V54.7**   Person on outside of pick-up truck or van injured in collision with heavy transport vehicle or bus in traffic accident

X● **V54.9**   Unspecified occupant of pick-up truck or van injured in collision with heavy transport vehicle or bus in traffic accident

CHAPTER 20 (V00-Y99)

● V55   **Occupant of pick-up truck or van injured in collision with railway train or railway vehicle**

The appropriate 7th character is to be added to each code from category V55

A	initial encounter
D	subsequent encounter
S	sequela

X● **V55.0**   Driver of pick-up truck or van injured in collision with railway train or railway vehicle in nontraffic accident

X● **V55.1**   Passenger in pick-up truck or van injured in collision with railway train or railway vehicle in nontraffic accident

X● **V55.2**   Person on outside of pick-up truck or van injured in collision with railway train or railway vehicle in nontraffic accident

X● **V55.3**   Unspecified occupant of pick-up truck or van injured in collision with railway train or railway vehicle in nontraffic accident

X● **V55.4**   Person boarding or alighting a pick-up truck or van injured in collision with railway train or railway vehicle

X● **V55.5**   Driver of pick-up truck or van injured in collision with railway train or railway vehicle in traffic accident

X● **V55.6**   Passenger in pick-up truck or van injured in collision with railway train or railway vehicle in traffic accident

X● **V55.7**   Person on outside of pick-up truck or van injured in collision with railway train or railway vehicle in traffic accident

X● **V55.9**   Unspecified occupant of pick-up truck or van injured in collision with railway train or railway vehicle in traffic accident

● V56   **Occupant of pick-up truck or van injured in collision with other nonmotor vehicle**

Includes	collision with animal-drawn vehicle, animal being ridden, streetcar

The appropriate 7th character is to be added to each code from category V56

A	initial encounter
D	subsequent encounter
S	sequela

X● **V56.0**   Driver of pick-up truck or van injured in collision with other nonmotor vehicle in nontraffic accident

X● **V56.1**   Passenger in pick-up truck or van injured in collision with other nonmotor vehicle in nontraffic accident

X● **V56.2**   Person on outside of pick-up truck or van injured in collision with other nonmotor vehicle in nontraffic accident

X● **V56.3**   Unspecified occupant of pick-up truck or van injured in collision with other nonmotor vehicle in nontraffic accident

X● **V56.4**   Person boarding or alighting a pick-up truck or van injured in collision with other nonmotor vehicle

X● **V56.5**   Driver of pick-up truck or van injured in collision with other nonmotor vehicle in traffic accident

X● **V56.6**   Passenger in pick-up truck or van injured in collision with other nonmotor vehicle in traffic accident

X● **V56.7**   Person on outside of pick-up truck or van injured in collision with other nonmotor vehicle in traffic accident

X● **V56.9**   Unspecified occupant of pick-up truck or van injured in collision with other nonmotor vehicle in traffic accident

● V57   **Occupant of pick-up truck or van injured in collision with fixed or stationary object**

The appropriate 7th character is to be added to each code from category V57

A	initial encounter
D	subsequent encounter
S	sequela

X● **V57.0**   Driver of pick-up truck or van injured in collision with fixed or stationary object in nontraffic accident

X● **V57.1**   Passenger in pick-up truck or van injured in collision with fixed or stationary object in nontraffic accident

X● **V57.2**   Person on outside of pick-up truck or van injured in collision with fixed or stationary object in nontraffic accident

X● **V57.3**   Unspecified occupant of pick-up truck or van injured in collision with fixed or stationary object in nontraffic accident

X● **V57.4**   Person boarding or alighting a pick-up truck or van injured in collision with fixed or stationary object

X● **V57.5**   Driver of pick-up truck or van injured in collision with fixed or stationary object in traffic accident

X● **V57.6**   Passenger in pick-up truck or van injured in collision with fixed or stationary object in traffic accident

X● **V57.7**   Person on outside of pick-up truck or van injured in collision with fixed or stationary object in traffic accident

X● **V57.9**   Unspecified occupant of pick-up truck or van injured in collision with fixed or stationary object in traffic accident

● V58   **Occupant of pick-up truck or van injured in noncollision transport accident**

Includes	overturning pick-up truck or van NOS
	overturning pick-up truck or van without collision

The appropriate 7th character is to be added to each code from category V58

A	initial encounter
D	subsequent encounter
S	sequela

X● **V58.0**   Driver of pick-up truck or van injured in noncollision transport accident in nontraffic accident

X● **V58.1**   Passenger in pick-up truck or van injured in noncollision transport accident in nontraffic accident

X● **V58.2**   Person on outside of pick-up truck or van injured in noncollision transport accident in nontraffic accident

X● **V58.3**   Unspecified occupant of pick-up truck or van injured in noncollision transport accident in nontraffic accident

X● **V58.4**   Person boarding or alighting a pick-up truck or van injured in noncollision transport accident

X● **V58.5**   Driver of pick-up truck or van injured in noncollision transport accident in traffic accident

X● **V58.6**   Passenger in pick-up truck or van injured in noncollision transport accident in traffic accident

X● **V58.7**   Person on outside of pick-up truck or van injured in noncollision transport accident in traffic accident

X● **V58.9**   Unspecified occupant of pick-up truck or van injured in noncollision transport accident in traffic accident

▶ New   ⟩⟩ Revised   ~~deleted~~ Deleted   Excludes 1   Excludes 2   Includes   Use additional   Code first   Code also   Key words

OGCR Official Guidelines   X Assign placeholder X   ● Use Additional Character(s)   ⟩ Manifestation Code   🐾 Hierarchical Condition Category   **Coding Clinic**

● **V59** Occupant of pick-up truck or van injured in other and unspecified transport accidents

The appropriate 7th character is to be added to each code from category V59

> A initial encounter
> D subsequent encounter
> S sequela

● **V59.0** Driver of pick-up truck or van injured in collision with other and unspecified motor vehicles in nontraffic accident

X● **V59.00** Driver of pick-up truck or van injured in collision with unspecified motor vehicles in nontraffic accident

X● **V59.09** Driver of pick-up truck or van injured in collision with other motor vehicles in nontraffic accident

● **V59.1** Passenger in pick-up truck or van injured in collision with other and unspecified motor vehicles in nontraffic accident

X● **V59.10** Passenger in pick-up truck or van injured in collision with unspecified motor vehicles in nontraffic accident

X● **V59.19** Passenger in pick-up truck or van injured in collision with other motor vehicles in nontraffic accident

● **V59.2** Unspecified occupant of pick-up truck or van injured in collision with other and unspecified motor vehicles in nontraffic accident

X● **V59.20** Unspecified occupant of pick-up truck or van injured in collision with unspecified motor vehicles in nontraffic accident

> Collision NOS involving pick-up truck or van, nontraffic

X● **V59.29** Unspecified occupant of pick-up truck or van injured in collision with other motor vehicles in nontraffic accident

X● **V59.3** Occupant (driver) (passenger) of pick-up truck or van injured in unspecified nontraffic accident

> Accident NOS involving pick-up truck or van, nontraffic
> Occupant of pick-up truck or van injured in nontraffic accident NOS

● **V59.4** Driver of pick-up truck or van injured in collision with other and unspecified motor vehicles in traffic accident

X● **V59.40** Driver of pick-up truck or van injured in collision with unspecified motor vehicles in traffic accident

X● **V59.49** Driver of pick-up truck or van injured in collision with other motor vehicles in traffic accident

● **V59.5** Passenger in pick-up truck or van injured in collision with other and unspecified motor vehicles in traffic accident

X● **V59.50** Passenger in pick-up truck or van injured in collision with unspecified motor vehicles in traffic accident

X● **V59.59** Passenger in pick-up truck or van injured in collision with other motor vehicles in traffic accident

● **V59.6** Unspecified occupant of pick-up truck or van injured in collision with other and unspecified motor vehicles in traffic accident

X● **V59.60** Unspecified occupant of pick-up truck or van injured in collision with unspecified motor vehicles in traffic accident

> Collision NOS involving pick-up truck or van (traffic)

X● **V59.69** Unspecified occupant of pick-up truck or van injured in collision with other motor vehicles in traffic accident

● **V59.8** Occupant (driver) (passenger) of pick-up truck or van injured in other specified transport accidents

X● **V59.81** Occupant (driver) (passenger) of pick-up truck or van injured in transport accident with military vehicle

X● **V59.88** Occupant (driver) (passenger) of pick-up truck or van injured in other specified transport accidents

X● **V59.9** Occupant (driver) (passenger) of pick-up truck or van injured in unspecified traffic accident

> Accident NOS involving pick-up truck or van

OCCUPANT OF HEAVY TRANSPORT VEHICLE INJURED IN TRANSPORT ACCIDENT (V60-V69)

Includes   18 wheeler
armored car
panel truck

Excludes1   bus
motorcoach

● **V60** Occupant of heavy transport vehicle injured in collision with pedestrian or animal

Excludes1 heavy transport vehicle collision with animal-drawn vehicle or animal being ridden (V66.-)

The appropriate 7th character is to be added to each code from category V60

> A initial encounter
> D subsequent encounter
> S sequela

X● **V60.0** Driver of heavy transport vehicle injured in collision with pedestrian or animal in nontraffic accident

X● **V60.1** Passenger in heavy transport vehicle injured in collision with pedestrian or animal in nontraffic accident

X● **V60.2** Person on outside of heavy transport vehicle injured in collision with pedestrian or animal in nontraffic accident

X● **V60.3** Unspecified occupant of heavy transport vehicle injured in collision with pedestrian or animal in nontraffic accident

X● **V60.4** Person boarding or alighting a heavy transport vehicle injured in collision with pedestrian or animal

X● **V60.5** Driver of heavy transport vehicle injured in collision with pedestrian or animal in traffic accident

X● **V60.6** Passenger in heavy transport vehicle injured in collision with pedestrian or animal in traffic accident

X● **V60.7** Person on outside of heavy transport vehicle injured in collision with pedestrian or animal in traffic accident

X● **V60.9** Unspecified occupant of heavy transport vehicle injured in collision with pedestrian or animal in traffic accident

● **V61** Occupant of heavy transport vehicle injured in collision with pedal cycle

The appropriate 7th character is to be added to each code from category V61

> A initial encounter
> D subsequent encounter
> S sequela

X● **V61.0** Driver of heavy transport vehicle injured in collision with pedal cycle in nontraffic accident

X● **V61.1** Passenger in heavy transport vehicle injured in collision with pedal cycle in nontraffic accident

X● **V61.2** Person on outside of heavy transport vehicle injured in collision with pedal cycle in nontraffic accident

X● **V61.3** Unspecified occupant of heavy transport vehicle injured in collision with pedal cycle in nontraffic accident

X● **V61.4** Person boarding or alighting a heavy transport vehicle injured in collision with pedal cycle while boarding or alighting

X● **V61.5** Driver of heavy transport vehicle injured in collision with pedal cycle in traffic accident

CHAPTER 20 (V00-Y99)

X● **V61.6** Passenger in heavy transport vehicle injured in collision with pedal cycle in traffic accident

X● **V61.7** Person on outside of heavy transport vehicle injured in collision with pedal cycle in traffic accident

X● **V61.9** Unspecified occupant of heavy transport vehicle injured in collision with pedal cycle in traffic accident

● **V62** Occupant of heavy transport vehicle injured in collision with two- or three-wheeled motor vehicle

The appropriate 7th character is to be added to each code from category V62

A	initial encounter
D	subsequent encounter
S	sequela

X● **V62.0** Driver of heavy transport vehicle injured in collision with two- or three-wheeled motor vehicle in nontraffic accident

X● **V62.1** Passenger in heavy transport vehicle injured in collision with two- or three-wheeled motor vehicle in nontraffic accident

X● **V62.2** Person on outside of heavy transport vehicle injured in collision with two- or three-wheeled motor vehicle in nontraffic accident

X● **V62.3** Unspecified occupant of heavy transport vehicle injured in collision with two- or three-wheeled motor vehicle in nontraffic accident

X● **V62.4** Person boarding or alighting a heavy transport vehicle injured in collision with two- or three-wheeled motor vehicle

X● **V62.5** Driver of heavy transport vehicle injured in collision with two- or three-wheeled motor vehicle in traffic accident

X● **V62.6** Passenger in heavy transport vehicle injured in collision with two- or three-wheeled motor vehicle in traffic accident

X● **V62.7** Person on outside of heavy transport vehicle injured in collision with two- or three-wheeled motor vehicle in traffic accident

X● **V62.9** Unspecified occupant of heavy transport vehicle injured in collision with two- or three-wheeled motor vehicle in traffic accident

● **V63** Occupant of heavy transport vehicle injured in collision with car, pick-up truck or van

The appropriate 7th character is to be added to each code from category V63

A	initial encounter
D	subsequent encounter
S	sequela

X● **V63.0** Driver of heavy transport vehicle injured in collision with car, pick-up truck or van in nontraffic accident

X● **V63.1** Passenger in heavy transport vehicle injured in collision with car, pick-up truck or van in nontraffic accident

X● **V63.2** Person on outside of heavy transport vehicle injured in collision with car, pick-up truck or van in nontraffic accident

X● **V63.3** Unspecified occupant of heavy transport vehicle injured in collision with car, pick-up truck or van in nontraffic accident

X● **V63.4** Person boarding or alighting a heavy transport vehicle injured in collision with car, pick-up truck or van

X● **V63.5** Driver of heavy transport vehicle injured in collision with car, pick-up truck or van in traffic accident

X● **V63.6** Passenger in heavy transport vehicle injured in collision with car, pick-up truck or van in traffic accident

X● **V63.7** Person on outside of heavy transport vehicle injured in collision with car, pick-up truck or van in traffic accident

X● **V63.9** Unspecified occupant of heavy transport vehicle injured in collision with car, pick-up truck or van in traffic accident

● **V64** Occupant of heavy transport vehicle injured in collision with heavy transport vehicle or bus

Excludes1 occupant of heavy transport vehicle injured in collision with military vehicle (V69.81)

The appropriate 7th character is to be added to each code from category V64

A	initial encounter
D	subsequent encounter
S	sequela

X● **V64.0** Driver of heavy transport vehicle injured in collision with heavy transport vehicle or bus in nontraffic accident

X● **V64.1** Passenger in heavy transport vehicle injured in collision with heavy transport vehicle or bus in nontraffic accident

X● **V64.2** Person on outside of heavy transport vehicle injured in collision with heavy transport vehicle or bus in nontraffic accident

X● **V64.3** Unspecified occupant of heavy transport vehicle injured in collision with heavy transport vehicle or bus in nontraffic accident

X● **V64.4** Person boarding or alighting a heavy transport vehicle injured in collision with heavy transport vehicle or bus while boarding or alighting

X● **V64.5** Driver of heavy transport vehicle injured in collision with heavy transport vehicle or bus in traffic accident

X● **V64.6** Passenger in heavy transport vehicle injured in collision with heavy transport vehicle or bus in traffic accident

X● **V64.7** Person on outside of heavy transport vehicle injured in collision with heavy transport vehicle or bus in traffic accident

X● **V64.9** Unspecified occupant of heavy transport vehicle injured in collision with heavy transport vehicle or bus in traffic accident

● **V65** Occupant of heavy transport vehicle injured in collision with railway train or railway vehicle

The appropriate 7th character is to be added to each code from category V65

A	initial encounter
D	subsequent encounter
S	sequela

X● **V65.0** Driver of heavy transport vehicle injured in collision with railway train or railway vehicle in nontraffic accident

X● **V65.1** Passenger in heavy transport vehicle injured in collision with railway train or railway vehicle in nontraffic accident

X● **V65.2** Person on outside of heavy transport vehicle injured in collision with railway train or railway vehicle in nontraffic accident

X● **V65.3** Unspecified occupant of heavy transport vehicle injured in collision with railway train or railway vehicle in nontraffic accident

X● **V65.4** Person boarding or alighting a heavy transport vehicle injured in collision with railway train or railway vehicle

X● **V65.5** Driver of heavy transport vehicle injured in collision with railway train or railway vehicle in traffic accident

X● **V65.6** Passenger in heavy transport vehicle injured in collision with railway train or railway vehicle in traffic accident

X● **V65.7** Person on outside of heavy transport vehicle injured in collision with railway train or railway vehicle in traffic accident

X● **V65.9** Unspecified occupant of heavy transport vehicle injured in collision with railway train or railway vehicle in traffic accident

● V66   **Occupant of heavy transport vehicle injured in collision with other nonmotor vehicle**

     Includes   collision with animal-drawn vehicle, animal being ridden, streetcar

     The appropriate 7th character is to be added to each code from category V66

A	initial encounter
D	subsequent encounter
S	sequela

X ● V66.0   Driver of heavy transport vehicle injured in collision with other nonmotor vehicle in nontraffic accident

X ● V66.1   Passenger in heavy transport vehicle injured in collision with other nonmotor vehicle in nontraffic accident

X ● V66.2   Person on outside of heavy transport vehicle injured in collision with other nonmotor vehicle in nontraffic accident

X ● V66.3   Unspecified occupant of heavy transport vehicle injured in collision with other nonmotor vehicle in nontraffic accident

X ● V66.4   Person boarding or alighting a heavy transport vehicle injured in collision with other nonmotor vehicle

X ● V66.5   Driver of heavy transport vehicle injured in collision with other nonmotor vehicle in traffic accident

X ● V66.6   Passenger in heavy transport vehicle injured in collision with other nonmotor vehicle in traffic accident

X ● V66.7   Person on outside of heavy transport vehicle injured in collision with other nonmotor vehicle in traffic accident

X ● V66.9   Unspecified occupant of heavy transport vehicle injured in collision with other nonmotor vehicle in traffic accident

● V67   **Occupant of heavy transport vehicle injured in collision with fixed or stationary object**

     The appropriate 7th character is to be added to each code from category V67

A	initial encounter
D	subsequent encounter
S	sequela

X ● V67.0   Driver of heavy transport vehicle injured in collision with fixed or stationary object in nontraffic accident

X ● V67.1   Passenger in heavy transport vehicle injured in collision with fixed or stationary object in nontraffic accident

X ● V67.2   Person on outside of heavy transport vehicle injured in collision with fixed or stationary object in nontraffic accident

X ● V67.3   Unspecified occupant of heavy transport vehicle injured in collision with fixed or stationary object in nontraffic accident

X ● V67.4   Person boarding or alighting a heavy transport vehicle injured in collision with fixed or stationary object

X ● V67.5   Driver of heavy transport vehicle injured in collision with fixed or stationary object in traffic accident

X ● V67.6   Passenger in heavy transport vehicle injured in collision with fixed or stationary object in traffic accident

X ● V67.7   Person on outside of heavy transport vehicle injured in collision with fixed or stationary object in traffic accident

X ● V67.9   Unspecified occupant of heavy transport vehicle injured in collision with fixed or stationary object in traffic accident

● V68   **Occupant of heavy transport vehicle injured in noncollision transport accident**

     Includes   overturning heavy transport vehicle NOS overturning heavy transport vehicle without collision

     The appropriate 7th character is to be added to each code from category V68

A	initial encounter
D	subsequent encounter
S	sequela

X ● V68.0   Driver of heavy transport vehicle injured in noncollision transport accident in nontraffic accident

X ● V68.1   Passenger in heavy transport vehicle injured in noncollision transport accident in nontraffic accident

X ● V68.2   Person on outside of heavy transport vehicle injured in noncollision transport accident in nontraffic accident

X ● V68.3   Unspecified occupant of heavy transport vehicle injured in noncollision transport accident in nontraffic accident

X ● V68.4   Person boarding or alighting a heavy transport vehicle injured in noncollision transport accident

X ● V68.5   Driver of heavy transport vehicle injured in noncollision transport accident in traffic accident

X ● V68.6   Passenger in heavy transport vehicle injured in noncollision transport accident in traffic accident

X ● V68.7   Person on outside of heavy transport vehicle injured in noncollision transport accident in traffic accident

X ● V68.9   Unspecified occupant of heavy transport vehicle injured in noncollision transport accident in traffic accident

● V69   **Occupant of heavy transport vehicle injured in other and unspecified transport accidents**

     The appropriate 7th character is to be added to each code from category V69

A	initial encounter
D	subsequent encounter
S	sequela

● V69.0   Driver of heavy transport vehicle injured in collision with other and unspecified motor vehicles in nontraffic accident

   X ● V69.00   Driver of heavy transport vehicle injured in collision with unspecified motor vehicles in nontraffic accident

   X ● V69.09   Driver of heavy transport vehicle injured in collision with other motor vehicles in nontraffic accident

● V69.1   Passenger in heavy transport vehicle injured in collision with other and unspecified motor vehicles in nontraffic accident

   X ● V69.10   Passenger in heavy transport vehicle injured in collision with unspecified motor vehicles in nontraffic accident

   X ● V69.19   Passenger in heavy transport vehicle injured in collision with other motor vehicles in nontraffic accident

● V69.2   Unspecified occupant of heavy transport vehicle injured in collision with other and unspecified motor vehicles in nontraffic accident

   X ● V69.20   Unspecified occupant of heavy transport vehicle injured in collision with unspecified motor vehicles in nontraffic accident

       Collision NOS involving heavy transport vehicle, nontraffic

   X ● V69.29   Unspecified occupant of heavy transport vehicle injured in collision with other motor vehicles in nontraffic accident

X ● **V69.3** **Occupant (driver) (passenger) of heavy transport vehicle injured in** unspecified nontraffic accident
  Accident NOS involving heavy transport vehicle, nontraffic
  Occupant of heavy transport vehicle injured in nontraffic accident NOS

● **V69.4** **Driver of heavy transport vehicle injured in collision with other and unspecified motor vehicles in** traffic accident

  X ● **V69.40** Driver of heavy transport vehicle injured in collision with unspecified motor vehicles in traffic accident

  X ● **V69.49** Driver of heavy transport vehicle injured in collision with other motor vehicles in traffic accident

● **V69.5** **Passenger in heavy transport vehicle injured in collision with other and unspecified motor vehicles in** traffic accident

  X ● **V69.50** Passenger in heavy transport vehicle injured in collision with unspecified motor vehicles in traffic accident

  X ● **V69.59** Passenger in heavy transport vehicle injured in collision with other motor vehicles in traffic accident

● **V69.6** Unspecified **occupant of heavy transport vehicle injured in collision with other and unspecified motor vehicles in** traffic accident

  X ● **V69.60** Unspecified occupant of heavy transport vehicle injured in collision with unspecified motor vehicles in traffic accident
    Collision NOS involving heavy transport vehicle (traffic)

  X ● **V69.69** Unspecified occupant of heavy transport vehicle injured in collision with other motor vehicles in traffic accident

● **V69.8** **Occupant (driver) (passenger) of heavy transport vehicle injured in other specified transport accidents**

  X ● **V69.81** Occupant (driver) (passenger) of heavy transport vehicle injured in transport accidents with military vehicle

  X ● **V69.88** Occupant (driver) (passenger) of heavy transport vehicle injured in other specified transport accidents

X ● **V69.9** **Occupant (driver) (passenger) of heavy transport vehicle injured in** unspecified traffic accident
  Accident NOS involving heavy transport vehicle

BUS OCCUPANT INJURED IN TRANSPORT ACCIDENT (V70-V79)

Includes	motorcoach
Excludes1	minibus (V50-V59)

● **V70** **Bus occupant injured in collision with pedestrian or animal**

  Excludes1 bus collision with animal-drawn vehicle or animal being ridden (V76.-)

  The appropriate 7th character is to be added to each code from category V70

A	initial encounter
D	subsequent encounter
S	sequela

X ● **V70.0** Driver **of bus injured in collision with pedestrian or animal in** nontraffic accident

X ● **V70.1** Passenger **on bus injured in collision with pedestrian or animal in** nontraffic accident

X ● **V70.2** Person on outside **of bus injured in collision with pedestrian or animal in** nontraffic accident

X ● **V70.3** Unspecified **occupant of bus injured in collision with pedestrian or animal in** nontraffic accident

X ● **V70.4** Person boarding or alighting **from bus injured in collision with pedestrian or animal**

X ● **V70.5** Driver **of bus injured in collision with pedestrian or animal in** traffic accident

X ● **V70.6** Passenger **on bus injured in collision with pedestrian or animal in** traffic accident

X ● **V70.7** Person on outside **of bus injured in collision with pedestrian or animal in** traffic accident

X ● **V70.9** Unspecified **occupant of bus injured in collision with pedestrian or animal in** traffic accident

● **V71** **Bus occupant injured in collision with pedal cycle**
  The appropriate 7th character is to be added to each code from category V71

A	initial encounter
D	subsequent encounter
S	sequela

X ● **V71.0** Driver **of bus injured in collision with pedal cycle in** nontraffic accident

X ● **V71.1** Passenger **on bus injured in collision with pedal cycle in** nontraffic accident

X ● **V71.2** Person on outside **of bus injured in collision with pedal cycle in** nontraffic accident

X ● **V71.3** Unspecified **occupant of bus injured in collision with pedal cycle in** nontraffic accident

X ● **V71.4** Person boarding or alighting **from bus injured in collision with pedal cycle**

X ● **V71.5** Driver **of bus injured in collision with pedal cycle in** traffic accident

X ● **V71.6** Passenger **on bus injured in collision with pedal cycle in** traffic accident

X ● **V71.7** Person on outside **of bus injured in collision with pedal cycle in** traffic accident

X ● **V71.9** Unspecified **occupant of bus injured in collision with pedal cycle in** traffic accident

● **V72** **Bus occupant injured in collision with two- or three-wheeled motor vehicle**
  The appropriate 7th character is to be added to each code from category V72

A	initial encounter
D	subsequent encounter
S	sequela

X ● **V72.0** Driver **of bus injured in collision with two- or three-wheeled motor vehicle in** nontraffic accident

X ● **V72.1** Passenger **on bus injured in collision with two- or three-wheeled motor vehicle in** nontraffic accident

X ● **V72.2** Person on outside **of bus injured in collision with two- or three-wheeled motor vehicle in** nontraffic accident

X ● **V72.3** Unspecified **occupant of bus injured in collision with two- or three-wheeled motor vehicle in** nontraffic accident

X ● **V72.4** Person boarding or alighting **from bus injured in collision with two- or three-wheeled motor vehicle**

X ● **V72.5** Driver **of bus injured in collision with two- or three-wheeled motor vehicle in** traffic accident

X ● **V72.6** Passenger **on bus injured in collision with two- or three-wheeled motor vehicle in** traffic accident

X ● **V72.7** Person on outside **of bus injured in collision with two- or three-wheeled motor vehicle in** traffic accident

X ● **V72.9** Unspecified **occupant of bus injured in collision with two- or three-wheeled motor vehicle in** traffic accident

▶ New   ⇒ Revised   ~~deleted~~ Deleted   Excludes 1   Excludes 2   Includes   Use additional   Code first   Code also   Key words
OGCR Official Guidelines   X Assign placeholder X   ● Use Additional Character(s)   ▷ Manifestation Code   🗪 Hierarchical Condition Category   **Coding Clinic**

● **V73**   **Bus occupant injured in collision with car, pick-up truck or van**

The appropriate 7th character is to be added to each code from category V73

> A   initial encounter
> D   subsequent encounter
> S   sequela

X● **V73.0**   Driver of bus injured in collision with car, pick-up truck or van in nontraffic accident

X● **V73.1**   Passenger on bus injured in collision with car, pick-up truck or van in nontraffic accident

X● **V73.2**   Person on outside of bus injured in collision with car, pick-up truck or van in nontraffic accident

X● **V73.3**   Unspecified occupant of bus injured in collision with car, pick-up truck or van in nontraffic accident

X● **V73.4**   Person boarding or alighting from bus injured in collision with car, pick-up truck or van

X● **V73.5**   Driver of bus injured in collision with car, pick-up truck or van in traffic accident

X● **V73.6**   Passenger on bus injured in collision with car, pick-up truck or van in traffic accident

X● **V73.7**   Person on outside of bus injured in collision with car, pick-up truck or van in traffic accident

X● **V73.9**   Unspecified occupant of bus injured in collision with car, pick-up truck or van in traffic accident

● **V74**   **Bus occupant injured in collision with heavy transport vehicle or bus**

> **Excludes1**   bus occupant injured in collision with military vehicle (V79.81)

The appropriate 7th character is to be added to each code from category V74

> A   initial encounter
> D   subsequent encounter
> S   sequela

X● **V74.0**   Driver of bus injured in collision with heavy transport vehicle or bus in nontraffic accident

X● **V74.1**   Passenger on bus injured in collision with heavy transport vehicle or bus in nontraffic accident

X● **V74.2**   Person on outside of bus injured in collision with heavy transport vehicle or bus in nontraffic accident

X● **V74.3**   Unspecified occupant of bus injured in collision with heavy transport vehicle or bus in nontraffic accident

X● **V74.4**   Person boarding or alighting from bus injured in collision with heavy transport vehicle or bus

X● **V74.5**   Driver of bus injured in collision with heavy transport vehicle or bus in traffic accident

X● **V74.6**   Passenger on bus injured in collision with heavy transport vehicle or bus in traffic accident

X● **V74.7**   Person on outside of bus injured in collision with heavy transport vehicle or bus in traffic accident

X● **V74.9**   Unspecified occupant of bus injured in collision with heavy transport vehicle or bus in traffic accident

● **V75**   **Bus occupant injured in collision with railway train or railway vehicle**

The appropriate 7th character is to be added to each code from category V75

> A   initial encounter
> D   subsequent encounter
> S   sequela

X● **V75.0**   Driver of bus injured in collision with railway train or railway vehicle in nontraffic accident

X● **V75.1**   Passenger on bus injured in collision with railway train or railway vehicle in nontraffic accident

X● **V75.2**   Person on outside of bus injured in collision with railway train or railway vehicle in nontraffic accident

X● **V75.3**   Unspecified occupant of bus injured in collision with railway train or railway vehicle in nontraffic accident

X● **V75.4**   Person boarding or alighting from bus injured in collision with railway train or railway vehicle

X● **V75.5**   Driver of bus injured in collision with railway train or railway vehicle in traffic accident

X● **V75.6**   Passenger on bus injured in collision with railway train or railway vehicle in traffic accident

X● **V75.7**   Person on outside of bus injured in collision with railway train or railway vehicle in traffic accident

X● **V75.9**   Unspecified occupant of bus injured in collision with railway train or railway vehicle in traffic accident

● **V76**   **Bus occupant injured in collision with other nonmotor vehicle**

> **Includes**   collision with animal-drawn vehicle, animal being ridden, streetcar

The appropriate 7th character is to be added to each code from category V76

> A   initial encounter
> D   subsequent encounter
> S   sequela

X● **V76.0**   Driver of bus injured in collision with other nonmotor vehicle in nontraffic accident

X● **V76.1**   Passenger on bus injured in collision with other nonmotor vehicle in nontraffic accident

X● **V76.2**   Person on outside of bus injured in collision with other nonmotor vehicle in nontraffic accident

X● **V76.3**   Unspecified occupant of bus injured in collision with other nonmotor vehicle in nontraffic accident

X● **V76.4**   Person boarding or alighting from bus injured in collision with other nonmotor vehicle

X● **V76.5**   Driver of bus injured in collision with other nonmotor vehicle in traffic accident

X● **V76.6**   Passenger on bus injured in collision with other nonmotor vehicle in traffic accident

X● **V76.7**   Person on outside of bus injured in collision with other nonmotor vehicle in traffic accident

X● **V76.9**   Unspecified occupant of bus injured in collision with other nonmotor vehicle in traffic accident

● **V77**   **Bus occupant injured in collision with fixed or stationary object**

The appropriate 7th character is to be added to each code from category V77

> A   initial encounter
> D   subsequent encounter
> S   sequela

X● **V77.0**   Driver of bus injured in collision with fixed or stationary object in nontraffic accident

X● **V77.1**   Passenger on bus injured in collision with fixed or stationary object in nontraffic accident

X● **V77.2**   Person on outside of bus injured in collision with fixed or stationary object in nontraffic accident

X● **V77.3**   Unspecified occupant of bus injured in collision with fixed or stationary object in nontraffic accident

X● **V77.4**   Person boarding or alighting from bus injured in collision with fixed or stationary object

X● **V77.5**   Driver of bus injured in collision with fixed or stationary object in traffic accident

X● **V77.6**   Passenger on bus injured in collision with fixed or stationary object in traffic accident

X● **V77.7**   Person on outside of bus injured in collision with fixed or stationary object in traffic accident

X● **V77.9**   Unspecified occupant of bus injured in collision with fixed or stationary object in traffic accident

● V78   Bus occupant injured in noncollision transport accident

Includes   overturning bus NOS
overturning bus without collision

The appropriate 7th character is to be added to each code from
category V78

> A   initial encounter
> D   subsequent encounter
> S   sequela

X● V78.0   Driver of bus injured in noncollision transport accident
in nontraffic accident

X● V78.1   Passenger on bus injured in noncollision transport
accident in nontraffic accident

X● V78.2   Person on outside of bus injured in noncollision
transport accident in nontraffic accident

X● V78.3   Unspecified occupant of bus injured in noncollision
transport accident in nontraffic accident

X● V78.4   Person boarding or alighting from bus injured in
noncollision transport accident

X● V78.5   Driver of bus injured in noncollision transport accident
in traffic accident

X● V78.6   Passenger on bus injured in noncollision transport
accident in traffic accident

X● V78.7   Person on outside of bus injured in noncollision
transport accident in traffic accident

X● V78.9   Unspecified occupant of bus injured in noncollision
transport accident in traffic accident

● V79   Bus occupant injured in other and unspecified transport
accidents

The appropriate 7th character is to be added to each code from
category V79

> A   initial encounter
> D   subsequent encounter
> S   sequela

● V79.0   Driver of bus injured in collision with other and
unspecified motor vehicles in nontraffic accident

X● V79.00   Driver of bus injured in collision with
unspecified motor vehicles in nontraffic
accident

X● V79.09   Driver of bus injured in collision with other
motor vehicles in nontraffic accident

● V79.1   Passenger on bus injured in collision with other and
unspecified motor vehicles in nontraffic accident

X● V79.10   Passenger on bus injured in collision with
unspecified motor vehicles in nontraffic
accident

X● V79.19   Passenger on bus injured in collision with other
motor vehicles in nontraffic accident

● V79.2   Unspecified bus occupant injured in collision with other
and unspecified motor vehicles in nontraffic accident

X● V79.20   Unspecified bus occupant injured in collision
with unspecified motor vehicles in nontraffic
accident
Bus collision NOS, nontraffic

X● V79.29   Unspecified bus occupant injured in collision
with other motor vehicles in nontraffic accident

X● V79.3   Bus occupant (driver) (passenger) injured in unspecified
nontraffic accident
Bus accident NOS, nontraffic
Bus occupant injured in nontraffic accident NOS

● V79.4   Driver of bus injured in collision with other and
unspecified motor vehicles in traffic accident

X● V79.40   Driver of bus injured in collision with
unspecified motor vehicles in traffic accident

X● V79.49   Driver of bus injured in collision with other
motor vehicles in traffic accident

● V79.5   Passenger on bus injured in collision with other and
unspecified motor vehicles in traffic accident

X● V79.50   Passenger on bus injured in collision with
unspecified motor vehicles in traffic accident

X● V79.59   Passenger on bus injured in collision with other
motor vehicles in traffic accident

● V79.6   Unspecified bus occupant injured in collision with other
and unspecified motor vehicles in traffic accident

X● V79.60   Unspecified bus occupant injured in collision
with unspecified motor vehicles in traffic
accident
Bus collision NOS (traffic)

X● V79.69   Unspecified bus occupant injured in collision
with other motor vehicles in traffic accident

● V79.8   Bus occupant (driver) (passenger) injured in other
specified transport accidents

X● V79.81   Bus occupant (driver) (passenger) injured in
transport accidents with military vehicle

X● V79.88   Bus occupant (driver) (passenger) injured in
other specified transport accidents

X● V79.9   Bus occupant (driver) (passenger) injured in unspecified
traffic accident
Bus accident NOS

OTHER LAND TRANSPORT ACCIDENTS (V80-V89)

● V80   Animal-rider or occupant of animal-drawn vehicle injured in
transport accident

The appropriate 7th character is to be added to each code from
category V80

> A   initial encounter
> D   subsequent encounter
> S   sequela

● V80.0   Animal-rider or occupant of animal drawn vehicle
injured by fall from or being thrown from animal or
animal-drawn vehicle in noncollision accident

● V80.01   Animal-rider injured by fall from or being
thrown from animal in noncollision accident

● V80.010   Animal-rider injured by fall from
or being thrown from horse in
noncollision accident

● V80.018   Animal-rider injured by fall from or
being thrown from other animal in
noncollision accident

X● V80.02   Occupant of animal-drawn vehicle injured by
fall from or being thrown from animal-drawn
vehicle in noncollision accident
Overturning animal-drawn vehicle NOS
Overturning animal-drawn vehicle without
collision

● V80.1   Animal-rider or occupant of animal-drawn vehicle
injured in collision with pedestrian or animal

Excludes1   animal-rider or animal-drawn vehicle
collision with animal-drawn vehicle
or animal being ridden (V80.7)

X● V80.11   Animal-rider injured in collision with
pedestrian or animal

X● V80.12   Occupant of animal-drawn vehicle injured in
collision with pedestrian or animal

● V80.2   Animal-rider or occupant of animal-drawn vehicle
injured in collision with pedal cycle

X● V80.21   Animal-rider injured in collision with pedal
cycle

X● V80.22   Occupant of animal-drawn vehicle injured in
collision with pedal cycle

● **V80.3** Animal-rider or occupant of animal-drawn vehicle injured in collision with two- or three-wheeled motor vehicle

   X● **V80.31** Animal-rider injured in collision with two- or three-wheeled motor vehicle

   X● **V80.32** Occupant of animal-drawn vehicle injured in collision with two- or three-wheeled motor vehicle

● **V80.4** Animal-rider or occupant of animal-drawn vehicle injured in collision with car, pick-up truck, van, heavy transport vehicle or bus

     Excludes1   animal-rider injured in collision with military vehicle (V80.910)

          occupant of animal-drawn vehicle injured in collision with military vehicle (V80.920)

   X● **V80.41** Animal-rider injured in collision with car, pick-up truck, van, heavy transport vehicle or bus

   X● **V80.42** Occupant of animal-drawn vehicle injured in collision with car, pick-up truck, van, heavy transport vehicle or bus

● **V80.5** Animal-rider or occupant of animal-drawn vehicle injured in collision with other specified motor vehicle

   X● **V80.51** Animal-rider injured in collision with other specified motor vehicle

   X● **V80.52** Occupant of animal-drawn vehicle injured in collision with other specified motor vehicle

● **V80.6** Animal-rider or occupant of animal-drawn vehicle injured in collision with railway train or railway vehicle

   X● **V80.61** Animal-rider injured in collision with railway train or railway vehicle

   X● **V80.62** Occupant of animal-drawn vehicle injured in collision with railway train or railway vehicle

● **V80.7** Animal-rider or occupant of animal-drawn vehicle injured in collision with other nonmotor vehicles

   ● **V80.71** Animal-rider or occupant of animal-drawn vehicle injured in collision with animal being ridden

     ● **V80.710** Animal-rider injured in collision with other animal being ridden

     ● **V80.711** Occupant of animal-drawn vehicle injured in collision with animal being ridden

   ● **V80.72** Animal-rider or occupant of animal-drawn vehicle injured in collision with other animal-drawn vehicle

     ● **V80.720** Animal-rider injured in collision with animal-drawn vehicle

     ● **V80.721** Occupant of animal-drawn vehicle injured in collision with other animal-drawn vehicle

   ● **V80.73** Animal-rider or occupant of animal-drawn vehicle injured in collision with streetcar

     ● **V80.730** Animal-rider injured in collision with streetcar

     ● **V80.731** Occupant of animal-drawn vehicle injured in collision with streetcar

   ● **V80.79** Animal-rider or occupant of animal-drawn vehicle injured in collision with other nonmotor vehicles

     ● **V80.790** Animal-rider injured in collision with other nonmotor vehicles

     ● **V80.791** Occupant of animal-drawn vehicle injured in collision with other nonmotor vehicles

● **V80.8** Animal-rider or occupant of animal-drawn vehicle injured in collision with fixed or stationary object

   X● **V80.81** Animal-rider injured in collision with fixed or stationary object

   X● **V80.82** Occupant of animal-drawn vehicle injured in collision with fixed or stationary object

● **V80.9** Animal-rider or occupant of animal-drawn vehicle injured in other and unspecified transport accidents

   ● **V80.91** Animal-rider injured in other and unspecified transport accidents

     ● **V80.910** Animal-rider injured in transport accident with military vehicle

     ● **V80.918** Animal-rider injured in other transport accident

     ● **V80.919** Animal-rider injured in unspecified transport accident

        Animal rider accident NOS

   ● **V80.92** Occupant of animal-drawn vehicle injured in other and unspecified transport accidents

     ● **V80.920** Occupant of animal-drawn vehicle injured in transport accident with military vehicle

     ● **V80.928** Occupant of animal-drawn vehicle injured in other transport accident

     ● **V80.929** Occupant of animal-drawn vehicle injured in unspecified transport accident

        Animal-drawn vehicle accident NOS

● **V81** Occupant of railway train or railway vehicle injured in transport accident

     Includes   derailment of railway train or railway vehicle

          person on outside of train

     Excludes1   streetcar (V82.-)

     The appropriate 7th character is to be added to each code from category V81

A	initial encounter
D	subsequent encounter
S	sequela

   X● **V81.0** Occupant of railway train or railway vehicle injured in collision with motor vehicle in nontraffic accident

     Excludes1   occupant of railway train or railway vehicle injured due to collision with military vehicle (V81.83)

   X● **V81.1** Occupant of railway train or railway vehicle injured in collision with motor vehicle in traffic accident

     Excludes1   occupant of railway train or railway vehicle injured due to collision with military vehicle (V81.83)

   X● **V81.2** Occupant of railway train or railway vehicle injured in collision with or hit by rolling stock

   X● **V81.3** Occupant of railway train or railway vehicle injured in collision with other object

        Railway collision NOS

   X● **V81.4** Person injured while boarding or alighting from railway train or railway vehicle

   X● **V81.5** Occupant of railway train or railway vehicle injured by fall in railway train or railway vehicle

   X● **V81.6** Occupant of railway train or railway vehicle injured by fall from railway train or railway vehicle

   X● **V81.7** Occupant of railway train or railway vehicle injured in derailment without antecedent collision

CHAPTER 20 (V00-Y99)

● **V81.8 Occupant of railway train or railway vehicle injured in other specified railway accidents**

X ● **V81.81 Occupant of railway train or railway vehicle injured due to explosion or fire on train**

X ● **V81.82 Occupant of railway train or railway vehicle injured due to object falling onto train**
Occupant of railway train or railway vehicle injured due to falling earth onto train
Occupant of railway train or railway vehicle injured due to falling rocks onto train
Occupant of railway train or railway vehicle injured due to falling snow onto train
Occupant of railway train or railway vehicle injured due to falling trees onto train

X ● **V81.83 Occupant of railway train or railway vehicle injured due to collision with military vehicle**

X ● **V81.89 Occupant of railway train or railway vehicle injured due to other specified railway accident**

X ● **V81.9 Occupant of railway train or railway vehicle injured in unspecified railway accident**
Railway accident NOS

● **V82 Occupant of powered streetcar injured in transport accident**

Includes interurban electric car
person on outside of streetcar
tram (car)
trolley (car)

Excludes1 bus (V70-V79)
motorcoach (V70-V79)
nonpowered streetcar (V76.-)
train (V81.-)

The appropriate 7th character is to be added to each code from category V82

A initial encounter
D subsequent encounter
S sequela

X ● **V82.0 Occupant of streetcar injured in collision with motor vehicle in nontraffic accident**

X ● **V82.1 Occupant of streetcar injured in collision with motor vehicle in traffic accident**

X ● **V82.2 Occupant of streetcar injured in collision with or hit by rolling stock**

X ● **V82.3 Occupant of streetcar injured in collision with other object**
Excludes1 collision with animal-drawn vehicle or animal being ridden (V82.8)

X ● **V82.4 Person injured while boarding or alighting from streetcar**

X ● **V82.5 Occupant of streetcar injured by fall in streetcar**
Excludes1 fall in streetcar:
while boarding or alighting (V82.4)
with antecedent collision (V82.0-V82.3)

X ● **V82.6 Occupant of streetcar injured by fall from streetcar**
Excludes1 fall from streetcar:
while boarding or alighting (V82.4)
with antecedent collision (V82.0-V82.3)

X ● **V82.7 Occupant of streetcar injured in derailment without antecedent collision**
Excludes1 occupant of streetcar injured in derailment with antecedent collision (V82.0-V82.3)

X ● **V82.8 Occupant of streetcar injured in other specified transport accidents**
Streetcar collision with military vehicle
Streetcar collision with train or nonmotor vehicles

X ● **V82.9 Occupant of streetcar injured in unspecified traffic accident**
Streetcar accident NOS

● **V83 Occupant of special vehicle mainly used on industrial premises injured in transport accident**

Includes battery-powered airport passenger vehicle
battery-powered truck (baggage) (mail)
coal-car in mine
forklift (truck)
logging car
self-propelled industrial truck
station baggage truck (powered)
tram, truck, or tub (powered) in mine or quarry

Excludes1 special construction vehicles (V85.-)
special industrial vehicle in stationary use or maintenance (W31.-)

The appropriate 7th character is to be added to each code from category V83

A initial encounter
D subsequent encounter
S sequela

X ● **V83.0 Driver of special industrial vehicle injured in traffic accident**

X ● **V83.1 Passenger of special industrial vehicle injured in traffic accident**

X ● **V83.2 Person on outside of special industrial vehicle injured in traffic accident**

X ● **V83.3 Unspecified occupant of special industrial vehicle injured in traffic accident**

X ● **V83.4 Person injured while boarding or alighting from special industrial vehicle**

X ● **V83.5 Driver of special industrial vehicle injured in nontraffic accident**

X ● **V83.6 Passenger of special industrial vehicle injured in nontraffic accident**

X ● **V83.7 Person on outside of special industrial vehicle injured in nontraffic accident**

X ● **V83.9 Unspecified occupant of special industrial vehicle injured in nontraffic accident**
Special-industrial-vehicle accident NOS

● **V84 Occupant of special vehicle mainly used in agriculture injured in transport accident**

Includes self-propelled farm machinery
tractor (and trailer)

Excludes1 animal-powered farm machinery accident (W30.8-)
contact with combine harvester (W30.0)
special agricultural vehicle in stationary use or maintenance (W30.-)

The appropriate 7th character is to be added to each code from category V84

A initial encounter
D subsequent encounter
S sequela

X ● **V84.0 Driver of special agricultural vehicle injured in traffic accident**

X ● **V84.1 Passenger of special agricultural vehicle injured in traffic accident**

X ● **V84.2 Person on outside of special agricultural vehicle injured in traffic accident**

X ● **V84.3 Unspecified occupant of special agricultural vehicle injured in traffic accident**

X ● **V84.4 Person injured while boarding or alighting from special agricultural vehicle**

X ● **V84.5 Driver of special agricultural vehicle injured in nontraffic accident**

X ● **V84.6 Passenger of special agricultural vehicle injured in nontraffic accident**

X ● **V84.7 Person on outside of special agricultural vehicle injured in nontraffic accident**

X ● **V84.9 Unspecified occupant of special agricultural vehicle injured in nontraffic accident**
Special-agricultural vehicle accident NOS

● **V85**   **Occupant of special construction vehicle injured in transport accident**

     Includes   bulldozer
                       digger
                       dump truck
                       earth-leveller
                       mechanical shovel
                       road-roller

     Excludes1   special industrial vehicle (V83.-)
                    special construction vehicle in stationary use or maintenance (W31.-)

The appropriate 7th character is to be added to each code from category V85

> A   initial encounter
> D   subsequent encounter
> S   sequela

X● **V85.0**   Driver of special construction vehicle injured in traffic accident

X● **V85.1**   Passenger of special construction vehicle injured in traffic accident

X● **V85.2**   Person on outside of special construction vehicle injured in traffic accident

X● **V85.3**   Unspecified occupant of special construction vehicle injured in traffic accident

X● **V85.4**   Person injured while boarding or alighting from special construction vehicle

X● **V85.5**   Driver of special construction vehicle injured in nontraffic accident

X● **V85.6**   Passenger of special construction vehicle injured in nontraffic accident

X● **V85.7**   Person on outside of special construction vehicle injured in nontraffic accident

X● **V85.9**   Unspecified occupant of special construction vehicle injured in nontraffic accident
     Special-construction-vehicle accident NOS

● **V86**   **Occupant of special all-terrain or other off-road motor vehicle, injured in transport accident**

     Excludes1   special all-terrain vehicle in stationary use or maintenance (W31.-)
                    sport-utility vehicle (V50-V59)
                    three-wheeled motor vehicle designed for on-road use (V30-V39)

The appropriate 7th character is to be added to each code from category V86

> A   initial encounter
> D   subsequent encounter
> S   sequela

● **V86.0**   Driver of special all-terrain or other off-road motor vehicle injured in traffic accident

   X● **V86.01**   Driver of ambulance or fire engine injured in traffic accident

   X● **V86.02**   Driver of snowmobile injured in traffic accident

   X● **V86.03**   Driver of dune buggy injured in traffic accident

   X● **V86.04**   Driver of military vehicle injured in traffic accident

   X● **V86.05**   Driver of 3- or 4-wheeled all-terrain vehicle (ATV) injured in traffic accident

   X● **V86.06**   Driver of dirt bike or motor/cross bike injured in traffic accident

   X● **V86.09**   Driver of other off-road special all-terrain or other off-road vehicle injured in traffic accident
     Driver of go cart injured in traffic accident
     Driver of golf cart injured in traffic accident

● **V86.1**   Passenger of special all-terrain or other off-road motor vehicle injured in traffic accident

   X● **V86.11**   Passenger of ambulance or fire engine injured in traffic accident

   X● **V86.12**   Passenger of snowmobile injured in traffic accident

   X● **V86.13**   Passenger of dune buggy injured in traffic accident

   X● **V86.14**   Passenger of military vehicle injured in traffic accident

   X● **V86.15**   Passenger of 3- or 4-wheeled all-terrain vehicle (ATV) injured in traffic accident

   X● **V86.16**   Passenger of dirt bike or motor/cross bike injured in traffic accident

   X● **V86.19**   Passenger of other off-road special all-terrain or other off-road off-road motor vehicle injured in traffic accident
     Passenger of go cart injured in traffic accident
     Passenger of golf cart injured in traffic accident

● **V86.2**   Person on outside of special all-terrain or other off-road motor vehicle injured in traffic accident

   X● **V86.21**   Person on outside of ambulance or fire engine injured in traffic accident

   X● **V86.22**   Person on outside of snowmobile injured in traffic accident

   X● **V86.23**   Person on outside of dune buggy injured in traffic accident

   X● **V86.24**   Person on outside of military vehicle injured in traffic accident

   X● **V86.25**   Person on outside of 3- or 4-wheeled all-terrain vehicle (ATV) injured in traffic accident

   X● **V86.26**   Person on outside of dirt bike or motor/cross bike injured in traffic accident

   X● **V86.29**   Person on outside of other special all-terrain or other off-road motor vehicle injured in traffic accident
     Person on outside of go cart in traffic accident
     Person on outside of golf cart injured in traffic accident

● **V86.3**   Unspecified occupant of special all-terrain or other off-road motor vehicle injured in traffic accident

   X● **V86.31**   Unspecified occupant of ambulance or fire engine injured in traffic accident

   X● **V86.32**   Unspecified occupant of snowmobile injured in traffic accident

   X● **V86.33**   Unspecified occupant of dune buggy injured in traffic accident

   X● **V86.34**   Unspecified occupant of military vehicle injured in traffic accident

   X● **V86.35**   Unspecified occupant of 3- or 4-wheeled all-terrain vehicle (ATV) injured in traffic accident

   X● **V86.36**   Unspecified occupant of dirt bike or motor/cross bike injured in traffic accident

   X● **V86.39**   Unspecified occupant of other special all-terrain or other off-road motor vehicle injured in traffic accident
     Unspecified occupant of go cart injured in traffic accident
     Unspecified occupant of golf cart injured in traffic accident

CHAPTER 20 (V00-Y99)

● V86.4   Person injured while boarding or alighting from special all-terrain or other off-road motor vehicle

     X● V86.41   Person injured while boarding or alighting from ambulance or fire engine

     X● V86.42   Person injured while boarding or alighting from snowmobile

     X● V86.43   Person injured while boarding or alighting from dune buggy

     X● V86.44   Person injured while boarding or alighting from military vehicle

     X● V86.45   Person injured while boarding or alighting from a 3- or 4-wheeled all-terrain vehicle (ATV)

     X● V86.46   Person injured while boarding or alighting from a dirt bike or motor/cross bike

     X● V86.49   Person injured while boarding or alighting from other special all-terrain or other off-road motor vehicle

         Person injured while boarding or alighting from go cart

         Person injured while boarding or alighting from golf cart

● V86.5   Driver of special all-terrain or other off-road motor vehicle injured in nontraffic accident

     X● V86.51   Driver of ambulance or fire engine injured in nontraffic accident

     X● V86.52   Driver of snowmobile injured in nontraffic accident

     X● V86.53   Driver of dune buggy injured in nontraffic accident

     X● V86.54   Driver of military vehicle injured in nontraffic accident

     X● V86.55   Driver of 3- or 4-wheeled all-terrain vehicle (ATV) injured in nontraffic accident

     X● V86.56   Driver of dirt bike or motor/cross bike injured in nontraffic accident

     X● V86.59   Driver of other off-road special all-terrain or other off-road motor vehicle injured in nontraffic accident

         Driver of go cart injured in nontraffic accident

         Driver of golf cart injured in nontraffic accident

● V86.6   Passenger of special all-terrain or other off-road motor vehicle injured in nontraffic accident

     X● V86.61   Passenger of ambulance or fire engine injured in nontraffic accident

     X● V86.62   Passenger of snowmobile injured in nontraffic accident

     X● V86.63   Passenger of dune buggy injured in nontraffic accident

     X● V86.64   Passenger of military vehicle injured in nontraffic accident

     X● V86.65   Passenger of 3- or 4-wheeled all-terrain vehicle (ATV) injured in nontraffic accident

     X● V86.66   Passenger of dirt bike or motor/cross bike injured in nontraffic accident

     X● V86.69   Passenger of other special all-terrain or other off-road vehicle injured in nontraffic accident

         Passenger of go cart injured in nontraffic accident

         Passenger of golf cart injured in nontraffic accident

● V86.7   Person on outside of special all-terrain or other off-road motor vehicle injured in nontraffic accident

     X● V86.71   Person on outside of ambulance or fire engine injured in nontraffic accident

     X● V86.72   Person on outside of snowmobile injured in nontraffic accident

     X● V86.73   Person on outside of dune buggy injured in nontraffic accident

     X● V86.74   Person on outside of military vehicle injured in nontraffic accident

     X● V86.75   Person on outside of 3- or 4-wheeled all-terrain vehicle (ATV) injured in nontraffic accident

     X● V86.76   Person on outside of dirt bike or motor/cross bike injured in nontraffic accident

     X● V86.79   Person on outside of other special all-terrain or other off-road motor vehicles injured in nontraffic accident

         Person on outside of go cart injured in nontraffic accident

         Person on outside of golf cart injured in nontraffic accident

● V86.9   Unspecified occupant of special all-terrain or other off-road motor vehicle injured in nontraffic accident

     X● V86.91   Unspecified occupant of ambulance or fire engine injured in nontraffic accident

     X● V86.92   Unspecified occupant of snowmobile injured in nontraffic accident

     X● V86.93   Unspecified occupant of dune buggy injured in nontraffic accident

     X● V86.94   Unspecified occupant of military vehicle injured in nontraffic accident

     X● V86.95   Unspecified occupant of 3- or 4-wheeled all-terrain vehicle (ATV) injured in nontraffic accident

     X● V86.96   Unspecified occupant of dirt bike or motor/cross bike injured in nontraffic accident

     X● V86.99   Unspecified occupant of other special all-terrain or other off-road motor vehicle injured in nontraffic accident

         Off-road motor-vehicle accident NOS

         Other motor-vehicle accident NOS

         Unspecified occupant of go cart injured in nontraffic accident

         Unspecified occupant of golf cart injured in nontraffic accident

         Unspecified occupant of race car injured in nontraffic accident

● V87   Traffic accident of specified type but victim's mode of transport unknown

     Excludes1   collision involving:
         pedal cycle (V10-V19)
         pedestrian (V01-V09)

     The appropriate 7th character is to be added to each code from category V87

A	initial encounter
D	subsequent encounter
S	sequela

     X● V87.0   Person injured in collision between car and two- or three-wheeled powered vehicle (traffic)

     X● V87.1   Person injured in collision between other motor vehicle and two- or three-wheeled motor vehicle (traffic)

     X● V87.2   Person injured in collision between car and pick-up truck or van (traffic)

     X● V87.3   Person injured in collision between car and bus (traffic)

     X● V87.4   Person injured in collision between car and heavy transport vehicle (traffic)

     X● V87.5   Person injured in collision between heavy transport vehicle and bus (traffic)

     X● V87.6   Person injured in collision between railway train or railway vehicle and car (traffic)

     X● V87.7   Person injured in collision between other specified motor vehicles (traffic)

     X● V87.8   Person injured in other specified noncollision transport accidents involving motor vehicle (traffic)

▶ New   ⇒ Revised   ~~deleted~~ Deleted   Excludes 1   Excludes 2   Includes   Use additional   Code first   Code also   Key words

OGCR Official Guidelines   X Assign placeholder X   ● Use Additional Character(s)   ▶ Manifestation Code   🅗 Hierarchical Condition Category   **Coding Clinic**

X● V87.9   Person injured in other specified (collision) (noncollision) transport accidents involving nonmotor vehicle (traffic)

● V88   Nontraffic accident of specified type but victim's mode of transport unknown

> **Excludes1**   collision involving:
> pedal cycle (V10-V19)
> pedestrian (V01-V09)

The appropriate 7th character is to be added to each code from category V88

> A   initial encounter
> D   subsequent encounter
> S   sequela

X● V88.0   Person injured in collision between car and two- or three-wheeled motor vehicle, nontraffic

X● V88.1   Person injured in collision between other motor vehicle and two- or three-wheeled motor vehicle, nontraffic

X● V88.2   Person injured in collision between car and pick-up truck or van, nontraffic

X● V88.3   Person injured in collision between car and bus, nontraffic

X● V88.4   Person injured in collision between car and heavy transport vehicle, nontraffic

X● V88.5   Person injured in collision between heavy transport vehicle and bus, nontraffic

X● V88.6   Person injured in collision between railway train or railway vehicle and car, nontraffic

X● V88.7   Person injured in collision between other specified motor vehicle, nontraffic

X● V88.8   Person injured in other specified noncollision transport accidents involving motor vehicle, nontraffic

X● V88.9   Person injured in other specified (collision) (noncollision) transport accidents involving nonmotor vehicle, nontraffic

● V89   Motor- or nonmotor-vehicle accident, type of vehicle unspecified

The appropriate 7th character is to be added to each code from category V89

> A   initial encounter
> D   subsequent encounter
> S   sequela

X● V89.0   Person injured in unspecified motor-vehicle accident, nontraffic
> Motor-vehicle accident NOS, nontraffic

X● V89.1   Person injured in unspecified nonmotor-vehicle accident, nontraffic
> Nonmotor-vehicle accident NOS (nontraffic)

X● V89.2   Person injured in unspecified motor-vehicle accident, traffic
> Motor-vehicle accident [MVA] NOS
> Road (traffic) accident [RTA] NOS

X● V89.3   Person injured in unspecified nonmotor-vehicle accident, traffic
> Nonmotor-vehicle traffic accident NOS

X● V89.9   Person injured in unspecified vehicle accident
> Collision NOS

WATER TRANSPORT ACCIDENTS (V90-V94)

● V90   Drowning and submersion due to accident to watercraft

> **Excludes1**   civilian water transport accident involving military watercraft (V94.81-)
> fall into water not from watercraft (W16.-)
> military watercraft accident in military or war operations (Y36.0-, Y37.0-)
> water-transport–related drowning or submersion without accident to watercraft (V92.-)

The appropriate 7th character is to be added to each code from category V90

> A   initial encounter
> D   subsequent encounter
> S   sequela

● V90.0   Drowning and submersion due to watercraft overturning

X● V90.00   Drowning and submersion due to merchant ship overturning

X● V90.01   Drowning and submersion due to passenger ship overturning
> Drowning and submersion due to ferry-boat overturning
> Drowning and submersion due to liner overturning

X● V90.02   Drowning and submersion due to fishing boat overturning

X● V90.03   Drowning and submersion due to other powered watercraft overturning
> Drowning and submersion due to hovercraft (on open water) overturning
> Drowning and submersion due to jet ski overturning

X● V90.04   Drowning and submersion due to sailboat overturning

X● V90.05   Drowning and submersion due to canoe or kayak overturning

X● V90.06   Drowning and submersion due to (nonpowered) inflatable craft overturning

X● V90.08   Drowning and submersion due to other unpowered watercraft overturning
> Drowning and submersion due to windsurfer overturning

X● V90.09   Drowning and submersion due to unspecified watercraft overturning
> Drowning and submersion due to boat NOS overturning
> Drowning and submersion due to ship NOS overturning
> Drowning and submersion due to watercraft NOS overturning

● V90.1   Drowning and submersion due to watercraft sinking

X● V90.10   Drowning and submersion due to merchant ship sinking

X● V90.11   Drowning and submersion due to passenger ship sinking
> Drowning and submersion due to ferry-boat sinking
> Drowning and submersion due to liner sinking

X● V90.12   Drowning and submersion due to fishing boat sinking

X● V90.13   Drowning and submersion due to other powered watercraft sinking
> Drowning and submersion due to hovercraft (on open water) sinking
> Drowning and submersion due to jet ski sinking

X ⬤ **V90.14** Drowning and submersion due to sailboat sinking

X ⬤ **V90.15** Drowning and submersion due to canoe or kayak sinking

X ⬤ **V90.16** Drowning and submersion due to (nonpowered) inflatable craft sinking

X ⬤ **V90.18** Drowning and submersion due to other unpowered watercraft sinking

X ⬤ **V90.19** Drowning and submersion due to unspecified watercraft sinking

Drowning and submersion due to boat NOS sinking

Drowning and submersion due to ship NOS sinking

Drowning and submersion due to watercraft NOS sinking

⬤ **V90.2** Drowning and submersion due to falling or jumping from burning watercraft

X ⬤ **V90.20** Drowning and submersion due to falling or jumping from burning merchant ship

X ⬤ **V90.21** Drowning and submersion due to falling or jumping from burning passenger ship

Drowning and submersion due to falling or jumping from burning ferry-boat

Drowning and submersion due to falling or jumping from burning liner

X ⬤ **V90.22** Drowning and submersion due to falling or jumping from burning fishing boat

X ⬤ **V90.23** Drowning and submersion due to falling or jumping from other burning powered watercraft

Drowning and submersion due to falling and jumping from burning hovercraft (on open water)

Drowning and submersion due to falling and jumping from burning jet ski

X ⬤ **V90.24** Drowning and submersion due to falling or jumping from burning sailboat

X ⬤ **V90.25** Drowning and submersion due to falling or jumping from burning canoe or kayak

X ⬤ **V90.26** Drowning and submersion due to falling or jumping from burning (nonpowered) inflatable craft

X ⬤ **V90.27** Drowning and submersion due to falling or jumping from burning water-skis

X ⬤ **V90.28** Drowning and submersion due to falling or jumping from other burning unpowered watercraft

Drowning and submersion due to falling and jumping from burning surf-board

Drowning and submersion due to falling and jumping from burning windsurfer

X ⬤ **V90.29** Drowning and submersion due to falling or jumping from unspecified burning watercraft

Drowning and submersion due to falling or jumping from burning boat NOS

Drowning and submersion due to falling or jumping from burning ship NOS

Drowning and submersion due to falling or jumping from burning watercraft NOS

⬤ **V90.3** Drowning and submersion due to falling or jumping from crushed watercraft

X ⬤ **V90.30** Drowning and submersion due to falling or jumping from crushed merchant ship

X ⬤ **V90.31** Drowning and submersion due to falling or jumping from crushed passenger ship

Drowning and submersion due to falling and jumping from crushed ferry-boat

Drowning and submersion due to falling and jumping from crushed liner

X ⬤ **V90.32** Drowning and submersion due to falling or jumping from crushed fishing boat

X ⬤ **V90.33** Drowning and submersion due to falling or jumping from other crushed powered watercraft

Drowning and submersion due to falling and jumping from crushed hovercraft

Drowning and submersion due to falling and jumping from crushed jet ski

X ⬤ **V90.34** Drowning and submersion due to falling or jumping from crushed sailboat

X ⬤ **V90.35** Drowning and submersion due to falling or jumping from crushed canoe or kayak

X ⬤ **V90.36** Drowning and submersion due to falling or jumping from crushed (nonpowered) inflatable craft

X ⬤ **V90.37** Drowning and submersion due to falling or jumping from crushed water-skis

X ⬤ **V90.38** Drowning and submersion due to falling or jumping from other crushed unpowered watercraft

Drowning and submersion due to falling and jumping from crushed surf-board

Drowning and submersion due to falling and jumping from crushed windsurfer

X ⬤ **V90.39** Drowning and submersion due to falling or jumping from crushed unspecified watercraft

Drowning and submersion due to falling and jumping from crushed boat NOS

Drowning and submersion due to falling and jumping from crushed ship NOS

Drowning and submersion due to falling and jumping from crushed watercraft NOS

⬤ **V90.8** Drowning and submersion due to other accident to watercraft

X ⬤ **V90.80** Drowning and submersion due to other accident to merchant ship

X ⬤ **V90.81** Drowning and submersion due to other accident to passenger ship

Drowning and submersion due to other accident to ferry-boat

Drowning and submersion due to other accident to liner

X ⬤ **V90.82** Drowning and submersion due to other accident to fishing boat

X ⬤ **V90.83** Drowning and submersion due to other accident to other powered watercraft

Drowning and submersion due to other accident to hovercraft (on open water)

Drowning and submersion due to other accident to jet ski

X ⬤ **V90.84** Drowning and submersion due to other accident to sailboat

X ⬤ **V90.85** Drowning and submersion due to other accident to canoe or kayak

X ⬤ **V90.86** Drowning and submersion due to other accident to (nonpowered) inflatable craft

X ⬤ **V90.87** Drowning and submersion due to other accident to water-skis

X ⬤ **V90.88** Drowning and submersion due to other accident to other unpowered watercraft

Drowning and submersion due to other accident to surf-board

Drowning and submersion due to other accident to windsurfer

X ⬤ **V90.89** Drowning and submersion due to other accident to unspecified watercraft

Drowning and submersion due to other accident to boat NOS

Drowning and submersion due to other accident to ship NOS

Drowning and submersion due to other accident to watercraft NOS

▶ New ⇒ Revised ~~deleted~~ Deleted | Excludes 1 | Excludes 2 | Includes | Use additional | Code first | Code also | Key words |
OGCR Official Guidelines X Assign placeholder X ⬤ Use Additional Character(s) ▶ Manifestation Code 🔖 Hierarchical Condition Category **Coding Clinic**

● V91 **Other injury due to accident to watercraft**
  Includes any injury except drowning and submersion as a result of an accident to watercraft
  Excludes1 civilian water transport accident involving military watercraft (V94.81-)
  military watercraft accident in military or war operations (Y36, Y37.-)
  Excludes2 drowning and submersion due to accident to watercraft (V90.-)

  The appropriate 7th character is to be added to each code from category V91

A	initial encounter
D	subsequent encounter
S	sequela

● V91.0 **Burn due to watercraft on fire**
  Excludes1 burn from localized fire or explosion on board ship without accident to watercraft (V93.-)
  X ● V91.00 **Burn due to merchant ship on fire**
  X ● V91.01 **Burn due to passenger ship on fire**
    Burn due to ferry-boat on fire
    Burn due to liner on fire
  X ● V91.02 **Burn due to fishing boat on fire**
  X ● V91.03 **Burn due to other powered watercraft on fire**
    Burn due to hovercraft (on open water) on fire
    Burn due to jet ski on fire
  X ● V91.04 **Burn due to sailboat on fire**
  X ● V91.05 **Burn due to canoe or kayak on fire**
  X ● V91.06 **Burn due to (nonpowered) inflatable craft on fire**
  X ● V91.07 **Burn due to water-skis on fire**
  X ● V91.08 **Burn due to other unpowered watercraft on fire**
  X ● V91.09 **Burn due to unspecified watercraft on fire**
    Burn due to boat NOS on fire
    Burn due to ship NOS on fire
    Burn due to watercraft NOS on fire

● V91.1 **Crushed between watercraft and other watercraft or other object due to collision**
    Crushed by lifeboat after abandoning ship in a collision
    Note: Select the specified type of watercraft that the victim was on at the time of the collision.
  X ● V91.10 **Crushed between merchant ship and other watercraft or other object due to collision**
  X ● V91.11 **Crushed between passenger ship and other watercraft or other object due to collision**
    Crushed between ferry-boat and other watercraft or other object due to collision
    Crushed between liner and other watercraft or other object due to collision
  X ● V91.12 **Crushed between fishing boat and other watercraft or other object due to collision**
  X ● V91.13 **Crushed between other powered watercraft and other watercraft or other object due to collision**
    Crushed between hovercraft (on open water) and other watercraft or other object due to collision
    Crushed between jet ski and other watercraft or other object due to collision
  X ● V91.14 **Crushed between sailboat and other watercraft or other object due to collision**
  X ● V91.15 **Crushed between canoe or kayak and other watercraft or other object due to collision**
  X ● V91.16 **Crushed between (nonpowered) inflatable craft and other watercraft or other object due to collision**

  X ● V91.18 **Crushed between other unpowered watercraft and other watercraft or other object due to collision**
    Crushed between surfboard and other watercraft or other object due to collision
    Crushed between windsurfer and other watercraft or other object due to collision
  X ● V91.19 **Crushed between unspecified watercraft and other watercraft or other object due to collision**
    Crushed between boat NOS and other watercraft or other object due to collision
    Crushed between ship NOS and other watercraft or other object due to collision
    Crushed between watercraft NOS and other watercraft or other object due to collision

● V91.2 **Fall due to collision between watercraft and other watercraft or other object**
    Fall while remaining on watercraft after collision
    Note: Select the specified type of watercraft that the victim was on at the time of the collision.
  Excludes1 crushed between watercraft and other watercraft and other object due to collision (V91.1-)
  drowning and submersion due to falling from crushed watercraft (V90.3-)
  X ● V91.20 **Fall due to collision between merchant ship and other watercraft or other object**
  X ● V91.21 **Fall due to collision between passenger ship and other watercraft or other object**
    Fall due to collision between ferry-boat and other watercraft or other object
    Fall due to collision between liner and other watercraft or other object
  X ● V91.22 **Fall due to collision between fishing boat and other watercraft or other object**
  X ● V91.23 **Fall due to collision between other powered watercraft and other watercraft or other object**
    Fall due to collision between hovercraft (on open water) and other watercraft or other object
    Fall due to collision between jet ski and other watercraft or other object
  X ● V91.24 **Fall due to collision between sailboat and other watercraft or other object**
  X ● V91.25 **Fall due to collision between canoe or kayak and other watercraft or other object**
  X ● V91.26 **Fall due to collision between (nonpowered) inflatable craft and other watercraft or other object**
  X ● V91.29 **Fall due to collision between unspecified watercraft and other watercraft or other object**
    Fall due to collision between boat NOS and other watercraft or other object
    Fall due to collision between ship NOS and other watercraft or other object
    Fall due to collision between watercraft NOS and other watercraft or other object

● V91.3 **Hit or struck by falling object due to accident to watercraft**
    Hit or struck by falling object (part of damaged watercraft or other object) after falling or jumping from damaged watercraft
  Excludes2 drowning or submersion due to fall or jumping from damaged watercraft (V90.2-, V90.3-)
  X ● V91.30 **Hit or struck by falling object due to accident to merchant ship**
  X ● V91.31 **Hit or struck by falling object due to accident to passenger ship**
    Hit or struck by falling object due to accident to ferry-boat
    Hit or struck by falling object due to accident to liner

X ● **V91.32** **Hit or struck by falling object due to accident to fishing boat**

X ● **V91.33** **Hit or struck by falling object due to accident to other powered watercraft**
> Hit or struck by falling object due to accident to hovercraft (on open water)
> Hit or struck by falling object due to accident to jet ski

X ● **V91.34** **Hit or struck by falling object due to accident to sailboat**

X ● **V91.35** **Hit or struck by falling object due to accident to canoe or kayak**

X ● **V91.36** **Hit or struck by falling object due to accident to (nonpowered) inflatable craft**

X ● **V91.37** **Hit or struck by falling object due to accident to water-skis**
> Hit by water-skis after jumping off of waterskis

X ● **V91.38** **Hit or struck by falling object due to accident to other unpowered watercraft**
> Hit or struck by surf-board after falling off damaged surf-board
> Hit or struck by object after falling off damaged windsurfer

X ● **V91.39** **Hit or struck by falling object due to accident to unspecified watercraft**
> Hit or struck by falling object due to accident to boat NOS
> Hit or struck by falling object due to accident to ship NOS
> Hit or struck by falling object due to accident to watercraft NOS

● **V91.8** **Other injury due to other accident to watercraft**

X ● **V91.80** **Other injury due to other accident to merchant ship**

X ● **V91.81** **Other injury due to other accident to passenger ship**
> Other injury due to other accident to ferry-boat
> Other injury due to other accident to liner

X ● **V91.82** **Other injury due to other accident to fishing boat**

X ● **V91.83** **Other injury due to other accident to other powered watercraft**
> Other injury due to other accident to hovercraft (on open water)
> Other injury due to other accident to jet ski

X ● **V91.84** **Other injury due to other accident to sailboat**

X ● **V91.85** **Other injury due to other accident to canoe or kayak**

X ● **V91.86** **Other injury due to other accident to (nonpowered) inflatable craft**

X ● **V91.87** **Other injury due to other accident to water-skis**

X ● **V91.88** **Other injury due to other accident to other unpowered watercraft**
> Other injury due to other accident to surf-board
> Other injury due to other accident to windsurfer

X ● **V91.89** **Other injury due to other accident to unspecified watercraft**
> Other injury due to other accident to boat NOS
> Other injury due to other accident to ship NOS
> Other injury due to other accident to watercraft NOS

● **V92** **Drowning and submersion due to accident on board watercraft, without accident to watercraft**

> **Excludes1** civilian water transport accident involving military watercraft (V94.81-)
> drowning or submersion due to accident to watercraft (V90-V91)
> drowning or submersion of diver who voluntarily jumps from boat not involved in an accident (W16.711, W16.721)
> fall into water without watercraft (W16.-)
> military watercraft accident in military or war operations (Y36, Y37)

The appropriate 7th character is to be added to each code from category V92

A	initial encounter
D	subsequent encounter
S	sequela

● **V92.0** **Drowning and submersion due to fall off watercraft**
> Drowning and submersion due to fall from gangplank of watercraft
> Drowning and submersion due to fall overboard watercraft

> **Excludes2** hitting head on object or bottom of body of water due to fall from watercraft (V94.0-)

X ● **V92.00** **Drowning and submersion due to fall off merchant ship**

X ● **V92.01** **Drowning and submersion due to fall off passenger ship**
> Drowning and submersion due to fall off ferry-boat
> Drowning and submersion due to fall off liner

X ● **V92.02** **Drowning and submersion due to fall off fishing boat**

X ● **V92.03** **Drowning and submersion due to fall off other powered watercraft**
> Drowning and submersion due to fall off hovercraft (on open water)
> Drowning and submersion due to fall off jet ski

X ● **V92.04** **Drowning and submersion due to fall off sailboat**

X ● **V92.05** **Drowning and submersion due to fall off canoe or kayak**

X ● **V92.06** **Drowning and submersion due to fall off (nonpowered) inflatable craft**

X ● **V92.07** **Drowning and submersion due to fall off water-skis**

> **Excludes1** drowning and submersion due to falling off burning water-skis (V90.27)
> drowning and submersion due to falling off crushed water-skis (V90.37)
> hit by boat while water-skiing NOS (V94.X)

X ● **V92.08 Drowning and submersion due to fall off other unpowered watercraft**
　　Drowning and submersion due to fall off surf-board
　　Drowning and submersion due to fall off windsurfer

> **Excludes1**　drowning and submersion due to fall off burning unpowered watercraft (V90.28)
> drowning and submersion due to fall off crushed unpowered watercraft (V90.38)
> drowning and submersion due to fall off damaged unpowered watercraft (V90.88)
> drowning and submersion due to rider of nonpowered watercraft being hit by other watercraft (V94.-)
> other injury due to rider of nonpowered watercraft being hit by other watercraft (V94.-)

X ● **V92.09 Drowning and submersion due to fall off unspecified watercraft**
　　Drowning and submersion due to fall off boat NOS
　　Drowning and submersion due to fall off ship
　　Drowning and submersion due to fall off watercraft NOS

● **V92.1 Drowning and submersion due to being thrown overboard by motion of watercraft**

> **Excludes1**　drowning and submersion due to fall off surf-board (V92.08)
> drowning and submersion due to fall off water-skis (V92.07)
> drowning and submersion due to fall off windsurfer (V92.08)

X ● **V92.10 Drowning and submersion due to being thrown overboard by motion of merchant ship**

X ● **V92.11 Drowning and submersion due to being thrown overboard by motion of passenger ship**
　　Drowning and submersion due to being thrown overboard by motion of ferry-boat
　　Drowning and submersion due to being thrown overboard by motion of liner

X ● **V92.12 Drowning and submersion due to being thrown overboard by motion of fishing boat**

X ● **V92.13 Drowning and submersion due to being thrown overboard by motion of other powered watercraft**
　　Drowning and submersion due to being thrown overboard by motion of hovercraft

X ● **V92.14 Drowning and submersion due to being thrown overboard by motion of sailboat**

X ● **V92.15 Drowning and submersion due to being thrown overboard by motion of canoe or kayak**

X ● **V92.16 Drowning and submersion due to being thrown overboard by motion of (nonpowered) inflatable craft**

X ● **V92.19 Drowning and submersion due to being thrown overboard by motion of unspecified watercraft**
　　Drowning and submersion due to being thrown overboard by motion of boat NOS
　　Drowning and submersion due to being thrown overboard by motion of ship NOS
　　Drowning and submersion due to being thrown overboard by motion of watercraft NOS

● **V92.2 Drowning and submersion due to being washed overboard from watercraft**
　　Code first any associated cataclysm (X37.0-)

X ● **V92.20 Drowning and submersion due to being washed overboard from merchant ship**

X ● **V92.21 Drowning and submersion due to being washed overboard from passenger ship**
　　Drowning and submersion due to being washed overboard from ferry-boat
　　Drowning and submersion due to being washed overboard from liner

X ● **V92.22 Drowning and submersion due to being washed overboard from fishing boat**

X ● **V92.23 Drowning and submersion due to being washed overboard from other powered watercraft**
　　Drowning and submersion due to being washed overboard from hovercraft (on open water)
　　Drowning and submersion due to being washed overboard from jet ski

X ● **V92.24 Drowning and submersion due to being washed overboard from sailboat**

X ● **V92.25 Drowning and submersion due to being washed overboard from canoe or kayak**

X ● **V92.26 Drowning and submersion due to being washed overboard from (nonpowered) inflatable craft**

X ● **V92.27 Drowning and submersion due to being washed overboard from water-skis**

> **Excludes1**　drowning and submersion due to fall off water-skis (V92.07)

X ● **V92.28 Drowning and submersion due to being washed overboard from other unpowered watercraft**
　　Drowning and submersion due to being washed overboard from surf-board
　　Drowning and submersion due to being washed overboard from windsurfer

X ● **V92.29 Drowning and submersion due to being washed overboard from unspecified watercraft**
　　Drowning and submersion due to being washed overboard from boat NOS
　　Drowning and submersion due to being washed overboard from ship NOS
　　Drowning and submersion due to being washed overboard from watercraft NOS

● **V93 Other injury due to accident on board watercraft, without accident to watercraft**

> **Excludes1**　civilian water transport accident involving military watercraft (V94.81-)
> other injury due to accident to watercraft (V91.-)
> military watercraft accident in military or war operations (Y36, Y37.-)

> **Excludes2**　drowning and submersion due to accident on board watercraft, without accident to watercraft (V92.-)

The appropriate 7th character is to be added to each code from category V93

A	initial encounter
D	subsequent encounter
S	sequela

● **V93.0 Burn due to localized fire on board watercraft**

> **Excludes1**　burn due to watercraft on fire (V91.0-)

X ● **V93.00 Burn due to localized fire on board merchant vessel**

X ● **V93.01 Burn due to localized fire on board passenger vessel**
　　Burn due to localized fire on board ferry-boat
　　Burn due to localized fire on board liner

CHAPTER 20 (VØØ-Y99)

X ● **V93.Ø2**   **Burn due to localized fire on board** fishing boat

X ● **V93.Ø3**   **Burn due to localized fire on board** other powered watercraft
     Burn due to localized fire on board hovercraft
     Burn due to localized fire on board jet ski

X ● **V93.Ø4**   **Burn due to localized fire on board** sailboat

X ● **V93.Ø9**   **Burn due to localized fire on board** unspecified watercraft
     Burn due to localized fire on board boat NOS
     Burn due to localized fire on board ship NOS
     Burn due to localized fire on board watercraft NOS

● **V93.1**   **Other burn on board watercraft**
     Burn due to source other than fire on board watercraft

     Excludes1   burn due to watercraft on fire (V91.Ø-)

X ● **V93.1Ø**   **Other burn on board** merchant vessel

X ● **V93.11**   **Other burn on board** passenger vessel
     Other burn on board ferry-boat
     Other burn on board liner

X ● **V93.12**   **Other burn on board** fishing boat

X ● **V93.13**   **Other burn on board** other powered watercraft
     Other burn on board hovercraft
     Other burn on board jet ski

X ● **V93.14**   **Other burn on board** sailboat

X ● **V93.19**   **Other burn on board** unspecified watercraft
     Other burn on board boat NOS
     Other burn on board ship NOS
     Other burn on board watercraft NOS

● **V93.2**   **Heat exposure on board watercraft**

     Excludes1   exposure to man-made heat not aboard watercraft (W92)
               exposure to natural heat while on board watercraft (X3Ø)
               exposure to sunlight while on board watercraft (X32)

     Excludes2   burn due to fire on board watercraft (V93.Ø-)

X ● **V93.2Ø**   **Heat exposure on board** merchant ship

X ● **V93.21**   **Heat exposure on board** passenger ship
     Heat exposure on board ferry-boat
     Heat exposure on board liner

X ● **V93.22**   **Heat exposure on board** fishing boat

X ● **V93.23**   **Heat exposure on board** other powered watercraft
     Heat exposure on board hovercraft

X ● **V93.24**   **Heat exposure on board** sailboat

X ● **V93.29**   **Heat exposure on board** unspecified watercraft
     Heat exposure on board boat NOS
     Heat exposure on board ship NOS
     Heat exposure on board watercraft NOS

● **V93.3**   **Fall on board watercraft**

     Excludes1   fall due to collision of watercraft (V91.2-)

X ● **V93.3Ø**   **Fall on board** merchant ship

X ● **V93.31**   **Fall on board** passenger ship
     Fall on board ferry-boat
     Fall on board liner

X ● **V93.32**   **Fall on board** fishing boat

X ● **V93.33**   **Fall on board** other powered watercraft
     Fall on board hovercraft (on open water)
     Fall on board jet ski

X ● **V93.34**   **Fall on board** sailboat

X ● **V93.35**   **Fall on board** canoe or kayak

X ● **V93.36**   **Fall on board** (nonpowered) inflatable craft

X ● **V93.38**   **Fall on board** other unpowered watercraft

X ● **V93.39**   **Fall on board** unspecified watercraft
     Fall on board boat NOS
     Fall on board ship NOS
     Fall on board watercraft NOS

● **V93.4**   **Struck by falling object on board watercraft**
     Hit by falling object on board watercraft

     Excludes1   struck by falling object due to accident to watercraft (V91.3)

X ● **V93.4Ø**   **Struck by falling object on** merchant ship

X ● **V93.41**   **Struck by falling object on** passenger ship
     Struck by falling object on ferry-boat
     Struck by falling object on liner

X ● **V93.42**   **Struck by falling object on** fishing boat

X ● **V93.43**   **Struck by falling object on** other powered watercraft
     Struck by falling object on hovercraft

X ● **V93.44**   **Struck by falling object on** sailboat

X ● **V93.48**   **Struck by falling object on** other unpowered watercraft

X ● **V93.49**   **Struck by falling object on** unspecified watercraft

● **V93.5**   **Explosion on board watercraft**
     Boiler explosion on steamship

     Excludes2   fire on board watercraft (V93.Ø-)

X ● **V93.5Ø**   **Explosion on board** merchant ship

X ● **V93.51**   **Explosion on board** passenger ship
     Explosion on board ferry-boat
     Explosion on board liner

X ● **V93.52**   **Explosion on board** fishing boat

X ● **V93.53**   **Explosion on board** other powered watercraft
     Explosion on board hovercraft
     Explosion on board jet ski

X ● **V93.54**   **Explosion on board** sailboat

X ● **V93.59**   **Explosion on board** unspecified watercraft
     Explosion on board boat NOS
     Explosion on board ship NOS
     Explosion on board watercraft NOS

● **V93.6**   **Machinery accident on board watercraft**

     Excludes1   machinery explosion on board watercraft (V93.4-)
               machinery fire on board watercraft (V93.Ø-)

X ● **V93.6Ø**   **Machinery accident on board** merchant ship

X ● **V93.61**   **Machinery accident on board** passenger ship
     Machinery accident on board ferry-boat
     Machinery accident on board liner

X ● **V93.62**   **Machinery accident on board** fishing boat

X ● **V93.63**   **Machinery accident on board** other powered watercraft
     Machinery accident on board hovercraft

X ● **V93.64**   **Machinery accident on board** sailboat

X ⊖ **V93.69**   **Machinery accident on board** unspecified watercraft
     Machinery accident on board boat NOS
     Machinery accident on board ship NOS
     Machinery accident on board watercraft NOS

● **V93.8**   **Other injury due to other accident on board watercraft**
     Accidental poisoning by gases or fumes on watercraft

X ● **V93.8Ø**   **Other injury due to other accident on board** merchant ship

X ● **V93.81**   **Other injury due to other accident on board** passenger ship
     Other injury due to other accident on board ferry-boat
     Other injury due to other accident on board liner

X ● **V93.82**   **Other injury due to other accident on board** fishing boat

X⬤ **V93.83** **Other injury due to other accident on board other powered watercraft**
   Other injury due to other accident on board hovercraft
   Other injury due to other accident on board jet ski

X⬤ **V93.84** **Other injury due to other accident on board sailboat**

X⬤ **V93.85** **Other injury due to other accident on board canoe or kayak**

X⬤ **V93.86** **Other injury due to other accident on board (nonpowered) inflatable craft**

X⬤ **V93.87** **Other injury due to other accident on board water-skis**
   Hit or struck by object while waterskiing

X⬤ **V93.88** **Other injury due to other accident on board other unpowered watercraft**
   Hit or struck by object while surfing
   Hit or struck by object while on board windsurfer

X⬤ **V93.89** **Other injury due to other accident on board unspecified watercraft**
   Other injury due to other accident on board boat NOS
   Other injury due to other accident on board ship NOS
   Other injury due to other accident on board watercraft NOS

⬤ **V94** **Other and unspecified water transport accidents**

Excludes1 military watercraft accidents in military or war operations (Y36, Y37)

The appropriate 7th character is to be added to each code from category V94

A	initial encounter
D	subsequent encounter
S	sequela

X⬤ **V94.0** **Hitting object or bottom of body of water due to fall from watercraft**

Excludes2 drowning and submersion due to fall from watercraft (V92.0-)

⬤ **V94.1** **Bather struck by watercraft**
   Swimmer hit by watercraft

X⬤ **V94.11** **Bather struck by powered watercraft**

X⬤ **V94.12** **Bather struck by nonpowered watercraft**

⬤ **V94.2** **Rider of nonpowered watercraft struck by other watercraft**

X⬤ **V94.21** **Rider of nonpowered watercraft struck by other nonpowered watercraft**
   Canoer hit by other nonpowered watercraft
   Surfer hit by other nonpowered watercraft
   Windsurfer hit by other nonpowered watercraft

X⬤ **V94.22** **Rider of nonpowered watercraft struck by powered watercraft**
   Canoer hit by motorboat
   Surfer hit by motorboat
   Windsurfer hit by motorboat

⬤ **V94.3** **Injury to rider of (inflatable) watercraft being pulled behind other watercraft**

X⬤ **V94.31** **Injury to rider of (inflatable) recreational watercraft being pulled behind other watercraft**
   Injury to rider of inner-tube pulled behind motor boat

X⬤ **V94.32** **Injury to rider of non-recreational watercraft being pulled behind other watercraft**
   Injury to occupant of dingy being pulled behind boat or ship
   Injury to occupant of life-raft being pulled behind boat or ship

X⬤ **V94.4** **Injury to barefoot water-skier**
   Injury to person being pulled behind boat or ship

⬤ **V94.8** **Other water transport accident**

⬤ **V94.81** **Water transport accident involving military watercraft**

⬤ **V94.810** **Civilian watercraft involved in water transport accident with military watercraft**
   Passenger on civilian watercraft injured due to accident with military watercraft

⬤ **V94.811** **Civilian in water injured by military watercraft**

⬤ **V94.818** **Other water transport accident involving military watercraft**

X⬤ **V94.89** **Other water transport accident**

X⬤ **V94.9** **Unspecified water transport accident**
   Water transport accident NOS

AIR AND SPACE TRANSPORT ACCIDENTS (V95-V97)

Excludes1 military aircraft accidents in military or war operations (Y36, Y37)

⬤ **V95** **Accident to powered aircraft causing injury to occupant**

The appropriate 7th character is to be added to each code from category V95

A	initial encounter
D	subsequent encounter
S	sequela

⬤ **V95.0** **Helicopter accident injuring occupant**

X⬤ **V95.00** **Unspecified helicopter accident injuring occupant**

X⬤ **V95.01** **Helicopter crash injuring occupant**

X⬤ **V95.02** **Forced landing of helicopter injuring occupant**

X⬤ **V95.03** **Helicopter collision injuring occupant**
   Helicopter collision with any object, fixed, movable or moving

X⬤ **V95.04** **Helicopter fire injuring occupant**

X⬤ **V95.05** **Helicopter explosion injuring occupant**

X⬤ **V95.09** **Other helicopter accident injuring occupant**

⬤ **V95.1** **Ultralight, microlight or powered-glider accident injuring occupant**

X⬤ **V95.10** **Unspecified ultralight, microlight or powered-glider accident injuring occupant**

X⬤ **V95.11** **Ultralight, microlight or powered-glider crash injuring occupant**

X⬤ **V95.12** **Forced landing of ultralight, microlight or powered-glider injuring occupant**

X⬤ **V95.13** **Ultralight, microlight or powered-glider collision injuring occupant**
   Ultralight, microlight or powered-glider collision with any object, fixed, movable or moving

X⬤ **V95.14** **Ultralight, microlight or powered-glider fire injuring occupant**

X⬤ **V95.15** **Ultralight, microlight or powered-glider explosion injuring occupant**

X⬤ **V95.19** **Other ultralight, microlight or powered-glider accident injuring occupant**

● **V95.2   Other private fixed-wing aircraft accident injuring occupant**

  X ● **V95.20   Unspecified accident to other private fixed-wing aircraft, injuring occupant**

  X ● **V95.21   Other private fixed-wing aircraft crash injuring occupant**

  X ● **V95.22   Forced landing of other private fixed-wing aircraft injuring occupant**

  X ● **V95.23   Other private fixed-wing aircraft collision injuring occupant**
        Other private fixed-wing aircraft collision with any object, fixed, movable or moving

  X ● **V95.24   Other private fixed-wing aircraft fire injuring occupant**

  X ● **V95.25   Other private fixed-wing aircraft explosion injuring occupant**

  X ● **V95.29   Other accident to other private fixed-wing aircraft injuring occupant**

● **V95.3   Commercial fixed-wing aircraft accident injuring occupant**

  X ● **V95.30   Unspecified accident to commercial fixed-wing aircraft injuring occupant**

  X ● **V95.31   Commercial fixed-wing aircraft crash injuring occupant**

  X ● **V95.32   Forced landing of commercial fixed-wing aircraft injuring occupant**

  X ● **V95.33   Commercial fixed-wing aircraft collision injuring occupant**
        Commercial fixed-wing aircraft collision with any object, fixed, movable or moving

  X ● **V95.34   Commercial fixed-wing aircraft fire injuring occupant**

  X ● **V95.35   Commercial fixed-wing aircraft explosion injuring occupant**

  X ● **V95.39   Other accident to commercial fixed-wing aircraft injuring occupant**

● **V95.4   Spacecraft accident injuring occupant**

  X ● **V95.40   Unspecified spacecraft accident injuring occupant**

  X ● **V95.41   Spacecraft crash injuring occupant**

  X ● **V95.42   Forced landing of spacecraft injuring occupant**

  X ● **V95.43   Spacecraft collision injuring occupant**
        Spacecraft collision with any object, fixed, moveable or moving

  X ● **V95.44   Spacecraft fire injuring occupant**

  X ● **V95.45   Spacecraft explosion injuring occupant**

  X ● **V95.49   Other spacecraft accident injuring occupant**

X ● **V95.8   Other powered aircraft accidents injuring occupant**

X ● **V95.9   Unspecified aircraft accident injuring occupant**
    Aircraft accident NOS
    Air transport accident NOS

● **V96   Accident to nonpowered aircraft causing injury to occupant**
    The appropriate 7th character is to be added to each code from category V96

A	initial encounter
D	subsequent encounter
S	sequela

● **V96.0   Balloon accident injuring occupant**

  X ● **V96.00   Unspecified balloon accident injuring occupant**

  X ● **V96.01   Balloon crash injuring occupant**

  X ● **V96.02   Forced landing of balloon injuring occupant**

  X ● **V96.03   Balloon collision injuring occupant**
        Balloon collision with any object, fixed, moveable or moving

  X ● **V96.04   Balloon fire injuring occupant**

  X ● **V96.05   Balloon explosion injuring occupant**

  X ● **V96.09   Other balloon accident injuring occupant**

● **V96.1   Hang-glider accident injuring occupant**

  X ● **V96.10   Unspecified hang-glider accident injuring occupant**

  X ● **V96.11   Hang-glider crash injuring occupant**

  X ● **V96.12   Forced landing of hang-glider injuring occupant**

  X ● **V96.13   Hang-glider collision injuring occupant**
        Hang-glider collision with any object, fixed, moveable or moving

  X ● **V96.14   Hang-glider fire injuring occupant**

  X ● **V96.15   Hang-glider explosion injuring occupant**

  X ● **V96.19   Other hang-glider accident injuring occupant**

● **V96.2   Glider (nonpowered) accident injuring occupant**

  X ● **V96.20   Unspecified glider (nonpowered) accident injuring occupant**

  X ● **V96.21   Glider (nonpowered) crash injuring occupant**

  X ● **V96.22   Forced landing of glider (nonpowered) injuring occupant**

  X ● **V96.23   Glider (nonpowered) collision injuring occupant**
        Glider (nonpowered) collision with any object, fixed, moveable or moving

  X ● **V96.24   Glider (nonpowered) fire injuring occupant**

  X ● **V96.25   Glider (nonpowered) explosion injuring occupant**

  X ● **V96.29   Other glider (nonpowered) accident injuring occupant**

X ● **V96.8   Other nonpowered-aircraft accidents injuring occupant**
    Kite carrying a person accident injuring occupant

X ● **V96.9   Unspecified nonpowered-aircraft accident injuring occupant**
    Nonpowered-aircraft accident NOS

● **V97   Other specified air transport accidents**
    The appropriate 7th character is to be added to each code from category V97

A	initial encounter
D	subsequent encounter
S	sequela

X ● **V97.0   Occupant of aircraft injured in other specified air transport accidents**
    Fall in, on or from aircraft in air transport accident

    Excludes1   accident while boarding or alighting aircraft (V97.1)

X ● **V97.1   Person injured while boarding or alighting from aircraft**

● **V97.2   Parachutist accident**

  X ● **V97.21   Parachutist entangled in object**
        Parachutist landing in tree

  X ● **V97.22   Parachutist injured on landing**

  X ● **V97.29   Other parachutist accident**

● **V97.3   Person on ground injured in air transport accident**

  X ● **V97.31   Hit by object falling from aircraft**
        Hit by crashing aircraft
        Injured by aircraft hitting house
        Injured by aircraft hitting car

  X ● **V97.32   Injured by rotating propeller**

  X ● **V97.33   Sucked into jet engine**

  X ● **V97.39   Other injury to person on ground due to air transport accident**

- **V97.8 Other air transport accidents, not elsewhere classified**
  - **Excludes1**   aircraft accident NOS (V95.9)
    - exposure to changes in air pressure during ascent or descent (W94.-)
  - **V97.81 Air transport accident involving military aircraft**
    - **V97.810 Civilian aircraft involved in air transport accident with military aircraft**
      - Passenger in civilian aircraft injured due to accident with military aircraft
    - **V97.811 Civilian injured by military aircraft**
    - **V97.818 Other air transport accident involving military aircraft**
  - X **V97.89 Other air transport accidents, not elsewhere classified**
    - Injury from machinery on aircraft

OTHER AND UNSPECIFIED TRANSPORT ACCIDENTS (V98-V99)

Excludes1   vehicle accident, type of vehicle unspecified (V89.-)

- **V98 Other specified transport accidents**

  The appropriate 7th character is to be added to each code from category V98

A	initial encounter
D	subsequent encounter
S	sequela

  - X **V98.0 Accident to, on or involving cable-car, not on rails**
    - Caught or dragged by cable-car, not on rails
    - Fall or jump from cable-car, not on rails
    - Object thrown from or in cable-car, not on rails
  - X **V98.1 Accident to, on or involving land-yacht**
  - X **V98.2 Accident to, on or involving ice yacht**
  - X **V98.3 Accident to, on or involving ski lift**
    - Accident to, on or involving ski chair-lift
    - Accident to, on or involving ski-lift with gondola
  - X **V98.8 Other specified transport accidents**

- X **V99 Unspecified transport accident**

  The appropriate 7th character is to be added to code V99

A	initial encounter
D	subsequent encounter
S	sequela

OTHER EXTERNAL CAUSES OF ACCIDENTAL INJURY (W00-X58)

SLIPPING, TRIPPING, STUMBLING AND FALLS (W00-W19)

Excludes1   assault involving a fall (Y01-Y02)
- fall from animal (V80.-)
- fall (in) (from) machinery (in operation) (W28-W31)
- fall (in) (from) transport vehicle (V01-V99)
- intentional self-harm involving a fall (X80-X81)

Excludes2   at risk for fall (history of fall) Z91.81
- fall (in) (from) burning building (X00.-)
- fall into fire (X00-X04, X08)

- **W00 Fall due to ice and snow**
  - **Includes**   pedestrian on foot falling (slipping) on ice and snow
  - **Excludes1**   fall on (from) ice and snow involving pedestrian conveyance (V00.-)
    - fall from stairs and steps not due to ice and snow (W10.-)

  The appropriate 7th character is to be added to each code from category W00

A	initial encounter
D	subsequent encounter
S	sequela

  - X **W00.0 Fall on same level due to ice and snow**
    - Coding Clinic: 2016, Q2, P5
  - X **W00.1 Fall from stairs and steps due to ice and snow**
  - X **W00.2 Other fall from one level to another due to ice and snow**
  - X **W00.9 Unspecified fall due to ice and snow**

- **W01 Fall on same level from slipping, tripping and stumbling**
  - **Includes**   fall on moving sidewalk
  - **Excludes1**   fall due to bumping (striking) against object (W18.0-)
    - fall in shower or bathtub (W18.2-)
    - fall on same level NOS (W18.30)
    - fall on same level from slipping, tripping and stumbling due to ice or snow (W00.0)
    - fall off or from toilet (W18.1-)
    - slipping, tripping and stumbling NOS (W18.40)
    - slipping, tripping and stumbling without falling (W18.4-)

  The appropriate 7th character is to be added to each code from category W01

A	initial encounter
D	subsequent encounter
S	sequela

  - X **W01.0 Fall on same level from slipping, tripping and stumbling without subsequent striking against object**
    - Falling over animal
  - **W01.1 Fall on same level from slipping, tripping and stumbling with subsequent striking against object**
    - X **W01.10 Fall on same level from slipping, tripping and stumbling with subsequent striking against unspecified object**
    - **W01.11 Fall on same level from slipping, tripping and stumbling with subsequent striking against sharp object**
      - **W01.110 Fall on same level from slipping, tripping and stumbling with subsequent striking against sharp glass**
      - **W01.111 Fall on same level from slipping, tripping and stumbling with subsequent striking against power tool or machine**
      - **W01.118 Fall on same level from slipping, tripping and stumbling with subsequent striking against other sharp object**
      - **W01.119 Fall on same level from slipping, tripping and stumbling with subsequent striking against unspecified sharp object**

● W01.19   **Fall on same level from slipping, tripping and stumbling with subsequent striking against other object**

    ● W01.190   Fall on same level from slipping, tripping and stumbling with subsequent striking against furniture

     Coding Clinic: 2021, Q1, P5

    ● W01.198   Fall on same level from slipping, tripping and stumbling with subsequent striking against other object

X ● W03   **Other fall on same level due to collision with another person**

    Fall due to non-transport collision with other person

    Excludes1   collision with another person without fall (W51)
         crushed or pushed by a crowd or human stampede (W52)
         fall involving pedestrian conveyance (V00-V09)
         fall due to ice or snow (W00)
         fall on same level NOS (W18.30)

    The appropriate 7th character is to be added to code W03

A	initial encounter
D	subsequent encounter
S	sequela

    Coding Clinic: 2015, Q1, P9-10; 2012, Q4, P108

X ● W04   **Fall while being carried or supported by other persons**

    Accidentally dropped while being carried

    The appropriate 7th character is to be added to code W04

A	initial encounter
D	subsequent encounter
S	sequel

● W05   **Fall from non-moving wheelchair, nonmotorized scooter and motorized mobility scooter**

    Excludes1   fall from moving wheelchair (powered) (V00.811)
         fall from moving motorized mobility scooter (V00.831)
         fall from nonmotorized scooter (V00.141)

    The appropriate 7th character is to be added to each code from category W05

A	initial encounter
D	subsequent encounter
S	sequela

   X ● W05.0   **Fall from non-moving wheelchair**
        Coding Clinic: 2019, Q2, P27

   X ● W05.1   **Fall from non-moving nonmotorized scooter**

   X ● W05.2   **Fall from non-moving motorized mobility scooter**

X ● W06   **Fall from bed**

    The appropriate 7th character is to be added to code W06

A	initial encounter
D	subsequent encounter
S	sequela

X ● W07   **Fall from chair**

    The appropriate 7th character is to be added to code W07

A	initial encounter
D	subsequent encounter
S	sequela

X ● W08   **Fall from other furniture**

    The appropriate 7th character is to be added to code W08

A	initial encounter
D	subsequent encounter
S	sequela

● W09   **Fall on and from playground equipment**

    Excludes1   fall involving recreational machinery (W31)

    The appropriate 7th character is to be added to each code from category W09

A	initial encounter
D	subsequent encounter
S	sequela

   X ● W09.0   Fall on or from playground slide
   X ● W09.1   Fall from playground swing
   X ● W09.2   Fall on or from jungle gym
   X ● W09.8   Fall on or from other playground equipment

● W10   **Fall on and from stairs and steps**

    Excludes1   fall from stairs and steps due to ice and snow (W00.1)

    The appropriate 7th character is to be added to each code from category W10

A	initial encounter
D	subsequent encounter
S	sequela

   X ● W10.0   Fall (on) (from) escalator
   X ● W10.1   Fall (on) (from) sidewalk curb
   X ● W10.2   Fall (on) (from) incline
        Fall (on) (from) ramp
   X ● W10.8   Fall (on) (from) other stairs and steps
   X ● W10.9   Fall (on) (from) unspecified stairs and steps

X ● W11   **Fall on and from ladder**

    The appropriate 7th character is to be added to code W11

A	initial encounter
D	subsequent encounter
S	sequela

X ● W12   **Fall on and from scaffolding**

    The appropriate 7th character is to be added to code W12

A	initial encounter
D	subsequent encounter
S	sequela

● W13   **Fall from, out of or through building or structure**

    The appropriate 7th character is to be added to each code from category W13

A	initial encounter
D	subsequent encounter
S	sequela

   X ● W13.0   Fall from, out of or through balcony
        Fall from, out of or through railing
   X ● W13.1   Fall from, out of or through bridge
   X ● W13.2   Fall from, out of or through roof
   X ● W13.3   Fall through floor
   X ● W13.4   Fall from, out of or through window
        ▶ **Excludes2**   fall with subsequent striking against sharp glass (W01.110-)
   X ● W13.8   Fall from, out of or through other building or structure
        Fall from, out of or through viaduct
        Fall from, out of or through wall
        Fall from, out of or through flag-pole
   X ● W13.9   Fall from, out of or through building, not otherwise specified
        Excludes1   collapse of a building or structure (W20.-)
                 fall or jump from burning building or structure (X00.-)

CHAPTER 20 (V00-Y99)

1512

▶ New   ▥ Revised   ~~deleted~~ Deleted   Excludes 1   Excludes 2   Includes   Use additional   Code first   Code also   Key words

OGCR Official Guidelines   X Assign placeholder X   ● Use Additional Character(s)   ▶ Manifestation Code   🏷 Hierarchical Condition Category   **Coding Clinic**

X ● **W14   Fall from tree**

     The appropriate 7th character is to be added to code W14

A	initial encounter
D	subsequent encounter
S	sequela

X ● **W15   Fall from cliff**

     The appropriate 7th character is to be added to code W15

A	initial encounter
D	subsequent encounter
S	sequela

● **W16   Fall, jump or diving into water**

     Excludes1   accidental non-watercraft drowning and submersion not involving fall (W65-W74)
                effects of air pressure from diving (W94.-)
                fall into water from watercraft (V90-V94)
                hitting an object or against bottom when falling from watercraft (V94.0)

     Excludes2   striking or hitting diving board (W21.4)

     The appropriate 7th character is to be added to each code from category W16

A	initial encounter
D	subsequent encounter
S	sequela

● **W16.0   Fall into swimming pool**

     Fall into swimming pool NOS

     Excludes1   fall into empty swimming pool (W17.3)

     ● **W16.01   Fall into swimming pool striking water surface**

         ● **W16.011   Fall into swimming pool striking water surface causing drowning and submersion**

                 Excludes1   drowning and submersion while in swimming pool without fall (W67)

         ● **W16.012   Fall into swimming pool striking water surface causing other injury**

     ● **W16.02   Fall into swimming pool striking bottom**

         ● **W16.021   Fall into swimming pool striking bottom causing drowning and submersion**

                 Excludes1   drowning and submersion while in swimming pool without fall (W67)

         ● **W16.022   Fall into swimming pool striking bottom causing other injury**

     ● **W16.03   Fall into swimming pool striking wall**

         ● **W16.031   Fall into swimming pool striking wall causing drowning and submersion**

                 Excludes1   drowning and submersion while in swimming pool without fall (W67)

         ● **W16.032   Fall into swimming pool striking wall causing other injury**

● **W16.1   Fall into natural body of water**

     Fall into lake
     Fall into open sea
     Fall into river
     Fall into stream

     ● **W16.11   Fall into natural body of water striking water surface**

         ● **W16.111   Fall into natural body of water striking water surface causing drowning and submersion**

                 Excludes1   drowning and submersion while in natural body of water without fall (W69)

         ● **W16.112   Fall into natural body of water striking water surface causing other injury**

     ● **W16.12   Fall into natural body of water striking bottom**

         ● **W16.121   Fall into natural body of water striking bottom causing drowning and submersion**

                 Excludes1   drowning and submersion while in natural body of water without fall (W69)

         ● **W16.122   Fall into natural body of water striking bottom causing other injury**

     ● **W16.13   Fall into natural body of water striking side**

         ● **W16.131   Fall into natural body of water striking side causing drowning and submersion**

                 Excludes1   drowning and submersion while in natural body of water without fall (W69)

         ● **W16.132   Fall into natural body of water striking side causing other injury**

● **W16.2   Fall in (into) filled bathtub or bucket of water**

     ● **W16.21   Fall in (into) filled bathtub**

         Excludes1   fall into empty bathtub (W18.2)

         ● **W16.211   Fall in (into) filled bathtub causing drowning and submersion**

                 Excludes1   drowning and submersion while in filled bathtub without fall (W65)

         ● **W16.212   Fall in (into) filled bathtub causing other injury**

     ● **W16.22   Fall in (into) bucket of water**

         ● **W16.221   Fall in (into) bucket of water causing drowning and submersion**

         ● **W16.222   Fall in (into) bucket of water causing other injury**

CHAPTER 20 (V00-Y99)

CHAPTER 20 (V00-Y99)

● **W16.3 Fall into other water**
    Fall into fountain
    Fall into reservoir
  ● **W16.31 Fall into other water striking water surface**
    ● **W16.311 Fall into other water striking water surface causing drowning and submersion**
        Excludes1 drowning and submersion while in other water without fall (W73)
    ● **W16.312 Fall into other water striking water surface causing other injury**
  ● **W16.32 Fall into other water striking bottom**
    ● **W16.321 Fall into other water striking bottom causing drowning and submersion**
        Excludes1 drowning and submersion while in other water without fall (W73)
    ● **W16.322 Fall into other water striking bottom causing other injury**
  ● **W16.33 Fall into other water striking wall**
    ● **W16.331 Fall into other water striking wall causing drowning and submersion**
        Excludes1 drowning and submersion while in other water without fall (W73)
    ● **W16.332 Fall into other water striking wall causing other injury**
● **W16.4 Fall into unspecified water**
  X ● **W16.41 Fall into unspecified water causing drowning and submersion**
  X ● **W16.42 Fall into unspecified water causing other injury**
● **W16.5 Jumping or diving into swimming pool**
  ● **W16.51 Jumping or diving into swimming pool striking water surface**
    ● **W16.511 Jumping or diving into swimming pool striking water surface causing drowning and submersion**
        Excludes1 drowning and submersion while in swimming pool without jumping or diving (W67)
    ● **W16.512 Jumping or diving into swimming pool striking water surface causing other injury**
  ● **W16.52 Jumping or diving into swimming pool striking bottom**
    ● **W16.521 Jumping or diving into swimming pool striking bottom causing drowning and submersion**
        Excludes1 drowning and submersion while in swimming pool without jumping or diving (W67)
    ● **W16.522 Jumping or diving into swimming pool striking bottom causing other injury**

● **W16.53 Jumping or diving into swimming pool striking wall**
  ● **W16.531 Jumping or diving into swimming pool striking wall causing drowning and submersion**
    Excludes1 drowning and submersion while in swimming pool without jumping or diving (W67)
  ● **W16.532 Jumping or diving into swimming pool striking wall causing other injury**
● **W16.6 Jumping or diving into natural body of water**
    Jumping or diving into lake
    Jumping or diving into open sea
    Jumping or diving into river
    Jumping or diving into stream
  ● **W16.61 Jumping or diving into natural body of water striking water surface**
    ● **W16.611 Jumping or diving into natural body of water striking water surface causing drowning and submersion**
        Excludes1 drowning and submersion while in natural body of water without jumping or diving (W69)
    ● **W16.612 Jumping or diving into natural body of water striking water surface causing other injury**
  ● **W16.62 Jumping or diving into natural body of water striking bottom**
    ● **W16.621 Jumping or diving into natural body of water striking bottom causing drowning and submersion**
        Excludes1 drowning and submersion while in natural body of water without jumping or diving (W69)
    ● **W16.622 Jumping or diving into natural body of water striking bottom causing other injury**
● **W16.7 Jumping or diving from boat**
  Excludes1 fall from boat into water - see watercraft accident (V90-V94)
  ● **W16.71 Jumping or diving from boat striking water surface**
    ● **W16.711 Jumping or diving from boat striking water surface causing drowning and submersion**
    ● **W16.712 Jumping or diving from boat striking water surface causing other injury**
  ● **W16.72 Jumping or diving from boat striking bottom**
    ● **W16.721 Jumping or diving from boat striking bottom causing drowning and submersion**
    ● **W16.722 Jumping or diving from boat striking bottom causing other injury**

● **W16.8 Jumping or diving into other water**
    Jumping or diving into fountain
    Jumping or diving into reservoir

    ● **W16.81 Jumping or diving into other water striking water surface**

        ● **W16.811 Jumping or diving into other water striking water surface causing drowning and submersion**

            Excludes1   drowning and submersion while in other water without jumping or diving (W73)

        ● **W16.812 Jumping or diving into other water striking water surface causing other injury**

    ● **W16.82 Jumping or diving into other water striking bottom**

        ● **W16.821 Jumping or diving into other water striking bottom causing drowning and submersion**

            Excludes1   drowning and submersion while in other water without jumping or diving (W73)

        ● **W16.822 Jumping or diving into other water striking bottom causing other injury**

    ● **W16.83 Jumping or diving into other water striking wall**

        ● **W16.831 Jumping or diving into other water striking wall causing drowning and submersion**

            Excludes1   drowning and submersion while in other water without jumping or diving (W73)

        ● **W16.832 Jumping or diving into other water striking wall causing other injury**

● **W16.9 Jumping or diving into unspecified water**

    X ● **W16.91 Jumping or diving into unspecified water causing drowning and submersion**

    X ● **W16.92 Jumping or diving into unspecified water causing other injury**

● **W17   Other fall from one level to another**

    The appropriate 7th character is to be added to each code from category W17

A	initial encounter
D	subsequent encounter
S	sequela

X ● **W17.0   Fall into well**

X ● **W17.1   Fall into storm drain or manhole**

X ● **W17.2   Fall into hole**
    Fall into pit

X ● **W17.3   Fall into empty swimming pool**
    Excludes1   fall into filled swimming pool (W16.0-)

X ● **W17.4   Fall from dock**

● **W17.8   Other fall from one level to another**

    X ● **W17.81   Fall down embankment (hill)**

    X ● **W17.82   Fall from (out of) grocery cart**
        Fall due to grocery cart tipping over

    X ● **W17.89   Other fall from one level to another**
        Fall from cherry picker
        Fall from lifting device
        Fall from mobile elevated work platform [MEWP]
        Fall from sky lift
        Coding Clinic: 2015, Q2, P6

● **W18   Other slipping, tripping and stumbling and falls**

    The appropriate 7th character is to be added to each code from category W18

A	initial encounter
D	subsequent encounter
S	sequela

● **W18.0   Fall due to bumping against object**
    Striking against object with subsequent fall
    Excludes1   fall on same level due to slipping, tripping, or stumbling with subsequent striking against object (W01.1-)

    X ● **W18.00   Striking against unspecified object with subsequent fall**

    X ● **W18.01   Striking against sports equipment with subsequent fall**

    X ● **W18.02   Striking against glass with subsequent fall**

    X ● **W18.09   Striking against other object with subsequent fall**

● **W18.1   Fall from or off toilet**

    X ● **W18.11   Fall from or off toilet without subsequent striking against object**
        Fall from (off) toilet NOS

    X ● **W18.12   Fall from or off toilet with subsequent striking against object**

X ● **W18.2   Fall in (into) shower or empty bathtub**
    Excludes1   fall in full bathtub causing drowning or submersion (W16.21-)

● **W18.3   Other and unspecified fall on same level**

    X ● **W18.30   Fall on same level, unspecified**

    X ● **W18.31   Fall on same level due to stepping on an object**
        Fall on same level due to stepping on an animal
        Excludes1   slipping, tripping and stumbling without fall due to stepping on animal (W18.41)

    X ● **W18.39   Other fall on same level**

● **W18.4   Slipping, tripping and stumbling without falling**
    Excludes1   collision with another person without fall (W51)

    X ● **W18.40   Slipping, tripping and stumbling without falling, unspecified**

    X ● **W18.41   Slipping, tripping and stumbling without falling due to stepping on object**
        Slipping, tripping and stumbling without falling due to stepping on animal
        Excludes1   slipping, tripping and stumbling with fall due to stepping on animal (W18.31)

    X ● **W18.42   Slipping, tripping and stumbling without falling due to stepping into hole or opening**

    X ● **W18.43   Slipping, tripping and stumbling without falling due to stepping from one level to another**

    X ● **W18.49   Other slipping, tripping and stumbling without falling**

X ● **W19   Unspecified fall**
    Accidental fall NOS
    The appropriate 7th character is to be added to code W19

A	initial encounter
D	subsequent encounter
S	sequela

Coding Clinic: 2021, Q2, P5; 2012, Q4, P95

EXPOSURE TO INANIMATE MECHANICAL FORCES (W20-W49)

Excludes1   assault (X92-Y09)
           contact or collision with animals or persons
                (W50-W64)
           exposure to inanimate mechanical forces
                involving military or war operations (Y36.-,
                Y37.-)
           intentional self-harm (X71-X83)
Coding Clinic: 2016, Q4, P129

● **W20   Struck by thrown, projected or falling object**

Code first any associated:
     cataclysm (X34-X39)
     lightning strike (T75.00)

Excludes1   falling object in machinery accident (W24,
                W28-W31)
           falling object in transport accident (V01-V99)
           object set in motion by explosion (W35-W40)
           object set in motion by firearm (W32-W34)
           struck by thrown sports equipment (W21.-)

The appropriate 7th character is to be added to each code from
category W20

A	initial encounter
D	subsequent encounter
S	sequela

X ● **W20.0   Struck by falling object in cave-in**
      Excludes2   asphyxiation due to cave-in (T71.21)
X ● **W20.1   Struck by object due to collapse of building**
      Excludes1   struck by object due to collapse of
                burning building (X00.2, X02.2)
X ● **W20.8   Other cause of strike by thrown, projected or falling
          object**
      Excludes1   struck by thrown sports equipment
                (W21.-)

● **W21   Striking against or struck by sports equipment**

Excludes1   assault with sports equipment (Y08.0-)
           striking against or struck by sports equipment
             with subsequent fall (W18.01)

The appropriate 7th character is to be added to each code from
category W21

A	initial encounter
D	subsequent encounter
S	sequela

● **W21.0   Struck by hit or thrown ball**
X ● **W21.00   Struck by hit or thrown ball, unspecified type**
X ● **W21.01   Struck by football**
X ● **W21.02   Struck by soccer ball**
X ● **W21.03   Struck by baseball**
X ● **W21.04   Struck by golf ball**
X ● **W21.05   Struck by basketball**
X ● **W21.06   Struck by volleyball**
X ● **W21.07   Struck by softball**
X ● **W21.09   Struck by other hit or thrown ball**
● **W21.1   Struck by bat, racquet or club**
X ● **W21.11   Struck by baseball bat**
X ● **W21.12   Struck by tennis racquet**
X ● **W21.13   Struck by golf club**
X ● **W21.19   Struck by other bat, racquet or club**
● **W21.2   Struck by hockey stick or puck**
● **W21.21   Struck by hockey stick**
● **W21.210   Struck by ice hockey stick**
● **W21.211   Struck by field hockey stick**

● **W21.22   Struck by hockey puck**
● **W21.220   Struck by ice hockey puck**
● **W21.221   Struck by field hockey puck**
● **W21.3   Struck by sports foot wear**
X ● **W21.31   Struck by shoe cleats**
         Stepped on by shoe cleats
X ● **W21.32   Struck by skate blades**
         Skated over by skate blades
X ● **W21.39   Struck by other sports foot wear**
X ● **W21.4   Striking against diving board**
         Use additional code for subsequent falling into water, if
         applicable (W16.-)
● **W21.8   Striking against or struck by other sports equipment**
X ● **W21.81   Striking against or struck by football helmet**
X ● **W21.89   Striking against or struck by other sports
            equipment**
X ● **W21.9   Striking against or struck by unspecified sports
       equipment**

● **W22   Striking against or struck by other objects**

Excludes1   striking against or struck by object with
             subsequent fall (W18.09)

The appropriate 7th character is to be added to each code from
category W22

A	initial encounter
D	subsequent encounter
S	sequela

● **W22.0   Striking against stationary object**
Excludes1   striking against stationary sports
             equipment (W21.8)
X ● **W22.01   Walked into wall**
X ● **W22.02   Walked into lamppost**
X ● **W22.03   Walked into furniture**
● **W22.04   Striking against wall of swimming pool**
● **W22.041   Striking against wall of swimming
               pool causing drowning and
               submersion**
             Excludes1   drowning and
                         submersion
                         while swimming
                         without striking
                         against wall
                         (W67)
● **W22.042   Striking against wall of swimming
               pool causing other injury**
X ● **W22.09   Striking against other stationary object**
● **W22.1   Striking against or struck by automobile airbag**
X ● **W22.10   Striking against or struck by unspecified
            automobile airbag**
X ● **W22.11   Striking against or struck by driver side
            automobile airbag**
X ● **W22.12   Striking against or struck by front passenger
            side automobile airbag**
X ● **W22.19   Striking against or struck by other automobile
            airbag**
X ● **W22.8   Striking against or struck by other objects**
         Striking against or struck by object NOS
      Excludes1   struck by thrown, projected or falling
                object (W20.-)

▶ New   ⇒ Revised   ~~deleted~~ Deleted   Excludes 1   Excludes 2   Includes   Use additional   Code first   Code also   Key words
OGCR Official Guidelines   X Assign placeholder X   ● Use Additional Character(s)   ▷ Manifestation Code   🏷 Hierarchical Condition Category   **Coding Clinic**

● W23 **Caught, crushed, jammed or pinched in or between objects**
　　Excludes1　injury caused by cutting or piercing instruments
　　　　　　　　　(W25-W27)
　　　　　　　　　injury caused by firearms malfunction (W32.1,
　　　　　　　　　W33.1-, W34.1-)
　　　　　　　　　injury caused by lifting and transmission devices
　　　　　　　　　(W24.-)
　　　　　　　　　injury caused by machinery (W28-W31)
　　　　　　　　　injury caused by nonpowered hand tools (W27.-)
　　　　　　　　　injury caused by transport vehicle being used as a
　　　　　　　　　means of transportation (V01-V99)
　　　　　　　　　injury caused by struck by thrown, projected or
　　　　　　　　　falling object (W20.-)
　　The appropriate 7th character is to be added to each code from
　　category W23

A	initial encounter
D	subsequent encounter
S	sequela

X ● W23.0 **Caught, crushed, jammed, or pinched between moving objects**

X ● W23.1 **Caught, crushed, jammed, or pinched between stationary objects**

● W24 **Contact with lifting and transmission devices, not elsewhere classified**
　　Excludes1　transport accidents (V01-V99)
　　The appropriate 7th character is to be added to each code from
　　category W24

A	initial encounter
D	subsequent encounter
S	sequela

X ● W24.0 **Contact with lifting devices, not elsewhere classified**
　　　　Contact with chain hoist
　　　　Contact with drive belt
　　　　Contact with pulley (block)

X ● W24.1 **Contact with transmission devices, not elsewhere classified**
　　　　Contact with transmission belt or cable

X ● W25 **Contact with sharp glass**
　　Code first any associated:
　　　injury due to flying glass from explosion or firearm discharge
　　　(W32-W40)
　　　transport accident (V00-V99)
　　➡**Excludes1**　fall on same level due to slipping, tripping and
　　　　　　　　stumbling with subsequent striking against
　　　　　　　　sharp glass (W01.110-)
　　　　　　　➡striking against sharp glass with subsequent fall
　　　　　　　　(W18.02-)
　　➡**Excludes2**　glass embedded in skin (W45.-)
　　The appropriate 7th character is to be added to code W25

A	initial encounter
D	subsequent encounter
S	sequela

● W26 **Contact with other sharp objects**
　　➡**Excludes2**　sharp object(s) embedded in skin (W45.-)
　　The appropriate 7th character is to be added to each code from
　　category W26

A	initial encounter
D	subsequent encounter
S	sequela

　　Coding Clinic: 2016, Q4, P73

X ● W26.0 **Contact with knife**
　　　　Excludes1　contact with electric knife (W29.1)

X ● W26.1 **Contact with sword or dagger**

X ● W26.2 **Contact with edge of stiff paper**
　　　　Paper cut
　　　　Coding Clinic: 2016, Q4, P73

X ● W26.8 **Contact with other sharp object(s), not elsewhere classified**
　　　　Contact with tin can lid
　　　　Coding Clinic: 2016, Q4, P73

X ● W26.9 **Contact with unspecified sharp object(s)**
　　　　Coding Clinic: 2016, Q4, P73

● W27 **Contact with nonpowered hand tool**
　　The appropriate 7th character is to be added to each code from
　　category W27

A	initial encounter
D	subsequent encounter
S	sequela

X ● W27.0 **Contact with workbench tool**
　　　　Contact with auger
　　　　Contact with axe
　　　　Contact with chisel
　　　　Contact with handsaw
　　　　Contact with screwdriver

X ● W27.1 **Contact with garden tool**
　　　　Contact with hoe
　　　　Contact with nonpowered lawn mower
　　　　Contact with pitchfork
　　　　Contact with rake

X ● W27.2 **Contact with scissors**

X ● W27.3 **Contact with needle (sewing)**
　　　　Excludes1　contact with hypodermic needle (W46.-)

X ● W27.4 **Contact with kitchen utensil**
　　　　Contact with fork
　　　　Contact with ice-pick
　　　　Contact with can-opener NOS

X ● W27.5 **Contact with paper-cutter**

X ● W27.8 **Contact with other nonpowered hand tool**
　　　　Contact with nonpowered sewing machine
　　　　Contact with shovel

X ● W28 **Contact with powered lawn mower**
　　Powered lawn mower (commercial) (residential)
　　　　Excludes1　contact with nonpowered lawn mower (W27.1)
　　　　Excludes2　exposure to electric current (W86.-)
　　The appropriate 7th character is to be added to code W28

A	initial encounter
D	subsequent encounter
S	sequela

● W29 **Contact with other powered hand tools and household machinery**
　　Excludes1　contact with commercial machinery (W31.82)
　　　　　　　　contact with hot household appliance (X15)
　　　　　　　　contact with nonpowered hand tool (W27.-)
　　　　　　　　exposure to electric current (W86)
　　The appropriate 7th character is to be added to each code from
　　category W29

A	initial encounter
D	subsequent encounter
S	sequela

X ● W29.0 **Contact with powered kitchen appliance**
　　　　Contact with blender
　　　　Contact with can-opener
　　　　Contact with garbage disposal
　　　　Contact with mixer

X ● W29.1 **Contact with electric knife**

X ● W29.2 **Contact with other powered household machinery**
　　　　Contact with electric fan
　　　　Contact with powered dryer (clothes) (powered) (spin)
　　　　Contact with washing-machine
　　　　Contact with sewing machine

X● **W29.3 Contact with powered garden and outdoor hand tools and machinery**
     Contact with chainsaw
     Contact with edger
     Contact with garden cultivator (tiller)
     Contact with hedge trimmer
     Contact with other powered garden tool
     Excludes1   contact with powered lawn mower (W28)

X● **W29.4 Contact with nail gun**

X● **W29.8 Contact with other powered hand tools and household machinery**
     Contact with do-it-yourself tool NOS

● **W30 Contact with agricultural machinery**
     Includes   animal-powered farm machine
     Excludes1   agricultural transport vehicle accident (V01-V99)
         explosion of grain store (W40.8)
         exposure to electric current (W86.-)

     The appropriate 7th character is to be added to each code from category W30

A	initial encounter
D	subsequent encounter
S	sequela

X● **W30.0 Contact with combine harvester**
     Contact with reaper
     Contact with thresher

X● **W30.1 Contact with power take-off devices (PTO)**

X● **W30.2 Contact with hay derrick**

X● **W30.3 Contact with grain storage elevator**
     Excludes1   explosion of grain store (W40.8)

● **W30.8 Contact with other specified agricultural machinery**

X● **W30.81 Contact with agricultural transport vehicle in stationary use**
     Contact with agricultural transport vehicle under repair, not on public roadway
     Excludes1   agricultural transport vehicle accident (V01-V99)

X● **W30.89 Contact with other specified agricultural machinery**

X● **W30.9 Contact with unspecified agricultural machinery**
     Contact with farm machinery NOS

● **W31 Contact with other and unspecified machinery**
     Excludes1   contact with agricultural machinery (W30.-)
         contact with machinery in transport under own power or being towed by a vehicle (V01-V99)
         exposure to electric current (W86)

     The appropriate 7th character is to be added to each code from category W31

A	initial encounter
D	subsequent encounter
S	sequela

X● **W31.0 Contact with mining and earth-drilling machinery**
     Contact with bore or drill (land) (seabed)
     Contact with shaft hoist
     Contact with shaft lift
     Contact with undercutter

X● **W31.1 Contact with metalworking machines**
     Contact with abrasive wheel
     Contact with forging machine
     Contact with lathe
     Contact with mechanical shears
     Contact with metal drilling machine
     Contact with milling machine
     Contact with power press
     Contact with rolling-mill
     Contact with metal sawing machine

X● **W31.2 Contact with powered woodworking and forming machines**
     Contact with band saw
     Contact with bench saw
     Contact with circular saw
     Contact with molding machine
     Contact with overhead plane
     Contact with powered saw
     Contact with radial saw
     Contact with sander
     Excludes1   nonpowered woodworking tools (W27.0)

X● **W31.3 Contact with prime movers**
     Contact with gas turbine
     Contact with internal combustion engine
     Contact with steam engine
     Contact with water driven turbine

● **W31.8 Contact with other specified machinery**

X● **W31.81 Contact with recreational machinery**
     Contact with roller-coaster

X● **W31.82 Contact with other commercial machinery**
     Contact with commercial electric fan
     Contact with commercial kitchen appliances
     Contact with commercial powered dryer (clothes) (powered) (spin)
     Contact with commercial washing-machine
     Contact with commercial sewing machine
     Excludes1   contact with household machinery (W29.-)
         contact with powered lawn mower (W28)

X● **W31.83 Contact with special construction vehicle in stationary use**
     Contact with special construction vehicle under repair, not on public roadway
     Excludes1   special construction vehicle accident (V01-V99)

X● **W31.89 Contact with other specified machinery**

X● **W31.9 Contact with unspecified machinery**
     Contact with machinery NOS

● **W32 Accidental handgun discharge and malfunction**
     Includes   accidental discharge and malfunction of gun for single hand use
         accidental discharge and malfunction of pistol
         accidental discharge and malfunction of revolver
         handgun discharge and malfunction NOS
     Excludes1   accidental airgun discharge and malfunction (W34.010, W34.110)
         accidental BB gun discharge and malfunction (W34.010, W34.110)
         accidental pellet gun discharge and malfunction (W34.010, W34.110)
         accidental shotgun discharge and malfunction (W33.01, W33.11)
         assault by handgun discharge (X93)
         handgun discharge involving legal intervention (Y35.0-)
         handgun discharge involving military or war operations (Y36.4-)
         intentional self-harm by handgun discharge (X72)
         Very pistol discharge and malfunction (W34.09, W34.19)

     The appropriate 7th character is to be added to each code from category W32

A	initial encounter
D	subsequent encounter
S	sequela

X● **W32.0 Accidental handgun discharge**

X● **W32.1 Accidental handgun malfunction**
     Injury due to explosion of handgun (parts)
     Injury due to malfunction of mechanism or component of handgun
     Injury due to recoil of handgun
     Powder burn from handgun

▶ New   ⇒ Revised   ~~deleted~~ Deleted   Excludes 1   Excludes 2   Includes   Use additional   Code first   Code also   Key words

OGCR Official Guidelines   X Assign placeholder X   ● Use Additional Character(s)   ▌ Manifestation Code   🐾 Hierarchical Condition Category   **Coding Clinic**

● **W33 Accidental rifle, shotgun and larger firearm discharge and malfunction**

Includes   rifle, shotgun and larger firearm discharge and malfunction NOS

Excludes1   accidental airgun discharge and malfunction (W34.010, W34.110)
accidental BB gun discharge and malfunction (W34.010, W34.110)
accidental handgun discharge and malfunction (W32.-)
accidental pellet gun discharge and malfunction (W34.010, W34.110)
assault by rifle, shotgun and larger firearm discharge (X94)
firearm discharge involving legal intervention (Y35.0-)
firearm discharge involving military or war operations (Y36.4-)
intentional self-harm by rifle, shotgun and larger firearm discharge (X73)

The appropriate 7th character is to be added to each code from category W33

> A   initial encounter
> D   subsequent encounter
> S   sequela

● **W33.0 Accidental rifle, shotgun and larger firearm discharge**

X ● **W33.00 Accidental discharge of unspecified larger firearm**
Discharge of unspecified larger firearm NOS

X ● **W33.01 Accidental discharge of shotgun**
Discharge of shotgun NOS

X ● **W33.02 Accidental discharge of hunting rifle**
Discharge of hunting rifle NOS

X ● **W33.03 Accidental discharge of machine gun**
Discharge of machine gun NOS

X ● **W33.09 Accidental discharge of other larger firearm**
Discharge of other larger firearm NOS

● **W33.1 Accidental rifle, shotgun and larger firearm malfunction**
Injury due to explosion of rifle, shotgun and larger firearm (parts)
Injury due to malfunction of mechanism or component of rifle, shotgun and larger firearm
Injury due to piercing, cutting, crushing or pinching due to (by) slide trigger mechanism, scope or other gun part
Injury due to recoil of rifle, shotgun and larger firearm
Powder burn from rifle, shotgun and larger firearm

X ● **W33.10 Accidental malfunction of unspecified larger firearm**
Malfunction of unspecified larger firearm NOS

X ● **W33.11 Accidental malfunction of shotgun**
Malfunction of shotgun NOS

X ● **W33.12 Accidental malfunction of hunting rifle**
Malfunction of hunting rifle NOS

X ● **W33.13 Accidental malfunction of machine gun**
Malfunction of machine gun NOS

X ● **W33.19 Accidental malfunction of other larger firearm**
Malfunction of other larger firearm NOS

● **W34 Accidental discharge and malfunction from other and unspecified firearms and guns**

The appropriate 7th character is to be added to each code from category W34

> A   initial encounter
> D   subsequent encounter
> S   sequela

● **W34.0 Accidental discharge from other and unspecified firearms and guns**

X ● **W34.00 Accidental discharge from unspecified firearms or gun**
Discharge from firearm NOS
Gunshot wound NOS
Shot NOS
Coding Clinic: 2015, Q1, P17

● **W34.01 Accidental discharge of gas, air or spring-operated guns**

● **W34.010 Accidental discharge of airgun**
Accidental discharge of BB gun
Accidental discharge of pellet gun

● **W34.011 Accidental discharge of paintball gun**
Accidental injury due to paintball discharge

● **W34.018 Accidental discharge of other gas, air or spring-operated gun**

X ● **W34.09 Accidental discharge from other specified firearms**
Accidental discharge from Very pistol [flare]

● **W34.1 Accidental malfunction from other and unspecified firearms and guns**

X ● **W34.10 Accidental malfunction from unspecified firearms or gun**
Firearm malfunction NOS

● **W34.11 Accidental malfunction of gas, air or spring-operated guns**

● **W34.110 Accidental malfunction of airgun**
Accidental malfunction of BB gun
Accidental malfunction of pellet gun

● **W34.111 Accidental malfunction of paintball gun**
Accidental injury due to paintball gun malfunction

● **W34.118 Accidental malfunction of other gas, air or spring-operated gun**

X ● **W34.19 Accidental malfunction from other specified firearms**
Accidental malfunction from Very pistol [flare]

X ● **W35 Explosion and rupture of boiler**

Excludes1   explosion and rupture of boiler on watercraft (V93.4)

The appropriate 7th character is to be added to code W35

> A   initial encounter
> D   subsequent encounter
> S   sequela

● **W36 Explosion and rupture of gas cylinder**

The appropriate 7th character is to be added to each code from category W36

> A   initial encounter
> D   subsequent encounter
> S   sequela

X ● **W36.1 Explosion and rupture of aerosol can**
X ● **W36.2 Explosion and rupture of air tank**
X ● **W36.3 Explosion and rupture of pressurized-gas tank**
X ● **W36.8 Explosion and rupture of other gas cylinder**
X ● **W36.9 Explosion and rupture of unspecified gas cylinder**

CHAPTER 20 (V00-Y99)

CHAPTER 20 (V00-Y99)

● W37   **Explosion and rupture of pressurized tire, pipe or hose**

The appropriate 7th character is to be added to each code from category W37

A	initial encounter
D	subsequent encounter
S	sequela

X ● **W37.0**   **Explosion of bicycle tire**

X ● **W37.8**   **Explosion and rupture of other pressurized tire, pipe or hose**

X ● **W38**   **Explosion and rupture of other specified pressurized devices**

The appropriate 7th character is to be added to code W38

A	initial encounter
D	subsequent encounter
S	sequela

X ● **W39**   **Discharge of firework**

The appropriate 7th character is to be added to code W39

A	initial encounter
D	subsequent encounter
S	sequela

● W40   **Explosion of other materials**

Excludes1   assault by explosive material (X96)
explosion involving legal intervention (Y35.1-)
explosion involving military or war operations (Y36.0-, Y36.2-)
intentional self-harm by explosive material (X75)

The appropriate 7th character is to be added to each code from category W40

A	initial encounter
D	subsequent encounter
S	sequela

X ● **W40.0**   **Explosion of blasting material**
Explosion of blasting cap
Explosion of detonator
Explosion of dynamite
Explosion of explosive (any) used in blasting operations

X ● **W40.1**   **Explosion of explosive gases**
Explosion of acetylene
Explosion of butane
Explosion of coal gas
Explosion in mine NOS
Explosion of explosive gas
Explosion of fire damp
Explosion of gasoline fumes
Explosion of methane
Explosion of propane

X ● **W40.8**   **Explosion of other specified explosive materials**
Explosion in dump NOS
Explosion in factory NOS
Explosion in grain store
Explosion in munitions

Excludes1   explosion involving legal intervention (Y35.1-)
explosion involving military or war operations (Y36.0-, Y36.2-)

X ● **W40.9**   **Explosion of unspecified explosive materials**
Explosion NOS

● W42   **Exposure to noise**

The appropriate 7th character is to be added to each code from category W42

A	initial encounter
D	subsequent encounter
S	sequela

X ● **W42.0**   **Exposure to supersonic waves**

X ● **W42.9**   **Exposure to other noise**
Exposure to sound waves NOS

● W45   **Foreign body or object entering through skin**

Includes   foreign body or object embedded in skin
nail embedded in skin

Excludes2   contact with hand tools (nonpowered) (powered) (W27-W29)
contact with other sharp object(s) (W26.-)
contact with sharp glass (W25.-)
struck by objects (W20-W22)

The appropriate 7th character is to be added to each code from category W45

A	initial encounter
D	subsequent encounter
S	sequela

X ● **W45.0**   **Nail entering through skin**

X ● **W45.8**   **Other foreign body or object entering through skin**
Splinter in skin NOS

● W46   **Contact with hypodermic needle**

The appropriate 7th character is to be added to each code from category W46

A	initial encounter
D	subsequent encounter
S	sequela

X ● **W46.0**   **Contact with hypodermic needle**
Hypodermic needle stick NOS

X ● **W46.1**   **Contact with contaminated hypodermic needle**

● W49   **Exposure to other inanimate mechanical forces**

Includes   exposure to abnormal gravitational [G] forces
exposure to inanimate mechanical forces NEC

Excludes1   exposure to inanimate mechanical forces involving military or war operations (Y36.-, Y37.-)

The appropriate 7th character is to be added to each code from category W49

A	initial encounter
D	subsequent encounter
S	sequela

● **W49.0**   **Item causing external constriction**

X ● **W49.01**   **Hair causing external constriction**

X ● **W49.02**   **String or thread causing external constriction**

X ● **W49.03**   **Rubber band causing external constriction**

X ● **W49.04**   **Ring or other jewelry causing external constriction**

X ● **W49.09**   **Other item causing external constriction**

X ● **W49.9**   **Exposure to other inanimate mechanical forces**

EXPOSURE TO ANIMATE MECHANICAL FORCES (W50-W64)

Excludes1   toxic effect of contact with venomous animals and plants (T63.-)

● W50   **Accidental hit, strike, kick, twist, bite or scratch by another person**

Includes   hit, strike, kick, twist, bite, or scratch by another person NOS

Excludes1   assault by bodily force (Y04)
struck by objects (W20-W22)

The appropriate 7th character is to be added to each code from category W50

A	initial encounter
D	subsequent encounter
S	sequela

X ● **W50.0**   **Accidental hit or strike by another person**
Hit or strike by another person NOS

X ● **W50.1**   **Accidental kick by another person**
Kick by another person NOS

▶ New   ⇒ Revised   ~~deleted~~ Deleted   Excludes 1   Excludes 2   Includes   Use additional   Code first   Code also   Key words
OGCR Official Guidelines   X Assign placeholder X   ● Use Additional Character(s)   ▌ Manifestation Code   🦠 Hierarchical Condition Category   **Coding Clinic**

X● **W50.2 Accidental twist by another person**
     Twist by another person NOS
     Coding Clinic: 2015, Q1, P8

X● **W50.3 Accidental bite by another person**
     Human bite
     Bite by another person NOS

X● **W50.4 Accidental scratch by another person**
     Scratch by another person NOS

X● **W51 Accidental striking against or bumped into by another person**

     Excludes1   assault by striking against or bumping into by
                another person (Y04.2)
                fall due to collision with another person (W03)

     The appropriate 7th character is to be added to code W51

A	initial encounter
D	subsequent encounter
S	sequela

X● **W52 Crushed, pushed or stepped on by crowd or human stampede**
     Crushed, pushed or stepped on by crowd or human stampede
        with or without fall

     The appropriate 7th character is to be added to code W52

A	initial encounter
D	subsequent encounter
S	sequela

● **W53 Contact with rodent**

     Includes   contact with saliva, feces or urine of rodent

     The appropriate 7th character is to be added to each code from
     category W53

A	initial encounter
D	subsequent encounter
S	sequela

   ● **W53.0 Contact with mouse**
     X● **W53.01 Bitten by mouse**
     X● **W53.09 Other contact with mouse**
   ● **W53.1 Contact with rat**
     X● **W53.11 Bitten by rat**
     X● **W53.19 Other contact with rat**
   ● **W53.2 Contact with squirrel**
     X● **W53.21 Bitten by squirrel**
     X● **W53.29 Other contact with squirrel**
   ● **W53.8 Contact with other rodent**
     X● **W53.81 Bitten by other rodent**
     X● **W53.89 Other contact with other rodent**

● **W54 Contact with dog**

     Includes   contact with saliva, feces or urine of dog

     The appropriate 7th character is to be added to each code from
     category W54

A	initial encounter
D	subsequent encounter
S	sequela

X● **W54.0 Bitten by dog**
X● **W54.1 Struck by dog**
     Knocked over by dog
X● **W54.8 Other contact with dog**

● **W55 Contact with other mammals**

     Includes   contact with saliva, feces or urine of mammal
     Excludes1   animal being ridden - see transport accidents
               bitten or struck by dog (W54)
               bitten or struck by rodent (W53.-)
               contact with marine mammals (W56.X-)

     The appropriate 7th character is to be added to each code from
     category W55

A	initial encounter
D	subsequent encounter
S	sequela

   ● **W55.0 Contact with cat**
     X● **W55.01 Bitten by cat**
     X● **W55.03 Scratched by cat**
     X● **W55.09 Other contact with cat**
   ● **W55.1 Contact with horse**
     X● **W55.11 Bitten by horse**
     X● **W55.12 Struck by horse**
     X● **W55.19 Other contact with horse**
   ● **W55.2 Contact with cow**
     Contact with bull
     X● **W55.21 Bitten by cow**
     X● **W55.22 Struck by cow**
         Gored by bull
     X● **W55.29 Other contact with cow**
   ● **W55.3 Contact with other hoof stock**
     Contact with goats
     Contact with sheep
     X● **W55.31 Bitten by other hoof stock**
     X● **W55.32 Struck by other hoof stock**
         Gored by goat
         Gored by ram
     X● **W55.39 Other contact with other hoof stock**
   ● **W55.4 Contact with pig**
     X● **W55.41 Bitten by pig**
     X● **W55.42 Struck by pig**
     X● **W55.49 Other contact with pig**
   ● **W55.5 Contact with raccoon**
     X● **W55.51 Bitten by raccoon**
     X● **W55.52 Struck by raccoon**
     X● **W55.59 Other contact with raccoon**
   ● **W55.8 Contact with other mammals**
     X● **W55.81 Bitten by other mammals**
     X● **W55.82 Struck by other mammals**
     X● **W55.89 Other contact with other mammals**

● **W56 Contact with nonvenomous marine animal**

     Excludes1   contact with venomous marine animal (T63.-)

     The appropriate 7th character is to be added to each code from
     category W56

A	initial encounter
D	subsequent encounter
S	sequela

   ● **W56.0 Contact with dolphin**
     X● **W56.01 Bitten by dolphin**
     X● **W56.02 Struck by dolphin**
     X● **W56.09 Other contact with dolphin**
   ● **W56.1 Contact with sea lion**
     X● **W56.11 Bitten by sea lion**
     X● **W56.12 Struck by sea lion**
     X● **W56.19 Other contact with sea lion**

CHAPTER 20 (V00–Y99)

● **W56.2 Contact with orca**
    Contact with killer whale
   X● **W56.21 Bitten by orca**
   X● **W56.22 Struck by orca**
   X● **W56.29 Other contact with orca**

● **W56.3 Contact with other marine mammals**
   X● **W56.31 Bitten by other marine mammals**
   X● **W56.32 Struck by other marine mammals**
   X● **W56.39 Other contact with other marine mammals**

● **W56.4 Contact with shark**
   X● **W56.41 Bitten by shark**
   X● **W56.42 Struck by shark**
   X● **W56.49 Other contact with shark**

● **W56.5 Contact with other fish**
   X● **W56.51 Bitten by other fish**
   X● **W56.52 Struck by other fish**
   X● **W56.59 Other contact with other fish**

● **W56.8 Contact with other nonvenomous marine animals**
   X● **W56.81 Bitten by other nonvenomous marine animals**
   X● **W56.82 Struck by other nonvenomous marine animals**
   X● **W56.89 Other contact with other nonvenomous marine animals**

X● **W57 Bitten or stung by nonvenomous insect and other nonvenomous arthropods**

> **Excludes1**   contact with venomous insects and arthropods (T63.2-, T63.3-, T63.4-)

The appropriate 7th character is to be added to code W57

A	initial encounter
D	subsequent encounter
S	sequela

● **W58 Contact with crocodile or alligator**

The appropriate 7th character is to be added to each code from category W58

A	initial encounter
D	subsequent encounter
S	sequela

● **W58.0 Contact with alligator**
   X● **W58.01 Bitten by alligator**
   X● **W58.02 Struck by alligator**
   X● **W58.03 Crushed by alligator**
   X● **W58.09 Other contact with alligator**

● **W58.1 Contact with crocodile**
   X● **W58.11 Bitten by crocodile**
   X● **W58.12 Struck by crocodile**
   X● **W58.13 Crushed by crocodile**
   X● **W58.19 Other contact with crocodile**

● **W59 Contact with other nonvenomous reptiles**

> **Excludes1**   contact with venomous reptile (T63.0-, T63.1-)

The appropriate 7th character is to be added to each code from category W59

A	initial encounter
D	subsequent encounter
S	sequela

● **W59.0 Contact with nonvenomous lizards**
   X● **W59.01 Bitten by nonvenomous lizards**
   X● **W59.02 Struck by nonvenomous lizards**
   X● **W59.09 Other contact with nonvenomous lizards**
     Exposure to nonvenomous lizards

● **W59.1 Contact with nonvenomous snakes**
   X● **W59.11 Bitten by nonvenomous snake**
   X● **W59.12 Struck by nonvenomous snake**
   X● **W59.13 Crushed by nonvenomous snake**
   X● **W59.19 Other contact with nonvenomous snake**

● **W59.2 Contact with turtles**

> **Excludes1**   contact with tortoises (W59.8-)

   X● **W59.21 Bitten by turtle**
   X● **W59.22 Struck by turtle**
   X● **W59.29 Other contact with turtle**
     Exposure to turtles

● **W59.8 Contact with other nonvenomous reptiles**
   X● **W59.81 Bitten by other nonvenomous reptiles**
   X● **W59.82 Struck by other nonvenomous reptiles**
   X● **W59.83 Crushed by other nonvenomous reptiles**
   X● **W59.89 Other contact with other nonvenomous reptiles**

X● **W60 Contact with nonvenomous plant thorns and spines and sharp leaves**

> **Excludes1**   contact with venomous plants (T63.X7-)

The appropriate 7th character is to be added to code W60

A	initial encounter
D	subsequent encounter
S	sequela

● **W61 Contact with birds (domestic) (wild)**

> **Includes**   contact with excreta of birds

The appropriate 7th character is to be added to each code from category W61

A	initial encounter
D	subsequent encounter
S	sequela

● **W61.0 Contact with parrot**
   X● **W61.01 Bitten by parrot**
   X● **W61.02 Struck by parrot**
   X● **W61.09 Other contact with parrot**
     Exposure to parrots

● **W61.1 Contact with macaw**
   X● **W61.11 Bitten by macaw**
   X● **W61.12 Struck by macaw**
   X● **W61.19 Other contact with macaw**
     Exposure to macaws

● **W61.2 Contact with other psittacines**
   X● **W61.21 Bitten by other psittacines**
   X● **W61.22 Struck by other psittacines**
   X● **W61.29 Other contact with other psittacines**
     Exposure to other psittacines

● **W61.3 Contact with chicken**
   X● **W61.32 Struck by chicken**
   X● **W61.33 Pecked by chicken**
   X● **W61.39 Other contact with chicken**
     Exposure to chickens

● **W61.4 Contact with turkey**
   X● **W61.42 Struck by turkey**
   X● **W61.43 Pecked by turkey**
   X● **W61.49 Other contact with turkey**

● **W61.5 Contact with goose**
   X● **W61.51 Bitten by goose**
   X● **W61.52 Struck by goose**
   X● **W61.59 Other contact with goose**

▶ New   ⇒ Revised   ~~deleted~~ Deleted   Excludes 1   Excludes 2   Includes   Use additional   Code first   Code also   Key words

OGCR Official Guidelines   X Assign placeholder X   ● Use Additional Character(s)   ▶ Manifestation Code   ℞ Hierarchical Condition Category   **Coding Clinic**

● **W61.6   Contact with duck**
   X● **W61.61   Bitten by duck**
   X● **W61.62   Struck by duck**
   X● **W61.69   Other contact with duck**
● **W61.9   Contact with other birds**
   X● **W61.91   Bitten by other birds**
   X● **W61.92   Struck by other birds**
   X● **W61.99   Other contact with other birds**
     Contact with bird NOS

● **W62   Contact with nonvenomous amphibians**

   Excludes1   contact with venomous amphibians
       (T63.81-R63.83)

The appropriate 7th character is to be added to each code from
   category W62

A	initial encounter
D	subsequent encounter
S	sequela

   X● **W62.0   Contact with nonvenomous frogs**
   X● **W62.1   Contact with nonvenomous toads**
   X● **W62.9   Contact with other nonvenomous amphibians**

X● **W64   Exposure to other animate mechanical forces**

   Includes   exposure to nonvenomous animal NOS
   Excludes1   contact with venomous animal (T63.-)

The appropriate 7th character is to be added to code W64

A	initial encounter
D	subsequent encounter
S	sequela

ACCIDENTAL NON-TRANSPORT DROWNING AND SUBMERSION (W65-W74)

   Excludes1   accidental drowning and submersion due to fall
       into water (W16.-)
       accidental drowning and submersion due to
       water transport accident (V90.-, V92.-)
   Excludes2   accidental drowning and submersion due to
       cataclysm (X34-X39)

X● **W65   Accidental drowning and submersion while in bathtub**

   Excludes1   accidental drowning and submersion due to fall
       in (into) bathtub (W16.211)

The appropriate 7th character is to be added to code W65

A	initial encounter
D	subsequent encounter
S	sequela

X● **W67   Accidental drowning and submersion while in swimming pool**

   Excludes1   accidental drowning and submersion due to fall
       into swimming pool (W16.011, W16.021,
       W16.031)
       accidental drowning and submersion due
       to striking into wall of swimming pool
       (W22.041)

The appropriate 7th character is to be added to code W67

A	initial encounter
D	subsequent encounter
S	sequela

X● **W69   Accidental drowning and submersion while in natural water**
     Accidental drowning and submersion while in lake
     Accidental drowning and submersion while in open sea
     Accidental drowning and submersion while in river
     Accidental drowning and submersion while in stream

   Excludes1   accidental drowning and submersion due to
       fall into natural body of water (W16.111,
       W16.121, W16.131)

The appropriate 7th character is to be added to code W69

A	initial encounter
D	subsequent encounter
S	sequela

X● **W73   Other specified cause of accidental non-transport drowning and submersion**
     Accidental drowning and submersion while in quenching tank
     Accidental drowning and submersion while in reservoir

   Excludes1   accidental drowning and submersion due to
       fall into other water (W16.311, W16.321,
       W16.331)

The appropriate 7th character is to be added to code W73

A	initial encounter
D	subsequent encounter
S	sequela

X● **W74   Unspecified cause of accidental drowning and submersion**
     Drowning NOS

The appropriate 7th character is to be added to code W74

A	initial encounter
D	subsequent encounter
S	sequela

EXPOSURE TO ELECTRIC CURRENT, RADIATION AND EXTREME AMBIENT AIR TEMPERATURE AND PRESSURE (W85-W99)

   Excludes1   exposure to:
       failure in dosage of radiation or temperature
         during surgical and medical care
         (Y63.2-Y63.5)
       lightning (T75.0-)
       natural cold (X31)
       natural heat (X30)
       natural radiation NOS (X39)
       radiological procedure and radiotherapy
         (Y84.2)
       sunlight (X32)

X● **W85   Exposure to electric transmission lines**
     Broken power line

The appropriate 7th character is to be added to code W85

A	initial encounter
D	subsequent encounter
S	sequela

● **W86   Exposure to other specified electric current**

The appropriate 7th character is to be added to each code from
   category W86

A	initial encounter
D	subsequent encounter
S	sequela

   X● **W86.0   Exposure to domestic wiring and appliances**
   X● **W86.1   Exposure to industrial wiring, appliances and electrical machinery**
       Exposure to conductors
       Exposure to control apparatus
       Exposure to electrical equipment and machinery
       Exposure to transformers

CHAPTER 20 (V00-Y99)

X ● **W86.8　Exposure to other electric current**
　　Exposure to wiring and appliances in or on farm (not farmhouse)
　　Exposure to wiring and appliances outdoors
　　Exposure to wiring and appliances in or on public building
　　Exposure to wiring and appliances in or on residential institutions
　　Exposure to wiring and appliances in or on schools

● **W88　Exposure to ionizing radiation**

　　Excludes1　exposure to sunlight (X32)

　　The appropriate 7th character is to be added to each code from category W88

A	initial encounter
D	subsequent encounter
S	sequela

X ● **W88.0　Exposure to X-rays**

X ● **W88.1　Exposure to radioactive isotopes**

X ● **W88.8　Exposure to other ionizing radiation**

● **W89　Exposure to man-made visible and ultraviolet light**

　　Includes　exposure to welding light (arc)

　　Excludes2　exposure to sunlight (X32)

　　The appropriate 7th character is to be added to each code from category W89

A	initial encounter
D	subsequent encounter
S	sequela

X ● **W89.0　Exposure to welding light (arc)**

X ● **W89.1　Exposure to tanning bed**

X ● **W89.8　Exposure to other man-made visible and ultraviolet light**

X ● **W89.9　Exposure to unspecified man-made visible and ultraviolet light**

● **W90　Exposure to other nonionizing radiation**

　　Excludes2　exposure to sunlight (X32)

　　The appropriate 7th character is to be added to each code from category W90

A	initial encounter
D	subsequent encounter
S	sequela

X ● **W90.0　Exposure to radiofrequency**

X ● **W90.1　Exposure to infrared radiation**

X ● **W90.2　Exposure to laser radiation**

X ● **W90.8　Exposure to other nonionizing radiation**

X ● **W92　Exposure to excessive heat of man-made origin**

　　The appropriate 7th character is to be added to code W92

A	initial encounter
D	subsequent encounter
S	sequela

● **W93　Exposure to excessive cold of man-made origin**

　　The appropriate 7th character is to be added to each code from category W93

A	initial encounter
D	subsequent encounter
S	sequela

　● **W93.0　Contact with or inhalation of dry ice**

　　X ● **W93.01　Contact with dry ice**

　　X ● **W93.02　Inhalation of dry ice**

● **W93.1　Contact with or inhalation of liquid air**

　X ● **W93.11　Contact with liquid air**
　　　Contact with liquid hydrogen
　　　Contact with liquid nitrogen

　X ● **W93.12　Inhalation of liquid air**
　　　Inhalation of liquid hydrogen
　　　Inhalation of liquid nitrogen

X ● **W93.2　Prolonged exposure in deep freeze unit or refrigerator**

X ● **W93.8　Exposure to other excessive cold of man-made origin**

● **W94　Exposure to high and low air pressure and changes in air pressure**

　　The appropriate 7th character is to be added to each code from category W94

A	initial encounter
D	subsequent encounter
S	sequela

X ● **W94.0　Exposure to prolonged high air pressure**

● **W94.1　Exposure to prolonged low air pressure**

　X ● **W94.11　Exposure to residence or prolonged visit at high altitude**

　X ● **W94.12　Exposure to other prolonged low air pressure**

● **W94.2　Exposure to rapid changes in air pressure during ascent**

　X ● **W94.21　Exposure to reduction in atmospheric pressure while surfacing from deep-water diving**

　X ● **W94.22　Exposure to reduction in atmospheric pressure while surfacing from underground**

　X ● **W94.23　Exposure to sudden change in air pressure in aircraft during ascent**

　X ● **W94.29　Exposure to other rapid changes in air pressure during ascent**

● **W94.3　Exposure to rapid changes in air pressure during descent**

　X ● **W94.31　Exposure to sudden change in air pressure in aircraft during descent**

　X ● **W94.32　Exposure to high air pressure from rapid descent in water**

　X ● **W94.39　Exposure to other rapid changes in air pressure during descent**

X ● **W99　Exposure to other man-made environmental factors**

　　The appropriate 7th character is to be added to code W99

A	initial encounter
D	subsequent encounter
S	sequela

EXPOSURE TO SMOKE, FIRE AND FLAMES (X00-X08)

Excludes1	arson (X97)
Excludes2	explosions (W35-W40)
	lightning (T75.0-)
	transport accident (V01-V99)

● **X00　Exposure to uncontrolled fire in building or structure**

　　Includes　conflagration in building or structure

　　Code first any associated cataclysm

　　Excludes2　exposure to ignition or melting of nightwear (X05)
　　　　exposure to ignition or melting of other clothing and apparel (X06.-)
　　　　exposure to other specified smoke, fire and flames (X08.-)

　　The appropriate 7th character is to be added to each code from category X00

A	initial encounter
D	subsequent encounter
S	sequela

X ● **X00.0　Exposure to flames in uncontrolled fire in building or structure**
　　Coding Clinic: 2016, Q2, P5-6; 2015, Q1, P19

X ● **X00.1　Exposure to smoke in uncontrolled fire in building or structure**

▶ New　　▶ Revised　　~~deleted~~ Deleted　　Excludes 1　　Excludes 2　　Includes　　Use additional　　Code first　　Code also　　Key words

OGCR Official Guidelines　　X Assign placeholder X　　● Use Additional Character(s)　　▶ Manifestation Code　　🔖 Hierarchical Condition Category　　**Coding Clinic**

w www

X● **X00.2** **Injury due to collapse** of burning building or structure in uncontrolled fire

 Excludes1 injury due to collapse of building not on fire (W20.1)

X● **X00.3** **Fall from** burning building or structure in uncontrolled fire

X● **X00.4** **Hit by object** from burning building or structure in uncontrolled fire

X● **X00.5** **Jump from** burning building or structure in uncontrolled fire

X● **X00.8** **Other** exposure to uncontrolled fire in building or structure

● **X01** **Exposure to uncontrolled fire, not in building or structure**

 Includes exposure to forest fire

The appropriate 7th character is to be added to each code from category X01

A	initial encounter
D	subsequent encounter
S	sequela

X● **X01.0** **Exposure to flames** in uncontrolled fire, not in building or structure

X● **X01.1** **Exposure to smoke** in uncontrolled fire, not in building or structure

X● **X01.3** **Fall due to** uncontrolled fire, not in building or structure

X● **X01.4** **Hit by object** due to uncontrolled fire, not in building or structure

X● **X01.8** **Other** exposure to uncontrolled fire, not in building or structure

● **X02** **Exposure to controlled fire in building or structure**

 Includes exposure to fire in fireplace exposure to fire in stove

The appropriate 7th character is to be added to each code from category X02

A	initial encounter
D	subsequent encounter
S	sequela

X● **X02.0** **Exposure to flames** in controlled fire in building or structure

X● **X02.1** **Exposure to smoke** in controlled fire in building or structure

X● **X02.2** **Injury due to collapse** of burning building or structure in controlled fire

 Excludes1 injury due to collapse of building not on fire (W20.1)

X● **X02.3** **Fall from** burning building or structure in controlled fire

X● **X02.4** **Hit by object** from burning building or structure in controlled fire

X● **X02.5** **Jump from** burning building or structure in controlled fire

X● **X02.8** **Other** exposure to controlled fire in building or structure

● **X03** **Exposure to controlled fire, not in building or structure**

 Includes exposure to bon fire exposure to camp fire exposure to trash fire

The appropriate 7th character is to be added to each code from category X03

A	initial encounter
D	subsequent encounter
S	sequela

X● **X03.0** **Exposure to flames** in controlled fire, not in building or structure

Coding Clinic: 2015, Q1, P19

X● **X03.1** **Exposure to smoke** in controlled fire, not in building or structure

X● **X03.3** **Fall due to** controlled fire, not in building or structure

X● **X03.4** **Hit by object** due to controlled fire, not in building or structure

X● **X03.8** **Other** exposure to controlled fire, not in building or structure

X● **X04** **Exposure to ignition of highly flammable material**

Exposure to ignition of gasoline
Exposure to ignition of kerosene
Exposure to ignition of petrol

 Excludes2 exposure to ignition or melting of nightwear (X05)
exposure to ignition or melting of other clothing and apparel (X06)

The appropriate 7th character is to be added to code X04

A	initial encounter
D	subsequent encounter
S	sequela

Coding Clinic: 2016, Q2, P4

X● **X05** **Exposure to ignition or melting of nightwear**

 Excludes2 exposure to uncontrolled fire in building or structure (X00.-)
exposure to uncontrolled fire, not in building or structure (X01.-)
exposure to controlled fire in building or structure (X02.-)
exposure to controlled fire, not in building or structure (X03.-)
exposure to ignition of highly flammable materials (X04.-)

The appropriate 7th character is to be added to code X05

A	initial encounter
D	subsequent encounter
S	sequela

● **X06** **Exposure to ignition or melting of other clothing and apparel**

 Excludes2 exposure to uncontrolled fire in building or structure (X00.-)
exposure to uncontrolled fire, not in building or structure (X01.-)
exposure to controlled fire in building or structure (X02.-)
exposure to controlled fire, not in building or structure (X03.-)
exposure to ignition of highly flammable materials (X04.-)

The appropriate 7th character is to be added to each code from category X06

A	initial encounter
D	subsequent encounter
S	sequela

X● **X06.0** **Exposure to ignition** of plastic jewelry

X● **X06.1** **Exposure to melting** of plastic jewelry

X● **X06.2** **Exposure to ignition** of other clothing and apparel

X● **X06.3** **Exposure to melting** of other clothing and apparel

● **X08** **Exposure to other specified smoke, fire and flames**

The appropriate 7th character is to be added to each code from category X08

A	initial encounter
D	subsequent encounter
S	sequela

● **X08.0** **Exposure to bed fire**

Exposure to mattress fire

X● **X08.00** **Exposure to bed fire due to unspecified** burning material

X● **X08.01** **Exposure to bed fire due to burning cigarette**

Coding Clinic: 2015, Q1, P19

X● **X08.09** **Exposure to bed fire due to other** burning material

● X08.1 **Exposure to sofa fire**
X ● X08.10 **Exposure to sofa fire due to** unspecified **burning material**
X ● X08.11 **Exposure to sofa fire due to burning** cigarette
X ● X08.19 **Exposure to sofa fire due to** other **burning material**
● X08.2 **Exposure to other furniture fire**
X ● X08.20 **Exposure to other furniture fire due to** unspecified **burning material**
X ● X08.21 **Exposure to other furniture fire due to burning** cigarette
X ● X08.29 **Exposure to other furniture fire due to** other **burning material**
X ● X08.8 **Exposure to other specified smoke, fire and flames**

CONTACT WITH HEAT AND HOT SUBSTANCES (X10-X19)

Excludes1 exposure to excessive natural heat (X30)
exposure to fire and flames (X00-X08)

● X10 **Contact with hot drinks, food, fats and cooking oils**
The appropriate 7th character is to be added to each code from category X10

A	initial encounter
D	subsequent encounter
S	sequela

X ● X10.0 **Contact with hot** drinks
X ● X10.1 **Contact with hot food**
X ● X10.2 **Contact with** fats and cooking oils

● X11 **Contact with hot tap-water**
Includes contact with boiling tap-water
contact with boiling water NOS
Excludes1 contact with water heated on stove (X12)
The appropriate 7th character is to be added to each code from category X11

A	initial encounter
D	subsequent encounter
S	sequela

X ● X11.0 **Contact with hot water in** bath or tub
Excludes1 contact with running hot water in bath or tub (X11.1)
X ● X11.1 **Contact with** running **hot water**
Contact with hot water running out of hose
Contact with hot water running out of tap
X ● X11.8 **Contact with** other **hot tap-water**
Contact with hot water in bucket
Contact with hot tap-water NOS

X ● X12 **Contact with other hot fluids**
Contact with water heated on stove
Excludes1 hot (liquid) metals (X18)
The appropriate 7th character is to be added to code X12

A	initial encounter
D	subsequent encounter
S	sequela

● X13 **Contact with steam and other hot vapors**
The appropriate 7th character is to be added to each code from category X13

A	initial encounter
D	subsequent encounter
S	sequela

X ● X13.0 Inhalation **of steam and other hot vapors**
X ● X13.1 Other **contact with steam and other hot vapors**

● X14 **Contact with hot air and other hot gases**
The appropriate 7th character is to be added to each code from category X14

A	initial encounter
D	subsequent encounter
S	sequela

X ● X14.0 **Inhalation** of hot air and gases
X ● X14.1 **Other contact with hot air and other hot gases**

● X15 **Contact with hot household appliances**
Excludes1 contact with heating appliances (X16)
contact with powered household appliances (W29.-)
exposure to controlled fire in building or structure due to household appliance (X02.8)
exposure to household appliances electrical current (W86.0)
The appropriate 7th character is to be added to each code from category X15

A	initial encounter
D	subsequent encounter
S	sequela

X ● X15.0 **Contact with hot** stove **(kitchen)**
X ● X15.1 **Contact with hot** toaster
X ● X15.2 **Contact with** hotplate
X ● X15.3 **Contact with hot** saucepan or skillet
X ● X15.8 **Contact with** other **hot household appliances**
Contact with cooker
Contact with kettle
Contact with light bulbs

X ● X16 **Contact with hot heating appliances, radiators and pipes**
Excludes1 contact with powered appliances (W29.-)
exposure to controlled fire in building or structure due to appliance (X02.8)
exposure to industrial appliances electrical current (W86.1)
The appropriate 7th character is to be added to code X16

A	initial encounter
D	subsequent encounter
S	sequela

X ● X17 **Contact with hot engines, machinery and tools**
Excludes1 contact with hot heating appliances, radiators and pipes (X16)
contact with hot household appliances (X15)
The appropriate 7th character is to be added to code X17

A	initial encounter
D	subsequent encounter
S	sequela

X ● X18 **Contact with other hot metals**
Contact with liquid metal
The appropriate 7th character is to be added to code X18

A	initial encounter
D	subsequent encounter
S	sequela

X ● X19 **Contact with other heat and hot substances**
Excludes1 objects that are not normally hot, e.g., an object made hot by a house fire (X00-X08)
The appropriate 7th character is to be added to code X19

A	initial encounter
D	subsequent encounter
S	sequela

▶ New ⇒ Revised ~~deleted~~ Deleted | Excludes 1 | Excludes 2 | Includes | Use additional | Code first | Code also | Key words
OGCR Official Guidelines X Assign placeholder X ● Use Additional Character(s) ▷ Manifestation Code 🔒 Hierarchical Condition Category **Coding Clinic**

EXPOSURE TO FORCES OF NATURE (X30-X39)

X● **X30**   **Exposure to excessive natural heat**
Exposure to excessive heat as the cause of sunstroke
Exposure to heat NOS

> **Excludes1**   excessive heat of man-made origin (W92)
> exposure to man-made radiation (W89)
> exposure to sunlight (X32)
> exposure to tanning bed (W89)

The appropriate 7th character is to be added to code X30

A	initial encounter
D	subsequent encounter
S	sequela

X● **X31**   **Exposure to excessive natural cold**
Excessive cold as the cause of chilblains NOS
Excessive cold as the cause of immersion foot or hand
Exposure to cold NOS
Exposure to weather conditions

> **Excludes1**   cold of man-made origin (W93.-)
> contact with or inhalation of dry ice (W93.-)
> contact with or inhalation of liquefied gas (W93.-)

The appropriate 7th character is to be added to code X31

A	initial encounter
D	subsequent encounter
S	sequela

X● **X32**   **Exposure to sunlight**

> **Excludes1**   man-made radiation (tanning bed) (W89)
>
> **Excludes2**   radiation-related disorders of the skin and subcutaneous tissue (L55-L59)

The appropriate 7th character is to be added to code X32

A	initial encounter
D	subsequent encounter
S	sequela

X● **X34**   **Earthquake**

> **Excludes2**   tidal wave (tsunami) due to earthquake (X37.41)

The appropriate 7th character is to be added to code X34

A	initial encounter
D	subsequent encounter
S	sequela

X● **X35**   **Volcanic eruption**

> **Excludes2**   tidal wave (tsunami) due to volcanic eruption (X37.41)

The appropriate 7th character is to be added to code X35

A	initial encounter
D	subsequent encounter
S	sequela

● **X36**   **Avalanche, landslide and other earth movements**

> **Includes**   victim of mudslide of cataclysmic nature
> **Excludes1**   earthquake (X34)
> **Excludes2**   transport accident involving collision with avalanche or landslide not in motion (V01-V99)

The appropriate 7th character is to be added to each code from category X36

A	initial encounter
D	subsequent encounter
S	sequela

X● **X36.0**   **Collapse of dam or man-made structure causing earth movement**

X● **X36.1**   **Avalanche, landslide, or mudslide**

● **X37**   **Cataclysmic storm**
The appropriate 7th character is to be added to each code from category X37

A	initial encounter
D	subsequent encounter
S	sequela

X● **X37.0**   **Hurricane**
   Storm surge   Typhoon

X● **X37.1**   **Tornado**
   Cyclone   Twister

X● **X37.2**   **Blizzard (snow) (ice)**

X● **X37.3**   **Dust storm**

● **X37.4**   **Tidalwave**

   X● **X37.41**   **Tidal wave due to earthquake or volcanic eruption**
       Tidal wave NOS
       Tsunami

   X● **X37.42**   **Tidal wave due to storm**

   X● **X37.43**   **Tidal wave due to landslide**

X● **X37.8**   **Other cataclysmic storms**
   Cloudburst
   Torrential rain

> **Excludes2**   flood (X38)

X● **X37.9**   **Unspecified cataclysmic storm**
   Storm NOS

> **Excludes1**   collapse of dam or man-made structure causing earth movement (X36.0)

X● **X38**   **Flood**
Flood arising from remote storm
Flood of cataclysmic nature arising from melting snow
Flood resulting directly from storm

> **Excludes1**   collapse of dam or man-made structure causing earth movement (X36.0)
> tidal wave NOS (X37.41)
> tidal wave caused by storm (X37.42)

The appropriate 7th character is to be added to code X38

A	initial encounter
D	subsequent encounter
S	sequela

● **X39**   **Exposure to other forces of nature**
The appropriate 7th character is to be added to each code from category X39

A	initial encounter
D	subsequent encounter
S	sequela

● **X39.0**   **Exposure to natural radiation**

> **Excludes1**   contact with and (suspected) exposure to radon and other naturally occurring radiation (Z77.123)
> exposure to man-made radiation (W88-W90)
> exposure to sunlight (X32)

   X● **X39.01**   **Exposure to radon**

   X● **X39.08**   **Exposure to other natural radiation**

X● **X39.8**   **Other exposure to forces of nature**

CHAPTER 20 (V00-Y99)

OVEREXERTION AND STRENUOUS OR REPETITIVE MOVEMENTS (X50)

●X50   Overexertion and strenuous or repetitive movements

The appropriate 7th character is to be added to each code from category X50

A	initial encounter
D	subsequent encounter
S	sequela

Coding Clinic: 2016, Q4, P73-74

X●X50.0   Overexertion from strenuous movement or load
Lifting heavy objects
Lifting weights
Coding Clinic: 2016, Q4, P74

X●X50.1   Overexertion from prolonged static or awkward postures
Prolonged bending
Prolonged kneeling
Prolonged reaching
Prolonged sitting
Prolonged standing
Prolonged twisting
Static bending
Static kneeling
Static reaching
Static sitting
Static standing
Static twisting

X●X50.3   Overexertion from repetitive movements
Use of hand as hammer
Excludes2   Overuse from prolonged static or awkward postures (X50.1)
Coding Clinic: 2016, Q4, P74

X●X50.9   Other and unspecified overexertion or strenuous movements or postures
Contact pressure
Contact stress

ACCIDENTAL EXPOSURE TO OTHER SPECIFIED FACTORS (X52, X58)

X●X52   Prolonged stay in weightless environment
Weightlessness in spacecraft (simulator)

The appropriate 7th character is to be added to code X52

A	initial encounter
D	subsequent encounter
S	sequela

X●X58   Exposure to other specified factors
Accident NOS
Exposure NOS

The appropriate 7th character is to be added to code X58

A	initial encounter
D	subsequent encounter
S	sequela

INTENTIONAL SELF-HARM (X71-X83)

Purposely self-inflicted injury
Suicide (attempted)

●X71   Intentional self-harm by drowning and submersion

The appropriate 7th character is to be added to each code from category X71

A	initial encounter
D	subsequent encounter
S	sequela

X●X71.0   Intentional self-harm by drowning and submersion while in bathtub A, D, S 🐾

X●X71.1   Intentional self-harm by drowning and submersion while in swimming pool A, D, S 🐾

X●X71.2   Intentional self-harm by drowning and submersion after jump into swimming pool A, D, S 🐾

X●X71.3   Intentional self-harm by drowning and submersion in natural water A, D, S 🐾

X●X71.8   Other intentional self-harm by drowning and submersion A, D, S 🐾

X●X71.9   Intentional self-harm by drowning and submersion, unspecified A, D, S 🐾

X●X72   Intentional self-harm by handgun discharge A, D, S 🐾
Intentional self-harm by gun for single hand use
Intentional self-harm by pistol
Intentional self-harm by revolver
Excludes1   Very pistol (X74.8)

The appropriate 7th character is to be added to code X72

A	initial encounter
D	subsequent encounter
S	sequela

●X73   Intentional self-harm by rifle, shotgun and larger firearm discharge
Excludes1   airgun (X74.01)

The appropriate 7th character is to be added to each code from category X73

A	initial encounter
D	subsequent encounter
S	sequela

X●X73.0   Intentional self-harm by shotgun discharge A, D, S 🐾

X●X73.1   Intentional self-harm by hunting rifle discharge A, D, S 🐾

X●X73.2   Intentional self-harm by machine gun discharge A, D, S 🐾

X●X73.8   Intentional self-harm by other larger firearm discharge A, D, S 🐾

X●X73.9   Intentional self-harm by unspecified larger firearm discharge A, D, S 🐾

●X74   Intentional self-harm by other and unspecified firearm and gun discharge

The appropriate 7th character is to be added to each code from category X74

A	initial encounter
D	subsequent encounter
S	sequela

●X74.0   Intentional self-harm by gas, air or spring-operated guns

X●X74.01   Intentional self-harm by airgun A, D, S 🐾
Intentional self-harm by BB gun discharge
Intentional self-harm by pellet gun discharge

X●X74.02   Intentional self-harm by paintball gun A, D, S 🐾

X●X74.09   Intentional self-harm by other gas, air or spring-operated gun A, D, S 🐾

X●X74.8   Intentional self-harm by other firearm discharge A, D, S 🐾
Intentional self-harm by Very pistol [flare] discharge

X●X74.9   Intentional self-harm by unspecified firearm discharge A, D, S 🐾

X●X75   Intentional self-harm by explosive material A, D, S 🐾

The appropriate 7th character is to be added to code X75

A	initial encounter
D	subsequent encounter
S	sequela

X●X76   Intentional self-harm by smoke, fire and flames A, D, S 🐾

The appropriate 7th character is to be added to code X76

A	initial encounter
D	subsequent encounter
S	sequela

▶ New   ⇒ Revised   ~~deleted~~ Deleted   Excludes 1   Excludes 2   Includes   Use additional   Code first   Code also   Key words

OGCR Official Guidelines   X Assign placeholder X   ● Use Additional Character(s)   ▶ Manifestation Code   🐾 Hierarchical Condition Category   **Coding Clinic**

● X77   **Intentional self-harm by steam, hot vapors and hot objects**

The appropriate 7th character is to be added to each code from category X77

A	initial encounter
D	subsequent encounter
S	sequela

X ● **X77.0**   Intentional self-harm by steam or hot vapors A, D, S 🔖

X ● **X77.1**   Intentional self-harm by hot tap water A, D, S 🔖

X ● **X77.2**   Intentional self-harm by other hot fluids A, D, S 🔖

X ● **X77.3**   Intentional self-harm by hot household appliances A, D, S 🔖

X ● **X77.8**   Intentional self-harm by other hot objects A, D, S 🔖

X ● **X77.9**   Intentional self-harm by unspecified hot objects A, D, S 🔖

● X78   **Intentional self-harm by sharp object**

The appropriate 7th character is to be added to each code from category X78

A	initial encounter
D	subsequent encounter
S	sequela

X ● **X78.0**   Intentional self-harm by sharp glass A, D, S 🔖

X ● **X78.1**   Intentional self-harm by knife A, D, S 🔖

X ● **X78.2**   Intentional self-harm by sword or dagger A, D, S 🔖

X ● **X78.8**   Intentional self-harm by other sharp object A, D, S 🔖

X ● **X78.9**   Intentional self-harm by unspecified sharp object A, D, S 🔖

X ● **X79**   **Intentional self-harm by blunt object A, D, S** 🔖

The appropriate 7th character is to be added to code X79

A	initial encounter
D	subsequent encounter
S	sequela

X ● **X80**   **Intentional self-harm by jumping from a high place A, D, S** 🔖
Intentional fall from one level to another

The appropriate 7th character is to be added to code X80

A	initial encounter
D	subsequent encounter
S	sequela

● X81   **Intentional self-harm by jumping or lying in front of moving object**

The appropriate 7th character is to be added to each code from category X81

A	initial encounter
D	subsequent encounter
S	sequela

X ● **X81.0**   Intentional self-harm by jumping or lying in front of motor vehicle A, D, S 🔖

X ● **X81.1**   Intentional self-harm by jumping or lying in front of (subway) train A, D, S 🔖

X ● **X81.8**   Intentional self-harm by jumping or lying in front of other moving object A, D, S 🔖

● X82   **Intentional self-harm by crashing of motor vehicle**

The appropriate 7th character is to be added to each code from category X82

A	initial encounter
D	subsequent encounter
S	sequela

X ● **X82.0**   Intentional collision of motor vehicle with other motor vehicle A, D, S 🔖

X ● **X82.1**   Intentional collision of motor vehicle with train A, D, S 🔖

X ● **X82.2**   Intentional collision of motor vehicle with tree A, D, S

X ● **X82.8**   Other intentional self-harm by crashing of motor vehicle A, D, S

● X83   **Intentional self-harm by other specified means**

Excludes 1   intentional self-harm by poisoning or contact with toxic substance - see Table of Drugs and Chemicals

The appropriate 7th character is to be added to each code from category X83

A	initial encounter
D	subsequent encounter
S	sequela

X ● **X83.0**   Intentional self-harm by crashing of aircraft A, D, S 🔖

X ● **X83.1**   Intentional self-harm by electrocution A, D, S 🔖

X ● **X83.2**   Intentional self-harm by exposure to extremes of cold A, D, S 🔖

X ● **X83.8**   Intentional self-harm by other specified means A, D, S 🔖

ASSAULT (X92-Y09)

Includes   homicide injuries inflicted by another person with intent to injure or kill, by any means

Excludes 1   injuries due to legal intervention (Y35.-)
injuries due to operations of war (Y36.-)
injuries due to terrorism (Y38.-)

● X92   **Assault by drowning and submersion**

The appropriate 7th character is to be added to each code from category X92

A	initial encounter
D	subsequent encounter
S	sequela

X ● **X92.0**   Assault by drowning and submersion while in bathtub

X ● **X92.1**   Assault by drowning and submersion while in swimming pool

X ● **X92.2**   Assault by drowning and submersion after push into swimming pool

X ● **X92.3**   Assault by drowning and submersion in natural water

X ● **X92.8**   Other assault by drowning and submersion

X ● **X92.9**   Assault by drowning and submersion, unspecified

X ● **X93**   **Assault by handgun discharge**
Assault by discharge of gun for single hand use
Assault by discharge of pistol
Assault by discharge of revolver

Excludes 1   Very pistol (X95.8)

The appropriate 7th character is to be added to code X93

A	initial encounter
D	subsequent encounter
S	sequela

● X94   **Assault by rifle, shotgun and larger firearm discharge**

Excludes 1   airgun (X95.01)

The appropriate 7th character is to be added to each code from category X94

A	initial encounter
D	subsequent encounter
S	sequela

X ● **X94.0**   Assault by shotgun

X ● **X94.1**   Assault by hunting rifle

X ● **X94.2**   Assault by machine gun

X ● **X94.8**   Assault by other larger firearm discharge

X ● **X94.9**   Assault by unspecified larger firearm discharge

CHAPTER 20 (V00-Y99)

● X95   **Assault by other and unspecified firearm and gun discharge**

The appropriate 7th character is to be added to each code from category X95

A	initial encounter
D	subsequent encounter
S	sequela

● X95.0   **Assault by gas, air or spring-operated guns**

X● X95.01   **Assault by airgun discharge**
Assault by BB gun discharge
Assault by pellet gun discharge

X● X95.02   **Assault by paintball gun discharge**

X● X95.09   **Assault by other gas, air or spring-operated gun**

X● X95.8   **Assault by other firearm discharge**
Assault by very pistol [flare] discharge

X● X95.9   **Assault by unspecified firearm discharge**
Coding Clinic: 2016, Q3, P24

● X96   **Assault by explosive material**

Excludes1   incendiary device (X97)
terrorism involving explosive material (Y38.2-)

The appropriate 7th character is to be added to each code from category X96

A	initial encounter
D	subsequent encounter
S	sequela

X● X96.0   **Assault by antipersonnel bomb**

Excludes1   antipersonnel bomb use in military or war (Y36.2-)

X● X96.1   **Assault by gasoline bomb**

X● X96.2   **Assault by letter bomb**

X● X96.3   **Assault by fertilizer bomb**

X● X96.4   **Assault by pipe bomb**

X● X96.8   **Assault by other specified explosive**

X● X96.9   **Assault by unspecified explosive**

X● X97   **Assault by smoke, fire and flames**
Assault by arson
Assault by cigarettes
Assault by incendiary device

The appropriate 7th character is to be added to code X97

A	initial encounter
D	subsequent encounter
S	sequela

● X98   **Assault by steam, hot vapors and hot objects**

The appropriate 7th character is to be added to each code from category X98

A	initial encounter
D	subsequent encounter
S	sequela

X● X98.0   **Assault by steam or hot vapors**

X● X98.1   **Assault by hot tap water**

X● X98.2   **Assault by hot fluids**

X● X98.3   **Assault by hot household appliances**

X● X98.8   **Assault by other hot objects**

X● X98.9   **Assault by unspecified hot objects**

● X99   **Assault by sharp object**

Excludes1   assault by strike by sports equipment (Y08.0-)

The appropriate 7th character is to be added to each code from category X99

A	initial encounter
D	subsequent encounter
S	sequela

X● X99.0   **Assault by sharp glass**

X● X99.1   **Assault by knife**

X● X99.2   **Assault by sword or dagger**

X● X99.8   **Assault by other sharp object**

X● X99.9   **Assault by unspecified sharp object**
Assault by stabbing NOS

X● Y00   **Assault by blunt object**

Excludes1   assault by strike by sports equipment (Y08.0)

The appropriate 7th character is to be added to code Y00

A	initial encounter
D	subsequent encounter
S	sequela

X● Y01   **Assault by pushing from high place**

The appropriate 7th character is to be added to code Y01

A	initial encounter
D	subsequent encounter
S	sequela

● Y02   **Assault by pushing or placing victim in front of moving object**

The appropriate 7th character is to be added to each code from category Y02

A	initial encounter
D	subsequent encounter
S	sequela

X● Y02.0   **Assault by pushing or placing victim in front of motor vehicle**

X● Y02.1   **Assault by pushing or placing victim in front of (subway) train**

X● Y02.8   **Assault by pushing or placing victim in front of other moving object**

● Y03   **Assault by crashing of motor vehicle**

The appropriate 7th character is to be added to each code from category Y03

A	initial encounter
D	subsequent encounter
S	sequela

X● Y03.0   **Assault by being hit or run over by motor vehicle**

X● Y03.8   **Other assault by crashing of motor vehicle**

● Y04   **Assault by bodily force**

Excludes1   assault by:
submersion (X92.-)
use of weapon (X93-X95, X99, Y00)

The appropriate 7th character is to be added to each code from category Y04

A	initial encounter
D	subsequent encounter
S	sequela

X● Y04.0   **Assault by unarmed brawl or fight**

X● Y04.1   **Assault by human bite**

X● Y04.2   **Assault by strike against or bumped into by another person**

X● Y04.8   **Assault by other bodily force**
Assault by bodily force NOS

▶ New   ⫸ Revised   ~~deleted~~ Deleted   Excludes 1   Excludes 2   Includes   Use additional   Code first   Code also   Key words

OGCR Official Guidelines   X Assign placeholder X   ● Use Additional Character(s)   ▶ Manifestation Code   🏷 Hierarchical Condition Category   **Coding Clinic**

OGCR Section I.C.19.f.

Adult and child abuse, neglect and other maltreatment

Sequence first the appropriate code from categories T74 or T76 for abuse, neglect and other maltreatment, followed by any accompanying mental health or injury code(s).

If the documentation in the medical record states abuse or neglect it is coded as confirmed (T74.-). It is coded as suspected if it is documented as suspected (T76.-).

For cases of confirmed abuse or neglect an external cause code from the assault section (X92-Y09) should be added to identify the cause of any physical injuries. A perpetrator code (Y07) should be added when the perpetrator of the abuse is known. For suspected cases of abuse or neglect, do not report external cause or perpetrator code.

If a suspected case of abuse, neglect or mistreatment is ruled out during an encounter code Z04.71, Encounter for examination and observation following alleged physical adult abuse, ruled out, or code Z04.72, Encounter for examination and observation following alleged adult rape, should be used, not a code from T76.

If a suspected case of alleged rape or sexual abuse is ruled out during an encounter code Z04.41, Encounter for examination and observation following alleged adult rape or code Z04.42, Encounter for examination and observation following alleged child rape should be used, not a code from T76.

● Y07   **Perpetrator of assault, maltreatment and neglect**

     Note: Codes from this category are for use only in cases of confirmed abuse (T74.-)

       Selection of the correct perpetrator code is based on the relationship between the perpetrator and the victim

       Includes   perpetrator of abandonment
                        perpetrator of emotional neglect
                        perpetrator of mental cruelty
                        perpetrator of physical abuse
                        perpetrator of physical neglect
                        perpetrator of sexual abuse
                        perpetrator of torture

     Coding Clinic: 2016, Q4, P129

● Y07.0   **Spouse or partner, perpetrator of maltreatment and neglect**
       Spouse or partner, perpetrator of maltreatment and neglect against spouse or partner

     Y07.01   **Husband, perpetrator of maltreatment and neglect**

     Y07.02   **Wife, perpetrator of maltreatment and neglect**

     Y07.03   **Male partner, perpetrator of maltreatment and neglect**

     Y07.04   **Female partner, perpetrator of maltreatment and neglect**

● Y07.1   **Parent (adoptive) (biological), perpetrator of maltreatment and neglect**

     Y07.11   **Biological father, perpetrator of maltreatment and neglect**

     Y07.12   **Biological mother, perpetrator of maltreatment and neglect**

     Y07.13   **Adoptive father, perpetrator of maltreatment and neglect**

     Y07.14   **Adoptive mother, perpetrator of maltreatment and neglect**

● Y07.4   **Other family member, perpetrator of maltreatment and neglect**

    ● Y07.41   **Sibling, perpetrator of maltreatment and neglect**

        Excludes1   stepsibling, perpetrator of maltreatment and neglect (Y07.435, Y07.436)

       Y07.410   **Brother, perpetrator of maltreatment and neglect**

       Y07.411   **Sister, perpetrator of maltreatment and neglect**

● Y07.42   **Foster parent, perpetrator of maltreatment and neglect**

     Y07.420   **Foster father, perpetrator of maltreatment and neglect**

     Y07.421   **Foster mother, perpetrator of maltreatment and neglect**

● Y07.43   **Stepparent or stepsibling, perpetrator of maltreatment and neglect**

     Y07.430   **Stepfather, perpetrator of maltreatment and neglect**

     Y07.432   **Male friend of parent (co-residing in household), perpetrator of maltreatment and neglect**

     Y07.433   **Stepmother, perpetrator of maltreatment and neglect**

     Y07.434   **Female friend of parent (co-residing in household), perpetrator of maltreatment and neglect**

     Y07.435   **Stepbrother, perpetrator or maltreatment and neglect**

     Y07.436   **Stepsister, perpetrator of maltreatment and neglect**

● Y07.49   **Other family member, perpetrator of maltreatment and neglect**

     Y07.490   **Male cousin, perpetrator of maltreatment and neglect**

     Y07.491   **Female cousin, perpetrator of maltreatment and neglect**

     Y07.499   **Other family member, perpetrator of maltreatment and neglect**

● Y07.5   **Non-family member, perpetrator of maltreatment and neglect**

     Y07.50   **Unspecified non-family member, perpetrator of maltreatment and neglect**

    ● Y07.51   **Daycare provider, perpetrator of maltreatment and neglect**

       Y07.510   **At-home childcare provider, perpetrator of maltreatment and neglect**

       Y07.511   **Daycare center childcare provider, perpetrator of maltreatment and neglect**

       Y07.512   **At-home adultcare provider, perpetrator of maltreatment and neglect**

       Y07.513   **Adultcare center provider, perpetrator of maltreatment and neglect**

       Y07.519   **Unspecified daycare provider, perpetrator of maltreatment and neglect**

    ● Y07.52   **Healthcare provider, perpetrator of maltreatment and neglect**

       Y07.521   **Mental health provider, perpetrator of maltreatment and neglect**

       Y07.528   **Other therapist or healthcare provider, perpetrator of maltreatment and neglect**
            Nurse perpetrator of maltreatment and neglect
            Occupational therapist perpetrator of maltreatment and neglect
            Physical therapist perpetrator of maltreatment and neglect
            Speech therapist perpetrator of maltreatment and neglect

       Y07.529   **Unspecified healthcare provider, perpetrator of maltreatment and neglect**

CHAPTER 20 (V00-Y99)

Y07.53   **Teacher or instructor, perpetrator of maltreatment and neglect**
     Coach, perpetrator of maltreatment and neglect

Y07.59   **Other non-family member, perpetrator of maltreatment and neglect**

Y07.6   **Multiple** perpetrators of maltreatment and neglect

Y07.9   **Unspecified** perpetrator of maltreatment and neglect

● Y08   Assault by other specified means

The appropriate 7th character is to be added to each code from category Y08

A	initial encounter
D	subsequent encounter
S	sequela

● Y08.0   Assault by strike by sport equipment

X● Y08.01   Assault by strike by hockey stick

X● Y08.02   Assault by strike by baseball bat

X● Y08.09   Assault by strike by other specified type of sport equipment

● Y08.8   Assault by other specified means

X● Y08.81   Assault by crashing of aircraft

X● Y08.89   Assault by other specified means

● Y09   Assault by unspecified means
Assassination (attempted) NOS
Homicide (attempted) NOS
Manslaughter (attempted) NOS
Murder (attempted) NOS

EVENT OF UNDETERMINED INTENT (Y21-Y33)

Undetermined intent is only for use when there is specific documentation in the record that the intent of the injury cannot be determined. If no such documentation is present, code to accidental (unintentional)

● Y21   Drowning and submersion, undetermined intent

The appropriate 7th character is to be added to each code from category Y21

A	initial encounter
D	subsequent encounter
S	sequela

X● Y21.0   Drowning and submersion while in bathtub, undetermined intent

X● Y21.1   Drowning and submersion after fall into bathtub, undetermined intent

X● Y21.2   Drowning and submersion while in swimming pool, undetermined intent

X● Y21.3   Drowning and submersion after fall into swimming pool, undetermined intent

X● Y21.4   Drowning and submersion in natural water, undetermined intent

X● Y21.8   Other drowning and submersion, undetermined intent

X● Y21.9   Unspecified drowning and submersion, undetermined intent

X● Y22   Handgun discharge, undetermined intent
Discharge of gun for single hand use, undetermined intent
Discharge of pistol, undetermined intent
Discharge of revolver, undetermined intent

Excludes2   very pistol (Y24.8)

The appropriate 7th character is to be added to code Y22

A	initial encounter
D	subsequent encounter
S	sequela

● Y23   Rifle, shotgun and larger firearm discharge, undetermined intent

Excludes2   airgun (Y24.0)

The appropriate 7th character is to be added to each code from category Y23

A	initial encounter
D	subsequent encounter
S	sequela

X● Y23.0   Shotgun discharge, undetermined intent

X● Y23.1   Hunting rifle discharge, undetermined intent

X● Y23.2   Military firearm discharge, undetermined intent

X● Y23.3   Machine gun discharge, undetermined intent

X● Y23.8   Other larger firearm discharge, undetermined intent

X● Y23.9   Unspecified larger firearm discharge, undetermined intent

● Y24   Other and unspecified firearm discharge, undetermined intent

The appropriate 7th character is to be added to each code from category Y24

A	initial encounter
D	subsequent encounter
S	sequela

X● Y24.0   Airgun discharge, undetermined intent
BB gun discharge, undetermined intent
Pellet gun discharge, undetermined intent

X● Y24.8   Other firearm discharge, undetermined intent
Paintball gun discharge, undetermined intent
Very pistol [flare] discharge, undetermined intent

X● Y24.9   Unspecified firearm discharge, undetermined intent

X● Y25   Contact with explosive material, undetermined intent

The appropriate 7th character is to be added to code Y25

A	initial encounter
D	subsequent encounter
S	sequela

X● Y26   Exposure to smoke, fire and flames, undetermined intent

The appropriate 7th character is to be added to code Y26

A	initial encounter
D	subsequent encounter
S	sequela

● Y27   Contact with steam, hot vapors and hot objects, undetermined intent

The appropriate 7th character is to be added to each code from category Y27

A	initial encounter
D	subsequent encounter
S	sequela

X● Y27.0   Contact with steam and hot vapors, undetermined intent

X● Y27.1   Contact with hot tap water, undetermined intent

X● Y27.2   Contact with hot fluids, undetermined intent

X● Y27.3   Contact with hot household appliance, undetermined intent

X● Y27.8   Contact with other hot objects, undetermined intent

X● Y27.9   Contact with unspecified hot objects, undetermined intent

● Y28   Contact with sharp object, undetermined intent

The appropriate 7th character is to be added to each code from category Y28

A	initial encounter
D	subsequent encounter
S	sequela

X● Y28.0   Contact with sharp glass, undetermined intent

X● Y28.1   Contact with knife, undetermined intent

▶ New   ⫸ Revised   ~~deleted~~ Deleted   Excludes 1   Excludes 2   Includes   Use additional   Code first   Code also   Key words

OGCR Official Guidelines   X Assign placeholder X   ● Use Additional Character(s)   ▷ Manifestation Code   🗲 Hierarchical Condition Category   **Coding Clinic**

X ● **Y28.2**   Contact with sword or dagger, undetermined intent

X ● **Y28.8**   Contact with other sharp object, undetermined intent

X ● **Y28.9**   Contact with unspecified sharp object, undetermined intent

X ● **Y29**   Contact with blunt object, undetermined intent

> The appropriate 7th character is to be added to code Y29

A	initial encounter
D	subsequent encounter
S	sequela

X ● **Y30**   Falling, jumping or pushed from a high place, undetermined intent

> Victim falling from one level to another, undetermined intent
>
> The appropriate 7th character is to be added to code Y30

A	initial encounter
D	subsequent encounter
S	sequela

X ● **Y31**   Falling, lying or running before or into moving object, undetermined intent

> The appropriate 7th character is to be added to code Y31

A	initial encounter
D	subsequent encounter
S	sequela

X ● **Y32**   Crashing of motor vehicle, undetermined intent

> The appropriate 7th character is to be added to code Y32

A	initial encounter
D	subsequent encounter
S	sequela

X ● **Y33**   Other specified events, undetermined intent

> The appropriate 7th character is to be added to code Y33

A	initial encounter
D	subsequent encounter
S	sequela

LEGAL INTERVENTION, OPERATIONS OF WAR, MILITARY OPERATIONS, AND TERRORISM (Y35-Y38)

● **Y35**   Legal intervention

> **Includes**   any injury sustained as a result of an encounter with any law enforcement official, serving in any capacity at the time of the encounter, whether on-duty or off-duty. Includes: injury to law enforcement official, suspect and bystander
>
> The appropriate 7th character is to be added to each code from category Y35

A	initial encounter
D	subsequent encounter
S	sequela

● **Y35.0**   Legal intervention involving firearm discharge

   ● **Y35.00**   Legal intervention involving unspecified firearm discharge

> Legal intervention involving gunshot wound
> Legal intervention involving shot NOS

     ● **Y35.001**   Legal intervention involving unspecified firearm discharge, law enforcement official injured

     ● **Y35.002**   Legal intervention involving unspecified firearm discharge, bystander injured

● **Y35.003**   Legal intervention involving unspecified firearm discharge, suspect injured

● **Y35.009**   Legal intervention involving unspecified firearm discharge, unspecified person injured

● **Y35.01**   Legal intervention involving injury by machine gun

   ● **Y35.011**   Legal intervention involving injury by machine gun, law enforcement official injured

   ● **Y35.012**   Legal intervention involving injury by machine gun, bystander injured

   ● **Y35.013**   Legal intervention involving injury by machine gun, suspect injured

   ● **Y35.019**   Legal intervention involving injury by machine gun, unspecified person injured

● **Y35.02**   Legal intervention involving injury by handgun

   ● **Y35.021**   Legal intervention involving injury by handgun, law enforcement official injured

   ● **Y35.022**   Legal intervention involving injury by handgun, bystander injured

   ● **Y35.023**   Legal intervention involving injury by handgun, suspect injured

   ● **Y35.029**   Legal intervention involving injury by handgun, unspecified person injured

● **Y35.03**   Legal intervention involving injury by rifle pellet

   ● **Y35.031**   Legal intervention involving injury by rifle pellet, law enforcement official injured

   ● **Y35.032**   Legal intervention involving injury by rifle pellet, bystander injured

   ● **Y35.033**   Legal intervention involving injury by rifle pellet, suspect injured

   ● **Y35.039**   Legal intervention involving injury by rifle pellet, unspecified person injured

● **Y35.04**   Legal intervention involving injury by rubber bullet

   ● **Y35.041**   Legal intervention involving injury by rubber bullet, law enforcement official injured

   ● **Y35.042**   Legal intervention involving injury by rubber bullet, bystander injured

   ● **Y35.043**   Legal intervention involving injury by rubber bullet, suspect injured

   ● **Y35.049**   Legal intervention involving injury by rubber bullet, unspecified person injured

● **Y35.09**   Legal intervention involving other firearm discharge

   ● **Y35.091**   Legal intervention involving other firearm discharge, law enforcement official injured

   ● **Y35.092**   Legal intervention involving other firearm discharge, bystander injured

   ● **Y35.093**   Legal intervention involving other firearm discharge, suspect injured

   ● **Y35.099**   Legal intervention involving other firearm discharge, unspecified person injured

CHAPTER 20 (V00-Y99)

● Y35.1   Legal intervention involving explosives
    ● Y35.10   Legal intervention involving unspecified explosives
        ● Y35.101   Legal intervention involving unspecified explosives, law enforcement official injured
        ● Y35.102   Legal intervention involving unspecified explosives, bystander injured
        ● Y35.103   Legal intervention involving unspecified explosives, suspect injured
        ● Y35.109   Legal intervention involving unspecified explosives, unspecified person injured
    ● Y35.11   Legal intervention involving injury by dynamite
        ● Y35.111   Legal intervention involving injury by dynamite, law enforcement official injured
        ● Y35.112   Legal intervention involving injury by dynamite, bystander injured
        ● Y35.113   Legal intervention involving injury by dynamite, suspect injured
        ● Y35.119   Legal intervention involving injury by dynamite, unspecified person injured
    ● Y35.12   Legal intervention involving injury by explosive shell
        ● Y35.121   Legal intervention involving injury by explosive shell, law enforcement official injured
        ● Y35.122   Legal intervention involving injury by explosive shell, bystander injured
        ● Y35.123   Legal intervention involving injury by explosive shell, suspect injured
        ● Y35.129   Legal intervention involving other explosives, unspecified person injured
    ● Y35.19   Legal intervention involving other explosives
          Legal intervention involving injury by grenade
          Legal intervention involving injury by mortar bomb
        ● Y35.191   Legal intervention involving other explosives, law enforcement official injured
        ● Y35.192   Legal intervention involving other explosives, bystander injured
        ● Y35.193   Legal intervention involving other explosives, suspect injured
        ● Y35.199   Legal intervention involving other explosives, unspecified person injured
● Y35.2   Legal intervention involving gas
      Legal intervention involving asphyxiation by gas
      Legal intervention involving poisoning by gas
    ● Y35.20   Legal intervention involving unspecified gas
        ● Y35.201   Legal intervention involving unspecified gas, law enforcement official injured
        ● Y35.202   Legal intervention involving unspecified gas, bystander injured
        ● Y35.203   Legal intervention involving unspecified gas, suspect injured
        ● Y35.209   Legal intervention involving unspecified gas, unspecified person injured

● Y35.21   Legal intervention involving injury by tear gas
    ● Y35.211   Legal intervention involving injury by tear gas, law enforcement official injured
    ● Y35.212   Legal intervention involving injury by tear gas, bystander injured
    ● Y35.213   Legal intervention involving injury by tear gas, suspect injured
    ● Y35.219   Legal intervention involving injury by tear gas, unspecified person injured
● Y35.29   Legal intervention involving other gas
    ● Y35.291   Legal intervention involving other gas, law enforcement official injured
    ● Y35.292   Legal intervention involving other gas, bystander injured
    ● Y35.293   Legal intervention involving other gas, suspect injured
    ● Y35.299   Legal intervention involving other gas, unspecified person injured
● Y35.3   Legal intervention involving blunt objects
      Legal intervention involving being hit or struck by blunt object
    ● Y35.30   Legal intervention involving unspecified blunt objects
        ● Y35.301   Legal intervention involving unspecified blunt objects, law enforcement official injured
        ● Y35.302   Legal intervention involving unspecified blunt objects, bystander injured
        ● Y35.303   Legal intervention involving unspecified blunt objects, suspect injured
        ● Y35.309   Legal intervention involving unspecified blunt objects, unspecified person injured
    ● Y35.31   Legal intervention involving baton
        ● Y35.311   Legal intervention involving baton, law enforcement official injured
        ● Y35.312   Legal intervention involving baton, bystander injured
        ● Y35.313   Legal intervention involving baton, suspect injured
        ● Y35.319   Legal intervention involving baton, unspecified person injured
    ● Y35.39   Legal intervention involving other blunt objects
        ● Y35.391   Legal intervention involving other blunt objects, law enforcement official injured
        ● Y35.392   Legal intervention involving other blunt objects, bystander injured
        ● Y35.393   Legal intervention involving other blunt objects, suspect injured
        ● Y35.399   Legal intervention involving other blunt objects, unspecified person injured
● Y35.4   Legal intervention involving sharp objects
      Legal intervention involving being cut by sharp objects
      Legal intervention involving being stabbed by sharp objects
    ● Y35.40   Legal intervention involving unspecified sharp objects
        ● Y35.401   Legal intervention involving unspecified sharp objects, law enforcement official injured
        ● Y35.402   Legal intervention involving unspecified sharp objects, bystander injured

● Y35.403   Legal intervention involving unspecified sharp objects, suspect injured

● Y35.409   Legal intervention involving unspecified sharp objects, unspecified person injured

● Y35.41   Legal intervention involving bayonet

    ● Y35.411   Legal intervention involving bayonet, law enforcement official injured

    ● Y35.412   Legal intervention involving bayonet, bystander injured

    ● Y35.413   Legal intervention involving bayonet, suspect injured

    ● Y35.419   Legal intervention involving bayonet, unspecified person injured

● Y35.49   Legal intervention involving other sharp objects

    ● Y35.491   Legal intervention involving other sharp objects, law enforcement official injured

    ● Y35.492   Legal intervention involving other sharp objects, bystander injured

    ● Y35.493   Legal intervention involving other sharp objects, suspect injured

    ● Y35.499   Legal intervention involving other sharp objects, unspecified person injured

● Y35.8   Legal intervention involving other specified means

    ● Y35.81   Legal intervention involving manhandling

       ● Y35.811   Legal intervention involving manhandling, law enforcement official injured

       ● Y35.812   Legal intervention involving manhandling, bystander injured

       ● Y35.813   Legal intervention involving manhandling, suspect injured

       ● Y35.819   Legal intervention involving manhandling, unspecified person injured

    ● Y35.83   Legal intervention involving a conducted energy device
       Electroshock device (taser)
       Stun gun

       ● Y35.831   Legal intervention involving a conducted energy device, law enforcement official injured

       ● Y35.832   Legal intervention involving a conducted energy device, bystander injured

       ● Y35.833   Legal intervention involving a conducted energy device, suspect injured

       ● Y35.839   Legal intervention involving a conducted energy device, unspecified person injured

    ● Y35.89   Legal intervention involving other specified means

       ● Y35.891   Legal intervention involving other specified means, law enforcement official injured

       ● Y35.892   Legal intervention involving other specified means, bystander injured

       ● Y35.893   Legal intervention involving other specified means, suspect injured
         Coding Clinic: 2018, Q1, P5

▶● Y35.899   Legal intervention involving other specified means, unspecified person injured

● Y35.9   Legal intervention, means unspecified

    X ● Y35.91   Legal intervention, means unspecified, law enforcement official injured

    X ● Y35.92   Legal intervention, means unspecified, bystander injured

    X ● Y35.93   Legal intervention, means unspecified, suspect injured

    X ● Y35.99   Legal intervention, means unspecified, unspecified person injured

● Y36   Operations of war

    Includes   injuries to military personnel and civilians caused by war, civil insurrection, and peacekeeping missions

    Excludes1   injury to military personnel occurring during peacetime military operations (Y37.-)
         military vehicles involved in transport accidents with non-military vehicle during peacetime (V09.01, V09.21, V19.81, V29.81, V39.81, V49.81, V59.81, V69.81, V79.81)

    The appropriate 7th character is to be added to each code from category Y36

A	initial encounter
D	subsequent encounter
S	sequela

● Y36.0   War operations involving explosion of marine weapons
     Weapons and military watercraft

    ● Y36.00   War operations involving explosion of unspecified marine weapon
       War operations involving underwater blast NOS

       ● Y36.000   War operations involving explosion of unspecified marine weapon, military personnel

       ● Y36.001   War operations involving explosion of unspecified marine weapon, civilian

    ● Y36.01   War operations involving explosion of depth-charge

       ● Y36.010   War operations involving explosion of depth-charge, military personnel

       ● Y36.011   War operations involving explosion of depth-charge, civilian

    ● Y36.02   War operations involving explosion of marine mine
       War operations involving explosion of marine mine, at sea or in harbor

       ● Y36.020   War operations involving explosion of marine mine, military personnel

       ● Y36.021   War operations involving explosion of marine mine, civilian

    ● Y36.03   War operations involving explosion of sea-based artillery shell

       ● Y36.030   War operations involving explosion of sea-based artillery shell, military personnel

       ● Y36.031   War operations involving explosion of sea-based artillery shell, civilian

    ● Y36.04   War operations involving explosion of torpedo

       ● Y36.040   War operations involving explosion of torpedo, military personnel

       ● Y36.041   War operations involving explosion of torpedo, civilian

CHAPTER 20 (V00-Y99)

● Y36.05   War operations involving accidental detonation of onboard marine weapons
     ● Y36.050   War operations involving accidental detonation of onboard marine weapons, military personnel
     ● Y36.051   War operations involving accidental detonation of onboard marine weapons, civilian
● Y36.09   War operations involving explosion of other marine weapons
     ● Y36.090   War operations involving explosion of other marine weapons, military personnel
     ● Y36.091   War operations involving explosion of other marine weapons, civilian

● Y36.1   War operations involving destruction of aircraft
   ● Y36.10   War operations involving unspecified destruction of aircraft
     ● Y36.100   War operations involving unspecified destruction of aircraft, military personnel
     ● Y36.101   War operations involving unspecified destruction of aircraft, civilian
   ● Y36.11   War operations involving destruction of aircraft due to enemy fire or explosives
     War operations involving destruction of aircraft due to air to air missile
     War operations involving destruction of aircraft due to explosive placed on aircraft
     War operations involving destruction of aircraft due to rocket propelled grenade [RPG]
     War operations involving destruction of aircraft due to small arms fire
     War operations involving destruction of aircraft due to surface to air missile
     ● Y36.110   War operations involving destruction of aircraft due to enemy fire or explosives, military personnel
     ● Y36.111   War operations involving destruction of aircraft due to enemy fire or explosives, civilian
   ● Y36.12   War operations involving destruction of aircraft due to collision with other aircraft
     ● Y36.120   War operations involving destruction of aircraft due to collision with other aircraft, military personnel
     ● Y36.121   War operations involving destruction of aircraft due to collision with other aircraft, civilian
   ● Y36.13   War operations involving destruction of aircraft due to onboard fire
     ● Y36.130   War operations involving destruction of aircraft due to onboard fire, military personnel
     ● Y36.131   War operations involving destruction of aircraft due to onboard fire, civilian
   ● Y36.14   War operations involving destruction of aircraft due to accidental detonation of onboard munitions and explosives
     ● Y36.140   War operations involving destruction of aircraft due to accidental detonation of onboard munitions and explosives, military personnel
     ● Y36.141   War operations involving destruction of aircraft due to accidental detonation of onboard munitions and explosives, civilian

   ● Y36.19   War operations involving other destruction of aircraft
     ● Y36.190   War operations involving other destruction of aircraft, military personnel
     ● Y36.191   War operations involving other destruction of aircraft, civilian

● Y36.2   War operations involving other explosions and fragments

> **Excludes1**   war operations involving explosion of aircraft (Y36.1-)
> war operations involving explosion of marine weapons (Y36.0-)
> war operations involving explosion of nuclear weapons (Y36.5-)
> war operations involving explosion occurring after cessation of hostilities (Y36.8-)

   ● Y36.20   War operations involving unspecified explosion and fragments
     War operations involving air blast NOS
     War operations involving blast NOS
     War operations involving blast fragments NOS
     War operations involving blast wave NOS
     War operations involving blast wind NOS
     War operations involving explosion NOS
     War operations involving explosion of bomb NOS
     ● Y36.200   War operations involving unspecified explosion and fragments, military personnel
     ● Y36.201   War operations involving unspecified explosion and fragments, civilian
   ● Y36.21   War operations involving explosion of aerial bomb
     ● Y36.210   War operations involving explosion of aerial bomb, military personnel
     ● Y36.211   War operations involving explosion of aerial bomb, civilian
   ● Y36.22   War operations involving explosion of guided missile
     ● Y36.220   War operations involving explosion of guided missile, military personnel
     ● Y36.221   War operations involving explosion of guided missile, civilian
   ● Y36.23   War operations involving explosion of improvised explosive device [IED]
     War operations involving explosion of person-borne improvised explosive device [IED]
     War operations involving explosion of vehicle-borne improvised explosive device [IED]
     War operations involving explosion of roadside improvised explosive device [IED]
     ● Y36.230   War operations involving explosion of improvised explosive device [IED], military personnel
     ● Y36.231   War operations involving explosion of improvised explosive device [IED], civilian
   ● Y36.24   War operations involving explosion due to accidental detonation and discharge of own munitions or munitions launch device
     ● Y36.240   War operations involving explosion due to accidental detonation and discharge of own munitions or munitions launch device, military personnel
     ● Y36.241   War operations involving explosion due to accidental detonation and discharge of own munitions or munitions launch device, civilian

▶ New   ⇒ Revised   ~~deleted~~ Deleted   Excludes 1   Excludes 2   Includes   Use additional   Code first   Code also   Key words
OGCR Official Guidelines   X Assign placeholder X   ● Use Additional Character(s)   ▷ Manifestation Code   🍥 Hierarchical Condition Category   **Coding Clinic**

● **Y36.25** War operations involving fragments from munitions

   ● **Y36.250** War operations involving fragments from munitions, military personnel

   ● **Y36.251** War operations involving fragments from munitions, civilian

● **Y36.26** War operations involving fragments of improvised explosive device [IED]

     War operations involving fragments of person-borne improvised explosive device [IED]

     War operations involving fragments of vehicle-borne improvised explosive device [IED]

     War operations involving fragments of roadside improvised explosive device [IED]

   ● **Y36.260** War operations involving fragments of improvised explosive device [IED], military personnel

   ● **Y36.261** War operations involving fragments of improvised explosive device [IED], civilian

● **Y36.27** War operations involving fragments from weapons

   ● **Y36.270** War operations involving fragments from weapons, military personnel

   ● **Y36.271** War operations involving fragments from weapons, civilian

● **Y36.29** War operations involving other explosions and fragments

     War operations involving explosion of grenade

     War operations involving explosions of land mine

     War operations involving shrapnel NOS

   ● **Y36.290** War operations involving other explosions and fragments, military personnel

   ● **Y36.291** War operations involving other explosions and fragments, civilian

● **Y36.3** War operations involving fires, conflagrations and hot substances

     War operations involving smoke, fumes, and heat from fires, conflagrations and hot substances

   Excludes1 war operations involving fires and conflagrations aboard military aircraft (Y36.1-)

         war operations involving fires and conflagrations aboard military watercraft (Y36.0-)

         war operations involving fires and conflagrations caused indirectly by conventional weapons (Y36.2-)

         war operations involving fires and thermal effects of nuclear weapons (Y36.53-)

● **Y36.30** War operations involving unspecified fire, conflagration and hot substance

   ● **Y36.300** War operations involving unspecified fire, conflagration and hot substance, military personnel

   ● **Y36.301** War operations involving unspecified fire, conflagration and hot substance, civilian

● **Y36.31** War operations involving gasoline bomb

     War operations involving incendiary bomb

     War operations involving petrol bomb

   ● **Y36.310** War operations involving gasoline bomb, military personnel

   ● **Y36.311** War operations involving gasoline bomb, civilian

● **Y36.32** War operations involving incendiary bullet

   ● **Y36.320** War operations involving incendiary bullet, military personnel

   ● **Y36.321** War operations involving incendiary bullet, civilian

● **Y36.33** War operations involving flamethrower

   ● **Y36.330** War operations involving flamethrower, military personnel

   ● **Y36.331** War operations involving flamethrower, civilian

● **Y36.39** War operations involving other fires, conflagrations and hot substances

   ● **Y36.390** War operations involving other fires, conflagrations and hot substances, military personnel

   ● **Y36.391** War operations involving other fires, conflagrations and hot substances, civilian

● **Y36.4** War operations involving firearm discharge and other forms of conventional warfare

   ● **Y36.41** War operations involving rubber bullets

     ● **Y36.410** War operations involving rubber bullets, military personnel

     ● **Y36.411** War operations involving rubber bullets, civilian

   ● **Y36.42** War operations involving firearms pellets

     ● **Y36.420** War operations involving firearms pellets, military personnel

     ● **Y36.421** War operations involving firearms pellets, civilian

   ● **Y36.43** War operations involving other firearms discharge

     War operations involving bullets NOS

     Excludes1 war operations involving munitions fragments (Y36.25-)

          war operations involving incendiary bullets (Y36.32-)

     ● **Y36.430** War operations involving other firearms discharge, military personnel

     ● **Y36.431** War operations involving other firearms discharge, civilian

   ● **Y36.44** War operations involving unarmed hand to hand combat

     Excludes1 war operations involving combat using blunt or piercing object (Y36.45-)

          war operations involving intentional restriction of air and airway (Y36.46-)

          war operations involving unintentional restriction of air and airway (Y36.47-)

     ● **Y36.440** War operations involving unarmed hand to hand combat, military personnel

     ● **Y36.441** War operations involving unarmed hand to hand combat, civilian

   ● **Y36.45** War operations involving combat using blunt or piercing object

     ● **Y36.450** War operations involving combat using blunt or piercing object, military personnel

     ● **Y36.451** War operations involving combat using blunt or piercing object, civilian

CHAPTER 20 (V00-Y99)

● Y36.46   War operations involving intentional restriction of air and airway
    ● Y36.460   War operations involving intentional restriction of air and airway, military personnel
    ● Y36.461   War operations involving intentional restriction of air and airway, civilian

● Y36.47   War operations involving unintentional restriction of air and airway
    ● Y36.470   War operations involving unintentional restriction of air and airway, military personnel
    ● Y36.471   War operations involving unintentional restriction of air and airway, civilian

● Y36.49   War operations involving other forms of conventional warfare
    ● Y36.490   War operations involving other forms of conventional warfare, military personnel
    ● Y36.491   War operations involving other forms of conventional warfare, civilian

● Y36.5   War operations involving nuclear weapons
    War operations involving dirty bomb NOS

● Y36.50   War operations involving unspecified effect of nuclear weapon
    ● Y36.500   War operations involving unspecified effect of nuclear weapon, military personnel
    ● Y36.501   War operations involving unspecified effect of nuclear weapon, civilian

● Y36.51   War operations involving direct blast effect of nuclear weapon
    War operations involving blast pressure of nuclear weapon
    ● Y36.510   War operations involving direct blast effect of nuclear weapon, military personnel
    ● Y36.511   War operations involving direct blast effect of nuclear weapon, civilian

● Y36.52   War operations involving indirect blast effect of nuclear weapon
    War operations involving being thrown by blast of nuclear weapon
    War operations involving being struck or crushed by blast debris of nuclear weapon
    ● Y36.520   War operations involving indirect blast effect of nuclear weapon, military personnel
    ● Y36.521   War operations involving indirect blast effect of nuclear weapon, civilian

● Y36.53   War operations involving thermal radiation effect of nuclear weapon
    War operations involving direct heat from nuclear weapon
    War operation involving fireball effects from nuclear weapon
    ● Y36.530   War operations involving thermal radiation effect of nuclear weapon, military personnel
    ● Y36.531   War operations involving thermal radiation effect of nuclear weapon, civilian

● Y36.54   War operation involving nuclear radiation effects of nuclear weapon
    War operation involving acute radiation exposure from nuclear weapon
    War operation involving exposure to immediate ionizing radiation from nuclear weapon
    War operation involving fallout exposure from nuclear weapon
    War operation involving secondary effects of nuclear weapons
    ● Y36.540   War operation involving nuclear radiation effects of nuclear weapon, military personnel
    ● Y36.541   War operation involving nuclear radiation effects of nuclear weapon, civilian

● Y36.59   War operation involving other effects of nuclear weapons
    ● Y36.590   War operation involving other effects of nuclear weapons, military personnel
    ● Y36.591   War operation involving other effects of nuclear weapons, civilian

● Y36.6   War operations involving biological weapons
    ● Y36.6X   War operations involving biological weapons
       ● Y36.6X0   War operations involving biological weapons, military personnel
       ● Y36.6X1   War operations involving biological weapons, civilian

● Y36.7   War operations involving chemical weapons and other forms of unconventional warfare
    Excludes 1   war operations involving incendiary devices (Y36.3-, Y36.5-)
    ● Y36.7X   War operations involving chemical weapons and other forms of unconventional warfare
       ● Y36.7X0   War operations involving chemical weapons and other forms of unconventional warfare, military personnel
       ● Y36.7X1   War operations involving chemical weapons and other forms of unconventional warfare, civilian

● Y36.8   War operations occurring after cessation of hostilities
    War operations classifiable to categories Y36.0-Y36.8 but occurring after cessation of hostilities
    ● Y36.81   Explosion of mine placed during war operations but exploding after cessation of hostilities
       ● Y36.810   Explosion of mine placed during war operations but exploding after cessation of hostilities, military personnel
       ● Y36.811   Explosion of mine placed during war operations but exploding after cessation of hostilities, civilian
    ● Y36.82   Explosion of bomb placed during war operations but exploding after cessation of hostilities
       ● Y36.820   Explosion of bomb placed during war operations but exploding after cessation of hostilities, military personnel
       ● Y36.821   Explosion of bomb placed during war operations but exploding after cessation of hostilities, civilian

▶ New   ⟹ Revised   ~~deleted~~ Deleted   Excludes 1   Excludes 2   Includes   Use additional   Code first   Code also   Key words
OGCR Official Guidelines   X Assign placeholder X   ● Use Additional Character(s)   ▷ Manifestation Code   ℚ Hierarchical Condition Category   **Coding Clinic**

● Y36.88   Other war operations occurring after cessation
           of hostilities
   ● Y36.880   Other war operations occurring after
              cessation of hostilities, military
              personnel
   ● Y36.881   Other war operations occurring after
              cessation of hostilities, civilian
● Y36.89   Unspecified war operations occurring after
           cessation of hostilities
   ● Y36.890   Unspecified war operations occurring
              after cessation of hostilities, military
              personnel
   ● Y36.891   Unspecified war operations occurring
              after cessation of hostilities, civilian
● Y36.9   Other and unspecified war operations
   X● Y36.90   War operations, unspecified
   X● Y36.91   War operations involving unspecified weapon
             of mass destruction [WMD]
   X● Y36.92   War operations involving friendly fire

● Y37   Military operations

   Includes   Injuries to military personnel and civilians
               occurring during peacetime on military
               property and during routine military
               exercises and operations

   Excludes1   military aircraft involved in aircraft accident with
               civilian aircraft (V97.81-)
               military vehicles involved in transport accident
                  with civilian vehicle (V09.01, V09.21, V19.81,
                  V29.81, V39.81, V49.81, V59.81, V69.81,
                  V79.81)
               military watercraft involved in water transport
                  accident with civilian watercraft (V94.81-)
               war operations (Y36.-)

   The appropriate 7th character is to be added to each code from
      category Y37

A	initial encounter
D	subsequent encounter
S	sequela

● Y37.0   Military operations involving explosion of marine
          weapons
   ● Y37.00   Military operations involving explosion of
             unspecified marine weapon
             Military operations involving underwater blast
                NOS
      ● Y37.000   Military operations involving
                 explosion of unspecified marine
                 weapon, military personnel
      ● Y37.001   Military operations involving
                 explosion of unspecified marine
                 weapon, civilian
   ● Y37.01   Military operations involving explosion of
             depth-charge
      ● Y37.010   Military operations involving
                 explosion of depth-charge, military
                 personnel
      ● Y37.011   Military operations involving
                 explosion of depth-charge, civilian
   ● Y37.02   Military operations involving explosion of
             marine mine
             Military operations involving explosion of
                marine mine, at sea or in harbor
      ● Y37.020   Military operations involving
                 explosion of marine mine, military
                 personnel
      ● Y37.021   Military operations involving
                 explosion of marine mine, civilian

● Y37.03   Military operations involving explosion of sea-
           based artillery shell
   ● Y37.030   Military operations involving
              explosion of sea-based artillery shell,
              military personnel
   ● Y37.031   Military operations involving
              explosion of sea-based artillery shell,
              civilian
● Y37.04   Military operations involving explosion of
           torpedo
   ● Y37.040   Military operations involving
              explosion of torpedo, military
              personnel
   ● Y37.041   Military operations involving
              explosion of torpedo, civilian
● Y37.05   Military operations involving accidental
           detonation of onboard marine weapons
   ● Y37.050   Military operations involving
              accidental detonation of onboard
              marine weapons, military personnel
   ● Y37.051   Military operations involving
              accidental detonation of onboard
              marine weapons, civilian
● Y37.09   Military operations involving explosion of
           other marine weapons
   ● Y37.090   Military operations involving
              explosion of other marine weapons,
              military personnel
   ● Y37.091   Military operations involving
              explosion of other marine weapons,
              civilian
● Y37.1   Military operations involving destruction of aircraft
   ● Y37.10   Military operations involving unspecified
             destruction of aircraft
      ● Y37.100   Military operations involving
                 unspecified destruction of aircraft,
                 military personnel
      ● Y37.101   Military operations involving
                 unspecified destruction of aircraft,
                 civilian
   ● Y37.11   Military operations involving destruction of
             aircraft due to enemy fire or explosives
             Military operations involving destruction of
                aircraft due to air to air missile
             Military operations involving destruction of
                aircraft due to explosive placed on aircraft
             Military operations involving destruction of
                aircraft due to rocket propelled grenade
                [RPG]
             Military operations involving destruction of
                aircraft due to small arms fire
             Military operations involving destruction of
                aircraft due to surface to air missile
      ● Y37.110   Military operations involving
                 destruction of aircraft due to enemy
                 fire or explosives, military personnel
      ● Y37.111   Military operations involving
                 destruction of aircraft due to enemy
                 fire or explosives, civilian
   ● Y37.12   Military operations involving destruction of
             aircraft due to collision with other aircraft
      ● Y37.120   Military operations involving
                 destruction of aircraft due to collision
                 with other aircraft, military personnel
      ● Y37.121   Military operations involving
                 destruction of aircraft due to collision
                 with other aircraft, civilian

● Y37.13   Military operations involving destruction of aircraft due to onboard fire
  ● Y37.130   Military operations involving destruction of aircraft due to onboard fire, military personnel
  ● Y37.131   Military operations involving destruction of aircraft due to onboard fire, civilian
● Y37.14   Military operations involving destruction of aircraft due to accidental detonation of onboard munitions and explosives
  ● Y37.140   Military operations involving destruction of aircraft due to accidental detonation of onboard munitions and explosives, military personnel
  ● Y37.141   Military operations involving destruction of aircraft due to accidental detonation of onboard munitions and explosives, civilian
● Y37.19   Military operations involving other destruction of aircraft
  ● Y37.190   Military operations involving other destruction of aircraft, military personnel
  ● Y37.191   Military operations involving other destruction of aircraft, civilian

● Y37.2   Military operations involving other explosions and fragments
  Excludes1   military operations involving explosion of aircraft (Y37.1-)
    military operations involving explosion of marine weapons (Y37.0-)
    military operations involving explosion of nuclear weapons (Y37.5-)

● Y37.20   Military operations involving unspecified explosion and fragments
  Military operations involving air blast NOS
  Military operations involving blast NOS
  Military operations involving blast fragments NOS
  Military operations involving blast wave NOS
  Military operations involving blast wind NOS
  Military operations involving explosion NOS
  Military operations involving explosion of bomb NOS
  ● Y37.200   Military operations involving unspecified explosion and fragments, military personnel
  ● Y37.201   Military operations involving unspecified explosion and fragments, civilian
● Y37.21   Military operations involving explosion of aerial bomb
  ● Y37.210   Military operations involving explosion of aerial bomb, military personnel
  ● Y37.211   Military operations involving explosion of aerial bomb, civilian
● Y37.22   Military operations involving explosion of guided missile
  ● Y37.220   Military operations involving explosion of guided missile, military personnel
  ● Y37.221   Military operations involving explosion of guided missile, civilian

● Y37.23   Military operations involving explosion of improvised explosive device [IED]
  Military operations involving explosion of person-borne improvised explosive device [IED]
  Military operations involving explosion of vehicle-borne improvised explosive device [IED]
  Military operations involving explosion of roadside improvised explosive device [IED]
  ● Y37.230   Military operations involving explosion of improvised explosive device [IED], military personnel
  ● Y37.231   Military operations involving explosion of improvised explosive device [IED], civilian
● Y37.24   Military operations involving explosion due to accidental detonation and discharge of own munitions or munitions launch device
  ● Y37.240   Military operations involving explosion due to accidental detonation and discharge of own munitions or munitions launch device, military personnel
  ● Y37.241   Military operations involving explosion due to accidental detonation and discharge of own munitions or munitions launch device, civilian
● Y37.25   Military operations involving fragments from munitions
  ● Y37.250   Military operations involving fragments from munitions, military personnel
  ● Y37.251   Military operations involving fragments from munitions, civilian
● Y37.26   Military operations involving fragments of improvised explosive device [IED]
  Military operations involving fragments of person-borne improvised explosive device [IED]
  Military operations involving fragments of vehicle-borne improvised explosive device [IED]
  Military operations involving fragments of roadside improvised explosive device [IED]
  ● Y37.260   Military operations involving fragments of improvised explosive device [IED], military personnel
  ● Y37.261   Military operations involving fragments of improvised explosive device [IED], civilian
● Y37.27   Military operations involving fragments from weapons
  ● Y37.270   Military operations involving fragments from weapons, military personnel
  ● Y37.271   Military operations involving fragments from weapons, civilian
● Y37.29   Military operations involving other explosions and fragments
  Military operations involving explosion of grenade
  Military operations involving explosions of land mine
  Military operations involving shrapnel NOS
  ● Y37.290   Military operations involving other explosions and fragments, military personnel
  ● Y37.291   Military operations involving other explosions and fragments, civilian

● **Y37.3 Military operations involving fires, conflagrations and hot substances**
    Military operations involving smoke, fumes, and heat from fires, conflagrations and hot substances
    Excludes1   military operations involving fires and conflagrations aboard military aircraft (Y37.1-)
           military operations involving fires and conflagrations aboard military watercraft (Y37.0-)
           military operations involving fires and conflagrations caused indirectly by conventional weapons (Y37.2-)
           military operations involving fires and thermal effects of nuclear weapons (Y36.53-)

  ● **Y37.30 Military operations involving unspecified fire, conflagration and hot substance**
    ● **Y37.300 Military operations involving unspecified fire, conflagration and hot substance, military personnel**
    ● **Y37.301 Military operations involving unspecified fire, conflagration and hot substance, civilian**

  ● **Y37.31 Military operations involving gasoline bomb**
    Military operations involving incendiary bomb
    Military operations involving petrol bomb
    ● **Y37.310 Military operations involving gasoline bomb, military personnel**
    ● **Y37.311 Military operations involving gasoline bomb, civilian**

  ● **Y37.32 Military operations involving incendiary bullet**
    ● **Y37.320 Military operations involving incendiary bullet, military personnel**
    ● **Y37.321 Military operations involving incendiary bullet, civilian**

  ● **Y37.33 Military operations involving flamethrower**
    ● **Y37.330 Military operations involving flamethrower, military personnel**
    ● **Y37.331 Military operations involving flamethrower, civilian**

  ● **Y37.39 Military operations involving other fires, conflagrations and hot substances**
    ● **Y37.390 Military operations involving other fires, conflagrations and hot substances, military personnel**
    ● **Y37.391 Military operations involving other fires, conflagrations and hot substances, civilian**

● **Y37.4 Military operations involving firearm discharge and other forms of conventional warfare**
  ● **Y37.41 Military operations involving rubber bullets**
    ● **Y37.410 Military operations involving rubber bullets, military personnel**
    ● **Y37.411 Military operations involving rubber bullets, civilian**

  ● **Y37.42 Military operations involving firearms pellets**
    ● **Y37.420 Military operations involving firearms pellets, military personnel**
    ● **Y37.421 Military operations involving firearms pellets, civilian**

  ● **Y37.43 Military operations involving other firearms discharge**
    Military operations involving bullets NOS
    Excludes1   military operations involving munitions fragments (Y37.25-)
           military operations involving incendiary bullets (Y37.32-)
    ● **Y37.430 Military operations involving other firearms discharge, military personnel**
    ● **Y37.431 Military operations involving other firearms discharge, civilian**

● **Y37.44 Military operations involving unarmed hand to hand combat**
    Excludes1   military operations involving combat using blunt or piercing object (Y37.45-)
           military operations involving intentional restriction of air and airway (Y37.46-)
           military operations involving unintentional restriction of air and airway (Y37.47-)
  ● **Y37.440 Military operations involving unarmed hand to hand combat, military personnel**
  ● **Y37.441 Military operations involving unarmed hand to hand combat, civilian**

● **Y37.45 Military operations involving combat using blunt or piercing object**
  ● **Y37.450 Military operations involving combat using blunt or piercing object, military personnel**
  ● **Y37.451 Military operations involving combat using blunt or piercing object, civilian**

● **Y37.46 Military operations involving intentional restriction of air and airway**
  ● **Y37.460 Military operations involving intentional restriction of air and airway, military personnel**
  ● **Y37.461 Military operations involving intentional restriction of air and airway, civilian**

● **Y37.47 Military operations involving unintentional restriction of air and airway**
  ● **Y37.470 Military operations involving unintentional restriction of air and airway, military personnel**
  ● **Y37.471 Military operations involving unintentional restriction of air and airway, civilian**

● **Y37.49 Military operations involving other forms of conventional warfare**
  ● **Y37.490 Military operations involving other forms of conventional warfare, military personnel**
  ● **Y37.491 Military operations involving other forms of conventional warfare, civilian**

● **Y37.5 Military operations involving nuclear weapons**
    Military operation involving dirty bomb NOS
  ● **Y37.50 Military operations involving unspecified effect of nuclear weapon**
    ● **Y37.500 Military operations involving unspecified effect of nuclear weapon, military personnel**
    ● **Y37.501 Military operations involving unspecified effect of nuclear weapon, civilian**

  ● **Y37.51 Military operations involving direct blast effect of nuclear weapon**
    Military operations involving blast pressure of nuclear weapon
    ● **Y37.510 Military operations involving direct blast effect of nuclear weapon, military personnel**
    ● **Y37.511 Military operations involving direct blast effect of nuclear weapon, civilian**

● Y37.52   **Military operations involving indirect blast effect of nuclear weapon**
  Military operations involving being thrown by blast of nuclear weapon
  Military operations involving being struck or crushed by blast debris of nuclear weapon
  ● Y37.520   **Military operations involving indirect blast effect of nuclear weapon, military personnel**
  ● Y37.521   **Military operations involving indirect blast effect of nuclear weapon, civilian**

● Y37.53   **Military operations involving thermal radiation effect of nuclear weapon**
  Military operations involving direct heat from nuclear weapon
  Military operation involving fireball effects from nuclear weapon
  ● Y37.530   **Military operations involving thermal radiation effect of nuclear weapon, military personnel**
  ● Y37.531   **Military operations involving thermal radiation effect of nuclear weapon, civilian**

● Y37.54   **Military operation involving nuclear radiation effects of nuclear weapon**
  Military operation involving acute radiation exposure from nuclear weapon
  Military operation involving exposure to immediate ionizing radiation from nuclear weapon
  Military operation involving fallout exposure from nuclear weapon
  Military operation involving secondary effects of nuclear weapons
  ● Y37.540   **Military operation involving nuclear radiation effects of nuclear weapon, military personnel**
  ● Y37.541   **Military operation involving nuclear radiation effects of nuclear weapon, civilian**

● Y37.59   **Military operation involving other effects of nuclear weapons**
  ● Y37.590   **Military operation involving other effects of nuclear weapons, military personnel**
  ● Y37.591   **Military operation involving other effects of nuclear weapons, civilian**

● Y37.6   **Military operations involving biological weapons**
  ● Y37.6X   **Military operations involving biological weapons**
    ● Y37.6X0   **Military operations involving biological weapons, military personnel**
    ● Y37.6X1   **Military operations involving biological weapons, civilian**

● Y37.7   **Military operations involving chemical weapons and other forms of unconventional warfare**
  Excludes 1   military operations involving incendiary devices (Y36.3-, Y36.5-)
  ● Y37.7X   **Military operations involving chemical weapons and other forms of unconventional warfare**
    ● Y37.7X0   **Military operations involving chemical weapons and other forms of unconventional warfare, military personnel**
    ● Y37.7X1   **Military operations involving chemical weapons and other forms of unconventional warfare, civilian**

● Y37.9   **Other and unspecified military operations**
  X ● Y37.90   **Military operations, unspecified**
  X ● Y37.91   **Military operations involving unspecified weapon of mass destruction [WMD]**
  X ● Y37.92   **Military operations involving friendly fire**

● Y38   **Terrorism**
  These codes are for use to identify injuries resulting from the unlawful use of force or violence against persons or property to intimidate or coerce a government, the civilian population, or any segment thereof, in furtherance of political or social objective
  Use additional code for place of occurrence (Y92.-)
  The appropriate 7th character is to be added to each code from category Y38

A	initial encounter
D	subsequent encounter
S	sequela

● Y38.0   **Terrorism involving explosion of marine weapons**
  Terrorism involving depth-charge
  Terrorism involving marine mine
  Terrorism involving mine NOS, at sea or in harbor
  Terrorism involving sea-based artillery shell
  Terrorism involving torpedo
  Terrorism involving underwater blast
  ● Y38.0X   **Terrorism involving explosion of marine weapons**
    ● Y38.0X1   **Terrorism involving explosion of marine weapons, public safety official injured**
    ● Y38.0X2   **Terrorism involving explosion of marine weapons, civilian injured**
    ● Y38.0X3   **Terrorism involving explosion of marine weapons, terrorist injured**

● Y38.1   **Terrorism involving destruction of aircraft**
  Terrorism involving aircraft burned
  Terrorism involving aircraft exploded
  Terrorism involving aircraft being shot down
  Terrorism involving aircraft used as a weapon
  ● Y38.1X   **Terrorism involving destruction of aircraft**
    ● Y38.1X1   **Terrorism involving destruction of aircraft, public safety official injured**
    ● Y38.1X2   **Terrorism involving destruction of aircraft, civilian injured**
    ● Y38.1X3   **Terrorism involving destruction of aircraft, terrorist injured**

● Y38.2   **Terrorism involving other explosions and fragments**
  Terrorism involving antipersonnel (fragments) bomb
  Terrorism involving blast NOS
  Terrorism involving explosion NOS
  Terrorism involving explosion of breech block
  Terrorism involving explosion of cannon block
  Terrorism involving explosion (fragments) of artillery shell
  Terrorism involving explosion (fragments) of bomb
  Terrorism involving explosion (fragments) of grenade
  Terrorism involving explosion (fragments) of guided missile
  Terrorism involving explosion (fragments) of land mine
  Terrorism involving explosion of mortar bomb
  Terrorism involving explosion of munitions
  Terrorism involving explosion (fragments) of rocket
  Terrorism involving explosion (fragments) of shell
  Terrorism involving shrapnel
  Terrorism involving mine NOS, on land
  Excludes 1   terrorism involving explosion of nuclear weapon (Y38.5)
  terrorism involving suicide bomber (Y38.81)
  ● Y38.2X   **Terrorism involving other explosions and fragments**
    ● Y38.2X1   **Terrorism involving other explosions and fragments, public safety official injured**
    ● Y38.2X2   **Terrorism involving other explosions and fragments, civilian injured**
    ● Y38.2X3   **Terrorism involving other explosions and fragments, terrorist injured**

▶ New   ⇒ Revised   ~~deleted~~ Deleted | Excludes 1 | Excludes 2 | Includes | Use additional | Code first | Code also | Key words |

OGCR Official Guidelines   X Assign placeholder X   ● Use Additional Character(s)   ▌ Manifestation Code   🔗 Hierarchical Condition Category   **Coding Clinic**

- **Y38.3** Terrorism involving fires, conflagration and hot substances
  - Terrorism involving conflagration NOS
  - Terrorism involving fire NOS
  - Terrorism involving petrol bomb
  - **Excludes1** terrorism involving fire or heat of nuclear weapon (Y38.5)
  - **Y38.3X** Terrorism involving fires, conflagration and hot substances
    - **Y38.3X1** Terrorism involving fires, conflagration and hot substances, public safety official injured
    - **Y38.3X2** Terrorism involving fires, conflagration and hot substances, civilian injured
    - **Y38.3X3** Terrorism involving fires, conflagration and hot substances, terrorist injured
- **Y38.4** Terrorism involving firearms
  - Terrorism involving carbine bullet
  - Terrorism involving machine gun bullet
  - Terrorism involving pellets (shotgun)
  - Terrorism involving pistol bullet
  - Terrorism involving rifle bullet
  - Terrorism involving rubber (rifle) bullet
  - **Y38.4X** Terrorism involving firearms
    - **Y38.4X1** Terrorism involving firearms, public safety official injured
    - **Y38.4X2** Terrorism involving firearms, civilian injured
    - **Y38.4X3** Terrorism involving firearms, terrorist injured
- **Y38.5** Terrorism involving nuclear weapons
  - Terrorism involving blast effects of nuclear weapon
  - Terrorism involving exposure to ionizing radiation from nuclear weapon
  - Terrorism involving fireball effect of nuclear weapon
  - Terrorism involving heat from nuclear weapon
  - **Y38.5X** Terrorism involving nuclear weapons
    - **Y38.5X1** Terrorism involving nuclear weapons, public safety official injured
    - **Y38.5X2** Terrorism involving nuclear weapons, civilian injured
    - **Y38.5X3** Terrorism involving nuclear weapons, terrorist injured
- **Y38.6** Terrorism involving biological weapons
  - Terrorism involving anthrax
  - Terrorism involving cholera
    - *A serious, often deadly, infectious disease of the small intestine*
  - Terrorism involving smallpox
  - **Y38.6X** Terrorism involving biological weapons
    - **Y38.6X1** Terrorism involving biological weapons, public safety official injured
    - **Y38.6X2** Terrorism involving biological weapons, civilian injured
    - **Y38.6X3** Terrorism involving biological weapons, terrorist injured
- **Y38.7** Terrorism involving chemical weapons
  - Terrorism involving gases, fumes, chemicals
  - Terrorism involving hydrogen cyanide
  - Terrorism involving phosgene
  - Terrorism involving sarin
  - **Y38.7X** Terrorism involving chemical weapons
    - **Y38.7X1** Terrorism involving chemical weapons, public safety official injured
    - **Y38.7X2** Terrorism involving chemical weapons, civilian injured
    - **Y38.7X3** Terrorism involving chemical weapons, terrorist injured

- **Y38.8** Terrorism involving other and unspecified means
  - **Y38.80** Terrorism involving unspecified means
    - Terrorism NOS
  - **Y38.81** Terrorism involving suicide bomber
    - **Y38.811** Terrorism involving suicide bomber, public safety official injured
    - **Y38.812** Terrorism involving suicide bomber, civilian injured
  - **Y38.89** Terrorism involving other means
    - Terrorism involving drowning and submersion
    - Terrorism involving lasers
    - Terrorism involving piercing or stabbing instruments
    - **Y38.891** Terrorism involving other means, public safety official injured
    - **Y38.892** Terrorism involving other means, civilian injured
    - **Y38.893** Terrorism involving other means, terrorist injured
- **Y38.9** Terrorism, secondary effects
  - **Note:** This code is for use to identify conditions occurring subsequent to a terrorist attack not those that are due to the initial terrorist attack.
  - **Y38.9X** Terrorism, secondary effects
    - **Y38.9X1** Terrorism, secondary effects, public safety official injured
    - **Y38.9X2** Terrorism, secondary effects, civilian injured categories

COMPLICATIONS OF MEDICAL AND SURGICAL CARE (Y62-Y84)

Includes complications of medical devices surgical and medical procedures as the cause of abnormal reaction of the patient, or of later complication, without mention of misadventure at the time of the procedure

MISADVENTURES TO PATIENTS DURING SURGICAL AND MEDICAL CARE (Y62-Y69)

Excludes1 surgical and medical procedures as the cause of abnormal reaction of the patient, without mention of misadventure at the time of the procedure (Y83-Y84)

- **Y62** Failure of sterile precautions during surgical and medical care
  - **Y62.0** Failure of sterile precautions during surgical operation
  - **Y62.1** Failure of sterile precautions during infusion or transfusion
  - **Y62.2** Failure of sterile precautions during kidney dialysis and other perfusion
  - **Y62.3** Failure of sterile precautions during injection or immunization
  - **Y62.4** Failure of sterile precautions during endoscopic examination
  - **Y62.5** Failure of sterile precautions during heart catheterization
  - **Y62.6** Failure of sterile precautions during aspiration, puncture and other catheterization
  - **Y62.8** Failure of sterile precautions during other surgical and medical care
  - **Y62.9** Failure of sterile precautions during unspecified surgical and medical care
- **Y63** Failure in dosage during surgical and medical care
  - **Excludes2** accidental overdose of drug or wrong drug given in error (T36-T50)
  - **Y63.0** Excessive amount of blood or other fluid given during transfusion or infusion
  - **Y63.1** Incorrect dilution of fluid used during infusion
  - **Y63.2** Overdose of radiation given during therapy

CHAPTER 20 (V00-Y99)

Y63.3   **Inadvertent exposure of patient to radiation during medical care**

Y63.4   **Failure in dosage in electroshock or insulin-shock therapy**

Y63.5   **Inappropriate temperature in local application and packing**

Y63.6   **Underdosing and nonadministration of necessary drug, medicament or biological substance**

Y63.8   **Failure in dosage during other surgical and medical care**

Y63.9   **Failure in dosage during** unspecified **surgical and medical care**

● Y64   **Contaminated medical or biological substances**

Y64.0   **Contaminated medical or biological substance, transfused or infused**

Y64.1   **Contaminated medical or biological substance, injected or used for immunization**

Y64.8   **Contaminated medical or biological substance administered by other means**

Y64.9   **Contaminated medical or biological substance administered by** unspecified **means**
     Administered contaminated medical or biological substance NOS

● Y65   **Other misadventures during surgical and medical care**

Y65.0   **Mismatched blood in transfusion**

Y65.1   **Wrong fluid used in infusion**

Y65.2   **Failure in suture or ligature during surgical operation**

Y65.3   **Endotracheal tube wrongly placed during anesthetic procedure**

Y65.4   **Failure to introduce or to remove other tube or instrument**

● Y65.5   **Performance of** wrong procedure **(operation)**

  ● Y65.51   **Performance of wrong procedure (operation) on correct patient**
       Wrong device implanted into correct surgical site

       Excludes1   performance of correct procedure (operation) on wrong side or body part (Y65.53)

  ● Y65.52   **Performance of procedure (operation) on patient not scheduled for surgery**
       Performance of procedure (operation) intended for another patient
       Performance of procedure (operation) on wrong patient

  ● Y65.53   **Performance of correct procedure (operation) on** wrong side or body part
       Performance of correct procedure (operation) on wrong side
       Performance of correct procedure (operation) on wrong site

Y65.8   **Other specified misadventures during surgical and medical care**
     Coding Clinic: 2019, Q2, P24

Y66   **Nonadministration of surgical and medical care**
     Premature cessation of surgical and medical care

     Excludes1   DNR status (Z66)
                palliative care (Z51.5)

Y69   Unspecified **misadventure during surgical and medical care**

MEDICAL DEVICES ASSOCIATED WITH ADVERSE INCIDENTS IN DIAGNOSTIC AND THERAPEUTIC USE (Y70-Y82)

Includes   breakdown or malfunction of medical devices (during use) (after implantation) (ongoing use)

Excludes2   later complications following use of medical devices without breakdown or malfunctioning of device (Y83-Y84)
misadventure to patients during surgical and medical care, classifiable to (Y62-Y69)
surgical and other medical procedures as the cause of abnormal reaction of the patient, or of later complication, without mention of misadventure at the time of the procedure (Y83-Y84)

● Y70   **Anesthesiology devices associated with adverse incidents**

Y70.0   **Diagnostic and monitoring anesthesiology devices associated with adverse incidents**

Y70.1   **Therapeutic (nonsurgical) and rehabilitative anesthesiology devices associated with adverse incidents**

Y70.2   **Prosthetic and other implants, materials and accessory anesthesiology devices associated with adverse incidents**

Y70.3   **Surgical instruments, materials and anesthesiology devices (including sutures) associated with adverse incidents**

Y70.8   **Miscellaneous anesthesiology devices associated with adverse incidents, not elsewhere classified**

● Y71   **Cardiovascular devices associated with adverse incidents**

Y71.0   **Diagnostic and monitoring cardiovascular devices associated with adverse incidents**

Y71.1   **Therapeutic (nonsurgical) and rehabilitative cardiovascular devices associated with adverse incidents**

Y71.2   **Prosthetic and other implants, materials and accessory cardiovascular devices associated with adverse incidents**

Y71.3   **Surgical instruments, materials and cardiovascular devices (including sutures) associated with adverse incidents**

Y71.8   **Miscellaneous cardiovascular devices associated with adverse incidents, not elsewhere classified**

● Y72   **Otorhinolaryngological devices associated with adverse incidents**

Y72.0   **Diagnostic and monitoring otorhinolaryngological devices associated with adverse incidents**

Y72.1   **Therapeutic (nonsurgical) and rehabilitative otorhinolaryngological devices associated with adverse incidents**

Y72.2   **Prosthetic and other implants, materials and accessory otorhinolaryngological devices associated with adverse incidents**

Y72.3   **Surgical instruments, materials and otorhinolaryngological devices (including sutures) associated with adverse incidents**

Y72.8   **Miscellaneous otorhinolaryngological devices associated with adverse incidents, not elsewhere classified**

● Y73   **Gastroenterology and urology devices associated with adverse incidents**

Y73.0   **Diagnostic and monitoring gastroenterology and urology devices associated with adverse incidents**

Y73.1   **Therapeutic (nonsurgical) and rehabilitative gastroenterology and urology devices associated with adverse incidents**

Y73.2   **Prosthetic and other implants, materials and accessory gastroenterology and urology devices associated with adverse incidents**

▶ New   ▦▶ Revised   ~~deleted~~ Deleted   Excludes 1   Excludes 2   Includes   Use additional   Code first   Code also   Key words

OGCR Official Guidelines   X Assign placeholder X   ● Use Additional Character(s)   ▶ Manifestation Code   🔖 Hierarchical Condition Category   **Coding Clinic**

Y73.3 Surgical instruments, materials and gastroenterology and urology devices (including sutures) associated with adverse incidents

Y73.8 Miscellaneous gastroenterology and urology devices associated with adverse incidents, not elsewhere classified

● **Y74** General hospital and personal-use devices associated with adverse incidents

Y74.0 Diagnostic and monitoring general hospital and personal-use devices associated with adverse incidents

Y74.1 Therapeutic (nonsurgical) and rehabilitative general hospital and personal-use devices associated with adverse incidents

Y74.2 Prosthetic and other implants, materials and accessory general hospital and personal-use devices associated with adverse incidents

Y74.3 Surgical instruments, materials and general hospital and personal-use devices (including sutures) associated with adverse incidents

Y74.8 Miscellaneous general hospital and personal-use devices associated with adverse incidents, not elsewhere classified

● **Y75** Neurological devices associated with adverse incidents

Y75.0 Diagnostic and monitoring neurological devices associated with adverse incidents

Y75.1 Therapeutic (nonsurgical) and rehabilitative neurological devices associated with adverse incidents

Y75.2 Prosthetic and other implants, materials and neurological devices associated with adverse incidents

Y75.3 Surgical instruments, materials and neurological devices (including sutures) associated with adverse incidents

Y75.8 Miscellaneous neurological devices associated with adverse incidents, not elsewhere classified

● **Y76** Obstetric and gynecological devices associated with adverse incidents

Y76.0 Diagnostic and monitoring obstetric and gynecological devices associated with adverse incidents ♀

Y76.1 Therapeutic (nonsurgical) and rehabilitative obstetric and gynecological devices associated with adverse incidents ♀

Y76.2 Prosthetic and other implants, materials and accessory obstetric and gynecological devices associated with adverse incidents ♀

Y76.3 Surgical instruments, materials and obstetric and gynecological devices (including sutures) associated with adverse incidents ♀

Y76.8 Miscellaneous obstetric and gynecological devices associated with adverse incidents, not elsewhere classified ♀

● **Y77** Ophthalmic devices associated with adverse incidents

Y77.0 Diagnostic and monitoring ophthalmic devices associated with adverse incidents

● **Y77.1** Therapeutic (nonsurgical) and rehabilitative ophthalmic devices associated with adverse incidents

    Y77.11 Contact lens associated with adverse incidents

        Rigid gas permeable contact lens associated with adverse incidents

        Soft (hydrophilic) contact lens associated with adverse incidents

    Y77.19 Other therapeutic (nonsurgical) and rehabilitative ophthalmic devices associated with adverse incidents

Y77.2 Prosthetic and other implants, materials and accessory ophthalmic devices associated with adverse incidents

Y77.3 Surgical instruments, materials and ophthalmic devices (including sutures) associated with adverse incidents

Y77.8 Miscellaneous ophthalmic devices associated with adverse incidents, not elsewhere classified

● **Y78** Radiological devices associated with adverse incidents

Y78.0 Diagnostic and monitoring radiological devices associated with adverse incidents

Y78.1 Therapeutic (nonsurgical) and rehabilitative radiological devices associated with adverse incidents

Y78.2 Prosthetic and other implants, materials and accessory radiological devices associated with adverse incidents

Y78.3 Surgical instruments, materials and radiological devices (including sutures) associated with adverse incidents

Y78.8 Miscellaneous radiological devices associated with adverse incidents, not elsewhere classified

● **Y79** Orthopedic devices associated with adverse incidents

Y79.0 Diagnostic and monitoring orthopedic devices associated with adverse incidents

Y79.1 Therapeutic (nonsurgical) and rehabilitative orthopedic devices associated with adverse incidents

Y79.2 Prosthetic and other implants, materials and accessory orthopedic devices associated with adverse incidents

Y79.3 Surgical instruments, materials and orthopedic devices (including sutures) associated with adverse incidents

Y79.8 Miscellaneous orthopedic devices associated with adverse incidents, not elsewhere classified

● **Y80** Physical medicine devices associated with adverse incidents

Y80.0 Diagnostic and monitoring physical medicine devices associated with adverse incidents

Y80.1 Therapeutic (nonsurgical) and rehabilitative physical medicine devices associated with adverse incidents

Y80.2 Prosthetic and other implants, materials and accessory physical medicine devices associated with adverse incidents

Y80.3 Surgical instruments, materials and physical medicine devices (including sutures) associated with adverse incidents

Y80.8 Miscellaneous physical medicine devices associated with adverse incidents, not elsewhere classified

● **Y81** General- and plastic-surgery devices associated with adverse incidents

Y81.0 Diagnostic and monitoring general- and plastic-surgery devices associated with adverse incidents

Y81.1 Therapeutic (nonsurgical) and rehabilitative general- and plastic-surgery devices associated with adverse incidents

Y81.2 Prosthetic and other implants, materials and accessory general- and plastic-surgery devices associated with adverse incidents

Y81.3 Surgical instruments, materials and general- and plastic-surgery devices (including sutures) associated with adverse incidents

Y81.8 Miscellaneous general- and plastic-surgery devices associated with adverse incidents, not elsewhere classified

● **Y82** Other and unspecified medical devices associated with adverse incidents

Y82.8 Other medical devices associated with adverse incidents

Y82.9 Unspecified medical devices associated with adverse incidents

CHAPTER 20 (V00–Y99)

SURGICAL AND OTHER MEDICAL PROCEDURES AS THE CAUSE OF ABNORMAL REACTION OF THE PATIENT, OR OF LATER COMPLICATION, WITHOUT MENTION OF MISADVENTURE AT THE TIME OF THE PROCEDURE (Y83-Y84)

Excludes1   misadventures to patients during surgical and medical care, classifiable to (Y62-Y69)

Excludes2   breakdown or malfunctioning of medical device (after implantation) (during procedure) (ongoing use) (Y70-Y82)

● Y83   **Surgical operation and other surgical** procedures as the cause of abnormal reaction of the patient, or of later complication, without mention of misadventure at the time of the procedure

    Y83.0   Surgical operation with transplant of whole organ as the cause of abnormal reaction of the patient, or of later complication, without mention of misadventure at the time of the procedure

    Y83.1   Surgical operation with implant of artificial internal device as the cause of abnormal reaction of the patient, or of later complication, without mention of misadventure at the time of the procedure

    Y83.2   Surgical operation with anastomosis, bypass or graft as the cause of abnormal reaction of the patient, or of later complication, without mention of misadventure at the time of the procedure

    Y83.3   Surgical operation with formation of external stoma as the cause of abnormal reaction of the patient, or of later complication, without mention of misadventure at the time of the procedure

    Y83.4   Other reconstructive surgery as the cause of abnormal reaction of the patient, or of later complication, without mention of misadventure at the time of the procedure

    Y83.5   Amputation of limb(s) as the cause of abnormal reaction of the patient, or of later complication, without mention of misadventure at the time of the procedure

    Y83.6   Removal of other organ (partial) (total) as the cause of abnormal reaction of the patient, or of later complication, without mention of misadventure at the time of the procedure

    Y83.8   Other surgical procedures as the cause of abnormal reaction of the patient, or of later complication, without mention of misadventure at the time of the procedure

    Y83.9   Surgical procedure, unspecified as the cause of abnormal reaction of the patient, or of later complication, without mention of misadventure at the time of the procedure

● Y84   **Other medical procedures** as the cause of abnormal reaction of the patient, or of later complication, without mention of misadventure at the time of the procedure

    Y84.0   Cardiac catheterization as the cause of abnormal reaction of the patient, or of later complication, without mention of misadventure at the time of the procedure

    Y84.1   Kidney dialysis as the cause of abnormal reaction of the patient, or of later complication, without mention of misadventure at the time of the procedure

    Y84.2   Radiological procedure and radiotherapy as the cause of abnormal reaction of the patient, or of later complication, without mention of misadventure at the time of the procedure
       Coding Clinic: 2019, Q1, P21; 2017, Q1, P34

    Y84.3   Shock therapy as the cause of abnormal reaction of the patient, or of later complication, without mention of misadventure at the time of the procedure

    Y84.4   Aspiration of fluid as the cause of abnormal reaction of the patient, or of later complication, without mention of misadventure at the time of the procedure

    Y84.5   Insertion of gastric or duodenal sound as the cause of abnormal reaction of the patient, or of later complication, without mention of misadventure at the time of the procedure

    Y84.6   Urinary catheterization as the cause of abnormal reaction of the patient, or of later complication, without mention of misadventure at the time of the procedure

    Y84.7   Blood-sampling as the cause of abnormal reaction of the patient, or of later complication, without mention of misadventure at the time of the procedure

    Y84.8   Other medical procedures as the cause of abnormal reaction of the patient, or of later complication, without mention of misadventure at the time of the procedure
       Coding Clinic: 2021, Q1, P5

    Y84.9   Medical procedure, unspecified as the cause of abnormal reaction of the patient, or of later complication, without mention of misadventure at the time of the procedure

SUPPLEMENTARY FACTORS RELATED TO CAUSES OF MORBIDITY CLASSIFIED ELSEWHERE (Y90-Y99)

Note: These categories may be used to provide supplementary information concerning causes of morbidity. They are not to be used for single-condition coding.

● Y90   **Evidence of alcohol involvement determined by blood alcohol level**
      Code first any associated alcohol related disorders (F10)

    Y90.0   Blood alcohol level of less than 20 mg/100 ml

    Y90.1   Blood alcohol level of 20-39 mg/100 ml

    Y90.2   Blood alcohol level of 40-59 mg/100 ml

    Y90.3   Blood alcohol level of 60-79 mg/100 ml

    Y90.4   Blood alcohol level of 80-99 mg/100 ml

    Y90.5   Blood alcohol level of 100-119 mg/100 ml

    Y90.6   Blood alcohol level of 120-199 mg/100 ml

    Y90.7   Blood alcohol level of 200-239 mg/100 ml

    Y90.8   Blood alcohol level of 240 mg/100 ml or more

    Y90.9   Presence of alcohol in blood, level not specified

OGCR Section I.C.20.b.

Place of Occurrence Guideline

Codes from category Y92, Place of occurrence of the external cause, are secondary codes for use after other external cause codes to identify the location of the patient at the time of injury or other condition.

Generally, a place of occurrence code is assigned only once, at the initial encounter for treatment. However, in the rare instance that a new injury occurs during hospitalization, an additional place of occurrence code may be assigned. No 7th characters are used for Y92. Only one code from Y92 should be recorded on a medical record.

Do not use place of occurrence code Y92.9 if the place is not stated or is not applicable.

● Y92   **Place of occurrence of the external cause**
      The following category is for use, when relevant, to identify the place of occurrence of the external cause. Use in conjunction with an activity code.
      Place of occurrence should be recorded only at the initial encounter for treatment

 ● Y92.0   **Non-institutional (private) residence** as the place of occurrence of the external cause

     Excludes1   abandoned or derelict house (Y92.89)
               home under construction but not yet occupied (Y92.6-)
               institutional place of residence (Y92.1-)

  ● Y92.00   Unspecified non-institutional (private) residence as the place of occurrence of the external cause

      Y92.000   Kitchen of unspecified non-institutional (private) residence as the place of occurrence of the external cause

      Y92.001   Dining room of unspecified non-institutional (private) residence as the place of occurrence of the external cause

Y92.002   **Bathroom** of unspecified non-institutional (private) residence as the place of occurrence of the external cause

Y92.003   **Bedroom** of unspecified non-institutional (private) residence as the place of occurrence of the external cause

Y92.007   **Garden or yard** of unspecified non-institutional (private) residence as the place of occurrence of the external cause

Y92.008   **Other place** in unspecified non-institutional (private) residence as the place of occurrence of the external cause

Y92.009   **Unspecified place** in unspecified non-institutional (private) residence as the place of occurrence of the external cause

> Home (NOS) as the place of occurrence of the external cause
> **Coding Clinic: 2021, Q2, P5**

● Y92.01   **Single-family non-institutional (private) house** as the place of occurrence of the external cause

> Farmhouse as the place of occurrence of the external cause

> **Excludes1**   barn (Y92.71)
>   chicken coop or hen house (Y92.72)
>   farm field (Y92.73)
>   orchard (Y92.74)
>   single family mobile home or trailer (Y92.02-)
>   slaughter house (Y92.86)

Y92.010   **Kitchen** of single-family (private) house as the place of occurrence of the external cause

Y92.011   **Dining room** of single-family (private) house as the place of occurrence of the external cause

Y92.012   **Bathroom** of single-family (private) house as the place of occurrence of the external cause

Y92.013   **Bedroom** of single-family (private) house as the place of occurrence of the external cause

Y92.014   **Private driveway** to single-family (private) house as the place of occurrence of the external cause

Y92.015   **Private garage** of single-family (private) house as the place of occurrence of the external cause

Y92.016   **Swimming pool** in single-family (private) house or garden as the place of occurrence of the external cause

Y92.017   **Garden or yard** in single-family (private) house as the place of occurrence of the external cause

Y92.018   **Other place** in single-family (private) house as the place of occurrence of the external cause

Y92.019   **Unspecified** place in single-family (private) house as the place of occurrence of the external cause

● Y92.02   **Mobile home** as the place of occurrence of the external cause

Y92.020   **Kitchen** in mobile home as the place of occurrence of the external cause

Y92.021   **Dining room** in mobile home as the place of occurrence of the external cause

Y92.022   **Bathroom** in mobile home as the place of occurrence of the external cause

Y92.023   **Bedroom** in mobile home as the place of occurrence of the external cause

Y92.024   **Driveway** of mobile home as the place of occurrence of the external cause

Y92.025   **Garage** of mobile home as the place of occurrence of the external cause

Y92.026   **Swimming pool** of mobile home as the place of occurrence of the external cause

Y92.027   **Garden or yard** of mobile home as the place of occurrence of the external cause

Y92.028   **Other place** in mobile home as the place of occurrence of the external cause

Y92.029   **Unspecified** place in mobile home as the place of occurrence of the external cause

● Y92.03   **Apartment** as the place of occurrence of the external cause

> Condominium as the place of occurrence of the external cause
> Co-op apartment as the place of occurrence of the external cause

Y92.030   **Kitchen** in apartment as the place of occurrence of the external cause

Y92.031   **Bathroom** in apartment as the place of occurrence of the external cause

Y92.032   **Bedroom** in apartment as the place of occurrence of the external cause

Y92.038   **Other place** in apartment as the place of occurrence of the external cause

Y92.039   **Unspecified** place in apartment as the place of occurrence of the external cause

● Y92.04   **Boarding-house** as the place of occurrence of the external cause

Y92.040   **Kitchen** in boarding-house as the place of occurrence of the external cause

Y92.041   **Bathroom** in boarding-house as the place of occurrence of the external cause

Y92.042   **Bedroom** in boarding-house as the place of occurrence of the external cause

Y92.043   **Driveway** of boarding-house as the place of occurrence of the external cause

Y92.044   **Garage** of boarding-house as the place of occurrence of the external cause

Y92.045   **Swimming pool** of boarding-house as the place of occurrence of the external cause

Y92.046   **Garden or yard** of boarding-house as the place of occurrence of the external cause

Y92.048 Other place in boarding-house as the place of occurrence of the external cause

Y92.049 Unspecified place in boarding-house as the place of occurrence of the external cause

● **Y92.09** Other non-institutional residence as the place of occurrence of the external cause

Y92.090 Kitchen in other non-institutional residence as the place of occurrence of the external cause

Y92.091 Bathroom in other non-institutional residence as the place of occurrence of the external cause

Y92.092 Bedroom in other non-institutional residence as the place of occurrence of the external cause

Y92.093 Driveway of other non-institutional residence as the place of occurrence of the external cause

Y92.094 Garage of other non-institutional residence as the place of occurrence of the external cause

Y92.095 Swimming pool of other non-institutional residence as the place of occurrence of the external cause

Y92.096 Garden or yard of other non-institutional residence as the place of occurrence of the external cause

Y92.098 Other place in other non-institutional residence as the place of occurrence of the external cause

Y92.099 Unspecified place in other non-institutional residence as the place of occurrence of the external cause

Coding Clinic: 2017, Q2, P10

● **Y92.1** Institutional (nonprivate) residence as the place of occurrence of the external cause

Y92.10 Unspecified residential institution as the place of occurrence of the external cause

● **Y92.11** Children's home and orphanage as the place of occurrence of the external cause

Y92.110 Kitchen in children's home and orphanage as the place of occurrence of the external cause

Y92.111 Bathroom in children's home and orphanage as the place of occurrence of the external cause

Y92.112 Bedroom in children's home and orphanage as the place of occurrence of the external cause

Y92.113 Driveway of children's home and orphanage as the place of occurrence of the external cause

Y92.114 Garage of children's home and orphanage as the place of occurrence of the external cause

Y92.115 Swimming pool of children's home and orphanage as the place of occurrence of the external cause

Y92.116 Garden or yard of children's home and orphanage as the place of occurrence of the external cause

Y92.118 Other place in children's home and orphanage as the place of occurrence of the external cause

Y92.119 Unspecified place in children's home and orphanage as the place of occurrence of the external cause

● **Y92.12** Nursing home as the place of occurrence of the external cause

Home for the sick as the place of occurrence of the external cause

Hospice as the place of occurrence of the external cause

Y92.120 Kitchen in nursing home as the place of occurrence of the external cause

Y92.121 Bathroom in nursing home as the place of occurrence of the external cause

Y92.122 Bedroom in nursing home as the place of occurrence of the external cause

Y92.123 Driveway of nursing home as the place of occurrence of the external cause

Y92.124 Garage of nursing home as the place of occurrence of the external cause

Y92.125 Swimming pool of nursing home as the place of occurrence of the external cause

Y92.126 Garden or yard of nursing home as the place of occurrence of the external cause

Y92.128 Other place in nursing home as the place of occurrence of the external cause

Y92.129 Unspecified place in nursing home as the place of occurrence of the external cause

Coding Clinic: 2017, Q2, P10

● **Y92.13** Military base as the place of occurrence of the external cause

Excludes1 military training grounds (Y92.83)

Y92.130 Kitchen on military base as the place of occurrence of the external cause

Y92.131 Mess hall on military base as the place of occurrence of the external cause

Y92.133 Barracks on military base as the place of occurrence of the external cause

Y92.135 Garage on military base as the place of occurrence of the external cause

Y92.136 Swimming pool on military base as the place of occurrence of the external cause

Y92.137 Garden or yard on military base as the place of occurrence of the external cause

Y92.138 Other place on military base as the place of occurrence of the external cause

Y92.139 Unspecified place military base as the place of occurrence of the external cause

● **Y92.14** Prison as the place of occurrence of the external cause

Y92.140 Kitchen in prison as the place of occurrence of the external cause

Y92.141 Dining room in prison as the place of occurrence of the external cause

Y92.142 Bathroom in prison as the place of occurrence of the external cause

Y92.143 Cell of prison as the place of occurrence of the external cause

▶ New   ➡ Revised   ~~deleted~~ Deleted   Excludes 1   Excludes 2   Includes   Use additional   Code first   Code also   Key words

OGCR Official Guidelines   X Assign placeholder X   ● Use Additional Character(s)   ▷ Manifestation Code   🞰 Hierarchical Condition Category   **Coding Clinic**

Y92.146   Swimming pool of prison as the place of occurrence of the external cause

Y92.147   Courtyard of prison as the place of occurrence of the external cause

Y92.148   Other place in prison as the place of occurrence of the external cause

Y92.149   Unspecified place in prison as the place of occurrence of the external cause

● Y92.15   Reform school as the place of occurrence of the external cause

Y92.150   Kitchen in reform school as the place of occurrence of the external cause

Y92.151   Dining room in reform school as the place of occurrence of the external cause

Y92.152   Bathroom in reform school as the place of occurrence of the external cause

Y92.153   Bedroom in reform school as the place of occurrence of the external cause

Y92.154   Driveway of reform school as the place of occurrence of the external cause

Y92.155   Garage of reform school as the place of occurrence of the external cause

Y92.156   Swimming pool of reform school as the place of occurrence of the external cause

Y92.157   Garden or yard of reform school as the place of occurrence of the external cause

Y92.158   Other place in reform school as the place of occurrence of the external cause

Y92.159   Unspecified place in reform school as the place of occurrence of the external cause

● Y92.16   School dormitory as the place of occurrence of the external cause

    Excludes1   reform school as the place of occurrence of the external cause (Y92.15-)
         school buildings and grounds as the place of occurrence of the external cause (Y92.2-)
         school sports and athletic areas as the place of occurrence of the external cause (Y92.3-)

Y92.160   Kitchen in school dormitory as the place of occurrence of the external cause

Y92.161   Dining room in school dormitory as the place of occurrence of the external cause

Y92.162   Bathroom in school dormitory as the place of occurrence of the external cause

Y92.163   Bedroom in school dormitory as the place of occurrence of the external cause

Y92.168   Other place in school dormitory as the place of occurrence of the external cause

Y92.169   Unspecified place in school dormitory as the place of occurrence of the external cause

● Y92.19   Other specified residential institution as the place of occurrence of the external cause

Y92.190   Kitchen in other specified residential institution as the place of occurrence of the external cause

Y92.191   Dining room in other specified residential institution as the place of occurrence of the external cause

Y92.192   Bathroom in other specified residential institution as the place of occurrence of the external cause

Y92.193   Bedroom in other specified residential institution as the place of occurrence of the external cause

Y92.194   Driveway of other specified residential institution as the place of occurrence of the external cause

Y92.195   Garage of other specified residential institution as the place of occurrence of the external cause

Y92.196   Pool of other specified residential institution as the place of occurrence of the external cause

Y92.197   Garden or yard of other specified residential institution as the place of occurrence of the external cause

Y92.198   Other place in other specified residential institution as the place of occurrence of the external cause
         Coding Clinic: 2017, Q2, P11

Y92.199   Unspecified place in other specified residential institution as the place of occurrence of the external cause
         Coding Clinic: 2017, Q2, P10

● Y92.2   School, other institution and public administrative area as the place of occurrence of the external cause
    Building and adjacent grounds used by the general public or by a particular group of the public

    Excludes1   building under construction as the place of occurrence of the external cause (Y92.6)
         residential institution as the place of occurrence of the external cause (Y92.1)
         school dormitory as the place of occurrence of the external cause (Y92.16-)
         sports and athletics area of schools as the place of occurrence of the external cause (Y92.3-)

● Y92.21   School (private) (public) (state) as the place of occurrence of the external cause

Y92.210   Daycare center as the place of occurrence of the external cause

Y92.211   Elementary school as the place of occurrence of the external cause
         Kindergarten as the place of occurrence of the external cause

Y92.212   Middle school as the place of occurrence of the external cause

Y92.213   High school as the place of occurrence of the external cause
         Coding Clinic: 2012, Q4, P108

Y92.214   College as the place of occurrence of the external cause
         University as the place of occurrence of the external cause

Y92.215   Trade school as the place of occurrence of the external cause

Y92.218   Other school as the place of occurrence of the external cause

Y92.219   Unspecified school as the place of occurrence of the external cause

Y92.22   **Religious institution** as the place of occurrence of the external cause
         Church as the place of occurrence of the external cause
         Mosque as the place of occurrence of the external cause
         Synagogue as the place of occurrence of the external cause

● Y92.23   **Hospital** as the place of occurrence of the external cause
         Excludes1   ambulatory (outpatient) health services establishments (Y92.53-)
                 home for the sick as the place of occurrence of the external cause (Y92.12-)
                 hospice as the place of occurrence of the external cause (Y92.12-)
                 nursing home as the place of occurrence of the external cause (Y92.12-)

    Y92.230   **Patient room** in hospital as the place of occurrence of the external cause
    Y92.231   **Patient bathroom** in hospital as the place of occurrence of the external cause
    Y92.232   **Corridor** of hospital as the place of occurrence of the external cause
    Y92.233   **Cafeteria** of hospital as the place of occurrence of the external cause
    Y92.234   **Operating room** of hospital as the place of occurrence of the external cause
    Y92.238   **Other place** in hospital as the place of occurrence of the external cause
    Y92.239   **Unspecified** place in hospital as the place of occurrence of the external cause

● Y92.24   **Public administrative building** as the place of occurrence of the external cause
    Y92.240   **Courthouse** as the place of occurrence of the external cause
    Y92.241   **Library** as the place of occurrence of the external cause
    Y92.242   **Post office** as the place of occurrence of the external cause
    Y92.243   **City hall** as the place of occurrence of the external cause
    Y92.248   **Other** public administrative building as the place of occurrence of the external cause

● Y92.25   **Cultural building** as the place of occurrence of the external cause
    Y92.250   **Art gallery** as the place of occurrence of the external cause
    Y92.251   **Museum** as the place of occurrence of the external cause
    Y92.252   **Music hall** as the place of occurrence of the external cause
    Y92.253   **Opera house** as the place of occurrence of the external cause
    Y92.254   **Theater** (live) as the place of occurrence of the external cause
    Y92.258   **Other** cultural public building as the place of occurrence of the external cause

  Y92.26   **Movie house** or cinema as the place of occurrence of the external cause

  Y92.29   **Other specified public building** as the place of occurrence of the external cause
         Assembly hall as the place of occurrence of the external cause
         Clubhouse as the place of occurrence of the external cause

● Y92.3   **Sports and athletics area** as the place of occurrence of the external cause
● Y92.31   **Athletic court** as the place of occurrence of the external cause
         Excludes1   tennis court in private home or garden (Y92.09)
    Y92.310   **Basketball** court as the place of occurrence of the external cause
    Y92.311   **Squash** court as the place of occurrence of the external cause
    Y92.312   **Tennis** court as the place of occurrence of the external cause
    Y92.318   **Other** athletic court as the place of occurrence of the external cause

● Y92.32   **Athletic field** as the place of occurrence of the external cause
    Y92.320   **Baseball** field as the place of occurrence of the external cause
    Y92.321   **Football** field as the place of occurrence of the external cause
    Y92.322   **Soccer** field as the place of occurrence of the external cause
    Y92.328   **Other** athletic field as the place of occurrence of the external cause
         Cricket field as the place of occurrence of the external cause
         Hockey field as the place of occurrence of the external cause

● Y92.33   **Skating rink** as the place of occurrence of the external cause
    Y92.330   **Ice** skating rink (indoor) (outdoor) as the place of occurrence of the external cause
    Y92.331   **Roller** skating rink as the place of occurrence of the external cause

  Y92.34   **Swimming pool** (public) as the place of occurrence of the external cause
         Excludes1   swimming pool in private home or garden (Y92.016)

  Y92.39   **Other specified** sports and athletic area as the place of occurrence of the external cause
         Golf-course as the place of occurrence of the external cause
         Gymnasium as the place of occurrence of the external cause
         Riding-school as the place of occurrence of the external cause
         Stadium as the place of occurrence of the external cause

● Y92.4   **Street, highway** and other paved roadways as the place of occurrence of the external cause
         Excludes1   private driveway of residence (Y92.014, Y92.024, Y92.043, Y92.093, Y92.113, Y92.123, Y92.154, Y92.194)

● Y92.41   **Street and highway** as the place of occurrence of the external cause
    Y92.410   **Unspecified** street and highway as the place of occurrence of the external cause
         Road NOS as the place of occurrence of the external cause
    Y92.411   **Interstate** highway as the place of occurrence of the external cause
         Freeway as the place of occurrence of the external cause
         Motorway as the place of occurrence of the external cause
    Y92.412   **Parkway** as the place of occurrence of the external cause
    Y92.413   **State road** as the place of occurrence of the external cause

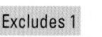

Y92.414   Local residential or business street as the place of occurrence of the external cause

Y92.415   Exit ramp or entrance ramp of street or highway as the place of occurrence of the external cause

● Y92.48   Other paved roadways as the place of occurrence of the external cause

Y92.480   Sidewalk as the place of occurrence of the external cause

Y92.481   Parking lot as the place of occurrence of the external cause

Y92.482   Bike path as the place of occurrence of the external cause

Y92.488   Other paved roadways as the place of occurrence of the external cause

● Y92.5   Trade and service area as the place of occurrence of the external cause

Excludes1   garage in private home (Y92.015)
schools and other public administration buildings (Y92.2-)

● Y92.51   Private commercial establishments as the place of occurrence of the external cause

Y92.510   Bank as the place of occurrence of the external cause

Y92.511   Restaurant or café as the place of occurrence of the external cause

Y92.512   Supermarket, store or market as the place of occurrence of the external cause

Y92.513   Shop (commercial) as the place of occurrence of the external cause

● Y92.52   Service areas as the place of occurrence of the external cause

Y92.520   Airport as the place of occurrence of the external cause

Y92.521   Bus station as the place of occurrence of the external cause

Y92.522   Railway station as the place of occurrence of the external cause

Y92.523   Highway rest stop as the place of occurrence of the external cause

Y92.524   Gas station as the place of occurrence of the external cause
Petroleum station as the place of occurrence of the external cause
Service station as the place of occurrence of the external cause

● Y92.53   Ambulatory health services establishments as the place of occurrence of the external cause

Y92.530   Ambulatory surgery center as the place of occurrence of the external cause
Outpatient surgery center, including that connected with a hospital as the place of occurrence of the external cause
Same day surgery center, including that connected with a hospital as the place of occurrence of the external cause

Y92.531   Health care provider office as the place of occurrence of the external cause
Physician office as the place of occurrence of the external cause

Y92.532   Urgent care center as the place of occurrence of the external cause

Y92.538   Other ambulatory health services establishments as the place of occurrence of the external cause
Coding Clinic: 2019, Q1, P21

Y92.59   Other trade areas as the place of occurrence of the external cause
Office building as the place of occurrence of the external cause
Casino as the place of occurrence of the external cause
Garage (commercial) as the place of occurrence of the external cause
Hotel as the place of occurrence of the external cause
Radio or television station as the place of occurrence of the external cause
Shopping mall as the place of occurrence of the external cause
Warehouse as the place of occurrence of the external cause

● Y92.6   Industrial and construction area as the place of occurrence of the external cause

Y92.61   Building [any] under construction as the place of occurrence of the external cause

Y92.62   Dock or shipyard as the place of occurrence of the external cause
Dockyard as the place of occurrence of the external cause
Dry dock as the place of occurrence of the external cause
Shipyard as the place of occurrence of the external cause

Y92.63   Factory as the place of occurrence of the external cause
Factory building as the place of occurrence of the external cause
Factory premises as the place of occurrence of the external cause
Industrial yard as the place of occurrence of the external cause

Y92.64   Mine or pit as the place of occurrence of the external cause
Mine as the place of occurrence of the external cause

Y92.65   Oil rig as the place of occurrence of the external cause
Pit (coal) (gravel) (sand) as the place of occurrence of the external cause

Y92.69   Other specified industrial and construction area as the place of occurrence of the external cause
Gasworks as the place of occurrence of the external cause
Power-station (coal) (nuclear) (oil) as the place of occurrence of the external cause
Tunnel under construction as the place of occurrence of the external cause
Workshop as the place of occurrence of the external cause

● Y92.7   Farm as the place of occurrence of the external cause
Ranch as the place of occurrence of the external cause

Excludes1   farmhouse and home premises of farm (Y92.01-)

Y92.71   Barn as the place of occurrence of the external cause

Y92.72   Chicken coop as the place of occurrence of the external cause
Hen house as the place of occurrence of the external cause

Y92.73   Farm field as the place of occurrence of the external cause

Y92.74   Orchard as the place of occurrence of the external cause

Y92.79   Other farm location as the place of occurrence of the external cause

CHAPTER 20 (V00-Y99)

- ● **Y92.8** **Other places** as the place of occurrence of the external cause
  - ● **Y92.81** **Transport vehicle** as the place of occurrence of the external cause

    Excludes1   transport accidents (V00-V99)

    - **Y92.810** **Car** as the place of occurrence of the external cause
    - **Y92.811** **Bus** as the place of occurrence of the external cause
    - **Y92.812** **Truck** as the place of occurrence of the external cause
    - **Y92.813** **Airplane** as the place of occurrence of the external cause
    - **Y92.814** **Boat** as the place of occurrence of the external cause
    - **Y92.815** **Train** as the place of occurrence of the external cause
    - **Y92.816** **Subway car** as the place of occurrence of the external cause
    - **Y92.818** **Other** transport vehicle as the place of occurrence of the external cause
  - ● **Y92.82** **Wilderness area**
    - **Y92.820** **Desert** as the place of occurrence of the external cause
    - **Y92.821** **Forest** as the place of occurrence of the external cause
    - **Y92.828** **Other wilderness area** as the place of occurrence of the external cause

      Swamp as the place of occurrence of the external cause

      Mountain as the place of occurrence of the external cause

      Marsh as the place of occurrence of the external cause

      Prairie as the place of occurrence of the external cause
  - ● **Y92.83** **Recreation area** as the place of occurrence of the external cause
    - **Y92.830** **Public park** as the place of occurrence of the external cause
    - **Y92.831** **Amusement park** as the place of occurrence of the external cause
    - **Y92.832** **Beach** as the place of occurrence of the external cause

      Seashore as the place of occurrence of the external cause
    - **Y92.833** **Campsite** as the place of occurrence of the external cause
    - **Y92.834** **Zoological garden** (zoo) as the place of occurrence of the external cause
    - **Y92.838** **Other recreation area** as the place of occurrence of the external cause
  - **Y92.84** **Military training ground** as the place of occurrence of the external cause
  - **Y92.85** **Railroad track** as the place of occurrence of the external cause
  - **Y92.86** **Slaughter house** as the place of occurrence of the external cause
  - **Y92.89** **Other specified places** as the place of occurrence of the external cause

    Derelict house as the place of occurrence of the external cause

OGCR Section I.C.20.b.

Do not use place of occurrence code Y92.9 if the place is not stated or is not applicable.

Y92.9 **Unspecified** place or not applicable

OGCR See Section I.C.20.c.

Activity Code

Assign a code from category Y93, Activity code, to describe the activity of the patient at the time the injury or other health condition occurred.

An activity code is used only once, at the initial encounter for treatment. Only one code from Y93 should be recorded on a medical record.

The activity codes are not applicable to poisonings, adverse effects, misadventures or sequela.

Do not assign Y93.9, Unspecified activity, if the activity is not stated.

A code from category Y93 is appropriate for use with external cause and intent codes if identifying the activity provides additional information about the event.

- ● **Y93** **Activity codes**

  Note: Category Y93 is provided for use to indicate the activity of the person seeking healthcare for an injury or health condition, such as a heart attack while shoveling snow, which resulted from, or was contributed to, by the activity. These codes are appropriate for use for both acute injuries, such as those from Chapter 19, and conditions that are due to the long-term, cumulative effects of an activity, such as those from Chapter 13. They are also appropriate for use with external cause codes for cause and intent if identifying the activity provides additional information on the event. These codes should be used in conjunction with codes for external cause status (Y99) and place of occurrence (Y92).

  This section contains the following broad activity categories:

  - Y93.0   Activities involving walking and running
  - Y93.1   Activities involving water and water craft
  - Y93.2   Activities involving ice and snow
  - Y93.3   Activities involving climbing, rappelling, and jumping off
  - Y93.4   Activities involving dancing and other rhythmic movement
  - Y93.5   Activities involving other sports and athletics played individually
  - Y93.6   Activities involving other sports and athletics played as a team or group
  - Y93.7   Activities involving other specified sports and athletics
  - Y93.A   Activities involving other cardiorespiratory exercise
  - Y93.B   Activities involving other muscle strengthening exercises
  - Y93.C   Activities involving computer technology and electronic devices
  - Y93.D   Activities involving arts and handcrafts
  - Y93.E   Activities involving personal hygiene and interior property and clothing maintenance
  - Y93.F   Activities involving caregiving
  - Y93.G   Activities involving food preparation, cooking and grilling
  - Y93.H   Activities involving exterior property and land maintenance, building and construction
  - Y93.I   Activities involving roller coasters and other types of external motion
  - Y93.J   Activities involving playing musical instrument
  - Y93.K   Activities involving animal care
  - Y93.8   Activities, other specified
  - Y93.9   Activity, unspecified
  - ● **Y93.0** **Activities involving walking and running**

    Excludes1   Activity, walking an animal (Y93.K1)

              Activity, walking or running on a treadmill (Y93.A1)

    - **Y93.01** **Activity, walking, marching and hiking**

      Activity, walking, marching and hiking on level or elevated terrain

      Excludes1   activity, mountain climbing (Y93.31)

    - **Y93.02** **Activity, running**

● **Y93.1** **Activities involving water and water craft**
Excludes 1   activities involving ice (Y93.2-)

Y93.11   **Activity, swimming**

Y93.12   **Activity, springboard and platform diving**

Y93.13   **Activity, water polo**

Y93.14   **Activity, water aerobics and water exercise**

Y93.15   **Activity, underwater diving and snorkeling**
Activity, SCUBA diving

Y93.16   **Activity, rowing, canoeing, kayaking, rafting and tubing**
Activity, canoeing, kayaking, rafting and tubing in calm and turbulent water

Y93.17   **Activity, water skiing and wake boarding**

Y93.18   **Activity, surfing, windsurfing and boogie boarding**
Activity, water sliding

Y93.19   **Activity, other involving water and watercraft**
Activity involving water NOS
Activity, parasailing
Activity, water survival training and testing

● **Y93.2** **Activities involving ice and snow**
Excludes 1   activity, shoveling ice and snow (Y93.H1)

Y93.21   **Activity, ice skating**
Activity, figure skating (singles) (pairs)
Activity, ice dancing
Excludes 1   activity, ice hockey (Y93.22)

Y93.22   **Activity, ice hockey**

Y93.23   **Activity, snow (alpine) (downhill) skiing, snowboarding, sledding, tobogganing and snow tubing**
Excludes 1   activity, cross country skiing (Y93.24)

Y93.24   **Activity, cross country skiing**
Activity, nordic skiing

Y93.29   **Activity, other activity involving ice and snow**
Activity, activity involving ice and snow NOS

● **Y93.3** **Activities involving climbing, rappelling and jumping off**
Excludes 1   activity, hiking on level or elevated terrain (Y93.01)
activity, jumping rope (Y93.56)
activity, trampoline jumping (Y93.44)

Y93.31   **Activity, mountain climbing, rock climbing and wall climbing**

Y93.32   **Activity, rappelling**

Y93.33   **Activity, BASE jumping**
Activity, building, Antenna, Span, Earth jumping

Y93.34   **Activity, bungee jumping**

Y93.35   **Activity, hang gliding**

Y93.39   **Activity, other activity involving climbing, rappelling and jumping off**

● **Y93.4** **Activities involving dancing and other rhythmic movement**
Excludes 1   activity, martial arts (Y93.75)

Y93.41   **Activity, dancing**
Coding Clinic: 2012, Q4, P108

Y93.42   **Activity, yoga**

Y93.43   **Activity, gymnastics**
Activity, rhythmic gymnastics
Excludes 1   activity, trampolining (Y93.44)

Y93.44   **Activity, trampolining**

Y93.45   **Activity, cheerleading**

Y93.49   **Activity, other involving dancing and other rhythmic movements**

● **Y93.5** **Activities involving other sports and athletics played individually**
Excludes 1   activity, dancing (Y93.41)
activity, gymnastic (Y93.43)
activity, trampolining (Y93.44)
activity, yoga (Y93.42)

Y93.51   **Activity, roller skating (inline) and skateboarding**

Y93.52   **Activity, horseback riding**

Y93.53   **Activity, golf**

Y93.54   **Activity, bowling**

Y93.55   **Activity, bike riding**

Y93.56   **Activity, jumping rope**

Y93.57   **Activity, non-running track and field events**
Excludes 1   activity, running (any form) (Y93.02)

Y93.59   **Activity, other involving other sports and athletics played individually**
Excludes 1   activities involving climbing, rappelling, and jumping (Y93.3-)
activities involving ice and snow (Y93.2-)
activities involving walking and running (Y93.0-)
activities involving water and watercraft (Y93.1-)

● **Y93.6** **Activities involving other sports and athletics played as a team or group**
Excludes 1   activity, ice hockey (Y93.22)
activity, water polo (Y93.13)

Y93.61   **Activity, American tackle football**
Activity, football NOS

Y93.62   **Activity, American flag or touch football**

Y93.63   **Activity, rugby**

Y93.64   **Activity, baseball**
Activity, softball

Y93.65   **Activity, lacrosse and field hockey**
Coding Clinic: 2015, Q1, P9

Y93.66   **Activity, soccer**

Y93.67   **Activity, basketball**
Coding Clinic: 2019, Q4, P18

Y93.68   **Activity, volleyball (beach) (court)**

Y93.6A   **Activity, physical games generally associated with school recess, summer camp and children**
Activity, capture the flag
Activity, dodge ball
Activity, four square
Activity, kickball

Y93.69   **Activity, other involving other sports and athletics played as a team or group**
Cricket

● **Y93.7** **Activities involving other specified sports and athletics**

Y93.71   **Activity, boxing**

Y93.72   **Activity, wrestling**

Y93.73   **Activity, racquet and hand sports**
Activity, handball
Activity, racquetball
Activity, squash
Activity, tennis

Y93.74   **Activity, frisbee**
Activity, ultimate frisbee

Y93.75   **Activity, martial arts**
Activity, combatives

Y93.79   **Activity, other specified sports and athletics**
Excludes 1   sports and athletics activities specified in categories Y93.0-Y93.6

● **Y93.A** Activities involving other cardiorespiratory exercise
Activities involving physical training

Y93.A1 Activity, exercise machines primarily for cardiorespiratory conditioning
Activity, elliptical and stepper machines
Activity, stationary bike
Activity, treadmill

Y93.A2 Activity, calisthenics
Activity, jumping jacks
Activity, warm up and cool down

Y93.A3 Activity, aerobic and step exercise

Y93.A4 Activity, circuit training

Y93.A5 Activity, obstacle course
Activity, challenge course
Activity, confidence course

Y93.A6 Activity, grass drills
Activity, guerilla drills

Y93.A9 Activity, other involving other cardiorespiratory exercise

> **Excludes1** activities involving cardiorespiratory exercise specified in categories Y93.0-Y93.7

● **Y93.B** Activity involving other muscle strengthening exercises

Y93.B1 Activity, exercise machines primarily for muscle strengthening

Y93.B2 Activity, push-ups, pull-ups, sit-ups

Y93.B3 Activity, free weights
Activity, barbells
Activity, dumbbells

Y93.B4 Activity, pilates

Y93.B9 Activity, other involving other muscle strengthening exercises

> **Excludes1** activities involving muscle strengthening specified in categories Y93.0-Y93.A

● **Y93.C** Activities involving computer technology and electronic devices

> **Excludes1** activity, electronic musical keyboard or instruments (Y93.J-)

Y93.C1 Activity, computer keyboarding
Activity, electronic game playing using keyboard or other stationary device

Y93.C2 Activity, hand held interactive electronic device
Activity, cellular telephone and communication device
Activity, electronic game playing using interactive device

> **Excludes1** activity, electronic game playing using keyboard or other stationary device (Y93.C1)

Y93.C9 Activity, other involving computer technology and electronic devices

● **Y93.D** Activities involving arts and handcrafts

> **Excludes1** activities involving playing musical instrument (Y93.J-)

Y93.D1 Knitting and crocheting

Y93.D2 Sewing

Y93.D3 Furniture building and finishing
Furniture repair

Y93.D9 Activity, other involving arts and handcrafts

● **Y93.E** Activities involving personal hygiene and interior property and clothing maintenance

> **Excludes1** activities involving cooking and grilling (Y93.G-)
> activities involving exterior property and land maintenance, building and construction (Y93.H-)
> activity involving caregiving (Y93.F-)
> activity, dishwashing (Y93.G1)
> activity, food preparation (Y93.G1)
> activity, gardening (Y93.H2)

Y93.E1 Activity, personal bathing and showering

Y93.E2 Activity, laundry

Y93.E3 Activity, vacuuming

Y93.E4 Activity, ironing

Y93.E5 Activity, floor mopping and cleaning

Y93.E6 Activity, residential relocation
Activity, packing up and unpacking involved in moving to a new residence

Y93.E8 Activity, other personal hygiene activity

Y93.E9 Activity, other household maintenance

● **Y93.F** Activities involving person providing caregiving
Activity involving the provider of caregiving

Y93.F1 Activity, caregiving involving bathing

Y93.F2 Activity, caregiving involving lifting
Coding Clinic: 2016, Q4, P74

Y93.F9 Activity, other caregiving

● **Y93.G** Activities involving food preparation, cooking and grilling

Y93.G1 Activity, food preparation and clean up
Activity, dishwashing

Y93.G2 Activity, grilling and smoking food

Y93.G3 Activity, cooking and baking
Activity, use of stove, oven and microwave oven

Y93.G9 Activity, other activity involving cooking and grilling

● **Y93.H** Activities involving property and land maintenance, building and construction

Y93.H1 Activity, digging, shoveling and raking
Activity, dirt digging
Activity, raking leaves
Activity, snow shoveling

Y93.H2 Activity, gardening and landscaping
Activity, pruning, trimming shrubs, weeding

Y93.H3 Activity, building and construction

Y93.H9 Activity, other activity involving property and land maintenance, building and construction

● **Y93.I** Activities involving roller coasters and other types of external motion

Y93.I1 Activity, rollercoaster riding

Y93.I9 Activity, other involving external motion

● **Y93.J** Activities involving playing musical instrument
Activity involving playing electric musical instrument

Y93.J1 Activity, piano playing
Activity, musical keyboard (electronic) playing

Y93.J2 Activity, drum and other percussion instrument playing

Y93.J3 Activity, string instrument playing

Y93.J4 Activity, winds and brass instrument playing

▶ New ⇒ Revised ~~deleted~~ Deleted Excludes 1 Excludes 2 Includes Use additional Code first Code also Key words

OGCR Official Guidelines X Assign placeholder X ● Use Additional Character(s) ▶ Manifestation Code 🐾 Hierarchical Condition Category Coding Clinic

● **Y93.K** **Activities involving animal care**

Excludes1 activity, horseback riding (Y93.52)

　　Y93.K1 **Activity, walking an animal**

　　Y93.K2 **Activity, milking an animal**

　　Y93.K3 **Activity, grooming and shearing an animal**

　　Y93.K9 **Activity, other activity involving animal care**

● **Y93.8** **Other activity**
Coding Clinic: 2016, Q4, P74

　　Y93.81 **Activity, refereeing a sports activity**

　　Y93.82 **Activity, spectator at an event**

　　Y93.83 **Activity, rough housing and horseplay**
　　　　Coding Clinic: 2015, Q1, P8

　　Y93.84 **Activity, sleeping**

　　Y93.85 **Activity, choking game**
　　　　Activity, blackout game
　　　　Activity, fainting game
　　　　Activity, pass out game
　　　　Coding Clinic: 2016, Q4, P74-76

　　Y93.89 **Activity, other specified**

OGCR See Section I.C.20.c.

Do not assign Y93.9, Unspecified activity, if the activity is not stated.

● **Y93.9** **Activity, unspecified**

Y95 **Nosocomial condition**

● **Y99** **External cause status**

Note: A single code from category Y99 should be used in conjunction with the external cause code(s) assigned to a record to indicate the status of the person at the time the event occurred.
Coding Clinic: 2016, Q4, P74

Y99.0 **Civilian activity done for income or pay**
　　Civilian activity done for financial or other compensation

Excludes1 military activity (Y99.1)
　　　　　　volunteer activity (Y99.2)

Y99.1 **Military activity**

Excludes1 activity of off duty military personnel (Y99.8)

Y99.2 **Volunteer activity**

Excludes1 activity of child or other family member assisting in compensated work of other family member (Y99.8)

Y99.8 **Other external cause status**
　　Activity NEC
　　Activity of child or other family member assisting in compensated work of other family member
　　Hobby not done for income
　　Leisure activity
　　Off-duty activity of military personnel
　　Recreation or sport not for income or while a student
　　Student activity

Excludes1 civilian activity done for income or compensation (Y99.0)
　　　　　　military activity (Y99.1)
Coding Clinic: 2012, Q4, P108

Y99.9 **Unspecified external cause status**

CHAPTER 20 (V00-Y99)

CHAPTER 21

FACTORS INFLUENCING HEALTH STATUS AND CONTACT WITH HEALTH SERVICES (Z00-Z99)

OGCR Chapter-Specific Coding Guidelines

21. **Chapter 21: Factors influencing health status and contact with health services (Z00-Z99)**
Note: The chapter specific guidelines provide additional information about the use of Z codes for specified encounters.

a. Use of Z codes in any healthcare setting
Z codes are for use in any healthcare setting. Z codes may be used as either a first-listed (principal diagnosis code in the inpatient setting) or secondary code, depending on the circumstances of the encounter. Certain Z codes may only be used as first-listed or principal diagnosis.

b. Z Codes indicate a reason for an encounter
Z codes are not procedure codes. A corresponding procedure code must accompany a Z code to describe any procedure performed.

c. Categories of Z Codes

1) Contact/Exposure
Category Z20 indicates contact with, and suspected exposure to, communicable diseases. These codes are for patients who do not show any sign or symptom of a disease but are suspected to have been exposed to it by close personal contact with an infected individual or are in an area where a disease is epidemic.

Category Z77, Other contact with and (suspected) exposures hazardous to health, indicates contact with and suspected exposures hazardous to health.

Contact/exposure codes may be used as a first-listed code to explain an encounter for testing, or, more commonly, as a secondary code to identify a potential risk.

2) Inoculations and vaccinations
Code Z23 is for encounters for inoculations and vaccinations. It indicates that a patient is being seen to receive a prophylactic inoculation against a disease. Procedure codes are required to identify the actual administration of the injection and the type(s) of immunizations given. Code Z23 may be used as a secondary code if the inoculation is given as a routine part of preventive health care, such as a well-baby visit.

3) Status
Status codes indicate that a patient is either a carrier of a disease or has the sequelae or residual of a past disease or condition. This includes such things as the presence of prosthetic or mechanical devices resulting from past treatment. A status code is informative, because the status may affect the course of treatment and its outcome. A status code is distinct from a history code. The history code indicates that the patient no longer has the condition.

A status code should not be used with a diagnosis code from one of the body system chapters, if the diagnosis code includes the information provided by the status code. For example, code Z94.1, Heart transplant status, should not be used with a code from subcategory T86.2, Complications of heart transplant. The status code does not provide additional information. The complication code indicates that the patient is a heart transplant patient.

For encounters for weaning from a mechanical ventilator, assign a code from subcategory J96.1, Chronic respiratory failure, followed by code Z99.11, Dependence on respirator [ventilator] status.

The status Z codes/categories are:
Z14   Genetic carrier
      Genetic carrier status indicates that a person carries a gene, associated with a particular disease, which may be passed to offspring who may develop that disease. The person does not have the disease and is not at risk of developing the disease.
Z15   Genetic susceptibility to disease Genetic susceptibility indicates that a person has a gene that increases the risk of that person developing the disease.
      Codes from category Z15 should not be used as principal or first-listed codes. If the patient has the condition to which he/she is susceptible, and that condition is the reason for the encounter, the code for the current condition should be sequenced first. If the patient is being seen for follow-up after completed treatment for this condition, and the condition no longer exists, a follow-up

code should be sequenced first, followed by the appropriate personal history and genetic susceptibility codes. If the purpose of the encounter is genetic counseling associated with procreative management, code Z31.5, Encounter for genetic counseling, should be assigned as the first-listed code, followed by a code from category Z15. Additional codes should be assigned for any applicable family or personal history.
Z16   Resistance to antimicrobial drugs
      This code indicates that a patient has a condition that is resistant to antimicrobial drug treatment. Sequence the infection code first.
Z17   Estrogen receptor status
Z18   Retained foreign body fragments
Z19   Hormone sensitivity malignancy status
Z21   Asymptomatic HIV infection status This code indicates that a patient has tested positive for HIV but has manifested no signs or symptoms of the disease.
Z22   Carrier of infectious disease Carrier status indicates that a person harbors the specific organisms of a disease without manifest symptoms and is capable of transmitting the infection.
Z28.3 Underimmunization status
Z33.1 Pregnant state, incidental This code is a secondary code only for use when the pregnancy is in no way complicating the reason for visit. Otherwise, a code from the obstetric chapter is required.
Z66   Do not resuscitate
This code may be used when it is documented by the provider that a patient is on do not resuscitate status at any time during the stay.
Z67   Blood type
Z68   Body mass index (BMI)
      BMI codes should only be assigned when the associated diagnosis (such as overweight or obesity) meets the definition of a reportable diagnosis (see Section III, Reporting Additional Diagnoses). Do not assign BMI codes during pregnancy. See Section I.B.14 for BMI documentation by clinicians other than the patient's provider.
Z74.01 Bed confinement status
Z76.82 Awaiting organ transplant status
Z78   Other specified health status
Code Z78.1, Physical restraint status, may be used when it is documented by the provider that a patient has been put in restraints during the current encounter. Please note that this code should not be reported when it is documented by the provider that a patient is temporarily restrained during a procedure.
Z79   Long-term (current) drug therapy
      Codes from this category indicate a patient's continuous use of a prescribed drug (including such things as aspirin therapy) for the long-term treatment of a condition or for prophylactic use. It is not for use for patients who have addictions to drugs. This subcategory is not for use of medications for detoxification or maintenance programs to prevent withdrawal symptoms in patients with drug dependence (e.g., methadone maintenance for opiate dependence). Assign the appropriate code for the drug dependence instead.
      Assign a code from Z79 if the patient is receiving a medication for an extended period as a prophylactic measure (such as for the prevention of deep vein thrombosis) or as treatment of a chronic condition (such as arthritis) or a disease requiring a lengthy course of treatment (such as cancer). Do not assign a code from category Z79 for medication being administered for a brief period of time to treat an acute illness or injury (such as a course of antibiotics to treat acute bronchitis).
Z88   Allergy status to drugs, medicaments and biological substances Except: Z88.9, Allergy status to unspecified drugs, medicaments and biological substances status
Z89   Acquired absence of limb
Z90   Acquired absence of organs, not elsewhere classified
Z91.0- Allergy status, other than to drugs and biological substances
Z92.82 Status post administration of tPA (rtPA) in a different facility within the last 24 hours prior to admission to a current facility Assign code Z92.82, Status post administration of tPA (rtPA) in a different facility within the last 24 hours prior to admission to current

facility, as a secondary diagnosis when a patient is received by transfer into a facility and documentation indicates they were administered tissue plasminogen activator (tPA) within the last 24 hours prior to admission to the current facility. This guideline applies even if the patient is still receiving the tPA at the time they are received into the current facility. The appropriate code for the condition for which the tPA was administered (such as cerebrovascular disease or myocardial infarction) should be assigned first. Code Z92.82 is only applicable to the receiving facility record and not to the transferring facility record.

Z93	Artificial opening status
Z94	Transplanted organ and tissue status
Z95	Presence of cardiac and vascular implants and grafts
Z96	Presence of other functional implants
Z97	Presence of other devices
Z98	Other postprocedural states

Assign code Z98.85, Transplanted organ removal status, to indicate that a transplanted organ has been previously removed. This code should not be assigned for the encounter in which the transplanted organ is removed. The complication necessitating removal of the transplant organ should be assigned for that encounter.

See Section I.C.19. for information on the coding of organ transplant complications.

Z99	Dependence on enabling machines and devices, not elsewhere classified

Note: Categories Z89-Z90 and Z93-Z99 are for use only if there are no complications or malfunctions of the organ or tissue replaced, the amputation site or the equipment on which the patient is dependent.

4) History (of)

There are two types of history Z codes, personal and family. Personal history codes explain a patient's past medical condition that no longer exists and is not receiving any treatment, but that has the potential for recurrence, and therefore may require continued monitoring.

Family history codes are for use when a patient has a family member(s) who has had a particular disease that causes the patient to be at higher risk of also contracting the disease.

Personal history codes may be used in conjunction with follow-up codes and family history codes may be used in conjunction with screening codes to explain the need for a test or procedure. History codes are also acceptable on any medical record regardless of the reason for visit. A history of an illness, even if no longer present, is important information that may alter the type of treatment ordered.

The history Z code categories are:

Z80	Family history of primary malignant neoplasm
Z81	Family history of mental and behavioral disorders
Z82	Family history of certain disabilities and chronic diseases (leading to disablement)
Z83	Family history of other specific disorders
Z84	Family history of other conditions
Z85	Personal history of malignant neoplasm
Z86	Personal history of certain other diseases
Z87	Personal history of other diseases and conditions
Z91.4-	Personal history of psychological trauma, not elsewhere classified
Z91.5	Personal history of self-harm
Z91.81	History of falling
Z91.82	Personal history of military deployment
Z92	Personal history of medical treatment Except: Z92.0, Personal history of contraception Except: Z92.82, Status post administration of tPA (rtPA) in a different facility within the last 24 hours prior to admission to a current facility

5) Screening

Screening is the testing for disease or disease precursors in seemingly well individuals so that early detection and treatment can be provided for those who test positive for the disease (e.g., screening mammogram).

The testing of a person to rule out or confirm a suspected diagnosis because the patient has some sign or symptom is a diagnostic examination, not a screening. In these cases, the sign or symptom is used to explain the reason for the test.

A screening code may be a first-listed code if the reason for the visit is specifically the screening exam. It may also be used as an additional code if the screening is done during an office visit for other health problems. A screening code is not necessary if the screening is inherent to a routine examination, such as a pap smear done during a routine pelvic examination.

Should a condition be discovered during the screening then the code for the condition may be assigned as an additional diagnosis.

The Z code indicates that a screening exam is planned. A procedure code is required to confirm that the screening was performed.

The screening Z codes/categories:

Z11	Encounter for screening for infectious and parasitic diseases
Z12	Encounter for screening for malignant neoplasms
Z13	Encounter for screening for other diseases and disorders Except: Z13.9, Encounter for screening, unspecified
Z36	Encounter for antenatal screening for mother

6) Observation

There are three observation Z code categories. They are for use in very limited circumstances when a person is being observed for a suspected condition that is ruled out. The observation codes are not for use if an injury or illness or any signs or symptoms related to the suspected condition are present. In such cases the diagnosis/symptom code is used with the corresponding external cause code.

The observation codes are to be used as principal diagnosis only. The only exception to this is when the principal diagnosis is required to be a code from category Z38, Liveborn infants according to place of birth and type of delivery. Then a code from category Z05, Encounter for observation and evaluation of newborn for suspected diseases and conditions ruled out, is sequenced after the Z38 code. Additional codes may be used in addition to the observation code but only if they are unrelated to the suspected condition being observed.

Codes from subcategory Z03.7 Encounter for suspected maternal and fetal conditions ruled out, may either be used as a first-listed or as an additional code assignment depending on the case. They are for use in very limited circumstances on a maternal record when an encounter is for a suspected maternal or fetal condition that is ruled out during that encounter (for example, a maternal or fetal condition may be suspected due to an abnormal test result). These codes should not be used when the condition is confirmed. In those cases, the confirmed condition should be coded. In addition, these codes are not for use if an illness or any signs or symptoms related to the suspected condition or problem are present. In such cases the diagnosis/symptom code is used.

Additional codes may be used in addition to the code from subcategory Z03.7, but only if they are unrelated to the suspected condition being evaluated.

Codes from subcategory Z03.7 may not be used for encounters for antenatal screening of mother. *See Section I.C.21. Screening.*

For encounters for suspected fetal condition that are inconclusive following testing and evaluation, assign the appropriate code from category O35, O36, O40 or O41.

The observation Z code categories:

Z03	Encounter for medical observation for suspected diseases and conditions ruled out
Z04	Encounter for examination and observation for other reasons Except: Z04.9, Encounter for examination and observation for unspecified reason
Z05	Encounter for observation and evaluation of newborn for suspected diseases and conditions ruled out

7) Aftercare

Aftercare visit codes cover situations when the initial treatment of a disease has been performed and the patient requires continued care during the healing or recovery phase, or for the long-term consequences of the disease. The aftercare Z code should not be used if treatment is directed at a current, acute disease. The diagnosis code is to be used in these cases.

Exceptions to this rule are codes Z51.0, Encounter for antineoplastic radiation therapy, and codes from subcategory Z51.1, Encounter for antineoplastic chemotherapy and immunotherapy. These codes are to be first-listed, followed by the diagnosis code when a patient's encounter is solely to receive radiation therapy, chemotherapy, or immunotherapy for the treatment of a neoplasm. If the reason for the encounter is more than one type of antineoplastic therapy, code Z51.0 and a code from subcategory Z51.1 may be assigned together, in which case one of these codes would be reported as a secondary diagnosis.

The aftercare Z codes should also not be used for aftercare for injuries. For aftercare of an injury, assign the acute injury code with the appropriate 7th character (for subsequent encounter).

The aftercare codes are generally first-listed to explain the specific reason for the encounter. An aftercare code may be used as an additional code when some type of aftercare is provided in addition to the reason for admission and no diagnosis code is applicable. An example of this would be the closure of a colostomy during an encounter for treatment of another condition.

Aftercare codes should be used in conjunction with other aftercare codes or diagnosis codes to provide better detail on the specifics of an aftercare encounter visit, unless otherwise directed by the classification. Should a patient receive multiple types of antineoplastic therapy during the same encounter, code Z51.0, Encounter for antineoplastic radiation therapy, and codes from subcategory Z51.1, Encounter for antineoplastic chemotherapy and immunotherapy, may be used together on a record. The sequencing of multiple aftercare codes depends on the circumstances of the encounter.

Certain aftercare Z code categories need a secondary diagnosis code to describe the resolving condition or sequelae. For others, the condition is included in the code title.

Additional Z code aftercare category terms include fitting and adjustment, and attention to artificial openings.

Status Z codes may be used with aftercare Z codes to indicate the nature of the aftercare. For example code Z95.1, Presence of aortocoronary bypass graft, may be used with code Z48.812, Encounter for surgical aftercare following surgery on the circulatory system, to indicate the surgery for which the aftercare is being performed. A status code should not be used when the aftercare code indicates the type of status, such as using Z43.0, Encounter for attention to tracheostomy, with Z93.0, Tracheostomy status.

The aftercare Z category/codes:

Z42	Encounter for plastic and reconstructive surgery following medical procedure or healed injury
Z43	Encounter for attention to artificial openings
Z44	Encounter for fitting and adjustment of external prosthetic device
Z45	Encounter for adjustment and management of implanted device
Z46	Encounter for fitting and adjustment of other devices
Z47	Orthopedic aftercare
Z48	Encounter for other postprocedural aftercare
Z49	Encounter for care involving renal dialysis
Z51	Encounter for other aftercare and medical care

8) Follow-up

The follow-up codes are used to explain continuing surveillance following completed treatment of a disease, condition, or injury. They imply that the condition has been fully treated and no longer exists. They should not be confused with aftercare codes, or injury codes with a 7th character for subsequent encounter, that explain ongoing care of a healing condition or its sequelae. Follow-up codes may be used in conjunction with history codes to provide the full picture of the healed condition and its treatment. The follow-up code is sequenced first, followed by the history code.

A follow-up code may be used to explain multiple visits. Should a condition be found to have recurred on the follow-up visit, then the diagnosis code for the condition should be assigned in place of the follow-up code.

The follow-up Z code categories:

Z08	Encounter for follow-up examination after completed treatment for malignant neoplasm
Z09	Encounter for follow-up examination after completed treatment for conditions other than malignant neoplasm
Z39	Encounter for maternal postpartum care and examination

9) Donor

Codes in category Z52, Donors of organs and tissues, are used for living individuals who are donating blood or other body tissue.

These codes are only for individuals donating for others, not for self-donations. They are not used to identify cadaveric donations.

10) Counseling

Counseling Z codes are used when a patient or family member receives assistance in the aftermath of an illness or injury, or when support is required in coping with family or social problems.

The counseling Z codes/categories:

Z30.0-	Encounter for general counseling and advice on contraception
Z31.5	Encounter for procreative genetic counseling
Z31.6-	Encounter for general counseling and advice on procreation
Z32.2	Encounter for childbirth instruction
Z32.3	Encounter for childcare instruction
Z69	Encounter for mental health services for victim and perpetrator of abuse
Z70	Counseling related to sexual attitude, behavior and orientation
Z71	Persons encountering health services for other counseling and medical advice, not elsewhere classified
Z76.81	Expectant mother prebirth pediatrician visit

11) Encounters for Obstetrical and Reproductive Services

See Section I.C.15. Pregnancy, Childbirth, and the Puerperium, for further instruction on the use of these codes.

Z codes for pregnancy are for use in those circumstances when none of the problems or complications included in the codes from the Obstetrics chapter exist (a routine prenatal visit or postpartum care). Codes in category Z34, Encounter for supervision of normal pregnancy, are always first listed and are not to be used with any other code from the OB chapter.

Codes in category Z3A, Weeks of gestation, may be assigned to provide additional information about the pregnancy. Category Z3A codes should not be assigned for pregnancies with abortive outcomes (categories O00-O08), elective termination of pregnancy (code Z33.2), nor for postpartum conditions, as category Z3A is not applicable to these conditions. The date of the admission should be used to determine weeks of gestation for inpatient admissions that encompass more than one gestational week.

The outcome of delivery, category Z37, should be included on all maternal delivery records. It is always a secondary code. Codes in category Z37 should not be used on the newborn record.

Z codes for family planning (contraceptive) or procreative management and counseling should be included on an obstetric record either during the pregnancy or the postpartum stage, if applicable.

Z codes/categories for obstetrical and reproductive services:

Z30	Encounter for contraceptive management
Z31	Encounter for procreative management
Z32.2	Encounter for childbirth instruction
Z32.3	Encounter for childcare instruction
Z33	Pregnant state
Z34	Encounter for supervision of normal pregnancy
Z36	Encounter for antenatal screening of mother
Z3A	Weeks of gestation
Z37	Outcome of delivery
Z39	Encounter for maternal postpartum care and examination
Z76.81	Expectant mother prebirth pediatrician visit

12) Newborns and Infants

See Section I.C.16. Newborn (Perinatal) Guidelines, for further instruction on the use of these codes.

Newborn Z codes/categories:

Z76.1	Encounter for health supervision and care of foundling
Z00.1-	Encounter for routine child health examination
Z38	Liveborn infants according to place of birth and type of delivery

13) Routine and administrative examinations

The Z codes allow for the description of encounters for routine examinations, such as, a general check-up, or, examinations for administrative purposes, such as, a pre-employment physical. The codes are not to be used if the examination is for diagnosis of a suspected condition or for treatment purposes. In such cases the diagnosis code is used. During a routine exam, should a diagnosis or condition be discovered, it should be coded as an additional code. Pre-existing and chronic conditions and history codes may also be included as additional codes as long as the examination is for administrative purposes and not focused on any particular condition.

Some of the codes for routine health examinations distinguish between "with" and "without" abnormal findings. Code assignment depends on the information that is known at the time the encounter is being coded. For example, if no abnormal findings were found during the examination, but the encounter is being coded before test results are back, it is acceptable to assign the code for "without abnormal findings." When assigning a code for "with abnormal findings," additional code(s) should be assigned to identify the specific abnormal finding(s).

Pre-operative examination and pre-procedural laboratory examination Z codes are for use only in those situations when a patient is being cleared for a procedure or surgery and no treatment is given.

The Z codes/categories for routine and administrative examinations:

Z00	Encounter for general examination without complaint, suspected or reported diagnosis
Z01	Encounter for other special examination without complaint, suspected or reported diagnosis
Z02	Encounter for administrative examination Except: Z02.9, Encounter for administrative examinations, unspecified
Z32.0-	Encounter for pregnancy test

14) Miscellaneous Z codes

The miscellaneous Z codes capture a number of other health care encounters that do not fall into one of the other categories. Certain of these codes identify the reason for the encounter; others are for use as additional codes that provide useful information on circumstances that may affect a patient's care and treatment.

Prophylactic Organ Removal

For encounters specifically for prophylactic removal of an organ (such as prophylactic removal of breasts due to a genetic susceptibility to cancer or a family history of cancer), the principal or first-listed code should be a code from category Z40, Encounter for prophylactic surgery, followed by the appropriate codes to identify the associated risk factor (such as genetic susceptibility or family history).

If the patient has a malignancy of one site and is having prophylactic removal at another site to prevent either a new primary malignancy or metastatic disease, a code for the malignancy should also be assigned in addition to a code from subcategory Z40.0, Encounter for prophylactic surgery for risk factors related to malignant neoplasms. A Z40.0 code should not be assigned if the patient is having organ removal for treatment of a malignancy, such as the removal of the testes for the treatment of prostate cancer.

Miscellaneous Z codes/categories:

Z28	Immunization not carried out Except: Z28.3, Underimmunization status
Z29	Encounter for other prophylactic measures
Z40	Encounter for prophylactic surgery
Z41	Encounter for procedures for purposes other than remedying health state Except: Z41.9, Encounter for procedure for purposes other than remedying health state, unspecified
Z53	Persons encountering health services for specific procedures and treatment, not carried out
Z55	Problems related to education and literacy
Z56	Problems related to employment and unemployment
Z57	Occupational exposure to risk factors
Z58	Problems related to physical environment
Z59	Problems related to housing and economic circumstances
Z60	Problems related to social environment
Z62	Problems related to upbringing
Z63	Other problems related to primary support group, including family circumstances
Z64	Problems related to certain psychosocial circumstances
Z65	Problems related to other psychosocial circumstances
Z72	Problems related to lifestyle Note: These codes should be assigned only when the documentation specifies that the patient has an associated problem
Z73	Problems related to life management difficulty

Z74	Problems related to care provider dependency Except: Z74.01, Bed confinement status
Z75	Problems related to medical facilities and other health care
Z76.0	Encounter for issue of repeat prescription
Z76.3	Healthy person accompanying sick person
Z76.4	Other boarder to healthcare facility
Z76.5	Malingerer [conscious simulation]
Z91.1-	Patient's noncompliance with medical treatment and regimen
Z91.83	Wandering in diseases classified elsewhere
Z91.84-	Oral health risk factors
Z91.89	Other specified personal risk factors, not elsewhere classified

See Section I.B.14 for Z55-Z65 Persons with potential health hazards related to socioeconomic and psychosocial circumstances, documentation by clinicians other than the patient's provider.

15) Nonspecific Z codes

Certain Z codes are so non-specific, or potentially redundant with other codes in the classification, that there can be little justification for their use in the inpatient setting. Their use in the outpatient setting should be limited to those instances when there is no further documentation to permit more precise coding. Otherwise, any sign or symptom or any other reason for visit that is captured in another code should be used.

Nonspecific Z codes/categories:

Z02.9	Encounter for administrative examinations, unspecified
Z04.9	Encounter for examination and observation for unspecified reason
Z13.9	Encounter for screening, unspecified
Z41.9	Encounter for procedure for purposes other than remedying health state, unspecified
Z52.9	Donor of unspecified organ or tissue
Z86.59	Personal history of other mental and behavioral disorders
Z88.9	Allergy status to unspecified drugs, medicaments and biological substances status
Z92.0	Personal history of contraception

16) Z Codes That May Only Be Principal/First-Listed Diagnosis

The following Z codes/categories may only be reported as the principal/first-listed diagnosis, except when there are multiple encounters on the same day and the medical records for the encounters are combined:

Z00	Encounter for general examination without complaint, suspected or reported diagnosis Except: Z00.6
Z01	Encounter for other special examination without complaint, suspected or reported diagnosis
Z02	Encounter for administrative examination
Z03	Encounter for medical observation for suspected diseases and conditions ruled out
Z04	Encounter for examination and observation for other reasons
Z33.2	Encounter for elective termination of pregnancy
Z31.81	Encounter for male factor infertility in female patient
Z31.83	Encounter for assisted reproductive fertility procedure cycle
Z31.84	Encounter for fertility preservation procedure
Z34	Encounter for supervision of normal pregnancy
Z39	Encounter for maternal postpartum care and examination
Z38	Liveborn infants according to place of birth and type of delivery
Z40	Encounter for prophylactic surgery
Z42	Encounter for plastic and reconstructive surgery following medical procedure or healed injury
Z51.0	Encounter for antineoplastic radiation therapy
Z51.1-	Encounter for antineoplastic chemotherapy and immunotherapy
Z52	Donors of organs and tissues Except: Z52.9, Donor of unspecified organ or tissue
Z76.1	Encounter for health supervision and care of foundling
Z76.2	Encounter for health supervision and care of other healthy infant and child
Z99.12	Encounter for respirator [ventilator] dependence during power failure

CHAPTER 21

FACTORS INFLUENCING HEALTH STATUS AND CONTACT WITH HEALTH SERVICES (Z00-Z99)

Note: Z codes represent reasons for encounters. A corresponding procedure code must accompany a Z code if a procedure is performed. Categories Z00-Z99 are provided for occasions when circumstances other than a disease, injury or external cause classifiable to categories A00-Y89 are recorded as "diagnoses" or "problems." This can arise in two main ways:

(a) When a person who may or may not be sick encounters the health services for some specific purpose, such as to receive limited care or service for a current condition, to donate an organ or tissue, to receive prophylactic vaccination (immunization), or to discuss a problem which is in itself not a disease or injury.

(b) When some circumstance or problem is present which influences the person's health status but is not in itself a current illness or injury.

This chapter contains the following blocks:

Z00-Z13	Persons encountering health services for examination
Z14-Z15	Genetic carrier and genetic susceptibility to disease
Z16	Resistance to antimicrobial drugs
Z17	Estrogen receptor status
Z18	Retained foreign body fragments
Z19	Hormone sensitivity malignancy status
Z20-Z29	Persons with potential health hazards related to communicable diseases
Z30-Z39	Persons encountering health services in circumstances related to reproduction
Z40-Z53	Encounters for other specific health care
Z55-Z65	Persons with potential health hazards related to socioeconomic and psychosocial circumstances
Z66	Do not resuscitate status
Z67	Blood type
Z68	Body mass index (BMI)
Z69-Z76	Persons encountering health services in other circumstances
Z77-Z99	Persons with potential health hazards related to family and personal history and certain conditions influencing health status

PERSONS ENCOUNTERING HEALTH SERVICES FOR EXAMINATIONS (Z00-Z13)

Note: Nonspecific abnormal findings disclosed at the time of these examinations are classified to categories R70-R94.

Excludes1 examinations related to pregnancy and reproduction (Z30-Z36, Z39.-)

● **Z00**   **Encounter for general examination without complaint, suspected or reported diagnosis**

    Excludes1 encounter for examination for administrative purposes (Z02.-)

    Excludes2 encounter for pre-procedural examinations (Z01.81-)
                special screening examinations (Z11-Z13)

● **Z00.0**   **Encounter for general adult medical examination**

    Encounter for adult periodic examination (annual) (physical) and any associated laboratory and radiologic examinations

    Excludes1 encounter for examination of sign or symptom - code to sign or symptom general health check-up of infant or child (Z00.12-)

    Coding Clinic: 2016, Q4, P131

    Z00.00   **Encounter for general adult medical examination without abnormal findings**   A
            Encounter for adult health check-up NOS
            Coding Clinic: 2017, Q4, P95; 2016, Q1, P37

    Z00.01   **Encounter for general adult medical examination with abnormal findings**   A
            Use additional code to identify abnormal findings
            Coding Clinic: 2016, Q1, P36

● **Z00.1**   **Encounter for newborn, infant and child health examinations**

    ● **Z00.11**   **Newborn health examination**
            Health check for child under 29 days old
            Use additional code to identify any abnormal findings

            Excludes1 health check for child over 28 days old (Z00.12-)

        Z00.110   **Health examination for newborn under 8 days old**   N
            Health check for newborn under 8 days old

        Z00.111   **Health examination for newborn 8 to 28 days old**   N
            Health check for newborn 8 to 28 days old
            Newborn weight check

    ● **Z00.12**   **Encounter for routine child health examination**
            Immunizations appropriate for age
            Health check (routine) for child over 28 days old
            Routine developmental screening of infant or child
            Routine vision and hearing testing

            Excludes1 health check for child under 29 days old (Z00.11-)
                  health supervision of foundling or other healthy infant or child (Z76.1-Z76.2)
                  newborn health examination (Z00.11-)

        Z00.121   **Encounter for routine child health examination with abnormal findings**   P
            Use additional code to identify abnormal findings
            Coding Clinic: 2017, Q4, P95; 2016, Q1, P34-35

        Z00.129   **Encounter for routine child health examination without abnormal findings**   P
            Encounter for routine child health examination NOS
            Coding Clinic: 2016, Q1, P34

   Z00.2   **Encounter for examination for period of rapid growth in childhood**   P

   Z00.3   **Encounter for examination for adolescent development state**   P
        Encounter for puberty development state

   Z00.5   **Encounter for examination of potential donor of organ and tissue**

   Z00.6   **Encounter for examination for normal comparison and control in clinical research program**
        Examination of participant or control in clinical research program

● **Z00.7**   **Encounter for examination for period of delayed growth in childhood**

    Z00.70   **Encounter for examination for period of delayed growth in childhood without abnormal findings**   P

    Z00.71   **Encounter for examination for period of delayed growth in childhood with abnormal findings**   P
        Use additional code to identify abnormal findings

   Z00.8   **Encounter for other general examination**
        Encounter for health examination in population surveys

▶ New   ⇢ Revised   ~~deleted~~ Deleted   Excludes 1   Excludes 2   Includes   Use additional   Code first   Code also   Key words

OGCR Official Guidelines   X Assign placeholder X   ● Use Additional Character(s)   ▶ Manifestation Code   🏷 Hierarchical Condition Category   **Coding Clinic**

● **Z01   Encounter for other special examination without complaint, suspected or reported diagnosis**

> **Includes**   routine examination of specific system

> **Note:** Codes from category Z01 represent the reason for the encounter. A separate procedure code is required to identify any examinations or procedures performed.

> **Excludes1**   encounter for examination for administrative purposes (Z02.-)
> encounter for examination for suspected conditions, proven not to exist (Z03.-)
> encounter for laboratory and radiologic examinations as a component of general medical examinations (Z00.0-)
> encounter for laboratory, radiologic and imaging examinations for sign(s) and symptom(s) - code to the sign(s) or symptom(s)

> **Excludes2**   screening examinations (Z11-Z13)

● **Z01.0   Encounter for examination of eyes and vision**

> **Excludes1**   examination for driving license (Z02.4)

> **Z01.00   Encounter for examination of eyes and vision without abnormal findings**
> > Encounter for examination of eyes and vision NOS

> **Z01.01   Encounter for examination of eyes and vision with abnormal findings**
> > Use additional code to identify abnormal findings
> > **Coding Clinic: 2016, Q4, P21**

> ● **Z01.02   Encounter for examination of eyes and vision following failed vision screening**
> > **➡Excludes1**   encounter for examination of eyes and vision with abnormal findings (Z01.01)
> > ➡encounter for examination of eyes and vision without abnormal findings (Z01.00)

> > ● **Z01.020   Encounter for examination of eyes and vision following failed vision screening without abnormal findings**

> > ● **Z01.021   Encounter for examination of eyes and vision following failed vision screening with abnormal findings**
> > > Use additional code to identify abnormal findings

● **Z01.1   Encounter for examination of ears and hearing**

> **Z01.10   Encounter for examination of ears and hearing without abnormal findings**
> > Encounter for examination of ears and hearing NOS
> > **Coding Clinic: 2016, Q4, P25**

> ● **Z01.11   Encounter for examination of ears and hearing with abnormal findings**
> > **Coding Clinic: 2016, Q3, P18**

> > **Z01.110   Encounter for hearing examination following failed hearing screening**
> > > **Coding Clinic: 2016, Q3, P18-19**

> > **Z01.118   Encounter for examination of ears and hearing with other abnormal findings**
> > > Use additional code to identify abnormal findings
> > > **Coding Clinic: 2016, Q3, P17**

> **Z01.12   Encounter for hearing conservation and treatment**

● **Z01.2   Encounter for dental examination and cleaning**

> **Z01.20   Encounter for dental examination and cleaning without abnormal findings**
> > Encounter for dental examination and cleaning NOS

> **Z01.21   Encounter for dental examination and cleaning with abnormal findings**
> > Use additional code to identify abnormal findings

● **Z01.3   Encounter for examination of blood pressure**

> **Z01.30   Encounter for examination of blood pressure without abnormal findings**
> > Encounter for examination of blood pressure NOS

> **Z01.31   Encounter for examination of blood pressure with abnormal findings**
> > Use additional code to identify abnormal findings

● **Z01.4   Encounter for gynecological examination**

> **Excludes2**   pregnancy examination or test (Z32.0-)
> routine examination for contraceptive maintenance (Z30.4-)

> ● **Z01.41   Encounter for routine gynecological examination**
> > Encounter for general gynecological examination with or without cervical smear
> > Encounter for gynecological examination (general) (routine) NOS
> > Encounter for pelvic examination (annual) (periodic)
> > Use additional code:
> > > for screening for human papillomavirus, if applicable (Z11.51)
> > > for screening vaginal pap smear, if applicable (Z12.72)
> > > to identify acquired absence of uterus, if applicable (Z90.71-)

> > **Excludes1**   gynecologic examination status-post hysterectomy for malignant condition (Z08)
> > screening cervical pap smear not a part of a routine gynecological examination (Z12.4)

> > **Z01.411   Encounter for gynecological examination (general) (routine) with abnormal findings ♀**
> > > Use additional code to identify any abnormal findings

> > **Z01.419   Encounter for gynecological examination (general) (routine) without abnormal findings ♀**

> **Z01.42   Encounter for cervical smear to confirm findings of recent normal smear following initial abnormal smear ♀**

● **Z01.8   Encounter for other specified special examinations**

> ● **Z01.81   Encounter for preprocedural examinations**
> > Encounter for preoperative examinations
> > Encounter for radiological and imaging examinations as part of preprocedural examination

> > **Z01.810   Encounter for preprocedural cardiovascular examination**

> > **Z01.811   Encounter for preprocedural respiratory examination**

> > **Z01.812   Encounter for preprocedural laboratory examination**
> > > Blood and urine tests prior to treatment or procedure
> > > **Coding Clinic: 2021, Q1, P38**

> > **Z01.818   Encounter for other preprocedural examination**
> > > Encounter for preprocedural examination NOS
> > > Encounter for examinations prior to antineoplastic chemotherapy

> **Z01.82   Encounter for allergy testing**
> > **Excludes1**   encounter for antibody response examination (Z01.84)

> **Z01.83   Encounter for blood typing**
> > Encounter for Rh typing

CHAPTER 21 (Z00-Z99)

Z01.84   Encounter for antibody response examination
Encounter for immunity status testing

> **Excludes1**   encounter for allergy testing (Z01.82)

Z01.89   Encounter for other specified special examinations

● **Z02   Encounter for administrative examination**

Z02.0   Encounter for examination for admission to educational institution
Encounter for examination for admission to preschool (education)
Encounter for examination for re-admission to school following illness or medical treatment

Z02.1   Encounter for pre-employment examination

Z02.2   Encounter for examination for admission to residential institution

> **Excludes1**   examination for admission to prison (Z02.89)

Z02.3   Encounter for examination for recruitment to armed forces

Z02.4   Encounter for examination for driving license

Z02.5   Encounter for examination for participation in sport

> **Excludes1**   blood-alcohol and blood-drug test (Z02.83)

Z02.6   Encounter for examination for insurance purposes

● **Z02.7   Encounter for issue of medical certificate**

> **Excludes1**   encounter for general medical examination (Z00-Z01, Z02.0-Z02.6, Z02.8-Z02.9)

Z02.71   Encounter for disability determination
Encounter for issue of medical certificate of incapacity
Encounter for issue of medical certificate of invalidity

Z02.79   Encounter for issue of other medical certificate

● **Z02.8   Encounter for other administrative examinations**

Z02.81   Encounter for paternity testing

Z02.82   Encounter for adoption services

Z02.83   Encounter for blood-alcohol and blood-drug test
Use additional code for findings of alcohol or drugs in blood (R78.-)

Z02.89   Encounter for other administrative examinations
Encounter for examination for admission to prison
Encounter for examination for admission to summer camp
Encounter for immigration examination
Encounter for naturalization examination
Encounter for premarital examination

> **Excludes1**   health supervision of foundling or other healthy infant or child (Z76.1-Z76.2)

Z02.9   Encounter for administrative examinations, unspecified

OGCR Section II.C.21.c.6.

Observation

There are three observation Z code categories. They are for use in very limited circumstances when a person is being observed for a suspected condition that is ruled out. The observation codes are not for use if an injury or illnesses or any signs or symptoms related to the suspected condition are present. In such cases the diagnosis/symptom code is used with the corresponding external cause code.

The observation codes are to be used as principal diagnosis only. The only exception to this is when the principal diagnosis is required to be a code from category Z38, Liveborn infants according to place of birth and type of delivery. Then a code from category Z05, Encounter for observation and evaluation of newborn for suspected diseases and conditions ruled out, is sequenced after the Z38 code. Additional codes may be used in addition to the observation code but only if they are unrelated to the suspected condition being observed.

Codes from subcategory Z03.7 Encounter for suspected maternal and fetal conditions ruled out, may either be used as a first listed or as an additional code assignment depending on the case. They are for use in very limited circumstances on a maternal record when an encounter is for a suspected maternal or fetal condition that is ruled out during that encounter (for example, a maternal or fetal condition may be suspected due to an abnormal test result). These codes should not be used when the condition is confirmed. In those cases, the confirmed condition should be coded. In addition, these codes are not for use if an illness or any signs or symptoms related to the suspected condition or problem are present. In such cases the diagnosis/symptom code is used.

Additional codes may be used in addition to the code from subcategory Z03.7, but only if they are unrelated to the suspected condition being evaluated.

Codes from subcategory Z03.7 may not be used for encounters for antenatal screening of mother. *See Section I.C.21. Screening.*

For encounters for suspected fetal condition that are inconclusive following testing and evaluation, assign the appropriate code from category O35, O36, O40 or O41.

The observation Z code categories:

Z03   Encounter for medical observation for suspected diseases and conditions ruled out

Z04   Encounter for examination and observation for other reasons Except: Z04.9, Encounter for examination and observation for unspecified reason

Z05   Encounter for observation and evaluation of newborn for suspected diseases and conditions ruled out

● **Z03   Encounter for medical observation for suspected diseases and conditions ruled out**
This category is to be used when a person without a diagnosis is suspected of having an abnormal condition, without signs or symptoms, which requires study, but after examination and observation, is ruled out. This category is also for use for administrative and legal observation status.

> **Excludes1**   contact with and (suspected) exposures hazardous to health (Z77.-)
> encounter for observation and evaluation of newborn for suspected diseases and conditions ruled out (Z05.-)
> person with feared complaint in whom no diagnosis is made (Z71.1)
> signs or symptoms under study - code to signs or symptoms

Z03.6   Encounter for observation for suspected toxic effect from ingested substance ruled out
Encounter for observation for suspected adverse effect from drug
Encounter for observation for suspected poisoning

▶ New   ⇒ Revised   ~~deleted~~ Deleted   Excludes 1   Excludes 2   Includes   Use additional   Code first   Code also   Key words
OGCR Official Guidelines   X Assign placeholder X   ● Use Additional Character(s)   ▶ Manifestation Code   🦋 Hierarchical Condition Category   **Coding Clinic**

● **Z03.7** Encounter for suspected maternal and fetal conditions ruled out

　　Encounter for suspected maternal and fetal conditions not found

　　Excludes1　known or suspected fetal anomalies affecting management of mother, not ruled out (O26.-, O35.-, O36.-, O40.-, O41.-)

Z03.71 Encounter for suspected problem with amniotic cavity and membrane ruled out ♀　　　　**M**

　　　Encounter for suspected oligohydramnios ruled out

　　　Encounter for suspected polyhydramnios ruled out

Z03.72 Encounter for suspected placental problem ruled out ♀　　　　　　　　　　　　**M**

Z03.73 Encounter for suspected fetal anomaly ruled out ♀　　　　　　　　　　　　**M**

　　　Coding Clinic: 2016, Q4, P6

Z03.74 Encounter for suspected problem with fetal growth ruled out ♀　　　　　　　**M**

Z03.75 Encounter for suspected cervical shortening ruled out ♀　　　　　　　　　**M**

Z03.79 Encounter for other suspected maternal and fetal conditions ruled out ♀　　　**M**

　　　Coding Clinic: 2016, Q4, P7

● **Z03.8** Encounter for observation for other suspected diseases and conditions ruled out

　● **Z03.81** Encounter for observation for suspected exposure to biological agents ruled out

　　　Z03.810 Encounter for observation for suspected exposure to anthrax ruled out

　　　Z03.818 Encounter for observation for suspected exposure to other biological agents ruled out

　● **Z03.82** Encounter for observation for suspected foreign body ruled out

　　　Excludes1　retained foreign body (Z18.-)
　　　　　　　　retained foreign body in eyelid (H02.81)
　　　　　　　　residual foreign body in soft tissue (M79.5)

　　　Excludes2　confirmed foreign body ingestion or aspiration including:
　　　　　　　　foreign body in alimentary tract (T18)
　　　　　　　　foreign body in ear (T16)
　　　　　　　　foreign body on external eye (T15)
　　　　　　　　foreign body in respiratory tract (T17)

　　　Z03.821 Encounter for observation for suspected ingested foreign body ruled out

　　　Z03.822 Encounter for observation for suspected aspirated (inhaled) foreign body ruled out

　　　Z03.823 Encounter for observation for suspected inserted (injected) foreign body ruled out

　　　　　Encounter for observation for suspected inserted (injected) foreign body in eye ruled out
　　　　　Encounter for observation for suspected inserted (injected) foreign body in orifice ruled out
　　　　　Encounter for observation for suspected inserted (injected) foreign body in skin ruled out

　Z03.89 Encounter for observation for other suspected diseases and conditions ruled out

● **Z04** Encounter for examination and observation for other reasons

　　Includes　encounter for examination for medicolegal reasons

　　　This category is to be used when a person without a diagnosis is suspected of having an abnormal condition, without signs or symptoms, which requires study, but after examination and observation, is ruled-out. This category is also for use for administrative and legal observation status.

Z04.1 Encounter for examination and observation following transport accident

　　Excludes1　encounter for examination and observation following work accident (Z04.2)

　　　Coding Clinic: 2019, Q2, P11

Z04.2 Encounter for examination and observation following work accident

Z04.3 Encounter for examination and observation following other accident

● **Z04.4** Encounter for examination and observation following alleged rape

　　Encounter for examination and observation of victim following alleged rape

　　Encounter for examination and observation of victim following alleged sexual abuse

　　Coding Clinic: 2016, Q4, P129

Z04.41 Encounter for examination and observation following alleged adult rape　　**A**

　　　Suspected adult rape, ruled out
　　　Suspected adult sexual abuse, ruled out

Z04.42 Encounter for examination and observation following alleged child rape　　**P**

　　　Suspected child rape, ruled out
　　　Suspected child sexual abuse, ruled out

Z04.6 Encounter for general psychiatric examination, requested by authority

● **Z04.7** Encounter for examination and observation following alleged physical abuse

Z04.71 Encounter for examination and observation following alleged adult physical abuse　　**A**

　　　Suspected adult physical abuse, ruled out

　　　Excludes1　confirmed case of adult physical abuse (T74.-)
　　　　　　　　encounter for examination and observation following alleged adult sexual abuse (Z04.41)
　　　　　　　　suspected case of adult physical abuse, not ruled out (T76.-)

Z04.72 Encounter for examination and observation following alleged child physical abuse　　**P**

　　　Suspected child physical abuse, ruled out

　　　Excludes1　confirmed case of child physical abuse (T74.-)
　　　　　　　　encounter for examination and observation following alleged child sexual abuse (Z04.42)
　　　　　　　　suspected case of child physical abuse, not ruled out (T76.-)

● **Z04.8** Encounter for examination and observation for other specified reasons

　　Encounter for examination and observation for request for expert evidence

Z04.81 Encounter for examination and observation of victim following forced sexual exploitation

Z04.82 Encounter for examination and observation of victim following forced labor exploitation

Z04.89 Encounter for examination and observation for other specified reasons

Z04.9 Encounter for examination and observation for unspecified reason

　　Encounter for observation NOS

CHAPTER 21 (Z00-Z99)

● **Z05   Encounter for observation and evaluation of newborn for suspected diseases and conditions ruled out**
This category is to be used for newborns, within the neonatal period (the first 28 days of life), who are suspected of having an abnormal condition, but without signs or symptoms, and which, after examination and observation, is ruled out.
Coding Clinic: 2019, Q2, P11; 2016, Q4, P54, 77, 126-127, 130

Z05.0   Observation and evaluation of newborn for suspected **cardiac** condition ruled out   N

Z05.1   Observation and evaluation of newborn for suspected **infectious** condition ruled out   N
Coding Clinic: 2019, Q2, P11

Z05.2   Observation and evaluation of newborn for suspected **neurological** condition ruled out   N

Z05.3   Observation and evaluation of newborn for suspected **respiratory** condition ruled out   N

● Z05.4   Observation and evaluation of newborn for suspected genetic, metabolic or immunologic condition ruled out

　　Z05.41   Observation and evaluation of newborn for suspected **genetic** condition ruled out   N
　　　　Coding Clinic: 2016, Q4, P55

　　Z05.42   Observation and evaluation of newborn for suspected **metabolic** condition ruled out   N

　　Z05.43   Observation and evaluation of newborn for suspected **immunologic** condition ruled out   N

Z05.5   Observation and evaluation of newborn for suspected **gastrointestinal** condition ruled out   N

Z05.6   Observation and evaluation of newborn for suspected **genitourinary** condition ruled out   N

● Z05.7   Observation and evaluation of newborn for suspected skin, subcutaneous, musculoskeletal and connective tissue condition ruled out

　　Z05.71   Observation and evaluation of newborn for suspected **skin and subcutaneous tissue** condition ruled out   N

　　Z05.72   Observation and evaluation of newborn for suspected **musculoskeletal** condition ruled out   N

　　Z05.73   Observation and evaluation of newborn for suspected **connective tissue** condition ruled out   N

Z05.8   Observation and evaluation of newborn for **other specified** suspected condition ruled out   N

Z05.9   Observation and evaluation of newborn for **unspecified** suspected condition ruled out   N

OGCR   See Section II.C.21.c.8.

The follow-up codes are used to explain continuing surveillance following completed treatment of a disease, condition, or injury. They imply that the condition has been fully treated and no longer exists. They should not be confused with aftercare codes, or injury codes with 7th character "D," that explain ongoing care of a healing condition or its sequelae. Follow-up codes may be used in conjunction with history codes to provide the full picture of the healed condition and its treatment. The follow-up code is sequenced first, followed by the history code.

A follow-up code may be used to explain multiple visits. Should a condition be found to have recurred on the follow-up visit, then the diagnosis code for the condition should be assigned in place of the follow-up code.

The follow-up Z code categories:

Z08   Encounter for follow-up examination after completed treatment for malignant neoplasm

Z09   Encounter for follow-up examination after completed treatment for conditions other than malignant neoplasm

Z39   Encounter for maternal postpartum care and examination

Z08   **Encounter for follow-up examination after completed treatment for malignant neoplasm**
Medical surveillance following completed treatment
Use additional code to identify any acquired absence of organs (Z90.-)
Use additional code to identify the personal history of malignant neoplasm (Z85.-)
Excludes1   aftercare following medical care (Z43-Z49, Z51)

Z09   **Encounter for follow-up examination after completed treatment for conditions other than malignant neoplasm**
Medical surveillance following completed treatment
⏩Use additional code to identify any applicable history of disease code (Z86.-, Z87.-)
Excludes1   aftercare following medical care (Z43-Z49, Z51)
　　　　surveillance of contraception (Z30.4-)
　　　　surveillance of prosthetic and other medical devices (Z44-Z46)
Coding Clinic: 2021, Q1, P33; 2017, Q1, P9; 2015, Q1, P8

OGCR   Section II.C.21.c.5.

Screening

Screening is the testing for disease or disease precursors in seemingly well individuals so that early detection and treatment can be provided for those who test positive for the disease (e.g., screening mammogram).

The testing of a person to rule out or confirm a suspected diagnosis because the patient has some sign or symptom is a diagnostic examination, not a screening. In these cases, the sign or symptom is used to explain the reason for the test.

A screening code may be a first listed code if the reason for the visit is specifically the screening exam. It may also be used as an additional code if the screening is done during an office visit for other health problems. A screening code is not necessary if the screening is inherent to a routine examination, such as a pap smear done during a routine pelvic examination.

Should a condition be discovered during the screening then the code for the condition may be assigned as an additional diagnosis.

The Z code indicates that a screening exam is planned. A procedure code is required to confirm that the screening was performed.

The screening Z codes/categories:

Z11   Encounter for screening for infectious and parasitic diseases

Z12   Encounter for screening for malignant neoplasms

Z13   Encounter for screening for other diseases and disorders
Except: Z13.9, Encounter for screening, unspecified

Z36   Encounter for antenatal screening for mother

● Z11   **Encounter for screening for infectious and parasitic diseases**
Screening is the testing for disease or disease precursors in asymptomatic individuals so that early detection and treatment can be provided for those who test positive for the disease.
Excludes1   encounter for diagnostic examination - code to sign or symptom

Z11.0   **Encounter for screening for intestinal infectious diseases**
Encounter for screening for active tuberculosis disease

Z11.1   **Encounter for screening for respiratory tuberculosis**

Z11.2   **Encounter for screening for other bacterial diseases**

Z11.3   **Encounter for screening for infections with a predominantly sexual mode of transmission**
Excludes2   encounter for screening for human immunodeficiency virus [HIV] (Z11.4)
　　　　encounter for screening for human papillomavirus (Z11.51)

Z11.4   **Encounter for screening for human immunodeficiency virus [HIV]**

▶ New   ⏩ Revised   ~~deleted~~ Deleted   Excludes 1   Excludes 2   Includes   Use additional   Code first   Code also   Key words
OGCR Official Guidelines   X Assign placeholder X   ● Use Additional Character(s)   ▶ Manifestation Code   🅒 Hierarchical Condition Category   Coding Clinic

● **Z11.5**   Encounter for screening for other viral diseases

> **Excludes2**   encounter for screening for viral intestinal disease (Z11.0)

   Z11.51   Encounter for screening for human papillomavirus (HPV)

   Z11.52   Encounter for screening for COVID-19
> Coding Clinic: 2021, Q1, P37, 42

   Z11.59   Encounter for screening for other viral diseases
> Coding Clinic: 2021, Q1, P37

Z11.6   Encounter for screening for other protozoal diseases and helminthiases
> *Diseases or infestations caused by parasitic worms*

> **Excludes2**   encounter for screening for protozoal intestinal disease (Z11.0)

Z11.7   Encounter for testing for latent tuberculosis infection

Z11.8   Encounter for screening for other infectious and parasitic diseases
> Encounter for screening for chlamydia
> Encounter for screening for rickettsial
> Encounter for screening for spirochetal
> Encounter for screening for mycoses

Z11.9   Encounter for screening for infectious and parasitic diseases, unspecified

● **Z12**   Encounter for screening for malignant neoplasms
> Screening is the testing for disease or disease precursors in asymptomatic individuals so that early detection and treatment can be provided for those who test positive for the disease.
>
> Use additional code to identify any family history of malignant neoplasm (Z80.-)

> **Excludes1**   encounter for diagnostic examination - code to sign or symptom

Z12.0   Encounter for screening for malignant neoplasm of stomach

● **Z12.1**   Encounter for screening for malignant neoplasm of intestinal tract

   Z12.10   Encounter for screening for malignant neoplasm of intestinal tract, unspecified

   Z12.11   Encounter for screening for malignant neoplasm of colon
> Encounter for screening colonoscopy NOS
> Coding Clinic: 2018, Q1, P7; 2017, Q1, P8-9

   Z12.12   Encounter for screening for malignant neoplasm of rectum

   Z12.13   Encounter for screening for malignant neoplasm of small intestine

Z12.2   Encounter for screening for malignant neoplasm of respiratory organs

● **Z12.3**   Encounter for screening for malignant neoplasm of breast

   Z12.31   Encounter for screening mammogram for malignant neoplasm of breast

> **Excludes1**   inconclusive mammogram (R92.2)
> Coding Clinic: 2015, Q1, P24

   Z12.39   Encounter for other screening for malignant neoplasm of breast

Z12.4   Encounter for screening for malignant neoplasm of cervix ♀
> Encounter for screening pap smear for malignant neoplasm of cervix

> **Excludes1**   when screening is part of general gynecological examination (Z01.4-)

> **Excludes2**   encounter for screening for human papillomavirus (Z11.51)

Z12.5   Encounter for screening for malignant neoplasm of prostate ♂

Z12.6   Encounter for screening for malignant neoplasm of bladder

● **Z12.7**   Encounter for screening for malignant neoplasm of other genitourinary organs

   Z12.71   Encounter for screening for malignant neoplasm of testis ♂

   Z12.72   Encounter for screening for malignant neoplasm of vagina ♀
> Vaginal pap smear status - post hysterectomy for non-malignant condition
> Use additional code to identify acquired absence of uterus (Z90.71-)

> **Excludes1**   vaginal pap smear status - post hysterectomy for malignant conditions (Z08)

   Z12.73   Encounter for screening for malignant neoplasm of ovary ♀

   Z12.79   Encounter for screening for malignant neoplasm of other genitourinary organs

● **Z12.8**   Encounter for screening for malignant neoplasm of other sites

   Z12.81   Encounter for screening for malignant neoplasm of oral cavity

   Z12.82   Encounter for screening for malignant neoplasm of nervous system

   Z12.83   Encounter for screening for malignant neoplasm of skin

   Z12.89   Encounter for screening for malignant neoplasm of other sites
> Coding Clinic: 2021, Q1, P15

Z12.9   Encounter for screening for malignant neoplasm, site unspecified

● **Z13**   Encounter for screening for other diseases and disorders
> Screening is the testing for disease or disease precursors in asymptomatic individuals so that early detection and treatment can be provided for those who test positive for the disease.

> **Excludes1**   encounter for diagnostic examination - code to sign or symptom

Z13.0   Encounter for screening for diseases of the blood and blood-forming organs and certain disorders involving the immune mechanism

Z13.1   Encounter for screening for diabetes mellitus

● **Z13.2**   Encounter for screening for nutritional, metabolic and other endocrine disorders

   Z13.21   Encounter for screening for nutritional disorder

   ● **Z13.22**   Encounter for screening for metabolic disorder

     Z13.220   Encounter for screening for lipoid disorders
> Encounter for screening for cholesterol level
> Encounter for screening for hypercholesterolemia
> Encounter for screening for hyperlipidemia

     Z13.228   Encounter for screening for other metabolic disorders

   Z13.29   Encounter for screening for other suspected endocrine disorder

> ~~Excludes1   encounter for screening for diabetes mellitus (Z13.1)~~

> ▶ **Excludes2**   encounter for screening for diabetes mellitus (Z13.1)

● **Z13.3**   Encounter for screening examination for mental health and behavioral disorders

   Z13.30   Encounter for screening examination for mental health and behavioral disorders, unspecified

   Z13.31   Encounter for screening for depression
> Encounter for screening for depression, adult
> Encounter for screening for depression for child or adolescent

Z13.32 Encounter for screening for maternal depression ♀
    Encounter for screening for perinatal depression

Z13.39 Encounter for screening examination for other mental health and behavioral disorders
    Encounter for screening for alcoholism
    Encounter for screening for intellectual disabilities

● **Z13.4** Encounter for screening for certain developmental disorders in childhood   P
    Encounter for development testing of infant or child
    Encounter for screening for developmental handicaps in early childhood
    Excludes2   encounter for routine child health examination (Z00.12-)

Z13.40 Encounter for screening for unspecified developmental delays

Z13.41 Encounter for autism screening

Z13.42 Encounter for screening for global developmental delays (milestones)
    Encounter for screening for developmental handicaps in early childhood

Z13.49 Encounter for screening for other developmental delays

Z13.5 Encounter for screening for eye and ear disorders
    Excludes2   encounter for general hearing examination (Z01.1-)
        encounter for general vision examination (Z01.0-)
    Coding Clinic: 2016, Q3, P17

Z13.6 Encounter for screening for cardiovascular disorders

● **Z13.7** Encounter for screening for genetic and chromosomal anomalies
    Excludes1   genetic testing for procreative management (Z31.4-)

Z13.71 Encounter for nonprocreative screening for genetic disease carrier status

Z13.79 Encounter for other screening for genetic and chromosomal anomalies

● **Z13.8** Encounter for screening for other specified diseases and disorders
    Excludes2   screening for malignant neoplasms (Z12.-)

● **Z13.81** Encounter for screening for digestive system disorders

    Z13.810 Encounter for screening for upper gastrointestinal disorder

    Z13.811 Encounter for screening for lower gastrointestinal disorder
        Excludes1   encounter for screening for intestinal infectious disease (Z11.0)

    Z13.818 Encounter for screening for other digestive system disorders

● **Z13.82** Encounter for screening for musculoskeletal disorder

    Z13.820 Encounter for screening for osteoporosis

    Z13.828 Encounter for screening for other musculoskeletal disorder

Z13.83 Encounter for screening for respiratory disorder NEC
    Excludes1   encounter for screening for respiratory tuberculosis (Z11.1)

Z13.84 Encounter for screening for dental disorders

● **Z13.85** Encounter for screening for nervous system disorders

    Z13.850 Encounter for screening for traumatic brain injury

    Z13.858 Encounter for screening for other nervous system disorders

Z13.88 Encounter for screening for disorder due to exposure to contaminants
    Excludes1   those exposed to contaminants without suspected disorders (Z57-Z77.-)

Z13.89 Encounter for screening for other disorder
    Encounter for screening for genitourinary disorders

Z13.9 Encounter for screening, unspecified

GENETIC CARRIER AND GENETIC SUSCEPTIBILITY TO DISEASE (Z14-Z15)

● **Z14** Genetic carrier

● **Z14.0** Hemophilia A carrier

    Z14.01 Asymptomatic hemophilia A carrier

    Z14.02 Symptomatic hemophilia A carrier

Z14.1 Cystic fibrosis carrier

Z14.8 Genetic carrier of other disease

● **Z15** Genetic susceptibility to disease
    Excludes1   chromosomal anomalies (Q90-Q99)
    Includes   confirmed abnormal gene
    Use additional code, if applicable, for any associated family history of the disease (Z80-Z84)

● **Z15.0** Genetic susceptibility to malignant neoplasm
    Code first if applicable, any current malignant neoplasm (C00-C75, C81-C96)
    Use additional code, if applicable, for any personal history of malignant neoplasm (Z85.-)

    Z15.01 Genetic susceptibility to malignant neoplasm of breast

    Z15.02 Genetic susceptibility to malignant neoplasm of ovary ♀

    Z15.03 Genetic susceptibility to malignant neoplasm of prostate ♂

    Z15.04 Genetic susceptibility to malignant neoplasm of endometrium ♀

    Z15.09 Genetic susceptibility to other malignant neoplasm
        Coding Clinic: 2021, Q1, P15

● **Z15.8** Genetic susceptibility to other disease

    Z15.81 Genetic susceptibility to multiple endocrine neoplasia [MEN]
        Excludes1   multiple endocrine neoplasia [MEN] syndromes (E31.2-)

    Z15.89 Genetic susceptibility to other disease

RESISTANCE TO ANTIMICROBIAL DRUGS (Z16)

● **Z16** Resistance to antimicrobial drugs
    Note: The codes in this category are provided for use as additional codes to identify the resistance and non-responsiveness of a condition to antimicrobial drugs.
    Code first the infection
    Excludes1   Methicillin resistant Staphylococcus aureus infection (A49.02)
        Methicillin resistant Staphylococcus aureus pneumonia (J15.212)
        Sepsis due to Methicillin resistant Staphylococcus aureus (A41.02)

CHAPTER 21 (Z00-Z99)

▶ New   ⇒ Revised   ~~deleted~~ Deleted   Excludes 1   Excludes 2   Includes   Use additional   Code first   Code also   Key words
OGCR Official Guidelines   X Assign placeholder X   ● Use Additional Character(s)   ▶ Manifestation Code   Hierarchical Condition Category   Coding Clinic

● **Z16.1   Resistance to beta lactam antibiotics**
Z16.10   Resistance to unspecified beta lactam antibiotics
Z16.11   Resistance to penicillins
Resistance to amoxicillin
Resistance to ampicillin
Z16.12   Extended spectrum beta lactamase (ESBL) resistance
Excludes2   Methicillin resistant Staphylococcus aureus infection in diseases classified elsewhere (B95.62)
Z16.19   Resistance to other specified beta lactam antibiotics
Resistance to cephalosporins

● **Z16.2   Resistance to other antibiotics**
Z16.20   Resistance to unspecified antibiotic
Resistance to antibiotics NOS
Z16.21   Resistance to vancomycin
Z16.22   Resistance to vancomycin related antibiotics
Z16.23   Resistance to quinolones and fluoroquinolones
Z16.24   Resistance to multiple antibiotics
Z16.29   Resistance to other single specified antibiotic
Resistance to aminoglycosides
Resistance to macrolides
Resistance to sulfonamides
Resistance to tetracyclines

● **Z16.3   Resistance to other antimicrobial drugs**
Excludes1   resistance to antibiotics (Z16.1-, Z16.2-)
Z16.30   Resistance to unspecified antimicrobial drugs
Drug resistance NOS
Z16.31   Resistance to antiparasitic drug(s)
Resistance to quinine and related compounds
Z16.32   Resistance to antifungal drug(s)
Z16.33   Resistance to antiviral drug(s)
● Z16.34   Resistance to antimycobacterial drug(s)
Resistance to tuberculostatics
Z16.341   Resistance to single antimycobacterial drug
Resistance to antimycobacterial drug NOS
Z16.342   Resistance to multiple antimycobacterial drugs
Z16.35   Resistance to multiple antimicrobial drugs
Excludes1   Resistance to multiple antibiotics only (Z16.24)
Z16.39   Resistance to other specified antimicrobial drug

ESTROGEN RECEPTOR STATUS (Z17)

● **Z17   Estrogen receptor status**
Code first malignant neoplasm of breast (C50.-)
Z17.0   Estrogen receptor positive status [ER+]
Z17.1   Estrogen receptor negative status [ER-]

RETAINED FOREIGN BODY FRAGMENTS (Z18)

● **Z18   Retained foreign body fragments**
Includes   embedded fragment (status)
embedded splinter (status)
retained foreign body status
Excludes1   artificial joint prosthesis status (Z96.6-)
foreign body accidentally left during a procedure (T81.5-)
foreign body entering through orifice (T15-T19)
in situ cardiac device (Z95.-)
organ or tissue replaced by means other than transplant (Z96.-, Z97.-)
organ or tissue replaced by transplant (Z94.-)
personal history of retained foreign body fully removed Z87.821
superficial foreign body (non-embedded splinter) - code to superficial foreign body, by site

● **Z18.0   Retained radioactive fragments**
Z18.01   Retained depleted uranium fragments
Z18.09   Other retained radioactive fragments
Other retained depleted isotope fragments
Retained nontherapeutic radioactive fragments

● **Z18.1   Retained metal fragments**
Excludes1   retained radioactive metal fragments (Z18.01-Z18.09)
Z18.10   Retained metal fragments, unspecified
Retained metal fragment NOS
Z18.11   Retained magnetic metal fragments
Z18.12   Retained nonmagnetic metal fragments
Z18.2   Retained plastic fragments
Acrylics fragments
Diethylhexylphthalates fragments
Isocyanate fragments

● **Z18.3   Retained organic fragments**
Z18.31   Retained animal quills or spines
Z18.32   Retained tooth
Z18.33   Retained wood fragments
Z18.39   Other retained organic fragments

● **Z18.8   Other specified retained foreign body**
Z18.81   Retained glass fragments
Z18.83   Retained stone or crystalline fragments
Retained concrete or cement fragments
Z18.89   Other specified retained foreign body fragments
Coding Clinic: 2016, Q3, P24
Z18.9   Retained foreign body fragments, unspecified material

HORMONE SENSITIVITY MALIGNANCY STATUS (Z19)

● **Z19   Hormone sensitivity malignancy status**
Code first malignant neoplasm —*see* Table of Neoplasms, by site, malignant
Coding Clinic: 2016, Q4, P129
Z19.1   Hormone sensitive malignancy status
Coding Clinic: 2016, Q4, P76
Z19.2   Hormone resistant malignancy status
Castrate resistant prostate malignancy status
Coding Clinic: 2016, Q4, P76

CHAPTER 21 (Z00-Z99)

PERSONS WITH POTENTIAL HEALTH HAZARDS RELATED TO COMMUNICABLE DISEASES (Z20-Z29)

● **Z20   Contact with and (suspected) exposure to communicable diseases**

    Excludes1   carrier of infectious disease (Z22.-)
                  diagnosed current infectious or parasitic disease - see Alphabetic Index

    Excludes2   personal history of infectious and parasitic diseases (Z86.1-)

    Coding Clinic: 2021, Q1, P37

  ● **Z20.0   Contact with and (suspected) exposure to intestinal infectious diseases**

      Z20.01   Contact with and (suspected) exposure to intestinal infectious diseases due to Escherichia coli (E. coli)

      Z20.09   Contact with and (suspected) exposure to other intestinal infectious diseases

  Z20.1   Contact with and (suspected) exposure to tuberculosis

  Z20.2   Contact with and (suspected) exposure to infections with a predominantly sexual mode of transmission

  Z20.3   Contact with and (suspected) exposure to rabies

  Z20.4   Contact with and (suspected) exposure to rubella

  Z20.5   Contact with and (suspected) exposure to viral hepatitis

  Z20.6   Contact with and (suspected) exposure to human immunodeficiency virus [HIV]

      Excludes1   asymptomatic human immunodeficiency virus [HIV]
                 HIV infection status (Z21)

  Z20.7   Contact with and (suspected) exposure to pediculosis, acariasis and other infestations

  ● **Z20.8   Contact with and (suspected) exposure to other communicable diseases**

    ● **Z20.81   Contact with and (suspected) exposure to other bacterial communicable diseases**

      Z20.810   Contact with and (suspected) exposure to anthrax

      Z20.811   Contact with and (suspected) exposure to meningococcus

      Z20.818   Contact with and (suspected) exposure to other bacterial communicable diseases

    ● **Z20.82   Contact with and (suspected) exposure to other viral communicable diseases**

      Z20.820   Contact with and (suspected) exposure to varicella

      Z20.821   Contact with and (suspected) exposure to Zika virus

      Z20.822   Contact with and (suspected) exposure to COVID-19
          Contact with and (suspected) exposure to SARS-CoV-2
          Coding Clinic: 2021, Q1, P37-39, 42

      Z20.828   Contact with and (suspected) exposure to other viral communicable diseases
          Coding Clinic: 2021, Q1, P37-39; 2016, Q4, P6-7, 121

    Z20.89   Contact with and (suspected) exposure to other communicable diseases

  Z20.9   Contact with and (suspected) exposure to unspecified communicable disease

● **Z21   Asymptomatic human immunodeficiency virus [HIV] infection status 🏷**

    HIV positive NOS

    Code first Human immunodeficiency virus [HIV] disease complicating pregnancy, childbirth and the puerperium, if applicable (O98.7-)

    Excludes1   acquired immunodeficiency syndrome (B20)
                  contact with human immunodeficiency virus [HIV] (Z20.6)
                  exposure to human immunodeficiency virus [HIV] (Z20.6)
                  human immunodeficiency virus [HIV] disease (B20)
                  inconclusive laboratory evidence of human immunodeficiency virus [HIV] (R75)

    Coding Clinic: 2019, Q1, P10-11

● **Z22   Carrier of infectious disease**

    Includes   colonization status
                suspected carrier

    Excludes2   carrier of viral hepatitis (B18.-)

  Z22.0   Carrier of typhoid

  Z22.1   Carrier of other intestinal infectious diseases

  Z22.2   Carrier of diphtheria

  ● **Z22.3   Carrier of other specified bacterial diseases**

    Z22.31   Carrier of bacterial disease due to meningococci

    ● **Z22.32   Carrier of bacterial disease due to staphylococci**

      Z22.321   Carrier or suspected carrier of Methicillin susceptible Staphylococcus aureus
          MSSA colonization

      Z22.322   Carrier or suspected carrier of Methicillin resistant Staphylococcus aureus
          MRSA colonization

    ● **Z22.33   Carrier of bacterial disease due to streptococci**

      Z22.330   Carrier of Group B streptococcus

          Excludes1   Carrier of streptococcus group B (GBS) complicating pregnancy, childbirth and the puerperium (O99.82-)

      Z22.338   Carrier of other streptococcus

    Z22.39   Carrier of other specified bacterial diseases

  Z22.4   Carrier of infections with a predominantly sexual mode of transmission

  Z22.6   Carrier of human T-lymphotropic virus type-1 [HTLV-1] infection

  Z22.7   Latent tuberculosis
    Latent tuberculosis infection (LTBI)

    Excludes1   nonspecific reaction to cell mediated immunity measurement of gamma interferon antigen response without active tuberculosis (R76.12)
                  nonspecific reaction to tuberculin skin test without active tuberculosis (R76.11)

  Z22.8   Carrier of other infectious diseases

  Z22.9   Carrier of infectious disease, unspecified

Z23   Encounter for immunization

    Code first any routine childhood examination

    Note: Procedure codes are required to identify the types of immunizations given.

    ▶Code also, if applicable, encounter for immunization safety counseling (Z71.85)

▶ New   ⬛▶ Revised   ~~deleted~~ Deleted   Excludes 1   Excludes 2   Includes   Use additional   Code first   Code also   Key words

OGCR Official Guidelines   X Assign placeholder X   ● Use Additional Character(s)   ▶ Manifestation Code   🏷 Hierarchical Condition Category   Coding Clinic

● **Z28 Immunization not carried out and underimmunization status**

    Includes   vaccination not carried out

    ▶Code also, if applicable, encounter for immunization safety counseling (Z71.85)

  ● **Z28.0 Immunization not carried out because of contraindication**

    Z28.01 Immunization not carried out because of acute illness of patient

    Z28.02 Immunization not carried out because of chronic illness or condition of patient

    Z28.03 Immunization not carried out because of immune compromised state of patient

    Z28.04 Immunization not carried out because of patient allergy to vaccine or component

    Z28.09 Immunization not carried out because of other contraindication

  Z28.1 Immunization not carried out because of patient decision for reasons of belief or group pressure
    Immunization not carried out because of religious belief

  ● **Z28.2 Immunization not carried out because of patient decision for other and unspecified reason**

    Z28.20 Immunization not carried out because of patient decision for unspecified reason

    Z28.21 Immunization not carried out because of patient refusal

    Z28.29 Immunization not carried out because of patient decision for other reason

  Z28.3 Underimmunization status
    Delinquent immunization status
    Lapsed immunization schedule status

  ● **Z28.8 Immunization not carried out for other reason**

    Z28.81 Immunization not carried out due to patient having had the disease

    Z28.82 Immunization not carried out because of caregiver refusal
      Immunization not carried out because of guardian refusal
      Immunization not carried out because of parent refusal

      Excludes1   immunization not carried out because of caregiver refusal because of religious belief (Z28.1)

    Z28.83 Immunization not carried out due to unavailability of vaccine
      Delay in delivery of vaccine
      Lack of availability of vaccine
      Manufacturer delay of vaccine

    Z28.89 Immunization not carried out for other reason

  Z28.9 Immunization not carried out for unspecified reason

● **Z29 Encounter for other prophylactic measures**

    Excludes1   desensitization to allergens (Z51.6)
          prophylactic surgery (Z40.-)
    Coding Clinic: 2016, Q4, P130

  ● **Z29.1 Encounter for prophylactic immunotherapy**
    Encounter for administration of immunoglobulin
    Coding Clinic: 2016, Q4, P78-79

    Z29.11 Encounter for prophylactic immunotherapy for respiratory syncytial virus (RSV)

    Z29.12 Encounter for prophylactic antivenin

    Z29.13 Encounter for prophylactic Rho(D) immune globulin
      Coding Clinic: 2019, Q3, P5

    Z29.14 Encounter for prophylactic rabies immune globin

  Z29.3 Encounter for prophylactic fluoride administration
    Coding Clinic: 2016, Q4, P79

  Z29.8 Encounter for other specified prophylactic measures
    Coding Clinic: 2016, Q4, P79

  Z29.9 Encounter for prophylactic measures, unspecified
    Coding Clinic: 2016, Q4, P79

PERSONS ENCOUNTERING HEALTH SERVICES IN CIRCUMSTANCES RELATED TO REPRODUCTION (Z30-Z39)

● **Z30 Encounter for contraceptive management**

  ● **Z30.0 Encounter for general counseling and advice on contraception**

    ● **Z30.01 Encounter for initial prescription of contraceptives**

      Excludes1   encounter for surveillance of contraceptives (Z30.4-)

      Z30.011 Encounter for initial prescription of contraceptive pills ♀

      Z30.012 Encounter for prescription of emergency contraception ♀
        Encounter for postcoital contraception

      Z30.013 Encounter for initial prescription of injectable contraceptive ♀

      Z30.014 Encounter for initial prescription of intrauterine contraceptive device ♀

        Excludes1   encounter for insertion of intrauterine contraceptive device (Z30.430, Z30.432)

      Z30.015 Encounter for initial prescription of vaginal ring hormonal contraceptive ♀
        Coding Clinic: 2016, Q4, P78

      Z30.016 Encounter for initial prescription of transdermal patch hormonal contraceptive device
        Coding Clinic: 2016, Q4, P78

      Z30.017 Encounter for initial prescription of implantable subdermal contraceptive
        Coding Clinic: 2016, Q4, P78

      Z30.018 Encounter for initial prescription of other contraceptives ♀
        Encounter for initial prescription of barrier contraception
        Encounter for initial prescription of diaphragm

      Z30.019 Encounter for initial prescription of contraceptives, unspecified ♀

    Z30.02 Counseling and instruction in natural family planning to avoid pregnancy

    Z30.09 Encounter for other general counseling and advice on contraception
      Encounter for family planning advice NOS

  Z30.2 Encounter for sterilization

  ● **Z30.4 Encounter for surveillance of contraceptives**

    Z30.40 Encounter for surveillance of contraceptives, unspecified

    Z30.41 Encounter for surveillance of contraceptive pills ♀
      Encounter for repeat prescription for contraceptive pill

    Z30.42 Encounter for surveillance of injectable contraceptive ♀

    ● **Z30.43 Encounter for surveillance of intrauterine contraceptive device**

      Z30.430 Encounter for insertion of intrauterine contraceptive device ♀

      Z30.431 Encounter for routine checking of intrauterine contraceptive device ♀

      Z30.432 Encounter for removal of intrauterine contraceptive device ♀

      Z30.433 Encounter for removal and reinsertion of intrauterine contraceptive device ♀
        Encounter for replacement of intrauterine contraceptive device

    Z30.44 Encounter for surveillance of vaginal ring hormonal contraceptive device ♀
      Coding Clinic: 2016, Q4, P78

N Newborn Age: 0   **P** Pediatric Age: 0–17   **M** Maternity DX: 9–64   **A** Adult Age: 15–124   ♀ Females Only   ♂ Males Only

1569

Z30.45   Encounter for surveillance of transdermal patch hormonal contraceptive device ♀
Coding Clinic: 2016, Q4, P78

Z30.46   Encounter for surveillance of implantable subdermal contraceptive ♀
Encounter for checking, reinsertion or removal of implantable subdermal contraceptive
Coding Clinic: 2016, Q4, P78

Z30.49   Encounter for surveillance of other contraceptives ♀
Encounter for surveillance of barrier contraception
Encounter for surveillance of diaphragm

Z30.8   Encounter for other contraceptive management
Encounter for postvasectomy sperm count
Encounter for routine examination for contraceptive maintenance

    Excludes1   sperm count following sterilization reversal (Z31.42)
                    sperm count for fertility testing (Z31.41)

Z30.9   Encounter for contraceptive management, unspecified

● Z31   Encounter for procreative management
~~Z31.001~~ ~~complications associated with artificial~~
~~fertilization (N98.-)~~
~~female infertility (N97.-)~~
~~male infertility (N46.-)~~

▶ Excludes2   complications associated with artificial fertilization (N98.-)
female infertility (N97.-)
male infertility (N46.-)

Z31.0   Encounter for reversal of previous sterilization

● Z31.4   Encounter for procreative investigation and testing
    Excludes1   postvasectomy sperm count (Z30.8)

Z31.41   Encounter for fertility testing
Encounter for fallopian tube patency testing
Encounter for sperm count for fertility testing

Z31.42   Aftercare following sterilization reversal
Sperm count following sterilization reversal

● Z31.43   Encounter for genetic testing of female for procreative management
Use additional code for recurrent pregnancy loss, if applicable (N96, O26.2-)
    Excludes1   nonprocreative genetic testing (Z13.7-)

Z31.430   Encounter for female for testing for genetic disease carrier status for procreative management ♀

Z31.438   Encounter for other genetic testing of female for procreative management ♀

● Z31.44   Encounter for genetic testing of male for procreative management
    Excludes1   nonprocreative genetic testing (Z13.7-)

Z31.440   Encounter for male for testing for genetic disease carrier status for procreative management ♂

Z31.441   Encounter for testing of male partner of patient with recurrent pregnancy loss ♂   A

Z31.448   Encounter for other genetic testing of male for procreative management ♂ A

Z31.49   Encounter for other procreative investigation and testing

Z31.5   Encounter for procreative genetic counseling

● Z31.6   Encounter for general counseling and advice on procreation

Z31.61   Procreative counseling and advice using natural family planning

Z31.62   Encounter for fertility preservation counseling
Encounter for fertility preservation counseling prior to cancer therapy
Encounter for fertility preservation counseling prior to surgical removal of gonads

Z31.69   Encounter for other general counseling and advice on procreation

Z31.7   Encounter for procreative management and counseling for gestational carrier ♀
    Excludes1   pregnant state, gestational carrier (Z33.3)
Coding Clinic: 2016, Q4, P78

● Z31.8   Encounter for other procreative management

Z31.81   Encounter for male factor infertility in female patient ♀

Z31.82   Encounter for Rh incompatibility status ♀
Coding Clinic: 2015, Q3, P40

Z31.83   Encounter for assisted reproductive fertility procedure cycle ♀
Patient undergoing in vitro fertilization cycle
Use additional code to identify the type of infertility
    Excludes1   pre-cycle diagnosis and testing - code to reason for encounter

Z31.84   Encounter for fertility preservation procedure
Encounter for fertility preservation procedure prior to cancer therapy
Encounter for fertility preservation procedure prior to surgical removal of gonads

Z31.89   Encounter for other procreative management

Z31.9   Encounter for procreative management, unspecified

● Z32   Encounter for pregnancy test and childbirth and childcare instruction

● Z32.0   Encounter for pregnancy test

Z32.00   Encounter for pregnancy test, result unknown ♀
Encounter for pregnancy test NOS

Z32.01   Encounter for pregnancy test, result positive ♀ M

Z32.02   Encounter for pregnancy test, result negative ♀

Z32.2   Encounter for childbirth instruction

Z32.3   Encounter for childcare instruction
Encounter for prenatal or postpartum childcare instruction

● Z33   Pregnant state

Z33.1   Pregnant state, incidental ♀   M
Pregnancy NOS
Pregnant state NOS
    Excludes1   complications of pregnancy (O00-O9A)
pregnant state, gestational carrier (Z33.3)

Z33.2   Encounter for elective termination of pregnancy ♀   M
    Excludes1   early fetal death with retention of dead fetus (O02.1)
late fetal death (O36.4)
spontaneous abortion (O03)
Coding Clinic: 2016, Q4, P130

Z33.3   Pregnant state, gestational carrier ♀
    Excludes1   encounter for procreative management and counseling for gestational carrier (Z31.7)
Coding Clinic: 2016, Q4, P78

Figure 21-1 Trimesters. (From Shiland, Betsy J. Medical Terminology & Anatomy for ICD-10 Coding, ed 2, Mosby, 2015)

First trimester (0 to 14 weeks)   Second trimester (14 to 28 weeks)   Third trimester (28 weeks to delivery)

● **Z34**   Encounter for supervision of normal pregnancy

    Excludes1   any complication of pregnancy (O00-O9A)
                encounter for pregnancy test (Z32.0-)
                encounter for supervision of high risk pregnancy (O09.-)

    Coding Clinic: 2016, Q4, P6

   ● **Z34.0**   Encounter for supervision of normal first pregnancy

      Z34.00   Encounter for supervision of normal first pregnancy, unspecified trimester ♀   M

      Z34.01   Encounter for supervision of normal first pregnancy, first trimester ♀   M

      Z34.02   Encounter for supervision of normal first pregnancy, second trimester ♀   M

      Z34.03   Encounter for supervision of normal first pregnancy, third trimester ♀   M

   ● **Z34.8**   Encounter for supervision of other normal pregnancy

      Z34.80   Encounter for supervision of other normal pregnancy, unspecified trimester ♀   M

      Z34.81   Encounter for supervision of other normal pregnancy, first trimester ♀   M

      Z34.82   Encounter for supervision of other normal pregnancy, second trimester ♀   M

      Z34.83   Encounter for supervision of other normal pregnancy, third trimester ♀   M

   ● **Z34.9**   Encounter for supervision of normal pregnancy, unspecified

      Z34.90   Encounter for supervision of normal pregnancy, unspecified, unspecified trimester ♀   M

      Z34.91   Encounter for supervision of normal pregnancy, unspecified, first trimester ♀   M

      Z34.92   Encounter for supervision of normal pregnancy, unspecified, second trimester ♀   M

      Z34.93   Encounter for supervision of normal pregnancy, unspecified, third trimester ♀   M

● **Z36**   Encounter for antenatal screening of mother ♀

    Includes   Encounter for placental sample (taken vaginally)
               Screening is the testing for disease or disease precursors in asymptomatic individuals so that early detection and treatment can be provided for those who test positive for the disease.

    Excludes1   diagnostic examination - code to sign or symptom
                encounter for suspected maternal and fetal conditions ruled out (Z03.7-)
                suspected fetal condition affecting management of pregnancy - code to condition in Chapter 15

    Excludes2   abnormal findings on antenatal screening of mother (O28.-)
                genetic counseling and testing (Z31.43-, Z31.5)
                routine prenatal care (Z34)

   Z36.0   Encounter for antenatal screening for chromosomal anomalies ♀   M

   Z36.1   Encounter for antenatal screening for raised alphafetoprotein level ♀   M
       Encounter for antenatal screening for elevated maternal serum alphafetoprotein level

   Z36.2   Encounter for other antenatal screening follow-up ♀   M
       Non-visualized anatomy on a previous scan

   Z36.3   Encounter for antenatal screening for malformations ♀   M
       Screening for a suspected anomaly

   Z36.4   Encounter for antenatal screening for fetal growth retardation ♀   M
       Intrauterine growth restriction (IUGR)/small-for-dates

   Z36.5   Encounter for antenatal screening for isoimmunization ♀   M

   ● **Z36.8**   Encounter for other antenatal screening

      Z36.81   Encounter for antenatal screening for hydrops fetalis ♀   M

      Z36.82   Encounter for antenatal screening for nuchal translucency ♀   M

      Z36.83   Encounter for fetal screening for congenital cardiac abnormalities ♀   M

      Z36.84   Encounter for antenatal screening for fetal lung maturity ♀   M

      Z36.85   Encounter for antenatal screening for Streptococcus B ♀   M

      Z36.86   Encounter for antenatal screening for cervical length ♀   M
          Screening for risk of pre-term labor

      Z36.87   Encounter for antenatal screening for uncertain dates ♀

      Z36.88   Encounter for antenatal screening for fetal macrosomia ♀   M
          Screening for large-for-dates

      Z36.89   Encounter for other specified antenatal screening ♀   M

      Z36.8A   Encounter for antenatal screening for other genetic defects ♀   M

   Z36.9   Encounter for antenatal screening, unspecified ♀   M

● **Z3A**   Weeks of gestation

    Note: Codes from category Z3A are for use, only on the maternal record, to indicate the weeks of gestation of the pregnancy, if known.

    ▶ Code first ~~complications of pregnancy, childbirth and the puerperium (O09-O9A)~~ obstetric condition or encounter for delivery (O09-O60, O80-O82)

    Coding Clinic: 2016, Q4, P130; 2013, Q2, P33

   ● **Z3A.0**   Weeks of gestation of pregnancy, unspecified or less than 10 weeks

      Z3A.00   Weeks of gestation not specified ♀   M

      Z3A.01   Less than 8 weeks gestation of pregnancy ♀   M

      Z3A.08   8 weeks gestation of pregnancy ♀   M

      Z3A.09   9 weeks gestation of pregnancy ♀   M

   ● **Z3A.1**   Weeks of gestation of pregnancy, weeks 10-19

      Z3A.10   10 weeks gestation of pregnancy ♀   M

      Z3A.11   11 weeks gestation of pregnancy ♀   M

      Z3A.12   12 weeks gestation of pregnancy ♀   M

      Z3A.13   13 weeks gestation of pregnancy ♀   M

      Z3A.14   14 weeks gestation of pregnancy ♀   M

      Z3A.15   15 weeks gestation of pregnancy ♀   M

      Z3A.16   16 weeks gestation of pregnancy ♀   M
          Coding Clinic: 2016, Q4, P5

      Z3A.17   17 weeks gestation of pregnancy ♀   M

      Z3A.18   18 weeks gestation of pregnancy ♀   M
          Coding Clinic: 2019, Q2, P11

      Z3A.19   19 weeks gestation of pregnancy ♀   M

   ● **Z3A.2**   Weeks of gestation of pregnancy, weeks 20-29

      Z3A.20   20 weeks gestation of pregnancy ♀   M
          Coding Clinic: 2016, Q4, P6

      Z3A.21   21 weeks gestation of pregnancy ♀   M

      Z3A.22   22 weeks gestation of pregnancy ♀   M
          Coding Clinic: 2016, Q4, P6

      Z3A.23   23 weeks gestation of pregnancy ♀   M

      Z3A.24   24 weeks gestation of pregnancy ♀   M

      Z3A.25   25 weeks gestation of pregnancy ♀   M

      Z3A.26   26 weeks gestation of pregnancy ♀   M

      Z3A.27   27 weeks gestation of pregnancy ♀   M

      Z3A.28   28 weeks gestation of pregnancy ♀   M

      Z3A.29   29 weeks gestation of pregnancy ♀   M

● **Z3A.3 Weeks of gestation of pregnancy, weeks 30-39**
    Z3A.30   30 weeks gestation of pregnancy ♀   M
    Z3A.31   31 weeks gestation of pregnancy ♀   M
    Z3A.32   32 weeks gestation of pregnancy ♀   M
              Coding Clinic: 2016, Q4, P6
    Z3A.33   33 weeks gestation of pregnancy ♀   M
    Z3A.34   34 weeks gestation of pregnancy ♀   M
    Z3A.35   35 weeks gestation of pregnancy ♀   M
    Z3A.36   36 weeks gestation of pregnancy ♀   M
    Z3A.37   37 weeks gestation of pregnancy ♀   M
    Z3A.38   38 weeks gestation of pregnancy ♀   M
              Coding Clinic: 2016, Q2, P34
    Z3A.39   39 weeks gestation of pregnancy ♀   M

● **Z3A.4 Weeks of gestation of pregnancy, weeks 40 or greater**
    Z3A.40   40 weeks gestation of pregnancy ♀   M
    Z3A.41   41 weeks gestation of pregnancy ♀   M
    Z3A.42   42 weeks gestation of pregnancy ♀   M
    Z3A.49   Greater than 42 weeks gestation of
                pregnancy ♀   M

● **Z37 Outcome of delivery**
    This category is intended for use as an additional code to
    identify the outcome of delivery on the mother's record. It
    is not for use on the newborn record.
    Excludes1   stillbirth (P95)
    Z37.0   **Single live birth** ♀   M
            Coding Clinic: 2016, Q2, P34
    Z37.1   **Single stillbirth** ♀   M
    Z37.2   **Twins, both liveborn** ♀   M
    Z37.3   **Twins, one liveborn and one stillborn** ♀   M
    Z37.4   **Twins, both stillborn** ♀   M
  ● Z37.5   **Other multiple births, all liveborn**
        Z37.50   Multiple births, unspecified, all liveborn ♀   M
        Z37.51   Triplets, all liveborn ♀   M
        Z37.52   Quadruplets, all liveborn ♀   M
        Z37.53   Quintuplets, all liveborn ♀   M
        Z37.54   Sextuplets, all liveborn ♀   M
        Z37.59   Other multiple births, all liveborn ♀   M
  ● Z37.6   **Other multiple births, some liveborn**
        Z37.60   Multiple births, unspecified, some liveborn ♀   M
        Z37.61   Triplets, some liveborn ♀   M
        Z37.62   Quadruplets, some liveborn ♀   M
        Z37.63   Quintuplets, some liveborn ♀   M
        Z37.64   Sextuplets, some liveborn ♀   M
        Z37.69   Other multiple births, some liveborn ♀   M
    Z37.7   **Other multiple births, all stillborn** ♀   M
    Z37.9   **Outcome of delivery, unspecified** ♀   M
            Multiple birth NOS
            Single birth NOS

● **Z38 Liveborn infants according to place of birth and type of delivery**
    This category is for use as the principal code on the initial record
    of a newborn baby. It is to be used for the initial birth
    record only. It is not to be used on the mother's record.
    Coding Clinic: 2017, Q2, P6-7; 2016, Q4, P126-127, 130; 2015, Q2, P15
  ● Z38.0   **Single liveborn infant, born in hospital**
        Single liveborn infant, born in birthing center or other
            health care facility
        Coding Clinic: 2017, Q2, P5-7
        Z38.00   Single liveborn infant, delivered vaginally   N
               Coding Clinic: 2018, Q4, P26; 2016, Q4, P7, 55
        Z38.01   Single liveborn infant, delivered by cesarean   N
               Coding Clinic: 2017, Q2, P7; 2016, Q3, P18
    Z38.1   **Single liveborn infant, born outside hospital**   N
    Z38.2   **Single liveborn infant, unspecified as to place of birth**   N
            Single liveborn infant NOS

● Z38.3   **Twin liveborn infant, born in hospital**
    Z38.30   Twin liveborn infant, delivered vaginally   N
    Z38.31   Twin liveborn infant, delivered by cesarean   N
  Z38.4   **Twin liveborn infant, born outside hospital**   N
  Z38.5   **Twin liveborn infant, unspecified as to place of birth**   N
● Z38.6   **Other multiple liveborn infant, born in hospital**
    Z38.61   Triplet liveborn infant, delivered vaginally   N
    Z38.62   Triplet liveborn infant, delivered by cesarean   N
    Z38.63   Quadruplet liveborn infant, delivered
               vaginally   N
    Z38.64   Quadruplet liveborn infant, delivered by
               cesarean   N
    Z38.65   Quintuplet liveborn infant, delivered
               vaginally   N
    Z38.66   Quintuplet liveborn infant, delivered by
               cesarean   N
    Z38.68   Other multiple liveborn infant, delivered
               vaginally   N
    Z38.69   Other multiple liveborn infant, delivered by
               cesarean   N
  Z38.7   **Other multiple liveborn infant, born outside hospital**   N
  Z38.8   **Other multiple liveborn infant, unspecified as to place of birth**   N

● **Z39 Encounter for maternal postpartum care and examination**
  Z39.0   **Encounter for care and examination of mother immediately after delivery** ♀   M
        Care and observation in uncomplicated cases when the
           delivery occurs outside a healthcare facility
        Excludes1   care for postpartum complication - see
               Alphabetic index
  Z39.1   **Encounter for care and examination of lactating mother** ♀   M
        Encounter for supervision of lactation
        Excludes1   disorders of lactation (O92.-)
  Z39.2   **Encounter for routine postpartum follow-up** ♀   M

ENCOUNTERS FOR OTHER SPECIFIC HEALTH CARE (Z40-Z53)

Categories Z40-Z53 are intended for use to indicate a reason
for care. They may be used for patients who have already been
treated for a disease or injury, but who are receiving aftercare or
prophylactic care, or care to consolidate the treatment, or to deal
with a residual state

    Excludes2   follow-up examination for medical surveillance
               after treatment (Z08-Z09)

● **Z40 Encounter for prophylactic surgery**
    Excludes1   organ donations (Z52.-)
               therapeutic organ removal - code to condition
    Coding Clinic: 2016, Q4, P79
  ● Z40.0   **Encounter for prophylactic surgery for risk factors related to malignant neoplasms**
        Admission for prophylactic organ removal
        Use additional code to identify risk factor
        Z40.00   Encounter for prophylactic removal of
               unspecified organ
        Z40.01   Encounter for prophylactic removal of breast
        Z40.02   Encounter for prophylactic removal of
               ovary(s) ♀
               Encounter for prophylactic removal of ovary(s)
               and fallopian tube(s)
        Z40.03   Encounter for prophylactic removal of fallopian
               tube(s) ♀
        Z40.09   Encounter for prophylactic removal of other
               organ
    Z40.8   **Encounter for other prophylactic surgery**
    Z40.9   **Encounter for prophylactic surgery, unspecified**

● **Z41   Encounter for procedures for purposes other than remedying health state**

Z41.1   Encounter for cosmetic surgery
Encounter for cosmetic breast implant
Encounter for cosmetic procedure

> **Excludes1**   encounter for plastic and reconstructive surgery following medical procedure or healed injury (Z42.-)
> encounter for post-mastectomy breast implantation (Z42.1)

Z41.2   Encounter for routine and ritual male circumcision ♂

Z41.3   Encounter for ear piercing

Z41.8   Encounter for other procedures for purposes other than remedying health state

Z41.9   Encounter for procedure for purposes other than remedying health state, unspecified

● **Z42   Encounter for plastic and reconstructive surgery following medical procedure or healed injury**

> **Excludes1**   encounter for cosmetic plastic surgery (Z41.1)
> encounter for plastic surgery for treatment of current injury - code to relevent injury

Z42.1   Encounter for breast reconstruction following mastectomy   A

> **Excludes1**   deformity and disproportion of reconstructed breast (N65.1-)

Z42.8   Encounter for other plastic and reconstructive surgery following medical procedure or healed injury
Coding Clinic: 2017, Q1, P42

● **Z43   Encounter for attention to artificial openings**

> **Includes**   closure of artificial openings
> passage of sounds or bougies through artificial openings
> reforming artificial openings
> removal of catheter from artificial openings
> toilet or cleansing of artificial openings

> **Excludes1**   complications of external stoma (J95.0-, K94.-, N99.5-)

> **Excludes2**   fitting and adjustment of prosthetic and other devices (Z44-Z46)

Z43.0   Encounter for attention to tracheostomy ✇

Z43.1   Encounter for attention to gastrostomy ✇

> **Excludes2**   artificial opening status only, without need for care (Z93.-)

Z43.2   Encounter for attention to ileostomy ✇
Coding Clinic: 2016, Q3, P5

Z43.3   Encounter for attention to colostomy ✇

Z43.4   Encounter for attention to other artificial openings of digestive tract ✇

Z43.5   Encounter for attention to cystostomy ✇

Z43.6   Encounter for attention to other artificial openings of urinary tract ✇
Encounter for attention to nephrostomy
Encounter for attention to ureterostomy
Encounter for attention to urethrostomy

Z43.7   Encounter for attention to artificial vagina

Z43.8   Encounter for attention to other artificial openings ✇

Z43.9   Encounter for attention to unspecified artificial opening ✇

● **Z44   Encounter for fitting and adjustment of external prosthetic device**

> **Includes**   removal or replacement of external prosthetic device

> **Excludes1**   malfunction or other complications of device - see Alphabetical Index presence of prosthetic device (Z97.-)

● **Z44.0   Encounter for fitting and adjustment of artificial arm**

● **Z44.00   Encounter for fitting and adjustment of unspecified artificial arm**

Z44.001   Encounter for fitting and adjustment of unspecified right artificial arm

Z44.002   Encounter for fitting and adjustment of unspecified left artificial arm

Z44.009   Encounter for fitting and adjustment of unspecified artificial arm, unspecified arm

● **Z44.01   Encounter for fitting and adjustment of complete artificial arm**

Z44.011   Encounter for fitting and adjustment of complete right artificial arm

Z44.012   Encounter for fitting and adjustment of complete left artificial arm

Z44.019   Encounter for fitting and adjustment of complete artificial arm, unspecified arm

● **Z44.02   Encounter for fitting and adjustment of partial artificial arm**

Z44.021   Encounter for fitting and adjustment of partial artificial right arm

Z44.022   Encounter for fitting and adjustment of partial artificial left arm

Z44.029   Encounter for fitting and adjustment of partial artificial arm, unspecified arm

● **Z44.1   Encounter for fitting and adjustment of artificial leg**

● **Z44.10   Encounter for fitting and adjustment of unspecified artificial leg**

Z44.101   Encounter for fitting and adjustment of unspecified right artificial leg ✇

Z44.102   Encounter for fitting and adjustment of unspecified left artificial leg ✇

Z44.109   Encounter for fitting and adjustment of unspecified artificial leg, unspecified leg ✇

● **Z44.11   Encounter for fitting and adjustment of complete artificial leg**

Z44.111   Encounter for fitting and adjustment of complete right artificial leg ✇

Z44.112   Encounter for fitting and adjustment of complete left artificial leg ✇

Z44.119   Encounter for fitting and adjustment of complete artificial leg, unspecified leg ✇

● **Z44.12   Encounter for fitting and adjustment of partial artificial leg**

Z44.121   Encounter for fitting and adjustment of partial artificial right leg ✇

Z44.122   Encounter for fitting and adjustment of partial artificial left leg ✇

Z44.129   Encounter for fitting and adjustment of partial artificial leg, unspecified leg ✇

● **Z44.2   Encounter for fitting and adjustment of artificial eye**

> **Excludes1**   mechanical complication of ocular prosthesis (T85.3)

Z44.20   Encounter for fitting and adjustment of artificial eye, unspecified

Z44.21   Encounter for fitting and adjustment of artificial right eye

Z44.22   Encounter for fitting and adjustment of artificial left eye

● **Z44.3   Encounter for fitting and adjustment of external breast prosthesis**

> **Excludes1**   complications of breast implant (T85.4-)
> encounter for adjustment or removal of breast implant (Z45.81-)
> encounter for initial breast implant insertion for cosmetic breast augmentation (Z41.1)
> encounter for breast reconstruction following mastectomy (Z42.1)

Z44.30   Encounter for fitting and adjustment of external breast prosthesis, unspecified breast

Z44.31   Encounter for fitting and adjustment of external right breast prosthesis

Z44.32   Encounter for fitting and adjustment of external left breast prosthesis

Z44.8 Encounter for fitting and adjustment of other external prosthetic devices

Z44.9 Encounter for fitting and adjustment of unspecified external prosthetic device

● **Z45** **Encounter for adjustment and management of implanted device**

> **Includes** removal or replacement of implanted device
>
> **Excludes1** malfunction or other complications of device - see Alphabetical Index
>
> **Excludes2** encounter for fitting and adjustment of non-implanted device (Z46.-)

● **Z45.0** Encounter for adjustment and management of cardiac device

● **Z45.01** Encounter for adjustment and management of cardiac pacemaker

Encounter for adjustment and management of cardiac resynchronization therapy pacemaker (CRT-P)

> **Excludes1** encounter for adjustment and management of automatic implantable cardiac defibrillator with synchronous cardiac pacemaker (Z45.02)

Z45.010 Encounter for checking and testing of cardiac pacemaker pulse generator [battery]

Encounter for replacing cardiac pacemaker pulse generator [battery]

Z45.018 Encounter for adjustment and management of other part of cardiac pacemaker

> **Excludes1** presence of other part of cardiac pacemaker (Z95.0)
>
> **Excludes2** presence of prosthetic and other devices (Z95.1-Z95.5, Z95.811-Z97)

Z45.02 Encounter for adjustment and management of automatic implantable cardiac defibrillator

Encounter for adjustment and management of automatic implantable cardiac defibrillator with synchronous cardiac pacemaker

Encounter for adjustment and management of cardiac resynchronization therapy defibrillator (CRT-D)

Z45.09 Encounter for adjustment and management of other cardiac device

Z45.1 Encounter for adjustment and management of infusion pump

Z45.2 Encounter for adjustment and management of vascular access device

Encounter for adjustment and management of vascular catheters

> **Excludes1** encounter for adjustment and management of renal dialysis catheter (Z49.01)

● **Z45.3** Encounter for adjustment and management of implanted devices of the special senses

Z45.31 Encounter for adjustment and management of implanted visual substitution device

● **Z45.32** Encounter for adjustment and management of implanted hearing device

> **Excludes1** encounter for fitting and adjustment of hearing aide (Z46.1)

Z45.320 Encounter for adjustment and management of bone conduction device

Z45.321 Encounter for adjustment and management of cochlear device

Z45.328 Encounter for adjustment and management of other implanted hearing device

● **Z45.4** Encounter for adjustment and management of implanted nervous system device

Z45.41 Encounter for adjustment and management of cerebrospinal fluid drainage device

Encounter for adjustment and management of cerebral ventricular (communicating) shunt

Z45.42 Encounter for adjustment and management of neuropacemaker

Encounter for adjustment and management of brain neurostimulator

Encounter for adjustment and management of gastric neurostimulator

Encounter for adjustment and management of peripheral nerve neurostimulator

Encounter for adjustment and management of sacral nerve neurostimulator

Encounter for adjustment and management of spinal cord neurostimulator

Encounter for adjustment and management of vagus nerve neurostimulator

Z45.49 Encounter for adjustment and management of other implanted nervous system device

● **Z45.8** Encounter for adjustment and management of other implanted devices

● **Z45.81** Encounter for adjustment or removal of breast implant

Encounter for elective implant exchange (different material) (different size)

➠ Encounter for removal of tissue expander with or without synchronous insertion of permanent implant

> **Excludes1** complications of breast implant (T85.4-)
>
> encounter for initial breast implant insertion for cosmetic breast augmentation (Z41.1)
>
> encounter for breast reconstruction following mastectomy (Z42.1)

Z45.811 Encounter for adjustment or removal of right breast implant

Z45.812 Encounter for adjustment or removal of left breast implant

Z45.819 Encounter for adjustment or removal of unspecified breast implant

Z45.82 Encounter for adjustment or removal of myringotomy device (stent) (tube)

Z45.89 Encounter for adjustment and management of other implanted devices

Z45.9 Encounter for adjustment and management of unspecified implanted device

● **Z46** **Encounter for fitting and adjustment of other devices**

> **Includes** removal or replacement of other device
>
> **Excludes1** malfunction or other complications of device - see Alphabetical Index
>
> **Excludes2** encounter for fitting and management of implanted devices (Z45.-)
>
> issue of repeat prescription only (Z76.0)
>
> presence of prosthetic and other devices (Z95-Z97)

Z46.0 Encounter for fitting and adjustment of spectacles and contact lenses

Z46.1 Encounter for fitting and adjustment of hearing aid

> **Excludes1** encounter for adjustment and management of implanted hearing device (Z45.32-)

▶ New   ⇒ Revised   ~~deleted~~ Deleted   Excludes 1   Excludes 2   Includes   Use additional   Code first   Code also   Key words

OGCR Official Guidelines   X Assign placeholder X   ● Use Additional Character(s)   ▶ Manifestation Code   🏷 Hierarchical Condition Category   **Coding Clinic**

Z46.2   Encounter for fitting and adjustment of other devices related to nervous system and special senses

    Excludes2   encounter for adjustment and management of implanted nervous system device (Z45.4-)
          encounter for adjustment and management of implanted visual substitution device (Z45.31)

Z46.3   Encounter for fitting and adjustment of dental prosthetic device

    Encounter for fitting and adjustment of dentures

Z46.4   Encounter for fitting and adjustment of orthodontic device

● **Z46.5**   Encounter for fitting and adjustment of other gastrointestinal appliance and device

    Excludes1   encounter for attention to artificial openings of digestive tract (Z43.1-Z43.4)

    Z46.51   Encounter for fitting and adjustment of gastric lap band

    Z46.59   Encounter for fitting and adjustment of other gastrointestinal appliance and device

Z46.6   Encounter for fitting and adjustment of urinary device

    Excludes2   attention to artificial openings of urinary tract (Z43.5, Z43.6)

● **Z46.8**   Encounter for fitting and adjustment of other specified devices

    Z46.81   Encounter for fitting and adjustment of insulin pump
          Encounter for insulin pump instruction and training
          Encounter for insulin pump titration

    Z46.82   Encounter for fitting and adjustment of non-vascular catheter

    Z46.89   Encounter for fitting and adjustment of other specified devices
          Encounter for fitting and adjustment of wheelchair

Z46.9   Encounter for fitting and adjustment of unspecified device

● **Z47**   Orthopedic aftercare

    Excludes1   aftercare for healing fracture - code to fracture with 7th character D

Z47.1   Aftercare following joint replacement surgery

    Use additional code to identify the joint (Z96.6-)
    Coding Clinic: 2020, Q1, P23-24

Z47.2   Encounter for removal of internal fixation device

    Excludes1   encounter for adjustment of internal fixation device for fracture treatment - code to fracture with appropriate 7th character
          encounter for removal of external fixation device - code to fracture with 7th character D
          infection or inflammatory reaction to internal fixation device (T84.6-)
          mechanical complication of internal fixation device (T84.1-)

● **Z47.3**   Aftercare following explantation of joint prosthesis

    Aftercare following explantation of joint prosthesis, staged procedure
    Encounter for joint prosthesis insertion following prior explantation of joint prosthesis
    Coding Clinic: 2020, Q1, P23; 2015, Q1, P17

    Z47.31   Aftercare following explantation of shoulder joint prosthesis

          Excludes1   acquired absence of shoulder joint following prior explantation of shoulder joint prosthesis (Z89.23-)
               shoulder joint prosthesis explantation status (Z89.23-)

    Z47.32   Aftercare following explantation of hip joint prosthesis

          Excludes1   acquired absence of hip joint following prior explantation of hip joint prosthesis (Z89.62-)
               hip joint prosthesis explantation status (Z89.62-)
          Coding Clinic: 2015, Q1, P17

    Z47.33   Aftercare following explantation of knee joint prosthesis

          Excludes1   acquired absence of knee joint following prior explantation of knee prosthesis (Z89.52-)
               knee joint prosthesis explantation status (Z89.52-)

● **Z47.8**   Encounter for other orthopedic aftercare

    Z47.81   Encounter for orthopedic aftercare following surgical amputation
          Use additional code to identify the limb amputated (Z89.-)

    Z47.82   Encounter for orthopedic aftercare following scoliosis surgery

    Z47.89   Encounter for other orthopedic aftercare
          Coding Clinic: 2015, Q1, P8

● **Z48**   Encounter for other postprocedural aftercare

    Excludes1   encounter for aftercare following injury - code to Injury, by site, with appropriate 7th character for subsequent encounter
          encounter for follow-up examination after completed treatment (Z08-Z09)

    Excludes2   encounter for attention to artificial openings (Z43.-)
          encounter for fitting and adjustment of prosthetic and other devices (Z44-Z46)

● **Z48.0**   Encounter for attention to dressings, sutures and drains

    Excludes1   encounter for planned postprocedural wound closure (Z48.1)

    Z48.00   Encounter for change or removal of nonsurgical wound dressing
          Encounter for change or removal of wound dressing NOS

    Z48.01   Encounter for change or removal of surgical wound dressing
          Coding Clinic: 2019, Q2, P33; 2015, Q4, P38

    Z48.02   Encounter for removal of sutures
          Encounter for removal of staples
          Coding Clinic: 2015, Q1, P6

    Z48.03   Encounter for change or removal of drains

Z48.1   Encounter for planned postprocedural wound closure

    Excludes1   encounter for attention to dressings and sutures (Z48.0-)

● **Z48.2**   Encounter for aftercare following organ transplant

    Z48.21   Encounter for aftercare following heart transplant 🦠

    Z48.22   Encounter for aftercare following kidney transplant

    Z48.23   Encounter for aftercare following liver transplant 🦠

    Z48.24   Encounter for aftercare following lung transplant 🦠

    ● **Z48.28**   Encounter for aftercare following multiple organ transplant

          Z48.280   Encounter for aftercare following heart-lung transplant 🦠

          Z48.288   Encounter for aftercare following multiple organ transplant

CHAPTER 21 (Z00-Z99)

● Z48.29   Encounter for aftercare following other organ transplant

     Z48.290   Encounter for aftercare following bone marrow transplant 🦠

     Z48.298   Encounter for aftercare following other organ transplant

Z48.3   Aftercare following surgery for neoplasm

     Use additional code to identify the neoplasm

● Z48.8   Encounter for other specified postprocedural aftercare

   ● Z48.81   Encounter for surgical aftercare following surgery on specified body systems

These codes identify the body system requiring aftercare. They are for use in conjunction with other aftercare codes to fully explain the aftercare encounter. The condition treated should also be coded if still present.

Excludes1   aftercare for injury - code the injury with 7th character D
aftercare following surgery for neoplasm (Z48.3)

Excludes2   aftercare following organ transplant (Z48.2-)
orthopedic aftercare (Z47.-)

     Z48.810   Encounter for surgical aftercare following surgery on the sense organs

     Z48.811   Encounter for surgical aftercare following surgery on the nervous system

Excludes2   encounter for surgical aftercare following surgery on the sense organs (Z48.810)

     Z48.812   Encounter for surgical aftercare following surgery on the circulatory system
Coding Clinic: 2012, Q4, P96

     Z48.813   Encounter for surgical aftercare following surgery on the respiratory system
Coding Clinic: 2019, Q2, P33

     Z48.814   Encounter for surgical aftercare following surgery on the teeth or oral cavity

     Z48.815   Encounter for surgical aftercare following surgery on the digestive system
Coding Clinic: 2015, Q4, P38

     Z48.816   Encounter for surgical aftercare following surgery on the genitourinary system

Excludes1   encounter for aftercare following sterilization reversal (Z31.42)

     Z48.817   Encounter for surgical aftercare following surgery on the skin and subcutaneous tissue
Coding Clinic: 2015, Q1, P6

   Z48.89   Encounter for other specified surgical aftercare

● Z49   Encounter for care involving renal dialysis

Code also associated end stage renal disease (N18.6)

● Z49.0   Preparatory care for renal dialysis

Encounter for dialysis instruction and training

   Z49.01   Encounter for fitting and adjustment of extracorporeal dialysis catheter 🦠
Removal or replacement of renal dialysis catheter
Toilet or cleansing of renal dialysis catheter

   Z49.02   Encounter for fitting and adjustment of peritoneal dialysis catheter 🦠

● Z49.3   Encounter for adequacy testing for dialysis

   Z49.31   Encounter for adequacy testing for hemodialysis 🦠

   Z49.32   Encounter for adequacy testing for peritoneal dialysis 🦠
Encounter for peritoneal equilibration test

● Z51   Encounter for other aftercare and medical care

Code also condition requiring care

Excludes1   follow-up examination after treatment (Z08-Z09)

Coding Clinic: 2017, Q1, P49; 2016, Q4, P130

Z51.0   Encounter for antineoplastic radiation therapy
Coding Clinic: 2017, Q4, P103

● Z51.1   Encounter for antineoplastic chemotherapy and immunotherapy

Excludes2   encounter for chemotherapy and immunotherapy for nonneoplastic condition-code to condition

   Z51.11   Encounter for antineoplastic chemotherapy
Coding Clinic: 2015, Q3, P19

   Z51.12   Encounter for antineoplastic immunotherapy

Z51.5   Encounter for palliative care
Coding Clinic: 2017, Q1, P48-49

Z51.6   Encounter for desensitization to allergens
Coding Clinic: 2016, Q4, P77-79

● Z51.8   Encounter for other specified aftercare

Excludes1   holiday relief care (Z75.5)

   Z51.81   Encounter for therapeutic drug level monitoring

Code also any long-term (current) drug therapy (Z79.-)

Excludes1   encounter for blood-drug test for administrative or medicolegal reasons (Z02.83)

   Z51.89   Encounter for other specified aftercare
Coding Clinic: 2012, Q4, P96-97

● Z52   Donors of organs and tissues

Includes   autologous and other living donors

Excludes1   cadaveric donor - omit code
examination of potential donor (Z00.5)

Coding Clinic: 2012, Q4, P100

● Z52.0   Blood donor

   ● Z52.00   Unspecified blood donor

     Z52.000   Unspecified donor, whole blood

     Z52.001   Unspecified donor, stem cells

     Z52.008   Unspecified donor, other blood

   ● Z52.01   Autologous blood donor

     Z52.010   Autologous donor, whole blood

     Z52.011   Autologous donor, stem cells

     Z52.018   Autologous donor, other blood

   ● Z52.09   Other blood donor
Volunteer donor

     Z52.090   Other blood donor, whole blood

     Z52.091   Other blood donor, stem cells

     Z52.098   Other blood donor, other blood

● Z52.1   Skin donor

   Z52.10   Skin donor, unspecified

   Z52.11   Skin donor, autologous

   Z52.19   Skin donor, other

● Z52.2   Bone donor

   Z52.20   Bone donor, unspecified

   Z52.21   Bone donor, autologous

   Z52.29   Bone donor, other

Z52.3   Bone marrow donor

Z52.4   Kidney donor

Z52.5   Cornea donor

Z52.6   Liver donor
Coding Clinic: 2012, Q4, P100

▶ New   ⇒ Revised   ~~deleted~~ Deleted   Excludes 1   Excludes 2   Includes   Use additional   Code first   Code also   Key words

OGCR Official Guidelines   X Assign placeholder X   ● Use Additional Character(s)   ▶ Manifestation Code   🦠 Hierarchical Condition Category   **Coding Clinic**

● **Z52.8**   **Donor of other specified organs or tissues**
   ● **Z52.81**   Egg (Oocyte) donor
     Z52.810   Egg (Oocyte) donor under age 35, anonymous recipient ♀
        Egg donor under age 35 NOS
     Z52.811   Egg (Oocyte) donor under age 35, designated recipient ♀
     Z52.812   Egg (Oocyte) donor age 35 and over, anonymous recipient ♀
        Egg donor age 35 and over NOS
     Z52.813   Egg (Oocyte) donor age 35 and over, designated recipient ♀
     Z52.819   Egg (Oocyte) donor, unspecified ♀
   Z52.89   Donor of other specified organs or tissues
  Z52.9   Donor of unspecified organ or tissue
     Donor NOS

● **Z53**   **Persons encountering health services for specific procedures and treatment, not carried out**
  ● **Z53.0**   Procedure and treatment not carried out because of contraindication
   Z53.01   Procedure and treatment not carried out due to patient smoking
   Z53.09   Procedure and treatment not carried out because of other contraindication
  Z53.1   Procedure and treatment not carried out because of patient's decision for reasons of belief and group pressure
  ● **Z53.2**   Procedure and treatment not carried out because of patient's decision for other and unspecified reasons
   Z53.20   Procedure and treatment not carried out because of patient's decision for unspecified reasons
   Z53.21   Procedure and treatment not carried out due to patient leaving prior to being seen by health care provider
   Z53.29   Procedure and treatment not carried out because of patient's decision for other reasons
  ● **Z53.3**   Procedure converted to open procedure
     Coding Clinic: 2016, Q4, P79
   Z53.31   Laparoscopic surgical procedure converted to open procedure
     Coding Clinic: 2016, Q4, P100
   Z53.32   Thoracoscopic surgical procedure converted to open procedure
   Z53.33   Arthroscopic surgical procedure converted to open procedure
   Z53.39   Other specified procedure converted to open procedure
  Z53.8   Procedure and treatment not carried out for other reasons
  Z53.9   Procedure and treatment not carried out, unspecified reason

---

PERSONS WITH POTENTIAL HEALTH HAZARDS RELATED TO SOCIOECONOMIC AND PSYCHOSOCIAL CIRCUMSTANCES (Z55-Z65)

● **Z55**   **Problems related to education and literacy**
   Excludes1   disorders of psychological development (F80-F89)
  Z55.0   Illiteracy and low-level literacy
  Z55.1   Schooling unavailable and unattainable
  Z55.2   Failed school examinations
  Z55.3   Underachievement in school
  Z55.4   Educational maladjustment and discord with teachers and classmates
  ▷ **Z55.5**   Less than a high school diploma
     ▷No general equivalence degree (GED)
  Z55.8   Other problems related to education and literacy
     Problems related to inadequate teaching
  Z55.9   Problems related to education and literacy, unspecified
     Academic problems NOS

● **Z56**   **Problems related to employment and unemployment**
   Excludes2   occupational exposure to risk factors (Z57.-)
     problems related to housing and economic circumstances (Z59.-)
  Z56.0   Unemployment, unspecified
  Z56.1   Change of job   A
  Z56.2   Threat of job loss
  Z56.3   Stressful work schedule
  Z56.4   Discord with boss and workmates
  Z56.5   Uncongenial work environment
     Difficult conditions at work
  Z56.6   Other physical and mental strain related to work
  ● **Z56.8**   Other problems related to employment
   Z56.81   Sexual harassment on the job
   Z56.82   Military deployment status
     Individual (civilian or military) currently deployed in theater or in support of military war, peacekeeping and humanitarian operations
   Z56.89   Other problems related to employment
  Z56.9   Unspecified problems related to employment
     Occupational problems NOS

● **Z57**   **Occupational exposure to risk factors**
  Z57.0   Occupational exposure to noise
  Z57.1   Occupational exposure to radiation
  Z57.2   Occupational exposure to dust
  ● **Z57.3**   Occupational exposure to other air contaminants
   Z57.31   Occupational exposure to environmental tobacco smoke
     Excludes2   exposure to environmental tobacco smoke (Z77.22)
   Z57.39   Occupational exposure to other air contaminants
  Z57.4   Occupational exposure to toxic agents in agriculture
     Occupational exposure to solids, liquids, gases or vapors in agriculture
  Z57.5   Occupational exposure to toxic agents in other industries
     Occupational exposure to solids, liquids, gases or vapors in other industries
  Z57.6   Occupational exposure to extreme temperature
  Z57.7   Occupational exposure to vibration
  Z57.8   Occupational exposure to other risk factors
  Z57.9   Occupational exposure to unspecified risk factor

▷● **Z58**   **Problems related to physical environment**
   ▷**Excludes2**   occupational exposure (Z57.-)
  ▷ **Z58.6**   Inadequate drinking-water supply
     ▷Lack of safe drinking water
     ▷**Excludes2**   deprivation of water (T73.1)

▷● **Z59**   **Problems related to housing and economic circumstances**
   Excludes2   problems related to upbringing (Z62.-)
  ▷● **Z59.0**   Homelessness
   ▷Z59.00 Homelessness unspecified
   ▷Z59.01 Sheltered homelessness
     ▷Doubled up
     ▷Living in a shelter such as: motel, scattered site housing, temporary or transitional living situation
   ▷Z59.02 Unsheltered homelessness
     ▷Residing in place not meant for human habitation such as: abandoned buildings, cars, parks, sidewalk
     ▷Residing on the street
  ● **Z59.1**   Inadequate housing
     Lack of heating
     Restriction of space
     Technical defects in home preventing adequate care
     Unsatisfactory surroundings
     Excludes1   problems related to the natural and physical environment (Z77.1-)

CHAPTER 21 (Z00-Z99)

Z59.2   Discord with neighbors, lodgers and landlord

Z59.3   Problems related to living in residential institution
Boarding-school resident
> **Excludes1**   institutional upbringing (Z62.2)

➡️● Z59.4   Lack of adequate food ~~and safe drinking water~~
~~Inadequate drinking water supply~~
~~**Excludes1**   effects of hunger (T73.0)~~
~~inappropriate diet or eating habits (Z72.4)~~
~~malnutrition (E40-E46)~~

> **Excludes2**   deprivation of food (T73.0)
> effects of hunger (T73.0)
> inappropriate diet or eating habits (Z72.4)
> malnutrition (E40-E46)

> **Z59.41 Food insecurity**

> **Z59.48 Other specified lack of adequate food**
> Inadequate food
> Lack of food

Z59.5   Extreme poverty

Z59.6   Low income

Z59.7   Insufficient social insurance and welfare support

➡️● Z59.8   Other problems related to housing and economic circumstances
~~Foreclosure on loan~~
~~Isolated dwelling~~
~~Problems with creditors~~

> ● **Z59.81 Housing instability, housed**
> Foreclosure on home loan
> Past due on rent or mortgage
> Unwanted multiple moves in the last 12 months

> > **Z59.811 Housing instability, housed, with risk of homelessness**
> > Imminent risk of homelessness

> > **Z59.812 Housing instability, housed, homelessness in past 12 months**

> > **Z59.819 Housing instability, housed unspecified**

> **Z59.89 Other problems related to housing and economic circumstances**
> Foreclosure on loan
> Isolated dwelling
> Problems with creditors

Z59.9   Problem related to housing and economic circumstances, unspecified

● **Z60   Problems related to social environment**

Z60.0   Problems of adjustment to life-cycle transitions
Empty nest syndrome
Phase of life problem
Problem with adjustment to retirement [pension]

Z60.2   Problems related to living alone

Z60.3   Acculturation difficulty
Problem with migration
Problem with social transplantation

Z60.4   Social exclusion and rejection
Exclusion and rejection on the basis of personal characteristics, such as unusual physical appearance, illness or behavior.
> **Excludes1**   target of adverse discrimination such as for racial or religious reasons (Z60.5)

Z60.5   Target of (perceived) adverse discrimination and persecution
> **Excludes1**   social exclusion and rejection (Z60.4)

Z60.8   Other problems related to social environment

Z60.9   Problem related to social environment, unspecified

● **Z62   Problems related to upbringing**
> **Includes**   current and past negative life events in childhood
> current and past problems of a child related to upbringing
> **Excludes2**   maltreatment syndrome (T74.-)
> problems related to housing and economic circumstances (Z59.-)

Z62.0   Inadequate parental supervision and control

Z62.1   Parental overprotection

● Z62.2   Upbringing away from parents
> **Excludes1**   problems with boarding school (Z59.3)

Z62.21   Child in welfare custody   P
Child in care of non-parental family member
Child in foster care
> **Excludes2**   problem for parent due to child in welfare custody (Z63.5)

Z62.22   Institutional upbringing
Child living in orphanage or group home

Z62.29   Other upbringing away from parents

Z62.3   Hostility towards and scapegoating of child   P

Z62.6   Inappropriate (excessive) parental pressure

● Z62.8   Other specified problems related to upbringing

● Z62.81   Personal history of abuse in childhood

Z62.810   Personal history of physical and sexual abuse in childhood
> **Excludes1**   current child physical abuse (T74.12, T76.12)
> current child sexual abuse (T74.22, T76.22)

Z62.811   Personal history of psychological abuse in childhood
> **Excludes1**   current child psychological abuse (T74.32, T76.32)

Z62.812   Personal history of neglect in childhood
> **Excludes1**   current child neglect (T74.02, T76.02)

Z62.813   Personal history of forced labor or sexual exploitation in childhood

Z62.819   Personal history of unspecified abuse in childhood
> **Excludes1**   current child abuse NOS (T74.92, T76.92)

● Z62.82   Parent-child conflict

Z62.820   Parent-biological child conflict
Parent-child problem NOS

Z62.821   Parent-adopted child conflict

Z62.822   Parent-foster child conflict

● Z62.89   Other specified problems related to upbringing

Z62.890   Parent-child estrangement NEC

Z62.891   Sibling rivalry

Z62.898   Other specified problems related to upbringing

Z62.9   Problem related to upbringing, unspecified

● **Z63   Other problems related to primary support group, including family circumstances**
> **Excludes2**   maltreatment syndrome (T74.-, T76)
> parent-child problems (Z62.-)
> problems related to negative life events in childhood (Z62.-)
> problems related to upbringing (Z62.-)

Z63.0   Problems in relationship with spouse or partner
Relationship distress with spouse or intimate partner
> **Excludes1**   counseling for spousal or partner abuse problems (Z69.1)
> counseling related to sexual attitude, behavior, and orientation (Z70.-)

Z63.1   Problems in relationship with in-laws

● Z63.3   Absence of family member
> **Excludes1**   absence of family member due to disappearance and death (Z63.4)
> absence of family member due to separation and divorce (Z63.5)

▶ New   ➡️ Revised   ~~deleted~~ Deleted   Excludes 1   Excludes 2   Includes   Use additional   Code first   Code also   Key words

OGCR Official Guidelines   X Assign placeholder X   ● Use Additional Character(s)   ▶ Manifestation Code   🐾 Hierarchical Condition Category   **Coding Clinic**

Z63.31   **Absence of family member due to military deployment**
       Individual or family affected by other family member being on military deployment
       Excludes1   family disruption due to return of family member from military deployment (Z63.71)

Z63.32   Other absence of family member

Z63.4   **Disappearance and death of family member**
     Assumed death of family member
     Bereavement

Z63.5   **Disruption of family by separation and divorce**
     Marital estrangement

Z63.6   **Dependent relative needing care at home**

● **Z63.7**   **Other stressful life events affecting family and household**

     Z63.71   **Stress on family due to return of family member from military deployment**
         Individual or family affected by family member having returned from military deployment (current or past conflict)

     Z63.72   **Alcoholism and drug addiction in family**

     Z63.79   **Other stressful life events affecting family and household**
         Anxiety (normal) about sick person in family
         Health problems within family
         Ill or disturbed family member
         Isolated family

Z63.8   **Other specified problems related to primary support group**
     Family discord NOS
     Family estrangement NOS
     High expressed emotional level within family
     Inadequate family support NOS
     Inadequate or distorted communication within family

Z63.9   **Problem related to primary support group, unspecified**
     Relationship disorder NOS

● **Z64**   **Problems related to certain psychosocial circumstances**

     Z64.0   **Problems related to unwanted pregnancy** ♀

     Z64.1   **Problems related to multiparity** ♀

     Z64.4   **Discord with counselors**
       Discord with probation officer
       Discord with social worker

● **Z65**   **Problems related to other psychosocial circumstances**

     Z65.0   **Conviction in civil and criminal proceedings without imprisonment**

     Z65.1   **Imprisonment and other incarceration**

     Z65.2   **Problems related to release from prison**

     Z65.3   **Problems related to other legal circumstances**
       Arrest
       Child custody or support proceedings
       Litigation
       Prosecution

     Z65.4   **Victim of crime and terrorism**
       Victim of torture

     Z65.5   **Exposure to disaster, war and other hostilities**
       Excludes1   target of perceived discrimination or persecution (Z60.5)

     Z65.8   **Other specified problems related to psychosocial circumstances**
       Religious or spiritual problem

     Z65.9   **Problem related to unspecified psychosocial circumstances**

DO NOT RESUSCITATE STATUS (Z66)

Z66   **Do not resuscitate**
     DNR status

BLOOD TYPE (Z67)

● **Z67**   **Blood type**
     Coding Clinic: 2015, Q3, P40

     ● **Z67.1**   Type A blood
         Z67.10   Type A blood, Rh positive
         Z67.11   Type A blood, Rh negative

     ● **Z67.2**   Type B blood
         Z67.20   Type B blood, Rh positive
         Z67.21   Type B blood, Rh negative

     ● **Z67.3**   Type AB blood
         Z67.30   Type AB blood, Rh positive
         Z67.31   Type AB blood, Rh negative

     ● **Z67.4**   Type O blood
         Z67.40   Type O blood, Rh positive
         Z67.41   Type O blood, Rh negative

     ● **Z67.9**   Unspecified blood type
         Z67.90   Unspecified blood type, Rh positive
         Z67.91   Unspecified blood type, Rh negative
         Coding Clinic: 2015, Q3, P40

BODY MASS INDEX [BMI] (Z68)

OGCR Section I.B.14.

> General Coding Guidelines
>
> 14. Documentation for BMI, Depth of Non-pressure ulcers, Pressure Ulcer Stages, Coma Scale, and NIH Stroke Scale
>
> For the Body Mass Index (BMI), depth of non-pressure chronic ulcers, pressure ulcer stage, coma scale, and NIH stroke scale (NIHSS) codes, code assignment may be based on medical record documentation from clinicians who are not the patient's provider (i.e., physician or other qualified healthcare practitioner legally accountable for establishing the patient's diagnosis), since this information is typically documented by other clinicians involved in the care of the patient (e.g., a dietitian often documents the BMI, a nurse often documents the pressure ulcer stages, and an emergency medical technician often documents the coma scale). However, the associated diagnosis (such as overweight, obesity, acute stroke, or pressure ulcer) must be documented by the patient's provider. If there is conflicting medical record documentation, either from the same clinician or different clinicians, the patient's attending provider should be queried for clarification.
>
> The BMI, coma scale, and NIHSS codes should only be reported as secondary diagnoses.

● **Z68**   **Body mass index [BMI]**
     Kilograms per meters squared
     Note: BMI adult codes are for use for persons 20 years of age or older.
         BMI pediatric codes are for use for persons 2-19 years of age.
         These percentiles are based on the growth charts published by the Centers for Disease Control and Prevention (CDC)
     Coding Clinic: 2018, Q4, P81; 2016, Q4, P129

     Z68.1   Body mass index [BMI] 19.9 or less, adult   A
         Coding Clinic: 2017, Q1, P39

     ● **Z68.2**   Body mass index [BMI] 20-29, adult
         Z68.20   Body mass index [BMI] 20.0-20.9, adult   A
         Z68.21   Body mass index [BMI] 21.0-21.9, adult   A
         Z68.22   Body mass index [BMI] 22.0-22.9, adult   A
         Z68.23   Body mass index [BMI] 23.0-23.9, adult   A
         Z68.24   Body mass index [BMI] 24.0-24.9, adult   A
         Z68.25   Body mass index [BMI] 25.0-25.9, adult   A
         Z68.26   Body mass index [BMI] 26.0-26.9, adult   A
         Z68.27   Body mass index [BMI] 27.0-27.9, adult   A
         Z68.28   Body mass index [BMI] 28.0-28.9, adult   A
         Z68.29   Body mass index [BMI] 29.0-29.9, adult   A

     ● **Z68.3**   Body mass index [BMI] 30-39, adult
         Z68.30   Body mass index [BMI] 30.0-30.9, adult   A
         Z68.31   Body mass index [BMI] 31.0-31.9, adult   A
         Z68.32   Body mass index [BMI] 32.0-32.9, adult   A

Z68.33	Body mass index [BMI] 33.0-33.9, adult	A
Z68.34	Body mass index [BMI] 34.0-34.9, adult	A
Z68.35	Body mass index [BMI] 35.0-35.9, adult	A
Z68.36	Body mass index [BMI] 36.0-36.9, adult	A
Z68.37	Body mass index [BMI] 37.0-37.9, adult	A
Z68.38	Body mass index [BMI] 38.0-38.9, adult	A
Z68.39	Body mass index [BMI] 39.0-39.9, adult	A

● **Z68.4 Body mass index [BMI] 40 or greater, adult**

Z68.41	Body mass index [BMI] 40.0-44.9, adult 🔶	A
Z68.42	Body mass index [BMI] 45.0-49.9, adult 🔶	A
Z68.43	Body mass index [BMI] 50.0-59.9, adult 🔶	A
Z68.44	Body mass index [BMI] 60.0-69.9, adult 🔶	A
Z68.45	Body mass index [BMI] 70 or greater, adult 🔶	A

● **Z68.5 Body mass index [BMI] pediatric**
Coding Clinic: 2018, Q4, P81

Z68.51 Body mass index [BMI] pediatric, less than 5th percentile for age
Coding Clinic: 2018, Q4, P82

Z68.52 Body mass index [BMI] pediatric, 5th percentile to less than 85th percentile for age

Z68.53 Body mass index [BMI] pediatric, 85th percentile to less than 95th percentile for age

Z68.54 Body mass index [BMI] pediatric, greater than or equal to 95th percentile for age

PERSONS ENCOUNTERING HEALTH SERVICES IN OTHER CIRCUMSTANCES (Z69-Z76)

● **Z69 Encounter for mental health services for victim and perpetrator of abuse**

Includes counseling for victims and perpetrators of abuse

● **Z69.0 Encounter for mental health services for child abuse problems**

● **Z69.01 Encounter for mental health services for parental child abuse**

Z69.010 Encounter for mental health services for victim of parental child abuse P
Encounter for mental health services for victim of child abuse by parent
Encounter for mental health services for victim of child neglect by parent
Encounter for mental health services for victim of child psychological abuse by parent
Encounter for mental health services for victim of child sexual abuse by parent

Z69.011 Encounter for mental health services for perpetrator of parental child abuse
Encounter for mental health services for perpetrator of parental child neglect
Encounter for mental health services for perpetrator of parental child psychological abuse
Encounter for mental health services for perpetrator of parental child sexual abuse

Excludes1 encounter for mental health services for non-parental child abuse (Z69.02-)

● **Z69.02 Encounter for mental health services for non-parental child abuse**

Z69.020 Encounter for mental health services for victim of non-parental child abuse P
Encounter for mental health services for victim of non-parental child neglect
Encounter for mental health services for victim of non-parental child psychological abuse
Encounter for mental health services for victim of non-parental child sexual abuse

Z69.021 Encounter for mental health services for perpetrator of non- parental child abuse
Encounter for mental health services for perpetrator of non-parental child neglect
Encounter for mental health services for perpetrator of non-parental child psychological abuse
Encounter for mental health services for perpetrator of non-parental child sexual abuse

● **Z69.1 Encounter for mental health services for spousal or partner abuse problems**

Z69.11 Encounter for mental health services for victim of spousal or partner abuse
Encounter for mental health services for victim of spouse or partner neglect
Encounter for mental health services for victim of spouse or partner psychological abuse
Encounter for mental health services for victim of spouse or partner violence, physical

Z69.12 Encounter for mental health services for perpetrator of spousal or partner abuse
Encounter for mental health services for perpetrator of spouse or partner neglect
Encounter for mental health services for perpetrator of spouse or partner psychological abuse
Encounter for mental health services for perpetrator of spouse or partner violence, physical
Encounter for mental health services for perpetrator of spouse or partner violence, sexual

● **Z69.8 Encounter for mental health services for victim or perpetrator of other abuse**

Z69.81 Encounter for mental health services for victim of other abuse
Encounter for mental health services for victim of non-spousal adult abuse
Encounter for mental health services for victim of spouse or partner violence, sexual
Encounter for rape victim counseling

Z69.82 Encounter for mental health services for perpetrator of other abuse
Encounter for mental health services for perpetrator of non-spousal adult abuse

● **Z70 Counseling related to sexual attitude, behavior and orientation**

Includes encounter for mental health services for sexual attitude, behavior and orientation

Excludes2 contraceptive or procreative counseling (Z30-Z31)

Z70.0 Counseling related to sexual attitude

Z70.1 Counseling related to patient's sexual behavior and orientation
Patient concerned regarding impotence
Patient concerned regarding non-responsiveness
Patient concerned regarding promiscuity
Patient concerned regarding sexual orientation

CHAPTER 21 (Z00-Z99)

▶ New ⇨ Revised ~~deleted~~ Deleted Excludes 1 Excludes 2 Includes Use additional Code first Code also Key words
OGCR Official Guidelines X Assign placeholder X ● Use Additional Character(s) ▶ Manifestation Code 🔶 Hierarchical Condition Category **Coding Clinic**

Z70.2   Counseling related to sexual behavior and orientation of third party
>Advice sought regarding sexual behavior and orientation of child
>Advice sought regarding sexual behavior and orientation of partner
>Advice sought regarding sexual behavior and orientation of spouse

Z70.3   Counseling related to combined concerns regarding sexual attitude, behavior and orientation

Z70.8   Other sex counseling
>Encounter for sex education

Z70.9   Sex counseling, unspecified

● **Z71**   Persons encountering health services for other counseling and medical advice, not elsewhere classified
>**Excludes2**   contraceptive or procreation counseling (Z30-Z31)
>sex counseling (Z70.-)

Z71.0   Person encountering health services to consult on behalf of another person
>Person encountering health services to seek advice or treatment for non-attending third party
>**Excludes2**   anxiety (normal) about sick person in family (Z63.7)
>expectant (adoptive) parent(s) pre-birth pediatrician visit (Z76.81)

Z71.1   Person with feared health complaint in whom no diagnosis is made
>Person encountering health services with feared condition which was not demonstrated
>Person encountering health services in which problem was normal state
>"Worried well"
>**Excludes1**   medical observation for suspected diseases and conditions proven not to exist (Z03.-)
>
>Coding Clinic: 2016, Q4, P7

Z71.2   Person consulting for explanation of examination or test findings

Z71.3   Dietary counseling and surveillance
>Use additional code for any associated underlying medical condition
>Use additional code to identify body mass index (BMI), if known (Z68.-)

● **Z71.4**   Alcohol abuse counseling and surveillance
>Use additional code for alcohol abuse or dependence (F10.-)

>**Z71.41**   Alcohol abuse counseling and surveillance of alcoholic

>**Z71.42**   Counseling for family member of alcoholic
>>Counseling for significant other, partner, or friend of alcoholic

● **Z71.5**   Drug abuse counseling and surveillance
>Use additional code for drug abuse or dependence (F11-F16, F18-F19)

>**Z71.51**   Drug abuse counseling and surveillance of drug abuser

>**Z71.52**   Counseling for family member of drug abuser
>>Counseling for significant other, partner, or friend of drug abuser

Z71.6   Tobacco abuse counseling
>Use additional code for nicotine dependence (F17.-)

Z71.7   Human immunodeficiency virus [HIV] counseling

● **Z71.8**   Other specified counseling
>**Excludes2**   counseling for contraception (Z30.0-)

Z71.81   Spiritual or religious counseling

Z71.82   Exercise counseling

Z71.83   Encounter for nonprocreative genetic counseling
>**Excludes1**   counseling for procreative genetics (Z31.5)
>counseling for procreative management (Z31.6)

Z71.84   Encounter for health counseling related to travel
>Encounter for health risk and safety counseling for (international) travel
>Code also, if applicable, encounter for immunization (Z23)
>**Excludes2**   encounter for administrative examination (Z02.-)
>encounter for other special examination without complaint, suspected or reported diagnosis (Z01.-)

▶ **Z71.85** Encounter for immunization safety counseling
>▶Encounter for vaccine product safety counseling
>▶Code also, if applicable, encounter for immunization (Z23)
>▶Code also, if applicable, immunization not carried out (Z28.-)
>▶**Excludes1**   encounter for health counseling related to travel (Z71.84)

Z71.89   Other specified counseling

Z71.9   Counseling, unspecified
>Encounter for medical advice NOS

● **Z72**   Problems related to lifestyle
>**Excludes2**   problems related to life-management difficulty (Z73.-)
>problems related to socioeconomic and psychosocial circumstances (Z55-Z65)
>Coding Clinic: 2016, Q4, P130

Z72.0   Tobacco use
>Tobacco use NOS
>**Excludes1**   history of tobacco dependence (Z87.891)
>nicotine dependence (F17.2-)
>tobacco dependence (F17.2-)
>tobacco use during pregnancy (O99.33-)

Z72.3   Lack of physical exercise

Z72.4   Inappropriate diet and eating habits
>**Excludes1**   behavioral eating disorders of infancy or childhood (F98.2.-F98.3)
>eating disorders (F50.-)
>⇢lack of adequate food (Z59.48)
>malnutrition and other nutritional deficiencies (E40-E64)

● **Z72.5**   High risk sexual behavior
>Promiscuity
>**Excludes1**   paraphilias (F65)

Z72.51   High risk heterosexual behavior

Z72.52   High risk homosexual behavior

Z72.53   High risk bisexual behavior

Z72.6   Gambling and betting
>**Excludes1**   compulsive or pathological gambling (F63.0)

● **Z72.8 Other problems related to lifestyle**
  ● **Z72.81 Antisocial behavior**
    Excludes1 conduct disorders (F91.-)
    Z72.810 Child and adolescent antisocial behavior P
      Antisocial behavior (child) (adolescent) without manifest psychiatric disorder
      Delinquency NOS
      Group delinquency
      Offenses in the context of gang membership
      Stealing in company with others
      Truancy from school
    Z72.811 Adult antisocial behavior A
      Adult antisocial behavior without manifest psychiatric disorder
  ● **Z72.82 Problems related to sleep**
    Z72.820 Sleep deprivation
      Lack of adequate sleep
      Excludes1 insomnia (G47.0-)
    Z72.821 Inadequate sleep hygiene
      Bad sleep habits
      Irregular sleep habits
      Unhealthy sleep wake schedule
      Excludes1 insomnia (F51.0-, G47.0-)
  Z72.89 Other problems related to lifestyle
    Self-damaging behavior
  Z72.9 Problem related to lifestyle, unspecified

● **Z73 Problems related to life management difficulty**
  Excludes2 problems related to socioeconomic and psychosocial circumstances (Z55-Z65)
  Z73.0 Burn-out
  Z73.1 Type A behavior pattern
  Z73.2 Lack of relaxation and leisure
  Z73.3 Stress, not elsewhere classified
    Physical and mental strain NOS
    Excludes1 stress related to employment or unemployment (Z56.-)
  Z73.4 Inadequate social skills, not elsewhere classified
  Z73.5 Social role conflict, not elsewhere classified
  Z73.6 Limitation of activities due to disability
    Excludes1 care-provider dependency (Z74.-)
  ● **Z73.8 Other problems related to life management difficulty**
    ● **Z73.81 Behavioral insomnia of childhood**
      Z73.810 Behavioral insomnia of childhood, sleep-onset association type P
      Z73.811 Behavioral insomnia of childhood, limit setting type P
      Z73.812 Behavioral insomnia of childhood, combined type P
      Z73.819 Behavioral insomnia of childhood, unspecified type P
    Z73.82 Dual sensory impairment
    Z73.89 Other problems related to life management difficulty
  Z73.9 Problem related to life management difficulty, unspecified

● **Z74 Problems related to care provider dependency**
  Excludes2 dependence on enabling machines or devices NEC (Z99.-)
  ● **Z74.0 Reduced mobility**
    Z74.01 Bed confinement status
      Bedridden
    Z74.09 Other reduced mobility
      Chairridden
      Reduced mobility NOS
      Excludes2 wheelchair dependence (Z99.3)

  Z74.1 Need for assistance with personal care
  Z74.2 Need for assistance at home and no other household member able to render care
  Z74.3 Need for continuous supervision
  Z74.8 Other problems related to care provider dependency
  Z74.9 Problem related to care provider dependency, unspecified

● **Z75 Problems related to medical facilities and other health care**
  Z75.0 Medical services not available in home
    Excludes1 no other household member able to render care (Z74.2)
  Z75.1 Person awaiting admission to adequate facility elsewhere
  Z75.2 Other waiting period for investigation and treatment
  Z75.3 Unavailability and inaccessibility of health care facilities
    Excludes1 bed unavailable (Z75.1)
  Z75.4 Unavailability and inaccessibility of other helping agencies
  Z75.5 Holiday relief care
  Z75.8 Other problems related to medical facilities and other health care
  Z75.9 Unspecified problem related to medical facilities and other health care

● **Z76 Persons encountering health services in other circumstances**
  Z76.0 Encounter for issue of repeat prescription
    Encounter for issue of repeat prescription for appliance
    Encounter for issue of repeat prescription for medicaments
    Encounter for issue of repeat prescription for spectacles
    Excludes2 issue of medical certificate (Z02.7)
      repeat prescription for contraceptive (Z30.4-)
  Z76.1 Encounter for health supervision and care of foundling
  Z76.2 Encounter for health supervision and care of other healthy infant and child P
    Encounter for medical or nursing care or supervision of healthy infant under circumstances such as adverse socioeconomic conditions at home
    Encounter for medical or nursing care or supervision of healthy infant under circumstances such as awaiting foster or adoptive placement
    Encounter for medical or nursing care or supervision of healthy infant under circumstances such as maternal illness
    Encounter for medical or nursing care or supervision of healthy infant under circumstances such as number of children at home preventing or interfering with normal care
  Z76.3 Healthy person accompanying sick person
  Z76.4 Other boarder to healthcare facility
    Excludes1 homelessness (Z59.0-)
  Z76.5 Malingerer [conscious simulation]
    Person feigning illness (with obvious motivation)
    Excludes1 factitious disorder (F68.1-, F68.A)
      peregrinating patient (F68.1-)
  ● **Z76.8 Persons encountering health services in other specified circumstances**
    Z76.81 Expectant parent(s) prebirth pediatrician visit
      Pre-adoption pediatrician visit for adoptive parent(s)
    Z76.82 Awaiting organ transplant status
      Patient waiting for organ availability
    Z76.89 Persons encountering health services in other specified circumstances
      Persons encountering health services NOS

▶ New   ⇒ Revised   ~~deleted~~ Deleted   Excludes 1   Excludes 2   Includes   Use additional   Code first   Code also   Key words
OGCR Official Guidelines   X Assign placeholder X   ● Use Additional Character(s)   ▌ Manifestation Code   ❝❞ Hierarchical Condition Category   **Coding Clinic**

PERSONS WITH POTENTIAL HEALTH HAZARDS RELATED TO FAMILY AND PERSONAL HISTORY AND CERTAIN CONDITIONS INFLUENCING HEALTH STATUS (Z77-Z99)

Code also any follow-up examination (Z08-Z09)

● **Z77**   Other contact with and (suspected) exposures hazardous to health

Includes	contact with and (suspected) exposures to potential hazards to health
Excludes2	contact with and (suspected) exposure to communicable diseases (Z20.-)

exposure to (parental) (environmental) tobacco smoke in the perinatal period (P96.81)

newborn affected by noxious substances transmitted via placenta or breast milk (P04.-)

occupational exposure to risk factors (Z57.-)

retained foreign body (Z18.-)

retained foreign body fully removed (Z87.821)

toxic effects of substances chiefly nonmedicinal as to source (T51-T65)

● **Z77.0**   Contact with and (suspected) exposure to hazardous, chiefly nonmedicinal, chemicals

   ● **Z77.01**   Contact with and (suspected) exposure to hazardous metals

      Z77.010   Contact with and (suspected) exposure to arsenic

      Z77.011   Contact with and (suspected) exposure to lead

      Z77.012   Contact with and (suspected) exposure to uranium

Excludes1	retained depleted uranium fragments (Z18.01)

      Z77.018   Contact with and (suspected) exposure to other hazardous metals

         Contact with and (suspected) exposure to chromium compounds

         Contact with and (suspected) exposure to nickel dust

   ● **Z77.02**   Contact with and (suspected) exposure to hazardous aromatic compounds

      Z77.020   Contact with and (suspected) exposure to aromatic amines

      Z77.021   Contact with and (suspected) exposure to benzene

      Z77.028   Contact with and (suspected) exposure to other hazardous aromatic compounds

         Aromatic dyes NOS

         Polycyclic aromatic hydrocarbons

   ● **Z77.09**   Contact with and (suspected) exposure to other hazardous, chiefly nonmedicinal, chemicals

      Z77.090   Contact with and (suspected) exposure to asbestos

      Z77.098   Contact with and (suspected) exposure to other hazardous, chiefly nonmedicinal, chemicals

         Dyes NOS

● **Z77.1**   Contact with and (suspected) exposure to environmental pollution and hazards in the physical environment

   ● **Z77.11**   Contact with and (suspected) exposure to environmental pollution

      Z77.110   Contact with and (suspected) exposure to air pollution

      Z77.111   Contact with and (suspected) exposure to water pollution

      Z77.112   Contact with and (suspected) exposure to soil pollution

      Z77.118   Contact with and (suspected) exposure to other environmental pollution

● **Z77.12**   Contact with and (suspected) exposure to hazards in the physical environment

      Z77.120   Contact with and (suspected) exposure to mold (toxic)

      Z77.121   Contact with and (suspected) exposure to harmful algae and algae toxins

         Contact with and (suspected) exposure to (harmful) algae bloom NOS

         Contact with and (suspected) exposure to blue-green algae bloom

         Contact with and (suspected) exposure to brown tide

         Contact with and (suspected) exposure to cyanobacteria bloom

         Contact with and (suspected) exposure to Florida red tide

         Contact with and (suspected) exposure to pfiesteria piscicida

         Contact with and (suspected) exposure to red tide

      Z77.122   Contact with and (suspected) exposure to noise

      Z77.123   Contact with and (suspected) exposure to radon and other naturally occurring radiation

Excludes2	radiation exposure as the cause of a confirmed condition (W88-W90, X39.0-)
	radiation sickness NOS (T66)

      Z77.128   Contact with and (suspected) exposure to other hazards in the physical environment

● **Z77.2**   Contact with and (suspected) exposure to other hazardous substances

      Z77.21   Contact with and (suspected) exposure to potentially hazardous body fluids

      Z77.22   Contact with and (suspected) exposure to environmental tobacco smoke (acute) (chronic)

         Exposure to second hand tobacco smoke (acute) (chronic)

         Passive smoking (acute) (chronic)

Excludes1	nicotine dependence (F17.-)
	tobacco use (Z72.0)

Excludes2	occupational exposure to environmental tobacco smoke (Z57.31)

      Z77.29   Contact with and (suspected) exposure to other hazardous substances

         Coding Clinic: 2016, Q2, P34

  Z77.9   Other contact with and (suspected) exposures hazardous to health

● **Z78**   Other specified health status

Excludes2	asymptomatic human immunodeficiency virus [HIV] infection status (Z21)
	postprocedural status (Z93-Z99)
	sex reassignment status (Z87.890)

  Z78.0   Asymptomatic menopausal state ♀   A

      Menopausal state NOS

      Postmenopausal status NOS

Excludes2	symptomatic menopausal state (N95.1)

  Z78.1   Physical restraint status

Excludes1	physical restraint due to a procedure - omit code

  Z78.9   Other specified health status

CHAPTER 21 (Z00-Z99)

● **Z79**   **Long term (current) drug therapy**

     Includes   long term (current) drug use for prophylactic purposes

     Code also any therapeutic drug level monitoring (Z51.81)

     Excludes2   drug abuse and dependence (F11-F19)

                    drug use complicating pregnancy, childbirth, and the puerperium (O99.32-)

● **Z79.0**   **Long term (current) use of anticoagulants and antithrombotics/antiplatelets**

     Excludes2   long term (current) use of aspirin (Z79.82)

     Coding Clinic: 2021, Q1, P12-13

     Z79.01   **Long term (current) use of anticoagulants**

              Coding Clinic: 2021, Q1, P5

     Z79.02   **Long term (current) use of antithrombotics/antiplatelets**

Z79.1   **Long term (current) use of non-steroidal anti-inflammatories (NSAID)**

     Excludes2   long term (current) use of aspirin (Z79.82)

Z79.2   **Long term (current) use of antibiotics**

Z79.3   **Long term (current) use of hormonal contraceptives**

     Long term (current) use of birth control pill or patch

Z79.4   **Long term (current) use of insulin**

     ~~Excludes1~~   ~~long term (current) use of oral antidiabetic drugs (Z79.84)~~

                ~~long term (current) use of oral hypoglycemic drugs (Z79.84)~~

     ▶ **Excludes2**   long term (current) use of oral hypoglycemic drugs (Z79.84)

            ▶long term (current) use of oral antidiabetic drugs (Z79.84)

● **Z79.5**   **Long term (current) use of steroids**

     Z79.51   **Long term (current) use of inhaled steroids**

     Z79.52   **Long term (current) use of systemic steroids**

● **Z79.8**   **Other long term (current) drug therapy**

     ● **Z79.81**   **Long term (current) use of agents affecting estrogen receptors and estrogen levels**

              Code first, if applicable:

                malignant neoplasm of breast (C50.-)

                malignant neoplasm of prostate (C61)

              Use additional code, if applicable, to identify:

                estrogen receptor positive status (Z17.0)

                family history of breast cancer (Z80.3)

                genetic susceptibility to malignant neoplasm (cancer) (Z15.0-)

                personal history of breast cancer (Z85.3)

                personal history of prostate cancer (Z85.46)

                postmenopausal status (Z78.0)

              Excludes1   hormone replacement therapy (Z79.890)

         Z79.810   **Long term (current) use of selective estrogen receptor modulators (SERMs)**

              Long term (current) use of raloxifene (Evista)

              Long term (current) use of tamoxifen (Nolvadex)

              Long term (current) use of toremifene (Fareston)

         Z79.811   **Long term (current) use of aromatase inhibitors**

              Long term (current) use of anastrozole (Arimidex)

              Long term (current) use of exemestane (Aromasin)

              Long term (current) use of letrozole (Femara)

         Z79.818   **Long term (current) use of other agents affecting estrogen receptors and estrogen levels**

              Long term (current) use of estrogen receptor downregulators

              Long term (current) use of fulvestrant (Faslodex)

              Long term (current) use of gonadotropin-releasing hormone (GnRH) agonist

              Long term (current) use of goserelin acetate (Zoladex)

              Long term (current) use of leuprolide acetate (leuprorelin) (Lupron)

              Long term (current) use of megestrol acetate (Megace)

     Z79.82   **Long term (current) use of aspirin**

     Z79.83   **Long term (current) use of bisphosphonates**

            Coding Clinic: 2016, Q4, P42

     Z79.84   **Long term (current) use of oral hypoglycemic drugs**

            Long term (current) use of oral antidiabetic drugs

            Excludes2   long term (current) use of insulin (Z79.4)

            Coding Clinic: 2016, Q4, P76, 121-122, 126

● **Z79.89**   **Other long term (current) drug therapy**

     Z79.890   **Hormone replacement therapy**

     Z79.891   **Long term (current) use of opiate analgesic**

            Long term (current) use of methadone for pain management

            Excludes1   methodone use NOS (F11.9-)

                  use of methodone for treatment of heroin addiction (F11.2-)

     Z79.899   **Other long term (current) drug therapy**

            Coding Clinic: 2015, Q4, P34, Q3, P21

● **Z80**   **Family history of primary malignant neoplasm**

     Z80.0   **Family history of malignant neoplasm of digestive organs**

            Conditions classifiable to C15-C26

            Coding Clinic: 2018, Q1, P7

     Z80.1   **Family history of malignant neoplasm of trachea, bronchus and lung**

            Conditions classifiable to C33-C34

     Z80.2   **Family history of malignant neoplasm of other respiratory and intrathoracic organs**

            Conditions classifiable to C30-C32, C37-C39

     Z80.3   **Family history of malignant neoplasm of breast**

            Conditions classifiable to C50.-

     ● **Z80.4**   **Family history of malignant neoplasm of genital organs**

            Conditions classifiable to C51-C63

         Z80.41   **Family history of malignant neoplasm of ovary**

         Z80.42   **Family history of malignant neoplasm of prostate**

         Z80.43   **Family history of malignant neoplasm of testis**

         Z80.49   **Family history of malignant neoplasm of other genital organs**

     ● **Z80.5**   **Family history of malignant neoplasm of urinary tract**

            Conditions classifiable to C64-C68

         Z80.51   **Family history of malignant neoplasm of kidney**

Z80.52   Family history of malignant neoplasm of bladder

Z80.59   Family history of malignant neoplasm of other urinary tract organ

Z80.6   Family history of leukemia
Conditions classifiable to C91-C95

Z80.7   Family history of other malignant neoplasms of lymphoid, hematopoietic and related tissues
Conditions classifiable to C81-C90, C96.-

Z80.8   Family history of malignant neoplasm of other organs or systems
Conditions classifiable to C00-C14, C40-C49, C69-C79

Z80.9   Family history of malignant neoplasm, unspecified
Conditions classifiable to C80.1

● Z81   Family history of mental and behavioral disorders

Z81.0   Family history of intellectual disabilities
Conditions classifiable to F70-F79

Z81.1   Family history of alcohol abuse and dependence
Conditions classifiable to F10.-

Z81.2   Family history of tobacco abuse and dependence
Conditions classifiable to F17.-

Z81.3   Family history of other psychoactive substance abuse and dependence
Conditions classifiable to F11-F16, F18-F19

Z81.4   Family history of other substance abuse and dependence
Conditions classifiable to F55

Z81.8   Family history of other mental and behavioral disorders
Conditions classifiable elsewhere in F01-F99

● Z82   Family history of certain disabilities and chronic diseases (leading to disablement)

Z82.0   Family history of epilepsy and other diseases of the nervous system
Conditions classifiable to G00-G99

Z82.1   Family history of blindness and visual loss
Conditions classifiable to H54.-

Z82.2   Family history of deafness and hearing loss
Conditions classifiable to H90-H91

Z82.3   Family history of stroke
Conditions classifiable to I60-I64

● Z82.4   Family history of ischemic heart disease and other diseases of the circulatory system
➧Conditions classifiable to I00-I5A, I65-I99

Z82.41   Family history of sudden cardiac death

Z82.49   Family history of ischemic heart disease and other diseases of the circulatory system

Z82.5   Family history of asthma and other chronic lower respiratory diseases
Conditions classifiable to J40-J47
Excludes2   family history of other diseases of the respiratory system (Z83.6)

● Z82.6   Family history of arthritis and other diseases of the musculoskeletal system and connective tissue
Conditions classifiable to M00-M99

Z82.61   Family history of arthritis

Z82.62   Family history of osteoporosis

Z82.69   Family history of other diseases of the musculoskeletal system and connective tissue

● Z82.7   Family history of congenital malformations, deformations and chromosomal abnormalities
Conditions classifiable to Q00-Q99

Z82.71   Family history of polycystic kidney

Z82.79   Family history of other congenital malformations, deformations and chromosomal abnormalities

Z82.8   Family history of other disabilities and chronic diseases leading to disablement, not elsewhere classified

● Z83   Family history of other specific disorders
Excludes2   contact with and (suspected) exposure to communicable disease in the family (Z20.-)

Z83.0   Family history of human immunodeficiency virus [HIV] disease
Conditions classifiable to B20

Z83.1   Family history of other infectious and parasitic diseases
Conditions classifiable to A00-B19, B25-B94, B99

Z83.2   Family history of diseases of the blood and blood-forming organs and certain disorders involving the immune mechanism
Conditions classifiable to D50-D89

Z83.3   Family history of diabetes mellitus
Conditions classifiable to E08-E13

● Z83.4   Family history of other endocrine, nutritional and metabolic diseases
Conditions classifiable to E00-E07, E15-E88

Z83.41   Family history of multiple endocrine neoplasia [MEN] syndrome

Z83.42   Family history of familial hypercholesterolemia
Coding Clinic: 2016, Q4, P77

● Z83.43   Family history of other disorder of lipoprotein metabolism and other lipidemias

Z83.430   Family history of elevated lipoprotein(a)
Family history of elevated Lp(a)

Z83.438   Family history of other disorder of lipoprotein metabolism and other lipidemia
Family history of familial combined hyperlipidemia

Z83.49   Family history of other endocrine, nutritional and metabolic diseases

● Z83.5   Family history of eye and ear disorders

● Z83.51   Family history of eye disorders
Conditions classifiable to H00-H53, H55-H59
Excludes2   family history of blindness and visual loss (Z82.1)

Z83.511   Family history of glaucoma

Z83.518   Family history of other specified eye disorder

Z83.52   Family history of ear disorders
Conditions classifiable to H60-H83, H92-H95
Excludes2   family history of deafness and hearing loss (Z82.2)

Z83.6   Family history of other diseases of the respiratory system
Conditions classifiable to J00-J39, J60-J99
Excludes2   family history of asthma and other chronic lower respiratory diseases (Z82.5)

● Z83.7   Family history of diseases of the digestive system
Conditions classifiable to K00-K93

Z83.71   Family history of colonic polyps
Excludes2   family history of malignant neoplasm of digestive organs (Z80.0)
Coding Clinic: 2021, Q1, P15

Z83.79   Family history of other diseases of the digestive system

● Z84   Family history of other conditions

Z84.0   Family history of diseases of the skin and subcutaneous tissue
Conditions classifiable to L00-L99

Z84.1   Family history of disorders of kidney and ureter
Conditions classifiable to N00-N29

Z84.2 Family history of other diseases of the genitourinary system
> Conditions classifiable to N30-N99
> **Coding Clinic: 2016, Q4, P77**

Z84.3 Family history of consanguinity

● **Z84.8** Family history of other specified conditions

Z84.81 Family history of carrier of genetic disease
> **Coding Clinic: 2021, Q1, P15**

Z84.82 Family history of sudden infant death syndrome
> Family history of SIDS

Z84.89 Family history of other specified conditions

● **Z85** Personal history of malignant neoplasm
> *Code first* any follow-up examination after treatment of malignant neoplasm (Z08)
>
> Use additional code to identify:
> alcohol use and dependence (F10.-)
> exposure to environmental tobacco smoke (Z77.22)
> history of tobacco dependence (Z87.891)
> occupational exposure to environmental tobacco smoke (Z57.31)
> tobacco dependence (F17.-)
> tobacco use (Z72.0)
>
> **Excludes2** personal history of benign neoplasm (Z86.01-)
> personal history of carcinoma-in-situ (Z86.00-)

● **Z85.0** Personal history of malignant neoplasm of digestive organs

Z85.00 Personal history of malignant neoplasm of unspecified digestive organ

Z85.01 Personal history of malignant neoplasm of esophagus
> Conditions classifiable to C15

● **Z85.02** Personal history of malignant neoplasm of stomach

Z85.020 Personal history of malignant carcinoid tumor of stomach
> Conditions classifiable to C7A.092

Z85.028 Personal history of other malignant neoplasm of stomach
> Conditions classifiable to C16

● **Z85.03** Personal history of malignant neoplasm of large intestine

Z85.030 Personal history of malignant carcinoid tumor of large intestine
> Conditions classifiable to C7A.022-C7A.025, C7A.029

Z85.038 Personal history of other malignant neoplasm of large intestine
> Conditions classifiable to C18

● **Z85.04** Personal history of malignant neoplasm of rectum, rectosigmoid junction, and anus

Z85.040 Personal history of malignant carcinoid tumor of rectum
> Conditions classifiable to C7A.026

Z85.048 Personal history of other malignant neoplasm of rectum, rectosigmoid junction, and anus
> Conditions classifiable to C19-C21

Z85.05 Personal history of malignant neoplasm of liver
> Conditions classifiable to C22

● **Z85.06** Personal history of malignant neoplasm of small intestine

Z85.060 Personal history of malignant carcinoid tumor of small intestine
> Conditions classifiable to C7A.01-

Z85.068 Personal history of other malignant neoplasm of small intestine
> Conditions classifiable to C17

Z85.07 Personal history of malignant neoplasm of pancreas
> Conditions classifiable to C25

Z85.09 Personal history of malignant neoplasm of other digestive organs

● **Z85.1** Personal history of malignant neoplasm of trachea, bronchus and lung

● **Z85.11** Personal history of malignant neoplasm of bronchus and lung

Z85.110 Personal history of malignant carcinoid tumor of bronchus and lung
> Conditions classifiable to C7A.090

Z85.118 Personal history of other malignant neoplasm of bronchus and lung
> Conditions classifiable to C34

Z85.12 Personal history of malignant neoplasm of trachea
> Conditions classifiable to C33

● **Z85.2** Personal history of malignant neoplasm of other respiratory and intrathoracic organs

Z85.20 Personal history of malignant neoplasm of unspecified respiratory organ

Z85.21 Personal history of malignant neoplasm of larynx
> Conditions classifiable to C32

Z85.22 Personal history of malignant neoplasm of nasal cavities, middle ear, and accessory sinuses
> Conditions classifiable to C30-C31

● **Z85.23** Personal history of malignant neoplasm of thymus

Z85.230 Personal history of malignant carcinoid tumor of thymus
> Conditions classifiable to C7A.091

Z85.238 Personal history of other malignant neoplasm of thymus
> Conditions classifiable to C37

Z85.29 Personal history of malignant neoplasm of other respiratory and intrathoracic organs

Z85.3 Personal history of malignant neoplasm of breast
> Conditions classifiable to C50.-

● **Z85.4** Personal history of malignant neoplasm of genital organs
> Conditions classifiable to C51-C63

Z85.40 Personal history of malignant neoplasm of unspecified female genital organ ♀

Z85.41 Personal history of malignant neoplasm of cervix uteri ♀

Z85.42 Personal history of malignant neoplasm of other parts of uterus ♀

Z85.43 Personal history of malignant neoplasm of ovary ♀

Z85.44 Personal history of malignant neoplasm of other female genital organs ♀

Z85.45 Personal history of malignant neoplasm of unspecified male genital organ ♂

Z85.46 Personal history of malignant neoplasm of prostate ♂

Z85.47 Personal history of malignant neoplasm of testis ♂

Z85.48 Personal history of malignant neoplasm of epididymis ♂

Z85.49 Personal history of malignant neoplasm of other male genital organs ♂

▶ New   ⇒ Revised   ~~deleted~~ Deleted   Excludes 1   Excludes 2   Includes   Use additional   Code first   Code also   Key words
OGCR Official Guidelines   X Assign placeholder X   ● Use Additional Character(s)   ▶ Manifestation Code   🅗 Hierarchical Condition Category   **Coding Clinic**

● **Z85.5**   **Personal history of malignant neoplasm of urinary tract**
     Conditions classifiable to C64-C68

   Z85.50   Personal history of malignant neoplasm of unspecified urinary tract organ

   Z85.51   Personal history of malignant neoplasm of bladder

●   **Z85.52**   Personal history of malignant neoplasm of kidney

     Excludes1   personal history of malignant neoplasm of renal pelvis (Z85.53)

     Z85.520   Personal history of malignant carcinoid tumor of kidney
       Conditions classifiable to C7A.093

     Z85.528   Personal history of other malignant neoplasm of kidney
       Conditions classifiable to C64

   Z85.53   Personal history of malignant neoplasm of renal pelvis

   Z85.54   Personal history of malignant neoplasm of ureter

   Z85.59   Personal history of malignant neoplasm of other urinary tract organ

Z85.6   **Personal history of leukemia**
     Conditions classifiable to C91-C95

     Excludes1   leukemia in remission C91.0-C95.9 with 5th character 1

● **Z85.7**   **Personal history of other malignant neoplasms of lymphoid, hematopoietic and related tissues**

   Z85.71   Personal history of Hodgkin lymphoma
     Conditions classifiable to C81

   Z85.72   Personal history of non-Hodgkin lymphomas
     Conditions classifiable to C82-C85

   Z85.79   Personal history of other malignant neoplasms of lymphoid, hematopoietic and related tissues
     Conditions classifiable to C88-C90, C96

     Excludes1   multiple myeloma in remission (C90.01)
       plasma cell leukemia in remission (C90.11)
       plasmacytoma in remission (C90.21)

● **Z85.8**   **Personal history of malignant neoplasms of other organs and systems**
     Conditions classifiable to C00-C14, C40-C49, C69-C75, C7A.098, C76-C79

●   **Z85.81**   Personal history of malignant neoplasm of lip, oral cavity, and pharynx
     Conditions classifiable to C00-C14

     Z85.810   Personal history of malignant neoplasm of tongue

     Z85.818   Personal history of malignant neoplasm of other sites of lip, oral cavity, and pharynx

     Z85.819   Personal history of malignant neoplasm of unspecified site of lip, oral cavity, and pharynx

●   **Z85.82**   Personal history of malignant neoplasm of skin

     Z85.820   Personal history of malignant melanoma of skin
       Conditions classifiable to C43

     Z85.821   Personal history of Merkel cell carcinoma
       Conditions classifiable to C4A

     Z85.828   Personal history of other malignant neoplasm of skin
       Conditions classifiable to C44

●   **Z85.83**   Personal history of malignant neoplasm of bone and soft tissue
     Conditions classifiable to C40-C41; C45-C49

     Z85.830   Personal history of malignant neoplasm of bone

     Z85.831   Personal history of malignant neoplasm of soft tissue

       Excludes2   personal history of malignant neoplasm of skin (Z85.82-)

●   **Z85.84**   Personal history of malignant neoplasm of eye and nervous tissue
     Conditions classifiable to C69-C72

     Z85.840   Personal history of malignant neoplasm of eye

     Z85.841   Personal history of malignant neoplasm of brain

     Z85.848   Personal history of malignant neoplasm of other parts of nervous tissue

●   **Z85.85**   Personal history of malignant neoplasm of endocrine glands
     Conditions classifiable to C73-C75

     Z85.850   Personal history of malignant neoplasm of thyroid

     Z85.858   Personal history of malignant neoplasm of other endocrine glands

   Z85.89   Personal history of malignant neoplasm of other organs and systems
     Conditions classifiable to C7A.098, C76, C77-C79

Z85.9   **Personal history of malignant neoplasm, unspecified**
     Conditions classifiable to C7A.00, C80.1

● **Z86**   **Personal history of certain other diseases**
     Code first any follow-up examination after treatment (Z09)

● **Z86.0**   **Personal history of in-situ and benign neoplasms and neoplasms of uncertain behavior**
     Excludes2   personal history of malignant neoplasms (Z85.-)

● **Z86.00**   **Personal history of in-situ neoplasm**
     Conditions classifiable to D00-D09

     Z86.000   Personal history of in-situ neoplasm of breast
       Conditions classifiable to D05

     Z86.001   Personal history of in-situ neoplasm of cervix uteri ♀
       Conditions classifiable to D06
       Personal history of cervical intraepithelial neoplasia III [CIN III]

     Z86.002   Personal history of in-situ neoplasm of other and unspecified genital organs
       Conditions classifiable to D07
       Personal history of high-grade prostatic intraepithelial neoplasia III [HGPIN III]
       Personal history of vaginal intraepithelial neoplasia III [VAIN III]
       Personal history of vulvar intraepithelial neoplasia III [VIN III]

     Z86.003   Personal history of in-situ neoplasm of oral cavity, esophagus and stomach
       Conditions classifiable to D00

CHAPTER 21 (Z00-Z99)

CHAPTER 21 (Z00-Z99)

Z86.004 **Personal history of in-situ neoplasm of other and unspecified digestive organs**
Conditions classifiable to D01
Personal history of anal intraepithelial neoplasia (AIN III)

Z86.005 **Personal history of in-situ neoplasm of middle ear and respiratory system**
Conditions classifiable to D02

Z86.006 **Personal history of melanoma in-situ**
Conditions classifiable to D03

　　Excludes2　sites other than skin - code to personal history of in-situ neoplasm of the site

Z86.007 **Personal history of in-situ neoplasm of skin**
Conditions classifiable to D04
Personal history of carcinoma in situ of skin

Z86.008 **Personal history of in-situ neoplasm of other site**
Conditions classifiable to D09

● **Z86.01** **Personal history of benign neoplasm**
Coding Clinic: 2017, Q1, P14

Z86.010 **Personal history of colonic polyps**
Coding Clinic: 2021, Q1, P15; 2017, Q1, P9, P14

Z86.011 **Personal history of benign neoplasm of the brain**

Z86.012 **Personal history of benign carcinoid tumor**

Z86.018 **Personal history of other benign neoplasm**
Coding Clinic: 2017, Q1, P14

Z86.03 **Personal history of neoplasm of uncertain behavior**

● **Z86.1** **Personal history of infectious and parasitic diseases**
Conditions classifiable to A00-B89, B99

　　Excludes1　personal history of infectious diseases specific to a body system sequelae of infectious and parasitic diseases (B90-B94)

Coding Clinic: 2016, Q4, P5

Z86.11 **Personal history of tuberculosis**

Z86.12 **Personal history of poliomyelitis**

Z86.13 **Personal history of malaria**

Z86.14 **Personal history of Methicillin resistant Staphylococcus aureus infection**
Personal history of MRSA infection

Z86.15 **Personal history of latent tuberculosis infection**

Z86.16 **Personal history of COVID-19**
Coding Clinic: 2021, Q1, P34-35, 40-42, 44, 46
▶ **Excludes1**　post COVID-19 condition (U09.9)

Z86.19 **Personal history of other infectious and parasitic diseases**
Coding Clinic: 2021, Q1, P34-35, 40-41

Z86.2 **Personal history of diseases of the blood and blood-forming organs and certain disorders involving the immune mechanism**
Conditions classifiable to D50-D89

● **Z86.3** **Personal history of endocrine, nutritional and metabolic diseases**
Conditions classifiable to E00-E88

Z86.31 **Personal history of diabetic foot ulcer**
　　Excludes2　current diabetic foot ulcer (E08.621, E09.621, E10.621, E11.621, E13.621)

Z86.32 **Personal history of gestational diabetes** ♀
Personal history of conditions classifiable to O24.4-
　　Excludes1　gestational diabetes mellitus in current pregnancy (O24.4-)

Z86.39 **Personal history of other endocrine, nutritional and metabolic disease**
Coding Clinic: 2020, Q1, P13

● **Z86.5** **Personal history of mental and behavioral disorders**
Conditions classifiable to F40-F59

Z86.51 **Personal history of combat and operational stress reaction**　　　　A

Z86.59 **Personal history of other mental and behavioral disorders**

● **Z86.6** **Personal history of diseases of the nervous system and sense organs**
Conditions classifiable to G00-G99, H00-H95

Z86.61 **Personal history of infections of the central nervous system**
Personal history of encephalitis
Personal history of meningitis

Z86.69 **Personal history of other diseases of the nervous system and sense organs**
Coding Clinic: 2016, Q4, P25

● **Z86.7** **Personal history of diseases of the circulatory system**
Conditions classifiable to I00-I99

　　Excludes2　old myocardial infarction (I25.2)
personal history of anaphylactic shock (Z87.892)
postmyocardial infarction syndrome (I24.1)

● **Z86.71** **Personal history of venous thrombosis and embolism**

Z86.711 **Personal history of pulmonary embolism**

Z86.718 **Personal history of other venous thrombosis and embolism**

Z86.72 **Personal history of thrombophlebitis**

Z86.73 **Personal history of transient ischemic attack (TIA), and cerebral infarction without residual deficits**
Personal history of prolonged reversible ischemic neurological deficit (PRIND)
Personal history of stroke NOS without residual deficits
　　Excludes1　personal history of traumatic brain injury (Z87.820)
sequelae of cerebrovascular disease (I69.-)
Coding Clinic: 2012, Q4, P3

Z86.74 **Personal history of sudden cardiac arrest**
Personal history of sudden cardiac death successfully resuscitated

Z86.79 **Personal history of other diseases of the circulatory system**
Coding Clinic: 2020, Q1, P13

● **Z87** **Personal history of other diseases and conditions**
Code first any follow-up examination after treatment (Z09)

● **Z87.0** **Personal history of diseases of the respiratory system**
Conditions classifiable to J00-J99

Z87.01 **Personal history of pneumonia (recurrent)**

Z87.09 **Personal history of other diseases of the respiratory system**

● **Z87.1** **Personal history of diseases of the digestive system**
Conditions classifiable to K00-K93

Z87.11 **Personal history of peptic ulcer disease**

Z87.19 **Personal history of other diseases of the digestive system**
Coding Clinic: 2017, Q1, P14

▶ New　　➡ Revised　　~~deleted~~ Deleted　　Excludes 1　　Excludes 2　　Includes　　Use additional　　Code first　　Code also　　Key words
OGCR Official Guidelines　　X Assign placeholder X　　● Use Additional Character(s)　　▷ Manifestation Code　　🔖 Hierarchical Condition Category　　Coding Clinic

Z87.2   Personal history of diseases of the skin and subcutaneous tissue
Conditions classifiable to L00-L99

> **Excludes2**   personal history of diabetic foot ulcer (Z86.31)

● Z87.3   Personal history of diseases of the musculoskeletal system and connective tissue
Conditions classifiable to M00-M99

> **Excludes2**   personal history of (healed) traumatic fracture (Z87.81)

● Z87.31   Personal history of (healed) nontraumatic fracture

Z87.310   Personal history of (healed) osteoporosis fracture
Personal history of (healed) fragility fracture
Personal history of (healed) collapsed vertebra due to osteoporosis

Z87.311   Personal history of (healed) other pathological fracture
Personal history of (healed) collapsed vertebra NOS

> **Excludes2**   personal history of osteoporosis fracture (Z87.310)

Z87.312   Personal history of (healed) stress fracture
Personal history of (healed) fatigue fracture

Z87.39   Personal history of other diseases of the musculoskeletal system and connective tissue

● Z87.4   Personal history of diseases of genitourinary system
Conditions classifiable to N00-N99

● Z87.41   Personal history of dysplasia of the female genital tract

> **Excludes1**   personal history of intraepithelial neoplasia III of female genital tract (Z86.001, Z86.008)
> personal history of malignant neoplasm of female genital tract (Z85.40-Z85.44)

Z87.410   Personal history of cervical dysplasia ♀

Z87.411   Personal history of vaginal dysplasia ♀

Z87.412   Personal history of vulvar dysplasia ♀

Z87.42   Personal history of other diseases of the female genital tract ♀

● Z87.43   Personal history of diseases of male genital organs

Z87.430   Personal history of prostatic dysplasia ♂

> **Excludes1**   personal history of malignant neoplasm of prostate (Z85.46)

Z87.438   Personal history of other diseases of male genital organs ♂

● Z87.44   Personal history of diseases of urinary system

> **Excludes1**   personal history of malignant neoplasm of cervix uteri (Z85.41)

Z87.440   Personal history of urinary (tract) infections

Z87.441   Personal history of nephrotic syndrome

Z87.442   Personal history of urinary calculi
Personal history of kidney stones

Z87.448   Personal history of other diseases of urinary system

● Z87.5   Personal history of complications of pregnancy, childbirth and the puerperium
Conditions classifiable to O00-O9A

> **Excludes2**   recurrent pregnancy loss (N96)

Z87.51   Personal history of pre-term labor ♀

> **Excludes1**   current pregnancy with history of pre-term labor (O09.21-)

Z87.59   Personal history of other complications of pregnancy, childbirth and the puerperium ♀
Personal history of trophoblastic disease

● Z87.7   Personal history of (corrected) congenital malformations
Conditions classifiable to Q00-Q89 that have been repaired or corrected

> **Excludes1**   congenital malformations that have been partially corrected or repair but which still require medical treatment - code to condition

> **Excludes2**   other postprocedural states (Z98.-)
> personal history of medical treatment (Z92.-)
> presence of cardiac and vascular implants and grafts (Z95.-)
> presence of other devices (Z97.-)
> presence of other functional implants (Z96.-)
> transplanted organ and tissue status (Z94.-)

● Z87.71   Personal history of (corrected) congenital malformations of genitourinary system

Z87.710   Personal history of (corrected) hypospadias ♂

Z87.718   Personal history of other specified (corrected) congenital malformations of genitourinary system

● Z87.72   Personal history of (corrected) congenital malformations of nervous system and sense organs

Z87.720   Personal history of (corrected) congenital malformations of eye

Z87.721   Personal history of (corrected) congenital malformations of ear

Z87.728   Personal history of other specified (corrected) congenital malformations of nervous system and sense organs

● Z87.73   Personal history of (corrected) congenital malformations of digestive system

Z87.730   Personal history of (corrected) cleft lip and palate

Z87.738   Personal history of other specified (corrected) congenital malformations of digestive system

Z87.74   Personal history of (corrected) congenital malformations of heart and circulatory system

Z87.75   Personal history of (corrected) congenital malformations of respiratory system

Z87.76   Personal history of (corrected) congenital malformations of integument, limbs and musculoskeletal system

● Z87.79   Personal history of other (corrected) congenital malformations

Z87.790   Personal history of (corrected) congenital malformations of face and neck

Z87.798   Personal history of other (corrected) congenital malformations

CHAPTER 21 (Z00-Z99)

● **Z87.8** **Personal history of other specified conditions**
▸ **Excludes2**   personal history of self harm (Z91.5-)

     Z87.81 **Personal history of (healed) traumatic fracture**
         Excludes2   personal history of (healed) nontraumatic fracture (Z87.31-)

●   **Z87.82** **Personal history of other (healed) physical injury and trauma**
         Conditions classifiable to S00-T88, except traumatic fractures

         Z87.820 **Personal history of traumatic brain injury**
            Excludes1   personal history of transient ischemic attack (TIA), and cerebral infarction without residual deficits (Z86.73)

         Z87.821 **Personal history of retained foreign body fully removed**

         Z87.828 **Personal history of other (healed) physical injury and trauma**

●   **Z87.89** **Personal history of other specified conditions**

         Z87.890 **Personal history of sex reassignment**

         Z87.891 **Personal history of nicotine dependence**
            Excludes1   current nicotine dependence (F17.2-)
            Coding Clinic: 2017, Q2, P27

         Z87.892 **Personal history of anaphylaxis**
            Code also allergy status such as: allergy status to drugs, medicaments and biological substances (Z88.-) allergy status, other than to drugs and biological substances (Z91.0-)

         Z87.898 **Personal history of other specified conditions**
            Coding Clinic: 2013, Q1, P21

● **Z88** **Allergy status to drugs, medicaments and biological substances**
     Excludes2   allergy status, other than to drugs and biological substances (Z91.0-)

     Z88.0 **Allergy status to penicillin**

     Z88.1 **Allergy status to other antibiotic agents**

     Z88.2 **Allergy status to sulfonamides**
         Coding Clinic: 2015, Q3, P23

     Z88.3 **Allergy status to other anti-infective agents**

     Z88.4 **Allergy status to anesthetic agent**

     Z88.5 **Allergy status to narcotic agent**

     Z88.6 **Allergy status to analgesic agent**

     Z88.7 **Allergy status to serum and vaccine**

     Z88.8 **Allergy status to other drugs, medicaments and biological substances**

     Z88.9 **Allergy status to unspecified drugs, medicaments and biological substances**

● **Z89** **Acquired absence of limb**
     Includes   amputation status postprocedural loss of limb post-traumatic loss of limb
     Excludes1   acquired deformities of limbs (M20-M21) congenital absence of limbs (Q71-Q73)

●   **Z89.0** **Acquired absence of thumb and other finger(s)**
●   **Z89.01** **Acquired absence of thumb**
         Z89.011 **Acquired absence of right thumb**
         Z89.012 **Acquired absence of left thumb**
         Z89.019 **Acquired absence of unspecified thumb**

●   **Z89.02** **Acquired absence of other finger(s)**
         Excludes2   acquired absence of thumb (Z89.01-)
         Z89.021 **Acquired absence of right finger(s)**
         Z89.022 **Acquired absence of left finger(s)**
         Z89.029 **Acquired absence of unspecified finger(s)**

●   **Z89.1** **Acquired absence of hand and wrist**
●   **Z89.11** **Acquired absence of hand**
         Z89.111 **Acquired absence of right hand**
         Z89.112 **Acquired absence of left hand**
         Z89.119 **Acquired absence of unspecified hand**

●   **Z89.12** **Acquired absence of wrist**
         Disarticulation at wrist
         Z89.121 **Acquired absence of right wrist**
         Z89.122 **Acquired absence of left wrist**
         Z89.129 **Acquired absence of unspecified wrist**

●   **Z89.2** **Acquired absence of upper limb above wrist**
●   **Z89.20** **Acquired absence of upper limb, unspecified level**
         Z89.201 **Acquired absence of right upper limb, unspecified level**
         Z89.202 **Acquired absence of left upper limb, unspecified level**
         Z89.209 **Acquired absence of unspecified upper limb, unspecified level**
            Acquired absence of arm NOS

●   **Z89.21** **Acquired absence of upper limb below elbow**
         Z89.211 **Acquired absence of right upper limb below elbow**
         Z89.212 **Acquired absence of left upper limb below elbow**
         Z89.219 **Acquired absence of unspecified upper limb below elbow**

●   **Z89.22** **Acquired absence of upper limb above elbow**
         Disarticulation at elbow
         Z89.221 **Acquired absence of right upper limb above elbow**
         Z89.222 **Acquired absence of left upper limb above elbow**
         Z89.229 **Acquired absence of unspecified upper limb above elbow**

●   **Z89.23** **Acquired absence of shoulder**
         Acquired absence of shoulder joint following explantation of shoulder joint prosthesis, with or without presence of antibiotic-impregnated cement spacer
         Z89.231 **Acquired absence of right shoulder**
         Z89.232 **Acquired absence of left shoulder**
         Z89.239 **Acquired absence of unspecified shoulder**

●   **Z89.4** **Acquired absence of toe(s), foot, and ankle**
●   **Z89.41** **Acquired absence of great toe**
         Z89.411 **Acquired absence of right great toe** 🦠
         Z89.412 **Acquired absence of left great toe** 🦠
         Z89.419 **Acquired absence of unspecified great toe** 🦠

●   **Z89.42** **Acquired absence of other toe(s)**
         Excludes2   acquired absence of great toe (Z89.41-)
         Z89.421 **Acquired absence of other right toe(s)** 🦠
         Z89.422 **Acquired absence of other left toe(s)** 🦠
         Z89.429 **Acquired absence of other toe(s), unspecified side** 🦠

▶ New   ⇒ Revised   ~~deleted~~ Deleted   Excludes 1   Excludes 2   Includes   Use additional   Code first   Code also   Key words

OGCR Official Guidelines   X Assign placeholder X   ● Use Additional Character(s)   ▷ Manifestation Code   🦠 Hierarchical Condition Category   **Coding Clinic**

- **Z89.43   Acquired absence of foot**
    - Z89.431   Acquired absence of right foot 🦶
    - Z89.432   Acquired absence of left foot 🦶
    - Z89.439   Acquired absence of unspecified foot 🦶
- **Z89.44   Acquired absence of ankle**
    Disarticulation of ankle
    - Z89.441   Acquired absence of right ankle 🦶
    - Z89.442   Acquired absence of left ankle 🦶
    - Z89.449   Acquired absence of unspecified ankle 🦶
- **Z89.5   Acquired absence of leg below knee**
    - **Z89.51   Acquired absence of leg below knee**
        - Z89.511   Acquired absence of right leg below knee 🦶
        - Z89.512   Acquired absence of left leg below knee 🦶
        - Z89.519   Acquired absence of unspecified leg below knee 🦶
    - **Z89.52   Acquired absence of knee**
        Acquired absence of knee joint following explantation of knee joint prosthesis, with or without presence of antibiotic-impregnated cement spacer
        - Z89.521   Acquired absence of right knee
        - Z89.522   Acquired absence of left knee
        - Z89.529   Acquired absence of unspecified knee
- **Z89.6   Acquired absence of leg above knee**
    - **Z89.61   Acquired absence of leg above knee**
        Acquired absence of leg NOS
        Disarticulation at knee
        - Z89.611   Acquired absence of right leg above knee 🦶
        - Z89.612   Acquired absence of left leg above knee 🦶
        - Z89.619   Acquired absence of unspecified leg above knee 🦶
    - **Z89.62   Acquired absence of hip**
        Acquired absence of hip joint following explantation of hip joint prosthesis, with or without presence of antibiotic-impregnated cement spacer
        Disarticulation at hip
        - Z89.621   Acquired absence of right hip joint
        - Z89.622   Acquired absence of left hip joint
        - Z89.629   Acquired absence of unspecified hip joint
    - **Z89.9   Acquired absence of limb, unspecified**
- **Z90   Acquired absence of organs, not elsewhere classified**
    - **Includes**   postprocedural or post-traumatic loss of body part NEC
    - **Excludes1**   congenital absence - see Alphabetical Index
    - **Excludes2**   postprocedural absence of endocrine glands (E89.-)
    - **Z90.0   Acquired absence of part of head and neck**
        - Z90.01   Acquired absence of eye
        - Z90.02   Acquired absence of larynx
        - Z90.09   Acquired absence of other part of head and neck
            Acquired absence of nose
            - **Excludes2**   teeth (K08.1)
    - **Z90.1   Acquired absence of breast and nipple**
        - Z90.10   Acquired absence of unspecified breast and nipple
        - Z90.11   Acquired absence of right breast and nipple
        - Z90.12   Acquired absence of left breast and nipple
        - Z90.13   Acquired absence of bilateral breasts and nipples

- Z90.2   Acquired absence of lung [part of]
- Z90.3   Acquired absence of stomach [part of]
- **Z90.4   Acquired absence of other specified parts of digestive tract**
    - **Z90.41   Acquired absence of pancreas**
        Code also exocrine pancreatic insufficiency (K86.81)
        Use additional code to identify any associated:
        diabetes mellitus, postpancreatectomy (E13.-)
        insulin use (Z79.4)
        - Z90.410   Acquired total absence of pancreas
            Acquired absence of pancreas NOS
        - Z90.411   Acquired partial absence of pancreas
    - Z90.49   Acquired absence of other specified parts of digestive tract
- Z90.5   Acquired absence of kidney
- Z90.6   Acquired absence of other parts of urinary tract
    Acquired absence of bladder
- **Z90.7   Acquired absence of genital organ(s)**
    - **Excludes1**   personal history of sex reassignment (Z87.890)
    - **Excludes2**   female genital mutilation status (N90.81-)
    - **Z90.71   Acquired absence of cervix and uterus**
        - Z90.710   Acquired absence of both cervix and uterus ♀
            Acquired absence of uterus NOS
            Status post total hysterectomy
        - Z90.711   Acquired absence of uterus with remaining cervical stump ♀
            Status post partial hysterectomy with remaining cervical stump
        - Z90.712   Acquired absence of cervix with remaining uterus ♀
    - **Z90.72   Acquired absence of ovaries**
        - Z90.721   Acquired absence of ovaries, unilateral ♀
        - Z90.722   Acquired absence of ovaries, bilateral ♀
    - Z90.79   Acquired absence of other genital organ(s)
- **Z90.8   Acquired absence of other organs**
    - Z90.81   Acquired absence of spleen
    - Z90.89   Acquired absence of other organs
- **Z91   Personal risk factors, not elsewhere classified**
    - **Excludes2**   contact with and (suspected) exposures hazardous to health (Z77.-)
        exposure to pollution and other problems related to physical environment (Z77.1-)
        female genital mutilation status (N90.81-)
        occupational exposure to risk factors (Z57.-)
        personal history of physical injury and trauma (Z87.81, Z87.82-)
    - **Z91.0   Allergy status, other than to drugs and biological substances**
        - **Excludes2**   allergy status to drugs, medicaments, and biological substances (Z88.-)
        - **Z91.01   Food allergy status**
            - **Excludes2**   food additives allergy status (Z91.02)
            - Z91.010   Allergy to peanuts
            - Z91.011   Allergy to milk products
                - **Excludes1**   lactose intolerance (E73.-)
            - Z91.012   Allergy to eggs
            - Z91.013   Allergy to seafood
                Allergy to shellfish
                Allergy to octopus or squid ink

CHAPTER 21 (Z00–Z99)

▶ **Z91.014 Allergy to mammalian meats**
  ▶ Allergy to beef
  ▶ Allergy to lamb
  ▶ Allergy to pork
  ▶ Allergy to red meats

Z91.018   Allergy to other foods
  Allergy to nuts other than peanuts

Z91.02   Food additives allergy status

● **Z91.03   Insect allergy status**

Z91.030   Bee allergy status

Z91.038   Other insect allergy status

● **Z91.04   Nonmedicinal substance allergy status**

Z91.040   Latex allergy status
  Latex sensitivity status

Z91.041   Radiographic dye allergy status
  Allergy status to contrast media used for diagnostic X-ray procedure

Z91.048   Other nonmedicinal substance allergy status

Z91.09   Other allergy status, other than to drugs and biological substances

● **Z91.1   Patient's noncompliance with medical treatment and regimen**

Z91.11   Patient's noncompliance with dietary regimen

● **Z91.12   Patient's intentional underdosing of medication regimen**
  Code first underdosing of medication (T36-T50) with fifth or sixth character 6
  Excludes1   adverse effect of prescribed drug taken as directed - code to adverse effect
    poisoning (overdose) - code to poisoning

Z91.120   Patient's intentional underdosing of medication regimen due to financial hardship

Z91.128   Patient's intentional underdosing of medication regimen for other reason

● **Z91.13   Patient's unintentional underdosing of medication regimen**
  Code first underdosing of medication (T36-T50) with fifth or sixth character 6
  Excludes1   adverse effect of prescribed drug taken as directed - code to adverse effect
    poisoning (overdose) - code to poisoning

Z91.130   Patient's unintentional underdosing of medication regimen due to age-related debility

Z91.138   Patient's unintentional underdosing of medication regimen for other reason

Z91.14   Patient's other noncompliance with medication regimen
  Patient's underdosing of medication NOS

Z91.15   Patient's noncompliance with renal dialysis 🝖

Z91.19   Patient's noncompliance with other medical treatment and regimen
  Nonadherence to medical treatment

● **Z91.4   Personal history of psychological trauma, not elsewhere classified**

● **Z91.41   Personal history of adult abuse**
  Excludes2   personal history of abuse in childhood (Z62.81-)

Z91.410   Personal history of adult physical and sexual abuse   A
  Excludes1   current adult physical abuse (T74.11, T76.11)
    current adult sexual abuse (T74.21, T76.11)

Z91.411   Personal history of adult psychological abuse   A

Z91.412   Personal history of adult neglect   A
  Excludes1   current adult neglect (T74.01, T76.01)

Z91.419   Personal history of unspecified adult abuse   A

Z91.42   Personal history of forced labor or sexual exploitation

Z91.49   Other personal history of psychological trauma, not elsewhere classified

⇒● **Z91.5   Personal history of self-harm**
  ~~Personal history of parasuicide~~
  ~~Personal history of self-poisoning~~
  ~~Personal history of suicide attempt~~
  ▶ Code also mental health disorder, if known

▶ **Z91.51 Personal history of suicidal behavior**
  ▶ Personal history of parasuicide
  ▶ Personal history of self-poisoning
  ▶ Personal history of suicide attempt

▶ **Z91.52 Personal history of nonsuicidal self-harm**
  ▶ Personal history of nonsuicidal self-injury
  ▶ Personal history of self-inflicted injury without suicidal intent
  ▶ Personal history of self-mutilation

● **Z91.8   Other specified personal risk factors, not elsewhere classified**

Z91.81   History of falling
  At risk for falling

Z91.82   Personal history of military deployment   A
  Individual (civilian or military) with past history of military war, peacekeeping and humanitarian deployment (current or past conflict)
  Returned from military deployment

▷ **Z91.83   *Wandering in diseases classified elsewhere***
  Code first underlying disorder such as:
    Alzheimer's disease (G30.-)
    autism or pervasive developmental disorder (F84.-)
    intellectual disabilities (F70-F79)
    unspecified dementia with behavioral disturbance (F03.9-)

● **Z91.84   Oral health risk factors**

Z91.841   Risk for dental caries, low

Z91.842   Risk for dental caries, moderate

Z91.843   Risk for dental caries, high

Z91.849   Unspecified risk for dental caries

Z91.89   Other specified personal risk factors, not elsewhere classified
  Coding Clinic: 2017, Q1, P46

▶ New   ⇒ Revised   ~~deleted~~ Deleted   Excludes 1   Excludes 2   Includes   Use additional   Code first   Code also   Key words

OGCR Official Guidelines   X Assign placeholder X   ● Use Additional Character(s)   ▷ Manifestation Code   🝖 Hierarchical Condition Category   Coding Clinic

● **Z92   Personal history of medical treatment**

   Excludes2   postprocedural states (Z98.-)

   Z92.0   Personal history of contraception

      Excludes1   counseling or management of current
      contraceptive practices (Z30.-)
      long term (current) use of contraception
      (Z79.3)
      presence of (intrauterine) contraceptive
      device (Z97.5)

● **Z92.2   Personal history of drug therapy**

      Excludes2   long term (current) drug therapy (Z79.-)

   **Z92.21   Personal history of antineoplastic
   chemotherapy**

   Z92.22   Personal history of monoclonal drug therapy

   Z92.23   Personal history of estrogen therapy

● **Z92.24   Personal history of steroid therapy**

      **Z92.240   Personal history of inhaled steroid
      therapy**

      **Z92.241   Personal history of systemic steroid
      therapy**
         Personal history of steroid therapy
         NOS

➡ **Z92.25   Personal history of immunosuppression
   therapy**

      Excludes2   personal history of steroid
      therapy (Z92.24)

   Z92.29   Personal history of other drug therapy

   Z92.3   Personal history of irradiation
      Personal history of exposure to therapeutic radiation

      Excludes1   exposure to radiation in the physical
      environment (Z77.12)
      occupational exposure to radiation
      (Z57.1)

● **Z92.8   Personal history of other medical treatment**
      Coding Clinic: 2016, Q4, P72

   **Z92.81   Personal history of extracorporeal membrane
   oxygenation (ECMO)**

   **Z92.82   Status post administration of tPA (rtPA) in a
   different facility within the last 24 hours prior
   to admission to current facility**

         *Code first condition requiring tPA administration,
         such as:*
         acute cerebral infarction (I63.-)
         acute myocardial infarction (I21.-, I22.-)

   Z92.83   Personal history of failed moderate sedation
      Personal history of failed conscious sedation

      Excludes2   failed moderate sedation during
      procedure (T88.52)

   **Z92.84   Personal history of unintended awareness
   under general anesthesia**

      Excludes2   unintended awareness under
      general anesthesia during
      procedure (T88.53)
      Coding Clinic: 2016, Q4, P72, 77

▶● **Z92.85 Personal history of cellular therapy**

   ▶ **Z92.850 Personal history of Chimeric Antigen
   Receptor T-cell therapy**
      ▶Personal history of CAR T-cell
      therapy

   ▶ **Z92.858 Personal history of other cellular
   therapy**

   ▶ **Z92.859 Personal history of cellular therapy,
   unspecified**

▶ **Z92.86 Personal history of gene therapy**

   Z92.89   Personal history of other medical treatment
      Coding Clinic: 2020, Q1, P18

● **Z93   Artificial opening status**

      Excludes1   artificial openings requiring attention or
      management (Z43.-)
      complications of external stoma (J95.0-, K94.-,
      N99.5-)

   Z93.0   Tracheostomy status 🦠

   Z93.1   Gastrostomy status 🦠

   Z93.2   Ileostomy status 🦠

   Z93.3   Colostomy status 🦠

   **Z93.4   Other artificial openings of gastrointestinal tract
   status** 🦠

● **Z93.5   Cystostomy status**

      Z93.50   Unspecified cystostomy status 🦠

      Z93.51   Cutaneous-vesicostomy status 🦠

      Z93.52   Appendico-vesicostomy status 🦠

      Z93.59   Other cystostomy status 🦠

   Z93.6   Other artificial openings of urinary tract status 🦠
      Nephrostomy status
      Ureterostomy status
      Urethrostomy status

   Z93.8   Other artificial opening status 🦠

   Z93.9   Artificial opening status, unspecified 🦠

● **Z94   Transplanted organ and tissue status**

      Includes   organ or tissue replaced by heterogenous or
      homogenous transplant

      Excludes1   complications of transplanted organ or tissue -
      see Alphabetical Index

      Excludes2   presence of vascular grafts (Z95.-)

   Z94.0   Kidney transplant status

   Z94.1   Heart transplant status 🦠

      Excludes1   artificial heart status (Z95.812)
      heart-valve replacement status
      (Z95.2-Z95.4)

   Z94.2   Lung transplant status 🦠

   Z94.3   Heart and lungs transplant status 🦠

   Z94.4   Liver transplant status 🦠

   Z94.5   Skin transplant status
      Autogenous skin transplant status

   Z94.6   Bone transplant status

   Z94.7   Corneal transplant status

● **Z94.8   Other transplanted organ and tissue status**

      Z94.81   Bone marrow transplant status 🦠

      Z94.82   Intestine transplant status 🦠

      Z94.83   Pancreas transplant status 🦠

      Z94.84   Stem cells transplant status 🦠

      Z94.89   Other transplanted organ and tissue status

   Z94.9   Transplanted organ and tissue status, unspecified

● **Z95   Presence of cardiac and vascular implants and grafts**

      Excludes2   complications of cardiac and vascular devices,
      implants and grafts (T82.-)

   Z95.0   Presence of cardiac pacemaker
      Presence of cardiac resynchronization therapy (CRT-P)
      pacemaker

      Excludes1   adjustment or management of cardiac
      device (Z45.0-)
      adjustment or management of cardiac
      pacemaker (Z45.0)
      presence of automatic (implantable)
      cardiac defibrillator with
      synchronous cardiac pacemaker
      (Z95.810)
      Coding Clinic: 2019, Q1, P33

CHAPTER 21 (Z00-Z99)

CHAPTER 21 (Z00-Z99)

Z95.1   Presence of aortocoronary bypass graft
         Presence of coronary artery bypass graft

Z95.2   Presence of prosthetic heart valve
         Presence of heart valve NOS

Z95.3   Presence of xenogenic heart valve

Z95.4   Presence of other heart-valve replacement

Z95.5   Presence of coronary angioplasty implant and graft
         Excludes1   coronary angioplasty status without
                          implant and graft (Z98.61)

● Z95.8 Presence of other cardiac and vascular implants and
         grafts
   ● Z95.81   Presence of other cardiac implants and grafts
        Z95.810   Presence of automatic (implantable)
                   cardiac defibrillator
                       Presence of automatic (implantable)
                           cardiac defibrillator with
                           synchronous cardiac pacemaker
                       Presence of cardiac
                           resynchronization therapy
                           defibrillator (CRT-D)
                       Presence of cardioverter-defibrillator
                           (ICD)
        Z95.811   Presence of heart assist device 🐾
        Z95.812   Presence of fully implantable
                   artificial heart 🐾
        Z95.818   Presence of other cardiac implants
                   and grafts
   ● Z95.82   Presence of other vascular implants and grafts
        Z95.820   Peripheral vascular angioplasty status
                   with implants and grafts
                       Excludes1   peripheral vascular
                                        angioplasty
                                        without implant
                                        and graft (Z98.62)
        Z95.828   Presence of other vascular implants
                   and grafts
                       Presence of intravascular prosthesis
                           NEC

Z95.9   Presence of cardiac and vascular implant and graft,
         unspecified

● Z96   Presence of other functional implants
         Excludes2   complications of internal prosthetic devices,
                          implants and grafts (T82-T85)
                          fitting and adjustment of prosthetic and other
                          devices (Z44-Z46)

Z96.0   Presence of urogenital implants

Z96.1   Presence of intraocular lens
         Presence of pseudophakia

● Z96.2 Presence of otological and audiological implants
        Z96.20   Presence of otological and audiological
                  implant, unspecified
        Z96.21   Cochlear implant status
        Z96.22   Myringotomy tube(s) status
        Z96.29   Presence of other otological and audiological
                  implants
                      Presence of bone-conduction hearing device
                      Presence of eustachian tube stent
                      Stapes replacement

Z96.3   Presence of artificial larynx

● Z96.4 Presence of endocrine implants
        Z96.41   Presence of insulin pump (external) (internal)
        Z96.49   Presence of other endocrine implants

Z96.5   Presence of tooth-root and mandibular implants

● Z96.6 Presence of orthopedic joint implants
        Z96.60   Presence of unspecified orthopedic joint
                  implant
   ● Z96.61   Presence of artificial shoulder joint
        Z96.611   Presence of right artificial shoulder
                   joint
        Z96.612   Presence of left artificial shoulder
                   joint
        Z96.619   Presence of unspecified artificial
                   shoulder joint
   ● Z96.62   Presence of artificial elbow joint
        Z96.621   Presence of right artificial elbow joint
        Z96.622   Presence of left artificial elbow joint
        Z96.629   Presence of unspecified artificial
                   elbow joint
   ● Z96.63   Presence of artificial wrist joint
        Z96.631   Presence of right artificial wrist joint
        Z96.632   Presence of left artificial wrist joint
        Z96.639   Presence of unspecified artificial wrist
                   joint
   ● Z96.64   Presence of artificial hip joint
             Hip-joint replacement (partial) (total)
        Z96.641   Presence of right artificial hip joint
                   Coding Clinic: 2016, Q3, P17
        Z96.642   Presence of left artificial hip joint
                   Coding Clinic: 2015, Q1, P16
        Z96.643   Presence of artificial hip joint,
                   bilateral
        Z96.649   Presence of unspecified artificial hip
                   joint
   ● Z96.65   Presence of artificial knee joint
        Z96.651   Presence of right artificial knee joint
        Z96.652   Presence of left artificial knee joint
                   Coding Clinic: 2019, Q3, P16
        Z96.653   Presence of artificial knee joint,
                   bilateral
        Z96.659   Presence of unspecified artificial knee
                   joint
   ● Z96.66   Presence of artificial ankle joint
        Z96.661   Presence of right artificial ankle joint
        Z96.662   Presence of left artificial ankle joint
        Z96.669   Presence of unspecified artificial
                   ankle joint
   ● Z96.69   Presence of other orthopedic joint implants
        Z96.691   Finger-joint replacement of right
                   hand
        Z96.692   Finger-joint replacement of left hand
        Z96.693   Finger-joint replacement, bilateral
        Z96.698   Presence of other orthopedic joint
                   implants

Z96.7   Presence of other bone and tendon implants
         Presence of skull plate

● Z96.8 Presence of other specified functional implants
        Z96.81   Presence of artificial skin
        Z96.82   Presence of neurostimulator
                      Presence of brain neurostimulator
                      Presence of gastric neurostimulator
                      Presence of peripheral nerve neurostimulator
                      Presence of sacral nerve neurostimulator
                      Presence of spinal cord neurostimulator
                      Presence of vagus nerve neurostimulator
        Z96.89   Presence of other specified functional implants

Z96.9   Presence of functional implant, unspecified

▶ New   ⇒ Revised   ~~deleted~~ Deleted   Excludes 1   Excludes 2   Includes   Use additional   Code first   Code also   Key words
OGCR Official Guidelines   X Assign placeholder X   ● Use Additional Character(s)   ❱ Manifestation Code   🐾 Hierarchical Condition Category   Coding Clinic

● Z97   Presence of other devices
    Excludes2   fitting and adjustment of prosthetic and other
        devices (Z44-Z46)
        presence of cerebrospinal fluid drainage device
        (Z98.2)

  Z97.0   Presence of artificial eye
● Z97.1   Presence of artificial limb (complete) (partial)
    Z97.10   Presence of artificial limb (complete) (partial),
        unspecified
    Z97.11   Presence of artificial right arm (complete)
        (partial)
    Z97.12   Presence of artificial left arm (complete)
        (partial)
    Z97.13   Presence of artificial right leg (complete)
        (partial)
    Z97.14   Presence of artificial left leg (complete) (partial)
    Z97.15   Presence of artificial arms, bilateral (complete)
        (partial)
    Z97.16   Presence of artificial legs, bilateral (complete)
        (partial)

  Z97.2   Presence of dental prosthetic device (complete) (partial)
    Presence of dentures (complete) (partial)
  Z97.3   Presence of spectacles and contact lenses
  Z97.4   Presence of external hearing-aid
  Z97.5   Presence of (intrauterine) contraceptive device ♀
    Excludes1   checking, reinsertion or removal of
        implantable subdermal contraceptive
        (Z30.46)
        checking, reinsertion or removal of
        intrauterine contraceptive device
        (Z30.43-)
  Z97.8   Presence of other specified devices

● Z98   Other postprocedural states
    Excludes2   aftercare (Z43-Z49, Z51)
        follow-up medical care (Z08-Z09)
        postprocedural complication - see Alphabetical
        Index

  Z98.0   Intestinal bypass and anastomosis status
    Excludes2   bariatric surgery status (Z98.84)
        gastric bypass status (Z98.84)
        obesity surgery status (Z98.84)
  Z98.1   Arthrodesis status
  Z98.2   Presence of cerebrospinal fluid drainage device
    Presence of CSF shunt
  Z98.3   Post therapeutic collapse of lung status
    Code first underlying disease
● Z98.4   Cataract extraction status
    Use additional code to identify intraocular lens implant
        status (Z96.1)
    Excludes1   aphakia (H27.0)
    Z98.41   Cataract extraction status, right eye
    Z98.42   Cataract extraction status, left eye
    Z98.49   Cataract extraction status, unspecified eye
● Z98.5   Sterilization status
    Excludes1   female infertility (N97.-)
        male infertility (N46.-)
    Z98.51   Tubal ligation status ♀
    Z98.52   Vasectomy status ♂   A
● Z98.6   Angioplasty status
    Z98.61   Coronary angioplasty status
        Excludes1   coronary angioplasty status with
            implant and graft (Z95.5)
    Z98.62   Peripheral vascular angioplasty status
        Excludes1   peripheral vascular angioplasty
            status with implant and
            graft (Z95.820)

● Z98.8   Other specified postprocedural states
    Coding Clinic: 2016, Q4, P76
  ● Z98.81   Dental procedure status
    Z98.810   Dental sealant status
    Z98.811   Dental restoration status
        Dental crown status
        Dental fillings status
    Z98.818   Other dental procedure status
  Z98.82   Breast implant status
    Excludes1   breast implant removal status
        (Z98.86)
  Z98.83   Filtering (vitreous) bleb after glaucoma surgery
    status
    Excludes1   inflammation (infection) of
        postprocedural bleb
        (H59.4-)
  Z98.84   Bariatric surgery status
    Gastric banding status
    Gastric bypass status for obesity
    Obesity surgery status
    Excludes1   bariatric surgery status
        complicating pregnancy,
        childbirth, or the
        puerperium (O99.84)
    Excludes2   intestinal bypass and
        anastomosis status (Z98.0)
    Coding Clinic: 2020, Q1, P12
  Z98.85   Transplanted organ removal status
    Transplanted organ previously removed due to
        complication, failure, rejection or infection
    Excludes1   encounter for removal of
        transplanted organ -
        code to complication of
        transplanted organ (T86.-)
  Z98.86   Personal history of breast implant removal
● Z98.87   Personal history of in utero procedure
    Z98.870   Personal history of in utero procedure
        during pregnancy ♀
        Excludes2   complications from in
            utero procedure
            for current
            pregnancy
            (O35.7)
            supervision of current
            pregnancy with
            history of in
            utero procedure
            during previous
            pregnancy
            (O09.82-)
    Z98.871   Personal history of in utero procedure
        while a fetus
● Z98.89   Other specified postprocedural states
    Coding Clinic: 2016, Q4, P76
    Z98.890   Other specified postprocedural
        states
        Personal history of surgery, not
        elsewhere classified
    Z98.891   History of uterine scar from previous
        surgery ♀
        Excludes1   Maternal care due to
            uterine scar from
            previous surgery
            (O34.2-)
        Coding Clinic: 2016, Q4, P52, P76

CHAPTER 21 (Z00-Z99)

CHAPTER 21 (Z00-Z99)

● **Z99** **Dependence on enabling machines and devices, not elsewhere classified**

> Excludes1   cardiac pacemaker status (Z95.0)

Coding Clinic: 2020, Q1, P11

Z99.0 **Dependence on aspirator**

● **Z99.1** **Dependence on respirator**
> Dependence on ventilator

> **Z99.11** **Dependence on respirator [ventilator] status** 🦠
> Coding Clinic: 2018, Q1, P14; 2015, Q1, P21

> **Z99.12** **Encounter for respirator [ventilator] dependence during power failure** 🦠
> > **Excludes1**   mechanical complication of respirator [ventilator] (J95.850)

Z99.2 **Dependence on renal dialysis** 🦠
> Hemodialysis status
> Peritoneal dialysis status
> Presence of arteriovenous shunt for dialysis
> Renal dialysis status NOS
> > **Excludes1**   encounter for fitting and adjustment of dialysis catheter (Z49.0-)
> > **Excludes2**   noncompliance with renal dialysis (Z91.15)

Coding Clinic: 2016, Q1, P13

Z99.3 **Dependence on wheelchair**
> Wheelchair confinement status
> *Code first cause of dependence, such as:*
> muscular dystrophy (G71.0-)
> obesity (E66.-)

● **Z99.8** **Dependence on other enabling machines and devices**

> **Z99.81** **Dependence on supplemental oxygen**
> > Dependence on long-term oxygen

> **Z99.89** **Dependence on other enabling machines and devices**
> > Dependence on machine or device NOS
> > Coding Clinic: 2020, Q1, P11

▶ New   ⇒ Revised   ~~deleted~~ Deleted   Excludes 1   Excludes 2   Includes   Use additional   Code first   Code also   Key words

OGCR Official Guidelines   X Assign placeholder X   ● Use Additional Character(s)   ▶ Manifestation Code   🦠 Hierarchical Condition Category   **Coding Clinic**

CHAPTER 22

CODES FOR SPECIAL PURPOSES (U00-U85)

Note: Codes from this chapter are for use on newborn records only, never on maternal records.

This chapter contains the following blocks:

U00-U49	Provisional assignment of new diseases of uncertain etiology or emergency use

PROVISIONAL ASSIGNMENT OF NEW DISEASES OF UNCERTAIN ETIOLOGY OR EMERGENCY USE (U00-U49)

U07   Emergency use of U07

U07.0   Vaping-related disorder

Dabbing related lung damage
Dabbing related lung injury
E-cigarette, or vaping, product use associated lung injury [EVALI]
Electronic cigarette related lung damage
Electronic cigarette related lung injury

Use additional code to identify manifestations, such as:
abdominal pain (R10.84)
acute respiratory distress syndrome (J80)
diarrhea (R19.7)
drug-induced interstitial lung disorder (J70.4)
lipoid pneumonia (J69.1)
weight loss (R63.4)

U07.1   COVID-19

Use additional code to identify pneumonia or other manifestations

Excludes1   coronavirus infection, unspecified (B34.2)
coronavirus as the cause of diseases classified elsewhere (B97.2-)
pneumonia due to SARS-associated coronavirus (J12.81)

Coding Clinic: 2021, Q1, P31-33, 36, 39-40, 47, 49

U09   Post COVID-19 condition

U09.9   Post COVID-19 condition, unspecified

Note: This code enables establishment of a link with COVID-19.

This code is not to be used in cases that are still presenting with active COVID-19. However, an exception is made in cases of re-infection with COVID-19, occurring with a condition related to prior COVID-19.

Post-acute sequela of COVID-19

Code first the specific condition related to COVID-19 if known, such as:
chronic respiratory failure (J96.1-)
loss of smell (R43.8)
loss of taste (R43.8)
multisystem inflammatory syndrome (M35.81)
pulmonary embolism (I26.-)
pulmonary fibrosis (J84.10)

Step One: Lear

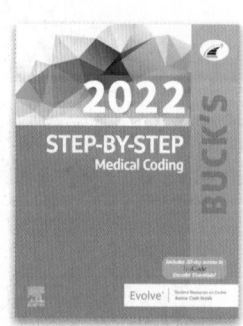

Buck's Step-by-Step Medical Coding, 2022 Editi
ISBN: 978-0-323-79038-3

Also available:
Buck's Workbook for Step-by-Step Medical Coding, 2022 Edition
ISBN: 978-0-323-79039-0

Buck's Medical Coding Online for Step-by-Step Medical Coding, 2022 Edition
ISBN: 978-0-323-79036-9

Step Two: Practic

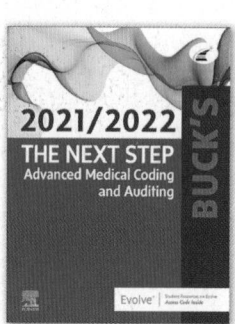

Buck's The Next Step: Advanced Medical Coding and Auditing, 2021/2022 Edition
ISBN: 978-0-323-76277-9

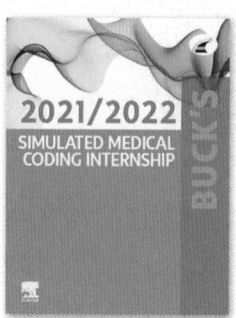

Buck's Simulated Medical Coding Internship, 2021/2022 Edition
ISBN: 978-0-323-76278-6

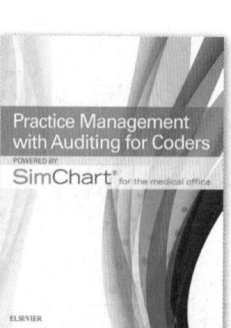

Practice Management with Auditing for Coders Powered by SimChart for the Medical Office
ISBN: 978-0-323-43011-1

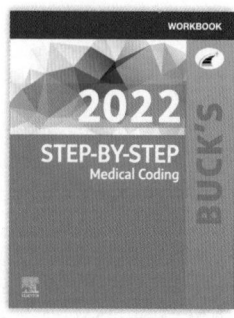

Buck's Workbook for Step-by-Step Medical Coding, 2022 Edition
ISBN: 978-0-323-79039-0